a LANGE medical book

CURRENT

Medical Diagnosis & Treatment 2001

40th Edition

Edited by

Lawrence M. Tierney, Jr., MD
Professor of Medicine
University of California, San Francisco
Associate Chief of Medical Services
Veterans Affairs Medical Center, San Francisco

Stephen J. McPhee, MD
Professor of Medicine
Division of General Internal Medicine
Department of Medicine
University of California, San Francisco

Maxine A. Papadakis, MD
Professor of Clinical Medicine
Associate Dean for Student Affairs
School of Medicine
University of California, San Francisco

With Associate Authors

Lange Medical Books/McGraw-Hill
Medical Publishing Division

New York St. Louis San Francisco Auckland Bogotá Caracas Lisbon London
Madrid Mexico City Milan Montreal New Delhi San Juan
Singapore Sydney Tokyo Toronto

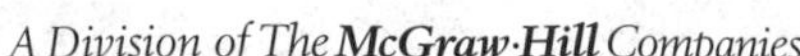

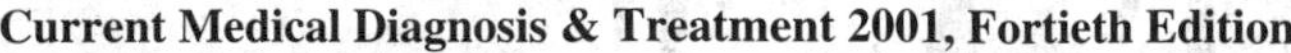

Current Medical Diagnosis & Treatment 2001, Fortieth Edition

1 2 3 4 5 6 7 8 9 0 DOW/DOW 0 9 8 7 6 5 4 3 2 1 0

ISBN 0-07-136466-8
ISSN 0092-8682

Notice

Medicine is an ever-changing science. As new research and clinical experience broaden our knowledge, changes in treatment and drug therapy are required. The authors and the publisher of this work have checked with sources believed to be reliable in their efforts to provide information that is complete and generally in accord with the standards accepted at the time of publication. However, in view of the possibility of human error or changes in medical sciences, neither the authors nor the publisher nor any other party who has been involved in the preparation or publication of this work warrants that the information contained herein is in every respect accurate or complete, and they disclaim all responsibility for any errors or omissions or for the results obtained from use of the information contained in this work. Readers are encouraged to confirm the information contained herein with other sources. For example and in particular, readers are advised to check product information sheet included in the package of each drug they plan to administer to be certain that the information contained in this work is accurate and that changes have not been made in the recommended dose or in the contraindications for administration. This recommendation is of particular importance in connection with new or infrequently used drugs.

The editors were Shelley Reinhardt, Jim Ransom, Isabel Nogueira, and Barbara Holton.
The production supervisor was Phil Galea.
The art manager was Charissa Baker.
The illustrator was Linda F. Harris.
The index was prepared by Kathy Pitcoff.

R.R. Donnelley and Sons, Inc. was printer and binder.

This book is printed on acid-free paper.

INTERNATIONAL EDITION ISBN 0-07-116332-8

Dedication

This volume of *Current Medical Diagnosis & Treatment* is dedicated with our deepest gratitude and respect to Dan Vaughan, who died this year after a brief illness. Long-time readers of this book know that Dr. Vaughan was the first author of the chapter on the eye and continued his contributions on every edition until this one—spanning decades of work. He held a similar position on the Lange series' textbook on ophthalmology, known as "The Yellow Book," used by thousands of physicians and students over the years to make a challenging subject both enjoyable and understandable. Those privileged to know Dan personally were fortunate indeed. He was a warm and gentle man and a superb physician whose opinion was sought by colleagues worldwide and who always considered the well-being of the entire patient even as he approached them through vision. His impact on the developing world was also enormous. As a member of the board of directors of the Proctor Foundation, associated with UCSF, he was instrumental in increasing our understanding of the pathogenesis, treatment, and epidemiology of ophthalmologic infections in many countries. One can only estimate how many human beings here and overseas owe their sight to him for this reason. This will be the last volume under his authorship, and he will be greatly missed by patients, family, and friends and by so many others who never knew him personally. He indeed was a giant in the Lange Medical Books community.

Contents

Preface

Current Medical Diagnosis & Treatment 2001 is the 40th annual volume of a general medical text designed as a single-source reference for practitioners in both hospital and ambulatory settings. *CMDT* covers all fields of internal medicine plus special topics of concern to primary care physicians and specialists who provide generalist care. It emphasizes the practical features of clinical diagnosis and patient management.

OUTSTANDING FEATURES

- Incorporates current advances up to time of publication
- Extensive coverage of all primary care topics, including gynecology, obstetrics, dermatology, ophthalmology, otolaryngology, psychiatry, neurology, toxicology, and urology
- Concise, readable format, facilitating efficient use in any practice setting
- More than 1000 diseases and disorders
- Only text including an annual update on HIV infection
- Brevity, conciseness, and easy accessibility of key information
- Emphasis on disease prevention and treatment costs
- Handy access to drug dosages; prices updated each edition
- Drug trade names indexed
- Annotated recent references, National Library of Medicine unique identifiers (NLM Cit ID) for all citations, and Web sites selected for clinical relevance
- Companion Web site featuring direct links to more than 450 selected Web sites
- Inexpensive

INTENDED AUDIENCE

House officers and medical students will find the concise, up-to-date descriptions of diagnostic and therapeutic procedures, with citations to the current literature, of daily usefulness in the care of patients.

Internists, family physicians, and other specialists who provide generalist care will appreciate CMDT as a ready reference and refresher text.

Physicians in other specialties, surgeons, and dentists will find the book a basic internal medicine reference.

Nurses, nurse practitioners, physician's assistants, and other health providers will welcome the concise format and broad scope of the book as a primary means of learning diagnostic principles and therapeutic procedures.

SPECIAL TO THIS EDITION

- New chapter on alternative medicine and complementary therapies
- New information on diagnosis and management of ischemic heart disease and pharmacologic treatment of congestive heart failure; separate chapter devoted to end-of-life care and end-of-life care information integrated throughout the text
- New recommendations for screening for gestational diabetes mellitus
- Up-to-date information regarding new dietary reference intakes and new drugs for obesity
- New developments in treatment of diabetes mellitus, asthma, and HIV infection
- Major revision of chapters on geriatric medicine, ear, nose and throat, the lung, the kidney, arthritis and musculoskeletal disorders, allergy-immunology, and information technology in patient care

- Drug information, bibliographies, and Web sites updated through June 2000
- An up-to-date chapter on HIV infection and approach to multidrug antiretroviral therapy
- An update on antibiotics
- Updated drug costs, including costs per unit dose and costs for 30 days of treatment
- Listing of key Internet addresses for peer-reviewed, current medical information, including:
  - Centers for Disease Control and Prevention traveler's and immunization information
  - National Institutes of Health Consensus Statements
  - The Agency for Health Care Quality of the United States Public Health Service Clinical Guidelines
  - Complete updated listing of USA Poison Control Centers with telephone numbers

COMPANION WEB SITE

CMDT's new companion Web site, Current-Med.com, contains additional information on the over 450 selected Internet sites referenced in the book. The Web site entries provide a brief description of each Internet site and rate them on a six-category scale. All linked Internet site addresses are updated monthly. The companion Web site address is now provided on the first page of each chapter in the book so that readers can access referenced Internet sites whose URLs have changed since publication.

ANNOUNCING *CMDT ON CD-ROM,* VERSION 2.0

In December 2000, a second version of *CMDT on CD-ROM* will be released. Besides the *CMDT 2001* text, the CD-ROM incorporates diagnostic test information from the *Pocket Guide to Diagnostic Tests,* 3rd edition, and drug information from the *Pocket Guide to Commonly Prescribed Drugs,* 3rd edition. Photographs of pills and capsules are also included. The *CMDT* CD-ROM incorporates a wide variety of multimedia illustrations, including color photographs, photomicrographs, electrocardiograms, echocardiograms, x-rays, and other diagnostic imaging procedures; graphs, algorithms, and nomograms; video footage of cardiac catheterizations, IUD insertions, and other procedures; heart sounds and lung sounds; patient education materials; and an extensive listing of Internet addresses for each chapter. Finally, links to MEDLINE abstracts are provided for all journal references in *CMDT*.

Visit your medical bookstore to purchase *CMDT on CD-ROM*, version 2.0. You may also return the enclosed postcard or call 1-800-262-4729.

ANNOUNCING ANNUAL SUBSCRIPTIONS TO *CMDT*

It is now possible to subscribe to the only annually updated textbook of medicine and its CD-ROM version simply by returning the enclosed postcards to McGraw-Hill. You will receive each annual edition of the text and/or CD-ROM automatically upon publication, and you will be billed when you are mailed your selection.

ACKNOWLEDGMENTS

We wish to thank our associate authors for participating once again in the annual updating of this important book. In particular, we wish to thank Dr. Ralph Gonzales of the University of Colorado Health Sciences Center for his editorial supervision of the CD-ROM project. Many students and physicians have contributed useful suggestions to this and previous editions, and we are grateful. We continue to welcome comments and recommendations for future editions in writing or via electronic mail. The editors' and authors' institutional and Internet e-mail addresses are given in the Authors section that follows.

Lawrence M. Tierney, Jr., MD
Stephen J. McPhee, MD
Maxine A. Papadakis, MD

San Francisco, California
September 2000

Bradly P. Jacobs, MD, MPH
Assistant Clinical Professor, Department of Medicine, and Medical Director, Clinical Programs, Osher Center for Integrative Medicine, University of California, San Francisco
Internet: bradlyj@itsa.ucsf.edu
Complementary & Alternative Medicine

Richard A. Jacobs, MD, PhD
Clinical Professor of Medicine and Clinical Pharmacy, University of California, San Francisco
Internet: jacobsd@medicine.ucsf.edu
General Problems in Infectious Diseases; Infectious Diseases: Spirochetal; Anti-infective Chemotherapeutic & Antibiotic Agents

C. Bree Johnston, MD, MPH
Assistant Clinical Professor of Geriatrics, Veterans Affairs Medical Center, San Francisco, California
Internet: bree526@itsa.ucsf.edu
Geriatric Medicine

Katherine Ann Julian, MD
Assistant Clinical Professor, University of California, San Francisco
Internet: kathyj@itsa.ucsf.edu
References

Michael J. Kaplan, MD
Associate Professor of Otolaryngology and Neurological Surgery, University of California, San Francisco
Internet: mjkaplan@orca.ucsf.edu
Ear, Nose & Throat

John H. Karam, MD
Professor of Medicine, Emeritus, University of California, San Francisco
Internet: bem69kar@aol.com
Diabetes Mellitus & Hypoglycemia

Mitchell H. Katz, MD
Associate Clinical Professor of Medicine, Epidemiology & Biostatistics, University of California, San Francisco; Director of Health, San Francisco Department of Public Health
Internet: mitch_katz@dph.sf.ca.us
HIV Infection

Jeffrey Lee Kishiyama, MD
Assistant Clinical Professor of Medicine, and Director, Clinical Allergy & Immunology, University of California, San Francisco
Internet: jkish@itsa.ucsf.edu
Allergic & Immunologic Disorders

Rick G. Kulkarni, MD
Resident, Harvard Affiliated Emergency Medicine Residency, Department of Emergency Medicine, Brigham & Women's Hospital, Harvard Medical School, Boston
Internet: kulkarni@secondvision.com
Information Technology in Patient Care: The Internet, Telemedicine, & Clinical Decision Support; Internet Resources

Kiyoshi Kurokawa, MD, MACP
Dean and Professor of Medicine, Tokai University School of Medicine, Isehara, Kanagawa, Japan
Internet: kurokawa@is.icc.u-tokai.ac.jp
Fluid & Electrolyte Disorders

Jonathan E. Lichtmacher, MD
Associate Director, Adult Psychiatry Clinic, Langley Porter Hospitals and Clinics, University of California, San Francisco
Internet: jonathanl@lppi.ucsf.edu
Psychistric Disorders

Charles A. Linker, MD
Clinical Professor of Medicine and Director, Adult Leukemia and Bone Marrow Transplantation Program, University of California, San Francisco
Internet: linkerc@medicine.ucsf.edu
Blood

William L. Lyons, MD
Assistant Clinical Professor, University of California, San Francisco
Internet: wlyons@itsa.ucsf.edu
Geriatric Medicine

H. Trent MacKay, MD, MPH
Associate Professor of Obstetrics and Gynecology, Uniformed Services, University of the Health Sciences, Bethesda, Maryland; Staff Physician, National Naval Medical Center, Bethesda, Maryland
Internet: mackayt@mail.nih.gov
Gynecology

Umesh Masharani, MB, BS, MRCP(UK)
Assistant Clinical Professor of Medicine, Department of Endocrinology and Metabolism, University of California, San Francisco
Internet: ubm@itsa.ucsf.edu
Diabetes Melitus & Hypoglycemia

Barry M. Massie, MD
Professor of Medicine, University of California, San Francisco; Chief, Cardiology Division, San Francisco Veterans Affairs Medical Center
Internet: barry.massie@med.va.gov
Heart; Systemic Hypertension

Stephen J. McPhee, MD
Professor of Medicine, Division of General Internal Medicine, Department of Medicine, University of California, San Francisco
Internet: smcphee@medicine.ucsf.edu
General Approach to the Patient; Health Maintenance & Disease Prevention; & Common Symptoms

Kenneth R. McQuaid, MD
Associate Professor of Clinical Medicine, University of California, San Francisco; Director of Gastrointestinal Endoscopy, San Francisco Veterans Affairs Medicine Center
Internet: krmcq@itsa.ucsf.edu
Alimentary Tract

Louis M. Messina, MD
Professor and Chief, Division of Vascular Surgery, Department of Surgery, University of California, San Francisco
Internet: messina@itsa.ucsf.edu
Blood Vessels & Lymphatics

Brent R. W. Moelleken, MD, FACS
Attending Surgeon, Plastic and Reconstructive Surgery, University of California, Los Angeles Medical Center; Private Practice, Beverly Hills, California
Internet: rijuv@aol.com
Disorders Due to Physical Agents

Gail Morrison, MD
Vice Dean for Education, Director of Academic Programs, and Professor of Medicine, School of Medicine, University of Pennsylvania, Philadelphia
Internet: morrisog@mail.med.upenn.edu
Kidney

C. Diana Nicoll, MD, PhD, MPA
Clinical Professor and Vice Chair, Department of Laboratory Medicine; Associate Dean, University of California, San Francisco; Chief of Staff and Chief, Laboratory Medicine Service, San Francisco Veterans Affairs Medical Center
Internet: nicoll.diana@sanfrancisco.va.gov
Diagnostic Testing & Medical Decision Making; Appendix: Therapeutic Drug Monitoring & Laboratory Reference Ranges

Kent R. Olson, MD
Clinical Professor of Medicine and Pharmacy, University of California, San Francisco; Medical Director, San Francisco Division, California Poison Control System, University of California, San Francisco
Internet: olson@itsa.ucsf.edu
Poisoning

Steven Z. Pantilat, MD
Assistant Clinical Professor of Medicine, University of California, San Francisco; Project on Death in America Faculty Scholar; Director, Comfort Care Suites and Attending Physician, Moffitt-Long Hospital, San Francisco
Internet: stevep@medicine.ucsf.edu
Care at the End of Life

Maxine A. Papadakis, MD
Professor of Clinical Medicine and Associate Dean for Student Affairs, School of Medicine, University of California, San Francisco
Internet: papadakm@medsch.ucsf.edu
Fluid & Electrolyte Disorders

Michael Pignone, MD, MPH
Assistant Professor of Medicine, University of North Carolina, Chapel Hill
Internet: pignone@med.unc.edu
Diagnostic Testing & Medical Decision-Making

William Plauth, MD
Medical Chief Resident, Moffitt-Long Hospital, San Francisco, California
Internet: wplauth@itsa.ucsf.edu
References

Thomas J. Prendergast, MD
Assistant Professor of Medicine, Dartmouth Medical School, Hanover, New Hampshire; Chief, Pulmonary Section, Veteran's Administration Medical Center, White River Junction, Vermont
Internet: thomas.j.prendergast@hitchcock.org
Lung

Joseph C. Presti, Jr., MD
Associate Professor; Director, Genitourinary Oncology Program, Department of Urology, Stanford University School of Medicine, Stanford, California
Internet: jpresti@stanford.edu
Urology

Reed E. Pyeritz, MD, PhD
Professor of Human Genetics, Medicine and Pediatrics, MCP Hahnemann University School of Medicine, Philadelphia
Internet: pyeritz@wpahs.org
Medical Genetics

Michael W. Rabow, MD
Assistant Clinical Professor of Medicine, Division of General Internal Medicine, University of California, San Francisco
Internet: mrabow@medicine.ucsf.edu
Care at the End of Life

Neil M. Resnick, MD
Professor of Medicine and Chief, Division of Geriatric Medicine, Univeristy of Pittsburgh, Pennsylvania
Internet: resnicknm@msx.dept-med.pitt.edu
Geriatric Medicine

Paul Riordan-Eva, FRCOphth
Consultant Ophthalmologist, King's College Hospital, London; Honorary Consultant Neuro-Ophthalmologist, National Hospital for Neurology and Neurosurgery, London, United Kingdom
Internet: paulreva@aol.com
Eye

Hope S. Rugo, MD
Associate Clinical Professor of Medicine, Comprehensive Cancer Center, University of California, San Francisco
Internet: hope.rugo@ucsfmedctr.org
Cancer

Steven A. Schroeder, MD
Clinical Professor of Medicine, University of Medicine and Dentistry of New Jersey, Robert Wood Johnson Medical School, New Brunswick; President and CEO, The Robert Wood Johnson Foundation, Princeton, New Jersey
Internet: ss@rwjf.org
General Approach to the Patient; Health Maintenance & Disease Prevention; & Common Symptoms

Wayne Xavier Shandera, MD
Assistant Professor of Internal Medicine, Baylor College of Medicine, Houston
Internet: shandera@bcm.tmc.edu
Infectious Diseases: Viral & Rickettsial

Marshall Leedy Stoller, MD
Professor, Department of Urology, University of California, San Francisco
Internet: mstoller@urol.ucsf.edu
Urology

John H. Stone, MD, MPH
Assistant Professor of Medicine, Division of Rheumatology, Johns Hopkins Hospital; Co-Director, Johns Hopkins Vasculitis Center, Baltimore
Internet: jstone@welch.jhu.edu
Arthritis & Musculoskeletal Disorders

Lawrence M. Tierney, Jr., MD
Professor of Medicine, University of California, San Francisco; Associate Chief of Medical Services, Veterans Affairs Medical Center, San Francisco
Internet: vaspa@itsa.ucsf.edu
Blood Vessels & Lymphatics

Paul D. Varosy, MD
Chief Resident, Department of Medicine, University of California, San Francisco
Internet: pvarosy@itsa.ucsf.edu
References

Daniel G. Vaughan, MD[†]
Clinical Professor of Ophthalmology, University of California, San Francisco; Governor, Francis I. Proctor Foundation for Research in Ophthalmology, San Francisco
Eye

Suzanne Watnick, MD
Nephrology Fellow, Yale University, Yale-New Haven Hospital, Connecticut
Internet: suzanne.watnick@yale.edu
Kidney

Jeffrey G. Wiese, MD
Assistant Clinical Professor of Medicine, University of California, San Francisco
Internet: jwieses@itsa.ucsf.edu
References

[†]Deceased

From inability to let alone; from too much zeal for the new and contempt for what is old; from putting knowledge before wisdom, and science before art and cleverness before common sense; from treating patients as cases; and from making the cure of the disease more grievous than the endurance of the same, Good Lord, deliver us.

—Sir Robert Hutchison

General Approach to the Patient; Health Maintenance & Disease Prevention; & Common Symptoms

1

See http://www.current-med.com/ch01.html for updated addresses of Web sites referenced in this chapter.

Stephen J. McPhee, MD, & Steven A. Schroeder, MD

GENERAL APPROACH TO THE PATIENT

The approach to diagnosis begins with the history and pertinent physical examination—both susceptible to errors of omission and commission. The medical interview serves three functions: to collect information, to respond to the patient's emotional state, and to educate the patient and influence patient behavior. Discussing psychosocial issues and forgoing clinician domination of the encounter increase patient satisfaction. Any diagnostic procedures ordered at this time should be chosen after consideration of the test characteristics (sensitivity and specificity), disease incidence and prevalence, potential risk, and cost-benefit profile (see Chapter 41). Successful treatment is reinforced by a confidently established and maintained doctor-patient relationship.

Patient Compliance

For many illnesses, treatment depends on fundamental behavioral changes—including alterations in diet, exercise, smoking, and drinking—which are difficult even for motivated patients. Compliance is a problem in every practice, with up to 50% of patients failing to achieve full compliance and a third never taking their medicines at all. Compliance rates for short-term, self-administered therapies are higher (about 75% initially) than for long-term therapies (< 25% for completion of antibiotic regimens). Compliance rates are inversely correlated with the number of interventions, their complexity and cost, and the patient's perception of overmedication.

Patients seem better able to recall instructions to take prescribed medications than to comply with recommendations to follow a diet, exercise regularly, or perform various self-care activities (such as monitoring blood glucose levels at home). Writing out advice to patients, including changes in medication, may be helpful. But where functional health illiteracy is endemic, over 40% of patients are unable to read and understand basic written instructions.

To help overcome noncompliance, clinicians can prescribe a simple dosage regimen for all medications (preferably one or two doses daily), help the patient devise cues to help in remembering to take doses (time of day, mealtime, alarms), provide ways to simplify dosing (medication boxes), and regularly monitor compliance. Single-unit doses supplied in foil-backed wrappers should be avoided for patients with difficulty opening them. Medication boxes with compartments (eg, Medisets) that are filled weekly by the patient, family member, or home health aid are useful. Microelectronic devices can provide feedback to show patients whether they have taken doses as scheduled or to notify patients within a day if doses are skipped.

Patient compliance is also improved when trusting doctor-patient relationships have been established. Clinicians can improve patient compliance by inquiring specifically about the behaviors in question and by reinforcement through family members. When asked, many patients admit to noncompliance with medication regimens, with advice about giving up cigarettes, or with engaging only in "safe sex" practices. The productivity requirements imposed by market pressures limit the time for individual patient encounters, but sufficient time must be made available for communication of health messages. Other direct ways of detecting medication noncompliance include pill counts and refill records; comparing dates on prescription labels with the number of pills remaining; monitoring serum, urine, or saliva levels of drugs or metabolites; or assessing predictable drug effects such as weight changes with diuretics or bradycardia from beta-blockers. Noncompliance is associated with a poorer prognosis. Even partial compliance, as with drug treatment of hypertension and diabetes mellitus, improves outcomes compared with noncompliance.

Guiding Principles

Ethical principles that guide the successful approach to diagnosis and treatment are honesty, beneficence, justice, avoidance of conflict of interest, and the pledge to do no harm. Increasingly, Western medicine involves patients in important decisions about medical care, including how far to proceed with treatment of patients with terminal illnesses (see Chapter 5).

The physician's role does not end with diagnosis and treatment. The importance of the empathic clinician in helping patients and their families bear the burden of serious illness and death cannot be overemphasized. "To cure sometimes, to relieve often, and to comfort always" is a French saying as apt today as it was five centuries ago—as is Francis Peabody's admonition: "The secret of the care of the patient is in caring for the patient."

Butler C et al: The practitioner, the patient and resistance to change: Recent ideas on compliance. Can Med Assoc J 1996;154:1357. [NLM Cit ID: 96208065] (Patients' resistance to change may stem partly from the way clinicians talk to them. The authors propose a patient-centered, negotiation-based framework that harnesses patients' intrinsic motivation to make their own decisions and promotes clinicians' acceptance of those decisions even if they run counter to current medical wisdom.)

Cramer JA: Enhancing patient compliance in the elderly. Role of packaging aids and monitoring. Drugs Aging 1998;12:7. [NLM Cit ID: 98128864] (Elderly patients are at risk of noncompliance because of common deficits in physical dexterity, cognitive skills and memory, and the number of medications they are typically prescribed.)

Roter DL et al: Effectiveness of interventions to improve patient compliance: A meta-analysis. Med Care 1998;36:1138. [NLM Cit ID: 98372293] (Comprehensive interventions combining cognitive, behavioral, and affective components were more effective than single-focus interventions.)

Wechsler H et al: The physician's role in health promotion revisited: A survey of primary care practitioners. N Engl J Med 1996;334:996. [NLM Cit ID: 96175227] (More clinicians now value and assume responsibility for health-promoting behaviors; notable exceptions are dietary counseling and available community resources.)

Williams MV et al: Inadequate functional health literacy among patients at two public hospitals. JAMA 1995;274:1677. [NLM Cit ID: 96088933] (High proportions of patients were unable to read and understand basic written instructions. Illiteracy was especially high among patients over 60 years of age [80%] and for Spanish-speaking patients [60%].)

HEALTH MAINTENANCE & DISEASE PREVENTION

Preventing disease is more important than treating it. Preventive medicine is categorized as primary, secondary, or tertiary. Primary prevention aims to remove or reduce disease risk factors (eg, immunization, giving up or not starting smoking). Secondary prevention techniques promote early detection of disease or precursor states (eg, routine cervical Papanicolaou screening to detect carcinoma of the cervix, or tuberculin skin testing to identify candidates for chemoprophylaxis of tuberculosis). Tertiary prevention measures are aimed at limiting the impact of established disease (eg, partial mastectomy and radiation therapy to remove and control localized breast cancer). Primary prevention is by far the most effective and economical; many clinicians are deficient in their counseling practices concerning preventable conditions.

Table 1–1 lists deaths from preventable causes in the USA—diseases which in 1990 accounted for 50% of all fatalities. These data will soon be updated and are expected to show the increased importance of obesity and inactivity. Clinicians can have a major role in reducing almost all of these risk factors.

Health maintenance and disease prevention usually begin with the office or clinic encounter. Table 1–2 compares and contrasts recommendations for periodic health examinations as developed by the United States Preventive Services Task Force, the American College of Physicians, and the Canadian Task Force on the Periodic Health Examination. Despite emerging consensus on many of the services, controversy persists for others.

[*Guide to Clinical Preventive Services,* 2nd ed]
http://158.72.20.10/pubs/guidecps/

Table 1–1. Deaths from preventable causes in the United States in 1990.[1]

Cause	Estimated Number of Deaths	Percentage of Total Deaths
Tobacco	400,000	19
Dietary factors and activity patterns	300,000	14
Alcohol	100,000	5
Microbial agents	90,000	4
Toxic agents	60,000	3
Firearms	35,000	2
High-risk sexual behavior	30,000	1
Motor vehicle injuries	25,000	1
Illicit use of drugs	20,000	< 1
TOTAL	1,060,000	≈50

[1]Reproduced, with permission, from McGinnis JM, Foege WH: Actual causes of death in the United States. JAMA 1993;270:2707.

Table 1–2. Expert recommendations for preventive care for asymptomatic, low-risk adults.

Preventive Service	United States Preventive Services Task Force			American College of Physicians			Canadian Task Force on the Periodic Health Examination		
	Sex	**Age**	**Minimum Frequency[1]**	**Sex**	**Age**	**Minimum Frequency**	**Sex**	**Age**	**Minimum Frequency[1]**
Physical examination									
Blood pressure	MF	18+	q 2 yrs	MF	18+	q 2 yrs	MF MF	25–64 65+	q 5 yrs q 2 yrs
Clinical breast examination	F	50–69[2]	q 1–2 yrs[3]	F	40+	Annually	F	50–69	Annually
Laboratory tests									
Papanicolaou smear	F	18[4]–65	q 3 yrs	F	20[4]–65[5]	q 3 yrs	F	18[4]–69	q 3 yrs[6]
Stool for occult blood	MF	50+	Annually	MF	50–70/80	Annually[7]	NR	NR	NR
Sigmoidoscopy	MF	50+	q ? yrs	MF	50–70	q 10 yrs	NR	NR	NR
Mammography	F	50–69[2]	q 1–2 yrs	F	50–75	q 2 yrs	F	50–69	Annually
Cholesterol	M F	35–65 45–65	q 5+ yrs	M F	35–65 45–65	Once	M	30–59	q ? yrs
Immunizations									
Tetanus-diphtheria booster	MF	18+	q 15–30 yrs	MF	18+	q 10 yrs or once at age 50	MF	18+	q 10 yrs
Influenza vaccination	MF	65+	Annually	MF	65+	Annually	MF	65+	Annually
Pneumococcal vaccination	MF	65+	Once[8]	MF	65+	Once[8]	NR	NR	NR
Counseling[9]	MF	18+	At routine visits	MF	18+	At routine visits	MF	18+	At routine visits

NR = no recommendation; ? = "periodic."
[1]Where question marks appear, the appropriate interval is left to clinical discretion because of lack of evidence.
[2]There is insufficient evidence to recommend for or against routine mammography or clinical breast examination for women age 40–49 or age ≥ 70, though recommendations for high-risk women in these age groups may be made on other grounds.
[3]Combined with mammography. There is insufficient evidence to recommend for or against clinical breast examination alone.
[4]Or following onset of sexual activity.
[5]There is insufficient evidence to recommend for or against an upper age limit for Papanicolaou testing after age 65 in women with regular previous normal smears.
[6]After two normal annual smears.
[7]For persons who decline screening sigmoidoscopy, barium enema, or colonoscopy.
[8]Reimmunize at age 65 those high-risk individuals who are 6 years or more after primary dose.
[9]Regarding tobacco use, nutrition, exercise, sexual behavior, substance abuse, injury prevention, and dental care.

Sox HC: Preventive health services in adults. N Engl J Med 1994;330:1589. [NLM Cit ID. 94232265]

US Preventive Services Task Force: *Guide to Clinical Preventive Services: A Report of the US Preventive Services Task Force,* 2nd ed. International Medical Publishing, 1997.

INFECTIOUS DISEASES

Much of the decline in the incidence and fatality rates of infectious diseases is attributable to public health measures—especially immunization, improved sanitation, and better nutrition.

Immunization remains the best means of preventing many infectious diseases. In the USA, immunization has contributed to an estimated 90% decline since 1900 in measles, mumps, rubella, poliomyelitis, diphtheria, pertussis, and tetanus. *Haemophilus influenzae* type b invasive disease has been reduced by more than 95% since introduction of the first conjugate vaccines. Opportunities still exist for reducing morbidity and mortality from vaccine-preventable diseases. For example, in adults in the USA, there are an estimated 50,000–70,000 deaths annually from influenza, hepatitis B, and invasive pneumococcal disease. Among targeted adult groups, only about 40% have had influenza vaccination, only 10% hepatitis B vaccination, and only 20% pneumococcal vaccination. The American College of Physicians recommends that clinicians should review each adult's immunization status at age 50; review risk factors that would indicate a need for pneumococcal vaccination and annual influenza immunizations; reimmunize at age 65 those who received an immunization against pneumococcus more than 6 years before; ensure that all adults have completed a primary diphtheria-tetanus immunization series, and administer a single booster at age 50; and assess the postvaccination serologic response to hepatitis B vaccination in all recipients who have ongoing risks of exposure to blood or body fluids (eg, sharp injuries, blood splashes).

Recommended immunization schedules for children and adults are set forth in Table 30–4. Persons traveling to countries where infections are endemic should take special precautions, as described in Chapter 30.

Skin testing for tuberculosis and then treating selected patients with isoniazid reduces the risk of reactivation tuberculosis (see Table 9–12). Attention to technique is particularly important for measurements close to the cutoff point separating negative from positive results. Drawing a skin line with a medium ballpoint pen, starting 1–2 cm away from the skin reaction and then stopping when resistance is felt, gives a more precise measurement of induration. Patients with HIV infection are at an especially high risk for tuberculosis. Approach to tuberculosis in HIV-infected patients is discussed in Chapter 31, as is the emerging concern about multidrug-resistant tuberculosis.

HIV infection is now the major infectious disease problem in the Western world. Since sexual contact is a common mode of transmission, prevention relies on eliminating unsafe sexual behavior by promoting abstinence, later onset of first sexual activity, decreased number of partners, and use of condoms. Appropriately used, condoms can reduce the rate of HIV transmission by nearly 70%. Couples who used condoms inconsistently had a considerable risk of infection: the rate of seroconversion was 4.8 per 100 persons per year, leading to an estimated cumulative incidence of 12.7% after 24 months. No seroconversions were noted with consistent condom use. Other approaches to prevent HIV infection include treatment of sexually transmitted diseases, behavioral interventions, development of vaginal microbicides, and vaccine development. Increasingly, cases of HIV infection are transmitted by intravenous drug use. HIV prevention activities should include provision of sterile injection equipment for these individuals.

Although live virus vaccines (such as MMR) are not generally recommended for immunocompromised patients, *asymptomatic* HIV-infected patients have not shown adverse consequences when given them. Thus, MMR and influenza vaccinations as well as tetanus, hepatitis B, *H influenzae* type b, and pneumococcal vaccinations should be given. However, if poliomyelitis immunization is required, the inactivated poliomyelitis vaccine is indicated. In *symptomatic* HIV-infected patients, live virus vaccines such as MMR should generally be avoided, but annual influenza vaccination is safe.

The last year for new reports of poliomyelitis cases in the Western Hemisphere was 1991. A goal has been established of worldwide eradication of poliomyelitis and dracunculiasis (dracontiasis; guinea worm disease) by the year 2000; if successful, their eradication will follow that of smallpox.

[Adult immunization schedule from the National Immunization Program of the CDC]
http://www.cdc.gov/nip/recs/adult-schedule.pdf

Coyle SL et al: Outreach-based HIV prevention for injecting drug users: A review of published outcome data. Public Health Rep 1998;113(Suppl 1):19. [NLM Cit ID: 98390031] (Outreach prevention programs can lead to lower HIV incidence rates among program participants.)

Des Jarlais DC et al: Maintaining low HIV seroprevalence in populations of injecting drug users. JAMA 1995; 274:1226. [NLM Cit ID: 96017572] (In low seroprevalence areas, early action and providing sterile injection equipment can limit transmission among intravenous drug users.)

Fingar AR et al: American College of Preventive Medicine Practice Policy Statement: Adult immunizations. Am J Prev Med 1998;14:156. [NLM Cit ID: 98294629]

Foege WH: Polio eradication—how near? (Editorial.) JAMA 1996;275:1682. [NLM Cit ID: 96245249] (The Pacific countries are now polio-free, but in more than 40 African countries, polio is still a public health problem.)

Marquardt D: Recommendations for immunizations in HIV-infected individuals. West J Med 1997;167:343. [NLM Cit ID: 98054693]

Pouchot J et al: Reliability of tuberculin skin test measurement. Ann Intern Med 1997;126:210. [NLM Cit ID: 97158930] (Ballpoint pen technique more reliable than palpation; readings close to cutoff point for positivity should be confirmed.)

Royce RA et al: Sexual transmission of HIV. N Engl J Med 1997;336:1072. [NLM Cit ID: 97224095]

Sisk JE et al: Cost-effectiveness of vaccination against pneumococcal bacteremia among elderly people. JAMA 1997;278:1333. [NLM Cit ID: 98001629] (Pneumococcal vaccination saves costs in prevention of bacteremia, yet is greatly underused among the elderly.)

CARDIOVASCULAR & CEREBROVASCULAR DISEASES

Impressive declines in age-specific mortality rates from heart disease and stroke have been achieved in all age groups in North America during the past 2 decades. The chief reasons for this favorable trend appear to be modification of risk factors, especially cigarette smoking and hypercholesterolemia, plus more aggressive detection and treatment of hypertension and heart disease.

Cigarette Smoking

Cigarette smoking remains the most important cause of preventable morbidity and early demise in developed countries. Nicotine is highly addictive and raises brain levels of dopamine. Brain changes during nicotine withdrawal are similar to those that occur during withdrawal from other drugs of abuse. Cigarettes are responsible for one in every five deaths in the USA, and even these figures underestimate the full hazards of tobacco. Alarmingly, smoking prevalence rates have been increasing among young people. For high school students it increased from 27% in 1991 to 40% in 1998; among college students, from 22% in 1993 to 25% in 1998. Recently, cigar smoking has also increased; there is also continued use of smokeless tobacco (chewing tobacco and snuff), particularly among young people. Tobacco dependence may have a genetic component. Racial differences in cotinine metabolism and intensity of nicotine uptake per cigarette result in black smokers having higher serum levels of cotinine—the principal metabolite of nicotine—than white smokers.

Smokers have twice the risk of fatal heart disease, ten times the risk of lung cancer, and several times the risk of cancers of the mouth, throat, esophagus, pancreas, kidney, bladder, and cervix; a two- to threefold higher incidence of stroke and peptic ulcers (which heal less well than in nonsmokers); a two- to fourfold greater risk of fractures of the hip, wrist, and vertebrae; four times the risk of invasive pneumococcal disease; and a twofold increase in developing cataracts. Both active and passive smoking are associated with deterioration of the elastic properties of the aorta and with progression of carotid artery atherosclerosis. Smoking has also been associated with increased risks of leukemia, of colon and prostate cancers, of breast cancer among postmenopausal women who are slow acetylators of *N*-acetyltransferase 2 enzymes, osteoporosis, and Alzheimer's disease. In cancers of the head and neck, lung, esophagus, and bladder, smoking is linked to mutations of the *P53* gene, the most common genetic change in human cancer. Patients with head and neck cancer who continue to smoke during radiation therapy have lower rates of response than those who do not smoke. Olfaction and taste are impaired in smokers, and facial wrinkles are increased. Diabetic patients who smoke may have an increased risk of proteinuria. Heavy smokers have a 2.5 greater risk of age-related macular degeneration. Smokers die 5–8 years earlier than never smokers.

The children of smokers have lower birth weights, are more likely to be mentally retarded, have more frequent respiratory infections, less efficient pulmonary function, and a higher incidence of chronic ear infections than children of nonsmokers and are more likely to become smokers themselves.

In addition, passive smoking by adults has been shown to increase the risk of cervical cancer, lung cancer, invasive pneumococcal disease, and heart disease, to promote endothelial damage and platelet aggregation, and to increase urinary excretion of tobacco-specific lung carcinogens. Of approximately 450,000 smoking-related deaths in the USA, as many as 53,000 are attributable to passive smoking.

Smoking cessation lessens the risks of death and of myocardial infarction in people with coronary artery disease; reduces the rate of death and acute myocardial infarction in patients who have undergone percutaneous coronary revascularization; lessens the risk of stroke; slows the rate of progression of carotid atherosclerosis; and is associated with reversal of chronic bronchitis and improved pulmonary function. Women smokers who quit smoking by age 35 add about 3 years to their life expectancy, and men more than 2 years to theirs. Smoking cessation can increase life expectancy even for those who stop after the age of 65.

The good news about cigarette smoking prevalence in the USA is that adult rates are now at an all-time low—23%. The bad news is that rates are climbing for young people, and for women more so than for men.

Although tobacco use constitutes the most serious common medical problem, access to effective treatment remains limited for most Americans. Over 70% of smokers see a physician each year, but only 20% of them receive any medical quitting advice or assistance. (Those whose physicians advise them to quit are 1.6 times as likely to attempt quitting.)

The five steps for helping smokers quit are summarized in Table 1–3. Common elements of supportive smoking cessation treatments are reviewed in Table 1–4. Most smokers who quit do so without recourse to nicotine replacement therapy, but guidelines for its use are summarized in Table 1–5. Suggestions for the nicotine patch are listed in Table 1–6 and for nicotine gum in Table 1–7. Both patch and gum are now available over-the-counter. Nicotine nasal spray is available by prescription. When the spray is combined with the use of the patch, cessation rates are substantially higher. The sustained-release antidepressant bupropion (150–300 mg/d) is an effective smoking cessation agent and is associated with minimal weight gain. It acts by boosting brain levels of dopamine and norepinephrine, mimicking the effect of nicotine. Bupropion, either alone or in combination with a nicotine patch, has been shown to produce significantly higher abstinence rates (30–35% at 1 year) than either a patch alone or placebo. Weight gain was less in the combined program.

Weight gain occurs in most patients (80%) following smoking cessation. For many it averages 2 kg, but for others (10–15%) major weight gain—over 13 kg—may occur.

Clinicians should not disapprove of patients who cannot stop smoking. Thoughtful admonition, family or social pressures, or the opportunity presented by an intercurrent illness such as acute bronchitis or acute myocardial infarction may enable even the most addicted smoker to quit or cut back. Such counseling is more cost-effective than treating hypertension. The clinician's role in smoking cessation is summarized in Table 1–4.

[AHCPR: Smoking Cessation]
http://text.nlm.nih.gov/ftrs/pick?dbName=smkc&ftrsK=43861&cp=1&t=928425611&collect=ahcpr

[CDC's Tobacco Information and Prevention Sourcepage]
http://www.cdc.gov/tobacco/index.htm

Ayanian JZ et al: Perceived risks of heart disease and cancer among cigarette smokers. JAMA 1999;281:1019. [NLM Cit ID: 99184241] (Only 29% and 40% of current smokers—respectively—believed they have a higher than average risk of myocardial infarction or cancer.)

Blonal T et al: Nicotine nasal spray with nicotine patch for

Table 1–3. Actions and strategies for the primary care clinician to help patients quit smoking.[1]

Action	Strategies for Implementation
	Step 1. Ask—Systematically Identify All Tobacco Users at Every Visit
Implement an officewide system that ensures that for *every* patient at *every* clinic visit, tobacco-use status is queried and documented[2]	Expand the vital signs to include tobacco use. Data should be collected by the health care team. The action should be implemented using preprinted progress note paper that includes the expanded vital signs, a vital signs stamp, or, for computerized records, an item assessing tobacco-use status. Alternatives to the vital signs stamp are to place tobacco-use status stickers on all patients' charts or to indicate smoking status using computerized reminder systems.
	Step 2. Advise—Strongly Urge All Smokers to Quit
In a *clear, strong,* and *personalized* manner, urge every smoker to quit	Advice should be *Clear:* "I think it is important for you to quit smoking now, and I will help you. Cutting down while you are ill is not enough." *Strong:* "As your clinician, I need you to know that quitting smoking is the most important thing you can do to protect your current and future health." *Personalized:* Tie smoking to current health or illness and/or the social and economic costs of tobacco use, motivational level/readiness to quit, and the impact of smoking on children and others in the household. Encourage clinic staff to reinforce the cessation message and support the patient's quit attempt.
	Step 3. Attempt—Identify Smokers Willing to Make a Quit Attempt
Ask every smoker if he or she is willing to make a quit attempt at this time	If the patient is willing to make a quit attempt at this time, provide assistance (see step 4). If the patient prefers a more intensive treatment or the clinician believes more intensive treatment is appropriate, refer the patient to interventions administered by a smoking cessation specialist and follow up with him or her regarding quitting (see step 5). If the patient clearly states he or she is not willing to make a quit attempt at this time, provide a motivational intervention.
	Step 4. Assist—Aid the Patient in Quitting
A. Help the patient with a quit plan	*Set a quit date.* Ideally, the quit date should be within 2 weeks, taking patient preference into account. *Help the patient prepare for quitting:* The patient must *Inform* family, friends, and coworkers of quitting and request understanding and support. *Prepare the environment* by removing cigarettes from it. Prior to quitting, the patient should avoid smoking in places where he or she spends a lot of time (eg, home, car). *Review* previous quit attempts. What helped? What led to relapse? *Anticipate* challenges to the planned quit attempt, particularly during the critical first few weeks.
B. Encourage nicotine replacement therapy except in special circumstances	Encourage the use of the nicotine patch or nicotine gum therapy for smoking cessation (see Tables 1–5 to 1–7 for specific instructions and precautions).
C. Give key advice on successful quitting	*Abstinence:* Total abstinence is essential. Not even a single puff after the quit date. *Alcohol:* Drinking alcohol is highly associated with relapse. Those who stop smoking should review their alcohol use and consider limiting or abstaining from alcohol use during the quit process. *Other smokers in the household:* The presence of other smokers in the household, particularly a spouse, is associated with lower success rates. Patients should consider quitting with their significant others and/or developing specific plans to maintain abstinence in a household where others still smoke.
D. Provide supplementary materials	*Source:* Federal agencies, including the National Cancer Institute and the Agency for Health Care Policy and Research; nonprofit agencies (American Cancer Society, American Lung Association, American Heart Association); or local or state health departments. *Selection concerns:* The material must be culturally, racially, educationally, and age appropriate for the patient. *Location:* Readily available in every clinic office.
	Step 5. Arrange—Schedule Follow-Up Contact
Schedule follow-up contact, either in person or via telephone[2]	*Timing:* Follow-up contact should occur soon after the quit date, preferably during the first week. A second follow-up contact is recommended within the first month. Schedule further follow-up contacts as indicated. *Actions during follow-up:* Congratulate success. If smoking occurred, review the circumstances and elicit recommitment to total abstinence. Remind the patient that a lapse can be used as a learning experience and is not a sign of failure. Identify the problems already encountered and anticipate challenges in the immediate future. Assess nicotine replacement therapy use and problems. Consider referral to a more intense or specialized program.

[1]Modified and reproduced, with permission, from: The Agency for Health Care Policy and Research. *Smoking Cessation Clinical Practice Guideline.* JAMA 1996;275:1270.

[2]Repeated assessment is not necessary in the case of the adult who has never smoked or not smoked for many years and for whom the information is clearly documented in the medical record.

Table 1–4. Common elements of supportive smoking treatments.[1]

Component	Examples
Encouragement of the patient in the quit attempt	Note that effective cessation treatments are now available. Note that half the people who have *ever* smoked have now quit. Communicate belief in the patient's ability to quit.
Communication of caring and concern	Ask how the patient feels about quitting. Directly express concern and a willingness to help. Be open to the patient's expression of fears of quitting, difficulties experienced, and ambivalent feelings.
Encouragement of the patient to talk about the quitting process	Ask about Reasons that the patient wants to quit. Difficulties encountered while quitting. Success the patient has achieved. Concerns or worries about quitting.
Provision of basic information about smoking and successful quitting	Inform the patient about The nature and time course of withdrawal. The addictive nature of smoking. The fact that any smoking (even a single puff) increases the likelihood of full relapse.

[1]Modified, with permission, from: The Agency for Health Care Policy and Research. *Smoking Cessation Clinical Practice Guideline.* JAMA 1996;275:1270.

Table 1–5. Clinical guidelines for prescribing nicotine replacement products.[1]

1. Who should receive nicotine replacement therapy?

Available research shows that nicotine replacement therapy generally increases rates of smoking cessation. Therefore, except in special circumstances, the clinician should encourage the use of nicotine replacement with patients who smoke. Little research is available on the use of nicotine replacement with light smokers (ie, those smoking ≤ 10–15 cigarettes/d). If nicotine replacement is to be used with light smokers, a lower starting dose of the nicotine patch or nicotine gum should be considered.

2. Should nicotine replacement therapy be tailored to the individual smoker?

Research does not support the tailoring of nicotine patch therapy (except with light smokers as noted above). Patients should be prescribed the patch dosages outlined in Table 1–6.

Research supports tailoring nicotine gum treatment. Specifically, research suggests that 4-mg gum rather than 2-mg gum be used with patients who are highly dependent on nicotine (eg, those smoking > 20 cigarettes/d, those who smoke immediately upon awakening, and those who report histories of severe nicotine withdrawal symptoms). Clinicians may also recommend the higher gum dose if patients request it or have failed to quit using the 2-mg gum.

3. Should patients be encouraged to use the nicotine patch or nicotine gum?

While both pharmacotherapies are efficacious, panel opinion is that nicotine patch therapy is preferable for routine clinical use. This preference is based on the following comparisons with nicotine gum therapy:

Nicotine patch therapy is associated with fewer compliance problems that interfere with effective use.

Nicotine patch therapy requires less clinician time and effort to train patients in its effective use.

The following factors would support the use of nicotine gum:

Patient preference.

Previous failure with the nicotine patch.

Contraindications specific to nicotine patch use (eg, severe skin reactions).

[1]Reproduced, with permission, from: The Agency for Health Care Policy and Research. *Smoking Cessation Clinical Practice Guideline.* JAMA 1996;275:1270.

smoking cessation: Randomized trial with six year follow-up. BMJ 1999;318:285. [NLM Cit ID: 99122873] (Patch plus spray better than patch alone.)

Hasdai D et al: Effect of smoking status on the long-term outcome after successful percutaneous coronary revascularization. N Engl J Med 1997;336:775. [NLM Cit ID: 97201368] (Patients who continued to smoke after successful revascularization were at greater risk for Q wave infarction and death than nonsmokers.)

Howard G et al: Cigarette smoking and progression of atherosclerosis. JAMA 1998;279:119. [NLM Cit ID: 98101611] (Active smoking, former smoking, and environmental tobacco smoke exposure are associated with accelerated irreversible carotid artery thickening.)

Hughes JR et al: Recent advances in the pharmacotherapy of smoking. JAMA 1999;281:72. [NLM Cit ID: 99107472] (Reviews nicotine gum and patch, nicotine nasal spray, nicotine inhaler, and bupropion.)

Hurt RD et al: A comparison of sustained-release bupropion and placebo for smoking cessation. N Engl J Med 1997;337:1195. [NLM Cit ID: 97465738] (Bupropion effective for smoking cessation and accompanied by reduced weight gain and minimal side effects.)

JAMA patient page: Secondhand smoke. JAMA 1998; 280:1968. [NLM Cit ID: 99066812]

Jorenby DE et al: A controlled trial of sustained-release bupropion, a nicotine patch, or both for smoking cessation. N Engl J Med 1999;340:685. [NLM Cit ID: 99150066] (Abstinence rates were 36% in the combined therapy group, 31% in the bupropion group, 16% in the nicotine patch group, and 16% in the placebo group. Weight gain at 7 weeks was significantly less in the combined-treatment group.)

Perez-Stable EJ et al: Nicotine metabolism and intake in black and white smokers. JAMA 1998;280:152. [NLM Cit ID: 98332451] (Slower metabolic clearance of cotinine and higher intake of nicotine per cigarette in blacks.)

Seidman DF et al: *Helping the Hardcore Smoker: A Clinician's Guide.* Lawrence Erlbaum Publishers, 1999.

Smoking Cessation Clinical Practice Guidelines Panel and Staff: The Agency for Health Care Policy and Research Smoking Cessation Guidelines. JAMA 1996;275:1270. [NLM Cit ID: 96186456] (Best single resource about smoking cessation.)

Stefanadis C et al: Unfavorable effects of passive smoking on aortic function in men. Ann Intern Med 1998;

Table 1–6. Suggestions for the clinical use of the nicotine patch.[1]

Parameter of Clinical Use	Suggestions
Patient selection	Appropriate as a primary pharmacotherapy for smoking cessation.
Precautions	*Pregnancy:* Pregnant smokers should first be encouraged to attempt cessation without pharmacologic treatment. The nicotine patch should be used during pregnancy only if the increased likelihood of smoking cessation, with its potential benefits, outweighs the risk of nicotine replacement and potential concomitant smoking. Similar factors should be considered in lactating women. *Cardiovascular diseases:* While not an independent risk factor for acute myocardial events, the nicotine patch should be used only after consideration of risks and benefits among particular cardiovascular patient groups: those in the immediate (within 4 weeks) post-myocardial infarction period, those with serious arrhythmias, and those with severe or worsening angina pectoris. *Skin reactions:* Up to 50% of patients using the nicotine patch will have a local skin reaction. Skin reactions are usually mild and self-limiting but may worsen over the course of therapy. Local treatment with hydrocortisone cream (2.5%) or triamcinolone cream (0.5%) and rotating patch sites may ameliorate such local reactions. In fewer than 5% of patients do such reactions require the discontinuation of nicotine patch treatment.
Dosage[2]	Treatment of 8 weeks or less has been shown to be as efficacious as longer treatment periods. Based on this finding, we suggest the following treatment schedules as reasonable for most smokers. Clinicians should consult the package insert for other treatment suggestions. Finally, clinicians should consider individualizing treatment based on specific patient characteristics such as previous experience with the patch, number of cigarettes smoked, and degree of addiction.
Prescribing instructions	Abstinence from smoking: The patient should refrain from smoking while using the patch. Location: At the start of each day, the patient should place a new patch on a relatively hairless location between the neck and the waist. Activities: There are no restrictions while using the patch. Time: Patches should be applied as soon as patients awaken on their quit day.

Brand	Duration (weeks)	Dosage (mg/h)
Nicoderm and Habitrol	4 then 2 then 2	21/24 14/24 7/24
Prostep	4 then 4	22/24 11/24
Nicotrol	4 then 2 then 2	15/16 10/16 5/16

[1]Reproduced, with permission, from: The Agency for Health Care Policy and Research. *Smoking Cessation Clinical Practice Guideline.* JAMA 1996;275:1270.
[2]These dosage recommendations are based on a review of the published research literature and do not necessarily conform to package insert information.

128:426. [NLM Cit ID: 98156406] (In a laboratory setting with human subjects, both passive and active smoking were associated with acute deterioration in the elastic properties of the aorta.)

Werner RM et al: What's so passive about passive smoking? Secondhand smoke as a cause of atherosclerotic disease. (Editorial.) JAMA 1998;279:157. [NLM Cit ID: 98101618] (One-third as much atherosclerotic progression as active smoking.)

Hypercholesterolemia

Serum cholesterol levels in the United States have declined impressively during the past 3 decades. Lowering elevated LDL cholesterol concentrations and raising low HDL levels reduce the risk from coronary heart disease, particularly in middle-aged men. Elevated plasma lipoprotein(a) is an independent risk factor for premature coronary heart disease in men but is not yet available as a routine test. Increases in life expectancy from modest decreases in blood cholesterol are low, especially in the absence of other risk factors such as smoking and hypertension. Screening and treatment for hypercholesterolemia may not be appropriate for older patients unless there is clinical evidence of atherosclerosis or other risk factors for death due to coronary heart disease. For high-risk patients, such as those with myocardial infarction or men with definite hypercholesterolemia, benefits from lowering cholesterol levels are greater.

Compliance with statin-type drugs is better than for the other classes of lipid-lowering agents. Statins

Table 1–7. Suggestions for the clinical use of nicotine gum.[1]

Parameter of Clinical Use	Suggestions
Patient selection	Appropriate as a primary pharmacotherapy for smoking cessation.
Precautions	*Pregnancy:* Pregnant smokers should first be encouraged to attempt cessation without pharmacologic treatment. Nicotine gum should be used during pregnancy only if the increased likelihood of smoking cessation, with its potential benefits, outweighs the risk of nicotine replacement and potential concomitant smoking. *Cardiovascular diseases:* Although not an independent risk factor for acute myocardial events, nicotine gum should be used only after consideration of risks and benefits among particular cardiovascular patient groups: those in the immediate (within 4 weeks) post-myocardial infarction period, those with serious arrhythmias, and those with serious or worsening angina pectoris. *Adverse effects:* Common adverse effects of nicotine chewing gum include mouth soreness, hiccups, dyspepsia, and jaw ache. These effects are generally mild and transient and can often be alleviated by correcting the patient's chewing technique (see "Prescribing instructions" below).
Dosage	*Dosage:* Nicotine gum is available in doses of 2 mg and 4 mg per piece. Patients should be prescribed the 2-mg gum initially. The 4-mg gum should be prescribed to patients who express a preference for it, have failed with the 2-mg gum but remain motivated to quit, and/or are highly dependent on nicotine. The gum is most commonly prescribed for the first few months of a quit attempt. Clinicians should tailor the duration of therapy to fit the needs of each patient. Patients using the 2-mg strength should use not more than 30 pieces per day, whereas those using the 4-mg strength should not exceed 20 pieces per day.
Prescribing instructions	*Abstinence from smoking:* The patient should refrain from smoking while using the gum. *Chewing technique:* The gum should be chewed slowly until a "peppery" taste emerges, then "parked" between cheek and gum to facilitate nicotine absorption through the oral mucosa. Gum should be slowly and intermittently chewed and parked for about 30 minutes. *Absorption:* Acidic beverages (eg, coffee, juices, soft drinks) interfere with the buccal absorption of nicotine, so eating and drinking anything except water should be avoided for 15 minutes before and during chewing. *Scheduling of dose:* A common problem is that patients do not use enough gum to get the maximum benefit: they chew too few pieces per day and do not use the gum for a sufficient number of weeks. Instructions to chew the gum on a fixed schedule (at least 1 piece every 1 to 2 hours) for at least 1 to 3 months may be more beneficial than ad lib use.

[1]Reproduced, with permission, from: The Agency for Health Care Policy and Research. *Smoking Cessation Clinical Practice Guideline.* JAMA 1996;275:1270.

appear to reduce the risk of stroke. In postmenopausal women with significant hypercholesterolemia, therapy with estrogen plus progestin has beneficial effects on lipoprotein levels—though somewhat less than statin therapy.

Guidelines for therapy are discussed in Chapter 28.

American College of Physicians: Guidelines for using serum cholesterol, high density lipoprotein cholesterol, and triglyceride levels as screening tests for preventing coronary heart disease in adults. Ann Intern Med 1996;124:515. [NLM Cit ID: 96169954] (Relatively conservative screening recommendations for primary prevention.)

Darling GM et al: Estrogen and progestin compared with simvastatin for hypercholesterolemia in postmenopausal women. N Engl J Med 1997;337:595. [NLM Cit ID: 97398283]

Hebert PR et al: Cholesterol lowering with statin drugs, risk of stroke, and total mortality: An overview of randomized trials. JAMA 1997;278:313. [NLM Cit ID: 97372174] (Patients given statin drugs had significant reductions in risk of stroke of 29%, cardiovascular disease deaths of 28%, and total mortality of 22%.)

JAMA patient page: Cholesterol. JAMA 1999;281:206. [NLM Cit ID: 99114164]

Shepherd J et al: Prevention of coronary heart disease with pravastatin in men with hypercholesterolemia. N Engl J Med 1995;333:1302. [NLM Cit ID: 96036646] (Coronary events, including fatal and nonfatal acute myocardial infarctions, were significantly less in the treatment group, and noncardiovascular deaths were not increased. Total and LDL cholesterol were both reduced.)

Woolf SH: The need for perspective in evidence-based medicine. JAMA 1999;282:2358. [NLM Cit ID:20077574] (Makes the case that primary prevention is more effective than treatment for cardiovascular disease.)

Hyperhomocysteinemia

Elevated plasma homocysteine may be a significant independent factor for coronary artery disease and imparts a risk similar to cigarette smoking or hyperlipidemia. It responds to treatment with folate and pyridoxine.

Bots ML et al: Homocysteine and short-term risk of myocardial infarction and stroke in the elderly: the Rotterdam Study. Arch Intern Med 1998;159:38. [NLM Cit ID: 99107346] (The risk of stroke and myocardial infarction increased by 6–7% for every 1 μmol/L increase in total plasma homocysteine.)

Folsom AR et al: Prospective study of coronary heart disease incidence in relation to fasting total homocysteine, related genetic polymorphisms, and B vitamins: the Atherosclerosis Risk in Communities (ARIC) study. Circulation 1998;98:204. [NLM Cit ID: 98361284] (Disputes the view that elevated plasma total homocysteine is a major independent causative risk factor for coronary heart disease.)

Wald NJ et al: Homocysteine and ischemic heart disease: results of a prospective study with implications regarding prevention. Arch Intern Med 1998;158:862. [NLM Cit ID: 98230096] (Serum homocysteine levels were significantly higher in men who died of ischemic heart disease than in men who did not, with risk increasing by 41% for each 5 μmol/L increase in the serum homocysteine level.)

Hypertension

Over 50 million adults in the USA have hypertension. In every adult age group—including those over 70 years old—higher values of systolic and diastolic blood pressure carry greater risks of stroke and congestive heart failure. Systolic blood pressure is a better predictor of morbid events than is diastolic blood pressure. Clinicians can apply specific blood pressure criteria, such as those of the Joint National Committee, to decide at what levels treatment should be considered in individual cases. Table 11–1 presents a classification of hypertension based on blood pressures. Primary prevention of hypertension can be accomplished by intervention strategies aimed at both the general population and special, high-risk populations. The latter include persons with high-normal blood pressure or a family history of hypertension, blacks, and individuals with various behavioral risk factors such as physical inactivity; excessive consumption of salt, alcohol, or calories; and deficient intake of potassium. Effective interventions for primary prevention of hypertension include reduced sodium and alcohol consumption, weight loss, and regular exercise. Interventions of unproved efficacy include pill supplementation of potassium, calcium, magnesium, fish oil, or fiber, macronutrient alteration, and stress management. A major cause of the recent impressive decline in stroke deaths has been improved diagnosis and treatment of hypertension. Diets rich in fruits and vegetables may also protect against stroke. Pharmacologic management of hypertension is discussed in Chapter 11.

Andersson OK et al: Survival in treated hypertension: follow up study after two decades. BMJ 1998;317:167. [NLM Cit ID: 98332662] (Treated hypertensive men had reduced overall survival and increased mortality from cardiovascular disease compared with nonhypertensive men of similar age.)

Perry HM Jr et al: Antihypertensive efficacy of treatment regimens used in Veterans Administration hypertension clinics. Department of Veterans Affairs Cooperative Study Group on Antihypertensive Agents. Hypertension 1998;31:771. [NLM Cit ID: 98154648] (The regimens of diuretic or diuretic plus beta-blocker gave the lowest average pressures and calcium antagonist the highest.)

Chemoprevention

As discussed in Chapters 10 and 24, aspirin is useful for the primary and secondary prevention of acute myocardial infarction and stroke. Tamoxifen as chemoprevention of breast cancer is discussed in Chapters 4 and 16. Fruit and vegetable consumption lowers the risk of ischemic stroke.

PHYSICAL INACTIVITY & SEDENTARY LIFESTYLE

Dietary factors and the lack of sufficient physical activity are the second most important contributors to preventable deaths, trailing only tobacco use. A sedentary lifestyle has been linked to 28% of deaths from leading chronic diseases. The CDC has recommended that every adult in the United States should engage in 30 minutes or more of moderate-intensity physical activity on most days of the week. This new guideline complements previous advice urging at least 20–30 minutes of more vigorous aerobic exercise three to five times a week.

Regular moderate to vigorous exercise lowers the risk of myocardial infarction, stroke, hypertension, type 2 diabetes mellitus, diverticular disease, and osteoporosis. The benefits of exercise appear to be dose-dependent, with a major difference in benefit between no and mild to moderate exercise and a smaller difference in benefit between moderate and vigorous exercise. The relative risk of stroke was found to be less than one-sixth in men who exercised vigorously compared with those who were inactive; the risk of type 2 diabetes mellitus was about half among men who exercised five or more times weekly compared with those who exercised once a week. Glucose control is improved in diabetics who exercise regularly, even at a modest level. Regular exercise is associated with a lower long-term risk of coronary events, including fatal myocardial infarctions; with elevated HDL cholesterol concentrations in both men and women; with improved coronary and endothelial and smooth muscle function; and with a decreased risk of hypertension. In older nonsmoking men, walking 2 miles per day or more is associated with an almost 50% reduction in overall mortality. Physical activity reduces the risk of colon cancer (though not rectal cancer) in men and women and of breast and reproductive organ cancer in women. Finally, weight-bearing exercise increases bone mineral content and retards development of osteoporosis in women.

Exercise may also confer benefits on those with chronic illness. Men and women with chronic symptomatic osteoarthritis of one or both knees benefited from a supervised walking program, with improved self-reported functional status and decreased use of pain medication. Exercise produces sustained lowering of both systolic and diastolic blood pressure in patients with mild hypertension. In addition, it can help patients maintain ideal body weight, and the risk of myocardial infarction is estimated to be 35–55% lower for individuals who maintain ideal body weight compared with those who are obese. Physical activity reduces depression and anxiety, improves adaptation to stress, improves sleep quality, and enhances mood, self-esteem, and overall performance.

However, physical exertion can also trigger the onset of acute myocardial infarction, particularly in persons who are habitually sedentary. The risk of infarction is considerably less among those reporting regular (at least five times per week), heavy physical exertion. Other potential complications of exercise include angina pectoris, arrhythmias, sudden death, and asthma. In insulin-requiring diabetics who undertake vigorous exercise, blood glucose levels should be carefully monitored to prevent hypoglycemia.

Only about 20% of adults in the USA are active at the moderate level—and only 8% currently exercise at the more vigorous level—recommended for health benefits. Instead, 60% report irregular or no leisure time physical activity. Generally, men are more active than women. Activity levels seem to increase with income and education and to decrease with age.

Clinicians should advise patients about the benefits and risks of exercise, prescribe an exercise program appropriate for each patient, and provide advice that will help to prevent injuries or complications. The value of routine electrocardiography or exercise electrocardiography remains controversial. Healthy individuals can exercise without supervision, but patients with ischemic heart disease or other cardiovascular disease require medically supervised, graded exercise programs. Exercise should not be prescribed for patients with decompensated congestive heart failure, complex ventricular arrhythmias, unstable angina pectoris, hemodynamically significant aortic stenosis, aortic aneurysm, or uncontrolled diabetes mellitus. Five- to 10-minute warm-up and cool-down periods, stretching exercises, and gradual increases in exercise intensity help to prevent musculoskeletal and cardiovascular complications.

Clinicians should educate their patients to understand that physical activity is something that can be incorporated into the daily routine. In fact, such "lifestyle" physical activity programs confer comparable benefits to more traditional structured programs—as measured by actual activity levels, fitness, body composition, and improvement in cardiovascular risk factors. For example, the clinician can advise the patient to take the stairs instead of the elevator, to walk or bike instead of driving, to do housework or yard work, to get off the bus one or two stops earlier and walk the rest of the way, to park at the far end of the parking lot, or to walk during the lunch hour. Table 29–2 shows energy expenditures of selected physical activities. The basic message must be: the more the better, and anything is better than nothing.

[Physical Activity and Health: A Report of the Surgeon General]
http://www.cdc.gov/nccdphp/sgr/sgr.htm

Blair SN et al: Influences of cardiorespiratory fitness and other precursors on cardiovascular disease and all-cause mortality in men and women. JAMA 1996;276:205. [NLM Cit ID: 96290594] (Highly and moderately fit persons had lower adjusted mortality rates than those with low fitness regardless of smoking status, systolic blood pressure, serum cholesterol, and general health.)

Dunn AL et al: Comparison of lifestyle and structured interventions to increase physical activity and cardiorespiratory fitness: A randomized trial. JAMA 1999;281:327. [NLM Cit ID: 99126165] (In previously sedentary healthy adults, a lifestyle of physical activity intervention is as effective as a structured exercise program in improving energy expenditure, cardiorespiratory fitness, and blood pressure.)

Ettinger WH et al: A randomized trial comparing aerobic exercise and resistance training to a health education program on physical disability in older adults with knee osteoarthritis. JAMA 1997;277:25. [NLM Cit ID: 97134646] (Exercise has beneficial but modest effect on pain, physical performance, and disability.)

Hakim AA et al: Effects of walking on mortality among nonsmoking retired men. N Engl J Med 1998;338:94. [NLM Cit ID: 98069967] (After adjusting for age, the mortality rate among men who walked more than 2 miles per day was almost half that of those who walked less than 1 mile.)

Hambrech R et al: Effect of exercise on coronary and endothelial function in patients with coronary artery disease. N Engl J Med 2000;342:454. [NLM Cit ID: 20125068]

Hu FB et al: Walking compared with vigorous physical activity and risk of type 2 diabetes in women. JAMA 1999;282:1433. [NLM Cit ID: 20004091] (Relative risk of developing type 2 diabetes was inversely proportionate to levels of activity even after adjusting for risk factors, including body mass index.)

JAMA patient page: Exercise. JAMA 1999;281:394. [NLM Cit ID: 99126177]

Kushi LH: Physical activity and mortality in postmenopausal women. JAMA 1997;277:1287. [NLM Cit ID: 97263551] (Among 40,417 postmenopausal women, those who reported regular physical activity had a significantly reduced risk of death at 7-year follow-up compared with women who did not [RR 0.77, 95% CI 0.66–0.90]. Increasing frequency of moderate exercise and of vigorous exercise were each associated with reduced risk of death.)

CANCER

Primary Prevention

Cigarette smoking is the most important preventable cause of cancer. Primary prevention of skin cancer consists of restricting exposure to ultraviolet light by wearing appropriate clothing and use of sunscreens. In the past 2 decades, there has been a threefold increase in the incidence of squamous cell carcinoma and a fourfold increase in melanoma in the United States. Regular physical exercise and avoidance of obesity has been associated with a significant reduction in breast and colon cancer risk. Prevention of occupationally induced cancers involves minimizing exposure to carcinogenic substances such as asbestos, ionizing radiation, and benzene compounds. Chemoprevention may be an important part of primary cancer prevention (see Chapter 4). For example, aspirin (in a dose as small as 325 mg four times weekly) and other NSAIDs (piroxicam, sulindac) may reduce the risk of colon cancer. Tamoxifen for breast cancer prevention is discussed in Chapters 4 and 16.

Secondary Prevention

Generally accepted techniques exist for secondary prevention of cancers of the breast, colon, and cervix through cancer screening procedures. Note that Table 1–8, derived from American Cancer Society guidelines, differs in many instances from the recommen-

Table 1–8. Screening for cancer: American Cancer Society (1999) guidelines for the early detection of cancer in people without symptoms.[1]

Test or Procedure	Sex	Age	Frequency
Sigmoidoscopy, flexible, or— Colonoscopy, or— Air contrast barium enema	MF	50 and over[2]	Every 5 years Every 10 years Every 5–10 years
Stool test for occult blood	MF	50 and over[2]	Every year
Digital rectal examination	MF	50 and over[2]	Every year
Prostate examination[3]	M	50 and over[4]	At the time of each screening sigmoidoscopy, colonoscopy, or barium enema
Papanicolaou test	F	Women who are or have been sexually active or have reached age 18 years	Annually until at least three consecutive satisfactory normal annual examinations, then less often at discretion of physician
Pelvic examination	F	18–40	Every 1–3 years with Papanicolaou test. Not indicated if cervix has been removed for a nonmalignant condition.
		Over 40	Every year
Endometrial tissue sample	F	At menopause; women at high risk[5]	At menopause and thereafter at the discretion of the physician
Breast self-examination	F	20 and over	Every month
Breast physical examination	F	20–40 40 and over	Every 3 years Every year
Mammography	F	40 and over	Every year
Health counseling and cancer checkup[6]	MF	Over 20 Over 40	Every 3 years Every year
Chest x-ray	Not recommended		
Sputum cytologic examination	Not recommended		

[1]From Update January 1992: The American Cancer Society Guidelines for the Cancer-Related Check-Up. CA Cancer J Clin 1992;42:44; and from the American Cancer Society 1999 update.

[2]People should begin colorectal cancer screening earlier or undergo screening more often (or both) if they have any of the following colorectal cancer risk factors: (1) a personal history of colorectal cancer or adenomatous polyps; (2) a strong family history of colorectal cancer or polyps (cancer or polyps in a first degree relative younger than 60 or in two first-degree relatives of any age); (3) families with hereditary colorectal cancer syndromes (familial adenomatous polyposis and hereditary nonpolyposis colon cancer).

[3]Digital rectal examination and serum prostate-specific antigen; if either is abnormal, further evaluation by transrectal ultrasound and biopsy as indicated.

[4]For men with ≥ 10-year life expectancy. Screening is recommended for younger men if at higher risk (blacks, strong family history of prostate cancer).

[5]History of infertility, obesity, failure of ovulation, abnormal uterine bleeding, or unopposed estrogen or tamoxifen therapy.

[6]To include examination for cancers of the thyroid, testicles, ovaries, lymph nodes, oral region, and skin.

dations of other authorities as shown previously in Table 1–2, which take a more conservative view of the efficacy of cancer screening maneuvers. For example, there is continuing controversy regarding the value of screening mammography for women aged 40–49, serum PSA testing for men, or fecal occult blood testing for men or women older than age 50. A federal consensus panel in 1997 was unable to agree on the advisability of routine mammography for women aged 40–49, leaving the decision instead to the discretion of individual patients and their clinicians. By contrast, the American Cancer Society mammography screening guidelines were changed to include annual mammograms for women in their 40s.

Single serum PSA measurements appear to offer relatively high sensitivity and specificity to detect prostate cancer. The sensitivity is about 67%, the specificity about 82%, and the positive predictive value for prostate cancer is about 43%. When both the digital rectal examination and serum PSA are abnormal, PSA specificity increases, but sensitivity falls (to 33%) and predictive value rises only slightly (to 49%). New tests that measure free PSA levels may yield greater specificity. Whether early detection and treatment alters the natural course of the disease remains to be seen. There are still no data on the morbidity and mortality benefits of such screening. Unlike the American College of Physicians, the American Cancer Society recommends annual PSA testing for men over age 50. Screening is not recommended for men who have estimated life expectancies of less than 10 years. Many clinicians remain ambivalent about recommending its routine use.

The risk of death from colon cancer among patients undergoing at least one sigmoidoscopic examination was reduced by 60–80% compared with that among those not having sigmoidoscopy. The finding of a 33% reduction in mortality rate from colorectal carcinoma in persons undertaking annual fecal occult blood testing (FOBT) has been more controversial. The predictive value of a positive FOBT was only 2.2%, and 38% of all patients screened underwent at least one follow-up colonoscopy during the 13-year study.

Screening for vaginal cancer with a Papanicolaou smear is not indicated in women who have undergone hysterectomies for benign disease with removal of the cervix.

Screening for other cancers in normal asymptomatic or even high-risk segments of the population is not recommended because adequate screening tests are not available.

[NCI: Physician's Data Query—Screening, Treatment, & Prevention Recommendations]
http://cancernet.nci.nih.gov/index.html

American College of Physicians: Screening for prostate cancer. Ann Intern Med 1997;126:480. [NLM Cit ID: 97208747] (Instead of routine screening, the ACP recommends that clinicians individualize the decision to screen.)

American College of Physicians: Suggested technique for fecal occult blood testing and interpretation in colorectal cancer screening: Clinical guideline: Part 1. Ann Intern Med 1997;126:808. [NLM Cit ID: 97282922]

Coley CM et al: Early detection of prostate cancer: Part II: estimating the risks, benefits, and costs. Ann Intern Med 1997;126:468. [NLM Cit ID: 97208746] (One-time digital rectal examination and PSA measurement may increase average life expectancy by approximately 2 weeks at a reasonable marginal cost for men aged 50–69.)

Elmore JG et al: Ten-year risk of false positive screening mammograms and clinical breast examinations. N Engl J Med 1998;338:1089. [NLM Cit ID: 98196615] (Over a 10-year period, one-third of women screened had a false-positive abnormal test result.)

Gabriel H et al: Breast cancer in women 65–74 years old: Earlier detection by mammographic screening. AJR Am J Roentgenol 1997;168:23. [NLM Cit ID: 97131261] (Screening revealed smaller and earlier stage tumors.)

Hartmann LC et al: Efficacy of bilateral prophylactic mastectomy in women with a family history of breast cancer. N Engl J Med 1999;340:77. [NLM Cit ID: 99091091] (Associated with a > 90% reduction in incidence of breast cancer in moderate-risk and high-risk women.)

Holmes MD et al: Association of dietary intake of fat and fatty acids with risk of breast cancer. JAMA 1999; 281:914. [NLM Cit ID: 99176374] (No evidence that lower intake of total fat or specific types of fat was associated with a decreased risk of breast cancer.)

Huang Z et al: Dual effects of weight and weight gain on breast cancer risk. JAMA 1997;278:1407. [NLM Cit ID: 98016075] (Avoiding weight gain may help prevent postmenopausal breast cancer, especially for women not receiving postmenopausal hormone replacement therapy.)

Kerlikowske K et al: Likelihood ratios for modern screening mammography: Risk of breast cancer based on age and mammographic interpretation. JAMA 1996;276:39. [NLM Cit ID: 96290398] (Based on the risk of breast cancer before mammography, which increases with age, the risk after mammography rose from 0.01 for ages 30–39 years to 0.05 for ages 50–59 years and to 0.07 for ages 70 years and older.)

Laya MB et al: Effect of estrogen replacement therapy on the specificity and sensitivity of screening mammography. J Natl Cancer Inst 1996;88:643. [NLM Cit ID: 96218816] (Current use of estrogen replacement therapy is associated with lower specificity and lower sensitivity of screening mammography.)

Muller AD et al: Prevention of colorectal cancer by flexible endoscopy and polypectomy: A case-control study of 32,702 veterans. Ann Intern Med 1995;123:904. [NLM Cit ID: 96072645] (Endoscopic polypectomies reduce the risk for colorectal cancer by 50% for periods lasting up to 6 years.)

Ransohoff DF et al: Screening for colorectal cancer with the fecal occult blood test: A background paper. Clinical guideline: Part II. Ann Intern Med 1997;126:811. [NLM Cit ID: 97282923] (Screening fecal occult blood tests are positive in 1–16% of cases depending on the age of the person being tested, whether the sample is rehydrated, and whether the test is used for initial screening or for rescreening. When persons who have positive test results are evaluated, colorectal cancer is found in about 2–17%. Early colorectal cancer [Dukes stage A or B] is found in about 2–14%.)

Read TE et al: Importance of adenomas 5 mm or less in diameter that are detected by sigmoidoscopy. N Engl J Med 1997;336:8. [NLM Cit ID: 97122456] (A substantial prevalence of proximal colonic neoplasms, including advanced lesions, in patients with rectosigmoid adenomas less than 5 mm in diameter justifies pancolonoscopy in these patients.)

Simon JB et al: Should all people over the age of 50 have regular fecal occult blood tests? N Engl J Med 1998;338:1151. [NLM Cit ID: 98196626] (Clinical debate.)

Smith-Warner SA et al: Alcohol and breast cancer in women: A pooled analysis of cohort studies. JAMA 1998;270:535. [NLM Cit ID: 98140734] (Breast cancer risk increases linearly with alcohol consumption.)

Thune I et al: Physical activity and the risk of breast cancer. N Engl J Med 1997;336;1269. [NLM Cit ID: 97258685] (Physical activity during leisure time and at work protects against breast cancer [RR 0.63]. Risk reduction was greater in younger [age under 45] than in older women.)

ACCIDENTS & VIOLENCE

Accidents remain the most important cause of loss of potential years of life before age 65 (Table 1–1), though there has been a steady decline in motor vehicle accident deaths per miles driven. Although seat belt use protects against serious injury and death in motor vehicle accidents, at least one-fourth of adults do not use seat belts routinely. Air bags are protective for adults but not for small children. In 1996, 64% of motorcyclists used helmets, an improvement from previous years. The rate approached 100% in states with helmet laws. In 1994 it was estimated that 20% of adults and 25% of children used bicycle helmets. The lowest rate—5%—was in the age group 18–24 years. Clinicians should try to educate their patients about seat belts, safety helmets, the risks of using cellular telephones while driving, drinking (or using other intoxicants or long-acting benzodiazepines) and driving, and the risks of having guns in the home. Chronic alcohol abuse adversely affects outcome from trauma and increases the risk of readmission for new trauma. Males aged 16–35 are at especially high risk for serious injury and death from accidents and violence, with blacks and Latinos at greatest risk. For 16- and 17-year-old drivers, the risk of fatal crashes increases with the number of passengers. Deaths from firearms have reached epidemic levels in the United States and will soon surpass in numbers deaths from motor vehicle accidents. Having a gun in the home increases the likelihood of homicide 2.7-fold and of suicide fivefold. Alcohol and illicit drug use are associated with an increased risk of violent death.

Finally, clinicians have a critical role in detection, prevention, and management of physical or sexual abuse—in particular, routine assessment of women for risk of domestic violence. Inclusion of a single question about domestic violence in the medical history—"At any time, has a partner ever hit you, kicked you, or otherwise physically hurt you?"—increased identification of this common problem from nil to 11.6%. Another screening device consists of three questions: (1) "Have you ever been hit, kicked, punched, or otherwise hurt by someone within the past year? If so, by whom?" (2) "Do you feel safe in your current relationship?" (3) "Is there a partner from a previous relationship who is making you feel unsafe now?" Use of these questions increased identification of domestic violence to 29.5% of women in an emergency department.

[National Center for Injury Prevention and Control] http://www.cdc.gov/ncipc/ncipchm.htm

Abbott J et al: Domestic violence against women: Incidence and prevalence in an emergency department population. JAMA 1995;273:1763. [NLM Cit ID: 95287569] (The incidence of acute domestic violence among 418 women with a current male partner was 11.7%; the cumulative lifetime prevalence of exposure to such violence was 54.2%.)

Chen LH et al: Carrying passengers as a risk factor for crashes fatal to 16- and 17-year-old drivers. JAMA 2000;283:1578. [NLM Cit ID: 20197441] (Risk steadily increases with increased number of passengers.)

Barrier PA: Domestic violence. Mayo Clin Proc 1998;73:271. [NLM Cit ID: 98172777]

Braver ER et al: Reductions in deaths in frontal crashes among right front passengers in vehicles equipped with passenger air bags. JAMA 1997;278:1437. [NLM Cit ID: 98016080] (Passenger air bags save lives of adults but not children; estimated reduction of fatality rates for adults was 18% for frontal crashes and 11% for all crashes.)

el-Bayoumi G et al: Domestic violence in women. Med Clin North Am 1998;82:391. [NLM Cit ID: 98193082]

Ferris LE et al: Guidelines for managing domestic abuse when male and female partners are patients of the same physician. JAMA 1997;278:851. [NLM Cit ID: 97438220]

Goodman P: Domestic violence resources on the Internet. JAMA 1998;280:477.

Hernmelgarn B et al: Use of long-half-life benzodiazepines in older persons was associated with increased risk for injurious motor vehicle accidents. JAMA 1997;278:27. [NLM Cit ID: 97350958]

JAMA patient page: Domestic violence. JAMA 1998;280:488. [NLM Cit ID: 98364820]

Lyznicki JM et al: Sleepiness, driving, and motor vehicle crashes. Council on Scientific Affairs, American Medical Association. JAMA 1998;279:1908. [NLM Cit ID: 98296021] (Driver sleepiness is a causative factor in at least 1–3% of all motor vehicle accidents in the United States.)

Reidelmeier DA et al: Association between cellular telephone calls and motor vehicle collisions. N Engl J Med 1997;336:453. [NLM Cit ID: 97160922] (Fourfold risk of a collision during the call period.)

Rivara FP et al: Alcohol and illicit drug abuse and the risk of violent death in the home. JAMA 1997;278:569. [NLM Cit ID: 97412165]

Rivara FP et al: Injury prevention. (Two parts.) N Engl J Med 1997;337:543, 613. [NLM Cit ID: 97398287] (Comprehensive review including magnitude of the problem, motor vehicle accidents, bicycling injuries, falls, poisoning, fires and scalding, drowning, injuries from firearms, and control strategies.)

Sherin KM et al: HITS: a short domestic violence screening tool for use in a family practice setting. Fam Med 1998;30:508. [NLM Cit ID: 98333771]

Teret SP et al: Support for new policies to regulate firearms. Results of two national surveys. N Engl J Med 1998;339:813. [NLM Cit ID: 98400649] (Strong public support, even among gun owners, for innovative strategies to regulate firearms, such as safety standards for new handguns, policies prohibiting gun sales to persons convicted of misdemeanors, and policies designed to reduce the illegal sale of guns.)

Thompson DC et al: Effectiveness of bicycle helmets in preventing head injuries: A case-control study. JAMA 1997;276:1968. [NLM Cit ID: 97126142] (Helmets provide substantial protection.)

SUBSTANCE ABUSE: ALCOHOL & ILLICIT DRUGS

Recent neurobiologic research emphasizes the common brain neurotransmitter changes following regular use of addictive substances such as alcohol, tobacco, and illicit drugs. Substance abuse is a major public health problem in the United States and is estimated to be a factor in 41% of highway fatality accidents. Approximately two-thirds of high school seniors are regular users of alcohol, and the lifetime prevalence of alcoholism is estimated to be between 12% and 16%. Underdiagnosis is substantial, both because of patient denial and lack of clinician alertness to historical and physical clues. The decline in alcohol-related traffic fatalities of 37% from 1982 to 1998 testifies to the success of educational and legal efforts to limit drinking and driving. Even so, alcohol-impaired driving remains prevalent, especially among men aged 18–34 years. Binge drinking among college students has recently increased.

As with cigarette use, clinician identification and counseling about alcoholism may improve the chances of recovery. Although about 10% of all adults seen in medical practices are problem drinkers, that fact is seldom recognized. An estimated 15–30% of hospitalized patients have problems with alcohol abuse or dependence, but the connection between patients' presenting complaints and their alcohol abuse is often missed. The CAGE test (see Table 1–9) is a simple screening test that is both sensitive and specific for chronic alcoholism. However, it is less sensitive in detecting heavy or binge drinking in elderly patients and has been criticized for being less applicable to minority groups or to women. Others recommend asking three questions: (1) How many days per week do you drink? (frequency.) (2) On a day when you drink alcohol, how many drinks do you have in one day? (quantity.) (3) On how many occasions in the last month did you drink more than five drinks? (binge drinking.) The Alcohol Use Disorder Identification Test (AUDIT) consists of questions on the quantity and frequency of alcohol consumption, on alcohol dependence symptoms, and on alcohol-related problems (Table 1–9). It has been found to accurately detect hazardous drinking, harmful drinking, and alcohol dependence and does not seem to be affected by ethnic or gender bias. Treatment is discussed in Chapter 25. The approach is complicated by the observation that moderate alcohol consumption appears to slightly reduce mortality rates in middle-aged and older adults. Choice of therapy remains controversial. However, use of screening procedures and brief intervention methods (see Table 1–10 and Chapter 25) can produce a 10–30% reduction in long-term alcohol use and alcohol-related problems.

Use of illegal drugs—including cocaine—either sporadically or episodically remains an important problem. A disturbing trend is the recent increase in use of marijuana and inhalants among eighth graders and high school students. Many drug users are employed, and many use drugs during pregnancy. Cocaine and tobacco use during early pregnancy substantially increase the risk of miscarriage. Abuse of anabolic-androgenic steroids has been associated with use of other illicit drugs, alcohol, and cigarettes and with violence and criminal behavior. As with alcohol abuse, the recognition of drug abuse presents special problems and requires that the clinician actively consider the diagnosis. Clinical aspects of substance abuse and treatment issues are discussed in Chapter 25.

[National Institute on Alcohol Abuse and Alcoholism Publications and Databases]
http://www.niaaa.nih.gov/

[National Institute on Drug Abuse Information on Common Drugs of Abuse]
http://www.nida.nih.gov/DrugAbuse.html

Bradley KA et al: Screening for problem drinking: Comparison of CAGE and AUDIT. J Gen Intern Med 1998;13:379. [NLM Cit ID: 98332230] (For identification of patients with heavy drinking or active alcohol abuse or dependence, the self-administered AUDIT was superior to the CAGE.)

Fleming MF et al: Brief physician advice for problem alcohol drinkers: A randomized, controlled trial in community-based primary care practices. JAMA 1997; 277:1039. [NLM Cit ID: 97238648] (Physicians provided two 10- to 15-minute counseling sessions using a scripted workbook that included advice, education, and contracting information. At 1-year follow-up, there were significant reductions in 7-day alcohol use, episodes of binge drinking, and frequency of excessive drinking.)

Friedmann PD et al: Management of adults recovering from alcohol or other drug problems: Relapse prevention in primary care. JAMA 1998;279:1227. [NLM Cit ID:

Table 1–9. Screening for alcohol abuse.

1. CAGE screening test[1]	
Have you ever felt the need to	Cut down on drinking?
Have you ever felt	Annoyed by criticism of your drinking?
Have you ever felt	Guilty about your drinking?
Have you ever taken a morning	Eye opener?
INTERPRETATION: Two "yes" answers are considered a positive screen. One "yes" answer should arouse a suspicion of alcohol abuse.	

2. The Alcohol Use Disorder Identification Test (AUDIT).[2] (Scores for response categories are given in parentheses. Scores range from 0 to 41, with a cutoff score of ≥ 5 indicating hazardous drinking, harmful drinking, or alcohol dependence.)

1. How often do you have a drink containing alcohol?
   (0) Never | (1) Monthly or less | (2) Two to four times a month | (3) Two or three times a week | (4) Four or more times a week
2. How many drinks containing alcohol do you have on a typical day when you are drinking?
   (0) 1 or 2 | (1) 3 or 4 | (2) 5 or 6 | (3) 7 to 9 | (4) 10 or more
3. How often do you have six or more drinks on one occasion?
   (0) Never | (1) Less than monthly | (2) Monthly | (3) Weekly | (4) Daily or almost daily
4. How often during the past year have you found that you were not able to stop drinking once you had started?
   (0) Never | (1) Less than monthly | (2) Monthly | (3) Weekly | (4) Daily or almost daily
5. How often during the past year have you failed to do what was normally expected of you because of drinking?
   (0) Never | (1) Less than monthly | (2) Monthly | (3) Weekly | (4) Daily or almost daily
6. How often during the past year have you needed a first drink in the morning to get yourself going after a heavy drinking session?
   (0) Never | (1) Less than monthly | (2) Monthly | (3) Weekly | (4) Daily or almost daily
7. How often during the past year have you had a feeling of guilt or remorse after drinking?
   (0) Never | (1) Less than monthly | (2) Monthly | (3) Weekly | (4) Daily or almost daily
8. How often during the past year have you been unable to remember what happened the night before because you had been drinking?
   (0) Never | (1) Less than monthly | (2) Monthly | (3) Weekly | (4) Daily or almost daily
9. Have you or has someone else been injured as a result of your drinking?
   (0) No | (2) Yes, but not in the past year | (4) Yes, during the past year
10. Has a relative or friend or a doctor or other health worker been concerned about your drinking or suggested you cut down?
   (0) No | (2) Yes, but not in the past year | (4) Yes, during the past year

[1]Modified from Mayfield D et al: The CAGE questionnaire: Validation of a new alcoholism screening instrument. Am J Psychiatry 1974;131:1121.

[2]From Piccinelli M et al: Efficacy of the alcohol use disorders identification test as a screening tool for hazardous alcohol intake and related disorders in primary care: A validity study. BMJ 1997;314:420.

98215049] (Summary of clinical approach to relapse prevention in the primary care setting.)

Fuchs CS et al: Alcohol consumption and mortality among women. N Engl J Med 1995;332:1245. [NLM Cit ID: 95223328] (Light-to-moderate alcohol consumption is associated with reduced mortality rates in women, largely among those at greatest risk for coronary heart disease.)

Garbutt JC et al: Pharmacologic treatment of alcohol dependency: a review of the evidence. JAMA 1999; 281:1318. [NLM Cit ID: 99222829] (Reviews use of naltrexone, acamprosate, and disulfiram.)

JAMA patient page: Alcohol. JAMA 1999;281:1352. [NLM Cit ID; 99222834.]

Ness RB et al: Cocaine and tobacco use and the risk of spontaneous abortion. N Engl J Med 1999;340:333. [NLM Cit ID: 99119164] (Both of these vasoconstrictive drugs increased the risk.)

O'Conner PG et al: Patients with alcohol problems. N Engl J Med 1998;338:592. [NLM Cit ID: 98129154] (Reviews criteria for diagnosis, epidemiology, screening and diagnostic procedures, available treatments, and clinician's role.)

Samet JH et al: Alcohol and other substance abuse. Med Clin North Am 1997;81:831. (Entire issue devoted to the subject. Articles cover general approaches, screening, pharmacologic and nonpharmacologic therapy, gender and geriatric issues, dual diagnosis, and clinician impairment.)

Schuckit MA: New findings in the genetics of alcoholism. JAMA 1999;281:1875. [NLM Cit ID: 99277380] (Brief review.)

Swift RM: Drug therapy for alcohol dependence. N Engl J Med 1999;340:1482. [NLM Cit ID: 99240030] (Comprehensive review of the condition and its treatments.)

Thun MJ et al: Alcohol consumption and mortality among middle-aged and elderly U.S. adults. N Engl J Med 1997;337:1705. [NLM Cit ID: 98041801] (Decreased cardiovascular death rates among moderate drinkers [at least one drink daily] versus nondrinkers were partly offset by increased rates of cirrhosis, alcoholism, cancers, breast cancer in women, and injuries.)

Table 1–10. Basic counseling steps for patients who abuse alcohol.[1]

Establish a therapeutic relationship
Make the medical office or clinic off-limits for substance abuse
Present information about negative health consequences
Emphasize personal responsibility and self-efficacy
Convey a clear message and set goals
Involve family and other supports
Establish a working relationship with community treatment resources
Provide follow-up

[1]From the United States Department of Health and Human Services, U.S. Public Health Service, Office of Disease Prevention and Health Promotion. *Clinician's Handbook of Preventive Services: Put Prevention Into Practice.* U.S. Government Printing Office, 1994.

Table 1–11. Recommended clinical approach to pain management.[1]

A. Ask about pain regularly. Assess pain systematically (quality, description, location, intensity or severity, aggravating and ameliorating factors, cognitive responses). Ask about goals for pain control, management preferences.
B. Believe the patient and family in their reports of pain and what relieves it.
C. Choose pain control options appropriate for the patient, family, and setting. Consider drug type, dosage, route, contraindications, side effects. Consider nonpharmacologic adjunctive measures.
D. Deliver interventions in a timely, logical, coordinated manner.
E. Empower patients and their families. Enable patients to control their course to the greatest extent possible.
F. Follow up to reassess persistence of pain, changes in pain pattern, development of new pain.

[1]Modified, with permission, from Jacox AK et al: Management of Cancer Pain: Quick Reference Guide No. 9. AHCPR Publication No. 94–0593. Rockville, MD: Agency for Health Care Policy and Research, Public Health Service, U.S. Department of Health and Human Services. March 1994.

COMMON SYMPTOMS

PAIN

Approach to the Patient

Pain is the most common symptom causing patients to seek medical attention. Information about the nature, location, timing, severity, and radiation of pain is crucial for proper treatment; the same is true for aggravating or alleviating factors.

Many emotional and cultural factors influence how pain is perceived. The primary cause (eg, trauma, infection), pathogenesis (eg, inflammation, ischemia), and contributory factors (eg, recent changes in life situation, symbolic attributes of pain) must all be sought. Fortunately, pain, whether due to trauma, surgery, cancer, or other diseases, can be managed effectively through relatively simple means.

The Agency for Health Care Policy and Research published two Clinical Practice Guidelines for *Management of Acute Pain* and *Management of Cancer Pain.* Table 1–11 gives the AHCPR's recommended approach to pain management. The AHCPR guidelines emphasize that although pain cannot always be entirely eliminated, appropriate use of drugs and other therapies can effectively relieve pain in the majority of patients. Unfortunately, pain is frequently undertreated, particularly in patients with cancer, AIDS, and previous substance abuse; and in minorities, women, children, and the elderly. Even patients in hospital intensive care units and nursing homes are frequently undertreated for pain.

Clinicians must be flexible to provide effective pain management, particularly in patients with cancer. Both clinicians and patients may hold negative misconceptions about cancer pain and its treatment that contribute to ineffective management. Patients differ not only in their diagnosis and stage of disease but also in their responses to pain; their capacity to achieve relief from pain management measures; and their personal preferences for measures to control pain. A team approach involving patients, their families, and other health professionals is essential for severe chronic pain. The clinician should discuss pain and its management explicitly with patients and their families, reassuring them that there are safe and effective methods to relieve the pain and encouraging them to be active partners in its management. Frequent reassessment for changes in pain pattern, development of new pain, or persistence of pain will enable the clinician to order appropriate diagnostic studies, modify the treatment plan, consider other causes (perhaps related to disease progression or treatment), and prescribe alternative, more invasive treatments. Standard pain management scales, based on patient self-report, can be used to assess pain and evaluate the response to interventions. In managing cancer pain, comprehensive pain assessment and algorithmic decision-making regarding analgesic use enhance pain control. Finally, effective management of pain includes efforts to improve the patient's quality of life and ability to work productively, to find pleasure in recreational activity, and to engage in normal social relationships.

Drug Therapy

Drug therapy for pain is effective, relatively low-risk, inexpensive, and rapid in onset. The World Health Organization recommends a three-step hierarchy for use of analgesics. Step 1 agents, used for mild to moderate pain, are nonopioids such as aspirin, acetaminophen, or NSAIDs given with or without adjunctive agents. If pain persists or increases, step 2 adds an opioid to the nonopioid, again with or without adjunctive agents (see below). If pain continues or intensifies, step 3 increases the opioid potency or dosage while continuing the nonopioid and adjunctive agents. Medication doses are scheduled regularly "around the clock" to maintain drug levels and prevent recurrence of pain rather than having to subdue it. Additional doses of rapid-onset, short-duration medication are administered on an "as-needed" basis for "breakthrough" pain.

A. Drugs for Mild to Moderate Pain: Most people can manage minor aches and pains with OTC analgesics, including aspirin, acetaminophen, and ibuprofen or naproxen in the 200 mg dosage formulation. For moderate pain, salicylates, NSAIDs, or acetaminophen in higher doses often suffice; if not, the clinician can prescribe drugs such as codeine or oxycodone.

1. Aspirin–Aspirin is often the drug of first choice for management of mild to moderate pain and is an effective antipyretic and anti-inflammatory agent. Analgesia is achieved with much lower doses and blood levels than are needed for anti-inflammatory action. Aspirin is available in many forms for oral administration—in a single 325 mg unit dose, as well as smaller (eg, 81 mg) and larger (eg, 500 mg) doses. The usual dose is one or two tablets (325–650 mg) every 4 hours as needed, taken with fluid. Gastrointestinal irritation can be reduced by ingestion with food or with an antacid. Enteric-coated aspirin, which is more expensive (Ecotrin; many others), essentially prevents gastric irritation, but absorption is delayed.

The main untoward effect of aspirin—especially in large doses or when taken chronically—is gastric irritation and microscopic blood loss from the gut. Rarely, there may be massive gastrointestinal hemorrhage, most commonly in heavy drinkers or patients with a history of peptic ulcer disease.

Aspirin allergy occurs infrequently and may be manifested as rhinorrhea, nasal polyps, asthma, and—very rarely—anaphylaxis. The incidence is less than 0.1%. Aspirin in high doses may produce a vitamin K-responsive prolongation of the prothrombin time.

Because of a possible association with Reye's syndrome, salicylates are avoided in children and teenagers with febrile viral illnesses such as influenza and chickenpox.

2. Acetaminophen–Acetaminophen in the same dosage as aspirin (650 mg orally every 4 hours) has comparable analgesic and antipyretic effects but lacks the anti-inflammatory property of aspirin. It is useful for people who cannot tolerate aspirin, for those with bleeding disorders, and for those at risk for Reye's syndrome. In very large doses (eg, > 4 g/d chronically, > 7 g/d acutely), acetaminophen can be hepatotoxic, manifested by hepatic necrosis with markedly elevated serum aminotransferase levels. Toxicity may occur at considerably lower doses in the chronic alcoholic.

See Chapter 39 for further details on salicylate and acetaminophen poisoning.

3. Nonsteroidal Anti-inflammatory Drugs (NSAIDs)–Table 1–12 lists the most commonly used NSAIDs along with dosages and pertinent comments. All NSAIDs are analgesic, antipyretic, and anti-inflammatory in a dose-dependent fashion. Their principal uses are in the control of moderate pain of various musculoskeletal disorders, menstrual cramps, and other—mainly self-limited—conditions, including moderate postoperative discomfort.

The activity of NSAIDs is mediated through inhibition of the biosynthesis of prostaglandins. Most of these drugs—to varying degrees—inhibit platelet aggregation and may cause gastric irritation (the risk of associated upper gastrointestinal bleeding is about 1.5 times normal and may be considerably higher than that in elderly patients); kidney damage (including acute renal failure, decreased glomerular filtration, nephrotic syndrome, papillary necrosis, interstitial nephritis, and type IV renal tubular acidosis); and bone marrow suppression, rashes, anorexia, and nausea. Kidney damage is more apt to occur in old men, diuretic users, and patients with heart disease. NSAIDs should generally not be prescribed to patients receiving oral anticoagulant therapy. The principal advantages of the other NSAIDs over aspirin are the longer duration of action—permitting less frequent dosing and better compliance—and the decreased frequency of gastrointestinal side effects. Low-dose ibuprofen appears to have the lowest gastrointestinal risk of the older NSAIDs except for enteric-coated aspirin. Patients susceptible to gastric or duodenal ulceration who must take NSAIDs regularly can be given misoprostol, a synthetic prostaglandin E_1 analog, in a dose of 200 μg orally three times daily. However, it is an abortifacient and thus contraindicated during pregnancy; side effects consist of diarrhea and crampy abdominal pain; the risk of gastric irritation is minimal. Enteric-coated aspirin is a reasonable alternative, as is omeprazole (20–40 mg daily) or high-dose famotidine (40 mg twice daily). NSAIDs may activate quiescent inflammatory bowel disease. Suicide attempts with overdoses of other NSAIDs are less serious and less often successful than attempts with aspirin.

Celecoxib and rofecoxib constitute a new class of NSAIDs which inhibit the enzyme cyclooxygenase-2 (COX-2) rather than cyclooxygenase-1, the enzyme inhibited by the older NSAIDs, in prostaglandin production. Clinical trials of celecoxib and rofecoxib in patients with osteoarthritis or rheumatoid arthritis have demonstrated a significantly lower incidence of gastrointestinal ulceration and bleeding, but these drugs are much more expensive (Table 1–12). Celecoxib and rofecoxib lack the antiplatelet effect of aspirin and many other NSAIDs.

B. Drugs for Moderate to Severe Pain: Opioid analgesics are indicated for moderate to severe pain

Table 1–12. Useful nonsteroidal anti-inflammatory drugs.[1]

Drug	Usual Dose for Adults ≥ 50 kg	Usual Dose for Adults < 50 kg[2]	Cost per Unit	Cost for 30 Days[3]	Comments[4]
Acetaminophen[5] (Tylenol, Datril, etc)	650 mg q4h or 975 mg q6h	10–15 mg/kg q4h (oral); 15–20 mg/kg q4h (rectal)	$0.01/325 mg (oral) OTC $0.28/325 mg (rectal) OTC	$3.60 (oral) $100.80 (rectal)	Not an NSAID because it lacks peripheral anti-inflammatory effects. Equivalent to aspirin as analgesic and antipyretic agent.
Aspirin[6]	650 mg q4h or 975 mg q6h	10–15 mg/kg q4h (oral); 15–20 mg/kg q4h (rectal)	$0.01/325 mg OTC $0.16/300 mg (rectal) OTC	$3.60 (oral) $57.60 (rectal)	Available also in enteric-coated form that is more expensive and more slowly absorbed but better tolerated.
Celecoxib[5] (Celebrex)	200 mg qd (osteoarthritis), 100–200 mg bid (rheumatoid arthritis)	100 mg qd–bid	$1.43/100 mg $2.42/200 mg	$72.60 OA; $145.20 RA	Cyclooxygenase 2 inhibitors. No antiplatelet effects. Lower doses for elderly who weigh < 50 kg. Lower incidence of endoscopic gastrointestinal ulceration. Not known if true lower incidence of gastrointestinal bleeding.
Rofecoxib[5] (Vioxx)	12.5–25 mg qd for OA	12 mg qd	$2.42/12.5 mg $2.42/25 mg	$72.60 OA	
Choline magnesium salicylate[7] (Trilasate)	1000–1500 mg tid	25 mg/kg tid	$0.34/500 mg	$91.80	Salicylates cause less gastrointestinal distress and renal impairment than NSAIDs but are probably less effective in pain management than NSAIDs.
Choline salicylate[7] (Arthropan)	870 mg q3–4h		$39.94/480 mL; 174 mg/mL	$60.00	Minimal antiplatelet effects.
Diclofenac (Voltaren, Cataflam, others)	50–75 mg bid–tid		$0.91/50 mg, $1.10/75 mg	$81.90 $99.00	May impose higher risk of hepatotoxicity. Low incidence of gastrointestinal side effects. Enteric-coated product, slow onset.
Diclofenac Sustained Release (Voltaren-XR)	100–200 mg qd		$3.12/100 mg	$187.20	
Diflunisal[8] (Dolobid)	500 mg q12h		$0.97/500 mg	$58.20	Fluorinated acetylsalicylic acid derivative.
Etodolac (Lodine)	200–400 mg q6–8h		$1.45/300 mg	$174.00	Perhaps less gastrointestinal toxicity.
Fenoprofen calcium (Nalfon)	300–600 mg q6h		$0.35/300 mg	$84.00	Perhaps more side effects than others, including tubulointerstitial nephritis.
Flurbiprofen (Ansaid)	50–100 mg tid–qid		$0.75/50 mg, $1.12/100 mg	$90.00 $100.80	Adverse gastrointestinal effects may be more common among elderly.
Ibuprofen (Motrin, Advil, Rufen, others)	400–800 mg q6h	10 mg/kg q6–8h	$0.12/400 mg Rx $0.18/600 mg Rx $0.06/200 mg OTC	$28.80 $21.60 $10.80	Relatively well tolerated. Less gastrointestinal toxicity.
Indomethacin (Indocin, Indometh, others)	25–50 mg bid–qid		$0.11/25 mg; $0.12/50 mg	$13.20 $14.40	Higher incidence of dose-related toxic effects, especially gastrointestinal and bone marrow effects.
Ketoprofen (Orudis, Oruvail, others)	25–50 mg q6–8h (max 300 mg/day)		$0.92/50 mg Rx; $1.02/75 mg Rx; $0.09/12.5 mg OTC	$165.60 $122.40 $16.20 OTC	Lower doses for elderly.

Table 1–12. Useful nonsteroidal anti-inflammatory drugs.[1] (continued)

Drug	Usual Dose for Adults ≥ 50 kg	Usual Dose for Adults < 50 kg[2]	Cost per Unit	Cost for 30 Days[3]	Comments[4]
Ketorolac tromethamine (Toradol)	10 mg q4–6h to a maximum of 40 mg/d		$1.13/10 mg	Not recommended	Short-term use (< 5 days) only; otherwise, increased risk of gastrointestinal side effects.
Ketorolac tromethamine[9] (Toradol)	60 mg initially, then 30 mg q6h IM		$8.72/60 mg	Not recommended	Intramuscular NSAID as alternative to opioid. Lower doses for elderly. Short-term use (< 5 days) only.
Magnesium salicylate (various)	650 mg q4h		$0.16/325 mg OTC	$38.40	
Meclofenamate sodium[10] (Meclomen)	50–100 mg q6h		$0.60/100 mg	$72.00	Diarrhea more common.
Mefenamic acid (Ponstel)	250 mg q6h		$1.09/250 mg	$130.80	
Nabumetone (Relafen)	500–1000 mg once daily (max dose 2,000 mg/day)		$1.27/500 mg $1.50/750 mg	$135.00	May be less ulcerogenic than ibuprofen, but overall side effects may not be less.
Naproxen (Naprosyn, Anaprox, Aleve [OTC], others)	200–500 mg q6–8h	5 mg/kg q8h	$1.14/500 mg Rx $0.09/220 mg OTC	$102.60 $8.10 OTC	Generally well tolerated. Lower doses for elderly.
Oxaprozin (Daypro)	600–1200 mg once daily		$1.53/600 mg	$91.80	Similar to ibuprofen. May cause rash, pruritus, photosensitivity.
Piroxicam (Feldene)	20 mg daily		$2.51/20 mg	$75.30	Single daily dose convenient. Long half-life. May cause higher rate of gastrointestinal bleeding and dermatologic side effects.
Sodium salicylate	325–650 q3–4h		$0.05/650 mg OTC	$12.00	
Sulindac (Clinoril)	150–200 mg bid		$0.94/150 mg; $1.15/200 mg	$56.40 $69.00	May cause higher rate of gastrointestinal bleeding. May have less nephrotoxic potential.
Tolmetin (Tolectin)	200–600 mg qid		$0.50/200 mg; $0.95/600 mg	$60.00 $114.00	Perhaps more side effects than others, including anaphylactic reactions.

OTC = over-the-counter; Rx = prescription; OA = osteoarthritis; RA = rheumatoid arthritis.

[1]Modified from Jacox AK et al: Management of Cancer Pain: Quick Reference Guide for Clinicians No. 9. AHCPR Publication No. 94–0593. Rockville, MD: Agency for Health Care Policy and Research, Public Health Service, U.S. Department of Health and Human Services. March 1994.

[2]Acetaminophen and NSAID dosages for adults weighing less than 50 kg should be adjusted for weight.

[3]Cost to pharmacist (average wholesale price, generic when possible) for quantity listed. Source: *Drug Topics Red Book,* March 2000; Vol. 19, No. 3.

[4]The adverse effects of headache, tinnitus, dizziness, confusion, rashes, anorexia, nausea, vomiting, gastrointestinal bleeding, diarrhea, nephrotoxicity, visual disturbances, etc, can occur with any of these drugs. Tolerance and efficacy are subject to great individual variations among patients. Note: All NSAIDs can increase serum lithium levels.

[5]Acetaminophen, celecoxib, and rofecoxib lack the antiplatelet activities of other NSAIDs.

[6]May inhibit platelet aggregation for 1 week or more and may cause bleeding.

[7]May have minimal antiplatelet activity.

[8]Administration with antacids may decrease absorption.

[9]Has the same gastrointestinal toxicities as oral NSAIDs.

[10]Coombs-positive autoimmune hemolytic anemia has been associated with prolonged use.

that cannot be relieved with other agents. Examples include the acute pain of severe trauma, burns, myocardial infarction, ureteral stone, and surgery and the chronic pain of progressive diseases such as cancer and AIDS. Opioids are effective, easily titrated, and have a favorable benefit-to-risk ratio. Large doses of opioids may be needed to control pain if it is severe, and extended courses may be necessary if the pain is chronic. Opioid analgesics can also be useful to treat selected patients with intractable pain due to causes other than malignancy, when efforts to remove its cause or to treat it in other ways have been unsuccessful. Continuation of opioid therapy in this circumstance should be based on the clinician's assessment of the results of treatment (degree of pain relief, changes in physical and psychologic functioning, number of prescription refills, telephone calls, clinic or emergency department visits, hospital stays, etc).

Long-term opioid administration may lead to **tolerance** (escalating opioid doses are needed for the same analgesic effect) and **physical dependence** (withdrawal symptoms occur upon sudden opioid discontinuation, though to varying degrees and after varying periods of use). Tolerance and physical dependence are normal physiologic consequences of extended opioid therapy and must not be confused with **addiction.** Addiction is psychologic dependence and is often manifested as drug abuse (variously defined as manipulative drug-seeking behavior or compulsive use of drugs for nonmedicinal purposes despite harmful effects). Patients and family members must be educated regarding the difference between tolerance, physical dependence, and addiction and about the low risk of addiction from long-term use or high doses of opioids for pain relief. Patients with chronic, severe pain must not consider themselves addicts because they are being treated with opioids. *Concerns about addiction should not prevent the appropriate use of opioids, especially in the management of terminal illness.*

Table 1–13 lists opioid analgesics with some of their characteristics. These drugs all have pharmacologic similarities to opium and suppress cough and gastrointestinal motility as well as relieve pain.

Opioids can be classified as full opioid agonists, partial agonists, or mixed agonist-antagonists depending on which specific central nervous system receptors they bind to and their actions at these receptors. Full agonists include morphine, hydromorphone, codeine, oxycodone, methadone, levorphanol, and fentanyl. Such agents are preferred in management of cancer pain, since their effectiveness is not generally limited by a "ceiling." Meperidine is an agonist also but generally should be avoided in severe, chronic pain (see below). Partial agonists such as buprenorphine are less effective analgesics because they are less active at the central nervous system opioid receptor and are limited by a dose-related "ceiling" effect. Mixed agonist-antagonists include pentazocine, butorphanol tartrate, and nalbuphine hydrochloride. Mixed agonist-antagonists block or are neutral at one type of opioid receptor while binding to and activating another. These agents also manifest a "ceiling" effect. In addition, mixed agonist-antagonists are contraindicated for use in patients already receiving opioid agonists because they may precipitate an acute withdrawal syndrome and cause increased pain.

C. Frequently Used Opioid Agonist Analgesics:

1. Morphine sulfate–Morphine is the most commonly prescribed opioid agent and is readily available in several forms. Morphine, 8–15 mg subcutaneously or intramuscularly, is effective for control of severe pain in many adults. The effects last 4–5 hours. In acute myocardial infarction or in acute pulmonary edema due to left ventricular failure, 2–6 mg may be injected slowly intravenously in 5 mL of saline solution. Patient-controlled administration of intravenous morphine is discussed below. Long-acting, sustained-release oral morphine preparations have an extended duration of action (8–12 hours) and allow less frequent dosing in chronic pain.

2. Morphine congeners–Examples of morphine congeners are hydromorphone and oxymorphone, 2–4 mg of either given orally every 4 hours or 1–3 mg of either given subcutaneously every 4 hours. These drugs give effects equivalent to 10 mg of morphine sulfate and have no specific advantages over morphine.

3. Methadone–Methadone, 15–20 mg orally every 6–8 hours, is most often used for treatment of addiction because of its long duration of action. Its side effects are similar to those of morphine (see below), but tolerance and physical dependence are slower to develop.

4. Codeine (sulfate or phosphate)–Codeine in doses of 15–60 mg orally or subcutaneously every 4–6 hours is somewhat less effective than morphine but also less habit-forming. It is often given together with aspirin or acetaminophen for enhanced analgesic effect. Codeine is a powerful cough suppressant in a dosage of 15–30 mg orally every 4 hours, but it is constipating.

5. Oxycodone and hydrocodone–These drugs are given orally and prescribed with another analgesic. The dosage is 5–7.5 mg every 4–6 hours in tablets that contain aspirin 325 mg (Percodan, Roxiprin) or acetaminophen 325 mg (Percocet, Roxicet) or 500 mg (Vicodin, Lortab, Zydone).

6. Meperidine–Meperidine, 50–150 mg orally or intramuscularly every 3–4 hours, provides analgesia similar to morphine in acute pain, but it should be avoided in severe chronic pain because of its short duration of action (2.5–3.5 hours) and in renal insufficiency because accumulation of its toxic metabolite (normeperidine) may predispose to seizures.

7. Fentanyl–Fentanyl transdermal patches also are long-acting (2–3 days). Four patch sizes are avail-

Table 1–13. Useful opioid agonist analgesics.[1]

Drug	Approximate Equianalgesic Dose[2] Oral	Approximate Equianalgesic Dose[2] Parenteral	Usual Starting Dose: Adults ≥ 50 kg Body Weight Oral	Usual Starting Dose: Adults ≥ 50 kg Body Weight Parenteral	Usual Starting Dose: Adults < 50 kg Body Weight Oral	Usual Starting Dose: Adults < 50 kg Body Weight Parenteral	Potential Advantages	Potential Disadvantages
OPIOID AGONISTS[3]								
Morphine[4]	30 mg q3–4h (repeat around-the-clock dosing); 60 mg q3–4h (single or intermittent dosing).	10 mg q3–4h	30 mg q3–4h $0.18/15 mg $86.40	10 mg q3–4h $1.18/10 mg $9.44/24 h $283.00	0.3 mg/kg q3–4h	0.1 mg/kg q3–4h	Standard of comparison; multiple dosage forms available.	No unique problems when compared with other opioids.
Morphine controlled-release[4] (MS Contin, Roxanol, Oramorph)	90–120 mg q12h	Not available	90–120 mg q12h $1.75/30 mg $315.00	Not available	Not available	Not available		
Hydromorphone[4] (Dilaudid)	7.5 mg q3–4h	1.5 mg q3–4h	2 mg q3–4h $0.46/2 mg $330.00	1.5 mg q3–4h $1.37/2 mg $329.00	0.06 mg/ q3–4h	0.015 mg/kg q3–4h	Similar to morphine. Available in injectable high-potency preparation, rectal suppository.	Short duration.
Levorphanol (Levo-Dromoran)	4 mg q6–8h	2 mg q6–8h	4 mg q6–8h $0.67/2 mg $161.00	2 mg q6–8h $3.54/2 mg $425.00	0.04 mg/kg q6–8h	0.02 mg q6–8h	Longer-acting than morphine sulfate.	
Meperidine[5] (Demerol)	300 mg q2–3h; normal dose, 50–150 mg q3–4h	100 mg q3h	Not recommended	100 mg q3h $0.68/50 mg	Not recommended	0.75 mg/kg q2–3h	May be useful for acute pain if the patient is intolerant to morphine.	Short duration. Metabolite in high concentrations may cause seizures.
Methadone (Dolophine, others)	20 mg q6–8h	10 mg q6–8h	20 mg q6–8h $0.14/10 mg $33.60 (80 mg/ 24 h)	10 mg q6–8h $1.60/10 mg $192.00 (40 mg/ 24h)	0.2 mg/kg q6–8h	0.1 mg/kg q6–8h	Somewhat longer-acting than morphine. Useful in cases of intolerance to morphine.	Analgesic duration shorter than plasma duration. May accumulate, requiring close monitoring during first weeks of treatment.
Oxymorphone[3] (Numorphan)	Not available	1 mg q3–4h	Not available	1 mg q3–4h $2.78/1 mg				
COMBINATION OPIOID-NSAID OR ANTIDEPRESSANT PREPARATIONS								
Codeine[6,7] (with aspirin or acetaminophen)[8]	180–200 mg q3–4h; normal dose, 15–60 mg q4–6h	130 mg q3–4h	60 mg q4–6h $0.19/60 mg $34.20	30 mg q4–6h $1.20/30 mg $216.00	0.5–1 mg/kg q4–6h	Not recommended	Similar to morphine.	Not useful for severe pain.

Table 1–13. Useful opioid agonist analgesics.[1] (continued)

Drug	Approximate Equianalgesic Dose[2] Oral	Approximate Equianalgesic Dose[2] Parenteral	Usual Starting Dose: Adults ≥ 50 kg Body Weight Oral	Usual Starting Dose: Adults ≥ 50 kg Body Weight Parenteral	Usual Starting Dose: Adults < 50 kg Body Weight Oral	Usual Starting Dose: Adults < 50 kg Body Weight Parenteral	Potential Advantages	Potential Disadvantages
COMBINATION OPIOID-NSAID OR ANTIDEPRESSANT PREPARATIONS								
Hydrocodone[6] (in Lorcet, Lortab, Vicodin, others)[8]	30 mg q3–4h	Not available	10 mg q3–4h $0.19/5 mg $45.60	Not available	0.2 mg/kg q3–4h	Not available		Combination with acetaminophen limits dosage titration.
Oxycodone[6] (Roxicodone, Percocet, Percodan, Tylox, others)[8]	30 mg q3–4h	Not available	10 mg q3–4h $0.24/5 mg $86.40	Not available	0.2 mg/kg q3–4h	Not available	Similar to morphine.	Combination with acetaminophen and aspirin limits dosage titration.
Tramadol (Ultram)		Not available	50–100 mg q4–6h $0.77/50 mg $184.80 maximum dose 400 mg/d	Not available	50–100 mg q4–6h maximum dose; 300 mg maximum dose for patients over 75 years of age	Not available	Novel agent. Both opioid and non-opioid (inhibits reuptake of noropinophrine and serotonin).	Withdrawal may occur if abruptly discontinued. Must reduce dose in elderly (age > 75); increase dosing interval in renal insufficiency.

[1]Modified from Jacox AK et al: Management of Cancer Pain: Quick Reference Guide for Clinicians No. 9. AHCPR Publication No. 94–0593. Rockville, MD. Agency for Health Care Policy and Research, Public Health Service, U.S. Department of Health and Human Services, March 1994. Reproduced in part from Hosp Formul 1994;29(8 Part 2)586. (Erstad BL: A rational approach to the management of acute pain states.) Copyright by Advanstar Communications, Inc.

[2]Published tables vary in the suggested doses that are equianalgesic to morphine. Clinical response is the criterion that must be applied for each patient; titration to clinical efficacy is necessary. Because there is not complete cross-tolerance among these drugs, it is usually necessary to use a lower than equianalgesic dose initially when changing drugs and to retitrate to response.

[3]***Caution:*** Recommended doses do not apply for adult patients with renal or hepatic insufficiency or other conditions affecting drug metabolism.

[4]***Caution:*** For morphine, hydromorphone, and oxymorphone, rectal administration is an alternative route for patients unable to take oral medications. Equianalgesic doses may differ from oral and parenteral doses. A short-acting opioid should normally be used for initial therapy.

[5]Not recommended for chronic pain. Doses listed are for brief therapy of acute pain only. Switch to another opioid for long-term therapy.

[6]***Caution:*** Doses of aspirin and acetaminophen in combination products must also be adjusted to the patient's body weight (Table 1–12).

[7]***Caution:*** Doses of codeine above 60 mg often are not appropriate because of diminishing incremental analgesia with increasing doses but continually increasing nausea, constipation, and other side effects.

[8]***Caution:*** Monitor total acetaminophen dose carefully, including any OTC use. Total acetaminophen dose maximum 4 g/d. If liver impairment or heavy alcohol use, maximum is 2 g/d.

Note: Cost to pharmacist (average wholesale price, generic when possible) for quantity listed. Source: *Drug Topics Red Book*, March 2000; Vol. 19, No. 3.

able (25 μg/h, 50 μg/h, 75 μg/h, and 100 μg/h) to provide flexibility in dosing. Doses above 25 μg/h are not used in opioid-naive patients. The maximum recommended daily dose is 300 μg/h. Each patch contains a 72-hour supply of the drug, but plasma levels rise slowly over 12–18 hours after initial patch placement. Thus, transdermal fentanyl is used mainly in patients with stable chronic pain who have infrequent episodes of "breakthrough" pain. The latter can be managed with oral transmucosal fentanyl citrate lozenges or with a supplemental oral or parenteral short-acting opioid agent. The fentanyl lozenges may actually have a faster onset of effectiveness (< 5 minutes) and produce more pain relief than the short-acting oral opioids (15–45 minutes). The most common adverse effects of fentanyl are nausea, mental clouding, dizziness, and skin irritation.

8. Tramadol–Tramadol is an atypical analgesic with both opioid and nonopioid features, contributing to a dual mode of action. Tramadol and its metabolite both bind moderately to opioid receptors; in addition, tramadol acts like the tricyclic and SSRI antidepressants to block reuptake of norepinephrine and serotonin. Adverse effects (central nervous system, gastrointestinal) are similar to those associated with opioids, but respiratory depression is less. While it does not interact with anticoagulants or oral hypoglycemic agents, tramadol should not be used in patients receiving monoamine oxidase inhibitors. Tramadol produces synergistic effects when used concurrently with NSAIDs and without increasing NSAID side effects. A reduced dose is recommended when administered with other agents that act upon the central nervous system, including opioid analgesic and sedative-hypnotic agents. Recommended doses are 50–100 mg every 4–6 hours up to a total dose of 400 mg/d (maximum 300 mg/d in patients age 75 or older). In patients with renal insufficiency (creatinine clearance < 30 mL/min), the dosage interval should be increased to every 12 hours and the maximum reduced to 200 mg daily. Abrupt cessation of the drug should be avoided to avoid possible withdrawal effects.

D. Other New Analgesic Agents: Gabapentin, an antiepileptic drug, has been shown in clinical trials to be effective for chronic neuropathic pain, such as diabetic neuropathy and postherpetic neuralgia. It targets a neurotransmitter that controls both nerve excitability and pain. It has desirable pharmacokinetic properties, acceptable side effects, and few interactions with other medications. Recommended doses are 900–1800 mg/d in three divided doses.

Dosing

Table 1–13 summarizes equianalgesic doses of commonly used opioids by patient body weight. The appropriate opioid dose is the amount required to control the pain without intolerable side effects. The need for increasing doses of opioids in patients with cancer often reflects progression of the disease rather than development of tolerance. If tolerance does develop, the same dose of drug can be taken more frequently. When a change in dosage is required, a reasonable titration strategy is to increase or decrease the next dose by one-quarter to one-half of the previous dose. If a change from oral to rectal route of administration is required, the oral dose is given first, and titrated upward. Parenteral administration of opioids starts with lower doses, which are similar for subcutaneous, intramuscular, and intravenous routes.

A. Schedule: A common error in management of chronic pain from cancer is to prescribe insufficient doses "prn" rather than adequate doses around-the-clock at specified intervals. Scheduling medication doses regularly "around the clock" maintains plasma drug levels and prevents recurrence of pain.

Patients can also achieve more reliable plasma opioid levels through the self-administration of small, repeated intravenous doses. Such **patient-controlled analgesia (PCA)** permits patients to maintain adequate pain control by allowing them to match drug delivery to the need for analgesia. The amount of medication is limited by preestablished dosing intervals and maximum doses within a defined period. Alternatively, continuous or basal delivery is also possible. Treatment starts with a bolus dose followed by a basal continuous rate to achieve desired baseline levels and to permit sleep. Additional doses are available on demand, within the limits established by the physician. A conventional intermittent dosing regimen is preferred, with a continuous infusion to be used only if pain relief is unsatisfactory. Adverse side effects occur less than half as often with PCA as with conventional therapy. Those who have experienced PCA overwhelmingly prefer it to conventional pain control regimens. Originally developed using a pump to deliver the opioid drug parenterally, the technique has been adapted to the oral route of medication delivery. In this use, oral opioids are kept at the bedside for charted patient self-administration.

B. Route: Given its convenience and low cost, oral administration of pain medications is generally preferred. In patients who cannot take oral agents (eg, those with intractable nausea and vomiting), rectal or transdermal routes of administration should be considered. Rectal administration is safe, inexpensive, and effective. However, the rectal route is inappropriate for the patient who has diarrhea, anal or rectal lesions, or mucositis; who is markedly neutropenic or thrombocytopenic; who cannot manage rectal suppositories; or who prefers other routes. The transdermal route (fentanyl) is not suitable for rapid titration of dosage and thus is generally used in situations of relatively stable pain when rapid increases or decreases of pain medication are unlikely to be required. However, oral fentanyl lozenges produce rapid transmucosal absorption and rapid onset of pain relief, both for acute postoperative pain and for breakthrough pain in chronic pain syndromes. Parenteral administration of pain medications is more invasive, more costly, and more demanding to administer. The intramuscular route should be avoided because of pain, inconvenience, and unreliable drug absorption. The intravenous route provides the most rapid onset of analgesia, but the duration of analgesia following a bolus dose is shorter. Continuous intravenous or epidural opioid infusion requires skill and expertise to manage a dedicated portable pump to deliver the drug safely. Epidural abscess and meningitis are complications of epidural catheters that can cause serious morbidity and even death. Therefore, epidural analgesia is most appropriate for cancer patients with a short life expectancy. An alternative is subcutaneous opioid infusion, which has proved practical in the hospital, hospice, or home.

Contraindications to Opioids

The opioid analgesics are relatively contraindicated in some acute illnesses. In patients with acute abdominal pain, for example, the pattern of pain may provide important diagnostic clues. However, some analgesia may be necessary in order to assess the history and perform an adequate physical examination. In head injuries, opioid drugs interfere with interpretation of neurologic findings.

Adverse Effects of Opioids

Patients with hypothyroidism, adrenal insufficiency, hypopituitarism, acute intermittent porphyria, reduced blood volume, and severe debility are particularly apt to suffer adverse effects from opioid analgesics. The side effects of all opioid narcotics are reversed by naloxone, but small doses must be employed to avoid reversal of analgesia and precipitation of acute withdrawal.

A. Respiratory Depression: Respiratory depression is a hazard of parenteral morphine administration. Morphine depresses the respiratory center in the brainstem. The respiratory rate decreases gradually, not abruptly. Severe respiratory depression is uncommon, occurring in 0.05–0.9% of treated patients. Although not usually a problem in patients with normal pulmonary function, dose-dependent respiratory depression may occur in patients with respiratory insufficiency, cardiac disease, thoracic or upper abdominal surgery, and age over 70 years. It may be more common in those who have not previously taken opioids and following epidural administration. It is less frequent in patients receiving long-term opioid analgesics for cancer pain, who generally develop tolerance to the respiratory depressant effects of these agents. Treatment of a mild decrease in respiratory rate can be accomplished by simple visual or auditory stimulation. A respiratory rate under 10/min may be treated by repeated bolus injections of naloxone (0.1–0.2 mg), by a continuous naloxone infusion, or (rarely) by endotracheal intubation and mechanical ventilation.

B. Central Nervous System Effects: Central nervous system effects include euphoria, mental clouding, and sedation. Antidepressants, antihistamines, phenothiazines, sedative-hypnotics, and alcohol can potentiate these effects. These central nervous system effects can be managed by withholding one or two doses, then reducing the dose by 25% but increasing the frequency of administration. Central nervous system stimulants such as caffeine, dextroamphetamine, pemoline, and methylphenidate are also effective.

C. Gastrointestinal Side Effects: Gastrointestinal side effects include constipation, nausea, and vomiting. Because constipation is an inevitable result of opioid administration, the clinician should attempt to prevent it by prescribing dietary fiber and regularly scheduled doses of a laxative. Severe constipation can be effectively treated with a stimulating cathartic (eg, bisacodyl, senna concentrate, lactulose, or sorbitol, orally or via suppository). Nausea and vomiting occurs in about one-third of patients given oral, parenteral, or epidural morphine. Nausea and vomiting occur because the opioid stimulates the chemoreceptor trigger zone in the central nervous system, decreases gastrointestinal motility and increases pyloric sphincter tone, and sensitizes the vestibular apparatus. Sometimes it can be controlled by reducing the dose or switching to another agent. Otherwise, trial of an antiemetic agent may be useful. In continuous nausea (often due to stimulation of the chemoreceptor trigger zone), a phenothiazine such as prochlorperazine may be useful. In postprandial nausea and vomiting (due to decreased gastrointestinal motility), metoclopramide may be helpful. In nausea and vomiting precipitated by ambulation or changes in head position (due to vestibular dysfunction), meclizine or transdermal scopolamine may be tried.

D. Urinary Retention: Urinary retention occurs because morphine inhibits parasympathetic outflow from the spinal cord, causing bladder spasm. It is more common following spinal (epidural) than parenteral or oral administration and more often a problem in older men with benign prostatic hyperplasia. Discontinuation of the narcotic may relieve the problem. If it does not, bethanechol 2.5 mg (dose titrated to effect) may be given subcutaneously, or naloxone 0.8 mg can be given intravenously.

E. Pruritus: Pruritus occurs commonly when morphine is administered via the epidural or intrathecal routes, less frequently with intravenous or intramuscular administration, and uncommonly following oral dosing. Its pathogenesis is unknown. If the pruritus is severe, naloxone is effective both for treatment (0.1 mg intravenous boluses every 30 minutes as needed) and for prophylaxis (0.4 mg/L by intravenous infusion over 24 hours). Doses of naloxone must be small to avoid reversal of analgesia. Droperidol 2.5 mg may decrease the incidence and severity of pruritus. Diphenhydramine, hydroxyzine, and cimetidine are also sometimes effective.

F. Hypersensitivity: Enhanced sensitivity to the opioid drugs occurs in patients with hepatic impairment; biliary spasm may cause severe biliary colic.

Special Circumstances

A history of substance abuse in the patient or family may complicate pain management. Interventions in such patients require extra care and monitoring, and consultation with experts in substance abuse or pain management is advisable.

Patients using opioids regularly (eg, patients using heroin, patients on methadone maintenance) or frequently (eg, patients with sickle cell disease) often have already developed some degree of tolerance; thus, they usually require higher starting doses and shorter dosing intervals.

In pain requiring chronic opioid therapy, asking patients to sign a formal pain medication "contract" may improve care by disseminating information, facilitating a mutually agreed-upon course, and enhancing compliance.

In advanced disease or terminal illness, clinicians are sometimes reluctant to give high enough doses of opioids to relieve the pain, fearing serious side effects. However, the clinician's primary ethical responsibility—to benefit patients by relieving their suffering—supports use of escalating doses even at the risk of side effects. Patients with cancer pain may become tolerant to opioids during long-term therapy but usually tolerate increasing opioid doses without unmanageable side effects, without development of dependency, and without shortening of their lives. Patients who are dying may require very large doses of opioids for control of pain (or dyspnea) at the risk of unintentional respiratory depression. However, most compassionate physicians are willing to accept this "double effect" and find that patients and families are grateful for the relief provided (see Chapter 5).

Several clinical strategies may be used to manage pain in patients who respond poorly to routine measures, including (1) opening the "therapeutic window" by more aggressive management of opioid side effects, (2) identifying an opioid with a more favorable balance between analgesia and side effects by opioid rotation, (3) introducing a pharmacologic intervention to reduce the systemic opioid requirement (either treatment with another nonopioid analgesic or a trial of intraspinal opioid therapy), or (4) offering a nonpharmacologic intervention (eg, nerve block) to reduce the systemic opioid requirement.

Adjuvant Drugs for Pain Control

Corticosteroids are helpful in management of cancer pain. Dexamethasone, 16–96 mg/d orally or intravenously, or prednisone, 40–100 mg/d orally, has potent anti-inflammatory activity and reduces cerebral and spinal cord edema. Because these agents have antiemetic activity and stimulate appetite, they are beneficial in management of cachexia and anorexia. They also can cause mood elevation.

Anticonvulsants (eg, phenytoin, 300–500 mg/d orally; carbamazepine, 200–1600 mg/d orally; gabapentin, 900–1800 mg/d orally), antidepressants (eg, amitriptyline or desipramine, 25–150 mg/d orally), and local anesthetics (eg, bupivacaine) are useful in management of neuropathic pain. Neuroleptics (eg, methotrimeprazine, 40–80 mg/d intramuscularly) help in chronic pain syndromes since they have antiemetic and anxiolytic effects and do not inhibit gastrointestinal motility or cause constipation. Hydroxyzine is an antihistamine with mild analgesic, anxiolytic, sedative, and antiemetic properties. Placebos should not be used in the management of severe, intractable pain such as that due to cancer or sickle cell crisis.

Physical, Psychologic, & Other Modalities

A variety of nonpharmacologic interventions assist in pain alleviation. Noninvasive physical and psychosocial modalities can be used concurrently with drugs. Physical measures include massage, cutaneous stimulation, heat, cold, exercise, repositioning, immobilization, and counterstimulation (transcutaneous electrical nerve stimulation and acupuncture). Psychologic modalities include patient education and reassurance; biofeedback, relaxation, and imagery techniques; cognitive distraction and framing; psychotherapy, support groups, and structured support; and prayer and pastoral counseling. For intractable chronic pain, such as occurs in metastatic cancer or neuropathic conditions, therapies such as nerve block or neurolysis, rhizotomy or ablative surgery, and neurosurgery may be useful in selected patients.

[AHCPR: Acute Pain Management]
http://text.nlm.nih.gov/ftrs/pick?dbName=apmc&ftrsK=44386&cp=1&t=928426386&collect=ahcpr

[AHCPR: Management of Cancer Pain]
http://text.nlm.nih.gov/ftrs/pick?dbName=capc&ftrsK=44386&cp=1&t=928426386&collect=ahcpr

Andersson GB et al: A comparison of osteopathic spinal manipulation with standard care for patients with low back pain. N Engl J Med 1999;341:1426. [NLM Cit ID: 20001874] (Randomized, controlled trial of 155 patients with subacute low back pain treated either with standard medical therapies or with osteopathic manual therapy. Results showed similar clinical outcomes but less use of medication and physical therapy with osteopathic treatment.)

Bernabei R et al: Management of pain in elderly patients with cancer. SAGE Study Group. Systematic Assessment of Geriatric Drug Use via Epidemiology. JAMA 1998;279:1877. [NLM Cit ID: 98296015] (Daily pain is prevalent among nursing home residents with cancer and is often untreated, particularly among older and minority patients.)

Cutson TM: Management of cancer pain. Prim Care 1998;25:407. [NLM Cit ID: 98294157]

Du Pen SL et al: Implementing guidelines for cancer pain management: results of a randomized controlled clinical trial. J Clin Oncol 1999;17:361. [NLM Cit ID: 99385437]

Farrar JT et al: oral transmucosal fentanyl citrate: randomized, double-binded, placebo-controlled trial for treatment of breakthrough pain in cancer patients. J Natl Cancer Inst 1998;90:611. [NLM Cit ID: 98213107] (Oral transmucosal fentanyl citrate provides effective relief in treatment of cancer-related breakthrough pain.)

Fishman SM et al: The opioid contract in the management of chronic pain. J Pain Symptom Manage 1999;18:27. [NLM Cit ID: 99368425]

Gottschalk A et al: Preemptive epidural analgesia and recovery from radical prostatectomy: a randomized controlled trial. JAMA 1998;279:1076. [NLM Cit ID: 98206642] (Epidural bupivacaine or fentanyl administered pre-, intra-, and postoperatively significantly decreased postoperative pain compared with postoperative epidural analgesia only.)

Hale ME et al: Efficacy and safety of controlled-release versus immediate-release oxycodone: randomized, double-blind evaluation in patients with chronic back pain. Clin J Pain 1999;15:179. [NLM Cit ID: 99452101]

(Controlled-release oxycodone given every 12 hours was comparable in efficacy and safety and more convenient than immediate-release oxycodone given four times daily for selected patients with persistent back pain that is inadequately controlled by nonopioids or as-needed opioid therapy.)
Hawkey CJ et al: Omeprazole compared with misoprostol for ulcers associated with nonsteroidal antiinflammatory drugs. N Engl J Med 1998;338:727. [NLM Cit ID: 98145773] (Omeprazole had a lower relapse rate and was better tolerated.)
Hays H et al: Using gabapentin to treat neuropathic pain. Can Fam Physician 1999;45:2109. [NLM Cit ID: 99438639]
Haythornthwaite JA et al: Outcome of chronic opioid therapy for non-cancer pain. J Pain Symptom Manage 1998;15:185. [NLM Cit ID: 98225280] (Patients receiving long-acting opioid medications showed significant reductions in anxiety, hostility, and perceived impairment in daily activities; definite improvements in psychomotor speed and sustained attention; and no declines in cognitive function.)
Henry D et al: Variability in risk of gastrointestinal complications with individual non-steroidal anti-inflammatory drugs: Results of a collaborative meta analysis. BMJ 1996;312:1563. [NLM Cit ID: 96268669] (Low-dose ibuprofen had by far the lowest risk for serious gastrointestinal complications requiring hospitalization.)
Langman MJ et al: Adverse upper gastrointestinal effects of rofecoxib compared with NSAIDs. JAMA 1999;282:1929. [NLM Cit ID: 20046403]
Mercadante SG: When oral morphine fails in cancer pain: the role of the alternative routes. Am J Hosp Palliat Care 1998;15:333. [NLM Cit ID: 99083688]
Mercadante S et al: Morphine versus methadone in the pain treatment of advanced-cancer patients followed up at home. J Clin Oncol 1998;16:3656. [NLM Cit ID: 99032200] (Methadone is an effective alternative.)
Moffett JK et al: Randomised controlled trial of exercise for low back pain: clinical outcomes, costs, and preferences. BMJ 1999;319:279. [NLM Cit ID: 99355662] (Demonstrating superiority of progressive exercise program compared with usual primary care management.)
Peng PW et al: A review of the use of fentanyl analgesia in the management of acute pain in adults. Anesthesiology 1999;90:576. [NLM Cit ID: 99135637]
Portenoy RK: Managing cancer pain poorly responsive to systemic opioid therapy. Oncology 1999;13(5 Suppl 2):25. [NLM Cit ID: 99285183]
Practice guidelines for acute pain management in the perioperative setting: A report by the American Society of Anesthesiologists Task Force on Pain Management, Acute Pain Section. Anesthesiology 1995;82:1071. [NLM Cit ID: 95233589]
Schiodt FV et al: Acetaminophen toxicity in an urban county hospital. N Engl J Med 1997;337:1112. [NLM Cit ID: 97457835] (It accounted for 12% of all patients hospitalized with overdoses and 40% of patients with acute liver failure during the study period.)
Sellick SM et al: Critical review of 5 nonpharmacologic strategies for managing cancer pain. Cancer Prev Control 1998;2:7. [NLM Cit ID: 98438898] (Assesses the effectiveness of acupuncture, massage therapy, hypnosis, therapeutic touch, and biofeedback; hypnosis can be efficacious, but evidence is less clear for the other therapies.)
Sharma S et al: Nonsteroidal anti-inflammatory drugs in the management of pain and inflammation: a basis for drug selection. Am J Ther 1999;6:3. [NLM Cit ID: 99354166]
Wolfe MM et al: Gastrointestinal toxicity of nonsteroidal antiinflammatory drugs. N Engl J Med 1999;340:1888. [NLM Cit ID: 99280043]

FEVER & HYPERTHERMIA

The average normal oral body temperature taken in mid-morning is 36.7 °C (range 36–37.4 °C). These ranges include 2 SD and thus encompass 95% of a normal population, measured in mid-morning. The normal rectal or vaginal temperature is 0.5 °C higher than the oral temperature, and the normal axillary temperature is correspondingly lower. Rectal temperature is more reliable than oral temperature, particularly in mouth-breathers or tachypnea.

The normal diurnal temperature variation is 0.5–1 °C, being lowest in the early morning and highest in the evening. There is a slight sustained temperature rise following ovulation during the menstrual cycle and in the first trimester of pregnancy.

Fever is a regulated rise to a new "set point" of body temperature. When proper stimuli act on appropriate monocyte-macrophages, these cells elaborate pyrogenic cytokines, causing elevation of the set point through effects in the hypothalamus. These cytokines include interleukin-1 (IL-1), tumor necrosis factor (TNF), interferon-gamma, and interleukin-6 (IL-6). The elevation in temperature results from either increased heat production (eg, shivering) or decreased loss (eg, peripheral vasoconstriction). Body temperature in cytokine-induced fever seldom exceeds 41.1 °C unless there is structural damage in the hypothalamus.

Hyperthermia—not mediated by cytokines—occurs when body metabolic heat production or environmental heat load exceeds normal heat loss capacity or when there is impaired heat loss; heat stroke is an example. Body temperature may rise to alarming levels (> 41.1 °C) capable of producing irreversible brain damage; no diurnal variation is observed.

Neuroleptic malignant syndrome (malignant hyperthermia) is a rare and potentially lethal idiosyncratic reaction to major tranquilizers, particularly haloperidol and fluphenazine. (See Chapters 25 and 39.)

Effect of Elevated Body Temperature

Fever as a symptom provides important information about the presence of illness, particularly infections, and about changes in the clinical status of the patient. The fever pattern, however, is of little or no use for specific diagnosis, except for the relapsing fever of malaria, borreliosis, and occasional cases of

Hodgkin's disease. Furthermore, the degree of temperature elevation does not necessarily correspond to the severity of the illness. In general, the febrile response tends to be greater in children than in adults; in elderly persons and neonates and those receiving certain medications (eg, NSAIDs, corticosteroids), a normal temperature or even hypothermia may be observed.

Markedly elevated body temperature may result in profound metabolic disturbances. High temperature during the first trimester of pregnancy may cause birth defects, such as anencephaly. Fever increases insulin requirements and alters the metabolism and disposition of drugs used for the treatment of the diverse diseases associated with fever.

Diagnostic Considerations

Most febrile illnesses are due to common infections, are short-lived, and are relatively easy to diagnose. In certain instances, however, the origin of the fever may remain obscure ("fever of undetermined origin"; FUO) after lengthy diagnostic examination. The term FUO has traditionally been reserved for cases of fever of over 38.3 °C on several occasions for 3 weeks in patients whose diagnosis is not apparent after 1 week or more of studies (see Chapter 30).

In a prospective case series of 199 consecutive cases of FUO patients from the 1980s, infections—especially tuberculosis, cytomegalovirus, and abscesses—accounted for 23% of cases; multisystem illnesses—such as giant cell arteritis and Still's disease—for 22%; malignant tumors—hematologic and solid—for 7%; drug-related fever for 3%; factitious fever for 4%; habitual hyperthermia for 3%; and miscellaneous causes—such as pulmonary embolism and Crohn's disease—for 15%. No diagnosis could be firmly established in 26% of cases. Diagnostic ultrasound and CT scans, often repeated after previous nondiagnostic studies, led to specific diagnoses in 8% and 15% of cases, respectively. Radionuclide agents currently available for investigating undiagnosed fever are labeled leukocytes, gallium-67, and radiolabeled human immunoglobulin.

The differential diagnosis of a febrile illness in the returned traveler is extensive but most commonly includes tropical infections such as malaria, dysentery, hepatitis, and dengue fever. A substantial number of febrile illnesses in travelers are never diagnosed.

Fever of unknown origin is commonly associated with AIDS and HIV-related infections, though HIV infection by itself is rarely a cause of prolonged fever. When FUO occurs in HIV-infected individuals, it usually occurs in the late stage of HIV infection. The most common causes are disseminated *Mycobacterium avium* infection, *Pneumocystis carinii* pneumonia, cytomegalovirus infection, disseminated histoplasmosis, and lymphoma.

Important Causes of Fever & Hyperthermia

A. Infections: Bacterial, viral, rickettsial, fungal, parasitic.

B. Autoimmune Diseases: Systemic lupus erythematosus, polyarteritis nodosa, rheumatic fever, polymyalgia rheumatica, giant cell arteritis, adult Still's disease, Wegener's granulomatosis, vasculitis, relapsing polychondritis; less prominent in dermatomyositis, adult rheumatoid arthritis.

C. Central Nervous System Disease: Cerebral hemorrhage, head injuries, brain and spinal cord tumors, degenerative central nervous system disease (eg, multiple sclerosis), spinal cord injuries. (This category represents interference with the thermal regulatory process rather than true "fever.")

D. Malignant Neoplastic Disease: Primary neoplasms (eg, colon and rectum, liver, kidney, neuroblastoma), tumors metastatic to the liver.

E. Hematologic Disease: Lymphomas, leukemias, hemolytic anemias.

F. Cardiovascular Disease: Myocardial infarction, thrombophlebitis, pulmonary embolism.

G. Gastrointestinal Disease: Inflammatory bowel disease, liver abscess, alcoholic hepatitis, granulomatous hepatitis.

H. Endocrine Disease: Hyperthyroidism or pheochromocytoma may raise temperature because of altered thermoregulation.

I. Diseases Due to Chemical Agents: Drug reactions (including serum sickness), neuroleptic malignant syndrome, malignant hyperthermia of anesthesia, serotonergic syndrome.

J. Miscellaneous Diseases: Sarcoidosis, familial Mediterranean fever, tissue injury, and hematoma.

K. Factitious fever.

Treatment

Most fever is well tolerated. When the temperature is greater than 40 °C, symptomatic treatment may be required. *Temperature over 41 °C is a medical emergency.* (See Heat Stroke, Chapter 38.)

A. Measures for Removal of Heat: Alcohol sponges, cold sponges, ice bags, ice-water enemas, and ice baths will lower body temperature and comfort patients.

B. Antipyretic Drugs: Antipyretic therapy is not needed except for patients with marginal hemodynamic status. Aspirin or acetaminophen, 325–650 mg every 4 hours, is quite effective in reducing fever. These drugs are best administered continuously rather than as needed, since "prn" dosing results in periodic chills and sweats due to fluctuations in temperature caused by varying levels of drug.

C. Antimicrobial Therapy: In many febrile patients, empirical antibiotic therapy can be deferred pending further evaluation. However, those patients in whom a clinically significant infection can be identified should be started on appropriate antibiotic therapy. Prompt empirical broad-spectrum antibiotic therapy is also indicated for febrile patients with potential serious infection, even before infection can be documented. This is particularly true for patients with hemodynamic instability, for patients with neutropenia (neutrophils less than 500/μL), and for those who are asplenic or immunosuppressed (including individuals taking systemic corticosteroids, azathioprine, cyclosporine, or other immunosuppressive medications, and those who are HIV-infected) (see Chapter 31). For treatment of fever during neutropenia following chemotherapy, outpatient parenteral antimicrobial therapy with an agent such as ceftriaxone can be provided effectively and safely. If a fungal infection is suspected in patients with prolonged fever and neutropenia, fluconazole is an equally effective but less toxic alternative to amphotericin B.

Armstrong WS et al: Human immunodeficiency virus-associated fever of unknown origin: a study of 70 patients in the United States and review. Clin Infect Dis 1999;28:341. [NLM Cit ID: 99162016]

Cunha BA: Fever of unknown origin. Infect Dis Clin North Am 1996;10:111. [NLM Cit ID: 96244915]

de Kleijn EM et al: Fever of unknown origin (FUO). II. Diagnostic procedures in a prospective multicenter study of 167 patients. The Netherlands FUO Study Group. Medicine 1997;76:401. [NLM Cit ID: 98075347] (Directed diagnostic workup using clues from repeated history taking and physical examination was the most efficient strategy.)

Knockaert DC et al: Long term follow up of patients with undiagnosed fever of unknown origin. Arch Intern Med 1996;156:618. [NLM Cit ID: 96205985] (A definitive diagnosis was established in 20%, usually within 2 months after discharge; 30% had persisting or recurring fever for months or even years; and half became symptom-free during hospitalization or shortly following discharge.

Mackowiak PA: Concepts of fever. Arch Intern Med 1998;158:1871. [NLM Cit ID: 98430482]

Magill AJ: Fever in the returned traveler. Infect Dis Clin North Am 1998;12:445. [NLM Cit ID: 98322389] (Causes include malaria, acute schistosomiasis, the enteric fevers, rickettsial diseases, leptospirosis, and dengue fever.)

Meller J et al: Clinical value of immunoscintigraphy in patients with fever of unknown origin. J Nuclear Med 1998;39:1248. [NLM Cit ID: 98332066] (High positive and negative predictive values of scans using radioimmunoglobulin bound to the surface of granulocytes.)

Pizzo PA: Fever in immunocompromised patients. N Engl J Med 1999;341:893. [NLM Cit ID: 99404889]

Suh KN et al: Evaluation of fever in the returned traveler. Med Clin North Am 1999;83:997. [NLM Cit ID: 99382632]

Volk EE et al: The diagnostic usefulness of bone marrow cultures in patients with fever of unknown origin. Am J Clin Pathol 1998;110:150. [NLM Cit ID: 98368310] (Among 61 patients with FUO, only one of 215 bone marrow cultures had a clinically significant isolate, *Mycobacterium avium* complex [MAC]; a small minority of biopsy specimens contained nonnecrotizing granulomas.)

WEIGHT LOSS

Involuntary weight loss is often an indication of serious physical or psychologic illness. When a patient complains of weight loss but appears to be adequately nourished, inquiry should be made about exact weight changes (with approximate dates) and about changes in clothing size. Family members may provide confirmation of weight loss, as may old documents such as driver's licenses.

Once the weight loss is established, the history, physical examination, and conventional laboratory and radiologic investigations such as chest x ray, upper gastrointestinal series, complete blood count, serum chemistries, and urinalysis usually reveal the cause. Involuntary weight loss is rarely due to "occult disease." Physical causes are usually evident during the initial evaluation. Cancer, gastrointestinal disorders, and depression are the most common causes. If the initial evaluation is unrevealing, follow-up is preferable to further diagnostic testing. Psychiatric consultation should be considered when there is evidence of depression, dementia, anorexia nervosa, or other psychologic problems. In approximately 25% of cases, no cause for the weight loss can be found.

A mild, gradual weight loss occurs in some older individuals. It is due to changes in body composition, including loss of height and lean body mass and lower basal metabolic rate, leading to decreased energy requirements. However, rapid unintentional weight loss is predictive of morbidity and mortality in any population. In addition to various disease states, causes in older individuals include loss of teeth and consequent difficulty with chewing, alcoholism, and social isolation.

Involuntary weight loss is a frequent complication of AIDS. Wasting is one element of the CDC's AIDS case definition (Table 31–1).

Bhasin S et al: Testosterone replacement and resistance exercise in HIV-infected men with weight loss and low testosterone levels. JAMA 2000;283:763. [NLM Cit ID: 20145260] (In HIV-infected men with weight loss and low testosterone levels, both testosterone replacement and resistance exercise promoted gains in body weight, muscle mass, muscle strength, and lean body mass.)

Gazewood JD et al: Diagnosis and management of weight loss in the elderly. J Fam Pract 1998;47:19. [NLM Cit ID: 98338391] (A loss of 4% of body weight over 1 year should trigger an investigation; clinicians should distinguish among anorexia, dysphagia, weight loss despite normal intake, or socioeconomic problems.)

Marton KI et al: Involuntary weight loss: Diagnostic and prognostic significance. Ann Intern Med 1981;95:568. [NLM Cit ID: 82044271] (Classic article on diagnostic approach to weight loss.)

Yaari S et al: Voluntary and involuntary weight loss: associations with long term mortality in 9,228 middle-aged and elderly men. Am J Epidemiol 1998;148:546. [NLM Cit ID: 98423931] (Both voluntary and involuntary weight loss were associated with a small increase in the risk of all-cause mortality.)

FATIGUE

Fatigue is one of the most common symptoms confronting the office practitioner. As an isolated symptom, it accounts for 1–3% of visits to generalists. The symptoms of fatigue may be less well defined and explained by patients than symptoms associated with specific functions. Fatigue or lassitude and the closely related complaints of weakness, tiredness, and lethargy are often explained by overexertion, poor physical conditioning, sleep disturbance, obesity, undernutrition, and emotional problems. A history of the patient's daily living and working habits may obviate the need for extensive and unproductive diagnostic studies.

Important diseases that can cause fatigue include hyperthyroidism and hypothyroidism, congestive heart failure, infections (endocarditis, hepatitis), COPD, sleep apnea, anemia, autoimmune disorders, and cancer. Alcoholism, drug side effects such as from sedatives and beta-blockers, and psychologic conditions such as insomnia, depression, and somatization disorder are other causes. The lifetime prevalence of significant fatigue (present for at least 2 weeks) is about 25%. Fatigue of unknown cause or related to psychiatric illness exceeds that due to physical illness, injury, medications, drugs, or alcohol. Psychiatric disorders associated with fatigue included depression, dysthymia, somatoform disorders, panic attack, and alcohol abuse.

Chronic Fatigue Syndrome

A working case definition of chronic fatigue syndrome (Figure 1–1) indicates that it is not a homogeneous abnormality, and there is no single pathogenic mechanism. No physical finding or laboratory test

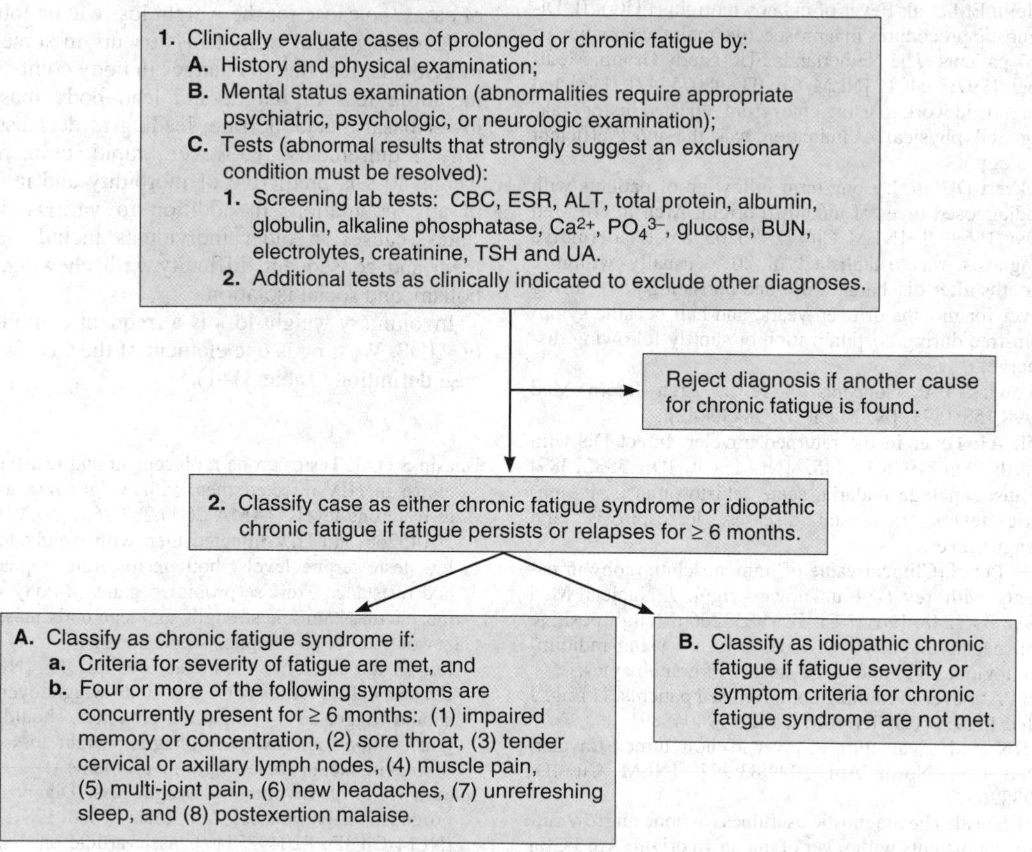

1. Clinically evaluate cases of prolonged or chronic fatigue by:
A. History and physical examination;
B. Mental status examination (abnormalities require appropriate psychiatric, psychologic, or neurologic examination);
C. Tests (abnormal results that strongly suggest an exclusionary condition must be resolved):
1. Screening lab tests: CBC, ESR, ALT, total protein, albumin, globulin, alkaline phosphatase, Ca^{2+}, PO_4^{3-}, glucose, BUN, electrolytes, creatinine, TSH and UA.
2. Additional tests as clinically indicated to exclude other diagnoses.
Reject diagnosis if another cause for chronic fatigue is found.
2. Classify case as either chronic fatigue syndrome or idiopathic chronic fatigue if fatigue persists or relapses for ≥ 6 months.
A. Classify as chronic fatigue syndrome if:
a. Criteria for severity of fatigue are met, and
b. Four or more of the following symptoms are concurrently present for ≥ 6 months: (1) impaired memory or concentration, (2) sore throat, (3) tender cervical or axillary lymph nodes, (4) muscle pain, (5) multi-joint pain, (6) new headaches, (7) unrefreshing sleep, and (8) postexertion malaise.
B. Classify as idiopathic chronic fatigue if fatigue severity or symptom criteria for chronic fatigue syndrome are not met.

Figure 1–1. Evaluation and classification of unexplained chronic fatigue. (ALT, alanine aminotransferase; BUN, blood urea nitrogen; CBC, complete blood count; ESR, erythrocyte sedimentation rate; Ca^{2+}, calcium; PO_4^{3-}, phosphate; TSH, thyroid-stimulating hormone; UA, urinalysis.) (Modified and reproduced, with permission, from Fukuda K et al: The chronic fatigue syndrome: A comprehensive approach to its definition and study. Ann Intern Med 1994;121:953.)

can be used to confirm the diagnosis of chronic fatigue syndrome.

Early theories postulated an infectious or immune dysregulation mechanism, and it appears that neurologic, affective, and cognitive symptoms also occur frequently. Neuropsychologic, neuroendocrine, and brain imaging studies have confirmed the occurrence of neurobiologic abnormalities in most patients. Sleep disorders have been reported in 33–80% of patients with chronic fatigue syndrome, but their treatment has provided only modest benefit, suggesting that it is an effect rather than a cause of the fatigue. MR imaging may show brain abnormalities on T2-weighted images—chiefly small, punctate, subcortical white matter hyperintensities, predominantly in the frontal lobes.

A standard investigation should include complete blood count, erythrocyte sedimentation rate, serum chemistries (BUN, serum electrolytes, glucose, creatinine, calcium; liver and thyroid function tests), antinuclear antibody, urinalysis, and tuberculin skin test, and screening questionnaires for psychiatric disorders. Other tests to be performed as clinically indicated are serum cortisol, rheumatoid factor, immunoglobulin levels, Lyme serology in endemic areas, and tests for HIV antibody. More extensive testing is usually unhelpful, including antibody to Epstein-Barr virus. There may be an abnormally high rate of postural hypotension; some of these patients report response to increases in dietary sodium as well as antihypotensive agents such as fludrocortisone, 0.1 mg/d.

A variety of treatments have been tried. Acyclovir, intravenous immunoglobulin, nystatin, and low-dose hydrocortisone do not improve symptoms. There is a greater prevalence of past and current psychiatric diagnoses in patients with this syndrome. Affective disorders are especially common, but fluoxetine alone, 20 mg daily, is not beneficial. Patients with chronic fatigue syndrome have benefited from a comprehensive multidisciplinary intervention, including optimal medical management, treating any ongoing affective or anxiety disorder pharmacologically, and implementing a comprehensive cognitive-behavioral treatment program. Cognitive behavior therapy, a form of nonpharmacologic treatment emphasizing self-help and aiming to change perceptions and behaviors that may perpetuate symptoms and disability, is helpful. Although few patients are cured, the treatment effect is substantial. At present, intensive individual cognitive behavioral therapy administered by a skilled therapist remains the treatment of choice for patients with chronic fatigue syndrome.

Finally, the clinician's sympathetic listening and explanatory responses can help overcome the patient's frustrations and debilitation by this still mysterious illness. All patients should be encouraged to engage in normal activities to the extent possible and should be reassured that full recovery is eventually possible in most cases.

Aaron LA et al: Overlapping conditions among patients with chronic fatigue syndrome, fibromyalgia, and temporomandibular disorder. Arch Intern Med 2000;160:221. [NLM Cit ID: 20112287] (Patients with chronic fatigue syndrome, fibromyalgia, and temporomandibular joint disorder share many clinical features, including myalgia, fatigue, sleep disturbances, and impairment in ability to perform activities of daily living.)

Jason LA et al: A community-based study of chronic fatigue syndrome. Arch Intern Med 1999;159:2129. [NLM Cit ID: 99454414] (The syndrome occurred in about 0.42% of randomly selected community-dwellers. It was most common among women, minority groups, and persons with lower levels of education and occupational status.)

Komaroff AL: A 56-year-old woman with chronic fatigue syndrome. JAMA 1997;278:1179. [NLM Cit ID: 97465788] (Excellent discussion of diagnostic approach and management of this often difficult clinical situation.)

Lee P: Recent developments in chronic fatigue syndrome. Am J Med 1998;105(Suppl 3A):1S. [NLM Cit ID: 99005134] (An entire journal issue devoted to chronic fatigue syndrome.)

Marlin RG et al: An evaluation of multidisciplinary intervention for chronic fatigue syndrome with long-term follow-up, and a comparison with untreated controls. Am J Med 1998;105(Suppl 3A):110S. [NLM Cit ID: 99005153] (About 10% remained disabled.)

Reid S et al: Chronic fatigue syndrome. BMJ 2000;320:292. [NLM Cit ID: 20115298]

Rowe PC et al: Neurally mediated hypotension and chronic fatigue syndrome. Am J Med 1998;105(Suppl 3A):15S. [NLM Cit ID: 99005138] (Patients with chronic fatigue syndrome have a high prevalence of neurally mediated hypotension, and its treatment has led to improvements in symptoms.)

Sharpe M: Cognitive behavior therapy for chronic fatigue syndrome: efficacy and implications. Am J Med 1998;105(Suppl 3A):104S. [NLM Cit ID: 99005152]

Tirelli U et al: Brain positron emission tomography (PET) in chronic fatigue syndrome: preliminary data. Am J Med 1998;105(Suppl 3A):54S. [NLM Cit ID: 99005144] (Brain stem hypometabolism was observed in chronic fatigue syndrome and not seen in either healthy controls or depressed patients.)

Wearden AJ et al: Randomised, double-blind, placebo-controlled treatment trial of fluoxetine and graded exercise for chronic fatigue syndrome. Br J Psychiatry 1998;172:485. [NLM Cit ID: 99046427] (Graded exercise produced improvements in functional work capacity and fatigue, while fluoxetine improved depression only.)

RELEVANT WORLD WIDE WEB SITES

[American College of Cardiology/American Heart Association Practice Guidelines]
http://www.acc.org/clinical/guidelines/index.html

[HSTAT: Health Services/Technology Assessment Text]
http://text.nlm.nih.gov/ftrs/gateway

[National Guideline Clearing House]
http://www.guideline.gov/index.asp

2 Preoperative Evaluation

See http://www.current-med.com/ch02.html for updated addresses of Web sites referenced in this chapter.

Joshua S. Adler, MD, & Lee Goldman, MD, MPH

Each year, tens of millions of patients in the United States undergo a surgical procedure requiring general or spinal-epidural anesthesia. A disproportionate number of these patients are over age 65. Most patients do not suffer complications as a result of the surgical procedure or the anesthetic. However, about 3–10% of patients do experience significant morbidity, most of which results from cardiac, pulmonary, or infectious complications.

The role of the medical consultant includes clearly defining the patient's medical conditions, evaluating the severity and stability of these conditions, providing a surgical risk assessment, and recommending perioperative measures to reduce surgical risk.

PHYSIOLOGIC EFFECTS OF ANESTHESIA & SURGERY

The complications of anesthesia and surgery are, for the most part, logical results of their known physiologic effects. Both general and spinal or epidural anesthetic agents usually cause peripheral vasodilation, and most of the commonly used general anesthetic regimens also decrease myocardial contractility. These effects often result in transient mild hypotension or, less frequently, prolonged or more severe hypotension. The decrease in tidal volume caused by general and spinal-epidural anesthesia can close small airways and lead to atelectasis. Epinephrine and norepinephrine levels increase during surgery and remain elevated for a day or two. The serum cortisol level is generally elevated for 1–3 days, and serum antidiuretic hormone levels may be elevated for up to 1 week postoperatively. There is some evidence that general anesthesia may be associated with a relative hypercoagulable state during the perioperative period. This does not occur with spinal or epidural anesthesia. The degree to which this hypercoagulability contributes to perioperative morbidity is not known.

There is no evidence that spinal or epidural anesthesia is preferable to general anesthesia in terms of cardiac outcomes or overall surgical outcomes. In general, the choice of anesthetic technique or agent should be left to the anesthesiologist.

EVALUATION OF THE ASYMPTOMATIC PATIENT

Patients without significant medical problems—especially those under age 50—are at very low risk for perioperative complications. The preoperative evaluation of these patients should include a complete history and physical examination. Special emphasis is placed on the assessment of functional status, exercise tolerance, and cardiopulmonary symptoms and signs in an effort to reveal previously unrecognized disease (especially cardiopulmonary disease) that may require further evaluation prior to surgery. Additionally, a directed bleeding history (Table 2–1) should be taken to uncover disorders of hemostasis that could contribute to excessive surgical blood loss.

Routine testing of patients whose history and physical examination does not disclose significant medical problems should include a 12-lead ECG for those over 50 years of age and for any patient with risk factors for coronary artery disease, specifically to look for evidence of silent myocardial ischemia or infarction. Additional testing of asymptomatic healthy patients has not been found to be helpful and is not recommended. However, the preoperative evaluation may provide an opportunity to perform other tests that are recommended as part of routine health maintenance (see Chapter 1).

Schein OD et al: The value of routine preoperative medical testing before cataract surgery. Study of Medical Testing for Cataract Surgery. N Engl J Med 2000;342:168. [NLM Cit ID: 20092361] (Randomized trial of preoperative laboratory testing versus no testing prior to cataract surgery showed no difference in outcomes.)

Tait AR et al: Evaluation of the efficacy of routine preoperative electrocardiograms. J Cardiothorac Vasc Anesth 1997;11:752. [NLM Cit ID: 97468202] (The preopera-

Table 2–1. A directed preoperative bleeding history.[1]

1. Have you ever bled for a long time or developed a swollen tongue or mouth after cutting or biting your tongue, cheek, or lip?
2. Do you develop bruises larger than a silver dollar without being able to remember when or how you injured yourself?
3. Has bleeding ever started up again the day after a tooth extraction?
4. Was bleeding after surgery ever hard to stop? Have you ever developed unusual bruising around an area of surgery or injury?
5. Has any blood relative had a problem with unusual bleeding or bleeding after surgery?

[1]Adapted, with permission, from Rapaport SI: Preoperative hemostatic evaluation: which tests, if any? Blood 1983; 61:229.

tive ECG in patients without risk factors for coronary artery disease is a poor predictor of perioperative cardiac outcomes.)

CARDIAC RISK ASSESSMENT

The cardiac complications of noncardiac surgery are perhaps the major cause of perioperative morbidity and demise. As such, this has been the most extensively studied area of perioperative medicine. The most important perioperative cardiac complications are myocardial infarction, congestive heart failure, and cardiac death. Older age, preexisting coronary artery disease, and congestive heart failure are the principal risk factors for development of these complications.

Coronary Artery Disease

Approximately one million patients undergoing surgery each year suffer a cardiac complication; 50,000 of these patients have a myocardial infarction. Patients without coronary artery disease are at extremely low risk (< 0.5%) for perioperative ischemic cardiac complications. Patients with known or suspected coronary artery disease, as defined in Table 2–2, have a five- to 50-fold increased risk of perioperative cardiac complications.

The estimated risk of cardiac complications in patients with coronary artery disease can be further refined through an assessment of the severity of anginal symptoms, the use of multifactorial indices, and the judicious use of noninvasive tests for ischemia. The severity of anginal symptoms is most accurately assessed using a standardized scale such as that shown in Table 2–3. Multifactorial indices combine several clinical parameters to estimate an overall risk of cardiac complications. A recently updated risk index is presented in Table 2–4. This index more accurately predicts perioperative outcomes using modern surgical techniques.

Table 2–2. Characteristics defining patients with known or suspected coronary artery disease.[1]

1. History of myocardial infarction
2. Angiographic evidence of coronary artery disease
3. Evidence of ischemia on prior noninvasive testing
4. Typical angina pectoris
5. Peripheral vascular disease

[1]Adapted, with permission, from Ashton CM et al: The incidence of perioperative myocardial infarction in men undergoing noncardiac surgery. Ann Intern Med 1993;118:504.

Preoperative Noninvasive Ischemia Testing

Noninvasive tests for myocardial ischemia such as exercise treadmill testing, dipyridamole-thallium scintigraphy, and dobutamine stress echocardiography have been shown to improve upon the clinical risk assessment and help to optimize preoperative management in selected patients. Most patients, however, can be accurately stratified through an assessment of anginal symptoms. Patients who have mild symptoms, defined as Canadian Cardiovascular Society (CCS) class 1 or 2 angina, and a low or intermediate score on one of the multifactorial indices are at low risk for cardiac complications. Patients with severe symptoms, CCS class 3 or 4 angina, or a high score on one of the multifactorial indices are likely to be at high risk for cardiac complications. Noninvasive ischemia testing in either of these groups of patients is unlikely to improve the accuracy of the clinical risk assessment. However, any patient who is considered a candidate for noninvasive ischemia testing independent of the planned noncardiac surgery should generally have such testing prior to surgery if the test result may lead to coronary revascularization. This is particularly true for patients found to be at high risk on clinical assessment.

Table 2–3. Canadian Cardiovascular Society angina class.[1]

I. Ordinary physical activity, such as walking and climbing stairs, does not cause angina. Angina occurs with strenuous or rapid or prolonged exertion at work or recreation.
II. Slight limitation of ordinary activity. Angina occurs with walking or climbing stairs rapidly, walking uphill, walking or stair climbing after meals, or only during the few hours after awakening. Angina occurs when walking more than two blocks on the level or climbing more than one flight of stairs at a normal pace and in normal conditions.
III. Marked limitation of ordinary physical activity. Angina occurs with walking one to two blocks on the level and climbing one flight of stairs in normal conditions and at a normal pace.
IV. Inability to carry on any physical activity without discomfort; angina may be present at rest.

[1]Reproduced, with permission, from Campeau L: Grading of angina pectoris. (Letter.) Circulation 1975;54:522.

been associated with the development of postoperative delirium (Table 2–8). Patients with three or more of these factors are at especially high risk. It may be important in high-risk patients to avoid the use of medications in the postoperative period that may increase the risk of developing delirium, including meperidine and most benzodiazepines.

Stroke may occur in up to 3% of patients undergoing cardiac surgery, carotid artery surgery, or peripheral vascular surgery, but it occurs in less than 1% of all other surgical procedures. Older age, symptomatic carotid stenoses (especially when > 50% occluded), and the occurrence of postoperative atrial fibrillation appear to be independent predictors of postoperative stroke. Most recent studies suggest that asymptomatic carotid bruits and asymptomatic carotid stenoses are associated with little or no increased risk of postoperative stroke. However, in coronary artery bypass graft surgery, an asymptomatic carotid occlusion or stenosis greater than 70% does appear to increase the risk of postoperative ipsilateral stroke. Prophylactic carotid endarterectomy in most patients with asymptomatic carotid artery disease is unlikely to be beneficial. On the other hand, patients with carotid disease who are candidates for carotid endarterectomy anyway (Chapter 12) should probably have the carotid surgery prior to the elective surgery. Some patients require both cardiac and carotid surgery. The ideal timing of these two procedures is not certain and must be decided individually for each patient. In general, the more symptomatic and threatening condition should be addressed first. Adverse neurologic outcomes are especially common after coronary artery bypass surgery. In a recent large multicenter study, the incidence of serious neurologic complications (neurologic death, nonfatal stroke, stupor or coma at discharge, deterioration in intellectual function, memory deficit, or seizures) was 6.1%. An adverse neurologic outcome was associated with a significantly increased mortality rate, a longer hospital stay, and an increased likelihood of discharge to a long-term care facility. The most important predictors of adverse neurologic outcomes after coronary artery bypass surgery were the presence of proximal aortic atherosclerosis, a history of neurologic disease, a history of pulmonary disease, and age over 70 years.

Table 2–8. Risk factors for the development of postoperative delirium.[1]

Preoperative factors
Age > 70 years
Alcohol abuse
Poor cognitive status
Poor physical function status
Markedly abnormal serum sodium, potassium, or glucose level[2]
Aortic aneurysm surgery
Noncardiac thoracic surgery
Postoperative factors
Use of meperidine or benzodiazepines

[1]Adapted, with permission, from Marcantonio ER et al: A clinical prediction rule for delirium after elective noncardiac surgery. JAMA 1994;271:134; and from Marcantonio ER et al: The relationship of postoperative delirium with psychoactive medications. JAMA 1994;272:1518.

[2]Defined as follows: sodium < 130 or > 150 mmol/L, potassium < 3 or > 6 mmol/L, glucose < 60 or > 300 mg/dL.

Dashe JF et al: Carotid occlusive disease and stroke risk in coronary artery bypass graft surgery. Neurology 1997;49:678. [NLM Cit ID: 97450334] (Asymptomatic carotid occlusion or high-grade stenosis increases the risk of stroke after CABG surgery.)

Marcantonio ER et al: A clinical prediction rule for delirium after elective noncardiac surgery. JAMA 1994;271: 134. [NLM Cit ID: 94087892]

Roach GW et al: Adverse cerebral outcomes after coronary bypass surgery. N Engl J Med 1996;325:1857. [NLM Cit ID: 97096835] (Prospective evaluation of neurologic outcomes after coronary bypass surgery.)

MANAGEMENT OF ENDOCRINE DISEASES

Diabetes Mellitus

Patients with diabetes are at increased risk for postoperative infections. Furthermore, diabetic patients are more likely to have cardiovascular disease and thus are at increased risk for postoperative cardiac complications. The most challenging issue in diabetics, however, is the maintenance of glucose control during the perioperative period.

The increased secretion of cortisol, epinephrine, glucagon, and growth hormone during surgery is associated with insulin resistance and hyperglycemia in diabetic patients. The goal of management is the prevention of severe hyperglycemia or hypoglycemia in the perioperative period.

Although the ideal blood glucose level during surgery is not known, a level between 100 and 250 mg/dL is usually recommended. In vitro studies have shown that cellular immunity may be impaired when the blood glucose level exceeds 250 mg/dL. However, it is not known whether blood glucose levels above 250 mg/dL are associated with more postoperative infections.

All diabetic patients should have serum electrolyte levels measured and abnormalities in any of these levels corrected prior to surgery. Blood urea nitrogen and serum creatinine levels should also be measured to assess renal function. The specific pharmacologic management of diabetes during the perioperative period depends on several factors, including the type of diabetes (insulin-dependent or not), the adequacy of preoperative glucose control, the preoperative diabetes therapy, and the type and length of surgery (Table 2–9).

All diabetic patients require careful management, including blood glucose monitoring to prevent hypoglycemia and to ensure prompt treatment of severe hyperglycemia (Table 2–10). For patients who require

Table 2–9. The need for intraoperative insulin.[1]

Insulin Generally Required	Insulin Generally Not Required
Type 1[2] patients undergoing any surgical procedure	Diet-controlled diabetics undergoing any surgical procedure
Type 2[3] patients on insulin undergoing any surgical procedure	Type 2 patients well controlled on oral agents undergoing minor surgery[4] requiring general or spinal anesthesia
Type 2 patients on oral agents undergoing major surgical procedures[5]	

[1]Adapted, with permission, from Schiff RL, Emanuele MA: The surgical patient with diabetes mellitus: Guidelines for management. J Gen Intern Med 1995;10:154.
[2]Type 1 = insulin-dependent diabetes mellitus.
[3]Type 2 = non-insulin-dependent diabetes mellitus.
[4]Minor surgery = procedures such as laparoscopic surgery and transurethral prostatectomy.
[5]Major surgery = thoracotomy, sternotomy, laparotomy, major vascular surgery.

intraoperative insulin, no single regimen has been found to be superior in comparative trials. Three commonly used insulin administration methods are shown in Table 2–11. The subcutaneous route is used most often because it is easier to implement and is less expensive. Intravenous insulin, which offers more rapid onset, shorter duration of action, and ease of dose titration, may be preferable in patients with poorly controlled diabetes.

Glucocorticoid Replacement

Perioperative complications (predominantly hypotension) resulting from primary or secondary adrenocortical insufficiency are rare. It is not known whether the administration of high-dose glucocorticoids during the perioperative period in patients at risk for adrenocortical insufficiency decreases the risk of these complications. In a trial comparing high-dose glucocorticoid therapy with simply administering chronic glucocorticoid medications in patients with secondary adrenal suppression, there were no differences in perioperative complications. Therefore, definitive recommendations regarding perioperative glucocorticoid therapy cannot be made. The most conservative approach would be to consider any patient to be at risk for having adrenocortical insufficiency who has received either the equivalent of 20 mg of prednisone daily for 1 week or the equivalent of 7.5 mg of prednisone daily for 1 month within the past year. A commonly used regimen is 100 mg of hydrocortisone given intravenously every 8 hours beginning on the morning of surgery and continuing for 48–72 hours. Tapering the dose is not necessary. Patients being maintained on chronic corticosteroids should then resume their usual dose.

Table 2–10. Management of patients who do not need insulin during surgery.

Patient	Recommended Management
Diabetes well controlled on diet alone	Avoid glucose-containing solutions during surgery Measure blood glucose level every 4–6 hours during surgery
Diabetes well controlled on an oral sulfonylurea or metformin	Discontinue oral agent the day before surgery Measure glucose every 6 hours in the perioperative period and give subcutaneous regular insulin as needed to maintain blood sugar below 250 mg/dL While the patient is fasting, infuse 5% glucose-containing solution at approximately 100 mL/h and continue until the patient is eating Measure blood glucose level every 4–6 hours (or more frequently as indicated) during surgery Resume oral hypoglycemic therapy when the patient returns to baseline diet

Hypothyroidism

Severe symptomatic hypothyroidism has been associated with several perioperative complications, including intraoperative hypotension, congestive heart failure, cardiac arrest, and death. Elective surgery should be delayed in patients with severe hypothyroidism until adequate thyroid hormone replacement can be achieved. Conversely, patients with asymptomatic or mild hypothyroidism generally tolerate surgery well, with only a slight increase in the incidence of intraoperative hypotension; surgery need not be delayed for the month or more required to ensure adequate thyroid hormone replacement.

Eldridge AJ et al: Perioperative management of diabetic patients, any changes for the better since 1985? Anesthesia 1996;51:45. [NLM Cit ID: 96246306] (Survey of anesthesiologist management of diabetes in the perioperative period and review of the relevant data regarding management strategies.)

Glowniak JV et al: A double blind study of perioperative steroid requirements in secondary adrenal insufficiency. Surgery 1997;121:123. [NLM Cit ID: 97188950]

Kroenke K et al: Chronic medications in the perioperative period. South Med J 1998;91:358. [NLM Cit ID: 98222892]

RENAL DISEASE

Although the mortality rate for elective major surgery is low (1–4%) in patients with dialysis-dependent chronic renal failure, the risk for perioperative complications, including postoperative hyperkalemia, pneumonia, fluid overload, and bleeding, is substantially increased. Postoperative hyperkalemia requiring emergent hemodialysis has been reported to occur in 20–30% of patients, and postoperative pneu-

Table 2–11. Intraoperative insulin administration methods

Method	Insulin Administration	Intravenous Glucose Administration	Blood Glucose Monitoring
Subcutaneous insulin	One-half to two-thirds of the usual dose of insulin is administered on the morning of surgery	Infuse 5% glucose-containing solution at a rate of at least 100 mL/h beginning on the morning of surgery and continuing until the patient begins eating	Every 2–4 hours beginning the morning of surgery
Continuous intravenous insulin infusion in glucose-containing solution	On the morning of surgery, infuse 5–10% glucose solution containing 5–15 units regular insulin per liter of solution at rate of 100 mL/h. This provides 0.5–1.5 units of insulin per hour. Additional insulin may be added as needed to keep blood sugar < 250 mg/dL		Every 2–4 hours during intravenous insulin infusion
Separate intravenous insulin and glucose infusions	Infuse intravenous regular insulin at a rate of 0.5–1.5 units/h, adjusting as needed to keep blood sugar < 250 mg/dL	Infuse 5–10% glucose-containing solution at a rate of 100 mL/h	Every 2–4 hours during intravenous insulin infusion

monia may occur in up to 20% of patients. Patients should be dialyzed preoperatively within 24 hours before surgery, and their serum electrolyte levels should be measured just prior to surgery and monitored closely during the postoperative period.

The risk for development of a significant reduction in renal function, including dialysis-requiring acute renal failure, after major surgery has been estimated to be between 2% and 20%. The mortality associated with the development of acute renal failure after general, vascular, or cardiac surgery exceeds 50%. Risk factors that have been associated with postoperative deterioration in renal function are shown in Table 2–12. It is especially important to maintain adequate intravascular volume during the perioperative period.

Chertow GM et al: Preoperative renal risk stratification. Circulation 1997;95:878. [NLM Cit ID: 97207452] (Risk factors for developing dialysis-requiring acute renal failure after cardiac surgery.)

ANTIBIOTIC PROPHYLAXIS OF SURGICAL WOUND INFECTIONS

The development of a postoperative wound infection is a common and extremely important cause of morbidity and prolonged hospital stays. There are an estimated 0.5–1 million postoperative wound infections annually in the United States. For most major procedures, the use of prophylactic antibiotics has been demonstrated to reduce the incidence of postoperative wound infections significantly. For example, antibiotic prophylaxis in colorectal surgery reduces the incidence of wound infection from 25–50% to below 9%. Prophylactic antibiotics are considered standard care for all but "clean" surgical procedures. Clean procedures are those that are elective, nontraumatic, and not associated with acute inflammation and that do not enter the respiratory, gastrointestinal, biliary, or genitourinary tract. The postoperative wound infection rate for clean procedures is thought to be roughly 2%. However, in certain clean procedures, such as those that involve the insertion of a foreign body, antibiotic prophylaxis is still recommended because the consequences of infection are serious.

Multiple studies have evaluated the effectiveness of different antibiotic regimens for various surgical procedures. In most cases, no single antibiotic regimen has been shown to be superior. Several general conclusions can be drawn from these data. First, there is substantial evidence to suggest that a single dose of an appropriate intravenous antibiotic—or combination of antibiotics—is as effective as multiple-dose regimens that extend into the postoperative period. For longer procedures, the dose should be repeated every 3–4 hours to ensure maintenance of a therapeutic serum level. One important exception is cardiac surgery, in which at least 24 hours of postoperative therapy is recommended. Second, for most procedures, a first-generation cephalosporin is as effective as later-generation agents. Third, with the exception of colorectal surgery, all prophylactic antibiotics should be given intravenously at induction of anesthesia or roughly 30 minutes prior to the skin incision. Although the type of procedure is the main fac-

Table 2–12. Risk factors for the development of postoperative acute renal failure.

Aortic surgery
Cardiac surgery
Peripheral vascular disease
Severe heart failure
Preoperative jaundice
Preoperative chronic renal insuffiency
Age > 70 years

Table 2–13. Recommended antibiotic prophylaxis for selected surgical procedures.

Procedure	Recommended Antibiotic	Adult Dose
Superficial cutaneous	None	
Head and neck	Cefazolin	1–2 g intravenously
Neurologic	Cefazolin	1–2 g intravenously
Thoracic	Cefazolin	1–2 g intravenously
Noncardiac vascular	Cefazolin	1–2 g intravenously
Orthopedic, clean, without implantation of foreign material	None	
Orthopedic, all other	Cefazolin	1–2 g intravenously
Cesarean delivery	Cefazolin	2 g intravenously
Hysterectomy	Cefazolin or Cefotetan	1–2 g intravenously
Gastroduodenal	Cefazolin (high risk only)[1]	1–2 g intravenously
Biliary	Cefazolin (high risk only)	1–2 g intravenously
Urologic	Cefazolin (high risk only)[2]	1–2 g intravenously
Appendectomy for uncomplicated appendicitis	Cefotetan or cefoxitin	1–2 g intravenously
Colorectal[3]	Neomycin sulfate plus erythromycin base –or– Cefotetan or cefoxitin	1 g of each agent given orally at 19, 18, and 9 hours before surgery 1–2 g intravenously
Breast and hernia	Cefazolin (high-risk only)[1]	1–2 g intravenously

[1]High risk defined as patients with risk factors for wound infection such as older age, diabetes, or multiple medical comorbidities.
[2]High risk defined as prolonged postoperative catheterization or positive urine cultures.
[3]All patients should have mechanical bowel preparation with polyethylene glycol, mannitol, or magnesium citrate.

tor determining the risk of developing a postoperative wound infection, certain patient factors have been associated with increased risk, including diabetes, older age, and multiple medical comorbidities. Current antibiotic prophylaxis recommendations for a variety of procedures are shown in Table 2–13.

The most promising new intervention to reduce the occurrence of postoperative wound infection may be the administration of supplemental oxygen during and immediately after surgery. In a recent study of patients undergoing colorectal surgery, the administration of 80% oxygen during and for 2 hours after surgery was associated with a 50% reduction in the development of postoperative wound infections compared with the use of 30% oxygen.

Greif R et al: Supplemental perioperative oxygen to reduce the incidence of surgical wound infections. N Engl J Med 2000;342:161. [NLM Cit ID: 20092360] (A randomized trial demonstrated that the perioperative administration of 80% oxygen reduces the incidence of postoperative wound infections compared with 30% oxygen.)

McDonald M et al: Single versus multiple-dose antimicrobial prophylaxis for major surgery; a systematic review. Aust N Z J Surg 1998;68:388. [NLM Cit ID: 98284914] (A systematic review of randomized trials comparing single-dose versus multiple-dose regimens. Concludes that single-dose regimens are as effective as multiple-dose regimens.)

Woods DK et al: Current guidelines for antibiotic prophylaxis of surgical wounds. Am Fam Physician 1998;57:2731. [NLM Cit ID: 98299965] (Review of literature and expert opinion.)

RELEVANT WORLD WIDE WEB SITES

[Preoperative Assessment and Premedication]
http://anesthesiology.mc.vanderbilt.edu/vpecguide/lab.htm

3 Geriatric Medicine

See http://www.current-med.com/ch03.html for updated addresses of Web sites referenced in this chapter.

William L. Lyons, MD, C. Bree Johnston, MD, Kenneth E. Covinsky, MD, & Neil M. Resnick, MD

Of all the people who have ever lived to age 65, more than two-thirds are currently alive. Although the implications of this statistic are usually viewed in demographic and economic terms, the impact of age on medical care is also substantial and requires significant alterations in the approach to the older patient.

GENERAL PRINCIPLES OF GERIATRIC MEDICINE

Human biologic aging is best characterized as the progressive constriction of each organ system's homeostatic reserve. This decline ("homeostenosis") begins in the fifth decade, is progressive, and varies among individuals. Each organ system's decline is largely independent of changes in other organ systems and is influenced by genetic factors, diet, environment, and personal habits.

Several principles follow from these facts: Individuals become more dissimilar as they age, rejecting any stereotype of aging; an abrupt decline in any system or function is almost certainly due to disease and not to "normal (or usual) aging"; "normal aging" can be attenuated to some extent by modification of risk factors (eg, increased blood pressure, smoking, sedentary lifestyle); and "healthy old age" is not an oxymoron. In the absence of disease, the decline in homeostatic reserve should not cause symptoms or impose restrictions on activities of daily living.

These facts may make it easier to understand the striking increases that have occurred in longevity (Table 3–1). The bulk of the years near the end of life is characterized by a lack of significant impairment—only 20% of people over age 85, for example, live in nursing homes, and about half of individuals in this age range are independent in their activities of self care. This has substantial implications for disease screening, patient counseling, and medical decision-making.

Still, as individuals age, they are more likely to suffer from disease, disability, and treatment side effects. Combined with the decrease in physiologic reserve, these added burdens (if present) make the older person more vulnerable to environmental, pathologic, or pharmacologic insults. Understanding these facts is crucial for optimal care of older patients.

The health problems and medical management of elderly patients differ from those of younger ones in important ways, explaining the development of specialized training in geriatrics. The following observations underlie this chapter and introduce common themes in the approach to the assessment of elderly patients, the choice of preventive measures, and the management of multifactorial geriatric syndromes:

(1) Disease presentation is often atypical in the elderly. A disorder in one organ system may lead to symptoms in another, especially one compromised by preexisting disease. Because these organ systems are often the brain, the lower urinary tract, or the cardiovascular or musculoskeletal system, a limited number of presenting symptoms predominate—confusion, depression, falling, incontinence, functional decline, and syncope—irrespective of the underlying disease. For example, whereas a 45-year-old may seek care for productive cough, fever, and dyspnea as manifestations of pneumonia, the same disease may cause an 80-year-old to present with a new problem with falls and difficulty following a conversation. Thus, regardless of the presenting symptom in older people, the differential diagnosis is often pretty much the same. The corollary is equally important: The organ system usually associated with a particular symptom is less likely to be the source of that symptom in older individuals than in younger ones. Thus, compared with middle-aged individuals, acute confusion in older patients is less often due to a new brain lesion, incontinence to a bladder disorder, falling to a neuropathy, or syncope to heart disease.

(2) Because of impaired compensatory mechanisms, disease in older patients often presents at an earlier stage (Figure 3–1). Heart failure may be precipitated by only mild hyperthyroidism, significant cognitive dysfunction by only mild hyperparathyroidism, urinary retention by only mild prostatic en-

Table 3–1. Median life expectancy, in years, of older women and men.

Age	Women	Men
70	15	13
75	12	10
80	9	7
85	7	5

largement, and nonketotic hyperosmolar coma by only mild glucose intolerance. Thus, treatment of the underlying disease can be easier in the elderly because it may be less advanced at the time of presentation. Similarly, drug side effects can occur with low doses of drugs that usually produce no side effects in younger people. For instance, a mild anticholinergic agent (eg, diphenhydramine) may cause confusion; diuretics may precipitate urinary incontinence; digoxin may induce anorexia even with normal serum levels; and over-the-counter sympathomimetics may result in urinary retention in older men with mild prostatic obstruction. The predisposition to develop symptoms at an earlier stage of disease is often offset by the change in illness behavior that occurs with age. The current cohort of elderly people may be less likely to seek attention until symptoms become disabling. Physicians must ask specific questions of their older patients in order to uncover problems in the early stages.

(3) Since many compensatory mechanisms are often compromised concurrently, there are usually multiple abnormalities amenable to treatment. Small improvements in each may yield dramatic benefits overall, at least in terms of quality of life. For instance, cognitive impairment in patients with Alzheimer's disease may respond much better to interventions that address comorbidity than to prescription of donepezil, as comorbid conditions may interfere with the ability to compensate for cognitive loss. Similar approaches apply to most other common geriatric syndromes, including falls, incontinence, depression, and syncope.

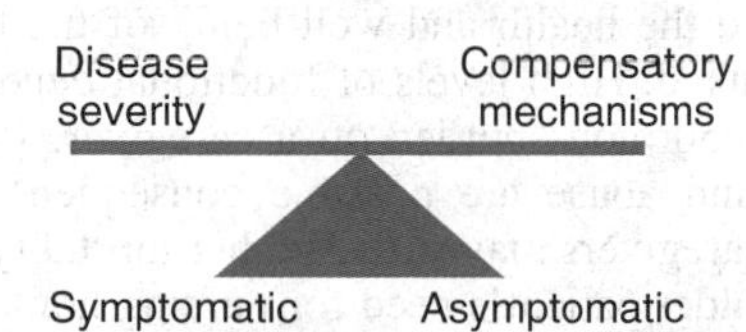

Figure 3–1. Most common symptoms result when the ability to compensate for organ system dysfunction is inadequate. Thus, even mild organ system dysfunction may cause symptoms if compensatory mechanisms are impaired. Because such impairments occur commonly in older patients, evaluation and therapy of most symptoms must extend beyond the organ system usually considered to be the cause. (Reproduced, with permission, from Resnick NM: An 89-year-old woman with urinary incontinence. JAMA 1996;276:1832.)

(4) Many abnormal findings in younger patients are relatively common in older people and may not be responsible for a particular symptom. Such findings include bacteriuria, premature ventricular contractions, impaired glucose tolerance, reduced vibratory sense in the toes, and involuntary bladder contractions. These may be only incidental findings resulting in missed diagnoses and misdirected therapy. For instance, finding bacteriuria should not end the search for a source of fever in an acutely ill older patient, nor should an elevated random blood sugar—especially in an acutely ill patient—be incriminated as the cause of neuropathy. On the other hand, some abnormalities must not be dismissed as due to old age. There is no anemia, impotence, depression, or confusion of old age.

(5) Symptoms in older people are often due to multiple causes, and the diagnostic "law of parsimony" often does not apply. Fever, anemia, retinal embolus, and a heart murmur are almost diagnostic of endocarditis in a younger patient but are more apt to reflect aspirin-induced blood loss, a cholesterol embolus, insignificant aortic sclerosis, and a viral illness in an older patient.

Moreover, even when the diagnosis is correct, treatment of a single disease in an older patient is unlikely to result in cure. In a younger patient, incontinence due to involuntary bladder contractions is treated effectively with a bladder relaxant medication. In an older patient whose incontinence is associated with fecal impaction, who is taking medications that cloud the sensorium, and who has impaired mobility and manual dexterity due to arthritis, treatment of the bladder abnormality is unlikely to restore continence. Disimpaction, discontinuation of the offending medications, and treatment of the arthritis are likely to restore continence without the need for a bladder relaxant.

(6) Because the older patient is more likely than a younger one to suffer the adverse consequences of disease, treatment—and even prevention—may be equally or even more effective. The benefits to survival of exercise, as well as beta-blocker therapy after myocardial infarction, appear to be at least as impressive in older patients as in younger ones; the relative benefits of immunization against influenza are even greater. Prevention in older patients must be viewed in a broader context. Although interventions to increase bone density may decrease fracture risk, this risk may be reduced further by strategies that improve balance, strengthen legs, ameliorate contributing medical conditions, replete nutritional deficits, and eliminate environmental hazards.

(7) In contrast to the care of younger patients, for whom cure of disease and prolongation of life are usu-

ally of paramount concern, the goals of care for older patients may well differ. Although some may seek a focus on life extension, others clearly want emphasis on improved function, comfort, and quality of life.

Palmer RM et al: When your patient is hospitalized: tips for primary care physicians. Geriatrics 1997;52:36. [NLM Cit ID: 97452781]

Resnick NM et al: How should clinical care of the aged differ? Lancet 1997;350:1157. [NLM Cit ID: 98003115] (Overview of differences required in approaching the elderly patient.)

GENERAL APPROACH TO THE OLDER PATIENT

Understanding the Patient's Values & Goals

An effective therapeutic encounter calls for a clear understanding of the patient's goals and preferences. Many older patients have definite ideas about what they want from a doctor and firm attitudes about screening, life prolongation, willingness to undergo medical testing, and use of medications or invasive procedures generally. Knowing about the patient's goals early will help the physician to focus the patient's visits appropriately. Some patients will not have clear-cut goals and are willing to be guided by the physician's judgment. Or goals made explicit at the outset may change after discussion with a physician. The patient's wishes regarding end-of-life care and attempts at resuscitation often flow from a frank discussion of these goals. If an advance directive has been executed, it should be reviewed and placed in the medical record. The clinician may ask if the patient has granted some individual a durable power of attorney for health, and that individual's name and contact information should be recorded as well. Goals and values for care should be discussed with the surrogate as well as with the patient.

Fischer GS et al: Can goals of care be used to predict intervention preferences in an advance directive? Arch Intern Med 1997;157:801. [NLM Cit ID: 97255101] (Discussions about overall goals are important but must be individualized.)

Tsevat J et al: Health values of hospitalized patients 80 years or older. HELP Investigators. Hospitalized Elderly Longitudinal Project. JAMA 1998;279:371. [NLM Cit ID: 98119558] (Elderly hospitalized patients, on average, valued 1 year at their current state of health to 9.7 months of excellent health; compared with surrogates, patients were willing to trade having less time for having better health. When possible, patients should be questioned directly about their preferences.)

Tulsky JA et al: Opening the black box: how do physicians communicate about advance directives? Ann Intern Med 1998;129:441. [NLM Cit ID: 98396840] (Physicians' discussions succeed in introducing patients to the concept of advance directives, but, as they rarely dealt with patients' values and attitudes toward uncertainty, discussions were of limited usefulness.)

Weighing Priorities

Optimal care for the older patient is facilitated when the clinician explicitly tries to set priorities, deciding what specific evaluations and therapies are most likely to provide benefit. Setting these priorities should be based upon the patient's goals for care, life expectancy, the prevalence of specific diseases, the performance of screening or diagnostic tests, and the effectiveness of therapeutic interventions.

Using this framework, the priorities for the elderly are likely to differ from those of younger people. Tight glucose control in an elderly diabetic might be sacrificed if it would call for initiation of insulin therapy with placement in a nursing facility. Colon cancer screening in 75-year-old men requires investigating about 300 men over their remaining lifetimes to prevent one death. But for men over 85 years of age, with average life expectancy of 5 years (Table 3–1), colon cancer screening is unlikely to increase life expectancy by finding screening-detectable cancers. In this same advanced age group, however, screening for falls requires questioning only two or three individuals to detect one at risk, and if standard interventions are taken, the number one must screen to prevent one fall would be about 20 over 1 year.

Some interventions produce almost immediate benefit, and those are useful at any age. Evidence supports the conclusion that even the oldest old can benefit from beginning an exercise program. Counseling patients on the benefits of physical activity is likely to be a good use of physician time at any age.

Caregiver Issues

Providing primary care for a frail elderly person requires attention to the caregiver as well as the patient, since the health and well-being of the two are closely linked. High levels of functional dependency place an enormous burden on a caregiver. Burnout, neglect, and abuse are possible consequences, and stressed caregivers may suffer higher mortality. Likewise, an older patient's need for nursing home placement is often better predicted from assessment of the caregiver characteristics and stress than the severity of the patient's illness. Direct questions to the caregiver about stress, burnout, anger, and guilt are often productive. For the stressed caregiver, a social worker may help identify programs such as caregiver support groups, respite programs, adult day care, or hired home health aids.

Direct questioning of the patient (Table 3–2) about abuse and neglect is also wise. Clues to the possibil-

Table 3–2. Questions that may elicit a history of elder abuse.

1. Has anyone ever hurt you?
2. Has anyone every touched you without your consent?
3. Has anyone ever made you do things you didn't want to do?
4. Has anyone taken anything of yours without asking?
5. Has anyone ever scolded or threatened you?
6. Have you signed any papers that you didn't understand?
7. Is there anyone at home you are fearful of?
8. Are you alone much?
9. Has anyone ever refused to help you take care of yourself when you needed help?

ity of elder abuse include behavioral changes in the presence of the caregiver, delays between injuries and sought treatment, inconsistencies between an observed injury and associated explanation, lack of appropriate clothing or hygiene, and not filling prescriptions. The elderly patient who is also a caregiver is at risk for depression and should be screened for it.

Lachs MS et al: The mortality of elder mistreatment. JAMA 1998;280:428. [NLM Cit ID: 98364807]

Schulz R et al: Caregiving as a risk factor for mortality: The Caregiver Health Effects Study. JAMA 1999;282:2215. [NLM Cit ID: 10071988] (Prospective cohort study suggests higher mortality in caregivers experiencing strain.)

Using Time Efficiently

Certain strategies can guide a physician in using time wisely with an elderly patient: (1) Identify the patient's goals and values for medical care early in your therapeutic relationship. (2) Use brief assessment instruments when appropriate, and train nonphysician personnel in their performance. (3) Employ portable amplifiers, large print information, and magnifying lenses. (4) Involve other professionals (nurses, social workers, dietitians, physical and occupational therapists, psychologists) in complex cases.

ASSESSMENT OF THE ELDERLY

Functional Assessment

Functional assessment gauges a patient's ability to manage tasks of self care, household management, and mobility.

About one-fourth of patients over 65 have impairments in their IADLs (instrumental activities of daily living: transportation, shopping, cooking, using the telephone, managing money, taking medications, housecleaning, laundry) or ADLs (activities of daily living: bathing, dressing, eating, transferring from bed to chair, continence, toileting). Fully one-half of those over 85 have these latter impairments. Persons who are unable to perform IADLs independently are 12 times more likely to have dementia than their independent counterparts.

Information about function can be used in a number of ways: (1) as baseline information; (2) as a measure of the patient's need for support services or placement; (3) as an indicator of possible caregiver stress; (4) as a potential marker of specific disease activity; and (5) to determine the need for therapeutic interventions.

In general, persons who need help only with IADLs may be aided by a chore worker, a day program, or placement in a board-and-care home or assisted living situation. While many persons who need help with ADLs may require a nursing home level of care, most live at home with caregivers.

Screening for Vision Impairment

An appreciable minority of elders have severe visual loss. Visual impairment is an independent risk factor for falls; it also has a significant impact on quality of life. Direct visual testing with a Snellen chart or Jaeger card is the most sensitive and specific approach to visual screening, though use of these instruments in the primary care setting is of uncertain validity. Referring all older people for optometric screening has the advantages of improving the quality of the examination and allowing for glaucoma screening, though costs and inconvenience may be barriers to this approach.

Screening for Hearing Impairment

Over one-third of those over 65 and half of those over 85 have some hearing loss. This deficit is correlated with social isolation and depression. Although the optimal screening method for hearing loss in the elderly is undetermined, the whispered voice test is easy to perform and has sensitivities and specificities ranging from 70% to 100%. To determine the degree to which the impairment interferes with functioning, the physician may ask if the patient becomes frustrated when conversing with family members, is embarrassed when meeting new people, has difficulty listening to the radio or watching TV, or has problems understanding conversations in noisy restaurants.

Compliance with hearing amplification can be a challenge because of the stigma associated with hearing aid use as well as the cost of such devices, which are not paid for under most Medicare plans. High compliance rates can be achieved with a proactive approach such as the use of loaner aids for low-income persons. In addition to standard hearing aids, pocket amplifiers as well as amplifiers to telephone, television, and radio may be useful.

Screening for Falls & Gait Impairment

Falls are the leading cause of nonfatal injuries in older persons, and their complications are the leading cause of death from injury in those over 65. Hip fractures are common precursors to functional impairment and nursing home placement. Furthermore, fear of falling may lead some elders to restrict their activities. About one-third of people over 65 fall each year, and the frequency increases markedly with advancing age.

Every older person should be asked about falls, as many will not volunteer such information. One should ask about home hazards that might be remediable. Because gait impairments commonly coexist with falls, gait assessment is performed in older people with a fall history and is likely to be more sensitive to abnormalities (commonly multifactorial, due to muscular weakness, arthritis, and neurologic impairments) than a neurologic examination.

Gait and balance can be assessed in a few minutes. The physician should pay attention to the following: Is the patient able to arise from a chair without use of his arms in a single, smooth attempt? Is there stability immediately upon standing, or does the patient stagger? Is balance maintained when the patient is pushed lightly on the sternum? Is there steadiness when standing with eyes closed? Can a 360 degree rotation be achieved in a smooth, continuous motion? How is walking initiated, and does each foot swing clear of the floor and pass the opposite foot? Are the steps equal? Is there stopping or discontinuity between steps, or sway of the trunk, flexion of knees or back, spreading out of the arms? Do the heels almost touch during the stride, or is there a wide-based gait? Is a walking aid (cane, walker) necessary?

Screening for Cognitive Impairment

The prevalence of dementia doubles every 5 years after age 60, so that by age 85 about 30–50% of individuals have some degree of impairment. Patients with mild or early dementia frequently remain undiagnosed because their social graces are retained.

Although there is no consensus at present on whether older patients should be screened for dementia, the benefits of early detection include the identification of reversible causes, planning for the future (including advance directives), and modification of interventions for other diseases as appropriate (eg, simplifying drug regimens, minimizing anticholinergic drug use).

The ideal screen would be simple, fast, cheap, sensitive, and specific. The combination of the clock draw (in which the patient is asked to sketch a clock face, with all the numerals placed properly, the two clock hands positioned at a specified time) and the three-item recall is fairly quick and has reasonable test characteristics. When the patient is able to recall all three items after 3 minutes, the likelihood ratio (see Chapter 41) for dementia is 0.06. Conversely, a markedly abnormally drawn clock is associated with a likelihood ratio of 24. When patients fall into an intermediate range, further testing with the Mini-Mental State Questionnaire (Figure 25–1) or other instruments can be used.

Manly JJ et al: Cognitive test performance among nondemented elderly African Americans and whites. Neurology 1998;50:1238. [NLM Cit ID: 98255408] (Clinicians must use culturally appropriate norms when evaluating ethnically diverse elderly patients for dementia.)

Robinson BE: Guideline for initial evaluation of the patient with memory loss. Geriatrics 1997;52:30. [NLM Cit ID: 98075171] (A useful guideline for early identification of Alzheimer's disease and related dementias.)

Screening for Incontinence

Incontinence in the elderly is common, and interventions can improve most patients. Many patients fail to tell their providers about it. A simple question about involuntary leakage of urine is a reasonable screen: "Do you have a problem with urine leaks or accidents?"

Screening for Depression

Although major depressive disorder has a slightly lower prevalence in the elderly than in younger populations, depressive symptomatology is actually more common. Its prevalence in ill and hospitalized elders is particularly high. A simple two-question screen (Table 3–3) has shown 96% sensitivity for detecting major depression in a general population. Positive responses can be followed up with more comprehensive, structured interviews, eg, Yesavage's Geriatric Depression Scale (Table 3–4).

Screening the High-Functioning Elder

Standard functional screening measures may not be useful in capturing subtle impairments in highly functional independent elders. One technique for these patients is to identify and regularly ask about a target activity, such as playing bridge, bowling, or practicing law. If the patient begins to have trouble with or drop such an "advanced activity of daily living," it may indicate early impairment, such as dementia, incontinence, or worsening hearing loss, which additional gentle questioning or assessment may uncover.

Assessment of Decision-Making Capacity

It is common for a cognitively impaired elder to face a serious medical decision and for the clinicians involved in his care to ascertain whether the capacity exists to make the choice. There are four components of a thorough assessment: (1) Ability to express a choice. (2) Ability to understand relevant information about the risks and benefits of planned therapy and the alternatives, including no treatment. (3) Ability to understand the situation and its possible consequences. (4) Ability to reason. A patient's choice should follow rationally from an understanding of the consequences.

In performing such assessments, it is to be remembered that decision-making capacity varies over time:

Table 3–3. Simple geriatric screen.

Assessment Procedure	Abnormal	Action
Do you have difficulty with eyesight? Jaeger Card or Snellen chart Test each eye (with glasses)	Yes Can't read 20/40	Refer
Whisper short sentence from 6–12 inches (out of view) or audiometry	Unable to hear	Cerumen check Refer
"Touch the back of your head with your hands" "Pick up the pencil"	Unable do do either	Further examination Consider occupational therapy?
"Rise from your chair (do not use arms to get up), walk 10 feet, walk back to the chair, and sit down"	Observed problem, or unable to perform in < 15 seconds	Formal balance and gait evaluation; further examination; home evaluation and physical therapy
"Have you had any falls in the last year?" "Do you have trouble with stairs, lighting, bathroom, or other home hazards?"	Yes Yes to any	Formal balance and gait evaluation Home evaluation, physical therapy
Body mass index < 21 or weight loss exceeding 5%	Yes to either	Nutrition evaluation
"Do you have a problem with urine leaks or accidents?"	Yes	Incontinence evaluation
"Over the past month, have you often been bothered by feeling sad, depressed, or hopeless?" "During the last month, have you often been bothered by little interest or pleasure in doing things?"	Yes to either	Geriatric Depression Scale or other depression assessment
Name three objects: ask again in three 3 minutes	Unable to recall	Mini-Mental State Examination

Do you have problems with any of the following areas? Who assists? Do you use devices to help you? (For "yes" answers, consider referral to occupational therapy, physical therapy, social services.)

–Strenuous activities (eg, fast walking, bicycling)	–Transferring out of bed
–Cooking	–Dressing
–Shopping	–Using the toilet
–Heavy housework (eg, washing windows)	–Eating
–Doing laundry	–Walking
–Transportation by driving or bus	–Bathing (sponge bath, tub, shower)
–Managing finances	

a delirious patient may regain his capacity after the infection is treated, and so reassessments are often appropriate. Furthermore, the capacity to make a decision is a function of the decision in question. A mildly demented woman may lack the capacity to consent to coronary artery bypass grafting yet retain the capacity to allow removal of a suspicious nevus.

Grisso T, Appelbaum PS: *Assessing Competence to Consent to Treatment: A Guide for Physicians and Other Health Professionals.* Oxford Univ Press, 1998. (A practical guide for conducting assessments of decision-making capacity.)

Functional Screening Instrument

Table 3–3 gives a simple functional screening list, based on earlier instruments developed by Lachs and Moore. In addition to ADL and IADL assessment, it looks for evidence of health problems that affect function: sensory impairment, limited upper extremity range of motion, mobility, falls, weight loss, incontinence, depressed mood, and cognitive impairment.

Kakaiya R et al: Evaluation of fitness to drive: the physician's role in assessing elderly or demented patients. Postgrad Med 2000;107:229. [NLM Cit ID: 20192391] (An approach to the evaluation and recommendations on how to advise some patients to stop driving.)

Moore AA et al: Screening for common problems in ambulatory elderly: clinical confirmation of a screening instrument. Am J Med 1996;100:438. [NLM Cit ID: 96194606] (A screening instrument that can be used by

Table 3–4. Yesavage Geriatric Depression Scale (short form).

1. Are you basically satisfied with your life? (no)
2. Have you dropped many of your activities and interests? (yes)
3. Do you feel that your life is empty? (yes)
4. Do you often get bored? (yes)
5. Are you in good spirits most of the time? (no)
6. Are you afraid that something bad is going to happen to you? (yes)
7. Do you feel happy most of the time? (no)
8. Do you often feel helpless? (yes)
9. Do you prefer to stay home at night, rather than go out and do new things? (yes)
10. Do you feel that you have more problems with memory than most? (yes)
11. Do you feel it is wonderful to be alive now? (no)
12. Do you feel pretty worthless the way you are now? (yes)
13. Do you feel full of energy? (no)
14. Do you feel that your situation is hopeless? (yes)
15. Do you think that most persons are better off than you are? (yes)

Score one point for each response that matches the yes-or-no answer after the question.
Scores: Normal 3 ± 2; Mildly depressed: 7 ± 3; Very depressed: 12 ± 2

office staff to screen for functional impairment in older persons.)

Sager MA et al: Functional outcomes of acute medical illness and hospitalization in older persons. Arch Intern Med 1996;156:645. [NLM Cit ID: 96205989] (Three key risk factors for functional decline associated with hospitalization: older age, Mini-Mental State Examination score under 22, and preexisting problems with IADLs.)

SELECTED PREVENTIVE MEASURES IN GERIATRIC PRACTICE

Exercise

Inactive elders are at greater risk of becoming functionally dependent than their more physically active counterparts. Physical activity is associated with reduced risks of developing diabetes mellitus and future disability. Even sedentary elders should be urged to increase their level of physical activity. By writing out an exercise prescription, a physician demonstrates the importance of the activity and may improve compliance. Components include strength training (isolated muscle group contractions), endurance training (walking, cycling, swimming), flexibility (static stretch of various muscle groups), and balance (tai chi, dance). The patient should aim for a total of 30 minutes of activity daily.

Hypertension

Treatment of hypertension is of substantial benefit in the elderly, and the absolute benefit of treatment may be greater in older than in younger patients. Antihypertensive treatment of patients over 80 reduces the incidence of strokes and other cardiovascular events as well as heart failure. Lifestyle modifications (weight loss for overweight patients, alcohol and sodium limitation, increased aerobic physical activity) are reasonable to recommend for all hypertensive patients for whom treatment is appropriate. For those who require pharmacologic treatment, thiazides are the drugs of choice unless a comorbid condition makes another choice preferable (eg, beta-blockers for coronary artery disease, angiotensin-converting enzyme inhibitors for systolic heart failure).

Stroke Prevention

The incidence of stroke in older adults roughly doubles with each 10 years of age. The single greatest risk factor is hypertension. Another is atrial fibrillation, the prevalence of which also increases with age. Many elderly patients with this arrhythmia are not anticoagulated because their physicians fear injuries due to falls. In patients not receiving anticoagulants, head injuries occur in about 1% of falls; anticoagulation provides an annual absolute risk reduction in stroke of 3–8%. It appears likely that the benefits of anticoagulation outweigh the risks of falling in most instances.

Cancer Screening

Screening elderly men for prostate cancer is not necessary since it does not prolong life and given the risk of incontinence or erectile dysfunction that may accompany surgical therapy or radiation. An older woman should undergo annual mammography and breast examinations until her life expectancy falls below 5–10 years (Table 3–1). Screening for colon cancer (either with colonoscopy every 10 years, or with annual fecal occult blood testing plus flexible sigmoidoscopy every 5 years) might also be reasonably stopped when a patient's life expectancy is less than 5–10 years.

Osteoporosis

Primary prevention of osteoporosis begins with identification of risk factors (older age, female gender, white or Asian race, low calcium intake, smoking, excessive alcohol use, and chronic glucocorticoid use). Calcium carbonate (500 mg three times daily at meals) and vitamin D (400–800 IU/d, contained in one or two multivitamin tablets) reduce the risk of osteoporotic fractures in both men and women. Measurement of bone mineral density (preferably using dual-energy x-ray absorptiometry of the proximal femur) of women with multiple risk factors may uncover asymptomatic osteoporosis; such women may also be offered hormone replacement therapy or alendronate.

Immunizations

Individuals over age 65—and health-care workers who are in contact with them—should receive annual influenza vaccination. Similarly, persons over 65 should receive at least one pneumococcal immunization; some experts recommend revaccination in those over 75 or with severe chronic disease and who were vaccinated more than 5 years previously. A single booster dose of tetanus and diphtheria vaccine should be given at age 65 or older.

PPD for Congregate Living

The elderly are a significant reservoir of tuberculosis, both primary and reactivation. Over 20% of elderly patients who develop the disease live in nursing homes. Long-term care facilities should routinely perform a tuberculin skin test (PPD) on all entering patients, using the two-step approach in which a second dose is administered to persons whose first was negative. If the second reaction is also negative, the patient is uninfected or anergic; if it is positive, a boosted response is likely, signifying a tuberculin reactor but not a recent converter. Whether these reactors need treatment is controversial, but their positive-PPD status should be noted on their active problem list. Prophylaxis and treatment regimens are described in Chapter 9. Skin testing should be repeated annually in congregate settings or if an active case is identified in the group.

Buchner DM: Physical activity and quality of life in older adults. (Editorial.) JAMA 1997;277:64. [NLM Cit ID: 97134653] (Summarizes results of exercise on insomnia and knee osteoarthritis.)

Clark F et al: Occupational therapy for independent-living older adults: Randomized controlled trial. JAMA 1997;278:1321. [NLM Cit ID: 98001627] (Self-reported benefits in a number of aspects of health, function, and quality of life compared with either a social activity control group or no intervention.)

Dawson-Hughes B et al: Effect of calcium and vitamin D supplementation on bone density in men and women 65 years of age or older. N Engl J Med 1997;337:670. [NLM Cit ID: 97407843] (Randomized study documented efficacy in reducing all fractures in older adults.)

Gueyffier F et al: Antihypertensive drugs in very old people: a subgroup meta-analysis of randomised controlled trials. Lancet 1999;353:793. [NLM Cit ID: 99387716] (Found treatment of hypertension reduced rate of strokes, other cardiovascular events, and heart failure in persons over 89, but effect on mortality was inconclusive.)

Psaty BM et al: Health outcomes associated with antihypertensive therapies used as first line agents: A systematic review and meta-analysis. JAMA 1997;277:739. [NLM Cit ID: 97195474] (Only thiazides and beta-blockers proved beneficial.)

COMMON PROBLEMS OF THE FRAIL ELDERLY

DEMENTIA

Older individuals experience occasional difficulty retrieving items from memory (usually manifested as word-finding complaints) and experience a slowing in their rate of information processing. By contrast, dementia is an acquired persistent and progressive impairment in intellectual function, with compromise in multiple cognitive domains at least one of which is memory. The demented patient's deficits must represent a significant decline in function and must be severe enough to interfere with work or social life.

Intellectual impairments in older patients are frequently the result of two other syndromes, each of which frequently coexists with dementia: depression and delirium. Depression is a common concomitant of dementia, but it can also masquerade as dementia. Moreover, a patient with depression and cognitive impairment whose intellectual function improves with treatment of the mood disorder has an almost fivefold greater risk of suffering irreversible dementia later in life. Delirium, characterized by acute confusion, occurs much more commonly in patients with underlying dementia. Depression and delirium are discussed in more detail below.

General Considerations

Dementia is the fourth leading cause of death in the United States and has a prevalence which doubles every 5 years in the senior population, reaching 30–50% at age 85. Women suffer disproportionately, both as patients (even after age adjustment) and as caregivers. Alzheimer's disease accounts for roughly two-thirds of cases in the USA, with vascular dementia (either alone or combined with Alzheimer's disease) accounting for much of the rest. Risk factors for Alzheimer's disease are older age, family history, and female gender. Risk factors for vascular dementia are those for stroke, ie, older age, male sex, black race, hypertension, cigarette use, previous myocardial infarction, atrial fibrillation, diabetes, and hyperlipidemia.

Causes of potentially reversible cognitive impairment include drug effect, depression, thyroid disease, vitamin B_{12} deficiency, hypercalcemia, subdural hematoma, and normal pressure hydrocephalus. Unfortunately, the prevalence of fully reversible dementias is well under 5%, and frequently the correction of these suspected causes leads only to partial improvement.

Clinical Features

Demented patients have memory impairment and at least one or more of the following: language im-

Causes of Falls

Balance and ambulation require a complex interplay of cognitive, neuromuscular, and cardiovascular function. With age, balance becomes impaired and sway increases. This predisposes the older person to a fall when challenged by an additional insult to any of these systems.

A fall may be the clinical manifestation of an occult problem, such as pneumonia or myocardial infarction, but much more commonly falls are due to the interaction between an impaired patient and an environmental risk factor. While a warped floorboard may pose little problem for a vigorous, unmedicated, cognitively intact person, it may be sufficient to precipitate a fall and hip fracture in the patient with impaired vision, balance, muscle tone, or cognition. Thus, falls in older people are rarely due to a single cause, and effective intervention entails a comprehensive assessment of the patient's intrinsic deficits (usually diseases and medications), the activity engaged in at the time of the fall, and environmental obstacles.

Intrinsic deficits are those that impair sensory input, judgment, blood pressure regulation, reaction time, and balance and gait. Although some of these may not be treatable, most are, and since the risk of falling is directly related to the number and severity of abnormalities, correction or amelioration of even a few contributory conditions may decrease the risk significantly. As for most geriatric conditions, medications and alcohol use are among the most common, significant, and reversible causes of falling. Long-acting benzodiazepines, opioids, phenothiazines, vasodilators, and diuretics particularly increase fall risk. Other often overlooked but treatable contributors include postprandial hypotension (which peaks 30–60 minutes after a meal), insomnia, urinary urgency, and peripheral edema (which can burden impaired leg strength and gait because of the additional weight).

Since most falls occur in or around the home, a visit by a visiting nurse, physical therapist, or physician reaps substantial benefits in identifying environmental obstacles and is generally reimbursed by third-party payers, including Medicare. Insufficient lighting is an underappreciated factor in many cases. In addition to the number and location of lamps, noting their wattage is also important; because of a loss of contrast sensitivity, older people often need twice the wattage to maximize visual acuity. Replacement of 60-watt bulbs with 100-watt bulbs may be cost-effective.

Complications of Falls

The most common fractures resulting from falls are of the wrist, hip, and vertebrae. There is a high mortality rate (approximately 20% in one year) in elderly women with hip fractures, particularly if they were debilitated prior to the time of the fracture.

Fear of falling again is a common, serious, but treatable factor in the elderly person's loss of confidence and independence. Referral to a physical therapist for gait training with special devices is often all that is required.

Chronic subdural hematoma is an easily overlooked complication of falls that must be considered in any elderly patient presenting with new neurologic symptoms or signs, particularly obtundation. Headache is uncommonly present. In many cases there is no history of trauma.

Dehydration, electrolyte imbalance, pressure sores, rhabdomyolysis, and hypothermia may all complicate a fall.

Prevention & Management

The risk of falling and consequent injury, disability, and potential institutionalization can be reduced by modifying those factors outlined in Table 3–5. Emphasis is placed on treating all contributory medical conditions, minimizing environmental hazards, and reducing the number of medications—particularly those that induce parkinsonism, orthostasis (eg, alpha-blockers, calcium channel blockers, nitrates, antiparkinsonism agents, antipsychotics, tricyclic antidepressants), peripheral edema, and confusion. Also important are strength, balance, and gait training as well as steps to improve bone density (with calcium and vitamin D supplementation).

Patients with repeated falls are often reassured by the availability of phones at floor level, a portable phone, or a lightweight radio call system. Their therapy should also include training in techniques for arising after a fall.

Table 3–5. Fall risk factors and targeted interventions.

Risk Factor	Targeted Intervention
Postural hypotension (> 20 mm Hg drop in systolic BP, or systolic BP < 90 mm Hg)	Behavioral recommendations, such as hand clenching, elevation of head of bed; discontinuation or substitution of high-risk medications
Use of benzodiazepine or sedative-hypnotic	Education about sleep hygiene, discontinuation or substitution of medications
Use of over three prescription medications	Review of medications
Environmental hazards	Appropriate changes; installation of safety equipment (eg, grab bars)
Gait impairment	Gait training, assistive devices, balance or strengthening exercises
Impairment in transfer or balance	Balance exercises, training in transfers, environmental alterations (eg, grab bars)
Impairment in leg or arm muscle strength or limb range of motion	Excercise with resistance bands or putty, with graduated increases in resistance

Campbell AJ et al: Randomised controlled trial of a general practice programme of home based exercise to prevent falls in elderly women. BMJ 1997;315:1065. [NLM Cit ID: 98033532] (Balance improved and the relative risk of falls and associated injuries was 30–40% lower among patients receiving program implemented by physiotherapists.)

Close J et al: Prevention of falls in the elderly trial: a randomised controlled trial. Lancet 1999;353:93. [NLM Cit ID: 99146498] (Risk of repeat falls was significantly reduced in the intervention group receiving medical and occupational therapy, with odds ratio 0.39.)

Cumming RG et al: Home visits by an occupational therapist for assessment and modification of environmental hazards: A randomized trial of falls prevention. J Am Geriatr Soc 1999;47:1397. [NLM Cit ID: 20057188] (Intervention consisting of a single home visit by an occupational therapist, with telephone follow-up to encourage adherence to recommendations, led to a significant reduction in falls in patient with a previous fall history.)

Gregg EW et al: Physical activity and osteoporotic fracture risk in older women. Study of Osteoporotic Fractures Research Group. Ann Intern Med 1998;129:81. [NLM Cit ID: 98318185]

Ray WA et al: A randomized trial of a consultation service to reduce falls in nursing homes. JAMA 1997;278:557. [NLM Cit ID: 97412163] (Interdisciplinary assessment and training of facility staff at each home reduced recurrent falls in residents not bed-bound from 54% to 44% and reduced injurious falls as well. Excellent accompanying editorial.)

Tinetti ME et al: Falls, injuries due to falls, and the risk of admission to a nursing home. N Engl J Med 1997; 337:1279. [NLM Cit ID: 97475839]

URINARY INCONTINENCE

Loss of bladder control has a major psychologic and social impact, and often contributes to institutionalization. Too often, the patient is simply labeled "incontinent," and no attempt is made to discern the type or to provide proper treatment. The problem is common and often not volunteered; clinicians should ask their patients about it.

Classification (Table 3–6)

Because continence requires adequate mobility, mentation, motivation, and manual dexterity, problems outside the bladder often result in geriatric incontinence. These are causes of transient incontinence, though they may cause prolonged incontinence if the problems are not identified and treated. Instances of new-onset incontinence often arise during hospitalization. In contrast to transient incontinence, causes of established, or persistent, incontinence generally can be found in the urinary tract itself.

A. Transient Causes: Use of the mnemonic "DIAPPERS" may help one remember the categories of transient incontinence.

Table 3–6. Classification of geriatric incontinence.

Transient
Delirium or confusional state
Infection, urinary (symptomatic)
Atrophic urethritis or vaginitis
Pharmaceuticals
Psychologic, especially severe depression
Excessive urine output (eg, congestive heart failure, hyperglycemia)
Restricted mobility
Stool impaction
Established
Detrusor overactivity (urge incontinence)
Detrusor underactivity (eg, neurogenic bladder)
Urethral obstruction
Urethral incompetence (stress incontinence)

1. Delirium–A clouded sensorium impedes recognition of both the need to void and the location of the nearest toilet. Delirium is the most common cause of incontinence in hospitalized patients; once it clears, incontinence resolves.

2. Infection–Symptomatic urinary tract infection commonly causes or contributes to incontinence. Asymptomatic bacteriuria does not.

3. Atrophic urethritis and vaginitis–Because it usually coexists with atrophic vaginitis, atrophic urethritis can be diagnosed presumptively by the presence of vaginal mucosal telangiectasia, petechiae, erosions, erythema, or friability. Urethral inflammation commonly contributes to incontinence in women and responds to treatment for several months with low-dose estrogen (eg, 0.3–0.6 mg conjugated estrogens by mouth; topical administration is more expensive and may be uncomfortable).

4. Pharmaceuticals–Drugs are one of the most common causes of transient incontinence. Typical offending agents include potent diuretics, anticholinergics, psychotropics, opioid analgesics, alpha blockers (in women), alpha agonists (in men), and calcium channel blockers.

5. Psychologic factors–Severe depression with psychomotor retardation may impede the ability or motivation to reach a toilet.

6. Excess urine output–Excess urine output may also overwhelm the ability of an older person to reach a toilet in time. In addition to diuretics, common causes include excess fluid intake; metabolic abnormalities (eg, hyperglycemia, hypercalcemia, diabetes insipidus); and disorders associated with peripheral edema, with its associated heavy nocturia when previously dependent legs assume a horizontal position in bed. Edema may be due to heart failure, venous insufficiency, malnutrition, cirrhosis, and use of calcium channel blockers or NSAIDs.

7. Restricted mobility–(See Immobility section, above.) If mobility cannot be improved, access to a urinal or commode (eg, at the bedside) may improve continence.

8. Stool impaction–This is a common cause of urinary incontinence in hospitalized or immobile patients. Although the mechanism is still unknown, a clinical clue to its presence is the onset of both urinary and fecal incontinence. Disimpaction restores urinary continence.

B. Established Causes: Causes of established incontinence (Figure 3–2) should be addressed after the transient causes have been uncovered and managed appropriately.

1. Detrusor overactivity (urge incontinence)–Detrusor overactivity refers to uninhibitable bladder contractions that cause leakage. It is the most common cause of established geriatric incontinence, accounting for two-thirds of cases. Women will complain of urinary leakage after the onset of an intense urge to urinate that cannot be forestalled. In men the symptoms are similar, but since detrusor overactivity may be due to coexisting urethral obstruction (typically from prostatic disease), urodynamic testing should be done if prescription of a bladder relaxant is planned, in order to avoid precipitating urinary retention. Because detrusor overactivity also may be due to bladder stones or tumor, the abrupt onset of otherwise unexplained urge incontinence—especially if accompanied by perineal or suprapubic discomfort or sterile hematuria—should be investigated by cystoscopy and cytologic examination of a urine specimen.

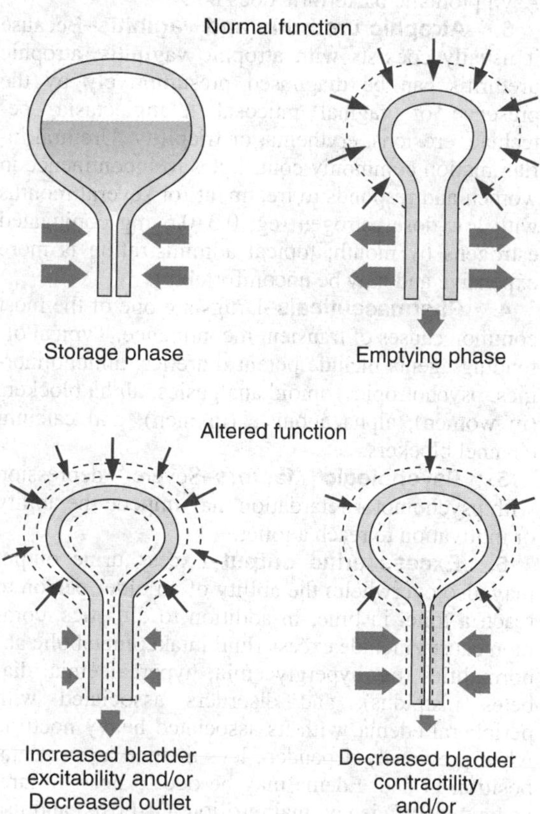

Figure 3–2. ***Top:*** Normal bladder physiology. ***Bottom:*** Pathophysiology underlying established causes of urinary incontinence.

2. Urethral incompetence (stress incontinence)–The second most common cause of established incontinence in older women (it is rare in men), stress incontinence is characterized by instantaneous leakage of urine in response to a stress maneuver. It commonly coexists with detrusor overactivity. Typically, urinary loss occurs with laughing, coughing, or lifting heavy objects. Leakage is worse, or occurs only during the day, unless another abnormality (eg, detrusor overactivity) is also present. To test for stress incontinence, have the patient relax her perineum and cough vigorously (a single cough) while standing with a full bladder. Instantaneous leakage indicates stress incontinence if urinary retention has been excluded by postvoiding residual determination using ultrasound. A delay of several seconds or persistent leakage suggests that the problem is instead caused by an uninhibited bladder contraction induced by coughing.

3. Urethral obstruction–Rarely present in women, urethral obstruction (due to prostatic enlargement, urethral stricture, bladder neck contracture, or prostatic cancer) is a common cause of established incontinence in older men. It can present as dribbling incontinence after voiding, urge incontinence due to detrusor overactivity (which coexists in two-thirds of cases), or overflow incontinence due to urinary retention. Renal ultrasound is required to exclude hydronephrosis in men whose postvoiding residual urine exceeds 150 mL. In older men for whom surgery is planned, urodynamic confirmation of obstruction is strongly advised.

4. Detrusor underactivity (overflow incontinence)–Detrusor underactivity is the least common cause of incontinence. It may be idiopathic or due to sacral lower motor nerve dysfunction ("neurogenic bladder"). When it causes incontinence, detrusor underactivity is associated with urinary frequency, nocturia, and frequent leakage of small amounts. The elevated postvoiding residual urine (generally over 450 mL) distinguishes it from detrusor overactivity and stress incontinence, but only urodynamic testing differentiates it from urethral obstruction in men. Such testing usually is not required in women, in whom obstruction is rarely present.

Treatment

A. Transient Causes: Each identified transient cause should be treated regardless of whether an established cause coexists. For patients with urinary retention induced by an anticholinergic agent, discontinuation of the drug should first be considered. If this is not feasible, substituting a less anticholinergic agent (eg, sertraline instead of desipramine for depression) may be useful.

B. Established Causes:

1. Detrusor overactivity–The cornerstone of treatment is behavioral therapy. Patients are instructed to void every 1–2 hours while awake. Once daytime continence is restored, the interval is increased by 30 minutes until the interval is 4–5 hours. Most patients who become continent during the day on this regimen become continent at night as well. For patients who are unable to manage on their own, caregivers should ask whether they need to void at suitable intervals.

Biofeedback can be extremely helpful in training cognitively intact, motivated patients to exercise their pelvic floor muscles and thus improve continence. Results superior to use of bladder relaxants are possible.

If behavioral approaches prove insufficient, drug therapy to relax the detrusor may be necessary. Regimens should be monitored to avoid inducing urinary retention. Use of oxybutynin (2.5–5 mg three or four times daily) or tolterodine (1–2 mg twice daily) may reduce episodes of incontinence, and the latter agent is less apt to cause dry mouth.

In refractory cases, where intermittent catheterization is feasible, the physician may choose intentionally to induce urinary retention with a bladder relaxant and have the patient empty the bladder three or four times daily. Clean but not sterile technique is required.

2. Urethral incompetence (stress incontinence)–Although a last resort, surgery is the most effective treatment for stress incontinence, resulting in a cure rate of 75–85% even in older women. For women who wish to avoid surgery and who can employ them indefinitely, pelvic muscle exercises are effective for mild to moderate stress incontinence; they can be combined, if necessary, with biofeedback or vaginal cones. Conjugated estrogens (0.3–0.6 mg daily) may be useful as well. Occasionally, a pessary or even a tampon (for women with vaginal stenosis) provides some relief, especially for frail women.

3. Urethral obstruction–Surgical decompression is the most effective treatment for obstruction, especially in the setting of urinary retention. A variety of newer, less invasive techniques make decompression feasible even for frail men. For the nonoperative candidate with urinary retention, intermittent or indwelling catheterization is used. For a man with prostatic obstruction who is not in retention and who wishes to defer surgery or is not a good surgical candidate, treatment with alpha-blocking agents (eg, terazosin 5–10 mg daily) may relieve symptoms. Finasteride may partially relieve symptoms in one-third of patients, but the onset of effect requires many months to a year.

4. Detrusor underactivity–For the patient with a poorly contractile bladder, augmented voiding techniques (eg, double voiding, suprapubic pressure) often prove effective. If further emptying is needed, intermittent or indwelling catheterization is the only option. Antibiotics should be used only for symptomatic upper urinary tract infection or as prophylaxis against recurrent symptomatic infections in a patient using intermittent catheterization; they should not be used as prophylaxis with an indwelling catheter.

Burgio KL et al: Behavioral vs drug treatment for urge urinary incontinence in older women: a randomized, controlled trial. JAMA 1998;280:1995. [NLM Cit ID: 99079554] (Episodes of incontinence were reduced over 80% on average with behavioral treatment, compared with 70% reduction from medication and 40% from placebo.)

Fantl JA et al: Urinary incontinence in adults: Acute and chronic management. Clinical Practice Guideline, No. 2, 1996 Update. Rockville, MD: US Dept of Health and Human Services. Public Health Service, AHCPR. Publication No. 96-0682.

Resnick NM: An 89-year-old woman with urinary incontinence. JAMA 1996;276:1832. [NLM Cit ID: 97102665] (Case conference discussion illustrating an effective multifactorial approach.)

Samsioe G: Urogenital aging—a hidden problem. Am J Obstet Gynecol 1998;178:S245. [NLM Cit ID: 98270762]

WEIGHT LOSS AND MALNUTRITION

Undernutrition affects substantial numbers of elderly persons and often precedes hospitalization for "failure to thrive." Unintended weight loss exceeding 5% in 1 month or 10% in 6 months deserves evaluation.

Table 3–7 lists causes of weight loss in older adults and may suggest points of history to explore. Useful laboratory and radiologic studies include com-

Table 3–7. Causes of unintended weight loss in the elderly.

Medical
Chronic heart, lung disease
Dementia
Oral problems (eg, poor denture fit)
Dysphagia
Mesenteric ischemia
Cancer
Diabetes
Hyperthyroidism
Psychosocial
Alcoholism
Depression
Social isolation
Limited funds
Problems with shopping or food preparation
Inadequate assistance with feeding
Drug-related
NSAIDs
Antiepileptics
Digoxin
Selective serotonin reuptake inhibitors

plete blood count, serum chemistries (including glucose, TSH, creatinine, calcium), urinalysis, and chest film. These studies are intended to uncover an occult metabolic or neoplastic cause but are not exhaustive.

Treatment with nutritional supplements may lead to weight gain, but they are expensive; use of instant breakfast powder in whole milk (for those who can tolerate dairy products) is a less costly alternative. Megestrol acetate has been employed as an appetite stimulant (primarily in cancer and AIDS patients) but has not been shown to increase body mass or lengthen life in the elderly population.

For those who have lost the ability to feed themselves, assiduous hand feeding may allow maintenance of weight. Although artificial nutrition and hydration ("tube feeding") may seem a more convenient alternative, it deprives the patient of the taste and texture of food as well as the social milieu typically associated with mealtime; before this option is chosen, the patient or his surrogate will wish to review the benefits and burdens of the treatment in light of overall goals of care. If the patient makes repeated attempts to pull out the tube during a trial of artificial nutrition, the treatment burden becomes substantial, and the utility of tube feeding should be reconsidered. Though commonly employed, there is no evidence that tube feeding prolongs life in patients with end-stage dementia.

"Failure to thrive" is a syndrome lacking a consensus definition but generally represents a constellation of weight loss (due to some combination of causes listed in Table 3–7), weakness, and progressive functional decline. The label is typically applied when some triggering event—loss of social support, a bout of depression or pneumonia, the addition of a new medication—pulls a struggling elderly person below the threshold of successful independent living. Ideally, use of the preventive measures recommended earlier in this chapter will reduce the patient's chances of reaching this stage of frailty.

Finucane TE et al: Tube feeding in patients with advanced dementia: a review of the evidence. JAMA 1999;282:1365. [NLM Cit ID: 99454308] (Authors found no data suggesting that tube feeding of advanced dementia patients reduced risk of pressure sores or infection nor that it improved function or provided palliation.)

Gazewood JD et al: Diagnosis and management of weight loss in the elderly. J Fam Pract 1998;47:19. [NLM Cit ID: 98338391]

Gurley RJ et al: Persons found in their homes helpless or dead. N Engl J Med 1996;334:1710. [NLM Cit ID: 96240533] (Alcohol and use of multiple medications contribute, as does acute illness; providing older and chronically ill patients with portable electronic alert devices is a potentially useful intervention.)

Sarkisian CA et al: "Failure to thrive" in older adults. Ann Intern Med 1996;124:1072. [NLM Cit ID: 96233417] (Authors suggest abandoning the term and assessing components instead, eg, impaired physical function, malnutrition, depression, and cognitive impairment.)

PHARMACOTHERAPY & POLYPHARMACY

There are several reasons for the greater incidence of iatrogenic drug reactions in the elderly population. Drug metabolism is often impaired in this group, due to a decrease in glomerular filtration rate, as well as reduced hepatic clearance. The latter is due to decreased activity of microsomal enzymes and reduced hepatic perfusion with aging. The volume of distribution of drugs is also affected. Since the elderly have a decrease in total body water and a relative increase in body fat, water-soluble drugs become more concentrated, and fat-soluble drugs have longer half lives. In addition, serum albumin levels decrease, especially in sick patients, so that there is reduction in protein binding of some drugs (eg, warfarin, phenytoin), leaving more free (active) drug available.

In addition, older individuals often have altered responses to a given serum drug level. Thus, they are more sensitive to some drugs (eg, opioids) and less sensitive to others (eg, beta-blocking agents).

Finally, the older patient with multiple chronic conditions is likely to be receiving many drugs, including nonprescribed agents. Thus, adverse drug reactions and dosage errors are more likely to occur, especially if the patient has visual, hearing, or memory deficits.

Precautions in Administering Drugs

The following suggestions are designed to reduce the risk of drug toxicity.

A. Drug Selection and Administration:

1. The symptom requiring treatment may be due to another drug, leading to a "prescribing cascade," in which adverse drug effects are attributed to new medical conditions, in time resulting in prescription of still more medications.

2. Nonpharmacologic means should be tried before drugs. Pharmacotherapy is not necessarily indicated in some common clinical situations. In asymptomatic bacteriuria, for example, antibiotics need not be given unless the disorder is associated with obstructive uropathy, other anatomic abnormalities, or stones. Ankle edema is often due to venous insufficiency, drugs (NSAIDs, calcium channel blockers), malnutrition, or inactivity in chair-bound patients and need not be treated with diuretics unless associated with heart failure. Leg elevation in the evening or fitted pressure-gradient stockings are often helpful.

3. Therapy is begun with less than the usual adult dosage and the dosage increased slowly, consistent with its pharmacokinetics in older patients. However, age-related changes in drug distribution and clearance are variable among individuals, and some require full doses. After determining acceptable measures of success and toxicity, the dose is increased until one or the other is reached.

Despite the importance of beginning new drugs in a slow, measured fashion, all too often an inadequate trial is permitted (in terms of duration of course, or ultimate dose) before they are discontinued. Angiotensin-converting enzyme inhibitors and antidepressants, in particular, are frequently stopped before therapeutic dosages are reached.

4. Steps are taken to improve adherence to the prescribed medical regimen. The following increase the odds of nonadherence: the patient lives alone; uses more than one pharmacy or provider; is prescribed medications with multiple daily doses; has a drug regimen that is changed frequently; is prescribed a large number of drugs; has difficulty reaching a pharmacy; and has poor cognition, vision, or dexterity. When possible, the physician should keep the dosing schedule simple, the number of pills low, and the medication changes infrequent.

5. A family member is asked to bring in all medications at each visit for reinforcing instructions regarding reasons for drug use, dosage, frequency of administration, and possible adverse effects.

6. Although serum drug levels may be useful for monitoring certain drugs with narrow therapeutic windows (eg, phenytoin, theophylline, lithium, tricyclic antidepressants), toxicity can still occur even with "normal" therapeutic levels of many drugs.

7. Trials of individual drug discontinuation should be considered (including antihypertensives, digoxin, antiepileptics), particularly in a controlled environment such as a nursing facility.

B. Considerations With Specific Drug Classes:

1. Anticoagulants–Many elderly patients with atrial fibrillation are not anticoagulated because physicians fear injuries and secondary bleeding due to falls. Head injuries due to falls are usually of greatest concern, and occur in about 1% of falls. Given that anticoagulation can result in an annual absolute risk reduction in stroke of 3–8%, the benefits of anticoagulation outweigh the risks of falling in most instances.

2. Glaucoma medications–Not only can topical beta-blockers cause systemic side effects (bradycardia, asthma, heart failure), but so too can oral carbonic anhydrase inhibitors. The latter may produce malaise, anorexia, and weight loss.

3. Analgesics–Meperidine is associated with an increased risk of delirium and seizures in the elderly, and should be avoided in this population. Of the NSAIDs, indomethacin carries the highest risk of causing confusion. For treatment of osteoarthritis, use of acetaminophen on a scheduled basis is safer than use of an NSAID, with comparable effectiveness.

4. Antihypertensives–In most instances, the first choice for treating hypertension in older people is a thiazide in low dosage, eg, hydrochlorothiazide 12.5 mg by mouth daily. Unfortunately, thiazides increase the risk of gout flares. Concomitant use of an NSAID can exacerbate hypertension.

5. Cold remedies–Over-the-counter cold remedies frequently cause adverse effects in elderly people. The anticholinergic properties of many can create confusion (even in nondemented persons), impair bladder emptying, or cause constipation, and decongestants not infrequently cause urinary hesitancy or retention in men.

6. Antiemetics–Prochlorperazine and metoclopramide both can cause drug-induced parkinsonism.

Beers MH: Explicit criteria for determining potentially inappropriate medication use by the elderly: An update. Arch Intern Med 1997;157:1531. [NLM Cit ID: 97379755]

McLeod PJ et al: Defining inappropriate practices in prescribing for elderly people: A national consensus panel. CMAJ 1997;156:385. [NLM Cit ID: 97185740]

RELEVANT WORLD WIDE WEB SITES

[Administration on Aging]
http://www.aoa.dhhs.gov

[AHCPR: Benign Prostatic Hyperplasia: Diagnosis and Treatment]
http://text.nlm.nih.gov/ftrs/pick?dbName=bphc&ftrsK=40746&cp=1&t=915077905&collect=ahcpr

[AHCPR: Cardiac Rehabilitation]
http://text.nlm.nih.gov/ftrs/pick?dbName=crpc&ftrsK=40746&cp=1&t=915078348&collect=ahcpr

[AHCPR: Cataracts in Adults: Management of Functional Impairment]
http://text.nlm.nih.gov/ftrs/pick?dbName=catc&ftrsK=40746&cp1&t=915077539&collect=ahcpr

[AHCPR: Depression in Primary Care]
http://text.nlm.nih.gov/ftrs/pick?dbName=dep1c&ftrsK=40746&cp=1&t=915077709&collect=ahcpr

[AHCPR: Pressure Ulcers in Adults: Prediction and Prevention]
http://text.nlm.nih.gov/ftrs/pick?dbName=ulcc&ftrsK=40746&cp=1&t=915077407&collect=ahcpr

[AHCPR: Post-stroke Rehabilitation]
http://text.nlm.nih.gov/ftrs/pick?dbName=psrc&ftrsK=40746&cp=1&t=915078090&collect=ahcpr

[AHCPR: Urinary Incontinence in Adults: Acute and Chronic Management]
http://text.nlm.nih.gov/ftrs/pick?dbName=cuic&ftrsK=40698&cp=1&t=915077055&collect=ahcpr

[Alzheimer's Association]
http://www.alz.org

[Geriatric Education Cases]
http://www.medinfo.ufl.edu/cme/geri

[Kansas Elder Law Network]
http://www.ink.org/public/keln/keln_index.html

[Medicare Publications]
http://www.medicare.gov/publications.html

[Multidisciplinary Education in Geriatrics and Aging]
http://cpmcnet.columbia.edu/dept/dental/Dental_Educational_Software/Gerontology_and_Geriatric_Dentistry/introduction.html#mainindex

4 Cancer

See http://www.current-med.com/ch04.html for updated addresses of Web sites referenced in this chapter.

Hope S. Rugo, MD

This chapter covers mainly the clinical aspects of cancer: prevention, diagnosis, primary treatment, management of complications, and paraneoplastic syndromes. Further information may be obtained by calling the NCI Cancer Information Service at 1-800-4CANCER or accessing NCI's comprehensive cancer information database "Physician Data Query" (PDQ) via the Internet. PDQ is also available on CD-ROM. The CANCERLIT feature of Medline is a familiar resource for articles about cancer that can be accessed by author or by subject words.

Many new Web sites are now available for both physician and patient use. Information includes statistics, treatment, and clinical trial information. Consultations can also be obtained. Web sites can be found by searching for the words "cancer" or "oncology."

[National Cancer Institute: Physician's Data Query]
http://cancernet.nci.nih.gov/pdq.htm

INCIDENCE & ETIOLOGY

Cancer is the second most common cause of death in the United States. It is estimated that over 1.2 million new cases of invasive cancer will be diagnosed in the year 2000, with over 500,000 deaths. One out of every two to three individuals in the United States will develop some type of invasive cancer during their lifetime. Table 4–1 summarizes current United States incidence and mortality figures for the ten leading types of cancer. Women have an approximately 1:7 lifetime chance of developing breast cancer, and men have an approximately 1:5 chance of developing prostate cancer. Cancers of the lung, prostate, and breast and of the colon and rectum account for about 54% of all new cancer diagnoses and for over 50% of cancer deaths in the United States. Table 4–2 summarizes the lifetime risk of being diagnosed with or dying from the five leading causes of cancer as well as from all types of cancer. The incidence of and the mortality from cancer has decreased an average of 1.3% per year from 1992 to 1997 in the United States, with variation by gender and race. This is the first sustained decline in the past 30 years and is attributed to changes in lifestyle as well as improved prevention, early detection, and treatment.

The cause of most cancers remains unknown. Recently, however, mutations in DNA sequences leading to abnormal or unregulated expression of protooncogenes or deletion of tumor suppressor genes—or both processes—have been linked to abnormal cellular proliferation. Oncogenes encode for cellular growth factor receptors, growth factors, or elements of the proliferative machinery of the cancer cell. Tumor suppressor genes govern regulatory proteins that normally suppress cellular proliferation. Cancer results from these and other mutations, which may be due to environmental exposure, genetic susceptibility, infectious agents, and other factors. Most tumors exhibit chromosomal abnormalities such as deletions, inversions, translocations, or duplications. Although usually nonspecific, certain genetic alterations are strongly associated with specific malignancies. In Burkitt's lymphoma, the *c-myc* oncogene is activated by translocation of genetic material from chromosome 8 to chromosome 14. In colon cancer, loss of the long arm of chromosome 18 predicts a poor outcome. A tumor suppressor termed *DCC* (deleted in colorectal cancer) is thought to be inactivated by this loss. When compared with colorectal cancers that express DCC, deletion of DCC is associated with a 30% reduction in the 5-year survival rate in stage II cancers and 20% in stage III. The *P53* gene appears to trigger programmed cell death (apoptosis) as a way of regulating uncontrolled cellular proliferation in the setting of aberrant growth signals. Mutations in the *P53* gene result in loss of the ability of the gene product to bind to DNA, thereby removing its suppressive effect. *P53* can also be inactivated by overexpression of an oncogene whose protein product binds to normal *P53* and pre-

Table 4–1. Incidence of and mortality from the ten most common cancers in the USA in males and females (all race

Rank		
		7
	7	2

Data obtained from the NCI SEER Program.
[1]Rates are per 100,000, 1990–1997, and are age-adjusted to the 1970 United States population.
[2]Uterus includes the cervix and corpus uteri.
[3]Both Hodgkin's disease and non-Hodgkin's lymphoma are included under lymphoma.
[4]Both oropharynx and larynx are included under oropharyngeal.

vents its action. This occurs in many soft tissue sarcomas. Another control against abnormal cellular proliferation also contributes to cellular aging. As a cell divides and ages, there is progressive shortening of the ends of the chromosomes, or telomeres. A striking correlation between cancer and the overexpression of telomerase (an enzyme capable of preventing the shortening of telomeres) suggests that it might be partially responsible for tumor cell immortality. Telomerase activity is present in about 85% of malignant tumors but absent in most normal somatic tissues. The stage and severity of neuroblastoma, breast cancer, and other cancers have been found to correlate with levels of telomerase activity, indicating a prognostic role of enzyme activity. Normal human cells transfected with the telomerase gene in vitro far exceeded their normal life span and ability to divide, thereby establishing a firmer causal relationship between telomere shortening and cellular senescence. This raises important possibilities for targeting telomerase activity as part of cancer therapy.

Table 4–2. Lifetime risks for the five most common cancers.[1]

Cancer	Risk of Diagnosis (%)	Risk of Death (%)
Prostate (men)	15.7	3.3
Breast (women)	13	3.3
Lung		
(men)	7.8	7.6
(women)	5.7	4.8
Colorectal		
(men)	5.8	2.5
(women)	5.5	2.4
Bladder (men)	3.3	0.7
Uterus[2]	3.5	0.8
Any cancer		
(men)	42.8	24
(women)	37.6	20.5

[1]Data obtained from the National Cancer Institute's SEER program, 1995–1997.
[2]Uterus includes the cervix and corpus uteri.

Autoimmune suppression may contribute to the development of cancer. Tumors are allowed to exist by virtue of tolerance—the ability of the tumor to escape the host immune system. The host immune system cannot recognize the tumor as foreign because of an absence of critical immunostimulatory molecules on the tumor itself, resulting in a state of anergy (deletion of tumor-specific lymphocytes) toward the growing cancer. Novel therapies aimed at correcting this immunodeficient state and stimulating the host immune response against tumor cells are now being developed and tested in the clinic. (See section on Novel Therapies at the end of this chapter.)

It is difficult to link exposures to carcinogens with the development of cancer, since latency is long and the nature of exposure poorly documented. Environmental carcinogens include chemical carcinogens such as benzene and asbestos, oncogenic viruses such as the human papillomavirus and the Epstein-Barr virus, and physical agents such as ionizing radiation and ultraviolet light.

Hereditary predisposition to some cancers has been linked to events within a gene and is manifested trong family history of a relatively rare cancer. nples include familial retinoblastoma, familial nomatous polyposis, multiple endocrine neoplasia ndromes, and the hereditary breast and ovarian ancer syndromes. Although familial adenomatous polyposis is a rare syndrome, somatic mutations in the affected gene (adenomatous polyposis coli; *APC*) also occur in more than 60% of patients with colonic carcinomas and in an equal proportion of patients with adenomas. Genetic mutations associated with an increased risk of developing breast and ovarian cancers appear to be much more common than previously thought and are strongly related to age at diagnosis of cancer. It is estimated that 5–10% of all breast cancers and more than 40% of breast cancers occurring in women under 30 are due to inheritance of an abnormal gene. The risk of ovarian and other cancers is also significantly increased in carriers of these susceptibility genes. A tumor suppressor gene termed *BRCA1* on chromosome 17 has been shown to be mutated in some families with early-onset breast and ovarian cancer. More than 100 mutations have been identified in the *BRCA1* gene, making identification of high-risk individuals difficult. Two recent population-based studies found that up to 20% of Jewish women with breast cancer at or before the age of 40 and approximately 10% of all women with breast cancer diagnosed before the age of 35 harbor mutations in the *BRCA1* gene. Inheritance of a mutated *BRCA1* gene confers a lifelong risk of 85% for breast cancer and 50% for ovarian cancer. Compared with sporadic ovarian cancers, those associated with the *BRCA1* mutation appeared to have a better clinical course, with a median survival of 77 months in women carrying the mutation compared with 29 months in controls. Inheritance of the *BRCA1* gene also appears to increase the risk of developing both colon and prostate cancers. Another gene, *BRCA2,* has been associated with an increased risk for male breast cancer as well. Many other less common genes have been identified that increase the risk of breast and other cancers.

With the discovery and cloning of cancer susceptibility genes such as *BRCA1,* commercial testing has been developed for "screening" using linked genetic markers. Tests for genes linked to familial cancer have raised concerns about the impact of positive results on patients. One study has evaluated indications for testing of the *APC* gene. Of the patients tested, 85% were felt to have valid indications for testing. However, only 20% received genetic counseling before the test; only 15% gave informed consent; and in 30% of cases the physicians misinterpreted the results. It is essential that physicians recognize the limitations of these tests and that genetic testing be made available in the appropriate setting. Educational programs and publications are available to help educate patients regarding genetic testing. Many cancer centers now have genetic screening and counseling programs. Patients with a strong family history of cancer should be referred to such programs before testing is performed. Early and regular cancer screening is recommended for affected members of the family, and aggressive but relatively effective preventive measures such as prophylactic mastectomy and oophorectomy should also be addressed.

Other familial clusterings of cancer have been described that have not yet been associated with inheritance of a particular gene. Evaluation of participants in a study of colonic polyps revealed an increased risk of colorectal cancer in the siblings and parents of patients with adenomatous polyps, particularly when the adenoma was diagnosed before age 60 or (for a sibling) when a parent had colorectal cancer. This syndrome, referred to as a hereditary nonpolyposis colorectal cancer (HNPCC), has been associated with a germ line mutation of DNA mismatch-repair genes. At least 2% of patients with colorectal cancer had these mutations in one European cohort. Testing for replication errors should be considered in patients under age 50 with colorectal cancer who have a family history of colorectal or endometrial cancer. Family members of patients with this syndrome may benefit from early screening. In addition to the germline mutations found in HNPCC, up to 10–15% of sporadic colorectal cancers have somatic mutations in DNA repair genes resulting in microsatellite instability (MSI) or alterations in the size of repetitive nucleotide sequences. These cancers are usually in the right side of the colon and have been associated both with a better prognosis and a striking sensitivity to adjuvant chemotherapy. The HER2/*neu* oncogene is overexpressed in about 25% of breast cancers; this phenotype is associated with more aggressive cancers, a worse prognosis, and enhanced anthracycline chemotherapy sensitivity. Identifying genetic factors that are associated with specific cancer phenotypes may allow effective tailoring of adjuvant chemotherapy.

Certain viral infections may increase the risk of cancer and clearly have a pathogenetic role, such as the association between Epstein-Barr virus infection and endemic Burkitt's lymphoma. Chronic hepatitis infection with hepatitis B or C viruses increases the risk of hepatocellular carcinoma. Largely owing to the increase in chronic hepatitis, the incidence of hepatocellular carcinoma has significantly increased during the 1990s compared with the 1970s. Infection with HIV has been associated with non-Hodgkin's lymphoma, Hodgkin's disease, Kaposi's sarcoma, and cervical and anal cancers. The finding of human herpesvirus-8 (HHV-8) DNA sequences in both AIDS-associated and non-AIDS-associated Kaposi's sarcoma and perhaps also in multiple myeloma supports a causative role of the herpesviruses in the development of some cancers. It appears that HHV-8 is sexually transmitted among men. Antibodies to HHV-8 correlate with the subsequent development of

Kaposi's sarcoma, supporting an etiologic role of HHV-8 in this malignancy. The sexually transmitted human papillomavirus (HPV) is a major risk factor for the development of cervical carcinoma and anal cancer. The prognosis of cervical cancer is dependent on the oncogenic potential of the associated HPV type, with the worst prognosis associated with HPV18. Typing of the virus strain in each cancer may allow risk-adjusted treatment planning.

An additional cause of cancer is chemotherapy or radiation therapy for a prior malignancy. More aggressive chemotherapeutic and radiation regimens—and especially those combining the two treatment modalities—have been associated with increased rates of both secondary leukemias and solid tumors. The latency period may be short (2–5 years for leukemia) or very long (10–20 years for solid tumors), but the prognosis is uniformly poor. Chemotherapeutic agents known to cause secondary malignancies include alkylating agents (busulfan, cyclophosphamide, mechlorethamine, etc) and topoisomerase II inhibitors (the epipodophyllotoxins: etoposide, teniposide). Secondary leukemias are usually associated with chromosomal aberrations involving chromosomes 5 and 7 in alkylator-induced leukemias and the long arm of chromosome 11 (11q23) in epipodophyllotoxin-induced leukemias. Abnormalities of 11q23 involve a specific breakpoint region thought to be involved in DNA transcription. An increase in the rate of secondary acute leukemia has been reported in breast cancer patients treated with dose intensification of cyclophosphamide in combination with doxorubicin (a topoisomerase II active drug) from 1992 to 1994. The incidence is approximately 0.3% in a multicenter study involving over 2500 women with positive axillary nodes, but the follow-up is still short. Platinum-based chemotherapy for ovarian cancer has been reported to increase the risk of leukemia twofold to eightfold, with larger doses and longer treatment courses associated with higher risks. This risk was significantly higher in women who had also received intravenous melphalan. The risk of certain secondary cancers may be age-dependent. Radiation therapy for Hodgkin's disease increases the risk of breast cancer if the radiation occurred in women under the age of 30. The relative risk of solid tumors and leukemias has been found to increase significantly with younger age at first chemotherapy treatment for Hodgkin's disease. This risk is especially high when chemotherapy and radiation are combined.

Recent data indicate that the combination of estrogen and progesterone given as long-term hormonal replacement therapy (HRT) to postmenopausal women may significantly increase the risk of breast cancer. Clearly, there is no increased risk associated with short-term (< 5 years) replacement, and cardiovascular and bone density benefits may outweigh these risks in the general population. Further prospective data will be needed to confirm this risk.

Aaltonen LA et al: Incidence of hereditary nonpolyposis colorectal cancer and the feasibility of molecular screening for the disease. N Engl J Med 1998;338:1481. [NLM Cit ID: 98242977] (By molecular analysis, 2% of 500 patients with colorectal cancer were found to have this syndrome.)

Buys CH: Telomeres, telomerase, and cancer. N Engl J Med 2000;342:1282. [NLM Cit ID: 20228766] (A brief but readable review of the role of telomerase in cancer and current research.)

Chang F et al: Implications of the *p53* tumor-suppressor gene in clinical oncology. J Clin Oncol 1995;13:1009. [NLM Cit ID: 95222299] (A summary of data on the alterations of the *P53* gene including implications for pathogenesis, diagnosis, prognosis, and therapy in cancers.)

Eisen A et al: Prophylactic surgery in women with a hereditary predisposition to breast and ovarian cancer. J Clin Oncol 2000;18:1980. [NLM Cit ID: 20247365] (A literature review of published retrospective trials and management recommendations.)

Fitzgerald MG et al: Germ-line *BRCA1* mutations in Jewish and non-Jewish women with early-onset breast cancer. N Engl J Med 1996;334:143. [NLM Cit ID: 96127978] (Two landmark population-based studies screening for this mutation found a 10–20% incidence in young women with breast cancer.)

Frisch M et al: Sexually transmitted infection as a cause of anal cancer. N Engl J Med 1997;337:1350. [NLM Cit ID: 98000004] (Human papillomavirus appears to cause both cervical and anal cancers and is transmitted sexually.)

Gryfe R et al: Tumor microsatellite instability and clinical outcome in young patients with colorectal cancer. N Engl J Med 2000;342:69. [NLM Cit ID: 20080316] (Microsatellite instability appears to be an independent predictor of favorable outcome and reduced incidence of metastatic disease.)

Lombard I et al: Human papillomavirus genotype as a major determinant of the course of cervical cancer. J Clin Oncol 1998;16:2613. [NLM Cit ID: 98368408] (Invasive cervical cancer with HPV18 or HPV16 sequences has a significantly poorer prognosis than does cancer associated with other HPV sequences.)

Martin JN et al: Sexual transmission and the natural history of human herpes virus 8 infection. N Engl J Med 1998;338:948. [NLM Cit ID: 98172957] (Antibodies to HHV-8 correlated with a history of sexually transmitted diseases, increased number of sexual partners, and the subsequent development of Kaposi's sarcoma.)

Schairer C et al: Menopausal estrogen and estrogen-progestin replacement therapy and breast cancer. JAMA 2000;283:485. [NLM Cit ID: 20123270] (Data from the Breast Cancer Detection Demonstration Project, a cohort study from 1980 to 1995, suggests that estrogen-progestin increases breast cancer risk over that associated with estrogen alone.)

Statement of the American Society of Clinical Oncology: Genetic Testing for Cancer Susceptibility. J Clin Oncol 1996;14:1730. [NLM Cit ID: 96208855] (Recommendations for screening.)

Travis LB et al: Risk of leukemia after platinum-based chemotherapy for ovarian cancer. N Engl J Med 1999;340:351. [NLM Cit ID: 99119167] (The risk of leukemia is increased in patients receiving platinum-based chemotherapy for ovarian cancer.)

Warmuth MA et al: A review of hereditary breast cancer: from screening to risk factor modification. Am J Med 1997;102:407. [NLM Cit ID: 97360660] (A review of genetic testing, risk factor modification, and screening.)

PREVENTION OF CANCER

PRIMARY PREVENTION

1. LIFESTYLE MODIFICATIONS

Population studies suggest that lifestyle—including tobacco use, diet, and alcohol consumption—accounts for a majority of avoidable cancer deaths in the United States. Other factors, including obesity, parity, and length of lactation, have also been associated with increased cancer risk. Although prostate and breast cancers are the most common malignancies in men and women, respectively, the most common cause of cancer death in both sexes is still lung cancer. Since 1973, there has been only a 10% increase in the incidence of lung cancer in men compared with a 124% increase in women, reflecting a marked increase in the number of women who smoke. Since tobacco-related cancers account for at least 29% of all fatal forms of cancer, smoking cessation is an important area for continued education and prevention efforts. Strategies for helping patients stop are described in Chapter 1. Programs directed both at cessation of smoking and at reversing the social acceptability of cigarette smoking have been more successful than programs encouraging cessation alone. In California and Massachusetts, increasing the excise tax on cigarettes combined with an antismoking campaign appears to have resulted in a 2–3% decrease in the prevalence of adult smoking. The molecular targets for carcinogens such as alcohol and tobacco have not yet been identified. However, an evaluation of tumor samples from over 100 patients with squamous cell carcinoma of the head and neck has associated cigarette smoking with genetic mutations in the *P53* gene, thought to result in the initiation or progression of this cancer. This supports the epidemiologic evidence that abstinence from smoking is important in preventing head and neck cancer.

Diet is an important area of intervention for primary cancer prevention. Epidemiologic studies suggest an inverse relationship between fruit and vegetable intake and the risk of common carcinomas, indicating a potential protective role of these dietary components. High intakes of fat and specific fatty acids had been postulated to increase the risk of breast, colon, prostate, and lung cancer. However, the Nurses' Health Study, which followed more than 88,000 women for 14 years with food frequency questionnaires every 4 years beginning in 1980, gathered no evidence that a lower intake of total fat or specific major types of fat decreased the risk of breast cancer. A meta-analysis published in 1999 evaluated dietary fat intervention studies (published from 1966 through 1998) of serum estradiol levels and fat consumption. These findings did not rule out the possibility that reducing fat consumption below 20% of calories might reduce breast cancer risk by lowering serum estradiol levels. Another study compared the dietary intake of saturated fat of 1665 men with prostate cancer to the diet of an equal number of men without the disease. A high intake of saturated fat increased the risk of prostate cancer in all four major ethnic groups evaluated. There was no increase in prostate cancer among men with the lowest intake of saturated fats.

A high intake of dietary fiber has long been thought to reduce the risk of colorectal cancer and adenomas. The Nurses' Health Study investigated the intake of dietary fiber in the same population specified above, and no association was found between the intake of dietary fiber and the risk of colorectal cancer or adenomas. A prospective study of over 10,000 men likewise did not find a significant association between fiber intake and the risk of developing adenomas. Two recent prospective, randomized trials tested the value of a high-fiber, low-fat diet or a high-fiber cereal supplement versus a standard diet in reducing the risk of recurrent colorectal adenomas in men and women with a recent prior diagnosis of adenoma and demonstrated no difference in the risk of recurrent adenoma based on dietary regimens. Other dietary factors such as folate may reduce the risk of colorectal malignancy, but this too will require further investigation.

The Women's Health Initiative, begun in 1993, is examining the effects of three distinct interventions: a low-fat eating pattern, hormone replacement therapy, and calcium supplementation on the prevention of cancer, cardiovascular disease, and osteoporosis in 64,500 women of all races. An additional 100,000 women will be enrolled in an observational study. This study will be completed in the year 2007.

Another lifestyle factor with important implications for primary prevention is exposure to ultraviolet light. Chronic cumulative exposure to solar ultraviolet radiation is the major risk factor for nonmelanomatous skin cancer. Regular use of sunscreen prevents the development of precancerous solar keratoses and results in regression of existing keratoses, although the effect of sunscreens on the incidence of melanoma is not clear. Protection from sunlight and the regular use of sunscreens should be recommended for the primary prevention of skin cancers.

Agency for Health Care Policy and Research: Smoking Cessation: Information for specialists. Clinical Practice

Guidelines. Quick Reference Guide for Clinicians 1996;18B:1. (A guide to the clinician.)

Alberts DS et al: Lack of effect of a high-fiber cereal supplement on the recurrence of colorectal adenomas. N Engl J Med 2000;342:1156. [NLM Cit ID: 20218601] (A dietary supplement of wheat-bran fiber does not protect against recurrent colorectal adenomas.)

Holmes MD et al: Association of dietary intake of fat and fatty acids with risk of breast cancer. JAMA 1999;281:914. [NLM Cit ID: 99176374] (Fat ingestion assessed by periodic dietary questionnaire did not contribute to the risk of breast cancer over a 14-year period.)

Osborne M et al: Cancer prevention. Lancet 1997; 348(Suppl 2):SII27. [NLM Cit ID: 97307232]

Schatzkin A et al: Lack of effect of a low-fat, high-fiber diet on the recurrence of colorectal adenomas. N Engl J Med 2000;342:1149. [NLM Cit ID: 20218600] (A diet low in fat and high in fiber, fruit, and vegetables does not influence the risk of recurrent colorectal adenomas.)

2. CHEMOPREVENTION

Chemoprevention focuses on the prevention of cancer by administering chemical compounds that interfere with the multistaged carcinogenic process. Better understanding of the biochemical and molecular mechanisms of carcinogenesis has made possible the identification of potential chemopreventive agents. Four risk groups have been identified for intervention: (1) previous cancer patients (to prevent second malignancies), (2) patients with preneoplastic lesions, (3) patients at high risk for malignancy (family history, lifestyle, occupation), and (4) the general population.

Chemicals used in chemoprevention must be nontoxic and well tolerated by otherwise asymptomatic individuals. Because of the long natural history of carcinogenesis, there must also be a method of evaluating the efficacy of chemopreventive agents other than waiting for the development of tumors. Biomarkers, including the premalignant markers such as leukoplakia, colonic polyps, and now aberrant crypt formation in the colon, are currently in clinical use. Molecular susceptibility markers may become useful; nuclear retinoic acid receptor agonists are under investigation in chemoprevention studies of patients with head and neck cancer.

Anticarcinogens under investigation include factors present within the diet (eg, vitamins), NSAIDs, and hormone-suppressing agents (eg, tamoxifen, finasteride). Retinoids, the natural derivatives and synthetic analogs of vitamin A, are the best-studied chemopreventive agents. Numerous additional investigations should reveal exciting new information—in particular, the role of the antihormonal agents tamoxifen and finasteride.

Beta-Carotene & Vitamin E

The carotenoids are plant pigments that protect plant cells from damage and were thought to have an antioxidant role in human tissues. Beta-carotene is a carotenoid found in high concentrations in human tissues; its importance as an antioxidant is controversial. A role for beta-carotene in the prevention of either premalignant or malignant disease has not been established. Vitamin E is another antioxidant that has been studied as a cancer prevention agent with interesting preliminary efficacy information.

Supplemental beta-carotene and vitamins C and E were not found to reduce the rate of colorectal adenomas by colonoscopy at 4 years of follow-up. Several randomized studies have evaluated the effect of beta-carotene and vitamin E on the prevention of cancer in high-risk populations. The Alpha-Tocopherol, Beta Carotene (ATBC) Cancer Prevention Study randomized 29,000 Finnish male smokers to receive beta-carotene, vitamin E, both agents, or neither agent for an average of 6 years. A minimal (2%) and statistically insignificant reduction in the incidence of lung cancer was seen in the men who received vitamin E. In contrast, there was an 18% higher incidence of lung cancer in the group taking beta-carotene. Vitamin E supplementation reduced prostate cancer incidence by 34% and colorectal cancer by 16%, though only the reduction in prostate cancer incidence was statistically significant. Men in the control group with higher levels of vitamin E or beta-carotene before the study was initiated developed fewer lung cancers, suggesting that other components of foods high in these vitamins may be responsible for some of the protective effects noted in epidemiologic studies.

The interim results of the Beta-Carotene and Retinal Efficacy Trial (CARET), a lung cancer chemoprevention study targeting high-risk populations, have been reported. This trial involved a total of 18,000 smokers, nonsmokers, and workers with extensive occupational exposure to asbestos. Participants were randomized to receive either a combination of 30 mg/d of beta-carotene (as an antioxidant) and 25,000 IU/d of retinol (vitamin A, as a tumor suppressor) or placebo. With an average of 4 years and 73,000 person-years of follow-up, the combination of beta-carotene and vitamin A had no benefit on the incidence of lung cancer. In fact, the active treatment group had a 28% higher incidence of lung cancer than the placebo group, and the mortality from all causes and the rate of death from cardiovascular disease were higher by 17% and 26%, respectively. On the basis of these results, this study was stopped in January 1996, though the participants will be followed for an additional 5 years beyond that time.

The Physician's Health Study investigated 22,000 United States male physicians randomized to receive beta-carotene (50 mg on alternate days) or placebo. The physicians were treated for an average of 12 years; 11% were current smokers and 39% were former smokers at the beginning of the study. In this trial, no evidence either of benefit or of increased risk for cancer was found, with a much longer follow-up than in the other two studies. There were no differences in the overall incidence of malignant neoplasms, cardiovascular disease, or overall mortality in the group as a whole or in the smokers. One additional randomized study in which a positive effect of beta-carotene supplementation was found evaluated a poorly nourished population group rather than the well-nourished populations described above. Linxian, China, is an area with one of the world's highest rates of esophageal and stomach cancer and a habitually low intake of several nutrients. In nearly 30,000 participants from the general population, the mortality rates from cancer were substantially lower among those who received daily supplementation with a combination of beta-carotene, alpha-tocopherol, and selenium over a 5-year period. A marked reduction in the cancer death rate (13%) was observed in the supplemented group, largely due to a 21% decrease in stomach cancer mortality. Over 85% of cancers arose in the esophagus or stomach, but 31 deaths were caused by lung cancer. The risk of death from lung cancer was reduced by 45% among those receiving supplements, though the numbers were very small (11 versus 20 lung cancer deaths), and only 30% of the group were cigarette smokers. The NCI is currently collaborating with agencies in China to pursue further chemoprevention studies in this unique population.

In summary, there is no evidence to support the use of beta-carotene in the primary prevention of cancer in well-nourished populations. The major criticism of the large studies conducted to date is that increasing one type of vitamin—even one stereoisomer of a vitamin—does not reflect the vitamin content of a diet high in vegetables. In addition, intake of beta-carotene is a marker of increased fruit and vegetable consumption. The balanced mixture of antioxidants found in a diet rich in fruit and vegetables may be more important and more effective in reducing cancer risk than beta-carotene supplementation. Other micronutrients such as vitamin E may prove more promising.

The Women's Health Study, begun in 1992, is a randomized, double-blind, placebo-controlled trial testing the risks and benefits of vitamin E, beta-carotene, and aspirin in the primary prevention of cancer and cardiovascular disease in 40,000 healthy female health professionals in the USA.

Isotretinoin & Acyclic Retinoids

Retinoids are modulators of epithelial cell differentiation both in vivo and in vitro that are thought to act on nuclear receptors to regulate both cellular growth and differentiation and cell apoptosis.

Isotretinoin has been shown to suppress leukoplakia, a premalignant lesion of the aerodigestive tract. Effectiveness and tolerability of low doses of isotretinoin have been demonstrated. Only patients with a demonstrated response to high-dose induction (1.5 mg/kg/d) were placed on low-dose maintenance therapy (0.5 mg/kg/d). The disease progression rate was only 8% compared with a rate of 55% in a separate group taking beta-carotene.

High doses of isotretinoin prevent the development of second primary tumors in patients with early squamous cell carcinoma of the head and neck. This information has led to the development of several trials investigating the role of isotretinoin in the prevention of second tumors following treatment of early-stage head and neck cancer or non-small-cell lung cancer. These trials are still under way. Because side effects were observed with high doses, the drug is now being given at a lower dose (30 mg/d) for a longer time after diagnosis (3 years). The major toxicity at higher doses includes skin dryness, cheilitis, hypertriglyceridemia, conjunctivitis, and leukoplakia. These toxicities require dose reduction or temporary discontinuation of the drug. Leukoplakia resolves when the medication is discontinued.

New retinoids have been synthesized that may also be potent chemopreventive agents. The acyclic retinoid polyprenoic acid inhibits chemically induced hepatocarcinogenesis in rats and spontaneous hepatomas in mice. In patients with hepatocellular carcinoma, the rate of recurrent and second primary tumors is high despite curative therapy with surgical resection and ethanol injection therapy. In one study, 89 patients who were free of disease after either method of treatment were randomized to receive either 600 mg/d of polyprenoic acid or placebo for 12 months. After a median follow-up of 38 months, 27% of patients in the polyprenoic acid group versus 49% of the patients in the placebo group had recurrent or new hepatocellular carcinomas, a result which was statistically significant. The difference was even greater in the groups that had secondary hepatomas. Longer follow-up has also shown a survival advantage. At a median of 62 months of follow-up, 75% of the treatment group versus 45% of the placebo group are alive. Toxicity was quite modest (headache, nausea), with none of the side effects usually described with isotretinoin. Three strategies that have been proved to prevent liver carcinogenesis are vaccination against hepatitis B, treatment of chronic active hepatitis C with interferon, and deletion of premalignant and latent malignant cells in the remnant livers of patients undergoing complete resection of hepatocellular carcinomas. A newer retinoid, fenretinide (4-HPR), is in early clinical trials for the chemoprevention of breast and prostate cancers.

Aspirin & Other NSAIDs

Aspirin and other NSAIDs inhibit tumor growth in experimental systems. Prostaglandin inhibitors can reduce the size and number of colon tumors in rats induced by chemicals or radiation. This effect is thought to be due to inhibition of cyclooxygenase activity (COX-1 and COX-2). Levels of COX-2 are elevated in some solid tumors, and COX-2 may act as a tumor promoter in the intestine. This is thought to be secondary to other initiating events, such as oncogene activation or mutation of a tumor suppressor gene. Regular aspirin administration at low doses (16 or more doses per month for at least 1 year) may reduce the risk of fatal colon cancer by as much as 40–50%. Low-dose aspirin may also protect against cancers of the esophagus, stomach, and rectum.

A study evaluating the use of sulindac versus placebo in patients with familial adenomatous polyposis showed reduction of both the number and the size of colorectal adenomas. The effect was incomplete, without complete regression of all polyps in any patient. After the sulindac was discontinued, both polyp size and polyp number increased. A large prospective cohort study was subsequently published evaluating aspirin use and the risk for both colorectal cancer and adenoma in 48,000 male health professionals over a 4-year period. The subsequent risk of developing colorectal cancer and adenomas was lower in men reporting regular use of aspirin (more than twice a week) on the study entry questionnaire even when multiple other variables were taken into account. In the Nurse's Health Study, 90,000 women were evaluated for the risk of colorectal cancer over a 12-year period according to the number of consecutive years of regular aspirin use (two or more tablets per week) reported on three consecutive questionnaires. There was a statistically significant decrease in the risk of colorectal cancer after 20 years of consistent aspirin use, with the maximal reduction seen in women who took four to six tablets per week. A slight reduction in risk was seen in women who took aspirin for 10–19 years as well. Known risk factors such as diet did not influence this risk reduction. Two ongoing investigations of aspirin in colorectal adenoma prevention should provide additional information. The effect of NSAIDs in prevention of other tumors is under investigation. A selective COX-2 enzyme inhibitor, celecoxib, has been shown to induce regression of polyps in patients with familial adenomatous polyposis. Celecoxib was recently approved for this purpose. The use of celecoxib and other selective COX-2 inhibitors in cancer prevention and treatment is being actively studied.

Calcium & Selenium

Dietary patterns continue to be associated with a risk of colorectal neoplasia. The changes in risk may be contributed to by alterations in bile acids. Calcium appears to bind bile acids in the bowel lumen, inhibiting bile-induced mucosal damage and perhaps carcinogenesis. A modest reduction in the incidence of adenomas in patients taking calcium supplementation has been shown in patients receiving it over a 4-year period. The Selenium and Vitamin E Cancer Prevention Trial (SELECT) is the largest chemoprevention study ever to be undertaken and is scheduled to begin in the latter half of 2000. This NCI-sponsored trial will randomize 32,400 men age 50–55 and older to selenium, vitamin E, both, or placebo for 7–12 years. This study is based on the results of the Alpha-Tocopherol Beta-Carotene Cancer Prevention Study, in which vitamin E reduced prostate cancer incidence by 32%, and the selenium and skin cancer trial, in which selenium reduced the incidence of prostate cancer by 63%.

Tamoxifen

Tamoxifen is an antiestrogen with an important role in the treatment of both early and advanced breast cancer. Studies of women taking tamoxifen as adjuvant therapy for unilateral breast cancer have shown a 30–40% reduction in the risk of developing a second primary in the opposite breast. The Breast Cancer Prevention Trial (BCPT) is a nationwide trial that randomized 13,400 women at high risk for breast cancer to receive either tamoxifen (20 mg/d) or placebo for 5 years. The trial was stopped at a median follow-up of 4 years due to a striking 50% reduction in the risk of breast cancer in the women taking tamoxifen—89 women taking tamoxifen developed breast cancer, compared with 175 taking placebo. This benefit was restricted solely to the development of estrogen-receptor-positive cancers. In addition to invasive cancer, there was a similar reduction in the risk of noninvasive breast cancer such as ductal or lobular carcinoma in situ. Tamoxifen also decreased the number of bone fractures. Two smaller European studies failed to confirm the chemopreventive role of tamoxifen. Not only were these studies smaller than the United States study, but the determination of risk used different parameters. Side effects of tamoxifen include a small increase in the risk of endometrial cancer, deep vein thrombosis, and pulmonary embolism. This effect was seen primarily in women over age 50.

The use of tamoxifen for this indication is controversial because of these secondary effects, primarily the increase in endometrial cancer. This risk is small when compared with the incidence of breast cancer in women on placebo in the trial. Even if the incidences of endometrial cancer and breast cancer are considered together, there was still a 30% reduction in the risk of cancer in the women receiving tamoxifen.

Raloxifene

Early results of the MORE (Multiple Outcomes of Raloxifene Evaluation) trial have provided more information regarding prevention of breast cancer. Raloxifene is a novel selective estrogen receptor modulator with estrogenic effects on bone and lipids and estrogen antagonist effects on the breast and uterus. Two different doses of raloxifene or placebo were administered to 7700 postmenopausal women to test the hypothesis that raloxifene would reduce the risk of bone fractures. After 2½ years, a 70% reduction in the risk of breast cancer was found in the women taking raloxifene compared to the women taking placebo. A suggestion of decreased risk of endometrial cancer was also found. The long-term safety and follow-up of raloxifene in these women is under continued study. The effects of raloxifene in women with breast cancer or in women at high risk for developing breast cancer has not been evaluated (see below).

Ongoing Trials in Breast Cancer

The Study of Tamoxifen and Raloxifene (STAR) starting in 1999 with a goal of randomizing 22,000 American and Canadian postmenopausal women (age 35 or older) at increased risk of breast cancer to either daily tamoxifen (20 mg/d) or raloxifene (60 mg/d) for 5 years, and 3100 women have been randomized as of January 2000. This study should answer the question of whether raloxifene is as effective as tamoxifen at reducing the chance of breast cancer—with additional benefits such as fewer side effects. Additional information regarding the STAR trial and eligibility criteria as well as other studies on breast cancer can be found at the NCI clinical trials Web site (http://cancertrials.nci.nih.gov) or by calling 800-4-CANCER.

Finasteride

Finasteride is a 5α-reductase inhibitor used to treat benign prostatic hyperplasia. This agent inhibits the enzyme responsible for converting testosterone to 5α-dihydrotestosterone, suppressing prostate cell and organ growth. In rats, finasteride prevented macroscopic but not microscopic prostate carcinogenesis—supporting the use of this agent in the prevention of conversion of latent prostate carcinoma to life-threatening disease. The Prostate Cancer Prevention Trial (PCPT) is evaluating the use of finasteride to prevent the development of prostate cancer in men with normal digital rectal examinations and prostate-specific antigen (PSA) concentrations. Eighteen thousand men have been randomized in this 7-year study to receive either finasteride or placebo. Results are expected in 2004.

Other Current Trials

Additional trials are under way investigating the effect of both diet and pharmacologic agents in the prevention of cancer. These include studies of soy isoflavones, folic acid, dietary fat and fish oils, raloxifene, retinoids, sulindac, and others. Dietary agents such as polyprenols in green tea are thought to play a role in chemoprevention and are under investigation.

Further information about ongoing chemoprevention trials can be obtained from the Chemoprevention Branch of the National Cancer Institute (301-496-8563).

Baron JA et al: Calcium supplements for the prevention of colorectal adenomas. N Engl J Med 1999;340:101. [NLM Cit ID: 99091094] (Calcium supplementation is associated with a moderate reduction in the risk of recurrent colorectal adenomas.)

Fisher G et al: Tamoxifen for the prevention of breast cancer: report of the National Surgical Adjuvant Breast and Bowel Project P-1 Study. J Natl Cancer Inst 1998;90:1371. [NLM Cit ID 98418640] (Results of the United States primary prevention trial.)

Garay CA et al: Chemoprevention of colorectal cancer: dietary and pharmacologic approaches. Oncology 1999; 13:89. [NLM Cit ID: 99151265] (Review of chemoprevention data for colorectal cancer.)

Kurie JM: The biologic basis of the use of retinoids in cancer prevention and treatment. Curr Opin Oncol 1999; 11:497. [NLM Cit ID: 20016207] (A summary of prevention and treatment trials as well as background on the molecular basis of using retinoids for cancer prevention.)

Prevention of cancer in the next millennium: Report of the chemoprevention working group to the American Association for Cancer Research. Cancer Res 1999;59:4743. [NLM Cit ID: 99446866] (A review of existing trials and evidence supporting chemoprevention.)

Tsukamoto S et al: A five-alpha reductase inhibitor or an antiandrogen prevents the progression of microscopic prostate carcinoma to macroscopic carcinoma in rats. Cancer 1998;82:531. [NLM Cit ID: 98112650] (Finasteride prevents the progression of prostate cancer in rats.)

Wu GD: A nuclear receptor to prevent colon cancer. N Engl J Med 2000;342:651. [NLM Cit ID: 20143082] (A readable review of the mechanism of the chemopreventive effects of nonsteroidal anti-inflammatory drugs.)

SECONDARY PREVENTION (Early Detection)

Given the inadequacy of current knowledge concerning the causes of cancer, effective prevention can be achieved for only a minority of malignancies. Other than primary prevention and perhaps chemoprevention, the most effective physician intervention is early diagnosis. Screening is used for early detection of cancer in otherwise asymptomatic populations. Detection of cancer may be achieved through observation (eg, skin, mouth, external genitalia, cervix), palpation (eg, breast, mouth, thyroid, rectum and anus, prostate, testes, ovaries and uterus, lymph nodes), and laboratory tests and procedures (eg, Papanicolaou smear, sigmoidoscopy, mammography). Effective screening requires that a test will specifically detect early cancers or premalignancies, be cost-effective, and result in improved therapeutic outcomes. Screening for breast and cervical cancer alone is projected to result in a 3% reduction in cancer deaths. For most cancers, stage at presentation is related to curability, with the highest cure rates reported when the tumor is small and there is no evidence of metastasis. However, for some tumors (eg, lung or ovarian cancer), distant metastases tend to occur early, even from a small primary. More sensitive detection methods such as tumor markers are being developed for many forms of cancer, and some tumor markers, such as PSA, are already a regular (though controversial) part of routine cancer screening (see section on tumor markers). Screening is not useful if no method of early detection exists (eg, cancer of the pancreas) or if there is no apparent localized stage (eg, leukemia).

Cancers for which screening or early detection has led to an improvement in outcome include cancers of the breast, cervix, colon, prostate, oral cavity, and skin. Techniques for early detection for breast cancer include self-examination, clinical examination, and mammography. There is strong evidence that regular mammography and clinical breast examination in women aged 40–69 or with a family history of breast cancer are effective in reducing the number of deaths. The reduction in mortality from screening in women aged 40–49 years is lower than in older women but still appears to be statistically significant, leading to higher cost per cancer discovered. The effect of screening on breast cancer mortality in women over age 70 is unknown. Both mammography and clinical examination of the breast are associated with a significant number of false-positive results, leading to further testing. Screening mammograms and clinical breast examinations in 2400 women over a 10-year period found that 24% and 13% (respectively) of women had at least one false-positive mammogram or false-positive clinical examination. Despite the sensitivity of mammography, about 10% of palpable breast cancers are not visible by this radiographic technique. All clinically suspicious lesions should be biopsied regardless of a negative mammogram.

Regular screening for cervical cancer (every 3 years in standard risk groups) with Papanicolaou tests has been found to decrease the mortality rate in women who are sexually active or are 18 years of age or older. Testing for HPV DNA in high-risk populations may improve early detection of cervical cancer. Self-collected vaginal swabs for DNA testing may improve screening in areas where cytology is not readily available or in populations where women are hesitant to undergo regular examinations. Routine screening with vaginal Pap smears in women who have previously undergone a hysterectomy for benign gynecologic disease is not as useful owing to the very low incidence of squamous cell cancers of the vagina. Annual fecal occult blood testing and screening with sigmoidoscopy every 5 years in people over age 50 decreases the mortality rate from colorectal cancer. In addition, removing polyps detected by colonoscopy reduces the risk of colorectal cancers. Even adenomatous polyps 5 mm or less in diameter detected in the rectosigmoid by sigmoidoscopy are markers for more advanced proximal neoplasms. These patients should undergo colonoscopy to evaluate the proximal bowel. Table 1–8 outlines the American Cancer Society's recommendations for cancer screening for standard-risk individuals. Unfortunately, screening for ovarian cancer with serum markers (eg, CA 125), transvaginal ultrasound, or pelvic examinations has not been shown to decrease the mortality rate from this disease. A multicenter trial is under way to test whether a multimodality screening program will be more effective than each of these methods alone. Screening for prostate cancer and hepatocellular cancer is discussed in the section on tumor markers.

Screening is underutilized in minority groups in the United States, especially in inner city and rural areas. This results in the diagnosis of cancers at more advanced stages. Educational and outreach programs should be directed at these underserved areas.

Elmore JG et al: Ten-year risk of false positive screening mammograms and clinical breast examinations. N Engl J Med 1998;338:1089. [NLM Cit ID: 98196615] (One-third of women screened who did not have breast cancer had an abnormal test result that required additional evaluation.)

Helm JF et al: Colorectal cancer screening. Med Clin North Am 1999;83:1403. [NLM Cit ID: 20051995] (Screening modalities and guidelines are reviewed.)

Read TE et al: Importance of adenomas 5 mm or less in diameter that are detected by sigmoidoscopy. N Engl J Med 1997;336:8. [NLM Cit ID: 97122456] (Even tiny distal polyps can predict advanced proximal tumors; these patients require colonoscopic evaluation.)

Smith RA et al: American Cancer Society Guidelines for the early detection of cancer. CA Cancer J Clin 2000;50:34. [NLM Cit ID: 20199189] (The current ACS guidelines and an explanation of how these guidelines were developed.)

Smith TJ et al: American Society of Clinical Oncology 1998 Update of Recommended Breast Cancer Surveillance Guidelines. J Clin Oncol 1999;17:1080. [NLM Cit ID: 99168861] (Recommendations for the detection of recurrent cancer based on impact on outcome.)

Wright TC Jr et al: HPV DNA testing of self-collected vaginal samples compared with cytologic screening to detect cervical cancer. JAMA 2000;283:81. [NLM Cit ID: 20096145] (HPV testing of self-collected vaginal swabs is less specific but as sensitive as Pap smears for detecting high-grade cervical disease and may be a way to increase screening in women from areas where cytology is not readily performed.)

SPECIAL TOPICS IN PREVENTION

Patients with a family history of colorectal cancer are at increased risk to develop this disease and should undergo regular screening, which clearly reduces the incidence and mortality from invasive cancer. Guidelines for patients with a risk of hereditary nonpolyposis colon cancer are referenced below. Approximately 10% of breast and ovarian cancers are hereditary, occurring primarily in women with mutations of *BRCA1* and *BRCA2*. Patients with a family history of breast or ovarian cancer are at higher risk to develop these cancers and require frequent monitoring for early detection, though screening is inadequate to detect early ovarian cancer. Prophylactic oophorectomy after completion of childbearing can decrease but not eliminate the risk of ovarian cancer in high-risk women; there is still a risk of peritoneal cystadenocarcinoma. Oral contraceptives appeared to decrease the risk of ovarian cancer by as much as 60% in women with a family history of ovarian cancer. Prophylactic mastectomy has been used for decades to reduce the risk of breast cancer in high-risk women and is associated with a substantial reduction in breast cancer risk. In women at both high and moderate risk of breast cancer based on family history, the incidence of breast cancer (and death from breast cancer) is reduced by at least 90%. Decisions about such prophylactic surgery in high-risk women must be made taking full account of many other factors—clearly, breast cancer would not have developed in all women undergoing the procedure. Any patient with a history of dysplasia or premalignant lesions is at high risk for development of invasive cancer and should undergo frequent and thorough screening for subsequent malignancy. Patients at a particularly high individual risk for cancer may require additional screening procedures. Screening for lung cancer in high-risk individuals with more sensitive radiographic techniques is being studied.

Burke W et al: Recommendations for follow-up care of individuals with an inherited predisposition to cancer. I. Hereditary nonpolyposis colon cancer. Cancer Genetics Studies Consortium. JAMA 1997;277:915. [NLM Cit ID: 97216041]

Burke W et al: Recommendations for follow-up care of individuals with an inherited predisposition to cancer. II. *BRCA1* and *BRCA2*. Cancer Genetics Studies Consortium. JAMA 1997;277:997. [NLM Cit ID: 97228039] (Suggestions for screening and prevention in these very high risk groups.)

Hartmann LC: Efficacy of bilateral prophylactic mastectomy in women with a family history of breast cancer. N Engl J Med 1999;340:77. [NLM Cit ID: 99091091] (Prophylactic mastectomy reduces incidence of breast cancer by about 90% in women at high and moderate risk.)

Narod SA et al: Oral contraceptives and the risk of hereditary ovarian cancer. N Engl J Med 1999;339:424. [NLM Cit ID: 98355342] (Oral contraceptives decrease the risk of ovarian cancer in women who carry the *BRCA1* and *BRCA2* mutations.)

STAGING OF CANCER

Standardized staging for tumor burden at the time of diagnosis is important both for determining prognosis and for making decisions about treatment. The American Joint Committee on Cancer (AJCC) has developed a simple classification scheme that can be incorporated into a form for staging and universally applied. This scheme is designed to encompass the life history of a tumor and is referred to as the TNM system. The untreated primary tumor (T) will gradually increase in size, leading to regional lymph node involvement (N) and, finally, distant metastases (M). The tumor is usually not clinically evident until local invasion or even spread to regional draining lymph nodes has occurred.

TNM staging is used clinically to indicate the extension of cancer before definitive therapy begins. The manner in which staging is accomplished—eg, by clinical examination or pathologic examination of a surgical specimen—must be carefully documented. Certain types of tumors, such as lymphomas and Hodgkin's disease, are usually staged by a different classification scheme that reflects the natural history of this type of tumor spread and helps to direct treatment decisions.

The TNM system allows a numerical assessment of the extent of primary tumor (T), the absence or presence and extent of regional lymph node metastases (N), and the absence or presence of distant metastases (M).

Traditional staging does not take into account the biology or aggressiveness of a particular tumor and may not allow differentiation of prognostic risk groups. For this reason, specific pathologic characteristics are added into the prognostic evaluation for certain tumors (eg, estrogen and progesterone receptors, grade and proliferative index for breast cancer; histologic grade for sarcoma). Overexpression or underproduction of oncogene products (eg, Her-2/*neu* in breast cancer), infection of cancer cells with specific viral genomes (eg, HPV18 in cervical cancer), and certain chromosomal translocations or deletions (eg, alteration of the retinoic acid receptor gene in acute promyelocytic leukemia) have important prognostic significance and may direct risk-adapted or cancer-specific therapy. As these characteristics become standardized and better understood, they may allow us to identify patients with a poorer prognosis early in the course of disease when the patient might benefit from more aggressive therapy.

AJCC Cancer Staging Manual/American Joint Committee on Cancer, 5th ed. Lippincott-Raven, 1997. (The bible of TNM staging.)

PRIMARY CANCER TREATMENT

The reader is referred to the NCCN Oncology Practice Guidelines Web site at the end of this chapter.

SURGERY & RADIATION THERAPY

Most cancers present initially as localized tumor nodules and cause local symptoms. Depending on the type of cancer, initial therapy may be directed locally in the form of surgery or radiation therapy. Surgical excision or local radiation (or both) is the treatment of choice for a variety of potentially curable cancers, including most gastrointestinal and genitourinary cancers, central nervous system tumors, and cancers arising from the breast, thyroid, or skin as well as most sarcomas.

Surgery at presentation has both diagnostic and therapeutic effectiveness, since it permits pathologic staging of the extent of local and regional invasion as well as an opportunity for removal of the primary neoplasm. CT and MRI play an increasing role in noninvasive tumor staging. However, it is often necessary for the surgeon to identify patients intraoperatively whose disease can perhaps be cured by local treatment alone. Although standard surgery for breast cancer has included excision of axillary nodes, this can result in chronic lymphedema, pain, and decreased range of motion of the arm. Sentinel axillary nodes can be detected by injection of radioactive colloid or blue dye into the breast around the tumor or the biopsy cavity. "Hot spots" are then identified with a gamma probe and resected. Biopsy of sentinel nodes can predict the presence or absence of axillary node metastases and direct more aggressive surgery with up to 97% accuracy. However, the procedure is technically challenging and the success rate thus varies with the surgeon. Surgery may also play an important role in the treatment of selected patients with limited metastatic cancer. Resection of isolated metastases has been used most commonly for breast cancer with single brain lesions or isolated liver or lung lesions. Removal of isolated liver metastases may result in long-term survival, with 20% of patients living more than 5 years. Additional surgery after subsequent limited recurrence may also result in long-term disease-free survival.

For certain tumor sites, complete surgical removal of the tumor can be disfiguring, disabling, or unachievable. Under those circumstances, primary local therapy with ionizing radiation may prove to be the treatment of choice. In other instances, surgery and radiation therapy are used in sequence. For stage I and stage II breast cancer, local incision or "lumpectomy" with axillary node dissection combined with radiation results in equivalent 10-year survivals when compared with the more disfiguring and extensive mastectomy procedure. Preoperative or "neoadjuvant" chemotherapy and radiation therapy allow limb-sparing surgery in osteosarcoma and organ preservation in oropharyngeal cancer, among others.

Radiation therapy is usually delivered as brachytherapy or teletherapy. In brachytherapy, the radiation source is placed close to the tumor. This intracavitary approach is used for many gynecologic or oral neoplasms. In teletherapy, supervoltage radiotherapy is usually delivered with a linear accelerator, as this instrument permits more precise beam localization and avoids the complication of skin radiation toxicity. Various beam-modifying wedges, rotational techniques, and other specific approaches are used to increase the radiation dosage to the tumor bed while minimizing toxicity to adjacent normal tissues.

Well-oxygenated tumors are more radiosensitive than hypoxic tumors. Hypoxic tumors are often bulky, implying a potential synergistic role of surgical debulking prior to radiotherapy. Radiation therapy is normally delivered in a fractionated fashion over 4–6 weeks, this method appearing to have radiobiologic superiority by permitting time for recovery of normal host tissues (but not the tumor) from sublethal damage during treatment.

For most tumor types, there is a sigmoid curve of increasing rate of control of the local tumor with increasing radiation dose. Radiosensitive tumors usually exhibit radiosensitivity over the dose range of 3500–5000 cGy.

Currently, more than half of all patients with cancer receive radiation therapy during the course of their illness. Radiation therapy is frequently the sole agent used with curative intent for tumors of the larynx (permitting cure without loss of the voice), oral cavity, pharynx, esophagus, uterine cervix, vagina, prostate, skin, Hodgkin's disease, and some tumors of the brain and spinal cord. For more extensive cancers, radiation is combined with surgery (eg, cancer of the breast, ovary, uterus, cervix, urinary bladder, rectum, lung, soft tissue sarcomas, and seminoma of the testis). Radiation therapy to the chest wall with or without chemotherapy for breast cancer allows limited resection of the primary tumor. Following mastectomy, radiation has been shown to reduce the risk of local recurrence from large or high-risk tumors and may increase overall survival by decreasing distant recurrence. Radiation given in combination with chemotherapy may improve long-term disease control. The combination of chemotherapy and radiation therapy for the treatment of invasive carcinoma of the cervix is significantly superior to radiation therapy alone. There is at least a 10% improvement in 3-year survival and a 30–50% reduction in the risk of death from cervical cancer with combination therapy. Twice-daily radiation given concurrently with combination chemotherapy for the treatment of limited small-cell lung cancer results in significantly improved 5-year survival rates compared with any prior treatment results. Twice-daily radiation also appears superior to once-daily treatment for this disease. Radiation combined with chemotherapy for cancer of the rectum or hormone therapy for cancer of the prostate improves survival over treatment with radiation alone. Radiation can also improve disease control when given as an adjuvant to chemotherapy for bulky lymphomas, for non-small-cell lung cancer, and for some cancers in children.

Occasionally, chemotherapy is used to sensitize tumor cells to the toxic effects of radiation. Radiation therapy for palliation of pain or dysfunction (eg, bone pain associated with advanced breast or other cancers) may improve the quality of life of patients suffering from incurable malignancies.

Various normal tissues (particularly skin, mucosa, myocardium, spinal cord, bone marrow, and lymphoid system) can exhibit early or late toxicity from radiation therapy. Acute toxicity may include generalized fatigue and malaise, anorexia, nausea and vomiting, local skin changes, diarrhea, and mucosal ulceration of the irradiated area. Radiation of large areas, especially the pelvis and proximal long bones, may result in bone marrow suppression. Radiation of the lungs, heart, and gastrointestinal tract must be approached with appropriate shielding to avoid toxicity such as radiation pneumonitis, congestive heart failure, or radiation gastroenteritis. Long-term toxicity from radiation therapy has significant long-term side effects that must be weighed against its possible benefits. Women under age 60 treated with left-sided adjuvant radiation for breast cancer with 10–15 years of follow-up have a significant increase in risk of death from myocardial infarction. Increased cardiac mortality has also been seen in patients who received radiation at a young age for Hodgkin's disease. Secondary leukemias and solid tumors can be seen after radiation therapy for a wide variety of cancers. This risk is particularly high in patients receiving a combination of both radiation and chemotherapy that includes alkylating agents. Treatment programs now combine less toxic chemotherapy with limited field radiation therapy to limit these fatal long-term side effects in long-term survivors from cancer. Other long-term toxicities include decreased function of the radiation organ (eg, decreased cognitive function after whole brain radiation), myelopathy, osteonecrosis, and hyperpigmentation of the involved skin.

Novel modalities are occasionally used to enhance penetrance into large tumors or to specifically target the site of radiation. Regional hyperthermia (40–42 °C) is an adjunct to ionizing irradiation for some tumor sites. The most useful application of hyperthermia to date has been in superficial or easily implantable tumors as well as in relatively bulky hypovascular tumors with some degree of hypoxia. Electron beam therapy has been used effectively to treat superficial tumors in the skin. Radiolabeled antibodies are currently under investigation as a means of delivering high levels of radiation locally to the tumor bed, thereby avoiding systemic toxicity (see section on Novel Therapy). Increasingly, the primary local therapy of cancer is integrated with systemic therapy, an approach that has proved to be superior for apparently localized tumor types with a high propensity for early metastatic spread and for which anticancer drugs are available.

D'Angelica M et al: Ninety-six five-year survivors after liver resection for metastatic colorectal cancer. J Am Coll Surg 1997;185:554. [NLM Cit ID: 98067383] (Surgical resection of isolated metastases may result in long-term survival.)

Dearnaley DP et al: Comparison of radiation side-effects of conformal and conventional radiotherapy in prostate cancer: a randomised trial. Lancet 1999;353:267. [NLM Cit ID: 99126098] (Conformational radiotherapy limits radiation to normal tissues and in this study significantly lowered the risk of late radiation-induced proctitis with excellent local tumor control.)

Dewhirst MW et al: Hyperthermic treatment of malignant diseases: Current status and a view toward the future. Semin Oncol 1997;24:616. [NLM Cit ID: 98082721]

Krag D et al: The sentinel node in breast cancer. N Engl J Med 1998;339:941. [NLM Cit ID: 98418644] (Biopsy of the sentinel node can predict the presence or absence of axillary node metastases in patients with breast cancer.)

Paszat L et al: Mortality from myocardial infarction after adjuvant radiotherapy for breast cancer in the surveillance, epidemiology and end-results cancer registries. J Clin Oncol 1998;16:2625. [NLM Cit ID: 98368410] (Left-sided adjuvant radiation therapy for breast cancer in women under age 60 increases the risk of fatal myocardial infarction.)

Ragaz J et al: Adjuvant radiotherapy and chemotherapy in node-positive premenopausal women with breast cancer. N Engl J Med 1997;337:956. [NLM Cit ID: 97441017] (Radiation therapy following mastectomy in node-positive women may reduce distant recurrence and improve survival.)

Thomas GM: Improved treatment for cervical cancer—concurrent chemotherapy and radiotherapy. N Engl J Med 1999;340:1198. [NLM Cit ID: 99200752] (An editorial summarizing the results of three of the five randomized studies in that issue shows that concurrent radiation and chemotherapy improves survival from invasive cervical cancer.)

SYSTEMIC CANCER THERAPY

Use of cytotoxic drugs, hormones, antihormones, and biologic agents has become a highly specialized and increasingly effective means of treating cancer. Therapy is usually administered by a medical oncologist. Selection of specific drugs or protocols for various types of cancer has traditionally been based on results of prior clinical trials. Many patients are treated on protocols to provide optimal therapy for refractory or poorly responsive malignancies. Treatment may be inadequate or ineffective because of drug resistance of the tumor cells. This has been attributed to spontaneous genetic mutations in subpopulations of cancer cells prior to exposure to chemotherapy. After chemotherapy has eliminated the sensitive cells, the resistant subpopulation grows to become the predominant cell type (Goldie-Coldman hypothesis). This has been the basis of alternating non-cross-resistant chemotherapy regimens.

Molecular mechanisms of drug resistance are now the subject of intense study. In many instances, specific drug resistance results from an amplification in the number of gene copies for an enzyme inhibited by a specific chemotherapeutic agent. A more general form of "multidrug resistance" (MDR) has been described in association with expression of a gene *(MDR1)* encoding a 170-kDa transmembrane glycoprotein (P-glycoprotein) on tumor cells. This protein is an energy-dependent transport pump that facilitates drug efflux from tumor cells and promotes resistance to a broad spectrum of unrelated cancer drugs. Acquired multidrug resistance in multiple myeloma and lymphoma has been reversed clinically by adding the calcium channel blocker verapamil to chemotherapy regimens. Unfortunately, the doses of verapamil required to overcome drug resistance are associated with cardiovascular side effects. High doses of cyclosporine appear to increase the cytotoxicity of etoposide both in vitro and in vivo, probably by inhibiting the function of P-glycoprotein. MDR modulators will need to be both less toxic and more potent to be clinically useful. PSC 833 is a cyclosporine analog with little of the immunosuppressive effects or renal toxicities of cyclosporine but with five- to tenfold greater MDR-modulating activity. PSC 833 is being used in conjunction with chemotherapy in a variety of cancers, including leukemias and solid tumors. Both improved response rates and improved survival with a tolerable toxicity profile using novel therapy such as this will have to be demonstrated to prove the effectiveness of this approach.

Chemotherapy is used primarily to cure a small percentage of malignancies, as adjuvant therapy to decrease the rate of relapse or improve the disease-free interval, and to palliate symptoms and prolong survival in some patients with incurable malignancies. In addition, chemotherapy may play a role as preoperative or "neoadjuvant" therapy to reduce the size and extent of the primary tumor, thereby allowing complete excision at the time of surgery. Neoadjuvant (preoperative) chemotherapy results in identical survival when compared with standard postsurgical chemotherapy for breast cancer and allows more limited or complete surgical excision of the primary tumor as well as giving important information about chemosensitivity. Chemotherapy was first shown to be curative in the treatment of advanced stages of choriocarcinoma in women. It is also curative in Hodgkin's disease, diffuse large-cell and some high-grade lymphomas (including Burkitt's), carcinoma of the testis, some cases of acute leukemia, and embryonal rhabdomyosarcoma. When combined with initial surgery—and in some instances with irradiation—chemotherapy increases the rate of long-term control and cure of breast cancer, cervical cancer, small-cell lung cancer, colon cancer, rectal cancer, and osteogenic sarcomas. Combination chemotherapy provides palliation and prolongation of survival in adults with non-Hodgkin's lymphoma, mycosis fungoides, multiple myeloma and Waldenström's macroglobulinemia, acute and chronic leukemias, and breast, ovarian, cervical, and small-cell lung carcinoma as well as carcinoid. Patients with incurable tumors who desire aggressive treatment should be referred for experimental protocol therapy. (See section on Novel Therapies at the end of this chapter.)

High-dose chemotherapy followed by bone marrow transplantation is curative therapy for various types of leukemia, high-risk or relapsed lymphoma, testicular cancer, and occasionally for multiple myeloma. Allogeneic or autologous bone marrow or peripheral blood stem cells with or without ex vivo purging is used depending on the disease. The use of growth factors and blood stem cells has decreased the toxicity and cost of bone marrow transplantation. Autologous transplantation may now be used with low morbidity and mortality on selected patients up to age 70. Dose-intense chemotherapy with autologous bone marrow or peripheral blood stem cell rescue has been intensely studied for the treatment of both high-risk and metastatic breast cancer for the past decade with unfortunately inconclusive or poor-quality data. Details of these studies are presented in the section on adjuvant therapy.

While most anticancer drugs are used systemically, there are selected indications for local or regional administration. Regional administration involves direct infusion of active chemotherapeutic agents into the tumor site (eg, intravesical therapy for bladder cancer, intraperitoneal therapy for ovarian cancer, hepatic artery infusion with or without embolization of the main blood supply of the tumor for cancers metastatic to the liver). These treatments can result in palliation and prolonged survival.

A summary of the types of cancer responsive to chemotherapy and the current treatments of choice is offered in Table 4–3. In some instances (eg, Hodgkin's disease, breast cancer, ovarian and lung cancers), optimal therapy may require a combination of therapeutic resources, eg, radiation plus chemotherapy rather than either modality alone. Patients with stage I or stage II Hodgkin's disease are often treated with radiation alone, avoiding the potential toxicity of systemic chemotherapy. A small percentage of these patients may require chemotherapy later for disease recurrence.

New drugs to treat cancer are under constant development and testing—with the aim of reducing toxicity to normal cells and increasing the toxicity to resistant cancer cells. Several of these newer agents developed over the last decade that are currently available are described in this section.

A purine analog, cladribine (2-chlorodeoxyadenosine; 2-CdA), is used as the primary agent to treat hairy cell leukemia. A 1-week course of therapy results in high and durable remission rates with modest and short-lived toxicity. Repeated courses for disease recurrence are also effective. Pentostatin (2-deoxycoformycin, an adenosine deaminase inhibitor) is also used to treat hairy cell leukemia.

Table 4–3. Treatment choices for cancers responsive to systemic agents.

Diagnosis	Current Treatment of Choice	Other Valuable Agents and Procedures
Acute lymphocytic leukemia	**Induction:** Combination chemotherapy. *Adults:* Vincristine, prednisone, daunorubicin, and asparaginase. **Consolidation:** Multiagent alternating chemotherapy. Allogeneic bone marrow transplant for young adults or high-risk disease or second remission. CNS prophylaxis with intrathecal methotrexate with or without whole brain radiation. **Remission maintenance:** Methotrexate, thioguanine.	Doxorubicin, cytarabine, cyclophosphamide, etoposide, teniposide (VM-26),[1] allopurinol,[2] autologous bone marrow transplantation
Acute myelocytic and myelomonocytic leukemia	**Induction:** Combination chemotherapy with cytarabine and an anthracycline (daunorubicin, idarubicin). Tretinoin with idarubicin for acute promyelocytic leukemia. **Consolidation:** High-dose cytarabine. Autologous (with or without purging) or allogeneic bone marrow transplantation for high-risk disease or second remission.	Mitoxantrone, idarubicin, etoposide, mercaptopurine, thioguanine, azacitidine,[1] amsacrine,[1] methotrexate, doxorubicin, tretinoin, allopurinol,[2] leukapheresis, prednisone
Chronic myelocytic leukemia	Hydroxyurea, alpha interferon. Allogeneic bone marrow transplantation for younger patients. Clinical trials: STI 541; Homoharringtonin	Busulfan, mercaptopurine, thioguanine, cytarabine, plicamycin, melphalan, autologous bone marrow transplantation, allopurinol[2]
Chronic lymphocytic leukemia	Chlorambucil and prednisone or fludarabine (if treatment is indicated).	Vincristine, cyclophosphamide, doxorubicin, cladribine (2-chlorodeoxyadenosine; CdA), allogeneic bone marrow transplant, androgens,[2] allopurinol[2]
Hairy cell leukemia	Cladribine (2-chlorodeoxyadenosine; CdA).	Pentostatin (deoxycoformycin), alpha interferon
Hodgkin's disease (stages III and IV)	**Combination chemotherapy:** doxorubicin (Adriamycin), bleomycin, vinblastine, dacarbazine (ABVD) or alternative combination therapy without mechlorethamine. Autologous bone marrow transplant for high-risk patients or relapsed disease.	Mechlorethamine, vincristine, prednisone, procarbazine (MOPP); carmustine, lomustine, etoposide, thiotepa, autologous bone marrow transplantation
Non-Hodgkin's lymphoma (intermediate to high grade)	**Combination therapy** depending on histologic classification but usually including cyclophosphamide, vincristine, doxorubicin, and prednisone (CHOP) with or without other agents. Autologous bone marrow transplantation in high-risk first remission or first relapse.	Bleomycin, methotrexate, etoposide, chlorambucil, fludarabine, lomustine, carmustine, cytarabine, thiotepa, amsacrine, mitoxantrone, allogeneic bone marrow transplantation
Non-Hodgkin's lymphoma (low-grade)	Chlorambucil and prednisone **or** Cyclophosphamide, vincristine, prednisone **or** Fludarabine	Rituximab, combination chemotherapy, autologous or allogeneic bone marrow transplantation
Cutaneous T cell lymphoma (mycosis fungoides)	Topical carmustine, electron beam radiotherapy, photochemotherapy	Interferon, combination chemotherapy, denileukin diftitox (ONTAK), targretin
Multiple myeloma	**Combination chemotherapy:** melphalan and prednisone or melphalan, cyclophosphamide, carmustine, vincristine, doxorubicin, and prednisone. Autologous bone marrow transplantation in first complete or partial remission. Allogeneic bone marrow transplantation for young patients with poor prognosis disease.	Etoposide, cytarabine, alpha interferon, dexamethasone, autologous bone marrow transplantation
Waldenström's macroglobulinemia	Fludarabine **or** chlorambucil **or** cyclophosphamide, vincristine, prednisone. Allogeneic bone marrow transplantation for high-risk young patients.	Cladribine, etoposide, alpha interferon, doxorubicin, dexamethasone, plasmapheresis, autologous bone marrow transplantation

(*continued*)

Table 4–3. Treatment choices for cancers responsive to systemic agents. (continued)

Diagnosis	Current Treatment of Choice	Other Valuable Agents and Procedures
Polycythemia vera Essential thrombocytosis	Hydroxyurea, phlebotomy for polycythemia	Busulfan, chlorambucil, cyclophosphamide, alpha interferon, radiophosphorus ^{32}P
Carcinoma of the lung Small cell	**Combination chemotherapy:** cisplatin and etoposide. Palliative radiation therapy.	Cyclophosphamide, doxorubicin, vincristine
Non-small cell[3]	**Advanced disease:** cisplatin, vinorelbine **Localized disease:** cisplatin, vinblastine	Doxorubicin, etoposide, mitomycin
Carcinoma of the head and neck[3]	**Combination chemotherapy:** cisplatin and fluorouracil	Methotrexate, bleomycin, hydroxyurea, doxorubicin, vinblastine
Carcinoma of the esophagus[3]	**Combination chemotherapy:** fluorouracil, cisplatin, mitomycin	Methotrexate, bleomycin, doxorubicin, mitomycin
Carcinoma of the stomach and pancreas[3]	**Stomach:** etoposide, leucovorin,[2] fluorouracil (ELF) **Pancreas:** fluorouracil or ELF, gemcitabine	Carmustine, mitomycin, lomustine, doxorubicin, gemcitabine. Doxorubicin, methotrexate, cisplatin, combinations for stomach.
Carcinoma of the colon and rectum[3]	**Colon:** fluorouracil plus levamisole (adjuvant) or with leucovorin and irinotecan (advanced) **Rectum:** fluorouracil with radiation therapy (adjuvant)	Irinotecan, methotrexate, mitomycin, carmustine, cisplatin, floxuridine
Carcinoma of the kidney[3]	Floxuridine, vinblastine, IL-2, alpha interferon	Alpha interferon, progestins, infusional FUDR, fluorouracil
Carcinoma of the bladder[3]	Intravesical BCG or thiotepa. Combination chemotherapy: methotrexate, vinblastine, doxorubicin (Adriamycin), cisplatin (M-VAC) or CMV alone	Cyclophosphamide, fluorouracil, intravesical valrubicin
Carcinoma of the testis[3]	**Combination chemotherapy:** etoposide and cisplatin. Autologous bone marrow transplantation for high-risk or relapsed disease.	Bleomycin, vinblastine, ifosfamide, mesna,[2] carmustine, carboplatin
Carcinoma of the prostate[3]	Estrogens or LHRH analog (leuprolide) plus an antiandrogen (flutamide)	Ketoconazole, doxorubicin, aminoglutethimide, progestins, cyclophosphamide, cisplatin, estramustine, vinblastine, etoposide, suramin[1]; PC-SPES; estramustine phosphate
Carcinoma of the uterus[3]	Progestins or tamoxifen	Doxorubicin, cisplatin, fluorouracil, ifosfamide
Carcinoma of the ovary[3]	**Combination chemotherapy:** paclitaxel and cisplatin/carboplatin	Docetaxel, doxorubicin, topotecan, cyclophosphamide, doxorubicin, etoposide
Carcinoma of the cervix[3]	**Combination chemotherapy:** methotrexate, doxorubicin, cisplatin, and vinblastine; or mitomycin, bleomycin, vincristine, and cisplatin with radiation therapy	Carboplatin, ifosfamide, lomustine
Carcinoma of the breast[3]	**Combination chemotherapy:** cyclophosphamide, doxorubicin, fluorouracil with sequential paclitaxel for node-positive disease, or cyclophosphamide, methotrexate, fluorouracil. Tamoxifen for estrogen/progesterone receptor-positive tumors.	Trastuzumab (Herceptin) with chemotherapy, paclitaxel, docetaxel, epirubicin, mitoxantrone, topotecan, capecitabine, vinorelbine, thiotepa, vincristine, vinblastine, carboplatin or cisplatin, plicamycin, anastrozole, letrozole, exemestane, toremifine, progestins, aminoglutethimide
Choriocarcinoma (trophoblastic neoplasms)[3]	Methotrexate or dactinomycin (or both) plus chlorambucil	Vinblastine, cisplatin, mercaptopurine, doxorubicin, bleomycin, etoposide
Carcinoma of the thyroid gland[3]	Radioiodine (^{131}I)	Doxorubicin, cisplatin, bleomycin, melphalan

(continued)

Table 4–3. Treatment choices for cancers responsive to systemic agents. (continued)

Diagnosis	Current Treatment of Choice	Other Valuable Agents and Procedures
Carcinoma of the adrenal gland[3]	Mitotane	Doxorubicin, suramin[1]
Carcinoid[3]	Fluorouracil plus streptozocin with or without alpha interferon	Doxorubicin, cyclophosphamide, octreotide, cyproheptadine,[2] methysergide[2]
Osteogenic sarcoma[3]	High-dose methotrexate, doxorubicin, vincristine	Cyclophosphamide, ifosfamide, bleomycin, dacarbazine, cisplatin, dactinomycin
Soft tissue sarcoma[3]	Doxorubicin, dacarbazine	Ifosfamide, cyclosphosphamide, etoposide, cisplatin, high-dose methotrexate, vincristine
Melanoma[3]	Dacarbazine, alpha interferon, IL-2	Carmustine, lomustine, melphalan, thiotepa, cisplatin, paclitaxel, tamoxifen, vincristine
Kaposi's sarcoma	Doxorubicin, vincristine alternating with vinblastine or vincristine alone. Palliative radiation therapy.	Alpha interferon, bleomycin, etoposide, doxorubicin
Neuroblastoma[3]	**Combination chemotherapy:** variations of cyclophosphamide, cisplatin, vincristine, doxorubicin, dacarbazine	Melphalan, ifosfamide, autologous or allogeneic bone marrow transplantation

[1]Investigational agent. Treatment is available through qualified investigators and centers authorized by the National Cancer Institute and Cooperative Oncology Groups.
[2]Supportive agent; not oncolytic.
[3]These tumors are generally managed initially with surgery with or without radiation therapy with or without adjuvant chemotherapy. For metastatic disease, the role of palliative radiation therapy is as important as that of chemotherapy.

Fludarabine phosphate, another purine analog, has shown improved response rates and progression-free survival compared with oral chlorambucil or combination chemotherapy for chronic lymphocytic leukemia (CLL). Fludarabine is now indicated as first-line therapy for most patients with CLL. Side effects include an increased risk of opportunistic infections as well as very rare problems such as hemolytic anemia and severe bone marrow suppression. Fludarabine is also effective therapy for low-grade lymphomas and Waldenström's macroglobulinemia. Cladribine and pentostatin are also used to treat CLL and the above disorders.

Paclitaxel (Taxol) is a novel agent isolated from the pacific yew tree that has replaced cyclophosphamide as front-line therapy (combined with carboplatin) for the treatment of ovarian cancer. Dose intensification as well as intraperitoneal instillation may also be helpful for advanced disease. Paclitaxel has also been shown to be one of the most effective agents against metastatic and early-stage breast cancer; it is also effective in AIDS-associated Kaposi's sarcoma and cancer. The primary toxicity of paclitaxel is hematologic and neurologic. Both are dose-dependent—the hematologic toxicity can be ameliorated by the use of myeloid growth factors.

Docetaxel (Taxotere) is a synthetic analog of paclitaxel that has also been shown to be effective in breast cancer as well as other advanced malignancies. Its toxicities include bone marrow suppression and significant peripheral edema. The edema can be treated and generally prevented with steroids.

Vinorelbine, a semisynthetic vinca alkaloid, has been shown to be effective in treating advanced non-small-cell lung cancer. Response rates of 30% have been observed when vinorelbine is used as a single agent against this poorly responsive tumor. Vinorelbine is also used to treat metastatic breast cancer as well as other tumors.

Capecitabine is an oral 5-FU prodrug that is now approved to treat anthracycline- and taxane-resistant breast cancers. Response rates range from 25% to 35%. Treatment can be complicated by a painful, red, and sometimes blistering rash on the palms and soles and severe diarrhea that resolves upon withholding therapy. A variety of other 5-FU prodrugs are in clinical trials but are not yet approved for use.

Gemcitabine, a pyrimidine analog for intravenous use, has been approved to treat pancreatic cancer and non-small-cell lung cancer but is active in other advanced malignancies, including breast cancer.

Topotecan was the first of a new class of drugs called camptothecans that inhibit the enzyme topoisomerase I to be FDA-approved for use. It is used to treat advanced ovarian cancer and has shown some efficacy in the treatment of several other tumors.

Irinotecan is now approved for the treatment of metastatic colorectal cancer. When compared with supportive care in resistant metastatic colorectal cancer, irinotecan has conferred a survival benefit of 1 year. Two recent randomized studies compared standard therapy (fluorouracil and leucovorin) to standard therapy with irinotecan in patients with untreated metastatic colorectal cancer. The use of irinotecan resulted in a significantly higher response rate, delayed time to progression, and, in one study, improved survival. Toxicity in the irinotecan arm was also significantly higher but reversible and included severe diarrhea and neutropenia. Antitumor responses have also been shown using irinotecan to treat non-small-cell lung cancer, small-cell lung cancer, ovarian cancer, gliomas, and others.

Novel inhibitors of thymidylate synthase are also under study for the treatment of advanced colorectal cancer. Raltitrexed is currently being used in Europe based on early data showing similar efficacy compared with fluorouracil and high-dose leucovorin. Liposomal encapsulation of active chemotherapeutic agents may improve drug delivery and decrease systemic toxicity. Two liposomally encapsulated drugs, doxorubicin and daunorubicin, are now available to treat Kaposi's sarcoma and have shown efficacy in treating many other diseases, including breast cancer and lymphoma.

Two monoclonal antibodies are used in cancer chemotherapy. Rituximab, a chimeric antibody against the B lymphocyte antigen CD20, is effective therapy for relapsed or resistant low-grade lymphomas and has shown limited usefulness in higher-grade lymphomas as well. Almost 50% of patients with low-grade lymphoma responded with shrinkage of lymph nodes to once-weekly dosing for 4 weeks. Responses lasted a median of over 1 year. Rituximab is now being evaluated in longer courses, earlier in the disease course, in combination with chemotherapy, and after bone marrow transplantation. Toxicities are generally quite mild, though anaphylaxis and infusion-related side effects have been reported. The HER2/*neu* oncogene (also called c-*erb*B-2), a gene that encodes a receptor tyrosine kinase, is known to be overexpressed in many human cancers and is associated with tumors with poorer prognoses. In breast cancer, overexpression of HER2/*neu* is seen in about 20–30% of women and is associated with a higher risk of metastatic disease and poorer survival. Trastuzumab (Herceptin) is a recombinant humanized monoclonal antibody directed against the HER2/*neu* gene product that is now approved for the treatment of metastatic breast cancer. When trastuzumab was used as a single agent to treat anthracycline-resistant breast cancer, the response rate was about 15%, with a median duration of response of over 8 months. However, when trastuzumab was added to first-line chemotherapy for metastatic breast cancer and compared with chemotherapy alone, patients receiving the combination therapy had response rate of almost 50% with improvement in both remission duration and survival. The most promising combination appears to be trastuzumab and paclitaxel (Taxol). The combination of trastuzumab and doxorubicin (Adriamycin) resulted in an increase in subclinical and clinical cardiac toxicity; combinations with anthracyclines should be avoided. Other toxicities of trastuzumab appear to be primarily infusion-related. Randomized trials starting in the year 2000 will test trastuzumab therapy as part of neoadjuvant or adjuvant therapy for node-positive breast cancer. In addition, trastuzumab is currently being tested for use in other HER2/*neu*-expressing tumors such as prostate and ovarian cancers.

Another exciting new agent approved for the treatment of cutaneous T cell lymphomas (CTCL) such as mycosis fungoides resistant to standard therapy is denileukin diftitox (ONTAK), a recombinant DNA-derived cytotoxic protein composed of amino acid sequences for diphtheria toxin fragments followed by the sequences for interleukin-2 (IL-2). This fusion protein was designed to direct the cytocidal action of diphtheria toxin to cells that express the IL-2 receptor, such as the tumor cells in CTCL. Cancer cells must be shown to express the IL-2 receptor, CD25. Thirty percent of patients with advanced CTCL responded to denileukin diftitox in a phase III randomized trial. Toxicity is significant, including acute hypersensitivity reactions—requiring administration of this agent in a close-observation setting—and delayed vascular leak syndrome.

Bisphosphonates are a class of agents that inhibit osteoclast activation. In addition to reducing bone pain, pamidronate reduces by approximately 50% the frequency of new skeletal events both in breast cancer metastatic to bone and in multiple myeloma. This effect will probably be demonstrated in metastatic prostate cancer as well. Pamidronate must be given intravenously on a monthly basis, with an estimated cost of $775 a month, and may worsen pain for the first few days following the infusion. For this reason, pamidronate therapy may be limited to patients with multiple lytic bone lesions or disease in weight-bearing bones or vertebrae.

Clodronate is an oral bisphosphonate that has been shown to reduce the number of new bone metastases in women with breast cancer. A study of women with a primary diagnosis of breast cancer and microscopic evidence of tumor cells in bone marrow randomized to receive either clodronate, 1600 mg/d for 2 years, or placebo—in addition to standard adjuvant therapy—showed a significant reduction of both osseous and visceral metastases. Mortality was also significantly reduced in the treatment group. Five-year follow-up shows continued reduction in new bone metastases but no longer any difference in the incidence of visceral metastases. Preliminary results of a larger study of women with operable breast cancer but no other specific high-risk features showed a reduction in the incidence of bone metastases but no difference in visceral metastases or survival. These observations suggest that clodronate may be useful primarily in a very high risk subset of women with primary breast cancer. Clodronate continues to be tested in clinical trials in Europe and is not yet available in the United States. A new intravenous bisphosphonate, zoledronic acid, is scheduled to be released in mid 2000 for the treatment of metastatic bone lesions. Its advantage compared with pamidronate is a much shorter infusion time (5–10 minutes compared with 2 or more hours). It is being tested in the United States in a national randomized study of node-positive women with breast cancer to see if the results of the clodronate study can be reproduced. Patients will not be selected on the basis of microscopic bone marrow metastases for this study.

Tretinoin is the first agent designed to target a specific fusion protein caused by a chromosome translocation. This oral agent induces differentiation and decreased proliferation without cytolysis of acute promyelocytic leukemia cells. Use of tretinoin combined with chemotherapy has been shown to improve disease-free and overall survival from this form of leukemia.

Retinoids modulate the growth and differentiation of a variety of epithelial cells. Bexarotene, a retinoid that selectively activates the retinoid X receptor (RXR), is now FDA-approved to treat cutaneous T cell lymphomas such as mycosis fungoides. Targretin is also in clinical trials for use in a variety of advanced solid tumors including breast cancer.

Several recombinant growth factors have been shown to be effective in the treatment of malignancy. Recombinant alpha interferon has marked antitumor effects in hairy cell leukemia and chronic myelogenous leukemia, moderate effects in lymphomas, in the epidemic (AIDS-associated) form of Kaposi's sarcoma, in multiple myeloma, and as adjuvant therapy for malignant melanoma. Alpha interferon has some utility also in metastatic melanoma, renal cell carcinoma, and carcinoid syndrome. Patients with chronic myelogenous leukemia may benefit from alpha interferon (especially when low doses of the chemotherapeutic agent cytarabine are also given) and achieve both a hematologic and a cytogenic remission. Patients with a cytogenic response to interferon (about 30% of treated patients) have a significantly longer survival than patients treated with standard oral chemotherapy. The addition of alpha interferon to systemic chemotherapy for multiple myeloma appears to enhance the degree of cytoreduction achieved as compared with chemotherapy alone; however, toxicity is additive. Use of alpha interferon for myeloma following chemotherapy or autologous bone marrow transplant has prolonged remission duration, though overall survival is not altered. Very high doses of interferon for approximately 1 year in patients with malignant melanoma and lymph node metastases may improve disease-free and overall survival, though newer data suggest that this benefit is probably not significant and the treatment is quite toxic. Another cytokine, interleukin-2, when administered alone or in combination with chemotherapy and interferon, exhibits marked antitumor activity in a minority of patients with metastatic melanoma or renal cancer, though its use is also associated with marked toxicity.

Newer experimental therapies are discussed briefly at the end of this chapter.

Hormonal therapy also plays an important role in cancer management. Hormonal therapy or ablation is important in treatment and palliation of breast and prostatic carcinoma, while added progestins are useful in suppression of endometrial carcinoma. Women with metastatic breast cancer who show objective improvement with hormonal therapy have tumors that contain cytoplasmic estrogen and progesterone receptors. Antiestrogens (eg, tamoxifen or letrazole) and aromatase inhibitors (eg, anastrazole or megestrol acetate) or aromatase inactivators (exemestane) that block peripheral conversion of adrenal androgens into estrogens obviate the need for oophorectomy in premenopausal women whose tumors are estrogen receptor-positive or progesterone receptor-positive. Newer hormonal agents with less toxicity are under investigation for the treatment of breast cancer. Hormonal approaches are also available to treat prostate cancer, though androgen receptors remain difficult to measure. These include the use of estrogen therapy, gonadotropin-releasing hormone agonists (eg, leuprolide), aromatase inhibitors (eg, aminoglutethimide), and antiandrogens (eg, flutamide). The use of leuprolide plus flutamide can be considered as an alternative to orchiectomy but also causes impotence. High-dose ketoconazole has been used to rapidly suppress adrenal production of steroids in crises such as cord compression. Use of this agent requires hydrocortisone supplementation.

Table 4–4 sets forth the currently used dosage schedules and toxicities of the most commonly used cancer chemotherapeutic agents. The dosage schedules given are for single-agent therapy. Combination therapy is used for most cancers. Hematologic or other toxicity may limit the therapeutic effectiveness of chemotherapy. It is possible to avoid the need for dose reductions or delay in therapy by using granulocyte colony-stimulating factor (G-CSF; filgrastim) or granulocyte-macrophage colony-stimulating factor (GM-CSF; sargramostim) to stimulate white blood cell recovery. Interleukin-11 is currently available to reduce the need for delay or dose reductions due to thrombocytopenia; however, the usefulness of this cytokine is quite limited because of its ineffective-

Table 4–4. Single-agent dosage and toxicity of anticancer drugs.

Drug	Dosage	Acute Toxicity	Delayed Toxicity
Alkylating agents			
Mechlorethamine	6–10 mg/m^2 IV every 3 weeks	Severe vesicant; severe nausea and vomiting	Moderate suppression of blood counts. Melphalan effect may be delayed 4–6 weeks. Excessive doses produce severe bone marrow suppression with leukopenia, thrombocytopenia, and bleeding. Alopecia and hemorrhagic cystitis occur with cyclophosphamide, while busulfan can cause hyperpigmentation, pulmonary fibrosis, and weakness (see text). Ifosfamide is always given with mesna to prevent cystitis. Acute leukemia may develop in 5–10% of patients receiving prolonged therapy with melphalan, mechlorethamine, or chlorambucil; all alkylators probably increase the risk of secondary malignancies with prolonged use. Most cause either temporary or permanent aspermia/amenorrhea.
Chlorambucil	0.1–0.2 mg/kg/d orally (6–12 mg/d) or 0.4 mg/kg pulse every 4 weeks	None	
Cyclophosphamide	100 mg/m^2/d orally for 14 days; 400 mg/m^2 orally for 5 days; 1–1.5 g/m^2 IV every 3–4 weeks	Nausea and vomiting with higher doses	
Melphalan	0.25 mg/kg/d orally for 4 days every 6 weeks	None	
Busulfan	2–8 mg/d orally; 150–250 mg/course	None	
Carmustine (BCNU)	200 mg/m^2 IV every 6 weeks	Local irritant	Prolonged leukopenia and thrombocytopenia. Rarely hepatitis. Acute leukemia has been observed to occur in some patients receiving nitrosoureas. Nitrosoureas can cause delayed pulmonary fibrosis with prolonged use.
Lomustine (CCNU)	100–130 mg orally every 6–8 weeks	Nausea and vomiting	
Procarbazine	100 mg/m^2/d orally for 14 days every 4 weeks	Nausea and vomiting	Bone marrow suppression, mental suppression, MAO inhibition, disulfiram-like effect.
Dacarbazine	250 mg/m^2/d IV for 5 days every 3 weeks; 1500 mg/m^2 IV as single dose	Severe nausea and vomiting; anorexia	Bone marrow suppression; flu-like syndrome.
Cisplatin	50–100 mg/m^2 IV every 3 weeks; 20 mg/m^2 IV for 5 days every 4 weeks	Severe nausea and vomiting	Nephrotoxicity, mild otic and bone marrow toxicity, neurotoxicity.
Carboplatin	360 mg/m^2 IV every 4 weeks	Severe nausea and vomiting	Bone marrow suppression, prolonged anemia; same as cisplatin but milder.
Structural analogs or antimetabolites			
Methotrexate	2.5–5 mg/d orally; 20–25 mg IM twice weekly; high-dose: 500–1000 mg/m^2 IV every 2–3 weeks; 12–15 mg intrathecally every week for 4–6 doses	None	Bone marrow suppression, oral and gastrointestinal ulceration, acute renal failure; hepatotoxicity, rash, increased toxicity when effusions are present. ***Note:*** Citrovorum factor (leucovorin) rescue for doses over 100 mg/m^2.
Mercaptopurine	2.5 mg/kg/d orally; 100 mg/m^2/d orally for 5 days for induction	None	Well tolerated. Larger doses cause bone marrow suppression.
Thioguanine	2 mg/kg/d orally; 100 mg/m^2/d IV for 7 days for induction	Mild nausea, diarrhea	Well tolerated. Larger doses cause bone marrow suppression.
Fluorouracil	15 mg/kg/d IV for 3–5 days every 3 weeks; 15 mg/kg weekly as tolerated; 500–1000 mg/m^2 IV every 4 weeks	None	Nausea, diarrhea, oral and gastrointestinal ulceration, bone marrow suppression, dacryocystitis.
Cytarabine	100–200 mg/m^2/d for 5–10 days by continuous IV infusion; 2–3 g/m^2 IV every 12 hours for 3–7 days; 20 mg/m^2 SC daily in divided doses	High-dose: nausea, vomiting, diarrhea, anorexia	Nausea and vomiting; cystitis; severe bone marrow suppression; megaloblastosis; CNS toxicity with high-dose cytarabine.

(*continued*)

Table 4–4. Single-agent dosage and toxicity of anticancer drugs. (continued)

Drug	Dosage	Acute Toxicity	Delayed Toxicity
Hormonal agents			
Testosterone propionate	100 mg IM 3 times weekly	None	Fluid retention, masculinization, leg cramps. Cholestatic jaundice in some patients receiving fluoxymesterone.
Fluoxymesterone	20–40 mg/d orally	None	
Flutamide	250 mg 3 times a day orally	None	Gynecomastia, hot flushes, decreased libido, mild gastrointestinal side effects.
Diethylstilbestrol	1–5 mg/d orally in divided doses	Occasional nausea and vomiting	Fluid retention, feminization, uterine bleeding, exacerbation of cardiovascular disease, painful gynecomastia, thromboembolic disease.
Ethinyl estradiol	3 mg/d orally	None	
Tamoxifen	20 mg/d orally in 2 divided doses	Transient flare of bone pain	?Increased risk of venous thrombosis; anovulation, endometrial cancer, cataracts.
Megestrol acetate	40 mg orally 4 times daily	None	Occasional fluid retention; rare thrombosis, weight gain, hot flushes.
Anastrazole	1 mg orally daily	None	
Letrozole	2.5 mg/d orally	None	
Exemestane	25 mg/d orally	None	
Toremifene	60 mg/d orally	None	
Medroxyprogesterone	100–200 mg/d orally; 200–600 mg orally twice weekly	None	
Adrenocorticosteroid			
Prednisone	20–100 mg/d orally or 50–100 mg every other day orally with systemic chemotherapy	Alteration in mood	Fluid retention, hypertension, diabetes, increased susceptibility to infection, "moon facies," osteoporosis, electrolyte abnormalities, gastritis.
Aromatase inhibitor			
Aminoglutethimide	500 mg/d orally, along with hydrocortisone, 40 mg/d orally	Initial drowsiness	Transient skin rash, which usually subsides with continued therapy; weight gain, fluid retention, leg cramps; cholestatic jaundice.
GnRH analogs			
Leuprolide	7.5 mg IM (depot) once a month; 1 mg/d SC	Local irritation, transient flare of symptoms	Hot flushes, decreased libido, impotence, gynecomastia, mild gastrointestinal side effects.
Goserelin acetate	3.6 mg SC monthly	Transient flare of symptoms	
Biologic response modifiers			
Interferon alfa-2a Interferon alfa-2b	3–5 million units SC 3 times weekly or daily	Fever, chills, fatigue, anorexia	General malaise, weight loss, confusion.
Aldesleukin (IL-2)	600,000 units/kg IV over 15 minutes every 8 hours for 14 doses, repeated after 9-day rest period. Some doses may be withheld or interrupted because of toxicity. ***Caution:*** High doses must be administered in an ICU setting by experienced personnel.	Hypotension, fever, chills, rigors, diarrhea, nausea, vomiting, pruritus, liver, kidney, and CNS toxicity, capillary leak (primarily at high doses), pruritic skin rash, infections (can be severe)	Hypoglycemia, anemia.
Peptide hormone inhibitor			
Octreotide acetate	100–600 μg/d SC in 2 divided doses	Local irritant; nausea and vomiting	Diarrhea, abdominal pain, hypoglycemia.
Natural products and miscellaneous agents			
Vinblastine	0.1–0.2 mg/kg or 6 mg/m² IV weekly	Mild nausea and vomiting; severe vesicant	Alopecia, peripheral neuropathy, bone marrow suppression, constipation, SIADH, areflexia.

(*continued*)

Table 4–4. Single-agent dosage and toxicity of anticancer drugs. (continued)

Drug	Dosage	Acute Toxicity	Delayed Toxicity
Vincristine	1.5 mg/m^2 (maximum: 2 mg weekly)	Severe vesicant	Areflexia, muscle weakness, peripheral neuropathy, paralytic ileus, alopecia (see text), SIADH.
Vinorelbine	30 mg/m^2 IV weekly	Mild nausea and vomiting, fatigue, severe vesicant	Granulocytopenia, constipation, peripheral neuropathy, alopecia.
Paclitaxel (Taxol)	135 mg/m^2 by continuous infusion over 24 hours every 3 weeks	Hypersensitivity reaction (premedicate with diphenhydramine and dexamethasone), mild nausea and vomiting	Peripheral neuropathy, bone marrow suppression, fluid retention.
Docetaxel (Taxotere)	60–100 mg/m^2 IV every 3 weeks		
Dactinomycin	0.04 mg/kg IV weekly	Nausea and vomiting; severe vesicant	Alopecia, stomatitis, diarrhea, bone marrow suppression.
Daunorubicin	30–60 mg/m^2 daily IV for 3 days, or 30–60 mg/m^2 IV weekly	Nausea, fever, red urine (not hematuria); severe vesicant; acute cardiotoxicity	Alopecia, stomatitis, bone marrow suppression, late cardiotoxicity. Risk of cardiotoxicity increases with radiation, cyclophosphamide.
Idarubicin	12 mg/m^2 daily IV for 3 days		
Doxorubicin	60 mg/m^2 IV every 3 weeks to a maximum total dose of 550 mg/m^2		
Epirubicin	60–100 mg/m^2 IV every 3 weeks		
Liposomal doxorubicin (Doxil)	20 mg/m^2 IV every 3 weeks		
Liposomal daunorubicin (DaunoXome)	40 mg/m^2 IV every 2 weeks		
Etoposide	100 mg/m^2/d IV for 5 days or 50–150 mg/d orally	Nausea and vomiting; occasionally hypotension	Alopecia, bone marrow suppression.
Plicamycin (mithramycin)	25–50 µg/kg IV every other day for up to 8 doses	Nausea and vomiting	Thrombocytopenia, diarrhea, hepatotoxicity, nephrotoxicity, stomatitis.
Mitomycin	10–20 mg/m^2 every 6–8 weeks	Severe vesicant; nausea	Prolonged bone marrow suppression, rare hemolytic-uremic syndrome.
Mitoxantrone	12–15 mg/m^2/d IV for 3 days with cytarabine; 8–12 mg/m^2 IV every 3 weeks	Mild nausea and vomiting	Alopecia, mild mucositis, bone marrow suppression.
Bleomycin	Up to 15 units/m^2 IM, IV, or SC twice weekly to a total dose of 200 units/m^2	Allergic reactions, fever, hypotension	Fever, dermatitis, pulmonary fibrosis.
Hydroxyurea	500–1500 mg/d orally	Mild nausea and vomiting	Hyperpigmentation, bone marrow suppression.
Mitotane	6–12 g/d orally	Nausea and vomiting	Dermatitis, diarrhea, mental suppression, muscle tremors.
Fludarabine	25 mg/m^2/d IV for 5 days every 4 weeks	Nausea and vomiting	Bone marrow suppression, diarrhea, mild hepatotoxicity, immune suppression.
Cladribine (CdA)	0.09 mg/kg/d by continuous IV infusion for 7 days	Mild nausea, rash, fatigue	Bone marrow suppression, fever, immune suppression.
Topotecan	1.5 mg/m^2 IV daily for 5 days every 3 weeks	Nausea, vomiting, diarrhea, headache, dyspnea	Alopecia, bone marrow suppression.

(*continued*)

Table 4–4. Single-agent dosage and toxicity of anticancer drugs. (continued)

Drug	Dosage	Acute Toxicity	Delayed Toxicity
Gemcitabine	1000 mg/m^2 every week up to 7 weeks, then 1 week off, then weekly for 3 out of 4 weeks	Nausea, vomiting, diarrhea, fever, dyspnea	Bone marrow suppression, rash, fluid retention, mouth sores, flu-like symptoms, paresthesias.
Estramustine phosphate	14 mg/kg orally in 3 or 4 divided doses	Nausea, vomiting, diarrhea	Thrombosis, thrombocytopenia, hypertension, glucose intolerance, edema.
Capecitabine	2500 mg/m^2 orally twice daily on days 1–14 every 3 weeks	Nausea, diarrhea	Hand and foot syndrome, mucositis.
Irinotecan	125 mg/m^2 weekly for 4 weeks, then a 2-week rest, then repeat	Flushing, salivation, lacrimation, bradycardia, abdominal cramps, diarrhea	Bone marrow suppression, diarrhea.
Novel therapeutic agents			
Tretinoin	45 mg/m^2 by mouth daily until remission or for 90 days	Retinoic acid syndrome (fever, dyspnea, pleural or pericardial effusion) must be treated emergently with dexamethasone, headache, dry skin rash, flushing.	
Trastuzimab (Herceptin)	Load: 4 mg/kg IV followed by 2 mg/kg weekly	Low-grade fever, chills, fatigue, constitutional symptoms with first infusion	Cardiac toxicity when given with anthracyclines.
Denileukin diftitox (ONTAK)	9–10 μg/kg/d IV for 5 days every 21 days	Hypersensitivity type reactions with first infusion	Vascular leak syndrome, low albumin, increased risk of infections, diarrhea, rash.
Rituximab	375 mg/m^2 IV weekly for 4–8 doses	Hypersensitivity type reactions with first infusion; fever, tumor lysis syndrome (can be life-threatening)	Mild cytopenias, rare red cell aplasia or aplastic anemia.
Targretin	300 mg/m^2 d/orally	Nausea	Hyperlipidemia, dry mouth, dry skin, constipation, leukopenia, edema.
Supportive agents			
Allopurinol	300–900 mg/d orally for prevention or relief of hyperuricemia	None	Rash, Stevens-Johnson syndrome; enhances effects and toxicity of mercaptopurine when used in combination.
Mesna	20% of ifosfamide dosage at the time of ifosfamide administration, then 4 and 8 hours after each dose of chemotherapy to prevent hemorrhagic cystitis	Nausea, vomiting, diarrhea	None.
Leucovorin	10 mg/m^2 every 6 hours IV or orally until serum methotrexate levels are below 5×10^{-8} mol/L with hydration and urinary alkalinization (about 72 hours)	None	Enhances toxic effects of fluorouracil.
Amifostine	910 mg/m^2 IV daily, 30 minutes prior to chemotherapy	Hypotension, nausea, vomiting, flushing	Decrease in serum calcium.
Dexrazoxane	10:1 ratio of anthracycline IV, before (within 30 minutes of) chemotherapy infusion	Pain on injection	Increased bone marrow suppression.

(*continued*)

Table 4–4. Single-agent dosage and toxicity of anticancer drugs. (continued)

Drug	Dosage	Acute Toxicity	Delayed Toxicity
Pilocarpine hydrochloride	5–10 mg orally 3 times daily	Sweating, headache, flushing; nausea, chills, rhinitis, dizziness, and urinary frequency at high dosage.	
Pamidronate	90 mg IV every month	Symptomatic hypoglycemia (rare), flare of bone pain, local irritation	None.
Epoetin alfa (erythropoietin)	100–300 units/kg IV or SC 3 times a week	Skin irritation or pain at injection site	Hypertension, headache, seizures in patients on dialysis (rare).
Filgrastim (G-CSF)	5 μg/kg/d SC or IV	Mild to moderate bone pain, mild hypotension (rare), irritation at injection sites (rare)	Unknown.
Sargramostim (GM-CSF)	250 μg/kg/d as a 2-hour IV infusion (can be given SC)	Fluid retention, dyspnea, capillary leak (rare), supraventricular tachycardia (rare), mild to moderate bone pain, irritation at injection sites	Unknown.
Neumega (IL-11)	50 μg/kg/d SC	Fluid retention, arrhythmias, headache, arthralgias, myalgias	Unknown.
Samarium-153 lexidronam (153Sm-EDTMP)	1 mCi/kg IV as single dose	None	Hematopoietic suppression.
Strontium-89	4 mCi every 3 months IV	None	Hematopoietic suppression.

ness in severe thrombocytopenia and its toxicity, which includes significant edema

Berkowitz RS et al: Chorionic tumors. N Engl J Med 1996;335:1740. [NLM Cit ID: 97072141] (Review of the clinical presentation and treatment of this curable tumor.)

Bolla M et al: Improved survival in patients with locally advanced prostate cancer treated with radiotherapy and goserelin. N Engl J Med 1997;337:295. [NLM Cit ID: 97365038] (Goserelin combined with radiation therapy is superior to radiation therapy alone for both local control and survival.)

Diel IJ et al: Reduction in new metastases in breast cancer with adjuvant clodronate treatment. N Engl J Med 1998;339:357. [NLM Cit ID 98346817] (An oral bisphosphonate available in Europe given as adjuvant therapy to women with high-risk breast cancer significantly reduced the risk of developing metastatic breast cancer in bone and viscera at 3 years of follow-up.)

Hartmann O et al: Peripheral blood stem cell and bone marrow transplantation for solid tumors and lymphomas: Hematologic recovery and costs. A randomized, controlled trial. Ann Intern Med 1997;126:600. [NLM Cit ID: 97243269]

Kaye SB: Multidrug resistance: clinical relevance in solid tumours and strategies for circumvention. Curr Opin Oncol 1998;10:S15. [NLM Cit ID: 88018662] (A general review of multidrug resistance and its clinical implications.)

Kemeny N et al: Hepatic arterial infusion of chemotherapy after resection of hepatic metastases from colorectal cancer. N Engl J Med 1999;341:2039. [NLM Cit ID: 20061996] (In this randomized study, hepatic arterial infusion of floxuridine with intravenous fluorouracil following liver resection resulted in improved 2-year survival compared with patients receiving intravenous therapy alone.)

McLaughlin P et al: Rituximab chimeric anti-CD-20 monoclonal antibody therapy for relapsed indolent lymphoma: half of patients respond to a four-dose regimen. J Clin Oncol 1998;16:2825. [NLM Cit ID 98368433] (This novel antibody therapy results in a high response rate in relapsed low-grade lymphoma with little toxicity.)

Negrier S et al: Recombinant human interleukin-2, recombinant human interferon alfa-2a, or both in metastatic renal-cell carcinoma. [NLM Cit ID: 98213297] N Engl J Med 1998;338:1272. (Cytokines are active in a few patients with metastatic disease but are very toxic, especially in combination.)

Tallman MS et al: All-*trans*-retinoic acid in acute promyelocytic leukemia. N Engl J Med 1997;337:1021. [NLM Cit ID: 97449069] (Tretinoin is superior to chemotherapy in the treatment of this leukemia.)

Trastuzumab and capecitabine for metastatic breast cancer. Med Lett Drugs Ther 1998;40:106. [NLM Cit ID: 99031912]

trointestinal tract can cause diarrhea that resolves gradually with cessation of therapy and healing of normal cells. Skin toxicity in the form of erythema and occasionally blistering and exfoliation of the area receiving radiation can also occur. Severe skin toxicity requires holding the radiation doses; the affected area is treated with local application of emollients.

Miscellaneous Drug-Specific Toxicities

The toxicities of individual drugs have been summarized in Table 4–4. Several of these warrant additional mention, since they occur with commonly administered agents, and special preventive measures are often indicated.

A. Hemorrhagic Cystitis Induced by Cyclophosphamide or Ifosfamide: Metabolic products of cyclophosphamide that retain cytotoxic activity are excreted into the urine. Some patients appear to metabolize more of the drug to these active excretory products. If their urine is concentrated, the toxic metabolite may cause severe bladder damage. Patients receiving cyclophosphamide must be advised to maintain a high fluid intake. Early symptoms of bladder toxicity include dysuria and frequency despite the absence of bacteriuria. If microscopic hematuria develops, it is advisable to stop the drug temporarily or switch to a different alkylating agent, increase fluid intake, and administer a urinary analgesic such as phenazopyridine. With severe cystitis, large segments of bladder mucosa may be shed and the patient may have prolonged gross hematuria. Such patients should be observed for signs of urinary obstruction and may require cystoscopy for removal of obstructing blood clots. The risk of developing hemorrhagic cystitis is dose-related and more common in patients who take the drug orally over a prolonged period of time. The cyclophosphamide analog ifosfamide or very high doses of cyclophosphamide can cause severe hemorrhagic cystitis when either is used alone. However, when they are used in conjunction with the neutralizing agent mesna, bladder toxicity can usually be prevented. Mesna is given with the chemotherapeutic agent and in a series of doses over the following 24 hours. Continuous bladder irrigation with 0.9% saline has been used with high-dose cyclophosphamide to prevent hemorrhagic cystitis. This appears to be less effective than mesna and may result in complications from Foley catheter trauma to the urethra, so it is used infrequently in high-risk situations—often in combination with mesna.

B. Neuropathy Induced by Vincristine and Other Agents: Neuropathy is a toxic side effect that is peculiar to the vinca alkaloid drugs, especially vincristine. A primarily sensory peripheral neuropathy is also commonly caused by two of the newer anticancer therapeutic agents, paclitaxel and vinorelbine. The peripheral neuropathy associated with vincristine can be sensory, motor, autonomic, or a combination of these effects. In its mildest form, it consists of paresthesias of the fingers and toes. Occasional patients develop acute jaw or throat pain after vincristine therapy. This may be a form of trigeminal or glossopharyngeal neuralgia. With continued vincristine therapy, the paresthesias may extend to the proximal interphalangeal joints, hyporeflexia can appear in the lower extremities, and weakness may develop in the quadriceps muscle group. At this point, it is wise to discontinue vincristine therapy until the neuropathy has subsided. In general, the neuropathy associated with paclitaxel and vinorelbine is mild, well-tolerated, and both dose-sensitive and schedule-sensitive. More frequent dosing of smaller amounts of chemotherapy can reduce this side effect; the neuropathy significantly improves when the chemotherapy is stopped. A useful means of judging whether peripheral motor neuropathy is severe enough to warrant stopping treatment is to have the patient attempt to do deep knee bends or rise from a chair without using the arm muscles.

Constipation is the most common symptom of autonomic neuropathy associated with vincristine therapy. Patients receiving vincristine should be started on stool softeners and mild cathartics when therapy is begun; otherwise, severe impaction may result as a consequence of an atonic bowel. More serious autonomic involvement can lead to acute intestinal ileus with signs indistinguishable from those of an acute abdomen.

Bladder neuropathies are uncommon but may be severe. Paralytic ileus and bladder atony are absolute contraindications to continued vincristine therapy. The majority of symptoms from vincristine are mild and resolve slowly after therapy has been completed. Docetaxel, cisplatin, carboplatin, and topotecan can also cause peripheral neuropathy, though in general symptoms improve gradually after treatment is stopped.

C. Methotrexate Toxicity and Leucovorin Rescue: In addition to standard uses of methotrexate for cancer chemotherapy, this drug is also used in very high doses that could lead to fatal bone marrow toxicity if given without an antidote. High-dose methotrexate therapy with leucovorin rescue is routinely used to treat osteogenic sarcoma, acute lymphocytic leukemia, some cases of non-Hodgkin's lymphoma, and primary lymphoma of the central nervous system.

The bone marrow and mucosal toxicity of methotrexate can be prevented by early administration of leucovorin (folinic acid). Serum levels of methotrexate are usually monitored and doses of leucovorin adjusted accordingly. Rescue is required for methotrexate doses over 80 mg/m^2 and is usually begun within 4 hours after completing treatment. Up to 100 mg/m^2 of leucovorin is given initially every 6 hours, with further doses adjusted for the serum methotrexate level. Rescue is usually continued orally for 3 days or longer until the serum methotrexate level is below 0.05 μmol/L. Asparaginase can be given as rescue for methotrexate in the treatment of lymphoblastic leukemia. If an overdose of methotrexate is administered accidentally, leucovorin therapy should be initiated as soon as possible, preferably within 1 hour. Intravenous infusion should be employed for larger overdosages to ensure adequate drug delivery. It is generally advisable to give leucovorin repeatedly in this situation.

Vigorous hydration and bicarbonate loading also appear to be important in preventing crystallization of high-dose methotrexate in the renal tubular epithelium. Serum creatinine is determined before beginning therapy and daily thereafter, since methotrexate excretion is slowed by renal insufficiency and toxicity will be enhanced. In high doses, methotrexate can itself cause renal injury. Methotrexate doses are reduced in renal insufficiency. Concomitant use of certain drugs will slow methotrexate excretion, and they are avoided during therapy. These drugs include aspirin, NSAIDs, penicillins, sulfonamides, and probenecid.

D. Busulfan Toxicity: The alkylating agent busulfan, occasionally used for the treatment of myeloproliferative diseases, has curious delayed toxicities, including increased skin pigmentation, a wasting syndrome similar to that seen in adrenal insufficiency, and progressive pulmonary fibrosis. Patients who develop either of the latter two problems should be switched to a different drug (eg, melphalan) when further therapy is needed. The pigmentary changes are innocuous and will usually regress slowly after treatment is discontinued. Long-term treatment with busulfan also results in an increased risk of secondary leukemias.

E. Bleomycin Toxicity: This antibiotic is used to treat squamous cell carcinoma, Hodgkin's disease, non-Hodgkin's lymphoma, and testicular cancer. Bleomycin can produce edema of the interphalangeal joints and hardening of the palmar and plantar skin. More serious toxicities include an anaphylactic or serum sickness-like reaction and a potentially fatal pulmonary fibrotic reaction (seen especially in elderly patients receiving a total dose of over 300 units). If a nonproductive cough, dyspnea, and pulmonary infiltrates develop, the drug is discontinued, and high-dose corticosteroids are instituted as well as empirical antibiotics pending cultures. Fever alone or with chills is an occasional complication of bleomycin treatment and is not an absolute contraindication to continued treatment. The fever may be avoided by hydrocortisone administration just prior to the injection. Fever alone is not predictive of pulmonary toxicity. About 1% of patients (especially those with lymphoma) may have a severe or even fatal hypotensive reaction after the initial dose of bleomycin. In order to identify and treat such patients, it is wise to administer a test dose of 5 units of bleomycin first and to have adequate monitoring and emergency facilities available. Patients exhibiting a hypotensive reaction should not receive further bleomycin therapy.

F. Anthracycline-Induced Cardiomyopathy: The anthracycline antibiotics doxorubicin, daunomycin, and idarubicin and the similar drug mitoxantrone both have acute and delayed cardiac toxicity. The problem is greater with doxorubicin because it has a major role and is used in repeated doses in the treatment of sarcomas, breast cancer, lymphomas, acute leukemia, and certain other solid tumors. Studies of left ventricular function and endomyocardial biopsies indicate that changes in cardiac dynamics occur in most patients by the time they have received 300 mg/m^2 of doxorubicin. The *mu*ltiple-*ga*ted ("MUGA") radionuclide cardiac scan is the most reproducible noninvasive test for assessing toxicity. Patients should not receive a total dose in excess of 450 mg/m^2, and 1–10% of patients who receive this dose develop cardiomyopathy. Doxorubicin should not be used in patients with intrinsic cardiac disease. Prior chest or mediastinal radiotherapy increases the risk of doxorubicin heart disease at lower total doses. The appearance of a high resting pulse may herald the appearance of cardiac toxicity. Unfortunately, the toxicity may be irreversible at dosage levels above 550 mg/m^2. At lower doses (eg, 350 mg/m^2), the symptoms and signs of cardiac failure generally respond well to medical therapy and cessation of doxorubicin.

Laboratory studies suggest that cardiac toxicity may be due to a mechanism involving the formation of intracellular free radicals in cardiac muscle. Pretreatment with dexrazoxane, an iron chelator that decreases free radical formation, appears to protect the myocardium from anthracycline-induced injury but may also reduce the anticancer efficacy of the anthracycline. Dexrazoxane is now approved for the prevention of cardiomyopathy in women with metastatic breast cancer receiving cumulative doxorubicin doses > 300 mg/m^2. Liposomally encapsulated doxorubicin and daunorubicin have been FDA-approved and appear to have minimal cardiac toxicity. Their main use to date has been to treat Kaposi's sarcoma, but they are also effective in the treatment of other anthracycline-sensitive cancers. The anthracycline analog idarubicin has shown efficacy against acute nonlymphocytic leukemia and breast cancer when used in combination with other agents. Idarubicin appears to have a similar potential for causing cardiotoxicity when compared with other anthracyclines, though a maximum lifetime dosage recommendation has not been made. Epirubicin, an anthracycline with perhaps lower cardiac toxicity than doxorubicin (but similar gastrointestinal toxicity), has recently been approved by the FDA for the treatment of breast cancer. There are no data comparing the effects of doxorubicin with epirubicin, which has been studied primarily in Europe and Canada.

G. Cisplatin Nephrotoxicity and Neurotoxic-

ity: Cisplatin is effective in the treatment of testicular, bladder, and ovarian cancer as well as in several other types of tumor. Nausea and vomiting are common, but nephrotoxicity and neurotoxicity are more serious. Vigorous hydration with or without mannitol diuresis may substantially reduce nephrotoxicity. Renal function must be carefully monitored during cisplatin therapy, as should serum magnesium, which may fall during therapy with this agent. Ototoxicity is a potentially serious neurotoxicity that can result in deafness. Other manifestations include peripheral neuropathy of mixed sensorimotor type that may be associated with painful paresthesias. The neurotoxicity of this drug is delayed and is more common after a total dose of 300 mg/m^2. The second-generation platinum analog carboplatin has been shown to be as effective as cisplatin in ovarian cancer. Carboplatin is less nephrotoxic and causes less severe nausea or vomiting, but it does induce significant myelosuppression along with neurotoxicity. Amifostine, an organic thiophosphate initially developed as a radioprotective agent, is effective in preventing renal toxicity from cisplatin. It is approved to reduce cumulative renal toxicity associated with repeat administration of cisplatin in advanced ovarian cancer. In addition, amifostine may reduce chemotherapy-induced hematologic toxicity and neurotoxicity. Glutathione also appears to be a promising agent in preventing cisplatin neurotoxicity. Glutathione has been given at a dose of 1.5 g/m^2 intravenously before cisplatin administration, then at a dose of 600 mg by intramuscular injection on days 2–5. These supportive measures do not appear to reduce the therapeutic effectiveness of platinum agents.

H. Alpha Interferon Toxicities: While alpha interferon is generally tolerated in the standard doses listed in Table 4–4, it has significant toxicity with the higher doses required to treat chronic myelogenous leukemia and malignant melanoma and is more toxic in elderly patients. Even standard doses may be intolerable to some patients. Fever and chills are initial side effects but are infrequent after continued treatment. These symptoms may be ameliorated or prevented by premedication with acetaminophen and bedtime dosing. However, anorexia, fatigue, and weight loss can be cumulative and with time may become severe. These symptoms may be dose- or treatment-limiting. Thirty percent or more of patients are intolerant of interferon therapy even at low doses. In some patients, central nervous system symptoms develop, usually manifested as confusion or somnolence. Interferon causes a reduction in blood counts, but this is usually not clinically important and is part of the desired effect in the treatment of chronic myelogenous leukemia. Interferon-induced side effects are sometimes confused with the symptoms of progressive cancer but usually clear within 1–2 weeks following cessation of interferon therapy.

Borden EC et al: A perspective on the clinical effectiveness and tolerance of interferon-alpha. Semin Oncol 1998;25:3. [NLM Cit ID: 98141638]

Ignoffo R et al (editors): *Cancer Chemotherapy Pocket Guide.* Lippincott-Raven, 1997.

EVALUATION OF TUMOR RESPONSE

Inasmuch as cancer chemotherapy can induce clinical improvement, serious toxicity, or both, it is important to critically assess the beneficial effects of treatment in patients with advanced cancer to determine that the net effect is favorable. The most valuable signs to follow during therapy include the following.

TUMOR SIZE

Shrinkage in tumor size can be demonstrated by physical examination, chest film or other x-ray, sonography, or a procedure such as radionuclide bone scanning (breast, lung, prostate cancer). CT scanning is important for the evaluation of tumor size and location and the extent of distant spread for a wide variety of tumors and sites. MRI is now the best noninvasive means of evaluating posterior fossa brain tumors, spinal cord tumors, spinal cord compression, and pelvic disease, but CT scanning remains useful and may provide additional information. Sonography is also helpful in the evaluation of pelvic neoplasms. Gallium scanning can be useful to detect residual disease in lymphomas, but some tumors are not gallium-avid, which limits the usefulness of this test. Positron emission tomography (PET scanning) is an emerging radiographic detection method that depends on metabolic activity for visualization. It appears to be very useful in detection of residual disease in lymphomas and in assessing the extent of disease in several solid tumors. A partial response (PR) is defined as a 50% or greater reduction in the original tumor mass. A complete response (CR) refers to the complete disappearance of detectable tumor. Progression is an increase of more than 25% in the size of the tumor or the appearance of any new lesions. New criteria for measuring responses of solid tumors have been established by the World Health Organization to avoid conflicts and inconsistency in measurements that influence reporting of tumor responses and to lead to more uniform reporting of outcomes of clinical trials. The RECIST criteria are based on measuring the largest single diameter of any tumor mass and include a minimum diameter for measurable lesions.

These criteria will be incorporated into all new cancer treatment protocols.

The effectiveness of any agent or combination of agents in the treatment of cancer is determined by the response rates (combination of CR, PR, and, for some aggressive neoplasms, stable disease), response duration, and survival. Treatment efficacy for metastatic or incurable disease is often measured by event free-survival (EFS) or time to progression (TTP). The usefulness of treatment given to prevent recurrence of potentially curable neoplasms is measured by relapse-free survival (RFS) or disease-free survival (DFS) as well as overall survival (OS).

TUMOR MARKERS

A decrease in the quantity of a tumor product or marker substance reflects a reduced amount of tumor in the body. Examples of such markers include paraproteins (abnormal immunoglobulins) in multiple myeloma and macroglobulinemia, human chorionic gonadotropin (hCG) in choriocarcinoma and testicular cancer, prostatic acid phosphatase and PSA in prostatic cancer, urinary steroids in adrenal carcinoma and paraneoplastic Cushing's syndrome, and 5-hydroxyindoleacetic acid (5-HIAA) in carcinoid syndrome.

Tumor-secreted fetal antigens are also used to follow the course and response to treatment of cancers. These include alpha$_1$-fetoprotein (AFP) in hepatoma, testicular cancer, teratoembryonal carcinoma, and in occasional cases of gastric carcinoma; ovarian tumor antigen (CA 125) in ovarian cancer; and carcinoembryonic antigen (CEA) in carcinomas of the colon, lung, breast, and pancreas. CA 15-3 (also referred to as CA 27.29) may become important in detecting early recurrence of breast cancer but is mainly used to follow response to therapy in metastatic disease. Monoclonal antibodies are now used for measurement of a number of tumor markers and offer the potential of delineating a number of additional markers for diagnostic purposes.

Tumor markers may play an important role in the early detection of some common tumors when combined with good physical examinations. PSA, an immunogenic glycoprotein produced solely by the prostate, is currently the only tumor marker with widespread (and very controversial) use in cancer screening. PSA was initially used to indicate tumor bulk and disease progression, but it is now sometimes used as a screening tool when paired with the digital rectal examination. The American Cancer Society National Prostate Cancer Detection Project is a multicenter study evaluating the use of PSA, digital rectal examination (DRE), and transrectal ultrasound (TRUS) in a large cohort of healthy men. In this and other studies, the combination of a monoclonal PSA greater than 4 ng/mL and an abnormal digital rectal examination was felt to produce a highly sensitive and specific method for detecting prostate cancer. The preliminary results of a large Canadian study have shown a significant reduction in death from prostate cancer in men undergoing regular screening. This study randomized more than 46,000 men aged 45–80 years to screening, with PSA (using 3 ng/mL as the upper limit of normal) and digital rectal examination followed by transrectal ultrasound for abnormal test results or for a 10% increase in PSA over 12 months. There was an almost threefold advantage of screening and early treatment to reduce mortality. The role of PSA screening must be carefully evaluated for each patient and the risks of screening (unnecessary biopsics and surgeries) discussed in detail.

An abnormal PSA or digital rectal examination requires further evaluation by transrectal ultrasound and possible biopsy, and this screening should be done regularly in men 45 years of age and older. The PSA may be elevated in benign prostatic hypertrophy and in prostatitis. Levels in benign disease are usually between 4 and 10 ng/mL; a level greater than 10 ng/mL increases the likelihood of finding cancer. In addition, 25–45% of patients with localized prostate cancer may have a normal PSA value. The increase in screening for prostate cancer over the last few years has markedly increased the reported incidence of this disease, though prostate cancer-specific mortality has been essentially stable. (See Table 4–1.)

Tumor markers may be useful to screen populations at high risk for a specific cancer. A recent study has shown that elevated and altered profiles of AFP can serve as predictive markers for the development of hepatocellular carcinoma in patients with cirrhosis. Most tumor markers are not specific or sensitive enough to be useful as screening tools owing to their frequent elevation in benign disease and their absence in some cases of malignancy.

In general, tumor markers are used to follow response to therapy of a specific cancer. In diseases where early treatment of recurrence can influence survival (eg, testicular cancer), tumor markers may be used to screen for recurrent disease before it becomes radiographically or clinically evident.

Coley CM et al: Early detection of prostate cancer. Part I: Prior probability and effectiveness of tests. Ann Intern Med 1997;126:394 [NLM Cit ID: 97192585]; and Part II: Estimating the risks, benefits, and costs. Ann Intern Med 1997;126:468. [NLM Cit ID: 97208746] (The lack of direct evidence showing a net benefit of screening in contrast to earlier detection of cancer mandates clinician-patient discussion about this procedure.)

Maggino T: Serum markers as prognostic factors in epithelial ovarian cancer: an overview. Eur J Gynaecol Oncol 2000;21:64. [NLM Cit ID: 20189157] (A review of the use of tumor markers in ovarian cancer.)

Prostate-specific antigen (PSA) best practice policy. American Urological Association. Oncology (Huntingt) 2000;14:267. [NLM Cit ID: 20201051] (Recommenda-

tions created by a multispecialty panel in the United States.)
Recommended breast cancer surveillance guidelines. J Clin Oncol 1997;15:2149. [NLM Cit ID: 97307015] (Clinical practice guidelines for surveillance strategy for the detection and treatment of recurrent breast cancer.)

GENERAL WELL-BEING, PERFORMANCE STATUS, & SUPPORTIVE CARE

The functional status of the cancer patient at diagnosis (or at the start of treatment) is a major prognostic factor and determinant of outcome with or without tumor-directed therapy. It is therefore important to assess functional status as well as tumor burden and symptoms before deciding on possible anticancer therapy. Functional status or performance status evaluates the patient's ability to perform activities of daily living and is clearly related to tumor burden, tumor site, and the patient's underlying physical condition.

Two scales are commonly used to measure performance status. The Karnofsky scale ranges from 100% (asymptomatic and fully functional) through 0% (dead) in steps of 10%. For example, a Karnofsky performance status of 40% implies a patient who is disabled and requires special care and assistance. This patient would be unable to work but would be able to live at home with special assistance. The more commonly used Eastern Cooperative Oncology Group (ECOG) scale is a five-point system that is simpler and easier to apply to clinical practice. The ECOG scoring system ranges from 0 to 4 as follows: 0, entirely asymptomatic; 1, symptomatic but fully ambulatory; 2, symptomatic and in bed less than 50% of the day; 3, symptomatic and in bed more than 50% of the day but not bedridden; and 4, bedridden. These two systems are often the basis for clinical decisions despite their obvious lack of precision. They are also useful in assessing the impact of therapy and disease progression.

The measures assessing functional status described above do not adequately assess quality of life, a major goal of cancer chemotherapy. Performance status is only one component of quality of life, which is a combination of subjective and objective factors. Factors included in the assessment of general well-being include improved appetite and weight gain and decreased pain as well as improved performance status. In general, cancer patients perceive that they receive inadequate analgesia and have impairment of function because of pain. The adequate use of pain medications is hampered by their sedating side effects. New guidelines for the management of pain and long-acting opioids delivered by a transdermal system may help (eg, fentanyl patch, changed every 3 days). In addition, a short-acting oral transmucosal fentanyl preparation is now available that may allow easier titration of analgesia. In addition, sedating effects can sometimes be avoided by adding nonsteroidal anti-inflammatory agents or antidepressants to opioid therapy. Occasionally, opioids may be given epidurally to relieve severe pain. As with the use of antiemetics, pain medications work better when given prophylactically on a regular schedule rather than as needed for chronic or severe pain. It is only by completely evaluating all of the factors described above that the physician is able to judge whether the net effect of chemotherapy is worthwhile palliation. See Chapters 1 and 5 for further discussions of pain management and care at the end of life.

In addition to opioids, agents that inhibit bone resorption may decrease bone pain and protect against skeletal complications (thereby improving quality of life) in women with breast cancer metastatic to bone, in men with prostate cancer metastatic to bone, and in patients with multiple myeloma and lytic bone lesions. The bisphosphonate pamidronate is well tolerated and is now considered standard therapy in these two groups of patients. Pamidronate is given at a dose of 90 mg intravenously over 2 hours once a month for about 1 year. Two radioactive agents are available for the palliation of bone pain. Strontium-89 and samarium-153 lexidronam are both given intravenously and have been shown to be effective in reducing bone pain from osteoblastic lesions. The major toxicity is hematopoietic suppression, which may limit the ability to give other palliative therapy. The use of agents such as pamidronate, dronabinol, growth factors such as erythropoietin, and appetite stimulants such as megestrol acetate (given in dosages ranging from 40 mg orally four times a day up to 800 mg once a day) can improve the quality of life for cancer patients.

As early detection of cancer increases and cancer therapy improves, a growing area of concern is the long-term care of cancer survivors. Careful attention must be paid to psychosocial as well as physical problems resulting from therapy. Chemotherapy often leads to early menopause, depression, sexual difficulties, and osteoporosis, among other problems. Physician awareness and referral to the appropriate resources is critical for maintaining quality of life in patients who are "survivors."

Cleeland CS et al: Pain and its treatment in outpatients with cancer. N Engl J Med 1994;330:592. [NLM Cit ID: 94134141] (Cancer patients do not receive adequate analgesia as outpatients.)
Foley KM: Advances in cancer pain. Arch Neurol 1999;56:413. [NLM Cit ID: 99213420] (An outline of medications and adjunctive therapy to treat cancer pain.)
Hortobagyi EN et al: Efficacy of pamidronate in reducing skeletal complications in patients with breast cancer and lytic bone metastases. N Engl J Med 1996;335:1785. [NLM Cit ID: 97081204] (Pamidronate as a supplement

to chemotherapy can protect against skeletal complications in women with breast cancer metastatic to bone.)

Kjaer M: The therapy of cancer pain and its integration into a comprehensive supportive care strategy. Ann Oncol 1997;8 Suppl 3:S15. [NLM Cit ID: 98001258]

Levy MH: Pharmacologic treatment of cancer pain. N Engl J Med 1996;335:1124. [NLM Cit ID: 96434829] (Review of the agents and guidelines for their use.)

Pfeilschifter J et al: Osteoporosis due to cancer treatment: pathogenesis and management. J Clin Oncol 2000; 18:1570. [NLM Cit ID: 20200511] (Pathogenesis, diagnostic tests, prevention, and treatment options are discussed in this review.)

CANCER COMPLICATIONS: DIAGNOSIS & MANAGEMENT

ONCOLOGIC EMERGENCIES

Cancer is a chronic disease, but acute emergencies may occur as a consequence of local involvement (spinal cord compression, superior vena cava syndrome, malignant effusions, etc) or generalized systemic effects (hypercalcemia, opportunistic infections, hypercoagulability, hyperuricemia, etc). These complications may be the presenting manifestation of cancer. Two relatively common complications covered elsewhere will not be discussed here: superior vena cava syndrome (Chapter 12) and hypercoagulability (Chapter 13).

Neilan BA: Oncologic emergencies: Treating acute problems resulting from cancer and chemotherapy. Postgrad Med 1994;95:131. [NLM Cit ID: 94105050]

1. SPINAL CORD COMPRESSION

Spinal cord compression by tumor mass is manifested by back pain, progressive weakness, and sensory loss (usually in the lower extremities). Less commonly, spinal cord disease may present as chest or abdominal pain or as signs of nerve root compression due to the epidural location of the tumor. Bowel and bladder dysfunction are late findings. Spinal cord compression may occur as a complication of metastatic solid tumor, lymphoma, or myeloma. Back pain at the level of the spinal cord lesion occurs in over 80% of cases and may be aggravated by lying down, weight-bearing, sneezing, or coughing. Because back pain may precede the development of neurologic symptoms or signs, it is important to investigate this complaint thoroughly in any patient with cancer.

If neurologic deficits are present at diagnosis, they are usually irreversible, though treatment immediately after symptoms develop may result in partial recovery. Neurologic impairment can progress rapidly. Treatment of early lesions may completely avoid significant compromise. Although patients who present with paralysis may not recover function, they should still be treated for pain relief and to limit the extent of progression. In addition, patients may respond to systemic therapy depending on the specific tumor type.

The diagnosis of spinal cord compression is made by MRI scan with contrast. With this noninvasive and sensitive test, it is possible to obtain detailed views of the area in question as well as sagittal images of the entire spinal cord and vertebral canal. A detailed examination is important for detection and treatment of multiple lesions. Bone radiographs and bone scans are useful for detecting vertebral metastases, but they do not aid in assessing spinal cord compromise.

Emergency Treatment

Radiation therapy to the area of spinal cord compression and two adjacent vertebrae above and below the lesion is the treatment of choice. High doses of glucocorticoids (usually dexamethasone, 10–100 mg intravenously) are administered as soon as the diagnosis is suspected or confirmed. A lower dose (eg, 4–6 mg every 6 hours intravenously or orally) is continued throughout the course of radiation therapy and tapered at or near the end of treatment.

Emergency surgery is indicated (1) for spinal cord compression in the absence of a diagnosis of malignancy, (2) for patients who have already received maximal doses of radiation to the involved area of the spine, and (3) for patients who develop progressive neurologic deficits during radiation whose prognosis warrants aggressive therapy. Chemotherapy is useful in treating lymphomas and multiple myeloma in conjunction with or following completion of radiation therapy.

Byrne TN: Spinal cord compression from epidural metastases. N Engl J Med 1992;327:614. [NLM Cit ID: 92350197] (Causes and pathogenesis.)

Coleman RE: Skeletal complications of malignancy. Cancer 1997;80:1588. [NLM Cit ID: 98026749] (A review of a variety of complications involving the skeleton, including spinal cord compression.)

Connelly C: Patients with low back pain: How to identify the few who need extra attention. Postgrad Med 1996;100:143. [NLM Cit ID: 97119192]

Helweg-Larsen S: Clinical outcome in metastatic spinal cord compression. A prospective study of 153 patients. Acta Neurol Scand 1996;94:269. [NLM Cit ID: 97091873]

Loblaw DA et al: Emergency treatment of malignant extradural spinal cord compression: an evidence-based guideline. J Clin Oncol 1998;16:1613. [NLM Cit ID: 98211800] (Canadian task force recommendations for emergency management.)

2. HYPERCALCEMIA

Hypercalcemia occurs in 10–20% of patients with cancer. Common causes include breast, lung, kidney, and head and neck carcinomas as well as multiple myeloma and lymphoma. Although the majority of cancers associated with hypercalcemia metastasize to the bones, approximately 20% of cases are not associated with bony lesions. The identification of a novel protein called parathyroid hormone-related protein (PTHrP) has revised some previously held views about the pathogenesis of hypercalcemia. Radioimmunoassays have identified this peptide in the serum of approximately two-thirds of cancer patients with hypercalcemia. High levels have been found in patients with hypercalcemia that was previously thought to be due solely to local osteolysis. PTHrP may become a useful tumor marker in normocalcemic patients. In addition, antibodies to PTHrP may be useful as treatment.

The symptoms and signs of hypercalcemia include nausea, vomiting, constipation, polyuria, muscular weakness and hyporeflexia, confusion, psychosis, tremor, and lethargy. Some patients may be asymptomatic. Electrocardiography often shows a shortening of the QT interval. The presence of hypercalcemia does not invariably indicate a dismal prognosis, especially in breast or prostate cancer and multiple myeloma or lymphoma. In the absence of signs or symptoms of hypercalcemia, a laboratory finding of elevated serum calcium should be rechecked to exclude the possibility of laboratory error.

Emergency Treatment

A. Hydration: Emergency treatment consists of aggressive intravenous hydration with 3–4 L/d of 0.9% saline followed by diuresis with 10–40 mg of intravenous furosemide. It is essential that the patient be well hydrated before beginning diuretic therapy and that hydration be maintained after diuresis is initiated. Although hydration alone is effective at slowly reducing the calcium level, it is rarely sufficient treatment and can lead to problems with fluid overload.

B. Drug Therapy: There are now several options for the emergent treatment of hypercalcemia used in conjunction with aggressive hydration.

1. Bisphosphonates–Bisphosphonates are potent inhibitors of osteoclast bone resorption and are currently the most important and least toxic agents for the treatment of cancer-related hypercalcemia. Pamidronate disodium is the most potent bisphosphonate currently available. A single 2-hour intravenous infusion of 90 mg with adequate hydration produces complete normalization of serum calcium within 3 days in 70–100% of patients. Pamidronate administrations can be repeated as necessary to control hypercalcemia. The most commonly reported side effects have been transient fever, myalgias, and an infusion site reaction. Pamidronate has also been found to reduce the incidence of new skeletal lesions and decrease pain from bone disease in multiple myeloma, prostate cancer, and breast cancer.

A new bisphosphonate, zoledronate, is scheduled to be released shortly. This agent is also highly effective in the treatment of cancer-related hypercalcemia and can be given as an intravenous infusion over 5–10 minutes. The side effects are identical to those of pamidronate.

2. Gallium nitrate–For treatment of hypercalcemia, gallium nitrate is given by continuous intravenous infusion at a dose of 100–200 mg/m^2/d for 5 days. Gallium nitrate is superior to calcitonin both in reducing calcium levels acutely and in keeping the levels low after treatment is completed. Renal function must be carefully monitored.

3. Calcitonin–Synthetic salmon calcitonin works immediately to inhibit bone resorption, whereas pamidronate may take 2–3 days to achieve its maximum effect. The usual dose of 4 IU/kg intramuscularly, subcutaneously, or intranasally every 12 hours may be increased to 8 IU/kg every 12 hours after 1–2 days. Skin testing is usually performed before the first dose to test for hypersensitivity reactions. Calcitonin alone is usually not effective at lowering serum calcium levels but can be added to pamidronate if necessary to achieve normal calcium levels. Repeated treatment with calcitonin is usually not as effective, and tachyphylaxis usually occurs after 1–3 days of treatment.

4. Other drugs–Prednisone has not been shown to be effective as a single agent to treat hypercalcemia, though it can be used in diseases that are responsive to steroids such as multiple myeloma or lymphoma. Refractory hypercalcemia may be treated with intravenous plicamycin, 25 μg/kg/d for 3 or 4 days. Although often effective, its effect may be short-lived, and its use is often associated with hepatic, renal, and bone marrow toxicity.

C. Chemotherapy: Patients with breast cancer may develop hypercalcemia as a "flare" associated with bone pain after initiation of estrogen or antiestrogen therapy. These patients often achieve excellent tumor response with continued therapy. Tumors may respond to chemotherapy or radiation therapy, leading to resolution of hypercalcemia. If chronic hypercalcemia persists and is refractory to chemotherapy, pamidronate, and aggressive oral hydration may be tried but are unfortunately rarely effective for long. When the more potent bisphosphonates become available in oral formulations, the management of chronic hypercalcemia may improve.

Berenson JR et al: Bisphosphonates in the treatment of malignant bone disease. Annu Rev Med 1999;50:237. [NLM Cit ID: 99172930] (An excellent overview.)

Kristensen B et al: Survival in breast cancer patients after the first episode of hypercalcemia. J Intern Med 1998;244:189. [NLM Cit ID: 98418513] (Median survival was 6 months after first diagnosis of hypercalcemia, with poorer prognosis correlating with severity of hypercalcemia.)

Mundy GR et al: Hypercalcemia of malignancy. Am J Med 1997;103:134. [NLM Cit ID: 97418821] (Management and biology of this disorder.)

3. HYPERURICEMIA & ACUTE URATE NEPHROPATHY

Hyperuricemia can occur both as a complication of rapidly proliferating malignancies or with treatment-associated tumor lysis of hematologic malignancies such as leukemia, lymphoma, and multiple myeloma. Neoplasms with a high nucleic acid turnover such as acute leukemia and lymphoma may present with elevated serum uric acid and associated renal insufficiency. This problem may be compounded by use of thiazide diuretics, which decrease urate excretion. If a patient presents with hyperuricemia, care must be taken to reduce the uric acid before institution of cancer therapy. Patients at risk for tumor lysis syndrome should be followed with twice-daily measurements of uric acid, phosphate, calcium, and creatinine for the first 2–3 days following initiation of chemotherapy. Rapid elevation of serum uric acid can result in acute urate nephropathy caused by uric acid crystallization in the distal tubules, collecting ducts, and renal parenchyma. A serum urate concentration above 15 mg/dL is associated with a high risk of uric acid nephropathy. Gouty arthritis is usually a problem only in patients with a history of gout.

Prophylactic therapy consists of decreasing the production and increasing the renal excretion of uric acid. Allopurinol is a competitive inhibitor of xanthine oxidase and prevents conversion of highly soluble hypoxanthine and xanthine to the relatively insoluble uric acid. Twelve to 24 hours before beginning chemotherapy, a dose of 600 mg is given, followed by 300 mg/d during the period of high risk. Higher doses (up to 900–1200 mg/d) are used when severe hyperuricemia is anticipated following chemotherapy. Patients receiving the purine antagonists mercaptopurine or azathioprine should be given only 25–35% of the calculated dose of chemotherapy if they are also receiving allopurinol, since the latter drug will potentiate both the therapeutic effects and the toxicity of these agents. Renal excretion of uric acid is enhanced by maintaining a high urine flow and by alkalinizing the urine to prevent uric acid crystallization, which occurs at acid pH. The urine can be alkalinized with 6–8 g of oral sodium bicarbonate per day or by adding two or three ampules of sodium bicarbonate to 1 liter of D_5W by infusion. Alkaline diuresis to maintain a urine pH near 7.0 is required only for prophylaxis in patients expected to have a rapid tumor response with marked hyperuricemia.

Emergency Treatment

Emergency therapy for established severe hyperuricemia consists of (1) hydration with 2–4 L of fluid per day; (2) alkalinization of the urine with 6–8 g of sodium bicarbonate per day; (3) allopurinol, 900–1200 mg/d; and (4) in severe cases, emergency hemodialysis. When severe hyperuricemia is present, adequate therapy may be impossible because of associated renal insufficiency and inadequate urine output. Intravenous allopurinol is available for use in patients unable to tolerate the oral form of this drug. Even if renal failure occurs and dialysis is required, renal function may return to normal after the acute tumor lysis has resolved.

4. MALIGNANT CARCINOID SYNDROME

Although tumors of argentaffin cells are uncommon, they are important because they secrete a variety of vasoactive materials. These include serotonin, histamine, catecholamines, prostaglandins, and vasoactive peptides. Carcinoid syndrome is usually associated with carcinoid tumors of the small bowel metastatic to the liver and, less commonly, with primary carcinoid tumors in other sites such as the lung or stomach. These tumors tend to metastasize early but have a relatively indolent course, making control of the syndrome important. Related syndromes occur in patients with pancreatic tumors secreting vasoactive peptides, which can cause severe watery diarrhea (pancreatic cholera).

The manifestations of carcinoid syndrome include facial flushing, edema of the head and neck (especially with bronchial carcinoid), abdominal cramps and diarrhea, bronchospasm, cardiac lesions (tricuspid or pulmonary stenosis or regurgitation), telangiectasias, and increased urinary 5-hydroxyindoleacetic acid (5-HIAA). The most common symptoms are flushing and diarrhea. The diagnosis is made by finding elevated levels of 5-HIAA in a 24-hour urine collection. Patients with symptomatic carcinoid usually excrete more than 25 mg of 5-HIAA per day in the urine. Ideally, all drugs and serotonin-rich foods such as bananas should be withheld for several days before beginning the urine collection.

Emergency Treatment

Emergency therapy for patients with symptomatic bronchial carcinoid includes prednisone, 15–30 mg/d. The associated abdominal cramping and diarrhea of intestinal carcinoids can often be managed by hydration and diphenoxylate with atropine. For severe diarrhea, the H_1 histamine receptor antagonist cyproheptadine (4 mg orally three times daily) or an antiserotonin agent such as methysergide maleate (2 mg orally three times daily until 16 mg has been given) may be effective. Other useful agents include cimetidine and the phenothiazines.

The synthetic peptide somatostatin agonist, octreotide acetate, is the most effective agent for reducing symptoms due to the carcinoid syndrome in association with achieving a reduction in levels of urinary 5-HIAA. The dose of octreotide in carcinoid syndrome is 100–600 μg/d in two to four divided doses by subcutaneous injection. Octreotide is also effective in the treatment of symptoms related to vasoactive intestinal peptide-secreting pancreatic tumors (VIPomas), markedly reducing the watery diarrhea syndrome associated with this neoplasm. The dose of octreotide used to treat patients with VIPomas is 200–300 μg/d in two to four divided doses.

Surgery is important in the treatment of localized carcinoid. Chemotherapy is moderately effective for patients with progressive advanced-stage disease. Active agents include fluorouracil, streptozocin, dacarbazine, cisplatin, doxorubicin, and alpha interferon.

Kulke MH et al: Carcinoid tumors. N Engl J Med 1999;340:858. [NLM Cit ID: 99165321] (Review of the disease and treatment of complications.)

Memon MA et al: Gastrointestinal carcinoid tumors: Current management strategies. Dis Colon Rectum 1997;40:349. [NLM Cit ID: 97438168] (Review of management of one of the most common sites of involvement.)

OTHER COMPLICATIONS

1. MALIGNANT EFFUSIONS

The development of effusions in the pleural, pericardial, and peritoneal spaces may be the presenting sign of some tumors or may cause diagnostic and therapeutic problems in patients with advanced neoplasms. Although the cause of an effusion can be elusive in a newly diagnosed asymptomatic patient, it is rarely difficult in the patient with advanced cancer. Approximately half of undiagnosed effusions in patients not known to have cancer will be malignant. The differential diagnosis includes congestive heart failure, pulmonary embolism, trauma, and infections such as tuberculosis. Direct involvement of the serous surface of the involved space with tumor appears to be the most frequent initiating factor, though many other mechanisms such as obstruction of lymphatic drainage that control the flow of fluid in the pleural space may play a role.

Most patients with pleural or pericardial effusions are symptomatic at presentation with chest pain, shortness of breath, or cough. The diagnosis is made by tapping the involved space. Pericardial effusions are aspirated under fluoroscopic guidance or direct vision through a subxiphoid incision. The fluid should be heparinized and sent for cell count and differential, protein content, lactate dehydrogenase level, and cytologic study. The gross appearance of the fluid is often helpful as well. Bloody effusions are usually due to cancer but occasionally are due to pulmonary embolism, tuberculosis, or trauma. Chylous effusions may be associated with thoracic duct obstruction or may result from enlarged mediastinal lymph nodes in lymphoma. If the cytologic smear is negative on two occasions but the suspicion of tumor is still high, closed pleural biopsy may be helpful.

The management of effusions should be appropriate to the severity of involvement. Treatment of the underlying neoplasm would be ideal but is often not effective in controlling local effusions. Treatment may result in palliation and improve short-term survival when there is substantial pulmonary or cardiac compromise. Diuretics are used as initial treatment for small to moderate-sized peritoneal effusions and as an adjunct to drainage of large effusions to minimize the possibility of reexpansion pulmonary edema that can occur after thoracentesis. Small or loculated effusions may require ultrasonographic localization, but drainage of a large pleural or peritoneal effusion can be accomplished rapidly using an intravenous catheter and phlebotomy tubing connected to a vacuum bottle. Thoracentesis alone controls fewer than 10% of effusions but may be useful in conjunction with systemic chemotherapy for sensitive tumors (eg, lymphoma, small-cell lung cancer, breast cancer). Pleural effusions may occasionally be managed by closed water-seal drainage with a chest tube for 3–4 days, though this procedure is usually performed in conjunction with chemosclerosis (see below). The aim of this procedure is to allow the pleural surfaces to come into close contact and become adherent.

Recurrent symptomatic effusions can often be controlled by drainage followed by chemosclerosis. In this procedure, a chemotherapeutic or nonchemotherapeutic agent is instilled with lidocaine into the involved space. The intended effect is local inflammation and sclerosis to encourage adherence of the serosal surfaces. Several drugs used in the past for this purpose have been abandoned because of severe pain or systemic toxicity, including myelosuppression. Agents currently in use include talc, bleomycin, and the anthracenedione compound mitoxantrone.

Talc poudrage has been used successfully to control malignant pleural effusions and appears to be relatively painless. For these reasons as well as cost considerations, talc is now the sclerosing agent of choice for malignant pleural effusions.

Bleomycin is more effective at controlling pleural effusions than tetracycline; when tetracycline was used, the recurrence rate 90 days after sclerosis was almost double, and the side effects were similar. Tetracycline is no longer manufactured or available for intracavitary instillation. The major side effects of bleomycin are pain, fever, and hypersensitivity reactions.

Mitoxantrone has been reported to be effective in controlling malignant pleural effusions, causing minimal fever and local pain. However, one trial evaluated the effectiveness of mitoxantrone versus chest tube alone and found no differences in response or in duration of response. The instillation of sclerosing agents may best be reserved for patients who fail pleural tube drainage alone.

Sclerosis is generally less useful for the management of malignant ascites, but success has been reported using bleomycin, doxorubicin, thiotepa, and other agents.

Before instilling the sclerosing agent, it is important that the space be drained as thoroughly as possible. For pleural effusions, a small-bore chest tube or pigtail catheter is usually placed and fluid is removed by negative suction until the drainage is under 100 mL per 24 hours and the lung has expanded. Sclerotherapy is ineffective if there is a large residual effusion. Talc is insufflated into the pleural space via a thoracoscope or instilled in a 5 g slurry with iodide via a chest tube. Talc instillation via a thoracoscope under anesthesia can be done quickly, has minimal complications, and appears highly effective. This is now the initial treatment of choice for malignant pleural effusions. To use chemotherapeutic agents, the patient is premedicated with an opioid, and 60 units of bleomycin or 30 mg of mitoxantrone in 50–100 mL of 0.9% saline is instilled directly into the chest tube. The chest tube is then clamped, and the patient is placed in different positions every 15 minutes for 4 hours to distribute the agent equally within the pleural space. At the end of this period, the clamp is removed and the chest tube is allowed to drain with suction. After 24 hours, the chest tube is removed from suction, and when the drainage is minimal, the tube is removed. The whole process takes 3–5 days. Occasionally, repeated doses of the sclerosing agent may be required to stop persistent reaccumulation of the effusion.

Surgery is infrequently used for patients with pleural or pericardial effusions who have failed sclerosis and who continue to have a long expected survival. Pleuroperitoneal shunting may have limited value in selected patients with high performance status who can participate actively in pumping the shunt the 100 times on five separate occasions each day required for adequate shunt function and fluid drainage. Pleurectomy has a high complication rate but offers excellent control of effusion in carefully selected patients. For malignant pericardial effusion, a pericardial window or stripping also offers good control with a lower complication rate and may also be performed for constrictive pericarditis following radiation therapy to the chest.

Burrows CM et al: Predicting survival in patients with recurrent symptomatic malignant pleural effusions: an assessment of the prognostic values of physiologic, morphologic, and quality of life measures of extent of disease. Chest 2000;117:73. [NLM Cit ID: 20098422] (The Karnofsky performance status was predictive of overall survival in patients with recurrent malignant pleural effusions.)

Erasmus JJ et al: Treatment of malignant pleural effusions. Curr Opin Pulm Med 1999;5:250. [NLM Cit ID: 99336034] (Review of the diagnosis and therapy of malignant pleural effusions.)

Girardi LN et al: Pericardiocentesis and intrapericardial sclerosis: effective therapy for malignant pericardial effusions. Ann Thorac Surg 1997;64:1422. [NLM Cit ID: 98047945] (Noncontrolled observation of equivalent outcomes with drainage of malignant pericardial effusions by percutaneous versus open approaches.)

Viallat JR et al: Thoracoscopic talc poudrage pleurodesis for malignant effusions: A review of 360 cases. Chest 1996;110:1387. [NLM Cit ID: 97143039] (An increasingly popular method of pleurodesis.)

2. INFECTIOUS COMPLICATIONS

The reader is referred also to the section on infections in the immunocompromised patient in Chapter 30.

Many patients with cancer have increased susceptibility to both bacterial and opportunistic infections. This may result from impaired host defense mechanisms (eg, Hodgkin's or non-Hodgkin's lymphoma, chronic lymphocytic leukemia, multiple myeloma, acute leukemia or preleukemia) or from the myelosuppressive and immunosuppressive effects of cancer chemotherapy. Impaired host defense mechanisms include defects in neutrophil function, abnormalities in antibody production, depressed cell-mediated function, impairment of mechanical barriers by indwelling intravenous catheters, and impairment of mucosal integrity. At least half of the infections seen in neutropenic patients are felt to be endogenous.

The bacterial organisms accounting for the majority of infections in cancer patients include Enterobacteriaceae (klebsiella, enterobacter, serratia, *Escherichia coli*), pseudomonas, staphylococcus, and streptococcus. Other important pathogens include corynebacterium, *Clostridium difficile,* mycobacterium, and legionella. Patients with prolonged neutropenia or those who have undergone bone marrow transplantation are at risk for infections with fungi such as candida, aspergillus, and pneumocystis and with viruses such as herpes zoster, cytomegalovirus, respiratory syncytial virus, and in-

knowledge of the molecular events responsible for disordered cellular growth and include antibodies directed against abnormal growth-enhancing factors and receptors as well as gene therapy to turn off signaling pathways or provide a missing tumor suppressor.

The goal of gene therapy for cancer is to inhibit the constitutive signals that drive tumor growth. Expanding knowledge about signal transduction has provided multiple possible attack points within this complicated multistep process involving a variety of somatic gene alterations. Although at present it is impossible to deliver therapeutic genes to every cancer cell, bystander effects or the cytotoxic effects produced by engineered cells on nonengineered cells may allow broad effects from a limited number of transduced cells. A variety of approaches are being investigated. These include enhancing the ability of the host immune system to respond to a specific tumor, sensitizing tumor cells to relatively nontoxic drugs or prodrugs, and selective replacement of altered or missing tumor suppressor genes or inactivation of oncogenes. Selective targeting of cells would allow either cell death or return of normal growth patterns without toxicity to nonneoplastic cells. One area of research in active clinical trial is replacement of the missing function of the mutated tumor suppressor gene, *P53,* or to inhibit the function of a dominant oncogene such as *ras.* One interesting approach is to create a vaccine directed against cells with mutant *P53* in order to generate a cytotoxic T cell response to tumor cells expressing the P53 protein. A vaccine made from a disabled adenovirus (the vector or carrier) and the *P53* gene and injected into the arterial circulation is delivered to tumors that have metastasized to the liver with subsequent expression of the *P53* gene. Another unique approach to tumor killing is the use of an adenovirus engineered to selectively kill tumor cells that are lacking *P53* but leave normal cells alone. This agent, ONYX-015, is also in clinical trials both with and without chemotherapy. It appears to be more effective when injected directly into tumors. Results from this and other agents are limited by a variety of problems, including difficulty delivering the agent, identifying tumors that lack *P53,* and production of the novel agent. Gene therapy is also being investigated in autologous stem cell transplantation for a variety of malignancies. In this setting, antitumor genes are added to cells that have been removed for transplantation following myeloablative chemotherapy. Trials are ongoing to study this form of therapy in chronic myelogenous leukemia. Multiple other trials, including the introduction of new genes that encode inhibitors of oncogene products or enhance tumor cell immunogenicity, are in progress.

Angiogenesis (the growth of new blood vessels) is thought to be an essential component of the ability of tumors to invade locally and to metastasize from the primary tumor site. Tumor angiogenesis is regulated by angiogenic stimulators such as vascular endothelial growth factor (VEGF) and newly described inhibitors of angiogenesis, angiostatin and endostatin. There is now intense interest in using inhibitors of angiogenesis to suppress tumor growth and metastases. This type of therapy might avoid the development of chemotherapy resistance and have less toxicity than standard cytotoxic therapy. A recombinant humanized antibody to the vascular endothelial growth factor (anti-VEGF, rhuMAb VEGF) has been tested alone and with chemotherapy in colon, breast, and lung cancers. The most promising results have been seen in patients with advanced colon cancer in conjunction with fluorouracil and leucovorin chemotherapy with improved response rates and survival in the anti-VEGF arm. Larger randomized trials using anti-VEGF in combination with chemotherapy versus chemotherapy alone in the treatment of advanced colon, lung, and breast cancers are scheduled to begin later this year. Endostatin and angiostatin are potent inhibitors of angiogenesis that appear to be very promising. A recent study showed that transfer of cells engineered to produce angiostatin into mice inhibited the growth of both the primary tumor and lung metastases from fibrosarcoma. Trials using endostatin to treat patients with advanced malignancy began in late 1999. More information about the endostatin trial and others using antiangiogenesis agents can be found at the NCI cancer trials Web site listed below. Another novel way to suppress angiogenesis is with antibodies to receptor tyrosine kinases (RTK inhibitors) that block VEGF-mediated receptor signaling. Several agents are in clinical trials treating advanced metastatic cancers of the colon and lung, usually in combination with chemotherapy, including SU5416 (Semoxind) and ZD1839 (Iressa). Phase II data suggest antitumor effects. Thalidomide has been shown to have antiangiogenic properties as well as other antitumor effects. Striking responses have been seen in advanced and resistant multiple myeloma. Clinical trials using thalidomide in combination with chemotherapy in multiple myeloma, prostate cancer, and other malignancies are ongoing. An interesting novel therapy now in clinical trials targets metalloproteases that are thought to be important in the ability of cancer cells to metastasize. Inhibiting the ability of these cells to cross endothelial barriers may help to control distant spread of cancer.

Immunotherapy is an exciting area of investigation of the treatment of cancer. The most extensively treated disease with immunotherapeutic modalities is malignant melanoma—for a variety of reasons, including easily identified immunogenic antigens, easy access to tumor cells, and the ability to grow these cells in vitro. Active specific immunotherapy with melanoma vaccines has been evaluated in phase II trials for advanced melanoma as well as in the adjuvant setting with encouraging results. The results of ongoing phase III trials should help to further define the role of vaccine therapy in the treatment of melanoma. The field of cancer vaccines is growing rapidly. One type of tumor vaccine in several clinical trials capitalizes on dendritic cells, which are antigen-presenting cells that enhance the response of the immune system to foreign antigens. Dendritic cells may be loaded with a particular abnormal protein to stimulate the immune response to a specific cancer. Early clinical trials in melanoma, multiple myeloma, and other cancers are ongoing. One interesting strategy is to target the dendritic cells to a known growth factor present on the tumor cell. A clinical trial using dendritic cells loaded with HER2/*neu* for the treatment of metastatic breast cancer is scheduled to begin later this year. This type of therapy might also be useful early in the disease course of an aggressive tumor. Other types of vaccines stimulate lymphocytes and dendritic cells ex vivo with immune stimulants or the tumor itself in order to enhance tumor cell death in vivo. This type of therapy can be used in conjunction with autologous stem cell transplantation; cells are removed at the time of stem cell harvesting, undergo in vitro stimulation, and are then returned to the patient after completion of chemotherapy and radiation therapy to eradicate bulk tumor. Both radiolabeled and toxin-linked antibodies have been used to treat lymphomas with very encouraging results and appear more effective than antibody (Bexxar) therapy alone. A large clinical study using a radiolabeled B cell antibody is under way. Antibodies linked to toxins, chemotherapeutic agents, and radiation have been used as a means of targeting therapy to reduce toxicity to normal tissues. An antibody against CD33 linked to the chemotherapeutic agent calicheamicin, has been effective and relatively nontoxic in the treatment of relapsed myeloid leukemia. Gemtuzumab zogamicin was recently FDA-approved for the treatment of relapsed AML in patients aged 60 and older. Clinical trials using ^{131}I linked to an antibody against CD20 (tositumomab) in patients with relapsed and early stage B cell lymphomas are ongoing with very encouraging early results. Many other antibody combinations are either under development or in preliminary clinical trials.

Other areas of investigation include discovery of novel agents that induce apoptosis (programmed cell death), stimulate differentiation, prevent tumor invasion or metastases, and specifically target hormone pathways that stimulate tumor growth. In addition, new antiproliferative agents with improved toxicity profiles and less cross-resistance to known agents are being evaluated or are already in use. Ongoing research is focusing on the identification of new growth factor receptors associated with malignant behavior that can be targeted to suppress cancer growth, such as HER2/*neu* and trastuzumab. The current explosion of clinical trials targeting various pathways of tumor growth as well as ongoing research to identify antigenic targets should lead to a new paradigm for cancer therapy in the coming decades. Several problems with vaccine therapy exist, including the difficulty of generating an immune response in an immunosuppressed cancer patient and the fact that an immune response does not necessarily correlate with tumor response. In order to enhance the immune response to vaccines, growth factors such as GM-CSF are given with the treatment.

Cao Y et al: Expression of angiostatin cDNA in murine fibrosarcoma suppresses primary tumor growth and produces long-term dormancy of metastases. J Clin Invest 1998;101:1055. [NLM Cit ID: 98153232] (Angiostatin appears to result in significant tumor regression in mice.)

Greten TF et al: Cancer vaccines. J Clin Oncol 1999; 17:1047. [NLM Cit ID: 99168858] (Timely review.)

Heise C et al: ONYX-015, an E1B gene-attenuated adenovirus, causes tumor-specific cytolysis and antitumoral efficacy that can be augmented by standard chemotherapeutic agents. Nat Med 1997;3:639. [NLM Cit ID: 97319587]

McDonnell WM et al: Molecular medicine: DNA vaccines. N Engl J Med 1996;334:42. [NLM Cit ID: 96105285]

Wilder RB et al: Radioimmunotherapy: Recent results and future directions. J Clin Oncol 1996;14:1383. [NLM Cit ID: 96243106] (A review of the literature on radiolabeled antibodies in cancer therapy.)

Zetter BR: Angiogenesis and tumor metastasis. Ann Rev Med 1998;49:407. [NLM Cit ID: 98170010] (Excellent review of this exciting area).

ALTERNATIVE & COMPLEMENTARY THERAPIES FOR CANCER

New areas of cancer therapy are rapidly expanding, and the next decade could bring important changes in the treatment of common malignancies. Many alternatives to traditional cancer therapy exist (one well-known example is shark cartilage, which is widely available and purported to have anti-angiogenic properties), but there is little evidence to support their efficacy or assess their potential toxicity, and at present there is no federal regulation of these products. Agents that are commonly used include green tea, echinacea, essiac tea, flaxseed, mistletoe, and coenzyme Q, as well as others.

It is critical that herbs be tested with the same rigorous standards as chemotherapeutic agents in scientifically based clinical trials. Most herbal preparations are available over the counter, and no information exists regarding the interaction of these herbs with other medications. Many interactions have recently been described between St. John's wort and critical medications such as antiretrovirals and cyclosporine that resulted in decreased drug levels due to enhanced metabolism.

A dietary supplement containing a combination of eight Chinese herbs with potent estrogenic activity, PC-SPES, has been tested in prostate cancer. All patients with hormone-sensitive and about 60% of patients with hormone-refractory prostate cancer responded with a decline in PSA; some patients also had improvement in bone scans. Toxicity was modest, including allergic reactions and thromboembolic events in about 4% of patients. Objective response rates and the duration of responses must be confirmed in larger randomized trials. More information about PC-SPES is available on the Web at http://cc.ucsf.edu/clinical/uro_pc-spes.html. Ongoing research is evaluating the effects of herbal combinations on side effects of adjuvant chemotherapy for breast cancer. The NCI is actively supporting research in the field of alternative therapies for cancer. Additional information on alternative treatment modalities can be found in Chapter 43.

There are now many Web sites devoted to providing information on alternative cancer therapies. The NIH National Center for Complementary and Alternative Medicine lists new research and research trials as well as an introduction to alternative medicine. There is also an extensive bibliography. This Web site may be reached at http://nccam.nih.gov. Additional resources can be found at the Cancer Guide Material on Alternative Medicine Web site http://cancerguide.org/alternative.html. The Center for Alternative Medicine Research in Cancer at the University of Texas-Houston Health Science Center (UT-CAM) maintains an excellent Web site with data pertaining to a wide variety of alternative medications and therapies. The Web site can be reached at http://www.sph.uth.tmc.edu/utcam/.

The American Society of Clinical Oncology: The physician and unorthodox cancer therapies. J Clin Oncol 1997;15:401. [NLM Cit ID: 97149359] (Nine percent of patients are estimated to use alternative cancer therapies. Physicians must be educated about these treatments and be able to discuss such issues with their patients.)

Ernst E: Second thoughts about safety of St John's wort. Lancet 1999;354:2014. [NLM Cit ID: 20100316] (A discussion of the enzyme-inducing properties of this herbal preparation.)

Jacobson JS et al: Research on complementary/alternative medicine for patients with breast cancer: a review of the biomedical literature. J Clin Oncol 2000;18:668. [NLM Cit ID: 20120886] (Many studies had encouraging results; none showed a difference in disease progression, though some modalities improved toxicities of therapy.)

Pfeifer BL et al: PC-SPES, a dietary supplement for the treatment of hormone-refractory prostate cancer. BJU Int 2000;85:481. [NLM Cit ID: 20157006] (A small study of the effects of PC-SPES in advanced prostate cancer showed a decline in PSA levels as well as reduction in pain and improvement in quality of life measures.)

RELEVANT WORLD WIDE WEB SITES

[American Society of Clinical Oncology]
http://www.asco.org
[NCCN Oncology Practice Guidelines]
http://www.cancernetwork.com
[START: State of the Art Oncology in Europe]
http://telescan.nki.nl/start/start.html
[National Cancer Institute—CancerLit]
http://cnetdb.nci.nih.gov/cancerlit.shtml
[National Cancer Institute—CancerNet]
http://cnetdb.nci.nih.gov/overview.html
[Talaria]
http://www.Talaria.org/
[American Alliance of Cancer Pain Initiatives]
http://www.fhcrc.org/cipr/aacpi/
[American Pain Society]
http://www.ampainsoc.org/
[Anal Cancer—American Cancer Society]
http://www3.cancer.org/cancerinfo/load_cont.asp?ct=47
[Anal Cancer—National Cancer Institute—CancerNet]
http://cancernet.nci.nih.gov/clinpdq/soa/Anal_cancer_Physician.html
[Bladder Cancer—National Cancer Institute—CancerNet]
http://cancernet.nci.nih.gov/clinpdq/soa/Bladder_cancer_Physician.html
[Transitional Cell Cancer of the Renal Pelvis and Ureter—National Cancer Institute—CancerNet]
http://cancernet.nci.nih.gov/clinpdq/soa/Transitional_cell_cancer_of_the_renal_pelvis_and_ureter_Physician.html
[Adult Brain Tumor—National Cancer Institute—CancerNet]
http://cancernet.nci.nih.gov/clinpdq/soa/Adult_brain_tumor_Physician.html
[Neuroblastoma—National Cancer Institute—CancerNet]
http://cancernet.nci.nih.gov/clinpdq/soa/Neuroblastoma_Physician.html
[Pituitary Tumor—National Cancer Institute—CancerNet]
http://cancernet.nci.nih.gov/clinpdq/soa/Pituitary_tumor_Physician.html
[Breast Cancer—American Cancer Society]
http://www3.cancer.org/cancerinfo/res_home.asp?ct=5
[Breast Cancer—National Cancer Institute—CancerNet]
http://cancernet.nci.nih.gov/cgi-bin/srchcgi.exe?DBID=pdq&TYPE=search&UID=208+00013&ZFILE=professional&SFMT=pdq_treatment/1/0/0
[Breast Cancer and Pregnancy—National Cancer Institute—CancerNet]
http://cancernet.nci.nih.gov/clinpdq/soa/Breast_cancer_and_pregnancy_Physician.html
[Breast Cancer Answers]

http://www.medsch.wisc.edu/bca
[Male Breast Cancer—National Cancer Institute—CancerNet]
http://cancernet.nci.nih.gov/clinpdq/soa/Male_breast_cancer_Physician.html
[Cervical Cancer—American Cancer Society]
http://www3.cancer.org/cancerinfo/load_cont.asp?ct=8
[Cervical Cancer—National Cancer Institute—CancerNet]
http://cancernet.nci.nih.gov/clinpdq/soa/Cervical_cancer_Physician.html
[Colorectal Cancer—American Cancer Society]
http://www3.cancer.org/cancerinfo/main_cont.asp?st=pr&ct=10
[Colon Cancer—National Cancer Institute—CancerNet]
http://cancernet.nci.nih.gov/clinpdq/soa/Colon_cancer_Physician.html
[Endometrial Cancer—American Cancer Society]
http://www3.cancer.org/cancerinfo/res_home.asp?st=wi&ct=11
[Endometrial Cancer—National Cancer Institute—Cancer—Net]
http://cancernet.nci.nih.gov/clinpdq/soa/Endometrial_cancer_Physician.html
[Esophageal Cancer—American Cancer Society
http://www3.cancer.org/cancerinfo/res_home.asp?st=wi&ct=12
[Esophageal Cancer—National Cancer Institute—CancerNet]
http://cancernet.nci.nih.gov/clinpdq/soa/Esophageal_cancer_Physician.html
[Laryngeal Cancer—American Cancer Society]
http://www3.cancer.org/cancerinfo/res_home.asp?st=wi&ct=23
[Laryngeal Cancer—National Cancer Institute—CancerNet]
http://cancernet.nci.nih.gov/clinpdq/soa/Laryngeal_cancer_Physician.html
[Adult Acute Lymphocytic Leukemia National Cancer Institute—CancerNet]
http://cancernet.nci.nih.gov/clinpdq/soa/Adult_acute_lymphocytic_leukemia Physician.html
[Adult Acute Myeloid Leukemia—National Cancer Institute—CancerNet]
http://cancernet.nci.nih.gov/clinpdq/soa/Adult_acute_myeloid_leukemia_Physician.html
[Chronic Lymphocytic Leukemia—National Cancer Institute—CancerNet]
http://cancernet.nci.nih.gov/clinpdq/soa/Chronic_lymphocytic_leukemia_Physician.html
[Chronic Myelogenous Leukemia—National Cancer Institute—CancerNet]
http://cancernet.nci.nih.gov/clinpdq/soa/Chronic_myelogenous_leukemia_Physician.html
[Liver Cancer—American Cancer Society]
http://www3.cancer.org/cancerinfo/res_home.asp?st=wi&ct=25
[Adult Primary Liver Cancer—National Cancer Institute—CancerNet]
http://cancernet.nci.nih.gov/clinpdq/soa/Adult_primary_liver_cancer_Physician.html
[Lung Cancer—American Cancer Society]
http://www3.cancer.org/cancerinfo/res_home.asp?st=wi&ct=26
[Non-Small Cell Lung Cancer—National Cancer Institute—CancerNet]
http://cancernet.nci.nih.gov/clinpdq/soa/Non-small_cell_lung_cancer_Physician.html
[Small Cell Lung Cancer—National Cancer Institute—CancerNet]
http://cancernet.nci.nih.gov/clinpdq/soa/Small_cell_lung_cancer_Physician.html
[Mesothelioma—American Cancer Society]
http://www3.cancer.org/cancerinfo/res_home.asp?st=wi&ct=29
[Malignant Mesothelioma—National Cancer Institute—CancerNet]
http://cancernet.nci.nih.gov/clinpdq/soa/Malignant_mesothelioma_Physician.html
[Osteosarcoma—American Cancer Society]
http://www3.cancer.org/cancerinfo/res_home.asp?st=wi&ct=52
[Osteosarcoma—National Cancer Institute—CancerNet]
http://cancernet.nci.nih.gov/clinpdq/soa/Osteosarcoma-malignant_fibrous_ histiocytoma_of_bone_Physician.html
[Ovarian Cancer—American Cancer Society]
http://www3.cancer.org/cancerinfo/res_home.asp?st=wi&ct=33
[Ovarian Epithelial Cancer—National Cancer Institute—CancerNet]
http://cancernet.nci.nih.gov/clinpdq/soa/Ovarian_epithelial_cancer_Physician.html
[Ovarian Germ Cell Tumor—National Cancer Institute—CancerNet]
http://cancernet.nci.nih.gov/clinpdq/soa/Ovarian_germ_cell_tumor_Physician.html
[Ovarian Low Malignant Potential Tumor—National Cancer Institute—CancerNet]
http://cancernet.nci.nih.gov/clinpdq/soa/Ovarian_low_malignant_potential_tumor_Physician.html
[Prostate Cancer—American Cancer Society]
http://www3.cancer.org/cancerinfo/res_home.asp?st=wi&ct=36
[Prostate Cancer—National Cancer Institute—CancerNet]
http://cancernet.nci.nih.gov/clinpdq/soa/Prostate_cancer_Physician.html
[Renal Cancer—American Cancer Society]
http://www3.cancer.org/cancerinfo/res_home.asp?st=wi&ct=22
[Renal Cell Cancer—National Cancer Institute—CancerNet]
http://cancernet.nci.nih.gov/clinpdq/soa/Renal_cell_cancer_Physician.html
[Salivary Gland Cancer—American Cancer Society]
http://www3.cancer.org/cancerinfo/res_home.asp?st=wi&ct=54
[Salivary Gland Cancer—National Cancer Institute—CancerNet]
http://cancernet.nci.nih.gov/clinpdq/soa/Salivary_gland_cancer_Physician.html
[Melanoma—National Cancer Institute—CancerNet]
http://cancernet.nci.nih.gov/clinpdq/soa/Melanoma_Physician.html
[Skin Cancer—American Academy of Dermatology]
http://www.aad.org/aadpamphrework/skincan.html
[Skin Cancer—National Cancer Institute—CancerNet]
http://cancernet.nci.nih.gov/clinpdq/soa/Skin_cancer_Physician.html
[Skin Cancer—American Academy of Dermatology]
http://www.aad.org/pamphlets/skincan.html
[Stomach Cancer—American Cancer Society]

http://www3.cancer.org/cancerinfo/res_home.asp?st=wi&ct=40

[Gastric Cancer—National Cancer Institute—CancerNet]
http://cancernet.nci.nih.gov/clinpdq/soa/Gastric_cancer_Physician.html

[Testicular Cancer—National Cancer Institute—CancerNet]
http://cancernet.nci.nih.gov/clinpdq/soa/Testicular_cancer_Physician.html

[Thyroid Cancer—National Cancer Institute—CancerNet]
http://cancernet.nci.nih.gov/clinpdq/soa/Thyroid_cancer_Physician.html

[Vaginal Cancer—National Cancer Institute—CancerNet]
http://cancernet.nci.nih.gov/clinpdq/soa/Vaginal_cancer_Physician.html

[Vulvar Cancer—National Cancer Institute—CancerNet]
http://cancernet.nci.nih.gov/clinpdq/soa/Vulvar_cancer_Physician.html

[Other Cancers—CancerNet]
http://cnetdb.nci.nih.gov/alphalist.html#ThePs

Care at the End of Life

5

See http://www.current-med.com/ch05.html for updated addresses of Web sites referenced in this chapter.

Michael W. Rabow, MD, Steven Z. Pantilat, MD, & Robert V. Brody, MD

THE END OF LIFE

DIAGNOSIS OF THE END OF LIFE

Eventually, everyone dies. In the United States, approximately 2.3 million people die each year. Despite all the successes of medical progress, death inevitably comes, and physicians battling to prolong life must recognize when life is ending in order to continue caring well for their patients. Unfortunately, end-of-life practices do not always meet the standards set by professional organizations. While death itself remains a mystery and while caring for the dying traditionally has not been well researched or adequately taught as part of medical training, caring for patients at the end of life is an important responsibility and a rewarding opportunity for physicians.

The terms "palliative care," "care of the dying," and "end-of-life care" imply a focus on care of the whole person who is approaching death rather than on an attempt to cure underlying disease. Since it emphasizes that the dying process is part of life, the expression "end-of-life care" is preferable and will be used here. From the medical perspective, the end of life may be defined as that time when death—whether due to terminal illness, acute or chronic illness, or age itself—is expected within weeks to months and can no longer be reasonably forestalled by medical intervention.

Physicians have an important role in helping patients understand that their lives are ending. This information influences patients' treatment decisions and changes how they may spend their remaining time. While certain diseases such as cancer are amenable to prognostic estimates regarding the time course to death, the other common causes of mortality in the United States—including heart disease, stroke, chronic lung disease, and dementia—have variable and difficult to predict prognoses. Even for patients with cancer, physician estimates of prognosis are often inaccurate. Nonetheless, clinical experience, epidemiologic data, guidelines from professional organizations,* and formal computer-based modeling and prediction tools† may be employed to help patients identify the end period of their lives. Recognizing that patients may have different levels of comfort with prognostic information, physicians can introduce the topic by simply saying, "I have information about the likely time course of your illness. Would you like to talk about it now?"

EXPECTATIONS ABOUT THE END OF LIFE

Patients' experiences of the end of life are influenced by their expectations about how they will die and the meaning of death. Many people fear how they will die more than death itself. Patients report fear of dying in pain or of suffocation, of loss of control, indignity, isolation, and being a burden to their families. All of these anxieties can be alleviated with good supportive care provided by an attentive group of caretakers.

For most of human history, death has been regarded as part of the natural process of life. However, with recent technologic advances that serve to forestall the end of life, death has become "medicalized." No longer seen clearly as a profound personal and spiritual event basic to the human condition, death is often regarded as a failure of medical science. The medicalization of death can create or heighten a sense of guilt about the failure to prevent dying. Both the general public and physicians are complicit in denying death, treating dying persons as patients and death as an enemy to be battled furiously in hospitals rather than as an inevitable outcome to be experi-

*For example, the National Hospice Organization.

†For example, the Acute Physiology and Chronic Health Evaluation (APACHE) system or the Study to Understand Prognoses and Preferences for Outcomes and Risks of Treatment (SUPPORT) model.

enced as a part of life at home. Currently in the United States, approximately 80% of people die in hospitals or long-term care facilities.

For most patients at the end of life, the physician should continue to pursue cure of potentially reversible disease, provide comfort, and in a sensitive way help the patient prepare for death. Patients at the end of life identify a number of elements as important to quality end-of-life care: adequate pain and symptom management; avoiding inappropriate prolongation of dying; achieving a sense of control; relieving the burden on others; and strengthening relationships with loved ones.

COMMUNICATION & THE ROLE OF THE PHYSICIAN AT THE END OF LIFE

Caring for patients at the end of life requires the same skills physicians employ in other tasks of doctoring: eliciting a complete history, examining for signs of physical disease, making careful diagnoses of treatable conditions, providing patient education, sharing in decision-making, and expressing understanding and caring. Communication skills are vitally important. In particular, physicians must become experts at delivering bad news and then dealing with its consequences (Table 5–1). Higher quality communication is associated with greater satisfaction and increased clinician knowledge of patient wishes.

Three further physician obligations are central to the physician's role at this time. First, physicians must work to identify, understand, and relieve patient suffering. Suffering is experienced by the person as a whole and may include physical, psychologic, social, or spiritual distress. Disease, disability, and disintegration at the end of life can threaten a person's sense of integrity or "intactness" and thereby cause suffering. In assisting with redirection and growth, providing support, assessing meaning, and fostering transcendence, physicians can help ameliorate their patients' suffering and help the patient and family live fully during this stage of life.

Second, physicians caring for patients at the end of life have an obligation to serve as a facilitator or catalyst for hope. While a particular outcome may be extremely unlikely (such as cure of advanced cancer following exhaustive conventional and experimental treatments), hope may be defined as the patient's belief in what is still possible. Although hope for a "miraculous cure" may be simplistic and even harmful, hope for relief of pain, for reconciliation with loved ones, for discovery of meaning in the life remaining, and for spiritual transformation is still quite supportable at the end of life. With questions such as "What is still possible for you?"—"What do you wish for before you die?"—"What good might come of this?" physicians can help patients uncover hope, explore meaningful and realistic goals, and develop strategies to realize them.

Third, patients' feelings of isolation and fear engendered by the prospect of dying demand that physicians communicate directly to patients that care will continue to be provided throughout the final stage of life. Perhaps the essential principle of care at the end of life is this promise of nonabandonment: a physician's pledge to an individual patient to serve as a caring partner, a resource for creative problem-solving and relief of suffering, a guide during uncertain times, and a witness to the patient's experiences—no matter what happens. Dying patients need their physicians to offer their presence—not necessarily the ability to solve all problems but rather a commitment to recognize and receive the patients' difficulties and experiences with respect and empathy. At its best, the patient-physician relationship can be a covenant of compassion and a recognition of common humanity.

Table 5–1. Suggestions for the delivery of bad news.

Prepare an appropriate place and time.
Address basic information needs.
Be direct; avoid jargon and euphemisms.
Allow for silence and emotional ventilation.
Assess and validate patient reactions.
Respond to immediate discomforts and risks.
Listen actively and express empathy.
Achieve a common perception of the problem.
Reassure about pain relief.
Ensure basic follow-up and make specific plans for the future.

CARING FOR THE FAMILY

In caring for patients at the end of life, physicians must appreciate the central role played by family, friends, and romantic partners and often must deal with strong emotions of fear, anger, shame, sadness, and guilt experienced by those individuals. While significant others may support and comfort a patient at the end of life, the threatened loss of a loved one may also create or reveal dysfunctional or painful family dynamics. Furthermore, physicians must be attuned to the potential impact of illness on the patient's family: substantial physical caregiving responsibilities and financial burdens as well as increased rates of anxiety, depression, chronic illness, and even mortality. Family caregivers commonly provide the bulk of care for patients at the end of life, yet their work is often not acknowledged or compensated.

Physicians can help families confront the imminent loss of a loved one (Table 5–2) and often must negotiate amid complex and changing family needs. Identifying a spokesperson for the family, conducting family meetings, allowing all to be heard, and providing time for consensus may help the physician work effectively with the family.

Table 5–2. Physician behaviors helpful to families of dying patients.[1]

Timely, frequent, and consistent communication
Adapting communication to need
Focusing on patient's wishes
Attending to the comfort of the patient
Being aware of family conflict
Accommodating family's grief
Refocusing hope
Encouraging planning
Remaining available
Following up with family after death

[1]Adapted, with permission, from Bascom PB, Tolle SW: Care of the family when the patient is dying. West J Med 1995;163:292.

THE LIMITS OF CARE AT THE END OF LIFE

Many physicians find caring for patients at the end of life to be one of the most rewarding aspects of practice. However, working with the dying requires tolerance of great uncertainty, ambiguity, and existential challenges. Physicians must recognize and respect their own limitations and attend to their own needs in order to avoid being overburdened, overly distressed, or emotionally depleted. Open recognition of their own feelings enables physicians to process their emotions and take steps to care for themselves: conferring and consulting with colleagues, retreating, relaxing and recuperating, obtaining informal or professional support, or even—under extraordinary circumstances—transferring the care of a patient to another physician when it is no longer possible to meet the patient's needs or comply with unreasonable requests. Moreover, care of patients at the end of life is not solely the responsibility of physicians. Ideally, physicians, nurses, social workers, psychologists, therapists (physical, occupational, recreational), dietitians, clergy, and volunteers can coordinate their efforts to care for patients and can support one another.

Physicians may be limited in caring for persons at the end of life not only by their emotional responses but by a sense of moral obligation as well. While the ethical, legal, and professional controversies over physician-assisted suicide are beyond the scope of this chapter, physicians should be aware of the growing "right to die" movement as an expression, at least in part, of patient dissatisfaction with how people are cared for at the end of life. In the United States, physician-assisted suicide is illegal in every state but Oregon—and legal there only with careful restrictions. While individual physicians must decide for themselves within the evolving legal context what their personal limits may be in caring for patients who request aid in dying (eg, physician-assisted suicide), all physicians can reclaim their long-privileged and universally accepted role of caring for the dying. They can do so by dedicating themselves not to abandon their patients and by providing appropriate attention to symptom management, sensitivity to psychologic and social stresses, and unconditional presence and openness to spiritual challenges at the end of life. Research has demonstrated that palliative care interventions can cause some patients who have requested physician-assisted suicide to withdraw their request.

Cassell EJ: Diagnosing suffering: a perspective. Ann Intern Med 1999;131:531. [NLM Cit ID: 99423361]

Emanuel EJ et al: Assistance from family members, friends, paid care givers, and volunteers in the care of terminally ill patients. N Engl J Med 1999;341:956. [NLM Cit ID: 99412079]

Fox E et al: Evaluation of prognostic criteria for determining hospice eligibility in patients with advanced lung, heart, or liver disease. JAMA 1999;282:1638. [NLM Cit ID: 20019218]

Ganzini L et al: Physicians experiences with the Oregon Death with Dignity Act. N Engl J Med 2000;342:557. [NLM Cit ID: 20132306]

Quill TE et al: Nonabandonment: A central obligation for physicians. Ann Intern Med 1995;122:368. [NLM Cit ID: 95150314]

Singer PA et al: Quality end-of-life care. JAMA 1999; 281:163. [NLM Cit ID: 99114158]

THE SETTING & STRUCTURE OF CARE

ETHICAL & LEGAL BACKGROUND

Physician care of patients at the end of life is guided by the same ethical and legal principles that inform other types of medical care. Foremost among these are the principles of truth-telling, nonmaleficence, beneficence, autonomy, proportionality, and distributive justice. These are the basic principles that must guide clinicians in helping patients make difficult decisions about care, including decisions about the withdrawal and withholding of support.

Three additional ethical considerations are relevant to care at the end of life. First, important ethical principles may be in conflict. For example, while a patient may desire a particular medical intervention, the physician may refuse to undertake the intervention if it is of no therapeutic benefit (ie, futile) or violates the physician's own moral code. In clinical practice, what constitutes a futile intervention is frequently a point of controversy. However, most disagreements can be resolved through repeated discussions between physicians and families.

Second, although physicians and family members often have very different emotional reactions to withholding versus withdrawing support, there is broad consensus among ethicists, supported by legal precedent, of their ethical equivalence. Patients have the same right to stop unwanted medical treatments once begun as they do to refuse those treatments in the first place, including artificial nutrition and hydration.

Third, the ethical principle of "double effect" argues that the potential to hasten imminent death is acceptable if it comes as the unintended consequence of a primary intention to provide comfort and relieve suffering. For example, sufficient doses of morphine should be provided to control pain even if there is the potential unintended secondary effect of depressing respiration. In practice, one can almost always find an effective pain regimen without hastening death.

ADVANCE DIRECTIVES

Well-informed, competent adults have a right to refuse medical intervention even if refusal is likely to result in death. Many people believe that there are fates worse than death and are willing to sacrifice some quantity of life in exchange for protecting a certain quality of life. In order to further patient autonomy, physicians are obligated to inform patients about the risks, benefits, alternatives, and expected outcomes of end-of-life medical interventions such as cardiopulmonary resuscitation, intubation and mechanical ventilation, vasopressor medication, hospitalization and ICU care, and artificial nutrition and hydration. Advance directives are oral or written statements made by patients when they are competent that are intended to guide care should they become incompetent. Advance directives allow patients to project their autonomy into the future to a time when they are incompetent. While oral statements about these matters are ethically binding, they are not legally binding in all states. Written advance directives are essential in order to give effect to the patient's wishes in these matters.

In addition to documenting patient preferences for care, the Durable Power of Attorney for Health Care (DPOA-HC) allows the patient to designate a surrogate decision-maker. The DPOA-HC is important since it is often difficult to anticipate what decisions will need to be made. The responsibility of the surrogate is to provide "substituted judgment"—to decide as the patient would, not as the surrogate wants. In the absence of an appropriate surrogate, physicians turn to family members or next of kin under the reasonable assumption that they know the patient's wishes. Unfortunately, surveys demonstrate that physicians and families often are no better than chance at predicting patient wishes, so it is imperative to have these discussions with all patients.

Physicians should educate all patients—ideally, well before the end of life—about the opportunity to formulate an advance directive. Research shows that most patients have already thought about end-of-life issues, want to discuss these issues with their physician, want the physician to bring up the subject, and feel better for having had the discussion. Chart reminders to physicians can increase the frequency of advance directive completions. It is especially important during discussions about end-of-life care that physicians reassure patients about the ability to control pain and other symptoms and make an explicit pledge not to abandon the patient. Despite regulations requiring physicians to inform patients of their rights to formulate an advance directive, only about 10% of people in the United States (including physicians) actually have executed advance directives, and studies have shown that physicians are often unaware of or actually ignore their patients' advance directives.

DNAR ORDERS

Physicians can encourage patients to express their preferences for the use of CPR. Unfortunately, most patients and many physicians are uninformed or misinformed about the nature and success of CPR. Despite the favorable portrayal of CPR in the popular media, only about 15% of all patients who undergo CPR in the hospital survive to hospital discharge. Moreover, among certain populations of patients—especially those with systemic noncardiac disease—the likelihood of survival to hospital discharge following CPR may be nil or extremely slight (Table 5–3).

Patients may ask their physician to write an order that CPR not be attempted on them. Although this order initially was referred to as a DNR ("do not resuscitate") order, many physicians now prefer the

Table 5–3. Survival to hospital discharge following cardiopulmonary resuscitation of patients with various underlying diseases.[1]

Conditions with highest survival rates:	
Ventricular fibrillation post-MI	26–46%
Drug reaction or overdose	22–28%
Ventricular arrhythmia	19–50%
Conditions with lowest survival rates:	
Malignancy[2]	0–3.5%
Neurologic disease	0–6.7%
Renal failure	0–10%
Respiratory disease	0–7%
Sepsis	0–7%
Nursing home residence	0–1.7%
Out-of-hospital cardiopulmonary arrest[3]	0.6%

[1]Modified, with permission, from Moss AH: Informing the patient about cardiopulmonary resuscitation: When the risks outweigh the benefits. J Gen Intern Med 1989;4:349.
[2]Survival was 0% in patients with metastatic disease in the first nine studies reported.
[3]If return of spontaneous circulation was not obtained after 25 minutes of standard advanced cardiac life support out-of-hospital.

term DNAR ("do not attempt resuscitation") to emphasize the low likelihood of successful resuscitation.

In addition to mortality statistics, patients deciding about CPR preferences should also be informed about the possible consequences of surviving a CPR attempt. CPR may result in fractured ribs, lacerated internal organs, and neurologic disability, and there is a high likelihood of requiring other aggressive interventions, such as ICU care, if CPR is successful.

For some patients at the end of life, decisions about CPR may be not about whether they will live or die but about how they will die. Physicians should correct the misconception that withholding CPR in appropriate circumstances is tantamount to "not doing everything" or "just letting someone die." Frequently, CPR will not improve the quality of a dying patient's life or alter the patient's underlying prognosis. While respecting the patient's right ultimately to make the decision—and keeping in mind their own biases and prejudices—physicians should offer explicit recommendations about DNAR orders and in that way protect dying patients and their families from feelings of guilt and from the sorrow associated with vain hopes. Finally, physicians should encourage patients and their families to make proactive decisions about what is wanted in end-of-life care rather than focusing only on what is not to be done.

HOSPICE CARE

While most patients die in hospitals and long-term care facilities, good care of the dying may not be the central goal of most hospitals and nursing homes. The hospice is a facility where the most urgent objective is to provide a caring environment for meeting the physical and emotional needs of the terminally ill. Hospice care focuses on the patient and family rather than the disease and on providing comfort and pain relief rather than on treating illness or prolonging life. Hospices provide intensive caring with the goal of helping people live well until they die.

The hospice philosophy emphasizes individualized attention, human contact, and an interdisciplinary team approach involving physicians, nurses, health aides, social workers, psychologists, therapists (physical, occupational, recreational), dietitians, chaplains, and volunteers. Hospice care can include arranging for respite for family caregivers and providing legal, financial, and other services. While some hospice care is provided in hospitals and institutional residences, about 80% of patients receiving hospice care remain at home where they can be cared for by the family and visiting hospice staff. Primary care physicians are strongly encouraged to continue caring for their patients during the time they are receiving hospice care.

Hospice care has been shown to increase patient satisfaction, to ease family anxiety, and even to reduce costs depending on when patients are referred to hospice care. While hospice care may be the appropriate standard of care for the dying, only about 15% of all patients who die receive hospice care, and 80% of these people have end-stage cancer. Hospice care tends to be utilized late in the course of the end of life. The average length of stay in hospices in the United States is just 36 days, with 15% of patients dying within 7 days after beginning hospice care.

Most hospice organizations require physicians to estimate the patient's probability of survival to be less than 6 months, since this is a criterion for eligibility to receive Medicare coverage (a benefit available since 1982). Unfortunately, as currently structured, the hospice benefit tends to be unavailable to people who are homeless, isolated, or with terminal prognoses that are difficult to quantify.

Many of the goals of hospice care, such as relief of suffering and attention to the patient as a person, are relevant to traditional medical care. However, the emphasis on patient well-being rather than on cure, the direct acknowledgment of death and dying issues, and the effort to care for people in their homes make hospice an important alternative to acute hospital care at the end of life. While the initiation of hospice care is often described as a transition from aggressive care to comfort care, hospice care too provides "aggressive" care, though not directed at achieving a cure. It is more appropriate to consider hospice care as one among many health care resources available to patients at the end of life. For the dying, it may be appropriate to "treat" pneumonia with morphine and antipyretics rather than with antibiotics. Helping patients decide when to avail themselves of the resources of hospice care is an important function even for physicians providing the most aggressive and intensive curative medical interventions.

CULTURAL ISSUES

The individual's experience of dying occurs in the context of a complex interaction of personal, philosophic, and cultural influences. Various religious, ethnic, gender, class, and cultural traditions inform patients' styles of communication, comfort in discussing particular topics, expectations about dying and medical interventions, and attitudes about the appropriate disposition of dead bodies. Studies have shown differences in knowledge and beliefs regarding advance directives, autopsy, organ donation, hospice care, and withdrawal of support among patients of different ethnic groups. While each patient must be considered an individual, understanding cultural assumptions and beliefs and respecting ethnic traditions are important responsibilities of the physician caring for a patient at the end of life, especially when the cultures of origin of the physician and patient differ.

[Five Wishes advance directive] http://www.comlab.fsu.edu/paul/index.htm

Council on Ethical and Judicial Affairs. Medical futility in end-of-life care. JAMA 1999;281:937. [NLM Cit ID: 99176378]

Dexter PR et al: Effectiveness of computer-generated reminders for increasing discussion about advance directives and completion of directive forms. Ann Intern Med 1998;128:102. [NLM Cit ID: 98085835] (Computer reminders increased discussion and completion of advance directives.)

Ebell MH et al: Survival after in-hospital cardiopulmonary resuscitation: a meta-analysis. J Gen Intern Med 1998;13:805. [NLM Cit ID: 99061867]

Johnston SC et al: Patient and physician roles in end-of-life decision making. J Gen Intern Med 1998;13:43. [NLM Cit ID: 98122326]

Mebane EW et al: The influence of physician race, age, and gender on physician attitudes toward advance care directives and preferences for end-of-life decision-making. J Am Geriatr Soc 1999;47:579. [NLM Cit ID: 99255252]

THE SPECIFIC TASKS OF CARING

SYMPTOM MANAGEMENT

For patients at the end of life, maximizing the quality of life—rather than postponing death—is the first priority of care. In this context, symptoms that cause disability and suffering must be considered medical emergencies and managed aggressively by frequent elicitation, continuous reassessment, and individualized treatment.

The relief of distressing symptoms at the end of life should not be withheld out of reluctance to use appropriate doses of opioids or sedatives. While physiologic dependence is expected with opioid use, at the end of life, the use of opioids for relief of pain and dyspnea is not associated with a risk of psychologic addiction and abuse (see Chapter 1). Furthermore, if properly informed, patients or their surrogates may decide to pursue aggressive symptom relief even if the treatments used inadvertently shorten life (ie, have a "double effect").

Pain

Pain is a common problem for patients at the end of life—up to 75% of patients dying of cancer experience pain—and is what many people say they fear most about dying. Pain may be a common complaint among patients with noncancer diagnoses as well. Pain is undertreated at the end of life. One study has documented that 50% of severely ill hospitalized patients spent half of their time during the last 3 days of life in moderate to severe pain.

The experience of pain also includes the patient's emotional reaction to it. Pain is subjective, and physicians cannot reliably detect or quantify pain without asking. A useful means of assessing pain and evaluating the effectiveness of analgesia is to ask the patient to rate the degree of pain along a numeric or visual pain scale (Table 5–4).

Recommendations for the use of analgesic, adjuvant, and nonpharmacologic pain management are reviewed in Chapter 1. The goal of pain management is most properly decided by the patient. While some patients may wish to be completely free of pain even if this entails significant sedation, most will wish to control pain at a level that still allows maximal functioning. Careful attention to pain relief and perseverance in achieving it is indicated for all patients. Hospice physicians regularly report a success rate higher than 90% in relieving pain in terminally ill patients. Chronic, severe pain, such as is often encountered at the end of life, should be treated around-the-clock.

There is no maximal allowable dose for opioid agonists such as morphine sulfate. The dose should be increased to whatever is necessary to relieve pain, remembering that certain types of pain (eg, neuropathic pain) may respond better to agents other than opioids. As dosages of opioids are increased, however, increasing difficulty with the three major side effects of opioids is to be expected. The management of constipation and nausea is outlined below. Sedation can be expected with opioids, though tolerance to the sedative effects of opioids may develop within 24–72 hours. Sedation typically appears well before significant respiratory depression. If treatment for sedation is desired, dextroamphetamine (2.5–7.5 mg orally every 6 hours) or methylphenidate (5–10 mg orally every 8–12 hours) may be given early in the day.

Dyspnea

Dyspnea is the subjective experience of difficulty in breathing and may be characterized by patients as tightness, shortness of breath, or a feeling of suffocation. Dyspnea is common among dying patients—up to one-half of severely ill patients may experience severe dyspnea.

Treatment of dyspnea is usually first directed at the underlying cause, which may be related to pneumonia, pulmonary embolism, pleural effusion, bronchospasm, tracheal obstruction, neuromuscular disease, restriction of movement of the chest or abdominal walls, cardiac ischemia, congestive heart failure, superior vena cava syndrome, or severe anemia.

At the end of life, dyspnea is often treated nonspecifically with opioids. Immediate-release morphine, preferably via the oral or buccal route, treats dyspnea effectively and typically at doses lower than would be necessary for the relief of moderate pain. Supplemental oxygen may be useful for the dyspneic patient who is hypoxic and may provide subjective benefit to other dyspneic patients as well. However, a nasal cannula and face mask are sometimes not well tolerated, and fresh air from a window or fan may

Table 5–4. Pain assessment scales.

A. Numeric Scale

No pain — Worst pain

1 2 3 4 5 6 7 8 9 10

B. Numeric Scale Translated into Word and Behavior Scales

Pain intensity	Word scale	Nonverbal behaviors
0	No pain	Relaxed, calm expression
1–2	Least pain	Stressed, tense expression
3–4	Mild pain	Guarded movement, grimacing
5–6	Moderate pain	Moaning, restless
7–8	Severe pain	Crying out
9–10	Excruciating pain	Increased intensity of above

C. Wong-Baker FACES Pain Rating Scale[1]

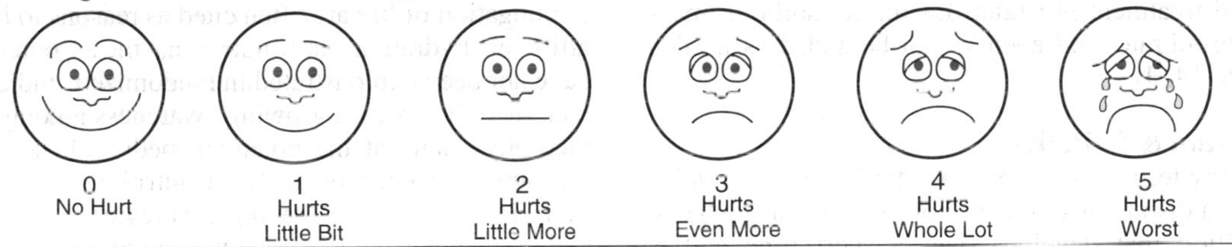

0	1	2	3	4	5
No Hurt	Hurts Little Bit	Hurts Little More	Hurts Even More	Hurts Whole Lot	Hurts Worst

[1]Especially useful for patients who cannot read English and for pediatric patients. Wong DL, Hockenberry-Eaton M, Wilson D, Winkelstein ML, Ahmann E, DeVito-Thomas PA: *Whaley and Wong's Nursing Care of Infants and Children*, ed. 6. St. Louis, 1999, Mosby p. 1153. Copyrighted by Mosby-Year Book, Inc. Reprinted by permission.

provide relief as well. Judicious use of nonpharmacologic relaxation techniques such as meditation and guided imagery may be beneficial for some patients. Anxiolytics may be useful for the anxiety associated with dyspnea but do not appear to act directly to relieve dyspnea

Nausea & Vomiting

Nausea and vomiting are common and distressing symptoms. As with pain, the management of nausea may be maximized by around-the-clock dosing. An understanding of the four major inputs to the vomiting center may help direct treatment. (See also Chapter 14.)

The chemoreceptor trigger zone may be stimulated by certain drugs (eg, morphine, NSAIDs), metabolic derangements, and chemotherapeutic agents. Vomiting associated with a particular opioid may be avoided by substitution with an equianalgesic dose of another opioid or a sustained-release formulation. In addition to the other dopamine antagonist antiemetics listed in Table 14–2 that block the trigger zone, haloperidol (0.5–5 mg orally every 4–6 hours) is commonly used.

Vomiting may be due to stimulation of peripheral afferent nerves. Offering patients small amounts of food only when they are hungry may prevent nausea and vomiting. Nasogastric suction may provide rapid relief for vomiting associated with constipation, gastroparesis, or gastric outlet obstruction, with the addition of laxatives, prokinetic agents (metoclopramide, 10–20 mg orally or intravenously four times a day; and high-dose corticosteroids as more definitive treatment. Treatment with high-dose corticosteroids (eg, dexamethasone, 20 mg orally or intravenously), ondansetron (8 mg orally three times daily), or cyclizine (5 mg orally every 8 hours) may be useful for nausea and vomiting due to disease of intra-abdominal or pelvic organs.

Increased intracranial pressure may cause vomiting and may be relieved with high-dose corticosteroids or palliative cranial radiation. Vomiting due to disturbance of the vestibular apparatus may be treated with anticholinergic and antihistaminic agents (see Table 14–2).

The beneficial effects of benzodiazepines for vomiting may derive mainly from their sedative and amnestic effects in the setting of anticipatory vomiting rather than as a primary antiemetic and should rarely be used alone for the relief of nausea. Many patients find dronabinol (2.5–20 mg orally every 4–6 hours) helpful in the management of nausea and vomiting as well.

discharge personal, professional, and business obligations. This might include completing important work or personal projects, distributing possessions, writing a will, and making funeral and burial arrangements.

The prospect of death often prompts patients to examine the quality of their interpersonal relationships, including their relationship with their physician. Dying may intensify the need for the patient to feel cared for by the doctor, highlighting the physician's obligation of nonabandonment and the need for physician empathy and compassion.

Concern about estranged relationships or "unfinished business" with significant others and interest in reconciliation may become paramount to people who are dying. At the end of life, even healthy interpersonal relationships must reach completion (Table 5–6).

Spiritual Challenges

Spirituality is the attempt to understand or accept the underlying meaning of life, one's relationships to oneself and other people, one's place in the universe, and the possibility of a "higher power" in the universe. Spirituality is distinguished from any particular religious practices or beliefs and is generally considered a universal human concern.

Perhaps because of an inappropriately exclusive attention to the biologic challenge of forestalling death or perhaps from feelings of discomfort or incompetence, physicians frequently ignore their patients' spiritual concerns or reflexively refer these important issues to psychiatrists or other caretakers (nurses, social workers, clergy).

However, the existential challenges of dying are central to the well-being of people at the end of life and are the proper concern of physicians. Within a biopsychosociospiritual model of medical care, physicians may work to provide more than simple physical comfort and control of bothersome symptoms. Physicians can help patients to die well by providing care to the whole person—by providing physical comfort and social support and by helping patients discover their own unique meaning in the world and an acceptance of death as a part of life.

Unlike physical ailments such as infections and fractures, which usually require a physician's intervention to be treated, the patient's spiritual concerns often require only a physician's attention, listening, and witness. Physicians should routinely inquire about the patient's spiritual concerns and ask whether the patient wishes to discuss them. For example, asking, "How are you within yourself?" communicates that the physician is interested in the patient's whole experience and provides an opportunity for the patient to share perceptions about his or her inner life. Questions that might constitute an existential "review of systems" are presented in Table 5–7.

Attending to the spiritual concerns of patients calls for listening carefully to their stories. Story-telling gives patients the opportunity to verbalize what is meaningful to them and to leave something of themselves behind—the promise of being remembered. Story-telling may be facilitated by suggesting that the patient share his or her life story with family members, record it on audio or video tape, assemble a photo album, organize a scrap book, or write an autobiography.

While dying may be a period of inevitable loss of physical functioning, the end of life also offers an opportunity for psychologic, interpersonal, and spiritual development. Individuals may grow—even achieve a heightened sense of well-being or transcendence—in the process of dying. Through listening, support, and presence, physicians may help foster this learning and be a catalyst for this transformation. Rather than thinking of dying simply as the termination of life, physicians and patients may be guided by a developmental model of dying that recognizes a series of lifelong developmental tasks and landmarks and allows for growth at the end of life.

American Thoracic Society: Dyspnea. Mechanisms, assessment, and management: a consensus statement. Am J Resp Crit Care Med 1999;159:321. [NLM Cit ID: 90991870]

Table 5–6. Five statements often necessary for the completion of important interpersonal relationships.[1]

(1) "Forgive me."	(An expression of regret)
(2) "I forgive you."	(An expression of acceptance)
(3) "Thank you."	(An expression of gratitude)
(4) "I love you."	(An expression of affection)
(5) "Good-bye."	(Leave-taking)

[1]Courtesy of Ira R. Byock, MD.

Table 5–7. An existential review of systems.

Intrapersonal
- How are you within yourself?[1]
- What does your illness/dying mean to you?
- What do you think caused your illness?
- How have you been healed in the past?
- What do you think is needed for you to be healed now?
- What is right with you now?
- What do you hope for?

Interpersonal
- Who is important to you?
- To whom does your illness/dying matter?
- Do you have any unfinished business with significant others?

Transpersonal
- What is your source of strength, help, or hope?
- Do you have spiritual concerns or a spiritual practice?
- If so, how does your spirituality relate to your illness/dying and how can I help integrate your spirituality into your health care?[1]
- What do you think happens after we die?
- What purpose might your illness/dying serve?
- What do you think is trying to happen here?[1]

[1]Courtesy of IR Byock, MD, DB Larson, MD, and AL Suchman., MD.

Brody H et al: Withdrawing intensive life-sustaining treatment: Recommendations for compassionate clinical management. N Engl J Med 1997;336:652. [NLM Cit ID: 97170831]

Ehman JW et al: Do patients want physicians to inquire about their spiritual or religious beliefs if they become gravely ill? Arch Intern Med 1999;159:1803. [NLM Cit ID: 99376015]

Finucane TE et al: Tube feeding in patients with advanced dementia: a review of the evidence. JAMA 1999;282: 1365. [NLM Cit ID: 99454308]

Prendergast TJ et al: A national survey of end-of-life care for critically ill patients. Am J Respir Crit Care Med 1998;158:1163. [NLM Cit ID: 98443311]

TASKS AFTER DEATH

After the death of a patient, the physician is called upon to perform a number of tasks, both required and recommended. The physician must plainly and directly inform the family of the death. Providing words of sympathy and reassurance, time for questions and initial grief, and a quiet private room for the family at this time are appropriate and much appreciated.

THE PRONOUNCEMENT & DEATH CERTIFICATE

In most states of the USA, physicians are legally required to confirm the death of a patient in a formal process called "pronouncement." The physician must verify the absence of spontaneous respirations and cardiac activity and the presence of fixed and dilated pupils. A note describing these findings and the time of death is entered in the patient's chart.

While the pronouncement may often seem like an awkward and unnecessary formality, physicians may use this time to reassure the patient's loved ones at the bedside that the patient died peacefully and that all appropriate care had been given. Both physicians and families may use the ritual of the pronouncement as an opportunity to process emotionally the death of the patient.

Accurately reporting the underlying cause of death on the death certificate is also legally required and important both for patients and their families (for insurance purposes and the need for an accurate family medical history) and for the epidemiologic study of disease and public health. Unfortunately, recent research has shown that physicians are untrained in and unskilled at correctly completing death certificates. The physician should be specific about the major cause of death (eg, "decompensated cirrhosis") and its contributory cause (eg, "hepatitis B and hepatitis C infections and chronic alcoholic hepatitis") as well as any associated conditions (eg, "acute renal failure")—and not simply put down "cardiac arrest" as the cause of death.

AUTOPSY & ORGAN DONATION

Discussing the options and obtaining consent for autopsy and organ donation with patients themselves prior to death is usually the best practice. This advances the principle of patient autonomy and lessens the responsibilities of distressed family members during the period immediately following the death of their loved one. Recent research demonstrates that after a patient dies, however, designated requestors are more successful than the treating physicians at obtaining consent for organ donation from surviving family members. Federal regulations now require that a designated representative of an organ procurement organization approach the family about organ donation. Most people in the United States support the donation of organs for transplants. Currently, however, organ transplantation is severely limited by the availability of donor organs. Many potential donors and the families of actual donors experience a sense of reward in contributing, even through death, to the lives of others.

Physicians must be sensitive to ethnic and cultural differences in attitudes about autopsy and organ donation. Patients or their families should be reminded of their right to limit autopsy or organ donation in any way they choose. Pathologists can perform autopsies without interfering with funeral plans or the appearance of the deceased.

The results of an autopsy may help surviving family members (and physicians) understand the exact cause of a patient's death and foster a sense of closure. A physician-family conference to review the results of the autopsy provides a good opportunity for physicians to assess how well families are grieving and to answer questions. Unfortunately, despite the advantages of conducting postmortem examinations, autopsy rates have fallen drastically to less than 15% today. Families report refusing autopsies out of fear of disfigurement of the body or delay of the funeral—or say they were simply not asked. They report allowing autopsies in order to advance medical knowledge, to identify the exact cause of their loved one's death, and to be reassured that appropriate care was given. Routinely addressing these issues when discussing autopsy may help increase the autopsy rate.

FOLLOW-UP & GRIEVING

Proper care of patients at the end of life includes following up with surviving family members after the patient has died. Following up enables the physician

Table 6–1. Useful topical dermatologic therapeutic agents.

	Formulations, Strengths, and Prices[1]	Apply	Potency Class	Common Indications	Comments
Corticosteroids Hydrocortisone acetate	Cream 1%: $3.22/30 g Ointment 1%: $3.34/30 g Lotion 1%: $15.31/120 mL	bid	Low	Seborrheic dermatitis. Pruritus ani. Intertrigo.	Not the same as hydrocortisone butyrate or valerate! Not for poison oak! OTC lotion (Aquinil HC). OTC solution (Scalpicin, T Scalp).
	Cream 2.5%: $8.84/30 g Ointment 2.5%: $8.84/30 g Lotion 2.5%: $29.68/60 mL	bid	Low	As for 1% hydrocortisone.	Perhaps better for pruritus ani. Not clearly better than 1%. More expensive. Not OTC.
Alclometasone dipropionate (Aclovate)	Cream 0.05%: $15.10/15 g Ointment 0.05%: $31.48/45 g	bid	Low	As for hydrocortisone.	More efficacious than hydrocortisone. Perhaps causes less atrophy.
Desonide	Cream 0.05%: $17.19/15 g Ointment 0.05%: $44.31/60 g Lotion 0.05%: $29.13/60 mL	bid	Low	As for hydrocortisone. For lesions on face or body folds resistant to hydrocortisone.	More efficacious than hydrocortisone. Can cause rosacea or atrophy. Not fluorinated.
Prednicarbate (Dermatop)	Emollient cream 0.1%: $15.42/15 g	bid	Medium	As for triamcinolone.	May cause less atrophy. No generic formulations. Preservative-free.
Triamcinolone acetonide	Cream 0.1%: $2.09/15 g Ointment 0.1%: $2.12/15 g Lotion 0.1%: $9.95/60 mL	bid	Medium	Eczema on extensor areas. Used for psoriasis with tar. Seborrheic dermatitis and psoriasis on scalp.	Caution in body folds, face. Economical in 0.5 lb and 1 lb sizes for treatment of large body surfaces. Economical as solution for scalp.
	Cream 0.025%: $1.82/15 g Ointment 0.025%: $1.52/15 g	bid	Medium	As for 0.1% strength.	Possibly less efficacy and few advantages over 0.1% formulation.
Fluocinolone acetonide	Cream 0.025%: $3.05/15 g Ointment 0.025%: $4.20/15 g	bid	Medium	As for triamcinolone.	
	Solution 0.01%: $10.80/60 mL	bid	Medium	As for triamcinolone solution.	
Mometasone furoate (Elocon)	Cream 0.1%: $20.03/15 g Ointment 0.1%: $20.03/15 g Lotion 0.1%: $41.45/60 mL	qd	Medium	As for triamcinolone.	Often used inappropriately on the face or in children. Not fluorinated.
Diflorasone diacetate (Florone, Maxiflor)	Cream 0.05%: $34.49/15 g Ointment 0.05%: $35.88/30 g	bid	High	Nummular dermatitis. Allergic contact dermatitis. Lichen simplex chronicus.	Only ultrapotent steroid that can be occluded (but with caution and not with gloves on the hands).
Amcinonide (Cyclocort)	Cream 0.1%: $18.13/15 g Ointment 0.1%: $18.13/15 g	bid	High	As for betamethasone.	
Fluocinonide	Cream 0.05%: $8.64/15 g Gel 0.05%: $12.00/15 g Ointment 0.05%: $17.92/15 g Solution 0.05%: $24.00/60 mL	bid	High	As for betamethasone. Gel useful for poison oak.	Economical generics. Lidex cream can cause stinging on eczema. Lidex emollient cream preferred.
Betamethasone dipropionate	Cream 0.05%: $5.57/15 g Ointment 0.05%: $5.57/15 g Lotion 0.05%: $14.23/60 mL	bid	Ultra-high	For lesions resistant to medium-potency steroids. Lichen planus. Insect bites.	Economical generics available.

(continued)

Table 6–1. Useful topical dermatologic therapeutic agents. (continued)

	Formulations, Strengths, and Prices[1]	Apply	Potency Class	Common Indications	Comments
Clobetasol propionate	Cream 0.05%: $19.92/15 g Ointment 0.05%: $19.92/15 g Lotion 0.05%: $47.54/50 mL	bid	Ultra-high	As for diflorasone.	Somewhat more potent than diflorasone. Limited to 2 continuous weeks of use. Limited to 50 g or less per week. Cream may cause stinging; use "emollient cream" formulation.
Halobetasol propionate (Ultravate)	Cream 0.05%: $27.25/15 g Ointment 0.05%: $27.25/15 g	bid	Ultra-high	As for clobetasol.	Marginally more effective than clobetasol in psoriasis. Same restrictions as clobetasol. Cream does not cause stinging.
Flurandrenolide (Cordran)	Tape: $33.04/large roll	q12h	Ultra-high	Lichen simplex chronicus.	Protects the skin and prevents scratching.
Antibiotics (for acne)					
Clindamycin phosphate	Solution 1%: $10.51/30 mL Gel 1%: $30.76/30 mL Lotion 1%: $42.80/60 mL Pledget 1%: $40.56/60	bid	N/A	Mild papular acne.	Lotion is less drying for patients with sensitive skin.
Erythromycin	Solution 2%: $7.04/60 mL Gel 2%: $19.73/30 g Pledget 2%: $21.31/60	bid	N/A	As for clindamycin.	Many different manufacturers. Economical.
Erythromycin/Benzoyl Peroxide (Benzamycin)	Gel $42.52/23.3 g Gel $81.16/46.6 g	bid	N/A	As for clindamycin. Can help treat comedonal acne.	No generics. More expensive. More effective than other topical antibiotics. Main jar requires refrigeration.
Antibiotics (for impetigo)					
Mupirocin (Bactroban)	Ointment 2%: $21.85/15 g	tid	N/A	Impetigo, folliculitis.	Stop after 10 days to prevent emergence of resistance. Used in the nose twice daily for 5 days to reduce staphylococcal carriage.
Antifungals					
Clotrimazole	Cream 1%: $13.20/15 g Solution 1%: $24.20/30 mL	bid	N/A	Dermatophyte and *Candida* infections.	Available OTC. Inexpensive generic cream available.
Miconazole	Cream 2%: $3.20/30 g	bid	N/A	As for clotrimazole.	As for clotrimazole.
Other imidazoles					
Econazole (Spectazole)	Cream 1%: $14.64/15 g	qd	N/A	As for clotrimazole.	No generic. Somewhat more effective than clotrimazole and miconazole.
Ketoconazole	Cream 2%: $17.44/15 g	qd	N/A	As for clotrimazole.	No generic. Somewhat more effective than clotrimazole and miconazole.
Oxiconazole (Oxistat)	Cream 1%: $17.08/15 g Lotion 1%: $26.84/30 mL	bid	N/A		
Sulconazole (Exelderm)	Cream 1%: $11.51/15 g Solution 1%: $24.77/30 mL	bid	N/A	As for clotrimazole.	No generic. Somewhat more effective than clotrimazole and miconazole.
Other antifungals					
Butenafine (Mentax)	Cream 1%: $29.56/15 g	qd	N/A	Dermatophytes	Fast response; high cure rate; expensive.
Ciclopirox (Loprox)	Cream 0.77%: $23.31/30 g Lotion 0.77%: $48.83/60 mL	bid	N/A	As for clotrimazole.	No generic. Somewhat more effective than clotrimazole and miconazole.

(*continued*)

Table 6–1. Useful topical dermatologic therapeutic agents. (continued)

	Formulations, Strengths, and Prices[1]	Apply	Potency Class	Common Indications	Comments
Naftifine (Naftin)	Cream 1%: $36.65/30 g Gel 1%: $57.82/60 mL	qd	N/A	Dermatophytes. Not FDA-approved for *Candida* but probably effective.	No generic. Somewhat more effective than clotrimazole and miconazole.
Terbinafine (Lamisil)	Cream 1%: $32.61/15 g	qd	N/A	For dermatophytes.	Fast clinical response. OTC.
Antipruritics					
Camphor/menthol	Compounded lotion (0.5% of each)	bid–tid	N/A	For mild eczema, xerosis, mild contact dermatitis.	
Pramoxine hydrochloride (Tronothane)	Cream 1%: $10.80/30 g	qid	N/A	As a cream for patients with dry skin, varicella, mild eczema, pruritus ani.	OTC formulations (Aveeno Anti-Itch Cream or Lotion; Itch-X Gel; Tronolane Cream for hemorrhoids). By prescription mixed with 1% or 2% hydrocortisone.
Doxepin (Zonalon)	Cream 5%: $23.57/30 g	qid	N/A	Topical antipruritic, best used in combination with appropriate topical steroid to enhance efficacy.	Can cause sedation.
Emollients					
Aveeno	Cream: $2.40/30 g Lotion: $5.40/120 mL	qd–tid	N/A	Xerosis, eczema.	Choice is most often based on personal preference by patient.
Aqua glycolic	Cream: $10.63/60 g, Lotion: $10.63/240 mL Shampoo: $5.63/240 mL	qd–tid	N/A	Xerosis. Ichthyosis, keratosis pilaris. Mild facial wrinkles. Mild acne or seborrheic dermatitis.	Contains 8% glycolic acid. Available from other makers, eg, Alpha Hydrox, or generic 8% glycolic acid lotion. May cause stinging on eczematous skin.
Aquaphor	Ointment: $13.20/454 g	qd–tid	N/A	Xerosis. Eczema. For protection of area in pruritus ani.	Not as greasy as petrolatum.
Complex 15	Lotion: $6.48/240 mL Cream: $4.82/75 g	qd–tid	N/A	Xerosis. Lotion or cream recommended for split or dry nails.	Active ingredient is a phospholipid.
DML	Cream, lotion, facial moisturizer	qd–tid	N/A	As for Complex 15.	Face cream has sunscreen.
Dermasil	Lotion, cream	qd–tid	N/A	Xerosis, eczema.	
Eucerin	Cream: $5.10/120 g Lotion: $5.10/240 mL	qd–tid	N/A	Xerosis, eczema.	Many formulations made. Eucerin Plus contains alphahydroxy acid and may cause stinging on eczematous skin. Facial moisturizer has SPF 25 sunscreen.
Lac-Hydrin	Lotion: $31.91/225 mL	bid	N/A	Xerosis, ichthyosis, keratosis pilaris.	Expensive, not OTC. May protect against corticosteroid-induced atrophy.
Lubriderm	Lotion: $5.28/300 mL	qd–tid	N/A	Xerosis, eczema.	Unscented usually preferred.
Neutrogena	Cream, lotion, facial moisturizer: $7.39/240 mL	qd–tid	N/A	Xerosis, eczema.	Face cream has titanium-based sunscreen.

[1]Cost to pharmacist (average wholesale price, generic when possible) for quantity listed. Source: *Drug Topics Red Book,* March 2000; Vol. 19, No. 3.

of specific dermatologic entities to follow; however, some basic principles of topical steroid therapy should be mentioned here. Topical steroids are divided into classes based on their potency. There is little (except price) to recommend one agent over another within the same class. For a given agent, an ointment is more potent than a cream because of its greater absorption; however, ointments are generally more greasy. The potency of a topical steroid may be dramatically increased by applying an occlusive dressing after application of the steroid. Such dressings may include gloves, plastic wrap, or plastic occlusive suits for patients with generalized erythroderma or atopy. Caution should be used in applying topical steroids to areas of thin skin (face, scrotum, vulva, skin folds). For patients using steroids on their eyelids, treatment should be limited to avoid the risk of glaucoma or cataracts. One may estimate the amount of topical steroid needed by using the "rule of nines" (as in burn evaluation; see Figure 38–4). In general, it takes an average of 20–30 g to cover the body surface of an adult once. Systemic absorption does occur, but adrenal suppression, diabetes, hypertension, osteoporosis, and other complications of systemic steroids are very rare with topical steroid therapy.

2. Emollients for dry skin ("moisturizers")– Many types of emollients are available. Petrolatum, mineral oil, Aquaphor, and Eucerin cream are the heaviest and best for very dry skin. Emollients are most effective when applied to wet skin immediately after a bath to trap the moisture. They should be applied with the "grain" of the hairs rather than by rubbing up and down to avoid folliculitis. If the skin is too greasy after application, pat dry again with the damp towel.

In some cases, lotions may be useful and are not as greasy as the creams and ointments listed above. The appearance of dry skin and ichthyosis may be improved by lactic acid products (Lac-Hydrin, Ulactin) or glycolic acid-containing lotions (Aquaglycolic) provided no inflammation (erythema) is present.

3. Drying agents for weepy dermatoses–If the skin is weepy from infection or inflammation, drying agents may afford relief. The best drying agent is water, and repeated compresses, with or without such agents as aluminum salts (Burow's solution, Domeboro tablets) or colloidal oatmeal (Aveeno) are a good first step. Shake lotions (eg, starch or calamine lotions) and powders (especially if the process is acute) may result in messy crusts and are seldom used by dermatologists.

4. Topical antipruritics–Lotions that contain 0.5% each of camphor and menthol (Sarna) are effective for mild pruritic dermatoses. Pramoxine hydrochloride, 1% cream or lotion, or pramoxine hydrochloride, 1%, with 0.5% menthol, as a surface anesthetic may be an effective antipruritic agent (Prax, PrameGel, Aveeno Anti-Itch lotion). Hydrocortisone, 1% or 2.5%, may be incorporated for its anti-inflammatory effect (Pramosone cream, lotion, or ointment). Doxepin cream 5% may reduce pruritus due to eczematous dermatoses. It appears most effective when applied together with a topical steroid of the appropriate class for the condition or site being treated. Like pramoxine, it is a steroid enhancer, improving response to a given strength of topical steroid. Drowsiness and dry mouth may occur. Monoamine oxidase inhibitors should be discontinued at least 2 weeks before treatment.

5. Systemic antipruritic drugs–

a. Antihistamines–H_1 blockers are the agents of choice for pruritus when due to histamine, such as in urticaria. Otherwise, they appear to relieve pruritus only by their sedating and not their antihistamine effects. Thus, less sedating antihistamines may be less effective in non-histamine-related pruritus. It should also be noted that though more expensive, the newer "nonsedating" antihistamines do not appear to be more potent than older, cheaper medications (ie, diphenhydramine). Except in the case of urticaria, nonsedating antihistamines are of little or no value in inflammatory skin diseases such as atopic dermatitis and are rarely indicated.

Traditional H_1 antihistamines are usually grouped into six classes (Table 19–1). Alkylamines (chlorpheniramine and dexchlorpheniramine) are the least sedating. Ethanolamines (diphenhydramine) are very sedating, as are phenothiazines (promethazine). Piperidines (cyproheptadine), piperazines (hydroxyzine), and ethylenediamines (tripelennamine) cause less sedation. The least sedating antihistamines are loratadine and famotidine. Cetirizine is also relatively nonsedating. Some tricyclic antidepressants, such as doxepin, have potent antihistaminic activity and are useful in urticaria and other forms of pruritus.

b. Systemic corticosteroids–(See Chapter 26.)

Greaves MW: Anti-itch treatments: Do they work? Skin Pharmacol 1997;10:225. [NLM Cit ID: 98110740]

Millikan LE: Treating pruritus: What's new in safe relief of symptoms? Postgrad Med 1996;99:173. [NLM Cit ID: 96133831]

Zuckerman E et al: Naloxone for intractable pruritus? (Letter.) Am J Gastroenterol 1997;92:183. [NLM Cit ID: 97149170]

Sunscreens

Protection from ultraviolet light should begin at birth but will reduce the incidence of actinic keratoses and some nonmelanoma skin cancers when initiated at any age. The best protection is shelter, but protective clothing, avoidance of direct sun exposure during the peak hours of the day, and the assiduous use of chemical sunscreens are important. Estimates are that if fair children were to use such sunscreens regularly, their lifetime incidence of skin cancer might be reduced by 75%.

A number of highly effective sunscreens are available in cream, lotion, and nongreasy gel and liquid formulations. Fair-complexioned persons should use a sunscreen with an SPF (sun protective factor) of at least 15 and preferably 30–40. For those who are sensitive to PABA (*p*-aminobenzoic acid), PABA-free formulations are available. Sunscreens with high SPF values (> 30) afford some protection against UVA as well as UVB light exposure and may be helpful in managing photosensitivity disorders. Many facial moisturizers contain a SPF 15–25 sunscreen in a nongreasy base suitable for daily use.

Physical blockers (titanium dioxide and zinc oxide [Blue Lizard]) are available in new vanishing formulations (Ti-Baby Natural, Ti Screen Natural, Neutrogena Chemical-Free Sun Blocker).

Cummings SR et al: Approaches to the prevention and control of skin cancer. Cancer Metastasis Rev 1997;16:309. [NLM Cit ID: 98095440] (Comprehensive review of pharmacologic and behavioral steps for primary and secondary prevention of skin cancer.)

Green AA et al: Daily sunscreen application and beta-carotene supplementation in prevention of basal-cell and squamous-cell carcinomas of the skin: a randomised controlled trial. Lancet 1999;354:723.

Naylor MF et al: The case for sunscreens: A review of their use in preventing actinic damage and neoplasia. Arch Dermatol 1997;133:1146. [NLM Cit ID: 97447142] (Review of literature discussing efficacy of sunscreen.)

Complications of Topical Dermatologic Therapy

Complications of topical therapy can be largely avoided. They fall into several categories:

A. Allergy: Of the topical antibiotics, neomycin has the greatest potential for sensitization. Diphenhydramine, benzocaine, and ethylenediamine are potential sensitizers in topical medications. Preservatives and even the topical steroids themselves can cause allergic contact dermatitis.

B. Irritation: Preparations of retinoic acid, benzoyl peroxide, and other acne medications should be applied sparingly to the skin when it is dry. Repeated use of lindane (Kwell, etc) and antiseptic soaps can be irritating. Podophyllum resin can be very irritating. Sunscreens may cause irritation or an acne-like eruption.

C. Absorption: Drugs may be absorbed through the skin, especially near mucous membranes, through broken or inflamed skin, or from under occlusive dressings. On average, the systemic dose absorbed by children is three times that of adults. The possibility of systemic absorption has special implications for pregnant women or women who may become pregnant while using the topical medication. A few notable examples of topical drugs that may be harmful to a fetus include podophyllum resin, lindane, and tretinoin (Retin-A). In most cases, substitutes are available (eg, permethrin or precipitated sulfur may be substituted for lindane). In general it is always prudent to consult a pharmacology textbook or pharmacist when prescribing medications for pregnant or nursing women. Agents containing phenol are contraindicated on open skin or mucous membranes of neonates.

D. Overuse: Fluorinated topical corticosteroids may induce acne-like lesions on the face (steroid rosacea) and atrophic striae in body folds.

Journe F et al: Sunscreen sensitization: a 5-year study. Acta Dermato-Venereologica 1999;79:211. [NLM Cit ID: 99311645] (A review of allergic reactions to sunscreen.)

Lutz ME et al: Allergic contact dermatitis due to topical application of corticosteroids: Review and clinical implications. Mayo Clinic Proc 1997;72:1141. [NLM Cit ID: 98075215]

I. COMMON DERMATOSES

Dermatologic diseases will be classified and discussed here, when possible, according to the types of lesions they cause. Therefore, in order to make a diagnosis, it is best to (1) focus on the type of individual lesion the patient exhibits; (2) choose the morphologic category the lesions seem to fit; and then (3) identify the specific features of the history, physical examination, and laboratory tests that will establish the working diagnosis.

The major morphologic types of skin lesion are listed in Table 6–2 along with the disorders with which they are most prominently associated. Miscellaneous skin, hair, and nail disorders and drug eruptions are discussed at the end of the chapter.

PIGMENTED LESIONS

Malignant melanoma accounts for the greatest number of deaths due to skin disease, and such deaths might be prevented by early diagnosis followed by excision. The nondermatologist physician must be able to evaluate pigmented lesions and appropriately refer for evaluation all potential malignant melanomas. In order to avoid missing some malignant melanomas, it is understood that many patients will be referred for what ultimately prove to be benign lesions.

In general, a **benign mole** is a small (< 5 mm), well-circumscribed lesion with a well-defined border and a

Table 6–2. Morphologic categorization of skin lesions and diseases.

Pigmented	Freckle, lentigo, seborrheic keratosis, nevus, blue nevus, halo nevus, dysplastic nevus, melanoma
Scaly	Psoriasis, dermatitis (atopic, stasis, seborrheic, chronic allergic contact or irritant contact), xerosis (dry skin), lichen simplex chronicus, tinea, tinea versicolor, secondary syphilis, pityriasis rosea, discoid lupus erythematosus, exfoliative dermatitis, actinic keratoses, Bowen's disease, Paget's disease, intertrigo
Vesicular	Herpes simplex, varicella, herpes zoster, dyshidrosis (vesicular dermatitis of palms and soles), vesicular tinea, dermatophytid, dermatitis herpetiformis, miliaria, scabies, photosensitivity
Weepy or encrusted	Impetigo, acute contact allergic dermatitis, any vesicular dermatitis
Pustular	Acne vulgaris, acne rosacea, folliculitis, candidiasis, miliaria, any vesicular dermatitis
Figurate (-shaped) erythema	Urticaria, erythema multiforme, erythema migrans, cellulitis, erysipelas, erysipeloid, arthropod bites
Bullous	Impetigo, blistering dactylitis, pemphigus, pemphigoid, porphyria cutanea tarda, drug eruptions, erythema multiforme, toxic epidermal necrolysis
Papular	Hyperkeratotic: warts, corns, seborrheic keratoses Purple-violet: lichen planus, drug eruptions, Kaposi's sarcoma Flesh-colored, umbilicated: molluscum contagiosum Pearly: basal cell carcinoma, intradermal nevi Small, red, inflammatory: acne, miliaria, candidiasis, scabies, folliculitis
Pruritus[1]	Xerosis, scabies, pediculosis, bites, systemic causes, anogenital pruritus
Nodular, cystic	Erythema nodosum, furuncle, cystic acne, follicular (epidermal) inclusion cyst
Photodermatitis (photodistributed rashes)	Drug, polymorphic light eruption, lupus erythematosus
Morbilliform	Drug, viral infection, secondary syphilis
Erosive	Any vesicular dermatitis, impetigo, aphthae, lichen planus, erythema multiforme
Ulcerated	Decubiti, herpes simplex, skin cancers, parasitic infections, syphilis (chancre), chancroid, vasculitis, stasis, arterial disease

[1]Not a morphologic class but included because it is one of the most common dermatologic presentations.

single shade of pigment from beige or pink to dark brown. Most or all of the individual patient's moles often are similar to each other with respect to size and color, or there may be two or three different types of moles on the same patient. The physical examination must take precedence over the history, though a reliable history that a lesion has been present without change for decades is obviously a comfort.

Suspicious moles have an irregular and asymmetric or fuzzy border where the pigment appears to be leaking into the normal surrounding skin; the topography may be irregular, ie, partly raised and partly flat. Color variegation is disturbing, and colors such as pink, blue, gray, white, and black are indications for referral. The American Cancer Society has proposed the mnemonic "ABCD = Asymmetry, Border irregularity, Color variegation, and Diameter greater than 6 mm." Bleeding and ulceration are ominous signs. A mole that stands out from the patient's other moles deserves special scrutiny. A patient with a large number of moles is statistically at increased risk for melanoma and deserves careful and periodic examination, particularly if the lesions are atypical.

The history of a changing mole (evolution) is the single most important historical reason for close evaluation and possible referral. Referral of suspicious pigmented lesions is always appropriate.

Moles have their own natural history. In the first decade of life, moles often appear as flat, small, brown lesions. They are called **junctional nevi** because the nevus cells are at the junction of the epidermis and dermis. Over the next 2 decades, these moles grow in size and often become raised, reflecting the appearance of a dermal component, giving rise to **compound nevi.** Moles may darken and grow during pregnancy. As Caucasian patients enter their seventh and eighth decades, most moles have lost their junctional component and dark pigmentation and undergo fibrosis or other degenerative changes. Still, at every stage of life, normal moles should be well-demarcated, symmetric, and uniform in contour and color.

Grob JJ et al: The "ugly duckling" sign. Arch Dermatol 1998;134:103. [NLM Cit ID: 98111574] (A mole that stands out or looks different than others should be carefully evaluated.)

prognostic factors for persistence into adulthood in atopic dermatitis include onset early in childhood, early generalized disease, and asthma. Only 40–60% of these patients have lasting remissions.

Berberian BJ et al: The addition of topical doxepin to corticosteroid therapy: an improved treatment regimen for atopic dermatitis. Int J Dermatol 1999;38:145. [NLM Cit ID: 99206387]

Hanifin JM et al: Update on therapy of atopic dermatitis. J Allergy Clin Immunol 1999;104(3 Part 2):S123. [NLM Cit ID: 99414190]

Landow K: Hand dermatitis: The perennial scourge. Postgrad Med 1998;103:141, 145, 151. [NLM Cit ID: 98110130]

Leung DY et al: Allergic and immunologic skin disorders. JAMA 1997;278:1914. [NLM Cit ID: 98057360] (Immunologic pathophysiology of eczema.)

LICHEN SIMPLEX CHRONICUS (Circumscribed Neurodermatitis)

Essentials of Diagnosis

- Chronic itching.
- Lichenified lesions with exaggerated skin lines overlying a thickened, well-circumscribed scaly plaque.
- Predilection for nape of neck, wrists, external surfaces of forearms, lower legs, popliteal and antecubital areas.

General Considerations

A traditional explanation for lichen simplex chronicus (circumscribed neurodermatitis) is that it represents a self-perpetuating scratch-itch cycle.

Clinical Findings

Intermittent itching incites the patient to scratch the lesions. Itching may be so intense as to interfere with sleep. Dry, leathery, hypertrophic, lichenified plaques appear on the neck, wrists, perineum, or almost anywhere. The patches are rectangular, thickened, and pigmented. The skin lines are exaggerated and divide the lesion into rectangular plaques.

Differential Diagnosis

This disorder can be differentiated from plaque-like lesions such as those of psoriasis (redder lesions having whiter scales on the elbows, knees, and scalp and nail findings), lichen planus (violaceous, usually smaller polygonal papules), and nummular (coin-shaped) dermatitis. Similar lesions are seen in chronic atopic dermatitis.

Treatment

Topical corticosteroids give relief. Clobetasol, halobetasol, diflorasone, and betamethasone dipropionate in augmented vehicle are effective without occlusion and are used twice daily for several weeks. In some patients, flurandrenolide (Cordran) tape may be more effective, since it prevents scratching and rubbing of the lesion. These superpotent steroids are probably the treatment of choice but must be used with careful follow-up to avoid local side effects. The injection of triamcinolone acetonide suspension (5–10 mg/mL) into the lesions may occasionally be curative. Use of tars, such as 10% LCD (coal tar, liquor carbonis detergens, Fototar) in triamcinolone 0.1% ointment, or continuous occlusion with DuoDerm (occlusive flexible hydrocolloid dressing) for 7 days at a time for 1–2 months, may also be helpful. The area should be protected and the patient encouraged to become aware of when he or she is scratching.

Prognosis

The disease tends to remit during treatment but may recur or develop at another site.

Jones RO: Lichen simplex chronicus. Clin Podiatr Med Surg 1996;13:47. [NLM Cit ID: 97002584]

PSORIASIS

Essentials of Diagnosis

- Silvery scales on bright red, well-demarcated plaques, usually on the knees, elbows, and scalp.
- Nail findings including pitting and onycholysis (separation of the nail plate from the bed).
- Mild itching (usually).
- May be associated with psoriatic arthritis.
- Histopathology is not often useful and can be confusing.

General Considerations

Psoriasis is a common benign, acute or chronic inflammatory skin disease that appears to be based upon a genetic predisposition. Injury or irritation of normal skin tends to induce lesions of psoriasis at the site (Koebner's phenomenon). Psoriasis has several variants—the most common is the plaque type. Eruptive (guttate) psoriasis consisting of myriad lesions 3–10 mm in diameter occurs occasionally in periods of stress or after streptococcal pharyngitis. Grave, occasionally life-threatening forms (generalized pustular and erythrodermic psoriasis) may rarely occur. Plaque type or extensive erythrodermic psoriasis with abrupt onset may accompany HIV infection.

Clinical Findings

There are often no symptoms, but itching may occur. Although psoriasis may occur anywhere, one should examine the scalp, elbows, knees, palms and soles, and nails. The lesions are red, sharply defined plaques covered with silvery scales. The glans penis and vulva may be affected. Occasionally, only the flexures (axillae, inguinal areas) are involved. Fine stippling ("pitting") in the nails is highly suggestive of psoriasis. Psoriatics often have a pink or red intergluteal fold. Not all patients have findings in all locations, but the occurrence of a few may help make the diagnosis when other lesions are not typical. Some patients present mainly with hand or foot dermatitis and only minimal findings elsewhere, posing a difficult diagnostic problem. There may be associated arthritis that can resemble the rheumatoid variety but with a negative rheumatoid factor; distal interphalangeal joints are frequently involved, especially if there are nail changes.

Differential Diagnosis

The combination of red plaques with silvery scales on elbows and knees, with scaliness in the scalp or nail findings, is diagnostic. Psoriasis lesions are well demarcated and affect extensor surfaces—in contrast to atopic dermatitis, with poorly demarcated plaques in flexural distribution. In body folds, scraping and culture for candida and examination of scalp and nails will distinguish psoriasis from intertrigo and candidiasis. Dystrophic changes in nails may simulate onychomycosis, but again, the general examination combined with a potassium hydroxide (KOH) or fungal culture will be valuable in diagnosis. The cutaneous features of Reiter's syndrome may mimic psoriasis.

Treatment

There are many therapeutic options in psoriasis, to be chosen according to the extent and severity of disease and with a clear understanding of the risks and benefits of therapy.

A. Limited Disease: For many patients, the easiest regimen is to use a high-potency to highest-potency topical steroid cream or ointment. It is best to restrict the highest potency steroids to 2–3 weeks of twice-daily use and then use them in a pulse fashion three or four times on weekends or switch to a midpotency corticosteroid. Topical corticosteroids rarely induce a lasting remission. They may induce tachyphylaxis or cause psoriasis to become unstable. Additional measures are therefore commonly added to topical steroid therapy. Tar preparations such as Estar or Psorigel or Fototar cream, LCD (liquor carbonis detergens) 10% in Nutraderm lotion, or mixed directly with triamcinolone 0.1% cream are useful adjuncts when applied twice daily. Occlusion alone has been shown to clear isolated plaques in 30–40% of patients. Occlusive dressings such as thin Duoderm are placed on the lesions and left undisturbed for as long as possible (a minimum of 5 days, up to 7 days) and then replaced. Responses may be seen within several weeks. Anthralin is another agent for localized disease, but it must be used properly, is irritating, and may stain the skin. Calcipotriene ointment 0.005%, a vitamin D analog, is used twice daily for treatment of moderate-plaque psoriasis. It has become the second most commonly used topical treatment for psoriasis (after topical steroids). Ten percent of patients have an adverse reaction, most often rash, erythema, pruritus, or burning. Initially, patients are treated with twice-daily steroids to rapidly improve the psoriasis. Calcipotriene is then substituted for one of the steroid applications for several weeks. Eventually the topical steroids are stopped, and once- or twice-daily calcipotriene is continued chronically. Calcipotriene usually cannot be applied to the groin or on the face because of irritation. Treatment of extensive psoriasis with calcipotriene may result in hypercalcemia. Calcipotriene ointment is very expensive.

Tazarotene gel, a topical retinoid, is useful for the treatment of mild to moderate plaque psoriasis. About 50% of patients obtained at least 75% improvement of their skin lesions with twice-daily application, though fewer than 10% of plaques completely clear with 8 weeks of treatment. Tazarotene gel is available in 0.05% and 0.1% formulations. There is no difference between once-daily and twice-daily applications of the 0.1% formulation, but the 0.05% formulation is less effective when used once-daily. This agent appears to be similar to calcipotriene in that it may be used to augment the benefits of other forms of treatment. It is more expensive than calcipotriene and more irritating.

For the scalp, start with a tar shampoo (Neutrogena T/Gel regular or extra strength or Ionil T Plus), used daily if possible. For thick scales, use 6% salicylic acid gel (eg, Keralyt), P & S solution (phenol, mineral oil, and glycerin), or fluocinolone acetonide 0.01% in oil (Derma-Smoothe/FS) under a shower cap at night, and shampoo in the morning. In order of increasing potency, triamcinolone 0.1%, or fluocinolone, betamethasone dipropionate, fluocinonide or amcinonide, and clobetasol are available in solution form for use on the scalp twice daily. For psoriasis in the body folds, treatment is much more difficult, since potent steroids cannot be used. When mild corticosteroids are not effective and involvement or itch is severe, some of the modalities described immediately below may be required.

B. Generalized Disease: If psoriasis involves more than 30% of the body surface, it is difficult to treat with topical agents. The treatment of choice is outpatient UVB light exposure three times weekly. Clearing occurs in an average of 7 weeks, and maintenance may be needed since relapses are frequent. Severe psoriasis unresponsive to outpatient ultraviolet light calls for treatment in a day care center with the Goeckerman regimen, which involves use of crude coal tar for many hours and exposure to UVB light. Such treatment may offer the best chance for prolonged remissions.

PUVA (psoralen plus ultraviolet A, ie, ultraviolet light in the 320- to 400-nm wavelength range) may be effective even in patients who have failed standard UVB treatment. Long-term use of PUVA is associated with an increased risk of skin cancer (especially squamous cell carcinoma and perhaps melanoma), particularly in persons with fair complexions or those who have received ionizing radiation. Thus, periodic examination of the skin is imperative. Atypical lentigines are common. There can be rapid aging of the skin in fair individuals. Cataracts are a threat but have not been reported with proper use of protective glasses. PUVA may be used in combination with other therapy, such as acitretin or methotrexate.

Parenteral corticosteroids should not be used because of the possibility of induction of pustular lesions. Methotrexate is very effective for severe psoriasis in doses up to 25 mg once weekly or in divided doses every 12 hours for three doses once a week. It should be used according to published protocols. Liver biopsy is performed initially after methotrexate has been used long enough by the patient to demonstrate that it is effective and well tolerated, and then at intervals depending on the cumulative dose, usually 1.5–2 g. Administration of folic acid, 1–5 mg daily, will eliminate nausea caused by methotrexate without compromising efficacy.

Acitretin, a synthetic retinoid, is most effective for pustular psoriasis in dosages of 0.5–1 mg/kg/d, but it also improves erythrodermic and plaque types and psoriatic arthritis. Liver enzymes and serum lipids must be checked periodically. Because acitretin is a teratogen and persists for long periods in fat, women of childbearing age must wait at least 3 years after completing acitretin treatment before considering pregnancy. When used as single agents, retinoids will flatten psoriatic plaques, but high doses may be required for complete clearing. Retinoids find their greatest use when combined with phototherapy—either UVB or PUVA, with which they are synergistic.

Cyclosporine dramatically improves psoriasis and may be used to control severe cases. Relapses are the rule after cessation of therapy, so another agent must be added if cyclosporine is stopped. Sulfasalazine in dosages of 1 g three times daily markedly improved about one-third of patients in a double-blinded study. Thus, sulfasalazine may be considered for patients who are not candidates for—or who cannot tolerate—more toxic drugs. Thioguanine is another effective alternative for severe disease and is used at doses of 40–80 mg for 2–7 days per week with frequent monitoring of the complete blood count.

Moderate to severe psoriasis in AIDS patients is best initially treated with acitretin, 25–50 mg/d, with the addition of UVB as needed. PUVA and methotrexate are not usually recommended as initial therapies.

Prognosis

The course tends to be chronic and unpredictable, and the disease may be refractory to treatment.

Cohen MR et al: Baseline relationships between psoriasis and psoriatic arthritis: analysis of 221 patients with active psoriatic arthritis. Department of Veterans Affairs Cooperative Study Group on Seronegative Spondyloarthropathies. J Rheumatol 1999;26:1752. [NLM Cit ID: 99378282]

Cuellar ML et al: Methotrexate use in psoriasis and psoriatic arthritis. Rheum Dis Clin North Am 1997;23:797. [NLM Cit ID: 98027019]

Federman DG et al: Topical psoriasis therapy. Am Fam Physician 1999;59:957. [NLM Cit ID: 99167842]

Koo J: Systemic sequential therapy of psoriasis: a new paradigm for improved therapeutic results. J Am Acad Dermatol 1999;41(3 Part 2):S25. [NLM Cit ID: 99412303]

Krueger GG et al: The safety and efficacy of tazarotene gel, a topical acetylenic retinoid in the treatment of psoriasis. Arch Dermatol 1998;134:57. [NLM Cit ID: 98111563]

Lauharanta J: Photochemotherapy. Clin Dermatol 1997;15:769. [NLM Cit ID: 97459200]

Lebwohl M et al: Cyclosporine consensus conference: with emphasis on the treatment of psoriasis. J Am Acad Dermatol 1998;39:464. [NLM Cit ID 98409163]

Lindelof B: Risk of melanoma with psoralen/ultraviolet A therapy for psoriasis. Do the known risks now outweigh the benefits? Drug Safety 1999;20:289. [NLM Cit ID: 99247194]

Stern RS: Psoriasis. Lancet 1997;350:349. [NLM Cit ID: 97395511]

PITYRIASIS ROSEA

Essentials of Diagnosis

- Oval, fawn-colored, scaly eruption following cleavage lines of trunk.
- Herald patch precedes eruption by 1–2 weeks.
- Occasional pruritus.

General Considerations

This is a common mild, acute inflammatory disease which is 50% more common in females. Young adults are principally affected, mostly in the spring or fall. Concurrent household cases have been reported. HHV-7 may be causative.

Clinical Findings

Itching is common but is usually mild. The diagnosis is made by finding one or more classic lesions. The lesions consist of oval, fawn-colored plaques up to 2 cm in diameter. The centers of the lesions have a crinkled or "cigarette paper" appearance and a collarette scale, ie, a thin bit of scale that is bound at the periphery and free in the center. Only a few lesions in the eruption may have this characteristic appearance, however. Lesions follow cleavage lines on the trunk (so-called Christmas tree pattern), and the proximal portions of the extremities are often involved. Variants that affect the flexures (axillae and groin), so called inverse pityriasis rosea, and papular variants, especially in black patients, also occur. An initial lesion ("herald patch") that is often larger than the later lesions often precedes the general eruption by 1–2 weeks. The eruption usually lasts 4–8 weeks and heals without scarring.

Differential Diagnosis

A serologic test for syphilis should be performed if at least a few perfectly typical lesions are not present, if the rash does not itch, and especially if there are palmar and plantar or mucous membrane lesions or adenopathy, features that are suggestive of secondary syphilis. For the nonexpert, an RPR test in all cases is not unreasonable. Tinea corporis may present with red, slightly scaly plaques, but rarely are there more than a few lesions of tinea corporis compared to the many lesions of pityriasis rosea. A scraping of scale for a KOH test will rapidly make the diagnosis. Seborrheic dermatitis on occasion presents on the body with poorly demarcated patches over the sternum, in the pubic area, and in the axillae. The classic lesions of pityriasis rosea are not present. Tinea versicolor lesions, viral exanthems, and drug eruptions may simulate pityriasis rosea.

Treatment

Pityriasis rosea often requires no treatment. In Asians, Hispanics, or blacks, in whom lesions may remain hyperpigmented for some time, more aggressive management may be indicated. The most effective management consists of daily UVB treatments for a week, or prednisone as used for contact dermatitis. Topical steroids of medium strength (triamcinolone 0.1%) may also be used if pruritus is bothersome.

Prognosis

Pityriasis rosea is usually an acute self-limiting illness that disappears in about 6 weeks.

Kempf W et al: Pityriasis rosea is not associated with human herpesvirus 7. Arch Dermatol 1999;135:1070. [NLM Cit ID: 99418643]

SEBORRHEIC DERMATITIS & DANDRUFF

Essentials of Diagnosis

- Dry scales and underlying erythema.
- Scalp, central face, presternal, interscapular areas, umbilicus, and body folds.

General Considerations

Seborrheic dermatitis is an acute or chronic papulosquamous dermatitis. Seborrheic dermatitis may represent an inflammatory reaction to *Malassezia furfur* yeasts present on the scalp of all humans.

Clinical Findings

Pruritus is an inconstant finding. The scalp, face, chest, back, umbilicus, eyelid margins, and body folds may be oily or dry, with dry scales or oily yellowish scurf. Fissuring and secondary infection are occasionally present. Patients with Parkinson's disease frequently develop moderately severe seborrheic dermatitis, as do patients who become acutely ill and are hospitalized for a variety of reasons. Patients with HIV infection often have seborrheic dermatitis.

Differential Diagnosis

There is often a clinical spectrum ranging from simple dandruff to seborrheic dermatitis to scalp psoriasis. On the scalp, the presence of well-demarcated red plaques usually is termed psoriasis, and general erythema without tight, thick, silvery scale is usually called seborrheic dermatitis. The presence of mild scaling without any erythema is often termed simple dandruff. Extensive seborrheic dermatitis may simulate intertrigo in flexural areas, but scalp, face, and sternal involvement suggests seborrheic dermatitis. Scaling of the scalp due to tinea capitis may simulate dandruff or seborrheic dermatitis, but alopecia is usually present in tinea capitis, a rare dermatophytosis in adults.

Treatment

A. Seborrhea of the Scalp: The clinician should suggest several shampoos and let the patient decide which is most acceptable. Shampoos that contain tar, zinc pyrithione, or selenium are used daily if possible, while ketoconazole shampoo is used twice weekly. Topical corticosteroid solutions or lotions are then added if necessary, and are used twice daily intermittently to avoid tachyphylaxis.

B. Facial Seborrheic Dermatitis: Mild soaps are usually used as described under atopic dermatitis so as not to further irritate the skin. Treatment of the scalp, if involved, is thought to decrease facial involvement. The mainstay of therapy is a mild corticosteroid (hydrocortisone 1%, alclometasone, desonide) used intermittently and not near the eyes. Potent fluorinated corticosteroids used on the face may produce steroid rosacea or atrophy and telangiectasia. These are rarely indicated for seborrheic dermatitis. If the disorder cannot be controlled with intermittent use of a topical steroid alone, ketoconazole (Nizoral) 2% cream is added twice daily.

C. Seborrheic Dermatitis of Nonhairy Areas: Low-potency steroid creams—ie, 1% or 2.5% hydrocortisone, desonide, or alclometasone dipropionate—are highly effective.

D. Seborrhea of Intertriginous Areas: Avoid greasy ointments. Apply low-potency steroid lotions or creams twice daily for 5–7 days and then once or twice weekly for maintenance as necessary. Ketoconazole shampoo may be a useful adjunct.

E. Involvement of Eyelid Margins: "Marginal blepharitis" usually responds to gentle cleaning of the lid margins nightly as needed, with undiluted Johnson and Johnson Baby Shampoo using a cotton swab.

Prognosis

The tendency is to lifelong recurrences. Individual outbreaks may last weeks, months, or years.

Janniger CK et al: Seborrheic dermatitis. Am Fam Physician 1995;52:149. [NLM Cit ID: 95328483]

Peter RJ et al: Successful treatment and prophylaxis of scalp seborrheic dermatitis and dandruff with 2% ketoconazole shampoo: Results of a multicentre, double-blind, placebo-controlled trial. Br J Dermatol 1995; 132:441. [NLM Cit ID: 95234554]

FUNGAL INFECTIONS OF THE SKIN

Mycotic infections are traditionally divided into two principal groups—superficial and deep. In this chapter, we will discuss only the superficial infections: tinea corporis and tinea cruris; dermatophytosis of the feet and dermatophytid of the hands; tinea unguium (onychomycosis); and tinea versicolor. See Chapter 36 for discussion of deep mycoses.

The diagnosis of fungal infections of the skin is usually based on the location and characteristics of the lesions and on the following laboratory examinations: (1) Direct demonstration of fungi in 10% KOH of scrapings from suspected lesions. "If it's scaly, scrape it" is a time-honored maxim. (2) Cultures of organisms on dermatophyte test medium (DTM); or one may use a microculture slide that produces color change and allows for direct microscopic identification. Histologic sections of nails stained with periodic acid-Schiff (Hotchkiss-McManus) technique may be diagnostic if cultures and scrapings are negative. Serologic and skin tests are of no value in the diagnosis of superficial fungal infections.

Principles of Treatment

In general, treatment follows a diagnosis confirmed by KOH preparation or culture, especially if systemic antifungal therapy is to be used. Many other diseases cause scaling, and use of an antifungal agent without a firm diagnosis makes subsequent diagnosis by a dermatologist more difficult. In general, fungal infections are treated topically except for those involving the scalp or nails or those deep in hair follicles on the face or body.

Griseofulvin is safe and effective for treating dermatophyte infections of the skin (except for the scalp and nails). It is more economical than the newer agents and may be used initially when systemic treatment is required for tinea cruris, tinea pedis, or tinea corporis.

Itraconazole, an azole antifungal, rapidly accumulates in the nail plate from the matrix and nail bed and persists for 6 months after oral administration is discontinued. Itraconazole suspension is better-absorbed and its use does not require the presence of gastric acid for optimal absorption.

Terbinafine is an allylamine oral antifungal. It has excellent activity against dermatophytes. In vitro activity against yeast forms is variable, but the drug is active against hyphal forms. It is well delivered to the nail plate and persists in the nail for 6–9 months after treatment has ended.

Fluconazole has excellent activity against yeasts and may be the treatment of choice for many forms of mucocutaneous candidiasis. It is not known whether fluconazole is selectively delivered to the keratin compartment, and there have not been sufficient studies to determine effective doses in treating dermatophytosis. Fluconazole appears to require longer treatment courses and so is more expensive than either itraconazole or terbinafine for the treatment of dermatophytosis.

Itraconazole, fluconazole, and terbinafine can all cause elevation of liver function tests and—though rarely in the dosing regimens used for the treatment of dermatophytosis—clinical hepatitis. Ketoconazole is no longer recommended for the treatment of dermatophytosis (except for tinea versicolor) because of the higher rate of hepatitis when it is used for more than a month.

General Measures & Prevention

The skin should be kept dry, since moist skin favors the growth of fungi. Dry the skin carefully after bathing or after perspiring heavily, and let it dry for 10–15 minutes before dressing, or use a hair dryer on low setting. Loose-fitting underwear is advisable. Socks should be changed frequently when moist from perspiration. Sandals or open-toed shoes should be worn if possible. Talc or other drying powders may be useful. The use of topical corticosteroids for other diseases may be complicated by intercurrent tinea or candidal infection, and topical antifungals are often used in intertriginous areas with steroids to prevent this.

Brennan B et al: Overview of topical therapy for common superficial fungal infections and the role of new topical agents. J Am Acad Dermatol 1997;36(2 Part 1):S3. [NLM Cit ID: 97191240]

Lesher JL Jr: Recent developments in antifungal therapy. Dermatol Clin 1996;14:163. [NLM Cit ID: 96418385]

Pierard GE et al: Treatment and prophylaxis of tinea infections. Drugs 1996;52:209. [NLM Cit ID: 96439408]

1. TINEA CORPORIS OR TINEA CIRCINATA (Body Ringworm)

Essentials of Diagnosis

- Ring-shaped lesions with an advancing scaly border and central clearing or scaly patches with a distinct border.
- On exposed skin surfaces or the trunk.

- Microscopic examination of scrapings or culture confirms the diagnosis.

General Considerations

The lesions are often on exposed areas of the body such as the face and arms. A history of exposure to an infected cat may occasionally be obtained, usually indicating microsporum infection. All species of dermatophytes may cause this disease, but *Trichophyton rubrum* is the most common pathogen, usually representing extension onto the trunk or extremities of tinea cruris, pedis, or manuum.

Clinical Findings

A. Symptoms and Signs: Itching may be present. In classic lesions, rings of erythema have an advancing scaly border and central clearing, occasionally with hyperpigmentation.

B. Laboratory Findings: Hyphae can be demonstrated by removing peripheral scale and examining it microscopically using KOH. The diagnosis may be confirmed by culture.

Differential Diagnosis

Positive fungal studies distinguish tinea corporis from other skin lesions with annular configuration, such as the annular lesions of psoriasis, lupus erythematosus, syphilis, erythema multiforme, and pityriasis rosea. Psoriasis has typical lesions on elbows, knees, scalp, and nails. Secondary syphilis is often manifested by characteristic palmar, plantar, and mucous membrane lesions. Erythema multiforme does not have peripheral scale, is mostly acral in distribution, and is often associated with recent herpes simplex infection. Tinea corporis rarely has the large number of lesions seen in pityriasis rosea. Granuloma annulare lacks scales.

Complications

Complications include extension of the disease down the hair follicles (in which case it becomes much more difficult to cure), pyoderma, and dermatophytid.

Prevention

Treat infected household pets (microsporum infections).

Treatment

A. Local Measures: The following applied topically are effective against dermatophyte infections other than those of the nails: miconazole, 2% cream; clotrimazole, 1% solution, cream, or lotion; ketoconazole, 2% cream; econazole, 1% cream or lotion; sulconazole, 1% cream; oxiconazole, 1% cream; ciclopirox, 1% cream; naftifine, 1% cream or gel; butenafine cream; and terbinafine, 1% cream. Miconazole, clotrimazole, and terbinafine are available OTC. A lylamines (naftifine, terbinafine, and butenafine) to the most rapid response. Treatment should be continued for 1–2 weeks after clinical clearing. Betamethasone dipropionate with clotrimazole is often overused by nondermatologists. In general, short-term use of betamethasone-clotrimazole (Lotrisone) does not justify the expense, and chronic improper use may result in side effects from the high-potency steroid component, especially in body folds. Cases of tinea that are clinically resistant to this combination have been reported.

B. Systemic Measures: Griseofulvin (ultramicrosize), 250–500 mg twice daily, is used. Typically, only 2–4 weeks of therapy are required. Itraconazole as a single week-long pulse of 200 mg once daily is also effective in tinea corporis. Terbinafine, 250 mg daily for 1 month, is an alternative.

Prognosis

Body ringworm usually responds promptly to conservative topical therapy or to griseofulvin by mouth within 4 weeks.

2. TINEA CRURIS (Jock Itch)

Essentials of Diagnosis

- Marked itching in intertriginous areas, usually sparing the scrotum.
- Peripherally spreading, sharply demarcated, centrally clearing erythematous lesions.
- May have associated tinea infection of feet or toenails.
- Laboratory examination with microscope or culture confirms diagnosis.

General Considerations

Tinea cruris lesions are confined to the groin and gluteal cleft. Intractable pruritus ani may occasionally be caused by a tinea infecti

Clinical Findings

A. Symptoms and ns: Itching may be se- ymptomatic. The lesions vere, or the rash may ared centers, and active, have sharp margins ies. Follicular pustules are spreading scaly pe . The area may be hyperpig- sometimes encour mented on resol

B. Labor Findings: Hyphae can be oscopically in potassium hydrox- demonstrate The organism may be cultured ide prepa readily.

Di l Diagnosis

ruris must be distinguished from other le- volving the intertriginous areas, such as can- is, seborrheic dermatitis, intertrigo, psoriasis of y folds ("inverse psoriasis"), erythrasma, and ely tinea versicolor. Candidiasis is generally bright red and marked by satellite papules and pustules outside of the main border of the lesion. Candida typically involves the scrotum. Tinea versicolor can be diagnosed by the KOH preparation. Seborrheic dermatitis of the inguinal area also often involves the face, sternum, and axillae. Intertrigo tends to be more red, less scaly, and present in obese individuals in moist body folds with less extension onto the thigh. Inverse psoriasis is characterized by distinct plaques. Other areas of typical psoriatic involvement should be checked, and the KOH examination will be negative. Erythrasma is best diagnosed with Wood's light—a brilliant coral-red fluorescence is seen.

Treatment

A. General Measures: Drying powder (eg, miconazole nitrate [Zeasorb-AF]) should be dusted into the involved area in patients with excessive perspiration or occlusion of skin due to obesity. Underwear should be loose-fitting.

B. Local Measures: Any of the preparations listed in the section on tinea corporis may be used. There is great variation in expense, with miconazole, clotrimazole, and terbinafine available OTC and usually at a lower price. Terbinafine cream is curative in over 80% of cases after twice-daily use for 7 days.

C. Systemic Measures: Griseofulvin ultramicrosize is reserved for severe cases. Give 250–500 mg orally twice daily for 1–2 weeks. One week of either itraconazole, 200 mg daily, or terbinafine, 250 mg daily, is also effective.

Prognosis

Tinea cruris usually responds promptly to topical or systemic treatment. It may leave behind postinflammatory hyperpigmentation.

Drake LA et al: [illegible]idelines of care for superficial mycotic infections of th[illegible]kin: Tinea corporis, tinea cruris, tinea faciei, tinea man[illegible]n, and tinea pedis. Guidelines/Outcomes Committee. [illegible]erican Academy of Dermatology. J Am Acad Dermat[illegible]996;34(2 Part 1):282. [NLM Cit ID: 96225801]

van Heerden JS et al: Ti[illegible]rporis/cruris: New treatment options. Dermatol 1997[illegible]Suppl 1):14. [NLM Cit ID: 97298993]

3. TINEA MANUUM & TI[illegible]EDIS (Dermatophytosis, Tine[illegible]alms & Soles, "Athlete's Foot")

Essentials of Diagnosis

- Most often presenting with asymp[illegible]
- May progress to fissuring or mac[illegible]caling. web spaces.
- Itching, burning, and stinging of interd[illegible]n toe palms, and soles seen occasionally; dee[illegible], in inflammatory cases.
- The fungus is shown in skin scrapings examined microscopically or by culture of scrapings.

General Considerations

Tinea of the feet is an extremely common acute or chronic dermatosis. Certain individuals appear to be more susceptible than others. Most infections are caused by trichophyton and epidermophyton species.

Clinical Findings

A. Symptoms and Signs: The presenting symptom may be itching, burning, or stinging. Pain may indicate secondary infection with complicating cellulitis. Interdigital tinea pedis is a common cause of leg cellulitis in healthy individuals. Tinea pedis has several presentations that vary with the location. On the sole and heel, tinea may appear as chronic noninflammatory scaling, occasionally with thickening and cracking of the epidermis. This may extend over the sides of the feet in a "moccasin" distribution. The KOH preparation is usually positive. Tinea pedis often appears as a scaling or fissuring of the toe webs, perhaps with denudation and sodden maceration. As the web spaces become more macerated, the KOH preparation and fungal culture are less often positive because bacterial species begin to dominate. Finally, there may also be grouped vesicles distributed anywhere on the soles or palms, generalized exfoliation of the skin of the soles, or nail involvement in the form of discoloration and thickening and crumbling of the nail plate.

B. Laboratory Findings: Hyphae can be demonstrated microscopically in skin scales treated with 10% potassium hydroxide. Culture does not always demonstrate pathogenic fungi from macerated areas.

Differential Diagnosis

Differentiate from other skin conditions involving the same areas, such as interdigital erythrasma (use Wood's light). Psoriasis may be a cause of chronic scaling on the palms or soles and may cause nail changes. Repeated fungal cultures should be negative, and the condition will not respond to antifungal therapy. Contact dermatitis (from shoes, powders, nail polish) will often involve the dorsal surfaces and will respond to topical or systemic corticosteroids. Vesicular lesions should be differentiated from pompholyx (dyshidrosis) and scabies by proper scraping of the roofs of individual vesicles. Rarely, gram-negative organisms may cause toe web infections in the setting of prior tinea or in its absence. Culture is not very specific, because gram-negative organisms can be cultured from normal toe webs. This entity is treated with aluminum salts (see below) and imidazole antifungal agents or ciclopirox.

Prevention

The essential factor in prevention is personal hygiene. Use of rubber or wooden sandals in community showers and bathing places is often recommended, though the effectiveness of this practice has not been studied. Careful drying between the toes after showering is essential. A hair dryer used on low setting may be used before dressing. Socks should be changed frequently. Apply dusting and drying powders as necessary. The use of powders containing antifungal agents (eg, Zeasorb-AF) or chronic use of antifungal creams may prevent recurrences of tinea pedis.

Treatment

A. Local Measures: *Caution:* Do not overtreat.

1. Macerated stage–Treat with aluminum subacetate solution soaks for 20 minutes twice daily. Broad-spectrum antifungal creams and solutions (containing imidazoles or ciclopirox instead of tolnaftate and haloprogin) will help combat diphtheroids and other gram-positive organisms present at this stage and alone may be adequate therapy.

2. Dry and scaly stage–Use any of the agents listed in the section on tinea corporis.

B. Systemic Measures: Griseofulvin should be used only for severe cases or those recalcitrant to topical therapy. If the infection is cleared by systemic therapy, the patient should be encouraged to begin maintenance with topical therapy, since recurrence is common.

Itraconazole, 200 mg daily for 2 weeks or 400 mg daily for 1 week, or terbinafine, 250 mg daily for 2–4 weeks, may be used in refractory cases.

Prognosis

For many individuals, tinea pedis is a chronic affliction, temporarily cleared by therapy only to recur.

Evans EG: Tinea pedis: Clinical experience and efficacy of short treatment. Dermatol 1997;194(Suppl 1):3. [NLM Cit ID: 97298990]

Gupta AK et al: Itraconazole for the treatment of tinea pedis: A dosage of 400 mg/day given for 1 week is similar in efficacy to 100 or 200 mg/day given for 2 to 4 weeks. J Am Acad Dermatol 1997;36(5 Part 1):789. [NLM Cit ID: 97292008]

Leyden JL: Tinea pedis pathophysiology and treatment. J Am Acad Dermatol 1994;31(3 Part 2):S31. [NLM Cit ID: 94358245] (Reviews fungal and bacterial microbiology and immune response.)

Tschen E et al: Treatment of interdigital tinea pedis with a 4-week once-daily regimen of butenafine hydrochloride 1% cream. J Am Acad Dermatol 1997;36(2 Part 1):S9. [NLM Cit ID: 97191241]

4. TINEA VERSICOLOR (Pityriasis Versicolor)

Essentials of Diagnosis

- Pale macules that will not tan, or hyperpigmented macules.
- Velvety, tan, pink, whitish, or brown macules that scale with scraping.
- Central upper trunk the most frequent site.
- Yeast observed on microscopic examination of scales.

General Considerations

Tinea versicolor is a mild, superficial *Malassezia furfur (Pityrosporum orbiculare)* infection of the skin (usually of the trunk). This yeast is a colonizer of all humans, which accounts for the high 2-year recurrence rate after treatment and initial cure. It is not understood why some patients manifest the spore and hyphal form of the organism and the clinical disease. The eruption is often called to patients' attention by the fact that the involved areas will not tan, and the resulting hypopigmentation may be mistaken for vitiligo. A hyperpigmented form is not uncommon.

Clinical Findings

A. Symptoms and Signs: Lesions are asymptomatic, but a few patients note itching. The lesions are velvety, tan, pink, white, or brown macules that vary from 4–5 mm in diameter to large confluent areas. The lesions initially do not look scaly, but scales may be readily obtained by scraping the area. Lesions may appear on the trunk, upper arms, neck, face, and groin.

B. Laboratory Findings: Large, blunt hyphae and thick-walled budding spores ("spaghetti and meatballs") may be seen under the 10× objective when skin scales have been cleared in 10% KOH. Fungal culture is not useful.

Differential Diagnosis

Hypopigmented lesions can be distinguished from vitiligo on basis of appearance. Vitiligo usually presents with periorificial lesions or lesions on the tips of the fingers. Vitiligo (and not tinea versicolor) is characterized by total depigmentation, not just a lessening of pigmentation. Pink and red-brown lesions on the chest are differentiated from seborrheic dermatitis of the same areas by the KOH preparation.

Treatment & Prognosis

Topical treatments include selenium sulfide lotion, which may be applied from neck to waist daily and left on for 5–15 minutes for 7 days; this treatment is repeated weekly for a month and then monthly for maintenance. Ketoconazole shampoo may also be used weekly chronically for maintenance. One must stress to the patient that the raised and scaly aspects of the rash are being treated; the alterations in pigmentation may take months to fade or fill in. One may also use equal parts of propylene glycol and water topically, diluting with water if there is irritation. Other choices are 3% salicylic acid in rubbing alcohol and Tinver lotion (contains sodium thiosul-

without a clear-cut prior history of skin disease or drug exposure, it may be impossible to make a specific diagnosis of the underlying condition even with skin biopsy, and diagnosis may require follow-up with time.

Clinical Findings

A. Symptoms and Signs: Symptoms may include itching, weakness, malaise, fever, and weight loss. Chills are prominent. Exfoliation may be generalized and sometimes includes loss of hair and nails. Generalized lymphadenopathy may be due to lymphoma or leukemia or may be part of the clinical picture of the skin disease (dermatopathic lymphadenitis). The mucosa is spared.

B. Laboratory Findings: A skin biopsy may show changes of a specific inflammatory dermatitis or cutaneous T cell lymphoma or leukemia. Peripheral leukocytes may show clonal rearrangements of the T cell receptor in Sézary syndrome.

Differential Diagnosis

It may be impossible to identify the cause of exfoliative dermatitis early in the course of the disease, so careful follow-up is necessary. Psoriasis, severe seborrheic dermatitis, and drug eruptions may have an erythrodermic phase.

Complications

Debility (protein loss) and dehydration may develop in patients with generalized inflammatory erythroderma; or sepsis may occur.

Treatment

A. Topical Therapy: Home treatment is with cool to tepid baths and application of mid-potency steroids under wet dressings or with the use of an occlusive plastic suit (Simmons Co., Chattanooga, Tennessee; or Sleep Sauna, Springhouse, Pennsylvania). If the erythroderma becomes chronic and is not manageable in an outpatient setting, hospitalize the patient. Keep the room at a constant warm temperature and provide the same topical treatment as for an outpatient.

B. Specific Measures: Stop all drugs, if possible. Systemic corticosteroids may provide spectacular improvement in severe or fulminant exfoliative dermatitis, but long-term therapy should be avoided (see Chapter 26). In addition, systemic corticosteroids must be used with caution because some patients with erythroderma have psoriasis and could develop pustular psoriasis. For cases of psoriatic erythroderma and pityriasis rubra pilaris, either acitretin or methotrexate may be indicated. Erythroderma secondary to lymphoma or leukemia requires specific topical or systemic chemotherapy. Suitable antibiotic drugs with coverage for staphylococcus should be given when there is evidence of bacterial infection.

Prognosis

Most patients recover completely or improve greatly over time but may require chronic therapy. Deaths are rare in the absence of cutaneous T cell lymphoma. A minority of patients will suffer from undiminished erythroderma for indefinite periods.

Karakayli G et al: Exfoliative dermatitis. Am Fam Physician 1999;59:625. [NLM Cit ID: 99154050]

MISCELLANEOUS SCALING DERMATOSES

Isolated scaly patches may represent actinic (solar) keratoses, nonpigmented seborrheic keratoses, or Bowen's or Paget's disease.

Actinic Keratoses

Actinic keratoses are small (0.2–1 mm) papules—flesh-colored, pink, or slightly hyperpigmented—that feel like sandpaper and are tender when the finger is drawn over them. They occur on sun-exposed parts of the body in persons of fair complexion. Actinic keratoses are considered premalignant, but only 1:1000 lesions per year progress to become squamous cell carcinomas.

Application of liquid nitrogen is a rapid and effective method of eradication. The lesions crust and disappear in 10–14 days. An alternative treatment is the use of 1–5% fluorouracil cream. This agent may be rubbed into the lesions morning and night until they become first red and sore and then crusted and eroded (usually 2–3 weeks), and then stopped. Similarly, 5% fluorouracil solution may be used two times a day on one or two consecutive days weekly for 7–10 weeks. Any lesions that persist should be evaluated for possible biopsy.

Callen JP et al: Actinic keratoses. J Am Acad Dermatol 1997;36:650. [NLM Cit ID: 97246525]

Epstein E: Does intermittent "pulse" topical 5-fluorouracil therapy allow destruction of actinic keratoses without significant inflammation? J Am Acad Dermatol 1998;38:77. [NLM Cit ID: 98107898] (Prospective study regarding a topic that influences patients interested in pursuing therapy.)

Bowen's Disease & Paget's Disease

Bowen's disease (intraepidermal squamous cell carcinoma) occurs either on sun-exposed or sun-protected cutaneous surfaces. The lesion is a small (1–3 cm), well-demarcated, slightly raised, pink to red, scaly plaque and may resemble psoriasis or a large actinic keratosis. While it may take some time, these lesions may progress to invasive squamous cell carcinoma. Excision or other definitive treatment is indicated.

Extramammary Paget's disease, considered by some to be a manifestation of apocrine sweat gland carcinoma, resembles chronic eczema and may involve apocrine areas such as the genitalia. There seems to be less likelihood of an underlying sweat gland carcinoma if the lesions are on the vulva than if they are on the perianal area. Mammary Paget's disease of the nipple, a unilateral or rarely bilateral red scaling plaque that may ooze, is associated with an underlying intraductal mammary carcinoma.

Burrows NP et al: Treatment of extramammary Paget's disease by radiotherapy. Br J Dermatol 1995;132:970. [NLM Cit ID: 95391560]

INTERTRIGO

Intertrigo is caused by the macerating effect of heat, moisture, and friction. It is especially likely to occur in obese persons and in humid climates. The symptoms are itching, stinging, and burning. The body folds develop fissures, erythema, and sodden epidermis, with superficial denudation. Candidiasis may complicate intertrigo. "Inverse psoriasis," tinea cruris, erythrasma, and candidiasis must be ruled out.

Maintain hygiene in the area, and keep it dry. Compresses may be useful acutely. Hydrocortisone 1% and an antifungal agent are effective. Recurrences are common.

VESICULAR DERMATOSES

HERPES SIMPLEX (Cold or Fever Sore; Genital Herpes)

Essentials of Diagnosis

- Recurrent small grouped vesicles on an erythematous base, especially in the orolabial and genital areas.
- May follow minor infections, trauma, stress, or sun exposure; regional lymph nodes may be swollen and tender.
- Tzanck smear is positive for multinucleated epithelial giant cells; viral cultures and direct fluorescent antibody tests are positive.

General Considerations

Over 85% of adults have serologic evidence of herpes simplex type 1 (HSV-1) infections, most often acquired asymptomatically in childhood. Occasionally, primary infections may be manifested as severe gingivostomatitis. Thereafter, the subject may have recurrent self-limited attacks, provoked by sun exposure, orofacial surgery, fever, or a viral infection.

About 25% of the United States population has serologic evidence of infection with herpes simplex type 2 (HSV-2). HSV-2 causes lesions whose morphology and natural history are similar to those caused by HSV-1 on the genitalia of both sexes. The infection is acquired by sexual contact. In monogamous heterosexual couples where one partner has HSV-2 infection, seroconversion of the noninfected partner occurs in 10% over a 1-year period. Up to 70% of such infections appeared to be transmitted during periods of asymptomatic shedding. Uninfected female partners are at greater risk than males. Owing to changes in sexual behavior, up to 40% of newly acquired cases of genital herpes are due to HSV-1.

Clinical Findings

A. Symptoms and Signs: The principal symptoms are burning and stinging. Neuralgia may precede or accompany attacks. The lesions consist of small, grouped vesicles that can occur anywhere but which most often occur on the vermilion border of the lips, the penile shaft, the labia, the perianal skin, and the buttocks. Regional lymph nodes may be swollen and tender. The lesions usually crust and heal in 1 week. Patients can be educated to recognize attacks that they previously did not identify as recurrences of herpes simplex. Herpes simplex is the most common cause of painful genital ulcerations in patients with HIV infection.

B. Laboratory Findings: Lesions of herpes simplex must be distinguished from chancroid, syphilis, pyoderma, or trauma. Direct immunofluorescent antibody slide tests offer rapid, sensitive diagnosis. Viral culture may also be helpful. The Tzanck smear, which demonstrates multinucleated cells, is the least sensitive test. Herpes simplex and varicella-zoster viruses cannot be distinguished on the Tzanck smear. Herpes serology is not used in the diagnosis of an acute genital ulcer.

Complications

Complications include pyoderma, eczema herpeticum, herpetic whitlow, herpes gladiatorum (epidemic herpes in wrestlers transmitted by contact), esophagitis, neonatal infection, keratitis, and encephalitis.

Prevention

Sunscreens are very useful adjuncts in preventing sun-induced recurrences. Prophylactic use of oral acyclovir may prevent recurrences. Acyclovir should be started at a dosage of 200 mg five times daily beginning 24 hours prior to ultraviolet light exposure, dental surgery, or orolabial cosmetic surgery.

Treatment

A. Systemic Therapy: Three systemic agents are available for the treatment of herpes infections: acyclovir, its valine analog valacyclovir, and famciclovir. All three agents are very effective and, when used properly, virtually nontoxic. Only acyclovir is available for intravenous administration. In general, with the exception of severe orolabial herpes, only genital disease is treated. For first clinical episodes (including primary) herpes simplex, the dosage of acyclovir is 200 mg orally five times daily (or 800 mg three times daily); of valacyclovir, 1000 mg twice daily; and of famciclovir, 250 mg three times daily. The duration of treatment is from 7 to 10 days depending on the severity of the outbreak. Most cases of recurrent herpes are mild and do not require therapy. In addition, pharmacotherapy is of limited benefit, with studies finding a reduction in the average outbreak by only 12–24 hours. If treatment is desired, recurrent herpes outbreaks may be treated with 5 days of acyclovir, 200 mg five times a day; valacyclovir, 500 mg twice daily; or famciclovir, 125 mg twice daily.

In patients with frequent or severe recurrences, suppressive therapy is most effective in controlling disease. Suppressive treatment will reduce outbreaks by 85% and reduces viral shedding by more than 90%. The recommended suppressive doses, taken continuously, are acyclovir, 400 mg twice daily; valacyclovir, 500 mg once daily; or famciclovir, 125–250 mg twice daily. Long-term suppression appears very safe, and after 5–7 years a substantial proportion of patients can discontinue treatment.

B. Local Measures: In general, topical therapy is not effective. It is strongly urged that 5% acyclovir ointment, if used at all, be limited to the restricted indications for which it has been approved, ie, initial herpes genitalis and mucocutaneous herpes simplex infections in immunocompromised patients. Penciclovir cream, to be applied at the first symptom every 2 hours while awake for 4 days for recurrent orolabial herpes, reduces the average attack duration from 5 days to 4.5 days.

Prognosis

Aside from the complications described above, recurrent attacks last several days, and patients recover without sequelae.

Baker DA et al: Once-daily valacyclovir hydrochloride for suppression of recurrent genital herpes. Obstet Gynecol 1999;94:103. [NLM Cit ID: 99316589]

Conant MA et al: Genital herpes: An integrated approach to management. J Am Acad Dermatol 1996;35:601. [NLM Cit ID: 97012475]

Sacks SL et al: Patient-initiated, twice-daily oral famciclovir for early recurrent genital herpes: A randomized, double-blind multicenter trial. Canadian Famciclovir Study Group. JAMA 1996;276:44. [NLM Cit ID: 96290399]

Stanberry L et al: New developments in the epidemiology, natural history and management of genital herpes. Antiviral Res 1999;42:1. [NLM Cit ID: 99263933]

Wald A: New therapies and prevention strategies for genital herpes. Clin Infect Dis 1999;28(Suppl 1):S4. [NLM Cit ID: 99152431]

HERPES ZOSTER (Shingles)

Essentials of Diagnosis

- Pain along the course of a nerve followed by painful grouped vesicular lesions.
- Involvement is unilateral; some lesions may occur outside the affected dermatome.
- Lesions are usually on face or trunk.
- Tzanck smear positive, especially in vesicular lesions.

General Considerations

Herpes zoster is an acute vesicular eruption due to the varicella-zoster virus. It usually occurs in adults. With rare exceptions, patients suffer only one attack. Dermatomal herpes zoster does not imply the presence of a visceral malignancy. Generalized disease, however, raises the suspicion of an associated immunosuppressive disorder such as Hodgkin's disease or HIV infection. HIV-infected patients are 20 times more likely to develop zoster, often before other clinical findings of HIV disease are present. A history of HIV risk factors and HIV testing when appropriate should be considered, especially in zoster patients under 55 years of age.

Clinical Findings

Pain usually precedes the eruption by 48 hours or more and may persist and actually increase in intensity after the lesions have disappeared. The lesions consist of grouped, tense, deep-seated vesicles distributed unilaterally along a dermatome. The commonest distributions are on the trunk or face. Up to 20 lesions may be found outside the affected dermatomes. Regional lymph glands may be tender and swollen.

Differential Diagnosis

Since poison oak and poison ivy dermatitis can occur unilaterally and in a streak by a single brush with the plant, it must be differentiated at times from herpes zoster. Allergic contact dermatitis is pruritic; zoster is painful. One must differentiate herpes zoster from lesions of herpes simplex, which occasionally occurs in a dermatomal distribution. One should use doses of antivirals appropriate for zoster in the absence of a clear diagnosis. Facial zoster may simulate erysipelas initially, but zoster is unilateral and shows vesicles after 24–48 hours. The pain of preeruptive herpes zoster may lead the clinician to diagnose migraine, myocardial infarction, acute abdomen, herniated nucleus pulposus, etc, depending on the dermatome involved.

Complications

Sacral zoster may be associated with bladder and bowel dysfunction. Persistent neuralgia, anesthesia or scarring of the affected area following healing, facial or other nerve paralysis, and encephalitis may occur. Postherpetic neuralgia is most common after involvement of the trigeminal region, and in patients over the age of 55. Early (within 72 hours after onset) and aggressive antiviral treatment of herpes zoster reduces the severity and duration of postherpetic neuralgia. Zoster ophthalmicus (V_1) can result in visual impairment.

Treatment

A. General Measures:

1. Immunocompetent host–Since early treatment of zoster reduces postherpetic neuralgia, those with a risk of developing this complication should be treated, ie, those over age 55. In addition, younger patients with acute moderate to severe pain may be benefited by effective antiviral therapy. Treatment can be given with oral acyclovir, 800 mg five times daily; famciclovir, 500 mg three times daily; or valacyclovir, 1 g three times daily—all for 7 days. For reasons of increased bioavailability and ease of dosing schedule, the preferred agents are those given three times daily. Patients should maintain good hydration, and elderly patients with reduced renal function should be followed closely. The dose of antiviral should be adjusted for renal function as recommended. Nerve blocks may be important in the management of initial severe pain. Ophthalmologic consultation is vital for involvement of the first branch of the trigeminal nerve. Systemic corticosteroids are effective in reducing acute pain, improving quality of life, and returning patients to normal activities much more quickly. They do not increase the risk of dissemination in immunocompetent hosts. If not contraindicated, a tapering 3-week course of prednisone, starting at 60 mg/d, should be considered for its adjunctive benefit in immunocompetent patients. Oral corticosteroids do not reduce the prevalence, severity, or duration of postherpetic neuralgia beyond that achieved by effective antiviral therapy.

2. Immunocompromised host–Given the safety and efficacy of currently available antivirals, most immunocompromised patients with herpes zoster are candidates for antiviral therapy. The dosage schedule is as listed above, but treatment should be continued until the lesions have completely crusted and are healed or almost healed (up to 2 weeks). Corticosteroids should not be given adjunctively in immunosuppressed hosts since they increase the risk of dissemination. Progression of disease may necessitate intravenous therapy with acyclovir, 10 mg/kg intravenously, three times daily. After 3–4 days, oral therapy may be substituted if there has been a good response to intravenous therapy. Adverse effects include decreased renal function from crystallization, nausea and vomiting, and abdominal pain.

Foscarnet, administered in a dosage of 40 mg/kg three times daily intravenously, is indicated for treatment of acyclovir-resistant varicella-zoster virus infections.

B. Local Measures: Calamine or starch shake lotions may be of some help.

C. Postherpetic Neuralgia: The most effective treatment is prevention with early and aggressive antiviral therapy. Once established, postherpetic neuralgia may be treated with capsaicin ointment, 0.025–0.075%. Chronic postherpetic neuralgia may be relieved by regional blocks (stellate ganglion, epidural, local infiltration, or peripheral nerve), with or without corticosteroids added to the injections. Amitriptyline, 25–75 mg as a single nightly dose, is the first-line oral therapy beyond simple analgesics. Gabapentin, up to 3600 mg daily (starting at 300 mg three times daily), may be added for additional pain relief.

Prognosis

The eruption persists 2–3 weeks and usually does not recur. Motor involvement in 2–3% may lead to temporary palsy.

Brody MB et al: Varicella-zoster virus infection. The complex prevention-treatment picture. Postgrad Med 1997;102:187, 192. [NLM Cit ID: 97367783]

Erlich KS: Management of herpes simplex and varicella-zoster virus infections. West J Med 1997;166:211. [NLM Cit ID: 97288219]

Johnson RW: Herpes zoster and postherpetic neuralgia: Optimal treatment. Drugs Aging 1997;10:80. [NLM Cit ID: 97214901]

Whitley RJ et al: Herpes zoster: risk categories for persistent pain. J Infect Dis 1999;179:9. [NLM Cit ID: 99059845]

POMPHOLYX (Dyshidrosis, Dyshidrotic Eczema)

Essentials of Diagnosis

- "Tapioca" vesicles of 1–2 mm on the palms, soles, and sides of fingers, associated with pruritus.
- Vesicles may coalesce to form multiloculated blisters.
- Scaling and fissuring may follow drying of the blisters.
- Appearance in the third decade, with lifelong recurrences.

General Considerations

"Dyshidrotic eczema" is a misnomer, suggesting that the vesicles of this condition are related to eccrine sweat ducts and sweating, which they are not. This is an extremely common form of hand dermatitis, preferably called pompholyx (Gr "bubble") or vesicular dermatitis of the palms and soles. Patients often have an atopic background and report flares with stress. Clues to a possible cause of pompholyx are suggested by the following observations. In Scandinavia, women with contact allergy to nickel and pompholyx appear to flare when given oral challenges with nickel. Nickel-free diets have given variable results. The chelator disulfiram has been reported to cause a 25% improvement in one controlled study in nickel-sensitive patients, and oral cromolyn sodium has also been shown to be of benefit. Patients with widespread dermatitis due to any cause may develop pompholyx-like eruptions as a part of an autoeczematization response.

Clinical Findings

Small clear vesicles stud the skin at the sides of the fingers and on the palms or soles. They look like the grains in tapioca. They may be associated with intense itching. Later, the vesicles dry and the area becomes scaly and fissured.

Differential Diagnosis

Unroofing the vesicles and scraping the blister roof for a KOH examination will reveal hyphae in cases of vesicular tinea. Blisters extending onto the dorsum of the hands may represent allergic contact dermatitis, and the culprit must be sought by history or by patch testing. Patients with inflammatory tinea pedis may have a vesicular dermatophytid of the palms. NSAIDs may produce an eruption very similar to that of dyshidrosis.

Prevention

There is no known way to prevent attacks.

Treatment

Topical and systemic corticosteroids help some patients dramatically. Since this is a chronic problem, systemic steroids are generally not appropriate therapy. A high-potency topical steroid used early in the attack may help abort the flare and ameliorate pruritus. Topical steroids are also important in treating the scaling and fissuring that are seen after the vesicular phase. It is essential that patients avoid anything that irritates the skin; they should wear cotton gloves inside vinyl gloves when doing dishes or other wet chores, use long-handled brushes instead of sponges, and use a hand cream after washing the hands. If a history of nickel allergy (rashes with costume jewelry or from watchbands) is obtained, nickel-free diets may be considered. Patients respond to PUVA therapy using topical psoralen and special UVA light sources designed to treat hands and feet.

Prognosis

For most patients, the disease is an inconvenience. Even with moderate to severe disease, flares can be controlled with scrupulous care. For some, pompholyx can be incapacitating.

DERMATOPHYTID (Allergy or Sensitivity to Fungi)

Essentials of Diagnosis

- Pruritic, grouped vesicular lesions involving the sides and flexor aspects of the fingers and the palms.
- Fungal infection elsewhere on the body, usually the feet.
- No fungus demonstrable in lesions.

General Considerations

Dermatophytid must be considered in the differential diagnosis of vesicles on the hands and feet. It is a hypersensitivity reaction to an active focus of inflammatory dermatophytosis elsewhere on the body, usually the feet. Fungi are present in the primary lesions but are not present in the lesions of dermatophytid. The hands are most often affected, but dermatophytid may occur on other areas also.

Clinical Findings

A. Symptoms and Signs: Itching is the only symptom. The lesions consist of grouped vesicles, often involving the thenar and hypothenar eminences. Lesions occasionally involve the backs of the hands or may even be generalized.

B. Laboratory Findings: This entity is best diagnosed morphologically and by response to treatment. The trichophytin skin test is positive, but it may also be positive with other disorders.

Differential Diagnosis

Dermatophytid must be distinguished from all diseases causing vesicular eruptions of the hands—especially contact dermatitis, pompholyx, and photosensitive drug eruptions and "id" reactions due to inflammatory rashes.

Treatment

The lesions should be treated according to type of dermatitis. The primary focus of tinea should be treated with an oral antifungal or by local measures as described for dermatophytosis (see above).

Prognosis

Dermatophytid may occur in an explosive series of episodes, and recurrences are not uncommon; however, it clears with adequate treatment of the primary infection elsewhere on the body.

Busch RF: Dermatophytid reaction and chronic otitis externa. Otolaryngol Head Neck Surg 1998;118(3 Part 1):420. [NLM Cit ID: 98186362]

PORPHYRIA CUTANEA TARDA

Essentials of Diagnosis

- Noninflammatory blisters on sun-exposed sites, especially the dorsal surfaces of the hands.

- Hypertrichosis, skin fragility.
- Associated liver disease.
- Elevated urine porphyrins.

General Considerations

Porphyria cutanea tarda is the most common type of porphyria. Cases are sporadic or hereditary. The disease is associated with ingestion of certain medications, and liver disease from alcoholism or hepatitis C. In patients with liver disease, hemosiderosis is often present.

Clinical Findings

A. Symptoms and Signs: Patients complain of painless blistering and fragility of the skin of the dorsal surfaces of the hands. Facial hypertrichosis and hyperpigmentation are common.

B. Laboratory Findings: Urinary uroporphyrins are elevated two- to fivefold above coproporphyrins. Patients may also have abnormal liver function tests, evidence of hepatitis C infection, and increased liver iron stores.

Differential Diagnosis

Skin lesions identical to those of porphyria cutanea tarda may be seen in patients being maintained on dialysis and with the ingestion of certain medications (tetracyclines and NSAIDs, especially naproxen). In this so-called pseudoporphyria, the biopsy results are identical to those associated with porphyria cutanea tarda, but urine porphyrins are normal.

Prevention

Although the lesions are triggered by sun exposure, the wavelength of light triggering the lesions is beyond that absorbed by sunscreens, which for that reason are ineffective. Barrier sun protection with clothing is required.

Treatment

Stopping all triggering medications and substantially reducing or stopping alcohol consumption may alone lead to improvement. Phlebotomy without oral iron supplementation at a rate of one unit every 2–4 weeks will gradually lead to improvement. Very low dose antimalarials (as low as 200 mg of hydroxychloroquine twice weekly) will increase the excretion of porphyrins, improving the skin disease. Treatment is continued until the patient is asymptomatic. Urine porphyrins may be monitored.

Prognosis

Most patients improve with treatment. Sclerodermoid skin lesions may develop on the trunk, scalp, and face.

Chuang TY et al: Porphyria cutanea tarda and hepatitis C virus: a case-control study and meta-analysis of the literature. J Am Acad Dermatol 1999;41:31. [NLM Cit ID: 99337214]

Rich JD et al: Highly active antiretroviral therapy leading to resolution of porphyria cutanea tarda in a patient with AIDS and hepatitis C. Dig Dis Sci 1999;44:1034. [NLM Cit ID: 99249694]

Rich MW: Porphyria cutanea tarda. Don't forget to look at the urine. Postgrad Med 1999;105:208. [NLM Cit ID: 99239603]

DERMATITIS HERPETIFORMIS

Dermatitis herpetiformis is an uncommon disease manifested by pruritic papules, vesicles, and papulovesicles mainly on the elbows, knees, buttocks, posterior neck, and scalp. It appears to have its highest prevalence in Scandinavia and is associated with HLA antigens -B8, -DR3, and -DQw2. The diagnosis is made by light microscopy, which demonstrates neutrophils at the dermal papillary tips. Direct immunofluorescence studies show granular deposits of IgA along the dermal papillae. Circulating anti-endomysium antibodies can be detected in all cases. Patients have gluten-sensitive enteropathy, but for the great majority it is subclinical. However, ingestion of gluten plays a role in the exacerbation of skin lesions, and strict long-term avoidance of dietary gluten has been shown to decrease the dose of dapsone (usually 100–200 mg/d) required to control the disease and may even eliminate the need for drug treatment. Although adherence to a gluten-free diet is difficult, the availability of many gluten-free foods makes this easier to accomplish. Patients with dermatitis herpetiformis are at increased risk for development of gastrointestinal lymphoma, and this risk is reduced by a gluten-free diet.

Egan CA et al: Dermatitis herpetiformis: A review of fifty-four patients. Ir J Med Sci 1997;166:241. [NLM Cit ID: 98055870]

Lewis HM et al: Protective effect of gluten-free diet against development of lymphoma in dermatitis herpetiformis. Br J Dermatol 1996;135:363. [NLM Cit ID: 97106678]

WEEPING OR ENCRUSTED LESIONS

IMPETIGO

Impetigo is a contagious and autoinoculable infection of the skin caused by staphylococci or streptococci (or both). Classically, two forms have been recognized: (1) a vesiculopustular type, with thick golden-crusted lesions caused by group A β-hemolytic streptococcus or *Staphylococcus aureus*; and

(2) a bullous type, associated with phage group II *S aureus.* However, most cases of impetigo of either presentation now appear to be due to staphylococci.

Clinical Findings

A. Symptoms and Signs: Itching is the only symptom. The lesions consist of macules, vesicles, bullae, pustules, and honey-colored gummy crusts that when removed leave denuded red areas. The face and other exposed parts are most often involved. **Ecthyma** is a deeper form of impetigo caused by staphylococci or streptococci, with ulceration and scarring. It occurs frequently on the legs and other covered areas, often as a complication of debility and local cutaneous trauma.

B. Laboratory Findings: Gram stain and culture confirm the diagnosis.

Differential Diagnosis

The main differential diagnosis is between impetigo and acute allergic contact dermatitis. Contact dermatitis may be suggested by the history or by linear distribution of the lesions, and culture should be negative for staphylococci and streptococci. Herpes simplex infection usually presents with grouped vesicles or discrete erosions and may be associated with a history of recurrences. Viral culture and Tzanck smears of the lesions are positive.

Treatment

Topical antibiotics are not as effective as systemic antibiotics. Two percent mupirocin ointment (Bactroban), dispensed as 15 g and used three times daily for 10 days, may be effective for limited disease. If the affected area is large or if there is fever or toxicity—or if there is any concern that a nephritogenic strain of streptococcus may be causative—systemic antibiotics should be given. Dicloxacillin, 250 mg four times daily, is usually effective, or one may use cephalexin, 50 mg/kg/24 h. Erythromycin, 250 mg four times daily, is a reasonable alternative depending on the prevalence of erythromycin-resistant staphylococci in the community and as determined by culture and sensitivity tests. Recurrent impetigo is associated with nasal carriage of *S aureus,* treated with rifampin, 600 mg daily, or intranasal mupirocin ointment twice daily for 5 days.

Crusts and weepy areas may be treated with compresses, and washcloths and towels must be segregated and washed separately.

Bass JW et al: Comparison of oral cephalexin, topical mupirocin and topical bacitracin for treatment of impetigo. Pediatr Infect Dis J 1997;16:708. [NLM Cit ID: 97383806]

Sadick NS: Current aspects of bacterial infections of the skin. Dermatol Clin 1997;15:341. [NLM Cit ID: 97253200]

ALLERGIC CONTACT DERMATITIS

Essentials of Diagnosis

- Erythema and edema, with pruritus, often followed by vesicles and bullae in an area of contact with a suspected agent.
- Later, weeping, crusting, or secondary infection.
- Often a history of previous reaction to suspected contactant.
- Patch test with agent usually positive.

General Considerations

Contact dermatitis is an acute or chronic dermatitis that results from direct skin contact with chemicals or allergens. Eighty percent of cases are due to excessive exposure to or additive effects of primary or universal irritants (eg, soaps, detergents, organic solvents) and are called irritant contact dermatitis. The minority are due to actual contact allergy such as poison ivy or poison oak. The most common topicals causing allergic rashes include antimicrobials (especially neomycin), antihistamines, anesthetics (benzocaine), hair dyes, preservatives (eg, parabens), latex, and adhesive tape. Occupational exposure is an important cause of allergic contact dermatitis. Weeping and crusting are typically due to allergic and not irritant dermatitis, which often appears red and scaly. With widespread precautions being taken against HIV infection, contact dermatitis due to latex rubber in gloves and condoms is being seen more frequently.

Clinical Findings

A. Symptoms and Signs: In allergic contact dermatitis, the acute phase is characterized by tiny vesicles and weepy and crusted lesions, whereas resolving or chronic contact dermatitis presents with scaling, erythema, and possibly thickened skin. Itching, burning, and stinging may be severe. The lesions, distributed on exposed parts or in bizarre asymmetric patterns, consist of erythematous macules, papules, and vesicles. The affected area is often hot and swollen, with exudation and crusting, simulating and at times complicated by infection. The pattern of the eruption may be diagnostic (eg, typical linear streaked vesicles on the extremities in poison oak or ivy dermatitis). The location will often suggest the cause: Scalp involvement suggests hair tints, sprays, or tonics; face involvement, creams, cosmetics, soaps, shaving materials, nail polish; neck involvement, jewelry, hair dyes, etc.

B. Laboratory Findings: Gram stain and culture will rule out impetigo or secondary infection (impetiginization). If itching is generalized and impetiginized scabies is considered, a scraping for mites should be done. During the acute episode, patch testing cannot be performed. After the episode has cleared, the patch test may be useful, but not all potential allergens are available for testing. In the event of a positive reaction, the clinical relevance of the chemical agent to the dermatitis must be determined. In suspected photocontact dermatitis—involvement of face, "V" of the upper chest, and hands, sparing the skin under the nose, chin, and inner upper eyelid—photopatch tests may be done by exposing the traditional patch test site to ultraviolet light after 24 hours.

Differential Diagnosis

Asymmetric distribution, blotchy erythema around the face, linear lesions, and a history of exposure help distinguish contact dermatitis from other skin lesions. The most commonly confused diagnosis is impetigo. Differentiation may be difficult if the area of involvement is consistent with that seen in other types of skin disorders such as scabies, dermatophytid, atopic dermatitis, pompholyx, and other eczemas.

Prevention

Prompt and thorough removal of allergens by prolonged washing with water or by dousing with solvents such as isopropyl alcohol or other chemical agents may be effective if done very shortly after exposure to poison oak or ivy. Recently, several barrier creams (eg, Stokogard, Ivy Shield) have been introduced that may offer some protection to patients at high risk for poison oak and ivy dermatitis. Iodoquinol cream (Vioform) may benefit nickel allergic patients in a similar manner. Ingestion of rhus antigen is of limited clinical value for the induction of tolerance.

The mainstay of prevention is identification of agents causing the dermatitis and avoidance of exposure or use of protective clothing and gloves. In industry-related cases, prevention may be accomplished by moving the worker to another part of the workplace with different responsibilities.

Treatment

A. Overview: While local measures are important, severe or widespread involvement is difficult to manage without systemic corticosteroids because even the highest-potency topical steroids seem not to work well on vesicular and weepy lesions. Localized involvement (except on the face) can often be managed solely with topical agents. Irritant contact dermatitis is treated by protection from the irritant and use of topical steroids as for atopic dermatitis (described above). The treatment of allergic contact dermatitis is detailed below.

B. Local Measures:

1. Acute weeping dermatitis–Compresses are most often used. It is unwise to scrub lesions with soap and water. Calamine or starch shake lotions may sometimes be used in intervals between wet dressings, especially for involvement of intertriginous areas or when oozing is not marked. Lesions on the extremities may be bandaged with wet dressings for 30–60 minutes several times a day. Potent topical corticosteroids in gel or cream form may help suppress acute contact dermatitis and relieve itching. In cases where weeping is marked or in intertriginous areas, ointments will make the skin even more macerated and should be avoided. Suggested preparations are fluocinonide gel, 0.05%, used two or three times daily with compresses, or clobetasol or halobetasol cream, used twice daily for a maximum of 2 weeks—not in body folds or on the face. This should be followed by tapering of the number of applications per day or use of a mid-potency steroid such as triamcinolone 0.1% cream to prevent rebound of the dermatitis. A soothing formulation is 0.1% triamcinolone acetonide in Sarna lotion (0.5% camphor, 0.5% menthol, 0.5% phenol). Frequent continued use may induce tachyphylaxis.

2. Subacute dermatitis (subsiding)–Mid-potency (triamcinolone 0.1%) to high-potency steroids (amcinonide, fluocinonide, desoximetasone) are the mainstays of therapy.

3. Chronic dermatitis (dry and lichenified)– High- to highest-potency steroids are used in ointment form if acceptable to the patient; creams if not.

C. Systemic Therapy: For acute severe cases, one may give prednisone orally for 12–21 days. Prednisone, 60 mg for 4–7 days, 40 mg for 4–7 days, and 20 mg for 4–7 days without a further taper is one useful regimen. Another is to dispense seventy-eight 5 mg pills to be taken 12 the first day, 11 the second day, and so on. The key is to use enough corticosteroid (and as early as possible) to achieve a clinical effect and to taper slowly enough to avoid rebound. A Medrol Dosepak (methylprednisolone) with 5 days of medication is inappropriate on both counts. Triamcinolone acetonide, 40–60 mg once intragluteally, with 0.5–1 mL of betamethasone for rapid onset of action, may be used instead. (See Chapter 26.)

Prognosis

Allergic contact dermatitis is self-limited if reexposure is prevented but often takes 2–3 weeks for full resolution. Sensitivity to industrial contactants may necessitate a change of occupation.

Bernstein DI: Allergic reactions to workplace allergens. JAMA 1997;278:1907. [NLM Cit ID: 98057359] (Discusses various workplace allergen exposures, including latex, nickel, and other industrial agents.)

Leung DY et al: Allergic and immunologic skin disorders. JAMA 1997;278:1914. [NLM Cit ID: 98057360]

Lutz ME et al: Allergic contact dermatitis due to topical application of corticosteroids: Review and clinical implications. Mayo Clinic Proc 1997;72:1141. [NLM Cit ID: 98075215]

PUSTULAR DISORDERS

ACNE VULGARIS

Essentials of Diagnosis

- Occurs often at puberty, though onset may be delayed into the third or fourth decade.
- Open and closed comedones are the hallmark of acne vulgaris.
- The most common of all skin conditions.
- Severity varies from purely comedonal to papular or pustular inflammatory acne to cysts or nodules.
- Face and trunk may be affected.
- Scarring may be a sequela of the disease or picking and manipulating by the patient.

General Considerations

Acne vulgaris is polymorphic. Open and closed comedones, papules, pustules, and cysts are found. The disease is of unknown cause and is apparently activated by androgens in those who are genetically predisposed.

Acne vulgaris is more common and more severe in males. It does not always clear spontaneously when maturity is reached. Twelve percent of women and 3% of men over age 25 have acne vulgaris. This rate does not decrease until after age 44. The skin lesions parallel sebaceous activity. Pathogenic events include plugging of the infundibulum of the follicles, retention of sebum, overgrowth of the acne bacillus *(Propionibacterium acnes)* with resultant release of and irritation by accumulated fatty acids, and foreign body reaction to extrafollicular sebum. The mechanism of antibiotics in controlling acne is not clearly understood, but they may work because of their antibacterial or anti-inflammatory properties. Relapse or resistance may occur after emergence of tetracycline- or erythromycin-resistant strains of *P acnes.* These strains are usually sensitive to minocycline, however.

When a resistant case of acne is encountered in a woman, hyperandrogenism may be suspected. This may or may not be accompanied by hirsutism, irregular menses, or other signs of virilism.

Clinical Findings

There may be mild soreness, pain, or itching. The lesions occur mainly over the face, neck, upper chest, back, and shoulders. Comedones are the hallmark of acne vulgaris. Closed comedones are tiny, flesh-colored, noninflamed bumps that give the skin a rough texture or appearance. Open comedones typically are a bit larger and have black material in them. Inflammatory papules, pustules, ectatic pores, acne cysts, and scarring are also seen.

Acne may have different presentations at different ages. Preteens often present with comedones as their first lesions. Some patients have primarily comedones, with few inflammatory lesions. Inflammatory lesions in young teenagers are often found in the middle of the face, extending outward as the patient becomes older. Women in their third and fourth decades (often with no prior history of acne) commonly present with papular lesions on the chin and around the mouth—so-called perioral dermatitis.

Differential Diagnosis

In adults, acne rosacea presents with papules and pustules in the middle third of the face, but telangiectasia, flushing, and perhaps rhinophyma distinguish this disease from acne vulgaris. A pustular eruption on the face in patients receiving antibiotics or with otitis externa should be investigated with culture to rule out an uncommon gram-negative folliculitis. Patients who use systemic steroids or topical fluorinated steroids on the face may develop acne. Acne may be exacerbated or caused by irritating creams or oils. Pustules on the face can also be caused by tinea infections. Lesions on the back are more problematic. When they occur alone, one should suspect staphylococcal folliculitis, miliaria ("heat rash"), or, uncommonly, malassezia folliculitis. Bacterial culture, trial of an antistaphylococcal antibiotic, and observing the response to therapy, will help in the differential diagnosis. In patients with HIV infection, folliculitis is common and often severe and may be either staphylococcal folliculitis or eosinophilic folliculitis.

Complications

Cyst formation, pigmentary changes in pigmented patients, severe scarring, and psychologic problems may result.

Treatment

A. General Measures:

1. Education of the patient–When scarring seems out of proportion to the severity of the lesions, one must suspect that the patient is manipulating the lesions. It is essential that the patient be educated in a supportive way about this complication. Although there are exceptions, it is wise to let the patient know that at least 4–6 weeks will be required to see improvement and that old lesions may take months to fade. Therefore, improvement will be judged according to the number of new lesions forming after 6–8 weeks of therapy. Additional time will be required to see improvement on the back and chest, as these areas are slowest to respond. If hair pomades are used, they should contain glycerin and not oil. Avoid topical exposure to oils, cocoa butter (theobroma oil), and greases.

2. Diet–Foods do not cause or exacerbate acne.

B. Comedonal Acne: Treatment of acne is based on the type and severity of lesions. Comedones require treatment different from that of pustules and cystic lesions. In assessing severity, one must also take the sequelae of the lesions into account. Therefore, one must treat an individual who gets only two new lesions per month that scar or leave postinflammatory hyperpigmentation much more aggressively than a comparable patient whose lesions clear without sequelae. Soaps play little role in acne treatment, and unless the patient's skin is exceptionally oily, a mild soap should be used to avoid irritation that will limit the usefulness of other topicals, all of which are themselves somewhat irritating.

1. Tretinoin (retinoic acid, Retin-A)–Tretinoin is very effective for comedonal acne or for treatment of the comedonal component of more severe acne, but its usefulness is limited by irritation. Start with 0.025% cream (not gel or liquid) and have the patient use it at first twice weekly at night, then build up to as often as nightly. A few patients cannot use even this low-strength preparation more than three times weekly, but even that may cause improvement. A pea-sized amount is sufficient to cover half the entire face. To avoid irritation, have the patient wait 20 minutes after washing to apply. Adapalene gel 0.1% (somewhat less effective) and reformulated 0.025% tretinoin (Renova) are other options for patients irritated by standard tretinoin preparations. Some patients—especially teenagers—do best on 0.01% gel. Although the absorption of tretinoin is minimal, its use during pregnancy is *not* recommended. Some patients report photosensitivity with tretinoin. Patients should be warned that they may flare in the first 4 weeks of treatment. Tazarotene (Tazorac), a topical retinoid approved for treatment of psoriasis and acne, may also be effective.

2. Benzoyl peroxide–Benzoyl peroxide products are available in concentrations of 2.5%, 4%, 5%, 8%, and 10%, but it appears that 2.5% is as effective as 10% and less irritating. In general, water-based and not alcohol-based gels should be used to decrease irritation. Benzoyl peroxide washes such as Desquam-X wash or Benzac W wash may also be used but should be stopped or limited if they are irritating.

3. Antibiotics–Use of topical antibiotics (see below) has been demonstrated to decrease comedonal lesions.

4. Comedo extraction–Open and closed comedones may be removed with a comedo extractor but will recur if not prevented by treatment.

C. Papular Inflammatory Acne: Antibiotics are the mainstay for treatment of inflammatory acne. They may be used topically or orally. The oral antibiotics of choice are tetracycline and erythromycin. Minocycline is often effective in acne unresponsive or resistant to treatment with these antibiotics but it is expensive. Doxycycline is effective, economical, and easy to take. Rarely, other antibiotics such as trimethoprim-sulfamethoxazole (one double-strength tablet twice daily) and clindamycin (150 mg twice daily) may be tried. Topical clindamycin phosphate and erythromycin are also used (see below). Topicals are probably the equivalent of about 500 mg/d of tetracycline given orally, which is half the usual starting dose. Topical antibiotics are used in three situations: for mild papular acne that can be controlled by topicals alone, for patients who refuse or cannot tolerate oral antibiotics, or to wean patients under good control from oral to topical preparations. It has been recommended that switching or rotating antibiotics be avoided to decrease resistance and that courses of benzoyl peroxide be used on occasion, since there is an increasing incidence of *P acnes* resistance.

1. Mild acne–The first choice of topical antibiotics in terms of efficacy and relative lack of induction of resistant *P acnes* is the combination of erythromycin with benzoyl peroxide topical gel (benzamycin). If this product is not tolerated, either clindamycin (Cleocin T) lotion (least irritating), gel, or solution, or one of the many brands of topical erythromycin gel, solution, or ointment may be used twice daily. The addition of tretinoin 0.025% cream or 0.01% gel at night may be effective, since it works via a different mechanism.

2. Moderate acne–Tetracycline, 500 mg twice daily, erythromycin, 500 mg twice daily, doxycycline, 100 mg twice daily, and minocycline, 50–100 mg twice daily, are all effective though minocycline is more expensive. When initiating minocycline therapy, start at 100 mg in the evening for 4–7 days, then 100 mg twice daily, to decrease the incidence of vertigo. Plan a return visit in 6 weeks and at 3–4 months after that. If the patient's skin is quite clear, instructions should be given for tapering the dose by 250 mg for tetracycline and erythromycin, by 100 mg for doxycycline, or by 50 mg for minocycline every 6–8 weeks—while treating with topicals—to arrive at the lowest systemic dose needed to maintain clearing. In general, lowering the dose to zero without other therapy results in prompt recurrence of acne. Tetracycline, minocycline, and doxycycline are contraindicated in pregnancy and in young children.

It is important to discuss the issue of contraceptive failure when prescribing antibiotics for women taking oral contraceptives. Case reports and studies of plasma and urinary hormones in women suggest a possible association between tetracycline or erythromycin therapy and oral contraceptive failure. Women may need to consider using barrier methods as well, and should report breakthrough bleeding.

3. Severe acne–

a. Isotretinoin (Accutane) is a vitamin A analog for treatment of severe cystic acne that has not responded to conventional therapy. Informed consent should be obtained before its use in women of childbearing age. A dosage of 0.5–1 mg/kg/d for 20 weeks for a cumulative dose of at least 120 mg/kg is usually adequate for severe cystic acne. Patients should be referred for isotretinoin therapy before they experience significant scarring if they are not promptly and adequately controlled by antibiotics. The drug is *absolutely contraindicated during pregnancy* because of its teratogenicity; serum pregnancy tests should be obtained before starting the drug in a female and every month thereafter. Sufficient medication for only 1 month should be dispensed. Effective contraception—some authorities say in two forms—must be used. Therapeutic abortion is an alternative for the patient who becomes pregnant during therapy, and the patient's feelings about this option should be discussed before starting therapy. Side effects occur in most patients, usually related to dry skin and mucous membranes (dry lips, nosebleed, and dry eyes). If headache occurs, pseudotumor cerebri must be considered. Depression has been reported. At higher dosage levels, about 25% of patients will develop hypertriglyceridemia, 15% hypercholesterolemia, and 5% a lowering of high-density lipoproteins. Some patients develop minor elevations of liver function tests. Fasting blood sugar may be elevated. Miscellaneous adverse reactions include decreased night vision, musculoskeletal or bowel symptoms, rash, thinning of hair, exuberant granulation tissue in lesions, and bony hyperostoses (seen only with very high doses or with long duration of therapy). Moderate to severe myalgias necessitate decreasing the dosage or stopping the drug. Laboratory tests to be performed in all patients before treatment and after 4 weeks on therapy include cholesterol, triglycerides, and liver function studies.

Elevations of liver enzymes and triglycerides return to normal upon conclusion of therapy. The drug may induce long-term remissions in 30–40%, or acne may recur that is more easily controlled with conventional therapy in 40–50%. Occasionally, acne does not respond or promptly recurs after therapy, but it may clear after a second course.

b. Intralesional injection–In otherwise moderate acne, intralesional injection of dilute suspensions of triamcinolone acetonide (2.5 mg/mL, 0.05 mL per lesion), will often hasten the resolution of deeper papules and occasional cysts.

c. Laser, dermabrasion–Cosmetic improvement may be achieved by excision and punch-grafting of deep scars and by abrasion of inactive acne lesions, particularly flat, superficial scars. The technique is not without untoward effects, since hyperpigmentation, hypopigmentation, grooving, and scarring have been known to occur. Dark-skinned individuals do poorly. Corrective surgery within 18 months after isotretinoin therapy may not be advisable.

Prognosis

Acne vulgaris eventually remits spontaneously, but when this will occur cannot be predicted. The condition may persist throughout adulthood and may lead to severe scarring if left untreated. Patients treated with antibiotics continue to improve for the first 3–6 months of therapy. Relapse during treatment may suggest the emergence of resistant *P acnes.* The disease is chronic and tends to flare intermittently in spite of treatment. Remissions following systemic treatment with isotretinoin may be lasting in up to 60% of cases. Relapses after isotretinoin usually occur within 3 years and require a second course in up to 20% of patients.

Burkhart CG et al: Acne: a review of immunologic and microbiologic factors. Postgrad Med J 1999;75:328. [NLM Cit ID: 99364023]

Goulden V et al: Prevalence of facial acne in adults. J Am Acad Dermatol 1999;41:577. [NLM Cit ID: 99426905]

Leyden JJ: Therapy for acne vulgaris. N Engl J Med 1997;336:1156. [NLM Cit ID: 97238758]

Miller DM et al: A practical approach to antibiotic treatment in women taking oral contraceptives. J Am Acad Dermatol 1994;30:1008. [NLM Cit ID: 94245951] (Reviews evidence relating antibiotic use to contraceptive failure and suggests an approach to the problem.)

Ortonne JP: Oral isotretinoin treatment policy: Do we all agree? Dermatology 1997;195(Suppl 1):34. [NLM Cit ID: 97456788]

ROSACEA

Essentials of Diagnosis

- A chronic facial disorder of middle-aged and older people.
- A vascular component (erythema and telangiectasis) and a tendency to flush easily.
- An acneiform component (papules and pustules) may also be present.
- A glandular component accompanied by hyperplasia of the soft tissue of the nose (rhinophyma).

General Considerations

No single factor adequately explains the pathogenesis of this disorder. A statistically significant incidence of migraine headaches accompanying rosacea has been reported.

Potent topical steroids can change trivial dermatoses of the face into **perioral dermatitis** and **steroid rosacea.** These occur predominantly in young women and may be confused with acne rosacea.

Clinical Findings

The cheeks, nose, and chin—at times the entire face—may have a rosy hue. One sees no comedones. Inflammatory papules are prominent, and there may be pustules. Associated seborrhea may be found. The patient often complains of burning or stinging with episodes of flushing. It is not uncommon for patients to have associated ophthalmic disease, including blepharitis and keratitis. This often requires systemic antibiotic therapy.

Differential Diagnosis

Rosacea is distinguished from acne by age, the presence of the vascular component, and the absence of comedones. The rosy hue of rosacea is due to inflammation and telangiectases and generally will pinpoint the diagnosis.

Treatment

Medical management is aimed only at the inflammatory papules and pustules and the erythema that surrounds them. The only satisfactory treatment for the telangiectasias is laser surgery. Rhinophyma (soft tissue and sebaceous hyperplasia of the nose) responds only to surgical debulking.

A. Local Therapy: Metronidazole, 0.75% gel applied twice daily or 1% cream once daily, is probably the topical treatment of choice. If metronidazole is not tolerated, topical clindamycin (solution, gel, or lotion) used twice daily is effective. Erythromycin as described above may be helpful (see Acne Vulgaris). Five to 8 weeks of treatment are needed for significant response.

B. Systemic Therapy: Tetracycline or erythromycin, 250 or 500 mg orally twice daily on an empty stomach, should be used when topical therapy is inadequate.

Isotretinoin may succeed where other measures fail. A dosage of 0.5–1 mg/kg/d orally for 12–28 weeks is recommended. See precautions above.

Metronidazole, 250 mg twice daily for 3 weeks, may be worth trying but is seldom required. Side effects are few, though metronidazole may produce a disulfiram-like effect when the patient ingests alcohol.

Prognosis

Rosacea tends to be a stubborn and persistent process. With the regimens described above, it can usually be controlled adequately.

Millikan L: Recognizing rosacea. Postgrad Med 1999;105: 149. [NLM Cit ID: 99150771]

FOLLICULITIS (Including Sycosis)

Essentials of Diagnosis

- Itching and burning in hairy areas.
- Pustules in the hair follicles.
- In sycosis, inflammation of surrounding skin.

General Considerations

Folliculitis has multiple causes. It may be caused by staphylococcal infection and may be more common in the diabetic. When the lesion is deep-seated, chronic, and recalcitrant on the head and neck, it is called sycosis. Sycosis is usually propagated by the autoinoculation and trauma of shaving. The upper lip is particularly susceptible to involvement in men.

Gram-negative folliculitis, which may develop during antibiotic treatment of acne, may present as a flare of acne pustules or nodules. Klebsiella, enterobacter, *E coli,* and proteus have been isolated from these lesions.

"Hot tub folliculitis," caused by *Pseudomonas aeruginosa,* is characterized by pruritic or tender follicular or pustular lesions occurring within 1–4 days after bathing in a hot tub, whirlpool, or public swimming pool. Rarely, systemic infections may result.

Nonbacterial folliculitis may also be caused by oils that are irritating to the follicle, and these may be encountered in the workplace (machinists) or at home (various cosmetics and cocoa butter or coconut oils).

Folliculitis may also be caused by occlusion, perspiration, and rubbing, such as that resulting from tight jeans and other heavy fabrics on the upper legs.

Folliculitis on the back that looks like acne but does not respond to acne therapy may be caused by the yeast *Malassezia furfur.* This infection may require biopsy for diagnosis.

Folliculitis—so called "steroid acne"—may be seen during topical or systemic corticosteroid therapy.

A form of sterile folliculitis consisting of urticarial papules with prominent eosinophilic infiltration is common in patients with AIDS.

Pseudofolliculitis is caused by ingrowing hairs in the beard area. In this entity, the papules and pustules are located at the side of and not in follicles. It may be treated by growing a beard or by using chemical depilatories or various proprietary shaving systems (eg, Moore Technique Shaving System).

Clinical Findings

The symptoms range from slight burning and tenderness to intense itching. The lesions consist of pustules of hair follicles. In sycosis, the surrounding skin becomes involved also and so resembles eczema, with redness and crusting.

Differential Diagnosis

It is important to differentiate bacterial from nonbacterial folliculitis. The history is important for pinpointing the causes of nonbacterial folliculitis, and a Gram stain and culture is indispensable. One must differentiate folliculitis from acne vulgaris or pustular miliaria (heat rash) and from infections of the skin such as impetigo or fungal infections. Pseudomonas folliculitis is often suggested by the history of hot tub use. Eosinophilic folliculitis in AIDS often requires biopsy for diagnosis.

Complications

Abscess formation is the major complication of bacterial folliculitis.

Prevention

Correct any predisposing local causes (eg, irritations of a mechanical or chemical nature, discharges). Control of blood glucose in diabetes may reduce the number of these infections. Be sure that the water in hot tubs and spas is treated properly with chlorine. If staphylococcal folliculitis is persistent, treatment of nasal or perineal carriage with rifampin, 600 mg daily for 5 days, or with topical mupirocin ointment 2% twice daily for 5 days, may help. The latter may cause stinging in some patients. Chronic oral clindamycin, 150–300 mg/d, is also effective in preventing recurrent staphylococcal folliculitis and furunculosis.

Treatment

A. Local Measures: Cleanse the area gently with chlorhexidine and apply saline or aluminum subacetate soaks or compresses to the involved area for 15 minutes twice daily if very exudative.

Anhydrous ethyl alcohol containing 6.25% aluminum chloride (Xerac AC), applied to lesions and environs and followed by an antibiotic ointment (see above), may be helpful, especially for chronic folliculitis of the buttocks.

B. Specific Measures: Systemic antibiotics may be tried if the skin infection is resistant to local treatment, if it is extensive or severe and accompanied by a febrile reaction, if it is complicated, or if it involves the nose or upper lip. Extended periods of treatment (4–8 weeks or more) with antistaphylococcal antibiotics are required in some cases.

Hot tub pseudomonas folliculitis virtually always resolves without treatment but may be treated in adults with ciprofloxacin, 500 mg twice daily for 5 days.

Gram-negative folliculitis in acne patients may be treated with isotretinoin in compliance with all precautions discussed above (see Acne Vulgaris).

Folliculitis due to *M furfur* is treated with topical 2.5% selenium sulfide, 15 minutes daily for 3 weeks, or with oral ketoconazole, 200 mg daily for 7–14 days.

Irritant folliculitis is best treated by protection from the offending substance and use of drying agents such benzoyl peroxide or Xerac AC.

Eosinophilic folliculitis may be treated initially by the combination of potent topical steroids and oral antihistamines. In more severe cases, treatment is with one of the following: topical permethrin (application for 12 hours every other night for 6 weeks); itraconazole, 200–400 mg daily (tablets) or 200–300 mg daily (suspension); UVB or PUVA phototherapy; or isotretinoin, 0.5 mg/kg/d for up to 5 months. A remission may be induced by some of these therapies, but chronic treatment may be required.

Prognosis

Bacterial folliculitis is occasionally stubborn and persistent, requiring prolonged or intermittent courses of antibiotics. Steroid folliculitis is treatable by acne therapy and resolves as steroids are discontinued.

Majors MJ et al: HIV-related eosinophilic folliculitis: A panel discussion. Semin Cutan Med Surg 1997;16:219. [NLM Cit ID: 97444101]

Sadick NS: Current aspects of bacterial infections of the skin. Dermatol Clin 1997;15:341. [NLM Cit ID: 97253200]

MILIARIA (Heat Rash)

Essentials of Diagnosis

- Burning, itching, superficial aggregated small vesicles, papules, or pustules on covered areas of the skin, usually the trunk.
- More common in hot, moist climates.
- Rare forms associated with fever and even heat prostration.

General Considerations

Miliaria is an acute dermatitis that occurs most commonly on the trunk and intertriginous areas. A hot, moist environment is the most frequent cause. Bedridden febrile patients are susceptible. Plugging of the ostia of sweat ducts occurs, with consequent ballooning and ultimate rupture of the sweat duct, producing an irritating, stinging reaction. Increase in numbers of resident aerobes, notably cocci, apparently plays a role.

Clinical Findings

The usual symptoms are burning and itching. In severe cases, fever, heat prostration, and even death may result. The lesions consist of small, superficial, reddened, thin-walled, discrete but closely aggregated vesicles (miliaria crystallina), papules (miliaria rubra), or vesicopustules or pustules (miliaria pustulosa). The reaction occurs most commonly on covered areas of the skin.

Differential Diagnosis

Miliaria is to be distinguished from drug rash and folliculitis.

Prevention

Use of an antibacterial preparation such as chlorhexidine prior to exposure to heat and humidity may help prevent the condition. Susceptible persons should avoid exposure to hot, humid environments.

Treatment

Triamcinolone acetonide, 0.1% in Sarna lotion, or a mid-potency corticosteroid in a lotion or cream—but not ointment—base, should be applied two to four times daily. Alternative measures that have been employed with varying success are drying shake lotions and antipruritic powders or other dusting powders. Secondary infections (superficial pyoderma) are treated with erythromycin or dicloxacillin, 250 mg four times daily by mouth. Anticholinergic drugs given by mouth may be very helpful in severe cases, eg, glycopyrrolate, 1 mg twice daily.

Prognosis

Miliaria is usually a mild disorder, but death may occur with the severe forms (tropical anhidrosis and asthenia) as a result of interference with the heat-regulating mechanism.

Wenzel FG et al: Nonneoplastic disorders of the eccrine glands. J Am Acad Dermatol 1998;38:1. [NLM Cit ID: 98107888]

MUCOCUTANEOUS CANDIDIASIS

Essentials of Diagnosis

- Severe pruritus of vulva, anus, or body folds.
- Superficial denuded, beefy-red areas with or without satellite vesicopustules.
- Whitish curd-like concretions on the oral and vaginal mucous membranes.
- Yeast on microscopic examination of scales or curd.

General Considerations

Mucocutaneous candidiasis is a superficial fungal infection that may involve almost any cutaneous or mucous surface of the body. It is particularly likely to occur in diabetics, during pregnancy, and in obese persons who perspire freely. Antibiotics and oral contraceptive agents may be contributory. Oral candidiasis may be the first sign of HIV infection. Esophageal candidiasis is a frequent AIDS-defining illness in HIV-infected persons (see Chapter 31).

Clinical Findings

A. Symptoms and Signs: Itching may be intense. Burning is reported, particularly around the vulva and anus. The lesions consist of superficially denuded, beefy-red areas in the depths of the body folds such as in the groin and the intergluteal cleft, beneath the breasts, at the angles of the mouth, and in the umbilicus. The peripheries of these denuded lesions are superficially undermined, and there may be satellite vesicopustules. Whitish, curd-like concretions may be present on the surface of the mucosal lesions. Paronychia and interdigital erosions may occur.

B. Laboratory Findings: Clusters of budding cells and hyphae can be seen under high power when skin scales or curd-like lesions have been cleared in 10% KOH. The organism may be isolated on Sabouraud's medium.

Differential Diagnosis

Intertrigo, seborrheic dermatitis, tinea cruris, "inverse psoriasis," and erythrasma involving the same areas may mimic mucocutaneous candidiasis.

Complications

Systemic invasive candidiasis with candidemia may be seen with immunosuppression and in patients receiving broad-spectrum antibiotic and hypertonic glucose solutions, as in hyperalimentation. There may or may not be clinically evident mucocutaneous candidiasis.

Treatment

A. General Measures: Affected parts should be kept dry and exposed to air as much as possible. If possible, discontinue systemic antibiotics. For treatment of systemic invasive candidiasis, see Chapter 36.

B. Local Measures:

1. Nails and skin–Apply ciclopirox cream, nystatin cream, 100,000 units/g, or miconazole, econazole, ketoconazole, or clotrimazole cream or lotion three or four times daily. Gentian violet, 1%, or carbolfuchsin paint (Castellani's paint) may be applied once or twice weekly as an alternative, but these preparations are messy.

2. Vulvar and anal mucous membranes–For vaginal candidiasis, use miconazole cream, one applicatorful vaginally at bedtime for 7 days; clotrimazole 10 mg, one suppository vaginally per day for 7 days; terconazole vaginal cream or suppositories; or nystatin, one tablet (100,000 units) vaginally twice daily for 7 days. Topical agents may not be as effective in women with recurrent vaginal candidiasis, and these "intractable" cases may require chronic suppressive therapy. Single-dose fluconazole (150 mg) is as effective as ketoconazole (200 mg twice daily for 5 days) for vaginal disease. Itraconazole suspension may be very useful in refractory oropharyngeal candidiasis since it may act locally (as it is held in the mouth and then swallowed) and then has a second systemic action. Even fluconazole-resistant candidiasis may respond to this treatment.

3. Balanitis–This is most frequent in uncircumcised men, and candida usually plays a role. Topical imidazole cream or nystatin ointment is the initial treatment if the lesions are mildly erythematous or superficially erosive. Soaking with dilute aluminum acetate for 15 minutes twice daily may quickly relieve burning or itching. Chronicity and relapses, especially after sexual contact, suggest reinfection from a sexual partner who should be treated. Severe purulent balanitis is usually due to bacteria. If it is so severe that phimosis occurs, oral antibiotics—some with activity against anaerobes—are required; if rapid improvement does not occur, urologic consultation is indicated.

Prognosis

Cases of cutaneous candidiasis range from the easily cured to the intractable and prolonged.

Guidelines of care for superficial mycotic infections of the skin: Mucocutaneous candidiasis. Guidelines/Outcome Committee. American Academy of Dermatology. J Am Acad Dermatol 1996;34:110. [NLM Cit ID: 96140331]

FIGURATE ERYTHEMAS

URTICARIA & ANGIOEDEMA

Essentials of Diagnosis

- Eruptions of evanescent wheals or hives.
- Itching is usually intense but may on rare occasions be absent.
- Special forms of urticaria have special features (dermographism, cholinergic urticaria, solar urticaria, or cold urticaria).
- Most incidents are acute and self-limited over a period of 1–2 weeks.
- Chronic urticaria (episodes lasting > 6 weeks) may defy the best efforts of the clinician to find and eliminate the cause.

General Considerations

Urticaria can result from many different stimuli on an immunologic or nonimmunologic basis. The most common immunologic mechanism is hypersensitivity mediated by IgE, seen for most patients with acute urticaria; another involves activation of the complement cascade. Some patients with chronic urticaria demonstrate autoantibodies directed against mast cell IgE receptors, with histamine-releasing activity. ACE inhibitor and angiotensin II receptor antagonist therapy may be complicated by urticaria or angioedema. In general, extensive costly workups are not indicated in patients who present with urticaria. A careful history and physical examination are more helpful.

Clinical Findings

A. Symptoms and Signs: Lesions are itchy red swellings of a few millimeters to many centimeters. For most types of urticaria, the erythema and the wheal are the same size. The morphology of the lesions may vary over a period of minutes to hours, resulting in geographic or bizarre patterns. Angioedema is involvement of deeper vessels, with swelling of the lips, eyelids, palms, soles, and genitalia in association with more typical lesions. Angioedema is no more likely than urticaria to be associated with systemic complications such as laryngeal edema or hypotension. In cholinergic urticaria, triggered by a rise in core body temperature (hot showers, exercise), wheals are 2–3 mm in diameter with a large surrounding red flare.

B. Laboratory Findings: Laboratory studies are not likely to be helpful in the evaluation of acute or chronic urticaria unless there are suggestive findings in the history and physical examination. The most common causes of acute urticaria are foods, viral and parasitic infections, and medications. The cause of chronic urticaria is often not found. In patients with individual slightly purpuric lesions that persist past 24 hours, a skin biopsy may help exclude urticarial vasculitis. Quantitative immunoglobulins, cryoglobulins, cryofibrinogens, and antinuclear antibodies are often sought in cold urticaria but are rarely found. Liver tests may be of interest, since a serum sickness-like prodrome, with urticaria, may be associated with hepatitis B, and hepatitis C may be found in cases of chronic urticaria.

Differential Diagnosis

Papular urticaria resulting from insect bites persists for days. A central punctum can usually be seen, as with flea or gnat bites. Streaked urticarial lesions may be seen in acute allergic plant dermatitis, eg, poison ivy, oak, or sumac. Contact urticaria may be caused by a host of substances, including chemicals, foods, and medications, and may be one type of reaction to latex. Contact urticaria is often limited to areas exposed to the contactant. Urticarial response to heat, sun, water, and pressure are quite rare. Urticaria may be seen as part of serum sickness, associated with fever and arthralgia.

In hereditary angioedema, there is generally a positive family history and gastrointestinal or respiratory symptoms, but urticaria is not part of the syndrome. Lesions are not pruritic.

Treatment

A. General Measures: A detailed search for a cause of acute urticaria should be undertaken, and treatment may then be tailored to include the provocative condition. The chief nonallergic causes are drugs, eg, atropine, pilocarpine, morphine, and codeine; arthropod bites, eg, insect bites and bee stings (though the latter may cause anaphylaxis as well as angioedema); physical factors such as heat, cold, sunlight, injury, and pressure; and, presumably, neurogenic factors such as in cholinergic urticaria induced by exercise, excitement, hot showers, etc.

Allergic causes may include penicillins, aspirin, and other medications; inhalants such as feathers and animal danders; ingestion of shellfish or strawberries; injections of sera and vaccines; external contactants, including various chemicals and cosmetics; and infections such as hepatitis.

B. Systemic Treatment: The mainstay of treatment initially includes H_1 antihistamines (see above). Hydroxyzine, 10 mg twice daily to 25 mg three times daily to even 100 mg three times daily, may be very useful if tolerated. Giving hydroxyzine as one dose of 50–75 mg at night may reduce sedation and other side effects. Cyproheptadine, 4 mg four times daily, may be especially useful for cold urticaria. "Nonsedating" or less sedating antihistamines are added if the generic sedating antihistamines are not effective. Loratadine in a dosage of 10 mg/d is similar to the other H_1 antihistamines in effectiveness. Cetirizine, a metabolite of hydroxyzine, is less sedating (13% of patients) and is given in a dosage of 10 mg/d. It has been studied in patients with chronic urticaria in doses of 5–20 mg daily, demonstrating efficacy similar to that of loratadine and hydroxyzine. Fexofenadine is given in a dosage of 60 mg twice a day.

Doxepin (a tricyclic antidepressant), 25 mg three times daily, or, more commonly, 25–75 mg at bedtime, appears to be effective in chronic urticaria. It has anticholinergic side effects.

H_2 antihistamines are rarely effective if used in combination with H_1 blockers in patients with chronic urticaria unresponsive to H_1 blockers alone. Symptomatic dermographism is the exception.

Other agents with some promise as adjuvants include calcium channel blockers (used for at least 4 weeks); terbutaline, 1.25–2.5 mg three times daily; colchicine, 0.6 mg twice daily; and attenuated androgens such as danazol. A few patients with chronic urticaria may respond to a salicylate- and tartrazine-free diet. Although salicylates are ubiquitous in nature, drugs and foods are the most obvious sources. One group has reported curing over 60% of chronic urticaria patients with an allergen elimination diet over a 3-month period. This diet proscribes milk products; beer, wine, and cider; mushrooms, soy sauce, canned tomatoes, pickled and smoked meats, shellfish, vinegar, soured breads, melon, dried fruit, diet soda, chocolate, nuts, peanut products, and strawberries. Systemic steroids in a dose of about 40 mg daily will usually suppress acute and chronic urticaria. However, the use of corticosteroids is rarely indicated, since properly selected combinations of agents with less toxicity are usually effective. Once steroids are withdrawn, the urticaria virtually always returns if it had been chronic. Rather than using systemic steroids in difficult cases, consultation should be sought from a dermatologist or allergist with experience in managing severe urticaria.

C. Local Treatment: Local treatment is rarely rewarding.

Prognosis

Acute urticaria usually lasts only a few days to 6 weeks. Half of patients whose urticaria persists for more than 6 weeks will have it for years.

Cha YJ et al: Angioedema due to losartan. Ann Pharmacother 1999;33:936. [NLM Cit ID: 99420243]

Friedmann PS: Assessment of urticaria and angio-oedema. Clin Exper Allergy 1999;29(Suppl 3):109. [NLM Cit ID: 99373289]

Heymann WR: Acquired angioedema. J Am Acad Dermatol 1997;36:611. [NLM Cit ID: 97246510]

Ishoo E et al: Predicting airway risk in angioedema: staging system based on presentation. Otolaryngol Head Neck Surg 1999;121:263. [NLM Cit ID: 99403177]

Sabroe RA et al: Angiotensin-converting enzyme (ACE) inhibitors and angio-oedema. Br J Dermatol 1997;136:153. [NLM Cit ID: 97221677]

ERYTHEMA MULTIFORME

Essentials of Diagnosis

- Sudden onset of symmetric erythematous skin lesions with history of recurrence.
- May be macular, papular, urticarial, bullous, or purpuric.
- "Target" lesions with clear centers and concentric erythematous rings or "iris" lesions may be noted in erythema multiforme minor. These are rare in drug-associated erythema multiforme major (Stevens-Johnson syndrome).
- Erythema multiforme minor on extensor surfaces, palms, soles, or mucous membranes. Erythema multiforme major favors the trunk.
- Herpes simplex, systemic infection or disease, and drug reactions are often associated.

General Considerations

Erythema multiforme is an acute inflammatory skin disease due to multiple causes. Erythema multiforme is divided clinically into minor and major types based on the clinical findings. Approximately 90% of cases of erythema multiforme minor follow outbreaks of herpes simplex. Erythema multiforme major (Stevens-Johnson syndrome) is marked by toxicity and involvement of two or more mucosal surfaces (often oral and conjunctival) and is most often caused by drugs, especially sulfonamides, nonsteroidal anti-inflammatory drugs, and anticonvulsants such as phenytoin. *Mycoplasma pneumoniae* may trigger erythema multiforme major. Erythema multiforme may also present as recurring oral ulceration, with skin lesions present in only half of the cases, and is diagnosed by oral biopsy. Since erythema multiforme may have its own prodrome, many medications taken for such symptoms have been implicated in its pathogenesis without definitive proof. As in all drug eruptions, the exposure to drugs associated with erythema multiforme may be systemic or topical; any agent should be considered a potential offender.

Clinical Findings

A. Symptoms and Signs: A classic target lesion, found most commonly in herpes-associated erythema multiforme, consists of three concentric zones of color change, most often found acrally on the hands and feet. Not all lesions will have this appearance. Drug-associated erythema multiforme is manifested by raised target-like lesions, with only two zones of color change and a central blister, or nondescript reddish or purpuric macules. In erythema multiforme major, mucous membrane ulcerations are present at two or more sites, causing pain on eating, swallowing, and urination.

B. Laboratory Findings: Blood tests are not useful for diagnosis. Skin biopsy is diagnostic. Direct immunofluorescence studies are negative.

Differential Diagnosis

Urticaria and drug eruptions are the chief entities that must be differentiated from erythema multiforme minor. Individual lesions of true urticaria itch, should come and go within 24 hours, are usually responsive to antihistamines, and do not affect the mucosa. In erythema multiforme major, the main differential diagnosis is toxic epidermal necrolysis, and some investigators regard these entities as variants of the same disease. The presence of blisters is always worrisome and dictates the need for consultation. The differential diagnosis of blisters includes pemphigus, pemphigoid, and bullous drug eruptions. Skin biopsy is the mainstay of diagnosis.

Complications

Visceral lesions are rare complications (eg, pneumonitis, myocarditis, nephritis). The tracheobronchial mucosa and conjunctiva may be involved in severe cases with resultant scarring (Stevens-Johnson syndrome).

Treatment

A. General Measures: Erythema multiforme major (Stevens-Johnson syndrome) with extensive denudation of skin is best treated in a burn unit. Otherwise, patients need not be admitted unless mucosal involvement interferes with hydration and nutrition. Patients who begin to blister should be seen daily.

B. Specific Measures: Although there are no good data to support the use of corticosteroids in erythema multiforme major, they are still often prescribed. There are retrospective studies showing that children with erythema multiforme treated with large doses of corticosteroids actually have a poorer outcome because of the complications of therapy. If corticosteroids are to be tried in more severe cases, they should be used early, before blistering occurs, and in moderate to high doses (prednisone, 100–250 mg) and stopped within days if there is no dramatic response. In one trial, IGIV (0.75 g/kg/d for 4 days) yielded dramatic benefit in severe cases. Oral and topical corticosteroids are useful in the oral variant of erythema multiforme. Oral acyclovir prophylaxis of herpes simplex infections may be effective in preventing recurrent herpes-associated erythema multiforme. Antistaphylococcal antibiotics are used for secondary infection, which is uncommon.

C. Local Measures: Topical therapy is not very effective in this disease. For oral lesions, 1% diphenhydramine elixir mixed with Kaopectate or with 1% dyclonine may be used as a mouth rinse several times daily.

Prognosis

Erythema multiforme minor usually lasts 2–6 weeks and may recur. Stevens-Johnson syndrome, in which visceral involvement may occur, may be serious or even fatal in the most severe cases.

Roujeau JC: Stevens-Johnson syndrome and toxic epidermal necrolysis are severity variants of the same disease which differs from erythema multiforme. J Dermatol 1997;24:726. [NLM Cit ID: 98094430]

Rzany B et al: Risk of Stevens-Johnson syndrome and toxic epidermal necrolysis during first weeks of antiepileptic therapy: a case-control study. Study Group of the International Case Control Study on Severe Cutaneous Adverse Reactions. Lancet 1999;353:2190. [NLM Cit ID: 99320154]

Viard I et al: Inhibition of toxic epidermal necrolysis by blockade of CD95 with human intravenous immunoglobulin. Science 1998;282:490.

ERYTHEMA MIGRANS (See also Chapter 34.)

Erythema migrans is a unique cutaneous eruption that characterizes the localized or generalized early stage of Lyme disease. Three to 32 days (median: 7 days) after a tick bite, there is gradual expansion of redness around the papule representing the bite site. The advancing border is usually slightly raised, warm, red to bluish-red, and free of any scale. Centrally, the site of the bite may clear, leaving only a rim of peripheral erythema, or it may become indurated, vesicular, or necrotic. The annular erythema usually grows to a median diameter of 15 cm (range: 3–68 cm, but virtually always > 5 cm). It is accompanied by a burning sensation in half of patients; rarely, it is pruritic or painful. Twenty percent of patients will develop multiple secondary annular lesions similar in appearance to the primary lesion but without indurated centers and generally of smaller size. In the southeastern USA, similar lesions are seen in patients without evidence of Lyme borreliosis. The etiology of these cases is unclear.

Without treatment, erythema migrans and the secondary lesions fade in a median of 28 days, though some may persist for months. Ten percent of untreated patients experience recurrences over the ensuing months. Treatment with systemic antibiotics (see Table 34–4) is necessary to prevent systemic involvement. However, only 60–70% of those with systemic involvement experience erythema migrans.

Luft BJ et al: Azithromycin compared with amoxicillin in the treatment of erythema migrans: A double-blind, randomized, controlled trial. Ann Intern Med 1996;124:785. [NLM Cit ID: 96188892]

Maraspin V et al: Treatment of erythema migrans in pregnancy. Clin Infect Dis 1996;22:788. [NLM Cit ID: 96309044]

Strle F et al: Comparison of culture-confirmed erythema migrans caused by *Borrelia burgdorferi sensu stricto* in New York State and by *Borrelia afzelii* in Slovenia. Ann Intern Med 1999;130:32. [NLM Cit ID: 99087458]

ERYSIPELAS

Essentials of Diagnosis

- Edematous, spreading, circumscribed, hot, erythematous area, with or without vesicle or bulla formation.
- Face frequently involved.
- Pain, chills, fever, and systemic toxicity may be striking.

General Considerations

Erysipelas is a superficial form of cellulitis that occurs classically on the cheek, caused by β-hemolytic streptococci.

Clinical Findings

A. Symptoms and Signs: The symptoms are pain, malaise, chills, and moderate fever. A bright red spot appears first, very often near a fissure at the angle of the nose. This spreads to form a tense, sharply demarcated, glistening, smooth, hot area. The margin characteristically makes noticeable advances in days or even hours. The lesion is somewhat edematous and can be pitted slightly with the finger. Vesicles or bullae occasionally develop on the surface. The lesion does not usually become pustular or gangrenous and heals without scar formation. The disease may complicate any break in the skin that provides a portal of entry for the organism.

B. Laboratory Findings: Leukocytosis and an increased sedimentation rate are almost invariably present but are not specific; blood cultures may be positive.

Differential Diagnosis

Erysipeloid is a benign bacillary infection producing redness of the skin of the fingers or the backs of the hands in fishermen and meat handlers.

Complications

Unless erysipelas is promptly treated, death may result from extension of the process and systemic toxicity, particularly in the very young and in the aged.

Treatment

Place the patient at bed rest with the head of the bed elevated. Intravenous antibiotics effective against group A beta-hemolytic streptococci and staphylococci are indicated for the first 48 hours in all but the mildest cases. A 7-day course is completed with penicillin VK, 250 mg, dicloxacillin, 250 mg, or a first-generation cephalosporin, 250 mg, orally four times a day. Either erythromycin, 250 mg four times daily for 7–14 days, or clarithromycin, 250 mg twice daily for 7–14 days, is a good alternative in penicillin-allergic patients. Quinolones have poor activity against streptococci and are not recommended.

Prognosis

Erysipelas formerly was a life-threatening infection. It can now usually be quickly controlled with systemic penicillin or erythromycin therapy.

Bisno AL et al: Streptococcal infections of skin and soft tissues. N Engl J Med 1996;334:240. [NLM Cit ID: 96132561]

Chartier C et al: Erysipelas: An update. Int J Dermatol 1996;35:779. [NLM Cit ID: 97072979]

CELLULITIS

Cellulitis, a diffuse spreading infection of the skin, usually on the lower leg, may be due to one of several organisms, usually gram-positive cocci, though gram-negative rods such as *Escherichia coli* may also be responsible. The lesion is hot and red. The major portal of entry for lower leg cellulitis is toe web tinea pedis with fissuring of the skin at this site. The toe webs should be carefully examined in all cases and any associated web space tinea pedis treated aggressively. Attempts to isolate the responsible organism by injecting and then aspirating saline are successful in 20% of cases. In cases of venous stasis, the only clue to cellulitis may be a new localized area of tenderness. Recurrent attacks may sometimes affect lymphatic vessels, producing a permanent swelling called "solid edema."

Two potentially life threatening entities that can mimic cellulitis (ie, present with a painful, red, swollen lower extremity) include deep venous thrombosis and necrotizing fasciitis. The presence of a positive Homans sign (pain in the calf on dorsiflexing the ankle of the affected limb) or palpable venous cord may suggest DVT, but these are insensitive signs. If clinical suspicion of DVT is high, the diagnosis should be pursued with lower extremity Doppler ultrasound, impedance plethysmography, or other available imaging modality. The diagnosis of necrotizing fasciitis should be suspected in a patient who has a very toxic appearance, bullae, crepitus or anesthesia of the involved skin, overlying skin necrosis, and laboratory evidence of rhabdomyolysis or DIC. While these findings may be present with severe cellulitis and bacteremia, it is essential to rule out necrotizing fasciitis because rapid surgical debridement is essential. Other skin lesions that may resemble cellulitis include lipodermatosclerosis, an acute, exquisitely tender red plaque on the medial lower legs above the malleolus in patients with venous stasis or varicosities, and acute severe contact dermatitis on a limb, which produces erythema, vesiculation, and edema as seen in cellulitis, but with itching instead of pain. The erythema and edema are also more superficial than in cellulitis.

Intravenous or parenteral antibiotics may be required for the first 24–72 hours. In mild cases or following the initial parenteral therapy, dicloxacillin or cephalexin, 250–500 mg four times daily for 7–10 days, is usually adequate. In patients in whom intravenous treatment is not instituted, the first dose of oral antibiotic can be increased to 750–1000 mg to achieve rapid high blood levels.

Basoglu M et al: Fournier's gangrene: Review of fifteen cases. Am Surg 1997;63:1019. [NLM Cit ID: 98023687]

Dupuy A et al: Risk factors for erysipelas of the leg (cellulitis): case-control study. BMJ 1999;318:1591. [NLM Cit ID: 99292635]

Lewis RT: Soft tissue infections. World J Surg 1998;22:146. [NLM Cit ID: 98113910]

Quartey-Papafio CM: Lesson of the week: importance of distinguishing between cellulitis and varicose eczema of the leg. BMJ 1999;318:1672. [NLM Cit ID: 99301838]

ERYSIPELOID

Erysipelothrix insidiosa infection must be differentiated from erysipelas and cellulitis. It is usually a benign infection, seen in fishermen and meat handlers, It is characterized by a well-demarcated, purplish, indurated plaque that extends peripherally with central clearing. Lesions are most common on a finger or the dorsal hand surface. Local joint symptoms may be present as the lesions slowly spread over several weeks.

Penicillin V potassium, 250–500 mg orally four times daily for 7–10 days, is usually promptly curative. Some strains are resistant to erythromycin but sensitive to ciprofloxacin. Penicillin G, 2–4 million units intravenously every 4 hours, may be used instead if the patient appears toxic, with arthritis or endocarditis.

BLISTERING DISEASES

PEMPHIGUS

Essentials of Diagnosis

- Relapsing crops of bullae.
- Often preceded by mucous membrane bullae, erosions, and ulcerations.
- Superficial detachment of the skin after pressure or trauma variably present (Nikolsky's sign).
- Acantholysis on biopsy.
- Immunofluorescence studies are confirmatory.

General Considerations

Pemphigus is an uncommon intraepidermal blistering disease occurring on skin and mucous membranes. It is caused by autoantibodies to adhesion molecules expressed in the skin and mucous membranes (desmoglein 3, sometimes desmoglein I and plakoglobin in pemphigus vulgaris), and to a complex containing desmosomal proteins, including desmoglein I (in pemphigus foliaceus). These autoantibodies cause acantholysis, the separation of epidermal cells from each other. The cause is unknown, and in the preantibiotic, presteroid era the condition, if untreated, was usually fatal within 5 years. The bullae appear spontaneously and are tender and painful when they rupture. If the lesions become extensive, the complications of the disease lead to great toxicity and debility. Drug-induced autoimmune pemphigus from drugs including penicillamine and captopril has been reported. More than 95% of patients with pemphigus vulgaris are positive for HLA-DR4/DQw3 or HLA-DRw6/DQw1, and in one series of 13 patients, all of whom were DQw1-positive, all had a single DQ_β allele designated $PV6_\beta$. Pemphigus may present with atypical features, and repeated reevaluation of clinical findings and changes shown by immunofluorescence and histopathologic studies may be necessary.

There are several forms of pemphigus: **pemphigus vulgaris** and its variant, **pemphigus vegetans;** and the more superficially blistering **pemphigus foliaceus** and its variant, **pemphigus erythematosus.** All forms may occur at any age but most commonly in middle age. The vulgaris form begins in the mouth in over 50% of cases. The foliaceus form is especially apt to be associated with other autoimmune diseases, or it may be drug-induced, eg, by exposure to penicillamine. Paraneoplastic pemphigus, a unique form of the disorder, is associated with numerous types of benign and malignant neoplasms.

Clinical Findings

A. Symptoms and Signs: Pemphigus is characterized by an insidious onset of flaccid bullae in crops or waves. In pemphigus vulgaris, lesions often appear first on the oral mucous membranes, and these rapidly become erosive. In some cases, erosions and crusts predominate over blisters. The scalp is another site of early involvement. Rubbing a cotton swab or finger laterally on the surface of uninvolved skin may cause easy separation of the epidermis **(Nikolsky's sign).**

B. Laboratory Findings: The diagnosis is made by light microscopy and by direct and indirect immunofluorescence microscopy. Microscopically, acantholysis is the hallmark of pemphigus, but in some patients there may be eosinophilic spongiosis initially. Immunofluorescence microscopy shows deposits of IgG intercellularly in the epidermis. C3 and other immunoglobulins and complement components may be present on occasion. Indirect immunofluorescence microscopy to detect circulating pemphigus antibodies is not necessary for the diagnosis, but antibody titers in some patients may correspond with disease activity and might help in management.

Differential Diagnosis

Blistering diseases include erythema multiforme, drug eruptions, bullous impetigo, contact dermatitis, dermatitis herpetiformis, and bullous pemphigoid, but flaccid blisters are not typical of these diseases, and acantholysis is not seen. In the early stages, pemphigus tends to be treated as impetigo, but bacterial cultures and clinical suspicion leading to early biopsy will clarify the diagnosis. All of these diseases have clinical characteristics and different immunofluorescence test results that distinguish them from pemphigus.

Paraneoplastic pemphigus is clinically, histologically, and immunologically distinct from other forms of the disease. Oral erosions and erythematous plaques resembling erythema multiforme are seen. Survival rates are low because of the underlying malignancy.

Complications

Secondary infection commonly occurs; this is a major cause of morbidity and mortality. Disturbances of fluid and electrolyte balance can occur owing to losses through the involved skin in severe cases.

Treatment

A. General Measures: When the disease is severe, hospitalize the patient at bed rest and provide antibiotics and intravenous feedings as indicated. Anesthetic troches used before eating ease painful oral lesions.

B. Systemic Measures: Pemphigus requires systemic therapy as early in its course as possible. However, the main morbidity in this disease today is generally due to the side effects of such therapy. Although high doses of prednisone have been advocated—180–360 mg/d for 6–10 weeks—most clinicians use doses of 80–120 mg to start and increase the dose for rapid progression of the disease or lack of response within a few weeks. A traditional next step has been to add immunosuppressive drugs, described below as "steroid-sparing" agents. However, tetracycline at a dosage of 1.5–2 g/d in divided doses with 500 mg of nicotinamide *(not nicotinic acid or niacin!)* twice to three times daily has been reported to be effective and is probably the preferred adjunctive measure in patients with stable pemphigus foliaceus. Of the immunosuppressive agents, mycophenolate mofetil (1 g twice daily) seems most predictably effective, with limited toxicity. Other options include azathioprine, 100–150 mg/d, given concurrently with prednisone or methotrexate, 25 mg/wk. When control is achieved, the prednisone is slowly tapered. Dapsone at 25–100 mg/d appears to be a useful agent that may allow the tapering of corticosteroids. Gold sodium thiomalate, given as for rheumatoid arthritis, is effective following initial prednisone. Pulse intravenous cyclophosphamide or IGIV may be tried in refractory cases.

C. Local Measures: In patients with limited disease, skin and mucous membrane lesions should be treated with topical corticosteroids. Complicating infection requires appropriate systemic and local antibiotic therapy.

Prognosis

The course tends to be chronic in most patients, though some appear to experience remission. Infection is the most frequent cause of death, usually from *Staphylococcus aureus* septicemia.

Enk AH et al: Mycophenolate is effective in the treatment of pemphigus vulgaris. Arch Dermatol 1999;135:54. [NLM Cit ID: 99120656]

Fleischli ME et al: Pulse intravenous cyclophosphamide therapy in pemphigus. Arch Dermatol 1999;135:57. [NLM Cit ID: 99120657]

Nousari HC et al: Pemphigus and bullous pemphigoid. Lancet 1999;354:667. [NLM Cit ID: 99394562]

Stanley JR: Therapy of pemphigus vulgaris. Arch Dermatol 1999;131:76. [NLM Cit ID: 9912066]

OTHER BLISTERING DISEASES

Many other skin disorders are characterized by formation of bullae, or blisters. These include bullous pemphigoid, cicatricial pemphigoid, dermatitis herpetiformis, herpes gestationis, and other less common bullous disorders, including the various forms of epidermolysis bullosa, which are due to genetic defects in epidermal keratin and various basement membrane zone components.

Bullous Pemphigoid

Bullous pemphigoid is a relatively benign pruritic disease characterized by tense blisters in flexural areas, usually remitting in 5 or 6 years, with a course characterized by exacerbations and remissions. Most affected persons are over the age of 60 (often in their 70s or 80s), and men are affected twice as frequently as women. The appearance of blisters may be preceded by urticarial or edematous lesions for months. Oral lesions are present in about one-third of affected persons. The disease may occur in various forms, including localized, vesicular, vegetating, erythematous, erythrodermic, and nodular. There is no statistical association with internal malignant disease.

The diagnosis is made by biopsy and direct immunofluorescence examination. Light microscopy shows a subepidermal blister. With direct immunofluorescence, IgG and C3 are found at the dermal-epidermal junction. Circulating anti-basement membrane antibodies can be found in the sera of patients in about 70% of cases.

If the patient has only a few blisters, ultrapotent steroids may be adequate. Prednisone at dosages of 60–80 mg/d is often used to achieve rapid control of more widespread disease. Although slower in onset of action, tetracycline or erythromycin, 1–1.5 g/d, alone or combined with nicotinamide—*not nicotinic acid!*—(up to 1.5 g/d), if tolerated, may control the disease in patients who cannot use corticosteroids or may allow decreasing or eliminating steroids after control is achieved. Dapsone is particularly effective in mucous membrane pemphigoid. If these drugs are not effective, methotrexate, 5–25 mg weekly, or azathioprine, 50 mg one to three times daily, may be used as steroid-sparing agents.

Bouscarat F et al: Treatment of bullous pemphigoid with dapsone: Retrospective study of thirty-six cases. J Am Acad Dermatol 1996;34:683. [NLM Cit ID: 96176738]

Ciarrocca KN et al: A retrospective study of the management of oral mucous membrane pemphigoid with dapsone. Oral Surg Oral Med Oral Pathol Oral Radiol Endod 1999;88:159. [NLM Cit ID: 99396562]

Heilborn JD et al: Low-dose oral pulse methotrexate as monotherapy in elderly patients with bullous pemphigoid. J Am Acad Dermatol 1999;40(5 Part 1):741. [NLM Cit ID: 99253520]

Nousari HC et al: Pemphigus and bullous pemphigoid. Lancet 1999;354:667. [NLM Cit ID: 99394562]

Herpes (Pemphigus) Gestationis

Herpes gestationis occurs in about one in 50,000–60,000 pregnancies. The vesicles and bullae often appear first in periumbilical distribution, and there may be erythematous papules and plaques. It usually begins in the fifth or sixth month of pregnancy, or the onset may be delayed to the postpartum period. The disease is self-limited, but it may recur in subsequent pregnancies. Use of estrogens or progesterone or the onset of menses may trigger flare-ups. The risks to mother and fetus appear to be less significant than was formerly thought but include an increase in prematurity and small-for-gestational-age infants. Blisters are subepidermal, with eosinophils present. Direct immunofluorescence shows C3 at the basement membrane zone in most cases. IgG is found less often.

Corticosteroids are the treatment of choice and are sometimes effective when used topically only.

Jenkins RE et al: Clinical features and management of 87 patients with pemphigoid gestationis. Clin Exp Dermatol 1999;24:255. [NLM Cit ID: 99388336]

PAPULES

WARTS

Essentials of Diagnosis

- Verrucous papules anywhere on the skin or mucous membranes, usually no larger than 1 cm in diameter.
- Prolonged incubation period (average 2–18 months). Spontaneous “cures” are frequent (50%).
- “Recurrences” (new lesions) are frequent.

General Considerations

Warts are caused by human papillomaviruses. The type of mucocutaneous surface infected and the morphology of the wart are closely related to the HPV type causing the infection. Especially in genital warts, simultaneous infection with numerous wart types is common. Genital HPVs are divided into low-risk and high-risk types depending on the likelihood of their association with cervical cancer.

Cervical warts may be transmitted to the newborn via passage through the infected birth canal, causing laryngeal papillomatosis.

Clinical Findings

There are usually no symptoms. Tenderness on pressure occurs with plantar warts; itching occurs with anogenital warts. Occasionally a wart will produce mechanical obstruction (eg, nostril, ear canal, urethra).

Warts vary widely in shape, size, and appearance. Flat warts are most evident under oblique illumination. Subungual warts may be dry, fissured, and hyperkeratotic and may resemble hangnails or other nonspecific changes. Plantar warts resemble plantar corns or calluses.

Differential Diagnosis

Some warty-looking lesions are actually hypertrophic actinic keratoses or squamous cell carcinomas. Some genital warty lesions may be due to secondary syphilis (condylomata lata). The lesions of molluscum contagiosum may be mistaken for warts, especially when they are very large in immunocompromised persons. Seborrheic keratosis may also be confused with warts. In AIDS, wart-like lesions may be caused by varicella-zoster virus.

Prevention

The use of condoms may reduce transmission of genital warts. A person with flat warts should be educated about the infectivity of warts and advised not to scratch or traumatize the areas. Using an electric shaver may prevent autoinoculation.

Treatment

Treatment is aimed at inducing "wart-free" intervals for as long as possible without scarring, since no treatment can guarantee a remission or prevent recurrences. In immunocompromised patients, the goal is even more modest, ie, to control the size and number of lesions present.

A. Removal: For common warts of the hands, patients are usually offered liquid nitrogen or keratolytic agents. The former may work in fewer treatments but requires office visits and is painful. Keratolytic agents are irritating but effective and usually painless if used correctly. They can be used at home but must be applied almost daily for 8–12 weeks for maximum effect.

1. Liquid nitrogen is applied to achieve a thaw time of 20–45 seconds. Two freeze-thaw cycles are given every 2–4 weeks for several visits. Scarring will occur if it is used incorrectly or too aggressively. For example, the face, dorsal hands, and legs are more sensitive than the palms. Improper use along the sides of the fingers has been reported to cause nerve damage and paresthesias. Liquid nitrogen may cause permanent depigmentation in darkly pigmented individuals. It is useful on dry penile warts and on filiform warts involving the face and body. Liquid nitrogen may be used for condylomas, but snipping of lesions followed by light electrodesiccation is more effective.

2. Keratolytic agents–Any of the following salicylic acid products may be used against common warts or plantar warts: Occlusal, Trans Ver-Sal, and Duofilm. Plantar warts may be treated by applying a 40% salicylic acid plaster (Mediplast) after paring. The plaster may be left on for 5–6 days, then removed, the lesion pared down, and another plaster applied. Although it may take weeks or months to eradicate the wart, the method is safe and effective with almost no side effects.

3. Podophyllum resin–Anogenital warts are often initially treated by painting them every 2–3 weeks with 25% podophyllum resin (podophyllin) in compound tincture of benzoin. Pregnant patients should not be so treated. The purified active component of the resin, podofilox, is available for use at home twice daily three consecutive days a week for cycles of 4–6 weeks. It is less irritating and more effective than podophyllum resin. After a single 4-week cycle, 45% of patients were wart-free; but of these, 60% relapsed at 6 weeks. Thus, multiple cycles of treatment are often necessary.

4. Imiquimod–A 5% cream of this local interferon inducer has moderate activity in clearing external genital warts. Seventy-seven percent of women and 40% of men with external genital warts had complete clearing of their lesions, and 90% and 74%, respectively, had greater than 50% reduction in their warts. The superior response in women may relate to enhanced penetration of the moist skin of the vulva as compared with the penile shaft. Treatment is once-daily on 3 alternate days per week. Response may be slow, with patients who eventually cleared having responses at 8 weeks (44%) or 12 weeks (69%). Once cleared, about 13% had recurrences in the short term. This low recurrence rate is encouraging.

There is less pregnancy risk than with podophyllum resin (category B versus category X with podophyllin). It is more expensive than podophyllotoxin, but given the high rate of response in women and its safety and low relapse rate, it appears to be the "patient-administered" treatment of choice in women. In men, the more rapid response, lower cost, and similar efficacy make podophyllotoxin the initial treatment of choice, with imiquimod used for recurrences or refractory cases. Anecdotally, this agent may also have efficacy in superficial flat warts.

5. Operative removal–Plantar warts may be removed by blunt dissection. Local anesthetic is injected into the base, and the wart is then removed with a curette or scissors or by shaving off at the base of the wart with a scalpel. Trichloroacetic acid or Monsel's solution on a tightly wound cotton-tipped applicator may be painted on the wound, or light electrocautery may be used. Excision of warts, however, may result in a permanent painful scar on the foot and is not recommended. For genital warts, snip biopsy (scissors) removal followed by light electrocautery is more effective than cryotherapy and does scar. It is often preferred by patients with pedunculated or large lesions that require multiple cryotherapy or podophyllin treatments for removal.

6. Laser therapy–The CO_2 laser is effective for treating recurrent warts, periungual warts, plantar warts, and condylomata acuminata. It leaves open wounds which must fill in with granulation tissue over 4–6 weeks and is best reserved for warts resistant to other modalities. Lasers with emissions of 585, 595, or 532 nm may also be used every 3–4 weeks to gradually ablate the wart. For genital warts, it has not been shown that laser therapy is more effective than electrosurgical removal.

7. Other agents–Bleomycin diluted to 1 unit/mL may be injected into warts. It has been shown to have a high cure rate for plantar and common warts. It should not be used on digital warts because of the potential complications of Raynaud's phenomenon, nail loss, and terminal digital necrosis.

B. Immunotherapy: Cimetidine in doses of 35–50 mg/kg daily may benefit younger patients with common warts. Squaric acid dibutylester may be effective for resistant warts but is not FDA-approved.

C. Retinoids: Tretinoin (Retin-A) cream or gel applied topically twice daily may be effective (anecdotally) for facial or beard flat warts. Extensive warts have been reported to disappear when oral retinoids are administered for 4–8 weeks.

D. Physical Modalities: Soaking warts in hot (42.2 °C) water for 10–30 minutes daily for 6 weeks has resulted in dramatic involution in some cases.

Prognosis

There is a striking tendency to the development of new lesions. Warts may disappear spontaneously or may be unresponsive to treatment.

Benton EC: Therapy of cutaneous warts. Clin Dermatol 1997;15:449. [NLM Cit ID: 97399323]

Beutner KR et al: Genital warts and their treatment. Clin Infect Dis 1999;28(Suppl 1):S37. [NLM Cit ID: 99152435]

Edwards L: Self-administered topical 5% imiquimod cream for external anogenital warts. Human Papilloma Virus Study Group. Arch Dermatol 1998;134:25. [NLM Cit ID: 98111559]

Kaiser JF et al: Squamous cell carcinoma in situ (Bowen's disease) mimicking subungual verruca vulgaris. J Fam Pract 1994;39:384. [NLM Cit ID: 95016481] (This case report reminds us that wart-like lesions, particularly around the nails and on the feet, that are somewhat atypical and resistant to therapy should be evaluated by biopsy to detect carcinoma.)

McMillan A: The management of difficult anogenital warts. Sex Transm Infect 1999;75:192. [NLM Cit ID: 99377511]

Tyring S et al: Safety and efficacy of 0.5% podofilox gel in the treatment of anogenital warts. Arch Dermatol 1998;134:33. [NLM Cit ID: 98111560]

CALLOSITIES & CORNS OF FEET OR TOES

Callosities and corns are caused by pressure and friction due to faulty weight-bearing, orthopedic deformities, improperly fitting shoes, or neuropathies.

Tenderness on pressure and "after-pain" are the only symptoms. The hyperkeratotic well-localized overgrowths always occur at pressure points. Dermatoglyphics are preserved over the surface. On paring, a glassy core is found (which differentiates these disorders from plantar warts, which have multiple capillary bleeding points or black dots when pared). A soft corn often occurs laterally on the proximal portion of the fourth toe as a result of pressure against the bony structure of the interphalangeal joint of the fifth toe.

Treatment consists of correcting mechanical abnormalities that cause friction and pressure. Shoes must be properly fitted and orthopedic deformities corrected. Callosities may be removed by careful paring of the callus after a warm water soak or with keratolytic agents as found in various brands of corn pads.

Plantar hyperkeratosis of the heels can be treated successfully by using 20% urea (Ureacin 20) nightly and a pumice stone after soaking in water or by applying equal parts of propylene glycol and water nightly and covering with thin polyethylene plastic film (Baggies).

Women who tend to form calluses and corns should not wear confining footgear and high-heeled shoes.

Singh D et al: Callosities, corns, and calluses. BMJ 1996;312:1403. [NLM Cit ID: 96243628]

MOLLUSCUM CONTAGIOSUM

Molluscum contagiosum, caused by a poxvirus, presents as single or multiple rounded, dome-shaped, waxy papules 2–5 mm in diameter that are umbilicated. Lesions at first are firm, solid, and flesh-colored but upon reaching maturity become softened, whitish, or pearly gray and may suppurate. The principal sites of involvement are the face, lower abdomen, and genitals.

The lesions are autoinoculable and spread by wet skin-to-skin contact. In sexually active individuals, they may be confined to the penis, pubis, and inner thighs and are considered a sexually transmitted disease.

Molluscum contagiosum is one of the common viral infections seen in patients with AIDS, usually with a helper T cell count < 100/μL. AIDS patients tend to develop extensive lesions over the face and neck as well as in the genital area.

The diagnosis is easily established in most instances because of the distinctive central umbilication of the dome-shaped lesion. The best treatment is by curettage or applications of liquid nitrogen as for warts—but more briefly, since molluscum contagiosum is more responsive to therapy than warts. When lesions are frozen, the central umbilication often becomes more apparent. Light electrosurgery with a fine needle is also effective. Imiquimod applied three to seven times weekly for 4–8 weeks may lead to clearing. It has been estimated that individual lesions persist for about 2 months. They are difficult to eradicate in patients with HIV infection unless immunity improves, in which case miraculous spontaneous clearing may occur.

Cattelan AM et al: A complete remission of recalcitrant molluscum contagiosum in an AIDS patient following highly active antiretroviral therapy (HAART). J Infect 1999;38:58. [NLM Cit ID: 99188924]

Ordoukhanian E et al: Warts and molluscum contagiosum: Beware of treatments worse than the disease. Postgrad Med 1997;101:223, 229, 235. [NLM Cit ID: 97198962]

BASAL CELL CARCINOMA

Basal cell carcinomas are the most common form of cancer. They occur on sun-exposed skin in otherwise normal fair-skinned individuals. The most common presentation is a papule or nodule that may have a central scab or erosion. Occasionally the nodules have a brown-gray color or have stippled pigment (pigmented basal cell carcinoma). Intradermal nevi without pigment on the face of older white individuals may resemble basal cell carcinomas. Basal cell carcinomas grow slowly, attaining a size of 1–2 cm or more in diameter, often after years of growth. There is a waxy, "pearly" appearance, with telangiectatic vessels easily visible. It is the pearly or translucent quality of these lesions that is most diagnostic, and that feature may be best appreciated if the skin is stretched. Less common types include morpheaform or scar-like lesions. These are hypopigmented, somewhat thickened plaques. On the back and chest, basal cell carcinomas appear as reddish, somewhat shiny, scaly plaques.

Clinicians should examine the skin routinely, looking for bumps, patches, and scabbed lesions. When examining the face, look at the eyelid margins and medial canthi, the nose and alar folds, the lips, and then around and behind the ears. While metastases almost never occur, therapy of basal cell carcinomas may cause significant cosmetic deformity in these areas, particularly for inadequately treated or recurrent lesions. Neglected lesions may ulcerate and produce great destruction. Basal cell carcinomas of the medial canthi are particularly dangerous. Recurrent lesions around the nose and ears may track along cartilage underneath the skin, requiring treatment of much more extensive areas than are apparent from inspection.

Lesions suspected to be basal cell carcinomas should be biopsied, by shave or punch biopsy. Therapy is then aimed at eradication with minimal cosmetic deformity, often by excision and suturing with recurrence rates of 5% or less. The technique of three cycles of curettage and electrodesiccation depends on the skill of the operator and is not recommended for head and neck lesions. After 4–6 weeks of healing, it leaves a broad, hypopigmented, at times hypertrophic scar. Radiotherapy is effective and often appropriate for older individuals (over 65), but recurrent tumors after radiation therapy are more difficult to treat and may be more aggressive. Mohs surgery—removal of the tumor followed by immediate frozen section histopathologic examination of margins with subsequent reexcision of tumor-positive areas and final closure of the defect—gives the highest cure rates (98%) and results in least tissue loss. It is appropriate therapy for tumors of the eyelids or for recurrent lesions, or where tissue sparing is needed for cosmesis. Sun avoidance, particularly in children, is essential to lower the incidence of new basal cell cancers. Patients with basal cell carcinomas must be followed for 5 years to detect new or recurrent lesions.

Frisch M et al: Risk for subsequent cancer after diagnosis of basal-cell carcinoma: A population-based, epidemiologic study (see comments). Ann Intern Med 1996;125:815. [NLM Cit ID: 97037755]

JAMA patient page: Skin cancer. JAMA 1999;281:676. [NLM Cit ID: 99151590]

Lear JT et al: Basal cell carcinoma. Postgrad Med J 1997;73:538. [NLM Cit ID: 98040922]

Schottenfeld D: Basal-cell carcinoma of the skin: A harbinger of cutaneous and noncutaneous multiple primary cancer. (Editorial and comment.) Ann Intern Med 1996;125:852. [NLM Cit ID: 97037761]

SQUAMOUS CELL CARCINOMA

Squamous cell carcinoma usually occurs on exposed parts in fair-skinned individuals who sunburn easily and tan poorly. It may arise from an actinic keratosis. The lesions appear as small red, conical, hard nodules that occasionally ulcerate. They are not as distinctive as basal cell carcinomas and are more easily misdiagnosed clinically. The frequency of metastasis is not precisely known, though metastatic spread is said to be less likely with squamous cell carcinoma arising out of actinic keratoses than with those that arise de novo. In actinically induced squamous cell cancers, rates of metastasis are estimated from retrospective studies to be 3–7%. Squamous cell carcinomas of the lip, oral cavity, tongue, and genitalia have much higher rates of metastasis and require special management.

Keratoacanthomas most often act in benign fashion but resemble squamous cell carcinoma histologically and for all practical purposes should be treated as though they were skin cancers.

Examination of the skin and therapy are essentially the same as for basal cell carcinoma. The preferred treatment of squamous cell carcinoma is excision. Electrodesiccation and curettage and x-ray radiation may be used for some lesions, and fresh tissue microscopically controlled excision (Mohs) is excellent treatment also. Some keratoacanthomas respond to intralesional injection of fluorouracil or methotrexate, but they must be excised if they do not. Follow-up for squamous cell carcinoma must be more frequent and thorough than for basal cell carcinoma, starting at every 3 months, with careful examination of lymph nodes. In addition, palpation of the lips is essential to detect hard or indurated areas that represent early squamous cell carcinoma. All such cases must be biopsied. Multiple squamous cell carcinomas are very common on the sun-exposed skin of organ transplant patients because of the host's immunosuppressed state. The tumors begin to appear after 5 years of immunosuppression. Biologic behavior may be aggressive, and careful management is required.

Bernstein SC et al: The many faces of squamous cell carcinoma. Dermatol Surg 1996;22:243. [NLM Cit ID: 96178087]

JAMA patient page: Skin cancer. JAMA 1999;281:676. [NLM Cit ID: 99151590]

Levi F et al: Incidence of invasive cancers following squamous cell skin cancer. Am J Epidemiol 1997;146:734. [NLM Cit ID: 98033416]

VIOLACEOUS TO PURPLE PAPULES & NODULES

LICHEN PLANUS

Essentials of Diagnosis

- Pruritic, violaceous, flat-topped papules with fine white streaks and symmetric distribution.
- Lacy lesions of the buccal mucosa.
- Commonly seen along linear scratch marks (Koebner phenomenon) on anterior wrists, penis, legs.
- Histopathologic examination is diagnostic.

General Considerations

Lichen planus is an inflammatory pruritic disease of the skin and mucous membranes characterized by distinctive papules with a predilection for the flexor surfaces and trunk. It is most often idiopathic. The three cardinal findings are typical skin lesions, mucosal lesions, and histopathologic features of band-like infiltration of lymphocytes and melanophages in the dermis. Drugs causing lichen planus-like reactions include gold, streptomycin, tetracycline, iodides, chloroquine, quinacrine, quinidine, NSAIDs, phenothiazines, and hydrochlorothiazide. Hepatitis C infection is found with greater frequency in lichen planus patients than in controls in Europe and the USA. Erosive lesions are more common in hepatitis C-associated lichen planus. Lichen planus has been seen after exposure to color film developing solutions.

Clinical Findings

Itching is mild to severe. The lesions are violaceous, flat-topped, angulated papules, 1–4 mm in diameter, discrete or in clusters, with very fine white streaks on the surface (Wickham's striae) on the flexor surfaces of the wrists and on the penis, lips, tongue, and buccal and vaginal mucous membranes. Mucosal lichen planus has been reported in the genital and anorectal areas, the gastrointestinal tract, the bladder, the larynx, and the conjunctiva. The papules may become bullous or ulcerated. The disease may be generalized. Mucous membrane lesions have a lacy white network overlying them that may be confused with leukoplakia. The Koebner phenomenon (appearance of lesions in areas of trauma) may be seen.

A special form of lichen planus is the erosive or ulcerative variety. On palms and soles, it can be disabling. It is a major problem in the mouth or vagina, and squamous cell carcinoma may develop.

Differential Diagnosis

Lichen planus must be distinguished from similar lesions produced by medications (see above) and other papular lesions such as psoriasis, lichen simplex chronicus, and syphilis. Lichen planus on the mucous membranes must be differentiated from leukoplakia. Erosive oral lesions require biopsy and often direct immunofluorescence for diagnosis since lichen planus may simulate other bullous diseases. Histologic examination may make the distinction from graft-versus-host disease and in some cases from lichen planus-like drug eruptions.

Treatment

A. Topical Therapy: Superpotent topical corticosteroids such as betamethasone dipropionate in optimized vehicle, diflorasone diacetate, clobetasol propionate, and halobetasol propionate ointments applied twice daily are most helpful for localized disease in nonflexural areas. Alternatively, high-potency corticosteroid cream or ointment may be used nightly under thin pliable plastic film.

Application of tretinoin cream 0.05% to mucosal lichen planus, followed by a corticosteroid ointment, may be helpful. For disabling hypertrophic lichen planus of the soles, tretinoin cream applied and covered with thin, pliable polyethylene film nightly is said to be effective.

B. Systemic Therapy: Corticosteroids (see Chapter 26) may be required in severe cases, or where the most rapid response to treatment is desired. Unfortunately, relapse almost always occurs as the steroids are tapered, making systemic corticosteroid therapy an impractical option for the management of chronic lichen planus.

Isotretinoin and acitretin by mouth appear to be effective in some cases of oral and cutaneous lichen planus.

Psoralens plus long-wave ultraviolet light (PUVA) may be effective treatment for lichen planus.

Prognosis

Lichen planus is a benign disease, but it may persist for months or years and may be recurrent. Hypertrophic lichen planus and oral lesions tend to be especially persistent, and neoplastic degeneration has been described in chronically eroded lesions. The oral retinoids appear to induce remissions and facilitate healing of erosive lesions in some patients.

Lewis FM et al: Vulval involvement in lichen planus: A study of 37 women. Br J Dermatol 1996;135:89. [NLM Cit ID: 96372551]

Lodi G et al: Hepatitis C virus infection and lichen planus: A short review. Oral Dis 1997;3:77. [NLM Cit ID: 98128452]

Lozada-Nur F et al: Oral lichen planus: Epidemiology, clinical characteristics, and associated diseases. Semin Cutan Med Surg 1997;16:273. [NLM Cit ID: 98081571]

Porter SR et al: Development of squamous cell carcinoma in hepatitis C virus-associated lichen planus. Oral Oncol 1997;33:58. [NLM Cit ID: 97328156]

KAPOSI'S SARCOMA

Before 1980 in the USA, this rare malignant skin lesion was seen mostly in elderly white men, had a chronic clinical course, and was rarely fatal. Kaposi's sarcoma occurs endemically in an often aggressive form in young black men of equatorial Africa, but it is rare in American blacks. Epidemic clusters of Kaposi's sarcoma, predominantly in homosexual men with AIDS, have been found in large cities of the USA. A novel herpesvirus, human herpes virus 8 (HHV-8) or Kaposi's sarcoma-associated herpes virus (KSHV), is universally present in all forms of Kaposi's sarcoma (endemic Kaposi's sarcoma in Africa, Kaposi's sarcoma in elderly males, and HIV associated Kaposi's sarcoma). The epidemiology of infection with this virus parallels the incidence of Kaposi's sarcoma in various risk groups and geographic regions. For example, it is a common infection in central Africa, is more common in Italy than in the USA, and is common in HIV-infected homosexual men and rare in HIV-infected hemophiliacs. The virus is present in the skin lesions and circulating B lymphocytes of persons with Kaposi's sarcoma, but uncommonly in their normal skin. A serologic test is available to detect infection with this virus, but its sensitivity is insufficient for commercial use at this time.

Red, purple, or dark plaques or nodules on cutaneous or mucosal surfaces should alert the clinician to the possibility of the disease. Kaposi's sarcoma commonly involves the gastrointestinal tract, but in asymptomatic patients these lesions are not sought or treated. Pulmonary Kaposi's sarcoma may be life-threatening and is managed aggressively. The incidence of AIDS-associated Kaposi's sarcoma appears to be diminishing.

For Kaposi's sarcoma in the elderly, palliative local therapy with intralesional chemotherapy or radiation is usually all that is required. In the setting of iatrogenic immunosuppression, the treatment of Kaposi's sarcoma is primarily reduction of doses of immunosuppressive medications. In AIDS-associated Kaposi's sarcoma, the patient should first be given effective anti-HIV antiretrovirals (including a protease inhibitor), because in some cases this treatment alone is associated with improvement. Other therapeutic options include cryotherapy or intralesional vinblastine (0.1–0.5 mg/mL) for cosmetically objectionable lesions; radiation therapy for accessible and space-occupying lesions; and laser surgery for certain intraoral and pharyngeal lesions. Systemic chemotherapy is indicated in patients with rapidly progressive skin disease (more than ten new lesions per month), with edema or pain, and with symptomatic visceral disease or pulmonary disease. Liposomal doxorubicin is highly effective in controlling these cases and has considerably less toxicity—and greater efficacy—than anthracycline monotherapy or combination chemotherapeutic regimens.

Brenner B et al: Tailoring treatment for classical Kaposi's sarcoma: comprehensive clinical guidelines. Int J Oncol 1999;14:1097. [NLM Cit ID: 99272785]

Jaffe HW et al: Human herpesvirus 8 and Kaposi's sarcoma—some answers, more questions. N Engl J Med 1999;340:1912. [NLM Cit ID: 99280046]

Northfelt DW et al: Efficacy of pegylated-liposomal doxorubicin in the treatment of AIDS-related Kaposi's sarcoma after failure of standard chemotherapy. J Clin Oncol 1997;15:653. [NLM Cit ID: 97178757]

PRURITUS (Itching)

Pruritus is a disagreeable sensation that provokes a desire to scratch. It is modulated by central factors, including cortical ones. Not all cases of pruritus are mediated by histamine.

Although many cases of generalized pruritus can be attributed to dry skin—whether naturally occurring and precipitated or aggravated by climatic conditions or arising from disease states—there are many other causes: scabies, dermatitis herpetiformis, atopic dermatitis, pruritus vulvae et ani, miliaria, insect bites, pediculosis, contact dermatitis, drug reactions, urticaria, urticarial eruptions of pregnancy, psoriasis, lichen planus, lichen simplex chronicus, exfoliative dermatitis, folliculitis, bullous pemphigoid, and fiberglass dermatitis.

Persistent pruritus not explained by cutaneous disease should prompt a staged workup for systemic causes. Perhaps the commonest cause of pruritus associated with systemic disease is uremia in conjunction with hemodialysis. Both this condition and the pruritus of obstructive biliary disease may be helped by phototherapy with ultraviolet B or PUVA. Naltrexone and nalmefene have been shown to relieve the pruritus of biliary cholestasis; naltrexone is effective also in management of other forms of pruritus. Endocrine disorders such as hypo- or hyperthyroidism, psychiatric disturbances, lymphoma, leukemia, and other internal malignant disorders, iron deficiency anemia, and certain neurologic disorders may also cause pruritus. Danazol, 400–800 mg daily, may be tried for pruritus associated with myeloproliferative disorders and other systemic illnesses.

Burning or itching involving the face, scalp, and genitalia may be manifestations of primary depression and treatable with antidepressant drugs such as amitriptyline, imipramine, or doxepin.

Prognosis

Elimination of external factors and irritating agents may give complete relief from pruritus. Pruritus accompanying specific skin disease will subside when the disease is controlled. Idiopathic pruritus and that accompanying serious internal disease may not respond to any type of therapy.

Bergasa NV et al: Oral nalmefene therapy reduces scratching activity due to the pruritus of cholestasis: a controlled study. J Am Acad Dermatol 1999;41(3 Part 1):431. [NLM Cit ID: 99389764]

Greaves MW: Anti-itch treatments: Do they work? Skin Pharmacol 1997;10:225. [NLM Cit ID: 96359646]

Gupta AK et al: Tinea capitis: an overview with emphasis on management. Pediatr Dermatol 1999;16:171. [NLM Cit ID: 99316048]

Kolodny L et al: Danazol relieves refractory pruritus associated with myeloproliferative disorders and other diseases. Am J Hematol 1996;51:112. [NLM Cit ID: 96160428]

Metze D et al: Efficacy and safety of naltrexone, an oral opiate receptor antagonist, in the treatment of pruritus in internal and dermatological diseases. J Am Acad Dermatol 1999;41:533. [NLM Cit ID: 99426897]

ANOGENITAL PRURITUS

Essentials of Diagnosis

- Itching, chiefly nocturnal, of the anogenital area.
- Examination is highly variable, ranging from no skin findings to excoriations and inflammation of any degree, including lichenification.

General Considerations

Most cases have no obvious cause, but multiple specific causes have been identified. Anogenital pruritus may be due to intertrigo, psoriasis, lichen simplex chronicus, or seborrheic or contact dermatitis (from soaps, colognes, douches, contraceptives, and perhaps scented toilet tissue), or it may be due to irritating secretions, as in diarrhea, leukorrhea, or trichomoniasis, or to local disease (candidiasis, dermatophytosis, erythrasma). Oxyuriasis (pinworm) is a rare cause in adults. Psychologic abnormalities are usually not evident. Lichen sclerosus et atrophicus may at times be the cause. Erythrasma is easily diagnosed by demonstration of coral-red fluorescence with Wood's light; it is easily cured with erythromycin orally and topically.

Uncleanliness may be at fault. In pruritus ani, hemorrhoids are often found, and leakage of mucus and bacteria from the distal rectum onto the perianal skin may be important in cases in which no other skin abnormality is found.

Many women experience pruritus vulvae. In women, pruritus ani by itself is rare, and pruritus vulvae does not usually involve the anal area, though anal itching will usually spread to the vulva. In men, pruritus of the scrotum is most commonly seen in the absence of pruritus ani. When all possible known causes have been ruled out, the condition is diagnosed as idiopathic or essential pruritus—by no means rare.

Clinical Findings

A. Symptoms and Signs: The only symptom is itching, which is chiefly nocturnal. Physical findings are usually not present, but there may be erythema, fissuring, maceration, lichenification, excoriations, or changes suggestive of candidiasis or tinea.

B. Laboratory Findings: Urinalysis and blood glucose testing may lead to a diagnosis of diabetes mellitus. Microscopic examination or culture of tissue scrapings may reveal yeasts or fungi. Stool examination may show pinworms.

Differential Diagnosis

The etiologic differential diagnosis consists of candida infection, parasitosis, local irritation from contact with drugs and irritants, and other primary skin disorders of the genital area such as psoriasis, seborrhea, intertrigo, or lichen sclerosus et atrophicus.

Prevention

Instruct the patient in proper anogenital hygiene after treating systemic or local conditions.

Treatment

A. General Measures: Treating constipation, preferably with high-fiber management (psyllium), may help. Instruct the patient to use very soft or moistened tissue or cotton after bowel movements and to clean the perianal area thoroughly with cool water if possible. Women should use similar precautions after urinating. Instruct the patient regarding the harmful and pruritus-inducing effects of scratching.

B. Local Measures: Pramoxine cream or lotion or hydrocortisone-pramoxine (Pramosone), 1% or 2.5% cream, lotion, or ointment, is helpful in managing pruritus in the anogenital area. The ointment or cream should be applied after a bowel movement. Iodochlorhydroxyquin-hydrocortisone creams are useful also but may stain underwear. Potent fluorinated topical corticosteroids may lead to atrophy and striae if used for more than a few days and should in general be avoided. This includes combinations with antifungals. The use of strong steroids on the scrotum may lead to persistent severe burning upon withdrawal of the drug. Soaks with aluminum subacetate solution, 1:20, are of value if the area is acutely inflamed and oozing. Underclothing should be changed daily. Affected areas may be painted with Castellani's solution. Balneol Perianal Cleansing Lotion or Tucks premoistened pads, ointment, or cream (all Tucks preparations contain witch hazel) may be very useful for pruritus ani.

Prognosis

Although benign, anogenital pruritus may be persistent and recurrent.

Vincent C: Anorectal pain and irritation: anal fissure, levator syndrome, proctalgia fugax, and pruritus ani. Prim Care 1999;26:53. [NLM Cit ID: 99121156]

SCABIES

Essentials of Diagnosis

- Generalized itching.
- Pruritic vesicles and pustules in "runs" or "galleries," especially on finger webs and the heels of the palms and in wrist creases.
- Mites, ova, and brown dots of feces visible microscopically.
- Red papules or nodules on the scrotum and on the penile glans and shaft are pathognomonic.

General Considerations

Scabies is caused by infestation with *Sarcoptes scabiei*. The infestation usually spares the head and neck (though even these areas may be involved in infants, in the elderly, and in patients with AIDS). Scabies is usually acquired by sleeping with or in the bedding of an infested individual or by other close contact. The entire household may be affected.

Clinical Findings

A. Symptoms and Signs: Itching is almost always present and can be quite severe. The lesions consist of more or less generalized excoriations with small pruritic vesicles, pustules, and "runs" or "burrows" on the sides of the fingers and the heels of the palms, wrists, elbows, and around the axillae. Often, burrows are found only on the feet, as they have been scratched off in other locations. The burrow appears as a short irregular mark, 2–3 mm long and the width of a hair. Characteristic lesions may occur on the nipples in females and as pruritic papules on the scrotum or penis in males. Pruritic papules may be seen over the buttocks.

B. Laboratory Findings: The diagnosis should be confirmed by microscopic demonstration of the organism, ova, or feces in a mounted specimen. The success of this procedure depends on choosing the best unexcoriated lesions from interdigital webs, wrists, elbows, or feet. A bit of immersion oil is placed on the lesion and a No. 15 blade is used to scrape the lesion until it is flat. Pinpoint bleeding may result from the scraping. The diagnosis can also be confirmed in most cases with the burrow ink test. Apply ink to the burrow and then do a very superficial shave biopsy by sawing off the burrow with a No. 15 blade, painlessly and bloodlessly. The mite, ova, and feces can be seen under the light microscope.

Differential Diagnosis

Scabies must be distinguished from the various forms of pediculosis and from other causes of pruritus.

Treatment & Prognosis

Treatment is aimed at killing scabies mites and controlling the dermatitis, which can persist for months after effective eradication of the mites, with midpotency topical steroids. Bedding and clothing should be laundered or cleaned or set aside for 14 days in plastic bags. Unless the lesions are complicated by severe secondary pyoderma, treatment consists primarily of disinfestation. If secondary pyoderma is present, it should be treated with systemic antibiotics. Unless treatment is aimed at all infected persons in a family or institutionalized group, reinfestations will probably occur. Resistance to 5% permethrin cream is rare.

Disinfestation with lindane (gamma benzene hexachloride), 1% in cream or lotion base, applied from the neck down overnight, may be used in adults. A warning has been issued by the FDA regarding potential neurotoxicity, and any use of lindane in infants and pregnant women or in any patient with widespread excoriations and open skin —as well as overuse in adults—is discouraged. This preparation can be used before secondary infection is controlled.

Permethrin 5% cream is highly effective and safe in the management of scabies. Treatment consists of a single application for 8–12 hours. It may be repeated in 1 week. The drug has been used safely in infants aged 2 months to 5 years and is the treatment of choice in children. An alternative drug is crotamiton cream or lotion, which may be applied in the same way as lindane but is used nightly for 4 nights. It is far less effective if used for only 48 hours.

Pregnant patients should be treated only if they have documented scabies themselves. Permethrin 5% cream once for 12 hours—or 5% or 6% sulfur in petrolatum applied nightly for 3 nights from the collarbones down—may be used.

Benzyl benzoate may be compounded as a lotion or emulsion in strengths from 20% to 35% and used as generalized applications (from collarbones down) overnight for two treatments 1 week apart. The USP formula is 275 mL benzyl benzoate (containing 5 g of triethanolamine and 20 g of oleic acid) in water to make 1000 mL. It is cosmetically acceptable, clean, and not overly irritating. Patients will continue to itch for several weeks after treatment. Use of triamcinolone 0.1% cream will help resolve the dermatitis. Scabies in nursing home patients, institutionalized or mentally impaired (especially Down's syndrome) patients, and AIDS patients may be much more difficult to treat. Failures with a single application of permethrin may be treated with repeated weekly applications or by the use of ivermectin, 200 μg/kg. While a single dose of ivermectin may be effective, a second dose 1 week later is superior

Persistent pruritic postscabietic papules may be treated with mid- to high-potency steroids or with intralesional triamcinolone acetonide (2.5–5 mg/mL).

Chouela EN et al: Equivalent therapeutic efficacy and safety of ivermectin and lindane in the treatment of human scabies. Arch Dermatol 1999;135:651. [NLM Cit ID: 99303184]

Meinking TL et al: Safety of permethrin vs lindane for the treatment of scabies. (Editorial and comment.) Arch Dermatol 1996;132:959. [NLM Cit ID: 96326147]

Taplin D et al: Treatment of HIV-related scabies with emphasis on the efficacy of ivermectin. Semin Cutan Med Surg 1997;16:235. [NLM Cit ID: 97444103]

PEDICULOSIS

Essentials of Diagnosis

- Pruritus with excoriation.
- Nits on hair shafts; lice on skin or clothes.
- Occasionally, sky-blue macules (maculae ceruleae) on the inner thighs or lower abdomen in pubic louse infestation.

General Considerations

Pediculosis is a parasitic infestation of the skin of the scalp, trunk, or pubic areas. Body lice usually occur among people who live in overcrowded dwellings with inadequate hygiene facilities. Pubic lice may be acquired by sexual transmission. Head lice may be transmitted by shared use of hats or combs and are epidemic among children of all socioeconomic classes in elementary schools. Head lice are very uncommon among black children. Adults contacting children with head lice frequently acquire the infestation.

There are three different varieties: (1) pediculosis pubis, caused by *Pthirus pubis* (pubic louse, "crabs"); (2) pediculosis corporis, by *Pediculus humanus* var *corporis* (body louse); and (3) pediculosis capitis, by *Pediculus humanus* var *capitis* (head louse).

Head and body lice are similar in appearance and are 3–4 mm long. The body louse can seldom be found on the body, because the insect comes onto the skin only to feed and must be looked for in the seams of the clothing. Trench fever, relapsing fever, and typhus are transmitted by the body louse in countries where those diseases are endemic.

Clinical Findings

Itching may be very intense in body louse infestations, and scratching may result in deep excoriations, especially over the upper shoulders, posterior flanks, and neck. In some cases, only itching is present, with few excoriations seen. Pyoderma may be the presenting sign in any of these infestations. Head lice can be found on the scalp or may be manifested as small nits resembling pussy willow buds on the scalp hairs close to the skin. They are easiest to see above the ears and at the nape of the neck. Pubic louse infestations are occasionally generalized, particularly in hairy individuals; the lice may even be found on the eyelashes and in the scalp.

Differential Diagnosis

Head louse infestation must be distinguished from seborrheic dermatitis, body louse infestation from scabies, and pubic louse infestation from anogenital pruritus and eczema.

Treatment

Body lice are treated by disposing of the infested clothing. For pubic lice, lindane lotion or cream (Kwell, Scabene) is used. A thin layer is applied to the infested and adjacent hairy areas. It is removed after 8 hours by thorough washing. Permethrin rinse 1% for 10 minutes and permethrin cream 5% applied for 8 hours are effective alternatives. Remaining nits may be removed with a fine-toothed comb or forceps. Sexual contacts should be treated. Clothes and bedclothes should be washed and dried at high temperature if possible.

Permethrin 1% cream rinse (Nix) is a topical OTC pediculicide and ovicide and is the treatment of choice for head lice. It is applied to the scalp and hair and left on for 30 minutes to 8 hours before being rinsed off. Treatment should be repeated in 1 week. Permethrin 1% cream (Nix) is more effective than synergized pyrethrins (RID), OTC products that are applied undiluted until the infested areas are entirely wet. After 10 minutes, the areas are washed thoroughly with warm water and soap and then dried. Nits may be treated as indicated above. For involvement of eyelashes, petrolatum is applied thickly twice daily for 8 days, and remaining nits are then plucked off. Adults with head lice virtually always acquire their infestation from elementary school-aged children, so a source of infection must always be sought. Head lice are extremely difficult to eradicate in the epidemic setting, probably because the currently available pediculicides are not uniformly ovicidal when applied as directed.

Drugs for head lice. Med Lett Drugs Ther 1997;39:6. [NLM Cit ID: 97161427]

Parish LC et al: The saga of ectoparasitoses: scabies and pediculosis. Int J Dermatol 1999;38:432. [NLM Cit ID: 99323710]

SKIN LESIONS DUE TO OTHER ARTHROPODS

Essentials of Diagnosis

- Localized rash with pruritus.
- Furuncle-like lesions containing live arthropods.
- Tender erythematous patches that migrate ("larva migrans").
- Generalized urticaria or erythema multiforme in some patients.

General Considerations

Some arthropods (eg, most pest mosquitoes and biting flies) are readily detected as they bite. Many others are not, eg, because they are too small, because there is no immediate reaction, or because they bite during sleep. Reactions may be delayed for many hours; many are allergic. Patients are most apt to consult a physician when the lesions are multiple and pruritus is intense.

Many persons will react severely only to their earliest contacts with an arthropod, thus presenting pruritic lesions when traveling, moving into new quarters, etc. Body lice, fleas, bedbugs, and mosquitoes should be considered. Spiders are often incorrectly believed to be the source of bites; they rarely attack humans, though the brown spider *(Loxosceles laeta, Loxosceles reclusa)* may cause severe necrotic reactions and death due to intravascular hemolysis, and the black widow spider *(Latrodectus mactans)* may cause severe systemic symptoms and death. (See also Chapter 39.)

In addition to arthropod bites, the most common lesions are venomous stings (wasps, hornets, bees, ants, scorpions) or bites (centipedes), furuncle-like lesions due to fly maggots or sand fleas in the skin, and a linear creeping eruption due to a migrating larva.

Clinical Findings

The diagnosis may be difficult when the patient has not noticed the initial attack but suffers a delayed reaction. Individual bites are often in clusters and tend to occur either on exposed parts (eg, midges and gnats) or under clothing, especially around the waist or at flexures (eg, small mites or insects in bedding or clothing). The reaction is often delayed for 1–24 hours or more. Pruritus is almost always present and may be all but intolerable once the patient starts to scratch. Secondary infection may follow scratching. Urticarial wheals are common. Papules may become vesicular. The diagnosis is aided by searching for exposure to arthropods and by considering the patient's occupation and recent activities.

The principal arthropods are as follows:

(1) Fleas: Fleas are bloodsucking ectoparasites that feed on dogs, cats, humans, and other species. Flea saliva produces papular urticaria in sensitized individuals. *Ctenocephalides felis* and *Ctenocephalides canis* are the most common species found on cats and dogs, and both species attack humans. The human flea is *Pulex irritans.*

To break the life cycle of the flea, one must treat the home, pets, and outside environment, using quick-kill insecticides, residual insecticides, and a growth regulator. Obviously, this is a repetitive job.

(2) Bedbugs: In crevices of beds or furniture; bites tend to occur in lines or clusters. Papular urticaria is a characteristic lesion of bedbug *(Cimex lectularius)* bites. The closely related kissing bug has a painful bite.

(3) Ticks: Usually picked up by brushing against low vegetation. Ticks may transmit Rocky Mountain spotted fever, Lyme disease, relapsing fever, and ehrlichiosis.

(4) Chiggers or red bugs: These are larvae of trombiculid mites. A few species confined to particular regions and locally recognized habitats (eg, berry patches, woodland edges, lawns, brush turkey mounds in Australia, poultry farms) attack humans, often around the waist, on the ankles, or in flexures, raising intensely itching erythematous papules after a delay of many hours. The red chiggers may sometimes be seen in the center of papules that have not yet been scratched.

(5) Bird and rodent mites: Larger than chiggers, bird mites infest pigeon lofts or nests of birds in eaves. Bites are multiple anywhere on the body. Room air conditioning units may suck in bird mites and infest the inhabitants of the room. Rodent mites from mice or rats may cause similar effects. The diagnosis of bird mites, rodent mites, or carpet mites may easily be overlooked and the patient treated for other dermatoses.

(6) Mites in stored products: These are white and almost invisible and infest products such as copra, vanilla pods, sugar, straw, cottonseeds, and cereals. Persons who handle these products may be attacked, especially on the hands and forearms and sometimes on the feet. Infested bedding may occasionally lead to generalized dermatitis.

(7) Caterpillars of moths with urticating hairs: The hairs are blown from cocoons or carried by emergent moths, causing severe and often seasonally recurrent outbreaks after mass emergence. The gypsy moth is a cause in the eastern USA.

(8) Tungiasis: Tungiasis is due to the burrowing flea known as *Tunga penetrans* and is found in Africa, the West Indies, and South and Central America. The female burrows under the skin, sucks blood, swells to 0.5 cm, and then ejects her eggs onto the ground. Ulceration, lymphangitis, gangrene, and septicemia may result, in some cases with lethal effect. Ethyl chloride spray will kill the insect when applied to the lesion, and disinfestation may be accomplished with insecticide applied to the terrain. Simple surgical excision is usually performed.

Differential Diagnosis

Arthropods should be considered in the differential diagnosis of skin lesions showing any of the above symptoms.

Prevention

Arthropod infestations are best prevented by avoidance of contaminated areas, personal cleanliness, and disinfection of clothing, bedclothes, and furniture as indicated. Chiggers, bedbugs, and mites

ficiency, either with obvious varicosities or with a past history of thrombophlebitis, or with immobility of the calf muscle group (paraplegics, etc). Red, pruritic patches of stasis dermatitis often precede ulceration. Because venous insufficiency is the most common cause of lower leg ulceration, testing of venous competence is still a required part of the evaluation even when no changes of venous insufficiency are present.

Clinical Findings

A. Symptoms and Signs: Classically, chronic edema is followed by a dermatitis, which is often pruritic. These changes are followed by hyperpigmentation, skin breakdown, and eventually sclerosis of the skin of the lower leg. The ulcer base may be clean, but it often has a yellow fibrin eschar that often requires surgical treatment. Ulcers that appear on the feet, toes, or above the knees should be approached with other diagnoses in mind.

B. Laboratory Findings: Thorough evaluation of the patient's vascular system (including measurement of the ankle/brachial index) is essential. Doppler and light rheography examinations as office procedures are usually sufficient (except in the diabetic) to elucidate the cause of most vascular cases of lower leg ulceration.

Differential Diagnosis

The differential includes vasculitis, pyoderma gangrenosum, arterial ulcerations, infection, trauma, insect bites (spiders) and sickle cell anemia. When the diagnosis is in doubt, a punch biopsy from the border (not base) of the lesion may be helpful.

Prevention

Compression stockings to reduce edema are the most important means of prevention. Compression should achieve a pressure of 30 mm Hg below the knee and 40 mm Hg at the ankle. The stockings should not be used in patients with arterial insufficiency with an ankle-brachial pressure index less than 0.7. Pneumatic sequential compression devices may be of great benefit.

Treatment

A. Local Measures: Institution of compression therapy is begun with cleaning of the ulcer. The patient is instructed to clean the base with saline or cleansers such as Saf-clens or Cara-klenz daily. A curette or small scissors can be used to remove the yellow fibrin eschar, under local anesthesia if the areas are very tender.

Once the base is clean, the ulcer is treated with metronidazole gel to reduce bacterial growth and odor. Any red dermatitic skin is treated with a medium- to high-potency steroid ointment. The ulcer is then covered with an occlusive hydroactive dressing (Duoderm or Cutinova) or a polyurethane foam (Allevyn) followed by an Unna zinc paste boot. This is changed weekly. The ulcer should begin to heal within weeks, and healing should be complete within 2–3 months. If the patient is diabetic, becaplermin (Regranex) may be applied to the ulcer along with good local treatment in those ulcers which are not becoming smaller or developing a granulating base. Some ulcerations require grafting. Full- or split-thickness grafts often do not take, and pinch grafts (small shaves of skin laid onto the bed) may be more effective. Cultured epidermal cell grafts—or Apligraf, a bilayered skin construct—may accelerate wound healing, but they are very expensive. They should be considered in refractory ulcers, especially those which have not healed after a year or more of conservative therapy.

B. Systemic Therapy: If cellulitis accompanies the ulcer, systemic antibiotics are recommended: both dicloxacillin, 250 mg orally four times a day, and ciprofloxacin, 500 mg orally twice a day, are effective.

Prognosis

The combination of compression stockings and newer dressings enables venous stasis ulcers to heal within weeks or months. Newer modalities appear to be effective in recalcitrant cases. Ongoing control of edema is essential to prevent recurrent ulceration.

Alguire PC et al: Chronic venous insufficiency and venous ulceration. J Gen Intern Med 1997;12:374. [NLM Cit ID: 97335590]

Choucair M et al: Compression therapy. Dermatol Surg 1998;24:141. [NLM Cit ID: 98125578]

Douglas WS et al: Guidelines for the management of chronic venous leg ulceration: Report of a multidisciplinary workshop. British Association of Dermatologists and the Research Unit of the Royal College of Physicians. Br J Dermatol 1995;132:446. [NLM Cit ID: 95234555]

Margolis DJ et al: Risk factors associated with the failure of a venous leg ulcer to heal. Arch Dermatol 1999;135:920. [NLM Cit ID: 99383243]

Weinzweig N et al: Free tissue transfer in treatment of the recalcitrant chronic venous ulcer. Ann Plast Surg 1997;38:611. [NLM Cit ID: 97332815]

II. MISCELLANEOUS DERMATOLOGIC DISORDERS*

PIGMENTARY DISORDERS

Although the color of skin may be altered by many diseases and agents, the vast majority of patients have either an increase or decrease in pigment sec-

*Hirsutism is discussed in Chapter 26.

ondary to some inflammatory disease such as acne or atopic dermatitis.

Other pigmentary disorders include those resulting from exposure to exogenous pigments such as carotenemia, argyria, deposition of other metals (such as gold when given chronically for rheumatoid arthritis), and tattooing. Other endogenous pigmentary disorders are attributable to metabolic substances—including hemosiderin (iron)—in purpuric processes; or to homogentisic acid in ochronosis; bile pigments; and carotenes.

Classification

One should first determine whether the disorder is hyper- or hypopigmentation, ie, an increase or decrease in normal skin colors. Each may be considered to be primary or to be secondary to other disorders.

A. Primary Pigmentary Disorders:

1. Hyperpigmentation–The disorders in this category are nevoid, congenital or acquired, and include pigmented nevi, mongolian spots, incontinentia pigmenti, ephelides (juvenile freckles), and lentigines (senile freckles). Hyperpigmentation occurs also in arsenical melanosis or in association with Addison's disease (due to lack of the inhibitory influence of cortisol on the production of MSH by the pituitary gland). Axillary freckling and café au lait spots may be seen in neurofibromatosis. **Melasma (chloasma)** occurs as patterned hyperpigmentation of the face, usually as a direct effect of estrogens and progesterones. It occurs not only during pregnancy but also in 30–50% of women taking oral contraceptives.

2. Hypopigmentation and depigmentation–The disorders in this category are vitiligo, albinism, and piebaldism. In vitiligo, pigment cells (melanocytes) are destroyed. The greater the pigment loss, the fewer the number of melanocytes. Vitiligo, present in approximately 1% of the population, may be associated with hyperthyroidism and hypothyroidism, pernicious anemia, diabetes mellitus, and Addison's disease. Albinism represents a number of different genetically determined traits, with different phenotypes. These often affect the eye and vision. Piebaldism, a localized hypomelanosis manifested by a white forelock, is an autosomal dominant trait that in some cases may be associated with neurologic abnormalities. Hypopigmented ash leaf spots may be seen in tuberous sclerosis. Hypopigmented halos are common around nevi and may occur around melanomas.

B. Secondary Pigmentary Disorders: Any damage to the skin (irritation, allergy, infection, excoriation, burns, or dermatologic therapy such as chemical peels and freezing with liquid nitrogen) may result in hyper- or hypopigmentation. Several disorders of clinical importance are as described below:

1. Hyperpigmentation–The most common type of secondary hyperpigmentation occurs after another dermatologic condition, such as acne, and is most commonly seen in dark-skinned persons. It is called postinflammatory hyperpigmentation.

Berloque hyperpigmentation is the pigmentation due to phototoxicity from essential oils in perfumes. Similar hyperpigmentation has been seen in phototoxic reactions to chemicals in the rinds of limes and other citrus fruits and to celery. Pigmentation may be produced by certain drugs, eg, chloroquine, chlorpromazine, minocycline, and amiodarone. Irritation from benzoyl peroxide and tretinoin can result in hyperpigmentation, as may topical fluorouracil. Fixed drug eruptions to phenolphthalein in laxatives, to trimethoprim-sulfamethoxazole, to NSAIDs, and to tetracyclines, for example, are further causes.

2. Hypopigmentation–Leukoderma is a disorder that may complicate atopic dermatitis, lichen planus, psoriasis, discoid lupus erythematosus, and lichen simplex chronicus. Physicians must exercise special care in using liquid nitrogen on any patient with olive or darker complexions, since doing so may result in hypopigmentation or depigmentation, at times permanent. Intralesional or intra-articular injections of high concentrations of corticosteroids may also cause localized temporary hypopigmentation.

Differential Diagnosis

One must distinguish true lack of pigment from pseudoachromia, such as occurs in tinea versicolor, pityriasis simplex, and seborrheic dermatitis. The evaluation of pigmentary disorders in Caucasians is helped by Wood's light, which accentuates epidermal pigmentation and highlights hypopigmentation.

Complications

Actinic keratoses and skin cancers are more likely to develop in persons with vitiligo and albinism. There may be severe emotional trauma in extensive vitiligo and other types of hypo- and hyperpigmentation, particularly when they occur in naturally dark-skinned persons.

Treatment & Prognosis

A. Hyperpigmentation: Therapeutic bleaching preparations generally contain hydroquinone. Hydroquinone has occasionally caused unexpected hypopigmentation, hyperpigmentation, or even secondary ochronosis and pigmented milia, particularly with prolonged use.

The role of exposure to ultraviolet light cannot be overstressed as a factor promoting or contributing to most disorders of hyperpigmentation, and such exposure should be minimized. Melasma, ephelides, and postinflammatory hyperpigmentation may be treated with varying success with 3–4% hydroquinone cream, gel, or solution and a sunscreen containing UVA photoprotectants (Avobenzone, zinc oxide, titanium dioxide). Solaquin Forte contains both hydroquinone and a sunscreen. Tretinoin cream, 0.025–0.05%, may be added. Superficial melasma responds well, but if there is predominantly dermal deposition of pigment (does *not* enhance with Wood's light), the prognosis is poor. Response to therapy takes months and requires avoidance of sunlight. Hyperpigmentation often recurs after treatment if the skin is exposed to ultraviolet light. Solar lentigines respond to liquid nitrogen application or to newer green light lasers. Controlled studies have demonstrated that tretinoin, 0.1% cream used over 10 months, will fade solar lentigines (liver spots), hyperpigmented facial macules in Asians, and postinflammatory hyperpigmentation in blacks. New laser systems for the removal of epidermal and dermal pigments are available, and referral should be considered for patients whose responses to medical treatment are inadequate.

B. Hypopigmentation: The pigment dilution is stable in various forms of albinism; spontaneous return of pigment is rare in vitiligo; in secondary hypopigmentation, repigmentation may occur spontaneously. Cosmetics such as Covermark and Dermablend are highly effective for concealing disfiguring patches. Therapy of vitiligo is long and tedious, and the patient must be strongly motivated. If less than 20% of the skin is involved (most cases), topical methoxsalen, 0.1% in ethanol and propylene glycol or in Acid Mantle cream or Unibase, is used, with cautious exposure to long-wavelength ultraviolet light (UVA), followed by thorough washing and sun avoidance. With 20–25% involvement, oral methoxsalen, 0.6 mg/kg 2 hours before UVA exposure, is best. Severe phototoxic response (sunburn) may occur with topical or oral psoralens plus UVA. The face and upper chest respond best, and the fingertips and the genital areas do not respond to this treatment. Years of treatment are often required. New techniques of using epidermal autografts and cultured epidermis combined with PUVA therapy give hope for surgical correction of vitiligo with a very low risk of scarring. Potent topical corticosteroids have been advocated for treatment of vitiligo, with daily use for 10 days followed by 10 days of rest, then repetition.

Grimes PE: Melasma: Etiologic and therapeutic considerations. Arch Dermatol 1995;131:1453. [NLM Cit ID: 96094883]

Kim NY et al: Pigmentary diseases. Med Clin North Am 1998;82:1185. [NLM Cit ID: 98441936]

Westerhof W et al: Left-right comparison study of the combination of fluticasone propionate and UV-A vs. either fluticasone propionate or UV-A alone for the long-term treatment of vitiligo. Arch Dermatol 1999;135:1061. [NLM Cit ID: 99418642]

BALDNESS (Alopecia)

Baldness Due to Scarring

Cicatricial baldness may occur following chemical or physical trauma, lichen planopilaris, severe bacterial or fungal infections, severe herpes zoster, chronic discoid lupus erythematosus, scleroderma, and excessive ionizing radiation. The specific cause is often suggested by the history, the distribution of hair loss, and the appearance of the skin, as in lupus erythematosus. Biopsy is useful in the diagnosis of scarring alopecia, but specimens must be taken from the active border and not from the scarred central zone.

Scarring alopecias are irreversible and permanent. It is important to diagnose and treat the scarring process as early in its course as possible.

Baldness Not Due to Scarring

Nonscarring alopecia may occur in association with various systemic diseases such as systemic lupus erythematosus, secondary syphilis, hyper- or hypothyroidism, iron deficiency anemia, and pituitary insufficiency. The only treatment necessary is prompt and adequate control of the underlying disorder, in which case hair loss may be reversible.

Androgenetic (pattern) baldness, the most common form of alopecia, is of genetic predetermination. The earliest changes occur at the anterior portions of the calvarium on either side of the "widow's peak." The extent of hair loss is variable and unpredictable. Rogaine Extra Strength, a solution containing 50 mg/mL of minoxidil, is available over the counter. The best results are achieved in persons with recent onset (< 5 years) and smaller diameters of alopecia. Approximately 40% of patients treated twice daily for a year will have moderate to dense growth. Finasteride (Propecia), 1 mg orally daily has similar efficacy and may be additive to minoxidil. As opposed to minoxidil, finasteride is used only in males.

Hair loss or thinning of the hair in women results from the same cause as common baldness in men (androgenetic alopecia) and may be treated with minoxidil (Rogaine). A workup consisting of determination of serum testosterone, DHEAS, iron, total iron binding capacity, and thyroid function tests and a complete blood count will identify most other causes of hair thinning in premenopausal women. Women who complain of thin hair but show little evidence of alopecia need follow-up, because more than 50% of the scalp hair can be lost before the clinician can perceive it.

Telogen effluvium is transitory increase in the number of hairs in the telogen (resting) phase of the hair growth cycle. This may occur spontaneously, may appear at the termination of pregnancy, may be precipitated by "crash dieting," high fever, stress from surgery or shock, or malnutrition, or may be provoked by hormonal contraceptives. Whatever the cause, telogen effluvium usually has a latent period of 2–4 months. The prognosis is generally good. The condition is diagnosed by the presence of large numbers of hairs with white bulbs coming out upon gentle tugging of the hair. Counts of hairs lost by the patient on combing or shampooing often exceed 150 per day, compared to an average of 70–100. In one study, a major cause of telogen effluvium was found to be iron deficiency, and the hair counts bore a clear relationship to serum iron levels.

Alopecia areata is of unknown cause but is believed to be an immunologic process. Typically, there are patches that are perfectly smooth and without scarring. Tiny hairs 2–3 mm in length, called "exclamation hairs," may be seen. Telogen hairs are easily dislodged from the periphery of active lesions. The beard, brows, and lashes may be involved. Involvement may extend to all of the scalp hair (alopecia totalis) or to all scalp and body hair (alopecia universalis). Severe forms may be treated by systemic corticosteroid therapy, although recurrences follow discontinuation of therapy. Alopecia areata is occasionally associated with Hashimoto's thyroiditis, pernicious anemia, Addison's disease, and vitiligo.

Intralesional corticosteroids are frequently effective for alopecia areata. Triamcinolone acetonide in a concentration of 2.5–10 mg/mL is injected in aliquots of 0.1 mL at approximately 1- to 2-cm intervals, not exceeding a total dose of 30 mg per month for adults. Alternatively, anthralin 0.5% ointment used daily, may help some patients. Alopecia areata is usually self-limiting, with complete regrowth of hair in 80% of patients, but some mild cases are resistant, as are the extensive totalis and universalis types. Both topical diphencyprone and squaric acid dibutylester, have been used to treat persistent alopecia areata. The principle is to sensitize the skin, then intermittently apply weaker concentrations to produce and maintain a slight dermatitis. Hair regrowth in 3–6 months in some patients has been reported to be remarkable. Long-term safety and efficacy have not been established. Support groups for patients with extensive alopecia areata are very beneficial. In **trichotillomania** (the pulling out of one's own hair), the patches of hair loss are irregular and growing hairs are always present, since they cannot be pulled out until they are long enough. The patches are often unilateral, occurring on the same side as the patient's dominant hand. The patient may be unaware of the habit.

Drug-induced alopecia is becoming increasingly important. Incriminated drugs include thallium, excessive and prolonged use of vitamin A, retinoids, antimitotic agents, anticoagulants, antithyroid drugs, oral contraceptives, trimethadione, allopurinol, propranolol, indomethacin, amphetamines, salicylates, gentamicin, and levodopa. While chemotherapy-induced alopecia is very distressing, it must be emphasized to the patient before treatment that it is invariably reversible.

Price VH: Treatment of hair loss. N Engl J Med 1999;341:964. [NLM Cit ID: 99412080]

Schwartz RA et al: Alopecia areata. Cutis 1997;59:238. [NLM Cit ID: 97312819]

Sperling LC et al: Hair diseases. Med Clin North Am 1998;82:1155. [NLM Cit ID: 98441934]

NAIL DISORDERS

1. MORPHOLOGIC ABNORMALITIES OF THE NAILS

Classification

Nail disorders may be classified as (1) local, (2) congenital or genetic, and (3) those associated with systemic or generalized skin diseases.

A. Local Nail Disorders:

1. Onycholysis (distal separation of the nail plate from the nail bed, usually of the fingers) is caused by excessive exposure to water, soaps, detergents, alkalies, and industrial keratolytic agents. Candidal infection of the nail folds and subungual area, nail hardeners, and drug-induced photosensitivity may cause onycholysis, as may hyper- and hypothyroidism and psoriasis.

2. Distortion of the nail occurs as a result of chronic inflammation of the nail matrix underlying the eponychial fold. Such changes may also be caused by warts, tumors, nevi, synovial and mucous cysts, etc, impinging on the nail matrix.

3. Discoloration and crumbly thickened nails are noted in dermatophyte infection and psoriasis.

4. Allergic reactions (to formaldehyde and resins in undercoats and polishes or to nail glues) are characterized by onycholysis or by grossly distorted, hypertrophic, and misshapen nails.

B. Congenital and Genetic Nail Disorders:

1. A longitudinal single nail groove may occur as a result of a genetic or traumatic defect in the nail matrix.

2. Nail atrophy may be congenital.

3. Clubbed fingers may be congenital.

C. Nail Changes Associated With Systemic or Generalized Skin Diseases:

1. Beau's lines (transverse furrows) may follow any serious systemic illness.

2. Atrophy of the nails may be related to trauma or to vascular or neurologic disease.

3. Clubbed fingers may be due to the prolonged hypoxemia associated with cardiopulmonary disorders. (See Chapter 9.)

4. Spoon nails may be seen in anemic patients.

5. Stippling or pitting of the nails is seen in psoriasis, alopecia areata, and hand eczema.

6. Nail hyperpigmentation may be caused by zidovudine, doxorubicin, cyclophosphamide, bleomycin, daunorubicin, fluorouracil, hydroxyurea, melphalan, mechlorethamine, and nitrosoureas.

Differential Diagnosis

It is important to distinguish congenital and genetic disorders from those caused by trauma and environmental disorders. Onychomycosis may cause nail changes identical to those seen in psoriasis. Careful examination for more characteristic lesions elsewhere on the body is essential to the diagnosis of the nail disorders. Cancer should be suspected (eg, Bowen's disease or squamous cell carcinoma) as the cause of any persistent solitary subungual or periungual lesion.

Complications

Secondary bacterial infection occasionally occurs in onychodystrophies and leads to considerable pain and disability and more serious consequences if circulation or innervation is impaired. Toenail changes may lead to an ingrown nail—in turn often complicated by bacterial infection and occasionally by exuberant granulation tissue. Poor manicuring and poorly fitting shoes may contribute to this complication. Cellulitis may result.

Treatment & Prognosis

Treatment consists usually of careful debridement and manicuring and, above all, reduction of exposure to irritants (soaps, detergents, alkali, bleaches, solvents, etc). Congenital or genetic nail disorders are usually uncorrectable. Longitudinal grooving due to temporary lesions of the matrix, such as warts, synovial cysts, and other impingements, may be cured by removal of the offending lesion. Intradermal triamcinolone acetonide suspension, 2.5 mg/mL, may be injected in the area of the nail matrix at intervals of 2–4 weeks for the successful management of various types of inflammatory nail dystrophies (psoriasis, lichen planus) but is painful.

If it is necessary to remove dystrophic nails for any reason (eg, fungal nails or severe psoriasis), a nonsurgical method is to apply urea 40%, anhydrous lanolin 20%, white wax 5%, white petrolatum 25%, and silica gel type H. The nail folds are painted with compound tincture of benzoin and covered with cloth adhesive tape. The urea ointment is applied generously to the nail surface and covered with plastic film, and then adhesive tape. The ointment is left on for 5–10 days; then the nail plate may be curetted off. Medication can then be applied that is appropriate for the condition being treated.

2. TINEA UNGUIUM (Onychomycosis)

Tinea unguium is a trichophyton infection of one or more (but rarely all) fingernails or toenails. The species most commonly found is *Trichophyton rubrum.* "Saprophytic" fungi may rarely (< 5%) cause onychomycosis.

The nails are lusterless, brittle, and hypertrophic, and the substance of the nail is friable. Irregular segments of the diseased nail may be broken. Laboratory diagnosis is mandatory. Portions of the nail should be cleared with 10% potassium hydroxide and examined under the microscope for hyphae. Fungi may also be cultured. Periodic acid-Schiff stain of a histologic section of the nail plate will also demonstrate the fungus readily.

Onychomycosis is difficult to treat because of the long duration of therapy required and the frequency of recurrences. Fingernails respond more readily than toenails. For toenails, it is in some situations best to discourage therapy and to control discomfort by paring the thickened nail plate.

Topical treatment has relatively low efficacy (10% or less), but in well-motivated patients with minimally thickened nails it can be useful. Naftifine gel 1% or ciclopirox lotion 8% applied twice daily may clear fingernails in 4–6 months and toenails in 12–18 months.

In general, systemic therapy is required for the treatment of nail onychomycosis. Fingernails can virtually always be cleared, whereas toenails respond in about 60% of cases. For fingernails, ultramicrosize griseofulvin, 750 mg or more daily for 6 months, is often effective. Treatment alternatives are itraconazole, 200 mg daily for 3 months; itraconazole, 400 mg the first 7 days of each month for 2 months; and terbinafine, 250 mg daily for 6 weeks. Once clear, fingernails often remain free of disease for years. The efficacy of griseofulvin for toenails is too low to be considered a therapeutic option in most cases. Ketoconazole, with its risk of hepatotoxicity with long-term use, is also not recommended. Itraconazole may be given as 200 mg daily for 3 months or 400 mg for the first 7 days of each month for 3 months for toenail onychomycosis. It is not FDA-approved for treatment of toenail onychomycosis. About 60% of patients will have substantial improvement, and 40% will be mycologically and clinically cured at 1 year. It interacts with numerous other medications and requires gastric acid to be absorbed.

In comparative trials, terbinafine, 250 mg daily for 3 months, has equal or superior efficacy. It is associated with fewer drug interactions (but may result in prolonged prothrombin times in patients taking warfarin) and is absorbed in patients with low gastric acid (those receiving H_2 blockers). More patients discontinue terbinafine therapy (8%) than itraconazole therapy (1%) due to adverse events. The rate of long-term recurrences following these forms of treatment is unknown. No matter which therapy is used, constant topical treatment for any coexistent tinea pedis is mandatory and should probably be continued for life to attempt to prevent recurrence.

Angello JT et al: A cost/efficacy analysis of oral antifungals indicated for the treatment of onychomycosis: griseofulvin, itraconazole, and terbinafine. Am J Manag Care 1997;3:443. [NLM Cit ID: 97418673]

Doncker PD et al: Itraconazole pulse therapy for onychomycosis and dermatomycoses: An overview. J Am Acad Dermatol 1997;37:969. [NLM Cit ID: 97437542]

Evans EG et al: Double blind, randomised study of continuous terbinafine compared with intermittent itraconazole in treatment of toenail onychomycosis. The LION Study Group. BMJ 1999;318:1031. [NLM Cit ID: 99221565]

Piraccini BM et al: Drug-induced nail disorders: incidence, management and prognosis. Drug Saf 1999;21:187. [NLM Cit ID: 99415338]

DERMATITIS MEDICAMENTOSA (Drug Eruption)

Essentials of Diagnosis

- Usually, abrupt onset of widespread, symmetric erythematous eruption.
- May mimic any inflammatory skin condition.
- Constitutional symptoms (malaise, arthralgia, headache, and fever) may be present.

General Considerations

As is well recognized, only a minority of cutaneous drug reactions result from allergy. True allergic drug reactions involve prior exposure, an "incubation" period, reactions to doses far below the therapeutic range, manifestations different from the usual pharmacologic effects of the drug, involvement of only a small portion of the population at risk, restriction to a limited number of syndromes (anaphylactic and anaphylactoid, urticarial, vasculitic, etc), and reproducibility.

Rashes are among the most common adverse reactions to drugs and occur in 2–3% of hospitalized patients. Amoxicillin, trimethoprim-sulfamethoxazole, and ampicillin or penicillin are the commonest causes of urticarial and maculopapular reactions. Toxic epidermal necrolysis and Stevens-Johnson syndrome are most commonly produced by sulfonamides and anticonvulsants. Phenolphthalein, pyrazolone derivatives, tetracyclines, NSAIDs, trimethoprim-sulfamethoxazole, and barbiturates are the major causes of fixed drug eruptions.

Clinical Findings

A. Symptoms and Signs: The onset is usually abrupt, with bright erythema and often severe itching, but may be delayed. Fever and other constitutional symptoms may be present. The skin reaction usually occurs in symmetric distribution.

Table 6–3 summarizes the types of skin reactions, their appearance and distribution, and the common offenders in each case.

B. Laboratory Findings: Routinely ordered blood work is of no value in the diagnosis of drug eruptions. However, skin biopsies may be helpful in making the diagnosis.

Differential Diagnosis

Observation after discontinuation, which may be a slow process, helps establish the diagnosis. Rechallenge, though of theoretical value, may pose a danger to the patient and is best avoided.

Complications

Some cutaneous drug reactions may be associated with a clinical complex involving other organs (complex drug reactions). The organ systems involved depend on the individual medication or drug class. Most common is an infectious mononucleosis-like illness and hepatitis associated with administration of anticonvulsants.

Treatment

A. General Measures: Systemic manifestations are treated as they arise (eg, anemia, icterus, purpura). Antihistamines may be of value in urticarial and angioneurotic reactions. Epinephrine 1:1000, 0.5–1 mL intravenously or subcutaneously, should be used as an emergency measure. In severe cases, corticosteroids may be used at doses similar to those used for acute contact dermatitis.

B. Local Measures: The varieties and stages of dermatitis are treated according to the major dermatitis present. Extensive blistering eruptions resulting in erosions and superficial ulcerations demand hospitalization and nursing care as for burn patients.

Prognosis

Drug rash usually disappears upon withdrawal of the drug and proper treatment.

Adcock BB et al: Ampicillin-specific rashes. Arch Fam Med 1996;5:301. [NLM Cit ID: 96212392]

deShazo RD et al: Allergic reactions to drugs and biologic agents. JAMA 1997;278:1895. [NLM Cit ID: 98057358]

Table 6–3. Skin reactions due to systemic drugs.

Reaction	Appearance	Distribution and Comments	Common Offenders
Toxic erythema	Morbilliform, maculopapular, exanthematous reactions.	The commonest skin reaction to drugs. Often more pronounced on the trunk than on the extremities. In previously exposed patients, the rash may start in 2–3 days. In the first course of treatment, the eruption often appears about the seventh to ninth days. Fever may be present.	Antibiotics (especially ampicillin and trimethoprim-sulfamethoxazole), sulfonamides and related compounds (including thiazide diuretics, furosemide, and sulfonylurea hypoglycemic agents), and barbiturates.
Erythema multiforme major	Target-like lesions. Bullae may occur. Mucosal involvement.	Mainly on the extensor aspects of the limbs.	Sulfonamides, penicillamine, barbiturates, and NSAIDs.
Erythema nodosum	Inflammatory cutaneous nodules.	Usually limited to the extensor aspects of the legs. May be accompanied by fever, arthralgias, and pain.	Oral contraceptives.
Allergic vasculitis	Inflammatory changes may present as urticaria that lasts over 24 hours, hemorrhagic papules ("palpable purpura"), vesicles, bullae, or necrotic ulcers.	Most severe on the legs.	Sulfonamides, indomethacin, phenytoin, allopurinol, and ibuprofen.
Purpura	Itchy, petechial macular rash.	Dependent areas. Results most typically from thrombocytopenia.	Thiazides, sulfonamides, sulfonylureas, barbiturates, quinine, and sulindac.
Eczema	Similar to contact dermatitis.	A rare epidermal reaction in patients previously sensitized by external exposure who are given the same or a related substance systemically.	Penicillin, neomycin, phenothiazines, and local anesthetics.
Exfoliative dermatitis and erythroderma	Red and scaly.	Entire skin surface.	Allopurinol, sulfonamides, isoniazid, gold, or carbamazepine.
Photosensitivity: Increased sensitivity to light, often of ultraviolet A wavelengths, but may be due to UVB or visible light as well	Sunburn, vesicles, papules in photodistributed pattern.	Exposed skin of the face, the neck, and the backs of the hands and, in women, the lower legs. Exaggerated response to ultraviolet light. On occasion, ultraviolet emission from fluorescent lighting may be sufficient.	Sulfonamides and sulfonamide-related compounds (thiazide diuretics, furosemide, sulfonylureas), tetracyclines (especially demeclocycline), phenothiazines, sulindac, amiodarone, and NSAIDs.
Drug-related lupus erythematosus	May present with a photosensitive rash accompanied by fever, polyarthritis, myalgia, and serositis.	Less severe than systemic lupus erythematosus, sparing the kidneys and central nervous system. Recovery often follows drug withdrawal.	Most commonly hydralazine and procainamide; less often, isoniazid and phenytoin.
Lichenoid and lichen planus-like eruptions	Pruritic, erythematous to violaceous polygonal papules that coalesce or expand to form plaques.	May be in photo- or nonphotodistributed pattern.	Bismuth, carbamazepine, chlordiazepoxide, chloroquine, chlorpropamide, dapsone, ethambutol, furosemide, gold salts, hydroxychloroquine, levamisole, meprobamate, methyldopa, paraphenylenediamine salts, penicillamine, phenothiazines, pindolol, propranolol, quinidine, quinine, quinacrine, streptomycin, sulfonylureas, tetracyclines, thiazides, and triprolidine.

(*continued*)

Table 6–3. Skin reactions due to systemic drugs. (continued)

Reaction	Appearance	Distribution and Comments	Common Offenders
Fixed drug eruptions	Single or multiple demarcated, round, erythematous plaques that often become hyperpigmented.	Recur at the same site when the drug is repeated. Hyperpigmentation, if present, remains after healing.	Numerous drugs, including antimicrobials, analgesics, barbiturates, cardiovascular drugs, heavy metals, antiparasitic agents, antihistamines, phenolphthalein, ibuprofen, and naproxen.
Toxic epidermal necrolysis	Large sheets of erythema, followed by separation, which looks like scalded skin.	Rare.	In adults, the eruption has occurred after administration of many classes of drugs, particularly barbiturates, phenytoin, sulfonamides, and NSAIDs.
Urticaria	Red, itchy wheals that vary in size from < 1 cm to many centimeters. May be accompanied by angioedema.	Chronic urticaria is rarely caused by drugs.	Acute urticaria: penicillins, NSAIDs, sulfonamides, opiates, and salicylates. Angioedema is common in patients receiving ACE inhibitors.
Pruritus	Itchy skin without rash.		Pruritus ani may be due to overgrowth of *Candida* after systemic antibiotic treatment. NSAIDs may cause pruritus without a rash.
Hair loss		Hair loss most often involves the scalp, but other sites may be affected.	A predictable side effect of cytotoxic agents and oral contraceptives. Diffuse hair loss also occurs unpredictably with a wide variety of other drugs, including anticoagulants, antithyroid drugs, newer antimicrobials, cholesterol-lowering agents, heavy metals, corticosteroids, androgens, NSAIDs, retinoids (isotretinoin, etretinate), and beta-blockers.
Pigmentary changes	Flat hyperpigmented areas.	Forehead and cheeks (chloasma, melasma). The most common pigmentary disorder associated with drug ingestion. Improvement is slow despite stopping the drug.	Oral contraceptives are the usual cause.
	Blue-gray discoloration.	Light-exposed areas.	Chlorpromazine and related phenothiazines.
	Brown or blue-gray pigmentation.	Generalized.	Heavy metals (silver, gold, bismuth, and arsenic). Arsenic, silver, and bismuth are not used therapeutically, but patients who receive gold for rheumatoid arthritis may show this reaction.
	Yellow color.	Generalized.	Usually quinacrine.
	Blue-black patches on the shins.		Minocycline, chloroquine.
	Blue-black pigmentation of the nails and palate and depigmentation of the hair.		Chloroquine.
	Slate-gray color.	Primarily in photoexposed areas.	Amiodarone.
	Brown discoloration of the nails.	Especially in more darkly pigmented patients.	Zidovudine (azidothymidine; AZT), hydroxyurea.

(*continued*)

Table 6–3. Skin reactions due to systemic drugs. (continued)

Reaction	Appearance	Distribution and Comments	Common Offenders
Psoriasiform eruptions	Scaly red plaques.	May be located on trunk and extremities. Palms and soles may be hyperkeratotic. May cause psoriasiform eruption or worsen psoriasis.	Chloroquine, lithium, beta-blockers, and quinacrine.
Pityriasis rosea-like eruptions	Oval, red, slightly raised patches with central scale.	Mainly on the trunk.	Barbiturates, bismuth, captopril, clonidine, gold salts, methopromazine, metoprolol, metronidazole, and tripelennamine.
Seborrheic dermatitis-like eruptions	Diffuse redness and loose scale.	On scalp, face, mid chest, axillae, groin.	Cimetidine, gold salts, and methyldopa.
Bullous eruptions	Tense blisters > 1 cm.	Hands, feet, genital areas common; other sites possible.	Aspirin, barbiturates, bromides, chlorpromazine, warfarin, phenytoin, sulfonamides and related compounds, and promethazine.

RELEVANT WORLD WIDE WEB SITES

[American Academy of Dermatology]
http://www.aad.org
[University of Iowa Department of Dermatology Homepage]
http://tray.dermatology.uiowa.edu/Home.html
[Cutaneous Drug Reaction Database]
gopher://gopher.dartmouth.edu:70/11/Research/BioSci/CDRD
[Dermatologic Image Database]
http://tray.dermatology.uiowa.edu/DermImag.htm
[Dermatology Differential Diagnosis by Morphology]
http://tray.dermatology.uiowa.edu/DDX-Morph.html
[Acne—American Academy of Dermatology]
http://www.aad.org/pamphlets/acnepamp.html
http://www.aad.org/pamphlets_spanish/acne.html
[AIDS—American Academy of Dermatology]
http://www.aad.org/pamphlets/aidspamp.html
[Athlete's Foot—American Academy of Dermatology]
http://www.aad.org/pamphlets/AthletFoot.html
[Black Skin—American Academy of Dermatology]
http://www.aad.org/pamphlets/black.html
[Cosmetics and Skin Care Products—American Academy of Dermatology]
http://www.aad.org/pamphlets/cosmetic.html
[Eczema/Atopic Dermatitis—American Academy of Dermatology]
http://www.aad.org/pamphlets/eczema.html
[Hair Loss—American Academy of Dermatology]
http://www.aad.org/pamphlets/hairloss.html
[Herpes Simplex—American Academy of Dermatology]
http://www.aad.org/pamphlets/herpes.html
[Mature Skin—American Academy of Dermatology]
http://www.aad.org/pamphlets/mature.html
http://www.aad.org/pamphlets/agingskin.html
[Moles—American Academy of Dermatology]
http://www.aad.org/pamphlets/Moles.html
[Nail Health—American Academy of Dermatology]
http://www.aad.org/pamphlets/nailhealth.html
[Pityriasis Rosea—American Academy of Dermatology]
http://www.aad.org/pamphlets/pityrias.html
[Poison Ivy—American Academy of Dermatology]
http://www.aad.org/pamphlets/PoisonIvy.html
[Psoriasis—American Academy of Dermatology]
http://www.aad.org/pamphlets/Psoriasis.html
[Scabies—American Academy of Dermatology]
http://www.aad.org/pamphlets/Scabies.html
[Seborrheic Dermatitis—American Academy of Dermatology]
http://www.aad.org/pamphlets/seborrhe.html
[Seborrheic Keratoses—American Academy of Dermatology]
http://www.aad.org/pamphlets/saborr_kera.html
[Skin Cancer—American Academy of Dermatology]
http://www.aad.org/pamphlets/skincan.html
[Spider Vein, Varicose Vein Therapy—American Academy of Dermatology]
http://www.aad.org/pamphlets/spiderve.html
[Sun Protection for Children—American Academy of Dermatology]
http://www.aad.org/pamphlets/ABCsFunSun.html
[The Sun and Your Skin—American Academy of Dermatology]
http://www.aad.org/pamphlets/SunSkin.html
[Tinea Versicolor—American Academy of Dermatology]
http://www.aad.org/pamphlets/tineav.html
[Ultraviolet Index—American Academy of Dermatology]
http://www.aad.org/pamphlets/UVIndex.html
[Urticaria Hives—American Academy of Dermatology]
http://www.aad.org/pamphlets/Urticaria.html
[Vascular Birthmarks—American Academy of Dermatology]
http://www.aad.org/pamphlets/VascBirthMk.html
[Vitiligo—American Academy of Dermatology]
http://www.aad.org/pamphlets/Vitiligo.html
[Warts—American Academy of Dermatology]
http://www.aad.org/pamphlets/warts.html
[What Is in a Scar?]
http://www.aad.org/pamphlets/whatsina.html

Table 7–1. The inflamed eye: Differential diagnosis of common causes.

	Acute Conjunctivitis	Acute Uveitis	Acute Glaucoma[1]	Corneal Trauma or Infection
Incidence	Extremely common	Common	Uncommon	Common
Discharge	Moderate to copious	None	None	Watery or purulent
Vision	No effect on vision	Often blurred	Markedly blurred	Usually blurred
Pain	Mild	Moderate	Severe	Moderate to severe
Conjunctival injection	Diffuse; more toward fornices	Mainly circumcorneal	Mainly circumcorneal	Mainly circumcorneal
Cornea	Clear	Usually clear	Steamy	Clarity change related to cause
Pupil size	Normal	Small	Moderately dilated and fixed	Normal
Pupillary light response	Normal	Poor	None	Normal
Intraocular pressure	Normal	Commonly low but may be elevated	Elevated	Normal
Smear	Causative organisms	No organisms	No organisms	Organisms found only in corneal ulcers due to infection

[1]Angle-closure glaucoma.

(Argyll Robertson pupils). Physiologic anisocoria is a common cause of unequal pupils that react normally.

A relative afferent pupillary defect, in which the pupillary light reaction is of reduced intensity when light is shined into the affected eye compared with the normal eye, is a sign indicating optic nerve disease. It is most easily detected with the "swinging light test," in which the pupillary light reactions are compared as a bright light is moved from one eye to the other.

Extraocular Movements

Examination of extraocular movements begins with an assessment of whether the two eyes are correctly aligned. A misalignment of the visual axes under binocular viewing conditions is known as a manifest deviation, or **tropia.** A deviation that becomes apparent only when binocular function is disrupted is known as a latent deviation, or **phoria.** A manifest deviation may be apparent by comparing the relative positions of the corneal light reflexes. A more reliable test is the **cover test,** in which the deviated eye moves to take up fixation when the other eye is occluded. The correctional movement is in the opposite direction to that of the original manifest deviation. If no manifest deviation is present, occlusion of one eye will elicit any latent deviation because binocular function will have been disrupted. As the occluder is removed **(uncover test),** latent deviation is then detected by any correctional movement that occurs to reestablish the normal alignment of the eyes. Latent deviation is common among normal individuals.

Horizontal diplopia indicates dysfunction of the medial and lateral rectus muscles; vertical diplopia results from dysfunction of the superior and inferior recti and the obliques. The false outer image arises from the affected eye. If a muscle is underacting, the image separation will be greatest in its normal direction of action. If a muscle is prevented from relaxing, image separation will be greatest in the direction opposite to its normal action. For example, a paretic lateral rectus or a tethered medial rectus of the right eye will cause maximal image separation on looking to the right.

Nystagmus in the primary position is always abnormal. Minor degrees of nystagmus at the extremes of gaze are normal. Other forms of physiologic nystagmus include optokinetic nystagmus and that induced by rotation or caloric stimulation. Exaggerated gaze-evoked nystagmus may be due to drugs or posterior fossa disease.

Proptosis (Exophthalmos)

Proptosis may be suspected by observing widening of the palpebral aperture, with exposure of sclera both superiorly and inferiorly. (Eyelid retraction generally causes more exposure superiorly than inferiorly.) By viewing from above while the patient is asked to look down and the upper lids are lifted by the examiner, a further estimate of the degree of proptosis can be made. Exophthalmometry should be performed for objective assessment. In nonaxial proptosis, there is also horizontal or vertical displace-

the aid of corrective (minus, concave) lenses. In **astigmatism,** the refractive errors in the horizontal and vertical axes differ.

Various surgical techniques are available for the correction of refractive errors, particularly myopia, including photorefractive keratectomy (PRK), in which the excimer laser is used to reshape the anterior cornea; radial keratotomy, in which radial incisions are made in the anterior cornea; laser-assisted in situ keratomileusis (LASIK), in which a portion of the corneal stroma undergoes laser remodeling and is then replaced under an anterior corneal flap; and extraction of the clear crystalline lens.

Presbyopia is the natural loss of accommodative capacity with age. Emmetropes usually notice inability to focus on objects at a normal reading distance at about age 45. Hyperopes experience symptoms at an earlier age. Presbyopia is corrected with plus lenses for near work.

Use of a pinhole will overcome most refractive errors and thus allows their exclusion as a cause of visual loss. Transient refractive errors occur in diabetes—typically when diabetic control is erratic—and may be the presenting feature. Autoinoculation of scopolamine from seasickness patches or atropine from vials for parenteral use leads to pupillary dilation and loss of accommodation.

Brahma A et al: Surgical correction of refractive errors. J R Soc Med 2000;93:118. [NLM Cit ID: 20205483] (General review of surgery for refractive errors.)

Colin J et al: Clear lensectomy and implantation of a low-power posterior chamber intraocular lens for correction of high myopia. A four-year follow-up. Ophthalmology 1997;104:73. [NLM Cit ID: 97174373] (Reasonable outcome in 49 eyes with myopia of 12 diopters or more undergoing clear lens extraction.)

El-Maghraby A et al: Randomized bilateral comparison of excimer laser in situ keratomileusis and photorefractive keratectomy for 2.50 to 8.00 diopters of myopia. Ophthalmology 1999;106:447. [NLM Cit ID: 99178284] (Thirty-three patients underwent LASIK in one eye and PRK in the other. LASIK produced less pain and quicker improvement in uncorrected visual acuity, but the final visual outcome was the same in the two groups.)

Contact Lenses

Contact lenses are used mostly for correction of refractive errors but also in the management of diseases of the cornea, conjunctiva, or lids. It has been estimated that there are 30 million contact lens wearers in the USA.

The various types of contact lenses are hard lenses made of polymethylmethacrylate (PMMA), rigid gas-permeable lenses made of cellulose acetate butyrate (CAB) or silicone acrylates, and soft or hydrogel lenses based on hydroxyethylmethacrylate (HEMA). Hard lenses are much more durable and easy to care for than soft lenses but are more difficult to tolerate. Rigid gas-permeable lenses are an effective compromise.

Contact lens care includes cleaning and sterilization whenever the lenses are removed and removal of protein deposits as required. Sterilization may involve thermal or chemical methods. For individuals developing reactions to preservatives in contact lens solutions, preservative-free systems are available. All contact lenses can be used on a daily-wear basis, ie, they are inserted in the morning and removed at night. Soft lenses are also available for extended wear. Disposable soft lenses to avoid the necessity for lens cleaning and sterilization are available for daily wear or extended wear.

The major risk from contact lens wear is corneal ulceration, potentially a blinding condition. Among the contact lens wearers in the USA, there are an estimated 12,000 corneal ulcers per year. Soft lenses present the major hazard, particularly with extended wear, for which there is an approximately eightfold greater risk of corneal ulceration compared with daily wear. The increased risk from extended wear begins with the first night of overnight wear and increases progressively thereafter. Disposable lenses do not overcome the risk of corneal ulceration.

Cosmetic contact lens wearers should be made aware of the risks they face and ways to minimize them, such as avoiding extended-wear soft lenses and maintaining meticulous lens hygiene. Whenever there is ocular discomfort or redness, contact lenses should be removed. Ophthalmologic care is sought if symptoms persist.

Stamler JF: The complications of contact lens wear. Curr Opin Ophthalmol 1998;9:66. [NLM Cit ID: 99260047] (Review of the complications that affect approximately 6% of contact lens wearers each year.)

Stern GA: Contact lens associated bacterial keratitis: Past, present, and future. CLAO J 1998;24:52. [NLM Cit ID: 98134796] (Personal review of the pathogenesis of contact lens-related corneal infections.)

DISORDERS OF THE LIDS & LACRIMAL APPARATUS

Hordeolum

Hordeolum is a common staphylococcal abscess that is characterized by a localized red, swollen, acutely tender area on the upper or lower lid. Internal hordeolum is a meibomian gland abscess that points onto the conjunctival surface of the lid; external hordeolum or sty is smaller and on the margin. The chief symptom is pain of an intensity directly related to the amount of swelling.

Warm compresses are helpful. Incision may be indicated if resolution does not begin within 48 hours. An antibiotic ointment (bacitracin or erythromycin) instilled into the conjunctival sac every 3 hours may be beneficial during the acute stage. Internal hordeolum may lead to generalized cellulitis of the lid.

Chalazion

Chalazion is a common granulomatous inflammation of a meibomian gland that may follow an internal hordeolum. It is characterized by a hard, nontender swelling on the upper or lower lid. The conjunctiva in the region of the chalazion is red and elevated. If the chalazion is large enough to impress the cornea, vision will be distorted.

Incision and curettage is done by an ophthalmologist.

Santa Cruz CS et al: Chalazion-induced hyperopia as a cause of decreased vision. Ophthalmic Surg Lasers 1997;28:683. [NLM Cit ID: 97414125] (Three cases of refractive visual loss due to chalazion.)

Tumors

Verrucae and papillomas of the skin of the lids can often be excised by the general physician if they do not involve the lid margin; otherwise, surgery should be performed by an ophthalmologist so as to avoid permanent notching of the lid. Cancer—including basal cell epithelioma, squamous cell carcinoma, meibomian gland carcinoma, and malignant melanoma—should be ruled out by microscopic examination of the excised material.

Kersten RC et al: Accuracy of clinical diagnosis of cutaneous eyelid lesions. Ophthalmology 1997;104:479. [NLM Cit ID: 97226432] (Two percent of eyelid lesions thought clinically to be benign were found to be malignant, mostly basal cell carcinoma, on histopathologic examination.)

Blepharitis

Blepharitis is a common chronic bilateral inflammation of the lid margins. Anterior blepharitis involves the eyelid skin, eyelashes, and associated glands. It may be ulcerative, because of infection by staphylococci; or seborrheic, and associated with seborrhea of the scalp, brows, and ears. Both types are commonly present. Posterior blepharitis is inflammation of the eyelids secondary to dysfunction of the meibomian glands. There may be bacterial infection, particularly with staphylococci, or a primary glandular dysfunction, in which there is a strong association with acne rosacea.

Symptoms are irritation, burning, and itching. In anterior blepharitis, the eyes are "red-rimmed," and scales or "granulations" can be seen clinging to the lashes. In posterior blepharitis, the lid margins are hyperemic with telangiectasias; the meibomian glands and their orifices are inflamed, with dilation of the glands, plugging of the orifices, and abnormal secretions. The lid margin is frequently rolled inward to produce a mild entropion, and the tears may be frothy or abnormally greasy.

Both anterior and, more particularly, posterior blepharitis may be complicated by hordeola or chalazions; abnormal lid or lash positions, producing trichiasis; recurrent conjunctivitis, epithelial keratitis of the lower third of the cornea, marginal corneal infiltrates, and inferior corneal vascularization and thinning.

In anterior blepharitis, cleanliness of the scalp, eyebrows, and lid margins is essential to effective local therapy. Scales must be removed from the lids daily with a damp cotton applicator and baby shampoo. An antistaphylococcal antibiotic eye ointment such as bacitracin or erythromycin is applied daily to the lid margins with a cotton-tipped applicator. Antibiotic sensitivity studies may be required in severe staphylococcal blepharitis.

In mild posterior blepharitis, regular meibomian gland expression may be sufficient to control symptoms. Inflammation of the conjunctiva and cornea indicates a need for more active treatment, including long-term low-dose systemic antibiotic therapy, usually with tetracycline (250 mg twice daily), doxycycline (100 mg daily), or erythromycin (250 mg three times daily), and short-term topical steroids, eg, prednisolone, 0.125% twice daily. Topical therapy with antibiotics such as ciprofloxacin 0.3% ophthalmic solution twice daily may be helpful but should be restricted to short courses.

Adenis JP et al: Ciprofloxacin ophthalmic solution in the treatment of conjunctivitis and blepharitis: A comparison with fusidic acid. Eur J Ophthalmol 1996;6:368. [NLM Cit ID: 97151594] (Ciprofloxacin as effective as fusidic acid in the treatment of blepharitis and conjunctivitis.)

Quarterman MJ et al: Ocular rosacea: Signs, symptoms, and tear studies before and after treatment with doxycycline. Arch Dermatol 1997;133:49. [NLM Cit ID: 97159031] (Suppression of meibomian gland dysfunction with doxycycline 100 mg daily for 12 weeks in 39 patients with ocular manifestations of acne rosacea.)

Entropion & Ectropion

Entropion (inward turning of usually the lower lid) occurs occasionally in older people as a result of degeneration of the lid fascia, or may follow extensive scarring of the conjunctiva and tarsus. Surgery is indicated if the lashes rub on the cornea. Botulinum toxin injections may also be used for temporary correction of the involutional lower eyelid entropion of older people.

Ectropion (outward turning of the lower lid) is fairly common in elderly people. Surgery is indicated if ectropion causes excessive tearing, exposure keratitis, or a cosmetic problem.

Elder MJ et al: Lid surgery: the management of cicatricial entropion and trichiasis. Dev Ophthalmol 1997;28:207. [NLM Cit ID: 98048184] (A general review of the management of entropion due to eyelid scarring.)

Steel DH et al: Botulinum toxin for the temporary treatment of involutional lower lid entropion: a clinical and morphological study. Eye 1997;11:472. [NLM Cit ID:

98086546] (Effective treatment of involutional lower lid entropion for a mean duration of 13 weeks in 30 patients.)

Dacryocystitis

Dacryocystitis is infection of the lacrimal sac due to obstruction of the nasolacrimal system. It may be acute or chronic and occurs most often in infants and in persons over 40. It is usually unilateral.

In acute dacryocystitis, the usual infectious organisms are *S aureus* and β-hemolytic streptococci; in chronic dacryocystitis, *S epidermidis,* anaerobic streptococci, or *Candida albicans.*

Acute dacryocystitis is characterized by pain, swelling, tenderness, and redness in the tear sac area; purulent material may be expressed. In chronic dacryocystitis, tearing and discharge are the principal signs, and mucus or pus may also be expressed.

Acute dacryocystitis responds well to systemic antibiotic therapy, but recurrences are common if the obstruction is not removed. The chronic form may be kept latent by using antibiotic drugs, but relief of the obstruction is the only cure. In adults, the standard procedure for obstruction of the lacrimal drainage system is dacryocystorhinostomy, which involves surgical exploration of the lacrimal sac and formation of a fistula into the nasal cavity. Laser-assisted endoscopic dacryocystorhinostomy and balloon dilation or probing of the nasolacrimal system are alternatives. Congenital nasolacrimal duct obstruction often resolves spontaneously but if necessary can be treated by probing of the nasolacrimal system.

Brook I et al: Aerobic and anaerobic microbiology of dacryocystitis. Am J Ophthalmol 1998;125:552. [NLM Cit ID: 98218645] (Aerobic bacteria isolated in 52% of cases of dacryocystitis, anaerobic in 32%, both aerobic and anaerobic in 11%, and fungi in 5%.)

Guinot-Saera A et al: Efficacy of probing as treatment of epiphora in adults with blocked nasolacrimal ducts. Br J Ophthalmol 1998;82:389. [NLM Cit ID: 98304368] (Probing of the nasolacrimal system under local anesthetic as an office procedure improved symptoms in 82% of patients.)

Sadiq SA et al: Endonasal laser dacryocystorhinostomy—medium term results. Br J Ophthalmol 1997;81:1089. [NLM Cit ID: 98158899] (Success rates at 12 months were much less than for conventional surgery.)

CONJUNCTIVITIS

Conjunctivitis is the most common eye disease. It may be acute or chronic. Most cases are due to bacterial (including gonococcal and chlamydial) or viral infection. Other causes include keratoconjunctivitis sicca, allergy, and chemical irritants. The mode of transmission of infectious conjunctivitis is usually direct contact via fingers, towels, handkerchiefs, etc, to the fellow eye or to other persons.

Conjunctivitis must be differentiated from acute uveitis, acute glaucoma, and corneal disorders (Table 7–1).

Morrow GL et al: Conjunctivitis. Am Fam Physician 1998;57:735. [NLM Cit ID: 98151696] (General review of management.)

Bacterial Conjunctivitis

The organisms found most commonly in bacterial conjunctivitis are staphylococci, streptococci (particularly *S pneumoniae*), *Haemophilus* spp, *Pseudomonas* spp, and *Moraxella* spp. All may produce a copious purulent discharge. There is no blurring of vision and only mild discomfort. In severe cases, examination of stained conjunctival scrapings and cultures are recommended.

The disease is usually self-limited, lasting about 10–14 days if untreated. A sulfonamide (eg, sulfacetamide, 10% ophthalmic solution or ointment) instilled locally three times daily will usually clear the infection in 2–3 days.

A. Gonococcal Conjunctivitis: Gonococcal conjunctivitis, usually acquired through contact with infected genital secretions, is manifested by a copious purulent discharge. It is an ophthalmologic emergency because corneal involvement may rapidly lead to perforation. The diagnosis should be confirmed by stained smear and culture of the discharge. If the cornea is not involved, a single intramuscular dose of ceftriaxone, 1 g, is effective. When the cornea is involved, a 5-day course of parenteral ceftriaxone, 1–2 g daily, is required. Topical antibiotics, such as erythromycin and bacitracin, may also be used. In such patients, other sexually transmitted diseases, including chlamydiosis, syphilis, and HIV infection, should be considered.

B. Chlamydial Keratoconjunctivitis:

1. Trachoma–(*Chlamydia trachomatis* serotypes A–C.) Trachoma is a major cause of blindness worldwide. Recurrent episodes of infection in childhood are manifest as bilateral follicular conjunctivitis, epithelial keratitis, and corneal vascularization (pannus). Cicatrization of the tarsal conjunctiva leads to entropion and trichiasis in adulthood, with secondary central corneal scarring.

The specific diagnosis can be made in Giemsa-stained conjunctival scrapings. Treatment should be started on the basis of clinical findings without waiting for laboratory confirmation. Oral tetracycline or erythromycin, 250 mg six times a day, or doxycycline, 100 mg twice a day, is given for 3–5 weeks. Single-dose therapy with azithromycin, 20 mg/kg, may also be effective. Local treatment is not necessary. Surgical treatment includes correction of eyelid deformities and corneal transplantation.

2. Inclusion conjunctivitis–(*C trachomatis* serotypes D–K.) The agent of inclusion conjunctivitis is a common cause of genital tract disease in adults.

The eye is usually involved following accidental contact with genital secretions. Adult inclusion conjunctivitis thus occurs most frequently in sexually active young adults. The disease starts with acute redness, discharge, and irritation. The eye findings consist of follicular conjunctivitis with mild keratitis. A nontender preauricular lymph node can often be palpated. Healing usually leaves no sequelae. Cytologic examination of conjunctival scrapings shows a picture similar to that of trachoma. Treatment is with oral tetracycline or erythromycin, 250–500 mg four times a day, or doxycycline, 300 mg initially followed by 100 mg once a day, for 2 weeks. Before treatment, all cases should be assessed for genital tract infection so that management can be adjusted accordingly.

Matters R et al: An outbreak of non-sexually transmitted gonococcal conjunctivitis in Central Australia and the Kimberley region. Commun Dis Intell 1998;22:52. [NLM Cit ID: 98244095] (Epidemic underlining the relationship between genital and ocular gonococcal infection.)

Nakagawa H: Treatment of chlamydial conjunctivitis. Ophthalmologica 1997;211(Suppl 1):25. [NLM Cit ID: 97218497] (Treatment of inclusion conjunctivitis in adults and neonates.)

Viral Conjunctivitis

One of the most common causes of viral conjunctivitis is adenovirus type 3. Conjunctivitis due to this agent is usually associated with pharyngitis, fever, malaise, and preauricular adenopathy (pharyngoconjunctival fever). Locally, the palpebral conjunctiva is red, and there is a copious watery discharge and scanty exudate. Children are more often affected than adults, and contaminated swimming pools are sometimes the source of infection. Epidemic keratoconjunctivitis is caused by adenovirus types 8 and 19. It is more likely to be complicated by visual loss due to corneal subepithelial infiltrates. Local sulfonamide therapy may prevent secondary bacterial infection, hot compresses reduce the discomfort of the associated lid edema, and weak topical steroids (eg, prednisolone, 0.125% four times daily) may be necessary to treat the corneal infiltrates. The disease usually lasts at least 2 weeks.

Azar MJ et al: Possible consequences of shaking hands with your patients with epidemic keratoconjunctivitis. Am J Ophthalmol 1996;121:711. [NLM Cit ID: 96243668] (A timely reminder of how hands and instruments so easily become contaminated with adenovirus.)

Keratoconjunctivitis Sicca (Dry Eyes)

This is a common disorder, particularly in elderly women. A wide range of conditions predispose to or are characterized by dry eyes. Hypofunction of the lacrimal glands, causing loss of the aqueous component of tears, may be due to aging, hereditary disorders, systemic disease (eg, Sjögren's syndrome), or systemic and topical drugs. Excessive evaporation of tears may be due to environmental factors (eg, a hot, dry, or windy climate) or abnormalities of the lipid component of the tear film, as in blepharitis. Mucin deficiency may be due to malnutrition, infection, burns, or drugs.

The patient complains of dryness, redness, or a scratchy feeling of the eyes. In severe cases there is persistent marked discomfort, with photophobia, difficulty in moving the eyelids, and often excessive mucus secretion. In many cases, gross examination reveals no abnormality, but on slitlamp examination there are subtle abnormalities of tear film stability and reduced volume of the tear film meniscus along the lower lid. In more severe cases, damaged corneal and conjunctival cells stain with 1% rose bengal. (Rose bengal staining should be avoided in severe cases because of the intense pain it may cause.) In the most severe cases there is marked conjunctival injection, loss of the normal conjunctival and corneal luster, epithelial keratitis that may progress to frank ulceration, and mucous strands. Schirmer's test, which measures the rate of production of the aqueous component of tears by the amount of wetting of filter paper strips during a 5-minute period, may be helpful when the diagnosis is in doubt, but false-positive and false-negative results are frequent.

Treatment depends upon the cause. In most early cases, the corneal and conjunctival epithelial changes are reversible. Aqueous deficiency can be treated by replacement of the aqueous component of tears with various types of artificial tears. The simplest preparations are physiologic (0.9%) or hypo-osmotic (0.45%) solutions of sodium chloride. Balanced salt solution is a more physiologic but also more expensive preparation. All these drop preparations can be used as frequently as every half-hour but in most cases are needed only three or four times a day. More prolonged duration of action can be achieved with drop preparations containing methylcellulose (eg, Isopto Plain) or polyvinyl alcohol (eg, Liquifilm Tears or Hypo Tears) or by using petrolatum ointment (Lacri-Lube). Such mucomimetics are particularly indicated when there is mucin deficiency. Artificial tear preparations are generally very safe and without side effects. However, the preservatives necessary to maintain their sterility are potentially toxic and allergenic and may cause keratitis and cicatrizing conjunctivitis in frequent users. Furthermore, the development of such reactions may be misinterpreted by both the patient and the doctor as a worsening of the dry eye state requiring more frequent use of the artificial tears and leading in turn to further deterioration, rather than being recognized as a need to change to a preservative-free preparation. If the mucus is tenacious, mucolytic agents (eg, acetylcysteine, 20% six times a day) may provide some relief. Blepharitis should be treated appropriately (see above).

Pflugfelder SC: Advances in the diagnosis and management of keratoconjunctivitis sicca. Curr Opin Ophthalmol 1998;9:50. [NLM Cit ID: 99260044] (Review of advances in diagnosis, pathogenesis, and therapy of keratoconjunctivitis.)

Schein OD et al: Prevalence of dry eye among the elderly. Am J Ophthalmol 1997;124:723. [NLM Cit ID: 98066521] (Among 2520 individuals aged 65–84 years, 15% had symptoms of dry eyes but only 3.5% also had confirmatory signs. There was no difference in prevalence of dry eye by race, sex, or age.)

Allergic Eye Disease

Allergic eye disease takes a number of different forms, but all are expressions of an atopic diathesis, which may also be manifested as atopic asthma, atopic dermatitis, or allergic rhinitis. Symptoms include itching, tearing, redness, stringy discharge, and, in the more severe forms, photophobia and visual loss.

Allergic conjunctivitis is a benign disease, occurring usually in late childhood and early adulthood. It may be seasonal (hay fever conjunctivitis), developing usually during the spring or summer, or perennial. Clinical signs are limited to conjunctival hyperemia and edema (chemosis), the latter occasionally being so marked and sudden in onset as to cause alarm. Vernal keratoconjunctivitis also tends to occur in late childhood and early adulthood. It is usually seasonal, with a predilection for the spring. The conjunctivitis is characterized by large "cobblestone" papillae on the upper tarsal conjunctiva. There may be lymphoid follicles at the limbus. Atopic keratoconjunctivitis is a more chronic disorder of adulthood. Both the upper and the lower tarsal conjunctiva exhibit a fine papillary conjunctivitis with fibrosis, resulting in forniceal shortening and entropion with trichiasis. Staphylococcal blepharitis is a frequent complicating factor. Corneal involvement, including refractory ulceration, is frequent during acute exacerbations of both vernal and atopic keratoconjunctivitis. They are also commonly complicated by herpes simplex keratitis.

Topical lodoxamide four times daily is the recommended treatment for mild and moderately severe allergic eye disease. It is a mast cell stabilizer and is thus better used as prophylaxis than for the treatment of acute episodes. Topical vasoconstrictors and antihistamines are advocated in hay fever conjunctivitis but are of limited efficacy and may produce rebound hyperemia and follicular conjunctivitis. Systemic antihistamines may be useful in prolonged, severe atopic keratoconjunctivitis. Topical corticosteroids are essential to the control of acute exacerbations of both vernal and atopic keratoconjunctivitis. Steroid-induced side effects, including cataracts, glaucoma, and exacerbation of herpes simplex keratitis, are major problems. Topical cyclosporine is a potential alternative treatment. Whether topical corticosteroid therapy is justifiable in allergic conjunctivitis is debatable. Systemic steroid therapy and even plasmapheresis may be required in severe atopic keratoconjunctivitis. In allergic conjunctivitis specific allergens may be identifiable and thus avoidable. In vernal keratoconjunctivitis, a cooler climate often provides significant benefit.

Friedlaender MH: The current and future therapy of allergic conjunctivitis. Curr Opin Ophthalmol 1998;9:54. (Review of treatment options for allergic conjunctivitis.)

Power WJ et al: Long-term follow-up of patients with atopic keratoconjunctivitis. Ophthalmology 1998;105:637. [NLM Cit ID: 98204195] (Corneal grafting required in 11 out of 20 patients with atopic keratoconjunctivitis.)

PINGUECULA & PTERYGIUM

Pinguecula is a yellow elevated nodule on either side of the cornea (more commonly on the nasal side) in the area of the palpebral fissure. It is common in persons over age 35.

Pterygium is a fleshy, triangular encroachment of the conjunctiva onto the nasal side of the cornea and is usually associated with constant exposure to wind, sun, sand, and dust. Pterygium may be either unilateral or bilateral. There may be a genetic predisposition, but no hereditary pattern has been described. Pterygium is fairly common in the southwestern USA.

Histologically, pinguecula and pterygium show similar features of which the most important is elastoid degeneration of the conjunctival substantia propria.

Pingueculae rarely grow, but inflammation (pingueculitis) may occur. No treatment is usually required for pingueculitis or episodes of inflammation of pterygium, but artificial tears are often beneficial, and short courses of topical nonsteroidal anti-inflammatory agents or weak steroids (prednisolone, 0.125% three times a day) may sometimes be necessary.

Excision of a pterygium is indicated if the growth threatens to interfere with vision by approaching the visual axis. Recurrences are frequent and often more aggressive than the primary lesion. Various forms of treatment are available to reduce the frequency of recurrence.

Manning CA et al: Intraoperative mitomycin in primary pterygium excision: A prospective, randomized trial. Ophthalmology 1997;104:844. [NLM Cit ID: 97303708] (Single intraoperative application of mitomycin found to be more effective than postoperative mitomycin or conjunctival autografting in preventing recurrence.)

Panchapakesan J et al: Prevalence of pterygium and pinguecula: the Blue Mountains Eye Study. Aust N Z J Ophthalmol 1998;26 Suppl 1:S2. [NLM Cit ID: 98348150] (Pingueculae identified in 70% and pterygium in 7% of 3564 individuals aged over 48 years.)

CORNEAL ULCER

Corneal ulcers are most commonly due to infection, which may involve bacteria, viruses, fungi, or amebas. Noninfectious causes—all of which may be complicated by infection—include neurotrophic keratitis (resulting from loss of corneal sensation), exposure keratitis (due to inadequate eyelid closure), severe dry eyes, severe allergic eye disease, and various inflammatory disorders that may be purely ocular or part of a systemic vasculitis. These noninfectious conditions will not be discussed further.

Delayed or ineffective treatment of corneal infection may lead to devastating consequences through intraocular infection or corneal scarring. Prompt effective treatment is essential, and for that reason patients must be referred immediately to an ophthalmologist.

Patients present with pain, photophobia, tearing, and reduced vision. The eye is red, with predominantly circumcorneal injection, and there may be purulent or watery discharge. The corneal appearance varies according to the organisms involved.

Parkin B et al: Bacterial keratitis in the critically ill. Br J Ophthalmol 1997;81:1060. [NLM Cit ID: 98158893] (Eight out of nine cases of bacterial keratitis affecting intensive care patients were due to respiratory tract *Pseudomonas aeruginosa.* Introduction of regular eye care, lid taping in eyes with corneal exposure, and tracheal suctioning from the side rather than over the patient's head led to a reduction in incidence of corneal infections.)

Rogers NK et al: Acoustic neuroma and the eye. Br J Neurosurg 1997;11:292. [NLM Cit ID: 97479274] (Postoperative corneal complications correlated closely with preoperative trigeminal sensory loss, confirming the particular risk of keratitis in the presence of both fifth and seventh cranial nerve dysfunction.)

Shiuey Y et al: Peripheral ulcerative keratitis and collagen vascular disease. Int Ophthalmol Clin 1998;38:21. [NLM Cit ID: 98193648] (Review of corneal disease associated with the systemic vasculitides.)

Bacterial Keratitis

Bacterial keratitis tends to pursue an aggressive course. Precipitating factors include contact lens wear, especially soft contact lenses worn overnight, and corneal trauma. The pathogens most commonly isolated are *Pseudomonas aeruginosa,* pneumococcus, moraxella species, and staphylococci. The cornea is hazy, with usually a central ulcer and adjacent stromal abscess. Hypopyon is often present. The ulcer should be scraped to recover material for Gram's stain and culture prior to starting treatment with high-concentration (fortified) topical antibiotics, given at least every hour night and day for the first 24 hours. The initial choice of antibiotics is based on the Gram stain result. For example, gram-positive cocci are treated with a cephalosporin, such as cefazolin, 100 mg/mL; and gram-negative bacilli are treated with an aminoglycoside, such as tobramycin, 15 mg/mL. If no organisms are seen, these two agents are used in parallel. A fluoroquinolone such as ciprofloxacin, 3 mg/mL, or ofloxacin, 3 mg/mL, may be used instead of an aminoglycoside.

Bennett HG et al: Antimicrobial management of presumed microbial keratitis: Guidelines for treatment of central and peripheral ulcers. Br J Ophthalmol 1998;82:137. [NLM Cit ID: 98276326] (Among 57 cases of presumed microbial keratitis, central ulcers were more frequently culture-positive than peripheral ulcers [73% versus 22%]. No factors could reliably predict whether a peripheral ulcer was likely to be culture-positive.)

Benson WH et al: Current diagnosis and treatment of corneal ulcers. Curr Opin Ophthalmol 1998;9:45. (A general review of the management of bacterial keratitis.)

Herpes Simplex Keratitis

Herpes simplex keratitis is an important cause of ocular morbidity in adults. The ability of the virus to colonize the trigeminal ganglion leads to recurrences that may be precipitated by fever, excessive exposure to sunlight, or immunodeficiency (eg, HIV infection).

The dendritic (branching) ulcer is the most characteristic manifestation of epithelial keratitis due to the herpes simplex virus. More extensive ("geographic") ulcers may also occur, particularly if topical corticosteroids have been used. These ulcers are most easily seen after instillation of sterile fluorescein and examination with a blue light. Epithelial disease in itself does not lead to corneal scarring. It responds well to simple debridement and patching. More rapid healing can be achieved by the addition of topical antivirals. Trifluridine drops or idoxuridine drops or ointment are used every 2 hours during the day. Acyclovir ophthalmic ointment may reduce the rates of recurrence and complications. Topical corticosteroids must not be used.

Stromal herpes simplex keratitis produces increasingly severe corneal opacity and irregularity with each recurrence. Topical antivirals alone are usually insufficient to control stromal disease. Thus, topical corticosteroids are frequently used in combination, but steroid dependence is a common consequence. Corticosteroids may also enhance viral replication, leading to severe epithelial disease. Oral acyclovir, 200–400 mg five times a day, may be helpful in the treatment of severe herpetic keratitis and for prophylaxis against recurrences, particularly in atopic or HIV-infected individuals. Corneal grafting is sometimes necessitated by severe stromal scarring, but the overall outcome is relatively poor. ***Caution:*** For patients with known or possible herpetic disease, topical corticosteroids should be prescribed only under strict ophthalmologic supervision.

A controlled trial of oral acyclovir for the prevention of stromal keratitis or iritis in patients with herpes simplex virus epithelial keratitis: The Epithelial Keratitis Trial. Arch Ophthalmol 1997;115:703. [NLM Cit ID: 97338158] (Oral acyclovir provided no apparent additional benefit over topical trifluridine in the prevention of stromal keratitis or iritis in patients with uncomplicated herpes simplex epithelial keratitis.)

Larkin DF: Corneal transplantation for herpes simplex keratitis. Br J Ophthalmol 1998;82:107. [NLM Cit ID: 98276321] (General review of the difficulties surrounding corneal grafting for herpes simplex keratitis.)

Fungal Keratitis

Fungal keratitis tends to occur after corneal injury involving plant material or in an agricultural setting and in immunocompromised patients. There is often an indolent course. The cornea characteristically has multiple stromal abscesses with relatively little epithelial loss. Intraocular infection is common. Corneal scrapings must be cultured on media suitable for fungi whenever the history or corneal appearance is suggestive of fungal disease.

Acanthamoeba Keratitis

Acanthamoeba has recently become a more commonly recognized cause of suppurative keratitis in contact lens wearers. Although severe pain and perineural and ring infiltrates in the corneal stroma are characteristic features, earlier forms of the disease with changes confined to the corneal epithelium are identifiable. Culture requires specialized media. Treatment is severely hampered by the organism's ability to encyst within the corneal stroma. Various agents have been used, including neomycin-polymyxin-gramicidin, chlorhexidine, the investigational agents propamidine isethionate and polyhexamethyl biguanide, and various oral and topical imidazoles such as ketoconazole, miconazole, and itraconazole. Epithelial debridement may be useful in early infections. Corneal grafting may be required in the acute stage to arrest the progression of infection or after resolution of the infection to restore vision.

Illingworth CD et al: Acanthamoeba keratitis. Surv Ophthalmol 1998;42:493. [NLM Cit ID: 98297823] (Review of management.)

Radford CF et al: Acanthamoeba keratitis: mulitcentre study in England, 1992–6. Br J Ophthalmol 1998;82:1387. [NLM Cit ID: 99129130] (Among 243 patients, diagnosis within 30 days of presentation was achieved in 72% compared with 49% in a previous study of cases presenting between 1984 and 1992.)

Herpes Zoster Ophthalmicus

Herpes zoster frequently involves the ophthalmic division of the trigeminal nerve. It presents with malaise, fever, headache, and burning and itching in the periorbital region. The rash is initially vesicular, quickly becoming pustular and then crusting. Involvement of the tip of the nose or the lid margins indicates a high likelihood of intraocular involvement. Ocular signs include conjunctivitis, keratitis, episcleritis, and anterior uveitis, often with elevated intraocular pressure. Recurrent anterior segment inflammation, neurotrophic keratitis, and posterior subcapsular cataract are possible long-term effects. Optic neuropathy, cranial nerve palsies, acute retinal necrosis, and cerebral angiitis are infrequent complications of the acute stage. HIV infection and AIDS are important risk factors for herpes zoster ophthalmicus and increase the chance of development of complications.

Treatment with high-dose oral acyclovir (800 mg five times a day for 10 days, started within 72 hours after eruption of the rash) reduces the incidence of ocular complications but not of postherpetic neuralgia. Anterior uveitis requires topical steroids and cycloplegics.

Margolis TP et al: Herpes zoster ophthalmicus in patients with human immunodeficiency virus infection. Am J Ophthalmol 1998;125:285. [NLM Cit ID: 98171096] (Although the incidence of sight-threatening complications was generally low among the 48 patients studied, those with retinitis or central nervous system disease were severely disabled and difficult to treat.)

ACUTE (ANGLE-CLOSURE) GLAUCOMA

Essentials of Diagnosis

- Rapid onset in older age groups, particularly hyperopes and Asians.
- Severe pain and profound visual loss.
- Red eye, steamy cornea, dilated pupil.
- Hard eye.

General Considerations

Primary acute angle-closure glaucoma can occur only with closure of a preexisting narrow anterior chamber angle, as is found in elderly persons (owing to physiologic enlargement of the lens), hyperopes, and Asians. About 1% of people over age 35 have narrow anterior chamber angles, but many of these never develop acute glaucoma; thus, the condition is uncommon. Angle closure is associated with pupillary dilation and thus might occur from sitting in a darkened movie theater, at times of stress (owing to increased circulating epinephrine), from pharmacologic mydriasis for ophthalmoscopic examination, or from systemic anticholinergic medications such as atropine (eg, preoperative medication), imipramine, or inhaled ipratropium bromide. Dilation of the pupil should be undertaken with caution if the anterior chamber is shallow (readily determined by oblique illumination of the anterior segment of the eye).

Acute angle-closure glaucoma may also occur secondary to long-standing anterior uveitis or dislocation of the lens. Symptoms are the same as in primary acute angle-closure glaucoma, but differentiation is important because of differences in management.

Clinical Findings

Patients with acute glaucoma usually seek treatment immediately because of extreme pain and blurred vision, though there are subacute cases in which presentation is delayed. The blurred vision is characteristically associated with halos around lights. Nausea and even abdominal pain may occur, and acute glaucoma must be remembered in the differential diagnosis of abdominal discomfort and vomiting. The eye is red, the cornea steamy, and the pupil moderately dilated and nonreactive to light. Tonometry (or palpation of the globe) reveals elevated intraocular pressure.

Differential Diagnosis

Acute glaucoma must be differentiated from conjunctivitis, acute uveitis, and corneal disorders (Table 7–1).

Treatment

A. Primary: In primary acute angle-closure glaucoma, laser peripheral iridotomy will usually result in permanent cure. Intraocular pressure must be lowered beforehand. A single 500 mg intravenous dose of acetazolamide, followed by 250 mg orally four times a day, is usually sufficient. Osmotic diuretics, such as oral glycerol and intravenous urea or mannitol—the dosage of all three being 1–2 g/kg—can be used if necessary. Once the intraocular pressure has started to fall, topical 4% pilocarpine, 1 drop every 15 minutes for 1 hour and then four times a day, is used to treat the underlying angle closure. The fellow eye should undergo prophylactic iridectomy.

B. Secondary: In secondary acute angle-closure glaucoma, systemic acetazolamide is also used, with or without osmotic agents, to control intraocular pressure. Further treatment is determined by the underlying pathogenesis.

Prognosis

Untreated acute glaucoma results in severe and permanent visual loss within 2–5 days after onset of symptoms.

Dayan M et al: Acute angle closure glaucoma masquerading as systemic illness. BMJ 1996;313:413. [NLM Cit ID: 96355701]

Erie JC et al: The incidence of primary angle-closure glaucoma in Olmsted County, Minnesota. Arch Ophthalmol 1997;115:177. [NLM Cit ID: 97198197] (The mean annual age- and sex-adjusted incidence of primary angle-closure glaucoma was only 8.3 per 100,000 people aged 40 years and older. Most patients blinded by the disease were blind at the time of diagnosis.)

OPEN-ANGLE GLAUCOMA

Essentials of Diagnosis

- Insidious onset in older age groups.
- No symptoms in early stages.
- Gradual loss of peripheral vision over a period of years, resulting in tunnel vision.
- Persistent elevation of intraocular pressure associated with pathologic cupping of the optic disks.
- "Halos around lights" are not present unless the intraocular tension is markedly elevated.

General Considerations

In open-angle glaucoma, the intraocular pressure is consistently elevated due to abnormal drainage of aqueous through the trabecular meshwork. Over a period of months or years, this results in excavation ("cupping") and pallor of the optic disk with loss of vision varying from slight constriction of the peripheral fields to complete blindness.

The cause of the decreased rate of aqueous outflow in primary open-angle glaucoma has not been clearly established. However a number of mutations, such as in the myocilin gene on chromosome 1, have been identified in a small proportion of cases. The disease is bilateral, and there is an increased prevalence in first-degree relatives of affected individuals and in diabetics. Primary open-angle glaucoma occurs at an earlier age, is more frequent in blacks, and may result in more severe optic nerve damage. There is increasing evidence that factors other than the level of intraocular pressure—particularly vascular abnormalities—may play a role in the pathogenesis of glaucomatous optic nerve damage. Open-angle glaucoma may also develop secondary to other eye disease, such as uveitis or the effects of trauma. Elevation of intraocular pressure is also a complication of steroid therapy, whether it be topical, systemic, inhaled, or administered by nasal spray.

In the USA, it is estimated that 1–2% of people over 40 have glaucoma; about 25% of these cases are undetected. Over 90% of all cases of glaucoma are of the open-angle type.

Clinical Findings

Patients with open-angle glaucoma have no symptoms initially. On examination, there may be slight cupping of the optic disk observed as an absolute increase—or an asymmetry between the two eyes—of the ratio of the diameter of the optic cup to the diameter of the whole optic disk (cup disk ratio). (Cup-disk ratio of greater than 0.3 or asymmetry of cup-disk ratio of 0.2 or more is suggestive of glaucoma.) Changes in the retinal nerve fiber layer may be observed as an earlier finding in some patients. The visual fields gradually constrict, but central vision remains good until late in the disease.

Tonometry, ophthalmoscopic visualization of the optic nerve, and central visual field testing are the three tests for the diagnosis and follow-up. The diagnosis of glaucoma generally depends upon identification of consistent abnormalities in at least two of these parameters. The normal range of intraocular pressure is 10–24 mm Hg. Except in acute cases, the diagnosis of glaucoma is not made on the basis of one tonometric measurement. Intraocular pressure is influenced by various factors, including posture and diurnal variation. In many individuals, elevated intraocular pressure is not associated with optic disk or visual field abnormalities. These ocular hypertensives are at increased risk of developing glaucomatous damage but may only need regular observation. Conversely, a significant proportion of patients with glaucoma have normal intraocular pressure when it is first measured, and it is only repeated measurement which identifies the abnormally high pressure. Furthermore, there are patients with normal tension glaucoma, in which the intraocular pressure is always within the normal range despite repeated measurement even though they have glaucomatous optic disk and visual field abnormalities. There are many other causes of optic disk abnormalities or visual field changes that mimic glaucomatous damage, and visual field testing may prove unreliable in some patients, particularly the elderly. Taken together, these factors mean that the diagnosis of glaucoma is not always straightforward, which greatly hampers the effectiveness of screening programs.

Prevention

All persons over age 40, particularly blacks, should have tonometric and ophthalmoscopic examinations every 3–5 years. In diabetics and in individuals with a family history of glaucoma, annual examination is indicated.

Treatment

Timolol, a β-adrenergic blocking agent, is an effective antiglaucoma agent in a dosage of 1 drop of 0.25% or 0.5% solution every 12 hours, possibly reducing to once daily after 3–6 weeks, or 1 drop of 0.25% or 0.5% gel once daily. Alternative agents are carteolol 1%, levobunolol, 0.5%, and metipranolol 0.3%, each used twice daily. They should be used cautiously if at all in patients with reactive airway disease or heart failure. Betaxolol, 0.25% or 0.5%, a β_1-receptor selective blocking agent, may be safer in patients with reactive airway disease, but its use is diminishing with the availability of other agents such as brimonidine and dorzolamide (see below). Epinephrine eye drops, 0.5–1%, or the prodrug dipivefrin, 0.1%, may be used twice a day either alone or in combination with betaxolol (to overcome the reduction in effect of betaxolol compared to the nonselective beta-blocking agents). Apraclonidine, 0.5–1%, an α_2 agonist administered three times a day, is helpful in controlling acute rises in intraocular pressure (such as after laser therapy) and for postponing the need for surgery in patients receiving maximal medical therapy. Its long-term use is limited by the high incidence of allergic reactions. Brimonidine, 0.2% solution used twice daily, is a more selective α_2 agonist. It may be used in addition to a β-blocker or as initial therapy when β-blockers are contraindicated. Pilocarpine, the standard drug for a century, is still used in 1–4% (and very occasionally higher) concentrations three or four times a day. Because of the induced myopia in younger patients and the pupillary constriction that compromises vision in patients with cataract, it is most often employed when additional therapy to either a beta-blocking agent, epinephrine, or dipivefrin is required. Latanoprost 0.005%, a prostaglandin analogue, used once daily, appears to be as effective as timolol, but permanent changes in iris color have been noted. The topical carbonic anhydrase inhibitor dorzolamide 2% is useful in patients resistant to beta-blockers, as adjunctive therapy twice a day, or when beta-blockers are contraindicated, three times a day as a single agent. Oral carbonic anhydrase inhibitors (eg, acetazolamide) may still be used if topical therapy is inadequate, but they are likely less frequently needed with the availability of dorzolamide. Laser trabeculoplasty is used as an adjunct to topical therapy to postpone the need for surgery. It has also been advocated as primary treatment. Surgical trabeculectomy is necessary for patients whose intraocular pressure remains elevated despite medical and laser therapy and may be used as primary treatment in some individuals. Adjunctive treatment with subconjunctival fluorouracil or mitomycin is used peri- or postoperatively in difficult cases to increase the chances of success of trabeculectomy.

Prognosis

Untreated chronic glaucoma that begins at age 40–45 will probably cause complete blindness by age 60–65. Early diagnosis and treatment will preserve useful vision throughout life in most cases.

Craig JE et al: Glaucoma genetics: Where are we? Where will we go? Curr Opin Ophthalmol 1999;10:126. [NLM Cit ID: 99307932] (A review of mutations so far identified in various types of glaucoma.)

Garbe E et al: Risk of ocular hypertension or open-angle glaucoma in elderly patients on oral glucocorticoids. Lancet 1997;350:979. [NLM Cit ID: 97470095] (Among 9739 patients with newly diagnosed ocular hypertension or glaucoma, the odds ratio for elevated intraocular pressure compared with controls was 1.26 for patients taking less than 40 mg of hydrocortisone per day and 1.88 for those taking 80 mg or more.)

Hattenhauer MG et al: The probability of blindness from open-angle glaucoma. Ophthalmology 1998;105:2099. [NLM Cit ID: 99033921] (Among 295 patients with glaucoma or ocular hypertension, 27% overall and 54% of the glaucoma patients were blind in at least one eye at 20 years follow-up and 9% overall were blind in both eyes.)

Katsushima H et al: Ocular hypertensive effects of corticosteroids applied to the skin. Ann Ophthalmol 1997;29: 128. (Glaucomatous visual loss was identified in 6% of 72 patients applying corticosteroids to the skin, but it only occurred in those treating the face.)

Tuck MW et al: The cost-effectiveness of various modes of screening for primary open angle glaucoma. Ophthalmic Epidemiol 1997;4:3. [NLM Cit ID: 97290765] (Glaucoma screening of people over age 40 years found to be justifiable as long as it is worth more than 850 dollars to detect a new case.)

UVEITIS

Uveitis means inflammation of the uveal tract, which is formed by the iris (iritis), ciliary body (cyclitis), and choroid (choroiditis). Inflammatory eye disease may also originate primarily in the retina (retinitis) or retinal blood vessels (retinal vasculitis).

Intraocular inflammation is classified as anterior uveitis, posterior uveitis, or panuveitis. Uveitis may also be categorized as acute or chronic and granulomatous or nongranulomatous. In most cases the pathogenesis of uveitis is primarily immunologic, but in AIDS or other immunodeficiency states, infection is the primary cause.

Clinical Findings

Anterior uveitis is characterized by inflammatory cells and flare within the aqueous. Cells may also be seen on the corneal endothelium as keratic precipitates (KPs). In granulomatous uveitis, these are large "mutton-fat" KPs, and iris nodules may be seen. In nongranulomatous uveitis, the KPs are smaller and iris nodules are not seen. Occasionally, granulomatous uveitis may initially masquerade as nongranulomatous disease. In severe anterior uveitis, there may be hypopyon (layered collection of white cells) and fibrin within the anterior chamber. In virtually all forms of anterior uveitis, the pupil is small, and with the development of posterior synechiae (adhesions between the iris and anterior lens capsule), it also becomes irregular.

Nongranulomatous anterior uveitis tends to present acutely with unilateral pain, redness, photophobia, and visual loss. Granulomatous anterior uveitis is more likely to present less acutely with blurred vision in a mildly inflamed eye.

In posterior uveitis, there are cells in the vitreous. Inflammatory lesions may be present in the retina or choroid. Fresh lesions are yellow, with indistinct margins, whereas older lesions have more definite margins and are commonly pigmented. Retinal vessel sheathing may occur adjacent to such lesions or more diffusely. In severe cases, vitreous opacity precludes visualization of retinal details.

Posterior uveitis tends to present with gradual visual loss in a relatively quiet eye. Bilateral involvement is common. Visual loss may be due to vitreous haze and opacities, inflammatory lesions involving the macula, macular edema, retinal vein occlusion, or, rarely, associated optic neuropathy.

Etiology

The systemic disorders associated with acute nongranulomatous anterior uveitis are the HLA-B27-related conditions sacroiliitis, ankylosing spondylitis, Reiter's syndrome, psoriasis, ulcerative colitis, and Crohn's disease. Behçet's syndrome produces both anterior uveitis with recurrent hypopyon and posterior uveitis with marked retinal vascular changes. Both herpes simplex and herpes zoster infections may cause nongranulomatous anterior uveitis.

Diseases producing granulomatous anterior uveitis also tend to be causes of posterior uveitis. These include sarcoidosis, which is commonly bilateral; tuberculosis; syphilis; toxoplasmosis; Vogt-Koyanagi-Harada syndrome (bilateral uveitis associated with alopecia, poliosis [depigmented eyelashes, eyebrows, or hair], vitiligo, and hearing loss); and sympathetic ophthalmia. Syphilis produces a characteristic "salt and pepper" fundus, often with surprisingly little visual loss unless there is also primary syphilitic optic atrophy. In congenital toxoplasmosis, there is usually evidence of previous episodes of retinochoroiditis. The principal agents responsible for ocular inflammation in AIDS and other immunodeficiency states are cytomegalovirus, herpes simplex and herpes zoster viruses, mycobacteria, cryptococcus, toxoplasma, and candida.

Autoimmune retinal vasculitis and pars planitis (intermediate uveitis) are idiopathic conditions that produce posterior uveitis.

Retinal detachment, intraocular tumors, and central nervous system lymphoma may all masquerade as uveitis.

Treatment

Anterior uveitis will usually respond to topical corticosteroids. Occasionally, periocular steroid injections or even systemic steroids may be required. Dilation of the pupil is important to relieve discomfort and prevent posterior synechiae.

Posterior uveitis more commonly requires systemic corticosteroid therapy and occasionally systemic immunosuppression with azathioprine or cyclosporine. Pupillary dilation is not usually necessary.

In all cases if an infectious cause is identified, specific chemotherapy may be indicated. In general, the prognosis for anterior uveitis, particularly the nongranulomatous type, is better than that for posterior uveitis.

Management of patients with uveitis must remain primarily in the hands of an ophthalmologist, but the cooperation of other physicians is essential for determining causes and in assisting in the administration of antimicrobials, high-dose systemic corticosteroids, and systemic immunosuppressants.

Akduman L et al: Prevalence of uveitis in an outpatient juvenile arthritis clinic: onset of uveitis more than a decade after onset of arthritis. J Pediatr Ophthalmol Strabismus 1997;34:101. [NLM Cit ID: 97476447] (Reiteration of the high risk of uveitis in girls with ANA-positive juvenile rheumatoid arthritis.)

Chan CC et al: Immunopathology of uveitis. Br J Ophthalmol 1998;82:91. [NLM Cit ID: 98197958] (A review of the pathogenesis of immune-mediated uveitis.)

Chatzistefanou K et al: Characteristics of uveitis presenting for the first time in the elderly. Ophthalmology 1998;105:347. [NLM Cit ID: 98139836] (The range of causes of uveitis presenting after age 60 was little different from that of uveitis presenting earlier.)

Dana MR et al: Prognosticators for visual outcome in sarcoid uveitis. Ophthalmology 1996;103:1846. [NLM Cit ID: 97098339] (Spectrum of disease and outcome in 60 patients.)

Power WJ et al: Outcomes in anterior uveitis associated with the HLA-B27 haplotype. Ophthalmology 1998;105: 1646. [NLM Cit ID: 98426780] (The HLA-B27 haplotype increased the incidence of complications, the need for greater levels of immunosuppression, and the prevalence of blindness.)

CATARACT

Essentials of Diagnosis

- Blurred vision, progressive over months or years.
- No pain or redness.
- Lens opacities (may be grossly visible).

General Considerations

A cataract is a lens opacity. Cataracts are usually bilateral. They may be congenital (owing to intrauterine infections such as rubella and cytomegalovirus, inborn errors of metabolism such as galactosemia); traumatic; or secondary to systemic disease (diabetes, myotonic dystrophy, atopic dermatitis), systemic or inhaled corticosteroid treatment, or uveitis. Senile cataract is by far the most common type; most persons over age 60 have some degree of lens opacity. Cigarette smoking increases the risk of cataract formation.

Clinical Findings

Even in its early stages, a cataract can be seen through a dilated pupil with an ophthalmoscope, a slitlamp, or an ordinary hand illuminator. As the cataract matures, the retina will become increasingly more difficult to visualize, until finally the fundus reflection is absent and the pupil is white.

The degree of visual loss depends on the type and density of the cataract.

Treatment

Functional visual impairment is the prime criterion for surgery. The cataract is usually removed by one of the techniques in which the delicate posterior lens capsule remains (extracapsular). This may, however, call for subsequent laser treatment if the posterior capsule opacifies. With the development of ultrasonic fragmentation (phacoemulsification) of the lens nucleus, it is now possible to perform cataract surgery through a small incision and without suturing the wound, thus reducing the postoperative complication rate and accelerating the patient's visual rehabilitation.

It is routine practice to implant an intraocular lens at the time of surgery. This dispenses with the need for heavy cataract glasses or contact lenses. With improved intraocular lenses, the success rate is high. Multifocal intraocular lenses have been used with some success to reduce the need for both distance and reading glasses.

Prognosis

If surgery is indicated, lens extraction improves visual acuity in 95% of cases. The remainder either have preexisting retinal damage or develop perioperative or postoperative complications.

[AHCPR: Cataracts In Adults: Management of Functional Impairment] http://text.nlm.nih.gov/ftrs/pick?dbName=catc&ftrsK=40746&cp=1&t=915077539&collect=ahcpr

Garbe E et al: Association of inhaled corticosteroid use with cataract extraction in elderly patients. JAMA 1998;280:539. [NLM Cit ID: 98370641] (More than 2 years of treatment with inhaled corticosteroids significantly increased the risk of undergoing cataract surgery.)

Hollick E: Posterior capsule opacification. Curr Med Literature 1998;8:99. (Review of the risk factors for posterior capsule opacification after cataract surgery.)

Javitt JC et al: Outcomes of cataract extraction with multifocal intraocular lens implantation—functional status and quality of life. Ophthalmology 1997;104:589. [NLM Cit ID: 97265313] (Fifty-nine percent of patients with bilateral multifocal implants still needed to wear spectacles.)

Klein BE et al: Incidence of age-related cataract: the Beaver Dam Eye Study. Arch Ophthalmol 1998;116:219. [NLM Cit ID: 98147599] (Nuclear sclerotic cataract in 40% of persons aged 75 years or older.)

Laidlaw DA et al: Randomised trial of effectiveness of second eye cataract surgery. Lancet 1998;352:925. [NLM Cit ID: 98423736] (Second eye cataract surgery had little influence on visual acuity or contrast sensitivity but produced major improvements in reported visual symptoms and quality of life.)

RETINAL DETACHMENT

Essentials of Diagnosis

- Blurred vision in one eye becoming progressively worse. ("A curtain came down over my eye.")
- No pain or redness.
- Detachment seen by ophthalmoscopy.

General Considerations

Detachment of the retina is usually spontaneous but may be secondary to trauma. Spontaneous detachment occurs most frequently in persons over 50 years of age. Cataract extraction and myopia are the two most common predisposing causes.

Clinical Findings

As soon as the retina is torn, fluid vitreous is able to pass through the tear and lodge behind the sensory retina. This, combined with vitreous traction and the pull of gravity, results in progressive detachment. The superior temporal area is the most common site of detachment. The area involved rapidly increases, causing corresponding progressive visual loss. Central vision remains intact until the macula becomes detached.

On ophthalmoscopic examination, the retina is seen hanging in the vitreous like a gray cloud. One or more retinal tears, usually crescent-shaped and red or orange, are usually present and can be seen by an experienced examiner.

Treatment

All cases of retinal detachment should be referred immediately to an ophthalmologist. During transportation, the patient's head should be positioned so that the detached portion of the retina will fall back with the aid of gravity.

Treatment is directed primarily at closing the retinal tears. A permanent adhesion between the neurosensory retina, the retinal pigment epithelium, and the choroid is produced in the region of the tears by applying cryotherapy to the sclera or laser photocoagulation to the retina. In order to achieve apposition of the neurosensory retina to the retinal pigment epithelium while this adhesion is developing, an indentation may be made in the sclera with a silicone sponge or buckle, the fluid between the neurosensory retina and the retinal pigment epithelium (subretinal fluid) may be drained via an incision in the sclera, and an expansile gas may be injected into the vitreous cavity. Certain types of uncomplicated retinal detachment may be treated by the technique of pneumatic retinopexy, in which an expansile gas is initially injected into the vitreous cavity followed by careful positioning of the patient's head to facilitate reattachment of the retina. Once the retina is repositioned, the retinal tear is sealed by laser photocoagulation or cryotherapy. All the stages of pneumatic retinopexy can be performed under local anesthesia as an office procedure. The last stage is the same as is used to seal retinal tears without associated detachment as prophylaxis against detachment.

In complicated retinal detachments—particularly those in which fibroproliferative tissue has developed on the surface of the retina or within the vitreous cavity—retinal reattachment can be accomplished only by removal of the vitreous, direct manipulation of the retina, and internal tamponade of the retina with air, expansile gases, or even silicone oil. (The presence of an expansile gas within the eye is a contraindication to air travel. Such gases may persist in the globe for weeks after surgery.) (See Chapter 38.)

Prognosis

About 80% of uncomplicated cases can be cured with one operation; an additional 15% will need repeated operations; and the remainder never reattach. The prognosis is worse if the macula is detached or if the detachment is of long duration. Without treatment, retinal detachment often becomes total within 6 months. Spontaneous detachments are ultimately bilateral in 2–25% of cases.

Nissen KR et al: Retinal detachment after cataract extraction in myopic eyes. J Cataract Refract Surg 1998; 24:772. [NLM Cit ID: 98306554] (Retinal detachment occurred in 2% of myopic eyes after extracapsular cataract surgery. The risk was increased to 6% by laser capsulotomy.)

Scott IU et al: Vitreoretinal surgery outcomes: Impact on bilateral visual function. Ophthalmology 1997;104:1041. [NLM Cit ID: 97329988] (Unilateral vitreoretinal surgery for a variety of retinal conditions provided a significant reduction in bilateral visual impairment in a sufficient proportion of patients to provide an overall cost saving. The potential for additional benefit in avoiding later loss of visual function was not included.)

VITREOUS HEMORRHAGE

Patients with vitreous hemorrhage complain of sudden visual loss, sudden onset of floaters that may progressively increase in severity, or, occasionally, "bleeding within the eye." Visual acuity ranges from 20/20 to light perception only. The eye is not inflamed, and the clue to diagnosis is the inability to see fundal details clearly despite the presence of a clear lens. Causes of vitreous hemorrhage include diabetic retinopathy, retinal tears (with or without retinal detachment), retinal vein occlusions, exudative age-related macular degeneration, blood dyscrasias, trauma, and subarachnoid hemorrhage (Terson's syndrome). In all cases, examination by an ophthalmologist is essential. Retinal tears and detachments necessitate urgent treatment (see above).

Spraul CW et al: Vitreous hemorrhage. Surv Ophthalmol 1997;42:3. [NLM Cit ID: 97410393] (Comprehensive review of the causes, presentation, outcome, and management of vitreous hemorrhage.)

AGE-RELATED MACULAR DEGENERATION

Age-related macular degeneration is the leading cause of permanent visual loss in the elderly. The exact cause is unknown, but the incidence increases with each decade over age 50 (to almost 30% by age

75). Other associations besides age include race (usually white), sex (slight female predominance), family history, and a history of cigarette smoking. Moderate wine consumption may be protective.

Age-related macular degeneration includes a broad spectrum of clinical and pathologic findings that can be classified into two groups: atrophic ("dry") and exudative ("wet"). Although both types are progressive and usually bilateral, they differ in manifestations, prognosis, and management. The precursor to age-related macular degeneration is age-related maculopathy, of which the hallmark is the development of retinal drusen. Hard drusen appear ophthalmoscopically as discrete yellow deposits, usually in the macular region. Soft drusen are larger, paler, and less distinct. Large, confluent soft drusen are particularly associated with the development of exudative age-related macular degeneration.

Atrophic degeneration is characterized by gradually progressive bilateral visual loss of moderate severity due to atrophy and degeneration of the outer retina, retinal pigment epithelium, Bruch's membrane, and choriocapillaris. In exudative degeneration, visual loss is of more rapid onset and greater severity, and the two eyes are frequently affected sequentially over a period of a few years. The exudative form accounts for about 90% of all cases of legal blindness due to this disorder. Impairment of the barrier function of Bruch's membrane (between the retinal pigment epithelium and the choriocapillaris) allows serous fluid or blood to leak into the retina to produce elevation of the retinal pigment epithelium from Bruch's membrane (retinal pigment epithelial detachment) or separation of the neurosensory retina from the retinal pigment epithelium (serous retinal detachment). These changes may resolve spontaneously, with variable visual outcome, but are often associated with neovascularization arising from the choroidal vessels and extending between the retinal pigment epithelium and Bruch's membrane (subretinal neovascular membrane). This membrane produces permanent visual loss.

Sudden visual loss in patients with exudative age-related macular degeneration occurs at the time of pigment epithelial or sensory retinal detachment or hemorrhage from a subretinal neovascular membrane. All these changes may occur in previously undiagnosed patients, in patients known to have atrophic changes, and in the other eye of patients with exudative disease. Laser photocoagulation of subretinal neovascular membranes may delay the onset of permanent visual loss but only when the membrane is far enough away from the fovea to permit such treatment. Conventional laser photocoagulation of subfoveal neovascular membranes is associated with an inevitable immediate reduction in vision because of associated retinal damage. Photodynamic laser therapy produces selective vascular damage, which may thus limit the degree of visual loss. Various surgical techniques to excise subfoveal neovascular membranes—or to reposition the macula away from them—are also being studied. The value of radiotherapy for subretinal neovascular membranes remains uncertain. Elderly patients developing sudden visual loss due to macular disease—particularly paracentral distortion or scotoma with preservation of central acuity—should be referred urgently to an ophthalmologist for assessment.

There is no specific treatment for atrophic age-related macular degeneration, but—as with the exudative form—patients often benefit from low vision aids. The disorder results in loss of central vision only. Peripheral fields and hence navigational vision are always maintained, though these may become impaired by cataract formation for which surgery may be helpful. Laser photocoagulation may reverse the development of soft drusen and reduce the risk of subsequent visual loss.

Ciulla TA et al: Age-related macular degeneration: a review of experimental treatments. Surv Ophthalmol 1998; 43:134. [NLM Cit ID: 98434102] (A review of novel laser, surgical, radiotherapeutic, and pharmacologic methods to treat subretinal neovascularization.)

Finger PT et al: Ophthalmic plaque radiotherapy for age-related macular degeneration associated with subretinal neovascularization. Am J Ophthalmol 1999;127:170. [NLM Cit ID: 99153630] (Radiotherapy treatment of subretinal neovascular membrane by application of a radioactive plaque directly to the globe, as used in the treatment of intraocular tumors.)

Lewis H et al: Macular translocation for subfoveal choroidal neovascularization in age-related macular degeneration: a prospective study. Am J Ophthalmol 1999;128:135. [NLM Cit ID: 99385350] (One of the various surgical techniques being tried to reposition the macula away from a subfoveal neovascular membrane.)

Pieramici DJ et al: Age-related macular degeneration and risk factors for the development of choroidal neovascularization in the fellow eye. Curr Opin Ophthalmol 1998;9:38. [NLM Cit ID: 98388482] (Review of the incidence rates and risk factors for choroidal neovascularization in the second eye of patients with age-related macular degeneration.)

Schmidt-Erfurth U et al: Photodynamic therapy of subfoveal choroidal neovascularization: clinical and angiographic examples. Graefes Arch Clin Exp Ophthalmol 1998;236:365. [NLM Cit ID: 98265031] (Absence of retinal damage in 61 patients with subfoveal neovascularization treated by laser photodynamic therapy.)

Wu L et al: Photodynamic therapy: a new approach to the treatment of choroidal neovascularization secondary to age-related macular degeneration. Curr Opin Ophthalmol 1999;10:217. [NLM Cit ID: 99309728] (Review of photodynamic therapy for subretinal neovascular membranes.)

CENTRAL & BRANCH RETINAL VEIN OCCLUSIONS

The severity of visual loss in central retinal vein occlusion is variable. The visual impairment is commonly first noticed upon waking in the morning. Ophthalmoscopic signs include disk swelling, venous dilation and tortuosity, retinal hemorrhages, and cotton-wool spots.

In those with initially good acuity (20/60 or better), the visual prognosis is good. In those with poor initial acuity (20/200 or worse), extensive hemorrhages and multiple cotton-wool spots indicate widespread retinal ischemia, which can be confirmed by demonstrating extensive areas of capillary closure on fluorescein angiography. These eyes are at high risk of developing neovascular (rubeotic) glaucoma, typically within 3 months after venous occlusion, and should be monitored by an ophthalmologist so that laser panretinal photocoagulation can be undertaken if neovascularization occurs. The visual prognosis in these cases is poor.

Branch retinal vein occlusions may present in a variety of ways. Sudden loss of vision may occur at the time of occlusion if the fovea is involved or some time afterward from vitreous hemorrhage due to retinal new vessels. More gradual visual loss may occur with development of macular edema or exudate. In a significant proportion, the occlusion is noted incidentally in patients with glaucoma, systemic hypertension, diabetes mellitus, or uveitis.

In acute branch retinal vein occlusion there are signs similar to those of central retinal vein occlusion but affecting only the retina drained by the obstructed vein. There is no specific treatment, but if retinal neovascularization develops, the area of retina affected by the initial occlusion should be laser-photocoagulated. Macular edema may also respond to laser treatment.

All patients with retinal vein occlusion should be referred urgently to an ophthalmologist and investigated for glaucoma, systemic hypertension, diabetes mellitus, and hyperlipidemia. In younger patients, levels of protein C, activated protein C resistance, protein S, and antithrombin III should be measured if there is a personal or family history of thrombotic disease. Hyperviscosity syndromes and other hematologic abnormalities are only rarely associated with retinal vein occlusions but may worsen their prognosis. Branch retinal vein occlusion is an important feature of Behçet's syndrome.

Gottlieb JL et al: Activated protein C resistance, factor V Leiden, and central retinal vein occlusion in young adults. Arch Ophthalmol 1998;116:577. [NLM Cit ID: 98255931] (Among 21 patients under 50 years of age with central retinal vein occlusion, only one had activated protein C resistance, also being the only patient with a family history of thrombotic disease.)

Natural history and clinical management of central retinal vein occlusion. Central Retinal Vein Occlusion Study Group. Arch Ophthalmol 1997;115:486. [NLM Cit ID: 97263885] (In a prospective study of 725 patients with central retinal vein occlusion, visual acuity at presentation generally predicted final visual outcome, and poor initial visual acuity and retinal ischemia were strong predictors of anterior segment neovascularization.)

Sperduto RD et al: Risk factors for hemiretinal vein occlusion: Comparison with risk factors for central and branch retinal vein occlusion: The Eye Disease Case-Control Study. Ophthalmology 1998;105:765. [NLM Cit ID: 98254205] (Principal risk factors for retinal vein occlusion were systemic hypertension, diabetes, and glaucoma.)

CENTRAL & BRANCH RETINAL ARTERY OCCLUSIONS

Central retinal artery occlusion presents as sudden profound visual loss. Visual acuity is reduced to counting fingers or worse, and visual field is commonly restricted to an island of vision in the temporal field. Ophthalmoscopy reveals pallid swelling of the retina, most obvious in the posterior segment, with a cherry-red spot at the fovea. The retinal arteries are attenuated, and "box-car" segmentation of blood in the veins may be seen. Occasionally, emboli are seen in the central retinal artery or its branches. The retinal swelling subsides over a period of 4–6 weeks, leaving a relatively normal retinal appearance but a pale optic disk and attenuated arterioles.

The patient should be referred as an emergency to an ophthalmologist. If seen within a few hours after onset, emergency treatment—including laying the patient flat, ocular massage, high concentrations of inhaled oxygen, intravenous acetazolamide, and anterior chamber paracentesis—may influence the visual outcome. Thrombolysis, particularly by local intra-arterial but also by peripheral intravenous injection, is being used more commonly.

The main management problem is identifying any treatable underlying disorder. Giant cell arteritis must be excluded in all older patients, especially because of the risk—highest in the first few days—of involvement of the other eye. If giant cell arteritis is diagnosed, either on the basis of associated symptoms (especially polymyalgia rheumatica or headache), with a high erythrocyte sedimentation rate, one should institute high-dose corticosteroids promptly and proceed immediately to temporal artery biopsy. Carotid and cardiac sources of emboli must also be considered in retinal artery occlusion and appropriate treatment given to reduce the risk of stroke (see Chapter 12).

Branch retinal artery occlusion may also present with sudden loss of vision if the fovea is involved, but more commonly sudden loss of visual field is the presenting complaint. Fundal signs of retinal swelling and adjacent cotton-wool spots are limited to the area of retina supplied by the occluded vessel. Embolic causes are proportionately more common than in central retinal artery occlusion. Migraine, oral contraceptives, and vasculitis must also be considered. Antiphospholipid antibodies have been associated with branch and central retinal artery occlusions in younger patients. Patients with branch retinal artery occlusions should be referred urgently to an ophthalmologist.

Hayreh SS et al: Giant cell arteritis: Validity and reliability of various diagnostic criteria. Am J Ophthalmol 1997;123:285. [NLM Cit ID: 97217216] (Jaw claudication, C-reactive protein > 24.5 mg/L, ESR > 46 mm/h, and age > 74 found to be the most useful predictors of giant cell arteritis.)

Schmidt D et al: Stage-dependent efficacy of intra-arterial fibrinolysis in central retinal artery occlusion (CRAO). Neuro-ophthalmology 1998;20:125. (Intra-arterial fibrinolysis produced complete recovery or marked improvement in 24% and partial improvement in 37% of 46 patients with central retinal artery occlusion, being most effective when administered within 14 hours after visual loss.)

Sharma S et al: Transthoracic echocardiographic findings in patients with acute retinal arterial obstruction. A retrospective review. Arch Ophthalmol 1996;114:1189. [NLM Cit ID: 97012261] (History or clinical signs of cardiac disease were found to be a reliable guide to the probable need for anticoagulation or cardiac surgery in 100 patients with retinal arterial occlusion.)

AMAUROSIS FUGAX

Amaurosis fugax ("fleeting blindness") is characteristically caused by retinal emboli from ipsilateral carotid disease. The visual loss is usually described as a curtain passing vertically across the visual field with complete monocular visual loss lasting a few minutes and a similar curtain effect as the episode passes. In order to reduce the risk of stroke, patients with high-grade stenosis (70–99%) of the ipsilateral internal carotid artery should be considered for carotid endarterectomy. Patients with medium-grade (30–69%) or low-grade (up to 29%) stenosis are better treated medically with aspirin or other antiplatelet drugs. The most reliable method of evaluating carotid stenosis is intra-arterial angiography, but this is associated with a number of complications including stroke. Developments in the noninvasive techniques of duplex ultrasonography and magnetic resonance angiography may soon lead to their becoming the methods of choice in most cases. Emboli from cardiac sources may also be responsible for amaurosis fugax. Echocardiography should be undertaken in young patients and in any patient with clinical evidence of a potential cardiac source of emboli. In younger patients without carotid or cardiac disease, amaurosis fugax may be due to choroidal or retinal vascular spasm, in which case calcium channel blockers such as slow-release nifedipine, 60 mg/d, appear to be effective.

Similar obscurations of vision may occur with poor ocular perfusion due to severe occlusive carotid disease or to aortic dissection. More transient obscurations (lasting only a few seconds to 1 minute) affecting both eyes occur in patients with raised intracranial pressure. In all cases of episodic visual loss, early ophthalmologic consultation is advisable.

Managing carotid stenosis. Drug Ther Bull 1998;36:9. (A comprehensive review of the role of surgical and medical treatment in the management of carotid stenosis.)

RETINAL DISORDERS ASSOCIATED WITH SYSTEMIC DISEASES

Many systemic diseases are associated with retinal manifestations. These include diabetes mellitus, essential hypertension, preeclampsia-eclampsia of pregnancy, blood dyscrasias, and AIDS. The retinal changes caused by these disorders can be easily observed with the aid of the ophthalmoscope.

Diabetic Retinopathy

Diabetic retinopathy is the leading cause of new blindness among US adults aged 20–65. It is broadly classified as nonproliferative and proliferative.

Nonproliferative retinopathy is characterized by dilation of veins, microaneurysms, retinal hemorrhages, retinal edema, and hard exudates. A major subgroup are those patients in which visual loss develops owing to edema, exudates, or ischemia at the macula (diabetic maculopathy). This is the most common cause of legal blindness in maturity-onset diabetes.

Proliferative retinopathy is characterized by neovascularization, arising either from the optic disk or the major vascular arcades. Vitreous hemorrhage is a common sequela. Proliferation into the vitreous of blood vessels, with their associated fibrous component, leads to tractional retinal detachment. Without treatment, the visual prognosis with proliferative retinopathy is generally much worse than that with nonproliferative retinopathy. Severe proliferative retinopathy is often complicated by maculopathy.

Nonproliferative retinopathy is occasionally present at the time of diagnosis in maturity-onset diabetes and may be the presenting feature. Treatment includes optimizing control of blood glucose and any associated systemic hypertension or hyperlipidemia. Institution of intensive insulin therapy can be associated with temporary exacerbation of retinopathy, particularly characterized by multiple cotton-wool spots. Laser photocoagulation is particularly helpful in the treatment of focal macular edema but may also be used when there is diffuse macular edema. The presence of macular edema can be detected only by stereoscopic examination of the retina or by fluorescein angiography. The level of visual acuity is a poor guide to the presence of treatable maculopathy—hence the need for regular ophthalmologic follow-up.

Proliferative retinopathy must be recognized early and treated by panretinal laser photocoagulation to prevent blindness. Neovascularization is all too often diagnosed only at the time of vitreous hemorrhage. In some patients, a "preproliferative" retinopathy may be identified. Whether panretinal laser photocoagulation should be undertaken at this time can be determined by the degree of retinal ischemia as assessed by fluorescein angiography.

Surgical treatment (vitrectomy) is being used increasingly either to remove vitreous hemorrhage and thus allow perioperative panretinal laser photocoagulation for the underlying retinal neovascularization, to deal with retinal detachments involving the macula, to manage rapidly progressive proliferative disease, or to treat persistent macular edema.

Patients with diabetes mellitus should have at least yearly ophthalmoscopic examination through dilated pupils. Examination by an ophthalmologist is usually advisable in juvenile-onset diabetes of more than 5 years' duration; at the time of diagnosis in maturity-onset diabetes; in early pregnancy, or prior to conception in women contemplating pregnancy, and every 4–8 weeks throughout pregnancy; if ocular symptoms develop; or if there are suspicious findings of retinopathy, especially neovascularization or macular exudates. Failure to diagnose diabetic retinopathy by ophthalmoscopic examination is common, particularly if the pupils are not dilated. The severity of diabetic retinopathy can be lessened by careful control of blood glucose levels, but good diabetic control is more important in preventing the development of retinopathy than in influencing its subsequent course. Proliferative diabetic retinopathy, especially after successful laser treatment, is not a contraindication to treatment with thrombolytic agents, aspirin, or warfarin unless there has been recent vitreous or preretinal hemorrhage.

Cordeiro MF et al: Relationship of diabetic microvascular complications to outcome in panretinal photocoagulation treatment of proliferative diabetic retinopathy. Eye 1997;11:531. [NLM Cit ID: 98086557] (Among 66 consecutively treated eyes, the number of retinal laser burns required to control proliferative diabetic retinopathy was almost 6000—much more than the 1600 burns recommended by the Diabetic Retinopathy Study.)

Davis MD et al: Risk factors for high-risk proliferative diabetic retinopathy and severe visual loss: Early Treatment Diabetic Retinopathy Study Report No. 18. Invest Ophthalmol Vis Sci 1998;39:233. [NLM Cit ID: 98138467] (Poor glycemic control once again found to be an important factor for poor outcome in diabetic retinopathy.)

Early worsening of diabetic retinopathy in the Diabetes Control and Complications Trial. Arch Ophthalmol 1998;116:874. [NLM Cit ID: 98347622] (Intensive insulin therapy was associated with worsening of retinopathy in 13% of patients, but the long-term outcome was better.)

Kohner EM et al: United Kingdom Prospective Diabetes Study, 30. Diabetic retinopathy at diagnosis of non-insulin dependent diabetes mellitus and associated risk factors. Arch Ophthalmol 1998;116:297. [NLM Cit ID: 98173417] (Thirty-five percent of men and 39% of women with newly diagnosed type 2 diabetes mellitus had diabetic retinopathy. Higher fasting plasma glucose, higher blood pressure, and lower serum insulin levels were risk factors for the presence of retinopathy.)

Neely KA et al: Diabetic retinopathy. Med Clin North Am 1998;82:847. [NLM Cit ID: 98371381] (Review of screening and management of diabetic retinopathy.)

Smiddy WE et al: Vitrectomy in the management of diabetic retinopathy. Surv Ophthalmol 1999;43:491. [NLM Cit ID: 99343181]

Hypertensive Retinochoroidopathy

Systemic hypertension affects both the retinal and choroidal circulations. The clinical manifestations vary according to the degree and rapidity of rise in blood pressure and the underlying state of the ocular circulation. The most florid disease occurs in young patients with abrupt elevations of blood pressure, such as may occur in pheochromocytoma, malignant essential hypertension, acute renal failure, or pre-eclampsia-eclampsia.

Chronic hypertension accelerates the development of atherosclerosis. The retinal arterioles become more tortuous and narrow and develop abnormal light reflexes ("silver-wiring" and "copper-wiring"). There is increased venous compression at the retinal arteriovenous crossings ("arteriovenous nicking"), which is an important factor predisposing to branch retinal vein occlusions. Flame-shaped hemorrhages occur in the nerve fiber layer of the retina.

Acute elevations of blood pressure result in loss of autoregulation in the retinal circulation, leading to the breakdown of endothelial integrity and occlusion of precapillary arterioles and capillaries. These pathologic changes are manifested as cotton-wool spots, retinal hemorrhages, retinal edema, and retinal exudates, often in a stellate appearance at the macula. In the choroid, vasoconstriction and ischemia result in serous retinal detachments and retinal pigment epithelial infarcts. These infarcts later develop into pigmented lesions that may be focal, linear, or wedge-shaped. The abnormalities in the choroidal circulation may also affect the optic nerve head, producing ischemic optic neuropathy with optic disk swelling. Malignant hypertensive retinopathy was the term previously used to describe the constellation of clinical signs resulting from the combination of abnormalities in the retinal, choroidal, and optic disk circulation. When there is such severe disease, there is likely to be permanent retinal, choroidal, or optic nerve damage. Precipitous reduction of blood pressure may exacerbate such damage.

Schubert HD: Ocular manifestations of systemic hypertension. Curr Opin Ophthalmol 1998;9:69. [NLM Cit ID: 99260071] (A general review of hypertensive retinochoroidopathy.)

Blood Dyscrasias

In conditions characterized by thrombocytopenia or severe anemia, various types of hemorrhages are present in both the retina and choroid and may lead to visual loss. If the dyscrasia is successfully treated and macular hemorrhages have not occurred, it is possible to regain normal vision.

Proliferative retinopathy (sickle cell retinopathy) is particularly common in hemoglobin SC disease but may also occur with other hemoglobin S variants. Severe visual loss is rare. Retinal photocoagulation reduces the frequency of vitreous hemorrhage. Surgery is occasionally needed for unresolving vitreous hemorrhage or tractional retinal detachment.

AIDS

Cotton-wool spots, retinal hemorrhages, and microaneurysms are the most common ophthalmic abnormalities in AIDS patients.

Cytomegalovirus retinitis occurs in many AIDS patients, generally when CD4 counts are below 50/μL. It is characterized by progressively enlarging yellowish-white patches of retinal opacification, which are accompanied by retinal hemorrhages; they usually begin adjacent to the major retinal vascular arcades. Patients are often asymptomatic until there is involvement of the fovea or optic nerve or until retinal detachment develops.

The agents effective in cytomegalovirus retinitis are ganciclovir, foscarnet, and the nucleotide analog cidofovir, formerly known as HPMPC, which has the significant advantage of a prolonged intracellular half-life such that no more than weekly administration is required. Major side effects are neutropenia with systemic ganciclovir due to bone marrow suppression, and limiting therapy with zidovudine (AZT), and nephrotoxicity with foscarnet and cidofovir. Dosage of both ganciclovir and foscarnet needs to be adjusted in renal failure. Oral probenecid and intravenous hydration are used to minimize nephrotoxicity from cidofovir. All three agents are only virostatic. Reactivation of disease and hence eventually complete loss of vision can only be delayed rather than prevented.

Initial therapy is either intravenous—ganciclovir, 5 mg/kg twice a day, foscarnet 60 mg/kg three times a day, or cidofovir 5 mg/kg once weekly, usually for 2 weeks—or by local administration, using either intravitreal injection of ganciclovir or foscarnet or the sustained-release ganciclovir intravitreal implant. Intravitreal cidofovir is effective, but there is a high incidence of uveitis, low intraocular pressure, and ciliary body necrosis. Maintenance therapy can be undertaken with lower-dose intravenous therapy (ganciclovir, 3.75 mg/kg/d, or foscarnet, 60 mg/kg/d, for 5 days each week; or cidofovir, 5 mg/kg once every 2 weeks), oral ganciclovir (3 g/d), or intravitreal therapy. Local therapy tends to be more effective than systemic therapy and avoids systemic side effects, but there is a risk of intraocular complications, and the incidences of retinitis in the fellow eye and of extraocular cytomegalovirus infection are higher. Unresponsive disease or reactivation during maintenance therapy can be managed by changing to a different agent or by use of combination therapy. Retinal detachment, either directly due to retinitis or as a complication of intravitreal therapy, generally requires vitrectomy and intravitreal silicone oil. The use of oral ganciclovir as prophylaxis against cytomegalovirus retinitis in patients with low CD4 counts or high CMV burdens has not been found to be worthwhile.

Antiretroviral therapy may result in reduction of HIV virus load and increase in CD4 counts, and even regression of CMV retinitis without the use of anticytomegalovirus therapy. If the CD4 count is maintained above 100/μL, it may be possible to discontinue maintenance anticytomegalovirus therapy.

Other opportunistic ophthalmic infections occurring in AIDS patients include herpes simplex retinitis, toxoplasmic and candidal chorioretinitis, and herpes zoster ophthalmicus. Kaposi's sarcoma of the conjunctiva and orbital lymphoma may also be seen on rare occasions.

Casado JL et al: Improved outcome of cytomegalovirus retinitis in AIDS patients after introduction of protease inhibitors. J Acquir Immune Defic Syndr Hum Retrovirol 1998;19:130. [NLM Cit ID: 98439557] (Protease inhibitor therapy increased by twofold the probability of remaining free from relapse of cytomegalovirus retinitis among 17 AIDS patients receiving anti-CMV therapy.)

Lalezari JP et al: Randomized, controlled study of the safety and efficacy of intravenous cidofovir for the treatment of relapsing cytomegalovirus retinitis in patients with AIDS. J Acquir Immune Defic Syndr Hum Retrovirol 1998;17:339. [NLM Cit ID: 98184347] (Intravenous induction cidofovir therapy—5 mg/kg weekly for 2 weeks—and then maintenance—5 mg/kg or 3 mg/kg weekly—delayed progression of cytomegalovirus retinitis that had relapsed on foscarnet or ganciclovir therapy.)

Robinson MR et al: Ocular manifestations of HIV infection. Curr Opin Ophthalmol 1999;10:431. [NLM Cit ID: 20064414] (Review of recent advances in the diagnosis and management of HIV-associated ocular disease.)

Tural C et al: Long-lasting remission of cytomegalovirus retinitis without maintenance therapy in human immunodeficiency virus-infected patients. J Infect Dis 1998; 177:1080. [NLM Cit ID: 98194610] (In seven AIDS patients with healed CMV retinitis and taking protease inhibitor therapy, with CD4 counts > 150/μL, HIV load of < 200/mL, and negative qualitative CMV PCR, withdrawal of anti-CMV therapy failed to result in any relapse of retinitis during a median follow-up of 9 months.)

ANTERIOR ISCHEMIC OPTIC NEUROPATHY

Anterior ischemic optic neuropathy—due to inadequate perfusion of the posterior ciliary arteries that

The primary clinical features are proptosis, lid retraction and lid lag, conjunctival chemosis and episcleral inflammation, and extraocular muscle abnormalities due to restriction of their actions. Resulting symptoms are cosmetic abnormalities, surface irritation, which usually responds to artificial tears, and diplopia, which should be treated conservatively (eg, with prisms) in the active stages of the disease and only by surgery when the disease has been static for at least 6 months.

The important complications are corneal exposure and optic nerve compression, both of which may lead to profound visual loss. Treatment is by urgent orbital decompression, either medically, with high-dose systemic steroids (prednisolone 80–100 mg/d)—although this is often of only short-term benefit—by radiotherapy, or by surgery, usually consisting of extensive removal of bone from the medial, inferior, and lateral walls of the orbit.

The optimal management of moderately severe dysthyroid eye disease without visual loss is controversial. Oral steroids, radiotherapy, and surgical decompression have all been advocated, but there is a risk of serious local or systemic side-effects from all three. Lateral tarsorrhaphy may be used for moderately severe corneal exposure. Other lid procedures are particularly useful for correcting lid retraction but should not be undertaken until the orbital disease is quiescent and orbital decompression or extraocular muscle surgery has been undertaken if necessary. Cigarette smoking adversely influences the course of dysthyroid eye disease and its response to treatment.

Bartalena L et al: Cigarette smoking and treatment outcomes in Graves ophthalmopathy. Ann Intern Med 1998;129:632. [NLM Cit ID: 98442933] (Cigarette smoking increased the risk of progression of dysthyroid eye disease after radioiodine therapy and reduced the rate of response to orbital radiotherapy and systemic steroid therapy.)

Bartalena L et al: Relation between therapy for hyperthyroidism and the course of Graves' ophthalmopathy. N Engl J Med 1998;338:73. [NLM Cit ID: 98069964] (Radioiodine compared with methimazole treatment for hyperthyroidism was associated with an increased rate of progression of orbital disease, which was prevented by prednisone therapy.)

Olver JM: Surgery for dysthyroid ophthalmopathy. Curr Medical Literature 1998;3:67. (Review of orbital, squint, and eyelid surgery for dysthyroid eye disease.)

ORBITAL CELLULITIS

Orbital cellulitis is manifested by an abrupt onset of fever, proptosis, restriction of extraocular movements, and swelling and redness of the lids, usually in a child. Infection of the paranasal sinuses is the usual underlying cause. Immediate treatment with intravenous antibiotics is necessary to prevent optic nerve damage and spread of infection to the cavernous sinuses—manifested as increased restriction of extraocular movements, impaired visual acuity, diminished pupillary reflexes, and papilledema, all of which may be bilateral—meninges, and brain. The response to antibiotics is usually excellent, but abscess formation may necessitate surgical drainage.

Donahue SP et al: Preseptal and orbital cellulitis in childhood: A changing microbiologic spectrum. Ophthalmology 1998;105:1902. [NLM Cit ID: 99003630] (Streptococcus species were the most frequently cultured organisms in cases of orbital or preseptal cellulitis.)

OCULAR TRAUMA

Conjunctival & Corneal Foreign Bodies

If a patient complains of "something in my eye" and gives a consistent history, a foreign body is usually present on the cornea or under the upper lid even though it may not be readily visible. Visual acuity should be tested before treatment is instituted, as a basis for comparison in the event of complications.

After a local anesthetic (eg, proparacaine, 0.5%) is instilled, the eye is examined with the aid of a hand flashlight, using oblique illumination, and loupe. Corneal foreign bodies may be made more apparent by the instillation of sterile fluorescein. They are then removed with a sterile wet cotton-tipped applicator. Polymyxin-bacitracin ophthalmic ointment should be instilled. It is not necessary to patch the eye, but the patient must be examined 24 hours later for secondary infection of the crater. If a corneal foreign body cannot be removed in this manner, the patient should be referred to an ophthalmologist.

Steel foreign bodies usually leave a diffuse rust ring. This requires excision of the affected tissue and is best done under local anesthesia using a slitlamp. ***Caution:*** Anesthetic drops should not be given to the patient for self-administration.

If there is no infection, a layer of corneal epithelial cells will line the crater within 24 hours. It should be emphasized that the intact corneal epithelium forms an effective barrier to infection, but once it is disturbed the cornea becomes extremely susceptible to infection. Early infection is manifested by a white necrotic area around the crater and a small amount of gray exudate. These patients should be referred immediately to an ophthalmologist, since untreated corneal infection may lead to loss of the eye.

In the case of a foreign body under the upper lid, a local anesthetic is instilled and the lid is everted by grasping the lashes gently and exerting pressure on the mid portion of the outer surface of the upper lid with an applicator. If a foreign body is present, it can easily be removed by passing a wet sterile cotton-tipped applicator across the conjunctival surface.

Intraocular Foreign Body

Intraocular foreign body requires emergency treatment by an ophthalmologist. Patients giving a history of "something hitting the eye"—particularly if it happens while hammering on metal or using grinding equipment—must be carefully assessed for the possibility of an intraocular foreign body, especially when no corneal foreign body is seen, a corneal or scleral wound is apparent, or there is marked visual loss or media opacity. Such patients must be treated as for corneal laceration (see below) and referred without delay to an ophthalmologist. Intraocular foreign bodies significantly increase the risk of intraocular infection.

Reynolds DS et al: Endophthalmitis after penetrating ocular trauma. Curr Opin Ophthalmol 1997;8:32. (Risk factors, including retained intraocular foreign body, and identification and management of intraocular infection complicating penetrating eye injury.)

Corneal Abrasions

A patient with a corneal abrasion complains of severe pain and photophobia. There is often a history of trauma to the eye, commonly involving a fingernail, piece of paper, or contact lens. Visual acuity is recorded, and the cornea and conjunctiva are examined with a light and loupe to rule out a foreign body. If an abrasion is suspected but cannot be seen, sterile fluorescein is instilled into the conjunctival sac: the area of corneal abrasion will stain a deeper green than the surrounding cornea.

Treatment includes polymyxin-bacitracin ophthalmic ointment and application of a bandage with firm pressure to prevent movement of the lid. The patient should rest at home, keeping the fellow eye closed, and should be observed the following day to be certain the cornea has healed. Recurrent corneal erosion may follow corneal abrasions.

Contusions

Contusion injuries of the eye and surrounding structures may cause ecchymosis ("black eye"), subconjunctival hemorrhage, edema or rupture of the cornea, hemorrhage into the anterior chamber (hyphema), rupture of the root of the iris (iridodialysis), paralysis of the pupillary sphincter, paralysis of the muscles of accommodation, cataract, dislocation of the lens, vitreous hemorrhage, retinal hemorrhage and edema (most common in the macular area), detachment of the retina, rupture of the choroid, fracture of the orbital floor ("blowout fracture"), or optic nerve injury. Many of these injuries are immediately obvious; others may not become apparent for days or weeks. Patients with moderate to severe contusions should be seen by an ophthalmologist.

Any injury severe enough to cause hyphema involves the danger of secondary hemorrhage, which may cause intractable glaucoma with permanent visual loss. Any patient with traumatic hyphema should be advised to rest quietly until complete resolution has occurred. Daily ophthalmologic assessment is essential. Aspirin and related drugs increase the risk of secondary hemorrhage and must be avoided.

Ashar A et al: Blindness associated with midfacial fractures. J Oral Maxillofac Surg 1998;56:1146. [NLM Cit ID: 98437929] (Ten out of 49 patients with midfacial fractures lost vision in one eye.)

Lacerations

A. Lids: If the lid margin is lacerated, the patient should be referred for specialized care, since permanent notching may result. Lacerations of the lower eyelid near the inner canthus often sever the lower canaliculus. Lid lacerations not involving the margin may be sutured just like any other skin laceration.

B. Conjunctiva: In superficial lacerations of the conjunctiva, sutures are not necessary. In order to prevent infection, sulfonamides or other antibiotics are instilled into the eye until the laceration is healed.

C. Cornea or Sclera: Patients with suspected corneal or scleral lacerations must be seen by an ophthalmologist as soon as possible. Manipulation is kept to a minimum, since pressure may result in extrusion of the intraocular contents. The eye is bandaged lightly and covered with a metal shield that rests on the orbital bones above and below. The patient should be instructed not to squeeze the eye shut and to remain as quiet as possible. The eye is routinely studied by x-ray, and CT scanning if necessary, to identify and localize any metallic intraocular foreign body. MRI is contraindicated owing to the risk of movement of the foreign body in the magnetic field.

Ultraviolet Keratitis (Actinic Keratitis)

Ultraviolet burns of the cornea are usually caused by use of a sunlamp without eye protection, exposure to a welding arc, or exposure to the sun when skiing ("snow blindness"). There are no immediate symptoms, but about 6–12 hours later the patient complains of agonizing pain and severe photophobia. Slitlamp examination after instillation of sterile fluorescein shows diffuse punctate staining of both corneas.

Treatment consists of binocular patching and instillation of 1–2 drops of 1% cyclopentolate (to relieve the discomfort of ciliary spasm). All patients recover within 24–48 hours without complications. Local anesthetics should not be prescribed.

Chemical Conjunctivitis & Keratitis

Chemical burns are treated by irrigation of the eyes with saline solution or plain water as soon as possible after exposure. Neutralization of an acid with an alkali or vice versa generates heat and may cause further damage. Alkali injuries are more serious and require prolonged irrigation, since alkalies are not precipitated by the proteins of the eye as are acids. It is important to remove any retained particulate matter such as is typically present in injuries involving cement and building plaster. This may require double eversion of the upper lid. The pupil should be dilated with 1% cyclopentolate, 1 drop twice a day, to relieve discomfort and prophylactic topical antibiotics should be started. In moderate to severe injuries, intensive topical corticosteroids and topical and systemic vitamin C are also necessary. Complications include mucus deficiency, scarring of the cornea and conjunctiva, symblepharon (adhesions between the tarsal and bulbar conjunctiva), tear duct obstruction, and secondary infection.

Wagner MD: Chemical injuries of the eye. Current concepts in pathophysiology and therapy. Surv Ophthalmol 1997;42:276. [NLM Cit ID: 97258293]

PRINCIPLES OF TREATMENT OF OCULAR INFECTIONS

Before one can determine the drug of choice, the causative organisms must be identified, but in most instances empirical treatment, based on clinical experience, is used in the first instance. In the treatment of conjunctivitis and for prophylaxis against ocular infection, it is preferable to use a drug that is not given systemically. Of the available local antibacterial agents, the sulfonamides are effective and inexpensive. Two reliable sulfonamides for ophthalmic use are sulfisoxazole and sodium sulfacetamide. The sulfonamides have the added advantages of low allergenicity and effectiveness against the chlamydial group of organisms. They are available in ointment or solution form. Combined bacitracin-polymyxin ointment is often used prophylactically after corneal foreign body removal for the protection it affords against both gram-positive and gram-negative organisms.

Among the most effective broad-spectrum antibiotics for ophthalmic use are gentamicin, tobramycin, neomycin, and ciprofloxacin. These drugs have some effect against gram-negative as well as gram-positive organisms but are generally not effective against the pneumococcus, for which penicillin G or nafcillin (if beta-lactamase resistance is present) is required. Allergic reactions to neomycin are common. Other antibiotics frequently used are erythromycin, the tetracyclines, and the cephalosporins.

Method of Administration

Most ocular anti-infective drugs are administered locally. Ointments have greater therapeutic effectiveness than solutions, since contact can be maintained longer. However, they do cause blurring of vision; if this must be avoided, solutions should be used.

Systemic administration is required for all intraocular infections, orbital cellulitis, dacryocystitis, gonococcal keratoconjunctivitis, inclusion conjunctivitis, and severe external infection that does not respond to local treatment.

TECHNIQUES USED IN THE TREATMENT OF OCULAR DISORDERS

Table 7–2 lists commonly used ophthalmic drugs and their indications and costs.

Instilling Medications

The patient is placed in a chair with head tilted back, both eyes open, and looking up. The lower lid is retracted slightly, and 2 drops of liquid are instilled into the lower cul-de-sac. The patient looks down while finger contact is maintained, so that the eyes are not squeezed shut. Ointments are instilled in the same general manner.

For self-medication, the same techniques are used except that medications are usually better instilled with the patient lying down.

Eye Bandage

Most eye bandages should be applied firmly enough to hold the lid securely against the cornea. An ordinary patch consisting of gauze-covered cotton is usually sufficient. Tape is applied from the cheek to the forehead.

PRECAUTIONS IN MANAGEMENT OF OCULAR DISORDERS

Use of Local Anesthetics

Unsupervised self-administration of local anesthetics is dangerous because the patient may further injure an anesthetized eye without knowing it. The drug may also interfere with the normal healing process.

Pupillary Dilation

Dilating the pupil can very occasionally precipitate acute glaucoma if the patient has a narrow anterior chamber angle and should be undertaken with caution if the anterior chamber is obviously shallow (readily determined by oblique illumination of the anterior segment of the eye). A short-acting mydriatic such as tropicamide should be used and the patient warned to report immediately if ocular discomfort or redness develops. Angle closure is probably more likely to occur if pilocarpine is used to overcome pupillary dilation than if the pupil is allowed to constrict naturally.

Local Corticosteroid Therapy

Repeated use of local corticosteroids presents several hazards: herpes simplex (dendritic) keratitis, fun-

Table 7–2. Topical ophthalmic agents.

Agent	Representative Cost/Size[1]	Sig	Indications
AGENTS FOR GLAUCOMA AND INTRAOCULAR HYPERTENSION			
Sympathomimetics			
Apraclonidine HCl 0.5% solution (Iopidine)	$47.52/5 mL	1 drop three times daily	Reduction of intraocular pressure. Expensive. Reserve for treatment of resistant cases.
Apraclonidine HCl 1% solution (Iopidine)	$7.03/unit dose 0.1 mL	1 drop 1 hour before and immediately after anterior segment laser surgery	To control or prevent elevations of intraocular pressure after laser trabeculoplasty or iridotomy.
Brimonidine tartrate 0.2% solution (Alphagan)	$27.18/5 mL	1 drop two or three times daily	Reduction of intraocular pressure.
Dipivefrin HCl 0.1% solution (various)[2]	$14.07/5 mL	1 drop every 12 hours	Open-angle glaucoma.
Epinephrine HCl 0.25%, 0.5% (Epifrin), 1% and 2% solution (various)[3]	1%: $37.23/15 mL 2%: $40.73/15 mL	1 drop twice daily	
Beta-adrenergic blocking agents			
Betaxolol HCl 0.5% solution (Betoptic) and 0.25% suspension (Betoptic S)[4]	0.5%: $46.00/10 mL	1 drop twice daily	Reduction of intraocular pressure.
Carteolol HCl 1% solution (Ocupress)[5]	$44.55/10 mL	1 drop twice daily	
Levobunolol HCl 0.25% and 0.5% solution (Betagan)[5]	0.5%: $32.29/10 mL	1 drop once or twice daily	
Metipranolol HCl 0.3% solution (OptiPranolol)[5]	$15.68/5 mL	1 drop twice daily	
Timolol 0.25% and 0.5% solution (Betimol)[5]	0.5%: $32.15/10 mL	1 drop once or twice daily	
Timolol maleate 0.25% and 0.5% solution (Timoptic) and 0.25% and 0.5% gel (Timoptic-XE)[5]	0.5% solution: $16.58/5 mL 0.5% gel: $29.94/5 mL	1 drop once or twice daily	
Miotics			
Pilocarpine HCl (various)[6] (1–4%, 6%, 8%, 10%)	2%: $10.03/15 mL	1 drop three or four times daily[8]	Reduction of intraocular pressure, treatment of acute or chronic angle-closure glaucoma, and pupillary constriction.
Pilocarpine HCl 4% gel (Pilopine HS)	$32.70/4 g	Apply 0.5-inch ribbon in lower conjunctival sac at bedtime.	
Pilocarpine 20 μg/h for 7 days, and 40 μg/h for 7 days ocular therapeutic system (Ocusert Pilo-20 and Ocusert Pilo-40)[7]	40 μg/h: $45.13/8 each	Replace each unit every 7 days.	
Carbonic anhydrase inhibitor			
Dorzolamide HCl 2% solution (Trusopt)	$24.10/5 mL $48.23/10 mL	1 drop three times daily	Reduction of intraocular pressure.
Brinzolamide 1% suspension (Azopt)	$21.90/5 mL $43.80/10 mL	1 drop three times daily	
Prostaglandin analog			
Latanoprost 0.005% solution (Xalaten)	$45.03/2.5 mL	1 drop once or twice daily in the evening	Reduction of intraocular pressure.

(continued)

Fraunfelder FT, Mayer SM: Ocular and systemic side effects of drugs. In: *General Ophthalmology,* 15th ed. Vaughan D, Asbury T, Riordan-Eva P (editors). Appleton & Lange, 1999.

RELEVANT WORLD WIDE WEB SITES

[Blind Links: Advocacy groups, training and assistance, and adaptive technology for the blind and their families]

http://www.seidata.com/~marriage/rblind.html

[Digital Ophthalmic Slide Collections: From the New York University Department of Ophthalmology and the Massachusetts Eye and Ear Infirmary]

http://mcrcr4.med.nyu.edu/Ophth/dosc

[EyeMax—Ocular Diseases: From the American Academy of Ophthalmology]

http://www.eyemax.com/eye_diseases_ocular_disease/index.html

[EyeNet—Eye Conditions and Diseases]

http://aa03.aaa.org/public/faqs

[Glaucoma Research Foundation]

http://www.glaucoma.org

[Ischemic Optic Neuropathy Module]

http://webeye.ophth.uiowa.edu/dept/AION/Ion_indx.htm

[University of Iowa, Department of Ophthalmology—Ischemic Optic Neuropathy]

http://webeye.ophth.uiowa.edu/dept/aion/ion_indx.htm

8

Ear, Nose, & Throat

See http://www.current-med.com/ch08.html for updated addresses of Web sites referenced in this chapter.

Robert K. Jackler, MD, & Michael J. Kaplan, MD

DISEASES OF THE EAR

HEARING LOSS

Classification

A. Conductive Hearing Loss: Conductive hearing loss results from dysfunction of the external or middle ear. There are four mechanisms, each resulting in impairment of the passage of sound vibrations to the inner ear: (1) obstruction (eg, cerumen impaction), (2) mass loading (eg, middle ear effusion), (3) stiffness effect (eg, otosclerosis), and (4) discontinuity (eg, ossicular disruption). Conductive hearing loss is generally correctable with medical or surgical therapy—or in some cases both.

B. Sensory Hearing Loss: Sensory hearing loss results from deterioration of the cochlea, usually due to loss of hair cells from the organ of Corti. Among the many common causes are noise trauma, ototoxicity, and aging (presbyacusis). Sensory hearing loss is not correctable with medical or surgical therapy but often may be prevented or stabilized.

C. Neural Hearing Loss: Neural hearing loss occurs with lesions involving the eighth nerve, auditory nuclei, ascending tracts, or auditory cortex. It is the least common clinically recognized cause of hearing loss. Examples include acoustic neuroma, multiple sclerosis, and cerebrovascular disease.

Weber PC et al: Hearing loss. Med Clin North Am 1999;83:125. [NLM Cit ID: 99126926] (A contemporary review of the subject.)

Epidemiology of Hearing Loss

Conductive losses in adults are most commonly due to cerumen impaction or transient auditory tube dysfunction associated with upper respiratory tract infection. Persistent conductive losses usually result from chronic ear infection, trauma, or otosclerosis.

Sensorineural losses in adults are common. A gradually progressive, predominantly high-frequency loss with advancing age is typical though not invariable. Other than aging effects, common causes of sensorineural loss include excessive noise exposure, head trauma, and systemic diseases such as diabetes mellitus.

Evaluation of Hearing (Audiology)

In a quiet room, the hearing level may be estimated by having the patient repeat aloud words presented in a soft whisper, a normal spoken voice, or a shout. Tuning forks are useful in differentiating conductive from sensorineural losses. A 512-Hz tuning fork is employed, since frequencies below this level elicit a tactile response. In the **Weber test,** the tuning fork is placed on the forehead or front teeth. In conductive losses, the sound appears louder in the poorer hearing ear, whereas in sensorineural losses it radiates to the better side. In the **Rinne test,** the tuning fork is placed alternately on the mastoid bone and in front of the ear canal. In conductive losses, bone conduction exceeds air conduction; in sensorineural losses, the opposite is true.

Formal audiometric studies are performed in a soundproofed room. Pure-tone thresholds in decibels (dB) are obtained over the range of 250–8000 Hz (the main speech frequencies are between 500 and 3000 Hz) for both air and bone conduction. Conductive losses create a gap between the air and bone thresholds, whereas in sensorineural losses both air and bone conduction are equally diminished. The threshold of normal hearing is from 0 to 20 dB, which corresponds to the loudness of a soft whisper. Mild hearing loss is indicated by a threshold of 20–40 dB (soft spoken voice), moderate loss by a threshold of 40–60 dB (normal spoken voice), severe loss by a threshold of 60–80 dB (loud spoken voice), and profound loss by a threshold of 80 dB (shout). The clarity of hearing is often impaired in sensorineural hearing loss. This is evaluated by speech discrimination testing, which is reported as percentage correct (90–100% is normal). The site of the lesion responsible for sensorineural loss—whether it lies in the cochlea or in the central auditory system—may be determined with auditory brain stem-evoked responses.

Every patient who complains of a hearing loss should be referred for audiologic evaluation unless the cause is easily remediable (eg, cerumen impaction, otitis media). Audiologic screening is not recommended for adults with apparently normal hearing unless they are exposed to potentially injurious levels of noise or have reached the age of 65, after which screening evaluations should be done every few years.

Burkey JM et al: Clinical utility of the 512-Hz Rinne tuning fork test. Am J Otol 1998;19:59. [NLM Cit ID: 98115485] (The continued value of tuning forks in the modern era.)

Ruth RA: Evaluation of sensorineural hearing loss. Compr Ther 1997;23:742. [NLM Cit ID: 98025278] (A review for the nonspecialist.)

Hearing Rehabilitation

Patients with hearing loss not correctable by medical therapy may benefit from hearing amplification. Contemporary hearing aids are comparatively free of distortion and have been miniaturized to the point where they often may be contained entirely within the ear canal. To optimize the benefit, a hearing aid must be carefully selected to conform to the nature of the hearing loss. Digitally programmable hearing aids are now becoming available that allow optimization of speech intelligibility and may be tuned to deal with difficult listening circumstances.

Aside from hearing aids, many assistive devices are available to improve comprehension in individual and group settings, to help with hearing television and radio programs, and for telephone communication. In individuals with profound sensory deafness, the cochlear implant—an electronic device that is surgically implanted to stimulate the auditory nerve—offers socially beneficial auditory rehabilitation to most adults with acquired deafness.

Clark GM: Cochlear implants in the third millennium. Am J Otol 1999;20:4. [NLM Cit ID: 99114695] (Futuristic view of high-technology innovations with potential use in the rehabilitation of deafness.)

Klein AJ, Weber PC: Hearing aids. Med Clin North Am 1999;83:139. [NLM Cit ID: 99126927] (Reviews new digital technology.)

Laszig R et al: Cochlear implants and electrical brainstem stimulation in sensorineural hearing loss. Curr Opin Neurol 1999;12:41. [NLM Cit ID: 99197956]

Osberger MJ, Koch DB (editors): Clinical results with the Clarion multistrategy cochlear implant. Ann Otol Rhinol Laryngol 1999;108(Suppl 177):1. [NLM Cit ID: 99229622] (Comprehensive review of electrical stimulation in the rehabilitation of deafness.)

DISEASES OF THE AURICLE

Disorders of the external ear are for the most part dermatologic. Skin cancers due to actinic exposure are common and may be treated with standard techniques. Traumatic auricular hematoma must be recognized and drained to prevent significant cosmetic deformity (cauliflower ear) resulting from dissolution of supporting cartilage. Similarly, cellulitis of the auricle must be treated promptly to prevent development of perichondritis and its resultant deformity. Relapsing polychondritis is a systemic disorder often associated with recurrent, frequently bilateral, painful episodes of auricular erythema and edema. Treatment with corticosteroids may help forestall cartilage dissolution. Respiratory compromise may occur as a result of progressive involvement of the tracheobronchial tree. Chondritis and perichondritis may be differentiated from auricular cellulitis by sparing of involvement of the lobule, which does not contain cartilage.

Chen S et al: Painful erythematous ear. Arch Dermatol 2000;136:418. [NLM Cit ID: 20186806]

DISEASES OF THE EAR CANAL

1. CERUMEN IMPACTION

Cerumen is a protective secretion produced by the outer portion of the ear canal. In most individuals, the ear canal is self-cleansing. Recommended hygiene consists of cleaning the external opening with a washcloth over the index finger without entering the canal itself. In most cases, cerumen impaction is self-induced through ill-advised attempts at cleaning the ear. It may be relieved with detergent ear drops (eg, 3% hydrogen peroxide; 6.5% carbamide peroxide), mechanical removal, suction, or irrigation. Irrigation is performed with water at body temperature to avoid a vestibular caloric response. The stream should be directed at the ear canal wall adjacent to the cerumen plug. Irrigation should be performed only when the tympanic membrane is known to be intact.

Use of jet irrigators designed for cleaning teeth (eg, WaterPik) for wax removal should be avoided since they may result in tympanic membrane perforations. Following irrigation, the ear canal should be thoroughly dried (eg, by instilling isopropyl alcohol or using a hair blow-dryer on low-power setting) to reduce the likelihood of inducing external otitis. Specialty referral for cleaning under microscopic guidance is indicated when the impaction has not responded to routine measures or if the patient has a history of chronic otitis media or tympanic membrane perforation.

Grossan M: Safe, effective techniques for cerumen removal. Geriatrics 2000;55:80. [NLM Cit ID: 20124301]

2. FOREIGN BODIES

Foreign bodies in the ear canal are more frequent in children than in adults. Firm materials may be removed with a loop or a hook, taking care not to displace the object medially toward the tympanic membrane; microscopic guidance is helpful. Aqueous irrigation should not be performed for organic foreign bodies (eg, beans, insects), because water may cause them to swell. Living insects are best immobilized before removal by filling the ear canal with lidocaine.

3. EXTERNAL OTITIS

External otitis presents with otalgia, frequently accompanied by pruritus and purulent discharge. There is often a history of recent water exposure or mechanical trauma (eg, scratching, cotton applicators). External otitis is usually caused by gram-negative rods (eg, pseudomonas, proteus) or fungi (eg, aspergillus), which grow in the presence of excessive moisture.

Examination reveals erythema and edema of the ear canal skin, often with a purulent exudate. Manipulation of the auricle often elicits pain. Because the lateral surface of the tympanic membrane is ear canal skin, it is often erythematous. However, in contrast to acute otitis media, it moves normally with pneumatic otoscopy. When the canal skin is very edematous, it may be impossible to visualize the tympanic membrane. Fundamental to the treatment of external otitis is protection of the ear from additional moisture and avoidance of further mechanical injury by scratching. Otic drops containing a mixture of aminoglycoside antibiotic and anti-inflammatory corticosteroid in an acid vehicle are generally very effective (eg, neomycin sulfate, polymyxin B sulfate, and hydrocortisone). Purulent debris filling the ear canal should be gently removed to permit entry of the topical medication. Drops should be used abundantly (5 or more drops three or four times a day) to penetrate the depths of the canal. When substantial edema of the canal wall prevents entry of drops into the ear canal, a wick is placed to facilitate entry of the medication. In recalcitrant cases—particularly when cellulitis of the periauricular tissue has developed—oral fluoroquinolones (eg, ciprofloxacin, 500 mg twice daily) are the drugs of choice because of their effectiveness against pseudomonas species.

Guthrie RM (editor): Diagnosis and treatment of acute otitis externa: An interdisciplinary update. Ann Otol Rhinol Laryngol 1999;108(Suppl 176):1.

4. PRURITUS

Pruritus of the external auditory canal, particularly at the meatus, is a common problem. While it may be associated with external otitis or with dermatologic conditions such as seborrheic dermatitis and psoriasis, most cases are self-induced either from excoriation or by overly zealous ear cleaning. To permit regeneration of the protective cerumen blanket, patients should be instructed to avoid use of soap and water or cotton swabs in the ear canal. Patients with excessively dry canal skin may benefit from application of mineral oil, which helps to counteract dryness and repel moisture. When an inflammatory component is present, topical application of a corticosteroid (eg, 0.1% triamcinolone) may be beneficial. It is axiomatic in persistent pruritus that the patient must cease scratching the ear. In stubborn cases, the fingernails must be kept short and the patient may need to wear cotton gloves at night to avoid manipulation during sleep. Symptomatic reduction of pruritus may be obtained by use of oral antihistamines (eg, diphenhydramine, 25 mg orally at bedtime). Topical application of isopropyl alcohol promptly relieves ear canal pruritus in many patients.

5. MALIGNANT EXTERNAL OTITIS

Persistent external otitis in the diabetic or immunocompromised patient may evolve into osteomyelitis of the skull base, often called malignant external otitis. Usually caused by *Pseudomonas aeruginosa,* osteomyelitis begins in the floor of the ear canal and may extend into the middle fossa floor, the clivus, and even the contralateral skull base. The patient usually presents with persistent foul aural discharge, granulations in the ear canal, deep otalgia, and progressive cranial nerve palsies involving nerves VI, VII, IX, X, XI, or XII. Diagnosis is confirmed by the demonstration of osseous erosion on CT and radionuclide scanning.

Treatment is chiefly medical, requiring prolonged antipseudomonal antibiotic administration, often for several months. Although intravenous therapy is often required, selected patients may be managed with the oral agent ciprofloxacin (500–1000 mg orally twice daily), which has proved effective against many of the causative pseudomonas strains. To avoid relapse, antibiotic therapy should be continued, even in the asymptomatic patient, until gallium scanning indicates a marked reduction in the inflammatory process. Surgical debridement of infected bone is reserved for cases of deterioration despite medical therapy.

6. EXOSTOSES & OSTEOMAS

Bony overgrowths of the ear canal are a frequent incidental finding and occasionally have clinical significance. Clinically, they present as skin-covered mounds in the medial ear canal obscuring the tympanic membrane to a variable degree. Solitary osteomas are of no significance as long as they do not cause obstruction or infection. Multiple exostoses, which are generally acquired from repeated exposure to cold water, often progress and require surgical removal.

Wong BJ et al: Prevalence of external auditory canal exostoses in surfers. Arch Otolaryngol Head Neck Surg 1999;125:969. [NLM Cit ID: 99417106] (Prolonged and frequent water exposure contributes to exostosis formation.)

7. NEOPLASIA

The most common neoplasm of the ear canal is squamous cell carcinoma. When an apparent otitis externa does not resolve on therapy, this should be suspected and biopsy performed. This disease carries a very high 5-year mortality rate and must be treated with wide surgical resection and radiation therapy. Adenomatous tumors, originating from the ceruminous glands, generally follow a more indolent course.

Pfreundner L et al: Carcinoma of the external auditory canal and middle ear. Int J Radiat Oncol Biol Phys 1999;44:777. [NLM Cit ID: 99313205] (A combination of aggressive surgery and radiotherapy is usually necessary.)

DISEASES OF THE AUDITORY TUBE

1. AUDITORY TUBE DYSFUNCTION

The tube that connects the middle ear to the nasopharynx—the auditory tube, or eustachian tube—provides ventilation and drainage for the middle ear cleft. It is normally closed, opening only during the act of swallowing or yawning. When auditory tube function is compromised, air trapped within the middle ear becomes absorbed and negative pressure results. The most common causes of auditory tube dysfunction are diseases associated with edema of the tubal lining, such as viral upper respiratory tract infections and allergy. The patient usually reports a sense of fullness in the ear and mild to moderate impairment of hearing. When the tube is only partially blocked, swallowing or yawning may elicit a popping or crackling sound. Examination reveals retraction of the tympanic membrane and decreased mobility on pneumatic otoscopy. Following a viral illness, this disorder is usually transient, lasting days to weeks. Treatment with systemic and intranasal decongestants (eg, pseudoephedrine, 60 mg orally every 4 hours; oxymetazoline, 0.05% spray every 8–12 hours) combined with autoinflation by forced exhalation against closed nostrils may hasten relief. Air travel, rapid altitudinal change, and underwater diving should be avoided. Autoinflation should not be recommended to patients with active intranasal infection, since this maneuver may precipitate middle ear infection. Allergic patients may also benefit from desensitization or intranasal corticosteroids (eg, beclomethasone dipropionate, two sprays in each nostril twice daily for 2–6 weeks).

An overly patent auditory tube is a relatively uncommon problem that may be quite distressing. Typical complaints include fullness in the ear and autophony, an exaggerated ability to hear oneself breathe and speak. A patulous auditory tube may develop during rapid weight loss, or it may commence without a discernible cause. In contrast to a hypofunctioning auditory tube, the aural pressure is often made worse by exertion and may diminish during an upper respiratory tract infection. Although physical examination is usually normal, respiratory excursions of the tympanic membrane may occasionally be detected during vigorous breathing. Treatment includes avoidance of decongestant products, insertion of a ventilating tube to reduce the outward stretch of the ear drum during phonation, and surgical narrowing of the auditory tube (rarely).

Derebery MJ et al: Allergic eustachian tube dysfunction: Diagnosis and treatment. Am J Otol 1997;18:160. [NLM Cit ID: 97247543] (Patients who do not respond well to conventional pharmacotherapy may benefit from specific allergic therapy.)

Monsell EM et al: Eustachian tube dysfunction. Otolaryngol Clin North Am 1996;29:437. [NLM Cit ID: 96336730] (Management of both hypo- and hyperfunction.)

2. SEROUS OTITIS MEDIA

When the auditory tube remains blocked for a prolonged period, the resultant negative pressure will result in transudation of fluid. This condition, known as serous otitis media, is especially common in children because their auditory tubes are narrower and more horizontal in orientation than adults. It is less common in adults, in whom it usually follows an upper respiratory tract infection or barotrauma. In an adult with persistent unilateral serous otitis media, nasopharyngeal carcinoma must be excluded. The tympanic membrane in serous otitis media is dull and hypomobile, occasionally accompanied by air bubbles in the middle ear and conductive hearing loss. The treatment of serous otitis media is similar to that for auditory tube dysfunction. A short course of oral corticosteroids (eg, prednisone, 40 mg/d for 7 days) has been advocated by some in the management of serous otitis media, as have oral antibiotics (eg, amoxicillin, 250 mg orally three times daily for 7 days)—or even a combination of the two. The role of these regimens remains controversial, but they are probably of little lasting benefit.

When medication fails to bring relief after several months, a ventilating tube placed through the tympanic membrane may restore hearing and alleviate the sense of aural fullness.

Morris MS: Tympanostomy tubes: types, indications, techniques, and complications. Otolaryngol Clin North Am 1999;32:385. [NLM Cit ID: 99322146]

Slack R et al: Current management of glue ear. Practitioner 1998;242:455. [NLM Cit ID: 99422627]

3. BAROTRAUMA

Individuals with auditory tube dysfunction due either to congenital narrowness or to acquired mucosal edema may be unable to equalize the barometric stress exerted on the middle ear by air travel, rapid altitudinal change, or underwater diving. The problem is generally most acute during airplane descent, since the negative middle ear pressure tends to collapse and lock the auditory tube. Several measures are useful to enhance auditory tube function and avoid otic barotrauma. The patient should be advised to swallow, yawn, and autoinflate frequently during descent, which may be painful if the auditory tube collapses. Systemic decongestants (eg, pseudoephedrine, 60–120 mg) should be taken several hours before anticipated arrival time so that they will be maximally effective during descent. Topical decongestants such as 1% phenylephrine nasal spray should be administered 1 hour before arrival.

The treatment of acute negative middle ear pressure that persists on the ground is with decongestants and attempts at autoinflation. Myringotomy provides immediate relief and is appropriate in the setting of severe otalgia and hearing loss. Repeated episodes of barotrauma in persons who must fly frequently may be alleviated by insertion of ventilating tubes.

Underwater diving represents even a greater barometric stress to the ear than flying. The problem occurs most commonly during the descent phase, when pain develops within the first 15 feet if inflation of the middle ear via the auditory tube has not occurred. Divers must descend slowly and equilibrate in stages to avoid the development of severely negative pressures in the tympanum that may result in hemorrhage (hemotympanum) or perilymphatic fistulization. In the latter, the oval or round window ruptures, resulting in sensory hearing loss and acute vertigo. Emesis due to acute labyrinthine dysfunction can be very dangerous during an underwater dive. Sensory hearing loss or vertigo, which develops during the ascent phase of a saturation dive, may be the first (or only) symptom of decompression sickness. Immediate recompression will return intravascular gas bubbles to solution and restore the inner ear microcirculation. Patients should be warned to avoid diving when they have upper respiratory infections or episodes of nasal allergy. Tympanic membrane perforation is an absolute contraindication to diving, as the patient will experience an unbalanced thermal stimulus to the semicircular canals and may experience vertigo, disorientation, and even emesis. Finally, individuals with only one hearing ear should be discouraged from diving because of the significant risk of otologic injury.

Clenney TL et al: Recreational scuba diving injuries. Am Fam Physician 1996;53:1761. [NLM Cit ID: 96209657] (Distinguishes between the otologic effects of barotrauma and decompression sickness.)

Jones JS et al: A double-blind comparison between oral pseudoephedrine and topical oxymetazoline in the prevention of barotrauma during air travel. Am J Emerg Med 1998;16:262. [NLM Cit ID: 98255867] (Taking pseudoephedrine 120 mg at least 30 minutes before flying appears to decrease the incidence of barotrauma, while oxymetazoline nasal spray alone is little more effective than placebo in reducing ear pain.)

DISEASES OF THE MIDDLE EAR

1. ACUTE OTITIS MEDIA

Acute otitis media is a bacterial infection of the mucosally lined air-containing spaces of the temporal bone. Purulent material forms not only within the middle ear cleft but also within the mastoid air cells and petrous apex when they are pneumatized. Acute otitis media is usually precipitated by a viral upper respiratory tract infection that causes auditory tube edema. This results in accumulation of fluid and mucus, which becomes secondarily infected by bacteria. The most common pathogens both in adults and in children are *Streptococcus pneumoniae, Haemophilus influenzae,* and *Streptococcus pyogenes.*

Acute otitis media is most common in infants and children, though it may occur at any age. The patient presents with otalgia, aural pressure, decreased hearing, and often fever. The typical physical findings are erythema and decreased mobility of the tympanic membrane. Occasionally, bullae will be seen on the tympanic membrane. Although it is taught that this represents infection with *Mycoplasma pneumoniae,* most cases involve more common pathogens.

Rarely, when middle ear empyema is severe, the tympanic membrane can be seen to bulge outward. In such cases, tympanic membrane rupture is imminent. Rupture is accompanied by a sudden decrease in pain, followed by the onset of otorrhea. With appropriate therapy, spontaneous healing of the tympanic

diluted 50:50 with bicarbonate), which is injected into the middle ear via a spinal needle. Results in patients with Meniere's disease have been impressive, with about 80–90% of patients relieved of severe episodic vertigo.

Antonelli PJ: Update on vertigo management. Compr Ther 1999;2:5. [NLM Cit ID: 99142060]

Cohen HS et al: Efficacy of treatments for posterior canal benign paroxysmal positional vertigo. Laryngoscope 1999;109:584. [NLM Cit ID: 99215928] (Excellent clinical results with either Epley maneuver or Sermont maneuver.)

Minor LB: Intratympanic gentamicin for control of vertigo in Meniere's disease: Vestibular signs that specify completion of therapy. Am J Otol 1999;20:209. [NLM Cit ID: 99198624] (Control of vertigo in 91% of patients with only a 3% incidence of hearing loss.)

Smith PF: Pharmacology of the vestibular system. Curr Opin Neurol 2000;13:31. [NLM Cit ID: 20184561]

Welling DB et al: Endolymphatic mastoid shunt: a reevaluation of efficacy. Otolaryngol Head Neck Surg 2000;122:340. [NLM Cit ID: 20164921] (Favorable results in selected medically refractory patients.)

DISEASES OF THE CENTRAL AUDITORY & VESTIBULAR SYSTEMS (Table 8–1)

Lesions of the eighth cranial nerve and central audiovestibular pathways produce neural hearing loss and vertigo. One characteristic of neural hearing loss is deterioration of speech discrimination out of proportion to the decrease in pure tone thresholds. Another is auditory adaptation, wherein a steady tone appears to the listener to decay and eventually disappear. Auditory evoked responses are useful in distinguishing cochlear from neural losses and may give insight into the site of lesion within the central pathways.

Vertigo arising from central lesions tends to be more chronic and debilitating than that seen in labyrinthine disease. The associated nystagmus is often nonfatigable, vertical rather than horizontal in orientation, without latency, and unsuppressed by visual fixation. Electronystagmography is useful in documenting these characteristics. The evaluation of central audiovestibular dysfunction usually requires imaging of the brain with CT scans or MRI. The paramagnetic contrast agent gadolinium-DTPA, when used with MRI scanning, substantially improves diagnostic sensitivity in the detection of central audiovestibular lesions.

Gates G et al: Central auditory dysfunction, cognitive dysfunction, and dementia in older people. Arch Otolaryngol Head Neck Surg 1996;122:16. [NLM Cit ID: 96223610] (Central auditory dysfunction often precedes dementia.)

Hirsch BE et al: Localizing retrocochlear hearing loss. Am J Otol 1996;17:537. [NLM Cit ID: 96439367] (Evaluation of patients with suspected eighth nerve and brainstem dysfunction.)

1. VESTIBULAR SCHWANNOMA (Acoustic Neuroma)

Eighth nerve schwannomas are among the most common of intracranial tumors. These benign lesions arise within the internal auditory canal and gradually grow to involve the cerebellopontine angle, eventually compressing the pons and resulting in hydrocephalus. Their typical auditory symptoms are unilateral hearing loss with a deterioration of speech discrimination exceeding that predicted by the degree of pure tone loss. Atypical presentations, such as sudden unilateral hearing loss, are fairly common. Any individual with a unilateral or asymmetric sensorineural hearing loss should be evaluated for an intracranial mass lesion. Vestibular dysfunction more often takes the form of continuous dysequilibrium than episodic vertigo. Other lesions of the cerebellopontine angle such as meningioma and epidermoids may have similar audiovestibular manifestations. Diagnosis is made by enhanced MRI, though auditory evoked responses may have a role in screening. Microsurgical excision is most often indicated, though small tumors in older individuals may be managed with stereotactic radiotherapy or simply followed with serial imaging studies.

Daniels RL et al: Causes of unilateral sensorineural hearing loss screened by high resolution fast spin echo magnetic resonance imaging: review of 1070 consecutive cases. Am J Otol 2000;21:173. [NLM Cit ID: 20195318] (Vestibular schwannoma identified in approximately 5% of those screened.)

Doyle KJ: Is there still a role for auditory brainstem response audiometry in the diagnosis of acoustic neuroma? Arch Otolaryngol 1999;125:232. [NLM Cit ID: 99154897] (Reduced role due to a high rate of both false-negative and false-positive responses. Enhanced MRI scans remain the gold standard for diagnosis.)

Rosenberg SI: Natural history of acoustic neuroma. Laryngoscope 2000;110:497. [NLM Cit ID: 20225064] (Older individuals with smaller tumors usually do not require intervention.)

2. VASCULAR COMPROMISE

Vertebrobasilar insufficiency is a common cause of vertigo in the elderly. It is often triggered by changes in posture or extension of the neck. Reduced flow in the vertebrobasilar system may be demonstrated noninvasively through magnetic resonance angiography. Empirical treatment is with vasodilators and aspirin.

Migraine may cause vertiginous attacks. The diagnosis is obvious when vertigo accompanies a typical headache pattern, but this is not always the case. In patients with a history of both migraine headaches and recurrent vertigo, a therapeutic trial of β-adrenergic blocking drugs (propranolol, 80–240 mg orally every 12–24 hours) and ergots (ergotamine, 1 mg orally every 4–6 hours) is reasonable.

Vascular loops that impinge upon the brain stem root entry zone of cranial nerves have been shown to cause dysfunction. Widely recognized examples are hemifacial spasm and tic douloureux. It has been suggested that hearing loss, tinnitus, and disabling positioning vertigo may result from such a loop abutting the eighth nerve.

Johnson GD: Medical management of migraine-related dizziness and vertigo. Laryngoscope 1998;108(1 Part 2 Suppl):1. [NLM Cit ID: 98090367] (Episodic vertigo is improved in 90% with drug treatment.)

Toursarkissian B et al: Surgical treatment of patients with symptomatic vertebrobasilar insufficiency. Ann Vasc Surg 1998;12:28. [NLM Cit ID: 98112372] (Over 50% of patients had dizziness; some were improved following revascularization.)

Welsh LW et al: Vertigo: analysis by magnetic resonance angiography. Ann Otol Rhinol Laryngol 2000;109:248. [NLM Cit ID: 20199565] (Abnormalities of the vertebrobasilar system were detected in 52% of older adults.)

3. MULTIPLE SCLEROSIS

Patients with multiple sclerosis may suffer from episodic vertigo and chronic imbalance. Hearing loss in this disease is most commonly unilateral and of rapid onset. Spontaneous recovery may occur.

Oznlli A et al: Multiple sclerosis: A cause of sudden hearing loss. Audiology 1998;37:528. [NLM Cit ID: 98134780] (Clinical, audiologic, and imaging findings.)

OTOLOGIC MANIFESTATIONS OF AIDS

The otologic manifestations of AIDS are protean. The pinna and external auditory canal may be affected by Kaposi's sarcoma as well as persistent and potentially invasive fungal infections, particularly due to *Aspergillus fumigatus*. The most common middle ear manifestation of AIDS is serous otitis media due to auditory tube dysfunction arising from adenoidal hypertrophy (HIV lymphadenopathy), recurrent mucosal viral infections, or an obstructing nasopharyngeal tumor (eg, lymphoma). Experience with middle ear effusion in AIDS patients suggests that ventilating tubes are seldom helpful and may trigger profuse watery otorrhea. Acute otitis media in the AIDS patient is usually caused by the typical bacterial organisms that occur in nonimmunocompromised patients, though *Pneumocystis carinii* otitis has been reported. Complaints referable to the inner ear are common in AIDS patients. Sensorineural hearing loss is common and in some cases appears to result from viral central nervous system infection. In cases of progressive hearing loss, it is important to evaluate for cryptococcal meningitis and syphilis. Acute facial paralysis due to herpes zoster infection (Ramsay Hunt's syndrome) is quite common and follows a clinical course similar to that in nonimmunocompromised patients. Treatment is primarily with high-dose acyclovir. Corticosteroids may also be effective.

Chandrasekhar SS et al: Otologic and audiologic evaluation of human immunodeficiency virus-infected patients. Am J Otolaryngol 2000;21:1. [NLM Cit ID: 20132104] (Ear disease affects up to 33% of HIV-infected patients. Otitis media is a frequent finding. Sensorineural hearing loss is more severe in patients with advanced HIV infection.)

Kohan D et al: Otologic surgery in patients with HIV-1 and AIDS. Otolaryngol Head Neck Surg 1999;121:355. [NLM Cit ID: 99436380] (Complications exceed those of healthier populations.)

Truitt TO et al: Otolaryngologic manifestations of human immunodeficiency virus infection. Med Clin North Am 1999;83:303. [NLM Cit ID: 99126937]

DISEASES OF THE NOSE & PARANASAL SINUSES

INFECTIONS OF THE NOSE & PARANASAL SINUSES

1. VIRAL RHINITIS (Common Cold)

The nonspecific symptoms of the ubiquitous common cold are present in the early phases of many diseases that affect the upper aerodigestive tract. Because there are numerous serologic types of rhinoviruses, adenoviruses, and other viruses, patients remain susceptible throughout life. Headache, nasal congestion, watery rhinorrhea, sneezing, and a scratchy throat accompanied by general malaise are typical in viral infections. Nasal examination usually shows reddened, edematous mucosa and a watery discharge. The presence of purulent nasal discharge suggests bacterial infection.

There is no proved specific treatment for a cold. There may, however, be misperceptions among members of some ethnic communities where nonprescription antibiotics are available that antibiotics are helpful. Supportive measures such as decongestants (pseudoephedrine, 30–60 mg every 4–6 hours or 120

Yohai RA et al: Survival factors in rhino-orbital-cerebral mucormycosis. Surv Ophthalmol 1994;39:3. [NLM Cit ID: 95064498] (A literature review and analysis of benefits of therapeutic options including aggressive surgery, intravenous amphotericin B, hyperbaric oxygen, and amphotericin B irrigation.)

ALLERGIC RHINITIS

The symptoms of "hay fever" are similar to those of viral rhinitis but are usually more persistent and show seasonal variation. Nasal symptoms are often accompanied by eye irritation, which causes pruritus, erythema, and excessive tearing. Numerous allergens may cause these symptoms: pollens are most common in the spring, grasses in the summer, and ragweed in the fall. Dust and household mites may produce year-round symptoms.

On physical examination, the mucosa of the turbinates is usually pale or violaceous because of venous engorgement—in contrast to the erythema of viral rhinitis. Nasal polyps, which are yellowish boggy masses of hypertrophic mucosa, may be seen.

Treatment of allergic and perennial rhinitis has definitely improved in recent years, but optimal specific management strategies that are evidence-based, cost-effective, and enjoy wide consensus have not been fully implemented. In addition to oral decongestants (such as pseudoephedrine, 60–120 mg orally, up to 240 mg/d), options include safer long-acting nonsedating histamine H_1 receptor antagonists and intranasal steroid sprays. Adjunctive options include intranasal anticholinergic agents such as ipratropium bromide 0.03% (42 μg per nostril three times daily) sprays when rhinorrhea is a major symptom, intranasal cromolyn spray prior to the onset of seasonal symptoms, and modifications in immunotherapy in selected patients when prior measures have proved inadequate. Antileukotrienes may possibly be shown to have efficacy as well. Numerous over-the-counter antihistamines, such as brompheniramine or chlorpheniramine (4 mg orally every 6–8 hours, or 8–12 mg orally every 8–12 hours as a sustained-release tablet) and clemastine (1.34–2.68 mg orally twice daily) offer the benefit of reduced cost though usually associated with higher rates of drowsiness compared with the newer prescription nonsedating antihistamines.

Oral H_1 receptor antagonist antihistamines are generally considered first-line management of allergic rhinitis. Numerous such medications are available that replace older drugs for which prolongation of QT_c intervals was an unacceptable risk. Widely available drugs include cetirizine (10 mg orally once daily), fexofenadine (60 mg orally twice daily or 120 mg once daily), and loratadine (10 mg orally once daily). Fexofenadine appears to be nonsedating; the other two minimally sedating. Also shown to be effective in randomized trials are ebastine (10–20mg orally once daily) and misolastine (10 mg once daily). Two H_1 receptor antagonist antihistamine nasal sprays have also been shown to be effective in randomized trials: levocabastine (0.2 mg twice daily) and azelastine (two sprays per nostril, 1.1 mg/d).

Intranasal corticosteroid sprays are also a mainstay of treatment in managing allergic rhinitis. Patients should be reminded that there may be a delay in onset of relief of 1–2 weeks. Steroid sprays may also shrink nasal polyps, thereby providing an improved nasal airway and delaying or eliminating the indications for endoscopic sinus surgery. Available preparations include beclomethasone (42 μg/spray twice daily each nostril), flunisolide (25 μg/spray twice daily each nostril), mometasone furoate (200 μg once daily per nostril), and fluticasone propionate (200 μg once daily per nostril). The latter two synthetic glucocorticoids appear to have higher topical potencies and lipid solubility and reduced systemic bioavailability, suggesting possible practical advantages.

Maintaining an allergen-free environment by covering pillows and mattresses with plastic covers, substituting synthetic materials (foam mattress, acrylics) for animal products (wool, horsehair), and removing dust-collecting household fixtures (carpets, drapes, bedspreads, wicker) is worth the attempt to help more troubled patients. Air purifiers and dust filters (such as Bionair models) may also aid in maintaining an allergen-free environment. When symptoms are extremely bothersome, a search for offending allergens may prove helpful. This can either be done by skin testing or by serum RAST testing. Desensitization by gradually increasing subdermal exposure to identified allergens may be tried in selected patients, with variable results.

Recent studies also suggest a possible role of sublingual-swallow immunotherapy or local specific nasal immunotherapy in seasonal and perennial rhinitis. Though not convenient for all patients and in the oral study less effective for rhinitis symptoms than for conjunctivitis and asthma symptoms, such intervention with oral drops and then tablets or using a nasal insufflator offers potential advantages compared with hyposensitization methods requiring injections.

Beckman DB et al: Pharmacotherapy to prevent the complications of allergic rhinitis. Allergy Asthma Proc 1999;20:215. [NLM Cit ID: 99405234] (A reminder that allergic rhinitis is more than a nuisance. It is a disease with potentially serious complications and side effects.)

Berger WE et al: Double-blind trials of azelastine nasal spray monotherapy versus combination therapy with loratadine tablets and beclomethasone nasal spray in patients with seasonal allergic rhinitis. Rhinitis Study Groups. Ann Allergy Asthma Immunol 1999;82:535. [NLM Cit ID: 99314637]

Berkowitz RB et al: Mometasone furoate nasal spray is rapidly effective in the treatment of seasonal allergic rhinitis in an outdoor (park), acute exposure setting. Allergy Asthma Proc 1999;20:167. [NLM Cit ID: 99317780]

Bousquet J et al: A 12-week, placebo-controlled study of the efficacy and safety of ebastine, 10 and 20 mg once daily, in the treatment of perennial allergic rhinitis. Multicentre Study Group. Allergy 1999;54:562. [NLM Cit ID: 99361822]

Casale TB et al: Safety and efficacy of once-daily fexofenadine HCl in the treatment of autumn seasonal allergic rhinitis. Allergy Asthma Proc 1999;20:193. [NLM Cit ID: 99317784)

Corren J: Intranasal corticosteroids for allergic rhinitis: how do different agents compare? J Allergy Clin Immunol 1999;104(4 Part 1):S144. [NLM Cit ID: 99449663] (Newer intranasal steroids such as mometasone and fluticasone appear to have practical advantages over older agents in terms of higher topical potencies and lipid solubilities and lower systemic bioavailabilities. All the available intranasal corticosteroids appear to be equally effective in controlling symptoms.)

Day J: Pros and cons of the use of antihistamines in managing allergic rhinitis. J Allergy Clin Immunol 1999;103(3 Part 2):S395. [NLM Cit ID: 99169162] (Reviews the pharmacology, clinical use, and side effect profiles of the commonly used H_1-receptor antagonists.)

Dockhorn R et al: Ipratropium bromide nasal spray 0.03% and beclomethasone nasal spray alone and in combination for the treatment of rhinorrhea in perennial rhinitis. Ann Allergy Asthma Immunol 1999;82:349. [NLM Cit ID: 99241872] (Ipratropium bromide nasal spray 0.03% is useful in troublesome rhinorrhea.)

Ferguson BJ et al: Allergic rhinitis and rhinosinusitis. Is there a connection between allergy and infection? Postgrad Med 1999;105:55. [NLM Cit ID: 99239592] (A basic introduction.)

Ferguson BJ: Cost-effective pharmacotherapy for allergic rhinitis. Otolaryngol Clin North Am 1998;31:91. [NLM Cit ID: 98191785] (Guidelines for use of antihistamines, decongestants, steroids, mast cell stabilizers, anticholinergic agents, and mucolytics.)

Hadley JA: Evaluation and management of allergic rhinitis. Med Clin North Am 1999;83:13. [NLM Cit ID: 99126918] (An overview.)

Hampel FC Jr et al: Efficacy and safety of levocabastine nasal spray for seasonal allergic rhinitis. Am J Rhinol 1999;13:55. [NLM Cit ID: 99188023] (More effective than placebo.)

Howarth PH et al: Double-blind, placebo-controlled study comparing the efficacy and safety of fexofenadine hydrochloride (120 and 180 mg once daily) and cetirizine in seasonal allergic rhinitis. J Allergy Clin Immunol 1999;104:927. [NLM Cit ID: 20020176] (Cetirizine had 9% drowsiness compared with 4% for fexofenadine and 5% for placebo. Both drugs relieved symptoms well.)

Kane KY et al: The best therapy for allergic rhinitis. J Fam Pract 1998;47:415. [NLM Cit ID: 99083891]

LaForce C: Use of nasal steroids in managing allergic rhinitis. J Allergy Clin Immunol 1999;103(3 Part 2):S388. [NLM Cit ID: 99169161] (Reviews the mechanism of action, the effects on chemical mediators of inflammation, and the risks and benefits associated with the use of nasal steroids.)

Lipworth BJ: Leukotriene-receptor antagonists. Lancet 1999;353:57. [NLM Cit ID: 99146571] (Leukotriene-receptor antagonists are effective in treating allergic rhinitis.)

Mabry RL: Allergy for rhinologists. Otolaryngol Clin North Am 1998;31:175. [NLM Cit ID: 98191790] (A review for the nonallergist.)

Mason J et al: The systemic safety of fexofenadine HCl. Clin Experimental Allergy 1999;29(Suppl 3):163. [NLM Cit ID: 99373298] (Unlike some other antihistamines, such as loratadine or cetirizine, the authors conclude fexofenadine is truly nonsedating.)

Meltzer EO et al: Impact of cetirizine on the burden of allergic rhinitis. Ann Allergy Asthma Immunol 1999; 83:455. [NLM Cit ID: 20047556]

Meltzer EO et al: Once-daily fexofenadine HCl improves quality of life and reduces work and activity impairment in patients with seasonal allergic rhinitis. Ann Allergy Asthma Immunol 1999;83:311. [NLM Cit ID: 20007436]

Mometasone furoate nasal spray for allergic rhinitis. Med Lett Drugs Therap 1999;41:16. [NLM Cit ID: 99159085]

Motta G et al: A multicenter trial of specific local nasal immunotherapy. Laryngoscope 2000;110:132. [NLM Cit ID: 20110649]

Naclerio RM: Pathophysiology of perennial allergic rhinitis. Allergy 1997;52(36 Suppl):7. [NLM Cit ID: 97356421] (A review of the early phase, largely mediated through mast cells, and late phase, involving cellular infiltration and mediator release.)

Ortolani C et al: A double-blind, placebo-controlled comparison of treatment with fluticasone propionate and levocabastine in patients with seasonal allergic rhinitis. FLNCO2 Italian Study Group. Allergy 1999;54:1173. [NLM Cit ID: 20068053]

Pradalier A et al: Sublingual-swallow immunotherapy (SLIT) with a standardized five-grass-pollen extract (drops and sublingual tablets) versus placebo in seasonal rhinitis. Allergy 1999;54:819. [NLM Cit ID: 99413395]

Pullerits T et al: Randomized placebo-controlled study comparing a leukotriene receptor antagonist and a nasal glucocorticoid in seasonal allergic rhinitis. Am J Respir Crit Care Med 1999;159:1814. [NLM Cit ID: 99280636] (Steroids were superior.)

Rachelefsky GS: National guidelines needed to manage rhinitis and prevent complications. Ann Allergy Asthma Immunol 1999;82:296. [NLM Cit ID: 99192035] (The optimal treatment of this common problem is debated. Practice guidelines that are evidence-based would be helpful, especially when allergic rhinitis coexists with asthma.)

Rachelefsky GS: Pharmacologic management of allergic rhinitis. J Allergy Clin Immunol 1998;101(2 Part 2): S367. [NLM Cit ID: 98160366]

Sabbah A et al: Comparison of the efficacy, safety, and onset of action of mizolastine, cetirizine, and placebo in the management of seasonal allergic rhinoconjunctivitis. MIZOCET Study Group. Ann Allergy Asthma Immunol 1999;83:319. [NLM Cit ID: 20007437]

Settipane RA: Complications of allergic rhinitis. Allergy Asthma Proc 1999;20:209. [NLM Cit ID: 99405233]

Sussman GL et al: The efficacy and safety of fexofenadine HCl and pseudoephedrine, alone and in combination, in seasonal allergic rhinitis. J Allergy Clin Immunol 1999;104:100. [NLM Cit ID: 99328928]

Tkachyk SJ: New treatments for allergic rhinitis. Can Fam Phys 1999;45:1255. [NLM Cit ID: 99278687] (Overview of newer treatments for allergic rhinitis, including newer antihistamines, intranasal steroid sprays, antileukotrienes, and short-course preseason six- to eleven-injection immunotherapy.)

Van Cauwenberge PB: Nasal sensitization. Allergy 1997; 52(33 Suppl):7. [NLM Cit ID: 97332778] (A review of the pathophysiology.)

Weber RW: Immunotherapy with allergens. JAMA 1997; 278:1881. [NLM Cit ID: 98057356] (The mechanism by which allergen immunotherapy improves clinical symptoms via decreased target organ hyperreactivity is still not entirely clear.)

OLFACTORY DYSFUNCTION

The physiology of olfaction is less well understood than that of the other special senses. In the past few years, however, discovery of the family of odor-receptor genes as well as inositol phosphate and cyclic nucleotide signaling pathways have led to a molecular basis of olfactory reception. Clinically, odorant molecules must traverse the nasal vault to reach the cribriform area and become soluble in the mucus overlying the exposed dendrites of receptor cells. Anatomic lack of access to the receptor cells of the first cranial nerve is the most common cause of olfactory dysfunction (hyposmia or anosmia). Polyps, septal deformities, and nasal tumors may all contribute to this inability of air to reach the area of the cribriform plate high in the nose where these receptors are located. Transient olfactory dysfunction often accompanies the common cold, nasal allergies, and perennial rhinitis. About 20% of impaired olfactory function is idiopathic, although it often follows a viral illness. Some have suggested administering large doses of vitamin A and zinc to such patients, although little evidence supports their use. Central nervous system neoplasms, especially those that involve the olfactory groove or temporal lobe, may affect olfaction. Head trauma accounts for less than 5% of cases of hyposmia. Absent, diminished, or distorted smell or taste has been reported in a wide variety of endocrine, nutritional, and nervous disorders. A great many medications have also been implicated.

Evaluation of olfactory dysfunction should include a thorough history of systemic illnesses and medication use as well as a physical examination focusing on the nose and nervous system. Most clinical offices are not set up to test olfaction, but such feats may at times be worthwhile if only to assess whether a patient possesses any sense of smell at all. Odor threshold should be tested in increasing concentrations. For example, use *n*-butyl alcohol (1-butanolol) in concentrations up to 4% in deionized water. Serial 3:1 dilutions in 12 steps produce an initial test of 46 ppm (v/v) and the maximum of 3055 ppm (at 4%). Odor identification can be tested using standardized choices (see references). In permanent hyposmia, counseling should be offered about seasoning foods with spices (eg, pepper) that stimulate the trigeminal as well as olfactory chemoreceptors and about safety issues such as the use of smoke alarms and electric rather than gas home appliances.

Axel R: The molecular logic of smell. Sci Am 1995; 273:154. [NLM Cit ID: 96066458]

Doty RL: Studies of human olfaction from the University of Pennsylvania Smell and Taste Center. Chem Senses 1997;22:565. [NLM Cit ID: 98029783] (A review of studies done since 1980 and a discussion of the olfactory vector hypothesis of neurodegenerative diseases.)

Henkin RI: Drug-induced taste and smell disorders: Incidence, mechanisms and management related primarily to treatment of sensory receptor dysfunction. Drug Saf 1994;11:318. [NLM Cit ID: 95177972] (Many drugs impair taste and smell.)

Keverne EB: Olfactory learning. Curr Opin Neurobiol 1995;5:482. [NLM Cit ID: 96051365] (Discovery of a huge family of odorant receptor genes is opening new avenues for study of olfaction and may lead to a molecular basis of olfactory perception.)

Schiffman SS: Taste and smell losses in normal aging and disease. JAMA 1997;278:1357. [NLM Cit ID: 98001633] (A review of a subject often minimized.)

EPISTAXIS

Bleeding from Kiesselbach's plexus, a vascular plexus on the anterior nasal septum, is by far the most common type of epistaxis encountered. Predisposing factors include nasal trauma (nose picking, foreign bodies, forceful nose blowing), rhinitis, drying of the nasal mucosa from low humidity, deviation of the nasal septum, alcohol use, and antiplatelet medications. Most cases of anterior epistaxis may be successfully treated by direct pressure on the bleeding site. The nasal alae should be firmly compressed for at least 10 minutes. Venous pressure is reduced in the sitting position, and leaning forward lessens the swallowing of blood. Short-acting topical nasal decongestants (eg, phenylephrine, 0.125–1% solution, one or two sprays), which act as vasoconstrictors, may also be helpful. When the bleeding does not readily subside, the nose should be examined, using good illumination and suction, in an attempt to locate the bleeding site. Topical 4% cocaine applied either as a spray or on a cotton strip serves both as an anesthetic and as a vasoconstricting agent. If cocaine is unavailable, a topical decongestant (eg, oxymetazoline) and a topical anesthetic (eg, tetracaine) provide equivalent results. When visible, the bleeding site may be cauterized with silver nitrate, diathermy, or electrocautery. A supplemental patch of Surgicel or Gelfoam may be helpful.

Occasionally, a site of bleeding may be inaccessible to direct control, or attempts at direct control may be unsuccessful. In such cases, nasal packing is necessary. A properly placed anterior pack requires several feet of half-inch iodoform packing lubricated with bacitracin or petroleum ointment. The packing is carefully and systematically placed along the floor and then the vault of the nose. If the equipment necessary to place a pack is not available, various manufactured nasal balloons may serve as either a temporizing or definitive solution.

About 5% of nasal bleeding originates in the posterior nasal cavity. This requires placement of a pack to occlude the choana before placement of a pack anteriorly. Because this is uncomfortable for the patient and because it requires oxygen supplementation to prevent hypoxia, hospitalization for several days is indicated. Narcotic analgesics are needed to reduce the considerable discomfort and elevated blood pressure caused by a posterior pack. Immediate ligation of the nasal arterial supply (internal maxillary artery and ethmoid arteries) is a possible alternative to posterior nasal packing, as is endovascular embolization of the internal maxillary artery. This is certainly necessary when packing fails to control life-threatening hemorrhage. On rare occasions, ligation of the external carotid artery may be necessary.

After control of epistaxis, the patient is advised to avoid vigorous exercise for several days. Avoidance of hot or spicy foods and tobacco is also advisable, as they may cause vasodilation. Avoiding nasal trauma, including digital self-trauma, is an obvious necessity. Lubrication with petroleum jelly or bacitracin ointment and increasing home humidity may be useful ancillary measures.

It is important in all patients with epistaxis to consider underlying causes of the bleeding. Laboratory assessment of bleeding parameters may be indicated, especially in recurrent cases. Other causes of recurrent epistaxis, such as hereditary hemorrhagic telangiectasia (Osler-Weber-Rendu syndrome), should also be considered. Similarly, once the acute episode has passed, careful examination of the nose and paranasal sinuses to rule out neoplasia is wise.

Patients presenting with epistaxis often have higher blood pressures than control patients. The majority will have sustained arterial hypertension, often without their knowledge. Continued management of patients with epistaxis and high blood pressure should therefore include follow-up investigation of possible sustained arterial hypertension.

Alvi A et al: Acute epistaxis: How to spot the source and stop the flow. Postgrad Med 1996;99:83. [NLM Cit ID: 96219038] (Cauterization, nasal packing, and intranasal tampon or balloon are often effective, but arterial ligation or angiographic embolization may be necessary.)

Cullen MM et al: Comparison of internal maxillary artery ligation versus embolization for refractory posterior epistaxis. Otolaryngol Head Neck Surg 1998;118:636. [NLM Cit ID: 98252559] (Internal maxillary artery ligation is more expensive, but embolization is usually unavailable in nonurban areas. Complication rates for ligation are the same or higher, but major complications of embolization are more serious.)

Herkner H et al: Hypertension in patients presenting with epistaxis. Ann Emerg Med 2000;35:126. [NLM Cit ID: 20117343] (Patients with epistaxis who have elevated blood pressure need follow-up to see if the hypertension is sustained and hence requires treatment.)

Leppanen M et al: Microcatheter embolization of intractable idiopathic epistaxis. Cardiovasc Intervent Radiol 1999;22:499. [NLM Cit ID: 20025795] (Embolization is safe and effective. It should be considered the primary treatment for intractable idiopathic epistaxis.)

Moreau S et al: Supraselective embolization in intractable epistaxis: review of 45 cases. Laryngoscope 1998;108: 887. [NLM Cit ID: 98290469] (Supraselective embolization in intractable epistaxis is successful in 97% of cases, with complications occurring in 8%.)

Pothula V et al: Nothing new under the sun: the management of epistaxis. J Laryngol Otol 1998;112:331. [NLM Cit ID: 98323677] (Historical review. The basis of many contemporary treatments was known and practiced by our ancient forebears.)

Tan LK et al: Epistaxis. Med Clin North Am 1999;83:43. [NLM Cit ID: 99126920] (In shifting management philosophy of epistaxis toward targeting the bleeding point, endoscopic evaluation may have a significant impact on decreasing length of stay and blood transfusion rates. Advances in interventional radiology have also reduced the risk of embolization. Patient education, especially teaching first-aid measures to patients at high risk for nosebleeds, also encourages more effective use of health care resources.)

NASAL TRAUMA

The nasal pyramid is the most frequently fractured bone in the body. Fracture is suggested by crepitance or palpably mobile bony segments. Epistaxis and pain are common, as are soft tissue hematomas ("black eye"). It is important to make certain that there is no palpable step-off of the infraorbital rim, which would indicate the presence of a zygomatic complex fracture. Radiologic confirmation may at times be helpful but is not necessary in uncomplicated nasal fractures.

Treatment is aimed at maintaining long-term nasal airway patency and nasal aesthetics. Closed reduction, using topical 4% cocaine and locally injected 1% lidocaine, should be attempted within 1 week of injury. In the presence of marked nasal swelling, it is best to wait several days for the edema to subside before undertaking reduction. Persistent functional or cosmetic defects may be repaired by delayed reconstructive nasal surgery.

Intranasal examination should be performed in all cases to rule out septal hematoma, which appears as a widening of the anterior septum, visible just posterior to the columella. The septal cartilage receives its only nutrition from its closely adherent mucoperichondrium. An untreated subperichondrial hematoma will result in loss of the nasal cartilage with resultant saddlenose deformity. Undrained septal hematomas may become infected, with *S aureus* the predominant organism. Treatment consists of incision and drainage via an intranasal septal mucosal incision. It is impor-

ronmental tobacco smoke on nasal and sinus disease: a review of the literature. Am J Rhinol 1999;13:435. [NLM Cit ID: 20096973]

Cantau G et al: Anterior craniofacial resection for malignant ethmoid tumors—a series of 91 patients. Head Neck 1999;21:185. [NLM Cit ID: 99223358]

Claus F et al: Postoperative radiotherapy of paranasal sinus tumours: a challenge for intensity modulated radiotherapy. Acta Otorhinolaryngol Belg 1999;53:263. [NLM Cit ID: 20101323] (Intensity-modulated radiotherapy is helpful in administering a high tumor dose while sparing surrounding organs in anatomically complex areas such as the paranasal sinuses and skull base.)

Fu KK: Combined radiotherapy and chemotherapy for nasopharyngeal carcinoma. Semin Radiat Oncol 1998;8:247. [NLM Cit ID: 99106072] (Reviews the results of randomized trials of combined chemotherapy and radiotherapy for nasopharyngeal carcinoma to date.)

Ho S et al: Staging and IgA VCA titre in patients with nasopharyngeal carcinoma: changes over a 12-year period. Oral Oncol 1998;34:491. [NLM Cit ID: 99129221] (The IgA VCA [viral capsid antigen to EBV] titer is often helpful in screening and monitoring nasopharyngeal carcinoma, but better serologic markers for screening are needed for early detection.)

Sanguineti G et al: Treatment of nasopharyngeal carcinoma: state of the art and new perspectives (review). Oncol Rep 1999;6:377. [NLM Cit ID: 99148168] (An overview of treatment advances.)

3. WEGENER'S GRANULOMATOSIS, NK CELL & T CELL EBV-POSITIVE LYMPHOMA, & SARCOIDOSIS

The nose and paranasal sinuses are involved in over 90% of cases of Wegener's granulomatosis. It is often not realized that involvement at these sites is more common than involvement of lungs or kidneys. Examination shows bloodstained crusts and friable mucosa. Biopsy classically shows necrotizing granulomas and vasculitis, but in practice the differential diagnosis may be more difficult. Sarcoidosis also commonly presents in the paranasal sinuses and is clinically similar to other chronic sinonasal inflammatory processes. Biopsy shows nonnecrotic granulomas.

Polymorphic reticulosis (midline malignant reticulosis, idiopathic midline destructive disease, lethal midline granuloma), as the multitude of apt descriptive terms suggest, is not well understood but appears to be a nasal lymphoma. In contrast to Wegener's granulomatosis, involvement is limited to the mid face, and there may be extensive bone destruction. Its progression in time to a lymphoma is being described with increasing frequency.

Many destructive lesions of the mucosa and structures of the nose once described by the terms in the previous paragraph are in fact non-Hodgkin's lymphoma of either NK cell or T cell origin. Immunophenotyping, especially for CD56 expression, is essential in the histologic evaluation of such a process. Even when they are apparently localized, the prognosis for these lymphomas is poor, with progression to distant relapse and death within a year the rule.

Wegener's granulomatosis may be treated with glucocorticoids and cyclophosphamide for remission induction, with consideration of methotrexate for remission maintenance. Alternatives include glucocorticoids and methotrexate as initial treatment (avoiding cyclophosphamide), but chronic disease courses are to be expected with this latter approach. Trimethoprim-sulfamethoxazole may be valuable in selected patients with limited forms of Wegener's granulomatosis.

Cheung MM et al: Primary non-Hodgkin's lymphoma of the nose and nasopharynx: Clinical features, tumor immunophenotype, and treatment outcome in 113 patients. J Clin Oncol 1998;16:70. [NLM Cit ID: 98101675] (As immunophenotype and stage correlate with prognosis, CD56 expression should be analyzed. NK and T cell lymphomas have a very poor prognosis.)

Courcoutsakis NA et al: Orbital involvement in Wegener granulomatosis: MR findings in 12 patients. J Comput Assist Tomogr 1997;21:452. [NLM Cit ID: 97281349] (A marked decrease in the T2 signal is characteristic. The unenhanced, non-fat-suppressed T1-weighted sequence is best for lesion detection and for definition of the anatomic extent.)

DeShazo RD et al: Diagnostic criteria for sarcoidosis of the sinuses. J Allergy Clin Immunol 1999;103(5 Part 1):789. [NLM Cit ID: 99262545]

Duffy M: Advances in diagnosis, treatment, and management of orbital and periocular Wegener's granulomatosis. Curr Opin Ophthalmol 1999;10:352. [NLM Cit ID: 99448289] (Trimethoprim-sulfamethoxazole or methotrexate may be useful in selected patients with limited forms of Wegener's granulomatosis.)

Hasni SA et al: Sarcoidosis presenting as necrotizing sinus destruction mimicking Wegener's granulomatosis. J Rheumatol 2000;27:512. [NLM Cit ID: 20148260]

Hausdorff J et al: Non-Hodgkin's lymphoma of the paranasal sinuses: Clinical and pathological features, and response to combined-modality therapy. Cancer J Sci Am 1997;3:303. [NLM Cit ID: 97468011] (Combined modality therapy with central nervous system prophylaxis improves outcome compared with radiotherapy, and autologous bone marrow transplantation as initial therapy is a consideration.)

Knecht K et al: More than a mouth ulcer. Oral ulcer due to Wegener's granulomatosis. Postgrad Med 1999;105:200. [NLM Cit ID: 99267811]

Krespi YP et al: Sarcoidosis of the sinonasal tract: A new staging system. Otolaryngol Head Neck Surg 1995; 112:221. [NLM Cit ID: 95140438] (A staging system to categorize severity and guide aggressiveness of therapy.)

Langford CA et al: A staged approach to the treatment of Wegener's granulomatosis: induction of remission with glucocorticoids and daily cyclophosphamide switching to methotrexate for remission maintenance. Arthritis Rheum 1999;42:2666. [NLM Cit ID: 20081762] (Median time to remission was 3 months; median time to discontinuation of glucocorticoids was 8 months. Sixteen percent of patients have had disease relapses at a median of 13 months after achieving remission.)

Magliulo G et al: Wegener's granulomatosis presenting as facial palsy. Am J Otolaryngol 1999;20:43. [NLM Cit ID: 99133611]

O'Devaney K et al: Wegener's granulomatosis of the head and neck. Ann Otol Rhinol Laryngol 1998;107(5 Part 1):439. [NLM Cit ID: 98255665] (Manifestations and differential diagnosis.)

Ohsawa M et al: Immunophenotypic and genotypic characterization of nasal lymphoma with polymorphic reticulosis morphology. Int J Cancer 1999;81:865. [NLM Cit ID: 99288977]

Perry SR et al: The clinical and pathologic constellation of Wegener granulomatosis of the orbit. Ophthalmology 1997;104:683. [NLM Cit ID: 97265327] (Reviews ophthalmologic symptoms such as decreased vision, redness, and ocular-facial pain; signs such as proptosis, scleritis, and lid inflammation; serologic tests; and treatment.)

Rinaldo A et al: Wegener's granulomatosis presenting with otologic manifestations. J Otolaryngol 1999;28:347. [NLM Cit ID: 20071832]

Stone JH et al: Treatment of non-life threatening Wegener's granulomatosis with methotrexate and daily prednisone as the initial therapy of choice. J Rheumatol 1999;26:1134. [NLM Cit ID: 99263775] (Effectively controls disease in selected cases, but a chronic disease course is the rule.)

DISEASES OF THE ORAL CAVITY & PHARYNX

LEUKOPLAKIA, ERYTHROPLAKIA, ORAL LICHEN PLANUS, & ORAL CANCER

Leukoplakia is any white lesion that, unlike oral candidiasis, cannot be removed by simply rubbing the mucosal surface. These areas are usually small but may be several centimeters in diameter. Histologically, they may be simple hyperkeratoses occurring in response to chronic irritation (eg, from dentures, tobacco); about 2–6%, however, represent either dysplasia or early invasive squamous cell carcinoma.

Erythroplakia is similar to leukoplakia except that it has a definite erythematous component. The distinction is important, since about 90% of cases of erythroplakia are either dysplasia or carcinoma. Squamous cell carcinoma accounts for 90% of oral cancer. Alcohol and tobacco are the major epidemiologic factors. The differential diagnosis may include oral candidiasis, necrotizing sialometaplasia, pseudoepitheliomatous hyperplasia, median rhomboid glossitis, and vesiculoerosive inflammatory disease such as erosive lichen planus. This should not be confused with the brown-black gingival melanin pigmentation—diffuse or speckled—common in nonwhites, blue-black embedded fragments of dental amalgam, or other systemic disorders associated with general pigmentation (neurofibromatosis, familial polyposis, Addison's disease). Intraoral melanoma is extremely rare.

Any erythroplakic or enlarging leukoplakic area should have an incisional biopsy or an exfoliative cytologic examination done by the clinician who will direct management of a cancer if one is discovered. Specialty referral should be sought early both for diagnosis and treatment. Intraoral staining with 1% toluidine blue may aid in selection of the most suspicious biopsy site. A systematic intraoral examination—including the lateral tongue, floor of the mouth, gingiva, buccal area, palate, and tonsillar fossae—and palpation of the neck for enlarged lymph nodes should be part of any general physical examination, especially in patients over 45 who smoke tobacco or drink immoderately. Indirect or fiberoptic examination of the nasopharynx, oropharynx, hypopharynx, and larynx should also be done by an otolaryngologist–head and neck surgeon or radiation oncologist. Fine-needle aspiration biopsy may be indicated if an enlarged lymph node is found.

Early detection of squamous cell carcinoma is the key to successful management. Lesions less than 4 mm in depth have a low propensity to metastasize. Most patients in whom the tumor is detected before it is 2 cm in diameter are cured. Small lesions are best treated with surgical excision, often with a laser. Radiation is an alternative but is associated with xerostomia, osteonecrosis of the mandible, and inability to use a curative dose again in the treatment field. Large tumors nevertheless are usually treated with a combination of resection and irradiation. Reconstruction, if required, is done at the time of resection and can involve the use of myocutaneous flaps or vascularized free flaps without bone.

Molecular analyses of premalignant and malignant tissues have produced strong evidence that clonal genetic alterations, such as loss of retinoic acid beta-receptor expression, occur during the early stage of aerodigestive tract carcinogenesis. These molecular and epidemiologic studies provide the foundation on which clinical trials have been designed to evaluate the role of retinoids and other compounds in the reversal of premalignancy and the possible reduction in the 4–7% annual rate of second primary tumors.

A number of clinical trials have suggested a role for beta-carotene, vitamin E, and retinoids in producing regression of leukoplakia and reducing the incidence of recurrent squamous cell carcinomas. Retinoids suppress head and neck and lung carcinogenesis in animal models and inhibit carcinogenesis in individuals with premalignant lesions. They also seem to reduce the incidence of second primary cancers in head and neck and lung cancer patients previously treated for a primary.

Carbone M et al: Topical corticosteroids in association with miconazole and chlorhexidine in the long-term management of atrophic-erosive oral lichen planus: a placebo-controlled and comparative study between clobetasol and fluocinonide. Oral Dis 1999;5:44. [NLM Cit ID: 99234664] (The topical steroid clobetasol propionate 0.05% in an adhesive medium of hydroxyethyl cellulose 4% gel was helpful in controlling oral lichen planus. The authors also used an antimycotic treatment consisting of miconazole gel and chlorhexidine 0.12% mouthwashes as prophylaxis against oropharyngeal candidiasis.)

Epstein JB et al: Topical application of vitamin A to oral leukoplakia: A clinical case series. Cancer 1999;86:921. [NLM Cit ID: 99423585] (Topical vitamin A had a minimal effect; topical 13-*cis*-retinoic acid may be more promising.)

Fantasia JE: Diagnosis and treatment of common oral lesions found in the elderly. Dent Clin North Am 1997;41:877. [NLM Cit ID: 98002967] (Reviews the wide variety of oral lesions seen in this population.)

Garewal HS et al: Beta-carotene produces sustained remissions in patients with oral leukoplakia: results of a multicenter prospective trial. Arch Otolaryngol Head Neck Surg 1999;125:1305. [NLM Cit ID: 20067896]

Geyer C et al: Chemoprevention in head and neck cancer: basic science and clinical application. Semin Radiat Oncol 1998;8:292. [NLM Cit ID: 99106077] (The rationale of retinoid chemoprevention of second head and neck cancers, based on the concepts of field cancerization and multistep carcinogenesis.)

Lotan R: Retinoids and chemoprevention of aerodigestive tract cancers. Cancer Metast Rev 1997;16:349. [NLM Cit ID: 98095442]

Martin GC et al: Oral leukoplakia status six weeks after cessation of smokeless tobacco use. J Am Dent Assoc 1999;130:945. [NLM Cit ID: 99351298] (Most leukoplakic lesions resolved clinically. If a young patient will stop using smokeless tobacco, delaying a biopsy of a minimally suspicious lesion may be reasonable.)

Miller WH Jr: The emerging role of retinoids and retinoic acid metabolism blocking agents in the treatment of cancer. Cancer 1998;83:1471. [NLM Cit ID: 98453201] (Although exogenous retinoids have not yet fulfilled their initial promise of chemoprevention, studies are ongoing. Modulation of endogenous retinoids may offer a significant new potential treatment for cancer.)

Papadimitrakopoulou VA et al: Retinoids in head and neck chemoprevention. Proc Soc Exp Biol Med 1997;216:283. [NLM Cit ID: 98007854] (Retinoids may be useful in chemoprevention. Current explorations of combinations with biologic response modifiers such as alpha interferon as well as new receptor-selective retinoids hold promise for the future.)

Piattelli A et al: *bcl*-2 expression and apoptotic bodies in 13-*cis*-retinoic acid (isotretinoin)-topically treated oral leukoplakia: a pilot study. Oral Oncol 1999;35:314. [NLM Cit ID: 20087733] (Topical treatment rather than oral ingestion of 13-*cis*-retinoic acid may also be effective.)

CANDIDIASIS

Oral candidiasis (thrush) is usually painful and looks like creamy-white curd-like patches overlying erythematous mucosa. Because these white areas are easily rubbed off (eg, by a tongue depressor)—unlike leukoplakia or lichen planus—only the underlying irregular erythema may be seen. Oral candidiasis is commonly encountered among denture wearers; in debilitation, diabetes, and anemia; in those undergoing chemotherapy or local irradiation; and in patients receiving corticosteroids or broad-spectrum antibiotics. Candidiasis is often seen prior to other manifestations of HIV infection in high-risk groups. Angular cheilitis is also a manifestation of candidiasis, though it is also seen in nutritional deficiencies.

The diagnosis is usually not difficult—painful intraoral white patches on an erythematous base in a patient at risk for candidiasis. A wet preparation of a smear with potassium hydroxide will confirm spores and may show nonseptate mycelia. Biopsy will show intraepithelial pseudomycelia of *Candida albicans*.

Effective antifungal therapy may be achieved with any of the following: fluconazole (100 mg daily for 7–14 days), ketoconazole (200–400 mg with breakfast [requires acidic gastric environment for absorption] for 7–14 days), clotrimazole troches (10 mg dissolved orally five times daily), or nystatin vaginal troches (100,000 units dissolved orally five times daily) or mouth rinses (500,000 units [5 mL of 100,000 units/mL] held in the mouth before swallowing three times daily). Shorter-duration therapy has also proved effective in many cases, using, for instance, fluconazole. In patients with HIV infection, however, longer courses may be needed, and itraconazole (200 mg orally daily) may be indicated in fluconazole-refractory cases. In addition, 0.12% chlorhexidine or half-strength hydrogen peroxide mouth rinses may provide local relief. Nystatin powder (100,000 units/g) applied to dentures three or four times daily for several weeks may help denture wearers.

Como JA et al: Oral azole drugs as systemic antifungal therapy. N Engl J Med 1994;330:263. [NLM Cit ID: 94097373] (Reviews the relative merits of use of ketoconazole, fluconazole, and itraconazole.)

Epstein JB et al: Oropharyngeal candidiasis: A review of its clinical spectrum and current therapies. Clin Ther 1998;20:40. [NLM Cit ID: 98182570] (In immunocompetent patients, topical agents often suffice in uncomplicated cases. Amphotericin B is now available as an oral suspension, adding another option, though systemic agents are often necessary in severe and recurrent cases.)

Graybill JR et al: Randomized trial of itraconazole oral solution for oropharyngeal candidiasis in HIV/AIDS patients. Am J Med 1998;104:33. [NLM Cit ID: 98187566] (There were few adverse reactions to either itraconazole or fluconazole. About half of patients in all groups relapsed by 1 month.)

Hedderwick S et al: Opportunistic fungal infections: superficial and systemic candidiasis. Geriatrics 1997;52:50. [NLM Cit ID: 97479153]

Kauffman CA et al: Antifungal agents in the 1990s: Current status and future developments. Drugs 1997;53:539. [NLM Cit ID: 97253215] (Reviews itraconazole and fluconazole as well as the emergence of drug resistance in

AIDS patients and shifts in the species of yeasts causing nosocomial infections. Discusses lipid-containing formulations of amphotericin B and new fungicidal agents in early trials.)

Laskaris G: Oral manifestations of infectious diseases. Dent Clin North Am 1996;40:395. [NLM Cit ID: 96252116] (Presents the clinical features of the most common and important oral infectious diseases.)

Mascarenhas AK et al: Factors associated with utilization of care for oral lesions in HIV disease. Oral Surg Oral Med Oral Pathol Oral Radiol Endod 1999;87:708. [NLM Cit ID: 99323792]

Saag MS et al: Treatment of fluconazole-refractory oropharyngeal candidiasis with itraconazole oral solution in HIV-positive patients. AIDS Res Hum Retroviruses 1999;15:1413. [NLM Cit ID: 20021574]

Smith D et al: A randomised, double-blind study of itraconazole versus placebo in the treatment and prevention of oral or oesophageal candidosis in patients with HIV infection. Int J Clin Pract 1999;53:349. [NLM Cit ID: 20159421] (Itraconazole, 200 mg daily, is effective and well-tolerated for treatment and subsequent prophylaxis.)

GLOSSITIS & GLOSSODYNIA

Inflammation of the tongue with loss of filiform papillae leads to a red, smooth-surfaced tongue (glossitis). Rarely painful, it may be secondary to nutritional deficiencies (eg, niacin, riboflavin, or vitamin E), drug reactions, dehydration, irritants, and possibly autoimmune reactions or psoriasis. Cultures may occasionally be helpful. If the primary cause cannot be identified and corrected, empirical nutritional replacement therapy may be of diagnostic value.

Glossodynia is burning and pain of the tongue; it may occur with or without glossitis. It has been associated with diabetes, drugs (eg, diuretics), tobacco, xerostomia, and candidiasis as well as the sometimes obscure causes of glossitis. Periodontal disease is not apt to be a factor. Treating possible underlying causes, changing chronic medications to alternative ones, and smoking cessation may resolve symptoms. Reassurance that there is no infection or tumor is likely to be appreciated. Anxiolytic medications and evaluation of possible psychologic status may be considered as well.

Bohmer T et al: The association between atrophic glossitis and protein-calorie malnutrition in old age. Age Aging 2000;29:47. [NLM Cit ID: 20152554] (Atrophic glossitis is common in elderly people and is a marker for malnutrition and reduced muscle function.)

Grinspan D et al: Burning mouth syndrome. Int J Dermatol 1995;34:483. [NLM Cit ID: 96067893] (After eliminating patients with local or systemic illnesses, this study reviews the definition of psychosomatic processes causing oral dysesthesia.)

Miyaoka H et al: A psychiatric appraisal of "glossodynia." Psychosomatics 1996;37:346. [NLM Cit ID: 96312085] (The psychopathology of patients felt to have these pain symptoms without a clear etiology may be more associated with personality trait characteristics than with neurotic or depressive symptoms.)

Osaki T et al: Candidiasis may induce glossodynia without objective manifestation. Am J Med Sci 2000;319:100. [NLM Cit ID: 20161920]

Wesselmann U et al: The dynias. Semin Neurol 1996;16:63. [NLM Cit ID: 97033312]

INTRAORAL ULCERATIVE LESIONS

1. NECROTIZING ULCERATIVE GINGIVITIS (Trench Mouth, Vincent's Infection)

Necrotizing ulcerative gingivitis, often caused by an infection of both spirochetes and fusiform bacilli, is common in young adults under stress (classically at examination time). Underlying systemic diseases may also predispose to this disorder. Clinically, there is painful acute gingival inflammation and necrosis, often with bleeding, halitosis, fever, and cervical lymphadenopathy. In addition to altering or removing, if possible, underlying factors and correcting dietary inadequacies, warm half-strength peroxide rinses and oral penicillin (250 mg three times daily for 10 days) may help. Dental gingival curettage may prove necessary.

Necrotizing ulcerative periodontitis is discussed later in this chapter in the section on AIDS.

Eng HL et al: Oral tuberculosis. Oral Surg Oral Med Oral Pathol Oral Radiol Endod 1996;81:415. [NLM Cit ID: 96288803] (Tuberculosis is in the differential diagnosis of an irregular ulceration or a discrete granular mass of the tongue or gingiva.)

Worle B et al. Chronic ulcerative stomatitis. Br J Dermatol 1997;137:262. [NLM Cit ID: 97437545] (Chronic ulcerative stomatitis has recently been described as an entity characterized by chronic ulceration of oral mucosa that responds to treatment with hydroxychloroquine.)

2. APHTHOUS ULCER (Canker Sore, Ulcerative Stomatitis)

Aphthous ulcers are very common and easy to recognize. Their cause remains uncertain, though one recent paper suggests an association with human herpesvirus 6. Found on nonkeratinized mucosa (eg, buccal and labial mucosa and not gingiva or palate), they may be single or multiple, are usually recurrent, and appear as painful small (usually 1–2 mm, but sometimes 1–2 cm) round ulcerations with yellow-gray fibrinoid centers surrounded by red halos. The painful stage lasts 7–10 days; healing is completed in 1–3 weeks.

Treatment is nonspecific. Topical steroids (triamcinolone acetonide, 0.1%, or fluocinonide ointment,

0.05%) in an adhesive base (Orabase Plain) do appear to provide symptomatic relief. Other topical therapies shown to be effective in controlled studies include diclofenac 3% in hyaluronan 2.5%, doxymycine-cyanoacrylate, mouthwashes containing the enzymes amyloglucosidase and glucose oxidase, and amlexanox 5% oral paste. A 1-week tapering course of prednisone (40–60 mg/d) has also been used successfully.

Large or persistent areas of ulcerative stomatitis may be secondary to erythema multiforme or drug allergies, acute herpes simplex, pemphigus, pemphigoid, bullous lichen planus, Behçet's disease, or inflammatory bowel disease. Squamous cell carcinoma may occasionally present in this fashion. When the diagnosis is not clear, incisional biopsy is indicated.

Chandrasekhar J et al: Oxypentifylline in the management of recurrent aphthous oral ulcers: an open clinical trial. Oral Surg Oral Med Oral Pathol Oral Radiol Endod 1999;87:564. [NLM Cit ID: 99276269] (Available in UK.)

Fridh G et al: Effect of a mouth rinse containing amyloglucosidase and glucose oxidase on recurrent aphthous ulcers in children and adolescents. Swed Dent J 1999;23:49. [NLM Cit ID: 99360009]

Ghodratnama F et al: Detection of serum antibodies against cytomegalovirus, varicella zoster virus and human herpesvirus 6 in patients with recurrent aphthous stomatitis. J Oral Pathol Med 1999;28:12. [NLM Cit ID: 99105457] (Suggests a possible etiologic role of HHV-6.)

Krause I et al: Recurrent aphthous stomatitis in Behçet's disease: clinical features and correlation with systemic disease expression and severity. J Oral Pathol Med 1999;28:193. [NLM Cit ID: 99243527]

MacPhail L: Topical and systemic therapy for recurrent aphthous stomatitis. Semin Cutan Med Surg 1997; 16:301. [NLM Cit ID: 98081575] (The most effective treatments involve systemic or topical steroids or thalidomide.)

Rogers RS 3rd: Recurrent aphthous stomatitis: Clinical characteristics and associated systemic disorders. Semin Cutan Med Surg 1997;16:278. [NLM Cit ID: 98081572] (Reviews associated systemic disorders or "correctable causes" for which treatment reduces disease activity.)

Ylikontiola L et al: Doxymycine-cyanoacrylate treatment of recurrent aphthous ulcers. Oral Surg Oral Med Oral Pathol Oral Radiol Endod 1997;83:329. [NLM Cit ID: 97237739] (In recurrent aphthous ulcers, a single application of topical doxymycine-cyanoacrylate reduces pain intensity remarkably for 6 days after a 1 day latency period.)

3. HERPETIC STOMATITIS

Herpetic gingivostomatitis is common, mild, and short-lived and requires no intervention in most adults. In immunocompromised individuals, however, reactivation of herpes simplex virus infection is frequent and may be severe. Clinically, there is initial burning, followed by typical small vesicles that rupture and form scabs. Acyclovir (200–800 mg five times daily for 7–14 days) may shorten the course and reduce postherpetic pain. Differential diagnosis includes ulcerative stomatitis (see above) as well as erythema multiforme, syphilitic chancre, and carcinoma. Coxsackievirus-caused lesions (grayish white tonsillar and palatal ulcers of herpangina or buccal and lip ulcers in hand-foot-and-mouth disease) are seen more commonly in children under age 6.

Woo SB, Lee SF: Oral recrudescent herpes simplex virus infection. Oral Surg Oral Med Oral Pathol Oral Radiol Endod 1997;83:239. [NLM Cit ID: 97184626] (Since acyclovir is available for treatment, the authors recommend all oral ulcers in immunocompromised patients be cultured for herpes simplex virus.)

PHARYNGITIS & TONSILLITIS

As common as respiratory tract infections are—and they account for over 10% of all office visits to primary care physicians and 50% of outpatient antibiotics used—one would think the most appropriate management would be a matter of agreement among physicians. However, the issues are deceptively complex. Controversy exists over when to culture an inflamed throat and how long to treat confirmed group A β-hemolytic streptococcal pharyngitis—and with what. Numerous well-conceived and well-controlled studies in the past few years as well as the increasing experience with rapid laboratory tests for detection of streptococci (eliminating the delay caused by culturing) appear to make a consensual approach more possible.

The clinical features suggestive of group A β-hemolytic streptococcal pharyngitis (GABHS) include fever over 38 °C, tender anterior cervical adenopathy, lack of a cough, and a pharyngotonsillar exudate. The sore throat may be severe, with odynophagia, tender adenopathy, and a scarlatiniform rash. An elevated white blood count and left shift are consistent with group A β-hemolytic streptococcal pharyngitis. Hoarseness, cough, and coryza are not suggestive of this disease. Marked lymphadenopathy and a shaggy white-purple tonsillar exudate, often extending into the nasopharynx, suggest mononucleosis, especially if present in a young adult. Hepatosplenomegaly and a positive heterophil agglutination test or elevated anti-EBV titer of course are corroborative. It should be kept in mind that about one-third of patients with infectious mononucleosis have secondary streptococcal tonsillitis, requiring treatment. (Ampicillin should be avoided if mononucleosis is suspected because it induces a rash in such patients.) Diphtheria (extremely rare today but described in the alcoholic population) presents with low-grade fever in an ill patient with a gray tonsillar pseudomembrane; it should be distinguished from the more common acute necrotizing ulcerative gingivitis and herpangina.

The most common pathogens other than group A β-hemolytic streptococci in the differential diagnosis of "sore throat" are viruses, *Neisseria gonorrhoeae,* mycoplasma, and *Chlamydia trachomatis.* Rhinorrhea would suggest a virus, as would lack of an exudate, but in practice the most reasonable assumption is that it is not possible to distinguish viral upper respiratory infection from group A β-hemolytic streptococcal infection on clinical grounds alone. Infections with *Corynebacterium diphtheriae,* anaerobic streptococci, and *Corynebacterium haemolyticum* (which responds better to erythromycin than penicillin) may also mimic pharyngitis due to group A β-hemolytic streptococci.

Treatment strategies for a sore throat range from "treat all comers" to "culture all comers, reserving treatment for positive cultures." Issues that affect this decision for an individual include the reliability of cultures and rapid tests for streptococci such as latex agglutination (LA) antigen tests and solid-phase enzyme immunoassays (ELISA), the incidence of pharyngitis not due to group A β-hemolytic streptococci, patient follow-up and medical compliance, and cost. The apparent advantage of the "treat all" approach is the initial short-term cost, savings from elimination of diagnostic tests, and prevention of most streptococcal complications, but such an approach necessarily causes the highest rate of antibiotic use and side effects and therefore overall the highest cost. At the other extreme is the "culture all" approach, which is associated with the fewest penicillin reactions but is more costly than an "antigen test and culture" approach and is also dependent on the excellent follow-up not routinely available in some busy city health clinics. With current sensitivity of rapid group A β-hemolytic streptococcal antigen tests between 80% and 85%, and specificity greater than 90%, the strategy of treating patients with positive antigen test results while culturing (and waiting for results) patients with negative test results appears to be an excellent option. As the sensitivity of newer LA tests, ELISA, or other immunoassays (such as an optical immunoassay for detection of group A streptococcal carbohydrate antigen reported to be 97% sensitive) appears to exceed 90%, the strategy of relying solely on such antigen tests to decide whether to treat is also most attractive. Webb and colleagues, using this approach, found no increase in rates of complications among 7500 patients annually, about 75% of whom had high-specificity antigen tests without culture confirmation of negative results. Individual decisions need to be based on the prevalence of streptococcal infection (seasonally and locally); patient allergic history, reliability, and compliance; availability of rapid group A β-hemolytic streptococcal antigen tests; and reliability of available bacteriology laboratories.

Thirty years ago, a single injection of benzathine penicillin or procaine penicillin was standard antibiotic treatment. This remains effective, but the injections are painful. If compliance is an issue, it may be the best choice. Oral treatment, however, is also effective. The controversy over choice of preparation revolves around reducing the already low (10–20%) incidence of treatment failures (positive culture after treatment despite symptomatic resolution) and recurrences. A review of recent controlled studies suggests that penicillin V potassium (250 mg orally three times daily or 500 mg twice daily for 10 days) or cefuroxime axetil (250 mg orally twice daily for 5–10 days) are both effective. Erythromycin (active against mycoplasma and chlamydia) is a reasonable alternative to penicillin in allergic patients. Several cephalosporins in their usual dosage schedules are somewhat more effective than penicillin in producing bacteriologic cures; 5-day administration has been successful for selected cephalosporins, such as cefpodoxime or cefuroxime. The macrolide antibiotics have also been reported to be successful in shorter-duration regimens. Azithromycin (500 mg once daily) because of its long half-life, need be taken for only 3 days.

Adequate antibiotic treatment usually avoids the streptococcal complications of scarlet fever, glomerulonephritis, rheumatic myocarditis, and local abscess formation. About 10% of the time, repeat cultures show persistent presence of group A streptococci.

Antibiotic choices for treatment failures are also somewhat controversial. Perhaps surprisingly, penicillin-tolerant strains are not necessarily isolated more frequently in those who fail to improve with treatment than in those treated successfully with penicillin. The reasons for failure appear to be complex, and a second course of treatment with the same drug is therefore not necessarily unreasonable. Alternatives to penicillin include cefuroxime and certain other cephalosporins, dicloxacillin (which is β-lactamase-resistant), and amoxicillin with clavulanate. In penicillin-allergic patients, the usual alternatives should be used, such as erythromycin and cephalosporins. When there is a history of possible penicillin allergy, the usual alternatives should be used, such as erythromycin or cephalosporin. Erythromycin resistance—with failure rates of about 25%—is becoming an increasing problem in many geographic areas. In cases of prior severe penicillin reaction, cephalosporins should probably be avoided as the cross-reaction is felt to be higher than the overall 8% rate.

Ancillary treatment of pharyngitis includes appropriate analgesics and anti-inflammatory agents, such as aspirin or acetaminophen. Some patients find that salt water gargling is soothing. In severe cases, anesthetic gargles and lozenges (eg, benzocaine) may provide additional symptomatic relief. Occasionally, odynophagia is so intense that hospitalization for intravenous hydration and antibiotics is warranted.

DiMatteo L: Managing streptococcal pharyngitis: a review of clinical decision-managing strategies, diagnostic evaluation, and treatment. J Am Acad Nurse Pract 1999;11:57. [NLM Cit ID: 99434545] (Penicillin remains the drug of choice.)

Esposito S et al: Clinical comparison of cefaclor twice daily versus amoxicillin-clavulanate or erythromycin three times daily in the treatment of patients with streptococcal pharyngitis. Clin Ther 1998;20:72. [NLM Cit ID: 98182572] (Cefaclor twice daily and amoxicillin-clavulanate three times daily achieve 90% cure, erythromycin three times daily 77%. No GABHS strain was resistant to cefaclor or to amoxicillin-clavulanate; 38% were resistant to erythromycin.)

Kaplan EL: Clinical guidelines for group A streptococcal throat infections. Lancet 1997;350:899. [NLM Cit ID: 97460481]

McIsaac WJ et al: A clinical score to reduce unnecessary antibiotic use in patients with sore throat. CMAJ 1998; 158:75. [NLM Cit ID: 98136392] (The proportion of patients receiving initial antibiotics would have been reduced 48% by following score-based recommendations.)

McIsaac WJ et al: Reconsidering sore throats. Part 1: Problems with current clinical practice. Can Fam Physician 1997;43:485. [NLM Cit ID: 97234922]

McIsaac WJ et al: Reconsidering sore throats. Part 2: Alternative approach and practical office tool. Can Fam Physician 1997;43:495. [NLM Cit ID: 97234923] (In this two-part article, the authors conclude as follows: "Four clinical characteristics [no cough, fever higher than 38 °C, exudate, and tender cervical nodes] linked to explicit management decisions form the basis for a sore throat score.")

Pacifico L et al: Comparative efficacy and safety of 3-day azithromycin and 10-day penicillin V treatment of group A beta-hemolytic streptococcal pharyngitis in children. Antimicrob Ag Chemother 1996;40:1005. [NLM Cit ID: 96254576] (Once-daily [10 mg/kg] 3-day oral regimen of azithromycin is as safe as a 10-day course of penicillin but not an effective alternative to penicillin for group A β-hemolytic streptococcal pharyngitis. Ten days of penicillin, taken at least twice daily, remains the gold standard.)

Perkins A: An approach to diagnosing the acute sore throat. Am Fam Physician 1997;55:131, 141. [NLM Cit ID: 97148706] (A review emphasizing symptoms, epidemiologic factors, and the appropriate place of laboratory tests.)

Pichichero ME et al: Variables influencing penicillin treatment outcome in streptococcal tonsillopharyngitis. Arch Pediatr Adolesc Med 1999;153:565. [NLM Cit ID: 99284187] (Penicillin 250 mg three times daily was equivalent to 500 mg twice daily. Earlier treatment did help.)

Pichichero ME: Sore throat after sore throat after sore throat. Are you asking the critical questions? Postgrad Med 1997;101:205, 209, 215. [NLM Cit ID: 97161442] (Possible causes of persistence and recurrence include noncompliance, bacterial resistance, repeated exposure, alteration of pharyngeal microbial ecology, suppression of antibody response due to prior antibiotics, and treatment failure. Treatment options include penicillin G benzathine [for noncompliance], macrolides, clindamycin, rifampin [in combination with a second agent], oral cephalosporins, and, for a patient with six or seven recurrences over 1 or 2 years despite antibiotics, tonsillectomy.)

Richardson MA: Sore throat, tonsillitis, and adenoiditis. Med Clin North Am 1999;83:75. [NLM Cit ID: 99126922]

Scaglione F et al: Optimum treatment of streptococcal pharyngitis. Drugs 1997;53:86. [NLM Cit ID: 97163895] (Oral penicillins and, alternatively, oral cephalosporins are the first-line agents for treatment of culture-confirmed group A beta-haemolytic streptococcal tonsillopharyngitis. Cephalosporins are useful especially for the treatment of recurrent streptococcal tonsillopharyngitis.)

Sonnad SS et al: Issues in the development, dissemination, and effect of an evidence-based guideline for managing sore throat in adults. Jt Comm J Qual Improv 1999;25:630. [NLM Cit ID: 20073586] (Had the guidelines been followed, the amount of testing would have been reduced by 17% and the appropriateness of testing improved for 32%.)

Webb KH et al: Use of a high-sensitivity rapid strep test without culture confirmation of negative results: 2 years' experience. J Fam Pract 2000;49:34. [NLM Cit ID: 20141806] (In two years' experience, use of a high-sensitivity antigen test without culture confirmation of all negative results was not associated with an increase in complications of group A beta-hemolytic streptococci.)

PERITONSILLAR ABSCESS & CELLULITIS

When infection penetrates the tonsillar capsule and involves the surrounding tissues, peritonsillar cellulitis results. Peritonsillar abscess and cellulitis present with severe sore throat, odynophagia, trismus, medial deviation of the soft palate and peritonsillar fold, and a "hot potato" voice. Following therapy, peritonsillar cellulitis usually either resolves over several days or evolves into peritonsillar abscess. The existence of an abscess may be confirmed by aspirating pus from the peritonsillar fold just superior and medial to the upper pole of the tonsil. A No. 19 or No. 21 needle should be passed no deeper than 1 cm, because the internal carotid artery passes posterior and deep to the tonsillar fossa. There is controversy about the best way to treat peritonsillar abscesses. Some incise and drain the area and continue with parenteral antibiotics, whereas others aspirate only and follow as an outpatient. At times it is appropriate to consider immediate tonsillectomy (quinsy tonsillectomy) both to drain the abscess and to avoid recurrence. Both approaches are rational and have support in the literature. Whichever approach is taken, one must be sure the abscess is adequately drained, since complications such as extension to the retropharyngeal, deep neck, and posterior mediastinal spaces are possible. Pus may also be aspirated into the lungs, resulting in pneumonia. While there is controversy about whether a single abscess is sufficient indication for tonsillectomy, most would agree that patients with recurrent abscesses should have their tonsils removed. Overall, about 30% of patients with peritonsillar abscess exhibit relative indications for tonsillectomy.

Herzon FS et al: Mosher Award thesis. Peritonsillar abscess: Incidence, current management practices, and a proposal for treatment guidelines. Laryngoscope 1995;105(8 Part 3 Suppl 74):1. [NLM Cit ID: 95356693] (An in-depth study, including meta-analysis; needle aspiration recommended for initial surgical drainage procedure unless indications for abscess tonsillectomy are present.)

Kieff DA et al: Selection of antibiotics after incision and drainage of peritonsillar abscesses. Otolaryngol Head Neck Surg 1999;120:57. [NLM Cit ID: 99114867] (Retrospective review. Penicillin was an excellent choice in cases requiring parenteral antibiotics.)

TONSILLECTOMY

Despite the frequency with which tonsillectomy is performed, the indications for the procedure remain controversial. Most would agree that airway obstruction causing sleep apnea or cor pulmonale is an absolute indication for tonsillectomy. Similarly, persistent marked tonsillar asymmetry should prompt an excisional biopsy to rule out lymphoma. Relative indications include recurrent streptococcal tonsillitis, causing considerable loss of time from school or work, recurrent peritonsillar abscess, and chronic tonsillitis.

Tonsillectomy is not an entirely benign procedure. Postoperative bleeding occurs in 1–8% of cases and on rare occasions can lead to laryngospasm and airway obstruction. Pain may be considerable, especially in the adult. The pros and cons of the procedure need to be discussed with each prospective patient. In addition, there is increasing economic pressure for these procedures to be done as outpatient surgery. Hemorrhage, protracted emesis, or fever appears to occur in about 1% of cases, and such immediate complications usually appear within 6 hours but continue to occur later within the once frequent 24-hour period of hospitalized observation. This topic will continue to receive attention; at present it seems clear that outpatient tonsillectomy is usually safe when followed by a 6-hour period of uneventful observation, but each decision rests on individual circumstances.

Although reports in the 1970s suggested an association of tonsillectomy with Hodgkin's disease, careful review of this literature reveals no conclusively causative association.

Boot H et al: Long-term results of uvulopalatopharyngoplasty for obstructive sleep apnea syndrome. Laryngoscope 2000;110(3 Part 1):469. [NLM Cit ID: 20181368] (The response to UPPP for obstructive sleep apnea syndrome decreases progressively over the years after surgery. UPPP in combination with tonsillectomy was more effective than UPPP alone.)

Peeters A et al: Tonsillectomy and adenotomy as a one day procedure? Acta Otorhinolaryngol Belg 1999;53:91. [NLM Cit ID: 99356367] (Because of a postoperative major bleeding frequency between 2.6% and 3%, the authors prefer an overnight postoperative stay.)

Pringle MB et al: Day-case tonsillectomy: Is it appropriate? Clin Otolaryngol 1996;21:504. [NLM Cit ID: 97179168] (Comprehensive review.)

Randall DA et al: Complications of tonsillectomy and adenoidectomy. Otolaryngol Head Neck Surg 1998;118:61. [NLM Cit ID: 98111306] (Review of common and rare potential complications.)

Smith I et al: Secondary tonsillectomy haemorrhage and non-steroidal anti-inflammatory drugs. J Laryngol Otol 1999;113:28. [NLM Cit ID: 99273461] (They may cause an increased secondary hemorrhage rate.)

DEEP NECK INFECTIONS

Deep neck abscesses usually present with marked neck pain and swelling in a toxic febrile patient. They are emergencies because they may rapidly compromise the airway. They may also spread to the mediastinum or cause septicemia. Most commonly, they originate from odontogenic infections. Other causes include suppurative lymphadenitis, direct spread of pharyngeal infection, penetrating trauma, pharyngoesophageal foreign bodies, cervical osteomyelitis, and intravenous injection of the internal jugular vein, especially in drug abusers. Recurrent deep neck infection may suggest an underlying congenital lesion such as a branchial cleft cyst. Fundamentals of treatment include securing the airway, intravenous antibiotics, and incision and drainage. The airway may be secured either by intubation or tracheotomy. Tracheotomy is preferable in the patients with substantial pharyngeal edema, since attempts at intubation may precipitate acute airway obstruction. Contrast-enhanced CT usually augments the clinical examination in defining the extent of the abscess. Bleeding in association with a deep neck abscess suggests the possibility of carotid artery or internal jugular vein involvement and requires prompt neck exploration both for drainage of pus and for vascular ligation.

Ludwig's angina is the most commonly encountered neck space infection. It is a cellulitis of the sublingual and submaxillary spaces, often arising from infection of the tooth roots that extend below the mylohyoid line of the mandible. Clinically, there is edema and erythema of the upper neck under the chin and often of the floor of the mouth. The tongue may be displaced upward and backward by the posterior spread of cellulitis. This may lead to occlusion of the airway and necessitate tracheotomy. Microbiologic isolates include streptococci, staphylococci, bacteroides, and fusobacterium. Hospitalization and intravenous antibiotics are necessary. Usual doses of penicillin plus metronidazole, ampicillin-sulbactam, clindamycin, or selective cephalosporins are good initial choices. Culture and sensitivity data will then refine the choice. Dental consultation is advisable. External drainage via bilateral submental incisions is required immediately if the airway is threatened and when medical therapy has not reversed the process.

Gidley PW et al: Contemporary management of deep neck space infections. Otolaryngol Head Neck Surg 1997; 116:16. [NLM Cit ID: 97170978] (Operative drainage, bacteriology, and complications.)

Kay DJ et al: Diagnosis and management of complications of self-injection injuries of the neck. Ear Nose Throat J 1996;75:670. [NLM Cit ID: 97097470] (Infectious complications as well as less common complications such as vocal cord paralysis and retained foreign bodies.)

Miller WD et al: A prospective, blinded comparison of clinical examination and computed tomography in deep neck infections. Laryngoscope 1999;109:1873. [NLM Cit ID: 20034713] (They complement each other in assessing suspected deep neck infection.)

Nusbaum AO et al: Recurrence of a deep neck infection: a clinical indication of an underlying congenital lesion. Arch Otolaryngol Head Neck Surg 1999;125:1379. [NLM Cit ID: 20067908]

Sakaguchi M et al: Characterization and management of deep neck infections. Int J Oral Maxillofac Surg 1997;26:131. [NLM Cit ID: 97295562] (Peritonsillar abscesses predominate, with submandibular and parapharyngeal spaces also commonly involved.)

Wong TY: A nationwide survey of deaths from oral and maxillofacial infections: the Taiwanese experience. J Oral Maxillofacial Surg 1999;57:1297. [NLM Cit ID: 20022719] (Two-thirds of deaths occurred in patients with diabetes. The death rate was about 1:150, usually associated with sepsis.)

DISEASES OF THE SALIVARY GLANDS

The salivary glands are divided into the two large parotid glands, two submandibular glands, several sublingual glands, and 600–1000 minor salivary glands located throughout the upper aerodigestive tract.

ACUTE INFLAMMATORY SALIVARY GLAND DISORDERS

1. SIALADENITIS

Acute bacterial sialadenitis in the adult most commonly affects either the parotid or submandibular gland. It typically presents with acute swelling of the gland, increased pain and swelling with meals, and tenderness and erythema of the duct opening. Pus often can be massaged from the duct. Sialadenitis often occurs in the setting of dehydration or in association with chronic illness. Underlying Sjögren's syndrome also predisposes. The pathogenesis is ductal obstruction, often by an inspissated mucous plug, followed by salivary stasis and secondary infection. The most common organism recovered from purulent draining saliva is *S aureus*. Treatment consists of intravenous antibiotics such as nafcillin (1 g intravenously every 4–6 hours) and measures to increase salivary flow, including hydration, warm compresses, sialagogues (eg, lemon drops), and massage of the gland. Failure of the process to resolve on this regimen suggests abscess formation, ductal stricture, stone, or tumor causing obstruction. Ultrasound or CT scan may be helpful in establishing the diagnosis. Sialography is best avoided in acute cases.

Bates D et al: Parotid and submandibular sialadenitis treated by salivary gland excision. Aust N Z J Surg 1998;68:120. [NLM Cit ID: 98153022] (In recurrent cases with prolonged symptoms, surgical excision of the affected gland is effective.)

Ellies M et al: Surgical management of nonneoplastic diseases of the submandibular gland: A follow-up study. Int J Oral Maxillofac Surg 1996;25:285. [NLM Cit ID: 97066633] (Extirpation of the affected gland proved effective in all.)

2. SIALOLITHIASIS

Calculus formation is more common in Wharton's duct (draining the submandibular glands) than in Stensen's duct (draining the parotid glands). Clinically, a patient may note postprandial pain and local swelling, often with a history of recurrent acute sialadenitis. Stones in Wharton's duct are usually large and radiopaque, whereas those in Stensen's duct are usually radiolucent and smaller. Those very close to the orifice of Wharton's duct may be palpated manually in the anterior floor of the mouth and removed intraorally by dilating or incising the distal duct. The duct proximal to the stone must be temporarily clamped (using, for instance, a single throw of a suture) to keep manipulation of the stone from pushing it back toward the submandibular gland. Those more than 1.5–2 cm from the duct are too close to the lingual nerve to be removed safely in this manner. Similarly, dilation of Stensen's duct, located on the buccal surface opposite the second maxillary molar, may relieve distal stricture or allow a small stone to pass. The location of the facial nerve makes intraoral retrieval of more proximal parotid stones unsafe.

Repeated episodes of sialadenitis invariably lead to stricture and chronic infection. If the obstruction cannot be safely removed or dilated, excision of the gland may be necessary. In recent years there has been increased success with endoscopic techniques both to diagnose and remove salivary stones, with success rates for calculus removal in excess of 80%.

Arzoz E et al: Endoscopic intracorporeal lithotripsy for sialolithiasis. J Oral Maxillofac Surg 1996;54:847. [NLM Cit ID: 96285518] (Pneumoballistic energy [Lithoclast] produced calculus fragmentation with more efficiency than lasertripsy [Dornier Impact] in this report of cases treated by forceps extraction, lithotripsy, or open extraction.)

Ellies M et al: Surgical management of nonneoplastic diseases of the submandibular gland: A follow-up study. Int J Oral Maxillofac Surg 1996;25:285. [NLM Cit ID: 97066633]

Ito H et al: Pulsed dye laser lithotripsy of submandibular gland salivary calculus. J Laryngol Otol 1996;110:942. [NLM Cit ID: 97132403] (Laser shock wave lithotripsy of salivary stones with endoscopic monitoring is successful.)

Nahlieli O et al: Endoscopic technique for the diagnosis and treatment of obstructive salivary gland diseases. J Oral Maxillofac Surg 1999;57:1394. [NLM Cit ID: 20061772] (Endoscopy was possible in 145 of 154, of which 112 were obstructed. The success rate was 82% for calculus removal. Thirty-two percent of the submandibular and 63% of the parotid sialoliths were undetected prior to the procedure.)

Ottaviani F et al: Extracorporeal electromagnetic shock-wave lithotripsy for salivary gland stones. Laryngoscope 1996;106:761. [NLM Cit ID: 96247354] (A report of 52 cases, with complications discussed.)

Ottaviani F et al: Salivary gland stones: US evaluation in shock wave lithotripsy. Radiology 1997;204:437. [NLM Cit ID: 97382528] (Among 80 patients in whom endoral calculi extraction was not indicated, favorable outcome after lithotripsy was associated with smaller stone diameter and, in the case of submandibular gland stones, with intraductal location.)

Williams MF: Sialolithiasis. Otolaryngol Clin North Am 1999;32:819. [NLM Cit ID: 99408931]

CHRONIC INFLAMMATORY & INFILTRATIVE DISORDERS OF THE SALIVARY GLANDS

Numerous infiltrative disorders may cause unilateral or bilateral parotid gland enlargement. Sjögren's disease and sarcoidosis are examples of lymphoepithelial and granulomatous diseases that may affect the salivary glands. Metabolic disorders, including alcoholism, diabetes mellitus, and vitamin deficiencies, may also cause diffuse enlargement. Several drugs have been associated with parotid enlargement, including thioureas, iodine, and drugs with cholinergic effects (eg, phenothiazines), which stimulate flow and cause more viscous saliva.

SALIVARY GLAND TUMORS

Approximately 80% of salivary gland tumors occur in the parotid gland. In adults, about 80% of these are benign. In the submandibular triangle, it is sometimes difficult to distinguish a primary submandibular gland tumor from a metastatic submandibular space node. Only 50–60% of primary submandibular tumors are benign. Tumors of the minor salivary glands are most likely to be malignant, with adenoid cystic carcinoma predominating.

Most parotid tumors present as an asymptomatic mass in the superficial part of the gland. Their presence may have been noted by the patient for months or years. Facial nerve involvement correlates strongly with malignancy. Tumors may extend deep to the plane of the facial nerve or may originate in the parapharyngeal space. In such cases, medial deviation of the soft palate is visible on intraoral examination. MRI and CT scans have largely replaced sialography in defining the extent of tumor.

When the clinician encounters a patient with an otherwise asymptomatic salivary gland mass where tumor is the most likely diagnosis, the choice is whether to simply excise the mass via a parotidectomy with facial nerve dissection or submandibular gland excision or to obtain a fine-needle aspiration (FNA) biopsy first. Although the accuracy of FNA biopsy for malignancy has been reported to be quite high, with rare misleading interpretations, results vary among institutions. If a negative FNA biopsy would lead to a decision not to proceed to surgery, then it should be considered. The overall health of the patient and the possibility of inflammatory disease as the cause of the mass would be examples where FNA biopsy might be helpful. Usually, however, in otherwise nonrecurrent straightforward cases, excision is indicated. In benign and small low-grade malignant tumors, no additional treatment is needed. Postoperative irradiation is required for larger and high-grade cancers.

Cajulis RS et al: Fine needle aspiration biopsy of the salivary glands: A five-year experience with emphasis on diagnostic pitfalls. Acta Cytol 1997;41:1412. [NLM Cit ID: 97450390] (Using histology as the definitive standard, sensitivity of FNA cytology was 91%, with a specificity of 96%. Noteworthy that all aspirates done by cytopathologists were diagnostic, whereas 23% of those by clinicians were not.)

Kaplan MJ: Benign parotid tumors. In: *Current Therapy in Otolaryngology–Head and Neck Surgery,* 6th ed. Gates GA (editor). Mosby, 1998.

Kaplan MJ, Johns ME: Malignant neoplasms (of the salivary glands): In: *Otolaryngology–Head and Neck Surgery,* 2nd ed. Cummings CW, Frederickson J (editors). Mosby, 1993. (Prognostic factors, treatment recommendations, and new developments in imaging and treatment.)

DISEASES OF THE LARYNX

DYSPHONIA, HOARSENESS, & STRIDOR

The primary symptoms of laryngeal disease are hoarseness and stridor. Hoarseness is caused by an abnormal flow of air past the vocal cords. The voice is "breathy" when too much air passes incompletely apposed vocal cords, as in unilateral vocal cord paralysis. The voice is harsh when turbulence is created by irregularity of the vocal cords, as in laryngitis or a mass lesion. Stridor, a high-pitched sound, is produced by lesions that narrow the airway. Airway impairment above the vocal cords produces predominantly inspiratory stridor. Lesions below the vocal cord level produce either expiratory or mixed stridor.

Evaluation of an abnormal voice begins with obtaining a history of the circumstances preceding its onset and an examination of the airway. This may include indirect or flexible laryngoscopy and at times videostrobolaryngoscopy. Especially when the patient has a history of tobacco use, laryngeal cancer or lung cancer (leading to paralysis of a recurrent laryngeal nerve) must be strongly considered. Laryngitis, voice abuse, and vocal cord nodules are among the most common causes of hoarseness.

Garrett CG et al: Hoarseness. Med Clin North Am 1999;83:115. [NLM Cit ID: 99126925] (Describes normal vocal anatomy and physiology and outlines a practical approach in evaluating patients with voice disorders.)

Hagen P et al: Dysphonia in the elderly: Diagnosis and management of age-related voice changes. South Med J 1996;89:204. [NLM Cit ID: 96165407]

Rosen CA et al: Evaluating hoarseness: keeping your patient's voice healthy. Am Fam Physician 1998;57:2775. [NLM Cit ID: 98299969] (In the absence of an upper respiratory tract infection, any patient with hoarseness persisting for more than 2 weeks requires evaluation. Voice therapy is helpful in many non-cancer-related cases of hoarseness.)

COMMON LARYNGEAL DISORDERS

1. EPIGLOTTITIS

Epiglottitis (or, more correctly, supraglottitis) in adults should be suspected when a patient presents with a rapidly developing sore throat or when odynophagia (pain on swallowing) is out of proportion to apparently minimal oropharyngeal findings on examination. It may be viral or bacterial in origin. Unlike the case of children, indirect laryngoscopy is generally safe and may demonstrate the swollen, erythematous epiglottis. Initial treatment is hospitalization for intravenous antibiotics—eg, ceftizoxime, 1–2 g intravenously every 8–12 hours; or cefuroxime, 750–1500 mg intravenously every 8 hours; and dexamethasone, usually 4–10 mg as initial bolus, then 4 mg intravenously every 6 hours—and observation of the airway. Steroids may be tapered as signs and symptoms resolve. Similarly, substitution of oral antibiotics may be appropriate to complete a 10-day course. When epiglottitis is recognized early in the adult, it is usually possible to avoid intubation. Indications for intubation are (1) dyspnea or (2) rapid pace of sore throat (where progression to airway compromise may occur before the effects of steroids and antibiotics take hold). If the patient is not intubated, prudence would suggest monitoring oxyhemoglobin saturation with continuous pulse oximetry and—though not all agree—initial admission to an intensive care unit.

Deeb ZE: Acute supraglottitis in adults: Early indicators of airway obstruction. Am J Ophthalmol 1997;18:112. [NLM Cit ID: 97228691] (The most reliable indicator of impending airway obstruction is a rapidly developing severe sore throat.)

Donnelly TJ et al: Acute supraglottitis: when a sore throat becomes severe. Geriatrics 1997;52:65. [NLM Cit ID: 97221578]

Ducic Y et al: Description and evaluation of the vallecula sign: a new radiologic sign in the diagnosis of adult epiglottitis. Ann Emerg Med 1997;30:1. [NLM Cit ID: 97352959] (Radiologic exclusion of epiglottitis may have merit compared with direct inspection in adults, but in children strong clinical suspicion should trigger a protocol that includes intraoperative inspection and airway control.)

Garpenholt O et al: Epiglottitis in Sweden before and after introduction of vaccination against *Haemophilus influenzae* type b. Pediatr Infect Dis J 1999;18:490. [NLM Cit ID: 99318060] (Interestingly, there was a tendency toward fewer cases of epiglottitis in adults even though only children were vaccinated. The incidence in children was reduced 20-fold.)

Hebert PC et al: Adult epiglottitis in a Canadian setting. Laryngoscope 1998;108(1 Part 1):64. [NLM Cit ID: 98092366] (Only the presence of dyspnea [noted in 29% of patients] at the time of admission predicted the need for intubation.)

Park KW et al: Airway management for adult patients with acute epiglottitis: a 12-year experience at an academic medical center (1984–1995). Anesthesiology 1998;88:254. [NLM Cit ID: 98107568]

2. LARYNGEAL PAPILLOMAS

Papillomas are common lesions of the larynx and other sites where ciliated and squamous epithelia meet. Unlike the oral cavity, in the larynx they are likely to be symptomatic, with hoarseness that progresses to stridor over weeks to months. The disease is more common in children but occurs also in adults. Repeated laser excisions via microdirect laryngoscopy are often needed to control the disease. Tracheotomy should be avoided, if possible, since it introduces an iatrogenic additional squamociliary junction where papilloma appear to preferentially grow. A possible role for interferon has been under investigation.

3. ACUTE LARYNGITIS

Acute laryngitis is probably the most common cause of hoarseness, which may persist for a week or so after other symptoms of upper respiratory infection have cleared. The patient should be warned to avoid vigorous use of the voice (singing, shouting) while laryngitis is present, since this may foster the formation of vocal nodules. Although thought to be usually viral in origin, both *Moraxella catarrhalis* and *Haemophilus influenzae* may be isolated from the nasopharynx at higher than expected frequencies, and erythromycin may reduce the severity of hoarseness and cough.

Kumazawa H et al: An increase in laryngeal aerosol deposition by ultrasonic nebulizer therapy with intermittent vocalization. Laryngoscope 1997;107:671. [NLM Cit ID: 97293119] (Fast inhalation with intermittent vocalization helps improve the deposition rate of aerosol particles into the upper airway with an ultrasonic nebulizer.)

4. GASTROESOPHAGEAL REFLUX & HOARSENESS

Gastroesophageal reflux into the larynx (laryngopharyngeal reflux) should be considered a possible cause of chronic hoarseness if other causes of abnormal laryngeal airflow (such as tumor) have been excluded by indirect or direct laryngoscopy. Gastroesophageal reflux disease (GERD) has also been implicated as a contributing factor to other symptoms such as throat clearing, throat discomfort, chronic cough, a sensation of postnasal drip, and esophageal spasm; as well as in many cases of posterior laryngitis and some cases of asthma. As less than half of patients with documented laryngopharyngeal reflux have typical symptoms of heartburn and regurgitation, the lack of such symptoms should not be construed as eliminating this cause. Management should initially exclude more serious laryngeal disease. Twenty-four-hour pH monitoring of the pharynx as well as the esophagus is the diagnostic tool that best documents reflux. A clinical trial of appropriate antireflux measures for a sufficient duration of time has been advocated as an alternative by some. If a clinical trial is to be used, recall that the effect of omeprazole and other proton pump inhibitors is more immediate than cimetidine or ranitidine and that proton pump inhibitors appear to be 90% clinically effective whereas H_2 antagonists are effective in about 70% of cases. Higher doses of omeprazole than are customary in typical gastroesophageal reflux are often needed; 40 mg/d should be the initial dose.

Ahuja V et al: Head and neck manifestations of gastroesophageal reflux disease. Am Fam Phys 1999;60:873. [NLM Cit ID: 99426401] (Reviews head and neck manifestations of GERD.)

Al-Sabbagh G et al: Supraesophageal manifestations of gastroesophageal reflux disease. Semin Gastrointest Dis 1999;10:113. [NLM Cit ID: 99362051] (Multiprobe ambulatory pH monitoring is the diagnostic test of choice. Response to antireflux therapy is less predictable than typical GERD.)

Beck IT et al: The Second Canadian Consensus Conference on the Management of Patients with Gastroesophageal Reflux Disease. Can J Gastroenterol 1997;11(Suppl B):7B. [NLM Cit ID: 98006722] (Although proton pump inhibitors may decrease symptoms, improvement alone is not diagnostic of the presence of GERD as the cause of the symptoms. Ambulatory pH studies may be useful in establishing causation.)

Fouad YM et al: Ineffective esophageal motility: the most common motility abnormality in patients with GERD-associated respiratory symptoms. Am J Gastroenterol 1999;94:1464. [NLM Cit ID: 99290676]

Giacchi RJ et al: Compliance with anti-reflux therapy in patients with otolaryngologic manifestations of gastroesophageal reflux disease. Laryngoscope 2000;110:19. [NLM Cit ID: 20110629] (A review of otolaryngologic symptoms of GERD, sore throat, throat clearing, sensation of postnasal drip, hoarseness, and esophageal spasm; with suggestions on management.)

Klinkenberg-Knol EC: Otolaryngologic manifestations of gastro-oesophageal reflux disease. Scand J Gastroenterol Suppl 1998;225:24. [NLM Cit ID: 98175499] (Documents that only 25% of patients with laryngopharyngeal symptoms felt to be secondary to GERD have esophagitis endoscopically—hence pH monitoring with a dual pH probe is necessary for diagnosis.)

Mujica VR et al: Recognizing atypical manifestations of GERD. Asthma, chest pain, and otolaryngologic disorders may be due to reflux. Postgrad Med 1999;105:53. [NLM Cit ID: 99123568] (Extraesophageal symptoms such as asthma, noncardiac chest pain, and hoarseness may be misdiagnosed and therefore poorly managed.)

Ulualp SO et al: Pharyngeal pH monitoring in patients with posterior laryngitis. Otolaryngol Head Neck Surg 1999;120:672. [NLM Cit ID: 99246436]

Woo P et al: Association of esophageal reflux and globus symptom: Comparison of laryngoscopy and 24-hour pH manometry. Otolaryngol Head Neck Surg 1996;115:502. [NLM Cit ID: 97124584] (Videolaryngoscopy and dual probe pH manometry were done in patients presenting with globus sensation. Over half of patients had some findings on either or both.)

TUMORS OF THE LARYNX

1. BENIGN TUMORS OF THE LARYNX

Vocal cord nodules are smooth, paired lesions that form at the junction of the anterior one-third and posterior two-thirds of the vocal cords. They are a common cause of hoarseness resulting from vocal abuse.

In adults, they are referred to as "singer's nodules"; in children, "screamer's nodules." Treatment requires modification of voice habits, and referral to a speech therapist is indicated. Recalcitrant nodules may require surgical excision.

Polypoid changes in the vocal cords may result from vocal abuse, smoking, or chemical industrial irritants or may be seen in hypothyroidism. Attention to the underlying problem may resolve the polypoid changes. Inhaled steroid spray (eg, beclomethasone, 42 μg/spray, or dexamethasone, 84 μg/spray, two or three times a day) may hasten resolution. At times, removal of the hyperplastic vocal cord mucosa may be indicated.

A common but often unrecognized cause of hoarseness is contact ulcers on the vocal processes of the arytenoid cartilages secondary to esophageal reflux. Treatment may be with H_2-receptor blockers or proton pump inhibitors (see Gastroesophageal Reflux and Hoarseness, above). Intubation granulomas may also be seen posteriorly between the vocal processes.

2. LARYNGEAL LEUKOPLAKIA

Leukoplakia is a frequent cause of hoarseness, most commonly arising in smokers. Direct laryngoscopy with biopsy is advised. Histologic examination usually demonstrates mild, moderate, or severe dysplasia. Cessation of smoking may reverse dysplastic changes. A certain percentage of patients—estimated to be less than 5% of those with mild dysplasia and about 35–60% of those with severe dysplasia—will subsequently develop squamous cell carcinoma. In some cases, invasive squamous cell carcinoma is present in the initial biopsy.

3. SQUAMOUS CELL CARCINOMA OF THE LARYNX

Squamous cell carcinoma is the most common cancer seen in the larynx. It occurs predominantly in heavy smokers, with alcohol an apparent cocarcinogen. It is most common between ages 50 and 70. Hoarseness is the usual presenting symptom. Any patient with hoarseness that has persisted beyond 2–3 weeks should be evaluated by indirect laryngoscopy. Odynophagia, hemoptysis, weight loss, referred otalgia, vocal cord immobility, and cervical adenopathy suggest more advanced disease.

Early squamous cell carcinoma is best treated with radiation, with cure rates in excess of 85–95%. Conservation surgery or total laryngectomy is necessary for radiation failures and for more advanced disease. Today, the use of tracheoesophageal valves following total laryngectomy restores useful speech for most laryngectomy patients.

VOCAL CORD PARALYSIS

Most cases of vocal cord paralysis result from involvement of a recurrent laryngeal nerve; others arise more proximally along the vagus nerve itself. Common causes of recurrent laryngeal nerve involvement include thyroid surgery (and occasionally thyroid cancer) or other neck surgery (anterior discectomy and carotid endarterectomy), and mediastinal or apical involvement by lung cancer. Not rarely, no cause can be identified. Skull base tumors often involve cranial nerves IX, X, and XI. When either no cause is found or the paresis follows surgical trauma in which the nerve was not divided, spontaneous recovery commonly occurs, usually within a year.

Unlike unilateral cord paralysis, which produces a breathy hoarseness, bilateral cord paralysis usually causes inspiratory and expiratory stridor if acute, in which case intervention to create an emergency airway may be needed. If insidious in onset, it may be asymptomatic at rest, including a normal voice, though there is usually dyspnea on exertion. Causes of bilateral cord paralysis include thyroid surgery, esophageal cancer, and ventricular shunt malfunction. The goal of intervention is creation of a safe airway with minimal reduction in voice quality and airway protection from aspiration. A number of cord lateralization procedures have been advocated as a means of removing the tracheotomy tube.

Unilateral or bilateral cord immobility may also be seen in cricoarytenoid arthritis secondary to advanced rheumatoid arthritis, intubation injuries, glottic and subglottic stenosis, and, of course, laryngeal cancer.

Surgical management of persistent or irrecoverable symptomatic unilateral vocal cord paralysis has evolved over the last several decades. The primary goal is medialization of the paralyzed cord in order to rehabilitate the voice. Additional goals include eliminating aspiration, improving diet, and aiding in the subsequent decannulation of individuals with glottic insufficiency. Success has been reported for years with injection medialization using predominantly Teflon, but other materials as well have been used, such as fat or Gelfoam, in selected circumstances. Laryngeal framework surgery in recent years has also been shown to be effective and more versatile. Procedures include medialization laryngoplasty or type I thyroplasty and arytenoid adduction—or both.

Carrau RL et al: Laryngeal framework surgery for the management of aspiration. Head Neck 1999;21:139. [NLM Cit ID: 99190403] (In addition to rehabilitation of the voice, medialization laryngoplasty with silicone with or without arytenoid adduction is usually helpful for aspiration as well.)

Espinoza FI et al: Vocal fold paralysis following carotid endarterectomy. J Laryngol Otol 1999;113:439. [NLM Cit ID: 99434782] (Ten percent noted hoarseness postoperatively; in 4%, examination confirmed vocal cord paralysis.)

Harries ML et al: Management of unilateral vocal cord paralysis by injection medialization with Teflon paste. Quantitative results. Ann Otol Rhinol Laryngol 1998; 107:332. [NLM Cit ID: 98216847] (Intracordal injection using Teflon instead of silicon has been used successfully as well.)

Harries ML: Unilateral vocal fold paralysis: A review of the current methods of surgical rehabilitation. J Laryngol Otol 1996;110:111. [NLM Cit ID: 96306221] (Assesses injection medialization, laryngeal framework surgery, and reinnervation procedures.)

Kraus DH et al: Arytenoid adduction as an adjunct to type I thyroplasty for unilateral vocal cord paralysis. Head Neck 1999;21:52. [NLM Cit ID: 99105357] (The authors conclude that arytenoid adduction as part of type I thyroplasty is safe and effective.)

Kraus DH et al: Vocal cord medialization for unilateral paralysis associated with intrathoracic malignancies. J Thorac Cardiovasc Surg 1996;111:334. [NLM Cit ID: 96160820] (Overall success rate of intervention was 90% among 63 patients. Intervention is helpful both in the acute and chronic settings, even for patients not likely to be cured.)

Lo CY et al: A prospective evaluation of recurrent laryngeal nerve paralysis during thyroidectomy. Arch Surg 2000;135:204. [NLM Cit ID: 20132366] (Of 33 cases of unilateral cord paralysis, only five had recognizable nerve damage intraoperatively. Complete recovery occurred in 26 of the remaining 28.)

Morpeth JF et al: Vocal fold paralysis after anterior cervical diskectomy and fusion. Laryngoscope 2000;110:43. [NLM Cit ID: 20110634] (Twenty-one [5%] of 441 developed vocal cord paralysis; 15 of 18 reviewed at 1 year had recovered.)

Ramadan HH et al: Outcome and changing cause of unilateral vocal cord paralysis. Otolaryngol Head Neck Surg 1998;118:199. [NLM Cit ID: 98141657] (Lung and skull base tumors and their surgical treatment are the most common causes today.)

Shindo ML et al: Autologous fat injection for unilateral vocal fold paralysis. Ann Otol Rhinol Laryngol 1996;105:602. [NLM Cit ID: 96332224] (The authors conclude that autologous fat injection is a method of temporary vocal fold medialization in patients in whom return of vocal fold function is expected. Gelfoam is also useful in this situation.)

TRACHEOTOMY & CRICOTHYROTOMY

There are two primary indications for tracheotomy: airway obstruction at or above the level of the larynx and respiratory failure requiring prolonged mechanical ventilation. In an acute emergency, cricothyrotomy secures an airway more rapidly than tracheotomy, with fewer potential immediate complications such as pneumothorax and hemorrhage. Although classically it has been recommended that one should change a cricothyrotomy to a tracheotomy as soon as convenient and safe, recent studies have questioned this if decannulation can be expected soon. Percutaneous dilation tracheotomy as an elective bedside (or ICU) procedure has undergone scrutiny in recent years as an alternative to tracheotomy. Advocates suggest that it is less costly and perhaps more convenient, as the main operating suites need not be used. The nonunanimous consensus appears to be that it is an alternative with an acceptably low rate of complications when performed by a surgeon experienced with the procedure and when a standard tracheotomy can be done immediately in case of an emergency. Especially in intubated patients in an ICU (where the airway is already controlled), percutaneous tracheotomy should be safe; in nonintubated patients, bronchoscopy may reduce complications.

The most common indication for elective tracheotomy is the need for prolonged mechanical ventilation. There is no firm rule about how many days a patient must be intubated before conversion to tracheotomy should be advised. The incidence of serious complications such as subglottic stenosis increases with extended endotracheal intubation. As soon as it is apparent that the patient will require protracted ventilatory support, tracheotomy should replace the endotracheal tube. Less frequent indications for tracheotomy are life-threatening aspiration pneumonia, the need to improve pulmonary toilet to correct problems related to insufficient clearing of tracheobronchial secretions, and sleep apnea.

Posttracheotomy care requires humidified air to prevent secretions from crusting and occluding the inner cannula of the tracheotomy tube. The tracheotomy tube should be cleaned several times daily. The most frequent early complication of tracheotomy is dislodgment of the tracheotomy tube. Surgical creation of an inferiorly based tracheal flap sutured to the inferior neck skin may make reinsertion of a dislodged tube easier. It should be recalled that the act of swallowing requires elevation of the larynx, which is prevented by tracheotomy. Therefore, frequent tracheal and bronchial suctioning is often required to clear the aspirated saliva as well as the increased tracheobronchial secretions. Care of the skin around the stoma is important to prevent maceration and secondary infection.

Berrouschot J et al: Perioperative complications of percutaneous dilational tracheostomy. Laryngoscope 1997;107 (11 Part 1):1538. [NLM Cit ID: 98034337] (Percutaneous dilational tracheostomy has replaced conventional tracheostomy for long-term intubated patients in many intensive care units. Simultaneous endoscopy may be warranted to reduce the severity of complications.)

Escarment J et al: Percutaneous tracheostomy by forceps dilation: report of 162 cases. Anaesthesia 2000;55:125. [NLM Cit ID: 20117328] (Appears to be a safe and convenient bedside procedure when done by surgeons experienced with the procedure. However, complications do occur, and further studies should address late sequelae such as tracheal stenosis.)

Fortune JB et al: Efficacy of prehospital surgical cricothyrotomy in trauma patients. J Trauma 1997;42:832. [NLM Cit ID: 97334998] (The authors conclude that prehospital cricothyrotomy by emergency medical technicians can be performed effectively with few complications after training on animal models; however, good neurologic outcome is rare when this has been necessary in the trauma patient prior to arrival at the hospital.)

Gysin C et al: Percutaneous versus surgical tracheostomy: a double-blind randomized trial. Ann Surg 1999;230:708. [NLM Cit ID: 20023752] (Both techniques are associated with a low rate of serious or intermediate complications when performed by surgeons experienced with the procedure.)

Henrich DE et al: Tracheotomy and the intensive care unit patient. Laryngoscope 1997;107:844. [NLM Cit ID: 97360089] (No complications associated with transport to surgery and a total of five complications in all—three minor and two pneumothoraces related to pressure control ventilation. Surgical tracheotomy in the controlled setting of the operating room should serve as the standard by which other procedures—such as percutaneous dilational tracheostomy—are judged.)

Law RC et al: Long-term outcome after percutaneous dilational tracheostomy: Endoscopic and spirometry findings. Anaesthesia 1997;52:51. [NLM Cit ID: 97166856] (Looks at outcomes at least 6 months from the procedure. Ten percent had > 10% tracheal stenosis, but none were symptomatic.)

Massick DD et al: Quantification of the learning curve for percutaneous dilatational tracheotomy. Laryngoscope 2000;110(2 Part 1):222. [NLM Cit ID: 20143155] (Identifiable learning curve is most prominent in the first 20 patients treated. Anyone doing this procedure must be prepared to perform an immediate emergency standard open tracheotomy.)

Maziak DE et al: The timing of tracheotomy: a systematic review. Chest 1998;114:605. [NLM Cit ID: 98393352] (Insufficient evidence that the timing of tracheotomy for critically ill patients in the ICU influences the duration of mechanical ventilation or the extent of airway injury.)

Moe KS et al: Percutaneous tracheostomy: a comprehensive evaluation. Ann Otol Rhinol Laryngol 1999;108:384. [NLM Cit ID: 99229600] (A relatively safe and expedient method of tracheostomy for selected intubated patients in an intensive care unit; no advantage for patients who must be taken to the operating room.)

Rosenbower TJ et al: The long-term complications of percutaneous dilatational tracheostomy. Am Surg 1998; 64:82. [NLM Cit ID: 98118159]

FOREIGN BODIES IN THE UPPER AERODIGESTIVE TRACT

FOREIGN BODIES OF THE TRACHEA & BRONCHI

Aspiration of foreign bodies occurs less frequently in adults than in children. The elderly and denture wearers appear to be at greatest risk. Wider familiarity with the Heimlich maneuver has reduced deaths. If the maneuver is unsuccessful, cricothyrotomy may be necessary. Plain chest radiographs may reveal a radiopaque foreign body. Detection of radiolucent foreign bodies may be aided by inspiration-expiration films that demonstrate air trapping distal to the obstructed segment. Atelectasis and pneumonia may occur later.

Tracheal and bronchial foreign bodies should be removed under general anesthesia by a skilled endoscopist working with an experienced anesthesiologist.

Burton EM et al: Tracheobronchial foreign body aspiration in children. South Med J 1996;89:195. [NLM Cit ID: 96165405] (Among 155 patients, 16 of whom had tracheal foreign bodies and the rest more distal, 85 had a cough and 60 were wheezing; radiologically, segmental hyperlucency [n = 59] and atelectasis [n = 38] were most common. If the chest x-ray was normal, the trachea was the site of the foreign body half the time.)

Cataneo AJ et al: Foreign body in the tracheobronchial tree. Clin Pediatr 1997;36:701. [NLM Cit ID: 98077679] (Two-thirds present with choking; atelectasis was seen in about 40%.)

Debeljak A et al: Bronchoscopic removal of foreign bodies in adults: experience with 62 patients from 1974–1998. Eur Respir J 1999;14:792. [NLM Cit ID: 20037893] (Flexible or rigid bronchoscopy is effective.)

Helmers RA et al: Rigid bronchoscopy: The forgotten art. Clin Chest Med 1995;16:393. [NLM Cit ID: 96087453] (Describes current indications in adults and children.)

Hughes CA et al: Pediatric tracheobronchial foreign bodies: Historical review from the Johns Hopkins Hospital. Ann Otol Rhinol Laryngol 1996;105:555. [NLM Cit ID: 96292397] (A review of 234 cases from 1939 to 1991.)

Oguzkaya F et al: Tracheobronchial foreign body aspirations in childhood: a 10-year experience. Eur J Cardiothorac Surg 1998;14:388. [NLM Cit ID: 99059276]

ESOPHAGEAL FOREIGN BODIES

Foreign bodies in the esophagus create urgent but not life-threatening situations as long as the airway is not compromised. It is a useful diagnostic sign of complete obstruction if the patient is drooling or cannot handle secretions. There is probably time to consult an experienced clinician for management. Patients are likely to have difficulty handling secretions and may be spitting out their saliva. They may often point to the exact level of the obstruction. Indirect laryngoscopy often shows pooling of saliva at the esophageal inlet. Plain films may detect radiopaque foreign bodies such as chicken bones. Coins tend to align in the coronal plane in the esophagus and sagittally in the trachea. If a foreign body is suspected but not certainly known to be present, barium swallow may help make the diagnosis or establish that a foreign body is not (or is no longer) present.

Some have suggested that a Foley catheter may be used to remove an esophageal foreign body. This method risks displacing it into the larynx with resultant airway obstruction. It should be used cautiously, with the patient prone, and only by experienced physicians, and only for proximally located blunt objects. Endoscopic removal with conscious sedation or under general anesthesia is safest. Flexible esophagoscopy is usually successful; right laryngoscopy or esophagoscopy is almost always successful. Highly selected patients with a prior history of food impaction may be treated with a likelihood of success by spasmolytic drugs, such as intravenous glucagon.

Harned RK 2nd et al: Esophageal foreign bodies: Safety and efficacy of Foley catheter extraction of coins. AJR Am J Roentgenol 1997;168:443. [NLM Cit ID: 97168631] (The authors conclude that fluoroscopically guided Foley catheter extraction of retained coins in pediatric patients who lack evidence of significant esophageal edema causing tracheal compromise is a safe and efficacious technique.)

Webb WA: Management of foreign bodies of the upper gastrointestinal tract: Update. Gastrointest Endosc 1995;41:39. [NLM Cit ID: 95212879] (Experience presented in the successful treatment of 242 foreign bodies of mainly the esophagus and pharynx; the forward-viewing flexible panendoscope has become the instrument of choice in most community and tertiary centers.)

DISEASES PRESENTING AS NECK MASSES

The differential diagnosis of neck masses is heavily dependent on the location in the neck, the age of the patient, and the presence of associated disease processes. Rapid growth and tenderness suggest an inflammatory process, while firm, painless, and slowly enlarging masses are often neoplastic. In young adults, most neck masses are benign (branchial cleft cyst, thyroglossal duct cyst, reactive lymphadenitis), though malignancy should always be considered (lymphoma, metastatic thyroid carcinoma, others). Lymphadenopathy is common in HIV-positive individuals, but a growing mass or a dominant mass may be lymphoma or squamous cell carcinoma metastasis. In adults over 40, cancer is the most common cause of persistent neck mass. A metastasis from squamous cell carcinoma arising within the mouth, pharynx, larynx, or upper esophagus should be suspected, especially if there is a history of tobacco or significant alcohol use. Among patients younger than 30 or older than 70, more consideration of a lymphoma should be given. Most important is a comprehensive otolaryngologic examination. Cytologic evaluation of the neck mass via fine-needle aspiration biopsy is likely to be the next step if an obvious primary tumor is not visible or palpable on physical examination.

CONGENITAL LESIONS PRESENTING AS NECK MASSES IN ADULTS

1. BRANCHIAL CLEFT CYSTS

Branchial cleft cysts usually present as a soft cystic mass along the anterior border of the sternocleidomastoid muscle. These lesions are usually recognized in the second or third decades of life, often when they suddenly swell or become infected. To prevent recurrent infection and possible carcinoma, they should be completely excised, along with their fistulous tracts.

First branchial cleft cysts present high in the neck, sometimes just below the ear. A fistulous connection with the floor of the external auditory canal may be present. Second cleft cysts, which are far more common, may communicate with the tonsillar fossa. Third cleft cysts, which may communicate with the piriform sinus, are rare.

Triglia JM et al: First branchial cleft anomalies: A study of 39 cases and a review of the literature. Arch Otolaryngol Head Neck Surg 1998;124:291. [NLM Cit ID: 98184425] (Three types of presentation are seen: chronic purulent drainage from the ear [n = 12], periauricular periparotid swelling [n = 18], and abscess or persistent fistula in the neck superior to the axial plane of the hyoid [n = 21]. There were four cases of membranous attachment between the floor of the external auditory canal and the tympanic membrane. Complications were 11 fistulas, 20 sinuses, and 8 cysts.)

2. THYROGLOSSAL DUCT CYSTS

Thyroglossal duct cysts are remnants occurring along the embryologic course of the thyroid's descent from the tuberculum impar of the tongue base to its usual position in the low neck. Although they may occur at any age, they are commonest before age 20. They present as a midline neck mass, often just below the hyoid bone, that moves with swallowing. Surgical excision is recommended to prevent recurrent infection. This requires removal of the entire fistulous tract along with the middle portion of the hyoid bone.

al-Dousary S: Current management of thyroglossal-duct remnant. J Otolaryngol 1997;26:259. [NLM Cit ID: 97409535] (Sistrunk's procedure continues to be the mainstay of treatment.)

Ghaneim A et al: The management of thyroglossal duct cysts. Int J Clin Pract 1997;51:512. [NLM Cit ID: 98197670] (In the rare instances when histologic examination of a thyroglossal duct cyst reveals a papillary carcinoma, total or near-total thyroidectomy should be done.)

Heshmati HM et al: Thyroglossal duct carcinoma: Report of 12 cases. Mayo Clinic Proc 1997;72:315. [NLM Cit ID: 97249235] (The frequency of papillary carcinoma among thyroglossal duct cyst excisions was 0.7%.)

Roback SA et al: Thyroglossal duct cysts and branchial cleft anomalies. Semin Pediatr Surg 1994;3:142. [NLM Cit ID: 95079188] (Once these congenital cysts become infected, surgical removal is very difficult, and the recurrence rate increases.)

INFECTIOUS & INFLAMMATORY NECK MASSES

1. REACTIVE CERVICAL LYMPHADENOPATHY

The normal cervical lymphatic chain is not palpable. Infections involving the pharynx, salivary glands, and scalp often cause tender enlargement of neck nodes. Enlarged nodes are common in HIV-infected persons. Except for the occasional node that suppurates and requires incision and drainage, treatment is directed against the underlying infection. An enlarged lymph node that persists may warrant fine-needle aspiration biopsy in order to confirm that it is reactive and allay concern about malignancy. An enlarging node unassociated with infection must be further evaluated.

2. TUBERCULOUS & NONTUBERCULOUS MYCOBACTERIAL LYMPHADENITIS

Granulomatous neck masses are not uncommon. The differential diagnosis includes cat-scratch disease (probably more common than realized), sarcoidosis, and mycobacterial adenitis. Atypical mycobacterial adenitis (scrofula) usually presents as persistent adenopathy and can become fixed to the skin and drain externally. Although fine-needle aspiration may suggest a granulomatous origin, demonstration of mycobacteria by acid-fast staining (of material taken by fine-needle aspiration or open excisional biopsy) or culture is necessary to confirm this diagnosis and address antibiotic sensitivity. Treatment of scrofula is most successful with total excision of the involved nodes and appropriate antituberculous antibiotics for at least 6 months. The antibiotics used will depend on sensitivity studies but are likely to include isoniazid, rifampin, and, for at least the first 2 months, ethambutol in standard doses (see Table 9–14). When total excision might pose formidable surgical risks (eg, facial nerve proximity), a trial of needle aspiration or incision and drainage (along with antituberculosis medication) is worthwhile.

Mycobacterial lymphadenitis is on the rise both in immunocompromised and immunocompetent individuals. Diagnosis of *Mycobacterium tuberculosis* by FNA polymerase chain reaction (PCR) from fine-needle aspirates is successful about 75% of the time. Open biopsy for histology and culture should be done if clinical suspicion remains high despite a negative PCR. A 6-month regimen consisting of an initial 4 months of streptomycin, isoniazid, rifampin, and pyrazinamide followed by 2 months of isoniazid and rifampin is recommended as the initial treatment of tuberculous lymphadenopathy.

Baek CH et al: Polymerase chain reaction detection of *Mycobacterium tuberculosis* from fine-needle aspirate for the diagnosis of cervical tuberculous lymphadenitis. Laryngoscope 2000;110:30. [NLM Cit ID: 20110631] (PCR successfully identified *M tuberculosis* in 13 of 17 proved cases.)

Benson-Mitchell R et al: Cervical lymphadenopathy secondary to atypical mycobacteria in children. J Laryngol Otol 1996;110:48. [NLM Cit ID: 96286847] (A discussion of diagnosis and treatment in immunocompetent individuals. See also reference by Kim on PCR diagnosis.)

Ellison E et al: Fine needle aspiration diagnosis of mycobacterial lymphadenitis. Sensitivity and predictive value in the United States. Acta Cytol 1999;43:153. [NLM Cit ID: 99197775] (Interpreting nondiagnostic granulomatous inflammation should be done with caution.)

Ersoz C et al: Fine needle aspiration (FNA) cytology in tuberculous lymphadenitis. Cytopathology 1998;9:201. [NLM Cit ID: 98302238] (Polymerase chain reaction successfully identified *M tuberculosis* in 19 of 23 cases where cytologic diagnoses were consistent with but not diagnostic of tuberculosis. If there is a discrepancy with the clinical impression, open biopsy is recommended.)

Gupta SK et al: Cytodiagnosis of tuberculous lymphadenitis: A correlative study with microbiologic examination. Acta Cytol 1993;37:329. [NLM Cit ID: 93269571] (One hundred and two cases of cytodiagnosis were examined. Acid-fast bacilli were seen in 20–32% of smears and cultured in 40–57%. In 8% of cases, the smears were positive when the cultures were negative.)

Hayase Y et al: Cervical tuberculous lymphadenitis in a frequent traveler to endemic areas of tuberculosis. Intern Med 1997;36:211. [NLM Cit ID: 97289093] (A reminder that scrofula—cervical tuberculous lymphadenitis—should be suspected in patients with a history of potential exposure to tuberculosis who present with cervical lymphadenopathy.)

Kim SS et al: Application of PCR from the fine needle aspirates for the diagnosis of cervical tuberculous lymphadenitis. J Korean Med Sci 1996;11:127. [NLM Cit ID: 96432707] (PCR is the most sensitive technique [60%] in the demonstration of *M tuberculosis* in patients with clinically suspected tuberculosis who have acid-fast bacilli on stains or culture-negative cytology.)

King AD et al: MRI of tuberculous cervical lymphadenopathy. J Comput Assist Tomogr 1999;23:244. [NLM Cit ID: 99193996] (Reviews the spectrum of findings.)

Lee KC et al: Tuberculous infections of the head and neck. Ear Nose Throat J 1995;74:395. [NLM Cit ID: 95354538]

van Loenhout-Rooyackers JH et al: Shortening the duration of treatment for cervical tuberculous lymphadenitis. Eur Respir J 2000;15:192. [NLM Cit ID: 20142113] (Six months is probably sufficient.)

Williams RG et al: *Mycobacterium* marches back. J Laryngol Otol 1995;109:5. [NLM Cit ID: 95182002] (Reviews the features of increasingly prevalent primary and secondary tuberculosis in various head and neck sites.)

3. LYME DISEASE

Lyme disease, caused by the spirochete *Borrelia burgdorferi* and transmitted by an *Ixodes ricinus* tick, may have protean manifestation, but over 75% of patients have symptoms involving the head and neck. Facial paralysis, dysesthesias, dysgeusia, or other cranial neuropathies are most common. Headache, pain, and cervical lymphadenopathy may occur. See Chapter 34 for a more thorough discussion.

Balcer LJ et al: Neuro-ophthalmic manifestations of Lyme disease. J Neuroophthalmol 1997;17:108. [NLM Cit ID: 97319895] (Overdiagnosis is common. Incorrect diagnoses suspected to be Lyme disease are reviewed as well as actual neuro-ophthalmologic manifestations.)

Dotevall L et al: Successful oral doxycycline treatment of Lyme disease-associated facial palsy and meningitis. Clin Infect Dis 1999;28:569. [NLM Cit ID: 99208423] (Doxycycline is an effective and convenient therapy for Lyme disease-associated facial palsy.)

Halperin JJ: Neuroborreliosis: Central nervous system involvement. Semin Neurol 1997;17:19. [NLM Cit ID: 97309540] (Diagnosis relies on a combination of demonstrated specific immune response and clinical judgment.)

Heir GM: Differentiation of orofacial pain related to Lyme disease from other dental and facial pain disorders. Dent Clin North Am 1997;41:243. [NLM Cit ID: 97287390] (Lyme disease may mimic dental and temporomandibular disorders: this differentiation may be difficult.)

Kaplan RF et al: Lyme encephalopathy: A neuropsychological perspective. Semin Neurol 1997;17:31. [NLM Cit ID: 97309542] (Mild chronic encephalopathy may be seen in late stage Lyme disease. Symptoms tend to be diffuse and nonspecific, with memory loss, sleep disturbance, fatigue, and depression. Abnormal cerebrospinal fluid is felt to confirm a neurologic basis to the illness in patients with these symptoms.)

Keenan GF: Lyme disease: diagnosis and management. Compr Ther 1998;24:147. [NLM Cit ID: 98220003]

Logigian EL: Peripheral nervous system Lyme borreliosis. Semin Neurol 1997;17:25. [NLM Cit ID: 97309541] (Reviews the fairly distinctive acute cranial neuritis or radiculoneuritis, with or without erythema migrans and meningeal signs, as well as the less severe and less distinct chronic radiculoneuropathies.)

Lotric-Furlan S et al: Lyme borreliosis and peripheral facial palsy. Wien Klin Wochenschr 1999;111:970. [NLM Cit ID: 20131463]

Nadelman RB et al: Lyme borreliosis. Lancet 1998; 352:557. [NLM Cit ID: 98379932]

Rahn DW et al: Lyme disease update. Current approach to early, disseminated, and late disease. Postgrad Med 1998;103:51, 57, 63. [NLM Cit ID: 98253211]

Treatment of Lyme disease. Med Lett Drugs Ther 1997; 39:47. [NLM Cit ID: 97295037]

Treib J et al: Clinical and serologic follow-up in patients with neuroborreliosis. Neurology 1998;51:1489. [NLM Cit ID: 99034202] (Persisting in over half of patients were nonspecific complaints resembling a chronic fatigue syndrome as well as positive immunoglobulin M serum titers for borrelia in Western blot analysis.)

Verdon ME et al: Recognition and management of Lyme disease. Am Fam Physician 1997;56:427, 439. [NLM Cit ID: 97408004]

Zaidman GW: The ocular manifestations of Lyme disease. Int Ophthalmol Clin 1997;37:13. [NLM Cit ID: 97414952] (Lyme disease may present with unusual forms of conjunctivitis, keratitis, cranial nerve palsies, optic nerve disease, uveitis, vitreitis, and other forms of posterior segment inflammatory disease. One of these along with history of exposure to endemic areas, rash, arthritis, or a known tick bite should trigger treatment for Lyme disease.)

TUMOR METASTASES

In older adults, 80% of firm, persistent, and enlarging neck masses are metastatic in origin. The great majority of these arise from squamous cell carcinoma of the upper aerodigestive tract. A complete head and neck examination may reveal the tumor of origin, but examination under anesthesia with direct laryngoscopy, esophagoscopy, and bronchoscopy is usually required to fully evaluate the tumor and exclude second primaries.

It is often helpful to obtain a cytologic diagnosis if initial head and neck examination fails to reveal the primary tumor. An open biopsy should be done only if physical examination fails to detect the primary tumor and fine-needle aspiration biopsy has also failed to yield a diagnosis.

Other than thyroid carcinoma, non-squamous cell metastases to the neck are infrequent. While tumors not involving the head and neck seldom metastasize to the middle or upper neck, the supraclavicular region is quite often involved by lung and breast tumors. Infradiaphragmatic tumors, with the exception of renal carcinoma, rarely metastasize to the neck.

LYMPHOMA

About 10% of lymphomas present in the head and neck. Multiple rubbery nodes, especially in the young adult, are suggestive of this disease. A thorough physical examination may demonstrate other sites of nodal or organ involvement. Needle aspiration may be diagnostic, but open biopsy is often required. Lymphoma arising in AIDS patients is an increasing concern.

OTOLARYNGOLOGIC MANIFESTATIONS OF HIV INFECTION (See also Chapter 31.)

ORAL CAVITY & PHARYNX

The evaluation of oral lesions is critically important in HIV-infected individuals and in patients suspected of being so. Necrotizing ulcerative periodontitis, hairy leukoplakia, oral candidiasis, and Kaposi's sarcoma are frequently the presenting signs of HIV infection. The course of candidiasis and hairy leukoplakia in known HIV-infected patients may correlate with immune suppression and overall disease progression, suggesting the subsequent development of AIDS. For these reasons, oral lesions are useful in staging HIV progression and in designing entry criteria and end points for antiretroviral clinical trials. The United States Department of Health Services Clinical Practice Guideline for Evaluation and Management of Early HIV Infection recommends examination of the oral mucosa with each physician visit as well as dental examination at least every 6 months.

When CD4 cell counts drop below 200/μL, the incidence of intraoral lesions rises dramatically. In the past few years, the severity of these lesions has slackened, but their incidence or reporting has increased. Candidiasis is common and may require treatment for longer than the usual 1-week course with fluconazole (100 mg daily) or ketoconazole (200–400 mg daily) for control, with clotrimazole or topical nystatin less effective. Itraconazole (200 mg daily) is often helpful in fluconazole-refractory cases, but some cases of resistance may be secondary to non-albicans species, which are frequently azole-unresponsive. Giant intraoral ulcers have been seen in some patients. Hairy leukoplakia occurring on the lateral border of the tongue is often an early finding. It may develop quickly and appears as slightly raised leukoplakic areas with a corrugated or "hairy" surface. Histologically, parakeratosis and koilocytes are seen with little or no underlying inflammation. Among HIV-positive patients with oral lesions, hairy leukoplakia was seen in 19% in one study. Although clinical response following administration of zidovudine or acyclovir has been reported, the success of treatment or even the need for treatment is under active investigation. The greater significance of the appearance of hairy leukoplakia among seropositive patients is that it may correlate positively with subsequent more ominous manifestations of AIDS.

Kaposi's sarcoma is most common on the hard palate but may be seen anywhere in the oral cavity and pharynx. It usually appears as a raised violaceous lesion beneath an intact mucosa, although it may be ulcerated, erythematous, and bleeding. Radiation therapy may control the tumor. A brisk mucositis can be expected following radiation therapy.

In addition to Kaposi's sarcoma, an increased incidence of non-Hodgkin's lymphoma is seen in AIDS. An increase in squamous cell carcinoma is also seen in the homosexual population, perhaps related to HIV infection.

Cartledge JD et al: Non-albicans oral candidosis in HIV-positive patients. J Antimicrob Chemother 1999;43:419. [NLM Cit ID: 99238117] (Ten percent of candidal cultures also included non-albicans species, predominantly from patients with low CD4 lymphocyte counts. About 90% of non-albicans isolates were resistant to fluconazole in vitro, and 60% of such patients treated with azole therapy failed to clear these isolates clinically.)

Cruz GD et al: The accurate diagnosis of oral lesions in human immunodeficiency virus infection: Impact on medical staging. Arch Otolaryngol Head Neck Surg 1996;122:68. [NLM Cit ID: 96133394] (Specific training and a comprehensive oral examination have a significant impact on the diagnoses of oral candidiasis and oral hairy leukoplakia and on the medical staging of individuals with HIV infection.)

Diz Dios P et al: Frequency of oropharyngeal candidiasis in HIV-infected patients on protease inhibitor therapy. Oral Surg Oral Med Oral Pathol Oral Radiol Endod 1999;87:437. [NLM Cit ID: 99240155] (Protease inhibitor therapy decreases the frequency of HIV-related oropharyngeal candidiasis.)

Graybill et al: Randomized trial of itraconazole oral solution for oropharyngeal candidiasis in HIV/AIDS patients. Am J Med 1998;104:33. [NLM Cit ID: 98187566] (Few adverse reactions to either drug.)

Greenspan D et al: HIV-related oral disease. Lancet 1996;348:729. [NLM Cit ID: 96399919]

Greenspan D et al: Management of the oral mucosal lesions seen in association with HIV infection. Oral Dis 1997;3(Suppl 1):S229. [NLM Cit ID: 98117811] (Discusses treatment of common oral lesions, including Kaposi's sarcoma, oral candidiasis, hairy leukoplakia, and recurrent oral ulcers associated with HIV disease.)

Greenspan JS: Sentinels and signposts: The epidemiology and significance of the oral manifestations of HIV disease. Oral Dis 1997;3(Suppl 1):S13. [NLM Cit ID: 98117766] (Hairy leukoplakia and pseudomembranous candidiasis are the commonest lesions in those with HIV infection and AIDS, with higher prevalence and incidence rates correlating with falling CD4 counts and disease progression.)

Lamster IB et al: Epidemiology and diagnosis of HIV-associated periodontal diseases. Oral Dis 1997;3(Suppl 1):S141. [NLM Cit ID: 98117794] (The authors note that the focus today is on the accelerated rate of chronic adult periodontitis occurring in seropositive patients. They also review HIV-associated gingivitis or linear gingival erythema and HIV-associated periodontitis or necrotizing ulcerative gingivitis.)

Margiotta V et al: HIV infection: oral lesions, CD4+ cell count and viral load in an Italian study population. J Oral Pathol Med 1999;28:173. [NLM Cit ID: 99249450] (Confirms correlation with CD4 depletion and high level of viral load. Monitoring oral lesions is a useful tool for identifying progression of HIV infection and is of possible value in monitoring antiretroviral therapy.)

Patton LL et al: Oral infections and other manifestations of HIV disease. Infect Dis Clin North Am 1999;13:879. [NLM Cit ID: 20046076] (An excellent overview of the importance of oral lesions in HIV disease.)

Ramirez-Amador VA et al: Prognostic value of oral candidosis and hairy leukoplakia in 111 Mexican HIV-infected patients. J Oral Pathol Med 1996;25:206. [NLM Cit ID: 96432764] (The presence of oral candidiasis, hairy leukoplakia, or both is an indicator of AIDS and calls for initiation of pharmacotherapy.)

Revankar SG et al: A randomized trial of continuous or intermittent therapy with fluconazole for oropharyngeal candidiasis in HIV-infected patients: clinical outcomes and development of fluconazole resistance. Am J Med 1998;105:7. [NLM Cit ID: 98351300] (Resistance occurred with both continuous and intermittent therapy; however, therapeutic responses with higher doses were excellent.)

Robinson PG et al: Gingival ulceration in HIV infection. A case series and case control study. J Clin Pharmacol 1998;25:260. [NLM Cit ID: 98202198] (Discusses necrotizing ulcerative gingivitis seen in HIV patients and gingival ulceration, which is seen in younger people, those with oral candidiasis, and those without AIDS.)

Robinson PG: Which periodontal changes are associated with HIV infection? J Clin Pharmacol 1998;25:278. [NLM Cit ID: 98224949]

Saag MS et al: Treatment of fluconazole-refractory oropharyngeal candidiasis with itraconazole oral solution in HIV-positive patients. AIDS Res Human Retroviruses 1999;15:1413. [NLM Cit ID: 20021574] (Over half such patients responded within 28 days, usually within 7 days. Side effects were predominantly gastrointestinal disturbances.)

Schuman P et al: Oral lesions among women living with or at risk for HIV infection. HIV Epidemiology Research Study (HERS) Group. Am J Med 1998;104:559. [NLM Cit ID: 98337476] (The high prevalence of oral lesions among HIV seropositive [40%] and at-risk seronegative [23%] women underscores the need for routine oral examination and targeted treatment of this population.)

Shiboski CH et al: Human immunodeficiency virus-related oral manifestations and gender: A longitudinal analysis. The University of California, San Francisco Oral AIDS Center Epidemiology Collaborative Group. Arch Intern Med 1996;156:2249. [NLM Cit ID: 97040512] (The occurrence of hairy leukoplakia and candidiasis was higher in men [22% and 24%, respectively] than in women [9% and 13%, respectively].)

Smith D et al: A randomised, double-blind study of itraconazole versus placebo in the treatment and prevention of oral or oesophageal candidosis in patients with HIV infection. Int J Clin Pract 1999;53:349. [NLM Cit ID: 20159421] (Itraconazole 200 mg daily is effective and well tolerated.)

Tsang PC et al: Oral manifestations of HIV infection in a group of predominantly ethnic Chinese. J Oral Pathol Med 1999;28:122. [NLM Cit ID: 99167070]

Webster-Cyriaque J et al: Epstein-Barr virus and human herpesvirus 8 prevalence in human immunodeficiency virus-associated oral mucosal lesions. J Infect Dis 1997;175:1324. [NLM Cit ID: 97323974] (Absence of HHV-8 DNA in both the EBV-associated hairy leukoplakia lesions and in the EBV-associated AIDS-related lymphomas strengthens the etiologic relationship of EBV to these pathologies and the etiologic role of HHV-8 in Kaposi's sarcoma.)

(See also references in Candidiasis section of this chapter.)

THE NECK

Persistent generalized lymphadenopathy is extremely common in HIV infection. In this setting, a tender or growing node may represent secondary infection, lymphoma, or other tumor. Fine-needle aspiration for culture and cytology is the best initial diagnostic step. Open biopsy will often be needed if granulomatous disease or lymphoma is suspected, though fine-needle aspiration biopsy may be diagnostic of *M tuberculosis* infection in seropositive patients.

Parotid cysts and benign lymphoepithelial lesions in HIV-positive patients may be seen, often in association with cervical adenopathy.

Carbone A et al: Morphologic patterns and molecular pathways of AIDS-related head and neck and other systemic lymphomas. Ann Otol Rhinol Laryngol 1996;105:495. [NLM Cit ID: 96228238] (Head and neck manifestations of HIV infection include lymph nodal and extranodal localization of non-Hodgkin's lymphoma. This article highlights the difficulties in defining HIV-related non-Hodgkin's lymphoma correctly.)

Craven DE et al: Response of lymphoepithelial parotid cysts to antiretroviral treatment in HIV-infected adults. Ann Intern Med 1998;128:455. [NLM Cit ID: 98156410] (In six of nine patients, cysts resolved completely with combination antiretroviral therapy. Surgical resection should be reserved for patients in whom medical therapy has failed or those who refuse or are poorly compliant with medical therapy.)

Hung CC et al: Etiology of lymphadenopathy in patients with AIDS in Taiwan. J Formos Med Assoc 1996; 95:119. [NLM Cit ID: 97076716] (Tuberculous lymphadenitis was among the more commonly identified causes of extrainguinal lymphadenopathy.)

Moazzez AH et al: Head and neck manifestations of AIDS in adults. Am Fam Physician 1998;57:1813. [NLM Cit ID: 98236233] (Common manifestations and current treatment recommendations.)

Schrot RJ et al: Cystic parotid gland enlargement in HIV disease. The diffuse infiltrative lymphocytosis syndrome. JAMA 1997;278:166. [NLM Cit ID: 97357185]

an electrocardiogram. Arterial blood gases, measurement of lung volumes, ventilation/perfusion scanning, echocardiography, and cardiopulmonary exercise testing are reserved for cases that elude diagnosis on initial evaluation.

Treatment

In patients with advanced lung disease, the responsible condition may be easily identified but treatment only partially effective. Oxygen improves survival in those who are hypoxemic and can improve the exercise training of all patients. Its effect on dyspnea is variable. Anxiety can play an important role in the distress caused by dyspnea and may be relieved by judicious use of benzodiazepines such as lorazepam, 0.5–1 mg orally every 4–6 hours. Pulmonary rehabilitation can improve respiratory function and train patients in energy conservation and breathing techniques that help moderate their sense of respiratory effort. Opioids reduce respiratory drive and blunt dyspnea. They can usually be titrated safely even in patients with advanced lung disease. Finally, fresh air or a fan may offer additional relief. Patients with progressive exertional dyspnea should know that they can limit future loss of function through smoking cessation.

Booth S et al: Does oxygen help dyspnea in patients with cancer? Am J Respir Crit Care Med 1996;153:1515. [NLM Cit ID: 96210194] (Oxygen and compressed air were compared, with no advantage in the oxygen group even in those hypoxemic at baseline.)

Campbell ML: Managing terminal dyspnea: Caring for the patient who refuses intubation or ventilation. Dimensions Crit Care Nurs 1996;15:41. [NLM Cit ID: 96232094] (A hospice nurse reviews strategies for managing dyspnea in dying patients.)

COUGH

Cough is one of the most common symptoms for which patients seek medical care. It is an important physiologic mechanism that helps to defend against pathogens and to clear the tracheobronchial tree of mucus, foreign particles, and noxious aerosols. Impairment of oxygenation may result from a reduced or absent cough, as in some postoperative patients or those with neuromuscular disorders, or from excessive cough, which disrupts not only respiration but also sleep and social functioning. Bronchospasm, syncope, rib fractures, and urinary incontinence are all potential complications of severe cough. Referrals for chronic cough may constitute up to one-third of a pulmonologist's outpatient practice.

Cough may be voluntary or involuntary. Involuntary cough is stimulated by vagal afferent receptors in the trachea, especially at the carina and the larynx, but also from others throughout the head and neck. Stimulation of cough receptors may be mechanical, as in cases of aspiration, or irritative.

Clinical Findings

It is important to distinguish acute (< 3 weeks) from chronic cough. Acute cough most commonly follows viral or bacterial upper respiratory tract infection. Within 2 days after onset of the common cold, 85% of untreated patients cough; 26% are still coughing 14 days later, and in a few it will persist for 6–8 weeks. Many patients with persistent cough following upper respiratory tract infection have underlying asthma. Other causes of acute cough include aspiration, pneumonia, pulmonary embolism, and pulmonary edema.

The most common cause of chronic cough is a low-grade chronic bronchitis secondary to exposure to tobacco smoke, though smokers do not commonly seek medical attention for this problem. Over 90% of cases of chronic cough in nonsmokers presenting for evaluation of cough are due to postnasal drip, gastroesophageal reflux disease, and asthma. Angiotensin-converting enzyme (ACE) inhibitors have become another common cause. In primary care settings, single causes predominate.

The character and timing of chronic cough and the presence or absence of sputum production do not permit an etiologic diagnosis and should not be used as the sole basis for empirical therapy. The history and physical examination should attempt to identify anatomic locations of the afferent limb of the cough reflex in light of the common causes listed above. A nasal discharge, frequent need to clear the throat, and mucoid or mucopurulent secretions in the posterior pharynx suggest postnasal drip. Sinus radiographs may be diagnostic of acute or chronic sinusitis. Wheezing on chest auscultation or airway obstruction on pulmonary function tests suggest asthma. In cough-variant asthma, methacholine bronchoprovocation testing may be positive in the absence of clinical findings of asthma. Gastroesophageal reflux disease is an important cause of chronic cough but is associated with the fewest clinical clues. Patients may complain of heartburn or regurgitation, but cough may be the only symptom. Barium swallow is specific but insensitive, and esophageal pH monitoring may be necessary. Chest radiographs are best reserved for cough in smokers and patients with hemoptysis or constitutional symptoms such as fever and weight loss.

Treatment

The first step is to eliminate irritant exposures such as tobacco smoke (primary or secondary) and occupational agents and to discontinue medications such as ACE inhibitors or beta-blockers, including eyedrops. Cough due to ACE inhibitors should subside within 1–4 days after discontinuing the medication, though it may take weeks to months. Angiotensin II receptor antagonists do not cause cough. Patients whose cough began after an upper respiratory tract infection usually respond to treatment with an antihistamine-decongestant combination or treatment for asthma, with inhaled bronchodilators and corticosteroids. Postnasal drip syndrome due to allergic rhinitis that does not respond to antihistamines should be treated with intranasal steroids. Chronic sinusitis may require prolonged antibiotics directed against *Haemophilus influenzae.* Cough caused by asthma that does not respond after 2 weeks of bronchodilators and corticosteroids suggests that another condition is contributing. Gastroesophageal reflux disease is difficult to treat, since H_2 blockers may not be adequate. Most practitioners now initiate antitussive therapy for gastroesophageal reflux disease with proton pump inhibitors.

Carney IK et al: A systematic evaluation of mechanisms in chronic cough. Am J Respir Crit Care Med 1997; 156:211. [NLM Cit ID: 97374301] (Found less gastroesophageal reflux disease and more somatization.)

Irwin RS et al: Chronic cough. Am Rev Respir Dis 1990;141:640. [NLM Cit ID: 90178836] (A classic article from the investigators who have developed and refined the anatomic diagnostic protocol approach to chronic cough.)

Mello CJ et al: Predictive values of the character, timing, and complications of chronic cough in diagnosing its cause. Arch Intern Med 1996;156:997. [NLM Cit ID: 96212400] (Clinical characteristics of a chronic cough in a referral population do not predict its cause.)

Philp EB: Chronic cough. Am Fam Physician 1997;56: 1395. [NLM Cit ID: 97479101] (Clinical approach to chronic cough from the perspective of a primary care physician.)

HEMOPTYSIS

Hemoptysis is the expectoration of blood that originates below the vocal cords. It is commonly classified as trivial, mild, or massive, the last defined as more than 200–600 mL in 24 hours. The dividing lines are arbitrary and difficult to draw, since the amount of blood is rarely quantified with precision. Massive hemoptysis can be usefully defined as any amount that is hemodynamically significant or threatens ventilation, in which case the initial management goal is not diagnostic but therapeutic.

The lungs are supplied with a dual circulation. The pulmonary arteries arise from the right ventricle to supply the pulmonary parenchyma in a low-pressure circuit. The bronchial arteries arise from the aorta or intercostal arteries and carry blood under systemic pressure to the airways, blood vessels, hila, and visceral pleura. The bronchial arterial circulation represents only 1–2% of total pulmonary blood flow but is frequently the source of hemoptysis: It is a high-pressure circuit; it provides the blood supply to the airways and lesions within those airways; and it can increase dramatically under conditions of chronic inflammation—eg, chronic bronchiectasis.

The causes of hemoptysis can be classified anatomically. Blood may arise from the airways in chronic bronchitis, bronchiectasis, and bronchogenic carcinoma; from the pulmonary vasculature in left ventricular failure, mitral stenosis, pulmonary emboli, and arteriovenous malformations; or from the pulmonary parenchyma in pneumonia, inhalation of crack cocaine, or autoimmune diseases such as Goodpasture's disease or Wegener's granulomatosis. Iatrogenic hemorrhage may follow transbronchial lung biopsies, anticoagulation, or pulmonary artery rupture due to distal placement of a balloon-tipped catheter.

Clinical Findings

Blood-tinged sputum in the setting of acute bronchitis in an otherwise healthy nonsmoker does not warrant an extensive diagnostic evaluation if the hemoptysis subsides with resolution of the infection. However, hemoptysis is frequently a sign of serious disease, especially in patients with a high prior probability of an underlying pulmonary condition. The goal of the history is to identify patients at risk for one of the disorders listed above. Pertinent features are tobacco use, duration of symptoms, and the presence of respiratory infection. Nonpulmonary sources of hemorrhage—from the nose or the gastrointestinal tract—should also be ruled out.

Laboratory evaluation should include a chest radiograph and complete blood count, including platelet count. Renal function tests, urinalysis, and coagulation studies are appropriate in specific circumstances. Flexible bronchoscopy will reveal endobronchial cancer in approximately 3–6% of patients with hemoptysis who have a normal (nonlateralizing) chest radiograph. Nearly all of these patients will be smokers over the age of 40, and most will have had symptoms for more than a week. Bronchoscopy is indicated in such patients; observation and follow-up is appropriate in patients without risk factors for cancer. High-resolution CT of the chest is complementary to bronchoscopy. It can diagnose unsuspected bronchiectasis and arteriovenous malformations and will show central endobronchial lesions in many cases. It is the test of choice for suspected small peripheral malignancies.

Treatment

The management of mild hemoptysis consists of identifying and treating the specific cause. Massive hemoptysis is life-threatening. The airway must be protected, ventilation ensured, and effective circulation maintained. If the locations of the bleeding sites are known, the patient should be placed in the decubitus position with the involved lung dependent. Uncontrollable hemorrhage warrants rigid bronchoscopy and surgical consultation. In stable patients, flexible bronchoscopy may localize the site of bleeding, and angiography can embolize the source. Embolization is effective initially in 85% of cases, though rebleeding may occur in up to 20% of patients over the following year. The anterior spinal artery arises from the bronchial artery in up to 5% of people, and paraplegia may result if it is inadvertently cannulated.

Colice GL: Hemoptysis. Three questions that can direct management. Postgrad Med 1996;100:227. [NLM Cit ID: 96283182] (Identify the site of bleeding, identify high-risk patients, and distinguish bronchial from pulmonary sources within the lung.)

Hirshberg B et al: Hemoptysis: Etiology, evaluation and outcome in a tertiary referral hospital. Chest 1997; 112:440. [NLM Cit ID: 97410167] (Bronchiectasis, bronchitis, lung cancer, and infections caused 73% of cases; bronchoscopy and CT were complementary.)

APPROACH TO THE PATIENT

PHYSICAL EXAMINATION

Examination of the patient with suspected pulmonary disease includes inspection, palpation, percussion, and auscultation of the chest. An efficient approach begins with observing the pattern of breathing, auscultation of the chest, and inspection for extrapulmonary signs of pulmonary disease. More detailed examination follows from initial findings.

The pattern of breathing refers to the respiratory rate and rhythm, the tidal volume, and the relative amount of time spent in inspiration and expiration. Normal values are a rate of 12–14 breaths per minute, tidal volumes of 5 mL/kg, and a ratio of inspiratory to expiratory time of 2:3. **Tachypnea** is an increased rate of breathing and is commonly associated with a decrease in tidal volume. The rhythm is normally regular, with a sigh (1.5–2 times normal tidal volume) every 90 breaths or so to recruit surfactant to maintain patency of alveoli. Alterations in the rhythm of breathing include rapid, shallow breathing, seen in restrictive lung disease and as a precursor to respiratory failure; Kussmaul breathing, rapid large-volume breathing indicating intense stimulation of the respiratory center, seen in metabolic acidosis; and Cheyne-Stokes respirations, a rhythmic waxing and waning of both rate and tidal volumes that includes regular periods of apnea. This pattern is seen in patients with end-stage left ventricular failure or neurologic disease and in many normal subjects at high altitude, especially during sleep.

During normal quiet breathing, the primary muscle of respiration is the diaphragm. Movement of the chest wall is minimal. The use of accessory muscles of respiration, the intercostal and sternocleidomastoid muscles, indicates high work of breathing. At rest, this is a sign of significant pulmonary impairment. As the diaphragm contracts, it pushes the abdominal contents down. Hence, the chest and abdominal wall normally expand simultaneously. Expansion of the chest but collapse of the abdomen on inspiration indicates weakness of the diaphragm. The thorax is normally symmetric. Asymmetric expansion suggests unilateral volume loss, as in atelectasis or pleural effusion, unilateral airway obstruction, asymmetric pulmonary or pleural fibrosis, or splinting from chest pain.

The examiner may palpate as follows: at the suprasternal notch, to detect shifts in the mediastinum; on the posterior chest wall, to gauge fremitus and the transmission through the lungs of vibrations of spoken words and to assess the cardiac impulse. All are characterized by low interobserver agreement.

Chest percussion identifies dull areas that correspond to lung consolidation or pleural effusion or hyperresonant areas of emphysema or pneumothorax. Percussion has a low sensitivity (10–20% in several studies) compared with chest radiographs to detect abnormalities. Specificity is high (85–99%), however, so percussion remains useful. Since an insensitive test is a poor screening examination, percussion and palpation are not necessary in every patient. These techniques do serve as important confirmatory tests in specific patients when the prior probability of a finding is increased. For example, in a patient with a suspected tension pneumothorax, the finding of tracheal shift and hyperresonance can be lifesaving, permitting immediate decompression of the affected side.

Auscultation of the chest depends on a reliable and consistent classification of auditory findings. Normal lung sounds heard over the periphery of the lung are called vesicular. They have a gentle, rustling quality heard throughout inspiration that fades during expiration. Normal sounds heard over the suprasternal notch are called tracheal or bronchial lung sounds. They are louder, higher-pitched, and have a hollow quality that tends to be louder on expiration. Bronchial lung sounds heard over the periphery of the lung are abnormal and imply consolidation. Globally diminished lung sounds are an important finding predictive of significant airflow obstruction.

Abnormal lung sounds ("adventitious" breath sounds) may be continuous (> 80 ms in duration) or discontinuous (< 20 ms). Continuous lung sounds are divided into wheezes, which are high-pitched, musical, and have a distinct whistling quality; and rhonchi, which are lower-pitched, sonorous, and may have a gurgling quality. Wheezes occur in the setting of bronchospasm, mucosal edema, or excessive secretions. In each, the airway is narrowed to the point where adjacent airway walls flutter as airflow is limited. Rhonchi originate in the larger airways when excessive secretions and abnormal airway collapsibility cause repetitive rupture of fluid films. Rhonchi frequently clear after cough.

Discontinuous lung sounds are called **crackles**—brief, discrete, nonmusical sounds with a popping quality. Fine crackles are soft, high-pitched, and crisp (< 10 ms in duration). They are formed by the explosive opening of small airways previously held closed by surface forces and are heard in interstitial diseases or early pulmonary edema. Coarse crackles are louder, lower-pitched, and slightly longer in duration (< 20 ms) and probably result from gas bubbling through fluid. Coarse crackles are heard in pneumonia, obstructive lung disease, and late pulmonary edema.

Interobserver agreement regarding auditory findings is good. The clinical usefulness of these findings is also well established. The presence of wheezes on physical examination is a powerful predictor of obstructive lung disease. The absence of wheezes is not helpful since patients may have significant airflow limitation without wheezing. Such patients will have globally diminished lung sounds as the clinical clue to their obstructive lung disease. Normal lung sounds exclude obstruction. The timing and character of crackles can reliably distinguish different pulmonary disorders. Fine, late inspiratory crackles suggest pulmonary fibrosis, while early coarse crackles suggest pneumonia or heart failure.

Extrapulmonary signs of intrinsic pulmonary disease include digital clubbing, cyanosis, elevation of central venous pressures, and lower extremity edema.

Digital clubbing refers to structural changes at the base of the nails that include softening of the nail bed and loss of the normal 150-degree angle between the nail and the cuticle. The distal phalanx is convex and enlarged: its thickness is equal to or greater than the thickness of the distal interphalangeal joint. Symmetric clubbing may be a normal variant but more commonly is a sign of underlying disease. Clubbing is seen in chronic infections of the lungs and pleura (lung abscess, empyema, bronchiectasis, cystic fibrosis), malignancies of the lungs and pleura, chronic interstitial lung disease (idiopathic pulmonary fibrosis), and arteriovenous malformations. It does not normally accompany asthma or COPD; when seen in the latter, one should suspect concomitant lung cancer. It is observed less often in small-cell cancer than in other histologic types. Clubbing is not specific to pulmonary disorders; it is also seen in cyanotic congenital heart disease, infective endocarditis, cirrhosis, and inflammatory bowel disease. Hypertrophic pulmonary osteoarthropathy is a syndrome of digital clubbing, chronic proliferative periostitis of the long bones, and synovitis. It is seen in the same conditions as digital clubbing but is particularly common in bronchogenic carcinoma. The cause of clubbing and hypertrophic osteoarthropathy is not known with certainty, but the disorder may reflect platelet clumping and local release of platelet-derived growth factor at the nail bed. Both clubbing and osteoarthropathy may resolve with appropriate treatment of the underlying disease.

Cyanosis is a blue or bluish-gray discoloration of the skin and mucous membranes caused by increased amounts (> 5 g/dL) of unsaturated hemoglobin in capillary blood. Since the oxygen saturation at which cyanosis becomes clinically apparent is a function of hemoglobin concentration, anemia may prevent cyanosis from appearing while polycythemia may lead to cyanosis in the setting of mild hypoxia. Cyanosis is therefore not a reliable indicator of hypoxemia but should always prompt direct measurement of arterial Po_2 or oxyhemoglobin saturation.

Estimation of **central venous pressure** (CVP) and assessment of lower extremity edema are indirect measures of pulmonary hypertension, the major cardiovascular complication of chronic lung disease. Estimation of CVP can be done with precision. Elevated CVP is a pathologic finding associated with impaired ventricular function, pericardial effusion or restriction, valvular heart disease, and chronic obstructive or restrictive lung disease. Peripheral edema is a nonspecific finding that, in the setting of COPD, suggests right ventricular failure.

Bettencourt PE et al: Clinical utility of chest auscultation in common pulmonary diseases. Am J Respir Crit Care Med 1994;150:1291. [NLM Cit ID: 95040288] (Acoustic analysis of crackles in COPD, congestive heart failure, idiopathic pulmonary fibrosis, and pneumonia demonstrates that the examination can identify specific diagnoses.)

Cook DJ et al: Does this patient have abnormal central venous pressure? JAMA 1996;275:630. [NLM Cit ID: 96174503] (Part of a series on the rational clinical examination.)

Holleman DR et al: Does the clinical examination predict airflow limitation? JAMA 1995;273:313. [NLM Cit ID: 95115252] (Part of a series on the rational clinical examination. The authors apply an evidence-based standard to the physical examination of the chest.)

Maitre B et al: Physical examination of the adult patient with respiratory diseases: Inspection and palpation. Eur Respir J 1995;8:1584. [NLM Cit ID: 96120046] (A neglected part of the physical examination.)

Pasterkamp H et al: Respiratory sounds. Advances beyond the stethoscope. Am J Respir Crit Care Med 1997; 156:974. [NLM Cit ID: 97455801]

PULMONARY FUNCTION TESTS

Routine pulmonary function tests measure airflow rates, lung volumes, and the ability of the lung to transfer gas across the alveolar-capillary membrane. Indications for pulmonary function testing include the following: assessment of the type and extent of lung dysfunction; diagnosis of causes of dyspnea and cough; detection of early evidence of lung dysfunction; longitudinal surveillance in occupational settings; follow-up of response to therapy; preoperative assessment; and disability evaluation.

Relative contraindications to pulmonary function testing include acute severe asthma, respiratory distress, angina aggravated by testing, pneumothorax, ongoing hemoptysis, and active tuberculosis. Many test results are effort-dependent, and some patients may be too impaired to make a maximal effort. Suboptimal effort limits validity and is a common cause of misinterpretation of results. All pulmonary function tests are measured against predicted values derived from large studies of healthy subjects. In general, these predictions vary with age, gender, height and, to a lesser extent, weight.

Spirometry (Table 9–1) and measurement of lung volumes allow measurement of the presence and severity of obstructive and restrictive pulmonary dysfunction. Obstructive dysfunction is marked by a reduction in airflow rates judged by a fall in the ratio of FEV_1 (forced expiratory volume in the first second) to FVC (forced vital capacity). Causes include asthma, COPD (chronic bronchitis and emphysema), bronchiectasis, bronchiolitis, and upper airway obstruction. Restrictive dysfunction is marked by a reduction in lung volumes. Severity is graded by the reduction in total lung capacity. A reduced FVC suggests pulmonary restriction but is not diagnostic. Causes include decreased lung compliance from infiltrative disorders such as pulmonary fibrosis; reduced muscle strength from phrenic nerve injury, diaphragm dysfunction, or neuromuscular disease; pleural disease, including large pleural effusion or marked pleural thickening; and prior lung resection. The flow-volume loop combines the maximal expiratory and inspiratory flow-volume curves and is especially helpful in determining the site of airway obstruction. (See Figure 9–1.)

Spirometry is adequate for evaluation of most patients with suspected respiratory disease. If airflow obstruction is evident, spirometry is repeated 10–20 minutes after an inhaled bronchodilator is administered. This doubles the cost of the study. The absence of improvement in spirometry after inhaled bronchodilator in the pulmonary function laboratory does *not* preclude a successful clinical response to bronchodilator therapy. Measurements of lung volumes and diffusing capacity are useful in selected patients, but these tests are expensive and should not be ordered routinely with spirometry.

Measurement of the single-breath **diffusing capacity** for carbon monoxide (D_LCO), which reflects the ability of the lung to transfer gas across the alveolar/capillary interface, is particularly helpful in evaluation of patients with diffuse infiltrative lung disease or emphysema. The total pulmonary diffusing capacity (D_L) depends upon the diffusion properties of the alveolar-capillary membrane and the amount of hemoglobin occupying the pulmonary capillaries. The

Table 9–1. Definitions of selected pulmonary function tests.

Tests	Definition
Tests derived from spirometry	
Forced vital capacity (FVC)	The volume of gas that can be forcefully expelled from the lungs after maximal inspiration
Forced expiratory volume in 1 second (FEV_1)	The volume of gas expelled in the first second of the FVC maneuver
Forced expiratory flow from 25% to 75% of the forced vital capacity ($FEF_{25–75}$)	The maximal midexpiratory airflow rate
Peak expiratory flow rate (PEFR)	The maximal airflow rate achieved in the FVC maneuver
Maximum voluntary ventilation (MVV)	The maximum volume of gas that can be breathed in 1 minute (usually measured for 15 seconds and multiplied by 4)
Lung volumes	
Slow vital capacity (SVC)	The volume of gas that can be slowly exhaled after maximal inspiration
Total lung capacity (TLC)	The volume of gas in the lungs after a maximal inspiration
Functional residual capacity (FRC)	The volume of gas in the lungs at the end of a normal tidal expiration
Residual volume (RV)	The volume of gas remaining in the lungs after maximal expiration
Expiratory reserve volume (ERV)	The volume of gas representing the difference between functional residual capacity and residual volume

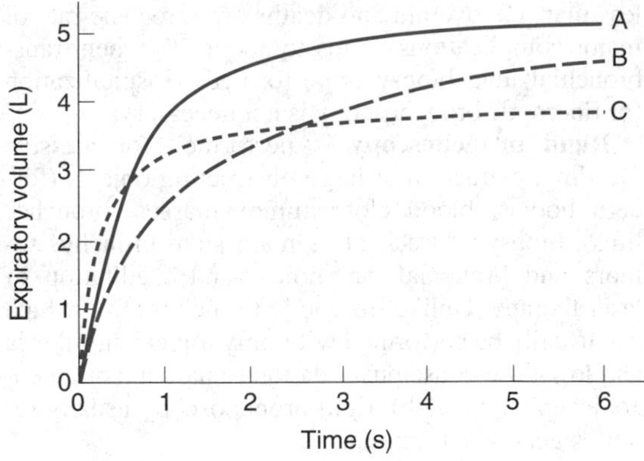

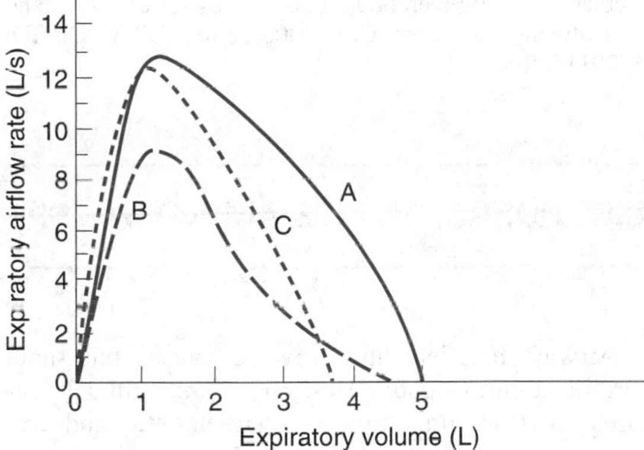

Figure 9–1. Representative spirograms (upper panel) and expiratory flow-volume curves (lower panel) for normal *(A)*, obstructive *(B)*, and restrictive *(C)* patterns.

diffusing capacity should therefore be corrected for the blood hemoglobin concentration.*

Elevated D_LCO is observed in pulmonary hemorrhage and may be seen in acute congestive heart failure and asthma due to an increase in pulmonary capillary blood volume. A diffusing capacity greater than 6 mL CO/mm Hg below the predicted value in women or 8.1 mL CO/mm Hg in men is considered abnormally low (Intermountain Thoracic Society guidelines). Reporting the ratio of measured diffusing capacity to alveolar volume (D_LCO/V_A) is helpful, because a diminished diffusing capacity may only reflect a reduction in lung volume. In patients with emphysema, the diffusing capacity is characteristically low, the alveolar volume normal or increased, and the D_LCO/V_A ratio is low. In patients with diffuse infiltrative lung disease, both the diffusing capacity and the alveolar volume are characteristically reduced, and the D_LCO/V_A ratio is normal or low.

*Corrected D_LCO = Measured $D_LCO \times \frac{[Hb] + 10.22}{1.7\,[Hb]}$ where [Hb] is the measured hemoglobin concentration (g/dL).

In patients with AIDS, D_LCO is a highly sensitive screening test for the presence of pulmonary disease, especially pneumocystis pneumonia, but it lacks specificity. A normal D_LCO in an AIDS patient is strong evidence against pneumocystis pneumonia. An abnormal result indicates the need for further diagnostic evaluation. Routine measurement of D_LCO and other pulmonary function tests in AIDS patients with pulmonary disease is not advised, because of expense and lack of specificity.

Arterial blood gas analysis is indicated whenever a clinically important acid-base disturbance, hypoxemia, or hypercapnia is suspected. **Oximetry** provides an inexpensive, noninvasive alternative means of monitoring oxyhemoglobin saturation with oxygen. Oximeters monitor oxygen saturation and not oxygen tension. Table 9–2 displays the normal relationship between oxyhemoglobin saturation and partial pressure of oxygen in blood. This relationship is not linear. The clinical accuracy of pulse oximeters is reduced in such conditions as severe anemia (< 5 g/dL hemoglobin), the presence of abnormal hemoglobin moictics (carboxyhemoglobin, methemoglobin, fetal hemoglobin), the presence of intravascular dyes, motion artifact, and lack of pulsatile arterial blood flow (hypotension, hypothermia, cardiac arrest, simultaneous use of a blood pressure cuff, and cardiopulmonary bypass). The normal arterial Po_2 falls with increasing altitude (Table 9–3).

Nonspecific bronchial provocation testing may aid the evaluation of suspected asthma, when baseline spirometry is normal, and in unexplained cough. The subject inhales a nebulized solution containing methacholine or histamine. These agents cause bronchial smooth muscle constriction in asthmatics at much lower doses than in nonasthmatics. If the FEV_1

Table 9–2. Relationship of oxyhemoglobin saturation and partial pressure of oxygen in blood.[1,2]

Saturation (%)	Partial Pressure (mm Hg)[3]
50	27
60	31
70	37
80	45
85	50
90	58
92	63
94	69
96	81
98	111
99	159

[1]Modified and reproduced, with permission, from Severinghaus JW: Values for a standard blood oxygen dissociation curve: Man. In: *Respiration and Circulation.* Altman PC, Dittmer DS (editors): Federation of American Societies for Experimental Biology, 1971.
[2]This relationship assumes a normal position of the oxyhemoglobin dissociation curve.
[3]Rounded to the nearest whole number.

Table 9–3. The effect of altitude on Po_2 in normals.

Altitude (feet)	Barometric Pressure (mm Hg)	Atmospheric[1] Po_2 (mm Hg)	Tracheal[2] Po_2 (mm Hg)	Arterial[3] Po_2 (mm Hg)
Sea level	760	159	149	99
2,000	707	148	138	88
4,000	656	137	127	77
6,000	609	127	118	68
8,000	564	118	108	58
10,000	523	109	100	50
15,000	426	90	80	30

[1]Dry gas.
[2]Saturated with water vapor.
[3]Actual values at altitude will be higher, depending on the degree of adaptation (ventilatory response to hypoxia).

falls by more than 20% at a dose of 16 mg/mL or less, the test is positive. Bronchial provocation testing is 95% sensitive for the diagnosis of asthma. A negative result therefore makes asthma unlikely. Specificity is lower—about 70%—since false positives may occur in several common conditions, including COPD, congestive heart failure, recent viral respiratory infection, cystic fibrosis, and sarcoidosis.

Crapo RO: Pulmonary-function testing. N Engl J Med 1994;331:25. [NLM Cit ID: 94261137]

James A et al: Testing airway responsiveness using inhaled methacholine or histamine. Respirology 1997;2:97. [NLM Cit ID: 98059573]

Cardiopulmonary Exercise Stress Testing

Cardiopulmonary exercise testing is usually performed to evaluate patients with unexplained exertional dyspnea. A bicycle ergometer or treadmill is used. Minute ventilation, expired oxygen and carbon dioxide tension, heart rate, blood pressure, and respiratory rate are monitored. The exercise protocol is determined by the indications for the test and the ability of the patient to exercise. Complications are rare.

Mottram CD: Exercise testing. Respir Care Clin N Am 1997;3:247. [NLM Cit ID: 98046499]

Bronchoscopy

Flexible fiberoptic bronchoscopy is an essential tool in the diagnosis and management of many pulmonary diseases. Bronchoscopy is indicated for evaluation of the airway, diagnosis and staging of bronchogenic carcinoma, evaluation of hemoptysis, biopsy of lung infiltrates, diagnosis of pulmonary infections, facilitation of bronchoalveolar lavage, and removal of retained secretions and foreign bodies from the airway. The procedure is contraindicated in severe bronchospasm and a bleeding diathesis. Complications include hemoptysis, fever, and a transient reduction in Po_2 (< 10 mm Hg). The rate of major complications is less than 1% overall, and deaths are rare. The rate of major complications jumps to about 7% when transbronchial lung biopsy is performed. Hospitalization for fiberoptic bronchoscopy is not necessary.

Rigid bronchoscopy is performed for massive bleeding, extraction of large obstructing objects (foreign bodies, blood clots, tumor masses, broncholiths), biopsy of tracheal or main stem bronchus tumors and bronchial carcinoids, and facilitation of laser therapy. Unlike fiberoptic bronchoscopy, which can usually be performed with only topical anesthesia and low-dose conscious sedation (a narcotic or a benzodiazepine, or both), rigid bronchoscopy usually requires general anesthesia.

Liebler JM et al: Fiberoptic bronchoscopy for diagnosis and treatment. Crit Care Clin 2000;16:83. [NLM Cit ID: 20116281]

DISORDERS OF THE AIRWAYS

Airway disorders have diverse causes but share certain common pathophysiologic and clinical features. Airflow limitation is characteristic and frequently causes dyspnea and cough. Other symptoms are often present and are typically disease-specific. Disorders of the airways can be classified as those which involve the upper airways—loosely defined as those above and including the vocal cords—and those which involve the lower airways.

DISORDERS OF THE UPPER AIRWAYS

Upper airway obstruction may occur acutely or present as a chronic condition. Acute upper airway obstruction can be immediately life-threatening and must be relieved promptly to avoid asphyxia. Causes of acute upper airway obstruction include foreign body aspiration, laryngospasm, laryngeal edema from airway burns or angioedema, trauma to the larynx or pharynx, various infections (Ludwig's angina, pharyngeal or retropharyngeal abscess, acute epiglottis), and acute allergic laryngitis.

Chronic obstruction of the upper airway may be caused by carcinoma of the pharynx or larynx, laryngeal or subglottic stenosis, laryngeal granulomas or webs, or bilateral vocal cord paralysis. Laryngeal or subglottic stenosis may become evident weeks or months following a period of translaryngeal endotracheal intubation. Inspiratory stridor, intercostal retractions on inspiration, a palpable inspiratory thrill over the larynx, and wheezing localized to the neck or trachea on auscultation are characteristic findings.

Flow-volume loops may show flow limitations characteristic of obstruction. Soft tissue radiographs of the neck may show supra- or infraglottic narrowing. CT and MRI scans can reveal exact sites of obstruction. Flexible endoscopy may be diagnostic, but caution is necessary to avoid exacerbating upper airway edema and precipitating critical airway narrowing.

Vocal cord dysfunction syndrome is a condition characterized by paradoxical vocal cord adduction, resulting in both acute and chronic upper airway obstruction. It can cause dyspnea and wheezing and may present as asthma and may be distinguished from asthma by the lack of response to bronchodilator therapy, normal spirometry immediately after an attack resolves, spirometric evidence of upper airway obstruction, a negative bronchial provocation test, or direct visualization of adduction of the vocal cords on both inspiration and expiration. Bronchodilators are of no therapeutic benefit. Treatment consists of speech therapy.

Morris MJ et al: Vocal cord dysfunction in patients with exertional dyspnea. Chest 1999;116:1676. [NLM Cit ID: 20062606] (Vocal cord abnormalities are a frequent occurrence in patients with symptoms of exertional dyspnea and should be strongly considered in their evaluation.)

Thomas PS et al: Pseudo-steroid resistant asthma. Thorax 1999;54:352. [NLM Cit ID: 99309111] (Diagnoses other than asthma, such as gastroesophageal reflux, hyperventilation, vocal cord dysfunction, and sleep apnea, should be considered as causes of "steroid-resistant" asthma.)

Wood RP et al: Vocal cord dysfunction. J Allergy Clin Immunology 1996;98:481. [NLM Cit ID: 96426229]

DISORDERS OF THE LOWER AIRWAYS

Tracheal obstruction may be intrathoracic (below the suprasternal notch) or extrathoracic. Fixed tracheal obstruction may be caused by acquired or congenital tracheal stenosis, primary or secondary tracheal neoplasms, extrinsic compression (tumors of the lung, thymus, or thyroid; lymphadenopathy; congenital vascular rings; aneurysms, etc), foreign body aspiration, tracheal granulomas and papillomas, and tracheal trauma.

Acquired **tracheal stenosis** is usually secondary to previous tracheostomy or endotracheal intubation. Dyspnea, cough, and inability to clear pulmonary secretions occur weeks to months after tracheal decannulation or extubation. Physical findings may be absent until tracheal diameter is reduced 50% or more, when wheezing, a palpable tracheal thrill, and harsh breath sounds may be detected. The diagnosis is usually confirmed by plain films or CT of the trachea. Complications include recurring pulmonary infection and life-threatening respiratory failure. Management is directed toward ensuring adequate ventilation and oxygenation and avoiding manipulative procedures that may increase edema of the tracheal mucosa. Surgical reconstruction, endotracheal stent placement, or laser photoresection may be required.

Bronchial obstruction may be caused by retained pulmonary secretions, aspiration, bronchogenic carcinoma, compression by extrinsic masses, and tumors metastatic to the airway. Clinical and radiographic findings vary depending on the location of the obstruction and the degree of airway narrowing. Symptoms include dyspnea, cough, wheezing, and, if infection is present, fever and chills. A history of recurrent pneumonia in the same lobe or segment or slow resolution (> 3 months) of pneumonia on successive radiographs suggests the possibility of bronchial obstruction and the need for bronchoscopy. Complete obstruction of a main stem bronchus may be obvious on physical examination (asymmetric chest expansion, mediastinal shift, absence of breath sounds on the affected side, and dullness to percussion), but partial obstruction is often difficult or impossible to detect. Prolonged expiration and localized wheezing may be the only clues. Segmental or subsegmental bronchial obstruction may produce no abnormalities on physical examination.

Roentgenographic findings range from **atelectasis** (lung collapse) to air trapping caused by unidirectional expiratory obstruction. CT scanning may demonstrate the nature and the exact location of obstruction of the central bronchi. MRI may be superior to CT for delineating the extent of the underlying disease in the hilum, but it is usually reserved for cases in which CT findings are equivocal. Bronchoscopy is the definitive diagnostic study, particularly if tumor or foreign body aspiration is suspected. The finding of tubular breath sounds on physical examination or an air bronchogram on chest radiograph in an area of atelectasis rules out complete airway obstruction. Bronchoscopy is unlikely to be of therapeutic benefit in this situation.

Right middle lobe syndrome is recurrent or persistent atelectasis of the right middle lobe. This collapse is related to the relatively long length and narrow diameter of the right middle lobe bronchus and the oval ("fish mouth") opening to the lobe, in the setting of impaired collateral ventilation. Fiberoptic bronchoscopy or CT scan is often necessary to rule out obstructing tumor. Foreign body or other benign causes are common.

Kwon KY et al: Middle lobe syndrome: A clinicopathological study of 21 patients. Hum Pathol 1995;26:302. [NLM Cit ID: 95197131] (Detailed description of clinical characteristics and pathologic findings in patients who had surgical resections.)

ASTHMA

Essentials of Diagnosis

- Episodic or chronic symptoms of airflow obstruction: breathlessness, cough, wheezing, and chest tightness.

- Symptoms frequently worse at night or in the early morning.
- Prolonged expiration and diffuse wheezes on physical examination.
- Limitation of airflow on pulmonary function testing or positive bronchial provocation challenge.
- Complete or partial reversibility of airflow obstruction, either spontaneously or following bronchodilator therapy.

General Considerations

Asthma is a common disease, affecting approximately 5% of the population. Men and women appear to be equally affected. Each year, approximately 470,000 hospital admissions and 5000 deaths in the USA are attributed to asthma. Hospitalization rates have been highest among blacks and children, and death rates for asthma are consistently highest among blacks aged 15–24 years.

Definition & Pathogenesis

Asthma is defined as a chronic inflammatory disorder of the airways. The histopathologic features include denudation of airway epithelium, collagen deposition beneath the basement membrane, airway edema, mast cell activation, and inflammatory cell infiltration with neutrophils, eosinophils, and lymphocytes (especially T lymphocytes). Hypertrophy of bronchial smooth muscle and hypertrophy of mucous glands with plugging of small airways with thick mucus can occur. This airway inflammation contributes to airway hyperresponsiveness, airflow limitation, respiratory symptoms (including recurrent episodes of wheezing, breathlessness, chest tightness, and cough, particularly during the night and the early morning), and disease chronicity.

A genetic predisposition to asthma is recognized. The strongest identifiable predisposing factor for the development of asthma is atopy. Exposure of sensitive patients to inhaled allergens increases airway inflammation, airway hyperresponsiveness, and symptoms. Patients may develop symptoms immediately (immediate asthmatic response) or 4–6 hours after their exposures (late asthmatic response). Common aeroallergens include house dust mites (often found in pillows, mattresses, upholstered furniture, carpets, and drapes), cockroaches, cats, and seasonal pollens. Substantially reducing exposure reduces these outcomes.

Nonspecific precipitants of asthma include exercise, upper respiratory tract infections, rhinitis, sinusitis, postnasal drip, aspiration, gastroesophageal reflux, changes in the weather, and stress. Exposure to environmental tobacco smoke also increases asthma symptoms and the need for medications and reduces lung function. Increased air levels of respirable particles, ozone, SO_2, and NO_2 precipitate asthma symptoms and increase emergency department visits and hospitalizations. Selected individuals may experience asthma symptoms after exposure to aspirin, nonsteroidal anti-inflammatory drugs, or tartrazine dyes. Certain other medications may also precipitate asthma symptoms (Table 9–28). Occupational asthma may be triggered by various agents in the workplace and occurs weeks to years after initial exposure and sensitization. Women may experience catamenial asthma at predictable times during the menstrual cycle. Exercise-induced bronchoconstriction usually begins within 3 minutes after the end of exercise, peaks within 10–15 minutes and then resolves by 60 minutes. This phenomenon is thought to be a consequence of the airways' attempt to warm and humidify an increased volume of expired air during exercise. "Cardiac asthma" is bronchospasm precipitated by uncompensated congestive heart failure.

Clinical Findings

Symptoms and signs vary widely from patient to patient as well as individually over time. General clinical findings in stable asthma patients are listed below; findings seen during asthma exacerbations are listed in Table 9–5.

A. Symptoms and Signs: Asthma is characterized by episodic wheezing, difficulty in breathing, chest tightness, and cough. The frequency of asthma symptoms is highly variable. Some patients may have only a chronic dry cough and others a productive cough. Some patients have infrequent, brief attacks of asthma and others may suffer nearly continuous symptoms. Asthma symptoms may occur spontaneously or may be precipitated or exacerbated by many different triggers as discussed above. Asthma symptoms are frequently worse at night; circadian variations in bronchomotor tone and bronchial reactivity reach their nadir between 3 and 4 AM, increasing symptoms of bronchoconstriction.

Some physical findings increase the probability of asthma. Nasal mucosal swelling, increased nasal secretions, and nasal polyps are often seen in patients with allergic asthma. Eczema, atopic dermatitis, or other manifestations of allergic skin disorders may also be present. Hunched shoulders and use of accessory muscles of respiration suggest an increased work of breathing. Wheezing during normal breathing or a prolonged forced expiratory phase correlates well with the presence of airflow obstruction. Wheezing during forced expiration does not. Chest examination may be normal between exacerbations in patients with mild asthma. During severe asthma exacerbations, airflow may be too limited to produce wheezing, and the only diagnostic clue on auscultation may be globally reduced breath sounds with prolonged expiration.

B. Pulmonary Function Testing: Clinicians are able to identify an obstructive ventilatory defect on examination, but they have limited ability to assess the degree of airflow obstruction or to predict whether obstruction is reversible. The evaluation for asthma should therefore include spirometry (FEV_1, FVC, FEV_1/FVC) before and after the administration of a short-acting bronchodilator. These measurements help determine whether there is airflow obstruction and whether it is immediately reversible. Airflow obstruction is indicated by a reduced FEV_1/FVC ratio (< 75%). In severe airflow obstruction with significant air trapping, the FVC may also be reduced, resulting in a pattern that suggests a restrictive ventilatory defect. Significant reversibility of airflow obstruction is defined by an increase of ≥ 12% and 200 mL in FEV_1 or ≥ 15% and 200 mL in FVC after inhaling a short-acting bronchodilator. However, the absence of improvement in airflow after administration of a bronchodilator is not proof of irreversible airflow obstruction.

Peak expiratory flow (PEF) meters are handheld devices designed as monitoring tools to be used at home. Their utility is limited by wide variability in PEF reference values and the lack of normative brand-specific reference values. However, PEF monitoring can establish peak flow variability and assist in the determination of asthma severity in patients with asthma symptoms and normal spirometry. PEF is generally lowest on first awakening and highest several hours before the midpoint of the waking day (diurnal variation). Ideally, PEF should be measured in the morning before the administration of a bronchodilator and in the afternoon after taking a bronchodilator; 20% variability in PEF values from morning to afternoon or over time suggests asthma. Predicted values for PEF vary with gender, age, and height. PEF values less than 200 L/min indicate severe airflow obstruction.

Bronchial provocation testing with histamine or methacholine—or exercise challenge testing—may be useful when asthma is suspected and spirometry is nondiagnostic. Bronchial provocation is not generally recommended if the FEV_1 is less than 65% of predicted. A positive test is defined as a decrease in FEV_1 of at least 20% at a dose of 16 mg/mL or less. A negative test has a negative predictive value for asthma of 95%.

Arterial blood gas measurements may be normal during a mild asthma exacerbation, but respiratory alkalosis and an increase in the alveolar-arterial oxygen difference (A-a DO_2) are common. During severe exacerbations, hypoxemia develops and the $PaCO_2$ returns to normal. The combination of an increased $PaCO_2$ and respiratory acidosis is a harbinger of respiratory failure and may indicate the need for mechanical ventilation.

C. Additional Testing: Routine chest radiographs in patients with asthma usually show only hyperinflation. Other findings include bronchial wall thickening and diminished peripheral lung vascular shadows. Chest radiographs are not necessary unless pneumonia, another disorder mimicking asthma, or a complication of asthma such as pneumothorax is suspected. The diagnostic usefulness of measurements of biologic markers of inflammation such as cell counts and mediator titers in blood and sputum is being investigated. Skin testing or in vitro testing to assess sensitivity to relevant environmental allergens may be useful in patients with persistent asthma. Evaluations for paranasal sinus disease or gastroesophageal reflux should be considered in patients with pertinent symptoms and in those who have severe refractory asthma.

Complications

Complications of asthma include exhaustion, dehydration, airway infection, cor pulmonale, and tussive syncope. Pneumothorax occurs but is rare. Acute hypercapnic and hypoxic respiratory failure occurs in severe disease.

Differential Diagnosis

Disorders that mimic asthma typically fall into one of three categories: upper and lower airway disorders, systemic vasculitides, and psychiatric disorders. It is prudent to consider these conditions in patients who have atypical asthma symptoms or response to therapy. Upper airway disorders that mimic asthma include vocal cord paralysis, vocal cord dysfunction syndrome, foreign body aspiration, laryngotracheal masses, tracheal narrowing, tracheomalacia, and airway edema as in the setting of angioedema or inhalation injury. Lower airway disorders include nonasthmatic chronic obstructive pulmonary disease (chronic bronchitis or emphysema), bronchiectasis, allergic bronchopulmonary mycosis, cystic fibrosis, eosinophilic pneumonia, and bronchiolitis obliterans. Systemic vasculitides that often have an asthmatic component include Churg-Strauss syndrome and other systemic vasculitides with pulmonary involvement. Psychiatric causes include conversion disorders, which have been variably referred to as functional asthma, emotional laryngeal wheezing, vocal cord dysfunction, or episodic laryngeal dyskinesis. Munchausen syndrome or malingering may rarely explain the patient's complaints.

Classification of Asthma Severity

The Expert Panel of the National Asthma Education and Prevention Program of the National Heart, Lung and Blood Institute has developed asthma classification schemes which are useful in directing asthma therapy and identifying patients at high risk of developing life-threatening asthma attacks. Table 9–4 is used to classify the severity of chronic, stable asthma, Table 9–5 to classify severity of asthma exacerbations. A patient's clinical features before treatment are used to classify the patient. The presence of only one of the severity features is sufficient to place a patient in that category; patients should be assigned to the most severe grade in which any feature occurs.

Table 9–4. Classification of asthma severity.[1]

	Symptoms	Nighttime Symptoms	Lung Function
Mild intermittent	Symptoms ≤ 2 times a week Asymptomatic and normal PEF between exacerbations Exacerbations brief (few hours to few days); intensity may vary	≤ 2 times a month	FEV_1 or PEF ≥ 80% predicted PEF variability ≤ 20%
Mild persistent	Symptoms > 2 times a week but < 1 time a day Exacerbations may affect activity	> 2 times a month	FEV_1 or PEF > 80% predicted PEF variability 20–30%
Moderate persistent	Daily symptoms Daily use of inhaled short-acting β_2-agonist Exacerbations affect activity Exacerbations ≥ 2 times a week; may last days	> 1 time a week	FEV_1 or PEF > 60% to < 80% predicted PEF variability > 30%
Severe persistent	Continual symptoms Limited physical activity Frequent exacerbations	Frequent	FEV_1 or PEF ≤ 60% predicted PEF variability > 30%

[1]Adapted from National Asthma Education and Prevention Program. Expert Panel Report 2: Guidelines for the Diagnosis and Management of Asthma. National Institutes of Health Pub No. 97-4051. Bethesda, MD, 1997.

Table 9–5. Classification of severity of asthma exacerbations[1]

	Mild	Moderate	Severe	Impending Respiratory Failure
Symptoms				
Breathlessness	With activity	With talking	At rest	At rest
Speech	Sentences	Phrases	Words	Mute
Signs				
Body position	Able to recline	Prefers sitting	Unable to recline	Unable to recline
Respiratory rate	Increased	Increased	Often > 30/min	> 30/min
Use of accessory respiratory muscles	Usually not	Commonly	Usually	Paradoxical thoracoabdominal movement
Breath sounds	Moderate wheezing at mid- to end-expiration	Loud wheezes throughout expiration	Loud inspiratory and expiratory wheezes	Little air movement without wheezes
Heart rate (beats/min)	< 100	100–120	> 120	Relative bradycardia
Pulsus paradoxus (mm Hg)	< 10	10–25	Often > 25	Often absent
Mental status	May be agitated	Usually agitated	Usually agitated	Confused or drowsy
Functional assessment				
PEF (% predicted or personal best)	> 80	50–80	< 50 or response to therapy lasts < 2 hours	< 50
SaO_2 (%, room air)	> 95	91–95	< 91	< 91
PaO_2 (mm Hg, room air)	Normal	> 60	< 60	< 60
$PaCO_2$ (mm Hg)	< 42	< 42	≥ 42	≥ 42

[1]Adapted from National Asthma Education and Prevention Program. Expert Panel Report 2: Guidelines for the Diagnosis and Management of Asthma. National Institutes of Health Pub No. 97-4051. Bethesda, MD, 1997.

Approach to Long-Term Treatment

The goals of asthma therapy are to minimize chronic symptoms that impair normal activity (including exercise), to prevent recurrent exacerbations, to minimize the need for emergency department visits or hospitalizations, and to maintain near-normal pulmonary function. These goals should be met while providing optimal pharmacotherapy with the fewest adverse effects and while meeting patients' and families' expectations of satisfaction with asthma care.

Current approaches to persistent asthma focus on daily anti-inflammatory therapy. Treatment algorithms are based on both the severity of a patient's baseline asthma and the severity of asthma exacerbations. Expert Panel Report 2 from the National Asthma Education and Prevention Program of the National Heart, Lung and Blood Institute recommends a stepwise approach to therapy (Table 9–6). The amount of medication and frequency of dosing are dictated by asthma severity and directed toward suppression of increasing airway inflammation. To establish prompt control, therapy should be initiated early at a higher level than anticipated for chronic therapy. Pharmacotherapy can then be cautiously stepped down once asthma control is achieved and sustained; this allows for identification of the minimum medication necessary to maintain long-term control.

Pharmacologic Agents for Asthma

Asthma medications can be divided into long-term control and quick-relief medications. Long-term control medications are taken daily to achieve and maintain control of persistent asthma. These agents—also known as maintenance, controller, or preventive medications—act primarily to attenuate airway inflammation. Quick-relief medications are taken to promote prompt reversal of acute airflow obstruction and relief of accompanying symptoms by direct relaxation of bronchial smooth muscle.

Many asthma medications can be administered orally or by inhalation. Inhalation of an appropriate agent offers the advantage of delivery of high concentrations of medication directly to the target organ. This results in a more rapid onset of pulmonary effects as well as less systemic effects compared with oral administration of the same dose. Metered-dose inhalers (MDIs) propelled by chlorofluorocarbons (CFCs) have been the most widely used delivery system, but non-CFC propellent systems and dry powder inhalers are becoming more widely available. These alternatives are effective and well tolerated. Proper MDI technique and the use of an inhalation chamber improve drug delivery to the lung and decrease oropharyngeal deposition. Nebulizer therapy is reserved for patients who cannot use MDIs because of difficulties with coordination or cooperation.

A. Long-Term Control Medications: Anti-inflammatory agents, long-acting bronchodilators, and leukotriene modifiers comprise the important medications in this group of agents (see Table 9–7). Other classes of agents are mentioned briefly below.

1. Corticosteroids–Corticosteroids are the most potent and consistently effective anti-inflammatory agents currently available. Their broad effects reduce both acute and chronic inflammation, resulting in fewer asthma symptoms, improvement in airflow, decreases in airway hyperresponsiveness, prevention of asthma exacerbations, and less airway remodeling. These agents may also potentiate the action of beta-adrenergic agonists.

Inhaled corticosteroids are preferred for the long-term control of asthma and are first-line agents for patients with persistent asthma. Patients with persistent symptoms and those with asthma exacerbations who are not taking inhaled corticosteroids should be started on an inhaled corticosteroid; patients already taking an inhaled corticosteroid should have the dose increased. Dosages for inhaled corticosteroids vary depending on the specific agent and delivery device. Because of limited data directly comparing the currently available inhaled corticosteroids and individual patient variability, the most important determinants of agent selection and appropriate dosing are the patient's status and response to treatment. For many patients, twice-daily dosing provides adequate control of asthma. Once-daily dosing may be sufficient in selected patients with mild persistent asthma. Maximum responses from inhaled corticosteroids may not be observed for months. The use of an inhalation chamber coupled with mouth washing after inhalation decreases local side effects (cough, dysphonia, oropharyngeal candidiasis) and systemic absorption. Systemic effects (adrenal suppression, osteoporosis, skin thinning, easy bruising, and cataracts) may occur with high-dose therapy, but the clinical significance of these effects has not been established.

Systemic corticosteroids are most effective in achieving prompt control of asthma during exacerbations or when initiating long-term asthma therapy. In patients with severe persistent asthma, systemic corticosteroids are often required for the long-term suppression of symptoms. Repeated efforts should be made to eliminate daily oral corticosteroids or to reduce the dose to the minimum needed to control symptoms. Alternate-day treatment is preferred to daily treatment. Rapid discontinuation of systemic corticosteroids after chronic use may precipitate adrenal insufficiency. Concurrent treatment with calcium supplements and vitamin D should be initiated to prevent steroid-induced bone mineral loss in long-term administration. Bisphosphonates may offer additional protection to these patients.

2. Long-acting bronchodilators–

a. Mediator inhibitors–Cromolyn sodium and nedocromil are long-term control medications that can be used to prevent asthma symptoms and improve airway function in patients with mild persistent

Table 9–6. Stepwise approach for managing asthma[1,2]

	Long-Term Control	Quick Relief	Education
Step 4: Severe persistent	Daily medication: Anti-inflammatory: inhaled corticosteroid (high dose) and Long-acting bronchodilator (long-acting inhaled β_2-agonist, sustained-release theophylline or long-acting β_2-agonist tablets) and Corticosteroid tablets or syrup (2 mg/kg/d, generally not to exceed 60 mg/d)	Short-acting bronchodilator: inhaled β_2-agonists as needed for symptoms. Intensity of treatment will depend on severity of exacerbation. Use of short-acting inhaled β_2-agonists on a daily basis, or increasing use, indicates the need for additional long-term control therapy.	Step 2 and 3 actions plus: Refer to individual education, counseling
Step 3: Moderate persistent	Daily medication: Either Anti-inflammatory: inhaled corticosteroid (medium dose) or Inhaled corticosteroid (low-medium dose) and a long-acting bronchodilator (long-acting inhaled β_2-agonist, sustained-release theophylline or long-acting β_2-agonist tablets) If needed: Anti-inflammatory: inhaled corticosteroid (medium-high dose) and Long-acting bronchodilator (long-acting inhaled β_2-agonist, sustained-release theophylline or long-acting β_2-agonist tablets)	Short-acting bronchodilator: inhaled β_2-agonists as needed for symptoms. Intensity of treatment will depend on severity of exacerbation. Use of short-acting inhaled β_2-agonists on a daily basis, or increasing use, indicates the need for additional long-term control therapy.	Step 1 actions plus: Teach self-monitoring Refer to group education if available Review and update self-management plan
Step 2: Mild persistent	One daily medication: Anti-inflammatory: either inhaled corticosteroid (low doses) or cromolyn or nedocromil Less desirable alternatives: sustained-release theophylline or leukotriene modifier	Short-acting bronchodilator: inhaled β_2-agonists as needed for symptoms. Intensity of treatment will depend on severity of exacerbation. Use of short-acting inhaled β_2-agonists on a daily basis, or increasing use, indicates the need for additional long-term control therapy.	Step 1 actions plus: Teach self-monitoring Refer to group education if available Review and update self-management plan
Step 1: Mild intermittent	No daily medication needed.	Short-acting bronchodilator: inhaled β_2-agonists as needed for symptoms. Intensity of treatment will depend on severity of exacerbation. Use of short-acting inhaled β_2-agonists > 2 times a week may indicate the need to indicate long-term control therapy.	Teach basic facts about asthma Teach inhaler/inhalation chamber technique Discuss roles of medications Develop self-management & action plans Discuss appropriate environmental control measures

Step down: Review treatment every 1–6 months; a gradual stepwise reduction in treatment may be possible.
Step up: If asthma control is not maintained, consider step up to next treatment level after reviewing medication technique, adherence, and environmental control.

[1]Modified from National Asthma Education and Prevention Program. Expert Panel Report 2: Guidelines for the Diagnosis and Management of Asthma. National Institutes of Health Pub No. 97-4051. Bethesda, MD, 1997.
[2]Preferred treatments are in bold print; however, specific medication plans should be tailored to individual patients.

Table 9–7. Long-term control medications for asthma.[1]

Drug	Important Formulations	Usual Adult Dosage	Cost[2]	Comments
Inhaled corticosteroids[3]				
Beclomethasone dipropionate (Beclovent, Vanceril)	MDI: 42 µg/puff; 200 puffs/inhaler 84 µg/puff; 120 puffs/inhaler	Two or three puffs four times a day, or four to six puffs twice daily Two puffs twice a day	$44.94/16.8 g	Chlorofluorocarbon propellant.
Budesonide (Pulmicort Turbuhaler)	Dry powder delivery system: 200 µg/puff; 200 puffs/inhaler	One inhalation twice a day	$119.10/inhaler	
Flunisolide (AeroBid)	MDI: 250 µg/puff; 100 puffs/inhaler	Two to four puffs twice a day	$63.22/7 g	Chlorofluorocarbon propellant.
Fluticasone (Flovent)	MDI: 44, 110 or 220 µg/puff; 120 puffs/inhaler	Two or three puffs (of 110 µg) twice a day	$62.16/13 g	Chlorofluorocarbon propellant.
(Flovent Rotadisk)	Dry powder delivery system: 44, 88, 220 µg/blister; 4 blisters/Rotadisk, 15 Rotadisks per tube	One or two puffs (of 88 µg) twice a day	$49.30/60 88 µg disks	
Triamcinolone acetonide (Azmacort)	MDI: 100 µg/puff; 240 puffs/inhaler	Two or three puffs four times a day, or four to six puffs twice daily	$53.18/20 g	Chlorofluorocarbon propellant.
Systemic corticosteroids				
Methylprednisolone (many)	Tablets: 4 mg	5–60 mg daily to every other day as needed	$0.54/4 mg	
Prednisolone (many)	Tablets, 5 mg	5–60 mg daily to every other day as needed	$0.05/5 mg	
Prednisone (many)	Tablets 1, 2.5, 5, 10, 20, 50 mg	5–60 mg daily to every other day as needed	$0.04/5 mg	
Cromolyn	MDI: 800 µg per puff: 200 puffs/inhaler	2–4 puffs 4 times a day	$69.30/14 g	Chlorofluorocarbon propellant.
	Nebulizer solution, 20 mg/2 mL ampule	20 mg (2 mL) four times a day	$1.02/2 mL	Administer with powered nebulizer.
Nedocromil	MDI: 1.75 mg/puff; 112 puffs/inhaler	Two puffs four times a day	$39.14/16 g	Chlorofluorocarbon propellant.
Long-acting β_2-agonists[4]				
Salmeterol (Serevent)	MDI: 21 µg/puff; 120 puffs/inhaler	Two puffs every 12 hours	$66.84/13 g	Chlorofluorocarbon propellant.
(Serevent Diskus)	Dry powder: 46 µg/blister; 60 blisters per pack	One blister every 12 hours	$69.78/60	
Sustained-release albuterol (Proventil Repetab)	Sustained-release tablet, 4 mg	One tablet every 12 hours	$0.78/4 mg	Usually reserved for nocturnal symptoms not improved with other therapies.
Theophylline (many)	Sustained-release tablets and capsules	Initially 10 mg/kg/d up to 300 mg maximum; then 200–600 mg every 8–24 hours	$0.34/200 mg	Maintenance dose guided by serum drug level. Absorption and dosing vary with brand.

(*continued*)

Table 9–7. Long-term control medications for asthma.[1] (continued)

Drug	Important Formulations	Usual Adult Dosage	Cost[2]	Comments
Leukotriene modifiers				
Montelukast (Singulair)	Tablet, 10 mg	One tablet each evening	\$2.37/10 mg \$71.17/mo	
Zafirlukast (Accolate)	Tablet, 20 mg	One tablet twice a day	\$1.04/20 mg \$62.40/mo	Administration with meals decreases bioavailability; take at least 1 hour before or 2 hours after meals
Zileuton (Zyflo)	Tablet, 600 mg	One tablet four times a day	\$0.81/600 mg \$97.20/mo	Monitor hepatic enzymes

[1]Only drugs available in the United States are listed.
[2]Cost to pharmacist (average wholesale price, generic when possible) for quantity listed. Source: *Drug Topics Red Book,* March 2000; Vol. 19, No. 3.
[3]Dosing should be individualized. See text.
[4]Not for acute relief of symptoms.

asthma or exercise-induced asthma. Both of these agents modulate mast cell mediator release and eosinophil recruitment and inhibit both early and late asthmatic responses to allergen challenge and exercise-induced bronchospasm. The clinical response to these agents is less predictable than the response to inhaled corticosteroids. Nedocromil may help reduce the dose requirements for inhaled corticosteroids. Both agents have excellent safety profiles.

b. Beta-adrenergic agents–Long-acting β_2-adrenergic agonists provide bronchodilation for up to 12 hours after a single dose. However, because their onset of action is delayed, they are not effective—and should not be used—in the treatment of acute bronchoconstriction. Salmeterol, the only agent of this class available in the USA, is indicated for long-term prevention of asthma symptoms—especially nocturnal symptoms—and the prevention of exercise-induced bronchospasm. Salmeterol should not be used in place of anti-inflammatory therapy and may provide more effective asthma control when added to standard doses of inhaled corticosteroids (compared with doubling the inhaled corticosteroid dose). A diminished bronchoprotective effect may occur early during chronic therapy, but the clinical significance of this phenomenon has not been established. Side-effects are limited at the standard dose of two puffs twice a day.

c. Phosphodiesterase inhibitors–Theophylline provides mild bronchodilation in asthmatics. This drug may also have important anti-inflammatory properties and enhance mucociliary clearance and diaphragmatic contractility. Sustained-release theophylline preparations are effective in controlling nocturnal asthma and are usually reserved for use as adjuvant therapy in patients with moderate or severe persistent asthma. They can also be used as alternative long-term preventive therapy in patients with mild persistent asthma. Theophylline serum concentrations need to be monitored closely owing to the drug's narrow toxic-therapeutic range, individual differences in metabolism, and the effects of many factors on drug absorption and metabolism. Decreases in theophylline clearance accompany the use of cimetidine, macrolide and quinolone antibiotics, and oral contraceptives. Increases in theophylline clearance are caused by rifampin, phenytoin, barbiturates, and tobacco.

Adverse effects at therapeutic doses include insomnia, upset stomach, aggravation of dyspepsia and gastroesophageal reflux symptoms, and urination difficulties in elderly men with prostatism. Dose-related toxicities are common and include nausea, vomiting, tachyarrhythmias, headache, seizures, hyperglycemia and hypokalemia.

3. Leukotriene modifiers–This is the newest class of medications for long-term control of asthma. Leukotrienes are potent biochemical mediators that contribute to airway obstruction and asthma symptoms by contracting airway smooth muscle, increasing vascular permeability and mucus secretion, and attracting and activating airway inflammatory cells. Zileuton is a 5-lipoxygenase inhibitor that decreases leukotriene production, and zafirlukast and montelukast are cysteinyl leukotriene receptor antagonists. They cause modest improvements in lung function and reductions in asthma symptoms and lessen the need for beta-agonist rescue therapy. These agents may be considered as alternatives to low-dose inhaled corticosteroids in patients with mild persistent asthma. Zileuton can cause reversible elevations in plasma aminotransferase levels, and a small number of patients who have taken montelukast or zafirlukast have been diagnosed with Churg-Strauss syndrome.

4. Desensitization–Immunotherapy for specific allergens may be considered in selected asthma patients who have exacerbations of asthma symptoms when exposed to allergens to which they are sensitive and who do not respond to environmental control measures and other forms of conventional therapy. Studies show a reduction in asthma symptoms in patients treated with single-allergen immunotherapy. Because of the risk of immunotherapy-induced bronchoconstriction in asthma patients, it should be administered only in a setting where such complications can be treated.

5. Miscellaneous agents–Oral sustained-release β_2-adrenergic agonists are reserved for patients with bothersome nocturnal asthma symptoms or moderate to severe persistent asthma who do not respond to other therapies. Corticosteroid-sparing anti-inflammatory agents such as troleandomycin, methotrexate, cyclosporine, intravenous immunoglobulin, and gold should be used only in selected severe asthmatics. These and other agents have variable benefit and worrisome toxicities.

B. Quick-Relief Medications: Short-acting bronchodilators and systemic corticosteroids comprise the important medications in this group of agents (Table 9–8).

1. Beta-adrenergic agents–Short-acting inhaled beta-adrenergic agonists are clearly the most effective bronchodilators during exacerbations and should be used in all patients to treat acute symptoms. These agents relax airway smooth muscle and cause a prompt increase in airflow and reduction of symptoms. Administration of one of these agents before exercise effectively prevents exercise-induced bronchoconstriction. There is no convincing evidence to support the use of one agent over another. However, β_2-selective agents produce less cardiac stimulation than those with mixed β_1 and β_2 activities. Currently available short-acting β_2-selective adrenergic agonists include albuterol, bitolterol, pirbuterol, and terbutaline.

Inhaled beta-adrenergic agonist therapy is as effective as oral or parenteral therapy in relaxing airway smooth muscle and improving acute asthma and offers the advantages of rapid onset of action (< 5 minutes) and less systemic side effects. In addition, repetitive administration produces incremental bronchodilation. Intravenous and subcutaneous routes of administration should be reserved for patients who because of age or mechanical factors are unable to inhale medications.

One or two inhalations of a short-acting inhaled beta-adrenergic agonist from a metered-dose inhaler is usually sufficient for mild to moderate symptoms; severe exacerbations may require up to four inhalations every few hours. Administration by wet nebulization does not offer more effective delivery than metered-dose inhalers; it is perceived to be more effective because it is given in higher doses. With most beta-adrenergic agonists, the recommended dose by nebulizer for acute asthma (albuterol, 2.5 mg) is 25–30 times that delivered by a single activation of the metered-dose inhaler (albuterol, 0.09 mg). This difference suggests that the standard use of inhalations from a metered-dose inhaler will often be insufficient. Equivalent bronchodilation can be achieved by either high doses (6–12 puffs) of a β_2-adrenergic agonist by metered-dose inhaler with an inhalation chamber or by nebulizer therapy. Nebulizer therapy may be more effective in patients who are unable to coordinate inhalation of medication from a metered-dose inhaler because of age, agitation, or severity of the exacerbation.

Regularly scheduled daily use is not generally recommended. Increased use (more than one canister a month) or lack of expected effect indicates diminished asthma control and dictates the need for additional long-term control therapy.

2. Anticholinergics–Anticholinergic agents reverse vagally mediated bronchospasm but not allergen- or exercise-induced bronchospasm. They may decrease mucus gland hypersecretion seen in asthma. Ipratropium bromide, a quaternary derivative of atropine free of atropine's side-effects, is the only available agent. This drug reverses acute bronchospasm and is an alternative for patients with intolerance to β_2-adrenergic agonists; it is the drug of choice for bronchospasm due to beta-blocker medications. Ipratropium bromide may be a useful adjunct to inhaled short-acting β_2-adrenergic agonists and considered in patients with moderate to severe asthma exacerbations. High doses of inhaled ipratropium bromide (0.5 mg) cause additional bronchodilation in some patients with severe airway obstruction, but the long-term role in management of asthma has not been clarified.

3. Phosphodiesterase inhibitors–Methylxanthines are not generally recommended for therapy of asthma exacerbations. Aminophylline has clearly been shown to be less effective than β_2-adrenergic agonists when used as single-drug therapy for acute asthma and adds little except toxicity to the acute bronchodilator effects achieved by nebulized metaproterenol alone. In patients currently taking a theophylline-containing preparation, the serum theophylline concentration should be determined to exclude theophylline toxicity.

4. Glucocorticoids–Systemic corticosteroids are effective primary treatment for patients with moderate to severe exacerbations or for patients who fail to respond promptly and completely to inhaled β_2-agonist therapy. They are one of the mainstays of the treatment of patients with severe asthma and are useful for patients with milder exacerbations. These medications speed the resolution of airflow obstruction and reduce the rate of relapse. Delays in administering corticosteroids may result in delayed benefits from these important agents. Therefore, oral corticosteroids should be available for early administration at home in many patients with moderate to severe asthma.

tance of a clinician. However, most such patients require a more comprehensive evaluation and treatment program such as that outlined below for severe asthma exacerbations. A course of oral corticosteroids is usually necessary.

Owing to the life-threatening nature of severe exacerbations of asthma, treatment should be started as soon as a severe asthma exacerbation is recognized and an assessment of lung function is made. All patients with a severe exacerbation should immediately receive oxygen, high doses of an inhaled short-acting β_2-adrenergic agonist, and systemic corticosteroids. A brief history pertinent to the exacerbation can be completed while treatment is given. More detailed assessments, including laboratory studies, usually add little in the early phase of evaluation and management and should be delayed until after initial therapy has been completed.

Asphyxia is a common cause of death, and oxygen therapy is therefore very important. Supplemental oxygen should be given to maintain an $SaO_2 > 90\%$ or a $PaO_2 > 60$ mm Hg. Oxygen-induced hypoventilation is very rare, and concern for hypercapnia should never delay correction of hypoxemia.

Frequent high-dose delivery of an inhaled short-acting β_2-adrenergic agonist is indicated and is usually well tolerated in the setting of severe airway obstruction. Some studies suggest that continuous therapy is more efficacious than intermittent administration of these agents, but there is no clear consensus as long as similar doses are administered. At least three metered-dose inhaler or nebulizer treatments should be given in the first hour of therapy. Thereafter, the frequency of administration varies according to the improvement in airflow and associated symptoms and the occurrence of side effects.

Systemic corticosteroids are administered as detailed above. Mucolytic agents (eg, acetylcysteine, potassium iodide) may worsen cough or airflow obstruction. Anxiolytic and hypnotic drugs are contraindicated in critically ill asthma patients because of their respiratory depressant effects.

Repeat assessment of patients with severe exacerbations should be made after the initial dose of inhaled bronchodilator and after three doses of inhaled bronchodilators (60–90 minutes after initiating treatment). The response to initial treatment is a better predictor of the need for hospitalization than is the severity of an exacerbation on presentation. The decision to hospitalize a patient should be based on the duration and severity of symptoms, severity of airflow obstruction, course and severity of prior exacerbations, medication use at the time of the exacerbation, access to medical care and medications, adequacy of social support and home conditions, and presence of psychiatric illness. In general, discharge to home is appropriate if the PEF or FEV_1 has returned to $\geq 70\%$ of predicted or personal best and symptoms are minimal or absent. Patients with a rapid response to treatment should be observed for 30 minutes after the most recent dose of bronchodilator to ensure stability of response before discharge to home.

A small minority of patients will not respond well to treatment and will show signs of impending respiratory failure due to a combination of worsening airflow obstruction and respiratory muscle fatigue (Table 9–5). Such patients can deteriorate rapidly and thus should be monitored in a critical care setting. Intubation of an acutely ill asthma patient is technically difficult and is best done semielectively, before the crisis of a respiratory arrest. At the time of intubation, close attention should be given to maintaining intravascular volume because hypotension commonly accompanies the administration of sedation and the initiation of positive-pressure ventilation in patients dehydrated due to poor recent oral intake and high insensible losses.

The main goals of mechanical ventilation are to ensure adequate oxygen and avoid barotrauma. Controlled hypoventilation with permissive hypercapnia is often required to limit airway pressures. Frequent high-dose delivery of inhaled short-acting β_2-adrenergic agonists should be continued along with anti-inflammatory agents as discussed above. Many questions remain regarding the optimal delivery of inhaled β_2-adrenergic agonists to intubated, mechanically ventilated patients. Further studies are needed to determine the comparative efficacy of metered-dose inhalers and nebulizers, optimal ventilator settings to use during drug delivery, ideal site along the ventilator circuit for introduction of the delivery system, and maximal acceptable drug doses. Unconventional therapies such as magnesium sulfate, helium-oxygen mixtures, and inhalational anesthetic agents may be beneficial in selected patients.

Assessment, Monitoring, & Prevention

Periodic assessments and ongoing monitoring of asthma are essential to determine if the goals of therapy are being met. Clinical assessment and patient self-assessment are the primary methods for monitoring asthma. Patients should be given a written action plan based on signs and symptoms or expiratory flow rates. An action plan is especially important for patients with moderate to severe asthma or those with a history of severe exacerbations. Patients should be taught to recognize symptoms—especially patterns indicating inadequate asthma control or predicting the need for additional therapy. The written asthma action plan should direct the asthma patient to adjust medications in response to particular signs, symptoms, and peak flow measurements and should state when to seek medical help.

Spirometry is recommended at the time of initial assessment, once treatment is initiated and symptoms and peak flows have stabilized, and at least every 1–2 years thereafter. Regular follow-up visits (at least every 6 months, or more frequently based on patient status) are essential to help maintain asthma control and to reevaluate medication requirements. Patients with persistent asthma should receive annual influenza vaccinations.

Drazen JM et al: Should antileukotriene therapies be used instead of inhaled corticosteroids in asthma? Yes. Am J Respir Crit Care Med 1998;158:1697. [NLM Cit ID: 99065640]

Kamada AK et al: Issues in the use of inhaled glucocorticoids. Am J Respir Crit Care Med 1996;153:1739. [NLM Cit ID: 96279757] (Controversial aspects of inhaled steroids for asthma.)

National Asthma Education and Prevention Program: Expert Panel Report 2: Guidelines for the diagnosis and management of asthma. National Institutes of Health, Pub No. 97-4051, Bethesda, MD, 1997. (Basic recommendations for the diagnosis and management of asthma based on exhaustive review of scientific literature and expert opinion.)

Wenzel SE: Should antileukotriene therapies be used instead of inhaled corticosteroids in asthma? No. Am J Respir Crit Care Med 1998;158:1699. [NLM Cit ID: 99065641] (Pro and con editorials that review the topic.)

CHRONIC OBSTRUCTIVE PULMONARY DISEASE (COPD)

Essentials of Diagnosis

- History of cigarette smoking.
- Chronic cough and sputum production (in chronic bronchitis) and dyspnea (in emphysema).
- Rhonchi, decreased intensity of breath sounds, and prolonged expiration on physical examination.
- Airflow limitation on pulmonary function testing.

General Considerations

Chronic obstructive pulmonary disease (COPD) is a disease state characterized by the presence of airflow obstruction due to chronic bronchitis or emphysema; the airflow obstruction is generally progressive, may be accompanied by airway hyperreactivity, and may be partially reversible (American Thoracic Society). Although emphysema and chronic bronchitis must be diagnosed and treated as specific diseases, most patients with COPD have features of both conditions. About 14 million Americans are affected. Grouped together, COPD and asthma now represent the fourth leading cause of death in the United States, with over 90,000 deaths reported annually. The death rate from COPD is increasing rapidly, especially among elderly men.

Chronic bronchitis is characterized by excessive secretion of bronchial mucus and is manifested by productive cough for 3 months or more in at least 2 consecutive years in the absence of any other disease that might account for this symptom. **Emphysema** denotes abnormal, permanent enlargement of air spaces distal to the terminal bronchiole, with destruction of their walls and without obvious fibrosis. It is worthwhile to note that chronic bronchitis is defined in clinical terms, whereas emphysema is defined in pathologic terms. Cigarette smoking is clearly the most important cause of COPD. Nearly all smokers suffer an accelerated decline in lung function that is dose- and duration-dependent. Fifteen percent develop progressively disabling symptoms. It is estimated that 80% of patients seen for COPD have significant exposure to tobacco smoke. Air pollution, airway infection, familial factors, and allergy have also been implicated in chronic bronchitis, and hereditary factors (deficiency of α_1-antiprotease) have been implicated in emphysema. The pathogenesis of emphysema may be excessive lysis of elastin and other structural proteins in the lung matrix by elastase and other proteases derived from lung neutrophils, macrophages, and mononuclear cells. Atopy and the tendency for bronchoconstriction to develop in response to nonspecific airway stimuli may be important risks for COPD.

Clinical Findings

A. Symptoms and Signs: Patients with COPD characteristically present in the fifth or sixth decade of life complaining of excessive cough, sputum production, and shortness of breath. Symptoms have often been present for 10 years or more. Dyspnea is noted initially only on heavy exertion, but as the condition progresses it occurs with mild activity. In severe disease, dyspnea occurs at rest. Frequent exacerbations of illness are common and result in absence from work and eventual disability. Pneumonia, pulmonary hypertension, cor pulmonale, and chronic respiratory failure characterize the late stage of COPD. Death usually occurs during an exacerbation of illness in association with acute respiratory failure. Hemoptysis occurs occasionally.

Clinical findings may be completely absent early in the course of COPD. As the disease progresses, two symptom patterns tend to emerge, historically referred to as "pink puffers" and "blue bloaters" (Table 9–9). These patterns have been thought to represent pure forms of emphysema and bronchitis, respectively, but this is a simplification of the anatomy and pathophysiology. Most COPD patients have pathologic evidence of both disorders, and their clinical course may reflect other factors such as central control of ventilation and concomitant sleep-disordered breathing.

B. Laboratory Findings: During exacerbations of illness, examination of the sputum may reveal *Streptococcus pneumoniae, Haemophilus influenzae,* or *Moraxella catarrhalis,* though these may be present in the carrier state between episodes of deterioration. The ECG may show sinus tachycardia, and in

Table 9–9. Patterns of disease in advanced COPD.

	Type A: Pink Puffer (Emphysema Predominant)	Type B: Blue Bloater (Bronchitis Predominant)
History and physical examination	Major complaint is dyspnea, often severe, usually presenting after age 50. Cough is rare, with scant clear, mucoid sputum. Patients are thin, with recent weight loss common. They appear uncomfortable, with evident use of accessory muscles of respiration. Chest is very quiet without adventitious sounds. No peripheral edema.	Major complaint is chronic cough, productive of mucopurulent sputum, with frequent exacerbations due to chest infections. Often presents in late 30s and 40s. Dyspnea usually mild, though patients may note limitations to exercise. Patients frequently overweight and cyanotic but seem comfortable at rest. Peripheral edema is common. Chest is noisy, with rhonchi invariably present; wheezes are common.
Laboratory studies	Hemoglobin usually normal (12–15 g/dL). PaO_2 normal to slightly reduced (65–75 mm Hg) but SaO_2 normal at rest. $PaCO_2$ normal to slightly reduced (35–40 mm Hg). Chest radiograph shows hyperinflation with flattened diaphragms. Vascular markings are diminished, particularly at the apices.	Hemoglobin usually elevated (15–18 g/dL). PaO_2 reduced (45–60 mm Hg) and $PaCO_2$ slightly to markedly elevated (50–60 mm Hg). Chest radiograph shows increased interstitial markings ("dirty lungs"), especially at bases. Diaphragms are not flattened.
Pulmonary function tests	Airflow obstruction ubiquitous. Total lung capacity increased, sometimes markedly so. D_LCO reduced. Static lung compliance increased.	Airflow obstruction ubiquitous. Total lung capacity generally normal but may be slightly increased. D_LCO normal. Static lung compliance normal.
Special evaluations		
V/Q matching	Increased ventilation to high V/Q areas, ie, high dead space ventilation.	Increased perfusion to low V/Q areas.
Hemodynamics	Cardiac output normal to slightly low. Pulmonary artery pressures mildly elevated and increase with exercise.	Cardiac output normal. Pulmonary artery pressures elevated, sometimes markedly so, and worsen with exercise.
Nocturnal ventilation	Mild to moderate degree of oxyhemoglobin desaturation not usually associated with obstructive sleep apnea.	Severe oxyhemoglobin desaturation, frequently associated with obstructive sleep apnea.
Exercise ventilation	Increased minute ventilation for level of oxygen consumption. PaO_2 tends to fall, $PaCO_2$ slightly.	Decreased minute ventilation for level of oxygen consumption. PaO_2 may rise; $PaCO_2$ may rise signficantly.

advanced disease, chronic pulmonary hypertension may produce electrocardiographic abnormalities typical of cor pulmonale. Supraventricular arrhythmias (multifocal atrial tachycardia, atrial flutter, and atrial fibrillation) and ventricular irritability also occur.

Arterial blood gas measurements characteristically show no abnormalities early in COPD other than an increased A-a DO_2. Indeed, they are unnecessary unless hypoxia or hypercapnia is suspected. Hypoxemia occurs in advanced disease, particularly when chronic bronchitis predominates. Compensated respiratory acidosis occurs in patients with chronic respiratory failure, particularly in chronic bronchitis, with worsening of acidemia during acute exacerbations. (See Chapter 21.)

Spirometry provides objective information about pulmonary function and assesses the results of therapy. Pulmonary function tests early in the course of COPD reveal only evidence of abnormal closing volume and reduced midexpiratory flow rate. Reductions in FEV_1 and in the ratio of forced expiratory volume to (FEV_1/FVC) occur later. In severe disease, the forced vital capacity is markedly reduced. Lung volume measurements reveal an increase in the total lung capacity (TLC), a marked increase in the residual volume (RV), and an elevation of the RV/TLC ratio, indicative of air trapping, particularly in emphysema.

C. Imaging: When emphysema is the main clinical feature, hyperinflation is apparent. Parenchymal bullae or subpleural blebs are pathognomonic of emphysema. Radiographs of patients with chronic bronchitis may show only nonspecific peribronchial and perivascular markings. Pulmonary hypertension becomes evident as enlargement of central pulmonary arteries in advanced disease. Doppler echocardiography is an effective way to estimate pulmonary artery pressure if pulmonary hypertension is suspected.

Differential Diagnosis

Clinical, roentgenographic, and laboratory findings should enable the clinician to distinguish COPD from other obstructive pulmonary disorders such as bronchial asthma, bronchiectasis, cystic fibrosis, bronchopulmonary mycosis, and central airway obstruction. Bronchiectasis is distinguished from COPD by features such as recurrent pneumonia and hemoptysis, digital clubbing, and radiographic abnormalities. Patients with severe α_1-antiprotease deficiency are recognized by the appearance of panacinar bibasilar emphysema early in life, usually in the third or fourth decade, and hepatic cirrhosis and hepatocellular carcinoma may occur. Cystic fibrosis occurs in children and younger adults. Rarely, mechanical obstruction of the central airways simulates COPD. Flow-volume loops may help separate patients with central airway obstruction from those with diffuse intrathoracic airway obstruction characteristic of COPD.

Complications

Acute bronchitis, pneumonia, pulmonary embolization, and concomitant left ventricular failure may worsen otherwise stable COPD. Pulmonary hypertension, cor pulmonale, and chronic respiratory failure are common in advanced COPD. Spontaneous pneumothorax occurs in a small fraction of patients with emphysema. Hemoptysis may result from chronic bronchitis or may signal bronchogenic carcinoma.

Prevention

COPD is largely preventable through elimination of chronic exposure to tobacco smoke. Smokers with early evidence of airflow limitation can alter their disease by smoking cessation. Smoking cessation slows the decline in FEV_1 in middle-aged smokers with mild airways obstruction. Vaccination against influenza and pneumococcal disease may also be of benefit.

Treatment

Standards for the management of patients with COPD have recently been published by the American Thoracic Society. See Chapter 38 for a discussion of air travel in patients with lung disease.

A. Ambulatory Patients: The single most important intervention in smokers with COPD is to encourage smoking cessation. Simply telling a patient to quit succeeds 5% of the time. The Lung Health Study reported 22% sustained abstinence at 5 years in their intervention group (behavior modification plus nicotine gum). Nicotine transdermal patch, nicotine gum, and buproprion increase cessation rates in motivated smokers (see Chapter 1).

The only drug therapy that is documented to alter the natural history of COPD is supplemental oxygen in those patients with resting hypoxemia. Requirements for Medicare coverage for a patient's home use of oxygen and oxygen equipment are listed in Table 9–10. Arterial blood gas analysis is preferable to ear or pulse oximetry to guide initial oxygen therapy. Hypoxemic patients with pulmonary hypertension, chronic cor pulmonale, erythrocytosis, impaired cognitive function, exercise intolerance, nocturnal restlessness, or morning headache are particularly likely to benefit from home oxygen therapy. Proved benefits of home oxygen therapy in advanced COPD include longer survival, reduced hospitalization needs, and better quality of life. Survival in hypoxemic patients with COPD treated with supplemental oxygen therapy is directly proportionate to the number of hours per day oxygen is administered. In such patients who are treated with continuous oxygen, the survival after 36 months is about 65%—significantly better than the survival rate of about 45% in those who are treated with only nocturnal oxygen.

Home oxygen may be supplied by liquid oxygen systems (LOX), compressed gas cylinders, or oxygen concentrators. Most patients benefit from having both stationary and portable systems. Oxygen by nasal prongs must be given at least 15 hours a day unless therapy is intended only for exercise or sleep. For most patients, a flow rate of 1–3 L/min achieves a PaO_2 greater than 55 mm Hg. The monthly cost of home oxygen therapy ranges from \$300.00 to \$500.00 or more, being higher for liquid oxygen systems. Medicare covers approximately 80% of home oxygen expenses. **Transtracheal oxygen** is an alternative method of delivery and may be useful for patients who require higher flows of oxygen than can be delivered via the nose or who are experiencing trou-

Table 9–10. Home oxygen therapy: requirements for Medicare coverage.[1]

Group I (any of the following):

1. $PaO_2 \le 55$ mm Hg or $SaO_2 \le 88\%$ taken at rest breathing room air, while awake.
2. During sleep (prescription for nocturnal oxygen use only):
   a. $PaO_2 \le 55$ mm Hg or $SaO_2 \le 88\%$ for a patient whose awake, resting, room air PaO_2 is ≥ 56 mm Hg or $SaO_2 \ge 89\%$,

   or

   b. Decrease in $PaO_2 > 10$ mm Hg or decrease in $SaO_2 > 5\%$ associated with symptoms or signs reasonably attributed to hypoxemia (eg, impaired cognitive processes, nocturnal restlessness, insomnia).
3. During exercise (prescription for oxygen use only during exercise):
   a. $PaO_2 \le 55$ mg Hg or $SaO_2 \le 88\%$ taken during exercise for a patient whose awake, resting, room air PaO_2 is ≥ 56 mm Hg or $SaO_2 \ge 89\%$.

   and

   b. There is evidence that the use of supplemental oxygen during exercise improves the hypoxemia that was demonstrated during exercise while breathing room air.

Group II:[2]

PaO_2 = 56–59 mm Hg or SaO_2 = 89% if there is evidence of any of the following:

1. Dependent edema suggesting congestive heart failure.
2. P pulmonale on ECG (P wave > 3 mm in standard leads II, III, or aVF).
3. Hematocrit > 56%.

[1]Health Care Financing Administration, 1989.
[2]Patients in this group must have a second oxygen test 3 months after the initial oxygen set-up.

are required for accurate diagnosis. A normal sweat chloride test does not exclude the diagnosis. Genotyping or other alternative diagnostic studies (such as measurement of nasal membrane potential difference, semen analysis, or assessment of pancreatic function) should be pursued if the test is repeatedly negative but there is a high clinical suspicion of cystic fibrosis. Standard genotyping is a limited diagnostic tool because it screens for only a fraction of the known cystic fibrosis mutations.

Treatment

Early recognition and comprehensive multidisciplinary therapy improve the chances of survival and amelioration of symptoms. Referral to a regional cystic fibrosis center is strongly recommended. Conventional treatment programs focus on the following areas: clearance and reduction of lower airway secretions, reversal of bronchoconstriction, treatment of respiratory tract infections and airway bacterial burden, pancreatic enzyme replacement, nutritional support, and psychosocial issues (including genetic and occupational counseling).

Clearance of lower airway secretions can be promoted by postural drainage and chest percussion or vibration techniques, positive expiratory pressure (PEP) or flutter valve breathing devices, directed cough, and other breathing techniques; these approaches require detailed patient instruction by experienced personnel. Sputum viscosity in cystic fibrosis is increased by the large quantities of extracellular DNA that result from chronic airways inflammation and the autolysis of neutrophils. Inhaled recombinant human deoxyribonuclease (rhDNase) cleaves extracellular DNA in sputum and when administered chronically at a daily nebulized dose of 2.5 mg leads to improved FEV_1 and reduces the risk of cystic fibrosis-related respiratory exacerbations and the need for intravenous antibiotics. Pharyngitis, laryngitis, and voice alterations are common adverse effects. The annual cost to the pharmacist exceeds $12,000. Antibiotics are used to treat active airway infections based on results of culture and susceptibility testing of sputum. *S aureus* (including methicillin-resistant strains) and a mucoid variant of *P aeruginosa* are commonly present. *Haemophilus influenzae, Stenotrophomonas maltophilia,* and *Burkholderia cepacia*—the latter a highly drug-resistant organism—are occasionally isolated. The use of aerosolized antibiotics (inhalational tobramycin solution and others) for prophylaxis or treatment of lower respiratory tract infections is sometimes helpful. Although some studies demonstrate reduced exacerbations and increases in FEV_1 in patients chronically infected with *P aeruginosa,* there is concern about the emergence of drug-resistant organisms, equipment contamination with *B cepacia,* and side effects such as bronchospasm.

Inhaled bronchodilators (eg, albuterol, two puffs every 4 hours as needed) should be considered in patients who demonstrate an increase of at least 10% in FEV_1 after an inhaled bronchodilator. Vaccination against pneumococcal infection and annual influenza vaccination are advised. Screening of family members for genetic counseling of a cystic fibrosis patient is suggested.

Lung transplantation is currently the only definitive treatment for advanced cystic fibrosis. Double-lung or heart-lung transplantation is required. A few transplant centers offer living lobar lung transplantation to selected patients. The 3-year survival rate following transplantation for cystic fibrosis is about 55%.

Investigational therapies for cystic fibrosis include anti-inflammatory agents (eg, ibuprofen, pentoxifylline, antiproteases), protein modification agents (eg, milrinone, phenylbutyrate), ion transport agents (eg, amiloride), and gene therapy.

Prognosis

The longevity of patients with cystic fibrosis is increasing, and the median survival age is now 31 years. Death occurs from pulmonary complications (eg, pneumonia, pneumothorax, or hemoptysis) or as a result of terminal chronic respiratory failure and cor pulmonale.

Campbell PW et al: Use of aerosolized antibiotics in patients with cystic fibrosis. Chest 1999;116:775. [NLM Cit ID: 99420035] (Comprehensive Cystic Fibrosis Foundation Consensus Conference Committee report.)

Davis PB et al: Cystic fibrosis. Am J Respir Crit Care Med 1996;154:1229. [NLM Cit ID: 97069751]

Ramsey BW: Management of pulmonary disease in patients with cystic fibrosis. N Engl J Med 1996;335:179. [NLM Cit ID: 96282472]

Ramsey BW et al: Intermittent administration of inhaled tobramycin in patients with cystic fibrosis. N Engl J Med 1999;340:23. [NLM Cit ID: 99090872] (Intermittent administration of inhaled tobramycin to patients with cystic fibrosis improves pulmonary function, decreases the density of *P aeruginosa* in sputum, and decreases the risk of hospitalization.)

Rosenstein BJ et al: The diagnosis of cystic fibrosis: a consensus statement. J Pediatr 1998;132:589. [NLM Cit ID: 98241855] (Cystic Fibrosis Foundation Consensus Panel guidelines for use of CF diagnostic tests.)

Rubin BK: Emerging therapies for cystic fibrosis lung disease. Chest 1999;115:1120. [NLM Cit ID: 99222899] (Comprehensive review article.)

BRONCHIOLITIS

Bronchiolitis is an acute, common, often severe respiratory illness of children under 2 years of age caused by respiratory syncytial virus, other viruses (occasionally), and *Mycoplasma pneumoniae*. An acute infectious bronchiolitis has not been recognized as a distinct entity in adults. However, **bronchiolitis obliterans** does occur in adults and is probably underrecognized. Cough, dyspnea, crackles on chest auscultation, and obstructive pulmonary dysfunction are characteristic.

Once classified as a type of chronic interstitial pneumonia, bronchiolitis obliterans has been reclassified. Five clinical types have been described: (1) toxic fume bronchiolitis obliterans, (2) postinfectious bronchiolitis obliterans, (3) bronchiolitis obliterans associated with connective tissue disease and organ transplantation, (4) bronchiolitis obliterans associated with localized lung lesions, and (5) idiopathic bronchiolitis obliterans with organizing pneumonia.

Toxic fume bronchiolitis obliterans follows 1–3 weeks after exposure to oxides of nitrogen, phosgene, and other noxious gases. The chest radiograph shows diffuse nonspecific alveolar or "ground-glass" densities.

Postinfectious bronchiolitis obliterans is a late response to mycoplasmal or viral lung infection in adults and has a highly variable radiographic appearance.

Bronchiolitis obliterans may occur in association with rheumatoid arthritis, polymyositis, and dermatomyositis. Penicillamine therapy has been implicated as a possible cause of bronchiolitis obliterans in patients with rheumatoid arthritis. Bronchiolitis obliterans is a common complication of heart-lung transplantation and a rare complication of allogeneic bone marrow transplantation, the latter occurring in the setting of chronic graft-versus-host disease.

Idiopathic bronchiolitis obliterans with organizing pneumonia (BOOP) affects men and women equally. Most patients are between the ages of 50 and 70. Dry cough, dyspnea, and a flu-like illness, ranging in duration from a few days to several months, are typical. Fever and weight loss are common. Physical examination demonstrates crackles in most patients, and wheezing is present in about a third. Clubbing is uncommon. Pulmonary function studies demonstrate restrictive dysfunction and hypoxemia. The chest radiograph typically shows patchy, bilateral, ground glass or alveolar infiltrates. Solitary pneumonia-like infiltrates and a diffuse interstitial pattern have also recently been described (see Table 9–20).

BOOP is usually a difficult diagnosis to make on clinical grounds alone. The presence of fever and weight loss, abrupt onset of symptoms (often with an upper respiratory tract infection), a relatively short duration of symptoms, the absence of clubbing, and the presence of alveolar infiltrates help the clinician distinguish this entity from idiopathic pulmonary fibrosis. However, open lung biopsy may be necessary. Buds of loose connective tissue and inflammatory cells fill alveoli and distal bronchioles. Corticosteroid therapy is effective in two-thirds of cases, often abruptly. Relapses are common if corticosteroids are stopped prematurely, and most patients require at least 6 months of therapy. Prednisone is usually given initially in doses of 1 mg/kg/d for 2–3 months. The dose is then tapered slowly to 20–40 mg/d, depending on response, and eventually to an alternate-day regimen.

Respiratory bronchiolitis is a disorder of small airways in cigarette smokers. Clinically and radiographically, this disorder resembles idiopathic pulmonary fibrosis. Cough, dyspnea, and crackles on chest auscultation are typical. However, the reduction in lung compliance seen in idiopathic pulmonary fibrosis is not found in this disorder. The condition may be recognized only on open lung biopsy, which demonstrates characteristic metaplasia of terminal and respiratory bronchioles and filling of respiratory and terminal bronchioles, alveolar ducts, and alveoli by pigmented alveolar macrophages.

Diffuse panbronchiolitis is an idiopathic disorder of respiratory bronchioles frequently diagnosed in Japan. The condition appears to be rare in the United States. Men are affected about twice as often as women and are most often between ages 20 and 80. About two-thirds of patients are nonsmokers. The large majority have a history of chronic pansinusitis. Marked dyspnea, cough, and sputum production are cardinal features. Crackles and rhonchi are noted on physical examination. Pulmonary function tests reveal obstructive abnormalities. The chest radiograph shows a distinct pattern of diffuse small nodular shadows and hyperinflation. Open lung biopsy is necessary for diagnosis.

Epler GR: Heterogeneity of bronchiolitis obliterans organizing pneumonia. Curr Opin Pulm Med 1998;4:93. [NLM Cit ID: 98275618] (An update of advances in the pathogenesis, radiographic features, clinical course, and categorization of the heterogeneity of BOOP.)

Lohr RH et al: Organizing pneumonia: Features and prognosis of cryptogenic, secondary, and focal variants. Arch Intern Med 1997;157:1323. [NLM Cit ID: 97344624] (Retrospective study of 74 patients seen at Mayo Clinic over 10 years.)

PULMONARY INFECTIONS

PNEUMONIA

Lower respiratory tract infections continue to be a major health problem despite advances in the identification of both old and new etiologic agents and the availability of potent antimicrobial drugs. In addition, there is still much controversy regarding diagnostic approaches and treatment choices for pneumonias.

Microorganisms gain access to the lower respiratory tract by aspiration of oropharyngeal secretions and associated bacterial flora, inhalation of infected aerosols, and hematogenous dissemination. The consequences of seeding the lower respiratory tract with microorganisms depends on the size of the inoculum, the virulence of the microorganism, and host susceptibility. The evaluation and management of otherwise normal immunocompetent hosts who may have pneumonia will be discussed separately from the approach to the evaluation and management of pulmonary infiltrates in immunocompromised hosts—defined as patients with HIV disease, absolute neutrophil counts < 100/μL, current or recent exposure to myelosuppressive or immunosuppressive drugs, or those currently taking prednisone in a dosage of over 5 mg/d. Characteristics of pneumonia caused by specific agents and appropriate antimicrobial therapy are presented in Table 9–11. Pneumonias are typically classified as being either community-acquired or hospital-acquired (nosocomial). Anaerobic pneumonias and lung abscess can occur in both settings and warrant separate consideration.

1. COMMUNITY-ACQUIRED PNEUMONIA

Essentials of Diagnosis

- Symptoms and signs of an acute lung infection: fever or hypothermia, cough with or without sputum, dyspnea, chest discomfort, sweats or rigors.
- Bronchial breath sounds or rales are frequent auscultatory findings.
- Parenchymal infiltrate on chest radiograph.
- Occurs outside of the hospital or less than 48 hours after admission in a patient who is not hospitalized or residing in a long-term care facility for more than 14 days before the onset of symptoms.

General Considerations

Community-acquired pneumonia is a common disorder, with approximately 3–4 million cases diagnosed each year in the United States. It is the most deadly infectious disease in the United States and the sixth leading overall cause of death. Mortality is estimated to be approximately 14% among hospitalized patients and less than 1% for patients who do not require hospitalization. Important risk factors for increased morbidity and mortality from community-acquired pneumonia include advanced age, alcoholism, comorbid medical conditions, altered mental status, respiratory rate ≥ 30/min, hypotension (defined by systolic blood pressure < 90 mm Hg or diastolic blood pressure < 60 mm Hg), and BUN > 30 mg/dL.

A predictor of patient risk and mortality from community-acquired pneumonia has been developed and validated by the Pneumonia Patient Outcomes Research Team (PORT). The PORT prediction scheme utilizes 19 clinical variables to stratify patients into five mortality risk classes. (See accompanying box.) Patients under 50 years of age without the comorbid conditions and specific physical examination abnormalities listed below are assigned to risk class I. All other patients are assigned to point-based risk classes II–V.

Condition	PORT Points Assigned
Cancer	30
Arterial pH < 7.35	30
Liver disease	20
Respiratory rate ≥ 30/min	20
Systolic blood pressure < 90 mm Hg	20
BUN ≥ 30 mg/dL	20
Serum sodium < 130 meq/L	20
Temperature < 35 °C or ≥ 40 °C	15
Congestive heart failure	10
Cerebrovascular disease	10
Renal disease	10
Pleural effusion	10
Nursing home residence	10
Heart rate ≥ 125 beats/min	10
Serum glucose ≥ 250 mg/dL	10
Hematocrit < 30%	10
PaO_2 < 60 mm Hg	10
Age, men	1 per yr
Age, women	1 per yr minus 10

Interpretation: Risk classes I–V are defined by the following number of points: I = no predictors, II = ≤ 70, III = 71–90, IV = 91–130, V = > 130. Risk class 30-day mortality rates are as follows: I = 0.1%, II = 0.6%, III = 2.8%, IV = 8.2%, V = 29.2%.

This model can be used along with clinician judgment to help make the initial decision about whether a patient with community-acquired pneumonia requires hospitalization.

Information from the history, physical examination, radiographs, and laboratory evaluations is not sensitive or specific for predicting a causative agent or for differentiating bacterial from viral causes or "typical" from "atypical" bacterial organisms as the cause of community-acquired pneumonia. Therefore, treatment of community-acquired pneumonia is often em-

Table 9–11. Characteristics and treatment of selected pneumonias.

Organism	Clinical Setting	Gram-Stained Smears of Sputum	Chest Radiograph[1]	Laboratory Studies	Complications	Antimicrobial Therapy[2,3]
Streptococcus pneumoniae (pneumococcus)	Chronic cardiopulmonary disease; follows upper respiratory tract infection.	Gram-positive diplococci.	Lobar consolidation.	Gram-stained smear of sputum; culture of blood, pleural fluid, sputum.	Bacteremia, meningitis, endocarditis, pericarditis, empyema.	Preferred:[4] Penicillin G or V, amoxicillin. Alternative: Macrolides, cephalosporins, doxycycline, fluoroquinolones, vancomycin.
Haemophilus influenzae	Chronic cardiopulmonary disease; follows upper respiratory tract infection.	Pleomorphic gram-negative coccobacilli.	Lobar consolidation.	Culture of sputum, blood, pleural fluid.	Empyema, endocarditis.	Preferred:[4] Cefotaxime ceftriaxone, or cefuroxime, doxycycline. Alternative: Cefuroxime, doxycycline, azithromycin, TMP-SMZ, fluoroquinolones[5]
Staphylococcus aureus	Residence in chronic care facility, nosocomial, influenza epidemics; cystic fibrosis, bronchiectasis, injection drug use.	Plump gram-positive cocci in clumps.	Patchy infiltrates.	Culture of sputum, blood, pleural fluid.	Empyema, cavitation.	For methicillin-susceptible strains: Preferred: A penicillinase-resistant penicillin. vancomycin. Alternative: A cephalosporin; clindamycin, fluoroquinolones, TMP-SMZ,[5] vancomycin. For methicillin-resistant strains: Vancomycin with or without gentamicin with or without rifampin.
Klebsiella pneumoniae	Alcohol abuse, diabetes mellitus; nosocomial,	Plump gram-negative encapsulated rods.	Lobar consolidation.	Culture of sputum, blood, pleural fluid.	Cavitation, empyema.	Preferred: Third-generation cephalosporin. For severe infections, add an aminoglycoside. Alternative: Aztreonam, imipenem, or beta-lactam/beta-lactamase inhibitor, or a fluoroquinolone.
Escherichia coli	Nosocomial; rarely, community-acquired.	Gram-negative rods.	Patchy infiltrates, pleural effusion.	Culture of sputum, blood, pleural fluid.	Empyema.	Same as for *Klebsiella pneumoniae*.
Pseudomonas aeruginosa	Nosocomial; cystic fibrosis, bronchiectasis.	Gram-negative rods.	Patchy infiltrates, cavitation.	Culture of sputum, blood.	Cavitation.	Preferred: An antipseudomonal beta-lactam plus an aminoglycoside. Alternative: Ciprofloxacin plus an aminoglycoside or an antipseudomonal beta-lactam.
Anaerobes	Aspiration, poor dental hygiene.	Mixed flora.	Patchy infiltrates in dependent lung zones.	Culture of pleural fluid or of material obtained by transtracheal or transthoracic aspiration.	Necrotizing pneumonia, abscess, empyema.	Preferred: Clindamycin, penicillin plus metronidazole, beta-lactam/beta-lactamase inhibitor.

(*continued*)

6 weeks or longer and is usually fastest in young patients, nonsmokers, and those with only single lobe involvement.

D. Special Examinations: Sputum induction is reserved for patients who cannot provide expectorated sputum samples and who may have *Pneumocystis carinii* or *Mycobacterium tuberculosis* pneumonia. Transtracheal aspiration, fiberoptic bronchoscopy, and transthoracic needle aspiration techniques to obtain samples of lower respiratory secretions or tissues are reserved for selected patients.

Thoracentesis with pleural fluid analysis (stains, cultures; glucose, lactate dehydrogenase, and total protein levels; leukocyte count with differential; pH determination) should be performed on most patients with pleural effusions to assist in diagnosis of the etiologic agent and assess for empyema or complicated parapneumonic process. Serologic assays, polymerase chain reaction tests, specialized culture tests, and other new diagnostic tests for organisms such as legionella, *Mycoplasma pneumoniae,* and *Chlamydia pneumoniae* are performed when these diagnoses are suspected. Selected specialized diagnostic tests are listed in Table 9–11. Limitations of many of these tests include delay in obtaining test results and variable sensitivity and specificity.

Treatment

Pathogen-directed antimicrobial therapy should be attempted and initiated promptly after the diagnosis of pneumonia is established and appropriate specimens are obtained, especially in patients who require hospitalization. Delays in obtaining diagnostic specimens or the results of testing should not preclude the early administration of antibiotics to acutely ill patients. Decisions regarding hospitalization should be based on prognostic criteria as outlined above in the section on general considerations. Treatment recommendations can be divided into those for patients who can be treated as outpatients and those for patients who require hospitalization.

Special consideration must be given to emerging resistance of *Streptococcus pneumoniae* strains to penicillin. Intermediate resistance to penicillin is defined as an MIC of 0.1–1 mg/mL. Strains with high-level resistance usually require an MIC $\geq$ 2 μg/mL for penicillin. Resistance to other antibiotics (beta-lactams, trimethoprim-sulfamethoxazole, macrolides, others) often accompanies resistance to penicillin. The prevalence of resistance varies by geographic region and over time, and local resistance pattern data should therefore guide empirical therapy of suspected or documented *S pneumoniae* infections until specific susceptibility test results are available.

A. Treatment of Outpatients: Empirical antibiotic options for patients with community-acquired pneumonia who do not require hospitalization include the following: (1) Macrolides (clarithromycin, 500 mg orally twice a day, or azithromycin, 500 mg orally as a first dose and then 250 mg once a day for 4 days). (2) Doxycycline (100 mg orally twice a day). (3) Fluoroquinolones (with enhanced activity against *S pneumoniae,* such as gatifloxacin, 400 mg orally once a day, levofloxacin 500 mg orally once a day, or moxifloxacin 400 mg orally once a day). Alternatives include amoxicillin-potassium clavulanate—especially for suspected aspiration pneumonia—500 mg orally three times a day or 875 mg orally twice a day, and some second- and third-generation cephalosporins such as cefuroxime axetil (250–500 mg orally twice a day), cefpodoxime (200 mg orally twice a day), proxetil (100–200 mg orally twice a day), or cefprozil, 250–500 mg orally twice a day).

There are limited data to guide recommendations for duration of treatment. The decision is influenced by the severity of illness, the etiologic agent, response to therapy, other medical problems, and complications. Therapy until the patient is afebrile for at least 72 hours is usually sufficient for pneumonia due to *S pneumoniae.* A minimum of 2 weeks of therapy is reasonable in *M pneumoniae, C pneumoniae,* or legionella pneumonias. Five days of therapy is usually sufficient if azithromycin is used.

B. Treatment of Hospitalized Patients: Empirical antibiotic options for patients with community-acquired pneumonia who require hospitalization can be divided into those for patients who can be cared for on a general medical ward and those for patients who require care in an intensive care unit. Patients who only require general medical ward care usually respond to a third-generation beta-lactam (such as ceftriaxone or cefotaxime) with or without a macrolide (clarithromycin or azithromycin is preferred if *H influenzae* infection is suspected) or a fluoroquinolone (with enhanced activity against *S pneumoniae*). Alternatives include cefuroxime with or without a macrolide or azithromycin alone. Patients requiring intensive care unit admission often require erythromycin, azithromycin, or a fluoroquinolone (with enhanced activity against *S pneumoniae*) plus ceftriaxone, cefotaxime, or a beta-lactam/beta-lactamase inhibitor (ampicillin-sulbactam, ticarcillin/potassium clavulanate, piperacillin-tazobactam). Patients with penicillin allergies can be treated with a fluoroquinolone (with enhanced activity against *S pneumoniae*) with or without clindamycin. Patients with suspected aspiration pneumonia receive a fluoroquinolone (with enhanced activity against *S pneumoniae*) plus clindamycin or a beta-lactam/beta-lactamase inhibitor. Patients with preexisting structural diseases of the lung such as bronchiectasis or cystic fibrosis benefit from empirical therapy with an antipseudomonal penicillin, carbapenem, or cefepime plus a macrolide or fluoroquinolone plus an aminoglycoside until sputum culture and sensitivity results are available. Expanded discussions of specific antibiotics are provided in Chapter 37. Antibiotic

empirical. Because of the high mortality rate, therapy must be started as soon as pneumonia is suspected. Initial regimens must be broad in spectrum and tailored to the specific clinical setting. There is no uniform consensus on the best regimens.

Recommendations for the treatment of hospital-acquired pneumonia have been proposed by the American Thoracic Society. Initial empirical therapy with antibiotics is determined by the severity of illness, risk factors, and the length of hospitalization. Empirical therapy for mild to moderate nosocomial pneumonia in a patient without unusual risk factors or a patient with severe early-onset (within 5 days after hospitalization) hospital-acquired pneumonia may consist of a second-generation cephalosporin, a nonantipseudomonal third-generation cephalosporin, or a combination of a beta-lactam and beta-lactamase inhibitor.

Empirical therapy for patients with severe, late-onset (≥ 5 days after hospitalization) hospital-acquired pneumonia or with ICU- or ventilator-associated pneumonia should be a combination of antibiotics directed against the most virulent organisms, particularly *P aeruginosa,* acinetobacter species, and enterobacter species. The antibiotic regimen should include an aminoglycoside or fluoroquinolone plus one of the following: an antipseudomonal penicillin, an antipseudomonal cephalosporin, imipenem-cilastatin, or aztreonam—aztreonam alone with an aminoglycoside will be inadequate if coverage for gram-positive organisms or *H influenzae* is required. Vancomycin is added if infection with methicillin-resistant *S aureus* infection is of concern (especially patients with coma, head trauma, diabetes mellitus, or renal failure or who are in the ICU). Anaerobic coverage with clindamycin or a beta-lactam/beta-lactamase inhibitor combination may be chosen or added for patients who have risk factors for anaerobic pneumonia, including aspiration, recent thoracoabdominal surgery, or an obstructing airway lesion. A macrolide is added when patients are at risk for legionella infection, such those receiving high-dose corticosteroids. After results of sputum, blood, and pleural fluid cultures have been obtained, it may be possible to switch to a regimen with a narrower spectrum. Duration of antibiotic therapy should be individualized based on the pathogen, severity of illness, response to therapy, and comorbid conditions. Therapy for gram-negative bacillary pneumonia should continue for at least 14–21 days.

Expanded discussions of specific antibiotics are provided in Chapter 37. Antibiotic dose suggestions are provided in Tables 37–4, 37–5, 37–7, 37–8 and 37–9.

Bruchhaus JD, McEachern R, Campbell GD Jr: Hospital-acquired pneumonia: Recent advances in diagnosis, microbiology and treatment. Curr Opin Pulm Med 1998;4:180. [NLM Cit ID: 98340121] (Highlights the recent literature with emphasis on significant publications and advances in the area of pneumonia pathogenesis, microbiology, diagnosis, and response to antimicrobial therapy.)

Kirtland SH et al: The diagnosis of ventilator-associated pneumonia: A comparison of histologic, microbiologic, and clinical criteria. Chest 1997;112:445. [NLM Cit ID: 97410168] (Discusses utility of tracheal aspirate and bronchoalveolar lavage fluid cultures for the diagnosis and treatment of ventilator pneumonia.)

3. ANAEROBIC PNEUMONIA & LUNG ABSCESS

Essentials of Diagnosis

- History of or predisposition to aspiration.
- Indolent symptoms, including fever, weight loss, malaise.
- Poor dental hygiene.
- Foul-smelling purulent sputum (in many patients).
- Infiltrate in dependent lung zone, with single or multiple areas of cavitation or pleural effusion.

General Considerations

Aspiration of small amounts of oropharyngeal secretions occurs during sleep in normal individuals and rarely causes disease. Sequelae of aspiration of larger amounts of material include nocturnal asthma, chemical pneumonitis, mechanical obstruction of airways by particulate matter, bronchiectasis, and pleuropulmonary infection. Individuals predisposed to disease induced by aspiration include those with depressed levels of consciousness due to drug or alcohol use, seizures, general anesthesia, or central nervous system disease; those with impaired deglutition due to esophageal disease or neurologic disorders; and those with tracheal or nasogastric tubes, which disrupt the mechanical defenses of the airways.

Periodontal disease and poor dental hygiene, which increase the number of anaerobic bacteria in aspirated material, is associated with a greater likelihood of anaerobic pleuropulmonary infection. Aspiration of infected oropharyngeal contents initially leads to pneumonia in dependent lung zones, such as the posterior segments of the upper lobes and superior and basilar segments of the lower lobes. Body position at the time of aspiration determines which lung zones are dependent. The onset of symptoms is insidious. By the time the patient seeks medical attention, necrotizing pneumonia, lung abscess, or empyema may be apparent.

Most aspiration patients with necrotizing pneumonia, lung abscess, and empyema are found to be infected with multiple species of anaerobic bacteria only. Most of the remainder are infected with both anaerobic and aerobic bacteria. *Prevotella melaninogenica,* peptostreptococcus, *Fusobacterium nuclea-*

tum, and bacteroides species are commonly isolated anaerobic bacteria.

Clinical Findings

A. Symptoms and Signs: Patients with anaerobic pleuropulmonary infection usually present with constitutional symptoms such as fever, weight loss, and malaise. Cough with expectoration of foul-smelling purulent sputum suggests anaerobic infection, though the absence of productive cough does not rule out such an infection. Dental hygiene is often poor. Patients are rarely edentulous, but if so, an obstructing bronchial lesion is nearly always present.

B. Laboratory Findings: Expectorated sputum is inappropriate for culture of anaerobic organisms because of contaminating mouth flora. Representative material for culture can be obtained only by transthoracic aspiration, thoracentesis, or bronchoscopy with a protected brush. Transthoracic aspiration is rarely indicated, because anaerobic pleuropulmonary infections usually respond well to empirical therapy.

C. Imaging: The different types of anaerobic pleuropulmonary infection are distinguished on the basis of their radiographic appearance. **Lung abscess** appears as a thick-walled solitary cavity surrounded by consolidation. An air-fluid level is usually present. Other causes of cavitary lung disease (tuberculosis, mycosis, cancer, infarction, Wegener's granulomatosis) should be excluded. **Necrotizing pneumonia** is distinguished by multiple areas of cavitation within an area of consolidation. **Empyema** is characterized by the presence of pleural fluid (purulent on thoracentesis) and may accompany either of the other two radiographic findings. Ultrasonography is of value in locating fluid and may also reveal pleural loculations.

Treatment

Penicillins have often been used as treatment for anaerobic pleuropulmonary infections. However, an increasing number of anaerobic organisms produce beta-lactamases, and up to 20% of patients do not respond to penicillins. Improved responses have been documented with clindamycin (600 mg intravenously every 8 hours until improvement, then 300 mg orally every 6 hours) or amoxicillin-clavulanate (875 mg orally every 12 hours). Penicillin (amoxicillin, 500 mg every 8 hours, or penicillin G, 1–2 million units intravenously every 4–6 hours) plus metronidazole (500 mg orally or intravenously every 8–12 hours) is another option. Antibiotic therapy should be continued until the chest radiograph improves, a process that may take a month or more; patients with lung abscesses should be treated until radiographic resolution of the abscess cavity is demonstrated. Anaerobic pleuropulmonary disease requires adequate drainage with tube thoracostomy for the treatment of empyema. Open pleural drainage is sometimes necessary because of the propensity of these infections to produce loculations in the pleural space.

PULMONARY INFILTRATES IN THE IMMUNOCOMPROMISED HOST

Pulmonary infiltrates in immunocompromised patients may be caused by infectious or noninfectious causes. Pneumonia may be due to bacterial, mycobacterial, fungal, protozoal, helminthic, or viral pathogens. Noninfectious processes such as pulmonary edema, alveolar hemorrhage, drug reactions, pulmonary thromboembolic disease, malignancy, and radiation pneumonitis may mimic infection.

Although almost any pathogen can cause pneumonia in a compromised host, two clinical tools help the clinician narrow the differential diagnosis. The first of these is knowledge of the underlying immunologic defect. Specific types of immunologic defects to particular infections—eg, defects in humoral immunity predispose mainly to bacterial infections; and defects in cellular immunity lead to infections with viruses, fungi, mycobacteria, and protozoa. Neutropenia and impaired granulocyte function predispose to infections from *S aureus,* aspergillus, gram-negative bacilli, and candida. The time course of infection also provides clues to the etiology of pneumonia in immunocompromised patients. A fulminant pneumonia is often caused by bacterial infection, whereas an insidious pneumonia is more apt to be caused by viral, fungal, protozoal, or mycobacterial infection; overlap occurs, however. Pneumonia occurring within 2–4 weeks after organ transplantation is usually bacterial, whereas several months or more after transplantation, infection caused by *P carinii,* viruses (CMV, others), and fungi (aspergillus, others) is encountered more often.

Chest radiography may be helpful in clarifying the differential diagnosis. Diffuse infiltrates are usually seen with pneumocystis or viral pneumonias. Bacterial and fungal infections are typically associated with more focal infiltrates. Examination of expectorated sputum for bacteria, fungi, mycobacteria, legionella, and *P carinii* is important and may preclude the need for an expensive, invasive diagnostic procedure. Sputum induction is often necessary for diagnosis. The sensitivity of induced sputum for detection of *P carinii* depends upon institutional expertise, number of specimens analyzed, and detection methods.

Frequently, routine evaluation fails to identify the causative organism. The clinician must then either begin empirical antimicrobial therapy or proceed to invasive procedures such as bronchoscopy, transthoracic needle aspiration, or open lung biopsy. Selection of the approach to management must be based on the severity of the pulmonary infection, the underlying disease, the risks of empirical therapy, and local expertise and experience with the diagnostic procedures. Bronchoalveolar lavage using the flexible bronchoscope is a safe and effective method for obtaining representative pulmonary secretions for microbiologic studies. It involves less risk of bleeding and other complications than bronchial brushing and transbronchial biopsy. Bronchoalveolar lavage is especially suitable for the diagnosis of *P carinii* pneumonia in patients with AIDS when induced sputum analysis is negative. Open lung biopsy, now often performed by video-assisted thoracoscopy, provides the best opportunity for diagnosis of pulmonary infiltrates in the immunocompromised host. However, information obtained uncommonly affects the outcome. Because a specific diagnosis is obtained in only about two-thirds of cases, empirical treatment is often preferred.

Shelhamer JH et al: The laboratory evaluation of opportunistic pulmonary infections. Ann Intern Med 1996; 124:585. [NLM Cit ID: 965175658] (Discussion of the appropriate specimens and tests for the diagnosis of lung infection in the immunosuppressed patient population.)

PULMONARY TUBERCULOSIS

Essentials of Diagnosis

- Fatigue, weight loss, fever, night sweats, and cough.
- Pulmonary infiltrates on chest radiograph, most often apical.
- Positive tuberculin skin test reaction (most cases).
- Acid-fast bacilli on smear of sputum or sputum culture positive for *Mycobacterium tuberculosis*.

General Considerations

Infection with *M tuberculosis* begins when aerosolized droplets containing viable organisms are inhaled by a person susceptible to the disease. When they reach the lungs, the organisms are ingested by macrophages and either die or persist and multiply. Widespread lymphatic and hematogenous dissemination of organisms occurs before development of an effective immune response. This stage of infection, called **primary tuberculosis,** is usually asymptomatic. Mycobacteria throughout the body are then walled off by granulomatous inflammation, with a few remaining viable in tissues with high oxygen content. At this time, pleural effusion commonly develops at the site of initial infection after droplet inhalation. Uncommonly, the immune response is inadequate, and progressive primary tuberculosis develops, accompanied by both pulmonary and constitutional symptoms. In these patients, hilar and mediastinal lymphadenopathy are prominent. Dormant but viable organisms persist for years, and reactivation of disease in any of these sites may occur if the host's defense mechanisms become impaired. In the past it has been customary to attribute about 90% of cases of tuberculosis in adults to reactivation of disease. However, recent reports of studies using DNA fingerprinting suggest that person-to-person transmission may account for as many as one-third of new cases of tuberculosis in large urban populations. The percentage of patients with atypical presentations—particularly elderly patients, patients with HIV infection, and those in nursing homes—has increased. Extrapulmonary tuberculosis is especially common in patients with HIV infection, who often display lymphadenitis or miliary disease.

Persons infected with the human immunodeficiency virus (HIV), with or without AIDS, are at increased risk of developing tuberculosis. HIV infection has emerged as the most important risk factor for the development of tuberculosis. The increase in the incidence of tuberculosis in the United States, beginning in 1986 but leveling off in the mid nineties, can be attributed to the HIV epidemic and to immigrants from Asia and Central America.

Strains of *M tuberculosis* resistant to one or more first-line antituberculous drugs are being encountered with increasing frequency. Risk factors for drug resistance include immigration from parts of the world with a high prevalence of drug-resistant tuberculosis, close and prolonged contact with individuals with drug-resistant tuberculosis, unsuccessful previous therapy, and patient noncompliance. Resistance to one or more antituberculosis drugs has been found in 15% of tuberculosis patients in the United States. New York City accounts for many of these cases. Outbreaks of multidrug-resistant tuberculosis in hospitals and correctional facilities in Florida and New York have been associated with mortality rates of 70–90% and median survival rates of 4–16 weeks.

Clinical Findings

A. Symptoms and Signs: The patient with reactivation tuberculosis typically presents with constitutional symptoms of fatigue, weight loss, anorexia, low-grade fever, and night sweats. Pulmonary symptoms include cough, which is initially dry but later productive of purulent sputum and often blood. Occasionally, there may be no symptoms. In 5%, the diagnosis is made at autopsy. On physical examination, patients often appear chronically ill and exhibit evidence of weight loss. Examination of the chest may be normal or may reveal findings such as posttussive apical rales.

B. Laboratory Findings: Definitive diagnosis depends on recovery of *M tuberculosis* from cultures or identification of the organism by DNA probe. Three consecutive morning sputum specimens are advised. Sputum induction may be helpful in patients who cannot voluntarily produce satisfactory specimens. The fluorochrome rhodamine-auramine stain of concentrated, digested sputum specimens is performed initially as a screening method, with confirmation by the Kinyoun or Ziehl-Neelsen stains. Demonstration of acid-fast bacilli on sputum smear does not confirm a diagnosis of tuberculosis, since saprophytic nontuberculous mycobacteria may colonize the airways or cause pulmonary disease.

In patients thought to have tuberculosis despite negative sputum smears, fiberoptic bronchoscopy can be considered. Bronchial washings are helpful; however, increased diagnostic yield may require transbronchial lung biopsies. Postbronchoscopy expectorated sputum specimens may also be useful. Early morning aspiration of gastric contents after an overnight fast is an alternative to bronchoscopy but is suitable only for culture and not for stained smear, because nontuberculous mycobacteria may be present in the stomach in the absence of tuberculous infection. *M tuberculosis* may also be cultured from blood. *M tuberculosis* bacteremia has been reported in 15% of patients with tuberculosis.

Cultures on solid media to identify *M tuberculosis* require 6–8 weeks. The polymerase chain reaction permits rapid detection of mycobacterial DNA and differentiation of *M tuberculosis* from other mycobacteria. A radiometric culture system (Bactec) allows detection of mycobacterial growth in several days. Susceptibility testing is now considered routine for the first isolate of *M tuberculosis,* when a treatment regimen is failing, and when sputum cultures remain positive after 3 months of therapy.

DNA fingerprinting using the restriction fragment length polymorphism analysis is available to identify individual strains of *M tuberculosis,* thereby revealing if infection has been transmitted from person to person. This methodology demonstrated that exogenous reinfection with multidrug-resistant tuberculosis has occurred during treatment for drug-susceptible tuberculosis in patients with HIV disease.

Needle biopsy of the pleura reveals granulomas in most patients with pleural effusions caused by *M tuberculosis.* Pleural fluid cultures for *M tuberculosis* are positive in less than 25% of cases of pleural tuberculosis, but culture of the biopsy specimen affords a much higher yield.

C. Imaging: Radiographic abnormalities in primary tuberculosis include small homogeneous infiltrates (usually in the upper lobe), hilar and paratracheal lymph node enlargement, and segmental atelectasis. Pleural effusion may be present, especially in adults, sometimes as the sole radiographic abnormality. Ghon (calcified primary focus) and Ranke (calcified primary focus and calcified hilar lymph node) complexes are detected as residual evidence of healed primary tuberculosis in a minority of patients.

Reactivation tuberculosis is associated with various radiographic manifestations, including fibrocavitary apical disease, nodules, and pneumonic infiltrates. The usual location is in the apical or posterior segments of the upper lobes or in the superior segments of the lower lobes; as many as 30% of patients may present with radiographic evidence of disease in other locations, however. This is especially true in elderly patients, in whom lower lobe infiltrates with or without pleural effusion are encountered with increasing frequency; these in fact may be primary infections. Lower lung tuberculosis, which may also occur with endobronchial tuberculosis, may masquerade as pneumonia or lung cancer. In HIV-infected patients who develop pulmonary tuberculosis, the radiographic features of tuberculosis may vary with the stage of HIV disease. In patients with early HIV infection, the radiographic features of tuberculosis resemble those in patients without HIV infection. In contrast, atypical radiographic features predominate in patients with late stage HIV infection. These patients often display lower lung zone, diffuse, or miliary infiltrates, pleural effusions, and involvement of hilar and, in particular, mediastinal lymph nodes.

D. Special Examinations: The **tuberculin skin test** identifies individuals who have been infected at some time with *M tuberculosis* but does not distinguish between current disease and past infection. The standard Mantoux test establishes exposure to tuberculosis in individuals, while the multiple puncture test is used for population screening. In the Mantoux test, 0.1 mL of standard purified protein derivative (PPD-S), containing 5 TU, is injected intradermally on the volar surface of the forearm using a 27-gauge needle on a tuberculin syringe. The transverse width (in millimeters) of the induration at the skin test site should be recorded after 48–72 hours. A negative reaction does not rule out the diagnosis of tuberculosis. Table 9–12 summarizes American Thoracic Society criteria for interpretation of the Mantoux tuberculin skin test.

Both false-positive and false-negative tuberculin reactions occur. False-positive reactions are due to infection with nontuberculous mycobacteria. False-negative reactions occur because of concurrent infection, malnutrition, old age, immunologic disorders, lymphoreticular malignancies, corticosteroid therapy, chronic renal failure, virus vaccinations or infections, fulminant tuberculosis, and improper testing technique. Patients with AIDS are commonly anergic.

"Boosting" of the skin test reaction by serial testing may cause a false impression of conversion, as dormant mycobacterial sensitivity is restored by the antigenic challenge of the initial skin test. This boosting phenomenon may increase the reaction size on a subsequent tuberculin test and is most commonly seen in those over age 55. A two-step testing procedure may identify a boosted tuberculin reaction. If the initial test is negative, it may be repeated a week later. If the second test result is negative, the person is uninfected or anergic. If it is positive, a boosted reaction is most likely. This effect may persist for at least 1 year. BCG (extract of *Mycobacterium bovis*) vaccination renders the PPD positive for at least 1 year. Thereafter, interpretation of the PPD skin test should be the same as for those who have not had BCG. An anergy skin test panel should be placed at the time of tuberculin testing if the patient is judged likely to be anergic for any reason.

Table 9–12. Classification of positive tuberculin skin test reactions.[1,2]

Reaction Size	Group
≥ 5 mm	1. Persons with HIV infection or those at risk for HIV infection, including injection drug users. 2. Close contacts of individuals with active tuberculosis. 3. Persons with chest x-rays suggestive of prior healed tuberculosis.
≥ 10 mm	1. From countries with a high prevalence of tuberculosis (eg, Asia, Africa, Latin America). 2. HIV-negative intravenous drug users. 3. Medically underserved, low income populations, including blacks, Hispanics, and Native Americans. 4. Long-term residents of correctional institutions, nursing homes, and mental institutions. 5. Persons with the following medical conditions that increase the risk of tuberculosis: gastrectomy, ≥ 10% below ideal body weight, jejunoileal bypass, diabetes mellitus, silicosis, chronic renal failure, corticosteroid or other immunosuppressive therapy, leukemia, lymphoma, and other malignancies.
≥ 15 mm	6. All other persons.

[1]Recommendations of American Thoracic Society: Am Rev Respir Dis 1990;142:725.

[2]A Mantoux skin test reaction is considered positive if the transverse diameter of the indurated area reaches the size required for the specific group. All other reactions are considered negative.

Treatment

All possible or proved cases of tuberculosis should be reported to local and state public health departments. Treatment of patients with tuberculosis should be conducted by physicians who are skilled and highly experienced in the management of this condition. This is especially important in cases of drug-resistant tuberculosis.

A. Hospitalization: Hospitalization for initial therapy of tuberculosis is not necessary in most patients, though it should be considered if a patient is incapable of self-care or is likely to expose new susceptible individuals to the risk of tuberculosis. Hospitalized patients with active disease require a private room with appropriate ventilation until they become sputum smear-negative for acid-fast bacilli.

B. Drug Therapy: (Tables 9–13 and 9–14.) (See also Chapter 33.) Standard therapy regimens for pulmonary infection due to *M tuberculosis* consider the increase in prevalence of drug-resistant tuberculosis in the United States. The treatment recommendations of the Centers for Disease Control and Prevention (CDC) for the initial empirical treatment of tuberculosis are summarized in Table 9–13, and recommended drug dosages are listed in Table 9–14. For patients without HIV infection, three options are suggested by the CDC:

1. The first option is a four-drug regimen consisting of isoniazid, rifampin, pyrazinamide, and either ethambutol or streptomycin. Therapy may be given daily or two or three times weekly if directly

Table 9–13. Recommended options for the initial treatment of tuberculosis.[1]

Tuberculosis Without HIV Infection			Tuberculosis With HIV Infection
Option 1	Option 2	Option 3	
Administer daily isoniazid, rifampin, and pyrazinamide for 8 weeks, followed by 16 weeks of isoniazid and rifampin daily or twice or three times weekly.[2] In areas where the isoniazid resistance rate is not documented to be < 4%, ethambutol or streptomycin should be added to the initial regimen until susceptibility to isoniazid and rifampin is demonstrated. Continue treatment for at least 6 months and 3 months beyond culture conversion. Consult a tuberculosis medical expert if the patient is symptomatic or if smear or culture is positive after 3 months.	Administer daily isoniazid, rifampin, pyrazinamide, and streptomycin or ethambutol for 2 weeks followed by twice-weekly[2] directly observed administration of the same drugs for 6 weeks, and subsequently with twice-weekly directly observed administration of isoniazid and rifampin for 16 weeks. Consult a tuberculosis medical expert if the patient is symptomatic or if smear or culture is positive after 3 months.	Treat by directly observed therapy three times a week[2] with isoniazid, rifampin, pyrazinamide, and ethambutol or streptomycin for 6 months.[3] Consult a tuberculosis medical expert if the patient is symptomatic or if the smear or culture is positive after 3 months.	Options 1, 2, or 3 can be used, but treatment regimens should continue for a total of 9 months and at least 6 months beyond culture conversion.

[1]Modified from: Initial therapy for tuberculosis in the era of multidrug resistance. Recommendations of the Advisory Council for the Elimination of Tuberculosis. MMWR Morbid Mortal Wkly Rep 1993;42(RR-7):1.

[2]All regimens administered twice or three times a week should be monitored by direct observation for the duration of therapy.

[3]The strongest evidence from clinical trials is for the effectiveness of all four drugs administered for the full 6 months. There is weaker evidence that streptomycin can be discontinued after 4 months if the isolate is susceptible to all drugs. The evidence for stopping pyrazinamide before the end of 6 months is equivocal for the thrice-weekly regimen, and there is no evidence for effectiveness of this regimen with ethambutol for less than the full 6 months.

taken an aggressive approach using a combination of agents, but these have been associated with a high incidence of drug-induced side effects. Adherence to such regimens is also difficult. Non-HIV-infected patients with MAC pulmonary disease usually receive a combination of daily clarithromycin or azithromycin, rifampin or rifabutin, and ethambutol. Streptomycin is considered for the first 2 months as tolerated. The optimal duration of treatment is unknown, but therapy should be continued for 12 months after sputum conversion. Medical treatment is initially successful in about two-thirds of cases, but relapses after treatment are common; long-term benefit is demonstrated in about half of all patients. Those who do not respond favorably generally have active but stable disease. Surgical resection is an alternative for the patient with progressive disease that responds poorly to chemotherapy; the success rate with surgical therapy is favorable.

A National Registry for Nontuberculous Mycobacterial Diseases has been established at the National Jewish Medical and Research Center in Denver (800-222-LUNG).

Diagnosis and treatment of disease caused by nontuberculous mycobacteria. Am J Respir Crit Care Med 1997;156(2 Part 2):S1. [NLM Cit ID: 97425234] (Reviews diagnostic criteria and treatment approaches for nontuberculous mycobacterial disease.)

French AL et al: Nontuberculous mycobacterial infections. Med Clin North Am 1997;81:361. [NLM Cit ID: 97247099] (Clinical syndromes and therapeutic options for nontuberculous mycobacterial disease.)

PULMONARY NODULES, MASSES, & TUMORS

SOLITARY PULMONARY NODULE

A solitary pulmonary nodule is a round or oval, more or less sharply circumscribed pulmonary lesion (up to 5 cm in diameter; larger lesions are termed "masses") surrounded by normal lung tissue. Central cavitation, calcification, or surrounding ("satellite") lesions may occur. Although mass population screening for lung cancer by chest radiograph is not advised, the finding of a solitary pulmonary nodule on chest radiograph in an individual patient is important. About 25% of cases of bronchogenic carcinoma present as solitary pulmonary nodules, and the 5-year survival rate for bronchogenic carcinoma that is detected in this form approaches 50%, which is considerably higher than the 10–15% 5-year survival rate of lung cancer overall.

In large surgical series, about 60% of solitary pulmonary nodules are benign lesions and 40% are malignant. Infectious granulomas account for most benign lesions, whereas primary lung cancer accounts for more than three-quarters of all malignant solitary pulmonary nodules. Solitary pulmonary nodules occasionally represent metastases from another primary tumor (see below).

Determining whether the lesion is likely to be benign or malignant preoperatively is more important than establishing other causes. Radiographic studies and *comparisons with old chest radiographs* are essential.

A lesion is almost certainly benign if the volume doubling time is less than 30 days or more than 500 days or if the lesion is calcified (central, "clustered," or laminated calcium pattern). Factors favoring a benign diagnosis are young age, absence of symptoms, small size (< 2 cm in diameter), smooth margins on CT, and presence of satellite lesions, but none of these criteria are foolproof. Malignant solitary pulmonary nodules are occasionally symptomatic, tend to occur in patients over 45 years of age, are usually larger than 2 cm, often have indistinct margins, and are rarely calcified. Typical features of solitary pulmonary metastases include smooth or lobulated margins, peripheral location, location in the lower lobe, and absence of satellite lesions.

Benign neoplasms of the lung typically present as asymptomatic solitary pulmonary nodules detected on routine chest radiography. They account for about 2% of all solitary pulmonary nodules. Hamartoma is the most common benign lung tumor. Fibromas, lipomas, leiomyomas, hemangiomas, and papillomas account for most of the remainder. The clustered ("popcorn") pattern of calcification on chest radiograph or CT scans is a helpful diagnostic clue to hamartoma. The medical history, physical examination, and radiographic studies do not permit reliable differentiation of malignant and benign lung tumors.

Skin tests and serologic studies for fungal infection are generally not helpful. Cytologic examination of sputum should be considered for evaluation of a large centrally located pulmonary nodule; a positive result might preclude the need for bronchoscopy or needle biopsy. However, sputum cytology is rarely diagnostic of malignancy in small or peripheral pulmonary nodules. CT scanning is particularly useful. High-resolution (1.5–5 mm) CT scanning is the preferred method for detection of calcification within the nodule. Investigations for primary cancer elsewhere in the body are not indicated unless abnormal symptoms, signs, and results of simple laboratory studies (complete blood count and differential, urinalysis, stool sample for occult blood) suggest an extrapulmonary cancer. Routine percutaneous needle aspiration of all solitary pulmonary nodules is not advised; it seldom changes subsequent therapy, and false negatives are common. A specific benign diagnosis from a percutaneous needle biopsy is obtained infrequently except in a few centers with great expertise in this procedure. Therefore, in most cases this procedure cannot be justified with the expectation that a specific benign diagnosis will be obtained. Furthermore, if the history, physical examination, and radiographic and laboratory studies indicate that the patient is a candidate for surgical resection, a separate preoperative fiberoptic bronchoscopic procedure for staging purposes is not necessary.

Treatment

The best approaches to this problem are watchful waiting, fiberoptic bronchoscopy, percutaneous needle aspiration, and resection. All solitary nodules in patients over age 35 should be considered potentially malignant and should be resected unless calcification typical of benign lesions or stability on radiography for 2 years is documented. Prospective evaluation is not appropriate if calcification is not present or if stability cannot be documented.

Strong indications of a benign diagnosis or contraindications to surgery justify a conservative approach. Otherwise, exploratory thoracotomy is advised. **Video-assisted thoracoscopy** is a safe and accurate way to perform a number of thoracic surgical procedures that previously required thoracotomy, including resection of solitary pulmonary nodules. The morbidity and mortality rates of this procedure are much less than those reported with standard thoracotomy.

Dholakia S, Rappaport DC: The solitary pulmonary nodule. Is it malignant or benign? Postgrad Med 1996;99:246. [NLM Cit ID: 96223918] (A brief review of diagnostic strategies.)

Lillington GA: Management of solitary pulmonary nodules: How to decide when resection is required. Postgrad Med 1997;101:145. [NLM Cit ID: 97228477] (Practical approach to management.)

BRONCHOGENIC CARCINOMA

Essentials of Diagnosis

- Cough, dyspnea, hemoptysis, anorexia, or weight loss.
- Enlarging mass, infiltrate, atelectasis, cavitation, or pleural effusion on chest radiograph or CT scan.
- Cytologic or histologic findings diagnostic of (primary) lung cancer in sputum, pleural fluid, or tissue.

General Considerations

Nearly 180,000 new cases of lung cancer are expected in the USA in 2001. Lung cancer accounts for 32% of cancer deaths in men and 25% of cancer deaths in women, and its incidence in women is rising rapidly. Most cases present between the ages of 50 and 70. Fewer than 5% of lung cancer patients are under 40 years of age. Cigarette smoking is the most important cause of lung cancer in both men and women in the USA. Secondhand smoke, ionizing radiation (indoor radon gas, therapeutic radiation), asbestos, heavy metals (nickel, chromium), and industrial carcinogens (chloromethyl ether) are established but less potent pulmonary carcinogens. Lung scars, air pollution, and genetic factors are also implicated, but the data supporting these associations are not conclusive. Chronic obstructive pulmonary disease may represent a risk factor for lung cancer even after controlling for cigarette smoking. Primary lung cancer in nonsmokers is uncommon.

More than 20 benign and malignant primary neoplasms of the lung have been identified and classified histologically. Ninety percent of malignant cancers belong to one of the four major cell types of bronchogenic carcinoma, a term denoting primary malignant tumors of the airway epithelium.

Squamous cell carcinoma and **adenocarcinoma** are the most common types of bronchogenic carcinoma and account for about 30–35% of primary tumors each. **Small cell carcinoma** and **large cell carcinoma** account for about 20–25% and 15%, respectively. Other malignant epithelial tumors of the lung include adenosquamous carcinoma, carcinoid tumor, bronchial gland carcinomas, and other rare tumors.

Squamous cell carcinoma of the lung tends to originate in the central bronchi as an intraluminal growth and is thus more amenable to early detection through cytologic examination of sputum than are the other types of carcinoma. Squamous cell carcinoma tends to metastasize to regional lymph nodes. About 10% cavitate. Small cell carcinoma also occurs centrally and tends to narrow bronchi by extrinsic compression; widespread metastases are common. Adenocarcinoma and large-cell carcinoma usually appear in the periphery of the lung and therefore are not amenable to early detection through examination of sputum. They typically metastasize to distant organs. **Bronchioloalveolar cell carcinoma,** a subtype of adenocarcinoma, is a low-grade carcinoma that represents about 2% of cases of bronchogenic carcinoma and presents as single or multiple pulmonary nodules or an alveolar infiltrate.

Early detection of lung cancer in an asymptomatic stage is feasible with cytologic examination of sputum and chest radiography. However, the mortality rate from lung cancer is not appreciably reduced by early detection except for peripheral coin lesions.

Clinical Findings

The clinical features of lung cancer depend on the primary cancer itself, its metastases, systemic effects of the cancer, and any coexisting paraneoplastic syndromes.

A. Symptoms and Signs: Only 10–25% of patients are asymptomatic at the time of diagnosis of lung cancer. Symptomatic lung cancer is generally advanced and often not resectable. Initial symptoms include nonspecific complaints such as cough, weight loss, dyspnea, chest pain, and hemoptysis. Physical findings vary and may be totally absent. Central tumors that obstruct segmental, lobar, or main stem bronchi may cause atelectasis and postobstructive pneumonitis with typical physical findings. Peripheral tumors may cause no abnormalities on physical examination. Extension of the tumor to the pleural surface may cause pleural effusion. Lymphadenopathy, hepatomegaly, and clubbing are present in about 20% of patients with lung cancer. Superior vena cava syndrome, **Horner's syndrome** (miosis, ptosis, enophthalmos, and loss of sweating on the affected side), **Pancoast's syndrome** (neurovascular complications of superior pulmonary sulcus tumor), recurrent laryngeal nerve palsy with hoarseness, phrenic nerve palsy with hemidiaphragm paralysis, and skin metastases are each seen in fewer than 5% of cases.

Paraneoplastic syndromes (extrapulmonary organ dysfunction not related to effects of the primary or metastases) occur in 15–20% of lung cancer patients (see Chapter 4). A number of tumor secretory products have been associated with lung cancer. The manifestations of paraneoplastic syndromes may precede, coincide with, or follow the diagnosis of lung cancer. Recognition of paraneoplastic syndromes in lung cancer is important, because treatment of the associated symptoms may improve the patient's well-being even though the primary tumor itself is not curable; occasionally, resection of the tumor is followed by immediate resolution of the paraneoplastic syndrome. Table 9–16 lists important paraneoplastic syndromes associated with lung cancer.

B. Laboratory Findings: Definitive diagnosis requires histologic evidence of cancer. Cytologic examination of expectorated sputum permits definitive diagnosis of lung cancer in up to 80% of centrally located tumors but less than 20% of peripheral nodules. A diagnosis of lung cancer by sputum cytologic examination may spare the patient the need for bronchoscopy or another invasive procedure. Examination of pleural fluid reveals cytologic findings positive for cancer in 40–50% of patients with malignant pleural effusion from lung cancer. Pleural biopsy yields a histologic diagnosis of cancer in about 55% of patients. Biopsy and cytologic study of pleural fluid combined establish a diagnosis of cancer in about 80% of patients with malignant pleural effusion.

Tissue for histologic confirmation of lung cancer may be obtained by various techniques, including bronchoscopy, percutaneous needle aspirate, mediastinoscopy, lymph node biopsy, or biopsy of other metastatic sites (eg, skin), and thoracotomy. Fine-needle aspiration of supraclavicular or cervical lymph nodes is useful if these nodes are enlarged on palpation. Thoracotomy is occasionally necessary to diagnose lung cancer when simpler cytologic and histologic evaluations are negative.

Table 9–16. Paraneoplastic syndromes in lung cancer.

Classification	Syndrome	Common Histologic Type of Cancer
Endocrine and metabolic	Cushing's syndrome	Small cell
	Inappropriate secretion of antidiuretic hormone (SIADH)	Small cell
	Hypercalcemia	Squamous cell
	Gynecomastia	Large cell
Connective tissue and osseous	Clubbing and hypertrophic pulmonary osteoarthropathy	Squamous cell, adenocarcinoma, large cell
Neuromuscular	Peripheral neuropathy (sensory, sensorimotor)	Small cell
	Subacute cerebellar degeneration	Small cell
	Myasthenia (Eaton-Lambert syndrome)	Small cell
	Dermatomyositis	All
Cardiovascular	Thrombophlebitis	Adenocarcinoma
	Nonbacterial verrucous (marantic) endocarditis	
Hematologic	Anemia	All
	Disseminated intravascular coagulation	
	Eosinophilia	
	Thrombocytosis	
Cutaneous	Acanthosis nigricans	All
	Erythema gyratum repens	

C. Imaging: Chest radiography demonstrates abnormal findings in nearly all patients with lung cancer. Comparison of old and current chest radiographs is especially important.

Radiographic abnormalities in primary lung cancer are not specific. Common abnormalities are hilar masses or enlargement, peripheral masses, atelectasis, infiltrates, cavitation, and pleural effusions. Multiple masses, consolidation, and chest wall involvement are unusual. Squamous cell and small cell carcinomas commonly produce a hilar mass and mediastinal widening. Cavitation suggests squamous cell carcinoma and is exceedingly rare in small cell carcinoma. Small peripheral masses usually are adenocarcinomas; larger lesions are more often large-cell tumors.

CT scanning, MRI, and ultrasound are useful imaging methods in selected patients with suspected or proved lung cancer. All depend upon initial detection of a suspicious lesion on the chest radiograph. CT scanning is particularly useful for evaluation of the lung parenchyma and pleura. MRI may be used for staging the mediastinum when use of an iodinated contrast agent is contraindicated.

D. Special Examinations: Staging of lung cancer utilizes the TNM international staging system for lung carcinoma, which was revised in 1996. In this system, T describes the primary tumor, N the nodal involvement, and M any distant metastases (Table 9–17). Small cell carcinoma is not evaluated by the TNM system but staged as limited (tumor confined to one hemithorax and hilar, mediastinal, and supraclavicular nodes) or extensive (spread to more distant sites). CT scan of the lungs, mediastinum, and upper abdomen (liver, adrenal glands, and periaortic lymph nodes) is usually helpful in staging lung cancer. In a patient with known lung cancer, the finding of mediastinal lymph nodes larger than 2 cm in diameter on CT scan is strong evidence of mediastinal spread of the tumor; however, occasional false-positive results occur with this technique. Nodes smaller than 1 cm have a low probability of tumor involvement. At least 85% of lung cancer patients with negative results on mediastinal CT scans have no evidence of mediastinal lymphadenopathy at the time of surgery.

History, physical examination, and simple laboratory studies are usually sufficient to detect metastases to distant sites such as liver, brain, bone, heart, abdomen, and skin. Patients with skeletal complaints should have bone radiographs. If these are negative, a radionuclide bone scan should be ordered. Radionuclide bone scanning for asymptomatic skeletal metastases is sensitive but lacks specificity. Those with abnormal central nervous system findings should have a CT scan or MRI of the brain. The latter is preferred for infratentorial lesions. Routine CT scanning of the brain is not indicated in lung cancer patients with no clinical features of brain metastases. In patients with adenocarcinoma of the lung, however, some authorities still advocate this procedure if the patient is a candidate for pulmonary resection.

Surgical exploration of the mediastinum from the suprasternal or parasternal approach should be strongly considered before thoracotomy if radiographic studies suggest significant mediastinal lymphadenopathy or direct extension of the lung cancer into the mediastinum. This approach reduces the number of thoracotomies that do not permit curative lung resection.

Complications

A. Superior Vena Cava Syndrome: See Chapter 12.

B. Phrenic Nerve Palsy: Tumor destruction of the phrenic nerve, which courses through the mediastinum to innervate the hemidiaphragm, occurs in about 1% of patients with lung cancer and results in hemidiaphragmatic paralysis.

C. Recurrent Laryngeal Nerve Palsy: Recurrent laryngeal nerve palsy due to destruction of the recurrent laryngeal nerve by tumor causes paralysis of the muscles of the larynx, resulting in hoarseness. This palsy almost always occurs on the left side and is seen in fewer than 3% of patients with lung cancer.

Treatment

The main treatment options in lung cancer include surgery, chemotherapy, and radiation therapy. Photoresection with the Nd:YAG laser is sometimes performed on obstructing central tumors to relieve obstruction, improve dyspnea and control hemoptysis.

Surgery remains the treatment of choice for patients with non-small cell carcinoma. Only about 25% of patients with lung cancer are appropriate candidates for surgery, and many of these are found to have unresectable disease at the time of thoracotomy. Contraindications to surgery include extrathoracic metastases; tumor involving the trachea, carina, or proximal main stem bronchi (< 2 cm from the carina); malignant pleural effusion; recurrent laryngeal nerve or phrenic nerve palsy; superior vena cava syndrome; tumor involving the esophagus or pericardium; spread to contralateral mediastinal lymph nodes; poor general health; markedly impaired pulmonary function (see below); and extensive involvement of the chest wall. Brain metastases of bronchogenic carcinoma have traditionally been considered unresectable and managed with radiation therapy and corticosteroids. However, there may be improved quality of life when selected patients with *solitary* brain metastases are treated with surgical resection followed by radiation therapy compared to those given radiation therapy alone. Survival was not affected.

Patients with lung cancer often have severe obstructive pulmonary dysfunction. Therefore, pulmonary function testing and measurement of arterial blood gases should be performed before lung resection. The preferred approach is to estimate the postresection FEV_1, using preoperative spirometry and a quantitative lung perfusion scan. The percentage of total perfusion that will remain after resection is estimated and multiplied by the optimal preoperative FEV_1. Values greater than 800 mL or 40% of predicted FEV_1 suggest that the patient will have adequate postoperative ventilatory function. However, the accuracy of such predictions has been questioned, and the cost of ventilation/perfusion lung scanning must be taken into consideration. Patients with hypercapnia ($Paco_2$ > 45 mm Hg) and those with significant pulmonary hypertension are in general not good candidates for lung resection. Older patients with severe COPD are especially likely to be functionally inoperable.

In patients with non-small cell carcinoma, adjuvant therapy (chemotherapy, radiation therapy, or both given in the postoperative period) has been disappointing. Single agent chemotherapy given postoperatively is of no value. In patients with stage II and stage III adenocarcinoma and large cell carcinoma, chemotherapy with a combination of three drugs for

Table 9–17. TNM staging for lung cancer.[1]

Stage	T	N	M
0	Tis		
IA	T1	N0	M0
IB	T2	N0	M0
IIA	T1	N1	M0
IIB	T2	N1	M0
	T3	N0	M0
IIIA	T3	N1	M0
	T1	N2	M0
	T2	N2	M0
	T3	N2	M0
IIIB	T4	N0	M0
	T4	N1	M0
	T4	N2	M0
	T1	N3	M0
	T2	N3	M0
	T3	N3	M0
	T4	N3	M0
IV	Any	Any	M1

Primary Tumor (T)

TX	Primary tumor cannot be assessed; or tumor proved by the presence of malignant cells in sputum or bronchial washings but not visualized by imaging or bronchoscopy.
T0	No evidence of primary tumor.
Tis	Carcinoma in situ.
T1	A tumor ≤ 3 cm in greatest dimension, surrounded by lung or visceral pleura, and without evidence of invasion proximal to a lobar bronchus at bronchoscopy.
T2	A tumor > 3.0 cm in greatest dimension, or a tumor of any size that either involves a main bronchus (but is ≥ 2 cm distal to the carina), invades the visceral pleura, or has associated atelectasis or obstructive pneumonitis extending to the hilar region. Any associated atelectasis or obstructive pneumonitis must involve less than an entire lung.
T3	A tumor of any size with direct extension into the chest wall (including superior sulcus tumors), the diaphragm, the mediastinal pleura, or the parietal pericardium; or a tumor in the main bronchus < 2 cm distal to the carina without involving the carina; or associated atelectasis or obstructive pneumonitis of the entire lung.
T4	A tumor of any size with invasion of the mediastinum, heart, great vessels, trachea, esophagus, vertebral body, or carina; or with a malignant pleural or pericardial effusion; or with satellite tumor nodules within the ipsilateral lobe of the lung containing the primary tumor.

Regional Lymph Nodes (N)

NX	Regional lymph nodes cannot be assessed.
N0	No demonstrable metastasis to regional lymph nodes.
N1	Metastasis to lymph nodes in the peribronchial or the ipsilateral hilar region, or both, including direct extension.
N2	Metastasis to ipsilateral mediastinal lymph nodes and/or subcarinal lymph nodes.
N3	Metastasis to contralateral mediastinal lymph nodes, contralateral hilar lymph nodes, ipsilateral or contralateral scalene or supraclavicular lymph nodes.

Distant Metastases (M)

MX	Presence of distant metastasis cannot be assessed.
M0	No (known) distant metastasis.
M1	Distant metastasis present.

[1]Adapted from Mountain CF: Revisions in the international system for staging lung cancer. Chest 1997;111:1710.

completely resected tumors apparently increases disease-free survival. In patients with incompletely resected non-small cell carcinoma, postoperative radiation therapy is frequently administered, and the disease-free survival may be further extended when postoperative radiation therapy is used with multidrug chemotherapy. Likewise, neoadjuvant therapy (combination chemotherapy given prior to surgical resection) may improve resectability and survival in patients with non-small cell carcinoma. Although tumor regression in non-small cell carcinoma is possible with combination chemotherapy, median survival is improved only modestly, often at the expense of considerable drug toxicity.

In unresectable non-small-cell carcinoma, radiation therapy combined with cisplatin-based chemotherapy appears to be superior to radiation therapy alone in regional control of tumor. Cisplatin is thought to increase sensitization to radiation.

Combination chemotherapy (see Chapter 4) is the treatment of choice for small cell carcinoma and results in considerable improvement in median survival. Single-agent chemotherapy has no proved value. Occasionally, posttreatment surgical debulking of primary lesions is carried out. Prophylactic cranial radiation is performed in patients with small cell carcinoma who have responded to chemotherapy.

Radiation therapy is often used to palliate symptoms of lung cancer such as cough, hemoptysis, pain due to bone metastases, and dyspnea from bronchial or tracheal obstruction. It is also employed to treat bronchial obstruction (atelectasis, pneumonia). Laser therapy is superior when the obstructing lesion is in a main stem bronchus. Radiation is also useful to treat superior vena cava syndrome resulting from non-small cell carcinoma; small cell carcinoma may be treated with chemotherapy or radiation. Symptomatic brain metastases are treated with radiation therapy and corticosteroids. Selected patients with unresectable lung cancer also receive external beam radiation to the primary tumor site. In patients with limited-stage small cell carcinoma, this improves complete response rates and survival when compared to chemotherapy alone. However, in non-small cell lung cancer, survival is not improved. Intraluminal radiation ("brachytherapy") is an alternative approach to relief of symptoms of recurrent endobronchial lung cancer.

Prognosis

The overall 5-year survival rate for lung cancer is 10–15%. Determinants of survival include the stage of disease at the time of presentation (Table 9–18), the patient's general health, age, histologic type of tumor, tumor growth rate, and type of therapy. Overall, the 5-year survival rate after "curative" resection of squamous cell carcinoma is 35–40%, compared with 25% for adenocarcinoma and large cell carcinoma. Patients with small cell carcinoma rarely live for 5 years after the diagnosis is made, regardless of therapy. As patients approach the end of life, meticulous efforts at palliative care are essential (see Chapter 5).

Table 9–18. Approximate 5-year survival rate of treated patients with lung cancer by TNM stage.

TNM Stage	Survival
Occult carcinoma	70–80%
0	No data available
I	50%
II	30%
IIIA	10–15%
IIIB	< 5%
IV	< 2%

Cook RM, Miller YE (editors): Lung cancer: Future directions. Semin Respir Crit Care Med 1996;17:283. (Tobacco control, smoking cessation, early detection, staging, treatment, and other topics.)

McVie JG (editor): NSCLC: Planning for the future. Chest 1996;109(Suppl):S79. [NLM Cit ID: 96256723] (A compendium of 14 articles on non-small-cell lung cancer.)

Mountain CF, Dresler CM: Regional lymph node classification for lung cancer staging. Chest 1997;111:1718. [NLM Cit ID: 97330740]

Mountain CF: Revisions in the international system for staging lung cancer. Chest 1997;111:1710. [NLM Cit ID: 97330739]

Strauss GM, Gleason RE, Sugarbaker DJ: Screening for lung cancer: Another look; a different view. Chest 1997;111:754. [NLM Cit ID: 97236155] (Review of prospective trials of lung cancer screening suggests that periodic chest radiograph screening may be appropriate for high-risk individuals.)

BRONCHIAL CARCINOID TUMORS

Carcinoid and bronchial gland tumors are sometimes termed bronchial adenomas, but this classification is a misnomer, because it implies that the lesions are benign, when in fact carcinoid tumors and bronchial gland carcinomas are low-grade malignant neoplasms.

Carcinoid tumors are about six times more common than bronchial gland carcinomas, and most of them occur as pedunculated or sessile growths in central bronchi. Men and women are equally affected. Most patients are under 60 years of age. Common symptoms of bronchial carcinoid tumors are hemoptysis, cough, wheezing, and recurrent pneumonia. Peripherally located bronchial carcinoid tumors are rare and present as asymptomatic solitary pulmonary nodules. Carcinoid syndrome (flushing, diarrhea, wheezing, hypotension, etc) is rare. Fiberoptic bronchoscopy reveals a pink or purple tumor in a central airway, and biopsy may be complicated by significant bleeding, because these lesions have a well-vascularized stroma. CT scanning is helpful to localize the lesion and to follow its growth over time. Octreotide scintigraphy is also available for localization of these tumors.

Bronchial carcinoid tumors grow slowly and rarely metastasize. Complications involve bleeding and airway obstruction rather than invasion by tumor and metastases. Surgical excision is necessary in some cases, and the prognosis is generally favorable. Most bronchial carcinoid tumors are resistant to radiation and chemotherapy.

Christin-Maitre S et al: Use of somatostatin analog for localization and treatment of ACTH secreting bronchial carcinoid tumor. Chest 1996;109:845. [NLM Cit ID: 96181832] (Octreotide scintigraphy.)

SECONDARY LUNG CANCER

Secondary lung cancers represent metastases from extrapulmonary malignant neoplasms that spread to the lungs through vascular or lymphatic channels or by direct extension. Almost any cancer can metastasize to the lung. Metastases usually occur via the pulmonary artery and are typically multiple masses on chest radiography. The radiographic differential diagnosis of multiple pulmonary nodules includes pulmonary arteriovenous malformation, pulmonary abscesses, granulomatous infection, sarcoidosis, rheumatoid nodules, and Wegener's granulomatosis in addition to malignancy. Metastases to the lungs are found in 20–55% of patients dying of various malignancies. Most are intraparenchymal. Endobronchial metastases occur in fewer than 5% of patients dying of nonpulmonary cancer; carcinoma of the kidney, breast, colon, and cervix and malignant melanoma are the most likely primary tumors.

Lymphangitic carcinoma denotes diffuse involvement of the pulmonary lymphatic network by secondary lung cancer, probably a result of extension of tumor from lung capillaries to the lymphatics. **Tumor embolization** from extrapulmonary cancer (renal cell carcinoma, hepatocellular carcinoma, choriocarcinoma) is an uncommon route for tumor spread to the lungs. Secondary lung cancer may also present as malignant pleural effusion (see below).

Clinical Findings

A. Symptoms and Signs: Symptoms are uncommon but include cough, hemoptysis, and, in advanced cases, dyspnea. Symptoms are more often referable to the site of the primary tumor.

B. Laboratory Findings: The diagnosis of secondary lung cancer is usually established by identifying a primary tumor. Appropriate studies should be ordered if there is a suspicion of any primary cancer, such as breast, thyroid, testis, or prostate, for which specific treatment is available. Mammography should be considered unless one has been performed recently. If the history and physical examination fail to reveal the site of the primary tumor, attention is better focused on the lung, where tissue samples obtained by bronchoscopy, needle biopsy, or thoracotomy establish the histologic diagnosis and suggest the most likely primary. Occasionally, cytologic studies of pleural fluid or pleural biopsy reveal the diagnosis. Sputum cytology is rarely helpful.

C. Imaging: Chest radiographs usually show multiple spherical densities with sharp margins. The size of metastatic lesions varies from a few millimeters (miliary densities) to large masses. Nearly all are less than 5 cm in diameter. The lesions are usually bilateral, pleural or subpleural in location, and more common in lower lung zones. Cavitation suggests primary squamous cell tumor; calcification suggests osteosarcoma. Conventional chest radiography is less sensitive than CT scan in detecting pulmonary metastases.

Lymphangitic spread and solitary pulmonary nodule are less common radiographic presentations of secondary lung cancer.

Treatment

Once the diagnosis has been established (usually by percutaneous needle biopsy or transbronchial biopsy), management consists of treatment of the primary neoplasm and any pulmonary complications. Surgical resection of a *solitary* pulmonary nodule is often prudent in the patient with known current or previous extrapulmonary cancer. Local resection of one or more pulmonary metastases is feasible in a few carefully selected patients with various sarcomas and carcinomas (breast, testis, colon, kidney, and head and neck). Surgical resection should be considered only if the primary tumor is under control, if the patient is a good surgical risk, if all of the metastatic tumor can be resected, if nonsurgical approaches are not available, and if there are no metastases elsewhere in the body. Relative contraindications to resection of pulmonary metastases include (1) malignant melanoma primary, (2) requirement for pneumonectomy, (3) pleural involvement, and (4) simultaneous appearance of two or more metastases. The overall 5-year survival rate in secondary lung cancer treated surgically is 20–35%. For patients with progressive disease, diligent attention to palliative care is essential (see Chapter 5).

MESOTHELIOMA

Mesotheliomas are primary tumors arising from the surface lining of the pleura (80% of cases) or peritoneum (20% of cases). About three-fourths of pleural mesotheliomas are diffuse (usually malignant) tumors, and the remaining one-fourth are localized (usually benign). Men outnumber women by a 3:1 ratio. Numerous studies have confirmed the association of **malignant pleural mesothelioma** with exposure to asbestos (particularly the crocidolite form). The lifetime risk to asbestos workers of developing malignant pleural mesothelioma is about 8%. The clinician should inquire about asbestos exposure through mining, milling, manufacturing, shipyard work, insulation, brake linings, building construction and demolition, roofing materials, and a variety of asbestos products (pipe, textiles, paint, tile, gaskets, panels). Sixty to 80 percent of patients with malignant mesothelioma report a history of asbestos exposure. Although cigarette smoking increases the risk of bronchogenic carcinoma in asbestos workers and aggravates asbestosis, there is no association between smoking and mesothelioma.

The mean age at onset of symptoms of malignant pleural mesothelioma is about 60 years. The latent period between exposure and onset of symptoms ranges from 20 to 40 years. Symptoms include the insidious onset of shortness of breath, nonpleuritic chest pain, and weight loss. Physical findings include dullness to percussion, diminished breath sounds, and, in some cases, finger clubbing. Radiographic abnormalities consist of nodular, irregular, unilateral pleural thickening and varying degrees of unilateral pleural effusion. CT scan helps demonstrate the extent of pleural involvement.

Pleural fluid is exudative and often hemorrhagic. Open pleural biopsy is usually necessary to obtain an adequate specimen for histologic diagnosis; even then, distinction from benign inflammatory conditions and from metastatic adenocarcinoma may be difficult. The histologic variants of malignant pleural mesothelioma are epithelial and fibrous (sarcomatous). Special stains and electron microscopy may be needed to confirm the diagnosis.

Malignant pleural mesothelioma progresses rapidly as the tumor spreads quickly along the pleural surface to involve the pericardium, mediastinum, and contralateral pleura. The tumor may eventually extend beyond the thorax to involve abdominal lymph nodes and organs. Progressive pain and dyspnea are characteristic. Median survival time from onset of symptoms ranges from 5 months in extensive disease to 16 months in localized disease, and about 75% of patients are dead within 1 year after diagnosis. Treatment with surgery, radiotherapy, chemotherapy, and a combination of methods has been attempted but is generally unsuccessful. Some surgeons believe that extrapleural pneumonectomy is the preferred surgical approach for patients with early stage disease. Drainage of pleural effusions, pleurodesis, radiation therapy, and even resectional surgery may offer palliative benefit in some patients.

Jett JR: Malignant pleural mesothelioma: A proposed new staging system. Chest 1995;108:895. [NLM Cit ID: 96010139] (A basis for future studies of a cancer with a very poor prognosis.)

Sugarbaker DJ, Norberto JJ: Multimodality management of malignant pleural mesothelioma. Chest 1998;113 (Suppl):61S. [NLM Cit ID: 98099530] (Extrapleural pneumonectomy plus combination chemotherapy.)

MEDIASTINAL MASSES

Various developmental, neoplastic, infectious, traumatic, and cardiovascular disorders may cause masses that appear in the mediastinum on chest radiograph. A useful convention arbitrarily divides the mediastinum into three compartments—anterior, middle, and posterior—in order to classify mediastinal masses and assist in differential diagnosis. Specific mediastinal masses have a predilection for one or more of these compartments; most are located in the anterior or middle compartment. The differential diagnosis of an anterior mediastinal mass includes thymoma, teratoma, thyroid lesions, lymphoma, and mesenchymal tumors (lipoma, fibroma). The differential diagnosis of a middle mediastinal mass includes lymphadenopathy, pulmonary artery enlargement, aneurysm of the aorta or innominate artery, developmental cyst (bronchogenic, enteric, pleuropericardial), dilated azygous or hemiazygous vein, and foramen of Morgagni hernia. The differential diagnosis of a posterior mediastinal mass includes hiatus hernia, neurogenic tumor, meningocele, esophageal tumor, foramen of Bochdalek hernia, thoracic spine disease, and extramedullary hematopoiesis. The neurogenic tumor group includes neurilemmoma, neurofibroma, neurosarcoma, ganglioneuroma, pheochromocytoma, and others.

Symptoms and signs of mediastinal masses are nonspecific and are usually caused by the effects of the mass on surrounding structures. Insidious onset of retrosternal chest pain, dysphagia, or dyspnea is often an important clue to the presence of a mediastinal mass. In about half of cases, symptoms are absent, and the mass is detected on routine chest radiograph. Physical findings vary depending upon the nature and location of the mass.

CT scanning is helpful in management; additional radiographic studies of benefit include barium swallow if esophageal disease is suspected, Doppler sonography or venography of brachiocephalic veins and the superior vena cava, and arteriography. MRI is useful; its advantages include distinction between vessels and masses, no need for contrast media, and better delineation of hilar structures. MRI also allows imaging in multiple planes, whereas CT permits only axial imaging. Tissue diagnosis is necessary if a neoplastic disorder is suspected. Treatment and prognosis depend on the underlying cause of the mediastinal mass.

Strollo DC et al: Primary mediastinal tumors. Part I. Tumors of the anterior mediastinum. Chest 1997;112:511. [NLM Cit ID: 97410177]

Strollo DC et al: Primary mediastinal tumors. Part II. Tumors of the middle and posterior mediastinum. Chest 1997;112:1344. [NLM Cit ID: 98033302]

INTERSTITIAL LUNG DISEASE (Diffuse Parenchymal Lung Disease)

Interstitial lung disease, or diffuse parenchymal lung disease, comprises a heterogeneous group of disorders that share a common response of the lung to injury: alveolitis, or inflammation, and fibrosis of the interalveolar septum. The term "interstitial" is misleading since the pathologic process begins with injury to the alveolar epithelial or capillary endothelial cells. Persistent alveolitis may lead to obliteration of alveolar capillaries and reorganization of the lung parenchyma, accompanied by irreversible fibrosis. The process does not affect the conducting airways proximal to the respiratory bronchioles. At least 180 disease entities may present as interstitial lung disease (Table 9–19). In the majority of patients, no specific cause can be identified. In the remainder, drugs and a variety of organic and inorganic dusts are the principal causes.

The clinical consequence of widespread lung fibrosis is diminished lung compliance, which presents as restrictive lung disease. Patients usually describe an insidious onset of exertional dyspnea and cough. Sputum production is minimal. Chest examination reveals fine, late inspiratory crackles at the lung bases. Digital clubbing is seen in 25–50% of patients on diagnosis. Pulmonary function testing shows a loss of lung volume with normal to increased airflow rates. The diffusing capacity for carbon monoxide is decreased, and hypoxemia with exercise is common. In advanced cases, resting hypoxemia may be present. The chest radiograph is normal on presentation in up to 10% of patients. More typically, it shows patchy distribution of ground-glass, reticular, or reticulonodular infiltrates. In advanced disease there are multiple small, thick-walled cystic spaces in the lung periphery ("honeycomb lung"). Honeycombing indicates the presence of locally advanced fibrosis with destruction of lung architecture. Conventional and high-resolution CT scanning (HRCT) reveal in greater detail the findings described on chest radiograph. In some cases, HRCT may be strongly suggestive of a specific pathologic process.

The history—particularly the occupational and medication history—may provide evidence of a specific cause. Serologic tests for antinuclear antibodies

Table 9–19. Differential diagnosis of interstitial lung disease.

Drug-related
- Antiarrhythmic agents (amiodarone)
- Antibacterial agents (nitrofurantoin, sulfonamides)
- Antineoplastic agents (bleomycin, cyclophosphamide, methotrexate, nitrosoureas)
- Antirheumatic agents (gold salts, penicillamine)
- Phenytoin
- Talc (injection drug users)

Environmental and occupational (inhalation exposures)
- Dust, inorganic
- Asbestos, silica, hard metals, beryllium
- Dust, organic
- Thermophilic actinomycetes, avian antigens, aspergillus species
- Gases, fumes, and vapors
- Chlorine, isocyanates, paraquat, sulfur dioxide
- Ionizing radiation

Infections
- Fungus, disseminated (*Coccidioides immitis, Blastocystis hominis, Histoplasma capsulatum*)
- Mycobacteria, disseminated
- *Pneumocystis carinii*
- Viral pneumonia

Primary pulmonary disorders
- Bronchiolitis obliterans-organizing pneumonia (BOOP)
- Idiopathic fibrosing interstitial pneumonia:
  - Acute interstitial pneumonitis, desquamative interstitial pneumonitis, nonspecific interstitial pneumonitis, usual interstitial pneumonitis
- Pulmonary alveolar proteinosis

Systemic disorders
- Acute respiratory distress syndrome (ARDS)
- Amyloidosis
- Ankylosing spondylitis
- Autoimmune disease: Dermatomyositis, polymyositis, rheumatoid arthritis, systemic sclerosis (scleroderma), systemic lupus erythematosus
- Chronic eosinophilic pneumonia
- Goodpasture's syndrome
- Idiopathic pulmonary hemosiderosis
- Inflammatory bowel disease
- Langerhans cell histiocytosis (eosinophilic granuloma)
- Lymphangitic spread of cancer (lymphangitic carcinomatosis)
- Lymphangioleiomyomatosis
- Pulmonary edema
- Pulmonary venous hypertension, chronic
- Sarcoidosis
- Wegener's granulomatosis

and rheumatoid factor are positive in 20–40% of patients but are rarely diagnostic. Antineutrophil cytoplasmic antibodies (ANCAs) may be diagnostic in some clinical settings. Invasive diagnostic testing is frequently necessary to make a specific diagnosis. Three diagnostic techniques are in common use: bronchoalveolar lavage, transbronchial biopsy through the flexible bronchoscope, and surgical lung biopsy, either through an open procedure or using video-assisted thoracoscopic surgery.

Bronchoalveolar lavage may provide a specific diagnosis in cases of infection, particularly with *Pneu-*

mocystis carinii or mycobacteria, or when cytologic examination reveals the presence of malignant cells. The findings may be suggestive if not diagnostic of eosinophilic pneumonia, Langerhans cell histiocytosis (eosinophilic granuloma), and alveolar proteinosis. Analysis of the cellular constituents of lavage fluid may suggest a specific disease, but these findings are not diagnostic.

Transbronchial biopsy using the flexible bronchoscope is easily performed in most patients. The risks of pneumothorax (5%) and hemorrhage (1–10%) are low. However, the tissue specimens recovered are small, sampling error is common, and crush artifact may complicate diagnosis. Transbronchial biopsy can make a definitive diagnosis of sarcoidosis, lymphangitic spread of carcinoma, pulmonary alveolar proteinosis, miliary tuberculosis, and Langerhans cell histiocytosis. Transbronchial biopsy cannot establish the diagnosis of idiopathic interstitial pneumonia. For patients in whom idiopathic interstitial pneumonia is suspected, patients may be better served by surgical lung biopsy than by nondiagnostic transbronchial biopsy.

Surgical lung biopsy is the standard for diagnosis of interstitial lung disease. Two or three biopsies taken from multiple sites in the same lung, including apparently normal tissue, may yield a specific diagnosis as well as prognostic information regarding the extent of fibrosis versus active inflammation. Patients under age 60 without a specific diagnosis generally should undergo surgical lung biopsy. In older patients, the decision must be weighed carefully for three reasons: (1) the morbidity of the procedure is significant; (2) a definitive diagnosis may not be possible even with surgical lung biopsy; and (3) when a specific diagnosis is made, there may be no effective treatment. Empirical therapy or no treatment may be preferable to surgical lung biopsy in some patients.

Known causes of interstitial lung disease are dealt with in their specific sections. The important idiopathic forms are discussed below.

IDIOPATHIC FIBROSING INTERSTITIAL PNEUMONIA (Formerly: Idiopathic Pulmonary Fibrosis)

The most common diagnosis among patients presenting with interstitial lung disease is idiopathic pulmonary fibrosis, known in Britain as cryptogenic fibrosing alveolitis. Historically, this diagnosis was based on clinical and radiographic criteria with only a minority of patients undergoing surgical lung biopsy. When biopsies were obtained, several histologic patterns were grouped together under the category idiopathic pulmonary fibrosis because of the common element of fibrosis. We now recognize that these distinct histopathologic features are associated with different natural histories and responses to therapy (see Table 9–20). Therefore, in the evaluation of patients with idiopathic interstitial lung disease, one should attempt to identify specific disorders and use the terms idiopathic pulmonary fibrosis or cryptogenic fibrosing alveolitis to denote only the histologic pattern of "usual interstitial pneumonitis."

Patients with idiopathic fibrosing interstitial pneumonia may present with any of the histologic patterns described in Table 9–20. The first step in evaluation is to identify patients whose disease is truly idiopathic. As indicated in Table 9–19, most identifiable causes of interstitial lung disease are either infectious, drug-related, or identifiable through a careful environmental and occupational history. Interstitial lung diseases associated with other medical conditions (pulmonary-renal syndromes, collagen-vascular disease) may be identified through a careful medical history. Apart from acute interstitial pneumonitis, the clinical presentations of the idiopathic interstitial pneumonias are sufficiently similar to preclude a specific diagnosis. Chest radiographs and CT scans are occasionally diagnostic. Ultimately, many patients with apparently idiopathic disease require surgical lung biopsy to make a definitive diagnosis. The importance of accurate diagnosis is twofold. First, it allows the clinician to provide accurate information about the cause and natural history of the illness. Second, accurate diagnosis helps to distinguish patients most likely to benefit from therapy. The role of surgical lung biopsy may be to identify patients with usual interstitial pneumonitis to spare them potentially morbid therapies.

The diagnosis of usual interstitial pneumonitis can be made on clinical grounds alone in selected patients. A diagnosis of usual interstitial pneumonitis can be made with 90% confidence in patients over 65 who present with idiopathic disease by history, demonstrate inspiratory crackles on physical examination and restrictive physiology on pulmonary function testing, characteristic radiographic evidence of progressive fibrosis over several years, and diffuse, patchy fibrosis with pleural-based honeycombing on high-resolution CT scan. Such patients do not need surgical lung biopsy. Note that the diagnosis cannot be confirmed on transbronchial lung biopsy since the histologic diagnosis requires a pattern of changes rather than a single pathognomonic finding.

Treatment of idiopathic fibrosing interstitial pneumonia is controversial. No randomized study has demonstrated that any treatment improves survival compared with no treatment. Clinical experience suggests that patients with desquamative interstitial pneumonitis, nonspecific interstitial pneumonitis, or bronchiolitis obliterans-organizing pneumonia (see Table 9–20) frequently respond to corticosteroids and should be given a trial of therapy—typically prednisone, 1–2 mg/kg/d for a minimum of 2 months. The same therapy is almost uniformly ineffective in patients with usual interstitial pneumonitis. Since this therapy carries significant morbidity, the pulmonary

Table 9–20. Idiopathic fibrosing interstitial pneumonias.

Name and Clinical Presentation	Histopathology	Radiographic Pattern	Response to Therapy and Prognosis
Usual interstitial pneumonitis (UIP) Age 55–60, slight male predominance. Insidious dry cough and exertional dyspnea of months' to years' duration. Clubbing present at diagnosis in 25–50%. Diffuse fine late inspiratory crackles on lung auscultation. Restrictive ventilatory deficit and reduced diffusing capacity on pulmonary function tests. ESR elevated. ANA and RF positive in 25% in the absence of collagen-vascular disease.	Patchy, nonuniform distribution of fibrosis, inflammation, honeycomb change, and normal lung. Type I pneumocytes are lost, and there is hyperproliferation of alveolar type II cells. There are "fibroblast foci" of actively proliferating fibroblasts and myofibroblasts. Inflammation is generally mild and consists of small lymphocytes. Intra-alveolar macrophage accumulation is present.	Diminished lung volume. Increased linear or reticular opacities at periphery and bases of both lungs. Unilateral disease is rare. CT shows variable amount of ground-glass and honeycomb change. Areas of normal lung may be adjacent to areas of advanced fibrosis. Between 2% and 10% have normal chest radiographs and CT scans on diagnosis.	No randomized study has demonstrated improved survival compared with untreated patients. Inexorably progressive. Response to corticosteroids and cytotoxic agents at best 15%, and these may represent misclassification of histopathology. Median survival approximately 3 years, depending on stage at presentation.
Desquamative interstitial pneumonitis (DIP)[1] Age 4–45. Presentation similar to that of UIP though in younger patients. Similar results on pulmonary function tests, but less severe abnormalities. Patients with respiratory bronchiolitis are invariably heavy smokers.	Increased numbers of macrophages evenly dispersed within the alveolar spaces. Rare fibroblast foci, little fibrosis, minimal honeycomb change. In RB-ILD the accumulation of macrophages is accentuated within the peribronchiolar air spaces.	May be distinguishable from UIP. More often presents with a nodular or reticulonodular pattern. Honeycombing rare.	Spontaneous remission occurs in up to 20% of patients, so natural history unclear. Prognosis clearly better than that of UIP: median survival over 10 years. No randomized study has demonstrated improved survival compared with untreated patients. Corticosteroids thought to be effective.
Acute interstitial pneumonitis (AIP) Clinically known as Hamman-Rich syndrome. Wide age range, many young patients. Acute onset of dyspnea followed by rapid development of respiratory failure. Half of patients report a viral syndrome preceding lung disease. Clinical course indistinguishable from that of ARDS.	Changes are uniform in time, presumably reflecting acute response to injury within days to weeks. Resembles organizing phase of diffuse alveolar damage. Fibrosis with minimal collagen deposition. May appear similar to UIP, but the process is more homogeneous and there is no honeycomb change—though this may appear if the process persists for more than a month in a patient on mechanical ventilation.	Diffuse bilateral airspace consolidation with areas of ground-glass attenuation on high-resolution CT scan.	Supportive care (mechanical ventilation) critical but effect of specific therapies unclear. High initial mortality: Fifty to 90 percent die within 2 months after diagnosis. Not progressive if patient survives. Lung function may return to normal or may be permanently impaired.
Nonspecific interstitial pneumonitis (NSIP) Age 45–55. Slight female predominance. Similar to UIP but onset of cough and dyspnea over months, not years.	Nonspecific in that histopathology does not fit into better-established categories. Varying degrees of inflammation and fibrosis, patchy in distribution but uniform in time, suggesting response to single injury. Most have lymphocytic and plasma cell inflammation without fibrosis. Honeycombing scant but not absent. Some have advocated division into cellular and fibrotic subtypes.	May be indistinguishable from UIP. Most typical picture is bilateral areas of ground-glass attenuation on CT scan. Honeycombing is rare.	Treatment thought to be effective, but no prospective clinical studies have been published. Prognosis overall good but depends on the extent of fibrosis at diagnosis. Median survival over 10 years.

(*continued*)

Table 9–20. Idiopathic fibrosing interstitial pneumonias. (continued)

Name and Clinical Presentation	Histopathology	Radiographic Pattern	Response to Therapy and Prognosis
Bronchiolitis obliterans organizing pneumonia (BOOP) Typically age 50–60 but wide variation. Abrupt onset, frequently weeks to a few months follwing a flu-like illness. Dyspnea and dry cough prominent, but constitutional symptoms are common: fatigue, fever, and weight loss. Pulmonary function tests usually show restriction, but up to 25% show concomitant obstruction.	Included in the idiopathic interstitial pneumonias on clinical grounds. Buds of loose connective tissue (Masson bodies) and inflammatory cells fill alveoli and distal bronchioles.	Lung volumes normal. Chest radiograph typically shows interstitial and parenchymal disease with discrete, peripheral alveolar and ground-glass infiltrates. Nodular opacities common. CT scan shows subpleural consolidation.	Rapid response to corticosteroids in two-thirds of patients. Relapses are common. Long-term prognosis generally good for those who respond.

[1]Includes respiratory bronchiolitis interstitial lung disease (RB-ILD).

community is shifting away from the use of corticosteroids in patients with usual interstitial pneumonitis. A recent small but well-designed clinical study has reported promising preliminary results with recombinant interferon gamma-1b.

Katzenstein AL et al: Idiopathic pulmonary fibrosis: Clinical relevance of pathologic classification. Am J Respir Crit Care Med 1998;157:1301. [NLM Cit ID: 98223243] (Focuses on clinical and pathologic characteristics of our distinct forms of idiopathic interstitial pneumonia formerly grouped together as pulmonary fibrosis.)

Lynch JP et al: Idiopathic pulmonary fibrosis: Is lung biopsy essential? J Respir Dis 2000;21:197. (A careful attempt to distinguish the specific clinical, radiographic, and pathologic features of the idiopathic interstitial pneumonias.)

Mason RJ et al: Pharmacological therapy for idiopathic pulmonary fibrosis. Past, present, and future. Am J Respir Crit Care Med 1999;160:1771. [NLM Cit ID: 20027712] (A detailed review of the current state of the art in treatment of the idiopathic interstitial pneumonias.)

Raghu G et al: The accuracy of the clinical diagnosis of new-onset idiopathic pulmonary fibrosis and other interstitial lung disease. Chest 1999;116:1168. [NLM Cit ID: 20025823] (A prospective assessment of selected referral patients comparing expert clinical and radiographic assessment with biopsy findings.)

Ryu JH et al: Idiopathic pulmonary fibrosis: Current concepts. Mayo Clin Proc 1998;73:1085. [NLM Cit ID: 99035406] (A thorough review arguing that idiopathic pulmonary fibrosis is a heterogeneous category that includes multiple clinicopathologic entities.)

Ziesche R et al: A preliminary study of long-term treatment with interferon gamma-1b and low dose prednisolone in patients with idiopathic pulmonary fibrosis. N Engl J Med 1999;341:1264. [NLM Cit ID: 99442270] (A prospective, randomized trial in 18 patients of low-dose prednisolone compared to prednisolone plus thrice-weekly subcutaneous interferon gamma-1b. The interferon patients showed improvements in lung volume and oxygenation.)

SARCOIDOSIS

Sarcoidosis is a systemic disease of unknown cause characterized in about 90% of patients by granulomatous inflammation of the lung. The incidence is highest in North American blacks and northern European whites; among blacks, women are more frequently affected than men. Onset of disease is usually in the third or fourth decade.

Patients may present with malaise, fever, and dyspnea of insidious onset. Alternatively, sarcoidosis symptoms referable to the skin, eyes, peripheral nerves, liver, kidney, or heart may cause the patient to seek care. Some individuals are asymptomatic and come to medical attention after abnormal findings (typically bilateral hilar and right paratracheal lymphadenopathy) on routine chest radiographs. Physical findings in the chest are not typical of those associated with interstitial lung involvement in that crackles are uncommon. Other findings may include erythema nodosum, parotid gland enlargement, hepatosplenomegaly, and lymphadenopathy.

Laboratory tests may show leukopenia, an elevated erythrocyte sedimentation rate, and hypercalcemia (about 5% of patients) or hypercalciuria (20%). Angiotensin-converting enzyme (ACE) levels are elevated in 40–80% of patients with active disease. This finding is neither sensitive nor specific enough to have diagnostic significance. Physiologic testing may reveal evidence of airflow obstruction, but restrictive changes of decreased lung volumes and diffusing capacity are more common signs. Skin test anergy is present in 70%.

Radiographic findings are variable and include bilateral hilar adenopathy alone (stage I), hilar adenopathy and parenchymal involvement (stage II), or parenchymal involvement alone (stage III). Parenchymal involvement is usually manifested radiographically by diffuse reticular infiltrates, but focal

case by eosinophilic pulmonary infiltrates, peripheral blood eosinophilia, and pulmonary symptoms such as dyspnea and cough. Many patients have constitutional symptoms, including fever. In **chronic eosinophilic pneumonia,** the pulmonary infiltrates are usually distinctly peripheral. It is predominantly a disorder of women and characterized by fever, night sweats, weight loss, and dyspnea. Therapy with oral prednisone (1 mg/kg daily for 1–2 weeks followed by a gradual taper over many months) usually results in dramatic improvement; however, most patients require at least 10–15 mg of prednisone every other day for a year or more (sometimes indefinitely) to prevent relapses.

Other eosinophilic pulmonary syndromes demonstrate a variety of patterns of pulmonary infiltrates associated with exposure to various drugs (common drugs include nitrofurantoin, phenytoin, ampicillin, acetaminophen, and ranitidine) or infection with helminths such as ascaris, hookworms, or strongyloides; Löffler's syndrome (if transient), or filariae (such as *Wuchereria bancrofti, Brugia malayi;* tropical pulmonary eosinophilia). Pulmonary eosinophilia can also be a feature of many other processes, including allergic bronchopulmonary aspergillosis, Churg-Strauss syndrome, systemic hypereosinophilic syndromes, eosinophilic granuloma of the lung (also referred to as pulmonary Langerhans cell granulomatosis or primary pulmonary histocytosis X), neoplasms, and numerous interstitial lung diseases. No precipitating cause may be apparent in as many as one-third of cases. If an extrinsic cause is identified, therapy consists of removal of the offending drug or treatment of the underlying parasitic infection. Corticosteroid treatment (prednisone, 1 mg/kg body weight orally per day) should be instituted if no treatable extrinsic cause is discovered. The response to corticosteroids is usually dramatic. Recurrences are common.

Pope-Harman AL et al: Acute eosinophilic pneumonia: A summary of 15 cases and review of the literature. Medicine 1996;75:334. [NLM Cit ID: 97136773] (Sixty references.)

DISORDERS OF THE PULMONARY CIRCULATION

PULMONARY THROMBOEMBOLISM

Essentials of Diagnosis

- Predisposition to venous thrombosis, usually of the lower extremities.
- Abrupt onset of dyspnea, chest pain, hemoptysis, or syncope.
- Tachypnea and a widened A-a Do_2 difference.
- Characteristic defects on ventilation/perfusion lung scan.
- Diagnostic findings on pulmonary angiogram or other imaging modality, especially spiral CT scan.

General Considerations

Pulmonary thromboembolism, often referred to as pulmonary embolism, is a common, serious and potentially fatal complication of thrombus formation within the venous circulation. Pulmonary thromboembolism is estimated to cause 50,000 deaths each year in the United States, making it the third leading cause of death among hospitalized patients. Despite this prevalence, the majority of cases are not recognized antemortem, and fewer than 10% of patients with fatal emboli have received specific treatment for the condition. Management demands a vigilant systematic approach to diagnosis and an understanding of risk factors so that appropriate preventive therapy can be given.

Many substances can embolize to the pulmonary circulation, including air (neurosurgery, central venous catheters), amniotic fluid (active labor), fat (long bone fractures), foreign bodies (talc in intravenous drug users), parasite eggs (schistosomiasis), septic emboli (acute infectious endocarditis), and tumor cells (renal cell carcinoma). The most common embolus is thrombus, which may arise anywhere in the venous circulation or heart but most often originates in the deep veins of the major calf muscles. Thrombi confined to the calf rarely embolize to the pulmonary circulation. However, about 20% of calf vein thrombi propagate proximally to the popliteal and ileofemoral veins, at which point they may break off and migrate to the pulmonary circulation. Fifty to 60 percent of patients with proximal deep venous thrombosis (DVT) will develop pulmonary emboli; half of these embolic events will be asymptomatic. Nearly 70% of patients who present with symptomatic pulmonary emboli will have DVT when evaluated.

Pulmonary embolism and deep venous thrombosis are two manifestations of the same disease: thrombus formation within the venous circulation, or venous thromboembolism. The risk factors for pulmonary emboli are the risk factors for deep venous thrombosis: venous stasis, injury to the vessel wall, and hypercoagulability. Venous stasis increases with immobility (bed rest—especially postoperative—obesity, stroke), hyperviscosity (polycythemia), and increased central venous pressures (low cardiac output states, pregnancy). Vessels may be damaged by prior episodes of thrombosis, orthopedic surgery, or trauma to the lower extremities. Hypercoagulability can be caused by medications (oral contraceptives) or disease (malignancy, extensive surgery) or can be inherited. The most common inherited cause in Caucasian populations is resistance to activated protein C, also known as factor V

Leiden. The trait is present in approximately 3% of healthy American men and in 20–40% of patients with idiopathic venous thrombosis. Other major risks for hypercoagulability include deficiencies in protein C, protein S, and antithrombin III.

Pulmonary thromboembolism has multiple physiologic effects. Physical obstruction of the vascular bed and vasoconstriction from neurohumoral reflexes both increase pulmonary vascular resistance. Massive thrombus may cause right ventricular failure. Vascular obstruction increases physiologic dead space (wasted ventilation) and leads to hypoxia through right to left shunting, decreased cardiac output, and surfactant depletion causing atelectasis. Reflex bronchoconstriction promotes wheezing and increased work of breathing.

Clinical Findings

A. Symptoms and Signs: The clinical diagnosis of pulmonary thromboembolism is notoriously difficult for two reasons. First, the clinical findings depend on both the size of the embolus and the patient's preexisting cardiopulmonary status. Second, common symptoms and signs of pulmonary emboli are not specific to this disorder (Table 9–21).

Indeed, no single symptom or sign or combination of clinical findings is specific to pulmonary thromboembolism. Some findings are fairly sensitive: dyspnea and pain on inspiration occur in 75–85% and 65–75% of patients, respectively. Tachypnea is the only sign reliably found in more than half of patients. A common clinical strategy is to use combinations of clinical findings to identify patients at low risk for pulmonary thromboembolism. For example, 97% of patients in the Prospective Investigation of Pulmonary Embolism Diagnosis (PIOPED) study with angiographically proved pulmonary emboli had one or more of three findings: dyspnea, chest pain with breathing, or tachypnea. Such a sensitive screen al-

Table 9–21. Frequency of specific symptoms and signs in patients at risk for pulmonary thromboembolism.

	UPET[1] PE+ (n = 327)	PIOPED[2] PE+ (n = 117)	PIOPED[2] PE– (n = 248)
Symptoms			
Dyspnea	84%	73%	72%
Respirophasic chest pain	74%	66%	59%
Cough	53%	37%	36%
Leg pain	nr	26%	24%
Hemoptysis	30%	13%	8%
Palpitations	nr	10%	18%
Wheezing	nr	9%	11%
Anginal pain	14%	4%	6%
Signs			
Respiratory rate ≥ 16 UPET, ≥ 20 PIOPED	92%	70%	68%
Crackles (rales)	58%	51%	40%[3]
Heart rate ≥ 100/min	44%	30%	24%
Fourth heart sound (S_4)	nr	24%	13%[3]
Accentuated pulmonary component of second heart sound (S_2P)	53%	23%	13%[3]
T ≥ 37.5 °C UPET, ≥ 38.5 °C PIOPED	43%	7%	12%
Homans' sign	nr	4%	2%
Pleural friction rub	nr	3%	2%
Third heart sound (S_3)	nr	3%	4%
Cyanosis	19%	1%	2%

[1]Data from the Urokinase-Streptokinase Pulmonary Embolism Trial, as reported in Bell WR, Simon TL, DeMets DL: The clinical features of submassive and massive pulmonary emboli. Am J Med 1977;62:355.
[2]Data from patients enrolled in the PIOPED Study, as reported in Stein PD et al: Clinical, laboratory, roentgenographic, and electrocardiographic findings in patients with acute pulmonary embolism and no preexisting cardiac or pulmonary disease. Chest 1991;100:598.
PE+ = confirmed diagnosis of pulmonary embolism; PE– = diagnosis of pulmonary embolism ruled out; nr = not reported.
[3]$p < .05$ comparing patients in the PIOPED Study.

Treatment

A. Anticoagulation: Anticoagulation is not definitive therapy but a form of secondary prevention. Heparin binds to and accelerates the ability of antithrombin III to inactivate thrombin, factor Xa, and factor IXa. It thus retards additional thrombus formation, allowing endogenous fibrinolytic mechanisms to lyse existing clot. The standard regimen of heparin followed by 6 months of oral warfarin results in an 80–90% reduction in the risk of both recurrent venous thrombosis and death from pulmonary thromboembolism.

Heparin has troublesome pharmacokinetics. Its clearance is dose-dependent; it is highly protein-bound; and a minimum or threshold level is necessary to achieve an antithrombotic effect. It is necessary to monitor the activated partial thromboplastin time (aPTT) and adjust dosing to maintain the aPTT 1.5–2.5 times control. In patients with a moderate to high clinical likelihood of pulmonary thromboembolism and no contraindications, full anticoagulation with heparin should begin with the diagnostic evaluation. Once the diagnosis of proximal DVT or pulmonary thromboembolism is established, it is critical to ensure adequate therapy. Failure to achieve therapeutic heparin levels within 24 hours is associated with a fivefold-increased risk of clot propagation. The weight-based regimen in Table 9–23 is superior to standard dosing. Because heparin causes immune-mediated thrombocytopenia, patients receiving it should have the platelet count measured daily.

Low-molecular-weight heparins are depolymerized preparations of heparin with multiple advantages over unfractionated heparin. They exhibit less binding to cells and proteins and have superior bioavailability, a longer plasma half-life, and more predictable dose-response characteristics. They appear to carry an equivalent or lower risk of hemorrhage, and thrombocytopenia is less common. LMW heparins appear to be at least as effective as unfractionated heparin in the treatment of venous thromboembolism. They are administered in dosages determined by body weight once or twice daily without the need for coagulation monitoring, and subcutaneous administration appears to be as effective as the intravenous route. This profile makes LMW heparins ideal for home-based therapy of venous thromboembolism. Home-based therapy appears safe and efficacious in a small number of selected patients. Table 9–24 lists agents available in the United States.

Table 9–23. Intravenous heparin dosing based on body weight.[1]

Initial dosing	
1. Load with 80 units/kg IV, then	
2. Initiate a maintenance infusion at 18 units/kg/h	
3. Check activated partial thromboplastin time (aPTT) in 6 hours	
Dose adjustment schedule based on aPTT results	
< 35 s (< 1.25 × control)	Rebolus with 80 units/kg; increase infusion by 4 units/kg/h
35–45 s (1.2–1.5 × control)	Rebolus with 40 units/kg; increase infusion by 2 units/kg/h
46–70 s (1.5–2.3 × control)	No change
71–90 s (2.3–3 × control)	Decrease infusion rate by 2 units/kg/h
> 90 s (> 3 × control)	Stop infusion for 1 hour, then decrease infusion by 3 units/kg/h

Repeat aPTT every 6 hours for the first 24 hours. If the aPTT is 46–70 s after 24 hours, then recheck once daily every morning. If the aPTT is outside this therapeutic range at 24 hours, continue checking every 6 hours until it is 46–70 s. Once it has been in the therapeutic range on two consecutive measurements after 24 hours, check once daily every morning.

[1]Adapted from Raschke RA et al: The weight-based heparin dosing nomogram compared with a "standard care" nomogram. Ann Intern Med 1993;119:874.

Anticoagulation therapy for venous thromboembolism is continued for a minimum of 3 months, so oral anticoagulant therapy with warfarin is usually initiated concurrently with heparin. Warfarin affects hepatic synthesis of vitamin K-dependent coagulant proteins. It usually requires 5–7 days to become therapeutic; therefore, intravenous heparin is generally continued for 5 days. Warfarin is safe if begun concurrently with heparin, initially at a dose of 5–10 mg/d. The lower dose is preferred in older patients. Maintenance therapy usually requires 2–15 mg/d. Adequacy of therapy must be monitored by following the prothrombin time, now most often adjusted for differences in reagents and reported as the international normalized ratio, or INR. The target INR is 2.5, with the acceptable range from 2.0 to 3.0; below 2.0, there is an increased risk of thrombosis; above 4.0, there is an increased risk of hemorrhage. Warfarin has interactions with many drugs. Meticulous attention to medications is part of the routine management of every patient receiving warfarin. Warfarin is a pregnancy category X medication, indicating known fetopathic and teratogenic effects. When oral anticoagulation with warfarin is contraindicated, LMW heparin is a convenient alternative.

The optimal duration of anticoagulation therapy for venous thromboembolism is unknown. There appears to be a protective benefit to continued anticoagulation in first-episode venous thromboembolism (twice the rate of recurrence in 6 weeks compared with 6 months of therapy) and recurrent disease (eightfold risk of recurrence in 6 months compared with 4 years of therapy). Studies do not distinguish patients with reversible risk factors, such as surgery or transient immobility, from patients who have a nonreversible hypercoagulable state such as factor V Leiden, inhibitor deficiency, antiphospholipid syndrome, or malignancy. Patients with idiopathic venous thromboembolism absent any risk factor may benefit most from prolonged therapy. For many patients, venous thrombosis is a recurrent disease, and

Table 9–24. Selected low-molecular-weight heparins and heparinoids.[1]

	Prophylactic Dose[2]	Treatment Dose[2]
Ardeparin (Normiflo)	50 anti-Xa units/kg twice daily	130 anti-Xa units/kg twice daily
Dalteparin (Fragmin)	2500–5000 anti-Xa units daily	120 anti-Xa units/kg twice daily, or 200 anti-Xa units/kg daily
Danaparoid (Orgaran)	750 anti-Xa units twice daily	2500 anti-Xa units by IV bolus, then 400 units per hour for 4 hours, 300 units per hour for 4 hours, and 150–200 units per hour to completion of treatment
Enoxaparin (Lovenox)	30 mg twice daily (orthopedic surgery); 40 mg daily (general surgery)	1–1.5 mg/kg twice daily, or 100 anti-Xa units/kg twice daily
Nadroparin (Fraxiparin)[3]	3100 anti-Xa units daily	180 anti-Xa units/kg daily
Tinzaparin (Innohep, Logiparin)[3]	3500 anti-Xa units daily	175 anti-Xa units/kg daily

[1]Adapted from Hyers TM: State of the Art: Venous thromboembolism. Am J Respir Crit Care Med 1999;159:1.
[2]Doses reflect data from multiple clinical trials. In the case of ardeparin, the number of treatment studies is small and the dose is not firmly established. Danaparoid is a heparinoid with a high anti-Xa/IIa ratio. Its units are not directly comparable to the LMWH preparations.
[3]Not available in the United States.

continued therapy will result in a lower rate of recurrence at the cost of an increased risk of hemorrhage. Therefore, the appropriate duration of therapy will need to take into consideration potentially reversible risk factors, the individual's age, the likelihood and potential consequences of hemorrhage, and preferences for continued therapy. It is reasonable to continue therapy for 6 months after a first episode when there is a reversible risk factor, 12 months after a first-episode idiopathic thrombus, and 6–12 months to indefinitely in patients with nonreversible risk factors or recurrent disease.

The major complication of anticoagulation is hemorrhage. Risk factors for hemorrhage include the intensity of the anticoagulant effect; the duration of therapy; concomitant administration of drugs such as aspirin that interfere with platelet function; and patient characteristics, particularly increased age, previous gastrointestinal hemorrhage, and coexistent renal insufficiency.

The reported incidence of major hemorrhage following intravenous administration of unfractionated heparin is nil to 7%; that of fatal hemorrhage is nil to 2%. The incidence with LMW heparins is not statistically different. There is no information comparing hemorrhage rates at different doses of heparin. The risk of subtherapeutic heparin administration in the first 24–48 hours after diagnosis is significant; it appears to outweigh the risk of short-term supratherapeutic heparin levels. The incidence of hemorrhage during therapy with warfarin is reported to be between 3% and 4% per patient year. The frequency varies with the target INR and is consistently higher when the INR exceeds 4.0. There is no apparent additional antithrombotic benefit in venous thromboembolism with a target INR above 2.0–3.0.

B. Thrombolytic Therapy: Streptokinase, urokinase, and recombinant tissue plasminogen activator (rt-PA; alteplase) increase plasmin levels and thereby directly lyse intravascular thrombi. In patients with established pulmonary thromboembolism, thrombolytic therapy accelerates resolution of emboli within the first 24 hours compared with standard heparin therapy. This is a consistent finding using angiography, V/Q scanning, echocardiography, and direct measurement of pulmonary artery pressures. However, at 1 week and 1 month after diagnosis, these agents show no difference in outcome compared with heparin and warfarin. There is no evidence that thrombolytic therapy improves mortality statistics. Subtle improvements in pulmonary function, including improved single-breath diffusing capacity and a lower incidence of exercise-induced pulmonary hypertension, have been observed. The reliability and clinical importance of these findings is unclear. The major disadvantages of thrombolytic therapy compared with heparin are its greater cost and a significant increase in major hemorrhagic complications. The incidence of intracranial hemorrhage in patients with pulmonary thromboemboli treated with alteplase is 2.1% compared with 0.2% of patients treated with heparin.

Current evidence supports thrombolytic therapy for pulmonary thromboembolism in patients at high risk for death in whom the more rapid resolution of thrombus may be lifesaving. Such patients are usually hemodynamically unstable despite heparin therapy. Absolute contraindications to thrombolytic therapy include active internal bleeding and stroke within the past 2 months. Major contraindications include hypertension and surgery or trauma within the past 6 weeks.

C. Additional Measures: In rare patients for whom thrombolytic therapy is contraindicated or unsuccessful, mechanical or surgical extraction of thrombus may be indicated. Pulmonary embolectomy is an emergency procedure of last resort with a very high mortality rate. It is now performed only in a few specialized centers. Several catheter devices to fragment and extract thrombus through a transvenous approach have been reported in small numbers of patients. Comparative outcomes with surgery, thrombolytic therapy, or heparin have not been studied.

Interruption of the inferior vena cava may be indicated in patients with major contraindications to anticoagulation; in those with recurrent pulmonary thromboemboli from the pelvis or lower extremities despite adequate medical therapy; in those with severe pulmonary hypertension in whom any thromboemboli would be life-threatening; and in those with paradoxical arterial embolism. Percutaneous transjugular placement of a mechanical filter is the preferred mode of inferior vena cava interruption. These devices reduce the short-term incidence of pulmonary thromboemboli in patients presenting with proximal lower extremity deep venous thrombosis. However, they are associated with a two-fold increased risk of recurrent venous thrombosis in the first 2 years following placement.

Prognosis

Pulmonary thromboembolism is estimated to cause more than 50,000 deaths annually. In the majority of deaths, pulmonary thromboembolism is not recognized antemortem or death occurs before specific treatment can be initiated. These statistics highlight the importance of preventive therapy in high-risk patients. The outlook for patients with diagnosed and appropriately treated pulmonary thromboembolism is generally good. Overall prognosis depends on the underlying disease that put the patient at risk for venous thromboembolism rather than the pulmonary thromboembolism itself. Death from recurrent thromboemboli is uncommon, occurring in less than 3% of cases. Perfusion defects resolve in most survivors. Approximately 1% of patients develop chronic thromboembolic pulmonary hypertension. These patients may benefit from pulmonary endarterectomy.

Clagett GP et al: Prevention of venous thromboembolism. Chest 1998;114(Suppl):531S. [NLM Cit ID: 99037856] (Exhaustive review of all aspects of prophylactic therapy, from the Fifth ACCP Consensus Conference on Antithrombotic Therapy.)

Dalen JE, Alpert JS, Hirsch J: Thrombolytic therapy for pulmonary embolism: Is it effective? Is it safe? When is it indicated? Arch Intern Med 1997;157:2550. [NLM Cit ID: 98189708] (Detailed, evidence-based approach to clinical trials of thrombolytic therapy in pulmonary embolism.)

Ginsberg JS et al: Sensitivity and specificity of a rapid whole-blood assay for D-dimer in the diagnosis of pulmonary embolism. Ann Intern Med 1998;129:1006. [NLM Cit ID: 99064841] (A normal simplified D-dimer test was useful in excluding pulmonary thromboembolism in patients with a low pretest probability of PE or a nondiagnostic lung scan.)

Goldhaber SZ: Pulmonary embolism. N Engl J Med 1998;339:93. [NLM Cit ID: 98307627] (In depth review by a noted researcher in the field.)

Hyers TM: State of the Art: Venous thromboembolism. Am J Respir Crit Care Med 1999;159:1. [NLM Cit ID: 99091824] (Detailed review, focusing on physiology and emerging directions for future research.)

Kearon C et al: A comparison of three months of anticoagulation with extended anticoagulation for a first episode of idiopathic venous thromboembolism. N Engl J Med 1999;340:901. [NLM Cit ID: 99173386] (Randomized, controlled, double-blinded study of 3 versus 24 months of anticoagulation therapy in first-episode venous thromboembolism. Trial halted early due to increased recurrence in control group.)

Muirn S et al: Hereditary thrombophilia and venous thromboembolism. Am J Respir Crit Care Med 1998;158:1369. [NLM Cit ID: 99034715] (The most common causes of hereditary thrombophilia are reviewed and the current status of laboratory testing for thrombophilia is discussed.)

Opinions regarding the diagnosis and management of venous thromboembolic disease. ACCP Consensus Committee on Pulmonary Embolism: American College of Chest Physicians. Chest 1998;113:499. [NLM Cit ID: 98140812] (Consensus report that addresses diagnosis and management of deep venous thrombosis.)

Rathbun SW et al: Sensitivity and specificity of helical computed tomography in the diagnosis of pulmonary embolism. A systematic review. Ann Intern Med. 2000; 132:227. [NLM Cit ID: 20104805] (An evidence-based review of clinical trials of HRCT in the diagnosis of pulmonary embolism.)

Tapson VF et al: The diagnostic approach to acute venous thromboembolism. Clinical practice guideline. American Thoracic Society. Am J Respir Crit Care Med 1999; 160:1043. [NLM Cit ID: 99403257]

Value of the ventilation/perfusion scan in acute pulmonary embolism. Results of the prospective investigation of pulmonary embolism diagnosis (PIOPED). The PIOPED Investigators. JAMA 1990;263:2753. [NLM Cit ID: 90238161] (Classic article defining the additive utility of clinical judgment with ventilation-perfusion scanning in the diagnostic evaluation of pulmonary embolism.)

Wells PS et al: Use of a clinical model for safe management of patients with suspected pulmonary embolism. Ann Intern Med 1998;129:997. [NLM Cit ID: 99064840] (Management of patients with suspected pulmonary embolism on the basis of pretest probability and results of ventilation-perfusion scanning was shown to be safe using the clinical model described.)

PULMONARY HYPERTENSION

Essentials of Diagnosis

- Dyspnea, fatigue, chest pain, and occasionally syncope on exertion.
- Narrow splitting of second heart sound with loud pulmonary component; findings of right ventricular hypertrophy and cardiac failure in advanced disease.
- Hypoxemia: wasted ventilation on pulmonary function tests.

- Electrocardiographic evidence of right ventricular strain or hypertrophy and right atrial enlargement.
- Enlarged central pulmonary arteries on chest radiograph.

General Considerations

The pulmonary circulation is unique because of its high blood flow, low pressure (normally 25/8 mm Hg, mean 12), and low resistance (normally 200–250 dynes/sec/cm^{-5}). It can accommodate large increases in blood flow during exercise with only modest increases in pressure because of its ability to recruit and distend blood vessels. The normal pulmonary circulation is also largely passive, since its pressures are determined mainly by the function of the right and left ventricles. Contraction of smooth muscle in the walls of pulmonary arteriolar resistance vessels becomes an important factor in numerous pathologic states. Pulmonary hypertension is present when pulmonary artery pressure rises to a high level inappropriate for a given level of cardiac output.

Primary (idiopathic) pulmonary hypertension (see Chapter 10) is a rare disorder of the pulmonary circulation occurring mostly in young and middle-aged women; it is characterized by progressive dyspnea, a rapid downhill course, and an invariably fatal outcome. This condition is also called plexogenic pulmonary arteriopathy, in reference to the characteristic histopathologic plexiform lesion found in muscular pulmonary arteries. It has been observed in occasional patients with HIV infection.

Selected mechanisms responsible for **secondary pulmonary hypertension** and examples of corresponding clinical conditions are set forth in Table 9–25. Pulmonary hypertension is usually caused by reduction of the cross-sectional area of the pulmonary vasculature at the arterial, capillary, or venous level. Hypoxia of any cause is the most important and potent stimulus of pulmonary arterial vasoconstriction. The mechanisms by which hypoxia causes pulmonary hypertension are poorly understood. Factors operating at the alveolar level and direct stimulation of arteriolar smooth muscle have been implicated. Interest has focused on the release of vasoactive substances from the endothelial cells of pulmonary arteries, such as endothelium-derived relaxing factor and endothelin-1, a potent vasoconstrictor peptide. Hypoxia is partially or fully responsible for the pulmonary hypertension observed in chronic bronchitis, infiltrative lung disease due to various causes, kyphoscoliosis, obesity-hypoventilation syndrome, chronic mountain sickness, obstructive sleep apnea, and neuromuscular disease. Acidosis is also a potent stimulus of pulmonary arterial vasoconstriction and exerts a synergistic vasoconstrictive effect with hypoxia.

Extensive obliteration and obstruction of the pulmonary arterial tree may cause pulmonary hypertension. Once present, pulmonary hypertension is self-perpetuating. It introduces secondary structural abnormalities in pulmonary vessels, including smooth muscle hypertrophy and intimal proliferation, and these may eventually stimulate atheromatous changes and in situ thrombosis, leading to further narrowing of the arterial bed.

Table 9–25. Mechanisms of pulmonary hypertension and examples of corresponding clinical conditions.

Reduction in cross-sectional area of pulmonary arterial bed
Vasoconstriction
Hypoxia from any cause
Acidosis
Loss of vessels
Lung resection
Emphysema
Vasculitis
Pulmonary fibrosis
Connective tissue disease
Obstruction of vessels
Pulmonary embolism (thromboemboli, tumor emboli, foreign body emboli, etc)
In situ thrombosis
Schistosomiasis
Narrowing of vessels
Secondary structural changes due to pulmonary hypertension
Increased pulmonary venous pressure
Constrictive pericarditis
Left ventricular failure or reduced compliance
Mitral stenosis
Left atrial myxoma
Pulmonary veno-occlusive disease
Mediastinal diseases compressing pulmonary veins
Increased pulmonary blood flow
Congenital left-to-right intracardiac shunts
Increased blood viscosity
Polycythemia
Miscellaneous
Pulmonary hypertension occurring in association with hepatic cirrhosis and portal hypertension

Increased pulmonary venous pressure, when sustained, may cause "postcapillary" pulmonary hypertension; left ventricular failure (systolic, diastolic, or both) is the most common cause.

Pulmonary veno-occlusive disease is a rare cause of postcapillary pulmonary hypertension occurring in children and young adults. The cause is unknown, but associations with various conditions such as viral infection, bone marrow transplantation, chemotherapy, and malignancy have been described. The disease is characterized by progressive fibrotic occlusion of pulmonary veins and venules, along with secondary hypertensive changes in the pulmonary arterioles and muscular pulmonary arteries. Nodular areas of pulmonary congestion, edema, hemorrhage, and hemosiderosis are found. Chest radiography reveals prominent, symmetric interstitial markings, Kerley B lines, pulmonary artery dilation, and normally sized left atrium and left ventricle. Premortem diagnosis is often difficult but is occasionally established by open lung biopsy. There is no effective therapy, and most

Table 9–28. Pulmonary manifestations of selected drug toxicities.

Asthma	**Pulmonary edema**
Beta-blockers	Noncardiogenic
Aspirin	Aspirin
Nonsteroidal anti-inflammatory drugs	Chlordiazepoxide
Histamine	Cocaine
Methacholine	Ethchlorvynol
Acetylcysteine	Heroin
Aerosolized pentamidine	Cardiogenic
Any nebulized medication	Beta-blockers
Chronic cough	**Pleural effusion**
Angiotensin-converting enzyme inhibitors	Bromocriptine
Pulmonary infiltration	Nitrofurantoin
Without eosinophilia	Any drug inducing systemic lupus erythematosus
Amitriptyline	Methysergide
Azathioprine	Chemotherapeutic agents
Amiodarone	**Mediastinal widening**
With eosinophilia	Phenytoin
Sulfonamides	Corticosteroids
L-Tryptophan	Methotrexate
Nitrofurantoin	**Respiratory failure**
Penicillin	Neuromuscular blockade
Methotrexate	Aminoglycosides
Crack cocaine	Succinylcholine
Drug-induced systemic lupus erythematosus	Gallamine
Hydralazine	Dimethyltubocurarine (metocurine)
Procainamide	Central nervous system depression
Isoniazid	Sedatives
Chlorpromazine	Hypnotics
Phenytoin	Opioids
Interstitial pneumonitis/fibrosis	Alcohol
Nitrofurantoin	Tricyclic antidepressants
Bleomycin	Oxygen
Busulfan	
Cyclophosphamide	
Methysergide	
Phenytoin	

ings are not specific. A high index of suspicion and a thorough medical history of drug usage are critical to establishing the diagnosis of drug-induced lung disease. The clinical response to cessation of the suspected offending agent is also helpful. Acute episodes of drug-induced pulmonary disease usually disappear 24–48 hours after the drug has been discontinued, but chronic syndromes may take longer to resolve. Challenge tests to confirm the diagnosis are risky and rarely performed.

Treatment of drug-induced lung disease consists of discontinuing the offending agent immediately and managing the pulmonary symptoms appropriately.

Inhalation of crack cocaine may cause a spectrum of acute pulmonary syndromes, including pulmonary infiltration with eosinophilia, pneumothorax and pneumomediastinum, bronchiolitis obliterans, and acute respiratory failure associated with diffuse alveolar damage and alveolar hemorrhage. Corticosteroids have been used with variable success to treat alveolar hemorrhage.

Copper JA Jr: Drug-induced lung disease. Adv Intern Med 1997;42:231. [NLM Cit ID: 97200186]

RADIATION LUNG INJURY

The lung is a radiosensitive organ that can be affected by external beam radiation therapy. The pulmonary response is determined by the volume of lung irradiated, the dose and rate of therapy, and potentiating factors, eg, concurrent chemotherapy, previous radiation therapy in the same area, and simultaneous withdrawal of corticosteroid therapy. Symptomatic radiation lung injury occurs in about 10% of patients treated with megavoltage therapy for carcinoma of the breast, 5–15% of patients treated for carcinoma of the lung, and 5–35% of patients treated for lymphoma. Two phases of the pulmonary response to radiation are apparent: an acute phase (radiation pneumonitis) and a chronic phase (radiation fibrosis).

Radiation Pneumonitis

Radiation pneumonitis usually occurs 2–3 months (range 1–6 months) after completion of radiotherapy and is characterized by insidious onset of dyspnea, intractable dry cough, chest fullness or pain, weakness, and fever. The pathogenesis of acute radiation pneumonitis is unknown, but there is speculation that hypersensitivity mechanisms are involved. The dominant histopathologic finding is that of a lymphocytic interstitial pneumonitis. Inspiratory crackles may be heard in the involved area. In severe disease, respiratory distress and cyanosis occur that are characteristic of acute respiratory distress syndrome (ARDS). An increased white blood cell count and elevated sedimentation rate are common. Pulmonary function studies reveal reduced lung volumes, reduced lung compliance, hypoxemia, reduced diffusing capacity, and reduced maximum voluntary ventilation. Chest radiograph, which correlates poorly with the presence of symptoms, usually demonstrates an alveolar or nodular infiltrate with a ground-glass opacification limited to the irradiated area. Air bronchograms are often observed. The sharp borders of the infiltrate help distinguish radiation pneumonitis from other conditions, eg, infectious pneumonia, lymphangitic spread of carcinoma, and recurrent tumor. Treatment consists of aspirin, cough suppressants, and bed rest. Acute respiratory failure, if present, is treated appropriately. Although there is no proof that corticosteroids are effective in radiation pneumonitis, prednisone (1 mg/kg/d orally) is usually given immediately for about 1 week. Thereafter, the dose is reduced and maintained at 20–40 mg/d for several weeks, then slowly tapered. Radiation pneumonitis usually resolves in 2–3 weeks. Death from ARDS is unusual.

Pulmonary Radiation Fibrosis

Pulmonary radiation fibrosis occurs in nearly all patients who receive a full course of radiation therapy for cancer of the lung and breast. Patients who experience radiation pneumonitis develop pulmonary fibrosis after an intervening period (6–12 months) of well-being. Most patients are asymptomatic, though slowly progressive dyspnea occurs in some. Radiation fibrosis may occur with or without antecedent radiation pneumonitis. Cor pulmonale and chronic respiratory failure are rare. Radiographic findings include obliteration of normal lung markings, dense interstitial and pleural fibrosis, reduced lung volumes, tenting of the diaphragm, and sharp delineation of the irradiated area. No specific therapy is necessary, and corticosteroids have no value.

Other Complications of Radiation Therapy

Other complications of radiation therapy directed to the thorax include pericardial effusion, constrictive pericarditis, tracheoesophageal fistula, esophageal candidiasis, radiation dermatitis, and rib fractures. Small pleural effusions, radiation pneumonitis outside the irradiated area, spontaneous pneumothorax, and complete obstruction of central airways are unusual occurrences.

Movsas B et al: Pulmonary radiation injury. Chest 1997;111:1061. [NLM Cit ID: 97260469] (Thorough review of radiation pneumonitis and radiation fibrosis, stressing the role of cytokines; 98 references.)

PLEURAL DISEASES

PLEURITIS

Pain due to acute pleural inflammation is caused by irritation of the parietal pleura. Such pain is localized, sharp, and fleeting and is made worse by cough, sneezing, deep breathing, or movement. When the central portion of the diaphragmatic parietal pleura is irritated, pain may be referred to the shoulder. There are numerous causes of pleuritis. The setting in which pleuritic pain develops helps to narrow the differential diagnosis; eg, in young, otherwise healthy individuals, pleuritis is usually caused by viral respiratory infections or pneumonia. The presence of pleural effusion, pleural thickening, or air in the pleural space requires further diagnostic and therapeutic measures. Simple rib fracture may cause severe pleurisy.

Treatment of pleuritis consists of treating the underlying disease. Analgesics and anti-inflammatory drugs (eg, indomethacin, 25 mg orally two or three times daily) are often helpful for pain relief. Codeine (30–60 mg orally every 8 hours) may be used to control cough associated with pleuritic chest pain if retention of airway secretions is not a likely complication. Intercostal nerve blocks are sometimes helpful.

PLEURAL EFFUSION

Essentials of Diagnosis

- Asymptomatic in many cases; pleuritic chest pain if pleuritis is present; dyspnea if effusion is large.
- Decreased tactile fremitus; dullness to percussion; distant breath sounds; egophony if effusion is large.
- Radiographic evidence of pleural effusion.
- Diagnostic findings on thoracentesis.

General Considerations

Pleural fluid is formed in the normal individual mostly on the parietal pleural surface at the rate of about 0.1 mL/kg body weight/h. Movement of fluid into and out of the pleural space is dependent on hydrostatic and osmotic forces in parietal and visceral pleural capillaries. Absorption of fluid occurs mostly through visceral pleural capillaries, while protein is recovered through parietal pleural lymphatics. The resultant homeostasis leaves 5–15 mL of fluid normally present in the pleural space. This amount is not detectable on conventional chest radiographs. **Pleural effusion** is an abnormal accumulation of fluid in the pleural space. The five major types of pleural effusion are transudates, exudates, empyema, hemorrhagic pleural effusion or hemothorax, and chylous or chyliform effusion.

Pleural effusions are classified as **transudates** or **exudates** to help in differential diagnosis. An exudate is a pleural fluid having *one or more* of the following features: (1) pleural fluid protein to serum protein ratio > 0.5; (2) pleural fluid LDH to serum LDH ratio > 0.6; and (3) pleural fluid LDH greater than two-thirds the upper limit of normal serum LDH. Transudates have none of these features.

Causes of transudates and exudates are listed in Table 9–29. Congestive heart failure accounts for most transudates and is the most common cause of pleural effusion. Mechanisms (and examples) leading to formation of transudates include increase in hydrostatic pressure (congestive heart failure), decreased oncotic pressure (hypoalbuminemia), and greater negative intrapleural pressure (acute atelectasis). Bacterial pneumonia and cancer are the commonest causes of exudative effusion. Exudates form as a result of disease of the pleura itself in association with increased capillary permeability (eg, pneumonia) or reduced lymphatic drainage (eg, carcinoma obstructing lymphatic drainage).

The gross appearance of pleural fluid helps to identify the other major types of pleural effusion. **Empyema** is an exudative pleural effusion caused by direct infection of the pleural space, causing the

Table 9–29. Causes of pleural fluid transudates and exudates.

Transudates	Exudates
Congestive heart failure (~90% of cases)	Pneumonia (parapneumonic effusion)
Cirrhosis with ascites	Cancer
Nephrotic syndrome	Pulmonary embolism
Peritoneal dialysis	Empyema
Myxedema	Tuberculosis
Acute atelectasis	Connective tissue disease
Constrictive pericarditis	Viral infection
Superior vena cava obstruction	Fungal infection
Pulmonary embolism	Rickettsial infection
	Parasitic infection
	Asbestos
	Meigs' syndrome
	Pancreatic disease
	Uremia
	Chronic atelectasis
	Trapped lung
	Chylothorax
	Sarcoidosis
	Drug reaction
	Post-myocardial infarction syndrome

pleural fluid to appear purulent or turbid. **Hemothorax** is the presence of gross blood in the pleural space, usually a result of chest trauma. **Hemorrhagic pleural effusion** is a mixture of blood and pleural fluid. About 10,000 red blood cells per microliter are necessary to create blood-tinged pleural fluid; 100,000 red blood cells per microliter make pleural fluid appear grossly bloody. If the hematocrit of pleural fluid is more than 50% of the hematocrit of peripheral blood, hemothorax is present. In the absence of trauma, grossly bloody pleural fluid suggests cancer or, less commonly, pulmonary embolism.

Pleural fluid milky in appearance should be centrifuged. Clearing of the milky appearance from the supernatant suggests empyema, whereas persistent cloudy or turbid supernatant signifies **chylous** or **chyliform pleural effusion.** Chylous pleural effusion occurs acutely in chylothorax as a result of disruption of the thoracic duct. Chyliform pleural effusion occurs in pseudochylothorax as a result of accumulation of cholesterol complexes in a chronically thickened pleural space, a phenomenon sometimes seen in cases of trapped lung (entrapment of lung by a fibrous peel on the visceral pleura), tuberculous pleuritis (especially with previous therapeutic pneumothorax), or rheumatoid pleural effusion. A chylous pleural effusion may have an acute or subacute onset. There is no associated pleural thickening on chest radiograph, and fluid analysis reveals chylomicrons and a high triglyceride level, usually above 100 mg/dL.

Clinical Findings

A. Symptoms and Signs: Small pleural effusions are usually asymptomatic, whereas large pleural effusions may cause dyspnea, particularly in the presence of underlying cardiopulmonary disease. Pleuritic chest pain and dry cough may occur; pleural fluid found in association with pleuritic chest pain is usually an exudate. Physical findings are absent if less than 200–300 mL of pleural fluid is present. Signs consistent with a larger pleural effusion include decrease in tactile fremitus, dullness to percussion, and diminution of breath sounds over the effusion. In large effusions that compress the lung, accentuation of breath sounds and egophony may be noted just above the effusion. A pleural friction rub indicates pleuritis. A massive pleural effusion with high intrapleural pressure may cause contralateral shift of the trachea and bulging of the intercostal spaces.

B. Laboratory Findings: Diagnostic thoracentesis should be performed whenever a pleural effusion is detected and no cause for the effusion is clinically apparent. Decubitus films are the preferred method to demonstrate free pleural fluid. Ultrasound examination is useful to find the site for thoracentesis of a small or a loculated pleural effusion.

Transudates occur in the setting of normal capillary integrity but altered hydrostatic and oncotic forces. Transudates therefore lack the distinguishing protein and LDH findings described above and often have other typical characteristics (white blood cell count < 1000/μL, predominance of mononuclear cells in the differential, glucose level in pleural fluid equal to that of serum, and normal pH). Transudates suggest the absence of local pleural disease; more than 90% are due to congestive heart failure. Laboratory findings in exudative pleural effusions are more variable and are summarized in Table 9–30. If an exudate is suspected, thoracentesis should be performed. The presence of malignant cells or positive results on smear or culture are definitive findings in pleural fluid; identification of other causes depends on a constellation of findings on gross examination and laboratory studies or on biopsy results. Laboratory tests of pleural fluid should include total and differential white blood cell count, protein, glucose, and LDH. Pleural fluid pH is helpful in narrowing the differential diagnosis of exudative effusions. A pH less than 7.30 indicates cancer, complicated parapneumonic effusion, lupus or rheumatoid effusion, tuberculosis, or esophageal rupture. A high percentage of lymphocytes in pleural fluid suggests tuberculosis (as does the absence of mesothelial cells) or cancer. Low levels of glucose in pleural fluid point toward cancer, empyema, tuberculosis, esophageal rupture, or connective tissue disease (rheumatoid pleuritis in particular). Elevated levels of amylase in pleural fluid suggest one of four diagnoses: pancreatitis, pancreatic pseudocyst, pancreatic cancer, or esophageal rupture.

Closed pleural biopsy with a Cope or Abrams needle should be considered whenever malignancy or tuberculosis is considered in the differential diagnosis of a pleural effusion that is unexplained after routine

Table 9–30. Characteristics of important exudative pleural effusions.

Etiology or Type of Effusion	Gross Appearance	White Blood Cell Count (cells/μL)	Differential[1]	Red Blood Cell Count (cells/μL)	Glucose	Comments
Malignant effusion	Turbid to bloody; occasionally serous	1000 to < 100,000	M	100 to several hundred thousand	Equal to serum levels; < 60 mg/dL in 15% of cases	Eosinophilia uncommon; positive results on cytologic examination
Uncomplicated parapneumonic effusion	Clear to turbid	5000–25,000	P	< 5000	Equal to serum levels	Tube thoracostomy unnecessary
Empyema	Turbid to purulent	25,000–100,000	P	< 5000	Less than serum levels; often very low	Drainage necessary; putrid odor suggests anaerobic infection
Tuberculosis	Serous to serosanguineous	5000–10,000	M	< 10,000	Equal to serum levels; occasionally < 60 mg/dL	Protein may exceed 5 g/dL; eosinophils (> 10%) or mesothelial cells (> 5%) make diagnosis unlikely
Rheumatoid effusion	Turbid; greenish-yellow	1000–20,000	M or P	< 1000	< 40 mg/dL	Secondary empyema common; high LDH, low complement, high rheumatoid factor, cholesterol crystals are characteristic
Pulmonary infarction	Serous to grossly bloody	1000–50,000	M or P	100 to > 100,000	Equal to serum levels	Variable findings; no pathognomonic features
Esophageal rupture	Turbid to purulent; red-brown	< 5000 to > 50,000	P	1000–10,000	Usually low	High amylase level (salivary origin); pneumothorax in 25% of cases; effusion usually on left side; pH < 6.0 strongly suggests diagnosis
Pancreatitis	Turbid to serosanguineous	1000–50,000	P	1000–10,000	Equal to serum levels	Usually left-sided; high amylase level

[1]M = mononuclear cell predominance; P = polymorphonuclear leukocyte predominance.

studies and thoracentesis. Contraindications include bleeding diathesis, poor respiratory reserve, empyema, and absence of pleural fluid. The expected yield of the procedure approximates 55% in pleural malignancy, somewhat less than with cytologic examination of pleural fluid, and over 75% in pleural tuberculosis if the tissue fragments are submitted for culture as well as histology. Open pleural biopsy is sometimes required to establish the diagnosis of pleural malignancy and is especially indicated for the diagnosis of malignant pleural mesothelioma. Thoracoscopy with a flexible or rigid instrument is an alternative procedure with excellent diagnostic accuracy in experienced hands.

C. Imaging: About 250 mL of pleural fluid must be present before effusion can be detected on conventional erect posteroanterior chest radiograph. Lateral decubitus views can detect much smaller amounts of free pleural fluid. CT scanning is sensitive in the detection of small amounts of pleural fluid. Free pleural fluid collects in the subpulmonary area. Larger amounts of fluid spill over into the costophrenic sulcus to form a meniscus. Thickening of major and minor fissures is common. Atypical collections of pleural fluid are frequently seen. Lateral displacement of the apex of the diaphragm and abrupt obliteration of lung markings at the level of the diaphragm are features of subpulmonary effusion. Pleural fluid may become trapped ("loculated") by pleural adhesions, forming unusual collections along the chest wall or in the lung fissures. Shadows with a broad base on the chest wall that point inward toward the hilum are characteristic of loculated effusions. Round or oval collections of loculated fluid in fissures resemble tumors ("pseudotumors"). Ultrasound is useful to locate loculated or small effusions.

Massive pleural effusion (opacification of an entire hemithorax) is commonly caused by cancer but has been observed in tuberculosis and other diseases.

Treatment

Treatment should address both the disease causing the pleural effusion and the effusion itself. A specific diagnosis can be established in most cases of pleural effusion.

A. Transudative Pleural Effusion: Transudative pleural effusions generally respond to treatment of the underlying condition; therapeutic thoracentesis is indicated only if massive effusion causes dyspnea. Pleurodesis and tube thoracostomy are rarely indicated. For example, when bilateral pleural effusions develop in a patient with congestive heart failure, neither diagnostic nor therapeutic thoracentesis is routinely indicated. Such effusions are likely to be transudates and will resolve with treatment of the underlying cardiac disease.

B. Malignant or Paramalignant Pleural Effusion: Pleural effusion in a patient with known cancer may be either malignant or paramalignant. In cancer patients with **malignant pleural effusion,** the pleural surface is directly invaded by malignant cells (pleural fluid cytology or pleural tissue biopsy reveals evidence of malignancy). In such cases the tumor causing the effusion is unresectable, and treatment with chemotherapy or radiotherapy is directed at the underlying cancer. Chemical **pleurodesis** (obliteration of the pleural space by producing fibrous adhesion between the visceral and the parietal pleura) is advised for selected patients with symptomatic malignant pleural effusion who fail to respond to chemotherapy or mediastinal radiation or who are not candidates for these forms of therapy. Chemical pleurodesis is usually performed by instilling bleomycin, mitoxantrone, or talc slurry into the pleural space (see Chapter 4). Repeated therapeutic thoracentesis, pleuroperitoneal shunting, and surgical pleurectomy are alternative approaches for certain patients with rapidly recurring malignant pleural effusion. The term **"paramalignant pleural effusion"** denotes a pleural effusion in a patient with cancer when the pleural space is not directly invaded by tumor and repeated thoracentesis and needle biopsy of the pleura give negative results. In this situation, the underlying tumor may or may not be resectable.

C. Parapneumonic Pleural Effusion: Pleural effusion in the setting of pneumonia ("parapneumonic effusion") usually responds to systemic antibiotic therapy. A common management decision is whether to drain a parapneumonic effusion via tube thoracostomy. The therapeutic intent of drainage is to avoid progression of the effusion from the exudative to subsequent (fibrinopurulent and organized) stages. The goal is to avoid formation of a thick pleural "peel" that may trap the lung and cause permanent loss of lung function. Effective therapy requires prompt intervention. Laboratory findings—especially the pH—are important guides to additional therapy. In "uncomplicated" parapneumonic effusion, no pleural infection is present, and the pleural fluid glucose and pH are normal. Such effusion is likely to resolve spontaneously, and chest tube drainage is not required. In "complicated" parapneumonic effusion, pleural fluid is either frank pus or has the potential to organize into a fibrous "peel." A low pH (< 7.2), low glucose (< 50 mg/dL), and high LDH (> 1000 units/L)—but not a high pleural fluid white blood cell count or protein concentration—help to separate complicated from uncomplicated parapneumonic effusions.

Tube thoracostomy is required for parapneumonic effusion if any of the following is present: (1) the fluid resembles frank pus or bacteria are seen on Gram stain, (2) pleural fluid glucose is < 40 mg/dL, or (3) pleural fluid pH is < 7.2. If the pleural fluid pH is between 7.2 and 7.3 or the LDH is > 1000 units/L, the physician should strongly consider chest tube placement or monitor the effusion carefully with serial thoracenteses. Serial thoracentesis is not an effective strategy for *treatment* of complicated parapneumonic effusions.

A parapneumonic effusion that does not respond to drainage within 24 hours may have become loculated. Intrapleural injection of streptokinase via the chest tube (250,000 units in 100 mL 0.9% saline daily for up to 10 days) may accelerate drainage. Localized pockets of empyema may be present in this circumstance, even though thoracentesis from another localized fluid collection did not reveal empyema. In such cases, ultrasound examination is required to guide placement of an additional chest tube in the proper location. Open surgical drainage may be necessary if these measures are ineffective. A thick pleural peel developing after treatment of complicated parapneumonic effusion may resolve slowly over several months.

D. Hemothorax: Hemothorax is generally managed by the immediate insertion of one or more large chest tubes in order to control bleeding by causing apposition of pleural surfaces; chest tubes help the physician determine the amount of bleeding and decrease the risk of complications such as empyema and eventual fibrothorax. As much blood as possible should be drained before the chest tube is removed. Thoracotomy is occasionally required to control bleeding, remove large volumes of blood clots, and treat coexisting complications of trauma such as bronchopleural fistula. A very small hemothorax that is stable or improving on chest radiograph can be managed without tube drainage.

E. Other Types of Pleural Effusion: Management of patients with exudative pleural effusion due to other causes consists mainly of treating the underlying disease. A low pleural fluid pH outside the setting of pneumonia is not an absolute indication for chest tube drainage. Patients with rheumatoid pleural effusions should be watched closely for the development of secondary empyema, though glucose levels less than 10 mg/dL are routinely observed without infection. Such patients invariably have seropositive rheumatoid arthritis and peripheral nodules.

Prognosis

The prognosis of patients with pleural effusion depends on the underlying disease.

Light RW et al: Management of parapneumonic effusions. Clin Chest Med 1998;19:373. [NLM Cit ID: 98310972] (Current concepts in management, including use of thrombolytic agents.)

Sasse SA: Parapneumonic effusions and empyema. Curr Opin Pulm Med 1996;2:320. [NLM Cit ID: 98029447] (Diagnosis, etiology, and treatment.)

SPONTANEOUS PNEUMOTHORAX

Essentials of Diagnosis

- Acute onset of ipsilateral chest pain and dyspnea.
- Minimal physical findings in mild cases; unilateral chest expansion, decreased tactile fremitus, hyper-resonance, diminished breath sounds, mediastinal shift, cyanosis in tension pneumothorax.
- Presence of pleural air on chest radiograph.

General Considerations

Pneumothorax, or accumulation of air in the pleural space, is classified as spontaneous (primary or secondary) or traumatic. Primary spontaneous pneumothorax occurs in the absence of an underlying lung disease, whereas secondary spontaneous pneumothorax is a complication of preexisting pulmonary disease. Traumatic pneumothorax results from penetrating or blunt trauma and is often iatrogenic. Iatrogenic pneumothorax may follow procedures such as thoracentesis, pleural biopsy, subclavian or internal jugular vein catheter placement, percutaneous lung biopsy, bronchoscopy with transbronchial biopsy, and positive-pressure mechanical ventilation. Tension pneumothorax usually occurs in the setting of penetrating trauma, lung infection, cardiopulmonary resuscitation, or positive-pressure mechanical ventilation. In tension pneumothorax, the pressure of air in the pleural space exceeds ambient pressure throughout the respiratory cycle. A check-valve mechanism allows air to enter the pleural space on inspiration and prevents egress of air on expiration.

Primary pneumothorax affects mainly tall, thin boys and men between the ages of 10 and 30 years. It is thought to occur from rupture of subpleural apical blebs in response to high negative intrapleural pressures. Family history and cigarette smoking may also be important factors.

Secondary pneumothorax occurs as a complication of COPD, asthma, cystic fibrosis, tuberculosis, and a wide variety of infiltrative lung diseases, including pneumocystis pneumonia. Aerosolized pentamidine and prior history of pneumocystis pneumonia are considered potential risk factors for the development of pneumothorax. One-half of patients with pneumothorax in the setting of recurrent pneumocystis pneumonia develop contralateral pneumothorax. The mortality rate of pneumothorax in pneumocystis pneumonia is high. Pneumothorax in association with menstruation (catamenial pneumothorax) is another well-established form of secondary pneumothorax.

Clinical Findings

A. Symptoms and Signs: Chest pain ranging from minimal to severe on the affected side and dyspnea occur in nearly all patients. Symptoms usually begin during rest and usually resolve within 24 hours even if the pneumothorax persists. Alternatively, pneumothorax may present with life-threatening respiratory failure if underlying COPD or asthma is present; this is true irrespective of the size of the pneumothorax.

If pneumothorax is small (less than 15% of a hemithorax), physical findings, other than mild tachycardia, are unimpressive. If pneumothorax is large, diminished breath sounds, decreased tactile fremitus, and decreased movement of the chest are often noted. Tension pneumothorax should be suspected in the presence of marked tachycardia, hypotension, and mediastinal or tracheal shift. Hyperresonance is more often observed in tension pneumothorax.

B. Laboratory Findings: Arterial blood gas analysis reveals hypoxemia and acute respiratory alkalosis in most patients but is often unnecessary. Left sided primary pneumothorax may produce QRS axis and precordial T wave changes on the ECG that may be misinterpreted as acute myocardial infarction.

C. Imaging: Demonstration of a visceral pleural line on chest radiograph is diagnostic and may only be revealed on an expiratory film. A few patients have secondary pleural effusion that demonstrates a characteristic air-fluid level on chest radiography. In supine patients, pneumothorax on a conventional chest radiograph may appear as an abnormally radiolucent costophrenic sulcus (the "deep sulcus" sign). In patients with tension pneumothorax, chest radiographs show a large amount of air in the affected hemithorax and contralateral shift of mediastinal structures.

Differential Diagnosis

If the patient is a young, tall, thin, cigarette-smoking man, the diagnosis of primary spontaneous pneumothorax is usually obvious and can be confirmed by

asleep during the evaluation. The oropharynx is frequently found to be narrowed by excessive soft tissue folds, large tonsils, pendulous uvula, or prominent tongue. Nasal obstruction by a deviated nasal septum, poor nasal air flow, and a nasal twang to the speech may be observed. A "bull neck" appearance is common. Facial deformities, retrognathia, and pharyngeal tumors are less frequently seen.

Erythrocytosis is common. A hemoglobin level and thyroid function tests should be obtained. Observation of the sleeping patient reveals loud snoring interrupted by episodes of increasingly strong ventilatory effort that fail to produce airflow. A loud snort accompanies the first breath following an apneic episode. Polysomnography reveals apneic episodes lasting as long as 1–2 minutes. Oxygen saturation falls, often to very low levels. Bradyarrhythmias such as sinus bradycardia, sinus arrest, or atrioventricular block may occur. Tachyarrhythmias, including paroxysmal supraventricular tachycardia, atrial fibrillation, and ventricular tachycardia, are common once airflow is reestablished.

Weight loss and strict avoidance of alcohol and hypnotic medications are the first steps in management. Weight loss may be curative, but most patients are unable to lose the 10–20% of body weight required. Nasal continuous positive airway pressure (nasal CPAP) at night is curative in many patients. Polysomnography is frequently necessary to determine the level of CPAP (usually 5–15 cm H_2O) necessary to abolish obstructive apneas. Unfortunately, only about 75% of patients continue to use nasal CPAP after 1 year. Pharmacologic therapy for obstructive sleep apnea is disappointing. Supplemental oxygen may lessen the severity of nocturnal desaturation but may also lengthen apneas. Polysomnography is necessary to assess the effects of oxygen therapy; it should not be routinely prescribed. Mechanical devices inserted into the mouth at bedtime to hold the jaw forward and prevent pharyngeal occlusion have modest effectiveness in relieving apnea, and patient compliance is not optimal.

Uvulopalatopharyngoplasty, a procedure consisting of resection of pharyngeal soft tissue and amputation of approximately 15 mm of the free edge of the soft palate and uvula, may be helpful in selected patients. It is more effective in eliminating snoring than apneic episodes. Only about half of these operations are successful. Uvulopalatopharyngoplasty may now be performed on an outpatient basis with a laser. **Nasal septoplasty** is performed if gross anatomic nasal septal deformity is present. **Tracheostomy** relieves upper airway obstruction and its physiologic consequences and represents the definitive treatment for obstructive sleep apnea. However, it has numerous adverse effects, including granuloma formation, difficulty with speech, and stoma and airway infection. Furthermore, the long-term care of the tracheostomy, especially in obese patients, can be difficult. Tracheostomy and other maxillofacial surgery approaches are reserved for patients with life-threatening arrhythmias or severe disability who have failed to respond to conservative therapy.

Exar EN et al: The upper airway resistance syndrome. Chest 1999;115:1127. [NLM Cit ID: 99222900] (Review of pathophysiology and diagnostic and therapeutic approaches.)

Loube DI et al: Indications for positive airway pressure treatment of adult obstructive sleep apnea patients: consensus statement. Chest 1999;115:863. [NLM Cit ID: 99181995]

Strohl KP et al: Recognition of obstructive sleep apnea. Am J Respir Crit Care Med 1996;154:279. [NLM Cit ID: 96328114] (State of the art review with 182 references.)

Wright J et al: Health effects of obstructive sleep apnoea and the effectiveness of continuous positive airway pressure: A systematic review of the research evidence. BJM 1997;314:851. [NLM Cit ID: 97246949]

HYPERVENTILATION SYNDROMES

Hyperventilation is an increase in alveolar ventilation that leads to hypocapnia. It may be caused by a variety of conditions, such as pregnancy, hypoxemia, obstructive and infiltrative lung diseases, sepsis, hepatic dysfunction, fever, and pain. The term "central neurogenic hyperventilation" denotes a monotonous, sustained pattern of rapid and deep breathing seen in comatose patients with brain stem injury of multiple causes. Functional hyperventilation may be acute or chronic. Acute hyperventilation presents with hyperpnea, paresthesias, carpopedal spasm, tetany, and anxiety. Chronic hyperventilation may present with various nonspecific symptoms, including fatigue, dyspnea, anxiety, palpitations, and dizziness. The diagnosis of chronic hyperventilation syndrome is established if symptoms are reproduced during voluntary hyperventilation. Once organic causes of hyperventilation have been excluded, treatment of acute hyperventilation consists of rebreathing expired gas from a paper bag held over the face in order to decrease respiratory alkalemia and its associated symptoms. Anxiolytic drugs are also useful.

Gardner WN: The pathophysiology of hyperventilation disorders. Chest 1996;109:516. [NLM Cit ID: 96187679] (Concise review.)

ACUTE RESPIRATORY FAILURE

Respiratory failure is defined as respiratory dysfunction resulting in abnormalities of oxygenation or ventilation (CO_2 elimination) severe enough to impair or threaten the function of vital organs. Arterial blood gas criteria for respiratory failure are not absolute but may be arbitrarily established as a Po_2 under 60 mm Hg and a Pco_2 over 50 mm Hg. Acute respiratory failure may occur in a variety of pulmonary and nonpulmonary disorders (Table 9–31). A complete discussion of treatment of acute respiratory failure is beyond the scope of this chapter. Only a few selected general principles of management will be reviewed here.

Clinical Findings

Symptoms and signs of acute respiratory failure are those of the underlying disease combined with those of hypoxemia and hypercapnia. The chief symptom of hypoxemia is dyspnea, though profound hypoxemia may exist in the absence of complaints. Signs of hypoxemia include cyanosis, restlessness, confusion, anxiety, delirium, tachypnea, tachycardia, hypertension, cardiac arrhythmias, and tremor. Dyspnea and headache are the cardinal symptoms of hypercapnia. Signs of hypercapnia include peripheral and conjunctival hyperemia, hypertension, tachycardia, tachypnea, impaired consciousness, papilledema, and asterixis. The symptoms and signs of acute respiratory failure are both insensitive and nonspecific; therefore, the physician must maintain a high index of suspicion and request an arterial blood gas analysis if respiratory failure is suspected.

Treatment

Treatment of the patient with acute respiratory failure consists of (1) specific therapy directed toward the underlying disease; (2) respiratory supportive care directed toward the maintenance of adequate gas exchange; and (3) general supportive care. Only the last two aspects are discussed below.

A. Respiratory Support: Respiratory support has both nonventilatory and ventilatory aspects.

1. Nonventilatory aspects–*The main therapeutic goal in acute hypoxemic respiratory failure is to ensure adequate oxygenation of vital organs.* Inspired oxygen concentration should be the lowest value that results in an oxygen saturation of ≥ 90% (Pao_2 about 60 mm Hg). Higher arterial oxygen tensions are of no benefit. Restoration of normoxia may cause hypoventilation in patients with chronic hypercapnia; however, *oxygen therapy should not be withheld for fear of causing progressive respiratory acidemia.* Hypoxemia in patients with obstructive airway disease is usually easily corrected by administering low-flow oxygen by nasal cannula (1–3 L/min) or Venturi mask (24–28%). Higher concentrations of oxygen are necessary to correct hypoxemia in patients with acute respiratory distress syndrome (ARDS), pneumonia, and other parenchymal lung diseases.

2. Ventilatory aspects–Ventilatory support consists of maintaining patency of the airway and ensuring adequate alveolar ventilation. Tracheal intubation and mechanical ventilation are often required.

a. Tracheal intubation–Indications for tracheal intubation are (1) hypoxemia which is not quickly reversed by supplemental oxygen, (2) upper airway obstruction, (3) impaired airway protection, (4) inadequate handling of secretions, and (5) facilitation of mechanical ventilation. In general, orotracheal intubation is preferred to nasotracheal intubation in urgent or emergency situations because it is easier, faster, and less traumatic. The position of the tip of the endotracheal tube at the level of the aortic arch should be verified by chest radiograph immediately following intubation, and auscultation should be performed to verify that both lungs are being inflated. Only tracheal tubes with high volume, low-pressure air-filled or foam cuffs should be used. Cuff inflation pressure should be kept below 20 mm Hg if possible to minimize tracheal mucosal injury.

b. Mechanical ventilation–Indications for mechanical ventilation include (1) apnea, (2) acute hypercapnia that is not quickly reversed by appropriate specific therapy, (3) severe hypoxemia, and (4) progressive patient fatigue despite appropriate treatment. In general, positive-pressure ventilators should be used to provide mechanical ventilatory support. Noninvasive positive-pressure ventilation using such approaches as nasal or face mask ventilation is an alternative in selected patients.

Several modes of positive-pressure ventilation are available. Assisted mechanical ventilation (AMV), or assist/control (A/C), is a ventilatory mode in which the ventilator is set to deliver a minimum number of

Table 9–31. Selected causes of acute respiratory failure in adults.

Airway disorders
Asthma
Chronic bronchitis or emphysema in acute exacerbation
Partial obstruction of pharynx, larynx, trachea, or lobar bronchi by edema, mucus, or foreign body
Parenchymal lung disorders
Acute respiratory distress syndrome
Congestive heart failure
Pneumonia
Hypersensitivity pneumonitis
Aspiration
Pulmonary vascular disorders
Pulmonary thromboembolism
Chest wall and pleural disorders
Flail chest
Pneumothorax
Pleural effusion
Neuromuscular disorders
Opioid or sedative-hypnotic overdose
Guillain-Barré syndrome
Botulism
Spinal cord injury
Myasthenia gravis
Poliomyelitis
Stroke
Traumatic brain injury

Tachypnea is also nonspecific, but pulmonary disease and heart failure should be considered when respiratory rates exceed 16/min under basal conditions. **Periodic breathing** (Cheyne-Stokes respiration) is not uncommon in severe heart failure.

Peripheral Pulses & Venous Pulsations

Diminished peripheral pulses most commonly result from arteriosclerotic peripheral vascular disease and may be accompanied by localized **bruits.** Asymmetry of pulses should also arouse suspicion of coarctation of the aorta or aortic dissection; previous cardiac catheterization may also be responsible. **Exaggerated pulses** may indicate aortic regurgitation, coarctation, patent ductus arteriosus, or other conditions that increase stroke volume. The carotid pulse is a valuable aid to assessment of left ventricular ejection. It has a **delayed upstroke** in aortic stenosis and a **bisferiens** quality (two palpable peaks) in mixed aortic stenosis and regurgitation or hypertrophic obstructive cardiomyopathy. **Pulsus paradoxus** (a decrease in systolic blood pressure during inspiration greater than the normal 10 mm Hg) is a valuable sign of pericardial tamponade, though it also occurs in asthma and chronic obstructive pulmonary disease. **Pulsus alternans,** in which the amplitude of the pulse alternates every other beat during sinus rhythm, occurs when cardiac contractility is very depressed or with large pericardial effusions.

Jugular venous pulsations provide insight into right atrial pressure. They indicate (1) **elevated central venous pressure** if they are more than 3 vertical centimeters above the angle of Louis, (2) increased central blood volume if they rise more than 1 cm with sustained (30 seconds) right upper quadrant abdominal pressure **(hepatojugular reflux)**, (3) tricuspid obstruction or pulmonary hypertension if the *a* wave is exaggerated, and (4) tricuspid regurgitation if **large** ***cv*** waves are seen. The latter may be associated with hepatic pulsations. Atrioventricular dissociation due to conduction block or ventricular arrhythmia can be recognized by intermittent **cannon *a* waves.**

McGee SR: Physical examination of venous pressure: a critical review. Am Heart J 1998;136:10. [NLM Cit ID: 98328149] (Precise estimation of venous pressure by bedside examination is difficult.)

Pulmonary Examination

Rales heard at the lung bases are a sign of congestive heart failure but may be caused by similarly localized pulmonary disease. **Wheezing** and **rhonchi** suggest obstructive pulmonary disease but may occur in left heart failure. **Pleural effusions** with bibasilar percussion dullness and reduced breath sounds are common in congestive heart failure.

Precordial Pulsations

A **parasternal lift** usually indicates right ventricular hypertrophy, pulmonary hypertension (pulmonary artery systolic pressure > 50 mm Hg), or left atrial enlargement; pulmonary artery pulsations may also be visible. The left ventricular **apical impulse,** if sustained and enlarged, suggests myocardial hypertrophy or dysfunction. If it is very prominent but not sustained, the apical impulse may indicate volume overload or high-output states. Additional precordial pulsations may reflect regional abnormalities of left ventricular contraction.

Heart Sounds & Murmurs

Auscultation is diagnostic of—or helpful in diagnosis of—many heart diseases, including cardiac failure. Specific findings are discussed under diagnostic headings.

The **first heart sound (S_1)** may be diminished with severe left ventricular dysfunction or accentuated with mitral stenosis or short PR intervals. **S_2** is usually split, with the two components (aortic preceding pulmonary) being separated more during inspiration; **splitting** is *fixed* in atrial septal defect, *wide* with right bundle branch block, and *absent* or *reversed* **(paradoxic splitting)** with aortic stenosis, left ventricular failure, or left bundle branch block. With normal splitting, an accentuated P_2 is an important sign of pulmonary hypertension. **Third and fourth heart sounds** (ventricular and atrial gallops, respectively) indicate ventricular volume overload or impaired compliance and may be heard over either ventricle. An apical S_3 is a normal finding in younger individuals and in pregnancy. Additional auscultatory findings include sharp, high-pitched sounds classified as **"clicks."** These may be early systolic and represent **ejection sounds** (as with a bicuspid aortic valve or pulmonary stenosis) or may occur in mid or late systole, indicating myxomatous changes in the mitral valve.

While many **murmurs** indicate valvular disease, a soft, short systolic murmur, usually localized along the left sternal border or toward the apex, may be innocent, reflecting pulmonary flow. **Innocent murmurs** often vary with inspiration, diminish in the upright position, and are most frequently heard in thin individuals. **Systolic murmurs** are **pansystolic (holosystolic)** when they merge with the first sound and persist through all of systole or **"ejection" murmurs** when they begin after the first sound and end before the second sound, with a peak in early or mid systole. The former represent mitral regurgitation if maximal at the apex or in the axilla and tricuspid regurgitation or ventricular septal defect if best heard at the sternal border. Short aortic ejection murmurs with a preserved A_2 are common in older individuals, especially when hypertension has been present, and even if they are moderately loud they usually reflect thickening (sclerosis) of the valve rather than stenosis. Association of murmurs with palpable vibrations (**"thrills"**) is always clinically significant, as are **diastolic murmurs.**

Etchells E et al: Does this patient have an abnormal systolic murmur? JAMA 1997;227:564. [NLM Cit ID: 97184362] (Literature review of useful techniques for determining causes of systolic murmurs.)

Edema

Subcutaneous fluid collections appear first in the lower extremities in ambulatory patients or in the sacral region of bedridden individuals. In heart disease, edema results from elevated right atrial pressures. Right heart failure most commonly results from left heart failure, although the right-sided signs may predominate. Other cardiogenic causes of edema include pericardial disease, right-sided valve lesions, and cor pulmonale. Edema may also be due to peripheral venous insufficiency, venous obstruction, nephrotic syndrome, cirrhosis, premenstrual fluid retention, drugs (especially vasodilators such as calcium channel blockers or salt-retaining medications such as nonsteroidal anti-inflammatory agents), or it may be idiopathic.

Brater DR: Diuretic therapy. N Engl J Med 1998;339:387. [NLM Cit ID: 98346823] (Clinical pharmacology and use in hepatic, renal, and cardiac disorders.)

Rasool A et al: Treatment of edematous disorders with diuretics. Am J Med Sci 2000;319:25. [NLM Cit ID: 20117167]

DIAGNOSTIC TESTING

The **chest x-ray** will provide information about heart size, the pulmonary circulation (with characteristic signs suggesting both pulmonary artery or pulmonary venous hypertension), primary pulmonary disease, and aortic abnormalities. The **echocardiogram** provides much more reliable information about chamber size, hypertrophy, pericardial effusions, valvular abnormalities, and congenital abnormalities, and where readily available this procedure has replaced the x-ray for evaluation of cardiac disease. The **electrocardiogram (ECG)** indicates cardiac rhythm, reveals conduction abnormalities, and provides evidence of ventricular hypertrophy, myocardial infarction, or ischemia. Nonspecific ST segment and T wave changes may reflect these processes but are also noted with electrolyte imbalance, drug effects, and many other conditions. Routine x-rays and ECGs are not recommended to screen for heart disease and have a limited role in the follow-up of patients with known heart disease. However, a baseline ECG is helpful in older patients.

NONINVASIVE DIAGNOSTIC TESTING

Noninvasive diagnostic procedures are growing in number and application. However, they are frequently overutilized. The clinician should carefully consider what question is being asked and how the results will alter patient management before ordering these tests. They have limited applicability in screening for asymptomatic disease and should not be substituted for a careful clinical evaluation.

The most versatile and generally informative noninvasive technique is **echocardiography,** which plays a crucial role in the evaluation of patients with most cardiac symptoms and conditions, including congenital, valvular, coronary, and cardiomyopathic heart disease. An overview of echocardiography and its applications is presented below. Other specialized noninvasive cardiac testing procedures, such as stress testing, ambulatory electrocardiography, and other imaging modalities are discussed in conjunction with their major applications.

Echocardiography

M-mode and **two-dimensional echocardiograms** provide measurements of left ventricular size, function, and thickness. Left ventricular segmental wall motion can be assessed, and the size of all four cardiac chambers can be determined. The morphology of the heart valves can be examined. Hypertrophic cardiomyopathy, pericardial effusion, mitral valve prolapse, valvular vegetations, and cardiac tumors may all be diagnosed. **Doppler ultrasound** provides a quantitative estimation of transvalvular gradients and pulmonary artery pressure and qualitative evaluation of valvular regurgitation and intraventricular shunts. **Color Doppler** visually demonstrates patterns and directionality of flow; it has been particularly useful in evaluating congenital heart disease. However, Doppler studies frequently detect *clinically insignificant* valvular regurgitation; care should be taken not to overinterpret those findings.

Transesophageal echocardiography is used to improve the quality of echocardiograms, to derive information about posterior structures (especially the atria and atrioventricular valves) and prosthetic valves, and to monitor patients during surgery. It is superior to surface echocardiography in diagnosing left atrial thrombi, valvular vegetations, and eccentric mitral regurgitant jets (especially with prosthetic valves). The absence of mural thrombi identifies patients in atrial fibrillation at low risk for embolization, thus facilitating early cardioversion. It is also quite sensitive in detecting aortic dissection and severe atherosclerosis of the ascending aorta, which may be the source for transient ischemic attacks or embolic strokes.

Stress echocardiography is being used increasingly to enhance the information available from ECGs and as an alternative to nuclear medicine procedures. Echocardiograms may be performed during or immediately following exercise. Transient depression of segmental wall motion during or following stress suggests ischemia. Improvement in wall motion during low-dose dobutamine infusions is an indicator of myocardial viability. Dobutamine infusions can also be utilized as a form of stress testing in patients unable to exercise.

ACC/AHA Guidelines for Clinical Applications of Echocardiography. J Am Coll Cardiol 1997;29:862. [NLM Cit ID: 97226403] (Extensive discussion and recommendations.)

Lewis JF: Current status of stress echocardiography. Clin Cardiol 2000;23:242. [NLM Cit ID: 20226280] (Review of indications and approaches.)

Stewart WJ et al: Echocardiography in emergency medicine: a policy statement by the American Society of Echocardiography and the American College of Cardiology. Task Force on Echocardiography in Emergency Medicine of the American Society of Echocardiography and the Echocardiography and Technology and Practice Executive Committees of the American College of Cardiology. J Am Coll Cardiol 1999;33:586. [NLM Cit ID: 99137329]

CARDIAC CATHETERIZATION & ANGIOGRAPHY

Although cardiac catheterization and angiography remain the standard tests for assessment of many hemodynamic and anatomic abnormalities of the heart, they have often been supplanted by echocardiography and other imaging modalities for the initial and serial evaluation of many conditions. Nonetheless, "invasive" procedures (ie, those involving the use of intravascular and intracardiac catheters), when appropriately employed, remain invaluable in the management of most patients with congenital, valvular, and coronary heart disease.

Right heart catheterization is convenient to perform and allows measurement of right atrial, right ventricular, pulmonary artery and pulmonary capillary wedge pressures (the latter an indicator of left atrial pressure), oxygen saturation, and cardiac output. These data may diagnose intracardiac shunts, physiologically significant pericardial disease, and right-sided valve lesions and can distinguish between cardiac and pulmonary disease. Balloon flotation catheters permit hemodynamic measurements and continuous monitoring at the bedside. These data can be critical in the evaluation and treatment of shock, heart failure, myocardial infarction, respiratory failure, postoperative hemodynamic instability, and many other situations. Bedside echocardiography can also be used in the evaluation and treatment of these entities when continuous monitoring is not required, and it is less invasive. Complications of right heart catheterization include bleeding, pneumothorax, arrhythmias, pulmonary emboli, pulmonary artery rupture, and sepsis. A recent study has suggested that the risk of right heart catheterization and resulting interventions may outweigh the benefits in many individuals.

Left heart catheterization permits quantitative assessment of mitral and aortic stenosis. With contrast angiography, valvular regurgitation and global and regional left ventricular function can be examined. Its main application is to produce selective coronary arteriograms. Since much of this information is available noninvasively, its main role is to confirm assessments of valvular abnormalities preoperatively and to obtain selective coronary arteriograms. Increasingly, the catheterization laboratory is being used for interventional procedures.

Chatterjee K et al: ACC expert consensus document. Present use of bedside right heart catheterization in patients with cardiac disease. J Am Coll Cardiol 1998;32:840. [NLM Cit ID: 98412566] (Consensus statement from the American College of Cardiology.)

Pepine CJ et al: *Diagnostic and Therapeutic Cardiac Catheterization,* 3rd ed. Williams & Wilkins, 1998. (Recently updated monograph.)

Scanlon PJ et al: ACC/AHA guidelines for coronary angiography. A report of the American College of Cardiology/American Heart Association Task Force on practice guidelines (Committee on Coronary Angiography). Developed in collaboration with the Society for Cardiac Angiography and Interventions. J Am Coll Cardiol 1999;33:1756. [NLM Cit ID: 99265625]

CONGENITAL HEART DISEASE

Congenital lesions account for only about 2% of heart disease in adults. Only the most common acyanotic lesions are discussed here.

Brickner ME et al: Congenital heart disease in adults. First of two parts. N Engl J Med 2000;342:256. [NLM Cit ID: 20098059] (Two-part series covering acyanotic and cyanotic conditions, surgical interventions, and late complications. Excellent diagrams accompany text.)

Brickner ME et al: Congenital heart disease in adults. Second of two parts. N Engl J Med 2000;342:334. [NLM Cit ID: 20106701] (Acyanotic and cyanotic conditions.)

Houston A et al: Echocardiography in adult congenital heart disease. Heart 1998;80(Suppl 1):S12. [NLM Cit ID: 99177797]

Perloff JK, Child JS: *Congenital Heart Disease in Adults.* Saunders, 1998.

PULMONARY STENOSIS

Essentials of Diagnosis

- No symptoms in patients with mild or moderately severe lesions.
- Severe cases may present with right-sided heart failure and cause sudden death.
- High-pitched systolic ejection murmur maximal in the second left interspace. S_2 delayed and soft or absent. Ejection click often present. Increased right ventricular impulse.
- Palpable thrill at second left intercostal space.
- Right ventricular hypertrophy on ECG; pulmonary artery dilation on x-ray. Echo-Doppler diagnostic.

General Considerations

Stenosis of the pulmonary valve or infundibulum increases the resistance to outflow, raises the right ventricular pressure, and limits pulmonary blood flow. In the absence of associated shunts, arterial saturation is normal, but severe stenosis causes peripheral cyanosis by reducing cardiac output. Clubbing and polycythemia do not develop unless a patent foramen ovale or atrial septal defect is present, permitting right-to-left shunting.

About two thirds of patients with Noonan's syndrome have pulmonary stenosis due to a dysplastic valve. Supravalvular stenosis occurs in the Williams syndrome along with hypercalcemia, elfin facies, and mental retardation.

Clinical Findings

A. Symptoms and Signs: Mild cases (right ventricular-pulmonary artery gradient < 30 mm Hg) are asymptomatic. Moderate to severe stenosis (gradients 50 to > 80 mm Hg) may cause dyspnea on exertion, syncope, chest pain, and eventually right ventricular failure.

There is a palpable parasternal lift. A loud, harsh systolic murmur and a prominent thrill are present in the left second and third interspaces parasternally; the murmur is in the third and fourth interspaces in infundibular stenosis. The second sound is obscured by the murmur in severe cases; the pulmonary component is diminished, delayed, or absent. Both components are audible in mild cases. A right-sided S_4 and a prominent *a* wave in the venous pulse are present in severe cases.

B. Electrocardiography and Chest X-Ray: Right axis deviation or right ventricular hypertrophy is noted; peaked P waves provide evidence of right atrial overload. Heart size may be normal on radiographs, or there may be a prominent right ventricle and atrium or gross cardiac enlargement, depending upon the severity. There is often poststenotic dilation of the main and left pulmonary arteries. Pulmonary vascularity is normal or diminished.

C. Diagnostic Studies: Echocardiography usually demonstrates the anatomic abnormality and assesses right ventricular size and function. Doppler ultrasound can estimate the gradient accurately; its findings are usually confirmed by cardiac catheterization.

Prognosis & Treatment

Patients with mild pulmonary stenosis may have a normal life expectancy. Severe stenosis is associated with sudden death and can cause heart failure in the 20s and 30s. Moderate stenosis may be asymptomatic in childhood and adolescence, but symptoms increase as patients grow older.

Symptomatic patients or those with evidence of right ventricular hypertrophy and resting gradients over 75–80 mm Hg require correction in most cases. Percutaneous balloon valvuloplasty has proved successful and is usually the treatment of choice. Surgery can be performed with an operative mortality rate of 2–4% and an excellent long-term result in most cases.

Gibbs JL: Interventional catheterisation. Opening up I: the ventricular outflow tracts and great arteries. Heart 2000;83:111. [NLM Cit ID: 20087441]

Rao PS: Long-term follow-up results after balloon dilatation of pulmonic stenosis, aortic stenosis, and coarctation of the aorta: a review. Prog Cardiovasc Dis 1999;42:59. [NLM Cit ID: 99433312] (Success rate about 80% for pulmonary stenosis in a series of children and adolescents.)

COARCTATION OF THE AORTA

Essentials of Diagnosis

- Infants may have severe heart failure; children and adults are usually asymptomatic, presenting with hypertension.
- Absent or weak femoral pulses.
- Systolic pressure higher in upper extremities than in lower extremities; diastolic pressures are similar.
- Harsh systolic murmur heard in the back.
- ECG shows left ventricular hypertrophy; chest x-ray shows rib notching; echo-Doppler is diagnostic.

General Considerations

Coarctation of the aorta consists of localized narrowing of the aortic arch just distal to the origin of the left subclavian artery. A bicuspid aortic valve is present in 25% of cases. Blood pressure is elevated in the aorta and its branches proximal to the coarctation and decreased distally. Collateral circulation develops through the intercostal arteries and branches of the subclavian arteries.

Clinical Findings

A. Symptoms and Signs: If cardiac failure does not occur in infancy, there are usually no symptoms until the hypertension produces left ventricular failure or cerebral hemorrhage; the latter may also occur from associated cerebral aneurysms. Strong arterial pulsations are seen in the neck and suprasternal notch. Hypertension is present in the arms, but the pressure is normal or low in the legs. This difference is exaggerated by exercise. Femoral pulsations are weak and are delayed in comparison with the brachial pulse. Patients with large collaterals may have relatively small gradients but still have severe coarctation. Late systolic ejection murmurs at the base are often heard better posteriorly, especially over the spinous processes. There may be an associated aortic insufficiency murmur due to a bicuspid aortic valve.

B. Electrocardiography and Chest X-Ray: The ECG usually shows left ventricular hypertrophy. Radiography shows scalloping of the ribs due to enlarged collateral intercostal arteries, dilation of the left subclavian artery and poststenotic aortic dilation, and left ventricular enlargement.

C. Diagnostic Studies: Measurement of the gradient across the lesion by catheterization and aortography remain the primary methods of diagnosis. MRI is a useful imaging adjunct, and Doppler ultrasound can also estimate the severity of obstruction.

Prognosis & Treatment

Cardiac failure is common in infancy and in older untreated patients; it is uncommon in late childhood and young adulthood. Most untreated patients with the adult form of coarctation die before age 50 from the complications of hypertension, rupture of the aorta, infective endarteritis, or cerebral hemorrhage (associated in some cases with congenital cerebral aneurysms). Aortic dissection also occurs with increased frequency in coarctation.

Resection of the coarcted site has a surgical mortality rate of 1–4%. The risks of the disease are such, however, that all coarctations in patients up to age 20 years should be resected. In patients under 40 years of age, surgery is advisable if the patient has refractory hypertension or significant left ventricular hypertrophy. The surgical mortality rate rises considerably in patients over age 50 and is of doubtful value. Balloon angioplasty of the stenosis has been accomplished successfully and may become the procedure of choice, but aortic tears have been described. About one-fourth of corrected patients continue to be hypertensive years after surgery and they have all the complications associated with hypertension.

Yetman AT et al: Balloon angioplasty for native aortic coarctation: A 12 year review. J Am Coll Cardiol 1997;30:811. [NLM Cit ID: 97429195]

ATRIAL SEPTAL DEFECT

Essentials of Diagnosis

- Usually asymptomatic until middle age.
- Right ventricular lift; S_2 widely split and fixed.
- Grade I–III/VI systolic ejection murmur at pulmonary area.
- ECG shows right ventricular conduction delay; x-ray shows dilated pulmonary arteries and increased vascularity; echo-Doppler usually diagnostic.

General Considerations

The most common form of atrial septal defect (80% of cases) is persistence of the ostium secundum in the mid septum; less commonly, the ostium primum (which is low in the septum) persists, in which case mitral or tricuspid abnormalities may also be present. A third form is the sinus venosus defect of the upper part of the septum. This is often associated with partial anomalous drainage of the pulmonary veins into the superior vena cava. In all cases, normally oxygenated blood from the left atrium passes into the right atrium, increasing right ventricular output and pulmonary blood flow.

Clinical Findings

A. Symptoms and Signs: Most patients with small or moderate defects are asymptomatic. With large shunts, exertional dyspnea or cardiac failure may develop, most commonly in the fourth decade or later. Prominent right ventricular and pulmonary artery pulsations are readily visible and palpable. A moderately loud systolic ejection murmur can be heard in the second and third interspaces parasternally as a result of increased pulmonary artery flow. S_2 is widely split and does not vary with breathing.

B. Electrocardiography and Chest X-Ray: Right axis deviation or right ventricular hypertrophy may be present in ostium secundum defects. Incomplete or complete right bundle branch block is present in nearly all cases of atrial septal defect, and superior axis deviation is noted in ostium primum defect. With sinus venosus defects, the P axis is leftward of +15 degrees. The chest radiograph shows large pulmonary arteries, increased pulmonary vascularity, an enlarged right atrium and ventricle, and a small aortic knob.

C. Diagnostic Studies: Echocardiography can demonstrate right ventricular volume overload with a large right ventricle and atrium, and sometimes the defect itself. Echocardiography with saline bubble contrast and Doppler flow studies can demonstrate shunting. A transesophageal echo is helpful when transthoracic echo quality is not optimal, and it improves the sensitivity for small shunts and patent foramen ovale. Radionuclide flow studies quantify left-to-right shunting, and MRI can also elucidate the anatomy. Cardiac catheterization remains the definitive diagnostic procedure, since it can demonstrate an increase in oxygen saturation between the venae cavae and right ventricle due to the admixture of oxygenated blood from the left atrium, quantify the shunt, and measure pulmonary vascular resistance. Right and left ventricular contrast angiography may demonstrate associated valvular abnormalities or anomalous pulmonary venous drainage.

Prognosis & Treatment

Patients with small shunts may live a normal life span. Large shunts cause disability by age 40. Raised pulmonary vascular resistance secondary to pulmonary hypertension rarely occurs in childhood or young adult life in secundum defects but is more common in primum defects; after age 40, pulmonary hypertension, cardiac arrhythmias (especially atrial fibrillation), and heart failure may occur in secundum defects. Paradoxic systemic arterial embolization is a concern, especially in patients with pulmonary hypertension or venous thrombosis. A patent foramen ovale is present in 20–30% of adults and is the lesion responsible for most paradoxic emboli. Infective endocarditis does not occur with increased frequency.

Small atrial septal defects do not require surgery. The risks are now sufficiently low so that patients with left-to-right shunts and pulmonary-to-systemic flow ratios between 1.5 and 2.0 may be operated on if the total clinical picture warrants. Ratios exceeding 2.0 are an indication for surgical closure of the defect.

Transcatheter techniques for closing atrial septal defects have been developed. These involve the deployment of an umbrella-like occlusion device from a femoral venous approach. The devices work best in patients with centrally located secundum defects.

Surgery should be withheld from patients with pulmonary hypertension with reversed (right-to-left) shunting (Eisenmenger's syndrome) because of the risk of acute right heart failure. Relocation of pulmonary veins is required in patients with partial anomalous venous drainage. In ostium primum defects, in addition to closure of the defect, suture of the valve clefts—especially those of the mitral valve—is advisable if mitral regurgitation of any significant degree is present. The surgical mortality rate is low (< 1%) in patients under age 45 who are not in cardiac failure and those who have systolic pulmonary artery pressures less than 60 mm Hg. It increases to 5–10% in patients over age 40 with cardiac failure or with systolic pulmonary artery pressures greater than 60 mm Hg.

Sievert H et al: Transcatheter closure of atrial septal defect and patent foramen ovale with the ASDOS device. Am J Cardiol 1998;82:1405. [NLM Cit ID: 99072748] (European trial demonstrated 87% procedural success, though almost 30% had some shunt present at 1 year.)

PATENT DUCTUS ARTERIOSUS

Essentials of Diagnosis

- Adults with small or moderately large patent ductus are usually asymptomatic at least until middle age.
- Widened pulse pressure; loud S_2.
- Continuous murmur over pulmonary area; thrill common.
- Echo-Doppler is helpful, but the lesion is best visualized by aortography.

General Considerations

The embryonic ductus arteriosus fails to close normally and persists as a shunt connecting the left pulmonary artery and aorta, usually near the origin of the left subclavian artery. Prior to birth, the ductus is kept patent by the effect of circulating prostaglandins; in early infancy, a patent ductus can often be closed by administration of intravenous indomethacin (0.2 mg/kg intravenously). If the defect is not closed, blood flows continuously from the aorta through the ductus into the pulmonary artery in both systole and diastole; the defect is a form of arteriovenous fistula, increasing the work of the left ventricle. If it remains open, obliterative changes in the pulmonary arterioles can cause pulmonary hypertension. Then the shunt is bidirectional or right-to-left (Eisenmenger's syndrome). This complication does not correlate with shunt size.

Clinical Findings

A. Symptoms and Signs: There are no symptoms unless left ventricular failure or pulmonary hypertension develops. The heart is of normal size or slightly enlarged, with a hyperdynamic apical impulse. The pulse pressure is wide, and diastolic pressure is low. A continuous rough "machinery" murmur, accentuated in late systole at the time of S_2, is heard best in the left first and second interspaces at the left sternal border. Thrills are common.

B. Electrocardiography and Chest X-Ray: A normal tracing or left ventricular hypertrophy is found, depending upon the magnitude of shunting. On chest radiographs, the heart is normal in size and contour, or there may be left ventricular and left atrial enlargement. The pulmonary artery, aorta, and left atrium are prominent.

C. Diagnostic Studies: Echocardiography quantifies left ventricular and atrial size. MRI can demonstrate the abnormality, and the magnitude of the shunt can also be determined by radionuclide flow studies. Cardiac catheterization establishes the presence and severity of a left-to-right shunt and whether pulmonary hypertension is present; angiography can define its anatomy.

Prognosis & Treatment

Large shunts cause a high mortality rate from cardiac failure early in life. Smaller shunts are compati-

Table 10–1. Differential diagnosis of valvular heart disease.

	Mitral Stenosis	Mitral Regurgitation	Aortic Stenosis	Aortic Regurgitation	Tricuspid Stenosis	Tricuspid Regurgitation
Inspection	Malar flush, precordial bulge, and diffuse pulsation in young patients.	Usually prominent and hyperdynamic apical impulse to left of MCL.	Sustained PMI, prominent atrial filling wave.	Hyperdynamic PMI to left of MCL and down. Visible carotid pulsations.	Giant *a* wave in jugular pulse with sinus rhythm. Often olive-colored skin (mixed jaundice and local cyanosis).	Large *v* wave in jugular pulse.
Palpation	"Tapping" sensation over area of expected PMI. Middiastolic or presystolic thrill at apex. Small pulse. Right ventricular pulsation left third to fifth ICS parasternally when pulmonary hypertension is present.	Forceful, brisk PMI; systolic thrill over PMI. Pulse normal, small, or slightly collapsing.	Powerful, heaving PMI to left and slightly below MCL. Systolic thrill over aortic area, sternal notch, or carotids. Small and slowly rising carotid pulse.	Apical impulse forceful and displaced significantly to left and down. Prominent carotid pulses. Rapidly rising and collapsing pulses.	Middiastolic thrill between lower left sternal border and PMI. Presystolic pulsation of liver (sinus rhythm only).	Right ventricular pulsation. Occasionally systolic thrill at lower left sternal edge. Systolic pulsation of liver.
Heart sounds, rhythm, and blood pressure	Loud snapping M_1. Opening snap following S_2 along left sternal border or at apex. Atrial fibrillation common. Blood pressure normal.	M_1 normal or buried in murmur. Prominent third heart sound. Atrial fibrillation common. Blood pressure normal. Midsystolic clicks may be present.	A_2 normal, soft, or absent. Paradoxic splitting of S_2 if A_2 is audible. Prominent S_4. Blood pressure normal, or systolic pressure normal with high diastolic.	S_1 normal or reduced, A_2 loud. Wide pulse pressure with diastolic pressure < 60 mm Hg.	S_1 often loud.	Atrial fibrillation is usually present.
Murmurs Location and transmission	Localized at or near apex. Rarely, short diastolic (Graham Steell) murmur along lower left sternal border in severe pulmonary hypertension.	Loudest over PMI; transmitted to left axilla, left infrascapular area. With posterior papillary muscle dysfunction, may transmit to base.	Right second ICS parasternally or at apex, heard in carotids and occasionally in upper interscapular area.	Louder along left sternal border in third to fourth interspace. Heard over aortic area and apex. May be associated with low-pitched middiastolic murmur at apex (Austin Flint) in nonrheumatic disease.	Third to fifth ICS along left sternal border out to apex.	As for tricuspid stenosis.
Timing	Onset at opening snap ("middiastolic") with presystolic accentuation if in sinus rhythm. Graham Steell begins with P_2 (early diastole).	Pansystolic: begins with M_1 and ends at or after A_2. May be late systolic in papillary muscle dysfunction.	Midsystolic: begins after M_1, ends before A_2, reaches maximum intensity in mid systole.	Begins immediately after aortic second sound and ends before first sound.	As for mitral stenosis.	As for mitral regurgitation.
Character	Low-pitched, rumbling; presystolic murmur merges with loud M_1 and ends at or after A_2. May be late systolic in papillary muscle dysfunction.	Blowing, high-pitched; occasionally harsh or musical.	Harsh, rough.	Blowing, often faint.	As for mitral regurgitation.	Blowing, coarse, or musical.

Murmurs (con't'd) Optimum auscultatory conditions	After exercise, left lateral recumbency. Bell chest piece lightly applied.	After exercise; diaphragm chest piece. In prolapse, findings most prominent while standing.	Patient resting, leaning forward, breath held in full expiration.	Patient leaning forward, breath held in expiration.	Murmur usually louder and at peak during inspiration. Patient recumbent.	Murmur usually becomes louder during inspiration.
X-ray	Straight left heart border. Large left atrium sharply indenting esophagus. Elevation of left main stem bronchus. Large right ventricle and pulmonary artery if pulmonary hypertension is present. Calcification occasionally seen in mitral valve.	Enlarged left ventricle and left atrium.	Concentric left ventricular hypertrophy. Prominent ascending aorta, small knob. Calcified valve common.	Moderate to severe left ventricular enlargement. Prominent aortic knob.	Enlarged right atrium only.	Enlarged right atrium and ventricle.
Electrocardiography	Broad P waves in standard leads; broad negative phase of diphasic P in V_1. If pulmonary hypertension is present, tall peaked P waves, right axis deviation, or right ventricular hypertrophy appears.	Left axis deviation or frank left ventricular hypertrophy. P waves broad, tall, or notched in standard leads. Broad negative phase of diphasic P in V_1.	Left ventricular hypertrophy.	Left ventricular hypertrophy.	Tall, peaked P waves. Normal axis.	Right axis usual.
Echocardiography M mode	Thickened, immobile mitral valve with anterior and posterior leaflets moving together. Slow early diastolic filling slope, left atrial enlargement, normal to small left ventricle.	Thickened mitral valve in rheumatic disease; mitral valve prolapse; flail leaflet or vegetations may be seen. Enlarged left ventricle with above-normal, normal, or decreased function.	Dense persistent echoes from the aortic valve with poor leaflet excursion, left ventricular hypertrophy with preserved contractile function.	Diastolic vibrations of the anterior leaflet of the mitral valve and septum, early closure of the mitral valve when severe, dilated left ventricle with normal or decreased contractility.	Tricuspid valve thickening, decreased early diastolic filling slope of the tricuspid valve. Mitral valve also usually abnormal.	Enlarged right ventricle, prolapsing valve, mitral valve often abnormal.
Two-dimensional	Maximum diastolic orifice size reduced, subvalvular apparatus foreshortened, variable thickening of other valves.	Same as M mode but more reliable.	Above plus poststenotic dilation of the aorta, restricted opening of the aortic leaflets, bicuspid aortic valve in about 30%.	Above plus may show vegetations in endocarditis, bicuspid valve, root dilation.	Above plus enlargement of the right atrium.	Same as above.
Doppler	Prolonged pressure half-time across mitral valve; indirect evidence of pulmonary hypertension.	Regurgitant flow mapped into left atrium; indirect evidence of pulmonary hypertension.	Increased transvalvular flow velocity, yielding calculated gradient. Valve area estimate using continuity equation.	Demonstrates regurgitation and qualitatively estimates severity.	Prolonged pressure half-time across tricuspid valve.	Regurgitant flow mapped into right atrium and venae cavae; right ventricular systolic pressure estimated.

A_2 = Aortic second sound
ICS = Intercostal space
M_1 = Mitral first sound
MCL = Midclavicular line
P_2 = Pulmonary second sound
PMI = Point of maximal impulse
S_2 = second heart sound
S_4 = fourth heart sound
V_1 = Chest ECG lead 1

Table 10–2. Effect of various interventions on systolic murmurs.[1]

Intervention	Hypertrophic Obstructive Cardiomyopathy	Aortic Stenosis	Mitral Regurgitation	Mitral Prolapse
Valsalva	↑	↓	↓ or ↔	↑ or ↓
Standing	↑	↑ or ↔	↓ or ↔	↑
Handgrip or squatting	↓	↓ or ↔	↑	↓
Supine position with legs elevated	↓	↑ or ↔	↔	↓
Exercise	↑	↑ or ↔	↓	↑
Amyl nitrite	↑↑	↑	↓	↑
Isoproterenol	↑↑	↑	↓	↑

Key: ↑ = increased; ↑↑ = markedly increased; ↓ = decreased; ↔ = unchanged
[1]Modified from Paraskos JA: Combined valvular disease. In: *Valvular Heart Disease.* Dalen JE, Alpert JS (editors). Little, Brown, 1987.

they persist throughout diastole when the lesion is severe or when the ventricular rate is rapid.

In mild cases, left atrial pressure and cardiac output may be essentially normal and the patient asymptomatic, but in moderate stenosis (valve area < 1.5 cm^2)—especially with tachycardia, which shortens diastole and increases mitral flow rate—dyspnea and fatigue appear as the left atrial pressure rises. With severe stenosis, the left atrial pressure is high enough to produce pulmonary venous congestion at rest and reduce cardiac output, with resulting dyspnea, fatigue, and right heart failure. Recumbency at night further increases the pulmonary blood volume, causing orthopnea and paroxysmal nocturnal dyspnea. Severe pulmonary congestion may also be initiated by any acute respiratory infection, excessive salt and fluid intake, endocarditis, or recurrence of rheumatic carditis. As a result of long-standing pulmonary venous hypertension, anastomoses develop between the pulmonary and bronchial veins in the form of bronchial submucosal varices. These often rupture, producing mild or severe hemoptysis. In a few patients, the pulmonary arterioles become narrowed; this greatly increases the pulmonary artery pressure and accelerates the development of right ventricular hypertrophy and failure. These patients have relatively little dyspnea but experience fatigue on exertion.

Fifty to 80 percent of patients develop paroxysmal or chronic atrial fibrillation that, until the ventricular rate is controlled, may precipitate dyspnea or pulmonary edema.

B. Diagnostic Studies: Echocardiography is the most valuable technique for assessing mitral stenosis. The valve is thickened, opens poorly, and closes slowly. The anterior and posterior leaflets are fixed and move together, rather than in opposite directions. Left atrial size can be determined by echocardiography: increased size denotes an increased likelihood of atrial fibrillation or systemic emboli. The mitral valve area can be measured, and the gradient and pulmonary artery pressure can be estimated by Doppler techniques. Echocardiography also detects atrial myxoma, which sometimes presents clinically in a fashion resembling mitral stenosis.

Because echocardiography and careful symptom evaluation provide most of the needed information, cardiac catheterization is employed primarily to detect associated valve, coronary, or myocardial disease—usually after the decision to intervene has been made.

Treatment & Prognosis

Mitral stenosis may be present for a lifetime with few or no symptoms, or it may become severe in a few years. In most cases, there is a long asymptomatic phase, followed by subtle limitation of activity. Pregnancy and its associated increase in cardiac output and the transmitral pressure gradient often precipitates symptoms. The onset of atrial fibrillation often precipitates more severe symptoms, although with return to sinus rhythm (using digoxin and, often, class I or III antiarrhythmic agents) or ventricular rate control, the patient may improve. Conversion to and subsequent maintenance of sinus rhythm is most commonly successful when the duration of atrial fibrillation is brief (< 6–12 months) and the left atrium is not severely dilated (diameter < 4.5 cm). Once atrial fibrillation occurs, the patient should receive warfarin anticoagulation therapy even if sinus rhythm is restored, since 20–30% of these patients will have systemic embolization if untreated. Systemic embolization in the presence of only mild to moderate disease is not an indication for surgery but should be treated with warfarin anticoagulation.

Indications for relieving the stenosis include the following: (1) uncontrollable pulmonary edema; (2) limiting dyspnea and intermittent pulmonary edema;

(3) evidence of pulmonary hypertension with right ventricular hypertrophy or hemoptysis; (4) limitation of activity despite ventricular rate control and medical therapy; and (5) recurrent systemic emboli despite anticoagulation with moderate or severe stenosis.

Open mitral commissurotomy may be effective in patients without substantial mitral regurgitation. Replacement of the valve is indicated when combined stenosis and insufficiency are present or when the mitral valve is so distorted and calcified that a satisfactory valvulotomy is not possible. Operative mortality rates are low: 1–3% in most institutions. Balloon valvuloplasty is effective in patients without accompanying regurgitation. Initial success rates are high, especially if valve calcification is not excessive. The rate of restenosis is lower than that with aortic stenosis. As a result, this option appears to be a suitable alternative to surgery for many patients in experienced centers.

Problems associated with prosthetic valves are thrombosis (especially at the mitral position), paravalvular leak, endocarditis, and degenerative changes in tissue valves. Warfarin anticoagulant therapy is mandatory with mechanical prostheses and is usually employed for at least the initial 3 months with bioprostheses, especially if the patient has significant left atrial enlargement. If atrial fibrillation persists postoperatively, ongoing anticoagulation is required.

Ben Farhat M et al: Percutaneous balloon versus surgical closed and open mitral commissurotomy: Seven-year follow-up results of a randomized trial. Circulation 1998;97:245. [NLM Cit ID: 98122357] (This prospective randomized controlled trial suggests that balloon commissurotomy should be the procedure of choice for correcting mitral stenosis. It is as efficacious as the open procedure, with less morbidity, and is superior to the closed procedure.)

Bruce CJ et al: Newer advances in the diagnosis and treatment of mitral stenosis. Curr Probl Cardiol 1998;23:130. [NLM Cit ID: 98229826] (Etiology, pathophysiology, and clinical examination are discussed. Diagnostic challenges using echo or invasive techniques are covered. Treatment algorithms include balloon valvotomy and surgical intervention.)

Hernandez R et al: Long-term clinical and echocardiographic follow-up after percutaneous mitral valvuloplasty with the Inoue balloon. Circulation 1999;99:1580. [NLM Cit ID: 99196869] (Follow-up of 561 patients showed nearly two-thirds in good clinical condition 7 years after valvuloplasty.)

MITRAL REGURGITATION (Mitral Insufficiency)

Essentials of Diagnosis

- Variable causes determine clinical presentation.
- May be asymptomatic for many years (or for life) or may cause left-sided heart failure.
- Pansystolic murmur at the apex, radiating into the axilla; associated with S_3.
- ECG shows left atrial abnormality or atrial fibrillation and left ventricular hypertrophy; x-ray shows left atrial and ventricular enlargement. Echo-Doppler confirms diagnosis and estimates severity.

General Considerations

Mitral regurgitation may result from many processes. Rheumatic disease is associated with a thickened valve with reduced mobility and often a mixed picture of stenosis and regurgitation. Rheumatic disease has been replaced as the commonest cause of mitral regurgitation in most developed countries by other processes, which include myxomatous degeneration (eg, **mitral valve prolapse** with or without connective tissue diseases such as Marfan's syndrome), infective endocarditis, and subvalvular dysfunction (due to papillary muscle dysfunction or ruptured chordae tendineae). Cardiac tumors, chiefly left atrial myxoma, are a rare cause of mitral regurgitation.

Clinical Findings

A. Symptoms and Signs: During left ventricular systole, the mitral leaflets do not close normally, and blood is ejected into the left atrium as well as through the aortic valve. The net effect is an increased volume load on the left ventricle, and the presentation depends on the rapidity with which the lesion develops. In acute regurgitation, left atrial pressure rises abruptly, leading to pulmonary edema if severe. When it is chronic, the left atrium enlarges progressively, but the pressure in pulmonary veins and capillaries rises only transiently during exertion. Exertional dyspnea and fatigue progress gradually over many years.

Mitral regurgitation, like mitral stenosis, predisposes to atrial fibrillation; but this arrhythmia is less likely to provoke acute pulmonary congestion, and fewer than 5% of patients have peripheral arterial emboli. Mitral regurgitation more often predisposes to infective endocarditis.

Clinically, mitral regurgitation is characterized by a pansystolic murmur maximal at the apex, radiating to the axilla and occasionally to the base; a hyperdynamic left ventricular impulse and a brisk carotid upstroke; and a prominent third heart sound. Left atrial enlargement is usually considerable in chronic mitral regurgitation; the degree of left ventricular enlargement usually reflects the severity of regurgitation. Calcification of the mitral valve is less common than in pure mitral stenosis. The same is true of enlargement of the main pulmonary artery on radiographs. Hemodynamically, left ventricular volume overload may ultimately lead to left ventricular failure and reduced cardiac output, but for many years the left ventricular end-diastolic pressure and the cardiac output may be normal at rest, even with considerable increase in left ventricular volume.

Nonrheumatic mitral regurgitation may develop abruptly, such as with papillary muscle dysfunction following myocardial infarction, valve perforation in infective endocarditis, or ruptured chordae tendineae in mitral valve prolapse. In acute mitral regurgitation, patients are in sinus rhythm rather than atrial fibrillation, have little or no enlargement of the left atrium, no calcification of the mitral valve, no associated mitral stenosis, and in many cases little left ventricular dilation.

Myxomatous mitral valve ("floppy" or "billowing" mitral valve, or mitral valve prolapse) is usually asymptomatic but may be associated with nonspecific chest pain, dyspnea, fatigue, or palpitations. Most patients are female, many are thin, and some have minor chest wall deformities. There are characteristic midsystolic clicks, which may be multiple, often but not always followed by a late systolic murmur. These findings are accentuated in the standing position. The diagnosis is primarily clinical but can be confirmed echocardiographically. Its significance is in dispute because of the frequency with which it is diagnosed in healthy young women (up to 10%) and men, but in occasional patients this lesion is not benign. Patients who have only a midsystolic click usually have no sequelae, but patients with a late or pansystolic murmur may develop significant mitral regurgitation, often due to rupture of chordae tendineae. The need for valve replacement is commonest in men and increases with aging, so that approximately 2% of patients with clinically significant regurgitation over age 60 will require surgery. Infective endocarditis may occur, chiefly in patients with murmurs; such patients should have antibiotic prophylaxis prior to dental work and surgical procedures. Sudden death is rare and is probably related to ventricular tachycardias; β-adrenergic blocking agents are often effective for supraventricular arrhythmias. If symptomatic ventricular tachycardia is present, antiarrhythmic therapy and, in many cases, electrophysiologic studies are indicated. An association between mitral prolapse and embolic cerebrovascular events has also been reported. Echocardiographic evidence of marked thickening or redundancy of the valve is associated with a higher incidence of most complications.

Papillary muscle dysfunction or infarction following acute myocardial infarction is less common. When mitral regurgitation is due to papillary dysfunction, it may subside as the infarction heals or left ventricular dilation diminishes. If severe regurgitation persists, these patients have a poor prognosis with or without surgery and a natural history that reflects their underlying heart disease. Transient—but sometimes severe—mitral regurgitation may occur during episodes of myocardial ischemia. Patients with dilated cardiomyopathies of any origin may have **secondary mitral regurgitation** due to papillary muscle dysfunction or dilation of the mitral annulus. In these, mitral valve replacement has been considered contraindicated because of the poor risk:benefit ratio and deterioration of left ventricular function postoperatively. However, several groups have reported good results with mitral valve repair in patients with left ventricular ejection fractions greater than 30% and secondary mitral insufficiency.

B. Diagnostic Studies: Echocardiography is useful in demonstrating the underlying pathologic process (rheumatic, prolapse, flail leaflet), and Doppler techniques provide qualitative and semiquantitative estimates of the severity of mitral regurgitation. It should be noted that Doppler also detects clinically insignificant regurgitation in many normal individuals, and this finding must be interpreted in the context of the clinical presentation. The accompanying information concerning left ventricular size and function, left atrial size, pulmonary artery pressure, and right ventricular function can be invaluable in planning treatment as well as in recognizing associated lesions. Transesophageal echocardiography may reveal the cause of regurgitation and identify candidates for valvular repair. Nuclear medicine techniques as well as MRI permit measurement of left ventricular function and estimation of the severity of regurgitation.

Cardiac catheterization provides accurate assessment of regurgitation and, additionally, of left ventricular function and pulmonary artery pressure. Coronary angiography is often indicated to determine the presence of coronary artery disease prior to valve surgery.

Treatment & Prognosis

Acute mitral regurgitation due to endocarditis, myocardial infarction, and ruptured chordae tendineae often requires emergency surgery. Some patients can be stabilized with vasodilators or intra-aortic balloon counterpulsation, which reduce the amount of regurgitant flow by lowering systemic vascular resistance. Patients with chronic lesions may remain asymptomatic for many years. Operation is usually necessary when patients develop symptoms. However, because progressive and irreversible deterioration of left ventricular function may occur prior to the onset of symptoms, early operation is indicated even in asymptomatic patients with a declining ejection fraction (< 50–55%) or marked left ventricular dilation (end-systolic dimension > 5 cm on echocardiography).

There has been growing success with valve repair in nonrheumatic lesions, which avoids the complications of prosthetic valves described earlier. In addition, left ventricular function is better preserved when the subvalvular structures can be maintained intact by valve repair. Selected patients with poor left ventricular function and severe mitral regurgitation may benefit from this intervention. Mitral valve surgery is increasingly being performed using the appreciably less invasive thoracoscopic approach.

Carabello BA: Mitral valve regurgitation. Curr Probl Cardiol 1998;23:200. [NLM Cit ID: 98251753] (Comprehensive review covering pathophysiology, diagnosis, and treatment. Various Doppler imaging techniques are covered, as well as newer surgical techniques including chordal preservation, valve repair, and the limited thoracotomy approach.)

Enriquez-Serano M et al: Mitral regurgitation: A new clinical perspective. Mayo Clin Proc 1997;72:1034. [NLM Cit ID: 98042410] (Reviews natural history and argues for early surgical intervention.)

Freed LA et al: Prevalence and clinical outcome of mitral-valve prolapse. N Engl J Med 1999;341:1. [NLM Cit ID: 99294363] (In the offspring cohort of the Framingham Heart Study, the prevalence of mitral valve prolapse was only 2.4%, considerably lower than previously reported.)

Gilon D et al: Lack of evidence of an association between mitral-valve prolapse and stroke in young patients. N Engl J Med 1999;341:8. [NLM Cit ID: 99294364] (Mitral valve prolapse is less common than previously reported and not clearly associated with ischemic neurologic events in young patients.)

AORTIC STENOSIS

Essentials of Diagnosis

- In adults, usually asymptomatic until middle or old age.
- Delayed and diminished carotid pulses.
- Soft, absent, or paradoxically split S_2.
- Harsh systolic murmur, sometimes with thrill along left sternal border, often radiating to the neck; may be louder at apex in older patients.
- ECG usually shows left ventricular hypertrophy; calcified valve on x-ray or fluoroscopy; echo-Doppler is diagnostic in most cases.

General Considerations

Aortic valvular stenosis may follow rheumatic fever but is more commonly caused by progressive valvular calcification superimposed upon a congenitally bicuspid valve, or in the elderly, a previously normal valve. In the latter group, the aortic valve becomes sclerotic and, with further calcification, stenotic. Approximately 25% of patients over age 65 and 35% of those over age 70 have echocardiographic evidence of sclerosis, with 2–3% of these exhibiting hemodynamic evidence of stenosis. Thus, aortic stenosis has become the most common surgical valve lesion in developed countries. Degenerative valve disease is three to four times more frequent in men than in women and is more common in smokers and hypertensives. Valvular stenosis must be distinguished from supravalvular obstruction and from outflow obstruction of the left ventricular infundibulum, both relatively rare.

Clinical Findings

A. Symptoms and Signs: Slightly narrowed, thickened, or roughened valves (aortic sclerosis) or aortic dilation may produce the typical murmur and thrill without causing significant hemodynamic effects. In mild or moderate cases, the characteristic signs are a systolic ejection murmur at the aortic area transmitted to the neck and apex; in severe cases, a palpable left ventricular heave or thrill, a weak to absent aortic second sound, or reversed splitting of the second sound are present (see Table 10–1). When the valve area is less than 0.8–1 cm^2 (normal, 3–4 cm^2), ventricular systole becomes prolonged and the typical carotid pulse pattern of delayed upstroke and low amplitude is present, but this may be an unreliable finding in older patients with extensive arteriosclerotic vascular disease. Left ventricular hypertrophy increases progressively, with resulting elevations in diastolic pressure. Cardiac output is maintained until the stenosis is severe (with a valve area < 0.8 cm^2). Patients may present with left ventricular failure, angina pectoris, or syncope.

Symptoms of failure may be sudden in onset or may progress gradually. Angina pectoris frequently occurs in aortic stenosis. One-half of patients with calcific aortic stenosis and angina have significant associated coronary artery disease, whereas coronary disease is noted at only half this rate in the absence of angina. Syncope is typically exertional and may be due to arrhythmias (usually ventricular tachycardia but sometimes sinus bradycardia), hypotension, or decreased cerebral perfusion resulting from increased blood flow to exercising muscle without compensatory increase in cardiac output. Sudden death may occur but is rarely the initial manifestation of aortic stenosis in previously asymptomatic patients.

B. Diagnostic Studies: The clinical assessment of aortic stenosis may be difficult, especially in older patients. The ECG reveals left ventricular hypertrophy or suggestive repolarization changes in most patients but may be normal in up to 10%. The chest radiograph may show a normal or enlarged cardiac silhouette, calcification of the aortic valve, and dilation and calcification of the ascending aorta. The echocardiogram provides useful data about aortic valve calcification and opening and left ventricular thickness and function, while Doppler can estimate the aortic valve gradient. These data can reliably exclude or diagnose severe stenosis. In patients with moderate obstruction, especially with low cardiac output or concomitant regurgitation, these evaluations may be inaccurate.

Cardiac catheterization is the definitive diagnostic procedure. The valve gradient is measured and the valve area calculated; a valve area below 0.8 cm^2 indicates severe stenosis. Aortic regurgitation can be quantified by aortic root angiography. Coronary arteriography should be performed in most adults with aortic stenosis to assess for concomitant coronary disease.

Prognosis & Treatment

Following the onset of heart failure, angina, or syncope, the prognosis without surgery is poor (50%

3-year mortality rate). Medical treatment may stabilize patients in heart failure, but surgery is indicated for all symptomatic patients, including those with left ventricular dysfunction, which often improves postoperatively. Valve replacement is usually not indicated in asymptomatic individuals. Exceptions are those with declining left ventricular function, very severe left ventricular hypertrophy, and very high gradients (> 80 mm Hg) or severely reduced valve areas (≤ 0.7 cm^2).

The surgical mortality rate for valve replacement is 2–5%, but it rises to 10% above the age of 75. Severe coronary lesions are usually bypassed at the same time. Anticoagulation with warfarin is required for mechanical prostheses but is not essential with bioprostheses. Although bioprosthetic valves have hitherto undergone degenerative changes and required replacement within 7–10 years (sometimes within 3 years), newer ones may be more durable. Some centers have begun performing the Ross procedure, which entails switching the patient's pulmonary valve to the aortic position and placing a bioprosthesis in the pulmonary position. Because bioprostheses do not deteriorate as fast on the right side of the heart, this procedure has produced excellent long-term results without anticoagulation.

Although percutaneous balloon valvuloplasty can produce short-term reductions in the severity of aortic stenosis, restenosis occurs rapidly in most adults who have calcified valves. Except in adolescents, balloon valvuloplasty should be reserved for individuals who are poor candidates for surgery or as an intermediate procedure to stabilize high-risk patients prior to surgery.

Lester J et al: The natural history and rate of progression of aortic stenosis. Chest 1998;113:1109. [NLM Cit ID: 98213375] (Focuses on symptoms and the question of when to operate.)

O'Rourke RA: Aortic valve stenosis: A common clinical entity. Curr Probl Cardiol 1998;23:429. [NLM Cit ID: 98423545] (Pathophysiology and clinical manifestations. Management principles include when to operate, what type of valve to choose, and follow-up considerations.)

Otto CM et al: Association of aortic-valve sclerosis with cardiovascular mortality and morbidity in the elderly. N Engl J Med 1999;341:142. [NLM Cit ID: 99316832] (An echocardiographic cohort study found that aortic valve sclerosis without stenosis is independently associated with a 50% increased risk of cardiovascular death and myocardial infarction.)

Sabet HY et al: Congenitally bicuspid aortic valves: a surgical pathology study of 542 cases (1991 through 1996) and a literature review of 2715 additional cases. Mayo Clin Proc 1999;74:14. [NLM Cit ID: 99142001] (Approximately 4 million United States citizens have bicuspid valves, and progression to calcific stenosis is common.)

Wang A et al: Balloon aortic valvuloplasty. Prog Cardiovasc Dis 1997;40:27. [NLM Cit ID: 97390696]

AORTIC REGURGITATION (Aortic Insufficiency)

Essentials of Diagnosis (Chronic Regurgitation)

- Usually asymptomatic until middle age; presents with left-sided failure or chest pain.
- Wide pulse pressure with associated peripheral signs.
- Hyperactive, enlarged left ventricle.
- Diastolic murmur along left sternal border.
- ECG shows left ventricular hypertrophy; x-ray shows left ventricular dilation. Echo-Doppler confirms diagnosis and estimates severity.

General Considerations

Rheumatic aortic regurgitation has become less common than in the preantibiotic era, but nonrheumatic causes are frequent and are the major cause of isolated aortic regurgitation. These include congenitally bicuspid valves, infective endocarditis, and hypertension. Many patients have aortic regurgitation secondary to aortic root diseases such as cystic medial necrosis (especially Marfan's syndrome), aortic dissection, ankylosing spondylitis, Reiter's syndrome, and syphilis.

Clinical Findings

A. Symptoms and Signs: The clinical presentation is determined by the rapidity with which regurgitation develops. In chronic regurgitation, the only sign for many years may be a soft aortic diastolic murmur. As the valve deformity increases, larger amounts regurgitate, diastolic blood pressure falls, and the left ventricle progressively enlarges. Most patients remain asymptomatic even at this point, and an often prolonged plateau phase, characterized by stable left ventricular dilation, occurs. Left ventricular failure is a late event and may be sudden in onset. Exertional dyspnea and fatigue are the most frequent symptoms, but paroxysmal nocturnal dyspnea and pulmonary edema may also occur. Angina pectoris or atypical chest pain may be present. Associated coronary artery disease and syncope are less common than in aortic stenosis.

Hemodynamically, because of compensatory left ventricular dilation, patients eject a large stroke volume which is adequate to maintain forward cardiac output until late in the course of the disease. Left ventricular diastolic pressure remains normal also but may abruptly rise when heart failure occurs. Abnormal left ventricular systolic function, as manifested by reduced ejection fraction and increasing end-systolic left ventricular volume, is a late sign.

The major physical findings relate to the wide arterial pulse pressure. The pulse has a rapid rise and fall (Corrigan's pulse), with an elevated systolic and low diastolic pressure, owing to the large stroke volume and rapid diastolic runoff back into the left ventricle, respectively. The large stroke volume is also responsible for characteristic findings such as Quincke's pulses (subungual capillary pulsations) and Duroziez's sign (diastolic murmur over a partially compressed peripheral artery, commonly the femoral). The apical impulse is prominent, laterally displaced, and usually hyperdynamic and may be sustained. The murmur itself may be quite soft and localized; the aortic diastolic murmur is high-pitched and decrescendo. A mid or late diastolic low-pitched mitral murmur (Austin Flint murmur) may be heard in advanced aortic regurgitation, owing to obstruction of mitral flow produced by partial closure of the mitral valve by the regurgitant jet.

When aortic regurgitation develops acutely (as in aortic dissection or infective endocarditis), left ventricular failure, manifested primarily as pulmonary edema, may develop rapidly, and surgery is urgently required. Patients with acute aortic regurgitation do not have the dilated left ventricle of chronic aortic regurgitation. In the same way, the diastolic murmur is shorter and may be minimal in intensity, and the pulse pressure may not be widened, making clinical diagnosis difficult.

B. Diagnostic Studies: The ECG usually shows moderate to severe left ventricular hypertrophy. Radiographs show cardiomegaly with left ventricular prominence.

Echocardiography can demonstrate whether the lesion involves the aortic root or if valvular disease is present. Serial assessments of left ventricular size and function are critical in determining the timing for valve replacement. Doppler techniques can qualitatively estimate the severity of regurgitation, though it should be noted that "mild" regurgitation is not uncommon and should not be overinterpreted. Scintigraphic studies can quantify left ventricular function and functional reserve during exercise—a useful predictor of prognosis.

Cardiac catheterization can help quantify severity and is used to evaluate the coronary and aortic root anatomy preoperatively.

Treatment & Prognosis

Aortic regurgitation that appears or worsens during or after an episode of infective endocarditis or aortic dissection may lead to acute severe left ventricular failure or subacute progression over weeks or months. The former usually presents as pulmonary edema; surgical replacement of the valve is indicated even during active infection. These patients may be transiently improved or stabilized by vasodilators.

Chronic regurgitation has a long natural history, but the prognosis without surgery becomes poor when symptoms occur. Vasodilators, such as hydralazine, nifedipine, and angiotensin-converting enzyme inhibitors, can reduce the severity of regurgitation, and prophylactic treatment may postpone or avoid surgery in asymptomatic patients with severe regurgitation and dilated left ventricles. Beta-blocker therapy may slow the rate of aortic dilation in Marfan's syndrome. Surgery is usually indicated once aortic regurgitation causes symptoms. Surgery is also indicated for those with few or no symptoms who present with significant left ventricular dysfunction (ejection fraction < 45–50%) or who exhibit progressive deterioration of left ventricular function, irrespective of symptoms. Although the operative mortality rate is higher when left ventricular function is severely impaired, valve replacement or repair is still indicated, since left ventricular function often improves somewhat and the long-term prognosis is thereby enhanced.

The operative mortality rate is usually in the 3–5% range. Surgeons are attempting valve repair more frequently in patients with leaflet prolapse (most frequently in individuals with bicuspid valves). Aortic regurgitation due to aortic root disease requires repair or replacement of the root, a more difficult operation. Following surgery, left ventricular size usually decreases and left ventricular function improves, except where dysfunction has been present chronically.

Dujardin KS et al: Mortality and morbidity of aortic regurgitation in clinical practice: a long term follow-up study. Circulation 1999;99:1851. [NLM Cit ID: 99216375] (Patients with low ejection fractions, dilated ventricles, or heart failure symptoms should undergo valve replacement surgery.)

Gaasch WH et al: Managing asymptomatic patients with chronic aortic regurgitation. Chest 1997;111:1702. [NLM Cit ID: 97330738] (Pathophysiology, natural history, medical and surgical therapy.)

TRICUSPID STENOSIS

Tricuspid stenosis is usually rheumatic in origin. It should be suspected when "right heart failure" appears in the course of mitral valve disease, marked by hepatomegaly, ascites, and dependent edema. The typical diastolic rumble along the lower left sternal border mimics mitral stenosis. In sinus rhythm, a presystolic liver pulsation may be found.

Hemodynamically, a diastolic pressure gradient of 5–15 mm Hg is found across the tricuspid valve in conjunction with raised pressure in the right atrium and jugular veins, with prominent *a* waves and with a slow *y* descent because of slow right ventricular filling.

Echocardiography usually demonstrates the lesion, and Doppler flow studies can measure the gradient; accompanying valve lesions can also be detected. Right heart catheterization is diagnostic.

Acquired tricuspid stenosis may be amenable to valvotomy under direct vision, but it usually requires a prosthetic valve replacement. Although experience is limited, balloon valvuloplasty may be the initial procedure of choice in many patients.

TRICUSPID REGURGITATION

Tricuspid regurgitation may occur in a variety of situations other than disease of the tricuspid valve itself. The most common is right ventricular overload resulting from left ventricular failure due to any cause. Tricuspid regurgitation occurs in association with right ventricular and inferior myocardial infarction. Tricuspid valve endocarditis and resulting regurgitation are common in intravenous drug users. Other causes include the carcinoid syndrome, lupus erythematosus, and myxomatous degeneration of the valve (associated with mitral valve prolapse). Ebstein's anomaly, a congenital defect of the tricuspid valve, often presents in adults as massive right-sided cardiomegaly due to tricuspid regurgitation.

The symptoms and signs of tricuspid regurgitation are identical to those resulting from right ventricular failure due to any cause. In the presence of mitral valve disease, the tricuspid valvular lesion can be suspected on the basis of early onset of right heart failure and a harsh systolic murmur along the lower left sternal border which is separate from the mitral murmur and which often increases in intensity during and just after inspiration.

Hemodynamically, tricuspid regurgitation is characterized by a prominent regurgitant systolic *(v)* wave in the right atrium and jugular venous pulse, with a rapid *y* descent and a small or absent *x* descent. The regurgitant wave, like the systolic murmur, is increased with inspiration, and its size depends upon the size of the right atrium. In tricuspid regurgitation, especially with right ventricular failure, an inspiratory S_3 may be present.

Tricuspid regurgitation secondary to severe mitral valve disease or other left-sided lesions may regress when the underlying disease is corrected. When surgery is required, valve repair or valvuloplasty of the tricuspid ring is often preferable to valve replacement. Replacement of the tricuspid valve is infrequently done now.

Singh JP et al: Prevalence and clinical determinants of mitral, tricuspid, and aortic regurgitation. Am J Cardiol 1999;83:897. [NLM Cit ID: 99204681] (Up to 20% of patients undergoing routine echo examination had some valve regurgitation, with age being the most common clinical predictor.)

CHOICE & MANAGEMENT OF PROSTHETIC VALVES

Valve repair may be useful for tricuspid, mitral, and occasionally aortic regurgitation. Likewise, percutaneous or open valvulotomy may be indicated in mitral, pulmonary, and tricuspid stenosis. Nonetheless, the number of valve replacement procedures continues to increase as a result of the aging of the population. The choice of a mechanical device versus a bioprosthesis is often a difficult one, balancing the risk of chronic anticoagulation and thromboembolism (mechanical) versus the need for eventual reoperation (bioprosthesis). In general, otherwise healthy patients below age 65 should receive mechanical valves unless anticoagulation is contraindicated because their life expectancy is greater than the durability of tissue prostheses. Furthermore, deterioration of bioprostheses is accelerated in younger patients. In patients with a small left ventricular cavity or aortic annulus, mechanical disk valves have significant hemodynamic advantages. Finally, patients who will require anticoagulation in any case, such as those in atrial fibrillation, should receive mechanical valves. Bioprostheses are preferable in older patients with life expectancies less than 10 years and when anticoagulation is contraindicated. However, hemodialysis patients should not receive tissue valves because they have a high failure rate. As noted previously, the Ross procedure offers another option in younger patients with aortic stenosis.

The identification of valve dysfunction may be difficult, but Doppler echocardiography, especially via the transesophageal approach, can identify regurgitation and stenosis in most cases. In patients with mechanical valves, careful anticoagulation is required with a target INR of 3.0–4.0. Anticoagulation should rarely be discontinued. For elective surgery, oral warfarin can be stopped 2–3 days preoperatively with heparin coverage until effective anticoagulation is resumed. In pregnant women, warfarin should be continued until 2 weeks before expected delivery, when heparin can be substituted, though the risk of fetal hemorrhage is increased somewhat. In one controlled study, aspirin, 100 mg daily, in addition to warfarin, reduced emboli and the mortality rate.

Tiede DJ et al: Modern management of prosthetic valve anticoagulation. Mayo Clin Proc 1998;73:665. [NLM Cit ID: 98327700] (Thorough review of anticoagulation in patients with prosthetic valves, including risks and benefits, dosing, and perioperative management.)

Vongpatanasin W et al: Prosthetic heart valves. N Engl J Med 1996;335:47. [NLM Cit ID: 96293372] (Concise review of the characteristics of various prosthetic heart valves, with discussion of complications and antithrombotic therapy.)

CORONARY HEART DISEASE (Arteriosclerotic Coronary Artery Disease; Ischemic Heart Disease)

Coronary atherosclerotic heart disease is the commonest cause of cardiovascular disability and death in the USA. Men are more often affected than women by an overall ratio of 4:1, but before age 40 the ratio is 8:1, and beyond age 70 it is 1:1. In men, the peak incidence of clinical manifestations is at age 50–60; in women, at age 60–70.

Risk Factors for Coronary Heart Disease

Epidemiologic studies have identified a number of important risk factors for premature coronary heart disease. These include a positive family history (particularly when onset is before age 50), age, male gender, blood lipid abnormalities, hypertension, physical inactivity, cigarette smoking, diabetes mellitus, elevated blood homocysteine levels, and hypoestrogenemia in women. Circumstantial evidence suggests that chronic infection may be involved. Overwhelming evidence indicates that abnormalities of lipid metabolism play a direct role in the pathophysiology of this condition. Risk increases progressively with higher levels of LDL cholesterol and declines with higher levels of HDL cholesterol. Therefore, the ratio of LDL to HDL cholesterol provides a composite marker of risk, with ratios below 3 indicating a lower risk and ratios above 5 indicating a higher risk. Patients with clinical manifestations of coronary disease before age 50 often have predisposing risk factors, though many do not. These risk factors are less closely linked to the onset of coronary disease in later years.

It is now apparent that other abnormalities of lipid metabolism may also play a role in the pathogenesis of coronary artery disease, and these should be sought in individuals with otherwise unexplained premature coronary atherosclerosis. Among the patterns associated with increased atherosclerosis are elevated levels of apolipoprotein(a) and of small, dense LDL lipoprotein particles. These lipoproteins and their accompanying lipids appear more likely to pass into the vessel wall and may be more difficult to clear. Accumulating evidence suggests that hypertriglyceridemia is an independent risk factor for coronary artery disease as well. Elevated triglyceride levels often occur in association with other lipid abnormalities, including low levels of HDL cholesterol and elevated concentrations of lipoprotein(a) and small, dense LDL particles.

Elevated levels of serum homocysteine and nonspecific markers of inflammation, such as cross-reactive protein (CRP), fibrinogen, and ferritin, correlate with the occurrence of coronary disease. Although hyperhomocysteinemia may increase the risk of thrombosis, it may also simply be a marker of inflammatory activity in coronary disease (see below).

Pathophysiology

Knowledge concerning the pathophysiology of atherosclerosis and the clinical presentations of coronary artery disease is accumulating rapidly. Abnormal lipid metabolism or excessive intake of cholesterol and saturated fats—especially when superimposed on a genetic predisposition—initiates the atherosclerotic process. The initial step is the "fatty streak," or subendothelial accumulation of lipids and lipid-laden monocytes (macrophages). Low-density lipoproteins (LDLs) are the major atherogenic lipid. High-density lipoproteins (HDLs), in contrast, are protective and probably assist in the mobilization of LDLs. The pathogenetic role of other lipids, including triglycerides, is less clear. LDLs undergo in situ oxidation, which makes them more difficult to mobilize as well as locally cytotoxic.

Macrophages migrate into the subendothelial space and take up lipids, giving them the appearance of "foam" cells. As the plaque progresses, smooth muscle cells also migrate into the lesion. At this stage, the lesion may be hemodynamically insignificant, but endothelial function is abnormal and its ability to limit the entry of lipoproteins into the vessel wall is impaired. If the plaque remains stable, a fibrous cap forms, the lesion becomes calcified, and the vessel lumen slowly becomes narrowed.

Although many atherosclerotic plaques remain stable or progress only gradually, others may rupture, with a resulting extrusion of lipids and tissue factors that result in a cascade of events culminating in intravascular thrombosis. The outcome of these events is determined by whether the vessel becomes occluded or whether thrombolysis occurs, either spontaneously or as the result of treatment, and whether the plaque subsequently becomes stabilized. The result may be partial or complete vessel occlusion (causing the symptoms of unstable angina or myocardial infarction), or the plaque may become restabilized, often with more severe stenosis.

Several features are associated with enhanced plaque vulnerability, including a higher lipid content, a higher concentration of macrophages, and a very thin fibrous cap. Lesions with these characteristics are often the culprit lesions in young individuals, in whom acute myocardial infarction or sudden death is the first manifestation of coronary disease; and this abrupt progression explains why most infarctions do not occur at the site of preexisting critical stenosis. Conversely, the relatively greater reduction in clinical events than in lesion severity in lipid-lowering treatment trials is probably explained by the regression or prevention of these early nonfibrotic lesions.

Recent observations have resurrected an old theory that atherosclerosis progresses as the result of an inflammatory response in the vessel wall, perhaps initiated or worsened by an infectious agent. A high circulating level of C-reactive protein, a nonspecific inflammatory marker, is associated with a higher rat of ischemic events. Agents as diverse as *Chlamyd pneumoniae*, cytomegalovirus, and *Helicobacter p lori* have been indirectly implicated.

Christen WG et al: Blood levels of homocysteine an increased risks of cardiovascular disease. Causal or casual.

Arch Intern Med 2000;160:422. [NLM Cit ID: 20158230] (Presents a strong case that homocysteine is elevated nonspecifically as an acute phase reactant.)

Hankey GJ et al: Homocysteine and vascular disease. Lancet 1999;354:407. [NLM Cit ID: 99364596] (There is a strong, independent correlation between homocysteine levels and atherothrombotic vascular events, suggesting a causal relationship. The effect of lowering homocysteine levels remains uncertain.)

He J et al: Passive smoking and the risk of coronary heart disease—a meta-analysis of epidemiologic studies. N Engl J Med 1999;340:920. [NLM Cit ID: 99173389] (A review of 18 studies suggests that passive smoking is associated with a small increase in the risk of coronary heart disease.)

Hennekens CH: Increasing burden of cardiovascular disease: Current knowledge and future directions for research on risk factors. Circulation 1998;97:1095. [NLM Cit ID: 98189744] (Thoughtful review of current knowledge of risk factors for coronary artery disease. Homocysteine, lipoprotein[a], and markers of inflammation may be added to the list of traditional risk factors.)

Hochman JS et al: Sex, clinical presentation, and outcome in patients with acute coronary syndromes. Global Use of Strategies to Open Occluded Coronary Arteries in Acute Coronary Syndromes IIb Investigators. N Engl J Med 1999;341:226. [NLM Cit ID: 99328493] (Women presenting with acute coronary syndromes have different risk profiles, clinical presentations, and outcomes compared with men.)

Kullo IJ et al: Vulnerable plaque: Pathobiology and clinical implications. Ann Intern Med 1998;129:1050. [NLM Cit ID: 99064848] (MEDLINE review of over 200 articles delineates pathophysiology and consequences of plaque rupture. Stresses the importance of developing techniques to identify and stabilize vulnerable plaque.)

Ross R: Atherosclerosis: An inflammatory disease. N Engl J Med 1999;340:115. [NLM Cit ID: 99091097] (Endothelial dysfunction and atherosclerosis are triggered by LDL, free radicals from cigarette smoke, hypertension, diabetes, homocysteine, herpesvirus, and *Chlamydia pneumoniae.*)

Primary & Secondary Prevention of Ischemic Heart Disease

Although many risk factors for coronary artery disease are not modifiable, it is now clear that interventions such as smoking cessation, treatment of dyslipidemia, and lowering of blood pressure can both prevent coronary disease and delay its progression and complications after it is manifest. Treatment of lipid abnormalities delays the progression of atherosclerosis and in some cases produces regression. Even in the absence of regression, fewer new lesions develop, endothelial function may be restored, and coronary event rates are markedly reduced in patients with clinical evidence of atherosclerosis.

A series of clinical trials has demonstrated the importance of elevated LDL cholesterol in the pathogenesis of coronary atherosclerosis—as well as stroke and peripheral arterial diseases—and the substantial benefit of treating hyperlipidemia in preventing these conditions. Trials have demonstrated improved outcomes in patients who have already experienced myocardial infarction (secondary prevention) treated with HMG-CoA reductase inhibitors, even when they have cholesterol levels previously considered satisfactory (LDL cholesterol levels as low as 125 mg/dL). These studies found reductions in cardiac events, cardiovascular deaths, and all-cause mortality. This occurred regardless of age, race, or the presence of hypertension. Aggressive lipid-lowering therapy should be implemented in all patients with dyslipidemia and coronary artery or peripheral vascular disease. There is now clear evidence that reduction of LDL cholesterol can prevent coronary events and stroke in patients without clinically manifest atherosclerosis (primary prevention) and LDL levels as low as 130 mg/dL. A European study enrolled high-risk patients with a mean LDL of 192 mg/dL and demonstrated a reduction of coronary death and nonfatal myocardial infarction with pravastatin. Another trial extended these findings to a less selected population with LDL levels between 130 and 190 mg/dL, again showing an impressive reduction in coronary and stroke events with lovastatin. Treatment of abnormally low HDL levels or elevations of lipoprotein(a) and small, dense LDL particles is more difficult, but oral niacin in high dosages (3 g/d or more) may be effective. A trial in postinfarction patients has demonstrated that an increase in HDL levels with gemfibrozil (600 mg twice daily) in patients with relatively low LDL levels prolongs reinfarction-free survival. The value of reducing elevated triglyceride levels is less clear, but since elevated triglycerides are often associated with other lipid abnormalities, treatment with niacin, gemfibrozil, or fenofibrate for levels above 400 mg/dL is appropriate.

Since LDL oxidation appears to play a role in the atherogenicity of lipid molecules that have passed into the vessel wall, antioxidant therapy has been advocated as a preventive measure. Thus far, however, there are few data to support this popular concept. Several large, well-controlled studies have failed to demonstrate a benefit with vitamin E therapy, and there have been no positive prospective trials with any antioxidant agent.

Elevated plasma homocysteine levels are associated with an increased risk of vascular events. Although homocysteine levels can be reduced with dietary supplements of folic acid (1 mg/d) in combination with vitamin B_6 and vitamin B_{12}, it is not clear that this reduces clinical events in individuals with coronary artery disease.

Another preventive measure is aspirin prophylaxis. Aspirin (325 mg every other day) in males over the age of 50 reduces the incidence of myocardial infarction. Whether this approach should be employed in the general population or only in those at higher risk is unclear, and the optimal dosage is not known. A prudent approach would be to administer 81–325 mg daily to men with multiple coronary risk factors or concomitant diabetes if no contraindication is present. The same approach is probably warranted for women, commencing 5–10 years later. It is of note that the previously mentioned GISSI Prevention Trial found a significant mortality reduction with omega-3 fatty acid administration (1 g daily) in postinfarction patients.

The effect of hormone replacement therapy in postmenopausal women is uncertain. Epidemiologic data suggest that estrogen protects against the development of coronary artery disease. However, the HERS trial, a prospective evaluation of estrogen use in women with coronary artery disease, showed no benefit in reducing mortality or preventing subsequent cardiac events. An early analysis from the Women's Health Initiative also suggested a possible early increase in coronary events with estrogen replacement, but this and other trials are ongoing, and this issue should be considered unresolved.

Control of blood pressure has now been shown to prevent infarctions in older patients. Although unproved, it seems likely that control of blood pressure in younger individuals also prevents subsequent coronary events. The role of exercise remains controversial. Although individuals who exercise for at least 30 minutes a week are at lower risk for subsequent coronary events, it is difficult to be certain that this outcome relates specifically to exercise rather than a generally healthy lifestyle.

The Heart Outcomes Prevention Evaluation (HOPE) trial demonstrated that the ACE inhibitor ramipril reduces fatal and nonfatal vascular events (cardiovascular deaths, nonfatal myocardial infarctions, and nonfatal strokes) by 20–25% in patients at high risk, including diabetics with additional risk factors or patients with clinical coronary, cerebral, or peripheral arterial atherosclerotic disease. Thus, the role of ACE inhibitors in secondary prevention appears to be expanding beyond patients with heart failure or left ventricular systolic dysfunction.

The decrease in number of coronary deaths over the last 2 decades may be due to a decrease in the prevalence of risk factors but probably also reflects improvements in medical therapy, the role of coronary care units, better treatment of angina, arrhythmias, and heart failure, and improved survival after coronary revascularization in some patient subsets.

Anderson JL et al: Randomized secondary prevention trial of azithromycin in patients with coronary artery disease and serological evidence for *Chlamydia pneumoniae* infection: The Azithromycin in Coronary Artery Disease: Elimination of Myocardial Infection with Chlamydia (ACADEMIC) study. Circulation 1999;99:1540. [NLM Cit ID: 99196863] (In a randomized, controlled trial, secondary prevention therapy for myocardial infarction with azithromycin resulted in reduced levels of markers for inflammation [C-reactive protein, IL-1, IL-6, and TNF-α], but unlike previous studies, there was no difference in clinical end points.)

Diaz MN et al: Antioxidants and atherosclerotic heart disease. N Engl J Med 1997;337:408. [NLM Cit ID: 97377707] (An unproved hypothesis.)

Downs JR et al: Primary prevention of acute coronary events with lovastatin in men and women with average cholesterol levels: Results of AFCAPS/TEXCAPS. JAMA 1998;279:1591. [NLM Cit ID: 98273991] (Important reduction in coronary events in what was formerly considered a low-risk group.)

Gould LA et al: Cholesterol reduction yields clinical benefit. Circulation 1998;97:946. [NLM Cit ID: 98188110] (Updated meta-analysis incorporating the results of eight recently published trials with statins confirms that cholesterol-lowering with these agents reduces coronary heart disease and mortality risk.)

Grundy SM et al: AHA/ACC scientific statement: Assessment of cardiovascular risk by use of multiple-risk-factor assessment equations: a statement for healthcare professionals from the American Heart Association and the American College of Cardiology. J Am Coll Cardiol 1999;34:1348. [NLM Cit ID: 99449130]

Grundy SM: Primary prevention of coronary heart disease: integrating risk assessment with intervention. Circulation 1999;100:988. [NLM Cit ID: 99398985] (Reviews strategies for detecting and modifying risk of coronary heart disease covering smoking cessation and treatment of diabetes, hypertension, and dyslipidemia.)

Hulley S et al: Randomized trial of estrogen plus progestin for secondary prevention of coronary heart disease in postmenopausal women. Heart and Estrogen/progestin Replacement Study (HERS) Research Group. JAMA 1998;280:605. [NLM Cit ID 98382151] (After 4.1 years of follow-up, study found no decrease in secondary prevention of coronary events with estrogen/progestins, and there were more thromboembolic events and gallbladder disease.)

JAMA patient page: Cholesterol. JAMA 1999;281:206. [NLM Cit ID: 99114164]

Jeppesen J et al: Triglyceride concentration and ischemic heart disease. Circulation 1998;97:1029. [NLM Cit ID: 98189735] (Eight-year follow up in nearly 3000 men identified elevated triglycerides as a strong independent risk factor for ischemic heart disease.)

Knopp IJ et al. Drug treatment of lipid disorders. N Engl J Med 1999;341:498. [NLM Cit ID: 99353507] (Excellent review of lipid metabolism, classification of lipid disorders, and treatment with statins, niacin, fibrates, and resins.)

Mosca L et al: AHA/ACC scientific statement: consensus panel statement. Guide to preventive cardiology for women. American Heart Association/American College of Cardiology. J Am Coll Cardiol 1999;33:1751. [NLM Cit ID: 99265624]

Rubins HB et al: Gemfibrozil for the secondary prevention of coronary heart disease in men with low levels of high-density lipoprotein cholesterol. Veterans Affairs High-Density Lipoprotein Cholesterol Intervention Trial Study Group. N Engl J Med 1999;341:410. [NLM Cit ID: 99345288] (Therapy with gemfibrozil reduced the risk of cardiovascular events in patients with low HDL and normal LDL.)

Tribble DL: AHA Science Advisory. Antioxidant consumption and risk of coronary heart disease: emphasis on vitamin C, vitamin E, and beta-carotene: A statement for healthcare professionals from the American Heart Association. Circulation 1999;99:591. [NLM Cit ID: 99126309]

Van den Hoogen PC et al: The relation between blood pressure and mortality due to coronary heart disease among men in different parts of the world. Seven Countries Study Research Group. N Engl J Med 2000;342:1. [NLM Cit ID: 20074112] (Relative increases in blood pressure resulted in increased risk of cardiovascular events in different parts of the world, but the same absolute blood pressures resulted in different risks in the various countries.)

Vaughan CJ et al: The evolving role of statins in the management of atherosclerosis. J Am Coll Cardiol 2000;35:1. [NLM Cit ID: 20100207]

Vitamin E supplementation and cardiovascular events in high-risk patients. The Heart Outcomes Prevention Evaluation Study Investigators. N Engl J Med 2000;342:154. [NLM Cit ID: 20092359] (In high-risk patients, treatment with vitamin E for a mean of 4.5 years had no effect on cardiovascular outcome.)

Welch GN et al: Homocysteine and atherothrombosis. N Engl J Med 1998;338:1042. [NLM Cit ID: 98181803] (Review of this newly appreciated pathogenic factor.)

Yusuf S et al: Effects of an angiotensin-converting-enzyme inhibitor, ramipril, on cardiovascular events in high-risk patients. The Heart Outcomes Prevention Evaluation Study Investigators. N Engl J Med 2000;342:145. [NLM Cit ID: 20092358] (In a placebo-controlled randomized trial, ramipril reduced the risk of death, myocardial infarction, and stroke in patients age 55 or older with known vascular disease or diabetes plus one other vascular risk factor. Of note is the accompanying article showing that vitamin E had no effect in the same population.)

Pathophysiology of Myocardial Ischemia & Acute Coronary Syndromes

Advanced coronary atherosclerosis and even complete occlusion may remain clinically silent. There is only a modest correlation between the clinical symptoms and the anatomic extent of disease. At present, the only means of determining the location and extent of narrowing is coronary arteriography, although ischemia can be recognized by other less invasive studies. Myocardial ischemia may be provoked by either increased myocardial oxygen requirements (exercise, mental stress, or spontaneous fluctuations in heart rate and blood pressure) or by decreased oxygen supply (caused by coronary vasospasm, platelet plugging, or partial thrombosis). Abnormal endothelial function appears to play a role in the fluctuating threshold for ischemia; impaired release of nitric oxide (endothelium-derived relaxing factor) may permit unopposed vasoconstriction and facilitate platelet adhesion.

Most studies indicate that in angina pectoris, increased oxygen demand is the most frequent mechanism. In contrast, the acute coronary syndromes of unstable angina and myocardial infarction are caused by plaque disruption, platelet plugging, and coronary thrombosis. Of interest is the predilection for these episodes to occur in the early morning or shortly after arising. The outcome of this series of events is determined by whether the vessel becomes occluded or whether thrombolysis occurs, either spontaneously or as a result of treatment, and whether the plaque subsequently becomes stabilized. Thus, therapy is primarily directed toward inhibition of platelet activity (aspirin) and thrombolysis in acute syndromes and toward minimizing myocardial oxygen requirements—as well as preventive measures—in chronic angina.

Some episodes of myocardial ischemia are painful, causing angina pectoris; others are completely silent. Many silent episodes are brought on by emotional and mental stress. In patients with diagnosed coronary disease, as evidenced by prior myocardial infarction or angina, silent ischemic episodes have the same prognostic import as painful ones. The prognosis for patients with only silent ischemia is not well established, nor is the potential benefit of preventing silent ischemia.

Arbustini E et al: From plaque biology to clinical setting. Am Heart J 1999;138:55. [NLM Cit ID: 99355533] (Inflammation, infection, and neointimal hyperplasia are reviewed. Predicting the culprit plaque is difficult.)

Falk E: Stable versus unstable atherosclerosis: clinical aspects. Am Heart J 1999;138:S421. [NLM Cit ID: 20007568] (Plaque vulnerability is a function of the state of the lipid core, the degree of inflammation, and the lack of smooth muscle cells.)

Myocardial Hibernation & Stunning

Areas of myocardium that are persistently underperfused but still viable may develop sustained contractile dysfunction. This phenomenon, which is termed myocardial hibernation, appears to represent an adaptive response but may lead to left ventricular failure. It is important to recognize this phenomenon, since this form of dysfunction is reversible following coronary revascularization. Hibernating myocardium can be identified with radionuclide testing, positron emission tomography, or its retained response to inotropic stimulation with dobutamine. A related phenomenon, termed myocardial stunning, is the occurrence of persistent contractile dysfunction following prolonged or repetitive episodes of myocardial ischemia.

Wijns W et al: Hibernating myocardium. N Engl J Med 1998;339:173. [NLM Cit ID: 98319551] (Mechanisms, diagnosis, and management.)

SUDDEN DEATH

Sudden death may be the first clinical manifestation of coronary disease in as many as one-fourth of patients but is more likely to occur in patients with prior infarction and moderate to severe left ventricular dysfunction. In addition, 20% of patients with acute myocardial infarction will die before reaching a hospital. Most of these deaths are caused by ventricular fibrillation. It is noteworthy that transient ischemia (as opposed to infarction or coronary occlusion) is rarely the cause of sudden death.

Note: See section on ventricular arrhythmias and evaluation of survivors of sudden death for management of patients at risk for sudden death and of survivors.

Burke AP et al: Coronary risk factors and plaque morphology in men with coronary disease who die suddenly. N Engl J Med 1997;336:1276. [NLM Cit ID: 97258686]

JAMA patient page: CPR. JAMA 1998;281:1244. [NLM Cit ID: 99213532]

Kannel WB et al: Sudden coronary death in women. Am Heart J 1998;136:205. [NLM Cit ID: 98368378] (Women have a lower sudden death rate than men at all ages but still account for one-third of all coronary fatalities.)

ANGINA PECTORIS

Essentials of Diagnosis

- Precordial chest pain, usually precipitated by stress or exertion, relieved rapidly by rest or nitrates.
- Electrocardiographic or scintigraphic evidence of ischemia during pain or stress testing.
- Angiographic demonstration of significant obstruction of major coronary vessels.

General Considerations

Angina pectoris is usually due to atherosclerotic heart disease. Coronary vasospasm may occur at the site of a lesion or, less frequently, in apparently normal vessels. Other unusual causes of coronary artery obstruction such as congenital anomalies, emboli, arteritis, or dissection may cause ischemia or infarction. Angina may also occur in the absence of coronary artery obstruction as a result of severe myocardial hypertrophy, severe aortic stenosis or regurgitation, or in response to increased metabolic demands, as in hyperthyroidism, marked anemia, or paroxysmal tachycardias with rapid ventricular rates. Rarely, angina occurs with angiographically normal coronary arteries and without other identifiable causes. This presentation has been labeled syndrome X and is most likely due to inadequate flow reserve in the resistance vessels (microvasculature). Although treatment is often not very successful in relieving symptoms, the prognosis of syndrome X is good.

Clinical Findings

A. History: The diagnosis of angina pectoris depends principally upon the history, which should specifically include the following information.

1. Circumstances that precipitate and relieve angina–Angina occurs most commonly during activity and is relieved by resting. Exertion that involves straining the thoracic or upper extremity muscles (eg, lifting) or walking rapidly uphill precipitates attacks most consistently. Patients prefer to remain upright rather than lie down. The amount of activity required to produce angina may be relatively consistent under comparable physical and emotional circumstances or may vary from day to day. It is usually less after meals, during excitement, or on exposure to cold. The threshold for angina is often lower in the morning or after strong emotion; the latter can provoke attacks in the absence of exertion. In addition, discomfort may occur during sexual activity, at rest, or at night as a result of coronary spasm.

2. Characteristics of the discomfort–Patients often do not refer to angina as "pain" but as a sensation of tightness, squeezing, burning, pressing, choking, aching, bursting, "gas," indigestion, or an ill-characterized discomfort. It is often characterized by clenching a fist over the mid chest. The distress of angina is rarely sharply localized and is not spasmodic.

3. Location and radiation–The distribution of the distress may vary widely in different patients but is usually the same for each patient unless unstable angina or myocardial infarction supervenes. In 80–90% of cases, the discomfort is felt behind or slightly to the left of the mid sternum. When it begins farther to the left or, uncommonly, on the right, it characteristically moves centrally substernally. Although angina may radiate to any dermatome from C8 to T4, it radiates most often to the left shoulder and upper arm, frequently moving down the inner volar aspect of the arm to the elbow, forearm, wrist, or fourth and fifth fingers. Radiation to the right shoulder and distally is less common, but the characteristics are the same. Occasionally, angina may be felt initially in the lower jaw, the back of the neck, the interscapular area, high in the left back, or in the volar aspect of the wrist. If the patient identifies the site of pain by pointing to the area of the apical impulse with one finger, angina is unlikely.

4. Duration of attacks–Angina is of short duration and subsides completely without residual discomfort. If the attack is precipitated by exertion and the patient promptly stops to rest, it usually lasts less than 3 minutes. Attacks following a heavy meal or brought on by anger often last 15–20 minutes. Attacks lasting more than 30 minutes are unusual and suggest the development of unstable angina, myocardial infarction, or an alternative diagnosis.

5. Effect of nitroglycerin–The diagnosis of angina pectoris is strongly supported if sublingual nitroglycerin invariably shortens an attack and if prophylactic nitrates permit greater exertion or prevent angina entirely.

6. Risk factors–The presence of risk factors described previously makes the diagnosis of angina more likely, but their absence does not exclude angina since most patients do not have a risk profile markedly different from that of the general population.

B. Signs: Examination during a spontaneous or induced attack frequently reveals a significant elevation in systolic and diastolic blood pressure, although hypotension may also occur; occasionally, a gallop rhythm and an apical systolic murmur due to transient mitral regurgitation from papillary muscle dysfunction are present during pain only. Supraventricular or ventricular arrhythmias may be present, either as the precipitating factor or as a result of ischemia.

It is important to detect signs of diseases that may contribute to or accompany atherosclerotic heart disease, eg, diabetes mellitus (retinopathy or neuropathy), xanthelasma, tendinous xanthomas, hypertension, thyrotoxicosis, myxedema, or peripheral vascular disease. Aortic stenosis or regurgitation, hypertrophic cardiomyopathy, and mitral valve prolapse should be sought, since they may produce angina or other forms of chest pain.

Differential Diagnosis

With an appropriate history, the diagnosis of angina pectoris is more than 90% certain. When atypical features are present—such as prolonged duration (hours or days); or darting, knifelike pains at the apex or over the precordium—ischemia is less likely.

Anterior chest wall syndrome is characterized by sharply localized tenderness of intercostal muscles. Inflammation of the chondrocostal junctions, which may be warm, swollen, and red, may result in diffuse chest pain that is also reproduced by local pressure (Tietze's syndrome). Intercostal neuritis (herpes zoster, diabetes mellitus, etc) also mimics angina.

Cervical or thoracic spine disease involving the dorsal roots produces sudden sharp, severe chest pain suggesting angina in location and "radiation" but related to specific movements of the neck or spine, recumbency, and straining or lifting. Pain due to cervical or thoracic disk disease involves the outer or dorsal aspect of the arm and the thumb and index fingers rather than the ring and little fingers.

Peptic ulcer, chronic cholecystitis, esophageal spasm, and functional gastrointestinal disease may produce pain suggestive of angina pectoris. Reflux esophagitis is characterized by lower chest and upper abdominal pain after heavy meals, occurring in recumbency or upon bending over. The pain is relieved by antacids, sucralfate, or H_2 receptor antagonists. The picture may be especially confusing because ischemic pain may also be associated with upper gastrointestinal symptoms, and esophageal motility disorders may be improved by nitrates and calcium channel blockers. Assessment of esophageal motility may be necessary.

Degenerative and inflammatory lesions of the left shoulder and thoracic outlet syndromes may cause chest pain due to nerve irritation or muscular compression; the symptoms are usually precipitated by movement of the arm and shoulder and are associated with paresthesias.

Spontaneous pneumothorax may cause chest pain as well as dyspnea and may create confusion with angina as well as myocardial infarction. Even the ECG may resemble infarction because of changes in voltage from the pneumothorax. The same is true of pneumonia and pulmonary embolization. Dissection of the thoracic aorta can cause severe chest pain that is commonly felt in the back; it is sudden in onset, reaches maximum intensity immediately, and may be associated with changes in pulses. Other cardiac disorders such as mitral valve prolapse, hypertrophic cardiomyopathy, myocarditis, pericarditis, aortic valve disease, or right ventricular hypertrophy may cause atypical chest pain or even myocardial ischemia. Noninvasive testing and, in many cases, cardiac catheterization may be required to establish the diagnosis.

Evaluation of Patients With Angina Pectoris

A. Laboratory Findings: Serum lipid levels should be determined in all patients with suspected angina. Anemia and diabetes may also be investigated if clinically appropriate.

B. Electrocardiography: The resting ECG is normal in about a quarter of patients with angina. In the remainder, abnormalities include old myocardial infarction, nonspecific ST–T changes, atrioventricular or intraventricular conduction defects, and changes of left ventricular hypertrophy. During anginal episodes, the characteristic electrocardiographic change is horizontal or downsloping ST segment depression that reverses after the ischemia disappears. T wave flattening or inversion may also occur. Less frequently, ST segment elevation is observed; this finding suggests severe (transmural) ischemia and often occurs with coronary spasm.

C. Exercise Electrocardiography: Exercise testing is the most useful noninvasive procedure for evaluating the patient with angina. Ischemia that is not present at rest is detected by precipitation of typical chest pain or ST segment depression (or, rarely, elevation). Exercise testing is often combined with scintigraphic studies or echocardiography (see below), but in patients without baseline ST segment abnormalities or in whom anatomic localization is not necessary, the exercise ECG should be the initial procedure because of considerations of cost and convenience.

Exercise testing can be done on a motorized treadmill or with a bicycle ergometer. A variety of exercise protocols are utilized, the most common being the Bruce protocol, which increases the treadmill speed and elevation every 3 minutes until limited by symptoms. At least two electrocardiographic leads should be monitored continuously.

1. Precautions and risks–The usually quoted risk of exercise testing is one infarction or death per 1000 tests, but individuals who continue to have pain at rest or minimal activity are at higher risk and should not be tested. Many of the traditional exclusions, such as recent myocardial infarction or congestive heart failure, are no longer employed *if the patient is stable and ambulatory*, but aortic stenosis remains a contraindication. While most tests are carried to a symptom-limited end point (except submaximal testing early postinfarction), the test should be terminated when hypotension, significant ventricular or supraventricular arrhythmias, more than mild to moderate angina, or more than 3- to 4-mm ST segment depression occurs.

2. Indications–Exercise testing is employed (1) to confirm the diagnosis of angina; (2) to determine the severity of limitation of activity due to angina; (3) to assess prognosis in patients with known coronary disease, including those recovering from myocardial infarction, by detecting groups at high or low risk; (4) to evaluate responses to therapy; and (5) less successfully, to screen asymptomatic populations for silent coronary disease. The latter application is controversial. Because false-positive tests often exceed true positives, leading to much patient anxiety and self-imposed or mandated disability, exercise testing of asymptomatic individuals should be done only for those at high risk (usually a strong family history of premature coronary disease or hyperlipidemia), those whose occupations place them or others at special risk (eg, airline pilots), and older individuals commencing strenuous activity.

3. Interpretation–The usual electrocardiographic criterion for a positive test is 1 mm (0.1 mV) horizontal or downsloping ST segment depression (beyond baseline) measured 80 ms after the J point. By this criterion, 60–80% of patients with anatomically significant coronary disease will have a positive test, but 10–30% of those without significant disease will also be positive. False-positives are uncommon when a 2-mm depression is present. Additional information is inferred from the time of onset and duration of the electrocardiographic changes, their magnitude and configuration, blood pressure and heart rate changes, the duration of exercise, and the presence of associated symptoms. In general, patients exhibiting more severe ST segment depression (> 2 mm) at low workloads (< 6 minutes on the Bruce protocol) or heart rates (< 70% of age-predicted maximum)—especially when the duration of exercise and rise in blood pressure are limited or when hypotension occurs during the test—have more severe disease and a poorer prognosis. Depending on symptom status, age, and other factors, such patients should be referred for coronary arteriography and possible revascularization. On the other hand, less impressive positive tests in asymptomatic patients are often "false-positives." Therefore, exercise testing results that do not conform to the clinical picture should be confirmed by stress scintigraphy or echocardiography.

D. Scintigraphic Assessment of Ischemia: Two nuclear medicine studies provide additional information about the presence, location, and extent of coronary artery disease.

1. Myocardial perfusion scintigraphy–This test provides images in which radionuclide uptake is proportionate to blood flow at the time of injection. Thallium-201 or technetium-99m sestamibi is most frequently used. Areas of diminished uptake reflect relative hypoperfusion (compared to other myocardial regions). If the radiotracer is injected during exercise or dipyridamole- or adenosine-induced coronary vasodilation, scintigraphic defects indicate a zone of ischemia or hypoperfusion that may represent either ischemia or scar. If the myocardium is viable, as relative blood flow equalizes over time or during a scintigram performed under resting conditions, these defects tend to "fill in" or reverse, indicating reversible ischemia. Defects observed when the radiotracer is injected at rest or still present 3–4 hours after an injection during exercise or pharmacologic vasodilation (intravenous adenosine or dipyridamole) usually indicate myocardial infarction (old or recent) but may be present with severe ischemia. Occasionally, other conditions, including infiltrative diseases (sarcoidosis, amyloidosis), left bundle branch block, and dilated cardiomyopathy, may produce resting or persistent perfusion defects.

In experienced laboratories, stress perfusion scintigraphy is positive in 75–90% of patients with anatomically significant coronary disease and in 20–30% of those without it. False-positive tests may occur as a result of diaphragmatic attenuation or, in women, attenuation through breast tissue. Tomographic imaging (SPECT) can reduce the severity of artifacts.

Myocardial scintigraphy is indicated (1) when the resting ECG makes an exercise ECG difficult to interpret (LBBB, baseline ST–T changes, low voltage, etc); (2) for confirmation of the results of the exercise ECG when they are contrary to the clinical impression (eg, a positive test in an asymptomatic patient); (3) to localize the region of ischemia; (4) to distinguish ischemic from infarcted myocardium; (5) to assess the completeness of vascularization following bypass surgery or coronary angioplasty; or (6) as a prognostic indicator in patients with known coronary disease.

2. Radionuclide angiography–This procedure images the left ventricle and measures its ejection fraction and wall motion. In coronary disease, resting abnormalities usually represent infarction, and those that occur with exercise usually indicate stress-induced ischemia. Normal subjects usually exhibit an increase in ejection fraction with exercise or no change; patients with coronary disease may exhibit a decrease. Exercise radionuclide angiography has approximately the same sensitivity as thallium-201 scintigraphy, but it is less specific in older individuals and those with other forms of heart disease. The indications are similar to those for thallium-201 scintigraphy.

3. Positron emission tomography (PET)–PET utilizes positron emitting agents to demonstrate either perfusion or metabolism of myocardium. PET can accurately distinguish transiently dysfunctional ("stunned") myocardium from scar by showing persistent glycolytic metabolism with the tracer fluorodeoxyglucose (FDG) in regions with reduced blood flow. A nearby cyclotron is required to produce this tracer, but the newer SPECT camera can provide acceptable images without the more expensive PET technology.

4. Technetium-99m–Technetium-99m pyrophosphate scintigraphy detects radiotracer uptake in areas of recent infarction. Its usefulness is limited by an 18- to 24-hour lag time after acute infarction before the test becomes positive and a limited sensitivity for small, especially nontransmural infarctions. Radiolabeled antimyosin antibodies have become available to detect myocardial necrosis following myocardial infarction. However, imaging must be performed 24–48 hours after injection. With the availability of assays of troponin T and troponin I, which are more specific for myocardial necrosis than creatine kinase and remain elevated for 5 days or longer, these imaging techniques do not have an important role.

E. Echocardiography: Echocardiography can image the left ventricle and reveal segmental wall motion abnormalities, which may indicate ischemia or prior infarction. It is a convenient technique for assessing left ventricular function, which is an important indicator of prognosis and determinant of therapy. Echocardiograms performed during supine exercise or immediately following upright exercise may demonstrate exercise-induced segmental wall motion abnormalities as an indicator of ischemia. This technique requires considerable expertise; however, in experienced laboratories, the increment in test accuracy is comparable to that obtained with scintigraphy—though a higher proportion of tests are technically inadequate. Pharmacologic stress with high-dose (20–40 μg/kg/min) dobutamine can be used as an alternative to exercise. Echo contrast agents are being developed that allow for perfusion imaging and may improve the diagnostic accuracy of this form of testing.

F. Newer Imaging Modalities: Many new imaging techniques have been developed, but their application in cardiovascular disease remains to be determined. **Computed tomography (CT scan)** can image the heart and, with contrast medium, the vascular system, but the relatively slow speed of most instruments limits its utility. The main application of CT is the evaluation of pericardial disease. **Ultrafast** or **cine CT** involves a specially designed instrument with high temporal resolution. Its availability is limited, but it provides excellent assessments of cardiac structure and function. Cine CT is increasingly being used to detect and quantify coronary artery calcification, but proper application of this highly sensitive test is uncertain. False-negative studies may occur in patients under 50 years of age, and positive studies in older patients do not necessarily provide a quantitative assessment of the severity of coronary arteriosclerosis. Thus, although this test can stratify patients into lower and higher risk groups, the appropriate management of individual patients with asymptomatic coronary artery calcification—beyond aggressive risk factors modification—is unclear.

Cardiac magnetic resonance imaging (MRI) is an evolving modality that provides high-resolution images of the heart and great vessels without radiation exposure or use of iodinated contrast media. It provides excellent anatomic definition, permitting assessment of pericardial disease, neoplastic disease of the heart, myocardial thickness, chamber size, and many congenital heart defects. It is the best noninvasive test for evaluating dissection of the aorta. Rapid acquisition sequences can produce excellent cine-mode images demonstrating left ventricular function and wall motion, and it is thus a useful alternative when the echocardiogram is suboptimal. Recent advances have been made in imaging the proximal coronary arteries and assessing myocardial perfusion with paramagnetic contrast agents, but these applications remain investigational.

G. Ambulatory Electrocardiographic Monitoring: With current ambulatory electrocardiographic recorders and with trained technicians, episodes of ischemic ST segment depression can be monitored. In patients with coronary artery disease, these episodes usually signify ischemia, even when asymptomatic ("silent"). In many, silent episodes are more frequent than symptomatic ones. In most cases, they occur in patients with other evidence of ischemia, and they respond to the same treatments, so that the role of ambulatory monitoring is unclear, as is the benefit of abolishing all such episodes in patients who are otherwise being managed properly.

H. Coronary Angiography: Selective coronary arteriography is the definitive diagnostic procedure for coronary artery disease. It can be performed with low mortality (about 0.1%) and morbidity (1–5%), but the cost is high, and with currently available noninvasive techniques it is usually not indicated solely for diagnosis.

Coronary arteriography should be performed in the following groups:

(1) Patients being considered for coronary artery revascularization because of limiting stable angina who have failed to improve on an adequate medical regimen.

(2) Patients in whom coronary revascularization is being considered because the clinical presentation (unstable angina, postinfarction angina, etc) or nonin-

vasive testing suggests high-risk disease (see Indications for Revascularization).

(3) Patients with aortic valve disease who also have angina pectoris, in order to determine whether the angina is due to accompanying coronary disease. Coronary angiography is also performed in asymptomatic older patients undergoing valve surgery so that concomitant bypass may be done if the anatomy is propitious.

(4) Patients who have had coronary revascularization with subsequent recurrence of symptoms, to determine whether bypass grafts or native vessels are occluded.

(5) Patients with cardiac failure in whom a surgically correctable lesion, such as left ventricular aneurysm, mitral regurgitation, or reversible ischemic dysfunction, is suspected.

(6) Patients surviving sudden death or with symptomatic or life-threatening arrhythmias in whom coronary artery disease may be a correctable cause.

(7) Patients with chest pain of uncertain cause or cardiomyopathy of unknown cause.

Coronary arteriography visualizes the location and severity of stenoses. Narrowing greater than 50% of the luminal diameter is considered clinically significant, although most lesions producing ischemia are associated with narrowing in excess of 70%. This information has important prognostic value, since mortality rates are progressively higher in patients with one-, two-, and three-vessel disease and those with left main coronary artery obstruction (ranging from 1% per year to 25% per year). Among stable patients, 20%, 30%, and 50% have one-, two-, and three-vessel involvement, respectively, while left main disease is present in 10%. In those with strongly positive exercise ECGs or scintigraphic studies, three-vessel or left main disease may be present in 75–95% depending upon the criteria employed. Coronary arteriography also shows whether the obstructions are amenable to bypass surgery or percutaneous transluminal coronary angioplasty (PTCA).

Coronary angiography may underestimate the degree of atherosclerosis because it images only the lumen of the vessel. If there is concentric plaque with arterial enlargement (remodeling), then the lumen may appear relatively normal. Intravascular ultrasound (IVUS) utilizes a small ultrasound transducer that can be positioned within the artery and image beneath the endothelial surface. This technique is useful when the angiogram is equivocal as well as for assessing the results of angioplasty or stenting.

I. Left Ventricular Angiography: Left ventricular angiography is usually performed at the same time as coronary arteriography. Global and regional left ventricular function are visualized, as well as mitral regurgitation if present. Left ventricular function is the major determinant of prognosis in stable coronary disease and of the risk of bypass surgery.

AHA Scientific Statement: Coronary artery calcification: Pathophysiology, epidemiology, imaging methods, and clinical applications. Circulation 1996;94:1175. [NLM Cit ID: 96382206] (Consensus statement concerning the evolving experience with this controversial approach to screening.)

Fleischmann KE et al: Exercise echocardiography or exercise SPECT imaging? JAMA 1998;280:913. [NLM Cit ID: 98410693] (Meta-analysis finds similar sensitivity for detecting coronary artery disease, but better specificity is achieved with echo.)

Geleijnse ML et al: Methodology, feasibility, safety and diagnostic accuracy of dobutamine stress echocardiography. J Am Coll Cardiol 1997;30:595. [NLM Cit ID: 97429164] (Based on about 2000 studies, dobutamine stress echocardiography has a sensitivity of 80% and specificity of 84% for detecting coronary artery disease, is better for three-vessel than one- or two-vessel disease, and is very safe—no deaths, and only one myocardial infarction or episode of ventricular fibrillation for every 2000 studies.)

Gibbons RJ et al: ACC/AHA Guidelines for exercise testing. J Am Coll Cardiol 1997;30:260. [NLM Cit ID: 97351370] (Extensively referenced consensus statement.)

Kaul S: Myocardial contrast echocardiography. Curr Probl Cardiol 1998;22:549. [NLM Cit ID: 98057521] (Basic principles and applications of the new technique.)

Merz CN et al: Imaging techniques for coronary artery disease: Current status and future directions. Clin Cardiol 1997;20:526. [NLM Cit ID: 97235209] (Review of sestamibi SPECT, PET, MRI, and contrast perfusion echo.)

Pilote L et al: Clinical yield and cost of exercise treadmill testing to screen for coronary artery disease in asymptomatic adults. Am J Cardiol 1998;81:219. [NLM Cit ID: 98252604] (Screening asymptomatic middle-aged patients with exercise treadmills is very low-yield: 15% were abnormal, 5% underwent coronary angiography, and only 0.5% overall had severe coronary artery disease at catheterization.)

Rumberger JA et al: Electron beam computed tomographic coronary calcium scanning: A review and guidelines for use in asymptomatic persons. Mayo Clin Proc 1999;74:243. [NLM Cit ID: 99189863] (Negative scan indicates low risk, and increasing calcium scores are associated with quantitatively greater coronary disease—but specificity for predicting future events remains relatively low.)

Schelbert HR: The usefulness of positron emission tomography. Curr Probl Cardiol 1998;23:69. [NLM Cit ID: 98162721] (Argues that PET is useful and potentially cost-effective in detection of coronary artery disease and assessment of myocardial viability.)

Schwaiger M et al: Cardiological applications of nuclear medicine. Lancet 1999:354:661. [NLM Cit ID: 99394561] (Reviews the clinical applications of radionuclide and PET imaging in cardiac disease.)

Skorton DJ et al (editors): *Cardiac Imaging,* 2nd ed. Saunders, 1996. (All aspects of invasive and noninvasive cardiac imaging.)

Coronary Vasospasm & Angina With Normal Coronary Arteriograms

Although most symptoms of myocardial ischemia result from fixed stenosis of the coronary arteries or

PTCA and stent procedures. Tirofiban (0.15 μg/kg/min) and eptifibatide (0.75 μg/kg/min) are small molecules that block the platelet receptor and have a shorter half-life and are less expensive than abciximab. Both have been shown to be effective in unstable angina and non-Q wave myocardial infarction. Low-molecular-weight heparin administered subcutaneously and without monitoring of the PTT appears to be at least as effective as and more convenient than intravenous heparin.

Since the vessel remains patent and the thrombi are undergoing continuous spontaneous formation and thrombolysis, thrombolytic therapy has had little effect on the outcome of unstable angina.

C. Nitroglycerin: The nitrates are first-line anti-ischemic therapy for unstable angina. Nonparenteral therapy with sublingual or oral agents or nitroglycerin ointment is usually sufficient. If pain persists or recurs, intravenous nitroglycerin should be started. The usual initial dosage is 10 μg/min. The dosage should be titrated to 1 μg/kg/min over 30–60 minutes and further increased as tolerated if pain recurs. Dosages up to 10 μg/kg/min or higher may be used. Tolerance to continuous nitrate infusion is common. Careful—usually continuous—blood pressure monitoring is required when intravenous nitroglycerin is used.

D. Beta-Blockers: These agents are also a part of the initial treatment of unstable angina unless otherwise contraindicated. If the patient has no history or physical findings of heart failure, these agents can usually be started without measurements of left ventricular function. Patients with evidence of large or multiple old infarctions are an exception. The pharmacology of these agents is discussed in Chapter 11 and summarized in Table 11–6. Use of agents with intrinsic sympathomimetic activity should be avoided in this setting. The goal of acute treatment is to reduce the heart rate below 60–70/min. Oral medication is adequate in most patients, but intravenous treatment with metoprolol, given as three 5 mg doses, or with esmolol (500 μg/kg followed by 50–200 μg/kg/min), is needed in patients with hemodynamic instability. Oral therapy should be aggressively titrated as blood pressure permits.

E. Calcium Entry Blockers: Calcium blockers have not been shown to favorably affect outcome in unstable angina, and they should be used primarily as third-line therapy in patients with continuing symptoms on nitrates and beta-blockers or those who are not candidates for these drugs. In the presence of nitrates and without accompanying beta-blockers, diltiazem or verapamil is preferred, since nifedipine and the other dihydropyridines are more likely to cause reflex tachycardia or hypotension. The initial dosage should be low, but upward titration should proceed rapidly.

F. Intra-aortic Balloon Counterpulsation (IABC): IABC can both reduce myocardial energy requirements (systolic unloading) and improve diastolic coronary blood flow. This approach is sometimes employed to stabilize patients prior to angiography or revascularization, but with modern techniques it is rarely necessary.

Prognosis & Indications for Revascularization

Over 90% of patients can be rendered pain-free with these measures. Patients who do not become ischemia-free on medical therapy should have early coronary arteriography and revascularization. Controlled trials have not shown any advantage in increased survival or lower infarction rates with CABG or PTCA compared to medical therapy, although many patients treated medically will need revascularization later for recurrent symptoms. Depending on the stringency of the definition of unstable angina, 10–30% of patients will have an early infarction, and the 1-year mortality rate is 10–20%. Elevated troponin T concentrations and "silent" ST segment shifts have both identified patients at higher risk for subsequent myocardial infarction or recurrence of severe ischemia.

Because recurrent episodes, infarction, and sudden death may occur following relief of unstable angina, additional evaluations should be performed in patients who have been stabilized, consisting of either (1) early exercise or pharmacologic stress testing to identify high-risk subsets for further invasive evaluation, or (2) coronary arteriography. The choice of approach should be individualized based on the patient's age and general health as well as the severity of symptoms and signs of ischemia. The artery responsible for the ischemia can usually be determined from electrocardiographic or scintigraphic changes during pain, and the lesion is often amenable to PTCA. If revascularization is not performed, long-term management is the same as that outlined for stable angina pectoris.

Ambrose JA et al: Unstable angina: current concepts of pathogenesis and treatment. Arch Intern Med 2000; 160:25. [NLM Cit ID: 20096163] (Review article covering pathogenesis and treatment with an emphasis on trials supporting the use of newer antithrombotic and antiplatelet therapy.)

Antman EM et al: Enoxaparin prevents death and cardiac ischemic events in unstable angina/non-Q-wave myocardial infarction: results of the thrombolysis in myocardial infarction (TIMI) 11B trial. Circulation 1999;100:1593. [NLM Cit ID: 99448154] (In nearly 4000 patients with unstable angina or non-Q wave myocardial infarction, low-molecular-weight heparin is more effective than unfractionated heparin in reducing death and serious cardiac ischemic events.)

Farkouh ME et al: A clinical trial of a chest-pain observation unit for patients with unstable angina. N Engl J Med 1998;339:1882. [NLM Cit ID: 99067152] (Randomized study of 424 patients managed in a chest pain unit versus routine hospital admission, showing that nearly half of the patients could be discharged from the emergency room without adverse consequences and with substantial cost savings.)

Invasive compared with non-invasive treatment in unstable coronary-artery disease: FRISC II prospective randomised multicentre study. FRagmin and Fast Revascularisation during InStability in Coronary artery disease Investigators. Lancet 1999;354:708. [NLM Cit ID: 99402166] (In a study of over 2400 patients in Scandinavian hospitals, patients with unstable coronary syndromes were randomized to either early coronary interventional procedures or medical management with 3 months of fragmin, a low-molecular-weight heparin. This is the first randomized study demonstrating an advantage to an early interventional strategy, but it should be noted that revascularization occurred at an average of 1 week post admission, after the patients were stabilized on medical therapy.)

Klootwijk P et al: Acute coronary syndromes: diagnosis. Lancet 1999;353(Suppl 2):SII10. [NLM Cit ID: 99301296]

Kong DF et al: Glycoprotein IIb/IIIa receptor antagonists in non-ST elevation acute coronary syndromes and percutaneous revascularisation: a review of trial reports. Drugs 1999;58:609. [NLM Cit ID: 20017595] (Concludes that treatment of 1000 patients is needed to prevent one death, 20 deaths or myocardial infarctions, and 30 deaths, myocardial infarctions, or revascularization procedures over a 30-day period.)

Yeghiazarians Y et al: Unstable angina pectoris. N Engl J Med 2000;342:101. [NLM Cit ID: 20080322] (Comprehensive review covering pharmacologic therapy, revascularization, and risk stratification.)

ACUTE MYOCARDIAL INFARCTION

Essentials of Diagnosis

- Sudden but not instantaneous development of prolonged (> 30 minutes) anterior chest discomfort (sometimes felt as "gas") that may produce arrhythmias, hypotension, shock, or cardiac failure.
- Rarely painless, masquerading as acute congestive heart failure, syncope, stroke, or shock.
- Electrocardiography: ST segment elevation or depression, evolving Q waves, symmetric inversion of T waves.
- Elevation of cardiac enzymes (CK-MB, troponin T, or troponin I).
- Appearance of segmental wall motion abnormality by imaging techniques.

General Considerations

Myocardial infarction results from prolonged myocardial ischemia, precipitated in most cases by an occlusive coronary thrombus at the site of a preexisting (though not necessarily severe) atherosclerotic plaque. More rarely, infarction may result from prolonged vasospasm, inadequate myocardial blood flow (eg, hypotension), or excessive metabolic demand. Very rarely, myocardial infarction may be caused by embolic occlusion, vasculitis, aortic root or coronary artery dissection, or aortitis. Cocaine is a cause of infarction, which should be considered in young individuals without risk factors.

The location and extent of infarction depend upon the anatomic distribution of the occluded vessel, the presence of additional stenotic lesions, and the adequacy of collateral circulation. Thrombosis in the anterior descending branch of the left coronary artery results in infarction of the anterior left ventricle and interventricular septum. Occlusion of the left circumflex artery produces anterolateral or posterolateral infarction. Right coronary thrombosis leads to infarction of the posteroinferior portion of the left ventricle and may involve the right ventricular myocardium and interventricular septum. The arteries supplying the atrioventricular node and the sinus node more commonly arise from the right coronary; thus, atrioventricular block at the nodal level and sinus node dysfunction occur more frequently during inferior infarctions. Individual variation in coronary anatomy and the presence of collateral vessels can make the prediction of coronary anatomy from infarct location inaccurate.

Infarctions are often classified as transmural, if the classic electrocardiographic evolution of ST segment elevation to Q waves was observed; or nontransmural or subendocardial, if pain, enzyme elevations, and ST–T wave changes occurred in the absence of new Q waves. However, on pathologic examination, most infarctions involve the subendocardium predominantly, and some transmural extension is common even in the absence of Q waves. Thus, a better classification is Q wave versus non-Q wave infarction. The latter generally results from incomplete occlusion or spontaneous lysis of the thrombus and often signifies the presence of additional jeopardized myocardium; it is associated with a higher incidence of reinfarction and recurrent ischemia.

The size and anatomic location of an infarction determine the acute course, the early complications, and the long-term prognosis. Hemodynamic stability is related to extent of necrosis. In small infarctions, cardiac function is normal, whereas with more extensive damage, early heart failure and hypotension (cardiogenic shock) may appear. Preventing extension of an infarct and subsequent myocardial injury is a major goal of early management. The complications of acute infarction are discussed below.

Marwick TH: The viable myocardium: Epidemiology, detection, and clinical implications. Lancet 1998;351:815. [NLM Cit ID: 98178795] (This review examines the pathogenesis of viable myocardium, techniques used to identify salvageable tissue, and clinical implications. Includes algorithms for investigation and intervention in patients with ventricular dysfunction and suspected viable myocardium.)

Ryan TJ et al: 1999 update: ACC/AHA guidelines for the management of patients with acute myocardial infarction. A report of the American College of Cardiology/

American Heart Association Task Force on Practice Guidelines (Committee on Management of Acute Myocardial Infarction). J Am Coll Cardiol 1999;34:890. [NLM Cit ID: 99411777] (Comprehensive and up-to-date guidelines. Available on the web at www.americanheart.org/Scientific/statements.)

Smith EA (editor): Myocardial infarction. Postgrad Med 1997;102:77. (Five-article symposium covering acute management, cardiac enzymes, and arrhythmias.)

Tavazzi L: Clinical epidemiology of acute myocardial infarction. Am Heart J 1999;138:548. [NLM Cit ID: 99355532] (The decline in mortality from acute myocardial infarction is due as much to primary and secondary prevention as to improved therapeutic intervention. Half of myocardial infarction survivors are rehospitalized within 1 year.)

Clinical Findings

A. Symptoms:

1. Premonitory pain–One-third of patients give a history of alteration in the pattern of angina, recent onset of typical or atypical angina, or unusual "indigestion" felt in the chest.

2. Pain of infarction–Most infarctions occur at rest unlike anginal episodes, and more commonly in the early morning. The pain is similar to angina in location and radiation but is more severe, and it builds up rapidly or in waves to maximum intensity over a few minutes or longer. Nitroglycerin has little effect; even opioids may not relieve the pain.

3. Associated symptoms–Patients may break out in a cold sweat, feel weak and apprehensive, and move about, seeking a position of comfort. They prefer not to lie quietly. Light-headedness, syncope, dyspnea, orthopnea, cough, wheezing, nausea and vomiting, or abdominal bloating may be present singly or in any combination.

4. Painless infarction–In a minority of cases, pain is absent or minor and is overshadowed by the immediate complications. As many as 25% of infarctions are detected on routine ECG without there having been any recallable acute episode.

5. Sudden death and early arrhythmias–Approximately 20% of patients with acute infarction will die before reaching the hospital; these deaths are usually in the first hour and are chiefly due to ventricular fibrillation.

B. Signs:

1. General–Patients usually appear anxious and are often sweating profusely. The heart rate may range from marked bradycardia (most commonly in inferior infarction) to tachycardia resulting from increased sympathetic nervous system activity, low cardiac output, or arrhythmia. The blood pressure may be high, especially in former hypertensives, or low in patients with shock. Respiratory distress usually indicates heart failure. Fever, usually low-grade, may appear after 12 hours and persist for several days.

2. Chest–Clear lung fields are a good prognostic sign, but basilar rales are common and do not necessarily indicate heart failure. More extensive rales or diffuse wheezing suggests pulmonary edema.

3. Heart–The cardiac examination may be unimpressive or very abnormal. An abnormally located ventricular impulse often represents the dyskinetic infarcted region. Jugular venous distention reflects right atrial hypertension, which may indicate right ventricular infarction or elevated left ventricular filling pressures. The absence of elevated central venous pressure, however, does not indicate normal left atrial or left ventricular diastolic pressures. Soft heart sounds may indicate left ventricular dysfunction. Atrial gallops (S_4) are the rule, whereas ventricular gallops (S_3) are less common and indicate significant left ventricular dysfunction. Mitral regurgitation murmurs are not uncommon and usually indicate papillary muscle dysfunction or, rarely, rupture. Pericardial friction rubs are uncommon in the first 24 hours but may appear later.

4. Extremities–Edema is usually not present. Cyanosis and cold temperature indicate low output. The peripheral pulses should be noted, since later shock or emboli may alter the examination.

C. Laboratory Findings: Leukocytosis of 10,000–20,000/μL often develops on the second day and disappears within a week. The most valuable diagnostic test is serial measurement of cardiac enzymes. A number of new assays have been developed, including quantitative determinations of CK-MB, troponin T, and troponin I. These are all quite specific for cardiac necrosis, though they may be elevated following severe ischemic episodes and with skeletal muscle damage. CK-MB isoforms may be positive within 6 hours after symptom onset, permitting better triage of patients with uncertain diagnoses. Circulating levels of troponin T and troponin I are more specific and remain elevated for 5–7 days or longer postinfarction. These should obviate the use of less specific LDH isoenzyme assays.

D. Electrocardiography: Most patients with acute infarction have ECG changes, and a normal tracing is rare. The extent of the electrocardiographic abnormalities provides only a crude estimate of the magnitude of infarction. The classic evolution of changes is from peaked ("hyperacute") T waves, to ST segment elevation, to Q wave development, to T wave inversion. This may occur over a few hours to several days. The evolution of new Q waves (> 30 ms in duration and 25% of the R wave amplitude) is diagnostic, but Q waves do not occur in 30–50% of acute infarctions (subendocardial or non-Q wave infarctions). If these patients have an appropriate clinical presentation, characteristic cardiac enzymes, and ST segment changes (usually depression) or T wave inversion lasting at least 48 hours, they are classified as having non-Q wave infarctions.

E. Chest X-Ray: The chest x-ray may demonstrate signs of congestive heart failure, but these changes often lag behind the clinical findings. Signs of aortic dissection should be sought as a possible alternative diagnosis.

F. Echocardiography: Echocardiography provides convenient bedside assessment of left ventricular global and regional function. This can help with the diagnosis and management of infarction; echocardiography has been used successfully to make judgments about admission and management of patients with suspected infarction, since normal wall motion makes an infarction unlikely. Doppler echocardiography is probably the most convenient procedure for diagnosing postinfarction mitral regurgitation or ventricular septal defect.

G. Scintigraphic Studies: Technetium-99m pyrophosphate scintigraphy can be used to diagnose acute myocardial infarction. When injected at least 18 hours postinfarction, the radiotracer complexes with calcium in necrotic myocardium to provide a "hot spot" image of the infarction. This test is insensitive to small infarctions, and false-positive studies occur, so its use is limited to patients in whom the diagnosis by electrocardiography and enzymes is not possible—principally those who present several days after the event or have intraoperative infarctions. Radiolabeled antimyosin antibody fragments are more sensitive and specific imaging agents, but scintigraphy must be performed 24 and 48 hours postinjection, so this test has limited clinical utility in the diagnosis of acute myocardial infarction.

Scintigraphy with thallium-201 or the newer technetium-based perfusion tracers will demonstrate "cold spots" in regions of diminished perfusion, which usually represent infarction when the radiotracer is administered at rest, but abnormalities do not distinguish recent from old damage.

Radionuclide angiography demonstrates akinesis or dyskinesis in areas of infarction and also measures ejection fraction, which can be valuable. Right ventricular dysfunction may indicate infarction of this chamber.

H. Hemodynamic Measurements: These can be invaluable in managing the complicated patient. Their use is described below and in Table 10–3.

Cannon CP et al: The electrocardiogram predicts one year outcomes of patients with unstable angina and non-Q-wave MI: Results of the TIMI III Registry ancillary study. J Am Coll Cardiol 1997;30:133. [NLM Cit ID: 97351352]

Hamm CW et al: Emergency room triage of patients with acute chest pain by means of rapid testing for cardiac troponin T or troponin I. N Engl J Med 1997;337:1648. [NLM Cit ID: 98035971] (Early normal troponin levels identify a low-risk group.)

Hathaway WR et al: Prognostic significance of the initial electrocardiogram in patients with acute myocardial infarction. JAMA 1998;279;387. [NLM Cit ID: 98119562] (ECG can predict 30-day risk.)

Nichol G et al: A critical pathway for management of patients with acute chest pain who are at low risk for myocardial ischemia. Ann Intern Med 1997;127:996. [NLM Cit ID: 98031970] (Identifying a low risk group can reduce resource use.)

Treatment

A. Thrombolytic Therapy: Thrombolytic therapy reduces mortality and limits infarct size. The greatest benefit occurs if treatment is initiated within the first 1–3 hours, when a 50% or greater reduction in mortality rate can be achieved. The magnitude of benefit declines rapidly thereafter, but a 10% mortality reduction can be achieved up to 12 hours after the onset of pain. The benefit is greatest in patients with potentially large infarcts, ie, those with anterior or multifocal electrocardiographic changes, but also occurs with inferior infarctions, which have a relatively good prognosis in any case. Patients with non-Q

Table 10–3. Hemodynamic subsets in acute myocardial infarction.

Category	CI or SWI	PCWP	Treatment	Comment
Normal	> 2.2, < 30	< 15	None	Mortality rate < 5%.
Hyperdynamic	> 3.0, > 40	< 15	Beta-blockers	Characterized by tachycardia; mortality rate < 5%.
Hypovolemic	< 2.5, < 30	< 10	Volume expansion	Hypotension, tachycardia, but preserved left ventricular function by echocardiography; mortality rate 4–8%.
Left ventricular failure	< 2.2, < 30	> 15	Diuretics	Mild dyspnea, rales, normal blood pressure; mortality rate 10–20%.
Severe failure	< 2.0, < 20	> 18	Diuretics, vasodilators	Pulmonary edema, mild hypotension; inotropic agents, IABC may be required; mortality rate 20–40%.
Shock	< 1.8, < 30	> 20	Inotropic agents, IABC	IABC early unless rapid reversal occurs; mortality rate > 60%.

CI = cardiac index (L/min/m^2); SWI = stroke work index (g-m/m^2, calculated as [mean arterial pressure − PCWP] × stroke volume index × 0.0136); PCWP = pulmonary capillary wedge pressure (in mm Hg; pulmonary artery diastolic pressure may be used instead); IABC = intra-aortic balloon counterpulsation.

wave infarctions generally have incomplete or partially recanalized occlusions and have not benefited as consistently from thrombolysis; thrombolytic therapy has not improved the prognosis of patients with prior CABG. Serious bleeding complications occur in 0.5–5% of patients. Contraindications include known bleeding diatheses, a history of any cerebrovascular disease, uncontrolled hypertension (> 190/110 mm Hg), pregnancy, and recent trauma or surgery of the head or spine. Relative contraindications include recent major thoracoabdominal surgery or biopsies, gastrointestinal or genitourinary bleeding, diabetic retinopathy, current oral anticoagulant therapy, prolonged cardiopulmonary resuscitation, and noncompressible puncture sites. Older patients have a higher complication rate but also a potentially greater benefit, since they have a much higher hospital mortality rate.

Therefore, the current recommendation is to administer thrombolytic therapy to patients up to age 80—or even older if the benefit-to-risk ratio seems favorable—with ST elevation, Q waves, or bundle branch block who present within 6–12 hours after onset of pain unless otherwise contraindicated. Adjunctive aspirin causes a further reduction in mortality rate and should therefore be administered concomitantly. Therapy can be initiated in the emergency room or ambulance if personnel are appropriately trained and equipped.

Prior to initiating thrombolytic therapy, a large-bore peripheral intravenous line should be established and not removed until 6 hours after the thrombolytic agent is discontinued. Arterial punctures and other invasive procedures should be avoided if possible. Samples should be drawn for baseline coagulation tests (prothrombin time, partial thromboplastin time, fibrinogen level, and platelet count), blood typing, and other blood tests. Automated blood pressure monitoring (preferably noninvasive) should be instituted.

Four thrombolytic agents have been evaluated extensively in acute infarction and are characterized in Table 10–4.

Recombinant tissue plasminogen activator (t-PA) is a naturally occurring thrombolytic factor that is theoretically thrombus-specific. However, bleeding complications have not been less frequent with t-PA, even though fibrinogen levels are better maintained,

Table 10–4. Thrombolytic therapy for acute myocardial infarction.

	Streptokinase	Alteplase; Tissue Plasminogen Activator (t-PA)	Reteplase	Anistreplase (APSAC)
Source	Group C streptococcus	Recombinant DNA	Recombinant DNA	Group C streptococcus
$T_{1/2}$	20 minutes	5 minutes	15 minutes	90 minutes
Usual dose	1.5 million units	100 mg	20 units	30 units
Administration	750,000 units over 20 minutes followed by 750,000 units over 40 minutes	Initial bolus of 15 mg, followed by 50 mg infused over next 30 minutes and 35 mg over the following 60 minutes	10 units as a bolus over 2 minutes, repeated after 30 minutes	Infuse over 2–5 minutes
Anticoagulation after infusion	Aspirin, 325 mg daily. There is no evidence that adjunctive heparin improves outcome following streptokinase.	Aspirin, 325 mg daily. Heparin, 5000 units as bolus, followed by 1000 units per hour infusion, subsequently adjusted to maintain PTT 1½–2 times control.	Aspirin, 325 mg; heparin as with t-PA	Aspirin, 325 mg daily
Clot selectivity	Low	High	High	Moderate
Fibrinogenolysis	+++	+	+	+
Bleeding	+	+	+	+
Hypotension	+++	+	+	+
Allergic reactions	++	0	0	+
Reocclusion	5–20%	10–30%	—	5–20%
Approximate cost[1]	$537.50	$2750.00	$2750.00	$2650.08

[1]Cost to pharmacist (average wholesale price, generic when possible) for quantity listed. Source: *Drug Topics Red Book,* March 2000; Vol. 19, No. 3.

and hemorrhagic strokes appear to be more frequent. In patients over age 70 or with elevated blood pressure, the rate of intracranial hemorrhage rises substantially, and t-PA should be avoided in these patients. t-PA produces faster reperfusion, especially when given in the first 4 hours. A regimen consisting of an initial bolus of 15 mg, 50 mg over the next 30 minutes, and 35 mg over the following 60 minutes, achieves higher early patency rates than previous dosing schedules. Reocclusion rates are higher with t-PA because of its shorter half-life, so intravenous heparin is recommended for at least 24 hours. **Reteplase** is a closely related thrombolytic agent made by recombinant technology that has been very effective in restoring patency of the infarct-related artery. Administration of reteplase is convenient—two 10-unit boluses are given 30 minutes apart, with adjunctive aspirin and heparin therapy. A large trial comparing outcomes with t-PA has shown that these agents are comparable.

Streptokinase is more likely to produce allergic reactions, including fever, chills, rashes, and anaphylaxis. This agent should be avoided if the patient has received it previously. Streptokinase also has a tendency to produce severe hypotension and therefore must be administered slowly. Hypotension should be treated by slowing or interrupting the infusion, placing the patient in the Trendelenburg position, and administering fluids. Unlike the experience with t-PA, there is no clear evidence that adjunctive heparin is beneficial in patients given streptokinase.

Anisoylated plasminogen streptokinase activator complex (anistreplase; APSAC) is a conjugate of streptokinase that is inactive until the anisoyl group is hydrolyzed, which occurs gradually after injection (half time, 90 minutes). The drug is concentrated at the site of the thrombus and is activated locally. Thus, it can be injected as a bolus but will provide continuing thrombolytic activity. This makes APSAC a convenient agent to administer out of the hospital or in a busy emergency room. Otherwise, it has many of the same features of streptokinase, including the potential to produce allergic reactions and hypotension, but it is far more expensive.

Selection of a thrombolytic agent: Although there is much debate over which agent to utilize, the overriding consideration is the early administration of any one of them. Three large international studies have compared the results with different thrombolytic therapies. The ISIS-3 trial compared three agents (t-PA, streptokinase, and anistreplase) in over 40,000 patients. No difference in mortality rates was observed between treatments, though cerebral hemorrhage was more common with t-PA. GISSI-2 compared the first two of these agents and also failed to show a difference. The GUSTO trial was the only one to use adjunctive intravenous heparin and also employed the accelerated regimen noted above for t-PA. Compared with streptokinase, t-PA produced a small improvement (one case per 100 patients treated) in 30-day and 6-month survival. Reteplase appears to have a similar modest advantage over streptokinase. Since t-PA and reteplase are significantly more expensive than streptokinase, and since intracranial hemorrhage is more frequent with these agents (especially in patients over age 70 and those with hypertension), and since the additional reduction in mortality is relatively small, many physicians limit the use of t-PA—and, by extension, reteplase—to patients in whom the greatest absolute benefits have been noted. These include patients under 70 years of age with anterior myocardial infarctions treated within 4 hours after onset and patients who show evidence of pump failure. Patients who have had streptokinase or APSAC within the past year or recent streptococcal infections and those with borderline blood pressure (systolic pressure < 100 mm Hg) are also better candidates for t-PA, while older patients, especially those with concomitant hypertension (systolic pressure ≥ 160 mm Hg) may be better candidates for streptokinase. The only apparent advantage of APSAC is convenience.

Postthrombolytic management: After completion of the thrombolytic infusion, aspirin should be continued. Anticoagulation with intravenous heparin is continued for at least 24 hours after t-PA and reteplase but is optional in patients receiving streptokinase. Prophylactic treatment with antacids and an H_2 blocker is indicated.

Reperfusion rates of 50–80% can be expected, determined primarily by the interval between onset of the infarction and treatment. Reperfusion is recognized clinically by the abrupt cessation of pain, the occurrence of ventricular arrhythmias (most characteristically accelerated idioventricular rhythm), the rapid evolution of the ECG to Q waves, and an early peak of CK (by 12 hours); however, all of these signs may be misleading. Even with anticoagulation, 10–20% of reperfused vessels will reocclude during hospitalization. This is usually recognized by the recurrence of pain and ST segment elevation and is treated by readministration of a thrombolytic agent or immediate angiography and PTCA.

The optimal management of myocardial infarction after thrombolysis is controversial but has been clarified considerably by the TIMI 2 trial. Patients with recurrent ischemic pain prior to discharge should undergo catheterization and, if indicated, revascularization. Asymptomatic, clinically stable patients should undergo predischarge evaluation to determine whether residual jeopardized myocardium is present. This can be accomplished by exercise or pharmacologic stress scintigraphy. Those with significantly positive tests or a low threshold for symptomatic ischemia should undergo angiography and revascularization where feasible. Patients with negative tests have an excellent prognosis without intervention, though they may require revascularization for symptoms at a later time.

B. Acute PTCA: A number of centers now manage acute myocardial infarction with primary PTCA (immediate angiography and PTCA of the "infarct-related" vessel), rather than thrombolysis. The results of this approach in specialized centers are excellent, exceeding those obtainable by thrombolytic therapy, but the experience may not be generalizable to centers with less experience or expertise. The use of stents in treating acute myocardial infarction is also under investigation. In the subgroup of patients with cardiogenic shock, early catheterization and PTCA or CABG is the preferred management, because thrombolysis has not improved the dismal prognosis of these individuals.

C. General Measures: CCU monitoring should be instituted as soon as possible. Uncomplicated patients can be transferred to less intensively monitored settings after 24–48 hours. Activity should initially be limited to bed rest, with the availability of a nearby toilet or commode in more stable patients. Progressive ambulation should be started after 24–72 hours if tolerated. Low-flow oxygen therapy (2–4 L/min) is usually given. A liquid diet is recommended during the initial 24 hours.

D. Analgesia: An initial attempt should be made to relieve pain with sublingual nitroglycerin. However, if no response occurs after two or three tablets, intravenous opioids provide the most rapid and effective analgesia. Morphine sulfate, 4–8 mg, or meperidine, 50–75 mg, should be given. Subsequent small doses can be given every 15 minutes until pain abates.

E. Beta-Adrenergic Blocking Agents: Several studies have shown modestly improved short-term survival when intravenous beta-blockers are given immediately after acute myocardial infarction. These agents reduce the duration of ischemic pain and the incidence of ventricular fibrillation. A favorable effect appears to persist even after thrombolytic therapy. However, the survival benefit is small, so beta-blockers should not be given to patients with relative contraindications. Long-term beta-blocker therapy is discussed below.

F. Nitrates: Nitroglycerin is the agent of choice for recurrent ischemic pain and is useful in lowering blood pressure or relieving pulmonary congestion. However, routine nitrate administration is not recommended, since no improvement in outcome has been observed in the ISIS-4 or GISSI-3 trials, in which a total of over 70,000 patients were randomized to nitrate treatment or placebo.

G. Angiotensin-Converting Enzyme (ACE) Inhibitors: A series of trials (SAVE, AIRE, SMILE, TRACE, GISSI-III, and ISIS-IV) have shown both short- and long-term improvement in survival with ACE inhibitor therapy. The benefits are greatest in patients with low ejection fractions, large infarctions, or clinical evidence of heart failure, and only these patients should receive chronic ACE inhibitor therapy for postinfarction indications. Acute short-term treatment may improve survival in a broader group of patients, but this is uncertain. Treatment should be commenced carefully in the first postinfarction day if the patient is not hypotensive. When there is no evidence of heart failure or when a very large infarction is not present, ACE inhibitors should be considered only after the administration of thrombolytic therapy, aspirin, beta-blockers, and, if the patient has evidence of continuing ischemia, nitrates.

H. Antiarrhythmic Prophylaxis: The incidence of ventricular fibrillation in hospitalized patients is approximately 5%, with 80% of episodes occurring in the first 12–24 hours. Prophylactic lidocaine infusions (1–2 mg/min) prevent most episodes, but this therapy has not reduced the mortality rate and it increases the risk of asystole, so this approach is no longer recommended except in patients with very frequent ectopic beats or nonsustained ventricular tachycardia. Intravenous magnesium sulfate has been effective in one study, but ISIS-4 did not report a benefit with routine magnesium administration.

I. Calcium Channel Blockers: There are no studies to support the use of calcium channel blockers in most acute myocardial infarction patients—and indeed, they have the potential to exacerbate ischemia and cause death from reflex tachycardia or myocardial depression. One exception is that diltiazem and verapamil appear to prevent reinfarction and ischemia in the subset of patients with non-Q wave infarction. The former agent is preferable because it causes less myocardial depression. The dosage is 240–360 mg daily. Otherwise, calcium channel blockers should be reserved for management of hypertension or ischemia as second- or third-line drugs after nitrates and beta-blockers.

J. Anticoagulation: With the exception of patients undergoing thrombolysis and subsequent heparin therapy, the use of full anticoagulation in the acute setting remains controversial. Patients who will be at bed rest or on limited activity status for some time should be given 5000 units of heparin subcutaneously every 8–12 hours unless contraindicated. Aspirin, 325 mg daily, should be given also unless contraindicated.

Antoniucci D et al: Current role of stenting in acute myocardial infarction. Am Heart J 1999;138:147. [NLM Cit ID: 99355547] (Five randomized trials demonstrate lower incidence of death, reinfarction, and revascularization compared with angioplasty.)

Boden WE et al: Outcomes in patients with acute non-Q-wave myocardial infarction randomly assigned to an invasive as compared with a conservative management strategy. N Engl J Med 1998;338:1785. [NLM Cit ID: 98283484] (Veterans Affairs study concludes that patients with non-Q myocardial infarction do not benefit from routine early intensive management consisting of coronary angiography and revascularization.)

Cairns JA et al: Coronary thrombolysis. Chest 1998;114: 634S. [NLM Cit ID: 99037862] (Review of recent thrombolytic trials with emphasis on subgroup analysis, adjuvant therapy and newer agents. Treatment recommendations are included.)

Cannon CP: Overcoming thrombolytic resistance: rationale and initial clinical experience combining thrombolytic therapy and glycoprotein IIb/IIIa receptor inhibition for acute myocardial infarction. J Am Coll Cardiol 1999;34:1395. [NLM Cit ID: 20017846] (Twenty-seven hundred patients have been enrolled in trials comparing angioplasty with fibrinolysis and suggest better short-term outcome with PTCA. Long-term clinical benefit is not as certain.)

Collins R et al: Aspirin, heparin, and fibrinolytic therapy in suspected acute myocardial infarction. N Engl J Med 1997;336:847. [NLM Cit ID: 97212613] (Review arguing for wider use of these therapies.)

Dries DL et al: Adjunctive therapy after reperfusion therapy in acute myocardial infarction. Clin Cardiol 1998; 21:379. [NLM Cit ID: 98294726] (Updated review covers beta blockers, nitrates, ACE inhibitors, and magnesium, focusing on the large clinical trials in the thrombolytic era. Nitrates and magnesium do not routinely reduce mortality.)

Nunn CM et al: Long-term outcome after primary angioplasty: report from the primary angioplasty in myocardial infarction (PAMI-I) trial. J Am Coll Cardiol 1999;33:640. [NLM Cit ID: 99178548] (The initial benefit of primary angioplasty is maintained over 2 years with reduced rate of reintervention and improved infarct-free survival.)

Ryan TJ et al: Primary PTCA versus thrombolytic therapy: an evidence-based summary. Am Heart J 1999;138:96. [NLM Cit ID: 99355540] (Combining thrombolytics with glycoprotein IIb/IIIa inhibitors may safely allow for more complete vessel patency in acute myocardial infarction. Large-scale trials are under way.)

White HD et al: Thrombolysis for acute myocardial infarction. Circulation 1998;97:1632. [NLM Cit ID: 98254401] (Review of thrombolysis covers eligibility, contraindications, and subgroup considerations. Newer agents are discussed.)

Zijlstra F et al: Long-term benefit of primary angioplasty as compared with thrombolytic therapy for acute myocardial infarction. N Engl J Med 1999;341:1413. [NLM Cit ID: 20001872] (Primary angioplasty is associated with improved clinical outcomes over 5 years when compared with streptokinase.)

Complications

A variety of complications can occur after myocardial infarction even when treatment is initiated promptly.

A. Infarct Extension and Postinfarction Ischemia: Recurrent infarction in the region of infarction (infarct extension) in the first 10–14 days occurs in approximately 10% of patients. It may be associated with prolonged or intermittent episodes of chest pain. In many cases, the process is relatively silent, being detected on routine ECG, by laboratory testing, or by onset or worsening of heart failure. Infarct extension is at least twice as common in non-Q wave infarcts and is more likely to occur after successful thrombolytic therapy owing to residual jeopardized myocardium. Diltiazem has been shown to reduce the rate of extension following non-Q wave infarction.

Approximately 30% of patients will have angina postinfarction. This is more common in patients with angina prior to infarction and in non-Q wave infarction. Postinfarction angina is associated with increased short- and long-term mortality. The underlying mechanism is usually inadequate blood flow through a recanalized vessel or reocclusion. Vigorous medical therapy should be instituted, including nitrates, beta-blockers, and calcium blockers, as well as aspirin and heparin. Most patients with postinfarction angina—and all who are refractory to medical therapy—should undergo early catheterization and revascularization by PTCA or CABG.

B. Arrhythmias: Abnormalities of rhythm and conduction are common.

1. Sinus bradycardia–This is most common in inferior infarctions or may be precipitated by medications. Observation or withdrawal of the offending agent is usually sufficient. If accompanied by signs of low cardiac output, atropine, 0.5–1 mg intravenously, is usually effective. Temporary pacing is rarely required.

2. Supraventricular tachyarrhythmias–Sinus tachycardia is common and may reflect either increased adrenergic stimulation or hemodynamic compromise due to hypovolemia or pump failure. In the latter, beta blockade is contraindicated. Supraventricular premature beats are common and may be premonitory for atrial fibrillation. Electrolyte abnormalities and hypoxia should be corrected and causative agents (especially aminophylline) stopped. Atrial fibrillation should be rapidly controlled or converted to sinus rhythm. Intravenous beta-blockers such as propranolol (1–2 mg), metoprolol (2.5–5 mg/h), or short-acting esmolol (50–200 μg/kg/min) are the agents of choice if cardiac function is adequate. Intravenous verapamil (2.5–5 mg administered as a slow bolus) or diltiazem (5–15 mg/h) may be used if beta-blockers are contraindicated or ineffective. Digoxin (0.5 mg as initial dose, then 0.25 mg every 90–120 minutes [up to 1–1.25 mg] for a loading dose, followed by 0.25 mg daily if renal function is normal) is preferable if heart failure is present with atrial fibrillation, but the onset of action is delayed. Electrical cardioversion (commencing with 100 J) may be necessary if atrial fibrillation is complicated by hypotension, heart failure, or ischemia, but the arrhythmia often recurs. A short course of a class Ia agent such as procainamide or quinidine may be required in addition to digoxin, a beta-blocker, or a calcium channel blocker to maintain sinus rhythm.

3. Ventricular arrhythmias–Ventricular arrhythmias are most common in the first few hours after infarction. Ventricular premature beats (VPBs) may be premonitory for ventricular tachycardia or fibrillation. Prophylactic lidocaine may be started (1 mg/kg bolus followed by an infusion of 2 mg/min) if more than 6 VPB/min, early (R on T wave) VPBs, couplets or nonsustained ventricular tachycardia are observed. Additional boluses of 0.5 mg/kg followed by an increased infusion rate (up to 4 mg/min) may be necessary, but toxicity (tremor, anxiety, confusion, seizures) is common, especially in older patients and those with hypotension, heart failure, or liver disease. The infusion rate should be reduced after 3–4 hours, since blood levels tend to rise, but generally, once initiated, lidocaine should be continued for at least 24 hours.

Ventricular tachycardia should be treated with a 1 mg/kg bolus of lidocaine if the patient is stable or by electrical cardioversion (100–200 J) if not. If the arrhythmia cannot be suppressed with lidocaine, procainamide should be initiated (100 mg boluses over 1–2 minutes every 5 minutes to a cumulative dose of 750–1000 mg, followed by an infusion of 20–80 μg/kg/min). Hypotension may occur acutely, and depression of myocardial function or conduction may complicate maintenance therapy. Refractory ventricular arrhythmias are most effectively treated with intravenous amiodarone (150 mg over 10 minutes, which may be repeated as needed, followed by 360 mg over 6 hours and then 540 mg over 18 hours). Intravenous amiodarone can be very effective. Bretylium tosylate (5 mg/kg intravenously over 3–5 minutes, repeated after 20 minutes if necessary, followed by an infusion of 1–2 mg/min) is an alternative. Ventricular fibrillation is treated electrically (300–400 J). Unresponsive ventricular fibrillation should be treated with additional amiodarone and repeat cardioversion while CPR is administered. Accelerated idioventricular rhythm is a regular, wide complex rhythm at a rate of 70–100/min. It often follows reperfusion and usually does not require specific therapy.

4. Conduction disturbances–All degrees of atrioventricular block may occur in the course of acute myocardial infarction. Block at the level of the atrioventricular node is more common than infranodal block and occurs in approximately 20% of inferior myocardial infarctions. First-degree block is the most common and requires no treatment. Second-degree block is usually of the Mobitz type I form (Wenckebach), is often transient, and requires treatment only if associated with a heart rate slow enough to cause symptoms. Complete atrioventricular block occurs in up to 5% of acute inferior infarctions, usually is preceded by second-degree block, and generally resolves spontaneously, though it may persist for hours to several weeks. The escape rhythm originates in the distal atrioventricular node or atrioventricular junction and hence has a narrow QRS complex and is reliable, albeit often slow (30–50 beats/min). Treatment is often necessary because of resulting hypotension and low cardiac output. Intravenous atropine (1 mg) usually restores atrioventricular conduction temporarily, but if the escape complex is wide or if repeated atropine treatments are needed, temporary ventricular pacing is indicated. The prognosis for these patients is only slightly worse than that of patients who do not develop atrioventricular block.

In anterior infarctions, the site of block is distal, below the atrioventricular node, and usually a result of extensive damage of the His-Purkinje system and bundle branches. New first-degree block (prolongation of the PR interval) is unusual in anterior infarction; Mobitz type II atrioventricular block or complete heart block may be preceded by intraventricular conduction defects or may occur abruptly. The escape rhythm, if present at all, is an unreliable wide-complex idioventricular rhythm. Urgent ventricular pacing is mandatory, but even with successful pacing, morbidity and mortality are high because of the extensive myocardial damage. New conduction abnormalities such as right or left bundle branch block or fascicular blocks may presage progression, often sudden, to second- or third-degree atrioventricular block. Temporary ventricular pacing is recommended for new-onset alternating bilateral bundle branch block, bifascicular block, or bundle branch block with worsening first-degree atrioventricular block. Patients with anterior infarction who progress to second- or third-degree block even transiently should be considered for insertion of a prophylactic permanent ventricular pacemaker before discharge.

C. Myocardial Dysfunction: The severity of cardiac dysfunction is proportionate to the extent of myocardial necrosis but is exacerbated by preexisting dysfunction and ongoing ischemia. Patients who have normal blood pressure, no signs of heart failure, and normal urine output have a good prognosis. Those with hypotension or evidence of more than mild heart failure should have bedside right heart catheterization and continuous measurements of arterial pressure. These measurements permit the accurate assessment of cardiac function, facilitate the correct choice of therapy, and provide important prognostic information. Table 10–3 categorizes patients based upon these hemodynamic findings.

1. Acute left ventricular failure–Basilar rales are common in acute myocardial infarction, but dyspnea, more diffuse rales, and arterial hypoxemia usually indicate left ventricular failure. Since both the physical examination and chest x-ray correlate poorly with hemodynamic measurements and since the central venous pressure does not correlate with the pulmonary capillary wedge pressure (PCWP), right heart catheterization may be essential in monitoring therapy. General measures include supplemental oxygen to increase arterial saturation to above 95% and elevation of the trunk. Diuretics are usually the initial therapy unless right ventricular infarction is present. Intravenous furosemide (10–40 mg) or bumetanide (0.5–1 mg) is preferred because of the reliably rapid onset and short duration of action of these drugs. Higher dosages can be given if an inadequate response occurs. Morphine sulfate (4 mg intravenously followed by increments of 2 mg) is valuable in acute pulmonary edema.

Diuretics are usually effective; however, since most patients with acute infarction are not volume overloaded, the hemodynamic response may be limited and may be associated with hypotension. Vasodilators will reduce PCWP and improve cardiac output by a combination of venodilation (increasing venous capacitance) and arteriolar dilation (reducing afterload and left ventricular wall stress). In mild heart failure, sublingual isosorbide dinitrate (2.5–10 mg every 2 hours) or nitroglycerin ointment (6.25–25 mg every 4 hours) may be adequate to lower PCWP. In more severe failure, especially if cardiac output is reduced, sodium nitroprusside is the preferred agent. It should be initiated only with hemodynamic monitoring; the initial dosage should be low (0.25 μg/kg/min) to avoid excessive hypotension, but the dosage can be increased by increments of 0.5 μg/kg/min every 5–10 minutes up to 5–10 μg/kg/min until the desired hemodynamic response (PCWP < 18 mm Hg, CI > 2.5) is obtained. Excessive hypotension (mean blood pressure < 65–75 mm Hg) or tachycardia (> 10/min increase) should be avoided. Combination of nitroprusside with inotropic agents may be necessary to preserve blood pressure or maximize benefit.

Intravenous nitroglycerin (starting at 10 μg/min) is usually less effective but may lower PCWP with less hypotension. Oral or transdermal vasodilator therapy with nitrates or angiotensin-converting enzyme inhibitors is often necessary after the initial 24–48 hours (see below).

Inotropic agents should be avoided if possible, because they often increase heart rate and myocardial oxygen requirements. Dobutamine has the best hemodynamic profile, increasing cardiac output and modestly lowering PCWP, usually without excessive tachycardia, hypotension, or arrhythmias. The initial dosage is 2.5 μg/kg/min, and it may be increased by similar increments up to 15–20 μg/kg/min at intervals of 5–10 minutes. Dopamine is more useful in the presence of hypotension (see below), since it produces peripheral vasoconstriction, but it has a less beneficial effect on PCWP. Amrinone is a positive inotrope and vasodilator that produces hemodynamic effects similar to those of dobutamine but with a greater decrease in PCWP. However, its longer duration of action makes it less useful in unstable situations. Milrinone is a more potent and newer congener of amrinone with fewer side effects. It should be commenced in a loading dose of 50 μg/kg over 10 minutes, followed by an infusion of 0.375–0.75 μg/kg/min. Digoxin has not been helpful in acute infarction except to control the ventricular response in atrial fibrillation, but it may be beneficial if chronic heart failure persists.

2. Hypotension and shock–Patients with hypotension (systolic blood pressure < 100 mm Hg, individualized depending on prior blood pressure) and signs of diminished perfusion (low urine output, confusion, cold extremities) should be hemodynamically monitored. Up to 20% will have findings indicative of intravascular hypovolemia (due to diaphoresis, vomiting, decreased venous tone, medications—such as diuretics, nitrates, morphine, beta-blockers, calcium channel blockers, and thrombolytic agents—and lack of oral intake). These should be treated with successive boluses of 100 mL of normal saline until PCWP reaches 15–18 mm Hg to determine whether cardiac output and blood pressure respond. Pericardial tamponade due to hemorrhagic pericarditis (especially after thrombolytic therapy or cardiopulmonary resuscitation) or ventricular rupture should be considered and excluded by echocardiography if clinically indicated. Right ventricular infarction, characterized by a normal PCWP but elevated right atrial pressure, can produce hypotension. This is discussed below.

Most hypotensive patients will have moderate to severe left ventricular dysfunction; pathologic studies indicate that more than 20% of the left ventricle is infarcted (> 40% in cardiogenic shock). If hypotension is only modest (systolic pressure > 90 mm Hg) and the PCWP is elevated, diuretics and an initial trial of nitroprusside (see above for dosing) are indicated. If the blood pressure falls, inotropic support will need to be added or substituted. Such patients may also be treated with IABC. This device unloads the left ventricle during systole and increases diastolic coronary artery filling pressure. It often facilitates the use of vasodilators in patients who previously did not tolerate them.

Dopamine is the most appropriate pressor for cardiogenic hypotension. It should be initiated at a rate of 2 μg/kg/min and increased at 5-minute intervals to the appropriate hemodynamic end point. At low dosages (< 5 μg/kg/min), it improves renal blood flow; at intermediate dosages (2.5–10 μg/kg/min), it stimulates myocardial contractility; at higher dosages (> 8 μg/kg/min), it is a potent α_1-adrenergic agonist. In general, blood pressure and cardiac index rise, but PCWP does not fall. Dopamine may be combined with nitroprusside or dobutamine (see above for dosing), or the latter may be used in its place if hypotension is not severe. Amrinone has hemodynamic effects similar to those of dobutamine, but its longer duration of action precludes rapid dosage adjustment. Norepinephrine (0.1–0.5 μg/kg/min) is the usual pressor of last resort, since isoproterenol and epinephrine produce less vasoconstriction, do not increase coronary perfusion pressure (aortic diastolic pressure), and tend to worsen the balance between myocardial oxygen delivery and utilization.

Patients with cardiogenic shock have a poor prognosis. If they do not respond rapidly, the previously described measure—IABC—should be instituted. Early PTCA may preserve enough viable myocardium to reverse the hypotension and should be attempted whenever feasible. Operation to repair mechanical defects (see below), revascularize ischemic myocardium, and resect aneurysms should be considered. Left ventricular assist devices as a bridge to early transplantation can be used in refractory patients under age 60–65 without other systemic illnesses.

D. Right Ventricular Infarction: Right ventricular infarction is present in one-third of patients with inferior wall infarction but is clinically significant in less than 50% of these. It presents as hypotension with relatively preserved left ventricular function and should be considered whenever patients with inferior infarction exhibit signs of low cardiac output and raised venous pressure. Hypotension is often exacerbated by medications that decrease intravascular volume or produce venodilation, such as diuretics, nitrates, and narcotics. Right atrial pressure and jugular venous pulsations are high, while PCWP is normal or low and the lungs are clear. The diagnosis is suggested by right precordial ST segment elevation using V_1 and leads to the right of the sternum corresponding to the location of V_3 and V_4. The diagnosis can be confirmed by echocardiography or hemodynamic measurements. When hypotension is present, hemodynamic measurements are necessary to monitor therapy. Treatment consists of fluid loading to improve left ventricular filling; inotropic agents may also be useful.

E. Mechanical Defects: Partial or complete rupture of a papillary muscle or of the interventricular septum occurs in less than 1% of acute myocardial infarctions and carries a poor prognosis. These complications occur in both anterior and inferior infarctions, usually 3–7 days after the acute event. They are detected by the appearance of a new systolic murmur and clinical deterioration, often with pulmonary edema. The two lesions are distinguished by the location of the murmur (apical versus parasternal) and by Doppler echocardiography. Hemodynamic monitoring is essential for appropriate management and demonstrates an increase in oxygen saturation between the right atrium and pulmonary artery in ventricular septal defect and, often, a large *v* wave with mitral regurgitation. Treatment by nitroprusside and, preferably, IABC reduces the regurgitation or shunt, but surgical correction is mandatory. In patients remaining hemodynamically unstable or requiring continuous parenteral pharmacologic treatment or counterpulsation, early surgery is recommended, though mortality rates are high (15% to nearly 100%, depending on residual ventricular function and clinical status). Patients who are stabilized medically can have delayed surgery with lower risks (10–25%).

F. Myocardial Rupture: Complete rupture of the left ventricular free wall occurs in less than 1% of patients and usually results in immediate death. It occurs 2–7 days postinfarction, usually involves the anterior wall, and is more frequent in older women. Incomplete or gradual rupture may be sealed off by the pericardium, creating a **pseudoaneurysm.** This may be recognized by echocardiography, radionuclide angiography, or left ventricular angiography, often as an incidental finding. It demonstrates a narrow-neck connection to the left ventricle. Early surgical repair is indicated, since delayed rupture is common.

G. Left Ventricular Aneurysm: Ten to 20 percent of patients surviving an acute infarction develop a left ventricular aneurysm, a sharply delineated area of scar that bulges paradoxically during systole. This usually follows anterior Q wave infarctions. Aneurysms are recognized by persistent ST segment elevation (beyond 4–8 weeks), and a wide neck from the left ventricle can be demonstrated by echocardiography, scintigraphy, or contrast angiography. They rarely rupture but may be associated with arterial emboli, ventricular arrhythmias, and congestive heart failure. Surgical resection may be performed for these indications if other measures fail. The best results (mortality rates of 10–20%) are obtained when the residual myocardium contracts well and when significant coronary lesions supplying adjacent regions are bypassed.

H. Pericarditis: The pericardium is involved in approximately 50% of infarctions, but pericarditis is often not clinically significant. Twenty percent of patients with Q wave infarctions will have an audible friction rub if examined repetitively. Pericardial pain occurs in approximately the same proportion after 2–7 days and is recognized by its variation with respiration and position (improved by sitting). Often, no treatment is required, but aspirin (650 mg every 4–6 hours) or indomethacin (25 mg three or four times daily) will usually relieve the pain. Anticoagulation should be avoided, since hemorrhagic pericarditis may result.

From 1 to 12 weeks after infarction, Dressler's syndrome (post-myocardial infarction syndrome) occurs in less than 5% of patients. This is an autoimmune phenomenon and presents as pericarditis with associated fever, leukocytosis, and, occasionally, pericardial or pleural effusion. It may recur over months. Treatment is the same as for other forms of pericarditis. A short course of corticosteroids may help if nonsteroidal agents do not relieve symptoms.

I. Mural Thrombus: Mural thrombi are common in large anterior infarctions but not in infarctions at other locations. Arterial emboli occur in approximately 2% of patients with known infarction, usually within 6 weeks. Anticoagulation with heparin followed by short-term (3-month) warfarin therapy prevents most emboli and should be considered in all patients with large anterior infarctions. Mural thrombi can be detected by echocardiography or CT scan (MRI has yielded frequent false-positive results) but with only moderate reliability, and only a small percentage (up to 25%) embolize, so these procedures should not be relied upon for determining the need for anticoagulation.

Anderson RD et al: Use of intraaortic balloon counterpulsation in patients presenting with cardiogenic shock: observations from the GUSTO-I Study. J Am Coll Cardiol 1997;30:708. [NLM Cit ID: 97429180] (Early intra-aortic balloon counterpulsation in patients with cardiogenic shock is associated with increased bleeding but a trend toward mortality benefit at 30 days and 1 year.)

Aronson D et al: Mechanisms determining the course and outcome of diabetic patients who have had acute myocardial infarction. Ann Intern Med 1997;126:296. [NLM Cit ID: 97172881] (The mechanism of increased mortality in diabetes and management of this increased risk are discussed.)

Becker RC et al: A composite view of cardiac rupture in the United States National Registry of Myocardial Infarction. J Am Coll Cardiol 1996;27:1321. [NLM Cit ID: 96228176] (Although the incidence of cardiac rupture was less than 1%, it accounted for 3% of hospital deaths and was less common in patients receiving thrombolytic therapy.)

Bowers TR et al: Effect of reperfusion on biventricular function and survival after right ventricular infarction. N Engl J Med 1998;338:933. [NLM Cit ID: 98172955] (Dramatic improvements in hemodynamics and outcomes with right coronary PTCA.)

Hochman JS et al: Early revascularization in acute myocardial infarction complicated by cardiogenic shock. SHOCK Investigators. Should We Emergently Revascularize Occluded Coronaries for Cardiogenic Shock. N Engl J Med 1999;341:625. [NLM Cit ID: 99383642] (In this trial, 152 patients with myocardial infarction and cardiogenic shock were randomized to early revascularization or initial medical stabilization prior to revascularization. There was a trend toward improved survival in the early revascularization group at 30 days, which was significant at 6 months in patients under 75 years of age. In patients 75 or older, there was a strong trend toward poorer outcomes with revascularization.)

Hollenberg SM et al: Cardiogenic shock. Ann Intern Med 1999;131:47. [NLM Cit ID: 99308808] (Practical review emphasizing need for early intervention and revascularization in appropriate patients.)

Postinfarction Management

Twenty percent of patients with acute myocardial infarction die before they reach the hospital. Mortality rates in hospitalized patients range from 5% to 15% and are determined chiefly by the size of the infarction and the age and general condition of the patient. Patients developing heart failure or hypotension have high early mortality rates. Several classification criteria have been developed to estimate early prognosis for survival. The most accurate is hemodynamic subsetting (Table 10–3). The prognosis after discharge is determined by three major factors: the degree of left ventricular dysfunction, the extent of residual ischemic myocardium, and the presence of ventricular arrhythmias. The mortality rate in the first year after discharge is approximately 6–8%, with over half of deaths occurring in the first 3 months, chiefly in patients with postinfarction heart failure. Subsequently, the mortality rate averages 4% per year.

A. Risk Stratification: A number of findings indicate increased risk after infarction. These include: (1) postinfarction angina; (2) non-Q wave infarction; (3) heart failure; (4) left ventricular ejection fraction less than 40%; (5) exercise-induced ischemia, diagnosed by electrocardiography or scintigraphy; and (6) ventricular ectopy (> 10 VPB/h). It is less certain whether this information should be collected and how it should be acted upon.

Patients with postinfarction angina should undergo coronary arteriography. Authorities differ about which tests should be performed routinely in other patients, but in most a noninvasive assessment of left ventricular function and residual ischemia is appropriate. Significant left ventricular dysfunction is most likely with anterior infarction or multiple infarctions. In such patients, noninvasive assessment of left ventricular function by echocardiography or scintigraphy will help assess prognosis and facilitate medical management. If the ejection fraction is less than 40%, coronary angiography may be indicated, as this is a high-risk subset in which revascularization may improve prognosis. ACE inhibitor therapy is also indicated. Submaximal exercise testing before discharge or a maximal test after 3–6 weeks (the latter being more sensitive for ischemia) helps patients and physicians plan the return to normal activity. Imaging in conjunction with stress testing adds additional sensitivity for ischemia and provides localizing information. Both exercise and pharmacologic stress imaging have successfully predicted subsequent outcome. One of these tests should usually be employed prior to discharge in patients who have received thrombolytic therapy as a means of selecting appropriate candidates for coronary angiography.

Ambulatory electrocardiographic monitoring for arrhythmias is of less clear value; though it has some prognostic value beyond measurements of left ventricular function, no benefit from antiarrhythmic therapy for asymptomatic patients has been demonstrated. Ischemia detected during ambulatory monitoring is an indicator of poor prognosis, but it is unclear how much additional information is obtained in patients who have also undergone exercise testing or scintigraphic studies. The role of other procedures such as assessment of heart rate variability or baroreceptor testing is uncertain.

A conservative approach to postinfarction evaluation would include measurement of left ventricular function in patients with signs of heart failure or large infarctions and a test for ischemia in patients without recurrent chest pain. The latter should occur before discharge if the patient has undergone thrombolytic therapy but may be delayed for 3–6 weeks in most other patients.

B. Prophylactic Therapy: Postinfarction management should begin with identification and modification of risk factors. Treatment of hyperlipidemia and smoking cessation both prevent recurrent infarction, and data now exist which confirm that aggressive lipid lowering improves survival in patients with clinical coronary artery disease. Recent guidelines suggest a target LDL cholesterol level below 100 mg/dL for patients with manifest coronary artery disease. Blood pressure control, weight loss, and exercise are recommended, though definite benefit on postinfarction prognosis has not been demonstrated.

Beta-blockers improve survival rates, primarily by reducing the incidence of sudden death in high-risk subsets of patients. Beta-blockers should be given to such individuals, except those with overt heart failure, but are of limited value in uncomplicated patients with small infarctions and normal exercise tests. No advantage of one preparation over another has been demonstrated except that those with intrinsic sympathomimetic activity have not proved beneficial in postinfarction patients.

Antiplatelet agents are beneficial; low-dose aspirin (325 mg daily) is recommended. Warfarin anticoagulation for 3 months reduces the incidence of arterial emboli after large anterior infarctions, and according to the results of at least one study it improves long-term prognosis, but after 6 months any benefit additive to aspirin has not been confirmed.

Calcium channel blockers have not been shown to improve prognoses overall and should not be prescribed purely for secondary prevention. However, these agents may be useful for managing hypertension or subsequent angina pectoris. Based on published studies, verapamil and diltiazem may be preferable to nifedipine (the only dihydropyridine studied) in the postinfarction patient.

Antiarrhythmic therapy other than with beta-blockers has not been shown to be effective except in patients with symptomatic arrhythmias and, in fact, class Ic agents increase the mortality rate in postinfarction patients. Although several small studies with amiodarone suggested some benefits, this has not been confirmed in two large trials conducted in postinfarct patients with either left ventricular dysfunction or frequent ventricular ectopy. However, amiodarone was not harmful, and it is therefore probably the agent of choice for individuals with symptomatic postinfarction arrhythmias, although emerging data suggest that implantable defibrillators may be a more effective option.

Cardiac rehabilitation programs and exercise training can be of considerable psychologic benefit, but it is not known whether they alter prognosis.

C. ACE Inhibitors in Patients With Left Ventricular Dysfunction: Patients who sustain substantial myocardial damage often experience subsequent progressive left ventricular dilation and dysfunction, leading to clinical heart failure and reduced long-term survival. In patients with ejection fractions less than 40%, captopril (25–50 mg three times daily commencing 3–16 days postinfarction) prevents left ventricular dilation and the onset of heart failure and also reduces the mortality rate. Similar data have been collected with several other ACE inhibitors. Although two large trials found a benefit from treating unselected patients beginning on admission, it is unclear if this accrues to patients without left ventricular dysfunction and whether there is any advantage to starting treatment while the patient may be hemodynamically unstable.

D. Revascularization: Because of the increasing use of thrombolytic therapy and accumulating experience with PTCA, the indications for revascularization are rapidly evolving. Postinfarction patients who appear likely to benefit from early revascularization if the anatomy is appropriate are (1) those who have undergone thrombolytic therapy and have residual symptoms or laboratory evidence of ischemia; (2) patients with left ventricular dysfunction (ejection fraction < 30–40%) and evidence of ischemia; (3) patients with non-Q wave infarction and evidence of more than mild ischemia; and (4) patients with markedly positive exercise tests and multivessel disease. The value of revascularization in the following groups is less clear: (1) patients treated with thrombolytic agents, with little evidence of reperfusion or residual ischemia; (2) patients with left ventricular dysfunction but no detectable ischemia; and (3) patients with preserved left ventricular function who have mild ischemia and are not symptom-limited. Patients who survive infarctions without complications, have preserved left ventricular function (ejection fraction > 50%), and have no exercise-induced ischemia have an excellent prognosis and do not require invasive evaluation.

Deedwania PC et al: Evidence-based, cost-effective risk stratification in management after myocardial infarction. Arch Intern Med 1997;157:273. [NLM Cit ID: 97192701] (Consensus panel review of relevant trials, providing recommendations for testing and treatment of infarct survivors.)

Gottlieb SS et al: Effect of beta-blockade on mortality among high-risk and low-risk patients after myocardial infarction. N Engl J Med 1998;339:489. [NLM Cit ID: 98363660] (Reinforces concept that patients with only relative contraindications to beta-blockers or those with non-Q wave myocardial infarction benefit from beta-blockers after infarction.)

JAMA patient page: Heart attack. JAMA 1998;280:1462. [NLM Cit ID: 99015629]

Michaels AD et al: Risk stratification after acute myocardial infarction in the reperfusion era. Prog Cardiovasc Dis 2000;42:273. [NLM Cit ID: 20125422]

Ryan TJ et al: 1999 update: ACC/AHA guidelines for the management of patients with acute myocardial infarction. A report of the American College of Cardiology/American Heart Association Task Force on Practice Guidelines (Committee on Management of Acute Myocardial Infarction). J Am Coll Cardiol 1999;34:890. [NLM Cit ID: 99411777]

Soumerai SB et al: Adverse outcomes of underuse of beta-blockers in elderly survivors of acute myocardial infarction. JAMA 1997;277:115. [NLM Cit ID: 97144568] (Review of Medicare data base, showing that only 21% of eligible patients were receiving beta-blocker therapy but that these had a 43% lower mortality rate and 22% lower rehospitalization rate. In contrast, an increasing number of elderly patients were receiving calcium channel blockers. These findings suggest a substantial frequency of inappropriate practices.)

DISTURBANCES OF RATE & RHYTHM

Abnormalities of cardiac rhythm and conduction can be lethal (sudden cardiac death), symptomatic (syncope, near syncope, dizziness, or palpitations), or asymptomatic. They are dangerous to the extent that they reduce cardiac output, so that perfusion of the brain or myocardium is impaired, or tend to deteriorate into more serious arrhythmias with the same consequences. Stable supraventricular tachycardia is generally well tolerated in patients without underlying heart disease but may lead to myocardial ischemia or congestive heart failure in patients with coronary disease, valvular abnormalities, and systolic or diastolic myocardial dysfunction. Ventricular tachycardia, if prolonged (lasting more than 10–30 seconds), often results in hemodynamic compromise and is more likely to deteriorate into ventricular fibrillation.

Whether slow heart rates produce symptoms at rest or on exertion depends upon whether cerebral perfusion can be maintained, which is generally a function of whether the patient is upright or supine and whether left ventricular function is adequate to maintain stroke volume. If the heart rate abruptly slows, as with the onset of complete heart block or sinus arrest, syncope or convulsions may result.

Arrhythmias are detected either because they present with symptoms or because they are detected during the course of monitoring. Arrhythmias causing sudden death, syncope, or near syncope require further evaluation and treatment unless they are related to conditions that are unlikely to recur (eg, electrolyte abnormalities or acute myocardial infarction). In contrast, there is controversy over when and how to evaluate and treat rhythm disturbances that are not symptomatic but are possible markers for more serious abnormalities (eg, nonsustained ventricular tachycardia). This uncertainty reflects two issues: (1) the difficulty of reliably stratifying patients into high-risk and low-risk groups; and (2) the lack of treatments which are both effective and safe. Thus, screening patients for these so-called "premonitory" abnormalities is often not productive.

A number of procedures are employed to evaluate patients with symptoms who are felt to be at risk for life-threatening arrhythmias, including in-hospital and ambulatory electrocardiographic monitoring, event recorders (instruments that can be worn for prolonged periods in order to record or transmit rhythm tracings when infrequent episodes occur), exercise testing, intracardiac electrophysiologic studies (to assess sinus node function, atrioventricular conduction, and inducibility of arrhythmias), signal-averaged ECGs, and tests of autonomic nervous system function (especially tilt-table testing). These are discussed below and in the subsequent sections on individual rhythm disturbance and symptomatic presentation. In general, these techniques are more successful in diagnosing symptomatic arrhythmias than in predicting the outcome of asymptomatic ones.

MECHANISMS OF ARRHYTHMIAS

Electrophysiologic studies have greatly increased our understanding of the mechanisms underlying most arrhythmias. These include (1) disorders of impulse formation or automaticity, (2) abnormalities of impulse conduction, (3) reentry, and (4) triggered activity.

Altered automaticity is the mechanism for sinus node arrest, many premature beats, and automatic rhythms as well as an initiating factor in reentry arrhythmias.

Abnormalities of impulse conduction can occur at the sinus or atrioventricular node, in the intraventricular conduction system, and within the atria or ventricles. These are responsible for sinoatrial exit block, for atrioventricular block at the node or below, and for establishing reentry circuits.

Reentry is the underlying mechanism for many arrhythmias, including premature beats, most paroxysmal supraventricular tachycardias, and atrial flutter. For reentry to occur, there must be an area of unidirectional block with an appropriate delay to allow repeat depolarization at the site of origin. Reentry is confirmed if the arrhythmia can be terminated by interruption of the circuit by a spontaneous or induced premature beat.

Triggered activity occurs when afterdepolarizations (abnormal electrical activity persisting after repolarization) reach the threshold level required to trigger a new depolarization. This may be the mechanism of ventricular tachycardia in the prolonged QT syndrome and in some cases of digitalis toxicity.

Priori SG et al: Genetic and molecular basis of cardiac arrhythmias: impact on clinical management. Parts I and II. Circulation 1999;99:518. [NLM Cit ID: 99126298]

(Consensus statement on the genetics of inherited arrhythmias and practical advice on the role of genetic testing in these syndromes.)

TECHNIQUES FOR EVALUATING RHYTHM DISTURBANCES

Electrocardiographic Monitoring

The ideal way of establishing a causal relationship between a symptom and a rhythm disturbance is to demonstrate the presence of the rhythm during the symptom. Unfortunately, this is not always easy because symptoms are usually sporadic.

Patients with aborted sudden death and recent or recurrent syncope are often monitored in the hospital. Those with less ominous symptoms may be monitored as outpatients. When episodes are infrequent, use of an event recorder is preferable to 24-hour continuous monitoring. Exercise testing may be helpful when the symptoms are associated with exertion or stress. If symptomatic bradyarrhythmias or supraventricular tachyarrhythmias are detected, therapy can usually be initiated without additional diagnostic studies. Further electrophysiologic studies may be useful in evaluating ventricular tachyarrhythmias.

Extreme caution is required before attributing a patient's symptom to rhythm or conduction abnormalities observed during monitoring without concomitant symptoms. In many cases, the symptoms are due to a different arrhythmia or to noncardiac causes. For instance, dizziness or syncope in older patients may be unrelated to concomitantly observed bradycardia, sinus node abnormalities, and ventricular ectopy. Ambulatory monitoring is frequently used to quantify ventricular ectopy and detect asymptomatic ventricular tachycardia in post-myocardial infarction or heart failure patients. Unfortunately, while asymptomatic ventricular arrhythmias have negative prognostic implications, there are few data to support specific therapeutic intervention. Thus, monitoring in asymptomatic individuals is usually not indicated.

Crawford MH at al: ACC/AHA Guidelines for Ambulatory Electrocardiography. A report of the American College of Cardiology/American Heart Association Task Force on Practice Guidelines (Committee to Revise the Guidelines for Ambulatory Electrocardiography). Developed in collaboration with the North American Society for Pacing and Electrophysiology. J Am Coll Cardiol 1999;34:912. [NLM Cit ID: 99411778] (Consensus statement on methodology and applications.)

Heart Rate Variability

Although it has long been appreciated that there are periodical fluctuations in heart rate even under basal conditions, considerable recent interest has been focused on measurements of **heart rate variability.** These measurements can be made under controlled conditions in the electrocardiography laboratory or from recordings obtained during ambulatory monitoring. Greater fluctuations in heart rate correspond to greater parasympathetic activity, and several studies have indicated that greater heart rate variability is associated with a better prognosis and fewer life-threatening arrhythmias in a variety of cardiac conditions. More recently, analyses have employed frequency transformation of RR cycle length variability to provide indices of the relative balance between parasympathetic and sympathetic activity, with the greater contribution of the parasympathetic system being considered to confer a better prognosis. In studies of postinfarction patients and patients with symptomatic arrhythmias, these indices have had some prognostic value. However, adequate data are not yet available to support routine use of this technique in clinical practice.

Heart rate variability: Standards of measurement, physiologic interpretation, and clinical use. Circulation 1996;93:1043. [NLM Cit ID: 96179036] (Comprehensive consensus document.)

Huikuri HV et al: Measurement of heart rate variability: a clinical tool or a research toy? J Am Coll Cardiol 1999;34:1878. [NLM Cit ID: 20053418] (Although there are significant associations between reduced heart rate variability and mortality, there is lack of consensus on what are the most useful measurements and how to utilize them in clinical practice.)

Signal-Averaged ECG

Another new technique is the **signal-averaged ECG.** Most commonly, an orthogonal three-lead system is employed to record 300 consecutive beats during basal conditions. Using appropriate electrical filtering and computer averaging of the signal, very low frequency signals called "late potentials" can be identified in the period following the QRS complex. Abnormal late potentials are considered markers for potential ventricular arrhythmias. Adequate data are not yet available to define the role of this technique with confidence, but it may be useful in detecting groups of patients at increased risk for arrhythmic events after myocardial infarction. Approximately one-third of these patients will have abnormal late potentials, and these individuals are at higher risk for arrhythmic events, though the positive predictive value of this finding is relatively low (10–15%). More importantly, the absence of late potentials identifies a group of patients at low risk for arrhythmic events, so post-myocardial infarction patients found to have frequent ventricular ectopy or nonsustained ventricular tachycardia in the absence of late potentials may not require further investigation or treatment. The prognostic value of late potentials in patients with chronic ischemic heart disease who are more than 6–12 months removed from myocardial infarction and in patients with other forms of heart disease is not yet known.

Kozer LM et al: Clinical significance of variability of ventricular late potentials detected before discharge in patients after myocardial infarction. Am Heart J 2000;139:134. [NLM Cit ID: 20086508] (In a series of 261 patients after myocardial infarction in whom two signal-averaged ECGs were obtained 10–12 hours apart, the investigators demonstrated that if both SAECGs were positive, this improved the positive predictive value for ventricular tachycardia and sudden cardiac death over the next year.)

Electrophysiologic Testing

Electrophysiologic testing employing intracardiac electrocardiographic recordings and programmed atrial or ventricular (or both) stimulation is useful in the diagnosis and management of complex arrhythmias. The primary indications for electrophysiologic testing are (1) evaluation of recurrent syncope of possible cardiac origin, when the ambulatory ECG has not provided the diagnosis; (2) differentiation of supraventricular from ventricular arrhythmias; (3) evaluation of therapy in patients with accessory atrioventricular pathways; (4) evaluation of the efficacy of pharmacotherapy in survivors of aborted sudden death or other patients with symptomatic or life-threatening ventricular tachycardia; and (5) evaluation of patients for catheter ablation procedures or antitachycardia devices.

Zipes DP et al: Guidelines for clinical intracardiac electrophysiological and catheter ablation procedures. A report of the American College of Cardiology/American Heart Association Task Force on Practice Guidelines (Committee on Clinical Intracardiac Electrophysiologic and Catheter Ablation Procedures), developed in collaboration with the North American Society of Pacing and Electrophysiology. J Am Coll Cardiol 1995;26:555. [NLM Cit ID: 95332634]

Autonomic Testing (Tilt Table Testing)

In many patients with recurrent syncope or near syncope, arrhythmias are not the cause. This is particularly true when the patient has no evidence of associated heart disease by history, examination, standard ECG, or noninvasive testing. Syncope may be neurocardiogenic in origin, mediated by excessive vagal stimulation or an imbalance between sympathetic and parasympathetic autonomic activity. With assumption of upright posture, there is venous pooling in the lower limbs. However, instead of the normal response, which consists of an increase in heart rate and vasoconstriction, a sympathetically mediated increase in myocardial contractility activates mechanoreceptors that trigger reflex bradycardia and vasodilation. Autonomic testing is an important component of the evaluation in these individuals and should usually precede invasive electrophysiologic procedures. Carotid sinus massage in patients who do not have carotid bruits or a history of cerebral vascular disease can precipitate sinus node arrest or atrioventricular block in patients with carotid sinus hypersensitivity. Head-up tilt-table testing can identify patients whose syncope may be on a vasovagal basis. Although different testing protocols are employed, passive tilting to at least 70 degrees for 10–40 minutes—in conjunction with isoproterenol infusion, if necessary—is typical. Syncope due to bradycardia, hypotension, or both will occur in approximately one-third of patients with recurrent syncope. Some recent studies have suggested that, at least with some of the more extreme protocols, false-positive responses may occur.

Antiarrhythmic Drugs (Table 10–5)

Antiarrhythmic drugs have limited efficacy and produce frequent side effects. They are often divided into four classes based upon their electropharmacologic actions.

Class I agents block membrane sodium channels. Three subclasses are further defined by the effect of agents on the Purkinje fiber action potential. Class Ia drugs slow the rate of rise of the action potential (V_{max}) and prolong its duration, thus slowing conduction and increasing refractoriness. Class Ib agents shorten action potential duration; they do not affect conduction or refractoriness. Class Ic agents prolong V_{max} and slow repolarization, thus slowing conduction and prolonging refractoriness, but more so than class Ia drugs.

Class II agents are the beta-blockers, which decrease automaticity, prolong atrioventricular conduction, and prolong refractoriness.

Class III agents block potassium channels and prolong repolarization, widening the QRS and prolonging the QT interval. They decrease automaticity and conduction and prolong refractoriness.

Class IV agents are the slow calcium channel blockers, which decrease automaticity and atrioventricular conduction.

Although the in vitro electrophysiologic effects of most of these agents have been defined, their use remains largely empirical. All can exacerbate arrhythmias (proarrhythmic effect), and most depress left ventricular function.

The risk of antiarrhythmic agents has been highlighted by the Coronary Arrhythmia Suppression Trial (CAST), in which two class Ic agents (flecainide, encainide) and a class Ia agent (moricizine) increased mortality rates in patients with asymptomatic ventricular ectopy after myocardial infarction. A similar result has been reported with D-sotalol, a class III agent without the beta-blocking activity of D,L-sotalol, the currently marketed formulation. Therefore, these agents (and perhaps any antiarrhythmic drug) should not be used except for life-threatening ventricular arrhythmias and symptomatic supraventricular tachyarrhythmias.

The use of antiarrhythmic agents for specific arrhythmias is discussed below.

Table 10–5. Antiarrhythmic drugs.

Agent	Intravenous Dosage	Oral Dosage	Therapeutic Plasma Level	Route of Elimination	Side Effects
Class Ia: Action: Sodium channel blockers: Depress phase 0 depolarization; slow conduction; prolong repolarization. **Indications:** Supraventricular tachycardia, ventricular tachycardia, prevention of ventricular fibrillation, symptomatic ventricular premature beats.					
Quinidine	6–10 mg/kg (IM or IV) over 20 min (rarely used parenterally)	200–400 mg every 4–6 h or every 8 h (long-acting)	2–5 mg/mL	Hepatic	GI, ↓LVF, ↑Dig
Procainamide	100 mg/1–3 min to 500–1000 mg; maintain at 2–6 mg/min	50 mg/kg/d in divided doses every 3–4 h or every 6 h (long-acting)	4–10 mg/mL; NAPA (active metabolite), 10–20 μg/mL	Renal	SLE, hypersensitivity, ↓LVF
Disopyramide		100–200 mg every 6–8 h	2–8 mg/mL	Renal	Urinary retention, dry mouth, markedly ↓LVF
Moricizine		200–300 mg every 8 h	***Note:*** Active metabolites	Hepatic	Dizziness, nausea, headache, ↓theophylline level, ↓LVF
Class Ib: Action: Shorten repolarization. **Indications:** Ventricular tachycardia, prevention of ventricular fibrillation, symptomatic ventricular beats.					
Lidocaine	1–2 mg/kg at 50 mg/min; maintain at 1–4 mg/min		1–5 mg/mL	Hepatic	CNS, GI
Mexiletine		100–300 mg every 6–12 h. Maximum: 1200 mg/d	0.5–2 mg/mL	Hepatic	CNS, GI, leukopenia
Phenytoin	50 mg/5 min to 1000 mg (12 mg/kg); maintain at 200–400 mg/d	200–400 mg every 12–24 h	5–20 mg/mL	Hepatic	CNS, GI
Class Ic: Action: Depress phase 0 repolarization; slow conduction. *Propafenone* is a weak calcium channel- and beta-blocker and prolongs action potential and refractoriness. **Indications:** Life-threatening ventricular tachycardia or fibrillation; refractory supraventricular tachycardia.					
Flecainide		100–200 mg twice daily	0.2–1 mg/mL	Hepatic	CNS, GI, ↓↓LVF, incessant VT, sudden death
Propafenone		150–300 mg every 8–12 h	***Note:*** Active metabolites	Hepatic	CNS, GI, ↓↓LVF, ↑Dig
Class II: Action: Beta-blocker, slows AV conduction. ***Note:*** Other beta-blockers may also have antiarrhythmic effects but are not yet approved for this indication in the USA. **Indications:** Supraventricular tachycardia; may prevent ventricular fibrillation.					
Esmolol	500 mg/kg over 1–2 min; maintain at 25–200 mg/kg/min	Other beta-blockers may be used	0.15–2 mg/mL	Hepatic	↓LVF, bronchospasm
Propranolol	1–5 mg at 1 mg/min	40–320 mg in 1–4 doses (depending on preparation)	Not established	Hepatic	↓LVF, bradycardia, AV block, bronchospasm
Metoprolol	2.5–5 mg	50–200 mg daily	Not established	Hepatic	↓LVF, bradycardia, positive ANA, lupus-like syndrome

(continued)

Table 10–5. Antiarrhythmic drugs. (continued)

Agent	Intravenous Dosage	Oral Dosage	Therapeutic Plasma Level	Route of Elimination	Side Effects
Class III: Action: Prolong action potential. **Indications:** *Amiodarone:* refractory ventricular tachycardia, supraventricular tachycardia, prevention of ventricular tachycardia, ventricular fibrillation; *dofetilide:* atrial fibrillation and flutter; *sotalol:* ventricular tachycardia; atrial fibrillation; *bretylium:* ventricular fibrillation, ventricular tachycardia; *ibutilide:* conversion of atrial fibrillation and flutter.					
Amiodarone	150 mg infused rapidly, followed by 1 mg/min infusion for 6 hours (360 mg) and then 0.5 mg/min. Additional 150 mg as needed	800–1600 mg/d for 7–21 days; maintain at 100–400 mg/d (higher doses may be needed)	1–5 mg/mL	Hepatic	Pulmonary fibrosis, hypothyroidism, hyperthyroidism, corneal and skin deposits, hepatitis, ↑Dig, neurotoxicity, GI
Sotalol		80–160 mg every 12 h (higher doses may be used for life-threatening arrhythmias)		Renal (dosing interval should be extended if creatinine clearance is < 60 mL/min)	Early incidence of torsade de pointes, ↓LVF, bradycardia, fatigue (and other side effects associated with beta-blockers)
Dofetilide		500 mg twice daily		Renal (dose must be reduced with renal dysfunction)	Torsade de pointes in 3%; interaction with cytochrome P450 inhibitors
Ibutilide	1 mg over 10 minutes, followed by a second infusion of 0.5–1 mg			Hepatic and renal	Torsade de pointes in up to 5% of patients within 3 hours after administration. Patients must be monitored with defibrillator nearby.
Bretylium	5–10 mg/kg over 5–10 min; maintain at 0.5–2 mg/min. Maximum: 30 mg/kg		0.5–1.5 mg/mL	Renal	Hypotension, nausea
Class IV: Action: Slow calcium channel blockers. **Indications:** Supraventricular tachycardia.					
Verapamil	10–20 mg over 2–20 min; maintain at 5 mg/kg/min	80–120 mg every 6–8 h; 240–360 mg once daily with sustained-release preparation	0.1–0.15 mg/mL	Hepatic	↓LVF, constipation, ↑Dig
Diltiazem	0.25 mg/kg over 2 min; second 0.35 mg/kg bolus after 15 min if response is inadequate; infusion rate, 5–15 mg/h	180–360 mg daily in 1–3 doses depending on preparation (oral forms not approved for arrhythmias)		Hepatic metabolism, renal excretion	Hypotension, ↓LVF

(*continued*)

Table 10–5. Antiarrhythmic drugs. (continued)

Agent	Intravenous Dosage	Oral Dosage	Therapeutic Plasma Level	Route of Elimination	Side Effects
Class V: Indications: Supraventricular tachycardia.					
Adenosine	6 mg rapidly followed by 12 mg after 1–2 min if needed			Adenosine receptor stimulation, metabolized in blood	Transient flushing, dyspnea, chest pain, AV block, sinus bradycardia; effect ↓ by theophylline, ↑ by dipyridamole
Digoxin	0.5 mg over 20 min followed by increment of 0.25 or 0.125 mg to 1–1.5 mg over 24 hours	1–1.5 mg over 24–36 hours in 3 or 4 doses; maintenance, 0.125–0.5 mg/d	0.7–2 mg/mL	Renal	AV block, arrhythmias, GI, visual changes

Key: AV = atrioventricular; CNS = central nervous system; ↑Dig = elevation of serum digoxin level; GI = gastrointestinal (nausea, vomiting, diarrhea); ↓LVF = reduced left ventricular function; SLE = systemic lupus erythematosus; VT = ventricular tachycardia

Connolly SJ: Evidence-based analysis of amiodarone efficacy and safety. Circulation 1999;100:2025. [NLM Cit ID: 20028344] (Review of pharmacology and utility of amiodarone in ventricular arrhythmias demonstrates efficacy in 13 trials. The drug is effective also in atrial fibrillation, but noncardiac toxicity may be limiting.)

Kowey PR: Pharmacological effects of antiarrhythmic drugs. Arch Intern Med 1998;158:325. [NLM Cit ID: 98148209]

McAlister FA et al: Antiarrhythmic therapies for the prevention of sudden cardiac death. Drugs 1997;54:235. [NLM Cit ID: 97401274] (Review of clinical trials covering class I agents, beta-blockers, and amiodarone.)

Nattel S et al: Evolution, mechanisms, and classification of antiarrhythmic drugs: focus on class III actions. Am J Cardiol 1999;84:11R. [NLM Cit ID: 20033303] (Focus on classification with respect to ion channel or receptor blockade.)

Roden DM: Mechanisms and management of proarrhythmia. Am J Cardiol 1998;82:49I. [NLM Cit ID: 98407672] (Reviews the recognition and management of the most common proarrhythmias.)

Radiofrequency Ablation for Cardiac Arrhythmias

Catheter ablation techniques have become the primary modality for treatment of many arrhythmias. This growing trend reflects the increasing ability to localize the origin or conduction pathways of many arrhythmias, the improved technology for delivering radiofrequency energy, and growing dissatisfaction with the efficacy and safety of pharmacologic therapy. Ablation has become the primary modality of therapy for many symptomatic supraventricular arrhythmias, including atrioventricular nodal reentry tachycardia, reentry tachycardias involving accessory pathways, paroxysmal atrial tachycardia, inappropriate sinus tachycardia, and automatic junctional tachycardia. Many laboratories have achieved reasonable success rates in preventing atrial flutter with radiofrequency techniques, and experience with atrial fibrillation is accumulating as well.

Catheter ablation of ventricular arrhythmias has proved more difficult. Three specific forms of ventricular tachycardia, however, have proved to be amenable to radiofrequency ablation. These include bundle-branch reentry, tachycardia originating in the right ventricular outflow tract, and some tachycardias originating in the left side of the interventricular septum. Other forms of ventricular tachycardia, particularly in patients with coronary artery disease, may be amenable to ablation, but experience thus far is limited.

These procedures are generally safe, though there is a low incidence of perforation of the atria or right ventricle that results in pericardial tamponade and sufficient damage to the atrioventricular node to require permanent cardiac pacing in up to 20% of patients. In addition, some procedures involve transseptal or retrograde left ventricular catheterization, with the attendant potential complications of aortic perforation, damage to the heart valves, or left-sided emboli.

Morady F: Radio-frequency ablation as treatment for cardiac arrhythmias. N Engl J Med 1999;340:534. [NLM Cit ID: 99134024] (Well-illustrated review discussing management of arrhythmias amenable to ablation.)

SUPRAVENTRICULAR ARRHYTHMIAS

1. SINUS ARRHYTHMIA, BRADYCARDIA, & TACHYCARDIA

Sinus arrhythmia is a cyclic increase in normal heart rate with inspiration and decrease with expiration. It results from reflex changes in vagal influence on the normal pacemaker and disappears with breath holding or increase of heart rate due to any cause. It has no clinical significance. It is common in both the young and the elderly.

Sinus bradycardia is a heart rate slower than 50/min due to increased vagal influence on the normal pacemaker or organic disease of the sinus node. The rate usually increases during exercise or administration of atropine. In healthy individuals, and especially in patients who are in excellent physical condition, sinus bradycardia to a rate of 50 or even lower is a normal finding. However, severe sinus bradycardia may be an indication of sinus node pathology (see below), especially in elderly patients and individuals with heart disease. It may cause weakness, confusion, or syncope if cerebral perfusion is impaired. Atrial and ventricular ectopic rhythms are more apt to occur with slow sinus rates. Pacing may be required if symptoms correlate with the bradycardia.

Sinus tachycardia is defined as a heart rate faster than 100 beats/min that is caused by rapid impulse formation from the normal pacemaker; it occurs with fever, exercise, emotion, pain, anemia, heart failure, shock, thyrotoxicosis, or in response to many drugs. Alcohol and alcohol withdrawal are common causes of sinus tachycardia and other supraventricular arrhythmias. The onset and termination are usually gradual, in contrast to paroxysmal supraventricular tachycardia due to reentry. The rate infrequently exceeds 160/min but may reach 180/min in young persons. The rhythm is basically regular, but serial 1-minute counts of the heart rate indicate that it varies five or more beats per minute with changes in position, with breath holding or with sedation. Rare individuals have persistent or episodic "inappropriate" sinus tachycardia that may be very symptomatic or may lead to left ventricular contractile dysfunction. Radiofrequency modification of the sinus node has mitigated this problem.

Mangrum JM et al. The evaluation and management of bradycardia. N Engl J Med 2000;342:703. [NLM Cit ID: 20155740] (Evaluation and management of sinus node dysfunction and AV node conduction block with a comprehensive differential diagnosis and electrocardiographic examples.)

2. ATRIAL PREMATURE BEATS (Atrial Extrasystoles)

Atrial premature beats occur when an ectopic focus in the atria fires before the next sinus node impulse or a reentry circuit is established. The contour of the P wave usually differs from the patient's normal complex. The subsequent R–R cycle length is usually unchanged or only slightly prolonged. Such premature beats occur frequently in normal hearts and are never a sufficient basis for a diagnosis of heart disease. Speeding of the heart rate by any means usually abolishes most premature beats. Early atrial premature beats may cause aberrant QRS complexes (wide and bizarre) or may be nonconducted to the ventricles because the latter are still refractory.

3. DIFFERENTIATION OF ABERRANTLY CONDUCTED SUPRAVENTRICULAR BEATS FROM VENTRICULAR BEATS

This distinction can be very difficult in patients with a wide QRS complex; it is important because of the differing prognostic and therapeutic implications of each type. Findings favoring a ventricular origin include (1) atrioventricular dissociation; (2) a QRS duration exceeding 0.14 s; (3) capture or fusion beats (infrequent); (4) left axis deviation with right bundle branch block morphology; (5) monophasic (R) or biphasic (qR, QR, or RS) complexes in V_1; and (6) a qR or QS complex in V_6. Supraventricular origin is favored by (1) a triphasic QRS complex, especially if there was initial negativity in leads I and V_6; (2) ventricular rates exceeding 170/min; (3) QRS duration longer than 0.12 s but not longer than 0.14 s; and (4) the presence of preexcitation syndrome.

The relationship of the P waves to the tachycardia complex is helpful. A 1:1 relationship usually means a supraventricular origin, except in the case of ventricular tachycardia with retrograde P waves. If the P waves are not clearly seen, Lewis leads (in which the right arm electrode is placed in the V_1 position two interspaces higher than usual and the left arm electrode is placed in the usual V_1 position) may be employed. This accentuates the size of the P waves. Esophageal leads, in which the electrode is placed directly posterior to the left atrium, achieve the same effect even more clearly. Right atrial electrograms may also help to clarify the diagnosis by accentuating the P waves.

4. PAROXYSMAL SUPRAVENTRICULAR TACHYCARDIA

This is the commonest paroxysmal tachycardia and often occurs in patients without structural heart disease. Attacks begin and end abruptly and may last a few seconds to several hours or longer. The heart rate may be 140–240/min (usually 160–220/min) and is perfectly regular (despite exercise or change in position). The P wave usually differs in contour from sinus beats. Patients may be asymptomatic except for awareness of rapid heart action, but some experience mild chest pain or shortness of breath, especially when episodes are prolonged, even in the absence of associated cardiac abnormalities. Paroxysmal supraventricular tachycardia may result from digitalis toxicity and then is commonly associated with atrioventricular block.

The most common mechanism for paroxysmal supraventricular tachycardia is reentry, which may be initiated or terminated by a fortuitously timed atrial or ventricular premature beat. The reentry circuit most commonly involves dual pathways (a slow and a fast pathway) within the atrioventricular node. This is referred to as AV nodal reentry tachycardia (AVNRT). Less commonly, reentry is due to an accessory pathway between the atria and ventricles (AVRT). Approximately one-third of patients have aberrant pathways to the ventricles. The pathophysiology and management of arrhythmias due to accessory pathways differs in important ways and is discussed separately below.

Treatment of the Acute Attack

In the absence of heart disease, serious effects are rare, and most attacks break spontaneously. Particular effort should be made to terminate the attack quickly if cardiac failure, syncope, or anginal pain develops or if there is underlying cardiac or (particularly) coronary disease. Because reentry is the most common mechanism for paroxysmal atrial tachycardia, effective therapy requires that conduction be interrupted at some point in the reentry circuit.

A. Mechanical Measures: A variety of methods have been used to interrupt attacks, and patients may learn to perform these themselves. These include Valsalva's maneuver, stretching the arms and body, lowering the head between the knees, coughing, and breath holding. Carotid sinus massage is often performed by physicians but should be avoided if the patient has carotid bruits or a history of transient cerebral ischemic attacks. Firm but gentle pressure and massage are applied first over the right carotid sinus for 10–20 seconds and, if unsuccessful, then over the left carotid sinus. *Pressure should not be exerted on both sides at the same time!* Continuous electrocardiographic or auscultatory monitoring of the heart rate is essential so that pressure can be relieved as soon as the rhythm is broken or if excessive bradycardia occurs. Carotid sinus pressure will interrupt up to half of the attacks, especially if the patient has received a digitalis glycoside or other agent (such as adenosine or a calcium channel blocker) that delays atrioventricular conduction. These maneuvers stimulate the vagus, delay atrioventricular conduction, and block the reentry mechanism, terminating the arrhythmias.

B. Drug Therapy: If mechanical measures fail, two rapidly acting intravenous agents will terminate more than 90% of episodes. Intravenous adenosine has a very brief duration of action and minimal negative inotropic activity. A 6-mg bolus is administered. If no response is observed after 1–2 minutes, a second and third 12-mg bolus should be given. Since the half-life of adenosine is less than 10 seconds, the drug must be given rapidly (in 1–2 seconds from a peripheral intravenous line). Adenosine is very well tolerated, but nearly 20% of patients will experience transient flushing, and some patients experience severe chest discomfort.

Calcium channel blockers also rapidly induce atrioventricular block and break most episodes of reentry supraventricular tachycardia. Intravenous verapamil may be given as a 2.5 mg-bolus, followed by additional doses of 2.5 mg to 5 mg every 1–3 minutes up to a total of 20 mg if blood pressure and rhythm are stable. If the rhythm recurs, further doses can be given. Oral verapamil, 80–120 mg every 4–6 hours, can be used as well in stable patients who are tolerating the rhythm without difficulty. Intravenous diltiazem (0.25 mg/kg over 2 minutes, followed by a second bolus of 0.35 mg/kg if necessary and then an infusion of 5–15 mg/h) may cause less hypotension and myocardial depression.

Esmolol, a short-acting beta-blocker, may also be effective; the initial dose is 500 μg/kg intravenously over 1 minute followed by an infusion of 25–200 μg/min. Parasympathetic stimulating drugs such as edrophonium, 5–10 mg intravenously, which delay atrioventricular conduction, may break the reentry mechanism. Because it frequently causes nausea and vomiting, it should be used only if the previously discussed agents fail. Metaraminol or phenylephrine, alpha-adrenergic stimulants that activate the baroreceptors by raising the blood pressure and causing vagal stimulation, can break attacks but should be used cautiously because they may provoke excessive hypertension. Digoxin is effective, but it often requires several hours to safely administer an adequate dose. An initial dose of 0.5–0.75 mg intravenously, followed by 0.25-mg or 0.125-mg increments every 2–4 hours up to a total of 1–1.25 mg, is used. Intravenous procainamide may terminate supraventricular tachycardia; however, since it facilitates atrioventricular conduction and an initial increase in rate may occur, it is usually not given until after digoxin, verapamil, or a beta-blocker has been administered. In patients with Wolff-Parkinson-White syndrome, in which an accessory pathway is involved, these agents may be contraindicated (see below).

C. Cardioversion: If the patient is hemodynamically stable or if adenosine and verapamil are contraindicated or ineffective, synchronized electrical cardioversion (beginning at 100 J) is almost universally successful. If digitalis toxicity is present or strongly suspected, as in the case of paroxysmal tachycardia with block, electrical cardioversion should be avoided.

Prevention of Attacks

A. Radiofrequency Ablation: Because of concerns about the safety and the intolerability of antiarrhythmic medications, radiofrequency ablation is the preferred approach to patients with recurrent symptomatic reentry supraventricular tachycardia, whether it is due to dual pathways within the atrial ventricular node or to accessory pathways.

B. Drugs: Digoxin orally is the usual drug of first choice because of its convenience and efficacy. Verapamil, alone or in combination with digitalis, is a second choice. (***Note:*** Verapamil increases digoxin serum levels.) Beta-blockers are also effective. Patients who do not respond to agents that increase refractoriness of the atrioventricular node may be treated with class Ia (disopyramide, quinidine, procainamide), class Ic (propafenone), or class III (sotalol, amiodarone) drugs. In patients with evidence of structural heart disease, either sotalol or amiodarone is probably a better choice because of the lower incidence of ventricular proarrhythmia during chronic therapy.

Bathina MN et al: Radiofrequency catheter ablation versus medical therapy for initial treatment of supraventricular tachycardia and its impact on quality of life and healthcare costs. Am J Cardiol 1998;82:589. [NLM Cit ID: 98401721] (As compared with medical therapy, ablation resulted in modest improvements in long-term quality of life, with a higher rate of complete amelioration of symptoms and similar long-term costs.)

Karas BJ et al: Reentrant tachycardias. Postgrad Med 1998;1:84. [NLM Cit ID: 98110126] (Mechanism, diagnosis, and treatment, with emphasis on radiofrequency ablation. This symposium also discusses ablation of atrial flutter, implantable defibrillators, and tilt table testing.)

Scheinman MM (editor): Advances in supraventricular tachycardia. Cardiol Clin 1997;15:517. (Mechanisms, diagnosis, and treatment for all forms of supraventricular tachycardia.)

5. SUPRAVENTRICULAR TACHYCARDIAS DUE TO ACCESSORY ATRIOVENTRICULAR PATHWAYS (Preexcitation Syndromes)

Pathophysiology & Clinical Findings

Accessory pathways between the atria and the ventricle which avoid the conduction delay of the atrioventricular node predispose to reentry tachycardias, such as AVRT and atrial flutter, and to atrial fibrillation. These may be wholly or partly within the node (Mahaim fibers), yielding a short PR interval and normal QRS morphology **(Lown-Ganong-Levine syndrome).** More commonly, they make direct connections between the atria and ventricle through Kent bundles **(Wolff-Parkinson-White syndrome).** This produces a short PR interval but an early delta wave at the onset of the wide, slurred QRS complex owing to early ventricular depolarization of the region adjacent to the pathway. While the morphology and polarity of the delta wave can suggest the location of the bypass tract, mapping by intracardiac recordings is required for precise anatomic localization.

Accessory pathways occur in 0.1–0.3% of the population and facilitate reentry arrhythmias owing to the disparity in refractory periods of the atrioventricular node and accessory pathway. Whether the tachycardia is associated with a narrow or wide QRS complex is determined by whether antegrade conduction is through the node (narrow) or the bypass tract (wide). Many patients with Wolff-Parkinson-White syndrome never conduct in an antegrade direction through the bypass tract which is therefore "concealed." Although reentry supraventricular tachycardias involving the atrioventricular node are commonest, 20–30% of patients with tachyarrhythmias have atrial fibrillation or flutter. Many have no arrhythmia. A minority of patients conduct antegrade through the accessory pathway, but these individuals may develop very fast rates, especially during atrial fibrillation. Patients with RR intervals less than 220 ms are at highest risk. Digoxin and, to a lesser extent, verapamil and beta-blockers may decrease accessory pathway refractoriness and increase ventricular response and should be avoided in atrial fibrillation with accessory pathways.

Treatment

Some patients have a delta wave found incidentally on electrocardiography. In the absence of palpitations, lightheadedness, or syncope, these patients do not require specific therapy. They should be advised to report the onset of any of these symptoms.

A. Radiofrequency Ablation: As with AVNRT, radiofrequency ablation has become the procedure of choice in patients with accessory pathways and recurrent symptoms. Patients with preexcitation syndromes who have episodes of atrial fibrillation or flutter should be tested by induction of atrial fibrillation in the electrophysiologic laboratory, noting duration of the RR cycle; if it is less than 220 ms, a short refractory period is present, and these individuals are at highest risk for sudden death, and prophylactic ablation is indicated. Success rates for ablation of accessory pathways with radiofrequency catheters exceed 90% in appropriate patients.

B. Pharmacologic Therapy: Narrow complex reentry rhythms can be managed as discussed for AVNRT other than atrial fibrillation or flutter. Adenosine has proved to be very effective; digoxin is best avoided in patients with known Wolff-Parkinson-White syndrome. The class Ia antiarrhythmics, as well as the newer class Ic and class III agents, will increase the refractoriness of the bypass tract and are the drugs of choice for wide-complex tachycardias. If hemodynamic compromise is present, electrical cardioversion is warranted.

Long-term therapy often involves a combination of agents that increase refractoriness in the bypass tract (class Ia or Ic agents) and in the atrioventricular node (verapamil, digoxin, and beta-blockers), provided that atrial fibrillation or flutter with short RR cycle lengths is not present (see above). Sotalol and amiodarone are effective in refractory cases. Patients who are difficult to manage should undergo electrophysiologic evaluation.

Al-Khatib SM et al: Clinical features of Wolff-Parkinson-White syndrome. Am Heart J 1999;138:403. [NLM Cit ID: 99397889] (History, pathology, epidemiology, genetics, and various dysrhythmias are reviewed. Asymptomatic patients may be treated conservatively unless there is family history of sudden death or they are in a high-risk profession.)

Gallagher JJ: Wolff-Parkinson-White syndrome: Surgery to radiofrequency catheter ablation. PACE 1997;20:512. [NLM Cit ID: 97211898] (Two-part review covering curative procedures.)

Goudevenos JA et al: Ventricular pre-excitation in the general population: a study on the mode of presentation and clinical course. Heart 2000;83:29. [NLM Cit ID: 20087421]

6. ATRIAL FIBRILLATION

Atrial fibrillation is the commonest chronic arrhythmia. It occurs in rheumatic heart disease, dilated cardiomyopathy, atrial septal defect, hypertension, mitral valve prolapse, and hypertrophic cardiomyopathy as well as in patients with no apparent cardiac disease; it may be the initial presenting sign in thyrotoxicosis. Atrial fibrillation often appears paroxysmally before becoming the established rhythm. Pericarditis, chest trauma or surgery, or pulmonary disease (as well as medications such as theophylline and beta-adrenergic agonists) may cause attacks in patients with normal hearts. Acute alcohol excess and alcohol withdrawal—and, in predisposed individuals, even consumption of small amounts of alcohol—may precipitate atrial fibrillation. This syndrome, which is often termed "holiday heart," is usually transient and self-limited. Short-term rate control with digoxin usually suffices as treatment.

Atrial fibrillation is the only common arrhythmia in which the ventricular rate is rapid and the rhythm very irregular. The atrial rate is 400–600/min, but most impulses are blocked at the atrioventricular node. The ventricular response is completely irregular, ranging from 80 to 180/min in the untreated state. Because of the varying stroke volumes resulting from varying periods of diastolic filling, not all ventricular beats produce a palpable peripheral pulse. The difference between the apical rate and the pulse rate is the "pulse deficit"; this deficit is greater when the ventricular rate is high.

Acute Management

Depending upon the ventricular rate and the status of left ventricular function, the initial presentation of atrial fibrillation may precipitate cardiac decompensation or may be an incidental asymptomatic finding. The short-term complications in atrial fibrillation are primarily hemodynamic. In patients with valvular heart disease or left ventricular diastolic or systolic dysfunction, rapid atrial fibrillation may lead to acute heart failure or pulmonary edema. Rapid ventricular rates may themselves cause progressive deterioration of left ventricular function, which is often reversible when the rate is controlled. These patients present with palpitations and a general feeling of discomfort.

The first consideration is to determine whether the patient is clinically stable, to ascertain whether there is a precipitating cause, and to estimate the duration of the arrhythmia. Atrial fibrillation may be present in patients with valvular heart disease (especially mitral stenosis or insufficiency), thyrotoxicosis, pulmonary embolism or decompensated pulmonary disease, and a variety of cardiac diseases. It may also be precipitated by alcohol, illicit drug use (stimulants, marijuana, cocaine), or medications (theophylline, adrenergic agonists, potent vasodilators). Atrial fibrillation without chest pain is an infrequent presentation of acute myocardial infarction, though it is not an uncommon finding in patients with coronary artery disease. In addition, patients without coronary disease may experience chest discomfort related to the rapid rate.

If the patient is hemodynamically unstable or experiencing myocardial ischemia, early electrical cardioversion is indicated. If these are not present, the choice is between a strategy of rate control with possible later cardioversion to sinus rhythm or early cardioversion. If there is a precipitating cause, cardioversion should generally be delayed until this is no longer present, since recurrence of atrial fibrillation is common if the underlying condition persists. Since the risk of systemic embolization from atrial thrombi increases when the duration of atrial fibrillation is greater than 24–48 hours, elective cardioversion should be delayed in such a patients until the patient has been adequately anticoagulated for 3–4 weeks or atrial thrombus has been excluded by transesophageal echocardiography. In this case, early rate control is the initial approach. Acute rate control can be obtained with intravenous beta-blockers (metoprolol administered as a series of 5 mg boluses, or esmolol if there is a concern for hemodynamic decompensation), intravenous verapamil or diltiazem, intravenous digoxin, or a combination of these approaches. The doses for these agents are given in the section on Paroxysmal Supraventricular Tachycardia.

Cardioversion should be the initial approach in unstable patients or when satisfactory rate control cannot be achieved. In addition, early cardioversion may be preferred in stable patients if the duration of atrial fibrillation is known to be less than 48 hours. There is some evidence that restoration to sinus rhythm becomes more difficult with time, and a strategy of early cardioversion may therefore be utilized if transesophageal echocardiogrpahy excludes atrial thrombus. Otherwise, elective cardioversion should be delayed until the patient has been anticoagulated for 3–4 weeks. Electrical cardioversion under conscious sedation is the approach most commonly employed, especially if it immediately follows a transesophageal echocardiogram. An initial shock with 100–200 joules is administered in synchrony with the R wave. If sinus rhythm is not restored, an additional attempt with 360 J is indicated. If this fails, cardioversion may be successful after loading with ibutilide (see below) or intravenous procainamide (500–1000 mg administered at rate of 100 mg per 5 minutes with careful monitoring of blood pressure).

Elective cardioversion can also be accomplished with pharmacologic agents. These include the oral administration of propafenone (300–600 mg), sotalol (160–320 mg), or flecainide (300–400 mg); the intravenous administration of procainamide (dose given above); or intravenous administration of the short-acting class III agent ibutilide. One milligram of the latter agent is infused over 10 minutes, followed by an additional 0.5–1 mg if sinus rhythm has not been restored in 10 minutes. The success rate of conversion to sinus rhythm is 40–50%. Ibutilide is associated with a 3–8% incidence of torsade de pointes, so it should not be given to patients who have prolonged QTc intervals (> 500 ms) or who have received other class I or III antiarrhythmics (with the exception of amiodarone). Patients should be monitored for at least 3 hours. Electrical cardioversion may be successful if pharmacotherapy fails.

Since atrial function returns only gradually following cardioversion, there continues to be an increased incidence of thromboembolic events. Therefore, beginning with heparin and converting to warfarin, anticoagulation is required for 4–6 weeks following cardioversion. Only about 25% of patients who are converted from atrial fibrillation will remain in sinus rhythm after 1 year, and this number can be increased to 40–60% with chronic antiarrhythmic therapy. However, the risks of chronic antiarrhythmic therapy may more than outweigh this small advantage.

Sotalol and dofetilide are class III anti-arrhythmic drugs that have been approved for the treatment of atrial fibrillation. Because they each carry a small risk of proarrhythmia, it is recommended that a patient be monitored on telemetry for initiation of therapy. In patients in whom there is a precipitating factor for the episode of atrial fibrillation or in whom there is no apparent cardiac disease, it may be worthwhile to withhold antiarrhythmic therapy or to utilize a beta-blocker or digoxin. Although these latter agents have not been proved to maintain sinus rhythm, they would at least limit the ventricular response of atrial fibrillation if it recurs.

If atrial fibrillation does return, a choice must be made between trying to maintain sinus rhythm or allowing the patient to remain in atrial fibrillation with rate control and chronic anticoagulation. Although there are no data to indicate improved outcomes with sinus rhythm (trials are ongoing to evaluate this question), some patients do not tolerate atrial fibrillation well because of palpitations, exercise intolerance, and fluctuating blood pressures. If recurrences are infrequent, they may be manageable by avoiding precipitating factors (alcohol, smoking, certain foods and activities) and by taking medications immediately following the onset of an episode. In such patients, propafenone 300–600 mg or flecainide 200–400 mg is often successful in restoring sinus rhythm in a short period of time.

In patients with more frequent or refractory episodes who do not have structural heart disease and are at low risk for the proarrhythmic effects of drug therapy, class I agents such as propafenone or flecainide or class III agents, including amiodarone, sotalol, or dofetilide, may be used chronically and initiated as outpatient therapy (see Table 10–5 for dosages). However, patients with structural heart disease have a higher risk of proarrhythmia with class I drugs. Amiodarone is often preferred because it has a very low risk of proarrhythmia, but many patients will not tolerate its noncardiac side effects and toxicity. Sotalol and dofetilide are alternatives, but because they may cause torsade de pointes early after initiation, they are usually started in hospital with telemetry monitoring in patients with underlying heart disease.

Treatment of Chronic Atrial Fibrillation

The problems posed by chronic atrial fibrillation are primarily two: symptoms related to the arrhythmias and the increased risk of thromboembolic phenomena. With adequate rate control, most patients are not particularly symptomatic, though exercise tolerance may be limited to some degree in active individuals. Rate control is usually obtained with a beta-blocker, a calcium channel blocker, or digoxin. Digoxin reduces the ventricular response at rest but is less effective in controlling the ventricular rate with exercise or activity. Thus, in active individuals, a beta-blocker or calcium blocker is probably the initial agent of choice; many patients with normally functioning atrioventricular nodes will require two agents for optimal rate control. In occasional individuals, when rate control cannot be achieved, one may add amiodarone, which at low doses effectively further reduces the ventricular response; or may perform radiofrequency modification of the atrioventricular node. This latter procedure is sometimes complicated by complete heart block and the requirement for a pacemaker, but in any case ventricular rate control can be achieved.

Atrial fibrillation is a major risk factor for stroke as a result of a severalfold increase in thromboembolic phenomena. The risk of stroke and other thrombotic events ranges from as low as 2–3% to as high as 20% per year. The factors that increase the risk of stroke include mitral valve disease, increasing age, reduced left ventricular function and heart failure, hypertension, and diabetes. Patients with "lone" atrial fibrillation (atrial fibrillation in the absence of cardiac disease, hypertension, or diabetes) below the age of 60 are at low risk for embolization and do not require anticoagulation, though many physicians would utilize aspirin 325 mg/d in such individuals. Antithrombotic therapy has been shown to reduce the risk of stroke in virtually all other subgroups of patients with chronic atrial fibrillation. In trials where warfarin and aspirin have been compared, warfarin has been consistently more effective in reducing thromboembolic events. However, the risk of bleeding, including hemorrhagic strokes, is higher with warfarin. Based on the experience of several large trials, it is recommended that patients at higher risk for strokes (patients with hypertension, heart failure, and left ventricular dysfunction, prior emboli, and diabetes) should be treated with warfarin. While even in the absence of these risk factors men above the age of 70 have an increased risk for stroke, the bleeding rate with warfarin makes aspirin a suitable alternative. As yet, the evidence is inadequate to show whether aspirin and warfarin are equivalent in women over age 75 without other risk factors for stroke.

Surgical and catheter-based treatments for atrial fibrillation have been developed. The Maze procedure is a surgical technique that involves numerous incisions in the interior surfaces of the atria to prevent propagation of fibrillatory waveforms. This may also be achieved with complex transvenous catheter ablation procedures, but success is variable. In some patients where atrial fibrillation is initiated by ectopic beats originating in the pulmonary veins, the specific focus can be ablated.

Blitzer M et al: Rhythm management in atrial fibrillation—with a primary emphasis on pharmacological therapy. PACE 1998;21:590. [NLM Cit ID: 98219387] (Three-part series extensively reviews strategies to control heart rate and to restore and maintain sinus rhythm.)

Calkins H et al: A new system for catheter ablation of atrial fibrillation. Am J Cardiol 1999;83:227D. [NLM Cit ID: 99189740] (A review of the surgical MAZE procedure and early results of a transvenous approach show high recurrence rate when only the right atrium is treated.)

Haissaguerre M et al: Spontaneous initiation of atrial fibrillation by ectopic beats originating in the pulmonary veins. N Engl J Med 1998;339:659. [NLM Cit ID: 98383828] (In a case series of 45 patients with refractory atrial fibrillation, the investigators found 69 foci of ectopic atrial firing. Sixty-five [94%] of these foci were in the pulmonary veins, and approximately half of those were in the left upper pulmonary vein. Ablation of these foci resulted in no recurrence over a mean follow-up of 8 months in 62% of these patients.)

Hart RG et al: Atrial fibrillation and thromboembolism: a decade of progress in stroke prevention. Ann Intern Med 1999;131:688. [NLM Cit ID: 99456452]

Klein AL et al: Cardioversion guided by transesophageal echocardiography: The Acute Pilot Study. Ann Intern Med 1997;126:200. [NLM Cit ID: 97158929] (Cardioversion can be accomplished more rapidly and without prior anticoagulation in patients without evidence of atrial thrombi on transesophageal echocardiography; anticoagulation for at least 1 month postconversion is essential.)

Laupacis A et al: Antithrombotic therapy in atrial fibrillation. Chest 1998;114:579S. [NLM Cit ID: 99037858]

McClellan KJ et al: Dofetilide: a review of its use in atrial fibrillation and flutter. Drugs 1999;58:1043. [NLM Cit ID: 20114812] (A new class III agent that has been effective in restoring and maintaining sinus rhythm. However, there is an early incidence of torsade de pointes, and care must be taken to avoid interactions with drugs that inhibit the cytochrome P450 system and to adjust the dose in patients with renal dysfunction.)

Murray KT: Ibutilide. Circulation 1998;97:493. [NLM Cit ID: 98140687] (The pharmacology and efficacy of this new class III drug is reviewed. It is most effective in recent-onset atrial flutter and may have a role after heart surgery.)

Roy D et al: Amiodarone to prevent recurrence of atrial fibrillation. Canadian Trial of Atrial Fibrillation Investigators. N Engl J Med 2000;30:913. [NLM Cit ID: 20183101]

Ryder KM et al: Epidemiology and significance of atrial fibrillation. Am J Cardiol 1999;84:131R. [NLM Cit ID: 20033320] (Atrial fibrillation affects over 2 million Americans with a median age of 75 years and increases the risk of stroke fivefold.)

Torp-Pedersen C et al: Dofetilide in patients with congestive heart failure and left ventricular dysfunction. Danish Investigations of Arrhythmia and Mortality on Dofetilide Study Group. N Engl J Med 1999;341:857. [NLM Cit ID: 99404883] (In patients with severe congestive heart failure and low left ventricular ejection fraction, the novel class III antiarrhythmic agent dofetilide reduced the risk of hospitalization for congestive heart failure. It also converted to sinus rhythm 11% of the patients in atrial fibrillation and reduced the risk of recurrence of atrial fibrillation. There was no difference in mortality between the groups, but 3.3% of the dofetilide group [versus none in the placebo group] developed polymorphous ventricular tachycardia.)

Tung F et al: Treatment strategies for atrial fibrillation. Am J Med 1998;104:272. [NLM Cit ID: 98211818]

7. ATRIAL FLUTTER

Atrial flutter is less common than fibrillation. It occurs most often in patients with COPD but may be seen also in those with rheumatic or coronary heart disease, congestive heart failure, atrial septal defect, or surgically repaired congenital heart disease. Ectopic impulse formation occurs at atrial rates of 250–350/min, with transmission of every second, third, or fourth impulse through the atrioventricular node to the ventricles. Ventricular rate control is accomplished using the same agents utilized in atrial fibrillation, but it is much more difficult with atrial flutter than with atrial fibrillation. Conversion of atrial flutter to sinus rhythm with class I antiarrhythmic agents is also difficult to achieve, and administration of these drugs has been associated with slowing of the atrial flutter rate to the point where 1:1 atrioventricular conduction can occur at rates in excess of 200/min, with subsequent hemodynamic collapse. The intravenous class III antiarrhythmic agent ibutilide has been significantly more successful in converting atrial flutter. About 50–70% of patients return to sinus rhythm within 60–90 minutes following the infusion of 1–2 mg of this agent. Electrical cardioversion is also very effective for atrial flutter, with approximately 90% of patients converting following shocks of as little as 25–50 J.

The persistence of atrial contractile function in this arrhythmia provides some protection against thrombus formation, though the risk of systemic embolization remains slightly increased. Precardioversion anticoagulation is usually not necessary for atrial flutter of short duration except in the setting of mitral valve disease. However, anticoagulation is prudent in chronic atrial flutter, particularly since transient periods of atrial fibrillation are common in these patients.

Chronic atrial flutter is often a difficult management problem, since rate control is difficult. Amiodarone is probably the pharmacologic agent of choice, since it has the potential of both maintaining sinus rhythm and helping with rate control when flutter recurs.

Atrial flutter can follow a typical or atypical reentry circuit around the atrium. The anatomy of this circuit has been well defined and allows for radiofrequency ablation within the atrium to interrupt the circuit and eliminate atrial flutter. This technique should be considered in patients refractory to drug therapy.

Chen PS et al: Mechanisms of atrial fibrillation and flutter and implications for management. Am J Cardiol 1999;84:125R. [NLM Cit ID: 20033319] (Discussion of the various theories of electrical activation of the atria in fibrillation and how this affects drug or ablation therapy.)

Shah DC et al: Atrial flutter: contemporary electrophysiology and catheter ablation. Pacing Clin Electrophysiol 1999;22:344. [NLM Cit ID: 99187515]

8. MULTIFOCAL (CHAOTIC) ATRIAL TACHYCARDIA

This is a rhythm characterized by varying P-wave morphology (by definition, three or more foci) and markedly irregular PP intervals. The rate is usually between 100 and 140/min, and atrioventricular block is unusual. Most patients have severe associated COPD. Treatment of the underlying condition is the most effective approach; verapamil, 240–480 mg daily in divided doses, is also of value in some patients.

McCord J et al: Multifocal atrial tachycardia. Chest 1998;113:203. [NLM Cit ID: 98101541] (Focus on patients with pulmonary disease; role for antiarrhythmic treatment unclear.)

9. ATRIOVENTRICULAR JUNCTIONAL RHYTHM

The atrial-nodal junction or the nodal-His bundle junctions may assume pacemaker activity for the heart, usually at a rate of 40–60/min. This may occur in patients with myocarditis, coronary artery disease, and digitalis toxicity as well as in individuals with normal hearts. The rate responds normally to exercise, and the diagnosis is often an incidental finding on electrocardiographic monitoring, but it can be suspected if the jugular venous pulse shows cannon *a* waves. Junctional rhythm is often an escape rhythm because of depressed sinus node function with sinoatrial block or delayed conduction in the atrioventricular node. **Nonparoxysmal junctional tachycardia** results from increased automaticity of the junctional tissues in digitalis toxicity or ischemia and is associated with a narrow QRS complex and a rate usually less than 120–130/min. It is usually considered benign when it occurs in acute myocardial infarction, but the ischemia that induces it may also cause ventricular tachycardia and ventricular fibrillation.

VENTRICULAR ARRHYTHMIAS

1. VENTRICULAR PREMATURE BEATS (Ventricular Extrasystoles)

Ventricular premature beats are characterized by wide QRS complexes that differ in morphology from the patient's normal beats. They are usually not preceded by a P wave, although retrograde ventriculoatrial conduction may occur. Unless the latter is present, there is a fully compensatory pause. Bigeminy and trigeminy are arrhythmias in which every second or third beat is premature; these patterns confirm a reentry mechanism for the ectopic beat. Exercise generally abolishes premature beats in normal hearts, and the rhythm becomes regular. The patient may or may not sense the irregular beat, usually as a skipped beat. Ambulatory electrocardiographic monitoring or monitoring during graded exercise may reveal more frequent and complex ventricular premature beats than occur in a single routine ECG.

tion system disease. Late potentials (after the QRS complex) on a signal-averaged surface ECG in patients with prior myocardial infarction may identify a group of patients at risk of ventricular arrhythmias and sudden death.

Unless ventricular fibrillation occurred shortly after myocardial infarction, is associated with ischemia, or is seen with an unusual correctable process (such as an electrolyte abnormality, drug toxicity, or aortic stenosis), surviving patients require evaluation and intervention since recurrences are frequent. Exercise testing or coronary arteriography should be performed to exclude coronary disease as the underlying cause, since revascularization may prevent recurrence. Conduction disturbances should be managed as described above. If prodromal supraventricular arrhythmias or ventricular arrhythmias, such as sustained or nonsustained ventricular tachycardia, are found by ambulatory electrocardiographic monitoring, their elimination by pharmacologic therapy or ablation may prevent further episodes. There is growing consensus that if myocardial infarction or ischemia, other precipitating causes, or bradyarrhythmias and conduction disturbances are not found to be the cause of the sudden death episode, an implantable defibrillator is the treatment of choice for appropriate patients.

AVID Investigators: The comparison of anti-arrhythmic drug therapy with implantable defibrillators in patients resuscitated from near fatal ventricular arrhythmias. N Engl J Med 1997;337:1576. [NLM Cit ID: 98026791]

Buxton AE et al: A randomized study of the prevention of sudden death in patients with coronary artery disease. Multicenter Unsustained Tachycardia Trial Investigators. N Engl J Med 1999;341:1882. [NLM Cit ID: 20046567] (In patients with coronary artery disease and a left-ventricular ejection fraction of less than 40% who also have nonsustained ventricular tachycardia inducible by electrophysiology study, antiarrhythmic therapy with implantable cardioverter-defibrillators but not with drug therapy reduces the risk of sudden death.)

JAMA patient page: CPR. JAMA 1998;281:1244. [NLM Cit ID: 99213532]

Klein H et al: New primary prevention trials of sudden cardiac death in patients with left ventricular dysfunction: SCD-HEFT and MADIT-II. Am J Cardiol 1999;83:91D. [NLM Cit ID: 99189718] (This article describes the rationale for two large ongoing trials studying the use of ICD for prevention of sudden death in patients with heart failure.)

Pinski SL et al: Implantable cardioverter-defibrillators. Am J Med 1999;106:446. [NLM Cit ID: 99239755] (Extensive review of clinical trials, indications, and future developments suggests that device therapy is more effective than antiarrhythmic drugs in patients with life-threatening ventricular tachyarrhythmias.)

Plaisance P et al: A comparison of standard cardiopulmonary resuscitation and active compression-decompression resuscitation for out-of-hospital cardiac arrest. N Engl J Med 1999;341:569. [NLM Cit ID: 99362123] (Active compression-decompression CPR resulted in improved outcomes for resuscitated patients when compared with standard CPR.)

Zipes DP et al: Sudden cardiac death. Circulation 1998;98:2334. [NLM Cit ID: 99043843] (Review of epidemiology, pathophysiology, and treatment of sudden death in a variety of acquired and congenital disease states. Treatment algorithm included.)

4. ACCELERATED IDIOVENTRICULAR RHYTHM

Accelerated idioventricular rhythm is a relatively regular wide complex rhythm with a rate of 60–120/min, usually with a gradual onset. Because the rate is often similar to the sinus rate, fusion beats and alternating rhythms are common. Two mechanisms have been invoked: (1) an escape rhythm due to suppression of higher pacemakers resulting from sinoatrial and atrioventricular block or from depressed sinus node function; and (2) slow ventricular tachycardia due to increased automaticity or, less frequently, reentry. It occurs commonly in acute infarction and following reperfusion after thrombolytic drugs. The incidence of associated ventricular fibrillation is much less than that of ventricular tachycardia with a rapid rate, and treatment is not indicated unless there is hemodynamic compromise or more serious arrhythmias. This rhythm also is common in digitalis toxicity.

Accelerated idioventricular rhythm must be distinguished from the idioventricular or junctional rhythm with rates less than 40–45/min that occurs in the presence of complete atrioventricular block. Atrioventricular dissociation—where ventricular rate exceeds sinus—but not atrioventricular block occurs in most cases of accelerated idioventricular rhythm.

5. LONG QT SYNDROME

Congenital long QT syndrome is an uncommon disease that is characterized by recurrent syncope, a long QT interval (usually 0.5–0.7 s), documented ventricular arrhythmias, and sudden death. The sympathetic nervous system (especially the left stellate ganglion) may be important in pathogenesis. Specific genetic mutations affecting membrane potassium and sodium channels have been identified and help delineate the mechanisms of susceptibility to arrhythmia.

Beta-blockers are the most effective therapy for congenital long QT syndrome, though phenytoin and the class Ib agents have also been beneficial. Agents that prolong the QT (classes Ia, Ic, and III) are contraindicated. ICDs are effective in patients who continue to have life-threatening ventricular arrhythmias while taking beta-blockers. Refractory acute arrhythmic episodes may be treated by local anesthetic block of the left stellate ganglion, and recurrent episodes

The prognosis of intraventricular block is generally that of the underlying myocardial process. Patients with no apparent heart disease have an overall survival rate similar to that of matched controls. However, left bundle branch block—but not right—is associated with a higher risk of development of overt cardiac disease and cardiac mortality. Even in bifascicular block, the incidence of occult complete heart block or progression to it is low, and pacing is not usually warranted. In patients with symptoms (eg, syncope) consistent with heart block and intraventricular block, pacing should be reserved for those with documented concomitant complete heart block on monitoring or those with a very prolonged HV interval (> 90 ms) with no other cause for symptoms. Even in the latter group, prophylactic pacing has not improved the prognosis significantly, probably because of the high incidence of ventricular arrhythmias in the same population.

PERMANENT PACING

The indications for permanent pacing have been discussed: symptomatic bradyarrhythmias, asymptomatic Mobitz II atrioventricular block, or complete heart block. The versatility of pacemaker generator units has increased markedly, and dual-chamber multiple programmable units are being implanted with increasing frequency. A standardized nomenclature for pacemaker generators is employed, usually consisting of four letters. The first letter refers to the chamber which is simulated (A = atrium, V = ventricle, D = dual, for both). The second letter refers to the chamber where sensing occurs (also A, V, or D). The third position refers to the sensory mode (I = inhibition by a sensed impulse, T = triggering by a sensed impulse, D = dual modes of response). The fourth letter refers to the programmability or rate modulation capacity (usually P for programming for two functions, M for programming more than two, and R for rate modulation).

Conceptually, a pacemaker that senses and paces in both chambers is the most physiologic approach to pacing patients who remain in sinus rhythm. However, because of the substantially greater cost and complexity of dual-chamber pacing and the shorter projected battery life, they should be used chiefly in patients in whom atrial contraction produces a substantial increment in stroke volume and in those in whom sensing the atrial rate to provide rate-responsive ventricular pacing is useful. Dual-chamber pacing is most useful for individuals with left ventricular systolic or—perhaps more importantly—diastolic dysfunction and for physically active individuals. In patients with single-chamber pacemakers, the lack of an atrial kick may lead to the so-called pacemaker syndrome, in which the patient experiences signs of low cardiac output while upright. Uncontrolled data suggest that chronic dual-chamber pacing is associated with a lower incidence of chronic atrial fibrillation than single-chamber ventricular pacing. However, patients in whom pacing is primarily prophylactic should undergo ventricular pacing.

Pulse generators are also available that can increase their rate in response to motion or respiratory rate when the atrial rate is not an indication of the optimal heart rate. These are most useful in active individuals. However, patients with intermittent or potential bradyarrhythmias or conduction disturbances in whom pacing is primarily prophylactic should undergo ventricular pacing. Follow-up after pacemaker implantation, usually by telephonic monitoring, is essential. All pulse generators and lead systems have an early failure rate that is now below 5% as well as a finite life expectancy varying from 4 to 10 years.

Gregoratos G et al: ACC/AHA Guidelines for Implantation of Cardiac Pacemakers and Arrhythmia Devices: Executive Summary—a report of the American College of Cardiology/American Heart Association Task Force on Practice Guidelines (Committee on Pacemaker Implantation). [NLM Cit ID: 98230132] Circulation 1998; 97:1325.

Lamas GA et al: Quality of life and clinical outcomes in elderly patients treated with ventricular pacing as compared with dual-chamber pacing. Pacemaker Selection in the Elderly Investigators. N Engl J Med 1998;338:1097. [NLM Cit ID: 98196616] (Placement of a pacemaker improved quality of life in elderly patients with indications for cardiac pacing. The group of patients with sinus-node dysfunction benefited from dual-chamber pacing, while patients with high-grade AV block had similar improvements in quality of life with both VVI and dual-chamber modes. One fourth of patients in the VVI mode arm, however, developed the "pacemaker syndrome," which improved with crossover to dual-chamber pacing.)

McComb JM et al: Effect of pacing mode on morbidity and mortality: update of clinical pacing trials. Am J Cardiol 1999;83:211D. [NLM Cit ID: 99189737] (A review of the literature on the effects of pacing mode. Retrospective studies suggest that there may be a mortality benefit to dual-chamber pacing, but they may be confounded by the possibility that older, sicker patients may selectively receive simpler VVI pacemakers. Prospective trials show that patients with sick sinus syndrome benefit from dual chamber pacing, while the data for patients with atrioventricular block are equivocal. Larger trials are currently ongoing.)

Morley-Davies A et al: Cardiac pacing. Lancet 1997;349: 41. [NLM Cit ID: 97141880]

EVALUATION OF SYNCOPE

Syncope, defined as a transient loss of consciousness and postural tone due to inadequate cerebral blood flow with prompt recovery without resuscitative measures, is a common clinical problem, especially in the elderly. Thirty percent of the adult population will experience at least one episode, and syncope accounts for approximately 3% of emergency room visits. Causes include cardiac abnormalities (either disturbances of rhythm or hemodynamics), vascular disorders, or neurologic processes. A specific cause is identified in about 50% of cases during the initial evaluation. The prognosis is relatively benign except when accompanying cardiac disease is present. Syncope is more likely to occur in patients with known heart disease, older men, and young women (who are prone to vasovagal episodes). Syncope is characteristically abrupt in onset, often resulting in injury, transient (lasting for seconds to a few minutes), and followed by prompt recovery or full consciousness.

Vasomotor syncope may be due to excessive vagal tone or impaired reflex control of the peripheral circulation. The most frequent type of vasodepressor syncope is vasovagal hypotension or the "common faint," which is often initiated by stressful, painful, or claustrophobic experience, especially in young women. Premonitory symptoms, such as nausea, diaphoresis, tachycardia, and loss of color, are usual. Episodes can be aborted by lying down or removing the inciting stimulus. Enhanced vagal tone with resulting hypotension is the cause of syncope in carotid sinus hypersensitivity and postmicturition syncope; vagal-induced sinus bradycardia, sinus arrest, and atrioventricular block are common accompaniments and may themselves be the cause of syncope. Carotid sinus massage under carefully monitored conditions or tilt-table testing may be diagnostic (see above under Autonomic Testing). Treatment consists largely of counseling patients to avoid predisposing situations. Paradoxically, beta-blockers may be helpful in patients with altered autonomic function uncovered by head-up tilt testing. Permanent pacing may benefit patients with documented bradycardiac responses.

Orthostatic (postural) hypotension is another common cause of vasomotor syncope, especially in the elderly, in diabetics or other patients with autonomic neuropathy, in patients with blood loss or hypovolemia, and in patients taking vasodilators, diuretics, and adrenergic blocking drugs. In addition, a syndrome of chronic idiopathic orthostatic hypotension exists primarily in older men. In most of these conditions, the normal vasoconstrictive response to assuming upright posture, which compensates for the abrupt decrease in venous return, is impaired. A greater than normal decline (20 mm Hg) in blood pressure immediately upon arising from the supine to the standing position is observed, with or without tachycardia depending on the status of autonomic (baroreceptor) function. Studying patients with a tilt table can establish the diagnosis with more certainty. Autonomic function can be assessed by observing blood pressure and heart rate responses to Valsalva's maneuver and by tilt testing. In older patients, vasoconstrictor abnormalities and autonomic insufficiency are perhaps the most common causes of syncope. Thus, tilt testing should be employed before proceeding to invasive studies unless clinical and ambulatory electrocardiographic evaluation suggests a cardiac abnormality.

Cardiogenic syncope can occur on a mechanical or arrhythmic basis. Mechanical problems that can cause syncope include aortic stenosis (where syncope may occur from autonomic reflex abnormalities or ventricular tachycardia), pulmonary stenosis, hypertrophic obstructive cardiomyopathy, congenital lesions associated with pulmonary hypertension or right-to-left shunting, and left atrial myxoma obstructing the mitral valve. Episodes are commonly exertional or postexertional. More commonly, cardiac syncope is due to disorders of automaticity (sick sinus syndrome), conduction disorders (atrioventricular block), or tachyarrhythmias (especially ventricular tachycardia and supraventricular tachycardia with rapid ventricular rate).

The evaluation for syncope depends on findings from the history and physical examination (especially orthostatic blood pressure evaluation, examination of carotid and other arteries, cardiac examination, and, if appropriate, carotid sinus massage). The resting ECG may reveal arrhythmias, evidence of accessory pathways, prolonged QT interval, and other signs of heart disease (such as infarction or hypertrophy). If the history is consistent with syncope, ambulatory electrocardiographic monitoring is essential. This may need to be repeated several times, since yields increase with longer periods of monitoring, at least up to 3 days. Event recorder and transtelephone electrocardiographic monitoring may be helpful in patients with intermittent presyncopal episodes. Electrophysiologic studies to assess sinus node function and atrioventricular conduction and to induce supraventricular or ventricular tachycardia are indicated in patients with recurrent episodes and nondiagnostic ambulatory ECGs. They reveal an arrhythmic cause in 20–50% of patients, depending on the study criteria, and are most often diagnostic when the patient has had multiple episodes and has identifiable cardiac abnormalities.

Benditt DG et al: Pharmacotherapy of neurally mediated syncope. Circulation 1999;100:1242. [NLM Cit ID: 99414137] (Discussion of mechanism and role of tilt table. Beta-blockers are the favored treatment although there is promise with vasoconstrictors such as midodrine and selective serotonin reuptake inhibitors.)

Henderson MC et al: Syncope: Current diagnosis and treatment. Curr Probl Cardiol 1997;22:239. [NLM Cit ID: 97294767] (Comprehensive review including pathophysiology, differential diagnosis, classification, appropriate testing, and treatment.)

Linzer M et al: Diagnosing syncope. Part 1: Value of history, physical examination, and electrocardiography. Ann Intern Med 1997;126:989. [NLM Cit ID: 97315720]

Part 2: Unexplained syncope. Ann Intern Med 1997; 127:76. [NLM Cit ID: 97339920] (Excellent evidence-based review.)

Martin TP et al: Risk stratification of patients with syncope. Ann Emergency Med 1997;29:459. [NLM Cit ID: 97249100] (An abnormal ECG or history of ventricular tachycardia or congestive heart failure placed patients at 75% risk of arrhythmia or death in the next year. Absence of those findings placed the risk at approximately 5%.)

RECOMMENDATIONS FOR RESUMPTION OF DRIVING

An important management problem in patients who have experienced syncope, symptomatic ventricular tachycardia, or aborted sudden death is to provide recommendations concerning automobile driving. According to a survey published in 1991, only eight states had specific laws dealing with this issue, whereas 42 had laws restricting driving in patients with seizure disorders. There are not adequate data to support driving restrictions in patients who have not experienced symptomatic arrhythmias, though patients with frequent nonsustained ventricular tachycardia, associated heart disease, and significant left ventricular dysfunction are at high enough risk to warrant cautioning. Patients with syncope or aborted sudden death thought to have been due to temporary factors (acute myocardial infarction, bradyarrhythmias subsequently treated with permanent pacing, drug effect, electrolyte imbalance) should be strongly advised after recovery not to drive for at least 1 month. Other patients with symptomatic ventricular tachycardia or aborted sudden death, whether treated pharmacologically, with antitachycardia devices, or with ablation therapy, should not drive for at least 6 months. Longer restrictions are warranted in many such patients if spontaneous arrhythmias persist. The physician should comply with local regulations and consult local authorities concerning individual cases.

Bansch D et al: Syncope in patients with an implantable cardioverter-defibrillator: Incidence, prediction and implications for driving restrictions. J Am Coll Cardiol 1998;31:608. [NLM Cit ID: 98161750] (Overall rate of syncope in patients with implantable cardioverter-defibrillators is about 15%, but those patients with ejection fractions > 40%, no inducible ventricular tachycardia, and no atrial fibrillation had much lower risk of syncope, implying that we may be able to risk-stratify patients with these devices and base driving recommendations on this stratification.)

Jung W et al: Recommendations for driving in patients with implantable cardioverter defibrillators. Eur Heart J 1997;18:1210. [NLM Cit ID: 98119996] (No driving for 6 months. If shocks occur, indefinite abstinence from driving recommended to determine whether incapacitating symptoms occur.)

CARDIAC FAILURE

Essentials of Diagnosis

- Left ventricular failure: Exertional dyspnea, cough, fatigue, orthopnea, paroxysmal nocturnal dyspnea, cardiac enlargement, rales, gallop rhythm, and pulmonary venous congestion.
- Right ventricular failure: Elevated venous pressure, hepatomegaly, dependent edema.
- Both: Combination of above.
- Diagnosis should be confirmed by noninvasive or hemodynamic measurements.

General Considerations

Systolic function of the heart is governed by four major determinants: the contractile state of the myocardium, the preload of the ventricle (the end-diastolic volume and the resultant fiber length of the ventricles prior to onset of the contraction), the afterload applied to the ventricles (the impedance to left ventricular ejection), and the heart rate.

Cardiac function may be inadequate as a result of alterations in any of these determinants. In most instances, the primary derangement is depression of myocardial contractility caused either by loss of functional muscle (due to myocardial infarction, etc) or by processes diffusely affecting the myocardium. However, the heart may fail as a pump because preload is excessively elevated, such as in valvular regurgitation, or when afterload is excessive, such as in aortic stenosis or in severe hypertension. Pump function may also be inadequate when the heart rate is too slow or too rapid. While the normal heart can tolerate wide variations in preload, afterload, and heart rate, the diseased heart often has limited reserve for such alterations. Finally, cardiac pump function may be supranormal but nonetheless inadequate when metabolic demands or requirements for blood flow are excessive. This situation is termed **high-output heart failure** and, though uncommon, tends to be specifically treatable. Causes of high output include thyrotoxicosis, beriberi, severe anemia, arteriovenous shunting, and Paget's disease of bone.

Manifestations of cardiac failure can also occur as a result of isolated or predominant **diastolic dysfunction** of the heart. In these cases, filling of the left or right ventricle is impaired because the chamber is noncompliant ("stiff") due to excessive hypertrophy or changes in composition of the myocardium. Even though contractility may be preserved, diastolic pressures are elevated and cardiac output may be reduced.

Pathophysiology

When the heart fails, a number of adaptations occur both in the heart and systemically. If the stroke volume of either ventricle is reduced by depressed contractility or excessive afterload, end-diastolic volume and pressure in that chamber will rise. This increases end-diastolic myocardial fiber length, resulting in a greater systolic shortening (Starling's law of the heart). If the condition is chronic, ventricular dilation will occur. While this may restore resting cardiac output, the resulting chronic elevation of diastolic pressures will be transmitted to the atria and to the pulmonary and systemic venous circulation. Ultimately, increased capillary pressure may lead to transudation of fluid with resulting pulmonary or systemic edema. Reduced cardiac output, particularly if associated with reduced arterial pressure or perfusion of the kidneys, will also activate several neural and humoral systems. Increased activity of the sympathetic nervous system will stimulate myocardial contractility, heart rate, and venous tone; the latter change results in a rise in the effective central blood volume, which serves to further elevate preload. Though these adaptations are designed to increase cardiac output, they may themselves be deleterious. Thus, tachycardia and increased contractility may precipitate ischemia in patients with underlying coronary artery disease, and the rise in preload may worsen pulmonary congestion. Sympathetic nervous system activation also increases peripheral vascular resistance; this adaptation is designed to maintain perfusion to vital organs, but when it is excessive it may itself reduce renal and other tissue blood flow. Peripheral vascular resistance is also a major determinant of left ventricular afterload, so that excessive sympathetic activity may further depress cardiac function.

One of the more important effects of lower cardiac output is reduction of renal blood flow and glomerular filtration rate, which leads to sodium and fluid retention. The renin-angiotensin-aldosterone system is also activated, leading to further increases in peripheral vascular resistance and left ventricular afterload as well as sodium and fluid retention. Heart failure is associated with increased circulating levels of arginine vasopressin, which also serves as a vasoconstrictor and inhibitor of water excretion. While release of atrial natriuretic peptide is increased in heart failure owing to the elevated atrial pressures, there is evidence of resistance to its natriuretic and vasodilating effects.

Hemodynamic Alterations

Myocardial failure is characterized by two hemodynamic derangements, and the clinical presentation is determined by their severity. The first is reduction in cardiac output, ie, the ability to increase cardiac output in response to increased demands imposed by exercise or even ordinary activity (cardiac reserve). The second abnormality, elevation of ventricular diastolic pressures, is primarily a result of the compensatory processes.

Heart failure may be right-sided or left-sided. Patients with the picture of **left heart failure** have symptoms of low cardiac output and elevated pulmonary venous pressure; dyspnea is the predominant feature. Signs of fluid retention predominate in **right heart failure,** with the patient exhibiting edema, hepatic congestion, and, on occasion, ascites. Most patients exhibit symptoms or signs of both right- and left-sided failure, and left ventricular dysfunction is the primary cause of right ventricular failure. Surprisingly, some individuals with severe left ventricular dysfunction will display few signs of left heart failure and appear to have isolated right heart failure. Indeed, they may be clinically indistinguishable from patients with cor pulmonale, who have right heart failure secondary to pulmonary disease.

Although this section primarily concerns cardiac failure due to systolic left ventricular dysfunction, patients with **diastolic dysfunction** experience many of the same symptoms and may be difficult to distinguish clinically. Diastolic pressures are elevated even though diastolic volumes are normal or small. These pressures are transmitted to the pulmonary and systemic venous systems, resulting in dyspnea and edema. The most frequent cause of diastolic cardiac dysfunction is left ventricular hypertrophy, commonly resulting from hypertension, but conditions such as hypertrophic or restrictive cardiomyopathy, diabetes, and pericardial disease can produce the same clinical picture. While diuretics are often useful in these patients, the other therapies discussed in this section (digitalis, vasodilators, inotropic agents) may be inappropriate.

Causes & Prevention of Cardiac Failure

The syndrome of cardiac failure can be produced by many diseases. In developed countries, coronary artery disease with resulting myocardial infarction and loss of functioning myocardium (ischemic cardiomyopathy) is the commonest cause. In the 4S study, aggressive lipid-lowering therapy in patients with known coronary disease reduced the incidence of heart failure by 30%. A number of processes may present with dilated or congestive cardiomyopathy, which is characterized by left ventricular or biventricular dilation and generalized systolic dysfunction. These are discussed elsewhere in this chapter, but the most common are alcoholic cardiomyopathy, viral myocarditis (including infections by HIV), and dilated cardiomyopathies with no obvious underlying cause (idiopathic cardiomyopathy). Rare causes of dilated cardiomyopathy include infiltrative diseases (hemochromatosis, sarcoidosis, amyloidosis, etc), other infectious agents, metabolic disorders, cardiotoxins, and drug toxicity.

Systemic hypertension remains an important cause of congestive heart failure and, even more commonly in the USA, an exacerbating factor in patients with cardiac dysfunction due to other causes. In several trials, antihypertensive therapy—particularly when directed to the systolic blood pressure—has been effective in reducing the incidence of new-onset heart failure by 40–60%. Valvular heart disease has become a less frequent cause of heart failure with the declining incidence and severity of rheumatic fever. However, aortic stenosis remains a common and reversible cause. Patients with chronic volume overload of the left ventricle, such as mitral or aortic regurgitation, may develop progressive myocardial dysfunction and have a picture of cardiomyopathy even after the underlying condition is corrected. This form of congestive heart failure is preventable by early diagnosis and treatment of the valvular lesion.

Baig MK et al: The pathophysiology of advanced heart failure. Am Heart J 1998;135:S216. [NLM Cit ID: 98292039] (The current understanding of the pathophysiology of congestive heart failure is reviewed.)

Bristow MR: Why does the myocardium fail? Insights from basic science. Lancet 1998;352(Suppl 1):8. [NLM Cit ID: 98405881] (Pathophysiology of myocardial dysfunction with thorough discussion of beta-adrenergic system.)

Dauterman KW et al: Heart failure with preserved systolic function. Am Heart J 1998;135:S310. [NLM Cit ID: 98292045] (Left ventricular function normal in 40%.)

Hunter JJ et al: Signaling pathways for cardiac hypertrophy and failure. N Engl J Med 1999;341:1276. [NLM Cit ID: 99442273] (In-depth review of the pathways involved in hypertrophy, apoptosis, and survival of myocytes and how these relate to treatment.)

Kostis JB: Prevention of heart failure by antihypertensive drug treatment in older persons with isolated systolic hypertension. JAMA 1997;278:212. [NLM Cit ID: 97361706] (Fifty percent of new cases can be prevented by aggressive control of systolic hypertension.)

Mann DL: Mechanisms and models in heart failure: A combinatorial approach. Circulation 1999;100:999. [NLM Cit ID: 99398986] (Cardiorenal, hemodynamic, and neurohormonal systems are discussed. Matrix metalloproteinases, tumor necrosis factor, and endothelin are relevant to these models.)

Massie BM et al: Evolving trends in the epidemiology of heart failure. Am Heart J 1997;133:703. [NLM Cit ID: 97343872]

Massie BM: Pathophysiology of heart failure. In: *Cecil Textbook of Medicine,* 21st ed. Saunders, 1999.

Schrier RW et al: Hormones and Hemodynamics in Heart Failure. N Engl J Med 1999;341:577. [NLM Cit ID: 99362125] (Physiologic review covers the role of the sympathetic nervous system, renin-angiotensin-aldosterone system, vasopressin, and natriuretic peptides.)

Williams RS: Apoptosis and heart failure. N Engl J Med 1999;341:759. [NLM Cit ID: 99383630] (Apoptosis—programmed cell death—may be triggered by ischemia, pressure overload, or other signals.)

Clinical Findings

A. Symptoms: The symptoms of cardiac failure have been discussed in part in earlier sections. The most common complaint is shortness of breath, chiefly exertional dyspnea at first and then progressing to orthopnea, paroxysmal nocturnal dyspnea, and rest dyspnea. A more subtle and often overlooked symptom of heart failure is a chronic nonproductive cough, which is often worse in the recumbent position. Nocturia due to excretion of fluid retained during the day and increased renal perfusion in the recumbent position is a common nonspecific symptom of heart failure. Patients with heart failure also complain of fatigue and exercise intolerance. These symptoms correlate poorly with the degree of cardiac dysfunction and result in part from changes in peripheral blood flow and blood flow to skeletal muscle which are part of the syndrome of heart failure. Patients with right heart failure may experience right upper quadrant pain due to passive congestion of the liver, loss of appetite and nausea due to edema of the gut or impaired gastrointestinal perfusion, and peripheral edema.

Cardiac failure may present acutely in a previously asymptomatic patient. Causes include myocardial infarction, myocarditis, and acute valvular regurgitation due to endocarditis or other conditions. These patients usually present with pulmonary edema. The management of acute heart failure has been discussed under myocardial infarction and centers around initial stabilization with diuretics and parenteral vasodilators or inotropic agents.

Patients with episodic symptoms may be having left ventricular dysfunction due to intermittent ischemia. This potentially reversible form of heart failure should be considered, especially in patients with angina pectoris and those with diabetes mellitus. Patients may also present with acute exacerbations of chronic, stable heart failure. Exacerbations are usually caused by alterations in therapy (or patient noncompliance), excessive salt and fluid intake, arrhythmias, excessive activity, pulmonary emboli, intercurrent infection, or progression of the underlying disease.

B. Signs: Many patients with heart failure, including some with severe symptoms, appear comfortable at rest. Others will be dyspneic during conversation or minor activity, and those with long-standing severe heart failure may appear cachectic or cyanotic. The vital signs may be normal, but tachycardia, hypotension, and reduced pulse pressure may be present. Patients often show signs of increased sympathetic nervous system activity, including cold extremities and diaphoresis. Important peripheral signs of heart failure can be detected by examination of the neck, the lungs, the abdomen, and the extremities. Right atrial pressure may be estimated through the height of the pulsations in the jugular venous system. In addition to the height of the venous pressure, abnormal pulsations such as regurgitant *v* waves should be sought. Examination of the carotid pulse allows estimation of pulse pressure as well as detection of aortic stenosis. The thyroid examination is important, since occult hyperthyroidism and hypothyroidism are readily treatable causes of heart failure. In the lungs, crackles at the bases reflect transudation of fluid into the alveoli. Pleural effusions may cause bibasilar dullness to percussion. Expiratory wheezing and rhonchi may be signs of heart failure. Patients with severe right heart failure may have hepatic enlargement—tender or nontender—due to passive congestion. Systolic pulsations may be felt in tricuspid regurgitation. Sustained moderate pressure on the liver may increase jugular venous pressure (a positive hepatojugular reflux is an increase of > 1 cm). Ascites may also be present. Peripheral pitting edema is a common sign in patients with right heart failure and may extend into the thighs and abdominal wall.

The cardiac examination has been discussed. Cardinal signs in heart failure are a parasternal lift, indicating pulmonary hypertension; an enlarged and sustained left ventricular impulse, indicating left ventricular dilation and hypertrophy; a diminished first heart sound, suggesting impaired contractility; and S_3 gallops originating in the left and sometimes the right ventricle. Murmurs should be sought to exclude primary valvular disease; secondary mitral regurgitation and tricuspid regurgitation murmurs are common in patients with dilated ventricles. In chronic heart failure, many of the expected signs of heart failure may be absent despite markedly abnormal cardiac function and hemodynamic measurements.

C. Laboratory Findings: A blood count may reveal anemia, a cause of high-output failure and an exacerbating factor in other forms of cardiac dysfunction. Biochemical studies may show renal insufficiency as a possible compounding factor. Renal function tests also determine whether cardiac failure is associated with prerenal azotemia. Electrolytes may disclose heightened neuroendocrine activity with resultant hyponatremia. Thyroid function in older patients should be assessed to detect occult thyrotoxicosis or myxedema. Appropriate biopsies may lead to a diagnosis of amyloidosis. Additional assessment in dilated cardiomyopathy should include iron studies to exclude hemochromatosis. Myocardial biopsy may exclude specific causes of dilated cardiomyopathy but rarely reveals specific reversible diagnoses.

D. Electrocardiography and Chest X-Ray: Electrocardiography may indicate an underlying or secondary arrhythmia, myocardial infarction, or nonspecific changes that often include low voltage, intraventricular conduction defects, left ventricular hypertrophy, and nonspecific repolarization changes. Chest radiographs provide information about the size and shape of the cardiac silhouette. Cardiomegaly is an important finding. Evidence of pulmonary venous hypertension includes relative dilation of the upper lobe veins, perivascular edema (haziness of vessel outlines), interstitial edema, and alveolar fluid. In acute heart failure, these findings correlate moderately well with pulmonary venous pressure, and when present in chronic failure they indicate elevated pressures. However, patients with chronic heart failure may show relatively normal pulmonary vasculature despite markedly elevated pressures. Pleural effusions are common and tend to be bilateral or right-sided.

E. Additional Studies: Many studies have indicated that the clinical diagnosis of systolic myocardial dysfunction is often inaccurate. The primary confounding conditions are diastolic dysfunction of the heart with decreased relaxation and filling of the left ventricle (particularly in hypertension and in hypertrophic states) and pulmonary disease. Since heart failure patients usually have significant resting electrocardiographic abnormalities, stress imaging procedures such as perfusion scintigraphy or dobutamine echocardiography are indicated.

The most useful test is the echocardiogram. This will reveal the size and function of both ventricles and of the atria. It will also allow detection of pericardial effusion, valvular abnormalities, intracardiac shunts, and segmental wall motion abnormalities suggestive of old myocardial infarction as opposed to more generalized forms of dilated cardiomyopathy.

Radionuclide angiography measures left ventricular ejection fraction and permits analysis of regional wall motion. This test is especially useful when echocardiography is technically suboptimal, such as in patients with severe pulmonary disease. When myocardial ischemia is suspected as a cause of left ventricular dysfunction, stress testing should be performed.

F. Cardiac Catheterization: In most patients with heart failure, clinical examination and noninvasive tests can determine left ventricular size and function well enough to confirm the diagnosis. Left heart catheterization is necessary when significant valvular disease must be excluded and when the presence and extent of coronary artery disease must be determined. The latter is particularly important when left ventricular dysfunction may be partially reversible by revascularization. The combination of angina or noninvasive evidence of significant myocardial ischemia with symptomatic heart failure is often an indication for coronary angiography if the patient is a potential candidate for revascularization. Right heart catheterization may be useful to select and monitor therapy in patients refractory to standard therapy.

Massie BM: Pathophysiology of heart failure. In: *Cecil Textbook of Medicine,* 21st ed. Goldman L, Bennett CJ (editors). Saunders, 2000.

Philbin EF et al: The relationship between cardiothoracic ratio and left ventricular ejection fraction in congestive heart failure. Arch Intern Med 1998;158:506. [NLM Cit ID: 98167653] (X-ray not very helpful in diagnosing congestive heart failure.)

Treatment

A. Correction of Reversible Causes: The major reversible causes of heart failure include valvular lesions, myocardial ischemia, arrhythmias (especially persistent tachycardias), alcohol- or drug-induced myocardial depression, intracardiac shunts, and high-output states. Calcium channel blockers, antiarrhythmic drugs, and nonsteroidal anti-inflammatory agents are important causes of worsening heart failure. Some metabolic and infiltrative cardiomyopathies may be partially reversible, or their progression may be slowed; these include hemochromatosis, sarcoidosis, and amyloidosis. Acute myocarditis may respond to immunosuppressive therapy and corticosteroids. Reversible causes of diastolic dysfunction include pericardial disease and left ventricular hypertrophy due to hypertension. Once it is established that there is no reversible component, the measures outlined below are appropriate.

B. Diet and Activity: Patients should routinely be under moderate salt restriction (2 g sodium or 5 g salt). More severe sodium restriction is usually difficult to achieve and unnecessary because of the availability of potent diuretic agents. In severe heart failure, restriction of activity may facilitate temporary recompensation. However, in stable angina patients, a prudent increase in activity or a regular exercise regimen can be encouraged. Indeed, a gradual exercise program is associated with diminished symptoms and substantial increases in exercise capacity.

C. Diuretic Therapy: Diuretics are the most effective means of providing symptomatic relief to patients with moderate to severe congestive heart failure. Few patients with symptoms or signs of fluid retention can be optimally managed without a diuretic. However, excessive diuresis can lead to electrolyte imbalance and neurohormonal activation. A combination of a diuretic and an ACE inhibitor should be the initial treatment in most symptomatic patients. When fluid retention is mild, thiazide diuretics or a similar type of agent (hydrochlorothiazide, 25–50 mg; metolazone, 2.5–5 mg; chlorthalidone, 25–50 mg; etc) may be sufficient. These agents block sodium reabsorption in the cortical diluting segment at the terminal portion of the loop of Henle and in the proximal portion of the distal convoluted tubule. The result is natriuresis and kaliuresis. These agents also have weak carbonic anhydrase inhibitor activity, which results in proximal tubule inhibition of sodium reabsorption.

The thiazides are generally ineffective when the glomerular filtration rate falls below 30 mL/min, a not infrequent occurrence in patients with severe heart failure. Metolazone maintains its efficacy down to a glomerular filtration rate of approximately 10–20 mL/min. Adverse reactions include hypokalemia and intravascular volume depletion with resulting prerenal azotemia, skin rashes, neutropenia and thrombocytopenia, hyperglycemia, hyperuricemia, and hepatic dysfunction.

Patients with more severe heart failure should be treated with one of the loop diuretics. These include furosemide (20–320 mg daily), bumetanide (1–8 mg daily), and torsemide (20–200 mg daily). These agents have a rapid onset and a relatively short duration of action. In patients with preserved renal function, two or more doses are preferable to a single larger dose. In acute situations or when gastrointestinal absorption is in doubt, they should be given intravenously. The loop diuretics inhibit chloride reabsorption in the ascending limb of the loop of Henle, which results in natriuresis, kaliuresis, and metabolic alkalosis. They are active even in severe renal insufficiency, but larger doses (up to 500 mg of furosemide or equivalent) may be required. The major adverse reactions include intravascular volume depletion, prerenal azotemia, and hypotension. Hypokalemia, particularly with accompanying digitalis therapy, is a major problem. Less common side effects include skin rashes, gastrointestinal distress, and ototoxicity (the latter more common with ethacrynic acid and possibly less common with bumetanide).

The potassium-sparing agents spironolactone, triamterene, and amiloride are often useful in combination with the loop diuretics and thiazides. Triamterene and amiloride act on the distal tubule to reduce potassium secretion. Their diuretic potency is only mild and not adequate for most patients with heart failure, but they may minimize the hypokalemia induced by more potent agents. Side effects include hyperkalemia, gastrointestinal symptoms, and renal dysfunction. Spironolactone is a specific inhibitor of aldosterone, which is often increased in congestive heart failure and has important effects beyond potassium retention (see below). Its onset of action is slower than the other potassium-sparing agents, and its side effects include gynecomastia. Combinations of potassium supplements or angiotensin converting enzyme inhibitors and potassium-sparing drugs can produce hyperkalemia but have been used with success in patients with persistent hypokalemia.

Patients with refractory edema may respond to combinations of a loop diuretic and thiazide-like agents. Metolazone, because of its maintained activity with renal insufficiency, is the most useful agent for such a combination. Extreme caution must be observed with this approach, since massive diuresis and electrolyte imbalances often occur; 2.5 mg of metolazone should be added to the previous dosage of loop diuretic. In many cases this is necessary only once or twice a week, but dosages up to 10 mg daily have been used in some patients.

D. Inhibitors of the Renin-Angiotensin-Aldosterone System: The renin-angiotensin-aldosterone system is activated early in the course of heart failure and plays an important role in the progression of this syndrome. Inhibition of this system with ACE inhibitors should be considered part of the initial therapy of this syndrome based on their favorable effects on prognosis.

1. Angiotensin-converting enzyme inhibitors–ACE inhibitors block the renin-angiotensin-aldosterone system by inhibiting the conversion of angiotensin I to angiotensin II, producing vasodilation by limiting angiotensin II-induced vasoconstriction, and decreasing sodium retention by reducing aldosterone secretion. Since angiotensin-converting enzyme is also involved in the degradation of bradykinin, ACE inhibitors result in higher bradykinin levels, which in turn stimulate the synthesis of prostaglandins and nitric oxide. Experimental data and hemodynamic studies in patients indicate that these latter actions may be important. Although the other vasodilators tend to stimulate the renin-angiotensin system and often lose part of their effect due to the resulting fluid retention, tolerance to the ACE inhibitors is uncommon.

A growing number of ACE inhibitors are becoming available (Table 11–7). Captopril and enalapril have been approved in the United States for the treatment of heart failure, both to prolong survival and alleviate symptoms. Several other ACE inhibitors have been approved based only on their ability to reduce symptoms, and it is likely that all agents of this class are effective.

Acute hemodynamic studies show that the ACE inhibitors reduce left ventricular filling pressure and right atrial pressure and moderately increase cardiac output. During long-term follow-up, these hemodynamic benefits are maintained or increased. ACE inhibitors lessen symptoms and increase exercise tolerance. They also correct the electrolyte abnormalities that characterize severe heart failure, such as hyponatremia and diuretic-induced hypokalemia, which may reduce the propensity to arrhythmias. Survival rates are improved by ACE inhibitor therapy in patients with mild, moderate, and severe heart failure. In addition, ACE inhibitors can delay the onset and progression of heart failure in patients with asymptomatic left ventricular dysfunction.

Because the ACE inhibitors may produce significant hypotension, particularly after the initial doses, they must be started with caution. Hypotension is most prominent in patients with hypovolemia, prerenal azotemia (especially if it is diuretic-induced), and hyponatremia (an indicator of activation of the renin-angiotensin system). In patients at high risk for hypotension, captopril is the preferred agent for beginning ACE inhibitor therapy because of its predictable onset and short duration of action (peak effect in 30–90 minutes). Treatment should be started with a low dose: either 12.5 mg or, in patients with hyponatremia or preexisting low blood pressure, 6.25 mg. The blood pressure should be monitored for the first 2 hours after dosing; if symptomatic or clinically significant hypotension does not occur, the patient may be sent home on a dosage of 12.5 mg three times daily. In most patients, longer-acting ACE inhibitors may be employed as initial therapy. Patients should be questioned about symptoms of hypotension, and renal function should be checked during the first week. The chronically effective dose of captopril appears to be 25–100 mg three times daily, although some patients will not tolerate this high a dose because of hypotension.

Enalapril has been utilized in many of the major trials of ACE inhibitors in heart failure. It should be initiated at 2.5 mg twice daily and titrated upward to 10 mg twice daily. It may be less well tolerated in patients with borderline blood pressure or underlying renal dysfunction. Other ACE inhibitors should be used similarly, starting at a low dosage and gradually titrating to dosages at the higher end of the antihypertensive range if tolerated. Most trials have employed much higher doses of ACE inhibitors than are generally used in clinical practice (total daily doses of enalapril 20 mg or captopril 150 mg or the equivalent). A recent trial comparing high and low doses of lisinopril (ATLAS) showed a lower incidence of morbidity and mortality at high doses and excellent tolerability. Therefore, patients should be titrated to high target doses—unless limited by major side effects such as symptomatic hypotension or progressive renal dysfunction (serum creatinine > 2.5–3 mg/dL).

The major limitation to ACE inhibitor therapy in heart failure is hypotension and renal insufficiency due to inadequate renal perfusion pressures. Other side effects such as dysgeusia, rash, cough, neutropenia, and proteinuria are less serious or very uncommon. Similarly uncommon but perhaps most serious, angioedema may develop at any time during the use of these agents. The ACE inhibitors tend to increase serum potassium concentrations. Potassium-sparing agents should be withdrawn before ACE inhibitor therapy is started; and although potassium supplements may be required in individuals receiving diuretics and digitalis, their dosage should be decreased and subsequently adjusted as needed.

2. Angiotensin II receptor blockers–Another approach to inhibiting the renin-angiotensin-aldosterone system is the use of specific angiotensin II receptor blockers (see Table 11–7), which will block or decrease most of the effects of the system. In addition, since there are alternative pathways of angiotensin II production in many tissues, the receptor blockers may provide more complete system blockade.

However, these agents do not share the effects of ACE inhibitors on other potentially important pathways that produce increases in bradykinin, prostaglandins, and NO in the heart, blood vessels, and other tissues. There are as yet no large clinical trials demonstrating improvement in clinical outcomes with angiotensin II receptor blockers in heart failure or other cardiovascular conditions, and the recently completed second Evaluation of Losartan in the Elderly (ELITE-2) trial failed to confirm the equivalence of the losartan with captopril. Indeed, there was an apparent trend toward poorer survival with losartan, indicating that angiotensin II receptor blockers should not be employed for congestive heart failure except in patients with proved intolerance to an ACE inhibitor due to cough.

3. Spironolactone–There is growing evidence that aldosterone may mediate some of the major effects of renin-angiotensin-aldosterone system activation, such as myocardial remodeling and fibrosis, as well as sodium retention and potassium loss at the distal tubules. Thus, spironolactone should be considered as a neurohormonal antagonist rather than narrowly as a potassium-sparing diuretic. The recently completed RALES trial compared spironolactone 25 mg daily with placebo in patients with advanced heart failure already receiving ACE inhibitors and diuretics and showed a 29% reduction in mortality as well as similar decreases in other clinical end points. Hyperkalemia was uncommon in this severe heart failure population, which was maintained on high doses of diuretic, but potassium levels should be monitored closely. However, neither the efficacy nor the safety of spironolactone has been established in the large majority of patients with mild or moderate heart failure who are taking low doses of diuretics, though this agent may be considered in patients who require potassium supplementation.

E. Beta-Blocker Therapy: Although beta-blockers have traditionally been considered contraindicated in patients with heart failure because they may block the compensatory actions of the sympathetic nervous system, there is now strong evidence that these agents have important beneficial effects in this patient population. The mechanism of this benefit remains unclear, but it is likely that chronic elevations of catecholamines and sympathetic nervous system activity cause progressive myocardial damage, leading to worsening left ventricular function and dilation. The primary evidence for this hypothesis is that over a period of 3–6 months, beta-blockers produce consistent substantial rises in ejection fraction (averaging 10% absolute increase) and reductions in left ventricular size and mass.

Clinical trial results have been reported in over 10,000 patients, primarily those with mild to moderate heart failure (NYHA class II and class III, ejection fraction < 35–40%) receiving ACE inhibitors and diuretics randomized to beta-blockers or placebo. Carvedilol, a nonselective β_1 and β_2 receptor blocker with additional weak alpha-blocking activity, was the first beta-blocker approved for heart failure in the United States after showing a reduction in death and hospitalizations in four smaller studies with a total of nearly 1100 patients. Subsequently, trials with two β_1-selective agents, bisoprolol (CIBIS II, with 2647 patients) and metoprolol (MERIT, with nearly 4000 patients), both showed 35% reductions in mortality as well as fewer hospitalizations. Recently, a trial using carvedilol in 2200 patients with severe (NYHA class III/IV) heart failure was terminated ahead of schedule because of an approximately 40% reduction in mortality. In these trials, there were reductions in sudden deaths and deaths from worsening heart failure, and benefits were seen in patients with underlying coronary disease and those with primary cardiomyopathies. In all these studies, the beta-blockers were generally well tolerated, with similar numbers of withdrawals in the active and placebo groups. This has led to a strong recommendation that *stable* patients (defined as having no recent deterioration or evidence of volume overload) with mild, moderate, and even severe heart failure should be treated with a beta-blocker unless there is a noncardiac contraindication. It is not known whether there are differences between beta-blockers, but a trial comparing carvedilol and metoprolol (COMET) is ongoing and should be completed in 2002 or earlier.

Since even apparently stable patients may deteriorate when beta-blockers are initiated, this must be done very gradually and with great care. Carvedilol is initiated at a dosage of 3.125 mg twice daily and may be increased to 6.25, 12.5, and 25 mg twice daily at intervals of approximately 2 weeks. The protocols for metoprolol use were starting at 12.5 or 25 mg four times daily and doubling at intervals of 2–4 weeks to a target dose of 200 mg four times daily (using the Toprol XL sustained-release preparation). Bisoprolol was administered at 1.25, 2.5, 3.75, 5, 7.5, and 10 mg four times daily, with increments at 1- to 4-week intervals.

Patients should be instructed to monitor their weights at home and to report any increase or change in symptoms immediately. Before each dose increase, the patient should be seen and examined to ensure that there has not been fluid retention or worsening of symptoms. If heart failure worsens, this can usually be managed by increasing diuretic doses and delaying further increases in beta-blocker doses, though downward adjustments or discontinuation is sometimes required. Carvedilol, because of its alpha-blocking activity, may cause dizziness or hypotension. This can usually be managed by reducing the doses of other vasodilators and by slowing the pace of dose increases.

F. Digitalis Glycosides: Digitalis is the only orally active positive inotropic agent currently available. It binds to the sodium-potassium ATPase on the sarcolemmal membrane, inhibiting the sodium pump and thereby increasing intracellular sodium. This facilitates sodium-calcium exchange, with a resultant increase in cytosolic calcium, which enhances contractile protein cross-bridge formation and force generation. The digitalis glycosides also have electrophysiologic effects that may be beneficial or deleterious in individual patients. The primary therapeutic effect is an enhancement of cardiac parasympathetic tone, which delays atrioventricular conduction and reduces sinus node automaticity, thereby decreasing the ventricular response in patients with atrial fibrillation. However, the increase in intracellular calcium and sodium may enhance automaticity of latent pacemakers, increasing the excitability of ventricular myocytes and inducing ventricular arrhythmias. Although these effects may be mitigated by maintaining intracellular potassium concentrations, they may enhance susceptibility to life-threatening arrhythmias in the setting of myocardial ischemia or hypokalemia.

Although the digitalis glycosides were once the mainstay of congestive heart failure treatment, their use in patients who are in sinus rhythm has declined because they lack the benefits of the neurohormonal antagonists on prognosis and because safety concerns persist. However, their efficacy in reducing the symptoms of heart failure has been established in at least four multicenter trials which have demonstrated that digoxin withdrawal is associated with worsening symptoms and signs of heart failure, more frequent hospitalizations for decompensation, and reduced exercise tolerance. This was also seen in the 6800-patient Digitalis Investigators Group (DIG) trial, though that study found no benefit (or harm) with regard to survival. A reduction in deaths due to progressive heart failure was balanced by an increase in deaths due to ischemic and arrhythmic events. In subgroup analyses, digoxin appeared more effective in patients with the worst heart failure symptoms, largest left ventricles, and lowest ejection fractions. Based on these results, digoxin should be used for patients who remain symptomatic when taking diuretics and ACE inhibitors as well as for heart failure patients who are in atrial fibrillation and require rate control.

Digoxin, the only widely employed digitalis preparation, has a half-life of 24–36 hours and is eliminated almost entirely by the kidneys. The oral maintenance dose may range from 0.125 mg three times weekly to 0.5 mg daily depending on renal function (lower with poor function), body size, age (lower in the elderly), gastrointestinal absorption (ordinarily 60–70% bioavailability), cardiac function (lower with low cardiac output), and thyroid function (lower with hypothyroidism). There are also a number of important drug interactions—including amiodarone, quinidine, propafenone, and verapamil—that increase digoxin levels; and bile acid sequestrants, oral antibiotics, and Kaopectate—that may reduce digoxin's gastrointestinal absorption. Although a loading dose of 0.75–1.25 mg (depending primarily on lean body size) over 24–48 hours may be given if an early effect is desired, in most patients with chronic heart failure it is sufficient to begin with the expected maintenance dose (usually 0.125–0.25 mg). Except when atrial fibrillation is present, where the ventricular rate is a marker of digoxin effect, it is prudent to measure a blood level after 7–14 days (and at least 6 hours after the last dose was administered). Most of the positive inotropic effect is apparent with serum digoxin levels between 0.7 ng and 1.2 ng/mL, and levels above this range may be associated with a higher risk of arrhythmias, though toxicity is rare below levels of 1.8 ng/mL. Once an appropriate maintenance dose is established, subsequent levels are usually not indicated unless there is a change in renal function or medications that affect digoxin levels or a significant deterioration in cardiac status that may be associated with reduced clearance.

Digoxin toxicity has become less frequent as there has been a better appreciation of its pharmacology, but the therapeutic-to-toxic ratio is quite narrow. Symptoms of digitalis toxicity include anorexia, nausea, headache, blurring or yellowing of vision, and disorientation. Cardiac toxicity may take the form of atrioventricular conduction or sinus node depression; junctional, atrial, or ventricular premature beats or tachycardias; or ventricular fibrillation. Potassium administration (following measurement, since severe toxicity may be associated with hyperkalemia) is usually indicated for the tachyarrhythmias even when levels are in the normal range, but may worsen conduction disturbances. Lidocaine or phenytoin may be useful for ventricular arrhythmias, as is overdrive pacing, but quinidine, amiodarone, and propafenone should be avoided because they will increase digoxin levels. Electrical cardioversion should be avoided if possible, since it may cause intractable ventricular fibrillation or cardiac standstill. First- and second-degree atrioventricular block can generally be observed, but pacing is indicated for higher degrees or for bradycardias. Digoxin immune fab (ovine) is available for life-threatening toxicity or large overdoses, but it should be remembered that their half-life is shorter than that of digoxin and so repeat administration may be required.

G. Vasodilators: Agents that dilate arteriolar smooth muscle and lower peripheral vascular resistance reduce left ventricular afterload. Medications that diminish venous tone and increase venous capacitance reduce the preload of both ventricles as their principal effect. Since most patients with moderate to severe heart failure have both elevated preload and reduced cardiac output, the maximum benefit of vasodilator therapy can be achieved by an agent or combination of agents with both actions. Many patients with heart failure have mitral or tricuspid regurgitation; agents that reduce resistance to ventricular outflow tend to redirect regurgitant flow in a forward direction.

Although vasodilators that are also neurohumoral antagonists—specifically, the ACE inhibitors—improve prognosis, such a benefit is less clear with the direct-acting vasodilators. The combination of hydralazine and isosorbide dinitrate has also improved survival, but to a lesser extent than ACE inhibitors.

The intravenous vasodilating drugs and their dosages have been discussed elsewhere in this chapter (in the section on complications in acute myocardial infarction).

1. Nitrates–Sodium nitroprusside is a potent dilator of both the arteriolar resistance and venous capacitance vessels, and it consistently increases cardiac output and reduces ventricular filling pressures. It is only occasionally employed in the management of chronic heart failure, usually during episodes of acute decompensation. In such cases it may produce excessive hypotension, and it has been combined with dopamine or dobutamine to produce optimal hemodynamic improvement. Intravenous nitroglycerin is less useful in chronic heart failure, since it produces only a limited increase in cardiac output.

Isosorbide dinitrate, 20–80 mg orally three times daily, has proved effective in several small studies. Nitroglycerin ointment, 12.5–50 mg (1–4 in) every 8 hours, appears to be equally effective although somewhat inconvenient for long-term therapy. The nitrates are moderately effective in relieving shortness of breath, especially in patients with mild to moderate symptoms, but less successful—probably because they have little effect on cardiac output—in advanced heart failure. Nitrate therapy is generally well tolerated, but headaches and hypotension may limit the dose of all agents. The development of tolerance to chronic nitrate therapy is now generally acknowledged. This is minimized by intermittent therapy, especially if a daily 8- to 12-hour nitrate-free interval is employed, but probably develops to some extent in most patients receiving these agents. Transdermal nitroglycerin patches have no sustained effect in patients with heart failure and should not be employed for this indication.

2. Hydralazine–Oral hydralazine is a potent arteriolar dilator and markedly increases cardiac output in patients with congestive heart failure. However, as a single agent, it has not been shown to improve symptoms or exercise tolerance during chronic treatment. The combination of nitrates and oral hydralazine produces greater hemodynamic and clinical effects.

Hydralazine therapy is frequently limited by side effects. Approximately 30% of patients are unable to tolerate the relatively high doses required to produce hemodynamic improvement in heart failure (200–400 mg daily in divided doses). The major side effect is gastrointestinal distress, but headaches, tachycardia, hypotension, and the drug-induced lupus syndrome are also relatively common.

3. Alpha-adrenergic blockers–These agents produce vasodilation by blocking postsynaptic alpha receptors. Although they cause short-term hemodynamic improvement, their efficacy is limited by the rapid development of tolerance. In a large trial in older hypertensives, the alpha-blocker doxazosin was associated with an increased incidence of heart failure hospitalizations compared with diuretics, so these agents should be avoided except when required for another indication.

H. Newer Positive Inotropic Agents: The digitalis derivatives are the only available oral inotropic agents at this time in the USA. However, a number of drugs that increase myocardial contractility in experimental preparations have been or are being investigated. These include beta-adrenergic agonists, dopaminergic agents, and a group of nondigitalis, noncatecholamine agents that increase myocardial contractility by inhibiting myocardial phosphodiesterase. Two of the latter class, milrinone and amrinone, have been approved for intravenous use. However, several trials with newer oral inotropic agents, including milrinone, xamoterol (a beta-adrenergic agonist), ibopamine (a dopaminergic agonist), and vesnarinone (an agent with multiple mechanisms of action) have demonstrated substantial increases in mortality. Further development of potent positive inotropic agents for chronic oral therapy is unlikely. Some physicians use intermittent or even continuous home infusions of dobutamine or milrinone in patients with severe heart failure. However, neither the safety nor the efficacy of these approaches has been demonstrated. If employed at all, they should be reserved for patients awaiting cardiac transplantation.

I. Calcium Channel Blockers: First-generation Ca^{2+} blockers may accelerate the progression of congestive heart failure. However, two trials with amlodipine in patients with severe heart failure showed that this agent was safe, though not superior to placebo. These agents should be avoided unless they are being utilized to treat associated angina or hypertension, and for these indications amlodipine is the drug of choice.

J. Anticoagulation: Patients with severe left ventricular failure are prone to development of systemic arterial emboli, particularly when they are in atrial fibrillation, although in prospective studies, the approximately two per 100 patient years of follow-up has been less than many expected. While these may be catastrophic, the routine use of anticoagulants is controversial, since these patients have short life expectancies and are taking multiple medications that may interfere with optimal regulation of anticoagulation. Most experts prescribe anticoagulants only to appropriate patients who have had embolic episodes or those with atrial fibrillation. Some also anticoagulate patients with severe dilated cardiomyopathy (ejection fraction < 20%) in normal sinus rhythm.

K. Antiarrhythmic Therapy: Patients with moderate to severe heart failure have a high incidence of both symptomatic and asymptomatic arrhythmias. Although fewer than 10% of patients have syncope or presyncope resulting from ventricular tachycardia, ambulatory monitoring reveals that up to 70% of patients have asymptomatic episodes of nonsustained ventricular tachycardia. These arrhythmias indicate a poor prognosis independent of the severity of left ventricular dysfunction, but many of the deaths are probably not arrhythmia-related. Beta-blockers, because of their marked favorable effect on prognosis in general and on the incidence of sudden death specifically, should be initiated in these as well as other heart failure patients. Several trials are addressing the question of whether amiodarone, the medication that appears to be both the most effective and least likely to be proarrhythmic, improves the prognosis in patients with frequent ventricular ectopia. Two large randomized controlled trials produced contradictory results, with one showing improved survival and the other no effect.

Patients with hemodynamically unstable ventricular arrhythmias or aborted sudden death require vigorous intervention. In general, if the patient has a reasonable life expectancy and stable, nonrefractory heart failure, an implantable defibrillator is the approach of choice (again in conjunction with beta blockade). There are not sufficient relevant data to make recommendations for the management of patients with asymptomatic nonsustained ventricular arrhythmias. Beta-blockers are the first line of therapy, but there is no evidence that antiarrhythmic drugs are beneficial, and they carry substantial risk (with the exception of amiodarone). Trials are ongoing that may elucidate the role of implantable defibrillators in this population.

L. Coronary Revascularization: Since underlying coronary artery disease is the cause of heart failure in the majority of patients, coronary revascularization may both improve symptoms and prevent progression. However, trials have not been performed in patients whose major symptom is heart failure. Nonetheless, patients with angina who are candidates for surgery should be evaluated for revascularization, usually by coronary angiography. Noninvasive testing for ischemic but viable myocardium may be a more appropriate first step in patients with known coronary disease but no current clinical evidence of ischemia. The benefit of evaluating patients with heart failure of new onset without angina or prior myocardial infarction is limited. In general, bypass surgery is preferable to PTCA in the setting of heart failure because it provides more complete revascularization.

Case Management

Thirty to 50 percent of patients who are hospitalized will be readmitted within 3–6 months. Strategies to prevent clinical deterioration, such as case management, home monitoring of weight and clinical status, and patient adjustment of diuretics, can prevent rehospitalizations and should be part of the treatment regimen of advanced heart failure.

Cardiac Transplantation

Because of the outlook in patients with advanced heart failure, cardiac transplantation has become widely used. Since the advent of cyclosporine immunosuppressive therapy and more careful screening of donor hearts, the survival of patients after cardiac transplantation has increased considerably. Many centers now have 1-year survival rates exceeding 80–90%, and 5-year survival rates above 70%. Infections, hypertension and renal dysfunction caused by cyclosporine, rapidly progressive coronary atherosclerosis, and immunosuppressant-related cancers have been the major complications. The high cost and limited number of donor organs require careful patient selection early in the course.

Other Surgical Treatment Options

Several surgical procedures for severe heart failure have received considerable publicity. Cardiomyoplasty is a procedure in which the latissimus dorsi muscle is wrapped around the heart and stimulated to contract synchronously with it. In ventricular reduction surgery, a large part of the anterolateral wall is resected to make the heart function more efficiently. Both procedures are too risky to perform in end-stage patients and have not been shown to improve prognosis or symptoms in controlled studies. Externally powered and implantable ventricular assist devices can be used in patients who require ventricular support either to allow the heart to recover or as a bridge to transplantation. The latest generation devices are small enough to allow patients unrestricted mobility and even discharge from the hospital. However, complications are frequent, including bleeding, thromboembolism, and infection, and the cost is very high, exceeding $150,000 in the initial 1–3 months.

Prognosis

Despite advances in treatment of patients with congestive heart failure, their prognosis remains poor, with annual mortality rates ranging from 5% in stable patients with mild symptoms to 30–50% in patients with advanced, progressive symptoms. Poorer prognosis is associated with severe left ventricular dysfunction (ejection fractions < 20%), prominent symptoms and limitation of exercise capacity (maximal oxygen consumption < 10 mL/kg/min), secondary renal insufficiency, hyponatremia, and elevated plasma catecholamine levels. About 40–50% of deaths in heart failure patients are sudden. Although many of these are due to ventricular arrhythmias, many others are the result of undiagnosed acute myocardial infarction or bradyarrhythmias. The remainder of deaths are due to progressive heart failure or comorbid conditions. Patients who develop end-stage heart failure may suffer severe dyspnea and require meticulous efforts at palliative care (see Chapter 5).

ACC/AHA Guidelines for the management of heart failure. J Am Coll Cardiol 1995;26:1396.

Brater DC: Diuretic therapy. N Engl J Med 1998;339:387. [NLM Cit ID: 98346823] (A clear presentation of pharmacology, with a focus on diuretic resistance.)

CIBIS-II Investigators: The cardiac insufficiency bisoprolol study II (CIBIS-II): A randomised trial. Lancet 1999;

353:9. [NLM Cit ID: 99146548] (Multicenter trial of 2647 patients with stable congestive heart failure demonstrates reduced mortality with bisoprolol.)

Frishman WH: Carvedilol. N Engl J Med 1998;339:1759. [NLM Cit ID: 99049890]

Gheorghiade M et al: Current medical therapy for advanced heart failure. Am Heart J 1998;135(6 Part 2 Suppl):S231. [NLM Cit ID: 98292040]

Goldstein DJ et al: Implantable left ventricular assist devices. N Engl J Med 1998;339:1522. [NLM Cit ID: 99025352] (Historical review, indications, complications, and future direction of these important devices used as a bridge to transplant.)

Hauptman PJ et al: Digitalis. Circulation 1999;99:1265. [NLM Cit ID: 99169054] (Review of the molecular and clinical pharmacology and focus on Digoxin Investigation Group data set still warrants the use of this drug in patients with heart failure.)

Hunt SA et al: Mechanical circulatory support and cardiac transplantation. Circulation 1998;97:2079. [NLM Cit ID: 98272071] (Review of currently available cardiac assist devices and summary of clinical experience with each. Selection, management, and alternatives to transplantation discussed.)

Hunt SA: Current status of cardiac transplantation. JAMA 1998;280:1692. [NLM Cit ID: 99048842] (Indications, patient selection, surgical technique, and immunosuppression are reviewed. Early and late limitations are outlined. Improved immunosuppression and better mechanical assist devices will improve future therapy.)

Massie BM: 15 years of heart-failure trials: What have we learned? Lancet 1998;352(Suppl 1):29. [NLM Cit ID: 98405884] (Brief review of all major clinical trials of vasodilators, ACE inhibitors, inotropes, and beta-blockers.)

McKelvie RS et al: Comparison of candesartan, enalapril, and their combination in congestive heart failure: randomized evaluation of strategies for left ventricular dysfunction (RESOLVD) pilot study. The RESOLVD Pilot Study Investigators. Circulation 1999;100:1056. [NLM Cit ID: 99406590] (In a randomized trial comparing candesartan, enalapril, and candesartan plus enalapril, the combination of both drugs resulted in greater improvements in aldosterone levels, left-ventricular ejection fraction, and end-diastolic volume than either drug alone. The other two drugs were comparable in safety and efficacy. There was no difference in quality of life, 6-minute walk, and NYHA functional class among the groups.)

MERIT-HF Study Group: Effect of metoprolol CR/XL in chronic heart failure: metoprolol CR/XL randomised intervention trial in congestive heart failure (MERIT-HF). Lancet 1999;353:2001. [NLM Cit ID: 99303107] (Study of nearly 4000 patients with congestive heart failure was stopped early because of reduction in all-cause mortality with metoprolol. This included reduction in sudden death and death from progressive heart failure.)

Myers J et al: Clinical, hemodynamic, and cardiopulmonary exercise test determinants of survival in patients referred for evaluation of heart failure. Ann Intern Med 1998;129:286. [NLM Cit ID: 98382169] (After 4 years of follow-up, actuarial survival was 73.4%; coronary artery disease was a strong determinant of death, and peak oxygen consumption was the variable that best predicted survival.)

Packer M et al: Consensus recommendations for the management of chronic heart failure. Am J Cardiol 1999;83:2A. [NLM Cit ID: 99170467] (Series of articles summarizing steering committee recommendations for evaluation and management of heart failure.)

Pitt B et al: Randomised trial of losartan versus captopril in patients over 65 with heart failure (Evaluation of Losartan in the Elderly Study, ELITE). Lancet 1997;349:747. [NLM Cit ID: 97228494] (In this randomized trial, patients treated with losartan had a lower mortality than patients treated with captopril. Losartan was tolerated better, as well.)

Pitt B et al: The effect of spironolactone on morbidity and mortality in patients with severe heart failure. Randomized Aldactone Evaluation Study Investigators. N Engl J Med 1999;341:709. [NLM Cit ID: 99383620] (In this randomized trial of over 1600 patients with severe congestive heart failure, spironolactone added to standard therapy for congestive heart failure resulted in a 30% decrease in mortality attributed to reductions in both sudden death and progression of heart failure. Morbidity was also decreased among patients treated with spironolactone. The effect was so pronounced that the trial was stopped after only 24 months of follow-up.)

Uretsky BF et al: Primary prevention of sudden cardiac death in heart failure: Will the solution be shocking? J Am Coll Cardiol 1997;30:1589. [NLM Cit ID: 94074106] (Review of drug trials with suggestion that implantable defibrillators will play a growing role.)

ACUTE PULMONARY EDEMA

Essentials of Diagnosis

- Acute onset or worsening of dyspnea at rest.
- Tachycardia, diaphoresis, cyanosis.
- Pulmonary rales, rhonchi; expiratory wheezing.
- X-ray shows interstitial and alveolar edema with or without cardiomegaly.
- Arterial hypoxemia.

General Considerations

Typical causes of cardiogenic pulmonary edema include acute myocardial infarction or severe ischemia, exacerbation of chronic heart failure, acute volume overload of the left ventricle (valvular regurgitation or ventricular septal defect), and mitral stenosis.

Clinical Findings

Acute pulmonary edema presents with a characteristic clinical picture of severe dyspnea, the production of pink, frothy sputum, and diaphoresis and cyanosis. Rales are present in all lung fields, as are generalized wheezing and rhonchi. Pulmonary edema may appear suddenly in the setting of chronic heart failure or may be the first manifestation of cardiac disease, usually acute myocardial infarction, which may be painful or silent.

A number of noncardiac conditions can also produce pulmonary edema. This occurs either because of imbalance in the Starling forces (either a decrease in plasma proteins or an increase in pulmonary venous pressure) or a functional or anatomic abnormality of the alveolar-capillary membrane. Causes include intravenous narcotics, increased intracerebral pressure, high altitude, sepsis, several medications, inhaled toxins, transfusion reactions, shock, and disseminated intravascular coagulation. These are distinguished from cardiogenic pulmonary edema by the clinical setting, the history, and the physical examination. Conversely, in most patients with cardiogenic pulmonary edema, an underlying cardiac abnormality can usually be detected clinically or by the ECG, chest x-ray, or echocardiogram.

The chest radiograph reveals signs of pulmonary vascular redistribution, blurriness of vascular outlines, increased interstitial markings, and, characteristically, the butterfly pattern of distribution of alveolar edema. The heart may be enlarged or normal in size depending on whether heart failure was previously present. Assessment of cardiac function by echocardiography or right heart catheterization is helpful in determining the cause. In cardiogenic pulmonary edema, the pulmonary capillary wedge pressure is invariably elevated, usually over 25 mm Hg. In noncardiogenic pulmonary edema, the wedge pressure may be normal or even low.

Treatment

The patient should be placed in a sitting position with legs dangling over the side of the bed; this facilitates respiration and reduces venous return. Oxygen is delivered by mask to obtain an arterial PO_2 greater than 60 mm Hg. Noninvasive pressure support ventilation may improve oxygenation and prevent severe CO_2 retention while pharmacologic interventions take effect. However, if respiratory distress remains severe, endotracheal intubation and mechanical ventilation may be necessary.

Morphine is highly effective in pulmonary edema. The initial dosage is 4–8 mg intravenously (subcutaneous administration is effective in milder cases) and may be repeated after 2–4 hours. Morphine increases venous capacitance, lowering left atrial pressure, and relieves anxiety, which can reduce the efficiency of ventilation. However, morphine may lead to CO_2 retention by reducing the ventilatory drive. It should be avoided in patients with narcotic-induced pulmonary edema, who may improve with narcotic antagonists, and in those with neurogenic pulmonary edema.

Intravenous diuretic therapy (furosemide, 40 mg, or bumetanide, 1 mg—or higher doses if the patient has been receiving chronic diuretic therapy) is usually indicated even if the patient has not exhibited prior fluid retention. These agents produce venodilation prior to the onset of diuresis. Other measures to help reduce left ventricular preload consist of the administration of sublingual or intravenous nitrates and phlebotomy of approximately 500 mL of blood or plasmapheresis. Bronchospasm may occur in response to pulmonary edema and may itself exacerbate hypoxemia and dyspnea. Treatment with inhaled beta-adrenergic agonists or intravenous aminophylline may be helpful, but both may also provoke tachycardia and supraventricular arrhythmias. Particularly in patients with elevated arterial pressures, vasodilators such as intravenous nitroprusside may be worthwhile. In patients with low-output states, particularly when hypotension is present, positive inotropic agents are indicated. These approaches to treatment have been discussed previously.

Sacchetti AD et al: Acute cardiogenic pulmonary edema. What's the latest in emergency treatment? Postgrad Med 1998;103:145. [NLM Cit ID: 98139851] (Clinical examples illustrate the use of drugs and noninvasive ventilatory support to treat acute pulmonary edema.)

MYOCARDITIS & THE CARDIOMYOPATHIES

ACUTE MYOCARDITIS

Acute myocarditis causes focal or diffuse inflammation of the myocardium. Most cases are infectious, caused by viral, bacterial, rickettsial, spirochetal, fungal, or parasitic agents; but toxins, drugs, and immunologic disorders can also cause myocarditis.

1. INFECTIOUS MYOCARDITIS

Essentials of Diagnosis

- Often follows an upper respiratory infection.
- May present with chest pain (pleuritic or nonspecific) or signs of heart failure.
- ECG may show sinus tachycardia, other arrhythmias, nonspecific repolarization changes, intraventricular conduction abnormalities.
- Echocardiogram documents cardiomegaly and contractile dysfunction.
- Myocardial biopsy, though not sensitive, may reveal a characteristic inflammatory pattern.

General Considerations

Viral myocarditis is the most common form and is usually caused by coxsackieviruses, but a host of other agents have also been responsible. Rickettsial myocarditis occurs with scrub typhus, Rocky Mountain spotted fever, and Q fever. Diphtheritic myocarditis is caused by the exotoxin and often is manifested by conduction abnormalities as well as heart failure.

Chagas' disease, caused by the insect-borne protozoan *Trypanosoma cruzi,* is a common form of myocarditis in Central and South America; the major clinical manifestations appear after a latent period of more than a decade. At this stage, patients present with cardiomyopathy, conduction disturbances, and sudden death. Associated gastrointestinal involvement (megaesophagus and megacolon) is the rule. Toxoplasmosis causes myocarditis that is usually asymptomatic but can lead to heart failure. Among parasitic infections, trichinosis is the most common cause of cardiac involvement. The potential for the HIV virus to cause myocarditis is now well recognized, though the prevalence of this complication is not known. In addition, other infectious myocarditides are more common in patients with AIDS.

Giant cell myocarditis is a rare idiopathic disorder characterized by giant cell and lymphocyte infiltration of the heart muscle. Patients usually die from ventricular arrhythmias or heart failure but occasionally respond to immunosuppressive therapy or early transplantation.

Clinical Findings

A. Symptoms and Signs: Patients may present several days to a few weeks after the onset of an acute febrile illness or a respiratory infection or with heart failure without antecedent symptoms. Pleural-pericardial chest pain is common. Examination reveals tachycardia, gallop rhythm, and other evidence of heart failure or conduction defect.

B. Electrocardiography and Chest X-Ray: Nonspecific ST–T changes and conduction disturbances are common. Ventricular ectopy may be the initial and only clinical finding. Chest x-ray is nonspecific, but cardiomegaly is frequent.

C. Diagnostic Studies: Echocardiography provides the most convenient way of evaluating cardiac function and can exclude many other processes. Gallium-67 scintigraphy has been reported to yield cardiac uptake in acute or subacute myocarditis. Paired serum viral titers and serologic tests for other agents may indicate the cause.

D. Endomyocardial Biopsy: Pathologic examinations may reveal a round cell inflammatory response with necrosis, but the patchy distribution of abnormalities makes the test relatively insensitive. This picture defines an "active" inflammatory stage and may persist for many months.

Treatment & Prognosis

Specific antimicrobial therapy is indicated when an infecting agent is identified. Immunosuppressive therapy with corticosteroids and other agents have been felt by some to improve the outcome when the process is acute (< 6 months) and if the biopsy suggests ongoing inflammation. However, controlled trials have not been positive, so the value of routine myocardial biopsies in patients presenting with an acute myocarditic picture is uncertain; immunosuppressive therapy without histologic confirmation is unwise. Otherwise, treatment is directed toward the manifestations of heart failure and arrhythmias.

Many cases resolve spontaneously, but in others cardiac function deteriorates progressively and may lead to dilated cardiomyopathy. Many cases of dilated cardiomyopathy may represent the end stage of viral myocarditis.

Cooper LT et al: Idiopathic giant-cell myocarditis: Natural history and treatment. N Engl J Med 1997;336:1860. [NLM Cit ID: 97324062]

Garg A et al: The ineffectiveness of immunosuppressive therapy in lymphocytic myocarditis: An overview. Ann Intern Med 1998;129:317. [NLM Cit ID: 98382174] (Prednisone, either alone or in combination with azathioprine or cyclosporine, did not improve survival or left ventricular function in patients with biopsy-proved lymphocytic myocarditis.)

Hager JM et al: Chagas' heart disease. Curr Probl Cardiol 1995;20:825. [NLM Cit ID: 96192409]

Kawai C: From myocarditis to cardiomyopathy: mechanisms of inflammation and cell death: learning from the past for the future. Circulation 1999;99:1091. [NLM Cit ID: 99160517] (This review summarizes clinical and experimental studies underlying viral pathogenesis of acute myocarditis and progression to dilated cardiomyopathy. Immunosuppressive and immunomodulating treatments may hold promise.)

McCarthy RE et al: Long-term outcome of fulminant myocarditis as compared with acute nonfulminant myocarditis. N Engl J Med 2000;342:690. [NLM Cit ID: 20155737] (Surprisingly, patients with acute myocarditis with rapid onset of symptoms and severe hemodynamic compromise fare better than those without such a dramatic presentation.)

Pisani B et al: Inflammatory myocardial diseases and cardiomyopathies. Am J Med 1997;102:459. [NLM Cit ID: 97360679] (Comprehensive review, including discussion of immunosuppressive therapy.)

Rerkpattanapipat P et al: Cardiac manifestations of acquired immunodeficiency syndrome. Arch Intern Med 2000; 160;602. [NLM Cit ID: 20186612] (Review of diverse presentations, including myocarditis, cardiomyopathy, and pericarditis.)

2. DRUG-INDUCED & TOXIC MYOCARDITIS

A variety of medications, illicit drugs, and toxic substances can produce acute or chronic myocardial injury; the clinical presentation varies widely. Doxorubicin and other cytotoxic agents, emetine, and catecholamines (especially with pheochromocytoma) can produce a pathologic picture of inflammation and necrosis together with clinical heart failure and arrhythmias; toxicity of the first two is dose-related. The phenothiazines, lithium, chloroquine, disopyramide, antimony-containing compounds, and arsenicals can also cause electrocardiographic changes, arrhythmias, or heart failure. Hypersensitivity reactions to sulfonamides, penicillins, and aminosalicylic acid as well as other drugs can result in cardiac dysfunction. Radiation can cause an acute inflammatory reaction as well as a chronic fibrosis of heart muscle, usually in conjunction with pericarditis.

The incidence of cocaine cardiotoxicity has increased markedly. Cocaine can cause coronary artery spasm, myocardial infarction, arrhythmias, and myocarditis. Because many of these processes are believed to be mediated by cocaine's inhibitory effect on norepinephrine reuptake by sympathetic nerves, beta-blockers have been used therapeutically. In coronary spasm, calcium channel blockers are more appropriate.

Chakko S et al: Cardiac complications of cocaine abuse. Clin Cardiol 1995;18:67. [NLM Cit ID: 95236697]

Frishman WH et al: Cardiovascular toxicity with cancer chemotherapy. Curr Probl Cardiol 1996;21:227. [NLM Cit ID: 96282241]

Singal PK et al: Doxorubicin-induced cardiomyopathy. N Engl J Med 1998;339:900. [NLM Cit ID: 98414375] (Mechanism, diagnosis, prevention, and treatment.)

THE CARDIOMYOPATHIES

The cardiomyopathies are a heterogeneous group of entities affecting the myocardium primarily and not associated with the major causes of cardiac disease, ie, ischemic heart disease, hypertension, valvular disease, or congenital defects. While some have specific causes, many cases are idiopathic. There is now general agreement on a classification based upon general features of presentation and pathophysiology (Table 10–6).

Eichhorn EJ (editor): New insights into dilated cardiomyopathy. Cardiol Clin 1998;16:603. (Monograph with articles on etiology, genetics, mechanisms of progression, and medical and surgical therapy.)

Richardson P et al: Report of the 1995 World Health Organization/International Society and Federation of Cardiology Task Force on the Definition and Classification of Cardiomyopathies. Circulation 1996;93:841. [NLM Cit ID: 96179010]

Role of Myocardial Biopsy

The indications for this procedure remain controversial, but it is essential for the early detection of transplant rejection. Biopsies have also been helpful in distinguishing restrictive cardiomyopathy from pericardial constriction, an often difficult problem. Occasionally, a specific diagnosis of amyloidosis, sarcoidosis, hemochromatosis, or an unusual infection can be made, but in most cases these conditions are suggested by other cardiac or systemic findings. Biopsies can reveal evidence of acute myocarditis and, if immunosuppressive therapy is contemplated, should be performed in appropriate patients.

1. PRIMARY DILATED CARDIOMYOPATHY

Essentials of Diagnosis

- Symptoms and signs of heart failure.
- ECG may show low QRS voltage, nonspecific repolarization abnormalities, intraventricular conduction abnormalities.

Table 10–6. Classification of the cardiomyopathies.

	Dilated	Hypertrophic	Restrictive
Frequent causes	Idiopathic, alcoholic, myocarditis, postpartum, doxorubicin, endocrinopathies, genetic diseases	Hereditary syndrome, possibly chronic hypertension	Amyloidosis, post radiation, post open heart surgery, diabetes, endomyocardial fibrosis
Symptoms	Left or biventricular congestive heart failure	Dyspnea, chest pain, syncope	Dyspnea, fatigue, right-sided congestive heart failure
Physical examination	Cardiomegaly, S_3, elevated jugular venous pressure, rales	Sustained point of maximal impulse, S_4, variable systolic murmur, bisferiens carotid pulse	Elevated jugular venous pressure, Kussmaul's sign
ECG	ST–T changes, conduction abnormalities, ventricular ectopy	Left ventricular hypertrophy, exaggerated septal Q waves	ST–T changes, conduction abnormalities, low voltage
Chest x-ray	Enlarged heart, pulmonary congestion	Mild cardiomegaly	Mild to moderate cardiomegaly
Echocardiogram, nuclear studies	Left ventricular dilation and dysfunction	Left ventricular hypertrophy, asymmetric septal hypertrophy, small left ventricular size, normal or supranormal function, systolic anterior mitral motion, diastolic dysfunction	Small or normal left ventricular size, normal or mildly reduced left ventricular function
Cardiac catheterization	Left ventricular dilation and dysfunction, high diastolic pressures, low cardiac output	Small, hypercontractile left ventricle, dynamic outflow gradient, diastolic dysfunction	High diastolic pressure, "square root" sign, normal or mildly reduced left ventricular function

- X-ray shows cardiomegaly.
- Echocardiogram confirms left ventricular dilation, thinning, and global dysfunction.

General Considerations

Dilated cardiomyopathies usually present with symptoms and signs of congestive heart failure (most commonly dyspnea). Occasionally, symptomatic ventricular arrhythmias are the presenting event. Left ventricular dilation and systolic dysfunction are essential for diagnosis. Often no cause can be identified, but chronic alcohol abuse and myocarditis are probably frequent causes. Histologically, the picture is one of extensive fibrosis.

Clinical Findings

A. Symptoms and Signs: In most patients, symptoms of heart failure develop gradually. They may be recognized because of asymptomatic cardiomegaly or electrocardiographic abnormalities, including arrhythmias. The initial presentation may be severe biventricular failure. The physical examination reveals cardiomegaly, S_3 gallop rhythm, and often a murmur of functional mitral regurgitation. Signs of left- and right-sided failure may be present on initial examination, a clue to a process involving the heart diffusely.

B. Electrocardiography and Chest X-Ray: The major findings are listed in Table 10–6.

C. Diagnostic Studies: An echocardiogram is indicated to exclude unsuspected valvular or other lesions and confirm the presence of dilated cardiomyopathy. Exercise thallium-201 scintigraphy may suggest the possibility of underlying coronary disease if a large reversible defect is found, but false-positives occur in cardiomyopathy. Cardiac catheterization is seldom of specific value unless myocardial ischemia or left ventricular aneurysm is suspected. The serum ferritin is an adequate screening study for hemochromatosis.

Treatment

Few cases of cardiomyopathy are amenable to specific therapy. Alcohol use should be discontinued. There is often marked recovery of cardiac function following a period of abstinence in alcoholic cardiomyopathy. Endocrine causes (thyroid dysfunction, acromegaly, pheochromocytoma) should be treated. Immunosuppressive therapy is not indicated in chronic dilated cardiomyopathy. The management of congestive heart failure is outlined in the section on heart failure.

Prognosis

The prognosis of dilated cardiomyopathy without clinical heart failure is variable, with some patients remaining stable, some deteriorating gradually, and others declining rapidly. Once heart failure is manifest, the natural history is similar to that of other causes of heart failure. Arterial and pulmonary emboli are more common in dilated cardiomyopathy than in ischemic cardiomyopathy; suitable candidates may benefit from chronic anticoagulation. Those patients whose disease progresses may require treatment for severe dyspnea (see above) and ultimately need high-quality palliative care (see Chapter 5).

Felker GM et al: Underlying causes and long-term survival in patients with initially unexplained cardiomyopathy. N Engl J Med 2000;342:1077. [NLM Cit ID: 20205681] (Series of 1230 patients with cardiomyopathy who underwent extensive work-up, including coronary angiography and endomyocardial biopsy, showing that the prognosis varies with the underlying cause.)

Koniaris LS et al: Anticoagulation in dilated cardiomyopathy. J Am Coll Cardiol 1998;31:745. [NLM Cit ID: 98184453] (A summary of the widely varying literature on the risk of thromboembolism in dilated cardiomyopathy and the subsequent benefit of anticoagulation. Still an unresolved issue.)

Leiden JM: The genetics of dilated cardiomyopathy—emerging clues to the puzzle. N Engl J Med 1997; 337:1080. [NLM Cit ID: 97449079] (Genes that encode structural proteins and transcription factors have been identified in patients with dilated cardiomyopathy.)

2. HYPERTROPHIC CARDIOMYOPATHY

Essentials of Diagnosis

- May present with dyspnea, chest pain, syncope.
- Examination shows sustained apical impulse, S_4, systolic ejection murmur.
- ECG shows left ventricular hypertrophy, occasionally septal Q waves in the absence of infarction.
- Echocardiogram shows hypertrophy, which may be asymmetric; usually shows normal or enhanced contractility and signs of dynamic obstruction.

General Considerations

Myocardial hypertrophy unrelated to any pressure or volume overload tends to impinge upon the left ventricular cavity. The interventricular septum may be disproportionately involved (asymmetric septal hypertrophy), but in some cases the hypertrophy is localized to the apex. The left ventricular outflow tract is often narrowed during systole between the bulging septum and an anteriorly displaced anterior mitral valve leaflet, causing a dynamic obstruction (hence the name idiopathic hypertrophic subaortic stenosis; IHSS). The obstruction is worsened by factors that increase myocardial contractility (sympathetic stimulation, digoxin, postextrasystolic beat) or that decrease left ventricular filling (Valsalva's maneuver, peripheral vasodilators).

Hypertrophic cardiomyopathy is in some cases inherited as an autosomal dominant trait with variable penetrance caused by mutations of a number of genes, most of which code for myosin heavy chains or proteins regulating calcium handling. It is becoming clear that the prognosis is related to the specific gene mutation. These patients usually present in early adulthood. Others are elderly, and many of those patients have a long history of hypertension. Some cases occur sporadically.

Except in late stages, hypertrophic cardiomyopathy is characterized by a small, hypercontractile left ventricle. Although dyspnea is a common symptom, it results mainly from markedly impaired diastolic compliance rather than systolic dysfunction or outflow obstruction.

Clinical Findings

A. Symptoms and Signs: The most frequent symptoms are dyspnea and chest pain. Syncope is also common and is typically postexertional, when diastolic filling diminishes and outflow obstruction increases. Arrhythmias are an important problem. Atrial fibrillation is a long-term consequence of chronically elevated left atrial pressures and is a poor prognostic sign. Ventricular arrhythmias are also common, and sudden death may occur, often in athletes after extraordinary exertion.

Features on physical examination are a bisferiens carotid pulse, triple apical impulse (due to the prominent atrial filling wave and early and late systolic impulses), and a loud S_4. In cases with outflow obstruction, a loud systolic murmur is present that increases with upright posture or Valsalva's maneuver and decreases with squatting.

B. Electrocardiography and Chest X-Ray: Left ventricular hypertrophy is nearly universal. Exaggerated septal Q waves inferolaterally may suggest myocardial infarction. The chest x-ray is often unimpressive.

C. Diagnostic Studies: The echocardiogram is diagnostic, revealing asymmetric left ventricular hypertrophy, systolic anterior motion of the mitral valve, early closing followed by reopening of the aortic valve, a small and hypercontractile left ventricle, and delayed relaxation and filling of the left ventricle during diastole. Doppler ultrasound reveals turbulent flow and a dynamic gradient across the aortic valve and, commonly, mitral regurgitation. Cardiac catheterization may confirm the gradient but adds little to echocardiographic studies.

Treatment

Beta-blockers should be the initial drug in symptomatic individuals, especially when dynamic outflow obstruction is noted on the echocardiogram. Dyspnea, angina, and arrhythmias respond in about 50% of patients. Calcium channel blockers, especially verapamil, have also been effective in symptomatic patients. Their effect may be due primarily to improved diastolic function, but their vasodilating actions may also increase outflow obstruction. Excision of part of the myocardial septum has been successful in patients with severe symptoms when performed by surgeons experienced with the procedure. Dual-chamber pacing may prevent the progression of hypertrophy and obstruction. Nonsurgical septal ablation has been performed by injection of alcohol into septal branches of the left coronary artery. Patients with malignant ventricular arrhythmias and unexplained syncope in the presence of a positive family history for sudden death are probably best managed with an implantable defibrillator.

Prognosis

The natural history of hypertrophic cardiomyopathy is highly variable. Several specific mutations are associated with a higher incidence of early malignant arrhythmias and sudden death, and definition of the genetic abnormality provides the best estimate of prognosis. Some patients remain asymptomatic for many years or for life. Sudden death, especially during exercise, may be the initial event. Indeed, hypertrophic cardiomyopathy is the pathologic feature most frequently associated with sudden death in athletes. Other patients have a history of gradually progressive symptoms. A final stage may be a transition into dilated cardiomyopathy.

Erwin JP et al: Dual chamber pacing for patients with hypertrophic obstructive cardiomyopathy. Mayo Clin Proc 2000;75:173. [NLM Cit ID: 20147281] (Little objective evidence of benefit, although some patients report improvement.)

Maron BJ et al: Assessment of permanent dual-chamber pacing as a treatment for drug-refractory symptomatic patients with obstructive hypertrophic cardiomyopathy. Circulation 1999;99:2927. [NLM Cit ID: 99289698] (This multicenter study of 48 patients failed to show consistent improvement in symptoms or outflow tract gradient demonstrated in previous trails and does not recommend pacing as primary therapy.)

Maron BJ et al: Efficacy of implantable cardioverter-defibrillators for the prevention of sudden death in patients with hypertrophic cardiomyopathy. N Engl J Med 2000;342:365. [NLM Cit ID: 20116951] (Ventricular tachycardia and ventricular fibrillation are the primary mechanisms of sudden death in patients with hypertrophic cardiomyopathy, and implantable cardioverter-defibrillators are effective for their treatment.)

Maron BJ: Hypertrophic cardiomyopathy. Lancet 1997; 350:127. [NLM Cit ID: 97372921]

Spirito P et al: The management of hypertrophic cardiomyopathy. N Engl J Med 1997;336:775. [NLM Cit ID: 97201372] (Review covering medical management and surgical intervention but with a particular focus on genetic mechanisms.)

Spirito P et al: Perspectives on the role of new treatment strategies in hypertrophic obstructive cardiomyopathy. J Am Coll Cardiol 1999;33:1071. [NLM Cit ID: 99190259] (A review of the natural history and pathophysiology of hypertrophic cardiomyopathy suggests that ethanol septal ablation and dual chamber pacing may be overutilized.)

3. RESTRICTIVE CARDIOMYOPATHY

Restrictive cardiomyopathy is characterized by impaired diastolic filling with preserved contractile function. This condition is relatively uncommon, with the most frequent causes being amyloidosis, radiation, and myocardial fibrosis after open heart surgery. In Africa, endomyocardial fibrosis, a specific entity in which there is severe fibrosis of the endocardium, often with eosinophilia (Löffler's syndrome) is common. Other causes of a restrictive picture are infiltrative cardiomyopathies (eg, sarcoidosis, hemochromatosis, carcinoid syndrome) and connective tissue diseases (eg, scleroderma).

Amyloidosis can affect the heart in several ways. Although it is a frequent cause of restrictive cardiomyopathy, it more often produces dilated cardiomyopathy with congestive heart failure. Almost invariably, conduction disturbances are present. Low voltages on the ECG combined with ventricular hypertrophy by echo are suggestive. Rectal, abdominal fat, or gingival biopsies—as well as myocardial biopsy—can be diagnostic.

The primary diagnostic problem with restrictive cardiomyopathy is differentiation from constrictive pericarditis. The clinical picture often strongly suggests the diagnosis, but the status of left ventricular function (usually normal with pericarditis, slightly depressed with restrictive cardiomyopathy) can be helpful, as can be evidence of a thickened pericardium. Myocardial biopsies are usually negative with pericarditis but not in restrictive cardiomyopathy. In some cases, only surgical exploration can make the diagnosis.

Unfortunately, little useful therapy is available for either the causative conditions or restrictive cardiomyopathy itself. Diuretics can help, but excessive diuresis can produce worsening symptoms. Steroids may be helpful in sarcoidosis but relieve conduction abnormalities more often than heart failure.

Falk RH et al: The systemic amyloidoses. N Engl J Med 1997;337:898. [NLM Cit ID: 97433009] (Review of most frequent cause of restrictive cardiomyopathy.)

Kushwaha SS et al: Restrictive cardiomyopathy. N Engl J Med 1997;336:267. [NLM Cit ID: 97136544] (Pathogenesis, diagnosis, and treatment of the diverse causes of restrictive cardiomyopathy.)

ACUTE RHEUMATIC FEVER & RHEUMATIC HEART DISEASE

Essentials of Diagnosis

- Uncommon in USA but may be overlooked.
- Peak incidence ages 5–15 years.
- Diagnosis based on Jones criteria and confirmation of streptococcal infection.
- May involve mitral and other valves acutely, rarely leading to heart failure.

General Considerations

Rheumatic fever is a systemic immune process which is a sequela to hemolytic streptococcal infection of the pharynx. Pyodermic infections are not associated with rheumatic fever. Signs of rheumatic fever usually commence 2–3 weeks after infection but may appear as early as 1 week or as late as 5 weeks. It had become quite uncommon in the USA, except in recent immigrants. However, there have been recent reports of new outbreaks in several regions of the USA. The peak incidence is between ages 5 and 15; rheumatic fever is rare before age 4 and after age 40. Rheumatic carditis and valvulitis may be self-limited or may lead to slowly progressive valvular deformity. The characteristic lesion is a perivascular granulomatous reaction with vasculitis. The mitral valve is attacked in 75–80% of cases, the aortic valve in 30% (but rarely as the sole valve), and the tricuspid and pulmonary valves in under 5%.

Clinical Findings

Diagnostic criteria first described by Jones are still employed. The presence of two major criteria—or one major and two minor criteria—establishes the diagnosis.

A. Major Criteria:

1. Carditis–Carditis is most likely to be evident in children and adolescents. Any of the following suggests the presence of carditis. (1) Pericarditis. (2) Cardiomegaly, detected by physical signs, radiography, or echocardiography. (3) Congestive failure, right- or left-sided—the former perhaps more prominent in children, with painful liver engorgement due to tricuspid regurgitation. (4) Mitral or aortic regurgitation murmurs, indicative of dilation of a valve ring with or without associated valvulitis. The Carey-Coombs short middiastolic mitral murmur may be present.

In the absence of any of the above definitive signs, the diagnosis of carditis depends upon the following less specific abnormalities. (1) Electrocardiographic changes: The most significant abnormality is PR prolongation greater than 0.04 s above the patient's normal. Changing contour of P waves or inversion of T waves is less useful. (2) Changing quality of heart sounds. (3) Sinus tachycardia persisting during sleep and markedly increased by slight activity. (4) Arrhythmias, shifting pacemaker, or ectopic beats.

2. Erythema marginatum and subcutaneous nodules–The former begin as rapidly enlarging macules that assume the shape of rings or crescents with clear centers. They may be raised, confluent, and either transient or persistent.

Subcutaneous nodules are uncommon except in children. They are small (≤ 2 cm in diameter), firm, and nontender and are attached to fascia or tendon sheaths over bony prominences. They persist for days or weeks, are recurrent, and are indistinguishable from rheumatoid nodules.

3. Sydenham's chorea–Sydenham's chorea—involuntary choreoathetoid movements primarily of the face, tongue, and upper extremities—may be the sole manifestation; only half of cases have other overt signs of rheumatic fever. Girls are more frequently affected, and occurrence in adults is rare. This is the least common (3% of cases) but most diagnostic of the manifestations of rheumatic fever.

4. Arthritis–This is a migratory polyarthritis that involves the large joints sequentially. In adults, only a single joint may be affected. The arthritis lasts 1–5 weeks and subsides without residual deformity. Prompt response of arthritis to therapeutic doses of salicylates or nonsteroidal agents is characteristic.

B. Minor Criteria: These include fever, polyarthralgias, reversible prolongation of the PR interval, rapid erythrocyte sedimentation rate, and evidence of an antecedent β-hemolytic streptococcal infection or a history of rheumatic fever.

C. Laboratory Findings: There is nonspecific evidence of inflammatory disease, as shown by a rapid sedimentation rate. High or increasing titers of antistreptococcal antibodies (antistreptolysin O and anti-DNAse B) are used to confirm recent infection; 10% of cases lack this serologic evidence.

Differential Diagnosis

Rheumatic fever may be confused with the following: rheumatoid arthritis, osteomyelitis, endocarditis, chronic meningococcemia, systemic lupus erythematosus, Lyme disease, sickle cell anemia, "surgical abdomen," and many other diseases.

Complications

Congestive heart failure occurs in severe cases. In the longer term, the development of rheumatic heart disease is the major problem. Other complications include arrhythmias, pericarditis with effusion, and rheumatic pneumonitis.

Treatment

A. General Measures: The patient should be kept at strict bed rest until the temperature returns to normal without medications, the sedimentation rate is normal, the resting pulse rate is normal (< 100/min in adults); and the ECG has returned to baseline.

B. Medical Measures:

1. Salicylates–The salicylates markedly reduce fever and relieve joint pain and swelling. They have no effect on the natural course of the disease. Adults may require aspirin, 0.6–0.9 g every 4 hours; children are treated with lower doses. Toxicity includes tinnitus, vomiting, and gastrointestinal bleeding.

2. Penicillin–Penicillin (benzathine penicillin, 1.2 million units intramuscularly once, or procaine penicillin, 600,000 units intramuscularly daily for 10 days) is employed to eradicate streptococcal infection if present. Erythromycin may be substituted.

3. Corticosteroids–There is no proof that cardiac damage is prevented or minimized by corticosteroids. A short course of corticosteroids (prednisone, 40–60 mg orally daily, with tapering over 2 weeks) usually causes rapid improvement and is indicated when response to salicylates has been inadequate.

Prevention of Recurrent Rheumatic Fever

The initial episode of rheumatic fever can usually be prevented by early treatment of streptococcal pharyngitis. (See Chapter 33.) Prevention of recurrent episodes is critical. Recurrences of rheumatic fever are most common in patients who have had carditis during their initial episode and in children, 20% of whom will have a second episode within 5 years. Recurrences are uncommon after 5 years and infrequent in patients over 25 years of age. Prophylaxis is usually discontinued after these times except in groups with a high risk of streptococcal infection—parents of young children, nurses, military recruits, etc.

A. Penicillin: The preferred method of prophylaxis is with benzathine penicillin G, 1.2 million units intramuscularly every 4 weeks. Oral penicillin (200,000–250,000 units twice daily) is less reliable.

B. Sulfonamides or Erythromycin: If the patient is allergic to penicillin, sulfadiazine (or sulfisoxazole), 1 g daily, or erythromycin, 250 mg orally twice daily, may be substituted.

Prognosis

Initial episodes of rheumatic fever may last months in children and weeks in adults. The immediate mortality rate is 1–2%. Persistent rheumatic carditis with cardiomegaly, heart failure, and pericarditis imply a poor prognosis; 30% of children thus affected die within 10 years after the initial attack. Eighty percent of affected children attain adult life, and half of these have little if any limitation of activity. After 10 years, two-thirds of patients will have detectable valvular disease. In adults, residual heart damage occurs in less than 20%, with mitral regurgitation the commonest; aortic insufficiency is more common than in children. In developing countries, acute rheumatic fever appears earlier in life, and the evolution to chronic valvular disease is accelerated.

Narula J et al: Diagnosis of active rheumatic carditis. Circulation 1999;100:1576. [NLM Cit ID: 99439697] (Argues for the incorporation of echocardiographic data into the classic Jones criteria for diagnosis of rheumatic carditis.)

Stollerman GH: Rheumatic fever. Lancet 1997;349:935. [NLM Cit ID: 97247129] (Clinical manifestations, pathogenesis, changing epidemiology, and prevention.)

RHEUMATIC HEART DISEASE

Chronic rheumatic heart disease results from single or repeated attacks of rheumatic fever that produce rigidity and deformity of valve cusps, fusion of the commissures, or shortening and fusion of the chordae tendineae. Stenosis or insufficiency results, and the two often coexist. The mitral valve alone is affected in 50–60% of cases; combined lesions of the aortic and mitral valves occur in 20%; pure aortic lesions are less common. Tricuspid involvement occurs only in association with mitral or aortic disease in about 10% of cases. The pulmonary valve is rarely affected. A history of rheumatic fever is obtainable in only 60% of patients with rheumatic heart disease.

The first clue to organic valvular disease is a murmur. Physical examination permits accurate diagnosis of most valve lesions. Echocardiography will reveal valve cusp thickening with decreased opening in stenosis, estimate the magnitude of regurgitation, and demonstrate the earliest stages of specific chamber enlargement.

Recurrences of acute rheumatic fever can be prevented (see above). The patient should also receive prophylactic antibiotics preceding dental extraction, urologic and surgical procedures, etc, to prevent endocarditis (Table 33–4). With mitral valve disease, it is important to identify the onset of atrial fibrillation in order to institute anticoagulation. The important findings in each of the major valve lesions are summarized in Table 10–1. The hemodynamic changes, symptoms, associated findings, and course have been discussed previously.

DISEASES OF THE PERICARDIUM

ACUTE PERICARDITIS

The pericardium consists of two layers: the inner visceral layer, which is attached to the epicardium; and an outer parietal layer. The pericardium stabilizes the heart in anatomic position and reduces contact between the heart and surrounding structures. It is composed of fibrous tissue, and while it will permit moderate changes in cardiac size, it cannot stretch rapidly enough to accommodate rapid dilation of the heart or accumulation of fluid without increasing intrapericardial (and, therefore, intracardiac) pressure.

The pericardium is often involved by processes that affect the heart, but it may also be affected by diseases of adjacent tissues and may itself be a primary site of disease.

INFLAMMATORY PERICARDITIS

Acute inflammation of the pericardium may be infectious in origin or may be due to systemic diseases (autoimmune syndromes, uremia), neoplasm, radiation, drug toxicity, hemopericardium, or contiguous inflammatory processes in the myocardium or lung. In many of these conditions, the pathologic process involves both the pericardium and the myocardium.

The presentation and course of inflammatory pericarditis depend on its cause, but all syndromes are often (not always) associated with chest pain, which is usually pleuritic and postural (relieved by sitting). The pain is substernal but may radiate to the neck, shoulders, back, or epigastrium. Dyspnea may also be present. A pericardial friction rub is characteristic, with or without evidence of fluid accumulation or constriction (see below). Fever and leukocytosis are often present. The ECG usually shows generalized ST and T wave changes and may manifest a characteristic progression beginning with diffuse ST elevation, followed by a return to baseline and then to T wave inversion. The chest x-ray may show cardiac enlargement if fluid has collected, as well as signs of related pulmonary disease. The echocardiogram may disclose pericardial effusions and indicate their hemodynamic significance, but it is often normal in inflammatory pericarditis.

Several of the specific pericarditis syndromes are discussed below.

Viral Pericarditis

Viral infections (especially infections with coxsackieviruses and echoviruses but also influenza, Epstein-Barr, varicella, hepatitis, mumps, and HIV viruses) are the commonest cause of acute pericarditis and probably are responsible for many cases classified as idiopathic. Males— usually under age 50— are most commonly affected. Pericardial involvement often follows upper respiratory infection. The diagnosis is usually clinical, but rising viral titers in paired sera may be obtained for confirmation. Cardiac enzymes may be slightly elevated, reflecting a myocarditic component. The differential diagnosis is primarily with myocardial infarction.

Treatment is generally symptomatic. Aspirin (650 mg every 3–4 hours) or other nonsteroidal agents (eg, indomethacin, 100–150 mg daily in divided doses) are usually effective. Corticosteroids may be beneficial in unresponsive cases. In general, symptoms subside in several days to weeks. The major early complication is tamponade, which occurs in fewer than 5% of patients. There may be recurrences in the first few weeks or months. Rare patients will continue to experience recurrences chronically, sometimes leading to constrictive pericarditis, when pericardial resection may be required.

Tuberculous Pericarditis

Tuberculous pericarditis has become rare in developed countries but remains common in other areas. It results from direct lymphatic or hematogenous spread; clinical pulmonary involvement may be absent or minor, although associated pleural effusions are common. The presentation tends to be subacute, but nonspecific symptoms (fever, night sweats, fatigue) may be present for days to months. Pericardial effusions are usually small or moderate but may be large. The diagnosis can be inferred if acid-fast bacilli are found elsewhere. The yield of organisms by pericardiocentesis is low; pericardial biopsy has a higher yield but may also be negative, and pericardiectomy may be required. Standard antituberculous drug therapy is usually successful (see Chapter 9), but constrictive pericarditis can occur.

Other Infectious Pericarditides

Bacterial pericarditis has become rare and usually results from direct extension from pulmonary infections. Symptoms and signs are similar to those of other types of inflammatory pericarditides, but patients appear toxic—often critically ill. *Borrelia burgdorferi,* the organism responsible for Lyme disease, can also cause myopericarditis.

Uremic Pericarditis

This syndrome is a common complication of renal failure whose pathogenesis is uncertain; it occurs both with untreated uremia and in otherwise stable dialysis patients. The pericardium is characteristically "shaggy," and the effusion is hemorrhagic and exudative. Uremic pericarditis can present with or without symptoms; fever is absent. The pericarditis usually resolves with the institution of—or with more aggressive—dialysis. Tamponade is fairly common, and partial pericardiectomy (pericardial window) may be necessary. While anti-inflammatory agents may relieve the pain and fever associated with uremic pericarditis, indomethacin and systemic glucocorticoids do not affect the natural history of uremic pericarditis.

Neoplastic Pericarditis

Spread of adjacent lung cancer as well as invasion by breast cancer, renal cell carcinoma, Hodgkin's disease, and lymphomas are the commonest neoplastic processes involving the pericardium and have become the most frequent cause of pericardial tamponade in many countries. Often the process is painless, and the presenting symptoms relate to hemodynamic compromise or the primary disease. The diagnosis can usually be made by cytologic examination of the effusion or by biopsy, but it may be difficult to establish clinically if the patient has received mediastinal radiation within the previous year. MRI and CT scan can visualize neighboring tumor when present. The prognosis with neoplastic effusion is dismal, with only a small minority surviving 1 year. If it is compromising the patient, the effusion is initially drained. Instillation of chemotherapeutic agents or tetracycline may also prevent recurrence. Pericardial windows are rarely effective, but partial pericardiectomy from a subxiphoid incision may be successful; patients may be too ill to tolerate this.

Postmyocardial Infarction or Postcardiotomy Pericarditis (Dressler's Syndrome)

Pericarditis may occur 2–5 days after infarction due to an inflammatory reaction to transmural myocardial necrosis. It usually presents as a recurrence of pain with pleural-pericardial features. A rub is often audible, and repolarization changes may be confused with ischemia. Large effusions are uncommon, and spontaneous resolution usually occurs in a few days. Aspirin or nonsteroidal agents in the dosages given in the section on viral pericarditis provide symptomatic relief.

Dressler's syndrome occurs weeks to several months after myocardial infarction or open heart surgery, may be recurrent, and probably represents an autoimmune syndrome. Patients present with typical pain, fever, malaise, and leukocytosis. The sedimentation rate is usually high. Large pericardial effusions and accompanying pleural effusions are frequent. Tamponade is rare with Dressler's syndrome after infarction but not when it occurs postoperatively. Nonsteroidal agents are given, but recurrences are common; corticosteroids are effective but may be difficult to withdraw without relapse.

Radiation Pericarditis

Radiation can initiate a fibrinous and fibrotic process in the pericardium, presenting as subacute pericarditis or constriction. The clinical onset is usually within the first year but may be delayed for many years. Radiation pericarditis usually follows treatments of more than 4000 cGy delivered to ports including more than 30% of the heart. Symptomatic therapy is the initial approach, but recurrent effusions and constriction often require surgery.

Other Causes of Pericarditis

These include connective tissue diseases, such as lupus erythematosus and rheumatoid arthritis, drug-induced pericarditis (minoxidil, penicillins), and myxedema.

Hoit BD: Pericardial heart disease. Curr Probl Cardiol 1997;22:353. [NLM Cit ID: 97391938] (An up-to-date review of pericardial disease, including acute and constrictive pericarditis, pericardial effusion, and tamponade.)

PERICARDIAL EFFUSION

Pericardial effusion can develop during any of the processes discussed in the preceding paragraphs. The speed of accumulation determines the physiologic importance of the effusion. Because the pericardium stretches, large effusions (> 1000 mL) that develop slowly may produce no hemodynamic effects. Smaller effusions that appear rapidly can cause tamponade. Tamponade is characterized by elevated intrapericardial pressure (> 15 mm Hg), which restricts venous return and ventricular filling. As a result, the stroke volume and pulse pressure fall, and the heart rate and venous pressure rise. Shock and death may result.

Clinical Findings

A. Symptoms and Signs: Pericardial effusions may be associated with pain if they occur as part of an acute inflammatory process or may be painless, as is often the case with neoplastic or uremic effusion. Dyspnea and cough are common, especially with tamponade. Other symptoms may result from the primary disease.

A pericardial friction rub may be present even with large effusions. In cardiac tamponade, tachycardia, tachypnea, a narrow pulse pressure, and a relatively preserved systolic pressure are characteristic. Pulsus paradoxus—a greater than 10 mm Hg decline in systolic pressure during inspiration due to further impairment of left ventricular filling—is the classic finding, but it may also occur with obstructive lung disease. Central venous pressure is elevated, and edema or ascites may be present; these signs favor a more chronic process.

B. Laboratory Findings: Laboratory tests tend to reflect the underlying processes.

C. Diagnostic Studies: Chest x-ray can suggest effusion by an enlarged cardiac silhouette with a globular configuration. The ECG often reveals nonspecific T wave changes and low QRS voltage. Electrical alternans is present uncommonly but is pathognomonic. Echocardiography is the primary method for demonstrating pericardial effusion. Tamponade presents a characteristic picture of inadequate ventricular filling (diastolic collapse of the right ventricle or right atrium). The echocardiogram readily discriminates pericardial effusion from congestive heart failure. MRI also demonstrates pericardial fluid and lesions. Diagnostic pericardiocentesis or biopsy is often indicated for microbiologic and cytologic studies; a pericardial biopsy may be performed relatively simply through a small subxiphoid incision.

Treatment

Small effusions can be followed clinically and with the aid of echocardiograms. When tamponade is present, urgent pericardiocentesis is required. Removal of a small amount of fluid often produces immediate hemodynamic benefit, but complete drainage with a catheter is preferable. Continued drainage may be indicated.

Additional therapy is determined by the nature of the primary process. Recurrent effusion in neoplastic disease and uremia, in particular, may require partial pericardiectomy.

Sagrista-Sauleda J et al: Long-term follow-up of idiopathic chronic pericardial effusion. N Engl J Med 1999; 341:2042. [NLM Cit ID: 20061998] (Large pericardial effusions are often well tolerated but may cause tamponade unexpectedly. Pericardiectomy should be considered in patients in whom effusion recurs after pericardiocentesis.)

Spodick DH: Pathophysiology of cardiac tamponade. Chest 1998;113:1372. [NLM Cit ID: 98255760] (Includes characteristic pressure wave forms.)

Tsang TS et al: Diagnosis and management of cardiac tamponade in the era of echocardiography. Clin Cardiol 1999;22:446. [NLM Cit ID: 99338476] (Role of the echocardiogram in diagnosing tamponade physiology and guiding treatment.)

CONSTRICTIVE PERICARDITIS

Inflammation can lead to a thickened, fibrotic, adherent pericardium that restricts diastolic filling and produces chronically elevated venous pressures. In the past, tuberculosis was the most common cause of constrictive pericarditis, but the process now more often occurs after radiation therapy, cardiac surgery, or viral pericarditis; histoplasmosis is another uncommon cause.

The principal symptoms are slowly progressive dyspnea, fatigue, and weakness. Chronic edema, hepatic congestion, and ascites are usually present. The examination reveals these signs and a characteristically elevated jugular venous pressure with a rapid *y* descent. Kussmaul's sign—an increase in jugular venous pressure during inspiration—occurs in constrictive pericarditis and restrictive cardiomyopathy. Pulsus paradoxus is unusual. Atrial fibrillation is common.

The chest x-ray may show normal heart size or cardiomegaly. Pericardial calcification is best seen on the lateral view and is common. Echocardiography can demonstrate a thick pericardium and small chambers. CT scans and MRI are helpful in revealing pericardial thickening and may be more sensitive than echocardiography.

The primary differential diagnoses are restrictive cardiomyopathy and tamponade. The former distinction can be difficult and is best made by evaluating left ventricular function (more consistently depressed in cardiomyopathy), measuring hemodynamics (which show more complete equalization of diastolic pressures in all four chambers in constrictive pericarditis), and demonstrating pericardial thickening and calcification.

Initial treatment consists of gentle diuresis. Surgical removal of the pericardium, which should be complete, is usually required in symptomatic patients but is associated with a relatively high mortality rate.

Myers RB et al: Constrictive pericarditis: clinical and pathophysiologic characteristics. Am Heart J 1999; 138:219. [NLM Cit ID: 99355504] (This article reviews constrictive pericarditis, including epidemiology, mechanism, clinical findings, diagnosis, and treatment, and offers a discussion of differentiation from restrictive cardiomyopathy.)

Osterberg L et al: Case presentation and review: Constrictive pericarditis. West J Med 1998;169:232. [NLM Cit ID: 99011685] (Pathophysiology, diagnosis, and treatment are reviewed. Etiology, physical findings, and hemodynamic waveforms are included. Surgical pericardiectomy is the treatment of choice.)

PULMONARY HYPERTENSION & HEART DISEASE

PRIMARY PULMONARY HYPERTENSION

Primary pulmonary hypertension is defined as pulmonary hypertension and elevated pulmonary vascular resistance in the absence of other disease of the lungs or heart. Pathologically, it is characterized by diffuse narrowing of the pulmonary arterioles. Circumstantial evidence suggests that unrecognized recurrent pulmonary emboli or in situ thrombosis may play a role in some cases. The latter may well be an exacerbating factor (precipitated by local endothelial injury) rather than a cause of the syndrome. Primary pulmonary hypertension must be distinguished from chronic pulmonary heart disease (cor pulmonale), recurrent pulmonary emboli, mitral stenosis, and congenital heart disease; cirrhosis of the liver is another cause. Exclusion of secondary causes by echocardiography and lung scanning—and, if necessary, pulmonary angiography—is essential.

The clinical picture is similar to that of pulmonary hypertension from other causes. Patients—characteristically young women—present with evidence of right heart failure that is usually progressive, leading to death in 2–8 years. Patients have manifestations of low cardiac output, with weakness and fatigue, as well as edema and ascites as right heart failure advances. Peripheral cyanosis is present, and syncope on effort may occur.

The chest x-ray shows enlarged main pulmonary arteries with reduced peripheral branches. The right ventricle is enlarged. The ECG shows right ventricular and atrial hypertrophy.

Some authorities advocate chronic oral anticoagulation. The efficacy of vasodilator drugs is controversial, in part because the responses are variable. For example, a response in the systemic circulation may worsen the problem by reducing venous return. The calcium channel blockers nifedipine and diltiazem appear to be the preferred agents. The best response may be in patients in the earlier stages of the disease, when a more reversible vasoconstrictive component is present.

The prognosis for patients with primary pulmonary hypertension is generally poor. Once symptoms develop, most patients pursue a downhill course. This outcome may be improved by chronic infusion of prostacyclin, a potent pulmonary vasodilator. This therapy often improves symptoms, sometimes dramatically, in patients who have not responded to other vasodilators. It is initiated only in individuals who have failed to respond to calcium channel blockers. The main application of this therapy may be as a bridge to heart-lung or single-lung transplantation. Without transplantation, symptoms usually progress, and many patients will require meticulous attention to relief of dyspnea and ultimately benefit from high-quality palliative care (see Chapter 5).

Gaine SP et al: Primary pulmonary hypertension. Lancet 1998;352:719. [NLM Cit ID: 98397221] (Epidemiology, pathology, diagnosis and treatment are covered with useful algorithms included. Intravenous prostacyclin and lung transplantation offer some promise.)

McLaughlin VV et al: Reduction in pulmonary vascular resistance with long-term epoprostenol (prostacyclin) therapy in primary pulmonary hypertension. N Engl J Med 1998;338:273. [NLM Cit ID: 98092071] (Multicenter trial of 27 patients demonstrated improvement in symptoms and hemodynamics, and this was sustained out to 16 months.)

PULMONARY HEART DISEASE (Cor Pulmonale)

Essentials of Diagnosis

- Symptoms and signs of chronic bronchitis and pulmonary emphysema.
- Elevated jugular venous pressure, parasternal lift, edema, hepatomegaly, ascites.
- ECG shows tall, peaked P waves (P pulmonale), right axis deviation, and right ventricular hypertrophy.
- Chest x-ray: Enlarged right ventricle and pulmonary artery.
- Echocardiogram or radionuclide angiography excludes primary left ventricular dysfunction.

General Considerations

The term "cor pulmonale" denotes right ventricular hypertrophy and eventual failure resulting from pulmonary disease and attendant hypoxia. Its clinical features depend upon both the primary disease and its effects on the heart.

Cor pulmonale is most commonly caused by chronic obstructive pulmonary disease. Rare causes include pneumoconiosis, pulmonary fibrosis, kyphoscoliosis, primary pulmonary hypertension, repeated episodes of subclinical or clinical pulmonary embolization, Pickwickian syndrome, schistosomiasis, and obliterative pulmonary capillary or lymphangitic infiltration from metastatic carcinoma.

Clinical Findings

A. Symptoms and Signs: The predominant symptoms of compensated cor pulmonale are related to the pulmonary disorder and include chronic productive cough, exertional dyspnea, wheezing respirations, easy fatigability, and weakness. When the pulmonary disease causes right ventricular failure, these symptoms may be intensified. Dependent edema and right upper quadrant pain may also appear. The signs of cor pulmonale include cyanosis, clubbing, distended neck veins, right ventricular heave or gallop (or both), prominent lower sternal or epigastric pulsations, an enlarged and tender liver, and dependent edema.

B. Laboratory Findings: Polycythemia is often present in cor pulmonale secondary to COPD. The arterial oxygen saturation is below 85%; PCO_2 may or may not be elevated.

C. Electrocardiography and Chest X-Ray: The ECG may show right axis deviation and peaked P waves. Deep S waves are present in lead V_6. Right axis deviation and low voltage may be noted in patients with pulmonary emphysema. Frank right ventricular hypertrophy is uncommon except in "primary pulmonary hypertension." The ECG often mimics myocardial infarction; Q waves may be present in leads II, III, and aVF because of the vertically placed heart, but they are rarely deep or wide, as in inferior myocardial infarction. Supraventricular arrhythmias are frequent and nonspecific.

The chest radiograph discloses the presence or absence of parenchymal disease and a prominent or enlarged right ventricle and pulmonary artery.

D. Diagnostic Studies: Pulmonary function tests usually confirm the underlying lung disease. The echocardiogram should show normal left ventricular size and function but right ventricular dilation. Perfusion lung scans are rarely of value, but, if negative, they help to exclude pulmonary emboli, an occasional cause of cor pulmonale. Pulmonary angiography is the most specific method of diagnosis for the pulmonary emboli, but it carries increased risk when performed in patients with pulmonary hypertension.

Differential Diagnosis

In its early stages, cor pulmonale can be diagnosed on the basis of radiologic, echocardiographic, or electrocardiographic evidence. Catheterization of the right heart will establish a definitive diagnosis but is usually performed to exclude left-sided heart failure, which may in some patients be an inapparent cause of right-sided failure. Differential diagnostic considerations relate chiefly to the specific pulmonary disease that has produced right ventricular failure (see above).

Treatment

The details of the treatment of chronic pulmonary disease (chronic respiratory failure) are discussed in Chapter 9. Otherwise, therapy is directed at the pulmonary process responsible for right heart failure. Oxygen, salt and fluid restriction, and diuretics are mainstays; digitalis has no place in right heart failure unless atrial fibrillation is present.

Prognosis

Compensated cor pulmonale has the same outlook as the underlying pulmonary disease. Once congestive signs appear, the average life expectancy is 2–5 years, but survival is significantly longer when uncomplicated emphysema is the cause.

MacNee W: Pathophysiology of cor pulmonale in chronic obstructive pulmonary disease. (Two parts.) Am J Respir Crit Care Med 1994;150:833, 1158. [NLM Cit IDs: 94373262, 95005665]

Vizza CD et al: Right and left ventricular dysfunction in patients with severe pulmonary disease. Chest 1998; 113:576. [NLM Cit ID: 98175580] (In patients with advanced pulmonary disease, left ventricular dysfunction is less common than right ventricular dysfunction, but problems with the left ventricle may be due in part to ventricular interdependence.)

NEOPLASTIC DISEASES OF THE HEART

Primary cardiac tumors are rare and constitute only a small fraction of all tumors that involve the heart or pericardium. Metastases from malignant tumors elsewhere are more frequent. Tumors involving the heart are bronchogenic carcinoma, carcinoma of the breast, malignant melanoma, the lymphomas, renal cell carcinoma, and, in patients with AIDS, Kaposi's sarcoma. These are often clinically silent but may lead to pericardial tamponade, arrhythmias and conduction disturbances, heart failure, and peripheral emboli. The diagnosis is often made by echocardiography, but MRI and CT scanning are also helpful. Electrocardiography may reveal regional Q waves. The prognosis is dismal; effective treatment is not available.

The commonest primary tumors of the heart are atrial myxomas. These tend to occur in middle age, more often in women than in men. They usually originate in the intraventricular septum, with over 80%

growing into the left atrium. Myxomas are benign tumors but can embolize systemically.

Patients with myxoma can present with a picture of a systemic illness, obstruction of blood flow through the heart, or signs of peripheral embolization. The characteristic picture includes fever, malaise, weight loss, leukocytosis, elevated sedimentation rate, and emboli (peripheral or pulmonary, depending on the location of the tumor). This picture is often confused with infective endocarditis, lymphoma, other cancers, or autoimmune diseases. In other cases, the tumor may grow to considerable size and produce symptoms by obstructing mitral flow. Episodic pulmonary edema (classically occurring when an upright posture is assumed) and signs of low output may result. Physical examination may reveal a diastolic sound related to motion of the tumor ("tumor plop") or a diastolic murmur similar to that of mitral stenosis. Right-sided myxomas may cause symptoms of right-sided failure. The diagnosis is established by echocardiography or by pathologic study of embolic material. MRI is also useful. Contrast angiography is usually not necessary. Surgical excision is usually curative.

Other primary cardiac tumors include rhabdomyomas, fibrous histiocytomas, hemangiomas, and a variety of unusual sarcomas. The diagnosis may be supported by an abnormal cardiac contour on x-ray. Echocardiography is usually helpful but may miss tumors infiltrating the ventricular wall. It is likely that MRI will be useful as well.

Reynen K: Cardiac myxomas. N Engl J Med 1995; 333:1610. [NLM Cit ID: 96072891]

Roberts WC: Primary and secondary neoplasms of the heart. Am J Cardiol 1997;80:671. [NLM Cit ID: 97439454] (Review of primary and metastatic cardiac tumors, including pathologic specimens.)

Roberts WC: A unique heart disease associated with a unique cancer: Carcinoid heart disease. Am J Cardiol 1997;80:251. [NLM Cit ID: 97373697] (Morphology, diagnosis, and surgical therapy discussed.)

CARDIAC INVOLVEMENT IN MISCELLANEOUS SYSTEMIC DISEASES

The heart may be involved in a number of systemic syndromes. Many of these have been mentioned briefly in prior subsections of this chapter. The pericardium, myocardium, heart valves, and coronary arteries may be involved either singly or in various combinations. In most cases the cardiac manifestations are not the dominant feature, but in some it is the primary cause of symptoms and may be fatal.

The most common type of myocardial involvement is an infiltrative cardiomyopathy, such as systemic amyloidosis, sarcoidosis, hemochromatosis, or glycogen storage disease. Cardiac calcinosis can occur in hyperparathyroidism (usually the secondary form) and in primary oxalosis. A number of muscular dystrophies can cause a cardiomyopathic picture (particularly Duchenne's, less frequently myotonic dystrophy, and several rarer forms). In addition to left ventricular dysfunction and heart failure, all of these conditions frequently cause conduction abnormalities, which may be the presenting or only feature. The myocardium may also be involved in inflammatory and autoimmune diseases. It is commonly affected in polymyositis and dermatomyositis, but usually this is subclinical. Systemic lupus erythematosus, scleroderma, and mixed connective tissue disease may cause myocarditis, but these commonly also involve the pericardium, coronary arteries, or valves. Several endocrinopathies, including acromegaly, thyrotoxicosis, myxedema, and pheochromocytoma, can produce cardiomyopathies, though again they are usually not isolated features.

Pericardial involvement is quite common in many of the connective tissue diseases. Systemic lupus erythematosus may present with pericarditis, and pericardial involvement is not uncommon (but is less frequently symptomatic) in active rheumatoid arthritis, systemic sclerosis, and mixed connective tissue disease. Endocardial involvement takes the form of patchy fibrous—predominantly on the right side—or inflammatory or sclerotic changes of the heart valves. Carcinoid heart disease typically is manifested as tricuspid regurgitation, and the same may be the case in systemic lupus erythematosus. The hypereosinophilic syndromes involve the endocardium, leading to restrictive cardiomyopathy. A variety of arthritic syndromes are associated with aortic valvulitis or aortitis, including ankylosing spondylitis, rheumatoid arthritis, and Reiter's syndrome, as is tertiary syphilis also. Disorders of elastic tissue (Marfan's syndrome is the most frequent) often affect the ascending aorta, with resulting aneurysmal dilation and aortic regurgitation.

Virtually any vasculitic syndrome can involve the coronary arteries, leading to myocardial infarction. This is most common with polyarteritis nodosa and systemic lupus erythematosus. Two vasculitic syndromes have a particular predilection for the coronary arteries—Kawasaki's disease and Takayasu's disease. In these, myocardial infarction may be the presenting symptom.

Moder KG et al: Cardiac involvement in systemic lupus erythematosus. Mayo Clin Proc 1999;74:275. [NLM Cit ID: 99189868] (SLE is the connective tissue disease that most frequently involves the heart [more than 50% of cases]. Pericarditis is most common, but myocarditis, endocarditis, and coronary arteritis all occur with moderate frequency.)

TRAUMATIC HEART DISEASE

Penetrating wounds to the heart are, of course, usually lethal unless surgically repaired. Stab wounds to the right ventricle occasionally lead to hemopericardium without progressing to tamponade. The clinical result may be constrictive pericarditis, so surgery is recommended even if the patient presents in an unstable condition.

Blunt trauma is a more frequent cause of cardiac injuries, particularly outside of the emergency room setting. This type of injury is quite frequent in motor vehicle accidents and may occur with any form of chest trauma. The most common injuries are myocardial contusions or hematomas. These may be asymptomatic (particularly in the setting of more severe injuries) or may present with chest pains of a nonspecific nature or, not uncommonly, with a pericardial component. A minority of patients will develop left or, less commonly, right ventricular aneurysm. Elevations of cardiac enzymes are frequent, and echocardiography may reveal an akinetic segment. Heart failure is uncommon if there are no associated cardiac or pericardial injuries, and conservative management is usually sufficient.

Severe trauma may also cause cardiac or valvular rupture. Cardiac rupture may involve any chamber, but survival is most likely if injury is to one of the atria or the right ventricle. Hemopericardium or pericardial tamponade is the usual clinical presentation, and surgery is almost always necessary. Mitral and aortic valve rupture may occur during severe blunt trauma—the former presumably if the impact occurs during systole and the latter if during diastole. Patients reach the hospital in shock or severe heart failure. Immediate surgical repair is essential. The same types of injuries may result in transection of the aorta, either at the level of the arch or distal to the takeoff of the left subclavian artery. Transthoracic and transesophageal echocardiography are the most helpful and immediately available diagnostic techniques.

Blunt trauma may also result in damage to the coronary arteries. Acute or subacute coronary thrombosis is the most common presentation. The clinical syndrome is one of acute myocardial infarction with attendant electrocardiographic, enzymatic, and contractile abnormalities. Emergent revascularization is sometimes feasible, either by the percutaneous route or by coronary artery bypass surgery. Left ventricular aneurysms are common outcomes of traumatic coronary occlusions. Coronary artery dissection or rupture may also occur in the setting of blunt cardiac trauma.

Link MS et al: An experimental model of sudden death due to low-energy chest-wall impact (commotio cordis). N Engl J Med 1998;338:1805. [NLM Cit ID: 98283487] (The occurrence of ventricular fibrillation following impact depends on the timing of the impact 15–30 ms prior to the peak of the T wave.)

Pretre R et al: Blunt trauma to the heart and great vessels. N Engl J Med 1997;336:626. [NLM Cit ID: 97170827]

THE CARDIAC PATIENT & SURGERY

Patients with known or suspected cardiac disease undergoing general surgery present a common management problem. Anesthesia and surgery are often associated with marked fluctuations of heart rate and blood pressure, changes in intravascular volume, myocardial ischemia or depression, arrhythmias, decreased oxygenation, increased sympathetic nervous system activity, and alterations in medical regimens and pharmacokinetics. Even with careful monitoring and management, the perioperative period can be very stressful to cardiac patients.

The risk of surgery in patients with heart disease depends primarily on three factors: the type of operation, the nature of the heart disease, and the degree of preoperative stability. The type of anesthesia is less important, though halothane, enflurane, and barbiturates are more severe myocardial depressants, while narcotics have little depressive effect. Spinal and epidural anesthesia were previously thought to be preferable in patients with heart disease, but this has not proved to be the case.

The highest-risk procedures are surgery of the aorta and vascular procedures, in part because these patients often have associated severe coronary disease but also because marked blood pressure and volume changes are common. Major abdominal and thoracic surgery are also associated with substantial cardiovascular risk, especially in older patients with associated cardiovascular disease.

Numerous studies have evaluated the excess risk of surgery in patients with various cardiac diseases. Recent (within 3 months) myocardial infarction, unstable angina, congestive heart failure, and significant aortic stenosis are associated with substantial increases in operative morbidity and mortality rates. Any degree of instability in these conditions magnifies the potential risk. Stable angina, especially in an inactive individual, is also associated with a higher operative risk. Although less common, cyanotic congenital heart disease and severe primary or secondary pulmonary hypertension pose great risks during major surgery. In patients with any of these problems, the risk-to-benefit ratio of the planned surgery should be carefully examined. If the procedure is necessary but elective, consideration should be given to delaying it until full recovery postinfarction and correction or optimal stabilization of the other conditions are achieved. Hypertension should be at least moderately controlled. Patients with severe angina should have increased medical therapy or be considered for revascularization before noncardiac surgery. Symptomatic arrhythmias, nonsustained ventricular tachycardia, or high-grade atrioventricular block and cardiac failure should be treated optimally.

Clinical assessment provides the most useful guidance in determining the risk of noncardiac surgery. Important indicators of high risk have been discussed above. Patients with known but clinically stable heart disease, such as angina pectoris or prior myocardial infarction, are at intermediate risk, particularly for major operations such as vascular surgery. If a history or symptoms of heart failure are present, assessment of left ventricular function can be very helpful in perioperative management. Although frequently advocated, further noninvasive testing for myocardial ischemia for the purpose of risk stratification is probably overutilized. Tests such as stress myocardial perfusion scintigraphy or dobutamine echocardiography should be reserved for situations in which the results may alter patient management. There is no evidence that prophylactic revascularization by either PTCA or coronary artery bypass surgery alters long-term outcome in patients undergoing noncardiac surgical procedures without the usual indications for PTCA or CABG. Only in the case of major vascular operations is perioperative mortality and morbidity high enough that prophylactic PTCA or CABG should be considered.

However, it should be noted that many patients undergoing surgery have not had recent medical follow-up, and this may be an appropriate opportunity to perform a more complete evaluation. Thus, stress testing may be indicated for selected patients with symptomatic angina or prior myocardial infarction with a view to instituting more comprehensive medical management or performing coronary revascularization to reduce long-term (rather than perioperative) mortality and morbidity. At the least, such patients should not be discharged without a plan for an appropriate follow-up and institution of antihyperlipidemic, aspirin, and beta-blocker therapy as indicated.

Once the decision to operate is made, careful management is essential. Most cardiac medications should be continued preoperatively and postoperatively. Institution of beta-blockers in patients who are known to have or be at high risk for developing coronary artery disease is a rational approach now supported by convincing evidence. Monitoring is an important prophylactic measure in high-risk individuals; hemodynamic monitoring can facilitate early intervention in patients with heart failure, severe valve disease, or easily induced myocardial ischemia. Excessive hypertension, hypotension, and myocardial ischemia should be identified and appropriately treated using rapidly acting agents. Transesophageal echocardiography can also be used for intraoperative monitoring of ischemia, but its value has never been established in well-designed studies. Ischemic events, whether symptomatic or silent, should be vigorously treated.

Eagle KA et al: Guidelines for perioperative cardiovascular evaluation for noncardiac surgery: An abridged version of the report of the American College of Cardiology/American Heart Association Task Force on Practice Guidelines. Mayo Clin Proc 1997;72:524. [NLM Cit ID: 97322646]

Guidelines for assessing and managing the perioperative risk from coronary artery disease associated with major noncardiac surgery. American College of Physicians. Ann Intern Med 1997;127:309. [NLM Cit ID: 97395387]

Lee TH et al: Derivation and prospective validation of a simple index for prediction of cardiac risk of major noncardiac surgery. Circulation 1999;100:1043. [NLM Cit ID: 99406588] (The authors propose a new cardiac-risk stratification tool for patients undergoing nonemergent noncardiac surgery. In their comparison, a simple list of six characteristics—high-risk type of surgery, history of ischemic heart disease, history of congestive heart failure, history of cerebrovascular disease, preoperative treatment with insulin, and serum creatinine > 2 mg/dL—predicted outcome with greater accuracy than several other well-known risk indices.)

Palda VA et al: Perioperative assessment and management of risk from coronary artery disease. Ann Intern Med 1997;127:313. [NLM Cit ID: 97395388] (Slightly different view from those of Eagle et al.)

Poldermans D et al: The effect of bisoprolol on perioperative mortality and myocardial infarction in high-risk patients undergoing vascular surgery. N Engl J Med 1999; 341:1789. [NLM Cit ID: 20055766] (Patients with abnormal dobutamine echo undergoing vascular surgery were ten times less likely to have a perioperative myocardial infarction or die if they were treated with a beta-blocker.)

THE CARDIAC PATIENT & PREGNANCY

The management of cardiac disease in pregnancy is discussed in detail in the references listed below. Only a few major points can be covered in this brief section.

CARDIOVASCULAR CHANGES DURING PREGNANCY

Normal physiologic changes during pregnancy can exacerbate symptoms of underlying cardiac disease even in previously asymptomatic individuals. Maternal blood volume rises progressively until the end of the sixth or seventh month. Stroke volume increases over the same time course as a result of the volume change and an increase in ejection fraction. The latter reflects predominantly a decline in peripheral resistance due to vasodilation and the low-resistance shunting through the placenta. The heart rate tends to rise in the third trimester. Overall, cardiac output increases by 30–50%; systolic blood pressure tends to rise slightly or remain unchanged, but diastolic pressure falls significantly.

High cardiac output causes alterations in the cardiac examination. A third heart sound is prominent and normal, and a pulmonary flow murmur is common. Electrocardiographic changes include rate-related decreases in PR and QT intervals, a leftward axis shift, inferior Q waves due to the more horizontal position of the heart, and nonspecific ST–T wave changes.

MANAGEMENT OF PREEXISTING CONDITIONS

The physiologic changes imposed by pregnancy can cause cardiac decompensation in patients with any significant cardiac abnormality, but the most severe problems are encountered in patients with valvular stenosis (especially mitral and aortic stenosis), congenital or acquired abnormalities associated with pulmonary hypertension or right-to-left shunting, congestive heart failure due to any cause, coronary heart disease, and hypertension. Valvular insufficiency or left-to-right shunting often diminishes because of the fall in peripheral resistance and is better tolerated.

Mitral stenosis becomes more hemodynamically severe owing to the increase in diastolic flow and the rate-related shortening of diastole. Left atrial pressures rise, and dyspnea or pulmonary edema can occur in previously asymptomatic individuals. The onset of atrial fibrillation often leads to acute decompensation. Patients with moderate to severe stenosis should have the condition corrected prior to becoming pregnant if possible. Patients who become symptomatic can undergo successful surgery, preferably in the third trimester. Balloon valvuloplasty is an attractive alternative, though radiation exposure to the fetus is unavoidable. Coarctation is usually well tolerated, but patients with symptoms should have corrective surgery before pregnancy. Patients with severe pulmonary hypertension and cyanotic congenital heart disease and those with severe aortic stenosis are at extremely high risk and should attempt to avoid pregnancy.

Asymptomatic arrhythmias should be closely observed unless underlying heart disease is present, in which case they should be treated with drugs. Paroxysmal supraventricular arrhythmias are quite common. Patients with Wolff-Parkinson-White syndrome may have more problems during pregnancy. Therapy is similar to that required for nonpregnant women.

Preexisting systemic hypertension is usually well tolerated and controllable, though the fetal morbidity rate is slightly increased. The incidence of preeclampsia and eclampsia (see Chapter 18) is increased.

Hydralazine and methyldopa are the antihypertensive agents for which there has been the greatest experience during pregnancy. Diuretics have also been used frequently, but concern has been raised that intravascular hypovolemia might impair uterine blood flow. Nonetheless, these agents are relatively safe. More recently, there has been considerable use of the combined alpha-beta-blocker labetalol and of calcium channel blockers, which have been proved effective and safe to both the mother and fetus. On the other hand, atenolol has been associated with lower fetal weights. ACE inhibitors and angiotensin II blockers are contraindicated in pregnancy because of the risk of fetal injury. Beta-blockers may retard fetal growth, but experience with them has been generally favorable. Little is known about the safety of most other antihypertensive agents.

CARDIOVASCULAR COMPLICATIONS OF PREGNANCY

Pregnancy-related hypertension (eclampsia and preeclampsia) is discussed in Chapter 18.

Cardiomyopathy of Pregnancy (Peripartum Cardiomyopathy)

In approximately one out of 4000–15,000 patients, dilated cardiomyopathy develops in the final month of pregnancy or within 6 months after delivery. The cause is unclear, but immune and viral causes have been postulated. The course of the disease is variable; many cases improve or resolve completely over several months, but others progress to refractory heart failure. Immunosuppressive therapy has been advocated, but few supportive data are available. Recently, beta-blockers have been administered judiciously to these patients, with at least anecdotal success. Recurrence in subsequent pregnancies has been reported.

Coronary Artery & Other Vascular Abnormalities

There have been a number of reports of myocardial infarction during pregnancy. It is known that pregnancy predisposes to dissection of the aorta and other arteries, perhaps because of the accompanying connective tissue changes. However, coronary artery dissection is responsible for only a minority of the infarctions, with the majority being caused by atherosclerotic coronary artery disease or coronary emboli. Most of the events occur near term or shortly following delivery. Clinical management is essentially similar to that of other patients with acute infarction.

SPECIAL PROBLEMS

Prophylaxis for Infective Endocarditis

Although there is not universal agreement, many authorities recommend antibiotic prophylaxis during labor for patients at risk for endocarditis, especially if forceps or an episiotomy is employed. Ampicillin (2 g intravenously or intramuscularly) plus gentamicin (1.5 mg/kg intravenously or intramuscularly [up to 80 mg]) followed by amoxicillin, 1.5 g orally every 6 hours, is the recommended regimen.

Management of Labor

While vaginal delivery is usually well tolerated, unstable patients (including patients with severe hypertension and worsening heart failure) should have cesarean section. An increased risk of aortic rupture has been noted during delivery in patients with coarctation of the aorta and severe aortic root dilation with Marfan's syndrome, and vaginal delivery should be avoided in these conditions.

Cardiovascular Drugs During Pregnancy

Experience during pregnancy with many drugs is limited, and the effect on the fetus is often not well defined. Drugs with known potential for teratogenicity or fetal injury include phenytoin and the ACE inhibitors. Warfarin also presents a risk, but—at least in patients with prosthetic heart valves—many recommend that it be continued until the final 2 weeks. Self-injected low-molecular-weight heparin may be a good alternative, but data regarding efficacy and safety are lacking. Other than antihypertensive agents, which have been discussed above, cardiac drugs that appear safe during pregnancy include the digitalis glycosides, quinidine, procainamide, lidocaine, and short-term verapamil.

Brown CS et al: Peripartum cardiomyopathy: a comprehensive review. Am J Obstet Gynecol 1998;178:409. [NLM Cit ID: 98160144]

Chan WS et al: Anticoagulation of pregnant women with mechanical heart valves. Arch Intern Med 2000;160:191. [NLM Cit ID: 20112283] (Literature review suggests the use of oral anticoagulation through most of pregnancy. Subcutaneous heparin may reduce the risk of fetal embryopathy during the first trimester but must be dose-adjusted.)

Chow T et al: Antiarrhythmic drug therapy in pregnancy and lactation. Am J Cardiol 1998;82:58I. [NLM Cit ID: 98407673] (Comprehensive review.)

Elkayam U, Glecher N (editors): *Cardiac Problems in Pregnancy: Diagnosis and Management of Maternal and Fetal Disease.* Saunders, 1998.

Lambert MB et al: Peri-partum cardiomyopathy. Am Heart J 1995;130:860. (Review covering definition, epidemiology, clinical presentation, treatment, and prognosis.)

Mosca L et al: Guide to preventive cardiology for women. AHA/ACC Scientific Statement Consensus panel statement. Circulation 1999;99:2480. [NLM Cit ID: 99252139]

CARDIOVASCULAR SCREENING OF ATHLETES

The sudden death of a competitive athlete inevitably becomes an occasion for local if not national publicity. On each such occasion, the public and the medical community ask whether such events could be prevented by more careful or complete screening. Although each such event is tragic, it must be appreciated that there are approximately 5 million competitive athletes at the high school level or above in any given year. The number of cardiac deaths occurring during athletic participation is unknown, but estimates at the high school level range from one in 300,000 to one in 100,000 participants. Death rates among more mature athletes increase as the prevalence of coronary artery disease rises. These numbers highlight the problem of how to screen individual participants. Even an inexpensive test such as an ECG would generate an enormous cost if required of all athletes, and it is likely that few at-risk individuals would be detected. Echocardiography, either as a routine test or as a follow-up examination for abnormal ECGs, would be prohibitively expensive.

Thus, the most feasible approach is that of a careful medical history and cardiac examination performed by personnel aware of the conditions responsible for most sudden deaths in competitive athletes. In a series of 158 athletic deaths in the United States between 1985 and 1995, hypertrophic cardiomyopathy (36%) and coronary anomalies (19%) were by far the most frequent underlying conditions. Left ventricular hypertrophy was present in another 10%, ruptured aorta (presumably due to Marfan's syndrome or cystic medial necrosis) in 6%, myocarditis or dilated cardiomyopathy in 6%, aortic stenosis in 4%, and arrhythmogenic right ventricular dysplasia in 3%.

It is likely that a careful family and medical history and cardiovascular examination will identify some individuals at risk. A family history of premature sudden death or cardiovascular disease or of any of these predisposing conditions should mandate further workup, including an echocardiogram and ECG. Symptoms of chest pain, syncope, or near-syncope also warrant further evaluation. A Marfan-like appearance, significant elevation of blood pressure or abnormalities of heart rate or rhythm, and pathologic heart murmurs or heart sounds should also be investigated before clearance for athletic participation is given. Such an evaluation is recommended before participation at the high school and college levels and every 2 years during athletic competition. Selective use of routine electrocardiography and stress testing is recommended in men above age 40 and women above age 50 who continue to participate in vigorous exercise and at earlier ages when there is a positive family history for premature coronary artery disease or multiple risk factors.

Corrado D et al: Screening for hypertrophic cardiomyopathy in young athletes. N Engl J Med 1998;339:364. [NLM Cit ID: 98346818] (Screening resulted in detection of hypertrophic cardiomyopathy in 0.07% of screened athletes, and its detection may have explained the relatively low incidence of sudden death due to that disorder in these young Italian athletes.)

Glover DW et al: Profile of preparticipation cardiovascular screening for high school athletes. JAMA 1998; 279:1817. [NLM Cit ID: 98290678] (Review of the practices of preparticipation cardiovascular screening for high school athletes finds that practices vary from state to state and that current practice may be severely limited in its ability to detect potentially lethal cardiac conditions.)

Maron BJ: Cardiovascular risks to young persons on the athletic field. Ann Intern Med 1998;129:379. [NLM Cit ID: 98398003] (Comprehensive review by a leading authority.)

RELEVANT WORLD WIDE WEB SITES

[American College of Cardiology/American Heart Association Practice Guidelines]
http://www.acc.org/clinical/statements.htm

[American Heart Association]
http://www.americanheart.org

[Auscultation Assistant!]
http://www.med.ucla.edu/wilkes/Intro.html

[Cardiac Arrhythmia Advisory System]
http://www.med-edu.com/htdocs/einthoven.html

[Clinical Trials Database]
http://www.cardiosource.com

[Cut to the Heart: Nova Heart Page]
http://www.pbs.org/wgbh/nova/heart/

[Emergency Medicine: Advance Cardiac Life Support]
http://www.vh.org/Providers/ClinRef/FPHandbook/Chapter01/01-1.html

[Healthfinder]
http://www.healthfinder.gov/default.htm

[Synapse HeartBeats]
http://www.medlib.com/spi/coolstuff2.htm

[HeartWeb Home Page]
http://www.heartweb.org/

[Index of Echocardiographic Images]
http://www2.umdnj.edu/~shindler/imgndx.html

[National Heart, Lung, and Blood Institute]
http://www.nhlbi.nih.gov/index.htm

[Pediatric Cardiology and Critical Care]
http://www.kumc.edu/kumopeds/cardiology/cardiology.html

[Right Atrial Myxoma Demonstration Case]
http://www.brighamrad.harvard.edu/Cases/bwh/hcache/46/full.html

[Synapse HeartBeats]
http://www.medlib.com/spi/coolstuff2.htm

[Urbana Atlas of Pathology—Cardiovascular Pathology]
http://www.med.uiuc.edu/PathAtlasf/titlePage.html#vol2contents

[Virtual Hospital: Pediatric Advanced Life Support]
http://www.vh.org/Providers/ClinRef/FPHandbook/Chapter01/03-1.html

11 Systemic Hypertension

See http://www.current-med.com/ch11.html for updated addresses of Web sites referenced in this chapter.

Barry M. Massie, MD

Fifty million Americans have elevated blood pressure (systolic blood pressure ≥ 140 mm Hg or diastolic blood pressure ≥ 90 mm Hg). Of these, 68% are aware of their diagnosis, 53% are receiving treatment, and only 27% are under control by the 140/90 mm Hg threshold. The proportion of individuals who are hypertensive increases with age and is greater in blacks than in whites. The mortality rates for stroke and coronary heart disease, the major complications of hypertension, have declined by up to 60% over the past 3 decades but have now leveled off. The incidence of end-stage renal disease and of heart failure, two other conditions in which hypertension plays a major causative role, continues to rise.

Cardiovascular morbidity and mortality increase as both systolic and diastolic blood pressures rise, but in individuals over age 50 the systolic blood pressure is a better predictor of complications. In a study of 18,700 physicians, borderline elevations of systolic blood pressure (140–159 mm Hg) were associated with a 42% increase in strokes and a 56% increase in cardiovascular deaths. As shown in Table 11–1, hypertension is now diagnosed based upon elevations of *either* the systolic or diastolic blood pressure, and the objective of management is to achieve normalization of both.

Blood pressure should be measured with well-calibrated sphygmomanometer with a cuff of proper size (the bladder width within the cuff should encircle at least 80% of the arm circumference) after the patient has been resting comfortably, back supported in the sitting or supine position, for a least 5 minutes and at least 30 minutes after smoking or coffee ingestion. Because blood pressure readings in many individuals are highly variable—especially in the office setting—the diagnosis of hypertension should be made only after elevation is noted on three readings on different occasions, over a period of several months unless the elevations are severe or associated with symptoms (see Table 11–1). Transient elevation of blood pressure caused by excitement or apprehension does not constitute hypertensive disease but may indicate a propensity toward its evolution. Ambulatory 24-hour blood pressure monitoring may be helpful in evaluating patients with borderline or variable office blood pressure ("white coat" hypertension), approximately 20% of whom will have no evidence of hypertension elsewhere, as well as in assessing resistant hypertension and possible treatment-related hypotensive symptoms. This technique has become convenient and increasingly available, but it should be employed only to address specific management problems because of cost ($200.00–$300.00).

Continued hypertension does not necessarily indicate the need for pharmacologic treatment. Nonpharmacologic approaches and individualized assessment of the benefit-to-risk ratio of drug therapy should precede pharmacologic management in patients with stage I hypertension (diastolic pressure < 100 mm Hg; systolic < 160 mm Hg). Some patients with pressure in these ranges do not require therapy if they have no evidence of target organ damage or concomitant cardiovascular disease or diabetes.

Feldman RD et al: Canadian recommendations for the management of hypertension. Task Force for the Development of the 1999 Canadian Recommendations for the Management of Hypertension. Can Med Assoc J 1999;161(Suppl 12):S1. [NLM Cit ID: 20089543] (Guidelines based on extensive literature review and expert opinion.)

He J et al: Epidemiology and prevention of hypertension. Med Clin North Am 1997;81:1077. [NLM Cit ID: 97453979]

JAMA patient page: Blood pressure. JAMA 1999;281:484. [NLM Cit ID: 99135686]

Kaplan NM: *Clinical Hypertension,* 7th ed. Williams & Wilkins, 1998. (Concise, practical monograph covering epidemiology, mechanisms, diagnosis, and treatment.)

O'Donnell CJ et al: Hypertension and borderline isolated systolic hypertension increase risks of cardiovascular disease and mortality in male physicians. Circulation 1997;95:1132. [NLM Cit ID: 97207548] (Prospective, randomized study of 18,682 male physicians demonstrating significantly increased risk of cardiovascular disease, stroke, and cardiovascular death in those with borderline isolated systolic hypertension.)

The sixth report of the Joint National Committee on prevention, detection, evaluation, and treatment of high blood pressure. Arch Intern Med 1997;157:2413. (Published erratum appears in Arch Intern Med 1997;157:2413.)

Table 11–1. Classification and follow-up of blood pressure measurements.[1]

Category[2]	Systolic Blood Pressure (mm Hg)	Diastolic Blood Pressure (mm Hg)	Follow-Up Recommended
Optional	< 120	< 80	Recheck in 2 years
Normal	< 130	< 85	Recheck in 2 years
High Normal	130–139	85–90	Recheck in 1 year[3]
Hypertension[4] Stage 1 (mild)	140–159	90–99	Confirm within 2 months.
Stage 2 (moderate)	160–179	100–109	Evaluate or refer within 1 month
Stage 3 (severe)	> 180	> 110	Evaluate or refer within 1 week.

[1]From: The sixth report of the Joint National Committee on detection, education, and treatment of high blood pressure (JNC VI). Arch Intern Med 1997;157:2413.
[2]When systolic and diastolic pressures fall into different categories, the higher category should be selected to classify the individual's blood pressure. Isolated systolic hypertension is defined as a systolic blood pressure of 140 mm Hg or more and a diastolic blood pressure of less than 90 mm Hg.
[3]Consider offering counseling about lifestyle modifications (Table 11–2).
[4]In individuals aged 18 years or older not taking antihypertensive drugs and not acutely ill. Based on the average of two or more readings on two or more occasions after initial screening.

[NLM Cit ID: 98046261] (Comprehensive, evidence-based guideline with special references to specific patient populations, with a focus on matching treatment decisions to individual patient risk and management of specific populations. Update expected in 2001.)

Staessen JA et al: Antihypertensive treatment based on conventional or ambulatory blood pressure measurement. A randomized controlled trial. Ambulatory Blood Pressure Monitoring and Treatment of Hypertension Investigators. JAMA 1997;278:1065. [NLM Cit ID: 97459804] (Multicenter, randomized study of 419 patients in whom ambulatory blood pressure monitoring compared with conventional blood pressure measurements led to less intensive drug treatment with preserved blood pressure control, general well-being, and inhibition of left ventricular enlargement but did not reduce the overall costs.)

Zanchetti A: The role of ambulatory blood pressure monitoring in clinical practice. Am J Hypertens 1997; 10:1069. [NLM Cit ID: 97464295] (Review of methods, results, and applications.)

MANAGEMENT OF HYPERTENSION

Etiology & Classification

A. Primary (Essential) Hypertension: In about 95% of cases, no cause can be established. The condition occurs in 10–15% of white adults and 20–30% of black adults in the USA. The onset of essential hypertension is usually between ages 25 and 55; it is uncommon before age 20. In young people, secondary hypertension resulting from renal insufficiency, renal artery stenosis, or coarctation of the aorta makes up a greater—but still relatively small—proportion of cases.

Elevations in pressure are often intermittent early in the course of the disease. Even in established cases, the blood pressure fluctuates widely in response to emotional stress and physical activity. Blood pressures taken by the patient at home or during daily activities using a portable apparatus are often lower than those recorded in the office, clinic, or hospital and may be more reliable in estimating prognosis. Patients with daytime average pressures less than 135/85 mm Hg have a low rate of cardiovascular complications and a low prevalence of left ventricular hypertrophy, suggesting that this is an appropriate ambulatory blood pressure criterion for diagnosing hypertension.

The pathogenesis of essential hypertension is multifactorial. Genetic factors play an important role. Children with one—and even more so with two—hypertensive parents have higher blood pressures. Environmental factors also are significant. Increased salt intake has long been incriminated as a pathogenic factor in essential hypertension. It alone is probably not sufficient to elevate blood pressure to abnormal levels; a combination of too much salt plus a genetic predisposition is required. Other factors that may be involved in the pathogenesis of essential hypertension are the following:

1. Sympathetic nervous system hyperactivity–Sympathetic nervous system hyperactivity is most apparent in younger hypertensives, who may exhibit tachycardia and an elevated cardiac output. However, correlations between plasma catecholamines and blood pressure are poor. Insensitivity of the baroreflexes may play a role in the genesis of adrenergic hyperactivity.

2. Renin-angiotensin system–Renin, a proteolytic enzyme, is secreted by the juxtaglomerular cells surrounding afferent arterioles in response to a number of stimuli, including reduced renal perfusion pressure, diminished intravascular volume, circulating catecholamines, increased sympathetic nervous system activity, increased arteriolar stretch, and hypokalemia. Renin acts on angiotensinogen to cleave off the ten-amino-acid peptide angiotensin I. This peptide is then acted upon by angiotensin-converting enzyme to create the eight-amino-acid peptide angiotensin II, a potent vasoconstrictor and a major stimulant of aldosterone release from the adrenal glands. Studies have suggested that the incidence of hypertension and its complications may be increased in individuals with the DD genotype of the allele coding for angiotensin-converting enzyme. Nonetheless, despite the important role of this system in the regulation of blood pressure, it probably does not play a primary role in the pathogenesis of essential hypertension in most individuals. Patients with low plasma renin activity may have higher intravascular volumes. Black hypertensives and older patients tend to have lower plasma renin activity. Plasma renin activity levels can be best classified in relation to dietary sodium intake or urinary sodium excretion. Approximately 10% of essential hypertension patients have high levels, 60% have normal levels, and 30% low levels. Although such measurements have contributed to our understanding of the pathophysiology of hypertension, there is little clinical utility to measuring plasma renin activity.

3. Defect in natriuresis–Normal individuals increase their renal sodium excretion in response to elevations in arterial pressure and to a sodium or volume load. Hypertensive patients, particularly when their blood pressure is normal, exhibit a diminished ability to excrete a sodium load. This defect may result in increased plasma volume and hypertension. However, during chronic hypertension, a sodium load is usually handled normally.

4. Intracellular sodium and calcium–Intracellular Na^+ is elevated in blood cells and other tissues in essential hypertension. This may result from abnormalities in Na^+-K^+ exchange and other Na^+ transport mechanisms. Circulating "digitalis-like" substances may be responsible. An increase in intracellular Na^+ may lead to increased intracellular Ca^{2+} concentrations as a result of facilitated exchange. This could explain the increase in vascular smooth muscle tone that is characteristic of established hypertension.

5. Exacerbating factors–A number of conditions elevate blood pressure, especially in predisposed individuals. The best-documented is **obesity,** which is associated with an increase in intravascular volume and an elevated cardiac output. Weight reduction lowers blood pressure modestly. The relationship between **sodium intake** and hypertension remains controversial, but it is clear that some—but by no means all—hypertensives respond to high salt intake with substantial blood pressure increases. Hypertensive patients should consume no more than 100 mmol/d of salt (2.4 g of sodium, 6 g of sodium chloride).

Excessive use of **alcohol** also raises blood pressure, perhaps by increasing plasma catecholamines. Hypertension can be difficult to control in patients who consume more than 40 g of ethanol (two drinks) daily or drink in "binges." **Cigarette smoking** acutely raises blood pressure, again by increasing plasma norepinephrine. Although the long-term effect of smoking on blood pressure is less clear, the synergistic effects of smoking and high blood pressure on cardiovascular risk are well documented. The relationship of **exercise** to hypertension is variable. Aerobic exercise lowers blood pressure in previously sedentary individuals, but increasingly strenuous exercise in already active subjects may have a lesser effect. The relationship between stress and hypertension is not clearly established. **Polycythemia,** whether primary or due to diminished plasma volume, increases blood viscosity and may raise blood pressure. **Nonsteroidal anti-inflammatory agents** produce significant increases in blood pressure, averaging 5 mm Hg, and should be avoided in patients with borderline or elevated blood pressures whenever possible. Low **potassium intake** is associated with higher blood pressure in some patients; an intake of 90 mmol/d is recommended.

B. Secondary Hypertension: Approximately 5% of patients with hypertension can be found to have specific causes. The history, examination, and routine laboratory tests may identify patients who are more likely to have secondary hypertension and warrant further evaluation. In particular, patients who develop hypertension at an early age without a positive family history, those who first exhibit hypertension when over age 50, or those who have previously been controlled but then become refractory to treatment are more likely to have secondary hypertension. Secondary causes include the following.

1. Estrogen use–A small increase in blood pressure occurs in most women taking oral contraceptives, but considerable rises are noted occasionally. This is caused by volume expansion due to increased activity of the renin-angiotensin-aldosterone system. The primary abnormality is an increase in the hepatic synthesis of renin substrate. Five percent of women taking oral contraceptives chronically will exhibit a rise in blood pressure above 140/90 mm Hg; this is twice the expected prevalence. Contraceptive-related hypertension is more common in women over 35 years of age, in those who have taken contraceptives for more than 5 years, and in obese individuals. It is less common in those taking low-dose estrogen tablets. In most, hypertension is reversible by discontinuing the contraceptive, but it may take several weeks. There is no evidence that postmenopausal estrogen use causes hypertension, perhaps because hormone replacement maintains endothelium-mediated vasodilation.

2. Renal disease–Any disease of the renal parenchyma can cause hypertension, and these conditions are the most common causes of secondary hypertension. Hypertension may result from glomerular diseases, tubular interstitial disease, and polycystic kidneys. Most cases are related to increased intravascular volume or increased activity of the renin-angiotensin-aldosterone system. Hypertension accelerates progression of renal insufficiency, and rigorous control to target blood pressure of 139/85 or even lower will retard this progression. Diabetic nephropathy is another cause of chronic hypertension. The progression of this process is exacerbated by intraglomerular hypertension, itself worsened by systemic hypertension. Dilation of the efferent arterioles by angiotensin-converting enzyme inhibition reduces the rate of progression.

3. Renal vascular hypertension–Renal artery stenosis is present in 1–2% of hypertensive patients. Its cause in most younger individuals is fibromuscular hyperplasia, which is most common in women under 50. The remainder of renal vascular disease is due to atherosclerotic stenoses of the proximal renal arteries. The mechanism of hypertension is excessive renin release due to reduction in renal blood flow and perfusion pressure. Renal vascular hypertension may occur when a single branch of the renal artery is stenotic, but in as many as 25% of patients both arteries are obstructed.

Renal vascular hypertension should be suspected in the following circumstances: (1) if the documented onset is below age 20 or after age 50; (2) if there are epigastric or renal artery bruits; (3) if there is atherosclerotic disease of the aorta or peripheral arteries (15–25% of patients with symptomatic lower limb atherosclerotic vascular disease have renal artery stenosis); or (4) if there is abrupt deterioration in renal function after administration of angiotensin-converting enzyme inhibitors. Additional evaluation is indicated in such patients, especially if hypertension is difficult to control.

There is no ideal "screening" test for renal vascular hypertension. If the suspicion of renal vascular hypertension is sufficiently high, renal arteriography, the definitive diagnostic test, is the best approach. Where suspicion is moderate to low, radioisotope renography before and after administration of an angiotensin-converting enzyme inhibitor is one standard approach. The baseline study may show a smaller kidney with diminished function on the side of the stenosis. Postdrug (captopril, 50 mg orally, or enalaprilat, 2.5 mg intravenously) uptake and clearance of the radiotracer are delayed. However, bilateral disease may be difficult to detect if both kidneys are equally affected, and this test becomes insensitive in the presence of renal insufficiency (serum creatinine > 20 mg/dL). Duplex Doppler flow studies and noninvasive angiograms using CT or MRI have proponents. Except when stenosis is critical (> 80–90%) and unifocal, its significance may be assessed by measuring differences in renin activity between the renal veins. If the lesion is not associated with an increase in renin activity, hypertension often persists despite correction.

The treatment of patients with renal vascular hypertension should be individualized. Young individuals and good-risk patients of any age who have not responded to medical therapy should have the lesion corrected. Percutaneous transluminal angioplasty or stent placement is now the preferred approach for fibromuscular hyperplasia and for discrete stenotic arteriosclerotic lesions that do not involve the renal artery ostium. In older individuals with arteriosclerosis, only a minority experience normalization without continued drug therapy. Thus, it is reasonable to manage these patients medically if renal function does not deteriorate. Although converting enzyme inhibitors have improved the success rate of medical therapy of hypertension due to renal artery stenosis, they have been associated with marked hypotension and renal dysfunction in individuals with bilateral renal artery stenosis. Thus, renal function and blood pressure should be closely monitored during the first weeks of therapy in patients in whom this is a consideration.

4. Primary hyperaldosteronism and Cushing's syndrome–Patients with excess aldosterone secretion make up less than 0.5% of all cases of hypertension. The usual lesion is an adrenal adenoma, though some patients have bilateral adrenal hyperplasia. The diagnosis should be suspected when patients present with hypokalemia prior to diuretic therapy associated with excessive urinary potassium excretion (usually > 40 meq/L on a spot specimen) and suppressed levels of plasma renin activity; serum sodium usually exceeds 140 meq/L. Aldosterone concentrations in urine and blood are elevated. The lesion can be demonstrated by CT scanning or MRI. Less commonly, patients with Cushing's syndrome (glucocorticoid excess) may manifest hypertension as a first sign of the disorder (see Chapter 26).

5. Pheochromocytoma–Although hypertension due to pheochromocytoma may be episodic, most patients have sustained elevations. The majority of patients have orthostatic falls in blood pressure, the converse of essential hypertension; some develop glucose intolerance. The diagnosis and treatment of this entity are discussed in Chapter 26.

6. Coarctation of the aorta–This uncommon cause of hypertension is discussed in Chapter 10.

7. Hypertension associated with pregnancy–Hypertension occurring de novo or worsening during pregnancy is one of the commonest causes of maternal and fetal morbidity and mortality (see Chapter 18).

8. Other causes of secondary hypertension–Hypertension has also been associated with hypercalcemia due to any cause, acromegaly, hyperthyroidism, hypothyroidism, and a variety of neurologic disorders causing increased intracranial pressure. A number of medications may cause or exacerbate hypertension—most importantly cyclosporine and NSAIDs.

Adcock BB et al: Secondary hypertension: a practical diagnostic approach Am Fam Physician 1997;55:1263. [NLM Cit ID: 97226077] (A comprehensive, practical review.)

Aitchison F et al: Diagnostic imaging of renal artery stenosis. J Hum Hypertens 1999;13:595. [NLM Cit ID: 99414260] (Review of the utility of intravenous urography, ultrasound, renal scintigraphy with angiotensin-converting enzyme inhibitors, angiography and CT and MRI imaging in the evaluation of renal artery stenosis.)

Dustan HP: Renal arterial disease and hypertension. Med Clin North Am 1997;81:1199. [NLM Cit ID: 97453985] (Diagnosis, treatment and effect on renal function.)

Ganguly A: Primary aldosteronism. N Engl J Med 1998; 339:1828. [NLM Cit ID: 99061028] (Pathology, diagnosis, and treatment.)

Januszewicz W et al: Secondary hypertension in the elderly. J Hum Hypertens 1998;12:603. [NLM Cit ID: 98454809] (Review highlighting the importance of considering secondary causes of hypertension in the elderly.)

Krijnen P et al: A clinical prediction rule for renal artery stenosis. Ann Intern Med 1998;129:705. [NLM Cit ID: 99008346] (Study provides a clinical prediction model to help select patients for further diagnostic procedures.)

Preston Y et al: Renal parenchymal hypertension: Current concepts of pathogenesis and management. Arch Intern Med 1996;156:602. [NLM Cit ID: 96205984] (Most frequent cause of secondary hypertension.)

Stewart PM: Mineralocorticoid hypertension. Lancet 1999;353:1341. [NLM Cit ID: 99232915] (A review emphasizing that hypertensive patients with hypokalemia, severe hypertension, or a family history of hypertension or stroke should be screened for mineralocorticoid excess.)

Zimmerman RS: Hormonal and humor considerations in hypertensive disease. Med Clin North Am 1997;81: 1213. [NLM Cit ID: 97453986] (Review of the evaluation of patients suspected of having hyperaldosteronism or a pheochromocytoma.)

Complications of Untreated Hypertension

Complications of hypertension are related either to sustained elevations of blood pressure, with consequent changes in the vasculature and heart, or to atherosclerosis that accompanies and is accelerated by long-standing hypertension. The excess morbidity and mortality related to hypertension are progressive over the whole range of systolic and diastolic blood pressures; the risk approximately doubles for each 6 mm Hg increase in diastolic blood pressure. However, target-organ damage varies markedly between individuals with similar levels of office hypertension. Ambulatory pressures are more closely related to end-organ damage. Specific complications include the following:

A. Hypertensive Cardiovascular Disease: Cardiac complications are the major causes of morbidity and mortality in essential hypertension, and preventing them is a major goal of therapy. Electrocardiographic evidence of left ventricular hypertrophy is found in 2–15% of chronic hypertensives. Once established, left ventricular hypertrophy is an indication of increased risk for morbidity and mortality; for any level of blood pressure, its presence is associated with incremental risk. Echocardiographic left ventricular hypertrophy is a powerful predictor of prognosis. Left ventricular hypertrophy may cause or facilitate many cardiac complications of hypertension, including congestive heart failure, ventricular arrhythmias, myocardial ischemia, and sudden death.

Left ventricular diastolic dysfunction, which may present with all of the signs and symptoms of congestive heart failure, is common in patients with long-standing hypertension. Hypertensive left ventricular hypertrophy regresses with therapy. Regression is most closely related to the degree of systolic blood pressure reduction and does not seem to be very dependent on the specific medication employed. Diuretics have produced equal or greater reductions of left ventricular mass when compared with other drug classes. Clinical trials are just beginning to show that effective blood pressure control can modify the risk or rate of progression of cognitive dysfunction.

B. Hypertensive Cerebrovascular Disease and Dementia: Hypertension is the major predisposing cause of stroke, especially intracerebral hemorrhage but also ischemic cerebral infarction. Cerebrovascular complications are more closely correlated with the systolic than the diastolic blood pressure. The incidence of these complications is markedly reduced by antihypertensive therapy. Preceding hypertension is associated with a higher incidence of subsequent dementia, both the vascular and the Alzheimer types.

C. Hypertensive Renal Disease: Chronic hypertension leads to nephrosclerosis, a common cause of renal insufficiency; it is diminished by aggressive blood pressure control. In patients with hypertensive nephropathy, the blood pressure should be 130/85 mm Hg or lower when proteinuria is present. Secondary renal disease is more common in blacks, particularly when accompanying diabetes is present. Hypertension also plays an important role in accelerating the progression of other forms of renal disease, most commonly diabetic nephropathy. Angiotensin-converting enzyme inhibitors have been shown to be particularly effective in preventing the latter complication, but these agents also appear to prevent the progression of other forms of nephropathy.

D. Aortic Dissection: Hypertension is a contributing factor in many patients with dissection of the aorta. Its diagnosis and treatment of aortic dissection are discussed in Chapter 12.

E. Atherosclerotic Complications: Most patients in the USA with hypertension die of complications of atherosclerosis, but the linkage between hypertension and atherosclerotic cardiovascular disease is much less close than that with the previously discussed complications. Effective antihypertensive therapy is thus less successful in preventing complications of coronary heart disease, but even coronary events can be reduced in high-risk patients.

Chobanian AV et al: Exacerbation of atherosclerosis by hypertension: Potential mechanisms and clinical implications. Arch Intern Med 1996;156:1952. [NLM Cit ID: 96420449] (Most of the complications of hypertension involve accelerated atherosclerosis. This paper discusses the mechanism for this interaction and the importance of treating both risk factors.)

Forette F et al: Prevention of dementia in randomised double-blind placebo-controlled Systolic Hypertension in Europe (Syst-Eur) trial. Lancet 1998;352:1347. [NLM Cit ID: 99017259] (Large, double-blind, placebo-controlled trial suggesting that the incidence of dementia may be reduced by controlling isolated systolic hypertension in the elderly.)

Kostis JD et al: Prevention of heart failure by anti-hypertensive drug treatment in older persons with isolated systolic hypertension. JAMA 1997;278:212. [NLM Cit ID: 97361706] (Treatment of isolated systolic hypertension reduced the incidence of congestive heart failure by nearly 50%.)

Maschio G et al: The effect of the angiotensin-converting-enzyme inhibitor benazepril on the progression of chronic renal insufficiency. N Engl J Med 1996;334: 939. [NLM Cit ID: 96175229] (ACE inhibitor therapy may prevent progressive renal insufficiency in a broad group of conditions.)

Srikanthan VS et al: Hypertension in coronary artery disease. Med Clin North Am 1997;81:1147. [NLM Cit ID: 97453983] (Myocardial ischemia and coronary events are responsible for much of morbidity and mortality related to hypertension.)

Clinical Findings

The clinical and laboratory findings are mainly referable to involvement of the target organs: heart, brain, kidneys, eyes, and peripheral arteries.

A. Symptoms: Mild to moderate essential hypertension is usually associated with normal health and well-being for many years. Suboccipital pulsating headaches, characteristically occurring early in the morning and subsiding during the day, are characteristic, but any type of headache may occur. Accelerated hypertension is associated with somnolence, confusion, visual disturbances, and nausea and vomiting (hypertensive encephalopathy).

Patients with pheochromocytomas that secrete predominantly norepinephrine usually have sustained hypertension but may have episodic hypertension. Attacks (lasting minutes to hours) of anxiety, palpitation, profuse perspiration, pallor, tremor, and nausea and vomiting occur; blood pressure is markedly elevated, and angina or acute pulmonary edema may occur. In primary aldosteronism, patients may have episodes of generalized muscular weakness or paralysis as well as paresthesias, polyuria, and nocturia due to hypokalemia; malignant hypertension is rare.

Chronic hypertension often leads to left ventricular hypertrophy, which may be associated with diastolic or, in late stages, systolic dysfunction. Exertional and paroxysmal nocturnal dyspnea may result. Severe left ventricular hypertrophy predisposes to myocardial ischemia (especially when concomitant coronary artery disease is present), ventricular arrhythmias, and sudden death.

Cerebral involvement causes (1) stroke due to thrombosis or (2) small or large hemorrhage from microaneurysms of small penetrating intracranial arteries. Hypertensive encephalopathy is probably caused by acute capillary congestion and exudation with cerebral edema. The findings are usually reversible if adequate treatment is given promptly. Although there is no strict correlation of diastolic blood pressure with hypertensive encephalopathy, it usually exceeds 130 mm Hg.

B. Signs: Physical findings depend upon the cause of hypertension, its duration and severity, and the degree of effect on target organs.

1. Blood pressure–On the initial observation, pressure should be examined in both arms and, if lower extremity pulses are diminished, in the legs to exclude coarctation of the aorta. An orthostatic drop is present in pheochromocytoma. Older patients may have falsely elevated readings by sphygmomanometry because of noncompressible vessels. This may be suspected in the presence of Osler's sign—a palpable brachial or radial artery when the cuff is inflated above systolic pressure. Occasionally, it may be necessary to make direct measurements of intra-arterial pressure, especially in patients with apparent severe hypertension who do not tolerate therapy.

2. Retinas–The Keith-Wagener (KW) classification of retinal changes in hypertension, in spite of deficiencies, presages a worse prognosis when stage II or higher changes are present (narrowing as defined by arterial diameter less than 50% of venous diameter, copper or silver wire appearance, exudates, hemorrhages, or papilledema).

3. Heart and arteries–A loud aortic second sound and an early systolic ejection click may occur. Left ventricular enlargement with a left ventricular heave indicates well-established disease. Older patients frequently have systolic ejection murmurs resulting from aortic sclerosis, and these may evolve to significant aortic stenosis in some individuals. Aortic insufficiency may be auscultated in up to 5% of patients, and hemodynamically insignificant aortic insufficiency can be detected by Doppler echocardiography in 10–20%. A presystolic (S_4) gallop due to decreased compliance of the left ventricle is quite common.

4. Pulses–The timing of upper and lower extremity pulses should be compared to exclude coarctation of the aorta. All major peripheral pulses should be evaluated to exclude aortic dissection and peripheral atherosclerosis, which may be associated with renal artery involvement.

C. Laboratory Findings: Recommended testing includes the following: hemoglobin; urinalysis and renal function studies, to detect hematuria, proteinuria, and casts, signifying primary renal disease or nephrosclerosis; serum K^+, since hypokalemia is typical of hyperaldosteronism; fasting blood sugar level, since hyperglycemia is noted in diabetes and pheochromocytoma; plasma lipids, as an indicator of atherosclerosis risk; and serum uric acid, since if elevated it is a relative contraindication to diuretic therapy.

D. Electrocardiography and Chest X-Ray: Electrocardiographic criteria are highly specific but not very sensitive for left ventricular hypertrophy. The "strain" pattern of ST–T wave changes is a sign of more advanced disease and is associated with a poor prognosis. A chest x-ray is not recommended in the routine evaluation of uncomplicated hypertension, since it usually does not yield additional information.

E. Echocardiography: The utility of echocardiography in individual patients is limited by the reproducibility of the technique. Although echocardiography has been advocated to determine the need for drug therapy in patients with borderline or mildly elevated pressures, it is unusual to find left ventricular mass readings above the upper 75% confidence limits in the absence of systolic hypertension. The primary role of echocardiography should be to evaluate patients with clinical symptoms or signs of cardiac disease.

F. Diagnostic Studies: Only if the clinical presentation or routine tests suggest secondary or complicated hypertension are additional diagnostic studies indicated. These may include blood and urine tests for endocrine causes of hypertension, renal ultrasound to diagnose primary renal disease (polycystic kidneys, obstructive uropathy) or renovascular abnormalities, and isotope renograms for the latter diagnosis. Further evaluation may include abdominal imaging studies (ultrasound, CT scan, or MRI) or renal arteriography.

G. Summary: Since most hypertension is "primary," few studies are necessary beyond those listed above. If conventional therapy is unsuccessful or if symptoms suggest a secondary cause, further studies are indicated.

Reeves RA: Does this patient have hypertension? How to measure blood pressure. JAMA 1995;273:1211. [NLM Cit ID: 95222862]

See also JNC VI and the Kaplan monograph cited at the beginning of this chapter.

Nonpharmacologic Therapy

Lifestyle modification may have a substantial impact on morbidity and mortality. A diet rich in fruits, vegetables, and low-fat dairy foods and low in saturated and total fats (DASH diet) has been shown to lower blood pressure. Additional measures can prevent or mitigate hypertension or its cardiovascular consequences as shown in Table 11–2.

Table 11–2. Lifestyle modifications for hypertension prevention and management.[1]

Lose weight if overweight.
Limit alcohol intake to no more than 1 oz (30 mL) of ethanol (eg, 24 oz [720 mL] of beer, 10 oz [300 mL] of wine, or 2 oz [60 mL] of 100-proof whiskey) per day or 0.5 oz (15 mL) of ethanol per day for women and lighter-weight people
Increase aerobic physical activity (30–45 minutes most days of the week)
Reduce sodium intake to no more than 100 mmol/d (2.4 g of sodium or 6 g of sodium chloride)
Maintain adequate intake of dietary potassium (approximately 90 mmol/d)
Maintain adequate intake of dietary calcium and magnesium for general health
Stop smoking and reduce intake of dietary saturated fat and cholesterol for overall cardiovascular health

[1]From: The sixth report of the Joint National Committee on detection, education, and treatment of high blood pressure (JNC VI). Arch Intern Med 1997;157:2413.

All patients with high normal or elevated blood pressures (as defined in Table 11–1), those who have a family history of cardiovascular complications of hypertension, and those who have multiple coronary risk factors should be counseled about nonpharmacologic approaches to lowering blood pressure. Approaches of proved but modest value include weight reduction, reduced alcohol consumption, and in some patients reduced salt intake. Gradually increasing activity levels should be encouraged in previously sedentary patients, but strenuous exercise training programs in already active individuals may have less benefit. Calcium and potassium supplements have been advocated, but their ability to lower blood pressure is limited.

Smoking cessation will reduce overall cardiovascular risk.

Burgess E et al: Lifestyle modifications to prevent and control hypertension. 6. Recommendations on potassium, magnesium and calcium. Canadian Hypertension Society, Canadian Coalition for High Blood Pressure Prevention and Control, Laboratory Centre for Disease Control at Health Canada, Heart and Stroke Foundation of Canada. CMAJ 1999;160:S35. [NLM Cit ID: 99266394] (Guidelines recommending a daily dietary intake of 60 mmol of potassium both for the prevention and for the treatment of hypertension. Further potassium supplementation, magnesium, and calcium supplementation is not recommended.)

Campbell NR et al: Lifestyle modifications to prevent and control hypertension. 3. Recommendations on alcohol consumption. Canadian Hypertension Society, Canadian Coalition for High Blood Pressure Prevention and Control, Laboratory Centre for Disease Control at Health Canada, Heart and Stroke Foundation of Canada. CMAJ 1999;160:S13. [NLM Cit ID: 99266391] (Guidelines recommending that alcohol consumption should not exceed 14 standard drinks per week for men and 9 standard drinks per week for women.)

Cleroux J et al: Lifestyle modifications to prevent and control hypertension. 4. Recommendations on physical exercise training. Canadian Hypertension Society, Canadian Coalition for High Blood Pressure Prevention and Control, Laboratory Centre for Disease Control at Health

Canada, Heart and Stroke Foundation of Canada. CMAJ 1999;160:S21. [NLM Cit ID: 99266392] (Recommendation that patients with mild hypertension should engage in 50–60 minutes of moderate exercise, such as brisk walking or cycling, three or four times per week.)

Fodor JD et al: Lifestyle modifications to prevent and control hypertension. 5. Recommendations on dietary salt. Canadian Hypertension Society, Canadian Coalition for High Blood Pressure Prevention and Control, Laboratory Centre for Disease Control at Health Canada, Heart and Stroke Foundation of Canada. CMAJ 1999;160:S29. [NLM Cit ID: 99266393]

Reisin E: Nonpharmacologic approaches to hypertension: Weight, sodium, alcohol, exercise, and tobacco cessation. Med Clin North Am 1997;81:1289. [NLM Cit ID: 98019412]

Spence JD et al: Lifestyle modifications to prevent and control hypertension. 7. Recommendations on stress management. Canadian Hypertension Society, Canadian Coalition for High Blood Pressure Prevention and Control, Laboratory Centre for Disease Control at Health Canada, Heart and Stroke Foundation of Canada. CMAJ 1999;160:S46. [NLM Cit ID: 99266395]

Whelton PK et al: Sodium reduction and weight loss in the treatment of hypertension in older persons: a randomized controlled trial of nonpharmacologic interventions in the elderly (TONE). TONE Collaborative Research Group. (Published erratum appears in JAMA 1998;279:1954.) JAMA 1998;279:839. [NLM Cit ID: 98175753] (Randomized, controlled trial of 975 elderly patients demonstrating that reduced sodium intake and weight loss may serve as a safe, effective nonpharmacologic therapy of hypertension in older persons.)

Who Should Be Treated With Medications? (Tables 11–3 and 11–4)

The objective of antihypertensive therapy is to prevent the morbidity and mortality related to this condition. Nearly 20 randomized control trials have shown that drug therapy of patients with stage II and III hypertension consistently reduces the incidence of stroke by 30–50%, congestive heart failure by 40–50%, and progression to accelerated hypertension syndromes. The decreases in fatal and nonfatal coronary heart disease and cardiovascular and total mortality have been less dramatic, ranging from 10% to 15%. This lesser decrease in coronary heart disease has generated controversy. Some have attributed the lesser benefit to characteristics of the drugs (primarily diuretics and beta-blockers), such as their adverse effect on lipid profiles and electrolyte balance. Others have attributed it to the more chronic and multifactorial nature of coronary artery disease, the generally low-risk populations included in trials, and the large number of crossovers from placebo to active therapy. Several trials in older persons with predominantly systolic hypertension have now confirmed that antihypertensive therapy prevents fatal and nonfatal myocardial infarction and overall cardiovascular mortality. These trials have also placed the focus on control of systolic blood pressure—in contrast to emphasis on diastolic blood pressures.

Table 11–3. Components of cardiovascular risk stratification in patients with hypertension.[1]

Major risk factors
Smoking
Dyslipidemia
Diabetes mellitus
Age > 60 years
Sex (men and postmenopausal women)
Family history of cardiovascular disease: women < 65 years or men < 55 years
Target organ damage/clinical cardiovascular disease
Heart diseases
Left ventricular hypertrophy
Angina or prior myocardial infarction
Prior coronary revascularization
Heart failure
Stroke or transient ischemic attack
Nephropathy
Peripheral arterial disease
Retinopathy

[1]From: The sixth report of the Joint National Committee on detection, education, and treatment of high blood pressure (JNC VI). Arch Intern Med 1997;157:2413.

Mulrow CD et al: Hypertension in the elderly: Implications and generalizability of randomized trials. JAMA 1994; 272:1932. [NLM Cit ID: 95082133] (Treatment of older persons is highly efficacious and cost-effective.)

Goals of Treatment

The decision to initiate drug therapy should be based upon the assessment of overall cardiovascular risk rather than the level of blood pressure alone. Table 11–3 lists the major risk factors for cardiovascular morbidity and mortality and the cardiovascular manifestations that predispose to further complications. These factors must be weighed together with the individual patient's blood pressure in determining whether to initiate therapy. Table 11–4 sets forth the criteria used in making this decision. Thus, patients with systolic blood pressure over 160 mm Hg with diastolic blood pressure over 90 mm Hg after repeated measurements should be treated to a goal blood pressure below 140 mm Hg systolic and below 90 mm Hg diastolic. Those with stage I hypertension and at least one additional indicator of increased risk should be treated also. Very high risk groups, such as diabetics, patients with nephropathy, and (most likely) patients with heart failure and coronary disease benefit from antihypertensive therapy even when their blood pressure is in the high normal range. There has been some concern that excessive lowering of diastolic blood pressures may induce myocardial ischemia (the so-called J curve), but the best data do not support this speculation. Indeed, it appears that a lower target blood pressure (130/85 mm Hg) is indicated in high-risk individuals such as diabetics and those with renal dysfunction.

Hansson L et al: Effects of intensive blood-pressure lowering and low-dose aspirin in patients with hypertension: princi-

Table 11–4. Risk stratification and treatment.[1,2]

Blood Pressure Stages (mm Hg)	Risk Group A (No Risk Factors; No TOD/CCD[3])	Risk Group B (At Least 1 Risk Factor, Not Including Diabetes; No TOD/CCD)	Risk Group C (TOD/CCD and/or Diabetes, With or Without Other Risk Factors)
High-normal (130–139/85–89)	Lifestyle modification	Lifestyle modification	Drug therapy[4]
Stage 1 (140–159/80–99)	Lifestyle modification (up to 12 mo)	Lifestyle modification[5] (up to 6 mo)	Drug therapy
Stages 2 and 3 (≥ 160/≥ 100)	Drug therapy	Drug therapy	Drug therapy

[1]From: The sixth report of the Joint National Committee on detection, education, and treatment of high blood pressure (JNC VI). Arch Intern Med 1997;157:2413.
[2]*Note:* For example, a patient with diabetes and blood pressure of 142/94 mm Hg plus left ventricular hypertrophy should be classified as having stage 1 hypertension with target organ disease (left ventricular hypertrophy) and with another major risk factor (diabetes). This patient would be categorized as "Stage 1, Risk Group C," and recommended for immediate initiation of pharmacologic treatment. Lifestyle modification should be adjunctive therapy for all patients recommended for pharmacologic therapy.
[3]TOD/CCD indicates target organ disease/clinical cardiovascular disease (see Table 11–3).
[4]For those with heart failure, renal insufficiency, or diabetes.
[5]For patients with multiple risk factors, clinicians should consider drugs as initial therapy plus lifestyle modifications.

pal results of the Hypertension Optimal Treatment (HOT) randomized trial. Lancet 1998;351:1755. [NLM Cit ID: 98297870] (Large study showing more intensive therapy reduced cardiovascular events, especially in diabetics.)

Lazarus JM et al: Achievement and safety of the low blood pressure goal in chronic renal disease. Hypertension 1997;29:641. [NLM Cit ID: 97192859] (Progressive renal failure dysfunction is slowed or even prevented by aggressive blood pressure reduction.)

Tight blood pressure control and risk of macrovascular and microvascular complications in type 2 diabetes. Prospective Diabetes Study Group. BMJ 1998;317:703. [NLM Cit ID: 98404064] (Aggressive control reduces end points; choice of drug may not be as important.)

DRUG THERAPY

General Principles

There are now eight to ten different classes of antihypertensive drugs (depending on how they are defined) of which five (diuretics, beta-blockers, ACE inhibitors, calcium channel blockers, and angiotensin II receptor antagonists) are suitable for initial or single drug therapy. A number of considerations enter into the selection of the initial drug for a given patient. These include the weight of evidence for beneficial effects on clinical outcomes, the safety and the tolerability of the drug, its cost, demographic differences in response, concomitant medical conditions, and lifestyle issues. The specific classes of antihypertensive medications are discussed below, and guidelines for the choice of the initial medications are offered thereafter.

Current Antihypertensive Agents (See Tables 11–5 to 11–9 for dosages.)

A. Diuretics: (Table 11–5.) Diuretics are the antihypertensives that have been most extensively studied and most consistently effective in clinical trials. Diuretics lower blood pressure initially by decreasing plasma volume (by suppressing tubular reabsorption of sodium, thus increasing the excretion of sodium and water) and cardiac output, but during chronic therapy their major hemodynamic effect is reduction of peripheral vascular resistance. Most of the antihypertensive effect of these agents is achieved at lower dosages than used previously (typically, 12.5 or 25 mg of hydrochlorothiazide or equivalent), but their biochemical effects are dose-related. The thiazide diuretics are the most widely used. During chronic therapy, hydrochlorothiazide may be administered every other day with undiminished efficacy. The loop diuretics (such as furosemide) may lead to electrolyte and volume depletion more readily than the thiazides and have short durations of action; therefore, they should not be used in hypertension except in the presence of renal dysfunction (serum creatinine above 2.5 mg/dL). Relative to the beta-blockers and the ACE inhibitors, diuretics are more potent in blacks, older individuals, the obese, and other subgroups with increased plasma volume or low plasma renin activity. Interestingly, they are relatively more effective in smokers than in nonsmokers. Chronic diuretic administration also mitigates the loss of bone mineral content in older women at risk for osteoporosis. Overall, diuretics administered alone control blood pressure in 50% of patients and can be used effectively in combination with all other agents. They are probably the most effective agents for lowering isolated or predominantly systolic hypertension.

The adverse effects of diuretics relate chiefly to the metabolic changes listed in Table 11–5. Impotence, skin rashes, and photosensitivity are less frequent side effects. Hypokalemia has been a concern but is uncommon at the recommended dosages (12.5–25 mg hydrochlorothiazide). The risk can be minimized by limiting salt intake or eating a high-

Table 11–5. Antihypertensive drugs: Diuretics.

Drug	Proprietary Name	Initial Dosage	Dosage Range	Cost per Unit	Cost for 30 Days' Treatment[1] (Average Dosage)	Adverse Effects	Comments
THIAZIDES AND RELATED DIURETICS							
Hydrochlorothiazide	Esidrix, Hydro-Diuril	12.5 or 25 mg once daily	12.5–50 mg once daily	\$0.03/50 mg	\$0.90	↓K^+, ↓Mg^{2+}, ↑Ca^{2+}, ↓Na^+, ↑uric acid, ↑glucose, ↑LDL cholesterol, ↑triglycerides; rash erectile dysfunction.	Low dosages effective in many patients without associated metabolic abnormalities; metolazone more effective with concurrent renal insufficiency; indapamide does not alter serum lipid levels.
Chlorthalidone	Hygroton, Thaliton	12.5 or 25 mg once daily	12.5–50 mg once daily	\$0.12/50 mg	\$3.60		
Metolazone	Diulo, Zaroxolyn Mykrox	1.25 or 2.5 mg once daily 0.5 mg once daily	1.25–5 mg once daily 0.5–1 mg once daily	\$0.73/5 mg \$0.85/0.5 mg	\$21.90 \$25.50		
Indapamide	Lozol	2.5 mg once daily	2.5–5 mg once daily	\$0.78/2.5 mg	\$23.40		
LOOP DIURETICS							
Furosemide	Lasix	20 mg bid	40–320 mg in 2 or 3 doses	\$0.14/40 mg	\$8.40	Same as thiazides, but higher risk of excessive diuresis and electrolyte imbalance. Increases calcium excretion.	**Furosemide:** Short duration of action a disadvantage; should be reserved for patients with renal insufficiency or fluid retention. Poor antihypertensive. **Torsemide:** Effective blood pressure medication at low dosage.
Bumetanide	Bumex	0.25 mg bid	0.5–10 mg in 2 or 3 doses	\$0.40/1 mg	\$24.00		
Torsemide	Demadex	2.5 mg once daily	5–10 mg once daily	\$0.58/10 mg	\$17.40		
COMBINATION PRODUCTS							
Hydrochlorothiazide and triamterene	Dyazide (25/50 mg) Maxzide (37.5/25 mg)	1 tab once daily	1 or 2 tabs once daily	\$0.35	\$10.50	Same as thiazides plus GI disturbances, hyperkalemia rather than hypokalemia, headache; triamterene can cause kidney stones and renal dysfunction; spironolactone causes gynecomastia. Hyperkalemia can occur if this combination is used in patients with renal failure or those taking ACE inhibitors.	Use should be limited to patients with demonstrable need for a potassium-sparing agent.
Hydrochlorothiazide and amiloride	Moduretic (50/5 mg)	½ tab once daily	1 or 2 tabs once daily	\$0.60	\$18.00		
Hydrochlorothiazide and spironolactone	Aldactazide (25/25 mg)	1 tab once daily	1 or 2 tabs once daily	\$0.43	\$12.90		

[1]Cost to pharmacist (average wholesale price, generic when possible) for quantity listed. Source: *Drug Topics Red Book,* March 2000; Vol. 19, No. 3.

potassium diet, and potassium replacement is usually not required to maintain serum K^+ at > 3.5 mmol/L. Higher serum levels are prudent in patients at special risk from intracellular potassium depletion (patients taking digoxin or having ventricular arrhythmias and diabetics in whom insulin release and insulin sensitivity are reduced by hypokalemia). Trials in which diuretic therapy proved most beneficial employed combinations of thiazide and potassium-sparing agents, such as triamterene or amiloride. Although these medications have additional side effects (primarily gastrointestinal), and may be dangerous in the presence of oliguria it is reasonable to use them in appropriate patients receiving higher doses of diuretics and in place of potassium supplements. Diuretics also increase serum uric acid and may precipitate gout. Increases in blood glucose, triglycerides, low-density lipoprotein cholesterol, and plasma insulin may occur but are relatively minor during long-term low-dose therapy.

B. Beta-Adrenergic Blocking Agents: (Table 11–6.) These drugs are effective in hypertension because they decrease the heart rate and cardiac output. Even after continued use of beta-blockers, cardiac output remains lower and systemic vascular resistance higher with agents that do not have intrinsic sympathomimetic or alpha-blocking activity. The beta-blockers also decrease renin release and are more efficacious in populations with elevated plasma renin activity, such as younger white patients. They neutralize the reflex tachycardia caused by vasodilators and are especially useful in patients with associated conditions that benefit from this mode of therapy. These include individuals with angina pectoris, patients with previous myocardial infarction, stable congenital heart failure, and those with migraine headaches and somatic manifestations of anxiety.

Although all beta-blockers appear to be similar in antihypertensive potency, controlling approximately 50% of patients, they differ in a number of pharmacologic properties (these differences are summarized in Table 11–6), including those relatively specific to the cardiac β_1 receptors (cardioselectivity) and whether they also block the β_2 receptors in the bronchi and vasculature; at higher dosages, however, all agents are nonselective. The beta-blockers also differ in their pharmacokinetics and lipid solubility—which determines whether they cross the blood-brain barrier and affect the incidence of central nervous system side effects—and route of metabolism. The effect on the pulse rate varies; agents with intrinsic sympathetic activity may be preferable in patients who develop more pronounced bradycardia (< 45/min) when given other beta-blockers. Labetalol is a combined alpha- and beta-blocker and, unlike most beta-blockers, decreases peripheral resistance.

The side effects of all beta-blockers include inducing or exacerbating bronchospasm in predisposed patients (asthmatics, some COPD patients); sinus node and atrioventricular conduction depression (resulting in bradycardia or AV block); precipitating or worsening left ventricular failure (although they are recommended for stable patients with underlying left ventricular systolic dysfunction); nasal congestion; Raynaud's phenomenon, especially in women; and central nervous system symptoms with nightmares, excitement, depression, and confusion. Fatigue, lethargy, and impotence may occur. All beta-blockers tend to increase plasma triglycerides. The nonselective and, to a lesser extent, the cardioselective (β_1-selective) beta-blockers tend to depress the protective HDL fraction of plasma cholesterol. This is not seen in agents with intrinsic sympathomimetic activity, and as with diuretics, the changes are blunted with time and dietary changes.

Beta-blockers have traditionally been considered contraindicated in patients with congestive heart failure. However, evolving experience suggests that they have a marked beneficial effect on the natural history of patients with chronic stable heart failure and reduced ejection fractions (see Chapter 10). Beta-blockers are relatively contraindicated in patients with type 1 diabetes, since they can mask the symptoms of hypoglycemia and prolong these episodes by inhibiting gluconeogenesis. Beta-blockers should also be used with caution in patients with advanced peripheral vascular disease associated with rest pain or nonhealing ulcers, but they are generally well tolerated in patients with mild claudication.

C. Angiotensin-Converting Enzyme (ACE) Inhibitors: (Table 11–7.) These drugs are being increasingly used as the initial medication in mild to moderate hypertension. Their primary mode of action is inhibition of the renin-angiotensin-aldosterone system, but they also inhibit bradykinin degradation, stimulate vasodilating prostaglandin synthesis, and, sometimes, reduce sympathetic nervous system activity. These latter actions may explain why they exhibit some effect even in patients with low plasma renin activity. The ACE inhibitors appear to be more effective in younger whites. They are relatively less effective in blacks and in the elderly and in predominantly systolic hypertension. While as single therapy they achieve adequate antihypertensive control in only about 40–50% of patients, the combination of an ACE inhibitor and a diuretic or calcium channel blocker is potent.

The ACE inhibitors are the agents of choice in type I diabetics with frank proteinuria or evidence of renal dysfunction, because they delay the progression to end-stage renal disease. Many authorities have extrapolated this indication to include type II diabetics and type I diabetics with microalbuminuria, even when they do not meet the usual criteria for antihypertensive therapy. The Heart Outcomes Prevention Evaluation (HOPE) trial demonstrated that the ACE inhibitor ramipril reduces the number of cardiovascular deaths, nonfatal myocardial infarctions and nonfa-

Table 11–6. Antihypertensive drugs: Beta-adrenergic blocking agents.

Drug	Proprietary Name	Initial Dosage	Dosage Range	Cost per Unit	Cost for 30 Days' Treatment (Based on Average Dosage)[1]	Special Properties					Comments[5]
						β_1 Selectivity[2]	ISA[3]	MSA[4]	Lipid Solubility	Renal vs Hepatic Elimination	
Acebutolol	Sectral	200 mg once daily	200–1200 mg in 1 or 2 doses	$1.64/400 mg	$49.20	+	+	+	+	H > R	Positive ANA; rare LE syndrome; also indicated for arrhythmias. Doses > 800 mg have β_1 and β_2 effects.
Atenolol	Tenormin	25 mg once daily	25–200 mg once daily	$0.67/50 mg	$20.10	+	0	0	0	R	Also indicated for angina pectoris and post-MI. Doses > 100 mg have β_1 and β_2 effects.
Betaxolol	Kerlone	10 mg once daily	10–40 mg once daily	$0.33/10 mg	$24.90	+	0	0	+	H > R	
Bisoprolol and hydrochlorothiazide	Ziac	5 mg/6.25 mg once daily	2.5–10 mg plus 6.25 mg	$1.19/2.5/6.25 mg	$35.70	+	0	0	0	R = H	Low-dose combination approved for initial therapy. Bisoprolol also effective for heart failure.
Carteolol	Cartrol	2.5 mg once daily	2.5–10 mg once daily	$1.06/5 mg	$31.80	0	+	0	+	R > H	
Carvedilol	Coreg	6.25 mg bid	12.5–100 mg in 2 doses	$1.59/25 mg	$95.40 (25 mg bid)	0	0	0	+++	H > R	α:β blocking activity 1:9; may cause orthostatic symptoms; effective for congestive heart failure.
Labetalo	Normodyne, Trandate	100 mg bid	200–1200 mg in 2 doses	$0.68/200 mg	$40.80	0	0/+	0	++	H	α:β blocking activity 1:3; more orthostatic hypotension, fever, hepatotoxicity.

(*continued*)

Table 11–6. Antihypertensive drugs: Beta-adrenergic blocking agents (continued).

Drug	Proprietary Name	Initial Dosage	Dosage Range	Cost per Unit	Cost for 30 Days' Treatment (Based on Average Dosage)[1]	Special Properties					Comments[5]
						β_1 Selectivity[2]	ISA[3]	MSA[4]	Lipid Solubility	Renal vs Hepatic Elimination	
Metoprolol	Lopressor	50 mg in 1 or 2 doses	50–200 mg in 1 or 2 doses	$0.46/50 mg	$27.60	+	0	+	+++	H	Also indicated for angina pectoris and post-MI. Effective for heart failure. Doses > 100 mg have β_1 and β_2 effects.
	Toprol XL (SR preparation)	50 mg once daily	50–200 mg once daily	$0.88/100 mg	$26.40						
Nadolol	Corgard	20 mg once daily	20–160 mg once daily	$1.00/40 mg	$30.00	0	0	0	0	R	
Penbutolol	Levatol	20 mg once daily	20–80 mg once daily	$1.30/20 mg	$39.00	0	+	0	++	R > H	
Pindolol	Visken	5 mg bid	10–60 mg in 2 doses	$0.68/5 mg	$40.80	0	++	+	+	H > R	In adults, 35% renal clearance.
Propranolol	Inderal	20 mg bid	40–320 mg in 2 doses	$0.19/40 mg	$11.40	0	0	++	+++	H	Once-daily SR preparation also available. Also indicated for angina pectoris and post-MI.
Timolol	Blocadren	5 mg bid	10–40 mg in 2 doses	$0.35/10 mg	$21.00	0	0	0	++	H > R	Also indicated post-MI. 80% hepatic clearance.

ISA = intrinsic sympathomimetic activity; MSA = membrane-stabilizing activity; 0 = no effect; +, ++, +++ = some, moderate, most effect.
[1]Cost to pharmacist (average wholesale price, generic when possible) for quantity listed. Source: *Drug Topics Red Book,* March 2000; Vol. 19, No. 3.
[2]Agents with β_1 selectivity are less likely to precipitate bronchospasm and decreased peripheral blood flow *in low doses,* but selectivity is only relative.
[3]Agents with ISA cause less resting bradycardia and lipid changes.
[4]MSA generally occurs at concentrations greater than those necessary for beta-adrenergic blockade. The clinical importance of MSA by beta-blockers has not been defined.
[5]Adverse effects of all beta-blockers: bronchospasm, fatigue, sleep disturbance and nightmares, bradycardia and atrioventricular block, worsening of congestive heart failure, cold extremities, gastrointestinal disturbances, impotence, ↑triglycerides, ↓HDL cholesterol, rare blood dyscrasias.

Table 11–7. Antihypertensive drugs: ACE inhibitors and angiotensin II blockers.

Drug	Proprietary Name	Initial Dosage	Dosage Range	Cost per Unit	Cost of 30 Days' Treatment (Average Dosage)[1]	Adverse Effects	Comments
ACE inhibitors							
Benazepril	Lotensin	10 mg once daily	5–40 mg in 1 or 2 doses	$0.83/20 mg	$24.90	Cough, hypotension, dizziness, renal dysfunction, hyperkalemia, angioedema; taste alteration and rash (may be more frequent with captopril); rarely, proteinuria, blood dyscrasia. Contraindicated in pregnancy.	More fosinopril is excreted by the liver in patients with renal dysfunction (dose reduction may or may not be necessary). Captopril and lisinopril are active without metabolism. Captopril, enalapril, lisinopril, and quinapril are approved for congestive heart failure.
Captopril	Capoten	25 mg bid	50–300 mg in 2 or 3 doses	$0.69/25 mg	$41.40		
Enalapril	Vasotec	5 mg once daily	5–40 mg in 1 or 2 doses	$1.63/20 mg	$48.90		
Fosinopril	Monopril	10 mg once daily	10–80 mg in 1 or 2 doses	$0.90/20 mg	$27.00		
Lisinopril	Prinivil, Zestril	5–10 mg once daily	5–40 mg once daily	$0.99/20 mg	$29.70		
Moexipril	Univasc	7.5 mg once daily	7.5–30 mg in 1 or 2 doses	$0.62/7.5 mg	$18.60		
Perindopril	Aceon	4 mg once daily	4–16 mg in 1 or 2 doses	$0.98/4 mg $1.40/8 mg	$42.00 (8 mg)		
Quinapril	Accupril	10 mg once daily	10–80 mg in 1 or 2 doses	$0.88/20 mg	$26.40		
Ramipril	Altace	2.5 mg once daily	2.5–20 mg in 1 or 2 doses	$1.00/5 mg	$30.00		
Trandolapril	Mavik	1 mg once daily	1–8 mg once daily	$0.72/4 mg	$21.60		
Angiotensin II blockers							
Candesartan cilexitil	Atacand	16 mg once daily	8–32 mg once daily	$1.24/16 mg	$37.20	Hyperkalemia, renal dysfunction, rare angioedema. Combinations have additional side effects. Contraindicated in pregnancy.	Losartan has a very flat dose-response curve. Valsartan and irbesartan have wider dose-response ranges and longer durations of action. Addition of low-dose diuretic (separately or as combination pills) increases the response.
Eprosartan	Micordis	40 mg once daily	40–80 mg once daily	$1.29/40 or 80 mg	$38.57		
Irbesartan	Avapro	150 mg once daily	150–300 mg once daily	$1.25/150 mg	$37.50		
Irbesartan and hydrochlorothiazide	Avalide	150 mg/ 12.5 mg once daily	150–300 mg irbesartan daily	$1.50/ tablet	$45.00		
Losartan	Cozaar	50 mg once daily	25–100 mg in 1 or 2 doses	$1.25/50 mg	$37.50 (50 mg once daily)		
Losartan and hydrochlorothiazide	Hyzaar	50 mg/ 12.5 mg once daily	One or 2 tablets once daily	$1.25/ tablet	$37.50 (1 tablet daily)		
Telmisartan	Teveten	600 mg once daily	400–500 mg in 1 or 2 doses	$0.94/ 400 mg tablet $1.25/600 600 mg caplet	$37.50 (600 mg once daily)		
Valsartan	Diovan	80 mg once daily	80–320 mg once daily	$1.34/160 mg	$40.20		

[1]Cost to pharmacist (average wholesale price, generic when possible) for quantity listed. Source: *Drug Topics Red Book,* March 2000; Vol. 19, No. 3.

tal strokes, and instances of new-onset heart failure in a population of patients at high risk for vascular events. This study included diabetics with at least one additional risk factor and patients with coronary artery disease, peripheral artery disease, and prior stroke. Although this was not specifically a hypertensive population, the results inferentially support the use of ACE inhibitors in similar hypertensive patients. ACE inhibitors may also delay the progression of other forms of renal disease. They are a drug of choice (usually in conjunction with a diuretic) in patients with congestive heart failure and are indicated also in asymptomatic patients with reduced ejection fractions, whether post myocardial infarction or from other causes.

An advantage of the ACE inhibitors is their relative freedom from troublesome side effects. Severe hypotension can occur in patients with bilateral renal artery stenosis; acute renal failure may ensue. Hyperkalemia may develop in patients with intrinsic renal disease and type IV renal tubular acidosis (commonly seen in diabetics) and in the elderly. A chronic dry cough due to bronchial or laryngeal irritation is seen, however, in 5–10% of patients and may require stopping the drug. Dizziness is also relatively common and may not be related to the degree of blood pressure lowering. Skin rashes may occur with any ACE inhibitor. Taste alterations are seen more often with captopril than with the non-sulfhydryl-containing agents (enalapril and lisinopril) but often disappear with continued therapy. Angioedema is an uncommon but potentially dangerous side effect of all agents of this class because of their secondary inhibition of kininase.

D. Angiotensin II Receptor Blocking Agents: (Table 11–7.) Although losartan, the first member of this group, was less potent in reducing blood pressure than the ACE inhibitors, the newer angiotensin II antagonists (valsartan, irbesartan, candesartan, telmisartan, and eprosartan) appear to be equipotent. It is still uncertain whether they share the efficacy of ACE inhibitors in patients with heart failure or asymptomatic left ventricular dysfunction or in diabetic or other forms of nephropathy. Unlike ACE inhibitors, the angiotensin II receptor blockers do not cause cough and are only infrequently associated with skin rashes, the most common side effects of the ACE inhibitors. However, they still present a risk of hypotension and renal failure in patients with bilateral renal stenosis and hyperkalemia. Rare cases of angioedema have been reported. Because of their higher costs, limited long-term experience, and unproved benefits in heart failure and diabetes, the angiotensin II blockers should be reserved primarily for patients who develop cough when taking ACE inhibitors.

E. Calcium Channel Blocking Agents: (Table 11–8.) All the agents of this class reduce blood pressure, and a number of new agents with a longer duration of action and perhaps less negative inotropic activity are available. They act by causing peripheral vasodilation, which is associated with less reflex tachycardia and fluid retention than other vasodilators. These agents are effective as single-drug therapy in approximately 60% of patients and appear to be effective in all demographic groups and all grades of hypertension. As a result, they may be preferable to beta-blockers and ACE inhibitors in blacks and older subjects. Calcium channel blockers and diuretics are less additive when given together than when either is combined with beta-blockers or ACE inhibitors. However, verapamil and diltiazem should be combined cautiously with beta-blockers because of their potential for depressing atrioventricular conduction and sinus node automaticity as well as contractility.

Concerns have been raised about increased risk of myocardial infarction in hypertensive patients and of higher mortality in acute coronary syndromes. Studies with long-acting calcium channel blockers have not confirmed early reports. In the Syst-Eur Trial, which evaluated the effects of a dihydropyridine, nitrendipine, in older patients with predominantly systolic hypertension, there was a reduction in stroke and other forms of cardiovascular morbidity and mortality equivalent to those seen with diuretic-based regimens. Based on these data, the long-acting calcium channel blockers appeared to be effective and safe in most hypertensives. However, an increased risk of myocardial infarction was observed in two trials comparing dihydropyridine calcium channel blockers (nisoldipine in one, amlodipine in another) with ACE inhibitors in diabetic patients with evidence of renal disease. Whether these outcomes reflect beneficial effects of ACE inhibitors or specific risks of calcium channel blockers is uncertain. Nonetheless, ACE inhibitors are the drugs of choice in this group of patients and current calcium channel blockers, despite their neutral metabolic effects, should not be used as initial therapy in diabetics.

The most common side effects of calcium channel blockers are headache, peripheral edema, bradycardia, and constipation (especially with verapamil in the elderly). The dihydropyridine agents—nifedipine, nicardipine, isradipine, felodipine, and amlodipine—are more likely to produce symptoms of vasodilation, such as headache, flushing, palpitations, and peripheral edema. Calcium channel blockers have negative inotropic effects and may cause or exacerbate heart failure in patients with cardiac dysfunction. This tendency may be less with amlodipine. Most of these agents are now available in preparations that can be administered once daily.

F. Alpha-Adrenoceptor Antagonists: (Table 11–9.) Prazosin, terazosin, and doxazosin block postsynaptic alpha receptors, relax smooth muscle, and reduce blood pressure by lowering peripheral vascular resistance. These agents are effective as single-drug therapy in some individuals, but tachyphylaxis may appear during long-term therapy and side effects

Table 11–8. Antihypertensive drugs: Calcium channel-blocking agents.

Drug	Proprietary Name	Initial Dosage	Dosage Range	Cost for 30 Days' Treatment (Average Dosage)[1]	Special Properties			Adverse Effects	Comments
					Peripheral Vasodilation	Cardiac Automaticity and Conduction	Contractility		
Nondihydropyridine agents									
Diltiazem	Cardizem SR	90 mg bid	180–360 mg in 2 doses	$87.00 (120 mg bid)	++	↓↓	↓↓	Edema, headache, bradycardia, GI disturbances, dizziness, AV block, congestive heart failure, urinary frequency.	Also approved for angina.
	Cardizem CD	180 mg qd	180–360 mg qd	$65.74 (240 mg qd)					
	Cartia XT	180 mg qd	120–300 mg qd	$55.81					
	Dilacor XR	180 or 240 mg qd	180–480 mg daily	$40.80 (240 mg qd)					
	Tiazac SA	240 mg qd	180–540 mg qd	$47.54 (240 mg qd)					
Verapamil	Calan SR Isoptin SR Verelan Covera-HS Generic Verapamil extended release	180 mg qd	180–480 mg in 1 or 2 doses	$48.90 $50.40 $47.70 $51.00 $37.20 (240 mg qd)	++	↓↓↓	↓↓↓	Same as diltiazem but more likely to cause constipation and congestive heart failure.	Also approved for angina and arrhythmias.

(*continued*)

Table 11–8. Antihypertensive drugs: Calcium channel-blocking agents (continued).

Drug	Proprietary Name	Initial Dosage	Dosage Range	Cost for 30 Days' Treatment (Average Dosage)[1]	Special Properties: Peripheral Vasodilation	Special Properties: Cardiac Automaticity and Conduction	Special Properties: Contractility	Adverse Effects	Comments
Dihydropyridines									
Amlodipine	Norvasc	5 mg qd	5–20 mg qd	$65.57 (10 mg qd)	+++	↓/0	↓/0	Edema, dizziness, palpitations, flushing, headache, hypotension, tachycardia, GI disturbances, urinary frequency, worsening of congestive heart failure (may be less common with felodipine, amlodipine).	Amlodipine, nicardipine, and nifedipine also approved for angina.
Felodipine	Plendil	5 mg qd	5–20 mg qd	$53.70 (10 mg qd)	+++	↓/0	↓/0		
Isradipine	DynaCirc	2.5 mg bid	2.5–5 mg bid	$64.80 (5 mg bid)	+++	↓/0	↓		
	DynaCirc CR	5 mg qd	5–10 mg qd	$58.20 (10 mg qd)					
Nicardipine	Cardene	20 mg tid	20–40 mg tid	$38.70 (20–40 mg tid)	+++	↓/0	↓		
	Cardene SR	30 mg bid	30–60 mg bid	$41.92					
Nifedipine	Adalat CC	30 mg qd	30–120 mg qd	$61.80 (60 mg qd)	+++	↓	↓↓		
	Procardia XL	30 mg qd	30–120 mg qd	$74.10 (60 mg qd)	+++	↓	↓↓		
Nisoldipine	Sular	20 mg/d	20–60 mg/d	$28.80 (40 mg qd)	+++	↓/0	↓		

[1]Cost to pharmacist (average wholesale price, generic when possible) for quantity listed. Source: *Drug Topics Red Book,* March 2000; Vol. 19, No. 3.

Table 11–9. Alpha-adrenoceptor blocking agents, sympatholytics, and vasodilators.

Drug	Proprietary Name	Initial Dosage	Dosage Range	Cost per Unit	Cost for 30 Days' Treatment (Average Dosage)[1]	Adverse Effects	Comments
ALPHA-ADRENOCEPTOR BLOCKERS							
Prazosin	Minipress	1 mg hs	2–20 mg in 2 or 3 doses	$0.64/5 mg	$38.40 (5 mg bid)	Syncope with first dose; postural hypotension, dizziness, palpitations, headache, weakness, drowsiness, sexual dysfunction, anticholinergic effects, urinary incontinence; first-dose effects may be less with doxazosin.	May ↑HDL and ↓LDL cholesterol. May provide short-term relief of obstructive prostatic symptoms. Tachyphylaxis may occur when used to treat congestive heart failure.
Terazosin	Hytrin	1 mg hs	1–20 mg in 1 or 2 doses	$1.60/1, 2, 5, 10 mg	$48.00 (5 mg qd)		
Doxazosin	Cardura	1 mg hs	1–16 mg qd	$1.08/4 mg	$32.40 (4 mg qd)		
CENTRAL SYMPATHOLYTICS							
Clonidine	Catapres	0.1 mg bid	0.2–0.6 mg in 2 doses	$0.18/0.1 mg	$10.80 (0.1 mg bid)	Sedation, dry mouth, sexual dysfunction, headache, bradyarrhythmias; side effects may be less with guanfacine. Contact dermatitis with clonidine patch. Methyldopa also causes hepatitis, hemolytic anemia, fever.	"Rebound" hypertension may occur even after gradual withdrawal. Methyldopa should be avoided in favor of safer agents.
	Catapres TTS	0.1 mg/d patch weekly	0.1–0.3 mg/d patch weekly	$15.30/0.2 mg	$61.20 (0.2 mg weekly)		
Guanabenz	Wytensin	4 mg bid	8–64 mg in 2 doses	$0.66/4 mg	$39.60 (4 mg bid)		
Guanfacine	Tenex	1 mg once daily	1–3 mg qd	$0.87/1 mg	$26.10 (1 mg qd)		
Methyldopa	Aldomet	250 mg bid	500–2000 mg in 2 doses	$0.44/500 mg	$26.40 (500 mg bid)		
PERIPHERAL NEURONAL ANTAGONISTS							
Guanethidine	Ismelin	10 mg once daily	10–100 mg qd	$1.18/25 mg	$35.42 (25 mg qd)	Orthostatic hypotension, diarrhea, exercise hypotension, sexual dysfunction, salt and water retention.	
Guanadrel	Hylorel	5 mg bid	10–70 mg in 2 doses	$1.65/10 mg	$99.00 (10 mg bid)		
Reserpine	Serpasil	0.05 mg once daily	0.05–0.25 mg qd	$0.13/0.1 mg	$3.90 (0.1 mg qd)	Depression (less likely at low dosages, ie, < 0.25 mg), night terrors, nasal stuffiness, drowsiness, peptic disease, gastrointestinal disturbances, bradycardia.	
DIRECT VASODILATORS							
Hydralazine	Apresoline	25 mg bid	50–300 mg in 2–4 doses	$0.05/25 mg	$3.00 (25 mg bid)	GI disturbances, tachycardia, headache, nasal congestion, rash, LE-like syndrome.	May worsen or precipitate angina.
Minoxidil	Loniten	5 mg once daily	5–40 mg qd	$0.55/10 mg	$16.50 (10 mg qd)	Tachycardia, fluid retention, headache, hirsutism, pericardial effusion, thrombocytopenia.	Should be used in combination with beta-blocker and diuretic.

[1]Cost to pharmacist (average wholesale price, generic when possible) for quantity listed. Source: *Drug Topics Red Book*, March 2000; Vol. 19, No. 3.

are relatively common. The major side effects are marked hypotension and syncope after the first dose, which, therefore, should be small and be given at bedtime. Postdosing palpitations, headache, and nervousness may continue to occur during chronic therapy. These side effects may be less frequent or severe with doxazosin because of its more gradual onset of action.

Unlike the beta-blockers and diuretics, the alpha-blockers have no adverse effect on serum lipid levels—in fact, they increase high-density lipoprotein cholesterol while reducing total cholesterol. Whether this is beneficial in the long term has not been established. Indeed, in the ongoing Antihypertensive Lipid Lowering Heart Attack Trial (ALLHAT), the limb involving doxazosin as initial therapy was discontinued because of a significant increase in heart failure hospitalizations and a higher incidence of stroke relative to the diuretic arm. This finding suggests that alpha-blockers should generally not be used as initial agents to treat hypertension—except perhaps in men with symptomatic prostatism.

G. Drugs With Central Sympatholytic Action: (Table 11–9.) Methyldopa, clonidine, guanabenz, and guanfacine lower blood pressure by stimulating alpha-adrenergic receptors in the central nervous system, thus reducing efferent peripheral sympathetic outflow. These agents are effective as single therapy in some patients, but they are usually employed as second- or third-line agents because of the high frequency of drug intolerance, including sedation, fatigue, dry mouth, postural hypotension, and impotence. An important concern is rebound hypertension following withdrawal. Methyldopa also causes hepatitis and hemolytic anemia and should be avoided except in individuals who have already tolerated chronic therapy. There is, however, considerable experience with methyldopa in pregnant women, so it is still used for this population. Clonidine is available in patches and may have particular value in patients in whom compliance is a troublesome issue.

H. Arteriolar Dilators: (Table 11–9.) Hydralazine and minoxidil relax vascular smooth muscle and produce peripheral vasodilation. When given alone, they stimulate reflex tachycardia, increase myocardial contractility, and cause headache, palpitations, and fluid retention. They are usually given in combination with diuretics and beta-blockers in resistant patients. Hydralazine produces frequent gastrointestinal disturbances and may induce a lupus-like syndrome. Minoxidil causes hirsutism and marked fluid retention; this agent is reserved for the most refractory of patients.

I. Peripheral Sympathetic Inhibitors: (Table 11–9.) These agents are now used infrequently. Reserpine remains a cost-effective antihypertensive agent. Its reputation for inducing mental depression and its other side effects—sedation, nasal stuffiness, sleep disturbances, and peptic ulcers—have made it unpopular, though these problems are uncommon at low dosages. Guanethidine and guanadrel inhibit catecholamine release from peripheral neurons but frequently cause orthostatic hypotension (especially in the morning or after exercise), diarrhea, and fluid retention. These agents are used chiefly in refractory hypertension.

Developing an Antihypertensive Regimen

Selection of the initial agent for treating an individual patient should follow the considerations discussed previously. Because the most extensive and most favorable experience in randomized control trials has been with diuretic-based and, to a lesser extent, beta-blocker-based regimens, these should be the initial agents for the majority of uncomplicated hypertensives. Figure 11–1 summarizes results achieved with these agents in clinical trials. However, many patients—perhaps the majority in middle-aged and older populations—will have associated medical conditions that become important determinants of drug selection. In some conditions (classified as "compelling indications" in the JNC VI report), specific medications have shown major benefits in randomized controlled trials and should therefore be the initial agents of choice for these populations. The favored agents include ACE inhibitors in patients with type 1 diabetes and proteinuria and perhaps in type 2 diabetics with microalbuminuria or atherosclerotic vascular disease; ACE inhibitors, beta-blockers, and diuretics in patients with congestive heart failure; beta-blockers in patients who have experienced a myocardial infarction; and ACE inhibitors in postinfarction patients with documented left ventricular systolic dysfunction (ejection fraction < 40%). The HOPE trial results indicate that ACE inhibitors prevent fatal and nonfatal vascular events, including myocardial infarction, stroke, and heart failure in normotensive or treated hypertensive patients at high risk for these complications. However, in the hypertensive population, it is not certain whether they are more effective in reducing these end points than diuretics or beta-blockers except perhaps in diabetics. In several trials in which ACE inhibitors have been compared with calcium antagonists in diabetic patients, there has been a lower incidence of myocardial infarction and heart failure with the ACE inhibitors.

Diuretics have consistently proved effective (even more so than beta-blockers) in trials of older patients with isolated or predominantly systolic hypertension, but the previously cited Syst-Eur Trial also showed that a calcium channel blocker could achieve similar benefits. Although the specific drug utilized in that trial, nitrendipine, is not available in the United States, it seems likely that other calcium channel blockers would share this benefit, and this class should therefore be considered a second-line alternative to diuretics in these patients. Table 11–10 also

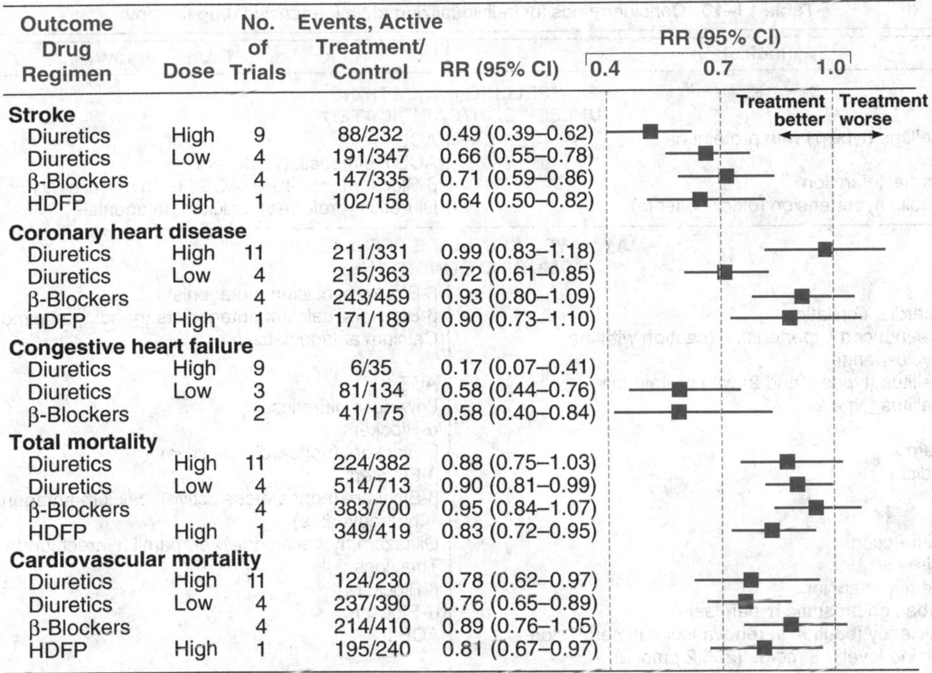

Outcome Drug Regimen	Dose	No. of Trials	Events, Active Treatment/ Control	RR (95% CI)
Stroke				
Diuretics	High	9	88/232	0.49 (0.39–0.62)
Diuretics	Low	4	191/347	0.66 (0.55–0.78)
β-Blockers		4	147/335	0.71 (0.59–0.86)
HDFP	High	1	102/158	0.64 (0.50–0.82)
Coronary heart disease				
Diuretics	High	11	211/331	0.99 (0.83–1.18)
Diuretics	Low	4	215/363	0.72 (0.61–0.85)
β-Blockers		4	243/459	0.93 (0.80–1.09)
HDFP	High	1	171/189	0.90 (0.73–1.10)
Congestive heart failure				
Diuretics	High	9	6/35	0.17 (0.07–0.41)
Diuretics	Low	3	81/134	0.58 (0.44–0.76)
β-Blockers		2	41/175	0.58 (0.40–0.84)
Total mortality				
Diuretics	High	11	224/382	0.88 (0.75–1.03)
Diuretics	Low	4	514/713	0.90 (0.81–0.99)
β-Blockers		4	383/700	0.95 (0.84–1.07)
HDFP	High	1	349/419	0.83 (0.72–0.95)
Cardiovascular mortality				
Diuretics	High	11	124/230	0.78 (0.62–0.97)
Diuretics	Low	4	237/390	0.76 (0.65–0.89)
β-Blockers		4	214/410	0.89 (0.76–1.05)
HDFP	High	1	195/240	0.81 (0.67–0.97)

Figure 11–1. Meta-analysis of randomized, placebo-controlled clinical trials in hypertension according to first-line treatment strategy. For these comparisons, the numbers of participants randomized to active treatment and placebo, respectively, were 7768 and 12,075 for high-dose diuretic therapy, 4305 and 5116 for low-dose diuretic therapy, and 6736 and 12,147 for beta-blocker therapy. Because the Medical Research Council trials included two active arms, the placebo group is included twice in these totals (for diuretic comparison and for beta-blocker comparison). The total number of participants randomized to active and control therapy were 24,294 and 23,926, respectively. RR indicates relative risk; CI, confidence interval; and HDFP, Hypertension Detection and Follow-up Program. (Data from Psaty et al. Reproduced, with permission, from: The sixth report of the Joint National Committee on prevention, detection, evaluation, and treatment of high blood pressure. Arch Intern Med 1997;157:2413. Copyright © 1997 by American Medical Association.)

lists a number of conditions for which there is evidence of an advantage of one class—as well as conditions in which certain antihypertensive drugs should be avoided.

When an initial agent is selected, the patient should be informed of common side effects and the need for diligent compliance. Treatment should start at a low dose, and unless the initial blood pressure is very high (> 180/110 mm Hg), follow-up visits should usually be at 4- to 6-week intervals to allow for full medication effects to be manifested (especially with diuretics) before further titration or adjustment. If, after titration to usual doses, the patient has shown a discernible but incomplete response and a good tolerance of the initial drug, the second agent should be added. If the initial medication was a diuretic or a calcium channel blocker, the second agent should generally be a beta-blocker, ACE inhibitor, or angiotensin II blocker, since these combinations are generally complementary. If the initial drug was a beta-blocker, ACE inhibitor, or angiotensin II blocker, the second drug should be a diuretic. On the other hand, if the initial agent showed no effect, another drug should be substituted. Again, if the first drug was a diuretic or a calcium channel blocker, the substituted drug should be a beta-blocker, ACE inhibitor, or angiotensin II blocker; if it was a beta-blocker, ACE inhibitor, or angiotensin II blocker, the substituted agent should be a diuretic or a calcium channel blocker. Low-dose combinations of complementary antihypertensive drugs are another approach to initial therapy.

Most patients with hypertension can be controlled with one-drug or two-drug regimens, which combine complementary agents. A minority of patients require three, four, or even more medications in combination. The need for multidrug regimens is more frequent in patients with high systolic pressures and in diabetics. Unless absolutely contraindicated, one of these components should be a diuretic. Particularly useful multidrug regimens are (1) a diuretic plus a beta-blocker plus a vasodilator or a calcium channel blocker; (2) a diuretic plus an ACE inhibitor plus either a calcium channel blocker or a sympatholytic (or both); and (3) a calcium channel blocker plus an ACE inhibitor plus either a sympatholytic or a beta-blocker (or both). Pa-

Table 11–10. Considerations for individualizing antihypertensive drug therapy.[1]

Indication	Drug Therapy
COMPELLING INDICATIONS UNLESS CONTRAINDICATED	
Diabetes mellitus (type 1) with proteinuria	ACE I
Heart failure	ACE I, diuretics, β-blockers
Post-myocardial infarction	β-Blockers (non-ISA), ACE I (with systolic dysfunction)
Isolated systolic hypertension (older patients)	Diuretics (preferred), calcium antagonists
MAY HAVE FAVORABLE EFFECTS ON COMORBID CONDITIONS[2]	
Angina	β-Blockers, calcium antagonists
Atrial tachycardia, fibrillation	β-Blockers, calcium antagonists (nondihydropyridine)
Cyclosporine-induced hypertension (caution with the dose of cyclosporine)	Calcium antagonists
Diabetes mellitus (types 1 and 2) with proteinuria	ACE I
Diabetes mellitus (type 2)	Low-dose diuretics
Dyslipidemia	α-Blockers
Essential tremor	β-Blockers (noncardioselective)
Hyperthyroidism	β-Blockers
Migraine	β-Blockers (noncardioselective), calcium antagonists (nondihydropyridine)
Myocardial infarction	Diltiazem hydrochloride, verapamil hydrochloride
Osteoporosis	Thiazides
Preoperative hypertension	β-Blockers
Prostatism (benign prostatic hyperplasia)	α-Blockers
Renal insufficiency (caution in renovascular hypertension and creatinine level ≥ 3 mg/dL [265.2 μmol/L]	ACE I
MAY HAVE UNFAVORABLE EFFECTS ON COMORBID CONDITIONS[2,3]	
Bronchospastic disease	β-Blockers[4]
Depression	β-Blockers, central α-agonists, reserpine[4]
Diabetes mellitus (types 1 and 2)	β-Blockers, high-dose diuretics
Dyslipidemia	β-Blockers (non-ISA), diuretics (high-dose)
Gout	Diuretics
Heart attack, primary or secondary	β-Blockers,[4] calcium antagonists (nondihydropyridine)[4]
Heart failure	Calcium antagonists (except amlodipine, perhaps felodipine)
Liver disease	Labetalol hydrochloride, methyldopa[4]
Peripheral vascular disease	β-Blockers
Pregnancy	ACE I,[4] angiotensin II receptor blockers[4]
Renal insufficiency	Potassium-sparing agents
Renovascular disease	ACE I, angiotensin II receptor blockers

Abbreviations: ACE I, angiotensin-converting enzyme inhibitors; ISA, intrinsic sympathomimetic activity.
[1]Modified from: The sixth report of the Joint National Committee on detection, education, and treatment of high blood pressure (JNC VI). Arch Intern Med 1997;157:2413.
[2]Conditions and drugs are listed in alphabetical order.
[3]These drugs may be used with special monitoring unless contraindicated.
[4]Contraindicated.

tients who are compliant with their medications and who do not respond to these combinations should usually be evaluated for secondary hypertension before proceeding to more complex regimens.

Blood Pressure Treatment Goals

Patients in whom antihypertensive therapy is indicated should generally be treated to normotensive levels (systolic pressure < 140 mm Hg and diastolic pressure < 90 mm Hg) unless these are not tolerated. Particular attention should be paid to systolic blood pressure control since this is the major determinant of cardiovascular mortality and morbidity. Individuals at high risk for cardiovascular complications, such as diabetics, patients with chronic renal insufficiency, and probably those with atherosclerotic vascular disease or heart failure, should be treated to 130/85 mm Hg or below.

Treatment of Additional Cardiovascular Risk Factors

Since the goal is to reduce cardiovascular morbidity and mortality, attention must be paid to the management of other risk factors. In particular, there is now overwhelming evidence that aggressive reduction of elevated LDL-cholesterol levels reduces the risk of myocardial infarction and death in patients with multiple risk factors. Thus, if LDL-cholesterol levels remain over 130 mg/dL following an attempt at dietary intervention, drug therapy is indicated in most hypertensives. Levels under 100 mg/dL should be achieved in patients with coronary artery disease, cerebrovascular disease, peripheral arterial disease, or diabetes. Smoking cessation, regular exercise, and weight loss when indicated are other important features of hypertension management.

Follow-Up of the Treated Hypertensive

Once blood pressure is controlled on a well-tolerated regimen, follow-up visits can be infrequent and laboratory testing should be limited to tests appropriate for the patient and the medications utilized. Yearly monitoring of blood lipids is recommended in patients with hypertension, and an ECG should be repeated at 2- to 4-year intervals depending on whether initial abnormalities are present, the presence of coronary risk factors, and age.

Patients who have had excellent blood pressure control for several years, especially if they have lost weight and initiated favorable lifestyle modifications, should be considered for "step-down" of therapy to determine if lower doses or discontinuing of medications is feasible.

Abernethy DR et al: Calcium-antagonist drugs. N Engl J Med 1999;341:1447. [NLM Cit ID: 20001878] (Review of mechanisms, pharmacology, and clinical indications, with special attention to the controversy over their safety.)

Bakris GL et al: Angiotensin-converting enzyme inhibitor-associated elevations in serum creatinine. Arch Intern Med 2000;160:685. (Elevations in serum creatinine often lead physicians to avoid or discontinue ACE inhibitors. This review demonstrates that patients with rises in creatinine up to 30% during the first 2 months of therapy are those that experience the greatest long-term preservation of renal function.)

Drugs for hypertension. Med Lett Drugs Ther 1999;41:23. [NLM Cit ID: 99192891] (Review of antihypertensive drugs.)

Effects of an angiotensin-converting-enzyme inhibitor, ramipril, on cardiovascular events in high-risk patients. The Heart Outcomes Prevention Evaluation Investigators. N Engl J Med 2000;342:145. [NLM Cit ID: 20092358] (Landmark trial in 9297 patients with vascular disease or diabetes in which ramipril prevented fatal and nonfatal events. Although many were not hypertensive, some extrapolation of these findings to the hypertensive population seems warranted.)

Giatras I et al: Effect of angiotensin-converting enzyme inhibitors on the progression of nondiabetic renal disease: A meta-analysis of randomized trials. Ann Intern Med 1997;127:337. [NLM Cit ID: 97410747] (Despite the initial worsening of renal function tests that sometimes occurs with ACE inhibitors, they appear to reduce the progression of renal disease in nondiabetic as well as diabetic patients.)

Gottdiener JS et al: Effect of single-drug therapy on reduction of left ventricular mass in mild to moderate hypertension: Comparison of 6 anti-hypertensive agents. Circulation 1997;95:227. [NLM Cit ID: 97278931] (Diuretic therapy was most effective in reducing left ventricular hypertrophy, perhaps because of its greater and more sustained effect on systolic blood pressure.)

Graves JW: Management of difficult to control hypertension. Mayo Clin Proc 2000;75:278. [NLM Cit ID: 20190154] (Practical step-by-step approach to the problem patient.)

Gueyffier F et al: Effect of anti-hypertensive drug treatment on cardiovascular outcomes in women and men: A meta-analysis of individual patient data from randomized controlled trials. Ann Intern Med 1997;126:761. [NLM Cit ID: 97282913] (Relative benefit does not differ between women and men, but the absolute benefit reflects the underlying risk of the population—frequently lower in women.)

Hansson L et al: Randomised trial of old and new antihypertensive drugs in elderly patients: The Swedish Trial in Old Patients with Hypertension-2. Lancet 1999; 354:1751. (Trial in 6,614 patients > 70 years of age comparing diuretic- and beta-blocker-based therapy with treatment with ACE inhibitors and calcium channel blockers. No difference was observed between older and newer drugs, but the incidence of myocardial infarction and heart failure was lower with ACE inhibitors than with calcium blockers.)

MacLeod MJ et al: Drug treatment of hypertension complicating diabetes mellitus. Drugs 1998;56:189. [NLM Cit ID: 98377323] (Review of this important problem; ACE inhibitors and low target blood pressures recommended.)

Sibai BM: Treatment of hypertension in pregnant women. N Engl J Med 1996;335:257. [NLM Cit ID: 96266389] (Practical review of therapy.)

The sixth report of the Joint National Committee on prevention, detection, evaluation, and treatment of high blood pressure. (Published erratum appears in Arch Intern Med 1998 Mar 23;158:573.) Arch Intern Med 1997;157:2413. [NLM Cit ID: 98046261] (Comprehensive, evidence-based guideline with recommendations for use of antihypertensive drugs.)

Weir MR et al: Diuretics and beta-blockers: is there a risk for dyslipidemia? Am Heart J 2000;139:174. [NLM Cit ID: 20086513] (A review of the minimal effects of low-dose thiazides or cardioselective beta-blockers on the lipid profile.)

HYPERTENSIVE URGENCIES & EMERGENCIES

Hypertensive emergencies have become less frequent in recent years but still require prompt recognition and aggressive but careful management. A spectrum of acute presentations exists, and the appropriate therapeutic approach varies accordingly.

Hypertensive urgencies are situations in which blood pressure must be reduced within a few hours. These include patients with asymptomatic severe hypertension (systolic blood pressure > 220 mm Hg, or diastolic pressure > 125 mm Hg that persist after a period of observation) and with optic disk edema, progressive target organ complications, and severe perioperative hypertension. Elevated blood pressure levels alone—in the absence of symptoms or new or progressive target organ damage—rarely require emergency therapy. Parenteral drug therapy is not usually required, and partial reduction of blood pressure with relief of symptoms is the goal.

Hypertensive emergencies require substantial reduction of blood pressure within 1 hour to avoid the risk of serious morbidity or death. Although blood pressure is usually strikingly elevated (diastolic pressure > 130 mm Hg), the correlation between pressure and end-organ damage is often poor. It is the latter that determines the seriousness of the emergency and the approach to treatment. Emergencies include hypertensive encephalopathy (headache, irritability, confusion, and altered mental status due to cerebrovascular spasm), hypertensive nephropathy (hematuria, proteinuria, and progressive renal dysfunction due to arteriolar necrosis and intimal hyperplasia of the interlobular arteries), intracranial hemorrhage, aortic dissection, preeclampsia-eclampsia, pulmonary edema, unstable angina, or myocardial infarction. **Malignant hypertension** is by historical definition characterized by encephalopathy or nephropathy with accompanying papilledema. Progressive renal failure usually ensues if treatment is not provided. The therapeutic approach is identical to that employed with other antihypertensive emergencies.

Parenteral therapy is indicated in most hypertensive emergencies, especially if encephalopathy is present. The initial goal in hypertensive emergencies is to reduce the pressure by no more than 25% (within minutes to 1 or 2 hours) and then toward a level of 160/100 mm Hg within 2–6 hours. Excessive reductions in pressure may precipitate coronary, cerebral, or renal ischemia. To avoid such declines, the use of agents that have a predictable, dose-dependent, transient, and not precipitous antihypertensive effect is preferable. In that regard, the use of sublingual or oral fast-acting nifedipine preparations is best avoided.

Pharmacologic Management

A. Parenteral Agents: A growing number of agents are available for management of acute hypertensive problems. (Table 11–11 lists drugs, dosages, and adverse effects.) Sodium nitroprusside is the agent of choice for the most serious emergencies because of its rapid and easily controllable action, but continuous monitoring is essential when this agent is used. In the presence of myocardial ischemia, intravenous nitroglycerin or an intravenous beta-blocker, such as labetalol or esmolol, is preferable.

1. Nitroprusside sodium–This agent is given by controlled intravenous infusion gradually titrated to the desired effect. It lowers the blood pressure within seconds by direct arteriolar and venous dilatation. Monitoring with an intra-arterial line avoids excessive blood pressure reductions. Nitroprusside—in combination with a beta-blocker—is especially useful in patients with aortic dissection.

2. Nitroglycerin, intravenous–This agent is a less potent antihypertensive than nitroprusside and should be reserved for patients with accompanying acute ischemic syndromes.

3. Labetalol–This combined beta- and alpha-adrenergic blocking agent is the most potent adrenergic blocker for rapid blood pressure reduction. Excessive blood pressure responses are unusual. Experience with this agent in hypertensive syndromes associated with pregnancy has been favorable.

4. Nicardipine–Intravenous nicardipine is the most potent and long-acting of the parenteral calcium channel blockers. As a primarily arterial vasodilator, it has the potential to precipitate reflex tachycardia, and for that reason it should not be used without a beta-blocker in patients with coronary artery disease.

5. Esmolol–This rapidly acting beta-blocker is approved only for treatment of supraventricular tachycardia. Though less potent than labetalol, it is useful in acutely lowering blood pressure, especially when combined with a vasodilator such as nitroprusside, nitroglycerin, or hydralazine; it is especially useful during myocardial ischemia.

6. Enalaprilat–This is the active form of the oral ACE inhibitor enalapril. The onset of action is usually within 15 minutes, but the peak effect may be delayed for up to 6 hours. Therefore, enalaprilat is useful primarily as an adjunctive agent.

7. Diazoxide–Diazoxide acts promptly as a vasodilator without decreasing renal blood flow. Because the magnitude of response is difficult to control and may be excessive, it is only infrequently used. To avoid hypotension, it should be given in small boluses or as an infusion rather than as the previously recommended large bolus. One use of diazoxide has been in preeclampsia-eclampsia. Hyperglycemia and sodium and water retention may occur. The drug should be used only for short periods and is best combined with a loop diuretic.

8. Hydralazine–Hydralazine can be given intravenously or intramuscularly, but its effect is less predictable than that of other drugs in this group. It produces reflex tachycardia and should not be given without beta-blockers in patients with possible coronary disease or aortic dissection. Based on historical experience, hydralazine is now used primarily in pregnancy and in children, but even in these situations, newer agents are supplanting it.

9. Trimethaphan–The ganglionic blocking agent trimethaphan is titrated with the patient sitting; its activity depends upon this. The patient can be placed supine if the hypotensive effect is excessive. The effect occurs within a few minutes and persists for the duration of the infusion. This agent has largely been supplanted by nitroprusside and newer medications.

10. Fenoldopam–Fenoldopam is a new peripheral dopamine-1 (DA_1) receptor agonist that causes a

Table 11–11. Drugs for hypertensive emergencies and urgencies.

Agent	Action	Dosage	Onset	Duration	Adverse Effects	Comments
PARENTERAL AGENTS (INTRAVENOUSLY UNLESS NOTED)						
Nitroprusside (Nipride)	Vasodilator	0.25–10 μg/kg/min	Seconds	3–5 minutes	GI, CNS; thiocyanate and cyanide toxicity, especially with renal and hepatic insufficiency; hypotension.	Most effective and easily titratable treatment. Use with beta-blocker in aortic dissection.
Nitroglycerin	Vasodilator	0.25–5 μg/kg/min	2–5 minutes	3–5 minutes	Headache, nausea, hypotension, bradycardia.	Tolerance may develop. Useful primarily with myocardial ischemia.
Labetalol (Normodyne, Trandate)	Beta- and alpha-blocker	20–40 mg every 10 minutes to 300 mg; 2 mg/min infusion	5–10 minutes	3–6 hours	GI, hypotension, bronchospasm, bradycardia, heart block.	Avoid in congestive heart failure, asthma. May be continued orally.
Esmolol (Brevibloc)	Beta-blocker	Loading dose 500 μg/kg over 1 minute; maintenance, 25–200 μg/kg/min	1–2 minutes	10–30 minutes	Bradycardia, nausea.	Avoid in congestive heart failure, asthma. Weak antihypertensive.
Nicardipine (Cardene)	Calcium channel blocker	5 mg/h; may increase by 1–2.5 mg/h every 15 minutes to 15 mg/h	1–5 minutes	3–6 hours	Hypotension, tachycardia, headache.	May precipitate myocardial ischemia.
Enalaprilat (Vasotec)	ACE inhibitor	1.25 mg every 6 hours	15 minutes	6 hours or more	Excessive hypotension.	Additive with diuretics; may be continued orally.
Furosemide (Lasix)	Diuretic	10–80 mg	15 minutes	4 hours	Hypokalemia, hypotension.	Adjunct to vasodilator.
Hydralazine (Apresoline)	Vasodilator	5–20 mg IV or IM (less desirable); may repeat after 20 minutes	10–30 minutes	2–6 hours	Tachycardia, headache, GI.	Avoid in coronary artery disease, dissection. Rarely used except in pregnancy.
Diazoxide (Hyperstat)	Vasodilator	50–150 mg repeated at intervals of 5–15 minutes, or 15–30 mg/min by IV infusion to a maximum of 600 mg	1–2 minutes	4–24 hours	Excessive hypotension, tachycardia, myocardial ischemia, headache, nausea, vomiting, hyperglycemia. Necrosis with extravasation.	Avoid in coronary artery disease and dissection. Use with beta-blocker and diuretic. Mostly obsolete.
Trimethaphan (Arfonad)	Ganglionic blocker	0.5–5 mg/min	1–3 minutes	10 minutes	Hypotension, ileus, urinary retention, respiratory arrest. Liberates histamine; use caution in allergic individuals.	Useful in aortic dissection. Otherwise rarely used.
ORAL AGENTS						
Nifedipine (Adalat, Procardia)	Calcium channel blocker	10 mg initially; may be repeated after 30 minutes	15 minutes	2–6 hours	Excessive hypotension, tachycardia, headache, angina, myocardial infarction, stroke.	Response unpredictable.
Clonidine (Catapres)	Central sympatholytic	0.1–0.2 mg initially; then 0.1 mg every hour to 0.8 mg	30–60 minutes	6–8 hours	Sedation.	Rebound may occur.
Captopril (Capoten)	ACE inhibitor	12.5–25 mg	15–30 minutes	4–6 hours	Excessive hypotension.	
Fenoldopam (Corlopam)	Dopamine receptor agonist	0.1–1.6 μg/kg/min	4–5 minutes	< 10 minutes	Reflex tachycardia, hypotension, ↑ intraocular pressure.	May protect renal function.

dose-dependent reduction in arterial pressure without evidence of tolerance, rebound or withdrawal, or deterioration of renal function. In higher dose ranges, tachycardia may occur.

11. Diuretics–Intravenous loop diuretics can be very helpful when the patient has signs of heart failure or fluid retention, but the onset of their hypotensive response is slow, making them an adjunct rather than a primary agent for hypertensive emergencies. Low dosages should be used initially (furosemide, 20 mg; or bumetanide, 0.5 mg). They facilitate the response to vasodilators, which often stimulate fluid retention.

B. Oral Agents: Patients with less severe acute hypertensive syndromes can often be treated with oral therapy. They should be closely monitored until a therapeutic end point is achieved. Abrupt blood pressure lowering is not usually necessary in asymptomatic individuals, and the frequent use of potent agents such as rapid-acting nifedipine probably causes more adverse effects than benefits.

1. Clonidine–Clonidine, 0.2 mg orally initially, followed by 0.1 mg every hour to a total of 0.8 mg, will usually lower blood pressure over a period of several hours. Sedation is frequent, and rebound hypertension may occur if the drug is stopped.

2. Captopril–Captopril, 12.5–25 mg orally, will also lower blood pressure in 15–30 minutes. The response is variable and may be excessive.

3. Nifedipine–Fast-acting nifedipine capsules are commonly employed in the emergency room or urgent care setting because they usually provide a rapid reduction in blood pressure. However, the nifedipine effect is unpredictable and may be excessive, resulting in hypotension and reflex tachycardia. Myocardial infarction and stroke have been reported in this setting.

C. Subsequent Therapy: When the blood pressure has been brought under control, combinations of oral antihypertensive agents can be added as parenteral drugs are tapered off over a period of 2–3 days. Most subsequent regimens should include a diuretic.

Grossman E et al: Should a moratorium be placed on sublingual nifedipine capsules given for hypertensive emergencies and pseudoemergencies? JAMA 1996;276:1328. [NLM Cit ID: 97015164] (See text for discussion.)

Kaplan NM: Management of hypertensive emergencies. Lancet 1994;344:1335. [NLM Cit ID: 95057610]

Zampaglione B et al: Hypertensive urgencies and emergencies. Prevalence and clinical presentation. Hypertension 1996;27:144. [NLM Cit ID: 96136738] (An observational study of the clinical presentations of hypertensive urgencies and emergencies.)

RELEVANT WORLD WIDE WEB SITES

[Treatment of Hypertension Teaching Module]
http://www-med.stanford.edu/school/DGIM/Teaching/Modules/HTN.html

Blood Vessels & Lymphatics

12

See http://www.current-med.com/ch12.html for updated addresses of Web sites referenced in this chapter.

Louis M. Messina, MD, & Lawrence M. Tierney, Jr., MD

Atherosclerosis is the cause of most degenerative arterial disease. It is a disease of the intima of the arterial wall characterized by smooth muscle migration and proliferation and extracellular lipid deposition. Features of complex lesions include a fibrous cap containing smooth muscle and inflammatory cells that overlie a central core of necrotic debris. These lesions can be complicated by calcification, intraplaque hemorrhage, and luminal thrombosis after cap rupture.

The incidence of atherosclerosis increases with age—people over age 40 are most commonly affected. Risk factors include hypercholesterolemia, diabetes mellitus, smoking, a positive family history, hypertension, and homocystinuria. Atherosclerosis is a systemic disease, with some degree of involvement of all major arteries, but it produces its clinical manifestations by critical involvement of a limited number of arteries. Narrowing and occlusion of the artery are the most common manifestations. Weakening of the arterial wall from loss of elastin and collagen may result in aneurysmal dilation. Aneurysms appear to result from an imbalance of tissue metalloproteinases and metalloproteinase inhibitors. Nonetheless, both processes may be present in the same individual. Less common arterial diseases include vasculitis (of both large and small arteries), thromboangiitis obliterans (Buerger's disease), fibrodysplasia of visceral arteries, syphilitic aortitis, and radiation arteritis.

Graham IM et al: Plasma homocysteine as a risk factor for vascular disease. The European Concerted Action Project. JAMA 1997;277:1775. [NLM Cit ID: 97322136] (Case-control study of 1750 patients showed that increased plasma homocysteine levels increased the relative risk of peripheral vascular disease to 2.2 compared with patients with normal homocysteine levels.)

DISEASES OF THE AORTA

ANEURYSMS OF THE ABDOMINAL AORTA

Essentials of Diagnosis

- Most aneurysms are asymptomatic, detected during a routine physical examination or sonography.
- Severe back or abdominal pain and hypotension indicate rupture.
- Concomitant atherosclerotic occlusive disease of lower extremities is present in 25%.

General Considerations

The infrarenal aorta is normally 2 cm in diameter; an aneurysm is considered present when the diameter exceeds 4 cm. Over 90% of abdominal aneurysms originate below the renal arteries, and many involve the common iliac arteries. Aneurysms of the proximal aorta are much less common.

Clinical Findings

A. Symptoms and Signs:

1. Asymptomatic–A pulsating abdominal mass may be discovered on a routine physical examination, most frequently in men over age 50. More often, sonography or abdominal CT scan done for other purposes detects asymptomatic aneurysms. Sonography is also the most cost-effective test for confirming a suspicion of aneurysm raised by physical examination. Peripheral pulses are often normal, but renal or lower extremity arterial occlusive disease is present in 25%. Aneurysms of the popliteal artery often coexist; indeed, detection of the latter should raise the suspicion of abdominal aneurysm, since one is present in more than one-third of patients with popliteal aneurysm.

2. Symptomatic–Chronic midabdominal or lower back pain (or both) may be present, often secondary to an inflammatory aortic aneurysm. Inflammatory aneurysms account for less than 5% of aortic aneurysms and are characterized by extensive periaortic and retroperitoneal inflammation of unknown cause. Peripheral emboli may occur, even from small aneurysms, and symptomatic arterial insufficiency in the legs may result.

3. Rupture–Patients who suffer rupture of an aortic aneurysm present with severe back, abdominal, or flank pain and hypertension. As many as 90% die either before they reach the hospital or after an attempted repair. Bleeding confined to the retroperitoneum can produce local tamponade and permit the patient to come to operation. Free peritoneal (anterior) rupture results in death within minutes if untreated.

B. Laboratory Findings: Electrocardiography and renal function studies should be obtained to assess concomitant dysfunction in those systems.

C. Imaging: Abdominal ultrasonography is the diagnostic study of choice and is also valuable for following aneurysm size in patients not immediately treated surgically. Curvilinear calcifications outlining portions of the aneurysm wall may be visible on plain films of the aortic area in approximately three-fourths of those with an aneurysm, but this study is less sensitive than ultrasonography. Contrast-enhanced CT scanning precisely defines the extent of the aneurysm. Aortography is helpful in planning repair when arterial occlusive disease of the visceral or lower extremity arteries is suspected but may underestimate the aneurysm's diameter if thrombus is present. MRI is as sensitive and specific as CT and does not require administration of contrast.

Treatment

A. Standard Therapy: Surgical excision and synthetic graft replacement is the treatment of choice for most aneurysms of the infrarenal abdominal aorta. Aneurysms may enlarge and rupture if left untreated. The diameter of the aneurysm correlates best with the risk of rupture. In asymptomatic good-risk patients, surgery is advised when the aneurysm exceeds 5 cm in diameter; in symptomatic patients, repair is indicated irrespective of size. Improving surgical techniques and postoperative care have led some to recommend surgical resection even for smaller aneurysms. Opinion differs about whether asymptomatic aneurysms in poor-risk patients should be repaired or followed closely by means of ultrasound measurements to detect signs of expansion. Long-term beta-blockade may be associated with a decreased rate of growth of aneurysms that are being followed. Patients with significant symptomatic coronary or carotid disease may be more likely to suffer myocardial infarction or stroke during and following aneurysm resection; coronary artery bypass grafting or coronary angioplasty to lessen this risk prior to elective aneurysm repair is advocated by some. However, overall mortality increases with each procedure. Prophylactic carotid endarterectomy has not been established as providing overall benefit given the considerations noted.

In general, individuals over age 80 with minimal preoperative risk factors can undergo elective surgery with an acceptable mortality rate; those with significant associated disease generally should not undergo operation without compelling indications.

B. Endovascular Repair: In the last decade, endovascular prostheses have been employed with increasing frequency. Consisting of synthetic grafts with endoluminal stents, these may be employed in any artery, including aneurysmal thoracic and abdominal aortas, iliac arteries, and more distal vessels. Operative time is reduced. Complications include leak around the prosthesis. Preoperative measurement of the diseased target vessels is essential to plan device insertion. Clinical trials have confirmed the safety and efficacy of endovascular repair of aortic aneurysms. Long-term durability of endovascular repair needs to be established before widespread application of this technique can be recommended.

Complications

The rate of complications after aortic aneurysm repair is usually between 5% and 10%. They include myocardial infarction, bleeding, respiratory insufficiency, ischemic colitis, limb ischemia, renal insufficiency, and stroke. Late complications include graft infection and graft-enteric fistula and are seen more frequently in cases where the initial surgery was performed on an emergent basis.

Prognosis

The mortality rate following elective surgical resection is 3–8%, though in certain centers it has recently approached 1%; clinicians must inquire into the surgical success rates in their own institutions before making the often difficult decision to recommend operation. Results of endovascular repair are now emerging. For high-risk patients, the results are promising. Of those who survive surgery, approximately 60% are alive 5 years later, and in those who die, myocardial infarction is the leading cause of death. Among unoperated patients, old studies indicate that less than 20% survive 5 years, and aneurysm rupture is the cause of 60% of the deaths; more recently, a less rapid rate of expansion has been reported, but some surgeons dispute this. In general, a patient with an aortic aneurysm has a three-fold greater chance of dying as a consequence of rupture of the aneurysm than of dying from surgical resection. If coronary or carotid artery surgery is done preoperatively, the added morbidity and mortality of these procedures must be considered in the overall approach to the patient.

Blum U et al: Endoluminal stent-graft for infrarenal abdominal aortic aneurysms. N Engl J Med 1997;336:13.

[NLM Cit ID: 97122457] (Early results showing safety and efficacy of endoluminal stent-grafts.)

Chuter TAM et al: Endovascular repair of abdominal aortic aneurysms: Getting out of trouble. Cardiovasc Surg 1998;6:232. [NLM Cit ID: 98368792]

Lederle F et al: The aneurysm detection and management study screening program. Validation cohort and final results. Arch Intern Med 2000;160:1425. [NLM Cit ID: 20284687] (Confirmation that the principal positive associations with abdominal aortic aneurysm are age, smoking, family history of this aneurysm, and atherosclerotic diseases. Female sex, diabetes, and black race remain principal negative associations.)

Rasmussen TE et al: Inflammatory aortic aneurysms: A clinical review with new perspectives in pathogenesis. Ann Surg 1997;225:155. [NLM Cit ID: 97188749]

van der Vliet JA et al: Abdominal aortic aneurysm. Lancet 1997;349:863. [NLM Cit ID: 97236874]

ANEURYSMS OF THE THORACIC AORTA

Aneurysms of the thoracic aorta account for less than 10% of aortic aneurysms. Thoracic aortic aneurysms are most commonly due to medial degeneration; syphilis is now a rare cause. Vasculitis and cystic medial necrosis, as occur in Marfan's syndrome, may also result in thoracic aneurysm. Traumatic aneurysms may occur at the ligamentum arteriosus just beyond the left subclavian artery when the wall of the aorta is incompletely torn as a result of a rapid-deceleration accident.

Clinical Findings

Manifestations depend largely on the size and position of the aneurysm and its rate of growth.

A. Symptoms and Signs: Most thoracic aneurysms are asymptomatic and are diagnosed during a diagnostic procedure done for other reasons. Substernal, back, or neck pain may occur, as well as symptoms and signs due to pressure on (1) the trachea (dyspnea, stridor, a brassy cough), (2) the esophagus (dysphagia), (3) the left recurrent laryngeal nerve (hoarseness), or (4) the superior vena cava (edema in the neck and arms, distended neck veins). Aortic regurgitation may be present.

B. Imaging: CT scan and MRI are the most sensitive and accurate means of imaging thoracic aneurysms. Aortography may be necessary to confirm the diagnosis and to delineate the precise location and extent of the aneurysm and its relation to the vessels arising from the arch. The coronary vessels and the aortic valve should also be studied if the ascending aorta is involved.

Differential Diagnosis

It may be difficult to determine on chest radiography whether a mass in the mediastinum is an aneurysm, a neoplasm, or a cyst. Radioactive isotope studies (^{125}I) may be helpful in diagnosing a substernal goiter.

Treatment

Indications for treatment of thoracic aneurysms include symptomatic or rapidly enlarging aneurysms and those whose greatest diameter exceeds 6 cm. Asymptomatic aneurysms in poor-risk patients are better treated only if progressive enlargement occurs. Control of hypertension may slow progression, and the use of beta-blockers makes empirical good sense. The overall morbidity and mortality rates of thoracic aneurysmectomy, however, are considerably higher than the rates for abdominal aneurysms.

If the aortic valve is involved, an aortic valve replacement may be necessary, and reattachment of the coronary arteries or aortocoronary bypass grafts may also be indicated. Paraplegia due to anterior spinal artery ischemia is a complication of excision and graft replacement in 5–30% of patients depending on the extent of aortic involvement.

Prognosis

The risk of rupture of thoracic aneurysms is related to their diameter. Elective repair is usually not considered until the maximum diameter exceeds 6 cm. Prognosis without repair is relatively poor, only 20–25% surviving for 5 years. Most deaths are due to rupture or to the complications of generalized atherosclerosis. Saccular aneurysms, those distal to the left subclavian artery, and those limited to the ascending aorta may be approached surgically in good-risk candidates, with the caveats cited above. Resection of aneurysms of the transverse aortic arch involves major technical challenges that can be dealt with only by skilled surgical teams using hypothermia to protect the nervous system.

Coselli JS et al: Results of contemporary surgical treatment of descending thoracic aortic aneurysms: Experience in 198 patients. Ann Vasc Surg 1996;10:131. [NLM Cit ID: 96315981]

Kouchoukos NT et al: Surgery of the thoracic aorta. N Engl J Med 1997;336:1876. [NLM Cit ID: 97324065]

PERIPHERAL ARTERY ANEURYSMS (Popliteal & Femoral)

Popliteal Aneurysms

Popliteal aneurysms account for approximately 85% of all peripheral artery aneurysms. Patients with peripheral artery aneurysms are thought to have a generalized disorder of the arterial wall. For example, in half of cases of popliteal and femoral aneurysms, the contralateral artery is involved as well. One-third of patients with popliteal aneurysms and two-thirds of those with femoral aneurysms harbor aortoiliac artery aneurysms as well. Peripheral aneurysms occur almost exclusively in men. More than half are symptomatic at the time of diagnosis. Symptoms are rarely due to rupture but result rather from thrombosis, peripheral embolization, or compression of adjacent structures with resultant venous thrombosis or neuropathy.

Ultrasound is the diagnostic study of choice to measure the diameter of the aneurysm as well as to search for other arterial aneurysms. Arteriography is required to define the anatomy of the outflow arteries in preparation for operative repair.

Repair of popliteal aneurysms is recommended for all asymptomatic aneurysms whose diameter exceeds 2 cm and for aneurysms less than 2 cm in diameter which become symptomatic.

A reversed saphenous vein bypass graft with proximal and distal ligation of the aneurysm is generally employed. In large aneurysms with manifestations of vein or nerve compression, resection of the aneurysm in addition to grafting is necessary.

Femoral Aneurysms

Femoral aneurysms present as pulsatile groin masses. They have the potential for the same complications as popliteal aneurysms. Because the incidence of these complications in asymptomatic patients is less than that for popliteal aneurysms, there is more reason to follow rather than operate on smaller, asymptomatic femoral aneurysms and to deal first with aortoiliac and then popliteal aneurysms in preference to femoral aneurysms when aneurysmal disease exists in all of these areas. Pseudoaneurysms often develop at distal anastomotic sites from previous aortic surgery and should be repaired when their diameter exceeds 2 cm.

Dawson I et al: Atherosclerotic popliteal aneurysm. Br J Surg 1997;84:293. [NLM Cit ID: 97232107]

AORTIC DISSECTION

Essentials of Diagnosis

- A history of hypertension or Marfan's syndrome is often present.
- Sudden severe chest pain with radiation to the back, occasionally migrating to the abdomen and hips.
- Patient appears to be in shock, but blood pressure is normal or elevated; pulse discrepancy in many patients.
- Acute aortic regurgitation may develop.

General Considerations

Aortic dissection is the most common aortic catastrophe requiring admission to a hospital. It originates at the site of an intimal tear and then propagates distally. Over 95% of intimal tears occur either in the ascending aorta just distal to the aortic valve (type A) or just distal to the left subclavian artery (type B). The initial intimal tear probably results from the shear forces applied to the ascending and proximal descending aorta occurring at these two points. Dissection occurs on rare occasions in an aorta without an apparent intimal tear; these aortas invariably show histologic abnormalities of the media. Proximal dissections are encountered more often in aortas involved with abnormalities of the smooth muscle, elastic tissue, or collagen; distal dissections occur in patients with long-standing hypertension. Pregnancy, bicuspid aortic valve, and coarctation are associated with an increased risk of type A and type B dissections; Marfan's syndrome makes a type A dissection more likely. Both hypertension and the rate of acceleration of pulsatile flow (dp/dt) are important in propagation of dissection, which may extend from the ascending aorta to the abdominal aorta or beyond. Alternatively, dissection may remain limited to the ascending aorta and the aortic valve area, especially if hypertension is not present or if it is controlled early; furthermore, dissection may progress not only distally but also proximally.

When not appropriately diagnosed and treated, aortic dissection is a lethal disease. Of untreated patients with type A dissections, 50% are dead within 48 hours and 90% at 1 month. Death is usually due to rupture of the aorta into the pericardial sac or pleural space or to acute aortic regurgitation with left ventricular failure. Deaths due to type B dissection are less common and usually secondary to free rupture in the pleural space, or they may occur as a consequence of acute mesenteric and renal ischemia.

Clinical Findings

A. Symptoms and Signs: Severe, persistent chest pain of sudden onset, nearly always anterior but often also posterior, later progressing to the abdominal and hip areas, is characteristic. Radiation down the arms or into the neck may or may not occur. Usually there is only a mild decrease in the level of blood pressure prior to rupture. Partial or complete occlusion of the arteries arising from the aortic arch or of the intercostal and lumbar arteries may lead to such nervous system findings as syncope, hemiplegia, or paralysis of the lower extremities. Peripheral pulses and blood pressures may be diminished or unequal. An aortic diastolic murmur may develop as a result of dissection close to the aortic valve, resulting in valvular regurgitation, heart failure, and cardiac tamponade.

B. Laboratory Findings: Electrocardiographic changes indicating left ventricular hypertrophy from long-standing hypertension are often present; acute changes may not develop unless the dissection involves the coronary ostium. In that case, inferior wall abnormalities predominate, since dissection leads to compromise of the right rather than the left coronary artery. In some, the ECG may be normal.

C. Imaging: Chest radiographs often reveal an abnormal aortic contour or a wide superior mediastinum, with changes in the configuration and thickness of the aortic wall in successive films. There may be findings of pleural or pericardial effusion. Diagnosis of dissection can be made by a variety of modalities, including dynamic CT scanning, angiography, MRI, and transesophageal echocardiography (TEE). The latter has been used with increasing frequency because of its high sensitivity (98%) and specificity (99%) and because it can be performed rapidly and relatively noninvasively. The best initial study is the one most readily available that can be interpreted accurately in a given hospital setting. MRI has not played a major role in the initial diagnosis but is ideal for serial follow-up.

Differential Diagnosis

Aortic dissection is most commonly confused with myocardial infarction (see Chapter 10) as well as other causes of chest pain, such as pulmonary embolization. However, it may simulate numerous neurologic lesions and even various abdominal conditions related to renal-visceral ischemia.

Treatment

A. Medical Measures: If hypertension is present, aggressive measures to lower the pressure should probably be initiated even before diagnostic studies have been completed, and while the need for surgery is being contemplated. Treatment generally includes the simultaneous reduction of the systolic blood pressure to 100 mm Hg and reduction of the pulsatile aortic flow (dp/dt) by means of the following:

(1) A rapid-acting antihypertensive agent as an intravenous infusion at a flow rate regulated by continuous blood pressure determinations. Nitroprusside or trimethaphan may be given as follows: (a) Nitroprusside (50 mg in 1000 mL of 5% dextrose in water) is started at a rate of 0.5 mL/min and the infusion rate increased by 0.5 mL every 5 minutes until adequate control of the pressure has been achieved. Thiocyanate levels should be obtained if treatment is continued for 48 hours, and the infusion should be stopped if the drug level reaches 10 mg/dL; (b) Trimethaphan (1 or 2 mg/mL) may be infused with the patient in the semi-Fowler position; or fenoldopam, 0.1–1.6 μg/kg/min, may be administered.

(2) Intravenous propranolol, 0.15 mg/kg given over a 5-minute period and repeated as necessary to maintain the pulse rate at 60/min. The rapid-acting beta-blocker esmolol may be tried first in patients in whom adverse effects are considered more likely to occur, although propranolol is believed by many to be more effective in this disorder. Intravenous reserpine (0.1–0.2 mg) may be used if beta-blockers are contraindicated.

All patients with type A dissection should undergo emergent surgical repair. Most patients with type B dissection can be managed successfully with aggressive drug therapy. Indications for surgical treatment of type B dissections are severe intractable pain, aortic rupture; mesenteric, renal, or limb ischemia; and progression of the dissection.

B. Surgical Measures: For type A dissection, the ascending aorta and, if necessary, the aortic valve and arch may be replaced with reattachment of the coronaries and brachiocephalic vessels. The mortality rate for such operations approaches 20% or more, but this is still less than the rate for untreated type A dissection.

Surgical treatment is increasingly popular for dissections arising in the descending thoracic aorta (type B); it may be delayed until the hypertension and dissection have been stabilized by medical means and oral antihypertensives instituted. The origin of the dissection is then removed; the false lumen is closed; and a graft is inserted to deliver all blood flow through the normal lumen, thus relieving the occlusive pressure on the aortic branches.

Since patients with type B dissections tend to be poor surgical risks, permanent medical therapy may be offered. Indeed, the surgical mortality rate is higher for this operation than for operation on the more technically challenging type A patient. Regimens should include beta-blockers and antihypertensive drugs; vasodilators are contraindicated unless used with beta-blockers.

Prognosis

Without treatment, the mortality rate of aortic dissection at 3 months exceeds 90%; of these, 20% die within a day and 60% die in less than 2 weeks. These figures may be somewhat worse for type A dissections. Although the surgical mortality rate is high in both groups, it is appreciably more so in type B patients because of co-morbid illnesses. Medical therapy of type A dissection is associated with a prohibitively high mortality rate (at least 30% in 24 hours, and up to 75% in 1 week). Intensive pharmacologic methods to lower dp/dt and blood pressure have led to healing of the type B dissected aorta in patients with acute dissection and will convert others to a subacute or chronic form. All unoperated patients should be followed with annual CT scans to detect progressive enlargement.

Braverman AC: Aortic dissection. Curr Opin Cardiol 1997;12:389. [NLM Cit ID: 97409262]

Hagan P et al: The international registry of acute aortic dissection (IRAD): New insights into an old disease. JAMA 2000;283:897. [NLM Cit ID: 201481150] (Classic findings at presentation are often absent. Aortic regurgitation and pulse deficit were noted in only 30% and 15% of patients, respectively. Twelve percent of initial chest X-rays showed no abnormalities.)

Pretre R et al: Aortic dissection. Lancet 1997;349:1461. [NLM Cit ID: 97307118]

Safi HJ et al: Operation for acute and chronic aortic dissection: Recent outcome with regard to neurological deficit and early death. Ann Thorac Surg 1998;66:402. [NLM Cit ID: 98391192]

Sommer T et al: Aortic dissection: A comparative study of diagnosis with spiral CT, multiplanar transesophageal echocardiography, and MR imaging. Radiology 1996; 199:347. [NLM Cit ID: 96202767]

Williams DM et al: The dissected aorta: percutaneous treatment of ischemic complications: principles and results. J Vasc Interv Radiol 1997;8:605. [NLM Cit ID: 97376468]

ATHEROSCLEROTIC OCCLUSIVE DISEASE*

Occlusive disease of the aorta and its branches is a common cause of disability. It is also a predictor of morbidity for patients with cardiac disease and those undergoing general surgery. It is essential for the primary physician to emphasize its prevention, particularly in light of what is known about etiologic factors. Discontinuance of smoking and dietary or pharmacologic management of elevated blood pressure, cholesterol, and glucose are important measures likely to reduce morbidity from atherosclerosis (see Chapters 1 and 28). Although peripheral occlusive disease is classified anatomically in the following sections, advances in therapy have made the approach to all such lesions similar irrespective of location.

OCCLUSIVE DISEASE OF THE AORTA & ILIAC ARTERIES

Occlusive disease of the aorta and the iliac arteries begins most frequently at the bifurcation of the aorta. Atherosclerotic changes occur in the intima and media, often with associated perivascular inflammation and calcified plaques in the media. The process may extend to cause occlusion of one or both common iliac arteries and then the abdominal aorta up to the segment just below the renal arteries. In general, two distinct patterns of occlusive disease occur, often referred to as type A and type B. In type A, the disease is localized to the aorta and common iliac arteries. In type B, the occlusive disease extends beyond the aortoiliac segments and encompasses the femoral and popliteal arteries. Less than 10% of patients present with the type A pattern. The main implication of these differences relates to the method of revascularization, which will be described below.

Clinical Findings

Intermittent claudication is pain or weakness in the muscles of the lower extremities brought on by walking and relieved after a few minutes of rest. It is almost always present in the calf muscles and often in the thighs and buttocks as well. Impotence is a common complaint in men. Vasculogenic impotence is often manifested by inability to sustain an erection. Rest pain, by which is meant pain even with the absence of exertion, is an infrequent but serious symptom. Rest pain is usually experienced as a nocturnal pain located in the region of the heads of the metatarsal bones of the feet. It is relieved by placing the legs in the dependent position, usually by hanging them over the side of the bed.

Femoral pulses are absent or weak, and distal pulses are often not palpable. A bruit may be heard over the aorta or over the iliac or femoral arteries. Systolic blood pressure, normally higher in the leg, is greater in the brachial artery than at the ankle; the difference is exaggerated by exercise. Atrophic changes of the skin, subcutaneous tissues, and muscles of the distal leg may be noted on physical examination. Dependent rubor and coolness of the skin are signs of more advanced ischemia. Aortography, including oblique views of the thigh and leg arteries, demonstrates the level and extent of the occlusion and the condition of the vessels distal to occlusive lesions. Aortography is not a diagnostic study and is undertaken only in preparation for therapeutic intervention. It may be replaced by MRI, which does not require contrast, or by Doppler ultrasonography. Lower extremity arterial Doppler studies permit noninvasive determination of the physiologic impact of the occlusive lesions on lower extremity blood flow. These studies provide an objective assessment of the degree of arterial insufficiency, the extent of progression or regression of lesions over time, and the effect of therapeutic intervention.

Treatment

Surgical or angioplastic treatment of claudication is indicated in good-risk patients whose claudication interferes appreciably with the patient's essential activities or work. Discontinuation of smoking is essential; some surgeons insist on it as a prerequisite to operation.

Because many of these patients have coexisting ischemic heart disease, their medical management should be maximized preoperatively. The roles of exercise testing and coronary angiography are discussed in Chapter 10 (in the section on the Cardiac Patient and Surgery). Some clinicians obtain these studies with an eye toward prophylactic bypass grafting or coronary angioplasty; this has not been conclusively

*Giant cell arteritis is discussed in Chapter 20. Arterial disease in diabetic patients is discussed in Chapter 27.

shown to be of benefit in this situation if patients are minimally symptomatic.

A. Conservative Care: A program of daily walking for fixed periods, stopping for claudication, increases pain-free walking distance in the majority of patients. Pentoxifylline, 400 mg three times daily, may help some patients. Many patients with claudication are receiving beta-blockers for angina or hypertension. Though in theory this may worsen symptoms by allowing unopposed alpha agonism, consensus holds that this is not a clinical problem.

The following therapies are best advanced for disabling symptoms, such as extremity pain at rest and skin ulceration. Both are harbingers of dry gangrene and potential limb loss.

B. Arterial Graft (Prosthesis): Aortobifemoral bypass using a synthetic prosthesis is effective treatment for complex aortoiliac occlusive disease. In general, the bifurcation graft extends from the infrarenal abdominal aorta, usually by means of an end-to-end anastomosis, to one or both common femoral arteries as end-to-side anastomoses. A patient may also be treated surgically with less risk but also less favorable results by means of a graft from the axillary artery to one or both femoral arteries or, in the case of unilateral iliac disease, from the femoral artery with normal blood flow to the contralateral femoral artery distal to the stenotic iliac vessel.

C. Thromboendarterectomy: This procedure, which avoids the use of a prosthesis, is reserved for patients who exhibit a type A pattern of occlusive disease, when the occlusion is limited to the aorta and common iliac arteries and when the external iliac and common femoral arteries are free of significant occlusive disease. Plaque is removed from arteries and flow restored, obviating the need for a synthetic graft and thereby avoiding the long-term risk of an infected prosthesis.

D. Endovascular Surgical Techniques: Occlusive lesions formerly treated as described in paragraphs B and C can under certain circumstances be repaired by percutaneous transluminal angioplasty and endoluminal stent. Atherectomy devices and laser probes have met with little success.

E. Pharmacotherapy: Until recently, drug therapy has had little impact on the management of claudication. Newer drugs such as cilostazol (100 mg orally twice daily) have been shown to increase pain-free walking distance. Sildenafil (Viagra) is a drug that has shown considerable promise in the treatment of the common complication of impotence. However, it should be used cautiously for impotence associated with aortoiliac occlusive disease because many of these patients have concomitant coronary artery disease and are receiving nitroglycerin. This combination is absolutely contraindicated because of an exaggerated fall in blood pressure. Moreover, given the mechanism of action of sildenafil (see Chapter 27), the drug may not prove to be maximally effective in patients with vascular disease.

Prognosis

The operative mortality rate is 2–5%—a great deal less for an endovascular procedure. The immediate and long-term benefits are often impressive. In patients with no distal occlusive disease, improvement is both subjective and objective, with relief of all or most of the claudication and, usually, return of all the pulses in the extremities. Long-term graft patency can be anticipated in more than 80% of patients 10 years after operation.

Dawson DL et al: Cilostazol has beneficial effects in treatment of intermittent claudication: Results from a multicenter, randomized, prospective double-blind trial. Circulation 1998;98:678. [NLM Cit ID: 98379718]

Drexel H et al: Predictors of the presence and extent of peripheral arterial occlusive disease. Circulation 1996;94(9 Suppl):II199. [NLM Cit ID: 97057407]

Ernst E: Chelation therapy for peripheral arterial occlusive disease: A systematic review. Circulation 1997;96:1031. [NLM Cit ID: 97407766]

Sildenafil: An oral drug for impotence. Med Lett Drugs Ther 1998;40:51. [NLM Cit ID: 98262297] (A succinct assessment emphasizing toxicity, especially drug-drug interactions, and cost.)

OCCLUSIVE DISEASE OF THE FEMORAL & POPLITEAL ARTERIES

In the region of the thigh and knee, the vessels most frequently blocked by occlusive disease are the superficial femoral artery and the popliteal artery. Atherosclerotic changes usually appear first at the most distal point of the superficial femoral artery, where it passes through the adductor magnus tendon into the popliteal space. In time, the whole superficial femoral artery may become occluded; the disease progresses into the popliteal artery less frequently. The common femoral and deep femoral arteries are usually patent and relatively free of disease, although the origin of the profunda femoris is sometimes narrowed. The distal popliteal and its three terminal branches may also be relatively free of occlusive disease.

Clinical Findings

A. Symptoms and Signs: Intermittent claudication of the calf is typical and is reported occasionally in the foot as well. Atrophic changes in the lower leg and foot are distinct, with loss of hair, thinning of the skin and subcutaneous tissues, and diminution in the size of the muscles. Dependent rubor and blanching on elevation of the foot are usually present if ischemia is advanced. When the leg is lowered after elevation, venous filling on the dorsal aspect of the foot may be slowed to 15–20 seconds or more. The foot is usually cool. The common femoral pulsations are usually normal, although a bruit may be heard. No popliteal or pedal pulses can be palpated. Pressure measurements in the distal leg, using Doppler ultrasound, will supply an objective functional assessment of the extent of arterial insufficiency. Angiography is indicated only when intervention is being considered.

B. Imaging: If revascularization is being considered, an arteriogram will show the location and extent of the blockages as well as the status of the distal vessels. Lateral or oblique views reveal whether the origin of the profunda femoris is narrow. It is important to know the condition of the aortoiliac vessels also, since a relatively normal inflow as well as an adequate distal "run-off" is important in determining the likelihood of success of an arterial procedure. Magnetic resonance angiography is now available as a less invasive way to acquire the same information.

Treatment

The cornerstone of conservative management is exercise as well as risk factor assessment and modification. A program of daily walking for a fixed distance, stopping after the onset of pain, and then resuming walking after resolution of the pain is an excellent strategy. Smoking must be discontinued.

Surgery is indicated (1) if intermittent claudication is progressive or incapacitating, interfering significantly with the patient's essential physical activities such as ability to work; or (2) if there is rest pain or pregangrenous or gangrenous lesions on the foot.

A. Arterial Graft: An autogenous vein graft using a reversed segment of the saphenous vein is the conduit of choice in the lower extremity to bypass the occluded segment. These bypass procedures are now performed routinely—with patency rates of 75–80% at 5 years—to the level of the dorsalis pedis or posterior tibial artery. Synthetic arterial prostheses provide substantially poorer long-term results except when used to bypass to the above-knee popliteal artery.

B. Thromboendarterectomy: Thromboendarterectomy may be successful if the occluded and stenotic segment is short.

When significant aortoiliac or common femoral occlusive disease exists as well as superficial femoral and popliteal occlusions, it is usually better to relieve the obstructions in the larger, proximal arteries and deliver more blood flow to the profunda femoris than to operate on the smaller distal vessels. If the origin of the profunda femoris is narrowed, a limited procedure at that site—a profundoplasty—may be successful in improving blood flow to the leg and foot and may be used, especially in poor surgical risk patients with rest pain.

C. Endovascular Surgery: As for aortoiliac disease, more distal lesions may be treated using one or more nonsurgical approaches, which include balloon angioplasty, mechanical atherectomy, and laser or thermal angioplasty. The results of these procedures remain inferior to open surgical revascularization.

Recurrent stenosis can often be re-treated by these techniques, or bypass surgery may be elected. Anticoagulants, antiplatelet drugs, and agents to counteract arterial spasm are also frequently employed acutely.

The most favorable lesions again include single, short discrete stenoses. Less favorable lesions are multiple stenoses in series, those longer than 5 cm, complete occlusions less than 5 cm long, lesions in the smaller arteries, and stenotic arterial anastomoses or grafts, particularly if the patient has diabetes or is a smoker.

After any of these procedures, the patient is generally maintained on permanent antiplatelet medication. A dosage of 80–325 mg/d of aspirin is usually employed, though the optimal amount is debated.

Prognosis

The risk of limb loss for patients with claudication is not as great as might be anticipated: only 7–10% of patients will require amputation. But this low amputation rate is due in part to a 5-year survival rate significantly lower than that of the normal population. Up to 50% die secondary to coronary artery disease. For this reason, operation is usually not recommended for mild or moderate claudication, and approximately 80% of these patients will have relatively stable symptoms and will go for years without much progression. Some may improve as collateral circulation develops. The 5-year overall patency rate for the saphenous vein bypass grafts is in the range of 60–80%. The 2-year patency rate after transluminal angioplasty is less, and this procedure is now reserved for poor surgical risk patients.

Pemberton M et al: Colour flow duplex imaging of occlusive arterial disease of the lower limb. Br J Surg 1997;84:912. [NLM Cit ID: 97384461]

OCCLUSIVE DISEASE OF THE ARTERIES IN THE LOWER LEG & FOOT

Occlusive processes in the lower leg and foot may involve, in order of incidence, the tibial and peroneal arteries, the pedal vessels, and occasionally the small digital vessels. Symptoms depend upon the vessels that are narrowed or thrombosed, the suddenness and extent of the occlusion, and the status of the proximal and collateral vessels. The clinical picture may be a rather stable or a slowly progressive form of vascular insufficiency that over months or years may ultimately result in atrophy, ischemic pain, and, occasionally, gangrene.

Clinical Findings

Although all of the possible manifestations of vascular disease in the lower leg and foot cannot be described here, there are certain significant clinical aspects that enter into the evaluation of these patients.

A. Symptoms and Signs: Intermittent claudication is the commonest presenting symptom. Aching fatigue during exertion usually appears first in the calf muscles; in more severe cases, a constant or cramping pain may be brought on by walking only a short distance. Less commonly, the feet are the site of most of the pain. The distance the patient can walk before onset of pain is indicative of the degree of circulatory inadequacy: two blocks (360–460 meters) or more is mild, one block is moderate, and one-half block or less is severe. Rest pain may occur at night and is a dull, persistent ache in the area of the heads of the metatarsals. As in the case of femoral and popliteal disease, rest pain implies severe arterial insufficiency and indeed suggests impending limb loss. A degree of relief can often be obtained by uncovering the foot and letting it hang over the side of the bed.

On examination, although the popliteal pulses may be present, pedal pulses are usually absent; exercise may make the latter disappear in some patients. Dependent rubor is prominent. The skin is cool, atrophic, and hairless. These findings may be indistinguishable from those of occlusive disease higher in the leg. The presence of a popliteal pulse points to more distal occlusion when these symptoms and signs are present.

B. Imaging: Radiographs of the lower leg and foot may show calcification of the vessels. If there is a draining sinus or an ulcer close to a bone or joint, osteomyelitis may be apparent on the film. Lower extremity Doppler studies may be misleading in patients with arterial wall calcification such as diabetics, patients with end-stage renal disease, and the elderly (> 80 years). In such patients, the digital arteries are usually free of calcification; under this condition, toe-brachial indices are of great value.

Treatment

A. Medical Measures: Low-dose aspirin (80–325 mg daily) has theoretical value and is given to all patients with severe peripheral vascular disease. Recently, clopidogrel (75 mg twice daily) has been shown to reduce vascular complications as well as death due to myocardial infarction or stroke. Pentoxifylline (400 mg three times daily) may have some usefulness in patients with chronic claudication.

B. Circulatory Insufficiency in the Foot and Toes: Historically, lumbar sympathectomy was indicated when ischemic or pregangrenous changes were present in the distal foot or when small ulcers were present in a foot with diminished circulation. Current techniques of arterial bypass allow a direct surgical approach. Successful arterial bypasses to the pedal vessels or their branches are now routine.

Sharis P et al: The antiplatelet effects of ticlopidine and clopidogrel. Ann Intern Med 1998:129:394. [NLM Cit ID: 98398005] (Useful review article.)

OCCLUSIVE CEREBROVASCULAR DISEASE

A transient ischemic attack (TIA) is defined as the sudden onset of a neurologic deficit that resolves completely within 24 hours. A stroke is a neurologic deficit that persists beyond 24 hours. Significant carotid artery stenosis or ulcerations releasing microemboli to the brain or the ipsilateral renal artery are responsible for many TIAs and often precede a complete stroke. The extracranial areas most often involved are (1) the common carotid bifurcation, including the origins of the internal and external carotid arteries (approximately 90%); (2) the origin of the vertebral artery; (3) the intrathoracic segments of the aortic arch branches; and (4) the aortic arch itself.

Clinical Findings

A. Symptoms: Transient ischemic attacks (TIAs) may be the earliest manifestation of carotid arterial stenosis or ulceration. Episodes usually last for only a few minutes but may continue for up to 24 hours. Significant carotid artery stenosis or ulcerations releasing microemboli to the brain or the ipsilateral retinal artery are responsible for many TIAs and precede a complete stroke in many of these patients. Typical manifestations include contralateral weakness or sensory changes, speech alterations, and visual disturbance (usually temporary partial or complete loss of vision in the ipsilateral eye). Vertebrobasilar TIAs are characterized by brain stem and cerebellar symptoms, including dysarthria, diplopia, vertigo, ataxia, and hemiparesis or quadriparesis.

Dizziness and unsteadiness, particularly when associated with a quick change in position, are nonspecific symptoms and more often the result of postural hypotension than of vertebrobasilar problems. Atypical neurologic symptoms or personality changes are not symptoms of cerebral ischemia.

B. Signs: Bruits in the neck, diminished or absent pulses in the neck or arms, and a blood pressure difference in the two arms of more than 10 mm Hg may be indications of occlusive disease in the brachiocephalic arteries. More significant than a brachiocephalic bruit is one sharply localized high in the lateral neck close to the angle of the jaw (overlying the common carotid bifurcation), but a major stenosis of 70% or more and thus sufficient to reduce the blood flow through the vessel is present in a minority of patients with these bruits. The murmur of aortic stenosis may be heard as a bruit over the subclavian and carotid arteries; when there is no such heart murmur, the bruit generally denotes disease in these arteries. Bruits are often present without symptoms, and the absence of a bruit does not exclude the possibility of carotid artery stenosis. Thus, bruits heard over the carotid arteries are neither sensitive nor specific enough to alter the diagnostic approach in this patient group. Microemboli can arise from ulcerations of arteries to the brain without stenosis or bruit, particularly if the ulcer is large. These emboli may be seen in the optic fundi at arteriolar branch points, appearing as shiny refractile objects referred to as Hollenhorst plaques. Regarding palpation, only the common carotid and superficial temporal pulses can be felt with accuracy; the internal carotid pulses cannot usually be appreciated.

Additional Studies

Studies of the cerebral circulation are both noninvasive and invasive. Of the former, duplex ultrasonography is now the investigation of choice. In duplex ultrasound, the clinician is provided with both physiologic and anatomic information. Most importantly, it provides an accurate assessment of the degree of stenosis present. It may also detect ulcerations and intraplaque hemorrhage, though with less precision. Results of duplex scanning are now so reliable that many patients can proceed directly to surgery. Magnetic resonance angiography provides detailed information when needed on the status of the intracranial circulation and the brain parenchyma. Catheter angiography is reserved for the purpose of resolving questions not answered by these modalities. Recently, plaques observed in the aortic arch by transesophageal echocardiography have been shown to be an independent risk for ischemic stroke.

Treatment

A. Medical Measures: Acute strokes, most progressive or evolving strokes, and those with major neurologic deficits are treated by medical means as discussed in the section on cerebrovascular accidents in Chapter 24. Patients with transient ischemic attacks may be treated with antiplatelet drugs (aspirin, 325 mg/d), ticlopidine (250 mg twice daily), or clopidogrel (75 mg twice daily).

B. Surgical Measures:

1. Transient ischemic attacks and stroke– Carotid endarterectomy plus optimal medical therapy is highly effective in preventing stroke and death in symptomatic patients with carotid stenosis greater than 70%. Recently, carotid endarterectomy has also been shown to be effective when the stenoses are between 50% and 69%, though the benefit is not as great as for patients with greater than 70% stenosis. Carotid endarterectomy is most effective when symptoms are specific for hemispheric ischemia of recent origin involving the anterior circulation, and it is essential that the vascular surgeon be one who performs carotid endarterectomies regularly with a mortality-complication rate of less than 5%. Primary care physicians are obliged to know this information prior to referral, since an increased risk of neurologic complications after carotid endarterectomy may outweigh the anticipated benefit.

2. Asymptomatic carotid stenosis–Asymptomatic carotid bruits are stronger predictors of death from coronary artery disease than from stroke. Nonetheless, in some patients they may signal the presence of a hemodynamically significant carotid stenosis. Many surgeons believe that with increasing accuracy of the noninvasive evaluation of carotid stenosis, it is possible to identify patients who might be helped by prophylactic endarterectomy. About 2% of patients per year with asymptomatic carotid stenosis suffer a stroke; this approximates 3% if the stenosis exceeds 75%. Thus, the risk of causing stroke from angiography and surgery should be less than 3% if surgery is offered. The American Heart Association has recommended upper limits of acceptable combined morbidity and mortality for carotid endarterectomy. These are 3% for asymptomatic patients and 5% for those with TIAs or stroke. These figures are 7% in patients with previous stroke and 10% in individuals with recurrent carotid stenosis. In 1995, a trial was reported comparing carotid endarterectomy with aspirin in patients with asymptomatic carotid stenosis exceeding 60%. Patients enrolled were under 80 years of age and were considered good surgical candidates, and the procedures were performed at centers with excellent staff. Despite an early mortality and morbidity disadvantage in the surgical group, projected 5-year data in these patients were considerably more favorable than the results achieved with aspirin alone. Thus, it now appears that this procedure may be offered to selected asymptomatic patients who are good surgical risks. The use of thromboendarterectomy for asymptomatic carotid stenoses remains controversial.

Endarterectomy may be indicated as an emergency procedure in patients with very early and fluctuating neurologic deficits with significant carotid stenosis. It is not useful in acute stroke, progressing stroke, or when there is also severe intracranial vascular disease.

Prognosis

The prognosis and results of therapy are related to the number of vessels involved, the degree of stenosis in each, and the collateral flow in the circle of Willis. Expertly performed surgery may have a 1–2% mortality rate and a 1–4% rate of permanent major or minor neurologic complications; there is wide institutional variation in these figures. Transient ischemic attacks known to be secondary to significant carotid artery stenosis or ulceration can often be eliminated by surgery, and although future strokes can occur in such patients, other arterial lesions, such as a contralateral carotid stenosis or intracranial arterial lesions, are often responsible. Concomitant coronary artery disease results in an overall mortality rate that is similar in operated and unoperated groups. In the best hands, the operative procedure in patients with transient ischemic attacks or stroke may reduce the chance of developing a permanent neurologic deficit within 5 years from 30% to 5%. The incidence of later stroke after uncomplicated endarterectomy is around 5–15%, and although restenosis may occur in the operated artery, it is usually not symptomatic. Significant carotid artery stenosis without symptoms entails no more than a 10–15% stroke risk over 3–5 years.

Amarenco P et al: Atherosclerotic disease of the aortic arch and the risk of ischemic stroke. N Engl J Med 1994; 331:1474. [NLM Cit ID: 95059251] (Plaques detected by transesophageal echo are an important risk factor.)

Barnett HJ et al: The dilemma of surgical treatment for patients with asymptomatic carotid disease. Ann Intern Med 1995;123:723. [NLM Cit ID: 96011282]

Brott T et al: Medical compared with surgical treatment of asymptomatic carotid artery stenosis. Ann Intern Med 1995;123:720. [NLM Cit ID: 96011281]

Executive Committee for the Asymptomatic Carotid Atherosclerosis Study: Endarterectomy for asymptomatic carotid artery stenosis. JAMA 1995;273:1421. [NLM Cit ID: 95239880] (Advantages for surgery in selected patients with stenoses greater than 60%.)

Moore WS et al: Guidelines for carotid endarterectomy: A multidisciplinary consensus statement from the Ad Hoc Committee, American Heart Association. Circulation 1995;91:566. [NLM Cit ID: 95103786] (Excellent review of the literature with guidelines.)

Sauve JS et al: Can bruits distinguish high-grade from moderate symptomatic carotid stenosis? The North American Symptomatic Carotid Endarterectomy Trial. Ann Intern Med 1994;120:633. [NLM Cit ID: 94182828] (Cervical bruits alone were not sufficiently predictive of high-grade symptomatic carotid stenosis to be useful in selecting patients for angiography; bruits were absent in over one-third of patients with high-grade stenosis.)

VISCERAL ARTERY INSUFFICIENCY

Chronic intestinal ischemia generally results from atherosclerotic occlusive lesions at or close to the origins of the superior mesenteric, celiac, and inferior mesenteric arteries, leading to a significant reduction of blood flow to the intestines. Symptoms consist of epigastric or periumbilical postprandial pains that last for 1–3 hours. To avoid pain, the patient limits oral intake, and weight loss results; pain at this stage of the process may be less prominent. Such a history in a person over 45 years of age who appears chronically ill and who has peripheral arterial disease is probably an indication for arteriography. Chronic intestinal ischemia is a diagnosis of exclusion, usually made after a negative workup, including upper and lower endoscopy and an abdominal CT scan. Asymptomatic visceral artery disease is common, not unlike asymptomatic coronary and carotid atherosclerosis. Angiography usually shows two of the three mesenteric arteries to have significant occlusive disease. Surgical management is directed toward restoration of antegrade visceral arterial flow by bypass or transaortic endarterectomy.

Acute intestinal ischemia results from (1) embolic occlusions of the visceral branches of the abdominal aorta, generally in patients with mitral valvular heart disease or especially with atrial fibrillation, or left ventricular mural thrombus; (2) thrombosis of one or more of the visceral vessels involved with atherosclerotic occlusive changes, sometimes in patients with a history of chronic intestinal ischemia as described above; or (3) nonocclusive mesenteric vascular insufficiency, generally in patients with congestive heart failure receiving recently instituted digitalis with diuretics or in those who are in shock. The acute onset of crampy or steady epigastric and periumbilical abdominal pain combined with minimal or no findings on abdominal examination and a high leukocyte count should suggest one of these three events in the superior mesenteric system. Pain may be more impressive than physical signs. The combination of lactic acidosis, hypotension, and abdominal distention suggests bowel infarction rather than ischemia. Angiography of the superior mesenteric artery is helpful for early diagnosis. Patients suspected of having acute mesenteric ischemia require emergent laparotomy. Mesenteric duplex scanning is a noninvasive technique for the anatomic and physiologic assessment of the visceral vessels and may be helpful in selecting patients with symptoms of chronic or acute mesenteric ischemia for arteriography. If occlusion is present, antibiotics specific for intestinal flora should be instituted (eg, ampicillin and aminoglycoside plus clindamycin or metronidazole), and laparotomy should be performed to reestablish blood flow to the intestine and remove necrotic bowel. The clinical picture of **acute mesenteric vein occlusion** is similar to that of arterial syndromes but may present in a more subacute manner. Patients should be treated with anticoagulation and surgery reserved for those suspected of having bowel infarction. Surgical management is usually confined to bowel resection and anticoagulation. In selected patients, venous thrombectomy may be considered. Patients at risk include those with systemic hypercoagulability such as is observed with paroxysmal nocturnal hemoglobinuria; protein C, protein S, or antithrombin III deficiency; factor V Leiden; and anti-phospholipid antibody syndrome.

Through early diagnosis and aggressive treatment, the very poor prognosis of the past should yield somewhat lower morbidity and mortality rates.

Patients who present with chronic mesenteric ischemia often appear ill; weight loss is a common feature.

Ischemic colitis develops when the diminished circulation is most prominent in the distribution of the inferior mesenteric artery. Because of the nature of the collaterals, infarction is uncommon in this instance. However, the patient may have episodic bouts of crampy lower abdominal pain associated with mild diarrhea, often bloody. This picture may be indistinguishable from inflammatory bowel disease. Colonoscopy may reveal segmental inflammatory changes, most often in the rectosigmoid and the splenic flexure where the collateral circulation is most active. Because adequate collateral circulation usually develops, the prognosis is better than when the vascular insufficiency involves the superior mesenteric circulation, and maintenance of hydration may be all that is necessary.

Klempnauer J et al: Long-term results after surgery for acute mesenteric ischemia. Surgery 1997;121:239. [NLM Cit ID: 97221618] (In 90 patients with acute mesenteric ischemia who went to surgery, the in-hospital mortality rate for acute mesenteric ischemia was 66%. Of the patients who were discharged alive, the 2- and 5-year mortality rates were 30% and 50%, respectively. Deaths were due mainly to cardiovascular comorbidity and malignant disease.)

Rapp JH et al: Durability of endarterectomy and antegrade grafts in the treatment of chronic visceral ischemia. J Vasc Surg 1986;3:799. [NLM Cit ID: 86200490] (Classic article describing the largest published clinical experience with the presentation and treatment of visceral ischemia.)

Toursarkissian B et al: Ischemic colitis. Surg Clin North Am 1997;77:461. [NLM Cit ID: 97292185]

ACUTE ARTERIAL OCCLUSION

Essentials of Diagnosis

- Symptoms and signs depend on the artery occluded, the organ or region supplied by the artery, and the adequacy of the collateral circulation to the area primarily involved.
- Occlusion in an extremity usually results in the six P's of acute arterial ischemia: pain, pallor, pulselessness, paresthesias, poikilothermia, and paralysis.
- Pulsations are absent in arteries distal to the occlusion. Occlusions in other areas result in such conditions as cerebrovascular accidents, intestinal ischemia and gangrene, and renal or splenic infarcts.

Differential Diagnosis

The primary differentiation is between arterial embolism and thrombosis. In an older individual with both arteriosclerotic vascular disease and cardiac disease, the differentiation may be very difficult, and in 10–20% a definitive diagnosis either cannot be made or turns out to be incorrect. Arterial trauma may result in either occlusion or spasm.

1. ARTERIAL EMBOLISM

Arterial embolism is generally a complication of heart disease; a minority of those with embolism have rheumatic heart disease, but most have ischemic heart disease, with or without myocardial infarction. Atrial fibrillation is often present. Other forms of heart disease and miscellaneous causes such as arterial embolism account for the rest. In 10%, there is more than one embolism, and recurrent emboli after initial successful treatment are common.

Emboli tend to lodge at the bifurcation of major arteries, with over half going to the aortic bifurcation or the vessels in the lower extremities; the carotid system is involved in 20%, and the upper extremity and the mesenteric arteries in the remainder. Emboli from arterial ulcerations are usually small, giving rise to transient symptoms in the toes or brain but occasionally to a systemic illness resembling vasculitis (see below).

Clinical Findings

In an extremity, the initial symptoms are usually pain (sudden or gradual in onset), numbness, coldness, and tingling. Signs include absence of pulsations in the arteries distal to the block, coldness, pallor or mottling, hypesthesia or anesthesia, and weakness, muscle spasm, or paralysis. The superficial veins are collapsed. Later, blebs and skin necrosis may appear, and gangrene can result.

Treatment

Immediate embolectomy is the treatment of choice in almost all early cases of emboli in extremities. It is best done within 4–6 hours after the embolic episode; it is occasionally successful after longer delays if the supplied tissue remains viable.

A. Emergency Preoperative Care:

1. Heparin–Heparin sodium should be given as soon as the diagnosis is made or suspected in an effort to prevent distal thrombosis and continued until the time of surgery, maintaining the partial thromboplastin time (PTT) at twice the normal level. It may also help relieve associated spasm.

2. Protect the part–The extremity is kept at or below the horizontal plane, and neither heat nor cold is applied. The limb must be protected from hard surfaces and overlying bedclothes.

3. Imaging–Arteriography is often of value either before or during surgery if the distinction between embolism and thrombosis cannot be made on clinical grounds. Echocardiography may confirm the source; the transesophageal approach increases the test's sensitivity for detection of left atrial thrombus.

B. Surgical Measures: Local anesthesia is generally used in high-risk patients if the occlusion is in an artery to an extremity. The embolus is removed through the arteriotomy by means of a specially designed catheter with a small inflatable balloon at the tip (Fogarty catheter). An embolus at the aortic bifurcation or in the iliac artery can often be removed under local anesthesia through common femoral arteriotomies with the use of these same catheters. Laparotomy is necessary for emboli to the mesenteric circulation. Heparinization for a week or more postoperatively is indicated, and lifelong anticoagulation is recommended because of the high frequency of recurrent emboli.

Delayed embolectomy carried out more than 12 hours following the embolism or when there is ischemia or necrosis—as evidenced by mottled cyanosis, muscle rigidity, anesthesia, or markedly elevated serum CK—involves a high risk of development of a compartment syndrome with attendant local risk of neurovascular occlusion and systemic consequences of acute respiratory distress syndrome and renal failure. Anticoagulation rather than surgery or catheter embolectomy may be the proper initial therapy under such circumstances, accepting urgent or elective amputation as the necessary lifesaving procedure in most instances. Myoglobinuria and renal failure can be minimized with aggressive hydration and sodium bicarbonate administered in doses sufficient to alkalinize the urine, thus diminishing the precipitation of myoglobin in the renal tubules. Mannitol and furosemide are used to maintain a brisk diuresis.

Prognosis

Arterial embolism is a threat not only to the limb (5–25% amputation rate) but also to the life of the patient (25–30% hospital mortality rate, with underlying heart disease responsible for over half of these deaths).

Emboli in the aortoiliac area are more dangerous than more peripheral emboli, and the mortality rate rises if there are multiple peripheral emboli or carotid or visceral emboli, approaching 100% if all three areas are involved. Emboli associated with ischemic heart disease have a poorer prognosis than those arising from rheumatic valvular disease.

In patients with atrial fibrillation, an attempt may be made to restore normal rhythm pharmacologically or by cardioversion after the patient has been anticoagulated; restoration of normal rhythm tends to be permanent only in patients with recent onset or transitory fibrillation. Long-term anticoagulant therapy diminishes the danger of further emboli and in the majority of patients is the only long-term prophylactic measure that can be instituted.

If no heart disease exists, arteriography may reveal an atherosclerotic ulcer or small aneurysm to be the origin of the embolus; depending upon location, these may be treated surgically. Three-fourths of the patients surviving the embolic episode and the associated hospital stay may then have a good quality of life.

2. ACUTE ARTERIAL THROMBOSIS

Acute arterial thrombosis generally occurs in an artery in which the lumen has become narrow as a result of atherosclerosis. Blood flowing through such a narrow, irregular, or ulcerated lumen may clot, leading to a sudden, complete occlusion of the narrow segment. The thrombosis may then propagate either up or down the artery to a point where the blood is flowing rapidly through a somewhat less diseased artery (usually to a significant arterial branch proximally or one or more functioning collateral vessels distally). Occasionally, the thrombosis is precipitated by the rupture of an arteriosclerotic plaque, blocking the lumen; trauma to the artery may precipitate a similar event. Inflammatory involvement of the arterial wall will also lead to thrombosis. Thrombosis in a diseased artery may be secondary to an episode of hypotension or cardiac failure. Polycythemia and dehydration also increase the chance of thrombosis, as do repeated arterial punctures. Finally, hypercoagulable states, such as anti-phospholipid antibody syndrome and hyperhomocysteinemia, can cause arterial thrombosis.

Chronic incomplete arterial obstruction usually results in the establishment of some collateral flow, and further flow will develop relatively rapidly through the collaterals once complete occlusion has developed. The extremity may be threatened for hours or days, however, while the additional collateral circulation develops around the block.

Clinical Findings

The local findings in the extremity are usually very similar to those described in the section on arterial embolism. The following differential points should be considered: (1) Are there manifestations of advanced occlusive arterial disease in other areas, especially the opposite extremity (bruit, absent pulses, secondary changes)? Is there a history of intermittent claudication? These clinical manifestations are suggestive but not diagnostic of thrombosis. (2) Is there a history or are there findings of rheumatic heart disease or of a recent episode of atrial fibrillation or myocardial infarction? If so, an embolism is more likely than a thrombosis. (3) Electrocardiography, echocardiography, and serum enzyme studies may give added information regarding the presence of a silent myocardial infarction and its likelihood as a source of an embolus. Ultimately, arteriography is necessary for accurate differential diagnosis and for planning therapy.

Treatment

Whereas emergency embolectomy is the usual approach in the case of an early occlusion from an embolus, a nonoperative approach is generally used in the case of thrombosis for two reasons: (1) The segment of thrombosed artery may be quite long, requiring extensive surgery (thromboendarterectomy or artery graft). The removal of a single embolus in a normal artery is, by comparison, relatively easy. (2) The extremity is more likely to survive without development of gangrene because some collateral circulation has usually formed during the slowly progressive stenosing phase before acute thrombosis. With an embolism, this is not usually the case; the block is most often at a major arterial bifurcation, occluding both branches, and the associated arterial spasm is usually more acute. Treatment—particularly if tissue necrosis is present—is as described for emergency preoperative care for arterial embolism. Thrombolytic therapy using streptokinase or the more expensive urokinase or tissue plasminogen activator (t-PA) may be tried in acute thrombosis if no signs of neurologic impairment or tissue necrosis exist; lysis may be achieved in 50–80% of cases, and direct arterial infusion into the thrombus has fewer bleeding complications than systemic therapy with these drugs since the dose given locally is much smaller. Owing to the relatively slow rate of thrombolysis and the inherent risks of the therapy itself, the rates of complications and amputation (20% and 5%, respectively) remain relatively high. If successful thrombolysis occurs, rethrombosis may be prevented by angioplasty. Otherwise, treatment is as outlined under emergency preoperative care for arterial embolism.

Prognosis

Limb survival usually occurs with acute thrombosis of the iliac or superficial femoral arteries; gangrene is more likely if the popliteal is suddenly occluded, especially if the period between occlusion and treatment is long or if there is considerable arterial spasm or proximal arterial occlusive disease. If the limb does survive the acute occlusion, significant functional recovery may occur gradually over a number of weeks. The later treatment and prognosis are outlined above in the section on occlusive disease of the iliac, femoral, and popliteal arteries.

Ouriel K et al: A comparison of recombinant urokinase with vascular surgery as initial treatment for acute arterial occlusion of the legs. Thrombolysis or Peripheral Arterial Surgery (TOPAS) Investigators. N Engl J Med 1998;338:1105. [NLM Cit ID: 98196617]

THROMBOANGIITIS OBLITERANS (Buerger's Disease)

Essentials of Diagnosis

- Almost always in young men who smoke.
- Extremities involved with inflammatory occlusions of the more distal arteries, resulting in circulatory insufficiency of the toes or fingers.
- Thromboses of superficial veins may also occur.
- Course is intermittent and amputation may be necessary, especially if smoking is not stopped.

General Considerations

Buerger's disease is an episodic and segmental inflammatory and thrombotic process of the arteries and veins, principally in the limbs. The cause is not known. It is seen most commonly in men under 40 who smoke and is especially common in Ashkenazi Jews of Eastern European background. The effects of the disease are almost solely due to occlusion of the arteries. The symptoms are primarily due to ischemia, complicated in the later stages by infection and tissue necrosis. The inflammatory process is intermittent, with quiescent periods lasting weeks, months, or years.

The arteries most commonly affected are the plantar and digital vessels in the foot and those in the lower leg. The arteries in the hands and wrists may also become involved. Different arterial segments may become occluded in successive episodes; a certain amount of recanalization occurs during quiescent periods. Superficial migratory thrombophlebitis is a common early indication of the disease.

Clinical Findings

The symptoms and signs are primarily those of arterial insufficiency, and the differentiation from arteriosclerotic peripheral vascular disease may be difficult; however, the following findings suggest Buerger's disease:

(1) The patient is a man under 40 who smokes.

(2) There is a history or finding of small, red, tender cords resulting from migratory superficial segmental thrombophlebitis, usually in the saphenous tributaries rather than the main vessel. A biopsy of such a vein provides suggestive evidence of Buerger's disease, though no finding is unambiguously pathognomonic.

(3) Intermittent claudication is common. Rest pain can be frequent and persistent. It tends to be more pronounced than in the patient with atherosclerosis. Numbness, diminished sensation, and pricking and burning pains may be present as a result of ischemic neuropathy.

(4) The digit or the entire distal portion of the foot may be pale and cold, or there may be rubor that may remain relatively unchanged by posture; the skin may not blanch on elevation, and on dependency the intensity of the rubor is often more pronounced than that seen in the atherosclerotic group. The distal vascular changes are often asymmetric, so that not all of the toes are affected to the same degree. Absence or impairment of pulsations in the dorsalis pedis, posterior tibial, ulnar, or radial artery is frequent.

(5) Trophic changes may be present, often with painful indolent ulcerations along the nail margins.

(6) There is usually evidence of disease in both legs and possibly also in the hands and lower arms. There may be a history or findings of Raynaud's phenomenon in the finger or distal foot.

(7) The course is usually intermittent, with acute and often dramatic episodes followed by rather definite remissions. When the collateral vessels as well as the main channels have become occluded, an exac-

erbation is more likely to lead to gangrene and amputation. The course in the patient with atherosclerosis tends to be less dramatic and more persistent.

Differential Diagnosis

Differences between thromboangiitis obliterans and atherosclerosis obliterans are discussed above.

Raynaud's disease causes symmetric bilateral color changes, primarily in young women. There is no impairment of arterial pulsations. Antiphospholipid antibody syndrome may include vasospasm and livedo reticularis, but arterial pulses are preserved, and the early blanching of the digits seen in Raynaud's disease does not occur. Likewise, cholesterol atheroembolic disease may mimic Buerger's disease, but it is most often observed in older patients with established atherosclerosis.

Treatment

The principles of therapy are the same as those outlined for atherosclerotic peripheral vascular disease, but the long-range outlook is better in patients with Buerger's disease, so that when possible the approach should be more conservative and tissue loss kept to a minimum.

A. General Measures: Smoking must be stopped; the physician must insist on it. The disease will progress if this advice is not followed.

B. Surgical Measures:

1. Sympathectomy–Sympathectomy may be useful in eliminating the vasospastic manifestations of the disease and aiding in the establishment of collateral circulation to the skin. It may also relieve the mild or moderate forms of rest pain. If amputation of a digit is necessary, sympathectomy may aid in healing of the surgical wound.

2. Amputation–The indications for amputation are similar in many respects to those outlined for the atherosclerotic group, although the approach should be more conservative from the point of view of preservation of tissue. Most patients with Buerger's disease who are managed carefully and who stop smoking do not require amputation of the fingers or toes. It is almost never necessary to amputate the entire hand, but amputation below the knee is occasionally necessary because of gangrene or severe pain in the foot.

Prognosis

Except in the case of the rapidly progressive form of the disease—and provided the patient stops smoking and takes good care of the feet—the prognosis for survival of the extremities is good.

Borner C et al: Long-term follow-up of thromboangiitis obliterans. Vasa 1998;27:80. [NLM Cit ID: 98275057]

The European TAO Study Group: Oral iloprost in the treatment of thromboangiitis obliterans (Buerger's disease): A double blind, randomized, placebo-controlled trial. Eur J Vasc Endovasc Surg 1998;15:300. [NLM Cit ID: 98273261]

Szuba A et al: Thromboangiitis obliterans. An update on Buerger's disease. West J Med 1998;168:255. [NLM Cit ID: 98245642]

IDIOPATHIC ARTERITIS OF TAKAYASU ("Pulseless Disease")

Pulseless disease, most frequent in young women, is an occlusive polyarteritis of unknown cause with a special predilection for the branches of the aortic arch. It occurs most commonly in Asians. Manifestations, depending upon the vessel or vessels involved, may include evidence of cerebrovascular insufficiency, with transient ischemic attacks and visual disturbances; and absent pulses in the arms, with a rich collateral flow in the shoulder, chest, and neck areas. The most common clinical finding, however, is a bruit. The extent of the vascular involvement may be defined by angiography.

Pulseless disease must be differentiated from vascular lesions of the aortic arch due to atherosclerosis, though in the latter instance concomitant lower extremity disease is invariably present. Histologically, the arterial lesions are indistinguishable from those of giant cell arteritis. In the early stage of the disease, the progression of the vascular stenosis may be reversed by corticosteroids; in the more advanced forms, bypass arterial grafts are necessary.

Kerr GS et al: Takayasu arteritis. Ann Intern Med 1994;120:919. [NLM Cit ID: 94226431] (A balanced clinical review.)

CHOLESTEROL ATHEROEMBOLIC DISEASE

In some patients with severe atherosclerosis involving the aorta and its branches, a distinct syndrome resulting from repeated microembolization from atherosclerotic plaques has been observed. Atheroembolism is the result of release of cholesterol-rich atheromatous debris from ulcerated atherosclerotic plaques. This syndrome occurs spontaneously after transfemoral aortographic procedures or as a consequence of surgical manipulation of an artery. Virtually any organ or extremity may be affected. History and physical findings are dependent on site of cholesterol embolization. These include transient ischemic attacks, amaurosis fugax, hypertension and progressive renal failure, abdominal pain, nausea, vomiting, melena, severe calf pain, livedo reticularis, purple toes, and normal pulses. Laboratory investigations disclose microhematuria, renal insufficiency, eosinophilia, and an elevated sedimentation rate, with hypocomplementemia during the first days of the clinical course. Biopsies of the kidney and other tissues show cholesterol clefts in the small vessels.

Misdiagnosis of systemic vasculitis may result in inappropriate use of immunomodulating drugs. The only treatment is identification of the responsible lesion by arteriography and its removal by endarterectomy or exclusion of the arterial segment by a bypass procedure. When atheroemboli are confined to the calf or foot, surgical treatment is a good option.

Bruno A et al: Vascular outcome in men with asymptomatic retinal cholesterol emboli: A cohort study. Ann Intern Med 1995;122:249. [NLM Cit ID: 95126304] (This case-control study of 140 patients with a mean follow-up of 3.4 years showed that stroke occurred at an annual rate of 8.5% among patients with retinal cholesterol emboli versus 0.8% among controls.)

Peat DS et al: Cholesterol emboli may mimic systemic vasculitis. BMJ 1996;313:546. [NLM Cit ID: 96382123]

Vidt DG: Cholesterol emboli: A common cause of renal failure. Annu Rev Med 1997;48:375. [NLM Cit ID: 97198994]

VASOMOTOR DISORDERS

RAYNAUD'S DISEASE & RAYNAUD'S PHENOMENON

Essentials of Diagnosis

- Paroxysmal bilateral symmetric pallor and cyanosis followed by rubor of the skin of the digits.
- Precipitated by cold or emotional upset; relieved by warmth.
- Primarily a disorder of young women.

General Considerations

Raynaud's disease is the primary, or idiopathic, form of paroxysmal digital cyanosis. Raynaud's phenomenon, which is more common than Raynaud's disease, may be due to a number of regional or systemic disorders. In Raynaud's disease the digital arteries respond excessively to vasospastic stimuli. The cause is not known, but some abnormality of the sympathetic nervous system seems to be active in this entity.

Clinical Findings

Raynaud's disease and Raynaud's phenomenon are characterized by intermittent attacks of pallor or cyanosis—or pallor followed by cyanosis—in the fingers (and rarely the toes), precipitated by cold or occasionally by emotional upsets. In early attacks of Raynaud's phenomenon, only 1–2 fingertips may be affected; as it progresses, all the fingers down to the distal palm may be involved. The thumbs are rarely affected. During recovery there may be intense rubor, throbbing, paresthesia, and slight swelling. Attacks usually terminate spontaneously or upon returning to a warm room or putting the extremity in warm water. Between attacks there are no abnormal findings. Sensory changes that often accompany vasomotor manifestations include numbness, stiffness, diminished sensation, and aching pain. The condition may progress to atrophy of the terminal fat pads and the digital skin, and gangrenous ulcers may appear near the fingertips; they may heal during warm weather.

Raynaud's disease appears first between ages 15 and 45, almost always in women. It tends to be progressive, and, unlike Raynaud's phenomenon (which may be unilateral and may involve only one or two fingers), symmetric involvement of the fingers of both hands is the rule. Spasm becomes more frequent and prolonged.

Raynaud's disease may be diagnosed if the phenomenon persists for greater than 3 years without evidence of an associated disease (see below). There are no specific laboratory abnormalities; the diagnosis is a clinical one, though studies to exclude the conditions associated with Raynaud's disease are warranted.

Differential Diagnosis

Raynaud's disease must be differentiated from the numerous disorders that may be associated with Raynaud's phenomenon. The history and examination lead to the diagnosis of rheumatoid arthritis, systemic sclerosis (including its more localized CREST variant), systemic lupus erythematosus, and mixed connective tissue disease, with which Raynaud's phenomenon is commonly associated. Raynaud's phenomenon is occasionally the first manifestation of these disorders.

The differentiation from thromboangiitis obliterans is usually not difficult, since thromboangiitis obliterans is generally a disease of men; peripheral pulses are often diminished or absent; and, when Raynaud's phenomenon occurs in association with thromboangiitis obliterans, it is usually in only one or two digits.

Raynaud's phenomenon may occur in patients with the thoracic outlet syndromes. In these disorders, involvement is generally unilateral, and symptoms referable to brachial plexus compression tend to dominate the clinical picture. Carpal tunnel syndrome should also be considered, and nerve conduction tests are appropriate in selected cases.

In acrocyanosis, cyanosis of the hands is permanent and diffuse. Frostbite may lead to chronic Raynaud's phenomenon. Ergot poisoning, particularly due to prolonged or excessive use of ergotamine, must also be considered.

A particularly severe form of Raynaud's phenomenon occurs in up to one-third of patients receiving bleomycin and vincristine in combination, often for testicular cancer. Treatment is unsuccessful, and the problem persists even with discontinuance of the drugs.

Finally, Raynaud's phenomenon may be mimicked by cryoglobulinemia, in which serum proteins aggregate in the cooler distal circulation. Cryoglobulinemia may be idiopathic or associated with multiple myeloma and other hyperglobulinemic states.

Treatment

A. General Measures: The body should be kept warm, and the hands especially should be protected from exposure to cold; gloves should be worn when out in the cold. The hands should be protected from injury at all times; wounds heal slowly, and infections are consequently hard to control. Softening and lubricating lotion to control the fissured dry skin should be applied to the hands frequently. Smoking should be stopped.

B. Vasodilators: Vasodilator drugs are of limited value but may be of some benefit in those patients who are not adequately controlled by general measures and when there is peripheral vasoconstriction without significant organic vascular disease. Shortening of temperature recovery time may occur with the use of transdermal nitroglycerin or a longer-acting oral nitrate. Low doses of nifedipine (sustained-release, 30 mg/d) have been employed with good effect in the treatment of Raynaud's phenomenon and disease.

C. Surgical Measures: Sympathectomy may be indicated when attacks have become frequent and severe, interfering with work and well-being—and particularly if trophic changes have developed and medical measures have failed. In the lower extremities, complete and permanent relief may result, whereas dorsal sympathectomies generally result in only temporary improvement in most patients treated with operation. Although vascular tone of the vessels in the hands usually ultimately reappears, the symptoms in the fingers that may thus recur in 1–5 years are usually milder and less frequent. Sympathectomies are of very limited value in far-advanced cases, particularly if significant digital artery obstructive disease with scleroderma is present.

Prognosis

Raynaud's disease is usually benign, causing mild discomfort on exposure to cold and progressing very slightly over the years. In a few cases rapid progression does occur, so that the slightest change in temperature may precipitate color changes. It is in this situation that sclerodactyly and small areas of gangrene may be noted, and such patients may become quite disabled by severe pain, limitation of motion, and secondary fixation of distal joints. The prognosis of Raynaud's phenomenon is that of the associated disease. Recently, a clinical study showed that *H pylori* eradication causes a significant decrease in clinical attacks of Raynaud's disease. The role of bacteria in the pathogenesis of this and other arterial disease continues to demand attention.

Gasbarrini A et al: *Helicobacter pylori* eradication ameliorates primary Raynaud's phenomenon. Dig Dis Sci 1998;43:1641. [NLM Cit ID: 98389537]

Spencer-Green G: Outcomes in primary Raynaud's phenomenon: A meta-analysis of the frequency, rates, and predictors of transition to secondary disease. Arch Intern Med 1998;158:595. [NLM Cit ID: 98180519]

LIVEDO RETICULARIS

Livedo reticularis is an uncommon vasospastic disorder of unknown cause that results in mottled discoloration on large areas of the extremities, generally in a fishnet pattern with reticulated cyanotic areas surrounding a paler central core. It occurs primarily in young women. It may be associated with an occult malignant neoplasm, polyarteritis nodosa, atherosclerotic microemboli to the skin, or antiphospholipid antibody syndrome.

Livedo reticularis is most apparent on the thighs and forearms and occasionally on the lower abdomen and is most pronounced in cold weather. The color may change to a reddish hue in warm weather but does not entirely disappear. A few patients complain of paresthesias, coldness, or numbness in the involved areas. Recurrent ulcers in the lower extremities may occur in severe cases.

Bluish mottling of the extremities is diagnostic. The peripheral pulses are normal. The extremity may be cold, with increased perspiration.

Treatment consists of protection from exposure to cold; use of vasodilators is seldom indicated. In most instances, livedo reticularis is entirely benign. In the rare patient who develops ulcerations or gangrene, underlying systemic disease should be considered.

See reference below.

ACROCYANOSIS

Acrocyanosis is an uncommon symmetric condition involving the skin of the hands and feet and, to a lesser degree, the forearms and legs. It is associated with arteriolar vasoconstriction combined with dilation of the subpapillary venous plexus of the skin, through which deoxygenated blood slowly circulates. It is worse in cold weather but does not completely disappear during the warm season. It occurs in either gender, is most common in the teens and 20s, and usually improves with advancing age or during pregnancy. It is characterized by coldness, sweating, slight edema, and cyanotic discoloration of the involved areas. Pain, trophic lesions, and disability do not occur, and the peripheral pulses are present. The individual may thus be reassured and encouraged to dress warmly in cold weather.

Naldi L et al: Cutaneous manifestations associated with antiphospholipid antibodies in patients with suspected primary antiphospholipid syndrome. Ann Rheum Dis 1993;52:219. [NLM Cit ID: 93249302] (Livedo reticularis and acrocyanosis were significantly associated with antiphospholipid antibodies.)

ERYTHROMELALGIA

Erythromelalgia is a paroxysmal bilateral vasodilatory disorder of unknown cause. Idiopathic (primary) erythromelalgia occurs in otherwise healthy persons and affects men and women equally. A secondary type is occasionally seen in patients with polycythemia vera, hypertension, gout, and neurologic diseases.

The chief symptom is bilateral burning pain that lasts minutes to hours, involving circumscribed areas on the soles or palms first and, as the disease progresses, the entire extremity. The attack occurs in response to stimuli producing vasodilation (eg, exercise, warm environment), especially at night when the extremities are warmed under bedclothes. Reddening or cyanosis as well as heat may be noted. Relief may be obtained by cooling the affected part and by elevation.

No findings are generally present between attacks. With onset of an attack, heat and redness are noted in association with the typical pain. Skin temperature and arterial pulsations are increased, and the involved areas may sweat profusely.

In primary erythromelalgia, aspirin, 650 mg every 4–6 hours, may give excellent relief. The patient should avoid warm environments. In severe cases, if medical measures fail, section of peripheral nerves may be necessary to relieve pain.

Primary idiopathic erythromelalgia is uniformly benign.

Kalgaard OM et al: A clinical study of 87 cases. J Intern Med 1997;242:191. [NLM Cit ID: 98011238]

van Genderen PH et al: Erythromelalgia: A pathognomonic microvascular thrombotic complication in essential thrombocytopenia and polycythemia vera. Semin Thromb Hemost 1997;23:357. [NLM Cit ID: 97408833]

REFLEX SYMPATHETIC DYSTROPHY

Essentials of Diagnosis

- Burning or aching pain of a severity greater than expected following trauma to an extremity.
- Manifestations of vasomotor instability are generally present and include alterations of temperature, color, and texture of the skin of the involved extremity.

General Considerations

Pain—usually burning or aching—in an injured extremity is the single most common finding, and the disparity between the severity of the inciting injury and the degree of pain experienced is the most characteristic feature. Crushing injuries with lacerations and soft tissue destruction are the most common causes, but closed fractures, simple lacerations, burns (especially electric), and elective operative procedures are also responsible for this syndrome. It may also involve the left upper extremity after intrathoracic diseases such as myocardial infarction. The manifestations of pain and the associated objective changes may be relatively mild or quite severe, and the initial manifestations often change if the condition proceeds to a chronic stage.

Clinical Findings

In the early stages, the pain, tenderness, and hyperesthesia may be strictly localized to the injured area, and the extremity may be warm, dry, swollen, and red or slightly cyanotic. The involved extremity is held in a splinted position by the muscles, and the nails may become ridged. In advanced stages, the pain is more diffuse and worse at night; the extremity becomes cool and clammy and intolerant of temperature changes (particularly cold); and the skin becomes glossy and atrophic. The joints become stiff, generally in a position that makes the extremity useless. Radiographs of the involved extremity reveal asymmetric severe osteopenia in excess of that anticipated due to disuse. The dominant concern of the patient may be to avoid the slightest stimuli to the extremity and especially to the trigger points that may develop.

Prevention

During operations on an extremity, peripheral nerves should be handled only when absolutely necessary and then with utmost gentleness. Splinting of an injured extremity for an adequate period during the early, painful phase of recovery, together with adequate analgesics, may help prevent this condition.

Treatment & Prognosis

A. Conservative Measures: It is most important that the condition be recognized and treated in the early stages, when the manifestations are most easily reversed and major secondary changes have not yet developed. In mild, early cases with minimal skin and joint changes, physical therapy involving active and passive exercises combined with diazepam, 2 mg twice daily, or alprazolam, 0.125–0.25 mg every 12 hours, may relieve symptoms. Protecting the extremity from irritating stimuli is important, and the use of nonaddicting analgesics may be necessary.

B. Surgical Measures: If the condition fails to respond to conservative treatment or if there are more severe or advanced objective findings, sympathetic blocks (stellate ganglion or lumbar) may be helpful. Intensive physical therapy may be used during the pain-free periods following effective blocks. Patients who achieve significant temporary relief of symptoms after sympathetic blocks but fail to obtain permanent relief by the blocks may be cured by sympathectomy. In the advanced forms—particularly in association with major local changes and emotional reactions—the prognosis for improvement is poor. The newer neurosurgical approaches using implantable electronic biostimulator devices to block pain impulses in the cervical spinal cord have met with some success.

Lopez RF: Reflex sympathetic dystrophy. Timely diagnosis and treatment can prevent severe contractures. Postgrad Med 1997;101:185. [NLM Cit ID: 97271260]

Paice E: Fortnightly review. Reflex sympathetic dystrophy. BMJ 1995;310:1645. [NLM Cit ID: 95315790]

VENOUS DISEASES

VARICOSE VEINS

Essentials of Diagnosis

- Dilated, tortuous superficial veins in the lower extremities.
- May be asymptomatic or may be associated with fatigue, aching discomfort, or pain.
- Edema, pigmentation, and ulceration of the skin of the distal leg may develop.
- Increased frequency after pregnancy.

General Considerations

Varicose veins develop predominantly in the lower extremities. They consist of abnormally dilated, elongated, and tortuous alterations in the saphenous veins and their tributaries. These vessels lie immediately beneath the skin and superficial to the deep fascia. An inherited defect seems to play a major role in the development of varicosities in many instances, but it is not known whether the basic valvular incompetence that exists is secondary to defective valves in the saphenofemoral veins or to a fundamental weakness of the walls of the vein, resulting in dilation of the vessel. Periods of high venous pressure related to prolonged standing or heavy lifting are contributing factors, and the highest incidence is in women who have been pregnant. Fifteen percent of adults develop varicosities.

Secondary varicosities can develop as a result of obstructive changes and valve damage in the deep venous system following thrombophlebitis, or occasionally as a result of proximal venous occlusion due to neoplasm. Congenital or acquired arteriovenous fistulas are also associated with varicosities.

The long saphenous vein and its tributaries are most commonly involved, but the short saphenous vein may also be affected. There may be one or many incompetent perforating veins in the thigh and lower leg, so that blood can reflux into the varicosities not only from above, by way of the saphenofemoral junction, but also from the deep system of veins through the incompetent perforators in the mid thigh or lower leg. Largely because of these valvular defects in the most proximal valve of the long saphenous vein or in the distal communicating veins, high venous pressures from within the deep system (> 300 mm Hg) that occur during calf compression of walking are transmitted to these superficial veins. Over the years, the veins progressively enlarge, and the surrounding tissue and skin may develop secondary changes such as fibrosis, chronic edema, and skin pigmentation and atrophy.

Clinical Findings

A. Symptoms: The severity of the symptoms caused by varicose veins is not necessarily correlated with the number and size of the varicosities; extensive varicose veins may produce no subjective symptoms, whereas minimal varicosities may produce symptoms. Dull, aching heaviness or a feeling of fatigue brought on by periods of standing is the most common complaint. Itching from an associated eczematoid dermatitis may occur above the ankle.

B. Signs: Dilated, tortuous, elongated veins beneath the skin in the thigh and leg are generally readily visible in the standing individual, although in very obese patients palpation may be necessary to detect their presence and location. Secondary tissue changes may be absent even in extensive varicosities; but if the varicosities are of long duration, brownish pigmentation and thinning of the skin above the ankle are often present. Swelling may occur, but signs of severe chronic venous stasis such as extensive swelling, fibrosis, pigmentation, and ulceration of the distal lower leg usually denote the postphlebitic state. Doppler ultrasonography or the duplex scanner is useful diagnostically in detecting the precise location of incompetent valves. These incompetent valves allow reflux of blood from the femoral, popliteal, or more peripheral deep veins into the superficial veins; such knowledge allows for more precise corrective surgery with better results. In this regard, the Trendelenburg test is useful to distinguish superficial venous insufficiency secondary to saphenofemoral valve incompetence from that due to perforator vein incompetence. The leg is elevated to reduce the blood volume in the leg. In the elevated position, an elastic tourniquet is placed around the distal thigh. If varicosities are due to saphenofemoral valve insufficiency, the varicosities will remain flat or undetectable when the patient stands. If upon standing the varicosities become immediately apparent, the major cause is perforator incompetence.

Differential Diagnosis

Primary varicose veins should be differentiated from those secondary to (1) chronic venous insufficiency of the deep system of veins (the postphlebitic syndrome); (2) retroperitoneal vein obstruction from extrinsic pressure or fibrosis; (3) arteriovenous fistula (congenital or acquired)—a bruit is present and a thrill is often palpable; and (4) congenital venous malformation. Pain or discomfort secondary to arthritis, radiculopathy, or arterial insufficiency should be distinguished from symptoms associated with coexistent varicose veins.

Complications

If thin, atrophic, pigmented skin has developed at or above the ankle, secondary ulcerations may occur—often as a result of little or no trauma. An ulcer will occasionally extend into the varix, and the resulting fistula will be associated with profuse hemorrhage unless the leg is elevated and local pressure is applied to the bleeding point.

Chronic stasis dermatitis with fungal and bacterial infection may be a problem.

Thrombophlebitis may develop in the varicosities, particularly in postoperative patients, pregnant or postpartum women, or those taking oral contraceptives. Local trauma or prolonged periods of sitting may also lead to superficial venous thrombosis. Extension of the thrombosis into the deep venous system by way of the perforating veins or through the saphenofemoral junction may occur, resulting in deep thrombophlebitis and the risk of pulmonary embolism.

Treatment

A. Nonsurgical Measures: The use of elastic graduated compression stockings (medium or heavy weight) to give external support to the veins of the proximal foot and leg up to but not including the knee is the best nonoperative approach to the management of varicose veins. (For most patients, a gradient of compression of 20–30 mm Hg is appropriate.) These may be useful in early varicosities as well, in preventing progression of disease. When elastic stockings are worn during the hours that involve much standing and when this is combined with the habit of elevation of the legs when possible, reasonably good control can be maintained and progression of the condition and the development of complications can often be avoided. This approach may be used in elderly patients, in those who refuse or wish to defer surgery, sometimes in women with mild or moderate varicosities who plan to have more children, and in those with mild asymptomatic varicosities.

B. Surgical Measures: The surgical treatment of varicose veins consists of excision of the varicosities and ligation of the saphenofemoral junction and its branches if indicated. Accurate delineation and division of the latter are required to prevent formation of recurrent varicosities in previously uninvolved veins. Venous segments that are not demonstrated to be incompetent and varicosed should not be ligated or removed; they may be needed as artery grafts later in the patient's life.

Varicose ulcers that are small generally heal with local care, frequent periods of elevation of the extremity, and compression bandages or some form of compression boot dressing for the ambulatory patient. It is best to defer a stripping procedure until healing has been achieved and stasis dermatitis has been controlled. Some ulcers require skin grafting.

C. Compression Sclerotherapy: Sclerotherapy to obliterate and produce permanent fibrosis of the involved veins is generally reserved for the treatment of residual small varicosities following definitive varicose vein surgery. The injection of the sclerosing solution into the varicosed vein is followed by a period of compression of the segment, resulting in obliteration of the vein. Complications such as phlebitis, tissue necrosis, or infection may occur, and vary in incidence with the skill of the operator.

Prognosis

Patients should be informed that even extensive and carefully performed surgery may not prevent the development of additional varicosities and that further (though usually more limited) surgery or sclerotherapy may become necessary. Good results with relief of symptoms are usually obtained in most patients. If extensive varicosities reappear after surgery, the completeness of the high ligation should be questioned, and reexploration of the saphenofemoral area may be necessary. Even after adequate treatment, secondary tissue changes may not regress.

Bergan JJ: New technology and recurrent varicose veins. Lancet 1996;348:210. [NLM Cit ID: 96304889]

Bergan JJ: Saphenous vein stripping and quality of outcome. Br J Surg 1996;83:1027. [NLM Cit ID: 97022937]

THROMBOPHLEBITIS

Thrombophlebitis is partial or complete occlusion of a vein by a thrombus with inflammatory changes in the wall of the vein. Virchow's triad of stasis, vessel damage, and hypercoagulability defines the clinical events that predispose a vein to the development of thrombophlebitis. Trauma to the endothelium of the vein wall resulting in exposure of subendothelial tissues to platelets in the venous blood may initiate thrombosis, especially if a degree of venous stasis also exists. Platelet aggregates form on the vein wall followed by the deposition of fibrin, leukocytes, and finally erythrocytes; a thrombus results that can then propagate along the veins as a free-floating clot. Within 7–10 days, this thrombus becomes adherent to the vein wall, and secondary inflammatory changes develop, although a free-floating tail may persist. The thrombus is ultimately invaded by fibroblasts, resulting in scarring of the vein wall and destruction of the valves. Central recanalization may occur later, with restoration of flow through the vein; however, because the valves do not recover function, directional flow is not reestablished, leading in turn to secondary functional and anatomic problems.

1. THROMBOPHLEBITIS OF THE DEEP VEINS

Essentials of Diagnosis

- Pain in the calf or thigh, often associated with edema; alternatively, there may be no symptoms.
- History of congestive heart failure, recent surgery, neoplasia, oral contraceptive use, or prolonged inactivity.
- Physical signs unreliable.
- Duplex ultrasound or venography is diagnostic.

General Considerations

Acute deep venous thrombosis is a common vascular disorder that is diagnosed in up to 800,000 new patients per year. The deep veins of the lower extremities and pelvis are most frequently involved. The process begins approximately 80% of the time in the deep veins of the calf, although it can arise in the femoral or iliac veins. When the process begins in the calf, propagation into the popliteal and femoral veins takes place in approximately 25% of these cases. About 3% of patients undergoing major general surgical procedures will develop clinical manifestations of thrombophlebitis, which may develop up to 2 weeks postoperatively; many others (up to 30%) develop asymptomatic deep vein thrombosis. Certain operations, such as total hip replacement, are associated with appreciably higher incidences of thromboembolic complications. Illnesses that involve periods of bed rest, such as cardiac failure or stroke, are associated with a high incidence of thrombophlebitis. Use of oral contraceptive drugs, especially by women over 30 and by those who smoke, may be associated with hypercoagulability, resulting in thrombophlebitis in some women. These drugs should not be prescribed for women with a history of phlebitis. Hypercoagulability is also observed in cancer, particularly adenocarcinoma and especially in tumors of the pancreas, prostate, breast, and ovary. Finally, rare conditions such as protein C and S deficiencies and antithrombin III deficiency should be considered in young patients with positive family histories and recurrent venous thrombosis. Homocystinuria, paroxysmal nocturnal hemoglobinuria, and a genetic abnormality, factor V Leiden, are also associated with venous hypercoagulability.

Clinical Findings

Approximately half of patients with thrombophlebitis have no symptoms or signs in the extremity in the early stages. The patient may suffer a pulmonary embolism, presumably from the leg veins, without symptoms or demonstrable abnormalities in the extremities.

A. Symptoms: The patient may complain of a dull ache, a tight feeling, or frank pain in the calf or, in more extensive cases, the whole leg, especially when walking.

B. Signs: Typical findings, though variable and unreliable and in about half of cases absent, are as follows: slight edema of the involved calf, distention of the superficial venous collaterals; and slight fever and tachycardia. Any of these signs may occur without deep vein thrombosis. When the femoral and iliac veins are also involved, there may be tenderness over these veins, and the edema of the extremity may be marked. The skin may be cyanotic if venous obstruction is severe, or pale and cool if a reflex arterial spasm is superimposed.

C. Diagnostic Techniques: Because of the difficulty in making a precise diagnosis by history and physical examination and because of the morbidity associated with treatment, diagnostic studies are essential. Duplex ultrasonography, because of its high sensitivity, specificity, and repeatability, has supplanted venography as the most widely used diagnostic test in the initial evaluation of patients suspected of having this disorder. (See Disorders of the Pulmonary Circulation in Chapter 9.)

1. Duplex Doppler ultrasonography and impedance plethysmography make it possible to examine noninvasively the major veins (ie, not the calf veins) in an extremity for thrombosis. Doppler ultrasound may be particularly helpful in detecting an extension of small thrombi in the calf veins into the popliteal and femoral veins on follow-up examinations. It is inexpensive but operator-dependent. Each venous segment is assessed for incompressibility of the vein during light probe pressure and the presence of abnormal Doppler flow signals, including absence of spontaneous flow, loss of flow variation with respiration, and failure to increase flow velocity with distal augmentation. An acute clot is usually anechoic (cannot be visualized directly), but its presence is inferred from a lack of compressibility. Incompetence of venous valves in the legs may also be inferred from this investigation. Impedance plethysmography may be used to detect the alteration of venous flow by obstruction of thrombi; in symptomatic patients, Doppler ultrasound is of superior sensitivity and may be used rather than phlebography to confirm positive or equivocal findings of plethysmography. These examinations may miss small thrombi in the calf veins when collateral channels are present; likewise, occasional false-positives are encountered.

2. Ascending contrast venography, the most accurate method of diagnosis, will define the location, extent, and degree of attachment of the thrombosis (thrombi in the profunda femoris and internal iliac veins will not be demonstrated). Because of the risk, expense, and discomfort involved, this test is not used as a screening study and is unsuitable for repeated monitoring. Venography is often not necessary since follow-up duplex Doppler ultrasonography can be used to determine whether deep vein thrombosis extension into (or above) the popliteal vein has occurred. However, venography is particularly useful when the clinical picture strongly suggests calf vein thromboses but noninvasive tests are equivocal. It may on occasion produce or exacerbate a thrombotic process, but this occurs in less than 5% of patients. It is the most accurate study for detection of deep vein thrombosis.

Differential Diagnosis

Calf muscle strain or contusion may be difficult to differentiate from thrombophlebitis; suspected deep vein thrombosis in the calf can be followed by serial duplex Doppler ultrasound examinations.

Cellulitis may be confused with thrombophlebitis; with infection, there is usually an associated wound, and inflammation of the skin is more marked.

Obstruction of the lymphatics or external compression of the iliac vein in the retroperitoneum by tumor or irradiation may lead to unilateral swelling. However, such obstruction or compression is more chronic and painless than with deep vein thrombosis.

An acute arterial occlusion is more painful, the distal pulses are absent, there is usually no swelling, and the superficial veins in the foot fill slowly when emptied.

Bilateral leg edema is more likely to be due to heart, kidney, or liver disease.

Occasionally, a ruptured Baker cyst may produce unilateral pain and swelling in the calf. A history of arthritis in the knee of the same leg is a clue to diagnosis, and the patient may report disappearance of the popliteal cyst at the time symptoms develop.

Complications

A. Pulmonary Thromboembolism: See Chapter 9.

B. Chronic Venous Insufficiency: Chronic venous insufficiency with or without secondary varicosities is a late complication of deep thrombophlebitis. (See Chronic Venous Insufficiency.)

Prevention

Prophylactic measures may diminish the incidence of venous thrombosis in hospitalized patients.

A. Nonpharmacologic Means: Venous stasis may be avoided by the following measures:

1. Elevation of the foot of the bed 15–20 degrees will encourage venous outflow from the legs. Slight flexion of the knees is desirable. This position is also maintained on the operating table and in the recovery room. Sitting in a chair for long periods in the early postoperative period should be avoided.

2. Early mobilization of the patient in the postoperative period remains the cornerstone of prophylaxis for deep vein thrombosis. Regular leg exercises, including ankle flexion and extension, are important as well. Intermittent pneumatic compression of the legs may be used prophylactically and may be the preventive measure of choice in patients in whom all anticoagulants are contraindicated, such as in patients undergoing neurosurgery. In addition, it is the most effective of all nonpharmacologic methods of prophylaxis.

3. Elastic antiphlebitic stockings may be employed, particularly in patients with varicose veins or a history of phlebitis who will require bed rest for a number of days. Walking for brief but regular periods postoperatively and during long airplane and automobile trips should be encouraged.

B. Anticoagulation: Low-dose heparin, 5000 units every 8–12 hours subcutaneously beginning 2 hours preoperatively and continuing during the postoperative period of bed rest and limited ambulation, appears to be effective in reducing the incidence of thromboembolic complications in moderate-risk patients. Its effectiveness in major pelvic and hip procedures has been disappointing. Adjusted-dose heparin to a PTT in the upper half of the normal range—or warfarin to an INR of 1.5–2.0—is recommended. LMW heparin is being used increasingly in this setting and is as effective as the standard formulation of heparin or warfarin. It is not necessary to follow clotting parameters in patients receiving low-molecular-weight heparin, and this may offset the greater cost of the drug in overall cost-benefit analysis. Likewise, there does not appear to be any increase in bleeding complications using this agent when compared with standard heparin or warfarin therapy. External pneumatic compression is significantly less effective than anticoagulation in this setting.

Treatment

A. Local Measures: When significant leg edema develops as a consequence of acute deep vein thrombosis, the legs should be elevated 15–20 degrees, the trunk should be kept horizontal, and the head and shoulders may be supported with pillows. The legs should be slightly flexed at the knees. The duration of bed rest now recommended is considerably less than the 7–14 days suggested in previous years and is largely dictated by the extent of leg edema.

B. Medical Measures (Anticoagulants): Therapy with anticoagulants is considered to be the preferred treatment in most cases of deep thrombophlebitis with or without pulmonary embolism. There is evidence that the incidence of fatal pulmonary embolism secondary to venous thrombosis is reduced by adequate anticoagulant therapy, and the incidence of death from additional emboli following an initial embolism is reduced. Progressive thrombosis with its associated morbidity is also reduced considerably, and the chronic secondary changes in the involved leg are probably also less severe. Heparin acts rapidly and must be considered the anticoagulant of choice for short-term therapy. LMW heparin has recently been shown to be effective in the treatment of deep vein thrombosis. Although more expensive than standard unfractionated heparin, it does not require monitoring of its anticoagulant effect. Furthermore, because it is administered subcutaneously, it can be used in the outpatient setting.

After the initial phase of therapy with heparin—and if a prolonged period of anticoagulation is advisable—warfarin can be used. Because warfarin also inhibits synthesis of protein C and protein S and because protein C has a short half-life, a hypercoagulable state can occur during the first few days of warfarin administration. Warfarin should be given after the patient is fully anticoagulated with heparin, and heparin is discontinued only after the prothrombin time has been prolonged by warfarin.

Treatment with heparin does not lyse thrombi but stops propagation and allows natural fibrinolysis to occur. The usual duration of therapy for uncomplicated deep vein thrombosis is 3 months. Most clinicians administer heparin for 7–10 days and oral anticoagulants for at least 11 weeks. Permanent anticoagulation may be considered if the stimulus to thrombosis is chronic—eg, congestive heart failure, postphlebitic syndrome—or if previous episodes have occurred. As experience with thrombolysis develops, it may replace heparin as the treatment of first choice; there is evidence that it reduces the incidence of postphlebitic syndrome.

Details on the use of heparin, oral anticoagulants, and thrombolytics may be found in Chapter 9.

Prognosis

With adequate treatment the patient usually returns to normal health and activity within 3–6 weeks. The prognosis in most cases is good once the period of danger of pulmonary embolism has passed. Occasionally, recurrent episodes of phlebitis will occur in spite of good local and anticoagulant management. Such cases may even have recurrent pulmonary emboli as well. Chronic venous insufficiency may result, with its associated complications; this is less likely when thrombolytics are used to treat acute phlebitis.

Brewer D: Should low-molecular weight heparins replace unfractionated heparin as the agent of choice for adults with deep vein thrombosis? J Fam Pract 1998;47:185. [NLM Cit ID: 98424937]

Haas SK: Treatment of deep venous thrombosis and pulmonary embolism. Current recommendations. Med Clin North Am 1998;82:495. [NLM Cit ID: 98310744] (The initial treatment regimens include thrombolysis, thrombectomy, inferior vena cava filters, and anticoagulation with either unfractionated heparin or low-molecular-weight heparins; thrombin inhibitors have been tried for initial treatment of thrombosis, but further investigation of efficacy, safety, and cost-effectiveness will be necessary to provide firm evidence of their superiority when compared with unfractionated or low-molecular-weight heparins.)

Howard AW et al: Low molecular weight heparin decreases proximal and distal deep venous thrombosis following total knee arthroplasty. A meta-analysis of randomized trials. Thromb Hemost 1998;79:902. [NLM Cit ID: 98270380] (Low-molecular-weight heparin is more effective than either adjusted-dose heparin or warfarin in preventing DVT following total knee arthroplasty.)

Kearon C et al: Management of anticoagulation before and after elective surgery. N Engl J Med 1997;336:1506. [NLM Cit ID: 97282679]

Low-molecular weight heparin in the treatment of patients with venous thromboembolism. The Columbus Investigators. N Engl J Med 1997;337:657. [NLM Cit ID: 97407841]

Thomas DP et al: Hypercoagulability in venous and arterial thrombosis. Ann Intern Med 1997;126:638. [NLM Cit ID: 97243275]

Weitz JI: Low-molecular-weight heparins. N Engl J Med 1997;337:688. [NLM Cit ID: 97407847] (Addresses use in every clinical situation currently requiring anticoagulation and provides a cautious assessment of safety profile.)

Wells PS et al: Expanding eligibility for outpatient treatment of deep venous thrombosis and pulmonary embolism with low-molecular-weight heparin: a comparison of patient self injection with homecare injection. Arch Intern Med 1998;158:1809. [NLM Cit ID: 98408991]

2. THROMBOPHLEBITIS OF THE SUPERFICIAL VEINS

Essentials of Diagnosis

- Induration, redness, and tenderness along a superficial vein.
- Often a history of recent intravenous line or trauma. No significant swelling of the extremity.

General Considerations

Superficial thrombophlebitis may occur spontaneously, as in pregnant or postpartum women or in individuals with varicose veins, thromboangiitis obliterans, or Behçet's disease; or it may be associated with trauma, as in the case of a blow to the leg or following intravenous therapy with irritating solutions. It may also be a manifestation of abdominal cancer such as carcinoma of the pancreas (Trousseau's sign) and may be the earliest sign of this cancer. The long saphenous vein is most often involved. Superficial thrombophlebitis is associated with occult deep vein thrombosis in about 20% of cases. Pulmonary emboli are rare.

Short-term plastic venous catheterization of superficial arm veins is now in routine use. The catheter should be observed daily for signs of local inflammation. It should be removed if a local reaction develops in the veins. Serious thrombotic or septic complications can occur if this policy is not followed. The steel intravenous needle with the anchoring flange (butterfly needle) is less likely to be associated with phlebitis and infection than the plastic catheter.

Clinical Findings

The patient usually experiences a dull pain in the region of the involved vein. Local findings consist of induration, redness, and tenderness along the course of a vein. The process may be localized, or it may involve most of the long saphenous vein and its tributaries. The inflammatory reaction generally subsides in 1–2 weeks; a firm cord may remain for a much longer period. Edema of the extremity and deep calf tenderness are absent unless deep thrombophlebitis has also developed. Chills and high fever suggest septic phlebitis and are often encountered when the phlebitis is secondary to an indwelling intravenous catheter.

Differential Diagnosis

The linear rather than circular nature of the lesion and the distribution along the course of a superficial vein serve to differentiate superficial phlebitis from cellulitis, erythema nodosum, erythema induratum, panniculitis, and fibrositis. Lymphangitis and deep thrombophlebitis must also be considered.

Treatment

If the process is well localized and not near the saphenofemoral junction, local heat and bed rest with the leg elevated are usually effective in limiting the thrombosis. Nonsteroidal anti-inflammatory drugs relieve symptoms.

If the process is very extensive or is progressing upward toward the saphenofemoral junction, or if it is in the proximity of the saphenofemoral junction initially, ligation and division of the saphenous vein at the saphenofemoral junction are indicated to prevent extension of clot into the deep venous system. Removal of the involved segment of vein may result in a more rapid recovery.

Anticoagulation therapy is not indicated unless the disease is rapidly progressing or if it extends into the deep system.

Septic thrombophlebitis requires excision of the involved vein up to its junction with an uninvolved vein in order to control the infection. Staphylococcus is the commonest pathogen, and antibiotics with antistaphylococcal activity should be instituted pending results of blood cultures. If cultures are positive, therapy should be continued for 7–10 days—or for 4–6 weeks if complicating endocarditis cannot be excluded. Other organisms, including fungi, may also be responsible.

Prognosis

The course is generally benign and brief, and the prognosis depends on the underlying pathologic process. Phlebitis of a saphenous vein occasionally extends to the deep veins, in which case pulmonary embolism may occur.

CHRONIC VENOUS INSUFFICIENCY

Essentials of Diagnosis

- History of phlebitis or leg injury.
- Ankle edema is the earliest sign.
- Stasis pigmentation, dermatitis, subcutaneous induration, and often varicosities occur later.
- Ulceration at or above the ankle is common (stasis ulcer).

General Considerations

Chronic venous insufficiency generally results from changes secondary to deep thrombophlebitis, although an unambiguous history of phlebitis is not obtainable in about 25% of these patients. There is often a history of leg trauma. It can also occur secondary to superficial venous insufficiency, as a result of neoplastic obstruction of the pelvic veins, or as a result of congenital or acquired arteriovenous fistula.

When insufficiency is secondary to deep thrombophlebitis (the postphlebitic syndrome), the valves in the deep venous channels of the lower leg have been damaged or destroyed by the thrombotic process. The recanalized deep veins are functionally inadequate because of the damaged valves in the deep and perforating veins. The antegrade venous flow ensured by the valves and the calf muscle pump is lost, resulting in bidirectional flow and abnormally high ambulatory venous pressures in the calf veins in particular. The high ambulatory venous pressure transmitted through the communicating veins to the subcutaneous veins and tissues of the calf and ankle areas results in a series of deleterious secondary changes, including edema, fibrosis of subcutaneous tissue and skin, pigmentation of skin, and, later, dermatitis, cellulitis, and ulceration. Dilation of the superficial veins may occur, leading to varicosities. Whereas superficial venous insufficiency with no abnormality of the deep venous system may be associated with some similar changes, the edema is more pronounced in the postphlebitic extremities, and the secondary changes are more extensive.

Clinical Findings

Chronic venous insufficiency is characterized first by progressive edema of the leg (particularly the lower leg) and later also by secondary changes in the skin and subcutaneous tissues. The usual symptoms are itching, a dull discomfort made worse by periods of standing, and pain if an ulceration is present. The skin is usually thin, shiny, atrophic, and cyanotic; and a brownish pigmentation often develops. Eczema may be present, with superficial weeping dermatitis. The subcutaneous tissues become thick and fibrous. Recurrent ulcerations may occur, usually just above the ankle, on the medial or anterior aspect of the leg; healing results in a thin scar on a fibrotic base that often breaks down with minor trauma. Varicosities frequently appear that are associated with incompetent perforating veins.

Differential Diagnosis

Congestive heart failure and chronic renal disease may result in bilateral edema of the lower extremities, but generally there are other clinical or laboratory findings of heart or kidney disease.

Lymphedema is associated with a brawny thickening in the subcutaneous tissue that does not respond readily to elevation; edema is particularly prominent on the dorsum of the feet and in the toes; varicosities are absent, and there is often a history of recurrent cellulitis.

Primary varicose veins may be difficult to differentiate from the secondary varicosities that often develop in this condition, as discussed above. It may be impossible to exclude superimposed acute phlebitis from chronic venous insufficiency without diagnostic tests.

Other conditions associated with chronic ulcers of the leg include autoimmune diseases (eg, Felty's syndrome), arterial insufficiency (often very painful), sickle cell anemia, erythema induratum (bilateral and usually on the posterior aspect of the lower part of the leg), and fungal infections (cultures specific; no chronic swelling or varicosities).

Prevention

Irreversible tissue changes and associated complications in the lower legs can be minimized through early and energetic treatment of acute thrombophlebitis with anticoagulants that may minimize the occlusive and valve damage, particularly in the calf, and specific measures to avoid chronic edema in subsequent years, as described in A, below. Thrombolytic therapies of acute phlebitis may be of greater value than other anticoagulants in prevention of chronic venous insufficiency.

Treatment

A. General Measures: Bed rest, with the legs elevated to diminish chronic edema, is fundamental in the treatment of the acute complications of chronic venous insufficiency. Measures to control the tendency toward edema include (1) intermittent elevation of the legs during the day and elevation of the legs at night (kept above the level of the heart with pillows under the mattress); (2) avoidance of long periods of sitting or standing; and (3) the use of well-fitting graduated compression stockings worn from the mid foot to just below the knee during the day and evening if there is any tendency for swelling to develop.

B. Stasis Dermatitis: Eczematous eruption may be acute or chronic; treatment varies accordingly.

1. Acute weeping dermatitis–

a. Wet compresses for 1 hour four times daily of solutions containing boric acid, buffered aluminum acetate (Burow's solution), or isotonic saline.

b. Compresses are followed with a local corticosteroid such as 0.5% hydrocortisone cream in a water-soluble base. (Neomycin and nystatin may be incorporated into this cream.)

c. Systemic antibiotics are indicated only if active infection is present.

2. Subsiding or chronic dermatitis–

a. Continue hydrocortisone cream for 1–2 weeks or until no further improvement is noted. Cordran tape, a plastic tape impregnated with flurandrenolide, is a convenient way to apply both medication and dressing.

b. Zinc oxide ointment with ichthammol, 3%, once or twice daily, cleaned off as desired with mineral oil.

c. Broad-spectrum antifungal such as clotrimazole cream (1%) or miconazole cream (2%) may be used.

3. Energetic treatment of chronic edema, as outlined in sections A and C, with almost complete bed rest is important during the acute phase of stasis dermatitis.

C. Ulceration: Ulcerations are preferably treated with compresses of isotonic saline solution, which aid the healing of the ulcer or may help prepare the base for a skin graft. A lesion can often be treated on an ambulatory basis by means of a semirigid boot applied to the leg after much of the swelling has been reduced by a period of elevation. The pumping action of the calf muscles on the blood flow out of the lower extremity is enhanced by a circumferential nonelastic bandage on the ankle and lower leg. The boot must be changed every 1–2 weeks, depending to some extent on the amount of drainage from the ulcer. The ulcer, tendons, and bony prominences must be adequately padded. Special ointments on the ulcer are not necessary. The semirigid boot may be made with Unna's paste (Gelocast, Medicopaste) or Gauztex bandage (impregnated with a nonallergenic self-adhering compound). After the ulcer has healed, heavy below-the-knee elastic stockings are used in an effort to prevent recurrent edema and ulceration. Occasionally, the ulcer is so large and chronic that total excision of the ulcer, with skin graft of the defect, is the best approach. This is often combined with ligation of all incompetent perforating veins.

D. Secondary Varicosities: Varicosities secondary to damage to the deep system of veins may in turn contribute to undesirable changes in the tissues of the lower leg. Varicosities should occasionally be removed and the incompetent veins connecting the superficial and deep system ligated, but the tendency toward edema will persist, because the chronic high venous pressure is usually not effectively lowered during walking by the procedure, and thus the measures outlined above (¶A) will be required for life. Varicosities can often be treated along with edema by elastic stockings and other nonoperative measures, and only about 15–20% require surgery. If the obstructive element in the deep system appears to be severe, B-mode ultrasonography, bidirectional Doppler velocity studies, or phlebography may be of value in mapping out the areas of venous obstruction or incompetence in the deep system as well as the number and location of the damaged perforating veins. A decision about whether to treat with surgery may be influenced by such a study; if the varicosities furnish the chief route of venous return, they should not be removed. Venous valvular reconstructive surgery is now in an investigative stage.

Prognosis

Individuals with chronic venous insufficiency often have recurrent problems, particularly if measures to counteract persistent venous hypertension, edema, and secondary tissue changes are not conscientiously adhered to throughout life. Additional episodes of acute thrombophlebitis may occur, and in reliable patients permanent anticoagulation is a reasonable therapeutic recommendation.

Alguire PC et al: Chronic venous insufficiency and venous ulceration. J Geriatr Intern Med 1997;12:374. [NLM Cit ID: 97335590]

Angle N et al: Chronic venous ulcer. BMJ 1997;314:1019. [NLM Cit ID: 97267518]

Kistner RL et al: Diagnosis of chronic venous disease of the lower extremities: The "CEAP" classification. Mayo Clin Proc 1996;71:338. [NLM Cit ID: 96197225] (Study of the specific facets of the clinical, etiologic, anatomic, and pathophysiologic [CEAP] classification provided precise information about the causes and the effects of venous abnormalities.)

SUPERIOR VENA CAVAL OBSTRUCTION

Partial or complete obstruction of the thin-walled superior vena cava is a relatively rare condition that is usually secondary to the neoplastic or inflammatory process in the superior mediastinum. The most frequent causes are (1) neoplasms, such as lymphomas, primary malignant mediastinal tumors, or carcinoma of the lung with direct extension (over 80%); (2) chronic fibrotic mediastinitis, either of unknown origin or secondary to tuberculosis, histoplasmosis, pyogenic infections, or drugs, especially methysergide; (3) thrombophlebitis, often by extension of the process from the axillary or subclavian vein into the innominate vein and vena cava and often associated with catheterization of these veins for central venous pressure measurements or for hyperalimentation; (4) aneurysm of the aortic arch; and (5) constrictive pericarditis.

Clinical Findings

A. Symptoms and Signs: The onset of symptoms is acute or subacute. Symptoms include swelling of the neck and face, headache, dizziness, visual disturbances, stupor, and syncope. There is progressive obstruction of the venous drainage of the head, neck, and upper extremities. The cutaneous veins of the upper chest and lower neck become dilated, and flushing of the face and neck develops. Brawny edema of the face, neck, and arms occurs later, and cyanosis of these areas then appears. Cerebral and laryngeal edema ultimately results in impaired function of the brain as well as respiratory insufficiency. Bending over or lying down accentuates the symptoms; sitting quietly is generally preferred. The manifestations are more severe if the obstruction develops rapidly and if the azygos junction or the vena cava between that vein and the heart is obstructed.

B. Laboratory Findings: The venous pressure is elevated in the arm and is normal in the leg. Since lung cancer is a common cause, bronchoscopy is often performed; transbronchial biopsy, however, is relatively contraindicated because of venous hypertension and the risk of bleeding.

C. Imaging: Chest radiographs and a CT scan will define the location and often the nature of the obstructive process, and phlebography will map out the extent and degree of the venous obstruction and the collateral circulation. Doppler ultrasound can demonstrate the presence of collaterals, and MRI may delineate the site of thrombosis as well as the nature of the cause. Brachial venography or radionuclide scanning following intravenous injection of technetium Tc 99m pertechnetate demonstrates a block to the flow of contrast material into the right heart and enlarged collateral veins. These techniques also allow estimation of blood flow around the occlusion as well as serial evaluation of the response to therapy.

Treatment

Though empirical therapy for neoplasm is occasionally warranted, the clinician should be aware of benign causes, especially histoplasmosis.

Urgent treatment for neoplasm consists of (1) cautious use of intravenous diuretics and (2) mediastinal irradiation, starting within 24 hours, with a treatment plan designed to give a high daily dose but a short total course of therapy to rapidly shrink the local tumor even further. Intensive combined therapy will palliate the process in up to 90% of patients. In patients with a subacute presentation, radiation therapy alone usually suffices. Chemotherapy is added if lymphoma or small-cell carcinoma is diagnosed.

Surgical procedures to bypass the obstruction are complicated by bleeding relating to high venous pressure. In cases secondary to mediastinal fibrosis or pericardial constriction, excision of the fibrous tissue around the great vessels may reestablish flow. Percutaneous angioplasty and stenting, when necessary, have played an increasingly important role in the management of these patients.

Prognosis

The prognosis depends upon the nature and degree of obstruction and its speed of onset. Slowly developing forms secondary to fibrosis may be tolerated for years. A high degree of obstruction of rapid onset secondary to cancer is often fatal in a few days or weeks because of increased intracranial pressure and cerebral hemorrhage, but treatment of the tumor with radiation and chemotherapeutic drugs may result in significant palliation.

Gross CM et al: Stent implantation in patients with superior vena cava syndrome. AJR Am J Roentgenol 1997; 169:429. [NLM Cit ID: 97386657] (Percutaneous implantation of Wallstent endoprostheses provided excellent palliation for 13 patients with superior vena cava syndrome.)

Kee ST et al: Superior vena cava syndrome: Treatment with catheter-directed thrombolysis and endovascular stent placement. Radiology 1998;206:187. [NLM Cit ID: 98085729]

DISEASES OF THE LYMPHATIC CHANNELS

LYMPHANGITIS & LYMPHADENITIS

Essentials of Diagnosis

- Red streak from wound or area of cellulitis toward regional lymph nodes, which are usually enlarged and tender.
- Chills, fever, and malaise may be present.

General Considerations

Lymphangitis and lymphadenitis are common manifestations of a bacterial infection that is usually caused by hemolytic streptococci or staphylococci (or by both organisms) and usually arises from an area of cellulitis, generally at the site of an infected wound. The wound may be very small or superficial, or an established abscess may be present, feeding bacteria into the lymphatics. The involvement of the lymphatics is often manifested by a red streak in the skin extending in the direction of the regional lymph nodes, which are, in turn, generally tender and enlarged. Systemic manifestations include fever, chills, tachycardia, and malaise. The infection may progress rapidly, often in a matter of hours, and may lead to septicemia and even death.

Clinical Findings

A. Symptoms and Signs: Throbbing pain is usually present in the area of cellulitis at the site of bacterial invasion. Malaise, anorexia, sweating, chills, and fever of 37.8–40 °C develop rapidly. The red streak, when present, may be definite or may be very faint and easily missed, especially in dark-skinned patients. It is not usually tender or indurated, as is the area of cellulitis. The involved regional lymph nodes may be significantly enlarged and are usually quite tender.

B. Laboratory Findings: Leukocytosis with a left shift is usually present. Later, a blood culture may be positive, most often for staphylococcal or streptococcal species. Culture and sensitivity studies on the wound exudate or pus may be helpful in treatment of the more severe or refractory infections but are often difficult to interpret because of skin contaminants.

Differential Diagnosis

Lymphangitis may be confused with superficial thrombophlebitis, but the erythematous reaction associated with thrombosis overlies the induration of the inflammatory reaction in and around the thrombosed vein. Venous thrombosis is not associated with lymphadenitis, and a wound of entrance with the secondary cellulitis is generally absent. Superficial thrombophlebitis frequently arises as a result of intravenous therapy, particularly when the needle or catheter is left in place for more than 2 days; if bacteria have also been introduced, suppurative thrombophlebitis may develop.

Cat-scratch fever should be considered when lymphadenitis is present in which the nodes, though often very large, are relatively nontender. Exposure to cats is common, but the scratch may be forgotten by the patient.

It is extremely important to differentiate cellulitis from soft tissue infections that require early and aggressive incision and often resection of necrotic infected tissue, eg, acute streptococcal hemolytic gangrene, necrotizing fasciitis, gram-negative anaerobic cutaneous gangrene, and progressive bacterial synergistic gangrene. These are deeper infections that are more anatomically extensive; patients appear more seriously ill, and subcutaneous crepitus may be palpated or auscultated using the diaphragm with light pressure over the involved area.

Treatment

A. General Measures: Prompt treatment should include heat (hot, moist compresses or heating pad), elevation when feasible, and immobilization of the infected area. Analgesics may be prescribed for pain.

B. Specific Measures: Antibiotic therapy should always be instituted when local infection becomes invasive, as manifested by cellulitis and lymphangitis. Because the causative organism is so frequently the streptococcus, penicillin G is usually the drug of choice, although antistaphylococcal penicillins (eg, nafcillin) or cephalosporins are favored by some. If the patient is allergic to penicillin, erythromycin may be substituted. (See Chapter 37.)

C. Wound Care: Drainage of pus from an infected wound should be carried out, generally after the above measures have been instituted and only when it is clear that there is an abscess associated with the site of initial infection.

Prognosis

With proper therapy and particularly with the use of an antibiotic effective against the invading bacteria, control of the infection can usually be achieved in a few days. Delayed or inadequate therapy can still lead to overwhelming infection with septicemia.

Sadick NS: Current aspects of bacterial infections of the skin. Dermatol Clin 1997;15:341. [NLM Cit ID: 98253200]

LYMPHEDEMA

Essentials of Diagnosis

- Painless edema of one or both lower extremities usually involves the dorsum of the foot and toes, primarily in young women.
- Initially, pitting edema, which becomes brawny and often nonpitting with time.
- Ulceration, varicosities, and stasis pigmentation do not occur. There may be episodes of lymphangitis and cellulitis.

General Considerations

The underlying mechanism in lymphedema is impairment of the flow of lymph from an extremity. When due to congenital developmental abnormalities consisting of hypo- or hyperplastic involvement of the proximal or distal lymphatics, it is referred to as the primary form. The obstruction may be in the pelvic or lumbar lymph channels and nodes when the disease is extensive and progressive. The secondary form results when an inflammatory or mechanical obstruction of the lymphatics occurs from trauma, regional lymph node resection or irradiation, or extensive involvement of regional nodes by malignant disease or filariasis. Secondary dilation of the lymphatics that occurs in both forms leads to incompetence of the valve system, disrupting the orderly flow along the lymph vessels, and results in progressive stasis of a protein-rich fluid, with secondary fibrosis. Episodes of acute and chronic inflammation may be superimposed, with further stasis and fibrosis. Hypertrophy of the limb results, with markedly thickened and fibrotic skin and subcutaneous tissue and diminution in the fatty tissue.

Lymphangiography and radioactive isotope studies are often useful in defining the specific lymphatic defect.

Treatment

The treatment of lymphedema is often not very satisfactory. The majority of patients can be treated conservatively with some of the following measures: (1) The flow of lymph out of the extremity, with a consequent decrease in the degree of stasis, can be aided through intermittent elevation of the extremity, especially during the sleeping hours (foot of bed elevated 15–20 degrees, achieved by placing pillows beneath the mattress); the constant use of graduated compression stockings (20–30 mm Hg) and massage toward the trunk—either by hand or by means of pneumatic pressure devices designed to milk edema out of an extremity. (The Wright linear pump delivers sequential pressure cycles that effectively milk fluid out of the foot and leg and then out of the thigh.) (2) Secondary cellulitis in the extremity should be avoided by means of good hygiene and treatment of any trichophytosis of the toes. Once an infection starts, it should be treated by adequate periods of rest, elevation, and antibiotics, with coverage of staphylococcus and streptococcus. Infection can be a serious and recurring problem and is often difficult to control. Intermittent prophylactic antibiotics may occasionally be necessary; dicloxacillin is a good choice. (3) Intermittent courses of diuretic therapy, especially in those with premenstrual or seasonal exacerbations. (4) In carefully selected cases, there are operative procedures that may give satisfactory functional results. Lymphaticovenous anastomosis using microsurgery has yielded some satisfactory cosmetic and functional results, particularly if lymph channels can be localized by lymphoscintigraphy and several lymphovenous anastomoses are made. This technique may replace the more deforming procedures and those aimed at introducing lymphatic bridges or lymphatic venous connections. Amputation is used as a last resort in very severe forms or when lymphangiosarcoma develops in the extremity.

Witte CL et al: Disorders of lymph flow. Acad Radiol 1995;2:324. [NLM Cit ID: 98080840]

HYPOTENSION & SHOCK

Essentials of Diagnosis

- Low systemic blood pressure and tachycardia.
- Peripheral hypoperfusion and, in most, vasoconstriction.
- Altered mental status.
- Oliguria or anuria.
- Metabolic acidosis in many.

General Considerations

Shock occurs when the circulation of arterial blood is inadequate to meet tissue metabolic needs. Treatment must be directed both at the manifestations of shock and at its cause.

Classification (Table 12–1)

A. Hypovolemic Shock: Decreased intravascular volume resulting from loss of blood, plasma, or fluids and electrolytes may be obvious (eg, external hemorrhage) or subtle (eg, sequestration in a "third space," as in pancreatitis). Compensatory vasoconstriction temporarily reduces the size of the vascular bed and may temporarily maintain the blood pressure, but if fluid is not replaced, hypotension occurs, peripheral resistance increases, capillary and venous beds collapse, and the tissues become progressively more hypoxic. Even a moderate sudden loss of circulating fluids can result in severe damage to vital organs.

B. Cardiogenic Shock: See discussion in Chapter 10.

C. Obstructive Shock: Obstruction of the systemic or pulmonary circulation, the aortic and mitral valves, or venous inflow, as in pericardial disease, may reduce cardiac output sufficiently to cause shock. Cardiac tamponade, tension pneumothorax, and massive pulmonary embolism are medical emergencies requiring prompt diagnosis and treatment. Tamponade calls for immediate echocardiography and pericardiocentesis. The prognosis for patients with massive pulmonary embolism is guarded despite therapy with anticoagulants or thrombolytics; surgical embolectomy adds little. A less common cause of obstructive shock is atrial myxoma with pulmonary hypertension.

D. Distributive Shock: Reduction in systemic vascular resistance from such diverse causes as sepsis, anaphylaxis, or acute adrenal insufficiency may result in inadequate cardiac output despite normal circulatory volume.

1. Septic shock–Most commonly, shock is due to gram-negative bacteremia (so-called septic shock). In overwhelming infection, there is an initial short period of vasoconstriction followed by vasodilation, with venous pooling of blood in the microcirculation.

Table 12–1. Classification of shock by mechanism and common causes.[1]

Hypovolemic shock
- Loss of blood (hemorrhagic shock)
  - External hemorrhage
    - Trauma
    - Gastrointestinal tract bleeding
  - Internal hemorrhage
    - Hematoma
    - Hemothorax or hemoperitoneum
- Loss of plasma
  - Burns
  - Exfoliative dermatitis
- Loss of fluid and electrolytes
  - External
    - Vomiting
    - Diarrhea
    - Excessive sweating
    - Hyperosmolar states (diabetic ketoacidosis, hyperosmolar nonketotic coma)
  - Internal ("third spacing")
    - Pancreatitis
    - Ascites
    - Bowel obstruction

Cardiogenic shock
- Dysrhythmia
  - Tachyarrhythmia
  - Bradyarrhythmia
- "Pump failure" (secondary to myocardial infarction or other cardiomyopathy)
- Acute valvular dysfunction (especially regurgitant lesions)
- Rupture of ventricular septum or free ventricular wall

Obstructive shock
- Tension pneumothorax
- Pericardial disease (tamponade, constriction)
- Disease of pulmonary vasculature (massive pulmonary emboli, pulmonary hypertension)
- Cardiac tumor (atrial myxoma)
- Left atrial mural thrombus
- Obstructive valvular disease (aortic or mitral stenosis)

Distributive shock
- Septic shock
- Anaphylactic shock
- Neurogenic shock
- Vasodilator drugs
- Acute adrenal insufficiency

[1]Reproduced, with permission, from Saunders CE, Ho MT (editors): *Current Emergency Diagnosis & Treatment,* 4th ed. Originally published by Appleton & Lange. Copyright © 1992 by The McGraw-Hill Companies, Inc.

The vasodilation of septic shock may be mediated by nitrous oxide. The mortality rate is high (40–80%). Responsible organisms are most commonly gram-negative rods (*Escherichia coli,* klebsiella, proteus, and pseudomonas) as well as gram-positive cocci (staphylococcus, streptococcus) and gram-negative anaerobes (eg, bacteroides). Septic shock occurs more often in the very young and the very old; in diabetes, hematologic cancers, and diseases of the genitourinary, hepatobiliary, and intestinal tracts; and in association with immunosuppressive therapy. Immediate precipitating factors may be urinary, biliary, or gynecologic manipulations.

Septic shock is suspected when a febrile patient has chills associated with hypotension. Early, the skin may be warm and the pulse full ("warm shock"). Hyperventilation results in respiratory alkalosis. The sensorium and urinary output are often initially normal, with classic signs of shock becoming manifest later. The symptoms and signs of the inciting infection are not invariably present.

2. Neurogenic shock–Neurogenic or psychogenic factors, eg, spinal cord injury, pain, trauma, fright, gastric dilation, or vasodilator drugs, may also cause distributive shock due to reflex vagal stimulation with decreased cardiac output, hypotension, and decreased cerebral blood flow.

Diagnosis of Shock & Impending Shock

Shock may be impending if the following signs are present.

A. Hypotension: Hypotension in adults is traditionally defined as a systolic blood pressure of 90 mm Hg or less. However, some normal adults may have levels that low without ill effects, and some hypertensive persons develop shock with what would ordinarily be considered normal blood pressures.

B. Orthostatic Changes in Vital Signs: Patients who are not clearly hypotensive when tested supine should have readings while sitting up with the legs dangling. If no change occurs, repeat the measurements with the patient standing. A drop in systolic pressure of more than 10–20 mm Hg with an increase in pulse of more than 15 suggests depleted intravascular volume. Some normovolemic patients with peripheral neuropathies or those taking certain medications (eg, some antihypertensive drugs) may demonstrate an orthostatic fall in blood pressure, but without associated increase in pulse rate.

C. Peripheral Hypoperfusion: Patients in shock often have cool or mottled extremities and weak or absent peripheral pulses.

D. Altered Mental Status: Patients may demonstrate normal mental status or may be restless, agitated, confused, lethargic, or comatose as a result of inadequate perfusion of the brain.

Treatment

Treatment depends upon prompt assessment of the cause, type, severity, and duration of shock as well as an accurate appraisal of underlying conditions that may influence the onset or maintenance of shock.

A. Position: The patient is placed in the Trendelenburg or supine position with legs elevated to maximize cerebral blood flow.

B. Oxygenation: Oxygen should be given because shock—especially septic shock—may result in hypoxia caused by pulmonary ventilation-perfusion mismatch or, in severe cases, by acute respiratory distress syndrome (see Chapter 9).

C. Analgesics: Severe pain is treated promptly with analgesic drugs. Morphine sulfate, 8–15 mg subcutaneously, is appropriate for severe pain; since subcutaneous absorption is poor in patients in shock, 4–8 mg slowly intravenously may be used as an alternative. Morphine should not be given to unconscious patients, to those who have head injuries, to those with severe hypotension or unstable blood pressure, or to those with respiratory depression.

D. Laboratory Studies: A complete blood count is obtained immediately, and a blood specimen is sent for typing and cross-matching. Electrolytes, blood glucose, serum creatinine, and urinalysis are also important diagnostically. Arterial blood gases (or finger oximeter oxygen saturation) are obtained routinely.

E. Urine Flow: Both oliguric and nonoliguric renal failure may occur in shock. In the patient without preexisting renal disease, urine output is a reliable indication of organ perfusion. An indwelling catheter to monitor urine flow (which should be kept above 0.5 mL/kg/h) may be indicated. Urine flow of less than 25 mL/h indicates inadequate renal perfusion, which, if not corrected, can result in renal tubular necrosis.

F. Monitor Cardiac Rhythm: Periodic electrocardiography or continuous automated monitoring will permit early detection and prompt treatment of myocardial ischemia from hypoperfusion, and arrhythmias from similar causes or from electrolyte and acid-base disturbances.

G. Central Venous Pressure (CVP) or Pulmonary Capillary Wedge Pressure (PCWP): Monitoring of central venous pressure or pulmonary capillary wedge pressure is helpful in treating shock. Central venous pressure determination is relatively simple but is not as reliable as the pulmonary capillary wedge pressure (PCWP) measured by the Swan-Ganz catheter technique, which theoretically provides a better index of left ventricular function. Determination of PCWP has been used traditionally in patients in whom there is uncertainty about the role of cardiac function in the genesis of shock or in myocardial infarction with shock. It is also useful in guiding volume resuscitation in shock patients with a history of heart disease or in such patients in whom pulmonary disease has produced high central venous pressure. Finally, it has a role in the therapy of right ventricular infarction. However, recent prospective studies have not shown benefit and provide some evidence of increased morbidity and mortality in patients receiving pulmonary artery catheters.

In central venous pressure determination, a catheter is inserted percutaneously (or by cutdown) through a major vein. Normal values range from 5 to 8 cm of water. A low central venous pressure suggests the need for fluid replacement. A high central venous pressure (above 15 cm of water) suggests volume overload, cardiac failure, pericardial tamponade, or pulmonary hypertension. The PCWP catheter is inserted in a similar fashion, with localization of its tip determined by monitoring the morphology of the pressure tracing as it is advanced. A PCWP over 14 mm Hg may serve as a warning of impending pulmonary edema. Catheter insertion requires a skilled and experienced physician and is expensive. Surveillance for complications of hemorrhage, sepsis, pneumothorax, arrhythmias, and pulmonary infarction is obligatory.

H. Volume Replacement: Initial or emergency needs may be determined by the history, general appearance, vital signs, and hematocrit. There is no simple technique by which to accurately judge the fluid requirements. An estimate of total fluid losses is an essential first step. Response to therapy—particularly the effect of carefully administered, gradually increasing amounts of intravenous fluids on the central venous pressure or PCWP—is a valuable index.

Selection of the proper fluid for restoration and maintenance of hemodynamic stability is often difficult and controversial. It will depend upon the type and electrolyte composition of fluid that has been lost (whole blood, plasma, water), associated medical problems, availability of the various replacement solutions, clinical and laboratory monitoring facilities, and, in some circumstances, expense. The most effective replacement fluid in case of hemorrhage is packed red cells with saline, but other available fluids should be given immediately pending return of laboratory studies.

Rapid volume replacement in blood loss will often prevent shock. If central venous pressure or PCWP is low and the hematocrit greater than 35%—and if there is no clinical evidence to suggest occult blood loss—blood volume should be supported with crystalloid solutions or colloids.

1. Crystalloid solutions–Isotonic (0.9%) sodium chloride solution 500–2000 mL, is given rapidly intravenously—ideally under central venous pressure or pulmonary capillary wedge pressure monitoring. The crystalloids are readily available for emergencies and mass casualties. They may obviate the need for blood or colloids. They are often effective, at least temporarily, when given in adequate doses.

2. Colloids–Colloids are high-molecular-weight substances that do not diffuse readily across normal capillary membranes. Colloidal solutions increase the plasma oncotic pressure and thus in theory can draw fluid from the interstitial space into the intravascular space to cause additional fluid volume expansion. However, capillary membranes in the lungs are often damaged in the patient in shock, so that larger molecules may leak from the intravascular space into the interstitium and have an adverse effect on pulmonary function (acute respiratory distress syndrome).

a. Blood–Packed or frozen red cells are preferred to whole blood, since remaining blood products may be used for other purposes. The amount of blood given depends on the clinical course, the hematocrit, and hemodynamic findings. Each unit raises the hematocrit by roughly 3%.

Screening of blood donors for hepatitis B and C infection and for HIV has reduced the frequency of those infections following transfusion. The risk of HIV infection from transfused blood is now estimated to be approximately 1:100,000 in industrialized countries that screen appropriately. The risk for contracting hepatitis B is 1:200,000 transfusions. Hepatitis C remains the commonest infectious complication of transfusion; with the advent of diagnostic tests for hepatitis C, the risk is diminishing but still of concern (1:3300 transfusions).

b. Plasma fractions–Group-specific frozen plasma is a satisfactory colloidal volume expander and occasionally can correct specific coagulation defects. Because of its expense, risk (same as blood transfusion), and relative ineffectiveness, however, its use should be limited. Single-donor plasma is preferable to pooled plasma. Albumin 5% in saline, albumin 25% in concentrate, or plasma protein fraction (containing 80–85% albumin) may be rapidly set up for emergencies, and blood typing is not required. These substances have been heat-treated to minimize the risk of infectious hepatitis, which in any case is trivial.

c. Dextrans–Dextrans are high-molecular-weight polysaccharide colloids that are fairly effective plasma expanders. Because they can impair blood coagulation and interfere with blood typing and because they may cause anaphylactoid reactions, dextrans are used very infrequently now.

I. Vasoactive Drugs: Some adrenergic drugs can be useful in the adjunctive therapy of shock. *The adrenergic drugs should not be considered a primary form of therapy in shock.* Simple blood pressure elevation produced by the vasopressor drugs has little beneficial effect on the underlying disturbance, and in many instances the effect may be detrimental. Pressors are given only when hypotension persists after volume deficits are corrected and obstructive causes excluded or remedied.

1. Dopamine hydrochloride has an advantage over other adrenergic drugs because it has a beneficial effect on renal blood flow (at low dose) and because it increases cardiac output and blood pressure. Dopamine hydrochloride, 200 mg in 500 mL of sodium chloride injection USP (400 μg/mL), is given initially at a rate of 1–2 μg/kg/min. This dosage stimulates both the dopaminergic receptors, which increase the renal blood flow and urinary output, and the β-adrenergic cardiac receptors, which increase the cardiac output. If shock persists, gradually increasing doses of dopamine may be required. If dopamine alone fails to maintain adequate perfusion pressure, it may sometimes be necessary to use it in combination with another appropriate adrenergic drug.

Adverse reactions include ventricular arrhythmias, anginal pain, nausea and vomiting, headache, hypotension, azotemia, and rare cases of peripheral gangrene. Special care should be exercised when dopamine is used in the treatment of shock following myocardial infarction, because the drug's inotropic effect may increase myocardial oxygen demand. Dopamine should not be used in patients with pheochromocytoma or uncorrected tachyarrhythmias or in those who are receiving monoamine oxidase inhibitors.

2. Dobutamine, a synthetic catecholamine similar to dopamine but with greater inotropic effect, may be useful when filling pressures are high because of fluid overload or heart failure. However, since dobutamine sometimes decreases systemic vascular resistance, dopamine may still be needed for blood pressure support.

J. Corticosteroids: Corticosteroids are lifesaving in the treatment of shock associated with acute adrenal insufficiency (see Chapter 26). In other types of shock, however, corticosteroids are of no benefit.

K. Diuretics: Diuretics are not employed until volume deficits are corrected or obstructive causes remedied. There is no evidence that diuretics reduce the overall incidence of renal failure, though some believe they may convert oliguric renal insufficiency to a nonoliguric type.

Barry WL et al: Cardiogenic shock: Therapy and prevention. Clin Cardiol 1998;21:72. [NLM Cit ID: 98150908]

Choi PT et al: Crystalloids vs colloids in fluid resuscitation: a systematic review. Crit Care Med 1999;27:200. [NLM Cit ID: 99131616]

Friedman G et al: Has the mortality with septic shock changed with time? Crit Care Med 1998;26:2078. [NLM Cit ID: 99091152]

Klosterhalfen B et al: Septic shock. Gen Pharmacol 1998;31:25. [NLM Cit ID: 98257629]

Parrillo JE: Pathogenetic mechanisms for septic shock. N Engl J Med 1993;328:1471. [NLM Cit ID: 93241234]

RELEVANT WORLD WIDE WEB SITES

[Carotid Artery Stenosis]
http://www.brighamrad.harvard.edu/Cases/bwh/hcache/6/full.html

[Partial Obstruction of the Superior Vena Cava]
http://www.brighamrad.harvard.edu/Cases/bwh/hcache/58/full.html

[3-D Visualization of Aortic Aneurysm]
http://everest.radiology.uiowa.edu/nlm/apps/aorta/aorta.html

Blood

13

See http://www.current-med.com/ch13.html for updated addresses of Web sites referenced in this chapter.

Charles A. Linker, MD

ANEMIAS

General Approach to Anemias

Anemia is present in adults if the hematocrit is less than 41% (hemoglobin < 13.5 g/dL) in males or 37% (hemoglobin < 12 g/dL) in females. Congenital anemia is suggested by the patient's personal and family history. Poor diet results in folic acid deficiency and contributes to iron deficiency. Bleeding should always be sought for in iron deficiency. Physical examination includes attention to signs of primary hematologic diseases (lymphadenopathy, hepatosplenomegaly, or bone tenderness). Mucosal changes such as a smooth tongue suggest megaloblastic anemia.

Anemias are classified according to their pathophysiologic basis, ie, whether related to diminished production or accelerated loss of red blood cells (Table 13–1); or according to cell size (Table 13–2). The diagnostic possibilities in microcytic anemia are iron deficiency, thalassemia, and anemia of chronic disease. A severely microcytic anemia (MCV < 70 fL) is due either to iron deficiency or thalassemia. Macrocytic anemia may be due to megaloblastic (folate or vitamin B_{12} deficiency) or nonmegaloblastic causes. A severely macrocytic anemia (MCV > 125 fL) is almost always megaloblastic; rare exceptions are the myelodysplastic syndromes, either before or after chemotherapy.

Williams WJ (editor): *Hematology,* 5th ed. McGraw-Hill, 1995.

IRON DEFICIENCY ANEMIA

Essentials of Diagnosis

- Both pathognomonic: absent bone marrow iron stores or serum ferritin < 12 μg/L.
- Nearly always caused by bleeding in adults.
- Response to iron therapy.

General Considerations

Iron deficiency is the most common cause of anemia worldwide. The causes are listed in Table 13–3. Iron is necessary for the formation of heme and other enzymes. Total body iron ranges between 2 g and 4 g: approximately 50 mg/kg in men and 35 mg/kg in women. Most (70–95%) of iron is present in hemoglobin in circulating red blood cells. One milliliter of packed red blood cells (not whole blood) contains approximately 1 mg of iron. In men, red blood cell volume is approximately 30 mL/kg. A 70-kg man will therefore have approximately 2100 mL of packed red blood cells and consequently 2100 mg of iron in his circulating blood. In women, the red cell volume is about 27 mL/kg; a 50-kg woman will thus have 1350 mg of iron circulating in her red blood cells. Only 200–400 mg of iron is present in myoglobin and nonheme enzymes. The amount of iron present in plasma is negligible. Aside from circulating red blood cells, the major location of iron in the body is the storage pool. Iron is deposited either as ferritin or as hemosiderin and is located in macrophages. The range for storage iron is wide (0.5–2 g); approximately 25% of women in the USA have none.

The average American diet contains 10–15 mg of iron per day. About 10% of this amount is absorbed. Absorption occurs in the stomach, duodenum, and upper jejunum. Dietary iron present as heme is efficiently absorbed (10–20%) but nonheme iron less so (1–5%), largely because of interference by phosphates, tannins, and other food constituents. Small amounts of iron—approximately 1 mg/d—are normally lost though exfoliation of skin and mucosal cells. There is no physiologic mechanism for increasing normal body iron losses.

Menstrual blood loss in women plays a major role in iron metabolism. The average monthly menstrual blood loss is approximately 50 mL, or about 0.7 mg/d. However, menstrual blood loss may be five times the average. In order to maintain adequate iron stores, women with heavy menstrual losses must absorb 3–4 mg of iron from the diet each day. This strains the upper limit of what may reasonably be ab-

Table 13–1. Classification of anemias by pathophysiology.

Decreased production
- Hemoglobin synthesis: iron deficiency, thalassemia, anemia of chronic disease
- DNA synthesis: megaloblastic anemia
- Stem cell: aplastic anemia, myeloproliferative leukemia
- Bone marrow infiltration: carcinoma, lymphoma
- Pure red cell aplasia

Increased destruction
- Blood loss
- Hemolysis (intrinsic)
  - Membrane: hereditary spherocytosis, elliptocytosis
  - Hemoglobin: sickle cell, unstable hemoglobin
  - Glycolysis: pyruvate kinase deficiency, etc
  - Oxidation: G6PD deficiency
- Hemolysis (extrinsic)
  - Immune: warm antibody, cold antibody
  - Microangiopathic: thrombotic thrombocytopenic purpura, hemolytic-uremic syndrome, mechanical cardiac valve, paravalvular leak
  - Infection: clostridial
  - Hypersplenism

sorbed, and women with menorrhagia of this degree will almost always become iron-deficient.

In general, iron metabolism is balanced between absorption of 1 mg/d and loss of 1 mg/d. Pregnancy may also upset the iron balance, since requirements increase to 2–5 mg of iron per day during pregnancy and lactation. Normal dietary iron cannot supply these requirements, and medicinal iron is needed during pregnancy and lactation. Repeated pregnancy (especially with breast feeding) is a common cause of iron deficiency if increased requirements are not met with supplemental medicinal iron. Decreased iron absorption can cause iron deficiency and is usually due to gastric surgery, though concomitant bleeding is frequent.

By far the most important cause of iron deficiency anemia is blood loss, especially gastrointestinal blood loss. Chronic aspirin use may cause chronic iron loss even without a documented structural lesion. Iron deficiency should prompt a search for a potential source of gastrointestinal bleeding if other sources of blood

Table 13–2. Classification of anemias by MCV.

- Microcytic
  - Iron deficiency
  - Thalassemia
  - Anemia of chronic disease
- Macrocytic
  - Megaloblastic
    - Vitamin B_{12} deficiency
    - Folate deficiency
  - Nonmegaloblastic
    - Myelodysplasia, chemotherapy
    - Liver disease
    - Increased reticulocytosis
    - Myxedema
- Normocytic
  - Many causes

Table 13–3. Causes of iron deficiency.

- Deficient diet
- Decreased absorption
- Increased requirements
  - Pregnancy
  - Lactation
- Blood loss
  - Gastrointestinal
  - Menstrual
  - Blood donation
- Hemoglobinuria
- Iron sequestration
  - Pulmonary hemosiderosis

loss (menorrhagia, other uterine bleeding, and repeated blood donations) are excluded.

Chronic hemoglobinuria may lead to iron deficiency, since more than 1 mg/d of iron can be lost by this route. The most common cause is traumatic hemolysis due to an abnormally functioning cardiac valve, usually mechanical and prosthetic. Other causes of intravascular hemolysis (eg, paroxysmal nocturnal hemoglobinuria) should also be considered if hemoglobinuria is documented.

Rare causes of iron deficiency include its sequestration in pulmonary macrophages in idiopathic pulmonary hemosiderosis.

Clinical Findings

A. Symptoms and Signs: As a rule, the only symptoms of iron deficiency anemia are those of the anemia itself (easy fatigability, tachycardia, palpitations and tachypnea on exertion). Severe deficiency causes skin and mucosal changes, including a smooth tongue, brittle nails, and cheilosis. Dysphagia because of the formation of esophageal webs (Plummer-Vinson syndrome) also occurs. Many iron-deficient patients develop pica, craving for specific foods (ice chips, lettuce, etc), often not rich in iron.

B. Laboratory Findings: Iron deficiency develops in stages. The first is depletion of iron stores. At this point, there is anemia and no changes in red blood cell size. The serum ferritin will become abnormally low. A ferritin value less than 30 μg/L nearly always indicates absent iron stores and is a highly reliable indicator of iron deficiency. The serum total iron-binding capacity (TIBC) rises.

After iron stores have been depleted, red blood cell formation will continue with deficient supplies of iron. Serum iron values will begin to fall to less than 30 μg/dL, and transferrin saturation will fall to less than 15%.

In the early stages, the MCV remains normal. Subsequently, the MCV falls and the blood smear shows hypochromic microcytic cells. With further progression, anisocytosis (variations in red blood cell size) followed by poikilocytosis (variation in shape of red cells) will develop. Severe iron deficiency will produce a bizarre peripheral blood smear, with severely hypochromic cells, target cells, hypochromic pencil-shaped cells, and occasionally small numbers of nucleated red blood cells. The platelet count is usually normal in mild iron deficiency anemia but is typically elevated in more severe cases.

Differential Diagnosis

Other causes of microcytic anemia include anemia of chronic disease, thalassemia, and (less commonly) sideroblastic anemia. Anemia of chronic disease is characterized by normal or increased iron stores in the bone marrow and a normal or elevated ferritin level. The TIBC is either normal or low. Thalassemia characteristically produces a greater degree of microcytosis for any given level of anemia than does iron deficiency. Red blood cell morphology on the peripheral smear becomes abnormal earlier in the evolution of anemia and shows numerous target cells at all stages.

Treatment

To make the diagnosis of iron deficiency anemia, one can either demonstrate an iron-deficient state or evaluate the response to a therapeutic trial of iron replacement.

Since the anemia itself is rarely life-threatening, the most important part of treatment is identification of the cause—especially a source of occult blood loss.

A. Oral Iron: There is no better treatment than ferrous sulfate, 325 mg three times daily, which provides 180 mg of iron daily of which up to 10 mg is absorbed (though absorption may exceed this amount in cases of severe deficiency). Compliance is often improved by introducing the medicine more slowly in a gradually escalating dose with food. An appropriate response is a return of the hematocrit level halfway toward normal within 3 weeks with full return to baseline after 2 months. Iron therapy should continue for 3–6 months after restoration of normal hematologic values in order to replenish iron stores. Failure of response to iron therapy is usually due to noncompliance, although occasional patients may absorb iron poorly. Other reasons for failure to respond include incorrect diagnosis (anemia of chronic disease, thalassemia) and ongoing gastrointestinal blood loss that exceeds the rate of new erythropoiesis.

B. Parenteral Iron: The indications are intolerance to oral iron, refractoriness to oral iron, gastrointestinal disease (usually inflammatory bowel disease) precluding the use of oral iron, and continued blood loss that cannot be corrected. Because of the possibility of severe hypersensitivity reactions, parenteral iron therapy should be used only in cases of clinically significant documented iron deficiency after every reasonable attempt has been made to use oral therapy.

The dose may be calculated by estimating the decrease in volume of red blood cell mass and then supplying 1 mg of iron for each milliliter of volume of red blood cells below normal. One should then add approximately 1 g for storage iron. The total dose is typically 1.5–2 g. The entire dose may be given as an intravenous infusion over 4–6 hours. A test dose of a dilute solution is given first, and the patient should be observed during the entire infusion in a setting in which anaphylaxis can be treated.

Andrews NC. Disorders of iron metabolism. N Engl J Med 1999;341:1986. [NLM Cit ID: 20057434]

Finch C: Regulators of iron balance in humans. Blood 1994;84:1697. [NLM Cit ID: 94362216]

Gordon S, Bensen S, Smith R: Long-term follow-up of older patients with iron deficiency anemia after a negative GI evaluation. Am J Gastroenterol 1996;91:885. [NLM Cit ID: 96212717] (Favorable prognosis of iron deficiency anemia in older patients after a negative gastrointestinal evaluation.)

Newton W: Laboratory diagnosis of iron deficiency anemia. J Fam Pract 1995;41:404. [NLM Cit ID: 96017590]

ANEMIA OF CHRONIC DISEASE

Many chronic systemic diseases are associated with mild or moderate anemia. Common causes include chronic infection or inflammation, cancer, and liver disease. The anemia of chronic renal failure is somewhat different in pathophysiology and is usually more severe.

Red blood cell survival is modestly reduced, and the bone marrow fails to compensate adequately by increasing red blood cell production. Failure to increase red cell production is largely due to sequestration of iron within the reticuloendothelial system. Decrease in erythropoietin is rarely an important cause of underproduction of red cells except in renal failure, when decreased erythropoietin is the rule except in polycystic disease.

Clinical Findings

A. Symptoms and Signs: The clinical features are those of the anemia, which is usually modest. The diagnosis should be suspected in patients with known chronic diseases; it is confirmed by the findings of low serum iron, low TIBC, and normal or increased serum ferritin (or normal or increased bone marrow iron stores). In cases of significant anemia (< 60% of baseline), coexistent iron deficiency or folic acid deficiency should be suspected. Decreased dietary intake of folate or iron is common in these ill patients, and many will also have ongoing gastrointestinal blood losses. Patients undergoing hemodialysis regularly lose both iron and folate during dialysis.

B. Laboratory Findings: The hematocrit rarely falls below 25% (except in renal failure). The MCV is usually normal or slightly reduced. Red blood cell morphology is nondiagnostic, and the reticulocyte count is neither strikingly reduced nor increased. Characteristically, both the serum iron values and the

TIBC are reduced. Serum iron values may be unmeasurable, and transferrin saturation may be extremely low. A mistaken diagnosis of iron deficiency anemia may be made if overemphasis is placed on the reduced serum iron. A low serum iron and percentage saturation are diagnostic of iron deficiency only when the TIBC is also increased. In contrast to iron deficiency, serum ferritin values should be normal or increased. A serum ferritin value of less than 30 μg/L should suggest coexistent iron deficiency.

Treatment

In most cases no treatment is necessary. In some, however, red blood cell transfusions are required for symptomatic anemia. Purified recombinant erythropoietin has been shown to be effective for treatment of the anemia of renal failure and other secondary anemias such as anemia related to cancer or inflammatory disorders (eg, rheumatoid arthritis). In renal failure, optimal response to erythropoietin requires adequate intensity of dialysis. Erythropoietin is commercially available as epoetin alfa; however, it must be injected subcutaneously three or more times weekly (usual dose 10,000 units) and is very expensive. This agent should be used to alleviate anemia only when the patient is transfusion-dependent or when the quality of life is clearly improved by the hematologic response.

Cazzola M: Use of recombinant human erythropoietin outside the setting of uremia. Blood 1997;89:4248. [NLM Cit ID: 97335952]

Gasché C: Intravenous iron and erythropoietin for anemia associated with Crohn's disease. Ann Intern Med 1997;126:782. [NLM Cit ID: 97282916]

Goodnough LT: Erythropoetin therapy. N Engl J Med 1997;336:933. [NLM Cit ID: 97209490]

THE THALASSEMIAS

Essentials of Diagnosis

- Microcytosis out of proportion to the degree of anemia.
- Positive family history or lifelong personal history of microcytic anemia.
- Abnormal red blood cell morphology with microcytes, acanthocytes, and target cells.
- In beta thalassemia, elevated levels of hemoglobin A_2 or F.

General Considerations

The thalassemias are hereditary disorders characterized by reduction in the synthesis of globin chains (alpha or beta). Reduced globin chain synthesis causes reduced hemoglobin synthesis and eventually produces a hypochromic microcytic anemia because of defective hemoglobinization of red blood cells. Thalassemias can be considered among the hypoproliferative anemias, the hemolytic anemias, and the anemias related to abnormal hemoglobin, since all of these factors may play a role in pathogenesis.

Normal adult hemoglobin is primarily hemoglobin A, which represents approximately 98% of circulating hemoglobin. Hemoglobin A is formed from a tetramer—two alpha chains and two beta chains—and can be designated $\alpha_2\beta_2$. Two copies of the α-globin gene are located on chromosome 16, and there is no substitute for α-globin in the formation of hemoglobin. The β-globin gene resides on chromosome 11 adjacent to genes encoding the beta-like globin chains, delta and gamma. The tetramer of $\alpha_2\delta_2$ forms hemoglobin A_2, which normally comprises 1–2% of adult hemoglobin. The tetramer $\alpha_2\gamma_2$ forms hemoglobin F, which is the major hemoglobin of fetal life but which comprises less than 1% of normal adult hemoglobin.

Alpha thalassemia is due primarily to gene deletion causing reduced α-globin chain synthesis (Table 13–4). Since all adult hemoglobins are alpha-containing, alpha thalassemia produces no change in the percentage distribution of hemoglobins A, A_2, and F. In severe forms of alpha thalassemia, excess beta chains may form a β_4 tetramer called hemoglobin H. Hemoglobin H has high oxygen affinity and delivers oxygen to tissues poorly. It is also unstable and subject to oxidative denaturation under conditions of infection or exposure to oxidative drugs (sulfonamides, etc).

Beta thalassemias are usually caused by point mutations rather than deletions (Table 13–5). These mutations result in premature chain termination or in problems with transcription of RNA and ultimately result in reduced or absent β-globin chain synthesis. The molecular defects leading to beta thalassemia are numerous and heterogeneous. Defects that result in absent globin chain expression are termed β^0, whereas those causing reduced synthesis are termed β^+. The reduced β-globin chain synthesis in beta thalassemia results in a relative increase in the percentages of hemoglobins A_2 and F compared to hemoglobin A, as the beta-like globins (gamma and delta) substitute for the missing beta chains. In the presence of reduced beta chains, the excess alpha chains are unstable and precipitate, leading to damage to red blood cell membranes. This damage causes marked intramedullary hemolysis (destruction of developing erythroid cells within the bone marrow) as well as he-

Table 13–4. Alpha thalassemia syndromes.

Alpha Globin Genes	Syndrome	Hematocrit	MCV
4	Normal	Normal	
3	Silent carrier	Normal	
2	Thalassemia minor	32–40%	60–75 fL
1	Hemoglobin H disease	22–32%	60–70 fL
0	Hydrops fetalis		

Table 13–5. Beta thalassemia syndromes.

	Beta Globin Genes	Hb A	Hb A_2	Hb F
Normal	Homozygous β	97–99%	1–3%	< 1%
	Homozygous $β^0$	0	4–10%	90–96%
	Homozygous $β^+$	0–10%	4–10%	90–96%
Thalassemia intermedia	Homozygous $β^+$ (mild)	0–30%	0–10%	6–100%
Thalassemia minor	Heterozygous $β^0$	80–95%	4–8%	1–5%
	Heterozygous $β^+$	80–95%	4–8%	1–5%

molysis in the peripheral blood. The bone marrow becomes markedly hyperplastic under the drive of severe anemia and the ineffective erythropoiesis that results from destruction of the developing erythroid cells. This marked expansion of the erythroid element in the bone marrow causes severe bony deformities, osteopenia, and pathologic fractures.

Clinical Findings

A. Symptoms and Signs: The alpha thalassemia syndromes are seen primarily in persons from southeast Asia and China, and, less commonly, in blacks. Normally, adults have four copies of the α-globin chain. When three α-globin genes are present, the patient is hematologically normal and is called a silent carrier. When two α-globin genes are present, the patient is said to have alpha thalassemia trait, one form of thalassemia minor. These patients are clinically normal and have normal life expectancy and performance status. They have a very mild microcytic anemia. When only one α-globin chain is present, the patient has hemoglobin H disease. This is a chronic hemolytic anemia of variable severity (thalassemia minor or intermedia). Physical examination will reveal pallor and splenomegaly. Although affected individuals do not usually require transfusions, they may do so during periods of hemolytic exacerbation caused by infection or other stresses. When all four α-globin genes are deleted, the affected fetus is stillborn as a result of hydrops fetalis.

Beta thalassemia affects persons of Mediterranean origin (Italian, Greek) and to a lesser extent Chinese, other Asians, and blacks. Patients homozygous for beta thalassemia have the syndrome of thalassemia major. Affected children are normal at birth but during the first year of life develop severe anemia requiring transfusion. Signs of thalassemia typically develop after 6 months of age, because this is the time when hemoglobin synthesis switches from hemoglobin F to hemoglobin A. Numerous clinical problems ensue, including growth failure, bony deformities (abnormal facial structure, pathologic fractures), hepatosplenomegaly, and jaundice. The clinical course is modified significantly by transfusion therapy, but the transfusional iron overload (hemosiderosis) results in a clinical picture similar to hemochromatosis, with heart failure, cirrhosis, and endocrinopathies. These problems develop because of the body's inability to excrete the iron (see above) in transfused red cells. Death from cardiac failure usually occurs between ages 20 and 30.

Patients homozygous for a milder form of beta thalassemia (allowing a higher rate of globin gene synthesis) have thalassemia intermedia. These patients have chronic hemolytic anemia but do not require transfusions except under periods of stress. These patients also develop iron overload because of periodic transfusion. They survive into adult life but with hepatosplenomegaly and bony deformities.

Patients heterozygous for beta thalassemia have thalassemia minor. These patients have a mild microcytic anemia that is not clinically significant.

Prenatal diagnosis is available for couples at risk of producing a child with one of the severe thalassemia syndromes. Genetic counseling should be offered and the opportunity for prenatal diagnosis discussed.

B. Laboratory Findings:

1. Alpha thalassemia trait–Patients with two α-globin genes have mild anemia, with hematocrits between 28% and 40%. The MCV is strikingly low (60–75 fL) despite the modest degree of anemia, and the red blood count is normal or increased. The peripheral blood smear shows mild abnormalities, including microcytes, hypochromia, occasional target cells, and acanthocytes (cells with irregularly spaced bulbous projections). The reticulocyte count and iron parameters are normal. Hemoglobin electrophoresis will show no increase in the percentage of hemoglobins A_2 or F and no hemoglobin H. Alpha thalassemia trait is usually diagnosed by exclusion in a patient with modest anemia, significant microcytosis, and no elevation of hemoglobins A_2 or F.

2. Hemoglobin H disease–These patients have a variably severe hemolytic anemia, with hematocrits between 22% and 32%. The MCV is strikingly low (60–70 fL). The peripheral blood smear is markedly abnormal, with hypochromia, microcytosis, target cells, and poikilocytosis. The reticulocyte count is elevated. Hemoglobin electrophoresis will show the presence of a fast migrating hemoglobin (hemoglobin H), which comprises 10–40% of the hemoglobin. A peripheral blood smear can be stained with supravital dyes to demonstrate the presence of hemoglobin H.

3. Beta thalassemia minor–Like patients with alpha thalassemia trait, these patients have a modest anemia with hematocrit between 28% and 40%. The MCV ranges from 55 to 75 fL, and the red blood cell count is normal or increased. The peripheral blood smear is mildly abnormal, with hypochromia, microcytosis, and target cells. In contrast to alpha thalassemia, basophilic stippling may be present. The reticulocyte count may be normal or slightly elevated. Hemoglobin electrophoresis (using quantitative techniques) may show an elevation of hemoglobin A_2 to 4–8% and occasional elevations of hemoglobin F to 1–5%.

4. Beta thalassemia major–Beta thalassemia major produces severe anemia, and without transfusion the hematocrit may fall to less than 10%. The peripheral blood smear is bizarre, showing severe poikilocytosis, hypochromia, microcytosis, target cells, basophilic stippling, and nucleated red blood cells. Little or no hemoglobin A is present. Variable amounts of hemoglobin A_2 are seen, and the major hemoglobin present is hemoglobin F.

Differential Diagnosis

Mild forms of thalassemia must be differentiated from iron deficiency. Compared to iron deficiency anemia, patients with thalassemia have a lower MCV, a more normal red blood count, and a more abnormal peripheral blood smear at modest levels of anemia. Iron studies are normal. Severe forms of thalassemia may be confused with other hemoglobinopathies. The diagnosis will be made by hemoglobin electrophoresis.

Treatment

Patients with mild thalassemia (alpha thalassemia trait or beta thalassemia minor) are clinically normal and require no treatment. Most importantly, patients with microcytosis should be identified so that they will not be subjected to repeated evaluations for iron deficiency and inappropriately given supplemental iron. Patients with hemoglobin H disease should take folate supplementation and avoid medicinal iron and oxidative drugs such as sulfonamides. Patients with severe thalassemia should be maintained on a regular transfusion schedule and receive folate supplementation. Splenectomy is performed if hypersplenism causes a marked increase in the transfusion requirement. Deferoxamine is routinely given as an iron-chelating agent to avoid or postpone hemosiderosis. Oral iron chelators are under investigation and appear to be effective, but toxicity (agranulocytosis) will probably limit their use.

Allogeneic bone marrow transplantation has been introduced as treatment for beta thalassemia major. Children who have not yet experienced iron overload and chronic organ toxicity do well, with long-term survival in more than 80% of cases.

Hoffbrand AV: Long-term trial of deferiprone in 51 transfusion-dependent iron overloaded patients. Blood 1998; 91:295. [NLM Cit ID: 98077542]

Lucarelli G: Bone marrow transplantation in adult thalassemia patients. N Engl J Med 1999;93:1164. [NLM Cit ID: 99135843]

Olivieri NF. The beta-thalassemias. N Engl J Med 1999; 341:99. [NLM Cit ID: 99305298]

Olivieri NF: Long-term safety and effectiveness of iron-chelation therapy with deferiprone for thalassemia major. N Engl J Med 1998;339:417. [NLM Cit ID: 98355341]

SIDEROBLASTIC ANEMIA

The sideroblastic anemias are a heterogeneous group of disorders in which hemoglobin synthesis is reduced because of failure to incorporate heme into protoporphyrin to form hemoglobin. Iron accumulates, particularly in the mitochondria. A Prussian blue stain of the bone marrow will reveal ringed sideroblasts, cells with iron deposits (in the mitochondria) encircling the red cell nucleus. The disorder is usually acquired. Sometimes it represents a stage in evolution of a generalized bone marrow disorder (myelodysplasia) that may ultimately terminate in acute leukemia. Other important causes include chronic alcoholism, drug toxicity (antituberculous agents, chloramphenicol), and lead poisoning.

Patients have no specific clinical features other than those related to anemia. The anemia is usually moderate, with hematocrits of 20–30%, but transfusions may occasionally be required. Although the MCV is usually normal or slightly increased, it may occasionally be low, leading to confusion with iron deficiency. The peripheral blood smear characteristically shows a dimorphic population of red blood cells, one normal and one hypochromic. In cases of lead poisoning, coarse basophilic stippling of the red cells is seen.

The diagnosis is made by examination of the bone marrow. Characteristically, there is marked erythroid hyperplasia, a sign of ineffective erythropoiesis (expansion of the erythroid compartment of the bone marrow that does not result in the production of reticulocytes in the peripheral blood). The iron stain of the bone marrow shows a generalized increase in iron stores and the presence of ringed sideroblasts. Other characteristic laboratory features include a high serum iron and a high transferrin saturation. In the presence of lead poisoning, serum lead levels will be elevated.

When lead toxicity is causative, it may be treated with chelation therapy. Occasional patients will respond to pharmacologic doses of pyridoxine (200 mg/d), but most patients do not respond to therapy. Anecdotal responses to chloroquine have been reported. Occasionally, the anemia is so severe that support with red cell transfusion is required. These patients usually do not respond to erythropoietin therapy.

VITAMIN B_{12} DEFICIENCY

Essentials of Diagnosis

- Macrocytic anemia.
- Macro-ovalocytes and hypersegmented neutrophils on peripheral blood smear.
- Serum vitamin B_{12} level less than 100 pg/mL.

General Considerations

Vitamin B_{12} belongs to the family of cobalamins and serves as a cofactor for two important reactions in humans. As methylcobalamin, it serves as a cofactor for methionine synthetase in the conversion of homocysteine to methionine. As adenosylcobalamin, it serves as a cofactor for the conversion of methylmalonyl-CoA to succinyl-CoA. All vitamin B_{12} comes from the diet, and vitamin B_{12} is present in all foods of animal origin. The daily absorption of vitamin B_{12} is 5 μg.

After being ingested, vitamin B_{12} becomes bound to intrinsic factor, a protein secreted by gastric parietal cells. Other cobalamin-binding proteins (called R factors) compete with intrinsic factor for vitamin B_{12}. Vitamin B_{12} bound to R factors cannot be absorbed. The vitamin B_{12}-intrinsic factor complex travels through the intestine and is absorbed in the terminal ileum by cells with specific receptors for the complex. It is then transported through plasma and stored in the liver. Three plasma transport proteins have been identified. Transcobalamins I and III (differing only in carbohydrate structure) are secreted by white blood cells. Although approximately 90% of plasma vitamin B_{12} circulates bound to these proteins, only transcobalamin II is capable of transporting vitamin B_{12} into cells. The liver contains 2000–5000 μg of stored vitamin B_{12}. Since daily losses are 3–5 μg/d, the body usually has sufficient stores of vitamin B_{12} so that vitamin B_{12} deficiency develops more than 3 years after vitamin B_{12} absorption ceases.

Since vitamin B_{12} is present in all foods of animal origin, dietary vitamin B_{12} deficiency is extremely rare and seen only in vegans—strict vegetarians who avoid all dairy products as well as meat and fish (Table 13–6). Abdominal surgery may lead to vitamin B_{12} deficiency in several ways. Gastrectomy will eliminate that site of intrinsic factor production; blind loop syndrome will cause competition for vitamin B_{12} by bacterial overgrowth in the lumen of the intestine; and surgical resection of the ileum will eliminate the site of vitamin B_{12} absorption. Rare causes of vitamin B_{12} deficiency include fish tapeworm (*Diphyllobothrium latum*) infection, in which the parasite uses luminal vitamin B_{12}, pancreatic insufficiency (with failure to inactivate competing cobalamin-binding proteins), and severe Crohn's disease, causing sufficient destruction of the ileum to retard vitamin B_{12} absorption.

Table 13–6. Causes of vitamin B_{12} deficiency.

Dietary deficiency (rare)
Decreased production of intrinsic factor
Pernicious anemia
Gastrectomy
Competition for vitamin B_{12} in gut
Blind loop syndrome
Fish tapeworm (rare)
Pancreatic insufficiency
Decreased ileal absorption of vitamin B_{12}
Surgical resection
Crohn's disease
Transcobalamin II deficiency (rare)

The most common cause of vitamin B_{12} deficiency is that associated with **pernicious anemia.** Although the disease is hereditary, it is rarely manifested before age 35. Pernicious anemia produces a number of clinical findings in addition to vitamin B_{12} deficiency. Atrophic gastritis is invariably present and results in histamine-fast achlorhydria. These patients may also have a number of other autoimmune diseases, including IgA deficiency, as well as polyglandular endocrine insufficiency. The atrophic gastritis is associated with an increased risk of gastric carcinoma.

Clinical Findings

A. Symptoms and Signs: The hallmark of vitamin B_{12} deficiency is megaloblastic anemia. The anemia may be severe, with hematocrits as low as 10–15%. The megaloblastic state also produces changes in mucosal cells, leading to glossitis, as well as other vague gastrointestinal disturbances such as anorexia and diarrhea. Vitamin B_{12} deficiency also leads to a complex neurologic syndrome. Peripheral nerves are usually affected first, and patients complain initially of paresthesias. The posterior columns next become impaired, and patients complain of difficulty with balance. In more advanced cases, cerebral function may be altered as well, and on occasion dementia and other neuropsychiatric changes may precede hematologic changes.

On examination, patients are usually pale and may be mildly icteric. Neurologic examination will reveal decreased vibration and position sense.

B. Laboratory Findings: The megaloblastic state produces an anemia of variable severity that on occasion may be very severe. The MCV is usually strikingly elevated, between 110 and 140 fL. However, it is possible to have vitamin B_{12} deficiency with a normal MCV. Occasionally, the normal MCV may be explained by coexistent thalassemia or iron deficiency, but in other cases the reason for the normal MCV is obscure. Patients with neurologic symptoms and signs that suggest possible vitamin B_{12} deficiency should be thoroughly evaluated for the possibility of that deficiency despite a normal MCV and the absence of anemia. The peripheral blood smear is usually strikingly abnormal, with anisocytosis and poikilocytosis. A characteristic finding is the macro-ovalocyte, but numerous other abnormal shapes are usually seen. The neutrophils are hypersegmented. Typical features include a mean lobe count greater than four or the finding of six-lobed neutrophils. The reticulocyte count is reduced. Because vitamin B_{12} deficiency affects all hematopoietic cell lines, in many cases the white blood cell count and platelet count are reduced, and pancytopenia is present.

Bone marrow morphology is characteristically abnormal. Marked erythroid hyperplasia is present as a response to defective red blood cell production (ineffective erythropoiesis). Megaloblastic changes in the erythroid series include abnormally large cell size and asynchronous maturation of the nucleus and cytoplasm—ie, cytoplasmic maturation continues while impaired DNA synthesis causes retarded nuclear development. In the myeloid series, giant metamyelocytes are characteristically seen.

Other laboratory abnormalities include elevated serum LDH and a modest increase in indirect bilirubin. These two findings are a reflection of intramedullary destruction of developing abnormal erythroid cells.

The diagnosis of vitamin B_{12} deficiency is made by finding an abnormally low vitamin B_{12} serum level. Whereas the normal vitamin B_{12} level is 150–350 pg/mL, most patients with overt vitamin B_{12} deficiency will have serum levels less than 100 pg/mL. The Schilling test is used to document the decreased absorption of oral vitamin B_{12} characteristic of pernicious anemia. Initially, a large intramuscular dose of vitamin B_{12} is given to saturate plasma transport proteins. Radiolabeled vitamin B_{12} is administered orally, and a 24-hour urine collection is performed to determine how much vitamin B_{12} is absorbed and subsequently excreted. Normally, more than 7% of a dose is present in the urine; most patients with impaired absorption will have less than 3% present in the urine. The second stage of the Schilling test is to give radiolabeled vitamin B_{12} together with intrinsic factor. If pernicious anemia (a lack of intrinsic factor) is the cause of vitamin B_{12} deficiency, the combined use of vitamin B_{12} and intrinsic factor should correct the abnormally low absorption. However, the full-blown megaloblastic state causes abnormalities in intestinal epithelium that may lead to generalized malabsorption. In these cases, the second stage of the Schilling test will remain abnormal until the intestinal mucosal defect is first corrected by vitamin B_{12} replacement (in approximately 2 months). The repeat evaluation should thus be deferred until there has been time for correction. If the deficiency is caused by bacterial overgrowth in a blind loop (eg, jejunal diverticula), a course of antibiotics will reverse the abnormal second stage of the Schilling test. If the deficiency has been produced by pancreatic insufficiency, a course of pancreatic enzymes will reverse the abnormality. If a tapeworm is responsible, an anthelmintic agent is indicated.

Differential Diagnosis

Vitamin B_{12} deficiency should be differentiated from folic acid deficiency, the other common cause of megaloblastic anemia, in which red blood cell folate is low while vitamin B_{12} levels are normal. The distinction between vitamin B_{12} deficiency and myelodysplasia (the other common cause of macrocytic anemia with abnormal morphology) is based on the characteristic morphology and the low vitamin B_{12} level. Neurologic symptoms or signs suggestive of vitamin B_{12} deficiency should be evaluated for that disorder even in the absence of anemia or macrocytosis.

Treatment

Patients with pernicious anemia are often treated with parenteral therapy. Intramuscular injections of 100 μg of vitamin B_{12} are adequate for each dose. Replacement is usually given daily for the first week, weekly for the first month, and then monthly for life. Pernicious anemia is a lifelong disorder, and if patients discontinue their monthly therapy, the vitamin deficiency will recur. Oral cobalamin may be used instead of parenteral therapy in a dose of 1000 μg/d and must be continued indefinitely.

Patients respond to therapy with an immediate improvement in their sense of well-being. Hypokalemia may complicate the first several days of therapy, particularly if the anemia is severe. A brisk reticulocytosis occurs in 5–7 days, and the hematologic picture normalizes in 2 months. Central nervous system symptoms and signs are reversible if they are of relatively short duration (less than 6 months), but they may be permanent if treatment is not initiated promptly.

Green R: Screening for vitamin B_{12} deficiency: Caveat emptor. (Editorial and comment.) Ann Intern Med 1996;124:509. [NLM Cit ID: 96169951]

Schilling RE, Williams WJ: Vitamin B_{12} deficiency: Underdiagnosed, overtreated? Hosp Pract (Off Ed) 1995 Jul;30:47. [NLM Cit ID: 95325377]

FOLIC ACID DEFICIENCY

Essentials of Diagnosis

- Macrocytic anemia.
- Macro-ovalocytes and hypersegmented neutrophils on peripheral blood smear.
- Normal serum vitamin B_{12} levels.
- Reduced folate levels in red blood cells or serum.

General Considerations

Folic acid is the term commonly used for pteroylmonoglutamic acid. In its reduced form of tetrahydrofolate, it serves as an important mediator of many reactions involving one-carbon transfers. Important reactions include the conversion of homocysteine to methionine and of deoxyuridylate to thymidylate, an important step in DNA synthesis.

Folic acid is present in most fruits and vegetables (especially citrus fruits and green leafy vegetables) and daily requirements of 50–100 μg/d are usually met in the diet. Total body stores of folate are approximately 5000 μg, enough to supply requirements for 2–3 months.

By far the most common cause of folate deficiency is inadequate dietary intake (Table 13–7). Alcoholics, anorectic patients, persons who do not eat fresh fruits and vegetables, and those who overcook their food are candidates for folate deficiency. Reduced folate absorption is rarely seen, since absorption occurs from the entire gastrointestinal tract. However, drugs such as phenytoin, trimethoprim-sulfamethoxazole, or sulfasalazine may interfere with folate absorption. Folic acid requirements are increased in pregnancy, hemolytic anemia, and exfoliative skin disease, and in these cases the increased requirements (five to ten times normal) may not be met by a normal diet. Patients with increased folate requirements should receive supplementation with 1 mg/d of folic acid.

Clinical Findings

A. Symptoms and Signs: The features are similar to those of vitamin B_{12} deficiency, with megaloblastic anemia and megaloblastic changes in mucosa. However, there are none of the neurologic abnormalities associated with vitamin B_{12} deficiency.

B. Laboratory Findings: The megaloblastic anemia is identical to that resulting from vitamin B_{12} deficiency (see above). However, the serum vitamin B_{12} level is normal. In contrast, the serum folic acid level is low, usually less than 3 ng/mL. The red blood cell folate level is more reliable and has replaced serum folate as the appropriate test. A red blood cell folate level of less than 150 ng/mL is diagnostic of folate deficiency.

Differential Diagnosis

The megaloblastic anemia of folate deficiency should be differentiated from vitamin B_{12} deficiency by the finding of a normal vitamin B_{12} level and a reduced red blood cell folate or serum folate level. Alcoholics, who often have folate deficiency, may also have anemia of liver disease. This latter macrocytic anemia does not cause megaloblastic morphologic changes but rather produces target cells in the peripheral blood. Patients with HIV-related illnesses being treated with zidovudine develop macrocytosis without megaloblastic morphology. Hypothyroidism is associated with mild macrocytosis but also with pernicious anemia.

Table 13–7. Causes of folate deficiency.

Dietary deficiency
Decreased absorption
Tropical sprue
Drugs: phenytoin, sulfasalazine, trimethoprim-sulfamethoxazole
Increased requirement
Chronic hemolytic anemia
Pregnancy
Exfoliative skin disease
Loss: dialysis
Inhibition of reduction to active form
Methotrexate

Treatment

Folic acid deficiency is treated with folic acid, 1 mg/d orally. The response is similar to that seen in the treatment of vitamin B_{12} deficiency, with rapid improvement and a sense of well-being, reticulocytosis in 5–7 days, and total correction of hematologic abnormalities within 2 months. Large doses of folic acid may produce hematologic responses in cases of vitamin B_{12} deficiency but will allow neurologic damage to progress.

PURE RED CELL APLASIA

Adult acquired pure red cell aplasia is rare. It appears to be an autoimmune disease mediated either by T lymphocytes or (less often) by an IgG antibody against erythroid precursors. In adults, the disease is usually idiopathic. However, cases have been seen in association with systemic lupus erythematosus, chronic lymphocytic leukemia, lymphomas, or thymoma. Some drugs (phenytoin, chloramphenicol) may cause red cell aplasia. Transient episodes of red cell aplasia are probably common in response to viral infections, especially parvovirus infections. However, these acute episodes will go unrecognized unless the patient has a chronic hemolytic disorder, in which case the hematocrit may fall precipitously.

Clinically, the only signs are those of anemia, unless the patient has an associated autoimmune or lymphoproliferative disorder. The anemia is often severe and is normochromic. Reticulocytes are very low or absent. Red blood cell morphology is normal, and the myeloid and platelet lines are unaffected. The bone marrow is normocellular. All elements present are normal, but erythroid precursors are markedly reduced or absent. In some cases, chest imaging studies will reveal a thymoma.

The disorder should be distinguished from aplastic anemia (in which the marrow is generally hypocellular and other cell lines are affected) and from myelodysplasia. This latter disorder is recognized by the presence of morphologic abnormalities that should not be present in pure red cell aplasia.

Possible offending drugs should be stopped. If a thymoma is present, resection results in amelioration of anemia in some instances. High-dose intravenous immune globulin has produced excellent responses in a small number of cases, especially in parvovirus-related cases. For most cases, the treatment of choice is immunosuppressive therapy with a combination of antithymocyte globulin and cyclosporine—similar to therapy of aplastic anemia.

Casadevall N et al: Autoantibodies against erythropoietin in a patient with pure red-cell aplasia. N Engl J Med 1996;334:630. [NLM Cit ID: 96172891]

Charles RJ et al: The pathophysiology of pure red cell aplasia: Implications for therapy. Blood 1996;87:4831. [NLM Cit ID: 96219665]

Lacy MQ, Kurtin PJ, Tefferi A: Pure red cell aplasia: Association with large granular lymphocyte leukemia and the prognostic value of cytogenetic abnormalities. Blood 1996;87:3000. [NLM Cit ID: 96219998]

HEMOLYTIC ANEMIAS

The hemolytic anemias are a group of disorders in which red blood cell survival is reduced, either episodically or continuously. The bone marrow has the ability to increase erythroid production up to eightfold in response to reduced red cell survival, so anemia will be present only when the ability of the bone marrow to compensate is outstripped. This will occur when red cell survival is extremely short or when the ability of the bone marrow to compensate is impaired for some second reason.

Since red blood cell survival is normally 120 days, in the absence of red cell production the hematocrit will fall at the rate of approximately 1/100 of the hematocrit per day, which translates to a decrease in the hematocrit reading of approximately 3% per week. For example, a fall of hematocrit from 45% to 36% over 3 weeks' time need not indicate hemolysis, since this rate of fall would result simply from cessation of red blood cell production. If the hematocrit is falling at a faster rate than that due to decreased production, blood loss or hemolysis is the cause.

Reticulocytosis is an important clue to the presence of hemolysis, since in most hemolytic disorders the bone marrow will respond with increased red blood cell production. However, hemolysis can be present without reticulocytosis when a second disorder (infection, folate deficiency) is superimposed on hemolysis; in these circumstances, the hematocrit will fall rapidly. However, reticulocytosis also occurs during recovery from hypoproliferative anemia or bleeding. Hemolysis is correctly diagnosed (when bleeding is excluded) if the hematocrit is either falling or stable despite reticulocytosis.

Hemolytic disorders are generally classified according to whether the defect is intrinsic to the red cell or due to some external factor (Table 13–8). Intrinsic defects have been described in all components of the red blood cell, including the membrane, enzyme systems, and hemoglobin. Most of these disorders are hereditary. Most hemolytic anemias due to external factors are the immune hemolytic anemias.

Table 13–8. Classification of hemolytic anemias.

Intrinsic
Membrane defects: hereditary spherocytosis, hereditary elliptocytosis, paroxysmal nocturnal hemoglobinuria
Glycolytic defects: pyruvate kinase deficiency, severe hypophosphatemia
Oxidation vulnerability: G6PD deficiency, methemoglobinemia
Hemoglobinopathies: sickle cell syndromes, unstable hemoglobins, methemoglobinemia
Extrinsic
Immune: autoimmune, lymphoproliferative disease, drug toxicity
Microangiopathic: thrombotic thrombocytopenic purpura, hemolytic-uremic syndrome, disseminated intravascular coagulation, valve hemolysis, metastatic adenocarcinoma, vasculitis
Infection: plasmodium, clostridium, borrelia
Hypersplenism
Burns

Certain laboratory features are common to all the hemolytic anemias. Haptoglobin, a normal plasma protein that binds and clears hemoglobin released into plasma, may be depressed in hemolytic disorders. However, haptoglobin levels are influenced by many factors and, by themselves, are not a reliable indicator of hemolysis. When intravascular hemolysis occurs, transient hemoglobinemia occurs. Hemoglobin is filtered through the glomerulus and usually reabsorbed by tubular cells. Hemoglobinuria will be present only when the capacity for reabsorption of hemoglobin by these cells is exceeded. In the absence of hemoglobinuria, evidence for prior intravascular hemolysis is the presence of hemosiderin in shed renal tubular cells (positive urine hemosiderin). With severe intravascular hemolysis, hemoglobinemia and methemalbuminemia may be present. Hemolysis increases the indirect bilirubin, and the total bilirubin may rise to 4 mg/dL. Bilirubin levels higher than this may indicate some degree of hepatic dysfunction. Serum LDH levels are strikingly elevated in cases of microangiopathic hemolysis (thrombotic thrombocytopenic purpura, hemolytic-uremic syndrome) and may be elevated in other hemolytic anemias. Chronic intravascular hemolysis will lead to iron deficiency due to the loss of iron in the urine; most hemolytic anemias are extravascular, allowing conservation and reuse of iron.

HEREDITARY SPHEROCYTOSIS

Essentials of Diagnosis

- Positive family history.
- Splenomegaly.
- Spherocytes and increased reticulocytes on peripheral blood smear.
- Microcytic, hyperchromic indices.

General Considerations

Hereditary spherocytosis is a disorder of the red blood cell membrane, leading to chronic hemolytic anemia. Normally, the red blood cell is a biconcave disk with a diameter of 7–8 μm. The red blood cells must be both strong and deformable—strong to withstand the stress of circulating for 120 days and deformable so as to pass through capillaries 3 μm in diameter and splenic fenestrations in the cords of the red pulp of approximately 2 μm. The red blood cell skeleton, made up primarily of the proteins spectrin and actin, gives the red cells these characteristics of strength and deformability.

The membrane defect in hereditary spherocytosis is most likely an abnormality in spectrin, the protein providing most of the scaffolding for the red blood cell membranes. The result is a decrease in surface-to-volume ratio that results in a spherical shape of the cell. These spherical cells are less deformable and unable to pass through 2-μm fenestrations in the splenic red pulp. Hemolysis takes place because of trapping of red blood cells within the spleen.

Clinical Findings

A. Symptoms and Signs: Hereditary spherocytosis is an autosomal dominant disease of variable severity. It is often diagnosed during childhood, but milder cases may be discovered incidentally late in adult life. Anemia may or may not be present, since the bone marrow may be able to compensate for shortened red cell survival. Severe anemia (aplastic crisis) may occur in folic acid deficiency or when bone marrow compensation is temporarily impaired by infection. Chronic hemolysis causes jaundice and pigment (calcium bilirubinate) gallstones, leading to attacks of cholecystitis. Examination may reveal icterus and a palpable spleen.

B. Laboratory Findings: The anemia is of variable severity, and the hematocrit may be normal. Reticulocytosis is always present. The peripheral blood smear shows the presence of spherocytes, small cells that have lost their central pallor. Spherocytes usually make up only a small percentage of red blood cells on the peripheral smear. Hereditary spherocytosis is the only important disorder associated with increased MCHC, often greater than 36 g/dL. As with other hemolytic disorders, there may be an increase in indirect bilirubin. The Coombs test is negative.

Because spherocytes are red cells that have lost some membrane surface, they are abnormally vulnerable to swelling induced by hypotonic media. Increased osmotic fragility merely reflects the presence of spherocytes and does not distinguish hereditary spherocytosis from other spherocytic hemolytic disorders such as autoimmune hemolytic anemia.

Treatment

These patients should receive uninterrupted supplementation with folic acid, 1 mg/d. The treatment of choice is splenectomy, which will not correct the membrane defect or correct the spherocytosis but will eliminate the site of hemolysis. In very mild cases discovered late in adult life, splenectomy may not be necessary.

Cynober T, Mohandas N, Tchernia G: Red cell abnormalities in hereditary spherocytosis: Relevance to diagnosis and understanding of the variable expression of clinical severity. J Lab Clin Med 1996;128:259. [NLM Cit ID: 96377824]

Hassoun H et al: Hereditary spherocytosis with spectrin deficiency due to an unstable truncated beta spectrin. Blood 1996;87:2538. [NLM Cit ID: 96203825]

PAROXYSMAL NOCTURNAL HEMOGLOBINURIA

Paroxysmal nocturnal hemoglobinuria is an acquired clonal stem cell disorder that results in abnormal sensitivity of the red blood cell membrane to lysis by complement. The defect involves both increased binding of C3b and increased vulnerability to lysis by complement, and is expressed as a deficiency in proteins normally linked to the cell by phosphoinositol. Paroxysmal nocturnal hemoglobinuria should be suspected in confusing cases of hemolytic anemia or pancytopenia. The best screening test is the sucrose hemolysis test.

Clinical Findings

A. Symptoms and Signs: Classically, patients report episodic hemoglobinuria resulting in reddish brown urine. Hemoglobinuria may be present in the first morning urine, since the mild respiratory acidosis of sleep leads to enhanced complement activity. In addition to anemia, these patients are prone to thrombosis, especially mesenteric and hepatic vein thromboses. This hypercoagulopathy may be related to platelet activation by complement. As this is a stem cell disorder, paroxysmal nocturnal hemoglobinuria may progress either to aplastic anemia, to myelodysplasia, or to acute myelogenous leukemia.

B. Laboratory Findings: Anemia is of variable severity, and reticulocytosis may or may not be present. Abnormalities on the blood smear are nondiagnostic and may include macro-ovalocytes. Since the episodic hemolysis in paroxysmal nocturnal hemoglobinuria is intravascular, the finding of urine hemosiderin is a useful test. Serum LDH is characteristically elevated. Iron deficiency is commonly present and is related to chronic iron loss from hemoglobinuria, since hemolysis is primarily intravascular.

The white blood cell count and platelet count may be decreased. A decreased leukocyte alkaline phosphatase– evidence for qualitative abnormality in the myeloid series—is good evidence for paroxysmal nocturnal hemoglobinuria. Bone marrow morphology is variable and may show either generalized hypoplasia or erythroid hyperplasia. Flow cytometric assays may confirm the diagnosis by demonstrating the absence of CD59.

Treatment

Iron replacement is often indicated for treatment of iron deficiency. This may improve the anemia but may also cause a transient increase in hemolysis. For unclear reasons, prednisone is effective in decreasing hemolysis, and some patients can be managed effectively with alternate-day steroids. In severe cases and cases of transformation to myelodysplasia, allogeneic bone marrow transplantation has been used to treat the disorder.

Hall SE, Rosse WF: The use of monoclonal antibodies and flow cytometry in the diagnosis of paroxysmal nocturnal hemoglobinuria. Blood 1996;87:5332. [NLM Cit ID: 96247538]

Hillmen P et al: Natural history of paroxysmal nocturnal hemoglobinuria. N Engl J Med 1995;333:1253. [NLM Cit ID: 96022135]

Kinoshita T, Inoue N, Takeda J: Role of phosphatidylinositol-linked proteins in paroxysmal nocturnal hemoglobinuria pathogenesis. Annu Rev Med 1996;47:1. [NLM Cit ID: 96266621]

GLUCOSE-6-PHOSPHATE DEHYDROGENASE DEFICIENCY

Essentials of Diagnosis

- X-linked recessive disorder seen commonly in American black men.
- Episodic hemolysis in response to oxidant drugs or infection.
- Minimally abnormal peripheral blood smear.
- Reduced levels of G6PD between hemolytic episodes.

General Considerations

Glucose-6-phosphate dehydrogenase (G6PD) deficiency is a hereditary enzyme defect that causes episodic hemolytic anemia because of decreased ability of red blood cells to deal with oxidative stresses. The hexose monophosphate shunt is not an important source of energy in red cells but is important in generating reduced glutathione, which protects hemoglobin from oxidative denaturation. The first step in this pathway is the production of NADPH by the action of G6PD on glucose 6-phosphate. NADPH serves as a cofactor for glutathione reductase in generating reduced glutathione, which detoxifies hydrogen peroxide. In the absence of reduced glutathione, hemoglobin may become oxidized. Oxidized hemoglobin denatures and forms precipitants called Heinz bodies. These Heinz bodies cause membrane damage, which leads to removal of these cells by the spleen.

Numerous types of G6PD enzymes have been described. The normal type found in Caucasians is designated G6PD-B. Most American blacks have G6PD-A, which is normal in function. Ten to 15 percent of American blacks have the variant G6PD designated A^-, in which there is only 15% of normal enzyme activity, and enzyme activity declines rapidly as the red blood cell ages past 40 days, a fact that explains many of the clinical findings in this disorder. Many other G6PD variants have been described, including some Mediterranean variants with extremely low enzyme activity.

Clinical Findings

G6PD deficiency is an X-linked recessive disorder affecting 10–15% of American black males. Female carriers are rarely affected—only when an unusually high percentage of cells producing the normal enzyme are inactivated.

A. Symptoms and Signs: Patients are usually healthy, without chronic hemolytic anemia or splenomegaly. Hemolysis occurs as a result of oxidative stress on the red blood cells, generated either by infection or exposure to certain drugs. Common drugs initiating hemolysis include dapsone, primaquine, quinidine, quinine, sulfonamides, and nitrofurantoin. Even with continuous use of the offending drug, the hemolytic episode is self-limited because older red blood cells (with low enzyme activity) are removed and replaced with a population of young red blood cells with adequate functional levels of G6PD. Severe G6PD deficiency (as in Mediterranean variants) may produce a chronic hemolytic anemia.

B. Laboratory Findings: Between hemolytic episodes, the blood is normal. During episodes of hemolysis, there is reticulocytosis and increased serum indirect bilirubin. The red blood cell smear is not diagnostic but may reveal a small number of "bite" cells—cells that appear to have had a bite taken out of their periphery. This indicates pitting of hemoglobin aggregates by the spleen. Heinz bodies may be demonstrated by staining a peripheral blood smear with crystal violet. (They are not visible on the usual Wright-stained blood smear.) Specific enzyme assays for G6PD may reveal a low level but may be misleading if they are performed shortly after a hemolytic episode when the enzyme-deficient cohort of cells has been removed. In these cases, the enzyme assays should be repeated weeks after hemolysis has resolved. In severe cases of G6PD deficiency, enzyme levels are always low.

Treatment

No treatment is necessary except to avoid known oxidant drugs.

Chang JG, Liu TC: Glucose-6-phosphate dehydrogenase deficiency. Crit Rev Oncol Hematol 1995;20:1. [NLM Cit ID: 96059485]

SICKLE CELL ANEMIA & RELATED SYNDROMES

Essentials of Diagnosis

- Irreversibly sickled cells on peripheral blood smear.
- Positive family history and lifelong history of hemolytic anemia.
- Recurrent painful episodes.
- Hemoglobin S is the major hemoglobin seen on electrophoresis.

General Considerations

Sickle cell anemia is an autosomal recessive disorder in which an abnormal hemoglobin leads to chronic hemolytic anemia with a variety of severe clinical consequences. The disorder is a classic example of disease caused by a point mutation. A single DNA base change leads to an amino acid substitution of valine for glutamine in the sixth position on the β-globin chain. The abnormal beta chain is designated β^s and the tetramer of $\alpha_2\beta^s{}_2$ is designated hemoglobin S.

When in the deoxy form, hemoglobin S forms polymers that damage the red blood cell membrane. Both polymer formation and early membrane damage are reversible. However, red blood cells that have undergone repeated sickling are damaged beyond repair and become irreversibly sickled cells.

The rate of sickling is influenced by a number of factors, most importantly by the concentration of hemoglobin S in the individual red blood cell. Red cell dehydration makes the cell quite vulnerable to sickling. Sickling is also strongly influenced by the presence of other hemoglobins within the cell. Hemoglobin F cannot participate in polymer formation, and its presence markedly retards sickling. Other factors that increase sickling are those which lead to formation of deoxyhemoglobin S, eg, acidosis and hypoxemia, either systemic or locally in tissues.

Prenatal diagnosis is now available for couples at risk of producing a child with sickle cell anemia. DNA from fetal cells can be directly examined, and the presence of the sickle cell mutation can be accurately and definitively diagnosed. Genetic counseling should be made available to such couples.

Clinical Findings

A. Symptoms and Signs: The hemoglobin S gene is carried in 8% of American blacks, and one birth out of 400 in American blacks will produce a child with sickle cell anemia. The disorder has its onset during the first year of life, when hemoglobin F levels fall as a signal is sent to switch from γ-globin to β-globin production.

Chronic hemolytic anemia produces jaundice, pigment (calcium bilirubinate) gallstones, splenomegaly, and poorly healing ulcers over the lower tibia. The chronic anemia may become life-threatening when severe anemia is produced by hemolytic or aplastic crises. The latter occur when the ability of the bone marrow to compensate is reduced by viral or other infection or by folate deficiency. Hemolytic crises may be related to splenic sequestration of sickled cells (primarily in childhood, before the spleen has been infarcted as a result of repeated sickling) or with coexistent disorders such as G6PD deficiency.

Acute painful episodes due to acute vaso-occlusion may occur spontaneously or be provoked by infection, dehydration, or hypoxia. Clusters of sickled red cells occlude the microvasculature of the organs involved. These episodes last hours to days and produce acute pain and low-grade fever. Common sites of acute painful episodes include the bones (especially the back and long bones) and the chest. Acute vaso-occlusion may also cause strokes due to sinus thrombosis and priapism. Vaso-occlusive episodes are not associated with increased hemolysis.

Repeated episodes of vascular occlusion affect a large number of organs, especially the heart and liver. Ischemic necrosis of bone occurs, rendering the bone susceptible to osteomyelitis due to staphylococci or (less commonly) salmonellae. Infarction of the papillae of the renal medulla causes renal tubular concentrating defects and gross hematuria, more often encountered in sickle cell trait than in sickle cell anemia. Retinopathy similar to that noted in diabetes is often present and may lead to blindness.

These patients are prone to delayed puberty. An increased incidence of infection is related to hyposplenism as well as to defects in the alternative pathway of complement.

On examination, patients are often chronically ill and jaundiced. There is hepatomegaly, but the spleen is not palpable in adult life. The heart is enlarged, with a hyperdynamic precordium and systolic murmurs. Nonhealing ulcers of the lower leg and retinopathy may be present.

Sickle cell anemia becomes a chronic multisystem disease, with death from organ failure. With improved supportive care, average life expectancy is now between ages 40 and 50.

B. Laboratory Findings: Chronic hemolytic anemia is present. The hematocrit is usually 20–30%. The peripheral blood smear is characteristically abnormal, with irreversibly sickled cells comprising 5–50% of red cells. Other findings include reticulocytosis (10–25%), nucleated red blood cells, and hallmarks of hyposplenism such as Howell-Jolly bodies and target cells. The white blood cell count is characteristically elevated to 12,000–15,000/μL, and thrombocytosis may occur. Indirect bilirubin levels are high.

Most clinical laboratories offer a screening test for sickle cell hemoglobin, and the diagnosis of sickle cell anemia is then confirmed by hemoglobin electrophoresis (Table 13–9). Hemoglobin S has an abnormal migration pattern on electrophoresis and will usually comprise 85–98% of hemoglobin. In ho-

Table 13–9. Hemoglobin distribution in sickle cell syndromes.

Genotype	Clinical Diagnosis	Hb A	Hb S	Hb A_2	Hb F
AA	Normal	97–99%	0	1–2%	< 1%
AS	Sickle trait	60%	40%	1–2%	< 1%
SS	Sickle cell anemia	0	86–98%	1–3%	5–15%
S β^0 thalassemia	Sickle β thalassemia	0	70–80%	3–5%	10–20%
S β^+ thalassemia	Sickle β thalassemia	10–20%	60–75%	3–5%	10–20%
AS, α thalassemia	Sickle trait	70–75%	25–30%	1–2%	< 1%

mozygous S disease, no hemoglobin A will be present. Hemoglobin F levels are variably increased, and high hemoglobin F levels are associated with a more benign clinical course.

Treatment

No specific treatment is available for the primary disease. Patients are maintained on folic acid supplementation and given transfusions for aplastic or hemolytic crises. Pneumococcal vaccination reduces the incidence of infections with this pathogen.

When acute painful episodes occur, precipitating factors should be identified and infections treated if present. The patient should be kept well hydrated, and oxygen should be given if the patient is hypoxic.

Acute vaso-occlusive crises can be treated with exchange transfusion. These are primarily indicated for the treatment of intractable pain crises, priapism, and stroke.

Cytotoxic agents such as hydroxyurea have been shown to increase hemoglobin F levels (by stimulating erythropoiesis in more primitive erythroid precursors). Hydroxyurea (500–750 mg/d) reduces the frequency of painful crises and is now indicated in patients whose quality of life is disrupted by frequent pain crises. Long-term safety is uncertain, and concern remains about the potential of secondary malignancies. Allogeneic bone marrow transplantation is being studied as a possible curative option for severely affected young patients.

Bunn FH: Pathogenesis and treatment of sickle cell disease. N Engl J Med 1997;337:762. [NLM Cit ID: 97413579]

Steinberg MH: Management of sickle cell disease. N Engl J Med 1999;340:1021. [NLM Cit ID: 99182218]

Vichinsky EP et al: Acute chest syndrome in sickle cell disease: Clinical presentation and course. Blood 1997; 89:1787. [NLM Cit ID: 97210591]

Walters MC: Collaborative multicenter investigation of marrow transplantation for sickle cell disease: Current results and future directions. Biol Blood Marrow Transplant 1997;3:30. [NLM Cit ID: 98161403]

SICKLE CELL TRAIT

Patients with the heterozygous genotype (AS) have sickle cell trait. These persons are clinically normal and have acute painful episodes only under extreme conditions such as vigorous exertion at high altitudes (or in unpressurized aircraft). The patients are hematologically normal, with no anemia and normal red blood cells on peripheral blood smear. They may, however, have a defect in renal tubular function, causing an inability to concentrate the urine, and experience episodes of gross hematuria. A screening test for sickle hemoglobin will be positive, and hemoglobin electrophoresis will reveal that approximately 40% of hemoglobin is hemoglobin S (Table 13–9).

No treatment is necessary. Genetic counseling is a reasonable strategy.

Brewer GJ: Risks in sickle cell trait. J Lab Clin Med 1993;122:354. [NLM Cit ID: 94045156]

SICKLE THALASSEMIA

Patients with homozygous sickle cell anemia and alpha thalassemia have a somewhat milder form of hemolysis because of a slower rate of sickling related to reduced hemoglobin concentration (MCHC) within the red blood cell.

Patients who are double heterozygotes for sickle cell anemia and beta thalassemia are clinically affected with sickle cell syndromes. Sickle β^0 thalassemia is clinically very similar to homozygous SS disease. Vaso-occlusive crises may be somewhat less severe, and the spleen is usually not infarcted. Hematologically, the MCV is usually low, in contrast to the normal MCV of sickle cell anemia. Hemoglobin electrophoresis (Table 13–9) reveals no hemoglobin A but will show an increase in hemoglobin A_2 which is not present in sickle cell anemia.

Sickle β^+ thalassemia is a milder disorder than homozygous SS disease, with fewer crises. The spleen is usually palpable. The hemolytic anemia is less severe, and the hematocrit is usually 30–38%, with reticulocytes of 5–10%. Hemoglobin electrophoresis shows the presence of some hemoglobin A.

HEMOGLOBIN C DISORDERS

Hemoglobin C is formed by a single amino acid substitution at the same site of substitution as in sickle hemoglobin but with lysine instead of valine substituted for glutamine at the β_6 position. Hemoglobin C is nonsickling but may participate in polymer formation in association with hemoglobin S. Homozygous hemoglobin C disease produces a mild hemolytic anemia with splenomegaly, mild jaundice, and pigment (calcium bilirubinate) gallstones. The peripheral blood smear shows generalized red cell targeting and occasional cells with rectangular crystals of hemoglobin C. Persons heterozygous for hemoglobin C are clinically normal.

Patients with hemoglobin SC disease are double heterozygotes for beta S and beta C. These patients, like those with sickle β^+ thalassemia, have a milder hemolytic anemia and milder clinical course than those with homozygous SS disease. There are fewer vaso-occlusive events, and the spleen remains palpable in adult life. However, persons with hemoglobin SC disease have more retinopathy and more ischemic necrosis of bone than those with SS disease. The hematocrit is usually 30–38%, with 5–10% reticulocytes and few irreversibly sickled cells on the blood smear. Target cells are more numerous than in SS disease. Hemoglobin electrophoresis will show approximately 50% hemoglobin C, 50% hemoglobin S, and no increase in hemoglobin F levels.

Olson JF et al: Hemoglobin C disease in infancy and childhood. J Pediatr 1994,125(5 Part 1):745. [NLM Cit ID: 95054779]

UNSTABLE HEMOGLOBINS

Unstable hemoglobins are prone to oxidative denaturation even in the presence of a normal G6PD system. The disorder is autosomal dominant and of variable severity. Most patients have a mild chronic hemolytic anemia with splenomegaly, mild jaundice, and pigment (calcium bilirubinate) gallstones. Less severely affected patients are not anemic except under conditions of oxidative stress.

The diagnosis is made by the finding of Heinz bodies and a normal G6PD level. Hemoglobin electrophoresis is usually normal, since these hemoglobins characteristically do not have a change in their migration pattern. These hemoglobins precipitate in isopropanol. Usually no treatment is necessary. Patients with chronic hemolytic anemia should receive folate supplementation and avoid known oxidative drugs. In rare cases, splenectomy may be required.

AUTOIMMUNE HEMOLYTIC ANEMIA

Essentials of Diagnosis

- Acquired anemia caused by IgG autoantibody.
- Spherocytes and reticulocytosis on peripheral blood smear.
- Positive Coombs test.

General Considerations

Autoimmune hemolytic anemia is an acquired disorder in which an IgG autoantibody is formed that binds to the red blood cell membrane. The antibody is most commonly directed against a basic component of the Rh system present on virtually all human red blood cells. When IgG antibodies coat the red blood cell, the Fc portion of the antibody is recognized by macrophages present in the spleen and other portions of the reticuloendothelial system. The interaction between splenic macrophage and the antibody-coated red blood cell results in removal of red blood cell membrane and the formation of a spherocyte because of the decrease in surface-to-volume ratio of the red blood cell. These spherocytic cells have decreased deformability and become trapped in the red pulp of the spleen because of their inability to squeeze through the 2-μm fenestrations. When large amounts of IgG are present on red blood cells, complement may be fixed. Direct lysis of cells is rare, but the presence of C3b on the surface of red blood cells allows Kupffer cells in the liver to participate in the hemolytic process because of the presence of C3b receptors on Kupffer cells.

Approximately half of all cases of autoimmune hemolytic anemia are idiopathic. The disorder may also be seen in association with systemic lupus erythematosus, chronic lymphocytic leukemia, or lymphomas. It must be distinguished from drug-induced hemolytic anemia. Methyldopa commonly stimulates the production of an autoantibody with the same specificity as that in idiopathic autoimmune hemolytic anemia. Other drugs (penicillin, quinidine) coat the red blood cell membrane, and the antibody is directed against the membrane-drug complex.

The Coombs antiglobulin test forms the basis for diagnosis of these immune hemolytic disorders. The Coombs reagent is a rabbit IgM antibody raised against human IgG or human complement. The direct Coombs test is performed by mixing the patient's red blood cells with the Coombs reagent and looking for agglutination, which indicates the presence of antibody on the red blood cell surface. The indirect Coombs test is performed by mixing the patient's serum with a panel of type O red blood cells. After incubation of the test serum and panel red blood cells, the Coombs reagent is added. Agglutination in this system indicates the presence of free antibody in the patient's serum. Because the traditional Coombs test relies on visible agglutination as an end point, the test is not very sensitive and will not detect immune hemolytic anemias in which only a small amount of IgG is present on red blood cells. More sensitive tests (micro-Coombs) are now available.

Clinical Findings

A. Symptoms and Signs: Autoimmune hemolytic anemia typically produces an anemia of rapid onset that may be life-threatening in severity. Patients complain of fatigue and may present with angina or congestive heart failure. On examination, jaundice and splenomegaly are usually present. If the patient has an underlying disorder such as systemic lupus erythematosus or chronic lymphocytic leukemia, features of these diseases may be present.

B. Laboratory Findings: The anemia is of variable severity but may be severe, with hematocrit of less than 10%. Reticulocytosis is usually present, and spherocytes are seen on the peripheral blood smear. In cases of severe hemolysis, the stressed bone marrow may also release nucleated red blood cells. As with other hemolytic disorders, indirect bilirubin is increased. Approximately 10% of patients with autoimmune hemolytic anemia have coincident immune thrombocytopenia (Evans's syndrome).

The direct Coombs test is positive, and the indirect Coombs test may or may not be positive. A positive indirect Coombs test indicates the presence of a large amount of autoantibody that has saturated binding sites in the red blood cell and consequently appears in the serum. A patient with acquired spherocytic hemolytic anemia that may be of the autoimmune variety who has a negative Coombs test should be tested with a micro-Coombs test (which is necessary to make the diagnosis in approximately 10% of cases). Because the patient's serum usually contains the autoantibody, it may be difficult to obtain a compatible cross-match with donor's cells. Suitable donors may be selected by special laboratory methods.

Treatment

Initial treatment consists of prednisone, 1–2 mg/kg/d in divided doses. Most transfused blood will survive no more poorly than the patient's own red blood cells. However, because of difficulty in performing the cross-match, it is possible that incompatible blood will be given, and patients must be monitored during transfusion. Decisions regarding transfusions should be made in consultation with a hematologist. If prednisone is ineffective or if the disease recurs on tapering the dose, splenectomy should be performed. Patients with autoimmune hemolytic anemia refractory to prednisone and splenectomy may be treated with a variety of immunosuppressive agents, including cyclophosphamide, azathioprine, or cyclosporine. Danazol, 600–800 mg/d, may be effective, though less often than in immune thrombocytopenia.

High-dose intravenous immune globulin (500 mg/kg daily for 1–4 days) may be highly effective in controlling hemolysis. However, the benefit is short-lived (1–3 weeks), and the drug is very expensive. Treatment with IGIV should be given only when prednisone is contraindicated.

The long-term prognosis for patients with this disorder is good. Splenectomy is often successful in controlling the disorder.

Jefferies LC: Transfusion therapy in autoimmune hemolytic anemia. Hematol Oncol Clin North Am 1994;8:1087. [NLM Cit ID: 95164340]

COLD AGGLUTININ DISEASE

Essentials of Diagnosis

- Increased reticulocytes and spherocytes on peripheral blood smear.
- Coombs test positive only for complement.
- Positive cold agglutinin test.

General Considerations

Cold agglutinin disease is an acquired hemolytic anemia due to an IgM autoantibody usually directed against the I antigen on red blood cells. These IgM autoantibodies characteristically will not react with cells at 37 °C but only at lower temperatures. Since the blood temperature (even in the most peripheral parts of the body) rarely goes lower than 20 °C, only antibodies active at higher temperatures than this will produce clinical effects. Hemolysis results indirectly from attachment of IgM, which in the cooler parts of the circulation (fingers, nose, ears) binds and fixes complement. When the red blood cell returns to a warmer temperature, the IgM antibody dissociates, leaving complement on the cell. Lysis of cells rarely occurs. Rather, C3b present on the red cells is recognized by Kupffer cells (which have receptors for C3b), and red blood cell sequestration ensues.

Most cases of chronic cold agglutinin disease are idiopathic. Others occur in association with Waldenström's macroglobulinemia, in which a monoclonal IgM paraprotein is produced. Acute postinfectious cold agglutinin disease occurs following mycoplasmal pneumonia or infectious mononucleosis (with antibody directed against antigen i rather than I).

Clinical Findings

A. Symptoms and Signs: In chronic cold agglutinin disease, symptoms related to red blood cell agglutination occur on exposure to cold, and patients may complain of mottled or numb fingers or toes. Hemolytic anemia is rarely severe, but episodic hemoglobinuria may occur on exposure to cold. The hemolytic anemia in acute postinfectious syndromes is rarely severe.

B. Laboratory Findings: Mild anemia is present with reticulocytosis and spherocytes. The direct Coombs test will be positive for complement only. Occasionally, a micro-Coombs test is necessary to reveal bound complement (low-titer cold agglutinin disease). A bedside cold agglutinin test may be performed by placing a glass slide in ice and then putting a few drops of heparinized blood on it. Inspection may reveal small clumps of agglutinated blood.

Treatment

Treatment is largely symptomatic, based on avoiding exposure to cold. Patients with severe involvement may be treated with alkylating agents such as chlorambucil. Splenectomy is ineffective, since hemolysis takes place in the liver. Prednisone is ineffective in reducing Kupffer cell function.

High-dose intravenous immunoglobulin (2 g/kg) may be effective temporarily, and interferon may be of benefit for some patients.

MICROANGIOPATHIC HEMOLYTIC ANEMIAS

The microangiopathic hemolytic anemias are a group of disorders in which red blood cell fragmentation takes place. The anemia is intravascular, producing hemoglobinemia, hemoglobinuria, and, in severe cases, methemalbuminemia. The hallmark of the disorder is the finding of fragmented red blood cells (schistocytes, helmet cells) on the peripheral blood smear.

These fragmentation syndromes can be caused by a variety of disorders (Table 13–8). Thrombotic thrombocytopenic purpura is the most important of these and is discussed below. Clinical features are variable and depend on the underlying disorder. Coagulopathy and thrombocytopenia are variably present.

Chronic microangiopathic hemolytic anemia (such as is present with a malfunctioning cardiac valve prosthesis) may cause iron deficiency anemia because of continuous low-grade hemoglobinuria.

Much-Pascual S, Samii K, Beris P: Microangiopathic hemolytic anemia complicating FK506 (tacrolimus) therapy. Am J Hematol 1996;52:310. [NLM Cit ID: 96319639]

APLASTIC ANEMIA

Essentials of Diagnosis

- Pancytopenia.
- No abnormal cells seen.
- Hypocellular bone marrow.

General Considerations

All hematopoietic cells are derived from a pluripotent stem cell that gives rise to precursors of erythroid, myeloid, and platelet forms. Injury to or suppression of this hematopoietic stem cell will result in pancytopenia. Aplastic anemia is a condition of bone marrow failure that arises from injury to or abnormal expression of the stem cell. The bone marrow becomes hypoplastic, and pancytopenia develops.

There are a number of causes of aplastic anemia (Table 13–10). Direct stem cell injury may be caused by radiation, chemotherapy, toxins, or pharmacologic agents. Systemic lupus erythematosus may rarely cause suppression of the hematopoietic stem cell by an IgG autoantibody directed against the stem cell. However, the most common pathogenesis of aplastic anemia appears to be autoimmune suppression of hematopoiesis by a T cell-mediated cellular mechanism.

Table 13–10. Causes of aplastic anemia.

Congenital (rare)
"Idiopathic" (probably autoimmune)
Systemic lupus erythematosus
Chemotherapy, radiotherapy
Toxins: benzene, toluene, insecticides
Drugs: chloramphenicol, phenylbutazone, gold salts, sulfonamides, phenytoin, carbamazepine, quinacrine, tolbutamide
Posthepatitis
Pregnancy
Paroxysmal nocturnal hemoglobinuria

Clinical Findings

A. Symptoms and Signs: Patients come to medical attention because of the consequences of bone marrow failure. Anemia leads to symptoms of weakness and fatigue; neutropenia causes vulnerability to bacterial infections; and thrombocytopenia results in mucosal and skin bleeding. Physical examination may reveal signs of pallor, purpura, and petechiae. Other abnormalities such as hepatosplenomegaly, lymphadenopathy, or bone tenderness should *not* be present, and their presence should lead one to question the diagnosis.

B. Laboratory Findings: The hallmark of aplastic anemia is pancytopenia. However, early in the evolution of aplastic anemia, only one or two cell lines may be reduced.

Anemia may be severe and is always associated with decreased reticulocytes. Red blood cell morphology is unremarkable. The MCV is usually normal but occasionally may be increased. Neutrophils and platelets are reduced in number, and no immature or abnormal forms are seen. The bone marrow aspirate and the bone marrow biopsy appear hypocellular, with only scant amounts of normal hematopoietic progenitors. No abnormal cells are seen.

Differential Diagnosis

The diagnosis of aplastic anemia is made in cases of pancytopenia with a hypocellular marrow biopsy containing no abnormal cells. Aplastic anemia must be differentiated from other causes of pancytopenia (Table 13–11). Myelodysplastic disorders or acute leukemia may occasionally be confused with aplastic anemia. These are differentiated by the presence of morphologic abnormalities or increased blasts. Hairy cell leukemia has been misdiagnosed as aplastic anemia and should be recognized by the presence of

Table 13–11. Causes of pancytopenia.

Bone marrow disorders
- Aplastic anemia
- Myelodysplasia
- Acute leukemia
- Myelofibrosis
- Infiltrative disease: lymphoma, myeloma, carcinoma, hairy cell leukemia

Megaloblastic anemia
- Nonmarrow disorders
- Hypersplenism
- Systemic lupus erythematosus
- Infection: tuberculosis, AIDS, leishmaniasis, brucellosis

splenomegaly and by abnormal lymphoid cells on the bone marrow biopsy. Pancytopenia with a normocellular bone marrow is usually due to systemic lupus erythematosus, disseminated infection, or hypersplenism. Isolated thrombocytopenia may occur early as aplastic anemia develops and be confused with immune thrombocytopenia.

Treatment

Mild cases of aplastic anemia may be treated with supportive care. Red blood cell transfusions and platelet transfusions are given as necessary, and antibiotics are used to treat infections.

Severe aplastic anemia is defined by the presence of neutrophils less than 500/μL, platelets less than 20,000/μL, reticulocytes less than 1%, and bone marrow cellularity less than 20%. When this constellation of features is present (or three of the four), the median survival without treatment is approximately 3 months, and only 20% of patients survive for 1 year. The treatment of choice for young adults (under age 50) who have HLA-matched siblings is allogeneic bone marrow transplantation. The best results are achieved in younger patients who have not had blood transfusions.

For adults over age 50 or those without HLA-matched siblings, the treatment of choice for severe aplastic anemia is immunosuppression with antithymocyte globulin (ATG) plus cyclosporine. ATG is given in the hospital in conjunction with transfusion and antibiotic support. A useful regimen is 40 mg/kg/d for 4 days in combination with cyclosporine, 6 mg/kg orally twice daily. ATG must be used in combination with corticosteroids (prednisone 1–2 mg/kg/d initially, followed by a rapid taper) to avoid complications of serum sickness. Responses usually occur in 4–12 weeks and are usually only partial, but the blood counts rise high enough to give patients a safe and transfusion-free life.

For patients in whom neutropenia is the dominant abnormality, the myeloid growth factors G-CSF (filgrastim), 5 μg/kg daily, or GM-CSF (sargramostim), 250 $\mu g/m^2/d$, may be effective in raising the neutrophil count and decreasing infections. However, they will not benefit other cell lines or provide definitive treatment.

Androgens have been widely used in the past, with a low response rate. However, a few patients can be maintained successfully with this form of treatment. One regimen is oxymetholone, 2–3 mg/kg orally daily. In the rare syndrome of systemic lupus erythematosus causing humorally mediated aplastic anemia, the combination of plasmapheresis and high-dose prednisone may be successful.

Course & Prognosis

Patients with severe aplastic anemia have a rapidly fatal illness if left untreated. Allogeneic bone marrow transplantation is highly successful in previously untransfused children and young adults with HLA-matched siblings. For this group of patients, the durable complete response rate exceeds 80%. For older adults or those who have previously been exposed to blood products, long-term survival rates are approaching 80% with new preparative regimens for transplantation giving the improved results due to a lower risk of graft rejection. ATG treatment leads to partial response in approximately 60% of adults, and the long-term prognosis of responders appears to be good. There is increasing evidence that some fraction (as many at 25%) of these nontransplanted patients may develop clonal hematologic disorders such as paroxysmal nocturnal hemoglobinuria or myelodysplasia after many years of follow-up.

Deeg HJ: Long-term outcome after marrow transplantation for severe aplastic anemia. Blood 1998;91:3637. [NLM Cit ID: 98241406]

Marsh J: Prospective randomized multicenter study comparing cyclosporin alone versus the combination of antithymocyte globulin and cyclosporin for treatment of patients with nonsevere aplastic anemia: a report from the European Blood and Marrow Transplant (EBMT) severe aplastic anemia working party. Blood 1999;93:2191. [NLM Cit ID: 99192433]

Tichelli A: Effectiveness of immunosuppressive therapy in older patients with aplastic anemia. Ann Intern Med 1999;130:193. [NLM Cit ID: 99149982]

Young NS: The pathophysiology of acquired aplastic anemia. N Engl J Med 1997;336:1365. [NLM Cit ID: 97263439]

NEUTROPENIA

Neutropenia exists when the neutrophil count falls below 1500/μL. However, blacks and other specific population groups may normally have neutrophil counts as low as 1200/μL. The neutropenic patient is increasingly vulnerable to infection by gram-positive and gram-negative bacteria and by fungi. The risk of infection is related to the severity of neutropenia. Patients with "chronic benign neutropenia" are free of infection for years despite very low neutrophil levels.

A variety of bone marrow disorders and nonmarrow conditions may cause neutropenia (Table 13–12). All the causes of aplastic anemia (Table 13–10) and pancytopenia (Table 13–11) may cause neutropenia. Isolated neutropenia is often due to an idiosyncratic reaction to a drug, and agranulocytosis (complete absence of neutrophils in the peripheral blood) is almost always due to a drug reaction. In these cases, examination of the bone marrow shows virtual absence of myeloid precursors, with other cell lines undisturbed. Pure white cell aplasia is a rare condition in which an autoantibody is formed against myeloid progenitors. **Felty's syndrome**—immune neutropenia associated with seropositive nodular rheumatoid arthritis and splenomegaly—is another cause. Neutropenia in the presence of a normal bone marrow may be due to immunologic peripheral destruction, sepsis, or hypersplenism. Severe neutropenia may be associated with clonal disorders of T lymphocytes, often with the morphology of large granular lymphocytes.

Clinical Findings

Neutropenia results in stomatitis and in infections due to gram-positive or gram-negative aerobic bacteria or to fungi such as candida or aspergillus. The most common infections are septicemia, cellulitis, and pneumonia. In the presence of severe neutropenia, the usual signs of inflammatory response to infection may be absent. Nevertheless, fever in the neutropenic patient should always be assumed to be of infectious origin.

Treatment

Potential causative drugs are discontinued. Infections are treated with many combinations of broad-spectrum antibiotics, but particular attention should be paid to enteric gram-negative bacteria. Third-generation cephalosporins such as ceftazidime, 2 g intravenously every 8 hours, are effective as single-agent therapy.

Table 13–12. Causes of neutropenia.

Bone marrow disorders
Aplastic anemia
Pure white cell aplasia
Congenital (rare)
Cyclic neutropenia
Drugs: sulfonamides, chlorpromazine, procainamide, penicillin, cephalosporins, cimetidine, methimazole, phenytoin, chlorpropamide, antiretrovirals
Benign chronic
Peripheral disorders
Hypersplenism
Sepsis
Immune
Felty's syndrome
HIV infection
Large granular lymphocytosis

When Felty's syndrome leads to repeated bacterial infections, splenectomy is the treatment of choice. It usually leads to healing of leg ulcers and to reduction in the rate of infection whether or not the neutrophil count rises.

The prognosis of patients with neutropenia depends on the underlying cause. Most patients with drug-induced agranulocytosis can be supported with broad-spectrum antibiotics and will recover completely. With improved antibacterial antibiotics, the prognosis of these patients has improved considerably. For selected low-risk patients, outpatient management with oral antibiotics or daily intravenous antibiotics may be feasible. The myeloid growth factors G-CSF (filgrastim) and GM-CSF (sargramostim) may be useful in shortening the duration of neutropenia associated with chemotherapy. The neutropenia associated with large granular lymphocytes has been reported to improve in response to cyclosporine therapy.

Pizzo PA: Fever in immunocompromised patients. N Engl J Med 1999;341:893. [NLM Cit ID: 99404889]

Sood R: Neutropenia associated with T-cell large granular lymphocyte leukemia: long-term response to cyclosporine therapy despite persistence of abnormal cells. Blood 1998;91:3372. [NLM Cit ID: 98226697]

Welte K, Dale D: Pathophysiology and treatment of severe chronic neutropenia. Ann Hematol 1996;72:158. [NLM Cit ID: 96210963]

LEUKEMIAS & OTHER MYELOPROLIFERATIVE DISORDERS

Myeloproliferative disorders are due to acquired clonal abnormalities of the hematopoietic stem cell. Since the stem cell gives rise to myeloid, erythroid, and platelet cells, one sees qualitative and quantitative changes in all these cell lines. In some disorders (chronic myelogenous leukemia), specific characteristic chromosomal changes are seen. In others, no characteristic cytogenetic abnormalities are seen.

Classically, the myeloproliferative disorders produce characteristic syndromes with well-defined clinical and laboratory features (Tables 13–13 and

Table 13–13. Classification of myeloproliferative disorders.

Myeloproliferative syndromes
Polycythemia vera
Myelofibrosis
Essential thrombocytosis
Chronic myeloid leukemia
Myelodysplastic syndromes
Acute myeloid leukemia

Table 13–14). However, these disorders are grouped together because the disease may evolve from one form into another and because hybrid disorders are commonly seen. All of the myeloproliferative disorders may progress to acute myelogenous leukemia.

POLYCYTHEMIA VERA

Essentials of Diagnosis

- Increased red blood cell mass.
- Splenomegaly.
- Normal arterial oxygen saturation.
- Usually elevated white blood count and platelet count.

General Considerations

Polycythemia vera is an acquired myeloproliferative disorder that causes overproduction of all three hematopoietic cell lines, most prominently the red blood cells. The hematocrit is elevated (at sea level) when values exceed 54% in males or 51% in females (Table 13–15).

When the hematocrit is elevated, the red blood cell mass should be measured to determine whether true polycythemia or relative polycythemia exists. Normal values for red blood cell mass are 26–34 mL/kg in men and 21–29 mL/kg in women. Relative ("spurious") polycythemia presents in middle-aged men who are overweight and hypertensive (often on diuretic therapy); the hematocrit is almost always less than 60%; they have a high normal red cell mass and a low-normal plasma volume.

If the red blood cell mass is increased, one must determine whether the increase is primary or secondary. Primary polycythemia (polycythemia vera) is a bone marrow disorder characterized by autonomous overproduction of erythroid cells. Erythroid production is independent of erythropoietin, and the serum erythropoietin level is low. In vitro, erythroid progenitor cells grow without added erythropoietin, a finding not seen in normal individuals.

Polycythemia vera is a relatively common disorder. Sixty percent of patients are male, and the median age at presentation is 60. Polycythemia rarely occurs under age 40.

Clinical Findings

A. Symptoms and Signs: Most patients present with symptoms related to expanded blood volume and increased blood viscosity. Common complaints include headache, dizziness, tinnitus, blurred vision, and fatigue. Generalized pruritus, especially that occurring following a warm shower or bath, may be a striking symptom and is related to histamine release from the increased number of basophils present. Patients may also initially complain of epistaxis. This is probably related to engorgement of mucosal blood vessels in combination with abnormal hemostasis due to qualitative abnormalities in platelet function.

Physical examination reveals plethora and engorged retinal veins. The spleen is palpable in 75% of cases but nearly always enlarged when imaged.

Thrombosis is the most common complication of polycythemia vera and the major cause of morbidity and death in this disorder. Thrombosis appears to be related to increased blood viscosity and abnormal platelet function. Uncontrolled polycythemia leads to a very high incidence of thrombotic complications of surgery, and elective surgery should be deferred until the condition has been treated. Paradoxically, in addition to thrombosis, increased bleeding also occurs. There is a high incidence of peptic ulcer disease as well as gastrointestinal bleeding. Overproduction of uric acid may lead to hyperuricemia.

B. Laboratory Findings: The hallmark of polycythemia vera is a hematocrit above normal, at times greater than 60%. Red blood cell morphology is normal. By definition, the red blood cell mass is elevated. The white blood count is elevated to 10,000–20,000/μL and the platelet count is variably increased, sometimes to counts exceeding 1,000,000/μL. Platelet morphology is usually normal. White blood cells are usually normal, but basophilia and eosinophilia are frequently present.

The bone marrow is hypercellular, with panhyperplasia of all hematopoietic elements. Iron stores are usually absent from the bone marrow, having been transferred to the increased circulating red blood cell mass. Iron deficiency may also result from chronic gastrointestinal blood loss. Bleeding may lower the hematocrit to the normal range (or lower), creating diagnostic confusion.

Vitamin B_{12} levels are strikingly elevated because of increased levels of transcobalamin III (secreted by white blood cells). The leukocyte alkaline phosphatase is elevated, and uric acid levels may be increased. There is no chromosomal abnormality in this disorder.

Table 13–14. Laboratory features of myeloproliferative disorders.

	White Count	Hematocrit	Platelet Count	Red Cell Morphology
Chronic myeloid leukemia	↑↑	N	N or ↑	N
Myelofibrosis	N or ↓ or ↑	N or ↓	↓ or N or ↑	Abn
Polycythemia vera	N or ↑	↑	N or ↑	N
Essential thrombocytosis	N or ↑	N	↑↑	N

Table 13–15. Causes of polycythemia.

Spurious polycythemia
Secondary polycythemia
Hypoxia: cardiac disease, pulmonary disease, high altitude
Carboxyhemoglobin: smoking
Renal lesions
Erythropoietin-secreting tumors (rare)
Abnormal hemoglobins (rare)
Polycythemia vera

Although red blood cell morphology is usually normal at presentation, microcytosis, hypochromia, and poikilocytosis may result from iron deficiency following treatment by phlebotomy (see below). Progressive hypersplenism may also lead to elliptocytosis.

Differential Diagnosis

Spurious polycythemia, in which an elevated hematocrit is due to contracted plasma volume rather than increased red cell mass, may be related to diuretic use or may occur without obvious cause.

A secondary cause of polycythemia should be suspected if splenomegaly is absent and the high hematocrit is not accompanied by increases in other cell lines. Arterial oxygen saturation should be measured to determine if hypoxia is the cause. A smoking history should be taken; carboxyhemoglobin levels may be elevated in smokers. A renal sonogram may be considered to look for an erythropoietin-secreting cyst or tumor. A positive family history should lead to investigation for congenital high-oxygen-affinity hemoglobin.

Polycythemia vera should be differentiated from other myeloproliferative disorders (Table 13–14). Marked elevation of the white blood count (above 30,000/μL) suggests chronic myelogenous leukemia. This disorder is confirmed by the presence of the Philadelphia chromosome. Abnormal red blood cell morphology and nucleated red blood cells in the peripheral blood are seen in myelofibrosis. This condition is diagnosed by bone marrow biopsy showing fibrosis of the marrow. Essential thrombocytosis is diagnosed when the platelet count is strikingly elevated and the red blood cell mass is normal.

Treatment

The treatment of choice is phlebotomy. One unit of blood (approximately 500 mL) is removed weekly until the hematocrit is less than 45%; the hematocrit is maintained at less than 45% by repeated phlebotomy as necessary. Because repeated phlebotomy worsens iron deficiency, the requirement for phlebotomy should gradually decrease. It is important to avoid medicinal iron supplementation, as this can thwart the goals of a phlebotomy program, and a diet low in iron may help. Maintaining the hematocrit at normal levels has been shown to decrease the incidence of thrombotic complications.

Occasionally, myelosuppressive therapy is indicated. Indications include a high phlebotomy requirement, thrombocytosis, and intractable pruritus. There is evidence that reduction of the platelet count to less than 700,000/μL will reduce the risk of thrombotic complications. Alkylating agents and radiophosphorus (^{32}P) have been shown to increase the risk of conversion of this disease to acute leukemia and should be avoided. Hydroxyurea is now being widely used when myelosuppressive therapy is indicated because of the established leukemogenic potential of alkylating agents. The usual dose is 500–1500 mg/d orally, adjusted to keep platelets < 500,000/μL without reducing the neutrophil count to < 2000/μL. Busulfan may also be used in a dose of 4–6 mg/d for 4–8 weeks, but care must be taken to avoid prolonged myelosuppression. Anagrelide is used in treatment of thrombocytosis and may prove valuable.

The role of antiplatelet agents such as aspirin in preventing thrombotic complications is controversial. High doses of aspirin (325 mg three times daily) plus dipyridamole (25 mg three times daily) cause a marked increase in gastrointestinal bleeding and should not be given routinely. However, antiplatelet treatment may be warranted in selected patients who have recurrent thromboses despite control of their platelet counts with myelosuppressive therapy. One aspirin tablet daily (325 mg) may be adequate.

Allopurinol may be indicated for hyperuricemia. Antihistamine therapy with diphenhydramine or other H_1 blockers may be helpful for control of pruritus.

Prognosis

Polycythemia is an indolent disease with median survival of 11–15 years. The major cause of morbidity and mortality is arterial thrombosis. Over time, polycythemia vera may convert to myelofibrosis or to chronic myelogenous leukemia. In approximately 5% of cases, the disorder progresses to acute myelogenous leukemia, which is usually refractory to therapy.

Lamy T: Inapparent polycythemia vera: An unrecognized diagnosis. Am J Med 1997;102:14. [NLM Cit ID: 97352938]

Najean Y: Treatment of polycythemia vera: The use of hydroxyurea and pipobroman in 292 patients under the age of 65 years. Blood 1997;90:3370. [NLM Cit ID: 98008100]

Najean Y: Treatment of polycythemia vera: Use of ^{32}P alone or in combination with maintenance therapy using hydroxyurea in 461 patients greater than 65 years of age. Blood 1997;89:2319. [NLM Cit ID: 97234675]

Nand S et al: Leukemogenic risk of hydroxyurea therapy in polycythemia vera, essential thrombocythemia, and myeloid metaplasia with myelofibrosis. Am J Hematol 1996;52.42. [NLM Cit ID: 96219907]

Polycythemia vera: The natural history of 1213 patients followed for 20 years. Gruppo Italiano Studio Policitemia. Ann Intern Med 1995;123:656. [NLM Cit ID: 96011273]

ESSENTIAL THROMBOCYTOSIS

Essentials of Diagnosis

- Elevated platelet count in absence of other causes.
- Normal red blood cell mass.
- Absence of Philadelphia chromosome.

General Considerations

Essential thrombocytosis is an uncommon myeloproliferative disorder of unknown cause in which marked proliferation of the megakaryocytes in the bone marrow leads to elevation of the platelet count.

Clinical Findings

A. Symptoms and Signs: The median age at presentation is 50–60 years, and there is a slightly increased incidence in women. Most commonly, the initial presentation is with thrombosis. Less commonly, the first finding is an elevated platelet count in an asymptomatic person without risk factors for vascular disease.

The most common clinical problem is thrombosis. The risk of thrombosis rises with age. Venous thromboses may occur in unusual sites such as the mesenteric, hepatic, or portal vein. Some patients experience erythromelalgia, painful burning of the hands accompanied by erythema; this symptom is reliably relieved by aspirin. Bleeding, typically mucosal, is less common and is related to a concomitant qualitative platelet defect. Splenomegaly is present in at least 25% of patients.

B. Laboratory Findings: An elevated platelet count is the hallmark of this disorder, and the count may be markedly elevated to over 2,000,000/μL. The white blood cell count is often mildly elevated, usually not above 30,000/μL, but with some immature myeloid forms. The hematocrit is normal. The peripheral blood smear reveals large platelets, but giant degranulated forms seen in myelofibrosis are not observed. Red blood cell morphology is normal. The bleeding time is prolonged in 20% of patients.

The bone marrow shows increased numbers of megakaryocytes but no other morphologic abnormalities. The Philadelphia chromosome is absent.

Differential Diagnosis

Essential thrombocytosis must be distinguished from secondary causes of an elevated platelet count. In reactive thrombocytosis, the platelet count seldom exceeds 1,000,000/μL. Inflammatory disorders such as rheumatoid arthritis and ulcerative colitis cause significant elevations of the platelet count, as may chronic infection. The thrombocytosis of iron deficiency is observed only when anemia is significant. The platelet count is temporarily elevated after splenectomy.

Regarding other myeloproliferative disorders, the lack of elevated hematocrit and red blood cell mass distinguishes it from polycythemia vera. Unlike myelofibrosis, red blood cell morphology is normal, nucleated red blood cells are absent, and giant degranulated platelets are not seen. In chronic myeloid leukemia, the Philadelphia chromosome establishes the diagnosis.

Treatment

The risk of thrombosis can be reduced by control of the platelet count, and one should aim to keep it less than 500,000/μL. Standard therapy has consisted of hydroxyurea in a dose of 0.5–2 g/d. In some cases this is not effective because of dose-limiting neutropenia. Anagrelide is highly effective in a dose of 2–4 mg/d but may cause headache, mild anemia, and peripheral edema, and in high doses congestive heart failure. Alpha interferon may control the platelet count but is often associated with bothersome symptoms of malaise and myalgias if the dose exceeds 2 million units three times weekly.

Vasomotor symptoms such as erythromelalgia and paresthesias respond well to control of the platelet count. In the unusual event of severe bleeding, the platelet count should be *lowered* emergently with plateletpheresis.

Course & Prognosis

Essential thrombocytosis is an indolent disorder and allows long-term survival. Average survival is longer than 15 years from diagnosis. The major source of morbidity—thrombosis—can be reduced by appropriate platelet control. Late in the course of the disease, the bone marrow may become fibrotic, and massive splenomegaly may occur, sometimes with splenic infarction. There is a 5% risk of transformation to acute leukemia over 20 years.

Harrison CN: A large proportion of patients with a diagnosis of essential thrombocytosis do not have a clonal disorder and may be at lower risk of thrombotic complications. Blood 1999;93:417. [NLM Cit ID: 99102371]

Sterkers Y: Acute myeloid leukemia and myelodysplastic syndromes following essential thrombocythemia treated with hydroxyurea: High proportion of cases with 17p deletion. Blood 1998;91:616. [NLM Cit ID: 98102444]

MYELOFIBROSIS

Essentials of Diagnosis

- Striking splenomegaly.
- Teardrop poikilocytosis on peripheral smear.
- Leukoerythroblastic blood picture; giant abnormal platelets.
- Hypercellular bone marrow with reticulin or collagen fibrosis.

General Considerations

Myelofibrosis (myelofibrosis with myeloid metaplasia, agnogenic myeloid metaplasia) is a myeloproliferative disorder characterized by fibrosis of the bone marrow, splenomegaly, and a leukoerythroblastic peripheral blood picture with teardrop poikilocytosis. It is widely believed that fibrosis occurs in response to increased secretion of platelet-derived growth factor (PDGF) and possibly other cytokines. In response to bone marrow fibrosis, extramedullary hematopoiesis takes place in the liver, spleen, and lymph nodes. In these sites, mesenchymal cells responsible for fetal hematopoiesis can be reactivated.

Clinical Findings

A. Symptoms and Signs: Myelofibrosis develops in adults over age 50 and is usually insidious in onset. Patients most commonly present with fatigue due to anemia or abdominal fullness related to splenomegaly. Uncommon presentations include bleeding and bone pain. On examination, splenomegaly is almost invariably present and is commonly massive. The liver is enlarged in more than half of cases.

Later in the course of the disease, progressive bone marrow failure takes place as it becomes progressively more fibrotic. Anemia becomes severe, requiring transfusion. Progressive thrombocytopenia leads to bleeding. The spleen continues to enlarge, which leads to early satiety. Painful episodes of splenic infarction may occur. Late in the course, the patient becomes cachectic and may experience severe bone pain, especially in the upper legs. Hematopoiesis in the liver leads to portal hypertension with ascites, esophageal varices, and occasionally transverse myelitis caused by myelopoiesis in the epidural space.

B. Laboratory Findings: Patients are almost invariably anemic at presentation. The white blood count is variable—either low, normal, or elevated—and may be increased to 50,000/μL. The platelet count is variable. The peripheral blood smear is dramatic, with significant poikilocytosis and numerous teardrop forms in the red cell line. Nucleated red blood cells are present and the myeloid series is shifted, with immature forms including a small percentage of promyelocytes or myeloblasts. Platelet morphology may be bizarre, and giant degranulated platelet forms (megakaryocyte fragments) may be seen. The triad of teardrop poikilocytosis, leukoerythroblastic blood, and giant abnormal platelets is highly suggestive of myelofibrosis.

The bone marrow usually cannot be aspirated (dry tap), though early in the course of the disease it is hypercellular, with a marked increase in megakaryocytes. Fibrosis at this stage is detected by a silver stain demonstrating increased reticulin fibers. Later, biopsy reveals more severe fibrosis, with eventual replacement of hematopoietic precursors by collagen. There is no characteristic chromosomal abnormality.

Differential Diagnosis

A leukoerythroblastic blood picture from other causes may be seen in response to severe infection, inflammation, or infiltrative bone marrow processes. However, teardrop poikilocytosis and giant abnormal platelet forms will not be present. Bone marrow fibrosis may be seen in metastatic carcinoma, Hodgkin's disease, and hairy cell leukemia. These disorders are diagnosed by characteristic morphology of involved tissues.

Concerning other myeloproliferative disorders, chronic myelogenous leukemia is diagnosed when there is marked leukocytosis, normal red blood cell morphology, and the presence of the Philadelphia chromosome. Polycythemia vera is characterized by an elevated red blood cell mass. Essential thrombocytosis shows predominant and consistent platelet count elevations.

Treatment

There is no specific treatment for this disorder. Anemic patients are supported with transfusion. Androgens such as oxymetholone, 200 mg orally daily, or testosterone reduce the transfusion requirement in one-third of cases but are poorly tolerated by women. Splenectomy is not routinely performed but is indicated for splenic enlargement causing recurrent painful episodes, severe thrombocytopenia, or an unacceptable transfusion requirement. Alpha interferon (2–5 million units subcutaneously three times weekly) leads to subjective and objective improvement in some cases. Allogeneic bone marrow transplantation has been performed successfully with 50% long-term survival.

Course & Prognosis

It is often hard to date the onset of myelofibrosis, but the median survival from time of diagnosis is approximately 5 years. End-stage myelofibrosis is a wasting illness characterized by generalized debility, liver failure, and bleeding from thrombocytopenia. Some cases may terminate in acute myelogenous leukemia.

Bourantas KL et al: Combination therapy with recombinant human erythropoietin, interferon-alpha-2b and granulocyte-macrophage colony-stimulating factor in idiopathic myelofibrosis. Acta Haematol 1996;96:79. [NLM Cit ID: 96328245]

Guardiola P: Allogeneic stem cell transplantation for agnogenic myeloid metaplasia: a European Group for Blood and Marrow Transplantation, Societé Française de Greffe de Moelle, Gruppo Italiano per il Trapianto del Midollo Osseo, and Fred Hutchinson Cancer Research Center collaborative study. Blood 1999;93:2831. [NLM Cit ID: 99233644]

Nand S et al: Leukemogenic risk of hydroxyurea therapy in polycythemia vera, essential thrombocythemia, and myeloid metaplasia with myelofibrosis. Am J Hematol 1996;52:42. [NLM Cit ID: 96219907]

CHRONIC MYELOGENOUS LEUKEMIA

Essentials of Diagnosis

- Strikingly elevated white blood count.
- Markedly left-shifted myeloid series but with a low percentage of promyelocytes and blasts.

- Presence of Philadelphia chromosome or *bcr-abl* gene.

General Considerations

Chronic myelogenous leukemia is a myeloproliferative disorder characterized by overproduction of myeloid cells. These myeloid cells retain the capacity for differentiation, and normal bone marrow function is retained during the early phases. The disease usually remains stable for years and then transforms to a more overtly malignant disease.

Chronic myelogenous leukemia is associated with a characteristic chromosomal abnormality, the Philadelphia chromosome, and was the first disease associated with a specific karyotypic abnormality. The Philadelphia chromosome is now recognized to be a reciprocal translocation between the long arms of chromosomes 9 and 22. A large portion of 22q is translocated to 9q, and a smaller piece of 9q is moved to 22q. The portion of 9q that is translocated contains *abl,* a proto-oncogene that is the cellular homolog of the Ableson murine leukemia virus. The *abl* gene is received at a specific site on 22q, the break point cluster (bcr). The fusion gene *bcr-abl* produces a novel protein that differs from the normal transcript of the *abl* gene in that it possesses tyrosine kinase activity (a characteristic activity of transforming genes). Evidence that the *bcr/abl* fusion gene is pathogenic is provided by transgenic mouse models in which introduction of the gene almost invariably leads to leukemia.

Usually at the time of diagnosis, the Philadelphia chromosome-positive clone dominates and may be the only one detected. However, a normal clone is present and may express itself either in vivo, after certain forms of therapy, or in vitro, in long-term bone marrow cultures. Approximately 5% of cases of chronic myelogenous leukemia are Philadelphia chromosome-negative at the level of light microscope cytogenetics, though molecular studies demonstrate the *bcr/abl* fusion gene. The entity formerly known as Philadelphia chromosome-negative CML is now recognized as chronic myelomonocytic leukemia (CMML), a subtype of myelodysplasia.

Early chronic myelogenous leukemia ("chronic phase") does not behave like a malignant disease. Normal bone marrow function is retained, white blood cells differentiate, and, despite some qualitative abnormalities (low leukocyte alkaline phosphatase), the neutrophils combat infection normally. However, chronic myelogenous leukemia is inherently unstable, and the disease progresses to accelerated phase and finally after several years, to blast crisis. This progression of the disease is often associated with added chromosomal defects superimposed on the Philadelphia chromosome. Blast crisis chronic myelogenous leukemia is morphologically indistinguishable from acute leukemia.

Clinical Findings

A. Symptoms and Signs: Chronic myelogenous leukemia is a disorder of middle age (median age at presentation is 42 years). Patients usually present with fatigue, night sweats, and low-grade fever related to the hypermetabolic state caused by overproduction of white blood cells. At other times, the patient complains of abdominal fullness related to splenomegaly, or an elevated white blood count is discovered incidentally. Rarely, the patient will present with a clinical syndrome related to leukostasis with blurred vision, respiratory distress, or priapism. The white blood count in these cases is usually greater than 500,000/μL.

On examination, the spleen is enlarged (often markedly so), and sternal tenderness may be present as a sign of marrow overexpansion.

Acceleration of the disease is often associated with fever in the absence of infection, bone pain, and splenomegaly. In blast crisis, patients may experience bleeding and infection related to bone marrow failure.

B. Laboratory Findings: The hallmark of chronic myelogenous leukemia is an elevated white blood count; the median white blood count at diagnosis is 150,000/μL. The peripheral blood is characteristic. The myeloid series is left-shifted, with mature forms dominating and with cells usually present in proportion to their degree of maturation. Blasts are usually less than 5%. Basophilia and eosinophilia of granulocytes may be present. At presentation, the patient is usually not anemic. Red blood cell morphology is normal, and nucleated red blood cells are rarely seen. The platelet count may be normal or elevated (sometimes to strikingly high levels). Platelet morphology is usually normal, but abnormally large forms may be seen.

The bone marrow is hypercellular, with left-shifted myelopoiesis. Myeloblasts comprise less than 5% of marrow cells.

The leukocyte alkaline phosphatase score is invariably low and is a sign of qualitative abnormalities in neutrophils. The vitamin B_{12} level is usually elevated because of increased secretion of transcobalamin III, and uric acid levels may be high. The Philadelphia chromosome may be detected in either the peripheral blood or the bone marrow. The *bcr-abl* gene may be reliably found in peripheral blood by molecular techniques.

With progression to the accelerated and blast phases, progressive anemia and thrombocytopenia occur, and the percentage of blasts in the blood and bone marrow increases. Blast phase chronic myelogenous leukemia is diagnosed when blasts comprise more than 30% of bone marrow cells.

Differential Diagnosis

Early chronic myelogenous leukemia must be differentiated from the reactive leukocytosis associated with infection. In such cases, the white blood count is usually less than 50,000/μL, splenomegaly is absent, the leukocyte alkaline phosphatase is increased, and the Philadelphia chromosome is not present.

Chronic myelogenous leukemia must be distinguished from other myeloproliferative disease (Table 13–14). The hematocrit should not be elevated, the red blood cell morphology is normal, and nucleated red blood cells are rare or absent. Definitive diagnosis is made by finding the Philadelphia chromosome or *bcr-abl*.

Treatment

Treatment is usually not emergent even with white blood counts over 200,000/μL, since the majority of circulating cells are mature myeloid cells that are smaller and more deformable than primitive leukemic blasts. In the rare instances in which symptoms result from extreme hyperleukocytosis (priapism, respiratory distress, visual blurring, altered mental status), emergent leukapheresis is performed in conjunction with myelosuppressive therapy.

Hydroxyurea was formerly the standard treatment for this disease. It has the advantages of being inexpensive, without side effects, and taken by mouth. The usual dose is 0.5–2.5 g/d, adjusted to keep the white blood cell count ideally near 5000/μL but in any case above 2000/μL. Hydroxyurea must be given without interruption, since the white blood count will rise within days after discontinuing this medication. The response is usually gratifying: the white count decreases, the spleen becomes smaller, and symptoms disappear. Most patients in the chronic phase of chronic myelogenous leukemia will have no symptoms either from the disease or their chemotherapy.

Recombinant alpha interferon has largely replaced hydroxyurea as the treatment of choice for chronic phase CML and should be offered to all motivated patients who are not proceeding directly to allogeneic bone marrow transplantation. In contrast to hydroxyurea, interferon prolongs the chronic phase of the disease and also prolongs survival. The combination of interferon with low doses of cytarabine may be even more effective than interferon alone. However, interferon has the disadvantages of being given by subcutaneous injection, expense, and side effects. These include fatigue, myalgias, and anorexia and can significantly impair quality of life. The best results are seen with the full dose of 5×10^6 units/m^2/d, continued for 5 years and then reduced to a lower dose. However, many patients will be unable to tolerate this dose because of constitutional symptoms. The survival benefit of interferon therapy appears to be limited to patients who achieve a cytogenetic response to the drug, ie, the appearance of Philadelphia-negative clones. This takes 12 (6–18) months to assess. Patients who achieve a complete cytogenetic response (10% of all patients) have an excellent prognosis, with 5-year survivals over 90%, and those who achieve a major response (< 35% Philadelphia-positive) also benefit with 5 year survivals over 60%. Cytogenetic nonresponders do not fare better than with hydroxyurea. Therefore, a trial of interferon therapy is usually warranted. One should determine the maximally tolerated dose and continue for at least 9 months, then assess cytogenetic response. At this point, the decision whether to continue interferon can be made.

The only available curative therapy is allogeneic bone marrow transplantation. This treatment is available for adults under age 60 who have HLA-matched siblings. Sixty percent of adults have long-term disease-free survival following bone marrow transplantation and appear to be cured of their disease. The best results (70–80% success rate) are obtained in patients who are transplanted within 1 year after initial diagnosis. All young patients should be offered allogeneic bone marrow transplantation in the chronic phase if they have suitable bone marrow donors. For young patients without sibling donors, HLA-matched unrelated donors may be located through registries of volunteer bone marrow donors (National Marrow Donors Program). Results are inferior to those achieved with matched sibling transplants but offer a cure rate of 40–60% for patients with an otherwise invariably fatal disease. We now know that allogeneic transplantation cures chronic myeloid leukemia by initial cytoreduction followed by long-term immunologic control mediated by the donor's immune system. This alloimmune phenomenon has been called the "graft-versus-leukemia" effect. The most compelling evidence for its importance is that chronic phase disease which has recurred after allogeneic transplantation can usually be reversed without additional chemotherapy by the infusion of T lymphocytes from the initial bone marrow donor. This procedure, called "donor lymphocyte infusion," can lead to long-term remission in 50–70% of cases.

Based on the appreciation of the importance of the graft-versus-leukemia effect, new and less toxic experimental forms of allogeneic transplantation have been developed that require much less initial cytoreductive therapy and rely exclusively on the immune effect for long-term disease control. If these modifications of allogeneic transplantation are validated, the role of transplantation in the management of chronic myeloid leukemia may be further expanded.

An experimental oral agent, STI 571, has recently been reported to produce remarkable results in this disease. The drug is a specifically designed inhibitor of the tyrosine kinase activity of the *bcr-abl* oncogene. Preliminary results of clinical trials appear to show excellent tolerability and low toxicity combined with nearly universal control of disease in the chronic phase. Excellent short-term results have also been seen in the more advanced phases of disease. If these results are confirmed, the therapeutic approach to chronic myeloid leukemia may undergo a significant change.

Course & Prognosis

In the past, median survival was 3–4 years. With interferon-based therapies, median survival has been increased to 5–6 years. It is possible that the investigational agent STI 571 will lead to further improvements in survival rates. At present, the only curative treatment is allogeneic bone marrow transplantation. This offers a 70% cure rate to young patients in early chronic phase.

Faderl S et al: The biology of chronic myeloid leukemia. N Engl J Med 1999;341:164. [NLM Cit ID: 99316836]

Gale RP: Survival with bone marrow transplantation versus hydroxyurea or interferon for chronic myelogenous leukemia. Blood 1998;91:1810. [NLM Cit ID: 98139479]

Lee SJ: Unrelated donor bone marrow transplantation for chronic myelogenous leukemia: A decision analysis. Ann Intern Med 1997;127:1080. [NLM Cit ID: 98049716]

Sacchi S: Early treatment decisions with interferon-alfa therapy in early chronic-phase chronic myelogenous leukemia. J Clin Oncol 1998;16:882. [NLM Cit ID: 98167594]

MYELODYSPLASTIC SYNDROMES

Essentials of Diagnosis

- Cytopenias with a hypercellular bone marrow.
- Morphologic abnormalities in two or more hematopoietic cell lines.

General Considerations

The myelodysplastic syndromes are a group of acquired clonal disorders of the hematopoietic stem cell. They are characterized by the constellation of cytopenias, a hypercellular marrow, and a number of morphologic and cytogenetic abnormalities. The disorders are usually idiopathic but may be seen after cytotoxic chemotherapy—especially mechlorethamine procarbazine for Hodgkin's disease and melphalan for multiple myeloma or ovarian carcinoma.

Despite the presence of adequate numbers of hematopoietic progenitor cells, "ineffective hematopoiesis" occurs, resulting in various cytopenias. Ultimately, the disorder may evolve into acute myelogenous leukemia, and the term "preleukemia" has been used to describe these disorders. Although no specific chromosomal abnormality is seen in myelodysplasia, there are frequently abnormalities involving the long arm of chromosome 5 (which contains a number of genes encoding both growth factors and receptors involved in myelopoiesis) as well as deletions of chromosomes 5 and 7.

Myelodysplasia encompasses several heterogeneous syndromes. Those without excess bone marrow blasts are termed "refractory anemia," with or without ringed sideroblasts. Those with excess blasts are diagnosed as "refractory anemia with excess blasts" (RAEB 5–19% blasts) and "refractory anemia with excess blasts in transition" (RAEB-T 20–29% blasts). Those with a proliferative syndrome including peripheral blood monocytosis greater than 1000/μL are termed chronic myelomonocytic leukemia (CMML).

Clinical Findings

A. Symptoms and Signs: Patients are usually over age 60. Many are diagnosed while asymptomatic because of the finding of abnormal blood counts. Patients usually present with fatigue, infection, or bleeding related to bone marrow failure. The course may be indolent, and the disease may present as a wasting illness with fever, weight loss, and general debility. On examination, splenomegaly may be present in combination with pallor, bleeding, and various signs of infection.

B. Laboratory Findings: Anemia may be marked and may require transfusion support. The MCV is normal or increased, and macro-ovalocytes may be seen on the peripheral blood smear. The reticulocyte count is usually reduced. The white blood cell count is usually normal or reduced, and neutropenia is common. The neutrophils may exhibit morphologic abnormalities, including deficient numbers of granules or a bilobed nucleus (Pelger-Huet). The myeloid series may be left-shifted, and small numbers of promyelocytes or blasts may be seen. The platelet count is normal or reduced, and hypogranular platelets may be present.

The bone marrow is characteristically hypercellular. Erythroid hyperplasia is common, and signs of abnormal erythropoiesis include megaloblastic features, nuclear budding, or multinucleated erythroid precursors. The Prussian blue stain may demonstrate ringed sideroblasts. The myeloid series is often left-shifted, with variable increases in blasts. Deficient or abnormal granules may be seen. A characteristic abnormality is the presence of dwarf megakaryoctyes with a unilobed nucleus.

Differential Diagnosis

In subtle cases, cytogenetic evaluation of the bone marrow may help distinguish this clonal disorder from other causes of cytopenias. As the number of blasts increases in the bone marrow, myelodysplasia is arbitrarily separated from acute myelogenous leukemia by the presence of less than 30% blasts.

Treatment

Patients affected primarily by anemia are supported with red blood cell transfusions. Those with severe neutropenia or thrombocytopenia or with marked constitutional symptoms may be treated with low-dose chemotherapy, although the results of therapy are often inadequate. Erythropoietin (epoetin alfa), 10,000 units subcutaneously three times weekly, reduces the red cell transfusion requirement in some patients. The response rate is 20% or less, but a 4-week trial of erythropoietin is reasonable since it will be of benefit and cost-effective for the subgroup of responders. The combination of myeloid growth factors and high doses of erythropoietin produces a higher response rate, but the cost is prohibitive. The myeloid growth factors G-CSF (filgrastim) and GM-CSF (sargramostim), 5 mg/kg/d, reliably raise the neutrophil count and reduce the incidence of infections. However, they do not usually benefit other cell types and appear not to change the course of the disease. The experimental drug azacitidine (5-azacytidine) has been reported to improve both symptoms and blood counts and appears to prolong the time to conversion to acute leukemia.

Patients under age 60 with matched sibling donors can be treated with ablative chemotherapy and allogeneic bone marrow transplantation. Cure rates are 30–50%.

Course & Prognosis

Myelodysplasia is an ultimately fatal disease. Patients most commonly succumb to infections or bleeding. The risk of transformation to acute myelogenous leukemia depends on the percentage of blasts in the bone marrow. Patients with refractory anemia may survive many years, and the risk of leukemia is low (< 10%). Those with excess blasts or CMML have short survivals (usually < 2 years) and have a higher (20–50%) risk of developing acute leukemia. The finding of deletions of chromosomes 5 and 7 is associated with a poor prognosis.

DeWitte T: Autologous bone marrow transplantation for patients with myelodysplastic syndrome (MDS) or acute myeloid leukemia following MDS. Blood 1997;90:3853. [NLM Cit ID: 98022776]

Greenberg P: International scoring system for evaluating prognosis in myelodysplastic syndromes. Blood 1997; 89:2079. [NLM Cit ID: 97211763]

Heaney ML: Myelodysplasias. N Engl J Med 1999;340: 1649.

Taylor KM et al: Myelodysplasia. Curr Opin Oncol 1994;6:32. [NLM Cit ID: 94264084] (Current biology, diagnosis, classification, and treatment options.)

ACUTE LEUKEMIA

Essentials of Diagnosis

- Short duration of symptoms, including fatigue, fever, and bleeding.
- Cytopenias or pancytopenia.
- More than 30% blasts in the bone marrow.
- Blasts in peripheral blood in 90%.

General Considerations

Acute leukemia is a malignancy of the hematopoietic progenitor cell. The malignant cell loses its ability to mature and differentiate. These cells proliferate in an uncontrolled fashion and replace normal bone marrow elements. Most cases arise with no clear cause. However, radiation and some toxins (benzene) are leukemogenic. In addition, a number of chemotherapeutic agents (especially procarbazine, melphalan, other alkylating agents, and etoposide) may cause leukemia. The leukemias seen after toxin or chemotherapy exposure often develop from a myelodysplastic prodrome and are associated with abnormalities in chromosomes 5 and 7.

Most of the clinical findings in acute leukemia are due to replacement of normal bone marrow elements by the malignant cell. Less common manifestations include organ infiltration (skin, gastrointestinal tract, meninges). Acute leukemia is now treatable and potentially curable with combination chemotherapy.

Acute lymphoblastic leukemia (ALL) comprises 80% of the acute leukemias of childhood. The peak incidence is between 3 and 7 years of age. It is also seen in adults, causing approximately 20% of adult acute leukemias. Acute myelogenous leukemia (AML; acute nonlymphocytic leukemia [ANLL]) is chiefly an adult disease with a median age at presentation of 50 years and an increasing incidence with advanced age.

Clinical Findings

A. Symptoms and Signs: Most patients have been ill for days or weeks. Bleeding (usually due to thrombocytopenia) occurs in the skin and mucosal surfaces, with gingival bleeding, epistaxis, or menorrhagia. Less commonly, widespread bleeding is seen in patients with disseminated intravascular coagulation (in acute promyelocytic leukemia and monocytic leukemia). Infection is due to neutropenia, with the risk of infection becoming high as the neutrophil count falls below 500/μL. Patients with neutrophil counts less than 100/μL almost invariably become infected within several days. The most common pathogens are gram-negative bacteria (*E coli*, klebsiella, pseudomonas) or fungi (candida, aspergillus). Common presentations include cellulitis, pneumonia, and perirectal infections. Septicemia in severely neutropenic patients can cause death within a few hours if treatment with appropriate antibiotics is delayed.

Patients may also seek medical attention because of gum hypertrophy and bone and joint pain. The most dramatic presentation is hyperleukocytosis, in which a markedly elevated circulating blast count (usually > 200,000/μL) leads to impaired circulation, presenting as headache, confusion, and dyspnea. Such patients require emergent leukapheresis and chemotherapy.

On examination, patients appear pale and have purpura, petechiae, and various signs of infection. Stomatitis and gum hypertrophy may be seen in patients with monocytic leukemia. There is variable enlargement of the liver, spleen, and lymph nodes. Bone tenderness may be present, particularly in the sternum, tibia, and femur.

B. Laboratory Findings: The hallmark of acute leukemia is the combination of pancytopenia with circulating blasts. However, blasts may be absent from the peripheral smear in as many as 10% of cases ("aleukemic leukemia").

The bone marrow is hypercellular and dominated by blasts. More than 30% blasts are required to make a diagnosis of acute leukemia.

A number of other laboratory abnormalities are noted. Hyperuricemia may be seen. If disseminated intravascular coagulation is present, the fibrinogen level will be reduced, the prothrombin time prolonged, and fibrin degradation products or fibrin D-dimers present. Patients with acute lymphoblastic leukemia (especially T cell) may have a mediastinal mass visible on chest radiograph. Patients with meningeal leukemia will have blasts present in the spinal fluid, as well as hypoglycorrhachia. This is seen in approximately 5% of cases at diagnosis and is more common in monocytic types of acute myelogenous leukemia.

Acute leukemia should be classified as either acute lymphoblastic or acute myelogenous leukemia, also called acute nonlymphocytic leukemia. Patients with acute myelogenous leukemia may have granules visible in the blast cells. The Auer rod, an eosinophilic needle-like inclusion in the cytoplasm, is pathognomonic of acute myelogenous leukemia. To confirm the myeloid nature of the cells, histochemical stains demonstrating myeloid enzymes such as peroxidase may be useful. Monocytic lineage can be demonstrated by the finding of butyrate esterase. Acute lymphoblastic leukemia should be considered when there is no morphologic or histochemical evidence of myeloid or monocytic lineage. The diagnosis is confirmed by demonstrating surface markers characteristic of primitive lymphoid cells. Terminal deoxynucleotidal transferase (TdT) is present in 95% of cases of acute lymphoblastic leukemia. A variety of monoclonal antibodies have been used to define other phenotypes of acute lymphoblastic leukemia. Primitive B lymphocyte antigens include CD10 and CD19. T cell acute lymphoblastic leukemia is diagnosed by the finding of CD2, CD5, and CD7.

Acute myelogenous leukemia is usually categorized on the basis of morphology and histochemistry as follows: Acute undifferentiated leukemia (M0), acute myeloblastic leukemia (M1), acute myeloblastic leukemia with differentiation (M2), acute promyelocytic leukemia (M3), acute myelomonocytic leukemia (M4), acute monoblastic leukemia (M5), erythroleukemia (M6), and megakaryoblastic leukemia (M7).

Acute lymphoblastic leukemia is most usefully classified by immunologic phenotype as follows: common, early B lineage, and T cell.

Cytogenetic studies have emerged as the most powerful prognostic factor in the acute leukemias. Favorable cytogenetics in acute myeloid leukemia include t(8;21), t(15;17), and inv(16)(p13;q22). These patients have a higher chance of achieving both short- and long-term disease control. Favorable cytogenetics in acute lymphoblastic leukemia are the hyperdiploid states. Unfavorable cytogenetics are monosomy 5 and 7, Philadelphia chromosome, and abnormalities of 11q23.

Differential Diagnosis

Acute myelogenous leukemia must be distinguished from other myeloproliferative disorders, chronic myelogenous leukemia, and myelodysplastic syndromes. Acute leukemia also resembles a left-shifted bone marrow recovering from a previous toxic insult. If the question is in doubt, a bone marrow study should be repeated in several days to see if maturation has taken place. Acute lymphoblastic leukemia must be separated from other lymphoproliferative disease such as chronic lymphocytic leukemia, lymphomas, and hairy cell leukemia. It may also be confused with the atypical lymphocytosis of mononucleosis. An experienced observer can distinguish these entities based on morphology.

Treatment

Most young patients with acute leukemia are treated with the objective of effecting a cure. The first step in treatment is to obtain complete remission, defined as normal peripheral blood with resolution of cytopenias, normal bone marrow with no excess blasts, and normal clinical status. The type of initial chemotherapy depends on the subtype of leukemia. Most patients with acute myeloid leukemia are treated with a combination of an anthracycline (daunorubicin or idarubicin) plus cytarabine. This therapy will produce complete remissions in 70–80% of patients under age 60 and in 40–60% of older patients. The treatment of patients with acute promyelocytic leukemia has been dramatically improved by the use of all-*trans* retinoic acid. This agent is an analog of vitamin A that leads to terminal differentiation of acute promyelocytic leukemia cells through an interaction with the abnormal retinoic acid receptor created by a specific chromosomal translocation which is the hallmark of the subtype of leukemia. Patients with acute promyelocytic leukemia should be treated with anthracyclines plus all-*trans* retinoic acid, and 90% will achieve complete remission. Adults with acute lymphoblastic leukemia are treated with combination chemotherapy, including daunorubicin, vincristine, prednisone, and asparaginase. This treatment produces complete remissions in 80–90% of patients.

Once a patient has entered remission, postremission therapy is given with curative intent. Options include standard chemotherapy and autologous and allogeneic transplantation. The optimal treatment strategy depends on the patient's age and clinical status and the risk factor profile of the leukemia. Acute promyelocytic leukemia is generally treated with chemotherapy plus retinoic acid, and approximately 60–70% of patients remain in long-term remission. For average-risk patients with acute myeloid leukemia, cure rates for postremission therapy are 25–30% for chemotherapy, 50% for autologous transplantation, and 50–60% for allogeneic transplantation.

Once leukemia has recurred after initial chemotherapy, the prognosis is much more guarded. For patients in second remission, transplantation (autologous or allogeneic) offers a 30–50% chance of cure. For those patients with acute promyelocytic leukemia who relapse, arsenic trioxide is a novel therapy which can produce second remissions.

Acute myelogenous leukemia is treated initially with intensive combination chemotherapy, including daunorubicin and cytarabine. Effective treatment produces aplasia of the bone marrow, which takes 2–3 weeks to recover. During this period, intensive supportive care, including transfusion and antibiotic therapy, is required. Once complete remission has been achieved, several different types of postremission therapy are potentially curative. Options include repeated intensive chemotherapy, high-dose chemoradiotherapy with allogeneic bone marrow transplantation, and high-dose chemotherapy with autologous bone marrow transplantation. Particular progress has been made in the treatment of acute promyelocytic leukemia (M3). The addition of all-*trans* retinoic acid to initial chemotherapy has improved the results of both initial treatment and long-term survival. Retinoic acid interacts with a unique fusion gene between the PML locus on chromosome 15 and the retinoic acid receptor on chromosome 17 formed in the t(15,17) translocation and appears to induce terminal differentiation in the malignant cell and hence to induce remission without cytotoxic effect. The experimental drug arsenic trioxide is an exciting new treatment that can produce remissions in patients with acute promyelocytic leukemia who have become resistant to other forms of therapy. Its role in the treatment of this subtype of leukemia is under study.

Acute lymphoblastic leukemia is treated initially with combination chemotherapy, including daunorubicin, vincristine, prednisone, and asparaginase. Remission induction therapy for acute lymphoblastic leukemia is less myelosuppressive than treatment for acute myelogenous leukemia and does not necessarily produce marrow aplasia. After achieving complete remission, patients receive central nervous system prophylaxis so that meningeal sequestration of leukemic cells does not develop. As with acute myelogenous leukemia, patients may be treated with either chemotherapy or high-dose chemotherapy plus bone marrow transplantation.

Prognosis

Approximately 70–80% of adults with acute myelogenous leukemia under age 60 achieve complete remission. High-dose postremission chemotherapy leads to cure in 30–40% of these patients, and high-dose cytarabine has been shown to be superior to therapy with lower doses. Allogeneic bone marrow transplantation (for younger adults with HLA-matched siblings) is curative in approximately 60% of cases. Autologous bone marrow transplantation is a promising new form of therapy that may cure 50–70% of patients in first remission; it may be superior to nonablative chemotherapy. Older adults with acute myelogenous leukemia reportedly achieve complete remission approximately 50% of the time.

Fenaux P et al: A randomized comparison of all trans-retinoic acid (ATRA) followed by chemotherapy and ATRA plus chemotherapy and the role of maintenance therapy in newly diagnosed acute promyelocytic leukemia. Blood 1999;94:1192. [NLM Cit ID: 99369665]

Grimwade D: The importance of diagnostic cytogenetics on outcome in AML: analysis of 1612 patients entered into the MRC AML 10 trial. Blood 1998;92:2322. [NLM Cit ID: 98421375]

Hiddemann W et al: Management of acute myeloid leukemia in elderly patients. J Clin Oncol 1999;17:3569. [NLM Cit ID: 200182373]

Kantarjian HM et al: Results of treatment with hyper-CVAD, a dose-intensive regimen, in adult acute lymphocytic leukemia. J Clin Oncol 2000;18:547. [NLM Cit ID: 20120873]

Linker CA et al: Autologous stem cell transplantation for acute myeloid leukemia in first remission. Biol Blood Marrow Transplant 2000;6:50. [NLM Cit ID: 20170272]

Lowenberg B et al: Acute myeloid leukemia. N Engl J Med 1999;341:1051. [NLM Cit ID: 99417084]

Pui C: Acute lymphoblastic leukemia. N Engl J Med 1998;339:605. [NLM Cit ID: 98361335]

Sievers EL et al: Selective ablation of acute myeloid leukemia using antibody-targed chemotherapy: a phase I study of anti-CD33 calicheamicin immunoconjugate. Blood 1999;93:3678. [NLM Cit ID: 99272410]

Soignet SL: Complete remission after treatment of acute promyelocytic leukemia with arsenic trioxide. N Engl J Med 1998;339:1341. [NLM Cit ID: 99006594]

CHRONIC LYMPHOCYTIC LEUKEMIA

Essentials of Diagnosis

- Lymphocytosis > 5000/μL.
- Mature appearance of lymphocytes.
- Co-expression of CD19, CD5.

General Considerations

Chronic lymphocytic leukemia (CLL) is a clonal malignancy of B lymphocytes (rarely T lymphocytes). The disease is usually indolent, with slowly progressive accumulation of long-lived small lymphocytes. These cells are immunoincompetent and respond poorly to antigenic stimulation.

Chronic lymphocytic leukemia is manifested clinically by immunosuppression, bone marrow failure, and organ infiltration with lymphocytes. Immunosuppression, bone marrow failure, and infiltration of organs account for most clinical manifestations. Immunodeficiency is also related to inadequate antibody production by the abnormal B cells. With advanced disease, chronic lymphocytic leukemia may cause damage by direct tissue infiltration.

Clinical Findings

A. Symptoms and Signs: Chronic lymphocytic leukemia is a disease of older patients, with 90% of cases occurring after age 50 and a median age at presentation of 65. Many patients will be incidentally discovered to have lymphocytosis. Others present with fatigue or lymphadenopathy. On examination, 80% of patients will have lymphadenopathy and half will have enlargement of the liver or spleen.

A prognostically useful staging system (Rai system) has been developed as follows: stage 0, lymphocytosis only; stage I, lymphocytosis plus lymphadenopathy; stage II, organomegaly; stage III, anemia; stage IV, thrombocytopenia.

Chronic lymphocytic leukemia usually pursues an indolent course but occasionally will present as a rapidly progressive disease. These patients usually have larger, less mature-appearing lymphocytes and are said to have "prolymphocytic" leukemia. In 5–10% of cases, chronic lymphocytic leukemia may be complicated by autoimmune hemolytic anemia or autoimmune thrombocytopenia. In approximately 5% of cases, while the systemic disease remains stable, an isolated lymph node will be transformed into an aggressive large cell lymphoma **(Richter's syndrome).**

B. Laboratory Findings: The hallmark of chronic lymphocytic leukemia is isolated lymphocytosis. The white blood count is usually greater than 20,000/μL and may be markedly elevated. Usually 75–98% of the circulating cells are lymphocytes. Lymphocytes appear small and mature, with condensed nuclear chromatin, and are morphologically indistinguishable from normal small lymphocytes. The hematocrit and platelet count are usually normal at presentation. The bone marrow is variably infiltrated with small lymphocytes. The malignant cells weakly express surface immunoglobulin, and the monoclonal nature of the cells can be demonstrated by the finding of a single light chain type on the surface. The immunophenotype of CLL is unique in that it co-expresses B lymphocyte lineage markers such as CD19 with the T lymphocyte marker CD5.

Hypogammaglobulinemia is present in half of cases and becomes more common with advanced disease. In some instances, a small amount of IgM paraprotein is present in the serum. Pathologic changes in lymph nodes are the same as in diffuse small cell lymphocytic lymphoma.

Differential Diagnosis

Few syndromes can be confused with chronic lymphocytic leukemia. Viral infections producing lymphocytosis should be obvious from the presence of fever and other clinical findings. Pertussis may cause a particularly high total lymphocyte count. Other lymphoproliferative diseases such as Waldenström's macroglobulinemia, hairy cell leukemia, or lymphoma in the leukemic phase are distinguished on the basis of the morphology of circulating lymphocytes and bone marrow.

Treatment

Most cases of early indolent chronic lymphocytic leukemia require no specific therapy. Indications for treatment include progressive fatigue, troublesome lymphadenopathy, or the development of anemia or thrombocytopenia. These patients have either symptomatic and progressive stage II disease or stage III/IV disease. The best initial treatment of CLL has become controversial. Standard treatment had been chlorambucil, 0.6–1 mg/kg orally every 3 weeks for approximately 6 months. This treatment is convenient, well tolerated, and usually effective. Fludarabine has been shown to produce a higher response rate and responses that are more complete and long-lasting. However, there is no improvement in overall survival with fludarabine as initial therapy as opposed to its use as second-line therapy for patients no longer responding to chlorambucil. Fludarabine requires intravenous infusion 5 days a week once a month for 4–6 months and causes immunosuppression that is often long-lasting. New treatments combining chemotherapy with antibodies directed against antigens expressed by CLL cells are being tested.

Complications such as autoimmune hemolytic anemia or immune thrombocytopenia may require treatment with prednisone or splenectomy. Fludarabine should be avoided in patients with autoimmune hemolytic anemia since it may markedly worsen this condition.

The rare young patient with aggressive CLL may be a candidate for allogeneic bone marrow transplantation, which may be curative.

Prognosis

Median survival is approximately 6 years, and 25% of patients live more than 10 years. Patients with stage 0 or I disease have a median survival of 10 years. It is important to reassure these patients that they can live a normal life for many years. Patients with stage III or IV disease have a median survival of less than 2 years.

Cheson BD et al: National Cancer Institute-sponsored Working Group guidelines for chronic lymphocytic leukemia: Revised guidelines for diagnosis and treatment. Blood 1996;87:4990. [NLM Cit ID: 96247500]

Dighiero G: Chlorambucil in indolent chronic lymphocytic leukemia. N Engl J Med 1998;338:1506. [NLM Cit ID: 98242980]

Keating MJ: Long-term follow-up of patients with chronic lymphocytic leukemia (CLL) receiving fludarabine regimens as initial therapy. Blood 1998;92:1165. [NLM Cit ID: 98361761]

Weiss RB: Hemolytic anemia after fludarabine therapy for chronic lymphocytic leukemia. J Clin Oncol 1998; 16:1885. [NLM Cit ID: 98246317]

HAIRY CELL LEUKEMIA

Essentials of Diagnosis

- Pancytopenia.
- Splenomegaly, often massive.
- Hairy cells present on blood smear and bone marrow biopsy.

General Considerations

Hairy cell leukemia, an uncommon form of leukemia, is an indolent cancer of B lymphocytes.

Clinical Findings

A. Symptoms and Signs: The disease characteristically presents in middle-aged men. The median age at presentation is 55 years, and there is a striking 5:1 male predominance. Most patients present with gradual onset of fatigue, others complain of symptoms related to markedly enlarged spleen, and some come to attention because of infection.

On physical examination, splenomegaly is almost invariably present and may be massive. The liver is enlarged in half of cases, but lymphadenopathy is uncommon.

Hairy cell leukemia is usually an indolent disorder whose course is dominated by pancytopenia and recurrent infections, including mycobacterial infections.

B. Laboratory Findings: The hallmark of hairy cell leukemia is pancytopenia. Anemia is nearly universal, and 75% of patients have thrombocytopenia and neutropenia as well. Nearly all patients have striking monocytopenia, which is encountered in almost no other condition. The "hairy cells" are usually present in small numbers on the peripheral blood smear and have a characteristic appearance with numerous cytoplasmic projections. Less commonly, a form of the disorder exists in which large numbers of hairy cells dominate the peripheral blood smear. The bone marrow is usually inaspirable (dry tap), and the diagnosis is made by characteristic morphology on bone marrow biopsy. The hairy cells have a characteristic histochemical staining pattern, with tartrate-resistant acid phosphatase (TRAP). On immunophenotyping, the cells co-express the antigens CD11c and CD22. Pathologic examination of the spleen shows marked infiltration of the red pulp with hairy cells. This is in marked contrast to the usual predilection of lymphomas to involve the white pulp of the spleen.

Differential Diagnosis

Hairy cell leukemia should be distinguished from other lymphoproliferative diseases such as Waldenström's macroglobulinemia and non-Hodgkin's lymphomas. It also may be confused with other causes of pancytopenia, including hypersplenism due to any cause.

Treatment

The treatment of hairy cell leukemia has been dramatically changed by the development of new effective agents. The treatment of choice is with cladribine (2-chlorodeoxyadenosine; CdA), 0.14 mg/kg daily for 7 days. This is a relatively nontoxic drug that produces benefit in 95% of cases and complete remission in more than 80%. Responses are long-lasting, with few patients relapsing in the first few years. Interferon and splenectomy are rarely used now.

Course & Prognosis

The development of new effective therapies appears to have changed the prognosis of this disease. Formerly, median survival was 6 years, and only one-third of patients survived longer than 10 years. Although longer follow-up will be required, it now appears that most patients with hairy cell leukemia will live longer than 10 years. With current trends in treatment, the prognosis appears open-ended at this time.

Hoffman MA: Treatment of hairy-cell leukemia with cladribine: Response, toxicity, and long-term follow-up. J Clin Oncol 1997;15:1138. [NLM Cit ID: 97213867]

Saven A: Long-term follow-up of patients with hairy cell leukemia after cladribine treatment. Blood 1998;92: 1918. [NLM Cit ID: 98402337]

LYMPHOMAS

NON-HODGKIN'S LYMPHOMAS

The non-Hodgkin's lymphomas are a heterogeneous group of cancers of lymphocytes. The disorders are variable in clinical presentation and course, varying from indolent disease to rapidly progressive devastating illnesses.

Molecular biology has provided clues to the pathogenesis of these disorders. The best-studied example is Burkitt's lymphoma, in which a characteristic cytogenetic abnormality of translocation between the long arms of chromosomes 8 and 14 has been identified. The proto-oncogene *c-myc* is translocated from its normal position on chromosome 8 to the heavy chain locus on chromosome 14. Cells committed to B cell differentiation are likely to have enhanced expression of this heavy chain locus, and it is likely that overexpression of *c-myc* (in its new anomalous position) is related to malignant transformation. In the follicular lymphomas, translocations of a possible oncogene *bcl*-2 from chromosome 8 to the heavy chain locus on chromosome 14 may play a similar role.

Classification of the lymphomas is a controversial area still undergoing evolution. The National Cancer Institute has sponsored a working formulation that characterizes these lymphomas according to their biologic behavior, whether indolent or aggressive (Table 13–16).

Clinical Findings

A. Symptoms and Signs: Patients with indolent lymphomas usually present with painless lymphadenopathy, which may be isolated or widespread. Involved lymph nodes may be present in the retroperitoneum, mesentery, and pelvis. The indolent lymphomas are often disseminated at the time of diagnosis, and bone marrow involvement is frequent.

Patients with intermediate and high-grade lymphomas may present with adenopathy or with constitutional symptoms such as fever, drenching night sweats, or weight loss. On examination, lymphadenopathy may be isolated, or extranodal sites of disease (skin, gastrointestinal tract) may be found. Patients with Burkitt's lymphoma frequently present with abdominal pain or abdominal fullness because of the predilection of the disease for the abdomen. Those with HIV disease also have an increased incidence of non-Hodgkin's lymphoma, which may be isolated to the central nervous system.

Once a pathologic diagnosis is established, the patient should be staged. Physical examination is supplemented by chest x-ray and CT scan of the abdomen and pelvis. The bone marrow should be biopsied, and—in selected cases with high-risk morphology—a lumbar puncture should be performed.

Table 13–16. Classification of lymphomas.

- Low-grade
  - Small lymphocytic
  - Small lymphocytic, plasmacytoid
  - Follicular small cleaved cell
  - Follicular mixed cell
- Intermediate-grade
  - Follicular large cell
  - Diffuse small cleaved cell
  - Diffuse mixed cell
  - Diffuse large cell
- High-grade
  - Immunoblastic
  - Small noncleaved (Burkitt's)
  - Small noncleaved (non-Burkitt's)
  - Lymphoblastic
  - True histiocytic
- Other
  - Cutaneous T cell (mycosis fungoides)
  - Adult T cell leukemia-lymphoma
  - Mantle cell
  - Marginal zone (MALT)
  - Peripheral T cell
  - Anaplastic large cell

B. Laboratory Findings: The peripheral blood is usually normal, but a number of lymphomas may present in a "leukemic" phase. In these situations, the distinction between leukemia and lymphoma is arbitrary, as the malignant cell has the same characteristics.

Bone marrow involvement is manifested as paratrabecular lymphoid aggregates. In some high-grade lymphomas, the meninges may be involved and the spinal fluid may contain malignant cells. The chest radiograph may show a mediastinal mass in lymphoblastic lymphoma. The serum LDH has been shown to be a useful prognostic marker and is now incorporated in risk stratification of treatment.

The diagnosis of lymphoma is made by tissue biopsy. Needle aspiration may yield suspicious results, but usually a lymph node biopsy (or biopsy of involved extranodal tissue) is required.

Treatment

The treatment of indolent lymphoma depends on the stage of disease and the clinical status of the patient. A small number of patients have limited disease with only one abnormal lymph node. These patients are treated with localized irradiation. Most patients with indolent lymphoma have disseminated disease at the time of diagnosis. If the disease is not bulky and the patient not symptomatic, no initial therapy may be required. Some patients will have spontaneous remissions and may defer treatment for 1–3 years. In the past, standard chemotherapy for patients requiring treatment has been based on alkylators such as chlorambucil, 0.6–1 mg/kg every 3 weeks, or combination therapy with cyclophosphamide, vincristine, and prednisone (CVP). However, chemotherapy with fludarabine may produce equivalent results. A monoclonal antibody (rituximab) directed against the B cell surface antigen CD20 is very effective as salvage therapy for relapsed low-grade B cell lymphomas and may improve outcomes when added to initial chemotherapy. Occasional young patients with clinically aggressive low-grade lymphomas may be appropriate candidates for allogeneic transplantation. The role of autologous transplantation remains controversial.

Patients with intermediate-grade lymphomas such as diffuse large cell lymphoma are treated with curative intent. Patients with localized disease are treated with short-course chemotherapy (such as three courses of cyclophosphamide, doxorubicin [Adriamycin], vincristine [Oncovin], and prednisone [CHOP]) plus localized radiation. Most patients who have more advanced disease are treated with six to eight cycles of chemotherapy such as CHOP. Some patients with high-risk lymphoma are best treated with autologous stem cell transplantation early in their course.

Patients with intermediate-grade lymphoma who relapse after initial chemotherapy may still be cured by autologous stem cell transplantation if their disease is still responsive to chemotherapy.

Patients with special forms of lymphoma require individualized therapy. Burkitt's lymphoma should be treated with intensive regimens specifically tailored for this histologic type. Those with lymphoblastic lymphoma should be treated with regimens similar to those used for T cell acute lymphoblastic leukemia. Mantle cell lymphoma is not effectively treated with standard chemotherapy regimens. The role of high-dose therapy with allogeneic or autologous transplantation is under study.

Prognosis

The median survival of patients with indolent lymphomas is 6–8 years. These diseases ultimately become refractory to chemotherapy. This often occurs at the time of histologic progression of the disease to a more aggressive form of lymphoma.

The International Prognostic Index is now widely used to categorize patients with intermediate grade lymphoma into risk groups. Factors that confer adverse prognosis are age over 60 years, elevated serum LDH, advanced stage disease (stage III or stage IV), and poor performance status. Patients with no risk factors or one risk factor have high complete response rates (80%) to standard chemotherapy, and most responses (80%) are durable. Patients with two risk factors have a 70% complete response rate, and 70% are long-lasting. Patients with higher-risk disease have lower response rates and poor survival with standard regimens, and alternative treatments are needed. Early treatment with high-dose therapy and autologous stem cell transplantation improves the outcome.

For patients who relapse after initial chemotherapy, the prognosis depends on whether the lymphoma is still partially sensitive to chemotherapy. If it is, autologous transplantation offers a 50% chance of long-term salvage.

The treatment of older patients with lymphoma has been difficult because of their poorer tolerance of aggressive chemotherapy. The use of myeloid growth factors to reduce neutropenic complications may improve outcomes.

Apostolidis J et al: High-dose therapy with autologous bone marrow support as consolidation of remission in follicular lymphoma: long-term clinical and molecular follow-up. J Clin Oncol 2000;18:527. [NLM Cit ID: 20120871]

Armitage JO: New approach to classifying non-Hodgkin's lymphomas: clinical features of the major histologic subtypes. J Clin Oncol 1998;16:2780. [NLM Cit ID: 98368429]

Harris NL et al: World health organization classification of neoplastic diseases of the hematopoietic and lymphoid tissues: report of the clinical advisory committee meeting-Airlie House, Virginia, November 1997. J Clin Oncol 1999;17:3835. [NLM Cit ID: 20044867]

Miller TP et al: Chemotherapy alone compared with chemotherapy plus radiotherapy for localized intermediate and high-grade non-Hodgkin's lymphoma. NEJM 1998;339:21. [NLM Cit ID: 98299382]

Shipp MA et al: International consensus conference on high-dose therapy with hematopoietic stem cell transplantation in aggressive non-hodgkin's lymphomas: report of the jury. J Clin Oncol 1999;17:423. [NLM Cit ID: 99385443]

Sweetenham JW et al: High-dose therapy and autologous stem-cell transplantation for adult patients with Hodgkin's disease who do not enter remission after induction chemotherapy: results in 175 patients reported to the European group for blood and marrow transplantation. J Clin Oncol 1999;17:3101. [NLM Cit ID: 99438175]

HODGKIN'S DISEASE

Essentials of Diagnosis

- Painless lymphadenopathy.
- Constitutional symptoms may be present.
- Pathologic diagnosis by lymph node biopsy.

General Considerations

Hodgkin's disease is a group of cancers characterized by Reed-Sternberg cells in an appropriate reactive cellular background. The nature of the malignant cell is a subject of controversy.

Clinical Findings

There is a bimodal age distribution, with one peak in the 20s and a second peak over age 50. Most patients present because of a painless mass, commonly in the neck. Others may seek medical attention because of constitutional symptoms such as fever, weight loss, or drenching night sweats, or because of generalized pruritus. An unusual symptom of Hodgkin's disease is pain in an involved lymph node following alcohol ingestion.

An important clinical feature of Hodgkin's disease is its tendency to arise within lymph node areas and to spread in an orderly fashion to contiguous areas of lymph nodes. Only late in the course of the disease will vascular invasion lead to widespread hematogenous dissemination.

The diagnosis is made by lymph node biopsy. Hodgkin's disease is divided into several subtypes: lymphocyte predominance, nodular sclerosis, mixed cellularity, and lymphocyte depletion. Hodgkin's disease should be distinguished pathologically from other malignant lymphomas and may occasionally be confused with reactive lymph nodes seen in infectious mononucleosis, cat-scratch disease, or drug reactions (eg, phenytoin).

Patients undergo a staging evaluation to determine the extent of disease. The staging nomenclature (Ann Arbor) is as follows: stage I, one lymph node region involved; stage II, involvement of two lymph node areas on one side of the diaphragm; stage III, lymph node regions involved on both sides of the diaphragm; stage IV, disseminated disease with bone marrow or liver involvement. In addition, patients are designated stage A if they lack constitutional symptoms and stage B if significant weight loss, fever, or night sweats are present.

Treatment

The treatment of Hodgkin's disease has evolved, with radiation therapy used as initial treatment only for patients with low-risk stage IA and IIA disease. Staging is usually clinical, and laparotomy is not routinely performed. The addition of limited chemotherapy for some patients treated with radiation is under study and appears promising.

Most patients with Hodgkin's disease (including all with stage IIIB and IV disease) are best treated with combination chemotherapy using doxorubicin (Adriamycin), bleomycin, vincristine, and dacarbazine (ABVD). This has been shown to be both more effective and less toxic than mechlorethamine, vincristine, procarbazine, and prednisone (MOPP). In particular, there is less reproductive sterility and less secondary leukemia. New shorter and more intensive regimens have produced promising preliminary results and may come to supplant ABVD in the treatment of advanced disease.

Prognosis

All patients with both localized and disseminated disease should be treated with curative intent. The prognosis of patients with stage IA or IIA disease treated by radiotherapy is excellent, with 10-year survival rates in excess of 80%. Patients with disseminated disease (IIIB, IV) have 5-year survival rates of 50–60%. Poorer results are seen in patients who are older, those who have bulky disease, and those with lymphocyte depletion or mixed cellularity on histologic examination. Patients whose disease recurs after initial radiotherapy treatment may still be curable with chemotherapy. The treatment of choice for patients who relapse after initial chemotherapy is high-dose chemotherapy with autologous stem cell transplantation. This offers a 35–50% chance of cure to patients whose disease is still chemotherapy-sensitive.

Aisenberg AC: Problems in Hodgkin's disease management. Blood 1999;93:761. [NLM Cit ID: 99120947]

Andre M: Comparison of high-dose therapy and autologous stem-cell transplantation with conventional therapy for Hodgkin's disease induction failures: a case-control study. J Clin Oncol 1999;17:222.

Diehl V: Clinical presentation, course, and prognostic factors in lymphocyte-predominant Hodgkin's disease and lymphocyte-rich classical Hodgkin's disease: report for the European task force on lymphoma project on lymphocyte-predominant Hodgkin's disease. J Clin Oncol 1999;17:776. [NLM Cit ID: 99168824]

Hasenclever D: A prognostic score for advanced Hodgkin's disease. N Engl J Med 1998;339:1506. [NLM Cit ID: 99025349]

MULTIPLE MYELOMA

Essentials of Diagnosis

- Bone pain, often in the lower back.
- Monoclonal paraprotein by serum or urine protein electrophoresis or immunoelectrophoresis.
- Replacement of bone marrow by malignant plasma cells.

General Considerations

Multiple myeloma is a malignancy of plasma cells characterized by replacement of the bone marrow, bone destruction, and paraprotein formation. There is evidence that a new herpesvirus may be implicated in pathogenesis. Myeloma causes clinical symptoms and signs through a variety of mechanisms.

Replacement of the bone marrow (and perhaps humoral suppression of myelopoiesis) leads initially to anemia and later to general bone marrow failure. Bone destruction causes bone pain, osteoporosis, lytic lesions, and pathologic fractures. Hypercalcemia is common and appears to be mediated by osteoclast activating factor (OAF) or similar lymphokines. The malignant plasma cells can form tumors (plasmacytomas) that may cause spinal cord compression.

The paraproteins secreted by the malignant plasma cells may cause problems in their own right. Very high paraprotein levels (either IgG or IgA) may cause the hyperviscosity syndrome, though this is more often caused by IgM in Waldenström's macroglobulinemia. The light chain component of the immunoglobulin may lead to renal failure (often aggravated by hypercalcemia). Light chain components may be deposited in tissues as amyloid, worsening renal failure and causing a vast array of systemic symptoms.

Myeloma patients are prone to recurrent infections for a number of reasons, including neutropenia and the immunosuppressive effects of chemotherapy. Additionally, there is a failure of antibody production in response to antigen challenge, and myeloma patients are especially prone to infections with encapsulated organisms such as *Streptococcus pneumoniae* and *Haemophilus influenzae*.

Clinical Findings

A. Symptoms and Signs: Myeloma is a disease of older adults (median age at presentation, 60 years). The most common presenting complaints are those related to anemia, bone pain, and infection. Bone pain is most common in the back or ribs or may present as a pathologic fracture, especially of the femoral neck. Patients may also come to medical attention because of renal failure; spinal cord compression, or the hyperviscosity syndrome (mucosal bleeding, vertigo, nausea, visual disturbances, alterations in mental status). Occasionally, patients are diagnosed as having myeloma because of initial laboratory findings of hypercalcemia, proteinuria, elevated sedimentation rate, or abnormalities on serum protein electrophoresis. A few patients come to medical attention because of amyloidosis.

Examination may reveal pallor, bone tenderness, and soft tissue masses. Patients may have neurologic signs related to neuropathy, spinal cord compression. Patients with amyloidosis may have an enlarged tongue, neuropathy, congestive heart failure, or hepatomegaly. Splenomegaly is absent unless amyloidosis is present.

B. Laboratory Findings: Anemia is nearly universal. Red blood cell morphology is normal, but rouleau formation is common and may be marked. The neutrophil and platelet counts are usually normal at presentation. Only rarely will plasma cells be visible on peripheral smear (plasma cell leukemia).

The hallmark of myeloma is the finding of a paraprotein on serum protein electrophoresis (SPEP). The majority of patients will have a monoclonal spike visible in the beta or gamma globulin region. Immunoelectrophoresis (IEP) will reveal this to be a monoclonal protein. Approximately 15% of patients will have no demonstrable paraprotein in the serum. In these, IEP of the urine will reveal either complete immunoglobulin or light chains. Overall, approximately 60% of myeloma patients will have an IgG paraprotein, 25% an IgA, and 15% light chains only.

The bone marrow will be infiltrated by variable numbers of plasma cells ranging from 5% to 100%. Occasionally, the plasma cells may be morphologically indistinguishable from normal cells but more commonly will appear abnormal. Bone radiographs are important in establishing the diagnosis of myeloma. Lytic lesions are most commonly seen in the axial skeleton: skull, spine, proximal long bones, and ribs. At other times, only generalized osteoporosis is seen. The radionuclide bone scan is not useful in detecting bone lesions in myeloma, as there is usually no osteoblastic component.

Other laboratory features include hypercalcemia, renal failure, and an elevated erythrocyte sedimentation rate; alkaline phosphatase is not elevated despite extensive bony involvement. Some patients have proximal renal tubular acidosis, with phosphaturia, glycosuria, and uricosuria. The urinalysis may reveal proteinuria, but the dipstick test (which detects primarily albumin) is unreliable for light chains. Often there is a narrow anion gap when the paraprotein is cationic (70% of cases). On occasion, the abnormal protein is cryoprecipitatable, resulting in positive studies for cryoglobulins.

Differential Diagnosis

When a patient is discovered to have a monoclonal paraprotein, the distinction between myeloma and monoclonal gammopathy of unknown significance (MGUS) must be made. MGUS is present in 1% of all adults and 3% of adults over age 70. Thus, if one considers all patients with paraproteins, MGUS is far more common than myeloma. Most commonly, patients with MGUS will have a monoclonal IgG spike less than 2.5 g/dL, and the height of the spike remains stable. In approximately 25% of cases, MGUS progresses to overt malignant disease, but this may take many years.

Myeloma is distinguished from MGUS by findings of replacement of the bone marrow, bone destruction, and progression. Although the height of the paraprotein spike should not be used by itself to distinguish benign from malignant disease, all patients with IgG spikes greater than 3.5 g/dL prove to have myeloma. An IgA spike of greater than 2 g/dL is almost always due to myeloma. If there is doubt about whether paraproteinemia is benign or malignant, the patient should be observed without therapy, since there is no advantage to early treatment of asymptomatic multiple myeloma.

Myeloma should be distinguished from polyclonal hypergammaglobulinemia seen in reactive states. The distinction is made by finding the polyclonal as opposed to the monoclonal spike. Myeloma may also need to be distinguished from other malignant lymphoproliferative diseases such as Waldenström's macroglobulinemia, lymphomas, and primary amyloidosis (with which it is commonly associated).

Treatment

The goal of treatment of myeloma is usually palliation. Patients with minimal disease or in whom the diagnosis of malignancy is in doubt should be observed without treatment. Most commonly, patients require treatment at diagnosis because of bone pain or other symptoms related to the disease. In the past, standard therapy has been melphalan plus prednisone; more recently, combination chemotherapy with alkylating agents has been used. The optimal chemotherapy regimen has not been determined.

The optimal initial therapy for younger patients (under 60) with myeloma is autologous stem cell transplantation. Early aggressive treatment prolongs both remission duration and overall survival. Autologous transplantation is also useful in management of patients with relapsed disease if the disease is still chemotherapy-sensitive. The height of the paraprotein spike on SPEP is a useful marker for monitoring response to therapy. Patients who fail to respond to standard therapy may be effectively salvaged with low-dose continuous infusion therapy, the VAD (vincristine, Adriamycin [doxorubicin], dexamethasone) regimen (see Chapter 4). Thalidomide has emerged as a promising new agent in the treatment of myeloma, and responses have been seen even in patients whose disease no longer responds to chemotherapy. The ultimate role of thalidomide remains to be determined.

Allogeneic transplantation is potentially curative in myeloma, but its role has been limited because of the unusually high mortality rate (40–50%) in myeloma patients. Newer and less toxic forms of allogeneic transplantation using nonmyeloablative regimens are being tested and may broaden the applications of the allogeneic approach.

A number of other ancillary measures are important in the treatment of myeloma. Localized radiotherapy may be useful for palliation of bone pain or for eradicating tumor at the site of pathologic fracture. Hypercalcemia should be treated aggressively and immobilization and dehydration avoided. The bisphosphonate pamidronate, 90 mg intravenously monthly, reduces pathologic fractures in patients with significant bony disease.

Prognosis

The median survival of patients with myeloma is 3 years. The prognosis is markedly affected by a number of prognostic features, with shorter survivals in those with high paraprotein spikes, renal failure, hypercalcemia, or extensive bony disease. Patients are said to have a "low tumor burden" if the IgG spike is less than 5 g/dL and there is no more than one lytic bone lesion and no evidence of hypercalcemia or renal failure. Such patients have a median survival of 5–6 years. Conversely, patients with a "high tumor burden" have an IgG spike greater than 7 g/dL, hematocrit less than 25%, calcium greater than 12 mg/dL, or more than three lytic bone lesions. Median survival for this group is approximately 1 year. Early intervention with autologous stem cell transplantation appears to prolong survival in these high-risk patients.

Barlogie B: Total therapy with tandem transplants for newly diagnosed multiple myeloma. Blood 1999;93:55. [NLM Cit ID: 99081602]

Bataille R: Multiple myeloma. N Engl J Med 1997;336:1657. [NLM Cit ID: 97301689]

Berenson JR: Long-term pamidronate treatment of advanced multiple myeloma patients reduces skeletal events. J Clin Oncol 1998;16:593. [NLM Cit ID: 98129249]

Singhal S et al: Antitumor activity of thalidomide in refractory multiple myeloma. N Engl J Med 1999;341:1565. [NLM Cit ID: 20014077]

WALDENSTRÖM'S MACROGLOBULINEMIA

Essentials of Diagnosis

- Symptoms nonspecific: splenomegaly common on examination.
- Monoclonal IgM paraprotein.
- Infiltration of bone marrow by plasmacytic lymphocytes.
- Absence of lytic bone disease.

General Considerations

Waldenström's macroglobulinemia is a malignant disease of B cells that appear to be a hybrid of lymphocytes and plasma cells. These cells characteristically secrete an IgM paraprotein, and many clinical manifestations of the disease are related to this macroglobulin.

Clinical Findings

A. Symptoms and Signs: This disease characteristically develops insidiously in patients in their 60s or 70s. Patients usually present with fatigue related to anemia. Hyperviscosity of serum may be manifested in a number of ways. Mucosal and gastrointestinal bleeding is related to engorged blood vessels and platelet dysfunction. Other complaints include nausea, vertigo, and visual disturbances. Alterations in consciousness vary from mild lethargy to stupor and coma. The IgM paraprotein may also cause symptoms of cold agglutinin disease or peripheral neuropathy.

On examination, there may be hepatosplenomegaly or lymphadenopathy. The retinal veins are engorged. Purpura may be present. There should be no bone tenderness.

B. Laboratory Findings: Anemia is nearly universal, and rouleau formation is common. The anemia is related in part to expansion of the plasma volume by 50–100% due to the presence of the paraprotein. Other blood counts are usually normal. The abnormal plasmacytic lymphocytes usually appear in small numbers on the peripheral blood smear. The bone marrow is characteristically infiltrated by the plasmacytic lymphocytes.

The hallmark of macroglobulinemia is the presence of a monoclonal IgM spike seen on serum protein electrophoresis (SPEP) in the beta or gamma globulin region. The serum viscosity is usually increased above the normal of 1.4–1.8 times that of water. Symptoms of hyperviscosity usually develop when the serum viscosity is over four times that of water, and marked symptoms usually arise when the viscosity is over six times that of water. Because paraproteins vary in their physicochemical properties, there is no strict correlation between the concentration of paraprotein and serum viscosity.

The IgM paraprotein may cause a positive Coombs test or have cold agglutinin or cryoglobulin properties. If one suspects macroglobulinemia but the SPEP shows only hypogammaglobulinemia, one should repeat the test while taking special measures to maintain the blood at 37 °C, since the paraprotein may precipitate out at room temperature if it is cryoprecipitatable.

Bone radiographs are normal, and there is no evidence of renal failure.

Differential Diagnosis

Waldenström's macroglobulinemia is differentiated from monoclonal gammopathy of unknown significance by the finding of bone marrow infiltration. It is distinguished from chronic lymphocytic leukemia and multiple myeloma by bone marrow morphology and the finding of the characteristic IgM spike, and also on clinical grounds.

Treatment

Patients who present with marked hyperviscosity syndrome (stupor or coma) should be treated on an emergency basis with plasmapheresis. On a chronic basis, some patients can be managed with periodic plasmapheresis alone. Others are treated with intermittent chemotherapy with chlorambucil or cyclophosphamide. New agents such as cladribine have produced encouraging results.

As with multiple myeloma, autologous stem cell transplantation is playing a more important role in management and should be considered in younger patients with more aggressive disease.

Prognosis

Waldenström's macroglobulinemia is an indolent disease with a median survival rate of 3–5 years. However, patients may survive 10 years or longer.

Dimopoulos MA et al: Waldenström's macroglobulinemia: clinical features, complications, and management. J Clin Oncol 2000;18:214. [NLM Cit ID: 20090991]

George JN: Drug-induced thrombocytopenia: a systematic review of published case reports. Ann Intern Med 1998;129:886. [NLM Cit ID. 99043213]

Leblond V: Activity of fludarabine in previously treated Waldenström's macroglobulinemia: a report of 71 cases. J Clin Oncol 1998;16:2060. [NLM Cit ID: 98249444]

DISORDERS OF HEMOSTASIS

Disorders of hemostasis may be due to defects in either platelet number or function or to problems in formation of a fibrin clot (coagulation). Bleeding due to platelet disorders is typically mucosal or dermatologic. Common problems include epistaxis, gum bleeding, menorrhagia, gastrointestinal bleeding, purpura, and petechiae. Petechiae are seen almost exclusively in conditions of thrombocytopenia and not platelet dysfunction. Bleeding due to coagulopathy may occur as deep muscle hematomas as well as skin bleeding. Spontaneous hemarthroses are seen only in severe hemophilia.

IDIOPATHIC (AUTOIMMUNE) THROMBOCYTOPENIC PURPURA

Essentials of Diagnosis

- Isolated thrombocytopenia.
- Other hematopoietic cell lines normal.
- No systemic illness.
- Spleen not palpable.
- Normal bone marrow with normal or increased megakaryocytes.

General Considerations

Idiopathic thrombocytopenic purpura is an autoimmune disorder in which an IgG autoantibody is formed that binds to platelets. It is not clear which antigen on the platelet surface is involved. Although the antiplatelet antibody may bind complement, platelets are not destroyed by direct lysis. Rather, destruction takes place in the spleen, where splenic macrophages with Fc receptors bind to antibody-coated platelets. Since the spleen is the major site both of antibody production and platelet sequestration, splenectomy is highly effective therapy.

Clinical Findings

A. Symptoms and Signs: Idiopathic thrombocytopenic purpura occurs commonly in childhood, frequently precipitated by viral infection and usually self-limited. In contrast, the adult form is usually a chronic disease and only infrequently follows a viral infection. It is a disease of young persons, with peak incidence between ages 20 and 50, and there is a 2:1 female predominance.

Patients are systemically well and not febrile. The presenting complaint is mucosal or skin bleeding. Common types of bleeding are epistaxis, oral bleeding, menorrhagia, purpura, and petechiae.

On examination, the patient appears well, and there are no abnormal findings other than those related to bleeding. An enlarged spleen should lead one to doubt the diagnosis. Common signs of bleeding are purpura, petechiae, and hemorrhagic bullae in the mouth.

B. Laboratory Findings: The hallmark of the disease is thrombocytopenia, which may be less than 10,000/μL. Other counts are usually normal except for occasional mild anemia, which can be explained by bleeding or associated hemolysis. Peripheral blood cell morphology is normal except that platelets are slightly enlarged (megathrombocytes). These larger platelets are young platelets produced in response to enhanced platelet destruction. Approximately 10% of patients will have coexistent autoimmune hemolytic anemia **(Evans's syndrome),** and in these cases one will see anemia, reticulocytosis, and spherocytes on peripheral smear. Red blood cell fragmentation should not be seen.

The bone marrow will appear normal, with a normal or increased number of megakaryocytes. Coagulation studies will be entirely normal. Tests now available to quantitate platelet-associated IgG may help in the diagnosis. At present, although these tests are highly sensitive (95%), they are very nonspecific, and 50% of all patients with thrombocytopenia from any cause may have increased levels of IgG on the platelet.

Differential Diagnosis

Thrombocytopenia may be produced either by abnormal bone marrow function or by peripheral destruction (Table 13–17). Although most bone marrow disorders produce abnormalities in addition to isolated thrombocytopenia, diagnoses such as myelodysplasia can only be excluded by examining the bone marrow. Most causes of thrombocytopenia resulting from peripheral destruction can be ruled out by initial evaluation. Disorders such as disseminated intravascular coagulation, thrombotic thrombocytopenic purpura, hemolytic-uremic syndrome, hypersplenism, and sepsis are easily excluded by the absence of systemic illness. Thus, patients with isolated thrombocytopenia with no other abnormal findings almost certainly have immune thrombocytopenia. Patients should be questioned regarding drug use, especially sulfonamides, quinine, thiazides, cimetidine, gold, and heparin. Heparin is now the most common cause of drug-induced thrombocytopenia in hospitalized patients. Systemic lupus erythematosus and chronic lymphocytic leukemia are common causes of secondary thrombocytopenic purpura, hematologically identical to idiopathic thrombocytopenic purpura.

Treatment

Few adults with idiopathic thrombocytopenic purpura will have spontaneous remissions, and most will require treatment. Initial treatment is with prednisone, 1–2 mg/kg/d. Prednisone works primarily by decreasing the affinity of splenic macrophages for antibody-coated platelets. High-dose prednisone therapy also reduces the binding of antibody to the platelet surface, and long-term therapy may decrease antibody production. Bleeding will often diminish within 1 day after beginning prednisone—even before the platelet count begins to rise. This effect has been attributed to enhanced vascular stability. The platelet count will usually begin to rise within a week, and responses are almost always seen within 3 weeks. About 80% of patients will respond, and the platelet count will usually return to normal. High-dose therapy should be continued until the platelet count is normal, and the dose should then be gradually tapered. In most, thrombocytopenia will recur if prednisone is completely withdrawn, and one aims to find a dose that will maintain an adequate platelet count. It is not necessary for the platelet count to be entirely normal; the risk of bleeding is small with platelet counts above 50,000/μL.

Table 13–17. Causes of thrombocytopenia.

- Bone marrow disorders
  - Aplastic anemia
  - Hematologic malignancies
  - Myelodysplasia
  - Megaloblastic anemia
  - Chronic alcoholism
- Nonmarrow disorders
  - Immune disorders
    - Idiopathic thrombocytopenic purpura
    - Drug-induced
    - Secondary (CLL, SLE)
    - Posttransfusion purpura
  - Hypersplenism
  - Disseminated intravascular coagulation
  - Thrombotic thrombocytopenic purpura
  - Hemolytic-uremic syndrome
  - Sepsis
  - Hemangiomas
  - Viral infections, AIDS
  - Liver failure

Splenectomy is the most definitive treatment for idiopathic thrombocytopenic purpura, and most adult patients will ultimately undergo splenectomy. High-dose prednisone therapy should not be continued indefinitely in an attempt to avoid surgery. Splenectomy is indicated if patients do not respond to prednisone initially or require unacceptably high doses to maintain an adequate platelet count. Other patients may be intolerant of prednisone or may simply prefer the surgical alternative. Splenectomy can be performed safely even with platelet counts less than 10,000/μL. Eighty percent of patients benefit from splenectomy with either complete or partial remission.

High-dose intravenous immunoglobulin, 400 mg/kg/d for 3–5 days, is highly effective in rapidly raising the platelet count. The response rate is 90%, and the platelet count rises within 1–5 days. However, this treatment is expensive, and the beneficial effect lasts only 1–2 weeks. Immunoglobulin treatment should be reserved for bleeding emergencies or situations such as preparing a severely thrombocytopenic patient for surgery.

For patients who fail to respond to prednisone and splenectomy, danazol, 600 mg/d, has been used, with responses obtained in about half of cases. Immunosuppressive agents employed in refractory cases include vincristine, vinblastine infusions, azathioprine, cyclosporine, and cyclophosphamide.

Platelet transfusions are rarely used in the treatment of idiopathic thrombocytopenic purpura, since exogenous platelets will survive no better than the patient's own and will survive less than a few hours. Platelet transfusion should be reserved for cases of life-threatening bleeding in which even fleeting hemostasis may be of benefit.

Prognosis

The prognosis for remission is good. In most cases, the disease is initially controlled with prednisone, and splenectomy offers definitive therapy. The major concern during the initial phases is cerebral hemorrhage, which becomes a risk when the platelet count is less than 5000/μL. These patients usually exhibit warning signs of mucosal bleeding. However, even at these very low platelet counts, fatal bleeding is rare.

George JN et al: Idiopathic thrombocytopenic purpura: A practice guideline developed by explicit methods for the American Society of Hematology. Blood 1996;88:3. [NLM Cit ID: 96290405]

Law C: High-dose intravenous immune globulin and the response to splenectomy in patients with idiopathic thrombocytopenic purpura. N Engl J Med 1997;336:1494. [NLM Cit ID: 97282676]

McMillan R: Therapy for adults with refractory chronic immune thrombocytopenic purpura. Ann Intern Med 1997;126:307. [NLM Cit ID: 97172882]

THROMBOTIC THROMBOCYTOPENIC PURPURA

Essentials of Diagnosis

- Microangiopathic hemolytic anemia.
- Thrombocytopenia, neurologic and renal abnormalities, fever.
- Normal coagulation tests.
- Elevated serum LDH.

General Considerations

Thrombotic thrombocytopenic purpura is an uncommon syndrome with microangiopathic hemolytic anemia, thrombocytopenia, and a markedly elevated serum LDH. Noninfectious fever, neurologic disorders, and renal abnormalities are less commonly seen. The cause is unknown. A platelet-agglutinating factor has been identified in the plasma of these patients. Its role in pathogenesis remains controversial.

Thrombotic thrombocytopenic purpura is seen primarily in young adults between ages 20 and 50, and there is a slight female predominance. The syndrome is occasionally precipitated by estrogen use or pregnancy, and is increasingly encountered in association with HIV disease.

Clinical Findings

A. Symptoms and Signs: Patients come to medical attention because of anemia, bleeding, or neurologic abnormalities. The neurologic symptoms and signs are unusual in that they may wax and wane over minutes. Neurologic symptoms include headache, confusion, aphasia, and alterations in consciousness from lethargy to coma. With more advanced disease, one may see hemiparesis and seizures.

On examination, the patient appears acutely ill and is usually febrile. One may detect pallor, purpura, petechiae, and signs of neurologic dysfunction. Patients may have abdominal pain and tenderness due to pancreatitis.

B. Laboratory Findings: Anemia is universal and may be marked. There is usually marked reticulocytosis and occasional circulating nucleated red blood cells. The hallmark is a microangiopathic blood picture with fragmented red blood cells (schistocytes, helmet cells, triangle forms) on the smear. One cannot make the diagnosis without significant red blood cell fragmentation. Thrombocytopenia is invariably present and may be severe. White blood cells may show increased band neutrophils.

Hemolysis may be manifested by increasing indirect bilirubin and occasionally hemoglobinemia and hemoglobinuria; methemalbuminemia may impart a brown color to the plasma. The LDH is markedly elevated in proportion to the severity of hemolysis; the Coombs test is negative.

Coagulation tests (prothrombin time, partial thromboplastin time, fibrinogen) are normal unless ischemic tissue damage causes secondary DIC. Elevated fibrin degradation products may be seen, as in other acutely ill patients. Renal insufficiency may be present, with an abnormal urinalysis.

Pathologically, one may see thrombi in capillaries and small arteries, with no evidence of inflammation.

Differential Diagnosis

The normal values of coagulation tests differentiate thrombotic thrombocytopenic purpura from disseminated intravascular coagulation (DIC). Other conditions causing microangiopathic hemolysis (Table 13–18) should be excluded. Evans's syndrome is the combination of autoimmune thrombocytopenia and autoimmune hemolytic anemia, but the peripheral smear will show spherocytes and not red blood cell fragments. Skin biopsy is usually not necessary for diagnosis but may be helpful when vasculitis is a consideration. Thrombotic thrombocytopenic purpura and hemolytic-uremic syndrome are not distinct disease entities—rather, there is a spectrum of disease, with thrombotic thrombocytopenic purpura characterized by more neurologic findings and more severe thrombocytopenia and hemolytic-uremic syndrome with more renal failure.

Treatment

Thrombotic thrombocytopenic purpura should be treated emergently with large-volume plasmapheresis. Sixty to 80 mL/kg of plasma should be removed and replaced with fresh-frozen plasma. Treatment should be continued daily until the patient is in complete remission. Prednisone and antiplatelet agents

Table 13–18. Causes of microangiopathic hemolytic anemia.

Thrombotic thrombocytopenic purpura
Hemolytic-uremic syndrome
Disseminated intravascular coagulation
Prosthetic valve hemolysis
Metastatic adenocarcinoma
Malignant hypertension
Vasculitis

(aspirin [325 mg three times daily] and dipyridamole [75 mg three times daily]) have been used in addition to plasmapheresis, but their role is unclear.

Patients who do not respond to plasmapheresis or who have rapid recurrences require splenectomy. The combination of splenectomy, corticosteroids, and dextran has been used with success. Splenectomy performed in remission may prevent subsequent relapses.

Prognosis

With the advent of plasmapheresis, the formerly dismal prognosis of thrombotic thrombocytopenic purpura has been dramatically changed. Eighty to 90 percent of patients now recover completely. Neurologic abnormalities are almost always completely reversed. Most complete responses are durable, but in 20% of cases the disease will be chronic and relapsing.

Furlan M: Von Willebrand factor-cleaving protease in thrombotic thrombocytopenic purpura and the hemolytic-uremic syndrome. N Engl J Med 1998;339:1578. [NLM Cit ID: 99275706]

Rock G et al: Cryosupernatant as replacement fluid for plasma exchange in thrombotic thrombocytopenic purpura. Members of the Canadian Apheresis Group. Br J Haematol 1996;94:383. [NLM Cit ID: 96326244]

Ruggenenti P, Remuzzi G: The pathophysiology and management of thrombotic thrombocytopenic purpura. Eur J Haematol 1996;56:191. [NLM Cit ID: 96222303]

HEMOLYTIC-UREMIC SYNDROME

Essentials of Diagnosis

- Microangiopathic hemolytic anemia.
- Thrombocytopenia and renal failure.
- Elevated serum LDH.
- Normal coagulation tests.
- Absence of neurologic abnormalities.

General Considerations

Hemolytic-uremic syndrome is an uncommon disorder consisting of microangiopathic hemolytic anemia, thrombocytopenia, and renal failure due to microangiopathy (with decreased glomerular filtration, proteinuria, and hematuria). The cause is unclear. The disease is similar to thrombotic thrombocytopenic purpura except that different vascular beds are involved. The pathogenesis of the two disorders is probably similar, and a platelet-agglutinating factor found in plasma may be involved. In children, hemolytic-uremic syndrome frequently occurs after a diarrheal illness secondary to infections with shigella, salmonella, *E coli* strain O157:H7, or viral agents. The mortality rate of this form is low (< 5%). In adults, this syndrome is often precipitated by estrogen use or by the postpartum state. Hemolytic-uremic syndrome may be seen as a delayed complication of high-dose corticosteroid therapy and autologous bone marrow or stem cell transplantation, or of the use of cyclosporine or tacrolimus as immunosuppression in allogeneic transplantation. A familial (hereditary) type has been identified in which members of a family have recurrent episodes over several years.

Clinical Findings

A. Symptoms and Signs: Patients present with anemia, bleeding, or renal failure. The renal failure may or may not be oliguric. In contrast to thrombotic thrombocytopenic purpura, there are no neurologic manifestations other than those due to the uremic state.

B. Laboratory Findings: As in thrombotic thrombocytopenic purpura, there is microangiopathic hemolytic anemia and thrombocytopenia, but the thrombocytopenia is often less severe. The peripheral blood smear should show striking red blood cell fragmentation, and the diagnosis is untenable without this finding. The LDH is usually elevated out of proportion to the degree of hemolysis, and the Coombs test is negative. Coagulation tests are normal with the exception of elevated fibrin degradation products.

Kidney biopsy will show endothelial hyaline thrombi in the afferent arterioles and glomeruli. Ischemic necrosis in the renal cortex may occur with obstruction from intravascular coagulation.

Differential Diagnosis

Disseminated intravascular coagulation is excluded by normal coagulation results. Other causes of microangiopathic hemolytic anemia (Table 13–18) should be entertained. Occasionally, vasculitis or acute glomerulonephritis is considered, and in these cases renal biopsy may be necessary to establish the diagnosis if the platelet count will allow it.

Hemolytic-uremic syndrome is arbitrarily distinguished from thrombotic thrombocytopenic purpura by the consistent presence of renal failure and the lack of neurologic findings.

Treatment

In children, hemolytic-uremic syndrome is almost always self-limited and requires only conservative management of acute renal failure. In adults, however, without treatment, there is a high rate of permanent renal insufficiency and death. The treatment of choice (as in thrombotic thrombocytopenic purpura) is large-volume plasmapheresis with fresh-frozen replacement (exchange of up to 80 mL/kg), repeated daily until remission is achieved.

Prognosis

The prognosis of hemolytic-uremic syndrome in adults remains unclear. Without effective therapy, up to 40% of patients have died, and 80% have had chronic renal insufficiency. Early institution of aggressive therapy with plasmapheresis promises to be beneficial. Survival and correction of hematologic abnormalities are the rule, but restoration of renal function requires that treatment be initiated early.

Matsumae T, Takebayashi S, Naito S: The clinico-pathological characteristics and outcome in hemolytic-uremic syndrome of adults. Clin Nephrol 1996;45:153. [NLM Cit ID: 96252043]

Melnyk AM, Solez K, Kjellstrand CM: Adult hemolytic-uremic syndrome: A review of 37 cases. Arch Intern Med 1995;155:2077. [NLM Cit ID: 96011566]

Slutsker L: *Escherichia coli* O157:H7 diarrhea in the United States: Clinical and epidemiologic features. Ann Intern Med 1997;126:505. [NLM Cit ID: 97230746]

CONGENITAL QUALITATIVE PLATELET DISORDERS

Bleeding disorders characterized by prolonged bleeding times despite a normal platelet count are called qualitative platelet disorders. Patients have a family history or lifelong personal history of the defect. The disorders may be classified as (1) von Willebrand's disease, a congenital disorder of a plasma protein necessary for platelet adhesion; and (2) congenital disorders intrinsic to the platelet (Table 13–19). When an intrinsic qualitative platelet disorder is suspected, platelet aggregation studies should be evaluated to make a specific diagnosis.

1. VON WILLEBRAND'S DISEASE

Essentials of Diagnosis

- Family history with autosomal dominant pattern of inheritance.
- Prolonged bleeding time, either at baseline or after challenge with aspirin.
- Reduced levels of factor VIII antigen or ristocetin cofactor.
- Reduced levels of factor VIII coagulant activity in some patients.

General Considerations

Von Willebrand's disease is the most common congenital disorder of hemostasis. It is transmitted in an autosomal dominant pattern. It is a group of disorders characterized by deficient or defective von Willebrand factor (vWF), a protein that mediates platelet adhesion. Adhesion is a process separate from platelet aggregation. Platelets adhere to the subendothelium via vWF, which is bound to a specific receptor on the platelet composed of glycoprotein Ib (and missing in Bernard-Soulier syndrome). Platelets aggregate via fibrinogen, which binds to a different receptor composed of glycoproteins IIb and IIIa (deficient in Glanzmann's thrombasthenia). The platelet aggregation system is entirely normal in von Willebrand's disease.

Table 13–19. Qualitative platelet disorders.

Congenital
Glanzmann's thrombasthenia
Bernard-Soulier syndrome
Storage pool disease
Acquired
Myeloproliferative disorders
Uremia
Drugs: aspirin, anti-inflammatory agents
Autoantibody
Paraproteins
Acquired storage pool disease
Fibrin degradation products
Von Willebrand's disease

Von Willebrand factor is synthesized in megakaryocytes and endothelial cells and circulates in plasma as multimers of varying size. Only the large multimeric forms are functional in mediating platelet adhesion. Von Willebrand factor has a separate function of binding the factor VIII coagulant protein and protecting it from degradation. The factor VIII coagulant protein (factor VIII:C), a protein encoded by a gene on the X chromosome, is the protein deficient in classic hemophilia. Any of the multimeric forms of vWF can bind and protect factor VIII:C. Von Willebrand's disease, although primarily a disorder of platelet function, may secondarily cause a coagulation disturbance because of deficient levels of factor VIII:C. However, this coagulopathy is rarely severe.

There are several subtypes of von Willebrand's disease. The most common type (type I, 80% of all cases) is caused by a quantitative decrease in vWF. Type IIa is caused by a qualitative abnormality in protein that prevents multimer formation. Only small multimers are present, and both intermediate and large forms that mediate platelet adhesion are missing. Type IIb von Willebrand's disease is caused by a qualitative abnormality in the protein that causes rapid clearance of the large multimeric forms. Type III von Willebrand's disease is a rare autosomal recessive disorder in which vWF is nearly absent. Pseudo-von Willebrand disease is a rare disorder manifested as an abnormal platelet membrane with excessive avidity for the large multimeric forms of vWF, causing their clearance from plasma.

Clinical Findings

A. Symptoms and Signs: Von Willebrand's disease is a common disorder affecting both men and women. Most cases are mild. Most bleeding is mucosal (epistaxis, gingival bleeding, menorrhagia), but gastrointestinal bleeding may occur. In most cases, incisional bleeding occurs after surgery or dental extractions. Von Willebrand's disease is rarely as severe as hemophilia, and spontaneous hemarthroses do not occur. The bleeding tendency is exacerbated by aspirin. Characteristically, bleeding decreases during pregnancy or estrogen use.

B. Laboratory Findings: Platelet number and morphology are normal, and the bleeding time is usually (not always) prolonged. The bleeding time should be ascertained whenever this diagnosis is considered; it correlates most closely with clinical bleeding. When the bleeding time is normal, it is prolonged markedly by aspirin. Normal persons will prolong their bleeding time to a minor extent with aspirin but rarely out of the normal range. In the most common form of von Willebrand's disease (type I), vWF levels in plasma are reduced. This may be measured by factor VIII antigen, which measures the immunologic presence of vWF, or by ristocetin cofactor activity, which measures functional properties of vWF in mediating platelet adhesion.

When factor VIII antigen is reduced, one may also see a decrease in factor VIII coagulant (factor VIII:C) levels. When factor VIII:C levels are less than 25%, the partial thromboplastin time (PTT) will be prolonged. Platelet aggregation studies with standard agonists (ADP, collagen, thrombin) are normal, but platelet aggregation in response to ristocetin may be subnormal.

In difficult cases, it may be helpful to assay directly the multimeric composition of vWF.

Differential Diagnosis

When patients present with a prolonged bleeding time, one must distinguish von Willebrand's disease from other qualitative platelet disorders (Table 13–19). Acquired qualitative disorders are suggested by recent onset of the bleeding tendency. Congenital intrinsic platelet disorders may present with a positive family history and lifelong history of bleeding episodes. Von Willebrand's disease is diagnosed by the finding of abnormal measurements of vWF and by normal results of platelet aggregation.

When patients present with a prolonged PTT, measurements of factor VIII:C will distinguish von Willebrand's disease from all disorders except hemophilia (Table 13–20). Hemophilia is diagnosed when factor VIII:C is reduced but all measurements of vWF (factor VIII antigen, ristocetin cofactor activity) are normal.

Patients with a suspicious bleeding history but with normal bleeding time and PTT pose a diagnostic problem. On occasion, the postaspirin bleeding time can be used to unmask a bleeding disorder. At other times, one must perform further plasma assays of vWF to make the diagnosis. Von Willebrand's disease waxes and wanes in severity and may be difficult to diagnose, especially in a woman taking estrogens, which raise vWF levels.

It is often useful to distinguish between subtypes of von Willebrand's disease (Table 13–21), because type I usually responds to desmopressin and type IIb may be aggravated by its use.

Table 13–20. Causes of prolonged partial thromboplastin time.

- Congenital factor deficiencies
  - Contact factors
  - Factor XII
  - Factor XI
  - Factor IX (hemophilia B)
  - Factor VIII
    - Hemophilia A
    - von Willebrand's disease
- Anticoagulants
  - Anti-VIII
  - Lupus
  - Heparin

Treatment

The bleeding disorder is characteristically mild, and no treatment is routinely given other than avoidance of aspirin. However, patients often need to be prepared for surgical or dental procedures. The bleeding time is probably the best indicator of the likelihood of bleeding, and prophylactic therapy may be reasonably withheld if the procedure is minor and the bleeding time is normal.

Desmopressin acetate is useful for mild type I von Willebrand's disease and should be considered first. The dose is 0.3 μg/kg, after which vWF levels usually rise two- to threefold in 30–90 minutes. Desmopressin acetate appears to cause release of stored vWF from endothelial cells. The treatment can be given only every 24 hours as stores of vWF become depleted. The drug is not effective in type IIa von Willebrand's disease, in which no endothelial stores are present, and may be harmful in type IIb, leading to thrombocytopenia and increased bleeding.

Factor VIII concentrates are available that replace cryoprecipitate as the treatment of choice for von Willebrand's disease if factor replacement is required. Some (not all) of these products now contain functional vWF and do not transmit HIV or hepatitis. One appropriate product is Humate-P (Armour). The dose is 20–50 units/kg depending on disease severity.

The antifibrinolytic agent tranexamic acid is useful as adjunctive therapy during dental procedures. After either cryoprecipitate or desmopressin acetate, the patient is given 25 mg/kg three times daily for 5–7 days to reduce the likelihood of bleeding.

Prognosis

The prognosis is excellent. In most cases, the bleeding disorder is mild, and in the more serious cases replacement therapy is effective.

Hemophilia and von Willebrand's disease: 1. Diagnosis, comprehensive care and assessment. Association of Hemophilia Clinic Directors of Canada. Can Med Assoc J 1995;153:19. [NLM Cit ID: 95316809]

Hemophilia and von Willebrand's disease: 2. Management. Association of Hemophilia Clinic Directors of Canada. Can Med Assoc J 1995;153:147. [NLM Cit ID: 95323851]

Mannucci P: Hemostatic drugs. N Engl J Med 1998; 339:245. [NLM Cit ID: 98328633]

Ruggeri ZM: Von Willebrand's disease and the mechanisms of platelet function. Ciba Found Symp 1995; 189:35. [NLM Cit ID: 96063309]

Table 13–21. Types of von Willebrand's disease.

	Bleeding Time	Factor VIII Antigen	Ristocetin Cofactor Activity	Factor VIII Coagulant Activity	Multimer
Type I	↑ or N[1]	↓ or N	↓ or N	↓ or N	N
Type IIa	↑	↓ or N	0	↓ or N	Abn
Type IIb	↑	↓ or N	↓ or N	↓ or N	Abn
Type III	↑	0	0	0	...
Pseudo-vW disease	↑	↓ or N	↓ or N	↓	Abn
Hemophilia A	N	N	N		N

[1]Increases with aspirin.

Tefferi A: Acquired von Willebrand's disease: Concise review of occurrence, diagnosis, pathogenesis, and treatment. Am J Med 1997;103:536. [NLM Cit ID: 98090512]

2. DISORDERS INTRINSIC TO THE PLATELETS

Glanzmann's Thrombasthenia

This is a rare autosomal recessive intrinsic platelet disorder causing bleeding. Platelets are unable to aggregate because of lack of receptors (containing glycoproteins IIb and IIa) for fibrinogen, which form the bridges between platelets during aggregation. Clinically, it is manifested chiefly as mucosal (epistaxis, gingival bleeding, menorrhagia) and postoperative bleeding. The defect is of variable severity but may be severe.

Platelet numbers and morphology are normal, but the bleeding time is markedly prolonged. Platelets fail to aggregate in response to typical agonists (ADP, collagen, thrombin) but aggregate normally in response to ristocetin, which causes platelet clumping by a separate mechanism.

Patients are treated with platelet transfusions when necessary. Platelet transfusion therapy is limited by the tendency of these patients to develop multiple alloantibodies.

Bernard-Soulier Syndrome

This is a rare autosomal recessive intrinsic platelet disorder causing bleeding. Platelets cannot adhere to subendothelium because they lack receptors (composed of glycoprotein Ib) for von Willebrand factor, which mediates platelet adhesion. This is often a severe bleeding disorder with mucosal and postoperative bleeding.

Thrombocytopenia may be present, and platelets on smear are abnormally large. The bleeding time is markedly prolonged. Platelet aggregation is normal in response to standard agonists (collagen, ADP, thrombin), but platelets fail to aggregate in response to ristocetin. Measurements of von Willebrand factor in the plasma are normal. Patients are treated with platelet transfusion when necessary.

Storage Pool Disease

This is a group of mild bleeding disorders characterized by defective secretion of platelet granule contents (especially ADP) that stimulate platelet aggregation. Most patients are mildly affected and have increased bruising and postoperative bleeding.

Platelets are normal in number and morphology, but the bleeding time is slightly prolonged. In some cases, the baseline bleeding time is normal, but it becomes markedly prolonged after aspirin. There are variable abnormalities in platelet aggregation studies.

Most patients do not require treatment but should avoid aspirin. Platelet transfusions transiently correct the bleeding tendency. Some patients respond to desmopressin acetate, 0.3 μg/kg every 24 hours.

Peretz H et al: Glanzmann's thrombasthenia associated with deletion-insertion and alternative splicing in the glycoprotein IIb gene. Blood 1995;85:414. [NLM Cit ID: 95111124]

ACQUIRED QUALITATIVE PLATELET DISORDERS

A number of acquired disorders lead to abnormal platelet function (Table 13–19).

Uremia

Uremia causes abnormal platelet function by unknown mechanisms. The severity of the bleeding tendency is roughly proportionate to the degree of renal insufficiency. Bleeding is most commonly mucosal and gastrointestinal and may occasionally be severe. Dialysis is effective in reducing the bleeding tendency but may not completely eliminate it. Patients respond to desmopressin acetate, 0.3 μg/kg every 24 hours.

Myeloproliferative Disorders

All the myeloproliferative disorders can produce abnormalities in platelet function. A number of biochemical abnormalities are present in these platelets, but the cause of the bleeding tendency is unclear. The severity of the bleeding tendency correlates roughly with the height of the platelet count, although conditions causing reactive thrombocytosis of normal platelets are not associated with abnormal function. Bleeding decreases when the platelet count is controlled with myelosuppressive therapy. In cases of life-threatening bleeding with high platelet counts, plateletpheresis may be necessary.

Other Disorders

Aspirin causes a mild bleeding tendency by irreversibly acetylating cyclooxygenase, an enzyme that participates in platelet aggregation. The effect lasts for the life of the platelet and may be manifest for 7–10 days, although the major effect lasts 3–5 days. The effect is not dose-dependent, and 65 mg of aspirin is sufficient.

Aspirin by itself does not cause significant bleeding, but it may unmask bleeding disorders such as mild von Willebrand's disease or mild thrombocytopenia. Certain antibiotics (ticarcillin, some cephalosporins) cause a mild bleeding tendency, presumably by coating the surface of platelets. Nonsteroidal anti-inflammatory drugs cause an aspirin-like effect that disappears when the drug leaves the system.

Patients with autoantibodies against platelets may have prolonged bleeding times even in the absence of thrombocytopenia. Platelet-associated IgG levels should be high, and the bleeding tendency responds quickly to modest doses of prednisone, eg, 20 mg/d. Acquired storage pool disease refers to the circulation of "exhausted platelets" that have been stimulated to release their granule contents and hence are no longer functional. Such granule release occurs in response to cardiopulmonary bypass and severe vasculitis.

Noris M et al: Uremic bleeding: closing the circle after 30 years of controversies? Blood 1999;94:2569. [NLM Cit ID: 99445365]

HEMOPHILIA A

Essentials of Diagnosis

- X-linked recessive pattern of inheritance with only males affected.
- Low factor VIII coagulant (VIII:C) activity.
- Normal factor VIII antigen.
- Spontaneous hemarthroses.

General Considerations

Hemophilia A (classic hemophilia, factor VIII deficiency hemophilia) is a hereditary disorder in which bleeding is due to deficiency of the coagulation factor VIII (VIII:C). In most cases, the factor VIII coagulant protein is quantitatively reduced, but in a small number of cases the coagulant protein is present by immunoassay but defective.

Hemophilia is an X-linked recessive disease, and as a rule only males are affected. In rare instances, female carriers are clinically affected if their normal X chromosomes are disproportionately inactivated. Females may also become affected if they are the offspring of a hemophiliac father and carrier mother.

Hemophilia is classified as severe if factor VIII:C levels are less than 1%, moderate if levels are 1–5%, and mild if levels are greater than 5%. Families tend to breed true in the severity of hemophilia produced.

Clinical Findings

A. Symptoms and Signs: Hemophilia A is the most common severe bleeding disorder and after von Willebrand's disease is the most common congenital bleeding disorder overall. Approximately one in 10,000 males is affected. The bleeding tendency is related to factor VIII:C levels. Bleeding may occur anywhere. The most common sites of bleeding are into joints (knees, ankles, elbows), into muscles, and from the gastrointestinal tract. Spontaneous hemarthroses are so characteristic of hemophilia that they are virtually diagnostic of the disorder. Patients with mild hemophilia bleed only after major trauma or surgery; those with moderately severe hemophilia bleed with mild trauma or surgery; and those with severe disease bleed spontaneously.

Many hemophiliacs are now seropositive for HIV infection transmitted via factor VIII concentrate, and many have already developed AIDS. HIV-associated immune thrombocytopenia may aggravate the bleeding tendency.

B. Laboratory Findings: The partial thromboplastin time (PTT) is prolonged, and other measures of coagulation, including prothrombin time, bleeding time, and fibrinogen level, are normal. Levels of factor VIII:C are reduced, but measurements of von Willebrand factor are normal (Table 13–21).

If one mixes plasma from a hemophiliac patient with normal plasma, the PTT will become normal. Failure of the PTT to normalize in such a mixing test is diagnostic of the presence of a factor VIII inhibitor.

A low platelet count should raise a suspicion of HIV-associated immune thrombocytopenia.

Differential Diagnosis

The finding of a reduced factor VIII:C level will distinguish this disorder from other causes of prolonged PTT (Table 13–20). Clinically, factor VIII hemophilia is indistinguishable from factor IX hemophilia, and only specific factor assays can distinguish these disorders. In cases of mild hemophilia, the disorder needs to be distinguished from von Willebrand's disease by VIII:A assay, which shows normal levels of factor VIII antigen in the former.

An important issue for the families of hemophiliac patients is identifying which females are carriers. They can usually be identified by the presence of low or normal levels of factor VIII:C with normal levels of factor VIII antigen.

Treatment

Standard treatment is based on infusion of factor VIII concentrates, now heat-treated to reduce the likelihood of transmission of HIV. Recombinant factor VIII appears safe and effective, though expensive, and should impose no risk of transmitting HIV or other viruses. The level of factor VIII one aims to achieve in plasma depends on the severity of the bleeding problem. In response to minor bleeding, it may be necessary only to raise factor VIII:C levels to 25% with one infusion. For moderate bleeding (such as deep muscle hematomas), it is adequate to raise the level initially to 50% and maintain the level at greater than 25% with repeated infusion for 2–3 days. When major surgery is to be performed, one raises the factor VIII:C level to 100% and then maintains the factor level at greater than 50% continuously for 10–14 days. Head injuries (with or without neurologic signs) should be emergently treated as though major bleeding were present.

The dose of factor VIII concentrate is calculated assuming that one unit of factor VIII is the amount present in 1 mL of plasma. Plasma volume is 40 mL/kg, and the volume of distribution of factor VIII:C is 1.5 times the plasma volume. Thus, to raise the level 100%, the dose should be $40 \times 1.5 = 60$ units/kg, or approximately 4000 units for a 70-kg individual. To raise the levels to 25% would require 1000 units. The half-life of factor VIII:C is approximately 12 hours. Thus, during major surgery, to achieve an initial level of 100% and maintain it continuously at greater than 50%, a dose of 60 units/kg (approximately 4000 units) initially followed by 30 units/kg (approximately 2000 units) every 12 hours should be adequate. During surgery, one should initially verify that these doses give the anticipated factor VIII levels. If factor VIII levels fail to rise as expected, one should suspect an inhibitor.

For mild hemophiliacs, desmopressin acetate, 0.3 μg/kg every 24 hours, may be useful in preparing for minor surgical procedures. Desmopressin acetate causes release of factor VIII:C and will raise the factor VIII:C levels two- to threefold for several hours. In the management of persistent bleeding following use of either desmopressin acetate or factor VIII concentrate, patients may be treated with aminocaproic acid (EACA; Amicar), 4 g orally every 4 hours for several days.

Aspirin should never be used.

Prognosis

The prognosis of patients with hemophilia has been transformed by the availability of factor VIII replacement. The major limiting factor is disability from recurrent joint bleeding. Viral infections (hepatitis B and C, HIV) from recurrent transfusion are diminishing in incidence. Approximately 15% of patients develop inhibitors to factor VIII, and these patents cannot be adequately supported with factor VIII.

Cohen AJ, Kessler CM: Treatment of inherited coagulation disorders. Am J Med 1995;99:675. [NLM Cit ID: 96106305]

ACQUIRED FACTOR VIII ANTIBODIES

Antibodies to factor VIII may develop either postpartum or with no underlying illness. Factor VIII antibodies also occur in 15% of patients with factor VIII hemophilia who have received infusions of plasma concentrates.

Factor VIII antibodies usually produce a severe bleeding disorder. The PTT is prolonged, and the fibrinogen level, prothrombin time, and platelet count are not affected. A plasma mixing test will usually reveal the presence of an inhibitor by the failure of normal plasma to correct the prolonged PTT. However, the mixing test may require incubation for 2–4 hours to reveal the inhibitor. Factor VIII coagulant levels are low.

Factor VIII antibodies should be suspected in any acquired severe bleeding disorder associated with a prolonged PTT. Factor VIII antibodies are distinguished from lupus anticoagulants both by the presence of clinical bleeding and more importantly by the reduced factor VIII:C level. The diagnosis is confirmed by mixing tests and in vivo by the failure of factor VIII concentrates to raise the factor VIII:C levels by the expected amount.

The treatment of choice is cyclophosphamide, usually combined with prednisone. In the interim, aggressive factor VIII replacement may be necessary. Plasmapheresis to reduce inhibitor levels may be useful.

The prognosis of these patients is variable; overwhelming bleeding may create difficult management problems.

Shaffer LG: Successful treatment of acquired hemophilia with oral immunosuppressive therapy. Ann Intern Med 1997;127:206. [NLM Cit ID: 97372759]

HEMOPHILIA B

Essentials of Diagnosis

- X-linked recessive inheritance, with only males affected.
- Low levels of factor IX coagulant activity.
- Spontaneous hemarthroses.

General Considerations

Hemophilia B (Christmas disease, factor IX hemophilia) is a hereditary bleeding disorder due to deficiency of coagulation factor IX. Most commonly, factor IX is quantitatively reduced, but in one-third of cases an abnormally functioning molecule is immunologically present. Factor IX deficiency is one-seventh as common as factor VIII deficiency hemophilia but is otherwise clinically and genetically identical.

The PTT is prolonged, and factor IX levels are reduced when measured by specific factor assays. Other laboratory features are the same as for factor VIII hemophilia.

Treatment

Factor IX hemophilia is managed with factor IX concentrates. Factor VIII concentrates are ineffective in this type of hemophilia; therefore it is imperative to distinguish between the two. The same dosing considerations apply as in factor VIII hemophilia, with the exception that the volume of distribution of factor IX is twice the plasma volume, so that 80 units/kg are necessary to achieve a 100% level. In addition, the half-life of factor IX is 18 hours. Thus, to maintain a patient through major surgery, the dosage should be 80 units/kg (approximately 6000 units) initially followed by 40 units/kg (3000 units) every 18 hours. Factor IX levels should be measured to ensure that expected levels are achieved and that an inhibitor is not present.

Unlike factor VIII concentrates, factor IX concentrates contain a number of other proteins, including activated coagulating factors that appear to contribute to a risk of thrombosis with recurrent usage of factor IX concentrates. Because of the risk of thrombosis, more care is needed in deciding to use these concentrates. Desmopressin acetate is not useful in this disorder, and patients should be cautioned to avoid aspirin.

Prognosis

The prognosis for these patients is the same as for those with factor VIII hemophilia.

Djulbegovic B et al: Safety and efficacy of purified factor IX concentrate and antifibrinolytic agents for dental extractions in hemophilia B. Am J Hematol 1996;51:168. [NLM Cit ID: 96160439]

Hemophilia and von Willebrand's disease: 1. Diagnosis, comprehensive care and assessment. Association of Hemophilia Clinic Directors of Canada. Can Med Assoc J 1995;153:19. [NLM Cit ID: 95316809]

Hemophilia and von Willebrand's disease: 2. Management. Association of Hemophilia Clinic Directors of Canada. Can Med Assoc J 1995;153:147. [NLM Cit ID: 95323851]

Scharrer I: The need for highly purified products to treat hemophilia B. Acta Haematol 1995;94(Suppl 1):2. [NLM Cit ID: 96024665]

OTHER CONGENITAL COAGULATION DISORDERS

Factor XI Deficiency

This disorder is seen primarily among Ashkenazi Jews and is autosomal recessive. The PTT may be markedly prolonged, and specific assays of factor XI will show reduced levels. This is usually a mild bleeding disorder manifested primarily by postoperative bleeding. Factor replacement is given with fresh-frozen plasma when necessary.

Afibrinogenemia

In this rare disorder, fibrinogen is absent and both prothrombin time and partial thromboplastin time are markedly prolonged. These patients may have a severe bleeding disorder similar to hemophilia. Fibrinogen is replaced with cryoprecipitate.

Other Coagulation Disorders

Bleeding disorders due to isolated deficiency of factors II, V, X, or VII are extremely rare. Deficiencies of factor XII and the contact pathway factors cause a markedly prolonged PTT but are not associated with any increased bleeding.

Factor XIII deficiency results in delayed bleeding after trauma or surgery. All coagulation tests are normal. The disorder is diagnosed by showing instability of the fibrin clot in 8-molar urea. Factor XIII is replaced with cryoprecipitate or plasma. A rare cause of bleeding is deficiency of the normal inhibitors of fibrinolytic activity: α_2-antiplasmin and plasminogen activator inhibitor.

Fay WP: Human plasminogen activator inhibitor-1 (PAI-1) deficiency: Characterization of a large kindred with a null mutation in the PAI-1 gene. Blood 1997;90:204. [NLM Cit ID: 97351078]

COAGULOPATHY OF LIVER DISEASE

Essentials of Diagnosis

- Prothrombin time more prolonged than PTT.
- No response to vitamin K.

General Considerations

The liver is the site of synthesis of all the coagulation factors except factor VIII. As hepatic insufficiency develops, the vitamin K-dependent factors (factors II, VII, IX, X) and factor V are the first to be affected. Because of its rapid turnover (half-life 6 hours), factor VII levels are the first to decline. Conversely, fibrinogen levels are remarkably well conserved, and decreased fibrinogen synthesis does not occur unless liver disease is very severe.

Liver disease has a number of other effects on the hemostatic system. Increased fibrinolysis occurs because the liver synthesizes α_2-antiplasmin (the main inhibitor of fibrinolysis), which is responsible for the clearance of plasminogen activator. Biliary tract disease may lead to malabsorption of vitamin K, and congestive splenomegaly may produce mild thrombocytopenia. A variety of chronic liver diseases cause abnormal posttranslation modification of fibrinogen with resultant dysfibrinogenemia. The majority of patients with cirrhosis have very low levels of thrombopoietin, and this may contribute to the thrombocytopenia.

Clinical Findings

A. Symptoms and Signs: The coagulopathy of liver disease may lead to bleeding at any site. Excessive fibrinolysis may lead to oozing at venipuncture sites. Most patients have clinically obvious serious liver disease.

B. Laboratory Findings: Hepatic coagulopathy produces a more marked abnormality in the prothrombin time (PT) than in the partial thromboplastin time (PTT). Early in the course of liver disease, only the PT will be affected. Fibrinogen levels should be normal, and the thrombin time should be normal unless dysfibrinogenemia is present. The platelet count is usually normal but may be reduced by low levels of thrombopoietin, by hypersplenism, or by bone marrow suppression by alcohol. The peripheral blood smear may show target cells.

Differential Diagnosis

Hepatic coagulopathy can be distinguished from vitamin K deficiency only by demonstrating the failure of vitamin K to correct the abnormal values. Liver disease is distinguished from disseminated intravascular coagulation by the normal fibrinogen level and lack of thrombocytopenia. End-stage liver disease almost invariably leads to some element of disseminated intravascular coagulation, and the disorders overlap (Tables 13–22 and 13–23).

Treatment

Long-term treatment of hepatic coagulopathy with factor replacement is usually ineffective. Fresh-frozen plasma is the treatment of choice, and volume overload will limit one's ability to maintain hemostatic factor levels. For example, to maintain factor levels greater than 25%, one must initially raise the level to 50% with 50% of the plasma volume (20 mL/kg) and then replace 10 mL/kg every 6 hours to maintain adequate factor VII levels. In average-sized persons, this will require transfusion of 1400 mL of plasma initially followed by 700 mL every 6 hours. Factor IX concentrates are contraindicated in liver disease because of their tendency to cause disseminated intravascular coagulation. If thrombocytopenia is present, platelet transfusion may be of some help, but platelet recovery is usually disappointing because of hypersplenism.

Table 13–22. Causes of isolated prolonged prothrombin time.

Liver disease
Vitamin K deficiency
Warfarin therapy
Factor VII deficiency

Table 13–23. Causes of prolonged prothrombin time and partial thromboplastin time.

Liver disease
Vitamin K deficiency
Disseminated intravascular coagulation
Heparin
Warfarin
Isolated factor deficiencies (rare): II, V, X, I

Prognosis

The prognosis is that of the underlying liver disease.

Martin TG: Thrombopoietin levels in patients with cirrhosis before and after orthotopic liver transplantation. Ann Intern Med 1997;127:285. [NLM Cit ID: 97395382]

Vadhan-Raj S: Stimulation of megakaryocyte and platelet production by a single dose of recombinant human thrombopoietin in patients with cancer. Ann Intern Med 1997;126:673. [NLM Cit ID: 97267476]

VITAMIN K DEFICIENCY

Essentials of Diagnosis

- Underlying dietary deficiency or antibiotic use.
- Prothrombin time more prolonged than PTT.
- Rapid correction with vitamin K replacement.

General Considerations

Vitamin K plays a role in coagulation by acting as a cofactor for the posttranslational γ-carboxylation of zymogens II, VII, IX, and X. The modified zymogens (with γ-carboxyglutamic acid residues) are able to bind to platelets in a calcium-dependent reaction and consequently better participate in the complex reactions that activate factors X and II. Without γ-carboxylation, these reactions on the platelet surface occur slowly and hemostasis is impaired.

Vitamin K is supplied in the diet primarily in leafy vegetables and endogenously from synthesis by intestinal bacteria. Factors that contribute to vitamin K deficiency include poor diet, malabsorption, and broad-spectrum antibiotics suppressing colonic flora. A characteristic setting for vitamin K deficiency is a postoperative patient who is not eating and who is receiving antibiotics. Body stores of vitamin K are small, and deficiency may develop in as little as 1 week.

Clinical Findings

A. Symptoms and Signs: There are no specific clinical features, and bleeding may occur at any site.

B. Laboratory Findings: The prothrombin time is prolonged to a greater extent than the PTT, and with mild vitamin K deficiency only the PT is defective (Tables 13–22 and 13–23). Fibrinogen level, thrombin time, and platelet count are not affected.

Differential Diagnosis

Vitamin K deficiency can be distinguished from hepatic coagulopathy only by assessing the response to vitamin K therapy. Surreptitious warfarin use will produce laboratory features indistinguishable from those of vitamin K deficiency.

Vitamin K deficiency is distinguished from disseminated intravascular coagulation by normal platelet count and fibrinogen levels in the former.

Treatment

Vitamin K deficiency responds rapidly to subcutaneous vitamin K, and a single dose of 15 mg will completely correct laboratory abnormalities in 12–24 hours.

Prognosis

The prognosis is excellent, as vitamin K deficiency can be completely corrected with replacement.

Lipsky JJ: Nutritional sources of vitamin K. Mayo Clin Proc 1994;65:462. [NLM Cit ID: 94223947] (Antibiotics do not cause hypoprothrombinemia except in those with renal failure, cancer, or poor oral intake; poor diet alone even with normal intestinal flora can produce vitamin K deficiency.)

DISSEMINATED INTRAVASCULAR COAGULATION (DIC)

Essentials of Diagnosis

- Underlying serious illness.
- Microangiopathic hemolytic anemia may be present.
- Hypofibrinogenemia, thrombocytopenia, fibrin degradation products, and prolonged prothrombin time.

General Considerations

Coagulation is usually confined to a localized area by the combination of blood flow and circulating inhibitors of coagulation, especially antithrombin III. If the stimulus to coagulation is too great, these control mechanisms can be overwhelmed, leading to the syndrome of disseminated intravascular coagulation. In pathophysiologic terms, disseminated intravascular coagulation can be thought of as the consequence of the presence of circulating thrombin (normally confined to a localized area). The effects of thrombin are to cleave fibrinogen to fibrin monomer, stimulate platelet aggregation, activate factors V and VIII, and release plasminogen activator, which generates plasmin. Plasmin in turn cleaves fibrin, generating fibrin degradation products, and further inactivates factors V and VIII. Thus, the excess thrombin activity produces hypofibrinogenemia, thrombocytopenia, depletion of coagulation factors, and fibrinolysis.

Disseminated intravascular coagulation can be caused by a number of serious illnesses, including sepsis (especially with gram-negative bacteria but possible with any widespread bacterial or fungal infection), severe tissue injury (especially burns and head injury), obstetric complications (amniotic fluid embolus, septic abortion, retained fetus), cancer (acute promyelocytic leukemia, mucinous adenocarcinomas), and major hemolytic transfusion reactions.

Clinical Findings

A. Symptoms and Signs: Disseminated intravascular coagulation leads to both bleeding and thrombosis. Bleeding is far more common than thrombosis, but the latter may dominate if coagulation is activated to a far greater extent than fibrinolysis. Bleeding may occur at any site, but spontaneous bleeding and oozing at venipuncture sites or wounds are important clues to the diagnosis. Thrombosis is most commonly manifested by digital ischemia and gangrene, but catastrophic events such as renal cortical necrosis and hemorrhagic adrenal infarction may occur. Disseminated intravascular coagulation may also secondarily produce microangiopathic hemolytic anemia.

Subacute disseminated intravascular coagulation is seen primarily in cancer patients and is manifested primarily as recurrent superficial and deep venous thromboses **(Trousseau's syndrome).**

B. Laboratory Findings: Disseminated intravascular coagulation produces a complex coagulopathy with the characteristic constellation of hypofibrinogenemia, elevated fibrin degradation products, thrombocytopenia, and a prolonged prothrombin time. Of the fibrin degradation products, the D-dimer is the most sensitive, since its cross-linking implies origin from fibrin in a clot. All fibrin degradation products are cleared by the liver and thus may be elevated in hepatic dysfunction. Hypofibrinogenemia is another important diagnostic laboratory feature, because only a few other disorders (congenital hypofibrinogenemia, severe liver disease) will lower the fibrinogen level. In some cases of disseminated intravascular coagulation, when the patient's baseline fibrinogen level is markedly elevated, the initial fibrinogen level may be normal. However, since the half-life of fibrinogen is approximately 4 days, a noticeably falling fibrinogen level will confirm the diagnosis of disseminated intravascular coagulation.

Other laboratory abnormalities are variably present. The partial thromboplastin time may or may not be prolonged. In approximately one-fourth of cases, a microangiopathic hemolytic anemia is present, and fragmented red blood cells are seen on the peripheral smear. Antithrombin III levels may be markedly depleted. When fibrinolysis is activated, levels of plasminogen and α_2-antiplasmin may be low.

Subacute disseminated intravascular coagulation produces a very different laboratory picture. Thrombocytopenia and elevated D-dimer are usually the only abnormalities. Fibrinogen levels are normal, and the PTT may be normal.

Differential Diagnosis

Liver disease may prolong both the PT and PTT, but fibrinogen levels are usually normal, and the platelet count is usually normal or only slightly reduced. However, severe liver disease may be difficult to distinguish from disseminated intravascular coagulation. Vitamin K deficiency will not affect the fibrinogen level or platelet count and will be completely corrected by vitamin K replacement.

Sepsis may produce thrombocytopenia and digital ischemia, and coagulopathy may be present because of vitamin K deficiency. However, in these cases, the fibrinogen level should be normal.

Thrombotic thrombocytopenic purpura may produce fever and microangiopathic hemolytic anemia. However, fibrinogen levels and other coagulation studies should be normal.

Treatment

The primary focus should be the diagnosis and treatment of the underlying disorder that has given rise to disseminated intravascular coagulation. In many cases, disseminated intravascular coagulation will produce laboratory abnormalities with only mild clinical manifestations, and in these cases no specific therapy is required.

When the underlying cause of disseminated intravascular coagulation is rapidly reversible (such as in obstetric cases), replacement therapy alone may be indicated. The role of heparin in the treatment of disseminated intravascular coagulation is controversial. In some cases, when any increase in bleeding is unacceptable (neurosurgical procedures), heparin therapy is contraindicated. However, when disseminated intravascular coagulation is producing serious clinical consequences and the underlying cause is not rapidly reversible, heparin may be necessary. Such therapy is routinely used in the treatment of acute promyelocytic leukemia.

In replacement therapy, platelet transfusion should be used to maintain a platelet count greater than 30,000/μL, and 50,000/μL if possible. Fibrinogen is replaced with cryoprecipitate, and one should aim for a plasma fibrinogen level of 150 mg/dL. One unit of cryoprecipitate usually raises the fibrinogen level by 6–8 mg/dL, so that 15 units of cryoprecipitate will raise the level from 50 to 150 mg/dL. Coagulation factor deficiency may require replacement with fresh-frozen plasma.

Heparin must be used in combination with replacement therapy, since heparin alone will lead to an unacceptable increase in bleeding. A dose of 500–750 units per hour is necessary. Heparin cannot be effective if antithrombin III levels are markedly depleted. Antithrombin III levels should be measured, and fresh-frozen plasma used to raise levels to greater than 50%. In using heparin, it is not necessary to prolong the PTT. Successful therapy is indicated by a rising fibrinogen level. Fibrin degradation products will decline over 1–2 days. Improvement in the platelet count may lag as much as 1 week behind control of the coagulopathy.

In some cases, when disseminated intravascular coagulation is complicated by excessive fibrinolysis, even the combination of heparin and replacement therapy may not be adequate to control bleeding. In these cases, aminocaproic acid, 1 g intravenously per hour, or tranexamic acid, 10 mg/kg intravenously every 8 hours, should be added to decrease the rate of fibrinolysis, raise the fibrinogen level, and control bleeding. Aminocaproic acid can *never* be used without heparin in disseminated intravascular coagulation because of the risk of thrombosis.

Prognosis

The prognosis is that of the underlying disease.

Bick RL: Disseminated intravascular coagulation: Objective clinical and laboratory diagnosis, treatment, and assessment of therapeutic response. Semin Thromb Hemost 1996;22:69. [NLM Cit ID: 96250037]

Baglin T: Disseminated intravascular coagulation: Diagnosis and treatment. BMJ 1996;312:683. [NLM Cit ID: 96182713]

HYPERCOAGULABLE STATES

In many cases, thrombosis is related to local factors causing stasis of blood flow or damage to a blood vessel. Common examples are deep venous thrombosis in the legs following prolonged sitting in one position and thrombosis in the femoral and iliac veins following hip surgery. However, in other cases a systemic disorder causes a general increase in the risk of thrombosis (Table 13–24).

Cancer is associated with an increased risk of both venous and arterial thrombosis. In some cases, low-grade disseminated intravascular coagulation appears to be responsible. In unusual cases, a unique cancer procoagulant stimulates the clotting system. Myeloproliferative disorders such as polycythemia vera, essential thrombocytosis, and paroxysmal nocturnal hemoglobinuria are associated with a high incidence of thrombosis, caused by qualitative platelet abnormalities. Venous thrombosis may occur in unusual locations such as the mesenteric, hepatic, or splenic venous beds. Arterial thrombosis occurs as well and

Table 13–24. Causes of hypercoagulability.

Acquired
Cancer
Inflammatory disorders: ulcerative colitis
Myeloproliferative disorders
Postoperative
Estrogens, pregnancy
Lupus anticoagulant
Heparin-induced thrombocytopenia
Anticardiolipin antibodies
Congenital
Antithrombin III deficiency
Factor V Leiden
Protein C deficiency
Protein S deficiency
Dysfibrinogenemia
Abnormal plasminogen

may be manifested as large vessel occlusion (stroke, myocardial infarction) or as microvascular events with painful burning in the hands and feet.

Heparin is an uncommon but important cause of hypercoagulability. Heparin has been associated with thrombocytopenia in about 10% of treatment courses. Often the thrombocytopenia is modest and resolves spontaneously. However, in some cases severe thrombocytopenia occurs. It is most often in this setting that arterial thrombosis occurs as a complication. The arteries involved are often large ones, such as the iliac artery or even the aorta. It is imperative that heparin be discontinued in this setting, since continuing the drug almost always leads to a fatal outcome.

A number of congenital biochemical defects have also been associated with hypercoagulability (Table 13–24). A family history is usually present. The thromboses are almost always venous and may occur in the large veins of the abdomen. Thromboses often occur during early adulthood rather than in childhood and are often precipitated by factors such as trauma or pregnancy. The most common of these disorders is an abnormal factor V (factor V Leiden), which is resistant to degradation by activated protein C. Dysfibrinogenemia is diagnosed by a prolonged reptilase time.

The syndrome of **warfarin-induced skin necrosis** may occur in patients with undiagnosed protein C deficiency. Protein C is vitamin K-dependent and has a shorter half-life than the coagulation proteins. Warfarin, by creating a vitamin K-dependent state, will transiently deplete protein C before it leads to anticoagulation. During the period of hypercoagulability due to unopposed protein C depletion, thrombosis of skin vessels may lead to infarction and necrosis. The syndrome can be prevented by the use of heparin for 5–7 days until warfarin induces anticoagulation.

Treatment

If a patient is recognized to be at increased risk of thrombosis, effective prophylactic therapy is usually available. Preoperatively, minidose heparin (5000 units every 8–12 hours) may be useful in reducing the risk of thrombosis in the perioperative period. The hypercoagulable state associated with cancer may benefit from treatment with heparin, 10,000 units subcutaneously every 12 hours. Low-molecular-weight heparin is a more convenient agent which is equally effective and requires less laboratory monitoring. Warfarin is usually ineffective in preventing thrombosis in this situation, most likely because low-grade disseminated intravascular coagulation is the cause. In patients with myeloproliferative disease who have had symptoms of thrombosis, antiplatelet therapy may be helpful. However, such therapy should not be used indiscriminately, because these patients are also at increased risk of bleeding. For patients with **erythromelalgia** (painful redness and burning of the hands), aspirin, 325 mg daily, is effective.

For patients with congenital biochemical defects such as deficiency of antithrombin III or the vitamin K-dependent proteins C and S, warfarin is effective and should probably be given for life. Family members should be screened for the presence of the defect so that their increased risk of thrombosis can be noted and acted upon.

De Stefano V et al: The risk of recurrent deep venous thrombosis among heterozygous carriers of both factor V Leiden and the G20210A prothrombin mutation. N Engl J Med 1999;341:801. [NLM Cit ID: 99393045]

Rosenberg RD: Vascular bed-specific hemostasis and hypercoagulable states. N Engl J Med 1999;340:1555. [NLM Cit ID: 99247678]

Thomas DP: Hypercoagulability in venous and arterial thrombosis. Ann Intern Med 1997;126:638. [NLM Cit ID: 97243275]

Toglia MR, Weg JG: Venous thromboembolism during pregnancy. N Engl J Med 1996;335:108. [NLM Cit ID: 96266362]

LUPUS ANTICOAGULANT

The lupus anticoagulant is an IgM or IgG immunoglobulin that produces a prolonged PTT by binding to the phospholipid used in the in vitro PTT assay. As such, it is a laboratory artifact and does not cause a clinical bleeding disorder. The "lupus anticoagulant" is seen in 5–10% of patients with systemic lupus erythematosus. More commonly, it is seen without an underlying disorder or in patients taking phenothiazines.

There is no bleeding defect unless a second disorder such as thrombocytopenia, hypoprothrombinemia, or a prolonged bleeding time is present. In fact, the lupus anticoagulant has been associated with an increased risk of thrombosis and of recurrent spontaneous abortions.

The PTT is prolonged and fails to correct when the patient's plasma is mixed in a 1:1 dilution with normal plasma. The PT is either normal or slightly prolonged. The fibrinogen level and thrombin time are normal. The Russell viper venom (RVV) time is a more sensitive assay and is specifically designed to demonstrate the presence of a lupus anticoagulant. An antiphospholipid, the lupus anticoagulant will cause a false-positive VDRL test for syphilis. A related autoantibody, anticardiolipin, can be detected by separate assays.

Lupus anticoagulant should be suspected in cases of a markedly prolonged PTT without clinical bleeding (other causes are factor XII or contact factor deficiency). The plasma mixing test will demonstrate the presence of an inhibitor by the failure of normal plasma to correct the PTT. When acquired factor VIII inhibitors are being considered, a factor VIII:C level may be measured; this will be normal in patients with lupus anticoagulant.

No specific treatment is necessary. Prednisone will usually rapidly eliminate the lupus anticoagulant, and it has been suggested that prednisone therapy reduces spontaneous abortions in this syndrome. It is not clear whether prednisone has any effect on the thrombotic tendency associated with lupus anticoagulant. Patients with thromboses should be treated with anticoagulation in standard doses. Because of the artificially prolonged PTT, heparin therapy is difficult to monitor properly, and low-molecular weight heparin may be preferred. The dose of warfarin administered may also be inadequate if the baseline PT is prolonged.

Ginsberg JS et al: Antiphospholipid antibodies and venous thromboembolism. Blood 1995;86:3685. [NLM Cit ID: 96068732]

Khamashta MA et al: The management of thrombosis in the antiphospholipid-antibody syndrome. N Engl J Med 1995;332:993. [NLM Cit ID: 95191634]

Shapiro SS: The lupus anticoagulant/antiphospholipid syndrome. Annu Rev Med 1996;47:533. [NLM Cit ID: 96266663]

BLOOD TRANSFUSIONS

RED BLOOD CELL TRANSFUSIONS

Red blood cell transfusions are given to raise the hematocrit levels in patients with anemia or to replace losses after acute bleeding episodes. Several types of components containing red blood cells are available.

(1) Fresh whole blood: The advantage of this component is the simultaneous presence of red blood cells, plasma, and fresh platelets. Fresh whole blood is never absolutely necessary, since all the above components are available separately. The major indications for use of whole blood are cardiac surgery or massive hemorrhage when more than ten units of blood are required in a 24-hour period.

(2) Packed red blood cells: Packed red cells are the component most commonly used to raise the hematocrit. Each unit has a volume of about 300 mL, of which approximately 200 mL consists of red blood cells. One unit of packed red cells will usually raise the hematocrit by approximately 4%. The expected rise in hematocrit can be calculated using an estimated red blood cell volume of 200 mL/unit and a total blood volume of about 70 mL/kg. For example, a 70-kg man will have a total blood volume of 4900 mL, and each unit of packed red blood cells will raise the hematocrit by 200 ÷ 4900 equals 4%.

(3) Leukopoor blood: Patients with severe leukoagglutinin reactions to packed red blood cells may require depletion of white blood cells and platelets from transfused units. White blood cells can be removed either by centrifugation or by washing. Preparation of leukopoor blood is expensive and leads to some loss of red cells.

(4) Frozen blood: Red blood cells can be frozen and stored for up to 3 years, but the technique is cumbersome and expensive, and frozen blood should be used sparingly. The major application is for the purpose of maintaining a supply of rare blood types. Patients with such types may donate units for autologous transfusion should the need arise. Frozen red cells are also occasionally needed for patients with severe leukoagglutinin reactions or anaphylactic reactions to plasma proteins, since frozen blood has essentially all white blood cells and plasma components removed.

(5) Autologous packed red blood cells: Patients scheduled for elective surgery may donate blood for autologous transfusion. These units may be stored for up to 35 days.

Compatibility Testing

Before transfusion, the recipient's and the donor's blood are cross-matched to avoid hemolytic transfusion reactions. Although many antigen systems are present on red blood cells, only the ABO and Rh systems are specifically tested prior to all transfusions. The A and B antigens are the most important, because everyone who lacks one or both red cell antigens has isoantibodies against the missing antigen or antigens in his or her plasma. These antibodies activate complement and can cause rapid intravascular lysis of the incompatible red cells. In emergencies, type O blood can be given to any recipient, but only packed cells should be given to avoid transfusion of donor plasma containing anti-A or anti-B antibodies.

The other important antigen routinely tested for is the D antigen of the Rh system. Approximately 15% of the population lack this antigen. In patients lacking the antigen, anti-D antibodies are not naturally present, but the antigen is highly immunogenic. A recipient whose red cells lack D and who receives D-positive blood may develop anti-D antibodies that can cause severe lysis of subsequent transfusions of D-positive red cells.

Blood typing includes assay of recipient serum for unusual antibodies by mixing the serum with panels of red cells representing commonly occurring weak antigens. The screening is particularly important if the recipient has had previous transfusions.

Hemolytic Transfusion Reactions

The most severe reactions are those involving mismatches in the ABO system. Most of these cases are due to clerical errors and mislabeled specimens. Hemolysis is rapid and intravascular, releasing free hemoglobin into the plasma. The severity of these reactions depends on the dose of red blood cells given. The most severe reactions are those seen in surgical patients under anesthesia.

Hemolytic transfusion reactions caused by minor antigen systems are typically less severe. The hemolysis usually takes place at a slower rate and is extravascular. Sometimes these transfusion reactions may be delayed for 5–10 days after transfusion. In such cases, the recipient has received blood containing an immunogenic action, and in the time since transfusion, a new alloantibody has been formed. The most common antigens involved in such reactions are Duffy, Kidd, Kell, and C and E loci of the Rh system.

A. Symptoms and Signs: Major hemolytic transfusion reactions cause fever and chills, with backache and headache. In severe cases, there may be apprehension, dyspnea, hypotension, and vascular collapse. *The transfusion must be stopped immediately.* In severe cases, disseminated intravascular coagulation, acute renal failure from tubular necrosis, or both can occur.

Patients under general anesthesia will not give such signs, and the first indication may be generalized bleeding and oliguria.

B. Laboratory Findings and Management: Identification of the recipient and of the blood should be checked. The donor transfusion bag with its pilot tube must be returned to the blood bank, and a fresh sample of the recipient's blood must accompany the donor bag for retyping of donor and recipient blood samples and for repeat of the cross-match.

The hematocrit will fail to rise by the expected amount. Coagulation studies may reveal evidence of renal failure and disseminated intravascular coagulation. Hemoglobinemia will turn the plasma pink and eventually result in hemoglobinuria. In cases of delayed hemolytic reactions, the hematocrit will fall and the indirect bilirubin will rise. In these cases, the new offending alloantibody is easily detected in the patient's serum.

C. Treatment: If a hemolytic transfusion reaction is suspected, the transfusion should be stopped at once. A sample of anticoagulated blood from the recipient should be centrifuged to detect free hemoglobin in the plasma. If hemoglobinemia is present, the patient should be vigorously hydrated to prevent acute tubular necrosis. Forced diuresis with mannitol may help prevent renal damage.

Leukoagglutinin Reactions

Most transfusion reactions are not hemolytic but represent reactions to antigens present on white blood cells in patients who have been sensitized to the antigens through previous transfusions or pregnancy. Most commonly, patients will develop fever and chills within 12 hours after transfusion. In severe cases, cough and dyspnea may occur and the chest x-ray may show transient pulmonary infiltrates. Because no hemolysis is involved, the hematocrit rises by the expected amount despite the reaction.

Leukoagglutinin reactions may respond to acetaminophen and diphenhydramine; corticosteroids are also of value. Removal of leukocytes by filtration before blood storage will reduce the incidence of these reactions.

Anaphylactic Reactions

Rarely, patients will develop urticaria or bronchospasm during a transfusion. These reactions are almost always due to plasma proteins rather than white blood cells. Patients who are IgA-deficient may develop these reactions because of antibodies to IgA. Patients with such reactions may require transfusion of washed or even frozen red blood cells to avoid future severe reactions.

Contaminated Blood

Rarely, blood is contaminated with gram-negative bacteria. Transfusion can lead to septicemia and shock from endotoxin. If this is suspected, the offending unit should be cultured and the patient treated with antibiotics as indicated.

Diseases Transmitted Through Transfusion

Despite the use of only volunteer blood donors and the routine screening of blood, transfusion-associated viral diseases remain a problem. All blood products (red blood cells, platelets, plasma, cryoprecipitate) can transmit viral diseases. All blood donors are screened with questionnaires designed to detect donors at high risk of transmitting diseases. All blood is now routinely screened with a variety of tests including hepatitis B surface antigen, antibody to hepatitis B core antigen, syphilis, p24 antigen and antibody to HIV, antibody to HCV, and antibody to HTLV.

With improved screening, the risk of posttransfusion hepatitis has steadily decreased. The risk of hepatitis B is 1:200,000 per unit and of HIV 1:250,000 per unit. The risk of seroconversion to HTLV is 1:70,000, but clinical sequelae when this occurs are rare. The major infectious risk of blood products is hepatitis C, with a seroconversion rate of 1:3300 per unit transfused. Most of these cases are clinically silent, but there is a high incidence of chronic hepatitis.

Platelet Transfusion

Platelet transfusions are indicated in cases of thrombocytopenia due to decreased platelet production. They are not useful in immune thrombocytopenia, since transfused platelets will last no longer than the patient's endogenous platelets. The risk of spontaneous bleeding rises when the platelet count falls to less than 10,000/μL, and the risk of life-threatening bleeding increases when the platelet count is less than 5000/μL. Because of this, prophylactic platelet transfusions are often given at these very low levels. Platelet transfusions are also given prior to invasive procedures or surgery, and the goal should be to raise the platelet count to over 50,000/μL.

Platelets are most commonly derived from donated blood units. One unit of platelets (derived from 1 unit of blood) usually contains 5–7 $\times$ 10^{10} platelets suspended in 35 mL of plasma. Ideally, 1 platelet unit will raise the recipient's platelet count by 10,000/μL, and transfused platelets will last for 2 or 3 days. However, responses are often suboptimal, with poor platelet increments and short survival times. This may be due to sepsis, splenomegaly, or alloimmunization. Most alloantibodies causing platelet destruction are directed at HLA antigens. Patients requiring long periods of platelet transfusion support should be monitored to document adequate responses to transfusions so that the most appropriate product can be used. Patients may benefit from HLA-matched platelets derived from either volunteer donors or family members, with platelets obtained by plateletpheresis. Techniques of cross-matching platelets have been developed and appear to identify suitable platelet donors (nonreactive with the patient's serum) without the need for HLA typing. Such single-donor platelets usually contain the equivalent of six units of random platelets, or 30–50 $\times$ 10^{10} platelets suspended in 200 mL of plasma. Ideally, these platelet concentrates will raise the recipient's platelet count by 60,000/μL. Leukocyte depletion of platelets has been shown to delay the onset of alloimmunization.

Granulocyte Transfusions

Granulocyte transfusions are seldom indicated and have largely been replaced by the use of myeloid growth factors (G-CSF and GM-CSF) that speed neutrophil recovery. However, they may be beneficial in patients with profound neutropenia (< 100/μL) who have gram-negative sepsis or progressive soft tissue infection despite optimal antibiotic therapy. In these cases, it is clear that progressive infection is due to failure of host defenses. In such situations, daily granulocyte transfusions should be given and continued until the neutrophil count rises to above 500/μL. Such granulocytes must be derived from ABO-matched donors. Although HLA matching is not necessary, it is preferred, since patients with alloantibodies to donor white blood cells will have severe reactions and no benefit.

The donor cells usually contain some immunocompetent lymphocytes capable of producing graft-versus-host disease in HLA-incompatible hosts whose immunocompetence may be impaired. Irradiation of the units of cells with 1500 cGy will destroy the lymphocytes without harm to the granulocytes or platelets.

Goodnough LT: Transfusion medicine. (Two parts.) N Engl J Med 1999;340:438, 525. [NLM Cit ID: 99122625 and 99134023]

Liang TJ: Pathogenesis, natural history, treatment, and prevention of hepatitis C. Ann Intern Med 2000;132:296. [NLM Cit ID: 20132334]

Sagmeister M: A restrictive platelet transfusion policy allowing long-term support of outpatients with severe aplastic anemia. Blood 1999;93:3124. [NLM Cit ID: 99233678]

TRANSFUSION OF PLASMA COMPONENTS

Fresh-frozen plasma is available in units of approximately 200 mL. Fresh plasma contains normal levels of all coagulation factors (about 1 unit/mL). Fresh frozen plasma is used to correct coagulation factor deficiencies and to treat thrombotic thrombocytopenic purpura. The risk of transmitting viral disease is comparable to that associated with transfusion of red blood cells.

Cryoprecipitate is made from fresh plasma. One unit has a volume of approximately 20 mL and contains approximately 250 mg of fibrinogen and between 80 and 100 units of factor VIII and von Willebrand factor. Cryoprecipitate is used to supplement fibrinogen in cases of congenital deficiency of fibrinogen or disseminated intravascular coagulation. One unit of cryoprecipitate will raise the fibrinogen level by about 8 mg/dL.

College of American Pathologists: Practice parameter for the use of fresh frozen plasma, cryoprecipitate, and platelets. JAMA 1994;271:777. [NLM Cit ID: 94158044]

RELEVANT WORLD WIDE WEB SITES

[Hemophilic Arthropathy Demonstration Case]
http://www.brighamrad.harvard.edu/Cases/bwh/hcache/164/full.html
[Introduction to Blood Morphology]
http://www.hslib.washington.edu/courses/blood/intro.html
[Leukemia Society of America]
http://www.leukemia.org
[Lymphoma Research Foundation]
http://www.lymphoma.org
[Plasma Cell Myeloma Demonstration Case]
http://www.brighamrad.harvard.edu/Cases/bwh/hcache/9/full.html
[Sickle Cell Anemia Demonstration Case]
http://www.brighamrad.harvard.edu/Cases/bwh/hcache/81/full.html

Alimentary Tract

14

See http://www.current-med.com/ch14.html for updated addresses of Web sites referenced in this chapter.

Kenneth R. McQuaid, MD

SYMPTOMS & SIGNS OF GASTROINTESTINAL DISEASE

DYSPEPSIA

"Dyspepsia" refers to a host of upper abdominal or epigastric symptoms such as pain, discomfort, fullness, bloating, early satiety, belching, heartburn, regurgitation, or, simply, "indigestion." It occurs in one-fourth of the adult population and accounts for 3% of general medical office visits.

Etiology

A wide variety of disorders may cause dyspepsia.

A. Drug Intolerance: Examples include aspirin, NSAIDs, antibiotics (metronidazole, erythromycin), corticosteroids, digoxin, theophylline, iron, narcotics, alcohol, and caffeine.

B. Luminal Gastrointestinal Tract Dysfunction: Of patients with dyspepsia who undergo endoscopy, gastroesophageal reflux disease is present in 5–15% and peptic ulcer disease in 15–25%. Gastric cancer is identified in 1% but is rare in persons under age 45 years. Other causes include gastroparesis (especially in diabetes mellitus), lactose intolerance and malabsorptive conditions, and parasitic infection (giardia, strongyloides). The role of chronic *Helicobacter pylori*-associated gastritis as a cause of dyspepsia remains controversial.

C. Pancreatic Disease: Pancreatic carcinoma, chronic pancreatitis.

D. Biliary Tract Disease: The abrupt onset of pain from biliary colic due to cholelithiasis or choledocholithiasis should be readily distinguishable from dyspepsia.

E. Other Conditions: Diabetes, thyroid disease, myocardial ischemia, autoimmune disease, intra-abdominal malignancy, and pregnancy.

F. Functional or "Nonulcer" Dyspepsia: This is the most common cause of chronic dyspepsia. Up to two-thirds of dyspeptic patients have no obvious organic or biochemical cause for their symptoms diagnosable by upper endoscopy or abdominal ultrasonography. Symptoms may arise from a complex interaction of increased visceral afferent sensitivity, delayed gastric emptying or impaired accommodation to food, or psychosocial stressors.

Clinical Findings

A. Symptoms and Signs: Given the nonspecific nature of dyspeptic symptoms, the history has limited diagnostic utility. It should clarify the chronicity, location, and quality of the discomfort. The presence of more specific symptoms should be elicited, such as weight loss, persistent vomiting, dysphagia, hematemesis, or melena. When present, they warrant endoscopy or abdominal imaging. Potentially offending medications and excessive alcohol use should be identified and discontinued if possible. The patient's reason for seeking care should be determined. Many patients report a fear of a serious underlying condition. Recent changes in employment, marital discord, physical and sexual abuse, anxiety, and depression may all contribute to the development and reporting of symptoms.

The symptom profile alone does not differentiate between nonulcer dyspepsia, peptic ulcer disease, and gastroesophageal reflux disease. Experienced clinicians are wrong as often as right in their initial clinical impression. Nevertheless, patients with peptic ulcer disease are more likely to be older (> 45 years), to smoke, and to have pain relieved by food or antacids. Patients with nonulcer dyspepsia are younger, report a variety of abdominal and extragastrointestinal complaints, show signs of anxiety or depression, or have a history of use of psychotropic medications. Heartburn as the predominant symptom is 90% specific for the diagnosis of gastroesophageal reflux disease. However, many patients with reflux disease have dyspepsia (ie, epigastric discomfort) in addition to heartburn.

The physical examination is rarely helpful. Signs of serious organic disease such as weight loss, organomegaly, abdominal mass, or fecal occult blood warrant further investigation. In patients over age 45, initial laboratory work should include a blood count, electrolytes, liver enzymes, calcium, and thyroid function tests.

Special Examinations: Upper endoscopy is the study of choice to diagnose gastroduodenal ulcers, erosive esophagitis, and upper gastrointestinal malignancy. Up to half of patients with gastroesophageal reflux disease will not have endoscopic evidence of esophagitis (erosions). Upper gastrointestinal barium radiography is inferior to endoscopy for the evaluation of dyspepsia.

The optimal cost-effective approach to dyspepsia is controversial. Upper endoscopy is indicated in all patients over age 45 years with new-onset dyspepsia and in all patients with weight loss, dysphagia, recurrent vomiting, evidence of bleeding, or anemia. It is also helpful for those patients who are concerned about serious underlying disease.

Recognition of the role of *H pylori* in peptic ulcer disease has altered the approach to younger patients with uncomplicated dyspepsia, in whom gastric cancer is rare. Consensus guidelines recommend an initial noninvasive test for *H pylori* (IgG serology or urea breath test) in most young, uncomplicated patients with dyspepsia. If negative in a patient not taking NSAIDs peptic ulcer disease is virtually excluded. The majority of these *H pylori*-negative patients have functional dyspepsia or gastroesophageal reflux disease and can be treated with either an antisecretory agent (H_2 antagonist or proton pump inhibitor) or a promotility agent (eg, cisapride) for 4–8 weeks. If symptoms fail to respond or rapidly recur after stopping treatment, endoscopy is recommended. In patients testing positive for *H pylori,* antibiotic therapy proves definitive for over 90% of peptic ulcers and conceivably may improve symptoms in a subset of patients with functional dyspepsia. Endoscopic evaluation is warranted when symptoms fail to respond.

Abdominal ultrasonography is indicated only when pancreatic or biliary tract disease is suspected. Gastric emptying studies are valuable only in patients with recurrent vomiting.

Treatment of Functional Dyspepsia

In patients with functional dyspepsia, the following should be considered.

A. General Measures: A stable physician-patient interaction is the most important aspect of therapy. Patients require reassurance that the condition is not serious but may be chronic. Alcohol and caffeine intake should be reduced or discontinued. A food diary, in which patients record their food intake, symptoms, and daily events, may reveal dietary or psychosocial precipitants of pain.

B. Pharmacologic Agents: Over half of patients derive relief from placebo. H_2 receptor antagonists (ranitidine, 150 mg twice daily; famotidine, 20 mg twice daily; or cimetidine, 400–800 mg twice daily) are slightly better than placebo but offer benefit to those with symptoms suggestive of gastroesophageal reflux. Prokinetic agents (cisapride, 10 mg, or metoclopramide, 10 mg, three to four times daily before meals) improve symptoms in 60–80% and are significantly better than placebo. Symptomatic improvement does not correlate with the presence or absence of gastric emptying delay. Drug treatment should be discontinued after 4–8 weeks and the patient observed for symptomatic relapse.

Anti-*H pylori* treatment: Eradication of *H pylori* has not been convincingly shown to improve symptoms in the majority of patients with functional dyspepsia, suggesting that *H pylori* is not a pathophysiologic factor in most cases. *H pylori* eradication is believed by some authorities to be more beneficial than antisecretory medication alone. Although the role of *H pylori* in functional dyspepsia remains uncertain, a trial of eradication therapy in patients with documented infection may be reasonable.

American Gastroenterological Association medical position statement: evaluation of dyspepsia. Gastroenterology 1998;114:579. [NLM Cit ID: 98156663] (An evidence-based review of evaluation and management of dyspepsia.)

Blum A et al: Lack of effect of treating *Helicobacter pylori* infection in patients with nonulcer dyspepsia. N Engl J Med 1998;339:1875. [NLM Cit ID: 99067151] (Symptom resolution was similar in two groups—one treated with eradication, the other with omeprazole—after a year.)

Fisher RS et al: Management of nonulcer dyspepsia. N Engl J Med 1998;339:1376. [NLM Cit ID: 99006600]

McColl K et al: Symptomatic benefit from eradicating *Helicobacter pylori* infection in patients with nonulcer dyspepsia. N Engl J Med 1998;339:1869. [NLM Cit ID: 99067150] (This is the first trial to show benefit of *H pylori* eradication for functional dyspepsia; similar in careful design to Blum paper cited above.)

NAUSEA & VOMITING

Nausea is a vague, intensely disagreeable sensation of sickness or "queasiness" that may or may not be followed by vomiting and is distinguished from anorexia. Vomiting often follows, as does retching (spasmodic respiratory and abdominal movements). Vomiting should be distinguished from regurgitation, the effortless reflux of liquid or food stomach contents.

Vomiting is controlled by a medullary center that coordinates the respiratory and vasomotor centers with the innervation of the gastrointestinal tract. The vomiting center may be stimulated by four different sources of afferent input: (1) Afferent vagal fibers (rich in serotonin 5-HT_3 receptors) and splanchnic fibers from the gastrointestinal viscera; these may be stimulated by biliary or gastrointestinal distention, mucosal or peritoneal irritation, or infections. (2) The vestibular system, which may be stimulated by motion or infections. These fibers have high concentrations of histamine H_1 and muscarinic cholinergic receptors. (3) Higher central nervous system centers; here, certain sights, smells, or emotional experiences may induce vomiting. For example, patients receiving chemotherapy may develop vomiting in anticipation of its administration. (4) The chemoreceptor trigger zone, located outside the blood-brain barrier in the area postrema of the medulla, which may be stimulated by drugs and chemotherapeutic agents, toxins, hypoxia, uremia, acidosis, and radiation therapy. This region is rich in serotonin 5-HT_3 and dopamine D_2 receptors. Although the causes of vomiting are many, a simplified list is provided in Table 14–1.

Complications of vomiting include dehydration, hypokalemia, metabolic alkalosis, aspiration, rupture of the esophagus (Boerhaave's syndrome), and bleeding secondary to a mucosal tear at the gastroesophageal junction (Mallory-Weiss syndrome).

Table 14–1. Causes of nausea and vomiting.

Visceral afferent stimulation	**Mechanical obstruction** Gastric outlet obstruction: peptic ulcer disease, malignancy Small intestinal obstruction: adhesions, hernias, volvulus, Crohn's disease, carcinomatosis **Dysmotility** Gastroparesis: diabetic, medications, postviral, postvagotomy Small intestine: scleroderma, amyloidosis, chronic intestinal pseudo-obstruction, familial myoneuropathies **Peritoneal irritation** Peritonitis: perforated viscus, appendicitis, spontaneous bacterial peritonitis **Infections** Viral gastroenteritis: Norwalk agent, rotavirus "Food poisoning": toxins from *B cereus, S aureus, C perfringens* Hepatitis A, B Acute systomic infections **Hepatobiliary or pancreatic disorders** Acute pancreatitis Cholecystitis or choledocholithiasis **Topical gastrointestinal irritants** Alcohol, NSAIDs, oral antibiotics **Other** Cardiac disease: acute myocardial infarction, congestive heart failure Urologic disease: stones, pyelonephritis
Central nervous system disorders	**Vestibular disorders** Labyrinthitis, Meniere's syndrome, motion sickness **Increased intracranial pressure** CNS tumors, subdural or subarachnoid hemorrhage **Infections** Meningitis, encephalitis **Psychogenic** Anticipatory vomiting, bulimia, psychiatric disorders
Irritation of chemoreceptor trigger zone	**Antitumor chemotherapy** **Medications** Opioids **Radiation therapy** **Systemic disorders** Diabetic ketoacidosis, uremia, adrenocortical crisis

Clinical Findings

A. Symptoms and Signs: Acute symptoms without abdominal pain are typically caused by food poisoning, infectious gastroenteritis, or drugs. Inquiry should be made into recent changes in medications, diet, other intestinal symptoms, or similar illnesses in family members. The acute onset of severe pain and vomiting suggests peritoneal irritation, acute intestinal obstruction, or pancreaticobiliary disease. Examination may reveal fever, focal tenderness or rigidity, guarding, or rebound tenderness. Persistent vomiting suggests pregnancy, gastric outlet obstruction, gastroparesis, intestinal dysmotility, psychogenic disorders, and central nervous system or systemic disorders. Vomiting immediately after meals strongly suggests bulimia or psychogenic causes. Vomiting of undigested food one to several hours after meals is characteristic of gastroparesis or a gastric outlet obstruction; physical examination may reveal a succussion splash. Patients with acute or chronic symptoms should be asked about neurologic symptoms such as headaches, stiff neck, vertigo, and focal paresthesias or weakness.

B. Special Examinations: In vomiting of acute onset, flat and upright abdominal radiographs are obtained in patients with severe pain or suspicion of mechanical obstruction to look for free intraperitoneal air or dilated loops of small bowel. If mechanical small intestinal or gastric obstruction is thought likely, a nasogastric tube is placed for relief of symptoms. Aspiration of more than 200 mL of residual material in a fasting patient suggests obstruction or gastroparesis. This may be confirmed by a saline load test showing more than 400 mL residual on gastric aspiration performed 30 minutes after nasogastric instillation of 750 mL of 0.9% saline. The cause of gastric outlet obstruction is best demonstrated by upper endoscopy. Gastroparesis is confirmed by nuclear scintigraphic studies, which show delayed gastric emptying and either upper endoscopy or barium upper GI series showing no evidence of mechanical gastric outlet obstruction. Abnormal liver function tests or elevated amylase suggests pancreaticobiliary disease, which may be investigated with an abdominal sonogram or CT scan.

Treatment

A. General Measures: Most causes of acute vomiting are mild, self-limited, and require no specific treatment. Patients should ingest clear liquids (broths, tea, soups, carbonated beverages) and small quantities of dry foods (soda crackers). For more severe acute vomiting, hospitalization may be required. Owing to inability to eat and loss of gastric fluids, patients may become dehydrated and develop hypokalemia with metabolic alkalosis. Intravenous 0.45% saline solution with 20 meq/L of potassium chloride is given in most cases to maintain hydration. A nasogastric suction tube for gastric decompression improves patient comfort and permits monitoring of fluid loss.

B. Antiemetic Medications: Medications may be given either to prevent or to control vomiting (see above). No single medication is effective in all patients. Combinations of drugs from different classes may provide better control of symptoms with less toxicity in some patients. All of these medications should be avoided in pregnancy. (For dosages, see Table 14–2.)

1. Serotonin 5-HT$_3$ receptor antagonists– Ondansetron, granisetron, and dolasetron, when initiated prior to treatment, are effective in the prevention of chemotherapy-induced emesis.

2. Dopamine antagonists–The phenothiazines, butyrophenones, and substituted benzamides have antiemetic properties which are due to dopaminergic blockade as well as to their sedative effects. High doses of these agents are associated with antidopaminergic side effects, including extrapyramidal reactions and depression. These agents are used in a variety of situations.

3. Antihistamines–These drugs (eg, meclizine) may be valuable in the prevention of vomiting due to motion sickness.

4. Sedatives–Benzodiazepines may be helpful in patients with psychogenic and anticipatory vomiting.

5. Corticosteroids–The corticosteroids are useful in combination with other agents in the treatment of chemotherapy-induced vomiting.

6. Cannabinoids–Marijuana has been used widely as an appetite stimulant and antiemetic. Pure Δ^9-tetrahydrocannabinol (THC) is the major active ingredient in marijuana and is available by prescription as dronabinol. In doses of 5–15 mg/m^2, oral dronabinol is effective in treating nausea associated with chemotherapy, but it is associated with central nervous system side effects in most patients.

Gralla RJ: Antiemetic therapy. Semin Oncol 1998;25:577. [NLM Cit ID: 98454918]

Voth EA et al: Medicinal applications of delta-9-tetrahydrocannabinol and marijuana. Ann Intern Med 1997;126: 791. [NLM Cit ID: 97282918]

Table 14–2. Common antiemetic dosing regimens.

	Dosage	Route
Serotonin 5-HT$_3$ antagonists		
Ondansetron	0.15 mg/kg 15 minutes before chemotherapy, then every 4 hours for two doses or 32 mg once	IV
	8 mg three times daily	PO
Granisetron	10 µg/kg once	IV
Dolasetron	1 mg twice daily	PO
	100 mg or 1.8 mg/kg	IV
Dopamine antagonists		
Prochlorperazine	5–10 mg every 4–6 hours	PO, IM
	25 mg suppository every 6 hours	PR
Promethazine	25 mg every 4–6 hours	PO, IM, PR
Droperidol	1–2.5 mg every 3–6 hours	IV
Metoclopramide	10–20 mg every 6 hours	PO
	30 mg or 0.5 mg/kg every 6–8 hours	IV
Antihistamine and anticholinergics		
Diphenhydramine	25–50 mg every 4–6 hours	PO, IM, IV
Scopolamine patch	1.5 mg every 3 days	Patch
Dimenhydrinate	50 mg every 4 hours	PO
Meclizine	25–50 mg every 24 hours	PO
Corticosteroids		
Dexamethasone	4–20 mg	PO
	8–20 mg before (or both before and after) chemotherapy for two to four total doses	IV
Sedatives		
Diazepam	2–5 mg every 4–6 hours	PO, IV
Lorazepam	1–2 mg every 4–6 hours	PO, IV

HICCUPS (Singultus)

Though usually a benign and self-limited annoyance, hiccups may be persistent and a sign of serious underlying illness. Reports that hiccups lead to exhaustion, weight loss, or death in otherwise healthy patients are unsubstantiated. In patients being maintained on mechanical ventilation, however, hiccups can trigger a full respiratory cycle and result in respiratory alkalosis.

Causes of benign, self-limited hiccups include gastric distention (carbonated beverages, air swallowing, overeating), sudden temperature changes (hot then cold liquids, hot then cold shower), alcohol ingestion, and states of heightened emotion (excitement, stress, laughing). There are over 100 causes of recurrent or persistent hiccups, grouped into the following categories:

(1) Central nervous system: Neoplasms, infections, cerebrovascular accident, trauma.

(2) Metabolic: Uremia, hypocapnia (hyperventilation).

(3) Irritation of the vagus or phrenic nerve: (a) Head, neck: Foreign body in ear, goiter, neoplasms. (b) Thorax: Pneumonia, empyema, neoplasms, myocardial infarction, pericarditis, aneurysm, esophageal obstruction, reflux esophagitis. (c) Abdomen: Subphrenic abscess, hepatomegaly, hepatitis, cholecystitis, gastric distention, gastric neoplasm, pancreatitis, or pancreatic malignancy.

(4) Surgical: General anesthesia, postoperative.

(5) Psychogenic and idiopathic.

Clinical Findings

Evaluation of the patient with persistent hiccups should include a detailed neurologic examination, serum creatinine, liver chemistry tests, and a chest radiograph. When the cause remains unclear, CT of the head, chest, and abdomen, echocardiography, bronchoscopy, and upper endoscopy may help. On occasion, hiccups may be unilateral; chest fluoroscopy will make the diagnosis.

Treatment

A number of simple remedies may be helpful in patients with acute benign hiccups. (1) Irritation of the nasopharynx by tongue traction, lifting the uvula with a spoon, catheter stimulation of the nasopharynx, and eating 1 tsp of dry granulated sugar. (2) Interruption of the respiratory cycle by breath holding, Valsalva's maneuver, sneezing, gasping (fright stimulus), or rebreathing into a bag. (3) Stimulation of the vagus, carotid massage. (4) Irritation of the diaphragm by holding knees to chest or by continuous positive airway pressure during mechanical ventilation. (5) Relief of gastric distention by belching or insertion of a nasogastric tube.

A number of drugs have been promoted as being useful in the treatment of hiccups, but none have been tested in a controlled fashion. Chlorpromazine, 25–50 mg orally or intramuscularly, is most commonly used. Other agents that have been reported to be effective in some cases include anticonvulsants (phenytoin, carbamazepine), benzodiazepines (lorazepam, diazepam), metoclopramide, baclofen, and occasionally general anesthesia.

Petroianu G et al: Idiopathic chronic hiccup: Combination therapy with cisapride, omeprazole, and baclofen. Clin Ther 1997;19:1031. [NLM Cit ID: 98046600]

Rousseau P: Hiccups. South Med J 1995;88:175. [NLM Cit ID: 95141089]

CONSTIPATION

Constipation is a term used variably by patients to refer to stools that are too hard, small, or infrequent or to excessive straining during defecation. Therefore, the first step in evaluating the patient is to determine what is meant by "constipation." In the general population, the "normal" frequency of bowel movements is broad, ranging from three to twelve per week. In many patients, the complaint may reflect a mistaken perception of what constitutes a normal bowel pattern. From a medical perspective, constipation is present when a patient has two or fewer bowel movements per week or excessive difficulty and straining at defecation. The many causes of constipation may be classified as discussed below and summarized in Table 14–3.

Common Identifiable Causes of Constipation

A. Poor Dietary and Behavioral Habits: The majority of constipated patients have mild symptoms that cannot be attributed to any structural abnormalities, intestinal motility disorders, or systemic disease. Dietary review will reveal that most of these patients do not consume adequate fiber and fluids. Ingestion of 10–12 g of fiber per day either by dietary changes or the addition or commercial fiber supplementation is often all that is needed. At least one or two glasses of fluid should be taken with meals. The elderly in particular are predisposed to constipation because of poor eating habits, a variety of medications that cause constipation, decreased colonic motility, and, in some cases, inability to sit on a toilet (bed-bound patients).

B. Structural Abnormalities: Colonic lesions that obstruct fecal passage must be excluded in patients with constipation. Particular concern is raised in patients with lifelong constipation (Hirschsprung's disease) and patients over age 50 with new-onset constipation, progressive thinning of stool, or associated weight loss or hematochezia (suggesting colon carcinoma).

C. Systemic Diseases: Medical diseases can cause constipation due to neurologic gut dysfunction, myopathies, endocrine disorders, and electrolyte abnormalities such as hypercalcemia or hypokalemia.

Table 14–3. Causes of constipation in adults.

Most common
Low-fiber diet
Poor bowel habits
Structural abnormalities
Perianal disease: fissure, abscess, thrombosed hemorrhoid
Colonic mass lesion with obstruction: adenocarcinoma
Colonic stricture: diverticulosis, radiation, ischemia
Hirschsprung's disease
Idiopathic megarectum
Systemic disease
Endocrine: hypothyroidism, hyperparathyroidism, diabetes mellitus
Metabolic: hypokalemia, hypercalcemia, uremia
Neurologic: paraplegia, Parkinson's disease, multiple sclerosis, prior pelvic surgery with disruption of pelvic nerves
Other: amyloidosis, scleroderma
Medications
Narcotics
Diuretics
Calcium channel blockers
Anticholinergics
Psychotropic agents
Antacids
Calcium and iron supplements
NSAIDs
Clonidine
Sucralfate
Levodopa
Anticholinergic medications (tricyclic antidepressants, antihistamines)
Slow colonic transit
Idiopathic: isolated to colon or part of generalized disorder
Psychogenic
Chronic intestinal pseudo-obstruction
Evacuation disorders
Rectocele
Rectal intussusception
Rectal prolapse
Perineal descent
Anismus (pelvic floor dysfunction)
Solitary rectal ulcer syndrome

D. Medications: Anticholinergic and opioid agents are common causes of constipation.

Causes of Severe or Refractory Constipation

Patients whose constipation cannot be attributed to the above causes and who do not respond to conservative dietary management present difficult management problems. Conceptually, these patients can be divided into two categories:

A. Colonic Inertia (Slow Colonic Transit): Some patients have an idiopathic delayed transit of stool through the large bowel. Normal colonic transit time is approximately 35 hours; more than 72 hours is significantly abnormal. Severe colonic inertia is more common in women, some of whom have a history of psychosocial problems or sexual abuse. Colonic inertia may be part of a more generalized gastrointestinal dysmotility syndrome. It may also be attributable to years of cathartic use.

B. Outlet Disorders: Patients with disorders of the rectum or pelvic floor—women more often than men—may have difficulty in moving stool out of the rectum. They may complain of excessive straining with a sense of incomplete evacuation, the need for digital pressure on the vagina or perineum, or even the need for digital disimpaction. Defecatory difficulties can be due to a variety of anatomic problems that impede or obstruct flow, some of which may benefit from surgery. In other patients, there is failure of the pelvic floor to relax during straining ("anismus").

Evaluation

A. First Level of Investigation: All patients should undergo a history and physical examination, including stool testing for occult blood. Laboratory studies should include a complete blood count, serum electrolytes including calcium, and serum TSH. In otherwise healthy patients with mild symptoms who are under age 45, a conservative trial of treatment with fiber is reasonable. In patients over age 45, those who have failed conservative treatment, or those with anemia or occult blood in the stools, colonoscopy or flexible sigmoidoscopy and barium enema are obtained to look for structural colonic lesions. Patients without evident structural, medical, or neurologic disease can be treated initially with fiber supplementation (and osmotic laxatives, if needed).

B. Second Level of Investigation: Patients with refractory constipation not responding to conservative measures may require further investigation.

1. Colonic transit study–To confirm that the patient truly has constipation and to measure the transit time, 24 radiopaque plastic markers are swallowed on 3 consecutive days. An abdominal radiograph is taken on days 4 and 7, and the total number of markers remaining in the colon is counted.

2. Studies of pelvic floor function–Defecography (a video study taken during straining and defecation) and anal manometry may assist in diagnosis.

Standard Treatment of Chronic Constipation

A. Dietary Measures: Proper dietary fluid and fiber intake should be emphasized. Fiber may be given by means of dietary alterations or fiber supplements. Increased dietary fiber may cause temporary distention and flatulence. Whereas fiber benefits the majority of patients with constipation, it normally does not benefit patients with severe colonic inertia or outlet disorders. Fiber supplements include the following.

1. Bran powder–One to 2 tbsp of bran powder twice daily, mixed with fluids or sprinkled over foods, is an excellent inexpensive means of providing 10–20 g/d of fiber. It may produce gas.

2. Pharmaceutical supplements–A variety of pharmaceutical fiber supplements are available, however, they are much more expensive than bran powder. They come in a variety of flavored powders, cookies, or tablets that are easy to ingest and may be less gas-producing than bran. Preparations include psyllium, 3.4 g, and methylcellulose, 2 g, one to three times daily (both are natural fibers derived from vegetable matter); and polycarbophil, 1 g one to four times daily (a synthetic fiber).

B. Osmotic Laxatives: These agents, used to soften stools, may be given alone or in combination with fiber supplements. They are commonly employed in elderly nonambulatory or institutionalized patients to prevent constipation and fecal impaction. They may be safely used long-term and do not induce dependency. The agents are typically titrated to a dose that results in soft to semiliquid stools.

1. Nonabsorbable sugars–Either sorbitol (70%) or lactulose, 15–60 mL daily, is efficacious, but sorbitol is less expensive. These malabsorbed sugars may result in increased bloating, cramps, and flatulence.

2. Magnesium salts–Either magnesium hydroxide or magnesium sulfate (15–30 mL daily) is effective. They should not be given to patients with renal insufficiency.

3. Polyethylene glycol solution–The solutions traditionally used for colonic lavage prior to colonoscopy (CoLyte, GoLYTELY, NuLytely) may be administered chronically in a dosage of 200–1000 mL daily.

C. Stool Surfactant Agents: Surfactant agents (docusate sodium, 50–200 mg/d; or mineral oil, 15–45 mL) may be given orally or rectally to promote softening of the stools.

Treatment of Chronic or Refractory Constipation

Most patients in this category will benefit from referral to a center with interest and expertise in these difficult problems.

A. Colonic Inertia: Many patients require chronic use of enemas and cathartic agents (see below). Patients with psychologic problems or a history of sexual abuse may benefit from psychiatric therapy. In particularly severe cases, subtotal colectomy may be necessary.

B. Outlet Disorders: Some anatomic problems (eg, rectal prolapse, vaginal rectocele) may benefit from surgical correction. Relaxation techniques and biofeedback are being used in patients with pelvic floor dysfunction.

Treatment of Acute Constipation (Table 14–4)

Normal people and patients with chronic constipation can become acutely constipated in response to acute medical or surgical illness, dietary changes, medications, travel, etc. If several days have passed since the last bowel movement, the therapies described above for chronic constipation will not be sufficient to induce prompt evacuation and relief of discomfort. In such cases, the following may be given. (***Caution:*** These agents should not be given to patients with a possible large bowel obstruction or fecal impaction.)

A. Cathartic Laxatives: These agents stimulate fluid secretion and colonic contraction, resulting in a bowel movement within 6–12 hours after oral ingestion or 15–60 minutes after rectal administration. They may cause severe cramps and diarrhea. Agents used in the medical setting include cascara sagrada, 4–8 mL orally; bisacodyl, 5–15 mg orally or 10 mg as suppository; and castor oil, 15–45 mL orally. Senna and phenolphthalein are common OTC laxatives. ***Note:*** Chronic use of any of these agents is discouraged and may result in loss of normal colonic neuromuscular function.

B. Osmotic Laxatives: Osmotic laxatives produce a prompt evacuation in 0.5–3 hours, generally with less discomfort than when cathartic laxatives are given. They are used in the medical setting for purgation prior to surgery or colonic examinations. Preparations include magnesium citrate, 18 g/10 oz; magnesium sulfate, 10–30 g (Epsom salts); sodium phosphate, 15–30 g (2–45 mL); and balanced polyethylene glycol lavage solution, 1–4 L over 1–4 hours (GoLYTELY, CoLyte, NuLytely).

C. Enemas: Enemas provide a simple and almost immediate means of relieving acute constipa-

Table 14–4. Pharmacologic management of constipation.

Bulk laxatives[1]	
Bran powder	1–2 tbsp orally at bedtime to twice daily
Psyllium fiber	3 g orally at bedtime to 3 times daily
Osmotic laxatives	
Lactulose	15–60 mL orally 1–3 times daily
Sorbitol	15–60 mL orally 1–3 times daily
Magnesium hydroxide	5–10 mL orally 1–4 times daily
Magnesium citrate	8 fluid oz orally daily
Sodium phosphate	30 mL orally daily, may repeat once
Detergent agents	
Docusate sodium	50–300 mg orally at bedtime to 3 times daily[2]
Stimulants	
Bisacodyl	5–15 mg orally at bedtime to 3 times daily or 10–20 mg rectally at bedtime
Senna	5–15 mg orally at bedtime to 3 times daily
Other inverventions	
Glycerine suppositories	
Enemas of saline, tap water, oil retention, soapsuds or milk and molasses	
Digital disimpaction[3]	

[1]Should be avoided in most ill patients and patients with bowel obstruction or impaction.
[2]Acts primarily as a stool softener.
[3]Should be preceded by oil retention enema, adequate lubrication, and premedication with an anxiolytic.

tion. In some cases of severe constipation, it is best to treat with an enema first in order to promote comfortable fecal movement prior to giving laxatives. Enemas vary in size and content: saline enemas, 120–240 mL (nonirritating); tap water enemas, 500–1000 mL (irritating); and oil retention enemas, 120 mL (useful for hard or impacted stool).

Treatment of Fecal Impaction

Severe impaction of stool in the rectal vault may result in obstruction of further fecal flow, leading to partial or complete large bowel obstruction. Predisposing factors include severe psychiatric disease, prolonged bed rest and debility, neurogenic diseases of the colon, and spinal cord disorders. Clinical presentation includes decreased appetite, nausea, vomiting, and abdominal pain and distention. There may be paradoxic "diarrhea" as liquid stool leaks around the impacted feces. Firm feces are palpable on digital examination in the rectal vault. Initial treatment is directed at relieving the impaction with enemas or digital disruption of the impacted fecal material. Care should be taken not to injure the anal sphincter. Rarely, spinal or general anesthesia is required as an aid to manual disimpaction. Long-term care is directed at maintaining soft stools and regular bowel movements (as above).

American Gastrointestinal Association Medical Position Statement on Anorectal Testing Techniques. Gastroenterology 1999;116:732. [NLM Cit ID: 99155291]

Mollen RMHG: The evaluation and treatment of functional constipation. Scan J Gastroenterol 1997;32(Suppl 223): 8. [NLM Cit ID: 97343777]

Prather CM et al: Evaluation and treatment of constipation and fecal impaction in adults. Mayo Clin Proc 1998; 73:881. [NLM Cit ID: 98407244]

GASTROINTESTINAL GAS

Belching

Belching (eructation) is the involuntary or voluntary release of gas from the stomach or esophagus. It occurs most frequently after meals, when gastric distention results in transient lower esophageal sphincter relaxation. Belching is a normal reflex and does not itself denote gastrointestinal dysfunction. Virtually all stomach gas comes from swallowed air. With each swallow, 2–5 mL of air are ingested, and excessive amounts may result in distention, flatulence, and abdominal pain. This may occur with rapid eating, gum chewing, smoking, and the ingestion of carbonated beverages. Some patients may consciously or unconsciously engage in forceful air swallowing (aerophagia). Chronic excessive belching is almost always caused by aerophagia, common in anxious individuals and institutionalized patients. Evaluation should be restricted to patients with other complaints such as dysphagia, heartburn, early satiety, or vomiting.

Belching and aerophagia may be reduced by behavioral changes that include chewing and eating food slowly, not drinking through a straw, and not chewing gum or drinking carbonated beverages. Once patients understand the relationship between aerophagia and belching, most can deal with the problem by behavioral modification. Physical defects that hamper normal swallowing (ill-fitting dentures, nasal obstruction) should be corrected. Antacids and simethicone are of no value.

Flatus

The rate and volume of expulsion of flatus is highly variable. Normal frequency ranges from six to twenty times a day, and normal volumes from 500 to 1500 mL/d. Flatus is derived from two sources: swallowed air and bacterial fermentation of undigested carbohydrate. The majority of swallowed air that is not belched passes through the gut and leaves as flatus. Swallowed air may contribute up to 500 mL of flatus per day (primarily nitrogen). Bacterial fermentation of undigested carbohydrates leads to the additional production of gas, particularly H_2, CO_2, and methane. Except for small intestine bacterial overgrowth, the majority of this fermentation takes place in the colon. Under normal circumstances, a small substrate of fermentable substrates reaches the colon. These substances include lactose, fructose, bean starch, and the complex carbohydrates of fiber, wheat, oats, corn, and potatoes. Gas production may be increased dramatically with diseases of malabsorption (eg, celiac sprue) or with the ingestion of poorly absorbed carbohydrates (eg, lactose, lactulose, or sorbitol). Gases derived from plant carbohydrates (hydrogen and methane) have relatively little odor. In contrast, hydrogen sulfide, derived in part from meat and other proteins, tends to be malodorous. Determining abnormal from normal amounts of flatus is difficult. Excessive amounts of flatus may suggest malabsorption, especially if accompanied by diarrhea or weight loss.

An initial trial of a lactose-free diet is recommended. Common gas-producing foods should be reviewed and the patient given an elimination trial. These commonly include brown beans, cauliflower, Brussels sprouts, broccoli, cabbage, onions, beer, red wine, and eggs. For patients with persistent complaints, fructose and complex carbohydrates may be eliminated, but such restrictive diets are unacceptable to most patients. The value of activated charcoal or simethicone is marginal. The nonprescription agent Beano (α-D-galactosidase enzyme) reduces gas production associated with cruciferous vegetables, legumes, and grains.

Complaints of chronic abdominal distention or bloating are common but do not correlate with increased intra-abdominal gas volumes. Many such patients have an underlying functional gastrointestinal disorder such as irritable bowel syndrome or nonulcer dyspepsia.

Levitt M et al: Evaluation of an extremely flatulent patient. Case report and proposed diagnostic and therapeutic approach. Am J Gastroenterol 1998;93:2276. [NLM Cit ID: 99036301] (Outstanding review by experts in the field.)

Suarez F et al: Bismuth subsalicylate markedly decreases hydrogen sulfide release in the human colon. Gastroenterology 1998;114:923. [NLM Cit ID: 98225122] (Bismuth subsalicylate [Pepto-Bismol], two tablets four times daily, dramatically reduced hydrogen sulfide release from human feces. This agent may be useful to treat malodorous flatus.)

DIARRHEA

Diarrhea is a common symptom that can range in severity from an acute self-limited annoyance to a severe, life-threatening illness. Patients may use the term "diarrhea" to refer to increased frequency of bowel movements, increased stool liquidity, a sense of fecal urgency, or fecal incontinence. To properly evaluate the complaint, the physician must determine the patient's normal bowel pattern and the nature of the current symptoms.

In the normal state, approximately 10 L of fluid enter the duodenum daily, of which all but 1.5 L are absorbed by the small intestine. The colon absorbs most of the remaining fluid, with only 100 mL lost in the stool. Diarrhea is defined medically as a stool weight of more than 250 g/24 h, but quantification of stool weight is necessary only in some patients with chronic diarrhea. In most cases, the physician's working definition of diarrhea is increased stool frequency (more than two or three bowel movements per day) or liquidity of feces.

The causes of diarrhea are myriad. In clinical practice, it is helpful to distinguish acute from chronic diarrhea, as the evaluation and treatment are entirely different (Tables 14–5 and 14–7).

1. ACUTE DIARRHEA

Etiology & Clinical Findings

Diarrhea that is acute in onset and persists for less than 3 weeks is most commonly caused by infectious agents, bacterial toxins (either ingested preformed in food or produced in the gut), or drugs. Epidemiologic information may provide clues to the etiologic agent (Table 30–3). Similar recent illness in family members suggests an infectious origin. Ingestion of improperly stored or prepared food implicates food poisoning, especially if other people were similarly affected. Exposure to unpurified water (camping, swimming) or contaminated produce may result in infection with giardia, cryptosporidium, or cyclospora. Recent travel abroad suggests "traveler's diarrhea" (see Chapter 30). Antibiotic administration within the preceding several weeks increases the likelihood of *Clostridium difficile* colitis. Finally, risk factors for HIV infection or sexually transmitted diseases should be determined. (AIDS-associated diarrhea is discussed in Chapter 31.) Persons practicing unprotected anal intercourse are at risk for a variety of infections that cause proctitis and rectal discharge, including gonorrhea, syphilis, lymphogranuloma venereum, and herpes simplex. A variety of medications may cause diarrhea through various mechanisms; these will not be discussed further here.

The nature of the diarrhea helps distinguish among different infectious causes (Table 14–5).

A. Noninflammatory Diarrhea: Watery, nonbloody diarrhea associated with periumbilical cramps, bloating, nausea, or vomiting (singly or in any combination) suggests small bowel enteritis caused by either a toxin-producing bacterium (enterotoxigenic *E coli* [ETEC], *Staphylococcus aureus, Bacillus cereus, Clostridium perfringens*) or other agents (viruses, giardia) that disrupt normal absorption and secretory processes in the small intestine. Prominent vomiting suggests viral enteritis or *S aureus* food poisoning. Though typically mild, the diarrhea (which originates in the small intestine) can be voluminous (ranging from 10 to 200 mL/kg/24 h) and result in dehydration with hypokalemia and meta-

Table 14–5. Causes of acute infectious diarrhea.

Noninflammatory Diarrhea	Inflammatory Diarrhea
Viral Norwalk virus Norwalk-like virus Rotavirus **Protozoal** *Giardia lamblia* Cryptosporidium **Bacterial** 1. Preformed enterotoxin production *Staphylococcus aureus* *Bacillus cereus* *Clostridium perfringens* 2. Enterotoxin production Enterotoxigenic *E coli* (ETEC) *Vibrio cholerae*	**Viral** Cytomegalovirus **Protozoal** *Entamoeba histolytica* **Bacterial** 1. Cytotoxin production Enterohemorrhagic *E coli* O157:H5 (EHEC) *Vibrio parahaemolyticus* *Clostridium difficile* 2. Mucosal invasion Shigella *Campylobacter jejuni* Salmonella Enteroinvasive *E coli* (EIEC) Aeromonas Plesiomonas *Yersinia enterocolitica* Chlamydia *Neisseria gonorrhoeae* *Listeria monocytogenes*

bolic acidosis due to loss of HCO_3^- in the stool (eg, cholera). Because tissue invasion does not occur, fecal leukocytes are not present.

B. Inflammatory Diarrhea: The presence of fever and bloody diarrhea (dysentery) indicates colonic tissue damage caused by invasion (shigellosis, salmonellosis, campylobacter or yersinia infection, amebiasis) or a toxin (*C difficile, E coli* O157:H7). Because these organisms involve predominantly the colon, the diarrhea is small in volume (< 1 L/d) and associated with left lower quadrant cramps, urgency, and tenesmus. Fecal leukocytes usually are present in infections with invasive organisms. *E coli* O157:H7 is a toxigenic noninvasive organism that may be acquired from contaminated meat or unpasteurized apple juice and has resulted in several outbreaks of an acute, often severe hemorrhagic colitis. In immunocompromised and HIV-infected patients, cytomegalovirus may result in intestinal ulceration with watery or bloody diarrhea.

Infectious dysentery must be distinguished from acute ulcerative colitis, which may also present acutely with fever, abdominal pain, and bloody diarrhea. Diarrhea that persists for more than 14 days is not attributable to bacterial pathogens (except for *C difficile*) and should be evaluated as chronic diarrhea.

C. Enteric Fever: A severe systemic illness manifested initially by prolonged high fevers, prostration, confusion, respiratory symptoms followed by abdominal tenderness, diarrhea, and a rash is due to infection with *Salmonella typhi* or *Salmonella paratyphi,* two pathogens that cause bacteremia and multiorgan dysfunction. In typhoid fever, constipation may be present before diarrhea ensues.

Evaluation

In over 90% of patients with acute diarrhea, the illness is mild and self-limited, responding within 5 days to simple rehydration therapy or antidiarrheal agents. In such cases, a laboratory investigation to determine the causative agent is unnecessary because it is costly, often unrevealing, and does not affect therapy or outcome. Indeed, the isolation rate of bacterial pathogens from stool cultures in patients with acute diarrhea is under 3%. Thus, the goal of initial evaluation is to distinguish patients with mild (and usually self-limited) disease from those with more serious illness. Such patients may be treated symptomatically without further initial evaluation. If diarrhea worsens or persists for more than 7–10 days, stool should be sent for fecal leukocyte determination, ovum and parasite evaluation, and bacterial culture.

Prompt medical evaluation is indicated in the following situations: (1) Patients with signs of inflammatory diarrhea manifested by any of the following require prompt medical attention: high fever (> 38.5 °C), bloody diarrhea, or abdominal pain. (2) Individuals who pass six or more unformed stools in 24 hours. (3) The presence of profuse watery diarrhea and dehydration (excessive thirst, dry mouth, oliguria). (4) The frail older patient. (5) Immunocompromised patients (AIDS, posttransplantation).

Physical examination pays particular note to mental status and the presence of abdominal tenderness or peritonitis. Peritoneal findings may be present in infection with *C difficile* or enterohemorrhagic *E coli.* Hospitalization is required in patients with severe dehydration, toxicity, or marked abdominal pain. Stool specimens should be sent in all cases for examination for fecal leukocytes and bacterial cultures (Table 14–6). The rate of positive bacterial cultures in such patients is 60–75%. A stool wet mount examination for amebiasis should be performed in patients who are sexually active homosexuals, those with a history of recent travel to amebiasis-endemic areas, and those whose bacterial cultures are negative. In patients with a history of antibiotic exposure, a stool sample should be tested for *C difficile* toxin. If *E coli*

Table 14–6. Fecal leukocytes in intestinal disorders.

Infectious			Noninfectious
Present	**Variable**	**Absent**	**Present**
Shigella Campylobacter Enteroinvasive *E coli* (EIEC)	Salmonella Yersinia *Vibrio parahaemolytica* *Clostridium difficile* Aeromonas	Norwalk virus Rotavirus *Giardia lamblia* *Entamoeba histolytica* Cryptosporidium "Food poisoning" *Staphylococcus aureus* *Bacillus cereus* *Clostridium perfringens* *Escherichia coli* Enterotoxigenic (ETEC) Enterohemorrhagic (EHEC)	Ulcerative colitis Crohn's disease Radiation colitis Ischemic colitis

O157:H7 is suspected, the laboratory is instructed to do specific serotyping. In patients with diarrhea that persists for more than 10 days, three stool examinations for ova and parasites should also be performed. Rectal swabs may be sent for culture of chlamydia, *Neisseria gonorrhoeae,* and herpes simplex virus in sexually active patients with suspected proctitis.

Sigmoidoscopy is warranted acutely in patients with symptoms of severe proctitis (tenesmus, discharge, rectal pain) and in patients with suspected *C difficile* colitis who appear ill. It may also be helpful in distinguishing infectious diarrhea from ulcerative colitis or ischemic colitis.

Treatment

A. Diet: The great majority of adults have mild diarrhea that will not lead to dehydration provided the patient takes adequate oral fluids containing carbohydrates and electrolytes. Patients will find it more comfortable to rest the bowel by avoiding high-fiber foods, fats, milk products, caffeine, and alcohol. Frequent feedings of fruit drinks, tea, "flat" carbonated beverages, and soft, easily digested foods (eg, soups, crackers) are encouraged.

B. Rehydration: In more severe diarrhea, dehydration can occur quickly, especially in children. Oral rehydration with fluids containing glucose, Na^+, K^+, Cl^-, and bicarbonate or citrate is preferred in most cases to intravenous fluids because it is inexpensive, safe, and highly effective in almost all awake patients. A convenient mixture is ½ tsp salt (3.5 g), 1 tsp baking soda (2.5 g $NaHCO_3$), 8 tsp sugar (40 g), and 8 oz orange juice (1.5 g KCl), diluted to 1 L with water. Alternatively, oral electrolyte solutions (eg, Pedialyte, Gatorade) are readily available. Fluids should be given at rates of 50–200 mL/kg/24 h depending on the hydration status. Intravenous fluids (lactated Ringer's injection) are preferred acutely in patients with severe dehydration.

C. Antidiarrheal Agents: Antidiarrheal agents may be used safely in patients with mild to moderate diarrheal illnesses to improve patient comfort. Opioid agents help decrease the stool number and liquidity and control fecal urgency. However, they should not be used in patients with bloody diarrhea, high fever, or systemic toxicity for fear of worsening the disease. Similarly, they should be discontinued in patients whose diarrhea is worsening despite therapy. With these provisos, such drugs provide excellent symptomatic relief. Loperamide is preferred, in a dosage of 4 mg initially, followed by 2 mg after each loose stool (maximum: 16 mg/24 h).

Bismuth subsalicylate (Pepto-Bismol), two tablets or 30 mL four times daily, reduces symptoms in patients with traveler's diarrhea by virtue of its anti-inflammatory and antibacterial properties. It is also useful to reduce vomiting associated with viral enteritis. Scores of other agents have undergone little or no controlled testing but appear to have minimal or no symptomatic benefit (lactobacilli, kaolin, pectin). Anticholinergic agents are contraindicated in acute diarrhea (eg, diphenoxylate with atropine) because of the rare development of toxic megacolon.

D. Antibiotic Therapy:

1. Empirical treatment–Because the majority of patients have mild, self-limited disease due to viruses or noninvasive bacteria, empirical antibiotic treatment of all patients with acute diarrhea is not warranted. Even patients with inflammatory diarrhea caused by invasive pathogens usually have mild disease that will resolve within several days without antimicrobials. Empirical treatment is recommended in patients in whom an invasive bacterial infection is suggested by the presence of moderate to severe fever, tenesmus, or bloody stools or the presence of fecal leukocytes while the stool bacterial culture is incubating. The drugs of choice are the fluoroquinolones (eg, ciprofloxacin, 500 mg twice daily) for 5–7 days. They provide good antibiotic coverage against most invasive bacterial pathogens, including shigella, salmonella, campylobacter, yersinia, and aeromonas. Alternatives include trimethoprim-sulfamethoxazole, 160/800 mg twice daily, or erythromycin, 250–500 mg four times daily. Empirical treatment with metronidazole (250 mg three times daily for 7 days) may also be given when giardia infection is suspected, because over half of stool specimens may be negative in infected patients.

2. Specific antimicrobial treatment–Antibiotics are not recommended in patients with nontyphoid salmonella, campylobacter, aeromonas, yersinia, or *E coli* O157:H7 infection except in severe or prolonged disease because they do not hasten recovery or reduce the period of fecal bacterial excretion. The infectious diarrheas for which treatment is recommended are shigellosis, cholera, extraintestinal salmonellosis, "traveler's" diarrhea, *C difficile* infection, giardiasis, amebiasis, and the sexually transmitted infections (gonorrhea, syphilis, chlamydiosis, and herpes simplex infection). Therapy of these infections and AIDS-related diarrhea are presented in other chapters of this book.

Dalton C et al: An outbreak of gastroenteritis and fever due to *Listeria monocytogenes* in milk. N Engl J Med 1997;336:100. [NLM Cit ID: 97130065]

Cody SH et al: An outbreak of *Escherichia coli* O157:H7 infection from unpasteurized commercial apple juice. Ann Intern Med 1999;130:202. [NLM Cit ID: 99149983]

Du Pont HC and the Practice Parameters Committee of the American College of Gastroenterology. Guidelines on acute infectious diarrhea in adults. Am J Gastroenterol 1997;92:1962. [NLM Cit ID: 98026497]

Herwaldt BL et al: The return of cyclospora in 1997; another outbreak of cyclosporiasis in North America associated with imported raspberries. Ann Intern Med 1999;130:210. [NLM Cit ID: 99149984] (Documenting the risks of infection from food sources and the need for increased safety measures from our federal food safety agencies. See also editorial by Osterholm M: Ann Intern Med 1999;130:233.)

2. CHRONIC DIARRHEA

Etiology

The causes of chronic diarrhea may be grouped into six major pathophysiologic categories (Table 14–7):

A. Osmotic Diarrheas: As stool leaves the colon, fecal osmolality is equal to the serum osmolality, ie, approximately 290 mosm/kg. Under normal circumstances, the major osmoles are Na^+, K^+, Cl^-, and HCO_3^-. The stool osmolality may be estimated by multiplying the stool ($Na^+ + K^+$) × 2. The **osmotic gap** is the difference between the *measured* osmolality of the stool (or serum) and the *estimated* stool osmolality and is normally less than 50 mosm/kg. An increased osmotic gap implies that the diarrhea is caused by ingestion or malabsorption of an osmotically active substance. The most common causes of osmotic diarrhea are disaccharidase deficiency (lactase deficiency), laxative abuse, and malabsorption syndromes (see below). Osmotic diarrheas resolve during fasting. Those caused by malabsorbed carbohydrates are characterized by abdominal distention, bloating, and flatulence due to increased colonic gas production.

Disaccharidase deficiencies are common and should be considered in all patients with chronic diarrhea. Lactase deficiency occurs in three-fourths of nonwhite adults and up to 25% of Caucasians. It may also be acquired after an episode of viral gastroenteritis, medical illness, or gastrointestinal surgery. Sorbitol is commonly used as a sweetener in gums, candies, and some medications that may cause diarrhea in some patients. The diagnosis of sorbitol or lactose malabsorption may be established by an elimination trial for 2–3 weeks. The diagnosis may be confirmed by measuring a rise in breath hydrogen of more than 20 ppm after lactose or sorbitol ingestion, but this is seldom necessary.

Ingestion of magnesium- or phosphate-containing compounds (laxatives, antacids) should be considered in enigmatic chronic diarrhea. Surreptitious use should be considered, especially in patients with possible eating disorders and psychiatric problems, a long history of undiagnosed medical ailments, or employment in the medical field. The fat substitute olestra is also believed to cause diarrhea and cramps in occasional patients.

B. Malabsorptive Conditions: The major causes of malabsorption are small mucosal intestinal diseases, intestinal resections, lymphatic obstruction, small intestinal bacterial overgrowth, and pancreatic insufficiency. The hallmarks of malabsorption are weight loss, osmotic diarrhea, and nutritional deficiencies. Significant diarrhea in the absence of weight loss is not likely to be due to malabsorption. The physical and laboratory abnormalities related to deficiencies of vitamins or minerals are discussed in

Table 14–7. Causes of chronic diarrhea.

Osmotic diarrhea
CLUES: Stool volume decreases with fasting; increased stool osmotic gap
1. Medications: antacids, lactulose, sorbitol
2. Disaccharidase deficiency: lactose intolerance
3. Factitious diarrhea: magnesium (antacids, laxatives)

Secretory diarrhea
CLUES: Large volume (> 1 L/d); little change with fasting; normal stool osmotic gap
1. Hormonally mediated: VIPoma, carcinoid, medullary carcinoma of thyroid (calcitonin), Zollinger-Ellison syndrome (gastrin)
2. Factitious diarrhea (laxative abuse); phenolphthalein, cascara, senna
3. Villous adenoma
4. Bile salt malabsorption (ileal resection; Crohn's ileitis; postcholecystectomy)
5. Medications

Inflammatory conditions
CLUES: Fever, hematochezia, abdominal pain
1. Ulcerative colitis
2. Crohn's disease
3. Microscopic colitis
4. Malignancy: lymphoma, adenocarcinoma (with obstruction and pseudodiarrhea)
5. Radiation enteritis

Malabsorption syndromes
1. Weight loss, abnormal laboratory values; fecal fat > 7–10 g/24 h, tropical sprue, Whipple's disease, eosinophilic gastroenteritis, Crohn's disease, small bowel resection (short bowel syndrome)
2. Lymphatic obstruction: lymphoma, carcinoid, infectious (TB, MAI), Kaposi's sarcoma, sarcoidosis, retroperitoneal fibrosis
3. Pancreatic disease: chronic pancreatitis, pancreatic carcinoma
4. Bacterial overgrowth: motility disorders (diabetes, vagotomy, scleroderma), fistulas, small intestinal diverticula

Motility disorders
CLUES: Systemic disease or prior abdominal surgery
1. Postsurgical: vagotomy, partial gastrectomy, blind loop with bacterial overgrowth
2. Systemic disorders: scleroderma, diabetes mellitus, hyperthyroidism
3. Irritable bowel syndrome

Chronic infections
1. Parasites: *Giardia lamblia, Entamoeba histolytica*
2. AIDS-related:
   Viral: Cytomegalovirus, HIV infection (?)
   Bacterial: *Clostridium difficile, Mycobacterium avium* complex
   Protozoal: Microsporida *(Enterocytozoon bieneusi)*, cryptosporidium, *Isospora belli*

Chapter 29. Briefly, they include anemia (microcytic or macrocytic), hypoalbuminemia, low serum cholesterol, hypocalcemia, and a prolonged prothrombin time.

C. Secretory Conditions: Increased intestinal secretion or decreased absorption results in a watery diarrhea that may be large in volume (1–10 L/d) but with a normal osmotic gap. There is little change in stool output during the fasting state, and dehydration and electrolyte imbalance may develop. Causes include endocrine tumors (stimulating intestinal or pancreatic secretion), bile salt malabsorption (stimulating colonic secretion), and laxative abuse.

D. Inflammatory Conditions: Diarrhea is present in most patients with inflammatory bowel disease (ulcerative colitis, Crohn's disease, microscopic colitis). A variety of other symptoms may be present, including abdominal pain, fever, weight loss, and hematochezia. (See Inflammatory Bowel Disease, below.)

E. Motility Disorders: Abnormal intestinal motility secondary to systemic disorders or surgery may result in diarrhea due to rapid transit or to stasis of intestinal contents with bacterial overgrowth, resulting in malabsorption.

F. Irritable Bowel: Probably the most common cause of chronic diarrhea is irritable bowel syndrome (see Irritable Bowel Syndrome, below). Although many of these patients complain of "diarrhea," the majority in fact have a normal stool weight.

G. Chronic Infections: Chronic parasitic infections may cause diarrhea through a number of mechanisms. Agents most commonly associated with diarrhea include the protozoans giardia, *Entamoeba histolytica,* and cyclospora as well as the intestinal nematodes.

Immunocompromised patients are susceptible to infectious agents that can cause acute or chronic diarrhea (see Chapter 31). Chronic diarrhea in AIDS is commonly caused by microsporida, cryptosporidium, cytomegalovirus, *Isospora belli,* cyclospora, and *Mycobacterium avium* complex.

H. Factitial Diarrhea: Approximately 15% of patients with chronic diarrhea have factitial diarrhea caused by surreptitious laxative abuse or dilution of stool.

Evaluation

Many tests are available for the evaluation of chronic diarrhea, but the history and physical examination suggest the underlying pathophysiologic category that guides the subsequent diagnostic workup (Figure 14–1). The following tests are commonly employed in the evaluation of chronic diarrhea. The evaluation of AIDS-associated diarrhea is discussed in Chapter 31.

A. Stool Analysis:

1. Twenty-four-hour stool collection for weight and quantitative fecal fat–A stool weight of more than 300 g/24 h confirms the presence of diarrhea. A weight greater than 1000–1500 g suggests a secretory process. A fecal fat determination in excess of 10 g/24 h indicates a malabsorptive disorder. (See Celiac Sprue and specific tests for malabsorption, below.)

2. Stool osmolality–An osmotic gap confirms osmotic diarrhea. Stool osmolality less than serum osmolality implies that water or urine has been added to the specimen (factitious diarrhea).

3. Stool laxative screen–In cases of suspected laxative abuse, stool magnesium, phosphate, and sulfate levels may be measured. Phenolphthalein, senna, and cascara are indicated by the presence of a bright red color after alkalinization of the stool or urine. Bisacodyl can be detected in the urine.

4. Fecal leukocytes–The presence of fecal leukocytes implies inflammatory diarrhea.

5. Stool for ova and parasites–The presence of giardia and *E histolytica* is detected in routine wet mounts. However, giardia may be absent in many patients with proved giardia infection; it is easier to detect with high-volume diarrhea. Cryptosporidium and cyclospora are found with modified acid-fast staining.

B. Blood Tests:

1. Routine laboratory tests–CBC, serum electrolytes, liver function tests, calcium, phosphorus, albumin, TSH, total T_4, beta-carotene, and prothrombin time may help. Anemia occurs in malabsorption syndromes (vitamin B_{12}, folate, and rarely iron deficiencies) and inflammatory conditions. Hypoalbuminemia is present in malabsorption, protein-losing enteropathies, and inflammatory diseases. Hyponatremia and non–anion gap metabolic acidosis may occur in profound secretory diarrheas.

2. Other laboratory tests–In patients with suspected secretory diarrhea, serum VIP (VIPoma), gastrin (Zollinger-Ellison syndrome), calcitonin (medullary thyroid carcinoma), cortisol (Addison's disease), and urinary 5-HIAA (carcinoid syndrome) levels should be obtained.

C. Proctosigmoidoscopy With Mucosal Biopsy: Examination may be helpful in detecting inflammatory bowel disease (including microscopic colitis) and melanosis coli, indicative of chronic use of anthraquinone laxatives.

D. Imaging: After the above studies have been completed, the cause of the diarrhea will generally be clear and further imaging studies ordered as indicated. Calcification on a plain abdominal radiograph confirms the diagnosis of chronic pancreatitis. An upper gastrointestinal series or enteroclysis study is helpful in evaluating Crohn's disease, lymphoma, or carcinoid syndrome. Colonoscopy identifies colonic inflammation due to inflammatory bowel disease. Upper endoscopy with small bowel biopsy is useful in suspected malabsorption due to mucosal diseases. Upper endoscopy with a duodenal aspirate and small bowel biopsy is also performed in patients with AIDS to document cryptosporidium, microsporida, and *M avium-intracellulare* infection. Abdominal CT re-

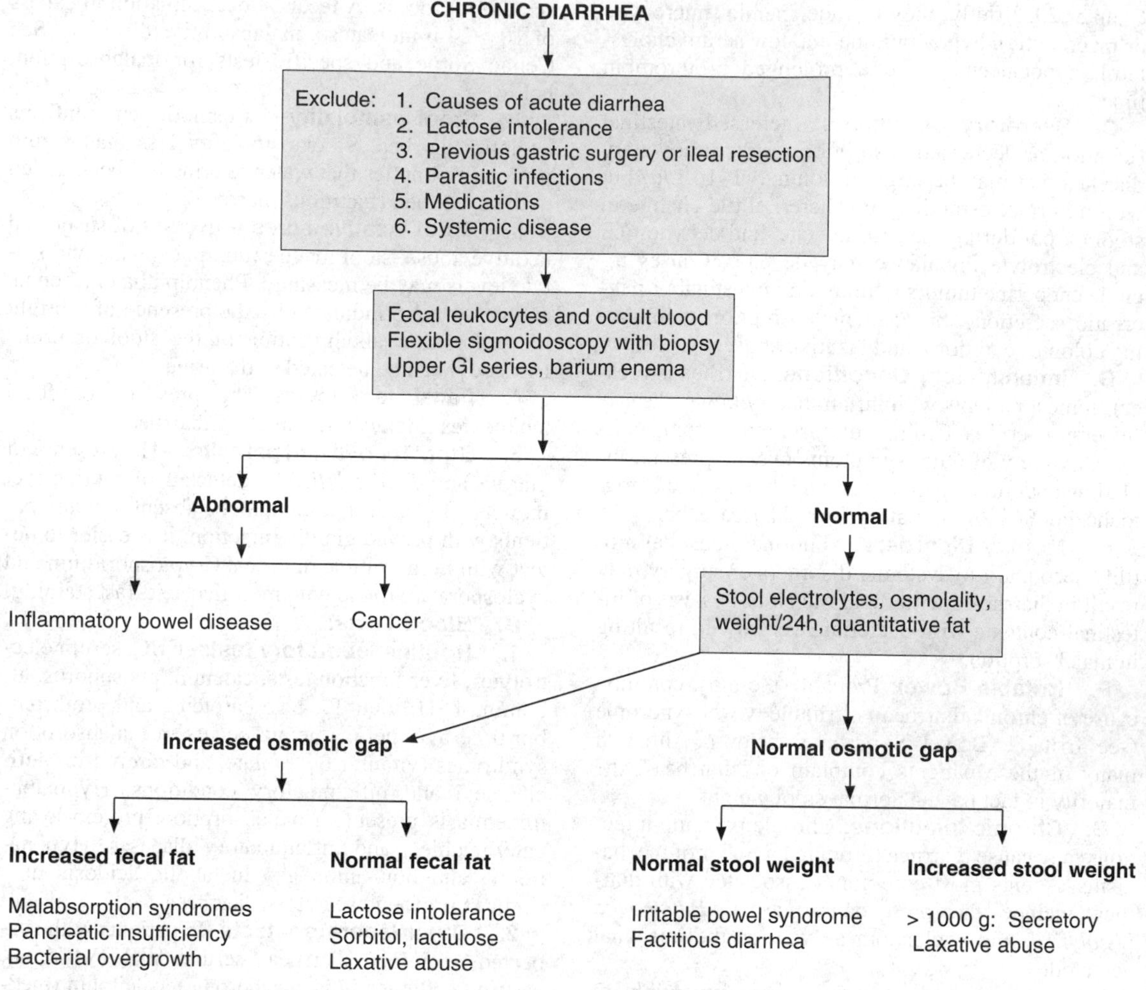

Figure 14–1. Decision diagram for diagnosis of causes of chronic diarrhea.

veals evidence of chronic pancreatitis or pancreatic endocrine tumors.

Treatment

A number of antidiarrheal agents may be used in certain patients with chronic diarrheal conditions and are listed below. Opioids may be used safely in most patients with chronic, stable symptoms.

A. Loperamide: 4 mg initially, then 2 mg after each loose stool (maximum: 16 mg/d).

B. Diphenoxylate With Atropine: One tablet three or four times daily as needed.

C. Codeine, Paregoric: Because of potential habituation, these drugs are generally avoided except in cases of chronic, intractable diarrhea. Codeine may be given in a dosage of 15–60 mg every 4 hours as needed; the dosage of paregoric is 4–8 mL after each liquid bowel movement.

D. Clonidine: α_2-Adrenergic agonists inhibit intestinal electrolyte secretion. A clonidine patch that delivers 0.1–0.2 mg/d for 7 days may help in some patients with secretory diarrheas, cryptosporidiosis, and diabetes.

E. Octreotide: This expensive somatostatin analog stimulates intestinal fluid and electrolyte absorption, and inhibits intestinal fluid secretion and the release of gastrointestinal peptides. It is given for secretory diarrheas due to VIPomas and carcinoid tumors and in some cases of diarrhea associated with AIDS. Effective doses range from 50 μg to 250 μg subcutaneously three times daily.

F. Cholestyramine: This bile salt-binding resin may be useful in patients with bile salt-induced diarrhea secondary to intestinal resection or ileal disease. A dosage of 4 g once daily to three times daily is recommended.

American Gastroenterological Association Medical Position Statement: Guidelines for the management of malnutrition and cachexia, chronic diarrhea, and hepatobiliary disease in patients with human immunodeficiency virus infection. Gastroenterology 1996;111:1722.

Donowitz M et al: Evaluation of patients with chronic diarrhea. (Current Concepts.) N Engl J Med 1995;332:725. [NLM Cit ID: 95157593]

Phillips S et al: Stool composition in factitial diarrhea: A 6-year experience with stool analysis. Ann Intern Med 1995;123:97. [NLM Cit ID: 95297761]

GASTROINTESTINAL BLEEDING

1. ACUTE UPPER GASTROINTESTINAL BLEEDING

Essentials of Diagnosis

- Hematemesis (bright red blood or "coffee grounds").
- Melena in most cases; hematochezia in massive upper gastrointestinal bleeds.
- Volume status to determine severity of blood loss; hematocrit is a poor early indicator of blood loss.
- Endoscopy diagnostic and may be therapeutic.

General Considerations

There are over 350,000 hospitalizations a year in the USA for acute upper gastrointestinal bleeding, with a mortality rate of 10%. Approximately half of patients are over 60 years of age, and in this age group the mortality rate is even higher. Patients seldom die of exsanguination but rather from complications of an underlying disease.

The most common presentation of upper gastrointestinal bleeding is with hematemesis or melena. Hematemesis may be either bright red blood or brown "coffee grounds" material. Melena develops after as little as 50–100 mL of blood in the upper gastrointestinal tract, whereas hematochezia develops with an acute loss of more than 1000 mL. Although hematochezia generally suggests a lower bleeding source (eg, colonic), upper gastrointestinal bleeding may present with hematochezia in as many as 10% of cases.

Upper gastrointestinal bleeding is self-limited in 80% of patients. In the remainder, urgent medical therapy and endoscopic evaluation are warranted. Patients with bleeding more than 48 hours prior to presentation have a low risk of recurrent bleeding.

Etiology

Acute upper gastrointestinal bleeding may originate from a number of sources. These are listed in order of the frequency and discussed in detail below.

A. Peptic Ulcer Disease: Peptic ulcers account for half of major upper gastrointestinal bleeding with an overall acute mortality rate of 6–10%.

B. Portal Hypertension: Portal hypertension may result in bleeding from varices (most commonly esophageal; rarely, gastric or duodenal) or portal hypertensive gastropathy. Less than one-third of patients with portal hypertension and varices will develop acute variceal bleeding. However, bleeding esophageal varices account for 10–20% of significant gastrointestinal hemorrhages, with a hospital mortality rate of 15–40%. If untreated, half will rebleed during hospitalization. A mortality rate of 60–80% is expected at 1–4 years. Bleeding from the gastric mucosa in portal hypertensive gastropathy may account for up to 20% of cases of upper gastrointestinal bleeding in patients with cirrhosis.

C. Mallory-Weiss Tears: Lacerations of the gastroesophageal junction account for 5–10% of cases of upper gastrointestinal bleeding. Most patients report a history of heavy alcohol use or retching. Less than 10% have continued or recurrent bleeding.

D. Vascular Anomalies: Vascular anomalies may be found throughout the gastrointestinal tract and may be the source of chronic or acute upper or lower gastrointestinal bleeding. They account for 7% of cases of acute upper tract bleeding. **Vascular ectasias** (angiodysplasias) have a bright red stellate appearance. They may be part of systemic conditions (hereditary hemorrhagic telangiectasia, CREST syndrome) or may occur sporadically. There is an increased incidence in patients with chronic renal failure.

E. Gastric Neoplasms: Gastric neoplasms account for 1% of significant upper gastrointestinal hemorrhages.

F. Erosive Gastritis: Because this process is superficial, it is a relatively unusual cause of severe gastrointestinal bleeding (< 5% of cases) and more commonly results in blood loss. Gastric mucosal erosions may be due to NSAIDs, alcohol, or severe medical or surgical illness ("stress gastritis").

G. Erosive Esophagitis: Severe erosive esophagitis due to chronic gastroesophageal reflux may rarely cause significant upper gastrointestinal bleeding.

H. Others: An aortoenteric fistula may complicate 2% of abdominal aortic grafts or can occur as the initial presentation of a previously untreated aneurysm. Usually located between the graft or aneurysm and the third portion of the duodenum, these fistulas characteristically present with a "herald" nonexsanguinating initial hemorrhage, with melena and hematemesis, or with chronic intermittent bleeding. The diagnosis may be confirmed by upper endoscopy or abdominal CT. Surgery is mandatory to prevent exsanguinating hemorrhage; patients are at very high risk, especially those with graft-enteric fistulas. Other rare causes of upper gastrointestinal bleeding include hemobilia (from hepatic tumor, angioma, penetrating trauma), pancreatic malignancy, pseudoaneurysm (hemosuccus pancreaticus), and Dieulafoy's lesion (aberrant gastric submucosal artery).

Initial Evaluation & Management

A. Stabilization: The first and most important step is assessment of the hemodynamic status by blood pressure and heart rate. A systolic blood pressure less than 100 mm Hg (irrespective of heart rate) identifies a high-risk patient with severe acute bleeding. A heart rate over 100/min with a systolic blood pressure over 100 mm Hg signifies moderate acute blood loss. A normal systolic blood pressure and heart rate suggests relatively minor hemorrhage. Postural hypotension and tachycardia are useful when present but may be due to causes other than blood loss. Because the hematocrit may take 24–72 hours to equilibrate with the extravascular fluid, it is not a reliable indicator of the severity of acute bleeding.

In patients with significant bleeding, two 18-gauge or larger intravenous lines should be started prior to further diagnostic tests. Blood is sent for complete blood count, prothrombin time with INR, serum creatinine, liver enzymes, and cross-matching for 2–4 units or more of packed red blood cells. In patients without hemodynamic compromise or overt active bleeding, aggressive fluid repletion can be delayed until the extent of the bleeding is further clarified. Patients with evidence of hemodynamic compromise should be given 0.9% saline or lactated Ringer's injection and crossmatched blood as soon as it becomes available. It is rarely necessary to administer type-specific or O-negative blood. Central venous pressure monitoring is desirable in some cases, but line placement should not interfere with rapid volume resuscitation.

A nasogastric tube should be placed in all patients with suspected upper tract bleeding. The finding of red blood or "coffee grounds" material on nasogastric aspirate confirms an upper gastrointestinal source of bleeding, though 10% of patients with confirmed upper tract sources of bleeding have nonbloody aspirates—especially when bleeding originates in the duodenum. An aspirate of bright red blood indicates active bleeding and is associated with the highest risk of further bleeding and complications, while a clear aspirate identifies patients at lower initial risk. Efforts to stop or slow bleeding by gastric lavage with large volumes of fluid are of no benefit and may expose the patient to an increased risk of aspiration. Periodic reaspiration of the nasogastric tube serves as an indicator of ongoing bleeding or rebleeding.

B. Blood Replacement: The amount of fluid and blood products required is based upon assessment of vital signs, evidence of active bleeding from nasogastric aspirate, and laboratory tests. Sufficient packed red blood cells should be given to maintain a hematocrit of 25–30%. In the absence of continued bleeding, the hematocrit should rise 3% for each unit of transfused packed red cells. Transfusion of blood should not be withheld from patients with brisk active bleeding regardless of the hematocrit. It is desirable to transfuse blood in anticipation of the nadir hematocrit. When the blood pressure and pulse rate have been restored to normal limits, the rate of transfusion can be slowed. In actively bleeding patients, platelets should be transfused if the platelet count is under 50,000/μL and considered if there is impaired platelet function due to aspirin use (regardless of the platelet count). Uremic patients (who also have dysfunctional platelets) with active bleeding are given one or two doses of desmopressin (DDAVP), 0.3 μg/kg intravenously, at 12- to 24-hour intervals. Fresh frozen plasma is administered for actively bleeding patients with a coagulopathy and an INR > 1.5. The INR is intended to guide warfarin therapy and is not a reliable marker of bleeding risk in the setting of liver disease. In the face of massive bleeding, 1 unit of fresh frozen plasma should be given for each 5 units of packed red blood cells transfused.

C. Initial Triage: Risk assessment and resuscitation proceed simultaneously when a patient presents with gastrointestinal hemorrhage. A preliminary assessment of risk based upon several clinical factors aids in the resuscitation as well as the rational triage of the patient.

1. Very low risk–Reliable patients without serious comorbid medical illnesses or advanced liver disease who have normal hemodynamics, no evidence of overt bleeding (hematemesis or melena) within 48 hours, a negative nasogastric lavage, and normal laboratory tests do not require hospital admission and can undergo further evaluation as outpatients as deemed necessary.

2. High risk–Patients with active bleeding manifested by hematemesis or bright red blood on nasogastric aspirate, an estimated loss of more than 5 units of blood, persistent hemodynamic derangement despite fluid resuscitation, serious comorbid medical illness, or evidence of advanced liver disease require ICU admission.

3. Low to moderate risk–All other patients should be admitted to a regular hospital unit after appropriate stabilization for further evaluation and treatment. In some centers, these patients undergo upper endoscopy either in the emergency room or in the endoscopy unit prior to hospital admission. Based upon the findings at endoscopy, patients deemed to be at low risk of rebleeding may be discharged and followed as outpatients, whereas patients at high risk are admitted to the hospital for further observation (see below).

Subsequent Evaluation & Treatment

Specific treatment of the various causes of upper gastrointestinal bleeding is discussed elsewhere in this chapter. The following general comments apply to most patients with bleeding:

A. History and Physical Examination: The physician's impression of the bleeding source is correct in only 40% of cases. Signs of chronic liver disease implicate bleeding due to portal hypertension, but a different lesion is identified in 25–50% of patients with cirrhosis. A history of dyspepsia, NSAID use, or peptic ulcer disease suggests peptic ulcer. Acute bleeding preceded by heavy alcohol ingestion or retching predicts a Mallory-Weiss tear, though most of these patients have neither.

B. Upper Endoscopy: Virtually all patients with upper tract bleeding should undergo upper endoscopy, performed after the patient is hemodynamically stable, usually within 12 hours after admission. Patients with continued active bleeding require more urgent endoscopic evaluation. The benefits of endoscopy in this setting are threefold.

1. To identify the source of bleeding–The appropriate acute and long-term medical therapy is determined by the underlying cause of bleeding. For example, patients with portal hypertension will be treated differently from those with ulcer disease. If surgery is required for uncontrolled bleeding, the source of bleeding as determined at endoscopy will determine the surgical approach.

2. To determine the risk of rebleeding– Patients with a nonbleeding Mallory-Weiss tear, esophagitis, gastritis, and ulcers that have a clean, white base have a very low risk of rebleeding. It may be safe and cost-effective to discharge such patients from the emergency room or endoscopy suite without hospital admission. Patients with ulcers that are actively bleeding or have a visible vessel or with variceal bleeding require initial management in an ICU setting.

3. To render endoscopic therapy–Hemostasis can be achieved in actively bleeding lesions with endoscopic modalities such as cautery or injection. About 90% of actively bleeding varices can be effectively treated acutely with injection of a sclerosant or application of a rubber band to the bleeding varix. Similarly, 90% of actively bleeding ulcers, angiomas, or Mallory-Weiss tears can be controlled with either injection of epinephrine or direct cauterization of the vessel by a heater probe or multipolar electrocautery probe. Certain nonbleeding lesions such as esophageal varices, ulcers with visible blood vessels, and angiomas are also treated with these therapies. Specific endoscopic therapy of varices, peptic ulcers, and Mallory-Weiss tears is dealt with elsewhere in this chapter.

C. Acute Pharmacologic Therapies:

1. H_2-receptor antagonists and proton pump inhibitors–H_2 receptor antagonists do not stop acute bleeding or reduce the incidence of rebleeding. High-dose proton pump inhibitors (omeprazole 40 mg or lansoprazole 60 mg, twice daily for 5 days) lower the risk of rebleeding in patients with peptic ulcers with high-risk features (active bleeding, visible vessel or adherent clot). Pending the results of endoscopic examination, it may be reasonable to initiate therapy with a proton pump inhibitor in patients with suspected peptic ulcer bleeding.

2. Octreotide–Continuous intravenous infusion of octreotide (100 μg bolus, followed by 50–100 μg/h) reduces splanchnic blood flow and portal blood pressures and is effective in the initial control of bleeding related to portal hypertension. It is administered promptly to all patients with active upper gastrointestinal bleeding and evidence of liver disease or portal hypertension until the source of bleeding can be determined by endoscopy.

3. Vasopressin–Because of its toxicity, intravenous vasopressin is not used in the treatment of patients with upper gastrointestinal bleeding. Octreotide has equivalent or superior efficacy but is virtually devoid of short-term side effects.

D. Other Treatment:

1. Intra-arterial embolization or vasopressin– Angiographic treatment is used rarely in patients with persistent bleeding from ulcers, angiomas, or Mallory-Weiss tears who have failed endoscopic therapy and are poor operative risks.

2. Transvenous intrahepatic portosystemic shunts (TIPS)–Placement of a wire stent from the hepatic vein through the liver to the portal vein provides effective decompression of the portal venous system and control of acute variceal bleeding. It is indicated in patients in whom endoscopic modalities have failed to control acute variceal bleeding.

Imperiale TF et al: Somatostatin or octreotide compared with H_2 antagonists and placebo in the management of acute nonvariceal upper gastrointestinal hemorrhage: A meta-analysis. Ann Intern Med 1997;127:1062. [NLM Cit ID: 98049714]

Khuroo M et al: A comparison of omeprazole and placebo for bleeding peptic ulcer. N Engl J Med 1997;336:1054. [NLM Cit ID: 97224091] (In patient with bleeding peptic ulcers, proton pump inhibitors reduced rebleeding from high-risk lesions from 36% to 10%.)

Longstreth GM et al: Successful outpatient management of acute upper gastrointestinal hemorrhage: use of practice guidelines in a large patient series. Gastrointest Endosc 1998;47:219. [NLM Cit ID: 98199940] (Clinical guidelines and endoscopic findings can be used to stratify patients with acute upper gastrointestinal bleeding, and low risk patients can be managed as outpatients.)

Steele R: The preprocedural care of the patient with gastrointestinal bleeding. Gastroenterol Clin North Am 1997;7:551. [NLM Cit ID: 98015830]

2. ACUTE LOWER GASTROINTESTINAL BLEEDING

Essentials of Diagnosis

- Hematochezia usually present.
- 10% of cases of hematochezia due to upper gastrointestinal source.
- Evaluation with colonoscopy in stable patients.
- Massive active bleeding calls for evaluation with sigmoidoscopy, upper endoscopy, and angiography or nuclear bleeding scan.

General Considerations

Lower gastrointestinal bleeding is defined as that arising below the ligament of Treitz, ie, the small intestine or colon; however, over 95% of cases arise from the colon. The severity of lower gastrointestinal bleeding ranges from mild anorectal bleeding to massive, large-volume hematochezia. Bright red blood that drips into the bowl after a bowel movement or is mixed with solid brown stool signifies mild bleeding, usually from an anorectosigmoid source, and can be evaluated in the outpatient setting. Serious lower gastrointestinal bleeding is more common in older men. In patients hospitalized with gastrointestinal bleeding, lower tract bleeding is one-fourth as common as upper gastrointestinal hemorrhage and tends to have a less severe clinical course. Patients hospitalized with lower gastrointestinal tract bleeding are less likely to present with shock or orthostasis (< 20%) or to require blood transfusions (< 40%). Spontaneous cessation of bleeding occurs in over 85% of cases, and hospital mortality is less than 3%.

Etiology

The cause of these lesions is dependent both upon the age of the patient and the severity of the bleeding. In patients under 50 years of age, the most common causes are infectious colitis, anorectal disease, and inflammatory bowel disease. In older patients, significant hematochezia is most often seen with diverticulosis, vascular ectasias, malignancy, or ischemia. Each of these entities is discussed in greater detail elsewhere in this chapter.

A. Diverticulosis: Hemorrhage occurs in 3–5% of all patients with diverticulosis and is the most common cause of major lower tract bleeding, accounting for 40% of cases. It most commonly presents as acute, painless, large-volume maroon or bright red hematochezia in patients over age 50. More than 95% of cases require less than 4 units of blood transfusion. Bleeding subsides spontaneously in 80% but may recur in up to 25% of patients.

B. Vascular Ectasias: Vascular ectasias (or angiodysplasias) may cause painless bleeding that ranges from acute hematochezia to chronic occult blood loss. They are responsible for 3–8% of cases of acute lower gastrointestinal bleeding. Bleeding is most common in patients over 70 years of age or in patients with chronic renal failure. Most commonly seen in the right colon, they occur throughout the upper and lower gastrointestinal tract. A murmur of aortic stenosis may be associated.

C. Neoplasms: Both benign polyps and carcinoma most commonly present with chronic occult blood loss or mild intermittent anorectal type hematochezia. However, colonic neoplasms may account for up to 10% of acute lower gastrointestinal hemorrhage. After endoscopic removal of colonic polyps, significant bleeding may occur up to 2 weeks later in 0.5% of patients. Delayed bleeding can be managed conservatively (ie, without repeat colonoscopy) in 70% of cases.

D. Inflammatory Bowel Disease: Patients with inflammatory bowel disease (especially ulcerative colitis) often have diarrhea with variable amounts of hematochezia. Bleeding may vary from occult blood loss to recurrent hematochezia which is usually mixed with stool. Symptoms of abdominal pain, tenesmus, and urgency are often present.

E. Anorectal Disease: Anorectal disease commonly results in small amounts of bright red blood noted on the toilet paper, streaking the stool, or dripping into the toilet bowl. The bleeding is usually slight and seldom results in significant blood loss. Painless bleeding is commonly caused by internal hemorrhoids. Bleeding associated with pain during bowel movements suggests an anal fissure.

F. Ischemic Colitis: This entity is seen in elderly patients, most of whom have known atherosclerotic disease. Acute ischemia results in hematochezia or bloody diarrhea, typically associated with mild cramps. In most cases, the bleeding is mild and self-limited.

G. Others: Radiation-induced colitis may result in intestinal bleeding that can occur years later. Acute infectious colitis due to shigella, campylobacter, and enterohemorrhagic *E coli* (see Acute Diarrhea, above) commonly causes bloody diarrhea. Rare causes of lower tract bleeding include vasculitis, solitary rectal ulcer syndrome, NSAID-induced ulcers in the small bowel, small bowel diverticula, and colonic varices.

Evaluation & Management

The color of the stool helps distinguish upper from lower gastrointestinal bleeding. Brown stools mixed or streaked with blood predict a source in the rectosigmoid or anus. Large volumes of bright red blood suggest a colonic source; maroon stools imply a lesion in the right colon or small intestine; and black stools (melena) predict a source proximal to the ligament of Treitz. Physicians should examine the stool themselves and not rely solely upon patients' subjective descriptions of stool color. Although 10% of patients admitted with self-reported hematochezia have an upper gastrointestinal source of bleeding (eg, peptic ulcer), true bright red blood per rectum occurs uncommonly with upper tract bleeding and almost always in the setting of massive hemorrhage with shock. Painless large-volume bleeding usually suggests diverticular bleeding or vascular ectasias. Bloody diarrhea associated with cramping abdominal pain, urgency, or tenesmus is characteristic of inflammatory bowel disease, infectious colitis, or ischemic colitis.

Important considerations include the following:

A. Exclusion of an Upper Tract Source: A nasogastric tube is inserted and lavage performed in all patients with massive hematochezia with orthostasis or shock. The presence of red blood or dark brown ("coffee grounds") guaiac-positive material strongly implicates an upper gastrointestinal source of bleeding. If blood is not seen and bile is aspirated, an upper source is found in only 1% of patients.

B. Anoscopy and Sigmoidoscopy: In otherwise healthy patients under age 45 with small-volume bleeding, anoscopy and sigmoidoscopy are performed to look for evidence of anorectal disease, inflammatory bowel disease, or infectious colitis. If a lesion is found, no further evaluation is needed immediately unless the bleeding persists or is recurrent. In patients over age 45 with small-volume hematochezia, the entire colon must be evaluated with either colonoscopy or sigmoidoscopy and barium enema, to exclude tumor.

C. Colonoscopy: An urgent colonoscopy should be performed in all patients with significant lower tract bleeding (ie, bleeding associated with a fall in hematocrit) when the bleeding has subsided or slowed (requiring less than 2 units of packed red blood cells per 24 hours). Colonoscopy is usually performed within 6–24 hours after admission once the colon has been cleansed with a standard oral lavage solution. A possible bleeding source is identified in over 70% of cases; however, active bleeding usually is not seen.

D. Nuclear Bleeding Scans and Angiography: Significant, continued active bleeding limits the diagnostic effectiveness of colonoscopy. In such patients, surgery may become necessary to control bleeding. It is important to attempt to localize the bleeding in order to guide the surgical approach. Although technetium-labeled red blood cell scanning can detect significant active bleeding and localize it to the small intestine, right colon, or left colon, its accuracy is only 78%. Furthermore, less than half of studies are diagnostic, either because the bleeding is intermittent or too slow. Tests are more likely positive in patients passing bright red or maroon stools at the time of the scan. Selective mesenteric angiography requires more brisk bleeding than technetium scans (0.5–1 mL/min) and can lead to major complications in up to 3% of patients. Accordingly, angiograms are performed only in patients with massive bleeding or positive technetium scans. Localization of an actively bleeding vessel is possible in up to 50%.

Treatment

The following general principles apply:

A. Discontinue Aspirin and Other NSAIDs: Over 80% of patients with lower gastrointestinal tract bleeding have evidence of recent aspirin ingestion. These agents potentiate bleeding through inhibition of platelet function.

B. Therapeutic Colonoscopy: Endoscopic electrocoagulation techniques are useful in treating vascular ectasias of the colon and postpolypectomy hemorrhage and for removal of bleeding colonic polyps.

C. Intra-arterial Vasopressin or Embolization: At angiography, the intra-arterial infusion of vasopressin, 0.2 units/min, may arrest bleeding in up to 90% of patients with active bleeding from a diverticulum or vascular ectasia. Embolization may be used in patients with continued bleeding who are poor operative candidates but is associated with intestinal infarction in 15% of cases.

D. Surgery: Surgery generally is indicated in patients with ongoing bleeding that requires more than 4–6 units of blood within 24 hours or more than 10 total units. Most such hemorrhages are caused by a bleeding diverticulum or vascular ectasia. Preoperative localization of the bleeding site by nuclear scan or angiography allows limited resection of the bleeding segment of small intestine or colon. When accurate localization is not possible or when emergency surgery is required for massive hemorrhage, total abdominal colectomy with ileorectal anastomosis usually is performed—with a significantly higher morbidity and mortality than limited resections. Surgery may also be indicated in patients with repeated hospitalizations for diverticular bleeding depending upon the severity of bleeding and the patient's other comorbid conditions.

Zuckerman GR et al: Acute lower intestinal bleeding. Part 1: Clinical presentation and diagnosis. Gastrointest Endosc 1998;48:606. [NLM Cit ID: 99069174]

Zuckerman GR et al: Acute lower intestinal bleeding. Part 2: Etiology, therapy and outcomes. Gastrointest Endosc 1999;49:228. [NLM Cit ID: 99124666]

3. OCCULT GASTROINTESTINAL BLEEDING

Essentials of Diagnosis

- No overt gastrointestinal bleeding (hematochezia, melena).
- Detected by fecal occult blood testing or iron deficiency anemia in an adult without other source of blood loss.
- Evaluation of colon with colonoscopy or barium enema mandatory.
- Evaluation of upper gastrointestinal tract with endoscopy or barium upper GI series guided by presence of symptoms.

General Considerations

Occult gastrointestinal bleeding is typically detected by a positive fecal occult blood test or the presence of iron deficiency anemia in an adult.

A. Fecal Occult Blood Testing (FOBT): Many patients over age 50 undergo annual routine testing of stool specimens for occult blood as a screen for colorectal neoplasms (see Colorectal Cancer Screening, below). From 1% to 2.7% of patients in screening programs will have a positive FOBT warranting investigation of the colon to exclude carcinoma. The positive predictive value of a nonrehydrated positive guaiac test is only 5–15%.

B. Iron Deficiency Anemia: In Western society, men and postmenopausal women with iron deficiency should be presumed to have occult gastrointestinal bleeding. Nutritional iron deficiency is rare. Potential gastrointestinal causes of blood loss can be identified in over 60% of patients with iron deficiency from both the upper and lower gastrointestinal tracts, and a malignancy is present in up to 15%. Celiac sprue may also present on rare occasions with iron deficiency.

Causes of Occult Blood Loss

The most common causes of occult gastrointestinal bleeding are similar to the causes of clinically apparent bleeding cited above. These include (1) neoplasms (colorectal cancers and polyps, gastric cancers, lymphomas), (2) infections (nematodes, especially hookworm; amebiasis, tuberculosis), (3) vascular abnormalities (vascular ectasias, portal hypertensive gastropathy), (4) acid-peptic lesions (peptic ulcer, reflux esophagitis, large hiatal hernias with erosions), (5) medications (especially NSAIDs, aspirin, or anticoagulants), and (6) other causes such as inflammatory bowel disease and malabsorption disorders.

Evaluation

A. Upper Endoscopy: Patients should be asked about symptoms such as heartburn, dyspepsia, nausea, vomiting, weight loss, early satiety, diarrhea, constipation, or change in bowel habits. In patients under age 45 years with obvious symptoms referable to the upper gastrointestinal tract, it is reasonable to proceed first with upper endoscopy to look for a source of acute or chronic bleeding. In asymptomatic patients with positive fecal occult blood tests whose colon evaluations are negative, the cost-effectiveness of evaluation of the upper tract is uncertain, and currently this procedure is not recommended. If iron deficiency anemia is also present, patients should undergo upper endoscopy after colonoscopy (see below). If no significant abnormality is found, a small bowel biopsy should be obtained during endoscopy to exclude celiac sprue and other malabsorptive disorders.

B. Colonoscopy Versus Barium Enema: In virtually all other patients with positive occult blood tests or iron deficiency anemia, the colon should be evaluated first with either colonoscopy or a combination of barium enema and sigmoidoscopy. (The latter is required to view the rectum and distal sigmoid adequately, since they are not well visualized by barium enema.) Colonoscopy detects over 95% of colorectal polyps or cancers and permits polypectomy, tumor biopsy, or endoscopic cautery of vascular ectasias. Barium enema examinations have only an 85–90% sensitivity for colorectal polyps, and up to 30–40% of patients with positive occult blood tests will have polyps detected on barium enema or sigmoidoscopy, which then necessitates colonoscopy to remove the polyps. Thus, although colonoscopy is more expensive than barium enema, the overall cost of these two diagnostic strategies is approximately the same.

C. Small Intestine Evaluation: Evaluation of the small intestine is unnecessary in most patients with positive fecal occult blood tests or iron deficiency anemia who have negative evaluation of the colon and upper gastrointestinal tract. With persistent chronic gastrointestinal blood loss that responds poorly to iron supplementation or requires transfusion, further evaluation for a small intestinal source of blood loss is needed. A small intestinal enteroclysis study is useful for detecting mucosal diseases such as Crohn's disease. Small bowel enteroscopy is now available at many centers and permits visualization of the upper one-third to one-half of the small intestine for vascular ectasias. Rarely, angiography or intraoperative endoscopy of the entire small intestine is necessary.

Ransohoff DF et al: Clinical guideline: Part 1. Suggested technique for fecal occult blood testing and interpretation in colorectal cancer screening. Ann Intern Med 1997;126:808. [NLM Cit ID: 97282922] Part 2. Screening for colorectal cancer with the fecal occult blood test: a background paper. Ann Intern Med 1997;126:811. [NLM Cit ID: 97282923] (Two papers provide a scholarly, evidence-based review of the indications and limitations of fecal occult blood testing and appropriate evaluation for positive results.)

Rockey DC et al: Relative frequency of upper gastrointestinal and colonic lesions in patients with positive fecal occult-blood tests. N Engl J Med 1998;339:153. [NLM Cit ID: 98319547] (Upper gastrointestinal lesions were identified more commonly than colonic lesions irrespective of symptoms in patients without anemia; upper endoscopy is warranted in patients with positive fecal occult blood tests who are symptomatic or who have iron deficiency anemia.)

DISEASES OF THE PERITONEUM

APPROACH TO THE PATIENT WITH ASCITES

Etiology of Ascites

The term "ascites" denotes the pathologic accumulation of fluid in the peritoneal cavity. Healthy men have little or no intraperitoneal fluid, but women normally may have up to 20 mL depending on the phase of the menstrual cycle. The causes of ascites may be classified into two broad pathophysiologic categories: that which is associated with a normal peritoneum and that which occurs due to a diseased peritoneum (Table 14–8). The most common cause of ascites is portal hypertension secondary to chronic liver disease, which accounts for over 80% of patients with ascites. The management of portal hypertensive ascites is discussed in Chapter 15. The most common causes of non-portal hypertensive ascites include infections (tuberculous peritonitis), intra-abdominal malignancy, inflammatory disorders of the peritoneum, and ductal disruptions (chylous, pancreatic, biliary).

Table 14–8. Causes of ascites.

NORMAL PERITONEUM
Portal hypertension (SAAG ≥ 1.1 g/dL)
1. Hepatic congestion[1]
Congestive heart failure
Constrictive pericarditis
Tricuspid insufficiency
Budd-Chiari syndrome
Veno-occlusive disease
2. Liver disease[2]
Cirrhosis
Alcoholic hepatitis
Fulminant hepatic failure
Massive hepatic metastases
Hepatic fibrosis
Acute fatty liver of pregnancy
3. Portal vein occlusion
Hypoalbuminemia (SAAG < 1.1 g/dL)
Nephrotic syndrome
Protein-losing enteropathy
Severe malnutrition with anasarca
Miscellaneous conditions (SAAG < 1.1 g/L)
Chylous ascites
Pancreatic ascites
Bile ascites
Nephrogenic ascites
Urine ascites
Myxedema (SAAG ≥ 1.1 g/dL)
Ovarian disease
DISEASED PERITONEUM (SAAG < 1.1 g/dL[2])
Infections
Bacterial peritonitis
Tuberculous peritonitis
Fungal peritonitis
HIV-associated peritonitis
Malignant conditions
Peritoneal carcinomatosis
Primary mesothelioma
Pseudomyxoma peritonei
Massive hepatic metastases
Hepatocellular carcinoma
Other conditions
Familial Mediterranean fever
Vasculitis
Granulomatous peritonitis
Eosinophilic peritonitis

SAAG = serum-ascites albumin gradient.
[1]Hepatic congestion usually associated with SAAG ≥ 1.1 g/dL and ascitic fluid total protein > 2.5 g/dL.
[2]There may be cases of "mixed ascites" in which portal hypertensive ascites is complicated by a secondary process such as infection. In these cases, the SAAG is ≥ 1.1 g/dL.

Clinical Features

A. Symptoms and Signs: The history usually is one of increasing abdominal girth, with the presence of abdominal pain depending on the cause. Because most ascites is secondary to chronic liver disease with portal hypertension, patients should be asked about risk factors for liver disease, especially ethanol consumption, blood transfusions, tattoos, intravenous drug use, a history of viral hepatitis or jaundice, and birth in an area endemic for hepatitis. A history of cancer or marked weight loss arouses suspicion of malignant ascites. Fevers may suggest infected peritoneal fluid, including bacterial peritonitis (spontaneous or secondary). Patients with chronic liver disease and ascites are at greatest risk of developing spontaneous bacterial peritonitis. In immigrants, immunocompromised hosts, or severely malnourished alcoholics, tuberculous peritonitis should be considered.

Physical examination should emphasize signs of portal hypertension and chronic liver disease. Elevated jugular venous pressure may suggest right-sided congestive heart failure or constrictive pericarditis. A large tender liver is characteristic of acute alcoholic hepatitis or Budd-Chiari syndrome. The presence of large abdominal wall veins with cephalad flow also suggests portal hypertension; inferiorly directed flow implies hepatic vein obstruction. Signs of chronic liver disease include palmar erythema, cutaneous spider angiomas, gynecomastia, and Dupuytren's contracture. Asterixis secondary to hepatic encephalopathy may be present. Anasarca may be due to cardiac failure or nephrotic syndrome with hypoalbuminemia. Finally, firm lymph nodes in the left supraclavicular region or umbilicus may suggest intra-abdominal malignancy.

The physical examination is relatively insensitive for detecting ascitic fluid. The most sensitive means of determining whether ascitic fluid is present is to test for "shifting dullness." In general, patients must have at least 1500 mL of fluid to be detected reliably by this method. In many cases, even the experienced clinician may find it difficult to distinguish between obesity and small-volume ascites. Abdominal ultrasound establishes the presence of fluid.

B. Laboratory Testing:

1. Abdominal paracentesis–Abdominal paracentesis is performed as part of the diagnostic evaluation in all patients with new onset of ascites and with any clinical alteration in patients with known ascites (fever, abdominal pain, sudden increase in the amount of ascites, or worsened encephalopathy).

a. Inspection–Cloudy fluid suggests infection. Milky fluid is seen with chylous ascites due to high triglyceride levels. Bloody fluid is most commonly attributable to a traumatic paracentesis, but up to 20% of cases of malignant ascites are bloody.

b. Routine studies–

(1) Cell count–A white blood cell count is the most important test. Normal ascitic fluid contains

< 500 leukocytes/μL and < 250 PMNs/μL. Any inflammatory condition can cause an elevated ascitic white blood count. A polymorphonuclear neutrophil count of > 250/μL (neutrocytic ascites) is highly suggestive of bacterial peritonitis, either spontaneous primary peritonitis or secondary peritonitis (ie, caused by an intra-abdominal source of infection, such as a perforated viscus or appendicitis). An elevated white count with a predominance of lymphocytes arouses suspicion of tuberculosis or peritoneal carcinomatosis.

(2) Albumin and total protein–The serum-ascites albumin gradient (SAAG) is the best single test for the classification of ascites into portal hypertensive and non-portal hypertensive causes (Table 14–8). Calculated by subtracting the ascitic fluid albumin from the serum albumin, the gradient correlates directly with the portal pressure. An SAAG ≥ 1.1 g/dL strongly suggests underlying portal hypertension, while gradients < 1.1 g/dL implicate non-portal hypertensive causes.

The accuracy of the SAAG exceeds 95% in classifying ascites. It should be recognized, however, that approximately 4% of patients have "mixed ascites," ie, underlying cirrhosis with portal hypertension complicated by a second cause for ascites formation (such as malignancy or tuberculosis). Thus, a high SAAG is indicative of portal hypertension but does not exclude concomitant malignancy.

The ascitic fluid total protein provides some additional clues to the cause. An elevated SAAG and a high protein level (> 2.5 g/dL) are seen in most cases of hepatic congestion secondary to cardiac disease or Budd-Chiari syndrome. However, an elevated ascitic fluid protein is also found in up to 20% of cases of uncomplicated cirrhosis. Two-thirds of patients with malignant ascites have a total protein level > 2.5 g/dL.

(3) Culture and Gram stain–The optimal technique for the culture of ascitic fluid consists of the inoculation of blood culture bottles with 5–10 mL of ascitic fluid at the patient's bedside, which increases the sensitivity for detecting bacterial peritonitis to over 85% in patients with neutrocytic ascites (> 250 PMNs/μL), compared with approximately 50% sensitivity by conventional agar plate or broth cultures.

c. Optional studies–Other laboratory tests are of utility in specific clinical situations but need not be ordered in the routine evaluation of ascites. Glucose and LDH may be helpful in distinguishing spontaneous from secondary bacterial peritonitis (see below). Glucose levels are reduced in patients with tuberculous peritonitis. An elevated amylase may suggest pancreatic ascites or a perforation of the gastrointestinal tract with leakage of pancreatic secretions into the ascitic fluid. Perforation of biliary origin is suspected with an ascitic bilirubin concentration that is greater than the serum bilirubin. An elevated ascitic creatinine suggests leakage of urine from the bladder or ureters. Ascitic fluid cytologic examination is required if intra-abdominal malignancy or peritoneal carcinomatosis is suspected.

C. Imaging: Abdominal ultrasound is useful in confirming the presence of ascites and in the guidance of paracentesis. Both ultrasound and CT imaging are useful in distinguishing between causes of portal and non-portal hypertensive ascites. Doppler ultrasound and CT can detect thrombosis of the hepatic veins (Budd-Chiari syndrome) or portal veins. In patients with non-portal hypertensive ascites, these studies are useful in detecting lymphadenopathy and masses of the mesentery and of solid organs such as the liver, ovaries, and pancreas. Furthermore, they permit directed percutaneous needle biopsies of these lesions. Ultrasound and CT are poor procedures for the detection of peritoneal carcinomatosis.

D. Laparoscopy: Laparoscopy is an important test in the evaluation of some patients with non-portal hypertensive ascites (low SAAG) or mixed ascites. It permits direct visualization and biopsy of the peritoneum, liver, and some intra-abdominal lymph nodes. Cases of suspected peritoneal tuberculosis or suspected malignancy with nondiagnostic CT imaging and ascitic fluid cytology are best evaluated by this method. At laparoscopy, up to three-fourths of patients with exudative ascites have peritoneal carcinomatosis.

Habeeb K et al: Management of ascites. Paracentesis as a guide. Postgrad Med 1997;101:191. [NLM Cit ID: 97161441]

Jaffe DL et al: Management of portal hypertension and its complications. Med Clin North Am 1996;80:1021. [NLM Cit ID: 96397479]

SPONTANEOUS BACTERIAL PERITONITIS

Essentials of Diagnosis

- Patient with chronic liver disease and ascites.
- Fever and abdominal pain.
- Neutrocytic ascites (> 250 PMNs/μL).
- Must be distinguished from secondary causes of peritonitis.

General Considerations

"Spontaneous" bacterial infection of ascitic fluid occurs in the absence of an apparent intra-abdominal source of infection. It is seen almost exclusively in patients with ascites caused by chronic liver disease. Translocation of enteric bacteria across the gut wall or mesenteric lymphatics leads to seeding of the ascitic fluid, as may bacteremia from other sites. Approximately 20–30% of cirrhotic patients with ascites develop spontaneous peritonitis; however, the incidence is greater than 40% in patients with ascitic fluid total protein < 1 g/dL, probably due to decreased ascitic fluid opsonic activity.

Virtually all cases of spontaneous bacterial peritonitis are caused by a monomicrobial infection. The most common pathogens are enteric gram-negative bacteria (*Escherichia coli, Klebsiella pneumoniae,* enterococcus species) or gram-positive bacteria (*Streptococcus pneumoniae,* viridans streptococci). Anaerobic bacteria are not associated with spontaneous bacterial peritonitis.

Clinical Findings

A. Symptoms and Signs: Eighty to 90 percent of patients with spontaneous bacterial peritonitis are symptomatic; however, in many cases the presentation is subtle. Spontaneous bacterial peritonitis may be present in 20% of patients hospitalized with chronic liver disease in the absence of any suggestive symptoms or signs.

The most common symptoms are fever and abdominal pain, present in one-half to two-thirds of patients. Spontaneous bacterial peritonitis may also present with a change in mental status due to exacerbation or precipitation of hepatic encephalopathy. Physical examination typically demonstrates signs of chronic liver disease with ascites. Significant abdominal tenderness is present in less than half of patients, and its presence suggests other processes.

B. Laboratory Findings: The most important diagnostic test is abdominal paracentesis. Ascitic fluid should be sent for cell count, and blood culture bottles should be inoculated at the bedside. Gram's stain is insensitive in the detection of spontaneous bacterial peritonitis. An ascitic fluid total protein of more than 1 g/dL is evidence against spontaneous bacterial peritonitis.

In the proper clinical setting, an ascitic fluid PMN count of > 250 cells/μL (neutrocytic ascites) is presumptive evidence of bacterial peritonitis. The percentage of PMNs is greater than 50–70% of the ascitic fluid white blood cells and commonly approximates 100%. Patients with neutrocytic ascites are presumed to be infected and should be started—regardless of symptoms—on antibiotics. Although 10–30% of patients with neutrocytic ascites have negative ascitic bacterial cultures ("culture-negative neutrocytic ascites"), it is presumed nonetheless that most of these patients have bacterial peritonitis, and they should all be treated empirically.

Differential Diagnosis

Spontaneous bacterial peritonitis must be distinguished from secondary bacterial peritonitis, in which ascitic fluid has become secondarily infected by an intra-abdominal infection. Even in the presence of perforation, clinical symptoms and signs of peritonitis may be lacking in up to 30% of patients owing to the separation of the visceral and parietal peritoneum by the ascitic fluid. Causes of secondary bacterial peritonitis include appendicitis, diverticulitis, perforated peptic ulcer, perforated bowel, and perforated gallbladder. Secondary bacterial infection may account for up to 15% of infected ascites.

Ascitic fluid total protein, LDH, and glucose are useful in distinguishing spontaneous bacterial peritonitis from secondary infection. Up to two-thirds of patients with secondary bacterial peritonitis have at least two of the following: decreased glucose level (< 50 mg/dL), an elevated LDH level (greater than serum), and total protein > 1 g/dL. Ascitic neutrophil counts > 10,000/μL also are suspicious; however, most patients with secondary peritonitis have neutrophil counts within the range of spontaneous peritonitis. The presence of multiple organisms on ascitic fluid Gram stain or culture is diagnostic of secondary peritonitis.

If secondary bacterial peritonitis is suspected, plain films, abdominal CT imaging, and water-soluble contrast studies of the upper and lower gastrointestinal tracts should be obtained to look for evidence of an intra-abdominal source of infection. If these studies are negative and secondary peritonitis still is suspected, repeat paracentesis should be performed after 48 hours of antibiotic therapy to confirm that the polymorphonuclear neutrophil count is decreasing. Secondary bacterial peritonitis should be suspected in patients in whom the polymorphonuclear neutrophil count is not below the pretreatment value at 48 hours.

Neutrocytic ascites may also be seen in some patients with peritoneal carcinomatosis, pancreatic ascites, or tuberculous ascites. In these circumstances, however, polymorphonuclear neutrophils account for less than 50% of the ascitic white blood cells.

Prevention

Up to 70% of patients who survive an episode of spontaneous bacterial peritonitis will have another episode within 1 year. Prophylactic therapy—with norfloxacin, 400 mg/d; ciprofloxacin, 750 mg weekly; or trimethoprim-sulfamethoxazole, one double-strength tablet daily—has been shown to reduce the rate of recurrent infections to less than 20% and is recommended. Prophylaxis should be considered also in patients who have not had prior bacterial peritonitis but are at increased risk of infection due to low-protein ascites (total ascitic protein < 1 g/dL). Although improvement in survival in cirrhotic patients with ascites treated with prophylactic antibiotics has not been shown, decision analytic modeling suggests that in patients with prior bacterial peritonitis or low ascitic fluid protein, the use of prophylactic antibiotics is a cost-effective strategy.

Treatment

Empirical therapy for spontaneous bacterial peritonitis should be initiated with a third-generation cephalosporin such as cefotaxime (dosage: 1 g every 12 hours to 2 g intravenously every 8 hours depending on renal function), which covers 98% of causative agents of this disorder. If enterococcus infection is suspected, ampicillin may be added. Because of a high risk of nephrotoxicity in patients with chronic liver disease, aminoglycosides should not be used. Although the optimal duration of therapy is unknown, a course of 5 days is sufficient in most patients, or until the ascites fluid polymorphonuclear neutrophil count decreases to < 250 cells/μL. Renal failure develops in up to 40% of patients and is a major cause of death. It has been suggested that in patients given intravenous albumin, 1.5 g/kg on day 1 and 1 g/kg on day 3, the incidence of renal failure and mortality were reduced significantly both during hospitalization and at follow-up, and it may be reasonable to administer intravenous albumin to these patients. Patients with suspected secondary bacterial peritonitis should be started on broad-spectrum coverage for enteric aerobic and anaerobic flora with a third-generation cephalosporin and metronidazole pending identification and definitive (usually surgical) treatment of the cause.

Prognosis

The mortality rate of spontaneous bacterial peritonitis exceeds 30%. However, if the disease is recognized and treated early, the rate is less than 10%. As the majority of patients have underlying severe liver disease, many may die of liver failure, hepatorenal syndrome, or bleeding complications from portal hypertension.

Guarner C et al: Risk of a first community-acquired spontaneous bacterial peritonitis in cirrhotics with low ascitic fluid protein levels. Gastroenterology 1999;117:414. [NLM Cit ID: 99350304]

Sorta P et al: Effect of intravenous albumin on renal impairment and mortality in patients with cirrhosis and spontaneous bacterial peritonitis. N Engl J Med 1999;341:403. [NLM Cit ID: 99345287]

Such J et al: Spontaneous bacterial peritonitis. Clin Infect Dis 1998;27:669. [NLM Cit ID: 99014747]

TUBERCULOUS PERITONITIS

Tuberculosis occurs in extrapulmonary sites in 10% of non-HIV-infected people and up to 70% of those infected with HIV. Although tuberculous involvement of the peritoneum accounts for less than 2% of all causes of ascites in the United States, it remains a significant problem in underdeveloped countries. In Western countries, its incidence is higher among those with HIV disease, immigrants from underdeveloped countries, the urban poor, and nursing home residents.

The presenting symptoms often are nonspecific, including low-grade fever, anorexia, and weight loss. The majority have abdominal swelling with clinically apparent ascites; over 95% have ascites evident on ultrasound examination. In patients without ascites, there may be a doughy consistency to the abdomen. In Western societies, half of patients have underlying cirrhosis and ascites from portal hypertension. In such patients, a diagnosis of tuberculous peritonitis may go unsuspected because symptoms are attributed to the underlying liver disease. A high index of suspicion is required for prompt diagnosis and treatment.

The diagnosis thus can be difficult to establish, particularly in patients with underlying cirrhosis with ascites. Chest radiographs are abnormal in over 70%, but active tuberculous pulmonary disease is evident in less than one-fourth of patients. Skin tests are positive in half. Smears of ascitic fluid for acid-fast bacilli are usually negative, and cultures are positive in only 20%. Other findings are an ascitic fluid total protein > 2.5 g/dL, LDH > 90 units/L, or mononuclear cell-predominant leukocytosis > 500/μL—each has a sensitivity of 70–80% but limited specificity. Although these values have excellent predictive value in patients with isolated tuberculous peritonitis, their accuracy declines in patients with underlying cirrhotic ascites, nephrogenous ascites, malignant ascites (in whom concomitant infection is rare), and pancreatic ascites. Ascitic fluid adenosine deaminase activity, initially believed to be a valuable study, has been shown to have limited predictive value in the presence of cirrhotic ascites.

In patients with suspected tuberculous peritonitis, laparoscopy establishes the diagnosis. In over 90% of patients, characteristic peritoneal nodules are visible, and granulomas are seen on peritoneal biopsy. Ascitic fluid cultures increase in sensitivity to about 85% with high-volume paracenteses. Peritoneal cultures require at least 4–6 weeks and are positive in less than two-thirds of patients.

Treatment of tuberculosis is discussed in Chapter 9.

Hillebrand DJ et al: Ascitic fluid adenosine deaminase insensitivity in detecting tuberculous peritonitis in the United States. Hepatology 1996;24:1408. [NLM Cit ID: 97092751]

Shakil AO et al: Diagnostic features of tuberculous peritonitis in the absence and presence of chronic liver disease: A case control study. Am J Med 1996;100:179. [NLM Cit ID: 96203000]

PERITONEAL CARCINOMATOSIS

Peritoneal involvement by the spread of primary neoplasms is common. The most common tumors are adenocarcinomas originating from tumors of the ovary, uterus, pancreas, stomach, colon, lung, or breast. Patients present with nonspecific abdominal discomfort and weight loss associated with increased abdominal girth owing to the development of malignant ascites. Acute nausea or vomiting may be caused by partial or complete intestinal obstruction. Paracentesis usually demonstrates a low SAAG (< 1.1 mg/dL) and an elevated white count (often both polymorphonuclear neutrophils and mononuclear cells) but with a lymphocyte predominance. Cytology is positive in the majority. Radiologic imaging studies are insensitive, and laparoscopy is required to confirm the diagnosis and to exclude tuberculous peritonitis, with which it may be confused. Malignant ascites does not respond to diuretic agents. Patients may be treated with periodic large-volume paracentesis for symptomatic relief from distention. Intraperitoneal chemotherapy is sometimes used to shrink the tumor. The overall prognosis is extremely poor, with only 10% survival at 6 months. Ovarian cancers represent an exception to this rule. With newer treatments consisting of surgical debulking and intraperitoneal chemotherapy, long-term survival from ovarian cancer is reported.

Parsons SL et al: Malignant ascites. Br J Surg 1996;83:6. [NLM Cit ID: 96264034]

FAMILIAL MEDITERRANEAN FEVER

This is a rare autosomal recessive disorder of unknown pathogenesis that almost exclusively affects people of Mediterranean ancestry, especially Sephardic Jews, Armenians, Turks, and Arabs. Most patients present with symptoms before the age of 20. It is characterized by episodic bouts of acute peritonitis that may be associated with serositis involving the joints and pleura. Peritoneal attacks are marked by the sudden onset of fever, severe abdominal pain, and abdominal tenderness with guarding or rebound tenderness. If left untreated, attacks resolve within 24–48 hours. Because symptoms resemble those of surgical peritonitis, patients may undergo unnecessary exploratory laparotomy. Colchicine, 0.6 mg two or three times daily, has been shown to decrease the frequency and severity of attacks. Interferon (3 million units) given at the start of an attack may also ameliorate symptoms. Secondary amyloidosis with renal or hepatic involvement may occur in 25% of cases. In the absence of amyloidosis, the prognosis is excellent. The gene responsible for familial Mediterranean fever has been identified and cloned, and the diagnosis can be established by genetic testing.

Babior B et al: The familial Mediterranean fever gene—cloned at last. N Engl J Med 1997;337:1548. [NLM Cit ID: 98026775]

Weekly Clinicopathological Exercises (Case 25–1999): A 16-year-old boy with recurrent abdominal pain. N Engl J Med 1999;341:593. [NLM Cit ID: 993632127]

MESOTHELIOMA

Primary malignant mesothelioma is a rare tumor. Over 70% of cases have a history of asbestos exposure. Patients present with abdominal pain or bowel obstruction, increased abdominal girth, and small to moderate ascites. The chest x-ray reveals pulmonary asbestosis in over 50%. The ascitic fluid is characteristically hemorrhagic, with a low serum-ascites albumin gradient. Cytology is often negative. Abdominal CT may reveal sheet-like masses involving the mesentery and omentum. Diagnosis is made at laparotomy or laparoscopy. The prognosis is extremely poor; however, long-term survivors have been described with a combination of radiation therapy and systemic or intraperitoneal chemotherapy.

Auerbach A et al: Peritoneal mesothelioma: Treatment approach based on natural history. Cancer Treat Res 1996;81:193. [NLM Cit ID: 96431504]

MISCELLANEOUS PERITONEAL DISEASES

Chylous ascites is the accumulation of lipid-rich lymph in the peritoneal cavity. The ascitic fluid is characterized by a milky appearance with a triglyceride level > 1000 mg/dL. The usual cause in adults is lymphatic obstruction or leakage caused by malignancy, especially lymphoma. Nonmalignant causes include postoperative trauma, cirrhosis, tuberculosis, pancreatitis, and filariasis.

Pancreatic ascites is the intraperitoneal accumulation of massive amounts of pancreatic secretions due either to disruption of the pancreatic duct or to a pancreatic pseudocyst. It is most commonly seen in patients with chronic pancreatitis and complicates up to 3% of cases of acute pancreatitis. Because the pancreatic enzymes are not activated, pain often is absent. The ascitic fluid is characterized by a high protein level (> 2.5 g/dL) but a low SAAG. Ascitic fluid amylase levels are in excess of 1000 units/L. In nonsurgical cases, initial treatment consists of bowel rest, total parenteral nutrition, and octreotide to decrease pancreatic secretion. Persistent leakage requires treatment with either endoscopic placement of stents into the pancreatic duct or surgical drainage.

Bile ascites is caused most commonly by complications of biliary tract surgery, percutaneous liver biopsy, or abdominal trauma. Unless the bile is infected, bile ascites usually does not cause abdominal pain, fever, or leukocytosis. Paracentesis reveals yellow fluid with a ratio of ascites bilirubin to serum bilirubin greater than 1.0. Treatment is dependent upon the location and rate of bile leakage. Postcholecystectomy cystic duct leaks may be treated with endoscopic sphincterotomy or biliary stent placement to facilitate bile flow across the sphincter of Oddi. Other leaks may be treated with percutaneous drainage by interventional radiologists or with surgical closure.

Kozarek R: Endoscopic therapy of complete and partial pancreatic duct disruptions. Gastroenterol Clin North Am 1998;8:39. [NLM Cit ID: 98070867]

Ryan M et al: Endoscopic intervention for biliary leaks after laparoscopic cholecystectomy: a multicenter review. Gastrointest Endosc 1998;47:261. [NLM Cit ID: 98199948]

DISEASES OF THE ESOPHAGUS

EVALUATION OF ESOPHAGEAL DISORDERS

Symptoms

Heartburn, dysphagia, and odynophagia virtually always indicate a primary esophageal disorder.

A. Heartburn: Heartburn (pyrosis) is the feeling of substernal burning, often radiating to the neck. Caused by the reflux of acidic (or, rarely, alkaline) material into the esophagus, it is highly specific for gastroesophageal reflux disease.

B. Dysphagia: Difficulties in swallowing may arise from problems in transferring the food bolus from the oropharynx to the upper esophagus (oropharyngeal dysphagia) or from impaired transport of the bolus through the body of the esophagus (esophageal dysphagia). The history usually leads to the correct diagnosis.

1. Oropharyngeal dysphagia–The oropharyngeal phase of swallowing is a complex process requiring elevation of the tongue, closure of the nasopharynx, relaxation of the upper esophageal sphincter, closure of the airway, and pharyngeal peristalsis. A brain stem medullary swallowing center integrates cranial nerves V, VII, IX, X, and XII. A variety of mechanical and neuromuscular conditions can disrupt this process (Table 14–9). Oropharyngeal dysphagia is characterized by coughing, choking, and regurgitation that occurs immediately upon initiating swallowing. Liquids are more difficult to swallow than soft foods. There may be associated dysphonia, dysarthria, or other neurologic symptoms.

Table 14–9. Causes of oropharyngeal dysphagia.

Neurologic disorders
Brain stem cerebrovascular accident, mass lesion
Pseudobulbar palsy
Amyotrophic lateral sclerosis, multiple sclerosis, poliomyelitis
Myasthenia gravis
Muscular disorders
Myopathies, polymyositis
Hypothyroidism
Motility disorders
Upper esophageal sphincter dysfunction
Structural defects
Zenker's diverticulum
Malignancy, surgery, radiation to oropharynx

2. Esophageal dysphagia–Esophageal dysphagia may be caused by **mechanical lesions** obstructing the esophagus or by **motility disorders** (Table 14–10). Patients with mechanical obstruction experience dysphagia, primarily for solids. This is recurrent, predictable, and, if the lesion progresses, will worsen as the lumen narrows. Patients with **motility disorders** have dysphagia for both solids and liquids. It is episodic, unpredictable, and nonprogressive.

C. Odynophagia: Odynophagia is sharp substernal pain on swallowing that may limit oral intake. It usually reflects severe erosive disease. It is most commonly associated with infectious esophagitis due to candida, herpesviruses, or cytomegalovirus, especially in immunocompromised patients. It may also be caused by corrosive injury due to caustic ingestions and by pill-induced ulcers.

Diagnostic Studies

A. Upper Endoscopy: Endoscopy is the study of choice for evaluating persistent heartburn, odynophagia, and structural abnormalities detected on barium esophagography. In addition to direct visualization, it allows biopsy of mucosal abnormalities and dilation of strictures.

B. Videoesophagography: Oropharyngeal dysphagia is best evaluated with rapid-sequence videoesophagography.

C. Barium Esophagography: Patients with esophageal dysphagia often are evaluated first with a radiographic barium study to differentiate between mechanical lesions and motility disorders, providing important information about the latter in particular. In patients in whom there is a high suspicion of a mechanical lesion, many clinicians will proceed first to endoscopic evaluation without a barium study. In patients with esophageal dysphagia and a suspected motility disorder, barium esophagoscopy should be obtained first.

D. Esophageal Manometry: Esophageal motility may be assessed using manometric techniques. A

Table 14–10. Causes of esophageal dysphagia.

Cause	Clues
Mechanical obstruction	**Solid foods worse than liquids**
Schatzki's ring	Intermittent dysphagia; not progressive
Peptic stricture	Chronic heartburn; progressive dysphagia
Esophageal cancer	Progressive dysphagia; age over 50
Motility disorder	**Solid and liquid foods**
Achalasia	Progressive dysphagia
Diffuse esophageal spasm	Intermittent; not progressive; may have chest pain
Scleroderma	Chronic heartburn; Raynaud's phenomenon

small pressure-sensing catheter assembly is passed nasally into the esophagus, allowing manometric assessment of the upper and lower esophageal sphincters and the esophageal body. It is indicated (1) to determine the location of the lower esophageal sphincter to allow precise placement of a pH probe; (2) to assess peristaltic function in the esophageal body in patients being considered for antireflux surgery; (3) to establish the diagnosis of achalasia or diffuse esophageal spasm in patients with dysphagia in whom these diagnoses have been first suggested by endoscopy or barium study.

E. Esophageal pH Recording: Esophageal pH may be monitored continuously by means of a small pH probe passed nasally and placed 5 cm above the lower esophageal sphincter. The probe is attached to a portable pH device capable of recording pH for up to 24 hours. The recording provides information about the amount of acid esophageal reflux and on the temporal correlations between symptoms and reflux. Its utility in the management of gastroesophageal reflux and related disorders is discussed below.

American Gastroenterological Association Medical Position Statement. Guidelines on the use of esophageal pH recording. Gastroenterology 1996;110:1981. [NLM Cit ID: 96239709]

American Gastroenterological Association Medical Position Statement on Management of Oropharyngeal Dysphagia. Gastroenterology 1999;116:452. [NLM Cit ID: 99122970]

Cohen S et al: Esophageal manometry in clinical practice: the need for evidence-based assessment of clinical efficacy. Am J Gastroenterol 1998;93:2319. [NLM Cit ID: 99075728]

INFLAMMATORY ESOPHAGEAL CONDITIONS

1. GASTROESOPHAGEAL REFLUX DISEASE

Essentials of Diagnosis

- Heartburn; may be exacerbated by meals, bending, or recumbency.
- Clinical diagnosis; typical uncomplicated cases do not require diagnostic studies.
- Endoscopy demonstrates abnormalities in < 50% of patients.
- Barium esophagography seldom helpful.

General Considerations

"Gastroesophageal reflux disease" affects 20% of adults, who report at least weekly episodes of heartburn, and up to 10% complain of daily symptoms. Though most patients have mild disease, a few develop esophageal mucosal damage (reflux esophagitis) or more severe complications. Several factors may contribute to gastroesophageal reflux disease.

A. Incompetent Lower Esophageal Sphincter: In most patients, reflux occurs during spontaneous, transient relaxations of the lower esophageal sphincter, even though the baseline lower esophageal sphincteric pressures (10–30 mm Hg) are adequate. Patients with more severe involvement (especially those with strictures or Barrett's esophagus) generally have an incompetent lower esophageal sphincter (< 10 mm Hg), resulting in free reflux or stress reflux during abdominal straining, lifting, or bending.

B. Irritant Effects of Refluxate: Esophageal mucosal damage is related to the potency of the refluxate and the amount of time it is in contact with the mucosa. Acidic gastric fluid (pH < 4.0) is extremely caustic to the esophageal mucosa and is the major injurious agent in the majority of cases. In some patients, reflux of bile or alkaline pancreatic secretions may be contributory.

C. Abnormal Esophageal Clearance: Acid refluxate normally is cleared and neutralized by esophageal peristalsis and salivary bicarbonate. During sleep, swallowing-induced peristalsis is infrequent, prolonging acid exposure to the esophagus. One-third of patients with severe gastroesophageal reflux disease also have diminished peristaltic clearance. Certain medical conditions such as scleroderma and its variants are frequently associated with diminished peristalsis. Conditions associated with impaired salivation such as Sjögren's syndrome, anticholinergic medications, and oral radiation therapy may exacerbate gastroesophageal reflux disease.

Hiatal hernias are common and of no significance in asymptomatic people. They are present in over 90% of patients with severe erosive esophagitis, especially when complicated by the development of strictures or Barrett's esophagus. The hernia sac may retard esophageal acid clearance.

D. Delayed Gastric Emptying: Impaired gastric emptying due to gastroparesis or partial gastric outlet obstruction potentiates gastroesophageal reflux disease.

Clinical Findings

A. Symptoms and Signs: The typical symptom of gastroesophageal reflux disease is heartburn. This most often occurs 30–60 minutes after meals and upon reclining. Patients often report relief from taking antacids or baking soda. When this symptom is dominant, the diagnosis is established with a high degree of reliability. Many patients, however, have less specific dyspeptic symptoms with or without heartburn. Overall, a clinical diagnosis of gastroesophageal reflux has a sensitivity of 80% but a specificity of only 70%. Severity is not correlated with the degree of tissue damage. In fact, some patients with severe esophagitis are almost asymptomatic. Patients may complain of regurgitation—the spontaneous reflux of sour or bitter gastric contents into the mouth. Less common symptoms include dysphagia, which may be due to abnormal peristalsis or the development of complications such as stricture or Barrett's metaplasia.

"Atypical" manifestations of gastroesophageal disease are being recognized with increasing frequency. These include asthma, chronic cough, chronic laryngitis, sore throat, and noncardiac chest pain. Gastroesophageal reflux may be either a causative or an exacerbating factor in up to 50% of these patients, especially those with refractory symptoms. Because many of these patients do not have heartburn or regurgitation, the diagnosis often is overlooked.

Physical examination and laboratory data are normal in uncomplicated disease.

B. Special Examinations: Uncomplicated patients with typical symptoms of heartburn and regurgitation may be treated empirically for 4 weeks for gastroesophageal reflux disease without the need for diagnostic studies. Further investigation is required in patients with complicated disease and those unresponsive to empirical therapy.

1. Upper endoscopy–Upper endoscopy with biopsy is the standard procedure for documenting the type and extent of tissue damage in gastroesophageal reflux disease. Approximately 50% of patients with proved acid reflux will have visible mucosal abnormalities such as erythema and friability of the squamocolumnar junction and erosions, known as reflux esophagitis. However, endoscopy is normal in up to half of symptomatic patients and does not exclude mild disease. Esophageal abnormalities are graded on a scale of I (mild) to IV (severe erosions, stricture, or Barrett's esophagus). Initial medical therapy for gastroesophageal reflux disease is guided by the presence of symptoms, not the endoscopic findings. Hence, endoscopy is not warranted for most patients with typical symptoms suggesting uncomplicated reflux disease. Endoscopy should be performed in patients whose symptoms have not responded after initial empirical therapy and patients with alarm symptoms suggesting complicated disease (dysphagia, odynophagia, occult or overt bleeding, or iron deficiency anemia). Endoscopy may be warranted in patients with long-standing symptoms (over 5 years) or patients requiring continuous maintenance therapy to look for Barrett's esophagus.

2. Barium esophagography–This study plays a limited role in the evaluation of gastroesophageal reflux disease in most centers because of its limited ability to identify reflux or mucosal abnormalities. In patients with severe dysphagia, it is sometimes obtained prior to endoscopy to identify a stricture.

3. Ambulatory esophageal pH monitoring–Ambulatory pH monitoring is the best study for documenting acid reflux, but it is unnecessary in most patients with gastroesophageal reflux disease. It is useful and indicated in the following situations: (1) to document abnormal esophageal acid exposure in a patient being considered for antireflux surgery who has a normal endoscopy (ie, no evidence of reflux esophagitis); (2) to evaluate patients with a normal endoscopy who have reflux symptoms unresponsive to therapy with a proton pump inhibitor; (3) to detect either abnormal amounts of reflux or an association between reflux episodes and atypical symptoms such as noncardiac chest pain, asthma, chronic cough, laryngitis, and sore throat. It is recommended, however, that most patients with atypical symptoms first be given an empirical trial of antireflux therapy with a proton pump inhibitor for at least 4 weeks.

4. Esophageal manometry–This study is indicated (1) to determine the location of the lower esophageal sphincter before placement of an esophageal pH probe, and (2) for the preoperative assessment of peristaltic function in patients being considered for antireflux surgery. It is not useful in the diagnosis or management of most patients with gastroesophageal reflux disease.

Differential Diagnosis

Symptoms of gastroesophageal reflux disease may be similar to those of other diseases such as esophageal motility disorders, peptic ulcer, cholelithiasis, nonulcer dyspepsia, and angina pectoris. Reflux erosive esophagitis may be confused with pill-induced damage, radiation esophagitis, or infections (CMV, herpes, candida).

Complications

A. Barrett's Esophagus: This is a condition in which the squamous epithelium of the esophagus is replaced by metaplastic columnar epithelium containing goblet and columnar cells (specialized intestinal metaplasia). Present in up to 10% of patients with chronic reflux, it is believed to arise from chronic reflux-induced injury to the esophageal squamous epithelium. Barrett's esophagus is suspected at endoscopy from the presence of orange, gastric type epithelium that extends upward from the stomach into the distal tubular esophagus in a tongue-like or circumferential fashion. Biopsies should be obtained at endoscopy to confirm the diagnosis. Three types of columnar epithelium may be identified: gastric cardiac, gastric fundic, and specialized intestinal metaplasia. Only the latter is believed to carry an increased risk of neoplasia and thus to be of clinical significance.

Barrett's esophagus does not provoke specific symptoms. Rather, symptoms are a consequence of gastroesophageal reflux disease. Most patients have a long history of reflux symptoms, such as heartburn and regurgitation. Dysphagia due to impaired motility is common. Paradoxically, one-third of patients report minimal or no symptoms of gastroesophageal reflux disease, suggesting decreased acid sensitivity of Barrett's epithelium. Indeed, over 90% of individuals with Barrett's esophagus in the general population do not seek medical attention and go unrecognized. Barrett's esophagus may be complicated by stricture formation or deep ulcerations, which can bleed.

Barrett's esophagus is indicative of severe gastroesophageal reflux disease and should be treated aggressively with long-term proton pump inhibitors. Surgical fundoplication may be desirable in some situations. Medical or surgical therapy may prevent progression of Barrett's esophagus, but there is no convincing evidence that regression occurs. Recently, endoscopic ablation of Barrett's epithelium with cautery probes or photodynamic therapy (using photosensitizers and laser energy) has resulted in partial or complete regression of columnar epithelium. Further studies are needed before such treatment can be recommended.

The most serious complication of Barrett's esophagus is esophageal adenocarcinoma, which has an estimated annual incidence of 0.8%, representing a 40-fold risk compared with patients without Barrett's esophagus. Virtually all adenocarcinomas of the esophagus and many such tumors of the gastric cardia arise from Barrett's metaplasia. Current guidelines suggest that patients with Barrett's esophagus who are reasonably good operative candidates undergo endoscopic surveillance with mucosal biopsies every 2–3 years. Patients with low-grade dysplasia should be treated with aggressive medical management and endoscopic surveillance every 6–12 months. The management of high-grade dysplasia is controversial. Because 30–40% may progress to (or already contain) invasive adenocarcinoma, surgery is usually recommended for good operative candidates. Photodynamic ablation may be considered for other patients.

It is now believed that Barrett's epithelium of any length carries an increased risk of neoplasia. Furthermore, specialized intestinal metaplasia is present at the gastroesophageal junction in up to 20% of patients undergoing endoscopy in the absence of visible Barrett's esophagus. In view of a rising incidence of adenocarcinoma of the distal esophagus and proximal stomach, the significance of specialized intestinal metaplasia of the gastroesophageal junction requires further study.

B. Peptic Stricture: Stricture formation occurs in about 10% of patients with esophagitis. It is manifested by the gradual development of solid food dysphagia, which progresses over months to years. Often there is a reduction in heartburn because the stricture acts as a barrier to reflux. Most strictures are located at the gastroesophageal junction. Strictures located above this level usually occur in the presence of Barrett's metaplasia. Endoscopy with biopsy is mandatory in all cases to differentiate peptic stricture from other benign or malignant causes of esophageal stricture (Schatzki's ring, esophageal carcinoma). Active erosive esophagitis is often present. Up to 90% of symptomatic patients are effectively treated with dilation. Dilation is continued over one to several sessions. A luminal diameter of 16–17 mm is usually sufficient to relieve dysphagia. Chronic therapy with a proton pump inhibitor (omeprazole or lansoprazole) is required to decrease the likelihood of stricture recurrence. Some patients require intermittent stricture dilation to maintain luminal patency. With the advent of proton pump inhibitors, operative management for strictures that do not respond to dilation is seldom required.

Treatment

A. Medical Treatment: The goal of treatment is to provide symptomatic relief, to heal esophagitis (if present), and to prevent complications. In the majority of patients with uncomplicated disease, empirical treatment is initiated based upon a compatible history without the need for further confirmatory studies. Patients not responding as predicted to empirical therapy and those with suspected complications should undergo further evaluation with upper endoscopy or esophageal pH recording.

Patients with known erosive esophagitis, complications (such as a peptic stricture or Barrett's esophagus), or suspected atypical manifestations (such as asthma or laryngitis) should be treated initially with a proton pump inhibitor (see below). In most other patients, treatment may proceed in the following stepwise fashion.

1. Mild, intermittent symptoms–Gastroesophageal reflux is a lifelong disease that requires lifestyle modifications as well as medical intervention. The single most important admonition is to avoid lying down within 3 hours after meals (the period of greatest reflux). Elevating the head of the bed on 6-inch blocks or a foam wedge to reduce reflux and enhance esophageal clearance is recommended, especially for patients with nocturnal and atypical symptoms. Patients should be advised to avoid acidic foods (tomato products, citrus fruits, spicy foods, coffee) and agents that relax the lower esophageal sphincter or delay gastric emptying (fatty foods, peppermint, chocolate, alcohol, and smoking). Weight loss, avoidance of bending after meals, and reduction of meal size may also be helpful.

Antacids are the mainstay for rapid relief of occasional heartburn; however, their duration of action is less than 2 hours. Commonly used formulations are Maalox TC or Mylanta II, either as a liquid (10–15 mL) or tablets (two to four). Gaviscon (two to four tablets) is an alginate-antacid combination that decreases reflux in the upright position and may be superior to other antacids.

All H_2 receptor antagonists are available in over-the-counter formulations: cimetidine 200 mg, ranitidine and nizatidine 75 mg, famotidine 10 mg—all of which are half of the typical prescription strength.

When taken for active heartburn, these agents have a delay in onset of at least 30 minutes, which means that antacids provide more immediate relief. However, once these agents take effect, they provide heartburn relief for up to 8 hours. When taken before meals known to provoke symptoms, these agents reduce the incidence of meal-induced heartburn.

2. Moderate symptoms–Uncomplicated patients with typical reflux symptoms that occur frequently (several times per week or daily) should be treated empirically with an H_2 receptor antagonist. Standard "prescription" doses of these agents are ranitidine or nizatidine 150 mg, famotidine 20 mg, or cimetidine 400–800 mg, twice daily. These agents reduce 24-hour acidity by over 60%. Ranitidine and cimetidine are available in less expensive generic formulations. Treatment twice daily affords improvement in up to two-thirds of patients. Given their superior efficacy and once-daily dosing, proton pump inhibitors increasingly are prescribed as first-line therapy for mild to moderate symptoms in preference to beginning with an H_2 receptor antagonist. However, generic H_2 receptor antagonists are significantly less expensive than proton pump inhibitors and provide effective symptomatic relief in most patients with mild to moderate reflux symptoms. Unless it is demonstrated to be a cost-effective approach, the use of proton pump inhibitors as first-line therapy for uncomplicated disease is not recommended.

For patients whose symptoms persist despite 6 weeks of standard doses of H_2 receptor antagonist therapy, continued therapy or an increase in dosage of H_2 receptor antagonists is seldom effective in providing symptom relief. Therefore, these patients should be treated with a proton pump inhibitor (omeprazole 20 mg, lansoprazole 30 mg, rabeprazole 20 mg, or pantoprazole 40 mg) once daily (see below). Although some authorities recommend that upper endoscopy be performed first to document the presence or absence of reflux esophagitis, the decision to prescribe proton pump inhibitors is based upon the presence of persistent symptoms, not the endoscopic findings.

In those who achieve good symptom relief with either an H_2 receptor antagonist or a proton pump inhibitor, therapy should be discontinued after 8–12 weeks. Patients whose symptoms relapse may be treated with either continuous or intermittent courses of therapy depending upon symptom frequency and patient preference. In general, the dosage should be reduced to the lowest level that maintains effective symptom control. Most patients are controlled adequately with intermittent courses of therapy rather than continuous maintenance treatment.

Promotility agents (metoclopramide, cisapride) reduce reflux by increasing lower esophageal sphincter tone and enhancing esophageal acid clearance and gastric emptying and appear to be comparable in efficacy to H_2 receptor antagonists for the treatment of mild to moderate reflux symptoms. However, side effects preclude the use of these agents for uncomplicated reflux disease. Cisapride (10 mg four times daily) may cause or exacerbate QT prolongation, leading rarely to serious cardiac arrhythmias. Hence, the use of this agent has recently been restricted by the FDA. It is metabolized by P450 3A4 and should not be taken with inhibitors of this enzyme (including many macrolide antibiotics, antifungal agents, and some protease inhibitors). Metoclopramide is a dopamine antagonist that may cause neuropsychiatric side effects in up to one-third of patients, limiting it to short-term use only.

3. Severe symptoms and erosive disease– For patients with severe symptoms and for patients who undergo endoscopy and have documented erosive esophagitis, the optimal initial therapy is a proton pump inhibitor (omeprazole 20 mg, lansoprazole 30 mg, rabeprazole 20 mg, pantoprazole 40 mg) once daily. Proton pump inhibitors given once daily provide symptom relief and healing of esophagitis in over 80% and given twice daily provide relief in over 95% of patients—compared with under 50% with standard doses of H_2 receptor antagonists—and are therefore the drugs of choice for severe or erosive disease. There appears to be little difference between these agents in efficacy or side effect profiles. Approximately 10–20% of patients fail to achieve symptom relief with a once-daily dose within 2–4 weeks and require a higher dosage (twice-daily) proton pump inhibitor. Therefore, some authorities recommend initiating therapy with a twice-daily dose of proton pump inhibitor, reducing therapy after 2–4 weeks to a once-daily dose. The initial course of therapy is usually 8–12 weeks. As tissue healing correlates well with symptom resolution, repeat endoscopy is warranted in patients only if they fail to respond to once-daily or twice-daily proton pump inhibitor therapy.

After discontinuation of proton pump inhibitor therapy, relapse of symptoms occurs in 80% of patients within 1 year—the majority of relapses occurring within the first 3 months. Therefore, chronic therapy to maintain symptom remission is required in most but not all patients. Patients with severe erosive esophagitis, Barrett's esophagus, or peptic stricture should be maintained on chronic therapy with a proton pump inhibitor at a dose sufficient to provide complete symptom relief. In other patients, a trial off proton pump inhibitors should be considered. Patients with prolonged symptomatic remissions (over 3 months) may be treated effectively with intermittent 4- to 8-week courses of acute proton pump inhibitor therapy. Patients with prompt recurrence of symptoms (within 3 months) require chronic maintenance therapy with either a proton pump inhibitor or an H_2 receptor antagonist. The therapy should be "stepped down" to the lowest dose that is effective in controlling reflux symptoms.

The maintenance doses of proton pump inhibitors may escalate over time, with over 20% of patients eventually requiring double or triple doses of proton pump inhibitors to control symptoms.

4. Extraesophageal reflux manifestations– Establishing a causal relationship between gastroesophageal reflux and extraesophageal symptoms (eg, asthma, hoarseness, cough) can be difficult as there is no standard diagnostic test. Although ambulatory esophageal pH testing can document the presence of increased acid esophageal reflux, it does not prove a causative connection. Most authorities recommend an empirical trial of a double-dose proton pump inhibitor (eg, omeprazole 40 mg) twice daily for 2–3 months to determine whether these symptoms improve after acid suppression.

5. Unresponsive disease– Approximately 10–20% of patients with gastroesophageal reflux symptoms do not respond to once-daily doses of proton pump inhibitors, and 5% do not respond to twice-daily doses. Patients with unresponsive symptoms should undergo endoscopy prior to escalation of therapy. Patients without endoscopically visible esophagitis should undergo esophageal pH monitoring to determine the amount of esophageal acid reflux and decide whether the refractory symptoms are truly acid-related. The presence of active erosive esophagitis usually is indicative of inadequate acid suppression and can almost always be treated successfully with higher proton pump inhibitor doses (eg, omeprazole 40 mg twice daily). Breakthrough acid production appears to occur at night in patients with severe disease. A twice-daily proton pump inhibitor (before breakfast and dinner) and a bedtime dose of an H_2 receptor antagonist may be more effective (and less expensive) in controlling nocturnal acid than a proton pump inhibitor given three times daily. Truly refractory esophagitis may be caused by gastrinoma with gastric acid hypersecretion (Zollinger Ellison syndrome), pill-induced esophagitis, resistance to proton pump inhibitors, and medical noncompliance.

C. Surgical Treatment: Surgical fundoplication affords good to excellent relief of symptoms and healing of esophagitis in over 85% of properly selected patients and may now be performed laparoscopically with low complication rates in most instances. Cost-effectiveness studies suggest that aggregate medical costs exceed surgical costs after 10 years. The longevity of the beneficial effects of fundoplication are debated. Reports from different surgical centers report 10-year success rates ranging from 60% to 90%. After fundoplication, over 30% of patients develop new symptoms of dysphagia, bloating, increased flatulence, or dyspepsia which can be difficult to manage. Surgical treatment should be considered for otherwise healthy patients (1) under age 50 with severe reflux who require chronic proton pump inhibitors; (2) with extraesophageal manifestations of reflux, as these symptoms often require high doses of proton pump inhibitors and may be more effectively controlled with antireflux surgery; and (3) with severe reflux disease who are unwilling to accept lifelong medical therapy due to its expense, inconvenience, or theoretical risks.

Bardhan K et al: Symptomatic gastroesophageal reflux disease: double blind controlled study of intermittent treatment with omeprazole or ranitidine. BMJ 1999;318:502. [NLM Cit ID: 99147883]

Chiba N et al: Speed of healing and symptom relief in grade II to IV gastroesophageal reflux disease: a meta-analysis. Gastroenterology 1997;112:1798. [NLM Cit ID: 97322015]

Gerson L et al: A cost-effectiveness analysis of prescribing strategies in the management of gastroesophageal reflux disease. Am J Gastroenterol 2000;95:395. [NLM Cit ID: 20148177] (This decision analysis suggests that initial therapy of moderate to severe reflux symptoms with a proton pump inhibitor for 8 weeks followed by intermittent 8 week courses of therapy "on demand" for symptom recurrence is most cost-effective treatment strategy.)

Gibson P et al: The effect of treatment for gastro-oesophageal reflux on asthma in adults and children. In: The Cochrane Library (Version 10 Feb 1999). Oxford: Update Software. (Meta-analysis of 256 studies finds no convincing evidence that medical treatment of GERD improves asthma outcomes.)

Irwin RS et al: Accurately diagnosing and treating chronic cough due to gastroesophageal reflux disease can be difficult. Am J Gastroenterol 1999;94:3095. [NLM Cit ID: 20030972] (Excellent review of relationship between cough and GERD; a failed response, however, does not exclude reflux of acid or non-acidic contents as potentiating mechanism of cough.)

Kahrilas P et al: High- versus standard-dose ranitidine for control of heartburn in poorly responsive acid reflux disease: a prospective controlled trial. Am J Gastroenterology 1999;94:92. [NLM Cit ID: 99131436] (Response rates were identical: 45% had mild symptoms or less.)

Lagergren J et al: Symptomatic gastroesophageal reflux as a risk factor for esophageal adenocarcinoma. N Engl J Med 1999;340:825. [NLM Cit ID: 99165315] (Endoscopy may be warranted in patients with chronic or severe heartburn to screen for Barrett's esophagus.)

Lightdale C: Ablation therapy for Barrett's esophagus: is it time to choose our weapons? Gastrointest Endosc 1999;49:122. [NLM Cit ID: 99088014]

Nandurkar S et al: Barrett's esophagus: the long and the short of it. Am J Gastroenterol 1999;94:30. [NLM Cit ID: 99131427]

Ormseth EJ et al: Reflux laryngitis: pathophysiology, diagnosis and management. Am J Gastroenterol 1999; 94:2812. [NLM Cit ID: 99449136]

INFECTIOUS ESOPHAGITIS

Essentials of Diagnosis

- Immunosuppressed patient.
- Odynophagia, dysphagia, and chest pain.
- Endoscopy with biopsy establishes diagnosis.

General Considerations

Infectious esophagitis occurs most commonly in immunosuppressed patients. Patients with AIDS, solid organ transplants, leukemia, lymphoma, and those receiving immunosuppressive drugs are at particular risk for opportunistic infections. *Candida albicans,* herpes simplex, and cytomegalovirus are the most common pathogens. Candida infection may occur also in patients who have uncontrolled diabetes and those being treated with systemic corticosteroids, radiation therapy, or systemic antibiotic therapy. Herpes simplex can affect normal hosts, in which case the infection is generally self-limited.

Clinical Findings

A. Symptoms and Signs: The most common symptoms are odynophagia and dysphagia. Substernal chest pain occurs in some patients. Patients with candidal esophagitis are sometimes asymptomatic. Oral thrush is present in only 75% of patients with candidal esophagitis and 25–50% of patients with viral esophagitis and is therefore an unreliable indicator of the cause of esophageal infection. Patients with esophageal CMV infection may have infection at other sites such as the colon and retina. Oral ulcers (herpes labialis) are often associated with herpes simplex esophagitis.

B. Special Examinations: Treatment may be empirical. For diagnostic certainty, endoscopy with biopsy and brushings (for microbiologic and histopathologic analysis) is preferred because of its high diagnostic accuracy. The endoscopic signs of candidal esophagitis are diffuse, linear, yellow-white plaques adherent to the mucosa. Cytomegalovirus esophagitis is characterized by one to several large, shallow, superficial ulcerations. Herpes esophagitis results in multiple small, deep ulcerations.

Treatment

A. Candidal Esophagitis: Treatment depends on the immune status of the patient and the severity of the illness. Topical therapy is used initially in patients with a normal immune system. Options include topical agents (nystatin, 500,000 units "swish and swallow" five times daily; clotrimazole troches, 10 mg dissolved in mouth five times daily) for 7–14 days. Initial therapy for immunocompromised patients (including AIDS) generally is with fluconazole, 100–200 mg/d orally. Ketoconazole should no longer be used because of its lower efficacy, unpredictable absorption, and greater risk of adverse effects. Patients not responding to oral therapy are treated with low-dose amphotericin B, 0.3–0.5 mg/kg/d. The duration of therapy is not standardized.

B. Cytomegalovirus Esophagitis: Initial therapy is with ganciclovir, 5 mg/kg intravenously every 12 hours for 3–6 weeks. Neutropenia is a frequent dose-limiting side effect. If resolution of symptoms occurs, the drug may be discontinued. If the condition has improved but not resolved, full-dose therapy may be continued for an additional 2–3 weeks. In some cases (especially in patients with AIDS), continuous ganciclovir, 5 mg/kg intravenously daily, is required for suppressive therapy. The role of oral ganciclovir in the maintenance treatment of CMV gastrointestinal disease is not established. Patients who either do not respond to or cannot tolerate ganciclovir are treated acutely with foscarnet, 90 mg/kg intravenously every 12 hours for 3–6 weeks. The principal toxicity is renal failure.

C. Herpetic Esophagitis: Immune-competent patients may be treated symptomatically and generally do not require specific antiviral therapy. Immunosuppressed patients may be treated with oral acyclovir, 200 mg orally five times daily, or 250 mg/m^2 intravenously every 8–12 hours, usually for 7–10 days. Famciclovir, 250 mg three times daily, and valacyclovir, 1 g twice daily, are effective but significantly more expensive than generic acyclovir. Nonresponders require therapy with foscarnet, 40 mg/kg intravenously every 8 hours for 21 days.

Prognosis

Most patients with infectious esophagitis can be effectively treated with complete symptom resolution. Depending on the patient's underlying immunodeficiency, relapse of symptoms off therapy can raise difficulties. Chronic suppressive therapy is sometimes required.

Darouiche RO: Oropharyngeal and esophageal candidiasis in immunocompromised patients: treatment issues. Clin Infect Dis 1998;26:259. [NLM Cit ID: 98161543]

Whitley RJ et al: Guidelines for the treatment of cytomegalovirus diseases in patients with AIDS in the era of potent retroviral therapy; recommendations of an international panel. Arch Intern Med 1998;158:957. [NLM Cit ID: 98247843]

Wilcox CM: Esophageal strictures complicating ulcerative esophagitis in patients with AIDS. Am J Gastroenterol 1999;94:339. [NLM Cit ID: 99145224]

PILL-INDUCED ESOPHAGITIS

A number of different medications may injure the esophagus, presumably through direct, prolonged mucosal contact. The most commonly implicated are the NSAIDs, potassium chloride pills, quinidine, zalcitabine, zidovudine, alendronate, iron, vitamin C, and antibiotics (doxycycline, tetracycline, clindamycin, trimethoprim-sulfamethoxazole). Because injury is most likely to occur if pills are swallowed without water or while supine, hospitalized or bed-bound patients are at greater risk. Symptoms include severe retrosternal chest pain, odynophagia, and dysphagia, often beginning several hours after taking a pill. These may occur suddenly and persist for days. Some patients (especially the elderly) have relatively little pain, presenting with dysphagia. Endoscopy may reveal one to several discrete ulcers that may be shallow or deep. Chronic injury may result in severe esophagitis with stricture, hemorrhage, or perforation. Healing occurs rapidly when the offending agent is eliminated. To prevent pill-induced damage, patients should take pills with 4 oz of water and remain upright for 30 minutes after ingestion. Known offenders should not be given to patients with esophageal dysmotility, dysphagia, or strictures.

Boyce HW: Drug-induced esophageal damage: diseases of medical progress. Gastrointest Endosc 1998;47:547. [NLM Cit ID: 99145224]

CAUSTIC ESOPHAGEAL INJURY

Caustic esophageal injury occurs from accidental (usually children) or deliberate (suicidal) ingestion of liquid or crystalline alkali (drain cleaners, etc) or acid. Ingestion is followed almost immediately by severe burning and varying degrees of chest pain, gagging, dysphagia, and drooling. Aspiration results in stridor and wheezing. Patients require urgent emergency room attention. Initial examination should be directed to circulatory status and to prompt assessment of airway patency, including laryngoscopy. Subsequently, there should be a careful examination of the oral cavity, chest, and abdomen. Chest and abdominal radiographs are obtained looking for pneumonitis or free perforation. Initial treatment is supportive, with intravenous fluids and analgesics. Nasogastric lavage and oral antidotes may be dangerous and should generally not be administered. Most patients may be managed medically. Endoscopy is usually performed within the first 24 hours to assess the extent of injury. Many patients are discovered to have no mucosal injury to the esophagus or stomach, allowing prompt discharge and psychiatric referral. Abnormal endoscopic appearance does not accurately predict the likelihood of transmural injury and perforation. All patients with mucosal damage must therefore be observed carefully in the first 72 hours for signs of deterioration. Circumferential injury to the esophagus portends an increased risk of stricture formation. Previously, antibiotics and corticosteroids were used acutely in an effort to decrease the incidence of stricture formation, but these have not been found to be effective. Surgery is indicated for sepsis, shock, perforation, or progressive deterioration.

Battle WM, Codella M: Caustic injury to the upper gastrointestinal tract. In: *Consultations in Gastroenterology.* Snape WM (editor). Saunders, 1996.

BENIGN ESOPHAGEAL LESIONS

1. MALLORY-WEISS SYNDROME (Mucosal Laceration of Gastroesophageal Junction)

Essentials of Diagnosis

- Hematemesis; usually self-limited.
- Prior history of vomiting, retching in 50%.
- Endoscopy establishes diagnosis.

General Considerations

Mallory-Weiss syndrome is characterized by a nonpenetrating mucosal tear at the gastroesophageal junction which is hypothesized to arise from events that suddenly raise transabdominal pressure, such as lifting, retching, or vomiting. Alcoholism is a strong predisposing factor. Mallory-Weiss tears are responsible for approximately 5% of cases of upper gastrointestinal bleeding.

Clinical Findings

A. Symptoms and Signs: Patients usually present with hematemesis with or without melena. A history of retching, vomiting, or straining is obtained in about 50% of cases.

B. Special Examinations: As with other causes of upper gastrointestinal hemorrhage, upper endoscopy should be performed after the patient has been appropriately resuscitated. The diagnosis is established by identification of a 0.5–4 cm linear mucosal tear usually located either at the gastroesophageal junction or, more commonly, just below the junction in the gastric mucosa.

Differential Diagnosis

At endoscopy, other potential causes of upper gastrointestinal hemorrhage are found in over 35% of patients with Mallory-Weiss tears, including peptic ulcer disease, erosive gastritis, arteriovenous malformations, and esophageal varices. Patients with underlying portal hypertension are at higher risk of continued or recurrent bleeding.

Treatment

Patients are initially treated as needed with fluid resuscitation and blood transfusions. Most patients stop bleeding spontaneously and require no therapy. Endoscopic hemostatic therapy is employed in patients who have continuing active bleeding. Injection with epinephrine (1:10,000) or cautery with a bipolar or heater probe coagulation device is effective in 90–95% of cases. Angiographic arterial embolization or operative intervention is required in patients who fail endoscopic therapy.

Bharucha AE et al: Clinical and endoscopic risk factors in the Mallory-Weiss syndrome. Am J Gastroenterol 1997;92:805. [NLM Cit ID: 97293136]

2. LOWER ESOPHAGEAL RING (Schatzki's Ring)

Schatzki's ring is a circumferential, thin, symmetric mucosal ring (< 4 mm in thickness) that occurs in the distal esophagus at the squamocolumnar junction. It is always associated with a hiatal hernia, but the cause is uncertain. Most are over 20 mm in diameter and are asymptomatic. Solid food dysphagia most often occurs with rings less than 13 mm in diameter. Characteristically, the dysphagia is intermittent and not progressive. Large, poorly chewed food boluses such as steak are most likely to cause dysphagia. Obstructing food boluses may pass by drinking extra liquids or are relieved by regurgitation. In some cases, an impacted bolus must be extracted endoscopically. Absence of gastroesophageal reflux symptoms and the nonprogressive nature of the dysphagia helps to distinguish Schatzki's ring from reflux-induced peptic strictures. Lower esophageal rings may be diagnosed by biopsy but are best visualized using a barium esophagogram with a solid radiopaque bolus (marshmallow or pill).

The majority of symptomatic patients can be effectively and permanently treated with the passage of large (17–20 mm) bougie dilators, which disrupt the mucosal ring. A single dilation session usually suffices, but repeat dilations are sometimes necessary.

AGA technical review on treatment of patients with dysphagia caused by benign disorders of the distal esophagus. Gastroenterology 1999;117:233. [NLM Cit ID: 99315574]

3. ESOPHAGEAL WEBS

Webs are thin, diaphragm-like membranes of squamous mucosa that typically occur in the mid or upper esophagus and may be multiple. They may be asymptomatic or cause intermittent solid food dysphagia. Though they may be congenital, they may also occur with graft-versus-host disease, pemphigoid, and epidermolysis bullosa, and, rarely, in association with iron deficiency anemia (Plummer-Vinson syndrome). The diagnosis is established by barium esophagography or upper endoscopy. Symptomatic webs are effectively treated with bougienage but may recur.

Longstreth GF et al: Multiple esophageal webs: Treatment and follow-up of seven patients. J. Clin Gastroenterol 1997;24:199. [NLM Cit ID: 97396676]

4. ESOPHAGEAL DIVERTICULA

Zenker's Diverticulum

Zenker's diverticulum is a protrusion of pharyngeal mucosa that develops at the pharyngoesophageal junction between the inferior pharyngeal constrictor and the cricopharyngeus. The cause is believed to be loss of elasticity of the upper esophageal sphincter, resulting in restricted opening during swallowing. Symptoms of dysphagia and regurgitation tend to develop insidiously over years in middle-aged to elderly patients. Initial symptoms include vague oropharyngeal dysphagia with coughing or throat discomfort. As the diverticulum enlarges and retains food, patients may note halitosis, spontaneous regurgitation of undigested food, nocturnal choking, gurgling in the throat, or a protrusion in the neck. Complications include aspiration pneumonia, bronchiectasis, and lung abscess. The diagnosis is best established by a barium esophagogram.

Symptomatic patients require upper esophageal myotomy and, in most cases, surgical diverticulectomy. Significant improvement occurs in over 90% of patients treated surgically. Small asymptomatic diverticula may be observed.

Bremner CG et al: Endoscopic treatment of Zenker's diverticulum. Gastrointest Endosc 1999;49:126. [NLM Cit ID: 99088015]

Esophageal Diverticula

Diverticula may occur in the mid or distal esophagus. These may arise secondary to motility disorders (diffuse esophageal spasm, achalasia) or may develop above esophageal strictures. Diverticula are seldom symptomatic, and treatment is directed at the underlying disorder.

Ferraro P et al: Esophageal diverticula. Chest Surg Clin North Am 1994;4:741. [NLM Cit ID: 95162626]

5. BENIGN ESOPHAGEAL NEOPLASMS

Benign tumors of the esophagus are quite rare. They are submucosal, the most common being leiomyoma. Most are asymptomatic and picked up incidentally on endoscopy or barium esophagography. Larger lesions can cause dysphagia. The major clinical importance of these lesions is to distinguish them from malignant neoplasms. At endoscopy, a smooth, sessile nodule is observed with normal overlying mucosa. Because the lesion is submucosal, endoscopic biopsies are generally nonrevealing. Endoscopic ultrasonography is extremely helpful to confirm the submucosal origin of the tumor.

6. ESOPHAGEAL VARICES

Essentials of Diagnosis

- Develop secondary to portal hypertension.
- Found in 50% of patients with cirrhosis.
- One-third of patients with varices develop upper gastrointestinal bleeding.
- Diagnosis established by upper endoscopy.

General Considerations

Esophageal varices are dilated submucosal veins that develop in patients with underlying portal hypertension and may result in serious upper gastrointestinal bleeding. The causes of portal hypertension are discussed elsewhere (Chapter 15). Under normal circumstances, there is a 2–6 mm Hg pressure gradient between the portal vein and the inferior vena cava. When the gradient exceeds 10 mm Hg, significant portal hypertension exists. Esophageal varices are the most common cause of important gastrointestinal bleeding due to portal hypertension, though gastric varices and, rarely, intestinal varices may also bleed. Bleeding from esophageal varices most commonly occurs in the distal 5 cm of the esophagus.

The most common cause of portal hypertension is cirrhosis. While approximately 50% of patients with cirrhosis have esophageal varices, only one-third of patients with varices develop serious bleeding from the varices. Bleeding esophageal varices have a higher morbidity and mortality rate than any other source of upper gastrointestinal bleeding. The mortality rate associated with acute bleeding episodes ranges from 15% to 40%, and over 60% of patients are dead within 5 years.

A number of factors have been identified that may portend an increased risk of bleeding from esophageal varices. The most important are (1) the size of the varices; (2) the presence at endoscopy of red wale markings on the varix (longitudinal markings that resemble whip marks); (3) the severity of liver disease (as assessed by Child scoring); and (4) active alcohol abuse—alcoholic cirrhotics who continue to drink have an extremely high risk of bleeding. The risk of bleeding correlates poorly with the absolute portosystemic pressure gradient, though bleeding almost never occurs with a gradient under 12 mm Hg.

Clinical Findings

A. Symptoms and Signs: Patients with bleeding esophageal varices present with symptoms and signs of acute gastrointestinal hemorrhage. (See Acute Upper Gastrointestinal Bleeding, above.) Most commonly, patients present with spontaneous emesis of either bright red blood or "coffee grounds" material that is typically accompanied by melena or hematochezia. Rarely, varices present with hematochezia or melena alone in the absence of hematemesis. In some cases, there may be preceding retching or dyspepsia attributable to alcoholic gastritis or withdrawal. Varices per se do not cause symptoms of dyspepsia, dysphagia, or retching. Variceal bleeding usually is severe, resulting in hypovolemia manifested by postural vital signs or shock. Twenty to 30 percent of patients with chronic liver disease who develop bleeding—despite findings such as spider angiomas, asterixis, and ascites—do so from some other source.

B. Laboratory Findings: A complete blood count, platelet count, prothrombin time, and partial thromboplastin time, liver function tests, serum electrolytes, and serum albumin should be obtained in all patients. The initial hematocrit is a poor indicator of the severity of acute blood loss. Patients with underlying chronic liver disease often have an abnormal bilirubin, AST, ALT, a prolonged prothrombin time, and a low serum albumin.

Initial Management

A. Acute Resuscitation: The initial management of patients with acute upper gastrointestinal bleeding is discussed in the section on acute upper gastrointestinal bleeding (see above). Variceal hemorrhage is life-threatening; rapid assessment and resuscitation with fluids or blood products are essential. Many patients with bleeding esophageal varices have coagulopathy due to underlying cirrhosis; fresh frozen plasma or platelets should be administered to patients with a prothrombin time greater than 1.5 times the normal range of control times, or platelet counts less than 50,000/μL in the presence of active bleeding. The INR should not be used in this setting as it is not a reliable marker of bleeding risk in patients with liver disease. Patients with advanced liver disease are at high risk of poor outcome regardless of the bleeding source and should be transferred to an ICU where constant monitoring can be provided. A nasogastric tube should be placed to evacuate the stomach (reducing nausea and vomiting) and to monitor for ongoing bleeding. Sixty to 80 percent of variceal bleeders will stop spontaneously; however, without therapy, over half of these will rebleed within 1 week.

B. Emergent Endoscopy: Emergent endoscopy should be performed after the patient's hemodynamic status has been appropriately stabilized (usually within 2–12 hours). In patients with active bleeding, endotracheal intubation is commonly performed to protect against aspiration during endoscopy. A vigorous gastric lavage through a large-bore tube is performed prior to endoscopy to facilitate visualization. An endoscopic examination is then performed to exclude other causes of upper gastrointestinal bleeding such as a Mallory-Weiss tear, peptic ulcer disease, and portal hypertensive gastropathy. In most patients, variceal bleeding has stopped spontaneously by the time of endoscopy, and the diagnosis of variceal bleeding is made presumptively. Acute endoscopic treatment of the varices is performed with either banding or sclerotherapy. These techniques can arrest active bleeding in 90% of patients. These techniques can reduce by half (from 70%) the chance of early recurrent bleeding, but their impact upon in-hospital mortality is less clear.

To perform banding (variceal ligation), a plastic hood encircled by small rubber bands is placed on the tip of the endoscope. The varix is drawn into the hood by suction, and a rubber band is released by a trip wire around the varix. Several bands may be applied near the gastroesophageal junction and up to 5 cm proximally. Repeat banding sessions are repeated at intervals of 1–2 weeks until the varices are obliterated or reduced to a small size. Banding achieves lower rates of rebleeding, complications, and death than sclerotherapy and should be considered the endoscopic treatment of choice for esophageal variceal bleeding.

Sclerotherapy is performed by advancing through the endoscope a disposable catheter with a retractable 25-gauge needle and injecting the variceal trunks with a sclerosing agent (eg, ethanolamine, tetradecyl sulfate). A repeat session is given at 3–7 days, followed by sessions at 1- to 3-week intervals, until the varices are obliterated. Complications occur in 20–30% and include chest pain, fever, bacteremia, esophageal ulceration, stricture, and perforation. However, sclerotherapy is still preferred by some endoscopists in the actively bleeding patient (in whom visualization for banding may be difficult) and by those with insufficient experience in banding.

C. Pharmacologic Therapy:

1. Antibiotic prophylaxis–Prophylactic antibiotics in cirrhotic patients with gastrointestinal hemorrhage reduce the incidence of infectious complications such as spontaneous bacterial peritonitis, bacteremia, pneumonia, and urinary tract infections. Administration of a quinolone (norfloxacin orally; ofloxacin or ciprofloxacin either intravenously or orally) for 3–10 days with a broad-spectrum antibiotic administered intravenously before endoscopy (amoxicillin-clavulanate or a third-generation cephalosporin) reduces the incidence of infections in this population from over 50% to less than 15%.

2. Octreotide–Somatostatin (not clinically available) and its long-acting synthetic analog octreotide (50 μg intravenous bolus followed by 50 μg/h) reduce splanchnic and hepatic blood flow and portal pressures in cirrhotic patients. These agents provide acute control of variceal bleeding in up to 80% of patients and may be comparable in efficacy to esophageal sclerotherapy. They are superior to vasopressin in the control of variceal bleeding and are without significant side effects. A combination of octreotide and endoscopic therapy resulted in a significant reduction in rebleeding and transfusion requirements compared with endoscopic treatment alone. In patients with advanced liver disease and upper gastrointestinal hemorrhage, it is reasonable to initiate therapy with octreotide on admission and continue for 5 days. If bleeding is determined by subsequent endoscopy not to be secondary to portal hypertension, the infusion can be discontinued.

Vasopressin is a nonselective vasoconstrictor that reduces splanchnic flow and portal pressures but achieves control of variceal hemorrhage in only 50% of cases. Side effects occur in up to one-fourth of patients and include abdominal pain, myocardial or mesenteric ischemia, stroke, bradycardia, hypertension, and hyponatremia. Given the superior efficacy and safety of octreotide, the use of vasopressin can no longer be recommended.

3. Vitamin K–In cirrhotic patients with an abnormal prothrombin time, vitamin K (10 mg) should be administered subcutaneously.

4. Lactulose–Encephalopathy may complicate an episode of gastrointestinal bleeding in patients with severe liver disease. Lactulose, 30 mL twice daily, may be given to prevent encephalopathy, increasing the dose as needed to induce two or three stools per day (see Chapter 15).

D. Balloon Tube Tamponade: Mechanical tamponade with specially designed nasogastric tubes containing large gastric and esophageal balloons (Minnesota or Sengstaken-Blakemore tubes) provides initial control of active variceal hemorrhage in 60–90% of patients; however, rebleeding occurs in 50%. The gastric balloon is inflated first, followed by the esophageal balloon if bleeding continues. After balloon inflation, tension is applied to the tube to directly tamponade the varices. Complications of prolonged balloon inflation include esophageal and oral ulcerations, perforation, aspiration, and airway obstruction (due to a misplaced balloon). Endotracheal intubation is recommended before placement. Given its high rate of complications, mechanical tamponade should be used as a temporizing measure only in patients with bleeding that cannot be controlled with pharmacologic or endoscopic techniques until more definitive decompressive therapy (eg, TIPS; see below) can be provided.

E. Portal Decompressive Procedures: In patients with variceal bleeding that cannot be controlled with pharmacologic or endoscopic therapy, emergency portal decompression is necessary.

1. Transvenous intrahepatic portosystemic shunts (TIPS)–A technique has been devised whereby angiographers pass via a transjugular route a needle-tip catheter into the hepatic vein, through the liver, and into the portal vein. Over a wire that is passed through the catheter, an expandable wire mesh stent (8–12 mm in diameter) is passed through the liver parenchyma, creating a portosystemic shunt from the portal vein to the hepatic vein. The rate of severe complications is only 1–2%. TIPS can control acute hemorrhage in over 90% of patients actively bleeding from gastric or esophageal varices. TIPS is indicated in the 10% of patients with acute variceal bleeding that cannot be controlled with pharmacologic and endoscopic therapy. It is not indicated as initial therapy to control variceal hemorrhage.

2. Emergency portosystemic shunt surgery–In most series, emergency portosystemic shunt surgery is associated with a 40–60% mortality rate. At centers where TIPS is available, that procedure has become the preferred means of providing emergency portal decompression.

Prevention of Rebleeding

Once the initial bleeding episode has been controlled, the risk of rebleeding is 60–80% without further therapy. The highest incidence of rebleeding is in the first six weeks. Several options are available to decrease the likelihood of rebleeding, though their relative merits are controversial. Use of these approaches varies in different medical centers.

A. Endoscopic Techniques: Multiple trials demonstrate that long-term treatment with sclerotherapy or band ligation reduces the incidence of rebleeding to 20–40%. Meta-analysis of these trials suggests that the mortality rate is also reduced. Band ligation of the varix appears to be equal or superior to sclerotherapy in preventing rebleeding and is associated with a significantly lower complication rate. In most patients, four to six treatment sessions are needed to eradicate the varices. Where expertise is available, endoscopic therapy is generally the preferred approach to long-term therapy of esophageal varices.

B. Beta-Blockers and Nitrates: Nonselective beta-adrenergic blockers (propranolol, nadolol) are effective in reducing the incidence of rebleeding from esophageal varices and portal hypertensive gastropathy compared with placebo. An improvement in mortality statistics has not been shown; the efficacy is comparable to that of sclerotherapy. Combination therapy with beta-blockers and sclerotherapy appears to be superior to sclerotherapy alone. Therefore, patients without contraindications to beta-blockers should be started on propranolol, 20 mg twice daily, or nadolol, 40 mg once daily. The dosage is increased gradually until the heart rate falls by 25% or reaches 55 beats/min. An average dose is propranolol or nadolol, 80 mg once daily.

Long-acting nitrates have also been shown to reduce portal pressures and the risk of variceal rebleeding. They may be given as monotherapy to patients who cannot tolerate beta-blockers. Isosorbide mononitrate is initiated at a dosage of 10 mg daily and gradually increased to 20–40 mg twice daily as tolerated. Side effects include hypotension or headache. Combination therapy with isosorbide mononitrate and beta-blockers has been shown to be more effective and better tolerated than beta-blockers alone in reducing portal pressures and rebleeding. At present, the merits of combination therapy versus monotherapy are still being defined.

C. Transvenous Intrahepatic Portosystemic Shunts (TIPS): In seven of nine randomized trials involving patients with a history of variceal bleeding, TIPS has resulted in a significant reduction in recurrent bleeding compared with endoscopic sclerotherapy or band ligation—either alone or in combination with beta-blocker therapy. At 1 year, rebleeding rates in patients treated with TIPS versus various endoscopic therapies average 20% and 40%, respectively. However, TIPS was also associated with a higher incidence of encephalopathy (35% versus 15%) and did not result in a decrease in mortality. Another limitation of TIPS is that stenosis and thrombosis of the stents occurs in the majority of patients over time with a consequent risk of rebleeding. Therefore, periodic monitoring with Doppler ultrasonography or hepatic venography is required. Stent patency usually can be maintained by balloon angioplasty or additional stent placement. Given these problems, TIPS should be reserved for patients who have recurrent (two or more) episodes of variceal bleeding that have failed endoscopic or pharmacologic therapies. TIPS is also useful in patients with recurrent bleeding from gastric varices or portal hypertensive gastropathy (for which endoscopic therapies cannot be used). TIPS should also be considered in patients who are noncompliant with other therapies or who live in remote locations (without access to emergency care).

D. Surgical Portosystemic Shunts: Shunt surgery has a significantly lower rate of rebleeding compared with endoscopic therapy but also a higher incidence of encephalopathy. Selective (distal splenorenal) shunts have a lower incidence of encephalopathy than portacaval shunts but are more difficult to perform. In most centers, shunt surgery has been reserved for patients who have failed sclerotherapy or for noncompliant patients. With the advent of TIPS, the role of surgical shunts is unclear.

E. Liver Transplantation: Candidacy for orthotopic liver transplantation should be assessed in all patients with chronic liver disease and bleeding due to portal hypertension. Transplant candidates should be treated with sclerotherapy or TIPS to control bleeding pretransplant.

Prevention of First Episodes of Variceal Bleeding

Because of the high mortality rate associated with variceal hemorrhage, prevention of the initial bleeding episode is desirable. Nonselective beta-adrenergic blockers (nadolol, propranolol) have been shown in multiple trials to decrease the long-term risk of bleeding to less than 15% (compared with about 25% in placebo-treated patients). Up to 15% of patients do not tolerate beta-blocker therapy and should instead be given a trial of therapy with isosorbide mononitrate, as discussed above. Because variceal bleeding occurs in only one-third of cirrhotics, it may be reasonable to use beta-blockers in compliant higher-risk patients, ie, patients with large varices or red color markings. Prophylactic sclerotherapy in those who have never had a variceal hemorrhage has been shown to result in a higher mortality rate than placebo or treatment with beta-blockers and should not be done. In contrast, recent studies report a reduction in the incidence of first episodes of variceal bleeding in patients treated with variceal ligation (banding). Large trials and cost-benefit analyses are required to determine how pharmacotherapy (beta-blockers, nitrates), variceal ligation, or a combination of both should be used in the prevention of first episodes of variceal bleeding.

Bernard B et al: Antibiotic prophylaxis for the prevention of bacterial infections in cirrhotic patients with gastrointestinal bleeding: a meta-analysis. Hepatology 1999;29:1655. [NLM Cit ID: 99278276]

Cello JP: Endoscopic management of esophageal variceal hemorrhage: injection, banding, glue, octreotide, or a combination? Semin Gastrointest Dis 1997;8:179. [NLM Cit ID: 98024599]

Sarin S et al: Comparison of endoscopic ligation and propranolol for the primary prevention of variceal bleeding. N Engl J Med 1999;340:988. [NLM Cit ID: 99182214] (The incidence of variceal bleeding at 18 months was significantly lower in a group treated with band ligation [15%] versus patients treated with propranolol [43%]. An accompanying editorial notes that the bleeding rate on propranolol is higher than previously reported and recommends for the time being that primary ligation therapy be reserved for patients with contraindications to beta-blockers.)

Shahi HM et al: Prevention of first variceal bleed: an appraisal of current therapies. Am J Gastroenterol 1998;93:2348. [NLM Cit ID: 99075734]

MALIGNANT ESOPHAGEAL LESIONS (Cancer of the Esophagus)

Essentials of Diagnosis

- Progressive solid food dysphagia.
- Weight loss common.
- Endoscopy with biopsy establishes diagnosis.

General Considerations

Esophageal cancer usually develops in persons between 50 and 70 years of age. The overall ratio of men to women is 3:1. There are two histologic types: squamous cell carcinoma and adenocarcinoma. In the United States, squamous cell cancer is much more common in blacks than in whites. Chronic alcohol and tobacco use are strongly associated with an increased risk of squamous cell carcinoma. The risk of squamous cell cancer is also increased in patients with tylosis (a rare disease transmitted by autosomal dominant inheritance and manifested by hyperkeratosis of the palms and soles), achalasia, caustic-induced esophageal stricture, and other head and neck cancers. Squamous cell cancer has a high incidence in certain regions of China and Southeast Asia. Approximately half of cases occur in the distal third of the esophagus and the other half in the proximal two-thirds. Adenocarcinoma is more common in whites. It is increasing dramatically in incidence and now is as common as squamous carcinoma. The great majority of adenocarcinomas develop as a complication of Barrett's metaplasia due to chronic gastroesophageal reflux. Thus, most adenocarcinomas arise in the distal third of the esophagus.

Clinical Findings

A. Symptoms and Signs: Most patients with esophageal cancer present with advanced, incurable disease. Over 90% have solid food dysphagia, which progresses over weeks to months. Odynophagia is sometimes present. Significant weight loss is common. Local tumor extension into the tracheobronchial tree may result in a tracheoesophageal fistula, characterized by coughing on swallowing or pneumonia. Chest or back pain suggests mediastinal extension. Recurrent laryngeal involvement may produce hoarseness. Physical examination is often unrevealing. The presence of supraclavicular or cervical lymphadenopathy or of hepatomegaly implies metastatic disease.

B. Laboratory Findings: Laboratory findings are nonspecific. Anemia related to chronic disease or occult blood loss is common. Elevated aminotransferase or alkaline phosphatase concentrations suggest hepatic or bony metastases. Hypoalbuminemia may result from malnutrition.

C. Imaging: Chest x-rays may show adenopathy, a widened mediastinum, pulmonary or bony metastases, or signs of tracheoesophageal fistula such as pneumonia. A barium esophagogram often is obtained as the first study to evaluate dysphagia. The appearance of a polypoid, infiltrative, or ulcerative lesion is suggestive of carcinoma and requires endoscopic evaluation. However, even lesions felt to be benign by radiography warrant endoscopic evaluation.

D. Upper Endoscopy: Endoscopy with biopsy establishes the diagnosis of esophageal carcinoma with a high degree of reliability. In some cases, significant submucosal spread of the tumor may yield nondiagnostic mucosal biopsies. Repeated biopsy may be necessary.

Differential Diagnosis

Esophageal carcinoma must be distinguished from other causes of progressive dysphagia, including peptic stricture, achalasia, and adenocarcinoma of the gastric cardia with esophageal involvement. Benign-appearing peptic strictures should be biopsied at presentation to exclude occult malignancy.

Staging of Disease

After confirmation of the diagnosis of esophageal carcinoma, the stage of the disease should be determined since doing so influences the choice of therapy. Patients should undergo evaluation with CT of the chest and liver to look for evidence of pulmonary or hepatic metastases, lymphadenopathy, and local tumor extension. If there is no evidence of distant metastases or extensive local spread on CT, endoscopic ultrasonography should be performed, which is superior to CT in demonstrating the level of local mediastinal extension and local lymph node involvement. Bronchoscopy is sometimes required in proximal esophageal cancer to exclude tracheobronchial extension. Apart from distant metastasis, the two most important predictors of poor survival are lymph node involvement and adjacent mediastinal spread.

Stages are determined by the TNM classification as set forth in the accompanying box.

STAGING CRITERIA FOR ESOPHAGEAL CANCER

Primary Tumor (T)

- **T1:** Invasion of lamina propria or submucosa
- **T2:** Invasion of muscularis propria
- **T3:** Invasion of adventitia
- **T4:** Invasion of adjacent structures

Regional Lymph Nodes (N)

- **N0:** No regional lymph node involvement
- **N1:** Regional lymph node involvement

Distant Metastasis (M)

- **M1:** Distant metastasis
- **M0:** No metastasis

Based upon these parameters, the tumor is classified as:

Stage I:	T1, N0, M0
Stage IIA:	T2 or T3, and N0, M0
Stage IIB:	T1 or T2, and N1, M0
Stage III:	T3, N1, M0 or T4, any N, M0
Stage IV:	Any T or N, M1

Treatment

The approach to esophageal cancer depends upon the tumor stage, patient preference, and the expertise of the attending surgeons, oncologists, and radiotherapists. There is no consensus about the optimal treatment approach. It is helpful, however, to classify patients into two general categories.

A. Palliative Therapy: Patients with extensive local tumor spread (T4) or distant metastases (M1) are incurable, ie, most patients with stage III and all with stage IV tumors. The goal in these patients is to provide relief from dysphagia and pain. The optimal palliative approach depends upon the patient's expected survival, patient preference, and local institutional experience. None of these modalities prolong survival, and many patients may prefer concerted efforts at pain relief (see Chapter 1) and care directed at symptom management (see Chapter 5).

1. Surgical resection–Palliative resection of the esophagus provides the most rapid and durable relief of dysphagia. For reasonably well-nourished patients without other serious comorbid medical problems (ie, suitable surgical candidates) who have an expected survival of more than 6–12 months, this may be recommended provided there is no significant involvement of mediastinal structures.

2. Radiation therapy–For patients with unresectable disease and for poor operative candidates, radiation therapy may afford significant short-term palliation of pain and dysphagia. During therapy, esophagitis may lead to worsening of dysphagia and odynophagia. Combined radiation therapy and chemotherapy may achieve palliation in two-thirds of patients.

3. Local tumor therapy–Patients with advanced esophageal cancer may be quite ill, with an average survival of less than 12 weeks from diagnosis. Palliation of dysphagia may be achieved by peroral placement of expandable, permanent wire stents or by application of endoscopic laser therapy. Although dysphagia and quality of life are improved significantly, patients can seldom eat normally. Complications of stents occur in 20–40% and include perforation, migration, and tumor ingrowth. These are most suitable for patients with a short life expectancy; patients with tracheoesophageal fistula; patients who have failed radiation therapy; or patients in locations where optimal surgical or radiation modalities are not available. A photosensitizing agent, porfimer sodium, has been approved for palliation of advanced esophageal cancer. Forty to 50 hours after porfimer administration, the tumor is illuminated with 630 nm laser light via a fiber passed through an endoscope. Clinical improvement in swallowing occurs in 65%.

B. "Curable" Disease: The approach to the remainder of patients is controversial and highly dependent upon institutional experience. Currently, there are three broad categories of therapy that may be considered.

1. Surgery alone–Patients with stage I and stage IIA cancer have high cure rates with surgery alone. There is controversy over the optimal surgical approach. The procedure with the lowest morbidity is transhiatal esophagectomy with anastomosis of the stomach to the cervical esophagus. Critics of this approach note that because it does not involve sampling or removal of mediastinal lymph nodes, it is not suitable as a "curative" approach for node-positive disease. Alternatively, many surgeons recommend transthoracic excision of the esophagus with nodal resection. Critics of this approach note that it has a higher morbidity and no better survival than the transhiatal approach. Regardless of the approach elected, overall 3-year survival after surgery is less than 15% in most series.

2. Chemotherapy plus radiation therapy–Combined therapy with chemotherapy and radiation therapy is superior to radiation therapy alone and has achieved overall survival rates that equal or exceed those of historical surgical cohorts, though there have been no trials specifically comparing these approaches. However, severe side effects occur commonly with combined therapy. The most promising chemotherapeutic agents have been cisplatin and fluorouracil.

3. Surgery with neoadjuvant chemotherapy and radiation therapy–If lymph node metastases have occurred (stage IIB and stage III), the rate of cure with surgery alone is markedly reduced to less than 10%. Trials of adjuvant (postoperative) or neoadjuvant (preoperative) radiation therapy or chemotherapy have not shown convincing benefits over surgery alone. In recent trials, patients have been treated with combination radiation therapy and chemotherapy (cisplatin and fluorouracil) prior to surgical resection. Several single-center trials have reported a complete pathologic remission (no evidence of tumor at the time of surgery) in up to 25% of patients treated with combination neoadjuvant therapy. However, a recent multicenter trial failed to demonstrate improvement in survival with neoadjuvant chemoradiotherapy in patients with squamous cell cancer but did report prolonged disease-free survival. Further comparisons of this multimodal treatment versus surgery are needed, and this approach currently should not be used outside of clinical trials.

Prognosis

The overall 5-year survival rate of esophageal carcinoma is less than 15%. Despite improvements in surgical mortality and increased surgical resectability rates, the prognosis of this disease has not changed for years, in part because most patients present with advanced disease. This suggests that surgical approaches alone are inadequate for most patients. For those patients whose disease progresses despite chemotherapy, meticulous effects at palliative care are essential (see Chapter 5).

[National Cancer Institute PDQ Internet Information for Esophageal Cancer]
http://cancernet.nci.nih.gov/cgi-bin/srchcgi.exe?DBID=pdq&TYPE=search&UID=208+00089

Bossett JF et al: Chemoradiotherapy followed by surgery compared with surgery alone in squamous-cell cancer of the esophagus. N Engl J Med 1997;337:161. [NLM Cit ID: 97347216]

Gossner L et al: KTP laser destruction of dysplasia and early cancer in columnar-lined Barrett's esophagus. Gastrointest Endosc 1999;49:8. [NLM Cit ID: 99087991]

Kelsen D: Multimodality therapy for adenocarcinoma of the esophagus. Gastroenterol Clin North Am 1997;26:635. [NLM Cit ID: 97455014]

Lightdale CJ: Esophageal cancer. Am J Gastroenterol 1999;94:20. [NLM Cit ID: 99131426]

Raijman I et al: Palliation of malignant dysphagia and fistulae with coated expandable metal stents: experience with 101 patients. Gastrointest Endosc 1998;48:172. [NLM Cit ID: 98381883]

ESOPHAGEAL MOTILITY DISORDERS

1. ACHALASIA

Essentials of Diagnosis

- Gradual, progressive dysphagia for solids and liquids.
- Regurgitation of undigested food.
- Barium esophagogram with "bird's beak" distal esophagus.
- Esophageal manometry confirms diagnosis.

General Considerations

Achalasia is an idiopathic motility disorder characterized by loss of peristalsis in the distal two-thirds (smooth muscle) of the esophagus and impaired relaxation of the lower esophageal sphincter. There appears to be denervation of the esophagus resulting from loss of ganglion cells in Auerbach's plexus and degeneration of the vagus nerve and dorsal motor nucleus.

Clinical Findings

A. Symptoms and Signs: There is a steady increase in the incidence of achalasia with age; however, it can be seen in individuals as young as 25 years. Patients complain of the gradual onset of dysphagia for solid foods and, in the majority, of liquids also. Symptoms at presentation may have persisted for months to years. Substernal discomfort or fullness may be noted after eating. Many patients eat more slowly and adopt specific maneuvers such as lifting the neck or throwing the shoulders back in order to enhance esophageal emptying. Regurgitation of undigested food is common and may occur during meals or up to several hours later. Nocturnal regurgitation can provoke coughing or aspiration. Up to half of patients report substernal chest pain that is unrelated to meals or exercise and may last up to hours. Weight loss is common. Physical examination is unhelpful.

B. Imaging: Chest x-rays may show an air-fluid level in the enlarged, fluid-filled esophagus. Barium esophagography discloses characteristic findings, including esophageal dilation, loss of esophageal peristalsis, poor esophageal emptying, and a smooth, symmetric "bird's beak" tapering of the distal esophagus. Without treatment, the esophagus may become markedly dilated ("sigmoid esophagus").

C. Special Examinations: After esophagography, endoscopy is always performed to evaluate the distal esophagus and gastroesophageal junction in order to exclude a distal stricture or a submucosal infiltrating carcinoma. The diagnosis is confirmed by esophageal manometry. The typical manometric features are as follows: (1) Complete absence of peristalsis; swallowing results in simultaneous waves which are usually of low amplitude. (2) Incomplete lower esophageal sphincteric relaxation with swallowing. Whereas the normal sphincter relaxes by over 90%, relaxation with most swallows in patients with achalasia is less than 50%. In many patients, the baseline lower esophageal sphincteric pressure is quite elevated. (3) Intraesophageal pressures are greater than gastric pressures due to a fluid- and food-filled esophagus.

Differential Diagnosis

Chagas' disease is associated with esophageal dysfunction that is indistinguishable from idiopathic achalasia and should be considered in patients from endemic regions (Central and South America). Primary or metastatic tumors can invade the gastroesophageal junction, resulting in a picture resembling that of achalasia, called "pseudoachalasia." Endoscopic ultrasonography and chest CT may be required to examine the distal esophagus in suspicious cases. Achalasia must be distinguished from other motility disorders such as diffuse esophageal spasm and scleroderma esophagus with a peptic stricture.

Treatment

A. Botulinum Toxin Injection: Endoscopically guided injection of botulinum toxin directly into the lower esophageal sphincter results in a marked reduction in lower esophageal sphincter pressure with initial improvement in symptoms in 85% of patients. However, symptom relapse occurs in over 50% of patients within 6–9 months. Approximately 25% of patients have a sustained response (lasting more than a year). Three-fourths of initial responders who relapse have improvement with repeated injections. The role of botulinum toxin injection relative to other therapies is debated. Because it is inferior to pneumatic dilation therapy and surgery in producing sustained symptomatic relief, this therapy may be most appropriate for elderly patients or those with multiple medical problems who are poor candidates for more invasive procedures.

B. Pneumatic Dilation: Over three-fourths of patients derive good to excellent relief of dysphagia after one or two sessions of pneumatic dilation of the lower esophageal sphincter. Under fluoroscopic guidance, 3- to 4-cm diameter balloons are inflated across the gastroesophageal junction in an effort to permanently disrupt the sphincter. Perforations occur in under 3% of dilations and may require operative repair.

C. Surgical Myotomy: A modified Heller cardiomyotomy of the lower esophageal sphincter and cardia results in good to excellent symptomatic improvement in over 85% of patients. Because gastroesophageal reflux may develop in up to 20% of patients after myotomy, most surgeons also perform an antireflux procedure (fundoplication). Myotomy is now performed with a laparoscopic approach. Because it is less invasive, reduces postoperative morbidity, and permits shorter hospital stay, laparoscopic myotomy is preferred to the open surgical approach.

Until recently, surgery has been performed most often in patients who have failed therapy with pneumatic dilation. However, the low morbidity of laparoscopic surgery has led some experts to recommend it for initial treatment. In experienced hands, the efficacy of pneumatic dilation and laparoscopic myotomy are nearly equivalent. Pneumatic dilation appears to be a more cost-effective strategy than either botulinum toxin injection or laparoscopic myotomy. The success of laparoscopic surgery does not appear to be compromised by prior therapy with either botulinum injection or pneumatic dilation. Pending further outcome studies, the risks and benefits of all three approaches should be discussed with the patient.

Eckardt VF et al: Chest pain in achalasia: patient characteristics and clinical course. Gastroenterology 1999;116: 1300. [NLM Cit ID: 99278242]

Prakash C et al: Botulinum toxin injections for achalasia symptoms can approximate the short term efficacy of single pneumatic dilation: a survival analysis approach. Am J Gastroenterol 1999;94:328. [NLM Cit ID: 99145222]

Vaezi M et al: Diagnosis and management of achalasia. Am J Gastroenterol 1999;94:3406. [NLM Cit ID: 2007231]

2. OTHER PRIMARY ESOPHAGEAL MOTILITY DISORDERS

Abnormalities in esophageal motility may cause dysphagia or chest pain. Dysphagia for liquids as well as solids tends to be intermittent and nonprogressive. Periods of normal swallowing may alternate with periods of dysphagia, which usually is mild though bothersome—rarely severe enough to result in significant alterations in lifestyle or weight loss. Dysphagia may be provoked by stress, large boluses of food, or hot or cold liquids. Some patients may experience anterior chest pain that may be confused with angina pectoris but usually is nonexertional. The pain generally is unrelated to eating. (See Chest Pain of Undetermined Origin, below.)

The evaluation of suspected esophageal motility disorders includes barium esophagography, upper endoscopy, and, in some cases, esophageal manometry. Barium esophagography is useful to exclude mechanical obstruction and to evaluate esophageal motility. The presence of simultaneous contractions (spasm), disordered peristalsis, or failed peristalsis supports a diagnosis of esophageal dysmotility. Upper endoscopy also is performed to exclude a mechanical obstruction (as a cause of dysphagia) and to look for evidence of erosive reflux esophagitis (a common cause of chest pain).

The further evaluation of noncardiac chest pain is discussed in a subsequent section. For patients with disabling symptoms of dysphagia, stationary esophageal manometry should be performed. Manometry should not be routinely used for mild to moderate symptoms because the findings seldom influence further medical management. Based upon the findings of esophageal manometry, patients may be diagnosed with the following conditions: (1) Diffuse esophageal spasm: normal primary peristalsis with more than 10% simultaneous contractions. (2) Nutcracker esophagus: normal peristalsis but increased duration and high amplitude of distal contractions (> 180 mm Hg). (3) Hypertensive lower esophageal sphincter: elevated lower esophageal sphincter pressure (> 45 mm

Hg) with normal peristalsis. (4) Nonspecific esophageal motility disorder: intermittent normal peristalsis with any of a number of abnormalities that do not allow classification into one of the above (> 20% nontransmitted peristaltic waves, prolonged duration of contractions, abnormal-appearing wave forms, low amplitude of peristaltic waves).

For patients with mild symptoms, therapy is directed at symptom reduction and reassurance. Patients with dysphagia should be instructed to eat more slowly and take smaller boluses of food. In some cases, a warm liquid at the start of a meal may facilitate swallowing. Treatment of more severe cases with nitrates (isosorbide, 10–30 mg four times daily) or nitroglycerin (0.4 mg sublingually as needed) and calcium channel blockers (nifedipine, 30–60 mg, or diltiazem, 60–90 mg, four times daily) may be tried; however, limited controlled data do not support their efficacy. For unclear reasons, dilation with esophageal Maloney bougies provides symptomatic relief in some cases. In debilitated patients, a long surgical myotomy (which may be performed via a thoracoscopic approach) may lead to improvement in 70–80% of cases.

Patti M et al: Evaluation and treatment of primary esophageal motility disorders. West J Med 1997;166:263. [NLM Cit ID: 97312243]

Triadafilopoulos G: Primary esophageal motility disorders: Incisive decisions. West J Med 1997;166:289. [NLM Cit ID: 97312253]

CHEST PAIN OF UNDETERMINED ORIGIN

Approximately 30% of patients with chest pain who undergo cardiac evaluation do not have an apparent cardiac cause of their symptoms. Patients with recurrent noncardiac chest pain can pose a difficult clinical problem. Because coronary artery disease is common and serious and can present in atypical fashion, it is imperative that it be excluded prior to evaluation for other noncardiac causes.

Causes of noncardiac chest pain may include the following.

A. Chest Wall and Thoracic Spine Disease: These are easily diagnosed by history and physical examination.

B. Gastroesophageal Reflux: Up to 25% of patients have increased amounts of gastroesophageal acid reflux. An empirical trial of acid suppressive therapy with a high-dose proton pump inhibitor (eg, omeprazole 40 mg in AM and 20 mg in PM) for 7 days is recommended, especially in patients with reflux symptoms. The sensitivity and specificity of this treatment are 78% and 86%, respectively, compared with therapy based on results of esophageal pH testing. In some cases, an ambulatory esophageal pH study is warranted in an effort to document a relationship between acid reflux episodes and chest pain events.

C. Heightened Visceral Sensitivity: Studies suggest that many patients with noncardiac chest pain report pain in response to a variety of minor noxious stimuli such as intraesophageal acid infusion, inflation of balloons within the esophageal lumen, injection of intravenous edrophonium (a cholinergic stimulus), or intracardiac catheter manipulation. Low doses of antidepressants such as trazodone 50 mg or imipramine 50 mg reduce chest pain symptoms. These agents are thought to reduce visceral afferent awareness.

D. Psychologic: A significant number of patients have underlying depression, anxiety, and panic disorder. Such patients may benefit from appropriate therapy. Patients reporting dyspnea, sweating, tachycardia, a sense of suffocation, dizziness, or fear of dying should be evaluated for panic disorder.

E. Esophageal Dysmotility: Esophageal motility abnormalities such as diffuse esophageal spasm or nutcracker esophagus are a rare cause of noncardiac chest pain. Stationary or ambulatory manometry is not recommended in the routine evaluation of this disorder because of the low specificity of these procedures and the unlikelihood of finding a clinically significant disorder. In patients with chest pain and dysphagia, barium swallow x-ray should be obtained initially to look for evidence of achalasia or diffuse esophageal spasm.

Achem SR et al: Unexplained chest pain at the turn of the century. Am J Gastroenterol 1999;94:5. [NLM Cit ID: 99131421]

Fass R et al: The clinical and economic value of a short course of omeprazole in patients with noncardiac chest pain. Gastroenterology 1998;115:222. [NLM Cit ID: 98323486] (In a double-blind crossover trial of patients with noncardiac chest pain, 62% were felt to have reflux-related chest pain based upon esophageal pH study. Of these, 80% had improved chest pain during omeprazole treatment, compared with 15% of patients without gastroesophageal reflux disease.)

Ofman J et al: The cost-effectiveness of the omeprazole test in patients with noncardiac chest pain. Am J Med 1999;107:219. [NLM Cit ID: 99420063] (An empirical trial of a high-dose proton pump inhibitor for 7 days may be more cost-effective than diagnostic strategies which employ invasive tests such as endoscopy and pH monitoring.)

DISEASES OF THE STOMACH & DUODENUM

GASTRITIS & GASTROPATHY

The term "gastritis" is beset by semantic confusion. Endoscopists employ the term to denote a number of gross mucosal features such as erythema, subepithelial hemorrhages, and erosions; to the pathologist, the term denotes histologic inflammation. The term "gastropathy" is used increasingly to denote conditions in which there is epithelial or endothelial damage without inflammation. Gastritis may be divided into three categories: (1) erosive and hemorrhagic gastritis; (2) nonerosive, nonspecific (histologic) gastritis; and (3) specific types of gastritis, characterized by distinctive histologic and endoscopic features that may be diagnostic of a disorder.

1. EROSIVE & HEMORRHAGIC GASTRITIS

Essentials of Diagnosis

- Most commonly seen in alcoholics, critically ill patients, or patients taking NSAIDs.
- Often asymptomatic; may cause epigastric pain, nausea, and vomiting.
- May cause hematemesis; usually not significant bleeding.

General Considerations

The most common causes of erosive gastritis are drugs (especially NSAIDs), alcohol, stress due to severe medical or surgical illness ("stress gastritis"), and portal hypertension ("portal gastropathy"). Uncommon causes include caustic ingestion and radiation. Erosive gastritis and hemorrhagic gastritis typically are diagnosed at endoscopy, often being performed because of dyspepsia or upper gastrointestinal bleeding. Endoscopic findings include subepithelial hemorrhages, petechiae, and erosions. These lesions are superficial, vary in size and number, and may be focal or diffuse. There usually is no significant inflammation on histologic examination, though gastropathy may be present.

Clinical Findings

A. Symptoms and Signs: Erosive gastritis is usually asymptomatic. Symptoms, when they occur, include anorexia, epigastric pain, nausea, and vomiting. There is poor correlation between symptoms and the number or severity of endoscopic abnormalities. The most common clinical manifestation of erosive gastritis is upper gastrointestinal bleeding, which presents as hematemesis, "coffee grounds" emesis, or bloody aspirate in a patient receiving nasogastric suction, or as melena. Because erosive gastritis is superficial, hemodynamically significant bleeding is rare.

B. Laboratory Findings: The laboratory findings are nonspecific. The hematocrit is low if significant bleeding has occurred.

C. Special Examinations: Upper endoscopy is the most sensitive method of diagnosis. Although bleeding from gastritis is usually insignificant, it cannot be distinguished on clinical grounds from more serious lesions such as peptic ulcers or esophageal varices. Hence, endoscopy is generally performed within 24 hours in patients with upper gastrointestinal bleeding to identify the source. An upper gastrointestinal series is sometimes obtained in lieu of endoscopy in patients with hemodynamically insignificant upper gastrointestinal bleeds to exclude serious lesions but is insensitive for the detection of gastritis.

Differential Diagnosis

Epigastric pain may be due to peptic ulcer, gastroesophageal reflux, gastric cancer, biliary tract disease, food poisoning, viral gastroenteritis, and functional dyspepsia. With severe pain, one should consider a perforated or penetrating ulcer, pancreatic disease, esophageal rupture, ruptured aortic aneurysm, gastric volvulus, and myocardial colic. Causes of upper gastrointestinal bleeding include peptic ulcer disease, esophageal varices, Mallory-Weiss tear, and arteriovenous malformations.

Specific Causes & Treatment

A. Stress Gastritis:

1. Prophylaxis—Stress-related mucosal erosions and subepithelial hemorrhages develop within 18 hours in the majority of critically ill patients. Clinically overt bleeding occurs in 6% but clinically important bleeding in less than 2–3%. Bleeding is associated with a higher mortality rate but is seldom the cause of death. Major risk factors include trauma, burns, hypotension, sepsis, central nervous system injury, coagulopathy, mechanical respiration, hepatic or renal failure, and multiorgan failure. The use of enteral nutrition reduces the risk of stress-related bleeding.

Pharmacologic prophylaxis with sucralfate or H_2 receptor antagonists in critically ill patients has been shown to reduce the incidence of clinically overt and significant bleeding by 50%. Prophylaxis should be routinely administered upon admission to critically ill patients with risk factors for significant bleeding. Two of the most important risk factors are coagulopathy and respiratory failure with the need for mechanical ventilation for over 48 hours. When these two risk factors are absent, the risk of significant bleeding is only 0.1%.

There is ongoing debate about whether sucralfate or an H_2 receptor antagonist is the preferred prophylactic agent. Meta-analyses of clinical trials suggest that sucralfate suspension (1 g orally every 4–6 hours) is comparable in efficacy to H_2 receptor antagonists in the prevention of stress-related bleeding but that it is associated with a 20% lower incidence of nosocomial pneumonia. However, a recent large multicenter trial in ICU patients requiring mechanical ventilation found that patients treated with ranitidine had significant reduction in clinically significant bleeding compared with patients treated with sucralfate (1.7% versus 3.8%). There was no difference in the incidence of ventilator-associated pneumonia. At this time, either sucralfate or infusions of H_2 receptor antagonists at a dose sufficient to maintain intragastric pH above 4.0 may be given as prophylactic therapy. Cimetidine (900–1200 mg), ranitidine (150 mg), or famotidine (20 mg) by continuous intravenous infusion over 24 hours is adequate to control pH in most patients. After 4 hours of infusion, the pH should be checked by nasogastric aspirate and the dose doubled if the pH is under 4.0. Oral proton pump inhibitors should not be used in the ICU for prophylaxis owing to their unpredictable absorption and the need for high doses in such patients. It is expected that an intravenous formulation of a proton pump inhibitor, pantoprazole, will become available soon. The role of intravenous proton pump inhibitors relative to less costly intravenous H_2 receptor antagonists in the prevention or treatment of stress gastritis at present is uncertain.

2. Treatment–Patients in whom stress gastritis results in clinically significant bleeding should receive continuous infusions of an H_2 receptor antagonist as well as sucralfate suspension. Because bleeding is diffuse, endoscopic hemostasis techniques are not helpful. Nevertheless, endoscopy is often performed in such patients to look for other treatable causes of upper gastrointestinal bleeding.

B. NSAID Gastritis: Although half of patients receiving NSAIDs on a chronic basis have gastritis at endoscopy, symptoms of dyspepsia develop in less than one-fourth. Furthermore, of patients with dyspepsia, up to half do not have significant mucosal abnormalities. Given the frequency of dyspeptic symptoms in patients taking NSAIDs, it is neither feasible nor desirable to investigate all such patients. Symptoms may improve with discontinuation of the agent, reduction to the lowest effective dose, or administration with meals. Patients with persistent symptoms despite conservative measures or patients at high risk for NSAID-induced ulcers (see section on peptic ulcer disease) should undergo diagnostic endoscopy. Those without significant NSAID ulceration may be treated symptomatically with sucralfate (1 g four times daily), with H_2 receptor antagonists given twice daily (cimetidine 400 mg, ranitidine 150 mg, or famotidine 20 mg), or with proton pump inhibitors once daily (omeprazole 20 mg, rabeprazole 20 mg, pantoprazole 40 mg, or lansoprazole 30 mg). Upper gastrointestinal bleeding due to NSAID gastritis is usually not severe.

C. Alcoholic Gastritis: Erosive gastritis and hemorrhagic gastritis account for 20% of episodes of upper gastrointestinal bleeding in chronic alcoholics. Therapy with H_2 receptor antagonists or sucralfate for 2–4 weeks often is prescribed. On occasion, bleeding may be severe.

D. Portal Hypertensive Gastropathy: Portal hypertension results in gastric mucosal and submucosal congestion of capillaries and venules. Bleeding from congestive gastropathy accounts for 25% of episodes of upper gastrointestinal bleeding in patients with portal hypertension. It may present suddenly with hematemesis or insidiously with iron deficiency anemia. Recurrent acute bleeding is common. Treatment with propranolol or nadolol reduces the incidence of recurrent acute bleeding by lowering portal pressures. Patients who fail propranolol therapy may be successfully treated with portal decompressive procedures (see section on treatment of esophageal varices).

Blendis L et al: Blocking the bleeding way. Gastroenterology 1998;115:120. [NLM Cit ID: 98323512] (Review of pharmacologic treatment of portal hypertension.)

Cook D et al: A comparison of sucralfate and ranitidine for the prevention of upper gastrointestinal bleeding in patients who required mechanical ventilation. N Engl J Med 1998;338:791. [NLM Cit ID: 98158033]

2. NONEROSIVE, NONSPECIFIC GASTRITIS

The diagnosis of nonerosive gastritis is based upon histologic assessment of mucosal biopsies. Endoscopic findings are normal in many cases and do not reliably predict the presence of histologic inflammation. The main types of nonerosive gastritis are those due to *H pylori* infection, those associated with pernicious anemia, and lymphocytic gastritis. (See Specific Types of Gastritis.)

Helicobacter pylori Gastritis

H pylori is a spiral gram-negative rod that resides beneath the gastric mucus layer adjacent to gastric epithelial cells. Although not invasive, it causes gastric mucosal inflammation with polymorphonuclear neutrophils and lymphocytes. The mechanisms of injury and inflammation may in part be related to the products of two genes, *vacA* and *cagA*.

In the United States, the prevalence of infection rises from less than 10% in Caucasians under age 30 to over 50% in those over age 60. The prevalence is higher in non-Caucasians and immigrants from developing countries and is correlated inversely with socioeconomic status. Transmission is from person to person, and an important mode of spread may be gastro-oral (ie, through exposure to vomitus). The majority of infections are probably acquired in childhood.

Acute infection with *H pylori* may cause a transient clinical illness characterized by nausea and abdominal pain that may last for several days and is associated with acute histologic gastritis with polymorphonuclear neutrophils. After these symptoms resolve, the majority progress to chronic infection with chronic, diffuse mucosal inflammation characterized by polymorphonuclear neutrophils and lymphocytes. Inflammation may be confined to the superficial gastric epithelium or may extend deeper into the gastric glands, resulting in varying degrees of gland atrophy (atrophic gastritis) and metaplasia of the gastric epithelium to intestinal type epithelium. Eradication of *H pylori* may be achieved with antibiotics in over 85% of patients and leads to resolution of the chronic gastritis (see section on peptic ulcer disease).

Although chronic *H pylori* infection with gastritis is present in 30–50% of the population, the vast majority are asymptomatic and suffer no sequelae. *H pylori* infection is strongly associated with peptic ulcer disease; however, only 15% of people with chronic infection develop a peptic ulcer (see section on peptic ulcer disease). Chronic *H pylori* gastritis is associated with a two- to sixfold increased risk of gastric adenocarcinoma and low-grade B cell gastric lymphoma (mucosa-associated lymphoid tissue lymphoma, or MALToma). There is little evidence that chronic *H pylori*-associated gastritis is a cause of dyspeptic symptoms. (See Dyspepsia at the beginning of this chapter.)

Investigation for *H pylori* infection is definitely indicated in patients with peptic ulcer disease and gastric MALToma, and increasingly also in patients with dyspepsia and a family history of gastric cancer. *H pylori* is detected by a variety of invasive and noninvasive means, all of which have greater than 90% sensitivity and specificity. At endoscopy, gastric mucosal biopsies can be assessed for urease activity by placing them in a pH-sensitive medium. Production of ammonia by the urease-secreting organism produces a color change in the medium within 3 hours—presumptive evidence of *H pylori*. This simple, inexpensive test is the preferred method of endoscopic diagnosis. Histologic assessment of gastric biopsies is more definitive but more expensive than the rapid urease test. The absence of chronic antral gastritis on histologic examination definitively excludes *H pylori*. *H pylori* cultures of mucosal biopsies are less sensitive and more expensive than other endoscopic tests and are seldom used.

Quantitative serum IgG antibodies to *H pylori* are detectable by ELISA. These laboratory-based tests have sensitivity and specificity of over 90% and cost 40–75 dollars. However, qualitative office-based kits (QuickVue; FlexSure) are now available that can be performed within 10 minutes at a cost of ten dollars. The qualitative tests have a slightly lower (80%) sensitivity and specificity.

Positive serologic tests do not necessarily denote ongoing, active infection. After successful *H pylori* eradication with antibiotics, antibody levels decline slowly over 6–12 months but may remain positive.

There are two noninvasive tests which indicate active *H pylori* infection: ^{14}C-urea or ^{13}C-urea breath tests (costs 60–300 dollars) and fecal antigen assay (cost 60 dollars), both of which have sensitivities and specificities of over 90%. These studies are the tests of choice for verifying eradication after antibacterial therapy.

Recommendations for noninvasive *H pylori* testing: Whole blood or serum serologic tests and the fecal antigen assay are recommended as the most cost-effective initial tests for *H pylori* infection. ^{13}C- and ^{14}C-urea breath tests are the tests of choice to confirm *H pylori* eradication when doing so is clinically indicated (complicated ulcer disease, recurrent dyspepsia, and MALT lymphoma). Although the urea breath tests are more accurate than serologic tests, their greater costs make them less attractive in most clinical settings. Of note, proton pump inhibitors reduce significantly the sensitivity of the urea breath tests, fecal antigen assay, and endoscopic biopsies (but not serologic tests) and should be discontinued at least 7–14 days prior to testing.

Howden C: Guidelines for the management of *Helicobacter pylori* infection. Am J Gastroenterol 1998;93:2330. [NLM Cit ID: 99075731]

Peek RM Jr et al: Pathophysiology of *Helicobacter pylori*-induced gastritis and peptic ulcer disease. Am J Med 1997;102:200. [NLM Cit ID: 97360607]

Rubin C: Are there three types of *Helicobacter pylori* gastritis? Gastroenterology 1997;112:2108. [NLM Cit ID: 97322051]

Pernicious Anemia Gastritis

Pernicious anemia gastritis is an autoimmune disorder involving the fundic glands with resultant achlorhydria and vitamin B_{12} malabsorption. Fundic histology is characterized by severe gland atrophy and intestinal metaplasia. Parietal cell antibodies directed against the H^+-K^+ ATPase pump are present in 90% of patients. Inflammation and autoimmune destruction of the acid-secreting parietal cells leads to secondary loss of fundic zymogen cells, which secrete intrinsic factor. Achlorhydria leads to pronounced hypergastrinemia (> 1000 pg/mL) due to loss of acid inhibition of gastrin G cells. Hypergastrinemia may induce hyperplasia of gastric enterochromaffin-like cells that may lead to the development of small, multicentric carcinoid tumors in 5% of patients. Metastatic spread is uncommon in lesions smaller than 2 cm. The risk of adenocarcinoma is increased threefold, with a prevalence of 1–3%. Endoscopy with biopsy is indicated in patients with pernicious anemia at the time of diagnosis. Patients with dysplasia or small carcinoids require periodic endoscopic surveillance. Pernicious anemia is discussed in detail in Chapter 13.

Toh BH et al: Pernicious anemia. N Engl J Med 1997;337:1441. [NLM Cit ID: 98010549]

3. SPECIFIC TYPES OF GASTRITIS

A number of disorders are associated with specific mucosal histologic features.

Infections

Acute bacterial infection of the gastric submucosa and muscularis with a variety of aerobic or anaerobic organisms produces a rare, rapidly progressive, life-threatening condition known as phlegmonous or necrotizing gastritis which requires emergency gastric resection and antibiotic therapy. Viral infection with CMV is commonly seen in patients with AIDS and after bone marrow or solid organ transplantation. Endoscopic findings include thickened gastric folds and ulcerations. Fungal infection with candida may occur in immunocompromised patients. Larvae of *Anisakis marina* ingested in raw fish or sushi may become embedded in the gastric mucosa, producing severe abdominal pain. Pain persists for several days until the larvae die. Endoscopic removal of the larvae provides rapid symptomatic relief.

Granulomatous Gastritis

Chronic granulomatous inflammation may be caused by a variety of systemic diseases, including tuberculosis, syphilis, fungal infections, sarcoidosis, or Crohn's disease. These may be asymptomatic or associated with a variety of gastrointestinal complaints.

Eosinophilic Gastritis

This is a rare disorder in which eosinophils infiltrate the antrum and sometimes the proximal intestine. Infiltration may involve the mucosa, muscularis, or serosa. Peripheral eosinophilia is prominent. Symptoms include anemia from mucosal blood loss, abdominal pain, early satiety, and postprandial vomiting. Treatment with corticosteroids is beneficial in the majority of patients.

Lymphocytic Gastritis

This is an idiopathic condition characterized by fluctuating abdominal pain, nausea, and vomiting. Endoscopic features include mucosal erosions and a varioliform ("pox-like") appearance. Biopsies reveal a diffuse lymphocytic gastritis. There is no established effective therapy.

Ménétrier's Disease (Hypertrophic Gastropathy)

This is an idiopathic entity characterized by giant thickened gastric folds involving predominantly the body of the stomach. Patients complain of nausea, epigastric pain, weight loss, and diarrhea. Because of chronic protein loss, patients may develop severe hypoproteinemia and anasarca. The cause is unknown. Treatment is directed at symptoms. Gastric resection is required in severe cases. There are case reports of resolution of symptoms and improvement in histologic appearance after *H pylori* eradication.

Kawasaki M et al: Ménétrier's disease associated with *Helicobacter pylori* infection: Resolution of enlarged gastric folds and hypoproteinemia after antibacterial treatment. Am J Gastroenterol 1997;92:1909. [NLM Cit ID: 98025775]

PEPTIC ULCER DISEASE

Essentials of Diagnosis

- History of nonspecific epigastric pain present in 80–90% of patients with variable relationship to meals.
- Ulcer symptoms characterized by rhythmicity and periodicity.
- 10–20% of patients present with ulcer complications without antecedent symptoms.
- Of NSAID-induced ulcers, 30–50% are asymptomatic.
- Upper endoscopy with antral biopsy for *H pylori* is diagnostic procedure of choice in most patients.
- Gastric ulcer biopsy or documentation of complete healing necessary to exclude gastric malignancy.

General Considerations

Peptic ulcer is a break in the gastric or duodenal mucosa that arises when the normal mucosal defensive factors are impaired or are overwhelmed by aggressive luminal factors such as acid and pepsin. By definition, ulcers extend through the muscularis mucosae and are usually over 5 mm in diameter. In the United States, there are about 500,000 new cases per year of peptic ulcer and 4 million ulcer recurrences; the lifetime prevalence of ulcers in the adult population is approximately 10%. Ulcers occur five times more commonly in the duodenum, where over 95% are in the bulb or pyloric channel. In the stomach, benign ulcers are located most commonly in the antrum (60%) and at the junction of the antrum and body on the lesser curvature (25%).

Ulcers occur slightly more commonly in men than in women (1.3:1). Although ulcers can occur in any age group, duodenal ulcers most commonly occur between the ages of 30 and 55, whereas gastric ulcers are more common between the ages of 55 and 70. Ulcers are more common in smokers and in patients taking NSAIDs on a chronic basis (see below). Alcohol and dietary factors do not appear to cause ulcer disease. The role of stress is uncertain. The incidence of duodenal ulcer disease has been declining dramatically for the past 30 years, but the incidence of gastric ulcers appears to be increasing, perhaps as a result of the widespread use of NSAIDs.

Etiology

Three major causes of peptic ulcer disease are now recognized: NSAIDs, chronic *H pylori* infection, and acid hypersecretory states such as Zollinger-Ellison syndrome. Evidence of *H pylori* infection or NSAID ingestion should be sought in all patients with peptic ulcer. NSAID- and *H pylori*-associated ulcers will be considered in the present section; Zollinger-Ellison syndrome will be discussed subsequently.

A. *H pylori*-Associated Ulcers: *H pylori* appears to be a necessary cofactor for the majority of duodenal and gastric ulcers not associated with NSAIDs. Prior studies indicated that 90% of cases of duodenal ulcer were associated with *H pylori* gastritis. However, it is now believed that the prevalence of *H pylori* infection in duodenal ulcer patients is somewhat lower—about 70–75%. It is not known precisely how chronic *H pylori* gastritis potentiates ulcers in the duodenum. Many *H pylori*-infected patients have increased gastric acid secretion. It is hypothesized that increased acid exposure can engender small islands of gastric metaplasia in the duodenal bulb. Colonization of these islands by *H pylori* may lead to duodenitis or duodenal ulcer. The association with gastric ulcers is lower, but *H pylori* is found in the majority in whom NSAIDs cannot be implicated. Overall, it is estimated that one in six infected patients will develop ulcer disease.

The natural history of peptic ulcer disease is well-defined. After standard therapies, 70–85% of patients will have an endoscopically documented recurrence within 1 year. Half of these will be asymptomatic. In international trials, successful eradication of *H pylori* was reported to decrease the ulcer recurrence rate to less than 5% per year. Analysis of trials from the United States suggest that the ulcer recurrence rate after *H pylori* eradication is substantially higher than reported in international studies—approximately 20% at 1 year. At least some of these recurrences are due to NSAID use. Notwithstanding these discrepancies, the importance of *H pylori* in the vast majority of cases of duodenal and gastric ulcers is undeniable.

B. NSAID-Induced Ulcers: There is a 10–20% prevalence of gastric ulcers and a 2–5% prevalence of duodenal ulcers in chronic NSAID users. The relative risk of gastric ulcers is increased 40-fold, but the risk of duodenal ulcers is only slightly increased. Users of NSAIDs are at least three times more likely than nonusers to suffer serious gastrointestinal complications from these ulcers such as bleeding, perforation, or death. It is noteworthy that gastric ulcers and duodenal ulcers cause about the same number of complications. Approximately 1–2% of chronic NSAID users will have a major complication within 1 year. Aspirin is the most ulcerogenic NSAID. The risk appears to be dose-related, with some risk even at doses as low as 81 mg every other day. The risk of NSAID complications is greater with higher NSAID dosage, during the first 3 months of administration, with advanced age, and with a prior history of ulcer disease, concomitant corticosteroid administration, or serious medical illness. Newer NSAIDs such as nabumetone, etodolac, and celecoxib are associated with a reduced incidence of ulcers because of relative sparing of gastric mucosal prostaglandin synthesis. Celecoxib and rofecoxib are the first of a new class of NSAIDs that selectively inhibits cyclooxygenase-2 (COX-2)—the principal enzyme involved in prostaglandin production at sites of inflammation—but spares cyclooxygenase-1 (COX-1), the principal enzyme involved with prostaglandin production in the gastric mucosa.

H pylori does not increase the likelihood of development of NSAID-associated ulcers. It is increasingly apparent that NSAIDs may cause small intestinal ulcerations and perforations, colitis, and colonic strictures.

Clinical Findings

A. Symptoms and Signs: Epigastric pain (dyspepsia), the hallmark of peptic ulcer disease, is present in 80–90% of patients. However, this complaint is not sensitive or specific enough to serve as a reliable diagnostic criterion for peptic ulcer disease. The clinical history cannot accurately distinguish duodenal from gastric ulcers. Less than one-fourth of patients with dyspepsia have ulcer disease at endoscopy. Up to 20% of patients with ulcer complications such as bleeding have no antecedent symptoms ("silent ulcers"). In patients with NSAID-induced ulcers, up to half are asymptomatic. Up to 60% of patients with complications do not have prior symptoms.

Pain is typically well localized to the epigastrium and not severe. It is described as gnawing, dull, aching, or "hunger-like." Classic features of peptic ulcer pain are rhythmicity and periodicity. Rhythmicity means that the pain fluctuates in intensity throughout the day and night. Approximately half of patients report relief of pain with food or antacids (especially duodenal ulcers) and a recurrence of pain 2–4 hours later. However, many patients deny any relationship to meals or report worsening of pain. Two-thirds of duodenal ulcers and one-third of gastric ulcers cause nocturnal pain that awakens the patient. A change from a patient's typical rhythmic discomfort to constant or radiating pain may reflect ulcer penetration or perforation. Most patients have symptomatic periods lasting up to several weeks with intervals of months to years in which they are pain-free (periodicity).

Nausea and anorexia may occur with gastric ulcers. Significant vomiting and weight loss are unusual with uncomplicated ulcer disease and suggest gastric outlet obstruction or gastric malignancy.

The physical examination is often unremarkable in uncomplicated peptic ulcer disease. Mild, localized epigastric tenderness to deep palpation may be present. Fecal occult blood testing is positive in one-third of patients.

B. Laboratory Findings: Laboratory tests are normal in uncomplicated peptic ulcer disease but are ordered to exclude ulcer complications or confounding disease entities. Anemia may occur with acute blood loss from a bleeding ulcer or less commonly from chronic blood loss. Leukocytosis suggests ulcer penetration or perforation. An elevated serum amylase in a patient with severe epigastric pain suggests ulcer penetration into the pancreas. A fasting serum gastrin level to screen for Zollinger-Ellison syndrome is obtained in some patients (see below). Because acid inhibition may raise serum gastrin levels, H_2 receptor antagonists should be withheld for 24 hours and proton pump inhibitors for 1 week before a gastrin level is measured.

C. Endoscopy: Upper endoscopy is the procedure of choice for the diagnosis of duodenal and gastric ulcers. Endoscopy provides better diagnostic accuracy than barium radiography and the ability to biopsy for the presence of malignancy and *H pylori* infection. In most cases of both gastric and duodenal ulcers, gastric mucosal biopsies are required to assess for the presence of *H pylori* (see below). Duodenal ulcers are virtually never malignant and do not require biopsy. Three to 5 percent of benign-appearing gastric ulcers prove to be malignant. Hence, cytologic brushings and biopsies of the ulcer margin are almost always performed. Provided that the gastric ulcer appears benign to the endoscopist and adequate biopsy specimens reveal no evidence of cancer, dyspepsia, or atypia, the patient may be followed without further endoscopy. If these conditions are not fulfilled, follow-up endoscopy should be performed 12 weeks after the start of therapy to document complete healing; nonhealing ulcers are suspicious for malignancy.

D. Imaging: Barium upper gastrointestinal series is an acceptable alternative to screening of uncomplicated patients with dyspepsia. However, because it has limited accuracy in distinguishing benign from malignant gastric ulcers, all gastric ulcers diagnosed by x-ray should be reevaluated with endoscopy after 8–12 weeks of therapy.

E. Testing for *H pylori*: Given the importance of *H pylori* in ulcer pathogenesis, testing for this organism should be performed in all patients with peptic ulcers (see section above on *H pylori* gastritis). In patients in whom an ulcer is diagnosed by endoscopy, gastric mucosal biopsies should be obtained both for a rapid urease test and for histologic examination. The specimens for histology are discarded if the urease test is positive.

In patients with a history of peptic ulcer or when an ulcer is diagnosed by upper gastrointestinal series, noninvasive assessment for *H pylori* with urea breath testing, fecal antigen assay, or serologic testing should be done. Proton pump inhibitors may cause false-negative urea breath tests and fecal antigen tests and should be withheld for at least 7 days before testing.

Differential Diagnosis

Peptic ulcer disease must be distinguished from other causes of epigastric distress (dyspepsia). Over half of patients with dyspepsia have no obvious organic explanation for their symptoms and are classified as having functional dyspepsia (see sections above on dyspepsia and functional dyspepsia). Atypical gastroesophageal reflux may be manifested by epigastric symptoms. Biliary tract disease is characterized by discrete, intermittent episodes of pain that should not be confused with other causes of dyspepsia. Severe epigastric pain is atypical for peptic ulcer disease unless complicated by a perforation or penetration. Other causes include acute pancreatitis, acute cholecystitis or choledocholithiasis, esophageal rupture, gastric volvulus, and ruptured aortic aneurysm.

Pharmacologic Agents

The pharmacology of several agents that enhance the healing of peptic ulcers is briefly discussed here. They may be divided into three categories: (1) acid-antisecretory agents, (2) mucosal protective agents, and (3) agents that promote healing through eradication of *H pylori*. Recommendations for their use are provided in subsequent sections.

A. Acid-Antisecretory Agents:

1. Proton pump inhibitors–Proton pump inhibitors covalently bind the acid-secreting enzyme H^+-K^+ ATPase, or "proton pump," permanently inactivating it. Restoration of acid secretion requires synthesis of new pumps, which have a half-life of 18 hours. Thus, although these agents have a serum half-life of less than 60 minutes, their duration of action exceeds 24 hours. The four available agents, omeprazole or rabeprazole 20 mg, lansoprazole 15–30 mg, and pantoprazole 40 mg, inhibit over 90% of 24-hour acid secretion, compared with under 65% for H_2 receptor antagonists in standard dosages. Proton pump inhibitors should be administered 30 minutes before meals (usually breakfast).

Each of the four proton pump inhibitors results in over 90% healing of duodenal ulcers after 4 weeks and 90% of gastric ulcers after 8 weeks when given once daily. Compared with H_2 receptor antagonists, proton pump inhibitors provide faster pain relief and more rapid ulcer healing. However, nearly equivalent overall healing rates may be achieved with longer courses of H_2 receptor antagonists.

The proton pump inhibitors are remarkably safe in short-term therapy. Serum gastrin levels rise significantly (> 500 pg/mL) in 10% of patients receiving chronic therapy, which is associated with the development of gastric enterochromaffin-like cell hyperplasia in humans and gastric carcinoid tumors in rats. Although the question of safety of long-term therapy with proton pump inhibitors is unresolved, clinical experience in patients taking these agents for up to 5 years has not demonstrated toxicity. Long-term use may lead to a mild decrease in vitamin B_{12} and iron absorption, but the clinical significance of this is unclear. Long-term use is unnecessary in peptic ulcer disease but is frequently required in gastroesophageal reflux disease.

2. H_2 receptor antagonists–Four H_2 receptor antagonists are available: cimetidine, ranitidine, famotidine, and nizatidine. These agents competitively inhibit histamine binding to the H_2 receptor on the gastric parietal cell, thereby reducing intracellular cAMP levels and acid secretion. They profoundly inhibit basal and nocturnal acid output but are less effective at inhibiting meal-stimulated acid secretion. Thus, administration of these agents two to four times daily markedly raises nocturnal intragastric pH but has only a modest impact upon the daytime pH profile. For uncomplicated peptic ulcers, H_2 receptor antagonists may be administered twice daily or once daily at bedtime with equivalent efficacy. Recommended doses (once daily at bedtime) for the treatment of acute peptic ulcers are as follows: cimetidine 800 mg; ranitidine and nizatidine 300 mg; and famotidine 40 mg. Complete ulcer symptom relief usually occurs within 2 weeks. Duodenal ulcer healing rates of 85–90% are obtained within 6–8 weeks of therapy. Gastric ulcer healing rates are delayed by 2–4 weeks compared with duodenal ulcers, but 8 weeks of therapy is sufficient in most patients.

The H_2 receptor antagonists are extremely well tolerated, and serious side effects are rare. Central nervous system symptoms of headache, confusion, and lethargy occur with all agents in 1% of patients, especially with intravenous administration. Cimetidine inhibits hepatic P450 drug metabolism, raising the serum concentration of warfarin, theophylline, lidocaine, and phenytoin. Ranitidine binds P450 with only one tenth the avidity of cimetidine; famotidine and nizatidine have negligible effects. Cimetidine inhibits estradiol metabolism and dihydrotestosterone metabolism and may cause gynecomastia or impotence, especially at higher doses.

B. Agents Enhancing Mucosal Defenses:

1. Sucralfate–Sucralfate is a complex salt of sucrose containing aluminum and sulfate. The negatively charged sulfate groups bind to positively charged proteins in the ulcer base, forming a protective barrier against acid, bile, and pepsin. In addition, sucralfate stimulates mucus and bicarbonate secretion, stimulates prostaglandin production, and binds fibroblast growth factor. Sucralfate is unabsorbed and virtually devoid of side effects except for constipation. Because it binds some medications and inhibits their absorption, it should not be administered within 2 hours of other medications.

Sucralfate, 1 g four times daily, is equivalent in efficacy to H_2 receptor antagonists in the treatment of duodenal ulcers. Its efficacy in gastric ulcers is less well established.

2. Bismuth–Bismuth compounds in a variety of formulations have been used to treat dyspepsia, peptic ulcer disease, and diarrhea. The only agents currently available in the United States are bismuth subsalicylate and a combination agent, ranitidine bismuth citrate. Bismuth promotes ulcer healing through stimulation of mucosal bicarbonate and prostaglandin production. In addition, it has direct antibacterial action against *H pylori,* eradicating the organism in up to one-third of patients. Less than 1% of bismuth is absorbed and renally excreted. Salicylate is freely absorbed but does not achieve excessive levels at standard doses. In short-term use, bismuth compounds have excellent safety profiles. Darkening of the feces is expected. Rare cases of encephalopathy are reported in overdoses or after protracted courses of high-dose therapy.

3. Prostaglandin analogs (misoprostol)–Prostaglandin analogs promote ulcer healing by stimulating mucus and bicarbonate secretion and modest inhibition of acid secretion. Misoprostol is the only clinically available agent. It is less effective than other antiulcer agents in the treatment of active ulcers (including NSAID-induced ulcers). It is used solely as a prophylactic agent to prevent NSAID-induced ulcers. Misoprostol causes a dose-related diarrhea in 10–20% of patients. It may also stimulate uterine contractions and induce abortion.

4. Antacids–Low-dose aluminum- and magnesium-containing antacid regimens (120–240 mmol/d) promote ulcer healing through stimulation of gastric mucosal defenses, not by neutralization of gastric acidity. Given the greater compliance and efficacy of other antiulcer regimens, antacids are no longer used as first-line agents in the treatment of acute ulcers. Because of the rapid relief of ulcer symptoms that they provide, they are commonly used as needed to supplement other antiulcer therapies. High-dose regimens are associated with diarrhea, hypophosphatemia, and hypermagnesemia, but at standard low doses these adverse effects are infrequent.

C. *H pylori* Eradication Therapy: Eradication of *H pylori* has proved difficult. The agents that have demonstrated the greatest efficacy against *H pylori* are clarithromycin, metronidazole, amoxicillin, tetracycline, proton pump inhibitors, and bismuth. These agents, however, fail to achieve acceptable rates of *H pylori* eradication when used as monotherapy. Furthermore, resistance rapidly develops to metronidazole and clarithromycin but not to amoxicillin or tetracycline. Combination regimens that employ two antibiotics with either bismuth or proton pump inhibitors are required to achieve adequate rates of eradication and to decrease failures due to antibiotic resistance. Although myriad regimens have been tested, there is no established optimal treatment. In the United States, up to 50% of strains of *H pylori* are resistant to metronidazole and 7% are resistant to clarithromycin. It may be advisable to use amoxicillin in most patients, reserving metronidazole for patients allergic to penicillin. All currently recommended regimens should achieve greater than 85–90% rates of eradication after 1–2 weeks of treatment. Treatment regimens may be divided into two categories:

1. Regimens using proton pump inhibitors– Combination therapy with a proton pump inhibitor and two antibiotics (clarithromycin plus either amoxicillin or metronidazole) is highly efficacious in *H pylori* eradication. The proton pump inhibitors have direct antimicrobial action against *H pylori.* Furthermore, by raising intragastric pH, they suppress bacterial growth and optimize antibiotic efficacy. The two treatment regimens that currently are favored are listed in Table 14–11. These regimens achieve eradication rates of over 85%. The amoxicillin-based regimen is preferable in areas in which there is high resistance of *H pylori* to metronidazole. Although a dual eradication therapy regimen of omeprazole and clarithromycin has been approved by the FDA, its efficacy is only 70% and it cannot be recommended.

2. Regimens using bismuth compounds– Combinations of bismuth subsalicylate plus two antibiotics (tetracycline plus either metronidazole or clarithromycin) also achieve eradication rates of over 85% after 2 weeks of therapy. However, these regimens require four times daily dosing and are associated with a higher incidence of side effects than proton pump inhibitor regimens. The addition of a twice-daily proton pump inhibitor to this regimen (ie, "quadruple" therapy) may further enhance eradication rates to over 95%. Recent trials suggest that triple therapy with ranitidine bismuth citrate, cla-

Table 14–11. Treatment options for peptic ulcer disease.

Active *Helicobacter pylori*-associated ulcer:

1. Treat with anti-*H pylori* regimen for 10–14 days. Treatment options:

   Proton pump inhibitor twice daily[1]
   Clarithromycin 500 mg twice daily
   Amoxicillin 1 g twice daily OR metronidazole 500 mg twice daily

   Proton pump inhibitor twice daily[1]
   Bismuth subsalicylate two tablets four times daily
   Tetracycline 500 mg four times daily
   Metronidazole 250 mg four times daily

   Ranitidine bismuth citrate 400 mg twice daily
   Clarithromycin 500 mg twice daily
   Amoxicillin 1g OR tetracycline 500 mg OR metronidazole 500 mg twice daily

   (Proton pump inhibitors administered before meals. Avoid metronidazole regimens in areas of known high resistance or in patients who have failed a course of treatment that included metronidazole).

2. After completion of 10–14 day course of *H pylori* eradication therapy, continue treatment with proton pump inhibitor[1] once daily or H_2 receptor antagonist (as below) for 4–8 weeks to promote healing.

Active ulcer not attributable to *H pylori:*

Consider other causes: NSAIDs, Zollinger-Ellision syndrome, gastric malignancy. Treatment options:

Proton pump inhibitors[1]:
  Uncomplicated duodenal ulcer: treat for 4 weeks
  Uncomplicated gastric ulcer: treat for 8 weeks
H_2 receptor antagonists:
  Uncomplicated duodenal ulcer: cimetidine 800 mg, ranitidine or nizatidine 300 mg, famotidine 40 mg, once daily at bedtime for 6 weeks
  Uncomplicated gastric ulcer: cimetidine 400 mg, ranitidine or nizatidine 150 mg, famotidine 20 mg, twice daily for 8 weeks
  Complicated ulcers: proton pump inhibitors are preferred drugs

Prevention of ulcer relapse:

1. NSAID-induced ulcer: prophylactic therapy for high-risk patients (prior ulcer disease or ulcer complications, use of corticosteroids or anticoagulants, age > 70 with serious comorbid illnesses).
   Treatment options:

   Proton pump inhibitor once daily
   COX-2 selective NSAID (rofecoxib, celecoxib)
   Misoprostol 100–200 μg four times daily

2. Chronic "maintenance" therapy indicated in patients with recurrent ulcers who either are *H pylori*-negative or who have failed attempts at eradication therapy: once daily proton pump inhibitor[1] or H_2 receptor antagonist at bedtime (cimetidine 400–800 mg, nizatidine or ranitidine 150–300 mg, famotidine 20–40 mg)

[1]Proton pump inhibitors: omeprazole 20 mg, rabeprazole 20 mg, lansoprazole 30 mg, pantoprazole 40 mg.

rithromycin, and amoxicillin results in over 90% eradication (compared with only 70% for ranitidine bismuth citrate and clarithromycin alone). This regimen (which is less expensive than proton pump inhibitor regimens) now may be recommended. The regimens that currently can be recommended are listed in Table 14–11. In areas in which there is high metronidazole resistance, clarithromycin, 500 mg three times daily, may be substituted.

Medical Treatment

Patients should be encouraged to eat balanced meals at regular intervals. There is no justification for bland or restrictive diets. Moderate alcohol intake is not harmful. Smoking retards the rate of ulcer healing and increases the frequency of recurrences and should be discouraged.

A. Treatment of *H pylori*-Associated Ulcers:

1. Treatment of active ulcer–The goals of treatment of active *H pylori*-associated ulcers are to relieve dyspeptic symptoms, to promote ulcer healing, and to eradicate *H pylori* infection. Uncomplicated *H pylori*-associated ulcers should be treated for the first 10–14 days with one of the proton pump inhibitor-based *H pylori* eradication regimens listed in Table 14–11. In addition to eliminating *H pylori,* the antisecretory effects of proton pump inhibitors provide rapid, effective symptom relief. It is recommended that an antisecretory agent be administered for an additional period after completion of antibiotic therapy for both gastric and duodenal ulcers to ensure symptom relief and ulcer healing. For duodenal ulcers, this is most conveniently done by continuing a proton pump inhibitor once daily for an additional 2 weeks (4 weeks total). For gastric ulcers, the proton pump inhibitor should be continued for 6 additional weeks (8 weeks total). Alternatively, after completion of the 2-week course of *H pylori* eradication therapy, H_2 receptor antagonists or sucralfate can be given for 6–8 weeks. Confirmation of *H pylori* eradication in patients with uncomplicated ulcers is not recommended.

2. Therapy to prevent recurrence–Prior to the recognition of the importance of *H pylori* in ulcer pathogenesis, the recurrence rate of peptic ulcers was over 80% per year. For that reason, patients with frequent ulcer recurrences or ulcer complications were maintained on continuous therapy with half-dose bedtime H_2 receptor antagonists (cimetidine 400 mg, ranitidine 150 mg, famotidine 20 mg). These "maintenance" regimens reduced the symptomatic ulcer recurrence rate to less than 15% per year and the rate of ulcer complications.

Since successful eradication reduces ulcer recurrence rates to less than 20%, all patients with a history of peptic ulcer disease (active or inactive) and *H pylori* infection should be given a course of eradication therapy. The most common cause of ulcer recurrence after antibiotic therapy is failure to achieve successful eradication, which should be evaluated. Once cure has been achieved, reinfection rates are less than 0.5% per year. Although *H pylori* eradication has dramatically reduced the need for maintenance H_2 receptor antagonist therapy, there remains a subset of patients who require chronic treatment. These include patients with *H pylori*-negative recurrent ulcers, patients with *H pylori*-positive recurrent ulcers who have failed eradication therapy, and patients with a history of *H pylori*-positive ulcers who have recurrent ulcers despite successful eradication. Surreptitious NSAID ingestion and hypersecretory states (such as gastrinoma) should be excluded in these patients.

C. Treatment of NSAID-Associated Ulcers:

1. Treatment of active ulcers–In patients with NSAID-induced ulcers, the offending agent should be discontinued whenever possible. Both gastric and duodenal ulcers respond rapidly to therapy with H_2 receptor antagonists, proton pump inhibitors, or sucralfate (Table 14–11) once NSAIDs are eliminated. In some patients with severe inflammatory diseases, it may not be feasible to discontinue NSAIDs. Although most uncomplicated ulcers will heal with twice-daily H_2 receptor antagonists or misoprostol, 200 μg four times daily, despite continued NSAID ingestion, ulcer healing is delayed. Therefore, patients with active ulcers or multiple erosions should be treated with proton pump inhibitors once daily, which result in ulcer healing rates of approximately 80% at 8 weeks versus 71% for misoprostol and 63% for H_2 receptor antagonists in patients continuing to take NSAIDs.

H pylori infection does not appear to increase the risk of NSAID-induced ulcers. Nevertheless, about half of patients who develop ulcers while using NSAIDs are infected with *H pylori,* and in such cases it is impossible to be certain which is the primary pathogenetic factor. Therefore, antibiotic eradication therapy should be given for NSAID-induced ulcers when *H pylori* tests are positive.

2. Prevention of NSAID-induced ulcers–The prostaglandin analog misoprostol is effective in the prevention of NSAID-induced gastric and duodenal ulcers and is the only agent approved by the FDA for this purpose. When coadministered with NSAIDs, misoprostol, 200 μg three or four times daily, reduces the incidence of endoscopically visualized peptic ulcers from 20% to less than 5%. Misoprostol has recently been demonstrated to reduce NSAID-induced ulcer complications by 40% in a clinical setting. Recent reports suggest that once-daily proton pump inhibitors are equivalent or superior to misoprostol for the prevention of endoscopically visible ulcers, but their impact upon NSAID-induced ulcer complications is untested. In two large multicenter trials of patients with a history of NSAID-induced ulcers, the incidence of recurrent ulcers at 6 months was 30–40% in patients treated with omeprazole 20 mg daily, 40%

with ranitidine 150 mg twice daily, and 50% with misoprostol 200 μg twice daily. Proton pump inhibitors have not been compared with misoprostol given three or four times daily (a more efficacious dosage regimen).

Determining the most cost-effective approach to the prevention of NSAID-induced complications is difficult. Although the incidence of NSAID-induced ulcers is high, most of these are clinically silent and of no consequence. The goal of prophylactic therapy is to prevent ulcer complications, which occur in only 1–2% of NSAID-treated patients per year. Therefore, prophylactic therapy should be reserved for patients at high risk of developing complications. Risk factors include a history of ulcer disease or complications, concurrent therapy with corticosteroids or anticoagulants, serious underlying medical illness, and age over 70 years. Such patients have a 5% or greater risk per year of developing a complicated ulcer on a traditional (nonselective NSAID). Whenever possible, NSAIDs should be avoided in this high-risk population. If NSAIDs must be given, either a COX-2 selective NSAID should be given or prophylactic therapy with a proton pump inhibitor or misoprostol. In data pooled from several large prospective trials, it appears that the relative risk of a clinically significant symptomatic ulcer or ulcer complication is approximately 0.5 in patients treated with COX-2 selective NSAIDs (celecoxib and rofecoxib) compared with conventional NSAIDs. However, this amounts to an absolute risk reduction from 2% to 1% per year, ie, for every 100 patients treated with a COX-2 selective inhibitor instead of a conventional NSAID, one clinically significant ulcer per year may be prevented. Alternatively, a traditional (nonselective) NSAID may be given with a once-daily proton pump inhibitor (omeprazole or rabeprazole 20 mg, lansoprazole 30 mg, pantoprazole 40 mg). Of note, the relative risks and benefits of COX-2 selective NSAIDs versus combination therapy with traditional NSAIDs and a proton pump inhibitor have not been evaluated in patients specifically deemed at high risk for NSAID complications. Thus, the optimal cost-effective approach to high-risk patients is unknown. The prescription costs of a COX-2 selective agent are slightly less than a combination of a generic nonselective NSAID and a proton pump inhibitor. Although prophylactic therapy with misoprostol 100–200 μg three or four times daily is effective in reducing NSAID-induced complications, the requirements for frequent dosing and the high incidence (10–20%) of gastrointestinal side effects have limited the clinical use of this agent. Patients with a history of ulcer disease should be screened for *H pylori* and treated if positive. Otherwise, there is no convincing evidence that screening for and treating *H pylori* reduces the incidence of endoscopic ulcers or ulcer complications in average or high-risk patients given NSAIDs.

D. Refractory Ulcers: Ulcers that are truly refractory to medical therapy are now uncommon. Less than 5% of ulcers are unhealed after 8 weeks of therapy with proton pump inhibitors. Noncompliance is the most common cause of ulcer nonhealing. Cigarettes retard ulcer healing and should be proscribed. NSAID and aspirin use, sometimes surreptitious, are commonly implicated in refractory ulcers and must be stopped. *H pylori* eradication enhances healing and decreases the high recurrence rates of refractory ulcers. Therefore, evidence of *H pylori* infection should be sought and the infection treated, if present, in all refractory ulcer patients. Fasting serum gastrin levels should be obtained to exclude gastrinoma with acid hypersecretion (Zollinger-Ellison syndrome). Nonhealing gastric ulcers raise concerns that an undiagnosed gastric malignancy may be masquerading as a benign gastric ulcer. Repeat ulcer biopsies are mandatory after 2–3 months of therapy in all nonhealed gastric ulcers, and they should be followed with serial endoscopies to verify complete healing. Almost all benign refractory ulcers heal within 8 weeks with a proton pump inhibitor twice daily (omeprazole or rabeprazole 20 mg twice daily, lansoprazole 30 mg twice daily). Patients with persistent nonhealing ulcers should be referred for surgical therapy after careful exclusion of NSAID use and persistent *H pylori* infection.

[CDC: *Helicobacter pylori* and Peptic Ulcer Disease] http://www.cdc.gov/ncidod/dbmd/hpylori.htm

Ciociola A et al: *Helicobacter pylori* infection rates in duodenal ulcer patients in the United States may be lower than previously estimated. Am J Gastroenterol 1999; 94:1834. [NLM Cit ID: 99332877]

Faigel D et al: Evaluation of rapid antibody tests for the diagnosis of *Helicobacter pylori* infection. Am J Gastroenterol 2000;95:72. [NLM Cit ID: 20102100]

Feldman M et al: Do cyclooxygenase-2 inhibitors provide benefits similar to those of traditional nonsteroidal anti-inflammatory drugs, with less gastrointestinal toxicity? Ann Intern Med 2000;132:134. [NLM Cit ID: 20092386]

Hawkey C et al: Omeprazole compared with misoprostol for ulcers associated with nonsteroidal anti-inflammatory drugs. N Engl J Med 1998;338:727. [NLM Cit ID: 98145773]

Houben M et al: A systematic review of *Helicobacter pylori* eradication therapy—the impact of antimicrobial resistance on eradication rates. Aliment Pharmacol Ther 1999;13:1047. [NLM Cit ID: 99398948]

Langman M et al: Adverse upper gastrointestinal effect of rofecoxib compared with NSAIDs. JAMA 1999;282: 1929. [NLM Cit ID: 20046403]

Proceedings of American Digestive Health Foundation International Update Conference on *Helicobacter pylori*. Gastroenterology 1997;113(6 Suppl):S1. (Outstanding review of epidemiology, pathogenesis, relationships to gastric cancer, relationship to dyspepsia, diagnosis, treatment, and research needs.)

Schoenfeld P et al: Nonsteroidal anti-inflammatory drug-associated gastrointestinal complications—guidelines for prevention and treatment. Aliment Pharmacol Ther 1999;13:1273. [NLM Cit ID: 20009940]

Yeomans N et al: A comparison of omeprazole with ranitidine for ulcers associated with nonsteroidal anti-inflammatory drugs. N Engl J Med 1998;338:719. [NLM Cit ID: 98145772]

COMPLICATIONS OF PEPTIC ULCER DISEASE

1. GASTROINTESTINAL HEMORRHAGE

Essentials of Diagnosis

- "Coffee grounds" emesis, hematemesis, melena, or hematochezia.
- Emergent upper endoscopy is diagnostic and therapeutic.

General Considerations

Approximately 50% of all episodes of upper gastrointestinal bleeding are due to peptic ulcer. Clinically significant bleeding occurs in 10–20% of ulcer patients. About 80% of patients stop bleeding spontaneously and generally have an uneventful recovery; the remainder have more severe bleeding. The overall mortality rate for ulcer bleeding is 6–10%, but it is higher in the elderly, in patients with comorbid medical problems, and in patients with nosocomial bleeding. Mortality is also higher in patients who present with persistent hypertension or shock, bright red blood in the vomitus or nasogastric lavage fluid, or severe coagulopathy.

Clinical Findings

A. Symptoms and Signs: Up to 20% of patients have no antecedent symptoms of pain; this is particularly true of patients receiving NSAIDs. Common presenting signs include melena and hematemesis. Massive upper gastrointestinal bleeding or rapid gastrointestinal transit may result in hematochezia rather than melena; this may be misinterpreted as signifying a lower tract bleeding source. Nasogastric lavage that demonstrates "coffee grounds" or bright red blood confirms an upper tract source. Recovered nasogastric lavage fluid that is negative for blood does not exclude active bleeding from a duodenal ulcer.

B. Laboratory Findings: The hematocrit may fall as a result of bleeding or expansion of the intravascular volume with intravenous fluids. The BUN may rise as a result of absorption of blood nitrogen from the small intestine and prerenal azotemia.

Treatment

The assessment and initial management of upper gastrointestinal tract bleeding is discussed elsewhere in this chapter. Specific issues pertaining to peptic ulcer bleeding are described below.

A. Medical Therapy: A number of pharmacologic agents, including acid inhibitory agents (H_2 receptor antagonists and proton pump inhibitors) and agents that reduce splanchnic blood flow (vasopressin, octreotide), have been used in patients with peptic ulcer bleeding in an attempt to arrest active bleeding and prevent recurrent bleeding. Since ulcer bleeding abates spontaneously in at least 80% of patients without any therapy, it is not surprising that the majority of these trials have been unable to demonstrate any benefit from pharmacologic therapy, in part due to inadequate sample sizes and in part because these agents were given to all patients admitted with ulcer bleeding rather than just those at highest risk of rebleeding.

Recently, four placebo-controlled trials have been reported in which either intravenous omeprazole (not available in the United States) or high-dose oral omeprazole (40 mg twice daily) was administered to patients with peptic ulcers whose appearance suggested a high risk for rebleeding (defined as active bleeding or oozing, visible vessels, or adherent clots). In two of these studies, appropriate endoscopic hemostasis treatment also was applied to the ulcers, but in two other studies standard endoscopic treatment was not applied. The four studies demonstrated a significant reduction in rebleeding, transfusions, and need for further endoscopic therapy. Although these studies require further confirmation, their potential benefits and relatively minimal cost supports the use of high-dose oral proton pump inhibitors (two capsules or pills twice daily for 5 days) in patients with bleeding ulcers whose endoscopic appearance suggests a high risk of rebleeding. Increasingly, many physicians choose to administer a high dose of a proton pump inhibitor (eg, omeprazole 40 mg or lansoprazole 60 mg) prior to endoscopy to all patients admitted to the hospital with a gastrointestinal bleed which is suspected to be caused by a peptic ulcer. Pantoprazole is less expensive and readily administered to most patients.

The efficacy of intravenous somatostatin or octreotide in the management of peptic ulcer bleeding has not been convincingly demonstrated in individual therapeutic trials. Nevertheless, a recent meta-analysis of 14 trials detected a significant risk reduction in rebleeding with these agents. If octreotide indeed is effective, it is not clear at this time what its therapeutic role should be. Whether octreotide should be administered after endoscopy to patients with high-risk ulcers or patients who rebleed despite endoscopic therapy requires further study.

One-third of patients with a history of bleeding ulcers develop recurrent ulcer hemorrhage within 3 years if no specific therapy is given. Chronic acid suppression with a bedtime maintenance dose of an H_2 antagonist (ranitidine, 150 mg daily) reduces the risk of ulcer rebleeding to less than 10%. Unblinded trials have demonstrated that in patients with bleeding ulcers who are *H pylori*-positive, successful eradication of *H pylori* effectively prevents recurrent ulcer bleeding in virtually all cases. It is therefore recommended that all patients with bleeding peptic ulcers be tested for *H pylori.* If positive, treatment should be initiated once patients resume oral feedings. Four to 8 weeks after completion of antibiotic therapy, testing should be done with a urea breath test or endoscopy to confirm successful eradication. In patients in whom *H pylori* infection persists, chronic H_2 antagonist or proton pump therapy should be prescribed.

B. Endoscopy: Endoscopy is the preferred diagnostic procedure in virtually all cases of upper gastrointestinal bleeding because of its high diagnostic accuracy, its ability to predict the likelihood of recurrent bleeding, and its availability for therapeutic intervention in high-risk lesions. Endoscopy should be performed within 12–24 hours in virtually all cases. In cases of severe active bleeding, endoscopy is performed as soon as patients have been appropriately resuscitated and are hemodynamically stable.

On the basis of clinical and endoscopic criteria, it is possible to predict which patients are at a higher risk of rebleeding and therefore to make more rational use of hospital resources. Nonbleeding ulcers under 2 cm in size with a base that is clean have a less than 5% chance of rebleeding. Most young (under age 60), otherwise healthy patients with clean-based ulcers may be monitored in the emergency room or on the hospital ward for 24 hours before discharge. Low-risk patients can be safely discharged from the hospital or emergency room immediately after endoscopy. Ulcers that have only a flat red or black spot have a less than 10% chance of significant rebleeding, and those with a firmly adherent clot have a 10–22% rebleeding risk. Patients who are hemodynamically stable with these findings should be admitted to a hospital ward for 48–72 hours and may begin immediate oral feedings and antiulcer (or anti-*H pylori*) medication.

By contrast, the risk of rebleeding or continued bleeding in ulcers with a nonbleeding visible vessel is 43%, and with active bleeding it is 70%. Endoscopic therapy with injection or thermocoagulation techniques now is the standard of care for such lesions because it reduces the risk of rebleeding, the number of transfusions, and the need for subsequent surgery. Injection is performed into and around the ulcer vessel with epinephrine (1:10,000). Thermocoagulation is achieved with contact cautery probes applied directly to the ulcer vessel. Using any of these techniques, successful hemostasis of actively bleeding lesions is achieved in 90%. For actively bleeding ulcers, a combination of epinephrine injection followed by thermocoagulation yields better control of bleeding than either modality alone. Significant rebleeding occurs in 10–20% of cases, of which over 70% can be managed successfully with repeat endoscopic treatment. After endoscopic therapy, the risk of rebleeding declines significantly over 3 days to less than 3%. Patients with these high-risk lesions should be monitored in an ICU setting for a minimum period of 24 hours and should remain hospitalized for at least 72 hours.

C. Surgical Treatment: Patients with high-risk endoscopic lesions and those whose condition warrants ICU admission should be evaluated by a surgeon. However, less than 10% of patients treated with hemostatic therapy require surgery for continued or recurrent bleeding. Overall surgical mortality for emergency ulcer bleeding is less than 6%. The prognosis is poorer for patients over age 60, those with serious underlying medical illnesses or chronic renal failure, and those who require more than 10 units of blood transfusion.

2. ULCER PERFORATION

Perforations develop in 5% of ulcer patients, usually from ulcers on the anterior wall of the stomach or duodenum. The incidence of perforations may be increasing, perhaps as a consequence of using NSAIDs or crack cocaine. Zollinger-Ellison disease should be considered in patients who present with ulcer perforation. Perforation results in a chemical peritonitis that causes sudden, severe generalized abdominal pain that prompts most patients to seek immediate attention. Elderly or debilitated patients and those receiving chronic steroid therapy may experience minimal initial symptoms, presenting late with bacterial peritonitis, sepsis, and shock. On physical examination, patients appear ill, with a rigid, quiet abdomen and rebound tenderness. Hypotension is not a feature of early ulcer perforation but develops later after bacterial peritonitis has developed. If hypotension is present early with the onset of pain, one should consider other abdominal catastrophes such as a ruptured aortic aneurysm, mesenteric infarction, or acute pancreatitis. Leukocytosis is almost always present. A mildly elevated serum amylase (less than twice normal) is sometimes seen. Upright or decubitus films of the abdomen reveal free intraperitoneal air in 75% of cases, and in most cases this establishes the diagnosis without need for further studies. The absence of free air may lead to a misdiagnosis of pancreatitis, cholecystitis, or appendicitis. Upper gastrointestinal radiography with water-soluble contrast may be useful in this setting. Barium studies are contraindicated in patients with possible perforation.

Traditional surgical dogma held that the majority of patients with perforated ulcers should undergo emergency laparotomy. Closure of the perforation was performed with an omental ("Graham") patch and, in stable patients, a proximal gastric vagotomy was performed to decrease the chance of ulcer recurrence. This approach is changing as a result of two factors. The first is minimally invasive surgical technique. Laparoscopic perforation closure can be performed in many centers, significantly reducing operative morbidity. Second is the recognition that *H pylori* infection is associated with most ulcers and ulcer perforations. Postoperative treatment of *H pylori* reduces the risk of ulcer recurrence, obviating the need for intraoperative vagotomy. The overall mortality rate in patients treated surgically is 5%.

Up to 40% of ulcer perforations seal spontaneously by the adherence of omentum or adjacent organs to the lesion and do not have significant intraperitoneal spillage. Thus, some centers advocate initial nonoperative management for patients whose onset of symptoms is less than 12 hours and whose upper gastrointestinal series with water-soluble contrast medium does not demonstrate leakage. At present, such conservative therapy is most appropriate for patients who are poor operative candidates. Patients should be monitored closely while receiving fluids, nasogastric suction, antisecretory agents, and broad-spectrum antibiotics. If their condition deteriorates over the first 12 hours (as evidenced by increasing pain, rising pulse or temperature, or worsening peritonitis), they should be taken to the operating room.

3. ULCER PENETRATION

An ulcer located along the posterior wall of the duodenum or stomach may perforate into contiguous structures such as the pancreas, liver, or biliary tree. Patients complain of a change in the intensity and rhythmicity of their ulcer symptoms. The pain becomes more severe and constant, may radiate to the back, and is unresponsive to antacids or food. Physical examination and laboratory tests are nonspecific. Mild amylase elevations may sometimes occur. Endoscopy and barium x-ray studies confirm the ulceration but are not diagnostic of an actual penetration. Patients should be given intravenous H_2 receptor antagonists (as above) or omeprazole, 40 mg/d, and followed closely. Those who fail to improve should be considered for surgical therapy.

4. GASTRIC OUTLET OBSTRUCTION

Gastric outlet obstruction occurs in 2% of patients with ulcer disease and is due to edema or cicatricial narrowing of the pylorus or duodenal bulb. Most patients have a prior known history of ulcer disease. Obstruction is less commonly caused by gastric neoplasms or extrinsic duodenal obstruction by intra-abdominal neoplasms. The most common symptoms are early satiety, vomiting, and weight loss. Early symptoms are epigastric fullness or heaviness after meals. Later, vomiting may develop that typically occurs one to several hours after eating and consists of partially digested food contents. Chronic obstruction may result in a grossly dilated, atonic stomach, severe weight loss, and malnutrition. Patients may develop dehydration, metabolic alkalosis, and hypokalemia. On physical examination, a succussion splash may be heard in the epigastrium. In most cases, nasogastric aspiration will result in evacuation of a large amount (> 200 mL) of foul-smelling fluid, which establishes the diagnosis. More subtle obstruction is diagnosed by a saline load test or by a nuclear gastric emptying study. Patients are treated initially with intravenous isotonic saline and KCl to correct fluid and electrolyte disorders, intravenous H_2 receptor antagonists (see treatment of stress gastritis, above), and nasogastric decompression of the stomach. Severely malnourished patients should receive total parenteral nutrition. Upper endoscopy is performed after 24–72 hours to define the nature of the obstruction and to exclude gastric neoplasm. At 72 hours, all patients should be evaluated with a saline load test. A positive test consists of more than 400 mL of residual volume 30 minutes after instillation of 750 mL of 0.9% saline into the stomach by nasogastric tube. Patients with a negative load test may be started on clear liquids and their diet advanced as tolerated. The remainder should remain on nasogastric suction for 5–7 days. Traditionally, patients unimproved after that time have been recommended for surgical treatment with vagotomy and either pyloroplasty or antrectomy. However, upper endoscopy with dilation of the gastric obstruction by hydrostatic balloons passed through the instrument has achieved success in two-thirds of patients. It may be reasonable to pursue dilation first in patients with milder symptoms, reserving surgery for those who fail to respond.

Chan F, Sung J: The medical care of patients with gastrointestinal bleeding after endoscopy. Gastrointest Endosc Clin North Am 1997;7:671. [NLM Cit ID: 98015837]

Donovan A et al: Perforated duodenal ulcer. Arch Surg 1998;133:1166. [NLM Cit ID: 99036231]

Lau JY et al: Endoscopic retreatment compared with surgery in patients with recurrent bleeding after initial endoscopic control of bleeding ulcers. N Engl J Med 1999;340:751. [NLM Cit ID: 99156341]

Lin HJ et al: A prospective randomized comparative trial showing that omeprazole prevents rebleeding in patients with bleeding peptic ulcers after successful endoscopic therapy. Arch Intern Med 1998;158:54. [NLM Cit ID: 98100025]

Longstreth G et al: Successful outpatient management of acute gastrointestinal hemorrhage: use of practice guidelines in a large patient series. Gastrointest Endosc 1998;47:219. [NLM Cit ID: 98199940]

ZOLLINGER-ELLISON SYNDROME (Gastrinoma)

Essentials of Diagnosis

- Peptic ulcer disease; may be severe and atypical.
- Gastric acid hypersecretion.

- Diarrhea common, relieved by nasogastric suction.
- Most cases are sporadic; 25% with MEN 1.

General Considerations

Zollinger-Ellison syndrome is caused by gastrin-secreting gut neuroendocrine tumors (gastrinomas), which result in hypergastrinemia and acid hypersecretion. Less than 1% of peptic ulcer disease is caused by gastrinomas. Primary gastrinomas may arise in the pancreas (25%), duodenal wall (45%), or lymph nodes (5–15%), and in other locations or of unknown primary in 20%. Approximately 80% arise within the "gastrinoma triangle" bounded by the porta hepatis, the neck of the pancreas, and the third portion of the duodenum. Most gastrinomas are solitary or multifocal nodules that are potentially resectable. Over two-thirds of gastrinomas are malignant, and one-third have already metastasized to the liver at initial presentation. Approximately 25% of patients have small multicentric gastrinomas associated with MEN 1 that are more difficult to resect.

Clinical Findings

A. Symptoms and Signs: Over 90% of patients with Zollinger-Ellison syndrome develop peptic ulcers. In most cases, the symptoms are indistinguishable from other causes of peptic ulcer disease and therefore may go undetected for years. Ulcers usually are solitary and located in the duodenal bulb, but they may be multiple or occur more distally in the duodenum. Isolated gastric ulcers do not occur. Gastroesophageal reflux symptoms occur often. Diarrhea occurs in one-third of patients, in some cases in the absence of peptic symptoms. Gastric acid hypersecretion can cause direct intestinal mucosal injury and pancreatic enzyme inactivation, resulting in diarrhea, steatorrhea, and weight loss; nasogastric aspiration of stomach acid stops the diarrhea. Screening for Zollinger-Ellison syndrome with fasting gastrin levels should be obtained in patients with ulcers that are refractory to standard therapies, giant ulcers (> 2 cm), ulcers located distal to the duodenal bulb, multiple duodenal ulcers, frequent ulcer recurrences, ulcers associated with diarrhea, ulcers occurring after ulcer surgery, and patients with ulcer complications. Ulcer patients with hypercalcemia or family histories of ulcers (suggesting MEN 1) should also be screened. Finally, patients with peptic ulcers who are *H pylori*-negative and who are not taking NSAIDs should be screened.

B. Laboratory Findings: The most sensitive and specific method for identifying Zollinger-Ellison syndrome is demonstration of an increased fasting serum gastrin concentration (> 150 pg/mL). Levels should be obtained with patients not taking H_2 receptor antagonists for 24 hours or omeprazole for 6 days. The median gastrin level is 500–700 pg/mL, and 60% have levels less than 1000 pg/mL. Hypochlorhydria with increased gastric pH is a much more common cause of hypergastrinemia than is gastrinoma. Therefore, a measurement of gastric pH (and, where available, gastric secretory studies) is performed in patients with fasting hypergastrinemia. Most patients have a basal acid output of over 15 meq/h. A gastric pH of > 3.0 implies hypochlorhydria and excludes gastrinoma. In a patient with a serum gastrin level of > 1000 pg/mL and acid hypersecretion, the diagnosis of Zollinger-Ellison syndrome is established. With lower gastrin levels (150–1000 pg/mL) and acid secretion, a secretin stimulation test is performed to distinguish Zollinger-Ellison syndrome from other causes of hypergastrinemia. Intravenous secretin (2 units/kg) produces a rise in serum gastrin of over 200 pg/mL within 2–30 minutes in 85% of patients with gastrinoma. Recently, the sole manufacturer of secretin in the United States ceased distribution, and as of mid 2000 the agent is not commercially available. An elevated serum calcium suggests hyperparathyroidism and MEN 1 syndrome. In all patients with Zollinger-Ellison syndrome, a serum PTH, prolactin, LH-FSH, and GH level should be obtained to exclude MEN 1.

C. Imaging: The approach to therapy is determined in large part by whether there is metastatic disease. Therefore, imaging studies are obtained in an attempt to determine whether there is metastatic disease and, if not, to identify the site of the primary tumor. Although conventional radiologic studies such as CT, MRI, and transabdominal ultrasound are commonly obtained, their sensitivity is less than 50–70% for hepatic metastases and 35% for primary tumors. These studies are being supplanted by somatostatin receptor scintigraphy (SRS) and endoscopic ultrasonography (EUS). The former should be the first study obtained because of its high sensitivity (> 90%) for detecting hepatic metastases, though its sensitivity for detecting the primary gastrinoma is much lower, particularly for primary tumors in the pancreas. If SRS is positive for tumor localization, further imaging studies are not necessary. In patients with negative SRS, endoscopic ultrasonography (EUS) is indicated in an effort to localize the primary tumor. This study has a sensitivity of > 90% for tumors of the pancreatic head and can visualize half of tumors in the duodenal wall or adjacent lymph nodes. With a combination of SRS and EUS, more than 90% of primary gastrinomas now can be localized preoperatively.

Differential Diagnosis

Gastrinomas are one of several gut neuroendocrine tumors that have similar histopathologic features and arise either from the gut or pancreas. These include carcinoid, insulinoma, VIPoma, glucagonoma, and somatostatinoma. These tumors usually are differentiated by the gut peptides that they secrete; however, poorly differentiated neuroendocrine tumors may not secrete any hormones. Gut neuroendocrine tumors may present in a number of ways. Functional symptoms arise from the effects of the secreted hormones (eg, Zollinger-Ellison syndrome, carcinoid syndrome). In other cases, patients may present with symptoms caused by tumor metastases (jaundice, hepatomegaly) rather than functional symptoms. Once a diagnosis of a neuroendocrine tumor is established from the liver biopsy, the specific type of tumor can subsequently be determined. Finally, both carcinoids and gastrinomas may be detected incidentally during endoscopy after biopsy of a submucosal nodule and must be distinguished by subsequent studies.

Hypergastrinemia due to gastrinoma must be distinguished from other causes of hypergastrinemia. Atrophic gastritis with decreased acid secretion is detected by gastric secretory analysis. Other conditions associated with hypergastrinemia (eg, gastric outlet obstruction, vagotomy, chronic renal failure) are associated with a negative secretin stimulation test.

Treatment

A. Metastatic Disease: The most important predictor of survival is the presence of hepatic metastases. In patients with multiple hepatic metastases, initial therapy should be directed at controlling hypersecretion. Proton pump inhibitors (omeprazole, rabeprazole, pantoprazole, or lansoprazole) are given at a dose of 40–120 mg/d, titrated to achieve a basal acid output of < 10 meq/h. At this level, there is complete symptomatic relief and ulcer healing. In patients with isolated hepatic metastases, surgical resection may decrease the need for antisecretory medications and may prolong survival. Owing to the slow growth of these tumors, 30% of patients with hepatic metastases have a survival of 10 years.

B. Localized Disease: Cure can be achieved only if the gastrinoma can be resected before hepatic metastatic spread has occurred. Lymph node metastases do not adversely affect prognosis. Laparotomy should be considered in all patients in whom preoperative studies fail to demonstrate hepatic or other distant metastases. A combination of preoperative studies and intraoperative palpation and sonography allows successful localization and resection in the majority of cases. The 15-year survival of patients who do not have liver metastases at initial presentation is over 80%.

Proye C et al: Noninvasive imaging of insulinomas and gastrinomas with endoscopic ultrasonography and somatostatin receptor scintigraphy. Surgery 1998;124:1143. [NLM Cit ID: 99071759]

BENIGN TUMORS OF THE STOMACH

Gastric epithelial polyps are usually detected incidentally at endoscopy. The majority are hyperplastic polyps, which are small, single or multiple, have no malignant potential, and do not require removal or endoscopic surveillance. Adenomatous polyps account for 10–20% of gastric polyps. They are usually solitary lesions. In rare instances they ulcerate, causing chronic blood loss. Because of their premalignant potential, endoscopic removal is indicated. Annual endoscopic surveillance is recommended to screen for further polyp development. Submucosal gastric polypoid lesions include leiomyoma and pancreatic rests.

MALIGNANT TUMORS OF THE STOMACH

1. GASTRIC ADENOCARCINOMA

Essentials of Diagnosis

- Dyspeptic symptoms with weight loss in patients over age 40.
- Iron deficiency anemia; occult blood in stools.
- Abnormality detected on upper gastrointestinal series or endoscopy.

General Considerations

Although gastric adenocarcinoma is the most common cancer (other than skin cancer) worldwide, its incidence in the United States has declined by two-thirds over the last 30 years to 20,000 cases annually. Gastric cancer is uncommon under age 40; the mean age at diagnosis is 63 years. Men are affected twice as often as women. The incidence is higher in Hispanics, African-Americans, and Asian Americans. Certain regions such as Chile, Colombia, Central America, and Japan have rates as high as 80 per 100,000 population. Although most gastric cancers arise in the antrum, the incidence of proximal tumors of the cardia and fundus is increasing dramatically.

Chronic *H pylori* gastritis is a strong risk factor for gastric carcinoma of the distal (but not proximal) stomach, increasing the relative risk four- to sixfold. It is estimated that 35–89% of cases of distal gastric carcinoma may be attributable to *H pylori*. Less than 1% of chronically infected individuals will develop carcinoma. Other risk factors for gastric cancer include chronic atrophic gastritis with intestinal metaplasia (often secondary to chronic *H pylori* infection), pernicious anemia, and a history of partial gastric resection more than 15 years previously.

Gastric cancer may occur in a variety of morphologic types: (1) polypoid or fungating intraluminal masses; (2) ulcerating masses; (3) diffusely spreading (linitis plastica), in which the tumor spreads through the submucosa, resulting in a rigid, atonic stomach with thickened folds (prognosis dismal); and (4) superficially spreading or "early" gastric cancer—confined to the mucosa or submucosa (with or without lymph node metastases) and associated with an excellent prognosis.

Clinical Findings

A. Symptoms and Signs: Gastric carcinoma is generally asymptomatic until the disease is quite advanced. Symptoms are nonspecific and are determined in part by the location of the tumor. Dyspepsia, vague epigastric pain, anorexia, early satiety, and weight loss are the presenting symptoms in most patients. Patients may derive initial symptomatic relief from over-the-counter remedies, further delaying diagnosis. Ulcerating lesions can lead to acute gastrointestinal bleeding with hematemesis or melena. Pyloric obstruction results in postprandial vomiting. Lower esophageal obstruction causes progressive dysphagia. Physical examination is rarely helpful. A gastric mass is palpated in less than one-fifth of patients. Signs of metastatic spread include a left supraclavicular lymph node (Virchow's node), an umbilical nodule (Sister Mary Joseph nodule), a rigid rectal shelf (Blumer's shelf), and ovarian metastases (Krukenberg tumor). Guaiac-positive stools may be detectable.

B. Laboratory Findings: Iron deficiency anemia due to chronic blood loss or anemia of chronic disease is common. Liver function test abnormalities may be present if there is metastatic liver spread. Other tumor markers are of no value.

C. Endoscopy: Upper endoscopy should be obtained in all patients over age 45 with new onset of epigastric symptoms (dyspepsia) and in anyone with dyspepsia that is persistent or fails to respond to a short trial of antisecretory therapy. Endoscopy with cytologic brushings and biopsies of suspicious lesions is highly sensitive for detecting gastric carcinoma. It can be difficult to obtain adequate biopsy specimens in linitis plastica lesions. Because of the high incidence of gastric carcinoma in Japan, screening upper endoscopy is performed to detect early gastric carcinoma. Approximately 40% of tumors detected by screening are early, with a 5-year survival rate of almost 90%. Screening programs are not recommended in the USA.

D. Imaging: A barium upper gastrointestinal series is an acceptable alternative when endoscopy is not readily available but may not detect small or superficial lesions and cannot reliably distinguish benign from malignant ulcerations. Any abnormalities detected with this procedure require endoscopic confirmation.

Once a gastric cancer is diagnosed, preoperative evaluation with abdominal CT and endoscopic ultrasonography is indicated to delineate the local extent of the primary tumor as well as nodal or distant metastases. Abdominal CT is valuable in identifying distant metastases and direct invasion of adjacent structures. Endoscopic ultrasound imaging is superior to CT in determining the depth of tumor penetration and nodal metastases.

E. Staging: Staging is defined according to the TNM system, in which T1 tumors invade to the submucosa, T2 invade the muscularis propria, T3 penetrate the serosa, and T4 invade adjacent structures. Nodes are graded as N0 if there is no involvement, N1 if there are metastases to perigastric nodes, and N2 if regional lymph nodes are involved. M1 signifies the presence of metastatic disease. The stages are defined as shown in the accompanying box.

STAGING CRITERIA FOR GASTRIC ADENOCARCINOMA

Stage I:	T1N0, T1N1, T2N0, all M0
Stage II:	T1N2, T2N1, T3N0, all M0
Stage III:	T2N2, T3N1, T4N0, all M0
Stage IV:	T4N2M0, any M1

Differential Diagnosis

Ulcerating gastric adenocarcinomas are distinguished from benign gastric ulcers by biopsies. Approximately 3% of gastric ulcers initially believed to be benign later prove to be malignant. To exclude malignancy, all gastric ulcers identified at endoscopy should be biopsied. Ulcers that are suspicious for malignancy to the endoscopist or that have atypia or dysplasia on histologic examination warrant repeat endoscopy in 2–3 months to verify healing and exclude malignancy. Nonhealing ulcers should be considered for resection. Infiltrative carcinoma with thickened gastric folds must be distinguished from lymphoma and other hypertrophic gastropathies such as Ménétrier's disease.

Treatment

A. Curative Surgical Resection: Surgical resection is the only therapy with curative potential. After preoperative staging, about two-thirds of patients will be found to have localized disease (ie, stages I–III) and should undergo surgical exploration. At surgery, approximately one-fourth of these patients will be found to have locally unresectable tumors or peritoneal, hepatic, or distant lymph node metastases for which "curative" surgical resection is not warranted (see below). The remaining patients with confirmed localized disease should undergo radical surgical resection with curative intent. For adenocarcinoma localized to the distal two-thirds of the stomach, a subtotal distal gastrectomy should be performed. For proximal gastric cancer or diffusely infiltrating disease, total gastrectomy is necessary. Although lymph node dissection should be performed for curative resections, there has been ongoing debate about whether an extended (perigastric and regional) lymph node dissection or a limited (perigastric) dissection is needed. A recent study has demonstrated greater short-term morbidity and no long-term survival advantage for extended lymph node dissection. Adjuvant therapy following curative resection has not conferred a survival benefit for postoperative chemotherapy.

B. Palliative Modalities: Many patients will be found either preoperatively or at the time of surgical exploration to have advanced disease that is not amenable to "curative" surgery due to peritoneal or distant metastases or local invasion of other organs. In many of these cases, palliative resection of the tumor nonetheless may be indicated. Such resection removes the risk of bleeding and obstruction, leads to improved quality of life, and improves survival. For patients with unresectable disease, gastrojejunostomy may be indicated to prevent obstruction. Bleeding or obstruction from unresected tumors may be treated with endoscopic laser or stent therapy, radiation therapy, or angiographic embolization. Although chemotherapy has not been shown to prolong life, single-agent or combination therapies with fluorouracil, doxorubicin, and cisplatin or mitomycin may provide palliation in up to 30%.

Prognosis

The long-term survival of gastric carcinoma is less than 15%. However, 5-year survival in patients who undergo successful curative resection is over 45%. Survival is related to tumor stage, location, and histologic features. Stage I and stage II tumors resected for cure have a greater than 50% long-term survival. Patients with stage III tumors have a poor prognosis (< 20% long-term survival) and should be considered for enrollment in clinical trials. Tumors of the diffuse and signet ring type have a worse prognosis than the intestinal type. Tumors of the proximal stomach (fundus and cardia) carry a far worse prognosis than distal lesions. Even with apparently localized disease, proximal tumors have a 5-year survival of less than 15%. For those whose disease progresses despite therapy, meticulous efforts at palliative care are essential (see Chapter 5).

[Gastric Cancer—National Cancer Institute–CancerNet] http://cancernet.nci.nih.gov/cgi-bin/srchcgi.exe?DBID=pdq&TYPE=search&UID=208+00025

Bonenkamp JJ et al: Extended lymph-node dissection for gastric cancer. N Engl J Med 1999;340:908. [NLM Cit ID: 99173387]

LYMPHOMA

Lymphoma is the second most common gastric malignancy, accounting for 3–6% of gastric cancers. More than 95% of these are non-Hodgkin's B cell lymphomas. Gastric lymphomas may be primary (arising from the gastric mucosa) or may represent a site of secondary involvement in patients with nodal lymphomas. Many primary gastric lymphomas are believed to arise from mucosa-associated lymphoid tissue (MALT). Distinguishing advanced primary gastric lymphoma with adjacent nodal spread from advanced nodal lymphoma with secondary gastric spread can be problematic. Because the prognosis and treatment of primary and secondary gastric lymphomas are entirely different, the distinction is important. Using a variety of B cell phenotypic markers, it now is possible to differentiate B cells of nodal origin from those derived from MALT (CD19- and CD20-positive).

Infection with *H pylori* may be an important risk factor for the development of primary gastric lymphoma. The normal gastric mucosa does not contain significant lymphoid tissue (ie, lymphoid aggregates or Peyer's patches). Chronic infection with *H pylori* causes an intense lymphocytic inflammatory response that may lead to the development of lymphoid follicles. Over 85% of low-grade primary gastric lymphomas and 40% of high-grade lymphomas are associated with *H pylori* infection. The risk of developing lymphoma is increased sevenfold in patients with chronic *H pylori* infection. It is hypothesized that chronic antigenic stimulation may result in a monoclonal lymphoproliferation that may culminate in a low-grade MALT lymphoma. At present, the relationship between high-grade primary lymphomas, MALT, and *H pylori* infection is unclear.

The clinical presentation and endoscopic appearance of gastric lymphoma are similar to those of adenocarcinoma. The majority of patients present with abdominal pain, weight loss, or bleeding. Night sweats are absent in primary lymphoma. At endoscopy, lymphoma may appear as an ulcer, mass, or diffusely infiltrating lesion. The diagnosis is established with endoscopic biopsy. All patients should undergo staging with abdominal and chest CT. Endoscopic ultrasonography is the most sensitive test for determining the presence of perigastric lymphadenopathy.

Nodal lymphomas with secondary gastrointestinal involvement usually present at an advanced stage with widely disseminated disease and are seldom curable. Their treatment is addressed in Chapter 13. By contrast, primary low-grade gastric lymphomas usually are localized to the stomach wall (stage IE) or adjacent lymph nodes (stage IIE) and have an excellent prognosis. Patients with primary low-grade gastric MALT-lymphoma should be tested for *H pylori* infection and treated if positive. Multiple studies have documented complete lymphoma regression after successful *H pylori* eradication in 75% of stage IE low-grade lymphoma. Remission may take as long as a year. Patients with stage IE high-grade lymphoma or stage I low grade lymphoma who either are not infected with *H pylori* or fail to respond to eradication therapy can be treated successfully with local radiation therapy. The optimal treatment of stage IIE primary gastric lymphomas (either low-grade or high-grade) is controversial. Radiation therapy (with or without chemotherapy) is widely used. Stage III and stage IV primary lymphomas are treated with combination chemotherapy. Because of a low risk of perforation with either radiation therapy or chemotherapy, surgical resection is no longer recommended. The long-term survival of primary gastric lymphoma for stage I is over 85% and for stage II is 35–65%.

Steinbach G et al: Antibiotic treatment of gastric lymphoma of mucosa-associated lymphoid tissue. Ann Intern Med 1999;131:88. [NLM Cit ID: 99333045] (Of 28 *H pylori*-positive patients with MALT lymphoma, 50% achieved complete remission after antibiotic therapy. Remission was 70% in patients with T1N0 disease.)

Zucca E et al: B-cell lymphoma of MALT type: a review with special emphasis on diagnostic and management problems of low-grade gastric tumors. Br J Haematol 1998;100:3. [NLM Cit ID: 98111260]

CARCINOID TUMORS

Gastric carcinoids are rare tumors that make up less than 1% of gastric neoplasms. They may occur sporadically or secondary to chronic hypergastrinemia that results in hyperplasia and transformation of enterochromaffin cells in the gastric fundus. Sporadic carcinoids account for 20% of gastric carcinoids. Most are solitary, over 2 cm in size, and have a strong propensity for metastatic spread. Most sporadic carcinoids already have carcinoid syndrome and hepatic or pulmonary metastatic involvement at initial presentation. Localized sporadic carcinoids should be treated with radical gastrectomy.

The majority of carcinoids caused by hypergastrinemia occur in association with either pernicious anemia (75%) or Zollinger-Ellison syndrome (5%). Carcinoids associated with Zollinger-Ellison syndrome occur almost exclusively in patients with MEN 1, in which loss of 11q13 has been reported. Carcinoids caused by hypergastrinemia tend to be multicentric, less than 1 cm in size, and have a low potential for metastatic spread or development of carcinoid syndrome. Small lesions may be successfully treated with endoscopic resection followed by periodic endoscopic surveillance. Antrectomy reduces serum gastrin levels and may lead to regression of small tumors. Patients with large or multiple carcinoids should undergo surgical tumor resection.

Kulke M et al: Carcinoid tumors. N Engl J Med 1999;340:858. [NLM Cit ID: 99165321]

DISEASES OF THE SMALL INTESTINE

MALABSORPTION

The term "malabsorption" denotes disorders in which there is a disruption of digestion and nutrient absorption. The clinical and laboratory manifestations of malabsorption are summarized in Table 14–12. Normal digestion and absorption may be divided into three phases:

Table 14–12. Clinical and laboratory manifestations of malabsorption.[1]

Manifestation	Laboratory Findings	Malabsorbed Nutrients
Steatorrhea (bulky, light-colored stools)	Increased fecal fat; decreased serum cholesterol	Fat
Diarrhea (increased fecal water)	Increased fecal fat or positive bile salt breath test	Fatty acids or bile salts
Weight loss; malnutrition (muscle wasting); weakness, fatigue, abdominal distention	Increased fecal fat and nitrogen; decreased glucose and xylose absorption	Calories (fat, protein, carbohydrates)
Iron deficiency anemia	Hypochromic anemia; low serum iron	Iron
Megaloblastic anemia	Macrocytosis; decreased vitamin B_{12} absorption (^{67}Co-labeled B_{12}); decreased serum vitamin B_{12} and red cell folate	Vitamin B_{12} or folic acid
Paresthesia; tetany; positive Trousseau and Chvostek signs	Decreased serum calcium, magnesium, and potassium	Calcium, vitamin D, magnesium, potassium
Bone pain; pathologic fractures; skeletal deformities	Osteoporosis on x-ray; osteomalacia on biopsy	Calcium, protein
Bleeding tendency (ecchymoses, melena, hematuria)	Prolonged prothrombin time	Vitamin K
Edema	Decreased serum albumin; increased fecal loss of α_1-antitrypsin (antiprotease)	Protein (or protein-losing enteropathy)
Nocturia; abdominal distention	Increased small bowel fluid on x-ray	Water
Milk intolerance (cramps, bloating, diarrhea)	Flat lactose tolerance test; decreased mucosal lactase levels	Lactose

[1]Modified from Bayless TM: Malabsorption in the elderly. Hosp Pract (Aug) 1979;14:67.

(1) Intraluminal phase: Dietary fats, proteins, and carbohydrates are hydrolyzed and solubilized by pancreatic and biliary secretions. Fats are broken down by pancreatic lipase to monoglycerides and fatty acids that form micelles with bile salts. Micelles are important for the solubilization and absorption of fat-soluble vitamins (A, D, E, K). Proteins are hydrolyzed by pancreatic proteases to di- and tripeptides and amino acids. Impaired intraluminal digestion may be caused by insufficient intraluminal concentrations of pancreatic enzymes or bile salts. These conditions will not be covered in detail here (see Chapter 15).

Pancreatic insufficiency may be caused by chronic pancreatitis, cystic fibrosis, or pancreatic cancer. Pancreatic enzymes may also be inactivated within the intestinal lumen by acid hypersecretion (Zollinger-Ellison syndrome). Significant pancreatic enzyme insufficiency generally results in significant steatorrhea (due to malabsorption of triglycerides)—often more than 20–40 g/24 h—resulting in weight loss, gaseous distention and flatulence, and large, greasy, foul-smelling stools. The digestion of proteins and carbohydrates is affected to a far lesser degree and is generally not clinically significant. Because micellar function and intestinal absorption are normal, signs of other nutrient or vitamin deficiencies are rare.

Decreased bile salt concentrations may be due to biliary obstruction or cholestatic liver diseases. Because bile salts are resorbed in the terminal ileum, resection or disease of this area (eg, Crohn's disease) can lead to insufficient intraluminal bile salts. Finally, destruction or loss of bile salts may be caused by bacterial overgrowth, massive acid hypersecretion, or medications that bind bile salts (eg, cholestyramine). (Bacterial overgrowth is discussed below.) Insufficient concentrations of intraluminal bile salts lead to mild steatorrhea (due to malabsorption of fatty acids and monoglycerides), though generally less than 20 g/d. Weight loss is minimal. Impaired absorption of fat-soluble vitamins (A, D, E, K) is common, resulting in bleeding tendencies, osteoporosis, and hypocalcemia (Table 14–12). Other nutrient absorption is intact. Intestinal loss of bile salts into the colon may cause a watery secretory diarrhea.

(2) Mucosal phase: The mucosal phase requires a sufficient surface area of intact small intestinal epithelium. Brush border enzymes are important in the hydrolysis of disaccharides and di- and tripeptides. Malabsorption of specific nutrients may occur as a result of deficiency in an isolated brush border enzyme. With the exception of lactase deficiency, these are rare congenital disorders that are evident in childhood. Malabsorption due to primary mucosal diseases, extensive intestinal resections (short bowel syndrome), or lymphoma is discussed below. These disorders result in malabsorption of all nutrients: fats, proteins, and amino acids. Depending upon the severity of malabsorption, patients may manifest a number of symptoms and signs, as outlined in Table 14–12.

(3) Absorptive phase: Obstruction of the lymphatic system results in impaired absorption of chylomicrons and lipoproteins. This may lead to steatorrhea and significant enteric protein losses or "protein-losing enteropathy," discussed below.

1. CELIAC SPRUE

Essentials of Diagnosis

- Weight loss.
- Distention, flatulence, greasy stools.
- Increased fecal fat (> 7 g/24 h).
- Abnormal small bowel biopsy.
- Clinical improvement on gluten-free diet.

General Considerations

Also known as gluten enteropathy or celiac disease, celiac sprue is characterized by diffuse damage to the proximal small intestinal mucosa that results in malabsorption of most nutrients. Although generally manifest in infancy, it may have its first clinical onset in the second to fourth decades, or even later. It occurs in 0.4% of whites of Northern European ancestry and is rare in Africans and Asians. It is strongly associated with selected HLA class II antigens: HLA-DR3 and HLA-DQw2. While the precise mechanism of damage is unknown, it is clear that removal of gluten from the diet results in resolution of symptoms and intestinal healing in most patients. Gluten is a storage protein that is present in certain grains such as wheat, rye, barley, and oats—but not rice or corn. It is hypothesized that in a genetically susceptible host, gluten—perhaps in conjunction with a viral infection—incites a humoral and cell-mediated inflammatory response that results in mucosal inflammation and destruction.

Clinical Findings

A. Symptoms and Signs: The symptoms and signs of malabsorption depend upon the length of small intestine that is involved. Most patients report diarrhea, marked flatulence (due to colonic bacterial digestion of malabsorbed nutrients), weight loss, and weakness. The stools are characteristically loose to soft, large, floating, oily or greasy, and foul-smelling. However, they may also be watery and frequent in number (up to 10–12 daily). Patients with minimal involvement of only the duodenum and proximal jejunum may have no diarrhea. Patients are often hyperphagic, and the severity of weight loss is highly variable. Physical examination may be normal in mild cases or may reveal signs of malabsorption, such as loss of muscle mass or subcutaneous fat, pallor due to anemia, easy bruising due to vitamin K deficiency, hyperkeratosis due to vitamin A deficiency, or bone pain due to osteomalacia. Abdominal examination may reveal distention with hyperactive bowel sounds.

Dermatitis herpetiformis, a characteristic skin rash, occurs in less than 10% of patients with celiac sprue. Pruritic papulovesicles occur over the extensor surfaces of the extremities and over the trunk, scalp, and neck. Of patients with dermatitis herpetiformis, over 85% have evidence of celiac disease on intestinal mucosal biopsy, though this may not be clinically evident.

B. Laboratory Findings:

1. Routine laboratory tests–Laboratory abnormalities depend upon the extent of intestinal involvement. A complete blood count, serum iron, red cell folate, vitamin B_{12} level, serum calcium, alkaline phosphatase, albumin, beta-carotene, and prothrombin time should be obtained in all patients with suspected malabsorption. Limited proximal involvement may result only in microcytic anemia due to iron deficiency. More extensive involvement results in a megaloblastic anemia due to folate deficiency. Low serum calcium or elevated alkaline phosphatase may reflect impaired calcium or vitamin D absorption with osteomalacia. Elevations of prothrombin time or a decreased serum beta-carotene reflect impaired fat-soluble vitamin absorption. Severe diarrhea may result in a non-anion gap acidosis and hypokalemia.

2. Specific tests for malabsorption–Steatorrhea is usually present but may be absent in mild disease. It may be detected by a qualitative (Sudan stain) or quantitative stool assessment for fecal fat. A positive Sudan stain is strong evidence of steatorrhea and usually obviates the need for quantitative analysis, but it is falsely negative in 25%. A quantitative 72-hour stool collection taken while patients are consuming a 100 g fat diet is a more sensitive means of detecting fat malabsorption. Excretion of more than 10 g/d of fat is abnormal and warrants further evaluation for malabsorption. Other tests of malabsorption such as the D-xylose test to provide evidence of mucosal malabsorption are no longer required with the availability of serologic screening for celiac disease.

3. Antibodies–A number of serologic tests can be used to screen for celiac disease and to monitor for patient adherence to the gluten-free diet. The IgA endomysial antibody has > 90% sensitivity and specificity in detecting untreated celiac sprue, making it the most useful screening test in patients with suspected malabsorption. IgG and IgA antigliadin antibodies are present in over 90% of patients with celiac sprue but are elevated also in other mucosal diseases. The IgG antibody is more sensitive, and the IgA antibody is more specific. A combination of the two tests provides a sensitivity and specificity of over 95%. A combination of all three tests has a greater than 99% positive and negative predictive value. Given this high degree of reliability, it is possible that mucosal biopsy will not be required in the future for confirmation of the diagnosis. IgA antiendomysial antibody may become undetectable after 6–12 months of gluten withdrawal, which may be a useful means of verifying dietary compliance.

C. Mucosal Biopsy: Mucosal biopsy of the distal duodenum or proximal jejunum is the standard method for the diagnosis of celiac sprue in patients with antiendomysial or antigliadin antibodies. The endoscopic biopsy has supplanted the use of a suction biopsy tube. At endoscopy, atrophy or scalloping of the duodenal folds may be observed. Histology reveals loss of intestinal villi, hypertrophy of the intestinal crypts, and extensive infiltration of the lamina propria with lymphocytes and plasma cells. An adequate normal biopsy excludes the diagnosis. Reversion of these abnormalities on repeat biopsy after a patient is placed on a gluten-free diet establishes the diagnosis. However, if a patient with a compatible biopsy demonstrates prompt clinical improvement on a gluten-free diet and a decrease in antigliadin antibodies, a repeat biopsy is unnecessary.

Differential Diagnosis

Celiac sprue must be distinguished from other causes of malabsorption, as outlined above. Severe panmalabsorption of multiple nutrients is almost always caused by mucosal disease. In a patient with steatorrhea, a normal D-xylose test points to pancreatic insufficiency, reduced bile salts, or lymphatic obstruction. If the D-xylose test, however, is also abnormal, it strongly implicates mucosal disorders or bacterial overgrowth. The histologic appearance of celiac sprue may resemble other mucosal diseases such as tropical sprue, bacterial overgrowth, cow's milk intolerance, viral gastroenteritis, eosinophilic gastroenteritis, and mucosal damage caused by acid hypersecretion associated with gastrinoma. Documentation of clinical response to gluten withdrawal therefore is essential to the diagnosis.

Treatment

Removal of all gluten from the diet is essential to therapy—all wheat, rye, and barley must be eliminated. Although oats previously were felt to be toxic to these patients, recent studies suggest that in adults moderate amounts of oats are without adverse effects. Rice, soybean, potato, and corn flours are safe. Because of the pervasive use of gluten products in manufactured foods and additives and by restaurants, it is imperative that patients and their families meet with a knowledgeable dietitian in order to comply satisfactorily with this lifelong diet. Several excellent dietary guides are available. Most patients with celiac disease also have lactose intolerance either temporarily or permanently and should avoid dairy products until the intestinal symptoms have improved on the gluten-free diet.

Improvement in symptoms should be evident within a few weeks on the gluten-free diet. The most common reason for failure is incomplete removal of gluten.

Prognosis & Complications

If appropriately diagnosed and treated, patients with celiac sprue have an excellent prognosis. Celiac disease may be associated with other autoimmune disorders, including Addison's disease, Graves' disease, type 1 diabetes mellitus, myasthenia gravis, scleroderma, Sjögren's syndrome, lupus erythematosus, and pancreatic insufficiency. Intestinal T cell lymphoma occurs in over 10% of patients with celiac sprue. The disorder should be suspected in patients previously responsive to the gluten-free diet who develop pain or new weight loss and malabsorption. Strict dietary compliance may reduce the risk of lymphoma development. In some patients, the disease may evolve and become refractory to the gluten-free diet. These patients generally have a poor prognosis, though some may respond to corticosteroids or immunosuppression with cyclosporine.

Celiac Disease Foundation, 13251 Ventura Blvd, Suite #1, Studio City, CA 91604-1838. http://www.celiac.org. (Excellent source for patient information, newsletters, dietary guidelines.)

Fine KD et al: The prevalence and causes of chronic diarrhea in patients with celiac sprue treated with a gluten-free diet. Gastroenterology 1997;112:1830. [NLM Cit ID: 97322019]

Trier JS: Diagnosis of celiac sprue. Gastroenterology 1998;115:211. [NLM Cit ID: 98323506]

2. WHIPPLE'S DISEASE

Essentials of Diagnosis

- Malabsorption.
- Multisystemic disease.
- Fever, lymphadenopathy, arthralgias.
- Duodenal biopsy with PAS-positive macrophages with characteristic bacillus.

General Considerations

Whipple's disease is a rare multisystemic illness caused by infection with the bacillus *Tropheryma whippelii.* It may occur at any age but most commonly affects white men in the fourth to sixth decades. The source of infection is unknown, but no cases of human-to-human spread have been documented.

Clinical Findings

A. Symptoms and Signs: The clinical manifestations are protean. Arthralgias or a migratory, nondeforming arthritis occur in 80% and are typically the first symptom experienced. Gastrointestinal symptoms occur in approximately 75% of cases. They include abdominal pain, diarrhea, and some degree of malabsorption with distention, flatulence, and steatorrhea. Weight loss, present in almost all patients, is the most common presenting symptom. Loss of protein due to intestinal or lymphatic involvement may result in protein-losing enteropathy with hypoalbuminemia and edema. In the absence of gastrointestinal symptoms, the diagnosis often is delayed for several years. Intermittent low-grade fever occurs in over 50% of cases. Chronic cough is common. There may be generalized lymphadenopathy that resembles sarcoidosis. Myocardial or valvular involvement may lead to congestive failure or valvular regurgitation. Ocular findings include uveitis, vitreitis, keratitis, retinitis, and retinal hemorrhages. Central nervous system involvement in approximately 10% of cases is manifested by a variety of findings such as dementia, lethargy, coma, seizures, myoclonus, or hypothalamic signs. Cranial nerve findings include ophthalmoplegia or nystagmus.

Physical examination may reveal hypotension (a late finding), low-grade fever, and evidence of malabsorption (see Table 14–12). Lymphadenopathy is present in 50%. Heart murmurs due to valvular involvement may be evident. Peripheral joints may be enlarged or warm, and peripheral edema may be present. Neurologic findings are cited above. Hyperpigmentation on sun-exposed areas is evident in up to 40%.

B. Laboratory Findings: If significant malabsorption is present, patients may have laboratory abnormalities as outlined in Table 14–12. There may be steatorrhea.

C. Histologic Evaluation: The diagnosis of Whipple's disease is established by histologic evaluation of the involved tissues. In most cases, the diagnosis is established by endoscopic biopsy of the duodenum, which demonstrates infiltration of the lamina propria with PAS-positive macrophages that contain gram-positive bacilli (which are not acid-fast) and dilation of the lacteals. The Whipple bacillus has a characteristic electron microscopic appearance. In some patients who present with nongastrointestinal symptoms, the duodenal biopsy may be normal, and biopsy of other involved organs or lymph nodes may be necessary. Because the PAS stain is less sensitive and specific for extraintestinal Whipple's disease, PCR is now used to confirm the diagnosis by demonstrating the presence of 16S ribosomal RNA of *T whippelii* in blood, cerebrospinal fluid, vitreous fluid, synovial fluid, or cardiac valves. The sensitivity of PCR is 97% and the specificity 100%.

Differential Diagnosis

Whipple's disease should be considered in patients who present with signs of malabsorption, fever of unknown origin, lymphadenopathy, seronegative arthritis, culture-negative endocarditis, or multisystemic disease. Small bowel biopsy readily distinguishes Whipple's disease from other mucosal malabsorptive disorders, such as celiac sprue. Patients with AIDS and infection of the small intestine with *Mycobacterium avium* complex may have a similar clinical and histologic picture; although both conditions are characterized by PAS-positive macrophages, they may be distinguished by the acid-fast stain, which is positive for MAC and negative for the Whipple bacillus. Other conditions that may be confused with Whipple's disease include sarcoidosis, Reiter's syndrome, familial Mediterranean fever, systemic vasculitides, Behçet's disease, intestinal lymphoma, and subacute infective endocarditis.

Treatment

Antibiotic therapy results in a dramatic clinical improvement within several weeks, even in some patients with neurologic involvement. The optimal regimen is unknown. Complete clinical response usually is evident within 1–3 months; however, relapse may occur in up to one-third of patients after discontinuation of treatment. Therefore, prolonged treatment for at least 1 year is required. Drugs that cross the blood-brain barrier are preferred. Trimethoprim-sulfamethoxazole (one double-strength tablet twice daily for 1 year) is recommended as first-line therapy. In patients allergic to sulfonamides, ceftriaxone or chloramphenicol may be reasonable. A patient with central nervous system disease refractory to antibiotics was recently treated successfully with interferon gamma. After treatment, repeat biopsies may be obtained for PCR. Negative results predict a low likelihood of clinical relapse.

Prognosis

If untreated, the disease is fatal. Because some neurologic signs may be permanent, the goal of treatment is to prevent this progression. Patients must be followed closely after treatment for signs of symptom recurrence.

Ramaiah C et al: Whipple's disease. Gastroenterol Clin North Am 1998;27:683. [NLM Cit ID: 99108852]

Raoult D et al: Cultivation of the bacillus of Whipple's disease. N Engl J Med 2000;342:620. [NLM Cit ID: 20143076] (The causative bacterium was cultivated from the mitral valve of a patient with endocarditis and propagated in a human fibroblast line. The authors were able to design an indirect antibody immunofluorescence assay that detected positive antibodies in seven of nine patients with proved Whipple's disease. The development of a commercial serologic test may be possible.)

3. BACTERIAL OVERGROWTH

The small intestine normally contains a small number of bacteria. Bacterial overgrowth in the small intestine of whatever cause may result in malabsorption via a number of mechanisms. Bacterial deconjugation of bile salts may lead to inadequate micelle formation, resulting in decreased fat absorption with steatorrhea. Microbial uptake of specific nutrients reduces absorption of vitamin B_{12} and carbohydrates. Bacterial proliferation also causes direct damage to intestinal epithelial cells and the brush border, further impairing absorption of proteins and carbohydrates. Passage of the malabsorbed bile acids and carbohydrates into the colon leads to an osmotic and secretory diarrhea.

Causes of bacterial overgrowth include the following: (1) gastric achlorhydria (especially if other predisposing conditions present); (2) anatomic abnormalities of the small intestine with stagnation (afferent limb of Billroth II gastrojejunostomy, small intestine diverticula, obstruction, blind loop, radiation enteritis); (3) small intestine motility disorders (scleroderma, diabetic enteropathy, chronic intestinal pseudo-obstruction); (4) gastrocolic or coloenteric fistula (Crohn's disease, malignancy, surgical resection); and (5) miscellaneous disorders (AIDS, chronic pancreatitis). Bacterial overgrowth is an important cause of malabsorption in the elderly, perhaps because of decreased gastric acidity or impaired intestinal motility.

Clinical Findings

Many patients with bacterial overgrowth are asymptomatic. Patients with severe overgrowth have symptoms and signs of malabsorption, including distention, weight loss, and steatorrhea (Table 14–12). Watery diarrhea is common. Megaloblastic anemia or neurologic signs due to vitamin B_{12} deficiency are common findings and may be manifest at presentation. In patients with vitamin B_{12} deficiency, the Schilling test is diagnostic of bacterial overgrowth if it is abnormal in phase I and II (without and with intrinsic factor) but normalizes after a course of antibiotics. Qualitative or quantitative fecal fat assessment typically is abnormal. D-Xylose absorption is also abnormal due to bacterial uptake of the carbohydrate.

Bacterial overgrowth should be considered in any patient with diarrhea, steatorrhea, weight loss, or macrocytic anemia, especially if the patient has a predisposing cause (such as prior gastrointestinal surgery). A stool collection should be obtained to corroborate the presence of steatorrhea. Small bowel barium radiography may be helpful to document conditions predisposing to intestinal stasis. Where indicated, a small intestinal biopsy may be necessary to exclude other mucosal malabsorptive conditions. A specific diagnosis can be established firmly only by an aspirate and culture of proximal jejunal secretion that demonstrates over 10^5 organisms/mL. However, this is an invasive and laborious test, not done in some clinical settings. A number of noninvasive breath tests have been developed but lack sufficient sensitivity and specificity to be of great utility. The ^{14}C-xylose breath test is the most reliable. In this test, bacterial uptake and degradation of the isotope lead to the release of $^{14}CO_2$, which can be measured in exhaled breath.

Owing to the lack of an optimal test for bacterial overgrowth, many clinicians employ an empirical antibiotic trial as a diagnostic and therapeutic maneuver in patients with predisposing conditions for bacterial overgrowth who develop unexplained diarrhea or steatorrhea.

Treatment

Where possible, the anatomic defect that has potentiated bacterial overgrowth should be corrected. In many cases, this is not possible. Empirical treatment as follows for 1–2 weeks with broad-spectrum antibiotics effective against enteric aerobes and anaerobes usually leads to dramatic improvement: twice daily ciprofloxacin 500 mg, norfloxacin 400 mg, or amoxicillin clavulanate 875 mg, or a combination of metronidazole 250 mg three times daily plus either trimethoprim-sulfamethoxazole (one double-strength tablet) twice daily or cephalexin 250 mg four times daily.

In patients in whom symptoms recur off antibiotics, cyclic therapy (eg, 1 week out of 4) may be sufficient. Continuous antibiotics should be avoided, if possible, to avoid development of bacterial antibiotic resistance.

In patients with severe intestinal dysmotility, treatment with small doses of octreotide has been shown to be of benefit in preliminary studies.

Attar A et al: Antibiotic efficacy in small intestinal bacterial overgrowth-related chronic diarrhea: a crossover randomized trial. Gastroenterology 1999;117:794. [NLM Cit ID: 99431900] (Symptoms and breath hydrogen were decreased after antibiotics but not after therapy with the probiotic bacteria.)

Bouhnik Y et al: Bacterial populations contaminating the upper gut in patients with small intestinal bacterial overgrowth syndrome. Am J Gastroenterol 1999;94:1327. [NLM Cit ID: 99249293]

4. SHORT BOWEL SYNDROME

Short bowel syndrome is the malabsorptive condition that arises secondary to removal of significant segments of the small intestine. The most common causes in adults are Crohn's disease, mesenteric infarction, radiation enteritis, and trauma. The type and degree of malabsorption depend upon the length and site of the resection and the degree of adaptation of the remaining bowel.

Terminal Ileal Resection

Resection of the terminal ileum results in malabsorption of bile salts and vitamin B_{12}, which are normally absorbed in this region. Patients with low serum vitamin B_{12} levels, an abnormal Schilling test, or resection of over 50 cm of ileum require monthly intramuscular vitamin B_{12} injections. In patients with less than 100 cm of ileal resection, bile salt malabsorption stimulates fluid secretion from the colon, resulting in watery diarrhea. This may be treated with bile salt binding resins (cholestyramine, 2–4 g three times daily with meals). Resection of over 100 cm of ileum leads to a reduction in the bile salt pool that results in steatorrhea and malabsorption of fat-soluble vitamins. Treatment is with a low-fat diet and vitamins supplemented with medium-chain triglycerides, which do not require micellar solubilization. Unabsorbed fatty acids bind with calcium, reducing its absorption and enhancing the absorption of oxalate. Oxalate kidney stones may develop. Calcium supplements should be administered to bind oxalate and increase serum calcium. Cholesterol gallstones due to decreased bile salts are common also. In patients with resection of the ileocolonic valve, bacterial overgrowth may occur in the small intestine, further complicating malabsorption (as outlined above).

Extensive Small Bowel Resection

Resection of 40–50% of the total length of small intestine usually is well tolerated. A more massive resection may result in nutrient and water and electrolyte malabsorption in addition to the deficits described above. After resection, the remaining intestine has a remarkable ability to adapt, increasing its absorptive capacity up to fourfold. As little as 100 cm of proximal jejunum may be sufficient to maintain adequate nutrition with oral feedings alone, though fluid and electrolyte losses still may be significant. Adaptation occurs gradually over 1 year. Patients with less than 100 cm of proximal jejunum remaining almost always require supplementation with either enteral supplements (elemental diets or polymeric) or total parenteral nutrition. Lactose should be eliminated. Duodenal resection may result in folate, iron, or calcium malabsorption. Levels of other minerals such as zinc and magnesium should be monitored. Parenteral vitamin supplementation may be necessary. Antidiarrheal agents (loperamide, 2–4 mg three times daily) slow transit and reduce diarrheal volume. Octreotide reduces intestinal transit time and fluid and electrolyte secretion. Gastric hypersecretion usually complicates intestinal resection and should be treated with H_2 receptor antagonists. Of patients who require chronic parenteral nutrition, the estimated annual mortality rate is 2–5% per year. Death is most commonly due to TPN-induced liver disease, sepsis, or loss of venous access. Small intestine transplantation is now being performed with reported 5-year survival rates of 60–70%. Currently, it is chiefly performed in patients requiring parenteral nutrition who develop irreversible liver disease.

Grant D: Current results of intestinal transplantation. The International Intestinal Transplant Registry. Lancet 1996;347:1801. [NLM Cit ID: 96281733] (Small bowel transplantation may be a lifesaving option for patients with short bowel syndrome who cannot tolerate TPN.)

5. LACTASE DEFICIENCY

Lactase is a brush border enzyme that hydrolyzes the disaccharide lactose into glucose and galactose. Congenital lactase deficiency is common in premature infants of less than 30 weeks' gestation. In full-term infants it is rare, usually inherited as an autosomal recessive trait. The concentration of lactase enzyme levels is high at birth but declines steadily in most people of non-European ancestry during childhood and adolescence and into adulthood. Thus, approximately 50 million people in the USA have partial to complete lactose intolerance. As many as 90% of Asian-Americans, 70% of African-Americans, 95% of Native Americans, 50% of Mexican-Americans, and 60% of Jewish Americans are lactose-intolerant compared with less than 25% of Caucasian adults. Lactase deficiency may also arise secondary to other gastrointestinal disorders that affect the proximal small intestinal mucosa. These include Crohn's disease, sprue, Whipple's disease, eosinophilic gastroenteritis, viral gastroenteritis, giardiasis, radiation enteritis, AIDS enteropathy (Microsporida infection, *Mycobacterium avium* complex infection, cryptosporidiosis), short bowel syndrome, and malnutrition. Malabsorbed lactose is fermented by intestinal bacteria, producing gas and organic acids. The nonmetabolized lactose and organic acids result in an increased stool osmotic load with an obligatory fluid loss.

Clinical Findings

A. Symptoms and Signs: Patients have great variability in clinical symptoms, depending both on the severity of lactase deficiency and the amount of lactose ingested. Because of the nonspecific nature of these symptoms, there is a tendency for both lactose-intolerant and lactose-tolerant individuals to mistakenly attribute a variety of abdominal symptoms to lactose intolerance. Most patients with lactose intolerance can drink one or two 8 oz glasses of milk daily without symptoms if taken with food at wide intervals, though rare patients have almost complete intolerance. With mild to moderate amounts of lactose malabsorption, patients may experience bloating, abdominal cramps, and flatulence. With higher lactose ingestions, an osmotic diarrhea will result. Isolated lactase deficiency does not result in other signs of malabsorption or weight loss. If these findings are present, other gastrointestinal disorders should be pursued. Diarrheal specimens reveal an increased osmotic gap and a pH of less than 6.0.

B. Laboratory Findings: The most widely available test for the diagnosis of lactase deficiency is the hydrogen breath test. After ingestion of 50 g of lactose, a rise in breath hydrogen of greater than 20 ppm within 90 minutes is a positive test, indicative of bacterial carbohydrate metabolism. In clinical practice, many physicians prescribe an empirical trial of a lactose-free diet for 2 weeks. Resolution of symptoms (bloating, flatulence, diarrhea) is highly suggestive of lactase deficiency (though a placebo response cannot be excluded) and may be confirmed, if necessary, with a breath hydrogen study.

Differential Diagnosis

The symptoms of late-onset lactose intolerance are nonspecific and may mimic a number of gastrointestinal disorders, such as inflammatory bowel disease, mucosal malabsorptive disorders, irritable bowel syndrome, and pancreatic insufficiency. Furthermore, lactase deficiency frequently develops secondary to other gastrointestinal disorders (as listed above). Concomitant lactase deficiency should always be considered in these gastrointestinal disorders.

Treatment

The goal of treatment in patients with isolated lactase deficiency is achieving patient comfort. Patients usually find their "threshold" of intake at which symptoms will occur. Foods that are high in lactose include milk (12 g/cup), ice cream (9 g/cup), and cottage cheese (8 g/cup). Aged cheeses have a lower lactose content (0.5 g/oz). Unpasteurized yogurt contains bacteria that produce lactase and is generally well tolerated.

Many patients will choose simply to restrict or eliminate milk products. By spreading dairy product intake throughout the day in quantities of less than 12 g of lactose (one cup of milk), most patients can take dairy products without symptoms and do not require lactase supplements. Calcium supplementation should be considered in susceptible patients to prevent osteoporosis. Most food markets provide milk that has been pretreated with lactase, rendering it 70–100% lactose-free. Lactase enzyme replacement is commercially available as a nonprescription formulation (Lactaid). Caplets of lactase may be taken with milk products, improving lactose absorption and eliminating symptoms. The number of caplets ingested depends upon the degree of lactose intolerance.

Briet F et al: Improved clinical tolerance to chronic lactose ingestion in subjects with lactose intolerance: a placebo effect? Gut 1997;41:632. [NLM Cit ID: 98076670]

ACUTE SMALL INTESTINAL OBSTRUCTION

Essentials of Diagnosis

- Cramping abdominal pain, vomiting.
- Tender distended abdomen.
- Radiographic evidence of dilated loops of small bowel; decreased air in colon.

General Considerations

Mechanical obstruction of the small intestine is a common surgical disorder that must be distinguished

Lymphoma

Gastrointestinal lymphomas may arise in the gastrointestinal tract or involve it secondarily with disseminated disease. In Western countries, primary gastrointestinal lymphomas account for 5% of lymphomas and up to one-third of small bowel malignancies. They occur most commonly in the distal small intestine. The majority are non-Hodgkin's B cell lymphomas. However, T cell lymphomas may arise in patients with celiac sprue. In the Middle East, lymphomas may arise also in the setting of immunoproliferative small intestinal disease (IPSID). In this condition, there is diffuse lymphoplasmacytic infiltration of the mucosa and submucosa that results in weight loss, diarrhea, and malabsorption which may lead to lymphomatous transformation. A characteristic feature of the disease is the presence of alpha heavy chains in the serum in 70%.

Presenting symptoms or signs of primary lymphoma include abdominal pain, weight loss, nausea and vomiting, distention, anemia, and occult blood in the stool. Fevers are unusual. Protein-losing enteropathy may result in hypoalbuminemia, but other signs of malabsorption are unusual. Barium radiography helps to localize the site of the lesion. The diagnosis requires endoscopic, percutaneous, or laparoscopic biopsy. In order to determine tumor stage, patients must undergo chest and abdominal CT, bone marrow biopsy, and, in some cases, lymphangiography.

Treatment depends on the stage of disease. Surgical resection of primary intestinal lymphoma (when possible) is usually recommended. Even in cases of stage III or stage IV disease, surgical debulking may improve survival. In patients with limited disease (stage IE) that is resected, the role of adjuvant chemotherapy is unclear. Most patients with more extensive disease are treated with systemic chemotherapy with or without radiation therapy (see Chapter 4).

Carcinoid Tumors

Carcinoids are the most common neuroendocrine tumors. Although many behave in an indolent fashion, the overall 5-year survival rate for patients with carcinoids is 50%, suggesting that most are malignant. Because many small carcinoids are detected incidentally at endoscopy or autopsy, it is likely that a significant percentage remain asymptomatic and undetected. Unfortunately, it is not possible by histologic examination to distinguish benign from malignant disease. The best indicator of prognosis is evidence of invasive growth and the presence of regional or distant metastasis.

Over 95% of gastrointestinal carcinoids occur in one of three sites: the rectum, the appendix, or the small intestine. Carcinoids account for up to one-third of small intestinal tumors. Rectal carcinoids are usually detected incidentally as submucosal nodules during proctoscopic examination. Similarly, appendiceal carcinoids are identified in 0.3% of appendectomies. Almost 80% of these tumors are less than 1 cm in size, and 90% are less than 2 cm. Rectal carcinoids less than 1 cm and appendiceal carcinoids less than 2 cm virtually never metastasize and are treated effectively with local excision or simple appendectomy. Tumors larger than 2 cm are associated with the development of metastasis in over 20% of appendiceal carcinoids and 10% of rectal carcinoids. Hence, in younger patients who are good operative risks, a more extensive cancer resection operation is warranted.

Small intestinal carcinoids most commonly arise in the ileum. Up to one-third are multicentric. Although 60% are less than 2 cm in size, even these small carcinoids may metastasize. Almost all tumors over 2 cm are associated with metastasis. Most smaller lesions are asymptomatic, though intussusception with obstruction occurs rarely. Carcinoids may extend locally into the muscularis, serosa, and mesentery, where they engender a fibroblastic reaction with contraction and kinking of the bowel. This may lead to symptoms of partial small bowel obstruction with intermittent abdominal pain. Small bowel barium studies may reveal kinking, but because the lesion is extraluminal the diagnosis may be overlooked for several years. Encasement of the mesenteric vessels can lead to bowel infarction. Further extension occurs to the local lymph nodes and to the liver. Abdominal CT may demonstrate a mesenteric mass with tethering of the bowel, lymphadenopathy, and hepatic metastasis. Carcinoid involvement of the heart (resulting in tricuspid regurgitation) is a late manifestation of metastatic disease. Carcinoid syndrome occurs in < 10% of patients (see Chapter 4) and only in patients with hepatic metastasis. Virtually all patients with carcinoid syndrome have obvious signs of cancer with liver metastasis on abdominal imaging. The optimal initial hepatic imaging study is somatostatin receptor scintigraphy, which is positive in over 90% of patients with metastatic carcinoid. A normal urinary 5-HIAA and serum serotonin excludes carcinoid syndrome with over 99% certainty.

Small intestinal carcinoids are extremely indolent tumors with slow spread. Patients with disease confined to the small intestine should have local excision, for which the cure rate exceeds 85%. In patients with resectable disease who have lymph node involvement, the 5-year disease-free survival is 80%; however, by 25 years, less than 25% remain disease-free. Even patients with hepatic metastases may have an indolent course with a median survival of 3 years. In patients with advanced disease, therapy should be deferred until the patient is symptomatic. Surgery should be directed toward palliation of obstructive symptoms. In patients with carcinoid syndrome or diarrhea, resection of hepatic metastases may provide dramatic improvement. The somatostatin analog octreotide (150–500 μg subcutaneously three times daily) inhibits hormone secretion from the carcinoid tumor, resulting in dramatic relief of diarrhea and symptoms of carcinoid syndrome in 90% of patients for a median period of 1 year. Thereafter, many patients escape from octreotide control. Hepatic artery occlusion and chemotherapy may provide symptomatic improvement in some patients with hepatic metastases.

Kulke M et al: Carcinoid tumors. N Engl J Med 1999; 340:858. [NLM Cit ID: 99165321]

Kaposi's Sarcoma

Kaposi's sarcoma is a common complication in AIDS, though the incidence appears to be declining. Recently, a newly recognized herpesvirus known as human herpesvirus 8 has been implicated as the infectious agent causing this disease. Kaposi's sarcoma is the most common intestinal tumor in HIV-infected patients. Lesions may be present anywhere in the intestinal tract. Visceral involvement usually is associated with cutaneous disease. Most lesions are clinically silent; however, large lesions may be symptomatic. Lesions of the gingiva, palate, and hypopharynx can lead to painful mastication and dysphagia. Lesions of the stomach or small intestine may lead to bleeding, obstruction, or even perforation. Obstruction of peritoneal lymph nodes can lead to protein-losing enteropathy and malabsorption. The diagnosis may be confirmed at endoscopy by the characteristic visual appearance and by biopsy. Oral complications can be treated with the CO_2 laser or radiation. Limited bleeding or obstructing lesions in the stomach or anus can be treated with the YAG laser or radiation therapy. Widespread involvement may be best treated by systemic chemotherapy using combinations of vincristine, bleomycin, or doxorubicin, to which the tumor is very responsive. Interferon-alfa, alone or in combination with reverse transcriptase inhibitors, has been reported to induce regression of Kaposi's sarcoma in up to one-third of patients.

Krown SE: Acquired immunodeficiency-associated Kaposi's sarcoma. Biology and management. Med Clin North Am 1997;81:471. [NLM Cit ID: 97247104]

APPENDICITIS

Essentials of Diagnosis

- Early: periumbilical pain; later: right lower quadrant pain and tenderness.
- Anorexia, nausea and vomiting, obstipation.
- Low-grade fever and leukocytosis.

General Considerations

Appendicitis is the most common abdominal surgical emergency, affecting approximately 10% of the population. It occurs most commonly between the ages of 10 and 30 years. It is initiated by obstruction of the appendix by a fecalith, inflammation, foreign body, or neoplasm. Obstruction leads to increased intraluminal pressure, venous congestion, infection, and thrombosis of intramural vessels. If untreated, gangrene and perforation develop within 36 hours.

Clinical Findings

A. Symptoms and Signs: Appendicitis usually begins with vague, often colicky periumbilical or epigastric pain. Within 12 hours the pain shifts to the right lower quadrant, manifested as a steady ache that is worsened by walking or coughing. Almost all patients have nausea with one or two episodes of vomiting. Protracted vomiting or vomiting that begins before the onset of pain suggests another diagnosis. A sense of constipation is typical, and some patients administer cathartics in an effort to relieve their symptoms—though some report diarrhea. Low-grade fever (< 38 °C) is typical; high fever or rigors suggest another diagnosis or appendiceal perforation.

On physical examination, localized tenderness with guarding in the right lower quadrant can be elicited with gentle palpation with one finger. When asked to cough, patients may be able to precisely localize the painful area, a sign of peritoneal irritation. Light percussion may also elicit pain. Although rebound tenderness is also present, it is unnecessary to elicit this finding if the above signs are present. The psoas sign (pain on passive extension of the right hip) and the obturator sign (pain with passive flexion and internal rotation of the right hip) are indicative of adjacent inflammation and strongly suggestive of appendicitis.

B. Laboratory Findings: Moderate leukocytosis (10,000–20,000/μL) with neutrophilia is common. Microscopic hematuria and pyuria are present in one-fourth of patients.

C. Imaging: No imaging studies are necessary in patients with typical appendicitis. Studies may be useful in patients in whom the diagnosis is uncertain. Abdominal or transvaginal ultrasound has a diagnostic accuracy of over 85% and is especially useful in the exclusion of adnexal disease in younger women. Abdominal CT is useful in cases of suspected appendiceal perforation to diagnose a periappendiceal abscess.

Atypical Presentations of Appendicitis

Owing to the variable location of the appendix, there are a number of "atypical" presentations. Because the retrocecal appendix does not touch the anterior abdominal wall, the pain remains less intense and poorly localized; abdominal tenderness is minimal and may be elicited in the right flank. The psoas sign may be positive. With pelvic appendicitis there is pain in the lower abdomen, often on the left, with an urge to urinate or defecate. Abdominal tenderness is absent, but tenderness is evident on pelvic or rectal examination; the obturator sign may be present. In the elderly, the diagnosis of appendicitis is often delayed because patients present with minimal, vague symptoms and mild abdominal tenderness. Appendicitis in pregnancy may present with pain in the right lower quadrant, periumbilical area, or right subcostal area owing to displacement of the appendix by the uterus.

Differential Diagnosis

Given its frequency and myriad presentations, appendicitis should be considered in the differential diagnosis of all patients with an acute abdominal problem. It can be extremely difficult to reliably diagnose appendicitis in some cases. Absence of the classic migration of pain (from the epigastrium to the right lower abdomen), right lower quadrant pain, fever, or guarding makes appendicitis less likely. Approximately 10–20% of patients with suspected appendicitis have either a negative examination at laparotomy or an alternative surgical diagnosis. The widespread use of ultrasonography and CT has reduced the number of incorrect diagnoses. Still, in some cases diagnostic laparotomy or laparoscopy is required. The most common causes of diagnostic confusion are gastroenteritis and gynecologic disorders. Viral gastroenteritis presents with nausea, vomiting, low-grade fever, and diarrhea and can be difficult to distinguish from appendicitis. The onset of vomiting before pain makes appendicitis less likely. As a rule, the pain of gastroenteritis is more generalized and the tenderness less well localized. Acute salpingitis or tubo-ovarian abscess should be considered in young, sexually active women with fever and bilateral abdominal or pelvic tenderness. A twisted ovarian cyst may also cause sudden severe pain. The sudden onset of lower abdominal pain in the middle of the menstrual cycle suggests mittelschmerz. Sudden severe abdominal pain with diffuse pelvic tenderness and shock suggests a ruptured ectopic pregnancy. A positive pregnancy test and pelvic ultrasonography are diagnostic. Retrocecal or retroileal appendicitis (often associated with pyuria or hematuria) may be confused with ureteral colic or pyelonephritis. Other conditions that may resemble appendicitis are diverticulitis, perforated colonic cancer, Crohn's ileitis, perforated peptic ulcer, cholecystitis, and mesenteric adenitis. It is virtually impossible to distinguish appendicitis from Meckel's diverticulitis; the distinction, however, is academic, as both require surgical treatment.

Complications

Perforation occurs in 20% of patients and should be suspected in patients with pain persisting for over 36 hours, high fever, diffuse abdominal tenderness or peritoneal findings, a palpable abdominal mass, or marked leukocytosis. Localized perforation results in a contained abscess, usually in the pelvis. A free perforation leads to suppurative peritonitis with toxicity. Septic thrombophlebitis (pylephlebitis) of the portal venous system is rare. It is suggested by high fever, chills, bacteremia, and jaundice.

Treatment

The treatment of uncomplicated appendicitis is surgical appendectomy. This may be performed through a laparotomy or by laparoscopy. Prior to surgery, patients should be given systemic antibiotics, which reduce the incidence of postoperative wound infections. Emergency appendectomy is also required in patients with perforated appendicitis with generalized peritonitis.

The optimal treatment of stable patients with perforated appendicitis and a contained abscess is controversial. Surgery in this setting can be difficult. Many recommend percutaneous CT-guided drainage of the abscess with intravenous fluids and antibiotics to allow the inflammation to subside. An interval appendectomy may be performed after 6 weeks to prevent recurrent appendicitis.

Prognosis

The mortality rate from uncomplicated appendicitis is extremely low. Even with perforated appendicitis, the mortality rate in most groups is only 0.2%, though it approaches 15% in the elderly.

Hale DA et al: Appendectomy: A contemporary appraisal. Ann Surg 1997;225:252. [NLM Cit ID: 97213891]

INTESTINAL TUBERCULOSIS

Intestinal tuberculosis is common in underdeveloped countries. Previously rare in the United States, its incidence has been rising in immigrant groups and patients with AIDS. It is caused by both *Mycobacterium tuberculosis* and *M bovis*. Active pulmonary disease is present in less than 50% of patients. The most frequent site of involvement is the ileocecal region; however, any region of the gastrointestinal tract may be involved. Intestinal tuberculosis may cause mucosal ulcerations or scarring and fibrosis with narrowing of the lumen. Patients may complain of chronic abdominal pain, obstructive symptoms, weight loss, and diarrhea. An abdominal mass may be palpable. Complications include intestinal obstruction, hemorrhage, fistula formation, and bacterial overgrowth with malabsorption. The PPD skin test may be negative, especially in patients with weight loss or AIDS. Barium radiography may demonstrate mucosal ulcerations, thickening, or stricture formation. The differential diagnosis includes Crohn's disease, carcinoma, and intestinal amebiasis. The diagnosis is established by either endoscopic or surgical biopsy revealing acid-fast bacilli within involved tissue.

Treatment with standard regimens is effective.

Leder RA et al: Tuberculosis of the abdomen. Radiol Clin North Am 1995;33:691. [NLM Cit ID: 95334568]

PROTEIN-LOSING ENTEROPATHY

Protein-losing enteropathy comprises a number of conditions that result in excessive loss of serum proteins into the gastrointestinal tract. The essential diagnostic features are hypoalbuminemia and an elevated fecal α_1-antitrypsin level.

The normal intact gut epithelium prevents the loss of serum proteins. Proteins may be lost through one of three mechanisms: (1) mucosal disease with ulceration, resulting in the loss of proteins across the disrupted mucosal surface; (2) lymphatic obstruction, resulting in the loss of protein-rich chylous fluid from mucosal lacteals; and (3) idiopathic change in permeability of mucosal capillaries and conductance of interstitium, resulting in "weeping" of protein-rich fluid from the mucosal surface (Table 14–13).

Hypoalbuminemia is the sine qua non of protein-losing enteropathy. However, a number of other serum proteins such as α_1-antitrypsin also are lost from the gut epithelium. In protein-losing enteropathy caused by lymphatic obstruction, loss of lymphatic fluid commonly results in lymphocytopenia (< 1000/μL), reduced serum gamma globulins, and reduced cholesterol.

In most cases, protein-losing enteropathy is recognized as a sequela of a known gastrointestinal disorder. In patients in whom the cause is unclear, evaluation is indicated and is guided by the clinical suspicion. Protein-losing enteropathy must be distinguished from other causes of hypoalbuminemia, which include liver disease and nephrotic syndrome; and from congestive heart failure. Protein-losing enteropathy is confirmed by determining the gut α_1-antitrypsin clearance (24-hour volume of feces × stool concentration of α_1-antitrypsin ÷ serum α_1-antitrypsin concentration). A clearance of more than 13 mL/24 h is abnormal.

Laboratory evaluation of protein-losing enteropathy consists of serum protein electrophoresis, lymphocyte count, and serum cholesterol to look for evidence of lymphatic obstruction. Serum ANA and C3 levels are useful to screen for collagen vascular disorders. Stool samples should be examined for ova and parasites. Evidence of malabsorption is evaluated by means of a stool qualitative fecal fat determination. Intestinal imaging is performed with an upper endoscopy with small bowel biopsy and a small bowel barium series. Colonic diseases are excluded with barium enema or colonoscopy. A CT scan of the abdomen is performed to look for evidence of neoplasms or lymphatic obstruction. Rarely, lymphangiography is helpful. In some situations, laparotomy with full-thickness intestinal biopsy is required to establish a diagnosis.

Treatment is directed at the underlying cause.

Table 14–13. Causes of protein-losing enteropathy.

Mucosal disease with ulceration
Chronic gastric ulcer
Gastric carcinoma
Lymphoma
Inflammatory bowel disease
Idiopathic ulcerative jejunoileitis
Lymphatic obstruction
Primary intestinal lymphangiectasia
Secondary obstruction
Cardiac disease: constrictive pericarditis, congestive heart failure
Infections: tuberculosis, Whipple's disease
Neoplasms: lymphoma, Kaposi's sarcoma
Retroperitoneal fibrosis
Sarcoidosis
Idiopathic mucosal transudation
Ménétrier's disease
Zollinger-Ellison syndrome
Acute viral gastroenteritis
Celiac sprue
Eosinophilic gastroenteritis
Allergic protein-losing enteropathy
Parasite infection: giardiasis, hookworm
Amyloidosis
Common variable immunodeficiency
Systemic lupus erythematosus

DISEASES OF THE COLON & RECTUM

IRRITABLE BOWEL SYNDROME

Essentials of Diagnosis

- Chronic functional disorder characterized by abdominal pain, alterations in bowel habits.
- Limited evaluation to exclude organic causes of symptoms.
- Symptoms usually begin in late teens to early 20s.

General Considerations

The functional gastrointestinal disorders are characterized by a variable combination of chronic or recurrent gastrointestinal symptoms *not explicable by the presence of structural or biochemical abnormalities.* Several clinical entities are included under this broad rubric, including chest pain of unclear origin (noncardiac chest pain), nonulcer dyspepsia, and biliary dyskinesia (sphincter of Oddi dysfunction). There is a large overlap between these entities. For example, over half of patients with noncardiac chest pain and over one-third with nonulcer dyspepsia also have symptoms compatible with irritable bowel syndrome. In none of these cases is there a definitive diagnostic process or test. Rather, the diagnosis is a subjective one based upon the presence of a compatible profile and the exclusion of other "organic" disorders.

Irritable bowel syndrome can be defined, therefore, as an idiopathic clinical entity characterized by some combination of chronic (more than 3 months) lower abdominal symptoms and bowel complaints that may be continuous or intermittent. A group of experts has met on two occasions in an effort to reach a consensus on the definition of functional gastrointestinal disorders, including irritable bowel syndrome, and to develop symptom-based diagnostic criteria that can be used in clinical care and research. The most recent or Rome II definition of irritable bowel syndrome is abdominal discomfort or pain that has two out of three features: (1) relieved with defecation; (2) onset associated with a change in frequency of stool; (3) onset associated with a change in form (appearance) of stool. Other symptoms supporting the diagnosis include abnormal stool frequency (more than three bowel movements per day or fewer than three per week); abnormal stool form (lumpy or hard or loose or watery); abnormal stool passage (straining, urgency, or feeling of incomplete evacuation); passage of mucus; bloating or feeling of abdominal distention.

Patients may have other somatic or psychologic complaints such as dyspepsia, heartburn, chest pain, fatigue, urologic dysfunction, gynecologic symptoms, anxiety, or depression.

The disorder is a common problem presenting to both gastroenterologists and primary care physicians. Up to 20% of the adult population have symptoms compatible with the diagnosis, but most never seek medical attention.

Pathogenesis

Irritable bowel syndrome probably represents a common clinical manifestation of a heterogeneous group of disorders. A number of pathophysiologic mechanisms have been identified and may have varying importance in different individuals.

A. Abnormal Motility: A variety of abnormal myoelectrical and motor abnormalities have been identified in the colon and small intestine. In some cases, these are temporally correlated with episodes of abdominal pain or emotional stress. Whether they represent a primary motility disorder or are secondary to psychosocial stress is debated. Differences between patients with constipation-predominant and diarrhea-predominant syndromes are reported.

B. Heightened Visceral Nociception: Patients often have a lower visceral pain threshold, reporting abdominal pain at lower volumes of colonic gas insufflation or colonic balloon inflation than controls. Although many patients complain of bloating and distention, washout studies have shown that their absolute intestinal gas volume is normal. Many patients report rectal urgency despite small rectal volumes of stool.

C. Psychosocial Abnormalities: More than half of patients with irritable bowel who seek medical attention have underlying depression, anxiety, or somatization. By contrast, those who do not seek medical attention are similar psychologically to normal individuals. Psychologic abnormalities may influence how the patient perceives or reacts to illness and minor visceral sensations.

Clinical Findings

A. Symptoms and Signs: Irritable bowel is a chronic lifelong condition. Symptoms usually begin in the late teens to twenties. Symptoms should be present for at least 3 months before the diagnosis can be considered. The diagnosis is established in the presence of compatible symptoms and after the exclusion of organic disease. Although patients report a variety of symptoms, four in particular are more common in this disorder than in organic disease: (1) abdominal distention, (2) abdominal pain relieved by defecation, (3) more frequent stools with the onset of abdominal pain, and (4) looser stools with the onset of pain. Over 90% of patients have two or more of these symptoms, compared with 30% with organic disorders. In patients over age 60, however, in whom organic disease is more common, the predictive value of these criteria is much lower.

Abdominal pain usually is intermittent, crampy, and in the lower abdominal region. It may be relieved by defecation, worsened by stress, and worse for 1–2 hours after meals. It does not usually occur at night or interfere with sleep. Patients may report predominant problems with constipation, diarrhea, or alternating constipation and diarrhea. It is important to clarify what the patient means by these complaints. The patient may use the term constipation to refer to hard or small stools, straining, or reduced stool frequency. Diarrhea may refer to loose stools, frequent stools, urgency, or fecal incontinence. Many patients report that they have a firm stool in the morning followed by progressively looser movements. Mucus is commonly seen. Complaints of visible distention and bloating are common, though these are not clinically evident.

The acute onset of symptoms raises the likelihood of organic disease. Nocturnal diarrhea, hematochezia, weight loss, and fever are incompatible with a diagnosis of irritable bowel syndrome and warrant investigation for underlying disease.

A thorough physical examination should be performed to look for evidence of organic disease and to allay the patient's anxieties. The physical examination usually is unremarkable. Abdominal tenderness, especially in the lower abdomen, is common but not pronounced. A new onset of symptoms in a patient over age 40 warrants further examination.

B. Laboratory Findings and Special Examinations: In a patient 20–50 years of age with a presumptive clinical diagnosis of irritable bowel syndrome, a limited series of examinations is warranted to screen for organic disease. The complete blood count, serologic tests, serum albumin, erythrocyte sedimentation rate, and stool occult blood test all should be normal. In patients with diarrhea, thyroid function tests and stool examination for ova and parasites should be performed. If diarrhea is predominant, a 24-hour stool collection is useful. Stool weight in excess of 300 g/d is atypical of irritable bowel and warrants further evaluation. In patients under age 40, flexible sigmoidoscopy should be performed. In patients over age 40 who have not had a previous evaluation, barium enema or colonoscopy should be considered.

Differential Diagnosis

These common symptoms may have multiple organic origins that should not be overlooked. Examples are colonic neoplasia, inflammatory bowel disease, causes of chronic constipation, causes of chronic diarrhea, endometriosis, and lactase deficiency. Psychiatric disorders such as depression and anxiety must be considered as well.

Treatment

A. General Measures: As with other functional disorders, the most important interventions the physician can offer are reassurance and a forthright explanation of the functional nature of the symptoms. Indeed, an ongoing therapeutic relationship may be the most important factor in successful management of this disorder. Patients should be told that their symptoms arise from either increased sensitivity to minor stimuli or increased reactivity resulting in spasm or abnormal motility. Although the "mind-gut" interaction should be mentioned, it should be emphasized that the symptoms are real, lest the patient conclude that the physician is implying that "it's all in my head." Physicians will earn the confidence of their patients by being nonjudgmental and attentive. Fears that the symptoms will progress, require surgery, or degenerate into serious illness should be allayed. The patient should understand that irritable bowel syndrome is a chronic disorder characterized by periods of exacerbation and quiescence. The physician can help but cannot "cure" such a disorder. The emphasis should be shifted from finding the cause of the symptoms to finding a way to cope with them. Physicians must resist the temptation to chase chronic complaints with new or repeated diagnostic studies.

B. Dietary Therapy: Patients commonly report dietary intolerances, though the role of dietary triggers in irritable bowel syndrome has never been convincingly proved. Nevertheless, the physician should be open to the idea that dietary changes—for whatever reason—may provide symptomatic benefit. In some patients, a food diary, in which symptoms, food intake, and life events are recorded, may reveal dietary or psychosocial factors that precipitate symptoms. Malabsorption of lactose, fructose, and sorbitol may cause bloating, distention, flatulence, and diarrhea. Lactose intolerance should be excluded in all patients with a trial of a lactose-free diet. Sorbitol is present in a number of artificially sweetened foods and some medications. A variety of foods are flatulogenic, producing pain and distention in some patients. These include brown beans, Brussels sprouts, cabbage, cauliflower, raw onions, grapes, plums, raisins, coffee, red wine, and beer. Caffeine is poorly tolerated by most patients with irritable bowel syndrome.

A trial of a high-fiber diet (20–30 g/d) should be recommended for most patients. This may be accomplished by giving 1 tbsp of bran powder two or three times daily with food or in 8 oz of liquid. Some patients report increased gas and distention from fiber supplementation with bran. Fiber supplements with psyllium, methylcellulose, or polycarbophil may be better tolerated (see section on constipation).

C. Pharmacologic Measures: More than two-thirds of patients with irritable bowel syndrome have mild symptoms that respond readily to education, reassurance, and dietary interventions. Drug therapy should be reserved for patients with more severe symptoms that do not respond to these conservative measures. These agents should be viewed as being adjunctive rather than curative. Given the wide spectrum of symptoms, no single agent is expected to provide relief in all or even most patients. Indeed, there is no convincing evidence that any of these agents are superior to placebo, which results in symptomatic improvement in up to 70% of patients. Nevertheless, therapy targeted at the specific dominant symptom (pain, constipation, or diarrhea) may be beneficial.

1. Antispasmodic agents–Anticholinergic agents may ameliorate postprandial abdominal pain when given 30–60 minutes before meals. Side effects include urinary retention, tachycardia, and dry mouth. Available agents include dicyclomine, 10–20 mg orally three or four times daily; hyoscyamine, 0.125 mg orally (or sublingually as needed), or sustained-release, 0.037 mg or 0.75 mg orally twice daily. Although calcium channel blockers relax gastrointestinal smooth muscle, they have not been well tested in patients with irritable bowel syndrome.

2. Antidiarrheal agents–Opioid and other antidiarrheal agents may be useful in patients with frequent loose stools (see section on chronic diarrhea). They may best be used "prophylactically" in situations where diarrhea is anticipated (such as stressful situations) or would be inconvenient (social engagements). Agents include loperamide, 2 mg orally three or four times daily, and diphenoxylate with atropine, 2.5 mg orally four times daily.

Serotonin 5-HT_3 receptors are involved in sensory, secretory, and motor processes in the gastrointestinal tract. Alosetron is a new 5-HT_3 receptor antagonist recently approved by the FDA for the treatment of women with diarrhea-predominant irritable bowel syndrome. Although its precise mechanisms of action are unknown, alosetron appears to slow colonic transit, enhance fluid absorption, and decrease visceral pain perception caused by colonic distention. In double-blind, placebo-controlled trials, alosetron 1 mg twice daily provided significant improvement in up to 50–60% of patients in abdominal pain and discomfort, urgency, and also resulted in a decreased stool frequency. For unexplained reasons, men with irritable bowel syndrome did not derive any benefit from this agent. Although the appropriate clinical role of this new agent is unclear, it may be useful in women with diarrhea-predominant symptoms who have failed conservative measures.

3. Anticonstipation agents–A trial of fiber supplementation with bran, psyllium, methylcellulose, or polycarbophil is beneficial in most cases. Patients who are unresponsive to fiber may be extremely difficult to manage.

4. Psychotropic agents–Some patients complain of chronic, unremitting abdominal pain. This small subset has a high incidence of underlying psychiatric disturbances and functional impairment and requires frequent office visits. These patients may benefit from antidepressants. Desipramine or imipramine may be started at a dosage of 25 mg at bedtime and increased gradually to 50 mg as tolerated. Serotonin reuptake inhibitors (sertraline 50–150 mg or fluoxetine 20–40 mg) are now commonly used because of their lower side effect profile and better safety than tricyclic antidepressants, though there are no controlled trials supporting their use. Improvement should be evident within 4 weeks.

5. Other agents–Anxiolytics and narcotics should not be used chronically in irritable bowel syndrome because they have addictive potential. Agents that reduce visceral afferent sensation (serotonin 5-HT_3 receptor antagonists) are currently under investigation.

D. Other Therapies: Behavioral modification with relaxation techniques and hypnotherapy may be beneficial in some patients. Patients with underlying psychologic abnormalities may benefit from evaluation by a psychiatrist or psychologist. Patients with severe disability should be referred to a pain treatment center.

Prognosis

The overwhelming majority of patients with irritable bowel syndrome learn to cope with their symptoms and lead productive lives.

Camilleri M et al: Improvement in pain and bowel function in female irritable bowel patients with alosetron, a 5-HT_3 receptor antagonist. Aliment Pharmacol Ther 1999; 13:1149. [NLM Cit ID: 99397956]

Camilleri M: Therapeutic approach to the patient with irritable bowel syndrome. Am J Med 1999;107(5A):27S. [NLM Cit ID: 20053391]

Drossman D et al: Rome II: a multinational consensus document on functional gastrointestinal disorders. Gut 1999;45(Suppl II):II1.

Drossman DA et al: Irritable bowel syndrome: A technical review for practice guideline development. Gastroenterology 1997;112:2120. [NLM Cit ID: 97322055]

ANTIBIOTIC-ASSOCIATED COLITIS

Essentials of Diagnosis

- Most cases of antibiotic-associated diarrhea are not attributable to *Clostridium difficile* and are usually mild and self-limited.
- Symptoms of antibiotic-associated colitis vary from mild to fulminant; almost all colitis is attributable to *C difficile.*
- Diagnosis in mild to moderate cases established by stool toxin assay.
- Flexible sigmoidoscopy provides most rapid diagnosis in severe cases.

General Considerations

Antibiotic-associated diarrhea is a common clinical occurrence. Characteristically, the diarrhea occurs during the period of antibiotic exposure, is dose-related, and resolves spontaneously after discontinuation of the antibiotic. In most cases, this diarrhea is mild, self-limited, and does not require any specific laboratory evaluation or treatment. Stool examination usually reveals no fecal leukocytes, and stool cultures reveal no pathogens. Although *C difficile* is identified in the stool of 15–25% of cases of antibiotic-associated diarrhea, it is also identified in 5–10% of patients treated with antibiotics who do not have diarrhea. Most cases of antibiotic-associated diarrhea are due to changes in colonic bacterial fermentation of carbohydrates and are not due to *C difficile.*

Antibiotic-associated colitis is a significant clinical problem almost always caused by *C difficile.* Hospitalized patients are most susceptible. This anaerobic bacterium colonizes the colon of 5% of healthy adults. In hospitalized patients, however, it is present in over 20% of patients, most of whom have received antibiotics that disrupt the normal bowel flora and thus allow the bacterium to flourish. Most of these patients are asymptomatic. Recently, patients receiving enteral tube feedings have been found to have a higher risk for acquisition of *C difficile* and the development of *C difficile*-associated diarrhea. The organism is spread in a fecal-oral fashion. It is found throughout hospitals in patient rooms and bathrooms and is readily transmitted from patient to patient by hospital personnel. Fastidious hand washing and use of disposable gloves are helpful in minimizing transmission.

In one-third of colonized patients, *C difficile*-induced colitis may develop. *C difficile* colitis is the major cause of diarrhea in patients hospitalized for more than 3 days, affecting 7:1000 patients. Although virtually all antibiotics have been implicated, colitis most commonly develops after use of ampicillin, clindamycin, and third-generation cephalosporins. Symptoms usually begin during or shortly after antibiotic therapy but may be delayed for up to 8 weeks. Thus, it is important to ask all patients with acute diarrhea about recent antibiotic exposure.

Clinical Findings

A. Symptoms and Signs: Most patients report mild to moderate greenish, foul-smelling watery diarrhea with lower abdominal cramps. Physical examination is normal or reveals mild left lower quadrant tenderness. With more serious illness, there is abdominal pain and profuse watery diarrhea with up to 30 stools per day. The stools may have mucus but seldom gross blood. There may be fever up to 40 °C, abdominal tenderness, and leukocytosis as high as 50,000/μL. In most patients, colitis is most severe in the distal colon and rectum. When colitis is more severe in the right side of the colon, there may be little or no diarrhea. In such cases, fever, abdominal distention, pain and tenderness, and leukocytosis suggest the presence of infection.

B. Special Examinations:

1. Stool studies–Pathogenic strains of *C difficile* produce two toxins: toxin A is an enterotoxin and toxin B a cytotoxin. In most patients, the diagnosis of antibiotic-associated colitis is established by the demonstration of *C difficile* toxins in the stool. A cytotoxin assay (toxin B) performed in cell cultures has a specificity of 90% and a sensitivity of 95%. This is the definitive test, but it takes 24 hours. Rapid enzyme immunoassays (EIA) (2–4 hours) for toxins A and B have been developed that have a 70–85% sensitivity. In a recent study, either the EIA or the cytotoxin assay was positive in only 81% of patients on the first stool sample and in 91% after two stool samples. Thus, one negative test does not exclude the diagnosis if the patient has typical symptoms and signs. Culture for *C difficile* is the most sensitive test, but 25% of isolates are not pathogenic. Because it is slower (2–3 days), more costly, and less specific than toxin assays, it is not used in most clinical settings. Fecal leukocytes are present in only 50% of patients with colitis.

2. Flexible sigmoidoscopy–Flexible sigmoidoscopy is performed in patients with more severe symptomatology when a rapid diagnosis is desired so that therapy can be initiated. In patients with mild to moderate symptoms, there may be no abnormalities or only patchy or diffuse, nonspecific colitis indistinguishable from other causes. In patients with severe illness, true **pseudomembranous colitis** is seen. This has a characteristic appearance, with yellow adherent plaques 2–10 mm in diameter scattered over the colonic mucosa interspersed with hyperemic mucosa. Biopsies reveal epithelial ulceration with a classic "volcano" exudate of fibrin and neutrophils. In 10% of cases, pseudomembranous colitis is confined to the proximal colon and may be missed at sigmoidoscopy.

3. Imaging studies–Abdominal radiographs are obtained in patients with fulminant symptoms to look for evidence of toxic dilation or megacolon but are of no value in mild disease. Mucosal edema or "thumbprinting" may be evident. Abdominal CT scan may be very useful in detecting colonic edema, especially in patients with predominantly right-sided colitis or abdominal pain without significant diarrhea (in whom the diagnosis may be unsuspected). CT is also useful in the evaluation of possible complications.

Differential Diagnosis

In the hospitalized patient who develops acute diarrhea after admission, the differential diagnosis includes simple antibiotic-associated diarrhea (not related to *C difficile*), enteral feedings, medications, and ischemic colitis. Other infectious causes are unusual in hospitalized patients who develop diarrhea more than 72 hours after admission, and it is not cost-effective to obtain stool cultures unless tests for *C difficile* are negative. Rarely, other organisms (staphylococci, *Clostridium perfringens*) have been associated with pseudomembranous colitis.

Complications

Fulminant disease may result in dehydration, electrolyte imbalance, toxic megacolon, perforation, and death. Chronic untreated colitis may result in weight loss and protein-losing enteropathy.

Treatment

A. Acute Therapy: If possible, antibiotic therapy should be discontinued. In patients with mild symptoms, doing so may result in prompt resolution of symptoms without specific treatment. If diarrhea is severe or persistent, specific therapy is warranted. The drug of choice is metronidazole, 500 mg orally three times daily. The duration of therapy is usually 10–14 days. However, in patients requiring long-term systemic antibiotics, it may be appropriate to continue metronidazole therapy until the antibiotics can be discontinued. Vancomycin, 125 mg orally four times daily, is equally effective as metronidazole but significantly more expensive, and it promotes the emergence of vancomycin-resistant nosocomial infections. Therefore, metronidazole is the preferred first-line therapy in most patients. Vancomycin should be reserved for patients who are intolerant of metronidazole, pregnant women, and children. Symptomatic improvement occurs in most patients within 72 hours. For patients with severe disease who do not respond rapidly to initial metronidazole therapy, therapy should be switched to vancomycin, 125 mg orally four times daily, escalating the dose to 500 mg four times daily if diarrhea and leukocytosis fail to improve. In patients who are unable to take oral medications and those with toxic megacolon, intravenous metronidazole, 500–750 mg every 6 hours, should be given; intravenous vancomycin does not penetrate the bowel and should not be used.

B. Treatment of Relapse: Up to 20% of patients have a relapse of diarrhea from *C difficile* within 1 or 2 weeks after stopping initial therapy. This may be due to reinfection or failure to eradicate the organism. Most relapses respond promptly to a second course of metronidazole therapy. Some patients have recurrent relapses that can be difficult to treat. The optimal treatment regimen for recurrent relapses is unknown. Many authorities recommend a 6-week tapering regimen of vancomycin (125 mg orally four times daily for 7 days; twice daily for 7 days; once daily for 7 days; every other day for 7 days; and every third day for 2 weeks). Oral administration of a live yeast, *Saccharomyces boulardii,* has been shown to reduce the incidence of relapse by 50% in one United States trial. However, this agent is not yet available in the United States.

Fekety R: Guidelines for the diagnosis and management of *Clostridium difficile*-associated diarrhea and colitis. Am J Gastroenterol 1997;92:739. [NLM Cit ID: 97293127]

Gorbach S: Antibiotics and *Clostridium difficile.* N Engl J Med 1999;341:1690. [NLM Cit ID: 20037753]

INFLAMMATORY BOWEL DISEASE

The term "inflammatory bowel disease" includes ulcerative colitis and Crohn's disease. Ulcerative colitis is a chronic, recurrent disease characterized by diffuse mucosal inflammation involving only the colon. Ulcerative colitis invariably involves the rectum and may extend proximally in a continuous fashion to involve part or all of the colon. Crohn's disease is a chronic, recurrent disease characterized by patchy transmural inflammation involving any segment of the gastrointestinal tract from the mouth to the anus.

Drug Therapies for Inflammatory Bowel Disease

Although ulcerative colitis and Crohn's disease appear to be distinct entities, the same pharmacologic agents are used to treat both. Despite extensive research, there are still no specific therapies for these diseases. The mainstays of therapy remain 5-aminosalicylic acid derivatives, corticosteroids, and mercaptopurine or azathioprine.

A. 5-Aminosalicylic Acid: 5-Aminosalicylic acid is a topically active agent that has a variety of anti-inflammatory effects. It is used in the active treatment of ulcerative colitis and Crohn's disease and during disease inactivity in order to maintain remission. It is readily absorbed from the small intestine but demonstrates minimal colonic absorption. A number of oral and topical compounds have been designed to target delivery of 5-aminosalicylic acid to the colon or small intestine while minimizing absorption. Formulations of 5-aminosalicylic acid currently available are sulfasalazine, olsalazine, and mesalamine.

1. Sulfasalazine–Sulfasalazine consists of 5-aminosalicylic acid linked by an azo bond to a sulfapyridine moiety. It is largely unabsorbed in the small intestine. In the colon, bacterial azoreductases cleave 5-aminosalicylic acid from the sulfapyridine group. It is unclear whether the sulfapyridine group has any anti-inflammatory effects. One gram of sulfasalazine contains 400 mg of 5-aminosalicylic acid. The 5-aminosalicylic acid works topically and is largely unabsorbed. The sulfapyridine group, however, is absorbed and may cause side effects in 15–30% of patients. Dose-related side effects include nausea, headaches, leukopenia, oligospermia, and impaired folate metabolism. Allergic and idiosyncratic side effects are fever, rash, hemolytic anemia, neutropenia, worsened colitis, hepatitis, pancreatitis, and pneumonitis. Sulfasalazine is significantly less expensive than other 5-aminosalicylic acid agents. It should always be administered in conjunction with folate.

2. Oral mesalamine agents–These 5-aminosalicylic acid agents are coated in various pH-sensitive resins (Asacol) or packaged in timed-release capsules (Pentasa). Mesalamine tablets dissolve at pH 7.0, releasing 5-aminosalicylic acid in the terminal small bowel and proximal colon. Pentasa releases 5-aminosalicylic acid slowly throughout the small intestine and colon. Side effects of these compounds are uncommon but include nausea, headache, pancreatitis, and nephropathy. Eighty percent of patients intolerant of sulfasalazine can tolerate 5-aminosalicylic acid.

3. Olsalazine–Olsalazine consists of two 5-aminosalicylic acid moieties linked by a diazo bond. Similar to sulfasalazine, it is not absorbed in the small intestine. A mild, dose-related secretory diarrhea occurs in 20% of patients. Since the advent of mesalamine, olsalazine is seldom used.

4. Topical mesalamine–5-Aminosalicylic acid is provided in the form of suppositories (500 mg) and enemas (Rowasa; 4 g/60 mL). These formulations can deliver much higher concentrations of 5-aminosalicylic acid to the distal colon than oral compounds. Side effects are extremely uncommon.

B. Corticosteroids: A variety of intravenous, oral, and topical steroid formulations have been used in inflammatory bowel disease. They have utility in the short-term treatment of moderate to severe disease. However, long-term use is associated with serious, potentially irreversible side effects and is to be avoided. The agents, route of administration, duration of use, and tapering regimens employed are based more upon personal bias and experience than upon data from rigorous clinical trials. The most commonly used intravenous formulations have been hydrocortisone or methylprednisolone, which are given by continuous infusion or every 6 hours. Oral formulations are prednisone or methylprednisolone. Topical preparations are provided as hydrocortisone suppositories (100 mg), foam (90 mg), and enemas (100 mg). Budesonide is a potent glucocorticoid with topical anti-inflammatory activity but low systemic activity due to high first-pass hepatic metabolism. An oral delayed-release formulation has been developed which delivers this agent to the ileum and colon, but it is not yet available in the United States.

C. Mercaptopurine and Azathioprine: Mercaptopurine and azathioprine are used in 10–15% of patients with refractory Crohn's disease and, increasingly, in ulcerative colitis. Side effects occur in 10%, including pancreatitis, bone marrow suppression, infections, hepatitis or cholestatic jaundice, allergies, and, potentially, a higher risk of neoplasm. After therapy is started, complete blood counts should be obtained weekly for 1 month and then once a month to monitor for myelosuppression. About one person in ten has a genetically acquired deficiency in the enzyme thiopurine methyltransferase (TPMT) that metabolizes these thiopurine medications, placing them at risk of profound immunosuppression. Levels of TPMT and mercaptopurine metabolites now are available clinically. Some studies have suggested that measurement of these levels may optimize drug dosing, improving efficacy and reducing toxicity of the agents. However, other studies report a limited correlation in individual patients between metabolite levels and clinical response. The proper role of these tests awaits further clinical testing.

Social Support for Patients With Inflammatory Bowel Disease

Inflammatory bowel disease is a lifelong illness that can have profound emotional and social impacts on the individual. Patients should be encouraged to become involved in the Crohn's and Colitis Foundation of America (CCFA). National headquarters may be contacted at 444 Park Avenue South, 11th Floor, New York, NY 10016-7374; phone 212-685-3440. Internet address: http://www.ccfa.org.

1. CROHN'S DISEASE

Essentials of Diagnosis

- Insidious onset.
- Intermittent bouts of low-grade fever, diarrhea, and right lower quadrant pain.
- Right lower quadrant mass and tenderness.
- Perianal disease with abscess, fistulas.
- Radiographic evidence of ulceration, stricturing, or fistulas of the small intestine or colon.

General Considerations

One-third of cases of Crohn's disease involve only the small bowel, most commonly the terminal ileum (ileitis). Half of cases involve the small bowel and colon, most often the terminal ileum and adjacent proximal ascending colon (ileocolitis). In 20% of cases, the colon alone is affected. Unlike ulcerative colitis, Crohn's disease is a transmural process that can result in mucosal inflammation and ulceration, stricturing, fistula development, and abscess formation.

Clinical Findings

A. Symptoms and Signs: Because of the variable location of involvement and severity of inflammation, Crohn's disease may present with a variety of symptoms and signs. In eliciting the history, the clinician should take particular note of fevers, the patient's general sense of well-being, the presence of abdominal pain, the number of liquid bowel movements per day, and prior surgical resections. Physical examination should focus upon the patient's temperature, weight, and nutritional status, the presence of abdominal tenderness or an abdominal mass, rectal examination, and extraintestinal manifestations. Most commonly, there is one or a combination of the following clinical constellations.

1. Chronic inflammatory disease–This is the most common presentation and is often seen in patients with ileitis or ileocolitis. Patients report low-grade fever, malaise, weight loss, and loss of energy. There may be diarrhea, which is nonbloody and often intermittent. Cramping or steady right lower quadrant or periumbilical pain is present. Physical examination reveals focal tenderness, usually in the right lower quadrant. A palpable, tender mass that represents thickened or matted loops of inflamed intestine may be present in the lower abdomen.

2. Intestinal obstruction–Narrowing of the small bowel may occur as a result of inflammation, spasm, or fibrotic stenosis. Patients report postprandial bloating, cramping pains, and loud borborygmi. This sometimes occurs in patients with active inflammatory symptoms (as above). More commonly, however, it occurs later in the disease from chronic fibrosis without other systemic symptoms or signs of inflammation.

3. Fistulization with or without infection–A subset of patients develop sinus tracts that penetrate through the bowel and form fistulas to a number of locations. Fistulas to the mesentery are usually asymptomatic but can result in intra-abdominal or retroperitoneal abscesses manifested by fevers, chills, a tender abdominal mass, and leukocytosis. Fistulas from the colon to the small intestine or stomach can result in bacterial overgrowth with diarrhea, weight loss, and malnutrition. Fistulas to the bladder or vagina produce recurrent infections. Enterocutaneous fistulas usually occur at the site of surgical scars.

4. Perianal disease–One-third of patients with either large or small bowel involvement develop perianal disease manifested by anal fissures, perianal abscesses, and fistulas. This can be a distressing problem.

5. Extraintestinal manifestations–The extracolonic manifestations (described in the section on ulcerative colitis) may also be seen with Crohn's disease, particularly Crohn's colitis. Other problems may also arise. Oral aphthous lesions are common. There is an increased prevalence of gallstones due to malabsorption of bile salts from the terminal ileum. Nephrolithiasis with urate or calcium oxalate stones may occur.

B. Laboratory Findings: There is a poor correlation between laboratory studies and the patient's clinical picture. Laboratory values may reflect inflammatory activity or nutritional complications of disease. A complete blood count and serum albumin should be obtained in all patients. Anemia may reflect chronic inflammation, mucosal blood loss, iron deficiency, or vitamin B_{12} malabsorption secondary to terminal ileal inflammation or resection. Leukocytosis may reflect inflammation or abscess formation or may be secondary to corticosteroid therapy. Hypoalbuminemia may be due to intestinal protein loss (protein-losing enteropathy), malabsorption, or chronic inflammation. The sedimentation rate or C-reactive protein level is elevated in many patients during active inflammation. Stool specimens are sent for examination for routine pathogens, ova and parasites, and *C difficile* toxin.

C. Special Diagnostic Studies: In most patients, the initial diagnosis of Crohn's disease is based upon a compatible clinical picture with supporting radiographic findings. An upper gastrointestinal series with small bowel follow-through is obtained in all patients. Suggestive findings include ulcerations, strictures, and fistulas. To evaluate the colon, a barium enema or colonoscopy is obtained. Colonoscopy offers the advantage of obtaining mucosal biopsies of the colon or terminal ileum. Typical endoscopic findings include aphthoid ulcers, linear or stellate ulcers, strictures, and segmental involvement with areas of normal-appearing mucosa adjacent to inflamed mucosa. In 10% of cases, it may be difficult to distinguish ulcerative colitis from Crohn's disease. When the diagnosis remains uncertain, two serologic tests may be useful in further distinguishing these two diseases. Antineutrophil cytoplasmic antibodies with perinuclear staining (pANCA) are found in 60–70% of patients with ulcerative colitis and 5–10% of patients with Crohn's disease. Antibodies to the yeast *S cerevisiae* (ASCA) are found in 60–70% of patients with Crohn's disease and 10–15% of patients with ulcerative colitis. A combination of pANCA negativity and ASCA positivity has been shown to have a 50% sensitivity and a 97% specificity for a diagnosis of Crohn's disease. Conversely, pANCA positivity and ASCA negativity has a 57% sensitivity and 97% specificity for a diagnosis of ulcerative colitis. The presence of granulomas on biopsy are seen in less than 25% of patients but are highly suggestive of Crohn's disease.

Complications

A. Abscess: The presence of a tender abdominal mass with fever and leukocytosis suggests an abscess. Emergent CT of the abdomen is necessary to confirm the diagnosis. Patients should be given broad-spectrum antibiotics and, if malnourished, maintained on TPN. Percutaneous drainage or surgery is usually required.

B. Obstruction: Small bowel obstruction may develop secondary to active inflammation or chronic fibrotic stricturing and is often acutely precipitated by dietary indiscretion. Patients should be given intravenous fluids with nasogastric suction for several days. Systemic steroids are indicated in patients with symptoms or signs of active inflammation but are unhelpful in patients with inactive, fixed disease. Patients unimproved on medical management require surgical resection of the stenotic area or strictureplasty.

C. Fistulas: The majority of enteromesenteric and enteroenteric fistulas are asymptomatic and require no specific therapy. Most symptomatic fistulas require surgical therapy, particularly when there is evidence of intestinal stricturing below the fistula. Medical therapy is effective in a subset of patients and is usually tried before surgery. Many fistulas close temporarily in response to TPN but recur when oral feedings are resumed. Azathioprine or mercaptopurine heals fistulas in 30–40% of patients but requires 3–6 months. The efficacy of an anti-TNF antibody, infliximab, in chronic fistulizing Crohn's disease was demonstrated in a recent multicenter trial. Fifty-five percent of patients given three infliximab injections (5 mg/kg) at zero, 2 and 6 weeks had rapid closure of their fistulas (both perianal and abdominal) for a median of 12 weeks. In patients treated with infliximab, it is recommended that mercaptopurine or azathioprine also be given to reduce the otherwise high likelihood of fistula recurrence. At this time, the optimal dosing regimen and the efficacy of repeated courses of infliximab for recurrent fistulous disease are unknown. Although cyclosporine has demonstrated some value for fistulous disease in small case series, high relapse rates and the risk of toxicity have limited use of this agent.

D. Perianal Disease: Patients with fissures, fistulas, and skin tags commonly have perianal discomfort. Severe pain should suggest a perianal abscess. The treatment of perianal problems can be very difficult. Initial conservative treatment with sitz baths, attempts to control diarrhea, and application of perianal cotton balls to absorb irritating drainage are warranted. Metronidazole, 250 mg three times daily, or ciprofloxacin, 500 mg twice daily, are commonly given but have not demonstrated any efficacy in controlled trials. Aminosalicylates are of no benefit. Steroids are of no value and may retard healing. The role of mercaptopurine or azathioprine and infliximab is discussed in the section on fistulas. Patients with abscesses require conservative incision and drainage. However, surgical fistulotomy can lead to incontinence and should be avoided. Patients with severe disease may sometimes benefit from placement of cutting seton drains by a colorectal surgeon.

E. Carcinoma: Patients with colonic Crohn's disease are at increased risk of developing colon carcinoma. Screening colonoscopy is recommended by most authorities.

F. Hemorrhage: Unlike ulcerative colitis, severe hemorrhage is unusual in Crohn's disease.

G. Malabsorption: Malabsorption may arise from bacterial overgrowth in patients with enterocolonic fistulas, strictures and stasis, extensive jejunal inflammation, and prior surgical resections.

Differential Diagnosis

Chronic cramping abdominal pain and diarrhea are typical of both irritable bowel syndrome and Crohn's disease, but x-ray examinations are normal in the former. Acute fever and right lower quadrant pain may resemble appendicitis or *Yersinia enterocolitica* enteritis. Intestinal lymphoma causes fever, pain, weight loss, and abnormal small bowel radiographs that may mimic Crohn's disease. Patients with undiagnosed AIDS may present with fever and diarrhea. Segmental colitis may be caused by tuberculosis, *Entamoeba histolytica,* chlamydia, or ischemic colitis. Diverticulitis with abscess formation may be difficult to distinguish acutely from Crohn's disease.

Treatment of Active Disease

Crohn's disease is a chronic lifelong illness characterized by exacerbations and periods of remission. As no specific therapy exists, current treatment is directed toward symptomatic improvement and controlling the disease process. The treatment must address the specific problems of the individual patient.

A. Nutrition:

1. Diet–Patients should eat a well-balanced diet with as few restrictions as possible. There is no convincing evidence of specific food allergy in disease pathogenesis. Because lactose intolerance is common, a trial off dairy products is warranted if flatulence or diarrhea is a prominent complaint. Patients with mainly colonic involvement benefit from fiber supplementation. Conversely, patients with obstructive symptoms should be placed on a low-roughage diet, ie, no raw fruits or vegetables, popcorn, nuts, etc. Resection of more than 100 cm of terminal ileum results in fat malabsorption. A low-fat diet with medium-chain triglyceride supplementation is used. Iron supplements may be necessary in patients with chronic intestinal blood loss. Parenteral vitamin B_{12} (100 μg intramuscularly per month) commonly is needed for patients with previous ileal resection or extensive terminal ileal disease.

2. Enteral therapy–Enteral therapy for 4 weeks is less effective than corticosteroids in inducing remission, and the relapse rate after return to a normal diet is high. Nevertheless, it may be considered in patients (especially children) who are refractory in an attempt to avoid chronic corticosteroids.

3. Total parenteral nutrition–TPN is used short-term in patients with active disease and progressive weight loss or those awaiting surgery who have malnutrition but cannot tolerate enteral feedings because of high-grade obstruction, high-output fistulas, severe diarrhea, or abdominal pain. It is required long-term in a small subset of patients with extensive intestinal resections resulting in short bowel syndrome with malnutrition.

B. Symptomatic Medications:

1. Symptomatic treatment of diarrhea–There are several potential mechanisms by which diarrhea may occur in Crohn's disease in addition to active Crohn's disease. A rational empirical treatment approach often yields therapeutic improvement that may obviate the need for corticosteroids or immunosuppressive agents. Involvement of the terminal ileum with Crohn's disease or prior ileal resection may lead to reduced absorption of bile acids that may induce secretory diarrhea from the colon. This diarrhea commonly responds to cholestyramine 2–4 g or colestipol 5 g two or three times daily before meals to bind the malabsorbed bile salts. Patients with extensive ileal disease or more than 100 cm of ileal resection have such severe bile salt malabsorption that steatorrhea may arise. Such patients may benefit from a low-fat diet; bile salt binding agents will exacerbate the diarrhea and should not be given. Patients with Crohn's disease are at risk for the development of small intestinal bacterial overgrowth due to enteral fistulas, ileal resection, and impaired motility and may benefit from a course of broad-spectrum antibiotics (see Bacterial Overgrowth, above). Other causes of diarrhea include lactase deficiency and short bowel syndrome (described in other sections). Use of antidiarrheals may provide benefit in some patients. Loperamide (2–4 mg), diphenoxylate with atropine (one tablet), or tincture of opium (5–15 drops) may be given as needed up to four times daily. Because of the risk of toxic megacolon, these drugs should not be used in patients with active severe colitis.

C. Specific Drug Therapy:

1. 5-Aminosalicylic acid agents–Sulfasalazine, 1.5–2 g twice daily, is effective in reducing clinical signs of disease activity in patients with colonic involvement but confers little benefit in small intestine disease. Although mesalamine (Asacol) and its slow-release form (Pentasa) are approved only for the treatment of ulcerative colitis, their release in the small intestine offers usefulness in the treatment of small bowel Crohn's disease. Several studies have confirmed remission rates of over 40% in patients with mild to moderate small bowel and ileocecal disease, particularly when these agents are used at high dosages (Pentasa 1 g four times daily; Asacol 0.8–1.2 g four times daily).

2. Antibiotics–For patients with mild disease who do not respond to aminosalicylates, antibiotic therapy with metronidazole (10 mg/kg/d) or ciprofloxacin (500 mg twice daily) appears to be as effective as aminosalicylates in controlled trials. Ciprofloxacin may be better for ileitis and metronidazole for ileocolitis or colitis.

3. Corticosteroids–Corticosteroids dramatically suppress the acute clinical symptoms or signs in most patients with both small and large bowel disease. However, steroids do not appear to alter the underlying disease. Prednisone, 40–60 mg/d, is generally administered to patients with an active flare-up of Crohn's disease. After improvement at 2–3 weeks, tapering proceeds at 5 mg/wk until a dosage of 20 mg/d is being given. Thereafter, very slow tapering of 2.5 mg/wk or every other week is recommended. Some patients cannot be completely withdrawn from steroids without experiencing a symptomatic flare-up. Chronic low steroid doses (2.5–10 mg/d) are often required. These may be associated with serious complications such as aseptic necrosis of the hips, osteoporosis, cataracts, diabetes, and hypertension. For these reasons, chronic steroids are to be avoided where possible. An ileal-release preparation of the oral topically active compound budesonide, 9 mg once daily, induces remission in 50–70% of patients with mild to moderate ileocolonic Crohn's disease. The efficacy of budesonide is superior to that of mesalamine and comparable to prednisone, with fewer steroid-related adverse effects. Budesonide is not yet available for oral use in the USA.

Patients with persisting symptoms despite oral steroids or those with high fever, persistent vomiting, evidence of intestinal obstruction, severe weight loss, severe abdominal tenderness, or suspicion of an abscess should be hospitalized. In patients with a tender, palpable inflammatory abdominal mass, CT scan of the abdomen should be obtained prior to administering steroids in order to rule out an abscess. If no abscess is identified, parenteral steroids should be administered (as described for ulcerative colitis). Nutritional support with enteral elemental feedings or parenteral nutrition is indicated for patients unable to tolerate an oral diet after 5 days.

4. Immunomodulatory drugs–Azathioprine (2–2.5 mg/kg) and mercaptopurine (1–1.5 mg/kg) are effective in the long-term treatment of Crohn's disease. They are most useful in the management of patients with unresponsive disease, those requiring chronic corticosteroids, and those with symptomatic fistulas. These agents permit elimination or reduction of steroids in over 75% and fistula closure in 30%. Blood counts should be monitored weekly for the first month, then monthly. Drug dosages should be monitored to maintain a white blood cell count > 3000/μL. Side effects requiring withdrawal of the drug occur in about 10%. The mean time to symptomatic response is 4 months, so these agents are not useful for acute exacerbations. Once patients achieve remission, these drugs reduce the 3-year relapse rate from over 60% to less than 25%. Other immunosuppressive agents have been investigated in the treatment of Crohn's disease, including cyclosporine and methotrexate; however, efficacy has been modest and toxicity greater than with the thiopurines.

A chimeric IgG anti-TNF antibody, infliximab, underwent expedited approval by the FDA for the treatment of active Crohn's disease. Improvement was demonstrated in 80% of patients with moderate to severe disease and remission in 33% after a single dose of 5 mg/kg intravenously. Maximal response is seen within 2 weeks in most patients and gradually diminishes over 3 months. Antinuclear antibodies and human antichimeric antibodies may develop, leading to a risk of infusion-related reactions, hypersensitivity reactions, and a lupus-like syndrome. At present, infliximab appears to be most useful in patients with severe Crohn's disease to promote rapid initial improvement while other immunosuppressives (azathioprine or mercaptopurine) are being initiated. Retreatment with infliximab every 8 weeks is required in some patients. Limited data suggest that efficacy is maintained during long-term treatment.

Maintenance of Remission

Crohn's disease is characterized by recurrent symptomatic flare-ups and remissions. All patients should be counseled firmly to stop smoking, as smokers appear to have a significantly higher recurrence rate. Although earlier trials of sulfasalazine (with or without corticosteroids) did not demonstrate efficacy of this agent in preventing disease recurrence, a recent meta-analysis of 15 randomized controlled trials confirms a modest (6.3%) but significant reduction in disease recurrence in patients treated with mesalamine (Asacol, 800 mg three times daily; or Pentasa, 500–750 mg four times daily). The benefit appears to be greatest in patients with ileal disease or recent surgical resection of active disease. Although chronic low doses of corticosteroids are often needed to control activity, they should not be used in patients with inactive disease to maintain remission. Alendronate should be considered to prevent osteoporosis in patients requiring chronic corticosteroids. The topically active steroid budesonide has not yet demonstrated convincing efficacy as maintenance therapy at 1 year. As discussed above, azathioprine and mercaptopurine have had a definite impact on maintaining remission and should be used in patients with frequent recurrences and patients who require chronic corticosteroids.

Indications for Surgery

Over half of patients will require at least one surgical procedure. The main indications for surgery are intractability to medical therapy, intra-abdominal abscess, massive bleeding, and obstruction with fibrous stricture. Patients with active inflammation who are unresponsive to medical therapy or who require chronic prednisone in doses exceeding 15 mg/d may achieve dramatic relief from limited surgical excision for 5–15 years before disease recurs.

Prognosis

With proper medical and surgical treatment, the majority of patients are able to cope with this chronic disease and its complications and lead productive lives. Few patients die as a direct consequence of the disease.

Colombel J et al: A controlled trial comparing ciprofloxacin with mesalamine for the treatment of active Crohn's disease. Am J Gastroenterol 1999;94:674. [NLM Cit ID: 99184454]

Pannaccione R et al: Is antibody testing for inflammatory bowel disease clinically useful? Gastroenterology 1999; 116:1001. [NLM Cit ID: 99192573]

Rutgeerts P et al: Efficacy and safety of retreatment with anti-tumor necrosis factor antibody (infliximab) to maintain remission in Crohn's disease. Gastroenterology 1999;117:761. [NLM Cit ID: 99431896]

Rutgeerts P: Clinical evaluation of the detection of antibodies in the serum for diagnosis and treatment of inflammatory bowel disease. Gastroenterology 1998;115:1006. [NLM Cit ID: 98456835]

2. ULCERATIVE COLITIS

Essentials of Diagnosis

- Bloody diarrhea.
- Lower abdominal cramps and fecal urgency.
- Anemia, low serum albumin.
- Negative stool cultures.
- Sigmoidoscopy is the key to diagnosis.

General Considerations

Ulcerative colitis is an idiopathic inflammatory condition that involves the mucosal surface of the colon, resulting in diffuse friability and erosions with bleeding. Approximately 50% of patients have disease confined to the rectosigmoid region (proctosigmoiditis); 30% extend to the splenic flexure (left-sided colitis); and less than 20% extend more proximally (extensive colitis). There is some correlation between disease extent and symptom severity. In the majority of patients, the extent of colonic involvement does not progress over time. In most patients, the disease is characterized by periods of symptomatic flare-ups and remissions.

Clinical Findings

A. Symptoms and Signs: The clinical profile in ulcerative colitis is highly variable. Bloody diarrhea is the hallmark. On the basis of several clinical and laboratory parameters, it is clinically useful to classify patients as having mild, moderate, or severe disease (Table 14–14). Patients should be asked about stool frequency, the presence and amount of rectal bleeding, cramps, abdominal pain, fecal urgency, and tenesmus. Physical examination should focus upon the patient's volume status as determined by orthostatic blood pressure and pulse measurements and by nutritional status. On abdominal examination, the clinician should look for tenderness and evidence of peritoneal inflammation. Red blood may be present on digital rectal examination.

1. Mild to moderate disease–Patients with mild disease have a gradual onset of infrequent diarrhea (less than five movements per day) with intermittent rectal bleeding and mucus. Stools may be formed too loose in consistency. Because of rectal inflammation, there is fecal urgency and tenesmus. Left lower quadrant cramps relieved by defecation are common, but there is no significant abdominal tenderness. Patients with moderate disease have more severe diarrhea with frequent bleeding. Abdominal pain and tenderness may be present but are not severe. There may be mild fever, anemia, and hypoalbuminemia.

2. Severe disease–Patients with severe disease have more than six to ten bloody bowel movements per day, resulting in severe anemia, hypovolemia, and impaired nutrition with hypoalbuminemia. Abdominal pain and tenderness are present. "Fulminant colitis" is a subset of severe disease characterized by rapidly worsening symptoms with signs of toxicity.

3. Extracolonic manifestations–Ulcerative colitis is associated with extraintestinal manifestations in 25% of cases. Some extracolonic signs are associated with disease activity. These include erythema nodosum, pyoderma gangrenosum, episcleritis, thromboembolic events, and an oligoarticular, nondeforming arthritis. In patients who are HLA B27-seropositive, there may be anterior uveitis or ankylosing spondylitis which is independent of colitis activity. Sclerosing cholangitis can occur in colitis patients even after total colectomy. Patients with this

Table 14–14. Ulcerative colitis: Assessment of disease activity.

	Mild	Moderate	Severe
Stool frequency (per day)	< 4	4–6	> 6 (mostly bloody)
Pulse (beats/min)	< 90	90–100	> 100
Hematocrit (%)	Normal	30–40	< 30
Weight loss (%)	None	1–10	> 10
Temperature (°F)	Normal	99–100	> 100
ESR (mm/h)	< 20	20–30	> 30
Albumin (g/dL)	Normal	3–3.5	< 3

entity are at higher risk of developing cholangiocarcinoma.

B. Laboratory Findings: The degree of abnormality of the hematocrit, sedimentation rate, and serum albumin reflect disease severity.

C. Endoscopy: In acute colitis, the diagnosis is readily established by sigmoidoscopy. The mucosal appearance is characterized by edema, friability, mucopus, and erosions. Colonoscopy should not be performed in patients with severe disease because of the risk of perforation. After patients have demonstrated improvement on therapy, colonoscopy is sometimes performed to determine the extent of disease, which will dictate the need for subsequent cancer surveillance.

D. Imaging: Plain abdominal radiographs are obtained in patients with severe colitis to look for significant colonic dilation. Barium enemas are of little utility in the evaluation of acute ulcerative colitis and may precipitate toxic megacolon in patients with severe disease.

Differential Diagnosis

The initial presentation of ulcerative colitis is indistinguishable from other causes of colitis, clinically as well as endoscopically. Thus, the diagnosis of idiopathic ulcerative colitis is reached after excluding other known causes of colitis. Infectious colitis should be excluded by sending stool specimens for routine bacterial cultures (to exclude salmonella, shigella, and campylobacter), ova and parasites (to exclude amebiasis), and stool toxin assay for *C difficile.* Mucosal biopsy can distinguish amebic colitis from ulcerative colitis. Enteroinvasive *E coli* and *E coli* O157:H7 will not be detected on routine bacterial cultures. CMV colitis occurs in immunocompromised patients (especially those with AIDS) and is diagnosed on mucosal biopsy. Gonorrhea, chlamydial infection, herpes, and syphilis are considerations in sexually active patients with proctitis. In elderly patients with cardiovascular disease, ischemic colitis may involve the rectosigmoid. A history of radiation to the pelvic region can result in proctitis months to years later. Crohn's disease involving the colon but not the small intestine may be confused with ulcerative colitis. In 10% of patients, a distinction between Crohn's disease and ulcerative colitis is difficult. The utility of ANCA and ASCA antibodies in these difficult patients is discussed in the section on Crohn's disease.

Treatment (Table 14–15)

There are two main treatment objectives: (1) to terminate the acute, symptomatic attack and (2) to prevent recurrence of attacks. The treatment of acute ulcerative colitis is dependent upon the extent of colonic involvement and the severity of illness.

Patients with mild to moderate disease should eat a regular diet but limit their intake of caffeine and gas-

Table 14–15. Treatment of ulcerative colitis.

Distal colitis
Proctitis
Mesalamine suppositories, 500 mg per rectum twice daily, or—
Hydrocortisone foam, 90 mg per rectum daily, or—
Hydrocortisone suppositories, 100 mg per rectum daily
Proctosigmoiditis
Mesalamine enema, 4 g per rectum daily, or—
Hydrocortisone enema, 100 mg per rectum daily
Extensive colitis
Mild to moderate
Sulfasalazine, 1.5–3 g orally twice daily, or—
Mesalamine tablets (delayed release), 2.4–4 g/d, or—
Olsalazine, 0.75–1.5 g orally twice daily
If no response after 2–4 weeks, add prednisone, 40–60 mg/d (taper by 5 mg/wk)
Severe
Methylprednisolone, 48–60 mg IV daily

producing vegetables. Fiber supplements decrease diarrhea and rectal symptoms (psyllium, 3.4 g twice daily; methylcellulose, 2 g twice daily; bran powder, 1 tbsp twice daily). Antidiarrheal agents should not be given in the acute phase of illness but are safe and helpful in patients with mild chronic symptoms. Loperamide (2 mg), diphenoxylate with atropine (one tablet), or tincture of opium (8–15 drops) may be given up to four times daily. Such remedies are particularly useful at nighttime and when taken prophylactically for occasions when patients may not have reliable access to toilet facilities.

A. Distal Colitis: Patients with disease confined to the rectum or rectosigmoid region generally have mild but distressing symptoms. Acute therapy is best approached with topical agents. Topical mesalamine is the drug of choice and is superior to topical corticosteroids. Mesalamine is administered as a suppository, 500 mg twice daily for proctitis, and as an enema, 4 g at bedtime for proctosigmoiditis, for 3–12 weeks, with 75% of patients improving. Topical steroids are a less expensive alternative to mesalamine but are also less effective. Hydrocortisone suppository or foam is prescribed for proctitis and hydrocortisone enema (80–100 mg) for proctosigmoiditis. Systemic effects from short-term use are very slight. It is not known whether combination therapy with mesalamine and hydrocortisone is advantageous. Patients with distal disease who fail to improve with topical therapy should be considered for systemic steroids or immunosuppressives as described below.

Patients whose acute symptoms resolve with acute therapy have an 80–90% chance of a symptomatic relapse within 1 year. Maintenance therapy with mesalamine suppositories (500 mg daily) or with oral agents (see below) reduce the relapse rate to less than 20% per year.

B. Mild to Moderate Colitis: Disease extending above the sigmoid colon is best treated with oral agents. The currently available agents—sulfasalazine and mesalamine—result in symptomatic improvement in 50–75% of patients. These drugs appear to be comparable in efficacy. To minimize side effects, sulfasalazine is begun at a dose of 500 mg twice daily and increased gradually over 1–2 weeks to 2 g twice daily. Most patients improve within 3 weeks, though some require 2–3 months. Total doses of 5–6 g/d may have greater efficacy but are poorly tolerated. Folic acid, 1 mg/d, should be administered to all patients taking sulfasalazine. Because of its greater cost, mesalamine should be reserved for patients who are intolerant of sulfasalazine. Mesalamine, 800 mg three times daily (Asacol) or 1 g four times daily (Pentasa), is approved for active disease. Higher doses (4–6 g daily) may be required in some patients. A recent controlled trial reported that the nicotine patch (22 mg) was more effective than placebo in symptom improvement in patients with mild to moderate ulcerative colitis. While this raises interesting questions related to disease pathogenesis, transdermal nicotine cannot yet be recommended for routine clinical use.

Patients with mild to moderate disease who fail to improve after 2–3 weeks of mesalamine therapy should have the addition of corticosteroid therapy. Topical therapy with hydrocortisone foam or enemas (80–100 mg twice daily) is tried first. Patients who fail to improve after 2 more weeks require systemic steroid therapy. Prednisone and methylprednisolone are most commonly used. Depending on the severity of illness, the initial oral dose of prednisone is 20–30 mg twice daily. Rapid improvement is observed in most cases. One can usually begin to taper prednisone after 2 weeks. Tapering of prednisone should proceed by no more than 5 mg/wk. After tapering to 15 mg/d, slower tapering is sometimes required. Complete tapering without symptomatic flare-ups is possible in the majority of patients.

C. Severe Colitis: About 10–15% of ulcerative colitis patients have a more severe course. Because they may deteriorate rapidly, hospitalization is generally required.

1. General measures–

a. Discontinue all oral intake. Total parenteral nutrition is indicated in patients with poor nutritional status.

b. Avoid all opiate or anticholinergic agents.

c. Restore circulating volume with fluids and blood as needed. Correct electrolyte abnormalities.

d. Perform frequent abdominal examinations to look for evidence of worsening distention or pain.

e. Obtain a plain abdominal radiograph on admission to look for evidence of colonic dilation.

f. Obtain surgical consultation in all patients with severe disease.

g. Send stools for bacterial (including *C difficile*) culture and examination for ova and parasites.

2. Corticosteroid therapy–Methylprednisolone, 48–64 mg, or hydrocortisone, 300 mg, is administered in four divided doses or by continuous infusion over 24 hours. Higher or "pulse" doses are of no benefit. Hydrocortisone enemas may also be administered twice daily as a drip, 100 mg over 30 minutes. In patients who have not previously received corticosteroids, administration of ACTH, 120 units/24 h, may be superior to corticosteroids. Approximately 50–75% of patients achieve remission with systemic steroids within 7–10 days. Once symptomatic improvement has occurred, oral fluids are reinstituted. If fluids are well tolerated, intravenous steroids are discontinued and the patient is started on oral prednisone (as described for moderate disease).

3. Cyclosporine–Intravenous cyclosporine benefits over 75% of patients with severe colitis who have not improved after 7–10 days of corticosteroids. This therapy may be considered in patients with severe steroid-resistant colitis who are reluctant to undergo colectomy. Of those who respond, over half will require colectomy within 6 months for recurrent disease.

4. Surgical therapy–Patients with severe disease who fail to improve after 7–10 days of corticosteroid therapy are unlikely to respond to continued steroids, and surgery is recommended. Patients with fulminant disease or toxic megacolon who worsen or fail to improve within 48–72 hours should undergo surgery to prevent perforation. If operation is performed before perforation, the mortality rate should be extremely low.

D. Fulminant Colitis and Toxic Megacolon: A subset of patients with severe disease have a more "fulminant" course with rapid progression of symptoms over 1–2 weeks and signs of severe toxicity. These patients appear quite ill, with prominent hypovolemia, hemorrhage requiring transfusion, and abdominal distention with tenderness. They are at a higher risk of perforation or development of toxic megacolon and must be followed closely. Broad-spectrum antibiotics should be administered to cover anaerobes and gram-negative bacteria.

Toxic megacolon develops in less than 2% of cases of ulcerative colitis. It is characterized by colonic dilation of more than 6 cm on plain films with signs of toxicity. In addition to the therapies outlined above, nasogastric suction should be initiated. Patients should be instructed to roll from side to side and onto the abdomen in an effort to decompress the distended colon. Serial abdominal plain films should be obtained to look for worsening dilation or ischemia.

Maintenance of Remission

Without chronic therapy, 75% of patients who initially go into remission on medical therapy will experience a symptomatic relapse within 1 year. Chronic maintenance therapy with sulfasalazine, 1–1.5 g twice daily; olsalazine, 500 mg twice daily; and mesalamine, 800 mg three times daily or 500 mg four times daily has been shown to reduce relapse rates to less than 33%.

Refractory Disease

A subset of patients either do not respond to aminosalicylates or corticosteroids or have symptomatic flares during attempts at steroid tapering. Surgical resection is traditionally recommended for patients with refractory disease. However, some patients may wish to avoid surgery and others have moderately severe disease for which surgery might not otherwise be warranted. Limited trials suggest that immunosuppressive therapy with mercaptopurine or azathioprine are of benefit in 60% of patients, allowing tapering of steroids and maintenance of remission. The risks of these agents and chronic immunosuppression must be weighed against the certainty of cure with surgical resection.

Risk of Colon Cancer

In ulcerative colitis patients with disease proximal to the sigmoid colon, there is a markedly increased risk of developing colon carcinoma. In patients who have had colitis for more than 10 years, the risk of developing colon cancer increases approximately 0.5–1% per year. Ingestion of folic acid, 1 mg/d, is associated with a decreased risk of cancer development. Colonoscopies are recommended every 1–2 years in patients with extensive colitis, beginning 8–10 years after diagnosis. At colonoscopy, multiple random biopsies are taken as well as biopsies of mass lesions to look for dysplasia or carcinoma. Because of the relatively high incidence of concomitant carcinoma in patients with dysplasia (either low- or high-grade), colectomy is recommended.

Surgery in Ulcerative Colitis

Surgery is required in 25% of patients. Severe hemorrhage, perforation, and documented carcinoma are absolute indications for surgery. Surgery is indicated also in patients with fulminant colitis or toxic megacolon that does not improve within 48–72 hours, in patients with dysplasia on surveillance colonoscopy; and in patients with refractory disease requiring chronic steroids to control symptoms.

Although total proctocolectomy (with placement of an ileostomy) provides complete cure of the disease, most patients seek to avoid it out of concern for the impact it may have upon their bowel function, their self-image, and their social interactions. After complete colectomy, patients may have a standard ileostomy with an external appliance, a continent ileostomy, or an internal ileal pouch which is anastomosed to the anal canal (ileoanal anastomosis). The latter maintains intestinal continuity, thereby obviating an ostomy. Under optimal circumstances, patients have five to seven loose bowel movements per day without incontinence. Inflammation in the ileal pouch develops in over one-fourth of patients but usually resolves with metronidazole. However, refractory cases of proctitis can be disabling and may require conversion to a standard ileostomy.

Prognosis

Ulcerative colitis is a lifelong disease characterized by exacerbations and remissions. For most patients, the disease is readily controlled by medical therapy without need for surgery. The majority never require hospitalization. A subset of patients with more severe disease will require surgery, which results in complete cure of the disease. Properly managed, most ulcerative colitis patients lead close to normal productive lives.

Han P et al: Nutrition and inflammatory bowel disease. Gastroenterol Clin North Am 1999;28:423. [NLM Cit ID: 99300863]

Meagher A et al: J ileal pouch-anal anastomosis for chronic ulcerative colitis: complications and long-term outcome in 1310 patients. Br J Surg 1998;85:800. [NLM Cit ID: 98330286]

Sands B: Novel therapies for inflammatory bowel disease. Gastroenterol Clin North Am 1999;28:323. [NLM Cit ID: 99300859]

Stein R et al: Medical therapy for inflammatory bowel disease. Gastroenterol Clin North Am 1999;28:297. [NLM Cit ID: 99300858]

VASCULAR ECTASIAS

Vascular ectasias, also called angiodysplasias and arteriovenous malformations, occur throughout the upper and lower intestinal tract. However, they most commonly occur in the cecum and ascending colon in elderly individuals (see sections on acute upper and lower gastrointestinal bleeding). They may be a cause of acute or chronic blood loss from the upper or lower gastrointestinal tract. Uncommonly, they are congenital, part of an inherited syndrome such as hereditary hemorrhagic telangiectasia, or related to autoimmune disorders such as scleroderma.

Most colonic ectasias are degenerative lesions that are hypothesized to arise from chronic colonic muscular contraction that obstructs the venous mucosal drainage. Over time, the mucosal capillaries dilate and become incompetent, and an arteriovenous communication forms. The cause of gastric and small intestine ectasias is unknown. Bleeding from vascular ectasias is commonly associated with a number of medical conditions, including valvular heart disease (especially aortic stenosis), chronic renal failure, and von Willebrand's disease.

Clinical Findings

Bleeding from vascular ectasias may present with acute or chronic gastrointestinal blood loss. Most patients are over age 70. Approximately 10% of patients have chronic or intermittent occult blood loss that may result in iron deficiency anemia. More commonly, patients develop recurrent, self-limited gastrointestinal bleeding that is not hemodynamically significant but is manifested by hematochezia, melena, or hematemesis. In a few patients, bleeding may be massive. Bleeding in younger patients is more apt to arise from the small intestine.

The evaluation and treatment of upper and lower gastrointestinal bleeding is discussed elsewhere. In patients with chronic or self-limited lower gastrointestinal bleeding, panendoscopy is the preferred means of identifying colonic, gastric, or duodenal vascular ectasias. They appear as flat red lesions (2–10 mm) with ectatic peripheral vessels radiating from a central vessel. However, ectasias can be identified in over 25% of subjects over age 60 and are multiple in over half of cases, which means that their mere presence does not *prove* that the lesion is the source of bleeding because active bleeding is uncommonly seen. Ectasias of the small intestine are extremely difficult to diagnose. Special long-push enteroscopes have been developed recently that permit evaluation of much of the jejunum. Even so, however, a large portion of the small intestine remains inaccessible to inspection. Patients with recurrent gastrointestinal hemorrhage may require laparotomy and intraoperative endoscopy in order to visualize the entire small bowel.

Treatment

A. Medical Management: Asymptomatic vascular ectasias discovered during routine endoscopy should not be treated, as the risk of subsequent bleeding is believed to be low. Patients with chronic gastrointestinal blood loss should receive iron supplementation. Some patients require intermittent transfusions. Uncontrolled trials have suggested that hormonal therapy with estrogen-progesterone (norethindrone, 1 mg, plus ethinyl estradiol, 0.05 mg) reduces the incidence of recurrent bleeding and the need for transfusions. A controlled trial, however, did not demonstrate any benefit from the conjugated estrogens, 0.625 mg/d, or birth control pills in patients with small intestine ectasias.

B. Endoscopic Therapies: Symptomatic gastric, duodenal, and colonic ectasias may be treated with endoscopic applications of cautery (bipolar cautery or heater probe) or with laser therapy. The incidence of subsequent bleeding episodes and the need for transfusions is reduced by these therapies but by less than 50%. Distal small intestinal ectasias are not accessible to these therapies.

C. Angiography: In patients with severe active lower gastrointestinal bleeding or bleeding from the distal jejunum or ileum, endoscopic therapy usually is not feasible. Selective superior mesenteric angiography may be able to identify the bleeding source and control hemorrhage in up to 80% of patients with vasopressin. Transcatheter embolization of the bleeding ectasia may also be used but is complicated by intestinal infarction in 15% of patients.

D. Surgery: Right hemicolectomy is performed in patients with recurrent bleeding attributed to colonic ectasias who have failed endoscopic ablation or in patients with severe bleeding that cannot be controlled with angiographic embolization. Where possible, it is highly desirable to localize the bleeding source to the right colon with angiography, scintigraphy, or colonoscopy prior to surgery. Because many of these patients are elderly and have concomitant medical problems, surgery has a significant risk. In up to 25% of patients, bleeding recurs after surgery from ectasias in the upper gastrointestinal tract. In patients with recurrent bleeding attributed to small intestinal ectasias, resection may be helpful if preoperative angiography can localize a single bleeding lesion. Alternatively, intraoperative endoscopy with resection or oversewing of identifiable ectasias may be necessary.

Barkin JS et al: Medical therapy for chronic gastrointestinal bleeding of obscure origin. Am J Gastroenterol 1998; 93:1250. [NLM Cit ID: 98370543] (Combination hormonal therapy [Ortho Novum 1/50] appeared to reduce the risk of rebleeding compared with estrogen alone in this uncontrolled observational study.)

Brandt L et al: Ability of naloxone to enhance the colonoscopic appearance of normal colon vasculature and colon vascular ectasias. Gastrointest Endosc 1999;49:79. [NLM Cit ID: 99088002] (Vascular ectasias can be difficult to visualize at colonoscopy. In this series of 114 patients, naloxone enhanced visualization of ectasias in 3%.)

Gordon R et al: Selective arterial embolization for the control of lower gastrointestinal bleeding. Am J Surg 1997;174:24. [NLM Cit ID: 97382956]

DIVERTICULAR DISEASE OF THE COLON

Colonic diverticulosis increases with age, ranging from 5% in those under age 40, to 30% at age 60, to more than 50% over age 80 in Western societies. In contrast, it is very uncommon in developing countries with much lower life expectancies. Most are asymptomatic, discovered incidentally at endoscopy or on barium enema. Complications in one-third include lower gastrointestinal bleeding and diverticulitis.

Colonic diverticula may vary in size from a few millimeters to several centimeters and in number from one to several dozen. Almost all patients with diverticulosis have involvement in the sigmoid colon; however, only 15% have proximal colonic disease.

In most patients, diverticulosis is believed to arise after many years of a diet deficient in fiber. The undistended, contracted segments of colon have higher intraluminal pressures. Over time, the contracted colonic musculature, working against greater pressures to move small, hard stools, develops hypertrophy, thickening, rigidity, and fibrosis. Diverticula may develop more commonly in the sigmoid because intraluminal pressures are highest in this region. The extent to which abnormal motility and hereditary factors contribute to diverticular disease is unknown. Patients with diffuse diverticulosis may have an inherent weakness in the colonic wall. Patients with abnormal connective tissue are also disposed to development of diverticulosis, including Ehlers-Danlos syndrome, Marfan's syndrome, and scleroderma.

1. UNCOMPLICATED DIVERTICULOSIS

More than two-thirds of patients with diverticulosis have uncomplicated disease and no specific symptoms. In some, diverticulosis may be an incidental finding detected during colonoscopic examination or barium enema examination. Some patients have nonspecific complaints of chronic constipation, abdominal pain, or fluctuating bowel habits. It is unclear whether these symptoms are due to alterations in the colonic musculature or underlying irritable bowel syndrome. Physical examination is usually normal but may reveal mild left lower quadrant tenderness with a thickened, palpable sigmoid and descending colon. Screening laboratory studies should be normal in uncomplicated diverticulosis.

There is no reason to perform imaging studies for the purpose of diagnosing uncomplicated disease. Diverticula are best seen on barium enema. Involved segments of colon may also be narrowed and deformed. Colonoscopy is a less sensitive means of detecting diverticula.

Asymptomatic patients in whom diverticulosis is discovered and patients with a history of complicated disease (see below) should be treated with a high-fiber diet or fiber supplements (bran powder, 1–2 tbsp twice daily; psyllium or methylcellulose) (see section on constipation). Retrospective studies suggest that such treatment may decrease the likelihood of subsequent complications.

2. DIVERTICULITIS

Essentials of Diagnosis

- Acute abdominal pain and fever.
- Left lower abdominal tenderness and mass.
- Leukocytosis.

Clinical Findings

A. Symptoms and Signs: Perforation of a colonic diverticulum results in an intra-abdominal infection that may vary from microperforation (most common) with localized paracolic inflammation to macroperforation with either abscess or generalized peritonitis. Thus, there is a range from mild to severe disease. Most patients with localized inflammation or infection report mild to moderate aching abdominal pain, usually in the left lower quadrant. Constipation or loose stools may be present. Nausea and vomiting are frequent. In many cases, symptoms are so mild that the patient may not seek medical attention until several days after onset. Physical findings include a low-grade fever, left lower quadrant tenderness, and a palpable mass. Stool occult blood is common, but hematochezia is rare. Leukocytosis is mild to moderate. Patients with free perforation present with a more dramatic picture of generalized abdominal pain and peritoneal signs.

B. Imaging: Plain abdominal films are obtained in all patients to look for evidence of free abdominal air (signifying free perforation), ileus, and small or large bowel obstruction. In patients with mild symptoms and a presumptive diagnosis of diverticulitis, empirical medical therapy is started without further imaging in the acute phase. Patients who respond to acute medical management should undergo sigmoidoscopy and barium enema after 7–10 days to corroborate the diagnosis and to exclude other disorders. If barium enema reveals a stricture or mass, colonoscopic evaluation should be performed to exclude malignancy. In patients who do not improve rapidly after 2–4 days of empirical therapy and in those with severe disease, CT scan of the abdomen is obtained to look for evidence of a free or contained abscess. Flexible sigmoidoscopy and barium enemas are contraindicated during the initial stages of an acute attack because there is a risk of free perforation.

Differential Diagnosis

Localized diverticulitis must be distinguished from perforated colonic carcinoma, Crohn's disease, appendicitis, ischemic colitis, and gynecologic disorders.

Complications

Fistula formation may involve the bladder, ureter, vagina, uterus, bowel, and abdominal wall. Diverticulitis may result in stricturing of the colon with partial or complete obstruction.

Treatment

A. Medical Management: Most patients can be managed with conservative measures. Patients with mild symptoms may be managed initially as outpatients on a low-residue diet and metronidazole, 500 mg three times daily, plus either ciprofloxacin, 500 mg twice daily, or trimethoprim-sulfamethoxazole, 160/800 mg twice daily orally for 14 days. Most cases of diverticulitis will require hospitalization acutely. Patients should be given nothing by mouth and should receive intravenous fluids. If ileus is present, a nasogastric tube should be placed. Intravenous antibiotics should be given to cover anaerobic and gram-negative bacteria. Single-agent therapy with ei-

higher than the expected prevalence in the adult population. (See section on colorectal cancer screening, below.) Thus, these tests are insensitive and nonspecific for adenomas.

C. Special Tests: Polyps are identified with barium enema examination, flexible sigmoidoscopy, or colonoscopy. Double contrast barium enema can detect up to 90% of polyps, especially those larger than 1 cm. Lesions identified on barium enema require colonoscopic removal or biopsy. Flexible sigmoidoscopy is commonly performed as part of colorectal cancer screening programs. Approximately one-half of colonic adenomas are within reach of a flexible sigmoidoscope. Polyps are seen in 10–20% of patients undergoing screening sigmoidoscopy and should be biopsied. Hyperplastic polyps require no further evaluation. Patients with "high-risk" adenomatous polyps at sigmoidoscopy (ie, those that are ≥ 1 cm in size, have villous histologic features, or have high-grade dysplasia) have an increased risk of harboring high-risk polyps or cancer in the proximal colon (8–10%) and therefore should undergo colonoscopy. Colonoscopy is the best means of detecting and removing these polyps, identifying 90% of polyps smaller than 8 mm and over 98% of larger polyps. The management of patients with small, low-risk adenomas (< 1 cm, no high-grade dyplasia or villous features) found at flexible sigmoidoscopy is controversial. Studies are conflicting as to whether such lesions are predictive of an increased prevalence of high-risk adenomas (> 1 cm or containing high-grade dysplasia or villous features) in the colon proximal to the splenic flexure. Therefore, while most clinicians recommend complete colonoscopy in all patients with adenomas detected on sigmoidoscopy in order to examine the proximal colon, there is debate about cost-effectiveness for colonoscopy in patients with single, small, distal adenomas.

Treatment

Most adenomatous polyps are amenable to safe colonoscopic removal. Large sessile lesions (> 2–3 cm) may be removed either in a piecemeal fashion or may require primary surgical resection. Once all adenomatous polyps have been removed, repeat "surveillance" colonoscopy is recommended in 3 years to look for missed polyps or new adenomas. If colonoscopy is negative after 3 years, subsequent surveillance may be increased to 5 years.

Malignant polyps may be considered to be adequately treated if (1) the polyp is completely excised and submitted for pathologic examination, (2) it is well differentiated, (3) the margin is not involved, or (4) there is no vascular or lymphatic involvement. The excision site of these "favorable" malignant polyps should be checked at 3 months for residual tissue. In patients with malignant polyps with unfavorable characteristics, surgical cancer resection is advised if the patient is a good operative candidate.

Prolonged regular use of aspirin (325 mg twice a week or oftener) or NSAIDs is associated with a 30–50% decrease in incidence of colorectal cancer and may reduce the number of colorectal adenomas. Pending results of aspirin chemoprevention trials, patients with colorectal adenomas may be advised to take aspirin 325 mg every other day prophylactically (see Chapter 1).

Prognosis

The results of a National Polyp Study involving over 1400 patients with adenomatous polyps treated with colonoscopic removal demonstrated a decline in the expected development of adenocarcinoma of almost 90% over a 13-year period. All but one of the cancers that did arise were Dukes A lesions.

Baron J et al: Calcium supplements for the prevention of colorectal adenomas. N Engl J Med 1999;340:101. [NLM Cit ID: 99091094] (Calcium carbonate resulted in a minimal [albeit significant] reduction in recurrent adenomas [OR 0.85; 95% CI 0.74–0.98]).

Levin TR et al: Predicting advanced colonic neoplasia with screening sigmoidoscopy. JAMA 1999;281:1611. [NLM Cit ID: 99249233]

Sandler R et al: Aspirin and nonsteroidal anti-inflammatory agents and the risk for colorectal adenomas. Gastroenterology 1998;114:441. [NLM Cit ID: 98156647] (Regular users of aspirin or NSAIDs were half as likely as nonusers [OR 0.56; 95% CI 0.34–0.92] to have adenomas at colonoscopy.)

Wallace MB et al: Is colonoscopy indicated for small adenomas found by screening flexible sigmoidoscopy? Ann Intern Med 1998;129:273. [NLM Cit ID: 98382167]

FAMILIAL POLYPOSIS SYNDROMES

Gastrointestinal polyposis syndromes are inherited conditions that result in the development of multiple polyps throughout the gastrointestinal tract and impose an increased risk of carcinoma. They are rare, accounting for less than 1% of colorectal cancers.

1. FAMILIAL ADENOMATOUS POLYPOSIS

Familial adenomatous polyposis is an autosomal dominant disease characterized by the development of hundreds to thousands of adenomas in the colon and by various extracolonic features. It is due to a defect in the adenomatous polyposis coli gene *(APC)*, which is located on the long arm of chromosome 5. Eighty percent of families have been found to have a genetic mutation in this gene. There is evidence that the location of the mutation affects the number of polyps and the risk of cancer development.

Polyps occur at a mean age of 16 years, and almost all affected individuals have adenomas by age 35 years. Colon cancer is inevitable by age 50 unless prophylactic colectomy is performed. Gastric fundic gland polyps occur in over 50% but have no malignant potential. In contrast, duodenal adenomatous polyps occur in over 90%. There is a 5% lifetime risk of malignancy in the duodenum, the pancreatic ampulla, and—less commonly—the stomach. Extraintestinal manifestations of familial adenomatous polyposis in some families include osteomas, soft tissue tumors of the skin, dermoid tumors, and congenital hypertrophy of the retina. The combination of familial adenomatous polyposis and extraintestinal lesions used to be called Gardner's syndrome. The distinction between familial adenomatous polyposis and Gardner's syndrome is now questionable, as the same genetic defects have been found in both. When central nervous system tumors are found with familial adenomatous polyposis, the condition has been called Turcot's syndrome. Two-thirds of these families have a defect in the *APC* gene. An attenuated variant of familial adenomatous polyposis has also been recognized in which affected family members form an average of only 30 polyps and therefore have a lower risk of cancer. These families appear to have a specific defect on the 5′ end of the *APC* gene.

In families known to be affected, screening sigmoidoscopy to detect the development of polyps should begin at age 10–12 and be repeated every 1–2 years. Genetic testing can now be offered, followed by appropriate counseling. Genetic testing is indicated to confirm the diagnosis in patients with a compatible clinical profile and in first-degree family members of affected patients with a proved gene mutation. The cost of genetic screening is 500–750 dollars per individual. Testing should not be performed in children under the age of 12. Affected family members should undergo total colectomy with either ileoanal or ileorectal anastomosis. Patients with the ileorectal anastomosis require frequent sigmoidoscopy for cancer surveillance and obliteration of rectal polyps. The risk of subsequent rectal cancer is over 10%. Sulindac, 150 mg twice daily, has been shown to decrease the number and size of adenomatous polyps in the rectal stump. Upper endoscopy should be performed every 1–3 years in affected family members to look for gastric and duodenal adenomas.

Giardiello F et al: Phenotypic expression of disease in families that have mutations in the 5′ region of the adenomatous polyposis coli gene. Ann Intern Med 1997;126:514. [NLM Cit ID: 97230747] (An attenuated phenotype of *APC* in which affected family members have an average of 30 adenomas and a more delayed development of colon cancer than classic *APC* families.)

Lindor N et al: The concise handbook of family cancer syndromes. J Natl Cancer Inst 1998;90:1039. [NLM Cit ID: 98335998]

2. OTHER POLYPOSIS SYNDROMES

Peutz-Jeghers syndrome is an autosomal dominant condition characterized by hamartomatous polyps throughout the gastrointestinal tract (most notably in the small intestine) as well as mucocutaneous pigmented macules on the lips, buccal mucosa, and skin. The hamartomas may become quite large, leading to bleeding, intussusception, or obstruction. Although hamartomas are not premalignant, up to 50% of these patients develop malignancies of the gastrointestinal tract (especially the stomach and duodenum) and nonintestinal organs (breasts, gonads, pancreas).

Familial juvenile polyposis is also autosomal dominant and characterized by several—more than ten—juvenile hamartomatous polyps, located most commonly in the colon. There is an increased risk of adenocarcinoma due to synchronous adenomatous polyps or mixed hamartomatous-adenomatous polyps.

Boardman L et al: Increased risk of cancer in patients with Peutz-Jeghers syndrome. Ann Intern Med 1998;128:896. [NLM Cit ID: 98285332]

COLORECTAL CANCER

Essentials of Diagnosis

- Symptoms or signs dependent upon tumor location.
- Proximal colon: fecal occult blood, anemia.
- Distal colon: change in bowel habits, hematochezia.
- Characteristic findings on barium enema.
- Diagnosis established with colonoscopy.

General Considerations

Colorectal cancer is the second leading cause of death due to malignancy in the United States. Approximately 5% of Americans will develop colorectal cancer and 40% of those will die of the disease. An estimated 134,000 new cases and 55,000 deaths occur annually. Colorectal cancers are almost all adenocarcinomas, which tend to form bulky exophytic masses or annular constricting lesions. Approximately half of cancers are located within the rectosigmoid region; one fourth are located proximally in the cecum and ascending colon. It is currently believed that the majority of colorectal cancers arise from malignant transformation of an adenomatous polyp.

Risk Factors

A number of factors increase the risk of developing colorectal cancer. Recognition of these has impact upon screening strategies. However, 75% of all new cases occur in people with no known predisposing factors.

A. Age: The incidence of colorectal cancer rises sharply after age 40, and 90% of cases occur in persons over age 50.

B. Personal History of Neoplasia: A history of adenomatous polyps (especially if multiple or > 1 cm) increases the risk of subsequent adenomas and

the size and depth of penetration, and the patient's overall condition. In carefully selected patients with small (< 3 cm), well-differentiated rectal tumors that are less than 7.5 cm from the anal verge and that appear on endosonography and CT imaging to be localized to the rectal wall, transanal excision may be performed. This approach avoids laparotomy and spares the rectum and anal sphincter, preserving normal bowel continence. All other patients will require either a low anterior resection with a colorectal anastomosis or an abdominoperineal resection with a colostomy, depending upon how far above the anal verge the tumor is located and the extent of local tumor spread. With unresectable rectal cancer, the patient may be palliated with a diverting colostomy, laser fulguration, or placement of an expandable wire stent.

A. Adjuvant Therapy for Colon Cancer: Adjuvant chemotherapy and radiotherapy have been demonstrated to improve overall and tumor-free survival in selected patients with colorectal cancer.

1. Stage I–Because of the excellent 5-year survival rate (80–100%), no adjuvant therapy is recommended.

2. Stage II (node-negative disease)–The expected 5-year survival rate is 50–75%. A benefit from adjuvant chemotherapy has not been demonstrated in controlled trials for stage II colon cancer. Patients with advanced local stage II disease (T3–T4) should be considered for study protocols looking at the role of adjuvant chemotherapy or radiotherapy for control of local recurrence.

3. Stage III (node-positive disease)–The expected 5-year survival rate is 30–50%. Adjuvant chemotherapy with fluorouracil and either levamisole or leucovorin has been shown to reduce mortality by up to 33%. Pending results of comparative trials of levamisole versus leucovorin, the combination of fluorouracil and levamisole is still considered the standard adjuvant regimen. Selected patients with locally advanced colon cancer (T3–T4) may benefit from radiotherapy to reduce the risk of local recurrence.

4. Stage IV (metastatic disease)–Approximately 20% of patients have metastatic disease at the time of initial diagnosis, and another 30% eventually develop distant metastasis. The long-term survival rate of these patients is only 5%. Resection or ablation (cryosurgery, embolization, ultrasound) of isolated (one to three) liver or lung metastases may result in long-term (> 5 years) survival in up to 20% of cases. Systemic chemotherapy with fluorouracil may offer palliation for some patients but does not prolong survival.

B. Adjuvant Therapy for Rectal Cancer: In the United States, combined postoperative adjuvant therapy with pelvic radiation and chemotherapy with fluorouracil is recommended for both stage II and stage III rectal cancers. Such therapy has been shown to improve both the overall and the disease-free survival rate and to decrease pelvic recurrences. In Europe, radiation is used preoperatively and chemotherapy typically is not used. The merits of these approaches are debated. Preoperative radiation may shrink tumor, permitting low anterior resection or transanal excision of some cases previously thought to need abdominoperineal resection with colostomy. However, it may lead to higher surgical complication rates and unnecessary treatment of some patients who are "over-staged" by clinical criteria. Postoperative therapy allows accurate staging but may lead to inadvertent radiation of small intestines as well as the surgical anastomosis. Pending further trials, therapy is individualized. Where possible, patients should be enrolled in clinical trials that seek to identify the optimal combined modality regimen.

Follow-Up After Surgery

Patients who have undergone resections for cure are followed closely to look for evidence of tumor recurrence. The optimal cost-effective strategy is not clear and varies in different medical centers. Two recent randomized trials reported that in the follow-up of colorectal cancer patients, intense follow-up with yearly colonoscopy, abdominal CT, and chest radiography did not improve overall outcome compared with most standard follow-up protocols. In the absence of consensus guidelines, the following may be recommended. Patients should be evaluated every 3–6 months for 3–5 years with history, physical examination, fecal occult blood testing, liver function tests, and CEA determinations. Colonoscopy is performed within 6–12 months after operation to look for evidence of recurrence and then every 3–5 years to look for metachronous polyps or cancer. A change in the patient's clinical picture, abnormal liver function tests, or a rising CEA warrant investigation with chest radiography and abdominal CT to look for recurrent or metastatic disease that may be amenable to therapy.

Prognosis

The stage of disease at presentation is the most important determinant of long-term survival: stage I, > 90%; stage II, > 70%; stage III with fewer than four positive lymph nodes, 67%; stage III with more than four positive lymph nodes, 33%; and stage IV, < 5%. For each stage, rectal cancers have a worse prognosis. Although molecular markers (eg, *P53* mutation, 18q deletion, Ki-*ras* mutation) may be independent risk factors for the development of metastatic disease, these are not yet used clinically to guide therapy or follow up. Tumors that have DNA replication errors due to inactivation of mismatch repair genes (HNPCC and 15% of sporadic cancers) appear to have a more favorable prognosis.

For those patients whose disease progresses despite therapy, meticulous efforts at palliative care are essential (see Chapter 5).

Screening for Colorectal Neoplasms

Because virtually all colorectal cancers arise from adenomas, it is theoretically possible to prevent colon cancer by the early detection and removal of adenomas or to improve survival from colon cancer by detecting it at an earlier, presymptomatic stage. Various strategies have been endorsed, including fecal occult blood testing, flexible sigmoidoscopy, and screening colonoscopy. At present, the optimal cost-effective strategy has not been agreed upon.

In 1996, the United States Preventive Services Task Force issued the following recommendation for colorectal cancer screening: "Screening for colorectal cancer is recommended for all persons aged 50 and older with annual fecal occult blood testing (FOBT), or sigmoidoscopy [periodicity unspecified], or both. There is insufficient evidence to determine which of these screening methods is preferable or whether the combination of FOBT and sigmoidoscopy produces greater benefits than does either test alone. There is also insufficient evidence to recommend for or against routine screening with digital rectal examination, barium enema, or colonoscopy, although recommendations against such screening in average-risk persons can be made on other grounds. Persons with a family history of hereditary syndromes associated with a high risk of colon cancer should be referred for diagnosis and management."

A. Fecal Occult Blood Testing (FOBT): The normal gastrointestinal tract loses less than 2 mL/d of blood. Most cancers and some adenomas result in increased chronic blood loss that may be detectable. A variety of tests have been developed that have varying sensitivities for fecal occult blood. A guaiac-based test (Hemoccult II) has undergone the most extensive testing and has had the greatest clinical use. Two slides should be prepared from each of three consecutive bowel movements. To reduce the likelihood of false-positive tests, patients should abstain from aspirin (in doses greater than 325 mg/d), NSAIDs, red meat, poultry, fish, and vegetables with peroxide activity (turnips, horseradish) for 72 hours. Vitamin C may cause a false-negative test. Slides should be developed within 7 days after preparation. When administered to the general population as part of a colorectal cancer screening program, 1–4.5% of tests are positive; if the slides are rehydrated, the incidence of positive tests rises to 10%.

Patients with positive fecal occult blood tests should undergo colonoscopy with removal of any polyps identified. If colonoscopy reveals no colorectal neoplasm or only a solitary small adenoma (< 1 cm), further screening for colorectal cancer may be deferred for 5 or more years. The sensitivity of nonrehydrated slides for colorectal cancer is 50–80%, and the specificity is 98%. Rehydrating slides increases the sensitivity to 80–90% but decreases the specificity to 90%. The positive predictive value for colorectal cancer of a positive test is 6–17% for unhydrated slides but only 2.2% for rehydrated slides. Because of the low specificity and positive predictive value, slides should not be rehydrated. The cancers that are detected are more likely to be earlier stage lesions (Dukes A or B). Adenomatous polyps are identified in 25–50% of patients with positive tests. The finding of these polyps in most instances is fortuitous, since most are < 1 cm in size and unlikely to cause bleeding.

The impact of fecal occult blood testing on the colorectal cancer mortality rate has been assessed in several large, prospective studies in which fecal occult blood testing was performed either yearly or biennially. Three studies have confirmed a reduction in colorectal cancer mortality of 15–33% after 8–13 years. Both annual and biennial screening have resulted in reduction in colon cancer mortality, but annual testing is recommended.

B. Flexible Sigmoidoscopy: Use of a flexible 60 cm sigmoidoscope permits visualization of the descending and rectosigmoid colon and identifies up to 60% of adenomatous polyps and colorectal cancers. At screening sigmoidoscopy, adenomatous polyps are identified in 10–20% and colorectal cancers in 1% of patients. Polyps less than 5–10 mm in diameter should be removed by biopsy. Patients found to have adenomatous polyps should undergo pancolonoscopy (to look for synchronous neoplasms in the proximal colon) with polypectomy. As discussed previously, the need for colonoscopy in the patient found to have a solitary small adenoma (< 10 mm in diameter) at sigmoidoscopy is controversial. In some studies, such patients have not been found to have a higher prevalence of proximal polyps.

Retrospective studies of populations in which sigmoidoscopy was performed have demonstrated a reduced incidence of subsequent rectosigmoid carcinoma. Prospective screening sigmoidoscopy studies are ongoing.

Although the optimal interval for sigmoidoscopy is unknown, the American Gastroenterological Association and the American Cancer Society recommend a 5-year interval and Medicare provides reimbursement every 4 years for average-risk patients. A combination of FOBT testing and sigmoidoscopy corrects some of the limitations of each method used alone; however, it is unclear whether the increased costs and risks result in improvements in outcome.

C. Screening Colonoscopy: Approximately 30% of significant neoplasms (cancer, large polyps, polyps with high-grade dysplasia) are located proximal to the splenic flexure, ie, above the reach of a flexible sigmoidoscopy examination. Up to 50–60% of such patients do not have an adenomatous polyp distal to the splenic flexure at sigmoidoscopy. Therefore, screening with flexible sigmoidoscopy will miss 20–30% of significant proximal neoplasms. Accordingly, colonoscopy—which examines the entire colon—increasingly is advocated as a screening modality even in average-risk patients. A Veterans Administration Cooperative study of screening colonoscopy in almost 3200 asymptomatic adults has demonstrated this to be a safe and effective modality.

The American Gastroenterological Association and the American Cancer Society have endorsed screening colonoscopy at an interval of 10 years. However, at present most private insurance carriers and Medicare do not provide coverage for screening colonoscopy in asymptomatic, average-risk individuals.

D. Virtual Colonoscopy: Using computer-assisted image reconstruction and rapid helical CT, three-dimensional views can be generated of the lumen that simulate the view of colonoscopy. This technique, known as "virtual colonoscopy," is performed rapidly, requires no sedation or intravenous contrast, and is without risk. Compared with conventional colonoscopy, the sensitivity of virtual colonoscopy for detection of polyps > 1 cm is > 90%. At present, virtual colonoscopy is costly and not available at most centers outside of clinical trials. Pending further large controlled trials, it cannot yet be recommended for screening of average-risk patients.

E. Summary: Screening in Average-Risk Patients: There is great debate among medical investigators, health care analysts, and insurance providers as to the optimal approach to population-based colorectal cancer screening. Even so, everyone agrees that screening of some kind should be offered to all average-risk patients over age 50. The cost per year of life saved is similar ($20,000 per year) with FOBT, sigmoidoscopy, a combination of FOBT and sigmoidoscopy, or colonoscopy. Therefore, all of these screening options have been widely endorsed. Pending further studies, the physician must weigh costs, risks, convenience, efficacy, and patient preference in recommending a screening method.

F. Screening in High-Risk Patients: The screening of patients with ulcerative colitis, patients from families with familial adenomatous polyposis and hereditary nonpolyposis colon cancer, and patients with prior histories of adenomatous polyps or cancer is discussed above.

Consensus recommendations for colorectal screening have been issued for patients with a family history of colon cancer. Patients with a single family member who developed colon cancer after age 55 should undergo routine screening with FOBT, sigmoidoscopy, or both but beginning at age 40. Patients with two or more first-degree relatives with colon cancer—or one first-degree member who developed colon cancer before age 55, or one first-degree member with an adenomatous polyp before age 60—should be considered for screening with colonoscopy. Patients with negative results at colonoscopy may defer further screening for 10 years.

[Colorectal Cancer—American Cancer Society]
http://www3.cancer.or/cancerinfo/maincont.asp?st=pr&ct=10

[Colon Cancer—National Cancer Institute—Cancer Net]
http://cancernet.nci.nih.gov/index.html

Aaltonen L et al: Incidence of hereditary nonpolyposis colorectal cancer and the feasibility of molecular screening for the disease. N Engl J Med 1998;338:1481. [NLM Cit ID: 98242977] (Recommendation that testing for DNA replication errors be performed in patients with colorectal cancer who are under 50 years of age, have a family history of colorectal or endometrial cancer, or have a history of multiple colorectal or endometrial cancers.)

Chung DC Molecular prognostic markers and colorectal cancer: the search goes on. Gastroenterology 1998; 114:1330. [NLM Cit ID: 98282373]

Fenlon H et al: A comparison of virtual and conventional colonoscopy for the detection of colorectal polyps. N Engl J Med 1999;341:1496. [NLM Cit ID: 20007498]

Lieberman D et al: Prevalence and location of serious neoplasia found at screening colonoscopy: preliminary results from the VA Colonoscopy screening trial. Gastroenterology 1999;116:G1996.

Lynch HT et al: Identifying hereditary nonpolyposis colorectal cancer. N Engl J Med 1998;338:1537. [NLM Cit ID: 98242985]

Smith TJ et al: Standard follow-up of colorectal cancer patients: Finally, we can make practice guidelines based on evidence. Gastroenterology 1998;114:211. [NLM Cit ID: 98089835]

Terdiman J et al: Genetic testing in hereditary colorectal cancer: indications and procedures. Am J Gastroenterol 1999;94:2344. [NLM Cit ID: 99411791]

Winawer S et al: Colorectal screening: clinical guidelines and rationale. Gastroenterology 1997;112:594. [NLM Cit ID: 97176776] (Consensus of an expert multidisciplinary panel convened to make recommendations regarding colorectal cancer screening and surveillance. A definitive work that summarizes all data through 1996.)

ANORECTAL DISEASES

HEMORRHOIDS

Essentials of Diagnosis

- Bright red blood per rectum
- Protrusion, discomfort
- Characteristic findings on external anal inspection and anoscopic examination

General Considerations

Internal hemorrhoids are a plexus of superior hemorrhoidal veins located above the dentate line which are covered by mucosa. They are a normal anatomic entity, occurring in all adults. Internal hemorrhoids form a vascular cushion in the lower rectum that may contribute to normal continence. They occur in three primary locations—right anterior, right posterior, and left lateral—though smaller hemorrhoids may occur between these primary locations. External hemorrhoids arise from the inferior hemorrhoidal veins located below the dentate line and are covered with squamous epithelium of the anal canal or perianal region.

Hemorrhoids may become symptomatic as a result of activities that increase venous pressure, resulting in distention and engorgement. Straining at stool, constipation, prolonged sitting, pregnancy, obesity, and low-fiber diets all may contribute. With time, redundancy and enlargement of the venous cushions may develop and result in bleeding or protrusion.

Clinical Findings

A. Symptoms and Signs: Patients often attribute a variety of perianal complaints to "hemorrhoids." However, the principal problems attributable to internal hemorrhoids are bleeding and mucoid discharge. Bleeding is manifested by bright red blood that may range from streaks of blood visible on toilet paper or stool to bright red blood that drips into the toilet bowl after a bowel movement. Rarely is bleeding severe enough to result in anemia. Initially, internal hemorrhoids are confined to the anal canal (stage I). Over time, the internal hemorrhoids may gradually enlarge and protrude from the anal opening. At first, this prolapse occurs during straining and reduces spontaneously (stage II). With progression over time, the prolapsed hemorrhoids may require manual reduction after bowel movements (stage III) or may remain chronically protruding (stage IV). Chronically prolapsed hemorrhoids may result in mucoid perianal discharge, resulting in irritation and soiling of underclothes. Discomfort and pain are unusual with internal hemorrhoids, occurring only when there is extensive inflammation and thrombosis of irreducible tissue or with thrombosis of an external hemorrhoid (see below)

B. Examination: External hemorrhoids are readily visible on perianal inspection. Nonprolapsed internal hemorrhoids are not visible but may protrude through the anus with gentle straining while the physician spreads the buttocks. Prolapsed hemorrhoids are visible as protuberant purple nodules covered by mucosa. The perianal region should also be examined for other signs of disease such as fistulas, fissures, skin tags, or dermatitis. On digital examination, uncomplicated internal hemorrhoids are neither palpable nor painful. Anoscopic evaluation, best performed in the prone jackknife position, provides optimal visualization of internal hemorrhoids.

Differential Diagnosis

Rectal bleeding may be caused by colorectal neoplasms, ulcerative colitis or Crohn's colitis, infectious proctitis, and diverticular disease. Rectal prolapse, in which a full thickness of rectum protrudes concentrically from the anus, is readily distinguished from mucosal hemorrhoidal prolapse. Proctosigmoidoscopy should be performed in all patients with hematochezia to exclude disease in the rectum or sigmoid colon that could be misinterpreted in the presence of hemorrhoidal bleeding. Patients with iron deficiency anemia should undergo colonoscopy or barium enema to exclude disease proximal to the sigmoid colon.

Treatment

A. Conservative Measures: Most patients with early (stage I and stage II) disease can be managed with conservative treatment. To decrease straining with defecation, patients should be given instructions for a high-fiber diet and told to increase fluid intake with meals. Dietary fiber may be supplemented with bran powder (1–2 tbsp twice daily added to food or in 8 oz of liquid) or with commercial psyllium bulk laxatives (eg, Metamucil, Citrucel). Suppositories and rectal ointments have no demonstrated utility in the management of mild disease. Mucoid discharge may be treated effectively by the local application of a cotton ball tucked next to the anal opening after bowel movements. For edematous, prolapsed hemorrhoids, gentle manual reduction may be supplemented by suppositories (Anusol) that have anesthetic and astringent properties and by warm sitz baths.

B. Surgical Treatment: Patients with stage I or stage II hemorrhoids and recurrent bleeding despite conservative measures may be treated with injection sclerotherapy or rubber band ligation. However, recurrence is common unless patients alter their dietary habits. Surgical excision (hemorrhoidectomy) is reserved for patients with chronic severe bleeding due to stage III or stage IV hemorrhoids or patients with acute thrombosed stage IV hemorrhoids.

Thrombosed External Hemorrhoid

Thrombosis of the external hemorrhoidal plexus results in a perianal hematoma. It most commonly occurs in otherwise healthy young adults and may be precipitated by coughing, heavy lifting, or straining at stool. The condition is characterized by the relatively acute onset of an exquisitely painful, tense and bluish perianal nodule covered with skin that may be up to several centimeters in size. Pain is most severe within the first few hours but gradually eases over 2–3 days as edema subsides. Symptoms may be relieved with warm sitz baths, analgesics, and ointments. If the patient is evaluated in the first 24–48 hours, removal of the clot may hasten symptomatic relief. With the patient in the lateral position, the skin around and over the lump is injected subcutaneously with 1% lidocaine. An ellipse of skin is then excised and the clot evacuated. A dry gauze dressing is applied for 12–24 hours, and daily sitz baths are then begun.

Salvati E: Nonoperative management of hemorrhoids. Dis Colon Rectum 1999;42:989. [NLM Cit ID: 99385301]

ANORECTAL INFECTIONS

A number of organisms can cause inflammation of the anal and rectal mucosa. Proctitis is defined as inflammation of the distal 15 cm of rectum and is characterized by anorectal discomfort, tenesmus, constipation, and discharge. Most cases of proctitis are sexually transmitted, especially by anal-receptive intercourse. Proctocolitis implies inflammation that extends above the rectum to the sigmoid colon or more proximally and is caused by entirely different organisms such as campylobacter, *Entamoeba histolytica,* shigella, and enteroinvasive *E coli.* These organisms are discussed earlier in the section on diarrhea. Symptoms include frequent, small-volume, bloody or watery diarrhea, urgency, cramps, and tenesmus.

Etiology & Management

Several organisms may cause infectious proctitis.

A. *Neisseria gonorrhoeae:* Gonorrhea may cause itching, burning, tenesmus, and a mucopurulent discharge. Blind swabs of the anal canal have a sensitivity of less than 60%. Swabs should be taken for Gram staining and culture during anoscopy, expressing mucopus from the anal crypts. Cultures should also be taken from the urethra and pharynx in men and from the cervix in women. Complications of untreated infections include strictures, fissures, fistulas, and perirectal abscesses.

B. *Treponema pallidum:* Anal syphilis may be asymptomatic or may lead to perianal pain and discharge. With primary syphilis, the chancre may be at the anal margin or within the anal canal and may mimic a fissure, fistula, or ulcer. Proctitis or inguinal lymphadenopathy may be present. With secondary syphilis, condylomata lata (pale-brown, flat verrucous lesions) may be seen, with secretion of foul-smelling mucus. The diagnosis is established with dark-field microscopy of scrapings from the chancre or condylomas. The VDRL test is positive in 75% of primary cases and in 99% of secondary cases.

C. *Chlamydia trachomatis:* Chlamydial infection may cause proctitis similar to gonorrheal proctitis or may cause lymphogranuloma venereum, characterized by proctocolitis with fever and bloody diarrhea, painful perianal ulcerations, anorectal strictures and fistulas, and inguinal adenopathy (buboes). The diagnosis is established by culture of rectal discharge or rectal biopsy, which is over 80% sensitive.

D. Herpes Simplex Type 2: HSV is a common cause of anorectal infection. Symptoms occur 4–21 days after exposure and include severe pain, itching, constipation, tenesmus, urinary retention, and radicular pain from involvement of lumbar or sacral nerve roots. Small vesicles or ulcers may be seen in the perianal area or anal canal. Sigmoidoscopy is not usually necessary but may reveal vesicular or ulcerative lesions in the distal rectum. Diagnosis is established by viral culture or antigen detection assays of vesicular fluid. Symptoms resolve within 2 weeks, but viral shedding may continue for several weeks. Patients may remain asymptomatic with or without viral shedding or may have recurrent mild relapses. Treatment of acute infection with acyclovir, 400 mg orally five times daily for 5–10 days, has been shown to reduce the duration of symptoms and viral shedding. Patients with AIDS and recurrent relapses may benefit from chronic suppressive therapy (see Chapter 32).

E. Venereal Warts: Venereal warts (condylomata acuminata) are a significant cause of anorectal symptoms. Caused by the human papillomavirus, they are seen in up to 50% of homosexual men. The warts are located on the perianal skin and extend within the anal canal up to 2 cm above the dentate line. Patients may have no symptoms or may report itching, bleeding, and pain. The warts may form a confluent mass that may obscure the anal opening. Treatment can be difficult. Topical application of podophyllum resin is effective for small perianal lesions. Anal lesions and large lesions may require CO_2 laser surgery or cryosurgery.

RECTAL PROLAPSE & SOLITARY RECTAL ULCER SYNDROME

Rectal prolapse is protrusion through the anus of some or all of the layers of the rectum. It is most commonly seen in the elderly. Although surgical and traumatic injuries are causative in some patients, in most cases rectal prolapse arises from chronic, excessive straining at stool in conjunction with weakening of pelvic support structures. Although prolapse initially reduces spontaneously after defecation, with time the rectal mucosa becomes chronically prolapsed, resulting in mucous discharge, bleeding, incontinence, and sphincteric damage. Patients with complete prolapse require surgical correction.

The term "solitary rectal ulcer syndrome" is a misnomer. The syndrome is characterized by anal pain, excessive straining at stool, and passage of mucus and blood. It is most commonly seen in young adults, especially women. Proctoscopic examination reveals either shallow ulcerations (single or multiple) or a nodular mass located anteriorly 6–10 cm above the anal verge. Biopsy is diagnostic. The disorder may be caused by rectal intussusception with straining. Treatment is directed at decreasing straining through education of the patient and use of bulking agents.

Eu K et al: Functional problems in adult rectal prolapse and controversies in surgical treatment. Br J Surg 1997;84:904. [NLM Cit ID: 97384460]

FECAL INCONTINENCE

Fecal incontinence is present in up to 10% of the elderly. There are five general requirements for bowel continence: (1) solid or semisolid stool (even healthy young adults have difficulty maintaining continence with liquid rectal contents); (2) a distensible rectal reservoir (as sigmoid contents empty into the rectum, the vault must expand to accommodate); (3) a sensation of rectal fullness (if the patient cannot sense this, overflow may occur before the patient can take appropriate action); (4) intact pelvic nerves and muscles; and (5) the ability to reach a toilet in a timely fashion.

Minor Incontinence

Many patients complain of slight soilage of undergarments that tends to occur after bowel movements or with straining or coughing. This may be due to local anal problems such as hemorrhoids and skin tags that make it difficult to form a tight anal seal, especially if stools are somewhat loose. Patients should be treated with fiber supplements to provide greater stool bulk. Loose application of a cotton ball near the anal opening may absorb small amounts of fecal leakage. Seepage may be improved by Kegel perineal strengthening exercises. Conditions such as ulcerative proctitis that cause tenesmus and urgency, chronic diarrheal conditions, and irritable bowel syndrome may result in difficulty in maintaining complete continence, especially if a toilet is not readily available. Similarly, the elderly may require more time or assistance to reach a toilet, which may lead to incontinence. Elderly patients with chronic constipation may develop stool impaction leading to "overflow" incontinence.

Major Incontinence

Complete uncontrolled loss of stool reflects a significant problem with sphincteric or neurologic damage. Causes of sphincteric damage include traumatic childbirth (especially forceps delivery), episiotomy, prolapse, prior anal surgery, and physical trauma. Neurologic disruption may be caused by obstetric trauma (with pudendal nerve damage), aging, diabetes mellitus, dementia, multiple sclerosis, spinal cord injury, and cauda equina syndrome.

Physical examination should include careful inspection of the perianal area for hemorrhoids, rectal prolapse, fissures, and fistulas. The perianal skin should be stimulated to confirm an intact anocutaneous reflex. Digital examination during relaxation and squeezing gives valuable information about resting tone (due to the internal sphincter) and external sphincter function and excludes fecal impaction. Anoscopy is required to evaluate for hemorrhoids, fissures, and fistulas. Proctosigmoidoscopy is useful to exclude rectal carcinoma or proctitis. Anal ultrasonography is the most reliable test for definition of anatomic defects in the external and internal anal sphincters. Anal manometry and surface electromyography may also be useful to define the severity of weakness, to diagnose nerve injury, and to predict response to biofeedback training.

Patients who are incontinent only of loose or liquid stools are treated with bulking agents and antidiarrheal drugs (eg, loperamide, 2 mg before meals and prophylactically before shopping trips). Patients with incontinence of solid stool benefit from scheduled toilet use after glycerin suppositories or tap water enemas. Biofeedback training with anal sphincter exercises is helpful in motivated patients to lower the threshold for awareness of rectal filling, or to improve anal sphincter squeeze function, or both. Operative management is seldom needed but should be considered in patients with major incontinence who have failed medical therapy.

Barnett JL et al: American Gastroenterological Association Medical Position Statement on Anorectal Testing Techniques. Gastroenterology 1999;116:732. [NLM Cit ID: 99155291]

Mavrontonis C et al: A clinical approach to fecal incontinence. J Clin Gastroenterol 1998;27:108. [NLM Cit ID: 98425766]

OTHER ANAL CONDITIONS

Anal Fissures

Anal fissures are linear or rocket-shaped ulcers that are usually less than 5 mm in length. They occur most commonly in the posterior midline, but 10% occur anteriorly. Fissures are believed to arise from trauma to the anal canal during defecation, perhaps caused by straining, constipation, or high internal sphincter tone. Patients complain of severe, tearing pain during defecation followed by throbbing discomfort that may lead to constipation due to fear of recurrent pain. There may be mild associated hematochezia, with blood on the stool or toilet paper. Anal fissures are confirmed by visual inspection of the anal verge while gently separating the buttocks. Acute fissures look like cracks in the epithelium. Chronic fissures result in fibrosis and the development of a skin tag at the outermost edge (sentinel pile). Digital and anoscopic examinations may cause severe pain and may not be possible. Medical management is directed at promoting effortless, painless bowel movements. Fiber supplements and sitz baths should be prescribed. Suppositories are of no benefit. Topical agents such as 1% hydrocortisone ointment may be helpful. Topical 0.2–0.5% nitroglycerin ointment applied by fingertip to the anus and anal canal twice daily for 6–8 weeks results in healing in up to 60% of patients. Injection of botulinum toxin (20 units) into the internal anal sphincter recently has been shown to cause healing in 90% of patients with chronic anal fissure. Chronic or recurrent fissures may benefit from partial lateral internal sphincterotomy; however, minor incontinence may complicate this procedure.

Perianal Abscess & Fistula

The anal glands located at the base of the anal crypts at the dentate line may become infected, leading to abscess formation. Other causes of abscess include anal fissure and Crohn's disease. Abscesses may extend upward or downward through the intersphincteric plane. Symptoms of perianal abscess are throbbing, continuous perianal pain. Erythema, fluctuance, and swelling may be found in the perianal region on external examination or in the ischiorectal fossa on digital rectal examination. Perianal abscesses are treated with local incision and drainage, while ischiorectal abscesses require drainage in the operating room. After drainage of an abscess, most patients are found to have a fistula in ano.

Fistula in ano most often arises in an anal crypt and is usually preceded by an anal abscess. In patients with fistulas that connect to the rectum, other disorders such as Crohn's disease, lymphogranuloma venereum, rectal tuberculosis, and cancer should be considered. Fistulas are associated with purulent discharge that may lead to itching, tenderness, and pain. Treatment is by surgical incision or excision under anesthesia. Care must be taken to preserve the anal sphincters.

Pruritus Ani

Pruritus ani is characterized by perianal itching and discomfort. It may be caused by poor anal hygiene associated with fistulas, fissures, prolapsed hemorrhoids, skin tags, and minor incontinence. Conversely, overzealous cleansing with soaps may contribute to local irritation or contact dermatitis. Pinworms, candidal infection (especially in diabetics), scabies, and condylomata acuminata must be excluded. In patients with idiopathic pruritus ani, examination may reveal erythema, excoriations, or lichenified, eczematous skin. Education is vital to successful therapy. After bowel movements, the perianal area should be cleansed with nonscented wipes premoistened with lanolin followed by gentle drying. A piece of cotton ball should be tucked next to the anal opening to absorb perspiration or fecal seepage. Anal ointments and lotions may exacerbate the condition and should be avoided.

Brisinda G et al: A comparison of injections of botulinum toxin and topical nitroglycerin ointment for the treatment of chronic anal fissure. N Engl J Med 1999;341:65. [NLM Cit ID: 99305292]

Metcalf A: Anorectal disorders. Five common causes of pain, itching, and bleeding. Postgrad Med 1995;98:81. [NLM Cit ID: 96063575]

Tsang CB et al: Rectovaginal fistulas: Therapeutic options. Surg Clin North Am 1997;77:95. [NLM Cit ID: 97226452]

SQUAMOUS (EPIDERMOID) CELL CARCINOMA OF THE ANUS

These tumors are relatively rare, comprising only 1–2% of all cancers of the anus and large intestine. Anal cancer is increased among people practicing receptive anal intercourse and those with a history of other sexually transmitted diseases. In over 80% of cases, human papillomavirus may be detected, suggesting that this virus may be a causal factor. Bleeding, pain, and local tumor are the commonest symptoms. The lesion is often confused with hemorrhoids or other common anal disorders. These tumors tend to become annular, invade the sphincter, and spread upward via the lymphatics into the perirectal mesenteric lymphatic nodes; they are encountered regularly in AIDS patients.

Treatment depends upon the tumor stage. CT scan and endoluminal ultrasound assist in determining the depth of penetration and local spread. Small superficial lesions may be treated by local excision. Larger tumors invading the sphincter or rectum are treated with combined modality therapy that includes external radiation with simultaneous chemotherapy (fluorouracil and either mitomycin or cisplatin). Local control is achieved in 80% of patients. Radical surgery (abdominoperineal resection) is now performed in patients who fail chemotherapy and radiation therapy. The 5-year survival rate is 60–70% for localized tumors and over 25% for metastatic (stage IV) disease.

Fuchshuber P et al: Anal canal and perianal epidermoid cancers. J Am Coll Surg 1997;185:494. [NLM Cit ID: 98019131]

RELEVANT WORLD WIDE WEB SITES

[Acute Appendicitis]
http://www.brighamrad.harvard.edu/Cases/bwh/hcache/112/full.html

[Acute Lower GI Bleeding]
http://www.brighamrad.harvard.edu/Cases/bwh/hcache/126/full.html

[American Gastroenterological Association]
http://www.gastro.org

[Atlas of Digestive Endoscopy]
http://www.luz.ve/ICA/Atlas_med/i_index.html

[Atlas of Gastrointestinal Endoscopy]
http://www.mindspring.com/~dmmmd/atlas_1.html

[Barrett's Esophagus]
http://www.brighamrad.harvard.edu/Cases/bwh/hcache/183/full.html

[Colonic Adenocarcinoma]
http://www.brighamrad.harvard.edu/Cases/bwh/hcache/85/full.html

[Diverticulitis]
http://www.brighamrad.harvard.edu/Cases/bwh/hcache/124/full.html

[Introduction to GERD]
http://www.gerd.com/intro/home.htm

[Jejunal Adenocarcinoma with Metastatic Disease to the Liver]
http://www.brighamrad.harvard.edu/Cases/bwh/hcache/60/full.html

[Lipomatous Hyperplasia of the Ileocecal Valve]
http://www.brighamrad.harvard.edu/Cases/bwh/hcache/48/full.html
[Meckel's Diverticulum]
http://www.brighamrad.harvard.edu/Cases/bwh/hcache/16/full.html
[Photography and Video of the Gastrointestinal Tract]
http://www.gastro.com/photo.htm
[Sigmoid Volvulus]
http://www.brighamrad.harvard.edu/Cases/bwh/hcache/5/full.html
[Lymphoma, Terminal Ileum]
http://www.brighamrad.harvard.edu/Cases/bwh/hcache/1/full.html
[Toxic Megacolon]
http://www.brighamrad.harvard.edu/Cases/bwh/hcache/178/full.html

15 Liver, Biliary Tract, & Pancreas

See http://www.current-med.com/ch15.html for updated addresses of Web sites referenced in this chapter.

Lawrence S. Friedman, MD

JAUNDICE (Icterus)

Jaundice results from the accumulation of bilirubin—a reddish pigment product of heme metabolism—in the body tissues; the cause may be hepatic or nonhepatic. Hyperbilirubinemia may be due to abnormalities in the formation, transport, metabolism, and excretion of bilirubin. Total serum bilirubin is normally 0.2–1.2 mg/dL, and jaundice may not be clinically recognizable until levels are about 3 mg/dL.

Pathophysiologically, jaundice may result from predominantly unconjugated or conjugated bilirubin in the serum (Table 15–1). Unconjugated hyperbilirubinemia may result from overproduction of bilirubin because of hemolysis; impaired hepatic uptake of bilirubin due to certain drugs; or impaired conjugation of bilirubin by glucuronide, as in Gilbert's syndrome, which is due to mild decreases in glucuronyl transferase, or Crigler-Najjar syndrome, due to moderate decreases or absence of glucuronyl transferase. In the absence of liver disease, hemolysis alone rarely elevates the serum bilirubin level to more than 7 mg/dL. Predominantly conjugated hyperbilirubinemia may result from impaired excretion of bilirubin from the liver due to hepatocellular disease, drugs, sepsis, hereditary disorders such as Dubin-Johnson syndrome, or extrahepatic biliary obstruction. Features of some hyperbilirubinemic syndromes are summarized in Table 15–2. The term "cholestasis" denotes retention of bile in the liver, and the term "cholestatic jaundice" is often used when conjugated hyperbilirubinemia results from impaired bile flow.

Manifestations of Diseases Associated With Jaundice

A. Unconjugated Hyperbilirubinemia: Stool and urine color are normal, and there is mild jaundice and indirect (unconjugated) hyperbilirubinemia with no bilirubin in the urine. Splenomegaly occurs in hemolytic disorders except in sickle cell anemia. Weakness or abdominal or back pain may occur with acute hemolytic crises.

B. Conjugated Hyperbilirubinemia:

1. Hereditary cholestatic syndromes or intrahepatic cholestasis–The patient may be asymptomatic; intermittent cholestasis is often accompanied by pruritus, light-colored stools, and, occasionally, malaise.

2. Hepatocellular disease–Malaise, anorexia, low-grade fever, and right upper quadrant discomfort are frequent. Dark urine, jaundice, and amenorrhea occur. An enlarged, tender liver; vascular spiders; palmar erythema; ascites; gynecomastia; sparse body hair; fetor hepaticus; and asterixis may be present, depending on the cause, severity, and chronicity of liver dysfunction.

C. Biliary Obstruction: There may be right upper quadrant pain, weight loss (suggesting carcinoma), jaundice, dark urine, and light-colored stools. Symptoms and signs may be intermittent owing to a stone or to carcinoma of the ampulla or junction of the hepatic ducts. Pain may be absent early in pancreatic cancer. Occult blood in the stools suggests cancer, particularly of the ampulla. Hepatomegaly, visible and palpable gallbladder (Courvoisier's sign), ascites, rectal (Blumer's) shelf, and weight loss also suggest cancer. Fever and chills suggest cholangitis.

Diagnostic Methods for Evaluation of Liver Disease & Jaundice (Table 15–3)

A. Laboratory Studies: Elevated serum aspartate and alanine aminotransferase levels (AST, ALT) result from hepatocellular necrosis or inflammation, as in hepatitis; ALT is more specific for the liver than AST, but an AST level at least twice that of the ALT is typical of alcoholic liver injury. In addition to signaling underlying liver disease, an isolated elevation of the serum ALT level may be the only clue to the diagnosis of celiac disease. Elevated alkaline phosphatase levels suggest cholestasis or infiltrative liver disease (eg, tumor, abscess, granulomas). Alkaline phosphatase elevations of hepatic rather than bone, intestinal, or placental origin are suggested by concomitant elevation of γ-glutamyl transpeptidase or 5′-nucleotidase levels.

Table 15–1. Classification of jaundice.

Type of Hyperbilirubinemia	Location and Cause
Unconjugated hyperbilirubinemia (predominant indirect-acting bilirubin)	Increased bilirubin production (eg, hemolytic anemias, hemolytic reactions, hematoma, infarction) Impaired bilirubin uptake and storage (eg, posthepatitis hyperbilirubinemia, Gilbert's syndrome, Crigler-Najjar syndrome, drug reactions)
Conjugated hyperbilirubinemia (predominant direct-acting bilirubin)	**HEREDITARY CHOLESTATIC SYNDROMES** Faulty excretion of bilirubin conjugates (eg, Dubin-Johnson syndrome, Rotor's syndrome) **HEPATOCELLULAR DYSFUNCTION** Biliary epithelial damage (eg, hepatitis, hepatic cirrhosis) Intrahepatic cholestasis (eg, certain drugs, biliary cirrhosis, sepsis, postoperative jaundice) Hepatocellular damage or intrahepatic cholestasis resulting from miscellaneous causes (eg, spirochetal infections, infectious mononucleosis, cholangitis, sarcoidosis, lymphomas, industrial toxins) **BILIARY OBSTRUCTION** Choledocholithiasis, biliary atresia, carcinoma of biliary duct, sclerosing cholangitis, choledochal cyst, external pressure on common duct, pancreatitis, pancreatic neoplasms

Table 15–2. Hyperbilirubinemic disorders.

	Nature of Defect	Type of Hyperbilirubinemia	Clinical and Pathologic Characteristics
Gilbert's syndrome	Glucuronyl transferase deficiency	Unconjugated (indirect) bilirubin	Benign, asymptomatic hereditary jaundice. Hyperbilirubinemia increased by 24- to 36-hour fast. No treatment required. Prognosis excellent.
Dubin-Johnson syndrome (familial chronic idiopathic jaundice)[1]	Faulty excretory function of hepatocytes	Conjugated (direct) bilirubin	Benign, asymptomatic hereditary jaundice. Gallbladder does not visualize on oral cholecystography. Liver darkly pigmented on gross examination. Biopsy shows centrilobular brown pigment. Prognosis excellent.
Rotor's syndrome			Similar to Dubin-Johnson syndrome, but liver is not pigmented and the gallbladder is visualized on oral cholecystography. Prognosis excellent.
Benign recurrent intrahepatic cholestasis[2]	Cholestasis, often on a familial basis	Unconjugated plus conjugated (total) bilirubin	Episodic attacks of jaundice, itching and malaise. Onset in early life and may persist for a lifetime. Alkaline phosphatase increased. Cholestasis found on liver biopsy. (Biopsy is normal during remission.) Prognosis excellent.
Recurrent jaundice of pregnancy			Benign cholestatic jaundice of unknown cause, usually occurring in the third trimester of pregnancy. Itching, gastrointestinal symptoms, and abnormal liver excretory function tests. Cholestasis noted on liver biopsy. Prognosis excellent, but recurrence with subsequent pregnancies or use of birth control pills is characteristic.

[1]The Dubin-Johnson syndrome is caused by a point mutation in the gene coding for an organic anion transporter in bile canaliculi on chromosome 10q23–24.

[2]Mutations in genes which control hepatocellular transport systems that are involved in the formation of bile and inherited as autosomal recessive traits are on chromosomes 18q21–22, 2q24, and 7q21 in families with progressive familial intrahepatic cholestasis. A gene mutation on chromosome 18q21–22 alters a P-type ATPase expressed in the small intestine and liver and causes benign recurrent intrahepatic cholestasis.

Table 15–3. Liver function tests: Normal values and changes in two types of jaundice.

Tests	Normal Values	Hepatocellular Jaundice	Uncomplicated Obstructive Jaundice
Bilirubin Direct Indirect	 0.1–0.3 mg/dL 0.2–0.7 mg/dL	 Increased Increased	 Increased Increased
Urine bilirubin	None	Increased	Increased
Serum albumin/total protein	Albumin, 3.5–5.5 g/dL Total protein, 6.5–8.4 g/dL	Albumin decreased	Unchanged
Alkaline phosphatase	30–115 units/L	Increased (+)	Increased (++++)
Prothrombin time	INR[1] of 1.0–1.4. After vitamin K, 10% increase in 24 hours	Prolonged if damage severe and does not respond to parenteral vitamin K	Prolonged if obstruction marked, but responds to parenteral vitamin K
ALT, AST	ALT, 5–35 units/L; AST, 5–40 units/L	Increased in hepatocellular damage, viral hepatitis	Minimally increased

[1]INR = International Normalized Ratio.

B. Liver Biopsy: Percutaneous liver biopsy is the definitive study for determining the cause and histologic severity of hepatocellular dysfunction or infiltrative liver disease. In patients with suspected metastatic disease or a hepatic mass, liver biopsy should be performed under ultrasound or CT guidance. A transjugular route can be used in patients with coagulopathy or ascites.

C. Imaging: Demonstration of dilated bile ducts by ultrasonography or CT scan indicates biliary obstruction (90–95% sensitivity). Ultrasonography, CT scan, and MRI can be used to demonstrate hepatomegaly, intrahepatic tumors, and changes of portal hypertension. The availability of helical, or spiral, arterial phase CT scanning, in which the liver is imaged during peak hepatic enhancement while the patient holds only one or two breaths, has improved diagnostic accuracy. CT arterial portography, in which imaging follows intravenous contrast infusion via a catheter placed in the superior mesenteric artery, and intraoperative ultrasonography are the most sensitive techniques for detection of individual small hepatic lesions in patients eligible for resection of metastases. MRI is the most accurate technique for identifying isolated liver lesions as hemangiomas, focal nodular hyperplasia, or focal fatty infiltration and for detecting hepatic iron overload. Because of its much lower cost, ultrasonography ($350) is preferable to CT ($1200–$1400) or MRI ($2000) as a screening test. Ultrasonography can detect gallstones with a sensitivity of 95%.

Endoscopic retrograde cholangiopancreatography (ERCP) or percutaneous transhepatic cholangiography (PTC) can identify the cause, location, and extent of biliary obstruction. ERCP requires a skilled endoscopist and may be utilized to demonstrate pancreatic or ampullary causes of jaundice, to carry out papillotomy and stone extraction, or to insert a stent through an obstructing lesion. Complications of ERCP include pancreatitis in 5% of cases and, less commonly, cholangitis, bleeding, or duodenal perforation after papillotomy. Severe complications of PTC occur in about 3% of cases and include fever, bacteremia, bile peritonitis, and intraperitoneal hemorrhage. Endoscopic ultrasonography, where available, is the most sensitive test for detecting small lesions of the ampulla or pancreatic head and for detecting portal vein invasion by pancreatic cancer. It is also accurate in detecting or excluding bile duct stones. Magnetic resonance cholangiopancreatography (MRCP) appears to be a sensitive, noninvasive method of detecting bile duct stones, strictures, and dilation, though without the therapeutic applications of ERCP.

Bezerra JA et al: Intrahepatic cholestasis: order out of chaos. Ganstroenterology 1999;117:1496. [NLM Cit ID: 20047887] (Terse review of recently identified molecular defects in hepatocellular membrane transporters that account for various genetic hyperbilirubinemic disorders.)

Brugge WR et al: Pancreatic and biliary endoscopy. N Engl J Med 1999;341:1808. [NLM Cit ID: 20055770] (Focuses on role of ERCP and endoscopic ultrasonography in the diagnosis and treatment of diseases of the pancreas and biliary tract.)

Grant A et al: Guidelines on the use of liver biopsy in clinical practice. Gut 1999;45(Suppl 4):IV1. [NLM Cit ID: 99436013] (Thorough review of indications, techniques, and complications.)

Ros PR et al: The incidental liver lesion: photon, proton, or needle? Hepatology 1998;27:1183. [NLM Cit ID: 98240801] (Compares imaging techniques for characterizing hepatic lesions.)

Whitehead MW et al: A prospective study of the causes of notably raised aspartate aminotransferase of liver origin. Gut 1999;45:129. [NLM Cit ID: 99298228] (Among hospitalized patients with a serum AST level greater than 400 units/L, 50% had ischemic hepatitis and 24% had pancreaticobiliary disease; only 3.6% had viral hepatitis.)

DISEASES OF THE LIVER

VIRAL HEPATITIS

Essentials of Diagnosis

- Prodrome of anorexia, nausea, vomiting, malaise, symptoms of upper respiratory infection or flu-like syndrome, aversion to smoking.
- Fever, enlarged and tender liver, jaundice.
- Normal to low white cell count; abnormal liver tests, especially markedly elevated aminotransferases early in the course.
- Liver biopsy shows characteristic hepatocellular necrosis and mononuclear infiltrate but is rarely indicated.

General Considerations

Hepatitis can be caused by many drugs and toxic agents as well as by numerous viruses, the clinical manifestations of which may be quite similar. The specific viruses causing viral hepatitis are (1) hepatitis A virus (HAV); (2) hepatitis B virus (HBV); (3) hepatitis C virus (HCV); (4) hepatitis D virus (delta agent); and (5) hepatitis E virus (an enterically transmitted hepatitis seen in epidemic form in Asia, North Africa, and Mexico). The designation hepatitis G virus (HGV; also known as the GB-C virus) has been applied to an agent that rarely, if ever, causes frank hepatitis. A DNA virus designated the TT virus (TTV) has been identified in up to 7.5% of blood donors and found to be transmitted readily by blood transfusions, but an association between this virus and liver disease has not been established. Recently, a new virus known as SEN-V has been reported to account for a substantial proportion of cases of transfusion-associated hepatitis. In immunocompromised hosts, cytomegalovirus, Epstein-Barr virus, and herpes simplex virus should be considered in the differential diagnosis of hepatitis. As yet unidentified agents account for a small percentage of cases of apparent acute viral hepatitis.

A. Hepatitis A: (Figure 15–1) HAV is a 27-nm RNA hepatovirus (in the picornavirus family) that may cause epidemics or sporadic cases of hepatitis. Transmission of the virus is usually by the fecal-oral route, and spread is favored by crowding and poor sanitation. Common source outbreaks may result from contaminated water or food. The incubation period averages 30 days. Excretion of hepatitis A virus (HAV) occurs up to 2 weeks prior to clinical illness. HAV is rarely demonstrated in feces after the first week of illness. The mortality rate for hepatitis A is low, and fulminant hepatitis A is uncommon except perhaps for rare instances in which acute hepatitis A occurs in a patient with chronic hepatitis C. Chronic

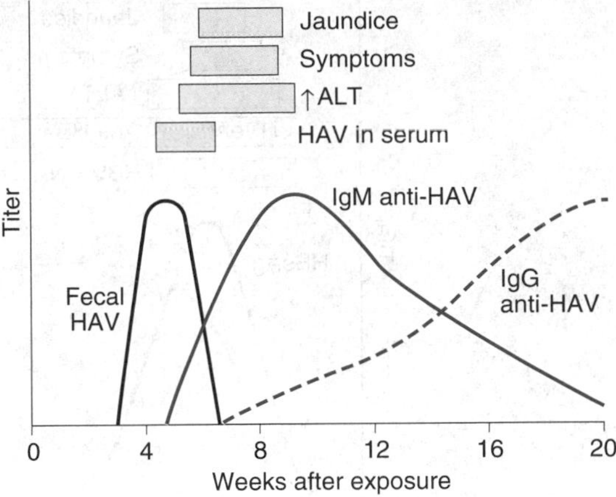

Figure 15–1. The typical course of acute type A hepatitis. (HAV, hepatitis A virus; anti-HAV, antibody to hepatitis A virus; ALT, alanine aminotransferase.) (Reproduced, with permission, from Schafer DF, Hoofnagle JH: View Dig Dis 1982;14:5.)

hepatitis A does not occur, and there is no carrier state. Clinical illness is more severe in adults than in children, in whom hepatitis A is often asymptomatic.

Antibody to hepatitis A (anti-HAV) appears early in the course of the illness. Both IgM and IgG anti-HAV are detectable in serum soon after the onset of the illness. Peak titers of IgM anti-HAV occur during the first week of clinical disease and usually disappear within 3–6 months. Detection of IgM anti-HAV is an excellent test for diagnosing acute hepatitis A. Titers of IgG anti-HAV peak after 1 month of the disease and may persist for years. The presence of IgG anti-HAV alone indicates previous exposure to HAV, noninfectivity, and immunity to recurring HAV infection. In the USA, about 33% of the population have serologic evidence of previous infection.

B. Hepatitis B: (Figure 15–2) Hepatitis B virus (HBV) is a 42-nm hepadnavirus with a partially double-stranded DNA genome, inner core protein (hepatitis B core antigen, HBcAg) and outer surface coat (hepatitis B surface antigen, HBsAg). HBV is usually transmitted by inoculation of infected blood or blood products or by sexual contact and is present in saliva, semen, and vaginal secretions. HBsAg-positive mothers may transmit HBV to their neonates at the time of delivery; the risk of chronic infection in the infant is as high as 90%. Hepatitis B virus (HBV) is highly prevalent in homosexuals and intravenous drug users, but most cases reported in the USA now result from heterosexual transmission. Other groups at high risk include patients and staff at hemodialysis centers, physicians, dentists, nurses, and personnel working in clinical and pathology laboratories and blood banks. The risk of HBV infection from a blood

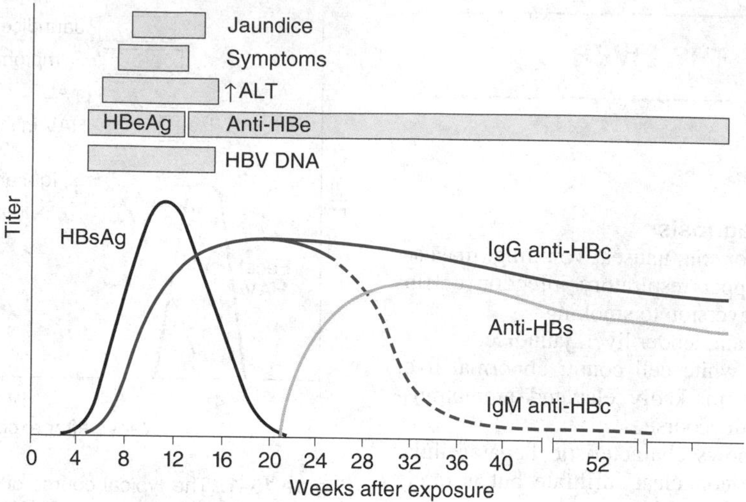

Figure 15–2. The typical course of acute type B hepatitis. (HBsAg, hepatitis B surface antigen; anti-HBs, antibody to HBsAg; HBeAg, hepatitis Be antigen; anti-HBe, antibody to HBeAg; anti-HBc, antibody to hepatitis B core antigen; ALT, alanine aminotransferase.) (Reproduced, with permission, from Hoofnagle JH, Schafer DF: Serologic markers of hepatitis B virus infection. Semin Liver Dis 1986;6:1.)

transfusion is less than one in 60,000 units transfused in the USA. The incubation period of hepatitis B is 6 weeks to 6 months (average 12–14 weeks).

Clinical features of hepatitis A and B are similar; however, the onset in hepatitis B tends to be more insidious and the aminotransferase levels higher. The risk of fulminant hepatitis is less than 1%, with a mortality rate of up to 60%. Following acute hepatitis B, HBV infection may persist in 1–2% of immunocompetent adults but a higher percentage of immunocompromised adults or children. Persons with chronic hepatitis B, particularly when HBV infection is acquired early in life and viral replication persists, are at substantial risk of cirrhosis and hepatocellular carcinoma (up to 25–40%). Infection caused by HBV may be associated with arthritis, glomerulonephritis, and polyarteritis nodosa.

There are three distinct antigen-antibody systems that relate to HBV infection and a variety of circulating markers that are useful in diagnosis. Interpretation of common serologic patterns is shown in Table 15–4.

1. HBsAg–The appearance of HBsAg is the first evidence of HBV infection, appearing before biochemical evidence of liver disease. HBsAg persists throughout the clinical illness. Persistence of HBsAg after the acute illness may be associated with clinical and laboratory evidence of chronic hepatitis for variable periods of time. The detection of HBsAg establishes infection with HBV and implies infectivity.

2. Anti-HBs–Specific antibody to HBsAg (anti-HBs) appears in most individuals after clearance of HBsAg and after successful vaccination against hepatitis B. The appearance of anti-HBs is occasionally delayed until after clearance of HBsAg. During this serologic gap (window period), infectivity has been demonstrated. Disappearance of HBsAg and the appearance of anti-HBs signals recovery from HBV infection, noninfectivity, and protection from recurrent HBV infection.

3. Anti-HBc–IgM anti-HBc appears shortly after HBsAg is detected. (HBcAg alone does not appear in serum.) Its presence in the setting of acute hepatitis indicates a diagnosis of acute hepatitis B, and it fills the serologic gap in patients who have cleared HBsAg but do not yet have detectable anti-HBs. IgM anti-HBc can persist for 3–6 months or more. IgM anti-HBc may also reappear during flares of previously inactive chronic hepatitis B. IgG anti-HBc also appears during acute hepatitis B but persists indefinitely, whether the patient recovers (with the appearance of anti-HBs in serum) or develops chronic hepatitis B (with persistence of HBsAg). In asymptomatic blood donors, an isolated anti-HBc with no other positive HBV serologic results may represent a falsely positive result or latent infection in which HBV DNA is detectable in serum only by polymerase chain reaction methodology.

4. HBeAg–HBeAg is a soluble protein found only in HBsAg-positive sera. It represents a secretory form of HBcAg that appears during the incubation period shortly after the detection of HBsAg. HBeAg indicates viral replication and infectivity. Persistence of HBeAg in serum beyond 3 months suggests an increased likelihood of chronic hepatitis B. Disappearance of HBeAg is often followed by the appearance

Table 15–4. Common serologic patterns in hepatitis B virus infection and their interpretation.

HBsAg	Anti-HBs	Anti-HBc	HBeAg	Anti-HBe	Interpretation
+	–	IgM	+	–	Acute hepatitis B
+	–	IgG[1]	+	–	Chronic hepatitis B with active viral replication
+	–	IgG	–	+	Chronic hepatitis B with low viral replication
+	+	IgG	+ or –	+ or –	Chronic hepatitis B with heterotypic anti-HBs (about 10% of cases)
–	–	IgM	+ or –	–	Acute hepatitis B
–	+	IgG	–	+ or –	Recovery from hepatitis B (immunity)
–	+	–	–	–	Vaccination (immunity)
–	–	IgG	–	–	False-positive; less commonly, infection in remote past

[1]Low levels of IgM anti-HBc may also be detected.

of anti-HBe, signifying diminished viral replication and decreased infectivity.

5. HBV DNA–The presence of HBV DNA in serum generally parallels the presence of HBeAg, though HBV DNA is a more sensitive and precise marker of viral replication and infectivity. Very low levels of HBV DNA, detectable only by polymerase chain reaction methodology, may persist in serum after a patient has recovered from acute hepatitis B, but the HBV DNA is bound to IgG and rarely infectious. In Mediterranean countries, a frequent variant form of HBV is characterized by severe chronic hepatitis and the presence of HBV DNA without HBeAg in serum because of a mutation that prevents synthesis of HBeAg in infected hepatocytes ("pre-core" mutant). The pre-core mutant may appear during the course of chronic "wild-type" HBV infection, presumably as a result of immune pressure.

C. Hepatitis D (Delta Agent): Hepatitis D virus (HDV) is a defective RNA virus that causes hepatitis only in association with hepatitis B infection and specifically only in the presence of HBsAg; it is cleared when the latter is cleared.

HDV may co-infect with HBV or may superinfect a person with chronic hepatitis B. When acute hepatitis D is coincident with acute HBV infection, the infection is generally similar in severity to acute hepatitis B alone. In chronic hepatitis B, superinfection by HDV appears to carry a worse short-term prognosis, often resulting in fulminant hepatitis or severe chronic hepatitis that progresses rapidly to cirrhosis. In the 1970s and early 1980s, HDV was endemic in some areas, such as the Mediterranean countries, where up to 80% of HBV carriers were superinfected with it, and occurred primarily among intravenous drug users in the USA. However, new cases of hepatitis D are now infrequent, and cases seen today are usually from cohorts infected years ago who survived the initial impact of hepatitis D and now have inactive cirrhosis. These patients have a threefold increased risk of hepatocellular carcinoma. Diagnosis is by detection of antibody to hepatitis D antigen (anti-HDV) or, where available, HDV RNA in serum.

Hepatitis D is best prevented by prevention of hepatitis B (eg, with HBV vaccine).

D. Hepatitis C (HCV): (Figure 15–3) The hepatitis C virus is a single-stranded RNA virus with properties similar to those of flavivirus. At least six major genotypes of HCV have been identified. In the past, HCV was responsible for over 90% of cases of posttransfusion hepatitis, yet only 4% of cases of hepatitis C were attributable to blood transfusions. Over 50% of cases are in fact attributable to past intravenous drug use. The risk of sexual and maternal-neonatal transmission is low and may be greatest in a subset of patients with high circulating levels of HCV RNA. Having multiple sexual partners may increase

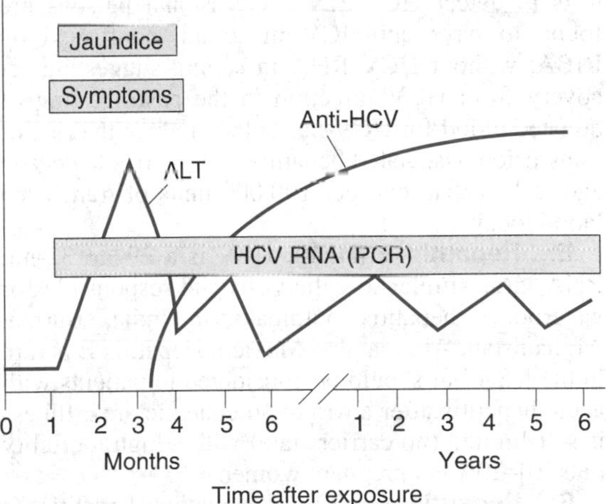

Figure 15–3. The typical course of acute and chronic hepatitis C. (ALT, alanine aminotransferase; Anti-HCV, antibody to hepatitis C virus by enzyme immunoassay; HCV RNA [PCR], hepatitis C viral RNA by polymerase chain reaction.)

the risk of HCV infection. Transmission via breast feeding has not been documented. An outbreak of hepatitis C in patients with immune deficiencies occurred in some recipients of intravenous immune globulin, and nosocomial transmission via multidose vials of saline used to flush Portacaths has been reported. In many patients, the source of infection is uncertain. There are about 2.7 million HCV carriers in the USA and another 1.3 million previously exposed persons.

The incubation period averages 6–7 weeks, and clinical illness is often mild, usually asymptomatic, and characterized by waxing and waning aminotransferase elevations and a high rate (> 80%) of chronic hepatitis. In pregnant patients, serum aminotransferase levels frequently normalize despite persistence of viremia, only to increase again after delivery. HCV may be a pathogenic factor in cryoglobulinemia, glomerulonephritis, autoimmune thyroiditis, lymphocytic sialadenitis, idiopathic pulmonary fibrosis, sporadic porphyria cutanea tarda, monoclonal gammopathies, and probably lymphoma.

Diagnosis of hepatitis C is based on an enzyme immunoassay that detects antibodies to HCV (anti-HCV). Anti-HCV is not a protective antibody, and in patients with acute or chronic hepatitis the presence of anti-HCV in serum generally signifies that HCV is the cause. Limitations of the enzyme immunoassay include moderate sensitivity (false-negatives) for the diagnosis of acute hepatitis C early in the course and in healthy blood donors and low specificity (false-positives) in some persons with elevated gamma globulin levels. In these situations, a diagnosis of hepatitis C may be confirmed by use of a supplemental recombinant immunoblot assay (RIBA). Most RIBA-positive persons are potentially infectious, as confirmed by use of polymerase chain reaction-based tests to detect HCV RNA. Occasional persons are found to have anti-HCV in serum, confirmed by RIBA, without HCV RNA in serum, suggesting recovery from HCV infection in the past. Testing of donated blood for HCV has helped reduce the risk of transfusion-associated hepatitis C from 10% a decade ago to less than one per 100,000 units of transfused blood today.

E. Hepatitis E (HEV): HEV is a 29- to 32-nm RNA virus similar to calicivirus and responsible for waterborne hepatitis outbreaks in India, Burma, Afghanistan, Algeria, and Mexico. Hepatitis E is rare in the USA but should be considered in patients with acute hepatitis after a trip to an endemic area. Illness is self-limited (no carrier state) with a high mortality rate (10–20%) in pregnant women.

F. Hepatitis G: The designation hepatitis G virus (HGV) has been applied to a flavivirus that is percutaneously transmitted and associated with chronic viremia lasting at least 10 years. HGV has been detected in 1.5% of blood donors, 50% of intravenous drug users, 30% of hemodialysis patients, 20% of hemophiliacs, and 15% of patients with chronic hepatitis B or C, but it does not appear to cause important liver disease or affect the response of patients with chronic hepatitis B or C to antiviral therapy.

Clinical Findings

The clinical picture of viral hepatitis is extremely variable, ranging from asymptomatic infection without jaundice to a fulminating disease and death in a few days.

A. Symptoms:

1. Prodromal phase–The onset may be abrupt or insidious, with general malaise, myalgia, arthralgia, easy fatigability, upper respiratory symptoms (nasal discharge, pharyngitis), and anorexia. A distaste for smoking, paralleling anorexia, may occur early. Nausea and vomiting are frequent, and diarrhea or constipation may occur. Skin rashes, arthritis, or serum sickness may be seen early in acute hepatitis B. Fever is generally present but is rarely over 39.5 °C save in occasional cases of hepatitis A. Defervescence often coincides with the onset of jaundice. Chills or chilliness may mark an acute onset.

Abdominal pain is usually mild and constant in the right upper quadrant or epigastrium and is often aggravated by jarring or exertion. (On rare occasions, upper abdominal pain may be severe enough to simulate cholecystitis or cholelithiasis.)

2. Icteric phase–Clinical jaundice occurs after 5–10 days but may appear at the same time as the initial symptomatology. Most patients never develop clinical icterus. With the onset of jaundice, there is often worsening of the prodromal symptoms, followed by progressive clinical improvement.

3. Convalescent phase–There is an increasing sense of well-being, return of appetite, and disappearance of jaundice, abdominal pain and tenderness, and fatigability.

4. Course and complications–The acute illness usually subsides over 2–3 weeks with complete clinical and laboratory recovery by 9 weeks in hepatitis A and by 16 weeks in hepatitis B. In 5–10% of cases, the course may be more protracted, and less than 1% will have an acute fulminant course. In some cases of acute hepatitis A, clinical, biochemical, and serologic recovery may be followed by one or two relapses, but ultimate recovery is the rule. Hepatitis B, D, and C (and G) may become chronic (see below).

B. Signs: Hepatomegaly—rarely marked—is present in over half of cases. Liver tenderness is usually present. Splenomegaly is reported in 15% of patients, and soft, enlarged lymph nodes—especially in the cervical or epitrochlear areas—may occur. Signs of general toxemia vary from minimal to severe.

C. Laboratory Findings: The white blood cell count is normal to low, especially in the preicteric phase. Large atypical lymphocytes, such as are found in infectious mononucleosis, may occasionally be seen. Rarely, aplastic anemia follows an episode of acute hepatitis not caused by any of the known hepatitis viruses. Mild proteinuria is common, and bilirubinuria often precedes the appearance of jaundice. Acholic stools are often present during the icteric phase. Blood studies reflect hepatocellular damage with often strikingly elevated AST or ALT values. Bilirubin and alkaline phosphatase are elevated and, in a minority of patients, remain so after aminotransferase levels have normalized. Cholestasis is occasionally marked in acute hepatitis A. Marked prolongation of the prothrombin time in severe hepatitis correlates with increased mortality.

Differential Diagnosis

The differential diagnosis of hepatitis includes other viral diseases such as infectious mononucleosis, cytomegalovirus infection, and herpes simplex virus infection; spirochetal diseases such as leptospirosis and secondary syphilis; brucellosis; rickettsial diseases such as Q fever; drug-induced liver disease; and shock liver (ischemic hepatitis). Occasionally, autoimmune hepatitis (see below) may have an acute onset mimicking acute viral hepatitis. Rarely, metastatic cancer of the liver may present with a hepatitis-like picture.

The prodromal phase of viral hepatitis must be distinguished from other infectious disease such as influenza, upper respiratory infections, and the prodromal stages of the exanthematous diseases. Occasionally, cholestasis may be prominent, particularly in hepatitis A, and mimic obstructive jaundice.

Prevention

Strict isolation of patients is not necessary, but hand washing after bowel movements is required. Thorough hand washing by medical attendants who come into contact with contaminated utensils, bedding, or clothing is essential. Careful handling of disposable needles—including not recapping used needles—is important for medical personnel. Screening of donated blood for HBsAg, anti-HBc, and anti-HCV has reduced the risk of transfusion-associated hepatitis markedly. Unnecessary transfusions and commercially obtained blood should be avoided. All pregnant women should undergo testing for HBsAg. HBV- and HCV-infected persons should practice "safe sex," but there is little evidence that HCV is spread easily by sexual contact. Vaccination against HAV and HBV is recommended for patients with chronic hepatitis C.

A. Hepatitis A: Immune globulin should be given routinely to all *close* (eg, household) personal contacts of patients with hepatitis A. The recommended dose of 0.02 mL/kg intramuscularly has been found to be protective for hepatitis A if administered during the incubation period. Two effective inactivated hepatitis A vaccines are available and recommended for persons living in or traveling to endemic areas, patients with chronic liver disease (preferably before decompensation), persons with clotting-factor disorders who are treated with concentrates, homosexual and bisexual men, animal handlers, illicit drug users, sewage workers, food handlers, and children and caregivers in day care centers and institutions. Routine vaccination of all children has been recommended in states with a high incidence of hepatitis A. The HAV vaccine has also been reported to be effective in the prevention of secondary spread to household contacts of primary cases. The recommended dose for adults is 1 mL (1440 ELISA units) of Havrix (SmithKline Beecham) or 0.5 mL (50 units) of Vaqta (Merck) intramuscularly with a booster dose at 6–12 months.

B. Hepatitis B: Hepatitis B immune globulin (HBIG) may be protective—or may at least attenuate the severity of illness—if given in large doses within 7 days after exposure (adult dose is 0.06 mL/kg body weight) followed by initiation of the HBV vaccine series (see below). At present, this approach is recommended for individuals exposed to hepatitis B surface antigen-contaminated material via the mucous membranes or through breaks in the skin and for persons who have had sexual contact with patients with HBV infection. HBIG is also indicated for newborn infants of HBsAg-positive mothers followed by initiation of the vaccine series (see below).

The currently used vaccines are recombinant-derived. Initially, the vaccine was targeted to persons at high risk, including renal dialysis patients and attending personnel, patients requiring repeated transfusions, spouses of HBsAg-positive individuals, male homosexuals, intravenous drug users, newborns of HBsAg-positive mothers, entering medical and nursing students, as well as all medical technologists. Because this strategy failed to lower the incidence of hepatitis B, the CDC recommended universal vaccination of infants and children in the USA. Over 90% of recipients of the vaccine mount protective antibody to hepatitis B. The standard regimen for adults is 10–20 μg initially (depending on the formulation) and again at 1 and 6 months, but alternative schedules have been approved; for greatest reliability of absorption, the deltoid muscle is the preferred site of injection. Vaccine formulations free of the mercury-containing preservative thimerosal are preferred in infants less than 6 months of age. When documentation of seroconversion is considered desirable, post-immunization anti-HBs titers may be checked. Protection appears to be excellent even if the titer wanes—at least for 10 years—and booster reimmunization is not routinely recommended but is advised for immunocompromised persons in whom anti-HBs titers fall below 10 mIU/mL. Universal vaccination of neonates in countries that are endemic for HBV reduces the incidence of hepatocellular carcinoma.

Treatment

Bed rest is recommended only on an as-needed basis during the acute initial phase of the disease, when symptoms are most severe. Return to normal activity during the convalescent period should be gradual. If nausea and vomiting are pronounced or if oral intake is substantially decreased, intravenous administration of 10% glucose solution is indicated. If the patient shows signs of encephalopathy or severe coagulopathy, acute hepatic failure should be suspected, and hospitalization is mandatory (see below).

In general, dietary management consists of giving palatable meals as tolerated, without overfeeding. Patients should avoid strenuous physical exertion, alcohol, and hepatotoxic agents. While the administration of small doses of oxazepam is safe (metabolism not affected by liver disease), morphine sulfate should be avoided.

In controlled studies, corticosteroids have demonstrated no benefit in patients with viral hepatitis, including those with fulminant hepatitis. Treatment of patients with acute hepatitis C with alpha interferon appears to decrease the risk of chronic hepatitis.

Prognosis

In most cases, clinical recovery is complete in 3–16 weeks. Laboratory evidence of liver dysfunction may persist for a longer period, but most patients recover completely. The overall mortality rate is less than 1%, but the rate is reportedly higher in older people.

Hepatitis A does not progress to chronic liver disease, though hepatitis A may persist for up to 1 year, and clinical and biochemical relapses may occur before full recovery. The mortality rate is less than 0.2%. The mortality rate for acute hepatitis B is 0.1–1%, and it is even higher for superimposed hepatitis D. Fulminant hepatitis C is rare in the USA. For unknown reasons, the mortality rate for hepatitis E is especially high in pregnant women (10–20%).

Chronic hepatitis, characterized by elevated aminotransferase levels for more than 6 months, develops in 1–2% of immunocompetent adult patients with acute hepatitis B but in as many as 90% of infected neonates and infants and a substantial proportion of immunocompromised adults with acute hepatitis B. Over 80% of all persons with acute hepatitis C develop chronic hepatitis, which in many cases progresses very slowly. Ultimately, cirrhosis may develop in up to 30% of those with chronic hepatitis C and 40% of those with chronic hepatitis B; the risk of cirrhosis is even higher in patients coinfected with both viruses or with HIV. Patients with cirrhosis are at risk (with a rate of 3–5% per year) of hepatocellular carcinoma.

JAMA patient page. Hepatitis C. JAMA 1998;280:2188. [NLM Cit ID: 99091090]

Koff RS: Hepatitis A. Lancet 1998;351:1643. [NLM Cit ID: 98282054]

Lee W (editor): Hepatitis B. Clin Liver Dis 1999;3:179. (Reviews of epidemiology, virology, immunopathogenesis, clinical features, natural history, treatment, and prevention.)

Liang TJ et al: Pathogenesis, natural history, treatment, and prevention of hepatitis C. Ann Intern Med 2000;132:296. [NLM Cit ID: 20132334]

Recommendations for prevention and control of hepatitis C virus (HCV) infection and HCV-related chronic disease. MMWR Morb Mortal Wkly Rep 1998;47(RR-19):1. [NLM Cit ID: 99004881] (Detailed review of epidemiology, natural history, and current guidelines for prevention and control.)

Rosina F et al: Changing pattern of chronic hepatitis D in southern Europe. Gastroenterology 1999;117:161. [NLM Cit ID: 99315564] (No longer epidemic in southern Europe, hepatitis D is now seen primarily in patients with cirrhosis who survived acute hepatitis D decades earlier; once cirrhosis is reached, HDV replication appears to subside, though in some cases HBV replication resumes.)

Zignego AL et al: Extrahepatic manifestations of HCV infection: Fact and controversies. J Hepatol 1999;31:369. [NLM Cit ID: 99381758] (Reviews evidence supporting an association between HCV infection and lymphoproliferative disorders, autoimmune thyroiditis, Sjögren's syndrome, idiopathic pulmonary fibrosis, and porphyria cutanea tarda.)

ACUTE HEPATIC FAILURE

Acute hepatic failure may be fulminant or subfulminant. Fulminant hepatic failure is characterized by the development of hepatic encephalopathy within 8 weeks after the onset of acute liver disease. Coagulopathy is invariably present. Subfulminant hepatic failure is the term used when encephalopathy occurs between 8 weeks and 6 months after the onset of acute liver disease and carries an equally poor prognosis.

Until recently about 70% of all cases of acute hepatic failure in the USA were caused by acute viral hepatitis, with up to 50% of cases due to hepatitis B—in some cases detectable only by polymerase chain reaction (PCR) methodology—and most of the remainder due to hepatitis A or unknown (non-ABCDE) viruses. In endemic areas, hepatitis D and hepatitis E may cause acute hepatic failure. Hepatitis C appears to be a rare cause of acute hepatic failure in the USA, but acute hepatitis A or B superimposed on chronic hepatitis C has been reported to be associated with a high risk of fulminant hepatitis. Recently, acetaminophen toxicity has been reported to be the most common cause of acute hepatic failure in the USA, as it has been in England for some time. Other causes of acute hepatic failure include idiosyncratic drug reactions, poisonous mushrooms, shock, hyper- or hypothermia, Budd-Chiari syndrome, malignancy (most commonly lymphomas), Wilson's disease, Reye's syndrome, fatty liver of pregnancy and other disorders of fatty acid oxidation, and parvovirus B19 infection.

In acute hepatic failure due to hepatitis, extensive necrosis of large areas of the liver gives the typical pathologic picture of acute liver atrophy. Toxemia, gastrointestinal symptoms, and hemorrhagic phenomena are common. Jaundice may be absent or minimal, but laboratory tests show severe hepatocellular damage. In acute hepatic failure due to microvesicular steatosis (eg, Reye's syndrome), serum aminotransferase elevations may be modest (< 300 units/L).

The treatment of acute hepatic failure is directed toward correcting metabolic abnormalities associated with severe liver cell dysfunction. These include coagulation defects; disordered fluid, electrolyte, and acid-base balance; renal failure; hypoglycemia; and encephalopathy. Prophylactic antibiotic therapy decreases the risk of infection, which is as high as 90%, but has no effect on survival and is not routinely recommended. For suspected sepsis, broad coverage is indicated pending culture results. The most frequent isolates are *Staphylococcus aureus,* streptococcus species, coliforms, and, later in the course, candida species. Early administration of acetylcysteine (140 mg/kg orally followed by 70 mg/kg orally every 4 hours for an additional 17 doses) is indicated for acetaminophen toxicity and has been reported to improve cerebral blood flow and oxygenation in patients with fulminant hepatic failure due to any cause. Early transfer to a liver transplantation center is essential. Extradural sensors may be placed to monitor intracranial pressure for the development of cerebral edema (thought to be mediated in part by high arterial ammonia concentrations) and decreased cerebral perfusion.

Mannitol 100–200 mL of a 20% solution by intravenous infusion over 10 minutes, may decrease cerebral edema but should be used with caution in patients with renal failure. The value of hyperventilation and of intravenous prostaglandin E_1 is uncertain. Hepatic-assist devices that use living hepatocytes and liver xenografts have shown promise in animal models and are undergoing clinical trials. The mortality rate of fulminant hepatitis with severe encephalopathy is as high as 80%. The outlook is especially poor in patients younger than 10 and older than 40 years of age and in those with an idiosyncratic drug reaction. Other adverse prognostic factors are a serum bilirubin level > 18 mg/dL, INR > 6.5, onset of encephalopathy more than 7 days after the onset of jaundice, and a low factor V level (< 20% of normal). For acetaminophen-induced fulminant hepatic failure, indicators of a poor outcome (which is uncommon) are acidosis (pH < 7.3), INR > 6.5, and azotemia (serum creatinine ≥ 3.4 mg/dL). Emergency liver transplantation should be considered for patients with stage II to stage III encephalopathy and has been associated with an 80% survival rate at 1 year. Compared with chronic hepatitis B, liver transplantation for fulminant hepatitis B is less likely to result in reinfection of the graft with HBV.

Rahman TM et al: Review article: liver support systems in acute hepatic failure. Aliment Pharmacol Ther 1999;13:1255. [NLM Cit ID: 20009939] (Discussion of technical aspects and preliminary results of emerging artificial liver support systems.)

Schiødt FV et al: Etiology and outcome for 295 patients with acute liver failure in the United States. Liver Transpl Surg 1999;5:29. [NLM Cit ID: 99091921] (Among patients with fulminant hepatic failure in the USA referred to a transplant center, acetaminophen overdose is now the most common cause [20%] but least likely to require liver transplantation [12% of cases].)

Shakil AO et al: Fulminant hepatic failure. Surg Clin North Am 1999;79:77. [NLM Cit ID: 99172838]

Vento S et al: Fulminant hepatitis associated with hepatitis A virus superinfection in patients with chronic hepatitis C. N Engl J Med 1998;338:286. [NLM Cit ID: 98092073] (Of 17 patients with chronic hepatitis C and acute hepatitis A, seven developed fulminant hepatic failure and six died.)

CHRONIC HEPATITIS

Chronic hepatitis is defined as a chronic inflammatory reaction of the liver of more than 3–6 months' duration, as demonstrated by persistently abnormal serum aminotransferase levels and characteristic histologic findings. The causes of chronic hepatitis include HBV, HCV, and HDV, autoimmune hepatitis, chronic hepatitis associated with certain medications (including methyldopa and isoniazid), Wilson's disease, and α_1-antiprotease (α_1-antitrypsin) deficiency. Traditionally, chronic hepatitis has been categorized histologically as chronic persistent hepatitis and chronic active hepatitis. However, with improved serologic and autoimmune markers, more precise categorization is preferred, based on etiology; the grade of portal, periportal, and lobular inflammation (minimal, mild, moderate, or severe); and the stage of fibrosis (none, mild, moderate, severe, cirrhosis).

Clinical Findings & Diagnosis

A. Autoimmune Hepatitis: This is generally a disease of young women but can occur in either sex at any age. Affected persons are often positive for HLA-B8 and -DR3 or, in older patients, HLA-DR4. The onset is usually insidious, but about 25% of cases present as an acute attack of hepatitis and some cases follow a viral illness such as hepatitis A, Epstein-Barr infection, or measles or exposure to a drug or toxin such as nitrofurantoin. The serum bilirubin is usually increased, but 20% of patients are anicteric. In classic cases, examination reveals a healthy-appearing young woman with multiple spider nevi, cutaneous striae, acne, hirsutism, and hepatomegaly. Amenorrhea may be a presenting feature. Extrahepatic features include arthritis, Sjögren's syndrome, thyroiditis, nephritis, ulcerative colitis, and Coombs-positive hemolytic anemia. In classic (type I) autoimmune hepatitis, antinuclear antibody (ANA) or smooth muscle antibody (either or both) is detected in serum. Serum gamma globulin levels are typically elevated (up to 5–6 g/dL). In patients with high gamma globulin levels, the enzyme immunoassay for antibody to HCV may be falsely positive. A second type (II), infrequently seen in the United States but more common in Europe, is characterized by circulating antibody to liver-kidney microsomes (anti-LKM1) without anti-smooth muscle antibody or ANA. Concurrent primary biliary cirrhosis or primary sclerosing cholangitis has been recognized in up to 13% of patients with autoimmune hepatitis.

B. Chronic Hepatitis B: Chronic hepatitis B chiefly affects males. It may be noted as a continuum of acute hepatitis or may be diagnosed on evaluation of persistently elevated aminotransferase levels. Chronic HBV infection afflicts nearly 400 million people worldwide and 1.25 million in the USA.

Early in the course, HBeAg and HBV DNA are present in serum, indicative of active viral replications. Low-level IgM anti-HBc is also present in about 70%. In some patients, clinical and biochemical improvement coincides with disappearance of HBeAg and HBV DNA from serum, appearance of anti-HBe, and integration of the HBV genome into the host genome in infected hepatocytes. Such patients may still be at increased risk for the development of cirrhosis and hepatocellular carcinoma. As discussed above, infection by a pre-core mutant of HBV or spontaneous mutation of the pre-core region of the HBV genome during the course of chronic hepatitis caused by wild-type HBV may result in particularly severe chronic hepatitis with rapid progression to cirrhosis, particularly when additional mutations in the core gene of HBV are present.

C. Hepatitis D: Acute hepatitis D infection superimposed on chronic HBV infection may result in severe chronic hepatitis, which may progress rapidly to cirrhosis and may be fatal. The diagnosis is confirmed by detection of anti-HDV in serum.

D. Chronic Hepatitis C: At least 80% of patients with acute hepatitis C develop chronic hepatitis C. It is clinically indistinguishable from chronic hepatitis due to other causes and may be the most common. In about 25% of cases, serum aminotransferase levels are persistently normal. The diagnosis is confirmed by detection of anti-HCV by enzyme immunoassy (EIA). In rare cases of suspected chronic hepatitis C but a negative EIA, the diagnosis may be confirmed by a positive recombinant immunoblot assay (RIBA) or detection of HCV RNA in serum by polymerase chain reaction. Progression to cirrhosis occurs in 20% of affected patients after 20 years, with an increased risk in men, those who drink more than 50 g of alcohol daily, and possibly those who acquire HCV infection after age 40. Immunosuppressed persons—including patients with hypogammaglobulinemia, with HIV infection and a low CD4 count, or with organ transplants and receiving immunosuppressants—appear to progress more rapidly to cirrhosis than immunocompetent persons with chronic hepatitis C.

Treatment

Activity should be modified according to the patient's symptoms, but strict bed rest is not necessary. The diet should be well balanced, without specific limitations other than sodium or protein restriction as dictated by fluid overload or encephalopathy.

A. Autoimmune Hepatitis: Prednisone with or without azathioprine has been shown to improve symptoms, decrease the serum bilirubin, aminotransferase, and gamma globulin levels, and reduce hepatic inflammation. Symptomatic patients with serum aminotransferase levels elevated tenfold (or fivefold if the serum globulins are elevated at least twofold) are optimal for therapy, and patients with more modest enzyme elevations may be considered for therapy depending on the clinical circumstances.

Prednisone or an equivalent drug is given initially in doses of 30 mg orally daily with azathioprine or mercaptopurine, 50 mg/d orally, which are generally well tolerated and permit the use of lower corticosteroid doses. Nevertheless, complete blood counts should be monitored weekly for the first 8 weeks of therapy and monthly thereafter because of the small risk of bone marrow suppression. The dose of prednisone is lowered from 30 mg/d after 1 week to 20 mg/d and again after 2 or 3 weeks to 15 mg/d. Ultimately, a maintenance dose of 10 mg/d is achieved. While symptomatic improvement is often prompt, biochemical improvement is more gradual, with normalization of serum aminotransferase levels after 6–12 months in many cases. Histologic resolution of inflammation may take up to 18–24 months, the time at which repeat liver biopsy is recommended. Failure of aminotransferase levels to normalize invariably predicts lack of histologic resolution.

The response rate to therapy with prednisone and azathioprine is 80–90%. Cirrhosis, however, does not reverse with therapy and may even develop after apparent biochemical and histologic remission (absence of inflammation). Once remission is achieved, therapy may be withdrawn, but the subsequent relapse rate is 50–90%. Relapses may again be treated in the same manner as the initial episode, with an expected remission rate again of 80–90%. After successful treatment of a relapse, the patient may be kept indefinitely on azathioprine up to 2 mg/kg and the lowest dose of prednisone needed to maintain aminotransferase levels as close to normal as possible. Nonresponders to prednisone and azathioprine may be considered for a trial of cyclosporine, tacrolimus, methotrexate, or budesonide. Liver transplantation may be required for treatment failures, and the disease has been recognized to recur in up to one-third of transplanted livers (and rarely to develop de novo) as immunosuppression is reduced.

B. Chronic hepatitis B: Patients with active viral replication (HBeAg and HBV DNA in serum; elevated aminotransferase levels) may be treated with recombinant human interferon alfa-2b in a dose of 5 million units a day or 10 million units three times a week intramuscularly for 4 months. About 40% of treated patients will respond with normalization of aminotransferase levels, disappearance of HBeAg and HBV DNA from serum, appearance of anti-HBe, and improved survival. A response is most likely in patients with an HBV DNA level under 200 pg/mL and high aminotransferase levels. Moreover, over 60% of these responders may eventually clear HBsAg from serum and liver, develop anti-HBs in serum, and thus be cured of the infection. Relapses are uncommon in such complete responders.

The nucleoside analog lamivudine, 100 mg orally daily as a single dose, may be used instead of interferon for the treatment of chronic hepatitis B and is much better tolerated. This agent reliably suppresses HBV DNA in serum, improves liver histology in 40% of patients, and leads to normal ALT levels in over 40% and HBeAg seroconversion in 20% of patients after 1 year of therapy. However, 15–30% of responders experience a mild relapse during therapy as a result of mutation in HBV DNA that confers resistance to lamivudine. Moreover, hepatitis activity may recur when the drug is stopped, and long-term, perhaps indefinite treatment may be required to suppress the disease when treatment does not result in HBeAg seroconversion. The drug is well tolerated even in patients with decompensated cirrhosis, and it may be effective in patients with rapidly progressive hepatitis B ("fibrosing cholestatic hepatitis") following organ transplantation. There is no evidence that combined use of interferon and lamivudine offers an advantage over the use of either drug alone.

Recombinant interferon alfa-2a (9 million units three times a week for 48 weeks) may lead to normalization of serum aminotransferase levels, histologic improvement, and elimination of HDV RNA from serum in about 50% of patients with chronic hepatitis D, but relapse is common after therapy is stopped. Lamivudine is not effective in chronic hepatitis D.

C. Chronic Hepatitis C: Treatment of chronic hepatitis C is generally considered in patients under age 70 with elevated serum aminotransferase levels and more than minimal inflammation or fibrosis on liver biopsy. Recombinant human interferon alfa-2b or alfa-2a in a dose of 3 million units three times a week for 24 weeks and "consensus" interferon (a synthetic recombinant interferon derived by assigning the most commonly observed amino acid at each position of several alpha interferon subtypes) in a dose of 9 mg three times a week have been shown to induce biochemical, virologic, and histologic improvement (return of ALT to normal, loss of HCV RNA from serum, decrease in hepatic inflammation, and occasionally regression of fibrosis) in up to 50% of patients. Most experience has been with interferon alfa-2b. Factors that predict an increased chance of responding to therapy include the absence of cirrhosis on liver biopsy, low serum HCV RNA levels, and infection by genotypes of HCV other than 1a and 1b. After stopping the medication at 24 weeks, only 30–50% of the treated responders will maintain the improvement. More prolonged treatment (eg, for 12–18 months) has been shown to increase the durability of remission and is now recommended. The use of higher doses of interferon alfa-2b (eg, 6 million units three times a week) increases toxicity and does not appear to increase the rate of sustained responses. Response rates among blacks appear to be lower than those for whites, for reasons that remain unclear. A slow-release, long-acting "pegylated" formulation of interferon taken only once a week is nearing commercial release.

Addition of the nucleoside analog ribavirin, 1000–1200 mg daily in two divided doses, results in higher sustained response rates and has been approved for previously untreated patients with chronic hepatitis C or patients who have had a relapse after an initial response to interferon-alfa alone. Sustained response rates are 40% and 50%, respectively, in these two groups following combination therapy. Patients taking ribavirin must be monitored for hemolysis, and, because of teratogenic effects in animals, women taking the drug must practice strict contraception (and men taking the drug should be cautioned against impregnating women) until they have been off the drug for at least 6 months.

Interferon alfa with ribavirin may be beneficial in the treatment of cryoglobulinemia associated with chronic hepatitis C. On the other hand, treatment of patients with chronic hepatitis C and persistently normal serum aminotransferase levels ("chronic carriers") is of uncertain benefit. Treatment with interferon alfa with ribavirin is costly ($8000 for a 24-week supply), and side effects, which include flu-like symptoms, are almost universal; more serious side effects—psychiatric symptoms (irritability, depression), thyroid dysfunction, and bone marrow suppression—are less common. Interferon is contraindicated in patients with decompensated cirrhosis, profound cytopenias, psychiatric disease, and autoimmune diseases. Ribavirin should be avoided in persons over age 65 or others in whom hemolysis could pose a risk of angina or stroke.

Prognosis

The course of chronic hepatitis is variable and unpredictable. Untreated autoimmune hepatitis has a 5-year mortality rate of 50%, which decreases markedly with treatment. The sequelae of chronic hepatitis secondary to hepatitis B include cirrhosis, liver failure, and hepatocellular carcinoma. Up to 40–50% of patients with chronic hepatitis B and cirrhosis die within 5 years after the onset of symptoms, though predictive models suggest that therapy with interferon improves the prognosis in responders. Chronic hepatitis C is an indolent, often subclinical disease that may lead to cirrhosis and hepatocellular carcinoma after decades. In one study, the mortality rate from transfusion-associated hepatitis C was no different from that of an age-matched control population. Nevertheless, mortality rates clearly rise once cirrhosis develops, and mortality from cirrhosis and hepatocellular carcinoma due to hepatitis C is expected to triple in the next 10–20 years. Recent data suggest that treatment with interferon has a beneficial effect on survival and quality of life, is cost-effective, and in responders may reduce the risk of hepatocellular carcinoma.

Alvarez F et al: International Autoimmune Hepatitis Group report: Review of criteria for diagnosis of autoimmune hepatitis. J Hepatol 1999;31:929. [NLM Cit ID: 20046538] (Detailed review of the clinical, biochemical, serologic, and histologic criteria for the diagnosis of autoimmune hepatitis.)

Baffis V et al: Use of interferon for prevention of hepatocellular carcinoma in cirrhotic patients with hepatitis B or hepatitis C virus infection. Ann Intern Med 1999; 131:691. [NLM Cit ID: 99456453] (Reviews evidence suggesting that interferon therapy may prevent hepatocellular carcinoma in patients with cirrhosis, particularly those infected with hepatitis C.)

Czaja AJ: Drug therapy in the management of type 1 autoimmune hepatitis. Drugs 1999;57:49. [NLM Cit ID: 99135433] (In-depth overview of indications for treatment, preferred drug regimens, complications, treatment results, and management of relapses and nonresponse.)

DeBisceglie AM (editor): Treatment advances in chronic hepatitis C. Semin Liver Dis 1999;19(Suppl 1):1. (Reviews of all aspects of drug therapy for chronic hepatitis C.)

Dienstag JL et al: Lamivudine as initial treatment for chronic hepatitis B in the United States. N Engl J Med 1999;341:1256. [NLM Cit ID: 99442269] (After 1 year of treatment, lamivudine, 100 mg orally daily, led to HBeAg seroconversion with loss of serum HBV DNA in 17%, sustained normalization of ALT levels in 41%, and histologic improvement in 52% of patients.)

Keeffe EB (editor): Treatment of chronic hepatitis C. Clin Liver Dis 1999;3:693. (Collection of reviews on various aspects of drug therapy for hepatitis C.)

McHutchinson JG et al: Interferon alfa-2b alone or in combination with ribavirin as initial treatment for chronic hepatitis C. N Engl J Med 1998;339:1485. [NLM Cit ID: 99025346] (Sustained virologic response after 48 weeks of therapy was achieved in 38% of patients given interferon and ribavirin compared with 13% of those given interferon alone.)

ALCOHOLIC HEPATITIS

Alcoholic hepatitis is characterized by acute or chronic inflammation and parenchymal necrosis of the liver induced by alcohol. While alcoholic hepatitis is often a reversible disease, it is the most common precursor of cirrhosis in the USA, and cirrhosis ranks among the most common causes of death of adults in this country.

The frequency of alcoholic cirrhosis is estimated to be about 8–15% among persons who consume over 50 g of alcohol (4 oz of 100-proof whiskey, 15 oz of wine, or four 12-oz cans of beer) daily for over 10 years. The risk of cirrhosis is even lower (approximately 5%) in the absence of other cofactors such as chronic viral hepatitis. Genetic factors may also account in part for differences in susceptibility. Women appear to be more susceptible than men, in part because of lower gastric mucosal alcohol dehydrogenase levels. Although alcoholic hepatitis may not develop in many patients even after several decades of alcohol abuse, it appears in a few individuals within a year after onset of excessive drinking. In general, over 80% of patients with alcoholic hepatitis have been drinking 5 years or more before developing any symptoms that can be attributed to liver disease; the longer the duration of drinking (10–15 or more years) and the larger the alcoholic consumption, the greater the probability of developing alcoholic hepatitis and cirrhosis. In individuals who drink alcohol excessively, the rate of ethanol metabolism can be sufficiently high to permit the consumption of large quantities of spirits without raising the blood alcohol level over 80 mg/dL, the concentration at which the conventional breath analyzer begins to detect ethanol.

The role of deficiencies in vitamins and calories in the development of alcoholic hepatitis or in the progression of this lesion to cirrhosis remains controversial but is at least contributory. Ethanol-induced elevation of circulating endotoxin levels is thought to play a critical role in the pathogenesis of alcoholic liver disease by inducing release of tumor necrosis factor-α and other cytokines by Kupffer cells. Concurrent HBV or HCV infection and heterozygosity for the *HFE* gene mutation for hemochromatosis increase the severity of alcoholic liver disease.

Clinical Findings

A. Symptoms and Signs: The clinical presentation of alcoholic hepatitis can vary from an asymptomatic patient with an enlarged liver to a critically ill individual who dies quickly. A recent period of heavy drinking, complaints of anorexia and nausea, and the demonstration of hepatomegaly and jaundice strongly suggest the diagnosis. Abdominal pain and tenderness, splenomegaly, ascites, fever, and encephalopathy may be present.

B. Laboratory Findings: Anemia (usually macrocytic) may be present. Leukocytosis with shift to the left is common in patients with severe disease. Leukopenia is occasionally seen and disappears after cessation of drinking. About 10% of patients have thrombocytopenia related to a direct toxic effect of alcohol on megakaryocyte production or to hypersplenism.

AST is usually elevated but rarely above 300 units/L. AST is almost invariably greater than ALT, often by a factor of 2 or more. Serum alkaline phosphatase is generally elevated, but rarely more than three times the normal value. Serum bilirubin is increased in 60–90% of patients. Serum GGTP, mean corpuscular volume, and carbohydrate-deficient transferrin may be elevated in alcoholics, but none of these tests have a sensitivity rate above 70%. Serum bilirubin levels greater than 10 mg/dL and marked prolongation of the prothrombin time (≥ 6 seconds above control) indicate severe alcoholic hepatitis with a mortality rate as high as 50%. The serum albumin is depressed, and the gamma globulin level is elevated in 50–75% of individuals with alcoholic hepatitis, even in the absence of cirrhosis. Increased transferrin saturation and hepatic iron stores may result from secondary iron overload, in some cases due to spur cell anemia.

C. Liver Biopsy: Liver biopsy is usually diagnostic and demonstrates macrovesicular fat, PMN infiltration with hepatic necrosis, and Mallory bodies (alcoholic hyaline). Micronodular cirrhosis may be present as well.

D. Other Studies: Ultrasound is often helpful in ruling out biliary obstruction or to assess for subclinical ascites. CT scanning with intravenous contrast or MRI may be indicated in selected cases to evaluate patients for collateral vessels, space-occupying lesions of the liver, or concomitant disease of the pancreas.

Differential Diagnosis

Alcoholic hepatitis may be closely mimicked by cholecystitis and cholelithiasis and by injury from certain drugs such as amiodarone. In selected cases, other causes of hepatitis or chronic liver disease may be excluded by serologic or biochemical testing, by imaging studies, or by liver biopsy. However, liver biopsy findings are identical to those of nonalcoholic steatohepatitis.

Treatment

A. General Measures: Abstinence from alcohol is essential and must be emphasized repeatedly. During periods of anorexia, every effort should be made to provide sufficient amounts of carbohydrates and calories to reduce endogenous protein catabolism and to promote gluconeogenesis and prevent hypoglycemia. Nutritional support (40 kcal/kg with 1.5–2 g/kg as protein) improves survival in patients with malnutrition. Use of liquid formulas rich in branched-chain amino acids does not improve survival beyond that achieved with less expensive caloric supplementation. The administration of vitamins, particularly folic acid and thiamin, is indicated, especially when deficiencies are noted.

B. Corticosteroids: Several studies have shown that methylprednisolone, 32 mg/d for 1 month or the equivalent, is beneficial in patients with alcoholic hepatitis and either encephalopathy or a greatly elevated bilirubin concentration and prolonged prothrombin time (specifically, when the patient's prothrombin time minus the control prothrombin time times 4.6 plus the total bilirubin in mg/dL is > 32).

Prognosis

A. Short-Term: When the prothrombin time is short enough to permit performance of liver biopsy without risk (< 3 seconds above control), the 1-year mortality rate is 7%, rising to 18% if there is progressive prolongation of the prothrombin time during hospitalization. Individuals in whom the prothrombin time is so prolonged that liver biopsy cannot be attempted have a 42% mortality rate at 1 year. Other unfavorable prognostic factors are a serum bilirubin greater than 10 mg/dL, hepatic encephalopathy, and azotemia.

B. Long-Term: In the USA, the 3-year mortality rate of persons who recover from acute alcoholic hepatitis is ten times greater than that of control individuals of comparable age. Histologically severe disease is associated with continued excessive mortality rates after 3 years, whereas the death rate is not increased after the same period in those whose liver biopsies show only mild alcoholic hepatitis. Complications of portal hypertension (ascites, variceal bleeding, hepatorenal syndrome), coagulopathy, and severe jaundice following recovery from acute alcoholic hepatitis also suggest a poor long-term prognosis.

The most important prognostic consideration is the indisputable fact that continued excessive drinking is associated with reduction of life expectancy in these individuals. The prognosis is indeed poor if the patient is unable to abstain from drinking, and liver transplantation is generally contraindicated without a 6-month period of abstinence.

Berlakovich GA et al: Carbohydrate-deficient transferrin for detection of alcohol relapse after orthotopic liver transplantation for alcoholic cirrhosis. Transplantation 1999;67:1231. [NLM Cit ID: 99271742] (In this prospective study, the sensitivity and specificity of carbohydrate-deficient transferrin as a marker for recurrent alcohol abuse after liver transplantation were 92% and 98%, respectively.)

Imperiale TF et al: Corticosteroids are effective in patients with severe alcoholic hepatitis. Am J Gastroenterol 1999;94:3066. [NLM Cit ID: 99449185] (Critical review of published randomized controlled trials and meta-analyses.)

McCullough AJ (editor): Alcoholic liver disease. Clin Liver Dis 1998;2:649. (Entire volume.)

McCullough AJ et al: Alcoholic liver disease: Proposed recommendations for the American College of Gastroenterology. Am J Gasteroenterol 1998;93:2022. [NLM Cit ID: 99036255] (Overview of diagnosis, risk factors, and prognosis with detailed guidelines for management.)

DRUG- & TOXIN-INDUCED LIVER DISEASE

The continuing synthesis, testing, and introduction of new drugs into clinical practice has resulted in an increase in toxic reactions of many types. Many widely used therapeutic agents, including over-the-counter "natural" products, may cause hepatic injury. Drug-induced liver disease can mimic viral hepatitis or biliary tract obstruction as well as any other type of liver disease. In any patient with liver disease, the clinician must inquire carefully about the use of potentially hepatotoxic drugs or exposure to hepatotoxins. In some cases, coadministration of a second agent may increase the toxicity of the first (eg, isoniazid and rifampin, acetaminophen and alcohol). Drug toxicity may be categorized on the basis of pathogenesis or histologic appearance.

Direct Hepatotoxic Group

The liver lesion caused by this group of drugs is characterized by (1) dose-related severity, (2) a latent period following exposure, and (3) susceptibility in all individuals. Examples include acetaminophen, alcohol, carbon tetrachloride, chloroform, heavy metals, mercaptopurine, niacin, plant alkaloids, phosphorus, tetracyclines, valproic acid, and vitamin A.

Idiosyncratic Reactions

Reactions of this type are sporadic, not related to dose, and occasionally associated with features suggesting an allergic reaction, such as fever and eosinophilia. In some cases, toxicity results directly from a metabolite that is produced only in certain individuals on a genetic basis. Examples include amiodarone, aspirin, carbamazepine, chloramphenicol, diclofenac, flutamide, halothane, isoniazid, ketoconazole, methyldopa, oxacillin, phenylbutazone, phenytoin, pyrazinamide, quinidine, streptomycin, troglitazone (withdrawn from the market in the United States), and perhaps tacrine.

Cholestatic Reactions

A. Noninflammatory: Direct effect of agent on bile secretory mechanisms: azathioprine, estrogens, or anabolic steroids containing an alkyl or ethinyl group at carbon 17, indinavir, mercaptopurine, methyltestosterone, and cyclosporine.

B. Inflammatory: Inflammation of portal areas with bile duct injury (cholangitis), often with allergic features such as eosinophilia: amoxicillin-clavulanic acid, chlorothiazide, chlorpromazine, chlorpropamide, erythromycin, penicillamine, prochlorperazine, semisynthetic penicillins (eg, cloxacillin), and sulfadiazine.

Acute or Chronic Hepatitis

Histologically and in some cases clinically indistinguishable from autoimmune hepatitis: aspirin, isoniazid, methyldopa, minocycline, nitrofurantoin, nonsteroidal anti-inflammatory drugs, propylthiouracil, ritonavir, sulfonamides, troglitazone (withdrawn from the market in the United States).

Other Reactions

A. Fatty Liver:

1. Macrovesicular–Alcohol, amiodarone, corticosteroids, methotrexate.

2. Microvesicular–Tetracyclines, valproic acid.

B. Granulomas: Allopurinol, quinidine, quinine, phenylbutazone, phenytoin.

C. Fibrosis and Cirrhosis: Methotrexate, vitamin A.

D. Peliosis Hepatis (Blood-Filled Cavities): Anabolic steroids, azathioprine, oral contraceptive steroids.

E. Neoplasms: Oral contraceptive steroids, estrogens (hepatic adenoma but not focal nodular hyperplasia); vinyl chloride (angiosarcoma).

Aithal PG et al: The natural history of histologically proved drug induced liver disease. Gut 1999;44:731. [NLM Cit ID: 99221695] (The drugs most commonly incriminated in hepatotoxicity are now antibiotics, such as amoxicillin-clavulanate, and nonsteroidal anti-inflammatory drugs, because of their widespread use.)

Black M (editor): Drug-induced liver disease. Clin Liver Dis 1998;2:457. (Entire volume.)

Schenker S et al: Antecedent liver disease and drug toxicity. J Hepatol 1999;31:1098. [NLM Cit ID: 20068086] (Underlying liver disease may predispose to greater dose-dependent drug toxicity but may also be protective, by reducing formation of a toxic metabolite. The frequency of idiosyncratic reactions is not increased by underlying liver disease.)

Selim K et al: Hepatotoxicity of psychotropic drugs. Hepatology 1999;29:1347. [NLM Cit ID: 99234111] (Hepatotoxicity is generally rare and idiosyncratic. The pattern of injury is cholestatic for chlorpromazine, haloperidol, and tricyclics and hepatitic for hydrazines, MAO inhibitors, cocaine, and ecstasy.)

Sulkowski MS et al: Hepatotoxicity associated with antiretroviral therapy in adults infected with human immunodeficiency virus and the role of hepatitis C and B virus infection. JAMA 2000;283:74. [NLM Cit ID: 20096144] (The risk of severe hepatotoxicity is highest [10%] with use of ritonavir; indinavir is associated with a risk of hyperbilirubinemia. Underlying chronic hepatitis C and B are associated with a slightly increased risk of drug hepatotoxicity.)

FATTY LIVER & NONALCOHOLIC STEATOHEPATITIS

Ethanol can cause hepatic steatosis (fatty liver) in the absence of malnutrition, although inadequate diets—specifically, those deficient in choline, methionine, and protein—can contribute to liver damage caused by ethanol. Other nonalcoholic causes of cirrhosis are "cryptogenic," and in many of these cases unrecognized steatohepatitis (NASH) may play a role. In advanced cases, hemochromatosis may be associated with "bronzing" of the skin, arthritis, heart failure, and diabetes mellitus; greater than 50% saturation of serum transferrin or serum ferritin level above the upper limit of normal, detection of the mutated *HFE* gene (see below), and special staining for iron and quantitation of the iron on liver biopsy are generally required to confirm the diagnosis. Other metabolic diseases that may lead to cirrhosis include Wilson's disease and α_1-antiprotease (α_1-antitrypsin) deficiency. Primary biliary cirrhosis occurs more frequently in women and is associated with pruritus, significant elevation of alkaline phosphatase, elevated immunoglobulin (IgM) and cholesterol levels, and antimitochondrial antibody. Secondary biliary cirrhosis may result from chronic biliary obstruction due to a stone, stricture, or neoplasm and is not associated with antimitochondrial antibody. Congestive heart failure and constrictive pericarditis may lead to hepatic fibrosis ("cardiac cirrhosis") complicated by ascites and may be mistaken for cirrhosis.

Complications

Upper gastrointestinal tract bleeding may occur from varices, portal hypertensive gastropathy, or gastroduodenal ulcer (see Chapter 14). Hemorrhage may be massive, resulting in fatal exsanguination or portosystemic encephalopathy. Varices may also result from portal vein thrombosis. Liver failure may be precipitated by alcoholism, surgery, and infection. Carcinoma of the liver occurs more frequently in patients with cirrhosis but is uncommon in the USA. Hepatic Kupffer cell (reticuloendothelial) dysfunction and decreased opsonic activity lead to an increased risk of systemic infection. Cardiomyopathy may result from alcohol abuse, impairment of cardiac β-adrenergic receptors, and altered hemodynamics due to portal hypertension.

Treatment

A. General Measures: The most important principle of treatment is abstinence from alcohol. The diet should be palatable, with adequate calories and protein (75–100 g/d) and, if there is fluid retention, sodium restriction. In the presence of hepatic encephalopathy, protein intake should be reduced to 60–80 g/d. Vitamin supplementation is desirable.

B. Complications:

1. Ascites and edema–Diagnostic paracentesis is usually indicated. Abdominal paracentesis is rarely associated with serious complications such as bleeding, infection, or bowel perforation even in patients with severe coagulopathy. In addition to a cell count and culture, the ascitic albumin level should be determined; a serum-ascites albumin gradient (serum albumin minus ascitic albumin) > 1.1 suggests portal hypertension. An elevated ascitic adenosine deaminase level is suggestive of tuberculous peritonitis, but the sensitivity of the test is reduced in patients with portal hypertension.

Ascites in patients with cirrhosis is thought to result from portal hypertension (increased hydrostatic pressure); hypoalbuminemia (decreased oncotic pressure); peripheral vasodilation, perhaps mediated by endotoxin-induced release of nitric oxide, with resulting increases in renin and angiotensin levels and sodium retention by the kidneys; impaired liver inactivation of aldosterone; and increased aldosterone secretion secondary to increased renin production. Free water excretion is also impaired in cirrhosis, and hyponatremia may develop.

In all patients with cirrhotic ascites, dietary sodium intake may initially be restricted to 400–800 mg/d; the intake of sodium may be liberalized slightly after diuresis ensues. Restriction of fluid intake (800–1000 mL/d) is required for patients with hyponatremia (serum sodium < 125 meq/L). In some patients, there is a rapid diminution of ascites on bed rest and dietary sodium restriction alone. In individuals with severe fluid retention or those who are considered to have "intractable" ascites, the urinary excretion of sodium is usually less than 10 meq/L.

a. Diuretics–Spironolactone should be used in patients who do not respond to salt restriction alone. After starting with 100 mg daily and monitoring the aldosterone antagonist effect, reflected by an increase in the urinary sodium concentration, the dose may be increased by 100 mg every 3–5 days (up to a maximal conventional single daily dose of 400 mg/d, though higher doses have been used) until diuresis is achieved, typically preceded by a rise in the urinary sodium concentration. Monitoring for hyperkalemia is important. In patients who cannot tolerate spironolactone because of side effects such as painful gynecomastia, amiloride, another potassium-sparing diuretic, may be used in a dose of 5–10 mg daily. Diuresis may be augmented by the addition of a loop diuretic such as furosemide. This potent diuretic, however, will maintain its effect even with a falling glomerular filtration rate, with resultant prerenal azotemia. The dose of furosemide ranges from 40 to 160 mg/d, and the drug should be administered with careful monitoring of blood pressure, urine output, mental status, and serum electrolytes, especially potassium.

The goal of weight loss in the ascitic patient without associated peripheral edema should be no more than 1–1.5 lb/d (0.5–0.7 kg/d).

b. Large-volume paracentesis–In patients with massive ascites and respiratory compromise, ascites refractory to diuretics, or intolerable diuretic side effects, large-volume paracentesis (4–6 L) is effective. When this is done, it is often the practice to give intravenous albumin concomitantly at a dosage of 10 g/L of ascites fluid removed to protect the intravascular volume, though this may not be necessary

cephalopathy. Five-year survival rates as high as 80% are now reported. Hepatocellular carcinoma, hepatitis B and C, and Budd-Chiari syndrome may recur in the transplanted liver. The incidence of recurrence of hepatitis B can be reduced by pre- and postoperative treatment with lamivudine and perioperative administration of hepatitis B immune globulin. Immunosuppression is achieved with cyclosporine or tacrolimus, corticosteroids, and azathioprine and may be complicated by infections, renal failure, and neurologic disorders as well as graft rejection, vascular occlusion, or bile leaks.

Prognosis

The prognosis of cirrhosis has shown little change over the years. Factors determining survival include the patient's ability to stop the intake of alcohol as well as the Child class (Table 15–5). Hematemesis, jaundice, and ascites are unfavorable signs. In established cases with severe hepatic dysfunction (serum albumin < 3 g/dL, bilirubin > 3 mg/dL, ascites, encephalopathy, cachexia, and upper gastrointestinal bleeding), only 50% survive 6 months. The risk of death in this subgroup of patients with advanced cirrhosis is associated with renal insufficiency, cognitive dysfunction, ventilatory insufficiency, age ≥ 65 years, and prothrombin time ≥ 16 seconds. For such patients, meticulous efforts at palliative care are essential (see Chapter 5). Liver transplantation has markedly improved the outlook for patients who are acceptable candidates and are referred for evaluation early.

Caldwell SH et al: Cryptogenic cirrhosis: Clinical characterization and risk factors for underlying disease. Hepatology 1999;29:664. [NLM Cit ID: 99162355] (Because diabetes and obesity were more common among patients with cryptogenic cirrhosis than among those with primary biliary cirrhosis or hepatitis C-related cirrhosis, the authors speculate that unrecognized NASH may play a role in many cases of cryptogenic cirrhosis.)

Carithers RL Jr: Liver transplantation. Liver Transplant 2000;6:122. [NLM Cit ID: 20167483] (Current practice guidelines, including indications, contraindications, timing, and prognostic tools.)

Gulberg V et al: Long-term therapy and retreatment of hepatorenal syndrome type 1 with ornipressin and dopamine. Hepatology 1999;30:870. [NLM Cit ID: 99428430]

Krowka MJ: Hepatopulmonary syndromes. Gut 2000;46:1. [NLM Cit ID: 20069487] (Whereas hepatopulmonary syndrome—the triad of liver disease, increased alveolar-arterial gradient, and intravascular pulmonary dilation—often reverses after liver transplantation, pulmonary hypertension [mean pulmonary artery pressure > 35 mm Hg] poses a high risk for posttransplantation mortality.)

Lazaridis KN et al: Hepatic hydrothorax: Pathogenesis, diagnosis, and management. Am J Med 1999;107:262. [NLM Cit ID: 99420069] (When conservative measures such as salt restriction, diuretics, and repeated thoracentesis fail, placement of a transjugular intrahepatic shunt may relieve hepatic hydrothorax.)

Ong JP et al: Transjugular intrahepatic portosystemic shunts: A decade later. J Clin Gastroenterol 2000;30:14. [NLM Cit ID: 20100161] (Reviews technical aspects, indications, contraindications, efficacy, and complications.)

Runyon BA: Management of adult patients with ascites caused by cirrhosis. Hepatology 1998;27:264. [NLM Cit ID: 98085915] (Current practice guidelines.)

Such J et al: Spontaneous bacterial peritonitis. Clin Infect Dis 1998;27:669. [NLM Cit ID: 99014747] (Reviews definition, variant forms, pathogenesis, clinical features, diagnosis, treatment, prevention, and prognosis.)

PRIMARY BILIARY CIRRHOSIS

Primary biliary cirrhosis is a chronic disease of the liver characterized by autoimmune destruction of intrahepatic bile ducts and cholestasis. It is insidious in onset, occurs usually in women aged 40–60, and is often detected by the chance finding of elevated alkaline phosphatase levels. The disease is progressive and may be complicated by steatorrhea, xanthomas, xanthelasma, osteoporosis, osteomalacia, and portal hypertension. It may be associated with scleroderma, Sjögren's syndrome, hypothyroidism, and celiac disease.

Table 15–5. Modified Child-Pugh classification for cirrhosis.

Parameter	Numerical Score 1	2	3
Ascites	None	Slight	Moderate to severe
Encephalopathy	None	Slight to moderate	Moderate to severe
Bilirubin (mg/dL)	< 2.0	2–3	> 3.0
Albumin (g/dL)	> 3.5	2.8–3.5	< 2.8
Prothrombin time (seconds increased)	1–3	4–6	> 6.0

Total numerical score	Child-Pugh class
5–6	A
7–9	B
10–15	C

Clinical Findings

A. Symptoms and Signs: Many patients are asymptomatic for years. The onset of clinical illness is insidious and is heralded by pruritus. As the disease progresses, physical examination reveals hepatosplenomegaly. Xanthomatous lesions may occur in the skin and tendons and around the eyelids. Jaundice and signs of portal hypertension are usually late findings.

B. Laboratory Findings: Blood counts are normal early in the disease. Liver function tests reflect cholestasis with elevation of alkaline phosphatase, cholesterol (especially high-density lipoproteins), and, in later stages, bilirubin. Antimitochondrial antibodies (directed against pyruvate dehydrogenase or other 2-oxo-acid enzymes in mitochondria) are present in 95% of patients, and serum IgM levels are elevated.

Diagnosis

The diagnosis of primary biliary cirrhosis is based on the detection of cholestatic liver chemistries (often an isolated elevation of the alkaline phosphatase) and antimitochondrial antibodies in serum in combination with characteristic histology on liver biopsy. Liver biopsy also permits histologic staging: I, portal inflammation with granulomas; II, bile duct proliferation, periportal inflammation; III, interlobular fibrous septa; and IV, cirrhosis.

Differential Diagnosis

The disease must be differentiated from chronic biliary tract obstruction (stone or stricture), carcinoma of the bile ducts, primary sclerosing cholangitis, sarcoidosis, drug toxicity (eg, chlorpromazine), and in some cases chronic hepatitis. Patients with a clinical and histologic picture of primary biliary cirrhosis but no antimitochondrial antibodies are said to have "autoimmune cholangitis," which in some studies has been associated with lower serum IgM levels and a greater frequency of smooth muscle and antinuclear antibodies. Some patients have overlappping features of primary biliary cirrhosis and autoimmune hepatitis.

Treatment

Treatment is primarily symptomatic. Cholestyramine (4 g) or colestipol (5 g) in water or juice three times daily may be beneficial for the pruritus. Rifampin, 150–300 mg orally twice daily, has been of benefit in some studies, but not others. Opioid antagonists (eg, naloxone, 0.2 μg/kg/min by intravenous infusion, or naltrexone, 50 mg/d by mouth) show promise in the treatment of pruritus. The 5-HT_3 serotonin receptor antagonist ondansetron may also provide some benefit. Deficiencies of vitamins A, K, and D may occur if steatorrhea is present and may be further aggravated when cholestyramine or colestipol is administered. Replacement dosages of these vitamins must be individualized. Calcium supplementation (500 mg three times daily) may help prevent osteomalacia but is of uncertain benefit in osteoporosis. Limited data suggest that oral bisphosphonates and estrogen may be of benefit in treating osteoporosis. Because of its lack of toxicity, ursodeoxycholic acid (10–15 mg/kg/d in one or two doses) is the preferred medical treatment and has been shown to slow the progression of disease, improve long-term survival, reduce the risk of developing esophageal varices, and delay the need for liver transplantation. Colchicine (0.6 mg twice daily) and methotrexate (15 mg/wk) have had some reported benefit in improving symptoms and serum levels of alkaline phosphatase and bilirubin. Methotrexate may also improve liver histology. Penicillamine, corticosteroids, and azathioprine have proved to be of no benefit. For patients with advanced disease, liver transplantation is the treatment of choice.

Prognosis

Without liver transplantation, survival averages 7–10 years once symptoms develop. In advanced disease, adverse prognostic markers are older age, high serum bilirubin, edema, low albumin, prolonged prothrombin time, and variceal hemorrhage. Among asymptomatic patients, about one-third will become symptomatic within 15 years. The risk of hepatobiliary malignancies appears to be increased in patients with primary biliary cirrhosis. Liver transplantation for advanced primary biliary cirrhosis is associated with a 1-year survival rate of 85–90%.

Angulo P et al: Long-term ursodeoxycholic acid delays histological progression in primary biliary cirrhosis. Hepatology 1999;29:644. [NLM Cit ID: 99162351] (Retrospective study showing that the risk of progression to cirrhosis in patients treated with ursodeoxycholic acid for a mean of 6.6 years is 13% compared with 49% for placebo recipients.)

Goulis J et al: Randomised controlled trials of ursodeoxycholic-acid therapy for primary biliary cirrhosis: a meta analysis. Lancet 1999;354:1053. [NLM Cit ID: 99437194] (Raises doubts about the value of ursodeoxycholic acid in delaying the progression of primary biliary cirrhosis.)

Leuschner M et al: Oral budesonide and ursodeoxycholic acid for treatment of primary biliary cirrhosis: Results of a prospective double-blind trial. Gastroenterology 1999;117:918. [NLM Cit ID: 99431915] (Preliminary trial suggesting that the addition of budesonide, a glucocorticoid with high first-pass metabolism and little toxicity, to therapy with ursodeoxycholic acid leads to greater biochemical and histologic improvement than therapy with ursodeoxycholic acid alone.)

Springer J et al: Asymptomatic primary biliary cirrhosis: A study of its natural history and prognosis. Am J Gastroenterol 1999;94:47. [NLM Cit ID: 99131429] (Patients who present with asymptomatic primary biliary cirrhosis have a shorter life span than the general population. One-third become symptomatic within 15 years.)

HEMOCHROMATOSIS

Hemochromatosis is an autosomal recessive disease with linkage in many cases to HLA-A3. The principal candidate genetic defect has been identified as a mutation in a newly recognized gene termed *HFE* on chromosome 6. The alteration leads to substitution of tyrosine for cysteine at position 282 *(C282Y)* in a region of the gene product involved in interaction with β_2-microglobulin. Presence of the mutation apparently reduces cell surface expression of an HFE-β_2 microglobulin complex on duodenal crypt cells, thereby impairing transferrin-mediated uptake of iron from the circulation into crypt cells and resulting in up-regulation of duodenal metal-transporter (DMT-1) expression on the luminal side of villous cells leading in turn to increased iron absorption from the intestine. About 85% of persons with well-established hemochromatosis are homozygous for the *C282Y* mutation. The frequency of the gene mutation averages 7% in Northern European and North American white populations, resulting in a 0.5% frequency of homozygotes (and of iron overload). By contrast, the gene mutation and hemochromatosis are uncommon in African-American and Asian-American populations. A second genetic mutation leading to substitution of aspartic acid for histidine at position 63 (H63D) of the same protein may contribute to the development of hemochromatosis in a small number of affected patients.

The disorder is characterized by increased accumulation of iron as hemosiderin in the liver, pancreas, heart, adrenals, testes, pituitary, and kidneys. Eventually the patient may develop hepatic, pancreatic, and cardiac insufficiency and hypogonadism. The disease is rarely recognized before the fifth decade. Heterozygotes do not develop cirrhosis in the absence of associated disorders such as viral hepatitis or nonalcoholic steatohepatitis.

Clinical Findings

The onset is usually after age 50. Clinical manifestations include arthropathy, hepatomegaly and evidence of hepatic insufficiency (late finding), occasional skin pigmentation (combination of slate gray due to iron and brown due to melanin, sometimes resulting in bronze color), cardiac enlargement with or without heart failure or conduction defects, diabetes mellitus with its complications, and impotence in the male. Bleeding from esophageal varices may occur, and in patients who develop cirrhosis, there is a 15–20% incidence of hepatocellular carcinoma. Affected patients are at increased risk of infection with *Vibrio vulnificus, Listeria monocytogenes, Yersinia enterocolitica,* and other iron-loving organisms. The disease should be considered in patients with a family history or otherwise unexplained mild liver test abnormalities. A variant presentation in patients around age 20 is characterized by cardiac dysfunction, hypogonadotropic hypogonadism, and a high mortality rate and is not associated with the *C282Y* mutation.

Laboratory findings include mildly abnormal liver tests (AST, alkaline phosphatase), an elevated plasma iron with greater than 50% saturation of the transferrin, and an elevated serum ferritin (although a normal ferritin does not exclude the diagnosis). CT and MRI may show changes consistent with iron overload of the liver, but these techniques are not sensitive enough for screening asymptomatic persons. Testing for *HFE* mutations is indicated in any patient with evidence of iron overload and in siblings of patients with confirmed hemochromatosis. In patients who are homozygous for *C282Y,* liver biopsy is often indicated to determine whether cirrhosis is present. Biopsy can be deferred, however, in patients in whom the serum ferritin level is < 1000 μg/L, serum AST level is normal, and hepatomegaly is absent on examination because of the low likelihood of cirrhosis in these individuals. Liver biopsy is also indicated when iron overload is suspected even though the patient is not homozygous for *C282Y.* In patients with hemochromatosis, the liver biopsy characteristically shows extensive iron deposition in hepatocytes and in bile ducts and the hepatic iron index—hepatic iron content per gram of liver converted to micromoles and divided by the patient's age—is generally greater than 1.9.

Treatment

Early diagnosis and treatment in the precirrhotic phase of hemochromatosis is of great importance. Affected patients should avoid red meat, alcohol, vitamin C, raw shellfish, and supplemental iron. Treatment consists initially of weekly phlebotomies of 500 mL of blood (about 250 mg of iron), continued for up to 2–3 years to achieve depletion of iron stores. This process is monitored by hematocrit and serum iron determinations. When iron store depletion is achieved, maintenance phlebotomies (every 2–4 months) are continued. The chelating agent deferoxamine, administered intravenously or subcutaneously in a dose of 40–50 mg/kg/d infused over 12 hours, can mobilize 30 mg of iron per day. The drug is indicated for patients with hemochromatosis and anemia or with secondary iron overload due to thalassemia who cannot tolerate phlebotomies. However, treatment is painful and not always practical. Complications of hemochromatosis—arthropathy, diabetes mellitus, heart disease, portal hypertension, and hypopituitarism—may require treatment.

The course of the disease is favorably altered by phlebotomy therapy. In precirrhotic patients, cirrhosis may be prevented. Cardiac conduction defects and insulin requirements improve with treatment. In patients with cirrhosis, varices may reverse, and the risk of bleeding declines. However, cirrhotic patients must be monitored for the development of hepatocellular carcinoma. Liver transplantation for advanced cirrhosis due to hemochromatosis is associated with lower survival rates than for other types of liver disease because of cardiac complications and an increased risk of infections. Genetic testing is recommended for all first-degree family members of the proband. Screening all white men over age 30 or all adults by measurement of the transferrin saturation has been recommended but requires further study.

Adams PC: Population screening for hemochromatosis. Hepatology 1999;29:1324. [NLM Cit ID: 99197117] (Hemochromatosis fulfills criteria established by the World Health Organization for population screening, which is cost-effective but may be impractical. The author recommends a more feasible goal of increasing public awareness and screening by primary care physicians.)

Adams PC et al: Genotypic/phenotypic correlations in genetic hemochromatosis: Evolution of diagnostic criteria. Gastroenterology 1998;114:319. [NLM Cit ID: 98114237] (The authors have observed occasional persons homozygous for the *HFE* gene mutation but with no biochemical evidence of iron overload as well as patients with iron overload but without the gene mutation.)

Andrews NC: Disorders of iron metabolism. N Engl J Med 1999;341:1986. [NLM Cit ID: 20057434] (Includes lucid discussions of the physiology of iron transport and disorders of iron overload.)

Bacon BR et al: Molecular medicine and hemochromatosis: At the crossroads. Gastroenterology 1999;116:193. [NLM Cit ID: 99087978] (Summary of a recent NIH workshop with discussions of pathogenesis, molecular genetics, epidemiology, clinical features, and management.)

El-Serag HB et al: Screening for hereditary hemochromatosis in siblings and children of affected patients: A cost-effectiveness analysis. Ann Intern Med 2000;132:261. [NLM Cit ID: 20132329] (Screening relatives of patients with C282Y homozygous hemochromatosis is cost-effective; siblings of an affected patient should undergo genetic testing, while children should undergo genetic testing if the patient's spouse is heterozygous for C282Y.)

Olynyk JK et al: A population based study of the clinical expression of the hemochromatosis gene. N Engl J Med 1999;341:718. [NLM Cit ID: 99383621] (Of 16 subjects homozygous for the C282Y mutation, only eight had clinical features of hemochromatosis; four had persistently normal serum ferritin levels over 4 years, illustrating the difficulty in detecting the disorder.)

WILSON'S DISEASE

Wilson's disease (hepatolenticular degeneration) is a rare autosomal recessive disorder that usually occurs between the first and third decades. The condition is characterized by excessive deposition of copper in the liver and brain. The genetic defect, localized to chromosome 13, has been shown to affect a copper-transporting adenosine triphosphatase (ATP7B) in the liver. Over 50 different mutations in the Wilson disease gene have been identified, making routine genetic diagnosis unlikely.

The major physiologic aberration in Wilson's disease is excessive absorption of copper from the small intestine and decreased excretion of copper by the liver, resulting in increased tissue deposition, especially in the liver, brain, cornea, and kidney. Serum ceruloplasmin, the plasma copper-carrying protein, is low. Urinary excretion of copper is high.

Clinical Findings

Wilson's disease tends to present as liver disease in adolescents and neuropsychiatric disease in young adults, but there is great variability. The diagnosis should always be considered in any child or young adult with hepatitis, splenomegaly with hypersplenism, hemolytic anemia, portal hypertension, and neurologic or psychiatric abnormalities. Wilson's disease should also be considered in persons under 40 years of age with chronic or fulminant hepatitis.

Hepatic involvement may range from elevated liver tests to cirrhosis and portal hypertension. The neurologic manifestations are related to basal ganglia dysfunction and include a resting, postural, or kinetic tremor and dystonia of the bulbar musculature with resulting dysarthria and dysphagia. Psychiatric features include behavioral and personality changes and emotional lability. The pathognomonic sign of the condition is the brownish or gray green Kayser-Fleischer ring, which represents fine pigmented granular deposits in Descemet's membrane in the cornea close to the endothelial surface. The ring is usually most marked at the superior and inferior poles of the cornea. It can frequently be seen with the naked eye and almost invariably by slit lamp examination. It may be absent in patients with hepatic manifestations only but is usually present in those with neuropsychiatric disease. Renal calculi, the Fanconi defect, renal tubular acidosis, and hypoparathyroidism may occur in patients with Wilson's disease.

The diagnosis is based on demonstration of increased urinary copper excretion (> 100 μg/24 h) or low serum ceruloplasmin levels (< 20 μg/dL), and elevated hepatic copper concentration (> 250 μg/g of dry liver). In equivocal cases, the diagnosis may require demonstration of low radiolabeled copper incorporation into ceruloplasmin. Liver biopsy may show acute or chronic hepatitis or cirrhosis.

Treatment

Early treatment to remove excess copper is essential before it can produce neurologic or hepatic damage. Early in the treatment phase, restriction of dietary copper (shellfish, organ foods, and legumes are rich in copper) may be of value. Oral penicillamine (0.75–2 g/d in divided doses) is the drug of choice, making possible urinary excretion of chelated copper. Pyridoxine, 50 mg per week, is added, since penicillamine is an antimetabolite of this vitamin. If penicillamine treatment cannot be tolerated because of gastrointestinal, hypersensitivity, or autoimmune reactions, consider the use of trientine, 250–500 mg three times a day. Oral zinc acetate, 50 mg three times a day, promotes fecal copper excretion and may be used as maintenance therapy after decoppering with a chelating agent or as first-line therapy in presymptomatic or pregnant patients. Ammonium tetrathiomolybdate has shown promise as initial therapy for neurologic Wilson's disease.

Treatment should continue indefinitely. The prognosis is good in patients who are effectively treated before liver or brain damage has occurred. Liver transplantation is indicated for fulminant hepatitis (often after plasma exchange as a stabilizing measure), end-stage cirrhosis, and, in selected cases, intractable neurologic disease. Family members, especially siblings, require screening with serum ceruloplasmin, liver function tests, and slitlamp examination.

Brewer GJ et al: Treatment of Wilson's disease with zinc. XVII: Treatment during pregnancy. Hepatology 2000; 31:364. [NLM Cit ID: 20122336] (In contrast to penicillamine, which is teratogenic in humans, and trientine, which is teratogenic in animals, zinc may be preferable in pregnant women with Wilson's disease.)

Gow PJ et al: Diagnosis of Wilson's disease: An experience over three decades. Gut 2000;46:415. [NLM Cit ID: 20138075] (In patients with nonfulminant presentations, the combination of a low serum ceruloplasmin and Kayser-Fleischer rings establishes the diagnosis but is present in only 55%; the rest require liver biopsy to demonstrate an elevated hepatic copper.)

Pfeil SA et al: Wilson's disease: Copper unfettered. J Clin Gastroenterol 1999;29:33. [NLM Cit ID: 99332137] (Lucid review of pathophysiology, clinical features, diagnosis, and treatment.)

HEPATIC VEIN OBSTRUCTION (Budd-Chiari Syndrome)

Occlusion of the hepatic veins may occur from a variety of causes. Many cases are associated with polycythemia vera or other myeloproliferative diseases, which may be subclinical. Hepatovenous obstructions may be associated with caval webs, right-sided heart failure or constrictive pericarditis, neoplasms causing hepatic vein occlusions, paroxysmal nocturnal hemoglobinuria, Behçet's syndrome, blunt abdominal trauma, use of birth control pills, and pregnancy. In some cases, an underlying predisposition to thrombosis (eg, hyperprothrombinemia, [factor II G20210A mutation], activated protein C resistance [factor V Leiden mutation], protein C or S or antithrombin deficiency, antiphospholipid antibodies, or lupus anticoagulant) can be identified. Some cytotoxic agents and pyrrolizidine alkaloids ("bush teas") may cause hepatic veno-occlusive disease (occlusion of terminal venules), which mimics Budd-Chiari syndrome clinically. Veno-occlusive disease, often associated with cardiopulmonary and renal failure, is common in patients who have undergone bone marrow transplantation, particularly those with pretransplant aminotransferase elevations or fever during cytoreductive therapy with cyclophosphamide, azathioprine, carmustine, busulfan, or etoposide or those receiving high-dose cytoreductive therapy or high-dose total body irradiation.

Clinical manifestations may include tender, painful hepatic enlargement; jaundice; splenomegaly; and ascites. With advanced disease, bleeding varices and hepatic coma may be evident. Hepatic imaging studies may show a prominent caudate lobe, since its venous drainage may not be occluded. The screening test of choice is duplex Doppler ultrasonography, which has a sensitivity of 85% for detecting evidence of hepatic venous or inferior vena caval thrombosis. Caval venography can delineate caval webs and occluded hepatic veins. Percutaneous liver biopsy frequently shows a characteristic centrilobular congestion.

Ascites should be treated with fluid and salt restriction and diuretics. Treatable causes of Budd-Chiari syndrome should be sought. Prompt recognition and treatment of an underlying hematologic disorder may avoid the need for surgery. Surgical decompression (mesocaval or mesoatrial shunt) of the congested liver may be required to relieve persistent hepatic congestion. In some cases, placement of a transjugular intrahepatic portosystemic shunt (TIPS) may be feasible. Balloon angioplasty, in some cases with placement of an intravascular metallic stent, is preferred in patients with an inferior vena caval web and may be feasible in patients with a short segment of thrombosis in the hepatic vein. Rarely, thrombolytic therapy may be attempted within 2 weeks of acute hepatic vein thrombosis. Liver transplantation is considered in patients with cirrhosis and hepatocellular dysfunction. Patients often require lifelong anticoagulation and treatment of the underlying myeloproliferative disease.

Denninger M-H et al: Cause of portal or hepatic venous thrombosis in adults: The role of multiple concurrent factors. Hepatology 2000;31:587. [NLM Cit ID: 20172008] (A coagulation disorder was found in 87% of patients with hepatic vein thrombosis and 72% of those with portal vein thrombosis. Causes in patients with hepatic vein thrombosis included a primary myeloproliferative disorder [50%], factor V Leiden mutation [22%], factor II G20210A mutation [6%], and protein C deficiency [20%].)

Ganguli SC et al: Budd-Chiari syndrome in patients with hematological disease: A therapeutic challenge. Hepatology 1998;27:1157. [NLM Cit ID: 98196805] (Concise review of management options.)

Okuda K et al: Proposal of a new nomenclature for Budd-Chiari syndrome: Hepatic vein thrombosis versus thrombosis of the inferior vena cava at its hepatic portion. Hepatology 1998;28:1191. [NLM Cit ID: 99013887] (In

derlying biliary malignancy or severe multiorgan dysfunction. Hepatic candidiasis often responds to intravenous amphotericin B (total dose of 2–9 g). Fungal abscesses are associated with mortality rates of up to 50% and are treated with intravenous amphotericin B and drainage.

Barakate MS et al: Pyogenic liver abscess: A review of 10 years' experience in management. Aust N Z J Surg 1999;69:205. [NLM Cit ID: 99173682] (The overall hospital mortality rate is still as high as 8%. Percutaneous drainage is usually successful for a single abscess, but laparotomy may be required for abscess rupture or incomplete percutaneous drainage.)

Dull JS et al: Non-surgical treatment of biliary liver abscesses: Efficacy of endoscopic drainage and local antibiotic lavage with nasobiliary catheter. Gastrointest Endosc 2000;51:55. [NLM Cit ID: 20092797] (Liver abscesses resulting from biliary obstruction can be treated by systemic antibiotics and drainage with antibiotic lavage via an endoscopically placed nasobiliary catheter.)

Lipsett PA et al: Fungal hepatic abscesses: Characterization and management. J Gastrointest Surg 1997;1:78. (Pure fungal abscesses are usually associated with hematologic malignancies, whereas mixed fungal and pyogenic abscesses are more likely to be associated with biliary or pancreatic malignancies; in either case, the mortality rate is as high as 50%.)

NEOPLASMS OF THE LIVER

1. HEPATOCELLULAR CARCINOMA

Malignant neoplasms of the liver that arise from parenchymal cells are called hepatocellular carcinomas; those that originate in the ductular cells are called cholangiocarcinomas.

Hepatocellular carcinomas are associated with cirrhosis in general and hepatitis B or C in particular. In Africa and most of Asia, hepatitis B is of major etiologic significance, whereas in western countries and Japan hepatitis C and alcoholic cirrhosis are the most common causes. Other associations include hemochromatosis, aflatoxin exposure (associated with mutation of the *P53* gene), α_1-antiprotease (α_1-antitrypsin) deficiency, and tyrosinemia. The fibrolamellar variant of hepatocellular carcinoma occurs in young women and is characterized by a distinctive histologic picture, absence of risk factors, and indolent course.

Histologically, hepatocellular carcinoma is made up of cords or sheets of cells that roughly resemble the hepatic parenchyma. Blood vessels such as portal or hepatic veins are commonly involved by tumor.

The presence of a hepatocellular carcinoma may be unsuspected until there is deterioration in the condition of a cirrhotic patient who was formerly stable. Cachexia, weakness, and weight loss are associated symptoms. The sudden appearance of ascites, which may be bloody, suggests portal or hepatic vein thrombosis by tumor or bleeding from the necrotic tumor.

Physical examination may show tender enlargement of the liver, with an occasionally palpable mass. In Africa, young patients typically present with a rapidly expanding abdominal mass. Auscultation may reveal a bruit over the tumor or a friction rub when the process has extended to the surface of the liver.

Laboratory tests may reveal leukocytosis, as opposed to the leukopenia that is frequently encountered in cirrhotic patients. Anemia is common, but a normal or elevated hematocrit may be found in up to one-third of patients owing to elaboration of erythropoietin by the tumor. Sudden and sustained elevation of the serum alkaline phosphatase in a patient who was formerly stable is a common finding. Hepatitis B surface antigen is present in a majority of cases in endemic areas, whereas in the United States anti-HCV is found in up to 40% of cases. Alpha-fetoprotein levels are elevated in up to 70% of patients with hepatocellular carcinoma in Western countries; however, mild elevations are also often seen in patients with chronic hepatitis. Cytologic study of ascitic fluid rarely reveals malignant cells.

Arterial phase helical CT scanning with and without intravenous contrast or MRI are the preferred imaging studies to characterize the location and vascularity of the tumor. Ultrasound is less sensitive but is used to screen for hepatic nodules in high-risk patients. Liver biopsy is diagnostic, though seeding of the needle tract by tumor is a potential risk (≤ 5%), and biopsy can be deferred if surgical resection is planned. Staging in the TNM classification includes the following definitions: T0: no evidence of primary tumor; T1: solitary tumor ≤ 2.0 cm; T2: solitary tumor ≤ 2.0 cm with vascular invasion or > 2.0 cm without vascular invasion or ≤ 2.0 cm and multiple in one lobe; T3: solitary tumor > 2.0 cm with vascular invasion or ≤ 2.0 cm and multiple in one lobe with vascular invasion or multiple in one lobe with any > 2.0 cm with or without vascular invasion; and T4: multiple tumors in more than one lobe or involving a major branch of the portal or hepatic veins.

Attempts at surgical resection are usually fruitless if concomitant cirrhosis is present and if the tumor is multifocal. Surgical resection of solitary hepatocellular carcinomas may result in cure if liver function is normal. Overall 5-year survival rates are up to 56% for patients with localized resectable disease (T1, T2, T3, selected T4; N0; M0) but virtually nil for those with localized unresectable or advanced disease. Liver transplantation may be appropriate for small unresectable tumors in a patient with advanced cirrhosis, with reported 5-year survival rates of up to 75%. Liver transplantation may achieve a better recurrence-free survival than resection in patients with well-compensated cirrhosis and small tumors but is often impractical because of the donor organ shortage. Chemotherapy has not been shown to prolong life, but chemoembolization via the hepatic artery may be palliative. Injection of absolute ethanol into, microwave ablation of, or cryotherapy of small tumors (< 3 cm) may prolong survival, and these are reasonable alternatives to surgical resection in some patients. For those patients whose disease progresses despite treatment, meticulous efforts at palliative care are essential (see Chapter 5). Such patients may develop severe pain due to expansion of the liver capsule by the tumor and require concerted efforts at pain management, including the use of opioids (see Chapter 1).

In the patient with chronic hepatitis B or cirrhosis caused by HCV or alcohol, surveillance for the development of hepatocellular carcinoma should be considered with regular (eg, every 6 months) alpha-fetoprotein testing and ultrasonography. The risk of hepatocellular carcinoma in a patient with cirrhosis is 3–5% a year.

2. BENIGN LIVER NEOPLASMS

Two distinct benign entities with characteristic clinical, radiologic, and histopathologic features have been described in women taking oral contraceptives. **Focal nodular hyperplasia** occurs at all ages but is questionably related to oral contraceptives. It is often asymptomatic and appears as a hypervascular mass, occasionally with a central hypodense "stellate" scar on CT scan or MRI. Microscopically, focal nodular hyperplasia consists of hyperplastic units of hepatocytes with a central stellate scar containing proliferating bile ducts. **Liver cell adenoma** occurs most commonly in the third and fourth decades of life; the clinical presentation is often one of acute abdominal pain due to necrosis of the tumor with hemorrhage. The tumor is hypovascular and reveals a cold defect on liver scan. Grossly, the cut surface appears structureless. As seen microscopically, the liver cell adenoma consists of sheets of hepatocytes without portal tracts or central veins. The only physical finding in focal nodular hyperplasia or liver cell adenoma is a palpable abdominal mass in a minority of cases. Liver function is usually normal.

Treatment of focal nodular hyperplasia is resection only in the symptomatic patient. The prognosis is excellent. Liver cell adenoma often undergoes necrosis and rupture, and resection is advised even in asymptomatic persons. In selected cases, laparoscopic resection may be feasible. Regression of benign hepatic tumors may follow cessation of oral contraceptives.

The most common benign neoplasm of the liver is the **cavernous hemangioma,** often an incidental finding on ultrasound or CT scan. This lesion must be differentiated from other space-occupying intrahepatic lesions, usually by MRI. Fine-needle biopsy may be necessary to differentiate these lesions and does not appear to carry an increased risk of bleeding. Cavernous hemangiomas rarely require treatment.

Badvie S: Hepatocellular carcinoma. Postgrad Med J 2000;76:4. [NLM Cit ID: 20160859] (Timely review emphasizing the spectrum of treatment options.)

Mathieu D et al: Oral contraceptive use and focal nodular hyperplasia of the liver. Gastroenterology 2000;118:560. [NLM Cit ID: 20167109] (In contrast to hepatic adenomas, neither the size nor the number of focal nodular hyperplasia lesions is influenced by oral contraceptive use.)

Okuda K et al (editors): Hepatocellular carcinoma. Semin Liver Dis 1999;19:233. (Issue includes discussions of molecular biology, pathogenesis, epidemiology, diagnosis, treatment, and prognosis.)

Schafer DF et al: Hepatocellular carcinoma. Lancet 1999;353:1253. [NLM Cit ID: 99231450] (Terse review of epidemiology, etiology, natural history, treatment, screening, and prevention.)

Yuen M-F et al: Early detection of hepatocellular carcinoma increases the chance of treatment: Hong Kong experience. Hepatology 2000;31:330. [NLM Cit ID: 20122331] (In a population of patients with cirrhosis due mainly to chronic hepatitis B, screening with serum alpha-fetoprotein testing and ultrasonography led to detection of tumors at an earlier stage than no screening.)

DISEASES OF THE BILIARY TRACT

CHOLELITHIASIS (Gallstones)

Gallstones are more common in women than in men and increase in incidence in both sexes and all races with aging. In the USA, over 10% of men and 20% of women have gallstones by age 65; the total exceeds 20 million people. Although cholesterol gallstones are less common in black people, cholelithiasis attributable to hemolysis occurs in over a third of individuals with sickle cell anemia. Native Americans of both the Northern and Southern Hemispheres have a high rate of cholesterol cholelithiasis, probably because of a genetic predisposition. As many as 75% of Pima women over the age of 25 years have cholelithiasis. Obesity is a risk factor for gallstones, especially in women, and rapid weight loss, particularly in obese persons or those who "cycle" between weight loss and weight gain, increases the risk of symptomatic gallstone formation. There is evidence that glucose intolerance and elevated serum insulin levels (insulin resistance syndrome) are risk factors for gallstones. A low-carbohydrate diet and physical activity may help prevent gallstones. The incidence of gallstones is high in individuals with Crohn's disease; approximately one-third of individuals with inflammatory involvement of the terminal ileum have gallstones due to disruption of bile salt resorption that results in decreased solubility of the bile. The incidence of cholelithiasis is also increased in patients with diabetes mellitus and in those with cirrhosis. Drugs such as clofibrate, octreotide, and ceftriaxone can cause gallstones. In contrast, aspirin and other nonsteroidal anti-inflammatory drugs may protect against gallstones. Prolonged fasting (over 5–10 days) can lead to formation of biliary "sludge" (microlithiasis), which usually resolves with refeeding but can lead to gallstones or biliary symptoms. Pregnancy is associated with an increased risk of gallstones and of symptomatic gallbladder disease.

Pathogenesis of Gallstones

Gallstones are classified according to chemical composition: stones containing predominantly cholesterol and those containing predominantly calcium bilirubinate. The latter comprise less than 20% of the stones found in Europe or the USA but 30–40% of stones found in Japan.

Three compounds comprise 80–95% of the total solids dissolved in bile: conjugated bile salts, lecithin, and cholesterol. Cholesterol is a neutral sterol, and lecithin is a phospholipid; both are almost completely insoluble in water. However, bile salts in combination with lecithin are able to form multimolecular aggregates (and micelles) or vesicles that solubilize cholesterol in an aqueous solution. Precipitation of cholesterol microcrystals may come about because of increased biliary secretion of cholesterol, defective formation of vesicles, an excess of factors promoting the nucleation of cholesterol crystals (or deficiency of antinucleating factors), or delayed emptying of the gallbladder.

Presentation (Table 15–6)

Cholelithiasis is frequently asymptomatic and is discovered fortuitously in the course of routine radiographic study, operation, or autopsy. There is generally no need for prophylactic cholecystectomy in an asymptomatic person unless the gallbladder is calcified or gallstones are over 3 cm in diameter. Ultimately, symptoms (biliary colic) develop in 10–25% of patients by 10 years. "Symptomatic" cholelithiasis usually means characteristic right upper quadrant discomfort or pain (biliary colic). Occasional patients present with small intestinal obstruction due to "gallstone ileus" as the initial manifestation of cholelithiasis.

Treatment

Laparoscopic cholecystectomy is the treatment of choice for symptomatic gallbladder disease. The minimal trauma to the abdominal wall makes it possible for patients to go home within 2 days after the procedure and to return to work within 7 days (instead of weeks for those undergoing standard open cholecystectomy). In selected cases, the procedure may even be performed on an outpatient basis. This procedure is suitable in most patients, including those with

Table 15–6. Diseases of the biliary tract.

	Clinical Features	Laboratory Features	Diagnosis	Treatment
Gallstones	Asymptomatic	Normal	Ultrasound	None
Gallstones	Biliary colic	Normal	Ultrasound	Laparoscopic cholecystectomy
Cholesterolosis of gallbladder	Usually asymptomatic	Normal	Oral cholecystography	None
Adenomyomatosis	May cause biliary colic	Normal	Oral cholecystography	Laparoscopic cholecystectomy if symptomatic
Porcelain gallbladder	Usually asymptomatic, high risk of gallbladder cancer	Normal	X-ray or CT	Laparoscopic cholecystectomy
Acute cholecystitis	Epigastric or right upper quadrant pain, nausea, vomiting, fever, Murphy's sign	Leukocytosis	Ultrasound, HIDA scan	Antibiotics, laparoscopic cholecystectomy
Chronic cholecystitis	Biliary colic, constant epigastric or right upper quadrant pain, nausea	Normal	Ultrasound (stones), oral cholecystography (nonfunctioning gallbladder)	Laparoscopic cholecystectomy
Choledocholithiasis	Asymptomatic or biliary colic, jaundice, fever; gallstone pancreatitis	Cholestatic liver function tests; leukocytosis and positive blood cultures in cholangitis; elevated amylase and lipase in pancreatitis	Ultrasound (dilated ducts), ERCP	Endoscopic sphincterotomy and stone extraction; antibiotics for cholangitis

ERCP = endoscopic retrograde cholangiopancreatography; HIDA = hepato-iminodiacetic acid

acute cholecystitis. If problems are encountered, the surgery can be converted to a conventional open cholecystectomy. Bile duct injuries occur in 0.1% of cases done by experienced surgeons. A conservative approach to biliary colic is advised in pregnant patients, but for patients with repeated attacks of biliary colic or acute cholecystitis, cholecystectomy can be performed—even by the laparoscopic route—preferably in the second trimester. Enterolithotomy alone is considered adequate treatment in most patients with gallstone ileus.

Persistence of symptoms after removal of the gallbladder (postcholecystectomy syndrome) implies either mistaken diagnosis, functional bowel disorder, technical error, retained or recurrent common bile duct stone, or spasm of the sphincter of Oddi (see below).

Cheno- and ursodeoxycholic acids are bile salts that when given orally for up to 2 years dissolve some cholesterol stones and may be considered in selected patients who refuse laparoscopic cholecystectomy. The dose is 7 mg/kg/d of each or 8–13 mg/kg of ursodeoxycholic acid in divided doses daily. They are most effective in patients with a functioning gallbladder, as determined by gallbladder visualization on oral cholecystography (representing not more than 15% of patients with gallstones), and multiple small "floating" gallstones. In half of patients, gallstones recur within 5 years after treatment is stopped.

Lithotripsy in combination with bile salt therapy for single radiolucent stones less than 20 mm in diameter was an option in the past but is no longer generally employed in the USA.

Bateson MC: Gallbladder disease. BMJ 1999;318:1745. [NLM Cit ID: 99310734] (Pathogenesis, epidemiology, diagnosis, and treatment.)

Everhart JE et al: Prevalence and ethnic differences in gallbladder disease in the United States. Gastroenterology 1999;117:632. [NLM Cit ID: 99394998] (More than 20 million persons have gallbladder disease in the USA, with estimated prevalence rates as follows: Mexican-American women 26.7%, non-Hispanic white women 16.6%, non-Hispanic black women 13.9%, Mexican-American men 8.9%, non-Hispanic white men 8.6%, and non-Hispanic black men 5.3%.)

Festi D et al: Clinical manifestations of gallstone disease: Evidence from the multicenter Italian study on cholelithiasis (MICOL). Hepatology 1999;30:839. [NLM Cit ID: 99428425] (Symptoms associated with cholelithiasis included pain in the right upper quadrant or epigastrium, often radiating to the right shoulder, and, to a lesser extent, intolerance to fried or fatty foods in the absence of heartburn.)

Leitzmann MF et al: Recreational physical activity and the risk of cholecystectomy in women. N Engl J Med 1999;341:777. [NLM Cit ID: 99393042] (Among 60, 290 asymptomatic women aged 40–65 followed for 10 years, increased recreational activity was associated with a significant reduction in the risk of cholecystectomy.)

ACUTE CHOLECYSTITIS

Essentials of Diagnosis

- Steady, severe pain and tenderness in the right hypochondrium or epigastrium.
- Nausea and vomiting.
- Fever and leukocytosis.

General Considerations

Cholecystitis is associated with gallstones in over 90% of cases. It occurs when a stone becomes impacted in the cystic duct and inflammation develops behind the obstruction. Acalculous cholecystitis should be considered when unexplained fever or right upper quadrant pain occurs within 2–4 weeks of major surgery or in a critically ill patient who has had no oral intake for a prolonged period. Primarily as a result of ischemic changes secondary to distention, gangrene may develop, resulting in perforation. Although generalized peritonitis is possible, the leak usually remains localized and forms a chronic, well-circumscribed abscess cavity. Acute cholecystitis caused by infectious agents (eg, cytomegalovirus, cryptosporidiosis, or microsporidiosis) may occur in patients with AIDS.

Clinical Findings

A. Symptoms and Signs: The acute attack is often precipitated by a large or fatty meal and is characterized by the relatively sudden appearance of severe, steady pain which is localized to the epigastrium or right hypochondrium and which in the uncomplicated case may gradually subside over a period of 12–18 hours. Vomiting occurs in about 75% of patients and in half of instances affords variable relief. Right upper quadrant abdominal tenderness is almost always present and is usually associated with muscle guarding and rebound pain. A palpable gallbladder is present in about 15% of cases. Jaundice is present in about 25% of cases and, when persistent or severe, suggests the possibility of choledocholithiasis. Fever is usually present.

B. Laboratory Findings: The white blood cell count is usually high (12,000–15,000/μL). Total serum bilirubin values of 1–4 mg/dL may be seen even in the absence of common duct obstruction. Serum aminotransferase and alkaline phosphatase are often elevated—the former as high as 300 units/mL, or even higher when associated with ascending cholangitis. Serum amylase may also be moderately elevated.

C. Imaging: Plain films of the abdomen may show radiopaque gallstones in 15% of cases. ^{99m}Tc hepatobiliary imaging (using iminodiacetic acid compounds), also known as the HIDA scan, is useful in demonstrating an obstructed cystic duct, which is the cause of acute cholecystitis in most patients. This test is reliable if the bilirubin is under 5 mg/dL (98% sensitivity and 81% specificity for acute cholecystitis).

Right upper quadrant abdominal ultrasound may show the presence of gallstones but is not specific for acute cholecystitis (67% sensitivity, 82% specificity).

Differential Diagnosis

The disorders most likely to be confused with acute cholecystitis are perforated peptic ulcer, acute pancreatitis, appendicitis in a high-lying appendix, perforated colonic carcinoma or diverticulum of the hepatic flexure, liver abscess, hepatitis, and pneumonia with pleurisy on the right side. Definite localization of pain and tenderness in the right hypochondrium, with radiation around to the infrascapular area, strongly favors the diagnosis of acute cholecystitis. True cholecystitis without stones raises the question of polyarteritis nodosa affecting the cystic artery (rarely).

Complications

A. Gangrene of the Gallbladder: Continuation or progression of right upper quadrant abdominal pain, tenderness, muscle guarding, fever, and leukocytosis after 24–48 hours suggests severe inflammation and possible gangrene of the gallbladder. Necrosis may occasionally develop without definite signs in the obese, diabetic, elderly, or immunosuppressed patient.

B. Cholangitis: Cholangitis classically presents with Charcot's triad, namely, fever and chills, right upper quadrant pain, and jaundice. Although 95% of patients who present with this picture will have common duct stones, only a minority of patients with acute cholecystitis have common duct stones that will present in this manner.

C. Chronic Cholecystitis and Other Complications: Chronic cholecystitis results from repeated episodes of acute cholecystitis or chronic irritation of the gallbladder wall by stones and is characterized pathologically by varying degrees of chronic inflammation of the gallbladder. Calculi are usually present. In about 4–5% of cases, the villi of the gallbladder undergo polypoid enlargement due to deposition of cholesterol that may be visible to the naked eye ("strawberry gallbladder," cholesterolosis). In other instances, adenomatous hyperplasia of all or part of the gallbladder wall may be so marked as to give the appearance of a myoma (pseudotumor). Hydrops of the gallbladder results when acute cholecystitis subsides but cystic duct obstruction persists, producing distention of the gallbladder with a clear mucoid fluid. Occasionally, a stone in the neck of the gallbladder may compress the bile duct and cause jaundice (Mirizzi's syndrome).

Cholelithiasis with chronic cholecystitis may be associated with acute exacerbations of gallbladder inflammation, common duct stone, fistulization to the bowel, pancreatitis, and, rarely, carcinoma of the gallbladder. Calcified (porcelain) gallbladder has a high association with gallbladder carcinoma and is an indication for cholecystectomy.

Treatment

Acute cholecystitis will usually subside on a conservative regimen (withholding of oral feedings, intravenous alimentation, analgesics, and antibiotics). Meperidine may be preferable to morphine for pain because of less spasm of the sphincter of Oddi. Because of the high risk of recurrent attacks (up to 10% by 1 month and over 30% by 1 year), cholecystectomy—generally laparoscopically—should generally be performed within 2–3 days after hospitalization. If nonsurgical treatment has been elected, the patient (especially if diabetic or elderly) should be watched carefully for recurrent symptoms, evidence of gangrene of the gallbladder, or cholangitis. In high-risk patients, ultrasound-guided aspiration of the gallbladder (percutaneous cholecystostomy) may postpone or even avoid the need for surgery. Cholecystectomy is mandatory when there is evidence of gangrene or perforation.

Surgical treatment of chronic cholecystitis is the same as for acute cholecystitis. If indicated, cholangiography can be performed during laparoscopic cholecystectomy. Choledocholithiasis can also be excluded by either pre- or postoperative ERCP or MRCP.

Prognosis

The overall mortality rate of cholecystectomy is less than 1%, but hepatobiliary tract surgery is a more formidable procedure in the elderly, in whom the mortality rate is 5–10%. A technically successful surgical procedure in an appropriately selected patient is generally followed by complete resolution of symptoms.

Borzellino G et al: Emergency cholecystostomy and subsequent cholecystectomy for acute gallstone cholecystitis in the elderly. Br J Surg 1999;86:1521. [NLM Cit ID: 20062421] (Among 84 patients over age 70 with ultrasonographically severe cholecystitis, cholecystostomy was successful in 83 and was followed by elective cholecystectomy in 70, with no mortality.)

Lai PB et al: Randomized trial of early versus delayed laparoscopic cholecystectomy for acute cholecystitis. Br J Surg 1998;85:764. [NLM Cit ID: 98330276] (Except for a shorter operating time, there was no difference in rates of conversion to open cholecystectomy or complications between patients randomized to laparoscopic cholecystectomy within 24 hours and those randomized to surgery 6–8 weeks later.)

PRE- & POSTCHOLECYSTECTOMY SYNDROMES

Precholecystectomy

In a small group of patients (mostly women) with biliary colic, conventional radiographic studies of the upper gastrointestinal tract and gallbladder—including cholangiography—are unremarkable. However, contraction and evacuation of the gallbladder does not take place on gallbladder scintigraphy following injection of cholecystokinin. Cholecystectomy is curative. Anatomic and histologic examination of the operative specimen may reveal obstruction of the cystic duct because of fibrotic stenosis or adhesions and kinking. Additional diagnostic considerations are ampullary spasm and biliary dyskinesia (see below).

Postcholecystectomy

Following cholecystectomy, some patients complain of continuing symptoms, ie, right upper quadrant pain, flatulence, and fatty food intolerance. The persistence of symptoms in this group of patients suggests the possibility of an incorrect diagnosis prior to cholecystectomy, eg, esophagitis, pancreatitis, radiculopathy, or functional bowel disease. It is important to rule out the possibility of choledocholithiasis or common duct stricture as a cause of persistent symptoms in the postoperative period.

Pain has been associated with dilation of the cystic duct remnant, neuroma formation in the ductal wall, foreign body granuloma, or traction on the common duct by a long cystic duct. The clinical presentation of colicky pain, chills, fever, or jaundice should suggest biliary tract disease. Biliary colic associated with elevated liver tests or amylase suggests the possibility of spasm or stenosis of the sphincter of Oddi. Abdominal or endoscopic ultrasonography or retrograde cholangiography may be necessary to demonstrate or exclude biliary tract disease. Biliary manometry may be useful in documenting elevated baseline sphincter of Oddi pressures typical of sphincter dysfunction. In some such cases, treatment with calcium channel blockers, long-acting nitrates, or possibly injection of the sphincter with botulinum toxin may be beneficial. Endoscopic sphincterotomy is most likely to relieve symptoms when they are associated with elevated liver chemistry tests, a dilated common duct, or an elevated sphincter of Oddi pressure. In some cases, surgical sphincteroplasty or removal of the cystic duct remnant may be necessary.

Corazziari E et al: Functional disorders of the biliary tract and pancreas. Gut 1999;45(Suppl 2):II48. [NLM Cit ID: 99388025] (Review of motor disorders of the gallbladder and sphincter of Oddi.)

Desautels SG et al: Postcholecystectomy pain syndrome: Pathophysiology of abdominal pain in sphincter of Oddi type III. Gastroenterology 1999;116:900. [NLM Cit ID: 99192559] (Postcholecystectomy biliary-like pain in the absence of liver enzyme or amylase elevations or biliary dilation may often be caused by increased sensitivity to duodenal distention [hyperalgesia] rather than sphincter of Oddi dysfunction.)

Tzovaras G et al: Diagnosis and treatment of sphincter of Oddi dysfunction. Br J Surg 1998;85:588. [NLM Cit ID: 98297724] (Definition, diagnostic studies including biliary manometry, and treatment options.)

CHOLEDOCHOLITHIASIS & CHOLANGITIS

Essentials of Diagnosis

- Often a history of biliary colic or jaundice.
- Sudden onset of severe right upper quadrant or epigastric pain, which may radiate to the right scapula or shoulder.
- Occasional patients present with painless jaundice.
- Nausea and vomiting.
- Fever, which may be followed by hypothermia and gram-negative shock, jaundice, and leukocytosis.
- Abdominal films may reveal gallstones.

General Considerations

About 15% of patients with gallstones have choledocholithiasis (common bile duct stones). The percentage rises with age, and the frequency in elderly people with gallstones may be as high as 50%. Common duct stones usually originate in the gallbladder but may also form spontaneously in the common duct postcholecystectomy. The stones are frequently "silent" as no symptoms result unless there is obstruction.

Clinical Findings

A. Symptoms and Signs: A history suggestive of biliary colic or prior jaundice may be obtained. Biliary colic results from rapid increases in common bile duct pressure due to obstructed bile flow. The additional features that suggest the presence of a common duct stone are (1) frequently recurring attacks of right upper abdominal pain that is severe and persists for hours; (2) chills and fever associated with severe colic; and (3) a history of jaundice associated with episodes of abdominal pain. The combination of pain, fever (and chills), and jaundice represents **Charcot's triad** and denotes the classic picture of cholangitis. The presence of altered sensorium, lethargy, and septic shock connotes acute suppurative cholangitis accompanied by pus in the obstructed duct and represents an endoscopic or surgical emergency.

Hepatomegaly may be present in calculous biliary obstruction, and tenderness is usually present in the right upper quadrant and epigastrium.

B. Laboratory Findings: Bilirubinuria and elevation of serum bilirubin are present if the common duct is obstructed; levels commonly fluctuate. Serum alkaline phosphatase elevation is especially suggestive of obstructive jaundice. Not uncommonly, serum amylase elevations are present because of secondary pancreatitis. On occasion, acute obstruction of the bile duct produces a transient striking increase in serum aminotransferase levels (> 1000 units/L). Prolongation of the prothrombin time occurs when there is prolonged interruption of the flow of bile to the intestine. When extrahepatic obstruction persists for more than a few weeks, differentiation of obstruction from chronic cholestatic liver disease becomes progressively more difficult.

C. Imaging: Ultrasonography, CT scan, and radionuclide imaging may demonstrate dilated bile ducts and impaired bile flow. Both endoscopic ultrasonography and MR cholangiography have been found to be accurate in demonstrating common duct stones. Endoscopic retrograde cholangiopancreatography (ERCP) or percutaneous transhepatic cholangiography provides the most direct and accurate means of determining the cause, location, and extent of obstruction. If the obstruction is thought to be due to a stone, ERCP is the procedure of choice because it permits papillotomy or balloon dilation of the papilla with stone extraction or stent placement.

Differential Diagnosis

The most common cause of obstructive jaundice is common duct stone. Next in frequency is carcinoma of the pancreas, ampulla of Vater, or common duct. Extrinsic compression of the common duct may result from metastatic carcinoma (usually from the gastrointestinal tract or breast) involving porta hepatis lymph nodes or, rarely, from a large duodenal diverticulum. Gallbladder cancer extending into the common duct often presents as obstructive jaundice. Chronic cholestatic liver diseases (primarily biliary cirrhosis, sclerosing cholangitis, drug-induced) must be considered. Hepatocellular jaundice can usually be differentiated by the history, clinical findings, and liver tests, but liver biopsy is necessary on occasion.

Complications

A. Biliary Cirrhosis: Common duct obstruction lasting longer than 30 days results in liver damage leading to cirrhosis. Hepatic failure with portal hypertension occurs in untreated cases.

B. Hypoprothrombinemia: Patients with obstructive jaundice or liver disease may bleed excessively as a result of prolonged prothrombin times. In contrast to hepatocellular dysfunction, hypoprothrombinemia due to obstructive jaundice will respond to 10 mg of parenteral vitamin K or water-soluble oral vitamin K (phytonadione, 5 mg) within 24–36 hours.

Treatment

Common duct stone in a patient with cholelithiasis is usually treated by endoscopic papillotomy and stone extraction followed by laparoscopic cholecystectomy. For the poor-risk patient, however, cholecystectomy may be deferred. ERCP should be performed before cholecystectomy in patients with gallstones and jaundice (serum total bilirubin > 2 mg/dL), a dilated common bile duct (> 7 mm), or stones in the bile duct seen on ultrasound or computed tomography. Although biliary pancreatitis results from choledocholithiasis, the stone has usually passed by the time of cholecystectomy, and preoperative ERCP is optional.

Choledocholithiasis discovered at laparoscopic cholecystectomy may be managed via laparoscopic removal or, if necessary, conversion to open surgery or by postoperative endoscopic sphincterotomy. In the postcholecystectomy patient with choledocholithiasis, endoscopic papillotomy with stone extraction is preferable to transabdominal surgery. Lithotripsy (endoscopic or external) or biliary stenting may be a therapeutic consideration for large stones. For the patient with a T tube and common duct stone, the stone may be extracted via the T tube (see below).

Emergency intervention for choledocholithiasis is rarely necessary unless severe ascending cholangitis is present. Liver function should be evaluated thoroughly. Prothrombin time should be restored to normal by parenteral administration of vitamin K (see above). Nutrition should be restored by a high-carbohydrate, high-protein diet and vitamin supplementation. Ciprofloxacin, 250 mg intravenously every 12 hours, penetrates into bile well and is effective treatment for cholangitis. An alternative regimen in severely ill patients is mezlocillin, 3 g intravenously every 4 hours, plus either metronidazole, 500 mg intravenously every 6 hours (if no prior manipulation of duct), or gentamicin, 2 mg/kg intravenously as loading dose, plus 1.5 mg/kg every 8 hours adjusted for renal function (if prior manipulation of duct), or both. Urgent decompression of the bile duct, generally by ERCP, may be required for patients who are septic or fail to improve on antibiotics within 12–24 hours.

At every operation for cholelithiasis, the advisability of operative cholangiography via the cystic duct should be considered. Operative findings of choledocholithiasis are palpable stones in the common duct, dilation or thickening of the wall of the common duct, and gallbladder stones small enough to pass through the cystic duct. If stones in the common duct are found, common duct exploration can be performed or a postoperative ERCP and sphincterotomy can be planned.

Following operative choledochostomy, a simple catheter or T tube is placed in the common duct for decompression. A properly placed tube should drain bile at the operating table and continuously thereafter; otherwise, it should be considered blocked or dislocated. The volume of bile drainage varies from 100 to 1000 mL daily (average, 200–400 mL). Above-average drainage may be due to obstruction at the ampulla (usually by edema).

Postoperative antibiotics are not administered routinely after biliary tract surgery. Cultures of the bile are always taken at operation. If biliary tract infection was present preoperatively or is apparent at operation, ampicillin (500 mg every 6 hours intravenously) with gentamicin (1.5 mg/kg every 8 hours) and metronidazole (500 mg every 6 hours) or ciprofloxacin (250 mg intravenously every 12 hours) or a third-generation cephalosporin (eg, cefoperazone, 1–2 g intravenous every 12 hours) is administered postoperatively until the results of sensitivity tests on culture specimens are available.

A T-tube cholangiogram should be done before the tube is removed, usually about 3 weeks after surgery. A small amount of bile frequently leaks from the tube site for a few days.

Carpenter HA: Bacterial and parasitic cholangitis. Mayo Clin Proc 1998;73:473. [NLM Cit ID: 98240668] (Review of epidemiology, pathology, clinical features, and management.)

Rhodes M et al: Randomised trial of laparoscopic exploration of common bile duct versus postoperative endoscopic retrograde cholangiography for common bile duct stones. Lancet 1998;351:159. [NLM Cit ID: 98111522] (In this study, both approaches resulted in a high rate of clearance of the bile duct of stones identified by intraoperative cholangiography. The hospital stay was shorter in patients who underwent initial laparoscopic exploration of the common bile duct.)

Soetikno RM et al: Endoscopic management of choledocholithiasis. J Clin Gastroenterol 1998;27:296. [NLM Cit ID: 99070899] (Discusses indications, techniques, complications, and approaches to difficult bile duct stones.)

Westphal J-F et al: Biliary tract infections: A guide to drug treatment. Drugs 1999;57:81. [NLM Cit ID:99135424] (On the basis of randomized controlled trials, mezlocillin or piperacillin are recommended for the treatment of acute cholangitis or cholecystitis of moderate severity. In severely ill patients, addition of metronidazole and an aminoglycoside is warranted, but use of the latter should not exceed a few days because the risk of aminoglycoside-induced nephrotoxicity is increased in cholestasis.)

BILIARY STRICTURE

Benign biliary strictures are the result of surgical trauma in about 95% of cases. The remainder are caused by blunt external injury to the abdomen, pancreatitis, or erosion of the duct by a gallstone.

Signs of injury to the duct may or may not be recognized in the immediate postoperative period. If complete occlusion has occurred, jaundice will develop rapidly; more often, however, a tear has been accidentally made in the duct, and the earliest manifestation of injury may be excessive or prolonged loss of bile from the surgical drains. Bile leakage may predispose to localized infection, which in turn accentuates scar formation and the ultimate development of a fibrous stricture.

Cholangitis is the most common complication of stricture. Typically, the patient experiences episodes of pain, fever, chills, and jaundice within a few weeks to months after cholecystectomy. Physical findings may include jaundice during an attack of cholangitis and right upper quadrant abdominal tenderness.

Serum alkaline phosphatase is usually elevated. Hyperbilirubinemia is variable, fluctuating during exacerbations and usually remaining in the range of 5–10 mg/dL. Blood cultures may be positive during an episode of cholangitis. Endoscopic retrograde cholangiopancreatography or percutaneous transhepatic cholangiography can be valuable in demonstrating the stricture, permitting biopsy and cytologic specimens, and allowing dilation and stent placement.

Differentiation from cholangiocarcinoma may require surgical exploration. Operative treatment of a stricture frequently necessitates performance of choledochojejunostomy or hepaticojejunostomy to reestablish bile flow into the intestine.

Significant hepatocellular disease due to secondary biliary cirrhosis will inevitably occur if a biliary stricture is not treated. The death rate for untreated stricture ranges from 10% to 15%.

Dumonceau J-M et al: Plastic and metal stents for postoperative benign bile duct strictures: The best and the worst. Gastrointest Endosc 1998;47:8. [NLM Cit ID: 98127935] (Benign bile duct strictures can be treated by temporary endoscopic placement of plastic stents with results comparable to those achieved with surgery; current metal stents caused extensive fibrosis of the bile duct and are less effective than plastic stents.)

PRIMARY SCLEROSING CHOLANGITIS

Primary sclerosing cholangitis is an uncommon disease characterized by a diffuse inflammation of the biliary tract leading to fibrosis and strictures of the biliary system. The disease is most common in men aged 20–40 and is closely associated with ulcerative colitis, which is present in approximately two-thirds of patients with primary sclerosing cholangitis; however, only 1–4% of patients with ulcerative colitis develop clinically significant sclerosing cholangitis. As for ulcerative colitis, smoking is associated with a decreased risk of primary sclerosing cholangitis. Primary sclerosing cholangitis is associated with the histocompatible antigens HLA-B8 and -DR3 or -DR4, suggesting that genetic factors may play an etiologic role. Antineutrophil cytoplasmic antibodies (ANCA), with fluorescent staining characteristics and target antigens distinct from those found in patients with Wegener's granulomatosis or vasculitis, are found in 70% of patients. In patients with AIDS, sclerosing cholangitis may result from infections caused by CMV, cryptosporidium, or microsporum.

The diagnosis of primary sclerosing cholangitis is made by endoscopic retrograde cholangiography;

preliminary observations suggest that magnetic resonance cholangiography is also a useful diagnostic test. Biliary obstruction by a stone or tumor should be excluded. The disease may be confined to small intrahepatic bile ducts, in which case ERCP is normal and the diagnosis is suggested by liver biopsy. Liver biopsy is also needed for staging, which is based on the degree of inflammation and fibrosis. In general, the diagnosis of primary sclerosing cholangitis is difficult to make after biliary surgery or intrahepatic artery chemotherapy, which may result in bile duct injury. Cholangiocarcinoma may complicate the course of primary sclerosing cholangitis in at least 10% of cases and may be difficult to diagnose by cytologic examination or biopsy because of false-negative results. A serum CA 19-9 level > 100 units/mL is suggestive but not diagnostic of cholangiocarcinoma.

Treatment with corticosteroids and broad-spectrum antimicrobial agents has been employed with inconsistent and unpredictable results. Episodes of acute bacterial cholangitis may be treated with ciprofloxacin. Ursodeoxycholic acid may improve liver function test results but does not appear to alter the natural history. Careful endoscopic evaluation of the biliary tree may permit balloon dilation of localized strictures. If there is a major stricture, short-term placement of a stent may relieve symptoms and improve biochemical abnormalities with sustained improvement after the stent is removed. In patients with ulcerative colitis, primary sclerosing cholangitis is an independent risk factor for the development of colorectal dysplasia and cancer, and strict adherence to a colonoscopic surveillance program is advisable. For patients with cirrhosis and clinical decompensation, liver transplantation is the procedure of choice.

Survival of patients with primary sclerosing cholangitis averages 10 years once symptoms appear. Adverse prognostic markers are older age, higher serum bilirubin and aspartate aminotransferase levels, lower albumin levels, and a history of variceal bleeding. Actuarial survival rates with liver transplantation are as high as 85% at 3 years, but rates are much lower once cholangiocarcinoma has developed. Following transplantation, patients have an increased risk of nonanastomotic biliary strictures and—in those with ulcerative colitis—colon cancer. Those patients who are unable to undergo liver transplantation will ultimately require high-quality palliative care (see Chapter 5).

Ahrendt SA et al: Primary sclerosing cholangitis: Resect, dilate, or transplant? Ann Surg 1998;227:412. [NLM Cit ID: 98186294] (Retrospective review of 146 cases suggesting that long-term survival is best with liver transplantation in patients with cirrhosis and that in noncirrhotic patients, surgical resection of a dominant bile duct stricture may lead to longer survival than endoscopic therapy by decreasing the subsequent risk of cholangiocarcinoma.)

Angulo P et al: Primary sclerosing cholangitis. Hepatology 1999;30:325. [NLM Cit ID: 99315772] (Concise review of pathogenesis, diagnosis, and management.)

Chalasani N et al: Cholangiocarcinoma in patients with primary sclerosing cholangitis: A multicenter case-control study. Hepatology 2000;31:7. [NLM Cit ID: 20080843] (A serum CA 19-9 level > 100 units/mL had 75% sensitivity and 80% specificity in identifying cholangiocarcinoma in patients with primary sclerosing cholangitis. Alcohol consumption was a risk factor for cholangiocarcinoma.)

CARCINOMA OF THE BILIARY TRACT

Carcinoma of the gallbladder occurs in approximately 2% of all people operated on for biliary tract disease. It is notoriously insidious, and the diagnosis is often made unexpectedly at surgery. Cholelithiasis (often large, symptomatic stones) is usually present. Other risk factors are chronic infection of the gallbladder with *Salmonella typhi,* gallbladder polyps over 1 cm in diameter, calcification of the gallbladder (porcelain gallbladder), and anomalous pancreaticobiliary ductal junction. Spread of the cancer—by direct extension into the liver or to the peritoneal surface—may be the initial manifestation. The TNM classification includes the following stages: Tis, carcinoma in situ; T1, invasion of mucosa (T1a) or muscle layer (T1b); T2, invasion of perimuscular connective tissue; T3, extension into serosa or into an adjacent organ; T4, invasion > 2 cm into liver or two or more adjacent organs; N1, metastasis in cystic duct, pericholedochal, or hilar nodes; N2, metastasis in peripancreatic head, periduodenal, periportal, celiac, or superior mesenteric nodes.

Carcinoma of the bile ducts, or cholangiocarcinoma, accounts for 3% of all cancer deaths in the USA. It affects both sexes equally but is more prevalent in individuals aged 50–70. Two-thirds arise at the confluence of the hepatic ducts (Klatskin tumors), and one-fourth arise in the distal extrahepatic bile duct; the remainder are intrahepatic. Staging is similar to that for carcinoma of the gallbladder. The frequency of carcinoma in persons with choledochal cysts has been reported to be over 14% at 20 years, and surgical excision is recommended. There is an increased incidence in patients with ulcerative colitis, especially those with primary sclerosing cholangitis. In southeast Asia, infection of the bile ducts with helminths *(Clonorchis sinensis, Opisthorchis viverrini, Fasciola hepatica)* is associated with chronic cholangitis and an increased risk of cholangiocarcinoma.

Clinical Findings

Progressive jaundice is the most common and usually the first sign of obstruction of the extrahepatic biliary system. Pain in the right upper abdomen with radiation into the back is usually present early in the course of gallbladder carcinoma, but this occurs later in the course of bile duct carcinoma. Anorexia and weight loss are common and often associated with fever and chills due to cholangitis. Rarely, hematemesis or melena results from erosion of tumor into a blood vessel (hemobilia). Fistula formation between the biliary system and adjacent organs may also occur. The course is usually one of rapid deterioration, with death occurring within a few months.

Physical examination reveals profound jaundice. A palpable gallbladder with obstructive jaundice usually is said to signify malignant disease (Courvoisier's law); however, this clinical generalization has been proved to be accurate only about 50% of the time. Hepatomegaly is usually present and is associated with liver tenderness. Ascites may occur with peritoneal implants. Pruritus and skin excoriations are common.

Laboratory examination reveals predominantly conjugated hyperbilirubinemia, with total serum bilirubin values ranging from 5 to 30 mg/dL. There is usually concomitant elevation of the alkaline phosphatase and serum cholesterol. AST is normal or minimally elevated. An elevated CA 19-9 level may help distinguish cholangiocarcinoma from a benign biliary stricture (in the absence of cholangitis).

Ultrasonography and CT may show a gallbladder mass in gallbladder carcinoma and intrahepatic mass or biliary dilation in carcinoma of the bile ducts. CT may also show involved regional lymph nodes. MRI permits visualization of the biliary tree and detection of vascular invasion and obviates the need for angiography. Preliminary observations suggest that positron emission tomography (PET) can detect cholangiocarcinomas as small as 1 cm. The most helpful diagnostic studies before surgery are either percutaneous transhepatic or endoscopic retrograde cholangiography with biopsy and cytologic specimens, though false-negative biopsy and cytology results are common.

Treatment

In young and fit patients, curative surgery may be attempted if the tumor is well localized. The 5-year survival rate for localized carcinoma of the gallbladder (stage 1, T1a, N0, M0) is as high as 80% with laparoscopic cholecystectomy but drops to 15%, even with a more extended open resection, if there is muscular invasion (T1b). If the tumor is unresectable at laparotomy, cholecystoduodenostomy or T-tube drainage of the common duct can be performed. Carcinoma of the bile ducts is curable by surgery in less than 10% of cases. Palliation can be achieved by placement of a self-expandable metal stent via the endoscopic or percutaneous transhepatic route. Preliminary experience supports a palliative role for photodynamic therapy. Radiotherapy may relieve pain and contribute to biliary decompression. In general, the prognosis is poor, with few patients surviving for more than 12 months after surgery. Although cholangiocarcinoma is generally considered to be a contraindication to liver transplantation because of rapid tumor recurrence, a 62% 5-year survival rate has been reported in patients with a single peripheral cholangiocarcinoma undergoing either transplantation or resection, with clear resection margins and no lymph node involvement.

For those patients whose disease progresses despite treatment, meticulous efforts at palliative care are essential (see Chapter 5).

de Groen PC et al: Biliary tract cancers. N Engl J Med 1999;341:1368. [NLM Cit ID: 99450917] (Reviews pathology, risk factors, molecular aspects, diagnosis, treatment, and prognosis.)

Ortner MA et al: Photodynamic therapy of nonresectable cholangiocarcinoma. Gastroenterology 1998;114:536. [NLM Cit ID: 98156658] (Photodynamic therapy using intraductal laser photoactivation of an intravenously administered hematoporphyrin derivative led to improved biliary drainage and in some cases resolution of jaundice in nine patients who had not improved after endoscopic insertion of a biliary stent.)

Prat F et al: Predictive factors for survival of patients with inoperable malignant distal biliary strictures: A practical management guideline. Gut 1998;42:76. [NLM Cit ID: 98166788] (The authors recommend endoscopic placement of a plastic stent for inoperable malignant bile duct strictures over 3 cm in diameter [median survival 3.2 months] but placement of a metal stent in those with a smaller tumor [median survival over 6 months].)

DISEASES OF THE PANCREAS

ACUTE PANCREATITIS

Essentials of Diagnosis

- Abrupt onset of deep epigastric pain, often with radiation to the back.
- Nausea, vomiting, sweating, weakness.
- Abdominal tenderness and distention, fever.
- Leukocytosis, elevated serum amylase, elevated serum lipase.
- History of previous episodes, often related to alcohol intake.

General Considerations

Acute pancreatitis is thought to result from "escape" of activated pancreatic enzymes from acinar cells into surrounding tissues. Most cases are related to biliary tract disease (a passed gallstone, usually < 5 mm in diameter) or heavy alcohol intake. The exact pathogenesis is not known but may include edema or obstruction of the ampulla of Vater, resulting in reflux of bile into pancreatic ducts, or direct injury to the acinar cells. Among the numerous other causes or associations are hypercalcemia, hyperlipidemias (chylomicronemia, hypertriglyceridemia, or both), abdominal trauma (including surgery), drugs (including azathioprine, mercaptopurine, asparaginase, pentamidine, didanosine, valproic acid, tetracyclines, estrogen, sulfonamides, and thiazides), vasculitis, viral infections (eg, mumps), peritoneal dialysis, and ERCP. In patients with pancreas divisum, a congenital anomaly in which the dorsal and ventral pancreatic ducts fail to fuse, acute pancreatitis may result from stenosis of the minor papilla with obstruction to flow from the accessory pancreatic duct. Apparently "idiopathic" acute pancreatitis is often caused by occult biliary microlithiasis.

Pathologic changes vary from acute edema and cellular infiltration to necrosis of the acinar cells, hemorrhage from necrotic blood vessels, and intra- and extrapancreatic fat necrosis. All or part of the pancreas may be involved.

Clinical Findings

A. Symptoms and Signs: Epigastric abdominal pain, generally abrupt in onset, is steady, boring, and severe and often made worse by walking and lying supine and better by sitting and leaning forward. The pain usually radiates into the back but may radiate to the right or left. Nausea and vomiting are usually present. Weakness, sweating, and anxiety are noted in severe attacks. There may be a history of alcohol intake or a heavy meal immediately preceding the attack, or a history of milder similar episodes or biliary colic in the past.

The abdomen is tender mainly in the upper abdomen, most often without guarding, rigidity, or rebound. The abdomen may be distended, and bowel sounds may be absent with associated paralytic ileus. Fever of 38.4–39 °C, tachycardia, hypotension (even true shock), pallor, and cool clammy skin are often present. Mild jaundice is common. Occasionally, an upper abdominal mass due to the inflamed pancreas or a pseudocyst may be palpated. Acute renal failure (usually prerenal) may occur early in the course of acute pancreatitis.

B. Assessment of Severity: Ranson's criteria are generally used in assessing the severity of acute alcoholic pancreatitis on presentation (pancreatitis due to other causes is assessed by similar criteria). When three or more of the following are present on admission, a severe course complicated by pancreatic necrosis can be predicted with a sensitivity of 60–80%.

1. Age over 55 years.
2. White blood cell count over 16,000/μL.
3. Blood glucose over 200 mg/dL.
4. Serum LDH over 350 units/L.
5. AST over 250 units/L.

Development of the following in the first 48 hours indicates a worsening prognosis:

1. Hematocrit drop of more than ten percentage points.
2. BUN rise greater than 5 mg/dL.
3. Arterial P_{O_2} of less than 60 mm Hg.
4. Serum calcium of less than 8 mg/dL.
5. Base deficit over 4 meq/L.
6. Estimated fluid sequestration of more than 6 L.

Mortality rates correlate with the number of criteria present:

Number of Criteria	Mortality Rate
0–2	1%
3–4	16%
5–6	40%
7–8	100%

The Acute Physiology and Chronic Health (APACHE) II scoring system may also be used to assess severity.

C. Laboratory Findings: Leukocytosis (10,000–30,000/μL), proteinuria, granular casts, glycosuria (10–20% of cases), hyperglycemia, and elevated serum bilirubin may be present. Blood urea nitrogen and serum alkaline phosphatase may be elevated and coagulation tests abnormal. Decrease in serum calcium may reflect saponification and correlates well with severity of disease. Levels lower than 7 mg/dL (when serum albumin is normal) are associated with tetany and an unfavorable prognosis. In patients with clear evidence of acute pancreatitis, a serum ALT level of more than 80 units/L suggests biliary pancreatitis.

Serum amylase and lipase are elevated, usually in excess of three times the upper limit of normal, within 24 hours in 90% of cases; their return to normal is variable depending on the severity of disease. Other tests that offer the possibility of simplicity, rapidity, ease of use, and low cost, including urinary trypsinogen-2 and carboxypeptidase B, are under study. In patients who develop ascites or left pleural effusions, fluid amylase content is high. An elevated C-reactive protein concentration after 48 hours suggests the development of pancreatic necrosis. Electrocardiography may show ST-T wave changes.

D. Imaging: Plain radiographs of the abdomen may show gallstones, a "sentinel loop" (a segment of air-filled small intestine most commonly in the left upper quadrant), the "colon cutoff sign"—a gas-filled segment of transverse colon abruptly ending at the area of pancreatic inflammation—or linear focal atelectasis of the lower lobe of the lungs with or without pleural effusion. CT scan is useful in demonstrating an enlarged pancreas when the diagnosis of pancreatitis is uncertain, in detecting pseudocysts, and in differentiating pancreatitis from other possible intra-abdominal catastrophes. Dynamic intravenous contrast-enhanced CT is of particular value after the first 3 days of severe acute pancreatitis to identify areas of necrotizing pancreatitis, though the use of intravenous contrast may increase the risk of renal failure and should be avoided when the serum creatinine level is greater than 1.5 mg/dL. The presence of a fluid collection in the pancreas correlates with an increased mortality rate. CT-guided needle aspiration of areas of necrotizing pancreatitis may disclose infection, usually by enteric organisms, which invariably leads to death unless surgical debridement is performed. The presence of gas bubbles on CT scan implies that infection by gas-forming organisms is present. Ultrasonography is less reliable, because the echoes are deflected by the gas-distended small intestine frequently associated with pancreatitis but is the initial imaging study required when pancreatitis is thought to be caused by gallstones.

Differential Diagnosis

Acute pancreatitis must be differentiated from an acutely perforated duodenal ulcer, acute cholecystitis, acute intestinal obstruction, leaking aortic aneurysm, renal colic, and acute mesenteric vascular insufficiency or thrombosis. Serum amylase may also be elevated in high intestinal obstruction, in mumps not involving the pancreas (salivary amylase), in ectopic pregnancy, after administration of narcotics, and after abdominal surgery.

Complications

Intravascular volume depletion secondary to leakage of fluids in the pancreatic bed and ileus with fluid-filled loops of bowel may result in prerenal azotemia and even acute tubular necrosis without overt shock. This usually occurs within 24 hours of the onset of acute pancreatitis and lasts 8–9 days. Some patients require peritoneal dialysis or hemodialysis.

As mentioned above, sterile or infected necrotizing pancreatitis may complicate the course of 5–10% of cases and accounts for most of the deaths. The risk of infection does not correlate with the extent of necrosis. Pancreatic necrosis is often associated with fever, leukocytosis, and, in some cases, shock and is associated with organ failure (eg, pulmonary, renal, gastrointestinal bleeding) in 50% of cases. Because infected pancreatic necrosis is an absolute indication for operative treatment, necrotic tissue should be aspirated under CT guidance for Gram stain and culture.

A serious complication of acute pancreatitis is acute respiratory distress syndrome (ARDS); cardiac dysfunction may be superimposed. It usually occurs 3–7 days after the onset of pancreatitis in patients who have required large volumes of fluid and colloid to maintain blood pressure and urine output. Most patients with ARDS require assisted respiration with positive end-expiratory pressure.

Pancreatic abscess is a suppurative process characterized by rising fever, leukocytosis, and localized tenderness and epigastric mass usually 6 or more weeks into the course of acute pancreatitis. This may be associated with a left-sided pleural effusion or an enlarging spleen secondary to splenic vein thrombosis. In contrast to infected necrosis, the mortality rate is low following drainage.

Pseudocysts, encapsulated fluid collections with high enzyme content, commonly appear in pancreatitis when CT scans are used to monitor the evolution of an acute attack. Although the natural history of pseudocysts is still not well delineated, it appears that those less than 6 cm in diameter often resolve spontaneously. They most commonly are within or adjacent to the pancreas but can present anywhere (eg, mediastinal, retrorectal), by extension along anatomic planes. Pseudocysts are multiple in 14% of cases. Pseudocysts may become secondarily infected, necessitating drainage as for an abscess. Erosion of the inflammatory process into a blood vessel can result in a major hemorrhage into the cyst.

Pancreatic ascites may present after recovery from acute pancreatitis as a gradual increase in abdominal girth and persistent elevation of the serum amylase level in the absence of frank abdominal pain. Marked elevations in the ascitic protein (> 3 g/dL) and amylase (> 1000 units/L) concentrations are typical. The condition results from rupture of the pancreatic duct or drainage of a pseudocyst into the peritoneal cavity.

Rare complications of acute pancreatitis include hemorrhage caused by erosion of a blood vessel to form a pseudoaneurysm and colonic necrosis. Chronic pancreatitis develops in about 10% of cases. Permanent diabetes mellitus and exocrine pancreatic insufficiency occur uncommonly after a single acute episode.

Treatment

A. Management of Acute Disease: In most patients, acute pancreatitis is a mild disease that subsides spontaneously within several days. The pancreatic rest program includes withholding food and liquids by mouth, bed rest, and, in patients with moderately severe pain or ileus and abdominal distention or vomiting, nasogastric suction. Pain is controlled with meperidine, up to 100–150 mg intramuscularly every 3–4 hours as necessary. In those with severe hepatic or renal dysfunction, the dose may need to be reduced. No fluid or foods should be given orally until the patient is largely free of pain and has bowel sounds. Clear liquids are then given, and gradual advancement to a regular low-fat diet is prescribed, guided by the patient's tolerance and by the absence of pain. Following recovery from acute biliary pancreatitis, laparoscopic cholecystectomy should be performed.

In more severe pancreatitis—particularly necrotizing pancreatitis—there may be considerable leakage of fluids, necessitating large amounts of intravenous fluids to maintain intravascular volume. Calcium gluconate must be given intravenously if there is evidence of hypocalcemia with tetany. Infusions of fresh frozen plasma or serum albumin may be necessary in patients with coagulopathy or hypoalbuminemia. With colloid solutions, there may be an increased risk of developing acute respiratory distress syndrome. If shock persists after adequate volume replacement (including packed red cells), pressors may be required. For the patient requiring a large volume of parenteral fluids, central venous pressure and blood gases should be monitored at regular intervals. Total parenteral nutrition (including lipids) should be considered in patients who have severe pancreatitis and ileus and will be without oral nutrition for at least 7–10 days. Enteral nutrition via a jejunal feeding tube is preferable in the absence of ileus. The role of intravenous somatostatin in severe acute pancreatitis is uncertain, but octreotide is thought to have no benefit. In preliminary trials, lexipafant, an antagonist of platelet-activating factor, was reported to reduce rates of multiple organ failure and mortality in patients with severe acute pancreatitis, but a subsequent trial was negative.

The patient with severe pancreatitis requires attention in an intensive care unit. Close follow-up of white blood count, hematocrit, serum electrolytes, serum calcium, serum creatinine, BUN, serum AST and LDH, and arterial blood gases is mandatory. Cultures of blood, urine, sputum, and pleural effusion (if present) and needle aspirations of areas of pancreatic necrosis (with CT guidance) should be obtained.

B. Treatment of Complications and Follow-Up: A surgeon should be consulted in all cases of severe acute pancreatitis. If the diagnosis is in doubt and investigations indicate a strong possibility of a serious surgically correctable lesion (eg, perforated peptic ulcer), exploration is indicated. When acute pancreatitis is unexpectedly found on exploratory laparotomy, it is usually wise to close without intervention of any kind. If the pancreatitis appears mild and cholelithiasis is present, cholecystostomy or cholecystectomy may be justified. When severe pancreatitis results from choledocholithiasis—particularly if jaundice (serum total bilirubin > 5 mg/dL) or cholangitis is present—ERCP with endoscopic sphincterotomy and stone extraction is indicated. The role of MRCP in this setting is evolving; eventually, MRCP may be useful in selecting patients for therapeutic ERCP.

Aggressive surgery may improve survival in patients with necrotizing pancreatitis and clinical deterioration or lack of resolution by 4–6 weeks and is always indicated for infected necrosis. Initially, enterostomy tubes and drainage are established. Subsequent surgery is performed to debride necrotic pancreas and surrounding tissue. In selected cases, nonsurgical drainage of necrotizing pancreatitis under radiologic or endoscopic guidance may be feasible depending on local expertise. Peritoneal lavage has not been shown to improve survival in severe acute pancreatitis, in part because late septic complications are unaffected.

The development of a pancreatic abscess is an indication for prompt percutaneous or surgical drainage. Chronic pseudocysts require endoscopic, percutaneous catheter, or surgical drainage when infected or associated with persisting pain, pancreatitis, or common duct obstruction. For pancreatic infections, imipenem, 500 mg every 8 hours intravenously, is a good antibiotic because it achieves bactericidal levels in pancreatic tissue for most causative organisms. Imipenem or cefuroxime (1.5 g intravenously three times daily, then 250 mg orally twice daily) administered to patients with sterile pancreatic necrosis may also reduce the risk of pancreatic infection.

Prognosis

The mortality rate for severe acute pancreatitis (more than three Ranson criteria) is high, especially when hepatic, cardiovascular, or renal impairment is present in association with pancreatic necrosis. Recurrences are common in alcoholic pancreatitis.

Baron TH et al: Acute necrotizing pancreatitis. N Engl J Med 1999;340:1412. [NLM Cit ID: 99228269] (Lucid review of definitions, clinical presentation, and management.)

Chang L et al: Preoperative versus postoperative endoscopic retrograde cholangiopancreatography in mild to moderate gallstone pancreatitis: A prospective randomized trial. Ann Surg 2000;231:82. [NLM Cit ID: 20100061] (Selective postoperative ERCP and common duct stone extraction is associated with a shorter hospital stay and less cost than routine preoperative ERCP.)

Dassopoulos T et al: Acute pancreatitis in human immunodeficiency virus-infected patients: A review. Am J Med 1999;107:78. [NLM Cit ID: 99330150] (In addition to the usual causes of acute pancreatitis, HIV-infected patients are at risk of pancreatitis caused by drugs [such as didanosine and pentamidine] and infections [such as cytomegalovirus and *Mycobacterium avium* complex].)

Enns R et al: Review article: The treatment of acute biliary pancreatitis. Aliment Pharmacol Ther 1999;13:1379. [NLM Cit ID: 20039957] (ERCP and sphincterotomy may be beneficial in patients with severe biliary pancreatitis and is indicated in patients who also have ascending cholangitis.)

Mergener K et al: Acute pancreatitis. BMJ 1998;316:44. [NLM Cit ID: 98113093] (Reviews pathophysiology, clinical presentation, diagnosis, prognostic indicators, complications, and treatment.)

CHRONIC PANCREATITIS

Chronic pancreatitis occurs most often in patients with alcoholism (70–80% of all cases). The risk of chronic pancreatitis increases with the duration and amount of alcohol consumed, but only 5–10% of heavy drinkers develop pancreatitis. Ethanol is thought to cause secretion of insoluble pancreatic proteins that calcify and occlude the pancreatic duct. Progressive fibrosis and destruction of functioning glandular tissue then occur, perhaps as a result of repeated episodes of necroinflammation and activation of pancreatic stellate cells. About 10–15% of patients with hyperparathyroidism develop pancreatitis. In tropical Africa and Asia, tropical pancreatitis, related in part to malnutrition, is the most common cause of chronic pancreatitis. A stricture, stone, or tumor obstructing the pancreas can lead to obstructive chronic pancreatitis. Rare cases of autoimmune chronic pancreatitis responsive to corticosteroids have been reported. About 10–20% of cases are idiopathic. Genetic factors may predispose to chronic pancreatitis in some of these cases. For example, a mutant trypsinogen gene for hereditary pancreatitis, transmitted as an autosomal dominant trait with variable penetrance, has been identified on chromosome 7. Furthermore, mutations of the cystic fibrosis transmembrane conductance regulator *(CFTR)* gene have been identified in up to 37% of patients with idiopathic chronic pancreatitis and no other clinical features of cystic fibrosis.

In many cases, chronic pancreatitis is a self-perpetuating disease characterized by chronic pain or recurrent episodes of acute pancreatitis and ultimately by pancreatic exocrine or endocrine insufficiency. After many years, chronic pain may resolve spontaneously or as a result of surgery tailored to the cause of pain.

Clinical Findings

A. Symptoms and Signs: Persistent or recurrent episodes of epigastric and left upper quadrant pain with referral to the upper left lumbar region are typical. Anorexia, nausea, vomiting, constipation, flatulence, and weight loss are common. Abdominal signs during attacks consist chiefly of tenderness over the pancreas, mild muscle guarding, and paralytic ileus. Attacks may last only a few hours or as long as 2 weeks; pain may eventually be almost continuous. Steatorrhea (as indicated by bulky, foul, fatty stools) may occur late in the course.

B. Laboratory Findings: Serum amylase and lipase may be elevated during acute attacks; normal amylase does not exclude the diagnosis, however. Serum alkaline phosphatase and bilirubin may be elevated owing to compression of the common duct. Glycosuria may be present. Excess fecal fat may be demonstrated on chemical analysis of the stool; pancreatic insufficiency may be confirmed by response to therapy with pancreatic enzyme supplements, by a bentiromide (NBT-PABA) test or secretin stimulation test if available. Where available, detection of decreased fecal chymotrypsin or elastase levels may be used to diagnose pancreatic insufficiency, though the tests lack sensitivity and specificity. Vitamin B_{12} malabsorption is detectable in about 40% of patients, but clinical deficiency of vitamin B_{12} and fat-soluble vitamins is rare.

C. Imaging: Plain films show calcifications due to pancreaticolithiasis in 30% of affected patients. CT may show calcifications not seen on plain films as well as ductal dilation and heterogeneity or atrophy of the gland. Endoscopic ultrasonography has shown promise in detecting changes of chronic pancreatitis. Endoscopic retrograde cholangiopancreatography is the diagnostic procedure of choice and may show dilated ducts, intraductal stones, strictures, or pseudocyst, but the results may be normal in patients with so-called minimal change pancreatitis. Magnetic resonance cholangiopancreatography is a promising alternative to endoscopic retrograde cholangiopancreatography.

Complications

Narcotic addiction is common. Other frequent complications include often brittle diabetes mellitus, pancreatic pseudocyst or abscess, cholestatic liver enzymes with or without jaundice, common bile duct stricture, steatorrhea, malnutrition, and peptic ulcer. Pancreatic cancer develops in 4% of patients after 20 years; the risk may relate to tobacco and alcohol use.

Treatment

Correctable coexistent biliary tract disease should be treated surgically.

A. Medical Measures: A low-fat diet should be prescribed. Alcohol is forbidden because it frequently precipitates attacks. Narcotics should be avoided if possible. Steatorrhea is treated with pancreatic supplements that are selected on the basis of their high lipase activity. A total dose of 30,000 units of lipase in capsules is given before, during, and after meals (Table 15–7). Concurrent administration of H_2 recep-

Table 15–7. Selected pancreatic enzyme preparations.[1]

Product	Enzyme Content Per Unit Dose		
	Lipase	Amylase	Protease
Conventional preparations			
Viokase	8,000	30,000	30,000
Ilozyme	11,000	≥ 30,000	≥ 30,000
Cotazym	8,000	30,000	30,000
Enteric-coated microencapsulated preparations			
Creon	8,000	30,000	13,000
Creon 10	10,000	33,200	37,500
Creon 20	20,000	66,400	75,000
Creon 25	25,000	74,700	62,500
Pancrease	4,500	20,000	25,000
Pancrease MT10	10,000	30,000	30,000
Pancrease MT16	16,000	48,000	48,000
Pancrease MT25	25,000	75,000	75,000
Cotazym-S	5,000	20,000	20,000

[1]Modified from *Drug Facts and Comparisons,* 2000.

tor antagonists (eg, ranitidine, 150 mg twice daily), or a proton pump inhibitor (eg, omeprazole, 20–60 mg daily), or sodium bicarbonate, 650 mg before and after meals, decreases the inactivation of lipase by acid and may thereby further decrease steatorrhea. In selected cases of alcoholic pancreatitis and in cystic fibrosis, enteric-coated microencapsulated preparations may offer an advantage. However, in patients with cystic fibrosis, high-dose pancreatic enzyme therapy has been associated with strictures of the ascending colon. Pain secondary to idiopathic chronic pancreatitis may be alleviated in some cases by the use of pancreatic enzymes (not enteric-coated) or octreotide, 200 μg subcutaneously three times daily. Associated diabetes should be treated (Chapter 27).

B. Surgical and Endoscopic Treatment: Surgery may be indicated in chronic pancreatitis to drain persistent pseudocysts, treat other complications, or attempt to relieve pain. The objectives of surgical intervention are to eradicate biliary tract disease, ensure a free flow of bile into the duodenum, and eliminate obstruction of the pancreatic duct. When obstruction of the duodenal end of the duct can be demonstrated by endoscopic retrograde cholangiopancreatography, dilation of the duct or resection of the tail of the pancreas with implantation of the distal end of the duct by pancreaticojejunostomy may be successful. When the pancreatic duct is diffusely dilated, anastomosis between the duct after it is split longitudinally and a defunctionalized limb of jejunum (modified Puestow procedure), in some cases combined with local resection of the head of the pancreas, is associated with relief of pain in 80% of cases. In advanced cases, subtotal or total pancreatectomy may be considered as a last resort but is associated with variable results and a high rate of pancreatic insufficiency and diabetes. Endoscopic or surgical drainage is indicated for symptomatic pseudocysts and, in many cases, those over 6 cm in diameter. Recent experience suggests that pancreatic ascites or pancreaticopleural fistulas due to a disrupted pancreatic duct can be managed by endoscopic placement of a stent across the disrupted duct. Fragmentation of stones in the pancreatic duct by lithotripsy and endoscopic removal of stones from the duct, pancreatic sphincterotomy, or pseudocyst drainage may relieve pain in selected patients. For patients with chronic pain and nondilated ducts, a percutaneous celiac plexus nerve block may be considered, but results are often disappointing.

Prognosis

This is a serious disease and often leads to chronic disability. The prognosis is best in patients with recurrent acute pancreatitis caused by a remediable condition such as cholelithiasis, choledocholithiasis, stenosis of the sphincter of Oddi, or hyperparathyroidism. Medical management of the hyperlipidemias frequently associated with the condition may also prevent recurrent attacks of pancreatitis. In alcoholic pancreatitis, pain relief is most likely when a dilated pancreatic duct can be decompressed. In patients with disease not amenable to decompressive surgery, addiction to narcotics is a frequent outcome of treatment.

Ammann RW et al: The natural history of pain in alcoholic chronic pancreatitis. Gastroenterology 1999;116:1132. [NLM Cit ID: 99238887] (Recurrent episodes of acute pancreatitis predominate early in the course. Chronic pain was typical later in the course and was associated with a complication such as a pseudocyst that could be treated surgically in two-thirds of cases.)

Apte MV et al: Chronic pancreatitis: Complications and management. J Clin Gastroenterol 1999;29:225. [NLM Cit ID: 99437648] (Thorough review of natural history, complications, and management.)

Barkin JS et al (editors): Pancreas update. Gastroenterol Clin North Am 1999;28:525. (Includes reviews of hereditary pancreatitis, medical and endoscopic therapy of chronic pancreatitis, and nutritional supplementation in pancreatitis as well as issues related to acute pancreatitis and pancreatic cancer.)

Cohn JA et al: Relation between mutations of the cystic fibrosis gene and idiopathic pancreatitis. N Engl J Med 1998;339:653. [NLM Cit ID: 98383827] (One of two preliminary studies showing a strong association between the *CTFR* gene and chronic pancreatitis.)

Layer P et al: Pancreatic enzymes: Secretion and luminal nutrient digestion in health and disease. J Clin Gastroenterol 1999;28:3. [NLM Cit ID: 99113695] (Lucid review of the physiology of digestion, pathophysiology of maldigestion, and enzyme treatment of pancreatic insufficiency.)

Warshaw AL et al: AGA technical review: Treatment of pain in chronic pancreatitis. Gastroenterology 1998;115:765. [NLM Cit ID: 98387856] (Comprehensive and critical review of various approaches to management, including supportive measures, pancreatic enzyme therapy, celiac nerve block, endoscopic treatment, and surgery.)

Whitcomb DC: Hereditary pancreatitis: New insights into acute and chronic pancreatitis. Gut 1999;45:317. [NLM Cit ID: 99376885] (Discussion of how mutations in the cationic trypsinogen gene may cause pancreatitis.)

CARCINOMA OF THE PANCREAS & THE PERIAMPULLARY AREA

Essentials of Diagnosis

- Obstructive jaundice (may be painless).
- Enlarged gallbladder (may be painful).
- Upper abdominal pain with radiation to back, weight loss, and thrombophlebitis are usually late manifestations.

General Considerations

Carcinoma is the commonest neoplasm of the pancreas. About 75% are in the head and 25% in the body and tail of the organ. Carcinomas involving the head of the pancreas, the ampulla of Vater, the distal common bile duct, and the duodenum are considered together, because they are usually indistinguishable clinically; of these, carcinomas of the pancreas constitute over 90%. They comprise 2% of all cancers and 5% of cancer deaths. About 7–8% of patients with pancreatic cancer have a family history of pancreatic cancer in a first-degree relative, compared with 0.6% of control subjects. Neuroendocrine tumors account for 2–5% of pancreatic neoplasms. Cystic neoplasms account for only 1% of pancreatic cancers, but they are important because they are often mistaken for pseudocysts. A cystic neoplasm should be suspected when a cystic lesion in the pancreas is found in the absence of a history of pancreatitis. Whereas serous cystadenomas are benign, mucinous cystadenomas, intraductal papillary mucinous tumors, and papillary cystic neoplasms are premalignant, though their prognoses are better than the prognosis of adenocarcinoma of the pancreas.

Clinical Findings

A. Symptoms and Signs: Pain is present in over 70% of cases and is often vague, diffuse, and located in the epigastrium or left upper quadrant when the lesion is in the tail. Radiation of pain into the back is common and sometimes predominates. Sitting up and leaning forward may afford some relief, and this usually indicates that the lesion has spread beyond the pancreas and is inoperable. Diarrhea, perhaps due to maldigestion, is an occasional early symptom. Migratory thrombophlebitis is a rare sign. Weight loss is a common but late finding and may be associated with depression. Occasionally a patient presents with acute pancreatitis in the absence of an alternative cause. Jaundice is usually due to biliary obstruction by a cancer in the pancreatic head. A palpable gallbladder is also indicative of obstruction by neoplasm (Courvoisier's law), but there are frequent exceptions. A hard, fixed, occasionally tender mass may be present.

B. Laboratory Findings: There may be mild anemia. Glycosuria, hyperglycemia, and impaired glucose tolerance or true diabetes mellitus are found in 10–20% of cases. The serum amylase or lipase level is occasionally elevated. Liver function tests may suggest obstructive jaundice. Steatorrhea in the absence of jaundice is uncommon. Occult blood in the stool is suggestive of carcinoma of the ampulla of Vater. CA 19-9, with a sensitivity of 70% and a specificity of 87%, has not proved sensitive enough for early detection; increased values are also found in acute and chronic pancreatitis and cholangitis. Point mutations in codon 12 of the K-*ras* oncogene are found in 70–100%, and inactivation of the tumor suppressor genes *P16* on chromosome 9, *P53* on chromosome 17, and *DCP4* on chromosome 18 are found in 95%, 50–70%, and 50% of pancreatic cancers, respectively.

C. Imaging: With carcinoma of the head of the pancreas, the upper gastrointestinal series may show a widening of the duodenal loop, mucosal abnormalities in the duodenum ranging from edema to invasion or ulceration, or spasm or compression. Ultrasound is not reliable because of interference by intestinal gas. Dual-phase spiral CT and MRI detect a mass in over 80% of cases and are helpful in delineating the extent of the tumor and allowing for percutaneous fine-needle aspiration for cytologic studies and tumor markers. Selective celiac and superior mesenteric arteriography may demonstrate vessel invasion by tumor, a finding that would interdict attempts at surgical resection, but it is less widely used since the advent of dual-phase spiral CT and endoscopic ultrasonography, which, if available, is the most accurate imaging test for diagnosing pancreatic cancer and for demonstrating venous or gastric invasion. Endoscopic ultrasonography may also be used to obtain a tissue diagnosis via fine-needle aspiration. ERCP may clarify an ambiguous CT or MRI study by delineating the pancreatic duct system or confirming an ampullary or biliary neoplasm. With obstruction of the splenic vein, splenomegaly or gastric varices are present, the latter delineated by endoscopy, endoscopic ultrasonography, or angiography.

Staging by the TNM classification includes the following definitions: T1: tumor limited to the pancreas (T1a if < 2 cm, T1b if > 2 cm); T2: extension into duodenum, bile duct, or peripancreatic tissues; T3: extension to stomach, spleen, colon, or adjacent large vessels.

Treatment

Abdominal exploration is usually necessary when cytologic diagnosis cannot be made or if resection is to be attempted, which includes about 30% of patients. In a patient with a localized mass in the head of the pancreas and without jaundice, laparoscopy may be used to detect tiny peritoneal or liver metastases and thereby avoid resection. Radical pancreaticoduodenal (Whipple) resection is indicated for lesions strictly limited to the head of the pancreas, periampullary zone, and duodenum (T1, N0, M0). Five-year survival rates are 20–25% in this group and as high as 40% in those with negative resection margins and without lymph node involvement. Adjuvant radiation therapy and fluorouracil-based chemotherapy or gemcitabine are of potential benefit. When resection is not feasible, cholecystojejunostomy or endoscopic stenting of the bile duct is performed to relieve jaundice. A gastrojejunostomy is also done if duodenal obstruction is expected to develop later; alternatively, endoscopic placement of a self-expandable duodenal stent may be feasible. Combined irradiation and chemotherapy may be used for palliation of unresectable cancer confined to the pancreas. Chemotherapy has been disappointing in metastatic pancreatic cancer, though improved results have been reported with gemcitabine. Celiac plexus nerve block or thoracoscopic splanchnicectomy may improve pain control.

Prognosis

Carcinoma of the pancreas, especially in the body or tail, has a poor prognosis. Reported 5-year survival rates range from 2% to 5%. Lesions of the ampulla have a better prognosis, with reported 5-year survival rates of 20–40% after resection. In carefully selected patients, resection of cancer of the pancreatic head is feasible and results in reasonable survival. In persons with a family history of pancreatic cancer, screening with spiral CT and endoscopic ultrasonography should be considered beginning 10 years before the age at which pancreatic cancer was diagnosed in a family member.

For those patients whose disease progresses despite treatment, meticulous efforts at palliative care are essential (see Chapter 5).

DiMagno E et al: AGA technical review on the epidemiology, diagnosis, and treatment of pancreatic ductal adenocarcinoma. Gastroenterology 1999;117:1464. [NLM Cit ID: 20047883] (Practice guidelines.)

Gress FG et al: Role of EUS in the preoperative staging of pancreatic cancer: A large single-center experience. Gastrointest Endosc 1999;50:786. [NLM Cit ID: 20040227] (One of several recent studies suggesting that endoscopic ultrasonography is more accurate than CT for staging pancreatic cancer, detecting vascular invasion, and predicting surgical resectability.)

Hawes RH et al: A multispecialty approach to the diagnosis and management of pancreatic cancer. Am J Gastroenterol 2000;95:17. [NLM Cit ID: 20102092] (Comprehensive review of epidemiology, molecular biology, natural history, clinical presentation, diagnosis, and treatment.)

LeBorgne J et al: Cystadenomas and cystadenocarcinomas of the pancreas: A multi-institutional retrospective study of 398 cases. Ann Surg 1999;230:152. [NLM Cit ID: 99377937] (Surgical resection is indicated for all mucinous cystic neoplasms, symptomatic serous cystadenomas, and cystic tumors that remain undefined after an evaluation that may include spiral CT, endoscopic ultrasonography, and diagnostic aspiration.)

RELEVANT WORLD WIDE WEB SITES

[Acalculous Cholecystitis]
http://www.brighamrad.harvard.edu/Cases/bwh/hcache/95/full.html

[Acute Acalculous Cholecystitis Demonstration Case]
http://www.brighamrad.harvard.edu/Cases/bwh/hcache/55/full.html

[Acute Cholecystitis Demonstration Case]
http://www.brighamrad.harvard.edu/Cases/bwh/hcache/96/full.html

[Acute Pancreatitis]
http://www.brighamrad.harvard.edu/Cases/bwh/hcache/187/full.html

[Alcoholics Anonymous]
http://www.alcoholics-anonymous.org

[Carcinoma of the Ampulla of Vater]
http://www.brighamrad.harvard.edu/Cases/bwh/hcache/43/full.html

[Choledocholithiasis]
http://www.brighamrad.harvard.edu/Cases/bwh/hcache/99/full.html

[Cystic and Papillary Epithelial Neoplasm of the Pancreas]
http://www.brighamrad.harvard.edu/Cases/bwh/hcache/159/full.html

[Diseases of the Liver]
http://cpmcnet.columbia.edu/dept/gi/disliv.html

[Hemorrhagic Gangrenous Cholecystitis]
http://www.brighamrad.harvard.edu/Cases/bwh/hcache/45/full.html

[Hepatic Venoocclusive Disease]
http://www.brighamrad.harvard.edu/Cases/bwh/hcache/192/full.html

[The Hepatitis Information Network]
http://www.hepnet.com

[Islet Cell Tumor of the Pancreas]
http://www.brighamrad.harvard.edu/Cases/bwh/hcache/184/full.html

[Liver Metastatic Disease Demonstration Case]
http://www.brighamrad.harvard.edu/Cases/bwh/hcache/60/full.html

[Liver Tutorials Visualization and Volume Measurement]
http://everest.radiology.uiowa.edu/nlm/app/livertoc/livertoc.html

[Pancreatic Carcinoma]
http://www.brighamrad.harvard.edu/Cases/bwh/hcache/27/full.html

16 Breast

See http://www.current-med.com/ch16.html for updated addresses of Web sites referenced in this chapter.

Armando E. Giuliano, MD

BENIGN BREAST DISORDERS

FIBROCYSTIC DISEASE

Essentials of Diagnosis

- Painful, often multiple, usually bilateral masses in the breast.
- Rapid fluctuation in the size of the masses is common.
- Frequently, pain occurs or increases and size increases during premenstrual phase of cycle.
- Most common age is 30–50. Rare in postmenopausal women not receiving hormonal replacement.

General Considerations

This disorder is the most frequent lesion of the breast. It is common in women 30–50 years of age but rare in postmenopausal women who are not taking hormonal replacement medications. Estrogen hormone is considered a causative factor. Fibrocystic disease encompasses a wide variety of pathologic entities. These lesions are always associated with benign changes in the breast epithelium, some of which are found so commonly in normal breasts that they are probably variants of normal breast histology but have nonetheless been termed a "disease."

The microscopic findings of fibrocystic disease include cysts (gross and microscopic), papillomatosis, adenosis, fibrosis, and ductal epithelial hyperplasia. Although fibrocystic disease has generally been considered to increase the risk of subsequent breast cancer, only the variants in which proliferation (especially with atypia) of epithelial components is demonstrated represent true risk factors.

Clinical Findings

A. Symptoms and Signs: Fibrocystic disease may produce an asymptomatic lump in the breast that is discovered by accident, but pain or tenderness often calls attention to the mass. There may be discharge from the nipple. In many cases, discomfort occurs or is increased during the premenstrual phase of the cycle, at which time the cysts tend to enlarge. Fluctuation in size and rapid appearance or disappearance of a breast mass are common in cystic disease. Multiple or bilateral masses are common, and many patients will give a history of a transient lump in the breast or cyclic breast pain.

B. Diagnostic Tests: Because a mass due to fibrocystic disease is frequently indistinguishable from carcinoma on the basis of clinical findings, suspicious lesions should be biopsied. Fine-needle aspiration cytology may be used, but if a suspicious mass that is nonmalignant on cytologic examination does not resolve over several months, it must be excised. Surgery should be conservative, since the primary objective is to exclude cancer. Simple mastectomy or extensive removal of breast tissue is rarely, if ever, indicated for mammary dysplasia.

Differential Diagnosis

Pain, fluctuation in size, and multiplicity of lesions are the features most helpful in differentiation from carcinoma. If a dominant mass is present, the diagnosis of cancer should be assumed until disproved by biopsy. Final diagnosis often depends on excisional biopsy. Mammography may be helpful, but the breast tissue in these young women is usually too radiodense to permit a worthwhile study. Sonography is useful in differentiating a cystic from a solid mass.

Treatment

When the diagnosis of fibrocystic disease has been established by previous biopsy or is likely because the history is classic, aspiration of a discrete mass suggestive of a cyst is indicated in order to alleviate pain and, more importantly, to confirm the cystic nature of the mass. The patient is reexamined at intervals thereafter. If no fluid is obtained or if fluid is bloody, if a mass persists after aspiration, or if at any time during follow-up a persistent lump is noted, biopsy is performed.

Breast pain associated with generalized fibrocystic disease is best treated by avoiding trauma and by wearing (night and day) a brassiere that gives good support and protection. Hormone therapy is not advisable, because it does not cure the condition and has undesirable side effects. Danazol (100–200 mg twice daily orally), a synthetic androgen, has been used for patients with severe pain. This treatment suppresses pituitary gonadotropins, but androgenic effects (acne, edema, hirsutism) usually make this treatment intolerable; in practice, it is rarely used.

The role of caffeine consumption in the development and treatment of fibrocystic disease is controversial. Some studies suggest that eliminating caffeine from the diet is associated with improvement. Many patients are aware of these studies and report relief of symptoms after giving up coffee, tea, and chocolate. Similarly, many women find vitamin E (400 IU daily) helpful. However, these observations remain anecdotal.

Prognosis

Exacerbations of pain, tenderness, and cyst formation may occur at any time until the menopause, when symptoms usually subside, except in patients receiving hormonal replacement therapy. The patient should be advised to examine her own breasts each month just after menstruation and to inform her physician if a mass appears. The risk of breast cancer in women with fibrocystic disease showing proliferative or atypical changes in the epithelium is higher than that of women in general. These women should be followed carefully with physical examinations and mammography.

Cady B et al: Evaluation of common breast problems: Guidance for primary care providers. CA Cancer J Clin 1998;48:49. [NLM Cit ID: 98111586]

Fitzgibbons PL et al: Benign breast changes and the risk for subsequent breast cancer: an update of the 1985 consensus statement. Cancer Committee of the College of American Pathologists Arch Pathol Lab Med 1998; 122:1053. [NLM Cit ID: 99086399] (A definition of the relative breast cancer risk associated with specific histologic abnormalities; includes data from recent case-control studies.)

Marchant DJ: Controversies in benign breast disease. Surg Oncol Clin N Am 1998;7:285. [NLM Cit ID: 98205103]

FIBROADENOMA OF THE BREAST

This common benign neoplasm occurs most frequently in young women, usually within 20 years after puberty. It is somewhat more frequent and tends to occur at an earlier age in black women. Multiple tumors are found in 10–15% of patients.

The typical fibroadenoma is a round or ovoid, rubbery, discrete, relatively movable, nontender mass 1–5 cm in diameter. It is usually discovered accidentally. Clinical diagnosis in young patients is generally not difficult. In women over 30, cystic disease of the breast and carcinoma of the breast must be considered. Cysts can be identified by aspiration or ultrasonography. Fibroadenoma does not normally occur after the menopause, but may occasionally develop after administration of hormones.

No treatment is usually necessary if the diagnosis can be made by needle biopsy or cytologic examination. Excision with pathologic examination of the specimen is performed if the diagnosis is uncertain.

Phyllodes tumor is a fibroadenoma-like tumor with cellular stroma that grows rapidly. It may reach a large size and if inadequately excised will recur locally. The lesion can be benign or malignant. If benign, phyllodes tumor is treated by local excision with a margin of surrounding breast tissue. The treatment of malignant phyllodes tumor is more controversial, but complete removal of the tumor with a rim of normal tissue avoids recurrence. Since these tumors may be large, simple mastectomy is sometimes necessary. Lymph node dissection is not performed, since the sarcomatous portion of the tumor metastasizes to the lungs and not the lymph nodes.

Alle KM et al: Conservative management of fibroadenoma of the breast. Br J Surg 1996;83:1798. [NLM Cit ID: 96408812]

Chilcote WA et al: Stereotactic breast biopsy: a less-invasive option. Cleve Clin J Med 1997;64:550. [NLM Cit ID: 98046852]

Greenberg R et al: Management of breast fibroadenomas. J Gen Intern Med 1998;13:640. [NLM Cit ID: 98425492] (Transformation of fibroadenoma is rare, and excision should be limited to fibroadenomas that fail to increase in size.)

Mangi AA et al: Surgical management of phyllodes tumors. Arch Surg 1999;134:487. [NLM Cit ID: 99254999] (Phyllodes tumors mimic fibroadenomas clinically; 1-cm excision margins recommended, or mastectomy for large lesions.)

Reinfuss M et al: The treatment and prognosis of patients with phyllodes tumors of the breast: An analysis of 170 cases. Cancer 1996;77:910. [NLM Cit ID: 96185370]

NIPPLE DISCHARGE

In order of decreasing frequency, the following are the commonest causes of nipple discharge in the nonlactating breast: duct ectasia, intraductal papilloma, and carcinoma. The important characteristics of the discharge and some other factors to be evaluated by history and physical examination are as follows:

(1) Nature of discharge (serous, bloody, or other).

(2) Association with a mass.

(3) Unilateral or bilateral.

(4) Single or multiple duct discharge.

(5) Discharge is spontaneous (persistent or intermittent) or must be expressed.

(6) Discharge produced by pressure at a single site or by general pressure on the breast.

(7) Relation to menses.

(8) Premenopausal or postmenopausal.
(9) Patient taking contraceptive pills or estrogen.

Unilateral, spontaneous serous or serosanguineous discharge from a single duct is usually caused by an intraductal papilloma or, rarely, by an intraductal cancer. A mass may not be palpable. The involved duct may be identified by pressure at different sites around the nipple at the margin of the areola. Bloody discharge is suggestive of cancer but is more often caused by a benign papilloma in the duct. Cytologic examination may identify malignant cells, but negative findings do not rule out cancer, which is more likely in women over age 50. In any case, the involved duct—and a mass if present—should be excised. Ductography is of limited value since excision of the bloody duct system is indicated regardless of findings.

In premenopausal women, spontaneous multiple duct discharge, unilateral or bilateral, most marked just before menstruation, is often due to mammary dysplasia. Discharge may be green or brownish. Papillomatosis and ductal ectasia are usually seen on biopsy. If a mass is present, it should be removed.

Milky discharge from multiple ducts in the nonlactating breast occurs in certain endocrine syndromes, as a result of hyperprolactinemia. Serum prolactin levels should be obtained to search for a pituitary tumor. TSH helps exclude causative hypothyroidism. Numerous antipsychotic agents and other drugs may also cause milky discharge that ceases on discontinuance of the of the medication.

Oral contraceptive agents or estrogen replacement therapy may cause clear, serous, or milky discharge from a single duct, but multiple duct discharge is more common. The discharge is more evident just before menstruation and disappears on stopping the medication. If it does not and is from a single duct, exploration should be considered.

Purulent discharge may originate in a subareolar abscess and require removal of the abscess and related lactiferous sinus.

When localization is not possible, no mass is palpable, and the discharge is nonbloody, the patient should be reexamined every 2 or 3 months for a year, and mammography should be done. Cytologic examination of nipple discharge for exfoliated cancer cells may rarely be helpful in diagnosis.

Jardines L: Management of nipple discharge. Am Surg 1996;62:119. [NLM Cit ID: 96146563]
Taber SW: The clinical challenge of nipple discharge. J Ky Med Assoc 1996;94:387. [NLM Cit ID: 97008474]

FAT NECROSIS

Fat necrosis is a rare lesion of the breast but is of clinical importance because it produces a mass, often accompanied by skin or nipple retraction, that is indistinguishable from carcinoma. Trauma is presumed to be the cause, though only about half of patients give a history of injury. Ecchymosis is occasionally present. If untreated, the mass effect gradually disappears. The safest course is to obtain a biopsy. Needle biopsy is often adequate, but frequently the entire mass must be excised, primarily to exclude carcinoma. Fat necrosis is common after segmental resection, radiation therapy, or flap reconstruction after mastectomy.

BREAST ABSCESS

During nursing, an area of redness, tenderness, and induration may develop in the breast. The organism most commonly found in these abscesses is *Staphylococcus aureus*. In the early stages, the infection can often be treated while nursing is continued from that breast by administering an antibiotic such as dicloxacillin or oxacillin, 250 mg four times daily for 7–10 days (see Puerperal Mastitis, Chapter 18). If the lesion progresses to form a localized mass with local and systemic signs of infection. Surgical drainage is performed, and nursing is discontinued.

A subareolar abscess may develop (rarely) in young or middle-aged women who are not lactating. These infections tend to recur after incision and drainage unless the area is explored during a quiescent interval, with excision of the involved lactiferous duct or ducts at the base of the nipple. Otherwise, infection in the breast is very rare unless the patient is lactating. In the nonlactating breast, inflammatory carcinoma is always considered. Thus, findings suggestive of abscess or cellulitis in the nonlactating breast are an indication for incision and biopsy of any indurated tissue. If the abscess can be percutaneously drained and completely resolves, the patient may be followed conservatively.

Schein M: Subareolar breast abscesses. Surgery 1996; 120:902. [NLM Cit ID: 97066048] (Highly successful nonoperative ultrasound-guided aspiration and antibiotic therapy of breast abscesses. This should probably be the first choice for treatment of small lesions.)

DISORDERS OF THE AUGMENTED BREAST

At least 4 million American women have had breast implants. Breast augmentation is performed by placing implants usually under the pectoralis muscle or, less desirably, in the subcutaneous tissue of the breast. Most implants are made of an outer silicone shell filled with a silicone gel, saline, or some combination of the two. About 15–25% of the patients develop capsule contraction or scarring around the implant, leading to a firmness and distortion of the breast that can be painful. Some require removal of the implant and capsule.

Implant rupture may occur in as many as 5–10% of women, and bleeding of gel through the capsule is noted even more commonly. While silicone gel may be an immunologic stimulant, there is no increase in autoimmune disorders in patients with such implants. The FDA has advised symptomatic women with ruptured implants to discuss possible surgical removal with their physicians. However, women who are asymptomatic and have no evidence of rupture of a silicone gel prosthesis should probably not undergo removal of the implant. Women with symptoms of autoimmune illnesses should address the possibility of removal.

Studies have failed to show any association between implants and an increased incidence of breast cancer. However, breast cancer may develop in a patient with a silicone gel prosthesis, as it does in women without them. Detection in patients with implants is made more difficult since mammography is less able to detect early lesions. However, local recurrence after breast reconstruction for cancer is usually cutaneous or subcutaneous and is easily palpated. If a cancer develops, it should be treated in the same manner as in women without implants. Such women should be offered the option of mastectomy or breast-conserving therapy, which may require removal or replacement of the implant. Adjuvant treatments should be given for the same indications as for women who have no implants.

Brinton LA et al: Breast implants and cancer. J Natl Cancer Inst 1997;89:1341. [NLM Cit ID: 97452289] (No apparent biologic basis for implants increasing cancer risk or worsening prognosis.)

Gabriel SE et al: Complications leading to surgery after breast implantation. N Engl J Med 1997;336:677. [NLM Cit ID: 97177205]

Gertzten PC: A formal risk assessment of silicone breast implants. Biomaterials 1999;20:1063. [NLM Cit ID: 99305152] (Review of scientific evidence for safety of silicone breast implants.)

Nyren O et al: Risk of connective tissue disease and related disorders among women with breast implants: A nationwide retrospective cohort study in Sweden. BMJ 1998;316:417. [NLM Cit ID: 98153540]

CARCINOMA OF THE FEMALE BREAST

Essentials of Diagnosis

- Risk factors include delayed childbearing, positive family history of breast cancer, and personal history of breast cancer or some types of mammary dysplasia.
- Most women with breast cancer do not have identifiable risk factors.
- Early findings: Single, nontender, firm to hard mass with ill-defined margins; mammographic abnormalities and no palpable mass.
- Later findings: Skin or nipple retraction; axillary lymphadenopathy; breast enlargement, redness, edema, pain; fixation of mass to skin or chest wall.

General Considerations

Breast cancer is the most-feared disease among American women The diagnosis forces a collision with reality, and the emotional impact is tremendous. Unlike many illnesses, breast cancer cannot be prevented, and an element of helplessness is thus associated with the disease.

The initial fear that accompanies the diagnosis of breast cancer is twofold: death and loss of a breast. Since breast cancer in its early stages does not cause physical pain, the only symptoms most women deal with from the time they discover a lump are anxiety and emotional mayhem. Emotions are raw and close to the surface; patients experience intense love, anger, fear, sadness, loss, courage, and desperation following the diagnosis.

While many think that a woman with breast cancer is facing death or disfigurement, more are in danger of being scarred by the psychologic impact of the disease. Breast cancer is devastating because the part of the body involved is the most prominent icon of womanhood. The impact of the disease, its treatment, and the attitudes of our culture toward women's breasts are stunning. Our culture worships the woman's body, and the female breast is the most famous body part in history. That which gives women their feeling of sexuality is also that which seriously threatens their health.

Like everyone in our society, surgeons are affected by our culture's attitudes. Many worry that they are destroying their patients psychologically by the surgery they must perform to save them physically. The truth is that most women who get breast cancer deal with it and go on to live normal, healthy lives.

It is important to know what a patient is or is not willing to risk. If a woman believes the treatment she and her physician have chosen gives her the best chance for recovery, her confidence will contribute to its efficacy. Optimism does not guarantee a good result, but even for those who do not recover it makes a positive difference. The psychologic aspect of dealing with breast cancer cannot be overstated—it is the physician's duty to provide emotional support as well as appropriate physical treatment. Medical management may come from the outside, but healing comes from within.

INCIDENCE & RISK FACTORS

Aside from skin cancer, the breast is the most common site of cancer in women, and cancer of the breast is second only to lung cancer as a cause of death from cancer among women. The probability of developing breast cancer increases throughout life. The mean and the median age of women with breast cancer is between 60 and 61 years.

There will be about 182,000 new cases of breast cancer and about 42,000 deaths from this disease in women in the USA in year 2000. An additional 40,000 cases of ductal carcinoma in situ will be detected, principally by screening mammography. One out of every eight or nine American women will develop breast cancer during her lifetime. Women whose mothers or sisters had breast cancer are three to four times more likely to develop the disease. Risk is further increased in patients whose mothers' or sisters' breast cancers occurred before menopause or was bilateral and in those with a family history of breast cancer in two or more first-degree relatives. However, there is no history of breast cancer among female relatives in over 75% of patients. Nulliparous women and women whose first full-term pregnancy was after age 35 have a 1.5 times higher incidence of breast cancer than multiparous women. Late menarche and artificial menopause are associated with a lower incidence, whereas early menarche (under age 12) and late natural menopause (after age 50) are associated with a slight increase in risk. Fibrocystic disease, when accompanied by proliferative changes, papillomatosis, or atypical epithelial hyperplasia, is associated with an increased incidence. A woman who has had cancer in one breast is at increased risk of developing cancer in the other breast. Such women develop a contralateral cancer at the rate of 1% or 2% per year. Women with cancer of the uterine corpus have a breast cancer risk significantly higher than that of the general population, and women with breast cancer have a comparably increased endometrial cancer risk. In the USA, breast cancer is more common in whites. The incidence of the disease among nonwhites (mostly blacks) is increasing, especially in younger women. In general, rates reported from developing countries are low, whereas rates are high in developed countries, with the notable exception of Japan. Some of the variability may be due to underreporting in the developing countries, but a real difference probably exists. Dietary factors, particularly increased fat consumption, may account for some differences in incidence. Oral contraceptives do not appear to increase the risk of breast cancer. There is evidence that administration of estrogens to postmenopausal women may result in a slightly increased risk of breast cancer, but only with higher, long-term doses of estrogens. Concomitant administration of progesterone and estrogen may markedly increase the incidence of breast cancer compared with the use of estrogen alone. Alcohol consumption increases the risk slightly. Some inherited breast cancers have been found to be associated with a gene on chromosome 17. This gene, *BRCA1,* is mutated in families with early-onset breast cancer and ovarian cancer. As many as 85% of women with *BRCA1* gene mutations will develop breast cancer in their lifetime. Other genes are associated with increased risk of breast and other cancers, such as *BRCA2,* ataxia-telangiectasia mutation, and *TP53,* the tumor suppressor gene. *TP53* mutations have been found in approximately 1% of breast cancers in women under 40 years of age. Genetic testing is now commercially available for women at high risk of breast cancer. Problems associated with management of patients with identified mutations, their insurability, and potential social conflicts are anticipated. Some states have enacted legislation to prevent insurance companies from considering mutations as "preexisting conditions" preventing insurability.

Women at greater than normal risk of developing breast cancer (Table 16–1) should be identified by their physicians, taught the techniques of breast self-examination, and followed carefully. Those with an exceptional family history should be counseled and given the option of genetic testing. Some of these high-risk women may consider prophylactic mastectomy or tamoxifen.

The NSABP conducted the Breast Cancer Prevention Trial (BCPT), which studied the efficacy of tamoxifen as a preventive agent in women who had never had breast cancer but were at high risk for developing the disease. Women who received tamoxifen for 5 years had about a 50% reduction in noninvasive and invasive cancers compared with women taking placebo. However, women above the age of 50 who received the drug had an increased incidence of endometrial cancer and deep venous thrombosis. Unfortunately, no survival data will be produced from this trial. The estrogen replacement raloxifene, effective in preventing osteoporosis, may also prevent breast cancer. Several large studies to examine this hypothesis are under way.

Audrain J et al: Genetic counseling and testing for breast-ovarian cancer susceptibility: What do women want? J Clin Oncol 1998;16:133. [NLM Cit ID: 98101684]

Table 16–1. Factors associated with increased risk of breast cancer.[1]

Race	White
Age	Older
Family history	Breast cancer in mother, sister, or daughter (especially bilateral or premenopausal)
Genetics	*BRCA1* or *BRCA2* mutation
Previous medical history	Endometrial cancer Proliferative forms of fibrocystic disease Cancer in other breast
Menstrual history	Early menarche (under age 12) Late menopause (after age 50)
Pregnancy	Nulliparous or late first pregnancy

[1]Normal lifetime risk in white women = 1 in 8 or 9.

Beckhardt S for the American Society of Clinical Oncology. Statement of the American Society of Clinical Oncology: Genetic testing for cancer susceptibility. J Clin Oncol 1996;14:1730. [NLM Cit ID: 96208855] (Summarizes the position of the American Society of Clinical Oncology on genetic testing for cancer susceptibility.)

Collaborative Group on Hormonal Factors in Breast Cancer (Radcliffe Infirmary, Oxford, England): Breast cancer and hormonal contraceptives: Collaborative reanalysis of individual data on 53,297 women with breast cancer and 100,239 women without breast cancer from 54 epidemiological studies. Lancet 1996;347:1713. [NLM Cit ID: 96256403] (The relationship appears more complex than previously appreciated.)

Fisher B et al: Tamoxifen for prevention of breast cancer: Report of the National Surgical Adjuvant Breast and Bowel Project P-1 Study. J Natl Cancer Inst 1998; 90:1371. [NLM Cit ID: 98418640]

Greely HT: Genetic testing for cancer susceptibility for creators of practice guidelines. Oncology (Huntingt) 1997;11(11A):171. [NLM Cit ID: 98092023]

Hartmann LC et al: Efficacy of bilateral prophylactic mastectomy in women with a family history of breast cancer. N Engl J Med 1999;340:77. [NLM Cit ID: 99091091]

JAMA patient page: Breast cancer. JAMA 1999;281:772. [NLM Cit ID: 99159816]

Klijn JG et al: Should prophylactic surgery be used in women with a high risk of breast cancer? Eur J Cancer 1997;33:2149. [NLM Cit ID: 98131576]

Kodish E et al: Genetic testing for cancer risk: How to reconcile the conflicts. JAMA 1998;279:179. [NLM Cit ID: 98099559]

Schairer C et al: Menopausal estrogen and estrogen-progestin replacement therapy and breast cancer risk. JAMA 2000;283:485. [NLM Cit ID: 20123270] (Estrogen-progestin hormone regimen increases breast cancer risk more than estrogen alone.)

Vassilopoulou-Sellin R et al: Estrogen replacement therapy after localized breast cancer: clinical outcome of 319 women followed prospectively. J Clin Oncol 1999; 17:1482. [NLM Cit ID: 99265703] (ERT does not increase breast cancer events in patients previously treated for localized breast cancer; randomized trials needed prior to changing standard of care, which is to avoid ERT after breast cancer.)

EARLY DETECTION OF BREAST CANCER

Screening Programs

A number of mass screening programs consisting of physical and mammographic examination of the breasts of asymptomatic women have been conducted. Such programs frequently identify about ten cancers per 1000 women older than age 50 and about two cancers per 1000 women younger than age 50. About 80% of these women have negative axillary lymph nodes at the time of surgery, whereas only 50% of nonscreened women found in the course of usual medical practice have uninvolved axillary nodes. Detecting breast cancer before it has spread to the axillary nodes greatly increases the chance of survival, and about 85% of such women will survive at least 5 years.

Both physical examination and mammography are necessary for maximum yield in screening programs, since about 35–50% of early breast cancers can be discovered only by mammography and another 40% can be detected only by palpation. About one-third of the abnormalities detected on screening mammograms will be found to be malignant when biopsy is performed. Women 20–40 years of age should have a breast examination as part of routine medical care every 2–3 years. Women over age 40 should have yearly breast examinations. The sensitivity of mammography varies from approximately 60% to 90%. This sensitivity depends on several factors, including patient age (breast density), tumor size, location, and mammographic appearance. In young women with dense breasts, mammography is less sensitive than in older woman with fatty breasts, in whom mammography can detect at least 90% of malignancies. Smaller tumors, particularly those without calcifications, are more difficult to detect, especially in dense breasts. The lack of sensitivity and the low incidence of breast cancer in young women has led to questions concerning the value of mammography for screening in women 40–50 years of age. The specificity of mammography in women under 50 varies from about 30% to 40% for nonpalpable mammographic abnormalities to 85% to 90% for clinically evident malignancies.

Doubt exists about the beneficial effect of screening in women under age 50. Questions such as the potential harmful effects of x-rays in a large population of young women and the general value of early detection were raised and largely ignored as various groups supported screening between ages 40 and 50. While the Health Insurance Plan Project study did show a beneficial effect of screening in such women, reducing breast cancer mortality 25% between 10 and 18 years after entry into the study, a Canadian trial demonstrated an unexplained shortening of survival from time of random assignment to death in the screening group. The small number of patients in this study experienced no beneficial effect, but the 95% confidence interval included a potential lifesaving effect as well as a potential harmful effect. A very large number of patients is necessary to show a beneficial effect of screening among patients age 40–49, where the incidence of breast cancer is low. In addition, the problems of crossover of patients in the control group with women undergoing physician examination and nonscreening mammograms, problems with mammography quality, and problems in recruitment, randomization, and compliance make the interpretation of such trials difficult. The beneficial effect of screening in women aged 50–69 is undisputed and has been confirmed by all clinical trials. The efficacy of screening in older women—those older than 70—is inconclusive and is difficult to determine because of the few women screened.

More recent studies showing a beneficial effect of screening young women and the recommendation of a Swedish consensus panel led the NCI to reconsider its position on screening mammography for women in their 40s. Two Swedish trials that had shown a 13% decrease in breast cancer mortality (not statistically significant) now showed a statistical advantage for screening women in their 40s, and a meta-analysis similarly revealed a statistical survival advantage for screened women with longer follow-up. In March 1997, the National Cancer Advisory Board recommended that women with average risk factors should have screening mammography every 1–2 years in their 40s and that women at higher risk should seek medical advice on when to begin screening. The American Cancer Society then recommended screening every year for asymptomatic women starting at age 40.

Self-Examination

All women over age 20 should be advised to examine their breasts monthly. Premenopausal women should perform the examination 7–8 days after the menstrual period. The breasts should be inspected initially while standing before a mirror with the hands at the sides, overhead, and pressed firmly on the hips to contract the pectoralis muscles. Masses, asymmetry of breasts, and slight dimpling of the skin may become apparent as a result of these maneuvers. Next, in a supine position, each breast should be carefully palpated with the fingers of the opposite hand. Some women discover small breast lumps more readily when their skin is moist while bathing or showering. Physicians should instruct women in the technique of self-examination and advise them to report a mass or other abnormality.

Mammography

Mammography is the most useful technique for the detection of early breast cancer. Film screen mammography delivers less than 0.4 cGy to the mid breast per view and has largely replaced the older xeromammographic technique, which delivers more radiation.

Mammography is the only reliable means of detecting breast cancer before a mass can be palpated. Slowly growing cancers can be identified by mammography at least 2 years before reaching a size detectable by palpation.

Calcifications are the most easily recognized mammographic abnormality. The most common findings associated with carcinoma of the breast are clustered polymorphic microcalcifications. Such calcifications are usually at least five to eight in number, aggregated in one part of the breast and differing from each other in size and shape, often including branched or V- or Y-shaped configurations. There may be an associated mammographic mass density or, at times, only a mass density with no calcifications. Such a density usually has irregular or ill-defined borders and may lead to architectural distortion within the breast. A small mass or architectural distortion, particularly in a dense breast, may be subtle and difficult to detect.

Indications for mammography are as follows: (1) to screen at regular intervals women at high risk for developing breast cancer (see above); (2) to evaluate each breast when a diagnosis of potentially curable breast cancer has been made, and at yearly intervals thereafter; (3) to evaluate a questionable or ill-defined breast mass or other suspicious change in the breast; (4) to search for an occult breast cancer in a woman with metastatic disease in axillary nodes or elsewhere from an unknown primary; (5) to screen women prior to cosmetic operations or prior to biopsy of a mass, to examine for an unsuspected cancer; and (6) to follow those women with breast cancer who have been treated with breast-conserving surgery and radiation.

Patients with a dominant or suspicious mass must undergo biopsy despite mammographic findings. The mammogram should be obtained prior to biopsy so that other suspicious areas can be noted and the contralateral breast can be checked. Mammography is never a substitute for biopsy, because it may not reveal clinical cancer in a very dense breast, as may be seen in young women with mammary dysplasia, and may not reveal medullary cancers.

Communication and documentation between the patient, the referring physician, and the interpreting physician are critical for high-quality screening and diagnostic mammography. The patient should be informed about *how* she will receive timely results of her mammogram, that mammography does not "rule out" cancer, and that she should expect a correlative examination at the mammography facility if referred for a suspicious lesion. She should also be aware of the technique and need for breast compression and that this may be uncomfortable. The mammography facility should be informed *in writing* of abnormal physical examination findings. It is strongly recommended in the AHCPR Clinical Practice Guidelines that all mammography reports be communicated with the patient as well as the health care provider in writing. Additional phone communication about any abnormal findings should take place between the interpreting and referring physicians. MRI and PET may play a role in imaging atypical lesions but only after diagnostic mammography has been performed.

Alberg AJ et al: Epidemiology, prevention, and early detection of breast cancer. Curr Opin Oncol 1997;9:505. [NLM Cit ID: 98037024]

Feig SA: Doubtful results in the Canadian national breast screening study. Breast Diseases 1996;6:354.

Gail M et al: Risk-based recommendations for mammographic screening for women in their forties. J Clin Oncol 1998;16:3105. [NLM Cit ID: 98408962] (Recommendations are based on individual risk factors and empirical assumptions.)

Kopans DB: Updated results of the trials of screening mammography. Surg Oncol Clin N Am 1997;6:233. [NLM Cit ID: 97281851]

Leitch AM et al: American Cancer Society guidelines for the early detection of breast cancer: Update 1997. CA Cancer J Clin 1997;47:150. [NLM Cit ID: 97296703] (Includes the most recent recommendations of the American Cancer Society, similar to but not identical with those of the National Cancer Institute.)

Obdeijn IM et al: MR lesion detection in a breast cancer population. J Magn Reson Imaging 1996;6:849. [NLM Cit ID: 97114378]

Clinical Clues to Early Detection of Breast Cancer

A. Symptoms and Signs: The presenting complaint in about 70% of patients with breast cancer is a lump (usually painless) in the breast. About 90% of breast masses are discovered by the patient herself. Less frequent symptoms are breast pain; nipple discharge; erosion, retraction, enlargement, or itching of the nipple; and redness, generalized hardness, enlargement, or shrinking of the breast. Rarely, an axillary mass or swelling of the arm may be the first symptom. Back or bone pain, jaundice, or weight loss may be the result of systemic metastases, but these symptoms are rarely seen on initial presentation.

The relative frequency of carcinoma in various anatomic sites in the breast is shown in Figure 16–1.

Inspection of the breast is the first step in physical examination and should be carried out with the patient sitting, arms at sides and then overhead. Abnormal variations in breast size and contour, minimal nipple retraction, and slight edema, redness, or retraction of the skin can be identified. Asymmetry of the breasts and retraction or dimpling of the skin can often be accentuated by having the patient raise her arms overhead or press her hands on her hips in order to contract the pectoralis muscles. Axillary and supraclavicular areas should be thoroughly palpated for enlarged nodes with the patient sitting (Figure 16–2). Palpation of the breast for masses or other changes should be performed with the patient both seated and supine with the arm abducted (Figure 16–3). Some authorities recommend palpation with a rotary motion of the examiner's fingers as well as a horizontal stripping motion.

Breast cancer usually consists of a nontender, firm or hard mass with poorly delineated margins (caused by local infiltration). Slight skin or nipple retraction is an important sign. Minimal asymmetry of the breast may be noted. Very small (1–2 mm) erosions of the nipple epithelium may be the only manifestation of Paget's carcinoma. Watery, serous, or bloody discharge from the nipple is an occasional early sign but is more often associated with benign disease.

A lesion smaller than 1 cm in diameter may be difficult or impossible for the examiner to feel and yet may be discovered by the patient. She should always be asked to demonstrate the location of the mass; if the physician fails to confirm the patient's suspicions, the examination should be repeated in 2–3 months, preferably 1–2 weeks after the onset of menses. During the premenstrual phase of the cycle, increased innocuous nodularity may suggest neoplasm or may obscure an underlying lesion. If there is any question regarding the nature of an abnormality under these circumstances, the patient should be asked to return

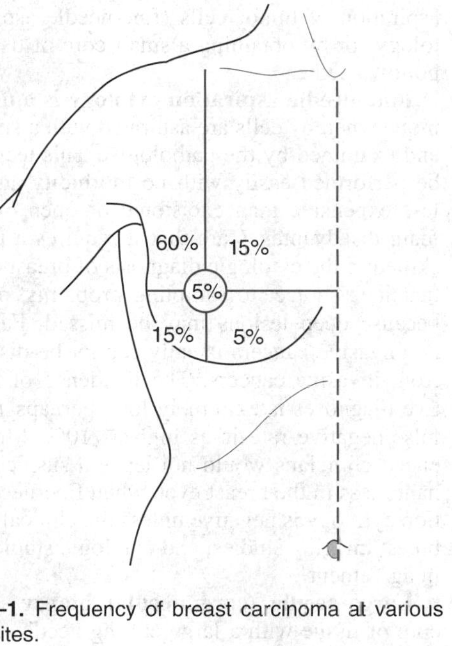

Figure 16–1. Frequency of breast carcinoma at various anatomic sites.

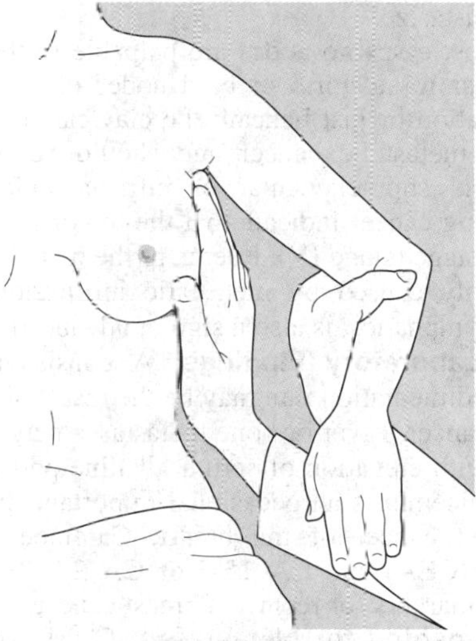

Figure 16–2. Palpation of axillary region for enlarged lymph nodes.

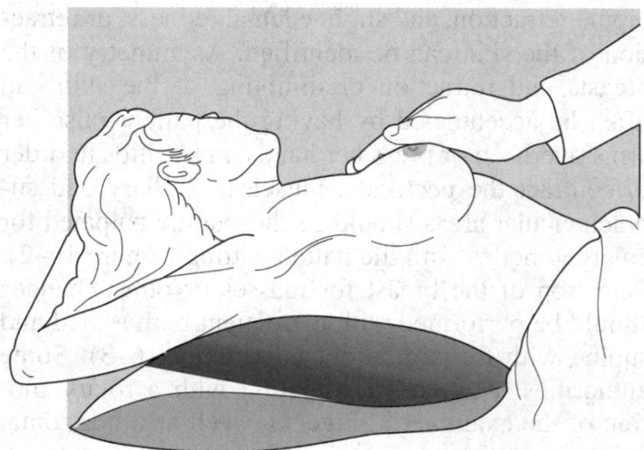

Figure 16–3. Palpation of breasts. Palpation is performed with the patient supine and arm abducted.

after her period. Ultrasound is often valuable and mammography essential when an area is felt by the patient to be abnormal but the physician feels no mass.

Metastases tend to involve regional lymph nodes, which may be palpable. One or two movable, nontender, not particularly firm axillary lymph nodes 5 mm or less in diameter are frequently present and are generally of no significance. Firm or hard nodes larger than 1 cm are typical of metastases. Axillary nodes that are matted or fixed to skin or deep structures indicate advanced disease (at least stage III). Microscopic metastases are present in about 30% of patients with clinically negative nodes. On the other hand, if the examiner thinks that the axillary nodes are involved, that impression will be borne out by histologic section in about 85% of cases. The incidence of positive axillary nodes increases with the size of the primary tumor. Noninvasive cancers do not metastasize.

In most cases no nodes are palpable in the supraclavicular fossa. Firm or hard nodes of any size in this location or just beneath the clavicle are suggestive of metastatic cancer and should be biopsied. Ipsilateral supraclavicular or infraclavicular nodes containing cancer indicate that the tumor is in an advanced stage (stage IV). Edema of the ipsilateral arm, commonly caused by metastatic infiltration of regional lymphatics, is also a sign of advanced cancer.

B. Laboratory Findings: A consistently elevated sedimentation rate may be the result of disseminated cancer. Liver or bone metastases may be associated with elevation of serum alkaline phosphatase. Hypercalcemia is an occasional important finding in advanced cancer of the breast. Carcinoembryonic antigen (CEA) and CA 15-3 or CA 27–29 may be used as markers for recurrent breast cancer.

C. Imaging for Metastases: Chest x-ray may show pulmonary metastases. CT scanning of the liver and brain is of value only when metastases are suspected in these areas. Bone scans utilizing technetium Tc 99m-labeled phosphates or phosphonates are more sensitive than skeletal x-rays in detecting metastatic breast cancer. Bone scanning has not proved to be of clinical value as a routine preoperative test in the absence of symptoms, physical findings, or abnormal alkaline phosphatase or calcium levels. The frequency of abnormal findings on bone scan parallels the status of the axillary lymph nodes on pathologic examination. Positron emission tomography (PET) may prove to be an effective single scan for bone and soft tissue or visceral metastases in patients with signs or symptoms of metastatic disease.

D. Diagnostic Tests:

1. Biopsy–The diagnosis of breast cancer depends ultimately upon examination of tissue or cells removed by biopsy. Treatment should never be undertaken without an unequivocal histologic or cytologic diagnosis of cancer. The safest course is biopsy examination of all suspicious masses found on physical examination and of suspicious lesions demonstrated by mammography. About 60% of lesions clinically thought to be cancer prove on biopsy to be benign, and about 30% of lesions believed to be benign are found to be malignant. These findings demonstrate the fallibility of clinical judgment and the necessity for biopsy. A breast mass should not be followed without histologic diagnosis, except perhaps in the premenopausal woman with a nonsuspicious mass presumed to be fibrocystic disease. A lesion such as this could be observed through one or two menstrual cycles. However, if the mass does not completely resolve during this time, it must be biopsied. Figures 16–4 and 16–5 present algorithms for management of breast masses in pre- and postmenopausal patients.

The simplest method is needle biopsy, either by aspiration of tumor cells (fine-needle aspiration cytology) or by obtaining a small core of tissue with a hollow needle.

Fine-needle aspiration cytology is a useful technique whereby cells are aspirated with a small needle and examined by the pathologist. This technique can be performed easily with no morbidity and is much less expensive than excisional or open biopsy. The main disadvantages are that it requires a pathologist skilled in the cytologic diagnosis of breast cancer and that it is subject to sampling problems, particularly because deep lesions may be missed. Furthermore, noninvasive cancers usually cannot be distinguished from invasive cancers. The incidence of false-positive diagnoses is extremely low, perhaps 1–2%. The false-negative rate is as high as 10%. Most experienced clinicians would not leave a suspicious dominant mass in the breast even when fine-needle aspiration cytology is negative unless the clinical diagnosis, breast imaging studies, and cytologic studies were all in agreement.

Large-needle (core needle) biopsy removes a core of tissue with a large cutting needle. Hand-held

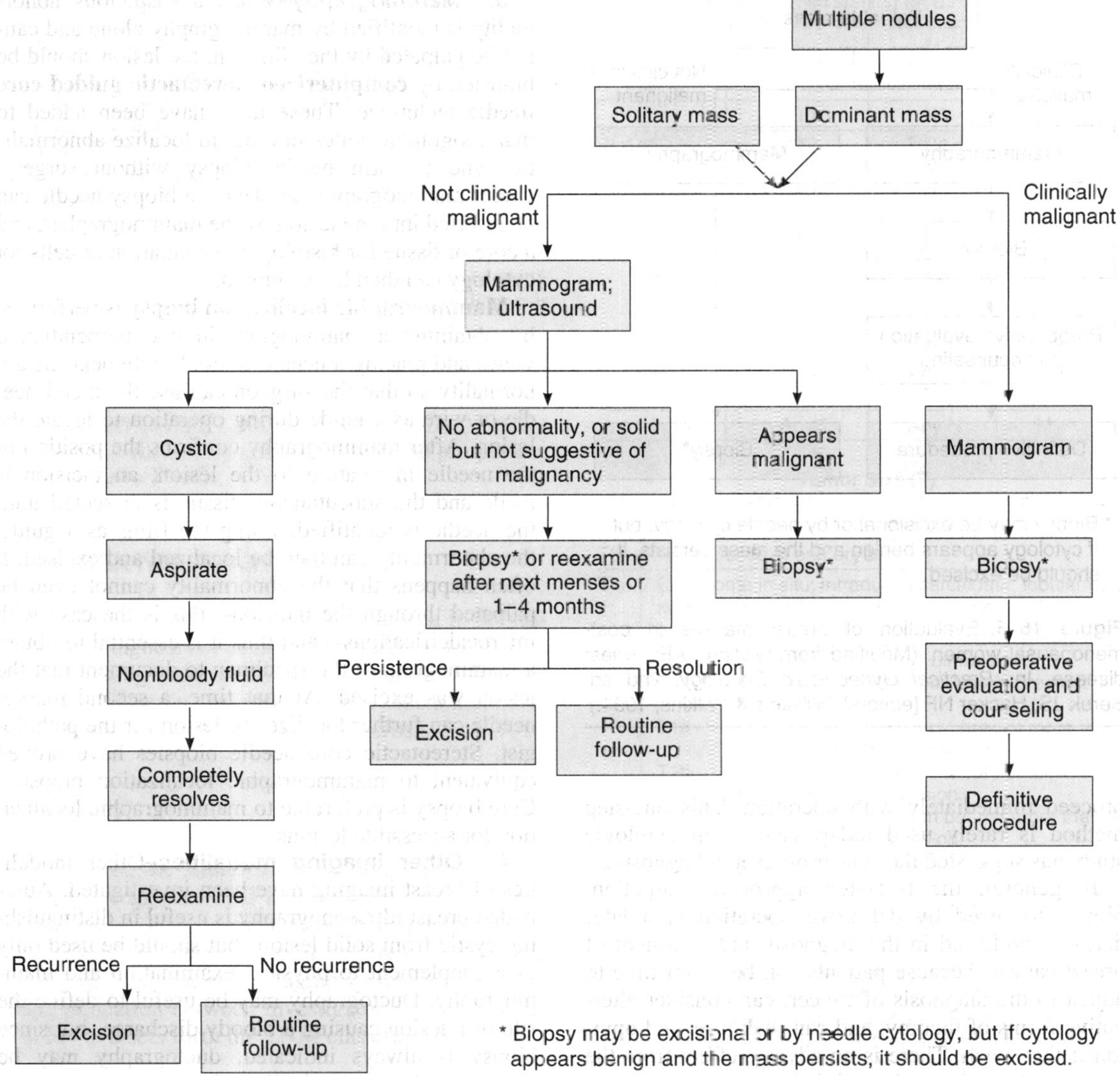

Figure 16–4. Evaluation of breast masses in premenopausal women. (Modified from Giuliano AE: Breast disease. In: *Practical Gynecologic Oncology,* 2nd ed. Berek JS, Hacker NF [editors]. Williams & Wilkins, 1994.)

biopsy devices make large-core needle biopsy of a palpable mass easy and cost-effective in the office with local anesthesia. As in the case of any needle biopsy, the main problem is sampling error due to improper positioning of the needle, giving rise to a false-negative test result.

Open biopsy under local anesthesia as a separate procedure prior to deciding upon definitive treatment is the most reliable means of diagnosis. Needle biopsy or aspiration, when positive, offers a more rapid approach with less expense and morbidity, but when nondiagnostic it must be followed by excisional biopsy.

Additional evaluation for metastatic disease and therapeutic options can be discussed with the patient after the histologic or cytologic diagnosis of cancer has been established. This approach has the advantage of avoiding unnecessary procedures, since cancer is found in the minority of patients biopsied for a breast lump. In situ cancers are not easily diagnosed cytologically and usually require excisional biopsy.

As an alternative in highly suspicious circumstances, the patient may be admitted to the hospital, where the diagnosis is made on frozen section of tissue obtained by open biopsy under general anesthesia. If the frozen section is positive, the surgeon can

Table 16–3. Histologic types of breast cancer.

Type	Frequency of Occurrence
Infiltrating ductal (not otherwise specified)	80–90%
Medullary	5–8%
Colloid (mucinous)	2–4%
Tubular	1–2%
Papillary	1–2%
Invasive lobular	6–8%
Noninvasive	4–6%
Intraductal	2–3%
Lobular in situ	2–3%
Rare cancers	< 1%
Juvenile (secretory)	
Adenoid cystic	
Epidermoid	
Sudoriferous	

lar). The cancer may be invasive or in situ. Most breast cancers arise from the intermediate ducts and are invasive (invasive ductal, infiltrating ductal), and most histologic types are merely subtypes of invasive ductal cancer with unusual growth patterns (colloid, medullary, scirrhous, etc). Ductal carcinoma that has not invaded the extraductal tissue is intraductal or in situ ductal. Lobular carcinoma may be either invasive or in situ.

Except for the in situ cancers, the histologic subtypes have only a slight bearing on prognosis when outcomes are compared after accurate staging. Various histologic parameters, such as invasion of blood vessels, tumor differentiation, invasion of breast lymphatics, and tumor necrosis have been examined, but they too seem to have little prognostic value.

The noninvasive cancers by definition are confined by the basement membrane of the ducts and lack the ability to spread. However, in patients whose biopsies show noninvasive intraductal cancer, associated invasive ductal cancers metastasize to lymph nodes in about 1–3% of cases. Lobular carcinoma in situ (LCIS) is a premalignant lesion that is not a true cancer but is a risk factor associated with subsequent development of invasive cancer in at least 20% of cases.

SPECIAL CLINICAL FORMS OF BREAST CANCER

Paget's Carcinoma

The basic lesion is usually an infiltrating ductal carcinoma, usually well differentiated, or a ductal carcinoma in situ (DCIS). The ducts of the nipple epithelium are infiltrated, but gross nipple changes are often minimal, and a tumor mass may not be palpable. The first symptom is often itching or burning of the nipple, with superficial erosion or ulceration. The diagnosis is established by biopsy of the erosion.

Paget's carcinoma is not common (about 1% of all breast cancers), but it is important because the nipple changes appear innocuous. These are frequently diagnosed and treated as dermatitis or bacterial infection, leading to delay in detection. When the lesion consists of nipple changes only, the incidence of axillary metastases is less than 5%, and the prognosis is excellent. When a breast mass is also present, the incidence of axillary metastases rises, with an associated marked decrease in prospects for cure by surgical or other treatment.

Inflammatory Carcinoma

This is the most malignant form of breast cancer and constitutes less than 3% of all cases. The clinical findings consist of a rapidly growing, sometimes painful mass that enlarges the breast. The overlying skin becomes erythematous, edematous, and warm. Often there is no distinct mass, since the tumor infiltrates the involved breast diffusely. The diagnosis should be made when the redness involves more than one-third of the skin over the breast and biopsy shows infiltrating carcinoma with invasion of the subdermal lymphatics. The inflammatory changes, often mistaken for an infection, are caused by carcinomatous invasion of the subdermal lymphatics, with resulting edema and hyperemia. If the physician suspects infection but the lesion does not respond rapidly (1–2 weeks) to antibiotics, biopsy is performed. Metastases tend to occur early and widely, and for this reason inflammatory carcinoma is rarely curable. Mastectomy is seldom indicated unless chemotherapy and radiation have resulted in clinical remission with no evidence of distant metastases. In these cases, residual disease in the breast may be eradicated. Radiation, hormone therapy, and chemotherapy are the measures most likely to be of value rather than operation.

Breast Cancer Occurring During Pregnancy or Lactation

Breast cancer complicates approximately one in 3000 pregnancies. The diagnosis is frequently delayed, because physiologic changes in the breast may obscure the lesion. This results in a tendency of both patients and physicians to misinterpret findings and to delay biopsy. When the cancer is confined to the breast, the 5-year survival rate after mastectomy is about 70%. Axillary metastases are already present in 60–70% of patients, and for them the 5-year survival rate after mastectomy is only 30–40%. Pregnancy (or lactation) is not a contraindication to operation, and treatment should be based on the stage of the disease as in the nonpregnant (or nonlactating) woman. Overall survival rates have improved, since cancers are now diagnosed in pregnant women earlier than in the past. Breast-conserving surgery may be performed—and radiation and chemotherapy given—even during the pregnancy.

Bilateral Breast Cancer

Clinically evident simultaneous bilateral breast cancer occurs in less than 1% of cases, but there is a

5–8% incidence of later occurrence of cancer in the second breast. Bilaterality occurs more often in familial breast cancer, in women under age 50, and when the tumor in the primary breast is lobular. The incidence of second breast cancers increases directly with the length of time the patient is alive after her first cancer—about 1% per year.

In patients with breast cancer, mammography should be performed before primary treatment and at regular intervals thereafter, to search for occult cancer in the opposite breast. Routine biopsy of the opposite breast is usually not warranted even for lobular cancer.

Noninvasive Cancer

Noninvasive cancer can occur within the ducts (ductal carcinoma in situ) or lobules (lobular carcinoma in situ). While ductal carcinoma in situ (DCIS) behaves as an early malignancy, lobular carcinoma in situ (LCIS) would perhaps better be called lobular neoplasia because it is not truly carcinoma. DCIS tends to be unilateral and most often progresses to invasive cancer if untreated. Approximately 40–60% of women who have DCIS treated with biopsy alone develop invasive cancer within the same breast. Lobular carcinoma in situ, however, appears to be a risk factor calling attention to the probability of developing invasive cancer in either breast. One in five women with lobular carcinoma in situ develop invasive cancer. This invasive cancer may occur in either breast regardless of the side of the original biopsy and is usually ductal.

The treatment of intraductal lesions is controversial. Ductal carcinoma can be treated with total mastectomy or by wide excision with or without radiation therapy. Lobular carcinoma in situ is well managed with observation, but patients unwilling to accept the increased risk of breast cancer may be offered bilateral total mastectomy. Another alternative is tamoxifen, which is effective in preventing invasive breast cancer from developing in both lobular cancer in situ and intraductal cancer in situ. Axillary metastases from in situ cancers should not occur unless there is an occult invasive cancer.

Colozza M et al: Induction chemotherapy with cisplatin, doxorubicin, and cyclophosphamide (CAP) in a combined modality approach for locally advanced and inflammatory breast cancer. Long-term results. Am J Clin Oncol 1996;19:10. [NLM Cit ID: 96152497]

Fish EB et al: Assessment of treatment for patients with primary ductal carcinoma in situ in the breast. Ann Surg Oncol 1998;5:724. [NLM Cit ID: 99084865] (Suggests high rate of recurrence and invasive disease for patients who underwent lumpectomies and did not receive adjuvant radiotherapy.)

Fisher ER et al: Pathologic findings from the National Surgical Adjuvant Breast Project (NSABP) eight-year update of protocol B-17: intraductal carcinoma. Cancer 1999;86:429. [NLM Cit ID: 99357320] (Degree of comedo necrosis is sufficient for defining high and low risk for second ipsilateral breast tumor after lumpectomy; low-risk patients benefit from radiotherapy.)

Silverstein MJ et al: The influence of margin width on local control of ductal carcinoma in situ of the breast. N Engl J Med 1999;340:1455. [NLM Cit ID: 99240025] (Patients with margins < 1 mm benefit from adjuvant radiotherapy; those with margins > 10 mm showed no benefit from postoperative radiotherapy.)

Solin LJ et al: Fifteen-year results of breast conserving surgery and definitive breast irradiation for the treatment of ductal carcinoma in situ of the breast. J Clin Oncol 1996;14:754. [NLM Cit ID: 96186199] (Showing that breast conservation is feasible in this group of patients.)

HORMONE RECEPTOR SITES

The presence or absence of estrogen and progesterone receptors in the cytoplasm of tumor cells is of paramount importance in managing patients with breast cancer. Patients whose primary tumors are receptor-positive have a more favorable course than those whose tumors are receptor-negative. Receptors are of value in determining adjuvant therapy and for treatment of advanced disease. Up to 60% of patients with metastatic breast cancer will respond to hormonal manipulation if their tumors contain estrogen receptors. Fewer than 5% of patients with metastatic, estrogen receptor-negative tumors can be treated successfully in this fashion.

Receptor status is valuable not only in management of metastatic disease but also helps select patients for adjuvant therapy. Adjuvant hormonal therapy (tamoxifen) with receptor-positive tumors and adjuvant chemotherapy with receptor-negative tumors improve survival rates even in the absence of lymph node metastases (see Adjuvant Therapy, below).

Progesterone receptors may be a more sensitive indicator than estrogen receptors of patients who may respond to hormonal manipulation. Up to 80% of patients with metastatic progesterone receptor-positive tumors improve with hormonal manipulation. Receptors have no relationship to response to chemotherapy.

Estrogen and progesterone receptor assays should be done routinely for every breast cancer at the time of initial diagnosis, either by quantitative assay or by immunohistochemistry. Receptor status may change after hormonal therapy, radiotherapy, or chemotherapy.

Carmeci C et al: Analysis of estrogen receptor messenger RNA in breast carcinomas from archival specimens is predictive of tumor biology. Am J Pathol 1997;150:1563. [NLM Cit ID: 97282949]

Raabe NK et al: Hormone receptor measurements and survival in 1335 consecutive patients with primary invasive breast carcinoma. Int J Oncol 1998;12:1091. [NLM Cit ID: 98207177] (Evaluation of relationship between ER and PR content to relapse and survival in patients without systemic adjuvant treatment.)

CURATIVE TREATMENT

Treatment may be curative or palliative. Curative treatment is advised for clinical stage I and stage II disease (Table 16–2). Patients with locally advanced (stage III) and even inflammatory tumors may be cured with multimodality therapy, but in most palliation is all that can be expected. Palliative treatment is appropriate for all patients with stage IV disease and for previously treated patients who develop distant metastases or who have unresectable local cancers.

The growth potential of tumors and host resistance factors vary widely from patient to patient and may be altered during the course of the disease. The doubling time of breast cancer cells ranges from several weeks in a rapidly growing lesion to a year in a slowly growing one. Assuming that the rate of doubling is constant and that the neoplasm originates in one cell, a carcinoma with a doubling time of 100 days may not reach clinically detectable size (1 cm) for about 8 years. Rapidly growing cancers have a much shorter preclinical course and a greater tendency to metastasize by the time a breast mass is discovered.

The long preclinical growth phase and the tendency of breast cancers to metastasize have led clinicians to believe that most breast cancer is a systemic disease at the time of diagnosis. Although it may be true that breast cancer cells are released from the tumor prior to diagnosis, variations in the host-tumor relationship prohibit the growth of disseminated disease in many patients. Clearly, not all breast cancer is systemic at the time of diagnosis. For this reason, a pessimistic attitude concerning the management of localized breast cancer is unwarranted, and many patients can be cured.

Controversy surrounds the timing of surgery with respect to the menstrual cycle. Some suggest that operation during the time of unopposed estrogen adversely affects survival, but most studies support no such effect. Several trials are currently examining this question.

Choice of Primary Therapy

The extent of disease and its biologic aggressiveness are the principal determinants of the outcome of primary therapy. Clinical and pathologic staging help in assessing extent of disease (Table 16–2), but each is to some extent imprecise. Other factors such as DNA flow cytometry, tumor grade, hormone receptor assays, and oncogene amplification may be of prognostic value but are not important in determining the type of local therapy. Since two-thirds of patients eventually manifest distant disease regardless of the form of primary therapy, there is a tendency to think of breast carcinoma as being systemic in most patients at the time of presentation.

Controversy surrounds the choice of primary therapy of stage I, II, and III breast carcinoma. A number of states require physicians to inform patients of alternative treatment methods in the management of breast cancer.

Breast-Conserving Therapy

Many nonrandomized trials, the Milan trial, and a large randomized trial conducted by the National Surgical Adjuvant Breast Project (NSABP) in the USA show that disease-free survival rates are similar for patients treated by partial mastectomy plus axillary dissection followed by radiation therapy and for those treated by modified radical mastectomy (total mastectomy plus axillary dissection). All patients whose axillary nodes contained tumor received adjuvant chemotherapy.

In the NSABP trial, patients were randomized to three treatment types: (1) "lumpectomy" (removal of the tumor with *confirmed* tumor-free margins) plus whole breast irradiation, (2) lumpectomy alone, and (3) total mastectomy. All patients underwent axillary lymph node dissection, and some had tumors as large as 4 cm with (or without) palpable axillary lymph nodes. The lowest local recurrence rate was among patients treated with lumpectomy and postoperative irradiation; the highest—nearly 40% at 8 years of follow-up—was among patients treated with lumpectomy alone. However, no statistically significant differences were observed in overall or disease-free survival among the three treatment groups. This study shows that lumpectomy and axillary dissection with postoperative radiation therapy is as effective as modified radical mastectomy for the management of patients with stage I and stage II breast cancer.

The results of these and other trials have demonstrated that much less aggressive surgical treatment of the primary lesion than has previously been thought necessary gives equivalent therapeutic results and may preserve an acceptable cosmetic appearance.

Tumor size is a major consideration in determining the feasibility of breast conservation. The lumpectomy trial of the NSABP randomized patients with tumors as large as 4 cm. To achieve an acceptable cosmetic result, the patient must have a breast of sufficient size to enable excision of a 4 cm tumor without considerable deformity. Therefore, large size is only a relative contraindication. Subareolar tumors are also difficult to excise without deformity, but this location is not a contraindication to breast conservation. Clinically detectable multifocality is a relative contraindication to breast-conserving surgery, as is fixation to the chest wall or skin or involvement of the nipple or overlying skin. The patient and not the surgeon should be the judge of what is cosmetically acceptable.

Axillary dissection is valuable in preventing axillary recurrences, in staging cancer, and in planning therapy. Intraoperative lymphatic mapping and sentinel node dissection identify lymph nodes most likely to harbor metastases if they are present in the axillary nodes. Numerous studies have confirmed the validity of this technique. Ongoing trials are examining the replacement of formal axillary dissection with sentinel node dissection. Results to date suggest that sentinel node biopsy may replace axillary dissection for staging and treatment in histopathologically node-negative women. A trial by the American College of Surgeons Oncology Group is examining the role of sentinel node dissection without axillary dissection for node-positive women. Bone marrow biopsy with examination by immunocytochemistry to detect early metastases may be as sensitive a staging procedure as axillary dissection and may identify patients at high risk for disseminating disease.

Current Recommendations

A 1990 NIH consensus statement asserts that breast-conserving surgery with radiation is the preferred form of treatment for patients with early-stage breast cancer. Despite the numerous randomized trials showing no survival benefit of mastectomy over breast-conserving partial mastectomy and irradiation, breast-conserving surgery appears underutilized and mastectomy remains the more common treatment. About 25% of patients in the United States with stage I or stage II breast cancer are treated with breast-conserving surgery and radiation therapy, compared with 75% treated with mastectomy. Use of breast-conserving surgery and radiation therapy varies by region of the country, ranging from 15% in the South Central United States to 30% in the Pacific Region.

Modified radical mastectomy (total mastectomy plus axillary lymph node dissection) has been the standard therapy for most patients with breast cancer. This operation removes the entire breast, overlying skin, nipple, and areolar complex as well as the underlying pectoralis fascia with the axillary lymph nodes in continuity. The major advantage of modified radical mastectomy is that radiation therapy is usually not necessary. The disadvantage, of course, is the psychologic trauma associated with breast loss. Radical mastectomy, which removes the underlying pectoralis muscle, should be performed rarely if at all. Axillary node dissection is not indicated for noninfiltrating cancers, because nodal metastases are rarely present. Radiotherapy after partial mastectomy consists of 5–6 weeks of five daily fractions to a total dose of 5000–6000 cGy. Some radiotherapists use a boost dose. Current studies suggest that radiotherapy after mastectomy may improve survival.

Preoperatively, full discussion with the patient regarding the rationale for operation and various alternative forms of treatment is essential. Breast-conserving surgery and radiation should be offered whenever possible, since most patients would prefer to save the breast. Breast reconstruction should be discussed with patients who choose or require mastectomy, and the option of simultaneous mastectomy with immediate reconstruction added. Time spent preoperatively in educating the patient and her family about these matters is well spent.

Adjuvant Systemic Therapy

Following surgery and radiation therapy, chemotherapy or hormonal therapy is advocated for most patients with curable breast cancer. The objective of adjuvant systemic therapy is to eliminate the occult metastases responsible for late recurrences while they are microscopic and most vulnerable to anticancer agents. In addition, adjuvant chemotherapy may decrease local recurrence in patients treated with breast conservation, and adjuvant tamoxifen decreases contralateral breast cancer occurrence.

Numerous clinical trials with various adjuvant chemotherapeutic regimens have been completed. The most extensive clinical experience is with the CMF (cyclophosphamide, methotrexate, and fluorouracil) regimen. Cyclophosphamide can be given either orally, in a dose of 100 mg/m^2 daily for 14 days; or intravenously, in a dose of 600 mg/m^2 on days 1 and 8. Methotrexate is given intravenously, 40 mg/m^2 on days 1 and 8; and fluorouracil is given intravenously, 600 mg/m^2 on days 1 and 8. This cycle is repeated every 4 weeks. Some clinicians prefer to give the drugs on 1 day only every 3 weeks. There appears to be no obvious advantage except that patient compliance is assured when the cyclophosphamide is given intravenously. The regimen is continued for 6 months in patients with axillary metastases. Premenopausal women with positive axillary nodes benefit from adjuvant chemotherapy. The recurrence rate in premenopausal patients who received no adjuvant chemotherapy is more than 1.5 times that of those who received such therapy. No therapeutic effect with CMF has been shown in postmenopausal women with positive nodes, perhaps because therapy was modified so often in response to side effects that the total amount of drugs administered was less than planned. Other trials with different agents support the value of adjuvant chemotherapy in postmenopausal women. There are many forms of combination chemotherapy that are effective. Most are variations of CMF or AC (Adriamycin [doxorubicin] plus cyclophosphamide). The addition of taxanes (docetaxel, paclitaxel) to AC improved survival in node-positive women.

Selection of patients to receive chemotherapy must take into account common health problems in older women and the effects of chemotherapy on the patient's overall health. Tamoxifen can be given with few side effects even in the elderly. It appears to increase bone density and favorably affect lipid and lipoprotein profiles, which may explain the observed decreased mortality rate from coronary artery disease seen in patients taking tamoxifen.

The addition of hormonal therapy, usually with tamoxifen, may improve the results of adjuvant therapy. It also has been shown to enhance the beneficial effects of melphalan and fluorouracil in postmenopausal women whose tumors are estrogen receptor (ER)-positive. Tamoxifen alone in a dosage of 10 mg orally twice a day has long been the recommended treatment for postmenopausal women with ER-positive tumors. Finally, an NSABP trial showed that tamoxifen plus chemotherapy (Adriamycin [doxorubicin] plus cyclophosphamide [AC] or prednisone plus Adriamycin plus fluorouracil [PAF]) lowered recurrence rates more than tamoxifen alone in postmenopausal women with ER-positive tumors.

The length of time adjuvant therapy must be administered remains uncertain. Shorter treatment periods may be as effective as longer ones. For example, one study compared 6 versus 12 cycles of postoperative CMF and found 5-year disease-free survival rates to be comparable. One of the earliest adjuvant trials used a 6-day perioperative regimen of intravenous cyclophosphamide alone; follow-up at 15 years shows a 15% improvement in disease-free survival rates for treated patients, suggesting that short-term therapy may be effective. An NSABP study shows that 5 years of treatment with tamoxifen may be superior to 10 years.

Several studies of adjuvant therapy in node-negative women reveal a beneficial effect of adjuvant chemotherapy or tamoxifen in delaying recurrence and improving survival. A number of protocols, including CMF with leucovorin rescue as well as tamoxifen alone, have increased disease-free survival. The magnitude of this improvement is about one-third, ie, a group of women with an estimated 30% recurrence rate would have a 20% recurrence rate after adjuvant systemic therapy. Quality of life while receiving chemotherapy does not appear to be greatly altered.

The current recommendations for adjuvant chemotherapy are summarized in Tables 16–4 and 16–5.

Previous recommendations from the NIH on early-stage breast cancer suggest (1) that all patients who are candidates for clinical trials be offered the opportunity to participate, and (2) that node-negative patients who are not candidates for clinical trials ". . . should be made aware of the benefits and risks of adjuvant systemic therapy. The decision to use adjuvant treatment should follow a thorough discussion with the patient regarding the likely risk of recurrence without adjuvant therapy, the expected reduction in risk with adjuvant therapy, toxicities of therapy, and its impact on quality of life." A new consensus conference is planned for the near future. In practice, most medical oncologists are currently using systemic adjuvant therapy for patients with node-negative and node-positive breast cancer. Other prognostic factors being used to determine the patient's risks are tumor size, estrogen and progesterone receptor status, nuclear grade, histologic type, proliferative rate, and oncogene expression (Table 16–6). The assumption is made that all patients with node-negative aggressive tumors should receive adjuvant therapy save those who have serious coexistent medical problems. Few patients cannot tolerate at least tamoxifen. The use of chemotherapy prior to resection of the primary tumor has also been examined. This "neoadjuvant" chemotherapy enables the assessment of in vivo chemosensitivity. A complete tumor response in vivo prior to operation appears to be associated with improvement in survival. Neoadjuvant chemotherapy also permits breast conservation by shrinking the primary tumor in women who would otherwise need mastectomy for local control.

Table 16–4. Adjuvant chemotherapy for premenopausal women.[1]

Nodal Involvement	Estrogen Receptors	Adjuvant Systemic Therapy
Yes	Positive	Combination chemotherapy
Yes	Negative	Combination chemotherapy
No	Positive	Tamoxifen
No	Negative	Combination chemotherapy

[1]Summary of NIH Consensus Conference, June 18–21, 1990.

Table 16–5. Adjuvant chemotherapy for postmenopausal women.[1]

Nodal Involvement	Estrogen Receptors	Adjuvant Systemic Therapy
Yes	Positive	Tamoxifen
Yes	Negative	Combination chemotherapy
No	Positive	Tamoxifen
No	Negative	Combination chemotherapy

[1]Summary of NIH Consensus Conference, June 18–21, 1990.

Table 16–6. Prognostic factors in node-negative breast cancer.

Prognostic Factor	Increased Recurrence	Decreased Recurrence
Size	T3, T2	T1, T0
Hormone receptors	Negative	Positive
DNA flow cytometry	Aneuploid	Diploid
Histologic grade	High	Low
Tumor labeling index	< 3%	> 3%
S phase fraction	> 5%	< 5%
Lymphatic or vascular invasion	Present	Absent
Cathepsin D	High	Low
HER-2/*neu* oncogene	High	Low
Epidermal growth factor receptor	High	Low

Important questions remaining to be answered are the timing and duration of adjuvant chemotherapy, which chemotherapeutic agents should be applied for which subgroups of patients, how best to coordinate adjuvant chemotherapy with postoperative radiation therapy, the use of combinations of hormonal therapy and chemotherapy, and the value of prognostic factors other than hormone receptors in predicting response to adjuvant therapy. Adjuvant systemic therapy is not generally used in patients with small tumors and those with negative lymph nodes who have favorable tumor markers. A small disease-free survival benefit even in patients with small favorable tumors has been suggested. It appears that adjuvant systemic therapy benefits all breast cancer patients, but the clinician must decide if the benefits outweigh the risks, complications, and expense.

Adjuvant systemic therapy for women with node-negative breast cancer. The Steering Committee on Clinical Practice Guidelines for the Care and Treatment of Breast Cancer. Can Med Assoc J 1998;10:158. [NLM Cit ID: 98145272]

Adjuvant systemic therapy for women with node-positive breast cancer. The Steering Committee on Clinical Practice Guidelines for the Care and Treatment of Breast Cancer. Can Med Assoc J 1998;10(Suppl):S52. [NLM Cit ID: 98145273]

Appelbaum FR: The use of bone marrow and peripheral blood stem cell transplantation in the treatment of cancer. CA Cancer J Clin 1996;46:142. [NLM Cit ID: 96219007]

Borden EC et al: Biological therapies for breast carcinoma: concepts for improvements in survival. Semin Oncol 1999;26(4 Suppl 12):28. [NLM Cit ID: 99409918] (Review of recent clinical and pre-clinical research in immune and cytotoxic cancer therapies.)

Braun S et al: Cytokeratin-positive cells in the bone marrow and survival of patients with stage I, II, or III breast cancer. N Engl J Med 2000;342:525. [NLM Cit ID: 20132301] (Presence of occult metastatic cells in bone marrow indicates increased risk of relapse in breast cancer patients.)

Clinical practice guidelines for the use of tumor markers in breast and colorectal cancer. J Clin Oncol 1996;14:2843. [NLM Cit ID: 97028333]

Dale PS et al: Nipple-areolar preservation during breast-conserving therapy for subareolar breast carcinomas. Ann Surg 1996;131:430. [NLM Cit ID: 96201511]

Giuliano AE et al: Sentinel lymphadenectomy in breast cancer. J Clin Oncol 1997;15:2345. [NLM Cit ID: 97339550] (SLND with frozen section and IHC is minimally invasive and an accurate method of intraoperative axillary staging.)

Haffty BG et al: Ipsilateral breast tumor recurrence as a predictor of distant disease: Implications for systemic therapy at the time of local relapse. J Clin Oncol 1996;14:52. [NLM Cit ID: 96140280]

Hillner BE et al: Trade-offs between survival and breast preservation for three initial treatments of ductal carcinoma-in-situ of the breast. J Clin Oncol 1996;14:70. [NLM Cit ID: 96140283]

Hudis CA et al: Adjuvant drug therapy for operable breast cancer. Semin Oncol 1996;23:475. [NLM Cit ID: 96347522]

Krag D et al: The sentinel node in breast cancer—a multicenter validation study. N Engl J Med 1998;339:941. [NLM Cit ID: 98418644] (Sentinel node biopsy is predictive of axillary lymph node metastases in breast cancer patients.)

Margolese RG: Surgical considerations for invasive breast cancer. Surg Clin North Am 1999;79:1031. [NLM Cit ID: 20038844] (Discussion of when breast-conserving surgery is and is not appropriate based on review of clinical data.)

Mehta K et al: Long-term outcome in patients with four or more positive lymph nodes treated with conservative surgery and radiation therapy. Int J Radiat Oncol Biol Phys 1996;35:679. [NLM Cit ID: 96305153] (For patients with four or more positive axillary lymph nodes, breast conserving surgery, radiotherapy to the breast, and adjuvant systemic therapy yield reasonable long-term survival with a high rate of local regional control.)

Ramirez AJ et al. Do patients with advanced breast cancer benefit from chemotherapy? Br J Cancer 1998;78:1488. [NLM Cit ID: 99052300] (Advanced breast cancer patients benefit from six cycles of first-line palliative treatment; factors predicting treatment failure or negative treatment outcomes are identified.)

Touboul E et al: Local recurrences and distant metastases after breast-conserving surgery and radiation therapy for early stage breast cancer. Int J Radiat Oncol Biol Phys 1999;43:25. [NLM Cit ID: 99142617] (Different factors predict local and metastatic recurrence.)

PALLIATIVE TREATMENT

This section covers palliative therapy of disseminated disease incurable by surgery (stage IV)

Radiotherapy

Palliative radiotherapy may be advised for locally advanced cancers with distant metastases in order to control ulceration, pain, and other manifestations in the breast and regional nodes. Irradiation of the breast and chest wall and the axillary, internal mammary, and supraclavicular nodes should be undertaken in an attempt to cure locally advanced and inoperable lesions when there is no evidence of distant metastases. A small number of patients in this group are cured in spite of extensive breast and regional node involvement. Neoadjuvant chemotherapy should be considered for such patients.

Palliative irradiation is of value also in the treatment of certain bone or soft tissue metastases to control pain or avoid fracture. Radiotherapy is especially useful in the treatment of isolated bony metastasis, chest wall recurrences, brain metastases, and acute spinal cord compression.

Hormone Therapy

Disseminated disease may shrink—or grow less rapidly—after endocrine therapy such as administration of hormones (eg, estrogens, androgens, progestins; see Table 16–7); ablation of the ovaries, adrenals, or pituitary; or administration of drugs that block hormone receptor sites (eg, antiestrogens) or drugs that block the synthesis of hormones (eg, aminoglutethimide). Hormonal manipulation is usually more successful in postmenopausal women even if they have received estrogen replacement therapy. If treatment is based on the presence of estrogen receptor protein in the primary tumor or metastases, however, the rate of response is nearly equal in premenopausal and postmenopausal women. A favorable response to hormonal manipulation occurs in about one-third of patients with metastatic breast cancer. Of those whose tumors contain estrogen receptors, the response is about 60% and perhaps as high as 80% for patients whose tumors contain progesterone receptors as well. Because only 5–10% of women whose tumors do not contain estrogen receptors respond, they should not receive hormonal therapy except in unusual circumstances, eg, in an older patient who cannot tolerate chemotherapy.

Since the quality of life during a remission induced by endocrine manipulation is usually superior to a remission following cytotoxic chemotherapy, it is usually best to try endocrine manipulation first in cases where the estrogen receptor status is unknown. When receptor status is unknown but the disease is progressing rapidly or involves visceral organs, however, endocrine therapy is rarely successful, and introducing it may waste valuable time.

In general, only one type of therapy should be given at a time unless it is necessary to irradiate a destructive lesion of weight-bearing bone while the patient is on another regimen. The regimen should be changed only if the disease is clearly progressing. This is especially important for patients with destructive bone metastases, since changes in the status of these lesions are difficult to determine radiographically. A plan of therapy that would simultaneously minimize toxicity and maximize benefits is often best achieved by hormonal manipulation.

The choice of endocrine therapy depends on the menopausal status of the patient. Women within 1 year of their last menstrual period are considered to be premenopausal, while women whose menstruation ceased more than a year ago are postmenopausal. If endocrine therapy is the initial choice, it is referred to as primary hormonal manipulation; subsequent endocrine treatment is called secondary or tertiary hormonal manipulation.

A. The Premenopausal Patient:

1. Primary hormonal therapy–The potent antiestrogen tamoxifen is the endocrine treatment of choice in the premenopausal patient. Tamoxifen is usually given orally in a dose of 20 mg daily. There is no significant difference in survival or response between tamoxifen therapy and bilateral oophorectomy. Tamoxifen is by far the most common and preferred method of hormonal manipulation for both pre- and postmenopausal women. The average remission is about 12 months. Tamoxifen can be given with little morbidity and few side effects. Controversy continues about whether a response to tamoxifen is predictive of probable success with other forms of endocrine manipulation. A new tamoxifen analog, toremifene, appears as effective as tamoxifen as primary hormonal therapy.

Bilateral oophorectomy is less desirable than primary hormonal manipulation in premenopausal women because tamoxifen is so well tolerated. Oophorectomy can be achieved rapidly and safely by surgery, however, or, if the patient is a poor operative risk, by irradiation of the ovaries. Ovarian radiation therapy should be avoided in otherwise healthy patients because of the high rate of complications and the longer time necessary to achieve results. Chemical ovarian ablation using a GnRH analog can also be utilized. Oophorectomy presumably works by eliminating estrogens, progestins, and androgens, which stimulate growth of the tumor.

2. Secondary or tertiary hormonal therapy–Although patients who do not respond to tamoxifen or oophorectomy should be treated with cytotoxic drugs, those who respond and then relapse may subsequently respond to another form of endocrine treatment (Table 16–7). The initial choice for secondary endocrine manipulation has not been clearly defined.

Patients who improve after oophorectomy but subsequently relapse should receive tamoxifen. If tamoxifen fails, aminoglutethimide or megestrol acetate

Table 16–7. Agents commonly used for hormonal management of metastatic breast cancer.

Drug	Action	Usual Oral Dose	Major Side Effects
Tamoxifen (Nolvadex)	Antiestrogen	10 mg twice daily	Hot flushes, uterine bleeding, thrombophlebitis, rash
Diethylstilbestrol (DES)	Estrogen	5 mg three times daily	Fluid retention, uterine bleeding, thrombophlebitis, nausea
Megestrol acetate (Megace)	Progestin	40 mg four times daily	Fluid retention
Aminoglutethimide (Cytadren)[1]	Aromatase inhibitor	250 mg four times daily	Adrenal suppression, skin rashes, neurologic reactions

[1]Used with hydrocortisone.

should be considered. Aminoglutethimide is an inhibitor of adrenal hormone synthesis and, when combined with a corticosteroid, provides a therapeutically effective "medical adrenalectomy." Megestrol is a progestational agent. Both drugs cause less morbidity and mortality than surgical adrenalectomy; can be discontinued once the patient improves; and are not associated with the many problems of postsurgical hypoadrenalism, so that patients who require chemotherapy are more easily managed. Adrenalectomy or hypophysectomy induces regression in 30–50% of patients who have previously responded to oophorectomy. Pharmacologic hormonal manipulation has in large part replaced these invasive procedures. Toremifene is not likely to be of value in women whose tumors no longer respond to tamoxifen.

B. The Postmenopausal Patient:

1. Primary hormonal therapy–Tamoxifen, 20 mg daily, is the initial therapy of choice for postmenopausal women with metastatic breast cancer amenable to endocrine manipulation. It has fewer side effects than diethylstilbestrol, the former therapy of choice, and is equally as effective. The main side effects of tamoxifen are nausea, vomiting, and skin rash. Rarely, it may induce hypercalcemia in patients with bony metastases.

2. Secondary or tertiary hormonal therapy– Postmenopausal patients who do not respond to tamoxifen should be given cytotoxic drugs such as cyclophosphamide, methotrexate, and fluorouracil (CMF) or Adriamycin (doxorubicin) and cyclophosphamide (AC). Postmenopausal women who respond initially to tamoxifen but later manifest progressive disease may be given diethylstilbestrol or megestrol acetate. Aromatase inhibitors (aminoglutethimide) have been available for the treatment of advanced breast cancer in postmenopausal women who fail tamoxifen treatment. Clinical trials have proved the efficacy of anastrozole for such purposes. Anastrozole, easily administered in daily doses of 1 mg, has few side effects. Androgens have many toxicities and should rarely be used. As in premenopausal patients, neither hypophysectomy nor adrenalectomy is still being performed.

Chemotherapy

Cytotoxic drugs should be considered for the treatment of metastatic breast cancer (1) if visceral metastases are present (especially brain or lymphangitic pulmonary); (2) if hormonal treatment is unsuccessful or the disease has progressed after an initial response to hormonal manipulation; or (3) if the tumor is ER-negative. The most useful single chemotherapeutic agent to date is doxorubicin (Adriamycin), with a response rate of 40–50%. Single agents are rarely used but rather given in combination with other cytotoxic drugs.

Combination chemotherapy using multiple agents has proved to be more effective, with objectively observed favorable responses achieved in 50–80% of patients with stage IV disease. Various combinations of drugs have been used, and clinical trials are continuing in an effort to improve results and reduce undesirable side effects. Nausea and vomiting are well controlled with drugs that directly affect the central nervous system, such as ondansetron and granisetron. These drugs are selective antagonists of serotonin receptors in the central nervous system and block nausea caused by cytotoxic chemotherapy. Doxorubicin (40 mg/m^2 intravenously on day 1) and cyclophosphamide (200 mg/m^2 orally on days 3–6) produce an objective response in about 85% of patients so treated. Other chemotherapeutic regimens have consisted of various combinations of drugs, including cyclophosphamide, vincristine, methotrexate, fluorouracil, and taxanes with response rates ranging up to 60–70%. Prior adjuvant chemotherapy does not seem to alter response rates in patients who relapse. Growth factors such as erythropoietin (epoetin alfa), which stimulates red blood cell production and mimics the effect of erythropoietin, and filgrastim (granulocyte colony-stimulating factor; G-CSF), which stimulates proliferation and differentiation of hematopoietic cells, prevent life-threatening anemia and neutropenia seen commonly with high doses of chemotherapy. These agents greatly diminish the incidence of infections that may complicate the use of myelosuppressive chemotherapy.

Paclitaxel, given by intravenous infusion in a dose of 135–175 mg/m^2, has been shown to be very effective for patients with breast cancer. It is usually given after failure of combination chemotherapy for metastatic disease or relapse shortly after completion of adjuvant chemotherapy. Paclitaxel has response rates of 30–40% in patients with metastatic disease and is used as both a first-line agent and as an adjuvant systemic agent, usually in combination with doxorubicin.

Docetaxel is another taxane (like paclitaxel) that shows promise for treatment of patients with anthracycline-resistant tumors. Both agents are currently being used after treatment with anthracyclines in patients with advanced disease as well as in adjuvant and neoadjuvant settings. Trastuzumab is a monoclonal antibody that binds to Her-2/neu receptors on the cancer cell and has been shown to be highly effective in Her-2/neu-expressive cancers. It appears superior to doxorubicin alone or doxorubucin and cyclophosphamide.

High-dose chemotherapy and autologous bone marrow or stem cell transplantation have aroused widespread interest for the treatment of metastatic breast cancer. With this technique, the patient receives high doses of cytotoxic agents, eradicating the marrow, for which the patient subsequently undergoes autologous bone marrow or stem cell transplantation. Complete response rates are as high as 30–35%—considerably better than what can be achieved with conventional chemotherapy. Most randomized trials, however, comparing high-dose chemotherapy with stem cell support show no improvement in survival over conventional chemotherapy. A study purporting to show an advantage to high-dose chemotherapy is South Africa was found to be falsified and discredited. Enthusiasm for high-dose chemotherapy with stem cell support has waned, but additional studies continue. The technique is extremely costly, and the treatment itself is associated with a mortality rate of about 3–7%.

Malignant Pleural Effusion

This condition develops at some time in almost half of patients with metastatic breast cancer (see Chapter 9).

Buzdar AU et al: A phase III trial comparing anastrozole (1–10 milligrams), a potent and selective aromatase inhibitor, with megestrol acetate in postmenopausal women with advanced breast carcinoma. Arimidex Study Group. Cancer 1997;79:730. [NLM Cit ID: 97177159]

Buzdar AU et al: Arimidex: A potent and selective aromatase inhibitor for the treatment of advanced breast cancer. J Steroid Biochem Mol Biol 1997;61:145. [NLM Cit ID: 98030466]

Clarke M: Tamoxifen for early breast cancer: an overview of the randomised trials. Lancet 1998;351:1451. [NLM Cit ID: 98266838] (Adjuvant tamoxifen yields significant improvement in 10-year survival rates in women with ER-positive tumors and in women with tumors of unknown ER status.)

Colmer R et al: Paclitaxel/gemcitabine administered every two weeks in advanced breast cancer: preliminary results of a phase II trial. Semin Oncol 2000;27(1 Suppl 2):20. [NLM Cit ID: 20160105] (Encouraging activity and low toxicity profile seen.)

Dhodapkar MV et al: Prognostic factors in elderly women with metastatic breast cancer treated with tamoxifen: An analysis of patients entered on four prospective clinical trials. Cancer 1996;77:683. [NLM Cit ID: 96186852]

Harvey HA: Issues concerning the role of chemotherapy and hormonal therapy of bone metastases from breast cancer. Cancer 1997;80(8 Suppl):1646. [NLM Cit ID: 98026754]

Pegram MD et al: Combination therapy with trastuzumab (Herceptin) and cisplatin for chemoresistant metastatic breast cancer: evidence for receptor-enhanced chemosensitivity. Semin Oncol 1999;26(4 Suppl 12):89. [NLM Cit ID: 99409925] (The combination yielded higher response rates than either single agent alone.)

Stadtmauer EA et al: Conventional-dose chemotherapy compared with high-dose chemotherapy plus autologous hematopoietic stem-cell transplantation for metastatic breast cancer. N Engl J Med 2000;342:1069. [NLM Cit ID: 20205680] (Randomized trial, high-dose chemotherapy given after induction of complete or partial remission with conventional-dose chemotherapy does not improve survival.)

Valero V: Combination docetaxel/cyclophosphamide in patients with advanced solid tumors. Oncology 1997; 11:34. [NLM Cit ID: 98031123]

PROGNOSIS

Stage of breast cancer is the most reliable indicator of prognosis (Table 16–8). Patients with disease localized to the breast and no evidence of regional spread after microscopic examination of the lymph nodes have by far the most favorable prognosis. Axillary lymph node status is the best-analyzed prognostic factor and correlates with survival at all tumor sizes. In addition, increased number of axillary nodes involved correlates directly with lower survival rates. Estrogen and progesterone receptors are prognostic variables because patients with hormone receptor-negative tumors and no evidence of metastases to the axillary lymph nodes have a much higher recurrence rate than do patients with hormone receptor-positive tumors and no regional metastases. The histologic subtype of breast cancer (eg, medullary, lobular, colloid) seems to have little significance in prognosis once these tumors are truly invasive. Flow cytometry of tumor cells to analyze DNA index and S-phase frequency aid in prognosis. Tumors with marked aneuploidy have a poor prognosis (Table 16–6). HER-2/*neu* oncogene amplification, epidermal growth factor receptors, and cathepsin D may have some prognostic value, but no markers are as significant as lymph node metastases in predicting outcome.

The mortality rate of breast cancer patients exceeds that of age-matched normal controls for nearly 20 years. Thereafter, the mortality rates are equal, though deaths that occur among breast cancer patients are often directly the result of tumor. Five-year statistics do not accurately reflect the final outcome of therapy.

When cancer is localized to the breast, with no evidence of regional spread after pathologic examination, the clinical cure rate with most accepted methods of therapy is 75–90%. Exceptions to this generalization may be related to the hormonal receptor content of the tumor, tumor size, host resistance, or associated illness. Patients with small mammographically detected estrogen and progesterone receptor-positive tumors and no evidence of axillary spread probably have a 5-year survival rate greater than 90%. When the axillary lymph nodes are in-

Table 16–8. Approximate survival (%) of patients with breast cancer by TNM stage.

TNM Stage	Five Years	Ten Years
0	95	90
I	85	70
IIA	70	50
IIB	60	40
IIIA	55	30
IIIB	30	20
IV	5–10	2
All	65	30

volved with tumor, the survival rate drops to 40–50% at 5 years and probably around 25% at 10 years. In general, breast cancer appears to be somewhat more malignant in younger than in older women, and this may be related to the fact that fewer younger women have ER-positive tumors.

For those patients whose disease progresses despite treatment, supportive group therapy has been shown to improve survival. As they approach the end of life, such patients will require meticulous efforts at palliative care (see Chapter 5).

Younes M et al: Stratified multivariate analysis of prognostic markers in breast cancer: a preliminary report. Anticancer Res 1997;17:1383. [NLM Cit ID: 97283370] (Discussion of a proposed integration of commonly used prognostic factors into prognostic scheme for use in making treatment decisions.)

FOLLOW-UP CARE

After primary therapy, patients with breast cancer should be followed for life for at least two reasons: to detect recurrences and to observe the opposite breast for a second primary carcinoma. Local and distant recurrences occur most frequently within the first 3 years. During this period, the patient should be examined every 6 months. Thereafter, examination is done annually. Special attention is paid to the remaining breast, because 10% of patients will develop a contralateral primary malignancy. The patient should examine her own breast monthly, and a mammogram should be obtained annually. In some cases, metastases are dormant for long periods and may appear 10–15 years or longer after removal of the primary tumor. Estrogen and progestational agents are rarely used for a patient free of disease after treatment of primary breast cancer, particularly if the tumor was hormone receptor-positive. Studies nevertheless have failed to show an adverse effect of hormonal agents in patients who are free of disease. Even pregnancy has not been clearly associated with shortened survival of patients rendered disease-free—yet most oncologists are reluctant to advise a young patient with breast cancer that she may become pregnant, and most are less than enthusiastic about prescribing hormone replacement therapy for the postmenopausal breast cancer patient. Estrogen replacement therapy may be prescribed for a woman with a history of breast cancer after discussion of the benefits and risks of such therapy for such conditions as osteoporosis and hot flushes. Raloxifene may prove to be appropriate replacement therapy to prevent osteoporosis after breast cancer, but as yet it has not been adequately studied.

Local Recurrence

The incidence of local recurrence correlates with tumor size, the presence and number of involved axillary nodes, the histologic type of tumor, the presence of skin edema or skin and fascia fixation with the primary, and the type of initial local (breast) therapy. About 8% of patients develop local recurrence on the chest wall after total mastectomy and axillary dissection. When the axillary nodes are not involved, the local recurrence rate is 5%, but the rate is as high as 25% when they are heavily involved. A similar difference in local recurrence rate was noted between small and large tumors. Factors affecting the rate of local recurrence in patients who have had partial mastectomies are not yet determined. Early studies show that factors such as multifocal cancer, in situ tumors, positive resection margins, chemotherapy, and radiotherapy are important.

Chest wall recurrences usually appear within the first 2 years but may occur as late as 15 or more years after mastectomy. Suspicious nodules and skin lesions should be biopsied. Local excision or localized radiotherapy may be feasible if an isolated nodule is present. If lesions are multiple or accompanied by evidence of regional involvement in the internal mammary or supraclavicular nodes, the disease is best managed by radiation treatment of the entire chest wall including the parasternal, supraclavicular, and axillary areas.

Local recurrence after mastectomy usually signals the presence of widespread disease and is an indication for bone scans, abdominal CT or liver ultrasound, posteroanterior and lateral chest x-rays, and other examinations as needed to search for evidence of metastases. Most patients with locally recurrent tumor will develop distant metastases within 2 years. When there is no evidence of metastases beyond the chest wall and regional nodes, irradiation for cure or complete local excision should be attempted. Patients with local recurrence may be cured with local resection and radiation. After partial mastectomy, local recurrence may not have as serious a prognostic significance as after mastectomy. However, those patients who do develop a breast recurrence have a worse prognosis than those who do not. It is speculated that the ability of a cancer to recur locally after radiotherapy is a sign of aggressiveness. Completion of the mastectomy should be done for local recurrence after partial mastectomy; some of these patients will survive for prolonged periods, especially if the breast recurrence is DCIS or more than 5 years after initial treatment. Systemic chemotherapy or hormonal treatment should be used for women who develop disseminated disease or those in whom local recurrence occurs.

Edema of the Arm

Significant edema of the arm occurs in about 10–30% of patients after radical mastectomy. It occurs more commonly if radiotherapy has been given or if there was postoperative infection. Partial mastectomy with radiation to the axillary lymph nodes is followed by chronic edema of the arm in 10–20% of patients. To avoid this complication, many authorities advocate axillary lymph node sampling rather than complete axillary dissection. However, since axillary dissection is a more accurate staging operation than axillary sampling, it is recommended that at least level I and II lymph nodes be removed, in combination with partial mastectomy. Sentinel lymph node dissection may offer accurate staging without the risk of lymphedema for node-negative patients. Judicious use of radiotherapy, with treatment fields carefully planned to spare the axilla as much as possible, can greatly diminish the incidence of edema, which will occur in only 5% of patients if no radiotherapy is given to the axilla after a partial mastectomy and lymph node dissection.

Late or secondary edema of the arm may develop years after treatment, as a result of axillary recurrence or of infection in the hand or arm, with obliteration of lymphatic channels. Infection in the arm or hand on the dissected side should be treated with antibiotics, rest, and elevation. When edema develops, careful examination of the axilla for recurrence should be done. If there is no sign of recurrence, the swollen extremity should be treated with rest and elevation. A mild diuretic may be helpful. If there is no improvement, a compressor pump decreases the swelling, and the patient is then fitted with an elastic glove or sleeve. Most patients are not bothered enough by mild edema to wear an uncomfortable glove or sleeve and will treat themselves with elevation alone. Benzopyrones have been reported to decrease lymphedema but are not approved for this use in the USA. Rarely, edema may be severe enough to interfere with use of the limb.

Breast Reconstruction

Breast reconstruction, with the implantation of a prosthesis, is usually feasible after standard or modified radical mastectomy. Reconstruction should be discussed with patients prior to mastectomy, because it offers an important psychologic focal point for recovery. Reconstruction is not an obstacle to the diagnosis of recurrent cancer. The most common breast reconstruction has been implantation of a silicone gel prosthesis in the subpectoral plane between the pectoralis minor and pectoralis major muscles. The FDA has placed a moratorium on the purely cosmetic use of silicone gel implants because of possible leakage of silicone and associated autoimmune phenomena. This remote possibility should not prevent the cancer patient from having a reconstruction, and breast cancer patients are exempt from the moratorium. Most plastic surgeons currently would place a saline-filled prosthesis rather than a silicone gel implant. Alternatively, autologous tissue can be used for reconstruction. Autologous tissue flaps are aesthetically superior to implant reconstruction in most patients. They also have the advantage of not feeling like a foreign body to the patient. The most popular autologous technique currently is the trans-rectus abdominis muscle flap (TRAM flap), which is done by rotating the rectus abdominis muscle with attached fat and skin cephalad to make a breast mound. The free TRAM flap is done by completely removing the rectus with overlying fat and skin and using microvascular surgical techniques reconstructing the vascular supply on the chest wall. A latissimus dorsi flap can be swung from the back but offers less fullness than the TRAM flap and is therefore less acceptable cosmetically. Reconstruction may be performed immediately (at the time of initial mastectomy) or may be delayed until later, usually when the patient has completed adjuvant therapy.

Risks of Pregnancy

Data are insufficient to determine whether interruption of pregnancy improves the prognosis of patients who are discovered during pregnancy to have potentially curable breast cancer and who receive definitive treatment. Theoretically, the increasingly high levels of estrogen produced by the placenta as the pregnancy progresses could be detrimental to the patient with occult metastases of hormone-sensitive breast cancer. Moreover, occult metastases are present in most patients with positive axillary nodes, and treatment by adjuvant chemotherapy could be potentially harmful to the fetus, although chemotherapy has been given to pregnant women. Under these circumstances, interruption of early pregnancy seems reasonable, with progressively less rationale for the procedure as term approaches. The decision is affected by many factors, including the patient's desire to have the baby and the generally poor prognosis when axillary nodes are involved.

Equally important is the advice regarding future pregnancy (or abortion in case of pregnancy) to be given to women of child-bearing age who have had definitive treatment for breast cancer. Under these circumstances, one must assume that pregnancy will be harmful if occult metastases are present, though this has not been demonstrated. Patients whose tumors are ER-negative probably would not be affected by pregnancy. To date, no adverse effect of pregnancy on survival of pregnant women who have had breast cancer has been demonstrated, though most oncologists advise against it.

In patients with inoperable or metastatic cancer (stage IV disease), induced abortion is usually advisable because of the possible adverse effects of hormonal treatment, radiotherapy, or chemotherapy upon the fetus.

Brennan MJ et al: Focused review: Postmastectomy lymphedema. Arch Phys Med Rehabil 1996;77(3 Suppl): SD74. [NLM Cit ID: 96183530]

Canty L: Breast cancer risk: Protective effect of an early first full-term pregnancy versus increased risk of induced abortion. Oncol Nurs Forum 1997;24:1025. [NLM Cit ID: 97387567]

Cummings P et al: Estimating the risk of breast cancer in relation to the interval since last term pregnancy. Epidemiology 1997;8:488. [NLM Cit ID: 97416999]

Price J et al: Prevention and treatment of lymphedema after breast cancer. Am J Nurs 1997;97:34. [NLM Cit ID: 97457527]

Schusterman MA et al: Advances in reconstruction for cancer patients. Cancer Treat Res 1997;90:71. [NLM Cit ID: 98033962]

Velentgas P et al: Pregnancy after breast carcinoma: outcomes and influence on mortality. Cancer 1999;85:2424. [NLM Cit ID: 99284305] (Findings indicate that pregnancy after breast cancer diagnosis does not have adverse effect on survival.)

Williams JK et al: The effects of radiation after TRAM flap breast reconstruction. Plast Reconstr Surg 1997;100:1153. [NLM Cit ID: 97467567]

CARCINOMA OF THE MALE BREAST

Essentials of Diagnosis

- A painless lump beneath the areola in a man usually over 50 years of age.
- Nipple discharge, retraction, or ulceration may be present.

General Considerations

Breast cancer in men is a rare disease; the incidence is only about 1% of that in women. The average age at occurrence is about 60—somewhat older than the commonest presenting age in women. The prognosis, even in stage I cases, is worse in men than in women. Blood-borne metastases are commonly present when the male patient appears for initial treatment. These metastases may be latent and may not become manifest for many years. As in women, hormonal influences are probably related to the development of male breast cancer. There is a high incidence of both breast cancer and gynecomastia in Bantu men, theoretically owing to failure of estrogen inactivation by a damaged liver by associated liver disease.

Clinical Findings

A painless lump, occasionally associated with nipple discharge, retraction, erosion, or ulceration, is the chief complaint. Examination usually shows a hard, ill-defined, nontender mass beneath the nipple or areola. Gynecomastia not uncommonly precedes or accompanies breast cancer in men. Nipple discharge is an uncommon presentation for breast cancer in men, as it is in women, but is an ominous finding associated with carcinoma in nearly 75% of cases.

Breast cancer staging is the same in men as in women. Gynecomastia and metastatic cancer from another site (eg, prostate) must be considered in the differential diagnosis. Biopsy settles the issue.

Treatment

Treatment consists of modified radical mastectomy in operable patients, who should be chosen by the same criteria as women with the disease. Irradiation is the first step in treating localized metastases in the skin, lymph nodes, or skeleton that are causing symptoms. Examination of the cancer for hormone receptor proteins may prove to be of value in predicting response to endocrine ablation. Adjuvant chemotherapy is used for the same indications as in breast cancer in women.

Since breast cancer in men is frequently a disseminated disease, endocrine therapy is of considerable importance in its management. Tamoxifen and castration are the main therapeutic resources for management of advanced breast cancer in men. Tamoxifen (20 mg daily) should be the initial treatment, though there is little experience. Castration in advanced breast cancer is a successful palliative measure and more beneficial than the same procedure in women. Objective evidence of regression may be seen in 60–70% of men who are castrated—approximately twice the proportion in women. The average duration of tumor growth remission is about 30 months, and life is prolonged. Bone is the most frequent site of metastases from breast cancer in men (as in women), and castration relieves bone pain in most patients so treated. The longer the interval between mastectomy and recurrence, the longer the tumor growth remission following castration. As in women, there is no correlation between the histologic type of the tumor and the likelihood of remission following castration.

Aminoglutethimide (250 mg orally four times a day) should replace adrenalectomy in men as it has in women. Corticosteroid therapy alone has been considered to be efficacious but probably has no value when compared with major endocrine ablation.

Estrogen therapy—5 mg of diethylstilbestrol three times daily orally—may be effective as secondary hormonal manipulation after medical adrenalectomy (with aminoglutethimide). Androgen therapy may exacerbate bone pain. Chemotherapy should be administered for the same indications and using the same dosage schedules as for women with metastatic disease.

Prognosis

The prognosis of breast cancer is poorer in men than in women. The crude 5- and 10-year survival rates for clinical stage I breast cancer in men are about 58% and 38%, respectively. For clinical stage II disease, the 5- and 10-year survival rates are approximately 38% and 10%. The survival rates for all stages at 5 and 10 years are 36% and 17%. For those patients whose disease progresses despite treatment, meticulous efforts at palliative care are essential (see Chapter 5).

Friedman LS et al: Mutation analysis of *BRCA1* and *BRCA2* in a male breast cancer population. Am J Hum Genet 1997;60:313. [NLM Cit ID: 97164597] (Reports *BRCA* genetic mutations in male breast cancer.)

Joshi MG et al: Male breast carcinoma: An evaluation of prognostic factors contributing to a poor outcome. Cancer 1996;77:490. [NLM Cit ID: 96230004]

Memon MA et al: Male breast cancer. Br J Surg 1997;84:433. [NLM Cit ID: 97267557]

Winchester DJ: Male breast cancer. Semin Surg Oncol 1996;12:364. [NLM Cit ID: 97027161] (Diagnosis, pathogenesis, and clinical course.)

RELEVANT WORLD WIDE WEB SITES

[Breast Tutorial]
http://www.surgery.wisc.edu/wolberg/

[Mammography Teaching File]
http://metalab.unc.edu/jksmith/UNC-Radiology-Webserver/Mammography.html

Gynecology 17

See http://www.current-med.com/ch17.html for updated addresses of Web sites referenced in this chapter.

H. Trent MacKay, MD, MPH

ABNORMAL PREMENOPAUSAL BLEEDING

Normal menstrual bleeding lasts an average of 4 days (range, 2–7 days), with a mean blood loss of 40 mL. Blood loss of over 80 mL per cycle is abnormal and frequently produces anemia. Excessive bleeding, often with the passage of clots, may occur at regular menstrual intervals **(menorrhagia)** or irregular intervals **(dysfunctional uterine bleeding).** When there are fewer than 21 days between the onset of bleeding episodes, the cycles are likely to be anovular. **Ovulation bleeding,** a single episode of spotting between regular menses, is quite common. Heavier or irregular intermenstrual bleeding warrants investigation.

Dysfunctional uterine bleeding is usually caused by overgrowth of endometrium due to estrogen stimulation without adequate progesterone to stabilize growth; this occurs in anovular cycles. Anovulation associated with high estrogen levels commonly occurs in teenagers, in women aged late 30s to late 40s, and in extremely obese women or those with polycystic ovary syndrome.

Clinical Findings

A. Symptoms and Signs: The diagnosis of the disorders underlying the bleeding usually depends upon the following: (1) A careful description of the duration and amount of flow, related pain, and relationship to the last menstrual period (LMP). The presence of blood clots or the degree of inconvenience caused by the bleeding may be more useful indicators. (2) A history of pertinent illnesses. (3) A history of all medications the patient has taken in the past month. (4) A careful pelvic examination to look for pregnancy, uterine myomas, adnexal masses, or infection.

B. Laboratory Studies: Cervical smears should be obtained as needed for cytologic and culture studies. Blood studies should include a complete blood count, sedimentation rate, and glucose levels to rule out diabetes. Diabetes may occasionally initially present with abnormal bleeding. A test for pregnancy and studies of thyroid function and blood clotting should be considered in the clinical evaluation. Tests for ovulation in cyclic menorrhagia include basal body temperature records, serum progesterone measured 1 week before the expected onset of menses, and analysis of an endometrial biopsy specimen for secretory activity shortly before the onset of menstruation.

C. Imaging: Ultrasound may be useful to evaluate endometrial thickness or to diagnose intrauterine or ectopic pregnancy or adnexal masses. Endovaginal ultrasound with saline infusion sonohysterography may be used to diagnose endometrial polyps or subserous myomas. MRI can definitively diagnose submucous myomas and adenomyosis.

D. Cervical Biopsy and Endometrial Curettage: Biopsy, curettage, or aspiration of the endometrium and curettage of the endocervix are often necessary to diagnose the cause of bleeding. These and other invasive gynecologic diagnostic procedures are described in Table 17–1. Polyps, endometrial hyperplasia, and submucous myomas are commonly identified in this way. If cancer of the cervix is a possibility, multiple quadrant biopsies (or colposcopically directed biopsies) and endocervical curettage are indicated as first steps.

E. Hysteroscopy: Hysteroscopy can visualize endometrial polyps, submucous myomas, and exophytic endometrial cancers. It is useful immediately before D&C.

Treatment

Premenopausal patients with abnormal uterine bleeding include those with submucous myomas, infection, early abortion, or pelvic neoplasms. The history, physical examination, and laboratory findings should identify such patients, who require definitive therapy depending upon the cause of the bleeding. A large group of patients remains, most of whom have dysfunctional uterine bleeding on a hormonal basis.

Dysfunctional uterine bleeding can usually be treated hormonally; progestins, which limit and stabilize endometrial growth, are generally effective. Office D&C is usually not necessary in women under age 40. Medroxyprogesterone acetate, 10 mg/d, or

Table 17–1. Common gynecologic diagnostic procedures.

Colposcopy
Visualization of cervical, vaginal, or vulvar epithelium under 5–50× magnification to identify abnormal areas requiring biopsy. Used to identify genital warts on males as well as females. An office procedure.

D&C
Dilation of the cervix and curettage of the entire endometrial cavity, using a metal curette or suction cannula and often using forceps for the removal of endometrial polyps. Performed to diagnose endometrial disease and to stop heavy bleeding. Can usually be done in the office under local anesthesia.

Endometrial biopsy
Removal of one or more areas of the endometrium by means of a curette or small aspiration device without cervical dilation. Less accurate diagnostically than D&C. An office procedure performed under local anesthesia.

Endocervical curettage
Removal of endocervical epithelium with a small curette for diagnosis of cervical dysplasia and cancer. An office procedure performed under local anesthesia.

Hysteroscopy
Visual examination of the uterine cavity with a small fiberoptic endoscope passed through the cervix. Biopsies, excision of myomas, and other procedures can be performed. Can be done in the office under local anesthesia or in the operating room under general anesthesia.

Hysterosalpingography
Injection of radiopaque dye through the cervix to visualize the uterine cavity and oviducts. Mainly used in investigation of infertility.

Laparoscopy
Visualization of the abdominal and pelvic cavity through a small fiberoptic endoscope passed through a subumbilical incision. Permits diagnosis, tubal sterilization, and treatment of many conditions previously requiring laparotomy. General anesthesia is usually used.

norethindrone acetate, 5 mg/d, should be given for 10–14 days starting on day 15 of the cycle, following which withdrawal bleeding (so-called medical curettage) will occur. The treatment is repeated for several cycles; it can be reinstituted if amenorrhea or dysfunctional bleeding recurs. In young women who are bleeding actively, any of the combination oral contraceptives can be given four times daily for one or 2 days followed by two pills daily through day 5 and then one pill daily through day 20; after withdrawal bleeding occurs, pills are taken in the usual dosage for three cycles. In cases of intractable heavy bleeding, danazol, 200 mg four times daily, is sometimes used to create an atrophic endometrium. Alternatively, a GnRH agonist such as depot leuprolide, 3.75 mg intramuscularly monthly, or nafarelin, 0.2–0.4 mg intranasally twice daily, can be used for up to 6 months to create a temporary cessation of menstruation by ovarian suppression. Symptoms of hypoestrinism are common and occur early in treatment, while use beyond 6 months is associated with significant osteopenia that is reversible after therapy is terminated.

In cases of heavy bleeding, intravenous conjugated estrogens, 25 mg every 4 hours for three or four doses, can be used, followed by oral conjugated estrogens, 2.5 mg daily, or ethinyl estradiol, 20 μg daily, for 3 weeks, with the addition of medroxyprogesterone acetate, 10 mg daily for the last 10 days of treatment, or a combination oral contraceptive daily for 3 weeks. This will thicken the endometrium and control the bleeding. If the abnormal bleeding is not controlled by hormonal treatment, a D&C is necessary to check for incomplete abortion, polyps, submucous myomas, or endometrial cancer. In women over age 40, a D&C or careful endometrial biopsy is generally indicated to rule out neoplasm before beginning hormonal therapy.

Endometrial ablation through the hysteroscope with laser photocoagulation or electrocautery is an option; this technique is designed to reduce or prevent any future menstrual flow.

Nonsteroidal anti-inflammatory drugs such as ibuprofen, naproxen, or mefenamic acid in the usual anti-inflammatory doses will often reduce blood loss in menorrhagia—even that associated with an IUD.

Prolonged use of a progestin, as in a minipill, in injectable contraceptives, or in the therapy of endometriosis, can also lead to intermittent bleeding, sometimes severe. In this instance, the endometrium is atrophic and fragile. If bleeding occurs, it should be treated with estrogen as follows: ethinyl estradiol, 20 μg/d for 7 days, or conjugated estrogens, 1.25 mg/d for 7 days.

It is useful for the patient and the physician to discuss stressful situations or life-styles that may contribute to anovulation and dysfunctional bleeding, such as prolonged emotional turmoil or excessive use of drugs or alcohol.

Brenner PF: Differential diagnosis of abnormal uterine bleeding. Am J Obstet Gynecol 1996;175:766. [NLM Cit ID: 96426265] (Brief but complete summary of causes.)

Farquhar CM et al: An evaluation of the risk factors for endometrial hyperplasia in premenopausal women with abnormal menstrual bleeding. Am J Obstet Gynecol 1999;181:525. [NLM Cit ID: 99417433] (Risk factors included body weight > 90 kg, age > 45 years, infertility, family history of colon cancer, and nulliparity.)

Goldstein SR et al: Ultrasonography-based triage for perimenopausal patients with abnormal uterine bleeding. Am J Obstet Gynecol 1997;177:102. [NLM Cit ID: 97382587] (An approach to diagnosis that limits the need for operation.)

POSTMENOPAUSAL VAGINAL BLEEDING

Vaginal bleeding that occurs 6 months or more following cessation of menstrual function should be investigated. The most common causes are atrophic endometrium, endometrial proliferation, hyperplasia, endometrial or cervical cancer, and administration of estrogens without added progestin. Other causes include atrophic vaginitis, trauma, endometrial polyps, trophic ulcers of the cervix associated with prolapse of the uterus, and blood dyscrasias. Uterine bleeding is usually painless, but pain will be present if the cervix is stenotic, if bleeding is severe and rapid, or if infection or torsion or extrusion of a tumor is present. The patient may report a single episode of spotting or profuse bleeding for days or months.

Diagnosis

The vulva and vagina should be inspected for areas of bleeding, ulcers, or neoplasms. A cytologic smear of the cervix and vaginal pool should be taken. An unstained wet mount of vaginal fluid in saline and potassium hydroxide may reveal white blood cells, infective organisms, or basal epithelial cells indicative of a low estrogen effect. Endocervical curettage and sampling by aspiration of the endometrium, preferably preceded by hysteroscopy, should be performed next, and careful search for endometrial polyps should be made. The tissue obtained in the course of the hysteroscopic examination may reveal atrophy, polyps, endometrial hyperplasia (with or without an atypical glandular pattern), or cancer.

Transvaginal sonography can be used to measure endometrial thickness (< 5 mm indicating atrophy).

Treatment

Aspiration curettage (with polypectomy if indicated) will frequently be curative. If simple endometrial hyperplasia is found, give cyclic progestin therapy (medroxyprogesterone acetate, 10 mg/d, or norethindrone acetate, 5 mg/d) for 21 days of each month for 3 months. A repeat D&C or endometrial biopsy can then be performed, and if tissues are normal and estrogen replacement therapy is reinstituted, a progestin should be prescribed (as above) for the last 10–14 days of each estrogen cycle, followed by 5 days with no hormone therapy, so that the uterine lining will be shed. If endometrial hyperplasia with atypical cells or carcinoma of the endometrium is found, hysterectomy is necessary.

Briley M et al: The role of transvaginal ultrasound in the investigation of women with post-menopausal bleeding. Clin Radiol 1998;53:502. [NLM Cit ID: 98378191] (A cohort of 182 women with postmenopausal bleeding were followed over 16 months with transvaginal ultrasound and endometrial biopsy with the finding of a negative predictive value of 95% for an endometrial stripe less than 5 mm on ultrasound.)

Gredmark T et al: Histopathological findings in women with postmenopausal bleeding. Br J Obstet Gynecol 1995;102:133. [NLM Cit ID: 95275765] (Among 457 women with postmenopausal bleeding, 8% had cancer and 7% significant hyperplasia.)

PREMENSTRUAL SYNDROME (Premenstrual Tension)

The premenstrual syndrome is a recurrent, variable cluster of troublesome physical and emotional symptoms that develop during the 7–14 days before the onset of menses and subside when menstruation occurs. The syndrome intermittently affects about one-third of all premenopausal women, primarily those 25–40 years of age. In about 10% of affected women, the syndrome may be severe. Although not every woman experiences all the symptoms or signs at one time, many describe bloating, breast pain, ankle swelling, a sense of increased weight, skin disorders, irritability, aggressiveness, depression, inability to concentrate, libido change, lethargy, and food cravings.

The pathogenesis of premenstrual syndrome is still uncertain. Psychosocial factors may play a role. Suppression of ovarian function with a GnRH agonist has been shown to diminish all symptoms during therapy. Add-back therapy with estrogen and progestin may allow extended use of a GnRH agonist. Suppression of ovulation with an oral contraceptive is sometimes helpful, but the patient often complains that she still has premenstrual syndrome.

Current treatment methods are mainly empirical. The physician should provide the best support possible for the patient's emotional and physical distress. This includes the following:

(1) Careful evaluation of the patient, with understanding, explanation, and reassurance, is of first importance.

(2) Advise the patient to keep a daily diary of all symptoms for 2–3 months, to help in evaluating the timing and characteristics of the syndrome. If her symptoms occur throughout the month rather than in the 2 weeks before menses, she may be depressed or may have other emotional problems in addition to premenstrual syndrome.

(3) A diet emphasizing complex carbohydrates can be recommended. Foods high in sugar content and alcohol should be avoided to minimize reactive hypoglycemia. Use of caffeine should be minimized whenever tension and irritability predominate.

(4) Vitamin B_6, up to 100 mg/d, may be beneficial in the treatment of premenstrual symptoms and premenstrual depression. At this dosage level, neurologic side effects are rare.

(5) A program of regular conditioning exercise, such as jogging, has been found to decrease depression, anxiety, and fluid retention premenstrually in several studies.

(6) Serotonin reuptake inhibitors such as fluoxetine, 20 mg/d, are effective in relieving tension, irritability, and dysphoria with few side effects. Short-acting benzodiazepines have also been used, but the potential for addiction to these drugs makes their use problematic in this recurrent disorder.

(7) Luteal phase administration of danazol, 200 mg/d on cycle days 14–28, is effective in reducing symptoms of mastalgia. Other symptoms are not affected by this low-dose therapy.

Freeman EW et al: Full- or half-cycle treatment of severe premenstrual syndrome with a serotonergic antidepressant. J Clin Psychopharmacol 1999;19:3. [NLM Cit ID: 97409321] (The SSRI sertraline, 50–100 mg/d, in the luteal phase is as effective as full-cycle treatment for the relief of severe premenstrual symptoms.)

Wyatt KM et al: Efficacy of vitamin B_6 in the treatment of premenstrual syndrome: systematic review. BMJ 1999; 318:1375. [NLM Cit ID: 99267356] (Review of nine published randomized clinical trials shows an OR = 2.32 [95% CI, 1.95–2.54] compared with placebo for improvement in overall PMS symptoms and an OR = 1.69 [95% CI, 1.39–2.06] for improvement in PMS depressive symptoms with vitamin B_6, 50–100 mg/d.)

DYSMENORRHEA

1. PRIMARY DYSMENORRHEA

Primary dysmenorrhea is menstrual pain associated with ovular cycles in the absence of pathologic findings. The pain usually begins within 1–2 years after the menarche and may become more severe with time. The frequency of cases increases up to age 20 and then decreases with age and markedly with parity. Fifty to 75 percent of women are affected at some time, and 5–6% have incapacitating pain.

Primary dysmenorrhea is low, midline, wave-like, cramping pelvic pain often radiating to the back or inner thighs. Cramps may last for 1 or more days and may be associated with nausea, diarrhea, headache, and flushing. The pain is produced by uterine vasoconstriction, anoxia, and sustained contractions mediated by prostaglandins.

Clinical Findings

The pelvic examination is normal between menses; examination during menses may produce discomfort, but there are no pathologic findings.

Treatment

Nonsteroidal anti-inflammatory drugs (ibuprofen, ketoprofen, mefenamic acid, naproxen) are generally helpful. Drugs should be started at the onset of bleeding to avoid inadvertent drug use during early pregnancy. Medication should be continued on a regular basis for 2–3 days. Ovulation can be suppressed and dysmenorrhea usually prevented by oral contraceptives.

2. SECONDARY DYSMENORRHEA

Secondary dysmenorrhea is menstrual pain for which an organic cause exists. It usually begins well after menarche, sometimes even as late as the third or fourth decade of life.

Clinical Findings

The history and physical examination commonly suggest endometriosis or pelvic inflammatory disease. Other causes may be submucous myoma, IUD use, cervical stenosis with obstruction, or blind uterine horn (rare).

Diagnosis

Laparoscopy is often needed to differentiate endometriosis from pelvic inflammatory disease. Submucous myomas can be detected most reliably by MRI but also by hysterogram, by hysteroscopy, or by passing a sound or curette over the uterine cavity during D&C. Cervical stenosis may result from induced abortion, creating crampy pain at the time of expected menses with no blood flow; this is easily cured by passing a sound into the uterine cavity after administering a paracervical block.

Treatment

A. Specific Measures: Periodic use of analgesics, including the nonsteroidal anti-inflammatory drugs given for primary dysmenorrhea, may be beneficial, and oral contraceptives may give relief, particularly in endometriosis. Danazol and GnRH agonists are effective in the treatment of endometriosis (see below).

B. Surgical Measures: If disability is marked or prolonged, laparoscopy or exploratory laparotomy is usually warranted. Definitive surgery depends upon the degree of disability and the findings at operation.

Coco AS: Primary dysmenorrhea. Am Fam Physician 1999;60:489. [NLM Cit ID 99392893] (Epidemiology, etiology, diagnosis, and treatment.)

VAGINITIS

Inflammation and infection of the vagina are common gynecologic problems, resulting from a variety of pathogens, allergic reactions to vaginal contraceptives or other products, or the friction of coitus. The normal vaginal pH is 4.5 or less, and lactobacillus is the predominant organism. At the time of the midcycle estrogen surge, clear, elastic, mucoid secretions from the cervical os are often profuse. In the luteal phase and during pregnancy, vaginal secretions are thicker, white, and sometimes adherent to the vaginal walls. These normal secretions can be confused with vaginitis by concerned women.

Clinical Findings

When the patient complains of vaginal irritation, pain, or unusual discharge, a careful history should be taken, noting the onset of the last menstrual period; recent sexual activity; use of contraceptives, tampons, or douches; and the presence of vaginal burning, pain, pruritus, or unusually profuse or malodorous discharge. The physical examination should include careful inspection of the vulva and speculum examination of the vagina and cervix. The cervix is cultured for gonococcus or chlamydia if applicable. A specimen of vaginal discharge is examined under the microscope in a drop of 0.9% saline solution to look for trichomonads or clue cells and in a drop of 10% potassium hydroxide to search for candida. The vaginal pH should be tested; it is frequently greater than 4.5 in infections due to trichomonads and bacterial vaginosis. A bimanual examination to look for evidence of pelvic infection should follow.

A. *Candida albicans:* Pregnancy, diabetes, and use of broad-spectrum antibiotics or corticosteroids predispose to candida infections. Heat, moisture, and occlusive clothing also contribute to the risk. Pruritus, vulvovaginal erythema, and a white curd-like discharge that is not malodorous are found. Microscopic examination with 10% potassium hydroxide reveals filaments and spores. Cultures with Nickerson's medium may be used if candida is suspected but not demonstrated.

B. *Trichomonas vaginalis:* This protozoal flagellate infects the vagina, Skene's ducts, and lower urinary tract in women and the lower genitourinary tract in men. It is transmitted through coitus. Pruritus and a malodorous frothy, yellow-green discharge occur, along with diffuse vaginal erythema and red macular lesions on the cervix in severe cases. Motile organisms with flagella are seen by microscopic examination of a wet mount with saline solution.

C. Bacterial Vaginosis: This condition is considered to be a polymicrobial disease which is not sexually transmitted. An overgrowth of gardnerella and other anaerobes is often associated with increased malodorous discharge without obvious vulvitis or vaginitis. The discharge is grayish and sometimes frothy, with a pH of 5.0–5.5. An amine-like ("fishy") odor is present if a drop of discharge is alkalinized with 10% potassium hydroxide. On wet mount in saline, epithelial cells are covered with bacteria to such an extent that cell borders are obscured (clue cells). Vaginal cultures are generally not useful in diagnosis.

D. Condylomata Acuminata (Genital Warts): Warty growths on the vulva, perianal area, vaginal walls, or cervix are caused by various types of the human papillomavirus. They are sexually transmitted. Pregnancy and immunosuppression favor growth. Vulvar lesions may be obviously wart-like or may be diagnosed only after application of 4% acetic acid (vinegar) and colposcopy, when they appear whitish, with prominent papillae. Fissures may be present at the fourchette. Vaginal lesions may show diffuse hypertrophy or a cobblestone appearance. Cervical lesions may be visible only by colposcopy after pretreatment with 4% acetic acid. These lesions may be related to dysplasia and cervical cancer. Vulvar cancer is also currently considered to be associated with the human papillomavirus.

Treatment

A. *Candida albicans:* Effective treatment can be given in several ways:

1. Three-day regimens–Butoconazole (2% cream, 5 g), clotrimazole (two 100 mg vaginal tablets), terconazole (0.8% cream, 5 g, or 80 mg suppository), or miconazole (200 mg vaginal suppository).

2. Seven-day regimens–Clotrimazole (1% cream or 100 mg vaginal tablet), miconazole (2% cream, 5 g, or 100 mg vaginal suppository), or terconazole (0.4% cream, 5 g).

3. Single-dose regimens–Clotrimazole (500 mg tablet) or ticconazole ointment (6.5%, 5 g). Fluconazole, 150 mg orally in a single dose, is also effective.

4. Fourteen-day regimens–Nystatin (100,000 unit vaginal tablet).

5. Recurrent vulvovaginitis–Ketoconazole, 100 mg orally once daily for up to 6 months.

B. *Trichomonas vaginalis:* Treatment of both partners simultaneously is necessary; metronidazole, 2 g as a single dose or 500 mg twice daily for 7 days, is usually employed. In the case of treatment failure, the patient should be retreated with metronidazole, 500 mg twice a day for 7 days. If repeated failure occurs in the absence of infection, treat with a single dose of 2 g of metronidazole once daily for 3–5 days. If this is not effective in eradicating the organisms, metronidazole susceptibility testing can be arranged with the CDC at 404-639-8315.

C. Bacterial Vaginosis: The recommended regimens are metronidazole, 500 mg twice daily for 7 days; clindamycin vaginal cream (2%, 5 g), once daily for 7 days; or metronidazole gel (0.75%, 5 g), twice daily for 5 days. Alternative regimens include metronidazole, 2 g orally as a single dose, or clindamycin, 300 mg orally twice daily for 7 days.

D. Condylomata Acuminata: Recommended treatments for vulvar warts include podophyllum resin 25% in tincture of benzoin (do not use during pregnancy or on bleeding lesions) or 80–90% trichloroacetic or bichloroacetic acid, carefully applied to avoid the surrounding skin. The pain of bi- or trichloroacetic acid application can be lessened by a sodium bicarbonate paste applied immediately after treatment. Podophyllum resin must be washed off after 2–4 hours. Freezing with liquid nitrogen or a cryoprobe and electrocautery are also effective. Patient-applied regimens include podofilox 0.5% solution or gel and imiquimod 5% cream. Vaginal warts may be treated with cryotherapy with liquid nitrogen, trichloroacetic acid, or podophyllum resin. Extensive warts may require treatment with CO_2 laser under local or general anesthesia. Interferon is not recommended for routine use because it is very expensive, associated with systemic side effects, and no more effective than other therapies. Routine examination of sex partners is not necessary for the management of genital warts since the risk of reinfection is probably minimal and curative therapy to prevent transmission is not available. However, partners may wish to be examined for detection and treatment of genital warts and other STDs.

1998 Guidelines for treatment of sexually transmitted diseases. MMWR Morb Mortal Wkly Rep 1998;47(RR-1):1. [NLM Cit ID: 98120951]

1998 Guidelines for the treatment of sexually transmitted diseases. Clin Infect Dis 1999;28(Suppl 1). [NLM Cit ID: 99152430–99152439] (Series of articles constituting the background information for the 1998 CDC STD Treatment Guidelines.)

CERVICITIS

Infection of the cervix must be distinguished from physiologic ectopy of columnar epithelium, which is common in young women. Mucopurulent cervicitis is characterized by a red edematous cervix with a purulent yellow discharge. The infection may result from a sexually transmitted pathogen such as *Neisseria gonorrhoeae,* chlamydia, or herpesvirus (which presents with vesicles and ulcers on the cervix during a primary herpetic infection), though in most cases none of these organisms can be isolated.

Mucopurulent cervicitis is an insensitive predictor of either gonorrheal or chlamydial infection and in addition has a low positive predictive value. Treatment should be based on microbiologic testing. Presumptive antibiotic treatment of mucopurulent cervicitis is not indicated unless there is a high prevalence of either *N gonorrhoeae* or chlamydia in the population or if the patient is unlikely to return for treatment. (See Chapter 33 for discussion.) Three months after treatment, approximately 20% of women will have persistent or recurrent mucopus in the cervix, not explained by relapse or reinfection.

Thorpe EM Jr et al: Chlamydial cervicitis and urethritis: Single dose treatment compared with doxycycline for seven days in community-based practices. Genitourin Med 1996;72:93. [NLM Cit ID: 96273394] (Single-dose azithromycin and doxycycline for 7 days are equally effective.)

CERVICAL POLYPS

Cervical polyps commonly occur after menarche and are occasionally noted in postmenopausal women. The cause is not known, but inflammation may play an etiologic role. The principal symptoms are discharge and abnormal vaginal bleeding. However, abnormal bleeding should not be ascribed to a cervical polyp without sampling the endocervix and endometrium. The polyps are visible in the cervical os on speculum examination.

Cervical polyps must be differentiated from polypoid neoplastic disease of the endometrium, small submucous pedunculated myomas, and endometrial polyps. Cervical polyps rarely contain malignant foci.

Treatment

Cervical polyps can generally be removed in the office by avulsion with a uterine packing forceps or ring forceps. If the cervix is soft, patulous, or definitely dilated and the polyp is large, surgical D&C is required (especially if the pedicle is not readily visible). Because of the possibility of endometrial disease, cervical polypectomy should be accompanied by endometrial sampling, and all tissue removed should be submitted for microscopic examination.

Pradhan S et al: Dilatation and curettage in patients with cervical polyps: A retrospective analysis. Br J Obstet Gynecol 1995;102:415. [NLM Cit ID: 95337011]

CYST & ABSCESS OF BARTHOLIN'S DUCT

Trauma or infection may involve Bartholin's duct, causing obstruction of the gland. Drainage of secretions is prevented, leading to pain, swelling, and abscess formation. The infection usually resolves and pain disappears, but stenosis of the duct outlet with distention often persists. Reinfection causes recurrent tenderness and further enlargement of the duct.

The principal symptoms are periodic painful swelling on either side of the introitus and dyspareunia. A fluctuant swelling 1–4 cm in diameter in the inferior portion of either labium minus is a sign of occlusion of Bartholin's duct. Tenderness is evidence of active infection.

Pus or secretions from the gland should be cultured for gonococci, chlamydiae, and other pathogens and treated accordingly (see Chapter 33); frequent warm soaks may be helpful. If an abscess develops, aspiration or incision and drainage are the simplest forms of therapy, but the problem may recur. Marsupialization, incision and drainage with the insertion of an indwelling Word catheter, or laser treatment will establish a new duct opening. An asymptomatic cyst does not require therapy.

EFFECTS OF EXPOSURE TO DIETHYLSTILBESTROL IN UTERO

Between 1947 and 1971, diethylstilbestrol (DES) was widely used in the USA for diabetic women during pregnancy and to treat threatened abortion. It is estimated that 2–3 million fetuses were exposed. A relationship between fetal DES exposure and clear cell carcinoma of the vagina was later discovered, and a number of other related anomalies have since been noted. In one-third of all exposed women, there are changes in the vagina (adenosis, septa), cervix (deformities and hypoplasia of the vaginal portion of the cervix), or uterus (T-shaped cavity).

At present, all exposed women are advised to have an initial colposcopic examination to outline vaginal and cervical areas of abnormal epithelium, followed by cytologic examination of the vagina (all four quadrants of the upper half of the vagina) and cervix at yearly intervals. Lugol's iodine stain of the vagina and cervix will also outline areas of metaplastic squamous epithelium.

Many women are not aware of having been exposed to DES. Therefore, in the age groups at risk (27–53 years), examiners should pay attention to structural changes of the vagina and cervix that may signal the possibility of DES exposure and indicate the need for follow-up.

The incidence of clear cell carcinoma is approximately one in 1000 exposed women, and the incidence of cervical and vaginal intraepithelial neoplasia (dysplasia and carcinoma in situ) is twice as high as in unexposed women. DES daughters have more difficulty conceiving and have an increased incidence of early abortion, ectopic pregnancy, and premature births. In addition, mothers treated with DES in pregnancy appear to have a small increase in the incidence of breast cancer, beginning 20 years after exposure.

Goldberg JM et al: Effect of diethylstilbestrol on reproductive function. Fertil Steril 1999;72:1. [NLM Cit ID: 99355093] (Review of published literature on in utero diethylstilbestrol exposure and the effects on rates of fertility, ectopic pregnancy, spontaneous abortion, and live births.)

CERVICAL INTRAEPITHELIAL NEOPLASIA (CIN; Dysplasia of the Cervix)

The squamocolumnar junction of the cervix is an area of active squamous cell proliferation. In childhood, this junction is located on the exposed vaginal portion of the cervix. At puberty, because of hormonal influence and possibly because of changes in the vaginal pH, the squamous margin begins to encroach on the single-layered, mucus-secreting epithelium, creating an area of metaplasia (transformation zone). Factors associated with coitus (see Prevention, below) may lead to cellular abnormalities, which over a period of time can result in the development of squamous cell dysplasia or cancer. There are varying degrees of dysplasia (Table 17–2), defined by the degree of cellular atypia; all types must be observed and treated if they persist or become more severe. At present, the malignant potential of a specific lesion cannot be predicted. Some lesions remain stable for long periods of time; some regress; and others advance.

Clinical Findings

There are no specific symptoms or signs of cervical intraepithelial neoplasia. The presumptive diagnosis is made by cytologic screening of an asymptomatic population with no grossly visible cervical changes. All visibly abnormal cervical lesions should be biopsied.

Diagnosis

A. Cytologic Examination (Papanicolaou Smear): Specimens should be taken from a nonmenstruating patient, spread on a single slide, and fixed or rinsed directly into preservative solution if a thin layer slide system (ThinPrep) is to be used. A specimen should be obtained from the squamocolumnar junction with a wooden or plastic spatula and from the endocervix with a cotton swab or nylon brush.

Cytologic reports from the laboratory may describe findings in one of several ways (see Table 17–2). While use of class I–IV is decreasing, the CIN classification continues to be used along with a description of abnormal cells, including evidence of human papillomavirus (HPV). The term "squamous intraepithelial lesions (SIL)," low-grade or high-grade, is increasingly used. Cytopathologists consider a Papanicolaou smear to be a medical consultation and will recommend further diagnostic procedures, treatment for infection, and comments on factors preventing adequate evaluation of the specimen. The role of HPV testing of cytologic smears remains undefined, and this procedure is not currently recommended for routine use.

Table 17–2. Classification systems for Papanicolaou smears.

Numerical	Dysplasia	CIN	Bethesda System
1	Benign	Benign	Normal
2	Benign with inflammation	Benign with inflammation	Normal
3	Mild dysplasia	CIN I	Low-grade SIL
3	Moderate dysplasia	CIN II	
3	Severe dysplasia	CIN III	High-grade SIL
4	Carcinoma in situ		
5	Invasive cancer	Invasive cancer	Invasive cancer

CIN = cervical intraepithelial neoplasia; SIL = squamous intraepithelial lesion.

B. Colposcopy: Viewing the cervix with 10–20× magnification allows for assessment of the size and margins of an abnormal transformation zone and determination of extension into the endocervical canal. The application of 3–5% acetic acid (vinegar) dissolves mucus, and the acid's desiccating action sharpens the contrast between normal and actively proliferating squamous epithelium. Abnormal changes include white patches and vascular atypia, which indicate areas of greatest cellular activity. Paint the cervix with Lugol's solution (strong iodine solution [Schiller's test]). Normal squamous epithelium will take the stain; nonstaining squamous epithelium should be biopsied. (The single-layered, mucus-secreting endocervical tissue will not stain either but can readily be distinguished by its darker pink, shinier appearance.)

C. Biopsy: Colposcopically directed punch biopsy and endocervical curettage are office procedures. If colposcopic examination is not available, the normal-appearing cervix shedding atypical cells can be evaluated by endocervical curettage and multiple punch biopsies of nonstaining squamous epithelium or biopsies from each quadrant of the cervix.

Data from both cervical biopsy and endocervical curettage are important in deciding on treatment.

Prevention

Current data suggest that cervical infection with the human papillomavirus (HPV) is associated with a high percentage of all cervical dysplasias and cancers. There are over 60 recognized HPV subtypes, of which types 6 and 11 tend to cause mild dysplasia, while types 16, 18, 31, and others cause higher grade cellular changes.

Cervical cancer almost never occurs in virginal women; it is epidemiologically related to the number of sexual partners a woman has had and the number of other female partners a male partner has had. Use of the diaphragm or condom has a protective effect. Long-term oral contraceptive users develop more dysplasias and cancers of the cervix than users of other forms of birth control, and smokers are also more at risk. Preventive measures include the following:

(1) Regular cytologic screening to detect abnormalities.

(2) Limiting the number of sexual partners.

(3) Using a diaphragm or condom for coitus.

(4) Stopping smoking.

Women with HIV infection appear to be at increased risk of the disease and of recurrent disease after treatment. Women with HIV infection should receive regular cytologic screening and should be followed closely after treatment for cervical intraepithelial neoplasia.

Treatment

Treatment varies depending on the degree and extent of cervical intraepithelial neoplasia. Biopsies should always precede treatment.

A. Cauterization or Cryosurgery: The use of either hot cauterization or freezing (cryosurgery) is effective for noninvasive small lesions visible on the cervix without endocervical extension.

B. CO_2 Laser: This well-controlled method minimizes tissue destruction. It is colposcopically directed and requires special training. It may be used with large visible lesions. In current practice it involves the vaporization of the transformation zone on the cervix and the distal 5–7 mm of endocervical canal.

C. Loop Resection: When the CIN is clearly visible in its entirety, a wire loop can be used for excisional biopsy. Cutting and hemostasis are effected with a low-voltage electrosurgical machine (Bovie). This office procedure with local anesthesia is quick and uncomplicated.

D. Conization of the Cervix: Conization is surgical removal of the entire transformation zone and endocervical canal. It should be reserved for cases of severe dysplasia or cancer in situ (CIN III), particularly those with endocervical extension. The procedure can be performed with the scalpel, the CO_2 laser, or by large-loop excision.

E. Follow-Up: Because recurrence is possible—especially in the first 2 years after treatment—and because the false-negative rate of a single cervical cytologic test is 20%, close follow-up is imperative. Vaginal cytologic examination should be repeated at 3-month intervals for at least 1 year.

Kaufmann RH et al: Relevance of human papillomavirus screening in management of cervical intraepithelial neoplasia. Am J Obstet Gynecol 1997;176:87. [NLM Cit ID: 97176556] (At present, HPV screening does not appear to be useful for identifying women with abnormal Papanicolaou smears who can be followed by cytology alone.)

Pearce KF et al: Cytopathological findings on vaginal Papanicolaou smears after hysterectomy for benign gynecologic disease. N Engl J Med 1996;335:1559. [NLM Cit ID: 97042244] (Because of the very low rate of abnormal Papanicolaou smears in women who have had a hysterectomy for benign disease, routine Papanicolaou smear screening is not justified in this population.)

Sawaya GF et al: Cervical cancer screening: Which techniques should be used and why? Clin Obstet Gynecol 1999;42:922. [NLM Cit ID: 20039000] (Existing data do not allow evidence-based recommendations for the use of liquid-based Pap smear methods. Pap smear reinterpretation technologies that review conventionally-read negative Pap smears are likely to be of minimal benefit, and women requesting such services should be informed of the risks and benefits to decide if the additional cost is justified.)

CARCINOMA OF THE CERVIX

Essentials of Diagnosis

- Abnormal uterine bleeding and vaginal discharge.
- Cervical lesion may be visible on inspection as a tumor or ulceration.

- Vaginal cytology usually positive; must be confirmed by biopsy.

General Considerations

Cancer appears first in the intraepithelial layers (the preinvasive stage, or carcinoma in situ). Preinvasive cancer (CIN III) is a common diagnosis in women 25–40 years of age and is etiologically related to infection with the human papillomavirus. Two to 10 years are required for carcinoma to penetrate the basement membrane and invade the tissues. After invasion, death usually occurs within 3–5 years in untreated or unresponsive patients.

Clinical Findings

A. Symptoms and Signs: The most common signs are metrorrhagia, postcoital spotting, and cervical ulceration. Bloody or purulent, odorous, nonpruritic discharge may appear after invasion. Bladder and rectal dysfunction or fistulas and pain are late symptoms.

B. Cervical Biopsy and Endocervical Curettage, or Conization: These procedures are necessary steps after a positive Papanicolaou smear to determine the extent and depth of invasion of the cancer. Even if the smear is positive, treatment is never justified until definitive diagnosis has been established through biopsy.

C. "Staging," or Estimate of Gross Spread of Cancer of the Cervix: The depth of penetration of the malignant cells beyond the basement membrane is a reliable clinical guide to the extent of primary cancer within the cervix and the likelihood of metastases. It is customary to stage cancers of the cervix under anesthesia as shown in Table 17–3. Further assessment may be carried out by abdominal and pelvic CT scanning or MRI.

Complications

Metastases to regional lymph nodes occur with increasing frequency from stage I to stage IV. Paracervical extension occurs in all directions from the cervix. The ureters are often obstructed lateral to the cervix, causing hydroureter and hydronephrosis and consequently impaired kidney function. Almost two-thirds of patients with untreated carcinoma of the cervix die of uremia when ureteral obstruction is bilateral. Pain in the back, in the distribution of the lumbosacral plexus, is often indicative of neurologic involvement. Gross edema of the legs may be indicative of vascular and lymphatic stasis due to tumor.

Vaginal fistulas to the rectum and urinary tract are severe late complications. Hemorrhage is the cause of death in 10–20% of patients with extensive invasive carcinoma.

Treatment

A. Emergency Measures: Vaginal hemorrhage originates from gross ulceration and cavitation in stage II–IV cervical carcinoma. Ligation and suturing of the cervix are usually not feasible, but ligation of the uterine or hypogastric arteries may be lifesaving when other measures fail. Styptics such as Monsel's solution or acetone are effective, although delayed sloughing may result in further bleeding. Wet vaginal packing is helpful. Emergency irradiation usually controls bleeding.

B. Specific Measures:

1. Carcinoma in situ (stage 0)–In women who have completed childbearing, total hysterectomy is the treatment of choice. In women who wish to re-

Table 17–3. International classification of cancer of the cervix.[1]

Stage	Description
Preinvasive carcinoma	
Stage 0	Carcinoma in situ, intraepithelial carcinoma.
Invasive carcinoma	
Stage I	Carcinoma strictly confined to the cervix (extension to the corpus should be disregarded).
IA	Invasive cancer diagnosed only by microscopy. All gross lesions, even with superficial invasion, are stage IB. Invasion is limited to maximum depth of 5 mm from the base of epithelium from which it originates and no wider than 7 mm. Vascular space involvement should not alter staging.
	IA1 Measured invasion of stroma no greater than 3 mm in depth and no wider than 7 mm.
	IA2 Measured invasion of stroma greater than 3 mm in depth and no greater than 5 mm in depth and no wider than 7 mm.
IB	Clinical lesions confined to the cervix or preclinical lesions greater than 1A.
	IB1 Clinical lesions no greater than 4 cm in size.
	IB2 Clinical lesions greater than 4 cm in size.
Stage II	Carcinoma extends beyond the cervix but has not extended to the pelvic wall. The carcinoma involves the vagina but not as far as the lower third.
IIA	No obvious parametrial involvement.
IIB	Obvious parametrial involvement.
Stage III	Carcinoma has extended either to the lower third of the vagina or to the pelvic sidewall. All cases of hydronephrosis or nonfunctioning kidney, unless known to be due to other causes.
IIIA	Involvement of lower third of vagina. No extension to pelvic sidewall.
IIIB	Extension onto the pelvic wall and/or hydronephrosis or nonfunctioning kidney.
Stage IV	Carcinoma extended beyond the true pelvis or clinically involving the mucosa of the bladder or rectum. Does not include edema of bladder mucosa.
IVA	Spread of growth to adjacent organs (ie, rectum or bladder with positive biopsy from those organs).
IVB	Spread of growth to distant organs.

[1]Shepherd JH: Staging announcement: FIGO staging of gynecologic cancers: cervical and vulva. Int J Gynecol Cancer 1995;5:319.

tain the uterus, acceptable alternatives include cervical conization or ablation of the lesion with cryotherapy or laser. Close follow-up with Papanicolaou smears every 3 months for 1 year and every 6 months for another year is necessary after cryotherapy or laser.

2. Invasive carcinoma–Microinvasive carcinoma (stage IA) is treated with simple, extrafascial hysterectomy. Stage IB and stage IIA cancers may be treated with either radical hysterectomy or radiation therapy. Stage IIB and stage III and IV cancers must be treated with radiation therapy. Because radical surgery results in fewer long-term complications than irradiation and may allow preservation of ovarian function, it may be the preferred mode of therapy in younger women without contraindications to major surgery.

Prognosis

The overall 5-year relative survival rate for carcinoma of the cervix is 68% in white women and 55% in black women in the United States. Survival rates are inversely proportionate to the stage of cancer: stage 0, 99–100%; stage IA, > 95%; stage IB-IIA, 80–90%; stage IIB, 65%; stage III, 40%; stage IV, < 20%.

[Cervical Cancer—American Cancer Society] http://www3.cancer.org/cancerinfo/main_cont.asp?st=pr&ct=8

[Cervical Cancer—National Cancer Institute-CancerNet] http://cancernet.nci.nih.gov/clinpdq/soa/Cervical_cancer_Physician.html

Cannistra SA et al: Cancer of the uterine cervix. (Medical Progress.) N Engl J Med 1996;334:1030. [NLM Cit ID: 96177835]

National Institutes of Health Consensus Development Conference statement on cervical cancer, April 1–3, 1996. Gynecol Oncol 1997;66:351. [NLM Cit ID: 97457833] (Guidelines for screening, prevention and treatment of cervical cancer.)

LEIOMYOMA OF THE UTERUS (Fibroid Tumor)

Essentials of Diagnosis

- Irregular enlargement of the uterus (may be asymptomatic).
- Heavy or irregular vaginal bleeding, dysmenorrhea.
- Acute and recurrent pelvic pain if the tumor becomes twisted on its pedicle or infarcted.
- Symptoms due to pressure on neighboring organs (large tumors).

General Considerations

Uterine leiomyomas are the most common benign neoplasm of the female genital tract. It is a discrete, round, firm, often multiple uterine tumor composed of smooth muscle and connective tissue. The most convenient classification is by anatomic location: (1) intramural, (2) submucous, (3) subserous, (4) intraligamentous, (5) parasitic (ie, deriving its blood supply from an organ to which it becomes attached), and (6) cervical. A submucous myoma may become pedunculated and descend through the cervix into the vagina.

Clinical Findings

A. Symptoms and Signs: In nonpregnant women, myomas are frequently asymptomatic. However, they can cause urinary frequency, dysmenorrhea, heavy bleeding (often with anemia), or other complications due to the presence of an abdominal mass. Occasionally, degeneration occurs, causing intense pain. Infertility may be due to a myoma that significantly distorts the uterine cavity.

B. Laboratory Findings: Hemoglobin levels may be decreased as a result of blood loss, but in rare cases polycythemia is present, presumably as a result of the production of erythropoietin by the myomas.

C. Imaging: Ultrasonography will confirm the presence of uterine myomas and can be used sequentially to monitor growth. When multiple subserous or pedunculated myomas are being followed, ultrasonography is important to exclude ovarian masses. MRI can delineate intramural and submucous myomas accurately. Hysterography or hysteroscopy can also confirm cervical or submucous myomas.

Differential Diagnosis

Irregular myomatous enlargement of the uterus must be differentiated from the similar but symmetric enlargement that may occur with pregnancy or adenomyosis (the presence of endometrial glands and stroma in the myometrium). Subserous myomas must be distinguished from ovarian tumors. Leiomyosarcoma is an unusual tumor occurring in 0.5% of women operated on for symptomatic myoma. It is very rare under the age of 40 and increases in incidence thereafter.

Treatment

A. Emergency Measures: If the patient is markedly anemic as a result of long, heavy menstrual periods, preoperative treatment with depot medroxyprogesterone acetate, 150 mg intramuscularly every 28 days, or danazol, 400–800 mg orally daily, will slow or stop bleeding, and medical treatment of anemia can be given prior to surgery. Emergency surgery is required for acute torsion of a pedunculated myoma. The only emergency indication for myomectomy during pregnancy is torsion; abortion is not an inevitable result.

B. Specific Measures: Women who have small asymptomatic myomas should be examined at 6-month intervals. If necessary, elective myomectomy can be done to preserve the uterus. Myomas do not require surgery on an urgent basis unless they cause significant pressure on the ureters, bladder, or bowel or severe bleeding leading to anemia or unless they are undergoing rapid growth. Cervical myomas larger than 3–4 cm in diameter or pedunculated myomas that protrude through the cervix must be removed. Submucous myomas can be removed using a hysteroscope and laser or resection instruments.

Because the risk of surgical complications increases with the increasing size of the myoma, preoperative reduction of myoma size is desirable. GnRH analogs such as depot leuprolide, 3.75 mg intramuscularly monthly, or nafarelin, 0.2–0.4 mg intranasally twice a day, are used preoperatively for 2- to 3-month periods to induce reversible hypogonadism, which temporarily reduces the size of myomas, suppresses their further growth, and reduces surrounding vascularity.

C. Surgical Measures: Surgical measures available for the treatment of myoma are myomectomy and total or subtotal abdominal, vaginal, or laparoscopy-assisted vaginal hysterectomy. Myomectomy is the treatment of choice during the child-bearing years. A recent development is transcatheter bilateral uterine artery embolization. While the approach is promising, additional data on long-term results are needed.

Prognosis

Surgical therapy is curative. Future pregnancies are not endangered by myomectomy, although cesarean delivery may be necessary after wide dissection with entry into the uterine cavity.

Chappatte O: Current fibroid management. Practitioner 1999;243:474. [NLM Cit ID: 99405481] (Summary of current diagnosis and management.)

CARCINOMA OF THE ENDOMETRIUM

Adenocarcinoma of the uterine corpus is the second most common cancer of the female genital tract. It occurs most often in women 50–70 years of age. Some patients will have taken unopposed estrogen in the past; their increased risk appears to persist for 10 or more years after stopping the drug. Obesity, nulliparity, diabetes, and polycystic ovaries with prolonged anovulation and the extended use of tamoxifen for the treatment of breast cancer are also risk factors.

Abnormal bleeding is the presenting sign in 80% of cases. Endometrial carcinoma may cause obstruction of the cervix with collection of pus (pyometra) or blood (hematometra) causing lower abdominal pain. However, pain generally occurs late in the disease, with metastases or infection.

Papanicolaou smears of the cervix occasionally show atypical endometrial cells but are an insensitive diagnostic tool. Endocervical and endometrial sampling is the only reliable means of diagnosis. Adequate specimens of each can usually be obtained during an office procedure performed following local anesthesia (paracervical block). Simultaneous hysteroscopy can be a valuable addition in order to localize polyps or other lesions within the uterine cavity. Vaginal ultrasonography may be used to determine the thickness of the endometrium as an indication of hypertrophy and possible neoplastic change.

Pathologic assessment is important in differentiating hyperplasias, which often can be treated with cyclic oral progestins.

Prevention

Prompt endometrial sampling for patients who report abnormal menstrual bleeding or postmenopausal uterine bleeding will reveal many incipient as well as clinical cases of endometrial cancer. Postmenopausal women taking estrogens or younger women with prolonged anovulation can be given oral progestins for 13 days at the end of each estrogen cycle in order to promote periodic shedding of the uterine lining; this has been associated with a decreased incidence of uterine adenocarcinoma.

Staging

Examination under anesthesia, endometrial and endocervical sampling, chest x-ray, intravenous urography, cystoscopy, sigmoidoscopy, transvaginal sonography, and MRI will help determine the extent of the disease and its appropriate treatment. The staging is based on the surgical and pathologic evaluation.

Treatment

Treatment consists of total hysterectomy and bilateral salpingo-oophorectomy. Peritoneal material for cytologic examination is routinely taken. Preliminary external irradiation or intracavitary radium therapy is indicated if the cancer is poorly differentiated or if the uterus is definitely enlarged in the absence of myomas. If invasion deep into the myometrium has occurred or if sampled preaortic lymph nodes are positive for tumor, postoperative irradiation is indicated.

Palliation of advanced or metastatic endometrial adenocarcinoma may be accomplished with large doses of progestins, eg, medroxyprogesterone, 400 mg intramuscularly weekly, or megestrol acetate, 80–160 mg daily orally.

Prognosis

With early diagnosis and treatment, the 5-year survival is 80–85%.

[Endometrial Cancer—National Cancer Institute—CancerNet]
http://cancernet.nci.nih.gov/clinpdq/soa/Endometrial_cancer_Physician.html

Ball HG et al: Endometrial cancer: Current concepts and management. Surg Oncol Clin N Am 1998;7:271. [NLM Cit ID: 98205102] (Review of current understanding of risk factors and current approaches to staging and treatment.)

Canavan TP et al: Endometrial cancer. Am Fam Physician 1999;59:3069. [NLM Cit ID: 99319761] (Diagnosis and treatment for primary care clinicians.)

CARCINOMA OF THE VULVA

Essentials of Diagnosis

- History of genital warts.
- History of prolonged vulvar irritation, with pruritus, local discomfort, or slight bloody discharge.
- Early lesions may suggest or include nonneoplastic epithelial disorders.
- Late lesions appear as a mass, an exophytic growth, or a firm, ulcerated area in the vulva.
- Biopsy is necessary to make the diagnosis.

General Considerations

The vast majority of cancers of the vulva are squamous lesions that classically have occurred in women over 50 years of age. Several subtypes (particularly 16, 18, and 31) of the human papillomavirus have been identified in some but not all vulvar cancers. As with squamous cell lesions of the cervix, a grading system of vulvar intraepithelial neoplasia (VIN) from mild dysplasia to carcinoma in situ has been established.

Differential Diagnosis

Biopsy is essential for the diagnosis of vulvar cancer and should be performed with any localized atypical vulvar lesion, including white patches. Multiple skin-punch specimens can be taken in the office under local anesthesia, with care to include tissue from the edges of each lesion sampled.

Benign vulvar disorders that must be excluded in the diagnosis of carcinoma of the vulva include chronic granulomatous lesions (eg, lymphogranuloma venereum, syphilis), condylomas, hidradenoma, or neurofibroma. Lichen sclerosus and other associated leukoplakic changes in the skin should be biopsied. The likelihood that a superimposed vulvar cancer will develop in a woman with a nonneoplastic epithelial disorder (vulvar dystrophy) ranges from 1% to 5%.

Treatment

A. General Measures: Early diagnosis and treatment of irritative or other predisposing or contributing causes to carcinoma of the vulva should be pursued. A 7:3 combination of betamethasone and crotamiton is particularly effective for itching. After an initial response, fluorinated steroids should be replaced with hydrocortisone because of their skin atrophying effect. Testosterone propionate (1–2% in petrolatum), applied to the vulva twice daily for 6 weeks, offers the best results in lichen sclerosus and can be used chronically in decreasing amounts and frequency.

B. Surgical Measures:

1. In situ squamous cell carcinoma of the vulva and small, invasive basal cell carcinoma of the vulva should be excised with a wide margin. If the squamous carcinoma in situ is extensive or multicentric, laser therapy or superficial surgical removal of vulvar skin may be required. In this way, the clitoris and uninvolved portions of the vulva may be spared. Skin grafting may be necessary, but mutilating vulvectomy is avoided.

2. Invasive carcinoma confined to the vulva without evidence of spread to adjacent organs or to the regional lymph nodes will necessitate radical vulvectomy and inguinal lymphadenectomy if the patient is able to withstand surgery. Debilitated patients may be candidates for palliative irradiation only.

Prognosis

Basal cell carcinomas very seldom metastasize, and carcinoma in situ by definition has not metastasized. With adequate excision, the prognosis for both lesions is excellent. Patients with invasive vulvar carcinoma 3 cm in diameter or less without inguinal lymph node metastases who can sustain radical surgery have about a 90% chance of a 5-year survival. If the lesion is greater than 3 cm and has metastasized, the likelihood of 5-year survival is less than 25%.

[Vulvar Cancer—National Cancer Institute—CancerNet] http://cancernet.nci.nih.gov/clinpdq/soa/Vulvar_cancer_Physician.html

Nash JD et al: Vulvar cancer. Surg Oncol Clin N Am 1998;7:335. [NLM Cit ID: 98205106] (A review of surgical and medical treatment of vulvar cancer.)

ENDOMETRIOSIS

Endometriosis is an aberrant growth of endometrium outside the uterus, particularly in the dependent parts of the pelvis and in the ovaries and is a common cause of abnormal bleeding and secondary dysmenorrhea. Its causes, pathogenesis, and natural course are poorly understood. The prevalence in the USA is 2% among fertile women and three- to fourfold greater than that in the infertile. Depending on the location and extent of the endometrial implants, infertility, dyspareunia, or rectal pain with bleeding may result. Aching pain tends to be constant, beginning 2–7 days before the onset of menses, and becomes increasingly severe until flow slackens. Pelvic examination may disclose tender indurated nodules in the cul-de-sac, especially if the examination is done at the onset of menstruation.

Endometriosis must be distinguished from pelvic inflammatory disease, ovarian neoplasms, and uterine myomas. In general, only in salpingitis and endometriosis are the symptoms aggravated by menstruation. Bowel invasion by endometrial tissue may produce clinical findings, including blood in the stool, that must be distinguished from bowel neoplasm. Differentiation in these instances depends upon proctosigmoidoscopy and biopsy.

Ultrasound examination will often reveal complex fluid-filled masses that cannot be distinguished from neoplasms. MRI is more sensitive and specific than ultrasound, particularly in the diagnosis of adnexal masses. However, the clinical diagnosis of endometriosis is presumptive and usually confirmed by laparoscopy or laparotomy.

Treatment

A. Medical Treatment: The goal of medical treatment is to preserve the fertility of women wanting future pregnancies, ameliorate symptoms, and simplify future surgery or make it unnecessary. Medications are designed to inhibit ovulation over 4–9 months and lower hormone levels, thus preventing cyclic stimulation of endometriotic implants and decreasing their size. The optimum duration of therapy is not clear, and the relative merits in terms of pregnancies, side effects, and long-term risks and benefits show insignificant differences when compared with each other, with surgery (including laser surgery), and, in mild cases, with placebo.

1. The GnRH analogs such as nafarelin nasal spray, 0.2–0.4 mg twice daily, or long-acting injectable leuprolide acetate, 3.75 mg intramuscularly monthly, used for 6 months, suppress ovulation. Side effects consisting of vasomotor symptoms and bone demineralization may be relieved by "add-back" therapy with norethindrone, 5–10 mg daily.

2. Danazol is used for 6–9 months in the lowest dose necessary to suppress menstruation, usually 200–400 mg twice daily. Side effects are androgenic and include decreased breast size, weight gain, acne, and hirsutism.

3. Any of the combination oral contraceptives may be given, one daily, without interruption, for 6–12 months. Breakthrough bleeding can be treated with conjugated estrogens, 1.25 mg daily for 1 week, or estradiol, 2 mg daily for 1 week.

4. Medroxyprogesterone acetate, 100 mg intramuscularly every 2 weeks for four doses; then 100 mg every 4 weeks; add oral estrogen or estradiol valerate, 30 mg intramuscularly, for breakthrough bleeding. Use for 6–9 months.

5. Low-dose oral contraceptives can also be given cyclically; prolonged suppression of ovulation will often inhibit further stimulation of residual endometriosis, especially if taken after one of the therapies mentioned above.

6. Analgesics, with or without codeine, may be needed during menses. Nonsteroidal anti-inflammatory drugs may be helpful.

B. Surgical Measures: The surgical treatment of moderately extensive endometriosis depends upon the patient's age and symptoms and her desire to preserve reproductive function. If the patient is under 35, resect the lesions, free adhesions, and suspend the uterus. At least 20% of patients so treated can become pregnant, although some must undergo surgery again if the disease progresses. If the patient is over 35 years old, is disabled by pain, and has involvement of both ovaries, bilateral salpingo-oophorectomy and hysterectomy will probably be necessary.

Foci of endometriosis can be treated at laparoscopy by bipolar coagulation or laser vaporization. Because pelvic endometriosis can take forms other than the classic powder burns and hemorrhagic cysts, a meticulous survey of the peritoneum is required.

Prognosis

The prognosis for reproductive function in early or moderately advanced endometriosis is good with conservative therapy. Bilateral ovariectomy is curative for patients with severe and extensive endometriosis with pain. Following hysterectomy and oophorectomy, estrogen replacement therapy is indicated.

Ling FW: Randomized controlled trial of depot leuprolide in patients with chronic pelvic pain and clinically suspected endometriosis. Pelvic Pain Study Group. Obstet Gynecol 1999;93:51. [NLM Cit ID: 99113994] (Empiric use of depot leuprolide in women with chronic pelvic pain suspected of having endometriosis is a cost-effective approach to nonsurgical diagnosis and treatment.)

Marcoux S et al: Laparoscopic surgery in infertile women with minimal or mild endometriosis. Canadian Collaborative Group on Endometriosis. N Engl J Med 1997;337:217. [NLM Cit ID: 97357242] (In infertile women with minimal or mild endometriosis, fertility was significantly enhanced by laparoscopic resection or ablation of endometriosis.)

Schenken RS (editor): Endometriosis. Clin Obstet Gynecol 1999;42:565. [NLM Cit ID 99381078–99381086] (Series of up-to-date review articles on pathogenesis and treatment of endometriosis.)

GENITAL PROLAPSE (Cystocele, Rectocele, Enterocele)

Cystocele, rectocele, and enterocele are vaginal hernias commonly seen in multiparous women. Cystocele is a hernia of the bladder wall into the vagina, causing a soft anterior fullness. Cystocele may be accompanied by urethrocele, which is not a hernia but a sagging of the urethra following its detachment from the pubic symphysis during childbirth. Rectocele is a herniation of the terminal rectum into the posterior vagina, causing a collapsible pouch-like fullness. Enterocele is a vaginal vault hernia containing small intestine, usually in the posterior vagina and resulting from a deepening of the pouch of Douglas. Enterocele may also accompany uterine prolapse or follow hysterectomy, when weakened vault supports or a deep unobliterated cul-de-sac containing intestine protrudes into the vagina. Two or all three types of hernia may occur in combination.

Supportive measures include a high-fiber diet. Weight reduction in obese patients and limitation of straining and lifting are helpful. Pessaries may reduce cystocele, rectocele, or enterocele temporarily and are helpful in women who do not wish surgery or are chronically ill.

The only cure for symptomatic cystocele, rectocele, or enterocele is corrective surgery. The prognosis following an uncomplicated procedure is good.

UTERINE PROLAPSE

Uterine prolapse most commonly occurs as a delayed result of childbirth injury to the pelvic floor (particularly the transverse cervical and uterosacral ligaments). Unrepaired obstetric lacerations of the levator musculature and perineal body augment the weakness. Attenuation of the pelvic structures with aging and congenital weakness can accelerate the development of prolapse.

In slight prolapse, the uterus descends only part way down the vagina; in moderate prolapse, the corpus descends to the introitus and the cervix protrudes slightly beyond; and in marked prolapse (procidentia), the entire cervix and uterus protrude beyond the introitus and the vagina is inverted. Inability to walk comfortably because of protrusion or discomfort from the presence of a vaginal mass is an indication that surgical treatment should be considered.

Treatment

The type of surgery depends upon the extent of prolapse and the patient's age and her desire for menstruation, pregnancy, and coitus. The simplest, most effective procedure is vaginal hysterectomy with appropriate repair of the cystocele and rectocele. If the patient desires pregnancy, a partial resection of the cervix with plication of the cardinal ligaments can be attempted. For elderly women who do not desire coitus, partial obliteration of the vagina is surgically simple and effective. Abdominal uterine suspension or ventrofixation will fail in the treatment of prolapse.

A well-fitted vaginal pessary (eg, inflatable doughnut type, Gellhorn pessary) may give relief if surgery is refused or contraindicated.

Morley GW: Treatment of uterine and vaginal prolapse. Clin Obstet Gynecol 1996;39:959. [NLM Cit ID: 97088107] (Review of diagnosis and surgical and nonsurgical treatment alternatives.)

Wu V et al: A simplified protocol for pessary management. Obstet Gynecol 1997;90:990. [NLM Cit ID: 98059266] (Pessaries may be a successful therapeutic approach in women with symptomatic genital prolapse, particularly those without stress incontinence.)

PELVIC INFLAMMATORY DISEASE (PID; Salpingitis, Endometritis)

Pelvic inflammatory disease is a polymicrobial infection of the upper genital tract associated with the sexually transmitted organisms *N gonorrhoeae* and *C trachomatis* as well as endogenous organisms, including anaerobes, *H influenzae,* enteric gram-negative rods, and streptococci. It is most common in young, nulliparous, sexually active women with multiple partners. Other risk markers include nonwhite race, douching, and smoking. The use of oral contraceptives or barrier methods of contraception may provide significant protection.

Tuberculous salpingitis is rare in the USA but more common in developing countries; it is characterized by pelvic pain and irregular pelvic masses not responsive to antibiotic therapy. It is not sexually transmitted.

Clinical Findings

A. Symptoms and Signs: Patients with pelvic inflammatory disease may have lower abdominal pain, chills and fever, menstrual disturbances, purulent cervical discharge, and cervical and adnexal tenderness. Right upper quadrant pain (Fitz-Hugh and Curtis syndrome) may indicate an associated perihepatitis. However, diagnosis of PID is complicated by the fact that many women may have subtle or mild symptoms, not readily recognized as PID.

B. Minimum Diagnostic Criteria: Women with lower abdominal, adnexal, or cervical motion tenderness should be considered to have PID and be treated with antibiotics unless there is a competing diagnosis such as ectopic pregnancy or appendicitis.

C. Additional Criteria: The following criteria may be used to enhance the specificity of the diagnosis: (1) oral temperature > 38.3 °C, (2) abnormal cervical or vaginal discharge, (3) elevated erythrocyte sedimentation rate, (4) elevated C-reactive protein, and (5) laboratory documentation of cervical infection with *N gonorrhoeae* or *C trachomatis.* Endocervical culture should be performed routinely, but treatment should not be delayed while awaiting results.

D. Definitive Criteria: In selected cases where the diagnosis based on clinical or laboratory evidence is uncertain, the following criteria may be used: (1) histopathologic evidence of endometritis on endometrial biopsy, (2) transvaginal sonography or other imaging techniques showing thickened fluid-filled tubes with or without free pelvic fluid or tubo-ovarian complex, and (3) laparoscopic abnormalities consistent with PID.

Differential Diagnosis

Appendicitis, ectopic pregnancy, septic abortion, hemorrhagic or ruptured ovarian cysts or tumors, twisted ovarian cyst, degeneration of a myoma, and acute enteritis must be considered. Pelvic inflammatory disease is more likely to occur when there is a history of pelvic inflammatory disease, recent sexual contact, recent onset of menses, or an IUD in place or if the partner has a sexually transmitted disease. Acute pelvic inflammatory disease is highly unlikely when recent intercourse has not taken place or an IUD is not being used. A sensitive serum pregnancy test should be obtained to rule out ectopic pregnancy. Culdocentesis will differentiate hemoperitoneum (ruptured ectopic pregnancy or hemorrhagic cyst) from pelvic sepsis (salpingitis, ruptured pelvic abscess, or ruptured appendix). Pelvic and vaginal ultrasound is helpful in the differential diagnosis of ectopic pregnancy of over 6 weeks. Laparoscopy is often utilized to diagnose pelvic inflammatory disease, and it is imperative if the diagnosis is not certain or if the patient has not responded to antibiotic therapy after 48 hours. The appendix should be visualized at laparoscopy to rule out appendicitis. Cultures obtained at the time of laparoscopy are often specific and helpful.

Treatment

A. Hospitalization: Patients with acute pelvic inflammatory disease should be admitted for intravenous antibiotic therapy if (1) surgical emergencies such as appendicitis cannot be ruled out; (2) the patient has a tubo-ovarian abscess; (3) the patient is pregnant; (4) the patient is unable to follow or tolerate an outpatient regimen; (5) the patient has failed to respond clinically to outpatient therapy; (6) the patient has severe illness, nausea and vomiting, or high fever; or (7) the patient is immunodeficient (ie, has HIV infection with low CD4 counts, is taking immunosuppressive therapy, or has another immunosuppressing disease). In the past, many experts recommended that all patients with PID be hospitalized for bed rest and supervised treatment with parenteral antibiotics. Outpatient parenteral therapy is available in some settings and may be an acceptable alternative, though data are lacking on the efficacy of this approach. Patients with tubo-ovarian abscesses should have direct inpatient observation for at least 24 hours prior to switching to outpatient parenteral therapy.

B. Antibiotics: Early treatment with appropriate antibiotics effective against *N gonorrhoeae, C trachomatis,* and the endogenous organisms listed above is essential to prevent long-term sequelae. The sexual partner should be examined and treated appropriately.

Two inpatient regimens have been shown to be effective in the treatment of acute pelvic inflammatory disease: (1) Cefoxitin, 2 g intravenously every 6 hours, or cefotetan, 2 g every 12 hours, plus doxycycline, 100 mg intravenously or orally every 12 hours. This regimen is continued for at least 24 hours after the patient shows significant clinical improvement. Doxycycline, 100 mg twice daily, should be continued to complete a total of 14 days therapy. (2) Clindamycin, 900 mg intravenously every 8 hours, plus gentamicin intravenously in a loading dose of 2 mg/kg followed by 1.5 mg/kg every 8 hours. This regimen is continued for at least 24 hours after the patient shows significant clinical improvement and is followed by either clindamycin, 450 mg four times daily, or doxycycline, 100 mg twice daily, to complete a total of 14 days of therapy.

Limited data exist on other parenteral regimens. Three regimens providing broad-spectrum coverage have been investigated in at least one clinical trial: (1) ofloxacin, 400 mg intravenously every 12 hours, plus metronidazole, 500 mg intravenously every 8 hours; (2) ampicillin-sulbactam, 3 g intravenously every 6 hours, plus doxycycline, 100 mg intravenously or orally every 12 hours; and (3) ciprofloxacin, 200 mg intravenously every 12 hours, plus doxycycline, 100 mg intravenously or orally every 12 hours, plus metronidazole, 500 mg intravenously every 8 hours.

Two outpatient regimens are recommended: (1) ofloxacin, 400 mg orally twice daily for 14 days, plus metronidazole, 500 mg orally twice daily, for 14 days; and (2) either a single dose of cefoxitin, 2 g intramuscularly, with probenecid, 1 g orally, or ceftriaxone, 250 mg intramuscularly, plus doxycycline, 100 mg orally twice daily, for 14 days.

C. Surgical Measures: Tubo-ovarian abscesses may require surgical excision or transcutaneous or transvaginal aspiration. Unless rupture is suspected, institute high-dose antibiotic therapy in the hospital, and monitor therapy with ultrasound. In 70% of cases, antibiotics are effective; in 30%, there is inadequate response in 48–72 hours, and intervention is required. Unilateral adnexectomy in the presence of unilateral abscess is acceptable. Hysterectomy and bilateral salpingo-oophorectomy may be necessary for overwhelming infection or in cases of chronic disease with intractable pelvic pain.

Prognosis

In spite of treatment, one-fourth of women with acute disease develop long-term sequelae, including repeated episodes of infection, chronic pelvic pain, dyspareunia, ectopic pregnancy, or infertility. The risk of infertility increases with repeated episodes of salpingitis: it is estimated at 10% after the first episode, 25% after a second episode, and 50% after a third episode.

1998 Guidelines for treatment of sexually transmitted diseases. MMWR Morb Mortal Wkly Rep 1998;47(RR-1):79. [NLM Cit ID: 98120951]

Paavonen J: Pelvic inflammatory disease: From diagnosis to prevention. Dermatol Clin 1998;16:747. [NLM Cit ID: 99108824] (Review of current approaches to diagnosis, management, and prevention.)

OVARIAN TUMORS

Essentials of Diagnosis

- Vague gastrointestinal discomfort.
- Pelvic pressure and pain.
- Many cases of early-stage cancer are asymptomatic.
- Pelvic examination, CA 125, and ultrasound are mainstays of diagnosis.

General Considerations

Ovarian tumors are common. Most are benign, but malignant ovarian tumors are the leading cause of death from reproductive tract cancer. The wide range of types and patterns of ovarian tumors is due to the complexity of ovarian embryology and differences in tissues of origin (Table 17–4).

In women with no family history of ovarian cancer, the lifetime risk is 1.6%, whereas a woman with one affected first-degree relative has a 5% lifetime risk. With two or more affected first-degree relatives, the risk is 7%. Approximately 3% of women with two or more affected first-degree relatives will have a hereditary ovarian cancer syndrome with a lifetime risk of 40%. Women with a *BRCA1* gene mutation have at least a 50% lifetime risk of ovarian cancer. These women should be screened annually with transvaginal sonography (TVS) and CA 125 testing, and prophylactic oophorectomy is recommended by age 35 or whenever childbearing is completed because of the high risk of disease. The benefits of such screening for women with one or no affected first-degree relatives are unproved, and the risks associated with unnecessary surgical procedures may outweigh the benefits in low-risk women. In women at increased risk of ovarian cancer, the long-term use of oral contraceptives may decrease the risk.

Clinical Findings

A. Symptoms and Signs: Unfortunately, most women with both benign and malignant ovarian neoplasms are either asymptomatic or experience only mild nonspecific gastrointestinal symptoms or pelvic pressure. Women with early disease are typically detected on routine pelvic examination. Women with advanced malignant disease may experience abdominal pain and bloating, and a palpable abdominal mass with ascites is often present.

B. Laboratory Findings: An elevated serum CA 125 (> 35 units) indicates a greater likelihood that an ovarian tumor is malignant. CA 125 is elevated in 80% of women with epithelial ovarian cancer overall but in only 50% of women with early disease. Furthermore, serum CA 125 may be elevated in premenopausal women with benign disease such as endometriosis.

C. Imaging Studies: TVS is useful for screening high-risk women and but has inadequate sensitivity for screening low-risk women. Ultrasound is helpful in differentiating ovarian masses that are benign and likely to resolve spontaneously from those with malignant potential. Color Doppler imaging may further enhance the specificity of ultrasound diagnosis.

Differential Diagnosis

Once an ovarian mass has been detected, it must be categorized as functional, benign neoplastic, or potentially malignant. Predictive factors include age, size of the mass, ultrasound configuration, CA 125 levels, the presence of symptoms, and whether the mass is unilateral or bilateral. In a premenopausal woman, an asymptomatic, mobile, unilateral, simple cystic mass less than 8–10 cm may be observed for 4–6 weeks. Most will resolve spontaneously. If the mass is larger or unchanged on repeat pelvic examination and TVS, surgical evaluation is required.

Most ovarian masses in postmenopausal women require surgical evaluation. However, a postmenopausal woman with an asymptomatic unilateral simple cyst less than 5 cm in diameter and a normal CA 125 level may be followed closely with TVS. All others require surgical evaluation.

Exploratory laparotomy has been the standard approach. Laparoscopy may be considered for a premenopausal woman with an ovarian mass small enough to be removed using a laparoscopic approach. If malignancy is suspected, preoperative workup should include chest x-ray, evaluation of liver and kidney function, and hematologic indices.

Treatment

If a malignant ovarian mass is suspected, surgical evaluation should be performed by a gynecologic oncologist. For benign neoplasms, tumor removal or unilateral oophorectomy is usually performed. For ovarian cancer in an early stage, the standard therapy is complete surgical staging followed by abdominal hysterectomy and bilateral salpingo-oophorectomy with omentectomy and selective lymphadenectomy. With more advanced disease, aggressive removal of all visible tumor improves survival. Except for women with low-grade ovarian cancer in an early stage, postoperative chemotherapy is indicated. Several chemotherapy regimens are effective, such as the combination of cisplatin and cyclophosphamide with or without doxorubicin, with clinical response rates of up to 60–70%.

Prognosis

Unfortunately, approximately 75% of women with ovarian cancer are diagnosed with advanced disease after regional or distant metastases have become established. The overall 5-year survival is approximately 17% with distant metastases, 36% with local spread, and 89% with early disease.

[Ovarian Cancer—American Cancer Society]
http://www3.cancer.org/cancerinfo/main_cont.asp?st=pr&ct=33

Table 17–4. Ovarian functional and neoplastic tumors.

Tumor	Incidence	Size	Consistency	Menstrual Irregularities	Endocrine Effects	Potential for Malignancy	Special Remarks
Follicle cysts	Rare in childhood; frequent in menstrual years; never in postmenopausal years.	< 6 cm, often bilateral.	Moderate	Occasional	Occasional anovulation with persistently proliferative endometrium	None	Often disappear after a 2-month regimen of oral contraceptives.
Corpus luteum cysts	Occasional, in menstrual years.	4–6 cm, unilateral.	Moderate	Occasional delayed period	Prolonged secretory phase	None	Functional cysts. Intraperitoneal bleeding occasionally.
Theca lutein cysts	Occurs with hydatidiform mole, choriocarcinoma; also with gonadotropin or clomiphene therapy.	To 4–5 cm, multiple, bilateral. (Ovaries may be ≥ 20 cm in diameter.)	Tense	Amenorrhea	hCG elevated as a result of trophoblastic proliferation	None	Functional cysts. Hematoperitoneum or torsion of ovary may occur. Surgery is to be avoided.
Inflammatory (tubo-ovarian abscess)	Concomitant with acute salpingitis.	To 15–20 cm, often bilateral.	Variable, painful	Menometrorrhagia	Anovulation usual	None	Unilateral removal indicated if possible.
Endometriotic cysts	Never in preadolescent or postmenopausal years. Most common in women aged 20–40 years.	To 10–12 cm, occasionally bilateral.	Moderate to softened	Rare	None	Very rare	Associated pelvic endometriosis. Medical treatment or conservative surgery recommended.
Teratoid tumors:							
Benign teratomas (dermoid cysts)	Childhood to postmenopause.	< 15 cm; 15% are bilateral.	Moderate to softened	None	None	Rare	Torsion can occur. Partial oophorectomy recommended.
Malignant teratomas	< 1% of ovarian tumors. Usually in infants and young adults.	> 20 cm, unilateral.	Irregularly firm	None	Occasionally, hCG elevated	All	Unresponsive to any therapy.

(continued)

Table 17–4. Ovarian functional and neoplastic tumors. (continued)

Tumor	Incidence	Size	Consistency	Menstrual Irregularities	Endocrine Effects	Potential for Malignancy	Special Remarks
Cystadenoma, cystadenocarcinoma	Common in reproductive years.	Serous: < 25 cm, 33% bilateral; mucinous: up to 1 cm, 10% bilateral.	Moderate to softened	None	None	> 50% for serous, about 5% for mucinous.	Peritoneal implants often occur with serous, rarely with mucinous. If mucinous tumor is ruptured, pseudomyxoma peritonei may occur.
Endometrioid carcinoma	15% of ovarian carcinomas.	Moderate, 13% bilateral.	Firm	None	None	All	Adenocarcinoma of endometrium coexists in 15–30% of cases.
Fibroma	< 5% of ovarian tumors.	Usually < 15 cm.	Very firm	None	None	Rare	Ascites in 20% (rarely, pleural fluid).
Arrhenoblastoma	Rare. Average age 30 years or more.	Often small (< 10 cm), unilateral.	Firm to softened	Amenorrhea	Androgens elevated.	< 20%	Recurrences are moderately sensitive to irradiation.
Theca cell tumor (thecoma)	Uncommon.	< 10 cm, unilateral.	Firm	Occasional irregularity	Estrogens or androgens elevated.	< 1%	
Granulosa cell tumor	Uncommon. Usually in prepubertal girls or women older than 50 years.	May be very small.	Firm to softened	Menometrorrhagia	Estrogens elevated.	15–20%	Recurrences are moderately sensitive to irradiation.
Dysgerminoma	About 1–2% of ovarian tumors.	< 30 cm, bilateral in 33%.	Moderate to softened	None	...	All	Very radiosensitive.
Brenner tumor	About 1% of ovarian tumors.	< 30 cm, unilateral.	Firm	None	...	Very rare	> 50% occur in postmenopausal years.
Secondary ovarian tumors	10% of fatal malignant disease in women.	Varies; often bilateral.	Firm to softened	Occasional	Very rare (thyroid, adrenocortical origin).	All	Bowel or breast metastases to ovary common.

Nahhas WA: Ovarian cancer: Current outlook on this deadly disease. Postgrad Med 1997;102:112. [NLM Cit ID: 97445032] (Comprehensive review article.)

NIH Consensus Conference: Ovarian cancer: Screening, treatment and followup. JAMA 1995:273:491. [NLM Cit ID: 95139174]

PERSISTENT ANOVULATION (Polycystic Ovary Syndrome)

Essentials of Diagnosis

- Chronic anovulation.
- Infertility.
- Elevated plasma testosterone and LH values and a reversed FSH/LH ratio.
- Hirsutism (in 70% of patients).

General Considerations

Polycystic ovary syndrome is a common endocrine disorder affecting 2–5% of women of reproductive age. The primary lesion is unknown. These patients have a relatively steady state of high estrogen, androgen, and LH levels rather than the fluctuating condition seen in ovulating women. Increased levels of estrone come from obesity (conversion of ovarian and adrenal androgens to estrone in body fat) or from excessive levels of androgens seen in some women of normal weight. The high estrogen levels are believed to cause suppression of pituitary FSH and a relative increase in LH. Constant LH stimulation of the ovary results in anovulation, multiple cysts, and theca cell hyperplasia with excess androgen output. The polycystic ovary has a thickened, pearly white capsule and may not be enlarged.

Women with Cushing's syndrome, congenital adrenal hyperplasia, and androgen-secreting adrenal tumors also tend to have high circulating androgen levels and anovulation with polycystic ovaries.

Clinical Findings

Polycystic ovary syndrome is manifested by hirsutism (70% of cases), obesity (40%), and virilization (20%). Fifty percent of patients have amenorrhea, 30% have abnormal uterine bleeding, and 20% have normal menstruation. Additionally, they show insulin resistance and hyperinsulinemia when infused with glucose, and these women are at increased risk of early-onset type 2 diabetes mellitus. The patients are generally infertile, although they may ovulate occasionally. They have an increased long-term risk of cancer of the breast and endometrium because of unopposed estrogen secretion.

Differential Diagnosis

Anovulation in the reproductive years may also be due to (1) premature menopause (high FSH and LH levels); (2) rapid weight loss, extreme physical exertion (normal FSH and LH levels for age), or obesity; (3) discontinuation of oral contraceptives (anovulation for 6 months or more occasionally occurs); (4) pituitary adenoma with elevated prolactin (galactorrhea may or may not be present); (5) hyper- or hypothyroidism. Always check FSH, LH, prolactin, TSH, testosterone, and dehydroepiandrosterone sulfate (DHEAS) levels when amenorrhea has persisted for 6 months or more without a diagnosis. A 10-day course of progestin (eg, medroxyprogesterone acetate, 10 mg/d) will cause withdrawal bleeding if estrogen levels are high. This will aid in the diagnosis and prevent endometrial hyperplasia. In long-term anovular patients over age 35, it is wise to search for an estrogen-stimulated cancer with mammography and endometrial aspiration.

Treatment

In obese patients with polycystic ovaries, weight reduction is often effective; a decrease in body fat will lower the conversion of androgens to estrone and thereby help to restore ovulation.

If the patient wishes to become pregnant, clomiphene or other drugs can be employed for ovulatory stimulation. The addition of dexamethasone 0.5 mg at bedtime to a clomiphene regimen may increase the likelihood of ovulation by suppression of ACTH and circulating adrenal androgens. For women who are unresponsive to clomiphene, 3- to 6-month courses of the oral hypoglycemic agent metformin, 500 mg three times daily, may bring resumption of regular cycles and ovulation. This agent reduces the hyperinsulinemia and hyperandrogenemia seen with polycystic ovary syndrome.

If the patient does not desire pregnancy, give medroxyprogesterone acetate, 10 mg/d for the first 10 days of each month. This will ensure regular shedding of the endometrium so that hyperplasia will not occur. If contraception is desired, a low-dose combination oral contraceptive can be used; this is also useful in controlling hirsutism, for which treatment must be continued for 6–12 months before results are seen.

Hirsutism may be managed with epilation and electrolysis. Dexamethasone, 0.5 mg each night, is helpful in women with excess adrenal androgen secretion. If hirsutism is severe, some patients will elect to have a hysterectomy and bilateral oophorectomy followed by estrogen replacement therapy. Spironolactone, an aldosterone antagonist, is also useful for hirsutism in doses of 25 mg three or four times daily.

Dunaif A (editor): Polycystic ovary syndrome. Endocrinol Metab Clin North Am 1999;28:247. [NLM Cit ID: 99281188–99281194] (Series of state-of-the-art articles on pathogenesis, diagnosis, and treatment.)

PAINFUL INTERCOURSE (Dyspareunia)

Questions related to sexual functioning should be asked as part of the reproductive history. Two helpful questions are, "Are you sexually active?" and "Are you having any sexual difficulties at this time?"

Painful intercourse may be caused by vulvovaginitis; vaginismus; an incompletely stretched hymen; insufficient lubrication of the vagina; vaginal atrophy; endometriosis; or tumors or other pathologic conditions. During the pelvic examination, the patient should be placed in a half-sitting position and given a hand-held mirror and then asked to point out the site of pain and describe the type of pain.

Etiology

A. Vulvovaginitis: Vulvovaginitis is inflammation or infection of the vagina. Areas of marked tenderness in the vulvar vestibule without visible inflammation occasionally show lesions resembling small condylomas on colposcopy (see Vaginitis, above).

B. Vaginismus: Vaginismus is voluntary or involuntary contraction of muscles around the introitus. It results from fear, pain, sexual trauma, or having learned negative attitudes toward sex during childhood.

C. Remnants of the Hymen: The hymen is usually adequately stretched during initial intercourse, so that pain does not occur subsequently. In some women, the pain of initial intercourse may produce vaginismus. In others, a thin or thickened rim or partial rim of hymen remains after several episodes of intercourse, causing pain.

D. Insufficient Lubrication of the Vagina: See Vaginal Atrophy, below.

E. Infection, Endometriosis, Tumors, or Other Pathologic Conditions: Pain occurring with deep thrusting during coitus is usually due to acute or chronic infection of the cervix, uterus, or adnexa; endometriosis; adnexal tumors; or adhesions resulting from prior pelvic disease or operation. Careful history taking and a pelvic examination will generally help in the differential diagnosis.

F. Vulvar Vestibulitis: This is the most frequent cause of dyspareunia in premenopausal women. It is characterized by pain on palpation of the vestibular area or on attempted vaginal entry. There are no physical findings other than minimal erythema, and biopsy shows only nonspecific inflammation. A subset of women with vulvar vestibulitis may experience continuous vulvar burning or pain.

Treatment

A. Vulvovaginitis: Lesions resembling warts on colposcopy or biopsy should be treated in the appropriate way (see Vaginitis). Irritation from spermicides may be a factor. The couple may be helped by a discussion of noncoital techniques to achieve orgasm until the infection subsides.

B. Vaginismus: Sexual counseling and education on anatomy and sexual functioning may be appropriate. The patient can be instructed in self-dilation, using a lubricated finger or test tubes of graduated sizes. Before coitus (with adequate lubrication) is attempted, the patient—and then her partner—should be able to easily and painlessly introduce two fingers into the vagina. Penetration should never be forced, and the woman should always be the one to control the depth of insertion during dilation or intercourse.

C. Remnants of the Hymen: In rare situations, manual dilation of a remaining hymen under general anesthesia is necessary. Surgery should be avoided.

D. Insufficient Lubrication of the Vagina: If inadequate sexual arousal is the cause, sexual counseling for the woman—and her partner if possible—is helpful. Lubricants may be used during sexual foreplay. For women with low plasma estrogen levels, use of a lubricant during coitus is sometimes sufficient. If not, use conjugated estrogen cream, one-eighth applicatorful daily for 10 days and then every other day. Using the applicator or a finger, the patient can apply the cream directly to the most tender area, usually the hymenal ring. Testosterone cream 1–2% in a water-soluble base is also helpful.

E. Infection, Endometriosis, Tumors, or Other Pathologic Conditions: Medical treatment of acute cervicitis, endometritis, or salpingitis and temporary abstention from coitus usually relieve pain. Hormonal or surgical treatment of endometriosis may be helpful. Dyspareunia resulting from chronic pelvic inflammatory disease or any condition causing extensive adhesions or fixation of pelvic organs is difficult to treat without extirpative surgery. Couples can be advised to try coital positions that limit deep thrusting and to use manual and oral sexual techniques.

F. Vulvar Vestibulitis: Since the cause of vulvar vestibulitis is unknown, management is difficult. Few treatment approaches have been subjected to methodologically rigorous trials. Surgery, usually consisting of vestibulectomy, has reportedly been the most consistently successful approach. A variety of specific (antiviral or antifungal) and nonspecific (corticosteroid or anesthetic) agents have been tried with varying degrees of success. Pain control through behavioral therapy, biofeedback, or acupuncture has also been tried. No single approach has been consistently shown to be effective. Patients with continuous genital burning or pain may benefit from treatment with a tricyclic antidepressant such as amitriptyline in gradually increasing doses from 10 mg/d to 75–100 mg/d.

Bergeron S et al: Vulvar vestibulitis syndrome: A critical review. Clin J Pain 1997;13:27. [NLM Cit ID: 97239288] (A comprehensive review of knowledge about etiology, clinical manifestations, and treatment.)

Davis GD et al: Clinical management of vulvodynia. Clin Obstet Gynecol 1999;42:221. [NLM Cit ID: 99298981] (Diagnosis and treatment of vulvar pain syndromes.)

INFERTILITY

A couple is said to be infertile if pregnancy does not result after 1 year of normal sexual activity without contraceptives. About 25% of couples experience infertility at some point in their reproductive lives; the incidence of infertility increases with age. The male partner contributes to about 40% of cases of infertility, and a combination of factors is common.

Diagnostic Survey

During the initial interview, the physician can present an overview of infertility and discuss a plan of study. Separate private consultations are then conducted, allowing appraisal of psychosexual adjustment without embarrassment or criticism. Pertinent details (eg, sexually transmitted disease or prior pregnancies) must be obtained. The ill effects of cigarettes, alcohol, and other recreational drugs on male fertility should be discussed. Prescription drugs that impair male potency should be discussed as well. The gynecologic history should include queries regarding the menstrual pattern. The present history includes use and types of contraceptives, douches, libido, sex techniques, frequency and success of coitus, and correlation of intercourse with time of ovulation. Family history includes repeated abortions and maternal DES use.

General physical and genital examinations are performed on both partners. Basic laboratory studies include complete blood count, urinalysis, cervical culture for chlamydia, serologic test for syphilis, rubella antibody determination, and thyroid function tests. Tay-Sachs screening should be offered if both parents are Jews and sickle cell screening if both parents are black.

The patient is instructed to chart her basal body temperature orally daily on arising and to record on a graph episodes of coitus and days of menstruation. Self-performed urine tests for the midcycle LH surge can be used to enhance temperature observations relating to ovulation. Couples should be advised that coitus resulting in conception occurs during the 6-day period ending with the day of ovulation.

The male partner is instructed to bring a complete ejaculate for analysis. Sexual abstinence for at least 3 days before the semen is obtained is emphasized. A clean, dry, wide-mouthed bottle for collection is preferred. Condoms should not be employed, as the protective powder or lubricant may be spermicidal. Semen should be examined within 1–2 hours after collection. Semen is considered normal with the following minimum values: volume, 3 mL; concentration, 20 million sperm per milliliter; motility, 50% after 2 hours; and normal forms, 60%. If the sperm count is abnormal, further evaluation includes a search for exposure to environmental and workplace toxins, alcohol or drug abuse, and hypogonadism.

A. First Testing Cycle: While the contribution of cervical factors to infertility is controversial, most gynecologists include a postcoital test in their workup. The test is scheduled for just before ovulation (eg, day 12 or 13 in an expected 28-day cycle). Preovulation timing can be enhanced by serial urinary LH tests. The patient is examined within 6 hours after coitus. The cervical mucus should be clear, elastic, and copious owing to the influence of the preovular estrogen surge. (The mucus is scantier and more viscid before and after ovulation.) A good spinnbarkeit (stretching to a fine thread 4 cm or more in length) is desirable. A small drop of cervical mucus should be obtained from within the cervical os and examined under the microscope. The presence of five or more active sperm per high-power field constitutes a satisfactory postcoital test. If no spermatozoa are found, the test should be repeated (assuming that active spermatozoa were present in the semen analysis). Sperm agglutination and sperm immobilization tests should be considered if the sperm are immotile or show ineffective tail motility.

The presence of more than three white blood cells per high-power field in the postcoital test suggests cervicitis in the woman or prostatitis in the man. When estrogen levels are normal, the cervical mucus dried on the slide will form a fern-like pattern when viewed with a low-power microscope. This type of mucus is necessary for normal sperm transport.

The serum progesterone level should be measured at the midpoint of the secretory phase (21st day); a level of 10–20 ng/mL confirms adequate luteal function.

B. Second Testing Cycle: Hysterosalpingography using an oil dye is performed within 3 days following the menstrual period. This x-ray study will demonstrate uterine abnormalities (septa, polyps, submucous myomas) and tubal obstruction. A repeat x-ray film 24 hours later will confirm tubal patency if there is wide pelvic dispersion of the dye. This test has been associated with an increased pregnancy rate by some observers. If the woman has had prior pelvic inflammation, give doxycycline, 100 mg twice daily, beginning immediately before and for 7 days after the x-ray study.

C. Further Testing:

1. Gross deficiencies of sperm (number, motility, or appearance) require repeat analysis. Zona-free hamster egg penetration tests are available to evaluate the ability of human sperm to fertilize an egg.

2. Obvious obstruction of the uterine tubes requires assessment for microsurgery or in vitro fertilization.

3. Absent or infrequent ovulation requires additional laboratory evaluation. Elevated FSH and LH levels indicate ovarian failure causing premature menopause. Elevated LH levels in the presence of normal FSH levels confirm the presence of polycystic ovaries. Elevation of blood prolactin (PRL) levels suggests pituitary microadenoma.

4. Major histocompatibility antigen typing of both partners will confirm human leukocyte antigen-

B locus homozygosity, which is found in greater than expected numbers among couples with unexplained infertility.

5. Ultrasound monitoring of folliculogenesis may reveal the occurrence of unruptured luteinized follicles.

6. Endometrial biopsy in the luteal phase associated with simultaneous serum progesterone levels will rule out luteal phase deficiency.

D. Laparoscopy: Approximately 25% of women whose basic evaluation is normal will have findings on laparoscopy explaining their infertility (eg, peritubal adhesions, endometriotic implants).

Treatment

A. Medical Measures: Fertility may be restored by appropriate treatment in many patients with endocrine imbalance, particularly those with hypo- or hyperthyroidism. Antibiotic treatment of cervicitis is of value. In women with abnormal postcoital tests and demonstrated antisperm antibodies causing sperm agglutination or immobilization, condom use for up to 6 months may result in lower antibody levels and improved pregnancy rates.

Women who engage in vigorous athletic training often have low sex hormone levels; fertility improves with reduced exercise and some weight gain.

B. Surgical Measures: Excision of ovarian tumors or ovarian foci of endometriosis can improve fertility. Microsurgical relief of tubal obstruction due to salpingitis or tubal ligation will reestablish fertility in a significant number of cases. In special instances of cornual or fimbrial block, the prognosis with newer surgical techniques has become much better. Peritubal adhesions or endometriotic implants often can be treated via laparoscopy or via laparotomy immediately following laparoscopic examination if prior consent has been obtained.

With varicocele in the male, sperm characteristics are often improved following surgical treatment.

C. Induction of Ovulation:

1. Clomiphene citrate–Clomiphene citrate stimulates gonadotropin release, especially LH. Consequently, plasma estrone (E_1) and estradiol (E_2) also rise, reflecting ovarian follicle maturation. If E_2 rises sufficiently, an LH surge occurs to trigger ovulation.

After a normal menstrual period or induction of withdrawal bleeding with progestin, give 50 mg of clomiphene orally daily for 5 days. If ovulation does not occur, increase the dose to 100 mg orally daily for 5 days. If ovulation still does not occur, repeat the course with 150 and then 200 mg daily for 5 days and add chorionic gonadotropin, 10,000 units intramuscularly, 7 days after clomiphene.

The rate of ovulation following this treatment is 90% in the absence of other infertility factors. The pregnancy rate is high. Twinning occurs in 5% of these patients, and three or more fetuses are found in rare instances (< 0.5% of cases). An increased incidence of congenital anomalies has not been reported. Painful ovarian cyst formation occurs in 8% of patients and may warrant discontinuation of therapy. Several recent studies have suggested a two- to threefold increased risk of ovarian cancer with the use of clomiphene for more than 1 year.

In the presence of increased androgen production (DHEA-S > 200 μg/dL), the addition of dexamethasone, 0.5 mg, or prednisone, 5 mg, at bedtime, improves the response to clomiphene. Dexamethasone should be discontinued after pregnancy is confirmed.

2. Bromocriptine–Use only if PRL levels are elevated and there is no withdrawal bleeding following progesterone administration (otherwise use clomiphene). To minimize side effects (nausea, diarrhea, dizziness, headache, fatigue), bromocriptine should be taken with meals. Begin with 2.5 mg once daily and increase to two or three times daily in increments of 1.25 mg. The drug is discontinued once pregnancy has occurred.

3. Human menopausal gonadotropins (hMG)–hMG is indicated in cases of hypogonadotropism and most other types of anovulation (exclusive of ovarian failure). Because of the complexities, laboratory tests, and expense associated with this treatment, patients who require hMG for the induction of ovulation should be referred to a specialist.

4. Gonadotropin-releasing hormone (GnRH)–Hypothalamic amenorrhea unresponsive to clomiphene will be reliably and successfully treated with subcutaneous pulsatile gonadotropin-releasing hormone (GnRH). Use of this substance will avoid the dangerous ovarian complications and the 25% incidence of multiple pregnancy associated with hMG, though the overall rate of ovulation and pregnancy is lower than when hMG is used.

D. Treatment of Endometriosis: See above.

E. Treatment of Inadequate Transport of Sperm: Intrauterine insemination of concentrated washed sperm has been used to bypass a poor cervical environment associated with scant or hostile cervical mucus. The sperm must be handled by sterile methods, washed in sterile saline or tissue culture solutions, and centrifuged. A small amount of fluid (0.5 mL) containing the sperm is then instilled into the uterus.

F. Artificial Insemination in Azoospermia: If azoospermia is present, artificial insemination by a donor usually results in pregnancy, assuming female function is normal. Both partners must consent to this method. The use of frozen sperm is currently preferable to fresh sperm because the frozen specimen can be held pending cultures and blood test results for sexually transmitted diseases, including AIDS.

G. Assisted Reproductive Technologies: Couples who have failed to respond to traditional infertility treatments, including those with tubal disease, severe endometriosis, oligospermia, and immunologic or unexplained infertility, may benefit from the newer technologies of in vitro fertilization (IVF), gamete intrafallopian transfer (GIFT), and zygote intrafallopian transfer (ZIFT). These techniques are complex and require a highly organized team of specialists. All of the procedures involve ovarian stimulation to produce multiple oocytes, oocyte retrieval by TVS-guided needle aspiration, and handling of the oocytes outside the body. With IVF, the eggs are fertilized in vitro and the embryos transferred to the uterine fundus. Extra embryos may be cryopreserved for subsequent cycles. The average delivery rate per retrieval for 281 programs in the USA and Canada in 1995 was 22.5%. Age is an important determinant of success; for couples under the age of 35, without additional infertility problems in the male partner, the average delivery rate per retrieval was 27.2%, while the rate for women over 40 was 8%. The use of donor oocytes will increase the likelihood of pregnancy for older women. In 1995, 36.6% of pregnancies were multiple. Ectopic pregnancy may occur in women with tubal disease.

GIFT involves the placement of sperm and eggs in the fallopian tube by laparoscopy or minilaparotomy. While GIFT is a more invasive procedure than IVF, the success rate is higher, 34.4% overall in 1995. For women under 35, the delivery rate per retrieval cycle without a male factor was 33.5%. For women over 39, the rate was 11.9%. GIFT is not appropriate for women with severe tubal disease and is less successful than IVF with male factor infertility, since fertilization cannot be documented. With ZIFT, fertilization occurs in vitro, and the early development of the embryo occurs in the natural site, the fallopian tube, after transfer by laparoscopy or minilaparotomy. The average delivery rate per retrieval in 1995 was 27.9%.

Prognosis

The prognosis for conception and normal pregnancy is good if minor (even multiple) disorders can be identified and treated; it is poor if the causes of infertility are severe, untreatable, or of prolonged duration (over 3 years).

It is important to remember that in the absence of identifiable causes of infertility, 60% of couples will achieve a pregnancy within 3 years. Couples with unexplained infertility who do not achieve pregnancy within 3 years should be offered ovulation induction or assisted reproductive technology. Also, offering appropriately timed information about adoption is considered part of a complete infertility regimen.

Bristow RE et al: Ovulation induction, infertility, and ovarian cancer risk. Fertil Steril 1996;66:499. [NLM Cit ID: 96413452] (Critical review of published data suggesting that association between ovulation induction and ovarian cancer is not necessarily causal and that infertility itself is an independent risk factor. There is no consistent dose-effect relationship, and latency is highly variable.)

Morell V: Basic infertility assessment. Prim Care 1997; 24:195. [NLM Cit ID: 97169323] (Summary of infertility management for the primary care provider.)

Society for Assisted Reproductive Technology, American Society for Reproductive Medicine: Assisted reproductive technology in the United States and Canada: 1995 results generated from the American Society for Reproductive Medicine/Society for Assisted Reproductive Technology Registry. Fertil Steril 1998;69:389. [NLM Cit ID: 98193015]

CONTRACEPTION

Voluntary control of childbearing benefits women, men, and the children born to them. Contraception should be available to all women and men of reproductive ages. Education about contraception and access to contraceptive pills or devices are especially important for sexually active teenagers and for women following childbirth or abortion.

1. ORAL CONTRACEPTIVES

Combined Oral Contraceptives

A. Efficacy and Methods of Use: Oral contraceptives have a theoretical failure rate of less than 0.5% if taken absolutely on schedule and a typical failure rate of 3%. Their primary mode of action is suppression of ovulation. The pills are initially started on the first or fifth day of the ovarian cycle and taken daily for 21 days, followed by 7 days of placebos or no medication, and this schedule is then continued for each cycle. The pills are often initially started on the first Sunday after the onset of menses, to help patients remember their starting day and to avoid menses on the weekend. If a pill is missed at any time, two pills should be taken the next day, and another method of contraception should be used for the rest of the cycle (eg, condoms or foam). A backup method should also be used during the first cycle if the pills are started later than the fifth day. Low-dose oral contraceptives is no longer contraindicated in women aged 35–50 who are nonsmokers and have no risk factors for cardiovascular disease.

B. Benefits of Oral Contraceptives: There are many noncontraceptive advantages to oral contraceptives. Menstrual flow is lighter, resultant anemia is less common, and dysmenorrhea is relieved for most women. Functional ovarian cysts generally disappear with oral contraceptive use, and new cysts do not occur. Pain with ovulation and postovulatory aching are relieved. The risk of ovarian and endometrial cancer is decreased. The risks of salpingitis and ectopic pregnancy may be diminished. Acne is usually improved. The frequency of developing myomas is lower in long-term users (> 4 years). There is a beneficial effect on bone mass.

C. Selection of an Oral Contraceptive: Any of the combination oral contraceptives containing less than 50 μg of estrogen are suitable for most women. Women taking pills containing 50 μg or more of estrogen should be switched to lower-dosage pills, since many of the adverse side effects are dose-related. There is some variation in potency of the various progestins in the pills, but there are essentially no clinically significant differences for most women among the progestins in the low-dose pills. Women who have acne or hirsutism may benefit from use of one of the pills containing the newer progestins, desogestrel or norgestimate, as they are the least androgenic. The dose of estrogen in oral contraceptives is four or more times higher than that in estrogen preparations used in menopause, and for that reason more side effects can be expected from oral contraceptives. The low-dose oral contraceptives commonly used in the United States are listed in Table 17–5.

D. Drug Interactions: Several drugs interact

Table 17–5. Commonly used low-dose oral contraceptives.

Name	Type	Progestin	Estrogen (Ethinyl Estradiol)	Cost per Month[1]
Alesse	Combination	0.1 mg levonorgestrel	20 μg	$28.68
Mircette	Combination	0.5 mg desogestrel	20 μg	$28.60
Loestrin 1/20	Combination	1 mg norethindrone acetate	20 μg	$29.67
Estrostep	Triphasic	1.0 mg norethindrone acetate (days 1–5)	20 μg	$29.67
		1.0 mg norethindrone acetate (days 6–12)	30 μg	
		1.0 mg norethindrone acetate (days 13–21)	35 μg	
Lo-Ovral	Combination	0.3 mg dl-norgestrel	30 μg	$30.61
Nordette and Levlen	Combination	0.15 mg levonorgestrel	30 μg	$29.50
Norinyl 1/35 [N] and Ortho-Novum 1/35 [O]	Combination	1 mg norethindrone	35 μg	$28.26 [N] $29.84 [O]
Loestrin 1.5/30	Combination	1.5 mg norethindrone acetate	30 μg	$29.81
Demulen 1/35	Combination	1 mg ethynodiol diacetate	35 μg	$31.16
Brevicon [B], Modicon [M], and Jenest [J]	Combination	0.5 mg norethindrone	35 μg	$26.57 [B] $32.71 [M] $21.52 [J]
Ovcon 35	Combination	0.4 mg norethindrone	35 μg	$31.53
Ortho-Cept [O] and Desogen [D]	Combination	0.15 mg desogestrel	30 μg	$29.98 [O] $24.88 [D]
Ortho-Cyclen	Combination	0.25 mg norgestimate	35 μg	$29.98
Ortho-Tricyclen	Triphasic	0.15 mg norgestimate (days 1–7) 0.215 mg norgestimate (days 8–14) 0.25 mg norgestimate (days 15–21)	35 μg	$29.98
Ortho-Novum 7/7/7	Triphasic	0.5 mg norethindrone (days 1–7) 0.75 mg norethindrone (days 8–14) 1 mg norethindrone (days 15–21)	35 μg	$29.98
Tri-Norinyl	Triphasic	0.5 mg norethindrone (days 1–7) 1 mg norethindrone (days 8–16) 0.5 mg norethindrone (days 17–21)	35 μg	$27.01
Triphasil [T] and Tri-Levlen [TL]	Triphasic	0.05 mg levonorgestrel (days 1–6) 0.0075 mg levonorgestrel (days 7–11) 0.125 mg levonorgestrel (days 12–21)	30 μg 40 μg 30 μg	$28.68 [T] $28.02 [TL]
Micronor [M] and Nor-QD [N]	Progestin-only minipill	0.35 mg norethindrone to be taken continuously	(None)	$34.82 [M] $29.55 [N]
Ovrette	Progestin-only minipill	0.075 mg dl-norgestrel to be taken continuously	(None)	$29.55

[1]Cost to pharmacist (average wholesale price, generic when possible) for quantity listed. Source: *Drug Topics Red Book*, March 2000; Vol. 19, No. 3.

with oral contraceptives to decrease their efficacy by causing induction of microsomal enzymes in the liver, by increasing sex hormone-binding globulin, and by other mechanisms. Some commonly prescribed drugs in this category are phenytoin, phenobarbital (and other barbiturates), primidone, carbamazepine, and rifampin. Women taking these drugs should use another means of contraception for maximum safety.

E. Contraindications and Adverse Effects: Oral contraceptives have been associated with many adverse effects; they are contraindicated in some situations and should be used with caution in others (Table 17–6).

1. Myocardial infarction–The risk of heart attack is higher with use of oral contraceptives, particularly with pills containing 50 μg of estrogen or more. Cigarette smoking, obesity, hypertension, diabetes, or hypercholesterolemia increases the risk. Young nonsmoking women have minimal increased risk. Smokers over age 40 and women with other cardiovascular risk factors should use other methods of birth control.

2. Thromboembolic disease–An increased rate of venous thromboembolism is found in oral contraceptive users, especially if the dose of estrogen is 50 μg or more. While the overall risk is very low (15 per 100,000 woman-years), several recent studies have reported a twofold increased risk in women using oral contraceptives containing the progestins gestodene (not available in the United States) or desogestrel compared with women using oral contraceptives with levonorgestrel and norethindrone. However, review of the data suggests that the results of these studies may have been biased by differences between users in underlying risk and in the likelihood of being diagnosed. Women who develop thrombophlebitis should stop using this method, as should those at risk of thrombophlebitis because of surgery, fracture, serious injury, or immobilization.

Table 17–6. Contraindications to use of oral contraceptives.

Absolute contraindications
Pregnancy
Thrombophlebitis or thromboembolic disorders (past or present)
Stroke or coronary artery disease (past or present)
Cancer of the breast (known or suspected)
Undiagnosed abnormal vaginal bleeding
Estrogen-dependent cancer (known or suspected)
Benign or malignant tumor of the liver (past or present)
Relative contraindications
Age over 35 years and heavy cigarette smoking (> 15 cigarettes daily)
Migraine or recurrent persistent severe headache
Hypertension
Cardiac or renal disease
Diabetes
Gallbladder disease
Cholestasis during pregnancy
Active hepatitis or infectious mononucleosis
Sickle cell disease (S/S or S/C type)
Surgery, fracture, or severe injury
Lactation
Significant psychologic depression

3. Cerebrovascular disease–Overall, a small increased risk of hemorrhagic stroke and subarachnoid hemorrhage and a somewhat greater increased risk of thrombotic stroke has been found; smoking, hypertension, and age over 35 years are associated with increased risk. Women who develop warning symptoms such as severe headache, blurred or lost vision, or other transient neurologic disorders should stop using oral contraceptives.

4. Carcinoma–A relationship between long-term (3–4 years) oral contraceptive use and occurrence of cervical dysplasia and cancer has been found in various studies. No confirmed relationship has been found between use of oral contraceptives and cancer of the breast. Combination oral contraceptives reduce the risk of endometrial carcinoma by 40% after 2 years of use and 60% after 4 or more years of use. The risk of ovarian cancer is reduced by 30% with pill use for less than 4 years, by 60% with use for 5–11 years, and by 80% after 12 or more years. Rarely, oral contraceptives have been associated with the development of benign or malignant hepatic tumors; this may lead to rupture of the liver, hemorrhage, and death. The risk increases with higher dosage, longer duration of use, and older age.

5. Metabolic disorders–A decrease in glucose tolerance and an increase in triglyceride levels is seen in pill takers, and women with diabetes using this method should be carefully monitored.

6. Hypertension–Oral contraceptives may cause hypertension in some women; the risk is increased with longer duration of use and older age. Women who develop hypertension while using oral contraceptives should use other contraceptive methods. However, with regular blood pressure monitoring, nonsmoking women under the age of 40 with well-controlled mild hypertension may use oral contraceptives.

7. Headache–Migraine or other vascular headaches may occur or worsen with pill use. If severe or frequent headaches develop while using this method, it should be discontinued.

8. Amenorrhea–Postpill amenorrhea lasting a year or longer occurs occasionally, sometimes with galactorrhea. PRL levels should be checked; if elevated, a pituitary prolactinoma may be present.

9. Disorders of lactation–Combined oral contraceptives can impair the quantity and quality of breast milk. While it is preferable to avoid the use of combination oral contraceptives during lactation, the effects on milk quality are small and are not associated with developmental abnormalities in infants. Combination oral contraceptives should be started no earlier than 6 weeks postpartum to allow for establishment of lactation. Progestin-only pills, levonorgestrel implants, and depot medroxyprogesterone acetate are alternatives with no adverse effects on milk quality.

10. Other disorders–Depression may occur or be worsened with oral contraceptive use. Fluid retention may occur. Patients who had cholestatic jaundice during pregnancy may develop it while taking birth control pills.

F. Minor Side Effects: Nausea and dizziness may occur in the first few months of pill use. A weight gain of 2–5 lb commonly occurs. Spotting or breakthrough bleeding between menstrual periods may occur, especially if a pill is skipped or taken late; this may be helped by switching to a pill of slightly greater potency (see ¶C, above). Missed menstrual periods may occur, especially with low-dose pills. A pregnancy test should be performed if pills have been skipped or if two or more menstrual periods are missed. Depression, fatigue, and decreased libido can occur. Chloasma may occur, as in pregnancy, and is increased by exposure to sunlight.

Progestin Minipill

A. Efficacy and Methods of Use: Formulations containing 0.35 mg of norethindrone or 0.075 mg of norgestrel are available in the USA. Their efficacy is slightly lower than that of combined oral contraceptives, with failure rates of 1–4% being reported. The minipill is believed to prevent conception by causing thickening of the cervical mucus to make it hostile to sperm, alteration of ovum transport (which may account for the higher rate of ectopic pregnancy with these pills), and inhibition of implantation. Ovulation is inhibited inconsistently with this method. The minipill is begun on the first day of a menstrual cycle and then taken continuously for as long as contraception is desired.

B. Advantages: The low dose and absence of estrogen make the minipill safe during lactation; it may increase the flow of milk. It is often tried by women who want minimal doses of hormones and by patients who are over age 35. The minipill can be used by women with uterine myomas or sickle cell disease (S/S or S/C). Like the combined pill, the minipill decreases the likelihood of pelvic inflammatory disease by its effect on cervical mucus.

C. Complications and Contraindications: Minipill users often have bleeding irregularities (eg, prolonged flow, spotting, or amenorrhea); such patients may need monthly pregnancy tests. Ectopic pregnancies are more frequent, and complaints of abdominal pain should be investigated with this in mind. The absolute contraindications and many of the relative contraindications listed in Table 17–6 apply to the minipill. Exceptions are mentioned in ¶E, above. Minor side effects of combination oral contraceptives such as weight gain and mild headache may also occur with the minipill.

Beral V et al: Mortality associated with oral contraceptive use: 25 year follow up of cohort of 46,000 women from Royal College of General Practitioners' oral contraceptive study. BMJ 1999;318:96. [NLM Cit ID: 99096741] (There was no difference in the overall rate of death among ever-users and never-users. Among current and recent [< 10 years] users, the relative risk of death from ovarian cancer was 0.2 [95% CI, 0.1–0.8], from cervical cancer, 2.5 [1.1–6.1], and from cerebrovascular disease, 1.9 [1.2–3.1].)

Chang CL et al: Migraine and stroke in young women: case-control study. The World Health Organization Collaborative Study of Cardiovascular Disease and Steroid Hormone Contraception. BMJ 1999;318:13. [NLM Cit ID: 99091458] (Overall, the odds ratios for thrombotic stroke were similar in women with both classic [with aura] and simple migraine [without aura]. Migraine in women of childbearing age increased the risk of thrombotic stroke but not hemorrhagic stroke. Although the absolute risk of stroke is low, oral contraceptive use, as well as smoking and hypertension, markedly increased the odds of thrombotic stroke in young women with migraine.)

DeCherney A: Bone-sparing properties of oral contraceptives. Am J Obstet Gynecol 1996;174:15. [NLM Cit ID: 96148661] (The most important benefit of oral contraceptives for women over 35 may be prevention of loss of bone mass.)

2. CONTRACEPTIVE INJECTIONS & IMPLANTS (Long-Acting Progestins)

The injectable progestin medroxyprogesterone acetate is approved for contraceptive use in the USA. There is extensive worldwide experience with this method over the past 3 decades. The medication is given as a deep intramuscular injection of 150 mg every 3 months and has a contraceptive efficacy of 99.7%. Common side effects include irregular bleeding, amenorrhea, weight gain, and headache. Bone mineral loss may occur. Users commonly have irregular bleeding initially and subsequently develop amenorrhea. Ovulation may be delayed after the last injection. Contraindications are similar to those for the minipill.

The other available long-acting progestin is the Norplant system, a contraceptive implant containing levonorgestrel. The system consists of six small Silastic capsules that are inserted subcutaneously in the inner aspect of the upper arm. They release daily and provide highly effective contraception for 5 years. In the first year of use, Norplant is 99.8% effective. Contraceptive effectiveness drops slightly in succeeding years, but even in the fifth year it is more effective than the combination pill. The most common side effects include irregular bleeding and spotting, amenorrhea, headache, acne, and weight gain. Irregular bleeding is the most common reason for discontinuation. Hormone levels drop rapidly after removal of the implants, and there is no delay in the return of fertility. Contraindications are similar to those for the minipill. Insertion of the implants requires a minor surgical procedure under local anesthesia. Removal is also done under local anesthesia and may be more difficult than insertion. Removal may be facilitated by the "U" technique, involving use of a modified vasectomy clamp through a 4 mm incision parallel to the implants between implants three and four.

Kaunitz AM: Injectable depot medroxyprogesterone acetate contraception: an update for U.S. clinicians. Int J Fertil Womens Med 1998;43:73. [NLM Cit ID: 98270369] (A review of the benefits and the disadvantages, including possible loss of bone mineral density.)

Rosenberg MJ et al: A comparison of "U" and standard techniques for Norplant removal. Obstet Gynecol 1997;89:168. [NLM Cit ID: 97167326] (This recently developed technique for Norplant removal is more easily performed than the standard technique, especially for inexperienced clinicians.)

3. INTRAUTERINE DEVICES (IUDs)

The only IUDs currently manufactured in the USA are the Progestasert (which secretes progesterone into the uterus) and the copper-bearing TCu380A; the mechanism of action is thought to be related to impaired fertilization due to effects on sperm motility and to abnormal development in the oviduct of those ova that may have been fertilized.

The TCu380A must be replaced every 10 years for maximum efficacy. The Progestasert must be replaced yearly but has the advantage of causing less cramping and menstrual flow.

The IUD is often an excellent contraceptive method for parous women in a mutually monogamous relationship. It is less desirable for young nulliparas because of the greater threat of pelvic inflammatory disease in young women and the possible impairment of future fertility.

Insertion

Insertion can be performed during or after the menses, at midcycle to prevent implantation, or later in the cycle if the patient has not become pregnant. Most clinicians wait for 6–8 weeks postpartum before inserting an IUD. When insertion is performed during lactation, there is greater risk of uterine perforation or embedding of the IUD. Insertion immediately following abortion is acceptable if there is no sepsis and if follow-up insertion a month later will not be possible; otherwise, it is wise to wait until 4 weeks postabortion.

Contraindications & Complications

Contraindications to use of IUDs are outlined in Table 17–7.

Table 17–7. Contraindications to IUD use.

Absolute contraindications
Pregnancy
Acute or subacute pelvic inflammatory disease or purulent cervicitis
Relative contraindications
History of pelvic inflammatory disease since the last pregnancy
History of ectopic pregnancy (progestin-containing IUD only)
Multiple sexual partners
Nulliparous woman concerned about future fertility
Lack of available follow-up care
Menorrhagia or severe dysmenorrhea
Cervical or uterine neoplasia
Abnormal size or shape of uterus, including myomas distorting cavity
Valvular heart disease

A. Pregnancy: An IUD can be inserted within 5 days following a single episode of unprotected midcycle coitus as a postcoital contraceptive. An IUD should not be inserted into a pregnant uterus. If pregnancy occurs as an IUD failure, there is a greater chance of spontaneous abortion if the IUD is left in situ (50%) than if it is removed (25%). Spontaneous abortion with an IUD in place is associated with a high risk of severe sepsis, and death can occur rapidly. Women using an IUD who become pregnant should have the IUD removed if the string is visible. It can be removed at the time of abortion if this is desired. If the string is not visible and the patient wants to continue the pregnancy, she should be informed of the serious risk of sepsis and, occasionally, death with such pregnancies. She should be informed that any flu-like symptoms such as fever, myalgia, headache, or nausea warrant immediate medical attention for possible septic abortion.

Since the ratio of ectopic to intrauterine pregnancies is increased among IUD wearers, clinicians should search for adnexal masses in early pregnancy and should always check the products of conception for placental tissue following abortion.

B. Pelvic Infection: There is an increased risk of pelvic infection during the first month following insertion. The subsequent risk of pelvic infection appears to be primarily related to the risk of acquiring sexually transmitted infections. The threat of sexually transmitted pelvic infection can be essentially eliminated by limiting the use of the IUD to parous women in a mutually monogamous relationship. The use of IUDs by young nulliparas is undesirable because of the increased risk of sexually transmitted disease and the threat to future fertility.

C. Menorrhagia or Severe Dysmenorrhea: The IUD can cause heavier menstrual periods, bleeding between periods, and more cramping, so it is generally not suitable for women who already suffer from these problems. However, progesterone-secreting IUDs can be tried in these cases, as they often cause decreased bleeding and cramping with menses.

Nonsteroidal anti-inflammatory drugs are also helpful in decreasing bleeding and pain in IUD users.

D. Complete or Partial Expulsion: Spontaneous expulsion of the IUD occurs in 10–20% of cases during the first year of use. Remove any IUD if the body of the device can be seen or felt in the cervical os.

E. Missing IUD Strings: If the transcervical tail cannot be seen, this may signify unnoticed expulsion, perforation of the uterus with abdominal migration of the IUD, or simply retraction of the string into the cervical canal or uterus owing to movement of the IUD or uterine growth with pregnancy. Once pregnancy is ruled out, one should probe for the IUD with a sterile sound or forceps designed for IUD removal, after administering a paracervical block. If the IUD cannot be detected, pelvic ultrasound will demonstrate the IUD if it is in the uterus. Alternatively, obtain anteroposterior and lateral x-rays of the pelvis with another IUD or a sound in the uterus as a marker, to confirm an extrauterine IUD. If the IUD is in the abdominal cavity, it should generally be removed by laparoscopy or laparotomy. Open-looped all-plastic IUDs such as the Lippes Loop can be left in the pelvis without danger, but ring-shaped IUDs may strangulate a loop of bowel and copper-bearing IUDs may cause tissue reaction and adhesions.

Perforations of the uterus are less likely if insertion is performed slowly, with meticulous care taken to follow directions applicable to each type of IUD.

Twelve years experience with the TCu380A and TCu220C. Contraception 1997;56:341. [NLM Cit ID: 98155871] (The TCu380A is highly efficacious and may be considered an alternative to surgical sterilization for women requiring long-term contraception.)

4. DIAPHRAGM & CERVICAL CAP

The diaphragm (with contraceptive jelly) is a safe and effective contraceptive method with features that make it acceptable to some women and not others. Failure rates range from 2% to 20%, depending on the motivation of the woman and the care with which the diaphragm is used. The advantages of this method are that it has no systemic side effects and gives significant protection against pelvic infection and cervical dysplasia as well as pregnancy. The disadvantages are that it must be inserted near the time of coitus and that pressure from the rim predisposes some women to cystitis after intercourse.

The cervical cap (with contraceptive jelly) is similar to the diaphragm but fits snugly over the cervix only (the diaphragm stretches from behind the cervix to behind the pubic symphysis). The cervical cap is more difficult to insert and remove than the diaphragm. The main advantages are that it can be used by women who cannot be fitted for a diaphragm because of a relaxed anterior vaginal wall or by women who have discomfort or develop repeated bladder infections with the diaphragm.

Because of the small risk of toxic shock syndrome, a cervical cap or diaphragm should not be left in the vagina for over 12–18 hours, nor should these devices be used during the menstrual period (see above).

5. CONTRACEPTIVE FOAM, CREAM, FILM, SPONGE, JELLY, & SUPPOSITORY

These products are available without prescription, are easy to use, and are fairly effective, with reported failure rates of 2–30%. All contain the spermicides nonoxynol 9 or octoxynol 9, which also have some virucidal and bactericidal activity. Nonoxynol-9 does not appear to adversely affect the vaginal colonization of hydrogen peroxide-producing lactobacilli. The products have the advantages of being simple to use and easily available. Their disadvantage is a slightly higher failure rate than the diaphragm or condom.

Richardson BA et al: Use of nonoxynol-9 and changes in vaginal lactobacilli. J Infect Dis 1998;178:441. [NLM Cit ID: 9697724] (A randomized controlled clinical trial demonstrated that daily use of nonoxynol-9 for 2 weeks reduced the likelihood of bacterial vaginosis.)

6. CONDOM

The male sheath of latex or animal membrane affords good protection against pregnancy—equivalent to that of a diaphragm and spermicidal jelly; latex (but not animal membrane) condoms also offer protection against sexually transmitted disease and cervical dysplasia. Men and women seeking protection against HIV transmission are advised to use a latex condom along with spermicide during vaginal or rectal intercourse. When a spermicide such as vaginal foam is used with the condom, the failure rate approaches that of oral contraceptives. Condoms coated with spermicide are available in the USA. The disadvantages of condoms are dulling of sensation and spillage of semen due to tearing, slipping, or leakage with detumescence of the penis.

A female condom made of polyurethane is now available in the USA. The reported failure rate in preventing pregnancy (26%) is somewhat higher than other barrier methods. However, it is the only female-controlled method that offers significant protection from both pregnancy and sexually transmitted diseases.

Rosen AD et al: Study of condom integrity after brief exposure to over-the-counter vaginal preparations. South

Med J 1999;92:305. [NLM Cit ID: 99192085] (Over-the-counter vaginal products that contain mineral oil or vegetable oil—as do some moisturizers, antipruritics, and antifungals—may weaken latex condoms and reduce their efficacy.)

Rosenberg MJ et al: Latex condom breakage and slippage in a controlled clinical trial. Contraception 1997;56:17. [NLM Cit ID: 97451051] (Monogamous couples using condoms for contraception had very low rates of breakage [0.28%] and slippage [0.63%].)

7. CONTRACEPTION BASED ON AWARENESS OF FERTILE PERIODS

There is renewed interest in methods to identify times of ovulation and avoidance of unprotected intercourse at that time as a means of family planning. These methods are most effective when the couple restricts intercourse to the postovular phase of the cycle or uses a barrier method at other times. Women benefit from learning to identify their fertile periods. Well-instructed, motivated couples may achieve low pregnancy rates with fertility awareness, but in many field trials, the pregnancy rates were as high as 20%.

"Symptothermal" Natural Family Planning

The basis for this approach is patient-observed increase in clear elastic cervical mucus, brief abdominal midcycle discomfort ("mittelschmerz"), and a sustained rise of the basal body temperature about 2 weeks after onset of menstruation. Unprotected intercourse is avoided from shortly after the menstrual period, when fertile mucus is first identified, until 48 hours after ovulation, as identified by a sustained rise in temperature and the disappearance of clear elastic mucus.

Calendar Method

After the length of the menstrual cycle has been observed for at least 8 months, the following calculations are made: (1) The first fertile day is determined by subtracting 18 days from the shortest cycle; (2) the last fertile day is determined by subtracting 11 days from the longest cycle. For example, if the observed cycles run from 24 to 28 days, the fertile period would extend from the sixth day of the cycle (24 minus 18) through the 17th day (28 minus 11).

Basal Body Temperature Method

This method indicates the safe time for intercourse after ovulation has passed. The temperature must be taken immediately upon awakening, before any activity. A slight drop in temperature often occurs 1–1½ days before ovulation, and a rise of about 0.4 °C occurs 1–2 days after ovulation. The elevated temperature continues throughout the remainder of the cycle. New data suggest that the risk of pregnancy increases starting 5 days prior to the day of ovulation, peaks on the day of ovulation, and then rapidly decreases to zero by the day after ovulation.

Frank-Herrmann P et al: Natural family planning with and without barrier method use in the fertile phase: efficacy in relation to sexual behavior: A German prospective long-term study. Adv Contracept 1997;13:179. [NLM Cit ID: 97434450] (Among 758 couples using natural family planning with and without barrier methods, "perfect use" of the method resulted in failure rates under 1%.)

Wilcox AJ et al: Timing of sexual intercourse in relation to ovulation. N Engl J Med 1995;333:1517. [NLM Cit ID: 96067433] (Among 221 women attempting conception, all pregnancies occurred with coitus during the 6-day period ending on the day of ovulation.)

8. EMERGENCY CONTRACEPTION

If unprotected intercourse occurs in midcycle and the woman is certain she has not inadvertently become pregnant earlier in the cycle, the following regimens are effective in preventing implantation. The failure rate is less than 1.5%. These methods should be started within 72 hours after coitus. (1) Ethinyl estradiol, 2.5 mg twice daily for 5 days. (2) Ovral (50 μg of ethinyl estradiol with 0.5 mg of norgestrel), two tablets at once followed by two tablets 12 hours later (also available prepackaged as Preven), or four pills twice, 12 hours apart, of Lo/Ovral, Nordette, Levlen, or the yellow pills in the Triphasil or Tri-Levlen regimens. Antinausea medication may be necessary with these regimens. Bleeding should occur within 3–4 weeks. If pregnancy occurs, abortion is advisable because of fetal exposure to possibly teratogenic doses of sex steroids. Levonorgestrel, 0.75 mg given in two doses 12 hours apart (available prepackaged as Plan B), starting within 72 hours after unprotected intercourse, is more effective and associated with less nausea and vomiting than the regimens described above. Mifepristone (RU 486), in a single 10 mg dose within 120 hours after unprotected intercourse, appears to be an excellent postcoital contraceptive with minimal side effects. Mifepristone is not currently available in the United States.

IUD insertion within 5 days after one episode of unprotected midcycle coitus will also prevent pregnancy; copper-bearing IUDs have been tested for this purpose. The disadvantage of this method is possible infection, especially in rape cases; the advantage is ongoing contraceptive protection if this is desired in a patient for whom the IUD is a suitable choice.

Information on clinics or individual clinicians providing emergency contraception in the United States may be obtained by calling 1-888-NOT-2-LATE.

Comparison of three single doses of mifepristone as emergency contraception: A randomized trial. Lancet 1999;

353:697. [NLM Cit ID: 99171519] (A single 10 mg dose of mifepristone was as effective as a 600 mg dose for emergency contraception.)

Piaggio G et al: Timing of emergency contraception with levonorgestrel or the Yuzpe regimen. Task Force on Postovulatory Methods of Fertility Regulation. Lancet 1999;353:721. [NLM Cit ID: 99171525] (There is a linear relationship between efficacy and time from intercourse to treatment with both regimens. The pregnancy rate increased from 0.5% when treatment was given within 12 hours to 4.1% when given between 61 and 72 hours after intercourse.)

Randomized controlled trial of levonorgestrel versus the Yuzpe regimen of combined oral contraceptives for emergency contraception. Lancet 1998;352:428. [NLM Cit ID: 98372481] (The levonorgestrel regimen was better tolerated and more effective than the current standard approach to hormonal emergency contraception.)

9. ABORTION

Since the legalization of abortion in the USA in 1973, the related maternal mortality rate has fallen markedly, because illegal and self-induced abortions have been replaced by safer medical procedures. Abortions in the first trimester of pregnancy are performed by vacuum aspiration under local anesthesia. A similar technique, dilation and evacuation, is often used in the second trimester, with general or local anesthesia. Techniques utilizing intra-amniotic instillation of hypertonic saline solution or prostaglandins are also occasionally used after 18 weeks from the LMP but are more difficult for the patient. Abortions are rarely performed after 20 weeks from the LMP. It is currently believed that fetal viability is established at about 24 weeks. Legal abortion has a mortality rate of 1:100,000. Rates of morbidity and mortality rise with length of gestation. Currently in the USA, 90% of abortions are performed before 12 weeks' gestation and only 3–4% after 17 weeks. Every effort should be made to continue the trend toward earlier abortion.

Complications resulting from abortion include retained products of conception (often associated with infection and heavy bleeding) and unrecognized ectopic pregnancy. Immediate analysis of the removed tissue for placenta can exclude or corroborate the diagnosis of ectopic pregnancy. Women presenting with fever, bleeding, or abdominal pain after abortion should be examined; use of broad-spectrum antibiotics and reaspiration of the uterus are frequently necessary. Hospitalization is advisable if acute salpingitis requires intravenous administration of antibiotics. Complications following illegal abortion often need emergency care for hemorrhage, septic shock, or uterine perforation.

Rh immune globulin should be given to all Rh-negative women following abortion. Contraception should be thoroughly discussed and contraceptive supplies or pills provided at the time of abortion. In women with a past history of pelvic inflammatory disease, prophylactic antibiotics are indicated: A one-dose regimen is doxycycline, 200 mg orally 1 hour before the procedure, or aqueous penicillin G, 1 million units intravenously 30 minutes before. In the second trimester, use cefazolin, 1 g intravenously 30 minutes before the procedure. Many clinics prescribe tetracycline, 500 mg four times daily for 5 days after the procedure for all patients.

Long-term sequelae of repeated induced abortions have been studied, but as yet there is no consensus on whether there are increased rates of fetal loss or premature labor. It is felt that such adverse sequelae can be minimized by performing early abortion with minimal cervical dilation or by the use of osmotic dilators to induce gradual cervical dilation. A recent population-based study showed no evidence of an increased risk of breast cancer in women who had undergone an induced abortion.

An oral abortifacient, mifepristone (RU 486), 600 mg as a single dose followed in 36–48 hours by a prostaglandin vaginally or orally, is 95% successful in spontaneously terminating pregnancies of up to 9 weeks' duration with minimum complications. The drug acts as an antihormone to progesterone and glucocorticoids without producing adrenal insufficiency. Currently available in some European countries, it is not approved for use in the USA. Although not approved by the FDA for this indication, a combination of intramuscular methotrexate, 50 mg/m^2 of body surface area, followed 7 days later by vaginal misoprostol, 800 μg, was 98% successful in terminating pregnancy at 8 weeks or less. Minor side effects such as nausea, vomiting, and diarrhea are common with these regimens. There is a 5–10% incidence of hemorrhage or incomplete abortion requiring curettage, but there are no known long-term complications.

Grimes DA: Medical abortion in early pregnancy: A review of the evidence. Obstet Gynecol 1997;89(5 Part 1):790. [NLM Cit ID: 97309132] (Medical abortion is safe and effective, but hemorrhage and gastrointestinal side effects are more common than with surgical abortion.)

Grimes DA: A 26-year-old woman seeking an abortion. JAMA 1999;282:1169. [NLM Cit ID: 99429229] (A thoughtful discussion of a number of aspects of induced abortion.)

Melbye M et al: Induced abortion and the risk of breast cancer. N Engl J Med 1997;336:81. [NLM Cit ID: 97130062] (A large population-based study demonstrating that induced abortion has no overall effect on the subsequent risk of breast cancer.)

10. STERILIZATION

In the USA, sterilization is the most popular method of birth control for couples who want no more children. Although sterilization is reversible in some instances, reversal surgery in both men and women is costly, complicated, and not always successful. Therefore, patients should be counseled carefully before sterilization and should view the procedure as final.

Vasectomy is a safe, simple procedure in which the vas deferens is severed and sealed through a scrotal incision under local anesthesia. Long-term follow-up studies on vasectomized men show no excess risk of cardiovascular disease. Several studies have shown a possible association with prostate cancer, but the evidence is weak and inconsistent.

Female sterilization is currently performed via laparoscopic bipolar electrocoagulation or plastic ring application on the uterine tubes or via minilaparotomy with Pomeroy tubal resection. The advantages of laparoscopy are minimal postoperative pain, small incisions, and rapid recovery. The advantages of minilaparotomy are that it can be performed with standard surgical instruments under local or general anesthesia. However, there is more postoperative pain and a longer recovery period. Failure rates after tubal sterilization are approximately 0.5%; this fact should be discussed with women preoperatively. Some studies have found an increased risk of menstrual irregularities as a long-term complication of tubal ligation, but findings in different studies have been inconsistent.

Peterson HB et al: The risk of pregnancy after tubal sterilization: Findings from the U.S. Collaborative Review of Sterilization. Am J Obstet Gynecol 1996;174:1161. [NLM Cit ID: 96199790] (The cumulative 10-year probabilities of pregnancy after clip sterilization, unipolar coagulation, and bipolar coagulation were 36.5/1000 procedures, 7.5/1000, and 54.3/1000, respectively.)

RAPE

Rape, or sexual assault, is legally defined in different ways in various jurisdictions. Physicians and emergency room personnel who deal with rape victims should be familiar with the laws pertaining to sexual assault in their own state. From a medical and psychologic viewpoint, it is essential that persons treating rape victims recognize the nonconsensual and violent nature of the crime. About 95% of reported rape victims are women. Penetration may be vaginal, anal, or oral and may be by the penis, hand, or a foreign object. The absence of genital injury does not imply consent by the victim. The assailant may be unknown to the victim or may be an acquaintance or even the spouse.

"Unlawful sexual intercourse," or statutory rape, is intercourse with a female before the age of majority even with her consent.

Rape represents an expression of anger, power, and sexuality on the part of the rapist. The rapist is usually a hostile man who uses sexual intercourse to terrorize and humiliate a woman. Women neither secretly want to be raped nor do they expect, encourage, or enjoy rape.

Rape involves severe physical injury in 5–10% of cases and is always a terrifying experience in which most victims fear for their lives. Consequently, all victims suffer some psychologic aftermath. Moreover, some rape victims may acquire sexually transmissible disease or become pregnant.

Because rape is a personal crisis, each patient will react differently. The rape trauma syndrome comprises two principal phases:

(1) Immediate or acute: Shaking, sobbing, and restless activity may last from a few days to a few weeks. The patient may experience anger, guilt, or shame or may repress these emotions. Reactions vary depending on the victim's personality and the circumstances of the attack.

(2) Late or chronic: Problems related to the attack may develop weeks or months later. The lifestyle and work patterns of the individual may change. Sleep disorders or phobias often develop. Loss of self-esteem can rarely lead to suicide.

Physicians and emergency room personnel who deal with rape victims should work with community rape crisis centers whenever possible to provide ongoing support and counseling.

General Office Procedures

The physician who first sees the alleged rape victim should be empathetic. Begin with a statement such as, "This is a terrible thing that has happened to you. I want to help."

(1) Secure written consent from the patient, guardian, or next of kin for gynecologic examination; and for photographs if they are likely to be useful as evidence. If police are to be notified, do so, and obtain advice on the preservation and transfer of evidence.

(2) Obtain and record the history in the patient's own words. The sequence of events, ie, the time, place, and circumstances, must be included. Note the date of the LMP, whether or not the woman is pregnant, and the time of the most recent coitus prior to the sexual assault. Note the details of the assault such as body cavities penetrated, use of foreign objects, and number of assailants.

Note whether the victim is calm, agitated, or confused (drugs or alcohol may be involved). Record whether the patient came directly to the hospital or whether she bathed or changed her clothing. Record findings but do not issue even a tentative diagnosis lest it be erroneous or incomplete.

(3) Have the patient disrobe while standing on a white sheet. Hair, dirt, and leaves; underclothing; and any torn or stained clothing should be kept as evidence. Scrape material from beneath fingernails and comb pubic hair for evidence. Place all evidence in

separate clean paper bags or envelopes and label carefully.

(4) Examine the patient, noting any traumatized areas that should be photographed. Examine the body and genitals with a Wood light to identify semen, which fluoresces; positive areas should be swabbed with a premoistened swab and air-dried in order to identify acid phosphatase. Colposcopy can be used to identify small areas of trauma from forced entry especially at the posterior fourchette.

(5) Perform a pelvic examination, explaining all procedures and obtaining the patient's consent before proceeding gently with the examination. Use a narrow speculum lubricated with water only. Collect material with sterile cotton swabs from the vaginal walls and cervix and make two air-dried smears on clean glass slides. Wet and dry swabs of vaginal secretions should be collected and refrigerated for subsequent acid phosphatase and DNA evaluation. Swab the mouth (around molars and cheeks) and anus in the same way, if appropriate. Label all slides carefully. Collect secretions from the vagina, anus, or mouth with a premoistened cotton swab, place at once on a slide with a drop of saline, and cover with a coverslip. Look for motile or nonmotile sperm under high, dry magnification, and record the percentage of motile forms.

(6) Perform appropriate laboratory tests as follows. Culture the vagina, anus, or mouth (as appropriate) for *N gonorrhoeae* and chlamydia. Perform a Papanicolaou smear of the cervix, a wet mount for *T vaginalis*, a baseline pregnancy test, and VDRL test. A confidential test for HIV antibody can be obtained if desired by the patient and repeated in 2–4 months if initially negative. Repeat the pregnancy test if the next menses is missed, and repeat the VDRL test in 6 weeks. Obtain blood (10 mL without anticoagulant) and urine (100 mL) specimens if there is a history of forced ingestion or injection of drugs or alcohol.

(7) Transfer clearly labeled evidence, eg, laboratory specimens, directly to the clinical pathologist in charge or to the responsible laboratory technician, in the presence of witnesses (never via messenger), so that the rules of evidence will not be breached.

Treatment

(1) Give analgesics or sedatives if indicated.

(2) Administer tetanus toxoid if deep lacerations contain soil or dirt particles.

(3) Give ceftriaxone, 125 mg intramuscularly, to prevent gonorrhea. In addition, give metronidazole, 2 g as a single dose, and doxycycline, 100 mg twice daily for 7 days to treat chlamydial infection. Incubating syphilis will probably be prevented by these medications, but the VDRL test should be repeated 6 weeks after the assault.

(4) Prevent pregnancy by using one of the methods discussed under Postcoital Contraception, if necessary (see above).

(5) Vaccinate against hepatitis B.

(6) Make sure the patient and her family and friends have a source of ongoing psychologic support.

Hampton HL: Care of the woman who has been raped. (Current Concepts.) N Engl J Med 1995;332:234. [NLM Cit ID: 95107364]

MENOPAUSAL SYNDROME

Essentials of Diagnosis

- Cessation of menses due to aging or to bilateral oophorectomy.
- Elevation of FSH and LH levels.
- Hot flushes and night sweats (in 80% of women).
- Decreased vaginal lubrication; thinned vaginal mucosa with or without dyspareunia.

General Considerations

The term "menopause" denotes the final cessation of menstruation, either as a normal part of aging or as the result of surgical removal of both ovaries. In a broader sense, as the term is commonly used, it denotes a 1- to 3-year period during which a woman adjusts to a diminishing and then absent menstrual flow and the physiologic changes that may be associated—hot flushes, night sweats, and vaginal dryness or soreness with coitus.

The average age at menopause in Western societies today is 51 years. Premature menopause is defined as ovarian failure and menstrual cessation before age 40; this often has a genetic or autoimmune basis. Surgical menopause due to bilateral oophorectomy is common and can cause more severe symptoms owing to the sudden rapid drop in sex hormone levels.

There is no objective evidence that cessation of ovarian function is associated with severe emotional disturbance or personality changes. However, mood changes toward depression and anxiety can occur at this time. Furthermore, the time of menopause often coincides with other major life changes, such as departure of children from the home, a midlife identity crisis, or divorce. These events, coupled with a sense of the loss of youth, may exacerbate the symptoms of menopause and cause psychologic distress.

Clinical Findings

A. Symptoms and Signs:

1. Cessation of menstruation–Menstrual cycles generally become irregular as menopause approaches. Anovular cycles occur more often, with irregular cycle length and occasional menorrhagia. Menstrual flow usually diminishes in amount owing to decreased estrogen secretion, resulting in less abundant endometrial growth. Finally, cycles become longer, with missed periods or episodes of spotting only. When no bleeding has occurred for one year, the menopausal transition can be said to have occurred. Any bleeding after this time warrants investigation by endometrial curettage or aspiration to rule out endometrial cancer.

2. Hot flushes–Hot flushes (feelings of intense heat over the trunk and face, with flushing of the skin and sweating) occur in 80% of women as a result of the decrease in ovarian hormones. Hot flushes can begin before the cessation of menses. An increase in pulsatile release of gonadotropin-releasing hormone from the hypothalamus is believed to trigger the hot flushes by affecting the adjacent temperature-regulating area of the brain. Hot flushes are more severe in women who undergo surgical menopause. Flushing is more pronounced late in the day, during hot weather, after ingestion of hot foods or drinks, or during periods of tension. Occurring at night, they often cause sweating and insomnia and result in fatigue on the following day.

3. Vaginal atrophy–With decreased estrogen secretion, thinning of the vaginal mucosa and decreased vaginal lubrication occur and may lead to dyspareunia. The introitus decreases in diameter. Pelvic examination reveals pale, smooth vaginal mucosa and a small cervix and uterus. The ovaries are not normally palpable after the menopause. Continued sexual activity will help prevent tissue shrinkage; use of lubricants, estrogen or testosterone cream, or oral estrogen therapy can prevent or relieve pain.

4. Osteoporosis–Osteoporosis may occur as a late sequela of menopause.

B. Laboratory Findings: Serum FSH and LH levels are elevated. Vaginal cytologic examination will show a low estrogen effect with predominantly parabasal cells, indicating lack of epithelial maturation due to hypoestrinism.

Treatment

A. Natural Menopause: Education and support from health providers, midlife discussion groups, and reading material will help most women having difficulty adjusting to the menopause. Physiologic symptoms can be treated as follows:

1. Vasomotor symptoms–Give conjugated estrogens, 0.3 mg or 0.625 mg; estradiol, 0.5 or 1 mg; or estrone sulfate, 0.625 mg; or estradiol can be given transdermally as skin patches that are changed once or twice weekly and secrete 0.05–0.1 mg of hormone daily. When either form of estrogen is used, add a progestin (medroxyprogesterone acetate) to prevent endometrial hyperplasia or cancer. The hormones can be given in several differing regimens. Give estrogen on days 1–25 of each calendar month, with 5–10 mg of medroxyprogesterone acetate added on days 14–25. Withhold hormones from day 26 until the end of the month, when the endometrium will be shed, producing a light, generally painless monthly period. Alternatively, give the estrogen along with 2.5 mg of medroxyprogesterone acetate daily, without stopping. This regimen causes some initial bleeding or spotting, but within a few months it produces an atrophic endometrium that will not bleed. If the patient has had a hysterectomy, a progestin need not be used. Explain to the patient that hot flushes will probably return if the hormone is discontinued. When women wish to stop hormone therapy, the dose should be tapered.

In women who cannot use estrogen, megestrol acetate, 20 mg twice daily, is effective in reducing the frequency of hot flushes. Clonidine given orally or transdermally. 100–150 μg daily, may also reduce the frequency of hot flushes, but its use is limited by side effects, including dry mouth, drowsiness, and hypotension.

2. Vaginal atrophy–This problem can be treated with hormone therapy as outlined above. Alternatively, topical use of hormone creams in small doses will often relieve pain with minimal systemic absorption. Use conjugated estrogens vaginal cream, one-eighth applicatorful (0.3 mg of conjugated estrogens) nightly for 7–10 nights. Thereafter, use every other night or twice weekly. Testosterone propionate 1–2%, 0.5–1 g, in a vanishing cream base used in the same manner is also effective if estrogen is contraindicated. A bland lubricant such as unscented cold cream or water-soluble gel can be helpful at the time of coitus.

3. Osteoporosis–Women should ingest at least 800 mg of calcium daily throughout life. Nonfat or low-fat milk products, calcium-fortified orange juice, green leafy vegetables, corn tortillas, and canned sardines or salmon consumed with the bones are good dietary sources. In addition, 1 g of elemental calcium should be taken as a daily supplement at the time of the menopause and thereafter; calcium supplements should be taken with meals to increase their absorption. Vitamin D, 400 units/d from food, sunlight, or supplements, is necessary to enhance calcium absorption. A daily program of energetic walking and exercise to strengthen the arms and upper body helps maintain bone mass.

Women most at risk for osteoporotic fractures should consider hormone replacement therapy. This includes Caucasian and Asian women, especially if they have a family history of osteoporosis; are thin, short, cigarette smokers, and physically inactive; or have had a low calcium intake in adult life.

B. Advantages and Risks of Hormone Therapy: Long-term estrogen therapy has been shown to decrease a woman's risk of fatal heart attack, probably by decreasing LDL cholesterol, increasing HDL cholesterol, and increasing the elasticity of blood vessel walls. However, a recent study showed no overall cardiovascular benefit with estrogen replacement therapy in a group of postmenopausal women with established coronary disease. Estrogen replacement therapy may prevent or delay the onset of

Alzheimer's disease. The dose of estrogen is much lower than that found in oral contraceptives, and side effects such as hypertension and other cardiovascular disorders are not seen. However, there may be a small increase in the risk of thromboembolic disease. Progestins counteract some but not all of these favorable effects. Estrogen helps to prevent osteoporosis, hot flushes, and dyspareunia and may elevate mood. The risks of estrogen include a probable small increase in breast cancer, especially in women with a close family history of the disease. Several recent studies have shown an increased risk of breast cancer in women using estrogen-progestin therapy, while estrogen therapy alone did not increase the risk. All of the studies have methodology flaws, and the implications for clinical practice are currently unclear. At the very least, clinicians should review with women the current or proposed use of estrogen-progestin therapy and carefully consider the risks and benefits in light of this new information. Endometrial cancer can occur unless adequate progestin is used. Estrogen may cause the growth of uterine myomas, which otherwise shrink after the menopause. (See also discussion of hormone replacement therapy in Chapter 26.)

C. Surgical Menopause: The abrupt hormonal decrease resulting from oophorectomy generally results in severe vasomotor symptoms and rapid onset of dyspareunia and osteoporosis unless treated. Estrogen replacement is generally started immediately after surgery. Conjugated estrogens 1.25 mg, estrone sulfate 1.25 mg, or estradiol 2 mg is given for 25 days of each month. After age 45–50 years, this dose can be tapered to 0.625 mg of conjugated estrogens or equivalent.

Greendale GA et al: The menopause. Lancet 1999;353:571. [NLM Cit ID: 99151457] (A review of current knowledge of the benefits and risks of hormone replacement therapy.)

Grodstein F et al: Postmenopausal estrogen and progestin use and the risk of cardiovascular disease. N Engl J Med 1996;335:453. [NLM Cit ID: 96295908] (Addition of a progestin to estrogen replacement therapy does not appear to reduce the cardioprotective effect of estrogen.)

Hulley S et al: Randomized trial of estrogen plus progestin for secondary prevention of coronary heart disease in postmenopausal women. Heart and Estrogen/Progestin Replacement Study (HERS) Research Group. JAMA 1998;280:605. [NLM Cit ID: 98382151] (A randomized secondary prevention trial of 2763 women with coronary disease found no significant difference between the placebo and hormone replacement therapy [HRT] group with respect to cardiovascular outcomes during an average of 4.1 years of follow-up despite beneficial lipid changes. There was a significant time trend, with more coronary heart disease events in the HRT group in year 1 and fewer in years 4 and 5.)

Schairer C et al: Menopausal estrogen and estrogen-progestin replacement therapy and breast cancer risk. JAMA 2000;283:485. [NLM Cit ID: 20123270] (In a cohort study of 46,355 postmenopausal women, the relative risk of breast cancer with estrogen and estrogen-progestin use for up to 4 years, compared with that of nonusers, was 1.2 [95% CI, 1.0–1.4] and 1.4 [1.1–1.8], respectively. The relative risk increased 0.01 for each year of estrogen use and 0.08 for each year of estrogen-progestin use.)

RELEVANT WORLD WIDE WEB SITES

[Cystic Teratoma]
http://www.brighamrad.harvard.edu/Cases/bwh/hcache/62/full.html

[Evaluation of Neoplasia of the Female Lower Genital Tract]
http://www.oncolink.upenn.edu/classroom/colp/

[Gynecologic Oncology Tutorials]
http://gynoncology.obgyn.washington.edu/Tutorials/Tutorials.html

[Hemorrhagic Corpus Luteum]
http://www.brighamrad.harvard.edu/Cases/bwh/hcache/26/full.html

[Hemorrhagic Torsion of a Left Ovarian Fibroma]
http://www.brighamrad.harvard.edu/Cases/bwh/hcache/44/full.html

[Salpingitis Isthmica Nodosa]
http://www.brighamrad.harvard.edu/Cases/bwh/hcache/56/full.html

Obstetrics*

18

See http://www.current-med.com/ch18.html for updated addresses of Web sites referenced in this chapter.

William R. Crombleholme, MD

DIAGNOSIS & DIFFERENTIAL DIAGNOSIS OF PREGNANCY

It is advantageous to diagnose pregnancy as promptly as possible when a sexually active woman misses a menstrual period or has symptoms suggestive of pregnancy. In the event of a desired pregnancy, prenatal care can begin early, and potentially harmful medications and activities, such as drug and alcohol use, smoking, and occupational chemical exposure, can be halted. In the event of an unwanted pregnancy, counseling about termination of the pregnancy or adoption can be provided at an early stage.

Pregnancy Tests

All urine or blood pregnancy tests rely on the detection of hCG produced by the placenta. hCG levels increase shortly after implantation, double approximately every 48 hours, reach a peak at 50–75 days, and fall to lower levels in the second and third trimesters. Laboratory and home pregnancy tests now use monoclonal antibodies specific for hCG. These tests are performed on urine or serum and are accurate at the time of the missed period or shortly after it.

Compared with intrauterine pregnancies, ectopic pregnancies may show lower levels of hCG, which level off or fall in serial determinations. Quantitative assays of hCG repeated at 48- to 72-hour intervals are used in the diagnosis of ectopic pregnancy, as well as in cases of molar pregnancy, threatened abortion, and missed abortion. Comparison of hCG levels between laboratories may be misleading in a given patient because different international standards may produce results that vary by a factor of two.

Manifestations of Pregnancy

The following symptoms and signs are usually due to pregnancy, but none are diagnostic. A record of the time and frequency of coitus is helpful for diagnosing and dating a pregnancy.

A. Symptoms: Amenorrhea, nausea and vomiting, breast tenderness and tingling, urinary frequency and urgency, "quickening" (noted at about the 18th week), weight gain.

B. Signs (in Weeks From LMP): Breast changes (enlargement, vascular engorgement, colostrum), abdominal enlargement, cyanosis of vagina and cervical portio (about the seventh week), softening of the cervix (seventh week), softening of the cervicouterine junction (eighth week), generalized enlargement and diffuse softening of the corpus (after eighth week).

The uterine fundus is palpable above the pubic symphysis by 12–15 weeks from the LMP and reaches the umbilicus by 20–22 weeks. Fetal heart tones can be heard by Doppler at 10–12 weeks of gestation and by 20 weeks with an ordinary fetoscope.

Differential Diagnosis

The nonpregnant uterus enlarged by myomas can be confused with the gravid uterus, but it is usually very firm and irregular. An ovarian tumor may be found midline, displacing the nonpregnant uterus to the side or posteriorly. Ultrasonography and a pregnancy test will provide accurate diagnosis in these circumstances.

ESSENTIALS OF PRENATAL CARE

The first prenatal visit should occur as early as possible after the diagnosis of pregnancy and should include the following.

History

Age, ethnic background, occupation. Onset of LMP and its normality, possible conception dates, bleeding after LMP, medical history, all prior pregnancies (duration, outcome, and complications), symptoms of present pregnancy. Use of drugs, alcohol, tobacco, caffeine, nutritional habits (Table 18–1).

*Parts of this chapter are reprinted from Brown JS, Crombleholme WR (editors): *Handbook of Gynecology/Obstetrics.* Originally published by Appleton & Lange. Copyright © 1993 by The McGraw-Hill Companies, Inc.

Table 18–1. Common drugs that are teratogenic or fetotoxic.[1]

ACE inhibitors	Estrogens
Alcohol	Griseofulvin
Amantadine	Hypoglycemics, oral
Aminopterin	Isotretinoin
Androgens	Lithium
Anticonvulsants	Methotrexate
Aminoglutethimide	Misoprostol
Carbamazepine	NSAIDs (third trimester)
Ethotoin	Opioids (prolonged use)
Phenytoin	Progestins
Valproic acid	Radioiodine (antithyroid)
Aspirin and other salicylates (third trimester)	Reserpine
Benzodiazepines	Ribavirin
Carbarsone (amebicide)	Sulfonamides (third trimester)
Chloramphenicol (third trimester)	Tetracycline (third trimester)
Cyclophosphamide	Thalidomide
Diazoxide	Tobacco smoking
Diethylstilbestrol	Trimethoprim (third trimester)
Disulfiram	Warfarin and other coumarin anticoagulants
Ergotamine	

[1]Many other drugs are also contraindicated during pregnancy. Evaluate any drug for its need versus its potential adverse effects. Further information can be obtained from the manufacturer or from any of several teratogenic registries around the country.

Family history of congenital anomalies and heritable diseases. History of childhood varicella. Prior STDs or risks for HIV infection.

Physical Examination

Height, weight, blood pressure, general physical examination. Abdominal and pelvic examination: (1) estimate uterine size or measure fundal height; (2) evaluate bony pelvis for symmetry and adequacy; (3) evaluate cervix for structural anatomy, infection, effacement, dilation; (4) detect fetal heart sounds by Doppler device after 10 weeks or fetoscope after 18 weeks.

Laboratory Tests

Urinalysis, culture of a clean-voided midstream urine sample, complete blood count with red cell indices, serologic test for syphilis, rubella antibody titer, blood group, Rh type, atypical antibody screening, and HBsAg evaluation. Human immunodeficiency virus (HIV) screening should be offered to all pregnant women. Cervical cultures are usually obtained for *Neisseria gonorrhoeae* and chlamydia, along with a Papanicolaou smear of the cervix. All black women should have sickle cell screening. Women of African, Asian, or Mediterranean ancestry with anemia or low MCV values should have hemoglobin electrophoresis performed to identify abnormal hemoglobins (Hb S, C, F, α-thalassemia, β-thalassemia). Tuberculosis skin testing is increasingly indicated for immigrant and inner city populations. Genetic counseling with the option of chorionic villus sampling or genetic amniocentesis should be offered to all women who will be 35 years of age or older at delivery and those who have had prior offspring with chromosomal abnormalities. Tay-Sachs blood screening is offered to Jewish women with Jewish partners. Screening for cystic fibrosis is offered based on the family history.

Pregnant women who work in medical-dental health care or the public safety field and those who are household contacts of a hepatitis B virus carrier or a hemodialysis patient and are HBsAg-negative at prenatal screening are at high risk of acquiring hepatitis B. They should be vaccinated during pregnancy.

Advice to Patients

A. Prenatal Visits: Prenatal care should begin early and maintain a schedule of regular prenatal visits: 0–28 weeks: every 4 weeks; 28–36 weeks: every 2 weeks; 36 weeks on: weekly.

B. Diet:

1. Eat a balanced diet containing the major food groups.

2. Take prenatal vitamins with iron and folic acid.

3. Expect to gain 20–40 lb. Do not diet to lose weight during pregnancy.

4. Decrease caffeine intake to 0–1 cup of coffee, tea, or cola daily.

5. Avoid eating raw or rare meat, and wash hands after handling raw meat.

6. Eat fresh fruits and vegetables and wash them before eating.

C. Medications: Do not take medications unless prescribed or authorized by your physician.

D. Alcohol and Other Drugs: Abstain from alcohol, tobacco, and all recreational ("street") drugs. No safe level of alcohol intake has been established for pregnancy. Fetal effects are manifest in the **fetal alcohol syndrome,** which includes growth restriction, facial abnormalities, and serious central nervous system dysfunction. These effects are thought to result from direct toxicity of ethanol itself as well as of its metabolites such as acetaldehyde. Characteristic findings include shortened palpebral fissures, low-set ears, midfacial hypoplasia, a smooth philtrum, a thin upper lip, microcephaly, mental retardation, and attention deficit disorder. Skeletal and cardiac abnormalities may also be seen.

Cigarette smoking results in fetal exposure to carbon monoxide and nicotine, which is thought to eventuate in a number of adverse pregnancy outcomes. An increased risk of abruptio placentae, placenta previa, and premature rupture of the membranes is documented among women who smoke. Premature delivery may occur 20% more frequently among smoking pregnant women, and the birth weights of their infants are on average 200 g lower than infants of nonsmokers. Women who smoke should quit or at least reduce the number of cigarettes smoked per day to as few as possible.

Sometimes compounding the above effects on pregnancy outcome are the independent adverse effects of illicit drugs. Cocaine use in pregnancy is associated with an increased risk of premature rupture of membranes, preterm delivery, placental abruption, intrauterine growth restriction, neurobehavioral deficits, and sudden infant death syndrome. Similar adverse pregnancy effects are associated with amphetamine use, perhaps reflecting the vasoconstrictive potential of both amphetamines and cocaine. Adverse effects associated with opioid use include intrauterine growth restriction, prematurity, stillbirth, and fetal death.

E. X-Rays and Noxious Exposures: Avoid x-rays unless essential and approved by a physician. Inform your dentist and your other physicians that you are pregnant. Avoid chemical or radiation hazards. Avoid excessive heat in hot tubs or saunas. Avoid handling cat feces or cat litter. Wear gloves when gardening.

F. Rest and Activity: Obtain adequate rest each day. Abstain from strenuous physical work or activities, particularly when heavy lifting or weight bearing is required. Exercise regularly at a mild to moderate level. Avoid exhausting or hazardous exercises or new athletic training programs during pregnancy. Heart rate should be kept below 140 beats/min during exercise.

G. Birth Classes: Enroll with your partner in a childbirth preparation class well before your due date.

Tests & Procedures

A. Each Visit: Weight, blood pressure, fundal height, fetal heart rate, urine specimen for protein and glucose. Review patient's concerns about pregnancy, health, and nutrition.

B. 6–12 Weeks: Confirm uterine size and growth by pelvic examination. Document fetal heart tones (audible at 10–12 weeks of gestation by Doppler). Chorionic villus sampling between 10 and 12 weeks when indicated.

C. 12–18 Weeks: Genetic counseling for women 35 years or older at EDC, or those with a family history of congenital anomalies, a previous child with a chromosomal abnormality, metabolic disease, or neural tube defect. Amniocentesis is performed as indicated and requested by the patient.

D. 12–24 Weeks: Fetal ultrasound examination to determine pregnancy dating and evaluate fetal anatomy. An earlier examination provides the most accurate dating, while a later examination demonstrates fetal anatomy in greater detail. The best compromise is at 18–20 weeks of gestation.

E. 16–20 Weeks: Maternal serum alpha-fetoprotein testing is offered to all women to screen for neural tube defects. In some states, such testing is mandatory. In some institutions, serum alpha-fetoprotein is combined with measurement of estriol and hCG (triple screen) for the detection of fetal Down's syndrome.

F. 20–24 Weeks: Instruct patient in symptoms and signs of preterm labor and rupture of membranes.

G. 24 Weeks to Delivery: Ultrasound examination is performed as indicated. Typically, fetal size and growth are evaluated when fundal height is 3 cm less than or more than expected for gestational age. In multiple pregnancies, ultrasound should be performed every 4 weeks to evaluate for discordant growth.

H. 26–28 Weeks: Screening for gestational diabetes by a 50-g glucose load (Glucola) and a 1-hour post-Glucola blood glucose determination. Abnormal values should be followed up with a 3-hour glucose tolerance test (see Table 18–4).

I. 28 Weeks: If initial antibody screen is negative, repeat antibody testing for Rh-negative patients, but result is not required before Rh_0 (D) immune globulin is administered.

J. 28–32 Weeks: Repeat the complete blood count to evaluate for anemia of pregnancy.

K. 28 Weeks to Delivery: Determination of fetal position and presentation. Question the patient at each visit for symptoms or signs of preterm labor or rupture of membranes. Assess maternal perception of fetal movement at each visit. Antepartum fetal testing is performed as medically indicated.

L. 36 Weeks to Delivery: Repeat syphilis and HIV testing, cervical cultures for *N gonorrhoeae* and chlamydia in at-risk patients. Discuss with the patient the indicators of onset of labor, admission to hospital, management of labor and delivery, and options for analgesia and anesthesia. Weekly cervical examinations are not necessary unless indicated to assess a specific clinical situation. Elective delivery (whether by induction or cesarean section) prior to 39 weeks of gestation requires confirmation of fetal lung maturity.

The CDC has recently approved two approaches—screening-based and risk factor-based—for management of group B streptococcal colonization in pregnancy:

1. In the screening-based approach, a single standard culture of the distal vagina and anorectum is collected at 35–37 weeks. No prophylaxis is needed if the screening culture is negative. Patients whose cultures are positive receive intrapartum penicillin prophylaxis with labor. Patients with risk factors such as a previous infant with invasive group B streptococcal disease, or group B streptococcal bacteriuria during the pregnancy, or delivery at less than 37 weeks of gestation also receive intrapartum prophylaxis. Patients whose cultures at 35–37 weeks were not done or whose results are not known receive prophylaxis only with the risk factors of intrapartum temperature greater than 38 °C or membrane rupture greater than 18 hours.

2. In the risk factor approach, no screening cultures are performed, and all patients with any of the risk factors noted above are treated.

3. The routine recommended regimen for prophylaxis is penicillin G, 5 million units intravenously as a loading dose and then 2.5 million units intravenously every 4 hours until delivery. In penicillin-allergic patients, clindamycin, 900 mg intravenously every 8 hours until delivery, is substituted.

M. 41 Weeks and Beyond: Cervical examination to determine probability of successful induction of labor. Based on this, induction of labor is undertaken if the cervix is favorable; if unfavorable, antepartum fetal testing is begun.

Haertsch M et al: What is recommended for healthy women during pregnancy? A comparison of seven prenatal clinical practice guideline documents. Birth 1999;26:24. [NLM Cit ID: 99280736]

Koren G et al: Drugs in pregnancy. N Engl J Med 1998; 338:1128. [NLM Cit ID: 98196621]

Leuzzi RA et al: Preconception counseling for the primary care physician. Med Clin North Am 1996;80:337. [NLM Cit ID: 96197389]

Macri J et al: Prenatal maternal dried blood screening with alpha-fetoprotein and free beta-human chorionic gonadotropin for open neural tube defect and Down syndrome. Am J Obstet Gynecol 1996;174:566. [NLM Cit ID: 96191857]

Prevention of perinatal group B streptococcal disease: A public health perspective. MMWR Morb Mortal Wkly Rep 1996;45(RR-7):1. [NLM Cit ID: 96256276]

NUTRITION IN PREGNANCY

Nutrition in pregnancy significantly affects maternal health and infant size and well-being. Pregnant women should have nutrition counseling early in prenatal care and access to supplementary food programs if they lack funds for adequate nutrition. Counseling should stress abstention from alcohol, smoking, and drugs. Caffeine and artificial sweeteners should be used only in small amounts. "Empty calories" should be avoided, and the diet should contain the following foods: protein foods of animal and vegetable origin, milk and milk products, whole-grain cereals and breads, and fruits and vegetables—especially green leafy vegetables.

Weight gain in pregnancy should be 20–40 lb, which includes the added weight of the fetus, placenta, and amniotic fluid and of maternal reproductive tissues, fluid, blood, increased fat stores, and increased lean body mass. Maternal fat stores are a caloric reserve for pregnancy and lactation; weight restriction in pregnancy to avoid developing such fat stores may affect the development of other fetal and maternal tissues and is not advisable. Obese women can have normal infants with less weight gain (15–20 lb) but should be encouraged to eat high-quality foods. Normally, a pregnant woman gains 2–5 lb in the first trimester and slightly less than 1 lb/wk thereafter. She needs approximately an extra 200–300 kcal/d (depending on energy output) and 30 g/d of additional protein for a total protein intake of about 75 g/d. Appropriate caloric intake in pregnancy helps prevent the problems associated with low birth weight.

Rigid salt restriction is not necessary. While the consumption of highly salted snack foods and prepared foods is not desirable, 2–3 g/d of sodium is permissible. The increased calcium needs of pregnancy (1200 mg/d) can be met with milk, milk products, green vegetables, soybean products, corn tortillas, and calcium carbonate supplements.

The increased need for iron and folic acid should be met from foods as well as vitamin and mineral supplements. (See section on anemia in pregnancy.) Megavitamins should not be taken in pregnancy, as they may result in fetal malformation or disturbed metabolism. However, a balanced prenatal supplement containing 30–60 mg of elemental iron, 0.5–0.8 mg of folate, and the recommended daily allowances of various vitamins and minerals is widely used in the USA and is probably beneficial to many women with marginal diets. There is evidence that periconceptional folic acid supplements can decrease the risk of neural tube defects in the fetus. For this reason, the United States Public Health Service recommends the consumption of 0.4 mg of folic acid per day for all women capable of becoming pregnant. Women with a prior neural tube defect-affected pregnancy may require higher supplemental doses as determined by their physician. Lactovegetarians and ovolactovegetarians do well in pregnancy; vegetarian women who eat neither eggs nor milk products should have their diets assessed for adequate calories and protein and should take oral vitamin B_{12} supplements during pregnancy and lactation.

Institute of Medicine, National Academy of Sciences: *Nutrition During Pregnancy.* Part I, *Weight Gain;* Part II, *Nutrient Supplements.* National Academy Press, 1990.

Kolasa KM et al: Nutrition during pregnancy. Am Fam Physician 1997;56:205. [NLM Cit ID: 97369188]

Locksmith GJ et al: Preventing neural tube defects: The importance of periconceptional folic acid supplements. Obstet Gynecol 1998;91:1027. [NLM Cit ID: 98272575] (Women of reproductive age should be advised to take multivitamin supplements containing 0.4 mg of folic acid daily. Women with previously affected offspring who intend to become pregnant should take daily supplementation containing 4 mg of folic acid in the periconceptional period to reduce the risk of recurrence.)

TRAVEL & IMMUNIZATIONS DURING PREGNANCY

During an otherwise normal low-risk pregnancy, travel can be planned most safely between the 18th and 32nd weeks. Commercial flying in pressurized cabins does not pose a threat to the fetus. An aisle seat will allow frequent walks. Adequate fluids should be taken during the flight.

It is not advisable to travel to endemic areas of yellow fever in Africa or Latin America or to areas of Africa or Asia where chloroquine-resistant falciparum malaria is a hazard, since complications of malaria are more common in pregnancy.

Ideally, all immunizations should precede pregnancy. Live virus products are contraindicated (measles, rubella, yellow fever). Inactivated poliovaccine (Salk) can be used instead of the oral vaccine. Vaccines against pneumococcal pneumonia, meningococcal meningitis, and hepatitis A can be used as indicated. Influenza vaccine is indicated in all pregnant women who will be in their second or third trimester during "flu season."

Pooled gamma globulin to prevent hepatitis A is safe and does not carry a risk of HIV transmission. Chloroquine can be used for malaria prophylaxis in pregnancy, and proguanil is also safe.

Water should be purified by boiling, since iodine purification may provide more iodine than is safe during pregnancy.

Do not use prophylactic antibiotics or bismuth subsalicylate during pregnancy to prevent diarrhea. Use oral rehydration fluids, and treat bacterial diarrhea with erythromycin or ampicillin if necessary.

Prevention and control of influenza: Recommendations of the Advisory Committee on Immunization Practices (ACIP). Morb Mortal Wkly Rep 1999;48(RR-4):1. [NLM Cit ID: 99292260]

Prevention of hepatitis A through active or passive immunization: Recommendations of the Advisory Committee on Immunization Practices (ACIP). MMWR Morb Mortal Wkly Rep 1996;45(RR-15):1. [NLM Cit ID: 97154733]

Rose SR: Pregnancy and travel. Emerg Med Clin N Am 1997;15:93. [NLM Cit ID: 97209272]

VOMITING OF PREGNANCY (Morning Sickness) & HYPEREMESIS GRAVIDARUM (Pernicious Vomiting of Pregnancy)

Morning or evening nausea and vomiting usually begin soon after the first missed period and cease after the fourth to fifth months of gestation. At least half of women, most of them primiparas, complain of nausea and vomiting during early pregnancy. This problem exerts no adverse effects on the pregnancy and does not presage other complications, though it is particularly common with multiple pregnancy and hydatidiform mole. The cause of vomiting during pregnancy is believed to be high estrogen levels.

Persistent, severe vomiting during pregnancy—hyperemesis gravidarum—can be disabling and require hospitalization. Dehydration, acidosis, and nutritional deficiencies may develop with protracted vomiting. Thyroid dysfunction can be associated with hyperemesis gravidarum, so it is advisable to determine TSH and free T_4 values in these patients.

Treatment

A. Mild Nausea and Vomiting of Pregnancy: Reassurance and dietary advice are all that is required in most instances. Because of possible teratogenicity, drugs used during the first half of pregnancy should be restricted to those of major importance to life and health. Antiemetics, antihistamines, and antispasmodics are generally unnecessary to treat nausea of pregnancy. Vitamin B_6 (pyridoxine), 50–100 mg/d orally, is nontoxic and may be helpful in some patients.

B. Hyperemesis Gravidarum: Hospitalize the patient in a private room at bed rest. Give nothing by mouth for 48 hours, and maintain hydration and electrolyte balance by giving appropriate parenteral fluids and vitamin supplements as indicated. Rarely, total parenteral nutrition may become necessary. As soon as possible, place the patient on a dry diet consisting of six small feedings daily with clear liquids 1 hour after eating. Prochlorperazine rectal suppositories may be useful. After in-patient stabilization, the patient can be maintained at home even if she requires intravenous fluids in addition to her oral intake.

Jacoby EB et al: *Helicobacter pylori* infection and persistent hyperemesis gravidarum. Am J Perinatol 1999; 16:85. [NLM Cit ID: 99282046]

Safari HR et al: Experience with oral methylprednisolone in the treatment of refractory hyperemesis gravidarum. Am J Obstet Gynecol 1998;178:1054. [NLM Cit ID: 98270746] (A short course of oral methylprednisolone appears to be a reasonable therapeutic alternative for intractable hyperemesis.)

SPONTANEOUS ABORTION

Abortion is defined as termination of gestation before the 20th week of pregnancy. About three-fourths of spontaneous abortions occur before the 16th week; of these, three-fourths occur before the eighth week. Almost 20% of all clinically recognized pregnancies terminate in spontaneous abortion.

More than 60% of spontaneous abortions result from chromosomal defects due to maternal or paternal factors; about 15% appear to be associated with maternal trauma, infections, dietary deficiencies, diabetes mellitus, hypothyroidism, or anatomic malformations. There is no reliable evidence that abortion may be induced by psychic stimuli such as severe fright, grief, anger, or anxiety. In about one-fourth of cases, the cause of abortion cannot be determined. There is no evidence that video display terminals or associated electromagnetic fields are related to an increased risk of spontaneous abortion.

It is important to differentiate women with a history of incompetent cervix from those with more typical early abortion and those with premature labor or rupture of the membranes. Characteristically, incompetent cervix presents as "silent" cervical dilation (ie, with minimal uterine contractions) between 16 and 28 weeks of gestation. Women with incompetent cervix often present with significant cervical dilation (2 cm or more) and minimal symptoms. When the cervix reaches 4 cm or more, active uterine contractions or rupture of the membranes may occur secondary to the degree of cervical dilation. This does not change the primary diagnosis. Factors that predispose to incompetent cervix are a history of incompetent cervix with a previous pregnancy; cervical conization or surgery; cervical injury; DES exposure; and anatomic abnormalities of the cervix. Prior to pregnancy or during the first trimester, there are no methods for determining whether the cervix will eventually be incompetent. After 14–16 weeks, ultrasound may be used to evaluate the internal anatomy of the lower uterine segment and cervix for the funneling and shortening abnormalities consistent with cervical incompetence.

Clinical Findings

A. Symptoms and Signs:

1. Threatened abortion–Bleeding or cramping occurs, but the pregnancy continues. The cervix is not dilated.

2. Inevitable abortion–The cervix is dilated and the membranes may be ruptured, but passage of the products of conception has not occurred. Bleeding and cramping persist, and passage of the products of conception is considered inevitable.

3. Complete abortion–The fetus and placenta are completely expelled. Pain ceases, but spotting may persist.

4. Incomplete abortion–Some portion of the products of conception (usually placental) remain in the uterus. Only mild cramps are reported, but bleeding is persistent and often excessive.

5. Missed abortion–The pregnancy has ceased to develop, but the conceptus has not been expelled. Symptoms of pregnancy disappear. There is a brownish vaginal discharge but no free bleeding. Pain does not develop. The cervix is semifirm and slightly patulous; the uterus becomes smaller and irregularly softened; the adnexa are normal.

B. Laboratory Findings: Pregnancy tests show low or falling levels of hCG. A complete blood count should be obtained if bleeding is heavy. Determine Rh type, and give Rh_o (D) immune globulin if the type is Rh-negative. All tissue recovered should be assessed by a pathologist and may be sent for genetic analysis in selected cases.

C. Ultrasonographic Findings: The gestational sac can be identified at 5–6 weeks from the LMP, a fetal pole at 6 weeks, and fetal cardiac activity at 6–7 weeks. Serial observations are often required to evaluate changes in size of the embryo. A small, irregular sac without a fetal pole with accurate dating is diagnostic of an abnormal pregnancy.

Differential Diagnosis

The bleeding that occurs in abortion of a uterine pregnancy must be differentiated from the abnormal bleeding of an ectopic pregnancy and anovular bleeding in a nonpregnant woman. The passage of hydropic villi in the bloody discharge is diagnostic of hydatidiform mole.

Treatment

A. General Measures:

1. Threatened abortion–Place the patient at bed rest for 24–48 hours followed by gradual resumption of usual activities, with abstinence from coitus and douching. Hormonal treatment is contraindicated. Antibiotics should be used only if there are signs of infection.

2. Missed or inevitable abortion–This calls for counseling regarding the fate of the pregnancy and planning for its elective termination at a time chosen by the patient and physician. Insertion of a laminaria to dilate the cervix followed by aspiration is the method of choice for a missed abortion. Prostaglandin vaginal suppositories are an effective alternative.

B. Surgical Measures:

1. Incomplete abortion–Prompt removal of any products of conception remaining within the uterus is required to stop bleeding and prevent infection. Analgesia and a paracervical block are useful, followed by uterine exploration with ovum forceps or uterine aspiration.

2. Cerclage and restriction of activities–These are the treatment of choice for incompetent cervix. A variety of suture materials including a 5 mm Mersilene band can be used to create a purse-string type of stitch around the cervix, using either the McDonald or Shirodkar method. Cerclage should be undertaken with caution when there is advanced cervical dilation or membranes are prolapsed into the vagina. Rupture of the membranes and infection are specific contraindications to cerclage. Cervical cultures for *N gonorrhoeae,* chlamydia, and group B streptococci should be obtained before or at the time of cerclage.

Hurd WW et al: Expectant management versus elective curettage for the treatment of spontaneous abortion. Fertil Steril 1997;68:601. [NLM Cit ID: 98000804]

Ness RB et al: Cocaine and tobacco use and the risk of spontaneous abortion. N Engl J Med 1999;340:333. [NLM Cit ID: 99119164]

RECURRENT (HABITUAL) ABORTION

Recurrent, or habitual, abortion has been defined for years as the loss of three or more previable (< 500 g) pregnancies in succession. Recurrent or chronic abortion occurs in about 0.4–0.8% of all pregnancies. Abnormalities related to repeated abortion can be identified in approximately half of the couples. If a woman has lost three previous pregnancies without identifiable cause, she still has a 70–80% chance of carrying a fetus to viability. If she has aborted four or five times, the likelihood of a successful pregnancy is 65–70%.

Recurrent abortion is a clinical rather than pathologic diagnosis. The clinical findings are similar to those observed in other types of abortion (see above).

Treatment

A. Preconception Therapy: Preconception therapy is aimed at detection of maternal or paternal defects that may contribute to abortion. A thorough general and gynecologic examination is essential. Polycystic ovaries should be ruled out. A random blood glucose test and thyroid function studies (including thyroid antibodies) should be done. Detection of lupus anticoagulant and other hemostatic abnormalities (proteins S and C and antithrombin III deficiency, hyperhomocysteinemia, anticardiolipin antibody, factor V Leiden mutation) and an antinuclear antibody test may be indicated. Endometrial tissue should be examined in the postovulation stage of the cycle to determine the adequacy of the response of the endometrium to hormones. The competency of the cervix must be determined and hysteroscopy or hysterography used to exclude submucous myomas and congenital anomalies. Chromosomal (karyotype) analysis of both partners rules out balanced translocations (found in 5% of infertile couples).

Recent experiments have focused on the major histocompatibility complex (MHC) of chromosome 6, which carries HLA loci and other genes that may influence reproductive success. Some women demonstrate a lack of maternal antibody response to paternal lymphocytes, which is customarily found in normal women after successful childbearing. However, several randomized controlled trials have found no benefit of IGIV therapy for recurrent spontaneous abortion.

B. Postconception Therapy: Provide early prenatal care and schedule frequent office visits. Complete bed rest is justified only for bleeding or pain. Empiric sex steroid hormone therapy is contraindicated.

Prognosis

The prognosis is excellent if the cause of abortion can be corrected.

Coumans AB et al: Haemostatic and metabolic abnormalities in women with unexplained recurrent abortion. Human Reprod 1999;14:211. [NLM Cit ID: 99302352]

Jablonowska B et al: Prevention of recurrent spontaneous abortion by intravenous immunoglobulin: A double-blind placebo-controlled study. Hum Reprod 1999; 14:838. [NLM Cit ID: 99236912]

Ridker PM et al: Factor V Leiden mutation as a risk factor for recurrent pregnancy loss. Ann Intern Med 1998; 128(12 Part 1):1000. [NLM Cit ID: 98273837]

ECTOPIC PREGNANCY

Any pregnancy arising from implantation of the ovum outside the cavity of the uterus is ectopic. Ectopic implantation occurs in about one out of 150 live births. About 98% of ectopic pregnancies are tubal. Other sites of ectopic implantation are the peritoneum or abdominal viscera, the ovary, and the cervix. Any condition that prevents or retards migration of the fertilized ovum to the uterus can predispose to an ectopic pregnancy, including a history of infertility, pelvic inflammatory disease, ruptured appendix, and prior tubal surgery. Combined intra- and extrauterine pregnancy (heterotopic) may occur rarely. In the USA, undiagnosed or undetected ectopic pregnancy is currently the most common cause of maternal death during the first trimester.

Clinical Findings

A. Symptoms and Signs: The cardinal symptoms and signs of tubal pregnancy are (1) amenorrhea or irregular bleeding and spotting, followed by (2) pelvic pain, and (3) pelvic (adnexal) mass formation. They may be acute or chronic.

1. Acute (40%)–Severe lower quadrant pain occurs in almost every case. It is sudden in onset, lancinating, intermittent, and does not radiate. Backache is present during attacks. Shock occurs in about 10%, often after pelvic examination. At least two-thirds of patients give a history of abnormal menstruation; many have been infertile.

2. Chronic (60%)–Blood leaks from the tubal ampulla over a period of days, and considerable blood may accumulate in the peritoneum. Slight but persistent vaginal spotting is reported, and a pelvic mass can be palpated. Abdominal distention and mild paralytic ileus are often present.

B. Laboratory Findings: Blood studies may show anemia and slight leukocytosis. Quantitative serum pregnancy tests will show levels generally lower than expected for normal pregnancies of the same duration. If pregnancy tests are followed over a few days, there may be a slow rise or a plateau rather than the near doubling every 2 days associated with normal early intrauterine pregnancy or the falling levels that occur with spontaneous abortion.

C. Imaging: Ultrasonography can reliably demonstrate a gestational sac 6 weeks from the LMP and a fetal pole at 7 weeks if located in the uterus. An empty uterine cavity raises a strong suspicion of extrauterine pregnancy, which can occasionally be revealed by endovaginal ultrasound. Specified levels of serum hCG have been reliably correlated with ultrasound findings of an intrauterine pregnancy. For example, an hCG level of 6500 mIU/mL with an empty uterine cavity by transabdominal ultrasound is virtually diagnostic of an ectopic pregnancy. Similarly, an hCG value of 2000 mIU/mL or more can be indicative of an ectopic pregnancy if no products of conception are detected within the uterine cavity by transvaginal ultrasound.

D. Special Examinations: With the advent of high-resolution transvaginal ultrasound, culdocentesis is rarely used in evaluation of possible ectopic pregnancy. Laparoscopy is the surgical procedure of choice to both confirm an ectopic pregnancy and in most cases to permit pelviscopic removal of the ectopic pregnancy without the need for exploratory laparotomy.

Differential Diagnosis

Clinical and laboratory findings suggestive or diagnostic of pregnancy will distinguish ectopic pregnancy from many acute abdominal illnesses such as acute appendicitis, acute pelvic inflammatory disease, ruptured corpus luteum cyst or ovarian follicle, and urinary calculi. Uterine enlargement with clinical findings similar to those found in ectopic pregnancy is also characteristic of an aborting uterine pregnancy or hydatidiform mole. Ectopic pregnancy should be suspected when postabortal tissue examination fails to reveal placenta. Steps must be taken for immediate diagnosis, including prompt microscopic tissue examination, ultrasonography, and serial hCG titers every 48 hours. Patients must be warned of possible ectopic pregnancy problems and followed very closely.

Treatment

The patient is hospitalized if there is a reasonable likelihood of ectopic pregnancy. Blood is typed and cross-matched. Ideally, diagnosis and operative treatment should precede frank rupture of the tube and intra-abdominal hemorrhage.

Surgical treatment is definitive. In a stable patient, diagnostic laparoscopy is the initial surgical procedure performed. Depending on the size of the ectopic pregnancy and whether or not it has ruptured, a salpingostomy with removal of the ectopic or a partial or complete salpingectomy can usually be performed pelviscopically through the laparoscope. Clinical conditions permitting, patency of the contralateral tube can be established by the injection of indigo carmine into the uterine cavity and flow through the contralateral tube confirmed visually by the surgeon.

Methotrexate (50 mg/m^2)—given systemically as single or multiple doses—is now acceptable medical therapy of early ectopic pregnancy. Favorable criteria are that the pregnancy should be less than 3.5 cm and unruptured, with no active bleeding.

Iron therapy for anemia may be necessary during convalescence. Give Rh_o (D) immune globulin (300 μg) to Rh-negative patients.

Prognosis

Repeat tubal pregnancy occurs in about 12% of cases. This should not be regarded as a contraindication to future pregnancy, but the patient requires careful observation and early ultrasound confirmation of an intrauterine pregnancy.

Buster J et al: Medical management of ectopic pregnancy. Clin Obstet Gynecol 1999;42:23. [NLM Cit ID: 99172951]

Job-Spira N et al: Ruptured tubal ectopic pregnancy: Risk factors and reproductive outcome: Results of a population-based study in France. Am J Obstet Gynecol 1999;180:938. [NLM Cit ID: 99221509]

Pisarska MD et al: Ectopic pregnancy. Lancet 1998; 351:1115. [NLM Cit ID: 98322034]

PREECLAMPSIA-ECLAMPSIA

Preeclampsia-eclampsia can occur any time after 20 weeks of gestation and up to 6 weeks postpartum. It is a disease unique to pregnancy, with the only cure being delivery of the fetus and placenta. Approximately 7% of pregnant women in the United States develop preeclampsia-eclampsia. Primiparas are most frequently affected; however, the incidence of preeclampsia-eclampsia is increased with multiple pregnancies, chronic hypertension, diabetes, renal disease, collagen-vascular and autoimmune disorders, and gestational trophoblastic disease. Five percent of women with preeclampsia progress to eclampsia. Uncontrolled eclampsia is a significant cause of maternal death.

The basic cause of preeclampsia-eclampsia is not known. Epidemiologic studies suggest an immunologic cause for preeclampsia, since it occurs predominantly in women who have had minimal exposure to sperm (having used barrier methods of contraception) or have new consorts; in primigravidas; and in women both of whose parents have similar HLA antigens. Preeclampsia is an endothelial disorder resulting from poor placental perfusion, which releases a factor that injures the endothelium, causing activation of coagulation and an increased sensitivity to pressors. Before the syndrome becomes clinically manifest in the second half of pregnancy, there has been vasospasm in various small vessel beds, accounting for the pathologic changes in maternal organs and the placenta with consequent adverse effects on the fetus.

The use of diuretics, dietary restriction or enhancement, sodium restriction, aspirin, and vitamin-mineral supplements such as calcium has not been shown to be useful in clinical studies. The only cure is termination of the pregnancy at a time as favorable as possible for fetal survival.

Definition

Preeclampsia is defined as the presence of the triad of elevated blood pressure, proteinuria, and edema during pregnancy. Eclampsia occurs with the addition of seizures to this triad. The three abnormalities of preeclampsia-eclampsia are defined as follows:

A. Blood Pressure: A sustained elevation of blood pressure of 140 mm Hg systolic or 90 mm Hg diastolic or more (in the absence of chronic hypertension) after 20 weeks of gestation. All abnormal blood pressure readings must be confirmed with two separate readings at least 6 hours apart.

B. Proteinuria: At least 0.3 g/24 h as determined by 24-hour urine collection.

C. Edema: Clinically apparent fluid retention, or increase in weight of 5 lb or more in 1 week. The edema should involve the upper extremities and face rather than just the lower extremities.

Classically, the presence of all three elements is required for the diagnosis of preeclampsia-eclampsia. Clinically, however, there is a great deal of variation in presentation. Hypertension occurs most frequently, but proteinuria or edema may be the dominant abnormality at presentation. The absence of one or two components does not exclude the diagnosis of preeclampsia-eclampsia, and many women with the disorder are asymptomatic early. Diagnosis at an early stage thus requires careful attention to details and a high index of suspicion.

Clinical Findings

Clinically, the severity of preeclampsia-eclampsia can be measured with reference to the six major sites in which it exerts its effects: the central nervous system, the kidneys, the liver, the hematologic and vascular systems, and the fetal-placental unit. By evaluating each of these areas for the presence of mild to moderate versus severe preeclampsia-eclampsia, the degree of involvement can be assessed, and an appropriate management plan can be formulated that is integrated with gestational age assessment (Table 18–2).

A. Preeclampsia:

1. Mild to moderate–Precise differentiation between mild and moderate preeclampsia-eclampsia is difficult because the abnormalities that define the disease are quite variable and fail to accurately predict progression to more severe disease. Symptoms are generally minimal or mild. With mild preeclampsia, patients usually have few complaints, and the diastolic blood pressure is less than 90–100 mm Hg. Edema is usually more pronounced with moderate disease, and diastolic blood pressures are in the range of 90–110 mm Hg. The platelet count is over 100,000/μL, antepartum fetal testing is reassuring, central nervous system irritability is minimal, epigastric pain is not present, and liver enzymes are not elevated.

2. Severe–Symptoms are more dramatic and persistent. The blood pressure is often quite high, with readings over 160/110 mm Hg. Thrombocytopenia (platelet counts < 100,000/μL) may be present and progress to disseminated intravascular coagulation. Severe epigastric pain may be present from hepatic subcapsular hemorrhage with significant stretch

Table 18–2. Indicators of mild to moderate versus severe preeclampsia-eclampsia.

Site	Indicator	Mild to Moderate	Severe
Central nervous system	Symptoms and signs	Hyperreflexia Headache	Seizures Blurred vision Scotomas Headache Clonus Irritability
Kidney	Proteinuria	0.3–5 g/24 h	> 5 g/24 h or catheterized urine with 4+ protein
	Urine output	> 20–30 mL/h	< 20–30 mL/h
Liver	AST, ALT, LDH	Normal	Elevated LFTs Epigastric pain Ruptured liver
Hematologic	Platelets Hemoglobin	> 100,000/μL Normal range	< 100,000/μL Elevated
Vascular	Blood pressure Retina	< 160/110 mm Hg Arteriolar spasm	> 160/110 mm Hg Retinal hemorrhages
Fetal-placental unit	Growth retardation Oligohydramnios Fetal distress	Absent May be present Absent	Present Present Present

AST, aspartate aminotransferase; ALT, alanine aminotransferase; LDH, lactate dehydrogenase; LFTs, liver function tests.

or rupture of the liver capsule. The HELLP syndrome (hemolysis, elevated liver enzymes, low platelets) is a form of severe preeclampsia.

B. Eclampsia: The occurrence of seizures defines eclampsia. It is a manifestation of severe central nervous system involvement. The other abnormal findings of severe preeclampsia are also observed with eclampsia.

Differential Diagnosis

Preeclampsia-eclampsia can mimic and be confused with many other diseases, including (among many others) chronic hypertension, chronic renal disease, primary seizure disorders, gallbladder and pancreatic disease, immune or thrombotic thrombocytopenic purpura, and hemolytic uremic syndrome. It must always be considered as a disease of exclusion in any pregnant woman beyond 20 weeks of gestation. It is particularly difficult to diagnose when preexisting disease such as hypertension is present. Uric acid values can be quite helpful in such situations, since hyperuricemia is uncommon in pregnancy except with gout, renal failure, or preeclampsia-eclampsia.

Treatment

A. Preeclampsia: Early recognition is the key to treatment. This requires careful attention to the details of prenatal care—especially subtle changes in blood pressure and weight. The objectives are to prolong pregnancy if possible to fetal lung maturity while preventing progression to severe disease and eclampsia. The critical factors are the gestational age of the fetus, fetal pulmonary maturity status, and the severity of maternal disease. Preeclampsia-eclampsia at 36 weeks or more of gestation is managed by delivery regardless of how mild the disease is judged to be. Prior to 36 weeks, severe preeclampsia-eclampsia requires delivery except in unusual circumstances associated with extreme fetal prematurity, in which case prolongation of pregnancy may be attempted. Epigastric pain, thrombocytopenia, and visual disturbances are strong indications for delivery of the fetus. For mild to moderate preeclampsia-eclampsia, bed rest is the cornerstone of therapy. This increases central blood flow to the kidneys, heart, brain, liver, and placenta and may stabilize or even improve the degree of preeclampsia-eclampsia for a period of time.

Bed rest may be attempted at home or in the hospital. Prior to making this decision, the physician should evaluate the six sites of involvement listed in Table 18–2 and make an assessment about the severity of disease.

1. Home management–Home management with bed rest may be attempted for patients with mild preeclampsia and a stable home situation. This requires homemaking assistance, rapid access to the hospital, a reliable patient, and the ability to obtain frequent blood pressure readings. A home health nurse can often provide frequent home visits and assessment.

2. Hospital care–Hospitalization is required for women with moderate or severe preeclampsia or those with unreliable home situations. Regular assessment of blood pressure, reflexes, urine protein, and fetal heart tones and activity are required. A complete blood count, platelet count, and electrolyte panel including liver enzymes should be checked every 1 or 2 days. A 24-hour urine collection for creatinine clearance and total protein should be obtained on admission and repeated as indicated. Sedatives and opioids should be avoided because the fetal central nervous system depressant effects interfere with fetal testing. Magnesium sulfate is not used until the diagnosis of severe preeclampsia-eclampsia is made or until labor occurs.

Fetal evaluation should be obtained as an integral part of the workup. If the patient is being admitted to the hospital, fetal testing must be performed on the same day to make certain that the fetus is safe. This may be done by fetal heart rate testing with nonstress or stress testing or by biophysical profile. A regular schedule of fetal surveillance must then be followed. Daily fetal kick counts can be recorded by the patient herself. Consideration should be given to amniocentesis to evaluate fetal lung maturity status if hospitalization occurs at 30–37 weeks of gestation. If immaturity is present, steroids (betamethasone 12 mg or dexamethasone 16 mg, two doses intramuscularly 12–24 hours apart) can be administered to the mother. Fetuses between 26 and 30 weeks of gestation can be presumed to be immature, and steroids should be given.

The method of delivery is determined by the maternal and fetal status. Cesarean section is reserved for the usual fetal indications.

B. Eclampsia:

1. Emergency care–If the patient is convulsing, she is turned on her side to prevent aspiration and to improve blood flow to the placenta. Fluid or food is aspirated from the glottis or trachea. The seizure may be stopped by giving an intravenous bolus of either magnesium sulfate, 4 g, or diazepam, 5–10 mg, over 4 minutes or until the seizure stops. A continuous intravenous infusion of magnesium sulfate is then started at a rate of 2–3 g/h unless the patient is known to have significantly reduced renal function. Magnesium blood levels are then checked every 4–6 hours and the infusion rate adjusted to maintain a therapeutic blood level. Urine output is checked hourly and the patient assessed for signs of possible magnesium toxicity such as loss of deep tendon reflexes or decrease in respiratory rate and depth, which can be reversed with calcium gluconate.

2. General care–The occurrence of eclampsia necessitates delivery once the patient is stabilized. It is important, however, that assessment of the status of the patient and fetus take place first. Continuous fetal monitoring must be performed and blood typed and cross-matched quickly. A urinary catheter is inserted to monitor urine output, and blood is sent for complete blood count, platelets, liver enzymes, uric acid, creatinine or urea nitrogen, and electrolytes. If hypertension is present with diastolic values over 110 mm Hg, antihypertensive medications should be administered to reduce the diastolic blood pressure to 90–100 mm Hg. Lower blood pressures than this may induce placental insufficiency through reduced perfusion. Hydralazine given in 5- to 10-mg increments intravenously every 20 minutes is frequently used to lower blood pressure. Nifedipine, 10 mg sublingually or orally, or labetalol, 10–20 mg intravenously, both every 20 minutes, can also be used.

3. Delivery–Except in unusual circumstances, delivery is mandated once eclampsia has occurred. Vaginal delivery may be attempted if the patient has already been in active labor or the cervix is quite favorable *and* the patient is clinically stable. The rapidity with which delivery must be achieved depends on the fetal and maternal status following the seizure and the availability of laboratory data on the patient. Oxytocin may be used to induce or augment labor. Regional analgesia or anesthesia is acceptable. Cesarean section is used for the usual obstetric indications or when rapid delivery is necessary for maternal or fetal indications.

4. Postpartum–Magnesium sulfate infusion (2–3 g/h) should be continued until preeclampsia-eclampsia has begun to resolve postpartum. This may take 1–7 days. The most reliable indicator of this is the onset of diuresis with urine output of over 100–200 mL/h. When this occurs, magnesium sulfate can be discontinued. Late-onset preeclampsia-eclampsia can occur during the postpartum period. It is usually manifested by either hypertension or seizures. Treatment is the same as prior to delivery—ie, with magnesium sulfate—though other antiseizure medications can be used since the fetus is no longer present.

Levine RJ et al: Trial of calcium to prevent pre-eclampsia. N Engl J Med 1997;337:69. [NLM Cit ID: 97337873]

North RA et al: Evaluation of a definition of pre-eclampsia. Br J Obstet Gynaecol 1999;106:767. [NLM Cit ID: 99381628]

Rajkovic A et al: Elevated homocysteine levels with pre-eclampsia. Obstet Gynecol 1997;90:168. [NLM Cit ID: 97385253]

Witlin A et al: Hypertension in pregnancy: Current concepts of pre-eclampsia. Annu Rev Med 1997;48:115. [NLM Cit ID: 97198975]

GESTATIONAL TROPHOBLASTIC NEOPLASIA (Hydatidiform Mole & Choriocarcinoma)

Gestational trophoblastic neoplasia is a spectrum of disease that includes hydatidiform mole, invasive mole, and choriocarcinoma. Partial moles generally show evidence of an embryo or gestational sac, are polypoid, slower-growing, and less symptomatic, and often present clinically as a missed abortion. Partial moles tend to follow a benign course, while complete moles have a greater tendency to become choriocarcinomas.

The highest rates of gestational trophoblastic neoplasia occur in some developing countries, with rates of 1:125 pregnancies in certain areas of Asia. In the USA, the frequency is 1:1500 pregnancies. Risk factors include low socioeconomic status, a history of mole, and age below 18 or above 40. Approximately 10% of women require further treatment after evacuation of the mole; 5% develop choriocarcinoma.

Clinical Findings

A. Symptoms and Signs: Excessive nausea and vomiting occur in over one-third of patients with hydatidiform mole. Uterine bleeding, beginning at 6–8 weeks, is observed in virtually all instances and is indicative of threatened or incomplete abortion. In about one-fifth of cases, the uterus is larger than would be expected in a normal pregnancy of the same duration. Intact or collapsed vesicles may be passed through the vagina. These grape-like clusters or enlarged villi are diagnostic. Bilaterally enlarged cystic ovaries are sometimes palpable. They are the result of ovarian hyperstimulation due to excess of hCG.

Preeclampsia-eclampsia, frequently of the fulminating type, may develop during the second trimester of pregnancy, but this is unusual.

Choriocarcinoma may be manifested by continued or recurrent uterine bleeding after evacuation of a mole or following a delivery, abortion, or ectopic pregnancy. The presence of an ulcerative vaginal tumor, pelvic mass, or evidence of distant metastatic tumor may be the presenting observation. The diagnosis is established by pathologic examination of curettings or by biopsy.

B. Laboratory Findings: A serum hCG β-subunit value above 40,000 mIU/mL or a urinary hCG value in excess of 100,000 units/24 h increases the likelihood of hydatidiform mole, though such values are occasionally seen with a normal pregnancy (eg, in multiple gestation).

C. Imaging: Ultrasound has virtually replaced all other means of preoperative diagnosis of hydatidiform mole. The multiple echoes indicating edematous villi within the enlarged uterus and the absence of a fetus and placenta are pathognomonic. A preoperative chest film is indicated to rule out pulmonary metastases of trophoblast.

Treatment

A. Specific (Surgical) Measures: Empty the uterus as soon as the diagnosis of hydatidiform mole is established, preferably by suction. Do not resect ovarian cysts or remove the ovaries; spontaneous regression of theca lutein cysts will occur with elimination of the mole.

If malignant tissue is discovered at surgery or during the follow-up examination, chemotherapy is indicated.

Thyrotoxicosis indistinguishable clinically from that of thyroid origin may occur. While hCG usually has minimal TSH-like activity, the very high hCG levels associated with moles can account for clinically significant TSH activity. Patients thyrotoxic on this basis should be stabilized with beta-blockers prior to induction of anesthesia for their surgical evacuation. Surgical removal of the mole promptly corrects the thyroid overactivity.

B. Follow-Up Measures: Effective contraception (preferably birth control pills) should be prescribed. Weekly quantitative hCG level measurements are initially required. Following successful surgical evacuation, moles show a progressive decline in hCG. After two negative weekly tests (< 5 mIU/mL), the interval may be increased to monthly for 6 months and then to every 2 months for a total of 1 year. If levels plateau or begin to rise, the patient should be evaluated by repeat chest film and D&C before the initiation of chemotherapy.

C. Antitumor Chemotherapy: For low-risk patients with a good prognosis, give methotrexate, 0.4 mg/kg intramuscularly over a 5-day period, or dactinomycin, 10–12 μg/kg/d intravenously over a 5-day period (see Chapter 4). Refer patients with a poor prognosis to a cancer center, where multiple-agent chemotherapy probably will be given. The side effects—anorexia, nausea and vomiting, stomatitis, rash, diarrhea, and bone marrow depression—usually are reversible in about 3 weeks and can be ameliorated by the administration of leucovorin (0.1 mg/kg). Repeated courses of methotrexate 2 weeks apart generally are required to destroy the trophoblast and maintain a zero chorionic gonadotropin titer, as indicated by hCG β-subunit determination.

D. Supportive Measures: Prescribe oral contraceptives (if acceptable) or another reliable birth control method to avoid the hazard and confusion of elevated hCG from a new pregnancy. hCG levels should be negative for a year before pregnancy is again attempted. In the pregnancy following a mole, the hCG level should be checked 6 weeks postpartum.

Prognosis

Five years' survival after courses of chemotherapy, even when metastases have been demonstrated, can be expected in at least 85% of cases of choriocarcinoma.

Burrows A et al: Regression pattern of beta human chorionic gonadotrophin in blood after chemotherapy for gestational trophoblastic neoplasia. Aust N Z J Obstet Gynaecol 1996;36:331. [NLM Cit ID: 97038169]

Newlands ES et al: Recent advances in gestational trophoblastic disease. Hematol Oncol Clin North Am 1999;13:225. [NLM Cit ID: 99179814]

THIRD-TRIMESTER BLEEDING

Five to ten percent of women have vaginal bleeding in late pregnancy. The physician must distinguish between placental causes (placenta previa, placental abruption, vasa previa) and nonplacental causes (infection, disorders of the lower genital tract, systemic disease). The approach to bleeding in late pregnancy should be conservative and expectant unless fetal distress or risk of maternal hemorrhage occurs.

The patient should be hospitalized and placed at bed rest with continuous fetal monitoring. A complete blood count should be obtained and two to four units of blood typed and cross-matched. If an ultrasound examination has been performed earlier in the pregnancy, it may be possible to exclude placenta previa as a cause. If not, one should be performed to determine placental location. A speculum and digital pelvic examination is done only after ultrasound study has ruled out placenta previa. Continuous electronic fetal monitoring is required to exclude fetal distress. While uterine contractions, pain, or tenderness often indicate associated abruptio placentae, an ultrasound negative for retroplacental clot does not exclude it. If vaginal bleeding is profuse and the uterus is painful or contracting, blood should be available before a vaginal examination is performed in case an emergency cesarean section is required.

If the patient is less than 36 weeks of gestation, continued hospitalization and bed rest may be necessary, especially with placenta previa during the initial 7–10 days following vaginal bleeding. If the patient has close proximity to the hospital and immediate access, can be on strict bed rest, and has complete resolution of bleeding and uterine contractions, home management may be considered. She must be well instructed and counseled regarding the risks. Patients with vaginal bleeding at less than 36 weeks of gestation should also be considered for amniocentesis to test for fetal lung maturity. Steroid therapy (betamethasone 12 mg intramuscularly, two doses 12–24 hours apart) is indicated if fetal lung immaturity is present.

Towers CV et al: Is tocolysis safe in the management of third-trimester bleeding? Am J Obstet Gynecol 1999; 180:1572. [NLM Cit ID: 99298116]

MEDICAL CONDITIONS COMPLICATING PREGNANCY

Anemia

Plasma volume increases 50% during pregnancy, while red cell volume increases 25%, causing lower hemoglobin and hematocrit values, which are maximally changed around the 24th to 28th weeks. Anemia in pregnancy is often defined as a hemoglobin measurement below 10 g/dL or hematocrit below 30%. Anemia is very common in pregnancy, causing fatigue, anorexia, dyspnea, and edema. Prevention through optimal nutrition and iron and folic acid supplementation is desirable.

A. Iron Deficiency Anemia: Many women enter pregnancy with low iron stores resulting from heavy menstrual periods, previous pregnancies, breast feeding, or poor nutrition. It is difficult to meet the increased requirement for iron through diet, and anemia often develops unless iron supplements are given. Red cells may not become hypochromic and microcytic until the hematocrit has fallen significantly. When this occurs, a serum iron level below 40 μg/dL and a transferrin saturation less than 10% suggest iron deficiency anemia (see Chapter 13). Treatment consists of a diet containing iron-rich foods and 60 mg of elemental iron (eg, 300 mg of ferrous sulfate) three times a day with meals. Iron is best absorbed if taken with a source of vitamin C (raw fruits and vegetables, lightly cooked greens). All pregnant women should take daily iron supplements.

B. Folic Acid Deficiency Anemia: Folic acid deficiency anemia is the main cause of macrocytic anemia in pregnancy, since vitamin B_{12} deficiency anemia is rare in the childbearing years. The daily requirement of folic acid doubles from 400 μg to 800 μg in pregnancy. Twin pregnancies, infections, malabsorption, and use of anticonvulsant drugs such as phenytoin can precipitate folic acid deficiency. The anemia may first be seen in the puerperium owing to the increased need for folate during lactation.

The diagnosis is made by finding macrocytic red cells and hypersegmented neutrophils in a blood smear (see Chapter 13). However, blood smears in pregnancy may be difficult to interpret, since they frequently show iron deficiency changes as well. Because the deficiency is hard to diagnose and folate intake is inadequate in some socioeconomic groups, 0.8–1 mg of folic acid is given as a supplement in pregnancy; the dose in established deficiency is 1–5 mg/d.

Good sources of folate in food are leafy green vegetables, orange juice, peanuts, and beans. Cooking and storage of food destroy folic acid. Strict vegetarians who eat no eggs or milk products should take vitamin B_{12} supplements during pregnancy and lactation.

C. Sickle Cell Anemia: Women with sickle cell anemia are subject to serious complications in pregnancy. The anemia becomes more severe, and crises may occur more frequently. Complications include infections, bone pain, pulmonary infarction, congestive heart failure, and preeclampsia. There is an increased rate of spontaneous abortion and higher maternal and perinatal mortality rates. Intensive medical treatment may improve the outcome for mother and fetus. Frequent indicated transfusions of packed cells or leukocyte-poor washed red cells lower the level of hemoglobin S and elevate the level of hemoglobin A; this minimizes the severity of anemia and the risk of sickle cell crises.

Genetic counseling should be offered to patients with sickle cell disease or sickle trait. They may wish to undergo first-trimester chorionic villus biopsy or second-trimester amniocentesis to determine whether the abnormality has been passed on to the fetus. IUDs and oral contraceptives are contraindicated, but progestin-only contraceptives may be used. Women with sickle cell trait alone usually have an uncomplicated gestation except for an increased risk of urinary tract infection. Sickle cell-hemoglobin C disease in pregnancy is similar to sickle cell anemia and is treated similarly.

Mason E et al: Medical problems during pregnancy. Med Clin North Am 1998;82:249. [NLM Cit ID: 98193076]

Smith J et al: Pregnancy in sickle cell disease: Experience of the Cooperative Study of Sickle Cell Disease. Obstet Gynecol 1996;87:199. [NLM Cit ID: 96148893]

Lupus Anticoagulant-Anticardiolipin-Antiphospholipid Antibody Syndrome

The presence of antibodies to phospholipids and a variety of clinical symptoms, including vascular thromboses, thrombocytopenia, and recurrent pregnancy loss, characterize the lupus anticoagulant-anticardiolipin-antiphospholipid antibody syndrome. Many of these patients have SLE-like symptoms but do not meet specific diagnostic criteria for that disease. The lupus anticoagulant and anticardiolipin nontreponemal antibody may occur in these patients, and both may cause arterial and venous thromboses. Detection of these antiphospholipid antibodies may require a combination of laboratory tests. The lupus anticoagulant will prolong both the partial thromboplastin time (PTT) and the Russell viper venom time. The latter is a more sensitive predictor of disease. Such patients should also be screened for the presence of the factor V Leiden mutation. Anticardiolipin antibody may be detected with ELISA testing. Either antibody may cause false-positive syphilis serologic tests.

This syndrome may require treatment with immunosuppressive or anticoagulant medications. In a small number of patients with recurrent pregnancy loss and a diagnosis of lupus anticoagulant syndrome, improved outcomes have been reported following treatment with daily high-dose prednisone (40 mg/d) and low-dose aspirin (81 mg) or heparin anticoagulation (8000–20,000 units in two or three doses daily) and low-dose aspirin begun before or early in pregnancy and continued until the postpartum period. Although complications have been reported with both regimens, current opinion seems to favor the heparin and low-dose aspirin combination.

Backos M et al: Pregnancy complications in women with recurrent miscarriage associated with antiphospholipid antibodies treated with low dose aspirin and heparin. Br J Obstet Gynecol 1999;106:102. [NLM Cit ID: 99353746].

Branch DW et al: Antiphospholipid antibodies other than lupus anticoagulant and anticardiolipin antibodies in women with recurrent pregnancy loss, fertile controls, and antiphospholipid syndrome. Obstet Gynecol 1997;89:549. [NLM Cit ID: 97236615]

Kutteh W: Antiphospholipid antibody-associated recurrent pregnancy loss: Treatment with heparin and low-dose aspirin is superior to low-dose aspirin alone. Am J Obstet Gynecol 1996;174:1584. [NLM Cit ID: 96240095] (The total daily dose of heparin given in two doses ranged from 8000 to 20,000 units.)

Asthma

The effect of pregnancy on asthma is unpredictable. About 50% of patients have no change, 25% improve, and 25% get worse. Management of acute and chronic asthma during pregnancy does not differ significantly from that of nonpregnant women. The goal is to maintain maternal $P_{O_2} > 80$ mm Hg to sustain normal fetal oxygenation (see Chapter 9).

Alexander S et al: Perinatal outcomes in women with asthma during pregnancy. Obstet Gynecol 1998;92:435. [NLM Cit ID: 98387240] (A retrospective cohort study included 817 asthmatic women and 13,709 nonasthmatic women.)

Dombrowski MP: Pharmacologic therapy of asthma during pregnancy. Obstet Gynecol Clin North Am 1997;24:559. [NLM Cit ID: 97411610]

AIDS During Pregnancy

Heterosexual acquisition (40%) is the commonest recognized mode of HIV infection among women, followed by injecting drug use (33%) and transfusion (2%). In 25%, no risk is reported or identified. Asymptomatic infection is not associated with a decreased pregnancy rate or increased risk of adverse pregnancy outcomes. There is no evidence that pregnancy causes AIDS progression.

Although some fetuses appear to acquire HIV infection antenatally by transplacental transmission, approximately two-thirds are infected close to or during the time of delivery. Zidovudine given to the mother antenatally (500 mg/d orally) and during labor (1 mg/kg/h intravenously) and then to the infant (2 mg/kg orally four times daily) for the first 6 weeks of life reduces the transmission rate from 25% to 8%. Pregnancy does not necessarily preclude the use of combinations of highly active antiretroviral agents (HAART). HIV-positive pregnant women should be assessed by CD4 count, plasma RNA levels, and prior or current antiretroviral use. In general, pregnant HIV-positive women should receive at least zidovudine but also HAART as appropriate for their HIV disease status after counseling regarding the potential impact of therapy on the fetus and infant after delivery. The use of prophylactic elective cesarean section before the onset of labor or rupture of the membranes to prevent vertical transmission of HIV infection from mother to fetus has been shown to reduce the transmission rate to 2% in infants of mothers taking zidovudine. There is no information on the impact of elective cesarean section on transmission rates in infants of mothers on HAART or with viral loads less than 1000 copies/mL. HIV-infected women should be advised not to breast-feed their infants.

ACOG Committee Opinion. Scheduled cesarean delivery and the prevention of vertical transmission of HIV infection. Number 219, August 1999. Committee on Obstetric Practice, American College of Obstetricians and Gynecologists. Int J Gynaecol Obstet 1999;66:305. [NLM Cit ID: 20046652]

International Perinatal HIV Group: The mode of delivery and the risk of vertical transmission of human immunodeficiency virus type 1. N Engl J Med 1999;340:977. [NLM Cit ID: 99182213]

Lindsay M: HIV infection in women. Clin Obstet Gynecol 1996;39:277.

Public Health Service Task Force recommendations for the use of antiretroviral drugs in pregnant women infected with HIV-1 for maternal health and for reducing perinatal HIV-1 transmission in the United States. MMWR Morb Mortal Wkly Rep 1998;47(RR-2):1. [NLM Cit ID: 98120942]

Diabetes Mellitus

Pregnancy is associated with increased tissue resistance to insulin, resulting in increased levels of blood insulin as well as glucose and triglycerides. These changes are due to placental lactogen and elevated circulating estrogens and progesterone. Although pregnancy does not appear to alter the long-term consequences of diabetes, retinopathy and nephropathy may first appear or become worse during pregnancy. The White classification (Table 18–3) summarizes the pathologic features of diabetes complicating pregnancy. It is also important to recognize the practical overlap between pregestational and gestational diabetes categorized as class A. Debate continues over whether gestational diabetics are women whose glucose intolerance is solely a function of their pregnant compared to their nonpregnant state. Alternatively, pregnancy may merely serve to unmask their underlying propensity for glucose intolerance, which will be evident even in the nonpregnant state at some time in the future if not in the immediate postpartum period. In part as an aid in the long-term management of such women, patients categorized as class A are commonly subdivided into A_1 and A_2 diabetes. A_1 diabetics are those patients whose fasting blood glucose is under 95 mg/dL but who have two abnormal

Table 18–3. Modified White classification of diabetes mellitus.[1]

Class A:	Chemical diabetes diagnosed *before* pregnancy; managed by diet alone; any age at onset, any duration
Class B:	Insulin treatment necessary *before* pregnancy; onset after age 20; duration of less than 10 years
Class C:	Onset at age 10–19, or duration of 10–19 years
Class D:	Onset before age 10, or duration of 20 years or more, or chronic hypertension, or background retinopathy
Class F:	Renal disease
Class H:	Coronary artery disease
Class R:	Proliferative retinopathy
Class T:	Renal transplant

[1]Reproduced, with permission, from DeCherney AH, Pernoll ML (editors): *Current Obstetric & Gynecologic Diagnosis & Treatment,* 8th ed. Appleton & Lange, 1994.

values among the remaining three glucose determinations on a glucose tolerance test. A_2 diabetics are those patients whose fasting blood glucose is 95 mg/dL or more and in addition have one or more elevations among the remaining three glucose determinations. A_1 diabetics typically can be managed by diet alone, while A_2 diabetics will most often require insulin therapy during their pregnancy.

Prepregnancy counseling and evaluation of diabetic women should include a complete chemistry panel, HbA_{1c} determination, 24-hour urine collection for total protein and creatinine clearance, funduscopic examination, and an ECG. Any medical problems should be addressed, and HbA_{1c} levels of less than 8% should be achieved before pregnancy. Euglycemia should be established before conception and maintained during pregnancy with daily home glucose monitoring by the patient. A well-planned dietary program is a key component, with an intake of 1800–2200 kcal/d divided into three meals and three snacks. Insulin is given subcutaneously in a split-dose regimen with frequent dosage adjustments. The use of continuous insulin pump therapy is currently limited to women with difficult (brittle) diabetes.

Congenital anomalies result from hyperglycemia during the first 4–8 weeks of pregnancy. They occur in 4–10% of diabetic pregnancies (two to three times the rate in nondiabetic pregnancies). Euglycemia in the early weeks of pregnancy, when organogenesis is occurring, reduces the rate of anomalies to near-normal levels. Even so, because few women with diabetes begin a rigorous program to achieve euglycemia until well after they have become pregnant, congenital anomalies are the principal cause of perinatal fetal deaths in diabetic pregnancies. All women with diabetes should receive counseling about pregnancy and, when the decision has been made to start a family, should receive prepregnancy management by physicians experienced in diabetic pregnancies.

Fasting and preprandial glucose values are lower during pregnancy in both diabetic and nondiabetic women. Euglycemia is considered to be 60–80 mg/dL while fasting and 30–45 minutes before meals and < 120 mg/dL 1 hour after meals. This is the target for good diabetic control during pregnancy. Glycosylated hemoglobin levels help determine the quality of glucose control both before and during pregnancy.

While perinatal problems for mother and baby are decreased by fastidious diabetic control, the incidence of hydramnios, preeclampsia-eclampsia, infections, and prematurity is increased even in carefully managed diabetic pregnancies. Diabetes is an inherently unstable disease characterized by fluctuations of blood glucose levels, particularly late in pregnancy. The risk of fetal demise in the third trimester (stillbirth) and neonatal death increases with the level of hyperglycemia. Consequently, pregnant women with type I diabetes must receive regular antepartum fetal testing (nonstress testing, contraction stress testing, biophysical profile) during the third trimester. The timing of delivery is dictated by the quality of diabetic control, the presence or absence of medical complications, and fetal status. The goal is to achieve 39 weeks (38 completed weeks) and then proceed with delivery. Confirmation of lung maturity is necessary only for delivery prior to 39 weeks. Cesarean sections are performed for obstetric indications.

Because 15% of patients with gestational diabetes require insulin during pregnancy and because the infants of gestational diabetics have some risks similar to those of infants of diabetic mothers (particularly macrosomia), screening of women for glucose intolerance has been recommended between the 24th and 28th weeks of pregnancy (Table 18–4). Patients with gestational diabetes should be evaluated 6–8 weeks postpartum by a 2-hour oral glucose tolerance test (75 g glucose load).

Metzger BE et al: Summary and recommendations of the Fourth International Workshop-Conference on Gestational Diabetes Mellitus. Diabetes Care 1998;21(Suppl 2):B161. [NLM Cit ID: 98369868]

Reece EA et al: The pathogenesis of diabetes associated congenital malformations. Diabetes in pregnancy. Obstet Gynecol Clin North Am 1996;23:29. [NLM Cit ID: 96247884]

Schwartz ML et al: The diagnosis and classification of gestational diabetes mellitus: is it time to change our tune? Am J Obstet Gynecol 1999;180:1560. [NLM Cit ID: 99298115]

Heart Disease

Most cases of heart disease complicating pregnancy in the USA are congenital, with 5% of maternal deaths due to heart disease. Normal pregnancy causes a faster pulse, an increase of cardiac output of more than 30%, and a rise in plasma volume greater than red cell mass with relative hemodilution. Both vital capacity and oxygen consumption rise only slightly.

Table 18–4. Screening and diagnostic criteria for gestational diabetes mellitus.

Screening for gestational diabetes

1. 50 g oral glucose load, administered between the 24th and 28th weeks, without regard to time of day or time of last meal. Recent recommendations suggest that universal blood glucose screening is appropriate for patients who are of Hispanic, African, Native American, South or East Asian, Pacific Island, or Indigenous Australian ancestry. Other patients who have no known diabetes in first-degree relatives, are under 25 years of age, have normal weight before pregnancy, and have no history of abnormal glucose metabolism or poor obstetric outcome do not require routine screening.
2. Venous plasma glucose measure 1 hour later.
3. Value of 130 mg/dL (7.2 mmol/L) or above in venous plasma indicates the need for a full diagnostic glucose tolerance test.

Diagnosis of gestational diabetes mellitus

1. 100 g oral glucose load, administered in the morning after overnight fast lasting at least 8 hours but not more than 14 hours, and following at least 3 days of unrestricted diet (> 150 g carbohydrate) and physical activity.
2. Venous plasma glucose is measured fasting and at 1, 2, and 3 hours. Subject should remain seated and should not smoke throughout the test.
3. Two or more of the following venous plasma concentrations must be equaled or exceeded for a diagnosis of gestational diabetes: fasting, 95 mg/dL (5.3 mmol/L); 1 hour, 180 mg/dL (10 mmol/L); 2 hours, 155 mg/dL (8.6 mmol/L); 3 hours, 140 mg/dL (7.8 mmol/L).

For practical purposes, the functional capacity of the heart is the best single measurement of cardiopulmonary status.

FUNCTIONAL CARDIAC ASSESSMENT

Class I	Ordinary physical activity causes no discomfort (perinatal mortality rate about 5%).
Class II	Ordinary activity causes discomfort and slight disability (perinatal mortality rate 10–15%).
Class III	Less than ordinary activity causes discomfort or disability; patient is barely compensated (perinatal mortality rate about 35%).
Class IV	Patient decompensated; any physical activity causes acute distress (perinatal mortality rate over 50%).

In general, patients with class I or class II functional disability (80% of pregnant women with heart disease) do well obstetrically, with four-fifths of maternal deaths due to heart disease occurring in women with class III or class IV disability. Congestive failure is the usual cause of death. Most deaths occur in the early puerperium. Pregnancy is contraindicated in Eisenmenger's complex; in primary pulmonary hypertension; in severe mitral stenosis with secondary pulmonary hypertension; and in Marfan's syndrome, in which the aorta is prone to dissection and rupture. In addition, pregnancy is poorly tolerated in patients with aortic stenosis, aortic coarctation, tetralogy of Fallot, and active rheumatic carditis.

Therapeutic abortion and elective sterilization should be offered to patients with significant cardiac disease. Cesarean section should be performed only for obstetric indications. Women with valvular heart disease, mitral valve prolapse associated with mitral insufficiency, or idiopathic hypertrophic subaortic stenosis should receive appropriate antibiotic prophylaxis against infective endocarditis during labor and delivery or termination of pregnancy.

Mendelson M: Congenital cardiac disease and pregnancy. Clin Perinatol 1997;24:467. [NLM Cit ID: 97353572]

Oakley CM: Pregnancy and heart disease. Br J Hosp Med 1996;55:423. [NLM Cit ID: 96290739]

Peripartum Cardiomyopathy

Cardiac failure that develops during pregnancy or during the first 6 months postpartum in a woman without a history of heart disease and with no cause for heart failure other than pregnancy is termed peripartum cardiomyopathy. The incidence varies from 1:4000 to 1:1000. It is higher in Africa. It occurs more often in older women, those with twins, and in patients with pregnancy-induced hypertension. The cause of peripartum cardiomyopathy is unknown. In patients who continue to have symptoms and signs of disease for more than 6 months postpartum, the mortality rate is high, and subsequent pregnancy is especially dangerous.

Symptoms of peripartum cardiomyopathy are those of congestive heart failure. An electrocardiogram may reveal tachycardia and atrial or ventricular arrhythmias. Death may occur as a result of arrhythmia or embolism. Autopsy usually reveals an enlarged, dilated heart, and mural thrombi (the source of pulmonary and systemic emboli) are often found.

The treatment of peripartum cardiomyopathy is that of congestive cardiomyopathy (see Chapter 10). Patients with persistent cardiomegaly or mural thrombi shown by echocardiography require anticoagulant therapy. The long-term prognosis in these patients depends on whether cardiomegaly resolves within 6 months after the onset of symptoms. If it does not resolve, the 5-year mortality rate is 35%. If it does resolve, the mortality rate is still about 15%. If cardiomegaly does not resolve and another pregnancy intervenes, cardiomyopathy recurs in 50% of cases, with an almost 100% mortality rate.

Heider AL et al: Peripartum cardiomyopathy: a review of the literature. Obstet Gynecol Surv 1999;54:526. [NLM Cit ID: 99363117]

Herpes Genitalis (See also Chapter 6.)

Infection of the lower genital tract by herpes simplex virus type 2 (HSV-2) is a common sexually transmitted disease of potential seriousness to pregnant women and their newborn infants. Although up to 20% of women in an obstetric practice may have antibodies to HSV-2, a history of the infection is unreliable and the incidence of neonatal infection is low (1:20,000–1:3000 live births). Most infected neonates are born to women with no symptoms, signs, or history of infection.

Women who have had *primary* herpes infection late in pregnancy are at high risk of shedding virus at delivery. Some authors suggest use of prophylactic acyclovir, 400 mg orally twice daily, to decrease the likelihood of active lesions at the time of labor and delivery.

Women with a history of *recurrent* genital herpes have a neonatal attack rate of 5% and should be followed by clinical observation and culture of any suspicious lesions. Since asymptomatic viral shedding is not predictable by antepartum cultures, current recommendations do not include routine cultures in individuals with a history of herpes without active disease. However, when labor begins, vulvar and cervical inspection and cultures should be performed, with prompt treatment of a newborn after a positive culture.

For treatment, see Chapter 32. The use of acyclovir in pregnancy is acceptable when there is significant fetal or neonatal risk.

Cesarean section is indicated at the time of labor if there are prodromal symptoms, active genital lesions, or a positive cervical culture obtained within the preceding week.

Brocklehurst P et al: A randomised placebo controlled trial of suppressive acyclovir in late pregnancy in women with recurrent genital herpes infection. Br J Obstet Gynaecol 1998;105:275. [NLM Cit ID: 98194180] (This randomized double blind placebo-controlled trial was unable to demonstrate that acyclovir can significantly decrease the number of cesarean deliveries; however, the number of clinical recurrences was significantly reduced.)

Brown ZA et al: The acquisition of herpes simplex virus during pregnancy. N Engl J Med 1997;337:509. [NLM Cit ID: 97390799]

Hensleigh PA et al: Genital herpes during pregnancy: Inability to distinguish primary and recurrent infections clinically. Obstet Gynecol 1997;89:891. [NLM Cit ID: 97314118]

Hypertensive Disease

Hypertensive disease in women of childbearing age is usually essential, but secondary causes should be considered: coarctation of the aorta, pheochromocytoma, hyperaldosteronism, and renovascular and renal hypertension.

Preeclampsia is superimposed on 20% of pregnancies in hypertensive women and appears earlier, is more severe, and is more often associated with intrauterine growth retardation. It may be difficult to determine whether or not hypertension in a pregnant woman precedes or derives from the pregnancy if she is not examined until after the 20th week. Serum uric acid can help differentiate, since it is elevated with preeclampsia and normal in chronic hypertension. If hypertension persists for 6–8 weeks postpartum, essential hypertension is likely.

Pregnant women with chronic hypertension require medication only if the diastolic pressure is sustained at or above 100 mm Hg. For initiation of treatment, methyldopa is still the drug of choice. Start with 250 mg orally twice daily and increase in divided doses as needed to as much as 3 g daily. The goal is to keep the diastolic pressure between 80 and 100 mm Hg.

If a hypertensive woman is being managed successfully by medical treatment when she registers for antenatal care, one may generally continue the antihypertensive medication. Diuretics may be continued in pregnancy. ACE inhibitors should be replaced with a drug of another class because of reports of fetal and neonatal renal failure with these compounds.

Use of antihypertensive medications in preeclampsia remains controversial. This should be attempted only with significant fetal prematurity, absence of fetal compromise, and close supervision of the patient.

Therapeutic abortion may be indicated in cases of severe hypertension during pregnancy. If pregnancy is allowed to continue, the risk to the fetus must be assessed periodically in anticipation of early delivery. An early second-trimester ultrasound examination will confirm the duration of pregnancy, and follow-up examinations after 28 weeks will evaluate intrauterine growth retardation.

Rey E et al: Report of the Canadian Hypertension Society Consensus Conference 3. Pharmacologic treatment of hypertensive disorders in pregnancy. Can Med Assoc J 1997;157:1245. [NLM Cit ID: 98027718]

Maternal Hepatitis B Carrier State

There are an estimated 200 million chronic carriers of hepatitis B virus worldwide. Among these people there is an increased incidence of chronic active hepatitis, cirrhosis, and hepatocellular carcinoma. The frequency of the hepatitis B carrier state varies from 1% in the USA and Western Europe to 35% in parts of Africa and Asia. All pregnant women should be screened for hepatitis B surface antigen (HBsAg). Transmission of the virus to the baby after delivery is likely if both surface antigen and e antigen are positive. Vertical transmission can be blocked by the immediate postdelivery administration to the newborn of 0.5 mL of hepatitis B immunoglobulin and hepatitis B vaccine intramuscularly. The vaccine dose is repeated at 1 and 6 months of age.

Hepatitis C virus infection is the most common chronic blood-borne infection in the United States. Risk factors for transmission include blood transfusion, injecting drug use, employment in patient care or clinical laboratory work, exposure to a sex partner or household member who has had a history of hepatitis, exposure to multiple sex partners, and low socioeconomic level. The average rate of HCV infection among infants born to HCV-positive, HIV-negative women is 5–6%. However, the average infection rate increases to 14% when mothers are coinfected with HCV and HIV. The principal factor associated with transmission is the presence of HCV RNA in the mother at the time of birth.

Kane M: Hepatitis viruses and the neonate. Clin Perinatol 1997;24:181. [NLM Cit ID: 97254274]

Recommendations for prevention and control of hepatitis C virus (HCV) infection and HCV-related chronic disease. MMWR Morb Mortal Wkly Rep 1998;47(RR-19):1. [NLM Cit ID: 99004881]

Thomas DL et al: Perinatal transmission of hepatitis C virus from human immunodeficiency virus type 1-infected mothers. Women and Infants Transmission Study. J Infect Dis 1998;177:1480. [NLM Cit ID: 98268839]

Acute Fatty Liver of Pregnancy

Acute fatty liver of pregnancy is a disorder limited to the gravid state. It occurs in the third trimester of pregnancy and involves acute hepatic failure. The mortality rate has been reported to be as high as 85%, but with improved recognition and immediate delivery, the mortality range is 20–30%. The disorder is usually seen after the 35th week of gestation and is more common in primigravidas and those with twins. The incidence is about 1:14,000 deliveries.

The cause of acute fatty liver of pregnancy is not known. Pathologic findings are unique to the disorder, with fatty engorgement of hepatocytes. Clinical onset is gradual, with flu-like symptoms that progress to the development of abdominal pain, jaundice, encephalopathy, disseminated intravascular coagulation, and death. On examination, the patient shows signs of hepatic failure.

Laboratory findings show marked elevation of alkaline phosphatase but only moderate elevations of ALT and AST. Prothrombin time and bilirubin are also elevated. The white blood cell count is elevated, and the platelet count is depressed. Hypoglycemia may be profound.

The differential diagnosis is that of fulminant hepatitis. However, liver aminotransferases for fulminant hepatitis are higher (> 1000 units/mL) than those for acute fatty liver of pregnancy (usually < 500 units/mL). It is also important to review the appropriate history and perform the appropriate tests for toxins that cause liver failure. Preeclampsia may involve the liver but typically does not cause jaundice. The elevations in liver function tests in patients with preeclampsia usually do not reach the levels seen in patients with acute fatty liver of pregnancy.

Diagnosis of acute fatty liver of pregnancy mandates immediate delivery. Supportive care during labor includes administration of glucose, platelets, and fresh frozen plasma as needed. Vaginal delivery is preferred. Resolution of encephalopathy occurs over days, and supportive care with a low-protein diet is needed.

Recurrence rates for this liver disorder are unclear. Most authorities advise against subsequent pregnancy, but there have been reported cases of successful outcomes in later pregnancies.

Castro MA et al: Reversible peripartum liver failure: a new perspective on the diagnosis, treatment, and cause of acute fatty liver of pregnancy, based on 28 consecutive cases. Am J Obstet Gynecol 1999;181:389. [NLM Cit ID: 99383852]

Seizure Disorders

Women contemplating pregnancy who have not had a seizure for 5 years should consider a prepregnancy trial of withdrawal from treatment. Those with recurrent epilepsy should use a single drug with blood level monitoring. Trimethadione and valproate are contraindicated during pregnancy; phenytoin and carbamazepine may be teratogenic in the first trimester and should not be used unless absolutely necessary. Newer antiepilepsy drugs have recently been introduced, but there is little information available on their safety in pregnancy and they should generally be avoided. Phenobarbital is considered the drug of choice. Serum levels should be measured in each trimester and dosage adjustments made to keep serum levels in the low normal therapeutic range. Pregnant women taking phenobarbital and phenytoin should receive vitamin supplements, including folic acid and vitamin D, throughout pregnancy. Vitamin K, 10–20 mg/d, is administered during the last month to help prevent bleeding problems in the newborn, who are at risk of bleeding tendencies due to decreased levels of clotting factors. Such infants should receive an injection of vitamin K_1, 1 mg given subcutaneously immediately after delivery, and should have clotting studies 2–4 hours later. Breast feeding is not contraindicated.

ACOG educational bulletin. Seizure disorders in pregnancy. Number 231, December 1996. Committee on Educational Bulletins of the American College of Obstetricians and Gynecologists. Int J Gynaecol Obstet 1997;56: 279. [NLM Cit ID: 97272458]

Syphilis, Gonorrhea, & *Chlamydia trachomatis* Infection (See also Chapters 33 and 34.)

These sexually transmitted diseases have significant consequences for mother and child. Untreated syphilis in pregnancy will cause late abortion, stillbirth, transplacental infection, and congenital syphilis. Gonorrhea will produce large-joint arthritis by hematogenous spread as well as ophthalmia neonatorum. Maternal chlamydial infections are largely asymptomatic but are manifested in the newborn by inclusion conjunctivitis and, at age 2–4 months, by pneumonia. The diagnosis of each can be reliably made by appropriate laboratory tests, which should be included in all prenatal care. The sexual partners of women with sexually transmitted diseases should be identified and treated also if that can be done.

Group B Streptococcal Infection

Group B streptococci frequently colonize the lower female genital tract, with an asymptomatic carriage rate in pregnancy of 5–30%. This rate depends on maternal age, gravidity, and geographic variation. Vaginal carriage is asymptomatic and intermittent, with spontaneous clearing in approximately 30% and recolonization in about 10% of women. Adverse perinatal outcomes associated with group B streptococcal colonization include urinary tract infection, intrauterine infection, premature rupture of membranes, preterm delivery, and postpartum endometritis.

Women with postpartum endometritis due to infection with group B streptococci, especially after cesarean section, develop fever, tachycardia, and abdominal distention, usually within 24 hours after delivery. Approximately 35% of these women are bacteremic.

Group B streptococcal infection is a common cause of neonatal sepsis. Transmission rates are high, yet the rate of neonatal sepsis is surprisingly low at less than 4:1000 live births. Unfortunately, the mortality rate associated with early-onset disease can be as high as 50% in premature infants and approaches 25% even in those at term. Moreover, these infections can contribute markedly to chronic morbidity, including mental retardation and neurologic disabilities. Late-onset disease develops through contact with hospital nursery personnel. Up to 45% of these health care workers can carry the bacteria on their skin and transmit the infection to newborns.

CDC recommendations for screening for and prophylaxis of group B streptococcal colonization are set forth above in the section on Tests and Procedures.

American Academy of Pediatrics Committee on Infectious Diseases and Committee on Fetus and Newborn: Revised guidelines for prevention of early-onset group B streptococcal (GBS) infection. Pediatrics 1997;99:489. [NLM Cit ID: 97193725]

Varicella

Commonly known as chickenpox, varicella-zoster virus (VZV) infection has a fairly benign course when incurred during childhood but may result in serious illness in adults, particularly during pregnancy. Infection results in lifelong immunity. Approximately 95% of women born in the USA have VZV antibodies by the time they reach reproductive age. The incidence of VZV infection during pregnancy has been reported as up to 7:10,000.

The incubation period for this infection is 10–20 days. A primary infection follows and is characterized by a flu-like syndrome with malaise, fever, and development of a pruritic maculopapular rash on the trunk which becomes vesicular and then crusts. Pregnant women are prone to the development of VZV pneumonia, often a fulminant infection sometimes requiring respiratory support. After primary infection, the virus becomes latent, ascending to dorsal root ganglia. Subsequent reactivation can occur as zoster, often under circumstances of immunocompromise, though this is rare during pregnancy.

Two types of fetal infection have been documented. The first is congenital VZV syndrome, which typically occurs in 2–3% of fetuses exposed to primary VZV infection during the first trimester. Anomalies include limb and digit abnormalities, microphthalmos, and microcephaly.

Infection during the latter two trimesters is less threatening. Maternal IgG crosses the placenta, protecting the fetus. The only infants at risk for severe infection are those born after maternal viremia but before development of maternal protective antibody. Maternal infection manifesting 5 days before or after delivery is the time period arbitrarily determined to be most hazardous for transmission to the fetus.

Diagnosis is commonly made on clinical grounds. Laboratory verification of recent infection is made most often by antibody detection techniques, including ELISA, fluorescent antibody, and hemagglutination inhibition. Serum obtained by cordocentesis may be tested for VZV IgM to document fetal infection.

Varicella zoster immune globulin (VZIG) has been shown to prevent or modify the symptoms of infection in some women. Treatment success depends on identification of susceptible women at or just following exposure. Women with a questionable or negative history of chickenpox should be checked for antibody, since the overwhelming majority will have been exposed previously. If the antibody is negative, VZIG (625 units intramuscularly) should be given within 96 hours after exposure. There are no known adverse effects of VZIG administration during pregnancy. Infants born within 5 days of onset of maternal infection should also receive VZIG (125 units).

Infected pregnant women should be closely observed and hospitalized at the earliest signs of pulmonary involvement. Intravenous acyclovir (10–15 mg/kg every 8 hours for 7–10 days) is recommended in the treatment of VZV pneumonia.

Chapman SJ: Varicella in pregnancy. Semin Perinatol 1998;22:339. [NLM Cit ID: 98409379]

Thyrotoxicosis

Thyrotoxicosis during pregnancy may result in fetal anomalies, late abortion, or preterm labor and fetal hyperthyroidism with goiter. Thyroid storm in late pregnancy or labor is a life-threatening emergency.

Radioactive isotope therapy must never be given during pregnancy. The thyroid inhibitor of choice is propylthiouracil, which acts to prevent further thyroxine formation by blocking iodination of tyrosine. There is a 2- to 3-week delay before the pretreatment hormone level begins to fall. The initial dose of propylthiouracil is 100–150 mg three times a day; the dose is lowered as the euthyroid state is approached. It is desirable to keep free T_4 in the high normal range during pregnancy. A maintenance dose of 100 mg/d minimizes the chance of fetal hypothyroidism and goiter.

Recurrent postpartum thyroiditis is a newly recognized entity occurring 3–6 months after delivery. A hyperthyroid state of 1–3 months' duration is followed by hypothyroidism, sometimes misdiagnosed as depression. Thyroperoxidase antibodies and thyroglobulin antibodies are present. Recovery is spontaneous in over 90% of cases after 3–6 months.

Glinoer D: The regulation of thyroid function in pregnancy: Pathways of endocrine adaptation from physiology to pathology. Endocr Rev 1997;18:404. [NLM Cit ID: 97326749]

Mestman J (editor): Thyroid diseases in pregnancy. Clin Obstet Gynecol 1997;40:3. [NLM Cit ID: 97257462]

Tuberculosis

The diagnosis of tuberculosis in pregnancy is made by history taking, physical examination, and skin testing, with special attention to women from ethnic groups with a high prevalence of the disease (such as women from southeast Asia). Chest films should not be obtained as a routine screening measure in pregnancy but should be used only in patients with a skin test conversion or with suggestive findings in the history and physical examination. Abdominal shielding must be used if a chest film is obtained.

If adequately treated, tuberculosis in pregnancy has an excellent prognosis. There is no increase in spontaneous abortion, fetal problems, or congenital anomalies.

Treatment is with isoniazid and ethambutol or isoniazid and rifampin (see Chapters 9 and 33). Because isoniazid therapy may result in vitamin B_6 deficiency, a supplement of 50 mg/d of vitamin B_6 should be given simultaneously. Streptomycin, ethionamide, and most other antituberculous drugs should be avoided in pregnancy.

Anderson GD: Tuberculosis in pregnancy. Semin Perinatol 1997;21:328. [NLM Cit ID: 97442173]

Urinary Tract Infection

The urinary tract is especially vulnerable to infections during pregnancy because the altered secretions of steroid sex hormones and the pressure exerted by the gravid uterus upon the ureters and bladder cause hypotonia and congestion and predispose to urinary stasis. Labor and delivery and urinary retention postpartum also may initiate or aggravate infection. *Escherichia coli* is the offending organism in over two-thirds of cases.

From 2% to 8% of pregnant women have asymptomatic bacteriuria, which some believe to be associated with an increased risk of prematurity. It is estimated that 20–40% of these women will develop pyelonephritis during pregnancy if untreated.

A first-trimester urine culture is indicated in women with a history of recurrent or recent episodes of urinary tract infection. If the culture is positive, treatment should be initiated as a prophylactic measure. Nitrofurantoin (100 mg twice daily), ampicillin (500 mg four times daily), and cephalexin (500 mg four times daily) are acceptable medications for 3–7 days. Sulfonamides should not be given in the third trimester because they interfere with bilirubin binding and thus impose a risk of neonatal hyperbilirubinemia and kernicterus. Fluoroquinolones are also contraindicated because of their potential teratogenic effects on fetal cartilage and bone. If bacteriuria returns, suppressive medication (one daily dose of an appropriate antibiotic) for the remainder of the pregnancy is indicated. Acute pyelonephritis requires hospitalization for intravenous administration of antibiotics until the patient is afebrile; this is followed by a full course of oral antibiotics.

MacLean AB: Urinary tract infection in pregnancy. Br J Urol 1997;80(Suppl 1):10. [NLM Cit ID: 97384550]

SURGICAL COMPLICATIONS DURING PREGNANCY

Elective major surgery should be avoided during pregnancy. Normal uncomplicated pregnancy does not alter operative risk except as it may interfere with the diagnosis of abdominal disorders and increase the technical problems of intra-abdominal surgery. Abortion is not a serious hazard after operation unless peritoneal sepsis or other significant complications occur. During the first trimester, congenital anomalies may be induced in the developing fetus by hypoxia. Thus, the second trimester is usually the optimal time for operative procedures.

Appendicitis

Appendicitis occurs in about one of 5000 pregnancies. Diagnosis is difficult, since the appendix is carried high and to the right, away from McBurney's point, as the uterus enlarges, and localization of pain does not usually occur. Nausea, vomiting, fever, and leukocytosis occur regularly. Any right-sided abdominal pain associated with these symptoms should arouse suspicion. In at least 20% of obstetric patients, the diagnosis of appendicitis is not made until rupture occurs and peritonitis has become established. Such a delay may lead to premature labor or abortion. With early diagnosis and appendectomy, the prognosis is good for mother and baby.

Carcinoma of the Breast

Cancer of the breast (see also Chapter 16) is diagnosed approximately once in 3500 pregnancies. Pregnancy may accelerate the growth of cancer of the breast, and delay in diagnosis affects the outcome of treatment. Inflammatory carcinoma is an extremely virulent type of breast cancer that occurs most commonly during lactation. Prepregnancy mammography should be encouraged for women over age 35 who are anticipating a pregnancy.

Breast enlargement during pregnancy obscures parenchymal masses, and breast tissue hyperplasia decreases the accuracy of mammography. Any discrete mass should be evaluated by aspiration to verify its cystic structure, with fine-needle biopsy if it is solid. A definitive diagnosis may require excisional biopsy under local anesthesia. If breast biopsy confirms the diagnosis of cancer, surgery should be done regardless of the stage of the pregnancy. If spread to the regional glands has occurred, irradiation or chemotherapy should be considered. Under these circumstances, the alternatives are termination of an early pregnancy or delay of therapy for fetal maturation.

Choledocholithiasis, Cholecystitis, & Idiopathic Cholestasis of Pregnancy

Severe choledocholithiasis and cholecystitis are not uncommon during pregnancy. When they do occur, it is usually in late pregnancy or in the puerperium. About 90% of patients with cholecystitis have gallstones; 90% of stones will be visualized by ultrasonography. Symptomatic relief may be all that is required.

Gallbladder surgery in pregnant women should be attempted only in extreme cases (eg, obstruction), because it increases the perinatal mortality rate to about 15%. Cholecystostomy and lithotomy may be all that is feasible during advanced pregnancy, cholecystectomy being deferred until after delivery. On the other hand, withholding surgery may result in necrosis and perforation of the gallbladder and peritonitis. Cholangitis due to impacted common duct stone requires surgical removal of gallstones and establishment of biliary drainage. Endoscopic retrograde cholangiopancreatography and endoscopic retrograde sphincterotomy can be performed safely in pregnant women if precautions are taken to minimize exposure to radiation.

Idiopathic cholestasis of pregnancy is due to a hereditary metabolic (hepatic) deficiency aggravated by the high estrogen levels of pregnancy. It causes intrahepatic biliary obstruction of varying degrees. The rise in bile acids is sufficient in the third trimester to cause severe, intractable, generalized itching and sometimes clinical jaundice. There may be mild elevations in blood bilirubin and alkaline phosphatase levels. The fetus is also threatened by this condition. An increased incidence of preterm delivery has been reported as well as unexplained intrauterine fetal demise. For this reason, antenatal surveillance of the fetus is mandatory in patients with this diagnosis. Resins such as cholestyramine (4 g three times a day) absorb bile acids in the large bowel and relieve pruritus but are difficult to take and may cause constipation. Their use requires vitamin K supplementation. The disorder is relieved once the infant has been delivered, but it recurs in subsequent pregnancies and sometimes with the use of oral contraceptives.

Ovarian Tumors

The most common adnexal mass in early pregnancy is the corpus luteum, which may become cystic and enlarge to 6 cm in diameter. Any persistent mass over 6 cm should be evaluated by ultrasound examination; unilocular cysts are likely to be corpus luteum cysts, whereas septated or semisolid tumors are likely to be neoplasms. The incidence of malignancy in ovarian masses over 6 cm in diameter is 2.5%. Ovarian tumors may undergo torsion and cause abdominal pain and nausea and vomiting and must be differentiated from appendicitis, other bowel disease, and ectopic pregnancy. Patients with suspected ovarian cancer should be referred to a tertiary perinatal center to determine whether the pregnancy can progress to fetal viability or whether treatment should be instituted without delay.

Coleman MT et al: Nonobstetric emergencies in pregnancy: trauma and surgical conditions. Am J Obstet Gynecol 1997;177:497. [NLM Cit ID: 97463912]

DiFronzo LA et al: Breast cancer in pregnancy and lactation. Surg Clin North Am 1996;76:267. [NLM Cit ID: 96192020]

PREVENTION OF HEMOLYTIC DISEASE OF THE NEWBORN (Erythroblastosis Fetalis)

The antibody anti-Rh_o (D) is responsible for most severe instances of hemolytic disease of the newborn (erythroblastosis fetalis). About 15% of whites and much lower proportions of blacks and Asians are Rh_o (D)-negative. If an Rh_o (D)-negative woman carries an Rh_o (D)-positive fetus, she may develop antibodies against Rh_o (D) when fetal red cells enter her circulation during small fetomaternal bleeding episodes in the early third trimester or during delivery, abortion, ectopic pregnancy, abruptio placentae, or other antepartum bleeding problems. This antibody, once produced, remains in the woman's circulation and poses the threat of hemolytic disease for subsequent Rh-positive fetuses.

Passive immunization against hemolytic disease of the newborn is achieved with Rh_o (D) immune globulin, a purified concentrate of antibodies against Rh_o (D) antigen. The Rh_o (D) immune globulin (one vial of 300 μg intramuscularly) is given to the mother within 72 hours after delivery (or spontaneous or induced abortion or ectopic pregnancy). The antibodies in the immune globulin destroy fetal Rh-positive cells so that the mother will not produce anti-Rh_o (D). During her next Rh-positive gestation, erythroblastosis will be prevented. An additional safety measure is the administration of the immune globulin at the 28th week of pregnancy. The passive antibody titer that results is too low to significantly affect an Rh-positive fetus. The maternal clearance of the globulin is slow enough that protection will continue for 12 weeks.

Hemolytic disease of varying degrees, from mild to serious, continue to occur in association with Rh subgroups (C, c, or E) or Kell, Kidd, and other factors. Therefore, atypical antibodies should be checked in the third trimester of all pregnancies.

ACOG practice bulletin. Prevention of Rh D alloimmunization. Number 4, May 1999. Clinical management guidelines for obstetrician-gynecologists. American College of Obstetrics and Gynecology. Int J Gynaecol Obstet 1999;66:63. [NLM Cit ID: 99385738]

PREVENTION OF PRETERM (PREMATURE) LABOR

Preterm (premature) labor is labor that begins before the 37th week of pregnancy; it is responsible for 85% of neonatal illnesses and deaths. The onset of labor is a result of a complex sequence of biologic events involving regulatory factors that are still poorly understood. Significant risk factors for the onset of preterm labor are a past history of preterm delivery, premature rupture of the membranes, urinary tract infection, or exposure to diethylstilbestrol. In addition, multiple gestation and abdominal or cervical surgery are especially important.

Low rates of preterm delivery are associated with success in educating patients to identify regular, frequent uterine contractions and in alerting medical and nursing staff to evaluate these patients early and initiate treatment if cervical changes can be identified. Cessation of work or physical activities that seem related to increased uterine activity is mandatory. Resting at home will often suffice to slow contractions. Despite initial promising findings, several prospective randomized controlled trials have failed to demonstrate a benefit of home uterine activity monitoring in preventing preterm birth.

In more acute situations, intravenous magnesium sulfate is effective, as are intravenous beta-adrenergic drugs. Magnesium sulfate is given as a 4- or 6-g bolus, followed by a continuous infusion of 2–3 g/h. The rate may be increased by 1 g/h every 1½–2 hours until contractions cease or a blood magnesium concentration of 6–8 mg/dL is reached. Magnesium levels are determined every 4–6 hours to monitor the therapeutic blood level. After contractions have ceased for 12–24 hours, magnesium can be stopped and the situation reassessed.

Uterine smooth muscle is largely under sympathetic nervous system control, and stimulation of β_2-adrenergic receptors relaxes the myometrium. Consequently, inhibition of uterine contractility often can be accomplished by the administration of beta-adrenergic drugs such as ritodrine or terbutaline.

Ritodrine is no longer manufactured. Terbutaline can be given as an intravenous infusion starting at 2.5 μg/min and increased by 2.5 μg/min every 20 minutes until contractions cease or to a maximum dose of 20 μg/min. Terbutaline can also be administered as subcutaneous injections of 250 μg every 3 hours. Oral terbutaline therapy following parenteral treatment is often elected and consists of giving 2.5–5 mg every 2–4 hours. With terbutaline, a dose-related elevation of heart rate of 20–40 beats/min may occur. An increase of systolic blood pressure up to 10 mm Hg is likely, and the diastolic pressure may fall 10–15 mm Hg during the infusion. Nifedipine has also been used in doses of 10–20 mg orally every 4–6 hours. Blood pressure may fall with nifedipine. Nonetheless, cardiac output increases considerably. Transient elevation of blood glucose, insulin, and fatty acids together with slight reduction of serum potassium have been reported with beta-adrenergics. Fetal tachycardia may be slight or absent. No drug-caused perinatal deaths have been reported with beta-agonists. Maternal side effects requiring dose limitation are tachycardia (≥ 120 beats/min), palpitations, and nervousness. Fluids should be limited to 2500 mL/24 h. Serious side effects (pulmonary edema, chest pain with or without electrocardiographic changes) are often idiosyncratic, not dose-related, and warrant termination of therapy.

One must identify cases in which untimely delivery is the sole threat to the life or health of the infant. An effort should be made to eliminate (1) maternal conditions that compromise the intrauterine environment and make premature birth the lesser risk, eg, preeclampsia-eclampsia; (2) fetal conditions that either are helped by early delivery or render attempts to stop premature labor meaningless, eg, severe erythroblastosis fetalis; and (3) clinical situations in which it is likely that an attempt to stop labor will be futile, eg, ruptured membranes with chorioamnionitis, cervix fully effaced and dilated more than 3 cm, strong labor in progress.

In pregnancies of less than 34 weeks' duration, betamethasone (12 mg intramuscularly repeated in 12–24 hours) is administered to hasten fetal lung maturation and permit delivery 48 hours after initial treatment when further prolongation of pregnancy is contraindicated.

Dyson D et al: Monitoring women at risk for preterm labor. N Engl J Med 1998;338:15. [NLM Cit ID: 98069940]

Gomez R et al: Pathogenesis of preterm labor and preterm premature rupture of membranes associated with intraamniotic infection. Infect Dis Clin North Am 1997;11:135. [NLM Cit ID: 97220628]

Mercer B et al: Preterm labor and preterm premature rupture of the membranes: Diagnosis and management. Infect Dis Clin North Am 1997;11:177. [NLM Cit ID: 97220629]

LACTATION

Breast feeding should be encouraged by educative measures throughout pregnancy and the puerperium. Mothers should be told the benefits of breast feeding—it is emotionally satisfying, promotes mother-infant bonding, is economical, and gives significant immunity to the infant. The period of amenorrhea associated with frequent and consistent breast feeding provides good birth control until menstruation begins at 6–12 months postpartum or the intensity of breast feeding diminishes. If the mother must return to work, even a brief period of nursing is beneficial. Transfer of immunoglobulins in colostrum and breast milk protects the infant against many systemic and enteric infections. Macrophages and lymphocytes transferred to the infant from breast milk play an immunoprotective role. The intestinal flora of breast-fed infants inhibits the growth of pathogens. Breast-fed infants have fewer bacterial and viral infections, less severe diarrhea, fewer allergy problems, and less subsequent obesity than bottle-fed infants.

Frequent breast feeding on an infant demand schedule enhances milk flow and successful breast feeding. Mothers breast feeding for the first time need help and encouragement from physicians, nurses, and other nursing mothers. Milk supply can be increased by increased suckling and increased rest.

Nursing mothers should have a fluid intake of over 2 L/d. The United States RDA calls for 21 g of extra protein (over the 44 g/d baseline for an adult woman) and 550 extra kcal/d in the first 6 months of nursing. Calcium intake should be 1200 mg/d. Continuation of a prenatal vitamin and mineral supplement is wise. Strict vegetarians who eschew both milk and eggs should always take vitamin B_{12} supplements during pregnancy and lactation.

Effects of Drugs in a Nursing Mother

Drugs taken by a nursing mother may accumulate in milk and be transmitted to the infant. The amount of a drug entering the milk depends on the drug's lipid solubility, mechanism of transport, and degree of ionization (Table 18–5).

Suppression of Lactation

A. Mechanical Suppression: The simplest and safest method of suppressing lactation after it has started is to gradually transfer the baby to a bottle or a cup over a 3-week period. Milk supply will decrease with decreased demand, and minimal discomfort ensues. If nursing must be stopped abruptly, the mother should avoid nipple stimulation, refrain from expressing milk, and use a snug brassiere. Ice packs and analgesics can be helpful. If suppression is desired before nursing has begun, use this same technique. Engorgement will gradually recede over a 2- to 3-day period.

B. Hormonal Suppression: Oral and long-acting injections of hormonal preparations were used at one time to suppress lactation. Because of their questionable efficacy and particularly because of associated side effects such as thromboembolic episodes and hair growth, their use for this purpose has largely been abandoned in recent years. Similarly, lactation suppression with bromocriptine is to be avoided because of reports of severe hypertension, seizures, strokes, and myocardial infarctions associated with its use.

Bailey B, Ito S: Breast-feeding and maternal drug use. Pediatr Clin North Am 1997;44:41. [NLM Cit ID: 97210719]

Neifert MR: Clinical aspects of lactation. Promoting breast-feeding success. Clin Perinatol 1999;26:281. [NLM Cit ID: 99322793]

PUERPERAL MASTITIS (See also Chapter 16.)

Postpartum mastitis occurs sporadically in nursing mothers shortly after they return home, or it may occur in epidemic form in the hospital. *Staphylococcus aureus* is usually the causative agent. Inflammation is generally unilateral, and women nursing for the first time are more often affected. Rarely, inflammatory carcinoma of the breast can be mistaken for puerperal mastitis.

Mastitis frequently begins within 3 months after delivery and may start with a sore or fissured nipple.

Table 18–5. Drugs or substances to be used cautiously or not at all by nursing mothers.[1] (Other drugs are also contraindicated during pregnancy and lactation. Evaluate any drug for its need versus its potential adverse effects.)

Drug or Substance	Effect on Nursing Infant
Alcohol	No harmful effects unless taken in excess, when it can be associated with decreased linear growth and sedation.
Antibiotics	
Aminoglycosides	Not advised. Will alter infant's bowel flora.
Nitrofurantoin	May cause hemolytic anemia in infant with glucose-6-phosphate dehydrogenase (G6PD) deficiency.
Tetracycline	Effects are dose-related. Amount infant receives from milk is too small to cause discoloration of teeth. Safe.
Chloramphenicol[2]	Neonate may be unable to conjugate the drug. Potential harm to bone marrow, leading to anemia, shock, and death.
Sulfonamides[2]	May cause jaundice in the neonatal period. May cause hemolytic anemia in infant with G6PD deficiency.
Metronidazole	Nursing may be resumed 48 hours after last dose.
Anticoagulants	
Phenindione[2]	Can use heparin or warfarin instead.
Antihistamines	Contraindicated because of increased sensitivity of newborns and infants to antihistamines.
Antineoplastics[2]	Suspend nursing if these drugs are taken.
Antithyroids	
Thiouracil,[2] methimazole[2]	Contraindicated. May cause goiter or agranulocytosis.
Propylthiouracil	Considered safe.
Cardiac drugs	
Quinidine[2]	Contraindicated. May cause arrhythmia in infant.
Cimetidine,[2] ranitidine	Concentrated in breast milk. May suppress gastric acidity and cause central nervous system stimulation.
Ergot alkaloids	
Ergotamine (in doses to treat migraine)[2]	Causes vomiting, diarrhea, convulsion. May suppress lactation.
Bromocriptine[2]	Suppresses lactation.
Gold salts[2]	Contraindicated.
Hormones	
Oral contraceptives (low-dose)	May cause reduction of milk supply. Progestin-only minipill may be used.
Laxatives	
Cascara, senna	Can cause diarrhea in infant.
Lithium carbonate[2]	Contraindicated because of toxicity.
Nicotine	Increased respiratory disease in infants exposed to smoke.
Radioactive materials for testing	
^{67}Ga	Insignificant amount excreted in milk. No nursing for 2 weeks.
^{125}I	Discontinue nursing for 48 hours.
^{131}I	After a test dose, nursing may be resumed after 24–36 hours. After a treatment dose, nursing may be resumed after 2–3 weeks.
^{99m}Tc	Discontinue nursing for 72 hours (half-life, 6 hours).
Sedatives and tranquilizers	Can cause sedation in infant. Benzodiazepines should be avoided.
Other drugs	
Caffeine	Irritability. Poor sleep pattern with large amounts.
Cannabis,[2] cocaine,[2] polyhalogenated biphenyls[2] (eg, PCBs, PBBs), D-lysergic acid[2] (LSD)	Contraindicated. May interfere with mother's caretaking abilities and nutrition.

[1]Modified and reproduced, with permission, from Sahu S: Drugs and the nursing mother. Am Fam Physician (Dec) 1981;24:137.
[2]Absolutely contraindicated.

occurs after a latent period of 1–2 days from the time of contact. Hypersensitivity pneumonitis (extrinsic allergic alveolitis) is a pulmonary T cell-mediated hypersensitivity disease.

ATOPIC DISEASE

Clinical manifestations resembling allergic hypersensitivity can also occur in the absence of an immunologic mechanism. Specific examples include nonallergic (intrinsic) asthma, which is triggered by the nonimmunologic effect of inhaled dusts and fumes, weather changes, viral respiratory infections, and stress rather than by aeroallergen-induced IgE-mediated mast cell degranulation; irritant dermatitis, which is the result of physical or chemical damage to skin rather than development of sensitized lymphocytes; and "anaphylactoid reactions" from nonimmunologic release of mast cell mediators, eg, "red man syndrome" secondary to vancomycin. Therefore, the diagnosis of allergy requires answers to the following questions: (1) What is the nature of the disease? (2) Is the disease caused by an IgE-mediated mechanism? (3) What specific allergens (one or several) are responsible?

The relevant history includes a survey of allergen exposure associated with home, work, hobbies, and habits as well as medications. Physical examination is most useful if performed during a period of allergen exposure. Demonstration of allergic hypersensitivity by in vivo or in vitro testing is essential for confirming clinical suspicions of allergic disease.

ALLERGIC RHINITIS

Essentials of Diagnosis

- Nasal pruritus, congestion, rhinorrhea, or paroxysms of sneezing, which may be associated with lower respiratory symptoms (chronic cough, wheezing, chest tightness, or dyspnea); eye irritation and pruritus; or eczematous dermatitis.
- Environmental allergen exposure.
- Confirmed by evidence of specific-IgE antibody to tested aeroallergens.

Clinical Findings

A. Symptoms and Signs: In addition to the symptoms listed above, the physical examination may reveal edematous or inflamed nasal mucosa. In severe cases, the affected mucosa may be pale, boggy, or blue-tinged from vascular engorgement and venous congestion.

B. Laboratory Findings:

1. Specific-IgE antibody tests–Allergy tests reveal an immune response to a particular allergen. To maximize the positive predictive value of allergy testing, a positive test result must be correlated with the history before one can conclude that the allergen caused the illness. The type of immune response must be consistent with the nature of the disease. For example, IgE antibody causes allergic rhinitis but not delayed-type allergic contact dermatitis. IgE antibodies are detected by in vivo (skin tests) or in vitro methods.

a. Skin tests–Epicutaneous or cutaneous allergen testing produces a localized pruritic wheal (induration) and flare (erythema) which is maximal at 15–20 minutes. It is used most commonly in the diagnosis of allergic respiratory disease (rhinitis and asthma) but can also be used in suspected cases of food or drug allergy and hymenoptera (bee, wasp, hornet or yellow jacket) venom hypersensitivity. Allergen extracts are available commercially for pollens, fungi, animal danders, and dust mites and should be selected appropriately for the patient's geographic area.

Skin testing is preferred to in vitro methods (discussed below) because it detects the presence of IgE antibody in tissue and shows biologic activity. For most applications, in vivo skin testing is more sensitive, more specific, more rapid, and less expensive than in vitro radioallergosorbent (RAST) testing. Any drug with antihistamine effects (H_1 antagonists, tricyclic antidepressants, phenothiazines) must be withdrawn prior to testing. Appropriate controls with a negative diluent and a positive histamine control are mandatory for valid results and accurate interpretation. Extensive active dermatitis may limit the availability of skin for testing. There is only a very small risk of inducing a systemic reaction. To avoid this, most allergists perform epicutaneous (prick) testing first, followed by selected intradermal tests to allergens negative by prick testing. Intradermal skin testing techniques are often employed for diagnostic confirmation of hymenoptera (insect venom) or penicillin hypersensitivity, as this method increases sensitivity of the assay for detection of IgE-mediated anaphylaxis. Skin testing with hymenoptera venom or a drug is performed by serial titration, starting with appropriately diluted solutions. Special allergenic extracts can be prepared for other allergens (food or latex) where indicated.

Skin testing for allergy to drugs is reliable for high-molecular-weight protein drugs (eg, heterologous serum, insulin) but not for low-molecular-weight compounds (most drugs), which must bind to larger proteins (haptenate) to become immunogenic. With the exception of penicillin, in vivo skin testing for low-molecular-weight drugs is limited in sensitivity and availability. Penicillin allergy skin testing is available because the immunochemistry has been delineated, identifying all haptenated molecules including the native drug and all metabolites that are potentially immunogenic. The combination of skin testing

response to allergen by stabilizing the mast cell, though the specific molecular mechanisms of action are unknown. Although unrelated, they have similar effects and, because of their poor bioavailability, they are effective only when applied directly to the involved organ. Furthermore, their action is short-lived, so that they must be given three or four times a day. Cromolyn is available as a bronchial inhaler, nasal spray, and ophthalmologic preparation; nedocromil is available in metered-dose inhalers. Not all patients respond, but the drugs have very few side effects and wide margins of safety. A high-dose oral form of cromolyn has been released for use in treating systemic mastocytosis, but poor oral absorption limits its effectiveness.

5. Anticholinergic agents–Ipratropium bromide is effective as a nasal topical agent for use in rhinitis. Mucous membrane glandular secretion is under cholinergic control and can be inhibited by anticholinergic agents. First-generation antihistamines have systemic anticholinergic activity, but ipratropium is preferred as adjunctive treatment of allergic rhinitis or as primary treatment for many types of nonallergic rhinitis. Ipratropium does not alleviate sneezing, pruritus, or nasal congestion but can be useful for treatment of postnasal drip and rhinorrhea.

C. Immunotherapy: Treatment of atopy—especially allergic rhinitis—by the repeated long-term injection of allergen has been shown in many controlled clinical trials to be an effective method for reducing or eliminating symptoms and signs of the allergic disorder.

1. Indications–This treatment is recommended for patients with severe allergic rhinitis who respond poorly to drug therapy and whose allergens are not avoidable. Immunotherapy is unequivocally effective in patients with allergic rhinitis and allergic conjunctivitis. Immunotherapy in allergic asthma has also shown proof of efficacy, but smaller trials with single-antigen treatment have reported conflicting results. The lower clinical response rates observed in asthma have been attributed to the multifactorial nature of the disease. There is no current evidence for an effect in atopic dermatitis. Food or drug hypersensitivity is treated by avoidance only, since immunotherapy is not currently available.

2. Immunologic effects–The term "allergen immunotherapy" is usually used instead of desensitization because the immunologic basis for this form of treatment is currently unknown. Nevertheless, certain immunologic changes can be induced by these injections. Circulating levels of IgE antibodies specific to the injected allergens increase slightly during the first few months, then decrease, eventually to substantially lower levels than before treatment. Seasonal rises in IgE antibodies to pollens are blunted or eliminated. IgG blocking antibody is produced. Changes in regulatory T cells favoring suppression of IgE antibody production have been reported. There is some evidence that TH2 cytokine responses are shifted toward TH1 responses in peripheral blood mononuclear cells. Higher thresholds for release of inflammatory mediators and decreases in late phase allergic reactions may be related to the reduction in biologic sensitivity of end organ systems (eyes, nose, bronchi, skin).

3. Clinical effects–Most patients with allergic rhinitis caused by aeroallergens become more tolerant to natural pollen exposure during successive seasons while on immunotherapy. A small minority become completely asymptomatic, but most patients enjoy a significant decrease in symptoms and medication usage. Only high-dose injected immunotherapy has been demonstrated to be effective in double-blind, placebo-controlled trials. A beneficial response may persist after treatment is stopped. The clinical effects and immunologic responses are antigen-specific.

4. Procedure–A sterile aqueous solution of the allergen or allergens responsible for the patient's disease is administered by subcutaneous injection in increasing doses once or twice a week until a maintenance dose is reached, at which time the interval is advanced to every 4 weeks. The maintenance dose is typically one to ten thousand times the starting dose. Ascending doses are used to minimize the risk of systemic allergic reactions during initial stages of immunotherapy. Three to 5 years is a typical course of therapy, but individual responses may prolong or shorten the duration of therapy.

5. Adverse effects–Reactions to treatment may be local or systemic. Localized immediate and late-phase skin reactions occur at injection sites. These are not harmful, but the dose must be adjusted to avoid excessively large or prolonged local reactions. Immediate systemic reactions or anaphylaxis are a potential problem with each injection and must be prevented by careful monitoring of dosage. The patient must remain at the treatment facility for at least 30 minutes after each injection so that drugs and equipment for treating anaphylaxis will be available if needed. No long-term adverse consequences of aqueous allergen extract immunotherapy are known to have occurred in immunocompetent individuals.

Abramson MJ, Puy RM, Weiner JM: Allergen immunotherapy and asthma. Am J Respir Crit Care Med 1995;151:969. [NLM Cit ID: 95211359] (Meta-analysis of randomized controlled trials of immunotherapy and asthma.)

Bousquet J, Lockey RF, Malling HF: WHO position paper. Allergen immunotherapy: Therapeutic vaccines for allergic diseases. Allergy 1998;S53:1. [NLM Cit ID: 99075374] (A comprehensive review from a consensus meeting of American and European allergy and immunology organizations.)

Demoly P, Michel FB, Bousquet J: In vivo methods for study of allergy skin tests, techniques, and interpretation.

In: *Allergy Principles and Practice,* 5th ed. Middleton E Jr et al (editors). Mosby, 1998.

Munir AKM, Kjellman N-IM, Bjorksten B: Exposure to indoor allergens in early infancy and sensitization. J Allergy Clin Immunol 1997;100:177. [NLM Cit ID: 97419061] (Looks at threshold levels of allergen exposure for sensitization.)

ANAPHYLAXIS, URTICARIA, ANGIOEDEMA

Essentials of Diagnosis

- Urticaria is characterized by large, irregularly shaped pruritic, erythematous wheals.
- Angioedema is painless, deeper, subcutaneous swelling, often involving periorbital, circumoral, and facial regions.
- Anaphylaxis is a systemic reaction with cutaneous symptoms, associated with dyspnea, visceral edema, and hypotension.
- These disorders may be diagnosed clinically, especially in the context of allergen exposure; detection of specific IgE or elevated serum tryptase can confirm diagnosis.

General Considerations

Certain allergens—especially drugs, insect venoms, and foods—may induce an IgE antibody response, causing a generalized release of mediators from mast cells and resulting in systemic anaphylaxis. This potentially fatal condition affects both nonatopic and atopic persons. Isolated urticaria and angioedema are more common cutaneous forms of anaphylaxis with a better prognosis.

Clinical Findings

A. Symptoms and Signs: The manifestations are (1) hypotension or shock from widespread vasodilation, (2) respiratory distress from bronchospasm or laryngeal edema, (3) gastrointestinal and uterine muscle contraction, and (4) urticaria and angioedema.

B. Laboratory Findings: In vivo allergy skin testing and in vitro RAST testing can detect allergen-specific IgE for a variety of foods, hymenoptera (bee, wasp, hornet, fire ant) venom, latex, and some medicines. Skin testing for food allergy is appropriate only if the patient has symptoms consistent with IgE-mediated allergy (eg, urticaria, angioedema, or anaphylaxis) within 2 hours after eating the suspect food.

Determination of serum tryptase can be used to identify recent anaphylactic reactions or other reactions due to systemic mast cell activation. Tryptase is a mast cell-derived neutral protease with a half-life of 60–90 minutes. Elevated tryptase levels have been associated with anaphylaxis, systemic mastocytosis, and non-IgE-mediated diseases characterized by mast cell degranulation ("anaphylactoid reactions"). Histamine is released during these disorders but has a very short serum half-life, making detection difficult even during symptomatic periods.

Treatment

A. Treatment of Anaphylaxis: At the first suspicion, aqueous epinephrine 1:1000 in a dose of 0.2–0.5 mL (0.2–0.5 mg) is injected subcutaneously or intramuscularly. Repeated injections can be given every 15–30 minutes when necessary. Essential is the rapid intravenous infusion of large volumes of fluids (saline, lactated Ringer's, plasma, colloid solutions, or plasma expanders) to replace loss of intravascular plasma into tissues. Other vasopressor drugs (high-dose dopamine, norepinephrine, phenylephrine) may be necessary if the patient remains hypotensive despite epinephrine.

Airway obstruction may be caused by edema of the larynx and hypopharynx or by bronchospasm. The former is treated by maintenance of an airway with endotracheal intubation or tracheostomy. Bronchospasm responds to subcutaneous epinephrine or terbutaline. Inhalation of selective β_2-adrenergic agonists such as albuterol or terbutaline and intravenous administration of theophylline are effective for bronchospasm.

Antihistamines (H_1 and H_2 receptor antagonists) may be useful as adjuvant therapy for alleviating the cutaneous manifestations of urticaria or angioedema and pruritus and for the gastrointestinal and uterine smooth muscle spasms. Corticosteroids will not reverse respiratory obstruction or shock. Long-term combined oral antihistamine and prednisone therapy has been shown to reduce the number and severity of attacks in patients with frequent life-threatening episodes of idiopathic anaphylaxis. Medical therapy does not reliably prevent true IgE-mediated hypersensitivity reactions.

There may be a clinical late-phase response in anaphylaxis, causing a recrudescence of symptoms hours (most commonly 6–12 hours) after exposure to the allergen. Since this may occur after subsidence of the immediate-phase response, all patients with anaphylaxis should be monitored for up to 24 hours.

Anaphylaxis in a patient being treated with β-adrenergic blocker drugs is a special problem because of refractoriness to epinephrine and selective β-adrenergic agonists. Higher doses of adrenergic drugs may be required for the desired effect; using glucagon in those patients taking beta-blockers may be additionally beneficial. Patients being treated with angiotensin-converting enzyme (ACE) inhibitors may suffer from more severe hypotension due to blockade of renin-angiotensin-dependent compensatory mechanisms.

B. Treatment of Urticaria and Angioedema: These disorders are discussed fully in Chapter 6.

Reisman RE: Insect stings. N Engl J Med 1994;331:523.

II. CLINICAL IMMUNOLOGY

CELLS INVOLVED IN IMMUNITY

Development of T & B Lymphocytes

The thymus-derived cells (T lymphocytes) are involved in cellular immune responses; the bone marrow-derived cells (B lymphocytes) are involved in humoral or antibody responses. Both T and B lymphocytes are derived from precursor or stem cells in the marrow. Precursors of T cells migrate to the thymus, where they develop some of the functional and cell surface characteristics of mature T cells. Through positive and negative selection, clones of autoreactive T cells are eliminated, and mature T cells migrate to the peripheral lymphoid tissues. There they enter the pool of long-lived lymphocytes that recirculate from the blood to the lymph.

B cell maturation proceeds in antigen-independent and antigen-dependent stages. Antigen-independent maturation includes development from precursor cells in the marrow through the naive B cell (a cell that has not been exposed to antigen previously) found in the peripheral lymphoid tissues. Antigen-dependent maturation occurs following the interaction of antigen with naive B cells. The final products of B cell development are circulating long-lived memory B cells and plasma cells found predominantly in primary follicles and germinal centers of the lymph nodes and spleen. Plasma cells are terminally differentiated B cells responsible for synthesis and secretion of immunoglobulin.

Subpopulations of T Cells

T lymphocytes are heterogeneous with respect to their cell surface features (Table 19–2) and functional characteristics. At least three subpopulations of T cells are now recognized.

A. Helper-Inducer T Cells: These cells help to amplify the production of antibody-forming cells from B lymphocytes after interaction with antigen. Helper (CD4) T cells also amplify the production of effector T cells that mediate cytotoxicity. Activated CD4 T cells regulate immune responses by two mechanisms:

Table 19–2. Selected surface antigens on immune cells detected by monoclonal antibodies.

Cluster of Differentiation	Primary Cellular Distribution	Function
CD2	T cells, NK cells	Adhesion molecule
CD3	Pan-T cell marker	T cell receptor
CD4	T helper-inducer cells, macrophage	Binds to MHC class II
CD5	T cells, B cell subset	
CD7	T cells	
CD8	T cytotoxic-suppressor cells	Binds MHC class I
CD10	Immature B cells	CALLA; Also found in ALL
CD11a CD11b CD11c	Leukocytes	Adhesion molecule
CD13/33	Granulocytes	Granulocyte marker
CD14	Monocytes	Monocyte marker
CD16/56	NK cells	NK cell markers; CD16 is low-affinity Fcγ receptor
CD19	Pan-B cell marker	Appears early in B cell maturation
CD20/21/22	B cell markers	Appear after CD19; CD21 is complement receptor (CR2)
CD23	Activated B cells, macrophages	Low-affinity Fcε receptor
CD25	Activated T, B cells and macrophages	IL-2 receptor; Activation marker
CD28	T cells	Costimulatory receptor
CD34	Hematopoietic progenitor cells	"Stem cell" marker
CD38	Plasma cells	
CD45	Leukocytes	Panleukocyte marker
CD45RA/RO	T cells	CD45RA on "naive" T cells; CD45RO on "memory" T cells

through cell-to-cell contact and through elaboration of soluble factors or cytokines. Two subsets of helper T cells can be identified on the basis of their pattern of cytokine production. The subsets are called type 1 T helper (TH1) cells, which produce interleukin (IL)-2 and gamma interferon; and type 2 T helper (TH2) cells, which produce interleukins-4, -5, and -6, among others. Both subsets produce IL-3 and GM-CSF. The TH1 subset of CD4 T cells provides cellular immune responses to intracellular pathogens and underlies the pathogenesis of delayed-type hypersensitivity.

TH2 helper T cells play a central role in immediate hypersensitivity and humoral immune responses, since IL-4 promotes IgE production and IL-5 is an eosinophil proliferation and differentiation factor (Table 19–3).

B. Cytotoxic or Killer T Cells: These cells are generated after mature T cells interact with certain foreign antigens. They are responsible for defense against intracellular pathogens (eg, viruses), tumor immunity, and organ graft rejection. Most killer T cells express the CD8 phenotype, though in certain circumstances CD4 T cells can be cytotoxic. Cytotoxic T cells may kill their target through osmotic lysis, by secretion of tumor necrosis factor (TNF), or by induction of apoptosis, ie, programmed cell death.

C. Suppressor T Cells: Suppressor T cells are regarded as CD8 regulatory cells that modulate antibody formation and cellular immunity in an antigen-specific manner. It is unclear, however, whether suppressor T cells are a distinct T cell phenotype or if their inhibitory functions merely reflect the profile of the factors they secrete.

B Lymphocytes

The majority of B cells express both IgM and IgD on the surface and are derived from pre-B cells found mainly in the bone marrow. Pre-B cells contain intracytoplasmic IgM but do not express surface immunoglobulin.

B cells have been commonly identified by other surface markers in addition to immunoglobulins. These include the receptor for the Fc portion of immunoglobulins, B cell-specific antigens CD19 and CD20, and surface antigens coded for by the HLA-D genetic region in humans. All mature B cells bear surface immunoglobulin that is the antigen-specific receptor. The major role of B cells is differentiation to antibody-secreting plasma cells. However, B cells may also release cytokines and function as antigen-presenting cells.

Other Cells Involved in Immune Responses

A. Macrophages: Macrophages are involved in the ingestion, processing, and presentation of antigens for interaction with lymphocytes. These CD14 cells play an important role in T and B lymphocyte cooperation in the induction of antibody responses. In addition, they are effector cells for certain types of tumor immunity.

B. NK (Natural Killer) Cells: These lymphocytic cells which are indirectly related to the T cell lineage, can kill a wide spectrum of target cells. They are recognized by the presence of specific surface antigens (CD16 or CD56) and Fc receptors. Many appear as large granular lymphocytes. Their role in host defense is probably the killing of virally infected cells and tumor cells in the absence of prior sensitization and without MHC restriction.

Cytokines

Many T cell functions are mediated by cytokines, which are humoral factors secreted by immunologi-

Table 19–3. Major activities of selected cytokines.

Cytokine	Primary Biologic Activity
IL-1	Major source is activated macrophages. Enhances T and B cell activation. Endogenous pyrogen and major inflammatory mediator.
IL-2	Autocrine and paracrine T cell activation and growth factor.
IL-3	Multilineage hematopoietic growth factor.
IL-4	T and B cell growth factor. Induces IgE isotype switching; TH2 CD4 cell and mast cell growth factor.
IL-5	Promotes eosinophil growth and differentiation and IgA synthesis.
IL-6	B cell differentiation factor; acute phase reactant.
IL-7	Growth factor for very early B and T lymphocytes.
IL-8	Chemotactic factor for neutrophils, lymphocytes. Up-regulates adhesion molecule expression.
IL-10	Down-regulates cellular activation. Inhibits production of proinflammatory cytokines by monocytes and macrophages.
IL-12	Augments IFN-γ production, enhances TH1 CD4 response.
IL-13	Functions overlap with those of IL-4.
TNF	Overlaps with activity with IL-1 but has more antitumor activity. Mediates host response to gram-negative bacteria and systemic toxicity of LPS.
IFN-α, -β, -γ	Antiviral and antitumor activities. Activates macrophages. Enhances cytotoxic lymphocyte and NK activity.
GM-CSF	Growth factor for granulocytes, macrophages, and eosinophils. Activates neutrophil phagocytosis. Enhances eosinophil-mediated cytotoxicity. Promotes basophil histamine release.
TGF-β	Major regulatory factor, inhibiting leukocyte growth, proliferation and proinflammatory cytokines.

cally active cells. Cytokines are secreted when cells are activated by antigens or other cytokines. Table 19–3 lists some examples of cytokines and their functions. The cytokines can be functionally organized into groups according to their major activities: (1) those that promote and mediate natural immunity, such as IL-1, IL-6, interferon (IFN)-γ, and IL-8; (2) those that support allergic inflammation, such as IL-4; promoters of IgE production, including IL-3, -4, -9, and -10; others that promote mast cell growth and IL-3, IL-5; and granulocyte-macrophage colony stimulating factor (GM-CSF), which stimulates the growth of eosinophils; (3) those controlling lymphocyte regulatory activity, such as IL-10, produced by the TH2 helper T cell, and IFN-γ, which is produced by the TH1 T helper cell; and (4) those that act as hematopoietic growth factors (IL-7 and GM-CSF). This complicated network of interacting cytokines functions to modulate and regulate cellular function in such a way that the host is able to survive in a hostile environment.

Ali H et al: Mechanisms of inflammation and leukocyte activation. Med Clin North Am 1997;81:1. [NLM Cit ID: 97164991]

Cohen MC, Cohen S: Cytokine function: A study in biologic diversity. Am J Clin Pathol 1996;105:589. [NLM Cit ID: 96202600]

Costa JJ, Weller PF, Galli SJ: The cells of the allergic response: Mast cells, basophils, and eosinophils. JAMA 1997;278:1815. [NLM Cit ID: 98057349]

Dutton RW: The regulation of the development of CD8 effector T cells. J Immunol 1996;157:4287. [NLM Cit ID: 97064182]

Favero J, Lafont V: Effector pathways regulating T cell activation. Biochem Pharmacol 1998;56:1539. [NLM Cit ID: 99137459]

Gretz JE et al: Sophisticated strategies for information encounter in the lymph node: The reticular network as a conduit of soluble information and a highway for cell traffic. J Immunol 1996;157:495. [NLM Cit ID: 96286021]

Liu CC, Young LH, Young JD: Lymphocyte-mediated cytolysis and disease. N Engl J Med 1996;335:1651. [NLM Cit ID: 97066825]

Wilson IA, Garcia KC: T-cell receptor structure and TCR complexes. Curr Opin Struct Biol 1997;7:839. [NLM Cit ID: 98096534]

TESTS FOR CELLULAR IMMUNITY

Leukocyte Immunophenotyping by Flow Cytometry

Utilizing fluorescent-labeled monoclonal antibodies directed against specific cell surface antigens, or clusters of differentiation (CD), leukocytes can be immunophenotyped and enumerated by flow cytometry. During lymphocyte development, different patterns of CD markers are expressed at various stages of maturation (Table 19–2). Flow cytometry segregates populations of leukocytes for analysis by cellular size and complexity. By these parameters, polymorphonuclear cells and monocytes can be enumerated and analyzed separately from peripheral blood lymphocyte populations.

In normal individuals, roughly 75% of circulating lymphocytes are T cells (CD3), two-thirds of which are CD4 T helper-inducer cells and one-third CD8 suppressor or cytotoxic T cells. CD19 B cells make up 7–24% of circulating lymphocytes, and the remainder are CD16/CD56 NK cells. Lymphocyte immunophenotyping can be utilized in suspected cases of immunodeficiency or lymphoproliferative syndromes or following organ transplantation.

Thymic hypoplasia (DiGeorge syndrome) is associated with a marked decrease in the number of T cells in the peripheral blood. On the other hand, the absence of B cells in the blood is frequently found in X-linked agammaglobulinemia. Marked reductions of both T and B cells occur in severe combined immunodeficiency disease (SCID). Patients with AIDS have reduced numbers of T cells and reduced CD4:CD8 ratios.

Many hematologic neoplasms can express aberrant CD markers or lose characteristic phenotypic patterns. For example, B cell lymphomas can express inappropriate maturational markers or even T cell- or granulocyte-associated clusters of differentiation. In lymphoproliferative diseases, the suspicious lymphocyte population may demonstrate a monoclonal pattern by bearing surface immunoglobulin of a single isotype (IgM, IgG or IgA) or a single immunoglobulin light chain (κ or λ). Immunophenotyping may be used in conjunction with histopathologic analysis of bone marrow biopsies and fine-needle aspirates from suspicious lymph nodes or peripheral blood. Immunophenotyping of poorly differentiated leukemias and lymphomas can also provide prognostic information and help optimize treatment regimens.

T Cell Antigen Receptors

The structure of T cell antigen receptors and the genes that encode these glycoproteins have been defined. The receptor structure is a complex of two molecules, one containing variable α/β or γ/δ chains and the other the monomorphic CD3 molecule. Genes encoding the β chain are homologous with immunoglobulin genes. Rearrangement of T cell receptor genes proceeds during T cell development to generate diversity for antigen recognition in a fashion similar to that of immunoglobulin genes in B cells. Lymphoid malignancies often feature chromosomal translocations that occur disproportionately in or near the T cell receptor genes. Identification of T cell receptor gene rearrangements have been used to distinguish clonal T cell leukemias and lymphomas from reactive processes.

Functional Testing of Cell-Mediated Immunity

A. Skin Testing: Cell-mediated immune function can be assessed qualitatively by evaluating skin reactivity following intradermal injection of a battery of recall antigens to which humans are frequently sensitized (ie, streptokinase, streptodornase, purified protein derivative, trichophyton, dermatophyton, mumps, tetanus, or candida). Intradermal injections of 0.1 mL of recommended test strengths are observed for maximal induration and erythema at 24 and 48 hours. A positive reaction varies in size with particular antigens but is generally at least 10 mm in diameter. Anergy or lack of skin reactivity to all of these substances usually indicates a depression of cell-mediated immunity. Delayed hypersensitivity skin tests depend on complex interactions of T cells, macrophages, and other immunoreactants; thus, failure to respond cannot identify the exact cellular defect.

Patch testing can be clinically indicated for the diagnosis of suspected allergic contact dermatitis. The patch test is performed by topical application of the suspected contactant allergen. A positive test at 48–72 hours consists of erythema, swelling, and papules. Concentrations of allergens for patch testing must be screened in nonallergic subjects to avoid false-positive irritant responses.

B. In Vitro Lymphocyte Proliferation After Stimulation With Mitogens or Antigens: T lymphocytes are transformed to blast cells upon short-term incubation with mitogens or recall antigens in vitro. Mitogens stimulate lymphocytes nonspecifically. Phytohemagglutinin (PHA), pokeweed mitogen (PWM), and concanavalin A (ConA) can all be used in clinical laboratory assays. T cell activation is determined quantitatively by following the cellular uptake and incorporation of [^{3}H]thymidine introduced into the culture medium. The uptake indicates T cell function and correlates well with other manifestations of cell-mediated immunity as measured by skin tests. These tests can detect abnormalities in T cells despite normal or slightly reduced cell counts, particularly following bone marrow transplantation or in congenital immunodeficiency diseases. Stimulation of recipients' lymphocytes or donor lymphocytes (the mixed lymphocyte reaction) is a critical test for determining histocompatibility, especially after renal and bone marrow transplantation.

Dutton RW, Bradley LM, Swain SL: T cell memory. Annu Rev Immunol 1998;16:201. [NLM Cit ID: 98259417]

Wulfing C, Sjzastad MD, Davis MM: Visualizing the dynamics of T cell activation. Proc Natl Acad Sci U S A 1998;95:6302. [NLM Cit ID: 98263351]

IMMUNOGLOBULIN STRUCTURE & FUNCTION

Disorders of immune function are the cause of many human illnesses. The basic unit of all immunoglobulins consists of four polypeptide chains linked by disulfide bonds. There are two identical heavy chains (MW 55,000–70,000) and two identical light chains (MW about 23,000). Both heavy and light chains have a carboxyl terminal constant (C) region and an amino terminal variable (V) region. A hypervariable portion of the V regions of heavy and light chains folded together in a three-dimensional conformation forms the combining site, which is responsible for the specific interaction with antigen.

Antibodies contain one of five classes of heavy chains (γ, α, μ, δ, and ε) and one of two types of light chains (κ and λ). About 10 million different antibody specificities are thought to exist in a given individual.

Immunoglobulin Classes

A. Immunoglobulin M (IgM): IgM is made up of five identical basic immunoglobulin units. These units are connected to one another by disulfide bonds and a small polypeptide known as the J chain. The molecular weight of IgM is about 900,000. The IgM molecule is found predominantly in the intravascular compartment and on the surface of B lymphocytes and does not normally cross the placenta. IgM antibody predominates in early, primary immune responses; carbohydrate antigens such as blood group substances stimulate IgM.

B. Immunoglobulin A (IgA): IgA is present in blood and in relatively high concentrations in saliva, colostrum, tears, and secretions of the bronchi and gastrointestinal tract. Serum IgA is a single immunoglobulin unit, whereas secretory IgA is made up of two units connected to each other by a J chain. A 70,000-MW molecule called secretory component is attached to the Fc portion. It is necessary to transport IgA into the ducts of exocrine glands, and it confers resistance to enzymatic destruction. Secretory IgA plays an important role in host defense against viral and bacterial infections by blocking transport of microbes across mucosa.

C. Immunoglobulin G (IgG): IgG is a single immunoglobulin unit of MW 150,000 that comprises about 85% of total serum immunoglobulins. IgG is distributed in the extracellular fluid and is the only immunoglobulin that normally crosses the placenta. Antigen-bound IgG fixes complement via the Fc region of the constant chain. Immune effector cells express Fc receptors and complement receptors that facilitate phagocytosis and cytolysis. Immune complex activation of the classic complement pathway also generates soluble factors that chemoattract neutrophils, increase vascular permeability, and amplify the inflammatory response.

D. Immunoglobulin E (IgE): IgE is present in serum in very low concentrations as a single immunoglobulin unit with ε heavy chains. Fifty percent of patients with allergic diseases have increased serum IgE levels. The specific interaction between antigen and mast cell-bound IgE results in the release of histamine, leukotrienes, proteases, chemotactic factors, and cytokines. These mediators can produce bronchospasm, vasodilation, increased vascular permeability, smooth muscle contraction, and chemoattraction of other inflammatory and immune cells.

E. Immunoglobulin D (IgD): IgD is present in the serum in very low concentrations. IgD is found on the surface of most B lymphocytes in association with IgM, where it probably serves as a receptor for antigen.

Tests for Immunoglobulins

In some diseases, particularly the gammopathies, increased serum immunoglobulins, especially monoclonal types, are critical for diagnosis. Chronic liver diseases, chronic infection, or idiopathic inflammatory states can cause polyclonal or oligoclonal increases in immunoglobulins which are incidental or of unknown significance. If immunodeficiency is suspected in the presence of recurrent bacterial infections, measurement of serum immunoglobulin levels provides an essential test of B cell and plasma cell function. In acquired immune deficiencies such as AIDS, paradoxical increases in immunoglobulins can occur.

Antibodies and immunoglobulins can be measured in three ways: (1) by quantitative and qualitative determinations of serum immunoglobulins; (2) by determination of isohemagglutinin and febrile agglutinin titers; and (3) by determination of antibody titers following immunization with tetanus toxoid, diphtheria toxoid, or pneumococcal polysaccharide vaccines. The first method tests for the presence of serum immunoglobulins but not for the functional adequacy of the immunoglobulins. The second tests for functional antibodies present in the serum of almost all individuals as a consequence of exposure to blood group antigens (ABO blood groups) or infection. The third method examines functional humoral immunity in the serum after intentional immunization.

Protein Electrophoresis & Immunoelectrophoresis

Serum protein electrophoresis is a test to measure semiquantitatively various proteins in serum or urine. Proteins are electrically separated on a strip of cellulose acetate on the basis of charge, into albumin, α_1, α_2, β, and γ globulins. This test is useful to screen for diseases with excess or deficiency of immunoglobulins.

Immunoelectrophoresis is used to identify the specific immunoglobulin class in a body fluid. Serum, for example, is separated electrophoretically and then reacted with appropriate antisera directed against IgG, IgA, or IgM. The resulting patterns allow identification of abnormal immunoglobulins such as myeloma (M) proteins. This method is also useful in differentiation of monoclonal from polyclonal increases in immunoglobulins. It is only semiquantitative and thus cannot be used to determine immunoglobulin levels precisely, eg, in Waldenström's macroglobulinemia.

A similar technique called immunofixation electrophoresis has to a large extent replaced immunoelectrophoresis. Serum proteins are separated electrophoretically in a gel and then immunoprecipitated in situ with monospecific antisera. This method has the advantages of more rapid results and slightly higher resolution of low levels of monoclonal immunoglobulin chains. If protein electrophoresis is normal despite suspicion of an M protein, immunoelectrophoresis or immunofixation electrophoresis of both serum and concentrated urine should be performed because of the greater sensitivity of these tests combined.

Quantitative Immunoglobulin Determinations

Quantitative determinations of total serum IgG, IgA, IgE, and IgM levels can be made rapidly and accurately by nephelometry. Nephelometry detects scattered light when specific antiserum immunoprecipitates soluble antigen. Antiserum is available for a variety of antigens, including all immunoglobulin isotypes. Measurement of serum IgD levels has no recognized clinical use, and antigen-specific IgE levels should be measured with more sensitive techniques such as in vitro radioallergosorbent testing (RAST) or in vivo allergy skin testing.

Functional Testing of Humoral Immunity

Laboratory evaluation of humoral function should include assessment of specific antibody responses. Isohemagglutinins are naturally occurring IgM antibodies against ABO blood groups and can be detected in most patients depending on blood type. Humoral responses can also be assessed by immunization with protein and carbohydrate antigens. This is most easily accomplished by measuring antitetanus, antidiphtheria, and antipneumococcal antibody titers before and 3–4 weeks after vaccination with diphtheria-tetanus (dT) and polyvalent pneumococcal vaccine. In this context, a fourfold increase in antibody titer is considered normal. In patients suspected to be suffering from humoral immunodeficiency, quantification of IgG subclasses may be appropriate, particularly when total IgG immunoglobulins are at the low end of the normal range.

Casali P, Schettino EW: Structure and function of natural antibodies. Curr Top Microbiol Immunol 1996;210:167. [NLM Cit ID: 96148122] (A comprehensive review of the emergence of antibodies in neonates from a cellular and molecular biology viewpoint.)

Huston DP: The biology of the immune system. JAMA 1997;278:1804. [NLM Cit ID: 98057348] (Provides a framework for understanding physiologic immune responses and the pathogenesis of immunologic disorders.)

Krause RM, et al: Summary of antibody workshop: The role of humoral immunity in the treatment and prevention of emerging and extant infectious diseases. J Infect Dis 1997;176:549. [NLM Cit ID: 97435076]

Rose NR et al (editors): *Manual of Clinical Laboratory Immunology,* 5th ed. American Society for Microbiology, 1997. (General reference for diagnostic laboratory immunology.)

Salkie ML: A retrospective study of the relative utility of electrophoresis, immunoelectrophoresis, immunofixation, and nephelometry in the investigation of serum proteins. Clin Biochem 1996;29:39. [NLM Cit ID: 97083248] (Except for quantitating monoclonal immunoglobulins, protein electrophoresis was unreliable as a quantitative procedure and nephelometry was preferred.)

IMMUNODEFICIENCY DISORDERS

The primary immunologic deficiency diseases include congenital and acquired disorders of humoral immunity (B cell function) or cell-mediated immunity (T cell function). Most of these diseases are rare, and since they are genetically determined, are seen primarily in children. Several immunodeficiency disorders affect adults, and are discussed below. The WHO classification of immunodeficiency disorders more often affecting adults is set forth in the accompanying box.

A. Primary immunodeficiency disorders:
1. Selective IgA deficiency.
2. Common variable immunodeficiency.
3. X-linked agammaglobulinemia
4. Immunodeficiency with normal serum globulins or hyperimmunoglobulinemia.
5. Immunodeficiency with thymoma.

B. Secondary immunodeficiency disorders (eg, AIDS).

Rosen FS, et al: The primary immunodeficiencies. N Engl J Med 1995;333:431. [NLM Cit ID: 95342196] (Review of primary immunodeficiency disorders with correlations to cellular ontogeny.)

Sicherer SH, et al: Primary immunodeficiency diseases in adults. JAMA 1998;279:58. [NLM Cit ID: 98084662] (A comprehensive review.)

SELECTIVE IMMUNOGLOBULIN A DEFICIENCY

Selective IgA deficiency is the most common primary immunodeficiency disorder and is characterized by the absence of serum IgA with normal levels of IgG and IgM; its prevalence is about 1:500 individuals. Most patients are asymptomatic because of compensatory increases in secreted IgG and IgM. Some affected patients have frequent and recurrent infections such as sinusitis, otitis, and bronchitis. Some cases of IgA deficiency may spontaneously remit. When IgG_2 subclass deficiency occurs in combination with IgA deficiency affected patients are more susceptible to encapsulated bacteria and the degree of immune impairment can be more severe. Patients with a combined IgA and IgG subclass deficiency should be assessed for functional antibody responses to glycoprotein antigen immunization.

Atopic disease and autoimmune disorders can be associated with IgA deficiency. Occasionally, a sprue-like syndrome with steatorrhea has been associated with an isolated IgA deficit. Treatment with commercial immune globulin is ineffective, since IgA and IgM are present only in trace quantities in these preparations. Frequent infusions of plasma (containing IgA) or unwashed blood transfusions are hazardous, since anti-IgA antibodies may develop, resulting in systemic anaphylaxis or serum sickness.

Burrows PD, et al: IgA deficiency. Adv Immunol 1997;65:245. [NLM Cit ID: 97381155]

COMMON VARIABLE IMMUNODEFICIENCY

Essentials of Diagnosis

- Frequent sinopulmonary infections secondary to humoral immune deficiency.
- Defect in terminal differentiation of B cells, with absent plasma cells and deficient synthesis of secreted antibody.
- Confirmation by evaluation of serum immunoglobulin levels and deficient functional antibody responses

General Considerations

The most common cause of panhypogammaglobulinemia in adults is common variable immunodeficiency, a heterogeneous immunodeficiency disorder clinically characterized by an increased incidence of recurrent infections, autoimmune phenomena, and neoplastic diseases. The onset generally is during adolescence or early adulthood but can occur at any age. The prevalence of common variable immunodeficiency is about 1:80,000 in the United States.

Clinical Findings

A. Symptoms and Signs: The pattern of immunoglobulin isotype deficiency is variable. Most patients present with significantly depressed IgG levels, but over time all antibody classes (IgG, IgA, and IgM) may be affected. Increased susceptibility to pyogenic infections is the hallmark of the disease. Virtually all patients suffer from recurrent sinusitis, with bronchitis, otitis, pharyngitis, and pneumonia also being common infections. Infections may be of prolonged duration or associated with unusual complications such as meningitis or sepsis.

Gastrointestinal disorders are commonly associated, and patients may develop a sprue-like syndrome, with diarrhea, steatorrhea, malabsorption, protein-losing enteropathy, and hepatosplenomegaly. Paradoxically, there is an increased incidence of autoimmune disease (20%), though patients may not display the usual serologic markers. Autoimmune cytopenias are most common, but also commonly seen are autoimmune endocrinopathies, seronegative rheumatic disease, and gastrointestinal disorders. Lymph nodes may be enlarged in these patients, yet biopsies show marked reduction in plasma cells. Noncaseating granulomas are frequently found in the spleen, liver, lungs, or skin. There is an increased propensity for the development of B cell neoplasms (50- to 400-fold increase risk of lymphoma), gastric carcinomas, and skin cancers.

B. Laboratory Findings: Diagnosis is confirmed in patients with recurrent infections by demonstration of functional or quantitative defects in antibody production. Serum IgG levels are usually less than 250 mg/dL; serum IgA and IgM levels are also subnormal. Decreased to absent functional antibody responses to protein antigen immunizations establish the diagnosis.

The cause of the panhypogammaglobulinemia in the majority of common variable immunodeficiency patients is an intrinsic B cell defect preventing terminal maturation into antibody-secreting plasma cells. In a small number, excessive suppressor T cell activity that inhibits B cells—or helper T cell activity inadequate to assist B cells to make antibody—has been identified. The absolute B cell count in the peripheral blood in most patients, despite the underlying cellular defect, is normal. A subset of these patients have concomitant T cell immunodeficiency with increased numbers of activated CD8 cells, splenomegaly, and decreased delayed-type hypersensitivity.

Treatment

Patients may be treated aggressively with antibiotics at the first sign of infection. Since antibody deficiency predisposes patients to high-risk pyogenic infections, antibiotic coverage should be sure to cover encapsulated bacteria. Only after the development of bronchiectasis or after sinus surgery do patients become significantly affected by more virulent organisms such as *Staphylococcus aureus* or *Pseudomonas aeruginosa.* Maintenance intravenous gamma globulin (IGIV) therapy is indicated, with infusions of 300–500 mg/kg of IGIV given at about monthly intervals. Adjustment of dosage or of the infusion interval is made on the basis of clinical responses and steady state trough serum IgG levels. Such therapy is effective in decreasing the incidence of potentially life-threatening infections and increasing quality of life. The yearly cost of monthly infusions can be in excess of $20,000–$30,000.

Spickett GP et al: Common variable immunodeficiency: How many diseases? Immunol Today 1997;18:325. [NLM Cit ID: 97381556]

DISEASES OF IMMUNOGLOBULIN OVERPRODUCTION (Gammopathies)

The monoclonal gammopathies include those diseases in which there is a proliferation of a single clone of immunoglobulin-forming cells that produce a homogeneous heavy chain, light chain, or complete molecule. The amino acid sequence of the variable (V) regions is fixed, and only one type (κ or λ) of light chain is produced. Polyclonal gammopathies result from proliferation of many B cell clones, resulting in a diffuse increase of immunoglobulins.

Monoclonal Gammopathy of Uncertain Significance (MGUS)

This diagnosis is made upon finding a monoclonal spike on serum protein electrophoresis, confirmed by immunoelectrophoresis to be a homogeneous immunoglobulin (with either κ or λ chains). The incidence of MGUS increases with age and may approach 3% in persons 70 years of age or older. As many as one-third of individuals with apparently benign monoclonal gammopathies will develop lymphoid malignancies, amyloidosis, or multiple myeloma. No specific therapy is necessary, but close observation is required. Risk for the development of a malignant disorder is 33% at 20 years. Parameters that suggest a favorable prognosis include (1) concentration of homogeneous immunoglobulin less than 2 g/dL, (2) no increase in concentration of the immunoglobulin from the time of diagnosis, (3) no decrease in the concentration of normal immunoglobulins, (4) absence of a homogeneous light chain in the urine, and (5) normal hematocrit and serum albumin.

Multiple Myeloma (See also Chapter 13.)

This disease is characterized by the overproduction and spread of neoplastic plasma cells throughout the bone marrow. Myeloma cells sometimes express molecules of early B cell or myelomonocytic lineages. Rarely, extraosseous plasmacytomas may be found. Anemia, hypercalcemia, increased susceptibility to infection, and bone pain are frequent. Diagnosis depends upon the presence of the following: (1) radiographic findings of osteolytic lesions or diffuse osteoporosis, (2) the presence of a homogeneous serum immunoglobulin (myeloma protein) or a single type of light chain in the urine (Bence Jones proteinuria), and (3) finding of an abnormal plasma cell infiltrate in the bone marrow biopsy (see Chapter 13). The presence of over 20% bone marrow plasma cells reliably differentiates early myeloma from MGUS. There is an approximate correlation between the incidence of immunoglobulin type in myeloma and the normal serum concentration of the immunoglobulin involved.

Waldenström's Macroglobulinemia

In Waldenström's macroglobulinemia, there is proliferation of abnormal lymphoid cells that have morphologic features of both B cells and plasma cells. These cells secrete a homogeneous macroglobulin (IgM) detectable by immunoelectrophoresis. Monoclonal light chains are present in 10% of cases. Clinical manifestations depend upon the physicochemical characteristics of the macroglobulin. Raynaud's phenomenon and peripheral vascular occlusions are associated with cold-insoluble proteins (cryoglobulins). Retinal hemorrhages, visual impairment, and transient neurologic deficits are common with high-viscosity serum. Bleeding diatheses or hemolytic anemia can occur when the macroglobulin complexes with coagulation factors or binds to the surface of red blood cells.

Amyloidosis

Amyloidosis is a group of disorders manifested by impaired organ function caused by infiltration of tissues with insoluble protein fibrils. Different fibril composition can be correlated with the clinical syndromes.

In primary amyloidosis (AL), the protein fibrils are monoclonal immunoglobulin light chains, whereas secondary amyloid (AA) proteins are derived from acute phase reactant apolipoprotein precursors. Other types of amyloidosis may also be hereditary.

Symptoms and signs of amyloid infiltration are related to malfunction of the organ involved (eg, nephrotic syndrome and renal failure, cardiomyopathy and cardiac conduction defects, intestinal malabsorption and pseudo-obstruction, carpal tunnel syndrome, macroglossia, peripheral neuropathy, end-organ insufficiency of endocrine glands, respiratory failure, and capillary damage with ecchymosis). Such widespread deposition is typical of primary amyloidosis; secondary amyloidosis more often is confined to liver, spleen, and adrenals. Familial syndromes commonly cause infiltrative neuropathies. Amyloidosis due to deposition of β_2-microglobulin in carpal ligaments occurs in chronic hemodialysis patients.

The diagnosis of primary amyloidosis is based on clinical suspicion, protein electrophoresis, and microscopic examination of biopsy specimens. In patients with systemic disease, rectal or gingival biopsies show a sensitivity of about 80%, bone-marrow biopsy about 50%, and abdominal fat aspiration between 70% and 80%. Fine-needle biopsy of subcutaneous abdominal fat is a simple and reliable method for diagnosing systemic amyloidosis.

Treatment of localized amyloid tumors is by surgical excision. There is no effective treatment of systemic amyloidosis, and death usually occurs within 1–3 years. Care is generally supportive, though hemodialysis and immunosuppressive therapy may be useful. When concomitant multiple myeloma is found, it is treated in the standard fashion (Chapter 13). Secondary disease is usually approached by aggressively treating the predisposing disease, but remission of fibril deposition does not occur.

Heavy Chain Disease (α, γ, μ)

These are rare disorders in which the abnormal serum and urine protein is a part of a homogeneous α, γ, or μ heavy chain. The clinical presentation is more typical of lymphoma than multiple myeloma, and there are no destructive bone lesions. Gamma chain disease presents as a lymphoproliferative disorder with autoimmune features. Alpha chain disease is frequently associated with severe diarrhea and infiltration of the lamina propria of the small intestine with abnormal plasma cells. Mu chain disease is associated with chronic lymphocytic leukemia.

Bataille R, Harcusseau JL: Multiple myeloma. N Engl J Med 1997;36:1657. [NLM Cit ID: 97301689]

Falk RH, Comenzo RL, Skinner M: The systemic amyloidoses. N Engl J Med 1997;337:898. [NLM Cit ID: 97433009]

Jorgensen C et al: Arthritis associated with monoclonal gammopathy: Clinical characteristics. Br J Rheumatol 1996;35:241. [NLM Cit ID: 96194182]

Samuels J et al: Familial Mediterranean fever at the millennium: Clinical spectrum, ancient mutations and a survey of 100 American referrals to the National Institutes of Health. Medicine 1998 77:268. [NLM Cit ID: 96148122]

Schiffer M: Molecular anatomy and the pathological expression of antibody light chains. Am J Pathol 1996;148:1339. [NLM Cit ID: 96208111]

AUTOIMMUNITY

Autoimmune diseases cannot be explained by a solitary cause or mechanism. Small amounts of autoantibodies are normally produced and may have physiologic roles in cellular interactions. The major theories regarding the development of autoimmune disease are (1) release of normally sequestered antigens; (2) escape from anergy or defective apoptosis (programmed cell death) leading to abnormal autoreactive cellular clones; (3) shared antigens between the host and microorganisms, ie, "molecular mimicry"; and (4) defects in helper or suppressor T cell function. A genetic susceptibility is also a likely determinant of autoimmune disease. In nearly all autoimmune diseases, multiple mechanisms of autoimmunity are operative.

Cell-Mediated Autoimmunity

Certain autoimmune diseases are mediated by T cells that have become specifically immunized to autologous tissues. Cytotoxic or killer T cells generated by this aberrant immune response injure specific organs in the absence of serum autoantibodies. Diminished suppressor T cell activity or loss of clonal anergy results in disordered regulation of immune function and consequent autoreactivity. The immune damage in systemic (non-organ-specific) diseases such as systemic lupus erythematosus may be due to such a mechanism.

Antibody-Mediated Autoimmunity

Several autoimmune diseases have been shown to be caused by autoantibodies in the absence of cell-mediated autoimmunity. The autoimmune hemolytic anemias, idiopathic thrombocytopenia, and Goodpasture's syndrome appear to be mediated solely by autoantibodies directed against autologous cell membrane constituents. In these diseases, antibody attaches to cell membranes and fixes complement; the ensuing inflammatory reaction injures the cells.

Anti-receptor antibodies that compete with or mimic physiologic agonists for cellular receptors cause several diseases. In Graves' disease, antibodies are present that bind to thyroid cells' TSH receptors and thereby stimulate thyroid hormone production. In rare instances of type 1 diabetes mellitus, anti-insulin receptor antibodies cause insulin resistance in peripheral target tissues. Antibodies to acetylcholine receptors of the myoneural junction in myasthenia gravis block neuromuscular transmission and produce muscle weakness.

Immune Complex Disease

In this group of diseases (systemic lupus erythematosus, lupus nephritis, rheumatoid arthritis, some drug-induced hemolytic anemias, and thrombocytopenias), autologous tissues are injured as "innocent bystanders." Autoantibodies are not directed against cellular components of the target organ but rather against autologous or heterologous antigens in the serum. The resultant antigen-antibody complexes bind nonspecifically to autologous membranes (eg, glomerular basement membrane) and fix complement. Fixation and subsequent activation of complement components produce a local inflammatory response resulting in tissue injury.

AUTOIMMUNE DISEASES (See also Chapter 20.)

The diagnosis and treatment of specific autoimmune diseases are described elsewhere in this book. Autoantibodies associated with certain autoimmune diseases may not be pathogenetic but are thought to be markers or by-products of the injury (eg, autoimmune thyroiditis and antithyroglobulin antibody). See Table 19–4 for autoantibody patterns in connective tissue diseases.

TESTS FOR AUTOANTIBODIES ASSOCIATED WITH AUTOIMMUNE DISEASE

Agglutination Assays

Red cells are incubated with purified specific antigen (eg, thyroglobulin), which is adsorbed to the cell surface. The antigen-coated cells are suspended in the patient's serum, and antibody is detected by red cell agglutination. Antigen-coated latex particles are substituted for red cells in latex fixation tests.

Enzyme-Linked Immunosorbent Assays (ELISA)

Antibodies to various tissue antigens can be readily detected by these tests. Extracted and purified antigens are fixed to a plastic microtiter well or beads. The patient's serum is added, and excess proteins are removed by washing and centrifugation. Adherent immunoglobulin is then detected when a second antibody coupled to an enzyme (eg, alkaline phosphatase) is added. Finally, the enzyme's substrate is added; color forms and is measured in a spectrophotometer. This test can also be adapted for antigen detection by placing the antibody on the plastic surface. ELISA assays are very sensitive and less cumbersome than radioimmunoassay techniques.

Immunofluorescence Microscopy

This technique is most frequently used for detection of antinuclear antibody (ANA). Frozen sections of mouse liver or other substrates are cut and placed on glass slides or, alternatively, monolayers of cultured cell lines may be used. A patient's serum is placed over the sections and incubated. Fluorescein-conjugated rabbit anti-human immunoglobulin is then applied and washed. Antinuclear antibody specifically binds to the nucleus, and the fluorescein conjugate binds to the human antibody. Fluorescence of the cell nucleus on microscopy indicates a positive test.

Complement Fixation

Specific antigen, unknown serum, and complement are combined. Sheep red blood cells coated with anti-sheep cell antibody are added for 30 minutes at 37 °C. If antigen-specific antibody is present

Table 19–4. Autoantibodies: Associations with connective tissue diseases.[1]

Suspected Disease State	Test	Primary Disease Association (Sensitivity, Specificity)	Other Disease Associations	Comments
CREST[2] syndrome	Anticentromere antibody	CREST (70–90%, high)	Scleroderma (10–15%), Raynaud's disease (10–30%).	Predictive value of a positive test is > 95% for scleroderma or related disease (CREST, Raynaud's). Diagnosis of CREST is made clinically.
Systemic lupus erythematosus (SLE)	Antinuclear antibody (ANA)	SLE (> 95%, low)	Rheumatoid arthritis (30–50%), discoid lupus, scleroderma (60%), drug-induced lupus (100%), Sjögren's syndrome (80%), miscellaneous inflammatory disorders.	Often used as a screening test; a negative test virtually excludes SLE; a positive test, while nonspecific, increases posttest probability of SLE. Titer does not correlate with disease activity.
	Anti-double-stranded-DNA (anti-ds-DNA)	SLE (60–70%, high)	Lupus nephritis, rarely rheumatoid arthritis, other connective tissue disease, usually in low titer.	Predictive value of a positive test is > 90% for SLE if present in high titer; a decreasing titer may correlate with worsening renal disease. Titer generally correlates with disease activity
	Anti-Smith antibody (anti-Sm)	SLE (30–40%, high)		SLE-specific. A positive test substantially increases posttest probability of SLE. Test rarely indicated.
Mixed connective tissue disease (MCTD)	Anti-ribonucleoprotein antibody (RNP)	Scleroderma (20–30%, low), MCTD (95–100%, low)	SLE (30%), Sjögren's syndrome, rheumatoid arthritis (10%), discoid lupus (20–30%).	A negative test essentially excludes MCTD a positive test in high titer, while nonspecific, increases posttest probability of MCTD.
Rheumatoid arthritis	Rheumatoid factor (RF)	Rheumatoid arthritis (50–90%)	Other rheumatic diseases, chronic infections, some malignancies, some healthy individuals, elderly patients.	Titer does not correlate with disease activity.
Scleroderma	Anti-Scl-70 antibody	Scleroderma (15–20%, low)		Predictive value of a positive test is > 95% for scleroderma.
Sjögren's syndrome	Anti-SS-A/Ro antibody	Sjögren's (60–70%, low)	SLE (30–40%), rheumatoid arthritis (10%), subacute cutaneous lupus, vasculitis.	Useful in counseling women of childbearing age with known connective tissue disease, since a positive test is associated with a small but real risk of neonatal SLE and congenital heart block
Wegener's granulomatosis	Anti-neutrophil cytoplasmic antibody (ANCA)	Wegener's granulomatosis (systemic necrotizing vasculitis) (56–96%, high)	Crescentic glomerulonephritis or other systemic vasculitis (eg, polyarteritis nodosa).	Ability of this assay to reflect disease activity remains unclear.

[1]Modified, with permission, from Harvey AM et al (editors): *The Principles and Practice of Medicine*, 22nd ed. Appleton & Lange, 1988; White RH, Robbins DL: Clinical significance and interpretation of antinuclear antibodies. West J Med 1987;147:210; and Tan EM: Autoantibodies to nuclear antigens (ANA): Their immunobiology and medicine. Adv Immunol 1982:33:167.
[2]CREST = calcinosis, Raynaud's phenomenon, esophageal dysmotility, sclerodactyly, and telangiectasia.

in the patient's serum, complement is bound and consumed, preventing lysis of sheep red cells.

Baker JR Jr: Autoimmune endocrine disease. JAMA 1997;278:1931. [NLM Cit ID: 98057362] (Autoimmune endocrine diseases include type 1 diabetes mellitus, thyroiditis, Graves' disease, Addison's disease, and polyglandular syndromes.)

Fleisher TA, Tomar RH: Introduction to diagnostic laboratory immunology. JAMA 1997;278:1823. [NLM Cit ID: 98057350] (Reviews diagnostic laboratory assays.)

Fox DA: The role of T cells in the immunopathogenesis of rheumatoid arthritis: New perspectives. Arthritis Rheum 1997;40:598. [NLM Cit ID: 97244292]

Miller-Blair DJ et al: Immunologic mechanisms in common rheumatologic diseases. Clin Orthop 1996;326:43. [NLM Cit ID: 96208078]

Rose NR et al (editors): *Manual of Clinical Laboratory Immunology,* 5th ed. American Society for Microbiology, 1997.

Winkelstein A, Kiss JE: Immunohematologic disorders. JAMA 1997;278:1982. [NLM Cit ID: 98057368] (Immune reactions can produce hemolytic anemia, thrombocytopenia, or neutropenia. Autoimmune phenomena and drug-induced reactions are the most common mechanisms.)

IMMUNOGENETICS & TRANSPLANTATION

GENETIC CONTROL OF THE IMMUNE RESPONSE

The ability to mount a specific immune response is under the direct control of genes closely associated on the same chromosome as the structural genes for the major transplantation antigens (major histocompatibility complex; MHC). The major transplantation antigens are the cell surface glycoproteins found on most cells of the body, which elicit the strongest transplantation rejection reaction when tissues are exchanged between two members of a particular species. These MHC molecules play a critical role in the process of antigen presentation between immunocompetent cells. In humans, this genetic region has been designated the **human leukocyte antigen (HLA)** complex because these antigens were first detected on peripheral blood lymphocytes. The complex includes antigens HLA-A, -B, -C, -DR, and others, each with many alleles.

The HLA region has been localized to chromosome 6. In nearly all instances, the HLA complex is inherited intact as two haplotypes (one from each parent), and within any particular family, therefore, the number of different combinations found is 25% (ie, siblings have a 1:4 chance of being HLA-identical). In contrast, the number of antigen combinations among unrelated individuals is enormous, resulting in probabilities of less than one in several thousand, depending upon the phenotype involved, of finding HLA-compatible individuals in a random donor pool. This is particularly important when compatible donors are needed for allosensitized patients requiring platelet transfusions or organ transplantation. Family members have the highest likelihood of being compatible donors, whereas compatibility between unrelated individuals has a low probability. HLA-A and -B typing or cross-matching is utilized for selection of compatible donors for platelet transfusions to allosensitized, thrombocytopenic recipients. Typing for these class I antigens as well as for HLA-D (class II) antigens is important in determining compatibility for organ transplantation. Typing for HLA markers is of value in studying associations between the HLA system and genetic control of disease susceptibility.

Pattison JM, Krensky AM: New insights into mechanisms of allograft rejection. Am J Med Sci 1997;313:257. [NLM Cit ID: 97290376] (Understanding of the molecular basis of organ allograft rejection has increased tremendously in the past decade, providing novel targets for immunotherapy.)

Polka MS: Histocompatibility antigens: Transplantation and HLA disease associations. Immunol Allergy Clin North Am 1994;14:323. (Reviews genetics, nomenclature, and molecular biology of HLA molecules as well as serologic typing and relevance to transplantation and association with diseases.)

VanBuskirk AM et al: Transplantation immunology. JAMA 1997;278:1993. [NLM Cit ID: 98057369] (This review discusses the three forms of graft rejection, each of which is addressed at the level of histopathology, pathobiology, incidence, and clinical strategies.)

ASSOCIATIONS BETWEEN HLA ANTIGENS & SPECIFIC DISEASES

In humans, very striking associations are observed between particular HLA antigens and specific diseases. Some of these are listed in Table 19–5. Major histocompatibility complex genes determine immune responses to various antigens.

The standard method for detecting HLA-A, -B, and -C antigens is that of lymphocyte microcytotoxicity. Lymphocytes isolated from peripheral blood or lymph nodes are added to each well of a typing tray filled with sera containing the appropriate cytotoxic alloantibody. When complement is added, cells to which antibody has been specifically bound will have complement activated at the cell surface, resulting in cell death or lysis. It is thus possible to type for all of the known HLA-A, -B, and -C specificities. An appreciable majority of typing serum samples are obtained from multiparous women since they form antibodies to fetal alloantigens.

Typing for the class II antigens HLA-DR and -DQ by serologic methods is technically more difficult. Antigens of the HLA-D, -DR, -DQ, and -DP series may also be detected by in vitro mixed lymphocyte culture (MLC). Lymphocytes of one individual (responder cells) will undergo proliferation upon encountering lymphocytes from another individual possessing foreign HLA-DR and -DQ antigens (stimulator cells). Lymphocyte proliferation can be readily measured by DNA incorporation of tritiated thymi-

Table 19–5. HLA and disease associations.

Disease	Antigen	Frequency		Relative Risk
		Patients (%)	Controls (%)	
Ankylosing spondylitis				
Caucasians	B27	89	4–13	69
Japanese	B27	85	< 1	207
Reiter's disease	B27	80	9	37
Salmonella arthritis	B27	60–92	8–14	30
Rheumatoid arthritis	DR4	68	25	3.8
Psoriasis vulgaris	Cw6	27	4	8.5
Graves' disease				
Caucasians	Dw3	56	25	3.7
Japanese	Dw12	48	6	5
Diabetes mellitus		DR3 heterozygotes		3
Diabetes mellitus		DR4 heterozygotes		3.6
Diabetes mellitus		DR3/DR4 heterozygotes		33
Acute lymphocytic leukemia	A2	83	44	6
Systemic lupus erythematosus	DR4	73	33	5
Narcolepsy	DR2	100	34	358

dine. Responders possessing matching -DR and -DQ antigens will remain nonreactive.

Increasingly, HLA class II typing is being performed by molecular technology. The DNA sequences for the HLA genes and their flanking sequences are known. Selected primers that amplify the gene of interest using the polymerase chain reaction (PCR) technique are known as sequence-specific primers. HLA typing by PCR provides better resolution than serologic identification because typing is done at the genetic level.

Apanius V et al: The nature of selection on the major histocompatibility complex. Crit Rev Immunol 1997;17:179. [NLM Cit ID: 97248224] (A comprehensive review of evidence for differing hypotheses on the mechanisms of gene diversity and immune responses.)

Colombe BW: Transplantation immunology: Histocompatibility testing and the HLA system in humans. In: *Manual of Allergy and Immunology,* 3rd ed. Lawlor GJ, Fischer TJ, Adelman DC (editors). Little, Brown, 1995.

Feltkamp TE, Khan MA, Lopez de Castro JA: The pathogenetic role of HLA-B27. Immunol Today 1996;17:5. [NLM Cit ID: 96226674]

CLINICAL TRANSPLANTATION

Organ transplants are in widespread use. Limitations include the scarcity of donor organs and expense. Failure to achieve successful grafts is primarily due to histoincompatibility and lack of safe and effective immunosuppressive regimens to halt rejection. Avoiding transmission of infectious agents (eg, HIV, HBV, HCV, CMV) from donor to recipient requires extensive pretransplant serologic testing.

Kidney Transplantation

End-stage renal disease is the indication for kidney transplantation. Factors that determine outcome include antigenic disparity (ABO blood groups and major histocompatibility or HLA) between donor and recipient, the type of immunologic response mounted by the host, and the immunosuppressive regimen used to prevent graft rejection.

Kidneys from living related donors who are HLA-identical and also red cell ABO-matched grafts have 90% survival at 1 year; grafts from less well matched relatives and from living unrelated donors have lower rates. Antigens are matched for HLA-A, -B and -DR loci, with -DR compatibility most important for long-term graft survival. Grafts from cadaver donors with zero HLA mismatches have a half-life of 11.3 years. Those with six mismatches have a half-life of 6.8 years, compared with those from HLA-identical siblings, which have a half-life of 23.6 years.

Some donors are highly sensitized to HLA antigens from previous transfusions, ie, possess high panel reactive antibody levels. It may be difficult to find a suitable donor, since a positive cross-match by cytotoxicity testing is likely and would be a contraindication to transplant. Donor screening is performed in all cases to assess suitability, rule out hypertension or anatomic anomalies, and avoid transmission of hepatitis viruses, HIV, and other infectious agents. Owing to the scarcity of related donors, living unrelated donors may be used in certain circumstances. Pretreatment of recipients with blood transfusions from the donor appears to extend graft survival even longer.

Delayed allograft function can be due to hyperacute graft rejection, post ischemic acute tubular necrosis, cyclosporine toxicity, or obstructive nephropathy. If conservative measures do not improve function or patients are at high risk of allograft rejection, renal biopsy should be performed for definitive diagnostic purposes. Renal allograft rejection may be due to hyperacute rejection from binding of cytotoxic antibodies and complement activation, acute rejection from cellular immune responses or chronic rejection with characteristic vasculopathy, and immune-mediated graft obliteration.

High-Dose Chemotherapy With Hematopoietic Progenitor Cell Transplantation

Transient myelosuppression after cancer chemotherapy is a well-established adverse effect of such treatments. For most regimens, it is rapidly reversible and requires no intervention. Some malignancies (eg, many leukemias, lymphomas, and chemotherapy-sensitive breast and small-cell lung carcinomas) may demonstrate a higher cure rate with higher-dose therapy; however, associated with this approach is an increase in hematologic toxicity. Administering the maximal tolerated chemotherapy dose and thus restoring all hematopoietic functions as rapidly as possible has led to evolution of the concept of hematopoietic progenitor cell (HPC) or "stem cell" transplant. HPC transplants have also expanded somewhat into the therapy of certain nonmalignant disorders of hematopoiesis and hematologic function; examples are aplastic anemia, sickle cell anemia, myelodysplasia, and paroxysmal nocturnal hemoglobinuria.

The sources of HPC are the bone marrow, peripheral blood, and cord blood. They comprise less than 0.5–1% of all nucleated bone marrow cells. Recently, it has become common practice to harvest HPCs from the peripheral blood by apheresis. As the peripheral blood has approximately one-fortieth the number of circulating HPCs as the bone marrow, these cells must be "mobilized" by the administration of cytotoxic chemotherapy (with the harvest being performed during the recovery phase) or enriched by the administration of hematopoietic growth factors. The cells are frozen and administered at a later date.

Because syngeneic transplants between identical (monozygotic) twins are rare, the two predominant transplants are autologous, where the HPCs are harvested from and returned to the patient; or allogeneic, where the source is an HLA-matched donor, ideally a sibling. The goals of the two procedures—and their associated adverse effects—are frequently different. Allogeneic transplants are most commonly offered to patients with malignant and nonmalignant disorders involving the bone marrow. Chemotherapy is given to ablate the marrow, resulting in maximal suppression or eradication of the recipient's native immune system. The bone marrow is repopulated by infusion of donor cells containing not only HPCs but also functional donor T lymphocytes. These T cells can cause graft-versus-host disease, in which the recipient's tissues are recognized as nonself. While this is occasionally desirable, as in the "graft-versus-leukemia" effect, it is the cause of considerable morbidity and can be fatal. There are two separate phases of graft-versus-host disease: acute, secondary to cytokine-mediated cytotoxicity against the cells of the liver, the mucosa of the gastrointestinal tract, and skin; and chronic, characterized by fibrosis and collagen deposition and resembling autoimmune disease such as scleroderma. The incidence of graft-versus-host disease can be decreased by depleting the donor marrow of T cells, but this is associated with a higher incidence of graft failure and, in the case of leukemia, a higher relapse rate. Though only a few allogeneic peripheral HPC transplants have been reported, graft-versus-host disease in such cases does not appear to be as severe, though experience is still very limited.

Autologous HPC transplants are performed solely for the treatment of malignancies. In these cases the chemotherapy is intensively myelosuppressive though not necessarily myeloablative. One prominent exception is patients with chronic myelogenous leukemia in blast crisis, who receive their autologous HPC in an effort to return their disease to the chronic phase. Since patients usually have some residual immune function and are receiving their own HPC—and thus do not require posttransplant immunosuppression—the risk of opportunistic infections and immunosuppression-related neoplasia is markedly reduced.

The success rates of HPC transplantation depend mostly upon the underlying disease and the associated risk of relapse (in cases of leukemia), the level of matching between donor and recipient (and thus the likelihood of graft-versus-host disease), the age of the recipient (over age 30, the incidence increases), and the complications associated with conditioning (veno-occlusive liver disease and infection). Overall, the survival rates at 1 year are about 60–70% in aplastic anemia and 40–75% in various forms of leukemia and other neoplasms such as non-Hodgkin's lymphomas and breast carcinomas.

Bhatia S et al: Malignant neoplasms following bone marrow transplantation. Blood 1996;87:3633. [NLM Cit ID: 96199399] (Bone marrow transplant recipients are at an increased risk of later malignancy, which may add significant morbidity and mortality to the transplant process.)

Duncombe A: ABC of clinical haematology: Bone marrow and stem cell transplantation. BMJ 1997;314:1179. [NLM Cit ID: 97291854]

Pattison JM, Krensky AM: New insights into mechanisms of allograft rejection. Am J Med Sci 1997;313:257. [NLM Cit ID: 97290376]

Peddi VR, First MR: Primary care of patients with renal

transplants. Med Clin North Am 1997;81:767. [NLM Cit ID: 97310490] (Outlines the management of renal transplant recipients and reviews the problems unique to this group of patients.)

Stadtmauer EA, Schneider CJ, Silberstein LE: Peripheral blood progenitor cell generation and harvesting. Semin Oncol 1995;22:291. [NLM Cit ID: 95296708] (Review of the current practice of HPC harvest techniques and outcomes.)

Terasaki PI et al: High survival rates of kidney transplants from spousal and living unrelated donors. N Engl J Med 1995;333:333. [NLM Cit ID: 95334041] (Excellent outcomes from use of spousal donors—equal to that of parental donors.)

MECHANISM OF ACTION OF IMMUNOSUPPRESSIVE DRUGS

The most frequently used immunosuppressive drugs and their modes of action are briefly summarized below.

Corticosteroids

This group of drugs has potent and direct anti-inflammatory effects on immunocompetent cells. Corticosteroids inhibit lymphocyte proliferation and cell-mediated immune responses more severely than they inhibit antibody responses. T helper cells, eosinophils, and monocytes are reduced in peripheral blood. Corticosteroids down-regulate cytokine gene expression through interference with transcription regulation. By inhibition of phospholipase A_2, synthesis of inflammatory arachidonic acid metabolites (prostaglandins and leukotrienes) is suppressed. Corticosteroids have been shown to block the activation of T cells by interleukin-1 (IL-1) derived from macrophages. They also inhibit the expression of class II histocompatibility antigens on the macrophage surface, thereby interfering with presentation of antigen to T cells. Cumulatively, these cellular changes result in reduced inflammatory responses.

Cytotoxic Drugs

The most frequently used cytotoxic drugs are the antimetabolites (see below) and cyclophosphamide. Cyclophosphamide is an alkylating agent that damages cells by cross-linking DNA. Although this cycle-specific drug is most effective in killing cells going through the mitotic cycle, it can also cause intermitotic cell injury and death. Cyclophosphamide can inhibit both T and B cell immunity as well as inflammation. Azathioprine and cyclophosphamide are effective inhibitors of the production of serum antibodies.

Antimetabolites

The most commonly used antimetabolites are methotrexate, an inhibitor of folic acid synthesis, and azathioprine, a structural analog of mercaptopurine, an antagonist of purine synthesis. Azathioprine is a phase-specific drug that kills rapidly replicating cells. It inhibits proliferation of both T and B cells as well as macrophages. Methotrexate inhibits rapidly proliferating cells in S phase and suppresses both cell-mediated and humoral immunity as well as inflammation. Without immunosuppression, the incidence of graft-versus-host disease after allogeneic HPC transplant is almost 100%; this can be reduced to 20–30% with immunosuppressive therapy, especially the combination of methotrexate and cyclosporine, in addition to corticosteroids. Cyclosporine prevents T cell activation, while methotrexate inhibits the function of T cells that are already activated.

Cyclosporine

This cyclic polypeptide derived from a fungus is used as an immunosuppressive drug in organ transplant recipients. Cyclosporine binds to cyclophilin, a cytoplasmic protein, thereby interfering with calcium-dependent events including secretion of interleukin-2 (IL-2) by T lymphocytes. Since IL-2 is necessary for T cell replication, this drug is a potent inhibitor of T cell proliferation and thereby inhibits T cell-mediated immune responses. Little effect has been shown on direct B cell immune responses or on inflammation. Its toxic effects are primarily on renal and, to a lesser extent, hepatic function. In addition to methotrexate, methylprednisolone has also been utilized with cyclosporine to treat graft-versus-host disease, though T cell-directed immunotoxins have not proved to be of any benefit. A recently developed microemulsion formulation offers improved oral bioavailability, safety, and efficacy.

Tacrolimus (FK506)

This drug was developed for use in transplantation and is a macrolide with potent anti-T cell properties and a mode of action similar to that of cyclosporine. Like cyclosporine, tacrolimus inhibits IL-2 and interferon-γ production and T cell activation. It has been approved for use in kidney and liver transplantation as a primary immunosuppressive agent or as rescue therapy. Both cyclosporine and tacrolimus block the intracellular pathway of calcineurin dephosphorylation of nuclear transcription factors.

Tacrolimus is approximately 100 times more potent than cyclosporine. Rates of graft-versus-host disease are lower for tacrolimus-based regimens. Tacrolimus appears to be at least as effective as cyclosporine, possibly better as prophylaxis of acute rejection. The major toxicities include hyperglycemia, nephrotoxicity, and neurotoxicity.

Mycophenolate Mofetil

Mycophenolate mofetil is used primarily as an adjunctive agent in kidney transplantation. By blocking lymphocyte production of guanine nucleotides, it inhibits T and B lymphocyte proliferation. Its use in combination with cyclosporine or tacrolimus has led to a lower incidence of acute graft rejection, reducing the need for high-dose corticosteroids or OKT3 (muromonab-CD3).

Humanized Anti-Interleukin-2 Receptor Antibody

A humanized monoclonal antibody directed to the low-affinity IL-2 receptor is approved for use in kidney transplantation. This antibody, administered for 8 weeks following the transplant, when added to standard immunosuppressive therapy, results in a reduction of the incidence of acute graft rejection to about 25%. Although the incidence of acute rejection is not substantially lower than that of other combinations of immunosuppressive agents, there appears to be a lower incidence and severity of side effects compared with antilymphocyte alternatives.

Muromonab-CD3

A murine monoclonal antibody, muromonab-CD3, is directed against human CD3, the T cell receptor. Indicated for acute graft rejection refractory to corticosteroids, large doses of the drug purge T cells from the systemic circulation. The drug has numerous side effects related to the release of cytokines, including fever, myalgias, dyspnea, and aseptic meningitis, and has also been associated with increased susceptibility to cytomegalovirus infection. Most patients are limited to a single course of therapy since recurrent courses may be associated with posttransplant lymphoproliferative disease.

IMMUNOMODULATING THERAPIES

Cytokine Therapy

The experimental and clinical applications of cytokines, as biologic response modifiers and therapeutic agents, have been greatly expanded in recent years. Some cytokines, such as tumor necrosis factor and interferon alfa, have direct antitumor activity. Other cytokines affect tumor immune responses by lymphokine-activated killer cells, tumor-infiltrating lymphocytes, and activated natural killer cells. Cytokines have been used to activate immune cells ex vivo prior to adoptive transfer or have been given concurrently with activated effector cells. Phase I and phase II trials of cellular adoptive therapy, with IL-2 activated killer cells, for the treatment of renal cell carcinoma and melanoma have demonstrated feasibility and regression of metastasis in some patients. To date, modest results, significant morbidity, and high cost have hampered widespread adoption of these techniques.

Interferon alfa is used in hairy cell leukemia, chronic myelogenous leukemia, Kaposi's sarcoma, and chronic active hepatitis B and C. Interferon beta is used for multiple sclerosis and interferon gamma for the treatment of chronic granulomatous disease. Constitutional symptoms are common with cytokine therapy, and in some instances the toxicity is considerable.

Intravenous Gamma Globulin

Immune globulin IV (IGIV) has numerous immunomodulatory and anti-inflammatory activities and is the standard of care for immunologically mediated disorders such as Kawasaki's syndrome and for antibody replacement in humoral immunodeficiency. When used in humoral immunodeficiency, serum IgG levels can become normal but the IGIV contains virtually no IgM and only traces of IgA.

Each lot of IGIV produced from donated serum contains millions of antibody specificities, reflecting the humoral immune repertoire from thousands of normal blood donors. Most current products undergo numerous purification and viral inactivation steps, including solvent-detergent treatment or pasteurization. The antibody reactivities can be directed against a wide range of foreign and self antigens. In addition to the above disorders, IGIV has been proved effective in Guillain-Barré syndrome, immune-mediated neuropathies, refractory acute idiopathic thrombocytopenic purpura, pediatric HIV infection, and post bone marrow transplantation. Many other potential indications have been supported only by anecdotal reports or uncontrolled trials.

Ballow M, Nelson R: Immunopharmacology: Immunomodulation and immunotherapy. JAMA 1997;278:2008. [NLM Cit ID: 98057371]

Spencer CM, Goa KL, Gillis JC: Tacrolimus. An update of its pharmacology and clinical efficacy in the management of organ transplantation. Drugs 1997;54:925. [NLM Cit ID: 98083475]

RELEVANT WORLD WIDE WEB SITES

[Allergy and Asthma Network/Mothers of Asthmatics, Inc.]
http://www.aanma.org

[Allergy, Asthma, and Immunology Online]
http://allergy.mcg.edu

[American Academy of Allergy, Asthma, and Immunology]
http://www.aaaai.org

[Asthma Management Handbook 1996]
http://www.NationalAsthma.org.au

[Asthma Tutorial for Patients]
http://www.med.virginia.edu/cmc/tutorials/asthma/asthma1.html

[Cytokines Online Pathfinder Encyclopedia]
http://www.copewithcytokines.de/

[The Cytokines Web]
http://www.psynix.co.uk/cytweb/

[JAMA Asthma Information Center]
http://www.ama-assn.org/special/asthma
[Medical Sciences Bulletin: Anti-inflammatory, Anti-allergic, and Immunologic Drug Reviews]
http://pharminfo.com/pubs/msb/msbanfl.html
[National Heart, Lung, and Blood Institute—Asthma]
http://www.nhlbi.nih.gov/
[National Institute of Allergy and Infectious Diseases]
http://www niaid.nih.gov
[National Psoriasis Foundation]
http://www psoriasis.org
[TransWeb]
http://www transweb.org

20 Arthritis & Musculoskeletal Disorders

See http://www.current-med.com/ch20.html for updated addresses of Web sites referenced in this chapter.

David B. Hellmann, MD, FACP, & John H. Stone, MD, MPH

DIAGNOSIS & EVALUATION

Examination of the Patient

The diagnosis of a rheumatic disease can often be made in the office or at the bedside by history and physical examination. In the patient with arthritis, the two clinical clues most helpful for diagnosis are the joint pattern and the presence or absence of extra-articular manifestations. The joint pattern is defined by answering three questions: (1) Is inflammation present? (2) How many joints are involved? and (3) What specific joints are affected? Joint inflammation is manifested by redness, warmth, swelling, and morning stiffness of at least 30 minutes' duration. Both the number of affected joints and the specific sites of involvement help determine the differential diagnosis (Table 20–1). Some diseases—gout, for example—are characteristically monarticular, whereas other diseases, such as rheumatoid arthritis, are chiefly polyarticular. The location of joint involvement can also be distinctive. Only two diseases cause prominent involvement of the distal interphalangeal joint (DIP): osteoarthritis and psoriatic arthritis. As will be detailed in the discussion of specific diseases, the presence or absence of extra-articular manifestations such as fever, rash, nodules, or neuropathy helps narrow the differential diagnosis (see Table 20–1). For patients who are chronically anticoagulated with warfarin, most joints can be readily aspirated provided that the INR is not greater than 3. In such patients, use of a small-gauge needle (eg, 22F or 25F) and application of firm pressure to the aspiration site following the procedure are prudent measures.

Laboratory procedures complete the evaluation, most commonly including sedimentation rate, tests for rheumatoid factor and antinuclear or other antibodies, synovial fluid analysis, and x-rays of affected joints. These studies are important for diagnosis and as a baseline for judging the results of therapy.

Arthrocentesis & Examination of Joint Fluid

Synovial fluid examination (Table 20–2) may provide specific diagnostic information in joint disease. Contraindications to arthrocentesis include infection of the overlying skin, bleeding disorder, or inability of the patient to cooperate. Most large joints are easily aspirated (Figure 20–1).

A. Types of Studies: When synovial fluid is examined, the following studies should be included:

1. Gross examination–If fluid is green or purulent, a Gram's stain is indicated. If grossly bloody, consider a bleeding disorder, trauma, or traumatic tap.

2. Microscopic examination–Compensated polarized light microscopy identifies and distinguishes monosodium urate (gout) and calcium pyrophosphate (pseudogout) crystals.

3. Culture–Routine bacterial cultures as well as special studies for gonococci, tubercle bacilli, or fungi when indicated.

B. Interpretation: (See Table 20–2.) Although synovial fluid analysis is diagnostic in infectious or microcrystalline arthritis, there is considerable overlap in the cytologic and biochemical values obtained in these and other diseases (Table 20–3). These studies do make possible, however, a differentiation according to severity of inflammation. Inflammatory joint fluids have more than 3000 white blood cells per microliter, of which 50% or more are polymorphonuclear neutrophils (Table 20–2). Noninflammatory disease fluids have fewer than 3000/μL and less than 25% polymorphonuclear neutrophils. Synovial fluid glucose and protein levels (Table 20–2) add little information and, therefore, should not be ordered.

Table 20–1. Diagnostic value of the joint pattern.

Characteristic	Status	Representative Disease
Inflammation	Present	Rheumatoid arthritis, systemic lupus erythematosus, gout
	Absent	Osteoarthritis
Number of involved joints	Monarticular	Gout, trauma, septic arthritis, Lyme disease
	Oligoarticular (2–4 joints)	Reiter's disease, psoriatic arthritis, inflammatory bowel disease
	Polyarticular (≥ 5 joints)	Rheumatoid arthritis, systemic lupus erythematosus
Site of joint involvement	Distal interphalangeal	Osteoarthritis, psoriatic arthritis (not rheumatoid arthritis)
	Metacarpophalangeal, wrists	Rheumatoid arthritis, systemic lupus erythematosus (not osteoarthritis)
	First metatarsal phalangeal	Gout, osteoarthritis

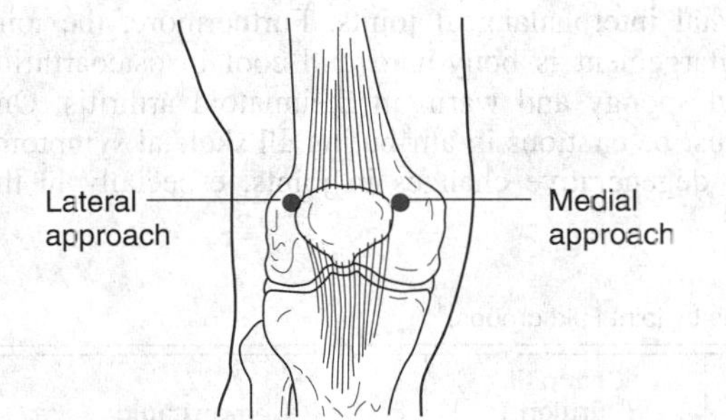

Figure 20–1. Aspiration of the knee joint. The knee joint—the most commonly aspirated joint—can be entered either medially or laterally. The patient should be supine, with the leg fully extended. Apply pressure on the side of the joint opposite to the puncture site to assist in directing the needle toward the bulging synovium. From the lateral approach, the needle (held parallel to the examining table) is directed medially, just beneath the patella, into the suprapatellar space. From the medial approach, the needle (held parallel to the examining table) is introduced between the patella and the medial condyle and advanced upward and laterally, beneath the patella and into the joint space. (Reproduced, with permission, from Nicoll D et al: *Pocket Guide to Diagnostic Tests,* 2nd ed. McGraw-Hill, 2000.)

DEGENERATIVE & CRYSTAL-INDUCED ARTHRITIS

DEGENERATIVE JOINT DISEASE (Osteoarthritis)

Essentials of Diagnosis

- A degenerative disorder without systemic manifestations.
- Pain relieved by rest; morning stiffness brief; articular inflammation minimal.
- X-ray findings: narrowed joint space, osteophytes, increased density of subchondral bone, bony cysts.
- Commonly secondary to other articular disease.

General Considerations

Osteoarthritis is the most common form of joint disease, sparing no age, race, or geographic area. At least 20 million adults in the USA suffer from the effects of this condition at any one time, and 90% of all people will have radiographic features of osteoarthritis in weight-bearing joints by age 40. Symptomatic disease also increases with age.

This arthropathy is characterized by degeneration of cartilage and by hypertrophy of bone at the articular margins. Inflammation is usually minimal. Hereditary and mechanical factors may be variably involved in the pathogenesis.

Degenerative joint disease is traditionally divided into two types: (1) primary, which most commonly affects some or all of the following: the terminal interphalangeal joints (Heberden's nodes) and less commonly the proximal interphalangeal joints (Bouchard's nodes), the metacarpophalangeal and carpometacarpal joints of the thumb, the hip, the knee, the metatarsophalangeal joint of the big toe, and the cervical and lumbar spine; and (2) secondary, which may occur in any joint as a sequela to articular injury resulting from either intra-articular (including rheumatoid arthritis) or extra-articular causes. The injury may be acute, as in a fracture; or chronic, as that due to occupational overuse of a joint, metabolic disease (eg, hyperparathyroidism, hemochromatosis, ochronosis), or neurologic disorders (tabes dorsalis; see below). Obesity is a risk factor for knee osteoarthritis and probably for the hip as well. Recreational running does not increase the incidence of osteoarthritis, but participation in competitive contact sports does. Jobs requiring frequent bending and carrying increase the risk of knee osteoarthritis.

Pathologically, the articular cartilage is first roughened and finally worn away, and spur formation and lipping occur at the edge of the joint surface. The synovial membrane becomes thickened, with hypertrophy of the villous processes; the joint cavity, how-

Table 20–2. Examination of joint fluid.

Measure	Normal	Group I (Noninflammatory)	Group II (Inflammatory)	Group III (Purulent)
Volume (mL) (knee)	< 3.5	Often > 3.5	Often > 3.5	Often > 3.5
Clarity	Transparent	Transparent	Translucent to opaque	Opaque
Color	Clear	Yellow	Yellow to opalescent	Yellow to green
WBC (per μL)	< 200	200–300	3000–50,000	> 50,000[1]
Polymorphonuclear leukocytes	< 25%	< 25%	50% or more	75% or more[1]
Culture	Negative	Negative	Negative	Usually positive
Glucose (mg/dL)	Nearly equal to serum	Nearly equal to serum	> 25, lower than serum	< 25, much lower than serum

[1]Counts are lower with infections caused by organisms of low virulence or if antibiotic therapy has been started.

ever, never becomes totally obliterated, and the synovial membrane does not form adhesions. Inflammation is prominent only in occasional patients with acute interphalangeal joint involvement.

Clinical Findings

A. Symptoms and Signs: The onset is insidious. Initially, there is articular stiffness, seldom lasting more than 15 minutes; this develops later into pain on motion of the affected joint and is made worse by activity or weight bearing and relieved by rest. Deformity may be absent or minimal; however, bony enlargement of the interphalangeal joints is occasionally prominent, and flexion contracture or varus deformity of the knee is not unusual. There is no ankylosis, but limitation of motion of the affected joint or joints is common. Coarse crepitus may often be felt in the joint. Joint effusion and other articular signs of inflammation are mild. There are no systemic manifestations.

B. Laboratory Findings: Elevated sedimentation rate and other laboratory signs of inflammation are not present.

C. Imaging: Radiographs may reveal narrowing of the joint space, sharpened articular margins, osteophyte formation and lipping of marginal bone, and thickened, dense subchondral bone. Bone cysts may also be present.

Differential Diagnosis

Because articular inflammation is minimal and systemic manifestations are absent, degenerative joint disease should seldom be confused with other arthritides. The distribution of joint involvement in the hands also helps distinguish osteoarthritis from rheumatoid arthritis. Osteoarthritis chiefly affects the distal and proximal interphalangeal joints and spares the wrist and metacarpophalangeal joints (except at the thumb); rheumatoid arthritis chiefly involves the wrists and metacarpophalangeal joints and spares the distal interphalangeal joints. Furthermore, the joint enlargement is bony-hard and cool in osteoarthritis but spongy and warm in rheumatoid arthritis. One must be cautious in attributing all skeletal symptoms to degenerative changes in joints, especially in the

Table 20–3. Differential diagnosis by joint fluid groups.[1]

Group 1 (Noninflammatory)	Group II (Inflammatory)	Group III (Purulent)	Hemorrhagic
Degenerative joint disease Trauma[2] Osteochondritis dissecans Osteochondromatosis Neuropathic arthropathy[2] Subsiding or early inflammation Hypertrophic osteoarthropathy[3] Pigmented villonodular synovitis[2]	Rheumatoid arthritis Acute crystal-induced synovitis (gout and pseudogout) Reiter's syndrome Ankylosing spondylitis Psoriatic arthritis Arthritis accompanying ulcerative colitis and regional enteritis Rheumatic fever[3] Systemic lupus erythematosus[3] Progressive systemic sclerosis (scleroderma)[3] Tuberculosis Mycotic infections	Pyogenic bacterial infections	Hemophilia or other hemorrhagic diathesis Trauma with or without fracture Neuropathic arthropathy Pigmented villonodular synovitis Synovioma Hemangioma and other benign neoplasms

[1]Reproduced from Rodnan GP (editor): Primer on the rheumatic diseases, 7th ed. JAMA 1973;224(Suppl):662.
[2]May be hemorrhagic.
[3]Group I or II.

spine, where metastatic neoplasia, osteoporosis, multiple myeloma, or other bone disease may coexist.

Prevention

Weight reduction has been shown in women to reduce the risk of developing symptomatic knee osteoarthritis. Several epidemiologic studies suggest that estrogen replacement therapy reduces the risk of knee and hip osteoarthritis. Similar studies suggest that maintaining normal vitamin D levels may reduce the occurrence and progression of osteoarthritis.

Treatment

A. General Measures: For patients with mild to moderate osteoarthritis of weight-bearing joints, a supervised walking program may result in clinical improvement of functional status without aggravating the joint pain. Weight loss can improve the symptoms of knee osteoarthritis.

B. Analgesic and Anti-inflammatory Drugs: For many patients, acetaminophen in doses of 2.6–4 g/d is as effective as and less toxic than NSAIDs. (See discussion of NSAID toxicity in the section on treatment of rheumatoid arthritis.) Patients who fail to improve with acetaminophen and nonpharmacologic therapies described above can be treated with salicylates or other NSAIDs (see Chapter 1). For patients at risk for upper gastrointestinal bleeding or who fail to respond adequately to acetaminophen, salicylates, or NSAIDs, COX-2 inhibitors may be useful. High doses of salicylates, as used in more inflammatory arthritides, are unnecessary. The need to continue any drug treatment for patients with osteoarthritis should be reviewed periodically. For many patients, it is possible eventually to reduce the dosage or limit use of the drug to periods of exacerbation. For patients with knee osteoarthritis and effusion, intra-articular injection of triamcinolone (20–40 mg) may obviate the need for analgesics or NSAIDs but usually should not be repeated more than two or three times in a year. Intra-articular injections of sodium hyaluronate have helped reduce symptoms moderately in some patients. Capsaicin cream 0.025% applied twice daily can also reduce knee pain without NSAIDs.

C. Surgical Measures: Total hip replacement provides excellent symptomatic and functional improvement when that joint is seriously afflicted, as indicated by severely restricted walking and pain at rest, particularly at night. Knee replacement is also usually effective. Although arthroscopic surgery for knee osteoarthritis is commonly performed, its long-term efficacy is unestablished. Experimental techniques to repair focal cartilage loss in the knee by autologous chondrocyte transplantation are promising. However, the precise indications for and limitations of this procedure require further definition in randomized trials.

Prognosis

Marked disability is less common than in rheumatoid arthritis, but symptoms may be quite severe and limit activity considerably (especially with involvement of the hips, knees, and cervical spine). Proper treatment may relieve symptoms and improve function.

Altman RD et al: Intraarticular sodium hyaluronate (Hyalgan) in the treatment of patients with osteoarthritis of the knee: A randomized clinical trial. J Rheumatol 1998;25:2203. [NLM Cit ID: 99033974] (Worked modestly well.)

Felson DT et al: An update on the epidemiology of knee and hip osteoarthritis with a view to prevention. Arthritis Rheum 1998;41:1343. [NLM Cit ID: 99368330] (Age, obesity, competitive athletics, female sex, estrogen deficiency, and low vitamin D levels are risk factors.)

Ettinger WH et al: A randomized trial comparing aerobic exercise and resistance exercise with a health education program in older adults with knee osteoarthritis. The fitness arthritis and seniors trial (FAST). JAMA 1997;277:25. [NLM Cit ID: 97134646] (Either walking or resistance exercise moderately reduces pain and disability.)

Lane NE et al: The relationship of running to osteoarthritis of the knee and hip and bone mineral density of the lumbar spine: A 9 year longitudinal study. J Rheumatol 1998;25:334. [NLM Cit ID: 98149474] (Runners have no higher prevalence of hip osteoarthritis and no more rapid progression of knee osteoarthritis compared with nonrunners.)

CRYSTAL DEPOSITION ARTHRITIS

1. GOUTY ARTHRITIS

Essentials of Diagnosis

- Acute onset, typically nocturnal and usually monarticular, often involving the first metatarsophalangeal joint.
- Postinflammatory desquamation and pruritus.
- Hyperuricemia in most; identification of urate crystals in joint fluid or tophi is diagnostic.
- Asymptomatic periods between acute attacks.
- Dramatic therapeutic response to NSAIDs or colchicine.
- With chronicity, urate deposits in subcutaneous tissue, bone, cartilage, joints, and other tissues.

General Considerations

Gout is a metabolic disease of heterogeneous nature, often familial, associated with abnormal amounts of urates in the body and characterized early by a recurring acute arthritis, usually monarticular, and later by chronic deforming arthritis. The associated hyperuricemia is due to overproduction or underexcretion of uric acid—sometimes both. The disease is especially common in Pacific islanders, eg, Filipinos and Samoans. It is rarely caused by a specifically determined genetic aberration (eg, Lesch-Nyhan syndrome). Secondary gout, which may have a heritable component, is related to acquired causes of hyperuricemia, eg, medication use (especially diuretics, cyclosporine, low-dose aspirin, and niacin), myeloproliferative disorders, multiple myeloma, hemoglobinopathies, chronic renal disease, hypothyroidism, psoriasis, sarcoidosis, and lead poisoning. Alcohol ingestion in any form promotes hyperuricemia by increasing urate production and decreasing the renal excretion of uric acid. Finally, hospitalized patients frequently suffer gout flares because of changes in diet (eg, inability to take oral feedings following abdominal surgery) or medications that lead either to rapid reductions or increases in the serum urate level.

About 90% of patients with primary gout are men, usually over 30 years of age. In women the onset is usually postmenopausal. The characteristic histologic lesion is the tophus, a nodular deposit of monosodium urate monohydrate crystals, with an associated foreign body reaction. These may be found in cartilage, subcutaneous and periarticular tissues, tendon, bone, the kidneys, and elsewhere. Urates have been demonstrated in the synovial tissues (and fluid) during acute arthritis; indeed, the acute inflammation of gout is believed to be activated by the phagocytosis by polymorphonuclear cells of urate crystals with the ensuing release from the neutrophils of chemotactic and other substances capable of mediating inflammation. The precise relationship of hyperuricemia to acute gouty arthritis is still obscure, since chronic hyperuricemia is found in people who never develop gout or uric acid stones (Table 20–4). Rapid fluctuations in serum urate levels, either increasing or decreasing, are important factors in precipitating acute gout. The mechanism of the late, chronic stage of gouty arthritis is better understood. This is characterized pathologically by tophaceous invasion of the articular and periarticular tissues, with structural derangement and secondary degeneration (osteoarthritis).

Uric acid kidney stones are present in 5–10% of patients with gout arthritis. Hyperuricemia correlates highly with the likelihood of developing stones, with the risk of stone formation reaching 50% in patients with a serum urate level above 13 mg/dL. Chronic urate nephropathy is caused by the deposition of monosodium urate crystals in the renal medulla and pyramids, which leads to mild albuminuria. Although progressive renal failure occurs in a substantial percentage of patients with chronic gout, the role of hyperuricemia in causing this outcome is controversial, because many patients with gout have numerous confounding risk factors for renal failure (eg, chronic lead exposure, hypertension, and other risk factors for vascular disease).

Unless there is a rapid breakdown of cellular nucleic acid following aggressive treatment of leukemia or lymphoma, uric acid-lowering drugs need not be instituted until arthritis, renal calculi, or tophi become apparent. Asymptomatic hyperuricemia should not be treated.

Table 20–4. Origin of hyperuricemia.[1]

Primary hyperuricemia
- A. Increased production of purine:
  1. Idiopathic.
  2. Specific enzyme defects (eg, Lesch-Nyhan syndrome, glycogen storage diseases).
- B. Decreased renal clearance of uric acid (idiopathic).

Secondary hyperuricemia
- A. Increased catabolism and turnover of purine:
  1. Myeloproliferative disorders.
  2. Lymphoproliferative disorders.
  3. Carcinoma and sarcoma (disseminated).
  4. Chronic hemolytic anemias.
  5. Cytotoxic drugs.
  6. Psoriasis.
- B. Decreased renal clearance of uric acid:
  1. Intrinsic kidney disease.
  2. Functional impairment of tubular transport:
     - a. Drug-induced (eg, thiazides, probenecid).
     - b. Hyperlacticacidemia (eg, lactic acidosis, alcoholism).
     - c. Hyperketoacidemia (eg, diabetic ketoacidosis, starvation).
     - d. Diabetes insipidus (vasopressin-resistant).
     - e. Bartter's syndrome.

[1]Modified from Rodnan GP: Gout and other crystalline forms of arthritis. Postgrad Med (Oct) 1975;58:6.

Clinical Findings

A. Symptoms and Signs: The acute arthritis is characterized by its sudden onset, frequently nocturnal, either without apparent precipitating cause or following rapid fluctuations in serum urate levels, such as from alcohol excess or medication changes (see above). The metatarsophalangeal joint of the great toe is the most susceptible joint ("podagra"), although others, especially those of the feet, ankles, and knees, are commonly affected. Hips and shoulders are rarely involved in gouty arthritis. More than one joint may occasionally be affected during the same attack; in such cases, the distribution of the arthritis is usually asymmetric. As the attack progresses, the pain becomes intense. The involved joints are swollen and exquisitely tender and the overlying skin tense, warm, and dusky red. Fever is common and may reach 39 °C. Local desquamation and pruritus during recovery from the acute arthritis are characteristic of gout but are not always present. Tophi may be found in the external ears, hands, feet, olecranon, and prepatellar bursas. They are usually seen only after several attacks of acute arthritis.

Asymptomatic periods of months or years commonly follow the initial acute attack. Later, gouty arthritis may become chronic, with symptoms of progressive functional loss and disability. Gross deformities, due usually to tophaceous invasion, are seen. Signs of inflammation may be absent or superimposed.

B. Laboratory Findings: The serum uric acid is elevated (> 7.5 mg/dL) in 95% of patients who have serial measurements during the course of an attack. However, a single uric acid determination is normal in up to 25% of cases, so a normal level does not exclude gout, especially in patients taking uricopenic drugs. During an acute attack, the erythrocyte sedimentation rate and white cell count are frequently elevated. Examination of the material aspirated from a tophus shows the typical crystals of sodium urate and confirms the diagnosis. Further confirmation is obtained by identification of sodium urate crystals by compensated polariscopic examination of wet smears prepared from joint fluid aspirates. Such crystals are negatively birefringent and needle-like and may be found free or in neutrophils.

C. Imaging: Early in the disease, radiographs show no changes. Later, punched-out erosions with an overhanging rim of cortical bone ("rat bite") develop. When these are adjacent to a soft tissue tophus, they are diagnostic of gout.

Differential Diagnosis

Acute gout is often confused with cellulitis. Appropriate bacteriologic studies should exclude acute pyogenic arthritis. Pseudogout is distinguished by the identification of calcium pyrophosphate crystals (strong positive birefringence) in the joint fluid, usually normal serum uric acid, the x-ray appearance of chondrocalcinosis, and the relative therapeutic ineffectiveness of colchicine.

Chronic tophaceous arthritis may rarely mimic chronic rheumatoid arthritis. In such cases, the diagnosis of gout is suggested by an earlier history of monarthritis and is established by the demonstration of urate crystals in a suspected tophus. Likewise, hips and shoulders are generally spared in tophaceous gout. Biopsy may be necessary to distinguish tophi from rheumatoid nodules. An x-ray appearance similar to that of gout may be found in rheumatoid arthritis, sarcoidosis, multiple myeloma, hyperparathyroidism, or Hand-Schüller-Christian disease. Chronic lead intoxication may result in attacks of gouty arthritis (saturnine gout); abdominal pain, peripheral neuropathy, renal insufficiency, and basophilic stippling of red cells are clues to the diagnosis.

Treatment

A. Acute Attack: The most common mistake in managing gout is starting drug treatment for both the acute arthritis and the hyperuricemia simultaneously. Treatment must be separated by treating the acute arthritis first and hyperuricemia later, if at all. Sudden reduction of serum uric acid often precipitates further episodes of gouty arthritis.

1. Nonsteroidal anti-inflammatory drugs– NSAIDs have become the treatment of choice for acute gout. Traditionally, indomethacin has been the most frequently used agent, but all of the other newer NSAIDs are probably equally effective. Indomethacin is initiated at a dosage of 25–50 mg every 8 hours and continued until the symptoms have resolved (usually 5–10 days). Active peptic ulcer disease, impaired renal function, and a history of allergic reaction to NSAIDs are contraindications to the use of these drugs. For patients at high risk for upper gastrointestinal bleeding, a COX-2 inhibitor may be an appropriate first choice for management of an acute gout attack.

2. Colchicine– Colchicine is also effective for acute gout but is less favored, since 80% of treated patients develop significant abdominal cramping, diarrhea, nausea, or vomiting. Colchicine is thought to work by inhibiting chemotaxis and thereby interfering with the inflammatory response to urate crystals; thus, it is most effective when given in the first few hours after onset of symptoms. The dose is 0.5 or 0.6 mg by mouth every hour until pain is relieved or until nausea or diarrhea appears; the drug is then stopped. The usual total dose required is 4–6 mg and should not exceed 8 mg. The incidence of gastrointestinal side effects of colchicine can be reduced by judicious use of intravenous administration. Toxicity, including local pain, tissue damage from extravasation, and marrow suppression, have been noted. The initial dose is 2 mg in 20–50 mL of saline solution given through an intravenous catheter. Two additional doses of 1 mg each can be administered at 6-hour intervals. The total dose should not exceed 4 mg; and no additional colchicine should be given by mouth for 3 weeks. Dosages must be reduced by at least 50% in the presence of renal or hepatic disease or old age. Combined renal and hepatic disease contraindicates the use of intravenous colchicine. Intravenous administration of colchicine is inadvisable if the oral route can be used. Oral colchicine should not be used in patients with inflammatory bowel disease.

3. Corticosteroids– Corticosteroids often give dramatic symptomatic relief in acute episodes of gout and will control most attacks. They are best reserved for patients unable to take oral NSAIDs. If the patient's gout is monarticular, intra-articular administration (eg, triamcinolone, 10–40 mg depending on the size of the joint) is most effective. For polyarticular gout, corticosteroids may be given intravenously (eg, methylprednisolone, 40 mg/d tapered off over 7 days) or orally (eg, prednisone, 40–60 mg/d tapered off over 7 days). It should be recognized that gouty and septic arthritis can coexist, albeit rarely. Therefore, joint aspiration and Gram stain of synovial fluid should be performed before corticosteroids are given.

4. Analgesics– At times the pain of an acute attack may require opioids. Aspirin should be avoided (see below).

5. Bed rest is important in the management of the acute attack and should be continued for about 24 hours after the acute attack has subsided. Early ambulation may precipitate a recurrence.

Physical therapy is of little value acutely, though hot compresses to or elevation of the affected joints makes some patients more comfortable.

B. Management Between Attacks: Treatment during symptom-free periods is intended to minimize urate deposition in tissues, which causes chronic tophaceous arthritis, and to reduce the frequency and severity of recurrences.

1. Diet–Potentially reversible causes of hyperuricemia are a high-purine diet, obesity, frequent alcohol consumption, and use of certain medications (see below). Although dietary purines usually contribute only 1 mg/dL to the serum uric acid level, moderation in eating foods with high-purine content is advisable (Table 20–5). Moderating alcohol use is particularly important, since alcohol is not only a source of purines but also inhibits the renal excretion of purines. A high liquid intake and, more importantly, a daily urinary output of 2 L or more will aid urate excretion and minimize urate precipitation in the urinary tract.

2. Avoidance of hyperuricemic medications–Thiazide and loop diuretics inhibit renal excretion of uric acid and should be avoided in patients with gout. Similarly, low doses of aspirin (< 3 g daily) aggravate hyperuricemia, as does niacin.

3. Colchicine–The decision to begin chronic pharmacologic treatment of gout should be based on an estimate of the likelihood of further attacks. Patients with a single episode of gout who are willing to lose weight and stop drinking alcohol are at low risk of another attack and therefore unlikely to benefit from chronic medical therapy. In contrast, older individuals with mild chronic renal failure who require diuretic use and have a history of multiple attacks of gout are more likely to benefit from pharmacologic treatment. In general, the higher the uric acid level and the more frequent the attacks, the more likely that chronic medical therapy will be beneficial.

There are two indications for daily colchicine administration: (1) It can be used to prevent future attacks. For the person who has mild hyperuricemia and occasional attacks of gouty arthritis, chronic colchicine prophylaxis may be all that is needed. The usual dose is 0.6 mg twice a day. Patients who have coexisting moderate renal insufficiency or heart failure should have the dose reduced to once a day in order to avoid the development of a mixed peripheral neuropathy and myositis that can complicate the use of higher doses. (2) It is also used when uricosuric drugs or allopurinol (see below) are started, to suppress the acute attacks that can be precipitated by abrupt changes in the serum uric acid level.

4. Reduction of serum uric acid–Indications include frequent acute arthritis not controlled by colchicine prophylaxis, tophaceous deposits, or renal damage. Hyperuricemia with infrequent attacks of arthritis may not require treatment; asymptomatic hyperuricemia should not be treated. If instituted, the goal of medical treatment is to maintain the serum uric acid below 6 mg/dL, which should prevent crystallization of urate.

Two classes of agents may be used to lower the serum uric acid—the uricosuric drugs and allopurinol (neither is of value in the treatment of acute gout). The choice of one or the other depends on the result of a 24-hour urine uric acid determination. A value under 800 mg/d indicates undersecretion of uric acid, which is amenable to uricosuric agents. Patients with more than 800 mg of uric acid in a 24-hour urine collection are overproducers of uric acid who require allopurinol.

a. Uricosuric drugs–These drugs, by blocking tubular reabsorption of filtered urate and reducing the metabolic pool of urates, prevent the formation of new tophi and reduce the size of those already present. Furthermore, when administered concomitantly with colchicine, they may lessen the frequency of recurrences of acute gout. The indication for uricosuric treatment is the increasing frequency or severity of acute attacks. Uricosuric agents are ineffective in patients with renal insufficiency, as manifested by a serum creatinine of more than 2 mg/dL.

The following uricosuric drugs may be employed: (1) Probenecid, 0.5 g daily initially, with gradual increase to 1–2 g daily; or (2) sulfinpyrazone, 50–100 mg twice daily initially, with gradual increase to 200–400 mg twice daily. Hypersensitivity to either uricosuric drug in the form of fever and rash occurs in 5% of cases; gastrointestinal complaints occur in 10%. Probenecid also inhibits the excretion of penicillin, indomethacin, dapsone, and acetazolamide.

Table 20–5. The purine content of foods.[1,2]

Low-purine foods
Refined cereals and cereal products, cornflakes, white bread, pasta, flour, arrowroot, sago, tapioca, cakes
Milk, milk products, and eggs
Sugar, sweets, and gelatin
Butter, polyunsaturated margarine, and all other fats
Fruit, nuts, and peanut butter
Lettuce, tomatoes, and green vegetables (except those listed below)
Cream soups made with low-purine vegetables but without meat or meat stock
Water, fruit juice, cordials, and carbonated drinks
High-purine foods
All meats, including organ meats, and seafood
Meat extracts and gravies
Yeast and yeast extracts, beer, and other alcoholic beverages
Beans, peas, lentils, oatmeal, spinach, asparagus, cauliflower, and mushrooms

[1]Reproduced, with permission, from Emmerson BT: The management of gout. N Engl J Med 1996;334:445.

[2]The purine content of a food reflects its nucleoprotein content and turnover. Foods containing many nuclei (eg, liver) have many purines, as do rapidly growing foods such as asparagus. The consumption of large amounts of a food containing a small concentration of purines may provide a greater purine load than consumption of a small amount of a food containing a large concentration of purines.

Precautions with uricosuric drugs. It is important to maintain a daily urinary output of 2000 mL or more in order to minimize the precipitation of uric acid in the urinary tract. This can be further prevented by giving alkalinizing agents (eg, potassium citrate, 30–80 meq/d) to maintain a urine pH of above 6.0. Uricosuric drugs are best avoided in patients with a history of uric acid lithiasis. Salicylates in low doses antagonize the action of uricosuric agents; doses greater than 3 g daily are themselves uricosuric, but low-dose aspirin should be avoided by patients with gout.

b. Allopurinol–The xanthine oxidase inhibitor allopurinol promptly lowers plasma urate and urinary uric acid concentrations and facilitates tophus mobilization. The drug is of special value in uric acid overproducers; in tophaceous gout; in patients unresponsive to the uricosuric regimen; and in gouty patients with uric acid renal stones. It should be used in low doses in patients with renal insufficiency and is not indicated in asymptomatic hyperuricemia. The most frequent adverse effect is the precipitation of an acute gouty attack. However, the commonest sign of hypersensitivity to allopurinol (occurring in 2% of cases) is a pruritic rash that may progress to toxic epidermal necrolysis. Vasculitis and hepatitis are other rare but serious complications.

The daily dose is determined by the serum uric acid response. The initial dose of allopurinol is 100 mg/d for 1 week; the dose is increased if the serum uric acid is still high. A normal serum uric acid level is often obtained with a daily dose of 200–300 mg. Occasionally (and in selected cases) it may be helpful to continue the use of allopurinol with a uricosuric drug. Neither of these drugs is useful in acute gout.

Allopurinol interacts with other drugs. The combined use of allopurinol and ampicillin causes a drug rash in 20% of patients. Allopurinol can increase the half-life of probenecid, while probenecid increases the excretion of allopurinol. Thus, a patient taking both drugs may need to use slightly higher than usual doses of allopurinol and lower doses of probenecid. Allopurinol potentiates the effect of azathioprine. If allopurinol cannot be avoided, the dose of azathioprine should be reduced by 75% before allopurinol is started.

C. Chronic Tophaceous Arthritis: Tophaceous deposits can be made to shrink and disappear altogether with allopurinol therapy. Resorption of extensive tophi may require maintaining a serum uric acid below 5 mg/dL, which may be achievable only with concomitant use of allopurinol and a uricosuric agent. Surgical excision of large tophi offers immediate mechanical improvement in selected deformities but is rarely required.

D. Gout in the Transplant Patient: Since many transplant patients have decreased renal function and require drugs that inhibit uric acid excretion (especially cyclosporine and diuretics), these patients commonly develop hyperuricemia and gout. Treating these patients is challenging: NSAIDs are usually contraindicated because of renal impairment; intravenous colchicine should be avoided for the same reason; and corticosteroids are already being used. Often the best approach for monarticular gout—after excluding infection—is injecting corticosteroids into the joint (see above). For polyarticular gout, increasing the dose of systemic corticosteroid may be the only alternative. Since transplant patients often have multiple attacks of gout, long-term relief requires lowering the serum uric acid with allopurinol. Renal impairment seen in many transplant patients would make uricosuric agents ineffective. Azathioprine must be stopped or reduced by 75% before allopurinol is started.

Prognosis

Without treatment, the acute attack may last from a few days to several weeks, but proper treatment quickly terminates the attack. The intervals between acute attacks vary up to years, but the asymptomatic periods often become shorter if the disease progresses. Chronic tophaceous arthritis occurs after repeated attacks of acute gout, but only after inadequate treatment. Although the deformities may be marked, only a small percentage of patients become bedridden. The younger the patient at the onset of disease, the greater the tendency to a progressive course. Destructive arthropathy is rarely seen in patients whose first attack is after age 50.

Patients with gout have an increased incidence of hypertension, renal disease (eg, nephrosclerosis, tophi, pyelonephritis), diabetes mellitus, hypertriglyceridemia, and atherosclerosis, although these relationships are not well understood.

Emmerson BT: The management of gout. N Engl J Med 1996;334:445. [NLM Cit ID: 96150235] (Annual incidence of gouty arthritis is 0.1–0.5% for serum urate < 7 mg/dL and about 5% for serum urate > 9 mg/dL.)

Feldman M et al: Do cyclooxygenase-2 inhibitors provide benefits similar to those of traditional nonsteroidal anti-inflammatory drugs, with less gastrointestinal toxicity? Ann Intern Med 2000;132:134. [NLM Cit ID: 20092386] (The early answer is, "Yes.")

2. CHONDROCALCINOSIS & PSEUDOGOUT (Calcium Pyrophosphate Dihydrate [CPPD] Deposition Disease)

The term chondrocalcinosis refers to the presence of calcium-containing salts in articular cartilage. It is most often first diagnosed radiologically. It may be familial and is commonly associated with a wide variety of metabolic disorders, eg, hemochromatosis, hyperparathyroidism, ochronosis, diabetes mellitus, hypothyroidism, Wilson's disease, and true gout.

Pseudogout, most often seen in persons age 60 or older, is characterized by acute, recurrent and rarely chronic arthritis that usually involves large joints (most commonly the knees and the wrists) and is almost always accompanied by chondrocalcinosis of the affected joints. Other joints frequently affected by CPPD are the metacarpophalangeal joints, hips, shoulders, elbows, and ankles. Involvement of the distal interphalangeal and proximal interphalangeal joints is no more common in CPPD deposition disease than in other age-matched controls. Pseudogout, like gout, frequently develops 24–48 hours after major surgery. Identification of calcium pyrophosphate crystals in joint aspirates is diagnostic of pseudogout. With light microscopy, the rhomboid-shaped pseudogout crystals can usually be distinguished from the needle-shaped gout crystals. A red compensator is used for positive identification, since pseudogout crystals are blue when parallel and yellow when perpendicular to the axis of the compensator. Urate crystals give the exact opposite color pattern. X-ray examination shows not only calcification (usually symmetric) of cartilaginous structures but also signs of degenerative joint disease (osteoarthritis). Unlike gout, pseudogout is usually associated with normal serum urate levels and is not dramatically improved by colchicine.

Treatment of chondrocalcinosis is directed at the primary disease, if present. Some of the nonsteroidal anti-inflammatory agents (salicylates, indomethacin, naproxen, and other drugs) are helpful in the treatment of acute episodes. Patients at increased risk for upper gastrointestinal bleeding may use a COX-2 inhibitor to treat acute attacks of pseudogout. Colchicine, 0.6 mg orally twice daily, appears to be more effective for prophylaxis than for acute attacks. Aspiration of the inflamed joint and intra-articular injection of triamcinolone, 10–40 mg, depending on the size of the joint, are also of value in resistant cases.

Handy JR: Pyrophosphate arthropathy in the knees of elderly persons. Arch Intern Med 1996;156:2426. [NLM Cit ID: 97100168]

PAIN SYNDROMES

CERVICOBRACHIAL PAIN SYNDROMES

A large group of articular and extra-articular disorders is characterized by pain that may involve simultaneously the neck, shoulder girdle, and upper extremity. Diagnostic differentiation is often difficult. Some of these entities and clinical syndromes represent primary disorders of the cervicobrachial region; others are local manifestations of systemic disease. The clinical picture is further complicated when two or more of these conditions occur coincidentally.

Clinical Findings

A. Symptoms and Signs: Neck pain may be limited to the posterior neck region or, depending upon the level of the symptomatic joint, may radiate segmentally to the occiput, anterior chest, shoulder girdle, arm, forearm, and hand. It may be intensified by active or passive neck motions. The general distribution of pain and paresthesias corresponds roughly to the involved dermatome in the upper extremity. Radiating pain in the upper extremity is often intensified by hyperextension of the neck and deviation of the head to the involved side. Limitation of cervical movements is the most common objective finding. Neurologic signs depend upon the extent of compression of nerve roots or the spinal cord. Compression of the spinal cord may cause long-tract involvement resulting in paraparesis or paraplegia.

B. Imaging: The radiographic findings depend on the cause of the pain; many plain x-rays are completely normal in patients who have suffered an acute cervical strain. Loss of the normal anterior convexity of the cervical curve (loss of cervical lordosis) is frequently seen but is a nonspecific result of paraspinal muscle spasm. In osteoarthritis, comparative reduction in height of the involved disk space is a frequent finding. The most common late x-ray finding is osteophyte formation anteriorly, adjacent to the disk; other late changes occur around the apophysial joint clefts, chiefly in the lower cervical spine. Use of advanced imaging techniques is indicated in the patient who has severe pain of unknown cause that fails to respond to conservative therapy or in the patient who has evidence of myelopathy. MRI is more sensitive than CT in detecting disk disease, extradural compression, and intramedullary cord disease.

Differential Diagnosis & Treatment

The causes of neck pain include acute and chronic cervical strain or sprains, herniated nucleus pulposus, osteoarthritis, ankylosing spondylitis, rheumatoid arthritis, osteomyelitis, neoplasms, spinal stenosis, compression fractures, and functional disorders.

A. Acute or Chronic Cervical Musculotendinous Strain: Cervical strain is generally caused by mechanical postural disorders, overexertion, or injury (eg, whiplash). Acute episodes are associated with pain, decreased cervical spine motion, and paraspinal muscle spasm, resulting in stiffness of the neck and loss of motion. Muscle trigger points can often be localized. Management includes neck and head immobilization by traction, a cervical collar, and administration of analgesics. Corticosteroid injection into cervical facet joints is ineffective. Gradual return to full activity is encouraged.

Patients with chronic symptoms often have few objective findings. Mechanical stress due to work or recreational activities is often implicated. Chronic pain, especially that radiating into the upper extremity, may require additional treatment such as bracing. Chronic pain in the zygapophysial joints resulting from whiplash injuries may benefit from percutaneous radiofrequency neurotomy.

B. Herniated Nucleus Pulposus: Rupture or prolapse of the nucleus pulposus of the cervical disks into the spinal canal causes pain that radiates to the arms at the level of C6–7. When intra-abdominal pressure is increased by coughing, sneezing, or other movements, symptoms are aggravated, and cervical muscle spasm may often occur. Neurologic abnormalities may include decreased reflexes of the deep tendons of the biceps and triceps and decreased sensation and muscle atrophy or weakness in the forearm or hand. Cervical traction, bed rest, and other conservative measures are usually successful. Radicular symptoms usually respond to conservative therapy, including NSAIDs, activity modification, intermittent cervical traction, and neck immobilization. Cervical epidural steroid injections may help those who fail. Surgery is indicated for unremitting pain and progressive weakness despite a full trial of conservative therapy and if a surgically correctable abnormality is identified by MRI or CT myelography. Surgical decompression achieves excellent results in 70–80% of such patients.

C. Arthritic Disorders: Cervical spondylosis (degenerative arthritis) is a collective term describing degenerative changes that occur in the apophysial joints and intervertebral disk joints, with or without neurologic signs. Osteoarthritis of the articular facets is characterized by progressive thinning of the cartilage, subchondral osteoporosis, and osteophytic proliferation around the joint margins. Degeneration of cervical disks and joints may occur in adolescents but is more common after age 40. Degeneration is progressive and is marked by gradual narrowing of the disk space, as demonstrated by x-ray. Osteocartilaginous proliferation occurs around the margin of the vertebral body and gives rise to osteophytic ridges that may encroach upon the intervertebral foramina and spinal canal, causing compression of the neurovascular contents.

Osteoarthritis of the cervical spine is often asymptomatic but may cause diffuse neck pain, radicular pain, or myelopathy. Myelopathy develops insidiously and is manifested by numb, clumsy hands. Some patients also complain of unsteady walking, urinary frequency and urgency, or electrical shock sensations with neck flexion or extension (Lhermitte's sign). Weakness, sensory loss, and spasticity with exaggerated reflexes develop below the level of spinal cord compression. Motor neuron disease, multiple sclerosis, syringomyelia, spinal cord tumors, and tropical spastic paresis from HTLV-1 infection can mimic myelopathy from cervical arthritis. The mainstay of conservative therapy is immobilizing the cervical spine with a collar. With moderate to severe symptoms, surgical treatment is indicated.

Ankylosing spondylitis is discussed below. Atlantoaxial subluxation may occur in patients with rheumatoid arthritis, regardless of the severity of disease. Inflammation of the synovial structures resulting from erosion and laxity of the transverse ligament can lead to neurologic signs of spinal cord compression. Treatment may vary from use of a cervical collar or more rigid bracing to operative treatment, depending on the degree of subluxation and neurologic progression. Surgical treatment may involve stabilization of the cervical spine.

D. Other Disorders: Osteomyelitis and neoplasms are discussed below. Osteoporosis is discussed in Chapter 26.

Lord SM et al: Percutaneous radio-frequency neurotomy for chronic cervical zygapophyseal-joint pain. N Engl J Med 1996;335:1721. [NLM Cit ID: 97072137] (In such patients, the procedure can provide lasting relief.)

McCormack BM et al: Cervical spondylosis: An update. West J Med 1996;165:43. [NLM Cit ID: 97008567] (Diagnosis and management.)

THORACIC OUTLET SYNDROMES

Thoracic outlet syndromes include those disorders that result in compression of the neurovascular structures supplying the upper extremity. Patients often have a history of trauma to the head and neck areas.

Symptoms and signs arise from intermittent or continuous pressure on elements of the brachial plexus and the subclavian or axillary vessels by a variety of anatomic structures of the shoulder girdle region. The neurovascular bundle can be compressed between the anterior or middle scalene muscles and a normal first thoracic rib or a cervical rib. Descent of the shoulder girdle may continue during adulthood and cause compression. Faulty posture, chronic illness, and occupation may be other predisposing factors. The components of the median nerve that encircle the axillary artery may cause compression and vascular symptoms. Sudden or repetitive strenuous physical activity may precipitate thrombosis of the axillary or subclavian vein.

Pain may radiate from the point of compression to the base of the neck, the axilla, the shoulder girdle region, arm, forearm, and hand. Paresthesias are frequently present and are commonly distributed to the volar aspect of the fourth and fifth digits. Sensory symptoms may be aggravated at night or by prolonged use of the extremities. Weakness and muscle atrophy are the principal motor abnormalities. Vascular symptoms consist of arterial ischemia characterized by pallor of the fingers on elevation of the extremity, sensitivity to cold, and, rarely, gangrene of the digits or venous obstruction marked by edema, cyanosis, and engorgement.

Deep reflexes are usually not altered. When the site of compression is between the upper rib and clavicle, partial obliteration of subclavian artery pulsation may be demonstrated by abduction of the arm to a right angle with the elbow simultaneously flexed and rotated externally at the shoulder so that the entire extremity lies in the coronal plane. Neck or arm position has no effect on the diminished pulse, which remains constant in the subclavian steal syndrome.

Chest x-ray will identify patients with cervical rib. MRI with the arms held in different positions is useful in identifying sites of impaired blood flow. Intraarterial or venous obstruction is confirmed by angiography. Determinations of the conduction velocities of the ulnar and other peripheral nerves of the upper extremity may help to localize the site of their compression.

Thoracic outlet syndrome must be differentiated from osteoarthritis of the cervical spine, tumors of the cervical spinal cord or nerve roots, and periarthritis of the shoulder.

Treatment is directed toward relief of compression of the neurovascular bundle. Overhead pulley exercises are useful to improve posture. Shoulder bracing, although uncomfortable, provides a constant stimulus to improve posture. When lying down, the shoulder girdle should be bolstered by arranging pillows in an inverted "V" position.

Symptoms may disappear spontaneously or may be relieved by conservative treatment. Operative treatment is more likely to relieve the neurologic rather than the vascular component that causes symptoms.

LOW BACK PAIN

Low back pain is exceedingly common, experienced at some time by up to 80% of the population. The differential diagnosis is broad and includes muscular strain, primary spine disease (eg, disk herniation, degenerative arthritis), systemic diseases (eg, metastatic cancer), and regional diseases (eg, aortic aneurysm). A precise diagnosis cannot be made in the majority of cases. Even when anatomic defects—such as vertebral osteophytes or a narrowed disk space—are present, clinical disease cannot be assumed since such defects are common in asymptomatic patients. The majority of patients will improve in 1–4 weeks and need no evaluation beyond the initial history and physical examination. The diagnostic challenge is to identify those patients who require more extensive or urgent evaluation.

In practice, this means identifying those patients with pain caused by (1) infection, (2) cancer, (3) inflammatory back disease such as ankylosing spondylitis, (4) or nonrheumatologic conditions, especially leaking aortic aneurysm. Significant or progressive neurologic deficits also require identification. If there is no evidence of these problems, conservative therapy is called for.

1. CLINICAL APPROACH TO DIAGNOSIS

General History & Physical Examination

Low back pain is a final common pathway of many processes; the pain of vertebral osteomyelitis, for example, is not very different in quality and intensity from the pain due to back strain of the weekend gardener. Historical factors of importance include smoking, weight loss, age over 50, and cancer, all of which are risk factors for vertebral body metastasis. Osteomyelitis most frequently occurs in adults with a history of recurrent urinary tract infections and is especially common in diabetics.

Previous peptic ulcer disease suggests that a patient's back pain is due to a penetrating ulcer. A history of cardiac murmurs should raise concern about endocarditis, since back pain is a not uncommon manifestation. A history of renal stones might indicate another cause of referred back pain.

History of the Back Pain

Certain qualities of a patient's pain can indicate a specific diagnosis. Low back pain radiating down the buttock and below the knee suggests a herniated disk causing nerve root irritation. Other conditions—including sacroiliitis, facet joint degenerative arthritis, spinal stenosis, or irritation of the sciatic nerve from a wallet—can also cause this pattern.

The diagnosis of disk herniation is further suggested by physical examination (see below) and confirmed by imaging techniques. Disk herniation can be asymptomatic, so its presence does not invariably link it to the symptom.

Low back pain at night, unrelieved by rest or the supine position, should suggest the possibility of malignancy, either vertebral body metastasis (chiefly from prostate, breast, lung, multiple myeloma, or lymphoma) or a cauda equina tumor. Similar pain can also be caused by compression fractures (from osteoporosis or myeloma).

Symptoms of large or rapidly evolving neurologic deficits identify patients who need urgent evaluation for possible cauda equina tumor, epidural abscess, or, rarely, massive disk herniation. Even with a herniated disk and nerve root impingement, pain is the most prominent symptom; numbness and weakness are less commonly reported and when present are of the magnitude consistent with compression of a single nerve root. Thus, symptoms of bilateral leg weakness (from multiple lumbar nerve root compressions) or of saddle area anesthesia, bowel or bladder incontinence, or impotence (indicating multiple sacral nerve root compressions) indicate a cauda equina process.

Low back pain that worsens with rest and improves with activity is characteristic of ankylosing spondylitis or other seronegative spondyloarthropathies, especially when the onset is insidious and begins before age 40. Most degenerative back diseases produce precisely the opposite pattern, with rest alleviating and activity aggravating the pain.

Low back pain causing the patient to writhe occurs in renal colic but can also indicate a leaking aneurysm.

Low back pain associated with pseudoclaudication from lumbar spinal stenosis is discussed below.

Physical Examination of the Back

Although examination of the back usually does not suggest a specific cause, several physical findings should be sought because they do help identify those few patients who need more than just conservative management.

Neurologic examination of the lower extremities will detect the small deficits produced by disk disease and the large deficits complicating such problems as cauda equina tumors. A positive straight leg raising test indicates nerve root irritation. The examiner performs the test on the supine patient by passively raising the patient's leg. The test is positive if radicular pain is produced with the leg raised 60 degrees or less. The test has a specificity of 40% but is 95% sensitive in patients with herniation at the L4–5 or L5–S1 level (the sites of 95% of disk herniations). It can be falsely negative, especially in patients with herniation above the L4–5 level.

The crossed straight leg sign is only 25% sensitive but is 90% specific for disk herniation and is positive when raising the contralateral leg reproduces the sciatica.

Detailed examination of the sacral and lumbar nerve roots, especially L5 and S1, is essential for detecting neurologic deficits associated with back pain. Disk herniation produces deficits predictable for the site involved (Table 20–6). Deficits of multiple nerve roots suggest a cauda equina tumor, an epidural abscess, or some other important process that requires urgent evaluation and treatment.

Table 20–6. Neurologic testing of lumbosacral nerve disorders.

Nerve Root	Motor	Reflex	Sensory Area
L4	Dorsiflexion of foot	Knee jerk	Medial calf
L5	Dorsiflexion of great toe	None	Medial forefoot
S1	Eversion of foot	Ankle jerk	Lateral foot

Measurement of spinal motion in the patient with acute pain is rarely of diagnostic utility and usually simply confirms that pain limits motion. An exception to this general rule is that evidence of decreased range of motion in multiple regions of the spine (cervical, thoracic, and lumbar) indicates a diffuse spinal disease such as ankylosing spondylitis. But by the time the patient has such limits, the diagnosis is usually not a mystery.

If back pain is not severe and does not itself limit motion, Schober's test of lumbar motion is helpful in early diagnosis of ankylosing spondylitis. To perform this test, two marks are made, one 10 cm above S1 and another 5 cm below. The patient then bends forward as far as possible, and the distance between the points is measured. Normally, the distance increases at least 5 cm. Anything less indicates reduced lumbar motion, which in the absence of severe pain is most commonly due to ankylosing spondylitis or other seronegative spondyloarthropathies.

Palpation of the spine usually does not yield diagnostic information. Point tenderness over a vertebral body is reported to suggest osteomyelitis, but this association is uncommon. A step-off noted between the spinous process of adjacent vertebral bodies may indicate spondylolisthesis, but the sensitivity of this finding is extremely low. Tenderness of the soft tissues overlying the greater trochanter of the hip is a manifestation of trochanteric bursitis.

Inspection of the spine is not often of value in identifying serious causes of low back pain. The classic posture of ankylosing spondylitis is a late finding. Scoliosis of mild degree is not associated with an increased risk of clinical back disease. Cutaneous neurofibromas can identify the very rare patient who has nerve root encasement.

Examination of the hips should be part of the complete examination. While hip arthritis usually produces groin pain, some patients have buttock or low back symptoms.

Further Examination

If the history and physical examination do not suggest the presence of infection, cancer, inflammatory back disease, major neurologic deficits, or pain referred from abdominal or pelvic disease, further evaluation can be eliminated or deferred while conservative therapy is tried. The great majority of patients will spontaneously improve with conservative care over 1–4 weeks.

Regular radiographs of the lumbosacral spine give 20 times the radiation dose of a chest x-ray and provide limited, albeit important, information. Oblique films double the radiation dose and are not routinely needed. X-rays can provide evidence of vertebral body osteomyelitis, cancer, fractures, or ankylosing spondylitis. Degenerative changes in the lumbar spine are ubiquitous in patients over 40 and do not prove clinical disease. Plain x-rays have very low sensitivity or specificity for disk disease. Thus, plain x-rays are warranted promptly for patients suspected of having infection, cancer, fractures, or inflammation; selected other patients who fail to improve after 2–4 weeks of conservative therapy are also candidates. The Agency for Health Care Policy and Research guidelines for obtaining lumbar radiographs are summarized in Table 20–7.

MRI provides exquisite anatomic detail but is reserved for patients in whom the information would change therapy. It is needed urgently in any patient suspected of having an epidural mass or cauda equina tumor but not if a patient is suspected of having a routine disk herniation, since most such patients will improve over 4–6 weeks of conservative therapy. Noncontrast CT does not image cauda equina tumors or other intradural lesions, and if used instead of MRI it must include intrathecal contrast.

Radionuclide bone scanning has limited utility. It is most useful for early detection of vertebral body osteomyelitis or metastases. The bone scan is often normal in multiple myeloma because lytic lesions do not take up isotope.

2. MANAGEMENT

While any management plan must be individualized, key elements of most conservative treatments for back pain include analgesia and education. Analgesia can usually be provided with NSAIDs, but severe pain may require opioids. Rarely does the need for opioids extend beyond 1–2 weeks, and they are contraindicated in the management of chronic low back pain.

Limited evidence supports the use of "muscle relaxants" such as diazepam, cyclobenzaprine, carisoprodol, and methocarbamol. These drugs should be reserved for patients who fail NSAIDs and should also be limited to courses of 1–2 weeks. Their use should be avoided in older patients, who are at risk of falling. All patients should be taught how to protect the back in daily activities—ie, not to lift heavy objects, to use the legs rather than the back when lifting, to use a chair with arm rests, and to rise from bed by first rolling to one side and then using the arms to push to an upright position. Back manipulation for benign, mechanical low back pain appears safe and as effective as therapies provided by physicians.

Rest and back exercises, once thought to be cornerstones of conservative therapy, are now known to be ineffective for acute back pain. Two days of bed rest gives better results than 7 days. Indeed, no bed rest with continuation of ordinary activities as tolerated is superior to either 2 days of bed rest or back mobilizing exercises. The value of corsets or traction is dubious. The efficacy of epidural corticosteroid injections in treating sciatica is still being debated. Corticosteroid injections into facet joints are ineffective for chronic low back pain.

Surgical consultation is needed urgently for any patient with a large or evolving neurologic deficit. Surgery for disk disease is indicated when there is documentation of herniation by some imaging procedure, a consistent pain syndrome, and a consistent neurologic deficit that has failed to respond to 4–6 weeks of conservative therapy. Percutaneous lumbar discectomy, performed under local anesthesia, is a safe and effective (up to 75%) alternative to laminectomy. The percutaneous procedure is contraindicated in the presence of tumor, infection, spondylolisthesis, foraminal stenosis, loose disk fragments, or severe facet joint arthritis.

Complaints without objective findings suggest a psychologic role in symptom formation. Treatment includes reassurance and nonopioid analgesics.

Table 20–7. AHCPR criteria for lumbar radiographs in patients with acute low back pain.[1]

Possible fracture
Major trauma
Minor trauma in patients > 50 years
Chronic steroid use
Osteoporosis
> 70 years
Possible tumor or infection
> 50 years
< 20 years
History of cancer
Constitutional symptoms
Recent bacterial infection
Intravenous drug use
Immunosuppression
Supine pain
Nocturnal pain

[1]Agency for Health Care Policy and Research (modified from JAMA 1997;277:1784).

LUMBAR SPINAL STENOSIS

Lumbar spinal stenosis may be congenital or (more commonly) acquired. Narrowing of the spinal canal most frequently results from enlarging osteophytes at the facet joints, hypertrophy of the ligamentum flavum, and protrusion or bulging of intervertebral disks. Exactly how spinal stenosis results in the pain syndromes described below is not defined, but ischemia from compression of nutrient arterioles is one possible mechanism.

Since age is the greatest risk factor for spinal degenerative changes, most patients with lumbar spinal stenosis are over 60 years old. Patients may present either with trouble walking or with back pain. Patients with gait disturbance notice the gradual onset of pain, weakness, or unsteadiness in both legs that is precipitated by walking or prolonged standing and relieved by sitting. The onset of symptoms with standing by itself, the location of the maximal discomfort to the thighs, and the preservation of pedal pulses help distinguish the "pseudoclaudication" of spinal stenosis from true claudication caused by vascular insufficiency. In some patients, unsteadiness of gait is most noticeable, prompting them to complain of having "spaghetti legs" or walking "like a drunken sailor." Because the lumbar spinal canal volume increases with back flexion and decreases with extension, some patients give the classic story that they have fewer symptoms walking uphill than down. When low back pain is the chief symptom, it is bilateral and often diffuse over the buttocks.

The back examination in patients with lumbar spinal stenosis is often unimpressive. Fewer than 10% have a positive straight leg raise sign, 25% have diminished deep tendon reflexes, and 60% have slight proximal weakness. Walking with the patient may reveal unsteadiness, though usually the patient's perception of gait disturbance is greater than that of any other observer. The diagnosis of spinal stenosis in a patient with symptoms is best confirmed by MRI. Weight loss and exercises aimed at reducing lumbar lordosis, which aggravates symptoms of spinal stenosis, can help. When disabling symptoms persist, decompressive laminectomy provides at least short-term relief in approximately 80%.

[AHCPR: Acute Low Back Problems in Adults] http://text.nlm.nih.gov/ftrs/pick?dbName=lbpc&ftrsK=46227&cp=1&t=928429185&collect=ahcpr

Andersson GB et al: A comparison of osteopathic spinal manipulation with standard care for patients with low back pain. N Engl J Med 1999;341:1426. [NLM Cit ID: 20001874] (Osteopathic manual care and one or more standard medical therapies—analgesics, NSAIDs, physical therapy, ultrasound, and TENS units—had comparable outcomes at 12 weeks.)

Carette S et al: Epidural corticosteroid injections for sciatica due to herniated nucleus pulposus. N Engl J Med 1997;336:1634. [NLM Cit ID: 97301685] (Epidural injections can provide short-term relief of sciatica but do not improve functional status or reduce need for surgery.)

Cherkin DC et al: A comparison of physical therapy, chiropractic manipulation, and provision of an educational booklet for the treatment of patients with low back pain. N Engl J Med 1998;339:1021. [NLM Cit ID: 98425646] (Chiropractic manipulation [$437], and physical therapy [$429] are more expensive and very slightly more effective than an education booklet [$153].)

Daltroy LH et al: A controlled trial of an educational program to prevent low back injuries. N Engl J Med 1997;337:322. [NLM Cit ID: 97365043] (Education did not prevent work-related low back injury.)

JAMA patient page: Low back pain. JAMA 1998;279:1846. [NLM Cit ID: 98290685]

Malanga GA et al: Nonoperative treatment of low back pain. Mayo Clin Proc 1999;74:1135 [NLM Cit ID: 20023259] (Thoughtful review of the available nonsurgical treatment approaches.)

Suarez-Almazor ME et al: Use of lumbar radiographs for the early diagnosis of low back pain. Proposed guidelines would increase utilization. JAMA 1997;277:1782. [NLM Cit ID: 97322137] (Argues that the AHCPR criteria lead to an excessive number of back x-rays.)

Vroomen PCAJ et al: Lack of effectiveness of bed rest for sciatica. N Engl J Med 1999;340:418. [NLM Cit ID: 99122621] (Title says it all.)

FIBROMYALGIA

Essentials of Diagnosis

- Chronic widespread musculoskeletal pain syndrome with multiple tender points.
- Fatigue, headaches, numbness common.
- Most frequent in women aged 20–50.
- Objective signs of inflammation absent; laboratory studies normal.
- Partially responsive to exercise, tricyclic antidepressants.

General Considerations

Fibromyalgia is one of the most common rheumatic syndromes in ambulatory general medicine affecting 3–10% of the general population. It shares many features with the chronic fatigue syndrome, namely, an increased frequency among women aged 20–50, absence of objective findings, and absence of diagnostic laboratory tests. While many of the clinical features of the two conditions overlap, musculoskeletal pain predominates in fibromyalgia whereas lassitude dominates the chronic fatigue syndrome.

The cause is unknown, but sleep disorders, depression, viral infections, and aberrant perception of normal stimuli have all been proposed. Fibromyalgia can be a complication of hypothyroidism, rheumatoid arthritis, or, in men, sleep apnea.

Clinical Findings

The patient complains of chronic aching pain and stiffness, frequently involving the entire body but with prominence of pain around the neck, shoulders, low back, and hips. Fatigue, sleep disorders, subjective numbness, chronic headaches, and irritable bowel symptoms are common. Even minor exertion aggravates pain and increases fatigue. Physical examination is normal except for "trigger points" of pain produced by palpation of various areas such as the trapezius, the medial fat pad of the knee, and the lateral epicondyle of the elbow.

Differential Diagnosis

Fibromyalgia is a diagnosis of exclusion. A detailed history and repeated physical examination can obviate the need for extensive laboratory testing. Rheumatoid arthritis and systemic lupus erythematosus virtually always present with objective physical findings or abnormalities on routine testing, including the erythrocyte sedimentation rate. Thyroid function tests are useful, since hypothyroidism can produce a secondary fibromyalgia syndrome. Polymyositis produces weakness rather than pain. The diagnosis of fibromyalgia probably should be made hesitantly in a patient over age 50 and should never be invoked to explain fever, weight loss, or any other objective signs. Polymyalgia rheumatica produces shoulder and girdle pain, is associated with anemia and an elevated sedimentation rate, and occurs after age 50.

Treatment

Patient education is of paramount importance. Patients can be comforted by the knowledge that they have a diagnosable syndrome that can be managed by means of specific though imperfect therapies and that the course is not progressive. Studies have demonstrated modest efficacy of amitriptyline, fluoxetine, chlorpromazine, or cyclobenzaprine. Amitriptyline is initiated at a dosage of 10 mg at bedtime and gradually increased to 40–50 mg depending on its efficacy and toxicity. Exercise programs are also beneficial. NSAIDs are generally ineffective. Opioids and corticosteroids are ineffective and should never be used to treat fibromyalgia.

Prognosis

Most patients have chronic symptoms. With treatment, however, many do eventually resume increased activities. Progressive or objective findings do not develop.

Bennett RM: Emerging concepts in the neurobiology of chronic pain: evidence of abnormal sensory processing in fibromyalgia. Mayo Clin Proc 1999;74:385. [NLM Cit ID: 99236658] (Review of the neurobiology of chronic pain, with particular reference to fibromyalgia.)

Goldenberg DL: Fibromyalgia syndrome a decade later: what have we learned? Arch Intern Med 1999;159:777. [NLM Cit ID: 99235329] (Acknowledges the existence of psychosocial factors in patients with fibromyalgia who seek medical care, compared with persons in the community who meet criteria for the syndrome who do not, and discusses the impact of such factors on therapy.)

Leventhal LJ: Management of fibromyalgia. Ann Intern Med 1999;131:850. [NLM Cit ID: 20043619] (Current opinion on the diagnosis and treatment of fibromyalgia.)

CARPAL TUNNEL SYNDROME

Carpal tunnel syndrome is a common painful disorder caused by compression of the median nerve between the carpal ligament and other structures within the carpal tunnel (entrapment neuropathy). The volume of the contents of the tunnel can be increased by organic lesions such as synovitis of the tendon sheaths or carpal joints, recent or malhealed fractures, tumors, and occasionally congenital anomalies. Even though no anatomic lesion is apparent, flattening or even circumferential constriction of the median nerve may be observed during operative section of the ligament. The disorder may occur in pregnancy, is seen in individuals with a history of repetitive use of the hands, and may follow injuries of the wrists. A familial type of carpal tunnel syndrome has been reported in which no etiologic factor can be identified.

Carpal tunnel syndrome can also be a feature of many systemic diseases: rheumatoid arthritis and other rheumatic disorders (inflammatory tenosynovitis); myxedema, amyloidosis, sarcoidosis, and leukemia (tissue infiltration); acromegaly; hyperparathyroidism, hypocalcemia, and diabetes mellitus.

Clinical Findings

Pain in the distribution of the median nerve, which may be burning and tingling (acroparesthesia), is the initial symptom. Aching pain may radiate proximally into the forearm and occasionally proximally to the shoulder, neck, and chest. Pain is exacerbated by manual activity, particularly by extremes of volar flexion or dorsiflexion of the wrist. It may be most bothersome at night. Impairment of sensation in the median nerve distribution may not be apparent. Subtle disparity between the affected and opposite sides can be demonstrated by testing for two-point discrimination or by requiring the patient to identify different textures of cloth by rubbing them between the tips of the thumb and the index finger. Tinel's or Phalen's sign may be positive. (Tinel's sign is tingling or shock-like pain on volar wrist percussion; Phalen's sign, pain or paresthesia in the distribution of the median nerve when the patient flexes both wrists to 90 degrees with the dorsal aspects of the hands held in apposition for 60 seconds.) The carpal compression test, performed by applying direct pressure on the carpal tunnel, may be more sensitive and specific than the Tinel and Phalen tests. Muscle weakness or atrophy, especially of the abductor pollicis brevis, appears later than sensory disturbances. Useful special examinations include electromyography and determinations of segmental sensory and motor conduction delay. Distal median sensory conduction delay may be evident before motor delay.

Differential Diagnosis

This syndrome should be differentiated from other cervicobrachial pain syndromes, from compression syndromes of the median nerve in the forearm or arm, and from mononeuritis multiplex. When left-sided, it may be confused with angina pectoris.

Treatment

Treatment is directed toward relief of pressure on the median nerve. When a primary lesion is discovered, specific treatment should be given. When soft tissue swelling is a cause, elevation of the extremity may relieve symptoms. Splinting of the hand and forearm at night may be beneficial. Injection of corticosteroid into the carpal tunnel can alleviate symptoms in some patients, particularly those with synovitis of the wrist. To reduce the chance of nerve injury, this injection should be performed by a physician thoroughly familiar with the anatomy of the carpal tunnel.

Operative division of the volar carpal ligament gives lasting relief from pain, which usually subsides within a few days. Muscle strength returns gradually, but complete recovery cannot be expected when atrophy is pronounced.

Atroshi I et al: Prevalence of carpal tunnel syndrome in a general population. JAMA 1999;282:153. [NLM Cit ID: 99336977] (In a population-based survey, nearly 15% of patients reported symptoms compatible with carpal tunnel syndrome. One in five symptomatic people had confirmation of the diagnosis by clinical examination and electrophysiologic testing.)

Franzblau A et al: What is carpal tunnel syndrome? JAMA 1999;282:186. [NLM Cit ID: 99336984] (Insightful discussion of the usefulness and limitations of clinical and laboratory tools used to diagnose carpal tunnel syndrome.)

DUPUYTREN'S CONTRACTURE

This relatively common disorder is characterized by hyperplasia of the palmar fascia and related structures, with nodule formation and contracture of the palmar fascia. The cause is unknown, but the condition has a genetic predisposition and occurs primarily in white men over 50 years of age. The incidence is higher among alcoholics and patients with chronic systemic disorders (eg, cirrhosis, diabetes, epilepsy, tuberculosis). It is also associated with systemic fibrosing syndrome, which includes Peyronie's disease, mediastinal and retroperitoneal fibrosis, and Riedel's struma. The onset may be acute, but slowly progressive chronic disease is more common.

Dupuytren's contracture manifests itself by nodular or cord-like thickening of one or both hands, with the fourth and fifth fingers most commonly affected. The patient may complain of tightness of the involved digits, with inability to satisfactorily extend the fingers, and on occasion there is tenderness. The resulting cosmetic problems may be unappealing, but in general the contracture is well tolerated since it exaggerates the normal position of function of the hand. Fasciitis involving other areas of the body may lead to plantar fibromatosis (10% of patients) or Peyronie's disease (1–2%).

If the palmar nodule is growing rapidly, injections of triamcinolone into the nodule may be of benefit. Surgical intervention is indicated in patients with significant flexion contractures, depending on the location, but recurrence is not uncommon.

Arkkila PE et al: Dupuytren's disease: Association with chronic diabetic complications. J Rheumatol 1997;24:153. [NLM Cit ID: 97155313] (Prevalence is 14% in both type 1 and type 2.)

REFLEX SYMPATHETIC DYSTROPHY

Reflex sympathetic dystrophy is a syndrome of pain and swelling of an extremity accompanied by signs of trophic skin changes in the extremity (eg, skin atrophy, hyperhidrosis) and signs and symptoms of vasomotor instability. Any extremity can be involved, but the disorder most commonly occurs in the hand and is associated with ipsilateral restricted shoulder motion (shoulder-hand syndrome). The swelling in reflex sympathetic dystrophy is diffuse ("catcher's mitt hand") and not restricted to joints. Pain is often described as burning in quality. The **shoulder-hand variant** of reflex sympathetic dystrophy is common after neck or shoulder injuries or following myocardial infarction. Direct trauma to the hand or foot can also provoke this syndrome. Reflex sympathetic dystrophy can also develop after a knee injury or after arthroscopic knee surgery. There are no systemic symptoms, and x-rays reveal severe generalized osteopenia. The severe osteoporosis occurring in the posttraumatic variant of reflex sympathetic dystrophy is known as Sudeck's atrophy. Bone scans also show increased uptake. In a significant minority of cases, symptoms and findings are bilateral.

This syndrome should be differentiated from other cervicobrachial pain syndromes, rheumatoid arthritis, polymyositis, scleroderma, and gout.

In addition to specific treatment of the underlying disorder, treatment is directed toward restoration of function. For most patients, physical therapy is the cornerstone of treatment. Patients who have restricted shoulder motion may benefit from the treatment described for scapulohumeral periarthritis. In resistant cases, prednisone, 30–40 mg/d for 2 weeks and then tapered off over 2 weeks, may be effective. Stellate ganglion block can also be effective for reflex sympathetic dystrophy.

The prognosis depends in part upon the stage in which the lesions are encountered and the extent and severity of associated organic disease. Early treatment offers the best prognosis for recovery.

BURSITIS

Inflammation of the synovium-like cellular membrane overlying bony prominences may be secondary to trauma, infection, or arthritic conditions such as gout, rheumatoid arthritis, or osteoarthritis. The most common locations are the subdeltoid, olecranon, ischial, trochanteric, semimembranous-gastrocnemius (Baker's cyst) and prepatellar bursae.

There are several ways to distinguish bursitis from arthritis. Bursitis is more likely than arthritis to begin abruptly and cause focal tenderness and swelling. Olecranon bursitis, for example, causes a "goose egg" swelling at the tip of the elbow, whereas elbow joint inflammation causes more diffuse swelling. Similarly, a patient with prepatellar bursitis has a small focus of swelling over the kneecap and no distention of the knee joint itself. Active and passive range of motion are usually much more limited in arthritis than in bursitis. A patient with trochanteric bursitis will have normal internal rotation of the hip, whereas a patient with hip arthritis will not. Bursitis caused by trauma responds to local heat, rest, immobilization, NSAIDs, and local corticosteroid injections.

Bursitis can result from infection. The two most common sites are the olecranon and prepatellar bursae. Acute swelling and redness at either of these two sites calls for aspiration to rule out infection. The absence of fever does not exclude infection, and one-third of those with septic olecranon bursitis have no fever. A bursal fluid white blood cell count of greater than 1000/μL indicates inflammation from infection, rheumatoid arthritis, or gout. In septic bursitis, the white cell count averages over 50,000/μL. Most cases are caused by *Staphylococcus aureus;* the Gram stain is positive in only two-thirds. Treatment involves antibiotics and repeated aspiration for tense effusions.

Chronic, stable olecranon bursa swelling unaccompanied by erythema or other signs of inflammation does not suggest infection and does not require aspiration. Aspiration of the olecranon bursa in rheumatoid arthritis and in gout runs the risk of creating a chronic drainage site. This risk can be reduced by using a small needle (25 gauge if possible) and pulling the skin over the bursa before introducing the needle so as to create a "zigzag" access route. Applying a pressure bandage may also help prevent chronic drainage. Surgical removal of the bursa is indicated only for cases in which repeated infections occur. Repetitive minor trauma to the olecranon bursa should be eliminated by avoiding resting the elbow on a hard surface or by wearing an elbow pad.

A bursa can also become symptomatic when it ruptures. This is particularly true for Baker's cyst, whose rupture can cause calf pain and swelling that mimic thrombophlebitis. The ruptured cyst can be imaged with sonography, MRI, or arthrography. In most cases, none of these tests are necessary because Baker's cyst or the frequently associated knee effusion is detectable on physical examination. Often it is more important to exclude thrombophlebitis than it is to visualize Baker's cyst. Treatment of a ruptured cyst includes rest, leg elevation, and injection of triamcinolone, 20–40 mg into the knee (which communicates with the cyst). Rarely, Baker's cyst can compress vascular structures and cause leg edema and true thrombophlebitis.

Shbeeb MI et al: Trochanteric bursitis (greater trochanter pain syndrome). Mayo Clin Proc 1996;71:565. [NLM Cit ID: 96232267]

SPORTS MEDICINE INJURIES

Musculoskeletal problems commonly occur as a result of both serious athletic pursuits and activities of daily living. For most such disorders, the diagnosis is made easily. Though not described in detail here, physical therapy is an important adjunct to the medical management of these disorders.

1. ROTATOR CUFF DISORDERS

A substantial majority of shoulder problems stem from disorders of the rotator cuff. The tendons of the rotator cuff form a musculotendinous unit near their insertions into the proximal humerus. As a result of years of cumulative irritation, attenuation of these tendons occurs with advancing age. Among the relevant muscles, the supraspinatus is the one most affected. Distinguishing between the various soft tissue disorders that cause shoulder pain may be difficult. Rotator cuff tendinitis, subacromial bursitis, partial and complete rotator cuff tears, and calcific tendinitis frequently cause similar symptoms. In addition, these disorders often occur together, though precise distinction is frequently unimportant for purposes of therapy.

Clinical Findings

Patients usually present with nonspecific pain localized to the shoulder, often noticed more at night when lying on the affected side. They experience locking sensations when moving the shoulder, particularly through abduction. Because of the shared innervation, symptoms are frequently referred down the proximal lateral arm. With rotator cuff tears, there may be an inability to abduct or flex the shoulder depending on the site of the tear.

The rotator cuff may be palpated just lateral to the head of the acromion. Maximum tenderness is usually noted over the supraspinatus insertion. The acromioclavicular joint may also be tender if there is accompanying degenerative arthritis in that joint. There may be prominent crepitus. Pain with range of motion is most pronounced between 60 and 120 degrees of abduction, the site of greatest impingement of the rotator cuff tissues between the humerus and coracoacromial arch.

For patients with partial rotator cuff tendon ruptures, the findings are identical to those of chronic tendinitis and bursitis. Patients with partial ruptures often demonstrate mild abduction weakness. With complete ruptures, weakness of abduction (and, to a lesser extent, flexion) is substantial, even though full range of motion may be maintained by the shoulder's accessory rotator muscles. Patients with complete tears usually have positive "drop" signs: inability to sustain passive abduction of the arm to 90 degrees.

Treatment

For most rotator cuff disorders, the central tenets of therapy are rest and abstention from the inciting activities. Temporary use of a sling is occasionally helpful in enforcing rest. NSAIDs and moist heat afford some symptomatic relief. For patients with symptoms that persist after 2 weeks of conservative management, injections of a corticosteroid preparation (eg, 1 mL of triamcinolone, 40 mg/mL) mixed with 2–3 mL of lidocaine hydrochloride (1–2%) may be useful. Tears or partial tears of the rotator cuff tendons that are believed to be chronic do not preclude a corticosteroid injection. Most patients obtain significant relief with one injection, but the procedure—along with continued rest—may be repeated after 2–3 weeks. Physical therapy is valuable for refractory cases—if the patient fails to maintain the shoulder's normal range of motion, stiffness and impaired function may ensue.

Aside from patients with complete rotator cuff tears, only those who fail to improve after months of conservative therapy are candidates for operation. Persistent symptoms may be a sign of complete tear, which may be diagnosed by MRI. Patients with symptoms that continue in the absence of a complete tear, however, sometimes require surgery to excise the inferolateral portion of the acromion, release obstructed soft tissue, and repair partial tendon tears. Depending on the degree of symptoms and functional status, complete tears may not always require surgical repair. Patients over 75 years of age rarely have symptoms or limitations that necessitate surgery. Moreover, surgical repairs are frequently less successful in the elderly because of the attrition of the rotator cuff that occurs with aging.

2. LATERAL & MEDIAL EPICONDYLITIS

These disorders are better known by their sports associations: "tennis elbow" and "golf elbow," respectively. Lateral epicondylitis is the more common of the two. The conditions are caused by overuse, and the pain results from minor tears in the tendons of the forearm's extensor and flexor muscles.

Clinical Findings

The patient presents with pain at the site of tendon insertion. Tasks that require grasping and squeezing, such as shaking hands or opening jars, are impaired.

The diagnoses are easily confirmed on physical examination by elicitation of point tenderness over the involved site. The characteristic pain may also be reproduced by extension or flexion of the wrist against pressure. Asking the patient to clench the fist and extend the wrist against the pressure of the examiner's palm is a useful maneuver for localizing lateral epicondylitis. Medial epicondylitis may be demonstrated by performing the same maneuver in flexion.

Treatment

Treatment is with rest and avoidance of activities that exacerbate the conditions. The use of "counterforce" straps (bands worn distal to the elbow, over the bulk of the forearm musculature), intended to decrease the forces transmitted to the elbow during activity, are inadequate substitutes for rest. NSAIDs are effective in mild cases. Symptoms that persist after 2 weeks of conservative therapy usually respond to infiltration of triamcinolone 10–20 mg mixed with 1–2 mL of 1% lidocaine around the involved epicondyle. After the pain and tenderness have subsided, patients may begin a physical therapy program involving daily stretching of the flexor and extensor tendons. There are anecdotal reports of dramatic relief with operative treatment.

3. PATELLO-FEMORAL SYNDROME

Patello-femoral syndrome is among the most common causes of knee complaints in primary care medicine, particularly among adolescent and young adult patients. The syndrome frequently gives rise to the chief complaint of anterior knee pain. The belief that furrowing and roughening of the cartilage on the patella's posterior surface cause the syndrome (chondromalacia patellae) is erroneous. It is now known that this finding is common, rarely leads to symptomatology, and requires no intervention. A variety of injuries or anatomic abnormalities predispose patients to irregular patellar movements, however, leading to the patello-femoral syndrome. Such predisposing conditions include imbalance of quadriceps strength, patella alta, recurrent patellar subluxation, direct trauma to the patella, and meniscal injuries. For most of these causes, the therapeutic approach is similar.

Clinical Findings

Patients frequently have difficulty localizing the source of their complaint but generally confirm that the pain is in the front of the knee, around or underneath the patella. Questions regarding specific precipitants of the pain may be useful in establishing the diagnosis. For example, because of the flexion load, patients have difficulty going up or down staircases. Another characteristic symptom is the positive "theater" sign: after remaining seated for a prolonged period, patients describe extreme discomfort with their first few steps after rising. The symptoms improve with further walking. Finally, patients with patello-femoral syndrome often complain of crepitus, joint locking, or sensations of joint instability, all of which lack anatomic explanations.

The physical examination is less useful than the history in establishing the diagnosis, but a significant number of patients have characteristic physical findings. In particular, when the knee is held in slight flexion, gentle pressure against the patella as the patient contracts the quadriceps muscles may reproduce the symptoms. In some cases, with the knee extended and the quadriceps relaxed, the typical pain may be reproduced by digital pressure under the medial or lateral border of the patella, with side-to-side movement of the bone. Inflammatory findings on examination are incompatible with the diagnosis of patellofemoral syndrome and suggest other disorders.

Treatment

Therapy includes avoidance of flexion loads and strengthening of the quadriceps. Referral to a physical therapist is helpful in educating the patient about home exercises. Many patients learn that the most effective therapy is bicycling, with the seat high enough to permit nearly full knee extension with each cycle. Although most cases respond to these interventions and even resolve altogether, some persist for years. Even in the latter, conservative therapy remains the rule; operation is rarely indicated.

4. OVERUSE SYNDROMES OF THE KNEE

Runners—particularly those who overtrain, fail to stretch prior to running, or do not attain the proper level of conditioning before starting a running program—may develop a variety of painful overuse syndromes of the knee. Most of these conditions are forms of tendinitis or bursitis that can be diagnosed on examination. The most common conditions include anserine bursitis, the iliotibial band syndrome, and popliteal and patellar tendinitis.

Clinical Findings

Symptoms resulting from all of these conditions worsen as the patient continues to run and often require cessation of the activity. Anserine bursitis results in pain medial and inferior to the knee joint over the medial tibia. The iliotibial band syndrome and popliteal tenosynovitis may be difficult to differentiate, because the popliteus tendon inserts into the lateral femoral condyle underneath the iliotibial band. Both conditions result in pain on the lateral side of the knee. Patellar tendinitis, a cause of anterior knee discomfort, typically occurs at the tendon's insertion into the patella rather than at its more inferior insertion.

All of these diagnoses are confirmed by palpation at the relevant sites around the knee. None is associated with joint effusions or other signs of synovitis.

Treatment

Rest and abstention from the associated physical activities for a period of days to weeks are essential. Once the acute pain from these conditions has subsided, a program of gentle stretching (particularly prior to resuming exercise) may prevent recurrence. Corticosteroid with lidocaine injections may be useful when intense discomfort is present, but caution must be employed when injecting corticosteroids into the region of a tendon.

5. MEDIAL MENISCUS INJURIES

Tears of the medial meniscus are the most common knee injuries encountered in primary care. Because the medial meniscus is firmly tethered to the underlying tibia, injuries to the medial meniscus occur ten times more commonly than injuries to the lateral meniscus. Both types of injury result from a twisting action exerted on the knee joint while the foot is in a weight-bearing position.

Clinical Findings

The injury is heralded by a tearing or popping sensation followed by severe pain. Occasionally, meniscal tears result from seemingly minor trauma. In contrast to ligamentous injuries, in which hemorrhage causes immediate swelling, effusions associated with meniscal injuries accumulate over hours and are typically worse on the day following the injury. Several days after resolution (full or partial), the patient may experience joint locking or instability, recurrent swelling with activity, and pain. The sensation of locking, which may result from mechanical blockage by a fragment of torn meniscus, more commonly results from "pseudolocking" caused by muscle spasm and swelling.

Joint effusion is usually present, frequently accompanied by a ballottable patella. Tenderness may be localized to the medial joint line, and range of motion in the knee may be restricted. In patients without an acutely painful, swollen knee, McMurray's test may suggest the diagnosis. This test is performed with the patient supine and the hip and knee in full flexion. The examiner has one hand on the involved knee and the other on the ipsilateral foot. As the foot is externally rotated, the examiner extends the patient's knee. The presence of a "snap" (palpable or audible) suggests a medial meniscus lesion. MRI is now the optimal test for confirming the diagnosis if plain films exclude other conditions.

Treatment

Initial management is conservative, with elevation of the joint and application of a compression dressing and ice. Weight bearing should be minimized for the first few days after the injury but may be resumed slowly thereafter. The patient should perform quadriceps-strengthening exercises under the instruction of a physical therapist. Surgery is reserved for patients with symptoms that recur upon resumption of normal activities or for patients with irreducible locking caused by mechanical problems.

6. ANKLE SPRAINS

Ankle sprains are among the most common of all sports injuries. Most sprains involve the lateral ligament complex, particularly the anterior talofibular ligament. In more severe injuries, the calcaneofibular ligament may also be involved. If both of these ligaments are ruptured, the injury results in significant joint instability and is classified as a grade III (severe) sprain. (Grades I and II correspond to mild and moderate injuries, respectively.) This section reviews only the type of ankle sprain resulting from inversion (varus) injuries, which account for 85% of all sprains.

Clinical Findings

Varus sprains include a spectrum of severity, ranging from slight loss of function to injuries in which the swelling is prompt, the pain prominent, and weight-bearing impossible. A history of hearing a "pop" at the time of injury is frequently associated with the latter.

Hemorrhage resulting from torn ligaments and damaged peroneal muscle tendons may cause substantial ecchymosis. Tenderness is typically present at the site of injury, and the associated swelling may be considerable. Stability of the anterior talofibular and calcaneofibular ligaments should be assessed with the "anterior drawer" sign: With the foot held in slight plantar flexion, the examiner cups the patient's heel with one hand and the patient's shin with the other. The examiner then applies gentle anterior force in the plane of the patient's foot. Excessive anterior motion of the foot constitutes a positive test (grade III sprain). Plain radiographs exclude associated bony injury.

Treatment

Most ankle sprains—even grade III sprains—usually are treated identically. The acronym "RICE" (rest, ice, compression, elevation) applies more accurately to ankle sprains than to any other injury. Early application of a compression dressing is essential to control swelling and provide stability to the traumatized joint. Weight bearing should be minimal, with liberal use of crutches. Elevation of the ankle for several days hastens functional recovery by diminishing pain and swelling, and ice is also helpful (alternating 30 minutes on, 30 minutes off). The ice should be applied on top of the compression dressing and not against the skin both because close apposition of the dressing to the skin is critical to control swelling and because direct application of ice is uncomfortable and even deleterious to the skin. Referral to a physical therapist may expedite recovery. Patients should be informed that symptoms from lateral ankle sprains may take weeks or months to resolve, and that this period will be prolonged by premature attempts to bear weight on the injured ankle. Surgical repairs of ruptured lateral ligaments provide excellent outcomes but are usually necessary only in cases of chronically unstable ankle joints.

7. PLANTAR FASCIITIS

The most common cause of foot pain in outpatient medicine is plantar fasciitis, which results from constant strain on the plantar fascia at its insertion into the medial tubercle of the calcaneus. Although certain inflammatory disorders such as the seronegative spondyloarthropathies predispose patients to enthesopathies, the majority of cases occur in patients with no associated disease. Most occur as the result of excessive standing and improper footwear.

Clinical Findings

Patients with plantar fasciitis report severe pain on the bottoms of their feet in the morning—the first steps out of bed in particular—but the pain subsides after a few minutes of ambulation.

The diagnosis may be confirmed by palpation over the plantar fascia's insertion on the medial heel. Radiographs have no role in the diagnosis of this condition—heel spurs frequently exist in patients without plantar fasciitis, and most symptomatic patients do not have heel spurs.

Treatment

Treatment consists of imposing an interval of days without prolonged standing and the use of arch supports. Arch supports give relief by requiring the arches to bear more of the patient's weight, thus unloading the plantar enthesis. NSAIDs may provide some relief. In severe cases, a corticosteroid with lidocaine injection (small volume—no more than a total of 1.5 mL) directly into the most tender area on the sole of the foot is helpful. Rare patients require release of the plantar fascia from its attachment site at the os calcis.

Anderson SJ: Evaluation and treatment of ankle sprains. Compr Ther 1996;22:30. [NLM Cit ID: 96233863] (Differential diagnosis of lateral sprains.)

Handy JR: Anserine bursitis: A brief review. South Med J 1997;90:376. [NLM Cit ID: 97269927] (Effectiveness of corticosteroid injections.)

Johnson RP: Anterior knee pain in adolescent and young adults. Curr Opin Rheumatol 1997;9:159. [NLM Cit ID: 97281614]

Speed CA et al: Calcific tendinitis of the shoulder. N Engl J Med 1999;340:1582. [NLM Cit ID: 99247682] (Concise review of the problem and an approach to therapy.)

Steinfeld R et al: A commonsense approach to shoulder problems. Mayo Clin Proc 1999;74:785. [NLM Cit ID: 99400534] (Well-written review of the anatomy, pathology, and differential diagnosis of common shoulder problems, directed at the primary care physician.)

AUTOIMMUNE DISEASES

The autoimmune disorders are a protean group of acquired diseases in which genetic factors appear to play a role. They have in common widespread immunologic and inflammatory alterations of connective tissue.

These illnesses share certain clinical features, and differentiation among them is often difficult because of this. Common findings include synovitis, pleuritis, myocarditis, endocarditis, pericarditis, peritonitis, vasculitis, myositis, skin rash, alterations of connective tissues, and nephritis. Laboratory tests may reveal Coombs-positive hemolytic anemia, thrombocytopenia, leukopenia, immunoglobulin excesses or deficiencies, antinuclear antibodies (which include antibodies to many nuclear constituents, including DNA and extractable nuclear antigen), rheumatoid factors, cryoglobulins, false-positive serologic tests for syphilis, elevated muscle enzymes, and alterations in serum complement.

Some of the laboratory alterations that occur in this group of diseases (eg, false-positive serologic tests for syphilis, rheumatoid factor) occur in asymptomatic individuals. These changes may also be demonstrated in certain asymptomatic relatives of patients with connective tissue diseases, in older persons, in patients using certain drugs, and in patients with chronic infectious diseases.

RHEUMATOID ARTHRITIS

Essentials of Diagnosis

- Prodromal systemic symptoms of malaise, fever, weight loss, and morning stiffness.
- Onset usually insidious and in small joints; progression is centripetal and symmetric; deformities common.
- Radiographic findings: juxta-articular osteoporosis, joint erosions, and narrowing of the joint spaces.
- Rheumatoid factor usually present.
- Extra-articular manifestations: subcutaneous nodules, pleural effusion, pericarditis, lymphadenopathy, splenomegaly with leukopenia, and vasculitis.

General Considerations

Rheumatoid arthritis is a chronic systemic inflammatory disease of unknown cause, chiefly affecting synovial membranes of multiple joints. The disease has a wide clinical spectrum with considerable variability in joint and extra-articular manifestations. The prevalence in the general population is 1–2%; female patients outnumber males almost 3:1. The usual age at onset is 20–40 years, although rheumatoid arthritis may begin at any age. Susceptibility to rheumatoid arthritis is genetically determined. Most patients have a class 2 human leukocyte antigen (HLA) with an identical five-amino-acid sequence. Although rheumatoid arthritis was once considered to be a relatively benign disorder that could be kept in check by slowly adding layers of treatment, it is now known to be a disease with such a strong tendency to shorten life and cause severe disability that early and aggressive treatment—often with drugs used in combination—has become the treatment of choice.

The pathologic findings in the joint include chronic synovitis with pannus formation. The pannus erodes cartilage, bone, ligaments, and tendons. In the acute phase, effusion and other manifestations of inflammation are common. In the late stage, organization may result in fibrous ankylosis; true bony ankylosis is rare. In both acute and chronic phases, inflammation of soft tissues around the joints may be prominent and is a significant factor in joint damage.

The microscopic findings most characteristic of rheumatoid arthritis are those of the subcutaneous nodule. This is a granuloma with a central zone of fibrinoid necrosis, a surrounding palisade of radially arranged elongated connective tissue cells, and a periphery of chronic granulation tissue. Pathologic alterations indistinguishable from those of the subcutaneous nodule are occasionally seen in the myocardium, pericardium, endocardium, heart valves, visceral pleura, lungs, sclera, dura mater, spleen, and larynx as well as in the synovial membrane, periarticular tissues, and tendons. Nonspecific pericarditis and pleuritis are found in 25–40% of patients at autopsy. Additional nonspecific lesions associated with rheumatoid arthritis include inflammation of small arteries, pulmonary fibrosis, mononuclear cell infiltration of skeletal muscle and perineurium, and hyperplasia of lymph nodes. Secondary amyloidosis may also be present.

Clinical Findings

A. Symptoms and Signs: The clinical manifestations of rheumatoid disease are highly variable. The onset of articular signs of inflammation is usually insidious, with prodromal symptoms of malaise, weight loss, and vague periarticular pain or stiffness. Less often, the onset is acute, apparently triggered by a stressful situation such as infection, surgery, trauma, emotional strain, or the postpartum period. There is characteristically symmetric joint swelling with associated stiffness, warmth, tenderness, and pain. Stiffness persisting for over 30 minutes is prominent in the morning and subsides during the day; its duration is a useful indicator of activity of disease. Stiffness may recur after daytime inactivity and may be much more severe after strenuous activity. Although any joint may be affected in rheumatoid arthritis, the proximal interphalangeal and metacarpophalangeal joints of the fingers as well as the wrists, knees, ankles, and toes are most often involved. Monarticular disease is occasionally seen early. Synovial cysts and rupture of tendons may occur. Entrapment syndromes are not unusual—particularly entrapment of the median nerve at the carpal tunnel of the wrist. Palmar erythema is noted occasionally, as are tiny hemorrhagic infarcts in the nail folds or finger pulps, which are signs of vasculitis. Twenty percent of patients have subcutaneous nodules, most commonly situated over bony prominences but also observed in the bursas and tendon sheaths; these nearly always occur in seropositive patients, as do most other extra-articular manifestations. A small number of patients have splenomegaly and lymph node enlargement. Low-grade fever, anorexia, weight loss, fatigue, and weakness often persist; chills are rare. After months or years, deformities may occur; the most common are ulnar deviation of the fingers, boutonnière deformity (hyperextension of the distal interphalangeal joint with flexion of the proximal interphalangeal joint), "swan-neck" deformity (flexion of the distal interphalangeal with extension of the proximal interphalangeal joint), and valgus deformity of the knee. Atrophy of skin or muscle is common. Dryness of the eyes, mouth, and other mucous membranes is found especially in advanced disease (see Sjögren's Syndrome). Other ocular manifestations include episcleritis and scleromalacia, often due to scleral nodules. Pericarditis and pleural disease, when present, are frequently silent clinically. Aortitis is a rare late complication that can result in aortic regurgitation or rupture and is usually associated with evidence of rheumatoid vasculitis elsewhere in the body.

B. Laboratory Findings: Serum protein abnormalities are often present. Rheumatoid factor, an IgM antibody directed against the Fc fragment of IgG, is present in the sera of more than 75% of patients. High titers of rheumatoid factor are commonly associated with severe rheumatoid disease. Titers may also be significantly elevated in a number of diverse conditions, including syphilis, sarcoidosis, infective endocarditis, tuberculosis, leprosy, and parasitic infections; in advanced age; and in asymptomatic relatives of patients with autoimmune diseases. Antinuclear antibodies are demonstrable in 20% of patients, though their titers are lower in rheumatoid arthritis than in systemic lupus erythematosus.

During both the acute and chronic phases, the erythrocyte sedimentation rate and the gamma globulins (most commonly IgM and IgG) are typically elevated. A moderate hypochromic normocytic anemia is common. The white cell count is normal or slightly elevated, but leukopenia may occur, often in the presence of splenomegaly (eg, Felty's syndrome). The platelet count is often elevated, roughly in proportion to the severity of overall joint inflammation. Joint fluid examination is valuable, reflecting abnormalities that are associated with varying degrees of inflammation. (See Tables 20–1 and 20–2.)

C. Imaging: Of all the laboratory tests, x-ray changes are the most specific for rheumatoid arthritis. X-rays, however, are not sensitive in that most of those taken during the first 6 months are read as normal. The earliest changes occur in the wrists or feet and consist of soft tissue swelling and juxta-articular demineralization. Later, diagnostic changes of uniform joint space narrowing and erosions develop. The erosions are often first evident at the ulnar styloid and at the juxta-articular margin, where the bony surface is not protected by cartilage. Diagnostic changes also occur in the cervical spine, with C1–2 subluxation, but these changes usually take several years to develop.

Differential Diagnosis

The differentiation of rheumatoid arthritis from other diseases of connective tissue can be difficult. However, certain clinical features are helpful. Rheumatic fever is characterized by the migratory nature of the arthritis, an elevated antistreptolysin titer, and a more dramatic and prompt response to aspirin; carditis and erythema marginatum may occur in adults, but chorea and subcutaneous nodules virtually never do. Butterfly rash, discoid lupus erythematosus, photosensitivity, alopecia, high titer to anti-DNA, renal disease, and central nervous system abnormalities point to the diagnosis of systemic lupus erythematosus. Degenerative joint disease (osteoarthritis) is not associated with constitutional manifestations, and the joint pain is characteristically relieved by rest, in contrast to the morning stiffness of rheumatoid arthritis. Signs of articular inflammation, prominent in rheumatoid arthritis, are usually minimal in degenerative joint disease. Osteoarthritis—in contrast to rheumatoid arthritis—spares the wrist and the metacarpophalangeal joints. While in the early years gouty arthritis is almost always intermittent and monarticular, in later years it can become a chronic polyarticular process that mimics rheumatoid arthritis. Gouty tophi can at times resemble rheumatoid nodules. The early history of intermittent monarthritis and the presence of synovial urate crystals are distinctive features of gout. Septic arthritis can be distinguished by chills and fever, demonstration of the causative organism in joint fluid, and the frequent presence of a primary focus elsewhere, eg, gonococcal arthritis. Septic arthritis can complicate rheumatoid arthritis and should be considered whenever a patient with rheumatoid arthritis has one joint inflamed out of proportion to the rest. Chronic Lyme disease typically involves only one joint, most commonly the knee, and is associated with positive serologic tests (see Chapter 34). Human parvovirus B19 infection in adults can occasionally mimic rheumatoid arthritis. The mean age at onset is 35–37; arthralgias are much more prominent than arthritis; and rash—on the cheeks, torso, or extremities—is common. The patients are rheumatoid factor-negative, do not have erosions, and have serologic evidence of recent human parvovirus B19 infection (ie, serum positive for anti-parvovirus B19 IgM antibody). Polymyalgia rheumatica occasionally causes polyarthritis in patients over age 50, but these patients remain rheumatoid factor-negative and have chiefly proximal muscle pain and stiffness. A variety of cancers produce paraneoplastic syndromes, including polyarthritis. One form is hypertrophic pulmonary osteoarthropathy most often produced by lung and gastrointestinal carcinomas, characterized by a rheumatoid-like arthritis associated with clubbing, periosteal new bone formation, and a negative rheumatoid factor. Diffuse swelling of the hands with palmar fasciitis has also been reported with a variety of cancers, especially ovarian carcinoma.

Treatment

A. Basic Program (Nonpharmacologic Management): The primary objectives in treating rheumatoid arthritis are reduction of inflammation and pain, preservation of function, and prevention of deformity. Patient satisfaction and the success of therapy depend on how effectively the clinician utilizes the nonpharmacologic measures outlined in the following paragraphs.

1. Education and emotional factors–The clinician should explain the disease, describe its fluctuations, and involve the patient in how decisions about therapy will be made. The concept of chronic disease control and empirical treatment employing different agents in series must be explained if the patient is to have confidence in the clinician. Education of the family is invaluable to the patient's long-term well-being.

2. Physical and occupational therapies– Physical and occupational therapists understand nonpharmacologic treatments of arthritis (described below) and can effectively teach them. The therapist can develop a program the patient can follow at home, with only periodic monitoring.

3. Systemic rest–The amount of systemic rest required depends upon the presence and severity of inflammation. Complete bed rest may be desirable in patients with profound systemic and articular inflammation, as can occur in rheumatoid arthritis, systemic lupus erythematosus, or psoriatic arthritis. With mild inflammation, 2 hours of rest each day may suffice. In general, rest should be continued until significant improvement is sustained for at least 2 weeks; thereafter, the program may be liberalized. However, the increase of physical activity must proceed gradually and with appropriate support for any involved weight-bearing joints.

4. Articular rest–Decrease of articular inflammation may be expedited by articular rest. Relaxation and stretching of the hip and knee muscles, to prevent flexion contractures, can be accomplished by having the patient lie in the prone position for 15 minutes several times daily. Sitting in a flexed position for prolonged periods is a poor form of joint rest. Appropriate adjustable supports provide rest for inflamed weight-bearing joints, relieve spasm, and may reduce deformities, soft tissue contracture, or instability of the ligaments. The supports must be removable to permit daily range of motion and exercise of the affected extremities (see below). When ambulation is started, care must be taken to avoid weight bearing, which may aggravate flexion deformities. This is accomplished with the aid of crutches or braces until the tendency toward contracture has subsided.

5. Exercise–Exercises are designed to preserve joint motion, muscular strength, and endurance. Initially, for inflammatory disease, passive range of motion and isometric exercises (such as straight leg raising) are best tolerated. The buoyancy of water permits maximum isotonic and isometric exercise with no more stress on joints than active range of motion exercises. Although ideal for arthritic patients, the cost of hydrotherapy often precludes its use. As tolerance for exercise increases and the activity of the disease subsides, progressive resistance exercises may be introduced. Patients should follow the general rule of eliminating any exercise that produces increased pain 1 hour after the exercise has ended.

6. Heat and cold–These are used primarily for their muscle-relaxing and analgesic effects. Radiant or moist heat is generally most satisfactory. The ambulatory patient will find warm tub baths convenient. Exercise may be better performed after exposure to heat. Some patients derive more relief of joint pain from local application of cold.

7. Assistive devices–Patients with significant hip or knee arthritis may benefit from having a raised toilet seat, a gripping bar, or a cane. Patients hold the cane in the hand opposite to the affected knee or hip, thus leaning away from the affected joint. Crutches or walkers may be needed for patients with more extensive disease.

8. Splints–Splints may provide joint rest, reduce pain, and prevent contracture, but certain principles should be adhered to.

a. Night splints of the hands or wrists (or both) should maintain the extremity in the position of optimum function. The elbow and shoulder lose motion so rapidly that other local measures and corticosteroid injections are usually preferable to splints.

b. The best "splint" for the hip is prone-lying for several hours a day on a firm bed. For the knee, prone-lying may suffice, but splints in maximum tolerated extension are frequently needed. Ankle splints are of the simple right-angle type.

c. Splints should be applied for the shortest period needed, should be made of lightweight materials for comfort, and should be easily removable for range-of-motion exercises once or twice daily to prevent loss of motion.

d. Corrective splints, such as those for overcoming knee flexion contractures, should be used under the guidance of a clinician familiar with their proper use.

Note: Avoidance of prolonged sitting or knee pillows may decrease the need for splints.

9. Weight loss–For overweight patients, achieving ideal body weight will reduce the wear and tear placed on arthritic joints of the lower extremities.

B. Nonsteroidal Anti-inflammatory Drugs (NSAIDs): The first drug used to treat rheumatoid arthritis is an NSAID. These agents have analgesic and anti-inflammatory effects but are believed not to be capable of preventing erosions or altering progression of the disease. A number of NSAIDs are available, including ibuprofen, fenoprofen, naproxen, tolmetin, sulindac, meclofenamate sodium, piroxicam, flurbiprofen, diclofenac, oxaprozin, nabumetone, etodolac, ketoprofen, celecoxib, and rofecoxib (see Table 1–11).

NSAIDs work in arthritis by the same mechanism that causes side effects: inhibition of cyclooxygenase, the enzyme that converts arachidonic acid to prostaglandins. Although prostaglandins play important roles in promoting inflammation and pain, they also help maintain homeostasis in several organs—especially the stomach, where prostaglandin E serves as a local hormone responsible for gastric mucosal cytoprotection. The discovery that cyclooxygenase (COX) exists in two isomers—COX-1 (which is expressed continuously in many cells and is responsible for the salutary effects of prostaglandins) and COX-2 (which is induced by cytokines and expressed in inflammatory tissues)—was initially of little practical consequence since all traditional NSAIDs inhibit both isomers. Recently, however, selective COX-2 inhibitors (celecoxib and rofecoxib) received FDA approval for the treatment of osteoarthritis. Celecoxib is also approved for rheumatoid arthritis. Short-term studies suggest that celecoxib has the efficacy of other NSAIDs in treating rheumatoid arthritis but—as would be expected given its COX-1-sparing effect—is less likely than traditional NSAIDs to cause endoscopically evident gastric ulcer. It is plausible but so far unproved that the reduced incidence of gastric ulcers with COX-2 inhibitors will translate into a reduced incidence of clinically important side effects such as gastrointestinal hemorrhage.

In terms of efficacy, all NSAIDs appear equivalent. Anecdotes more than data suggest that indomethacin is more effective than other NSAIDs for ankylosing spondylitis (see below). But for rheumatoid arthritis, no NSAID is convincingly more effective than another.

For traditional NSAIDs that inhibit both COX-1 and COX-2, gastrointestinal side effects, such as gastric ulceration, perforation, and gastrointestinal hemorrhage, are the most common serious side effects. The overall rate of bleeding with NSAID use is low (1:6000 users or less) but is increased by chronic use, concomitant corticosteroids or anticoagulants, the presence of rheumatoid arthritis, history of peptic ulcer disease or alcoholism, and age over 70. Approximately 25% of all hospitalizations and deaths from peptic ulcer disease result from traditional NSAID therapy. Some reports suggest that each year 1:1000 patients with rheumatoid arthritis will require hospitalization for NSAID-related gastrointestinal bleeding or perforation. Although all traditional NSAIDs can cause massive gastrointestinal bleeding, the risk may be higher with indomethacin and piroxicam, probably because these drugs preferentially inhibit COX-1 in the stomach.

There are two approaches to reducing the gastrointestinal toxicity of NSAIDs. One approach is to use a COX-2 inhibitor, either celecoxib (100–200 mg twice daily for rheumatoid arthritis or 100 mg twice daily for osteoarthritis) or rofecoxib (12.5–25 mg once daily for osteoarthritis). The other approach is to use a traditional NSAID and add either omeprazole 20 mg daily, famotidine 40 mg twice daily, or misoprostol. The expense of these medications dictates that their use should be reserved for patients with risk factors for NSAID-induced gastrointestinal toxicity (noted above). Carafate, antacids, and ranitidine either do not work or do not work as well as omeprazole. The efficacy of misoprostol is limited by its poor tolerance. For example, 20% of patients cannot tolerate the diarrhea and bloating associated with full doses (200 μg four times daily). Giving smaller amounts of misoprostol (eg, 100 μg four times daily) or using less frequent dosing (eg, 200 μg twice daily) improves tolerance while reducing efficacy only modestly. Misoprostol is an abortifacient and is contraindicated in patients who are or might become pregnant.

NSAIDs can also affect the lower intestinal tract, causing perforation or aggravating inflammatory bowel disease.

Acute liver injury from NSAIDs is rare, occurring in about one out of every 25,000 patients using these agents. Having rheumatoid arthritis or taking sulindac may increase the risk. Minor transient increases in aminotransferase levels do not predict risk for NSAID-associated hepatotoxicity.

All of the NSAIDs, including aspirin, can produce renal toxicity, resulting in interstitial nephritis, nephrotic syndrome, reversible renal failure, and aggravation of baseline hypertension. Hyperkalemia due to hyporeninemic hypoaldosteronism may also be seen. The risk of renal toxicity is low but is increased by age over 60, a history of renal disease, congestive heart failure, ascites, and diuretic use. Whether celecoxib has less renal toxicity than traditional NSAIDs is not yet established.

All NSAIDs except the nonacetylated salicylates and the COX-2 inhibitors interfere with platelet function and prolong bleeding time. For all older NSAIDs except aspirin, the effect on bleeding time resolves as the drug is cleared. Aspirin irreversibly inhibits platelet function, so the bleeding time effect resolves only as new platelets are made. Indomethacin is probably no more effective than the salicylates in rheumatoid arthritis, and its untoward effects are greater. Phenylbutazone is not advised for chronic therapy because of its toxicity.

Although groups of patients with rheumatoid arthritis respond similarly to NSAIDs, individuals may respond differently—an NSAID that works for one patient may not work for another. Thus, if the first NSAID chosen is not effective after 2–3 weeks of use, another should be tried.

C. Additional Drugs: If the patient fails to respond to the basic regimen with a reduction in morning stiffness, fatigue, and joint swelling, additional medications are added. They should be added early and used aggressively to maximize the chance of achieving a good outcome.

1. Methotrexate–Many now believe that methotrexate is the treatment of choice for patients with rheumatoid arthritis who fail to respond to NSAIDs. Methotrexate is generally well-tolerated and often produces a beneficial effect in 2–6 weeks—compared with the 2- to 6-month onset of action for drugs such as gold, penicillamine, and antimalarials. The usual initial dose is 7.5 mg of methotrexate orally once weekly. If the patient has tolerated methotrexate but has not responded in 1 month, the dose can be increased to 15 mg orally once per week. The maximal dose is approximately 20 mg/wk. The most frequent side effects are gastric irritation and stomatitis. If needed to minimize gastrointestinal toxicity, methotrexate can be administered by subcutaneous or intramuscular injection. A severe, potentially life-threatening interstitial pneumonitis occurs rarely and usually responds to cessation of the drug and institution of corticosteroids. Hepatotoxicity with fibrosis and cirrhosis is another important toxic effect of methotrexate that fortunately appears to be very rare, with a risk of approximately 1:1000 after 5 years of methotrexate therapy. Still, methotrexate is contraindicated in a patient with any form of chronic hepatitis. Diabetes, obesity, and renal disease appear to increase the risk of hepatotoxicity. Liver function tests should be monitored every 4–8 weeks, along with the CBC, serum creatinine, and serum albumin. Heavy alcohol use increases the hepatotoxicity, so patients should be advised not to drink. In a patient with no risk factors for hepatotoxicity, liver biopsy is not needed initially but is performed if aminotransferase levels are elevated, despite dosage reduction, in 6 out of 12 monthly determinations or if the serum albumin falls below normal. Cytopenia due to bone marrow suppression and infection are other important potential problems. The risk of developing cytopenia is much higher in patients with a serum creatinine of 2 mg/dL or higher. Side effects, including hepatotoxicity, may be reduced by prescribing either daily folate (1 mg) or weekly leucovorin calcium (2.5–5 mg taken 24 hours after the dose of methotrexate). To date, methotrexate has not been proved to increase the risk of malignancy. The combination of methotrexate and other folate antagonists, such as trimethoprim-sulfamethoxazole, should be used cautiously, since pancytopenia can result. Probenecid should also be avoided since it increases methotrexate drug levels and toxicity.

2. Tumor necrosis factors inhibitors–For years it has been hoped that biologic therapies with designer monoclonal antibodies and anticytokines would provide effective and more specific treatment for rheumatoid arthritis. Inhibitors of tumor necrosis factor (TNF) are at last fulfilling that hope and are now frequently added to the treatment of patients who have not responded adequately to methotrexate. TNF has been targeted because it is a cytokine that activates lymphocytes and leukocytes and is greatly increased in the synovial fluid of patients with rheumatoid arthritis. Two inhibitors of TNF have been released. The first is etanercept, a soluble recombinant TNF receptor:Fc fusion protein (administered at a dosage of 25 mg subcutaneously twice weekly). The second is infliximab, an anti-TNF antibody that is administered at a dosage of 3–10 mg/kg intravenously initially and then repeated after 2, 6, 10, and 14 weeks. Both drugs produce substantial improvement in over 60% of patients. Etanercept is very well tolerated, causing only minor irritation at injection sites. Infliximab is usually well tolerated but can cause anaphylaxis and can induce anti-DNA antibodies. Concomitant use of methotrexate appears to enhance the clinical response to infliximab and to prevent development of neutralizing antibodies to the drug (which is a hybrid human-mouse antibody). Because both drugs cost more than $10,000 per year, many insurers do not cover their cost unless the patient has a definite diagnosis of rheumatoid arthritis and has failed methotrexate.

3. Antimalarials–Hydroxychloroquine sulfate is the antimalarial agent most often used against rheumatoid arthritis. It should be reserved for patients with mild disease, since only 25–50% will respond and in some of those cases only after 3–6 months of therapy. The advantage of hydroxychloroquine is its comparatively low toxicity. A dosage of 200–400 mg/d minimizes the likelihood of toxic reactions. The most important reaction, pigmentary retinitis causing visual loss, is fortunately rare when the dosage is kept low. Ophthalmologic examinations every 6–12 months are required when this drug is employed for long-term therapy. Other reactions include neuropathies and myopathies of both skeletal and cardiac muscle, which usually improve when the drug is withdrawn.

4. Corticosteroids–Although corticosteroids usually produce an immediate and dramatic anti-inflammatory effect in rheumatoid arthritis, they do not alter the natural progression of the disease; furthermore, clinical manifestations of active disease commonly reappear when the drug is discontinued. The serious problem of untoward reactions resulting from prolonged corticosteroid therapy greatly limits its long-term use. Another disadvantage that might stem from the use of steroids lies in the tendency of the patient and the physician to neglect the less spectacular but proved benefits derived from general supportive treatment, physical therapy, and orthopedic measures.

Corticosteroids may be used on a short-term basis to tide patients over acute disabling episodes, to facilitate other treatment measures (eg, physical therapy), or to manage serious extra-articular manifestations (eg, pericarditis, perforating eye lesions). Corticosteroids may also be indicated for active and progressive disease that does not respond favorably to conservative management and when there are contraindications to or therapeutic failure of methotrexate, gold salts, or other disease-modifying agents.

The least amount of steroid that will achieve the desired clinical effect should be given, but not more than 10 mg of prednisone or equivalent per day is appropriate for articular disease. Many patients do reasonably well on 5–7.5 mg daily. (The use of 1 mg tablets is to be encouraged.) When the steroids are to be discontinued, they should be phased out gradually on a planned schedule appropriate to the duration of treatment. All patients receiving chronic corticosteroid therapy should take measures to prevent osteoporosis.

Intra-articular corticosteroids may be helpful if one or two joints are the chief source of difficulty. Intra-articular triamcinolone, 10–40 mg depending on the size of the joint to be injected, may be given for symptomatic relief, but no more often than four times a year.

5. Gold salts (chrysotherapy)–For patients who fail to improve on or who cannot tolerate methotrexate, treatment with gold salts may be effective. About 60% of patients may be expected to benefit from gold therapy, although complete remissions are uncommon. Their mode of action is not known.

a. Indications–Disease responding unfavorably to conservative management; erosive disease.

b. Contraindications–Previous gold toxicity; significant renal, hepatic, or hematopoietic dysfunction.

c. Preparations of choice–Intramuscular gold sodium thiomalate or aurothioglucose; oral auranofin. Intramuscular gold is used most often because it is more effective than oral gold.

d. Dosage–Intramuscular gold is given as a 10 mg test dose the first week and a 25 mg dose the second week before reaching the maintenance dose of 50 mg weekly, which is then continued (for up to 20 weeks) unless toxic reactions appear. If there is no response after 800 mg has been administered, the drug should be discontinued. If the response is good, a total dose of 1 g should be given, followed by a regimen of 50 mg every 2 weeks and, with continued improvement, every 3 and then every 4 weeks for an indefinite period.

The oral dose of auranofin is 3 mg twice daily until benefit or toxicity occurs.

e. Toxic reactions–About one-third of patients (range: 4–50%) experience toxic reactions to gold therapy; the mortality rate is less than 0.4%. The manifestations of toxicity are similar to those of poisoning by other heavy metals (notably arsenic) and include dermatitis (mild to exfoliative, and pruritic), stomatitis, neutropenia, proteinuria, and nitritoid reactions (especially to gold thiomalate and presumably due to its vehicle). Auranofin causes side effects less frequently than intramuscular gold, though diarrhea is common. In order to prevent or reduce the severity of toxic reactions, gold should not be given to patients with any of the contraindicating disorders listed above. Periodic urinalyses and complete blood counts should be obtained.

Severe toxicity may require corticosteroids for control, and failure to respond might then be an indication for the cautious use of penicillamine or dimercaprol (BAL) as chelating agents for the gold. Worsening of articular symptoms after the initial dose is often temporary and is not an indication for withdrawal of the drug. Patients so affected may ultimately respond favorably if treatment is continued.

6. Sulfasalazine–This drug has become established as a second-line agent for rheumatoid arthritis, with an efficacy similar to that of gold and penicillamine. Sulfasalazine is usually introduced at a dosage of 0.5 g twice daily and then increased each week by 0.5 g until the patient improves or the daily dose reaches 3 g. Side effects, particularly neutropenia and thrombocytopenia occur in 10–25% and are serious in 2–5%. Sulfasalazine also causes hemolysis in patients with glucose-6-phosphate dehydrogenase (G6PD) deficiency. Patients taking sulfasalazine should have complete blood counts monitored every 2–4 weeks for the first 3 months, then every 3 months.

7. Azathioprine–This agent, like methotrexate, is an antimetabolite that is effective for severe rheumatoid arthritis not responsive to gold or antimalarials. The usual initial dose is 1 mg/kg, gradually increased as needed to a maximum of 2.5–3 mg/kg. Its potential for severe toxicity, including immunosuppression complicated by opportunistic infection, restricts its use.

8. Penicillamine–Penicillamine is very rarely used nowadays. It is no more effective than gold and is more toxic. Careful monitoring for toxicity is essential.

9. Minocycline–Minocycline has been shown to be more effective than placebo for rheumatoid arthritis. This agent should be reserved for mild cases, since its efficacy is modest. The mechanism of action is not clear, but tetracyclines do have antiinflammatory properties, including the ability to inhibit destructive enzymes such as collagenase. The dose of minocycline is 200 mg/d. Adverse effects are uncommon except for dizziness, which occurs in about 10%.

10. Combination therapy–Combination therapy can be considered for patients who have failed to respond to individual agents. The combination of methotrexate, hydroxychloroquine, and sulfasalazine appears more effective than methotrexate alone. The combination of cyclosporine (2.5–5 mg/kg/d) plus methotrexate also appears more effective than methotrexate alone. However, regimens should be considered experimental until the long-term effects have been assessed.

D. Other Therapies: Leflunomide, a pyrimidine synthesis inhibitor, has also received FDA approval for treatment of rheumatoid arthritis. Leflunomide is begun at a dose of 100 mg/d for 3 days followed by a maintenance dose of 20 mg daily. The most frequent side effects are diarrhea, rash, reversible alopecia, and hepatotoxicity. The drug is carcinogenic, teratogenic, and has a half-life of 2 weeks. Thus, it is contraindicated in women who can get pregnant or in men who wish to father children.

The efficacy of removing rheumatoid factor by performing apheresis and passing the patient's plasma over a Prosorba column containing staphylococcal protein A (which binds rheumatoid factor) has been demonstrated in short-term studies.

Dietary modification, especially supplementation with n-3 fatty acids in doses of 2.5–3 g/d, has been helpful to some patients, as has oral administration of collagen from articular cartilage.

E. Surgical Measures: See below.

Course & Prognosis

Determining the best initial treatment is difficult because patients suspected of having rheumatoid arthritis can follow two widely divergent courses. Of all patients who present with polyarthritis that appears to be (but probably is not) rheumatoid arthritis, 50–75% experience remission within 2 years. These patients are often negative for rheumatoid factor, have good functional status even during disease activity, and are commonly seen in community practices but rarely in academic centers. Clearly, conservative therapy makes good sense for this patient population.

For patients whose joint symptoms persist beyond 2 years the outcome is not so favorable. Patients in this group die, on average, 10–15 years earlier than people without rheumatoid arthritis. In fact, for patients who have persistent symptoms and poor functional status, the mortality curve resembles that for stage IV Hodgkin's disease or triple-vessel coronary artery disease. The most common causes of death are infection, heart disease, respiratory failure, renal failure, and gastrointestinal disease. Factors that identify those at particular risk of early death include positive rheumatoid factor, poor functional status, more than 30 inflamed joints, and extra-articular manifestations (eg, rheumatoid lung disease). These patients, then, need aggressive therapy and probably need it early, since extensive bone damage can occur during the first 2 years.

Since some patients with polyarthritis will remit and others will sustain substantial damage within the first 2 years, a guidepost for early decisions about aggressive treatment is needed. Recent studies suggest that patients who have polyarthritis lasting more than 12 weeks are those at greatest risk of having persistent disease and are appropriate candidates for whom aggressive therapy should be considered. Although genetic risk factors for developing rheumatoid arthritis have been identified, it has not been possible in this way to consistently identify those patients needing aggressive therapy.

Feldman M et al: Do cyclooxygenase-2 inhibitors provide benefits similar to those of traditional nonsteroidal antiinflammatory drugs, with less gastrointestinal toxicity? Ann of Intern Med 2000;132:134. [NLM Cit ID: 20092386] (The early answer is, "Yes.")

Levy GD et al: Incidence of hydroxychloroquine retinopathy in 1,207 patients in a large multicenter outpatient practice. Arthritis Rheum 1997;40:1482. [NLM Cit ID: 97402365] (Retinal toxicity rare and did not occur when the hydroxychloroquine dose was less than 6.5 mg/kg/d.)

O'Dell JR et al: Treatment of rheumatoid arthritis with methotrexate alone, sulfasalazine and hydroxychloroquine, or a combination of all three medications. N Engl J Med 1996;334:1287. [NLM Cit ID: 96200568] (Combination therapy with methotrexate, sulfasalazine, and hydroxychloroquine is more effective than either methotrexate alone or a combination of sulfasalazine and hydroxychloroquine.)

Taha AS et al: Famotidine for the prevention of gastric and duodenal ulcers caused by nonsteroidal antiinflammatory drugs. N Engl J Med 1996;334:1435. [NLM Cit ID: 96218827] (Famotidine 40 mg orally twice daily significantly reduces the risk of ulcers caused by NSAIDs.)

van der Heide A et al: The effectiveness of early treatment with "second-line" antirheumatic drugs: A randomized, controlled trial. Ann Intern Med 1996;124:699. [NLM Cit ID: 96213850] (Compared with delayed use of second-line agents, early and aggressive treatment improves disability, pain, joint score, and ESR—but not x-ray findings—after 1 year.)

Weinblatt ME et al: A trial of etanercept, a recombinant tumor necrosis factor receptor:Fc fusion protein, in patients with rheumatoid arthritis receiving methotrexate. N Engl J Med 1999;340:253. [NLM Cit ID: 99110540] (Over 70% of patients responded.)

Wolfe MM et al: Gastrointestinal toxicity of nonsteroidal antiinflammatory drugs. N Engl J Med 1999;340:1888. [NLM Cit ID: 99280043] (Extensive review.)

ADULT STILL'S DISEASE

Still's disease is considered a variant of rheumatoid arthritis in which high spiking fevers are much more prominent, especially at the outset, than arthritis. This syndrome also occurs in adults. Most adults are in their 20s or 30s, and onset after age 60 is rare. The fever is dramatic, often spiking to 40 °C, associated with sweats and chills, and then plunging to several degrees below normal. Many patients initially complain of sore throat. An evanescent salmon-colored nonpruritic rash, chiefly on the chest and abdomen, is a characteristic feature. However, the rash can easily be missed since it often appears only with the fever spike. Many patients also have lymphadenopathy and pericardial effusions. Joint symptoms are mild or absent in the beginning, but a destructive arthritis, especially of the wrists, may develop months later. Anemia and leukocytosis, with white blood counts sometimes exceeding 40,000/μL, are the rule. Although the diagnosis requires exclusion of other causes of fever, the diagnosis of adult Still's disease is strongly suggested by the fever pattern, sore throat, and the classic rash. About half of the patients respond to high-dose aspirin (eg, 1 g three times daily) or other NSAIDs, and half require prednisone, sometimes in doses greater than 60 mg/d. About one-third of patients have recurrent episodes.

Fautrel B et al: Corticosteroid sparing effect of low dose methotrexate treatment in adult Still's disease. J Rheumatol 1999;26:373. [NLM Cit ID: 99137257] (Methotrexate is an effective second-line drug.)

Nguyen KHY et al: Severe sore throat as a presenting symptom of adult-onset Still's disease: A case series and review of the literature. J Rheumatol 1997;24:592. [NLM Cit ID: 97211705] (Sixty-nine percent of patients with Still's disease present with sore throat.)

SYSTEMIC LUPUS ERYTHEMATOSUS

Essentials of Diagnosis

- Occurs mainly in young women.
- Rash over areas exposed to sunlight.
- Joint symptoms in 90% of patients. Multiple system involvement.
- Depression of hemoglobin, white blood cells, platelets.
- Serologic findings: antinuclear antibody with high titer to native DNA.

General Considerations

Systemic lupus erythematosus (SLE) is an inflammatory autoimmune disorder that may affect multiple organ systems. Many of its clinical manifestations are secondary to the trapping of antigen-antibody complexes in capillaries of visceral structures or to autoantibody-mediated destruction of host cells (eg, thrombocytopenia). The clinical course is marked by spontaneous remission and relapses. The severity may vary from a mild episodic disorder to a rapidly fulminant, life-threatening illness.

The prevalence of SLE is influenced by many factors, including gender, race, and genetic inheritance. About 85% of patients are women. Sex hormones appear to play some role, since most cases develop after menarche and before menopause. Among the patients who develop SLE during childhood or after the age of 50, the gender distribution is more equal. Race is also a factor, as SLE occurs in 1:1000 white women but in 1:250 black women. Familial occurrence of SLE has been repeatedly documented, and the disorder is concordant in 25–70% of identical twins. If a mother has SLE, her daughters' risk of developing the disease is 1:40 and her sons' risk is 1:250. Aggregation of serologic abnormalities (positive antinuclear antibody) is seen in asymptomatic family members, and the prevalence of other rheumatic diseases is increased among close relatives of patients. The importance of specific genes in SLE is emphasized by the high frequency of certain HLA haplotypes, especially DR2 and DR3, and null complement alleles.

Before making a diagnosis of SLE, it is imperative to ascertain that the condition has not been induced by a drug. A host of pharmacologic agents have been implicated as causing a lupus-like syndrome, but only a few cause the disorder with appreciable frequency (Table 20–8). Procainamide, hydralazine, and isoniazid are the best-studied drugs. While antinuclear antibody tests and other serologic findings become positive in many persons receiving these agents, clinical manifestations occur in only a few.

Table 20–8. Drugs associated with lupus erythematosus.[1]

Definite association	
Chlorpromazine	Methyldopa
Hydralazine	Procainamide
Isoniazid	Quinidine
Possible association	
Beta-blockers	Methimazole
Captopril	Nitrofurantoin
Carbamazepine	Penicillamine
Cimetidine	Phenytoin
Ethosuximide	Propylthiouracil
Hydrazines	Sulfasalazine
Levodopa	Sulfonamides
Lithium	Trimethadione
Unlikely association	
Allopurinol	Penicillin
Chlorthalidone	Phenylbutazone
Gold salts	Reserpine
Griseofulvin	Streptomycin
Methysergide	Tetracyclines
Oral contraceptives	

[1]Modified and reproduced, with permission, from Hess EV, Mongey AB: Drug-related lupus. Bull Rheum Dis 1991;40:1.

Four features of drug-induced lupus separate it from SLE: (1) the sex ratio is nearly equal; (2) nephritis and central nervous system features are not ordinarily present; (3) hypocomplementemia and antibodies to native DNA are absent; and (4) the clinical features and most laboratory abnormalities often revert toward normal when the offending drug is withdrawn.

The diagnosis of SLE should be suspected in patients having a multisystem disease with serologic positivity (eg, antinuclear antibody, false-positive serologic test for syphilis). Differential diagnosis includes rheumatoid arthritis, vasculitis, scleroderma, chronic active hepatitis, acute drug reactions, polyarteritis, and drug-induced lupus.

The diagnosis of SLE can be made with reasonable probability if 4 of the 11 criteria set forth in Table 20–9 are met. These criteria should be viewed as rough guidelines that do not supplant clinical judgment in the diagnosis of SLE.

Clinical Findings

A. Symptoms and Signs: The systemic features include fever, anorexia, malaise, and weight loss. Most patients have skin lesions at some time; the characteristic "butterfly" rash affects fewer than half of patients. Other cutaneous manifestations are discoid lupus, typical fingertip lesions, periungual erythema, nail fold infarcts, and splinter hemorrhages. Alopecia is common. Mucous membrane lesions tend to occur during periods of exacerbation. Raynaud's phenomenon, present in about 20% of patients, often antedates other features of the disease.

Table 20–9. Criteria for the classification of SLE.[1] (A patient is classified as having SLE if any 4 or more of 11 criteria are met.)

1. Malar rash
2. Discoid rash
3. Photosensitivity
4. Oral ulcers
5. Arthritis
6. Serositis
7. Renal disease
   a. > 0.5 g/d proteinuria, or—
   b. ≥ 3+ dipstick proteinuria, or—
   c. Cellular casts
8. Neurologic disease
   a. Seizures, or—
   b. Psychosis (without other cause)
9. Hematologic disorders
   a. Hemolytic anemia, or—
   b. Leukopenia (< 4000/μL), or—
   c. Lymphopenia (< 1500/μL), or—
   d. Thrombocytopenia (< 100,000/μL)
10. Immunologic abnormalities
   a. Positive LE cell preparation, or—
   b. Antibody to native DNA, or—
   c. Antibody to Sm, or—
   d. False-positive serologic test for syphilis
11. Positive antinuclear antibody (ANA)

[1]Modified and reproduced, with permission, from Tan EM et al: The 1982 revised criteria for the classification of systemic lupus erythematosus. Arthritis Rheum 1982;25:1271.

Joint symptoms, with or without active synovitis, occur in over 90% of patients and are often the earliest manifestation. The arthritis is seldom deforming; erosive changes are almost never noted on radiographs. Subcutaneous nodules are rare.

Ocular manifestations include conjunctivitis, photophobia, transient or permanent monocular blindness, and blurring of vision. Cotton-wool spots on the retina (cytoid bodies) represent degeneration of nerve fibers due to occlusion of retinal blood vessels.

Pleurisy, pleural effusion, bronchopneumonia, and pneumonitis are frequent. Restrictive lung disease is often demonstrated.

The pericardium is affected in the majority of patients. Cardiac failure may result from myocarditis and hypertension. Cardiac arrhythmias are common. Atypical verrucous endocarditis of Libman-Sacks is usually clinically silent but occasionally can produce acute or chronic valvular incompetence—most commonly mitral regurgitation—and can serve as a source of emboli.

Mesenteric vasculitis occasionally occurs in SLE and may closely resemble polyarteritis nodosa, including the presence of aneurysms in medium-sized blood vessels. Abdominal pain (particularly postprandial), ileus, peritonitis, and perforation may result.

Neurologic complications of SLE include psychosis, organic brain syndrome, seizures, peripheral and cranial neuropathies, transverse myelitis, and strokes. Severe depression and psychosis are sometimes exacerbated by the administration of large doses of corticosteroids.

Several forms of glomerulonephritis may occur, including mesangial, focal proliferative, diffuse proliferative, and membranous (see Chapter 22). Some patients may also have interstitial nephritis. With appropriate therapy, the survival rate even for patients with serious renal disease (proliferative glomerulonephritis) is favorable.

Other clinical features include arterial and venous thrombosis, lymphadenopathy, splenomegaly, Hashimoto's thyroiditis, hemolytic anemia, and thrombocytopenic purpura.

B. Laboratory Findings: (Tables 20–10 and 20–11.) SLE is characterized by the production of many different autoantibodies, some of which produce specific laboratory abnormalities (eg, hemolytic anemia). Antinuclear antibody tests are sensitive but not specific for systemic lupus—ie, they are positive in virtually all patients with lupus but are positive also in many patients with nonlupus conditions such as rheumatoid arthritis, various forms of hepatitis, and interstitial lung disease. Antibodies to double-stranded DNA and to Sm are specific for systemic lupus but not sensitive, since they are present in only

Table 20–10. Frequency (%) of autoantibodies in rheumatic diseases.

	ANA	Anti-Native DNA	Rheumatoid Factor	Anti-Sm	Anti-SS-A	Anti-SS-B	Anti-SCL-70	Anti-Centromere	Anti-Jo-1	ANCA
Rheumatoid arthritis	30–60	0–5	72–85	0	0–5	0–2	0	0	0	0
Systemic lupus erythematosus	95–100	60	20	10–25	15–20	5–20	0	0	0	0–1
Sjögren's syndrome	95	0	75	0	60–70	60–70	0	0	0	0
Diffuse scleroderma	80–95	0	25–33	0	0	0	1	1	0	0
Limited scleroderma (CREST syndrome)	80–95	0	25–33	0	0	0	50	50	0	0
Polymyositis/dermatomyositis	80–95	0	33	0	0	0	0	0	20–30	0
Wegener's granulomatosis	0–15	0	50	0	0	0	0	0	0	93–96[1]

ANA = antinuclear antibodies; ANCA = anti-neutrophil cytoplasmic antibody.
[1]Frequency for generalized, active disease.

60% and 30% of patients, respectively. Depressed serum complement—a finding suggestive of disease activity—often returns toward normal in remission. Anti-double-stranded DNA antibody levels also correlate with disease activity; anti-Sm levels do not.

Three types of antiphospholipid antibodies occur (Table 20–11). The first causes the biologic false-positive tests for syphilis; the second is the lupus anticoagulant, which despite its name is a risk factor for venous and arterial thrombosis and miscarriage. It is most commonly identified by prolongation of the activated partial thromboplastin time, an in vitro phenomenon related to antibody reacting to phospholipid in the test materials. Anticardiolipin antibodies are the third type of antiphospholipid antibodies. In many cases, the "anticardiolipin antibody" appears to be directed at a serum cofactor (β_2-glycoprotein-I) rather than at phospholipid itself. A primary **antiphospholipid antibody syndrome** is diagnosed in patients who have recurrent venous or arterial occlusions, recurrent fetal loss, or thrombocytopenia in the presence of antiphospholipid antibodies but without features of SLE. Livedo reticularis, skin ulcers, mental status changes, and mitral regurgitation are also noted.

Table 20–11. Frequency of laboratory abnormalities in systemic lupus erythematosus.[1]

Anemia	60%
Leukopenia	45%
Thrombocytopenia	30%
Biologic false-positive tests for syphilis	25%
Lupus anticoagulant	7%
Anti-cardiolipin antibody	25%
Direct Coombs-positive	30%
Proteinuria	30%
Hematuria	30%
Hypocomplementemia	60%
ANA	95–100%
Anti-native DNA	50%
Anti-Sm	20%

[1]Modified and reproduced, with permission, from Hochberg MC et al: Systemic lupus erythematosus: A review of clinicolaboratory features and immunologic matches in 150 patients with emphasis on demographic subsets. Medicine 1985; 64:285.

Abnormality of urinary sediment is almost always found in association with renal lesions. Showers of red blood cells, with or without casts, and mild proteinuria are frequent during exacerbation of the disease; these usually abate with remission.

Treatment

Some patients with SLE have a benign form of the disease requiring only supportive care and need little or no medication. Emotional support, as described for rheumatoid arthritis, is especially important for patients with lupus. Patients with photosensitivity should be cautioned against sun exposure and should apply a protective lotion to the skin while out of doors. Skin lesions often respond to the local administration of corticosteroids. Minor joint symptoms can usually be alleviated by rest and NSAIDs. Every drug that may have precipitated the condition should be withdrawn if possible.

Antimalarials (hydroxychloroquine) may be helpful in treating lupus rashes or joint symptoms that do not respond to NSAIDs. When these are used, the dose should not exceed 400 mg/d, and biannual monitoring for retinal changes is recommended. Drug-induced neuropathy and myopathy may be erroneously ascribed to the underlying disease.

Corticosteroids are required for the control of certain serious complications. These include thrombocytopenic purpura, hemolytic anemia, myocarditis, pericarditis, convulsions, and nephritis. Forty to 60 mg of prednisone is often needed initially; however, the lowest dose of corticosteroid that controls the condition should be employed. Central nervous system lupus may require higher doses of corticosteroids than are usually given; however, steroid psychosis may mimic lupus cerebritis, in which case reduced doses are appropriate. In lupus nephritis, sequential studies of serum complement and antibodies to DNA often permit early detection of disease exacerbation and thus prompt increase in corticosteroid therapy. Such studies also allow for lowering the dosage of the drugs and withdrawing them when they are no longer needed. Immunosuppressive agents such as cyclophosphamide, chlorambucil, and azathioprine are used in cases resistant to corticosteroids. The exact role of immunosuppressive agents is controversial. Cyclophosphamide improves renal survival. Overall patient survival, however, is no better than in the prednisone-treated group. Very close follow-up is needed to watch for potential side effects when immunosuppressants are employed; these agents should be given by physicians experienced in their use. The androgenic steroid danazol may be effective therapy for thrombocytopenia not responsive to corticosteroids. Dehydroepiandrosterone (DHEA) appears to have a therapeutic role comparable to that of the antimalarial agents in the treatment of SLE, but its side effects (particularly acne) may be troubling to some patients. Anticoagulation, most commonly with warfarin to achieve an INR > 3, is prescribed for patients who have antiphospholipid antibodies and clotting of the arterial or venous systems. Systemic steroids are not usually given for minor arthritis, skin rash, leukopenia, or the anemia associated with chronic disease. Positive serologic findings in asymptomatic patients are not an indication for treatment.

Course & Prognosis

The prognosis for patients with systemic lupus appears to be considerably better than older reports implied. From both community settings and university centers, 10-year survival rates exceeding 85% are routine. In most patients, the illness pursues a relapsing and remitting course. Corticosteroids, often needed in doses of 40 mg/d or more during severe flares, can usually be tapered to low doses (10–15 mg/d) during disease inactivity. However, there are some in whom the disease pursues a virulent course, leading to serious impairment of vital structures such as lung, heart, brain, or kidneys, and the disease may lead to death. With improved control of lupus activity and with increasing use of corticosteroids and immunosuppressive drugs, the mortality and morbidity patterns in lupus have changed. Infections—especially with opportunistic organisms—have become the leading cause of death, followed by active SLE, chiefly due to renal or central nervous system disease. Although such manifestations are more likely to be seen in the early phases of the illness, one must be alert to the possibility of their occurrence at any time. Accelerated atherosclerosis attributed, in part, to corticosteroid use, has been responsible for a rise in late deaths due to myocardial infarction. With more patients living longer, it has become evident that avascular necrosis of bone, affecting most commonly the hips and knees, is responsible for substantial morbidity. Still, it must be emphasized that the outlook for most patients with SLE has become increasingly favorable.

American College of Rheumatology Ad Hoc Committee on Systemic Lupus Erythematosus Guidelines: Guidelines for referral and management of systemic lupus erythematosus in adults. Arthritis Rheum 1999;42:1785. [NLM Cit ID: 99441949] (Useful algorithm for the diagnosis, referral, and treatment of SLE, with discussion of difficult clinical questions such as when to perform renal biopsy.)

Gomez-Pacheco L et al: Serum anti-beta$_2$-glycoprotein I anticardiolipin antibodies during thrombosis in systemic lupus erythematosus patients. Am J Med 1999;106:417. [NLM Cit ID: 99239750] (Beta$_2$-glycoprotein-I antibodies are strongly associated with thrombosis in SLE.)

Pisetsky DS et al: Systemic lupus erythematosus: Diagnosis and treatment. Med Clin North Am 1997;81:113. [NLM Cit ID: 97164995] (Comprehensive review of the topic.)

Tan EM et al: Range of antinuclear antibodies in "healthy" individuals. Arthritis Rheum 1997;40:1601. [NLM Cit ID: 97464193] (Frequency of positive ANA in normal people was 31.7% at 1:40 serum dilution, 13.3% at 1:80, 5% at 1:160, and 3.3% at 1:320. Age did not influence the positive rate.)

Wilson WA et al: International consensus statement on preliminary classification criteria for definite antiphospholipid syndrome: report of an international workshop. Arthritis Rheum 1999;42:1309. [NLM Cit ID: 99330050] (Concise discussion of the clinical and laboratory criteria for the diagnosis of antiphospholipid syndrome.)

SYSTEMIC SCLEROSIS (Scleroderma; SSc)

Essentials of Diagnosis

- Diffuse thickening of skin, with telangiectasia and areas of increased pigmentation and depigmentation.
- Raynaud's phenomenon in 90% of patients.
- Systemic features of dysphagia, hypomotility of gastrointestinal tract, pulmonary fibrosis, and cardiac and renal involvement.
- Positive test for antinuclear antibodies nearly universal.

General Considerations

Systemic sclerosis is a chronic disorder characterized by diffuse fibrosis of the skin and internal organs. The causes of systemic sclerosis are not known, but autoimmunity, fibroblast dysregulation, graft-versus-host disease from fetal lymphocytes retained in the maternal circulation, and occupational exposure to silica have been implicated. Symptoms usually appear in the third to fifth decades, and women are affected two to three times as frequently as men.

Two forms of systemic sclerosis are generally recognized: limited (80% of patients) and diffuse (20%).

Two bedside clues help distinguish the two subsets. First, in the CREST syndrome, hardening of the skin (scleroderma) is limited to the face and hands, whereas in diffuse scleroderma the skin changes also involve the trunk and proximal extremities. Second, tendon friction rubs, especially frequent over the wrists, ankles, and knees, occur uniquely (but not universally) in diffuse scleroderma. Patients with CREST syndrome have a much better prognosis than those with diffuse disease, in large part because patients with limited disease do not develop renal failure or interstitial lung disease. Curiously, patients with limited disease are more liable to develop digital ischemia and pulmonary hypertension. Gastrointestinal and cardiac disease also tend to be more severe and more rapidly progressive in diffuse scleroderma.

Clinical Findings

A. Symptoms and Signs: Most frequently, the disease makes its appearance in the skin, although visceral involvement may precede cutaneous alteration. Polyarthralgia and Raynaud's phenomenon (present in 90% of patients) are early manifestations. Subcutaneous edema, fever, and malaise are common. With time the skin becomes thickened and hidebound, with loss of normal folds. Telangiectasia, pigmentation, and depigmentation are characteristic. Ulceration about the fingertips and subcutaneous calcification are seen. Dysphagia due to esophageal dysfunction is common and results from abnormalities in motility and later from fibrosis. Fibrosis and atrophy of the gastrointestinal tract cause hypomotility, and malabsorption results from bacterial overgrowth. Large-mouthed diverticula occur in the jejunum, ileum, and colon. Diffuse pulmonary fibrosis and pulmonary vascular disease are reflected in low diffusing capacity and decreased lung compliance. Cardiac abnormalities include pericarditis, heart block, myocardial fibrosis, and right heart failure secondary to pulmonary hypertension. Systemic sclerosis renal crisis, resulting from obstruction of smaller renal blood vessels, indicates a grave prognosis.

B. Laboratory Findings: Mild anemia is often present, and it is occasionally hemolytic because of mechanical damage to red cells from diseased small vessels. Elevation of the sedimentation rate is unusual. Proteinuria and cylindruria appear in association with renal involvement. Antinuclear antibody tests are nearly always positive, frequently in high titers (Table 20–9). The scleroderma antibody (SCL-70) directed against topoisomerase III is found in one-third of patients with diffuse systemic sclerosis and in 20% of those with CREST syndrome; an anticentromere antibody is seen in 50% of those with CREST syndrome and in 1% of individuals with diffuse systemic sclerosis (Table 20–9). Although present in only a minority of patients with diffuse systemic sclerosis, anti-Scl-70 antibodies may portend a poor prognosis, with a high likelihood of serious internal organ involvement (eg, interstitial lung disease). Anticentromere antibodies are highly specific for limited systemic sclerosis, but they also occur occasionally in overlap syndromes.

Differential Diagnosis

Several conditions classified as "localized" sclerosis may mimic systemic morphea and limited systemic sclerosis. These disorders are generally limited to the skin (typically in a localized fashion) and are associated with excellent prognoses. Linear scleroderma is occasionally associated with atrophy of underlying muscle and bone and may cause deformities that are both cosmetically and functionally disabling.

Eosinophilic fasciitis is a rare disorder presenting with skin changes that resemble diffuse systemic sclerosis. The inflammatory abnormalities, however, are limited to the fascia rather than the dermis and epidermis. Patients with eosinophilic fasciitis are further distinguished from those with systemic scleroderma by the presence of peripheral blood eosinophilia, the absence of Raynaud's phenomenon, the good response to prednisone, and an increased risk of developing aplastic anemia.

The eosinophilia-myalgia syndrome was first noted in patients who ingested tryptophan, an essential amino acid that was sold as an over-the-counter remedy for insomnia and premenstrual symptoms—until banned by the Food and Drug Administration. Weeks to months after beginning ingestion, affected patients developed a syndrome of severe generalized myalgias, and cutaneous abnormalities ranging from hives to generalized swelling and induration of the arms and legs. Peripheral eosinophilia (> 1000/μL) is characteristic. Other common clinical manifestations have included pulmonary symptoms, fever, myopathy, lymphadenopathy, and ascending polyneuropathy. Besides eosinophilia, laboratory features include mild elevations of aldolase with normal creatine kinase levels and, frequently, positive ANA tests. Full-thickness biopsies may reveal features of systemic sclerosis, evidence of fasciitis or myositis, or small vessel vasculitis. While some patients improve after discontinuing tryptophan, others progress and require corticosteroid therapy, which is not always effective. Deaths have been reported, especially from neurologic involvement. Patients presenting with systemic sclerosis or an eosinophilic fasciitis-like syndrome should be asked about tryptophan use.

Case reports have suggested that silicone breast implants can cause scleroderma or other rheumatic diseases, including SLE and undifferentiated autoimmune diseases. Population studies have failed to detect a link between silicone breast implants and any defined rheumatic disease.

Treatment

Treatment of systemic sclerosis is symptomatic and supportive. Severe Raynaud's syndrome may respond to calcium channel blockers, eg, long-acting nifedipine, 30–120 mg/d, or to losartan, 50 mg/d. Intravenous iloprost, a prostacyclin analog that causes vasodilation and platelet inhibition, is moderately effective in healing digital ulcers. Patients with esophageal disease should take medications in liquid or crushed form. Esophageal reflux can be reduced and scarring prevented by avoiding late-night meals, elevating the head of the bed, and using antacids and H_2 blockers. Proton pump inhibitors (eg, omeprazole, 20–40 mg/d) are the only drugs that achieve near-complete inhibition of gastric acid production, and they are remarkably effective for refractory esophagitis. Patients with delayed gastric emptying maintain their weight better if they eat small, frequent meals and remain upright for at least 2 hours after eating. Prokinetic drugs (eg, cisapride) infrequently produce a meaningful improvement in gastric emptying and are ineffective in promoting esophageal emptying. Octreotide, a somatostatin analog, has helped a few patients with bacterial overgrowth and pseudo-obstruction. Malabsorption due to bacterial overgrowth also responds to antibiotics, eg, tetracycline, 500 mg four times daily. The hypertensive crises associated with systemic sclerosis renal crisis must be treated early and aggressively (in the hospital) with angiotensin-converting enzyme inhibitors, eg, captopril, 37.5–75 mg/d in three divided doses. Prednisone has little or no role in the treatment of scleroderma. Cyclophosphamide, a drug with many important side effects, may improve severe interstitial lung disease.

The prognosis tends to be worse in blacks, in males, and in older patients. In most cases, death results from renal, cardiac, or pulmonary failure. Breast and lung cancer may be more common in patients with scleroderma.

Bryan C et al: Prediction of five-year survival following presentation with scleroderma. Arthritis Rheum 1999;42:2660. [NLM Cit ID: 20081761] (Proteinuria > trace, ESR ≥ 25 mm/h, and D_LCO < 70% independently predict increased risk of death.)

Dziadzio M et al: Losartan therapy for Raynaud's phenomenon and scleroderma. Arthritis Rheum 1999;42:2646. [NLM Cit ID: 20081759] (Losartan 50 mg/d works better in primary Raynaud's than in scleroderma.)

Yee AM et al: Adventitial stripping: a digit saving procedure in refractory Raynaud's phenomenon. J Rheumatol 1998;25:269. [NLM Cit ID: 98149462] (Digital sympathectomy and stripping of the adventitia of digital arteries improved ischemia long-term.)

IDIOPATHIC INFLAMMATORY MYOPATHIES (Polymyositis & Dermatomyositis)

Essentials of Diagnosis

- Bilateral proximal muscle weakness.
- Characteristic cutaneous manifestations in dermatomyositis (Gottron's papules, heliotrope rash).
- Diagnostic tests: elevated creatine kinase and other muscle enzymes, muscle biopsy, electromyography.
- Increased risk of malignancy, particularly in adult dermatomyositis.

General Considerations

Polymyositis and dermatomyositis are systemic disorders of unknown cause whose principal manifestation is muscle weakness. Although their clinical presentations (aside from the presence of certain skin findings in dermatomyositis, some of which are pathognomonic) and treatments are similar, the two diseases are pathologically quite distinct. They affect persons of any age group, but the peak incidence is in the fifth and sixth decades of life. Women are affected twice as commonly as men, and the diseases (particularly polymyositis) also occur more often among blacks than whites. There is an increased risk of malignancy, particularly in adult patients with dermatomyositis. Indeed, up to one patient in four with dermatomyositis has an occult malignancy. Malignancies may be evident at the time of presentation with the muscle disease but may not be detected until months afterward in some cases. Some patients with dermatomyositis have skin disease without overt muscle involvement, a condition termed "dermatomyositis sine myositis."

Clinical Findings

A. Symptoms and Signs: Polymyositis may begin abruptly, but the usual presentation is one of gradual and progressive muscle weakness. The weakness chiefly involves proximal muscle groups of the upper and lower extremities as well as the neck. Leg weakness (eg, difficulty in rising from a chair or climbing stairs) typically precedes arm symptoms. Pain and tenderness of affected muscles occur in one-fourth of cases, but these are rarely the chief complaints. Muscle atrophy and contractures occur as late complications of advanced disease. Clinically significant myocarditis is uncommon even though there is often CK-MB elevation.

In dermatomyositis, the characteristic rash is dusky red and may appear in malar distribution mimicking the classic rash of SLE. Erythema also occurs over other areas of the face, neck, shoulders, and upper chest and back ("shawl sign"). Periorbital edema and a purplish (heliotrope) suffusion over the eyelids are typical signs. Periungual erythema, dilations of nailbed capillaries, and scaly patches over the dorsum of proximal interphalangeal and metacarpophalangeal joints (Gottron's sign) are highly suggestive.

A subset of patients with polymyositis and dermatomyositis develop the "antisynthetase syndrome," a group of findings including inflammatory arthritis, Raynaud's phenomenon, interstitial lung disease, and often severe muscle disease that is associated with certain autoantibodies (eg, anti-Jo1 antibodies).

B. Laboratory Findings: Measurement of serum levels of muscle enzymes, especially creatine phosphokinase and aldolase, is most useful in diagnosis and in assessment of disease activity. Anemia is uncommon. The sedimentation rate is not appreciably elevated in half of the patients. Rheumatoid factor is found in a minority of patients. Antinuclear antibodies are present in many patients, and anti-Jo-1 antibodies are seen in the subset of patients who have associated interstitial lung disease (Table 20–9). Chest radiographs are usually normal, though interstitial fibrosis is occasionally seen. Electromyographic abnormalities consisting of polyphasic potentials, fibrillations, and high-frequency action potentials are helpful in establishing the diagnosis. None of the studies are specific. The search for an occult malignancy should begin with a history and physical examination and include the cancer screening tests that would be routine for that patient based on age, gender, and special risk factors, eg, smoking (see Chapter 1). If these evaluations are unrevealing, then a more invasive or extensive laboratory evaluation is probably not cost-effective. Since women with dermatomyositis have an increased risk of occult ovarian carcinoma, pelvic ultrasonography and serum CA-125 levels may be useful. No matter how extensive the initial screening, some malignancies will not become evident for months after the initial presentation.

C. Muscle Biopsy: Biopsy of clinically involved muscle is the only specific diagnostic test. The pathology findings in polymyositis and dermatomyositis are distinct. Although both include lymphoid inflammatory infiltrates, the findings in dermatomyositis are localized to perivascular regions and there is evidence of humoral and complement-mediated destruction of microvasculature associated with the muscle. In addition to its vascular orientation, the inflammatory infiltrate in dermatomyositis centers on the interfascicular septa and is located around, rather than in, muscle fascicles. In contrast, the pathology of polymyositis characteristically includes endomysial infiltration of the inflammatory infiltrate. Owing to the sometimes patchy distribution of pathologic abnormalities, however, false-negative biopsies sometimes occur in both disorders.

Differential Diagnosis

Muscle inflammation may occur as a component of SLE, systemic sclerosis, or Sjögren's syndrome. In those cases, associated findings usually permit the precise diagnosis of the primary condition.

Inclusion body myositis, because of its tendency to mimic polymyositis, is a common cause of "treatment-resistant polymyositis." In contrast to the epidemiologic features of polymyositis, however, the typical inclusion body myositis patient is white, male, and over the age of 50. The onset of inclusion body myositis is even more insidious than that of polymyositis or dermatomyositis (eg, occurring over years rather than months), and asymmetric distal motor weakness is common in inclusion body myositis. Inclusion body myositis is less likely to respond to therapy and is associated with characteristic pathologic findings evident on frozen section or electron microscopy.

Most endocrine diseases can be associated with proximal muscle weakness. This is particularly true for hyper- and hypothyroidism, and the latter is associated also with elevations of creatinine phosphokinase. Patients with polymyalgia rheumatica are over the age of 50 and—in contrast to patients with polymyositis—have pain but no objective weakness. Disorders of the peripheral and central nervous systems (eg, chronic inflammatory polyneuropathy, multiple sclerosis, myasthenia gravis, Eaton-Lambert disease and amyotrophic lateral sclerosis) can produce weakness but are distinguished by characteristic symptoms and neurologic signs and often by distinctive electromyographic abnormalities. Many drugs, including corticosteroids, alcohol, clofibrate, penicillamine, tryptophan, and hydroxychloroquine, can produce proximal muscle weakness. Chronic use of colchicine at doses as low as 0.6 mg twice a day in elderly patients with mild to moderate renal insufficiency can produce a mixed neuropathy-myopathy that mimics polymyositis. The weakness and muscle enzyme elevation reverse with cessation of the drug. Lovastatin, a drug increasingly used to treat hypercholesterolemia, also can rarely produce myositis, especially when used in combination with gemfibrozil. Polymyositis can occur as a complication of HIV or HTLV-I infection and with zidovudine therapy as well.

Treatment

Most patients respond to corticosteroids. Often a daily dose of 40–60 mg or more of prednisone is required initially The dose is then adjusted downward according to the response of sequentially observed serum levels of muscle enzymes. Long-term use of steroids is often needed, and the disease may recur or reemerge when they are withdrawn. Patients with an associated neoplasm have a poor prognosis, although remission may follow treatment of the tumor; steroids may or may not be effective in these patients. In patients resistant or intolerant to corticosteroids, therapy with methotrexate or azathioprine may be helpful, but these agents should be used with caution in view of their adverse effects. Intravenous immune globulin has also been shown to be effective for dermatomyositis resistant to prednisone, but leukapheresis and plasma exchange are not.

Vazquez-Abad D et al: Sensitivity and specificity of anti-Jo-1 antibodies in autoimmune diseases with myositis. Arthritis Rheum 1996;39:292. [NLM Cit ID: 96197015] (Jo-1 antibody 20% sensitive and 100% specific for polymyositis and dermatomyositis.)

OVERLAP (OR MIXED) CONNECTIVE TISSUE DISEASE

Not infrequently, patients have features of more than one rheumatic disease. Special attention has been drawn to patients who have overlapping features of SLE, systemic sclerosis, and polymyositis. Initially, these patients were thought to have a distinct entity ("mixed connective tissue disease") defined by a specific autoantibody to ribonuclear protein (RNP). With time in many patients, the manifestations evolve to one predominant disease, such as scleroderma, and many patients with antibodies to RNP have clear-cut SLE. Therefore, "overlap connective tissue disease" is the preferred designation for patients having features of different rheumatic diseases.

SJÖGREN'S SYNDROME

Essentials of Diagnosis

- 90% of patients are women; the average age is 50 years.
- Dryness of eyes and dry mouth (sicca components) are the most common features; they occur alone or in association with rheumatoid arthritis or other connective tissue disease.
- Rheumatoid factor and other autoantibodies common.
- Increased incidence of lymphoma.

General Considerations

Sjögren's syndrome, an autoimmune disorder, is the result of chronic dysfunction of exocrine glands in many areas of the body. It is characterized by dryness of the eyes, mouth, and other areas covered by mucous membranes and is frequently associated with a rheumatic disease, most often rheumatoid arthritis. The disorder is predominantly a disease of women, in a ratio of 9:1, with greatest incidence between age 40 and 60 years.

Disorders with which Sjögren's syndrome is frequently associated include rheumatoid arthritis, SLE, primary biliary cirrhosis, scleroderma, polymyositis, Hashimoto's thyroiditis, polyarteritis, and interstitial pulmonary fibrosis. When Sjögren's syndrome occurs without rheumatoid arthritis, HLA-DR2 and -DR3 antigens are present with increased frequency.

Clinical Findings

A. Symptoms and Signs: Keratoconjunctivitis sicca results from inadequate tear production caused by lymphocyte and plasma cell infiltration of the lacrimal glands. Symptoms include burning, itching, ropy secretions, and impaired tear production during crying. Parotid enlargement, which may be chronic or relapsing, develops in one-third of patients. Dryness of the mouth (xerostomia) leads to difficulty in speaking and swallowing and to severe dental caries. There may be loss of taste and smell. Desiccation may involve the nose, throat, larynx, bronchi, vagina, and skin.

Systemic manifestations include dysphagia, pancreatitis, pleuritis, obstructive lung disease (in the absence of smoking), neuropsychiatric dysfunction, and vasculitis; they may be related to the associated diseases noted above. Renal tubular acidosis (type I, distal) occurs in 20% of patients. Chronic interstitial nephritis, which may result in impaired renal function, may be seen. A glomerular lesion is rarely observed but may occur secondary to associated cryoglobulinemia.

A spectrum of lymphoproliferation ranging from benign to malignant may be found. Malignant lymphomas and Waldenström's macroglobulinemia occur nearly 50 times more frequently than can be explained by chance alone in primary Sjögren's syndrome.

B. Laboratory Findings: Laboratory findings include mild anemia, leukopenia, and eosinophilia. Rheumatoid factor is found in 70% of patients. Heightened levels of gamma globulin, antinuclear antibodies, and antibodies against RNA, salivary gland, lacrimal duct, and thyroid may be noted. Antibodies against the cytoplasmic antigens SS-A and SS-B (also called Ro and La, respectively) are often present in Sjögren's syndrome (Table 20–10). When SS-A antibodies are present, extraglandular manifestations of Sjögren's syndrome are far more common.

Useful ocular diagnostic tests include the Schirmer test, which measures the quantity of tears secreted. Lip biopsy, a simple procedure, is the only specific diagnostic technique and has minimal risk; if lymphoid foci are seen in accessory salivary glands, the diagnosis is confirmed. Biopsy of the parotid gland should be reserved for patients with atypical presentations such as unilateral gland enlargement.

Treatment & Prognosis

Treatment is symptomatic and supportive. Artificial tears applied frequently will relieve ocular symptoms and avert further desiccation. The mouth should be kept well lubricated. Atropinic drugs and decongestants decrease salivary secretions and should be avoided. A program of oral hygiene is essential in order to preserve dentition. If there is an associated rheumatic disease, its treatment is not altered by the presence of Sjögren's syndrome.

The disease is usually benign and may be consistent with a normal life span; it is influenced mainly by the nature of the associated disease. The patients (3–10% of the total Sjögren's population) at greatest risk of developing lymphoma have severe dryness, marked parotid gland enlargement, splenomegaly, vasculitis, peripheral neuropathy, anemia, and mixed monoclonal cryoglobulinemia.

Kruize AA et al: Long-term followup of patients with Sjögren's syndrome. Arthritis Rheum 1996;39:297. [NLM Cit ID: 96197016] (Primary Sjögren's syndrome usually followed a stable and mild course over 10 years except that 10% died of lymphoma.)

Voulgarelis M et al: Malignant lymphoma in primary Sjögren's syndrome. Arthritis Rheum 1999;42:1765. [NLM Cit ID: 99374545] (Patients with lymphoma have lymphadenopathy [66%], skin vasculitis [33%], peripheral neuropathy [24%], low grade fever [25%], anemia [48%], and lymphopenia [79%]. Lymphoma both nodal and extranodal in 45%, exclusively nodal in 18%, and exclusively extranodal [parotid glands] in 36%).

RHABDOMYOLYSIS

Defined strictly, rhabdomyolysis is necrosis of skeletal muscle and may be encountered in a wide variety of clinical settings, alone or in concert with other disorders of muscle. One of the latter is myopathy, or objective weakness of muscle; another is myalgia, or pain in the muscle. In some conditions, such as polymyositis, all three processes may coexist, as in a patient with proximal muscle weakness, pain, and an elevated creatine kinase (the biochemical indicator of skeletal muscle necrosis). The myopathies are dealt with elsewhere in this chapter, and myalgias are sufficiently nonspecific and widespread so that they need not be discussed separately—the exception being polymyalgia rheumatica. When the term "rhabdomyolysis" is employed without being otherwise defined, physicians ordinarily think of the syndrome of crush injury to muscle, associated with myoglobinuria, renal insufficiency, markedly elevated creatine kinase levels, and, frequently, multiorgan failure as a consequence of other complications of the trauma. Renal insufficiency in myoglobinuria is caused by tubular damage resulting from filtered myoglobin post-injury and is nearly always associated with hypovolemia. Experimental models of severe rhabdomyolysis in which blood volume and pressure are maintained ordinarily are not associated with acute tubular necrosis. From a practical point of view, however, many patients who suffer crush injuries are indeed volume-contracted, and oliguric renal failure is encountered routinely.

Vigorous fluid resuscitation, mannitol, and urine alkalinization are suggested early in the course, but it is not clear that the outcome is affected by these measures. On occasion, oliguric tubular necrosis may be converted to a nonoliguric variety, and—though the prognosis for recovery of renal function and mortality is the same—many clinicians believe it is easier to care for nonoliguric disease, since hyperkalemia and pulmonary edema are less important concerns.

In addition to crush injuries, prolonged immobility, particularly after drug overdose or intoxication and commonly associated with exposure hypothermia, may be associated with rhabdomyolysis. Often there is little evidence for muscle injury on external examination of these patients—and specifically, neither myalgia nor myopathy present. The clue to muscle necrosis in such individuals may be a urinary dipstick testing positive for blood in the absence of red cells in the sediment. This false positive finding is due to myoglobinuria, which results in a positive reading for blood. Such an abnormality is investigated by serum creatine kinase determination. Other studies elevated in rhabdomyolysis include ALT and LDH—and once again, these studies may be obtained for other reasons. such as suspected liver disease or hemolysis. When disproportionately elevated, it is prudent to make certain they are not of muscle origin by confirming them with CK determination.

A number of other causes of rhabdomyolysis are encountered, and the statin group of drugs for treatment of hyperlipidemia are common offenders. A simple intramuscular injection may cause some elevation of CK, and acute alcoholic intoxication is also culpable on rare occasions. For the most part, however, rhabdomyolysis is seen with concomitant myopathy, though the term rhabdomyolysis refers only to a test abnormality. Certain types of myopathies—notably the endocrine myopathies associated with hyperthyroidism and hypercortisolism—are not found with elevated muscle enzymes. The same is true of polymyalgia rheumatica. If these conditions are thought to be present but the CK is elevated, alternative explanations need to considered.

Patel DK et al: Muscle aches and fatigue in a man with elevated creatine kinase. Hosp Pract 1998;33:115. [NLM Cit ID: 98383213]

Slater MS et al: Rhabdomyolysis and myoglobinuric renal failure in trauma and surgical patients: a review. J Am Coll Surg 1998;186:693. [NLM Cit ID: 98293949]

VASCULITIS SYNDROMES

The vasculitis syndromes are a heterogeneous group of disorders characterized by the pathologic features of inflammation and necrosis of blood vessels. The cause of most forms of vasculitis is not known. Infection is important in the pathogenesis of some forms of vasculitis. In polyarteritis nodosa, 30–50% of patients have evidence of hepatitis B or C. Most patients with mixed cryoglobulinemia are infected with hepatitis C. Infective endocarditis and syphilis can be associated with vasculitis, and cases of herpes zoster are rarely followed by central nervous system vasculitis. Drug reactions—especially to penicillins, sulfonamides, and allopurinol—can produce serum sickness associated with vasculitis. No common pathogenic link has been identified for these disorders, though the deposition of immune complexes in the vascular system occurs in many.

Although vasculitis is seen in multiple disorders, only the major vasculitides will be discussed here.

POLYARTERITIS NODOSA & MICROSCOPIC POLYANGIITIS

Essentials of Diagnosis

- Microscopic polyangiitis may involve small blood vessels (capillaries, arterioles, venules) as well as medium-sized vessels. Classic polyarteritis nodosa involves only medium-sized vessels, but substantial overlap occurs.
- Clinical findings depend on the arteries involved.
- Common symptoms of both disorders include fever and other constitutional symptoms, abdominal pain, livedo reticularis, mononeuritis multiplex, anemia, and an elevated sedimentation rate.
- Classic polyarteritis nodosa is often associated with hypertension but spares the lung.
- Twenty to 30 percent of polyarteritis nodosa are associated with hepatitis B or C.
- Microscopic polyangiitis is frequently associated with antineutrophil cytoplasmic antibodies (ANCAs), pulmonary hemorrhage, and glomerulonephritis.

General Considerations

Polyarteritis nodosa was the first form of vasculitis recognized (in 1866). For many years, all forms of inflammatory vascular disease were termed "polyarteritis nodosa." In recent decades, numerous subtypes of vasculitis have been recognized, greatly narrowing the spectrum of vasculitis called polyarteritis nodosa. Currently, the term is reserved for a medium-sized necrotizing arteritis that has a predilection for involving peripheral nerves, mesenteric vessels (including renal arteries), heart, and brain but the capability of involving most organs. Microscopic polyangiitis, as its name implies, is the term given to nongranulomatous vasculitis involving small blood vessels. It is often associated with ANCAs that produce a pANCA pattern on immunofluorescence testing and are directed against myeloperoxidase, a constituent of neutrophil granules. Because microscopic polyangiitis may involve medium-sized as well as small blood vessels, its spectrum overlaps that of polyarteritis nodosa.

Clinical Findings

A. Symptoms and Signs: The clinical onset is usually insidious, with fever, malaise, weight loss, and other symptoms developing over weeks to months. Extremity pain is often a prominent early feature caused by arthralgia, myalgia (particularly affecting the calves), or neuropathy. In fact, the combination of mononeuritis multiplex (with the most common lesion being foot-drop) and features of a systemic illness is one of the earliest specific clues to the presence of an underlying vasculitis in the spectrum of polyarteritis nodosa–microscopic polyangiitis.

A wide variety of findings suggesting vasculitis of small blood vessels may develop in microscopic polyangiitis. These include palpable purpura and numerous other signs of cutaneous vasculitis; hematuria, proteinuria, and red blood cell casts in the urine; and pulmonary hemorrhage. The renal lesion is a segmental, necrotizing glomerulonephritis with extracapillary proliferation, often with localized intravascular coagulation. The pathologic findings in the lung are typically those of capillaritis.

In polyarteritis nodosa, the classic findings reflect the involvement of deeper, medium-sized blood vessels. Skin findings often include livedo reticularis, subcutaneous nodules, and skin ulcers. Digital gangrene is not an unusual occurrence. Involvement of the renal arteries leads to a renin-mediated hypertension (much less characteristic of vasculitides involving smaller blood vessels). For unclear reasons, classic polyarteritis nodosa seldom involves the lung.

Abdominal pain—particularly diffuse pain beginning about 30 minutes after meals ("abdominal angina")—is common to both polyarteritis nodosa and microscopic polyangiitis. Nausea and vomiting are frequently associated. Infarction compromises the function of major viscera and may lead to acalculous cholecystitis or appendicitis. Some patients present dramatically with an acute abdomen caused by mesenteric vasculitis and gut perforation or with hypotension resulting from rupture of a microaneurysm in the liver, kidney, or bowel.

Subclinical cardiac involvement is common in polyarteritis nodosa, and overt cardiac dysfunction occasionally occurs (eg, myocardial infarction secondary to coronary vasculitis, or myocarditis).

B. Laboratory Findings: The sedimentation rate is almost always elevated, often strikingly so. Most patients have a slight anemia, and leukocytosis is common. With the exception of ANCAs, present in three-fourths of patients with microscopic polyangiitis, serologic tests are typically negative in these forms of vasculitis. (However, the presence of pANCAs often causes a positive ANA.) Serologic tests for hepatitis B or C are positive in 20–30% of patients with polyarteritis nodosa.

C. Biopsy and Angiography: The diagnosis of both of these disorders requires confirmation with either biopsy of an involved tissue or, in the case of polyarteritis nodosa, an angiogram. Biopsies of symptomatic sites (eg, nerve, muscle, lung, or kidney) have high sensitivities and specificities. They should be performed in the order of least invasive to most invasive, but if performed by experienced physicians the tests normally have high benefit-risk ratios because of the importance of establishing the diagnosis. Patients suspected of having polyarteritis nodosa—eg, on the basis of mesenteric ischemia or new-onset hypertension occurring in the setting of a systemic illness—may be diagnosed by the angiographic finding of aneurysmal dilations in the renal, mesenteric, or hepatic arteries. Angiography must be performed cautiously in patients with baseline renal dysfunction.

Treatment

For polyarteritis nodosa, corticosteroids in high doses (up to 60 mg of prednisone daily) may control fever and constitutional symptoms and heal vascular lesions. Pulse methylprednisolone (eg, 1 g intravenously daily for 3 days) may be necessary for patients who are critically ill at presentation. Immunosuppressive agents, especially cyclophosphamide, appear to improve the survival of patients when given with steroids. Some patients who have polyarteritis nodosa associated with viral hepatitis may respond to a short course of prednisone followed by antiviral treatment and plasmapheresis.

In microscopic polyangiitis, patients are more likely to require cyclophosphamide because of the urgency in treating pulmonary hemorrhage and necrotizing glomerulonephritis. Cyclophosphamide may be administered either in an oral daily fashion or via intermittent (usually monthly) intravenous pulses.

Prognosis

Without treatment, the 5-year survival rate in these disorders is poor—on the order of 20%. With appropriate therapy, remissions are possible in many cases and the 5-year survival rate has improved to 60–90%. Poor prognostic factors are renal insufficiency, proteinuria, gastrointestinal ischemia, central nervous system disease, and cardiac involvement. Relapses following disease remissions may occur in both disorders—approximately 35% among patients with microscopic polyangiitis and perhaps less in those with idiopathic polyarteritis nodosa. For polyarteritis nodosa associated with hepatitis B or C, the likelihood of chronic disease may be higher.

Guillevin L et al: Microscopic polyangiitis: Clinical and laboratory findings in 85 patients. Arthritis Rheum 1999;42:421. [NLM Cit ID: 99186624]

Guillevin L et al: Prognostic factors in polyarteritis nodosa and Churg-Strauss syndrome. A prospective study in 342 patients. Medicine 1996;75:17. [NLM Cit ID: 96160345] (Argues that patients with idiopathic polyarteritis nodosa and a good prognosis should be treated with prednisone alone; those with cardiac, central nervous system, renal, or gastrointestinal involvement with prednisone and cyclophosphamide; and those with hepatitis B-associated polyarteritis nodosa with prednisone followed by plasmapheresis and antiviral agents.)

Guillevin L et al: Treatment of polyarteritis nodosa and microscopic polyangiitis. Arthritis Rheum 1998;41:2100. [NLM Cit ID: 99086413]

Jennette JC et al: Small vessel vasculitis. N Engl J Med 1997;337:1512. [NLM Cit ID: 98026769] (Excellent review of the approach to vasculitic syndromes.)

POLYMYALGIA RHEUMATICA & GIANT CELL ARTERITIS

Essentials of Diagnosis

- Giant cell arteritis is characterized by headache, jaw claudication, polymyalgia rheumatica, visual abnormalities, and a markedly elevated ESR.
- The hallmark of polymyalgia rheumatica is pain and stiffness in shoulders and hips.

General Considerations

Polymyalgia rheumatica and giant cell arteritis probably represent a spectrum of one disease: Both affect the same population (patients over the age of 50), show preference for the same HLA haplotypes, and show similar patterns of cytokines in blood and arteries. Polymyalgia rheumatica and giant cell arteritis also frequently coexist. Clinically, the important difference between the two conditions is that polymyalgia rheumatica alone does not cause blindness and responds to low-dose (10–20 mg/d) prednisone therapy, whereas giant cell arteritis can cause blindness and requires high-dose therapy (40–60 mg/d).

Clinical Findings

A. Polymyalgia Rheumatica: Polymyalgia rheumatica is a clinical diagnosis based on pain and stiffness of the shoulder and pelvic girdle areas, frequently in association with fever, malaise, and weight loss. It can occur in the absence of giant cell arteritis. Anemia and a markedly elevated sedimentation rate are almost always present. Because of the shoulder and pelvic area stiffness and pain, patients have trouble combing their hair, putting on a coat, or getting up out of a chair. In contrast to polymyositis, polymyalgia rheumatica does not cause muscular weakness. A few patients have joint swelling, particularly of the knees, wrists, and sternoclavicular joints. The differential diagnosis of malaise, anemia, and a markedly elevated sedimentation rate includes multiple myeloma, other malignant disorders, and chronic infections such as bacterial endocarditis.

B. Giant Cell Arteritis: Giant cell arteritis is a systemic panarteritis affecting medium-sized and large vessels in patients over the age of 50. The condition is also called temporal arteritis, since that artery is frequently involved, as are other extracranial branches of the carotid artery. About 50% of patients with giant cell arteritis also have polymyalgia rheumatica. The classic symptoms suggesting that a patient has arteritis are headache, scalp tenderness, visual symptoms, jaw claudication, or throat pain. The temporal artery is usually normal on physical examination but may be nodular, enlarged, tender, or pulseless. Blindness results from occlusive arteritis of the posterior ciliary branch of the ophthalmic artery. The ischemic optic neuropathy of giant cell arteritis may produce no funduscopic findings for the first 24–48 hours after the onset of blindness. Asymmetry of pulses in the arms, a murmur of aortic regurgitation, or bruits heard near the clavicle resulting from subclavian artery stenoses identify patients in whom giant cell arteritis has affected the aorta or its major branches. Large vessel involvement, particularly thoracic aortic aneurysms, occurs in approximately 15% of patients with giant cell arteritis, sometimes years after the diagnosis. Forty percent of patients with giant cell arteritis have nonclassic symptoms at presentation, chiefly respiratory tract problems (most frequently dry cough), mononeuritis multiplex (most frequently with painful paralysis of a shoulder), or fever of unknown origin. Giant cell arteritis accounts for 15% of all cases of fever of unknown origin in patients over the age of 65. The fever can be as high as 40 °C and is frequently associated with rigors and sweats. In contrast to patients with infection, patients with giant cell arteritis and fever almost always have a normal white blood count (before prednisone is started). Thus, in an older patient with fever of unknown origin, a very high erythrocyte sedimentation rate, and a normal white blood count, giant cell arteritis must be considered even in the absence of specific features such as headache or jaw claudication. In some cases, instead of having the well-known symptom of jaw claudication, patients complain of vague pain affecting other locations, including the tongue, nose, or ears. Indeed, unexplained head or neck pain in an older patient may signal the presence of giant cell arteritis.

Treatment

A. Polymyalgia Rheumatica: Patients with polymyalgia rheumatica by itself are treated with prednisone, 10–20 mg/d. If the patient fails to experience a dramatic improvement within 72 hours, the diagnosis should be doubted. Within 1–2 months after beginning treatment, the patient's symptoms and laboratory abnormalities will resolve. Slow tapering of the prednisone reduces the likelihood of relapse. The total duration of treatment varies considerably but ranges from 6 months to more than 2 years.

B. Giant Cell Arteritis: The urgency of early diagnosis and treatment in giant cell arteritis relates to the prevention of blindness. Once blindness develops, it is usually permanent. Therefore, when a patient has symptoms and findings suggestive of temporal arteritis, therapy with prednisone, 60 mg daily, is initiated immediately, and temporal artery biopsy is promptly obtained. Although it is prudent to obtain a temporal artery biopsy as soon as possible after instituting treatment, diagnostic findings of giant cell arteritis may still be present 2 weeks (or even considerably longer) after starting corticosteroids. Typically, a positive biopsy shows inflammatory infiltrate in the media and adventitia with lymphocytes, histiocytes, plasma cells, and giant cells. An adequate biopsy specimen (3–5 cm in length) is essential, because the disease tends to be segmental. Unilateral temporal artery biopsies are positive in approximately 80–85% of patients; bilateral biopsies add 10–15% to the yield. Prednisone should be continued in a dosage of 60 mg/d for 1–2 months before tapering. When only the symptoms of polymyalgia rheumatica are present, temporal artery biopsy is not necessary.

In adjusting the dosage of steroid, the erythrocyte sedimentation rate is a useful but not absolute guide to disease activity. Blindness rarely occurs when the ESR has reached the normal range. The drug may be slowly tapered when disease activity ceases, although the disorder may recur and in some patients remains active for years. Thoracic aortic aneurysms occur 17 times more frequently in patients with giant cell arteritis than in normal individuals. The aneurysms can develop at any time but typically occur 7 years after the diagnosis of giant cell arteritis is made.

Blockmans D et al: Positron emission tomography in giant cell arteritis and polymyalgia rheumatica: evidence for inflammation of the aortic arch. Am J Med 2000;108:246. [NLM Cit ID: 20186529] (Abnormal PET scan of the thoracic aorta and branches for the diagnosis of giant cell arteritis or polymyalgia rheumatica is 56% sensitive and 98% specific.)

Cid MC et al: Association between strong inflammatory response and low risk of developing visual loss and other cranial ischemic complications in giant cell (temporal) arteritis. Arthritis Rheum 1998;41:26. [NLM Cit ID: 98093955] (Patients with fever, weight loss, anemia, and very high ESRs were *less* likely to develop visual loss.)

Gonzalez-Gay MA et al: Polymyalgia rheumatica without significantly increased erythrocyte sedimentation rate. A more benign syndrome. Arch Intern Med 1997;157:317. [NLM Cit ID: 97192707] (Suggests that polymyalgia rheumatica with an ESR < 40 mm/h is more common than previously thought, especially in men.)

Schmidt WA et al: Color duplex ultrasonography in the diagnosis of temporal arteritis. N Engl J Med 1997;337:1336. [NLM Cit ID: 98000002] (Abnormalities of the temporal artery are identified by color duplex ultrasonography in 93% of patients with temporal arteritis.)

WEGENER'S GRANULOMATOSIS

Essentials of Diagnosis

- Originally defined by the triad of upper respiratory tract disease, lower respiratory disease, and glomerulonephritis.
- Suspect this diagnosis whenever mundane respiratory systems (eg, nasal congestion, sinusitis) are refractory to usual treatment.
- Pathology defined by the triad of small vessel vasculitis, granulomatous inflammation, and necrosis.

- cANCA relatively sensitive and specific.
- Renal disease often rapidly progressive without treatment.

General Considerations

Wegener's granulomatosis is a rare disorder (prevalence of three per 100,000) characterized by vasculitis of small arteries, arterioles, and capillaries, necrotizing granulomatous lesions of both upper and lower respiratory tract, and glomerulonephritis. Without treatment it is invariably fatal, most patients surviving less than a year after diagnosis. It occurs most commonly in the fourth and fifth decades of life and affects men and women with equal frequency.

Clinical Findings

A. Symptoms and Signs: The disorder usually develops over 4–12 months, with 90% of patients presenting with upper or lower respiratory tract symptoms or both. Upper respiratory tract symptoms can include nasal congestion, sinusitis, otitis media, mastoiditis, gum hypertrophy, or stridor due to subglottic stenosis. Since many of these symptoms are common, the underlying disease is not often suspected until the patient develops systemic symptoms or the original problem is refractory to treatment. The lung is affected initially in 40% and eventually in 80%, with symptoms including cough, dyspnea, and hemoptysis. Other early symptoms can include unilateral proptosis (from pseudotumor), red eye from scleritis, arthritis, purpura, and dysesthesia due to neuropathy. Renal involvement, which develops in three-fourths of the cases, usually does not cause symptoms before the diagnosis is established. Fever, malaise, and weight loss are common.

Physical examination can be remarkable for congestion, crusting, ulceration, bleeding, and even perforation of the nasal mucosa. Destruction of the nasal cartilage with "saddle nose" deformity occurs late. Otitis media, proptosis, and scleritis are other common findings. Newly acquired hypertension, a frequent feature of polyarteritis, is rare in Wegener's granulomatosis.

Although limited forms of Wegener's granulomatosis have been described in which the kidney is spared initially, most untreated patients will develop renal disease. In such cases the urinary sediment invariably contains red cells, with or without white cells, and red cell casts. Renal biopsy discloses a segmental necrotizing glomerulonephritis with multiple crescents; this is characteristic but not diagnostic. Granulomas are observed in only 10% of renal biopsy specimens but are found much more commonly on lung biopsy.

B. Laboratory Findings: Most patients have slight anemia, mild leukocytosis, and an elevated erythrocyte sedimentation rate. Chest CT is more sensitive than chest radiography; lesions include infiltrates, nodules, masses, and cavities. Often the radiographs prompt concern about lung cancer. Hilar adenopathy is very rare in Wegener's granulomatosis; if present, sarcoidosis, tumor, or infection is more likely. Other common laboratory or radiographic abnormalities include hematuria, red blood cell casts, and sinus destruction.

Histologic features of Wegener's granulomatosis include vasculitis, granulomatous inflammation, geographic necrosis, and acute and chronic inflammation. The full range of pathologic changes are usually evident only on thoracoscopic lung biopsy. Nasal biopsies often do not show vasculitis but may show other changes which, interpreted by an experienced pathologist, can serve as convincing evidence of the diagnosis.

Serum tests for antineutrophil cytoplasmic antibodies (ANCA) help in the diagnosis of Wegener's granulomatosis and related forms of vasculitis. Several different types of ANCA are recognized. The cytoplasmic pattern (cANCA), caused by antibodies to proteinase-3, a constituent of neutrophil granules, has a high specificity (> 90%) for Wegener's granulomatosis. In the setting of active disease, the sensitivity of cANCA is also reasonably high (≥ 70%). Although ANCA testing may be very helpful when used properly, it does not eliminate the need in most cases for confirmation of the diagnosis by tissue biopsy. Furthermore, ANCA levels correlate erratically with disease activity, and changes in titer should not dictate changes in therapy in the absence of supporting clinical data. The perinuclear (pANCA) pattern is caused by antibodies to myeloperoxidase and is much less specific for Wegener's granulomatosis. Approximately 10–25% of patients with classic Wegener's granulomatosis have pANCA. Owing to involvement of the same types of blood vessels, similar patterns of organ involvement, and the possibility of failing to identify granulomatous pathology on tissue biopsies because of sampling error, Wegener's granulomatosis is often difficult to differentiate from microscopic polyangiitis.

Atypical patterns of ANCA occur frequently in patients with systemic lupus erythematosus and inflammatory bowel disease.

Treatment

It is essential that the diagnosis of Wegener's granulomatosis be made early, since treatment may be lifesaving. Early treatment is also crucial in preventing renal failure. While Wegener's granulomatosis may involve the sinuses or lung for months, once proteinuria or hematuria develops, progression to renal failure can be rapid (over several weeks). Remissions have been induced in up to 75% of patients treated with cyclophosphamide and prednisone, though half of such patients have a recurrence of the disease. The cyclophosphamide is best given daily by mouth; intermittent high-dose intravenous cyclophosphamide is less effective. Unfortunately, the traditional therapy of oral cyclophosphamide continued for 12 months after the patient achieves remission has resulted in severe toxicity, including a 2.4 times increased risk of all malignancies, a 33-fold increase in bladder cancer, and a 60% chance of ovarian failure. Methotrexate, 20 mg/wk, is a reasonable substitute for oral cyclophosphamide in patients who do not have immediately life-threatening disease. Another strategy to limit cyclophosphamide use is to employ the drug for about 3 months in order to induce remission and then switch to methotrexate. Trimethoprim-sulfamethoxazole (one double-strength tablet twice daily) is ineffective for life-threatening Wegener's disease; however, the drug has been shown to be effective in helping to keep patients in remission. Trimethoprim-sulfamethoxazole and methotrexate are both folate antagonists; the combination can cause aplastic anemia and should be used with great care.

De Groot K et al: Induction of remission in Wegener's granulomatosis with low dose methotrexate. J Rheumatol 1998;25:492. [NLM Cit ID: 98176948] (Suggests that methotrexate is an acceptable alternative to cyclophosphamide in patients whose disease is not immediately life-threatening.)

Langford CA et al: A staged approach to the treatment of Wegener's granulomatosis. Arthritis Rheum 1999; 42:2666. [NLM Cit ID: 20081762] (Three months of cyclophosphamide followed by methotrexate induced remission in 31 of 31 patients. Only 6% withdrew because of toxicity.)

Stegeman CA et al: Trimethoprim-sulfamethoxazole (co-trimoxazole) for the prevention of relapses of Wegener's granulomatosis. N Engl J Med 1996;335:16. [NLM Cit ID: 96249129] (TMP-SMZ given twice daily to patients in remission helps prevent relapses; 20% of patients stopped the drug because of toxicity.)

Stone JH et al: Treatment of non-life threatening Wegener's granulomatosis with methotrexate and daily prednisone as the initial therapy of choice. J Rheumatol 1999; 26:1134. [NLM Cit ID: 99263775] (Eighty-nine percent improve; however, the relapse rate is high when drugs are tapered.)

Talar-Williams C et al: Cyclophosphamide-induced cystitis and bladder cancer in patients with Wegener granulomatosis. Ann Intern Med 1996;124:477. [NLM Cit ID: 96169945] (Incidence of bladder cancer was 5% at 10 years and 15% at 15 years; nonglomerular hematuria identified group at high risk.)

CRYOGLOBULINEMIA

Vasculitis secondary to cryoglobulinemia is uncommon but should be considered when patients present with palpable purpura on the lower extremities, glomerulonephritis (reflected by hematuria, proteinuria, and red blood cell casts), and peripheral neuropathy. Abnormal liver function tests, abdominal pain, cardiac disease, and pulmonary disease may also occur. The diagnosis is based on a compatible clinical picture and a positive serum test for cryoglobulins. Type II (monoclonal antibody with rheumatoid factor activity) and type III (polyclonal antibody with rheumatoid factor activity) cryoglobulins are most common in patients with vasculitis. Type I cryoglobulin (a monoclonal protein that does not have rheumatoid factor activity) is more commonly seen in lymphoproliferative disease associated with a hyperviscosity syndrome. Although the cause of cryoglobulinemia in vasculitis is unknown, the majority of patients have evidence of hepatitis C infection. Prednisone and immunosuppressive drugs are, at best, moderately effective for visceral complications such as renal insufficiency and neuropathy.

Lamprecht P et al: Cryoglobulinemic vasculitis. Arthritis Rheum 1999;42:2507. [NLM Cit ID: 20081741] (Extensive, up-to-date review.)

HENOCH-SCHÖNLEIN PURPURA

Henoch-Schönlein purpura is the most common systemic vasculitis in children, and it occurs in adults as well. Typical features are nonthrombocytopenic purpura, abdominal pain, arthritis, and hematuria. Pathologic features include leukocytoclastic vasculitis with IgA deposition. The disorder often remits spontaneously. The cause is not known.

Hypersensitivity to aspirin and food and drug additives has been reported. The purpuric skin lesions are typically located on the lower extremities but may also be seen on the hands, arms, and trunk. Localized areas of edema, especially common on the dorsal surfaces of the hands, are frequently observed. Joint symptoms are present in the majority of patients, the knees and ankles being most commonly involved. Abdominal pain secondary to vasculitis of the intestinal tract is often associated with gastrointestinal bleeding. Hematuria signals the presence of a renal lesion that is usually reversible, although it occasionally may progress to renal insufficiency. Children tend to have more frequent and more serious gastrointestinal vasculitis, whereas adults more often suffer from renal disease. Biopsy of the kidney reveals segmental glomerulonephritis with crescents and mesangial deposition of IgA and, sometimes, IgG. Aside from an elevated sedimentation rate, most laboratory findings are noncontributory; the platelet count is normal or elevated.

The disease is usually self-limited, lasting 1–6 weeks, and subsides without sequelae if renal involvement is not severe. The efficacy of treatment is not well established. In a small number of patients, high-dose immunoglobulin therapy has been reported to stabilize patients whose nephritis had been progressive.

Blanco R et al: Henoch-Schönlein purpura in adulthood and childhood: two different expressions of the same syndrome. Arthritis Rheum 1997;40:859. [NLM Cit ID: 97297915]

Tancrede-Bohin E et al: Schönlein-Henoch purpura in adult patients. Predictive factors for IgA glomerulonephritis in a retrospective study of 57 cases. Arch Dermatol 1997;133:438. [NLM Cit ID: 97271055]

RELAPSING POLYCHONDRITIS

This is a rare disease of unknown cause characterized by inflammatory destructive lesions of cartilaginous structures, principally the ears, nose, trachea, and larynx. It may be associated either with other immunologic disorders such as SLE, rheumatoid arthritis, or Hashimoto's thyroiditis or with cancers, especially multiple myeloma. The disease, which is usually episodic, affects males and females equally. The cartilage is painful, swollen, and tender during an attack and subsequently becomes atrophic, resulting in permanent deformity. Biopsy of the involved cartilage shows inflammation and chondrolysis. Noncartilaginous manifestations of the disease include fever, episcleritis, uveitis, deafness, aortic insufficiency, and rarely glomerulonephritis. In 85% of patients, a migratory, asymmetric, and seronegative arthropathy occurs, affecting both large and small joints and the costochondral junctions.

Prednisone, 0.5–1 mg/kg/d, is often effective. Dapsone (100–200 mg/d) may also be effective, sparing the need for chronic high-dose corticosteroid treatment. Involvement of the tracheobronchial tree, leading to its collapse, may cause death if tracheostomy is not done promptly.

Trentham DE et al: Relapsing polychondritis. Ann Intern Med 1998;129:114. [NLM Cit ID: 98318191] (Comprehensive review.)

BEHÇET'S SYNDROME

Named after the Turkish dermatologist who first described it, this disease of unknown cause is characterized by recurrent oral and genital ulcers, uveitis, seronegative arthritis, and central nervous system abnormalities. Other features include ulcerative skin lesions, erythema nodosum, thrombophlebitis, and vasculitis. Arthritis occurs in about two-thirds of patients, most commonly affecting the knees and ankles. Keratitis, retinal vasculitis, anterior uveitis (often with hypopyon—pus in the anterior chamber), and optic neuritis are observed. The ocular involvement is often fulminant and may result in blindness. Involvement of the central nervous system often results in serious disability or death. Findings include cranial nerve palsies, convulsions, encephalitis, mental disturbances, and spinal cord lesions. Leukocytosis and a rapid sedimentation rate are common.

The clinical course may be chronic but is often characterized by remissions and exacerbations. Corticosteroids, azathioprine, chlorambucil, pentoxifylline, and cyclosporine have been used with beneficial results. Oral base corticosteroids may be of some help for oral ulcerations.

Hamuryudan V et al: Azathioprine in Behçet's syndrome: effects on long-term prognosis. Arthritis Rheum 1997; 40:769. [NLM Cit ID: 97244313] (Early therapy with azathioprine improves prognosis.)

Sakane T et al: Behçet's disease. N Engl J Med 1999;341:1284. [NLM Cit ID: 99442274]

SERONEGATIVE SPONDYLOARTHROPATHIES

The seronegative spondyloarthropathies are ankylosing spondylitis, psoriatic arthritis, Reiter's syndrome (also called reactive arthritis), and colitic arthritis. These disorders are noted for onset usually before age 40, inflammatory arthritis of the spine or the large peripheral joints (or both), uveitis in a significant minority, the absence of autoantibodies in the serum, and a striking association with HLA-B27. Present in only 8% of normal Caucasians and 3% of normal blacks, HLA-B27 is positive in 90% of patients with ankylosing spondylitis and 75% with Reiter's syndrome. HLA-B27 also occurs in 50% of the psoriatic and colitic arthritis patients who have sacroiliitis; patients with only peripheral arthritis in these two syndromes do not show an increase in HLA-B27.

That HLA-B27 itself and not some other nearby gene confers susceptibility to these diseases has been demonstrated by experiments with transgenic rats. When the human HLA-B27 gene is expressed in rats, the animals develop a spinal and peripheral arthritis, psoriasiform nail and skin changes, and bowel inflammation. Thus, HLA-B27 is an important risk factor for the spondyloarthropathies. Because some patients with these disorders are HLA-B27-negative and because the great majority of HLA-B27-positive individuals do not develop spondyloarthropathies, the gene is neither necessary nor sufficient to cause spondyloarthropathies.

Infection also appears to play a key role in some of the spondyloarthropathies, especially Reiter's syndrome, which characteristically develops days to weeks after bacterial dysentery or a nongonococcal sexually transmitted infection (see below). The interplay of susceptibility genes and environmental infections is demonstrated by the fact that the risk of developing Reiter's syndrome is 0.2% in the general population, 2% in the HLA-B27 individuals, and 20% in patients with HLA-B27 who become infected with salmonella, shigella, or enteric organisms. The importance of infection in the pathogenesis of spondyloarthropathies is also demonstrated by the transgenic rats expressing human HLA-B27; rats raised in germ-free environments do not develop arthritis. Despite these gains in our understanding of the importance of HLA-B27 and infection, the precise mechanism by which genes and infection cause spondyloarthropathy is not yet known.

ANKYLOSING SPONDYLITIS

Essentials of Diagnosis

- Chronic low backache in young adults.
- Progressive limitation of back motion and of chest expansion.
- Transient (50%) or permanent (25%) peripheral arthritis.
- Uveitis in 20–25%.
- Diagnostic x-ray changes in sacroiliac joints.
- Accelerated erythrocyte sedimentation rate and negative serologic tests for rheumatoid factor. HLA-B27 usually positive.

General Considerations

Ankylosing spondylitis is a chronic inflammatory disease of the joints of the axial skeleton, manifested clinically by pain and progressive stiffening of the spine. The age at onset is usually in the late teens or early 20s. The incidence is greater in males than in females, and symptoms are more prominent in men, with ascending involvement of the spine more likely to occur.

Clinical Findings

A. Symptoms and Signs: The onset is usually gradual, with intermittent bouts of back pain that may radiate down the thighs. As the disease advances, symptoms progress in a cephalad direction and back motion becomes limited, with the normal lumbar curve flattened and the thoracic curvature exaggerated. Chest expansion is often limited as a consequence of costovertebral joint involvement. Radicular symptoms due to cauda equina fibrosis may occur years after onset of the disease. In advanced cases, the entire spine becomes fused, allowing no motion in any direction. Transient acute arthritis of the peripheral joints occurs in about 50% of cases, and permanent changes in the peripheral joints—most commonly the hips, shoulders, and knees—are seen in about 25%.

Spondylitic heart disease, characterized chiefly by atrioventricular conduction defects and aortic insufficiency, occurs in 3–5% of patients with long-standing severe disease. Nongranulomatous anterior uveitis is associated in as many as 25% of cases and may be a presenting feature. Pulmonary fibrosis of the upper lobes, with progression to cavitation and bronchiectasis mimicking tuberculosis, may occur, characteristically long after the onset of skeletal symptoms. Constitutional symptoms similar to those of rheumatoid arthritis are absent in most patients.

B. Laboratory Findings: The erythrocyte sedimentation rate is elevated in 85% of cases, but serologic tests for rheumatoid factor are characteristically negative. Anemia may be present but is often mild.

HLA-B27 is found in 90% of patients with ankylosing spondylitis. Because this antigen occurs in 8% of the normal population, it is not a specific diagnostic test. Persons with other rheumatic diseases such as rheumatoid arthritis, degenerative joint disease (osteoarthritis), and gout do not show a higher than normal incidence of HLA-B27.

C. Imaging: The earliest radiographic changes are usually in the sacroiliac joints. In the first few months of the disease process, the sacroiliac changes may be detectable only by CT scanning. Later, erosion and sclerosis of these joints are evident on plain radiographs. Involvement of the apophysial joints of the spine, ossification of the annulus fibrosus, calcification of the anterior and lateral spinal ligaments, and squaring and generalized demineralization of the vertebral bodies may occur in more advanced stages. The term "bamboo spine" has been used to describe the late radiographic appearance of the spinal column.

Additional x-ray findings include periosteal new bone formation on the iliac crest, ischial tuberosities and calcanei, and alterations of the pubic symphysis and sternomanubrial joint similar to those of the sacroiliacs. Radiologic changes in peripheral joints, when present, tend to be asymmetric and lack the demineralization and erosions seen in rheumatoid arthritis.

Differential Diagnosis

In contrast to ankylosing spondylitis, rheumatoid arthritis predominantly affects multiple, small, peripheral joints of the hands and feet, spares the sacroiliac joint, has little effect on the rest of the spine except for C1–C2, causes rheumatoid nodules, is associated with rheumatoid factor, and is not associated with HLA-B27. The history and physical findings of ankylosing spondylitis serve to distinguish this disorder from other causes of low back pain such as disk disease, osteoporosis, soft tissue trauma, and tumors. The single most valuable distinguishing radiologic sign of ankylosing spondylitis is the appearance of the sacroiliac joints, although a similar pattern may be seen in Reiter's syndrome and in the arthritis associated with inflammatory intestinal diseases and psoriasis. A spondyloarthropathy associated with hidradenitis suppurativa has been described in blacks. In ankylosing hyperostosis (diffuse idiopathic skeletal hyperostosis [DISH], Forestier's disease), there is exuberant osteophyte formation. The osteophytes are thicker and more anterior than the syndesmophytes of ankylosing spondylitis, and the sacroiliac joints are not affected. The x-ray appearance of the sacroiliac joints in spondylitis should be distinguished from that in osteitis condensans ilii. In some geographic areas and in persons with appropriate occupations, brucellosis and fluoride poisoning may be important in the differential diagnosis.

Treatment

A. Basic Program: The general principles of managing chronic arthritis (see above) apply equally well to ankylosing spondylitis. The importance of postural and breathing exercises should be stressed.

B. Drug Therapy: The nonsteroidal anti-inflammatory agents are employed in the treatment of this disorder. Of these, indomethacin appears to be the most effective, though it can be quite toxic. The dosage of indomethacin is usually 25–50 mg three times a day, but the smallest effective dose should be used. Indomethacin may produce a variety of untoward reactions, including headache, giddiness, nausea and vomiting, peptic ulcer, renal insufficiency, depression, and psychosis. Newer NSAIDs are valuable alternatives and may be used as primary therapy. Sulfasalazine (see above) is sometimes useful for the peripheral arthritis in patients with spondyloarthropathies but has little symptomatic effect on spinal and sacroiliac joint disease.

C. Physical Therapy: See above.

Prognosis

Almost all patients have persistent symptoms over decades; rare individuals experience long-term remissions. The severity of disease varies greatly, with about 10% of patients having work disability after 10 years. Developing hip disease within the first 2 years of disease onset presages a worse prognosis.

Bergfeldt L: HLA-B27-associated cardiac disease. Ann Intern Med 1997;127:621. [NLM Cit ID: 97460342] (Men, but not women, with HLA-B27 have a 6.7 increased risk of needing a permanent pacemaker; many patients with HLA-B27-associated heart disease do not have clinically evident ankylosing spondylitis.)

Clegg DO et al: Comparison of sulfasalazine and placebo in the treatment of ankylosing spondylitis: A Department of Veterans Affairs Cooperative Study. Arthritis Rheum 1996;39:2004. [NLM Cit ID: 97121239] (Sulfasalazine 2000 mg/d is effective for peripheral arthritis but not for long-standing spinal disease.)

PSORIATIC ARTHRITIS

Essentials of Diagnosis

- Psoriasis precedes onset of arthritis in 80% of cases.
- Arthritis usually asymmetric, with "sausage" appearance of fingers and toes; resembles rheumatoid arthritis; rheumatoid factor is negative.
- Sacroiliac joint involvement common; ankylosis of the sacroiliac joints may occur.
- X-ray findings: osteolysis; pencil-in-cup deformity; relative lack of osteoporosis; bony ankylosis; asymmetric sacroiliitis and atypical syndesmophytes.

General Considerations

In 15–20% of patients with psoriasis, arthritis coexists. The patterns or subsets of arthritis that may accompany psoriasis include the following:

(1) Joint disease that resembles rheumatoid arthritis in which polyarthritis is symmetric. Usually, fewer joints are involved than in rheumatoid arthritis.

(2) An oligoarticular form that may lead to considerable destruction of the affected joints.

(3) A pattern of disease in which the distal interphalangeal joints are primarily affected. Early, this may be monarticular, and often the joint involvement is asymmetric. Pitting of the nails and onycholysis are frequently associated.

(4) A severe deforming arthritis (arthritis mutilans) in which osteolysis is marked.

(5) A spondylitic form in which sacroiliitis and spinal involvement predominate; 50% of these patients are HLA-B27-positive.

Clinical Findings

A. Symptoms and Signs: Although psoriasis usually precedes the onset of arthritis, arthritis precedes or occurs simultaneously with the skin disease in approximately 20% of cases. Arthritis is at least five times more common in patients with severe skin disease than in those with only mild skin findings. Occasionally, however, patients may have a single patch of psoriasis (typically hidden in the scalp, gluteal cleft, or umbilicus) and are unaware of its connection to the arthritis. Thus, a detailed search for cutaneous lesions is essential in patients with arthritis of new onset. Also, the psoriatic lesions may have cleared when arthritis appears—in such cases, the history is most useful in diagnosing previously unexplained cases of mono- or oligoarthritis. Nail pitting, a residue of previous psoriasis, is sometimes the only clue.

B. Laboratory Findings: Laboratory studies show an elevation of the sedimentation rate, but rheumatoid factor is not present. Uric acid levels may be high, reflecting the active turnover of skin affected by psoriasis. There is a correlation between the extent of psoriatic involvement and the level of uric acid, but gout is no more common than in patients without psoriasis. Desquamation of the skin may also reduce iron stores.

C. Imaging: Radiographic findings are most helpful in distinguishing the disease from other forms of arthritis. There are marginal erosions of bone and irregular destruction of joint and bone, which, in the phalanx, may give the appearance of a sharpened pencil. Fluffy periosteal new bone may be marked, especially at the insertion of muscles and ligaments into bone. Such changes will also be seen along the shafts of metacarpals, metatarsals, and phalanges. Paravertebral ossification occurs, which may be distinguished from ankylosing spondylitis by the absence of ossification in the anterior aspect of the spine.

Treatment

Treatment regimens are symptomatic. Nonsteroidal anti-inflammatory drugs are usually sufficient for mild cases. Corticosteroids are less effective in psoriatic arthritis than in other forms of inflammatory arthritis. In addition, they may exacerbate the skin disease during tapers. Antimalarials may also exacerbate psoriasis. Sulfasalazine and gold may be beneficial. In resistant cases, methotrexate may be helpful. Successful treatment of the skin lesions commonly—though not invariably—is accompanied by an improvement in peripheral articular symptoms.

Clegg DO et al: Comparison of sulfasalazine and placebo in the treatment of psoriatic arthritis: A Department of Veterans Affairs Cooperative Study. Arthritis Rheum 1996;39:2013. [NLM Cit ID: 97121240] (Sulfasalazine 2000 mg/d moderately more effective than placebo.)

REITER'S SYNDROME (Reactive Arthritis)

Essentials of Diagnosis

- Fifty to 80 percent of patients are HLA-B27-positive.
- Oligoarthritis, conjunctivitis, urethritis, and mouth ulcers most common features.
- Usually follows dysentery or a sexually transmitted infection.

General Considerations

Reiter's syndrome, also called "reactive arthritis," is a clinical tetrad of urethritis, conjunctivitis (or, less commonly, uveitis), mucocutaneous lesions, and aseptic arthritis. It occurs most commonly in young men, is associated with HLA-B27 in 80% of white patients and 50–60% of blacks, and often follows infection (see above).

Clinical Findings

A. Symptoms and Signs: Most cases of Reiter's syndrome develop within days or weeks after either a dysenteric infection (with shigella, salmonella, yersinia, campylobacter) or a sexually transmitted infection (with *Chlamydia trachomatis* or perhaps *Ureaplasma urealyticum*). Whether the inciting infection is sexually transmitted or dysenteric does not affect the subsequent manifestations but does influence the sex ratio: The ratio is 1.0 after enteric infections but 9:1 with male predominance after sexually transmitted infections.

Although affected joints are culture-negative, fragments of putative organisms have been identified in swollen joints. The exact role of infection remains unclear.

The arthritis is most commonly asymmetric and frequently involves the large weight-bearing joints (chiefly the knee and ankle); sacroiliitis or ankylosing spondylitis is observed in at least 20% of patients, especially after frequent recurrences. Systemic symptoms including fever and weight loss are common at the onset of disease. The mucocutaneous lesions may include balanitis, stomatitis, and keratoderma blennorrhagicum, indistinguishable from pustular psoriasis. Involvement of the fingernails in Reiter's syndrome may also mimic psoriatic changes. Carditis and aortic regurgitation may occur. While most signs of the disease disappear within days or weeks, the arthritis may persist for several months or even years. Recurrences involving any combination of the clinical manifestations are common and are sometimes followed by permanent sequelae, especially in the joints.

B. Imaging: X-ray signs of permanent or progressive joint disease may be seen in the sacroiliac as well as the peripheral joints.

Differential Diagnosis

Gonococcal arthritis can initially mimic Reiter's syndrome, but the marked improvement after 24–48 hours of antibiotic administration and the culture results distinguish the two disorders. Rheumatoid arthritis, idiopathic ankylosing spondylitis, and psoriatic arthritis must also be considered.

The association of Reiter's syndrome and HIV has been debated, but evidence now indicates Reiter's syndrome is equally common in sexually active men regardless of HIV status.

Treatment

NSAIDs have been the mainstay of therapy. Antibiotics may also have some role. Antibiotics given at the time of a nongonococcal sexually transmitted infection reduce the chance that the individual will develop Reiter's syndrome. Tetracycline (250 mg four times daily) given for 3 months to patients with Reiter's syndrome associated with *C trachomatis* reduces the duration of symptoms. Tetracyclines have anti-inflammatory properties, so the response need not be attributed solely to an antimicrobial effect. Patients with enteric Reiter's syndrome do not respond to antibiotics. Patients who fail NSAIDs and antibiotics may respond to sulfasalazine, 1000 mg twice daily.

Clegg DO et al: Comparison of sulfasalazine and placebo in the treatment of reactive arthritis (Reiter's syndrome): A Department of Veterans Affairs Cooperative Study. Arthritis Rheum 1996;39:2021. [NLM Cit ID: 97121241] (Sulfasalazine 2000 mg/d is well tolerated and effective.)

Gaston JS et al: Identification of 2 *Chlamydia trachomatis* antigens recognized by synovial fluid T cells from patients with *Chlamydia* induced reactive arthritis. J Rheumatol 1996;23:130. [NLM Cit ID: 96435635] (That Reiter's syndrome may be caused by an immune response to chronic joint infections is suggested by finding synovial T cells that respond to chlamydial antigens.)

Wakefield D et al: Ciprofloxacin treatment does not influence course or relapse rate of reactive arthritis and anterior uveitis. Arthritis Rheum 1999;42:1894. [NLM Cit ID: 99441962] (Double-blind, randomized study showing ciprofloxacin ineffective for reactive arthritis or anterior uveitis.)

ARTHRITIS & INFLAMMATORY INTESTINAL DISEASES

One-fifth of patients with inflammatory bowel disease have arthritis, making it second only to anemia as the most common extraintestinal manifestation. Arthritis complicates Crohn's disease somewhat more frequently than it does ulcerative colitis. In both diseases, two distinct forms of arthritis occur. The first is peripheral arthritis—usually a nondeforming asymmetric oligoarthritis of large joints—in which the activity of the joint disease parallels that of the bowel disease. The arthritis usually begins months to years after the bowel disease, but occasionally the joint symptoms develop earlier and may be prominent enough to cause the patient to overlook intestinal symptoms. The second form of arthritis is a spondylitis that is indistinguishable by symptoms or x-ray from ankylosing spondylitis and follows a course independent of the bowel disease. About 50% of these patients are HLA-B27-positive.

Controlling the intestinal inflammation usually eliminates the peripheral arthritis. The spondylitis often requires NSAIDs, which need to be used cautiously since these agents may activate the bowel disease in a few patients. Range-of-motion exercises as prescribed for ankylosing spondylitis can be helpful.

About two-thirds of patients with Whipple's disease experience arthralgia or arthritis, most often an episodic, large-joint polyarthritis. The arthritis usually precedes the gastrointestinal manifestations by years. In fact, the arthritis resolves as the diarrhea develops. Thus, Whipple's disease should be considered in the differential diagnosis of unexplained episodic arthritis.

About 15% of patients who have jejunoileal bypass surgery for morbid obesity develop an inflammatory symmetric polyarticular disorder. The arthritis is usually acute in onset and nonmigratory and may affect the small as well as the large joints. The sedimentation rate is elevated, and antinuclear antibody and rheumatoid factor tests may be positive. Nonsteroidal anti-inflammatory agents are often effective, although some patients require prednisone.

INFECTIOUS ARTHRITIS*

NONGONOCOCCAL ACUTE BACTERIAL (SEPTIC) ARTHRITIS

Essentials of Diagnosis

- Sudden onset of acute arthritis, usually monarticular, most often in large weight-bearing joints and wrists.
- Previous joint damage or intravenous drug abuse common risk factors.
- Infection with causative organisms commonly found elsewhere in body.
- Joint effusions are usually large, with white blood counts commonly > 50,000/µL.

General Considerations

Nongonococcal acute bacterial arthritis is a disease of an abnormal host. The key risk factors are persistent bacteremia (eg, intravenous drug abuse, endocarditis) and damaged joints (eg, rheumatoid arthritis). *Staphylococcus aureus* is the most common cause of nongonococcal septic arthritis, followed by group A and group B streptococci. Gram-negative septic arthritis, once rare, has become more common, especially in intravenous drug abusers and in other immunocompromised hosts. *Escherichia coli* and *Pseudomonas aeruginosa* are the most common gram-negative isolates in adults.

The widespread use of arthroscopy and prosthetic joint surgery has also increased the frequency of septic arthritis. In the latter conditions, *Staphylococcus epidermidis* is the usual offending organism. Pathologic changes include varying degrees of acute inflammation, with synovitis, effusion, abscess formation in synovial or subchondral tissues, and, if treatment is not adequate, articular destruction.

Clinical Findings

A. Symptoms and Signs: The onset is usually sudden, with acute pain, swelling, and heat of one joint—most frequently the knee. Other commonly affected sites are the hip, wrist, shoulder, and ankle. Unusual sites, such as the sternoclavicular or sacroiliac joint, can be involved in intravenous drug abusers. Chills and fever are common but are absent

*Lyme disease is discussed in Chapter 34.

in up to 20% of patients. Infection of the hip usually does not produce apparent swelling but results in groin pain greatly aggravated by walking.

B. Laboratory Findings: Blood cultures are positive in approximately 50% of patients. The leukocyte count of the synovial fluid exceeds 50,000 and often 100,000/μL, with 90% or more polymorphonuclear cells. Synovial fluid glucose is usually low. Gram stain of the synovial fluid is positive in 75% of staphylococcal infections and in 50% of gram-negative infections.

C. Imaging: Radiographs are usually normal early in the disease, but evidence of demineralization may be present within days of onset. Bony erosions and narrowing of the joint space followed by osteomyelitis and periostitis may be seen within 2 weeks.

Differential Diagnosis

The septic course with chills and fever, the acute systemic reaction, the joint fluid findings, evidence of infection elsewhere in the body, and the evidence of response to appropriate antibiotics are diagnostic of bacterial arthritis. Gout and pseudogout are excluded by the failure to find crystals on synovial fluid analysis. Acute rheumatic fever and rheumatoid arthritis commonly involve many joints; Still's disease may mimic septic arthritis, but laboratory evidence of infection is absent. Pyogenic arthritis may be superimposed on other types of joint disease, notably rheumatoid arthritis, and must be excluded (by joint fluid examination) in any apparent acute relapse of the primary disease, particularly when a joint has been needled or when one is more strikingly inflamed than the others.

Treatment

Prompt systemic antibiotic therapy of any septic arthritis should be based on the best clinical judgment of the causative organism and the results of smear and culture of joint fluid, blood, urine, or other specific sites of potential infection. If the organism cannot be determined clinically, treatment should be started with bactericidal antibiotics effective against staphylococci, pneumococci, and gram-negative organisms.

Frequent (even daily) local aspiration is indicated when synovial fluid rapidly reaccumulates and causes symptoms. Immediate surgical drainage is reserved for septic arthritis of the hip, because that site is inaccessible to repeated aspiration. For most other joints, surgical drainage is used only if medical therapy fails over 2–4 days to improve the fever and the synovial fluid volume, white blood count, and culture results. Pain can be relieved with local hot compresses and by immobilizing the joint with a splint or traction. Rest, immobilization, and elevation are used at the onset of treatment. Early active motion exercises within the limits of tolerance will hasten recovery.

Prognosis

With prompt antibiotic therapy and no serious underlying disease, functional recovery is usually good. Five to 10 percent of patients with an infected joint die, chiefly from respiratory complications of sepsis. The mortality rate is 30% for patients with polyarticular sepsis. Bony ankylosis and articular destruction commonly also occur if treatment is delayed or inadequate.

Kaandorp CJ et al: The outcome of bacterial arthritis: a prospective community-based study. Arthritis Rheum 1997;40:884. [NLM Cit ID: 97297918] (Risk factors for poor prognosis were older age, preexisting joint disease, and infected prosthetic joints.)

GONOCOCCAL ARTHRITIS

Essentials of Diagnosis

- Prodromal migratory polyarthralgias.
- Tenosynovitis most common sign.
- Purulent monarthritis in 50%.
- Characteristic skin rash.
- Most common in young women during menses or pregnancy.
- Symptoms of urethritis frequently absent.
- Dramatic response to antibiotics.

General Considerations

Disseminated gonococcal infection is the most common cause of infectious arthritis in large urban areas. In contrast to nongonococcal bacterial arthritis, gonococcal arthritis chiefly occurs in otherwise healthy individuals. Host factors, however, influence the expression of the disease: gonococcal arthritis is two to three times more common in women than in men, is especially common during menses and pregnancy, and is rare after age 40. Gonococcal arthritis is also common in male homosexuals, whose high incidence of asymptomatic gonococcal pharyngitis and proctitis predisposes them to disseminated gonococcal infection. Some of the signs of disseminated gonococcal infection may result from an immunologic reaction to nonviable fragments of the organism's cell wall; this may explain the frequent inability to culture organisms from skin and joint lesions. Recurrent disseminated gonococcal infection should prompt evaluation for a congenital deficiency of complement components, especially C7 and C8.

Clinical Findings

A. Symptoms and Signs: One to 4 days of migratory polyarthralgias involving the wrist, knee, ankle, or elbow is the most common initial course. Thereafter, two patterns emerge, one (60% of patients) characterized by tenosynovitis and the other (40%) by purulent monarthritis, most frequently involving the knee. Less than half of patients have fever, and less than one-fourth have any genitourinary symptoms. Most patients will have asymptomatic but highly characteristic skin lesions that usually consist of two to ten small necrotic pustules distributed over the extremities, especially the palms and soles.

B. Laboratory Findings: The peripheral blood leukocyte count averages about 10,000 cells/μL and is elevated in less than one-third of patients. The synovial fluid white blood cell count, however, is typically over 50,000 cells/μL. The synovial fluid Gram stain is positive in one-fourth of cases and culture in less than half. Positive blood cultures are seen in 40% of patients with tenosynovitis and virtually never in patients with suppurative arthritis. Urethral, throat, and rectal cultures should be done in all patients, since they are often positive in the absence of local symptoms. Culturing *Neisseria gonorrhoeae* is facilitated by rapid transport to the microbiology laboratory, inoculation on appropriate media, and incubation in carbon dioxide.

C. Imaging: Radiographs are usually normal or show only soft tissue swelling.

Differential Diagnosis

Reiter's syndrome can also produce acute monarthritis in a young person but is distinguished by negative cultures, sacroiliitis, and failure to respond to antibiotics. Lyme disease involving the knee is less acute, does not show positive cultures, and may be preceded by known tick exposure and characteristic rash. The synovial fluid analysis will exclude gout, pseudogout, and nongonococcal bacterial arthritis. Rheumatic fever and sarcoidosis can produce migratory tenosynovitis but have other distinguishing features. Infective endocarditis with septic arthritis can mimic disseminated gonococcal infection.

Treatment

In most cases, patients suspected of having gonococcal arthritis should be admitted to the hospital to confirm the diagnosis, to exclude endocarditis, and to start treatment. While outpatient treatment has been recommended in the past, the rapid rise in gonococci resistant to penicillin makes initial inpatient treatment advisable. Approximately 4–5% of all gonococcal isolates produce a β-lactamase that confers penicillin resistance. An additional 15–20% of gonococcal species have chromosomal mutations that result in relative resistance to penicillin. Therefore, the current recommendations for initial treatment of gonococcal arthritis are to give ceftriaxone, 1 g intravenously daily (or cefotaxime, 1 g intravenously every 8 hours; or ceftizoxime, 1 g intravenously every 8 hours; or spectinomycin, 2 g intramuscularly every 12 hours, for patients with beta-lactam allergy). Once improvement from parenteral antibiotics has been achieved for 24–48 hours, patients can be switched to oral cefixime, 400 mg orally twice daily, or ciprofloxacin, 500 mg orally twice daily, to complete a 7- to 10-day course.

Prognosis

Generally, gonococcal arthritis responds dramatically in 24–48 hours after initiation of antibiotics so that daily joint aspirations are rarely needed. Complete recovery is the rule.

RHEUMATIC MANIFESTATIONS OF HIV INFECTION

Infection with human immunodeficiency virus (HIV) has been associated with various rheumatic disorders, most commonly arthralgias or Reiter's syndrome. More rarely myositis, psoriatic arthritis, Sjögren's syndrome, or vasculitis occur (see Chapter 31). It is possible that these disorders stem directly from HIV infection itself or from the many other infections that occur in immunodeficient patients. The rheumatic syndromes may follow the diagnosis of AIDS or may precede it by several months. Thus, coexistent HIV infection must be considered in patients presenting with Reiter's syndrome. The lower extremity joints, especially the knees and ankles, are most commonly affected. Often, as in classic Reiter's syndrome, Achilles tendon inflammation (enthesopathy) or knee periarthritis is a prominent and distinguishing feature. Many patients respond to NSAIDs, though a few are unresponsive and develop progressive deformities. The use of immunosuppressive agents, however, is contraindicated in these immunodeficient patients.

VIRAL ARTHRITIS

Arthritis may be a manifestation of many viral infections. It is generally mild and of short duration, terminating without lasting ill effects. Mumps arthritis may occur in the absence of parotitis. Rubella arthritis, which occurs more commonly in adults than in children, may appear immediately before, during, or soon after the disappearance of the rash. Its usual polyarticular and symmetric distribution mimics that of rheumatoid arthritis. However, the seronegative tests for rheumatoid factor and the rising rubella titers in convalescent serum help to confirm the diagnosis. Post-rubella vaccination arthritis may have its onset as long as 6 weeks following vaccination and occurs in all age groups. In adults, arthritis may follow infection with human parvovirus B19.

Transient polyarthritis may be associated with type B hepatitis and typically occurs before the onset of jaundice; it may occur in anicteric hepatitis as well. Urticaria or other types of skin rash may be present. Indeed, the clinical picture may be indistinguishable from that of serum sickness. Serum transaminase levels are elevated, and hepatitis B surface antigen is most often present. Serum complement levels are usually low during active arthritis and become normal after remission of arthritis. False-positive tests for rheumatoid factor, when present, disappear within several weeks. The arthritis is mild; it rarely lasts more than a few weeks and is self-limiting and without deformity. Hepatitis C infection may be associated with chronic polyarthralgia or polyarthritis that mimics rheumatoid arthritis.

Ray P et al: Risk of chronic arthropathy among women after rubella vaccination. JAMA 1997;278:551. [NLM Cit ID: 97412162] (Risk of chronic arthritis not seen with RA 27/3 rubella vaccine.)

INFECTIONS OF BONES

Direct microbial contamination of bones results from open fracture, surgical procedures, gunshot wounds, diagnostic needle aspirations, and therapeutic or self-administered drug injections.

Indirect or secondary infections are first noticed in other areas of the body and extend to bones by hematogenous routes.

ACUTE PYOGENIC OSTEOMYELITIS

Essentials of Diagnosis

- Fever and chills associated with pain and tenderness of involved bone.
- Aspiration of involved bone is usually diagnostic.
- Culture of blood or lesion tissue is essential for precise diagnosis.
- Radiographs early in the course are typically negative.

General Considerations

Osteomyelitis is a serious infection that is often difficult to diagnose and treat. Infection of bone occurs as a consequence of (1) hematogenous dissemination of bacteria, (2) invasion from a contiguous focus of infection, and (3) skin breakdown in the setting of vascular insufficiency.

Clinical Findings

A. Symptoms and Signs:

1. Hematogenous osteomyelitis–Osteomyelitis resulting from bacteremia is a disease associated with sickle cell disease, intravenous drug users, or the elderly. Patients with this form of osteomyelitis often present with sudden onset of high fever, chills, and pain and tenderness of the involved bone. The site of osteomyelitis and the causative organism depend on the host. Among patients with hemoglobinopathies such as sickle cell anemia, osteomyelitis is caused by salmonellae ten times as often as by other bacteria. Intravenous drug users develop osteomyelitis most commonly in the spine. Although in this setting *S aureus* is most common, gram-negative infections, especially *P aeruginosa* and serratia species, are also frequent pathogens. Rapid progression to epidural abscess causing fever, pain, and sensory and motor loss is not uncommon. In older patients with hematogenous osteomyelitis, the most common sites are the thoracic and lumbar vertebral bodies. Risk factors for these patients include diabetes, intravenous catheters, and indwelling urinary catheters. These patients often have more subtle presentations, with low-grade fever and gradually increasing bone pain.

2. Osteomyelitis from a contiguous focus of infection–Prosthetic joint replacement, decubitus ulcer, neurosurgery, and trauma most frequently cause soft tissue infections that can spread to bone. *S aureus* and *S epidermidis* are the most common organisms. Localized signs of inflammation are usually evident, but high fever and other signs of toxicity are usually absent.

3. Osteomyelitis associated with vascular insufficiency–Patients with diabetes and vascular insufficiency are susceptible to developing a very challenging form of osteomyelitis. The foot and ankle are the most commonly affected sites. Infection originates from an ulcer or other break in the skin that is usually still present when the patient presents but may appear disarmingly unimpressive. Bone pain is often absent or muted by the associated neuropathy. Fever is also commonly absent. One of the best bedside clues that the patient has osteomyelitis is the ability to easily advance a sterile probe through a skin ulcer to bone.

B. Imaging and Laboratory Findings: The plain film is the most readily available imaging procedure to establish the diagnosis of osteomyelitis, but it can be falsely negative early. Early radiographic findings may include soft tissue swelling, loss of tissue planes, and periarticular demineralization of bone. About 2 weeks after onset of symptoms, erosion of bone and alteration of cancellous bone appear, followed by periostitis.

MRI, CT, and nuclear medicine bone scanning are more sensitive than conventional radiography. MRI is believed to be the most sensitive and is particularly helpful in demonstrating the extent of soft tissue involvement. Radionuclide bone scanning is most valuable when osteomyelitis is suspected but no site is obvious.

Identifying the offending organism is a crucial step in selection of antibiotic therapy. Bone biopsy for culture is required except in those with hematogenous osteomyelitis, who have positive blood cultures. Cultures from overlying ulcers, wounds, or fistulas are unreliable.

Differential Diagnosis

Acute hematogenous osteomyelitis should be distinguished from suppurative arthritis, rheumatic fever, and cellulitis. More subacute forms must be differentiated from tuberculosis or mycotic infections of bone and Ewing's sarcoma or, in the case of vertebral osteomyelitis, from metastatic tumor. When osteomyelitis involves the vertebrae, it commonly traverses the disk—a finding not observed in tumor.

Complications

Inadequate treatment of bone infections results in chronicity of infection, and this possibility is increased by delaying diagnosis and treatment. Extension to adjacent bone or joints may complicate acute osteomyelitis. Recurrence of bone infections often results in anemia, a markedly elevated erythrocyte sedimentation rate, weight loss, weakness, and, rarely, amyloidosis or nephrotic syndrome. Pseudoepitheliomatous hyperplasia, squamous cell carcinoma, or fibrosarcoma may occasionally arise in persistently infected tissues.

Treatment

Most patients require both debridement of necrotic bone and prolonged administration of antibiotics. Patients with vertebral body osteomyelitis and epidural abscess require urgent neurosurgical decompression. Depending on the site and extent of debridement, surgical procedures to stabilize, fill in, cover, or revascularize may be needed. Traditionally, in adults, antibiotics have been administered parenterally for at least 4–6 weeks. Oral therapy with quinolones (eg, ciprofloxacin, 750 mg twice daily) for 6–8 weeks has been shown to be as effective as standard parenteral antibiotic therapy for chronic osteomyelitis in adults with susceptible organisms. When treating osteomyelitis caused by *S aureus,* quinolones are usually combined with rifampin, 300 mg twice daily.

Prognosis

If sterility of the lesion is achieved within 2–4 days, a good result can be expected in most cases if there is no compromise of the patient's immune system. However, progression of the disease to a chronic form may occur. It is especially common in the lower extremities and in patients in whom circulation is impaired (eg, diabetics).

Lew DP et al: Osteomyelitis. N Engl J Med 1997;336:999. [NLM Cit ID: 97222384]

MYCOTIC INFECTIONS OF BONES & JOINTS

Fungal infections of the skeletal system are usually secondary to a primary infection in another organ, frequently the lungs (see Chapter 36). Although skeletal lesions have a predilection for the cancellous portions of long bones and vertebral bodies, the predominant lesion—a granuloma with varying degrees of necrosis and abscess formation—does not produce a characteristic clinical picture.

Differentiation from other chronic focal infections depends upon culture studies of synovial fluid or tissue obtained from the local lesion. Serologic tests provide presumptive support of the diagnosis.

1. CANDIDIASIS

Candidal osteomyelitis most commonly develops in debilitated, malnourished patients undergoing prolonged hospitalization for cancer, neutropenia, trauma, complicated abdominal surgical procedures, or intravenous drug use. Infected intravenous catheters frequently serve as a hematogenous source.

For susceptible candida species, fluconazole, 200 mg orally twice daily, is probably as effective as amphotericin B.

2. COCCIDIOIDOMYCOSIS

Coccidioidomycosis of bones and joints is usually secondary to primary pulmonary infection. Arthralgia with periarticular swelling, especially in the knees and ankles, occurring as a nonspecific manifestation of systemic coccidioidomycosis, should be distinguished from actual bone or joint infection. Osseous lesions commonly occur in cancellous bone of the vertebrae or near the ends of long bones at tendinous insertions. These lesions are initially osteolytic and thus may mimic metastatic tumor or myeloma.

The precise diagnosis depends upon recovery of *Coccidioides immitis* from the lesion or histologic examination of tissue obtained by open biopsy. Rising titers of complement-fixing antibodies also provide evidence of the disseminated nature of the disease.

Itraconazole, 200 mg twice daily for 6–12 months, has become the treatment of choice for bone and joint coccidioidomycosis. Chronic infection is rarely cured with antifungal agents and may require operative excision of infected bone and soft tissue; amputation may be the only solution for stubbornly progressive infections. Immobilization of joints by plaster casts and avoidance of weight bearing provide benefit. Synovectomy, joint debridement, and arthrodesis are reserved for more advanced joint infections.

Stevens DA: Coccidioidomycosis. N Engl J Med 1995; 332:1077. [NLM Cit ID: 95206336] (Disseminated disease most commonly affects bones of skull, hands, feet, spine, and tibia. Most common joints are ankles and knees.)

3. HISTOPLASMOSIS

Focal skeletal or joint involvement in histoplasmosis is rare and generally represents dissemination from a primary focus in the lungs. Skeletal lesions may be single or multiple and are not characteristic.

TUBERCULOSIS OF BONES & JOINTS

Essentials of Diagnosis

- A disease of children, the elderly, or those with HIV infection.
- In most cases, a single site of bone or joint is infected.
- Spine—especially lower thoracic—or knee most common sites.
- Chest x-ray abnormal in less than half.

General Considerations

Most tuberculous infections in the USA are caused by the human strain of *Mycobacterium tuberculosis* (see Chapter 9). Infection of the musculoskeletal system is caused by hematogenous spread from a primary lesion of the respiratory tract; it may occur shortly after primary infection or may be seen years later as a disease reactivation. Tuberculosis of the thoracic or lumbar spine (Pott's disease) usually occurs in the absence of extraspinal infection. It is a disease of children in developing nations and of the elderly in the United States. Tuberculosis of peripheral joints is almost always monarticular, with the knee the most common site. Extra-articular tuberculosis occurs in only 20%.

Clinical Findings

A. Symptoms and Signs: The onset of symptoms is generally insidious and not accompanied by general manifestations of fever, sweating, toxicity, or prostration. Pain may be mild at onset, is usually worse at night, and may be accompanied by stiffness. As the disease process progresses, limitation of joint motion becomes prominent because of muscle contractures and joint destruction. The knee is the most commonly involved peripheral joint. Symptoms of pulmonary tuberculosis may also be present.

Local findings during the early stages may be limited to tenderness, soft tissue swelling, joint effusion, and increase in skin temperature about the involved area. As the disease progresses without treatment, muscle atrophy and deformity become apparent. Abscess formation with spontaneous drainage externally leads to sinus formation. Progressive destruction of bone in the spine may cause a gibbus, especially in the thoracolumbar region.

B. Laboratory Findings: The precise diagnosis rests upon recovery of the acid-fast organism from joint fluid, pus, or tissue specimens. Biopsy of the bony lesion, synovium, or a regional lymph node may demonstrate the characteristic histopathologic picture of caseating necrosis and giant cells.

C. Imaging: There is a latent period between the onset of symptoms and the initial positive radiographic finding. The earliest changes of tuberculous arthritis are those of soft tissue swelling and distention of the capsule by effusion. Subsequently, bone atrophy causes thinning of the trabecular pattern, narrowing of the cortex, and enlargement of the medullary canal. As joint disease progresses, destruction of cartilage, both in the spine and in peripheral joints, is manifested by narrowing of the joint cleft and focal erosion of the articular surface, especially at the margins. Where the lesion is limited to bone, especially in the cancellous portion of the metaphysis, radiography may demonstrate single or multilocular cysts surrounded by sclerotic bone. With spinal tuberculosis, CT scanning is helpful in demonstrating paraspinal soft tissue extensions of the infection (eg, psoas abscess, epidural extension).

Differential Diagnosis

Tuberculosis of the musculoskeletal system must be differentiated from all subacute and chronic infections, rheumatoid arthritis, gout, and, occasionally, osseous dysplasia. In the spine, metastatic tumor may be suggested.

Complications

Destruction of bones or joints may occur in a few weeks or months if adequate treatment is not provided. Deformity due to joint destruction, abscess formation with spread into adjacent soft tissues, and sinus formation are common. Paraplegia is the most serious complication of spinal tuberculosis. As healing of severe joint lesions takes place, spontaneous fibrous or bony ankylosis follows.

Treatment (See also Chapter 33.)

A. General Measures: General care is especially important when prolonged recumbency is necessary; skillful nursing care must be provided.

B. Chemotherapy: Because of the rise of resistant organisms, the new recommendation for treating bony tuberculosis is to begin with four drugs: isoniazid, 300 mg/d; rifampin, 600 mg/d; pyrazinamide, 25 mg/kg/d; and ethambutol, 15 mg/kg/d. If the isolate is sensitive to isoniazid and rifampin, the ethambutol can be stopped, with the pyrazinamide maintained for 2 months. Isoniazid and rifampin are continued for a total of 6 months. Cure without need for surgical intervention may be effected in most cases, even with extensive disease.

C. Surgical Measures: In acute infections where synovitis is the predominant feature, treatment can be conservative, at least initially. Immobilization by splint or plaster, aspiration, and chemotherapy may suffice to control the infection. Synovectomy may be valuable for less acute hypertrophic lesions that involve tendon sheaths, bursae, or joints.

A 15-year assessment of controlled trials of the management of tuberculosis of the spine in Korea and Hong Kong. Thirteenth Report of the Medical Research Council Working Party on Tuberculosis of the Spine. J Bone Joint Surg Br 1998;80:456. [NLM Cit ID: 98281235]

ARTHRITIS IN SARCOIDOSIS

The frequency of arthritis among patients with sarcoidosis is variously reported between 10% and 35%. It is usually acute in onset, but articular symptoms may appear insidiously and often antedate other manifestations of the disease. Knees and ankles are most commonly involved, but any joint may be affected. Distribution of joint involvement is usually polyarticular and symmetric. The arthritis is commonly self-limited, resolving after several weeks or months and rarely resulting in chronic arthritis, joint destruction, or significant deformity. Sarcoid arthropathy is often associated with erythema nodosum, but the diagnosis is contingent upon the demonstration of other extra-articular manifestations of sarcoidosis and, notably, biopsy evidence of noncaseating granulomas. In chronic arthritis, radiographs show typical changes in the bones of the extremities with intact cortex and cystic changes.

Treatment of arthritis in sarcoidosis is usually symptomatic and supportive. Colchicine may be of value. A short course of corticosteroids may be effective in patients with severe and progressive joint disease.

Mana J et al: Periarticular ankle sarcoidosis: A variant of Lofgren's syndrome. J Rheumatol 1996;23:874. [NLM Cit ID: 96315748] (Periarticular ankle inflammation with bilateral hilar adenopathy is an acute form of sarcoidosis that follows a benign course.)

TUMORS & TUMOR-LIKE LESIONS OF BONE

Essentials of Diagnosis

- Persistent pain, swelling, or tenderness of a skeletal part.
- Pathologic ("spontaneous") fractures.
- Suspicious areas of bony enlargement, deformity, radiodensity, or radiolucency on x-ray.
- Histologic evidence of bone neoplasm on biopsy specimen.

General Considerations

Primary tumors of bone are relatively uncommon in comparison with secondary or metastatic neoplasms. They are, however, of great clinical significance because some grow rapidly and metastasize widely.

Although tumors of bone have been categorized classically as primary or secondary, there is some disagreement about which tumors are primary to the skeleton. Tumors of mesenchymal origin that reflect skeletal tissues (eg, bone, cartilage, and connective tissue) and tumors developing in bones that are of hematopoietic, nerve, vascular, fat cell, and notochordal origin should be differentiated from secondary malignant tumors that involve bone by direct extension or hematogenous spread. Because of the great variety of bone tumors, it is difficult to establish a satisfactory simple classification of bone neoplasms.

Clinical Findings

Persistent skeletal pain and swelling, with or without limitation of motion of adjacent joints or spontaneous fracture are indications for prompt clinical, radiographic, laboratory, and possibly biopsy examination. Radiographs may reveal the location and extent of the lesion and certain characteristics that may suggest the specific diagnosis. The so-called classic radiographic findings of certain tumors (eg, punched-out areas of the skull in multiple myeloma, "sun ray" appearance of osteogenic sarcoma, and "onion peel" effect of Ewing's sarcoma), although suggestive, are not pathognomonic. Even a bone tumor's histologic characteristics, considered in isolation, provide incomplete information about the nature of the disease. The age of the patient, the duration of complaints, the site of involvement and the number of bones involved, and the presence or absence of associated systemic disease—as well as the histologic characteristics—must all be considered for proper management.

The possibility of benign developmental skeletal abnormalities, metastatic neoplastic disease, infections (eg, osteomyelitis), posttraumatic bone lesions, or metabolic disease of bone must always be kept in mind. If bone tumors occur in or near the joints, they may be confused with the various types of arthritis, especially monarticular arthritis.

Specific Bone Tumors

Tumors arising from osteoblastic connective tissue include osteoid osteoma and osteosarcoma. Osteoid osteomas are benign tumors of children and adolescents that should be surgically removed. Osteosarcoma, the most common malignancy of bone, typically occurs in an adolescent who presents with pain or swelling in a bone or joint (especially in or around the knee). Since the symptoms often appear to begin following a sports-related injury, accurate diagnosis may be delayed. Osteosarcoma can also develop in patients with Paget's disease of bone, enchondromatosis, fibrous dysplasia, or hereditary multiple exostoses. Osteosarcomas are treated by resection and chemotherapy, with 5-year survival rates improving from 15% in 1965 to 60% at this time. Fibrosarcomas, which are derived from nonosteoblastic connective tissue, have a prognosis similar to that of the osteogenic sarcomas. Tumors derived from cartilage include enchondromas, chondromyxoid fibromas, and chondrosarcomas. Histologic examination is confirmatory in this group, and the prognosis with appropriate curettement or surgery is generally good.

Other bone tumors include giant cell tumors (osteoclastomas), chondroblastomas, and Ewing's sarcoma. Of these, chondroblastomas are almost always benign. About 50% of giant cell tumors are benign, while the rest may be frankly malignant or recur after excision. Ewing's sarcoma, which affects children, adolescents, and young adults, has a 50% mortality rate in spite of chemotherapy, irradiation, and surgery.

Treatment

Although prompt action is essential for optimal treatment of certain bone tumors, accurate diagnosis is required because of the great potential for harm that may result from temporization, radical or ablative operations, or unnecessary irradiation.

Arndt C et al: Common musculoskeletal tumors of childhood and adolescence. N Engl J Med 1999;341:342. [NLM Cit ID: 99336993] (Review of rhabdomyosarcoma, osteosarcoma, and Ewing's sarcoma.)

NEUROGENIC ARTHROPATHY (Charcot's Joint)

Neurogenic arthropathy is joint destruction resulting from loss or diminution of proprioception, pain, and temperature perception. Although traditionally associated with tabes dorsalis, it is more frequently seen in diabetic neuropathy, syringomyelia, spinal cord injury, pernicious anemia, leprosy, and peripheral nerve injury. Prolonged administration of hydrocortisone by the intra-articular route may also cause Charcot's joint. As normal muscle tone and protective reflexes are lost, secondary degenerative joint disease ensues, resulting in an enlarged, boggy, painless joint with extensive cartilage erosion, osteophyte formation, and multiple loose joint bodies. Radiographic changes may be degenerative or hypertrophic in the same patient.

Treatment is directed against the primary disease; mechanical devices are used to assist in weight bearing and prevention of further trauma. In some instances, amputation becomes unavoidable.

OTHER RHEUMATIC DISORDERS

RHEUMATIC MANIFESTATIONS OF CANCER

Rheumatologic syndromes may be the presenting manifestations for a variety of cancers (Table 4–6). Dermatomyositis in adults, for example, is associated with cancer. Middle-aged or older patients with polyarthritis that mimics rheumatoid arthritis but is associated with new onset of clubbing and periosteal new bone formation should be suspected of having hypertrophic pulmonary osteoarthropathy, a disorder commonly associated with both malignant diseases (eg, lung and intrathoracic cancers) and nonmalignant ones (eg, cyanotic heart disease, cirrhosis, and lung abscess). Palmar fasciitis is characterized by bilateral palmar swelling and finger contraction and may be the first indication of cancer, particularly ovarian carcinoma. Palpable purpura due to leukocytoclastic vasculitis may be the presenting complaint in myeloproliferative disorders. Hairy cell leukemia can be associated with medium-sized vessel vasculitis such as polyarteritis nodosa. Acute leukemia can produce joint pains that are disproportionately severe in comparison to the minimal swelling and heat that are present. Leukemic arthritis complicates approximately 5% of cases. Rheumatic manifestations of myelodysplastic syndromes include cutaneous vasculitis, lupus-like syndromes, neuropathy, and episodic intense arthritis. Erythromelalgia, a painful warmth and redness of the extremities that (unlike Raynaud's) improves with cold exposure or with elevation of the extremity, is often associated with myeloproliferative diseases.

Jacobson AF: Musculoskeletal pain as an indicator of occult malignancy: Yield of bone scintigraphy. Arch Intern Med 1997;157:105. [NLM Cit ID: 97149239] (Bone scan useful in detecting occult malignancy in patients over 50 with enigmatic diffuse musculoskeletal pain or in patients with focal pain out of proportion to plain x-ray findings.)

PALINDROMIC RHEUMATISM

Palindromic rheumatism is a disease of unknown cause characterized by frequent recurring attacks (at irregular intervals) of acutely inflamed joints. Periarticular pain with swelling and transient subcutaneous nodules may also occur. The attacks cease within several hours to several days. The knee and finger joints are most commonly affected, but any peripheral joint may be involved. Systemic manifestations other than fever do not occur. Although hundreds of attacks may take place over a period of years, there is no permanent articular damage. Laboratory findings are usually normal. Palindromic rheumatism must be distinguished from acute gouty arthritis and an atypical, acute onset of rheumatoid arthritis. In some patients, palindromic rheumatism is a prodrome of rheumatoid arthritis.

Symptomatic treatment with NSAIDs is usually all that is required during the attacks. Hydroxychloroquine may be of value in preventing recurrences.

AVASCULAR NECROSIS OF BONE

Avascular necrosis of bone is a complication of corticosteroid use, trauma, SLE, pancreatitis, alcoholism, gout, sickle cell disease, and infiltrative diseases (eg, Gaucher's disease). The most commonly affected sites are the proximal and distal femoral heads, leading to hip or knee pain. Many patients with hip disease actually first present with pain referred to the knee. Physical examination will reveal that it is internal rotation of the hip—not movement of the knee—that is painful. Other commonly affected sites include the ankle, shoulder, and elbow. Initially, radiographs are often normal; MRI, CT scan, and bone scan are all more sensitive techniques. Treatment involves avoidance of weight bearing on the affected joint for at least several weeks. The value of surgical core decompression is controversial. Unfortunately, the natural history of avascular necrosis is usually progression of the bony infarction to cortical collapse, resulting in significant joint dysfunction. Total hip replacement is the usual outcome for all patients who are candidates for that procedure.

Plancher KD et al: Management of osteonecrosis of the femoral head. Orthop Clin North Am 1997;28:461. [NLM Cit ID: 97354454] (Presentation, diagnosis, and management.)

SOME ORTHOPEDIC PROCEDURES FOR ARTHRITIC JOINTS

Synovectomy

This procedure attempts to eliminate inflammation at a joint by surgically removing as much of the synovium as possible. The procedure has been performed most commonly in patients with rheumatoid arthritis who, despite medical therapy, have a persistent pannus of inflamed synovium (usually around a wrist or a knee). Patients with degenerative diseases do not have marked synovial inflammation and are not candidates for this procedure.

Unfortunately, synovium can regrow. Even in patients with rheumatoid arthritis, the long-term benefits of synovectomy remain unproved.

Arthroplasty

Realigning arthritic joints (arthroplasty) generally does not work as well as complete joint replacement, but it can defer the need for joint replacement. The typical candidate is an adult under 50 years of age who has severe osteoarthritis of one compartment of the knee (typically the medial compartment). Excising a wedge of femur will realign the patient's knee so as to shift weight to the compartment with normal cartilage and thereby eliminate or reduce the patient's pain.

Tendon Rupture

This is a fairly common complication in rheumatoid arthritis and requires immediate orthopedic referral. The most common sites are the finger flexors and extensors, the patellar tendon, and the Achilles tendon.

Arthrodesis

Arthrodesis (fusion) is being used less now than formerly, but a chronically infected, painful joint may be an indication for this surgical procedure.

Total Joint Arthroplasty

In the last 3 decades, remarkable progress has been made in the replacement of severely damaged joints with prosthetic materials. Although many different joints can be replaced, the largest experience and greatest success have been with hip and knee replacement. Indication for total joint arthroplasty is severe pain (usually including pain at rest) accompanied by loss of function and severe destruction of the joint on x-ray. Age is also a consideration, as the durability of artificial joints beyond 10–15 years is limited with older surgical techniques and unproved with newer techniques. Thus, patients over 65 are less likely than younger ones to face the challenge of revision.

Whatever the patient's age, success of the replacement depends upon the amount of physical stress to which the prosthetic components are subjected. Vigorous impact activity, even with the most advanced biomaterials and design, will result in failure of the prosthesis with time. Revision operations are technically more difficult, and the results may not be as good as with the primary procedure. The patient, therefore, must understand the limitations of joint replacement and the consequences of unrestrained joint usage.

A. Total Hip Arthroplasty: Hip replacement was originally designed for use in patients over 65 years of age with severe osteoarthritis. In these patients—usually less active physically—the prosthesis not only functioned well but outlasted the patients. Severe arthritis that fails to respond to conservative measures remains the principal indication for hip arthroplasty. Hip arthroplasty may also be indicated in younger patients severely disabled by painful hip disease (eg, rheumatoid arthritis), since in such cases it can be assumed that stress on the prosthetic joint will not be great. Contraindications to the operation include active infection and neurotrophic joint disease. Obesity is a relative contraindication. Serious complications may occur in about 1% of patients and include thrombophlebitis, pulmonary embolization, infection, and dislocation of the joint. Extensive experience has now been accumulated, and the short-term results are highly successful in properly selected patients. The long-term success has been limited by loosening of the prosthesis, a complication seen in 30–50% of patients 10 years after replacement with "first generation" techniques. Although loosening and periprosthetic osteolysis were blamed on the cement, second-generation cementing techniques for prosthetic hips have proved more durable than cementless hips in one out of four cases.

B. Total Knee Arthroplasty: The indications and contraindications for total knee arthroplasty are similar to those for hip arthroplasty. Results are slightly better in osteoarthritis patients than in those with rheumatoid arthritis. Complications are similar to those with hip arthroplasty. The failure rate of knee arthroplasty is slightly higher than that of hip arthroplasty.

Lynch NM et al: Complications after concomitant bilateral total knee arthroplasty in elderly patients. Mayo Clin Proc 1997;72:799. [NLM Cit ID: 97440217] (Cardiovascular and neurologic complications more common with concomitant bilateral knee replacement in elderly patients.)

Mahomed N et al: Revision total hip arthroplasty: Indications and outcomes. Arthritis Rheum 1996;39:1939. [NLM Cit ID: 97121232] (Patients with loosening should be considered for revision.)

RELEVANT WORLD WIDE WEB SITES

[Arthritis Foundation]
http://www.arthritis.org

[Enchondroma With Pathologic Fracture]
http://www.brighamrad.harvard.edu/Cases/bwh/hcache/163/full.html

[Juxtacortical Chondrosarcoma]
http://www.brighamrad.harvard.edu/Cases/bwh/hcache/53/full.html

[Orthopedic 3-Dimensional Imaging of the Knee]
http://everest.radiology.uiowa.edu/nlm/app/ortho/knee.html

[Osteogenesis Imperfecta]
http://www.brighamrad.harvard.edu/Cases/bwh/hcache/76/full.html

[Osteoid Osteoma]
http://www.brighamrad.harvard.edu/Cases/bwh/hcache/91/full.html

[Osteoid Osteoma]
http://www.brighamrad.harvard.edu/Cases/bwh/hcache/54/full.html

[Osteomyelitis of Cervical Spine]
http://www.brighamrad.harvard.edu/Cases/bwh/hcache/119/full.html

[Thoracic Outlet Syndrome]
http://www.brighamrad.harvard.edu/Cases/bwh/hcache/170/full.html

[Wheeless' Textbook of Orthopaedics]
http://www.medmedia.com

Fluid & Electrolyte Disorders

21

See http://www.current-med.com/ch21.html for updated addresses of Web sites referenced in this chapter.

Masafumi Fukagawa, MD, PhD, Kiyoshi Kurokawa, MD, MACP, & Maxine A. Papadakis, MD

DIAGNOSIS OF FLUID & ELECTROLYTE DISORDERS

Approach to the Patient

A. History and Physical Examination:

1. Alterations in body fluid volume–Causes of changes in body fluid volume can usually be determined by the history and physical examination. **Volume overload** is manifested by an increase in weight and peripheral edema or ascites. Edema from local obstruction of venous return must be differentiated from systemic processes (congestive heart failure, cirrhosis, and nephrotic syndrome). A history of increased dietary sodium intake and use of medications that affect the renin-angiotensin system (converting enzyme inhibitors, prostaglandin synthesis inhibitors, mineralocorticoids, calcium channel blockers) should be sought. **Volume depletion** is characterized by weight loss, excessive thirst, and dry mucous membranes. The term **dehydration,** pure water deficit, should be distinguished from volume depletion, in which both water and salt are lost. There may be resting tachycardia, orthostatic hypotension, or shock. Causes include vomiting or diarrhea, diuretic use, renal disease, diabetes mellitus or diabetes insipidus, inadequate oral intake associated with altered mental status, and excessive insensible losses from sweating or fever.

B. Further Evaluation: Treatment of fluid and electrolyte disorders is based on (1) assessment of total body water and its distribution, (2) electrolyte concentrations, and (3) serum osmolality. Serial changes in body weight constitute the best way of knowing if there has been an acute change in body water balance.

1. Body water–Table 21–1 shows the sex difference in total body water and the decrease in total body water that occurs with aging.

2. Electrolytes–Table 21–2 shows the normal values for serum electrolytes.

3. Serum osmolality–Serum osmolality (normally 285–295 mosm/kg) can be calculated from the following formula:

$$\text{Osmolality} = 2(\text{Na}^+\text{meq/L}) + \frac{\text{Glucose mg/dL}}{18} + \frac{\text{BUN mg/dL}}{2.8}$$

(1 mosm of glucose equals 180 mg/L, and 1 mosm of urea nitrogen equals 28 mg/L.)

Solute concentration is usually expressed in terms of osmolality. The number of particles in solution (ie, osmolytes; either molecules or ions) determines the number of milliosmoles. Each particle has a unit value of 1, so if a substance ionizes, each ion contributes the same amount as a nonionizable molecule. More importantly, permeability of the particle across the cell membrane determines if it acts as a physiologically active osmolyte. Only impermeable particles contribute to tonicity, and it is tonicity, not osmolality, that stimulates both thirst and ADH release. Substances that easily permeate cell membranes (eg, urea, ethanol) are not effective osmolytes and therefore do not cause shifting of fluid in body fluid compartments. For example, glucose in solution is nonionizable. Therefore, 1 mmol of glucose has an osmole concentration of 1 mosm/kg H_2O. One millimole of NaCl, however, forms two ions in water (one Na^+ and one Cl^-) and has an osmole concentration of roughly 2 mosm/kg H_2O. "Osmoles per kilogram of water" is *osmolality;* "osmoles per liter of solution" is *osmolarity.* At the solute concentration of body fluids, the two measurements correspond so closely that they are interchangeable.

C. Clinical Implications: In many instances, electrolyte disorders are asymptomatic. However, patients may develop lethargy, weakness, confusion, delirium, and seizures, especially in the presence of an abnormal serum sodium concentration. Often these symptoms are mistaken for primary neurologic or metabolic disorders. Muscle weakness occurs in patients with severe hypokalemia, hyperkalemia, and hypophosphatemia; confusion, seizures, and coma may develop in those with severe hypercalcemia.

Table 21–1. Total body water (as percentage of body weight) in relation to age and sex.

Age	Male	Female
18–40	60%	50%
41–60	60–50%	50–40%
Over 60	50%	40%

Measurement of electrolytes (sodium, potassium, chloride, bicarbonate, calcium, magnesium, and phosphorus) is indicated for any patient with even vague neuromuscular symptoms.

TREATMENT OF SPECIFIC FLUID, ELECTROLYTE, & ACID-BASE DISORDERS

DISORDERS OF SODIUM CONCENTRATION

1. HYPONATREMIA

Hyponatremia (defined as a serum sodium concentration less than 130 meq/L) is the most common electrolyte abnormality observed in a general hospitalized population, seen in about 2% of patients. The initial approach to its investigation is the determination of serum osmolality (Figure 21–1).

The Urine Sodium

Measurement of urine sodium helps distinguish renal from nonrenal causes of hyponatremia. Urine sodium exceeding 20 meq/L is consistent with renal salt wasting (diuretics, ACE inhibitors, mineralocorticoid deficiency, salt-losing nephropathy). Urine sodium less than 10 meq/L or fractional excretion of sodium less than 1% (unless diuretics have been given) implies avid sodium retention by the kidney to compensate for extrarenal fluid losses from vomiting, diarrhea, sweating, or third-spacing, as with ascites. Fractional excretion (FE) of sodium or urea is calculated using a random urine sample with simultaneously obtained plasma samples for sodium (or urea) and creatinine (Cr):

$$FE_{Na}\ (\%) = \frac{Urine_{sodium} / Plasma_{sodium}}{Urine_{creatinine} / Plasma_{creatinine}} \times 100$$

Table 21–2. Normal values and mass conversion factors.[1]

	Normal Plasma Values	Mass Conversion
Na^+	135–145 meq/L	23 mg = 1 meq
K^+	3.5–5 meq/L	39 mg = 1 meq
Cl^-	98–107 meq/L	35 mg = 1 meq
HCO_3^-	22–28 meq/L	61 mg = 1 meq
Ca^{2+}	8.5–10.5 mg/dL	40 mg = 1 mmol
Phosphorus	2.5–4.5 mg/dL	31 mg = 1 mmol
Mg^{2+}	1.6–3 mg/dL	24 mg = 1 mmol
Osmolality	280–295 mosm/kg	. . .

[1]Modified and reproduced, with permission, from Cogan MG: *Fluid and Electrolytes: Physiology and Pathophysiology.* Originally published by Appleton & Lange. Copyright © 1991 by The McGraw-Hill Companies, Inc.

Isotonic Hyponatremia

In hyperlipidemia and hyperproteinemia, the marked increases in lipids (chylomicrons and triglycerides, but not cholesterol) and proteins (> 10 g/dL) occupy a disproportionately large portion of the plasma volume. Plasma osmolality remains normal because its measurement is unaffected by the lipids or proteins. A decreased volume of water results, so that the sodium concentration in total plasma volume is decreased. Because the sodium concentration in the plasma water is normal, hyperlipidemia and hyperproteinemia cause pseudohyponatremia. Most United States laboratories now measure serum electrolytes using ion-specific electrodes and thus avoid misdiagnosis.

Hypotonic Hyponatremia

Hypotonic hyponatremia is true hyponatremia in a physiologic sense. Since the capacity of the kidney to excrete electrolyte-free water is potentially great—up to 20–30 L/d—in the presence of a normal GFR (100 L/d), electrolyte-free water intake must theoretically exceed 30 L/d for hyponatremia to develop. Thus, impairment of electrolyte-free water excretion (renal failure, inappropriate ADH excess, etc) is nearly always observed in hyponatremia.

A. Hypovolemic Hypotonic Hyponatremia: Hyponatremia with decreased extracellular fluid volume occurs in the setting of renal or extrarenal volume loss (Figure 21–1). Total body sodium is decreased. To maintain intravascular volume, antidiuretic hormone (ADH) secretion increases, and free water is retained. The drive to replenish intravascular volume overrules the need to sustain normal osmolality; losses of salt and water are replaced by water alone. The combination of low fractional excretion of sodium (< 0.5%) and low fractional urea clearance (< 55%) is the best way to predict improvement with saline therapy. Hyponatremia has been shown to develop in patients with intracranial diseases through renal sodium wasting. Unlike those with SIADH, these patients are hypovolemic, though plasma levels of ADH are inappropriately high for the osmolality. Observations in patients with subarachnoid hemorrhage suggest that the cerebral salt-wasting syndrome is

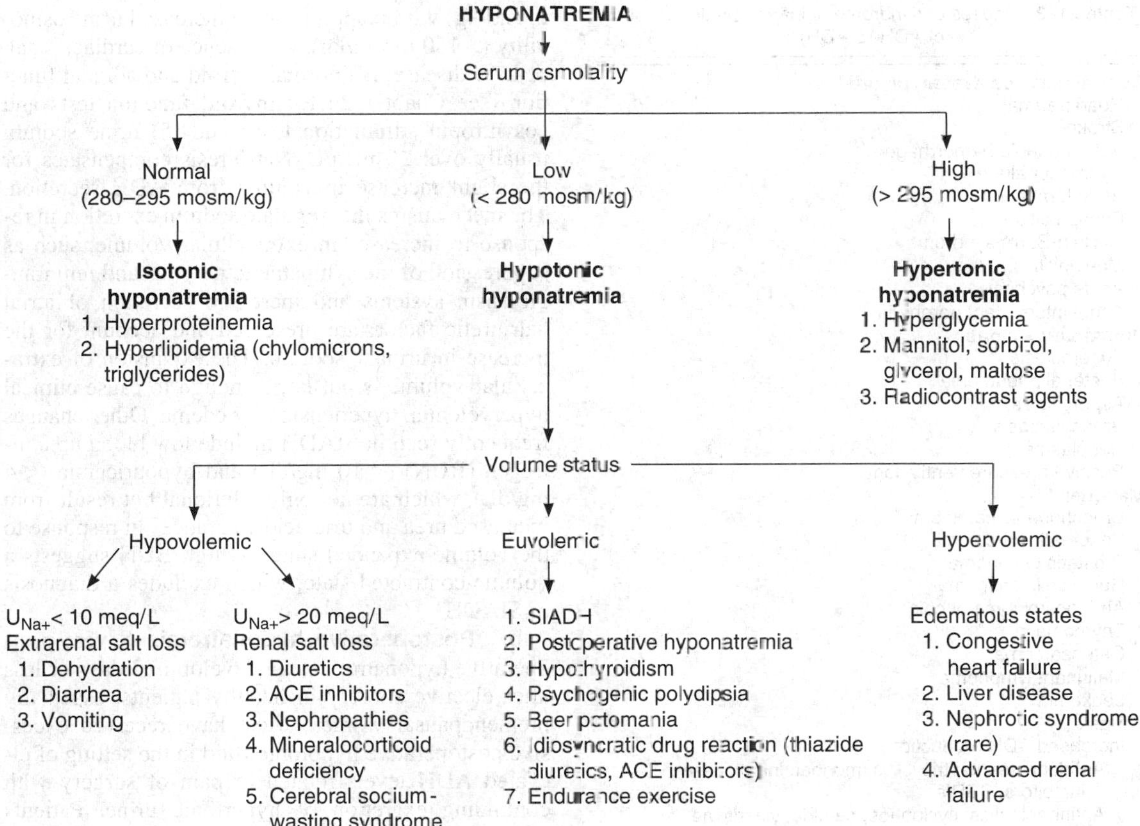

Figure 21–1. Evaluation of hyponatremia using serum osmolality and extracellular fluid volume status. (Adapted, with permission, from Narins RG et al: Diagnostic strategies in disorders of fluid, electrolyte and acid-base homeostasis. Am J Med 1982;72:496).

caused by increased secretion of brain natriuretic peptide with suppression of aldosterone secretion.

Treatment consists of replacement of lost volume with isotonic or half-normal (0.45%) saline or lactated Ringer's infusion. The rate of correction must be adjusted to prevent permanent cerebral damage (see below). Corticosteroids can be used empirically if hypocortisolism is considered in the differential diagnosis. See Adrenocortical Hypofunction in Chapter 26 for diagnosis (by means of the cosyntropin stimulation test) and treatment of hypocortisolism.

B. Euvolemic Hypotonic Hyponatremia: In this setting, determinations of urine osmolality (Figure 21–1) along with urine sodium are useful for appropriate diagnosis.

1. Clinical syndromes–

a. Syndrome of inappropriate ADH secretion (SIADH)–(Table 21–3.) Hypovolemia physiologically stimulates ADH secretion, so the diagnosis of SIADH is made only if the patient is euvolemic. In SIADH, increased ADH release occurs without osmolality-dependent or volume-dependent physiologic stimulation. Normal regulation of ADH release occurs from both the central nervous system and the chest via baroreceptors and neural input. It follows that the causes of SIADH are disorders affecting the central nervous system—structural, metabolic, psychiatric, or pharmacologic—or the lungs. Furthermore, some carcinomas, such as small cell lung carcinoma, synthesize ADH. Other states associated with SIADH include administration of drugs that either increase ADH secretion or potentiate its action. SIADH induced by selective serotonin (or epinephrine) reuptake inhibitors such as fluoxetine is fairly common in geriatric patients.

(1) Patterns of abnormal ADH secretion–

(a) Random secretion–ADH release is unrelated to osmoregulation. This pattern is seen in carcinomas and central nervous system diseases.

(b) Reset osmostat–This variant is characterized by ADH secretion appropriately suppressed at very low serum osmolalities but with ADH osmoregulation downset to a lower level of "normal." Therefore, ADH is secreted at a subnormal serum osmolality threshold (< 280 mosm/kg). Appropriate urinary dilution can be attained but at low serum osmolalities. This pattern is

Table 21–3. Causes of syndrome of inappropriate secretion of ADH (SIADH).

Central nervous system disorders
Head trauma
Stroke
Subarachnoid hemorrhage
Hydrocephalus
Brain tumor
Encephalitis
Guillain-Barré syndrome
Meningitis
Acute psychosis
Acute intermittent porphyria
Pulmonary lesions
Tuberculosis
Bacterial pneumonia
Aspergillosis
Bronchiectasis
Neoplasms
Positive pressure ventilation
Malignancies
Bronchogenic carcinoma
Pancreatic carcinoma
Prostatic carcinoma
Renal cell carcinoma
Adenocarcinoma of colon
Thymoma
Osteosarcoma
Malignant lymphoma
Leukemia
Drugs
Increased ADH production
Antidepressants: tricyclics, monoamine oxidase inhibitors, SSRIs
Antineoplastics: cyclophosphamide, vincristine
Carbamazepine
Methylenedioxymethamphetamine (MDMA; Ecstasy)
Clofibrate
Neuroleptics: thiothixene, thioridazine, fluphenazine, haloperidol, trifluoperazine
Potentiated ADH action
Carbamazepine
Chlorpropamide, tolbutamide
Cyclophosphamide
NSAIDs
Somatostatin and analogs
Others
Postoperative
Pain
Stress
AIDS
Pregnancy (physiologic)
Hypokalemia

seen in the elderly, in patients with pulmonary processes, tuberculosis, or malnutrition. During pregnancy, the physiologic reset osmostat may suppress osmolality by about 10 mmol/kg of water.

(c) Leak of ADH–In conditions such as basilar skull fractures, low levels of ADH are "leaked" despite hypo-osmolality. If serum osmolality rises to normal, ADH secretion increases appropriately and then continues to respond normally if osmolality further increases.

(2) Clinical features–SIADH is characterized by (1) hyponatremia; (2) decreased osmolality (< 280 mosm/kg) with inappropriately increased urine osmolality (> 150 mosm/kg); (3) absence of cardiac, renal, or liver disease; (4) normal thyroid and adrenal function (see Chapter 26 for thyroid function tests and cosyntropin stimulation test); and (5) urine sodium usually over 20 meq/L. Natriuresis compensates for the slight increase in volume from ADH secretion. The mechanisms that regulate sodium excretion in response to increases in extracellular volume, such as suppression of the sympathetic nervous and renin-angiotensin systems and increased secretion of atrial natriuretic factor, are preserved and account for the increase in urinary sodium. The expansion of extracellular volume is not large enough to cause clinical hypervolemia, hypertension, or edema. Other changes frequently seen in SIADH include low blood urea nitrogen (BUN) (< 10 mg/dL) and hypouricemia (< 4 mg/dL), which are not only dilutional but result from increased urea and uric acid clearances in response to the volume-expanded state. A high BUN suggests a volume-contracted state, which excludes a diagnosis of SIADH.

b. Postoperative hyponatremia–Severe postoperative hyponatremia can develop in 2 days or less after elective surgery in healthy patients, especially premenopausal women. Most have received excessive postoperative hypotonic fluid in the setting of elevated ADH levels related to pain of surgery with continuing excretion of hypertonic urine. Patients awake normally from general anesthesia but within 2 days develop nausea, headache, seizures, and even respiratory arrest. Serum sodium levels may be less than 110 meq/L. Premenopausal women who develop hyponatremic encephalopathy are about 25 times more likely than menopausal women to die or to suffer permanent brain damage, suggesting a hormonal role in the pathophysiology of this disorder. Hyponatremia may result from direct absorption of hypotonic irrigating fluids through veins during endometrial ablation or transurethral prostate resection. These patients can be symptomatic intraoperatively, with tremulousness, hypothermia, or hypoxia, or upon awakening from anesthesia, with headache, nausea, and vomiting.

c. Hypothyroidism–Hyponatremia is not commonly caused by hypothyroidism, but it can occur on occasion with serum sodium levels as low as 105 meq/L. Water retention is the cause, probably both from inappropriately elevated ADH levels and from nonhormonal alterations in the handling of water by the kidneys.

d. Psychogenic polydipsia and beer potomania–Marked excess free water intake (generally > 10 L/d) may produce hyponatremia. Euvolemia is maintained through the renal excretion of sodium. Urine sodium is therefore generally elevated (> 20 meq/L), but unlike SIADH, levels of ADH are suppressed. Urine osmolality is appropriately low (< 300 mosm/kg) as the increased free water is excreted. Hyponatremia from bursts of ADH occurs in manic-depressive patients with excess free water intake. Psychogenic polydipsia is observed in patients with psychologic problems, and these patients frequently take drugs interfering with water excretion. Similarly, excessive intake of beer, which contains very small amounts of sodium (< 5 meq/L), can cause severe hyponatremia in cirrhotic patients, who have elevated ADH and often decreased GFR. Very low solute intake may also be associated with disturbed water excretion leading to hyponatremia.

e. Idiosyncratic diuretic reaction–In addition to hyponatremia developing from volume contraction due to diuretic therapy (see above), a less common diuretic-induced hyponatremia can occur in euvolemic patients, typically from thiazides. This syndrome is most often seen in healthy older women (over 70 years of age) often after a few days of therapy. The mechanism for the hyponatremia appears to be a combination of excessive renal sodium loss and water retention.

f. Idiosyncratic ACE inhibitor reactions– ACE inhibitors can cause central polydipsia and increased antidiuretic hormone secretion, both of which result in severe, symptomatic hyponatremia. Patients given ACE inhibitors who develop polydipsia should have their serum Na^+ levels checked.

g. Endurance exercise hyponatremia–Hyponatremia after endurance exercise (eg, triathlon events) may be caused by a combination of excessive fluid overload and continued ADH secretion. Reperfusion of the exercise-induced ischemic splanchnic bed causes delayed absorption of excessive quantities of hypotonic fluid ingested during exercise. Sustained elevation of ADH prevents water excretion in this setting. The retention of hypotonic fluid may be further exacerbated by NSAIDs frequently used by athletes.

2. Treatment–

a. Symptomatic hyponatremia–Symptomatic hyponatremia is usually seen in patients with serum sodium levels less than 120 meq/L. If there are central nervous system symptoms, hyponatremia should be rapidly treated at any level of serum sodium concentration.

(1) Rate and degree of correction–Central pontine myelinolysis may occur from osmotically induced demyelination due to overly rapid correction of serum sodium (an increase of more than 1 meq/L/h, or 25 meq/L within the first day of therapy). Hypoxic-anoxic episodes during hyponatremia may contribute to the demyelination. A reasonable approach is to increase the serum sodium concentration by no more than 1–2 meq/L/h and not more than 25–30 meq/L in the first 2 days; the rate should be reduced to 0.5–1 meq/L/h as soon as neurologic symptoms improve. The initial goal is to achieve a serum sodium concentration of 125–130 meq/L, guarding against overcorrection.

(2) Saline plus furosemide–Hypertonic (eg, 3%) saline with furosemide is indicated for symptomatic hyponatremic patients. If one administers 3% saline without a diuretic to a patient with SIADH, the serum sodium concentration increases temporarily, but euvolemic patients excrete the excess sodium. If one adds furosemide (0.5–1 mg/kg intravenously), however, the kidney cannot concentrate urine even in the presence of high levels of ADH. Infusion of 3% saline is accompanied by excretion of isotonic urine with a net loss of free water. The sodium concentration of 3% saline is 513 meq/L. In order to determine how much 3% saline to administer, a spot urinary Na^+ is determined after a furosemide diuresis has begun. The excreted Na^+ is replaced with 3% saline, empirically begun at 1–2 mL/kg/h and then adjusted based on urinary output and urinary sodium. For example, after administration of furosemide, urine volume may be 400 mL/h and sodium plus potassium excretion 100 meq/L. The excreted Na^+ plus K^+ is 40 meq/h, which is replaced with 78 mL/h of 3% saline (40 meq/h divided by 513 meq/L). Free water loss is about 1% of total body water. Therefore, an approximately 1% rise in plasma sodium concentration (1–1.5 meq/L/h) can be expected. Measurements of plasma sodium should be done approximately every 4 hours and the patient observed closely.

b. Asymptomatic hyponatremia–In asymptomatic hyponatremia, the correction rate of hyponatremia need be no more than 0.5 meq/L/h. No specific treatment is needed for patients with reset osmostats.

(1) Water restriction–Water intake should be restricted to 0.5–1 L/d. Gradual increase of serum sodium will occur over days.

(2) 0.9% saline–0.9% saline with furosemide may be used in asymptomatic patients whose serum sodium is less than 120 meq/L. Urinary sodium and potassium losses are replaced as above.

(3) Demeclocycline–Demeclocycline (300–600 mg twice daily) is useful for patients who cannot adhere to water restriction or need additional therapy; it inhibits the effect of ADH on the distal tubule. Onset of action may require 1 week, and concentrating may be permanently impaired. Therapy with demeclocycline in cirrhosis appears to increase the risk of renal failure.

(4) Fludrocortisone–Hyponatremia occurring as part of the cerebral salt-wasting syndrome can be treated with fludrocortisone.

C. Hypervolemic Hypotonic Hyponatremia: Hyponatremia with increased extracellular fluid volume is seen when hyponatremia is accompanied by edema-associated disorders such as congestive heart failure, cirrhosis, nephrotic syndrome, and advanced renal disease (Figure 21–1). In congestive heart failure, hyponatremia carries a poor prognosis, presaging death within a year for over half of patients. Total body sodium is increased, yet effective circulating volume is sensed as inadequate by baroreceptors. Increased ADH and aldosterone results, with retention of water and sodium.

The **urine sodium** concentration is generally less than 10 meq/L unless the patient has been taking diuretics.

Treatment

A. Water Restriction: The treatment of hyponatremia is that of the underlying condition (eg, improving cardiac output in congestive heart failure) and water restriction (to < 1–2 L of water daily).

B. Diuretics: To hasten excretion of water and salt, use of diuretics may be indicated. Since diuretics may worsen hyponatremia, the patient must be cautioned not to increase free water intake.

C. Hypertonic (3%) Saline: Hypertonic saline administration is dangerous in volume-overloaded states and is not routinely recommended. In patients with severe hyponatremia (serum sodium < 110 meq/L) and central nervous system symptoms, judicious administration of small amounts (100–200 mL) of 3% saline with diuretics may be necessary. Emergency dialysis should also be considered.

Hypertonic Hyponatremia

Hypertonic hyponatremia is most commonly seen with hyperglycemia. When blood glucose becomes acutely elevated, water is drawn from the cells to the extracellular space, diluting the serum sodium. The plasma sodium level falls 1.6 meq/L for every 100 mg/dL rise when the glucose concentration is between 200 and 400 mg/dL. If the glucose concentration is above 400 mg/dL, the plasma sodium concentration falls 4 meq/L for every 100 mg/dL rise in glucose. This dilutional hyponatremia is not pseudohyponatremia, since the sodium concentration does indeed fall. Infusion of hypertonic solutions containing osmotically active osmoles (eg, mannitol) may also cause hypertonic hyponatremia by drawing water to the extracellular space.

Adrogue HJ et al: Hyponatremia. N Engl J Med 2000;342:1581. [NLM Cit ID: 20267493]

Berendes E et al: Secretion of brain natriuretic peptide in patients with aneurysmal subarachnoid haemorrhage. Lancet 1997;349:245. [NLM Cit ID: 97167223]

Bouman WP et al: Incidence of selective serotonin reuptake inhibitor (SSRI) induced hyponatremia due to the syndrome of inappropriate antidiuretic hormone (SIADH) secretion in the elderly. Int J Geriatr Psychiatry 1998;13:12. [NLM Cit ID: 98149219]

Fried LF et al: Hyponatremia and hypernatremia. Med Clin North Am 1997;81:585. [NLM Cit ID: 97310480]

Hillier TA et al: Hyponatremia: Evaluating the correction factor for hyperglycemia. Am J Med 1999;106:399. [NLM Cit ID: 99239747]

Hirshberg B et al: The syndrome of inappropriate antidiuretic hormone secretion in the elderly. Am J Med 1997;103:270. [NLM Cit ID: 98026442] (SIADH in the elderly is usually idiopathic and follows a benign course; an exhaustive diagnostic workup is not warranted in most cases.)

Kumar S et al: Sodium. Lancet 1998;352:220. [NLM Cit ID: 98346757] (Up-to-date review of the pathogenesis of and practical treatment recommendations for sodium imbalance.)

Laureno R et al: Myelinolysis after correction of hyponatremia. Ann Intern Med 1997;126:57. [NLM Cit ID: 97127952]

Oster JR et al: Hyponatremia, hyposmolality, and hypotonicity: tables and fables. Arch Intern Med 1999;159: 333. [NLM Cit ID: 99153376] (An insightful review of the interpretation of hyponatremia.)

Steele A et al: Postoperative hyponatremia despite near-isotonic saline infusion: A phenomenon of desalination. Ann Intern Med 1997;126:20. [NLM Cit ID: 97127947]

Thaler SM et al: "Beer potomania" in non-beer drinkers: effect of low dietary solute intake. Am J Kidney Dis 1998;31:1028. [NLM Cit ID: 98293610] (Low solute intake as a cause of free water excretion defect.)

Hyponatremia in AIDS

Hyponatremia is seen in up to 50% of patients hospitalized for AIDS and in 20% of ambulatory AIDS patients, often associated with pneumonia and central nervous system processes. If hyponatremia is present at the time of hospital admission, it is just as likely to be due to hypovolemic gastrointestinal loss as to euvolemic SIADH. However, if hyponatremia develops after hospital admission, most patients have euvolemic SIADH. Infrequently, hypovolemic hyponatremia is due to adrenal insufficiency, isolated mineralocorticoid deficiency with hyporeninemic hypoaldosteronism, or an HIV-specific impairment in renal sodium conservation. Hyponatremia from adrenal insufficiency may coexist with hypokalemia if the patient also has diarrhea. Adrenal function can be tested with corticotropin stimulation to determine the adequacy of serum cortisol response (see Chapter 26). Patients with isolated hyporeninemic hypoaldosteronism have normal cortisol responses to corticotropin but have decreased serum aldosterone levels.

2. HYPERNATREMIA

An intact thirst mechanism usually prevents hypernatremia (> 145 meq/L). Thus, whatever the underlying disorder (eg, dehydration, lactulose or mannitol therapy, central and nephrogenic diabetes insipidus), excess water loss can cause hypernatremia only when appropriate water intake is not possible. This situation frequently occurs with inappropriate fluid therapy, especially in unconscious patients. Rarely, excessive sodium intake may cause hypernatremia. Hypernatremia in primary aldosteronism is mild and usually does not cause symptoms. Hypernatremia in the presence of salt and water overload is uncommon but has been reported in very ill patients in the course of therapy.

Clinical Findings

A. Symptoms and Signs: When dehydration exists, orthostatic hypotension and oliguria are typical findings. Hyperthermia, delirium, and coma may be seen with severe hyperosmolality.

B. Laboratory Findings:

1. Urine osmolality > 400 mosm/kg–Renal water-conserving ability is functioning.

a. Nonrenal losses–Hypernatremia will develop if water ingestion fails to keep up with hypotonic losses from excessive sweating, exertional losses from the respiratory tract, or through stool water. Lactulose causes an osmotic diarrhea with loss of free water.

b. Renal losses–While diabetic hyperglycemia can cause pseudohyponatremia (see above), progressive volume depletion from the osmotic diuresis of glycosuria can result in true hypernatremia. Osmotic diuresis can occur with the use of mannitol or urea.

2. Urine osmolality < 250 mosm/kg–A dilute urine with osmolality less than 250 mosm/kg with hypernatremia is characteristic of central and nephrogenic diabetes insipidus. Nephrogenic diabetes insipidus, seen with lithium or demeclocycline therapy, after relief of prolonged urinary tract obstruction, or with interstitial nephritis, results from renal insensitivity to ADH. Hypercalcemia and hypokalemia may be contributing factors when present.

Treatment

Treatment of hypernatremia is directed toward correcting the cause of the fluid loss and replacing water and, as needed, electrolytes. In response to increases in plasma osmolality, brain cells synthesize solutes—or idiogenic osmoles—which increase osmotic flow of water back into the brain cells to regulate their volume. This begins 4–6 hours after dehydration and takes several days to reach a steady state. If hypernatremia is too rapidly corrected, the osmotic imbalance may cause water to preferentially enter brain cells, causing cerebral edema and potentially severe neurologic impairment. Fluid therapy should be administered over a 48-hour period, aiming for a decrease in serum sodium of 1 meq/L/h (1 mmol/L/h). Potassium and phosphate may be added as indicated by serum levels; other electrolytes are also monitored frequently.

A. Choice of Type of Fluid for Replacement:

1. Hypernatremia with hypovolemia–Severe hypovolemia should be treated with isotonic (0.9%) saline to restore the volume deficit and to treat the hyperosmolality, since the osmolality of isotonic saline (308 mosm/kg) is often lower than that of the plasma. This should be followed by 0.45% saline to replace any remaining free water deficit. Milder volume deficit may be treated with 0.45% saline and 5% dextrose in water.

2. Hypernatremia with euvolemia–Water drinking or 5% dextrose and water intravenously will result in excretion of excess sodium in the urine. If GFR is decreased, diuretics will increase urinary sodium excretion but may impair renal concentrating ability, increasing the quantity of water that needs to be replaced.

3. Hypernatremia with hypervolemia–Treatment consists of providing water as 5% dextrose in water to reduce hyperosmolality, but this will expand vascular volume. Thus, loop diuretics such as furosemide (0.5–1 mg/kg) should be administered intravenously to remove the excess sodium. In severe renal insufficiency, hemodialysis may be necessary.

B. Calculation of Water Deficit: When calculating fluid replacement, both the deficit and the maintenance requirements should be added to each 24-hour replacement regimen.

1. Acute hypernatremia–In acute dehydration without much solute loss, free water loss is similar to the weight loss. Initially, 5% dextrose in water may be employed. As correction of water deficit progresses, therapy should continue with 0.45% saline with dextrose.

2. Chronic hypernatremia–Water deficit is calculated to restore normal osmolality for total body water. Total body water (TBW) (Table 21–1) correlates with muscle mass and therefore decreases with advancing age, cachexia, and dehydration and is lower in women than in men. Current TBW equals 0.4–0.6 of current body weight.

$$\text{Volume (in L) to be replaced} = \text{Current TBW} \times \frac{[Na^+] - 140}{140}$$

Adrogue HJ et al: Hypernatremia. N Engl J Med 2000; 342:1493. [NLM Cit ID: 20256709]

Kahn T: Hypernatremia with edema. Arch Intern Med 1999;159:93. [NLM Cit ID: 99107355]

DISORDERS OF POTASSIUM CONCENTRATION

1. HYPOKALEMIA

The total potassium content of the body is 50 meq/kg, more than 95% of which is intracellular. The plasma potassium concentration is maintained in a narrow range (Table 21–2) through two main regulating mechanisms: potassium shift between intracellular and extracellular compartments and modulation of renal potassium excretion. A deficit of 4–5 meq/kg occurs for each 1 meq/L decrement in serum potassium concentration below a level of 4 meq/L.

Clinical Findings

A. Symptoms and Signs: Muscular weakness, fatigue, and muscle cramps are frequent complaints in mild to moderate hypokalemia. Smooth muscle involvement may result in constipation or ileus. Flaccid paralysis, hyporeflexia, hypercapnia, tetany, and rhabdomyolysis may be seen with severe hypokalemia (< 2.5 meq/L).

B. Laboratory Findings: The ECG shows decreased amplitude and broadening of T waves, prominent U waves, premature ventricular contractions, and depressed ST segments. Hypokalemia also increases the likelihood of digitalis toxicity.

Pathophysiology & Diagnosis

Hypokalemia can occur as a result of shift of potassium from outside to inside the cell, extrarenal potassium loss (or insufficient potassium intake), or renal potassium loss (Table 21–4). Potassium uptake by the cell is stimulated by insulin in the presence of glucose. It is also facilitated by adrenergic beta-stimulation, whereas adrenergic alpha-stimulation blocks it. All of these effects are transient. Self-limited hypokalemia occurs in 50–60% of trauma patients, perhaps related to enhanced release of epinephrine. Aldosterone, which facilitates urinary potassium excretion through enhanced potassium secretion at the distal renal tubules, is the most important regulator of body potassium content. Urinary potassium concentration is low (< 20 meq/L) as a result of extrarenal fluid loss (eg, diarrhea, vomiting) and inappropriately high (> 40 meq/L) with urinary losses (eg, mineralocorticoid excess, Bartter's syndrome, Liddle's syndrome). Various genetic mutations that affect fluid and electrolyte metabolism, including disorders of potassium metabolism, have been reported recently (Table 21–5). Licorice-induced hypokalemia results from inhibition of 11β-hydroxysteroid dehydrogenase, which inactivates cortisol. Cortisol thus escapes degradation, binds to aldosterone receptors, and exerts aldosterone-like effects.

Table 21–4. Causes of hypokalemia.

Decreased intake

Potassium shift into the cell
- Increased secretion of insulin, postprandial
- Alkalosis
- Trauma (via beta-adrenergic stimulation?)
- Periodic paralysis (hypokalemic)

Renal potassium loss
- Increased aldosterone (mineralocorticoid) effects
  - Primary aldosteronism
  - Secondary aldosteronism (dehydration, heart failure)
  - Renovascular hypertension
  - Malignant hypertension
  - Ectopic ACTH-producing tumor
  - Bartter's syndrome
  - Cushing's syndrome
  - Licorice (European)
  - Renin-producing tumor
  - Congenital abnormality of steroid metabolism (eg, adrenogenital syndrome, 17α-hydroxylase defect, apparent mineralocorticoid excess)
- Increased flow of distal nephron
  - Diuretics (furosemide, thiazides)
  - Salt-losing nephropathy
- Hypomagnesemia
  - Unreabsorbable anion
  - Carbenicillin, penicillin
- Renal tubular acidosis (type I or II)
  - Fanconi's syndrome
  - Interstitial nephritis
  - Metabolic alkalosis (bicarbonaturia)
- Congenital defect of distal nephron
  - Liddle's syndrome

Extrarenal potassium loss
- Vomiting, diarrhea, laxative abuse
- Villous adenoma, Zollinger-Ellison syndrome

Table 21–5. Genetic disorders associated with electrolyte metabolism disturbances.

Disease	Site of Mutation
Potassium	
Hypokalemia	
Hypokalemic periodic paralysis	Dihydropyridine-sensitive skeletal muscle voltage-gated calcium channel
Bartter's syndrome	Na-K-2Cl cotransporter, K^+ channel (ROMK), or Cl^- channel of thick ascending limb of Henle (hypofunction)
Liddle's syndrome	β or γ subunit of amiloride-sensitive Na^+ channel (hyperfunction)
Apparent mineralocorticoid excess	11β-Hydroxysteroid dehydrogenase (failure to inactivate cortisol)
Glucocorticoid-remediable aldosteronism	Regulatory sequence of 11β-hydroxylase controls aldosterone synthase inappropriately
Hyperkalemia	
Hyperkalemic periodic paralysis	α subunit of calcium channel
Pseudohypoaldosteronism type I	β or γ subunit of amiloride-sensitive Na^+ channel (hypofunction)
Calcium	
Familial hypocalciuric hypercalcemia	Ca^{2+}-sensing protein (hypofunction)
Familial hypocalcemia	Ca^{2+}-sensing protein (hyperfunction)
Phosphate	
Hypophosphatemic rickets	*PEX* gene
Water	
X-linked (type I) nephrogenic diabetes insipidus	Vasopressin receptor

Treatment

The safest way to treat mild to moderate deficiency is with oral potassium, which is rapidly absorbed. Liquid potassium chloride has an unpleasant taste and may be better tolerated if added to fruit juice. Rarely, enteric-coated or slow-release tablets or capsules of potassium chloride can cause ulcers of the small intestine.

Intravenous potassium replacement is indicated for patients with severe hypokalemia and for those who cannot take oral supplementation. For severe deficiency, potassium may be given through a peripheral intravenous line in a concentration that should not exceed 40 meq/L at rates of up to 40 meq/L/h. Continuous electrocardiographic monitoring is indicated, and the serum potassium level should be checked every 3–6 hours.

Occasionally, hypokalemia may be refractory to potassium replacement. Magnesium deficiency may make potassium correction more difficult. Concomitant magnesium repletion avoids this problem.

Gennari FJ: Hypokalemia. N Engl J Med 1998;339:451. [NLM Cit ID: 98355347] (Comprehensive review.)

Halperin ML et al: Potassium. Lancet 1998;352:135. [NLM Cit ID: 98336038] (Pathophysiologic review of potassium disorders.)

Scheinmann SJ et al: Genetic disorders of renal electrolyte transport. N Engl J Med 1999;340:1177. [NLM Cit ID: 99200750] (A comprehensive review of the molecular pathogenesis of several genetic disorders, including Bartter's syndrome and Liddle's syndrome.)

Stewart OM: Mineralocorticoid hypertension. Lancet 1999;353:1341. [NLM Cit ID: 99232915]

Table 21–6. Causes of hyperkalemia.

Spurious
Leakage from erythrocytes when separation of serum from clot is delayed (plasma K^+ normal)
Marked thrombocytosis or leukocytosis with release of K^+ (plasma K^+ normal)
Repeated fist clenching during phlebotomy, with release of K^+ from forearm muscles
Specimen drawn from arm with K^+ infusion
Decreased excretion
Renal failure, acute and chronic
Renal secretory defects (may or may not have frank renal failure): renal transplant, interstitial nephritis, systemic lupus erythematosus, sickle cell disease, amyloidosis, obstructive uropathy
Hyporeninemic hypoaldosteronism (often in diabetic patients with mild to moderate nephropathy) or selective hypoaldosteronism (some patients with AIDS)
Heparin (regardless of molecular size; suppresses aldosterone secretion)
Drugs that inhibit potassium excretion (spironolactone, triamterene, ACE inhibitors, trimethoprim, NSAIDs)
Shift of K^+ from within the cell
Massive release of intracellular K^+ in burns, rhabdomyolysis, hemolysis, severe infection, internal bleeding vigorous exercise
Metabolic acidosis (in the case of organic acid accumulation—eg, lactic acidosis—a shift of K+ does not occur since organic acid can easily move across the cell membrane)
Hypertonicity (solvent drag)
Insulin deficiency (metabolic acidosis may not be apparent)
Hyperkalemic periodic paralysis
Drugs: succinylcholine, arginine, digitalis toxicity, beta-adrenergic antagonists
Alpha-adrenergic stimulation?
Excessive intake of K^+

2. HYPERKALEMIA

Many cases of hyperkalemia are spurious or associated with acidosis (Table 21–6). The common practice of repeatedly clenching and unclenching a fist during venipuncture may raise the potassium concentration by 1–2 meq/L by causing acidosis and consequent potassium loss from cells.

Intracellular potassium shifts to the extracellular fluid in hyperkalemia associated with acidosis. Serum potassium concentration rises about 0.7 meq/L for every decrease of 0.1 pH unit during acidosis. Potassium movement out of cells occurs primarily in metabolic acidosis due to the accumulation of minerals such as NH_4Cl or HCl. The inability of the chloride anion to permeate the cell membrane results in the transcellular exchange of H^+ for K^+. Metabolic acidosis from organic acids (keto acids and lactic acid) does not induce hyperkalemia. Unlike the minerals, these organic acids easily permeate cell membranes and retard Na^+-K^+ ATPase. The hyperkalemia frequently observed in diabetic ketoacidosis is not due to the acidosis but to a combination of the hyperosmolality (the intracellular K^+ concentration of the dehydrated cell increases and K^+ diffuses extracellularly) and deficiencies of insulin, catecholamines, and aldosterone. In the absence of acidosis, serum potassium concentration rises about 1 meq/L when there is a total body potassium excess of 1–4 meq/kg. However, the higher the serum potassium concentration, the smaller the excess necessary to raise the potassium levels further.

Trimethoprim is structurally related to amiloride and triamterene, and all three drugs inhibit renal potassium excretion through suppression of sodium channels in the distal nephron. Serum potassium levels rise progressively over 4–5 days in patients treated with standard or high-dose trimethoprim (combined with sulfamethoxazole or dapsone), especially if there is concurrent renal insufficiency. Over half of inpatients taking this drug have potassium levels over 5 meq/L, and 20% have marked hyperkalemia (> 5.5 meq/L). The potassium concentration returns to baseline after drug discontinuation.

Hyperkalemia is commonly seen in patients with AIDS and has been attributed to impaired renal excretion of potassium due to the use of pentamidine or trimethoprim-sulfamethoxazole or to hyporeninemic hypoaldosteronism. An abnormality in the redistribution between the intracellular and extracellular compartments may also play a role.

Clinical Findings

An elevated K^+ concentration interferes with normal neuromuscular function to produce muscle weakness and, rarely, flaccid paralysis; abdominal distention and diarrhea may occur. Electrocardiography is not a sensitive method for detecting hyperkalemia, since nearly half of patients with a serum potassium level greater than 6.5 meq/L will not manifest electrocardiographic changes. Electrocardiographic changes in hyperkalemia include peaked T waves of increased amplitude, widening of the QRS, and biphasic QRS–T complexes. An interesting rhythm is caused by inhibition of atrial depolarization despite normal conduction through usual pathways. This sinoventricular rhythm resembles a junctional mechanism and occurs because of greater sensitivity of atrial myocytes to hyperkalemia than is the case for ventricular muscle cells. The heart rate may be slow; ventricular fibrillation and cardiac arrest are terminal events.

Treatment (Table 21–7)

One first confirms that the elevated level of serum K^+ is genuine. Potassium concentration can be measured in plasma rather than in serum to avoid leakage of potassium out of cells into the serum of the blood sample in the course of clotting, which may be observed in thrombocytosis.

Treatment consists of withholding potassium and giving cation exchange resins by mouth or enema. Sodium polystyrene sulfonate, 40–80 g/d in divided doses, is usually effective. Emergent treatment of hyperkalemia is indicated if cardiac toxicity or muscular paralysis is present or if the hyperkalemia is severe (serum potassium > 6.5–7 meq/L) even in the absence of electrocardiographic changes. Insulin plus 10–50% glucose (5–10 g of glucose per unit of insulin) may be employed to deposit K^+ with glycogen in the liver. Calcium may be given intravenously as an antagonist ion—but not when digoxin toxicity is suspected, since calcium may augment the deleterious effects of digoxin on the heart. Transcellular shifts of potassium can also be mediated by β_2-adrenergic stimulation. Albuterol, a nebulized β_2 agonist, is effective in decreasing serum potassium in patients on hemodialysis. For such patients, one or two standard doses of nebulized albuterol can reduce serum K^+ 0.5–1 meq/L within 30 minutes after administration, and this effect is sustained for at least 2 hours. Albuterol and insulin are probably equally efficacious in lowering potassium in uremic patients, and the hypokalemic effects of coadministration of the two drugs (with glucose) are additive and appear not to constitute a hazard. Sodium bicarbonate can be given intravenously as an emergency measure in severe hyperkalemia; the increase in blood pH results in a shift of K^+ into cells. Hemodialysis or peritoneal dialysis may be required to remove K^+ in the presence of protracted renal insufficiency. Therapy of the precipitating event proceeds concurrently.

Alappan R et al: Hyperkalemia in hospitalized patients treated with trimethoprim-sulfamethoxazole. Ann Intern Med 1996;124:316. [NLM Cit ID: 96148640] (Marked hyperkalemia [> 5.5 meq/L] occurred in 20% of patients.)

Caramelo C et al: Hyperkalemia in patients infected with the human immunodeficiency virus: involvement of a systemic mechanism. Kidney Int 1999;56:198. [NLM Cit ID: 99340507]

DuBose T Jr: Hyperkalemic hyperchloremic metabolic acidosis: Pathophysiologic insights. Kidney Int 1997;51: 591. [NLM Cit ID: 97179459]

Reardon LC et al: Hyperkalemia in outpatients using angiotensin-converting enzyme inhibitors. How much should we worry? Arch Intern Med 1998;158:26. [NLM Cit ID: 98100021] (Serious hyperkalemia is uncommon in ACE-treated patients under 70 who have normal renal function.)

DISORDERS OF CALCIUM CONCENTRATION

Calcium constitutes about 2% of body weight, but only about 1% of the total body calcium is in solution in body fluid. In the plasma, only 50% of calcium is present as ionized calcium; the remainder forms a complex with protein—mostly albumin (40%)—or anions, including citrate, bicarbonate, and phosphate (10%). The normal total plasma (or serum) calcium concentration is 9–10.3 mg/dL. It is ionized calcium (normal: 4.7–5.3 mg/dL) which, under physiologic regulation, is necessary for muscle contraction and nerve function. Calcium-sensing protein, a receptor-like protein with the special function of detecting extracellular calcium ion concentrations, has been identified in parathyroid cells and in the kidney. Some diseases (eg, familial hypocalcemia and familial hypocalciuric hypercalcemia) associated with disturbed calcium metabolism are due to functional defects of this protein (Table 21–5).

1. HYPOCALCEMIA

Important causes of hypocalcemia are listed in Table 21–8.

The most common cause of hypocalcemia is renal failure, in which decreased production of active vitamin D_3 and hyperphosphatemia both play a role. Some cases of primary hypoparathyroidism are due to mutation of calcium-sensing protein in which inappropriate suppression of PTH release leads to

Table 21–7. Treatment of hyperkalemia.[1]

Modality	Mechanism of Action	Onset	Duration	Prescription	K^+ Removed From Body
EMERGENCY					
Calcium	Antagonizes cardiac conduction abnormalities	0–5 minutes	1 hour	Calcium gluconate 10%, 5–30 mL IV; or calcium chloride 5%, 5–30 mL IV	0
Bicarbonate	Distributes K^+ into cells	15–30 minutes	1–2 hours	$NaHCO_3$, 44–88 meq (1–2 ampules) IV	0
Insulin	Distributes K^+ into cells	15–60 minutes	4–6 hours	Regular insulin, 5–10 units IV, plus glucose 50%, 25 g (1 ampule) IV	0
Albuterol	Distributes K^+ into cells	15–30 minutes	2–4 hours	Nebulized albuterol, 10–20 mg in 4 mL normal saline, inhaled over 10 minutes	0

Modality	Mechanism of Action	Duration of Treatment	Prescription	K^+ Removed From Body
NONEMERGENCY				
Loop diuretic	↑ Renal K^+ excretion	0.5–2 hours	Furosemide, 40–160 mg IV or orally with or without $NaHCO_3$, 0.5–3 meq/kg daily	Variable
Sodium polystyrene sulfonate (Kayexalate)	Ion exchange resin binds K^+	1–3 hours	Oral: 15–30 g in 20% sorbitol (50–100 mL) Rectal: 50 g in 20% sorbitol	0.5–1 meq/g
Hemodialysis	Extracorporeal K^+ removal	48 hours	Blood flow ≥ 200–300 mL/min. Dialysate [K^+] ~ 0.	200–300 meq
Peritoneal dialysis	Peritoneal K^+ removal	48 hours	Fast exchange, 3–4 L/h	200–300 meq

[1]Modified and reproduced, with permission, from Cogan MG: *Fluid and Electrolytes: Physiology and Pathophysiology*. Originally published by Appleton & Lange. Copyright © 1991 by The McGraw-Hill Companies, Inc.

hypocalcemia. Hypocalcemia in pancreatitis is also a marker for severe disease (see Chapter 15).

Clinical Findings

A. Symptoms and Signs: Hypocalcemia increases excitation of nerve and muscle cells, primarily affecting the neuromuscular and cardiovascular systems. Extensive spasm of skeletal muscle causes cramps and tetany. Laryngospasm with stridor can obstruct the airway. Convulsions can occur as well as paresthesias of lips and extremities and abdominal pain. Chvostek's sign (contraction of the facial muscle in response to tapping the facial nerve anterior to the ear) and Trousseau's sign (carpal spasm occurring after occlusion of the brachial artery with a blood pressure cuff for 3 minutes) are usually readily elicited. Prolongation of the QT interval (due to lengthened ST segment) predisposes to the development of ventricular arrhythmias. In chronic hypoparathyroidism, cataracts and calcification of basal ganglia of the brain may appear. (See Hypoparathyroidism, Chapter 26.)

B. Laboratory Findings: Serum Ca^{2+} is low (< 9 mg/dL). The depressed level of serum Ca^{2+} must be correlated with the simultaneous concentration of serum albumin: When albumin is low, serum Ca^{2+} concentration is depressed in a ratio of 0.8–1 mg of Ca^{2+} to 1 g of albumin. Serum phosphate is usually elevated in hypoparathyroidism or end-stage renal failure, whereas it is suppressed in early stage renal failure or vitamin D deficiency. Serum Mg^{2+} is commonly low, and hypomagnesemia reduces both parathyroid hormone release and tissue responsiveness to parathyroid hormone, causing hypocalcemia. In respiratory alkalosis, total serum calcium is normal but ionized calcium is low, which can be measured by use of a Ca^{2+}-sensitive electrode. The ECG shows a prolonged QT interval.

Treatment*

A. Severe, Symptomatic Hypocalcemia: In the presence of tetany, arrhythmias, or seizures, calcium gluconate 10% (10–20 mL) administered intra-

*See also Chapter 26 for discussion of the treatment of hypoparathyroidism.

Table 21–8. Causes of hypocalcemia.

Decreased intake or absorption
Malabsorption
Small bowel bypass, short bowel
Vitamin D deficit (decreased absorption, decreased production of 25-hydroxyvitamin D or 1,25-dihydroxyvitamin D)
Increased loss
Alcoholism
Chronic renal insufficiency
Diuretic therapy
Endocrine disease
Hypoparathyroidism (genetic, acquired; including hypo- and hypermagnesemia)
Sepsis
Pseudohypoparathyroidism
Calcitonin secretion with medullary carcinoma of the thyroid
Familial hypocalcemia
Physiologic causes
Associated with decreased serum albumin[1]
Decreased end-organ response to vitamin D
Hyperphosphatemia
Induced by aminoglycoside antibiotics, plicamycin, loop diuretics, foscarnet

[1]Calcium ion concentration is normal.

Table 21–9. Causes of hypercalcemia.

Increased intake or absorption
Milk-alkali syndrome
Vitamin D or vitamin A excess
Endocrine disorders
Primary hyperparathyroidism (adenoma, hyperplasia, carcinoma)
Secondary hyperparathyroidism (renal insufficiency, malabsorption)
Acromegaly
Adrenal insufficiency
Neoplastic diseases
Tumors producing PTH-related proteins (ovary, kidney, lung)
Multiple myeloma (elaboration of osteoclast-activating factor)
Miscellaneous causes
Thiazide diuretic-induced
Sarcoidosis
Paget's disease of bone
Hypophosphatasia
Immobilization
Familial hypocalciuric hypercalcemia
Complications of renal transplantation
Iatrogenic

venously over 10–15 minutes is indicated. Because of the short duration of action, calcium infusion is usually required. Ten to 15 milligrams of calcium per kilogram body weight, or six to eight 10-mL vials of 10% calcium gluconate (558–744 mg of calcium), is added to 1 L of D_5W and infused over 4–6 hours. By monitoring the serum calcium level frequently (every 4–6 hours), the infusion rate is adjusted to maintain the serum calcium level at 7–8.5 mg/dL.

B. Asymptomatic Hypocalcemia: Oral calcium (1–2 g) and vitamin D preparations (Table 26–10) are used. Calcium carbonate is well tolerated and less expensive than many other calcium tablets. The low serum Ca^{2+} associated with low serum albumin concentration does not require replacement therapy. If serum Mg^{2+} is low, therapy must include replacement of magnesium, which by itself usually will correct hypocalcemia.

Bushinsky DA et al: Calcium. Lancet 1998;352:306. [NLM Cit ID: 98352735] (Pathophysiology, differential diagnosis, and treatment of hypocalcemia and hypercalcemia.)

2. HYPERCALCEMIA

Important causes of hypercalcemia are listed in Table 21–9. Primary hyperparathyroidism is the most common cause of hypercalcemia in ambulatory patients as well as the commonest paraneoplastic endocrine syndrome, accounting for most cases of hypercalcemia in inpatients. The neoplasm is clinically apparent in nearly all cases when the hypercalcemia is detected, and the prognosis is poor. Chronic hypercalcemia (over 6 months) or some manifestation such as nephrolithiasis suggests a benign course. Primary hyperparathyroidism and malignancy account for 90% of all cases of hypercalcemia.

The milk-alkali syndrome, which had become rare with the advent of nonabsorbable antacid therapy for ulcer disease, should be considered as a cause of hypercalcemia with the current popularity of calcium ingestion for osteoporosis prevention. In the milk-alkali syndrome, massive calcium and vitamin D ingestion can cause hypercalcemic nephropathy. Because of the decreased GFR, retention of the alkali in the calcium antacid occurs and causes metabolic alkalosis, which can be worsened by the vomiting associated with this disorder.

Clinical Findings

A. Symptoms and Signs: Symptoms of hypercalcemia irrespective of cause are constipation and polyuria. The focus of the history and physical examination should be on the duration of the process hypercalcemia and evidence for a neoplasm. Symptoms usually occur if the serum calcium is above 12 mg/dL and tend to be more severe if hypercalcemia develops acutely.

Interestingly, polyuria is absent in hypercalcemia in familial hypocalciuric hypercalcemia, in which function of calcium-sensing protein is altered in the kidney as well. A variety of neurologic symptoms also are observed. Stupor, coma, and azotemia may develop in severe hypercalcemia. Ventricular extrasystoles and idioventricular rhythm occur and can be accentuated by digitalis.

B. Laboratory Findings: A significant elevation of serum Ca^{2+} is seen; the level must be interpreted in relation to the serum albumin level (see Hypocalcemia). The highest serum calcium levels (> 15 mg/dL) generally occur in malignancy. More than 200 mg/d of urinary calcium excretion suggests hypercalciuria; less than 100 mg/d, hypocalciuria. Serum phosphate may or may not be low, depending on the cause. The ECG shows a shortened QT interval. Measurement of plasma PTH-related protein is useful to diagnose malignancy-associated hypercalcemia.

Treatment

Until the primary disease can be brought under control, renal excretion of calcium with resultant decrease in serum Ca^{2+} concentration is promoted. Excretion of Na^+ is accompanied by excretion of Ca^{2+}; therefore, establishing euvolemia and inducing natriuresis by giving saline with furosemide is the emergency treatment of choice. In dehydrated patients with normal cardiac and renal function, 0.45% saline or 0.9% saline can be given rapidly (250–500 mL/h). Intravenous furosemide (20–40 mg every 2 hours) prevents volume overload and enhances Ca^{2+} excretion. Thiazides can actually worsen hypercalcemia (as can furosemide if inadequate saline is given). In the treatment of hypercalcemia of malignancy, bisphosphonates are safe and effective in more than 95% of patients and are the mainstay of treatment. See Chapter 4 for a discussion of the treatment of hypercalcemia of malignancy; and see Chapter 26 for a discussion of the treatment of hypercalcemia of hyperparathyroidism.

Mundy GR et al: Hypercalcemia of malignancy. Am J Med 1997;103:134. [NLM Cit ID: 97418821]

Strewler GL: The physiology of a parathyroid hormone-related protein. N Engl J Med 2000;342:177. [NLM Cit ID: 20092363] (An updated review on the action of PTHrP.)

DISORDERS OF PHOSPHORUS CONCENTRATION

Phosphate is important in the body as a constituent of bone and is crucial in cellular energy transfer and metabolism. Phosphate occupies 1% of body weight, and 80% of it is combined with calcium in bones and teeth. Only 10% is incorporated into a variety of organic compounds, and 10% is combined with proteins, lipids, carbohydrates, and other compounds in muscle and blood. Organic phosphate is the principal intracellular anion. In plasma, phosphate is mainly present as inorganic phosphate, and this fraction is very small (< 0.2% of total phosphate). However, body phosphate metabolism is regulated through plasma inorganic phosphate. Important determinants of plasma inorganic phosphate concentration are its intestinal absorption, renal excretion, and shift between the intracellular and extracellular spaces. Intestinal absorption of phosphate is facilitated by active vitamin D. Parathyroid hormone stimulates phosphate release from bone and suppresses proximal tubular reabsorption of phosphate, leading to hypophosphatemia and to bone phosphate store depletion if hypersecretion continues. Renal proximal tubular reabsorption of phosphate is attenuated by volume expansion, glucocorticoid administration, and proximal tubular dysfunction, such as occurs in Fanconi's syndrome due to myeloma or other diseases. Growth hormone, on the other hand, augments proximal tubular reabsorption of phosphate.

Cellular phosphate uptake is stimulated by various factors and conditions, including alkalemia, insulin, epinephrine, feeding, hungry bone syndrome, and accelerated cell proliferation.

Phosphorus metabolism and homeostasis are intimately related to calcium metabolism. See sections on metabolic bone disease in Chapter 26.

1. HYPOPHOSPHATEMIA

Hypophosphatemia may occur in the presence of normal phosphate stores. Serious depletion of body phosphate stores may exist with low, normal, or high concentrations of phosphorus in serum. Leading causes of hypophosphatemia are listed in Table 21–10.

In the presence of severe hypophosphatemia (1 mg/dL or less), affinity of hemoglobin for oxygen is increased through a decrease in the erythrocyte 2,3-diphosphoglycerate concentration. This impairs tissue oxygenation and thus cell metabolism, which underlies the effects of hypophosphatemia such as muscle weakness or even rhabdomyolysis.

Severe hypophosphatemia is common in alcoholic patients, both because of prior phosphate depletion due to poor dietary intake and accompanying respiratory alkalosis. Magnesium depletion may also exacerbate hypophosphatemia.

Hypophosphatemia is a potent stimulator of 1α-hydroxylation of vitamin D in the kidney to form active vitamin D. However, in oncogenic osteomalacia, which accompanies various mesenchymal tumors, activation of vitamin D is suppressed in spite of hypophosphatemia. This suppression may be due to overproduction of phosphatonin, a poorly understood factor that stimulates phosphaturia.

Clinical Findings

A. Symptoms and Signs: Acute, severe hypophosphatemia (0.1–0.2 mg/dL) can lead to acute hemolytic anemia with increased erythrocyte fragility, increased susceptibility to infection from impaired chemotaxis of leukocytes, and platelet dys-

Table 21–10. Causes of hypophosphatemia.

Diminished supply or absorption
Starvation
Parenteral alimentation with inadequate phosphate content
Malabsorption syndrome, small bowel bypass
Absorption blocked by oral aluminum hydroxide or bicarbonate
Vitamin D-deficient and vitamin D-resistant osteomalacia
Increased loss
Phosphaturic drugs: theophylline, diuretics, bronchodilators, corticosteroids
Hyperparathyroidism (primary or secondary)
Hyperthyroidism
Renal tubular defects permitting excessive phosphaturia (congenital, induced by monoclonal gammopathy, heavy metal poisoning)
Hypokalemic nephropathy
Inadequately controlled diabetes mellitus
Alcoholism
Hypophosphatemic rickets
Oncogenic osteomalacia
Intracellular shift of phosphorus
Administration of glucose, fructose (transient)
Anabolic steroids, estrogen, oral contraceptives
Respiratory alkalosis
Salicylate poisoning
Electrolyte abnormalities
Hypercalcemia
Hypomagnesemia
Metabolic alkalosis
Abnormal losses followed by inadequate repletion
Diabetes mellitus with acidosis, particularly during aggressive therapy
Recovery from starvation or prolonged catabolic state
Chronic alcoholism, particularly during restoration of nutrition; associated with hypomagnesemia
Respiratory alkalosis
Recovery from severe burns

function with petechial hemorrhages. Rhabdomyolysis, encephalopathy (irritability, confusion, dysarthria, seizures, and coma), and heart failure are uncommon but serious manifestations.

Chronic severe depletion may be manifested by anorexia, pain in muscles and bones, and fractures.

B. Laboratory Findings: In addition to hypophosphatemia, evidence of anemia due to hemolysis may be present (eg, elevated serum lactate dehydrogenase). Rhabdomyolysis results in elevated serum creatine kinase (which contains mostly the MM fraction but also some MB fraction) and, in many cases, myoglobin in the urine. Other values vary according to the cause. Renal glycosuria and hypouricemia together with hypophosphatemia indicate Fanconi's syndrome. In chronic depletion, radiographs and biopsies of bones show changes resembling those of osteomalacia.

Treatment

Treatment is best directed toward prophylaxis by including phosphate in repletion and maintenance fluids. A rapid decline in calcium levels can occur with parenteral administration of phosphate; therefore, when possible, oral replacement of phosphate is preferable. For parenteral alimentation, 620 mg (20 mmol) of phosphorus is required for every 1000 nonprotein kcal to maintain phosphate balance and to ensure anabolic function. A daily ration for prolonged parenteral fluid maintenance is 620–1240 mg (20–40 mmol) of phosphorus. For asymptomatic hypophosphatemia (serum phosphorus 0.7–1 mg/dL), an infusion should provide 279–310 mg (9–10 mmol)/12 h until the serum phosphorus exceeds 1 mg/dL. Since the response to phosphate supplementation is not predictable, frequent monitoring of plasma and urine phosphate is necessary. A magnesium deficit often coexists and should be treated simultaneously. In administering phosphate-containing solutions, serum creatinine and calcium must be monitored to guard against hypocalcemia.

For oral use, phosphate salts are available in skim milk (approximately 1 g [33 mmol]/L). Tablets or capsules of mixtures of sodium and potassium phosphate may be given to provide 0.5–1 g (18–32 mmol) per day.

Contraindications to therapy with phosphate salts include hypoparathyroidism, renal insufficiency, tissue damage and necrosis, and hypercalcemia. When hyperglycemia due to any cause is treated, phosphate accompanies glucose into cells, and hypophosphatemia may ensue.

Barak V et al: Prevalence of hypophosphatemia in sepsis and infection: The role of cytokines. Am J Med 1998;104:40. [NLM Cit ID: 98187567] (Hypophosphatemia observed in sepsis may be related to overproduction of cytokines.)

Subramian R et al: Severe hypophosphatemia: Pathophysiologic implications, clinical presentations, and treatment. Medicine 2000;79:1. [NLM Cit ID: 20135301]

2. HYPERPHOSPHATEMIA

Causes of hyperphosphatemia are given in Table 21–11. Growing children normally have serum phosphate levels higher than those of adults.

Clinical Findings

A. Symptoms and Signs: The clinical manifestations are those of the underlying disorders (eg, chronic renal failure, hypoparathyroidism). Hyperphosphatemia in chronic renal failure leads to secondary hyperparathyroidism and renal osteodystrophy.

B. Laboratory Findings: In addition to elevated phosphate, other blood chemistry values are those characteristic of the underlying disease.

Treatment

Treatment is that of the underlying disease and of associated hypocalcemia if present. In acute and

Table 21–11. Causes of hyperphosphatemia.

Massive load of phosphate into the extracellular fluid
From outside the body
Hypervitaminosis D
Laxatives or enemas containing phosphate
Intravenous phosphate supplement
From inside the body
Rhabdomyolysis (especially if renal insufficiency coexists)
Cell destruction by chemotherapy of malignancy, particularly lymphoproliferative diseases
Metabolic acidosis (lactic acidosis, ketoacidosis)
Respiratory acidosis (phosphate incorporation into cells is disturbed)
Decreased excretion into urine
Renal failure (acute, chronic)
Hypoparathyroidism
Pseudohypoparathyroidism
Excessive growth hormone (acromegaly)
Pseudohyperphosphatemia
Multiple myeloma, hypertriglyceridemia, cell lysis

chronic renal failure, dialysis will reduce serum phosphate. Absorption of phosphate can be reduced by administration of calcium carbonate, 0.5–1.5 g three times daily with meals (500 mg tablets). This approach is preferred to the traditional use of aluminum hydroxide because of concerns about aluminum toxicity. Another phosphate binder is sevelamer hydrochloride. Since this agent does not contain calcium or aluminum, it may be especially useful for patients with hypercalcemia or uremia.

Slatopolsky EA et al: Renagel, a nonabsorbed calcium- and aluminum-free phosphate binder, lowers serum phosphorus and parathyroid hormone. Kidney Int 1999;55:299. [NLM Cit ID: 99111492]

Weisinger JR et al: Magnesium and phosphorus. Lancet 1998;352:391. [NLM Cit ID: 98382044] (Review of the significance of abnormal levels of magnesium and phosphorus.)

DISORDERS OF MAGNESIUM CONCENTRATION

About 50% of total body magnesium exists in the insoluble state in bone. Only 5% is present as extracellular cation; the remaining 45% is contained in cells as intracellular cation. The normal plasma concentration is 1.5–2.5 meq/L, with about one-third bound to protein and two-thirds existing as free cation. Excretion of magnesium ion is via the kidney. Normally, about 3% of magnesium filtered by the glomerulus is excreted in urine.

Magnesium is an important activator ion, participating in the function of many enzymes involved in phosphate transfer reactions. Magnesium exerts physiologic effects on the nervous system resembling those of calcium. Magnesium acts directly upon the myoneural junction.

Altered concentration of Mg^{2+} in the plasma usually provokes an associated alteration of Ca^{2+}. Hypermagnesemia suppresses secretion of parathyroid hormone with consequent hypocalcemia. Severe and prolonged magnesium depletion impairs secretion of PTH with consequent hypocalcemia. Hypomagnesemia may impair end-organ response to PTH as well.

1. HYPOMAGNESEMIA

Causes of hypomagnesemia are given in Table 21–12. Nearly half of hospitalized patients in whom serum electrolytes are ordered have unrecognized hypomagnesemia. Common causes include use of large volumes of intravenous fluids, diuretics, cisplatin in cancer patients (with concomitant hypokalemia), and administration of nephrotoxic agents such as aminoglycosides and amphotericin B.

Clinical Findings

A. Symptoms and Signs: Common symptoms are weakness, muscle cramps, and tremor. There is marked neuromuscular and central nervous system hyperirritability, with tremors, athetoid movements, jerking, nystagmus, and a positive Babinski response. There may be hypertension, tachycardia, and ventricular arrhythmias. Confusion and disorientation may be prominent features.

B. Laboratory Findings: Urinary excretion of magnesium exceeding 10–30 mg/d or a fractional excretion more than 2% indicates renal magnesium wasting. In calculating fractional excretion of magnesium, since only 30% is protein-bound, it follows that 70% of circulating magnesium is filtered by the

Table 21–12. Causes of hypomagnesemia.

Diminished absorption or intake
Malabsorption, chronic diarrhea, laxative abuse
Prolonged gastrointestinal suction
Small bowel bypass
Malnutrition
Alcoholism
Total parenteral alimentation with inadequate Mg^{2+} content
Increased renal loss
Diuretic therapy (loop diuretics, thiazide diuretics)
Hyperaldosteronism, Bartter's syndrome
Hyperparathyroidism, hyperthyroidism
Hypercalcemia
Volume expansion
Tubulointerstitial diseases
Transplant kidney
Drugs (aminoglycoside, cisplatin, amphotericin B, pentamidine)
Others
Diabetes mellitus
Post parathyroidectomy (hungry bone syndrome)
Respiratory alkalosis
Pregnancy

glomerulus. In addition to hypomagnesemia, hypocalcemia and hypokalemia are often present. The ECG shows a prolonged QT interval, due to lengthening of the ST segment. Parathyroid hormone secretion is often suppressed (see Hypocalcemia, above).

Treatment

Treatment consists of the use of intravenous fluids containing magnesium as chloride or sulfate, 240–1200 mg/d (10–50 mmol/d) during the period of severe deficit, followed by 120 mg/d (5 mmol/d) for maintenance. Magnesium sulfate may also be given intramuscularly in a dosage of 200–800 mg/d (8–33 mmol/d) in four divided doses. Serum levels must be monitored and dosage adjusted to keep the concentration from rising above 2.5 mmol/L. K^+ and Ca^{2+} may be required as well. Magnesium oxide, 250–500 mg by mouth two to four times daily, is useful for repleting stores in those with chronic hypomagnesemia. Hypokalemia and hypocalcemia of hypomagnesemia do not recover without magnesium supplementation.

Argus ZS: Hypomagnesemia. J Am Soc Nephrol 1999; 10:1616. [NLM Cit ID: 99332130]

Quamme GA: Renal magnesium handling: New insights in understanding old problems. Kidney Int 1997;52:1180. [NLM Cit ID: 98011743] (Physiologic overview.)

Tosiello L: Hypomagnesemia and diabetes mellitus: A review of clinical implications. Arch Intern Med 1996; 156:1143. [NLM Cit ID: 96235056] (Hypomagnesemia has been correlated with both poor diabetic control and insulin resistance in elderly patients.)

2. HYPERMAGNESEMIA

Magnesium excess is almost always the result of renal insufficiency and the inability to excrete what has been taken in from food or drugs, especially antacids and laxatives.

Clinical Findings

A. Symptoms and Signs: Muscle weakness, decreased deep tendon reflexes, mental obtundation, and confusion are characteristic manifestations. Weakness—even flaccid paralysis—and hypotension are noted. There may be respiratory muscle paralysis or cardiac arrest.

B. Laboratory Findings: Serum Mg^{2+} is elevated. In the common setting of renal insufficiency, concentrations of BUN and of serum creatinine, phosphate, and uric acid are elevated; serum K^+ may be elevated. Serum Ca^{2+} is often low. The ECG shows increased PR interval, broadened QRS complexes, and peaked T waves, probably related to associated hyperkalemia.

Treatment

Treatment is directed toward alleviating renal insufficiency. Calcium acts as an antagonist to Mg^{2+} and may be given intravenously as calcium chloride, 500 mg or more at a rate of 100 mg (4.5 mmol)/min. Hemodialysis or peritoneal dialysis may be indicated.

Weisinger JR et al: Magnesium and phosphorus. Lancet 1998;352:391. [NLM Cit ID: 98382044] (Review of the significance of abnormal levels of magnesium and phosphorus.)

HYPEROSMOLAR DISORDERS & OSMOLAR GAPS

1. HYPEROSMOLALITY WITH ONLY TRANSIENT OR NO SIGNIFICANT SHIFT IN WATER

Urea and alcohol are two substances that readily cross cell membranes and can produce hyperosmolality. Because of its permeant nature, urea has little effect on the shift of water across the cell membrane. Alcohol quickly equilibrates between intracellular and extracellular water, adding 22 mosm/L for every 1000 mg/L. This measured hyperosmolality does not produce symptoms by itself because of the equilibrium described, but in any case of stupor or coma in which measured osmolality exceeds that calculated from values of serum Na^+ and glucose and BUN, ethanol intoxication should be considered as a possible explanation of the discrepancy (osmolar gap). Toxic alcohol ingestion, particularly methanol or ethylene glycol, also causes an osmolar gap characterized by anion gap metabolic acidosis (Chapter 39).

The combination of anion gap metabolic acidosis and an osmolar gap exceeding 10 mosm/kg is not specific for toxic alcohol ingestion. Nearly half of patients with alcoholic ketoacidosis or lactic acidosis have similar findings, caused in part by elevations of endogenous glycerol, acetone, and acetone metabolites.

Glaser OS: Utility of the serum osmol gap in the diagnosis of methanol or ethylene glycol ingestion. Ann Emerg Med 1996;27:343. [NLM Cit ID: 96178198] (Limitations of the test.)

Osterloh JD et al: Discrepancies in osmolal gaps and calculated alcohol concentrations. Arch Pathol Lab Med 1996;120:637. [NLM Cit ID: 96340182] (Describes the common discrepancy of the unexplained osmolal gap in ethanol intoxication and discusses the potential causes.)

2. HYPEROSMOLALITY ASSOCIATED WITH SIGNIFICANT SHIFTS IN WATER

Increased concentrations of solutes that do not readily enter cells produce a shift of water from the intracellular space to effect a true intracellular dehydration. Sodium and glucose are the solutes commonly involved. In these instances, the hyperosmolality does produce symptoms.

Clinical symptoms are mainly referred to the central nervous system. The severity of symptoms depends on the degree of hyperosmolality and rapidity of development. In acute hyperosmolality, symptoms of somnolence and confusion can appear when the osmolality exceeds 320–330 mosm/L, and coma, respiratory arrest, and death when it exceeds 340–350 mosm/L.

ACID-BASE DISORDERS

About 1 meq/L/kg/d of nonvolatile acid (H^+) is newly produced, together with volatile acid (CO_2), by whole body metabolism. Body fluid pH, however, remains relatively constant at about 7.40. This constancy of body fluid pH is achieved by removal of CO_2 and H^+ through lung and kidney, respectively.

In order to assess a patient's acid-base status, measurement of arterial pH, partial pressure of carbon dioxide (P_{CO_2}), and plasma bicarbonate (HCO_3^-) is needed. Blood gas analyzers directly measure pH and P_{CO_2}, and the HCO_3^- value is calculated from the Henderson-Hasselbalch equation:

$$\text{pH} = 6.1 + \log \frac{HCO_3^-}{0.03 \times P_{CO_2}}$$

The total venous CO_2 measurement is a more direct determination of HCO_3^-. Because of the dissociation characteristics of carbonic acid (H_2CO_3) at body pH, dissolved CO_2 is almost exclusively in the form of HCO_3^-, and for clinical purposes the total carbon dioxide content is equivalent (± 3 meq/L) to the HCO_3^- concentration:

$$H^+ + HCO_3^- \leftrightarrow H_2CO_3 \leftrightarrow CO_2 + H_2O$$

If precise measurements of oxygenation are not needed or if oxygen saturation obtained from the pulse oximeter is adequate, venous blood gases generally provide useful information for assessment of acid-base balance and can be used interchangeably with arterial blood gases since the arteriovenous differences in pH and P_{CO_2} are small and relatively constant. Venous blood pH is usually 0.03–0.04 units lower than that of arterial blood, and venous blood P_{CO_2} is 7 or 8 mm Hg higher. Calculated HCO_3^- concentration in venous blood is at most 2 meq/L higher than that of arterial blood. An important exception to the rule of interchangeability between arterial and venous blood gases for determination of acid-base balance is during cardiopulmonary arrest. In this setting arterial pH may be 7.41 and venous pH 7.15, and arterial blood P_{CO_2} can be 32 mm Hg with a venous blood P_{CO_2} of 74 mm Hg.

Types of Acid-Base Disorders

There are two types of acid-base disorders: respiratory and metabolic. Primary respiratory disorders affect blood acidity by causing changes in P_{CO_2}, and primary metabolic disorders are caused by disturbances in the HCO_3^- concentration. The primary disturbances are usually accompanied by compensatory changes; however, even though these changes attenuate a pH shift from the normal value (7.40), they do not fully compensate for the primary acid-base disorders even if the disorders are chronic. Therefore, if the pH is less than 7.40, the primary process is acidosis (either respiratory or metabolic). If the pH is higher than 7.40, the primary process is either respiratory or metabolic alkalosis. The presence of one disorder with its appropriate compensatory change is a simple disorder.

Mixed Acid-Base Disorders

The presence of more than one simple disorder (not compensatory) is a mixed disorder. Double or triple disorders can coexist but not quadruple ones, since simultaneous respiratory acidosis and alkalosis are not possible.

Clinicians frequently find it difficult to decide if a mixed disorder is present. One useful scheme is to determine if the degree of compensation for the primary disorder is appropriate (Table 21–13). In respiratory disorders, if the magnitude of compensation in HCO_3^- level differs from that which is predicted, the patient has a mixed disorder. Therefore, superimposed metabolic acidosis will decrease HCO_3^- to lower than the predicted level, and a metabolic alkalosis will increase HCO_3^- over the predicted value. For example, a patient with chronic respiratory acidosis and P_{CO_2} of 60 mm Hg should have a HCO_3^- of 31 meq/L (assuming that normal HCO_3^- is 24 meq/L). If the HCO_3^- is 25 meq/L, a superimposed metabolic acidosis exists, and if the HCO_3^- is 45 meq/L, there is a superimposed metabolic alkalosis. Using data from Table 21–13, similar calculations can be made for primary metabolic disorders.

Furthermore, corrected bicarbonate ($cHCO_3^-$), calculated from measured HCO_3^- plus the increase in anion gap (see below), is useful to assess the superimposed metabolic alkalosis or normal anion gap metabolic acidosis. In increased anion gap acidosis, there must be a mole for mole decrease in HCO_3^- as anion gap decreases. Therefore, an HCO_3^- value higher or lower than normal (24 meq/L) indicates the concomitant presence of metabolic alkalosis or normal anion gap acidosis, respectively.

Table 21–13. Primary acid-base disorders and expected compensation.

Disorder	Primary Defect	pH	Compensatory Response	Magnitude of Compensation
Respiratory				
Acidosis				
Acute	↑P_{CO_2}	↓pH	↑HCO_3^-	↑HCO_3^- 1 meq/L per 10 mm Hg ↑P_{CO_2}
Chronic	↑P_{CO_2}	↓pH	↑HCO_3^-	↑HCO_3^- 3.5 meq/L per 10 mm Hg ↑P_{CO_2}
Alkalosis				
Acute	↓P_{CO_2}	↑pH	↓HCO_3^-	↓HCO_3^- 2 meq/L per 10 mm Hg ↓P_{CO_2}
Chronic	↓P_{CO_2}	↑pH	↓HCO_3^-	↓HCO_3^- 5 meq/L per 10 mm Hg ↓P_{CO_2}
Metabolic				
Acidosis	↓HCO_3^-	↓pH	↓P_{CO_2}	↓P_{CO_2} 1.3 mm Hg per 1 meq/L ↓HCO_3^-
Alkalosis	↑HCO_3^-	↑pH	↑P_{CO_2}	↑P_{CO_2} 0.7 mm Hg per 1 meq/L ↑HCO_3^-

STEP-BY-STEP ANALYSIS OF ACID-BASE STATUS

Step 1: Determine the primary (or main) disorder—whether it is metabolic or respiratory—from blood pH, HCO_3^-, and P_{CO_2} values.
Step 2: Determine the presence of mixed acid-base disorders by calculating the range of compensatory responses (Table 21–13).
Step 3: Calculate the anion gap (Table 21–15).
Step 4: Calculate the HCO_3^- concentration if the anion gap is increased (see above).
Step 5: Examine the patient to determine whether the clinical signs are compatible with the acid-base analysis thus obtained.

Gluck SL: Acid-base. Lancet 1998;352:474. [NLM Cit ID: 98372510] (A clinical approach to diagnosis and management.)

Laski ME et al: Acid-base disorders in medicine. Dis Mon 1996;42:51. [NLM Cit ID: 96231831]

Williamson JC: Acid-base disorders: Classification and management strategies. Am Fam Physician 1995;52:584. [NLM Cit ID: 95351253]

1. RESPIRATORY ACIDOSIS

Respiratory acidosis results from decreased alveolar ventilation and subsequent hypercapnia. Pulmonary as well as nonpulmonary disorders can cause hypoventilation. The clinician must be mindful of readily reversible causes of respiratory acidosis, especially opioid-induced central nervous system depression.

Acute respiratory failure is associated with severe acidosis and only a small increase in the plasma bicarbonate. After 6–12 hours, the primary increase in P_{CO_2} evokes a renal compensatory response to generate more HCO_3^-, which tends to ameliorate the respiratory acidosis. This usually takes several days to complete.

Chronic respiratory acidosis is generally seen in patients with underlying lung disease, such as chronic obstructive disease. Urinary excretion of acid in the form of NH_4^+ and Cl^- ions results in the characteristic hypochloremia of chronic respiratory acidosis. When chronic respiratory acidosis is corrected suddenly, especially in patients who receive mechanical ventilation, there is a 2- to 3-day lag in renal bicarbonate excretion, resulting in posthypercapnic metabolic alkalosis.

Clinical Findings

A. Symptoms and Signs: With acute onset, there is somnolence and confusion, and myoclonus with asterixis may be seen. Coma from CO_2 narcosis ensues. Severe hypercapnia increases cerebral blood flow and cerebrospinal fluid pressure. Signs of increased intracranial pressure (papilledema, pseudotumor cerebri) may be seen.

B. Laboratory Findings: Arterial pH is low, and P_{CO_2} is increased. Serum HCO_3^- is elevated, but not enough to completely compensate for the hypercapnia. If the disorder is chronic, hypochloremia is seen.

Treatment

Since drug overdose is an important reversible cause of acute respiratory acidosis, administration of naloxone, 0.04–2 mg intravenously (see Chapter 39) is given to all such patients if no obvious cause for respiratory depression is present. In all forms of respiratory acidosis, treatment is directed at the underlying disorder to improve ventilation.

2. RESPIRATORY ALKALOSIS

Respiratory alkalosis, or hypocapnia, occurs when hyperventilation reduces the P_{CO_2}, which increases the pH. The most common cause of respiratory alkalosis is hyperventilation syndrome (Table 21–14), but bacterial septicemia and cirrhosis are other common causes. Symptoms in acute respiratory alkalosis are related to decreased cerebral blood flow induced by the disorder. Pregnancy is another cause of chronic respiratory alka-

Table 21–14. Causes of respiratory alkalosis.[1]

Hypoxia
Decreased inspired oxygen tension
High altitude
Ventilation/perfusion inequality
Hypotension
Severe anemia
CNS-mediated disorders
Voluntary hyperventilation
Anxiety-hyperventilation syndrome
Neurologic disease
Cerebrovascular accident (infarction, hemorrhage)
Infection
Trauma
Tumor
Pharmacologic and hormonal stimulation
Salicylates
Nicotine
Xanthines
Pregnancy (progesterone)
Hepatic failure
Gram-negative septicemia
Recovery from metabolic acidosis
Heat exposure
Pulmonary disease
Interstitial lung disease
Pneumonia
Pulmonary embolism
Pulmonary edema
Mechanical overventilation

[1]Adapted from Gennari FJ: Respiratory acidosis and alkalosis. In: *Maxwell and Kleeman's Clinical Disorders of Fluid and Electrolyte Metabolism,* 5th ed. Narins RG (editor). McGraw-Hill, 1994.

losis, probably from progesterone stimulation of the respiratory center, with an average P_{CO_2} of 30 mm Hg.

Determination of appropriate compensatory changes in the HCO_3^- is useful to sort out the presence of an associated metabolic disorder (see above under Mixed Acid-Base Disorders). As in respiratory acidosis, the changes in HCO_3^- values are greater if the respiratory alkalosis is chronic (Table 21–13). While serum HCO_3^- is frequently below 15 meq/L in metabolic acidosis, it is unusual to see such a low level in respiratory alkalosis, and its presence would imply a superimposed (noncompensatory) metabolic acidosis.

Clinical Findings

A. Symptoms and Signs: In acute cases (hyperventilation), there is light-headedness, anxiety, paresthesias, numbness about the mouth, and a tingling sensation in the hands and feet. Tetany occurs in more severe alkalosis from a fall in ionized calcium. In chronic cases, findings are those of the responsible condition.

B. Laboratory Findings: Arterial blood pH is elevated, and P_{CO_2} is low. Serum bicarbonate is decreased in chronic respiratory alkalosis.

Treatment

Treatment is directed toward the underlying cause. In acute hyperventilation syndrome from anxiety, rebreathing into a paper bag will increase the P_{CO_2}. The processes are usually self-limited since muscle weakness caused by hyperventilation-induced alkalemia will suppress ventilation. Sedation may be necessary if the process persists. Rapid correction of chronic respiratory alkalosis may result in metabolic acidosis as P_{CO_2} is increased in the setting of previous compensatory decrease in HCO_3^-.

3. METABOLIC ACIDOSIS

The hallmark of metabolic acidosis is decreased HCO_3^-, seen also in respiratory alkalosis (see above), but the pH distinguishes between the two disorders. Calculation of the anion gap is useful in determining the cause of the metabolic acidosis (Table 21–15). The anion gap represents the difference between readily measured anions and cations.

In plasma,

$$Na^+ + \text{Unmeasured cations} = HCO_3^- + Cl^- + \text{Unmeasured anions}$$

$$\text{Anion gap} = (Na^+) - (HCO_3^- + Cl^-)$$

Table 21–15. Abnormal anion gap.[1]

Decreased (< 6 meq)
Hypoalbuminemia (decreased unmeasured anion)
Plasma cell dyscrasias
Monoclonal protein (cationic paraprotein) (accompanied by chloride and bicarbonate)
Bromide intoxication
Increased (>12 meq)
Metabolic anion
Diabetic ketoacidosis
Alcoholic ketoacidosis
Lactic acidosis
Renal insufficiency (PO_4^{3-}, SO_4^{2-})
Starvation
Metabolic alkalosis (increased number of negative charges on protein)
Drug or chemical anion
Salicylate intoxication
Sodium carbenicillin therapy
Methanol (formic acid)
Ethylene glycol (oxalic acid)
Normal (6–12 meq)
Loss of HCO_3^-
Diarrhea
Recovery from diabetic ketoacidosis
Pancreatic fluid loss ileostomy (unadapted)
Carbonic anhydrase inhibitors
Chloride retention
Renal tubular acidosis
Ileal loop bladder
Administration of HCl equivalent or NH_4Cl
Arginine and lysine in parenteral nutrition

[1]Reference ranges for anion gap may vary based on differing laboratory methods.

The major unmeasured cations are calcium (1 meq/L), magnesium (2 meq/L), gamma globulins, and potassium (4 meq/L). The major unmeasured anions are negatively charged albumin (2 meq/L per g/dL), phosphate (2 meq/L), sulfate (1 meq/L), lactate (1–2 meq/L), and other organic anions (3–4 meq/L). Traditionally, the normal anion gap has been 12 ± 4 meq/L. With the new generation of autoanalyzers, the reference range may be lower (6 ± 1 meq/L), primarily from an increase in Cl^- values. Despite its usefulness, the serum anion gap can be misleading. Non-acid-base disorders that may contribute to an error in anion gap interpretation include hypoalbuminemia (see below), antibiotic administration (eg, carbenicillin is an unmeasured anion; polymyxin is an unmeasured cation), hypernatremia, or hyponatremia.

Decreased Anion Gap

A decreased anion gap can occur because of a reduction in unmeasured anions or an increase in unmeasured cations.

A. Decreased Unmeasured Anions: If the sodium concentration remains normal but HCO_3^- and Cl^- increase, the anion gap will decrease. This is seen when there are decreased unmeasured anions, especially in hypoalbuminemia. For every 1 g/dL decline in serum albumin, a 2 meq/L decrease in anion gap will occur.

B. Increased Unmeasured Cations: If the sodium concentration falls because of addition of unmeasured cations but HCO_3^- and Cl^- remain unchanged, the anion gap will decrease. This is seen in (1) severe hypercalcemia, hypermagnesemia, or hyperkalemia; (2) IgG myeloma, where the immunoglobulin is cationic in 70% of cases; and (3) lithium toxicity.

Jurado RL et al: Low anion gap. South Med J 1998;91:624. [NLM Cit ID: 98335553] (Differential diagnosis of the low anion gap and the importance of this clue in the diagnosis of occult myeloma or intoxications.)

Increased Anion Gap Acidosis (Increased Unmeasured Anions)

The hallmark of this disorder is that metabolic acidosis (thus low HCO_3^-) is associated with normal serum Cl^-, so that the anion gap increases. Normochloremic metabolic acidosis generally results from addition to the blood of nonchloride acids such as lactate, acetoacetate, β-hydroxybutyrate, and exogenous toxins. An exception is uremia, with underexcretion of organic acids and anions.

A. Lactic Acidosis: Lactic acid is formed from pyruvate in anaerobic glycolysis. Therefore, most of the lactate is produced in tissues with high rates of glycolysis, such as gut (responsible for over 50% of lactate production), skeletal muscle, brain, skin, and erythrocytes. Normally, lactate levels remain low (1 meq/L) because of metabolism of lactate principally by the liver through gluconeogenesis or oxidation via the Krebs cycle. Furthermore, the kidneys metabolize about 30% of lactate.

In lactic acidosis, lactate levels are at least 4–5 meq/L but commonly 10–30 meq/L. The mortality rate exceeds 50%. There are two basic types of lactic acidosis, both associated with increased lactate production and decreased lactate utilization. Type A is characterized by hypoxia or decreased tissue perfusion, whereas in type B there is no clinical evidence of hypoxia. Type A (hypoxic) lactic acidosis is the more common type, resulting from poor tissue perfusion; cardiogenic, septic, or hemorrhagic shock; and carbon monoxide or cyanide poisoning. These conditions not only cause lactic acid production to increase peripherally but, more importantly, hepatic metabolism of lactate to decrease as liver perfusion declines. In addition, severe acidosis impairs the ability of the liver to extract the perfused lactate.

Type B lactic acidosis may be due to metabolic causes, such as diabetes, ketoacidosis, liver disease, renal failure, infection, leukemia, or lymphoma; or may occur as a result of toxicity from ethanol, methanol, salicylates, or isoniazid. AIDS without AIDS-related lymphoma is associated with type B lactic acidosis.

Idiopathic lactic acidosis, usually in debilitated patients, has an extremely high mortality rate. (For treatment of lactic acidosis, see below and Chapter 27.)

B. Diabetic Ketoacidosis: This metabolic abnormality is characterized by hyperglycemia and metabolic acidosis (pH < 7.25 or plasma bicarbonate < 16 meq/L). Anion gap metabolic acidosis is the acid-base disturbance generally ascribed to diabetic ketoacidosis:

$$H^+ + B^- + NaHCO_3 \leftrightarrow CO_2 + NaB + H_2O$$

where B^- is β-hydroxybutyrate or acetoacetate.

The anion gap should be calculated from the serum electrolytes as measured, since correction of the serum sodium for the dilutional effect of hyperglycemia will incorrectly exaggerate the anion gap. The increased anion gap is due to hyperketonemia (acetoacetate and β-hydroxybutyrate) and at times to an increase in serum lactate secondary to reduced tissue perfusion and increased anaerobic metabolism. If a rise in anion gap from normal is equal to a fall in HCO_3^-, a diagnosis of simple metabolic acidosis can be made. However, the presence of concurrent metabolic alkalosis or normal anion gap metabolic acidosis is suggested if the value of the measured HCO_3^- plus the increase in anion gap ($cHCO_3^-$) is higher or lower than the normal value for HCO_3^-, respectively.

During the recovery phase of diabetic ketoacidosis, anion gap acidosis can be transformed into hyperchloremic non-anion gap acidosis. The mechanism for this is as follows: As GFR increases from NaCl therapy of diabetic ketoacidosis, the retention of Cl^- causes a mild decrease in the anion gap from dilution. More importantly, the increased GFR causes the urinary excretion of ketone salts (NaB), which are formed as bicarbonate is consumed:

$$HB + NaHCO_3^- \rightarrow NaB + H_2CO_3$$

The kidney reabsorbs ketone anions poorly but can compensate for the loss of anions (and therefore Na^+) by increasing the reabsorption of Cl^-. Conversely, even on presentation, patients with diabetic ketoacidosis and normal renal perfusion may have marked ketonuria, severe metabolic acidosis, and only a mildly increased anion gap. Again, the variable relationship between the rise in the anion gap and the fall in the HCO_3^- can occur with the urinary loss of Na^+ or K^+ salts of β-hydroxybutyrate, which will lower the anion gap without altering the H^+ excretion or the severity of the acidosis.

Since Ketostix reacts to acetoacetate, less to acetone, and not at all to the predominant keto acid, β-hydroxybutyrate, the test may become more positive even as the patient improves owing to the metabolism of hydroxybutyrate. Thus, the patient's clinical status and the reduction of the anion gap are better markers of improvement than monitoring the serum acetone test. Conversely, in the presence of concomitant lactic acidosis, a shift in the redox state can increase β-hydroxybutyrate and decrease the readily detectable acetoacetate, thus lowering the nitroprusside reaction.

C. Alcoholic Ketoacidosis: This is a common disorder of chronically malnourished patients who consume large quantities of alcohol daily. Most of these patients have mixed acid-base disorders (10% have a triple acid-base disorder). While decreased HCO_3^- is usual, half the patients may have normal or alkalemic pH. The three types of metabolic acidosis seen in alcoholic ketoacidosis are the following: (1) Ketoacidosis due to β-hydroxybutyrate and acetoacetate excess. (2) Lactic acidosis: Alcohol metabolism increases the NADH:NAD ratio, causing increased production and decreased utilization of lactate. Accompanying thiamin deficiency, which inhibits pyruvate carboxylase, further enhances lactic acid production in many cases. Moderate to severe elevations of lactate (> 6 mmol/L) are seen with concomitant disorders such as sepsis, pancreatitis, or hypoglycemia. (3) Hyperchloremic acidosis from bicarbonate loss in the urine associated with ketonuria (see above). Metabolic alkalosis occurs from volume contraction and vomiting. Respiratory alkalosis results from alcohol withdrawal, pain, or associated disorders such as sepsis or liver disease. Half of the patients have either hypoglycemia or hyperglycemia. When serum glucose levels are greater than 250 mg/dL, the distinction from diabetic ketoacidosis is difficult. The diagnosis of alcoholic ketoacidosis is supported by absence of a diabetic history and by no evidence of glucose intolerance after initial therapy.

D. Toxins: (See also Chapter 39.) Multiple toxins and drugs can increase the anion gap by increasing endogenous acid production. Examples include methanol (metabolized to formic acid), ethylene glycol (glycolic and oxalic acid), and salicylates (salicylic acid and lactic acid), which can cause a mixed disorder of metabolic acidosis with respiratory alkalosis.

E. Uremic Acidosis: At glomerular filtration rates below 20 mL/min, the inability to excrete H^+ with retention of acid anions such as PO_4^{3-} and SO_4^{2-} result in an increased anion gap acidosis, which rarely is severe. The unmeasured anions "replace" HCO_3^- (which is consumed as a buffer). Hyperchloremic normal anion gap acidosis may be seen in milder cases of renal insufficiency.

Normal Anion Gap Acidosis (Table 21–16)

The hallmark of this disorder is that the low HCO_3^- of metabolic acidosis is associated with hyperchloremia, so that the anion gap remains normal. The most common causes are gastrointestinal HCO_3^- loss and defects in renal acidification (renal tubular acidoses). The urinary anion gap can differentiate between these two common causes (see below).

A. Gastrointestinal HCO_3^- Loss: Bicarbonate is secreted in multiple areas in the gastrointestinal tract. Small bowel and pancreatic secretions contain large amounts of HCO_3^-. Therefore, massive diarrhea or pancreatic drainage can result in HCO_3^- loss because of increased HCO_3^- secretion and decreased absorption. Hyperchloremia occurs because the ileum and colon secrete HCO_3^- in a one-to-one exchange for Cl^- by countertransport. The resultant volume contraction causes increased Cl^- retention by the kidney in the setting of decreased anion, HCO_3^-. Patients with ureterosigmoidostomies can develop hyperchloremic metabolic acidosis because the colon secretes HCO_3^- in the urine in exchange for Cl^-.

B. Renal Tubular Acidosis: In renal tubular acidosis, the defect is either inability to excrete H^+ (inadequate generation of new HCO_3^-) or inappropriate reabsorption of HCO_3^-. Four discrete types can be differentiated by the clinical setting, urinary pH, urinary anion gap (see below), and serum K^+ level.

1. Classic distal renal tubular acidosis (type I)–This disorder is characterized by hypokalemic hyperchloremic metabolic acidosis and is due to selective deficiency in H^+ secretion in the distal nephron. Despite acidosis, urinary pH cannot be acidified and is always above 5.5, which retards the

Table 21–16. Hyperchloremic, normal anion gap metabolic acidoses.[1]

	Renal Defect	Serum $[K^+]$	Distal H^+ Secretion: Minimal Urine pH	Distal H^+ Secretion: Urinary NH_4^+ Plus Titratable Acid	Urinary Anion Gap	Treatment
Gastrointestinal HCO_3^- loss	None	↓	< 5.5	↑↑	Negative	Na^+, K^+, and HCO_3^- as required
Renal tubular acidosis						
I. Classic distal	Distal H^+ secretion	↓	> 5.5	↓	Positive	$NaHCO_3$ (1–3 meq/kg/d)
II. Proximal	Proximal H^+ secretion	↓	< 5.5	Normal	Positive	$NaHCO_3$ or $KHCO_3$ (10–15 meq/kg/d), thiazide
III. Glomerular insufficiency	NH_3 production	Normal	< 5.5	↓	Positive	$NaHCO_3$ (1–3 meq/kg/d)
IV. Hyporeninemic hypoaldosteronism	Distal Na^+ reabsorption, K^+ secretion, and H^+ secretion	↑	< 5.5	↓	Positive	Fludrocortisone (0.1–0.5 mg/d), dietary K^+ restriction, furosemide (40–160 mg/d), $NaHCO_3$ (1–3 meq/kg/d)

[1]Modified and reproduced, with permission, from Cogan MG: *Fluid and Electrolytes: Physiology and Pathophysiology.* Originally published by Appleton & Lange.

binding of H^+ to phosphate ($H^+ + HPO_4^{2-} \rightarrow H_2PO_4$), and thus inhibits titratable acid excretion. Furthermore, urinary excretion of $NH_4^+Cl^-$ is decreased, and the urinary anion gap is positive (see below). Enhanced K^+ excretion occurs probably because there is less competition from H^+ in the distal nephron transport system. Furthermore, as a response to renal salt wasting, hyperaldosteronism occurs. Nephrocalcinosis and nephrolithiasis frequently accompany this disorder.

2. Proximal renal tubular acidosis (type II)–Proximal renal tubular acidosis is a hypokalemic hyperchloremic metabolic acidosis due to a selective defect in the proximal tubule's ability to adequately reabsorb filtered HCO_3^-. Carbonic anhydrase inhibitors (acetazolamide) can cause proximal renal tubular acidosis. About 90% of filtered HCO_3^- is absorbed by the proximal tubule. The distal nephron has a limited ability to absorb HCO_3^- but becomes overwhelmed and does not function adequately when there is increased delivery. Eventually, distal delivery of filtered HCO_3^- declines because the plasma HCO_3^- level has dropped as a result of progressive urinary HCO_3^- wastage. When the plasma HCO_3^- level drops to 15–18 meq/L, delivery of HCO_3^- drops to the point where the distal nephron is no longer overwhelmed and can regain function. At that point, bicarbonaturia disappears, and urinary pH can be acidic. Thiazide-induced volume contraction can be used to enhance proximal HCO_3^- reabsorption, leading to the decrease in distal HCO_3^- delivery and improvement of bicarbonaturia and renal acidification. The increased delivery of HCO_3^- to the distal nephron also increases K^+ secretion, and hypokalemia results if a patient is loaded with excess HCO_3^- and K^+ is not adequately supplemented. Proximal renal tubular acidosis often exists with other defects of absorption in the proximal tubule, resulting in glucosuria, aminoaciduria, phosphaturia, and uricaciduria. Causes include multiple myeloma with Fanconi's syndrome and nephrotoxic drugs.

3. Renal tubular acidosis of glomerular insufficiency (type III)–When GFR decreases to 20–30 mL/min, ability to generate adequate NH_3 is impaired, with subsequent decreased $NH_4^+Cl^-$ excretion. A normokalemic, hyperchloremic metabolic acidosis ensues. Further reduction in GFR results in increased anion gap acidosis of uremia (see above).

4. Hyporeninemic hypoaldosteronemic renal tubular acidosis (type IV)–Type IV is the only type characterized by hyperkalemic, hyperchloremic acidosis. The defect is aldosterone deficiency or antagonism, which impairs distal nephron Na^+ reabsorption and K^+ and H^+ excretion. Renal salt wasting is frequently present. Relative hypoaldosteronism from hyporeninemia is most commonly found in diabetic nephropathy, tubulointerstitial renal diseases, hypertensive nephrosclerosis, and AIDS. In patients with these disorders, caution must be taken when using drugs that can exacerbate the hyperkalemia, such as angiotensin-converting enzyme inhibitors (which will further reduce aldosterone levels), aldosterone receptor blockers such as spironolactone, and NSAIDs.

C. Dilutional Acidosis: Rapid dilution of plasma volume by 0.9% NaCl may cause a mild hyperchloremic acidosis.

D. Recovery From Diabetic Ketoacidosis: See above.

E. Posthypocapnia: In prolonged respiratory alkalosis, HCO_3^- decreases and Cl^- increases from decreased renal $NH_4^+Cl^-$ excretion. If the respiratory alkalosis is corrected quickly, P_{CO_2} will increase acutely but HCO_3^- will remain low until the kidneys can generate new HCO_3^-, which generally takes several days. In the meantime, the increased P_{CO_2} with low HCO_3^- causes metabolic acidosis.

F. Hyperalimentation: Hyperalimentation fluids may contain amino acid solutions that acidify when metabolized, such as arginine hydrochloride and lysine hydrochloride.

Urinary Anion Gap to Assess Hyperchloremic Metabolic Acidosis

Increased renal $NH_4^+Cl^-$ excretion to enhance H^+ removal is a normal physiologic response to metabolic acidosis. NH_3 reacts with H^+ to form NH_4^+, which is accompanied by the anion Cl^- for excretion. The normal daily urinary excretion of NH_4Cl of about 30 meq can be increased up to 200 meq in response to acid load.

Urinary anion gap from a random urine sample ($[Na^+ + K^+] - Cl^-$) reflects the ability of the kidney to excrete NH_4Cl as in the following equation:

$$Na^+ + K^+ + NH_3^+ = Cl^- + 80$$

where 80 is the average value for the difference in the urinary anions and cations other than Na^+, K^+, NH_3^+, and Cl^-.

Therefore, urinary anion gap is equal to ($80 - NH_3^+$), and thus aids in the distinction between gastrointestinal and renal causes of hyperchloremic acidosis. If the cause of the metabolic acidosis is gastrointestinal HCO_3^- loss (diarrhea), renal acidification ability remains normal and NH_4Cl excretion increases in response to the acidosis. The urinary anion gap is negative (eg, −30 meq/L). If the cause is distal renal tubular acidosis, the urinary anion gap is positive (eg, +25 meq/L), since the basic lesion in the disorder is inability of the kidney to excrete H^+ and thus inability to increase NH_4Cl excretion. Urinary pH may not as readily differentiate between the two causes. Despite acidosis, if volume depletion from diarrhea causes inadequate Na^+ delivery to the distal nephron and therefore decreased exchange with H^+, urinary pH may not be lower than 5.3. In the presence of this relatively high urine pH, however, H^+ excretion continues due to buffering of NH_3 to NH_4^+, since the pK of this reaction is as high as 9.1. Potassium depletion, which can accompany diarrhea (and surreptitious laxative abuse), may also impair renal acidification. Thus, when volume depletion is present, the urinary anion gap is a better measurement of ability to acidify the urine than urinary pH.

Clinical Findings

A. Symptoms and Signs: Symptoms of metabolic acidosis are mainly those of the underlying disorder. Compensatory hyperventilation is an important clinical sign and may be misinterpreted as a primary respiratory disorder; when severe, Kussmaul respirations (deep, regular, sighing respirations) are seen.

B. Laboratory Findings: Blood pH, serum HCO_3^-, and P_{CO_2} are decreased. Anion gap may be normal (hyperchloremic) or increased (normochloremic). Hyperkalemia may be seen (see above).

Treatment

A. Increased Anion Gap Acidosis: Treatment is aimed at the underlying disorder, such as insulin and fluid therapy for diabetes and appropriate volume resuscitation to restore tissue perfusion. The metabolism of lactate will produce HCO_3^- and increase pH. The use of supplemental HCO_3^- is indicated for treatment of hyperkalemia (Table 21–7) and some forms of normal anion gap acidosis but has been controversial for treatment of increased anion gap metabolic acidosis. Administration of large amounts of HCO_3^- may have deleterious effects, including hypernatremia and hyperosmolality. Furthermore, intracellular pH may decrease because administered HCO_3^- is converted to CO_2, which easily diffuses into cells. There, it combines with water to create additional hydrogen ions and worsening of intracellular acidosis. Theoretically, this could impair cellular function, but the clinical significance of this phenomenon is uncertain. In addition, alkali administration is known to stimulate phosphofructokinase activity, thus exacerbating lactic acidosis via enhanced lactate production. Ketogenesis is also augmented by alkali therapy. In salicylate intoxication, however, alkali therapy must be started unless blood pH is already alkalinized by respiratory alkalosis, since the increment in pH converts salicylate to more impermeable salicylic acid and thus prevents central nervous system damage. In alcoholic ketoacidosis, thiamine should be given together with glucose to avoid the development of Wernicke's encephalopathy. The amount of HCO_3^- deficit can be calculated as follows:

$$\text{Amount of } HCO_3^- \text{ deficit} = 0.5 \times \text{Body weight} \times (24 - HCO_3^-)$$

Half of the calculated deficit should be administered within the first 3–4 hours to avoid overcorrection and volume overload.

B. Normal Anion Gap Acidosis: (Table 21–16.) In distal renal tubular acidosis, supplementation of bicarbonate is necessary since acid accumulates systemically in this disorder. However, in proximal renal tubular acidosis, correction of low serum bicarbonate is sometimes hazardous and unnecessary except in severe cases. If the blood bicarbonate concentration is elevated in response to its administration, and the concentration in the glomerular filtrate exceeds the capacity of the proximal tubule to reabsorb it, a large quantity of bicarbonate is excreted into the urine accompanied by potassium, exacerbating hypokalemia. Thus, potassium should also be given when bicarbonate therapy is indicated in proximal renal tubular acidosis.

Adrogue HJ et al: Management of life threatening acid base disorders. (Part 1.) N Engl J Med 1998;338:26. [NLM Cit ID: 98069943]

Galla JH: Metabolic alkalosis. J Am Soc Nephrol 2000;11:369. [NLM Cit ID: 20127711]

Hood VL et al: Protection of acid-base balance by pH regulation of acid production. N Engl J Med 1998;339:819. [NLM Cit ID: 98400650] (Systemic pH regulates acid production in a negative feedback manner.)

Okuda Y et al: Counterproductive effects of sodium bicarbonate in diabetic ketoacidosis. J Clin Endocrinol Metab 1996;81:314. [NLM Cit ID: 96142006] (Bicarbonate therapy in diabetic ketoacidosis may be deleterious because the exogenous alkali augments ketone production.)

Smulders YM et al: Renal tubular acidosis: Pathophysiology and diagnosis. Arch Intern Med 1996;156:1629. [NLM Cit ID: 96316793]

4. METABOLIC ALKALOSIS

Classification

Metabolic alkalosis is characterized by high HCO_3^-. The high HCO_3^- is seen also in chronic respiratory acidosis (see above), but pH differentiates the two disorders. It is useful to classify the causes of metabolic alkalosis into two groups based on "saline responsiveness" or urinary Cl^-, which are markers for volume status (Table 21–17). Saline-responsive metabolic alkalosis is a sign of extracellular volume contraction, and saline-unresponsive alkalosis implies a volume-expanded state. It is rare for a compensatory increase in P_{CO_2} to exceed 55 mm Hg. A higher value implies a superimposed respiratory acidosis.

A. Saline-Responsive Metabolic Alkalosis: Saline-responsive metabolic alkalosis is by far the more common disorder. It is characterized by normotensive extracellular volume contraction and hypokalemia. Less frequently, hypotension or orthostatic hypotension may be seen. In vomiting or nasogastric suction, for example, loss of acid (HCl) initiates the alkalosis, but volume contraction from loss of Cl^- sustains the alkalosis because the decline in GFR causes avid renal Na^+ and HCO_3^- reabsorption. Since there is Cl^- depletion from loss of HCl, NaCl, and KCl from the stomach, the available anion is HCO_3^-, whose reabsorption is increased proximally, and urine pH may remain acidic despite alkalemia (paradoxical aciduria). Renal Cl^- reabsorption

Table 21–17. Metabolic alkalosis.[1]

Saline-Responsive (U_{Cl} < 10 meq/d)	Saline-Unresponsive (U_{Cl} > 10 meq/d)
Excessive body bicarbonate content	**Excessive body bicarbonate content**
Renal alkalosis	Renal alkalosis
Diuretic therapy	Normotensive
Poorly reabsorbable anion therapy: carbenicillin, penicillin, sulfate, phosphate	Bartter's syndrome (renal salt wasting and secondary hyperaldosteronism)
Posthypercapnia	Severe potassium depletion
Gastrointestinal alkalosis	Refeeding alkalosis
Loss of HCl from vomiting or nasogastric suction	Hypercalcemia and hypoparathyroidism
Intestinal alkalosis: chloride diarrhea	Hypertensive
Exogenous alkali	Endogenous mineralocorticoids
$NaHCO_3$ (baking soda)	Primary aldosteronism
Sodium citrate, lactate, gluconate, acetate	Hyperreninism
Transfusions	Adrenal enzyme deficiency: 11- and 17-hydroxylase
Antacids	Liddle's syndrome
Normal body bicarbonate content	Exogenous mineralocorticoids
"Contraction alkalosis"	Licorice

[1]Modified and reproduced, with permission, from Narins RG et al: Diagnostic strategies in disorders of fluid, electrolyte and acid-base homeostasis. Am J Med 1982;72:496.

(as well as Na^+) reabsorption is high, and the urinary Cl^- is therefore low (< 10–20 meq/L). In alkalosis, bicarbonaturia may force Na^+ excretion as the accompanying cation even if volume depletion is present. Therefore, urinary Cl^- is preferred to urinary Na^+ as a measure of extracellular volume. An exception to the usefulness of urinary Cl^- is in patients who have recently received diuretics. Their urine may contain high Na^+ and Cl^- despite extracellular volume contraction. If diuretics are discontinued, the urinary Cl^- will decrease.

Metabolic alkalosis is generally associated with hypokalemia. This is due partly to the direct effect of alkalosis per se on renal potassium excretion and partly to secondary hyperaldosteronism from volume depletion. Hypokalemia induced in this fashion further worsens the metabolic alkalosis by increasing bicarbonate reabsorption in the proximal tubule and hydrogen ion secretion in the distal tubule. Administration of KCl will correct the disorder. Repletion of KCl is important to reverse the disorder.

1. Contraction alkalosis–Diuretics can acutely decrease extracellular volume from urinary loss of NaCl and water. There is no associated bicarbonaturia, so that body HCO_3^- content remains normal. However, plasma HCO_3^- increases because of extracellular fluid contraction—the reverse of what occurs in dilutional acidosis.

2. Posthypercapnia alkalosis–In chronic respiratory acidosis, compensatory increases in HCO_3^- occur (Table 21–13). Hypercapnia also directly affects the proximal tubule to decrease NaCl reabsorption, which can cause extracellular volume depletion. If PCO_2 is corrected rapidly, as with mechanical ventilation, metabolic alkalosis will ensue until adequate bicarbonaturia occurs. Hypovolemia will inhibit bicarbonaturia until Cl^- is repleted. Many patients with chronic respiratory acidosis receive diuretics, which further exacerbates the metabolic alkalosis.

B. Saline-Unresponsive Alkalosis:

1. Hyperaldosteronism–Primary hyperaldosteronism causes expansion of extracellular volume with hypertension. Metabolic alkalosis with hypokalemia results from the renal mineralocorticoid effect. In an attempt to decrease extracellular volume, high levels of NaCl are excreted, and for that reason the urinary Cl^- is high (> 20 meq/L, often higher). Therapy with NaCl will only increase volume expansion and hypertension and will not treat the underlying problem of mineralocorticoid excess.

2. Alkali administration with decreased GFR–Despite large ingestions of HCO_3^-, enhanced bicarbonaturia almost always prevents a patient with normal renal function from developing metabolic alkalosis. However, with renal insufficiency, urinary excretion of bicarbonate is inadequate. If large amounts of HCO_3^- or metabolizable salts of organic acids such as sodium lactate, sodium citrate, or sodium gluconate are consumed, as with intensive antacid therapy, metabolic alkalosis will occur. In milk-alkali syndrome, large and sustained ingestion of absorbable antacids and milk causes renal insufficiency from hypercalcemia. Decreased GFR prevents appropriate bicarbonaturia from the ingested alkali, and metabolic alkalosis occurs. Volume contraction from renal hypercalcemic effects further exacerbates the alkalosis.

Clinical Findings

A. Symptoms and Signs: There are no characteristic symptoms or signs. Orthostatic hypotension may be encountered. Weakness and hyporeflexia occur if serum K^+ is markedly low. Tetany and neuromuscular irritability occur rarely.

B. Laboratory Findings: The arterial blood pH and bicarbonate are elevated. The arterial PCO_2 is increased. Serum potassium and chloride are decreased. There may be an increased anion gap.

Treatment

Mild alkalosis is generally well tolerated. Severe or symptomatic alkalosis (pH > 7.60) requires urgent treatment.

A. Saline-Responsive Metabolic Alkalosis: Therapy for saline-responsive metabolic alkalosis is aimed at correction of extracellular volume deficit. Depending on the degree of hypovolemia, adequate amounts of 0.9% NaCl and KCl should be administered. Discontinuation of diuretics and administration of H_2-blockers in patients whose alkalosis is due to nasogastric suction can be useful. If impaired pulmonary or cardiovascular status prohibits adequate volume repletion, acetazolamide, 250–500 mg intravenously every 4–6 hours, can be used. One must be alert to the possible development of hypokalemia, since potassium depletion can be induced by forced kaliuresis via bicarbonaturia. Administration of acid can be used as emergency therapy. HCl, 0.1 mol/L, is infused via a central vein (the solution is sclerosing). Dosage is calculated to decrease the HCO_3^- level by one-half over 2–4 hours, assuming a HCO_3^- volume of distribution (L) of 0.5 × body weight (kg). Patients with marked renal insufficiency may require dialysis.

B. Saline-Unresponsive Metabolic Alkalosis: Therapy for saline-unresponsive metabolic alkalosis includes surgical removal of a mineralocorticoid-producing tumor and blockage of aldosterone effect with an angiotensin-converting enzyme inhibitor or with spironolactone. Metabolic alkalosis in primary aldosteronism can be treated only with potassium repletion.

Adrogue HJ et al: Management of life threatening acid base disorders. (Part 2.) N Engl J Med 1998;338:107. [NLM Cit ID: 98069970]

Laski ME et al: Acid-base disorders in medicine. Dis Mon 1996;42:51. [NLM Cit ID: 96231831]

Table 21–18. Replacement guidelines for sweat and gastrointestinal fluid losses.

	Average Electrolyte Composition				Replacement Guidelines per Liter Lost				
	Na^+ (meq/L)	K^+ (meq/L)	Cl^- (meq/L)	HCO_3^- (meq/L)	0.9% saline (mL)	0.45% saline (mL)	D_5W (mL)	KCl (meq/L)	7.5% $NaHCO_3$ (45 meq HCO_3^-/amp)
Sweat	30–50	5	50			500	500	5	
Gastric secretions	20	10	10			300	700	20	
Pancreatic juice	130	5	35	115		400	600	5	2 amps
Bile	145	5	100	25	600		400	5	0.5 amp
Duodenal fluid	60	15	100	10		1000		15	0.25 amp
Ileal fluid	100	10	60	60		600	400	10	1 amp
Colonic diarrhea	140[1]	10	85	60		1000		10	1 amp

[1]In the absence of diarrhea, colonic fluid Na^+ levels are low (40 meq/L).

FLUID MANAGEMENT

Most of those who require water and electrolyte intravenously are relatively normal people who cannot take orally what they require for maintenance. The range of tolerance for water and electrolytes (homeostatic limits) permits reasonable latitude in therapy provided normal renal function exists to accomplish the final regulation of volume and concentration.

An average adult whose entire intake is parenteral would require for maintenance 2500–3000 mL of 5% dextrose in 0.2% saline solution (34 meq Na^+ plus 34 meq Cl^-/L). To each liter, 30 meq of KCl could be added. In 3 L, the total chloride intake would be 192 meq, which is easily tolerated. Guidelines for gastrointestinal fluid losses are shown in Table 21–18.

In situations requiring maintenance or maintenance plus replacement of fluid and electrolyte by parenteral infusion, the total daily ration should be administered continuously over the 24-hour period in order to ensure the best utilization by the patient.

If parenteral fluids are the only source of water, electrolytes, and calories for longer than a week, more complex fluids containing amino acids, lipid, trace metals, and vitamins may be indicated. (See Total Parenteral Nutrition, Chapter 29.)

RELEVANT WORLD WIDE WEB SITES

[Renal Tubular Acidosis]
http://www.niddk.nih.gov/health/kidney/pubs/rta.htm
[Hyperparathyroidism]
http://www.niddk.nih.gov/health/endo/pubs/hyper/hyper.htm

Kidney

22

See http://www.current-med.com/ch22.html for updated addresses of Web sites referenced in this chapter.

Suzanne Watnick, MD, & Gail Morrison, MD

APPROACH TO RENAL DISEASE

A patient will present with renal disease in one of two ways: discovered incidentally during a routine medical evaluation or with evidence of renal dysfunction such as hypertension, edema, nausea, and hematuria. The initial approach in both situations should be to assess the cause and severity of renal abnormalities. In all cases this evaluation includes (1) an estimation of disease duration, (2) a careful urinalysis, and (3) an assessment of the glomerular filtration rate (GFR). The history and physical examination, though equally important, are variable among renal syndromes—thus specific symptoms and signs are discussed under each disease entity. Further diagnostic categorization is according to anatomic distribution: prerenal disease, postrenal disease, and intrinsic renal disease. Intrinsic renal disease can further be divided into glomerular, tubular, interstitial, and vascular abnormalities.

DISEASE DURATION

Renal disease may be acute or chronic. Acute renal failure is worsening of renal function over hours to days, resulting in the retention of nitrogenous wastes (such as urea nitrogen) and creatinine in the blood. Retention of these substances is called azotemia. Chronic renal failure results from a loss of renal function over months to years. Differentiating between the two is important for diagnosis, treatment, and outcome. Oliguria is unusual in chronic renal insufficiency. Anemia (from low renal erythropoietin production) is rare in acute renal failure. Small kidneys are most consistent with chronic renal failure, whereas normal size can be seen with both.

URINALYSIS

A urinalysis has been likened to "a poor man's renal biopsy." The urine is collected in midstream or, if that is not feasible, by bladder catheterization. The urine should be examined within 1 hour after collection. Urinalysis includes a dipstick examination followed by microscopic assessment if the dipstick has positive findings. The dipstick examination measures urinary specific gravity, pH, protein, hemoglobin, glucose, ketones, bilirubin, nitrites, and leukocyte esterase. Microscopy searches for all formed elements—crystals, cells, casts, and infecting organisms.

Various findings on the urinalysis are indicative of certain patterns of renal disease (Table 22–1). A bland urinary sediment is common, especially in chronic renal disease and prerenal and postrenal disorders. Red blood cells are misshapen during passage from the capillary through the glomerular basement membrane into the urinary space of Bowman's capsule. The presence of hematuria with dysmorphic red blood cells, red blood cell casts, and mild proteinuria is indicative of glomerulonephritis. Casts are composed of Tamm-Horsfall urinary mucoprotein in the shape of the nephron segment where they were formed. Heavy proteinuria and lipiduria are consistent with the nephrotic syndrome. Pigmented granular casts and renal tubular epithelial cells alone or in casts suggest acute tubular necrosis. White blood cells, including neutrophils and eosinophils, white blood cell casts, red blood cells, and small amounts of protein can be found in interstitial nephritis; Wright's stain is required to detect eosinophilia. Pyuria alone can indicate a urinary tract infection. Hematuria and proteinuria are discussed more thoroughly below.

Proteinuria

Significant proteinuria is a sign of an underlying renal abnormality, usually glomerular in origin. It is usually accompanied by other clinical abnormalities—elevated BUN and serum creatinine levels, abnormal urinary sediment, or evidence of systemic illness (eg, fever, rash, vasculitis).

There are four primary reasons for development of proteinuria.

(1) Functional proteinuria is a benign process stemming from stressors such as acute illness, exercise, and "orthostatic proteinuria." The latter condi-

Table 22–1. Significance of specific urinary casts.

Type	Significance
Hyaline casts	Concentrated urine, febrile disease, after strenuous exercise, in the course of diuretic therapy (not indicative of renal disease)
Red cell casts	Glomerulonephritis
White cell casts	Pyelonephritis, interstitial nephritis (indicative of infection or inflammation)
Renal tubular cell casts	Acute tubular necrosis, interstitial nephritis
Coarse, granular casts	Nonspecific; can represent acute tubular necrosis
Broad, waxy casts	Chronic renal failure (indicative of stasis in collecting tubule)

tion, generally found in people under age 30, results in the excretion of abnormal amounts of urinary protein, typically less than 1 g/d.

(2) Proteinuria can result from overproduction of circulating, filterable plasma proteins, such as Bence Jones proteins associated with multiple myeloma. Urinary protein electrophoresis will exhibit a discrete protein peak.

(3) Glomerular proteinuria results from abnormalities in the glomerular basement membrane (GBM) or, less commonly, from changes in the glomerular capillary pressure. All glomerular diseases exhibit some degree of proteinuria. The urinary electrophoresis will have a pattern exhibiting a large albumin spike indicative of increased permeability of albumin across a damaged GBM.

(4) Tubular proteinuria occurs as a result of damaged reabsorption of normally filtered proteins in the proximal tubule. Causes include acute tubular necrosis, toxic injury (lead, aminoglycosides), drug-induced interstitial nephritis, and hereditary metabolic disorders (Wilson's disease and Fanconi's syndrome).

Evaluation of proteinuria by urinary dipstick primarily detects albumin and intact globulins, while overlooking light chains of immunoglobulins. These proteins can be detected by the addition of sulfosalicylic acid to the urine specimen. The lack of precipitation indicates no paraproteins.

The next step—and the most reliable way to quantify proteinuria—is a 24-hour urine collection. A finding of > 165 mg/24 h is abnormal, and > 3.5 g/24 h is consistent with nephrotic-range proteinuria. A simpler and less accurate method is to collect a random urine sample. The ratio of the urinary protein concentration to the urinary creatinine concentration ($U_{protein}/U_{creatinine}$) correlates with 24-hour urine protein collection (< 0.2 is normal and corresponds to excretion of less than 200 mg/d). If a patient has proteinuria with loss of renal function, renal biopsy may be indicated, particularly if the renal insufficiency is acute in onset. The clinical consequences of proteinuria are discussed in the section on the nephrotic syndrome.

In some instances, notably diabetes mellitus, therapy aimed at reducing proteinuria may also reduce progression of renal disease. ACE inhibitors are effective by lowering efferent arteriolar resistance out of proportion to afferent arteriolar resistance, thereby reducing glomerular capillary pressure and lowering urinary protein excretion. ACE inhibitors are best used in patients whose GFRs are not markedly impaired, because of worsening renal failure and hyperkalemia. The consequences of dietary restrictions in patients with proteinuria are discussed in the section on chronic renal failure.

Hematuria

Hematuria is significant if there are more than three to five red cells per high-power field. It is usually detected incidentally by the urine dipstick examination or by an episode of macroscopic hematuria. The diagnosis must be confirmed via microscopic examination, as false-positive dipstick tests can be caused by vitamin C, beets and rhubarb, bacteria, and myoglobin. Transient hematuria is common, but in patients under 40 it is less often of clinical significance.

Hematuria may be due to renal or extrarenal causes. Extrarenal causes are addressed in Chapter 23. Renal causes account for approximately 10% of cases and are best considered anatomically as glomerular or nonglomerular. The most common extraglomerular sources include cysts, calculi, interstitial nephritis, and renal neoplasia. Glomerular causes include IgA nephropathy, thin GBM disease, postinfectious glomerulonephritis, membranoproliferative glomerulonephritis, and the systemic nephritic syndromes.

See Chapter 23 for evaluation of hematuria.

ESTIMATION OF GFR

The glomerular filtration rate (GFR) provides a useful index of overall renal function. The GFR measures the amount of plasma ultrafiltered across the glomerular capillaries and correlates with the ability of the kidneys to filter fluids and various substances. Daily GFR in normal individuals is variable, with a range of 150–250 L/24 h or 100–120 mL/min/1.73 m^2 of body surface area. GFR can be measured indirectly by determining the renal clearance of plasma substances which are not bound to plasma proteins, are freely filterable across the glomerulus, and are neither secreted nor reabsorbed along the renal tubules.

The formula used to determine the renal clearance of a substance is

$$C = \frac{U \times \dot{V}}{P}$$

where C is the clearance, U and P are the urine and plasma concentrations of the substance (mg/dL), and $\dot{V}$ is the urine flow rate (mL/min). Inulin and creatinine clearance are used as markers of GFR. Inulin clearance following a continuous infusion is the most accurate method for measurement of GFR. The cost and the complexity of the administration and analysis of inulin preclude its routine use. In clinical practice, the clearance rate of endogenous creatinine, the creatinine clearance (C_{cr}), is the usual means of estimating GFR.

Creatinine is a product of muscle metabolism produced at a relatively constant rate and cleared by renal excretion. It is freely filterable by the glomerulus and not reabsorbed by the renal tubules. With stable renal function, creatinine production and excretion are equal, thus, plasma creatinine concentrations remain constant. However, it is not a perfect indicator of GFR for the following reasons: (1) a small amount is normally eliminated by tubular secretion, and the fraction secreted progressively increases as GFR declines (overestimating GFR); (2) with severe renal failure, gut microorganisms degrade creatinine, (3) an individual's meat intake and muscle mass affect baseline plasma creatinine levels; (4) commonly used drugs such as cimetidine, probenecid, and trimethoprim reduce tubular secretion of creatinine, increasing the plasma creatinine concentration and falsely indicating renal dysfunction; and (5) the accuracy of the measurement necessitates a stable plasma creatinine concentration over a 24-hour period, so that during the development of and recovery from acute renal failure, the C_{cr} is a questionable value (see Table 22–2).

To measure creatinine clearance, collect a 24-hour urine sample and determine the plasma creatinine level on the same day. An incomplete or prolonged urine collection is a common source of error. One way of estimating the completeness of the collection is to calculate a 24-hour creatinine excretion; the amount should be constant:

$$U_{cr} \times V = 15\text{–}20 \text{ mg/kg for healthy young women}$$
$$U_{cr} \times V = 20\text{–}25 \text{ mg/kg for healthy young men}$$

The creatinine clearance is approximately 100 mL/min/1.73 m^2 in healthy young women and 120 mL/min/1.73 m^2 in healthy young men. The C_{cr} declines by 1 mL/min/yr after age 40 as part of the aging process.

Since urine collection may be difficult, creatinine clearance can be estimated from the formula of Cockcroft and Gault, which incorporates age, sex, and weight to estimate creatinine clearance from plasma creatinine levels without any urinary measurements:

$$C_{cr} = \frac{(140 - \text{Age}) \times \text{Weight (kg)}}{P_{cr} \times 72}$$

For women, the estimated GFR is multiplied by 0.85 because muscle mass is less.

Urea is another index helpful in assessing renal function. It is synthesized mainly in the liver and is the end product of protein catabolism. Urea is freely filtered by the glomerulus, and about 30–70% is reabsorbed in the nephron. Unlike creatinine clearance, which overestimates GFR, urea clearance underestimates GFR. Urea reabsorption may be decreased in well-hydrated patients, whereas dehydration causes increased reabsorption, increasing blood urea nitrogen (BUN). A normal BUN:creatinine ratio is 10:1. With dehydration, the ratio can increase to 20:1 or higher. Other causes of increased BUN include increased catabolism (gastrointestinal bleeding, cell lysis, and steroid usage), increased dietary protein, and decreased renal perfusion (congestive heart failure, renal artery stenosis (Table 22–3). Reduced BUN is seen in liver disease and in the syndrome of inappropriate antidiuretic hormone secretion (SIADH).

Table 22–2. Conditions affecting serum creatinine independently of GFR.

Condition	Mechanism
Conditions causing elevation	
Ketoacidosis	Noncreatinine chromogen
Cephalothin, cefoxitin	Noncreatinine chromogen
Other drugs: aspirin, cimetidine, trimethoprim	Inhibition of tubular creatinine secretion
Conditions causing decrease	
Advanced age	Physiologic decrease in muscle mass
Cachexia	Pathologic decrease in muscle mass
Liver disease	Decreased hepatic creatine synthesis and cachexia

IMAGING STUDIES

Radionuclide Studies

Radionuclide studies can measure renal function. Technetium diethylenetriamine pentaacetic acid (^{99m}Tc-DTPA) is freely filtered by the glomerulus and not reabsorbed and is used to estimate GFR. Technetium dimercaptosuccinate (^{99m}Tc-DMSA) is bound to the tubules and provides an assessment of functional renal mass. Radioiodinated (^{131}I) orthoiodohippurate is secreted into the renal tubules and assesses renal plasma flow (RPF). The indications for nuclear renography are to measure function and flow; to determine the contribution of each kid-

Table 22–3. Conditions affecting BUN independently of GFR.

Increased BUN
Reduced effective circulating blood volume (prerenal azotemia)
Catabolic states
High-protein diets
Gastrointestinal bleeding
Glucocorticoids
Tetracycline
Decreased BUN
Liver disease
Malnutrition
Sickle cell anemia
SIADH

ney to overall renal function; to demonstrate the presence or absence of functioning renal tissue in mass lesions; to detect obstruction; and to evaluate renovascular disease.

Poor flow along with poor function is consistent with acute tubular necrosis or end-stage renal disease. Decreased flow to one kidney suggests arterial occlusion of that kidney. To further investigate renal artery stenosis, the test is done both with and without captopril (see Chapter 11).

Ultrasonography

Ultrasonography can identify the renal cortex, medulla, pyramids, and a distended collection system or ureter. Kidney size can be determined; a kidney less than 9 cm in length indicates significant irreversible renal disease. A difference in size of more than 1.5 cm between the two kidneys is observed in unilateral renal disease. Renal ultrasound is also performed to search for hydronephrosis, characterize renal mass lesions, screen for autosomal dominant polycystic kidney disease, evaluate the perirenal space, localize the kidney for a percutaneous invasive procedure, and assess postvoiding bladder residual.

Intravenous Urography

The intravenous pyelogram (IVP) has been for many years the standard imaging procedure for evaluating the urinary tract since it provides an assessment of the kidneys, ureters, and bladder. The dye is filtered and secreted by the renal tubules in normal kidneys, resulting in a nephrogram formed by opacification of the renal parenchyma. The density of the nephrogram is dependent on the GFR. Filling of the pelvicaliceal system produces the pyelogram. The IVP can demonstrate differential function between the right and left kidneys by the rate of appearance of the nephrogram phase.

An IVP necessitates the injection of contrast and is relatively contraindicated in patients with an increased risk for developing acute renal failure (eg, diabetes mellitus with serum creatinine > 2 mg/dL, severe volume contraction, or prerenal azotemia), chronic renal failure with serum creatinine greater than 5 mg/dL, and multiple myeloma. IVP is performed to obtain a detailed view of the pelvicaliceal system, assess renal size and shape, detect and localize renal stones, and assess renal function. Ultrasonography has replaced it in many clinical situations.

Computed Tomography

Computed tomography (CT) is required for further investigation of abnormalities detected by ultrasound or IVP. Although the routine study requires radiographic contrast administration, no contrast is necessary if the reason for the study is to demonstrate hemorrhage or calcifications in the kidneys. Since contrast is filtered by the glomeruli and concentrated in the tubules, there is enhancement of parenchymal tissue, making abnormalities such as cysts or neoplasms easily identified and allowing good visualization of renal vessels and ureters. CT is especially useful for evaluation of solid or cystic lesions in the kidney or the retroperitoneal space, particularly if the ultrasound results are suboptimal.

Magnetic Resonance Imaging (MRI)

MRI can easily distinguish renal cortex from medulla. Loss of corticomedullary function, which can be seen in a variety of disorders (glomerulonephritis, hydronephrosis, renal vascular occlusion, and renal failure) will be evident on MRI. Renal cysts seen on a CT scan can also be identified by MRI. For some solid lesions, MRI may be superior to CT scanning. MRI is indicated as an addition or alternative to CT for staging renal cell cancer and as a substitute for CT in the evaluation of a renal mass, especially for patients in whom contrast is contraindicated; in addition, the adrenals are well imaged.

Arteriography & Venography

Renal arteriography is useful in the evaluation of atherosclerotic or fibrodysplastic stenotic lesions, aneurysms, vasculitis, and renal mass lesions. Venography is useful to diagnose renal vein thrombosis, though CT and MRI are less invasive for this purpose.

RENAL BIOPSY

Indications for percutaneous needle biopsy include (1) unexplained acute renal failure or chronic renal insufficiency; (2) acute nephritic syndromes; (3) unexplained proteinuria; (4) previously identified and treated lesions to plan future therapy; (5) systemic diseases associated with kidney dysfunction, such as systemic lupus erythematosus, Goodpasture's syndrome, and Wegener's syndrome, to confirm the extent of renal involvement and to guide management; and (6) suspected transplant rejection, to differentiate it from other causes of acute renal failure and to guide treatment. Contraindications include a solitary or ectopic kidney (exception: transplant allografts), horseshoe kidney, uncorrected bleeding disorder, severe uncontrolled hypertension, renal infection, renal neoplasm, hydronephrosis, end-stage renal disease, congenital anomalies, multiple cysts, or an uncooperative patient.

Percutaneous kidney biopsies are generally safe. One percent of patients will experience significant bleeding and 0.1% will require blood transfusions. Risk of nephrectomy and mortality are each about 0.06%. When a percutaneous needle biopsy is technically not feasible and renal tissue is deemed clinically essential, open renal biopsy under general anesthesia can be done.

Ahmed Z et al: Asymptomatic urinary abnormalities. Hematuria and proteinuria. Med Clin North Am 1997; 81:641. [NLM Cit ID: 97310482] (A guide for the evaluation of hematuria and proteinuria.)

Andreucci VE et al: Role of renal biopsy in the diagnosis and prognosis of acute renal failure. Kidney Int 1998;66(Suppl):S91. [NLM Cit ID: 98234665]

Mucelli RP et al: Imaging techniques in acute renal failure. Kidney Int 1998;66(Suppl):S102. [NLM Cit ID: 98234667]

Ruggenenti P et al: Cross sectional longitudinal study of spot morning urine protein:creatinine ratio, 24 hour urine protein excretion rate, glomerular filtration rate, and end stage renal failure in chronic renal disease in patients without diabetes. BMJ 1998;316:504. [NLM Cit ID: 98162332] (Cross-sectional study of 177 nondiabetic outpatients with chronic renal disease. When compared with 24-hour urinary protein collection, the protein:creatinine ratio in a spot urine sample is a precise indicator of proteinuria.)

ACUTE RENAL FAILURE

Essentials of Diagnosis

- Sudden increase in BUN or serum creatinine.
- Oliguria often associated.
- Symptoms and signs depend on cause.

General Considerations

Five percent of hospital admissions and 30% of ICU admissions have acute renal failure, and 2–5% of hospitalized patients will develop it. Acute renal failure is defined as a sudden decrease in renal function, resulting in an inability to maintain fluid and electrolyte balance and to excrete nitrogenous wastes. Serum creatinine is a convenient marker. In the absence of functioning kidneys, serum creatinine concentration will increase daily by as much as 1–1.5 mg/dL.

Clinical Findings

A. Symptoms and Signs: When symptoms are present, they are often due to azotemia and the underlying cause of acute renal failure. Azotemia can cause nausea, vomiting, malaise, and altered sensorium. Hypertension is rare, but fluid homeostasis is often altered. Hypovolemia can cause prerenal failure, whereas hypervolemia can result from intrinsic renal failure or postrenal failure. Pericardial effusions can occur with azotemia, and a pericardial friction rub can be present. Effusions may result in cardiac tamponade. Arrhythmias occur especially with hyperkalemia. The pulmonary examination may show rales in the presence of hypervolemia. Acute renal failure can cause nonspecific diffuse abdominal pain and ileus as well as platelet dysfunction; thus, bleeding is more common in these patients. The neurologic examination reveals encephalopathic changes with asterixis and confusion; seizures may ensue.

B. Laboratory Findings: Elevated BUN and creatinine are present, though these elevations do not in themselves distinguish acute from chronic renal failure (Table 22–4). Hyperkalemia often occurs from impaired potassium excretion and the ECG can reveal peaked T waves and a long QT segment from hypocalcemia. Anion gap metabolic acidosis (due to decreased organic acid clearance) frequently is noted. Hyperphosphatemia occurs when phosphorus cannot be secreted by damaged tubules either with or without increased cell catabolism. Hypocalcemia with metastatic calcium phosphate deposition may be observed when the product of calcium and phosphorus exceeds 70 mg/dL. Anemia is common as a result of decreased erythropoietin production, and associated platelet dysfunction is typical.

Classification & Etiology

Acute renal failure can be divided into three categories: prerenal azotemia, intrinsic renal failure, and postrenal azotemia. Identifying the cause is the first step toward managing the patient. (See Table 22–4.)

A. Prerenal Azotemia: Prerenal azotemia is the most common cause of acute renal failure. It is due to renal hypoperfusion. If this can be immediately reversed with restoration of renal blood flow, renal parenchymal damage does not occur. If hypoperfusion persists, ischemia can result, causing intrinsic renal failure.

Decreased renal perfusion can occur in one of three ways: a decrease in intravascular volume, a change in vascular resistance, or low cardiac output. Causes of volume depletion include hemorrhage, gas-

Table 22–4. Classification and differential diagnosis of renal failure.

	Prerenal Azotemia	Postrenal Azotemia	Intrinsic Renal Disease: Acute Tubular Necrosis (Oliguric or Polyuric)	Intrinsic Renal Disease: Acute Glomerulonephritis	Intrinsic Renal Disease: Acute Interstitial Nephritis
Etiology	Poor renal perfusion	Obstruction of the urinary tract	Ischemia, nephrotoxins	Poststreptococcal; collagen-vascular disease	Allergic reaction; drug reaction
Urinary indices Serum BUN:Cr ratio	> 20:1	> 20:1	< 20:1	> 20:1	< 20:1
U_{Na} (meq/L)	< 20	Variable	> 20	< 20	Variable
FE_{Na} (%)	< 1	Variable	> 1	< 1	< 1; > 1
Urine osmolality (mosm/kg)	> 500	< 400	250–300	Variable	Variable
Urinary sediment	Benign, or hyaline casts	Normal or red cells, white cells, or crystals	Granular casts, renal tubular casts	Dysmorphic red cells and red cell casts	White cells, white cell casts, with or without eosinophils

trointestinal losses, dehydration, excessive diuresis, extravascular space sequestration, pancreatitis, burns, trauma, and peritonitis.

Changes in vascular resistance can occur systemically with sepsis, anaphylaxis, anesthesia, and afterload-reducing drugs. ACE inhibitors prevent efferent renal arteriolar constriction out of proportion to the afferent arteriole; thus, GFR will decrease. NSAIDs prevent afferent arteriolar vasodilation by inhibiting prostaglandin-mediated signals. Thus, in cirrhosis and congestive heart failure, when prostaglandins are recruited to increase renal blood flow, NSAIDs will have particularly deleterious effects. Epinephrine, norepinephrine, anesthetic agents, and cyclosporine also can cause renal vasoconstriction. Renal artery stenosis causes increased resistance and decreased perfusion.

Low cardiac output is a state of effective hypovolemia. This occurs in states of cardiogenic shock, congestive heart failure, pulmonary embolus, and pericardial tamponade. Arrhythmias and valvular disorders can also reduce cardiac output. In the ICU setting, positive-pressure ventilation will decrease venous return, also decreasing cardiac output.

When GFR falls acutely, it is important to determine whether acute renal failure is due to prerenal or intrinsic renal causes. The history and physical examination are important, and urinalysis can be helpful. The BUN:creatinine ratio will typically exceed 20:1 owing to increased urea reabsorption. Another useful index is the fractional excretion of sodium. With decreased GFR, the kidney will reabsorb salt and water avidly if there is no intrinsic tubular dysfunction. Thus, patients with prerenal failure should have a low fractional excretion percent of sodium (< 1%). The FE_{Na} is calculated as follows: Fractional excretion of Na^+ (FE_{Na}) = clearance of Na^+/GFR = Clearance of Na^+/creatinine clearance (C_{Cr}):

$$FE_{Na^+} = \frac{Urine_{sodium} / Plasma_{sodium}}{Urine_{creatinine} / Plasma_{creatinine}} \times 100\%$$

The causes of oliguric states are more accurately assessed with this formula than the causes of nonoliguric states because the kidneys do not avidly reabsorb water and sodium in nonoliguric states. (Oliguria is defined as urine output < 500 mL/d.) Diuretics can cause increased sodium excretion. Thus, if the FE_{Na} is high within 12–24 hours after diuretic administration, the cause of acute renal failure may not be accurately predicted. Acute renal failure due to glomerulonephritis can have a low FE_{Na} because sodium reabsorption and tubular function are not compromised.

Treatment of prerenal azotemia depends entirely on its cause, but maintenance of euvolemia, attention to serum potassium, and avoidance of nephrotoxic drugs are the benchmarks of therapy. This involves careful assessment of volume status, drug usage, and cardiac function.

B. Postrenal Azotemia: Postrenal azotemia is the least common cause of acute renal failure, accounting for approximately 5% of cases, but is perhaps the most important cause because of its reversibility. It occurs when urinary flow from both kidneys is obstructed. Each nephron has an elevated intraluminal pressure, causing a decrease in GFR.

Causes include urethral obstruction, bladder dysfunction or obstruction, and obstruction of both ureters or renal pelves. In men, benign prostatic hyperplasia is the most common cause. Patients taking anticholinergic drugs are particularly at risk. Bladder, prostate, and cervical cancers as well as retroperitoneal processes and neurogenic bladder can also cause obstruction. Less common causes are bilateral ureteral stones, urethral stones or stricture, and bilateral papillary necrosis. In patients with a single functioning kidney, obstruction of a solitary ureter can cause postrenal azotemia.

Patients may be anuric or polyuric and may complain of lower abdominal pain. Obstruction can be constant or intermittent. On examination, the patient may have an enlarged prostate, distended bladder, or a mass detected on pelvic examination.

Laboratory examination may initially reveal high urine osmolality, low urine sodium, high BUN:creatinine ratio, and low FE_{Na}. These indices are similar to a prerenal picture because extensive intrinsic renal damage has not occurred. After several days, the urine sodium increases as the kidneys fail and are unable to concentrate the urine—thus, isosthenuria is present. The urine sediment is generally benign.

Patients with acute renal failure and suspected postrenal azotemia should undergo bladder ultrasonography and bladder catheterization if hydroureter and hydronephrosis are present along with an enlarged bladder. These patients often undergo a postobstructive diuresis, and care should be taken to avoid dehydration. Rarely, the presence of obstruction is not seen via ultrasonography. For example, patients with retroperitoneal fibrosis from tumor or radiation may not show dilation of the urinary tract. If suspicion does exist, a CT scan or MRI can establish the diagnosis. Promptly treated obstruction with catheters or stents can result in complete reversal of the acute process.

C. Intrinsic Renal Failure: Intrinsic renal disorders account for half of all cases of acute renal failure. Intrinsic (or parenchymal) dysfunction is considered after prerenal and postrenal causes have been excluded. The sites of injury are the tubules, the interstitium, the vasculature, and the glomeruli.

ACUTE TUBULAR NECROSIS

Essentials of Diagnosis

- Acute renal insufficiency.
- $FE_{Na} > 1\%$.
- Urine sediment with pigmented granular casts and renal tubular epithelial cells.

General Considerations

Acute renal failure due to tubular damage is termed acute tubular necrosis and accounts for 85% of intrinsic acute renal failure. The two major causes of acute tubular necrosis are ischemia and toxin exposure. Ischemia causes tubular damage from states of low perfusion and is often preceded by a state of prerenal azotemia. Ischemic acute renal failure is characterized not only by inadequate GFR but also by renal blood flow inadequate to maintain parenchymal cellular formation. This occurs in the setting of prolonged hypotension or hypoxemia such as dehydration, shock, and sepsis. Major surgical procedures can involve prolonged periods of hypoperfusion which are exacerbated by vasodilating anesthetic agents.

The other major cause of acute tubular necrosis is nephrotoxin exposure. Exogenous nephrotoxins more commonly cause damage than endogenous toxins.

A. Exogenous Nephrotoxins: Up to 25% of hospitalized patients receiving therapeutic levels of aminoglycosides sustain some degree of acute tubular necrosis. Nonoliguric renal failure typically occurs after 5–10 days of exposure. Predisposing factors include underlying renal damage, dehydration, and advanced age. Monitoring of peak and trough levels is important, but trough levels are more helpful in predicting renal toxicity. Gentamicin is the most and tobramycin the least nephrotoxic. Amphotericin B is typically nephrotoxic after a dose of 2–3 g. This causes severe vasoconstriction with distal tubular damage and can lead to distal renal tubular acidosis with hypokalemia and nephrogenic diabetes insipidus. Vancomycin, acyclovir, and several cephalosporins have been known to cause acute tubular necrosis.

Radiographic contrast media can be directly nephrotoxic. Predisposing factors include advanced age, preexisting renal disease (serum creatinine > 5 mg/dL), volume depletion, diabetes mellitus with renal insufficiency (serum creatinine > 2 mg/dL), repeated doses of contrast, and recent exposure to other nephrotoxic agents. The combination of diabetes mellitus and renal dysfunction poses the greatest risk for contrast nephropathy. Toxicity usually occurs 24–48 hours after the radiocontrast study. Nonionic contrast media may be less toxic, but this has never been proved. Prevention should be the goal when using these agents. Patients should be hydrated with 1 L of 0.45% saline over 12 hours both before and after the contrast administration—cautiously to patients with preexisting cardiac dysfunction. Neither mannitol nor furosemide offers benefit over saline hydration. Other nephrotoxic agents should be avoided during the day before and after administration.

Cyclosporine toxicity is usually dose-dependent. It causes distal tubular dysfunction from severe vasoconstriction. Regular blood level monitoring is important to prevent nephrotoxicity. With patients who are taking cyclosporine for renal transplant rejection, kidney biopsy is often necessary to distinguish transplant rejection from cyclosporine toxicity. Renal function usually improves after reducing the dose or stopping the drug.

Other exogenous nephrotoxins include antineoplastics such as cisplatin and heavy metals such as mercury, cadmium, and arsenic.

B. Endogenous Nephrotoxins: Endogenous nephrotoxins include heme-containing products, uric acid, and paraproteins. Myoglobinuria as a consequence of rhabdomyolysis leads to acute tubular necrosis. Necrotic muscle releases large amounts of myoglobin, which is freely filtered across the glomerulus. The myoglobin is reabsorbed by the renal tubules, and direct damage can occur. Distal tubular obstruction from pigmented casts can also cause damage. This type of renal failure occurs in the setting of crush injury, muscle necrosis from prolonged unconsciousness, seizures, cocaine, and alcohol abuse. Dehydration and acidosis predisposes to the development of myoglobinuric acute renal failure. Patients may complain of muscular pain and often have signs of muscle injury. Rhabdomyolysis of clinical importance commonly occurs with a serum creatine kinase of > 50,000–100,000 IU/L. The globin moiety will cause the urine dipstick to read falsely positive for hemoglobin: the urine appears dark brown, but no red cells are present. With lysis of muscle cells, patients also become hyperkalemic, hyperphosphatemic, and hyperuricemic. The mainstay of treatment is hydration. Other adjunctive treatments include mannitol for free radical clearance and diuresis as well as alkalinization of the urine. These modalities have not been proved to change outcomes in human trials.

Hemoglobin can cause a similar form of acute renal tubular necrosis. Massive intravascular hemolysis is seen in transfusion reactions and in certain hemolytic anemias. Reversal of the underlying disorder and hydration are the mainstays of treatment.

Hyperuricemia can occur in the setting of rapid cell turnover and lysis. Chemotherapy for germ cell neoplasms and leukemia and lymphoma are the primary causes. Acute renal failure occurs with intratubular deposition of uric acid crystals; serum uric acid levels are often > 20 mg/dL and urine uric acid levels > 600 mg/24 h. A urine uric acid to urine creatinine ratio > 1.0 indicates risk for acute renal failure.

Bence Jones protein seen in conjunction with multiple myeloma can cause direct tubular toxicity and tubular obstruction. Other renal complications from multiple myeloma include hypercalcemia and proximal renal tubular acidosis.

Clinical Findings

A. Symptoms and Signs: See Acute Renal Failure, above.

B. Laboratory Findings: Urinalysis may show evidence of acute tubular damage. The urine may be brown. On microscopic examination, an active sediment may show pigmented granular casts or "muddy brown" casts. Renal tubular epithelial cells and epithelial cell casts are often present as well. Hyperkalemia and hyperphosphatemia are commonly encountered.

Treatment

Treatment is aimed at hastening recovery and avoiding complications. Preventive measures should be taken to avoid volume overload and hyperkalemia. Loop-blocking diuretics may be used in large doses (eg, furosemide in doses ranging from 20 mg to 160 mg orally or intravenously twice daily) to effect adequate diuresis, and may help convert oliguric to nonoliguric renal failure. Side effects of supranormal dosing include deafness. This is mainly due to peak furosemide levels and can be avoided by the use of a furosemide drip. A starting dose of 0.4–0.6 mg/kg/h is appropriate, increasing to a maximum of 1 mg/kg/h. A bolus of the hourly dose should be administered at the beginning of treatment. Intravenous thiazide diuretics can be used to augment urine output; chlorothiazide, 500 mg intravenously every 8–12 hours, is a reasonable choice. Nutritional support should maintain adequate intake while preventing excessive catabolism. Dietary protein restriction of 0.6 g/kg/d helps to prevent metabolic acidosis. Hypocalcemia and hyperphosphatemia can be improved with diet and phosphate-binding agents such as aluminum hydroxide (500 mg orally three times daily) over the short term and calcium carbonate (500–1500 mg orally three times daily). Hypermagnesemia can occur because of reduced magnesium excretion by the renal tubules, so magnesium-containing antacids and laxatives should be avoided in these patients. Dosages must be adjusted according to the estimated degree of renal impairment for drugs eliminated by the kidney.

Indications for dialysis in acute renal failure from acute tubular necrosis or other intrinsic disorders are as follows: life-threatening electrolyte disturbances (such as hyperkalemia), volume overload unresponsive to diuresis, worsening acidosis, and uremic complications (eg, encephalopathy, pericarditis, and seizures).

Course & Prognosis

The clinical course of acute tubular necrosis is often divided into three phases: initial injury, maintenance, and recovery. The maintenance phase is expressed as either oliguric (urine output < 400 mL/d) or nonoliguric. Nonoliguric acute tubular necrosis has a better outcome—conversion from oliguric to nonoliguric states is desired. Drugs such as dopamine and diuretics are sometimes used for this purpose but have not been shown to improve overall outcomes. Average duration of this period is 1–3 weeks but may be several months. Cellular repair and removal of tubular debris occur during the maintenance phase. The recovery phase is heralded by diuresis. GFR begins to rise; BUN and serum creatinine fall.

The mortality rate from acute renal failure is 20–50% in medical illness and up to 70% in a surgical setting. Increased mortality is associated with advanced age, severe underlying disease, and multisystem organ failure. Leading causes of death are infections, fluid and electrolyte disturbances, and worsening of underlying disease. Mortality rates have not changed significantly over 20 years, making prevention of acute renal failure a high priority.

INTERSTITIAL NEPHRITIS

Essentials of Diagnosis

- Fever.
- Transient maculopapular rash.
- Acute renal insufficiency.
- Pyuria (including eosinophiluria), white blood cell casts, and hematuria.

General Considerations

Acute interstitial nephritis accounts for 10–15% of cases of intrinsic renal failure. An interstitial inflammatory response with edema and possible tubular cell damage is the typical pathologic finding. Cell-mediated immune reactions prevail over humoral responses. T lymphocytes can cause direct cytotoxicity or release lymphokines that recruit monocytes and inflammatory cells.

Although drugs account for over 70% of cases, acute interstitial nephritis also occurs in infectious diseases or immunologic disorders or may be idiopathic. The most common drugs are penicillins and cephalosporins, sulfonamides and sulfonamide-containing diuretics, NSAIDs, rifampin, phenytoin, and allopurinol. Infectious causes include streptococcal infections, leptospirosis, CMV, histoplasmosis, and Rocky Mountain spotted fever. Immunologic entities are more commonly associated with glomerulonephritis, but systemic lupus erythematosus, Sjögren's syndrome, sarcoidosis, and cryoglobulinemia have been seen with interstitial nephritis.

Clinical Findings

Clinical features can include fever (> 80%), rash (25–50%), arthralgias, and peripheral blood eosinophilia (80%). The urine often contains red cells (95%), white cells, and white cell casts. Proteinuria can be a feature, particularly in NSAID-induced interstitial nephritis but is usually modest. Eosinophiluria can be detected by Wright's stain.

Treatment & Prognosis

Acute interstitial nephritis often carries a good prognosis. Recovery occurs over weeks to months, but acute dialytic therapy may be necessary in up to one-third of all patients before resolution. (See indications for dialysis, above.) Patients rarely progress to end-stage renal disease. Those with prolonged courses of oliguric failure and advanced age have a worse prognosis. Treatment consists of supportive measures and removal of the inciting agent. Short-term, high dose methylprednisolone (0.5–1 g/d for 1–4 days) or prednisone (60 mg/d for 1–2 weeks) followed by a prednisone taper can be used in the more severe cases of drug-induced interstitial nephritis.

GLOMERULONEPHRITIS

Essentials of Diagnosis

- Hematuria, dysmorphic red cells, red cell casts, and mild proteinuria.
- Dependent edema and hypertension.
- Acute renal insufficiency.

General Considerations

Acute glomerulonephritis is a relatively uncommon cause of acute renal failure, accounting for about 5% of cases of intrinsic renal failure. Pathologically, inflammatory glomerular lesions are seen. These include mesangioproliferative, focal and diffuse proliferative, and crescentic lesions. The larger the percentage of glomeruli involved and the more severe the lesion, the more likely it is that the patient will have a poor clinical outcome.

Categorization of acute glomerulonephritis can be done by serologic analysis. Markers include antineutrophil cytoplasmic autoantibodies (ANCA), antiglomerular basement membrane (GBM) autoantibodies, and other immune markers of disease.

Immune complex deposition usually occurs when moderate antigen excess over antibody production occurs. Complexes formed with marked antigen excess tend to remain in the circulation. Antibody excess with large antigen-antibody aggregates usually results in phagocytosis and clearance of the precipitates by the mononuclear phagocytic system in the liver and spleen. Causes include IgA nephropathy (Berger's disease), peri- or postinfectious glomerulonephritis, lupus nephritis, cryoglobulinemic glomerulonephritis (often associated with hepatitis C virus), and membranoproliferative glomerulonephritis

Anti-GBM-associated acute glomerulonephritis is either confined to the kidney or associated with pulmonary hemorrhage. The latter is termed Goodpasture's syndrome. Injury is related to autoantibodies aimed against type IV collagen in the glomerular basement membrane rather than to immune complex deposition.

ANCA-associated acute glomerulonephritis is a form of small-vessel vasculitis, causing primary and secondary renal diseases that do not have direct immune complex deposition or antibody binding. Tissue injury is believed to be due to cell-mediated immune processes. An example is Wegener's granulomatosis, a systemic necrotizing vasculitis of small arteries and veins associated with intravascular and extravascular granuloma formation. In addition to glomerulonephritis, these patients can have upper airway, pulmonary, and skin manifestations of disease.

Cytoplasmic ANCA (cANCA) is both specific (88%) and sensitive (95%) for this entity. Microscopic polyangiitis is another pauci-immune vasculitis causing acute glomerulonephritis. Perinuclear staining (pANCA) is the common pattern. ANCA-associated and anti-GBM-associated acute glomerulonephritis can evolve to crescentic glomerulonephritis and often have poor outcomes unless treatment is started early. Both are described more fully below.

Other vascular causes of acute glomerulonephritis include malignant hypertension and the thrombotic microangiopathies such as hemolytic-uremic syndrome (Chapter 11) and thrombotic thrombocytopenic purpura (Chapter 13).

Clinical Findings

A. Symptoms and Signs: Patients with acute glomerulonephritis are often hypertensive, edematous, and have an abnormal urinary sediment. The edema is found first in body parts with low tissue tension such as the periorbital and scrotal regions.

B. Laboratory Findings: Dipstick and microscopic evaluation will reveal evidence of hematuria, moderate proteinuria (usually < 2 g/d), and cellular elements such as red cells, red cell casts, and white cells. Red cell cases are specific for glomerulonephritis, and a detailed search is warranted. Twenty-four hour urine for protein excretion and creatinine clearance quantifies the amount of proteinuria and documents the degree of renal dysfunction. FE_{Na} is usually low unless renal dysfunction is marked.

Further tests include complement levels (C3, C4, CH50), ASO titer, anti-GBM antibody levels, ANCAs, ANA titers, cryoglobulin and hepatitis panels, C3 nephritic factor, renal ultrasound, and renal biopsy.

Treatment

Depending on the nature and severity of disease, treatment can consist of high-dose steroids and cytotoxic agents such as cyclophosphamide. Plasma exchange can be used in Goodpasture's disease. Treatment and prognosis for specific diseases are more fully discussed below.

Albers FJ: Clinical characteristics of atherosclerotic renovascular disease. Am J Kidney Dis 1994;24:636. [NLM Cit ID: 95029343]

Bellomo R et al: Indications and criteria for initiating renal replacement therapy in the intensive care unit. Kidney Int 1998;66(Suppl):S106. [NLM Cit ID: 98234668] (Addresses the question why a more aggressive approach to dialysis may be warranted in patients in the ICU compared with those with near end-stage renal failure.)

Chertow GM et al: Is the administration of dopamine associated with adverse or favorable outcomes in acute renal failure? Auriculin Anaritide Acute Renal Failure Study Group. Am J Med 1996;101:49. [NLM Cit ID: 96302159] (Randomized study concludes that the routine use of low-dose dopamine should be discouraged until a prospective, randomized, placebo-controlled trial establishes its safety and efficacy.)

Choudhury D et al: Drug-induced nephrotoxicity. Med Clin North Am 1997;81:705. [NLM Cit ID: 973104861] (The spectrum of presentations.)

Forni LG et al: Continuous hemofiltration in the treatment of acute renal failure. N Engl J Med 1997;336:1303. [NLM Cit ID: 97258691] (A review of the basic principles and practical aspects of hemodialysis and hemofiltration for the generalist.)

Michel DM et al: Acute interstitial nephritis. J Am Soc Nephrol 1998;9:506. [NLM Cit ID: 98175102]

Nissenson AR: Acute renal failure: Definition and pathogenesis. Kidney Int 1998;66(Suppl):S7. [NLM Cit ID: 98234649] (Review of four main pathophysiologic mechanisms of acute renal failure.)

Parker RA et al: Prognosis of patients with acute renal failure requiring dialysis: Results of a multicenter study. Am J Kidney Dis 1998;32:432. [NLM Cit ID: 98410876] (A multicenter controlled trial found that APACHE scores and the presence of oliguria in patients with acute renal failure were predictive of outcome after hemodialysis.)

Perazella MA: Crystal-induced acute renal failure. Am J Med 1999;106:459. [NLM Cit ID: 99239756]

Rudnick MR et al: Contrast media-associated nephrotoxicity. Semin Nephrol 1997;17:15. [NLM Cit ID: 97153256] (A clinical update on the topic.)

Thadhani R et al: Acute renal failure. N Engl J Med 1996;334:1448. [NLM Cit ID: 96218830] (Diagnosis and management.)

CHRONIC RENAL DISEASE

Essentials of Diagnosis

- Progressive azotemia over months to years.
- Prolonged symptoms and signs of uremia.
- Hypertension in the majority.
- Isosthenuria and broad casts in urinary sediment are common.
- Bilateral small kidneys on ultrasound are diagnostic.
- Radiologic evidence of renal osteodystrophy confirms the diagnosis.

General Considerations

Over 50% of cases of chronic renal failure are due to diabetes mellitus and hypertension. Glomerulonephritis, cystic diseases, and other urologic diseases account for another 20–25%, and nearly one-sixth of patients have unknown causes. The major causes of chronic renal failure are listed in Table 22–5.

Chronic renal disease is rarely reversible and leads to progressive decline in renal function. This occurs even after an inciting event has been removed. Re-

Table 22–5. Major causes of chronic renal failure.

Glomerulopathies
- Primary glomerular diseases:
  1. Focal and segmental glomerulosclerosis
  2. Membranoproliferative glomerulonephritis
  3. IgA nephropathy
  4. Membranous nephropathy
- Secondary glomerular diseases:
  1. Diabetic nephropathy
  2. Amyloidosis
  3. Post infectious glomerulonephritis
  4. HIV-associated nephropathy
  5. Collagen vascular diseases
  6. Sickle cell nephropathy
  7. HIV-associated membranoproliferative glomerulonephritis

Tubulointerstitial nephritis
- Drug hypersensitivity
- Heavy metals
- Analgesic nephropathy
- Reflux/chronic pyelonephritis
- Idiopathic

Hereditary diseases
- Polycystic kidney disease
- Medullary cystic disease
- Alport's syndrome

Obstructive nephropathies
- Prostatic disease
- Nephrolithiasis
- Retroperitoneal fibrosis/tumor
- Congenital

Vascular diseases
- Hypertensive nephrosclerosis
- Renal artery stenosis

Table 22–6. Symptoms and signs of uremia.

Organ System	Symptoms	Signs
General	Fatigue, weakness	Sallow-appearing, chronically ill
Skin	Pruritus, easy bruisability	Pallor, ecchymoses, excoriations, edema, xerosis
ENT	Metallic taste in mouth, epistaxis	Urinous breath
Eye		Pale conjunctiva
Pulmonary	Shortness of breath	Rales, pleural effusion
Cardiovascular	Dyspnea on exertion, retrosternal pain on inspiration (pericarditis)	Hypertension, cardiomegaly, friction rub
Gastrointestinal	Anorexia, nausea, vomiting, hiccup	
Genitourinary	Nocturia, impotence	Isosthenuria
Neuromuscular	Restless legs, numbness and cramps in legs	
Neurologic	Generalized irritability and inability to concentrate, decreased libido	Stupor, asterixis, myoclonus, peripheral neuropathy

duction in renal mass leads to hypertrophy of the remaining nephrons with hyperfiltration, and the glomerular filtration rate in these nephrons transiently returns to normal levels. These adaptations place a burden on the remaining nephrons and lead to progressive glomerular sclerosis and interstitial fibrosis, suggesting that hyperfiltration may worsen renal function. Decreased renal function in patients who have donated kidneys, however, has not been shown to lead to chronic renal failure.

Clinical Findings

A. Symptoms and Signs: The symptoms of chronic renal failure often develop slowly and are nonspecific (Table 22–6). Individuals can remain asymptomatic until renal failure is far-advanced (GFR < 10–15 mL/min). Manifestations include fatigue, weakness, and malaise. Gastrointestinal complaints such as anorexia, nausea, vomiting, a metallic taste in the mouth, and hiccups are common. Neurologic problems include irritability, difficulty in concentrating, insomnia, restless legs, and twitching. Pruritus is common and difficult to treat. As uremia progresses, decreased libido, menstrual irregularities, chest pain from pericarditis, and paresthesias can develop. Symptoms of drug toxicity—especially for drugs eliminated by the kidney—increase as renal clearance worsens. (See Table 22–7 for antimicrobial dosages.)

On physical examination, the patient appears chronically ill. Hypertension is common. The skin may be yellow, with signs of easy bruisability. Rarely seen in the dialysis era is uremic frost, a cutaneous reflection of end-stage renal disease. Uremic fetor is the characteristic fishy odor of the breath. Cardiopulmonary signs may include rales, cardiomegaly, edema, and a pericardial friction rub. Mental status can vary from decreased concentration to confusion, stupor, and coma. Myoclonus and asterixis are additional signs of uremic encephalopathy.

The term "uremia" is used for this clinical syndrome, but the exact cause remains unknown. BUN and serum creatinine are believed to be markers for unknown toxins, with urea believed to play a partial role in the syndrome.

In any patient with renal failure, it is important to identify and correct all possibly reversible causes. Urinary tract infections, obstruction, extracellular volume depletion, nephrotoxins, hypertension, and congestive heart failure should be excluded (Table 22–8). Any one can worsen underlying chronic renal failure.

B. Laboratory Findings: The diagnosis of renal failure is made by documenting elevations of the BUN and serum creatinine concentrations. Further evaluation is needed to differentiate between acute and chronic renal failure. Evidence of previously elevated BUN and creatinine, abnormal prior urinalyses, and

Table 22–7. Antimicrobial dosages in renal failure.[1]

	No Change	Moderate Reduction	Marked Reduction	Avoid
Aminoglycoside				
Amikacin			✓	
Gentamicin			✓	
Netilmicin			✓	
Tobramycin			✓	
Amphotericin B			✓	
Cephalosporins				
First-generation:				
Cefadroxil			✓	
Cephradine			✓	
Cephalexin	✓			
Cephalothin		✓		
Cephapirin		✓		
Cefazolin			✓	
Second-generation:				
Cefaclor	✓			
Cefonicid			✓	
Cefotetan			✓	
Cefoxitin			✓	
Cefuroxime			✓	
Third-generation:				
Cefoperazone	✓			
Cefotaxime			✓	
Ceftazidime			✓	
Ceftizoxime			✓	
Ceftriaxone	✓			
Chloramphenicol	✓			
Clindamycin	✓			
Erythromycin	✓			
Monobactams (aztreonam)			✓	
Nitrofurantoin				✓
Penicillins				
Amoxicillin		✓		
Ampicillin		✓		
Azlocillin			✓	
Carbenicillin	✓			
Dicloxacillin		✓		
Methicillin		✓		
Mezlocillin	✓			
Nafcillin	✓			
Penicillin G		✓		
Piperacillin			✓	
Ticarcillin			✓	
Quinolones				
Ciprofloxacin		✓		
Norfloxacin		✓		
Trimethoprim-sulfamethoxazole			✓	
Tetracyclines				
Doxycycline	✓			
Tetracycline				✓
Vancomycin			✓	

[1]GFR = < 10 mL/min

Table 22–8. Reversible causes of renal failure.

Reversible Factors	Diagnostic Clues
Infection	Urine culture and sensitivity tests
Obstruction	Bladder catheterization, then renal ultrasound
Extracellular fluid volume depletion	Orthostatic blood pressure and pulse: ↓BP and ↑pulse upon sitting up from a supine position
Hypokalemia, hypercalcemia, and hyperuricemia (usually > 15 mg/dL)	Serum electrolytes, calcium, phosphate, uric acid
Nephrotoxic agents	Drug history
Pericarditis	Echocardiography, chest x-ray
Hypertension	Blood pressure, chest x-ray
Congestive heart failure	Physical examination, chest x-ray

stable but abnormal serum creatinine on successive days is most consistent with a chronic process. It is helpful to plot the inverse of serum creatinine ($1/S_{cr}$) versus time if three or more prior measurements are available; this estimates time to end-stage renal disease (Figure 22–1). If the slope of the line acutely declines, new causes of renal failure should be excluded as outlined above. Anemia, metabolic acidosis, hyperphosphatemia, hypocalcemia, and hyperkalemia can occur with both acute and chronic renal failure. The urinalysis shows isosthenuria if tubular concentrating and diluting ability are impaired. The urinary sediment can show broad waxy casts as a result of dilated, hypertrophic nephrons.

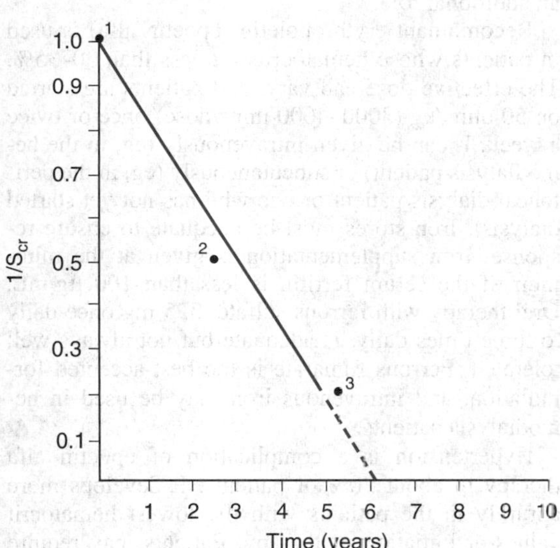

Figure 22–1. Decline in renal function plotted against time to end-stage renal disease. The solid line indicates the linear decline in renal function over time. The dotted line indicates the approximate time to end-stage renal disease.

C. Imaging: The findings of small echogenic kidneys bilaterally (< 10 cm) by ultrasonography supports a diagnosis of chronic renal failure, though normal or even large kidneys can be seen with chronic renal failure caused by adult polycystic kidney disease, diabetic nephropathy, HIV-associated nephropathy, multiple myeloma, amyloidosis, and obstructive uropathy. Radiologic evidence of renal osteodystrophy is another helpful finding, since x-ray changes of secondary hyperparathyroidism do not appear unless parathyroid levels have been elevated for at least 1 year. Evidence of subperiosteal reabsorption along the radial sides of the digital bones of the hand confirms hyperparathyroidism.

Complications

A. Hyperkalemia: Potassium balance generally remains intact in chronic renal failure until the GFR is less than 10 mL/min. However, certain states pose an increased risk of hyperkalemia at higher GFRs. Endogenous causes include any type of cellular destruction such as hemolysis and trauma, the hyporeninemic hypoaldosteronism (type IV renal tubular acidosis, seen particularly in diabetes mellitus), and acidemic states (0.6 meq/L elevation in K^+ for each 0.1 unit decrease in pH). Exogenous causes include diet (eg, salt substitutes containing potassium) and drugs that block K^+ secretion (amiloride, triamterene, spironolactone, NSAIDs, ACE inhibitors) or block cellular uptake (beta-blockers).

Treatment of acute hyperkalemia involves cardiac monitoring, calcium chloride, insulin administration with glucose, bicarbonate, and an orally or rectally administered ion exchange resin (sodium polystyrene sulfate). The resin exchanges sodium for potassium and can administer a significant sodium load to a patient (see Chapter 21). Chronic hyperkalemia is best treated with dietary potassium restriction and sodium polystyrene sulfonate when necessary. The usual dose is 15–30 g once a day in juice or sorbitol.

B. Acid-Base Disorders: Damaged kidneys are unable to excrete the 1 meq/kg/d of acid generated by metabolism of dietary proteins. The resultant metabolic acidosis is primarily due to loss of renal mass. This limits production of ammonia (NH_3) and limits buffering of H^+ in the urine. (Other causes include decreased filtration of titratable acids such as sulfates and phosphates and decreased renal tubular hydrogen ion secretion.) Although patients with chronic renal failure are in positive hydrogen ion balance, the arterial blood pH is maintained at 7.33–7.37 and serum bicarbonate concentration rarely falls below 15 meq/L.

The excess hydrogen ions are buffered by the large calcium carbonate and calcium phosphate stores in bone. This contributes to the renal osteodystrophy of chronic renal failure described below.

The serum bicarbonate level should be maintained at > 20 meq/L. Base supplements include sodium bicarbonate, calcium bicarbonate, and sodium citrate. Administration should begin with 20–30 mmol/d of alkali divided into two doses per day and titrated as needed.

C. Cardiovascular Complications:

1. Hypertension–As renal failure progresses, hypertension due to salt and water retention usually develops. Hyperreninemic states and exogenous erythropoietin administration can also exacerbate hypertension. Hypertension is the most common complication of end-stage renal disease and must be meticulously controlled. Failure to do so can accelerate the progression of renal damage.

Control of hypertension can be achieved with salt and water restriction, weight loss if indicated, and pharmacologic therapy. The ability of the kidney to adjust to variations in sodium and water intake becomes limited as renal failure progresses. An elevated sodium chloride intake leads to congestive heart failure, edema, and hypertension, whereas low salt intake leads to volume contraction and hypotension. A mildly decreased salt diet (4–6 g/d) can be started, and salt intake should be reduced to 2 g/d if hypertension persists. Initial drug therapy can include ACE inhibitors or angiotensin II receptor blockers (if serum potassium and GFR permit), calcium channel-blocking agents, diuretics, and beta-blocking agents. The adjunctive drugs that are often needed (clonidine, hydralazine, minoxidil, etc) reflect the difficulty of achieving and maintaining hypertensive control in these patients.

2. Pericarditis–With uremia, pericarditis may develop. The cause is believed to be retention of metabolic toxins. Symptoms include chest pain and fever. Pulsus paradoxus can be present. A friction rub may be auscultated, but the lack of a rub does not rule out a significant pericardial effusion. Chest radiography will show an enlarged cardiac silhouette, and electrocardiography will show characteristic findings as explained in Chapter 10. Cardiac tamponade can occur; these patients have signs of poor cardiac output, with jugular venous distention and lungs clear to auscultation. Pericarditis is an absolute indication for initiation of hemodialysis.

3. Congestive heart failure–Patients with end-stage renal disease tend toward a high cardiac output. They often have extracellular fluid overload, shunting of blood through an arteriovenous fistula for dialysis, and anemia. In addition to hypertension, these abnormalities cause increased myocardial work and oxygen demand. Patients with chronic renal failure may also have accelerated rates of atherosclerosis. All of these factors contribute to left ventricular hypertrophy and dilation. Parathyroid hormone may also play a role in the pathogenesis of the cardiomyopathy of renal failure.

Water and salt intake should be controlled in patients who are oliguric or anuric. Diuretics are of value, though thiazides are ineffective when the GFR is less than 10–15 mL/min. Loop diuretics are commonly used, and higher doses are required as renal function declines. Digoxin should be used with caution since it is excreted by the kidney. The proved efficacy of ACE inhibitors in congestive heart failure holds true for patients with chronic renal failure. However, they are typically not used with a serum creatinine greater than 3 mg/dL without close supervision because of the risks of hyperkalemia and worsening renal function. Nonetheless, ACE inhibitors are increasingly employed at higher levels of stable serum creatinines with the desire of prolonging time to initiation of dialysis. Once a patient is on dialysis, these risks become less relevant. When an ACE inhibitor is initiated, patients should have serum creatinine and potassium checked within 2–3 days.

D. Hematologic Complications:

1. Anemia–The anemia of chronic renal failure is characteristically normochromic and normocytic. It is due primarily to decreased erythropoietin production, which becomes clinically significant when GFR falls below 20–25 mL/min. Many patients are iron-deficient as well. Low-grade hemolysis and blood loss from platelet dysfunction or hemodialysis play an additional role.

Recombinant erythropoietin (epoetin alfa) is used in patients whose hematocrits are less than 30–35%. The effective dose can vary, and patients are started on 50 units/kg (3000–4000 units/dose) once or twice a week. It can be given intravenously (eg, in the hemodialysis patient) or subcutaneously (eg, in the peritoneal dialysis patient or one who has not yet started dialysis). Iron stores must be adequate to ensure response. Iron supplementation is given at the minimum if the serum ferritin is less than 100 μg/mL. Oral therapy with ferrous sulfate, 325 mg once daily to three times daily, is adequate but not always well tolerated. Ferrous fumarate is the best-accepted formulation, and intravenous iron may be used in hemodialysis patients.

Hypertension is a complication of epoetin alfa therapy in about 20% of patients. It develops more abruptly in the patients with the lowest hematocrit values at initiation of therapy. Patients may require dosage adjustment or may have to be started on antihypertensive drugs.

2. Coagulopathy–The coagulopathy of chronic renal failure is mainly caused by platelet dysfunction. Platelet counts are only mildly decreased, but the bleeding time is prolonged. Platelets show abnormal adhesiveness and aggregation. Clinically, patients can have petechiae, purpura, and an increased tendency for bleeding during surgery.

Treatment is required only in patients who are symptomatic. Raising the hematocrit to 30% can reduce bleeding time in many patients. Desmopressin (25 μg intravenously every 8–12 hours for 2 doses) is effective and often used in preparation for surgery. It causes release of factor VIII von Willebrand's factor from endothelial cells. Conjugated estrogens, 0.6 mg/kg diluted in 50 mL of 0.9% sodium chloride infused over 30–40 minutes daily, or 2.5–5 mg orally for 5–7 days, have an effect for several weeks. Dialysis improves the bleeding time but does not normalize it. Peritoneal dialysis is preferable to hemodialysis because the latter requires heparin use to prevent clotting in the dialyzer. Cryoprecipitate (10–15 bags) is rarely used and lasts less than 24 hours.

E. Neurologic Complications: Uremic encephalopathy does not occur until GFR falls below 10–15 mL/min. Parathyroid hormone is believed to be one of the uremic toxins. Patients can develop markedly elevated intact PTH levels from tertiary hyperparathyroidism. When calcium levels exceed 12–15 mg/dL, mental status changes often follow. Symptoms begin with difficulty in concentrating and can progress to lethargy, confusion, and coma. Physical findings include nystagmus, weakness, asterixis, and hyperreflexia. These symptoms and signs may improve after initiation of dialysis.

Neuropathy is found in 65% of patients on dialysis but not until GFR is 10% of normal. Peripheral neuropathies manifest themselves as sensorimotor polyneuropathies (stocking and glove distribution) and isolated or multiple isolated mononeuropathies. Patients can have restless legs, loss of deep tendon reflexes, and distal pain. The earlier initiation of dialysis may prevent peripheral neuropathies, and the response to dialysis is variable. Other neuropathies result in impotence and autonomic dysfunction.

F. Disorders of Mineral Metabolism: The disorders of calcium, phosphorus, and bone are referred to as renal osteodystrophy. The most common disorder is osteitis fibrosa cystica—the bony changes of secondary hyperparathyroidism. As GFR decreases below 25% of normal, phosphorus excretion is impaired. Hyperphosphatemia leads to hypocalcemia, stimulating secretion of parathyroid hormone, which has a phosphaturic effect and normalizes serum phosphorus. This continuous process leads to markedly elevated parathyroid hormone levels and high bone turnover with osteoclastic bone resorption and subperiosteal lesions. Clinically, patients experience bony pain and proximal muscle weakness. Metastatic calcifications can occur. Radiographically, lesions are most prominent in the phalanges and lateral ends of the clavicles.

Osteomalacia is a form of renal osteodystrophy with low bone turnover. With worsening renal function, there is decreased renal conversion of 25-hydroxycholecalciferol to the 1,25-dihydroxy form. Gut absorption of calcium is diminished, leading to hypocalcemia and abnormal bone mineralization. Deposition of aluminum in bone can also lead to osteomalacia. Elevated aluminum levels are seen in patients after years of chronic aluminum hydroxide administration for phosphorus binding. This entity is seen with decreasing frequency because aluminum-based binders are used less in the chronic setting and water used for hemodialysis is now cleared of aluminum.

Both of the above entities can cause bony pain and proximal muscle weakness. Spontaneous bone fractures can occur which are slow to heal. When the calcium-phosphorus product (serum calcium [mg/dL] × serum phosphate [mg/dL]) is above 60–70, metastatic calcifications are commonly seen in blood vessels, soft tissues, lungs, and myocardium. Treatment should begin with dietary phosphorus restriction. Oral phosphorus binding agents such as calcium carbonate or calcium acetate act in the gut and are given in divided doses three or four times daily with meals. These should be titrated to a serum calcium of 10 mg/dL (preventing hypercalcemia) and serum phosphorus of 4.5 mg/dL. Aluminum hydroxide is another effective phosphorus binder but can cause osteomalacia and neurologic complications. It can be used in the acute setting; however, chronic use should be avoided. If aluminum levels are high, chelation with deferoxamine can be effective. Vitamin D should be given with hyperparathyroidism (iPTH more than two to three times normal) if phosphorus levels are < 7 mg/dL and calcium < 11 mg/dL. Vitamin D suppresses PTH and increases serum calcium and phosphorus levels; oral or parenteral calcitriol is the preferred agent once phosphorus levels are controlled. The dose should be 0.25–0.5 μg daily or every other day initially.

G. Endocrine Disorders: Circulating insulin levels are higher because of decreased renal insulin clearance. Glucose intolerance can occur in chronic renal failure when GFR is less than 10–20 mL/min. Primarily, this is due to peripheral insulin resistance. Fasting glucose levels are usually normal or only slightly elevated. Therefore, patients can be either hyperglycemic or hypoglycemic depending on the predominant disturbance. Most commonly, diabetic patients require decreased doses of antihyperglycemic agents.

Decreased libido and impotence are common in chronic renal failure. Men have decreased testosterone levels; women are often anovulatory. Despite a high degree of infertility, pregnancy can occur—particularly in women who are well dialyzed and well nourished. Therefore, contraception is advisable for women who do not wish to become pregnant.

Thyroid, pituitary, and adrenal function are often normal despite abnormalities in thyroxine, growth hormone, aldosterone, and cortisol levels.

Treatment

A. Dietary Management: Every patient with chronic renal failure should be evaluated by a renal nutritionist. Specific recommendations should be made concerning protein, salt, water, potassium, and phosphorus intake.

1. Protein restriction–Experimental models have shown that protein restriction slows the progression to end-stage renal disease; however, clinical trials have not consistently proved this. The Modification of Diet in Renal Disease (MDRD) Study was meant to clarify the issue, but the results were inconclusive. A subsequent meta-analysis of five clinical trials did show a significant benefit but did not control for certain effects such as ACE inhibitor therapy. Protein intake should not exceed 1 g/kg/d, and if protein restriction proves to be beneficial, it should not exceed 0.6 g/kg/d.

2. Salt and water restriction–In advanced renal failure, the kidney is unable to adapt to large changes in sodium intake. Intake greater than 3–4 g/d can lead to edema, hypertension, and congestive heart failure, whereas intake of less than 1 g/d can lead to volume depletion and hypotension. For the nondialysis patient approaching end-stage renal disease, 2 g/d of sodium is an initial recommendation. A daily intake of 1–2 L of fluid maintains water balance.

3. Potassium restriction–Restriction is needed once the GFR has fallen below 10–20 mL/min. Patients should receive detailed lists concerning potassium content of foods and should limit their intake to less than 60–70 meq/d. (Normal intake is about 100 meq/d.)

4. Phosphorus restriction–Phosphorus levels should be kept below 4.5 mg/dL. Foods rich in phosphorus such as eggs, dairy products, and meat should be limited. Renal failure patients with a GFR > 10–20 mL/min should restrict phosphorus intake to 5–10 mg/kg/d. Below this GFR, phosphorus binders are usually required. The treatment of hyperphosphatemia is discussed in the section on disorders of mineral metabolism.

5. Magnesium restriction–Magnesium is excreted primarily by the kidneys. Dangerous hypermagnesemia is rare unless the patient ingests medications high in magnesium or receives it parenterally. All magnesium-containing laxatives and antacids are relatively contraindicated in renal failure.

B. Dialysis: When conservative management of end-stage renal disease is inadequate, hemodialysis, peritoneal dialysis, and kidney transplantation are alternatives (see below). Indications for dialysis include the following: (1) uremic symptoms such as pericarditis, encephalopathy, or coagulopathy; (2) fluid overload unresponsive to diuresis; (3) refractory hyperkalemia; (4) severe metabolic acidosis (pH < 7.20); and (5) neurologic symptoms such as seizures or neuropathy. According the Dialysis Outcomes Quality Initiative (DOQI) guidelines, dialysis should be started when a patient has a GFR of 10 mL/min or serum creatinine of 8 mg/dL. Diabetics should start when the GFR reaches 15 mL/min or serum creatinine is 6 mg/dL.

Preparation for dialysis requires a team approach. Dietitians, social workers, psychiatrists, and transplant surgeons should be involved as well as primary care physicians and nephrologists. The patient and family need early counseling regarding the risks and benefits of therapy. The option of not starting therapy or withdrawing therapy should be discussed openly.

1. Hemodialysis–Hemodialysis requires a constant flow of blood along one side of a semipermeable membrane with a cleansing solution, or dialysate, on the other. Diffusion and convection allow the dialysate to remove unwanted substances from the blood while adding back needed components. Vascular access for hemodialysis can be accomplished by an arteriovenous fistula or prosthetic shunt. Native fistulae typically last longer than prosthetic shunts but require longer (6–8 weeks or more after surgical construction) before they can be used. Infection, thrombosis, and aneurysm formation are complications seen more often in shunts than fistulae. *Staphylococcus aureus* is the most common infecting agent.

Patients typically require hemodialysis three times a week. Sessions last 3–5 hours depending on patient size, type of dialyzer used, and other factors. Home hemodialysis is an option that is becoming less popular because of the need for a trained helper, large equipment, and costs.

2. Peritoneal dialysis–With peritoneal dialysis, the peritoneal membrane is the "dialyzer." Fluids and solutes move across the capillary bed that lies between the (visceral and parietal) layers of the membrane into the dialysate. Dialysate enters the peritoneal cavity through a catheter. The most common kind of peritoneal dialysis is continuous ambulatory peritoneal dialysis (CAPD). Patients exchange the dialysate four to six times a day. Continuous cyclic peritoneal dialysis (CCPD) utilizes a cycler machine to automatically perform exchanges at night. The dialysate remains in the peritoneal cavity between exchanges.

The percentage of dialysis patients using peritoneal dialysis has been relatively constant over the past 10 years. Peritoneal dialysis permits greater patient autonomy; its continuous nature minimizes the symptomatic swings observed in hemodialysis patients; and poorly dialyzable compounds such as phosphates are better cleared, which permits less dietary restriction.

The most common complication of peritoneal dialysis is peritonitis. Rates are as high as 0.8 episodes per patient year. The patient can experience nausea and vomiting, abdominal pain, diarrhea or constipation, and fever. The dialysate will be cloudy and contain > 100 white cells per microliter of which over 50% should be polymorphonuclear neutrophils. *S aureus* is the most common infecting organism.

The total costs of peritoneal dialysis and hemodialysis are approximately the same. Equipment expenses are less for peritoneal dialysis, but the costs of peritonitis are high. Patients treated with both modalities more often prefer peritoneal to hemodialysis.

Survival rates on dialysis depend on the underlying disease process. Five-year Kaplan-Meier survival rates vary from 18% for diabetics to 40% for patients with glomerulonephritis. Overall 5-year survival is currently estimated at 30%. Patients undergoing dialysis have an average life expectancy of 3–4 years, but survival for as long as 25 years is seen depending on the disease entity.

C. Kidney Transplantation: Up to one-half of all patients with end-stage renal disease are suitable for transplantation. Age is becoming less of a barrier. Two-thirds of kidney transplants come from cadaveric donors; the remainder from living related or unrelated donors. Immunosuppressive drugs include corticosteroids, azathioprine, mycophenolate mofetil, tacrolimus, and cyclosporine. A patient with a cadaveric renal transplant typically requires stronger immunosuppression than patients with living related kidney transplants. However, this depends to a great extent on the degree of HLA-type matching. The 1- and 5-year kidney graft survival rates are approximately 93% and 82%, respectively, for living related and living unrelated donor transplants and 85% and 74%, respectively, for cadaveric donor transplants. The median wait for a cadaveric transplant is 2 years. Aside from medication use, the life of a transplanted patient can return to nearly normal.

D. Prognosis: Mortality is higher for patients with end-stage renal disease than for age-matched controls. Yearly mortality is 17.6 deaths per 100 patient years. The expected remaining lifetime for the age group 55–64 is 22 years, whereas that of the end-stage renal disease population is 5 years. The most common cause of death is cardiac dysfunction (48%). Other causes include infection (15%), cerebrovascular disease (6%), and malignancy (4%). Diabetes, age, a low serum albumin, lower socioeconomic status, and inadequate dialysis are all significant predictors of mortality.

For those who require dialysis to sustain life but elect not to undergo dialysis, death ensues within days to weeks. In general, patients develop uremia and lose consciousness prior to death. Arrhythmias can occur as a result of electrolyte imbalance. Volume overload and dyspnea can be managed by volume restriction and opioids as described in Chapter 5. Meticulous efforts at palliative care are essential.

Barrett BJ et al: Clinical practice guidelines for the management of anemia coexistent with chronic renal failure. J Am Soc Nephrol 1999;10(Suppl 13):S292. [NLM Cit ID: 99354344]

Drueke TB: Medical management of secondary hyperparathyroidism in uremia. Am J Med Sci 1999;317:383. [NLM Cit ID: 99300053]

Gaede P et al: Intensified multifactorial intervention in patients with type 2 diabetes mellitus and microalbuminuria: the Steno type 2 randomised study. Lancet 1999;353:617. [NLM Cit ID: 99153397] (Randomized trial demonstrating that intensified multifactorial treatment of risk factors in diabetic patients with microalbuminuria can slow the progression of nephropathy, retinopathy, and neuropathy.)

Mackenzie HS et al: Current strategies for retarding progression of renal disease. Am J Kidney Dis 1998;31:161. [NLM Cit ID: 98088745] (A review of the mechanisms of renal disease progression and clinical trials to prevent disease progression, with a particular focus on protein restriction, ACE inhibitor use, antihypertensive therapy, and glycemic control.)

McCarthy JR: A practical approach to the management of patients with chronic renal failure. Mayo Clin Proc 1999;74:269. [NLM Cit ID: 99189867] (Review of the predialysis care of patients with renal failure.)

Rahman M et al: Chronic renal insufficiency: a diagnostic and therapeutic approach. Arch Intern Med 1998;158:1743. [NLM Cit ID: 98408983]

Rao VK: Posttransplant medical complications. Surg Clin North Am 1998;78:113. [NLM Cit ID: 98193090] (Medical, surgical, and psychosocial problems.)

US Renal Data System: *USRDS 1997 Annual Report*. The National Institutes of Health, National Institute of Diabetes and Digestive and Kidney Diseases, Bethesda, MD, 1997. (Epidemiology of end-stage renal disease.)

RENAL ARTERY STENOSIS

The two most common forms of renal artery stenosis are atherosclerotic ischemic renal disease and fibromuscular dysplasia. The prevalence of this condition has only been estimated by autopsy and angiographic studies. Approximately 5% of Americans with hypertension suffer from renal artery stenosis.

Atherosclerotic ischemic renal disease accounts for 67–95% of all cases of renal artery stenosis. It occurs most commonly in those over 45 years of age with a history of atherosclerotic disease. Other risk factors include renal insufficiency, diabetes mellitus, tobacco use, and hypertension.

Clues to diagnosis include refractory hypertension, new-onset hypertension in an older patient, pulmonary edema with poorly controlled blood pressure, and acute renal failure upon starting an angiotensin-converting enzyme inhibitor. In addition to hypertension, physical examination may reveal an audible abdominal bruit on the affected side. Laboratory values can show elevated BUN and creatinine levels in the setting of significant renal ischemia, and abdominal ultrasound discloses asymmetric kidney size.

Three prevailing methods used for screening are doppler ultrasonography, captopril renography, and magnetic resonance angiography (MRA). Doppler ultrasonography is highly sensitive and specific (> 90% with an experienced ultrasonographer) and relatively inexpensive. However, this method is extremely operator- and patient-dependent. Measurements of blood flow must be made at the aorta and along each third of the renal artery in order to assess the disease. This test is a poor choice for patients who are obese, unable to lie supine, or have interfering bowel gas patterns.

Captopril renography capitalizes on the difference in renal perfusion with and without ACE inhibitors. A kidney distal to a significant stenosis requires high angiotensin II levels to maintain adequate perfusion. With an ACE inhibitor, perfusion is markedly diminished. The affected kidney enhances less, whereas the unaffected one enhances more in the setting of a captopril challenge. Specificity ranges from 75% to 100% and specificity from 60% to 90%. This procedure is not accurate in moderate to severe renal insufficiency.

MRA is an excellent but expensive way to screen for renal artery stenosis. Sensitivity is 99–100%. Specificity ranges from 71% to 96%. Turbulent blood flow can cause falsely positive results.

Renal angiography is the standard procedure for diagnosis. CO_2 subtraction angiography can be used in place of dye when the risk of dye nephropathy exists—eg, in diabetic patients with renal insufficiency. Lesions are most commonly found in the proximal third or ostial region of the renal artery.

Treatment is controversial. Options include medical management, angioplasty with or without stenting, and surgical bypass. Angioplasty appears to reduce the number of antihypertensive medications but does not significantly change outcome in comparison to patients medically managed. Stenting produces significantly better angioplastic results. However, blood pressure is equally improved, and serum creatinines are similar at 6 months of observation. Angioplasty is equally as effective as and safer than surgical revision.

Fibromuscular dysplasia primarily affects young women. Unexplained hypertension in a young woman is reason to screen for this disorder. The noninvasive tests mentioned above should be used for detection. This disorder has a characteristic "beads-on-a-string" appearance on angiography. Treatment with percutaneous transluminal angioplasty is often curative.

Greco B et al: Atherosclerotic ischemic renal disease. Am J Kidney Dis 1997;29:167. [NLM Cit ID: 97169080]

Plouin P et al: Management of the patient with atherosclerotic renal artery stenosis. New information from randomized trials. Nephrol Dial Transplant 1999;14:1623. [NLM Cit ID: 99362245]

GLOMERULONEPHROPATHIES

Abnormalities of glomerular function can be caused by damage to the major components of the glomerulus: the epithelium (podocytes), the basement membrane, the capillary endothelium, or the mesangium. The damage is often manifested as an inflammatory process. A specific histologic pattern of glomerular injury can be seen on renal biopsy, one of the most helpful techniques available for defining the cause of glomerular disease. Clinically, hematuria, proteinuria, hypertension, and a reduced GFR are typical findings of glomerular diseases presenting as *nephritic* syndromes; heavy proteinuria (> 3.5 g/24 h) and hypoalbuminemia, hyperlipidemia, and edema are typical findings of glomerular diseases presenting as *nephrotic* syndromes.

Classification

Glomerular diseases generally can be classified into one of three major syndromes: nephritic syndrome, nephrotic syndrome, and asymptomatic renal disease. Specific glomerular diseases usually exhibit characteristics of one of the above syndromes, though some can have varying components of all three.

Glomerular diseases can also be classified according to whether they cause only renal abnormalities (primary renal disease) or whether the renal abnormalities result from a systemic disease (secondary renal disease).

NEPHRITIC SYNDROME

Essentials of diagnosis

- Edema.
- Hypertension.
- Hematuria (with or without dysmorphic red cells, red blood cell casts).

General Considerations

Acute glomerulonephritis usually signifies an inflammatory process causing renal dysfunction over days to weeks that may or may not resolve. If the inflammatory process is severe, the glomerulonephritis may lead to a greater than 50% loss of nephron function over the course of just weeks to months. Such a process, called rapidly progressive acute glomerulonephritis, causes permanent damage to glomeruli. Prolonged inflammatory changes can result in chronic glomerulonephritis with persistent renal abnormalities that progress to end-stage renal disease.

Clinical Findings

A. Symptoms and Signs: Edema is first seen in regions of low tissue pressure such as the periorbital and scrotal areas. Hypertension, if present, is due to volume overload rather than vasoactive substances such as angiotensin II, whose levels are low.

B. Laboratory Findings:

1. Serum chemistries–There are no serum chemistries characteristic of nephritic syndrome, but certain special tests are often performed depending on the history and the results of the preliminary evaluation. These include complement levels, antinuclear antibodies (ANA), cryoglobulins, hepatitis panels, serum IgA, ANCA, anti-GBM antibodies, ASO titers, and C3 nephritic factor. (See Figure 22–2.)

2. Urinalysis–The urinalysis shows red blood cells. These may be misshapen from traversing a damaged capillary membrane—so-called dysmorphic red blood cells. Red blood cell casts and moderate degrees of proteinuria are also characteristic of the urinary sediment. Placing the patient in a lordotic position for an hour increases sensitivity for finding red cell casts in the next urine specimen.

3. Biopsy–Renal biopsy should be considered if there are no other contraindications to biopsy (eg, bleeding disorders, thrombocytopenia, uncontrolled hypertension). Rapidly progressive glomerulonephritis is likely when over 50% of glomeruli contain crescents. The type of disease can be categorized according to the immunofluorescent pattern and appearance on electron microscopy (see Table 22–9).

Treatment

Treatment includes aggressive reduction of hypertension and fluid overload, and uremia and specific therapeutic maneuvers aimed at the underlying cause. Salt and water restriction, diuretic therapy, and possibly dialysis are needed. The inflammatory glomerular injury may require corticosteroids and cytotoxic agents. (See specific diseases discussed below.)

GLOMERULAR DISEASES WITH NEPHRITIC PRESENTATIONS

1. POSTINFECTIOUS GLOMERULONEPHRITIS

Postinfectious glomerulonephritis is most often associated with poststreptococcal infection due to nephritogenic group A beta-hemolytic streptococci, especially type 12. It can occur sporadically or in clusters and during epidemics can account for up to 10% of known streptococcal infections. It commonly appears after pharyngitis or impetigo. Onset occurs within 1–3 weeks after infection (average, 7–10 days).

Other causes of postinfectious glomerulonephritis include bacteremic states such as systemic *Staphylococcus aureus* infection. Infective endocarditis and shunt infections cause similar lesions. These are referred to as peri-infectious glomerulonephritis. Viral, fungal, and parasitic causes include hepatitis B, cytomegalovirus infection, infectious mononucleosis, coccidioidomycosis, malaria, and toxoplasmosis.

Clinical Findings

A. Symptoms and Signs: The patient is oliguric, edematous, and variably hypertensive.

B. Laboratory Findings: Serum complement levels are low; antistreptolysin O (ASO) titers can be high unless the immune response has been blunted with previous antibiotic treatment. Classically, the urine is described as cola-colored. Urinary red blood cells, red cell casts, and proteinuria under 3.5 g/d is present. On microscopy, this entity appears as a diffuse proliferative glomerulonephritis. Immunofluorescence shows IgG and C3 in a granular pattern in the mesangium and along the capillary basement membrane. Electron microscopy shows large, dense subepithelial deposits or "humps."

Treatment

Treatment for this entity is supportive. Antihypertensives, salt restriction, and diuretics should be employed if needed. Corticosteroids have not been shown to improve outcome. Prognosis in children is very favorable, but adults are more prone to crescentic formation and chronic renal insufficiency. Less than 5% of adults will develop a rapidly progressive glomerulonephritis, and a smaller percentage will progress to end-stage renal disease.

2. IgA NEPHROPATHY & HENOCH-SCHÖNLEIN PURPURA

IgA Nephropathy

IgA nephropathy (Berger's disease) is a primary renal disease of IgA deposition in the glomerular mesangium. The inciting cause is unknown, but the same lesion is seen in Henoch-Schönlein purpura.

IgA nephropathy is the most common form of acute glomerulonephritis in the United States and is even more prevalent worldwide, particularly in Asia. It is most commonly seen in children and young adults, with males affected two to three times more commonly than females.

An episode of gross hematuria is the commonest presenting complaint. Frequently this is associated with an upper respiratory infection (50%), gastrointestinal symptoms (10%), or a flu-like illness (15%). The urine becomes red or cola-colored 1–2 days after onset. In contrast to postinfectious glomerulonephritis, this feature has been called "synpharyngitic hematuria" since there is no significant latent period. Other findings include asymptomatic microscopic hematuria as an incidental finding and the nephrotic syndrome (see below). Approximately one-third of patients will experience a clinical remission. Forty to 50 percent of patients will have progressive renal insufficiency. The remainder will show chronic microscopic hematuria and a stable serum creatinine. Hypertension and proteinuria of more than 3 g/d are poor prognostic factors.

The serum IgA level is increased in up to 50% of patients, and for that reason a normal serum IgA does not rule out the disease. Serum complement levels are usually normal, and renal biopsy is the standard for diagnosis. Glomeruli show a focal glomeru-

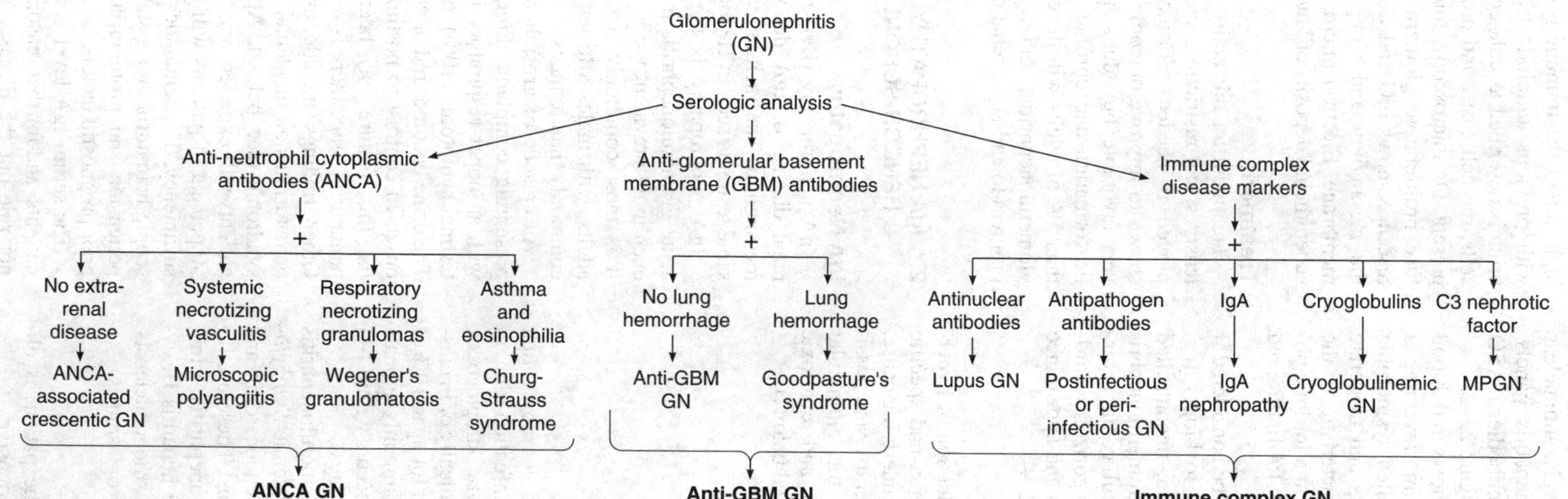

Figure 22–2. Serologic analysis of patients with glomerulonephritis. ANCA, anti-neutrophil cytoplasmic antibodies; GBM, glomerular basement membrane; GN, glomerulonephritis; MPGN, membranoproliferative glomerulonephritis. (Reproduced, with permission, from Jennette JC, Falk RJ: *Primer on Kidney Diseases.* Academic Press, 1994.)

Table 22–9. Classification and findings in glomerulonephritis: Nephritic syndromes.

	Etiology	Histopathology	Pathogenesis
Acute (postinfectious) glomerulonephritis	Streptococci, other bacteria	Light: Diffuse proliferative glomerulonephritis Immunofluorescence: IgG; C3, granular pattern Electron microscopy: Subepithelial deposits or "humps"	Trapped immune complexes
IgA nephropathy (Berger's disease and Henoch-Schönlein purpura)	In association with viral upper respiratory tract infections; gastrointestinal infection or flu-like syndrome	Light: Mesangioproliferative glomerulonephritis Immunofluorescence: IgA +/– IgG, C3) Electron microscopy: Mesangial deposits	Unknown
Rapidly progressive glomerulonephritis	Lupus erythematosus, mixed cryoglobulinemia, subacute infective endocarditis, shunt infections	Light: Crescentic glomerulonephritis Immunofluorescence: IgG, IgA; C3 granular pattern Electron microscopy: Deposits in subepithelium, subendothelium, or mesangium	Trapped immune complexes
	Goodpasture's syndrome or idiopathic	Light: Crescentic glomerulonephritis Immunofluorescence: IgG; C3, linear pattern Electron microscopy: Widening of basement membrane	Anti-GBM antibodies
	Wegener's granulomatosis, polyarteritis, idiopathic	Light: Crescentic glomerulonephritis Immunofluorescence: No immunoglobulins Electron microscopy: No deposits	Unknown

lonephritis with diffuse mesangial IgA deposits and proliferation of mesangial cells. IgG and C3 can also be seen in the mesangium of all glomeruli. Skin biopsy often reveals granular deposits of IgA in dermal capillaries of affected patients.

If nephrotic syndrome is present, treatment with glucocorticoids (prednisone, 60 mg orally daily for 4–6 weeks) may cause a remission but often will not halt the progression of renal disease. A daily dose of 12 g of fish oil may retard the rate of loss of renal function—particularly in patients with mildly impaired renal function. Renal transplantation is an excellent option for patients with end-stage renal disease, but recurrent disease has been documented in 30% of patients 5–10 years posttransplant.

Henoch-Schönlein Purpura (Anaphylactoid Purpura)

This disease is a leukocytoclastic vasculitis of unknown cause. It is most common in children and has a male predominance. It classically presents with palpable purpura, arthralgias, and abdominal symptoms such as nausea, colic, and melena. Purpuric skin lesions are most often found on the lower extremities. Renal insufficiency is common with a nephritic presentation. The renal lesions are identical to those found in IgA nephropathy. Most patients will recover fully over several weeks.

Further details about Henoch-Schönlein purpura are provided in Chapter 20.

3. PAUCI-IMMUNE GLOMERULONEPHRITIS (ANCA-Associated)

Pauci-immune glomerular lesions are seen with Wegener's granulomatosis and microscopic polyangiitis. Both are small-vessel vasculitides. Wegener's granulomatosis also involves granulomatous inflammation of the respiratory tract with a necrotizing vasculitis of small and medium-sized vessels. Microscopic polyangiitis (polyarteritis) is similar to Wegener's granulomatosis without granulomatous inflammation, but both commonly exhibit a necrotizing glomerulonephritis. ANCA-associated glomerulonephritis can also present as a primary renal lesion. The pathogenesis of these entities is unknown, but more than 80% of pauci-immune glomerulonephritis is associated with antineutrophil cytoplasmic autoantibodies.

Clinical Findings

A. Symptoms and Signs: Patients can present with symptoms of a systemic inflammatory disease, including fever, malaise, and weight loss. In addition to hematuria and proteinuria from glomerular inflammation, some patients exhibit purpura from dermal capillary involvement and mononeuritis multiplex from nerve arteriolar involvement. Ninety percent of patients with Wegener's will have upper or lower respiratory tract symptoms with nodular lesions that can cavitate and bleed.

B. Laboratory Findings: Serologically, ANCA subtype analysis is useful. A cytoplasmic pattern (cANCA) is specific for antiproteinase 3 antibodies, while a perinuclear pattern (pANCA) is specific for antimyeloperoxidase antibodies. Over 90% of patients with Wegener's syndrome will have cANCA; the remainder can have a pANCA pattern. Microscopic angiitis will have either a pANCA or cANCA pattern about 80% of the time. Pathologically, the small vessels and glomeruli will lack immune deposits (pauci-immune); however, a cell-mediated immune response is often seen. Necrotizing lesions and crescents signify a rapidly progressive glomerulonephritis.

Treatment

Treatment should be instituted early if aggressive disease is suspected. High doses of corticosteroids (methylprednisolone, 1–2 g/d for 3 days, followed by prednisone, 1 mg/kg for 1 month, with a slow taper over the next 6 months) and cytotoxic agents (cyclophosphamide, 2 mg/kg orally for 3 months, tapered over 1 year) are recommended for controlling end-organ damage. Without treatment, prognosis is extremely poor, but with the above regimen complete remission can be achieved in up to 75% of patients. Prognosis depends mainly on the extent of glomerular involvement before treatment is started. ANCA levels can be followed to help determine the efficacy of treatment.

4. ANTI-GBM GLOMERULONEPHRITIS & GOODPASTURE'S SYNDROME

Goodpasture's syndrome is defined by the clinical constellation of glomerulonephritis and pulmonary hemorrhage; injury to both is mediated by anti-glomerular basement membrane (anti-GBM) antibodies. Up to one-third of patients with anti-GBM glomerulonephritis have no evidence of lung injury. Anti-GBM-associated glomerulonephritis accounts for about 5% of patients with rapidly progressive acute glomerulonephritis. The incidence in males is approximately six times that in females, and the disease occurs most commonly in the second and third decades but has a wide range. It has been associated with influenza A infection, hydrocarbon solvent exposure, and HLA-DR2 and -B7 antigens.

Clinical Findings

A. Symptoms and Signs: Patients experience hemoptysis, dyspnea, and possible respiratory failure. Hypertension and edema are seen as components of the nephritic syndrome.

B. Laboratory Findings: Laboratory evaluation can show iron deficiency anemia, and complement levels are normal. Sputum contains hemosiderin-laden macrophages. Chest x-rays can show shifting pulmonary infiltrates due to pulmonary hemorrhage. The diffusion capacity of carbon monoxide is markedly increased. Diagnosis is confirmed by finding circulating anti-GBM antibodies.

Treatment

The treatment of choice is a combination of plasma exchange therapy to remove circulating antibodies and immunosuppressive drugs. Steroids are given initially in pulse doses of prednisone or methylprednisolone, 1–2 g/d for 3 days, then 1 mg/kg/d. Cyclophosphamide is administered at a dosage of 2–3 mg/kg/d. A poorer prognosis exists in patients with oliguria and a serum creatinine greater than 6–7 mg/dL. Anti-GBM antibody levels should decrease as the clinical course improves.

5. CRYOGLOBULIN-ASSOCIATED GLOMERULONEPHRITIS

Essential (mixed) cryoglobulinemia is a disorder associated with cold-precipitable immunoglobulins (cryoglobulins). Glomerular disease results from the precipitation of cryoglobulins in glomerular capillaries. The cause is typically an underlying infection such as hepatitis B and C or other occult viral, bacterial, and fungal infections.

Patients exhibit necrotizing skin lesions in dependent areas, arthralgias, fever, and hepatosplenomegaly. Serum complement levels are depressed. Rapidly progressive glomerulonephritis is seen on pathologic examination with the presence of crescents.

Treatment consists of aggressively treating the underlying infection. Pulse steroids, plasma exchange, and cytotoxic agents can be used. Alfa-interferon has been shown to benefit patients with hepatitis C-related cryoglobulinemia.

Other important examples of glomerulonephritis include systemic lupus erythematosus and membranoproliferative glomerulonephritis. These are described below under the heading of diseases exhibiting manifestations of nephritic and nephrotic syndrome.

Hricik DE et al: Glomerulonephritis. N Engl J Med 1998;339:888. [NLM Cit ID: 98414374]

Kallenberg CG: Laboratory findings in the vasculitides. Baillieres Clinic Rheumatol 1997;11:395. [NLM Cit ID: 97363791] (Review of antineutrophil cytoplasmic antibodies in these disorders.)

Nolin L et al: Management of IgA nephropathy: evidence-based recommendations. Kidney Int 1999;70(Suppl): S56. [NLM Cit ID: 99295870] (Review of the evidence for the use of steroids, fish oils, and control of hypertension.)

Ritz E et al: Nephropathy in patients with type 2 diabetes mellitus. N Engl J Med 1999;341:1127. [NLM Cit ID: 99426588] (Review of renal complications of diabetes with an emphasis on prevention and control of disease.)

NEPHROTIC SYNDROME

Essentials of Diagnosis

- Urine protein excretion > 3.5 g/1.73 m^2 per 24 hours.
- Hypoalbuminemia (albumin < 3 g/dL).
- Peripheral edema.

General Considerations

In adults, about one-third of patients with nephrotic syndrome have a systemic renal disease such as diabetes mellitus, amyloidosis, or systemic lupus erythematosus. The remainder have idiopathic nephrotic syndrome. The four most common are minimal change disease, focal glomerular sclerosis, membranous nephropathy, or membranoproliferative glomerulonephritis.

Clinical Findings

A. Symptoms and Signs: Peripheral edema is a hallmark of the nephrotic syndrome, occurring when the serum albumin concentration is less than 3 g/dL. Edema is most likely due to sodium retention (from renal disease), not from arterial underfilling from low plasma oncotic pressure. Initially this presents in the dependent areas of the body such as the lower extremities; however, this can become generalized. Patients can experience dyspnea due to pulmonary edema, pleural effusions, and diaphragmatic compromise with ascites. Complaints of abdominal fullness may also be present in patients with ascites.

Patients may show signs and symptoms of infection more frequently than the general population owing to loss of immunoglobulins and certain complement moieties in the urine.

B. Laboratory Findings:

1. Urinalysis–Proteinuria occurs as a result of an alteration of the negative charge in the GBM. The screening test for proteinuria is the urinary dipstick analysis; however, one must bear in mind that this test indicates albumin only. The addition of sulfosalicylic acid to the urine sediment can detect the presence of abnormal paraproteins. Urine dipstick testing can detect as little as 15 mg/dL of protein, but the results must be interpreted along with the urine specific gravity. Trace protein seen on highly concentrated specimens may be insignificant, while trace protein on dilute specimens may indicate true renal disease.

Microscopically, the urinary sediment has relatively few cellular elements or casts. However, if marked hyperlipidemia is present, patients can have oval fat bodies in the urine. These represent lipid deposits in sloughed renal tubular epithelial cells. They appear as "grape clusters" under light microscopy and "Maltese crosses" under polarized light.

2. Blood chemistries–Characteristic blood chemistries include a decreased serum albumin (< 3 g/dL) and total serum protein < 6 g/dL. Hyperlipidemia occurs in about one-half of those with early nephrotic syndrome. As patients excrete larger amounts of protein per day, the frequency of hyperlipidemia increases. There is increased hepatic production of lipids owing to a fall in oncotic pressure (apoprotein B lipoproteins) and decreased clearance of VLDLs (hypertriglyceridemia). Patients can also have an elevated erythrocyte sedimentation rate as a result of alterations in some plasma components such as increased levels of fibrinogen.

Other less common tests may be necessary depending on the patient's clinical presentation, including complement levels, serum and urine protein electrophoresis, ANA, and serologic tests for hepatitis. Patients may become deficient in vitamin D, zinc, and copper from loss of binding proteins in the urine.

3. Renal biopsy–Specific classification and findings are set forth in Table 22–10. Specimens

Table 22–10. Classification and findings in glomerulonephritis: Nephrotic syndromes.

	Etiology	Histopathology	Pathogenesis
Minimal change disease (nil disease; lipoid nephrosis)	Associated with allergy, Hodgkin's disease, NSAIDs	Light: Normal (+/– mesangial proliferation) Immunofluorescence: No immunoglobulins Electron microscopy: Fusion foot processes	Unknown
Focal and segmental glomerulosclerosis	Associated with heroin abuse, HIV infection, reflux nephropathy, obesity	Light: Focal segmental sclerosis Immunofluorescence: IgM and C3 in sclerotic segments Electron microscopy: Fusion foot processes	Unknown
Membranous nephropathy	Associated with non-Hodgkin's lymphoma, carcinoma (gastrointestinal, renal, bronchogenic, thyroid), gold therapy, penicillamine, lupus erythematosus	Light: Thickened GBM and spikes Immunofluorescence: Granular IgG and C3 along capillary loops Electron microscopy: Dense deposits in subepithelial area	In situ immune complex formation
Membranoproliferative glomerulonephropathy	Type I associated with upper respiratory infection	Light: Increase mesangial cells and matrix with splitting of basement membrane Immunofluorescence: Granular C3, C1q, C4 with IgG and IgM Electron microscopy: Dense deposits in subendothelium	Unknown
	Type II	Light: Same as type I Immunofluorescence: C3 only Electron microscopy: Dense material in GBM	Unknown

are examined by light microscopy, with immunofluorescent stains, and by electron microscopy. Renal biopsy is often performed in adults with new-onset idiopathic nephrotic syndrome if one suspects a primary renal disease that may require drug therapy (eg, corticosteroids, cytotoxic agents) for a possibly treatable lesion. Significantly elevated creatinine levels may indicate irreversible renal disease mitigating the need for renal biopsy. Disease due to amyloid or diabetes mellitus often does not need to be biopsied, since nephrotic range proteinuria in these diseases represents irreversible damage, although bone marrow transplant with high-dose chemotherapy can be considered in some patients with amyloid. The role of biopsy for other systemic renal diseases is debated. An occasional unexpected diagnosis is made, such as membranous nephropathy due to lupus erythematosus without serologic evidence of that illness.

Management of Nephrotic Syndrome

A. Protein Loss: Moderate protein restriction (0.5–0.6 g/kg/d) is often employed. Restriction is often advocated since increased protein intake may have an adverse effect on renal function in some diseases. The daily total dietary protein intake should replace the daily urinary protein losses so as to avoid negative nitrogen balance. Protein malnutrition often occurs with urinary protein losses greater than 10 g/d.

B. Edema: Dietary salt restriction is essential for managing edema; however, most patients also require diuretic therapy. Commonly used diuretics include thiazide and loop diuretics. Both are highly protein-bound. With hypoalbuminemia, diuretic delivery to the kidney is reduced, and patients often require large doses. The combination of loop and thiazide diuretics can potentiate the diuretic effect. This may be needed for patients with refractory fluid retention associated with pleural effusions and ascites.

C. Hyperlipidemia: Hypercholesterolemia and hypertriglyceridemia occur as outlined above. Dietary management in patients with nephrotic syndrome is of little value; however, dietary modification and exercise should be advocated. Pharmacologic treatment is discussed in Chapter 28.

D. Hypercoagulable State: Patients with serum albumin less than 2 g/dL can become hypercoagulable. Nephrotic patients have urinary losses of antithrombin III, protein C, and protein S and increased platelet activation. Patients are prone to renal vein thrombosis and other venous thromboemboli, especially with membranous glomerulopathy. Anticoagulation therapy is warranted for at least 3–6 months in patients with evidence of thrombosis. Patients with renal vein thrombosis and recurrent thromboemboli require indefinite anticoagulation.

NEPHROTIC DISEASE IN PRIMARY RENAL DISORDERS

1. MINIMAL CHANGE DISEASE

Minimal change disease is most commonly seen in children but is occasionally present in adults. In patients over 40 with primary nephrotic syndrome, the incidence of minimal change disease is 20–25%, with equal distribution between men and women. In younger patients, there is a male predominance. Minimal change disease can be idiopathic but also occurs following viral upper respiratory infections, in association with tumors such as Hodgkin's disease, and with hypersensitivity reactions (especially with NSAIDs and bee stings).

Clinical Findings

A. Symptoms and Signs: Patients can exhibit the manifestations of nephrotic syndrome. They are more susceptible to infection, especially with gram-positive organisms, have a tendency toward thromboembolic events, develop severe hyperlipidemia, and experience protein malnutrition.

B. Histologic Findings: Glomeruli show no changes on light microscopy or immunofluorescence. On electron microscopy, there is a characteristic fusion of epithelial foot processes. A subgroup of patients also show mesangial cell proliferation. These people have more hematuria and hypertension and respond poorly to steroid treatment.

Treatment

Treatment is with prednisone, 1 mg/kg/d. Response is excellent, but about 10% of patients become steroid-resistant after 4–6 weeks. A significant number of patients will relapse and require further steroid treatment. Patients with frequent relapses and steroid resistance may need cyclophosphamide or chlorambucil to induce subsequent remissions. Complications most often arise from prolonged steroid use.

2. MEMBRANOUS NEPHROPATHY

Membranous nephropathy is the most common cause of primary nephrotic syndrome in adults. It is an immune-mediated disease characterized by immune complex deposition in the subepithelial portion of glomerular capillary walls. The antigens in primary disease are not known. Secondary disease is associated with infections such as hepatitis B, endocarditis, and syphilis; autoimmune disease such as systemic lupus erythematosus, mixed connective tissue disease, and thyroiditis; carcinoma; and certain drugs such as gold, penicillamine, and captopril. Membranous nephropathy occurs most commonly in adults in their fifth and sixth decades and almost always after age 30.

Clinical Findings

A. Symptoms and Signs: Patients exhibit the signs of nephrotic syndrome and have a higher incidence of renal vein thrombosis than most nephrotic patients. A higher incidence of occult neoplasms of lung, stomach, and colon are found in people over 50. The course of disease is variable, with about 50% of patients progressing to end-stage renal disease over 3–10 years. Poorer outcome is associated with concomitant tubulointerstitial fibrosis, male gender, elevated serum creatinine, hypertension, and heavy proteinuria (> 10 g/d).

B. Laboratory Findings: By light microscopy, capillary wall thickness is increased without inflammatory changes or cellular proliferation. When stained with silver methenamine, a "spike and dome" pattern may be observed owing to projections of excess basement membrane between the subepithelial deposits. Immunofluorescence shows IgG and C3 uniformly along capillary loops. Electron microscopy shows a discontinuous pattern of dense deposits along the subepithelial surface of the basement membrane.

Treatment

Treatment is controversial. After underlying causes are excluded or treated, a 3-month course of prednisone, 2 mg/kg/d, may induce remission. Cytotoxic agents are added only if there is renal dysfunction. Patients are excellent candidates for transplant.

3. FOCAL SEGMENTAL GLOMERULAR SCLEROSIS

This lesion can present as idiopathic disease or secondary to conditions such as heroin use, morbid obesity, and HIV infection. Clinically, patients show evidence of nephrotic syndrome, but they also have more nephritic features than membranous nephropathy or minimal change disease. Eighty percent of patients have microscopic hematuria at presentation, and many are hypertensive. Decreased renal function is present in 25–50% at time of diagnosis.

Diagnosis requires renal biopsy. Light microscopy shows the lesions of focal segmental glomerular sclerosis. It is thought that these lesions occur first in the juxtamedullary glomeruli and are then seen in the superficial renal cortex. IgM and C3 are seen in the sclerotic lesions on immunofluorescence. Electron microscopy shows fusion of epithelial foot processes as seen in minimal change disease (Table 22–10).

Treatment is controversial, though supportive care should be given as outlined above for the nephrotic syndrome. Prednisone, 1–1.5 mg/kg/d for 4 weeks followed by 1 mg/kg every other day for 4 weeks, is used in patients with frank nephrotic syndrome because up to 40% of patients respond. Cytotoxic drug therapy should be considered in refractory patients. Despite treatment, most patients progress to end-stage renal disease in 5–10 years.

Eddy AA et al: The nephrotic syndrome: From the simple to the complex. Semin Nephrol 1998;18:304. [NLM Cit ID: 98279521] (Pathophysiology and consequences.)

Orth SR et al: The nephrotic syndrome. N Engl J Med 1998;338:1202. [NLM Cit ID: 98209526] (Etiology, pathogenesis, and treatment.)

NEPHROTIC DISEASE FROM SYSTEMIC DISORDERS

Amyloidosis

Amyloidosis consists of extracellular deposition of the fibrous protein amyloid in one or more sites in the body. This may occur in the absence of systemic disease or associated with an inflammatory process or multiple myeloma. This usually occurs in older age groups and displays a benign urinary sediment. The degree of proteinuria is not associated with the extent of renal lesions. Kidneys can be enlarged as a result of amyloid deposition. Pathologically, glomeruli are filled with amorphous deposits that stain positive with Congo red and show green birefringence.

Treatment options are few. Remissions can occur in secondary amyloidosis if the inciting agent is removed. Primary amyloidosis of the kidney progresses to end-stage renal disease in an average of 2–3 years. Five-year overall survival is less than 20%, with death occurring from end-stage renal disease and heart disease. Renal transplant is an option in these patients, but bone marrow transplant may prove more effective in attenuating progression.

Diabetic Nephropathy

Diabetic nephropathy is the most common cause of end-stage renal disease in the United States (about 4000 cases a year). Type 1 diabetes mellitus carries a 30–40% chance of nephropathy after 20 years, whereas Type 2 has a 15–20% chance after 20 years. Patients at higher risk include males, African-Americans, and Native Americans.

Patients at risk for nephropathy progress to develop the nephrotic syndrome. Diabetic retinopathy is invariably present in these patients. Initial screening of diabetics should always include urine examination for microalbuminuria. Dipstick examination may not be sensitive enough; therefore, 24-hour urine collection or an early morning spot urine albumin:creatinine ratio should be ordered. (A ratio < 3.5 is normal; > 10 is abnormal; and values between 3.5 and 10 need reevaluation.) In patients prone to nephropathy, microalbuminuria will develop within 10–15 years after onset of diabetes and progress over the next 3–7 years to overt proteinuria. During the onset of subclinical proteinuria, aggressive treatment is called for. Strict glycemic control and treatment of hypertension may slow progression of disease. In particular, ACE inhibitors lower the rate of progression to clinical proteinuria. This may reduce intraglomerular pressure as well as treat hypertension. Once a patient has progressed to clinical proteinuria, strict glycemic control and antihypertensive treatment are not as effective.

The most common lesion is diffuse glomerulosclerosis, but nodular glomerulosclerosis (Kimmelstiel-Wilson nodules) is pathognomonic for this entity. The kidneys in these patients are usually enlarged as a result of cellular hypertrophy and proliferation. At the onset of diabetic nephropathy, glomerular disease will cause an increase in GFR. As the nephropathy progresses, with the development of macroalbuminuria, the GFR returns to normal and continues to decrease.

Patients with diabetes are prone to other renal disease. These include papillary necrosis, chronic interstitial nephritis, and type IV renal tubular acidosis (hyporeninemic hypoaldosteronemic type). Patients are more susceptible to acute renal failure from contrast material and have a poor prognosis once dialysis is begun.

HIV-Associated Nephropathy

HIV-associated nephropathy can present as the nephrotic syndrome in patients with HIV infection. Most patients are young black men. In these patients, the more common mode of acquisition of HIV is through intravenous drug use.

Patients can have a nephrotic picture with normal complement levels. Light microscopy shows focal segmental glomerulosclerosis as described above, but these patients have more collapsing glomerular lesions.

Highly active antiretroviral therapy (HAART) for a prolonged course may be beneficial. Occasionally, corticosteroid treatment has been used with variable success at dosages of 1 mg/kg/d.

DISEASES DEMONSTRATING NEPHRITIC & NEPHROTIC COMPONENTS

Systemic Lupus Erythematosus

Systemic lupus erythematosus is a systemic autoimmune disease in which renal involvement is common. In various series, clinical renal involvement ranges from 35% to 90%.

Patients present with nephritic or nephrotic syndromes. All patients with systemic lupus erythematosus should have routine urinalyses to monitor for the appearance of hematuria or proteinuria. If urinary abnormalities are detected, renal biopsy is often performed. The type of glomerular injury depends on the site of immune complex deposition. Five patterns of renal histology are seen on biopsy: type I, normal; type II, mesangial proliferative; type III, focal and segmental proliferative; type IV, diffuse proliferative; and type V, membranous nephropathy.

Individuals with type I and type II patterns require no treatment. Transformation of these types to a more active lesion is usually accompanied by an increase in lupus serologic activity and evidence of deteriorating renal function (eg, rising serum creatinine, increasing proteinuria). Repeat biopsy to confirm the transformation in these patients is standard. Patients with extensive type III lesions and all type IV lesions should receive aggressive immunosuppressive therapy. Indications for treatment of type V disease are unclear; however, if superimposed proliferative lesions exist, aggressive therapy should be instituted.

Corticosteroids are the mainstay of treatment (methylprednisolone 1 g intravenously daily for 3 days followed by prednisone, 60 mg orally daily for 4–6 weeks) but are associated with many side effects and may not prevent progression of chronic lesions. Cyclophosphamide can be added for patients with inadequate renal response or aggressive lesions. Cytotoxic agents appear to improve long-term renal survival in those with type IV nephritis. They are typically used for 18–24 months. The return of serologic measurements to normal can be useful in monitoring treatment. Markers include dsDNA antibodies, C3, C4, CH50, and serum creatinine. Urinary protein and sediment are also helpful markers. Systemic lupus erythematosus patients on dialysis have a favorable prospect for long-term survival. Patients with kidney transplants have recurrent renal disease in 8% of cases.

Membranoproliferative Glomerulonephritis

Membranoproliferative glomerulonephritis in its primary form is an idiopathic syndrome that can present with nephritic or nephrotic features. (The secondary form can be seen in all of the immune complex glomerulonephritides discussed above.) Most patients are under 30 years of age. At least two major subgroups are recognized: type I and type II.

Patients with type I membranoproliferative glomerulonephritis present with a history of recent upper respiratory tract infection about a third of the time. Patients typically have a nephrotic picture, and complement levels are low. Histologically, the GBM is thickened because of immune complex deposition and abnormal mesangial cell proliferation between the GBM and the endothelial cells. This gives a characteristic "splitting" appearance to the capillary wall. Immunofluorescence shows IgG, IgM, and granular deposits of C3, C1q, and C4 (Table 22–10).

Type II membranoproliferative glomerulonephritis often presents with a nephritic picture and is less common than type I. Light microscopy is similar to type I. Serologically, type II is associated with C3 nephritic factor, which is a circulating IgG antibody. EM shows a characteristic dense deposit of homogeneous material that replaces part of the glomerular basement membrane.

Treatment is controversial in this disorder: it consists of steroid therapy (there is no standard dosage for adults) and antiplatelet drugs (aspirin, 500–975 mg/d, plus dipyridamole 225 mg/d). The rationale for antiplatelet therapy is that platelet consumption is increased in membranoproliferative glomerulonephritis and may play a role in glomerular injury. Most patients progress to end-stage renal disease within 10 years. Less favorable prognostic findings include type II disease, early renal insufficiency, hypertension, and persistent nephrotic syndrome. Both types of membranoproliferative glomerulonephritis will recur after renal transplantation; however, type II recurs more commonly.

Agati V et al: Renal pathology of human immunodeficiency virus infection. Semin Nephrol 1998;18:406. [NLM Cit ID: 98355081] (Review of the diverse array of the renal complications of HIV infection, including glomerular, tubulointerstitial, and vascular disease.)

Daghestani L et al: Renal manifestations of hepatitis C infection. Am J Med 1999;106:347. [NLM Cit ID: 99204660] (Includes review of hepatitis C-associated renal disease, with or without cryoglobulinemia.)

Jennette JC et al: Diagnosis and management of glomerular diseases. Med Clin North Am 1997;81:653. [NLM Cit ID: 97310483] (Glomerular disease as a spectrum from nephritic to nephrotic lesions with diagnosis and management of major clinical entities.)

Mallick NP et al: Minimal change nephropathy and focal segmental glomerulosclerosis. Kidney Int 1997;51 (Suppl):S80. [NLM Cit ID: 97220789] (Differences associated with minimal change nephropathy and focal glomerular sclerosis.)

Mojcik CF et al: End-stage renal disease and systemic lupus erythematosus. Am J Med 1996;101:100. [NLM Cit ID 96302166] (Review article stressing that patients with lupus have decreased disease activity once end-stage lupus nephropathy occurs and are good candidates for dialysis and renal transplantation.)

Rao TK: Acute renal failure syndromes in human immunodeficiency virus infection. Semin Nephrol 1998;18:378. [NLM Cit ID: 98355079] (In-depth review of acute renal failure in patients with human immunodeficiency virus.)

TUBULOINTERSTITIAL DISEASES

Tubulointerstitial disease may be acute or chronic. Acute disease is most commonly associated with toxins and ischemia. Interstitial edema, infiltration with polymorphonuclear neutrophils, and tubular cell necrosis can be seen. (See Acute Renal Failure, above, and Table 22–11.) Chronic disease is associated with insult from an acute factor or progressive insult without any obvious acute cause. Interstitial fibrosis and tubular atrophy are present, with a mononuclear cell predominance. The chronic disorders are described below.

CHRONIC TUBULOINTERSTITIAL DISEASES

Essentials of Diagnosis

- Kidney size: small and contracted.
- Decreased urinary concentrating ability.
- Hyperchloremic metabolic acidosis.
- Hyperkalemia.
- Reduced GFR.

General Considerations

There are four main causes of chronic tubulointerstitial disease. Other causes include multiple myeloma and gout, which are discussed in the section on multisystem disease with variable kidney involvement.

A. Obstructive Uropathy: The most common cause of chronic tubulointerstitial disease is pro-

Table 22–11. Causes of acute tubulointerstitial nephritis.

Drug reactions
Antibiotics
Beta-lactam antibiotics: methicillin, penicillin, ampicillin, cephalosporins
Ciprofloxacin
Erythromycin
Sulfonamides
Tetracycline
Vancomycin
Trimethoprim-sulfamethoxazole
Ethambutol
Rifampin
Nonsteroidal anti-inflammatory drugs
Diuretics
Thiazides
Furosemide
Miscellaneous
Allopurinol
Cimeticine
Phenytoin
Systemic Infections
Bacteria
Streptococcus
Corynebacterium diphtheriae
Legionella
Viruses
Epstein-Barr virus
Others
Mycoplasma
Rickettsia rickettsii
Leptospira icterohaemorrhagiae
Toxoplasma
Idiopathic
Tubulointerstitial nephritis-uveitis (TIN–U)

longed obstruction of the urinary tract. In partial obstruction, urine output alternates between polyuria (due to vasopressin insensitivity) and oliguria (due to decreased GFR). Azotemia and hypertension (due to increased renin-angiotensin production) are usually present. The major causes are prostatic disease in men; bilateral ureteral calculi; carcinoma of the cervix, colon, and bladder; and involvement of the retroperitoneum with other tumors or fibrosis.

Abdominal, rectal, and genitourinary examinations are helpful. Urinalysis can show hematuria, pyuria, and bacteriuria but is often benign. Abdominal ultrasound may detect mass lesions, hydroureter, and hydronephrosis. CT scanning and MRI provide more detailed information.

B. Vesicoureteral Reflux: Reflux nephropathy is primarily a disorder of childhood and occurs when urine passes retrograde from the bladder to the kidneys during voiding. It is the second most common cause of chronic tubulointerstitial disease. It occurs as a result of an incompetent vesicoureteral sphincter. Urine can extravasate into the interstitium; an inflammatory response develops, and fibrosis occurs. The inflammatory response is due to either bacteria or the normal urinary components.

Patients present as adolescents or young adults with hypertension, renal insufficiency, and a history of urinary tract infections as a child. Focal glomerulosclerosis is often seen. This is a cause of substantial proteinuria, unusual in most tubular diseases. Renal ultrasound or IVP can show renal scarring and hydronephrosis. Although most damage occurs before age 5, progressive renal deterioration to end-stage renal disease continues as a result of the early insults.

C. Analgesics: Analgesic nephropathy is most commonly seen in patients who ingest large quantities of analgesic combinations. The drugs of concern are phenacetin metabolites such as acetaminophen and paracetamol, aspirin, and NSAIDs. Chronic ingestion of 1 g/d for 3 years is the minimal amount needed for renal dysfunction. This disorder occurs most frequently in individuals who are using analgesics for chronic headaches, muscular pains, and arthritis. Most patients grossly underestimate their analgesic use.

Tubulointerstitial inflammation and papillary necrosis are seen on pathologic examination. Papillary tip and inner medullary concentrations of some analgesics are tenfold higher than in the renal cortex. Acetaminophen is metabolized in the papillae by the prostaglandin hydroperoxidase pathway to reactive intermediates that bind covalently to interstitial cell macromolecules, causing necrosis. Aspirin and other NSAIDs may worsen the damage by decreasing medullary blood flow (via inhibition of prostaglandin synthesis) and decreasing glutathione levels (which are necessary for detoxification).

Patients can exhibit hematuria, mild proteinuria, polyuria (from tubular damage), anemia (from gastrointestinal bleeding) and sterile pyuria. As a result of papillary necrosis, sloughed papillae can be found in the urine. An IVP may be helpful for detecting these—contrast will fill the area of the sloughed papillae, leaving a "ring shadow" sign at the papillary tip.

D. Heavy Metals: Environmental exposure to heavy metals—such as lead and cadmium—is seen less frequently now in the United States. Chronic lead exposure can lead to tubulointerstitial disease. Individuals at risk are those with occupational exposure (eg, among welders who work with lead-based paint) and drinkers of alcohol distilled in automobile radiators (moonshine users). Lead is filtered by the glomerulus and is transported across the proximal convoluted tubules, where it accumulates and causes cell damage. Fibrosed arterioles and cortical scarring also lead to damaged kidneys. Proximal tubular damage leads to decreased secretion of uric acid, resulting in hyperuricemia and saturnine gout. Patients commonly are hypertensive. Diagnosis is most reliably performed with a calcium disodium edetate (EDTA) chelation test. Urinary excretion of more than 600 mg of lead in 24 hours following 1 g of EDTA indicates excessive lead exposure.

Occupational exposure to cadmium also causes proximal tubular dysfunction. Hypercalciuria and nephrolithiasis can be seen. Other heavy metals that can cause tubulointerstitial disease include mercury and bismuth.

Clinical Findings

A. Symptoms and Signs: Polyuria is common because tubular damage leads to inability to concentrate the urine. Dehydration can also occur as a result of salt-wasting defect in some individuals.

B. Laboratory Findings: Patients are hyperkalemic because the distal tubules become aldosterone-resistant. A hyperchloremic renal tubular acidosis is characteristic. The cause of the renal tubular acidosis is threefold: (1) reduced ammonia production, (2) inability to acidify the distal tubules, and (3) proximal tubular bicarbonate wasting. The urinalysis is nonspecific, as opposed to that seen in acute interstitial nephritis. Proteinuria is typically less than 2 g/d (owing to inability of the proximal tubule to reabsorb freely filterable proteins); a few cells may be seen; and broad waxy casts are often present.

Treatment

Treatment depends first upon identifying the disorder responsible for renal dysfunction. The degree of interstitial fibrosis that has developed can help to predict recovery of renal function. Once there is evidence for loss of parenchyma (small shrunken kidneys or interstitial fibrosis on biopsy), nothing can prevent the progression toward end-stage renal disease. Treatment is then directed at medical management. Tubular dysfunction may require potassium and phosphorus restriction and sodium, calcium, or bicarbonate supplements.

If hydronephrosis is present, relief of obstruction should be accomplished promptly. Prolonged obstruction leads to further tubular damage—particularly in the distal nephron—which may be irreversible despite relief of obstruction. Neither surgical correction of reflux nor medical therapy with antibiotics can prevent deterioration toward end-stage renal disease once renal scarring has occurred.

Those suspected of having lead nephropathy should continue chelation therapy with EDTA if there is no evidence of irreversible renal damage (eg, renal scarring or small kidneys). Continued exposure should be avoided.

Treatment of analgesic nephropathy requires withdrawal of all analgesics. Stabilization or improvement of renal function may occur if significant interstitial fibrosis is not present. Hydration during exposure to analgesics may also have some beneficial effects.

Bennett WM et al: The renal effects of nonsteroidal anti-inflammatory drugs: summary and recommendations. Am J Kidney Dis 1996;28:S56. [NLM Cit ID: 96279696] (Review with special emphasis on the clinical features, pathophysiologic mechanism, and risk factors for acute renal failure.)

De Broe ME et al: Analgesic nephropathy. N Engl J Med 1998;338:446. [NLM Cit ID: 98117073]

Michel DM et al: Acute interstitial nephritis. J Am Soc Nephrol 1998;9:506. [NLM Cit ID: 981751021] (Causes and management.)

Rastegar A et al: The clinical spectrum of tubulointerstitial nephritis. Kidney Int 1998;54:313. [NLM Cit ID 98354655]

CYSTIC DISEASES OF THE KIDNEY

Renal cysts are epithelium-lined cavities filled with fluid or semisolid material. They develop primarily from renal tubular elements. One or more simple cysts are found in 50% of individuals over the age of 50. They are rarely symptomatic and have little clinical significance. In contrast, generalized cystic diseases are associated with cysts scattered throughout the cortex and medulla of both kidneys and can progress to end-stage renal disease (Table 22–12).

SIMPLE OR SOLITARY CYSTS

Simple cysts account for 65–70% of all renal masses. They are generally found at the outer cortex and contain fluid that is consistent with an ultrafiltrate of plasma. Most are found incidentally on ultrasonographic examination. Simple cysts are typically asymptomatic but can become infected.

The main concern with simple cysts is to differentiate them from malignancy, abscess, or polycystic kidney disease. Ultrasound and CT scanning are the recommended procedures for evaluating these masses. Simple cysts must meet three sonographic criteria to be considered benign: (1) echo-free, (2) sharply demarcated mass with smooth walls, and (3) an enhanced back wall (indicating good transmission through the cyst). Complex cysts can have thick walls, calcifications, solid components, and mixed echogenicity. On CT scan, the simple cyst should have a smooth thin wall which is sharply demarcated.

Table 22–12. Clinical features of renal cystic disease.

	Simple Renal Cysts	Acquired Renal Cysts	Autosomal Dominant Polycystic Kidney Disease	Medullary Sponge Kidney	Medullary Cystic Kidney
Prevalence	Common	Dialysis patients	1:1000	1:5000	Rare
Inheritance	None	None	Autosomal dominant	None	Autosomal dominant
Age at onset	...	...	20–40	40–60	Adulthood
Kidney size	Normal	Small	Large	Normal	Small
Cyst location	Cortex and medulla	Cortex and medulla	Cortex and medulla	Collecting ducts	Cortico-medullary junction
Hematuria	Occasional	Occasional	Common	Rare	Rare
Hypertension	None	Variable	Common	None	None
Associated complications	None	Adenocarcinoma in cysts	Urinary tract infections, renal stones, cerebral aneurysms 10–15%, hepatic cysts 40–60%	Renal stones, urinary tract infections	Polyuria, salt wasting
Renal failure	Never	Always	Frequently	Never	Always

It should not enhance with contrast media. A renal cell carcinoma will enhance but typically is of lower density than the rest of the parenchyma. Arteriography can also be used to evaluate a mass preoperatively. A renal cell carcinoma is hypervascular in 80%, hypovascular in 15%, and avascular in 5% of cases.

If a cyst meets the criteria for being benign, periodic reevaluation is the standard of care. If the lesion is not consistent with a simple cyst, surgical exploration is recommended.

AUTOSOMAL DOMINANT POLYCYSTIC KIDNEY DISEASE

This disorder is among the most common hereditary disease in the United States, affecting 1:1000 to 1:400 individuals. Fifty percent of patients will have end-stage renal disease by age 60. The disease has variable penetrance but accounts for 10% of dialysis patients in the USA. At least two genes account for this disorder: *ADPKD1* on the short arm of chromosome 16, and *ADPKD2*.

Clinical Findings

Most patients present with abdominal or flank pain and microscopic or gross hematuria. A history of urinary tract infections and nephrolithiasis is common. A family history is positive in 75% of cases, and more than 50% of patients have hypertension (see below) that may antedate the disease. Patients have large kidneys that may be palpable on abdominal examination. The combination of hypertension and an abdominal mass should suggest the disease. Forty to 50 percent have concurrent hepatic cysts, and pancreatic and splenic cysts occur also. Hemoglobin and hematocrit tend to be maintained as a result of erythropoietin production by the cysts. The urinalysis may show hematuria and mild proteinuria. Ultrasonography confirms the diagnosis—more than five cysts should be found scattered in the cortex and medulla of each kidney. If sonographic results are unclear, CT scan is recommended and highly sensitive.

Complications & Treatment

A. Pain: Abdominal or flank pain is caused by infection, bleeding into cysts, and nephrolithiasis. Bed rest and analgesics are recommended. Cyst decompression can help with chronic pain.

B. Hematuria: Gross hematuria is most commonly due to rupture of a cyst into the renal pelvis, but it can also be caused by a renal stone or urinary tract infection. Hematuria typically resolves within 7 days with bed rest and hydration. Recurrent bleeding should suggest the possibility of underlying renal cell carcinoma, particularly in men over age 50.

C. Renal Infection: Patients presenting with flank pain, fever, and leukocytosis should be suspected of having an infected renal cyst. Blood cultures may be positive, and urinalysis may be normal because the cyst does not communicate directly with the urinary tract. CT scans can be helpful because an infected cyst may have an increased wall thickness. Bacterial cyst infections are difficult to treat. Antibiotics with cystic penetration should be used, eg, fluoroquinolones, trimethoprim-sulfamethoxazole, and chloramphenicol. Treatment may require 2 weeks of parenteral therapy followed by long-term oral therapy.

D. Nephrolithiasis: Up to 20% of patients have kidney stones, primarily calcium oxalate. Hydration (2–3 L/d) is recommended.

E. Hypertension: Fifty percent of patients have hypertension at time of presentation, and most will develop it during the course of the disease. Cyst-induced ischemia appears to cause activation of the renin-angiotensin system, and cyst decompression can lower blood pressure temporarily. Hypertension should be treated aggressively, as this may prolong the time to end-stage renal disease. (Diuretics should be used cautiously since the effect on renal cyst formation is unknown.)

F. Cerebral Aneurysms: About 10–15% of these patients have arterial aneurysms in the circle of Willis. Screening arteriography is not recommended unless the patient has a family history of aneurysms or is undergoing elective surgery with a high risk of developing hypertension.

G. Other Complications: Vascular problems include mitral valve prolapse in up to 25% of patients, aortic aneurysms, and aortic valve abnormalities. Colonic diverticula are more common in this population.

Prognosis

No medical therapy has been shown to prevent the development of renal failure, though treatment of hypertension and a low-protein diet may slow the progression of disease.

MEDULLARY SPONGE KIDNEY

This disease is a relatively common and benign disorder that is present at birth and not usually diagnosed until the fourth or fifth decade. Kidneys have a marked irregular enlargement of the medullary and interpapillary collecting ducts. This is associated with medullary cysts that are diffuse, giving a "Swiss cheese" appearance in these regions.

Clinical Findings

Medullary sponge kidney presents with gross or microscopic hematuria, recurrent urinary tract infections, or nephrolithiasis. Common abnormalities are a decreased urinary concentrating ability and nephrocalcinosis; less common is incomplete type I distal renal tubular acidosis. The diagnosis is confirmed with intravenous pyelography, which shows striations in the papillary portions of the kidney produced by the accumulation of contrast in dilated collecting ducts.

Treatment

There is no known therapy. Adequate fluid intake (2 L/d) helps to prevent stone formation. If hypercalciuria is present, thiazide diuretics are recommended because they decrease calcium excretion. Alkali therapy is recommended if renal tubular acidosis is present.

Prognosis

Renal function is well maintained unless there are complications from recurrent urinary tract infections and nephrolithiasis.

JUVENILE NEPHRONOPHTHISIS-MEDULLARY CYSTIC DISEASE

This is a rare disorder associated with almost universal progression to end-stage renal disease. The childhood type—juvenile nephronophthisis—is an autosomal recessive disorder; the type appearing in adulthood—medullary cystic disease—is autosomal dominant. Both types are manifested by multiple small renal cysts at the corticomedullary junction and medulla. The cortex becomes fibrotic, and as the disease progresses, interstitial inflammation and glomerular sclerosis appear.

Clinical Findings

Patients with both forms exhibit polyuria, pallor, and lethargy. Hypertension occurs at the later stages of disease. The juvenile form causes growth retardation and end-stage renal disease before age 20. Patients require large amounts of salt and water as a result of renal salt wasting. Ultrasound and CT scan show small, scarred kidneys, and an open renal biopsy may be necessary to recover tissue from the corticomedullary junction.

Treatment & Prognosis

There is no medical therapy that will prevent progression to renal failure. Adequate salt and water intake are essential to replenish renal losses.

Hwang DY et al: Unilateral renal cystic disease in adults. Nephrol Dial Transplant 1999;14:1999. [NLM Cit ID: 99389380] (Case reports and review emphasizing the lack of a genetic background or progressive renal failure in patients with unilateral renal cystic disease compared with those with autosomal dominant polycystic kidney disease.)

Levine E et al: Current concepts and controversies in imaging of renal cystic diseases. Urol Clin North Am 1997;24:523. [NLM Cit ID: 97421860] (Overview of current concepts regarding the pathophysiology, management, and malignant potentials of eight renal cystic diseases.)

MULTISYSTEM DISEASES WITH VARIABLE KIDNEY INVOLVEMENT*

MULTIPLE MYELOMA

Multiple myeloma is a malignancy of plasma cells (see Chapter 13). Renal involvement occurs in about one-fourth of all patients. "Myeloma kidney" is the presence of light chain immunoglobulins (Bence Jones protein) in the urine causing renal toxicity. Bence Jones protein causes direct renal tubular toxicity and results in tubular obstruction by precipitating in the tubules. The earliest tubular damage results in Fanconi's syndrome (a type II proximal renal tubular acidosis). The proteinuria seen with multiple myeloma is primarily due to light chains which are not detected on urine dipstick, which mainly detects albumin. Patients with multiple myeloma can also develop glomerular amyloidosis; in these patients, dipstick protein determinations are positive. Hypercalcemia and hyperuricemia are frequently seen. Other conditions resulting in renal dysfunction include plasma cell infiltration of the renal parenchyma and a hyperviscosity syndrome compromising renal blood flow.

SICKLE CELL DISEASE

Renal dysfunction associated with sickle cell disease is most commonly due to sickling of red blood cells in the renal medulla because of low oxygen tension and hypertonicity. Congestion and stasis lead to hemorrhage, interstitial inflammation, and papillary infarcts. Clinically, hematuria is common. Damage to renal capillaries also leads to diminished concentrating ability. Isosthenuria (urine osmolality equal to that of serum) is routine, and patients can easily become dehydrated. Papillary necrosis occurs as well. These abnormalities are commonly encountered in sickle cell trait. Sickle cell glomerulopathy is less common but will inexorably progress to end-stage

*Other diseases with variable renal involvement described elsewhere in this chapter include systemic lupus erythematosus, diabetes mellitus, and the vasculitides such as Wegener's granulomatosis and Goodpasture's disease.

renal disease. Its primary clinical manifestation is proteinuria.

TUBERCULOSIS

The classic renal manifestation of tuberculosis is the presence of microscopic pyuria with a sterile urine culture—or "sterile pyuria." More often, other bacteria are present in addition. Microscopic hematuria is often present with pyuria. Urine cultures may demonstrate tubercle bacilli, and cavitation of the renal parenchyma occurs. Adequate drug therapy can result in resolution of renal involvement.

GOUT & THE KIDNEY

The kidney is the primary organ for excretion of uric acid. Depending on the pH and uric acid concentration, deposition can occur in the tubules, the interstitium, or the urinary tract. The more alkaline pH of the interstitium causes urate salt deposition, whereas the acidic environment of the tubules and urinary tract causes uric acid crystal deposition at high concentrations.

Three disorders are commonly seen: (1) uric acid nephrolithiasis, (2) acute uric acid nephropathy, and (3) chronic urate nephropathy. Renal dysfunction with uric acid nephrolithiasis stems from obstructive nephropathy. Acute uric acid nephropathy presents similarly to acute tubulointerstitial nephritis with direct toxicity from uric acid crystals. Chronic nephropathy is caused by deposition of urate crystals in the alkaline medium of the interstitium; this can lead to fibrosis and atrophy.

Treatment between gouty attacks involves avoidance of food and drugs causing hyperuricemia, aggressive hydration, and pharmacotherapy aimed at reducing serum uric acid levels. These disorders are seen in both "overproducers" and "underexcretors" of uric acid. The latter situation may seem counterintuitive; however, these patients have hyperacidic urine, which explains the deposition of relatively insoluble uric acid crystals.

THE KIDNEY & AGING

Renal mass declines progressively after the fourth decade. The renal medulla is spared in comparison to the cortex. Renal blood flow decreases with a resultant increase in arteriolar resistance. This allows for an increased filtration fraction and a relative sparing of the glomerular filtration rate (GFR). After the age of 40, GFR declines at a rate of approximately 0.8 mL/min/1.73 m^2/yr (though some older patients show little or no change). Serum creatinine values remain relatively constant because of decreased muscle mass along with the decrease in GFR. GFR impairment is partially due to thickening of the glomerular basement membrane, leading to glomerulosclerosis.

Renal tubular changes include impaired sodium handling, decreased concentration and dilutional ability, and impaired acidification. Thus, older patients are more prone to volume overload, hypo- and hypernatremia, and acidosis. Decreased renin synthesis and 1α-hydroxylase activity is also observed. These abnormalities can result in hyperkalemia, hypocalcemia, and elevated parathyroid hormone activity.

More adverse drug reactions occur in older patients. Three main pharmacokinetic changes occur: (1) altered volume of distribution, (2) altered drug half-life, and (3) altered elimination. The latter two are directly related to impaired renal clearance of drug.

Over one-third of the dialysis population in recent years have been over 65. Hemodialysis is the modality of choice for those with functional impairment. Peritoneal dialysis is tolerated much better in those with cardiovascular disease. Sudden fluid and electrolyte shifts can cause hypotension, ischemia, and arrhythmias.

Renal transplantation is being offered to more older individuals as it seems to benefit even those over 65. The main complications in this population are infection and cardiovascular disease. A reduced steroid requirement with the introduction of steroid-sparing agents such as cyclosporine has diminished infection rates.

Rodriguez-Puyol D: The aging kidney. Kidney Int 1998; 54:2247. [NLM Cit ID: 99070406]

RELEVANT WORLD WIDE WEB SITES

[Horseshoe Kidney]
http://www.brighamrad.harvard.edu/Cases/bwh/hcache/18/full.html

[Hypertension, Dialysis, and Clinical Nephrology, Renal Disease Electronic Journal]
http://www.hdcn.com/

[Medullary Nephrocalcinosis Secondary to Parathyroid Adenoma]
http://www.brighamrad.harvard.edu/Cases/bwh/hcache/186/full.html

[Pyonephrosis]
http://www.brighamrad.harvard.edu/Cases/bwh/hcache/4/full.html

[RenalNet]
http://www.renalnet.org/renalnet/renalnet.cfm

[Renal Osteodystrophy Case Study]
http://www.med.harvard.edu:80/JPNM/BoneTF/Case21/WriteUp21.html

[Renal Trauma]
http://www.brighamrad.harvard.edu/Cases/bwh/hcache/127/full.html

Urology

23

See http://www.current-med.com/ch23.html for updated addresses of Web sites referenced in this chapter.

Marshall L. Stoller, MD, Joseph C. Presti, Jr., MD, & Peter R. Carroll, MD, FACS

UROLOGIC EVALUATION

HISTORY

Pain

Pain in the genitourinary tract is usually associated with distention of a hollow viscus (ureteral obstruction, urinary retention) or the capsule of an organ (acute prostatitis, acute pyelonephritis). Pain may be local or referred. Pain associated with malignancy is usually a late manifestation and indicative of advanced disease.

A. Renal Pain: Pain of renal origin is usually located in the ipsilateral costovertebral angle. It may radiate to the umbilicus and may be referred to the ipsilateral testicle in men or the labium in women. In infection, the pain is typically constant, whereas in obstruction it may come and go. Nausea and vomiting may result from reflex stimulation of the celiac ganglion. Patients with intraperitoneal pathology will typically lie motionless to avoid pain, while patients with renal disease will move about to try to find a more comfortable position.

B. Ureteral Pain: Ureteral pain is usually acute and a result of obstruction. Distention of the ureter along with hyperperistalsis and spasm of the smooth muscle of the ureter may result in two different pain patterns. Distention may cause a constant dull ache, while the spasms result in colic. The site of obstruction is often predicted by the site of pain. Upper ureteral obstruction may result in pain referred to the scrotum in males or to the labium in females. Midureteral obstruction may cause pain in the lower quadrant and thus may be confused with appendicitis in right-sided ureteral obstruction or diverticulitis in left-sided ureteral obstruction. Lower ureteral obstruction may cause inflammation of the ureteral orifice and thus be associated with symptoms of vesical irritability.

C. Vesical Pain: Acute urinary retention results in severe suprapubic discomfort. Chronic urinary retention is usually painless despite tremendous vesical distention. Suprapubic pain not related to the act of micturition is rarely vesical in origin. Acute cystitis pain is usually referred to the distal urethra and is associated with micturition.

D. Prostatic Pain: Prostatic pain is associated with inflammation and is located in the perineum. Pain radiates to the lumbosacral spine, inguinal canals, or lower extremities. Because of its location near the bladder neck, inflammatory processes of the prostate result in irritative voiding complaints.

E. Penile Pain: Pain in the flaccid penis is secondary to inflammatory processes caused by sexually transmitted diseases or paraphimosis, a condition of the uncircumcised male in which the retracted foreskin is trapped behind the glans penis, resulting in vascular congestion and painful swelling of the glans. Pain in the erect penis may be due to Peyronie's disease (fibrous plaque of the tunica albuginea, resulting in painful curvature of the erect penis) or to priapism (prolonged painful erection).

F. Testicular Pain: Acute conditions such as trauma, torsion of the testis or one of its appendices, or epididymo-orchitis cause acute pain within the scrotum with radiation to the ipsilateral groin. Chronic pain may persist for months following successful treatment of acute epididymitis. Chronic pain produced by a varicocele or hydrocele results in "heaviness" without radiation. Disorders of the kidney, retroperitoneal structures, or inguinal canal may result in pain referred to the testis.

Hematuria

Gross hematuria in adults is considered a sign of malignancy until proved otherwise.

The character of the hematuria may give a clue to the site of origin. **Initial hematuria,** the presence of blood at the beginning of the urinary stream that clears during the stream, implies an anterior (penile) urethral source. **Terminal hematuria,** the presence of blood at the end of the urinary stream, implies a bladder neck or prostatic urethral source. **Total hematuria,** the presence of blood throughout the urinary stream, implies a bladder or upper tract source.

Associated symptoms give clues to the cause. Hematuria associated with renal colic suggests ureteral stone, but the passage of blood clots from a bleeding tumor mimics this scenario. Irritative voiding symptoms in a young woman may suggest acute bacterial infection and associated hemorrhagic cystitis, yet the same picture in an older woman or in any male raises concerns about neoplasm. In any situation, if cultures are negative or symptoms persist after therapy, further evaluation is warranted. Absent other symptoms, gross hematuria may be more indicative of tumor, but staghorn calculi, glomerulonephropathies, and polycystic kidney disease are in the differential.

Irritative Voiding Symptoms

Urgency is the sudden desire to void. It is observed in inflammatory conditions such as cystitis or in hyperreflexic neuropathic conditions such as neurogenic bladders resulting from upper motor neuron lesions. **Dysuria** (painful urination) is usually associated with inflammation. The pain is typically referred to the tip of the penis in men or to the urethra in women. **Frequency** is the increased number of voids during the daytime, and **nocturia** is nocturnal frequency. Adults normally void five or six times a day and once at most during the nighttime hours. Increased numbers of voidings may result from increased urinary output or decreased functional bladder capacity. Diabetes mellitus, diabetes insipidus, excess fluid ingestion, and diuretics (including caffeine and alcohol) are a few of the causes of increased urinary output. Decreased functional bladder capacities may result from bladder outlet obstruction (increased residual urine volume results in a lower functional capacity), neurogenic bladder disorders (spasticity and reduced compliance), extrinsic bladder compression (uterine fibroids, radiation-induced fibrosis, pelvic neoplasms), or psychologic factors (anxiety).

Obstructive Voiding Symptoms

Hesitancy is a delay in the initiation of micturition. It results from the increased time required for the bladder to attain the high pressure necessary to exceed that of the urethra in the obstructed setting. **Decreased force of stream** results from the high resistance the bladder faces and is often associated with a decrease in caliber of the stream. **Intermittency** and **postvoid dribbling** are interruption of the urinary stream and the uncontrolled release of the terminal few drops of urine, respectively. Obstructive symptoms are most commonly due to benign prostatic hyperplasia, urethral stricture, or neurogenic bladder disorders. Prostatic or urethral carcinoma and foreign body are other causes.

Incontinence

Urinary incontinence is the involuntary loss of urine. The history permits subclassification into one of four categories of incontinence. Such a distinction is necessary, as the workup and treatment vary with each of the categories. With **total incontinence,** patients lose urine at all times and in all positions. **Stress incontinence** is the loss of urine associated with activities that result in an increase in intra-abdominal pressure (coughing, sneezing, lifting, exercising). Uncontrolled loss of urine preceded by a strong urge to void is known as **urge incontinence.** Chronic urinary retention may result in **overflow incontinence.**

Systemic Manifestations

Fever when associated with other symptoms of a urinary tract infection (see below) helps to localize the site of infection. In women, high fevers occur in acute pyelonephritis. Fevers are not typical of uncomplicated cystitis. In men, a febrile urinary tract infection implies acute pyelonephritis, acute prostatitis, or acute epididymitis. Fever may also be seen associated with malignancy of the kidney, bladder, or testis.

Weight loss and malaise also may be associated with tumor or disease states associated with chronic renal failure.

Other Symptoms

Hematospermia, the presence of blood in the ejaculate, results from inflammation of the prostate or seminal vesicles. Blood in the initial portion of the ejaculate implicates the prostate, whereas terminal hematospermia implies a seminal vesicle origin. Workup should include urinalysis, digital rectal examination with prostate massage, and microscopic evaluation of the expressed prostatic secretions. More invasive procedures such as cystoscopy or transrectal ultrasound with prostate biopsy are reserved for patients with hematuria or abnormal rectal examinations, respectively. Persistent hematospermia warrants similar testing. The risk of malignancy with isolated hematospermia, normal urinalysis, and normal digital rectal examination is low.

Pneumaturia, the presence of gas in the urine, is usually secondary to a fistula between the bladder and the gastrointestinal tract. Diverticulitis is the most common cause, followed by colonic carcinoma, Crohn's disease, and radiation enteritis. The patient reports bubbles or particulate matter in the urine.

Urethral discharge is the most common symptom of sexually transmitted diseases. Dysuria and urethral itching are seen in association with the discharge. A bloody urethral discharge, especially in an elderly patient, suggests urethral carcinoma.

Cloudy urine may be secondary to a urinary tract infection, yet in the absence of infection it can be a result of an alkaline urinary pH. Such conditions result in phosphate crystal precipitation. Chyluria, the presence of lymph in the urine, results from a fistula between the urinary tract and the lymphatic system.

Filariasis, tuberculosis, and retroperitoneal tumors are some of the possible causes of this rare symptom.

PHYSICAL EXAMINATION

General Examination

The pallor of anemia and cachexia may be seen in malignancy. Gynecomastia occurs in testicular carcinomas or as a complication of hormonal therapy in prostatic cancer. Hypertension can be a result of renovascular disease or adrenal cancer.

Detailed Examination

A. Kidney: Because of the liver, the right kidney is lower than the left. The lower pole of the right kidney may be palpable in thin patients, yet the left kidney is usually not palpable unless abnormally enlarged. To palpate the kidney, one hand is placed posteriorly in the costovertebral angle to push the kidney anteriorly, while the second hand is placed anteriorly under the costal margin. With inspiration, the kidney may be palpated between the two hands.

Auscultation of the upper abdominal quadrants in hypertensive patients may reveal a systolic bruit associated with renal artery stenosis or an arteriovenous malformation; however, aortic bruits or transmitted heart murmurs may give similar findings.

Patients with flank pain should be tested for hyperesthesia of the overlying skin by pin testing, as this may be secondary to nerve root irritation and radiculitis rather than being of renal origin.

B. Bladder: The normal adult bladder is not palpable unless filled with at least 150 mL of urine. Percussion is better than palpation in diagnosing the distended bladder. Dullness is appreciated over the full bladder and changes to tympany if the air-filled bowel is anterior to the bladder.

Bimanual examination under anesthesia is helpful in the evaluation of patients with suspected bladder neoplasms. In the male, the bladder is palpated between the abdominal wall and the rectum while in the female it is palpated between the abdominal wall and the vagina. This is the best means of assessing vesical mobility and thus resectability.

C. Penis: The foreskin must be retracted in the uncircumcised male to permit inspection of the urethral meatus and glans. The position of the urethral meatus, the presence of urethral discharge, inflammation, penile tumor, and skin lesions must be noted. In **phimosis,** the foreskin cannot be retracted over the glans. In **paraphimosis,** the foreskin has been left retracted behind the glans, resulting in painful engorgement and edema of the glans. If not attended to, this may result in glandular ischemia. Congenital anomalies of position of the urethral meatus are called **hypospadias** when the meatus is located on the ventral aspect of the penis, scrotum, or perineum and **epispadias** when it is located on the dorsal aspect of the penis. A thick yellow urethral discharge is seen in gonococcal urethritis, whereas a thin clear or white discharge is noted in nongonococcal urethritis. Palpation of the dorsal penile shaft for plaques of Peyronie's disease and of the ventral surface for urethral tumors should be performed.

D. Scrotum and Its Contents: The most common referral to the urologist concerning the scrotum is for evaluation of a mass. It is important to determine whether the lesion resides within the testicle or is related to the epididymis or cord structures. The testes are palpated between the fingertips of both hands. Normal testes measure 6 × 4 cm and are rubbery in consistency. The epididymis rests posterolateral to the testis and varies in its degree of testicular attachment. Masses arising from within the testes are usually malignant; those from the epididymis and spermatic cord structures are usually benign. Transillumination will distinguish solid and cystic lesions.

The history and physical examination can make the diagnosis in the majority of cases. Tumors of the testis are usually painless, firm, solid lesions within the substance of the testis. These lesions do not transilluminate.

Acute epididymitis is an acute infectious process and is associated with painful enlargement of the epididymis. Fever and irritative voiding symptoms are common. In advanced states, the infection can spread to the testis, making the distinction between the epididymis and the testicle difficult on physical examination. The entire scrotal contents may be painful on palpation, yet relief may be offered to the supine patient by elevation of the scrotum above the pubic symphysis (Prehn's sign).

A **hydrocele** is a collection of fluid between the two layers of the tunica vaginalis. The diagnosis is readily made by transillumination. Evaluation of the testis is necessary, as approximately 10% of testicular tumors may have an associated hydrocele.

A **varicocele** is engorgement of the internal spermatic veins above the testis. These almost always occur on the left side as the left spermatic vein empties into the left renal vein while the right empties into the inferior vena cava. Varicoceles should diminish in size or disappear with the patient in the supine position. The sudden onset of a right varicocele should raise the question of a retroperitoneal malignancy resulting in obstruction of the right spermatic vein; a left varicocele suggests obstruction of the left renal vein, as in renal cell carcinoma.

Torsion of the testis typically occurs in the 10- to 20-year age group and presents with acute onset of pain and swelling within the testis. Examination reveals a painful testis that may have a "high lie" in relation to the other testis. The acute onset, lack of voiding symptoms, and the different age distribution may help distinguish it from epididymitis.

Torsion of the appendices of the testis or epididymis may be indistinguishable from torsion of the testis and affects a similar age group as torsion of the testis. On occasion a small palpable lump on the superior pole of the testis or epididymis is discernible that may appear blue when the skin is pulled tautly over it ("blue dot sign").

E. Rectal Examination in the Male: Inspection for anal pathology (fissures, warts, carcinoma, hemorrhoids) should be performed first. Upon insertion of the finger, anal tone can be estimated and a bulbocavernosus reflex can be elicited. As the anal and urinary sphincter derive from a common innervation, clues to neurogenic disorders may be obtained. The entire prostate is then examined, with attention being directed toward size and consistency. The normal prostate is approximately 4 × 4 cm and weighs 25 g. Normal consistency is that of the contracted thenar eminence with the thumb opposed to the little finger. Rubbery enlargement of the prostate is noted in benign prostatic hyperplasia. Induration may be perceived with carcinoma but also with chronic inflammation. The remainder of the rectum is then examined to exclude primary rectal disease.

F. Pelvic Examination in the Female: Examination of the introitus should include inspection for atrophic changes, ulcers, discharge, and warts. The urethral meatus can be inspected for caruncles and palpated for tumors or diverticula. Bimanual examination of the bladder, uterus, and adnexa should be performed with two fingers in the vagina and one hand on the abdomen, and attention is directed toward abnormal masses.

URINALYSIS

Collection of Specimens

In the male, a clean-catch urine is obtained in separate aliquots. Such a scheme may permit localization of disease. The first 5–10 mL is collected and represents the urethral specimen; a midstream specimen reflects conditions in the bladder and upper urinary tracts. If necessary, the prostate is then massaged and the expressed secretions collected. If no fluid is obtained, the next 2–3 mL of urine are collected, which reflects prostatic pathology. (See also Hematuria.)

Dipstick Urinalysis

A. pH: There is no role for dipstick urinalysis screening for urinary tract disorders in asymptomatic adults except for pregnant women. Urinary pH (range 5.0–9.0) may be helpful in the diagnosis and treatment of some urologic conditions. Alkaline urine in a patient with a urinary tract infection suggests the presence of a urea-splitting organism, most commonly *Proteus mirabilis,* though some strains of klebsiella, pseudomonas, providencia, and staphylococcus may also produce urease. Acidic urine in a patient with urolithiasis suggests uric acid or cystine stones. Failure to acidify the urine below a pH of 5.5 despite a metabolic acidosis suggests a distal renal tubular acidosis.

B. Protein: Dipsticks using bromphenol blue can detect protein in concentrations exceeding 10 mg/dL. It measures albumin and is not sensitive for the light chain of immunoglobulins (Bence Jones proteins). False-positive results are seen in urine containing numerous leukocytes or epithelial cells. (See Proteinuria in Chapter 22.)

C. Urobilinogen and Bilirubin: Urobilinogen is formed from the catabolism of conjugated bilirubin in the gut by bacteria, and the majority is cleared by the liver. Normally, only 1–4 mg of urobilinogen is excreted in the urine per day. Hemolytic processes or hepatocellular disease can lead to increased urinary levels, while complete biliary obstruction or broad-spectrum antibiotics that alter the gut bacterial flora may result in absent urinary urobilinogen. Unconjugated bilirubin is not filtered by the glomerulus, while only 1% of conjugated bilirubin is filtered. Normally no bilirubin is detected by urinary dipstick, since only concentrations greater than 0.4 mg/dL are detectable. Conditions manifesting elevated conjugated bilirubin in the serum will result in higher urinary levels. Ascorbic acid may cause false-negative results, while phenazopyridine may cause false-positive results.

D. Glucose and Ketones: Only small amounts of glucose are normally excreted in the urine, and these levels are below the sensitivity of the dipstick. Any positive finding requires evaluation for diabetes. The test is specific for glucose and does not cross-react with any other sugars. Ascorbic acid or elevated ketones may result in false-negative results.

Ketones are not normally found in the urine, but fasting, postexercise states, and pregnancy may result in elevated urinary ketones. Diabetics often demonstrate elevated urinary ketone levels prior to an elevation in serum levels. False-positive results occur in dehydration or in the presence of levodopa metabolites, mesna (sodium mercaptoethanesulfonate), and other sulfhydryl-containing compounds.

E. Nitrites: Normally, the urine does not contain nitrites. Many gram-negative bacteria can reduce nitrate to nitrite, which is thus an indicator of bacteriuria. However, the low sensitivity of the test requires clarification. Adequate numbers of bacteria must be present (10^5 organisms/mL), nitrates must be available in the urine, and the bacteria must be in contact with the urine for a sufficient time (usually 4 hours). Therefore, the first morning voided sample is preferable. False-negative results may be due to non-nitrate-reducing organisms, frequent urination, dilute or acidic urine (pH < 6.0), and the presence of urobilinogen. False-positive results are usually secondary to contaminated specimens, so that bacteria are indeed present in the sample yet not present in the urinary tract.

F. Leukocyte Esterase: Leukocyte esterase is an enzyme produced by white cells. The dipstick detects leukocytes in the urine, which is thus suggestive but not diagnostic for bacteria. False-positive tests result from specimen contamination. False-negative tests result from high specific gravity, glycosuria, the presence of urobilinogen, and medications, including rifampin, phenazopyridine, and ascorbic acid.

G. Blood: The urinary dipstick for blood measures intact erythrocytes, free hemoglobin, and myoglobin. False-positive results in women may occur as a result of contamination at collection with menstrual blood. Concentrated urine may also cause a false-positive result, as patients normally excrete 1000 erythrocytes per milliliter of urine. Vigorous exercise and vitamins or foods associated with high oxidant levels may also give a false-positive result. High ascorbic acid levels may give a false-negative result.

Microscopic Urinalysis

A. Leukocytes: The presence of more than five leukocytes per high-power field is considered significant pyuria. Leukocytes in the urine are indicative of injury to the urinary tract, which may or may not be due to infection. Other causes of pyuria include calculous disease, strictures, neoplasm, glomerulonephropathy, or interstitial cystitis. Leukocyte counts will vary by the state of hydration, method of collection, and degree of injury to the urinary tract.

B. Erythrocytes: The presence of more than five erythrocytes per high-power field is considered significant and warrants further investigation. (See Evaluation of Hematuria, below.) The appearance of the red cells sometimes gives a clue to their origin within the urinary tract. Dysmorphic (irregularly shaped) cells have an uneven distribution of hemoglobin and cytoplasm, and usually indicate glomerular disease. Red cells that are round, with evenly distributed hemoglobin, suggest disease along the epithelial lining of the urinary tract. All patients with hematuria require further diagnostic workup (see below); morphology, though of interest, is not of sufficient accuracy to allow firm diagnostic conclusions.

C. Epithelial Cells: The presence of squamous epithelial cells in the urinary sediment is indicative of contamination and thus requires a repeat collection. Transitional epithelial cells are occasionally noted in normal urinary sediment, but if present in large numbers or clumps they cause concern about possible neoplasm. Cytologic examination may be necessary to confirm the finding.

D. Bacteria and Yeasts: The identification of organisms in an uncontaminated specimen implies infection, which must be confirmed by culture. The presence of several organisms per high-power field usually correlates with a culture count of 10^5 organisms per milliliter. Gram staining may further aid in characterizing the organism. *Candida albicans* is the most common yeast seen in the urine, and characteristic budding and clumps are typically observed.

E. Casts: Casts are formed in the distal tubules and collecting ducts as a result of Tamm-Horsfall mucoprotein precipitation. They congregate near the edges of the coverslip and are detected best in a fresh specimen viewed under low power. If the urine is devoid of cells, hyaline casts are formed. Casts with entrapped red cells are indicative of glomerulonephritis or vasculitis. Leukocyte casts are suggestive of pyelonephritis. Epithelial casts in small numbers are normal, but in large numbers they suggest intrinsic renal disease. Granular casts result from degeneration of other cellular casts and also suggest intrinsic renal disease.

F. Crystals: Uric acid, oxalate, and cystine crystals are more often precipitated in acid urine, while phosphate crystals are more commonly seen in alkaline urine. The presence of uric acid, phosphate, and oxalate crystals can be seen in normal patients as well as in stone-formers. Cystine crystals, with a characteristic hexagonal benzene ring shape, are seen only in patients with cystinuria and are thus pathologic.

Bove P et al: Reexamining the value of hematuria testing in patients with acute flank pain. J Urol 1999;162(3 Part 1):685. [NLM Cit ID: 99385524] (Fourteen percent of patients presenting with ureterolithiasis had a negative dipstick for blood and fewer than two red cells per high-power field.)

EVALUATION OF HEMATURIA

If gross hematuria occurs, a description of the timing (initial, terminal, total) may give a clue to the localization of disease. Associated symptoms (ie, renal colic, irritative voiding symptoms, constitutional symptoms) should be investigated. Drug ingestion and associated medical problems may also provide diagnostic clues. Anticoagulants, analgesic abuse (papillary necrosis), cyclophosphamide (chemical cystitis), antibiotics (interstitial nephritis), diabetes mellitus, sickle cell trait or disease (papillary necrosis), a history of stone disease, or malignancy should all be investigated. The presence of hematuria in patients on anticoagulation therapy warrants a complete evaluation consisting of upper tract imaging, cystoscopy, and urine cytology.

Physical examination should emphasize signs of systemic disease (fever, rash, lymphadenopathy, abdominal or pelvic masses) as well as signs of medical renal disease (hypertension, volume overload). Urologic evaluation may demonstrate an enlarged prostate, flank mass, or urethral disease.

Initial laboratory investigations include a urinalysis and urine culture. Proteinuria and casts suggest renal origin. Irritative voiding symptoms, bacteriuria, and a positive urine culture in the female suggest urinary tract infection, but follow-up urinalysis is important after treatment to ensure resolution of the hematuria.

Further evaluation includes urinary cytology, upper tract imaging, and cystoscopy. Cytology especially assists in the diagnosis of bladder neoplasm, and three voided samples are recommended to maximize sensitivity. Upper tract imaging (usually an intravenous urogram) may identify neoplasms of the kidney or ureter as well as identifying benign conditions such as urolithiasis, obstructive uropathy, papillary necrosis, medullary sponge kidney, or polycystic kidney disease. The role of ultrasonographic evaluation of the urinary tract for hematuria is unclear. While it may provide adequate information for the kidney, its sensitivity in detecting ureteral disease may be lower. In addition, its higher degree of operator dependence may further confound the issue. Cystoscopy can assess for bladder or urethral neoplasm, benign prostatic enlargement, and radiation or chemical cystitis. For gross hematuria, cystoscopy is ideally performed while the patient is actively bleeding to allow better localization (ie, lateralize to one side of the upper tracts, bladder, or urethra).

In patients with gross or microscopic hematuria, an upper tract source (kidneys and ureters) can be identified in 10% of cases. For upper tract sources, stone disease accounts for 40%, medical renal disease (medullary sponge kidney, glomerulonephritis, papillary necrosis) for 20%, renal cell carcinoma for 10%, and transitional cell carcinoma of the ureter or renal pelvis for 5%. In the absence of infection, gross hematuria from a lower tract source is most commonly from transitional cell carcinoma of the bladder. Microscopic hematuria in the male is most commonly from benign prostatic hyperplasia. In patients with negative evaluations, repeat evaluations are warranted to avoid a missed malignancy; however, the ideal frequency of such evaluations is not defined. Urinary cytology can be repeated in 3–6 months, and cystoscopy and upper tract imaging after a year.

Angulo JC et al: The value of comparative volumetric analysis of urinary and blood erythrocytes to localize the source of hematuria. J Urol 1999;162:119. [NLM Cit ID: 99306421] (Red cells originating from the kidney and going through the glomerulus are smaller than those originating from other nonrenal sources of the genitourinary collecting system.)

GENITOURINARY TRACT INFECTIONS

Urinary tract infections are among the most common entities encountered in medical practice. In acute infections, a single pathogen is usually found, whereas two or more pathogens are often seen in chronic infections. Coliform bacteria are responsible for most nonnosocomial, uncomplicated urinary tract infections, with *E coli* being the most common. Such infections typically are sensitive to a wide variety of orally administered antibiotics and respond quickly. Nosocomial infections often are due to more resistant pathogens and may require parenteral antibiotics. Renal infections are of particular concern because if they are inadequately treated, loss of renal function may result. Previously, a colony count > 10^5/mL was considered the criterion for urinary tract infection. However, it is now recognized that up to 50% of women with symptomatic infections have lower counts. In addition, the presence of pyuria correlates poorly with the diagnosis of urinary tract infection, and thus urinalysis alone is not adequate for diagnosis. With respect to treatment, soft tissue infections (pyelonephritis, prostatitis) require intensive therapy for 3–4 weeks, while mucosal infections (cystitis) may require 1–3 days of therapy.

Classification & Pathogenesis

First infections—ie, first documented infections—in young women tend to be uncomplicated. **Unresolved bacteriuria** occurs when the urinary tract is never sterilized during therapy. This may result from bacterial resistance to therapy, noncompliance, mixed infections with organisms having different susceptibilities, renal insufficiency, or the rapid emergence of resistance from an initially sensitive organism. **Persistent bacteriuria** occurs when the urinary tract is initially sterilized during therapy but a persistent source of infection in contact with the urinary tract remains. This may result from infected stones, chronic pyelonephritis or prostatitis, vesicoenteric or vesicovaginal fistulas, obstructive uropathy, foreign bodies, or urethral diverticula. **Reinfections** occur when new infections with new pathogens occur following successful treatment.

Ascending infection from the urethra is the most common route. Women are particularly at risk for urinary tract infections because the female urethra is short and the vagina becomes colonized with bacteria. Sexual intercourse is a major precipitating factor in young women, and the use of diaphragms and spermicidal creams (alters normal vaginal bacterial flora) further increases the risk for cystitis. Pyelonephritis most commonly results from ascent of infection up the ureter. **Hematogenous spread** to the urinary tract is uncommon, the exceptions being tuberculosis and cortical renal abscesses. **Lymphogenous spread** is rare. **Direct extension** from other organs may occur, especially from intraperitoneal abscesses in inflammatory bowel disease or pelvic inflammatory disease.

Susceptibility Factors

A. Bacterial Virulence Factors: Over 90% of first infections are caused by *E coli.* While there are over 150 strains of *E coli,* most infections are caused by only five serogroups (O1, O4, O6, O18, and O75). It appears that strains implicated in infection have a higher degree of bacterial adherence, which is mediated by the bacterial fimbriae or pili. A relationship between the type of fimbriae and the type of infection exists. P-fimbriated strains of *E coli* are associated with pyelonephritis in normal urinary tracts, whereas strains without P fimbriae are associated with pyelonephritis only when vesicoureteral reflux is present.

B. Host Susceptibility Factors:

1. Bladder and upper tract factors–Intrinsic defense mechanisms in the bladder include efficient emptying of the bladder with voiding, which decreases colony counts; a protective glycosaminoglycan layer, which interferes with bacterial adherence; and the antimicrobial properties of urine (high osmolality and extremes of pH). The presence of vesicoureteral reflux, diminished renal blood flow, or intrinsic renal disease may increase the likelihood of upper tract involvement.

2. Female-specific factors–The anatomically short female urethra facilitates the ascent of organisms from the introitus into the bladder. Women with recurrent urinary tract infections have more adhesin receptors on their genitourinary mucosa and therefore have more binding sites for pathogens. Women whose mucosal secretions lack fucosyltransferase activity ("nonsecretors") are more prone to urinary tract infections. The lack of this enzyme results in lack of expression of the A, B, and H blood group antigens that normally may mask some of the bacterial adhesin receptors, making these receptors more available for pathogen binding.

3. Male-specific factors–A higher incidence of urinary tract infections in the uncircumcised male in comparison to the circumcised male has been observed. The mucosal surface of the foreskin has a propensity for colonization with P-fimbriated bacteria in a fashion analogous to that of the female introitus. The prostate in normal males secretes zinc, which is a potent antibacterial agent and thus prevents ascending infection. Lower zinc levels are seen in prostatic secretions of men with bacterial prostatitis.

Prevention of Reinfections

Prophylactic antibiotic therapy is given to prevent recurrence after treatment of urinary tract infection.

Women who have more than three episodes of cystitis per year are considered candidates for prophylaxis. Prior to institution of therapy, a thorough urologic evaluation is warranted to exclude any anatomic abnormality (stones, reflux, fistula, etc). Only selected antimicrobial agents are effective in prophylaxis. To be successful, the agent must eliminate pathogenic bacteria from the fecal or introital reservoirs and not cause bacterial resistance. Single dosing at bedtime or at the time of intercourse is the recommended schedule. The three most commonly used agents for prophylaxis are trimethoprim-sulfamethoxazole (40 mg/200 mg), nitrofurantoin (100 mg), and cephalexin (250 mg).

Melekos MD et al: Post-intercourse versus daily ciprofloxacin prophylaxis for recurrent urinary tract infections in premenopausal women. J Urol 1997;157:935. [NLM Cit ID: 97188831] (Long term post-intercourse prophylaxis equally as effective as daily prophylaxis in dramatically reducing incidence of UTI.)

Proceedings of the 5th International Symposium on Clinical Evaluation of Drug Efficacy in Urinary Tract Infection and of the Urinary Tract Infections Symposia of the Commission for Treatment of Urinary Tract Infection of the International Society of Chemotherapy. 29 June–3 July 1997. Sydney, Australia. Int J Antimicrob Agents 1999;11:183. [NLM Cit ID: 99388826]

Semeniuk H et al: Evaluation of the leukocyte esterase and nitrite urine dipstick screening tests for detection of bacteriuria in women with suspected uncomplicated urinary tract infections. J Clin Microbiol 1999;37:3051. [NLM Cit ID: 99380336] (A urine dipstick screen for leukocyte esterase or nitrite may be negative in 19% of patients with significant bacteriuria.)

ACUTE CYSTITIS

Essentials of Diagnosis

- Irritative voiding symptoms.
- Patient usually afebrile.
- Positive urine culture; blood cultures may also be positive.

General Considerations

Acute cystitis is an infection of the bladder most commonly due to the coliform bacteria (especially *E coli*) and occasionally gram-positive bacteria (enterococci). The route of infection is typically ascending from the urethra. Viral cystitis due to adenovirus is sometimes seen in children but is rare in adults.

Clinical Findings

A. Symptoms and Signs: Irritative voiding symptoms (frequency, urgency, dysuria) and suprapubic discomfort are common. Women may experience gross hematuria, and symptoms in women may often appear following sexual intercourse. Physical examination may elicit suprapubic tenderness, but examination is often unremarkable. Systemic toxicity is absent.

B. Laboratory Findings: Urinalysis shows pyuria and bacteriuria and varying degrees of hematuria. The degree of pyuria and bacteriuria does not necessarily correlate with the severity of symptoms. Urine culture is positive for the offending organism, but colony counts exceeding 10^5/mL are not essential for the diagnosis.

C. Imaging: Follow-up imaging is warranted only if pyelonephritis, recurrent infections, or anatomic abnormalities are suspected.

Differential Diagnosis

In women, infectious processes such as vulvovaginitis and pelvic inflammatory disease can usually be distinguished by pelvic examination and urinalysis. In men, urethritis and prostatitis may be distinguished by physical examination (urethral discharge or prostatic tenderness). Cystitis in men is rare and implies a pathologic process such as infected stones, prostatitis, or chronic urinary retention requiring further investigation.

Noninfectious causes of cystitis-like symptoms include pelvic irradiation, chemotherapy (cyclophosphamide), bladder carcinoma, interstitial cystitis, voiding dysfunction disorders, and psychosomatic disorders.

Treatment

Uncomplicated cystitis in women can be treated with short-term antimicrobial therapy, which consists of single-dose therapy or 1–3 days of therapy. Trimethoprim-sulfamethoxazole can be ineffective in significant numbers of patients because of the emergence of resistant organisms. Nitrofurantoin and fluoroquinolones are now the drugs of choice for un-

Table 23–1. Empirical therapy for urinary tract infections.

Diagnosis	Antibiotic	Route	Duration	Cost per Duration Noted[1]
Acute pyelonephritis	Ampicillin, 1 g every 6 hours, and gentamicin, 1 mg/kg every 8 hours	IV	21 days	$348.18 not including IV supplies
	Ciprofloxacin, 750 mg every 12 hours	Orally	21 days	$174.50
	Ofloxacin, 200–300 mg every 12 hours	Orally	21 days	$197.00
	Trimethoprim-sulfamethoxazole, 160/800 mg every 12 hours[2]	Orally	21 days	$7.56
Chronic pyelonephritis	Same as for acute pyelonephritis, but duration of therapy is 3–6 months			
Acute cystitis	Cephalexin, 250–500 mg every 6 hours	Orally	1–3 days	$11.88/3 days (500 mg)
	Ciprofloxacin, 250–500 mg every 12 hours	Orally	1–3 days	$24.93/3 days (500 mg)
	Nitrofurantoin (Macrocrystals), 100 mg every 12 hours	Orally	7 days	$22.54
	Norfloxacin, 400 mg every 12 hours	Orally	1–3 days	$20.40/3 days
	Ofloxacin, 200 mg every 12 hours	Orally	1–3 days	$23.65/3 days
	Trimethoprim-sulfamethoxazole, 160/800 mg, two tablets[2]	Orally	Single dose	$0.36
Acute bacterial prostatitis	Same as for acute pyelonephritis		21 days	
	Ciprofloxacin, 250–500 mg every 12 hours	Orally	1–3 months	$249.00/1 month (500 mg)
	Ofloxacin, 200–400 mg every 12 hours	Orally	1–3 months	$297.00/1 month (400 mg)
	Trimethoprim-sulfamethoxazole, 160/800 mg every 12 hours[2]	Orally	1–3 months	$10.80/month
Acute epididymitis Sexually transmitted	Ceftriaxone, 250 mg as single dose, plus: Doxycycline, 100 mg every 12 hours	IM Orally	 10 days	$15.42/250 mg $7.75
Non-sexually transmitted	Same as for chronic bacterial prostatitis	Orally	3 weeks	

[1]Cost to pharmacist (average wholesale price, generic when possible) for quantity listed. Source: *Drug Topics Red Book,* March 2000; Vol. 19, No. 3.
[2]Increasing resistance noted (up to 20%)

complicated cystitis. (Table 23–1). Because uncomplicated cystitis is rare in men, elucidation of the underlying problem with appropriate investigations is warranted. Hot sitz baths or urinary analgesics (phenazopyridine, 200 mg orally three times daily) may provide symptomatic relief.

Prognosis

Infections typically respond rapidly to therapy, and failure to respond suggests resistance to the selected drug or anatomic abnormalities requiring further investigation.

Chew LD et al: Recurrent cystitis in nonpregnant women. West J Med 1999;170:274. [NLM Cit ID: 99307891] (Continuous or postcoital antibiotic prophylaxis with nitrofurantoin, fluoroquinolones, or TMP-SMZ can reduce infection rates in women with recurrent cystitis.)

Gupta K et al: The prevalence of antimicrobial resistance among uropathogens causing acute uncomplicated cystitis in young women. Int J Antimicrob Agents 1999;11:305. [NLM Cit ID: 99320911] (Increasing resistance to many antibiotics is noted. *E coli,* the most common species isolated, was resistant to ampicillin [25% of the time], tetracycline [24%], and TMP-SMZ [11%].)

Gupta K et al: Increasing prevalence of antimicrobial resistance among uropathogens causing acute uncomplicated cystitis in women. JAMA 1999;281:736. [NLM Cit ID: 99159809] (Resistance of *E coli* in women with uncomplicated cystitis increased from 9% in 1992 to 18% in 1996 and from 8% to 16% among all isolates combined.)

Hooton TM: Diagnosis and treatment of uncomplicated urinary tract infection. Infect Dis Clin North Am 1997; 11:551. [NLM Cit: ID: 98017683]

ACUTE PYELONEPHRITIS

Essentials of Diagnosis

- Fever.
- Flank pain.
- Irritative voiding symptoms.
- Positive urine culture.

General Considerations

Acute pyelonephritis is an infectious inflammatory disease involving the kidney parenchyma and renal pelvis. Gram-negative bacteria are the most common causative agents including *E coli,* proteus, klebsiella, enterobacter, and pseudomonas. Gram-positive bacteria are less commonly seen but include *Enterococcus faecalis* and *Staphylococcus aureus.* The infection usually ascends from the lower urinary tract—with the exception of *S aureus,* which usually is spread by a hematogenous route.

Clinical Findings

A. Symptoms and Signs: Symptoms include fever, flank pain, shaking chills, and irritative voiding symptoms (urgency, frequency, dysuria). Nausea and vomiting and diarrhea are not uncommon. Signs include fever and tachycardia. Costovertebral angle tenderness is usually pronounced.

B. Laboratory Findings: Complete blood count shows leukocytosis and a left shift. Urinalysis shows pyuria, bacteriuria, and varying degrees of hematuria. White cell casts may be seen. Urine culture demonstrates heavy growth of the offending agent, and blood culture may also be positive.

C. Imaging: In complicated pyelonephritis, renal ultrasound may show hydronephrosis from a stone or other source of obstruction.

Differential Diagnosis

Acute intra-abdominal disease such as appendicitis, cholecystitis, pancreatitis, or diverticulitis must be distinguished from pyelonephritis. A normal urinalysis is usually seen in gastrointestinal disorders; however, on occasion, inflammation from adjacent bowel (appendicitis or diverticulitis) may result in hematuria or pyuria. Abnormal liver function tests or elevated amylase levels may assist in the differentiation. Lower lobe pneumonia is distinguishable by the abnormal chest radiograph.

In males, the main differential diagnosis for a febrile urinary tract infection includes acute epididymitis, acute prostatitis, and acute pyelonephritis. Physical examination and the location of the pain should permit this distinction.

Complications

Sepsis with shock can occur with acute pyelonephritis. In diabetics, emphysematous pyelonephritis resulting from gas-producing organisms may be life-threatening if not adequately treated. Healthy adults usually recover complete renal function, yet if coexistent renal disease is present, scarring or chronic pyelonephritis may result. Inadequate therapy could result in abscess formation.

Treatment

Severe infections or complicating factors require hospital admission. Urine and blood cultures are obtained to identify the causative agent and to determine antimicrobial sensitivity. Intravenous ampicillin and an aminoglycoside are initiated prior to obtaining sensitivity results (Table 23–1). In the outpatient setting, quinolones or nitrofurantoin may be initiated (Table 23–1). Antibiotics are adjusted according to sensitivities. Fevers may persist for up to 72 hours; failure to respond warrants radiographic imaging (ultrasound) to exclude complicating factors that may require intervention. Catheter drainage may be necessary in the face of urinary retention and nephrostomy drainage if there is ureteral obstruction. In inpatients, intravenous antibiotics are maintained for 24 hours after the patient defervesces, and oral antibiotics are then given to complete a 3-week course of therapy. Follow-up urine cultures are mandatory several weeks following the completion of treatment.

Prognosis

With prompt diagnosis and appropriate treatment, acute pyelonephritis carries a good prognosis. Complicating factors, underlying renal disease, and increasing patient age may lead to a less favorable outcome.

Behr MA et al: Fever duration in hospitalized acute pyelonephritis patients. Am J Med 1996;101:277. [NLM Cit ID: 97027350] (Fever in treated pyelonephritis can take 4 days to resolve, and routine urologic investigation after 2–3 days of fever may be unwarranted.)

Weidner W et al: Rational diagnostic steps in acute pyelonephritis with special reference to ultrasonography and computed tomography scan. Int J Antimicrob Agents 1999;11:257. [NLM Cit ID: 99320903] (Ultrasonography is an excellent modality to rule out urinary tract obstruction. Patients who respond poorly to antibiotic therapy should have CT of the kidney with and without contrast.)

ACUTE BACTERIAL PROSTATITIS

Essentials of Diagnosis

- Fever.
- Irritative voiding symptoms.
- Perineal or suprapubic pain; exquisite tenderness common on rectal examination.
- Positive urine culture.

General Considerations

Acute bacterial prostatitis is usually caused by gram-negative rods, especially *E coli* and pseudomonas species and less commonly by gram-positive organisms (eg, enterococcus). The most likely routes of infection include ascent up the urethra and reflux of infected urine into the prostatic ducts. Lymphatic and hematogenous routes are probably rare.

Clinical Findings

A. Symptoms and Signs: Perineal, sacral, or suprapubic pain, fever, and irritative voiding complaints are common. Varying degrees of obstructive symptoms may occur as the acutely inflamed prostate swells, which may lead to urinary retention. High fevers and a warm and often exquisitely tender prostate are detected on examination. Care should be taken in performing a gentle rectal examination, as vigorous manipulations may result in septicemia. Prostatic massage is contraindicated.

B. Laboratory Findings: Complete blood count shows leukocytosis and a left shift. Urinalysis shows pyuria, bacteriuria, and varying degrees of hematuria. Urine cultures will demonstrate the offending pathogen.

Differential Diagnosis

Acute pyelonephritis or acute epididymitis should be distinguishable by the location of pain as well as by physical examination. Acute diverticulitis is occasionally confused with acute prostatitis; however, the history and urinalysis should permit clear distinction. Urinary retention from benign or malignant prostatic enlargement is distinguishable by initial or follow-up rectal examination.

Treatment

Hospitalization may be required, and parenteral antibiotics (ampicillin and aminoglycoside) should be initiated until organism sensitivities are available (Table 23–1). After the patient is afebrile for 24–48 hours, oral antibiotics (quinolones) are used to complete 4–6 weeks of therapy. If urinary retention develops, urethral catheterization or instrumentation is contraindicated, and a percutaneous suprapubic tube is required. Follow-up urine culture and examination of prostatic secretions should be performed after the completion of therapy to ensure eradication.

Prognosis

With effective treatment, chronic bacterial prostatitis is rare.

CHRONIC BACTERIAL PROSTATITIS

Essentials of Diagnosis

- Irritative voiding symptoms.
- Perineal or suprapubic discomfort, often dull and poorly localized.
- Positive expressed prostatic secretions and culture.

General Considerations

Although chronic bacterial prostatitis may evolve from acute bacterial prostatitis, many men have no history of acute infection. Gram-negative rods are the most common etiologic agents, but only one gram-positive organism (enterococcus) is associated with chronic infection. Routes of infection are the same as discussed for acute infection.

Clinical Findings

A. Symptoms and Signs: Clinical manifestations are variable. Some patients are asymptomatic, but most have varying degrees of irritative voiding symptoms. Low back and perineal pain is not uncommon. Many patients report a history of urinary tract infections. Physical examination is often unremarkable, though the prostate may feel normal, boggy, or indurated.

B. Laboratory Findings: Urinalysis is normal unless a secondary cystitis is present. Expressed prostatic secretions demonstrate increased numbers of leukocytes (> 10/hpf), especially lipid-laden macrophages. However, this finding is consistent with inflammation and is not diagnostic of bacterial prostatitis. Culture of the secretions or the post-prostatic massage urine specimen is necessary to make the diagnosis.

C. Imaging: Imaging tests are not necessary,

though pelvic radiographs or transrectal ultrasound may demonstrate prostatic calculi.

Differential Diagnosis

Chronic urethritis may mimic chronic prostatitis, though cultures of the fractionated urine may localize the source of infection. Cystitis may be secondary to prostatitis, but fractionated urine samples should localize the infection. Anal disease may share some of the symptoms of prostatitis, but physical examination should permit a distinction between the two.

Treatment

Few antimicrobial agents attain therapeutic intraprostatic levels in the absence of acute inflammation. Trimethoprim does diffuse into the prostate, and trimethoprim-sulfamethoxazole is associated with the best cure rates (Table 23–1). Other effective agents include carbenicillin, erythromycin, cephalexin, and the quinolones. The optimal duration of therapy remains controversial, ranging from 6 to 12 weeks. Symptomatic relief may be provided by anti-inflammatory agents (indomethacin, ibuprofen) and hot sitz baths.

Prognosis

Chronic bacterial prostatitis is difficult to cure, but its symptoms and tendency to cause recurrent urinary tract infections can be controlled by suppressive antibiotic therapy.

NONBACTERIAL PROSTATITIS

Essentials of Diagnosis

- Irritative voiding symptoms.
- Perineal or suprapubic discomfort, similar to that of chronic bacterial prostatitis.
- Positive expressed prostatic secretions, but culture is negative.

General Considerations

Nonbacterial prostatitis is the most common of the prostatitis syndromes, and its cause is unknown. Speculation implicates chlamydiae, mycoplasmas, ureaplasma, and viruses, but no substantial proof exists. In some cases, nonbacterial prostatitis may represent a noninfectious inflammatory disorder. Some investigators have postulated an autoimmune origin. Because the cause of nonbacterial prostatitis remains unknown, the diagnosis is usually one of exclusion.

Clinical Findings

A. Symptoms and Signs: The clinical presentation is identical to that of chronic bacterial prostatitis; however, no history of urinary tract infections is present.

B. Laboratory Findings: Increased numbers of leukocytes are seen on expressed prostatic secretions, but all cultures are negative.

Differential Diagnosis

The major distinction is from chronic bacterial prostatitis. The absence of a history of urinary tract infection and of positive cultures makes the distinction (Table 23–2). In older men with irritative voiding symptoms and negative cultures, the possibility of bladder cancer must be excluded. Urinary cytologic examination and cystoscopy are warranted.

Treatment

Because of the uncertainty regarding the etiology of nonbacterial prostatitis, a trial of antimicrobial therapy directed against ureaplasma, mycoplasma, or chlamydia is warranted. Erythromycin (250 mg orally four times daily) can be initiated for 14 days yet should only be continued (for 3–6 weeks) if a favorable clinical response ensues. Some symptomatic relief may be obtained with anti-inflammatory agents or sitz baths. Dietary restrictions are not necessary unless the patient relates a history of symptom exacerbation by certain substances such as alcohol, caffeine, and perhaps certain foods.

Prognosis

Annoying, recurrent symptoms are common, but serious sequelae have not been identified.

Table 23–2. Clinical characteristics of prostatitis and prostatodynia syndromes.

Findings	Acute Bacterial Prostatitis	Chronic Bacterial Prostatitis	Nonbacterial Prostatitis	Prostatodynia
Fever	+	–	–	–
Urinalysis	+	–	–	–
Expressed prostatic secretions	Contraindicated	+	+	–
Bacterial culture	+	+	–	–

Litwin MS et al: The National Institutes of Health chronic prostatitis symptom index: development and validation of a new outcome measure. Chronic Prostatitis Collaborative Research Network. J Urol 1999;162:369. [NLM Cit ID: 99336822]

Nickel JC et al: Research guidelines for chronic prostatitis: consensus report from the first National Institutes of Health International Prostatitis Collaborative Network. Urology 1999;54:229. [NLM Cit ID: 99371316]

PROSTATODYNIA

Prostatodynia is a noninflammatory disorder that affects young and middle-aged men and has variable causes, including voiding dysfunction and pelvic floor musculature dysfunction. The term "prostatodynia" is a misnomer, as the prostate is actually normal.

Clinical Findings

A. Symptoms and Signs: Symptoms are the same as those seen with chronic prostatitis, yet there is no history of urinary tract infection. Additional symptoms may include hesitancy and interruption of flow. Patients may relate a lifelong history of voiding difficulty. Physical examination is unremarkable, but increased anal sphincter tone and periprostatic tenderness may be observed.

B. Laboratory Findings: Urinalysis is normal. Expressed prostatic secretions show normal numbers of leukocytes. Urodynamic testing may show signs of dysfunctional voiding (detrusor contraction without urethral relaxation, high urethral pressures, spasms of the urinary sphincter) and is indicated in patients failing empiric trials of alpha-blockers or anticholinergics.

Differential Diagnosis

Normal urinalysis will distinguish it from acute infectious processes. Examination of expressed prostatic secretions will distinguish this entity from prostatitis syndromes (Table 23–2).

Treatment

Bladder neck and urethral spasms can be treated by α-blocking agents (terazosin, 1–10 mg orally once a day; or doxazosin, 1–8 mg orally once a day). Pelvic floor muscle dysfunction may respond to diazepam and biofeedback techniques. Sitz baths may contribute to symptomatic relief.

Prognosis

Prognosis is variable depending upon the specific cause.

Pewitt EB et al: Urinary tract infection in urology, including acute and chronic prostatitis. Infect Dis Clin North Am 1997;11:623. [NLM Cit ID: 98017687]

Roberts RO et al: A review of clinical and pathological prostatitis syndromes. Urology 1997;49:809. [NLM Cit ID: 97331352]

ACUTE EPIDIDYMITIS

Essentials of Diagnosis

- Fever.
- Irritative voiding symptoms.
- Painful enlargement of epididymis.

General Considerations

Most cases of acute epididymitis are infectious and can be divided into one of two categories that have different age distributions and etiologic agents. Sexually transmitted forms typically occur in men under age 40, are associated with urethritis, and result from *C trachomatis* or *N gonorrhoeae.* Non-sexually transmitted forms typically occur in older men, are associated with urinary tract infections and prostatitis, and are caused by gram-negative rods. The route of infection is probably via the urethra to the ejaculatory duct and then down the vas deferens to the epididymis. Amiodarone has been associated with self-limited epididymitis.

Clinical Findings

A. Symptoms and Signs: Symptoms may follow acute physical strain (heavy lifting), trauma, or sexual activity. Associated symptoms of urethritis (pain at the tip of the penis and urethral discharge) or cystitis (irritative voiding symptoms) may occur. Pain develops in the scrotum and may radiate along the spermatic cord or to the flank. Fever and scrotal swelling are usually apparent. Early in the course, the epididymis may be distinguishable from the testis; however, later the two may appear as one enlarged, tender mass. The prostate may be tender on rectal examination.

B. Laboratory Findings: Complete blood count shows leukocytosis and a left shift. In the sexually transmitted variety, Gram staining of a smear of urethral discharge may be diagnostic of gram-negative intracellular diplococci *(N gonorrhoeae).* White cells without visible organisms on urethral smear represent nongonococcal urethritis, and *C trachomatis* is the most likely pathogen. In the non-sexually transmitted variety, urinalysis shows pyuria, bacteriuria, and varying degrees of hematuria. Urine cultures will demonstrate the offending pathogen.

C. Imaging: Scrotal ultrasound may aid in the diagnosis if examination is difficult because of the presence of a large hydrocele or because questions exist regarding the diagnosis.

Differential Diagnosis

Tumors generally cause painless enlargement of the testis. Urinalysis is negative, and examination reveals a normal epididymis. Scrotal ultrasound is helpful to define the pathology. Testicular torsion usually occurs in prepubertal males but is occasionally seen in young adults. Acute onset of symptoms and a negative urinalysis favor testicular torsion or torsion of one of the testicular or epididymal appendages. Prehn's sign (elevation of the scrotum above the pubic symphysis improves pain from epididymitis) may be helpful but is not reliable.

Treatment

Bed rest with scrotal elevation is important in the acute phase. Treatment is directed toward the identified pathogen (Table 23–1). The sexually transmitted variety is treated with 10–21 days of antibiotics, and the sexual partner must be treated as well. Non-sexually transmitted forms are treated for 21–28 days with appropriate antibiotics, at which time evaluation of the urinary tract is warranted to identify underlying disease.

Prognosis

Prompt treatment usually results in a favorable outcome. Delayed or inadequate treatment may result in epididymo-orchitis, decreased fertility, or abscess formation.

Barloon TJ et al: Diagnostic imaging of patients with acute scrotal pain. Am Fam Physician 1996;53:1734. [NLM Cit ID: 96209655] (Doppler ultrasound can be useful in distinguishing between epididymitis [increased blood flow] and testicular torsion [decreased blood flow].)

Joly-Guillou ML et al: Practical recommendations for the drug treatment of bacterial infections of the male genital tract including urethritis, epididymitis and prostatitis. Drugs 1999;57:743. [NLM Cit ID: 99279739] (Men less than 35 years usually have infections caused by sexually transmitted bacteria, while those over 35 usually have infections related to Enterobacteriaceae.)

URINARY STONE DISEASE

Urinary stone disease is exceeded in frequency as a urinary tract disorder only by infections and prostatic disease and is estimated to afflict 240,000–720,000 Americans per year. Men are more frequently affected by urolithiasis than women, with a ratio of 4:1. Initial presentation predominates in the third and fourth decades. The ratio of men to women approaches parity in the sixth and seventh decades.

Urinary calculi are polycrystalline aggregates composed of varying amounts of crystalloid and a small amount of organic matrix. Stone formation requires saturated urine that is dependent upon pH, ionic strength, solute concentration, and complexation. There are five major types of urinary stones: calcium oxalate, calcium phosphate, struvite, uric acid, and cystine. The most common types are composed of calcium, and for that reason most urinary stones (85%) are radiopaque. Uric acid stones can be radiolucent yet frequently are composed of a combination of uric acid and calcium oxalate and thus are radiopaque. Cystine stones frequently have a smooth-edged ground-glass appearance.

Geographic factors contribute to the development of stones. Areas of high humidity and elevated temperatures appear to be contributing factors, and the incidence of symptomatic ureteral stones is greatest during hot summer months.

Diet and fluid intake may be important factors in the development of urinary stones. Those afflicted with recurrent urinary stone disease are encouraged to maintain a diet restricted in sodium and protein intake. Sodium should be restricted to 100 meq/d. Increased sodium intake will increase sodium and calcium excretion and increase monosodium urate saturation (that can act as a nidus for stone growth), and increase the relative saturation of calcium phosphate, and a decrease in urinary citrate excretion. All of these factors encourage stone growth. Protein intake should be limited to 1 g/kg/d. An increased protein load can also increase calcium, oxalate, and uric acid excretion and can also decrease urinary citrate excretion. Carbohydrates and fats have not been proved to have any impact on urinary stone disease. Bran can significantly decrease urinary calcium by increasing bowel transit time and mechanically binding to calcium. Excess intake of oxalate and purines can increase the incidence of stones in predisposed individuals. Although a reduction in dietary calcium results in reduced urinary calcium, the concurrent increase in urinary oxalate may promote stone formation. Only type II absorptive hypercalciuric patients (see below) benefit from a low-calcium diet. Persons in sedentary occupations have a higher incidence of stones than manual laborers.

Genetic factors may contribute to urinary stone formation. Cystinuria is an autosomal recessive disorder. Homozygous individuals have markedly increased excretion of cystine and frequently have numerous recurrent episodes of urinary stones despite attempts to optimize medical treatment. Distal renal tubular acidosis may be transmitted as a hereditary trait, and urolithiasis occurs in up to 75% of patients affected with this disorder.

Clinical Findings

A. Symptoms and Signs: Obstructing urinary stones usually present with colic. Pain usually occurs suddenly and may awaken patients from sleep. It is localized to the flank, is usually severe, and may be associated with nausea and vomiting. Patients are constantly moving—in sharp contrast to those with an acute abdomen. The pain may occur episodically and may radiate anteriorly over the abdomen. As the stone progresses down the ureter, the pain may be referred into the ipsilateral testis or labium. If the stone becomes lodged at the ureterovesical junction, patients will complain of marked urinary urgency and frequency. Stone size does not correlate with the severity of the symptoms.

B. Metabolic Evaluation: Stone analysis should be performed on recovered stones. Controversy exists in deciding which patients need a thorough metabolic evaluation for stone disease. Uncomplicated first-time stone-formers should probably undergo blood screening for abnormalities of serum calcium, phosphate, electrolytes, and uric acid as a baseline.

More extensive evaluation is required in recurrent stone-formers or patients with a family history of stone disease. A 24-hour urine collection on a random diet should ascertain volume, urinary pH, and calcium, uric acid, oxalate, phosphate, and citrate excretion. A second collection on a restricted calcium (400 mg/d) and sodium (100 meq/d) diet is undertaken to subcategorize patients, if necessary. Serum PTH and calcium load tests can be performed at a third visit. A calcium load test is performed as follows: After a patient has been on a restricted calcium diet for at least 1 week, the patient is told to fast from 9 PM. The patient discards his early morning voided specimen (7 AM). While still fasting, the patient voids at 9 AM, which is the fasting sample. The patient then ingests 1 g of calcium gluconate, and all urine is collected from 9 AM to 1 PM, the calcium load sample. Table 23–3 demonstrates the diagnostic criteria for the hypercalciuric states. (See discussion below.)

C. Laboratory Findings: Urinalysis usually reveals microscopic or gross (≈ 10%) hematuria. However, the absence of microhematuria does not exclude urinary stones. Infection must be excluded, because the combination of infection and urinary tract obstruction requires prompt intervention as described below. Urinary pH is a valuable clue to the cause of the possible stone. Normal urine pH is 5.85. There is a normal postprandial urinary alkaline tide. Numerous dipstick measurements are valuable in the complete workup of a stone patient. Persistent urinary pH below 5.0 is suggestive of uric acid or cystine stones, both relatively radiolucent as seen on plain films of the abdomen. In contrast, a persistent pH above 7.5 is suggestive of a struvite infection stone, radiopaque on plain films.

D. Imaging: A plain film of the abdomen and renal ultrasound examination will diagnose most stones. Spiral CT has emerged as a useful tool in evaluating flank pain with sensitivities for kidney stones in some trials exceeding those of ultrasound and intravenous urography. Stones suspected of being located at the ureterovesical junction can be imaged with abdominal ultrasonography with the aid of the acoustic window of a full bladder. Alternatively, transvaginal or transrectal ultrasonography will help identify calculi near the ureterovesical junction. When the diagnosis remains uncertain, intravenous urography is indicated.

Medical Treatment & Prevention

To reduce the recurrence rate of urinary stones, one must attempt to achieve a stone-free status. Small stone fragments may serve as a nidus for future stone development. Selected patients must be thoroughly evaluated to reduce stone recurrence rates. Uric acid stone-formers may have recurrences within months if appropriate therapy is not initiated. If no medical treatment is provided after surgical stone removal, stones will generally recur in 50% of patients within 5 years. Of greatest importance in reducing stone recurrence is an increased fluid intake. Absolute volumes are not established, but doubling previous fluid intake is recommended. Patients are encouraged to ingest fluids during meals, 2 hours after each meal (when the body is most dehydrated), and prior to going to sleep in the evening—enough to awaken the patient to void and to ingest additional fluids during the night. Increasing fluids only during daylight hours may not dilute a supersaturated urine and thus initiate a new stone.

A. Calcium Nephrolithiasis:

1. Hypercalciuric–Hypercalciuric calcium nephrolithiasis (> 200 mg/24 h) can be caused by absorptive, resorptive, and renal disorders.

Absorptive hypercalciuria is secondary to increased absorption of calcium at the level of the small bowel, predominantly in the jejunum, and can be further subdivided into types I, II, and III. Type I ab-

Table 23–3. Diagnostic criteria of different types of hypercalciuria.

	Absorptive Type I	Absorptive Type II	Absorptive Type III	Resorptive	Renal
Serum					
Calcium	N	N	N	↑	N
Phosphorus	N	N	↓	↓	N
PTH	N	N	N	↑	↑
Vitamin D	N	N	↑	↑	↑
Urinary calcium					
Fasting	N	N	↑	↑	↑
Restricted	↑	N	↑	↑	↑
After calcium load	↑	↑	↑	↑	↑

Key: ↑ = elevated, ↓ = low, N = normal

sorptive hypercalciuria is independent of calcium intake. There is increased urinary calcium on a regular or even a calcium-restricted diet. Treatment is centered upon decreasing bowel absorption of calcium. Cellulose phosphate, a chelating agent, is an effective form of therapy. An average dose is 10–15 g in three divided doses. It binds to the calcium and impedes small bowel absorption due to its increased bulk. Cellulose phosphate does not change the intestinal transport mechanism. It should be given with meals so it will be available to bind to the calcium. Taking this chelating agent prior to bedtime is ineffective. Postmenopausal women should be treated with caution. It is interesting, however, that there is no enhanced decline in bone density after long-term use. Inappropriate use without an initial metabolic evaluation (see above) may result in a negative calcium balance and a secondary parathyroid stimulation. Long-term use without follow-up metabolic surveillance may result in hypomagnesemia and secondary hyperoxaluria and recurrent calculi. Routine follow-up every 6–8 months will help encourage medical compliance and permit adjustments in medical therapy based upon repeat metabolic studies.

Thiazide therapy is an alternative to cellulose phosphate in the treatment of type I absorptive hypercalciuria. Thiazides decrease renal calcium excretion but have no impact on intestinal absorption. This therapy results in increased bone density of approximately 1% per year. Thiazides have limited long-term utility (< 5 years) as they lose their hypocalciuric effect with continued therapy.

Type II absorptive hypercalciuria is diet-dependent. Decreasing calcium intake by 50% (approximately 400 mg/d) will decrease the hypercalciuria to normal values (150–200 mg/24 h). There is no specific medical therapy.

Type III absorptive hypercalciuria is secondary to a renal phosphate leak. This results in increased vitamin D synthesis and secondarily increased small bowel absorption of calcium. This can be readily reversed by orthophosphates (0.5 g three times per day). Orthophosphates do not change intestinal absorption but rather inhibit vitamin D synthesis.

Resorptive hypercalciuria is secondary to hyperparathyroidism. Hypercalcemia, hypophosphatemia, hypercalciuria, and an elevated parathyroid hormone value are found. Appropriate surgical resection of the adenoma cures the disease and the urinary stones. Medical management is invariably a failure.

Renal hypercalciuria occurs when the renal tubules are unable to efficiently reabsorb filtered calcium, and hypercalciuria results. Spilling calcium in the urine results in secondary hyperparathyroidism. Serum calcium is normal. Thiazides are effective long-term therapy in patients with this disorder.

2. Hyperuricosuric–Hyperuricosuric calcium nephrolithiasis is secondary to dietary excesses or uric acid metabolic defects. Both disorders can be treated with purine dietary restrictions or allopurinol therapy (or both). In contrast to uric acid nephrolithiasis, patients with hyperuricosuric calcium stones will maintain a urinary pH greater than 5.5. Monosodium urates absorb inhibitors and promote heterogeneous nucleation. Hyperuricosuric calcium nephrolithiasis is probably secondary to epitaxy, or heterogeneous nucleation. In such situations, similar crystal structures (ie, uric acid and calcium oxalate) can grow together with the aid of a protein matrix infrastructure.

3. Hyperoxaluric–Hyperoxaluric calcium nephrolithiasis is usually due to primary intestinal disorders. Patients usually present with a history of chronic diarrhea frequently associated with inflammatory bowel disease or steatorrhea. Increased bowel fat combines with intraluminal calcium to form a soap-like product. Calcium is therefore unavailable to bind to oxalate, which is then freely and rapidly absorbed. A small increase in oxalate absorption will significantly increase stone formation. If the diarrhea or steatorrhea cannot be effectively curtailed, oral calcium supplements should be given with meals. It remains controversial whether excess ascorbic acid increases urinary oxalate levels. Emphasis on encouraging increased fluid intake is required for these patients as for all stone-formers.

Any condition that results in metabolic acidosis (including prolonged fasting, hypomagnesemia, and hypokalemia) will decrease urinary citrate excretion, since it will be consumed by the citric acid cycle within the mitochondria of renal cells.

4. Hypocitraturic–Hypocitraturic calcium nephrolithiasis may be secondary to chronic diarrhea, type I (distal) renal tubular acidosis, chronic hydrochlorothiazide treatment, and, in rare cases, is idiopathic. It is frequently associated with other forms of calcium stone formation. Citrate appears to bind to calcium in solution, thereby decreasing available calcium for stone formation. Potassium citrate supplements are usually effective. Urinary citrate is decreased in acidosis and is increased during alkalosis. The potassium will supplement the frequent hypokalemic states, and citrate will help to correct the acidosis. A typical dose is 20 meq three times a day (available in solution or in 5 and 10 meq tablets or in crystal formulations).

B. Uric Acid Calculi: The average urinary pH is 5.85. Uric acid stone-formers frequently have urinary pH values less than 5.5. The pK of uric acid is 5.75, at which point half of the uric acid is ionized as a urate salt and is soluble, while the other half is insoluble. Increasing the pH above 6.5 dramatically increases solubility and can effectively dissolve large calculi. Potassium citrate is the most frequently used medication to increase urinary pH. It can be given in liquid preparation, as crystals that need to be taken with fluids, or as tablets (10 meq), two by mouth three or four times daily. Compliant urinary alkalinization may dissolve uric acid calculi at a rate of 1 cm of stone per month. Patients with uric acid calculi should be given Nitrazine pH paper with which to monitor the effectiveness of their urinary alkalinization. Other contributing factors include hyperuricemia, myeloproliferative disorders, malignancy with increased uric acid production, abrupt and dramatic weight loss, and uricosuric medications. If hyperuricemia is present, allopurinol (300 mg/d) may be given. Although pure uric acid stones are relatively radiolucent, most have some calcium components and can be visualized on plain abdominal radiographs. Renal ultrasonography is a helpful adjunct for appropriate diagnosis and long-term management.

C. Struvite Calculi: Struvite stones are synonymous with magnesium-ammonium-phosphate stones. They are commonly seen in women with recurrent urinary tract infections recalcitrant to appropriate antibiotics. They rarely form as ureteral stones without prior upper tract endourologic intervention. Frequently they are discovered as a large staghorn calculus forming a cast of the renal collecting system. These stones are radiodense. Urinary pH is high, usually above 7.0–7.5. These stones are formed secondary to urease-producing organisms, including proteus, pseudomonas, providencia, and, less commonly, klebsiella, staphylococci, and mycoplasma. An *E coli* urinary tract infection is not consistent with an infectious reservoir originating from a struvite calculus. These frequently large stones are relatively soft and amenable to percutaneous nephrolithotomy. Appropriate perioperative antibiotics are required. They can recur rapidly, and efforts should be taken to render the patient stone-free. Postoperative irrigation through nephrostomy tubes can eliminate small fragments. Acetohydroxamic acid is an effective urease inhibitor, but it is poorly tolerated by most patients because of its gastrointestinal toxicity.

D. Cystine Calculi: Cystine stones are a result of abnormal excretion of cystine, ornithine, lysine, and arginine. Cystine is the only amino acid that becomes insoluble in urine. These stones are particularly difficult to manage medically. Prevention is centered around increased fluid intake, alkalinization of the urine above pH 7.5 (monitored with Nitrazine pH paper), and a variety of medications including penicillamine and tiopronin.

Surgical Treatment

Forced intravenous fluids will not push stones down the ureter. Effective peristalsis directing a bolus of urine down the ureter requires opposing ureteral walls to approach each other and touch, which large dilated systems cannot do. In fact, diuresis is counterproductive and will exacerbate the pain. Associated fever may represent infection, a medical emergency requiring prompt drainage by a ureteral catheter or a percutaneous nephrostomy tube. Antibiotics alone are inadequate unless obstruction is released.

A. Ureteral Stones: Impediment to urine flow by ureteral stones usually occurs at three sites: (1) at the ureteropelvic junction, (2) at the crossing of the ureter over the iliac vessels, and finally (3) as the ureter enters the bladder at the ureterovesical junction. Prediction of spontaneous stone passage is difficult. Stones less than 6 mm in diameter as seen on a plain abdominal radiograph will usually pass spontaneously. Conservative observation with appropriate pain medications is appropriate for the first 6 weeks. If spontaneous stone passage has failed, therapeutic intervention is required. Distal ureteral stones are best managed either with ureteroscopic stone extraction or in situ extracorporeal shock wave lithotripsy (ESWL). Ureteroscopic stone extraction involves placement of a small endoscope through the urethra and into the ureter. Under direct vision, basket extraction or fragmentation followed by extraction is performed. Complications during endoscopic retrieval increase as the duration of conservative observation increases beyond 6 weeks. Indications for earlier intervention include severe pain unresponsive to medications, fever, persistent nausea and vomiting requiring intravenous hydration, social requirements requiring return to work, or anticipated travel. Most upper tract stones that enter the bladder can exit the urethra with minimal discomfort.

In situ ESWL, an alternative, utilizes an external energy source that is focused upon the stone. This focused energy is additive, resulting in minimal tissue insult except at the focus where the stone is positioned with the aid of fluoroscopy or ultrasonography. This can be performed under anesthesia as an outpatient procedure and usually results in stone fragmentation. Most stone fragments will pass uneventfully within 2 weeks, but those that have not passed within 3 months are unlikely to pass without intervention. Women of childbearing age are best not treated with ESWL for a stone in the lower ureter, as the impact upon the ovary is unknown.

Proximal and midureteral stones—those above the inferior margin of the sacroiliac joint—can be treated with ESWL or ureteroscopy. ESWL is delivered directly to the stone (in situ), or the stones can be pushed back into the renal pelvis (via a retrograde ureteral catheter) to allow for a more capacious surrounding space and more efficient fragmentation. To help ensure adequate drainage after ESWL, a double J ureteral stent is frequently placed. Double J stents do not ensure passage of stone fragments after ESWL. Occasionally, stone fragments will obstruct the ureter after ESWL. Conservative management will usually result in spontaneous resolution with eventual passage of the stone fragments. If this is unsuccessful, adequate proximal drainage through a percutaneous nephrostomy tube will facilitate passage. In rare instances, ureteroscopic extraction will be required.

B. Renal Stones: Patients with renal calculi presenting without pain, urinary tract infections, or obstruction need not be treated. They should be followed with serial abdominal radiographs or renal ultrasonographic examinations. If calculi are growing or become symptomatic, intervention should be undertaken. Renal stones less than 3 cm in diameter are best treated with ESWL. Stones located in the inferior calix frequently result in suboptimal stone-free rates as measured at 3 months by x-ray. Such stones and others of larger diameter are best treated via percutaneous nephrolithotomy. Perioperative antibiotic coverage should be given on the basis of preoperative urine cultures.

Denton ER et al: Unenhanced helical CT for renal colic—is the radiation dose justifiable? Clin Radiol 1999;54:444. [NLM Cit ID: 99364383] (Noncontrast CT avoids the risks of intravenous contrast associated with an intravenous pyelography but exposes the patient to three times the radiation.)

Fielding JR et al: Spiral computerized tomography in the evaluation of acute flank pain: A replacement for excretory urography. J Urol 1997;157:2071. [NLM Cit ID: 97292042] (Among 100 patients presenting to the emergency room with flank pain, spiral CT had sensitivity of 98%, specificity of 100%, and 97% negative predictive value.)

Kosar A et al: Comparative study of long-term stone recurrence after extracorporeal shock wave lithotripsy and open stone surgery for kidney stones. Int J Urol 1999;6:125. [NLM Cit ID: 99243409] (Stone burden is a key determinant of recurrent urinary stone disease after ESWL or open stone surgery.)

Larkin GL et al: Efficacy of ketorolac tromethamine versus meperidine in the ED treatment of acute renal colic. Am J Emerg Med 1999;17:6. [NLM Cit ID: 99125767] (Ketorolac was more effective than meperidine in reducing renal colic.)

Parivar F et al: The influence of diet on urinary stone disease. J Urol 1996;155:432. [NLM Cit ID: 96134266] (In an extensive literature review, dietary manipulation was beneficial in the prevention of recurrent urolithiasis in only a selected group of patients.)

URINARY INCONTINENCE

Urinary incontinence is most common in older patients. Its prevalence varies from 5% to 15% in the community to perhaps more than 50% in long-term care facilities. The normal urinary bladder can store relatively large volumes of urine at low pressures. Continence is dependent upon a compliant reservoir and sphincteric efficiency that has two components: the involuntary smooth muscle of the bladder neck and the voluntary skeletal muscle of the external sphincter. (See also discussion in Chapter 3.)

Classification

Urinary incontinence occurs when urine leaks involuntarily and can be classified into one of four categories.

A. Total Incontinence: With total incontinence, patients lose urine at all times and in all positions. This results when sphincteric efficiency is lost (previous surgery, nerve damage, cancerous infiltration) or when an abnormal connection between the urinary tract and the skin exists that bypasses the urinary sphincter (vesicovaginal or ureterovaginal fistulas).

B. Stress Incontinence: Stress incontinence is the loss of urine associated with activities that result in an increase in intra-abdominal pressure (coughing, sneezing, lifting, exercising). Patients do not leak in the supine position. Laxity of the pelvic floor musculature—most commonly seen in the multiparous woman or in patients who have undergone pelvic surgery—results in urethral sphincteric insufficiency.

C. Urge Incontinence: The uncontrolled loss of urine that is preceded by a strong, unexpected urge to void is known as urge incontinence. It is unrelated to position or activity and is indicative of detrusor hyperreflexia or sphincter dysfunction. Inflammatory conditions or neurogenic disorders of the bladder are commonly associated with urge incontinence.

D. Overflow Incontinence: Chronic urinary retention may result in overflow incontinence. Incontinence results from the chronically distended bladder receiving an additional increment of urine, so that intravesical pressure just exceeds the outlet resistance, allowing a small amount of urine to dribble out.

Clinical Findings

A. Symptoms and Signs: The history is the most important step in the evaluation of urinary incontinence. It may be supplemented with a voiding diary prepared by the patient. Physical examination is important to exclude fistula for cases of total incontinence, neurologic abnormalities in cases of urge incontinence (spasticity, flaccidity, rectal sphincter tone), or the distended bladder in cases of overflow incontinence. Rectal examination will reveal the general function of the pelvic floor. Normal anal tone suggests an intact external sphincter. A tender levator ani suggests an overfacilitated pelvic floor. A lax sphincter suggests a lower motor neuron lesion. The bulbocavernosus reflex further confirms the integrity of the lower motor neurons. This reflex is confirmed by feeling an anal contraction in response to pressure on the glans penis or the clitoris.

B. Laboratory Findings: Urinalysis and urine culture are important to exclude urinary tract infection in cases of urge incontinence. Abnormal renal function may be detected in cases of overflow incontinence. Cystograms may demonstrate fistula sites. Lateral stress cystograms may show descensus of the bladder neck (descent of bladder neck more than 1.5 cm on straining view) in cases of stress incontinence.

Those suspected of overflow incontinence can have postvoid residual urine volume assessed by urethral catheterization or ultrasonography.

C. Special Tests: Urinary continence depends upon both bladder and sphincteric mechanisms; dysfunction of either component may result in incontinence. Urodynamic evaluation can assess both bladder and sphincteric function. Such testing is indicated in patients with moderate to severe incontinence, those suspected of having neurologic disease, and those with urge incontinence when infection and neoplasm have been excluded.

Bladder capacity, accommodation, sensation, voluntary control, contractility, and response to pharmacologic intervention can be assessed by cystometry. Cystometry is performed by filling the bladder with water or CO_2 and simultaneously recording intravesical pressure.

During filling, the normal bladder has the ability to maintain a low pressure. As volume increases, compliance increases. Normal sensation is first appreciated with volumes less than 150 mL. There is a strong sensation prior to micturition. Normal capacity in an adult bladder is 350–500 mL. Micturition is consciously initiated starting with pelvic floor relaxation followed by a sustained bladder contraction. Normal bladder function will empty the bladder completely. Uninhibited contractions during the normal filling phase are abnormal and are usually associated with a strong urge to void. Causes of decreased urinary capacity include incontinence, infections, interstitial cystitis, radiation damage, upper motor neuron lesions, and postoperative changes. Increased bladder capacity is seen with chronic urinary tract obstruction, lower motor neuron lesions, and sensory neuropathies.

Responses to routine medications during cystometry will help confirm a diagnosis and facilitate appropriate therapy. Lack of an appropriate detrusor contraction may be secondary to poor bladder muscle function or inadequate filling. Myogenic function can be assessed with bethanechol chloride, a parasympathomimetic drug. Lack of response to intravenous bethanechol suggests intrinsic muscle damage. In contrast, an exaggerated response is suggestive of a lower motor neuron lesion.

Sphincteric function assessment is necessary in the evaluation of urinary incontinence. More formal evaluation of the urinary sphincter may be performed using urethral profilometry, electromyography, or combined video studies.

Treatment

A. Total Incontinence: True incontinence is due to anatomic abnormalities, either congenital or acquired. Congenital defects, including bladder exstrophy, ectopic ureteral orifices, and urethral diverticula, and acquired lesions such as vesicovaginal fistulas require surgical correction. Sphincter injuries following prostatectomy may be managed by surgical reconstruction (bladder neck reconstruction), periurethral collagen injections, or placement of an artificial urinary sphincter.

B. Stress Incontinence: In patients with stress urinary incontinence, the bladder neck will descend below the midportion of the pubic symphysis when viewed on a lateral stress cystogram. Urodynamic investigations usually reveal a shortened functional urethral length, decreased urethral closure pressure, minimal augmentation of closure pressure with stress activities, decreased urethral pressure and length when assuming an upright position, and decreased closure pressure with bladder filling.

If hypoestrogenism of the vagina or urethra is discovered, topical estrogen creams applied locally are indicated. Mild cases can be treated medically with agents directed at increasing urethral resistance (phenylpropanolamine, 50 mg orally daily). Surgical treatment is centered upon placing the bladder neck into an appropriate anatomic location, allowing increased intra-abdominal pressure to be transmitted to both the bladder and the bladder neck. These procedures also lengthen the urethra. Transvaginal or suprapubic (culpocystourethropexy) approaches can pull the bladder neck into proper position. Surgery is usually corrective.

C. Urge Incontinence: The etiology of urge urinary incontinence includes urethral or detrusor instability or a combination of these mechanisms. Treatment is medical rather than surgical. Effective agents include antispasmodic medication (oxybutinin, 5 mg orally three times daily), anticholinergic medication (propantheline 15 mg orally three times daily), or tricyclic antidepressants (imipramine, 25–75 mg orally at bedtime). Sacral nerve stimulation can be effective in treating refractory urinary urge incontinence.

D. Overflow Incontinence: Placement of a urethral catheter is both diagnostic and therapeutic in the acute setting. Further treatment must address the underlying disease. Men with benign prostatic hyperplasia can be treated with medical therapy, prostatectomy, or newer less invasive procedures (see below). Patients with urethral strictures can be treated with a direct internal urethrotomy or open urethroplasty. Neurogenic causes (external sphincteric spasticity) may be managed with intermittent catheterization regimens with or without pharmacotherapy.

[Urinary Incontinence in Adults: 1996 Update (Clinical Guide)]
http://text.nlm.nih.gov/ftrs/pick?collect=ahcpr&dbName=cuic&cd=1&t=948686686

Butler RN et al: Urinary incontinence: keys to diagnosis of the older woman. 1. Geriatrics 1999;54:22, 29. [NLM Cit ID: 20010571] (The topic of urinary incontinence should be addressed, especially in older patients.)

Jackson S et al: The effect of oestrogen supplementation on post-menopausal urinary stress incontinence: a double-blind placebo-controlled trial. Br J Obstet Gynaecol 1999;106:711. [NLM Cit ID: 99355483] (Estrogen supplementation is ineffective in treating postmenopausal stress urinary incontinence.)

JAMA patient page: Incontinence. JAMA 1998;280:2054. [NLM Cit ID: 99079565]

Knapp PM Jr: Identifying and treating urinary incontinence: The crucial role of the primary care physician. Postgrad Med 1998;103:279. [NLM Cit ID: 998214217] (General review.)

Ouslander JG et al: Does eradicating bacteriuria affect the severity of chronic urinary incontinence in nursing home residents? Ann Intern Med 1995;122:749. [NLM Cit ID: 95233644]

Resnick NM: Urinary incontinence. Lancet 1995;346:94. [NLM Cit ID: 95326822] (General review.)

Schmidt RA et al: Sacral nerve stimulation for treatment of refractory urinary urge incontinence. Sacral Nerve Stimulation Study Group. J Urol 1999;162:352. [NLM Cit ID: 99336818] (Sacral nerve stimulation is a treatment option for refractory urge urinary incontinence.)

Swami SK et al: Urge incontinence. Urol Clin North Am 1996;23:417. [NLM Cit ID: 96323074] (Entire volume dedicated to urinary incontinence.)

INTERSTITIAL CYSTITIS

Essentials of Diagnosis

- Pain with a full bladder or urinary urgency.
- Submucosal petechiae on cystoscopic examination.
- Diagnosis of exclusion.

General Considerations

Interstitial cystitis is characterized by pain with bladder filling that is relieved by emptying and is often associated with urgency and frequency. This is a diagnosis of exclusion, and patients must have a negative urine culture and cytology and no other obvious cause such as radiation cystitis, chemical cystitis (cyclophosphamide), vaginitis, urethral diverticulum, or genital herpes.

Population-based studies have demonstrated a prevalence of between 18 and 40 per 100,000 people. Both sexes are involved, but the majority of patients are women with a mean age of 40 years at onset. Patients with interstitial cystitis are more likely to report bladder problems in childhood, and there appears to be a higher prevalence in Jewish women. Up to 50% of patients may experience spontaneous remission of symptoms, with a mean duration of 8 months without treatment.

The etiology of interstitial cystitis is unknown, and it is most likely not a single disease but rather several diseases with similar symptomatology. Associated diseases include severe allergies, irritable bowel syndrome, or inflammatory bowel disease. Theories regarding the cause of interstitial cystitis include increased epithelial permeability, neurogenic causes (sensory nervous system abnormalities), and autoimmunity.

Clinical Findings

A. Symptoms and Signs: Pain with bladder filling that is relieved with urination or urgency, frequency, and nocturia are the most common symptoms. Exposures such as pelvic radiation or prior cyclophosphamide should be inquired about. Examination should exclude genital herpes, vaginitis, or a urethral diverticulum.

B. Laboratory Findings: Urinalysis and urine culture are obtained to exclude infectious causes. Urinary cytology is obtained to exclude bladder malignancy. Urodynamic testing assesses bladder sensation and compliance and excludes detrusor instability.

C. Cystoscopy: The bladder is distended with fluid (hydrodistention) to detect glomerulations (submucosal hemorrhage), which must be present in at least three quadrants of the bladder. Biopsy should be performed to exclude other causes such as carcinoma, eosinophilic cystitis, and tuberculous cystitis. The presence of submucosal mast cells is not needed to make the diagnosis of interstitial cystitis.

Differential Diagnosis

Exposures to radiation or cyclophosphamide are obtained by the history. Bacterial cystitis, genital herpes, or vaginitis can be excluded by urinalysis, culture, and physical examination. A urethral diverticulum may be suspected if palpation of the urethra demonstrates an indurated mass that results in the expression of pus from the urethral meatus. Urethral carcinoma presents as a firm mass on palpation.

Treatment

There is no cure for interstitial cystitis, but most patients achieve symptomatic relief from one of several approaches, including hydrodistention, which is usually done as part of the diagnostic evaluation. Approximately 20–30% of patients will notice symptomatic improvement following this maneuver. Also of importance is the measurement of bladder capacity during hydrodistention, since patients with very small bladder capacities (< 200 mL) are unlikely to respond to medical therapy.

Amitriptyline is often used as first-line medical therapy in patients with interstitial cystitis. Both central and peripheral mechanisms may contribute to its activity. Nifedipine and other calcium channel blockers have also demonstrated some activity in interstitial cystitis patients. Pentosan polysulfate sodium (Elmiron) is an oral synthetic sulfated polysaccharide that helps restore integrity to the epithelium of the bladder in a few patients.

The mainstay of therapy for interstitial cystitis is intravesical instillation of dimethyl sulfoxide (DMSO). Other agents, including heparin and BCG, are being investigated, with the latter achieving up to 60% response rates.

Other treatment modalities include transcutaneous electric nerve stimulation (TENS) and acupuncture. Surgical therapy for interstitial cystitis should only be considered as a last resort and may require cystourethrectomy with urinary diversion.

Hanno PM et al: The diagnosis of interstitial cystitis revisited: lessons learned from the National Institutes of Health Interstitial Cystitis Database study. J Urol 1999; 161:553. [NLM Cit ID: 99112653] (Initial criteria used to diagnose interstitial cystitis may be too restrictive.)

Jepsen JV et al: Long-term experience with pentosanpolysulfate in interstitial cystitis. Urology 1998;51:381. [NLM Cit ID: 98169159] (Ninety-seven patients followed for up to 116 months demonstrated a response rate between 6% and 18%.)

Peters KM et al: The efficacy of intravesical bacillus Calmette-Guérin in the treatment of interstitial cystitis. J Urol 1998;159:1483. [NLM Cit ID: 98213000] (After a mean follow-up of 8 months in this prospective, double-blind, placebo-controlled study, the BCG group demonstrated a 60% response rate compared with a 27% rate for placebo.)

Sant GR et al: Interstitial cystitis. Curr Opin Urol 1999;9:297. [NLM Cit ID: 99388756] (Interstitial cystitis is a common inflammatory condition of the bladder.)

MALE ERECTILE DYSFUNCTION & SEXUAL DYSFUNCTION

Erectile dysfunction is defined as the consistent inability to maintain an erect penis with sufficient rigidity to allow sexual intercourse. This condition is thought to affect 10 million American men, and its incidence is age-related. Approximately 25% of all men older than age 65 suffer from this disorder. Most cases of male erectile disorders have an organic rather than a psychogenic cause. Normal male erection is a neurovascular phenomenon relying on an intact autonomic and somatic nerve supply to the penis, smooth and striated musculature of the corpora cavernosa and pelvic floor, and arterial inflow supplied by the paired pudendal arteries. Erection is precipitated and maintained by an increase in arterial flow, active relaxation of the smooth muscle elements of the sinusoids within the corporal bodies of the penis, and an increase in venous resistance. Contraction of the bulbocavernosus and ischiocavernosus muscles results in further rigidity of the penis. The neurotransmitters that initiate the process have not been identified with certainty, though nitric oxide, vasoactive intestinal peptide, acetylcholine, and prostaglandins have all been postulated to initiate or contribute to male erection.

Male sexual dysfunction may be manifested in a variety of ways, and the history is critical to the proper classification and subsequent treatment. Androgens have a strong influence on the sexual desire of men. A **loss of libido** may indicate androgen deficiency on the basis of either hypothalamic, pituitary or testicular disease. Serum testosterone and gonadotropin levels may help localize the site of disease. **Loss of erections** may result from arterial, venous, neurogenic, or psychogenic causes. Concurrent medical problems may damage one or more of the mechanisms. In addition, many medications, especially antihypertensives, are associated with erectile dysfunction. Centrally acting sympatholytics (methyldopa, clonidine, reserpine) can result in loss of erection, while vasodilators, alpha-blockers, and diuretics rarely alter erections. Beta-blockers and spironolactone may result in loss of libido. It is important to determine whether the patient ever had any normal erections, such as early morning or during sleep. If normal erections do occur, an organic cause is unlikely. The gradual loss of erections over a period of time is more suggestive of an organic cause. The **loss of emission** (lack of antegrade seminal fluid during ejaculation) may result from several underlying disorders. **Retrograde ejaculation** may occur as a result of mechanical disruption of the bladder neck, especially following transurethral resection of the prostate or sympathetic denervation as a result of medications (alpha-blockers), diabetes mellitus, or radical pelvic or retroperitoneal surgery. Androgen deficiency may also result in lack of emission by decreasing the amount of prostatic and seminal vesicle secretions. If libido and erection are intact, the **loss of orgasm** is usually of psychologic origin. **Premature ejaculation** is usually an anxiety-related disorder and rarely has an organic cause. The history may elucidate the presence of a new partner, unreasonable expectations about performance, or emotional disorders.

Clinical Findings

A. Symptoms and Signs: Erectile dysfunction should be clearly distinguished from problems of ejaculation, libido, and orgasm. The degree of the dysfunction (whether chronic, occasional, or situational) as well as its timing should be noted. The history should include inquiries about hyperlipidemia, hypertension, neurologic disease, diabetes mellitus, renal failure, and adrenal and thyroid disorders. Trauma to the pelvis or pelvic or peripheral vascular surgery also identifies patients at increased risk of impotence. A complete recording of drug use should be made, since about 25% of all cases of sexual dysfunction may be drug-related. The use of alcohol, tobacco, and recreational drugs should be recorded as well, since each is associated with an increased risk of sexual dysfunction.

During the physical examination, secondary sexual characteristics should be assessed. Neurologic and peripheral vascular examination should be performed. Motor and sensory examination should be performed as well as palpation and quantification of lower extremity vascular pulsations. The genitalia should be examined, noting the presence of penile scarring or plaque formation (Peyronie's disease) and any abnormalities in size or consistency of either testicle. Examination of the prostate is essential.

B. Laboratory Findings: Laboratory evaluation is limited and should consist of a complete blood count, urinalysis, lipid profile, determination of serum testosterone, glucose, and prolactin. Patients with abnormalities of testosterone or prolactin require further evaluation with measurement of serum FSH and LH, and endocrinologic consultation is advised.

C. Special Tests: Further testing is based on the patient's goals. Patients who will accept only noninvasive forms of therapy may be offered medical therapy or a vacuum constriction device, as described below. Most patients undergo further evaluation with direct injection of vasoactive substances into the penis. Such substances (prostaglandin E_1, papavarine, or a combination of drugs) will induce erections in men with intact vascular systems. Patients who respond with a rigid erection require no further vascular evaluation. However, organic and psychogenic impotence can be differentiated by use of nocturnal penile tumescence testing, where the frequency as well as the rigidity of erections are recorded by a simple device attached to the penis before sleep. Patients with psychogenic impotence will have nocturnal erections of adequate frequency and rigidity.

Additional vascular testing is indicated in patients who fail to achieve an erection with injection of vasoactive substances on serial attempts using increasing doses or combination of drugs and who would consider vascular reconstructive surgery. The diameter and flow in the cavernous arteries can be assessed using duplex ultrasound. Patients with poor arterial inflow in the absence of known peripheral vascular disease (as in patients who have sustained pelvic trauma) are candidates for pelvic arteriography before planned arterial reconstruction. Patients with normal arterial inflow should be suspected of suffering from venous leak. Further testing in this group would include cavernosometry (measurement of flow required to maintain erection) and cavernosography (contrast study of the penis to determine site and extent of venous leak).

Treatment

The vast majority of men suffering from erectile dysfunction can be managed successfully with one of the approaches outlined below. Men who do not suffer from organic dysfunction will probably benefit from behaviorally oriented sex therapy.

A. Hormonal Replacement: Testosterone injections (200 mg intramuscularly every 3 weeks) or topical patches (2.5–6 mg/d) are offered to men with documented androgen deficiency who have undergone endocrinologic evaluation as described and in whom prostatic cancer has been excluded by PSA screening and digital rectal examination.

B. Vacuum Constriction Device: The vacuum constriction device is a cylindric device that draws the penis into an erect state by inducing a vacuum within the cylinder. Once adequate tumescence has been achieved, a rubber constriction device or band is placed around the proximal penis to prevent loss of erection, and the cylinder is removed. Such devices are suitable for patients with venous disorders of the penis and those who fail to achieve an adequate erection with injection of vasoactive substances. Complications are rare.

C. Vasoactive Therapy: Direct injection of vasoactive prostaglandins into the penis is an acceptable form of treatment for most men with impotence. These injections are performed using a tuberculin syringe. The base and lateral aspect of the penis is used as the injection site to avoid injury to the superficial blood supply located anteriorly. Complications are rare and include dizziness, local pain, fibrosis, and infection. A prolonged erection requiring aspiration of blood and injection of epinephrine and phenylephrine to achieve detumescence occurs very rarely. A mechanism of delivering vasoactive prostaglandins (alprostadil) via a urethral suppository has been developed, and results are good. Pellet sizes are 125, 250, 500, and 1000 μg.

Sildenafil (Viagra) inhibits phosphodiesterase 5—itself an inhibitor of erection—and allows cGMP to function unopposed. Ordinarily, nitric oxide-mediated release from parasympathetic nerves and endothelium generates this compound, and prolongation of its half-life results in sustained inflow of blood into the erect penis. Fifty milligrams taken 1 hour prior to anticipated sexual activity is recommended, with peak action at 2 hours. There is no effect on libido, nor is priapism a problem, but the additive effect on nitrates may lead to exaggerated cardiac preload reduction and hypotension. Thus, the drug is contraindicated in patients receiving nitroglycerin. All patients being evaluated for acute chest pain should be asked if they are taking sildenafil before administering nitroglycerin. Fixed atherosclerotic disease in the aortoiliac system is associated with diminished efficacy.

D. Penile Prostheses: Prosthetic devices may be implanted directly into the paired corporal bodies. Such prostheses may be rigid, malleable, hinged, or inflatable. Each is manufactured in a variety of sizes and diameters. Inflatable models may result in a more cosmetic appearance but may be associated with a greater likelihood of mechanical failure.

E. Vascular Reconstruction: Patients with disorders of the arterial system are candidates for various forms of arterial reconstruction, including endarterectomy and balloon dilation for proximal arterial occlusion and arterial bypass procedures utilizing arterial (epigastric) or venous (deep dorsal vein) segments for distal occlusion. Patients with disorders of venous occlusion may be managed with ligation of certain veins (deep dorsal or emissary veins) or the crura of the corpora cavernosa. Experience with vascular reconstructive procedures is still limited, and many patients so treated still fail to achieve a rigid erection.

[NIH Consensus Statement: Impotence]
http://text.nlm.nih.gov/nih/cdc/www/91txt.html

Boolell M et al: Sildenafil, a novel effective oral therapy for male erectile dysfunction. Br J Urol 1996;78:257. [NLM Cit ID: 96408939] (Sildenafil is a well-tolerated and effective oral therapy for male erectile dysfunction with no established organic cause.)

Goldstein I et al: Oral sildenafil in the treatment of erectile dysfunction. Sildenafil Study Group. N Engl J Med 1998;338:1397. [NLM Cit ID: 98234126] (Sildenafil is an effective, well-tolerated treatment for erectile dysfunction due to organic, psychogenic, and mixed causes.)

JAMA patient page: Sexual dysfunction. JAMA 1999; 281:584. [NLM Cit ID: 99144715]

Padma-Nathan H et al: Treatment of men with erectile dysfunction with transurethral alprostadil. Medicated Urethral System for Erection (MUSE) Study Group. N Engl J Med 1997;336:1. [NLM Cit ID: 97122455] (Alprostadil was delivered transurethrally in a double-blind, placebo-controlled study of 1511 men who had chronic erectile dysfunction from various organic causes. Sixty-six percent of patients had erections sufficient for intercourse. The most common side effect was mild penile pain, which occurred in 11%.)

MALE INFERTILITY

Primary infertility affects 15–20% of married couples. Approximately one-third of cases result from male factors, one-third from female factors, and one-third from combined factors. It is thus critical to have simultaneous evaluation of the female partner. Clinical evaluation is warranted following 6 months of unprotected intercourse. Endocrinologic profiles and detailed semen analyses are the cornerstones of laboratory investigations after the history and physical examination. **Oligospermia** is the presence of less than 20 million sperm/mL of the ejaculate; **azoospermia** is the absence of sperm. As spermatogenesis takes approximately 74 days, it is thus important to review events from the past 3 months.

Clinical Findings

A. Symptoms and Signs: The history should include prior testicular insults (torsion, cryptorchism, trauma), infections (mumps orchitis, epididymitis), environmental factors (excessive heat, radiation, chemotherapy), medications (anabolic steroids, cimetidine, and spironolactone may affect spermatogenesis; phenytoin may lower FSH; sulfasalazine and nitrofurantoin affect sperm motility), and drugs (alcohol, marijuana). Sexual habits, frequency and timing of intercourse, use of lubricants, and each partner's previous fertility experiences are important. Loss of libido and headaches or visual disturbances may indicate a pituitary tumor. The past medical or surgical history may reveal thyroid or liver disease (abnormalities of spermatogenesis), diabetic neuropathy (retrograde ejaculation), radical pelvic or retroperitoneal surgery (absent seminal emission secondary to sympathetic nerve injury), or hernia repair (damage to the vas deferens or testicular blood supply).

Physical examination should pay particular attention to features of hypogonadism: underdeveloped secondary sexual characteristics, diminished male pattern hair distribution (axillary, body, facial, pubic), eunuchoid skeletal proportions (arm span 2 inches > height; upper to lower body ratio < 1.0), gynecomastia. The scrotal contents should be carefully evaluated. Testicular size should be noted (normal size approximately 4.5 × 2.5 cm, volume 18 mL). Varicoceles should be looked for in the standing position and on occasion may only be appreciated with the Valsalva maneuver. The vas deferens, epididymis, and prostate should be palpated.

B. Laboratory Findings: Semen analysis should be performed after 72 hours of abstinence. The specimen should be analyzed within 1 hour after collection. Abnormal sperm concentrations are less than 20 million/mL. Normal semen volumes range between 1.5 and 5 mL (volumes < 1.5 mL may result in inadequate buffering of the vaginal acidity and may be due to retrograde ejaculation or androgen insufficiency). Normal sperm motility and morphology demonstrate 50–60% motile cells and more than 60% normal morphology. Abnormal motility may result from antisperm antibodies or infection. Abnormal morphology may result from a varicocele, infection, or exposure history.

Endocrinologic evaluation is warranted if sperm counts are low or if there is a clinical basis (from the history and physical examination) for suspecting an endocrinologic origin. Testing should include serum FSH, LH, and testosterone. Elevated FSH and LH and low testosterone (hypergonadotropic hypogonadism) are associated with primary testicular failure, which is usually irreversible. Low FSH and LH associated with low testosterone occur in secondary testicular failure (hypogonadotropic hypogonadism) and may be of hypothalamic or pituitary origin. Such defects may be correctable. In such cases, serum prolactin should be checked to exclude pituitary prolactinoma.

C. Imaging: Scrotal ultrasound may detect a subclinical varicocele. Vasography may be required in patients with suspected ductal obstruction.

D. Special Tests: Azoospermic patients should have postmasturbation urine samples centrifuged and analyzed for sperm to exclude retrograde ejaculation.

Azoospermic patients and patients with ejaculate volumes less than 1 mL should have fructose levels determined on the ejaculate. Fructose is produced in the seminal vesicles and if absent in the ejaculate implies obstruction of the ejaculatory ducts.

Treatment

A. General Measures: Education with respect to the proper timing for intercourse in relation to the female's ovulatory cycle as well as the avoidance of spermicidal lubricants should be discussed. In cases of toxic exposure or medication-related factors, the offending agent should be removed. Patients with active genitourinary tract infections should be treated with appropriate antibiotics.

B. Endocrine Therapy: Hypogonadotropic hypogonadism may be treated with chorionic gonadotropin once primary pituitary disease has been excluded or treated. Dosage is usually 2000 IU intramuscularly three times a week. If sperm counts fail to rise after 12 months, FSH therapy should be initiated. Menotropins (Pergonal) is available as a premixed vial of 75 IU of FSH and 75 IU of LH. The usual dosage ranges from one-half to one vial intramuscularly three times per week.

C. Retrograde Ejaculation Therapy: Oligospermic patients with retrograde ejaculation may benefit from alpha-adrenergic agonists (pseudoephedrine, 60 mg orally three times a day) or imipramine (25 mg orally three times a day). Medical failures may require the collection of postmasturbation urine for intrauterine insemination or electroejaculation in the case of absent emission.

D. Varicocele: Surgical approaches to varicoceles may be accomplished via a scrotal, inguinal, or laparoscopic approach. More recently, percutaneous venographic approaches have been developed, obviating the need for an anesthetic.

E. Ductal Obstruction: The level of obstruction must be delineated via a vasogram prior to operative treatment. Mechanical obstruction of the ejaculatory duct may be corrected by transurethral resection and unroofing of the ducts in the prostatic urethra. Obstruction of the vas deferens is best managed by a microsurgical approach, and a vasovasostomy or vasoepididymostomy may be required.

F. Assisted Reproductive Techniques: Advances in reproductive technology may provide alternatives to patients who have failed other means of treating reduced sperm counts and motility. Such measures include intrauterine insemination, in vitro fertilization, and gamete intrafallopian transfer.

Bartoov B et al: Quantitative ultramorphological analysis of human sperm: fifteen years of experience in the diagnosis and management of male factor infertility. Arch Androl 1999;43:13. [NLM Cit ID: 99374127] (The utility of quantitative ultramorphological sperm analysis in the diagnosis and treatment of male infertility is presented.)

McClure RD: Male infertility—realistic treatment options [editorial; comment]. J Urol 1999;161:1166. [NLM Cit ID: 99179899]

BENIGN PROSTATIC HYPERPLASIA

Essentials of Diagnosis

- Obstructive or irritative voiding symptoms.
- May have enlarged prostate on rectal examination.
- Absence of urinary tract infection, neurologic disorder, stricture disease, prostatic or bladder malignancy.

General Considerations

Benign prostatic hyperplasia is the most common benign tumor in men, and its incidence is age-related. The prevalence of histologic benign prostatic hyperplasia in autopsy studies rises from approximately 20% in men aged 41–50 years, to 50% in men aged 51–60 and to over 90% in men over 80 years of age. Although clinical evidence of disease occurs less commonly, symptoms of prostatic obstruction are also age-related. At age 55, approximately 25% of men report obstructive voiding symptoms. At age 75 years, 50% of men report a decrease in the force and caliber of the urinary stream.

Risk factors for the development of benign prostatic hyperplasia are poorly understood. Some studies have suggested a genetic predisposition and some have noted racial differences. Approximately 50% of men under age 60 who undergo surgery for benign prostatic hyperplasia may have a heritable form of the disease. This form is most likely an autosomal dominant trait, and first-degree male relatives of such patients carry an increased relative-risk of approximately fourfold.

Etiology

The etiology is not completely understood, but the disorder seems to be multifactorial and under endocrine control. The prostate is composed of both stromal and epithelial elements, and each, either alone or in combination, can give rise to hyperplastic nodules and the symptoms associated with benign prostatic hyperplasia. Each element may be targeted in medical management schemes.

Laboratory and clinical studies have identified two factors necessary for the development of benign prostatic hyperplasia: dihydrotestosterone (DHT) and aging. Animal studies have demonstrated that the aging prostate becomes more sensitive to androgens. Prostatic growth in aging dogs appears to be related more to a decrease in cell death than to an increase in cell proliferation. Laboratory studies have suggested several theories in this area, including the following: (1) stromal-epithelial interactions (stroma cell may regulate growth of epithelial cell or other stromal cells via a paracrine or autocrine mechanism by secreting growth factors such as basic fibroblast growth factor or transforming growth factor-β); and (2) aging may result in stem cells undergoing a block in the maturation process, preventing them from entering into programmed cell death (apoptosis). The impact of aging in animal studies appears to be mediated via estrogen synergism. In canines, estrogens induce the androgen receptor; alter steroid metabolism, resulting in higher levels of intraprostatic DHT; inhibit cell death when given in the presence of androgens; and stimulate stroma collagen production.

Studies have demonstrated that benign prostatic hyperplasia is under endocrine control. Castration results in the regression of established disease and improvement in urinary symptoms. Administration of a luteinizing hormone-releasing hormone (LHRH) analog in men reversibly shrinks established benign prostatic hyperplasia, resulting in objective improvement in flow rate and subjective improvement in symptoms. Further investigations have demonstrated a positive correlation between levels of free testosterone and estrogen and the volume of the gland. The latter may suggest that the association between aging and benign prostatic hyperplasia might reflect increasing estrogen levels of aging, resulting in induction of the androgen receptor and thus sensitizing the prostate to free testosterone. However, no studies to date have been able to demonstrate elevated estrogen receptor levels in humans with the disease.

Pathology

Benign prostatic hyperplasia is truly a hyperplastic process, resulting from an increase in cell numbers. Microscopic evaluation reveals a nodular growth pattern consisting of varying amounts of stroma or epithelium. Stroma is composed of varying amounts of collagen and smooth muscle. The differential representation of various histologic components of benign prostatic hyperplasia in part explains the potential responsiveness to medical therapy. Thus, alpha-blocker therapy may result in excellent responses in patients with benign prostatic hyperplasia when there is a significant component of smooth muscle, while hyperplasia composed predominantly of epithelium might respond better to 5α-reductase inhibitors. Patients with significant components of collagen in the stroma may not respond to either form of medical therapy. One cannot reliably predict responsiveness to specific therapy (see below).

As benign prostatic hyperplasia nodules in the transition zone enlarge, they compress the outer zones of the prostate, resulting in the formation of a "surgical capsule." This boundary separates the transition zone from the peripheral zone of the gland and serves as a cleavage plane for open enucleation of the prostate during simple prostatectomies.

Pathophysiology

One can relate the symptoms of benign prostatic hyperplasia either to the obstructive component of the prostate or to the secondary response of the bladder to the outlet resistance. The obstructive component can be subdivided into mechanical obstruction and dynamic obstruction.

As prostatic enlargement occurs, mechanical obstruction may result from intrusion into the urethral lumen or bladder neck, resulting in a higher bladder outlet resistance. Prostatic size on digital rectal examination (DRE) correlates poorly with symptoms.

The dynamic component of prostatic obstruction explains the variable nature of the symptoms. The prostatic stroma is composed of smooth muscle and collagen and is rich in adrenergic nerve supply. The level of autonomic stimulation thus sets a "tone" to the prostatic urethra. Alpha-blocker therapy decreases this tone, resulting in a decrease in outlet resistance.

The irritative voiding complaints (see below) of benign prostatic hyperplasia result from the secondary response of the bladder to the increased outlet resistance. Bladder outlet obstruction results in detrusor muscle hypertrophy and hyperplasia as well as collagen deposition. The latter is most likely responsible for a decrease in bladder compliance, but detrusor instability also occurs. On gross inspection, thickened detrusor muscle bundles are seen as trabeculation on cystoscopic examination. If left unchecked, mucosal herniation between detrusor muscle bundles ensues, resulting in diverticulum formation ("false" diverticula composed of mucosa and serosa only).

Clinical Findings

A. Symptoms: The symptoms of benign prostatic hyperplasia can be divided into obstructive and irritative complaints. Obstructive symptoms include hesitancy, decreased force and caliber of the stream, sensation of incomplete bladder emptying, double voiding (urinating a second time within 2 hours), straining to urinate, and postvoid dribbling. Irritative symptoms include urgency, frequency, and nocturia.

The American Urological Association (AUA) has developed a self-administered questionnaire that is reliable in identifying patients who need therapy and in monitoring the response to therapy. The AUA symptom index (Table 23–4) is perhaps the single most important tool used in the evaluation of patients with this disorder and should be calculated for all patients before starting therapy. The answers to seven questions quantitate the severity of obstructive or irritative complaints on a scale of 0–5. Thus, the score can range from 0 to 35, in increasing severity of symptoms.

Table 23–4. American Urological Association symptom index for benign prostatic hyperplasia.[1,2]

Questions to Be Answered	Not at All	Less Than One Time in Five	Less Than Half the Time	About Half the Time	More Than Half the Time	Almost Always
1. Over the past month, how often have you had a sensation of not emptying your bladder completely after you finish urinating?	0	1	2	3	4	5
2. Over the past month, how often have you had to urinate again less than 2 hours after you finished urinating?	0	1	2	3	4	5
3. Over the past month, how often have you found you stopped and started again several times when you urinated?	0	1	2	3	4	5
4. Over the past month, how often have you found it difficult to postpone urination?	0	1	2	3	4	5
5. Over the past month, how often have you had a weak urinary stream?	0	1	2	3	4	5
6. Over the past month, how often have you had to push or strain to begin urination?	0	1	2	3	4	5
7. Over the past month, how many times did you most typically get up to urinate from the time you went to bed at night until the time you got up in the morning?	0 (None)	1 (1 time)	2 (2 times)	3 (3 times)	4 (4 times)	5 (5 times)

[1]Sum of seven circled numbers equals the symptom score. See text for explanation.
[2]Reproduced, with permission, from Barry MJ et al: The American Urological Association symptoms index for benign prostatic hyperplasia. J Urol 1992;148:1549.

A detailed history focusing on the urinary tract should be obtained to exclude other possible causes of symptoms such as prostate cancer or disorders unrelated to the prostate such as urinary tract infection, neurogenic bladder, or urethral stricture.

B. Signs: A physical examination, digital rectal examination (DRE), and a focused neurologic examination should be performed on all patients. The size and consistency of the prostate should be noted, but prostate size does not correlate with the severity of symptoms or the degree of obstruction. Benign prostatic hyperplasia usually results in a smooth, firm, elastic enlargement of the prostate. Induration, if detected, must alert the physician to the possibility of cancer, and further evaluation is needed (ie, PSA, transrectal ultrasound, and biopsy). Examination of the lower abdomen should be performed to assess for a distended bladder.

C. Laboratory Findings: Urinalysis should be done to exclude infection or hematuria, and serum creatinine should be measured to assess renal function. Renal insufficiency may be observed in 10% of patients with prostatism and if observed warrants upper tract imaging. Patients with renal insufficiency are at an increased risk of developing complications following operative treatment for benign prostatic hyperplasia. A serum PSA is considered optional, yet most physicians will include it in the initial evaluation. PSA certainly increases the ability to detect prostate cancer over DRE alone, yet because there is much overlap between levels seen in benign prostatic hyperplasia and prostate cancer, its use remains controversial (see below in the section on screening for prostate cancer).

D. Imaging: Upper tract imaging (intravenous pyelogram or renal ultrasound) is only recommended in the presence of concomitant urinary tract disease or complications from benign prostatic hyperplasia (ie, hematuria, urinary tract infection, renal insufficiency, history of stone disease).

E. Cystoscopy: Cystoscopy is not recommended to determine the need for treatment but may assist in determining the surgical approach in patients opting for invasive therapy.

F. Additional Tests: Cystometrograms and urodynamic profiles should be reserved for patients with suspected neurologic disease or those who have failed prostate surgery. Flow rates, postvoid residual urine determination, and pressure-flow studies are considered optional.

Differential Diagnosis

Other obstructive conditions of the lower urinary tract such as urethral stricture, bladder neck contracture, bladder stone, or carcinoma of the prostate must be considered when evaluating men with presumptive benign prostatic hyperplasia. A history of prior urethral instrumentation, urethritis, or trauma should be elucidated to exclude urethral stricture or bladder neck contracture. Hematuria and pain are commonly associated with bladder stones. Carcinoma of the prostate may be detected by abnormalities on the DRE or an elevated PSA (see below). A urinary tract infection can mimic the irritative symptoms of benign prostatic hyperplasia and can be readily identified by urinalysis and culture, however, a urinary tract infection can also be a complication of benign prostatic hyperplasia. Carcinoma of the bladder, especially carcinoma in situ, may also present with irritative voiding complaints; however, urinalysis usually shows evidence of hematuria. Patients with neurogenic bladder may also have many of the same signs and symptoms as those with benign prostatic hyperplasia; however, a history of neurologic disease, stroke, diabetes mellitus, or back injury may be obtained, and diminished perineal or lower extremity sensation or alterations in rectal sphincter tone or the bulbocavernosus reflex might be observed on examination. Simultaneous alterations in bowel function (constipation) might also alert one to the possibility of a neurologic disorder.

Treatment

Clinical practice guidelines exist for the evaluation and treatment of patients with benign prostatic hyperplasia (Figure 23–1). Following evaluation as outlined above, patients should be offered various forms of therapy for benign prostatic hyperplasia. Patients are advised to consult with their primary care physicians and make an educated decision on the basis of the relative efficacy and side effects of the treatment options (Table 23–5).

Patients with mild symptoms (scores 0–7) should be managed by watchful waiting only. Absolute surgical indications are refractory urinary retention (failing at least one attempt at catheter removal), large bladder diverticula, or any of the following sequelae of benign prostatic hyperplasia: recurrent urinary tract infection, recurrent gross hematuria, bladder stones, or renal insufficiency.

A. Watchful Waiting: The risk of progression or complications is uncertain. However, in men with symptomatic disease, it is clear that progression is

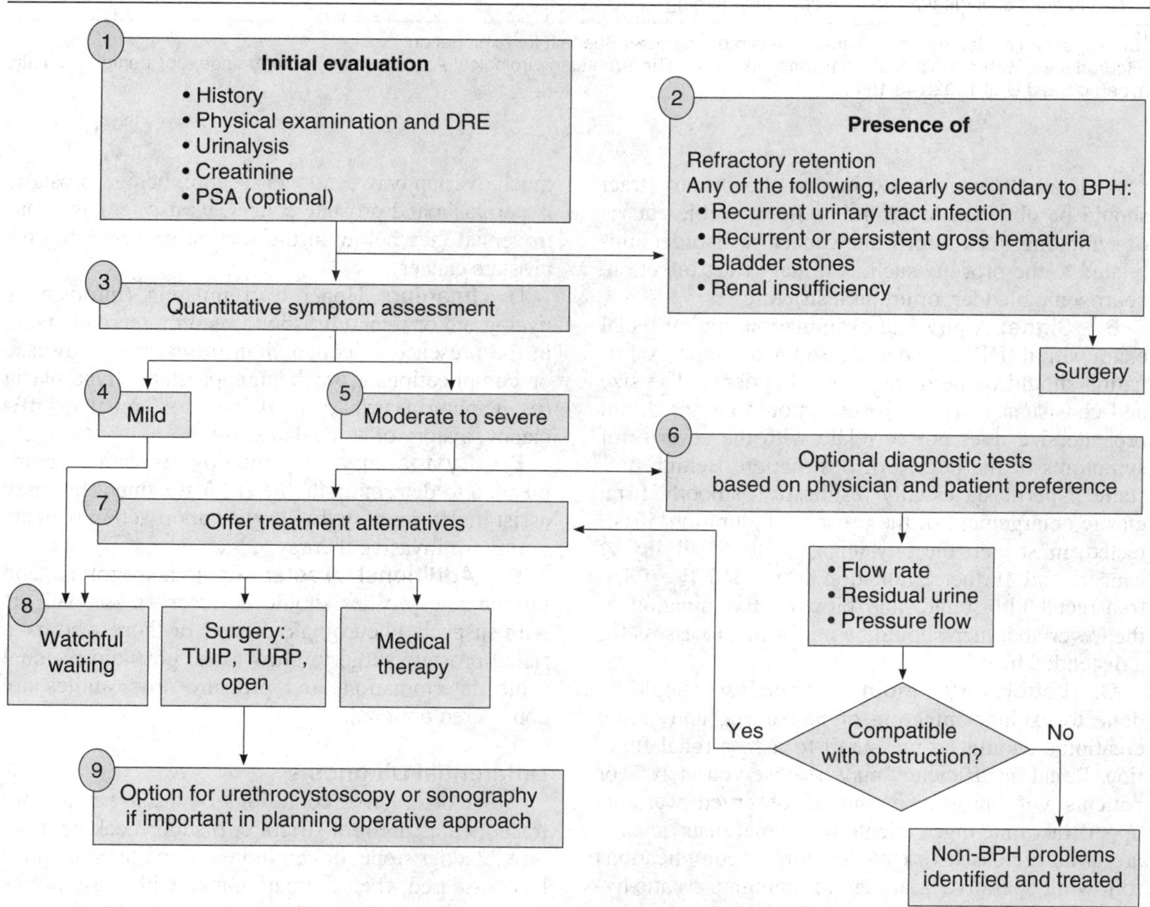

Figure 23–1. Benign prostatic hyperplasia decision diagram. (PSA, prostate-specific antigen; BPH, benign prostatic hyperplasia; DRE, digital rectal examination; TUIP, transurethral incision of the prostate; TURP, transurethral resection of the prostate.)

Table 23–5. Balance sheet for benign prostatic hyperplasia treatment outcomes.[1]

Outcome	TUIP	Open Surgery	TURP	Watchful Waiting	Alpha Blockers	Finasteride[2]
Chance for improvement[1]	78–83%	94–99.3%	75–96%	31–55%	59–86%	54–78%
Degree of symptom improvement (% reduction in symptom score)	73%	79%	85%	Unknown	51%	31%
Morbidity and complications[1]	2.2–33.3%	7–42.7%	5.2–30.7%	1–5%	2.9–43.3%	13.6–18.8%
Death within 30–90 days[1]	0.2–1.5%	1–4.6%	0.5–3.3%	0.8%	0.8%	0.8%
Total incontinence[1]	0.1–1.1%	0.3–0.7%	0.7–1.4%	2%	2%	2%
Need for operative treatment for surgical complications[1]	1.3–2.7%	0.6–14.1%	0.7–10.1%	0	0	0
Impotence[1]	3.9–24.5%	4.7–39.2%	3.3–34.8%	3%	3%	2.5–5.3%
Retrograde ejaculation	6–55%	36–95%	25–99%	0	4–11%	0
Loss of work in days	7–21	21–28	7–21	1	3.5	1.5
Hospital stay in days	1–3	5–10	3–5	0	0	0

TUIP = transurethral incision of the prostate; TURP = transurethral resection of the prostate

[1]90% confidence interval.

[2]Most of the data reviewed for finasteride is derived from three trials that have required an enlarged prostate for entry. The chance of improvement in men with symptoms yet minimally enlarged prostates may be much less, as noted from the VA Cooperative Trial.

not inevitable and that some men undergo spontaneous improvement or resolution of their symptoms.

Retrospective studies on the natural history of benign prostatic hyperplasia are inherently subject to bias, relating in part to patient selection and also to the type and extent of follow-up. Very few prospective studies addressing the natural history have been reported. One small series demonstrated that approximately 10% of symptomatic men may progress to urinary retention while half of patients demonstrate marked improvement or resolution of symptoms. Recently, a large randomized study was reported comparing finasteride with placebo in men with moderate to severely symptomatic disease and enlarged prostates on DRE. Patients in the placebo arm demonstrated a 7% risk of developing urinary retention over 4 years.

Men with moderate or severe symptoms can be managed also in this fashion if they so choose. The optimal interval for follow-up is not defined, nor are the specific end points for intervention.

B. Medical Therapy:

1. Alpha blockers–The human prostate and bladder base contains α_1 adrenoceptors, and the prostate will show a contractile response to such agonists. The contractile properties of the prostate and bladder neck seem to be mediated primarily by α_{1a} receptors. Alpha blockade has been shown to result in both objective and subjective degrees of improvement in the symptoms and signs of benign prostatic hyperplasia in some patients. Alpha-blockers can be classified according to their receptor selectivity as well as their half-life (Table 23–6). The efficacies of phenoxybenzamine and prazosin are comparable with respect to symptomatic relief; however, the higher side effect profile of phenoxybenzamine, resulting from its lack of alpha-receptor specificity, precludes its use in benign prostatic hyperplasia patients. Dose titration is necessary with prazosin, with typical therapy starting at 1 mg orally at bedtime for 3 nights, then increasing to 1 mg orally twice daily and then titrating up to 2 mg orally twice daily if necessary. Little additional symptomatic improvement is observed at higher doses, and side effects increase. Typical side effects include orthostatic hypotension, dizziness, tiredness, retrograde ejaculation, rhinitis, and headache.

Long-acting alpha-blockers allow for once-a-day dosing, but dose titration is still necessary. Terazosin is started at a dosage of 1 mg orally daily for 3 days,

Table 23–6. Alpha blockade for benign prostatic hyperplasia.

Agent	Action	Dose
Phenoxybenzamine	α_1 and α_2 blockade	5–10 mg twice daily
Prazosin	α_1 blockade	1–5 mg twice daily
Terazosin	α_1 blockade	1–10 mg daily
Doxazosin	α_1 blockade	1–8 mg daily
Tamsulosin	α_{1a} blockade	0.4 or 0.8 mg daily

increased to 2 mg orally daily for 11 days, then 5 mg orally daily. Additional dose escalation to 10 mg orally daily can be performed if necessary. Doxazosin is started at a dosage of 1 mg orally daily for 7 days, increased to 2 mg orally daily for 7 days, then 4 mg orally daily. Additional dose escalation to 8 mg orally daily can be performed if necessary. Side effects are similar to those described above for prazosin.

The most recent advance in alpha-blocker therapy has been the identification of subtypes of α_1 receptors. The α_{1a} receptors are those localized to the prostate and bladder neck, and selective blockade results in fewer systemic side effects (orthostatic hypotension, dizziness, tiredness, rhinitis, and headache), thus obviating the need for dose titration. Tamsulosin is started at a dosage of 0.4 mg orally daily and can be increased to 0.8 mg orally daily if necessary.

Several randomized, double-blind, placebo-controlled trials have been performed comparing terazosin, doxazosin, or tamsulosin with placebo. All agents have demonstrated safety and efficacy. Comparative trials between different alpha-blockers are ongoing.

2. 5α-Reductase inhibitors–Finasteride is a 5α-reductase inhibitor that blocks the conversion of testosterone to dihydrotestosterone. This drug impacts upon the epithelial component of the prostate, resulting in reduction in size of the gland and improvement in symptoms. Six months of therapy are required for maximum effects on prostate size (20% reduction) and symptomatic improvement.

Several randomized, double-blind, placebo-controlled trials have been performed comparing finasteride with placebo. Efficacy, safety, and durability are well established. However, symptomatic improvement is seen only in men with enlarged prostates (> 40 mL). Side effects include decreased libido, decrease in volume of ejaculate, and impotence. Serum PSA is reduced by approximately 50% in patients receiving finasteride therapy. However, individual values may vary, thus complicating cancer detection.

A recent report suggests that finasteride therapy may decrease the incidence of urinary retention and the need for operative treatment in men with enlarged prostates and moderate to severe symptoms. However, optimal identification of appropriate patients for prophylactic therapy remains to be determined.

3. Combination therapy–The first randomized, double-blind, placebo-controlled study investigating combination therapy of an alpha-blocker and a 5α-reductase inhibitor was recently reported. This was a four-arm Veterans Administration Cooperative Trial comparing placebo, finasteride alone, terazosin alone, and combination of finasteride and terazosin. Over 1200 patients participated, and significant decreases in symptom scores and increases in urinary flow rates were seen only in the arms containing terazosin. However, one must note that enlarged prostates were not an entry criterion, and in fact prostate size in this study was much smaller than in previous controlled trials using finasteride (32 versus 52 mL). Additional combination therapy trials are ongoing.

4. Phytotherapy–Phytotherapy is the use of plants or plant extracts for medicinal purposes. Its use in benign prostatic hyperplasia has been popular in Europe for years, and its use in the United States is growing as a result of patient-driven enthusiasm. Several plant extracts have been popularized, including the saw palmetto berry, the bark of *Pygeum africanum,* the roots of *Echinacea purpurea* and *Hypoxis rooperi,* pollen extract, and the leaves of the trembling poplar. The mechanisms of action of these agents are unknown, and their efficacy and safety has not been tested in multicenter, randomized, double-blind, placebo-controlled studies.

C. Conventional Surgical Therapy:

1. Transurethral resection of the prostate (TURP)–Ninety-five percent of simple prostatectomies can be performed endoscopically. Most of these procedures are performed under a spinal anesthetic and require a 1- to 2-day hospital stay. Symptom scores and flow rate improvement are superior following TURP relative to any minimally invasive therapy; however, the length of the hospital stay is greater. Much controversy revolves around possible higher rates of morbidity and mortality associated with TURP in comparison with open surgery, but the higher rates observed in one study probably related to more significant comorbidities in the TURP patients compared with the patients who received open surgical treatment. Several other studies could not confirm the difference in mortality when controlling for age and comorbidities. The risks of TURP include retrograde ejaculation (75%), impotence (5–10%), and urinary incontinence (< 1%). Complications include bleeding, urethral stricture or bladder neck contracture, perforation of the prostate capsule with extravasation, and, if severe, transurethral resection syndrome, a hypervolemic, hyponatremic state resulting from absorption of the hypotonic irrigating solution. Clinical manifestations of the syndrome include nausea, vomiting, confusion, hypertension, bradycardia, and visual disturbances. The risk of transurethral resection syndrome increases with resection times over 90 minutes. Treatment includes diuresis and, in severe cases, hypertonic saline administration.

2. Transurethral incision of the prostate (TUIP)–Men with moderate to severe symptoms and small prostates often have posterior commissure hyperplasia or an "elevated bladder neck." These patients will often benefit from incision of the prostate. The procedure is more rapid and less morbid than TURP. Outcomes in well-selected patients are comparable, though a lower rate of retrograde ejaculation has been reported (25%). The technique involves two incisions using the Collins knife at the 5 and 7 o'clock positions. The incisions are started just distal to the ureteral orifices and extended outward to the verumontanum.

3. Open simple prostatectomy–When the prostate is too large to remove endoscopically, open enucleation is necessary. What size is "too large" depends upon the surgeon's experience with TURP. Glands over 100 g are usually considered for open enucleation. In addition to size, other relative indications for open prostatectomy include concomitant bladder diverticulum or bladder stone and whether dorsal lithotomy positioning is or is not possible.

Open prostatectomies can be performed with either a suprapubic or retropubic approach. Simple suprapubic prostatectomy is performed transvesically and is the operation of choice if there is concomitant bladder pathology. After the bladder is opened, a semicircular incision is made in the bladder mucosa distal to the trigone. The dissection plane is initiated sharply, and blunt dissection with the finger is then performed to deliver the adenoma. The apical dissection should be performed sharply to avoid injury to the distal sphincteric mechanism. After the adenoma is removed, hemostasis is attained with suture ligatures and both a urethral and a suprapubic catheter are inserted prior to closure.

In simple retropubic prostatectomy, the bladder is not entered but rather a transverse incision is made in the surgical capsule of the prostate and the adenoma is enucleated as described above. Only a urethral catheter is needed at the end of the case.

D. Minimally Invasive Therapy:

1. Laser therapy–Many techniques of laser surgery for the prostate have been described. Two main energy sources of lasers have been utilized—neodymium:yttrium-aluminum-garnet (Nd:YAG) and Holmium-YAG.

Several different coagulation necrosis techniques have been described. TULIP (transurethral laser-induced prostatectomy) is performed under transrectal ultrasound guidance. The instrument is placed in the urethra and transrectal ultrasound is used to direct the device as it is slowly pulled from the bladder neck to the apex. The depth of treatment is monitored with ultrasound.

Most urologists prefer to use visually directed laser techniques. Visual coagulative necrosis is performed under cystoscopic control, and the laser fiber is pulled through the prostate at several designated areas depending upon the size and configuration of the gland. Four-quadrant and sextant approaches have been described for lateral lobes, with additional treatments directed at enlarged median lobes. Coagulative techniques do not create an immediate visual defect in the prostatic urethra—tissue is sloughed over the course of several weeks up to 3 months following the procedure.

Visual contact ablative techniques take longer in the operating room because the fiber is placed in direct contact with the prostate tissue, which is vaporized. An immediate defect is obtained in the prostatic urethra, similar to that seen during TURP.

Interstitial laser therapy places fibers directly into the prostate, usually under cystoscopic control. At each puncture, the laser is fired, resulting in submucosal coagulative necrosis. Irritative voiding symptoms may be less in these patients as the urethral mucosa is spared and prostate tissue is resorbed by the body rather than sloughed.

Advantages to laser surgery include minimal blood loss, rare occurrence of transurethral resection syndrome, the ability to treat patients while on anticoagulation therapy, and outpatient surgery. Disadvantages are that no tissue is recovered for pathologic examination, the postoperative catheterization time is longer, there are more irritative voiding complaints, and the expense of laser fibers and generators.

Large multicenter, randomized studies with long-term follow-up are needed in comparing laser prostate surgery with TURP and other forms of minimally invasive surgery.

2. Transurethral electrovaporization of the prostate–This technique uses the standard resectoscope but replaces a conventional loop with a variation of a grooved rollerball. High current densities result in heat vaporization of tissue, creating a cavity in the prostatic urethra. Because the device requires slower sweeping speeds over the prostatic urethra and the depth of vaporization is approximately one-third of a standard loop, this procedure usually takes longer than a standard TURP. Long-term comparative data are needed.

3. Hyperthermia–Microwave hyperthermia is most commonly delivered with a transurethral catheter. Some devices cool the urethral mucosa to decrease the risk of injury. However, if temperatures do not go above 45 °C, cooling is unnecessary. Symptom score and flow rate improvement are obtained, but (as with laser surgery) large randomized studies with long-term follow-up are needed to assess durability and cost-effectiveness.

4. Transurethral needle ablation of the prostate (TUNA)–This procedure uses a specially designed urethral catheter that is passed into the urethra. Interstitial radiofrequency needles are then deployed from the tip of the catheter, piercing the mucosa of the prostatic urethra. Radiofrequencies are then used to heat the tissue, resulting in coagulative necrosis. Bladder neck and median lobe enlargement are not well treated by TUNA. Subjective and objective improvement in voiding occurs. In randomized trials comparing TUNA to transurethral resection of the prostate (TURP), similar improvement was seen when comparing pre- and postoperative AUA symptom scores, bother and quality-of-life scores, peak urinary flow rates, and postvoid residual urine.

5. High-intensity focused ultrasound (HIFU)– HIFU is another means of performing thermal tissue ablation. A specially designed dual-function ultrasound probe is placed in the rectum. This probe allows transrectal imaging of the prostate and also delivers short bursts of high-intensity focused ultrasound energy, which heats the prostate tissue and causes coagulative necrosis. Bladder neck and median lobe enlargement are not well treated by HIFU. Ongoing clinical trials demonstrate some improvement in symptom score and flow rate, but the durability of the response is not known.

6. Intraurethral stents–Intraurethral stents endoscopically are placed in the prostatic fossa to keep the prostatic urethra patent. They are usually covered by urothelium within 4–6 months following insertion. These devices are typically used for patients with limited life expectancies who are not deemed good surgical or anesthetic candidates; however, with the advent of other minimally invasive techniques requiring minimal anesthesia (conscious sedation, or prostatic blocks), their application has become more limited.

7. Transurethral balloon dilation of the prostate–Balloon dilation of the prostate is performed with specially designed catheters that permit dilation of the prostatic fossa alone or dilation of the prostatic fossa and bladder neck. The technique is most effective in small prostates (< 40 mL), and while it may result in improvement in symptom score and flow rates, the effects are transient. This technique is rarely used today.

Djavan B et al: Prospective randomized comparison of high energy transurethral microwave thermotherapy versus alpha-blocker treatment of patients with benign prostatic hyperplasia. J Urol 1999;161:139. [NLM Cit ID: 99154990] (Alpha blockade resulted in rapid improvement in symptoms. Transurethral microwave therapy was associated with superior outcomes at 12 weeks to 6 months.)

Fawzy A et al: Long-term (4 year) efficacy and tolerability of doxazosin for the treatment of concurrent benign prostatic hyperplasia and hypertension. Int J Urol 1999; 6:346. [NLM Cit ID: 99372476] (Doxazosin is well-tolerated and effective long-term therapy for concurrent benign prostatic hyperplasia and hypertension.)

Lepor H et al: The efficacy of terazosin, finasteride, or both in benign prostatic hyperplasia. N Engl J Med 1996; 335:533. [NLM Cit ID: 96310759] (This was a four-arm, randomized, placebo-controlled study with 1200 men. In men with symptoms of BPH, treatment with alpha-blockers resulted in significant improvement in symptom score and urinary flow rates compared with placebo. No significant improvement in symptom score or urinary flow rates were seen in men treated with finasteride. Results of men receiving both drugs looked similar to those of men receiving alpha-blockers alone. However, since prostatic enlargement was not an entry criteria in this study, the study design was biased to favor alpha-blockers.)

McConnell JD et al: The effect of finasteride on the risk of acute urinary retention and the need for surgical treatment among men with benign prostatic hyperplasia. N Engl J Med 1998;338:557. [NLM Cit ID: 98129148] (3040 men with moderate to severe urinary symptoms and prostatic enlargement were randomized to receive placebo or finasteride. After 4 years, significant decreases in the incidence of acute urinary retention was seen in the finasteride group compared with the placebo group [7% versus 3%], and fewer men in the finasteride group underwent surgery for BPH [5% versus 10%]. Economic analysis is needed to determine whether use of the medication in this aspect is cost-effective.)

Medina JJ et al: Benign prostatic hyperplasia (the aging prostate). Med Clin North Am 1999;83:1213. [NLM Cit ID: 99432679]

Wasson JH et al: A comparison of transurethral surgery with watchful waiting for moderate symptoms of benign prostatic hyperplasia. The Veterans Affairs Cooperative Study Group on Transurethral Resection of the Prostate. N Engl J Med 1995;332:75. [NLM Cit ID: 95082881] (Surgery is more effective than watchful waiting in men with moderate symptoms of benign prostatic hyperplasia.)

Wilde MI et al: Finasteride: an update of its use in the management of symptomatic benign prostatic hyperplasia. Drugs 1999;57:557. [NLM Cit ID: 99249772] (Finasteride reduces disease progression and decreases the incidence of acute urinary retention. It is a therapeutic option for patients unable or unwilling to undergo more definitive operative management.)

MALIGNANT GENITOURINARY TRACT DISORDERS

PROSTATE CANCER

Essentials of Diagnosis

- Prostatic induration on digital rectal examination or elevation of PSA.
- Most often asymptomatic.
- Systemic symptoms (weight loss, bone pain) in 20% of patients.

General Considerations

Prostatic cancer is the most common cancer detected in American men. In the United States in 2000, over 179,000 new cases of prostate cancer will be diagnosed, and over 37,000 deaths will result. However, the clinical incidence of the disease does not match the prevalence noted at autopsy, where more than 40% of men over 50 years of age are found to have prostatic carcinoma. Most such occult cancers are small and contained within the prostate gland. Few are associated with regional or distant disease. The incidence of prostatic cancer increases with age.

Whereas 30% of men age 60–69 will have the disease, autopsy incidence increases to 67% in men aged 80–89 years. Although the prevalence of prostatic cancer in autopsy specimens around the world varies little, the clinical incidence is considerably different (high in North America and European countries, intermediate in South America, and low in the Far East), suggesting that environmental or dietary differences among populations may be important for prostatic cancer growth. A 50-year-old American man has a lifetime risk of 40% for latent cancer, 9.5% for developing clinically apparent cancer, and a 2.9% risk of death due to prostatic cancer. Blacks, men with a family history of prostatic cancer or a history of high dietary fat intake, and perhaps men who have undergone vasectomy are at an increased risk of developing it.

Clinical Findings

A. Symptoms and Signs: Most prostatic cancers are detected in asymptomatic men who are found to have focal nodules or areas of induration within the prostate at the time of digital rectal examination.

Rarely, patients present with signs of urinary retention (palpable bladder) or neurologic symptoms as a result of epidural metastases and cord compression. Obstructive voiding symptoms are most often due to benign prostatic hyperplasia, which occurs in the same age group. However, large or locally extensive prostatic cancers can cause obstructive voiding symptoms. Lymph node metastases can lead to lower extremity lymphedema. As the axial skeleton is the most common site of metastases, patients may present with back pain or pathologic fractures.

B. Laboratory Findings:

1. Serum tumor markers–Prostate-specific antigen (PSA) is a glycoprotein produced only in the cytoplasm of benign and malignant prostate cells. The serum level correlates with the volume of both benign and malignant prostatic tissue. Measurement of PSA may be useful in detecting and staging prostatic cancer, monitoring response to treatment, and detecting recurrence before it becomes obvious clinically. As a first-line screening test, PSA will be elevated in approximately 10–15% of men self-referred for screening. Approximately 20–25% of men with intermediate degrees of elevation (4.1–10 ng/mL; normal < 4 ng/mL) will be found to have prostatic cancer. Almost two-thirds of those with elevations greater than 10 ng/mL will have prostatic cancer. (See age-specific PSA reference ranges under Screening for Prostatic Cancer, below.) Patients with intermediate levels of PSA will usually have localized and therefore potentially curable cancers. However, it should be remembered that approximately 20% of patients who undergo radical prostatectomy for localized prostatic cancer will have normal levels of PSA.

In untreated patients with prostatic cancer, the level of PSA correlates with the volume and stage of the disease. Whereas most organ-confined cancers are associated with PSA levels less than 10 ng/mL, more advanced disease (seminal vesicle invasion, lymph node involvement, or occult distant metastases) is more common in patients with PSA levels in excess of 40 ng/mL. Approximately 98% of patients with metastatic prostatic cancer will have elevated PSA. However, there are occasional cancers which are localized despite substantial elevations in PSA. Therefore, treatment decisions in patients with untreated cancers cannot be made on the basis of PSA testing alone. A rising level of PSA after treatment is consistent with progressive disease whether it be locally recurrent or metastatic.

Until the advent of PSA testing, serum acid phosphatase was the standard serum tumor marker used in the evaluation of patients with localized and metastatic prostatic cancer. Because PSA is more sensitive than serum acid phosphatase, it has largely replaced its use. However, an elevated serum acid phosphatase is more predictive of metastatic disease than an elevated PSA, and for this reason it is still used by some. Serum acid phosphatase levels will be normal in approximately 25% of patients with metastatic disease.

2. Miscellaneous laboratory testing–Patients in urinary retention or those with ureteral obstruction due to locally or regionally advanced prostatic cancers may present with elevations in serum urea nitrogen or creatinine. Patients with bony metastases may have elevations in alkaline phosphatase or hypercalcemia. Laboratory and clinical evidence of disseminated intravascular coagulation can occur in patients with advanced prostatic cancers.

3. Prostatic biopsy–Transrectal ultrasound-guided biopsy seems to be a better method for detection of prostatic cancer than finger-guided biopsy. The use of a spring-loaded, 18-gauge biopsy needle has allowed transrectal biopsy to be performed with little patient discomfort and low attendant morbidity. The specimen preserves glandular architecture and allows for accurate grading as described below. Taking biopsy specimens from the apex, midportion, and base of the prostate is recommended by some and should be considered in patients with significant elevations in PSA but a normal digital rectal examination. Patients with abnormalities of the seminal vesicles can have guided biopsies of these structures performed to allow for detection of local tumor invasion. Aspiration biopsies of the prostate, though accurate and associated with low morbidity, have been used rarely since the introduction of the spring-loaded biopsy device but should be considered in patients at an increased risk of bleeding.

C. Imaging: Modern transrectal ultrasound instrumentation provides high-definition images of the prostate. Transrectal ultrasonography has been used largely for the staging of prostatic carcinomas. In addition, transrectal ultrasound-guided—rather than digitally guided—biopsy of the prostate may be a more accurate way to investigate suspicious lesions. Most prostatic cancers are hypoechoic.

MRI of the prostate allows for evaluation of the prostatic lesion as well as regional lymph nodes. The positive predictive value for detection of both capsular penetration and seminal vesicle invasion is similar for both transrectal ultrasound and MRI. CT scanning plays little role in evaluation because of its inability to accurately identify or stage prostatic cancers.

Radionuclide bone scan is superior to conventional plain skeletal x-rays in detecting bony metastases. Most prostatic cancer metastases are multiple and are most commonly localized to the axial skeleton. Because of the high frequency of abnormal scans in patients in this age group resulting from degenerative joint disease, plain films are often useful in evaluating patients with indeterminate radionuclide findings. Intravenous urography and cystoscopy are not routinely used to evaluate patients with prostatic cancer.

Imaging can be tailored to the likelihood of advanced disease in newly diagnosed patients. Asymptomatic patients with well to moderately well differentiated cancers—thought to be localized to the prostate on digital rectal examination and transurethral ultrasound and associated with normal or only modest elevations of PSA (ie, < 10 ng/mL)—need no further evaluation.

Those with more advanced local lesions, symptoms of metastases (ie, bone pain), and elevations in PSA greater than 10 ng/mL should undergo radionuclide bone scan. Cross-sectional imaging of the prostate is usually indicated only in those patients in the latter group who have negative bone scans in an attempt to detect lymph node metastases. Patients found to have enlarged pelvic lymph nodes are candidates for fine-needle aspiration. Despite application of modern and sophisticated imaging, understaging of prostatic cancer is common.

Screening for Prostatic Cancer

The incidence of prostate cancer is rising in this country, partly due to wider application of detection techniques (transrectal ultrasound and PSA testing). The goal of a screening effort should be to detect and effectively treat only those prostatic carcinomas most likely to cause morbidity or mortality if left untreated. Detection of latent, nonprogressive cancers would expose patients to unnecessary treatment and its attendant complications and costs. Whether screening for prostatic cancer will result in a decrease in yearly mortality rates due to the disease is the subject of much current debate.

The screening tests currently available include digital rectal examination, PSA testing, and transrectal ultrasound. Depending on the patient population being evaluated, detection rates using digital rectal examination alone will vary from 1.5% to 7%. Unfortunately, most cancers detected in this way are advanced (stages T3 or greater). Transrectal ultrasound should not be used as a first-line screening tool because of its expense, its low specificity (and therefore high biopsy rate), and the fact that it increases the detection rate very little when compared with the combined use of digital rectal examination and PSA testing.

PSA testing will increase the detection rate of prostatic cancers compared with digital rectal examination. Approximately 2–2.5% of men older than age 50 will be found to have prostatic cancer using PSA testing compared with a rate of approximately 1.5% using digital rectal examination alone. PSA is not specific for cancer, and there is considerable overlap of values between men with benign prostatic hyperplasia and those with prostatic cancers. The sensitivity, specificity, and positive predictive value of PSA and digital rectal examination are listed in Table 23–7. PSA-detected cancers are more likely to be localized compared with those detected with digital rectal examination alone.

In order to improve the performance of PSA as a screening test, several investigators have developed alternative methods for its use. The serial measurement of PSA (PSA velocity) may increase specificity for cancer detection with little loss in sensitivity. A rate of change in PSA greater than 0.75 ng/mL per year is associated with an increased likelihood of cancer detection. In a patient with a normal digital rectal examination, an elevated PSA, and a normal transrectal ultrasound, the indications for prostate biopsy may be refined by calculating PSA density (serum PSA/volume of the prostate as measured by ultrasound). Patients with high PSA density are more likely to have disease in spite of a normal digital rectal examination and normal transrectal ultrasound. As PSA concentration is directly related to patient age, establishment of age-specific reference ranges would increase specificity (fewer older men with benign

Table 23–7. Screening for prostatic cancer: Test performance.[1]

Test	Sensitivity	Specificity	Positive Predictive Value
Abnormal PSA (> 4 ng/mL)	0.67	0.97	0.43
Abnormal DRE	0.50	0.94	0.24
Abnormal PSA or DRE	0.84	0.92	0.28
Abnormal PSA *and* DRE	0.34	0.995	0.49

Key: DRE = digital rectal examination; PSA = prostate-specific antigen.

[1]Modified from Kramer BS et al: Prostate cancer screening: What we know and what we need to know. Ann Intern Med 1993;119:914.

prostatic hyperplasia would undergo evaluation) and increase sensitivity (more younger men with cancer would undergo evaluation). Age-specific reference ranges have been established: men 40–49, < 2.5 ng/mL; men 50–59, < 3.5 ng/mL; men 60–69, < 4.5 ng/mL; men 70–79, < 6.5 ng/mL (based on a previously normal serum PSA of < 4 ng/mL). However, age-specific reference ranges for PSA need to be validated in larger patient populations, including various ethnic groups. The most recent attempt at refining PSA has been the measurement of free serum and protein-bound levels (cancer patients have a lower percentage of free serum PSA). Numerous centers are analyzing this assay to define an optimal cutoff level. Early reports using cutoffs of 18–20% of free PSA resulted in 5–10% lost sensitivity for 15–40% gains in specificity.

Pathology & Staging

The majority of prostatic cancers are adenocarcinomas. Most arise in the periphery of the prostate (peripheral zone), though a small percentage arise in the central (5–10%) and transition zones (20%) of the gland. Most pathologists employ the Gleason grading system whereby a "primary" grade is applied to the architectural pattern of cancerous glands occupying the largest area of the specimen and a "secondary" pattern is assigned to the next largest area of cancerous growth. Grading is based on architectural (rather than histologic) criteria, and five possible "grades" are possible. Adding the score of the primary and secondary patterns gives a Gleason score. Grade correlates well with tumor volume, stage, and prognosis. The TNM classification of the American Joint Cancer Committee for prostatic cancer is shown in Table 23–8.

The patterns of prostatic cancer progression have been well defined. The likelihood of both local invasion and metastases is greater in larger or less well differentiated cancers. Small and well-differentiated cancers (grades 1 and 2) are usually confined within the prostate, whereas large-volume (> 4 mL) or poorly differentiated (grades 4 and 5) cancers are more commonly locally extensive or metastatic to regional lymph nodes or bone. Penetration of the prostatic capsule by cancer is common and often occurs along perineural spaces. Seminal vesicle invasion is associated with a high likelihood of regional or distant disease. Lymphatic metastases are most often identified in the obturator lymph node chain. The axial skeleton, as mentioned previously, is the most common site of distant metastases.

Table 23–8. TNM staging system for prostate cancer.

T: Primary tumor	
Tx	Cannot be assessed
T0	No evidence of primary tumor
Tis	Carcinoma in situ (CIS)
T1a	Carcinoma in 5% or less of tissue resected; normal DRE
T1b	Carcinoma in more than 5% of tissue resected; normal DRE
T1c	Detected from elevated PSA alone; normal DRE
T2a	Tumor in one lobe
T2b	Tumor in both lobes
T3a	Extracapsular extension
T3b	Seminal vesicle involvement
T4	Adjacent organ involvement
N: Regional lymph nodes	
Nx	Cannot be assessed
N0	No regional lymph node metastasis
N1	Metastasis in one or more regional lymph nodes
M: Distant metastasis	
Mx	Cannot be assessed
M0	No distant metastasis
M1	Distant metastasis present

DRE = digital rectal examination; PSA = prostate-specific antigen.

Treatment

A. Localized Disease: What constitutes the optimal form of treatment for patients with clinically localized cancers remains controversial. Treatment decisions are at present made on the basis of tumor grade and stage and the age and health of the patient. Although selected patients may be candidates for surveillance based on age or health and the presence of small-volume or well-differentiated cancers, most patients with an anticipated survival in excess of 10 years should be considered for treatment with irradiation or surgery. Both radiation therapy and radical prostatectomy allow for acceptable levels of local control. A randomized trial comparing watchful waiting and radical prostatectomy in men with clinically localized prostate cancer is currently under way in the United States (PIVOT: Prostate Cancer Intervention Versus Observation Trial). This trial will randomize 1000 patients and will run for 15 years. Patients need to be advised of all treatment options (including surveillance) along with their particular benefits, risks, and limitations.

B. Radical Prostatectomy: In radical prostatectomy, the seminal vesicles, prostate, and ampullae of the vas deferens are removed. Refinements in technique have allowed maintenance of urinary continence in most patients and erectile function in selected patients. However, the procedure should be used selectively. As capsular penetration is a common finding in patients with presumed localized prostatic cancer, preservation of the neurovascular bundle contiguous with a prostatic cancer may increase the likelihood of local tumor recurrence. Local recurrence is uncommon after radical prostatectomy, and its incidence is related to pathologic stage. Organ-confined cancers rarely recur (2% local, 1% distant). However, cancers found to be locally extensive (capsular penetration, seminal vesicle invasion) are associated with higher local (10–25%) and distant (20–25%) relapse rates.

Ideal candidates for the procedure include healthy patients with stages T1 and T2 prostatic cancers. Patients with advanced local tumors (T3 and T4) and those with lymph node metastases are rarely candidates for this procedure.

Patients with positive surgical margins are at an increased risk for local and distant tumor relapse. Such patients are often considered candidates for adjuvant therapy (radiation for positive margins or androgen deprivation for lymph node metastases). Although adjuvant radiation seems to be associated with fewer local recurrences (0–5% with radiation versus 15–30% without), it has little or no impact on distant failure rates (30–35% with radiation versus 30–45% without).

C. Radiation Therapy: Radiation can be delivered by a variety of techniques including use of external beam radiotherapy and transperineal implantation of radioisotopes. Morbidity is limited, and the survival of patients with localized cancers (T1, T2, and selected T3) approaches 65% at 10 years. As with surgery, the likelihood of local failure correlates with technique and tumor stage. The likelihood of a positive prostatic biopsy more than 18 months after surgery varies between 20% and 60% in selected series. Patients with local recurrence are at an increased risk of cancer progression and cancer death compared with those who have negative biopsies. Ambiguous target definitions, inadequate radiation doses, and understaging of patients may be responsible for the failure noted in some series. Newer techniques of radiation (implantation, conformal therapy using three-dimensional reconstruction of CT-based tumor volumes, heavy particle, charged particle, and heavy charged particle) may improve local control rates.

D. Surveillance: A positive impact of localized prostatic cancer treatment with regard to survival has not been conclusively demonstrated. Surveillance alone may be an appropriate form of management for selected patients with prostatic cancer. However, many patients in such series are older and have very small and well-differentiated cancers. Even in such a selected population, cancer death rates approach 10%. In addition, end points for intervention in patients on surveillance regimens have not been defined.

E. Locally and Regionally Advanced Disease: Prostatic cancers associated with minimal degrees of capsular penetration are candidates for standard irradiation or surgery. Those with locally extensive cancers, including those with seminal vesicle and bladder neck invasion, are at increased risk of both local and distant relapse despite conventional therapy. Currently, a variety of investigational regimens are being tested in an effort to improve local and distant relapse rates in such patients. Combination therapy (androgen deprivation combined with surgery or irradiation), cryosurgery, newer forms of irradiation, and hormonal therapy alone are being tested in such patients. Neoadjuvant androgen deprivation therapy combined with external beam radiation therapy have demonstrated improved survival over external beam radiation therapy alone. Similarly, patients with lymph node metastases may benefit little from aggressive local therapy and are best treated with androgen deprivation because of the inevitability of distant relapse in the majority of such patients.

F. Metastatic Disease: Since death due to prostatic carcinoma is almost invariably a result of failure to control metastatic disease, research has emphasized efforts to improve control of distant disease. It is well known that most prostatic carcinomas are hormone-dependent, and approximately 70–80% of men with metastatic prostatic carcinoma will respond to various forms of androgen deprivation. Testosterone, the major circulating androgen, is produced by Leydig cells in the testes (95%), with a smaller amount being produced by peripheral conversion of other steroids. Although 98% of serum testosterone is protein-bound, free testosterone enters prostate cells and is converted to dihydrotestosterone, the major intracellular androgen. Dihydrotestosterone binds a cytoplasmic receptor protein, and the complex moves to the cell nucleus, where it modulates transcription. Androgen deprivation may be induced at several levels along the pituitary-gonadal axis using a variety of methods or agents (Table 23–9). Use of LHRH agonists (leuprolide, goserelin)—drugs delivered in monthly or 3-monthly depot—has allowed induction of androgen deprivation without orchiectomy or administration of diethylstilbestrol. Presently, administration of LHRH agonists and orchiectomy are the most common forms of primary androgen blockade used. Because of its rapid onset of action, ketoconazole should be considered in patients with advanced prostatic cancer who present with spinal cord compression, bilateral ureteral obstruction, or disseminated intravascular coagulation. Although testosterone is the major circulating androgen, the adrenal gland secretes the androgens dehydroepiandrosterone, dehydroepiandrosterone sulfate, and androstenedione. Some investigators believe that suppressing both testicular and adrenal androgens will allow for a better initial and longer response than methods which inhibit production of only testicular androgens. Complete androgen blockade can be achieved by combining an antiandrogen with use of an LHRH agonist or orchiectomy. Flutamide is a nonsteroidal antiandrogen that appears to act by competitively binding the receptor for dihydrotestosterone, the intracellular androgen responsible for prostatic cell growth and development. When patients with metastatic prostatic cancer are stratified with regard to extent of disease and performance status, those patients with limited disease and a good performance status treated with combined androgen blockade (LHRH agonist and flutamide) seem to sur-

Table 23–9. Androgen ablation for prostatic cancer.

Level	Agent	Dose	Sequelae
Pituitary, hypothalamus	Estrogens	1–3 mg daily	Gynecomastia, hot flushes, thromboembolic disease, erectile dysfunction
	LHRH agonists	Monthly or 3-monthly depot injection	Erectile dysfunction, hot flushes, gynecomastia, rarely anemia
Adrenal	Ketoconazole	400 mg three times daily	Adrenal insufficiency, nausea, rash, ataxia
	Aminoglutethimide	250 mg four times daily	Adrenal insufficiency, nausea, rash, ataxia
	Glucocorticoids	Prednisone: 20–40 mg daily	Gastrointestinal bleeding, fluid retention
Testis	Orchiectomy		Gynecomastia, hot flushes, erectile dysfunction
Prostate cell	Antiandrogens	Flutamide: 250 mg three times daily Bicalutamide: 50 mg daily	No erectile dysfunction when used alone; nausea, diarrhea

vive longer than those treated with an LHRH agonist alone. However, a recent trial has demonstrated no benefit from the addition of an antiandrogen in patients treated with orchiectomy. Additional trials examining the potential benefits of intermittent androgen deprivation are ongoing, and new antiandrogens are being tested.

Although androgen deprivation is effective, most patients with advanced disease so treated will experience disease relapse, usually within 3 years. In patients on complete androgen blockade, withdrawal of the antiandrogen can result in a secondary response in 20% of patients. The mechanism of this response remains unclear, yet both serologic (PSA) and clinical responses (improvement in bone scan and pain) have been reported. Once relapse has been identified, survival is limited. Palliative care including adequate pain control and focal irradiation of symptomatic or unstable bone disease should be instituted in patients who have failed standard hormonal therapy. Secondary therapy with chemotherapeutic agents has had limited results but should be considered in patients with a reasonable performance status. Preliminary trials of suramin, a growth factor antagonist, suggest that it may have some activity in patients with hormone-refractory prostatic cancer, and dose-escalation studies are currently ongoing. Other agents being investigated include ketoconazole and mitoxantrone.

[Prostate Cancer]
http://cancernet.nci.nih.gov/Cancer_Types/Prostate_Cancer.shtml

Bolla M et al: Improved survival in patients with locally advanced prostate cancer treated with radiotherapy and goserelin. N Engl J Med 1997;337:295. [NLM Cit ID: 97365038] (415 patients with locally advanced prostate cancer were randomized to receive radiation therapy alone or in conjunction with LHRH agonists. Improved local control and survival was seen in patients receiving neoadjuvant hormonal therapy.)

Fried RM et al: Prostate cancer screening and management. Med Clin North Am 1997;81:801. [NLM Cit ID: 97310492]

JAMA patient page: Prostate cancer. JAMA 1998; 280:1030 [NLM Cit ID: 98419918]

Klutke JJ et al: Long-term results after antegrade collagen injection for stress urinary incontinence following radical retropubic prostatectomy. Urology 1999;53:974. [NLM Cit ID: 99238003] (Collagen injection cured or improved 45% of patients with stress urinary incontinence after radical prostatectomy.)

Labrie F et al: Screening decreases prostate cancer death: first analysis of the 1988 Quebec prospective randomized controlled trial. Prostate 1999;38:83. [NLM Cit ID: 99137378]

Oh WK et al: Management of hormone refractory prostate cancer: Current standards and future prospects. J Urol 1998;160:1220. [NLM Cit ID: 98421943]

Presti JC Jr et al: Local staging of prostatic carcinoma: Comparison of transrectal sonography and endorectal MR imaging. AJR Am J Roentgenol 1996;166:103. [NLM Cit ID: 96110507] (Both imaging modalities had comparable predictive values for the detection of extracapsular extension.)

Rietbergen JB et al: The changing pattern of prostate cancer at the time of diagnosis: characteristics of screen detected prostate cancer in a population based screening study. J Urol 1999;161:1192. [NLM Cit ID: 99179905]

Rodriguez RR, et al: High dose rate brachytherapy in the treatment of prostate cancer. Hematol Oncol Clin North Am 1999;13:503. [NLM Cit ID: 99360990]

Walsh PC: Treatment with finasteride preserves usefulness of prostate-specific antigen in the detection of prostate cancer: results of a randomized, double-blind, placebo-controlled clinical trial. J Urol 1999;161:350. [NLM Cit ID: 99155040]

BLADDER CANCER

Essentials of Diagnosis

- Irritative voiding symptoms.
- Gross or microscopic hematuria.

- Positive urinary cytology in most patients.
- Filling defect within bladder noted on imaging.

General Considerations

Bladder cancer is the second most common urologic cancer, occurs more commonly in men than women (2.7:1), and the mean age at diagnosis is 65 years. Cigarette smoking and exposure to industrial dyes or solvents are risk factors for the disease and account for approximately 60% and 15% of new cases, respectively.

Clinical Findings

A. Symptoms and Signs: Hematuria—gross or microscopic, chronic or intermittent—is the presenting symptom in 85–90% of patients with bladder cancer. Irritative voiding symptoms (urinary frequency and urgency) will occur in a small percentage of patients as a result of the location or size of the cancer. Most patients with bladder cancer will fail to have signs of the disease because of its superficial nature. Masses detected on bimanual examination may be present in patients with large-volume or deeply infiltrating cancers. Hepatomegaly or supraclavicular lymphadenopathy may be present in patients with metastatic disease, and lymphedema of the lower extremities may be present as a result of locally advanced cancers or metastases to pelvic lymph nodes.

B. Laboratory Findings: Urinalysis will reveal hematuria in the majority of cases. On occasion, it may be accompanied by pyuria. Azotemia may be present in a small number of cases associated with ureteral obstruction. Anemia may occasionally be due to chronic blood loss or to bone marrow metastases. Exfoliated cells from normal and abnormal urothelium can be readily detected in voided urine specimens. Cytology may be useful in detecting the disease at the time of initial presentation or to detect recurrence. Cytology is very sensitive in detecting cancers of higher grade and stage (80–90%) but less so in detecting superficial or well-differentiated lesions (50%). Sensitivity of detection using exfoliated cells may be enhanced by flow cytometry.

C. Imaging: Bladder cancers may be detected using intravenous urography, ultrasound, CT, or MRI where filling defects within the bladder are noted. However, the presence of cancer is confirmed by cystoscopy and biopsy, so imaging is useful primarily for evaluating the upper urinary tract and in staging the more advanced lesions.

D. Cystourethroscopy and Biopsy: The diagnosis and staging of bladder cancers is made by cystoscopy and transurethral resection. If cystoscopy—performed usually under local anesthesia—confirms the presence of bladder cancer, the patient is scheduled for transurethral resection under general or regional anesthesia. A careful bimanual examination is performed initially and at the end of the procedure, noting the size, position, and degree of fixation of a mass, if present. Any suspicious lesions are resected using electrocautery. Resection is carried down to the muscular elements of the bladder wall so as to allow complete staging. Random bladder and, on occasion, prostatic urethral biopsies are performed to detect occult disease elsewhere in the bladder and, therefore, identify patients at high risk of recurrence and progression.

Pathology & Selection of Treatment

Ninety-eight percent of primary bladder cancers are epithelial malignancies, with the majority being transitional cell carcinomas (90%). These latter cancers most often appear as papillary growths, but higher-grade lesions are often sessile and ulcerated. Grading is based on histologic architecture: size, pleomorphism, mitotic rate, and hyperchromatism. The frequency of recurrence and progression is strongly correlated with grade. Whereas progression may be noted in few grade I cancers (19–37%), it is common with poorly differentiated lesions (33–67%). Carcinoma in situ is recognizable as a flat, nonpapillary, anaplastic epithelium and may occur focally or diffusely, but it is most often found in association with papillary bladder cancers. Its presence identifies a patient at increased risk of recurrence and progression.

Adenocarcinomas and squamous cell cancers account for approximately 2% and 7% (respectively) of all bladder cancers detected in the USA. The latter is often associated with schistosomiasis, vesical calculi, or chronic catheter use.

Bladder cancer staging is based on the extent of bladder wall penetration and the presence of either regional or distant metastases. The TNM classification of the American Joint Cancer Committee for bladder cancer is shown in Table 23–10.

The natural history of bladder cancer is based on two separate but related processes: tumor recurrence and progression to higher stage disease. Both are related to tumor grade and stage. At initial presentation, approximately 50–80% of bladder cancers will be superficial: Ta, Tis, T1. Lymph node metastases and progression are uncommon in such patients when they are properly treated, and survival is excellent at 81%. Patients with superficial cancers (Ta, T1) are treated with complete transurethral resection and the selective use of intravesical chemotherapy. The latter is used to prevent or delay recurrence. Patients who present with large, high-grade, recurrent Ta lesions, T1 cancers, and those with carcinoma in situ are good candidates for intravesical chemotherapy. Patients with more invasive (T2, T3) but still localized cancers are at risk of both nodal metastases and progression, and they require more aggressive surgery, irradiation, or the combination of chemotherapy and selective surgery or irradiation due to the much higher risk of progression compared to patients with

Table 23–10. TNM staging system for bladder cancer.

T: Primary tumor	
Tx	Cannot be assessed
T0	No evidence of primary tumor
Tis	Carcinoma in situ (CIS)
Ta	Noninvasive papillary carcinoma
T1	Invasion into lamina propria
T2a	Invasion into superficial layer of muscularis propria
T2b	Invasion into deep layer of muscularis propria
T3	Invasion through serosa into perivesical fat
T4a	Invasion into adjacent organs
T4b	Invasion into pelvic sidewall
N: Regional lymph nodes	
Nx	Cannot be assessed
N0	No regional lymph node metastasis
N1	Metastasis in a single lymph node 2 cm or less
N2	Metastasis in a single lymph node > 2 cm and < 5 cm or multiple nodes none > 5 cm
N3	Metastasis in lymph node > 5 cm
M: Distant metastasis	
Mx	Cannot be assessed
M0	No distant metastasis
M1	Distant metastasis present

lower-stage lesions. Patients with evidence of lymph node or distant metastases should undergo systemic chemotherapy initially.

Treatment

A. Intravesical Chemotherapy: Immuno- or chemotherapeutic agents can be delivered directly into the bladder by a urethral catheter. They can be used to eradicate existing disease or to reduce the likelihood of recurrence in those who have undergone complete transurethral resection. Such therapy is more effective in the latter situation. Most agents are administered weekly for 6–12 weeks. The use of maintenance therapy after the initial induction regimen may be beneficial. Efficacy may be increased by prolonging contact time to 2 hours. Common agents include thiotepa, mitomycin, doxorubicin, and BCG, the latter being the most effective agent when compared with the others. Side effects of intravesical chemotherapy include irritative voiding symptoms and hemorrhagic cystitis. Systemic effects are rare. Patients who develop symptoms from BCG may require antituberculous therapy.

B. Surgical Treatment: Although transurethral resection is the initial form of treatment for all bladder cancers as it is diagnostic, allows for proper staging, and will control superficial cancers, muscle infiltrating cancers will require more aggressive treatment. Partial cystectomy may be indicated in patients with solitary lesions and those with cancers in a bladder diverticulum. Radical cystectomy entails removal of the bladder, prostate, seminal vesicles, and surrounding fat and peritoneal attachments in men and in women also the uterus, cervix, urethra, anterior vaginal vault, and usually the ovaries. Bilateral pelvic lymph node dissection is performed simultaneously.

Urinary diversion can be performed using a conduit of small or large bowel. However, continent forms of diversion have been developed that avoid the necessity of an external appliance.

C. Radiotherapy: External beam radiotherapy delivered in fractions over a 6- to 8-week period is generally well tolerated, but approximately 10–15% of patients will develop bladder, bowel, or rectal complications. Unfortunately, local recurrence is common after radiotherapy (30–70%). Increasingly, radiotherapy is being combined with systemic chemotherapy in an effort to improve local and distant relapse rates.

D. Chemotherapy: Fifteen percent of patients with newly diagnosed bladder cancer will present with metastatic disease, and 40% of those thought to have localized disease at the time of cystectomy or definitive radiotherapy will develop metastases usually within 2 years after the start of treatment. Cisplatin-based combination chemotherapy will result in partial or complete responses in 15–35% and 15–45% of patients, respectively.

Combination chemotherapy has been integrated into trials of surgery and radiotherapy. It has been used before each in an attempt to preserve the bladder and decrease recurrence rates. Alternatively, it has been employed postoperatively in patients who have undergone cystectomy and have been found to be at high risk of recurrence. In current practice, adjuvant chemotherapy when indicated—ie, when the primary tumor invades perivesical fat or adjacent organs or when lymph nodes are found to have metastatic disease—is being offered mainly to patients being treated with radical cystectomy. It is used less often for patients with unresectable disease (extension to pelvic side wall).

Carroll PR: Urothelial carcinoma: Cancers of the bladder, ureter and renal pelvis. In: *Smith's General Urology,* 15th ed. Tanagho EA, McAninch JW (editors). McGraw-Hill, 2000.

Ozen H: Bladder cancer. Curr Opin Oncol 1998;10:273. [NLM Cit ID: 98283124] (General review with discussion of several new tumor markers and implications for therapy.)

Smith JA Jr et al: Bladder cancer clinical guidelines panel summary report on the management of nonmuscle invasive bladder cancer (stages Ta, T1 and Tis). The American Urological Association. J Urol 1999;162:1697. [NLM Cit ID: 99452540]

Sternberg CN: Neoadjuvant and adjuvant chemotherapy in locally advanced bladder cancer. Semin Oncol 1996; 23:621. [NLM Cit ID: 97049143] (Patients with high-stage or unresectable disease are appropriate candidates for neoadjuvant chemotherapy. Bladder preservation after neoadjuvant chemotherapy is a controversial issue that will require validation in randomized trials. Adjuvant chemotherapy may prolong disease-free survival in patients at high risk for relapse after cystectomy.)

CANCERS OF THE URETER & RENAL PELVIS

Cancers of the renal pelvis and ureter are rare and occur more commonly in smokers, in those with Balkan nephropathy, in those exposed to Thorotrast (a contrast agent with radioactive thorium in use until the 1960s), or those with a long history of analgesic abuse. The majority are transitional cell carcinomas. Gross or microscopic hematuria occurs in most patients, and flank pain secondary to bleeding and obstruction occurs less commonly. Like primary bladder cancers, urinary cytology is often positive. The most common signs identified at the time of intravenous pyelography include an intraluminal filling defect, unilateral nonvisualization of the collecting system, and hydronephrosis. Ureteral and renal pelvic tumors must be differentiated from calculi, blood clots, papillary necrosis, or inflammatory or infectious lesions. On occasion, such lesions are accessible to direct biopsy, fulguration, or resection using a ureteroscope. Treatment is based on the site, size, depth of penetration, and number of tumors present. Most such cancers are excised with nephroureterectomy (renal pelvic and upper ureteral lesions) or segmental excision of the ureter (distal ureteral lesions). Endoscopic resection may be indicated in patients with limited renal function and in the management of focal, low-grade, upper tract cancers.

[Transitional Cell Cancer of Renal Pelvis and Ureter]
http://cancernet.nci.nih.gov/Cancer_Types/Transitional_Cell_Cancer.shtml

PRIMARY TUMORS OF THE KIDNEY

1. RENAL CELL CARCINOMA

Essentials of Diagnosis

- Gross or microscopic hematuria.
- Flank pain or mass in some patients.
- Systemic symptoms such as fever, weight loss may be prominent.
- Solid renal mass on imaging.

General Considerations

Renal cell carcinoma accounts for 2.3% of all adult cancers. In the United States in 1999, approximately 30,900 cases of renal cell carcinoma will be diagnosed and 11,900 deaths will result. Renal cell carcinoma has a peak incidence in the sixth decade of life and a male-to-female ratio of 2:1.

The cause is unknown. Cigarette smoking is the only significant environmental risk factor that has been identified. Familial settings for renal cell carcinoma have been identified (von Hippel-Lindau syndrome) as well as an association with dialysis-related acquired cystic disease, but sporadic tumors are far more common.

Renal cell carcinoma originates from the proximal tubule cells. Various cell types (clear, granular, spindle) and histologic patterns (acinar, papillary, solid) are observed. However, cell type and histologic pattern do not affect treatment. The TNM classification of the American Joint Cancer Committee for kidney cancer is shown in Table 23–11.

Clinical Findings

A. Symptoms and Signs: Historically, 60% of patients presented with gross or microscopic hematuria. Flank pain or an abdominal mass was detected in approximately 30% of cases. The triad of flank pain, hematuria, and mass was found in only 10–15% of patients and is often a sign of advanced disease. Symptoms of metastatic disease (cough, bone pain) occur in 20–30% of patients at presentation. Because of the more widespread use of ultrasound and CT scanning for diverse indications, renal tumors are being detected incidentally in patients with no urologic symptoms.

B. Laboratory Findings: Hematuria is present in 60% of patients. Paraneoplastic syndromes are not uncommon in renal cell carcinoma. Erythrocytosis from increased erythropoietin production occurs in 5%, though anemia is far more common; hypercalcemia may be present in up to 10% of patients. Stauf-

Table 23–11. TNM staging system for kidney cancer.

T: Primary tumor	
Tx	Cannot be assessed
T0	No evidence of primary tumor
T1	Tumor ≤ 7 cm limited to kidney
T2	Tumor > 7 cm limited to kidney
T3a	Tumor invades adrenal gland or perinephric tissue
T3b	Tumor extends into renal vein or vena cava
T3c	Tumor extends into renal vein or vena cava above diaphragm
T4	Tumor invades outside of Gerota's fascia
N: Regional lymph nodes	
Nx	Cannot be assessed
N0	No regional lymph node metastasis
N1	Metastasis in a single lymph node
N2	Metastasis in multiple nodes
N3	Metastasis in lymph node > 5 cm
M: Distant metastasis	
Mx	Cannot be assessed
M0	No distant metastasis
M1	Distant metastasis present

fer's syndrome is a reversible syndrome of hepatic dysfunction in the absence of metastatic disease.

C. Imaging: Renal masses are often first detected by intravenous urography. Further evaluation requires ultrasound to determine whether it is solid or cystic. CT scanning is the most valuable imaging test for renal cell carcinoma. It confirms the character of the mass and further stages the lesion with respect to regional lymph nodes, renal vein, or hepatic involvement. It also gives valuable information on the contralateral kidney (function, bilaterality of neoplasm). Chest radiographs exclude pulmonary metastases, and bone scans should be performed for large tumors and in patients with bone pain or elevated alkaline phosphatase levels. MRI and duplex Doppler ultrasonography are excellent methods of assessing for the presence and extent of tumor thrombus within the renal vein or vena cava in selected patients.

Differential Diagnosis

Solid lesions of the kidney are renal cell carcinoma until proved otherwise. Other solid masses include angiomyolipomas (fat density usually visible by CT); transitional cell cancers of the renal pelvis (more centrally located, involvement of the collecting system, positive urinary cytology reports); adrenal tumors (supero-anterior to the kidney) and oncocytomas (indistinguishable from renal cell carcinoma preoperatively); and renal abscesses.

Treatment & Prognosis

Radical nephrectomy is the primary treatment for localized renal cell carcinoma. Tumors confined to the renal capsule (T1–T2) demonstrate 5-year disease-free survivals of 90–100%. Tumors extending beyond the renal capsule (T3 or T4) and node-positive tumors have 50–60% and 0–15% 5-year disease-free survivals, respectively.

No effective chemotherapy is available for metastatic renal cell carcinoma. Vinblastine is the single most effective agent, with short-term partial response rates of 15%. Biologic response modifiers have received much attention, including alpha interferon and interleukin-2. Partial response rates of 15–20% and 15–35%, respectively, have been reported. Responders tend to have lower tumor burdens, metastatic disease confined to the lung, and a high performance status. Because of these low response rates, new investigations are ongoing with tumor vaccines and gene therapy.

One subgroup of metastatic patients has demonstrated long-term survival, namely, those with solitary resectable metastases. In this setting, radical nephrectomy with resection of the metastasis has resulted in 5-year disease-free survival rates of 15–30%.

[Renal Cell Cancer]
http://cancernet.nci.nih.gov/cancer_types/bladder_cancer.shtml

Figlin RA: Renal cell carcinoma: management of advanced disease. J Urol 1999;161:381. [NLM Cit ID: 99112614] (IL-2 can produce durable complete remissions.)

Gleave ME et al: Interferon gamma-1b compared with placebo in metastatic renal cell carcinoma. Canadian Urologic Oncology Group. N Engl J Med 1998;338:1265. [NLM Cit ID: 98213296] (Treatment with interferon gamma no better than placebo in patients with metastatic renal cell carcinoma.)

Guinan PD et al: Renal cell carcinoma: Tumor size, stage and survival. Members of the Cancer Incidence and End Results Committee. J Urol 1995;153:901. [NLM Cit ID: 95156668] (Tumor size correlated with tumor stage and survival.)

Javidan J et al: Prognostic significance of the 1997 TNM classification of renal cell carcinoma. J Urol 1991;62:1277. [NLM Cit ID: 99419928]

Negrier S et al: Recombinant human interleukin-2, recombinant human interferon alfa-2a, or both in metastatic renal cell carcinoma. Groupe Français d'Immunothérapie. N Engl J Med 1998;338:1272. [NLM Cit ID: 98213297] (Response rates of 6.5% and 7.5% with interferon or IL-2 alone and a statistically significant 18.6% response rate with combination therapy, though there was substantial treatment-related morbidity.)

2. OTHER PRIMARY TUMORS OF THE KIDNEY

Oncocytomas account for 3–5% of renal tumors and are indistinguishable from renal cell carcinoma by all imaging modalities. The biologic potential of these lesions is not well defined. These tumors are seen in other organs, including the adrenals, the salivary glands, and the thyroid and parathyroid glands.

Angiomyolipomas are rare benign tumors composed of fat, smooth muscle, and blood vessels. They are most commonly seen in patients with tuberous sclerosis (often multiple and bilateral) or in young to middle-aged women. CT scanning may identify the fat component, which is diagnostic for angiomyolipoma. Asymptomatic lesions less than 5 cm in diameter usually do not require intervention.

Dechet CB et al: Renal oncocytoma: multifocality, bilateralism, metachronous tumor development and coexistent renal cell carcinoma. J Urol 1999;162:40. [NLM Cit ID: 99306403] (Oncocytomas are benign. Renal cell carcinoma may coexist in 10% of these tumors.)

SECONDARY TUMORS OF THE KIDNEY

The kidney is not an infrequent site for metastatic disease. Of the solid tumors, the lung is the most common (20%), followed by breast (10%), stomach (10%), and the contralateral kidney (10%). Lymphoma, both Hodgkin's and non-Hodgkin's, may also involve the kidney, though it tends to be a diffusely infiltrative process resulting in renal enlargement rather than a discrete mass.

PRIMARY TUMORS OF THE TESTIS

Essentials of Diagnosis

- Commonest neoplasm in men aged 20–35.
- Typical presentation as a patient-identified painless nodule.
- Orchiectomy necessary for diagnosis.

General Considerations

Malignant tumors of the testis are rare, with approximately two to three new cases per 100,000 males being reported in the United States each year. Ninety to 95 percent of all primary testicular tumors are germ cell tumors (seminoma and nonseminoma), while the remainder are nongerminal neoplasms (Leydig cell, Sertoli cell, gonadoblastoma). The lifetime probability of developing testicular cancer is 0.2% for an American white male. For the purposes of this review, we will only consider germ cell tumors. Survival in testicular cancer has improved dramatically in recent years as a result of the development and application of effective combination chemotherapy.

Testicular cancer is slightly more common on the right than on the left, which parallels the increased incidence of cryptorchism on the right side. One to 2 percent of primary testicular tumors are bilateral, and up to 50% of these men have a history of unilateral or bilateral cryptorchism. Primary bilateral testicular tumors may occur synchronously or asynchronously but tend to be of the same histology. Seminoma is the most common histologic finding in bilateral *primary* testicular tumors, while malignant lymphoma is the most common bilateral testicular tumor.

While the cause of testicular cancer is unknown, both congenital and acquired factors have been associated with tumor development. Approximately 5% of testicular tumors develop in a patient with a history of cryptorchism, with seminoma being the most common. However, 5–10% of these tumors occur in the contralateral, normally descended testis. The relative risk of development of malignancy is highest for the intra-abdominal testis (1:20) and lower for the inguinal testis (1:80). Placement of the cryptorchid testis into the scrotum (orchiopexy) does not alter the malignant potential of the cryptorchid testis; however, it does facilitate examination and tumor detection.

In animal models, exogenous estrogen administration during pregnancy has been associated with an increased relative risk for testicular tumors ranging from 2.8 to 5.3. Other acquired factors such as trauma and infection-related testicular atrophy have been associated with testicular tumors; however, a causal relationship has not been established.

Histopathology & Clinical Staging

From a treatment standpoint, testicular carcinoma can be divided into two major categories: (1) nonseminomas, which include embryonal cell carcinomas (20%), teratomas (5%), choriocarcinomas (< 1%), and mixed cell types (40%); and (2) seminomas (35%). In a commonly used staging system for nonseminoma germ cell tumors, a stage A lesion is confined to the testis; stage B demonstrates regional lymph node involvement in the retroperitoneum; and stage C indicates distant metastasis. For seminoma, the M.D. Anderson system is commonly used. In this system, a stage I lesion is confined to the testis, a stage II lesion has spread to the retroperitoneal lymph nodes, and a stage III lesion has supradiaphragmatic nodal or visceral involvement. The TNM classification of the American Joint Cancer Committee for testis cancer is shown in Table 23–12.

Clinical Findings

A. Symptoms and Signs: The most common symptom of testicular cancer is painless enlargement of the testis. Sensations of heaviness are not unusual. Patients are usually the first to recognize an abnormality, yet the typical delay in seeking medical attention ranges from 3 to 6 months. Acute testicular pain resulting from intratesticular hemorrhage occurs in approximately 10% of cases. Ten percent of patients are asymptomatic at presentation, and 10% manifest symptoms relating to metastatic disease such as back pain (retroperitoneal metastases), cough (pulmonary metastases), or lower extremity edema (vena cava obstruction).

Table 23–12. TNM staging system for testicular cancer.

T: Primary tumor	
Tx	Cannot be assessed
T0	No evidence of primary tumor
Tis	Intratubular cancer (CIS)
T1	Limited to testis without vascular invasion
T2	Invades beyond tunica albuginea or into epididymis, or limited to testis with vascular invasion
T3	Invades spermatic cord
T4	Invades scrotum
N: Regional lymph nodes	
Nx	Cannot be assessed
N0	No regional lymph node metastasis
N1	Metastasis in a single lymph node 2 cm or less
N2	Metastasis in a single lymph node > 2 cm and < 5 cm or multiple nodes none > 5 cm
N3	Metastasis in lymph node > 5 cm
M: Distant metastasis	
Mx	Cannot be assessed
M0	No distant metastasis
M1	Distant metastasis present

A testicular mass or diffuse enlargement of the testis is found in the majority of cases on physical examination. Secondary hydroceles may be present in 5–10% of cases. In advanced disease, supraclavicular adenopathy may be detected, and abdominal examination may palpate a retroperitoneal mass. Gynecomastia is seen in 5% of germ cell tumors.

B. Laboratory Findings: Several biochemical markers are important in the diagnosis and treatment of testicular carcinoma, including human chorionic gonadotropin (hCG), alpha-fetoprotein, and LDH. Alpha-fetoprotein is never elevated in seminomas, and while hCG is occasionally elevated in seminomas, levels tend to be lower than those seen in nonseminomas. LDH may be elevated in either type of tumor. Liver function tests may be elevated in the presence of hepatic metastases, and anemia may be present in advanced disease. In patients with advanced disease who will receive chemotherapy, renal function is assessed with a 24-hour creatinine clearance urine collection.

C. Imaging: Scrotal ultrasound can readily determine whether the mass is intra- or extratesticular in origin. Once the diagnosis of testicular cancer has been established by inguinal orchiectomy, clinical staging of the disease is accomplished by chest radiograph and abdominal and pelvic CT scanning.

Differential Diagnosis

An incorrect diagnosis is made at the initial examination in up to 25% of patients with testicular tumors. The differential diagnosis of scrotal masses has been discussed previously in this chapter. Scrotal ultrasonography should be performed if any uncertainty exists with respect to the diagnosis. Although most intratesticular masses are malignant, one benign lesion, an epidermoid cyst, may rarely been seen. Epidermoid cysts are usually very small benign nodules located just underneath the tunica albuginea; on occasion, however, they can be large.

Treatment

Inguinal exploration with early vascular control of the spermatic cord structures is the initial intervention to exclude neoplasm. If cancer cannot be excluded by examination of the testis, radical orchiectomy is warranted. Scrotal approaches and open testicular biopsies should be avoided. Further therapy is dependent upon the histology of the tumor as well as the clinical stage.

The 5-year disease-free survival rates for stage I and IIa (retroperitoneal disease < 10 cm in diameter) seminomas treated by radical orchiectomy and retroperitoneal irradiation are 98% and 92–94%, respectively. High-stage seminomas of stage IIb (> 10 cm retroperitoneal involvement) and stage III receive primary chemotherapy (etoposide and cisplatin or cisplatin, etoposide, and bleomycin). Ninety-five percent of patients with stage III disease will attain a complete response following orchiectomy and chemotherapy. Surgical resection of residual retroperitoneal masses is warranted only if the mass is larger than 3 cm in diameter, under which circumstances 40% will harbor residual carcinoma.

Up to 75% of stage A nonseminomas are cured by orchiectomy alone. Currently, such patients may be treated by modified retroperitoneal lymph node dissections designed to preserve the sympathetic innervation for ejaculation. Selected patients who meet specific criteria may be offered surveillance. These criteria are as follows: (1) tumor is confined within the tunica albuginea; (2) tumor does not demonstrate vascular invasion; (3) tumor markers normalize after orchiectomy; (4) radiographic imaging shows no evidence of disease (chest x-ray and CT); and (5) the patient is reliable. Surveillance should be considered an active process both by the physician and by the patient. Patients are followed monthly for the first 2 years and bimonthly in the third year. Tumor markers are obtained at each visit, and chest x-ray and CT scans are obtained every 3–4 months. Follow-up continues beyond the initial 3 years; however, the majority of relapses will occur within the first 8–10 months. With rare exceptions, patients who relapse can be cured by chemotherapy or surgery. The 5-year disease-free survival rate for patients with stage A disease ranges from 96% to 100%. For low-volume stage B disease, 90% 5-year disease-free survival is attainable.

Patients with bulky retroperitoneal disease (> 3 cm nodes) or metastatic nonseminomas are treated with primary cisplatin-based combination chemotherapy following orchiectomy (etoposide and cisplatin or cisplatin, etoposide, and bleomycin). If tumor markers normalize and a residual mass greater than 3 cm is apparent on imaging studies, resection of that mass is mandatory because 20% of the time it will harbor residual cancer and 40% of the time it will be teratoma. Even if patients have a complete response to chemotherapy, retroperitoneal lymphadenectomy is advocated by some as 10% of patients may harbor residual carcinoma and 10% may have teratoma in the retroperitoneum. If tumor markers fail to normalize following primary chemotherapy, salvage chemotherapy is required (cisplatin etoposide, bleomycin, ifosfamide).

Prognosis

Patients with bulky retroperitoneal or disseminated disease treated with primary chemotherapy followed by surgery have a 5-year disease-free survival rate of 55–80%.

[Testis Cancer]
http://cancernet.nci.nih.gov/cancer_types/testicular_cancer.shtml

Carroll PR et al: Testis cancer. Urol Clin North Am 1998;25. (Entire volume.)

Nichols CR et al: Defining new standards for adjuvant therapy of testis cancer [editorial]. J Clin Oncol 1995;13: 2681. [NLM Cit ID: 96067223]

Puc HS et al: Management of residual mass in advanced seminoma: Results and recommendations from the Memorial Sloan-Kettering Cancer Center. J Clin Oncol 1996;14:454. [NLM Cit ID: 96223401] (Patients with advanced seminoma who have normal radiographs or residual masses less than 3 cm after chemotherapy can be observed without further intervention.)

SECONDARY TUMORS OF THE TESTIS

Secondary tumors of the testis are rare. Lymphoma is the most common testis tumor in a patient over the age of 50 and is the most common secondary neoplasm of the testis, accounting for 5% of all testicular tumors. It may be seen in three clinical settings: (1) as a late manifestation of widespread lymphoma; (2) as the initial presentation of clinically occult disease; and (3) as primary extranodal disease. Radical orchiectomy is indicated to make the diagnosis. Prognosis is related to the stage of disease.

Metastasis to the testis is rare. The most common primary site is the prostate, followed by the lung, gastrointestinal tract, melanoma, and kidney.

RELEVANT WORLD WIDE WEB SITES

[Chronic Prostatitis]
http://www.parsec.it/summit/p0.htm

[Digital Urology Journal]
http://www.duj.com

[Testicular Torsion]
http://www.brighamrad.harvard.edu/Cases/bwh/hcache/125/full.html

[Obstructive Hydroureteronephrosis]
http://www.brighamrad.harvard.edu/Cases/bwh/hcache/188/full.html

[Testicular Torsion]
http://www.brighamrad.harvard.edu/Cases/bwh/hcache/80/full.html

[Left Renal Obstruction]
http://www.brighamrad.harvard.edu/Cases/bwh/hcache/2/full.html

[Transitional Cell Carcinoma of the Bladder]
http://www.brighamrad.harvard.edu/Cases/bwh/hcache/79/full.html

Nervous System

24

See http://www.current-med.com/ch24.html for updated addresses of Web sites referenced in this chapter.

Michael J. Aminoff, MD, FRCP

HEADACHE

Headache is such a common complaint and can occur for so many different reasons that its proper evaluation may be difficult. Although underlying structural lesions are not present in most patients presenting with headache, it is nevertheless important to bear this possibility in mind. About one-third of patients with brain tumors, for example, present with a primary complaint of headache.

The intensity, quality, and site of pain—and especially the duration of the headache and the presence of associated neurologic symptoms—may provide clues to the underlying cause. The onset of severe headache in a previously well patient is more likely than chronic headache to relate to an intracranial disorder such as subarachnoid hemorrhage or meningitis. Headaches that disturb sleep, exertional headaches, and late-onset paroxysmal headaches are also more suggestive of an underlying structural lesion, as are headaches accompanied by neurologic symptoms such as drowsiness, visual or limb problems, seizures, or altered mental status. Chronic headaches are commonly due to migraine, tension, or depression, but they may be related to intracranial lesions, head injury, cervical spondylosis, dental or ocular disease, temporomandibular joint dysfunction, sinusitis, hypertension, and a wide variety of general medical disorders. Depending on the initial clinical impression, the need for such investigations as CT scan or MRI of the head, electroencephalography, and lumbar puncture must be assessed on an individual basis. The diagnosis and treatment of primary neurologic disorders associated with headache are considered separately under these disorders.

Tension Headache

Patients frequently complain of poor concentration and other vague nonspecific symptoms, in addition to constant daily headaches that are often vise-like or tight in quality and may be exacerbated by emotional stress, fatigue, noise, or glare. The headaches are usually generalized, may be most intense about the neck or back of the head, and are not associated with focal neurologic symptoms.

When treatment with simple analgesics is not effective, a trial of antimigrainous agents (see Migraine, below) is worthwhile. Techniques to induce relaxation are also useful and include massage, hot baths, and biofeedback. Exploration of underlying causes of chronic anxiety is often rewarding.

Depression Headache

Depression headaches are frequently worse on arising in the morning and may be accompanied by other symptoms of depression. Headaches are occasionally the focus of a somatic delusional system. Tricyclic antidepressant drugs are often helpful, as may be psychiatric consultation.

Migraine

Classic migrainous headache is a lateralized throbbing headache that occurs episodically following its onset in adolescence or early adult life. In many cases, however, the headaches do not conform to this pattern, although their associated features and response to antimigrainous preparations nevertheless suggest that they have a similar basis. In this broader sense, migrainous headaches may be lateralized or generalized, may be dull or throbbing, and are sometimes associated with anorexia, nausea, vomiting, photophobia, phonophobia, and blurring of vision. They usually build up gradually and may last for several hours or longer. They have been related to dilation and excessive pulsation of branches of the external carotid artery. Focal disturbances of neurologic function may precede or accompany the headaches and have been attributed to constriction of branches of the internal carotid artery. Visual disturbances occur quite commonly and may consist of field defects; of luminous visual hallucinations such as stars, sparks, unformed light flashes (photopsia), geometric patterns, or zigzags of light; or of some combination of field defects and luminous hallucinations (scintillating scotomas). Other focal disturbances such as aphasia or numbness, tingling, clumsiness, or weakness in a circumscribed distribution may also occur.

Patients often give a family history of migraine. Attacks may be triggered by emotional or physical stress, lack or excess of sleep, missed meals, specific foods (eg, chocolate), alcoholic beverages, menstruation, or use of oral contraceptives.

An uncommon variant is **basilar artery migraine,** in which blindness or visual disturbances throughout both visual fields are initially accompanied or followed by dysarthria, disequilibrium, tinnitus, and perioral and distal paresthesias and are sometimes followed by transient loss or impairment of consciousness or by a confusional state. This, in turn, is followed by a throbbing (usually occipital) headache, often with nausea and vomiting.

In **ophthalmoplegic migraine,** lateralized pain—often about the eye—is accompanied by nausea, vomiting, and diplopia due to transient external ophthalmoplegia. The ophthalmoplegia is due to third nerve palsy, sometimes with accompanying sixth nerve involvement, and may outlast the orbital pain by several days or even weeks. The ophthalmic division of the fifth nerve has also been affected in some patients. Ophthalmoplegic migraine is rare; more common causes of a painful ophthalmoplegia are internal carotid artery aneurysms and diabetes.

In rare instances, the neurologic or somatic disturbance accompanying typical migrainous headaches becomes the sole manifestation of an attack ("migraine equivalent"). Very rarely, the patient may be left with a permanent neurologic deficit following a migrainous attack.

The pathophysiology of migraine probably relates to the neurotransmitter serotonin. Headache may result from release of neuropeptides acting as neurotransmitters at trigeminal nerve branches, leading to an inflammatory process; another possible mechanism involves activation of the dorsal raphe nucleus.

Management of migraine consists of avoidance of any precipitating factors, together with prophylactic or symptomatic pharmacologic treatment if necessary.

During acute attacks, many patients find it helpful to rest in a quiet, darkened room until symptoms subside. A simple analgesic (eg, aspirin) taken right away often provides relief, but treatment with extracranial vasoconstrictors or other drugs is sometimes necessary. Cafergot, a combination of ergotamine tartrate (1 mg) and caffeine (100 mg), is often particularly helpful; one or two tablets are taken at the onset of headache or warning symptoms, followed by one tablet every 30 minutes, if necessary, up to six tablets per attack and ten tablets per week. Because of impaired absorption or vomiting during acute attacks, oral medication sometimes fails to help. Cafergot given rectally as suppositories (one-half to one suppository containing 2 mg of ergotamine); ergotamine tartrate given by inhalation (0.36 mg per puff; up to six puffs per attack) or sublingually (2 mg tablets; not more than three tablets per 24 hours); or dihydroergotamine mesylate (0.5–1 mg intravenously or 1–2 mg subcutaneously or intramuscularly) may be useful in such cases. Alternatively, prochlorperazine administered rectally (25 mg suppository) or intravenously (10 mg) may be prescribed. Ergotamine-containing preparations may affect the gravid uterus and thus should be avoided during pregnancy. Sumatriptan is a rapidly effective agent for aborting attacks when given subcutaneously by an autoinjection device. It has a high affinity for $serotonin_1$ receptors. It should probably be avoided in pregnancy. Sumatriptan can also be taken in a nasal form, but absorption is limited and a bitter aftertaste may be disturbing; an oral preparation is available but is poorly absorbed. Zolmitriptan, another selective $serotonin_1$ receptor agonist, has high bioavailability after oral administration and is also effective for the acute treatment of migraine. The optimal initial dose is 2.5 mg, and relief usually occurs within 1 hour.

Prophylactic treatment may be necessary if migrainous headaches occur more frequently than two or three times a month. Some of the more common drugs used for this purpose are listed in Table 24–1. Their mode of action is unclear and may involve both an effect on extracerebral vasculature and a cerebral effect, eg, by stabilizing serotonergic neurotransmission. Several drugs may have to be tried in turn before the headaches are brought under control. Once a drug has been found to help, it should be continued for several months. If the patient remains headache-free, the dose can then be tapered and the drug eventually withdrawn.

Calcium channel antagonist drugs may decrease the frequency of attacks after an interval of several weeks, but the severity and duration of attacks are not influenced. They should not be used with beta-blockers.

Cluster Headache (Migrainous Neuralgia)

Cluster headache affects predominantly middle-aged men. Its cause is unclear but may relate to a vascular headache disorder or a disturbance of serotonergic mechanisms. There is often no family history of headache or migraine. Episodes of severe unilateral periorbital pain occur daily for several weeks and are often accompanied by one or more of the following: ipsilateral nasal congestion, rhinorrhea, lacrimation, redness of the eye, and Horner's syndrome. Episodes usually occur at night, awaken the patient, and last for less than 2 hours. Spontaneous remission then occurs, and the patient remains well for weeks or months before another bout of closely spaced attacks occurs. During a bout, many patients report that alcohol triggers an attack; others report that stress, glare, or ingestion of specific foods occasionally precipitates attacks. In occasional patients, typical attacks of pain and associated symptoms recur at intervals without remission. This variant has been referred to as chronic cluster headache.

Examination reveals no abnormality apart from Horner's syndrome that either occurs transiently dur-

Table 24–1. Prophylactic treatment of migraine.

Drug	Usual Adult Daily Dose	Common Side Effects
Aspirin	650–1950 mg	Dyspepsia, gastrointestinal bleeding.
Propranolol	80–240 mg	Fatigue, lassitude, depression, insomnia, nausea, vomiting, constipation.
Amitriptyline	10–150 mg	Sedation, dry mouth, constipation, weight gain, blurred vision, edema, hypotension, urinary retention.
Imipramine	10–150 mg	Similar to those of amitriptyline (above).
Sertraline	50–200 mg	Anxiety, insomnia, sweating, tremor, gastrointestinal disturbances.
Fluoxetine	20–60 mg	Similar to those of sertraline (above).
Ergonovine maleate	0.6–2 mg	Nausea, vomiting, abdominal pain, diarrhea.
Cyproheptadine	12–20 mg	Sedation, dry mouth, epigastric discomfort, gastrointestinal disturbances.
Clonidine	0.2–0.6 mg	Dry mouth, drowsiness, sedation, headache, constipation.
Methysergide	4–8 mg	Nausea, vomiting, diarrhea, abdominal pain, cramps, weight gain, insomnia, edema, peripheral vasoconstriction. Retroperitoneal and pleuropulmonary fibrosis and fibrous thickening of cardiac valves may occur.
Verapamil[1]	80–160 mg	Headache, hypotension, flushing, edema, constipation. May aggravate atrioventricular nodal heart block and congestive heart failure.

[1]Other calcium channel antagonists (eg, nimodipine, nifedipine, and diltiazem) may also be used.

ing an attack or, in long-standing cases, remains as a residual deficit between attacks.

Treatment of an individual attack with oral drugs is generally unsatisfactory, but subcutaneous sumatriptan (6 mg) or dihydroergotamine (1–2 mg) or use of ergotamine tartrate aerosol or inhalation of 100% oxygen (7 L/min for 15 minutes) may be effective. Butorphanol tartrate, a synthetic opioid agonist-antagonist, may also be helpful when administered by nasal spray. The dose is 1 mg (one spray in one nostril), repeated after 60–90 minutes if necessary. Ergotamine tartrate is an effective prophylactic and can be given as rectal suppositories (0.5–1 mg at night or twice daily), by mouth (2 mg daily), or by subcutaneous injection (0.25 mg three times daily for 5 days per week). Various prophylactic agents that have been found to be effective in individual patients are propranolol, amitriptyline, valproate, cyproheptadine, lithium carbonate (monitored by plasma lithium determination), prednisone (20–40 mg daily or on alternate days for 2 weeks, followed by gradual withdrawal), verapamil (240–480 mg daily), and methysergide (4–6 mg daily).

Giant Cell (Temporal or Cranial) Arteritis

The superficial temporal, vertebral, ophthalmic, and posterior ciliary arteries are often the most severely affected pathologically. Most patients are elderly. The major symptom is headache, often associated with or preceded by myalgia, malaise, anorexia weight loss, and other nonspecific complaints. Loss of vision is the most feared manifestation and occurs quite commonly. Clinical examination often reveals tenderness of the scalp and over the temporal arteries. Further details, including approaches to treatment, are given in Chapter 20.

Posttraumatic Headache

A variety of nonspecific symptoms may follow closed head injury, regardless of whether consciousness is lost. Headache is often a conspicuous feature. Some authorities believe that psychologic factors may be important because there is no correlation of severity of the injury with neurologic signs.

The headache itself usually appears within a day or so following injury, may worsen over the ensuing weeks, and then gradually subsides. It is usually a constant dull ache, with superimposed throbbing that may be localized, lateralized, or generalized. It is sometimes accompanied by nausea, vomiting, or scintillating scotomas.

Disequilibrium, sometimes with a rotatory component, may also occur and is often enhanced by postural change or head movement. Impaired memory, poor concentration, emotional instability, and increased irritability are other common complaints and occasionally are the sole manifestations of the syndrome. The duration of symptoms relates in part to the severity of the original injury, but even trivial injuries are sometimes followed by symptoms that persist for months.

Special investigations are usually not helpful. The electroencephalogram may show minor nonspecific changes, while the electronystagmogram sometimes suggests either peripheral or central vestibulopathy. CT scans or MRI of the head usually show no abnormal findings.

Treatment is difficult, but optimistic encouragement and graduated rehabilitation, depending upon the occupational circumstances, are advised. Headaches often respond to simple analgesics, but severe headaches may necessitate treatment with amitriptyline, propranolol, or ergot derivatives.

pending on response and tolerance, up to 2400 mg/d is given in divided doses.

In the past, alcohol injection of the affected nerve, rhizotomy, or tractotomy was recommended if pharmacologic treatment was unsuccessful. More recently, however, posterior fossa exploration has frequently revealed some structural cause for the neuralgia (despite normal findings on CT scans, MRI, or arteriograms), such as an anomalous artery or vein impinging on the trigeminal nerve root. In such cases, simple decompression and separation of the anomalous vessel from the nerve root produce lasting relief of symptoms. In elderly patients with a limited life expectancy, radiofrequency rhizotomy is sometimes preferred because it is easy to perform, has few complications, and provides symptomatic relief for a period of time. Gamma radiosurgery to the trigeminal root is another noninvasive approach that appears to be successful in 80% of patients, with essentially no side effects other than facial paresthesias in a few instances. Surgical exploration generally reveals no abnormality and is inappropriate in patients with trigeminal neuralgia due to multiple sclerosis.

Khan OA: Gabapentin relieves trigeminal neuralgia in multiple sclerosis patients. Neurology 1998;51:611. [NLM Cit ID: 98373824] (Clinical experience in seven patients.)

Kondziolka D et al: Gamma knife radiosurgery for trigeminal neuralgia: Results and expectations. Arch Neurol 1998;55:1524. [NLM Cit ID: 99081394] (Clinical trial.)

Atypical Facial Pain

Facial pain without the typical features of trigeminal neuralgia is generally a constant, often burning pain that may have a restricted distribution at its onset but soon spreads to the rest of the face on the affected side and sometimes involves the other side, the neck, or the back of the head as well. The disorder is especially common in middle-aged women, many of them emotionally depressed, but it is not clear whether depression is the cause of or a reaction to the pain. Simple analgesics should be given a trial, as should tricyclic antidepressants, carbamazepine, and phenytoin; the response is often disappointing. Opioid analgesics pose a danger of addiction in patients with this disorder. Attempts at surgical treatment are not indicated.

Glossopharyngeal Neuralgia

Glossopharyngeal neuralgia is an uncommon disorder in which pain similar in quality to that in trigeminal neuralgia occurs in the throat, about the tonsillar fossa, and sometimes deep in the ear and at the back of the tongue. The pain may be precipitated by swallowing, chewing, talking, or yawning and is sometimes accompanied by syncope. In most instances, no underlying structural abnormality is present. Carbamazepine is the treatment of choice and should be tried (in daily doses up to 1200 mg) before any surgical procedures are considered. Microvascular decompression is generally preferred over destructive surgical procedures such as partial rhizotomy in medically refractory cases and is often effective without causing severe complications.

Kondo A: Follow-up results of using microvascular decompression for treatment of glossopharyngeal neuralgia. J Neurosurg 1998;88:221. [NLM Cit ID: 98112606] (Follow-up study of 16 patients.)

Postherpetic Neuralgia

Herpes zoster (shingles) is due to infection of the nervous system by varicella-zoster virus. About 15% of patients who develop shingles suffer from postherpetic neuralgia. This complication seems especially likely to occur in the elderly, when the rash is severe, and when the first division of the trigeminal nerve is affected. A history of shingles and the presence of cutaneous scarring resulting from shingles aid in the diagnosis. Severe pain with shingles correlates with the intensity of postherpetic symptoms.

The incidence of postherpetic neuralgia may be reduced by the treatment of shingles with oral acyclovir or famciclovir but not with systemic corticosteroids. Management of the established complication is essentially medical. If simple analgesics fail to help, a trial of a tricyclic drug (eg, amitriptyline, up to 100–150 mg/d) in conjunction with a phenothiazine (eg, perphenazine, 2–8 mg/d) is often effective. Other patients respond to carbamazepine (up to 1200 mg/d), phenytoin (300 mg/d), or gabapentin (up to 3600 mg/d) Topical application of capsaicin cream (eg, Zostrix, 0.025%) may also be helpful, perhaps because of depletion of pain-mediating peptides from peripheral sensory neurons.

Dworkin RH et al: Postherpetic neuralgia: impact of famciclovir, age, rash severity, and acute pain in herpes zoster patients. J Infect Dis 1998;178(Suppl 1):S76. [NLM Cit ID: 99070082] (Famciclovir reduces the prevalence and duration of postherpetic neuralgia.)

Kost RG et al: Postherpetic neuralgia: Pathogenesis, treatment and prevention. N Engl J Med 1996;335:32. [NLM Cit ID: 96249133]

Rowbotham M et al: Gabapentin for the treatment of postherpetic neuralgia: a randomized controlled trial. JAMA 1998;280:1837. [NLM Cit ID: 99061235]

Facial Pain Due to Other Causes

Facial pain may be caused by temporomandibular joint dysfunction in patients with malocclusion, abnormal bite, or faulty dentures. There may be tenderness of the masticatory muscles, and an association between pain onset and jaw movement is sometimes noted. Treatment consists of correction of the underlying problem.

A relationship of facial pain to chewing or temperature changes may suggest a dental disturbance. The cause is sometimes not obvious, and diagnosis requires careful dental examination and x-rays. Pain on mastication may also occur in giant cell arteritis. Sinusitis and ear infections causing facial pain are usually recognized by the history of respiratory tract infection, fever, and, in some instances, aural discharge. There may be localized tenderness. Radiologic evidence of sinus infection or mastoiditis is confirmatory.

Glaucoma is an important ocular cause of facial pain, usually localized to the periorbital region.

On occasion, pain in the jaw may be the principal manifestation of angina pectoris. Precipitation by exertion and radiation to more typical areas establish the cardiac origin.

EPILEPSY

Essentials of Diagnosis

- Recurrent seizures.
- Characteristic electroencephalographic changes accompany seizures.
- Mental status abnormalities or focal neurologic symptoms may persist for hours postictally.

General Considerations

The term epilepsy denotes any disorder characterized by recurrent seizures. A seizure is a transient disturbance of cerebral function due to an abnormal paroxysmal neuronal discharge in the brain. Epilepsy is common, affecting approximately 0.5% of the population in the USA.

Etiology

Epilepsy has several causes. Its most likely cause in individual patients relates to the age at onset.

A. Idiopathic or Constitutional Epilepsy: Seizures usually begin between 5 and 20 years of age but may start later in life. No specific cause can be identified, and there is no other neurologic abnormality.

B. Symptomatic Epilepsy: There are many causes for recurrent seizures.

1. Congenital abnormalities and perinatal injuries may result in seizures presenting in infancy or childhood.

2. Metabolic disorders–Withdrawal from alcohol or drugs is a common cause of recurrent seizures, and other metabolic disorders such as uremia and hypoglycemia or hyperglycemia may also be responsible.

3. Trauma is an important cause of seizures at any age, but especially in young adults. Posttraumatic epilepsy is more likely to develop if the dura mater was penetrated and generally becomes manifest within 2 years following the injury. However, seizures developing in the first week after head injury do not necessarily imply that future attacks will occur. There is suggestive evidence that prophylactic anticonvulsant drug treatment reduces the incidence of posttraumatic epilepsy.

4. Tumors and other space-occupying lesions may lead to seizures at any age, but they are an especially important cause of seizures in middle and later life, when the incidence of neoplastic disease increases. The seizures are commonly the initial symptoms of the tumor and often are partial (focal) in character. They are most likely to occur with structural lesions involving the frontal, parietal, or temporal regions. Tumors must be excluded by appropriate laboratory studies in all patients with onset of seizures after 30 years of age, focal seizures or signs, or a progressive seizure disorder.

5. Vascular diseases become increasingly frequent causes of seizures with advancing age and are the most common cause of seizures with onset at age 60 years or older.

6. Degenerative disorders such as Alzheimer's disease are a cause of seizures in later life.

7. Infectious diseases must be considered in all age groups as potentially reversible causes of seizures. Seizures may occur with an acute infective or inflammatory illness, such as bacterial meningitis or herpes encephalitis, or in patients with more long-standing or chronic disorders such as neurosyphilis or cerebral cysticercosis. In patients with AIDS, they may result from central nervous system toxoplasmosis, cryptococcal meningitis, secondary viral encephalitis, or other infective complications. Seizures are a common sequela of supratentorial brain abscess, developing most frequently in the first year after treatment.

Classification of Seizures

Seizures can be categorized in various ways, but the descriptive classification proposed by the International League Against Epilepsy is clinically the most useful. Seizures are divided into those that are generalized and those affecting only part of the brain (partial seizures).

A. Partial Seizures: The initial clinical and electroencephalographic manifestations of partial seizures indicate that only a restricted part of one cerebral hemisphere has been activated. The ictal manifestations depend upon the area of the brain involved. Partial seizures are subdivided into simple seizures, in which consciousness is preserved, and complex seizures, in which it is impaired. Partial seizures of either type sometimes become secondarily generalized, leading to a tonic, clonic, or tonic-clonic attack.

1. Simple partial seizures–Simple seizures may be manifested by focal motor symptoms (convulsive jerking) or somatosensory symptoms (eg, paresthesias or tingling) that spread (or "march") to different parts of the limb or body depending upon their cortical representation. In other instances, special sensory symptoms (eg, light flashes or buzzing) indicate involvement of visual, auditory, olfactory, or gustatory regions of the brain, or there may be autonomic symptoms or signs (eg, abnormal epigastric sensations, sweating, flushing, pupillary dilation). When psychic symptoms occur, they are usually accompanied by impairment of consciousness, but the sole manifestations of some seizures are phenomena such as dysphasia, dysmnesic symptoms (eg, déjà vu, jamais vu), affective disturbances, illusions, or structured hallucinations.

2. Complex partial seizures–Impaired consciousness may be preceded, accompanied, or followed by the psychic symptoms mentioned above, and automatisms may occur. Such seizures may also begin with some of the other simple symptoms mentioned above.

B. Generalized Seizures: There are several different varieties of generalized seizures, as outlined below. In some circumstances, seizures cannot be classified because of incomplete information or because they do not fit into any category.

1. Absence (petit mal) seizures–These are characterized by impairment of consciousness, sometimes with mild clonic, tonic, or atonic components (ie, reduction or loss of postural tone), autonomic components (eg, enuresis), or accompanying automatisms. Onset and termination of attacks are abrupt. If attacks occur during conversation, the patient may miss a few words or may break off in mid sentence for a few seconds. The impairment of external awareness is so brief that the patient is unaware of it. Absence seizures almost always begin in childhood and frequently cease by the age of 20 years, although occasionally they are then replaced by other forms of generalized seizure. Electroencephalographically, such attacks are associated with bursts of bilaterally synchronous and symmetric 3-Hz spike-and-wave activity. A normal background in the electroencephalogram and normal or above-normal intelligence imply a good prognosis for the ultimate cessation of these seizures.

2. Atypical absences–There may be more marked changes in tone, or attacks may have a more gradual onset and termination than in typical absences.

3. Myoclonic seizures–Myoclonic seizures consist of single or multiple myoclonic jerks.

4. Tonic-clonic (grand mal) seizures–In these seizures, which are characterized by sudden loss of consciousness, the patient becomes rigid and falls to the ground, and respiration is arrested. This tonic phase, which usually lasts for less than a minute, is followed by a clonic phase in which there is jerking of the body musculature that may last for 2 or 3 minutes and is then followed by a stage of flaccid coma. During the seizure, the tongue or lips may be bitten, urinary or fecal incontinence may occur, and the patient may be injured. Immediately after the seizure, the patient may either recover consciousness, drift into sleep, have a further convulsion without recovery of consciousness between the attacks **(status epilepticus),** or after recovering consciousness have a further convulsion **(serial seizures).** In other cases, patients will behave in an abnormal fashion in the immediate postictal period, without subsequent awareness or memory of events **(postepileptic automatism).** Headache, disorientation, confusion, drowsiness, nausea, soreness of the muscles, or some combination of these symptoms commonly occurs postictally.

5. Tonic, clonic, or atonic seizures–Loss of consciousness may occur with either the tonic or clonic accompaniments described above, especially in children. Atonic seizures **(epileptic drop attacks)** have also been described.

Clinical Findings

A. Symptoms and Signs: Nonspecific changes such as headache, mood alterations, lethargy, and myoclonic jerking alert some patients to an impending seizure hours before it occurs. These prodromal symptoms are distinct from the aura which may precede a generalized seizure by a few seconds or minutes and which is itself a part of the attack, arising locally from a restricted region of the brain.

In most patients, seizures occur unpredictably at any time and without any relationship to posture or ongoing activities. Occasionally, however, they occur at a particular time (eg, during sleep) or in relation to external precipitants such as lack of sleep, missed meals, emotional stress, menstruation, alcohol ingestion (or alcohol withdrawal; see below), or use of certain drugs. Fever and nonspecific infections may also precipitate seizures in known epileptics. In a few patients, seizures are provoked by specific stimuli such as flashing lights or a flickering television set **(photosensitive epilepsy),** music, or reading.

Clinical examination between seizures shows no abnormality in patients with idiopathic epilepsy, but in the immediate postictal period, extensor plantar responses may be seen. The presence of lateralized or focal signs postictally suggests that seizures may have a focal origin. In patients with symptomatic epilepsy, the findings on examination will reflect the underlying cause.

B. Imaging: MRI is indicated for patients with focal neurologic symptoms or signs, focal seizures, or electroencephalographic findings of a focal disturbance; some physicians routinely order imaging studies for all patients with new-onset seizure disorders. Such studies should certainly be performed in patients with clinical evidence of a progressive disorder and in those presenting with new onset of seizures after the age of 20 years, because of the possibility of an underlying neoplasm. A chest radiograph should also be obtained in such patients, since the lungs are a common site for primary or secondary neoplasms.

C. Laboratory and Other Studies: Initial investigations should always include a full blood count, blood glucose determination, liver and renal function tests, and serologic tests for syphilis. The hematologic and biochemical screening tests are important both in excluding various causes of seizures and in providing a baseline for subsequent monitoring of long-term effects of treatment.

Electroencephalography may support the clinical diagnosis of epilepsy (by demonstrating paroxysmal abnormalities containing spikes or sharp waves), may provide a guide to prognosis, and may help classify the seizure disorder. Classification of the disorder is important for determining the most appropriate anticonvulsant drug with which to start treatment. For example, absence (petit mal) and complex partial seizures may be difficult to distinguish clinically, but the electroencephalographic findings and treatment of choice differ in these two conditions. Finally, by localizing the epileptogenic source, the electroencephalographic findings are important in evaluating candidates for surgical treatment.

Differential Diagnosis

The distinction between the various disorders likely to be confused with generalized seizures is usually made on the basis of the history. The importance of obtaining an eyewitness account of the attacks cannot be overemphasized.

A. Differential Diagnosis of Partial Seizures:

1. Transient ischemic attacks–These attacks are distinguished from seizures by their longer duration, lack of spread, and symptomatology. Level of consciousness, which is unaltered, does not distinguish them. There is a loss of motor or sensory function (eg, weakness or numbness) with transient ischemic attacks, whereas positive symptomatology (eg, convulsive jerking or paresthesias) characterizes seizures.

2. Rage attacks–Rage attacks are usually situational and lead to goal-directed aggressive behavior.

3. Panic attacks–These may be hard to distinguish from simple or complex partial seizures unless there is evidence of psychopathologic disturbances between attacks and the attacks have a clear relationship to external circumstances.

B. Differential Diagnosis of Generalized Seizures:

1. Syncope–Syncopal episodes usually occur in relation to postural change, emotional stress, instrumentation, pain, or straining. They are typically preceded by pallor, sweating, nausea, and malaise and lead to loss of consciousness accompanied by flaccidity; recovery occurs rapidly with recumbency, and there is no postictal headache or confusion. Serum creatine kinase measured about 3 hours after the event is generally normal after syncopal episodes but markedly elevated after tonic-clonic seizures.

2. Cardiac dysrhythmias–Cerebral hypoperfusion due to a disturbance of cardiac rhythm should be suspected in patients with known cardiac or vascular disease or in elderly patients who present with episodic loss of consciousness. Prodromal symptoms are typically absent. A relationship of attacks to physical activity and the finding of a systolic murmur is suggestive of aortic stenosis. Repeated Holter monitoring may be necessary to establish the diagnosis; monitoring initiated by the patient ("event monitor") may be valuable if the disturbances of consciousness are rare.

3. Brainstem ischemia–Loss of consciousness is preceded or accompanied by other brainstem signs. Basilar artery migraine and vertebrobasilar vascular disease are discussed elsewhere in this chapter.

4. Pseudoseizures–The term pseudoseizures is used to denote both hysterical conversion reactions and attacks due to malingering when these simulate epileptic seizures. Many patients with pseudoseizures also have true seizures or a family history of epilepsy. Although pseudoseizures tend to occur at times of emotional stress, this may also be the case with true seizures.

Clinically, the attacks superficially resemble tonic-clonic seizures, but there may be obvious preparation before pseudoseizures occur. Moreover, there is usually no tonic phase; instead, there is an asynchronous thrashing of the limbs, which increases if restraints are imposed and which rarely leads to injury. Consciousness may be normal or "lost," but in the latter context the occurrence of goal-directed behavior or of shouting, swearing, etc, indicates that it is feigned. Postictally, there are no changes in behavior or neurologic findings.

Laboratory studies may aid in recognition of pseudoseizures. There are no electrocerebral changes, whereas the electroencephalogram changes during organic seizures accompanied by loss of consciousness. The serum level of prolactin has been found to increase dramatically between 15 and 30 minutes after a tonic-clonic convulsion in most patients, whereas it is unchanged after a pseudoseizure.

Treatment

A. General Measures: For patients with recurrent seizures, drug treatment is prescribed with the goal of preventing further attacks and is usually continued until there have been no seizures for at least 3 years. Epileptic patients should be advised to avoid situations that could be dangerous or life-threatening if further seizures should occur. State legislation may require physicians to report to the state department of public health any patients with seizures or other episodic disturbances of consciousness.

1. Choice of medication–The drug with which treatment is best initiated depends upon the type of seizures to be treated (Table 24–2). The dose of the selected drug is gradually increased until seizures are controlled or side effects prevent further increases. If seizures continue despite treatment at the maximal tolerated dose, a second drug is added and the dose increased depending on tolerance; the first drug is then gradually withdrawn. In treatment of partial and secondarily generalized tonic-clonic seizures, the success rate is higher with carbamazepine, phenytoin, or valproic acid than with phenobarbital or primidone. Gabapentin, topiramate, and lamotrigine are newer antiepileptic drugs that are effective adjunctive therapy for partial or secondarily generalized seizures. Felbamate is also effective for such seizures but, because it may cause aplastic anemia or fulminant hepatic failure, it should be used only in selected patients unresponsive to other measures. Tiagabine is another adjunctive agent that has recently been approved for partial seizures. In most patients with seizures of a single type, satisfactory control can be achieved with a single anticonvulsant drug. Treatment with two drugs may further reduce seizure frequency or severity, but usually only at the cost of greater toxicity. Treatment with more than two drugs is almost always unhelpful unless the patient is having seizures of different types.

2. Monitoring–Monitoring serum drug levels has led to major advances in the management of seizure disorders. The same daily dose of a particular drug leads to markedly different blood concentrations in different patients, and this will affect the therapeutic response. In general, the dose of an antiepileptic agent is increased depending on the clinical response regardless of the serum drug level. The trough drug level is then measured to provide a reference point for the maximum tolerated dose. Dosing should not be based simply on serum levels because many patients require levels that exceed the therapeutic range ("toxic levels") but tolerate these without ill effect. Steady-state drug levels in the blood should be measured after treatment is initiated, dosage is changed, or another drug is added to the therapeutic regimen and when seizures are poorly controlled. Dose adjustments are then guided by the laboratory findings. The most common cause of a lower concentration of drug than expected for the prescribed dose is poor patient compliance. Compliance can be improved by limiting to a minimum the number of daily doses. Recurrent seizures or status epilepticus may result if drugs are taken erratically, and in some circumstances noncompliant patients may be better off without any medication.

All anticonvulsant drugs have side effects, and some of these are shown in Table 24–2. In most patients, a complete blood count should be performed at least annually because of the risk of anemia or blood dyscrasia. Treatment with certain drugs may require more frequent monitoring or use of additional screening tests. For example, periodic tests of hepatic function are necessary if valproic acid, carbamazepine, or felbamate is used, and serial blood counts are important with carbamazepine, ethosuximide, or felbamate.

3. Discontinuance of medication–Only when patients have been seizure-free for several (at least 3) years should withdrawal of medication be considered. Unfortunately, there is no way of predicting which patients can be managed successfully without treatment, although seizure recurrence is more likely in patients who initially failed to respond to therapy, those with seizures having focal features or of multiple types, and those with continuing electroencephalographic abnormalities. Dose reduction should be gradual over a period of weeks or months, and drugs should be withdrawn one at a time. If seizures recur, treatment is reinstituted with the same drugs used previously. Seizures are no more difficult to control after a recurrence than before.

4. Surgical treatment–Patients with surgically remediable epilepsy or seizures refractory to pharmacologic management may be candidates for operative treatment, which is best undertaken in specialized centers.

5. Vagal nerve stimulation–Treatment by chronic vagal nerve stimulation for adults and adolescents with medically refractory partial-onset seizures is approved in the USA and provides an alternative approach for patients who are not optimal candidates for surgical treatment. The mechanism of therapeutic action is unknown. Adverse effects consist mainly of transient hoarseness during stimulus delivery.

B. Special Circumstances:

1. Solitary seizures–In patients who have had only one seizure, investigation should exclude an underlying cause requiring specific treatment. An EEG should also be performed, preferably within 24 hours after the seizure, because the findings may influence management—especially when focal abnormalities are present. Prophylactic anticonvulsant drug treatment is generally not required unless further attacks occur or investigations reveal some underlying pathology that itself is untreatable. The risk of seizure recurrence varies in different series between about 30% and 70%. Epilepsy should not be diagnosed on the basis of a solitary seizure. If seizures occur in the context of transient, nonrecurrent systemic disorders such as acute cerebral anoxia, the diagnosis of epilepsy is inaccurate, and long-term prophylactic anticonvulsant drug treatment is unnecessary.

2. Alcohol withdrawal seizures–One or more generalized tonic-clonic seizures may occur within 48 hours or so of withdrawal from alcohol after a period of high or chronic intake. If the seizures have consistently focal features, the possibility of an associated structural abnormality, often traumatic in origin, must be considered. Head CT scan should be performed in patients with new onset of generalized seizures and whenever there are focal features associated with any seizures. Treatment with anticonvulsant drugs is generally not required for alcohol withdrawal seizures, since they are self-limited. Status epilepticus may rarely follow alcohol withdrawal and is managed along conventional lines (see below).

Further attacks will not occur if the patient abstains from alcohol.

3. Tonic-clonic status epilepticus–Poor compliance with the anticonvulsant drug regimen is the most common cause; others include alcohol withdrawal, intracranial infection or neoplasms, metabolic disorders, and drug overdose. The mortality rate may be as high as 20%, and among survivors the incidence of neurologic and mental sequelae may be high. The prognosis relates to the length of time between onset of status epilepticus and the start of effective treatment.

Status epilepticus is a medical emergency. Initial management includes maintenance of the airway and 50% dextrose (25–50 mL) intravenously in case hypoglycemia is responsible. If seizures continue, 10 mg of diazepam is given intravenously over the course of 2 minutes, and the dose is repeated after 10 minutes if necessary. Alternatively, a 4 mg intravenous bolus of lorazepam, repeated once after 10 minutes if necessary, is given in place of diazepam. This is usually effective in halting seizures for a brief period but occasionally causes respiratory depression.

Regardless of the response to diazepam or lorazepam, phenytoin (18–20 mg/kg) is given intravenously at a rate of 50 mg/min; this provides initiation of long-term seizure control. The drug is best injected directly but can also be given in saline; it precipitates, however, if injected into glucose-containing solutions. Because arrhythmias may develop during rapid administration of phenytoin, electrocardiographic monitoring is prudent. Hypotension may complicate phenytoin administration, especially if diazepam has also been given. In the United States, injectable phenytoin has been replaced by fosphenytoin, which is rapidly and completely converted to phenytoin following intravenous administration. No dosing adjustments are necessary because fosphenytoin is expressed in terms of phenytoin equivalents (PE); fosphenytoin is less likely to cause reactions at the infusion site, can be given with all common intravenous solutions, and may be administered at a faster rate (150 mg PE/min). It is also more expensive.

If seizures continue, phenobarbital is then given in a loading dose of 10–20 mg/kg intravenously by slow or intermittent injection. Respiratory depression and hypotension are common complications and should be anticipated; they may occur also with diazepam alone, though less commonly. If these measures fail, general anesthesia with ventilatory assistance and neuromuscular junction blockade may be required. Alternatively, intravenous midazolam may provide control of refractory status epilepticus; the suggested loading dose is 0.2 mg/kg, followed by 0.05–0.2 mg/kg/h.

After status epilepticus is controlled, an oral drug program for the long-term management of seizures is started, and investigations into the cause of the disorder are pursued.

4. Nonconvulsive status epilepticus–Absence (petit mal) and complex partial status epilepticus are characterized by fluctuating abnormal mental status, confusion, impaired responsiveness, and automatism. Electroencephalography is helpful both in establishing the diagnosis and in distinguishing the two varieties. Initial treatment with intravenous diazepam is usually helpful regardless of the type of status epilepticus, but phenytoin, phenobarbital, carbamazepine, and other drugs may also be needed to obtain and maintain control in complex partial status epilepticus.

Delanty N et al: Medical causes of seizures. Lancet 1998;352:383. [NLM Cit ID: 98382043] (Most ill patients with secondary seizures do not have epilepsy, and only those patients with recurrent seizures and predisposing factors need long-term treatment with anticonvulsant medication.)

Devinsky O: Patients with refractory seizures. N Engl J Med 1999;340:1565. [NLM Cit ID: 99247679] (Review of diagnostic evaluation, therapy, and psychosocial burdens.)

Lowenstein DH et al: Status epilepticus. N Engl J Med 1998;338:970. [NLM Cit ID: 98172961]

King MA et al: Epileptology of the first-seizure presentation: A clinical, electroencephalographic, and magnetic resonance imaging study of 300 consecutive patients. Lancet 1998;352:1007. [NLM Cit ID: 98430542]

Mattson RH: Medical management of epilepsy in adults. Neurology 1998;51(Suppl 4):515. [NLM Cit ID: 99034228]

SYNCOPE & DYSAUTONOMIA

Dysautonomia may occur as a result of central or peripheral pathologic processes. It is manifested by a variety of symptoms that may occur in isolation or in various combinations and relate to abnormalities of blood pressure regulation, thermoregulatory sweating, gastrointestinal function, sphincter control, sexual function, respiration, and ocular function. Such symptoms include syncope, postural hypotension, paroxysmal hypertension, persistent tachycardia without other cause, facial flushing, hypo- or hyperhidrosis, vomiting, constipation, diarrhea, dysphagia, abdominal distention, disturbances of micturition or defecation, apneic episodes, and declining night vision.

Syncope is characterized by a transient loss of consciousness, usually accompanied by hypotension and bradycardia. It may occur in response to emotional stress, postural hypotension, vigorous exercise in a hot environment, obstructed venous return to the heart, acute pain or its anticipation, fluid loss, and a variety of other circumstances. A prodrome of malaise, nausea, headache, diaphoresis, pallor, visual disturbance, loss of postural tone, and a sense of weakness and impending loss of consciousness is followed by actual loss of consciousness. Although the patient is usually flaccid, some motor activity is not uncommon, and urinary (and, rarely, fecal) incontinence may also occur, thereby simulating a seizure. Recovery is rapid once the patient becomes recumbent, but headache, nausea, and fatigue are common postictally.

Evaluation of the Patient

Clinical evaluation is important to exclude reversible, nonneurologic causes of symptoms. Testing of autonomic function helps to establish the diagnosis, exclude other causes of symptoms, assess the severity of involvement, and guide prognostication. Such testing includes evaluating the cardiovascular response to the Valsalva maneuver, startle, mental stress, postural change, and deep respiration, and the sudomotor responses to warming or a deep inspiratory gasp. Tilt-table testing may reproduce syncopal or presyncopal symptoms. Pharmacologic studies to evaluate the pupillary responses, radiologic studies of the bladder or gastrointestinal tract, uroflowmetry and urethral pressure profiles, and recording of nocturnal penile tumescence may also be necessary in selected cases.

Neurologic Causes

A. Central Causes: Disease at certain sites in the central nervous system, regardless of its nature, may lead to dysautonomic symptoms. Postural hypotension, which is usually the most troublesome and disabling symptom, may result from spinal cord transection and other myelopathies (eg, due to tumor or syringomyelia) above the T6 level or from brain stem lesions such as syringobulbia and posterior fossa tumors. Sphincter or sexual disturbances may result from cord lesions below T6. Certain primary degenerative disorders are responsible for dysautonomia occurring in isolation (**pure autonomic failure**) or in association with more widespread abnormalities (**multisystem atrophy** or **Shy-Drager syndrome**) that may include parkinsonian, pyramidal symptoms, and cerebellar deficits.

B. Peripheral Causes: A pure autonomic neuropathy may occur acutely or subacutely after a viral infection or as a paraneoplastic disorder related usually to small cell lung cancer. Patients typically present with postural hypotension, impaired thermoregulatory sweating, xerostomia or xerophthalmia, abnormal gastrointestinal motility, dilated pupils, or acute urinary retention. Dysautonomia is often conspicuous in patients with Guillain-Barré syndrome, manifesting with marked hypotension or hypertension or cardiac arrhythmias that may have a fatal outcome. It may also occur with diabetic, uremic, amyloidotic, and various other metabolic or toxic neuropathies; in association with leprosy or Chagas' disease; and as a feature of certain hereditary neuropathies. Autonomic symptoms are prominent in the crises of hepatic porphyria. Patients with botulism or the Lambert-Eaton myasthenic syndrome may have constipation, urinary retention, and a sicca syndrome as a result of impaired cholinergic function.

Treatment

The most disabling symptom of dysautonomia is usually postural hypotension and syncope. Abrupt postural change, prolonged recumbency, and other precipitants should be avoided. Treatment may include wearing waist-high elastic hosiery, salt supplementation, sleeping in a semierect position (which minimizes the natriuresis and diuresis that occur during recumbency), and fludrocortisone (0.1–0.2 mg daily). Vasoconstrictor agents may be helpful and include midodrine (2.5–10 mg three times daily) and ephedrine (15–30 mg three times daily). Other agents that have been used occasionally or experimentally are dihydroergotamine, yohimbine, and clonidine; refractory cases may respond to erythropoietin (epoetin alfa) or desmopressin. Patients must be monitored for recumbent hypertension. Postprandial hypotension is helped by caffeine. There is no satisfactory treatment for disturbances of sweating, but an air-conditioned environment is helpful in avoiding extreme swings in body temperature.

Kaufmann H: Neurally mediated syncope and syncope due to autonomic failure: Differences and similarities. J Clin Neurophysiol 1997;14:183. [NLM Cit ID: 97386309] (Pathophysiology, diagnosis, and treatment.)

SENSORY DISTURBANCES

Patients may complain of either lost or abnormal sensations. The term "numbness" is often used by patients to denote loss of feeling, but the word also has other meanings and the patient's intention must be clarified. Abnormal spontaneous sensations are generally called paresthesias, and unpleasant or painful sensations produced by a stimulus that is usually painless are called dysesthesias.

Sensory symptoms may be due to disease located anywhere along the peripheral or central sensory pathways. The character, site, mode of onset, spread, and temporal profile of sensory symptoms must be established and any precipitating or relieving factors identified. These features—and the presence of any associated symptoms—help identify the origin of sensory disturbances, as do the physical signs as well. Sensory symptoms or signs may conform to the territory of individual peripheral nerves or nerve roots. Involvement of one side of the body—or of one limb in its entirety—suggests a central lesion. Distal involvement of all four extremities suggests polyneuropathy, a cervical cord or brainstem lesion, or—when symptoms are transient—a metabolic disturbance such as hyperventilation syndrome. Short-lived sensory complaints may be indicative of sensory seizures or cerebral ischemic phenomena as well as metabolic disturbances. In patients with cord lesions, there may be a transverse sensory level. "Dissociated sensory loss" is characterized by loss of some sensory modalities with preservation of others. Such findings may be encountered in patients with either peripheral or central disease and must therefore be interpreted in the clinical context in which they are found.

The absence of sensory signs in patients with sensory symptoms does not mean that symptoms have a nonorganic basis. Symptoms are often troublesome before signs of sensory dysfunction have had time to develop.

WEAKNESS & PARALYSIS

Loss of muscle power may result from central disease involving the upper or lower motor neurons; from peripheral disease involving the roots, plexus, or peripheral nerves; from disorders of neuromuscular transmission; or from primary disorders of muscle. The clinical findings help to localize the lesion and thus reduce the number of diagnostic possibilities.

Weakness due to upper motor neuron lesions is characterized by selective involvement of certain muscle groups and is associated with spasticity, increased tendon reflexes, and extensor plantar responses. The site of upper motor neuron (pyramidal) involvement may be indicated by the presence of other clinical signs or by the distribution of the motor deficit. Lower motor neuron lesions lead to muscle wasting as well as weakness, with flaccidity and loss of tendon reflexes, but no change in the plantar responses unless the neurons subserving them are directly involved. Fasciculations may be evident over affected muscles. In distinguishing between a root, plexus, or peripheral nerve lesion, the distribution of the motor deficit and of any sensory changes is of particular importance. In patients with disturbances of neuromuscular transmission, weakness is patchy in distribution, often fluctuates over short periods of time, and is not associated with sensory changes. In myopathic disorders, weakness is usually most marked proximally in the limbs, is not associated with sensory loss or sphincter disturbance, and is not accompanied by muscle wasting or loss of tendon reflexes—at least not until an advanced stage.

TRANSIENT ISCHEMIC ATTACKS

Essentials of Diagnosis

- Risk factors for vascular disease often present.
- Focal neurologic deficit of acute onset.
- Clinical deficit resolves completely within 24 hours.

General Considerations

Transient ischemic attacks are characterized by focal ischemic cerebral neurologic deficits that last for less than 24 hours (usually less than 1–2 hours). About 30% of patients with stroke have a history of transient ischemic attacks, and proper treatment of the attacks is an important means of prevention. The incidence of stroke does not relate to either the number or the duration of individual attacks but is increased in patients with hypertension or diabetes. The risk of stroke is highest in the month after a transient ischemic attack and progressively declines thereafter.

Etiology

An important cause of transient cerebral ischemia is embolization. In many patients with these attacks, a source is readily apparent in the heart or a major extracranial artery to the head, and emboli sometimes are visible in the retinal arteries. Moreover, an embolic phenomenon explains why separate attacks may affect different parts of the territory supplied by the same major vessel. Cardiac causes of embolic ischemic attacks include rheumatic heart disease, mitral valve disease, cardiac arrhythmia, infective endocarditis, atrial myxoma, and mural thrombi complicating myocardial infarction. Atrial septal defects and patent foramen ovale may permit emboli from the veins to reach the brain ("paradoxical emboli"). An ulcerated plaque on a major artery to the brain may serve as a source of emboli. In the anterior circulation, atherosclerotic changes occur most commonly in the region of the carotid bifurcation extracranially, and these changes may cause a bruit. In some patients with transient ischemic attacks or strokes, an acute or recent hemorrhage is found to have occurred into this atherosclerotic plaque, and this finding may have pathologic significance. Patients with AIDS have an increased risk of developing transient ischemic deficits or strokes.

Other (less common) abnormalities of blood vessels that may cause transient ischemic attacks include fibromuscular dysplasia, which affects particularly the cervical internal carotid artery; inflammatory arterial disorders such as giant cell arteritis, systemic lupus erythematosus, polyarteritis, and granulomatous angiitis and meningovascular syphilis. Hypotension may cause a reduction of cerebral blood flow if a major extracranial artery to the brain is markedly stenosed, but this is a rare cause of transient ischemic attack.

Hematologic causes of ischemic attacks include polycythemia, sickle cell disease, and hyperviscosity syndromes. Severe anemia may also lead to transient focal neurologic deficits in patients with preexisting cerebral arterial disease.

The **subclavian steal syndrome** may lead to transient vertebrobasilar ischemia. Symptoms develop when there is localized stenosis or occlusion of one subclavian artery proximal to the source of the vertebral artery, so that blood is "stolen" from this artery. A bruit in the supraclavicular fossa, unequal radial pulses, and a difference of 20 mm Hg or more between the systolic blood pressures in the arms should suggest the diagnosis in patients with vertebrobasilar transient ischemic attacks.

Clinical Findings

A. Symptoms and Signs: The symptoms of transient ischemic attacks vary markedly among patients; however, the symptoms in a given individual tend to be constant in type. Onset is abrupt and without warning, and recovery usually occurs rapidly, often within a few minutes.

If the ischemia is in the carotid territory, common symptoms are weakness and heaviness of the contralateral arm, leg, or face, singly or in any combination. Numbness or paresthesias may also occur either as the sole manifestation of the attack or in combination with the motor deficit. There may be slowness of movement, dysphasia, or monocular visual loss in the eye contralateral to affected limbs. During an attack, examination may reveal flaccid weakness with pyramidal distribution, sensory changes, hyperreflexia or an extensor plantar response on the affected side, dysphasia, or any combination of these findings. Subsequently, examination reveals no neurologic abnormality, but the presence of a carotid bruit or cardiac abnormality may provide a clue to the cause of symptoms.

Vertebrobasilar ischemic attacks may be characterized by vertigo, ataxia, diplopia, dysarthria, dimness or blurring of vision, perioral numbness and paresthesias, and weakness or sensory complaints on one, both, or alternating sides of the body. These symptoms may occur singly or in any combination. Drop attacks due to bilateral leg weakness, without headache or loss of consciousness, may occur, sometimes in relation to head movements.

The natural history of attacks is variable. Some patients will have a major stroke after only a few attacks, whereas others may have frequent attacks for weeks or months without having a stroke. Attacks may occur intermittently over a long period of time, or they may stop spontaneously. In general, carotid ischemic attacks are more liable than vertebrobasilar ischemic attacks to be followed by stroke.

B. Imaging: CT scan of the head will exclude the possibility of a small cerebral hemorrhage or a cerebral tumor masquerading as a transient ischemic attack. A number of noninvasive techniques, such as ultrasonography, have been developed for studying the cerebral circulation and imaging the major vessels to the head. Carotid duplex ultrasonography is useful for detecting significant stenosis of the internal carotid artery, but arteriography remains important for demonstrating the status of the cerebrovascular system. MR angiography may reveal stenotic lesions of large vessels but is less sensitive than conventional arteriography. Accordingly, if findings on CT scan are normal, if there is no cardiac source of embolization, and if age and general condition indicate that the patient is a good operative risk, bilateral carotid arteriography should be considered in the further evaluation of carotid ischemic attacks, although the ultrasound findings may help in selecting patients for study.

C. Laboratory and Other Studies: Clinical and laboratory evaluation must include assessment for hypertension, heart disease, hematologic disorders, diabetes mellitus, hyperlipidemia, and peripheral vascular disease. It should include complete blood count, fasting blood glucose and serum cholesterol determinations, serologic tests for syphilis, and an ECG and chest x-ray. Echocardiography with bubble contrast is performed if a cardiac source is likely, and blood cultures are obtained if endocarditis is suspected. Holter monitoring is indicated if a transient, paroxysmal disturbance of cardiac rhythm is suspected.

Differential Diagnosis

Focal seizures usually cause abnormal motor or sensory phenomena such as clonic limb movements, paresthesias, or tingling, rather than weakness or loss of feeling. Symptoms generally spread ("march") up the limb and may lead to a generalized tonic-clonic seizure.

Classic migraine is easily recognized by the visual premonitory symptoms, followed by nausea, headache, and photophobia, but less typical cases may be hard to distinguish. The patient's age and medical history (including family history) may be helpful in this regard. Patients with migraine commonly have a history of episodes since adolescence and report that other family members have a similar disorder.

Focal neurologic deficits may occur during periods of hypoglycemia in diabetic patients receiving insulin or oral hypoglycemic agent therapy.

Treatment

When arteriography reveals a surgically accessible high-grade stenosis (70–99% in luminal diameter) on the side appropriate to carotid ischemic attacks and there is relatively little atherosclerosis elsewhere in the cerebrovascular system, operative treatment (carotid thromboendarterectomy) reduces the risk of ipsilateral carotid stroke, especially when transient ischemic attacks are of recent onset (< 2 months). Surgery is not indicated for mild stenosis (< 30%); its benefits are unclear with severe stenosis plus diffuse intracranial atherosclerotic disease. See Chapter 12 for additional discussion.

In patients with carotid ischemic attacks who are poor operative candidates (and thus have not undergone arteriography) or who are found to have extensive vascular disease, medical treatment should be instituted. Similarly, patients with vertebrobasilar ischemic attacks are treated medically and are not subjected to arteriography unless there is clinical evidence of stenosis or occlusion in the carotid or subclavian arteries.

Medical treatment is aimed at preventing further attacks and stroke. Cigarette smoking should be stopped, and cardiac sources of embolization, hypertension, diabetes, hyperlipidemia, arteritis, or hematologic disorders should be treated appropriately. If anticoagulants are indicated for the treatment of embolism from the heart, they should be started immediately, provided there is no contraindication to their use. There is no advantage in delay, and the common fear of causing hemorrhage into a previously infarcted area is misplaced, since there is a far greater risk of further embolism to the cerebral circulation if treatment is withheld. Treatment is initiated with intravenous heparin (in a loading dose of 5000–10,000 units of standard molecular weight heparin, and maintenance infusion of 1000–2000 units per hour depending on the partial thromboplastin time) while warfarin sodium is introduced in a daily dose of 5–15 mg orally, depending on the INR. Alternatively, aspirin (325 mg daily) may be used in patients with nonrheumatic atrial fibrillation to reduce the risk of stroke.

In patients with presumed or angiographically verified atherosclerotic changes in the extracranial or intracranial cerebrovascular circulation, antithrombotic medication is prescribed. Treatment depends upon the patient's age, the likelihood of compliance in taking the drug, and the ready availability of medical and laboratory services. Some physicians use anticoagulant drugs (eg, warfarin, with temporary heparinization until the dose of warfarin is adequate) unless they are medically contraindicated, continuing them for 3–6 months before they are tapered and ultimately replaced with aspirin, which is continued for another year. However, there is no convincing evidence that anticoagulant drugs are of value. Other physicians therefore prefer aspirin from the onset.

The evidence supporting a therapeutic role for aspirin to suppress platelet aggregation is convincing. Platelets adhere to and aggregate around an atherosclerotic plaque and release various substances including thromboxane A_2. Treatment with aspirin significantly reduces the frequency of transient ischemic attacks and the incidence of stroke or myocardial infarcts in high-risk patients. A daily dose of 325 mg is adequate; higher doses may provide added benefit but are associated with a higher incidence of gastrointestinal side effects. Dipyridamole is not as effective, and when added to aspirin does not offer any advantage over aspirin alone for stroke prevention. In patients intolerant of aspirin, ticlopidine (another platelet aggregation inhibitor) may be used in a dose of 250 mg twice daily, but patients must be monitored closely for the development of neutropenia or agranulocytosis.

In recent years, many patients with transient ischemic attacks associated with stenotic lesions of the distal internal carotid or the proximal middle cerebral arteries have undergone surgical extracranial-intracranial arterial anastomosis. However, no benefit of surgical treatment could be demonstrated in a large controlled prospective study.

Feinberg WM et al: Guidelines for the management of transient ischemic attacks. From the Ad Hoc Committee on Guidelines for the Management of Transient Ischemic Attacks of the Stroke Council of the American Heart Association. Circulation 1994;89:2950. [NLM Cit ID: 94265365]

Kucey DS et al: Determinants of outcome after carotid endarterectomy. J Vasc Surg 1998;28 1051. [NLM Cit ID: 99061886]

STROKE

Essentials of Diagnosis

- Sudden onset of characteristic neurologic deficit.
- Patient often has history of hypertension, diabetes mellitus, valvular heart disease, or atherosclerosis.
- Distinctive neurologic signs reflect the region of the brain involved.

General Considerations

In the USA, stroke remains the third leading cause of death, despite a general decline in the incidence of stroke in the last 30 years. The precise reasons for this decline are uncertain, but increased awareness of risk factors (hypertension, diabetes, hyperlipidemia, cigarette smoking, cardiac disease, AIDS, recreational drug abuse, heavy alcohol consumption, family history of stroke) and improved prophylactic measures and surveillance of those at increased risk have been contributory. Elevation of the blood homocysteine level is also a risk factor for stroke, but it is unclear whether this risk is reduced by treatment to lower the level. A previous stroke makes individual patients more susceptible to further strokes.

For years, strokes have been subdivided pathologically into infarcts (thrombotic or embolic) and hemorrhages, and clinical criteria for distinguishing between these possibilities have been emphasized. However, it is often difficult to determine on clinical grounds the pathologic basis for stroke.

1. LACUNAR INFARCTION

Lacunar infarcts are small lesions (usually < 5 mm in diameter) that occur in the distribution of short penetrating arterioles in the basal ganglia, pons, cerebellum, anterior limb of the internal capsule, and, less commonly, the deep cerebral white matter. Lacunar infarcts are associated with poorly controlled hypertension or diabetes and have been found in several clinical syndromes, including contralateral pure motor or pure sensory deficit, ipsilateral ataxia with crural paresis, and dysarthria with clumsiness of the hand. The neurologic deficit may progress over 24–36 hours before stabilizing.

Lacunar infarcts are sometimes visible on CT scans as small, punched-out, hypodense areas, but in other patients no abnormality is seen. In some instances, patients with a clinical syndrome suggestive of lacunar infarction are found on CT scanning to have a severe hemispheric infarct.

The prognosis for recovery from the deficit produced by a lacunar infarct is usually good, with partial or complete resolution occurring over the following 4–6 weeks in many instances.

2. CEREBRAL INFARCTION

Thrombotic or embolic occlusion of a major vessel leads to cerebral infarction. Causes include the disorders predisposing to transient ischemic attacks (see above) and atherosclerosis of cerebral arteries. The resulting deficit depends upon the particular vessel involved and the extent of any collateral circulation. Cerebral ischemia leads to release of excitatory and other neuropeptides that may augment calcium flux into neurons, thereby leading to cell death and increasing the neurologic deficit.

Clinical Findings

A. Symptoms and Signs: Onset is usually abrupt, and there may then be very little progression except that due to brain swelling. Clinical evaluation always includes examination of the heart and auscultation over the subclavian and carotid vessels to determine whether there are any bruits.

1. Obstruction of carotid circulation–Occlusion of the ophthalmic artery is probably symptomless in most cases because of the rich orbital collaterals, but its transient embolic obstruction leads to amaurosis fugax—sudden and brief loss of vision in one eye.

Occlusion of the anterior cerebral artery distal to its junction with the anterior communicating artery causes weakness and cortical sensory loss in the contralateral leg and sometimes mild weakness of the arm, especially proximally. There may be a contralateral grasp reflex, paratonic rigidity, and abulia (lack of initiative) or frank confusion. Urinary incontinence is not uncommon, particularly if behavioral disturbances are conspicuous. Bilateral anterior cerebral infarction is especially likely to cause marked behavioral changes and memory disturbances. Unilateral anterior cerebral artery occlusion proximal to the junction with the anterior communicating artery is generally well tolerated because of the collateral supply from the other side.

Middle cerebral artery occlusion leads to contralateral hemiplegia, hemisensory loss, and homonymous hemianopia (ie, bilaterally symmetric loss of vision in half of the visual fields), with the eyes deviated to the side of the lesion. If the dominant hemisphere is involved, global aphasia is also present. It may be impossible to distinguish this clinically from occlusion of the internal carotid artery. With occlusion of either of these arteries, there may also be considerable swelling of the hemisphere, leading to drowsiness, stupor, and coma in extreme cases. Occlusions of different branches of the middle cerebral artery cause more limited findings. For example, involvement of the anterior main division leads to a predominantly expressive dysphasia and to contralateral paralysis and loss of sensations in the arm, the face, and, to a lesser extent, the leg. Posterior branch occlusion produces a receptive (Wernicke's) aphasia and a homonymous visual field defect. With involvement of the nondominant hemisphere, speech and comprehension are preserved, but there may be a confusional state, dressing apraxia, and constructional and spatial deficits.

2. Obstruction of vertebrobasilar circulation–Occlusion of the posterior cerebral artery may lead to a thalamic syndrome in which contralateral hemisensory disturbance occurs, followed by the development of spontaneous pain and hyperpathia. There is often a macular-sparing homonymous hemianopia and sometimes a mild, usually temporary, hemiparesis. Depending on the site of the lesion and the collateral circulation, the severity of these deficits varies and other deficits may also occur, including involuntary movements and alexia. Occlusion of the main artery beyond the origin of its penetrating branches may lead solely to a macular-sparing hemianopia.

Vertebral artery occlusion distally, below the origin of the anterior spinal and posterior inferior cerebellar arteries, may be clinically silent because the circulation is maintained by the other vertebral artery. If the remaining vertebral artery is congenitally small or severely atherosclerotic, however, a deficit similar to that of basilar artery occlusion is seen unless there is good collateral circulation from the anterior circulation through the circle of Willis. When the small paramedian arteries arising from the vertebral artery are occluded, contralateral hemiplegia and sensory deficit occur in association with an ipsilateral cranial nerve palsy at the level of the lesion. An obstruction of the posterior inferior cerebellar artery or an obstruction of the vertebral artery just before it branches to this vessel leads ipsilaterally to spinothalamic sensory loss involving the face, ninth and tenth cranial nerve lesions, limb ataxia and numbness, and Horner's syndrome, combined with contralateral spinothalamic sensory loss involving the limbs.

Occlusion of both vertebral arteries or the basilar artery leads to coma with pinpoint pupils, flaccid quadriplegia and sensory loss, and variable cranial nerve abnormalities. With partial basilar artery occlusion, there may be diplopia, visual loss, vertigo, dysarthria, ataxia, weakness or sensory disturbances in some or all of the limbs, and discrete cranial nerve palsies. In patients with hemiplegia of pontine origin, the eyes are often deviated to the paralyzed side, whereas in patients with a hemispheric lesion, the eyes commonly deviate from the hemiplegic side.

Occlusion of any of the major cerebellar arteries produces vertigo, nausea, vomiting, nystagmus, ipsilateral limb ataxia, and contralateral spinothalamic sensory loss in the limbs. If the superior cerebellar artery is involved, the contralateral spinothalamic loss also involves the face; with occlusion of the anterior inferior cerebellar artery, there is ipsilateral spinothalamic sensory loss involving the face, usually in conjunction with ipsilateral facial weakness and deafness. Massive cerebellar infarction may lead to coma, tonsillar herniation, and death.

3. Coma–Infarction in either the carotid or vertebrobasilar territory may lead to loss of consciousness. For example, an infarct involving one cerebral hemisphere may lead to such swelling that the function of the other hemisphere or the rostral brainstem is disturbed and coma results. Similarly, coma occurs with bilateral brainstem infarction when this involves the reticular formation, and it occurs with brainstem compression after cerebellar infarction.

B. Imaging: Radiography of the chest may reveal cardiomegaly or valvular calcification; the presence of a neoplasm would suggest that the neurologic deficit is due to metastasis rather than stroke. A CT scan of the head (without contrast) is important in excluding cerebral hemorrhage, but it may not permit distinction between a cerebral infarct and tumor. CT scanning is preferable to MRI in the acute stage because it is quicker and because intracranial hemorrhage is not easily detected by MRI within the first 48 hours after a bleeding episode. In selected patients, carotid duplex studies, MRI and MR angiography, and conventional angiography may also be necessary. Diffusion-weighted MRI is more sensitive than standard MRI in detecting cerebral ischemia.

C. Laboratory and Other Studies: Investigations should include a complete blood count, sedimentation rate, blood glucose determination, and serologic tests for syphilis. Antiphospholipid antibodies (lupus anticoagulants and anticardiolipin antibodies) promote thrombosis and are associated with an increased incidence of stroke. Similarly, elevated serum cholesterol and lipids and serum homocysteine may indicate an increased risk of thrombotic stroke. Electrocardiography will help exclude a cardiac arrhythmia or recent myocardial infarction that might be serving as a source of embolization. Blood cultures should be performed if endocarditis is suspected, echocardiography if heart disease is suspected, and Holter monitoring if paroxysmal cardiac arrhythmia requires exclusion. Examination of the cerebrospinal fluid is not always necessary but may be helpful if there is diagnostic uncertainty; it should be delayed until after CT scanning.

Treatment

If the neurologic deficit progresses over the following minutes or hours, heparinization may be of value in limiting or arresting further deterioration. Since the signs of progressing stroke may be simulated by an intracerebral hematoma, the latter must be excluded by immediate CT scanning or angiography before the patient is heparinized.

Intravenous thrombolytic therapy with recombinant tissue plasminogen activator (0.9 mg/kg to a maximum of 90 mg, with 10% given as a bolus over 1 minute and the remainder over 1 hour) is effective in reducing the neurologic deficit in selected patients without CT evidence of intracranial hemorrhage when administered within 3 hours after onset of ischemic stroke, but later administration has not been proved effective or safe. Recent hemorrhage, increased risk of hemorrhage (eg, treatment with anticoagulants), arterial puncture at a noncompressible site, and systolic pressure above 185 mm Hg or diastolic pressure above 110 mm Hg are among the contraindications to this treatment. Early management of a completed stroke otherwise consists of attention to general supportive measures. During the acute stage, there may be marked brain swelling and edema, with symptoms and signs of increasing intracranial pressure, an increasing neurologic deficit, or herniation syndrome. Corticosteroids have been prescribed in an attempt to reduce vasogenic cerebral edema. Prednisone (up to 100 mg/d) or dexamethasone (16 mg/d) has been used, but the evidence that corticosteroids are of any benefit is conflicting. Dehydrating hyperosmolar agents have also been prescribed in efforts to reduce brain swelling, but there is little evidence of any lasting benefit. Likewise, clinical benefit from treatment with vasodilators such as papaverine is minimal. Neither hypercapnia nor hypocapnia has been shown to have any benefit. Barbiturates are known to decrease neuronal metabolism and energy requirements and have been reported to improve functional recovery in experimental stroke models; their use in humans, however, is experimental. Attempts to lower the blood pressure of hypertensive patients during the acute phase of a stroke should be avoided, since there is loss of cerebral autoregulation and lowering the blood pressure may further compromise ischemic areas.

Anticoagulant drugs have no role in the management of patients with a completed stroke, except when there is a cardiac source of embolization. Treatment is then started with intravenous heparin while warfarin is introduced. The target is an INR of 2–3 for the prothrombin time. If the CT scan shows no evidence of hemorrhage and the cerebrospinal fluid is clear, anticoagulant treatment may be started without delay. Some physicians prefer to wait for 2 or 3 days before initiating anticoagulant treatment; the CT scan is then repeated and anticoagulant therapy is initiated if it again shows no evidence of hemorrhagic transformation.

Preliminary studies suggest that calcium channel blocking drugs such as nimodipine (30 mg orally every 6 hours for 4 weeks) reduce the deficit produced by cerebral ischemia and the morbidity and mortality rates from stroke. Blockage of glutamate, an excitatory neurotransmitter, reduces the sensitivity of central neurons to ischemia. The *N*-methyl-D-aspartate (NMDA) type of glutamate receptors is linked to calcium-permeable channels, and studies in animals have shown that specific NMDA-receptor antagonists reduce stroke size, deficits, and the percentage of severely ischemic neurons. The role of these therapeutic approaches in humans is currently under study.

Physical therapy has an important role in the management of patients with impaired motor function. Passive movements at an early stage will help prevent contractures. As cooperation increases and some recovery begins, active movements will improve strength and coordination. In all cases, early mobilization and active rehabilitation are important. Occupational therapy may improve morale and motor skills, while speech therapy may be beneficial in patients with expressive dysphasia or dysarthria. When there is a severe and persisting motor deficit, a device such as a leg brace, toe spring, frame, or cane may help the patient move about, and the provision of other aids to daily living may improve the quality of life.

Prognosis

The prognosis for survival after cerebral infarction is better than after cerebral or subarachnoid hemorrhage. The only proved effective therapy for acute stroke requires initiation within 3 hours after stroke onset, and the prognosis therefore depends on the time that elapses before arrival at the hospital. Loss of consciousness after a cerebral infarct implies a poorer prognosis than otherwise. The extent of the infarct governs the potential for rehabilitation. Patients who have had a cerebral infarct are at risk for further strokes and for myocardial infarcts. Patients with massive strokes from which meaningful recovery is unlikely should receive palliative care (Chapter 5).

Adams HP Jr et al: Guidelines for Thrombolytic Therapy for Acute Stroke: A Supplement to the Guidelines for the Management of Patients with Acute Ischemic Stroke. A statement for healthcare professionals from a Special Writing Group of the Stroke Council, American Heart Association. Stroke 1996;27:1711. [NLM Cit ID: 96378594]

Albers GW et al: Antithrombotic and thrombolytic therapy for ischemic stroke. Chest 1998;114:683S. [NLM Cit ID: 99037865]

Albers GW et al: Intravenous tissue-type plasminogen activator for treatment of acute stroke: the Standard Treatment with Alteplase to Reverse Stroke (STARS) study. JAMA 2000;283:1145. [NLM Cit ID: 20166516]

American Academy of Neurology, Quality Standards Subcommittee: Thrombolytic therapy for acute ischemic stroke—summary statement. Neurology 1996;47:835. [NLM Cit ID: 96390506] (Practice advisory.)

Brickner ME: Cardioembolic stroke. Am J Med 1996; 100:465. [NLM Cit ID: 96194611] (Review.)

Easton JD: Current advances in the management of stroke. Neurology 1998;51(Suppl 3):S1. [NLM Cit ID: 98416071]

JAMA patient page: Stroke. JAMA 1999;281:1146. [NLM Cit ID: 99202552]

Lutsep HL et al: Clinical utility of diffusion-weighted magnetic resonance imaging in the assessment of ischemic stroke. Ann Neurol 1997;41:574. [NLM Cit ID: 97297886]

Sacco RL: Identifying patient populations at high risk for stroke. Neurology 1998;51(3 Suppl 3):S27. [NLM Cit ID: 98416078]

3. INTRACEREBRAL HEMORRHAGE

Spontaneous intracerebral hemorrhage in patients with no angiographic evidence of an associated vascular anomaly (eg, aneurysm or angioma) is usually due to hypertension. The pathologic basis for hemorrhage is probably the presence of microaneurysms that are now known to develop on perforating vessels of 100–300 μm in diameter in hypertensive patients. Hypertensive intracerebral hemorrhage occurs most frequently in the basal ganglia and less commonly in the pons, thalamus, cerebellum, and cerebral white matter. Hemorrhage may extend into the ventricular system or subarachnoid space, and signs of meningeal irritation are then found. Hemorrhages usually occur suddenly and without warning, often during activity.

In addition to its association with hypertension, nontraumatic intracerebral hemorrhage may occur with hematologic and bleeding disorders (eg, leukemia, thrombocytopenia, hemophilia, or disseminated intravascular coagulation), anticoagulant therapy, liver disease, cerebral amyloid angiopathy, and primary or secondary brain tumors. Bleeding is primarily into the subarachnoid space when it occurs from an intracranial aneurysm or arteriovenous malformation (see below), but it may be partly intraparenchymal as well. In some cases, no specific cause for cerebral hemorrhage can be identified.

Clinical Findings

A. Symptoms and Signs: With hemorrhage into the cerebral hemisphere, consciousness is initially lost or impaired in about one-half of patients. Vomiting occurs very frequently at the onset of bleeding, and headache is sometimes present. Focal symptoms and signs then develop, depending on the site of the hemorrhage. With hypertensive hemorrhage, there is generally a rapidly evolving neurologic deficit with hemiplegia or hemiparesis. A hemisensory disturbance is also present with more deeply placed lesions. With lesions of the putamen, loss of conjugate lateral gaze may be conspicuous. With thalamic hemorrhage, there may be a loss of upward gaze, downward or skew deviation of the eyes, lateral gaze palsies, and pupillary inequalities.

Cerebellar hemorrhage may present with sudden onset of nausea and vomiting, disequilibrium, headache, and loss of consciousness that may terminate fatally within 48 hours. Less commonly, the onset is gradual and the course episodic or slowly progressive—clinical features suggesting an expanding cerebellar lesion. In yet other cases, however, the onset and course are intermediate, and examination shows lateral conjugate gaze palsies to the side of the lesion; small reactive pupils; contralateral hemiplegia; peripheral facial weakness; ataxia of gait, limbs, or trunk; periodic respiration; or some combination of these findings.

B. Imaging: CT scanning (without contrast) is important not only in confirming that hemorrhage has occurred but also in determining the size and site of the hematoma. It is superior to MRI for detecting intracranial hemorrhage of less than 48 hours duration. If the patient's condition permits further intervention, cerebral angiography may be undertaken thereafter to determine if an aneurysm or arteriovenous malformation is present (see below).

C. Laboratory and Other Studies: A complete blood count, platelet count, bleeding time, prothrombin and partial thromboplastin times, and liver and renal function tests may reveal a predisposing cause for the hemorrhage. Lumbar puncture is contraindicated because it may precipitate a herniation syndrome in patients with a large hematoma, and CT scanning is superior in detecting intracerebral hemorrhage.

Treatment

Neurologic management is generally conservative and supportive, regardless of whether the patient has a profound deficit with associated brainstem compression, in which case the prognosis is grim, or a more localized deficit not causing increased intracranial pressure or brainstem involvement. Decompression is helpful, however, when a superficial hematoma in cerebral white matter is exerting a mass effect and causing incipient herniation. In patients with cerebellar hemorrhage, prompt surgical evacuation of the hematoma is appropriate, because spontaneous unpredictable deterioration may otherwise lead to a fatal outcome and because operative treatment may lead to complete resolution of the clinical deficit. The treatment of underlying structural lesions or bleeding disorders depends upon their nature.

Hill MD et al: Rate of stroke recurrence in patients with primary intracerebral hemorrhage. Stroke 2000;31:123. [NLM Cit ID: 20093022] (Clinical study.)

4. SUBARACHNOID HEMORRHAGE

Between 5% and 10% of strokes are due to subarachnoid hemorrhage. Although hemorrhage is usually from rupture of an aneurysm or arteriovenous malformation, no specific cause can be found in 20% of cases.

Clinical Findings

A. Symptoms and Signs: Subarachnoid hemorrhage has a characteristic clinical picture. Its onset is with sudden headache of a severity never experienced previously by the patient. This may be followed by nausea and vomiting and by a loss or impairment of consciousness that can either be transient or progress inexorably to deepening coma and death. If consciousness is regained, the patient is often confused and irritable and may show other symptoms of an altered mental status. Neurologic examination generally reveals nuchal rigidity and other signs of meningeal irritation, except in deeply comatose patients. A focal neurologic deficit is occasionally present and may suggest the site of the underlying lesion.

B. Imaging: A CT scan should be performed immediately to confirm that hemorrhage has occurred and to search for clues regarding its source. It is preferable to MRI because it is faster and more sensitive in detecting hemorrhage in the first 24 hours. CT findings sometimes are normal in patients with suspected hemorrhage, and the cerebrospinal fluid must then be examined for the presence of blood or xanthochromia before the possibility of subarachnoid hemorrhage is discounted.

Cerebral arteriography may be undertaken to determine the source of bleeding; it is not performed unless or until the patient's condition has stabilized and is good enough so that operative treatment is feasible. In general, bilateral carotid and vertebral arteriography are necessary because aneurysms are often multiple, while arteriovenous malformations may be supplied from several sources. MR angiography may also permit these vascular anomalies to be visualized but is less sensitive than conventional arteriography.

Treatment

The measures outlined in the section on stupor and coma are applied to comatose patients. Conscious patients are confined to bed, advised against any exertion or straining, treated symptomatically for headache and anxiety, and given laxatives or stool softeners. If there is severe hypertension, the blood pressure can be lowered gradually, but not below a diastolic level of 100 mm Hg. Phenytoin is generally prescribed routinely to prevent seizures. Further comment concerning the specific operative management of arteriovenous malformations and aneurysms follows.

Johnston SC et al: The burden, trends, and demographics of mortality from subarachnoid hemorrhage. Neurology 1998;50:1413. [NLM Cit ID: 98255436]

5. INTRACRANIAL ANEURYSM

Saccular aneurysms ("berry" aneurysms) tend to occur at arterial bifurcations, are considerably more common in adults than in children, are frequently multiple (20% of cases), and are usually asymptomatic. They may be associated with polycystic kidney disease and coarctation of the aorta. Most aneurysms are located on the anterior part of the circle of Willis—particularly on the anterior or posterior communicating arteries, at the bifurcation of the middle cerebral artery, and at the bifurcation of the internal carotid artery.

Clinical Findings

A. Symptoms and Signs: Aneurysms may cause a focal neurologic deficit by compressing adjacent structures. However, most are asymptomatic or produce only nonspecific symptoms until they rupture, at which time subarachnoid hemorrhage results. There is often a paucity of focal neurologic signs in patients with subarachnoid hemorrhage, but when present, such signs may relate either to a focal hematoma or to ischemia in the territory of the vessel with the ruptured aneurysm. Hemiplegia or other focal deficit sometimes occurs after a delay of 4–14 days and is due to focal arterial spasm in the vicinity of the ruptured aneurysm. This spasm is of uncertain, probably multifactorial, cause, but it sometimes leads to significant cerebral ischemia or infarction, and it may further aggravate any existing increase in intracranial pressure. Subacute hydrocephalus due to interference with the flow of cerebrospinal fluid may occur after 2 or more weeks, and this leads to a delayed clinical deterioration that is relieved by shunting.

In some patients, "warning leaks" of a small amount of blood from the aneurysm precede the major hemorrhage by a few hours or days. They lead to headaches, sometimes accompanied by nausea and neck stiffness, but the true cause of these symptoms is often not appreciated until massive hemorrhage occurs.

B. Imaging: The CT scan generally confirms that subarachnoid hemorrhage has occurred, but occasionally it is normal. Angiography (bilateral carotid and vertebral studies) generally indicates the size and site of the lesion, sometimes reveals multiple aneurysms, and may show arterial spasm. If subarachnoid hemorrhage is confirmed by lumbar puncture or CT scanning but arteriograms show no abnormality, the examination should be repeated after 2 weeks, because vasospasm may have prevented detection of an aneurysm during the initial study.

C. Laboratory and Other Studies: The cerebrospinal fluid is bloodstained. The electroencephalogram sometimes indicates the side or site of hemorrhage but frequently shows only a diffuse abnormality. Electrocardiographic evidence of arrhythmias or myocardial ischemia has been well described and probably relates to excessive sympathetic activity. Peripheral leukocytosis and transient glycosuria are also common findings.

Treatment

The major aim of treatment is to prevent further hemorrhages. Definitive treatment requires a surgical approach to the aneurysm and ideally consists of clipping of its base. Alternatively, endovascular treatment (coil embolization) by interventional radiologists may be undertaken and is sometimes feasible even for inoperable aneurysms. Otherwise, medical management as outlined above for subarachnoid hemorrhage is continued for about 6 weeks and is followed by gradual mobilization.

The risk of further hemorrhage is greatest within a few days of the first hemorrhage; approximately 20% of patients will have further bleeding within 2 weeks and 40% within 6 months. Attempts have been made to reduce this risk pharmacologically. Treatment with an antifibrinolytic agent such as aminocaproic acid during the first 14 days reduces the risk of recurrent hemorrhage but is associated with such an increase in cerebral ischemic complications that the mortality rate and the degree of disability among survivors are unchanged. Thus, early operation (ie, within about 2 days of hemorrhage) is preferred for good operative candidates.

Calcium channel-blocking agents have helped to reduce or reverse experimental vasospasm, and nimodipine has been shown to reduce, in neurologically normal patients, the incidence of ischemic deficits from arterial spasm without producing any side effects. The dose of nimodipine is 60 mg every 4 hours for 21 days. After surgical obliteration of any aneurysms, symptomatic vasospasm may also be treated by intravascular volume expansion, induced hypertension, or transluminal balloon angioplasty of involved intracranial vessels.

With regard to unruptured aneurysms, those that are symptomatic merit prompt treatment, either surgically or by endovascular coil embolization, whereas small asymptomatic ones discovered incidentally are often followed arteriographically and corrected surgically only if they increase in size to over 10 mm. The natural history of unruptured aneurysms is not clearly defined.

Connolly ES et al: Management of symptomatic and asymptomatic unruptured aneurysms. Neurosurg Clin North Am 1998;9:509. [NLM Cit ID: 98338797] (Literature review.)

International Study of Unruptured Intracranial Aneurysms Investigators: Unruptured intracranial aneurysms: Risks of rupture and risks of surgical intervention. N Engl J Med 1998;339:1725. [NLM Cit ID: 99049884] (Multicenter study.)

Johnston SC et al: Which unruptured cerebral aneurysms should be treated? A cost-utility analysis. Neurology 1999;52:1806. [NLM Cit ID: 99297937] (Cost-utility analysis.)

Lanzino G et al: Surgical treatment of the ruptured aneurysm: Timing. Neurosurg Clin North Am 1998;9: 541. [NLM Cit ID: 98338799] (Literature review.)

Schievink WI: Intracranial aneurysms. N Engl J Med 1997; 336:28. [NLM Cit ID: 97122460]

6. ARTERIOVENOUS MALFORMATIONS

Arteriovenous malformations are congenital vascular malformations that result from a localized maldevelopment of part of the primitive vascular plexus and consist of abnormal arteriovenous communications without intervening capillaries. They vary in size, ranging from massive lesions that are fed by multiple vessels and involve a large part of the brain to lesions so small that they are hard to identify at arteriography, surgery, or autopsy. In approximately 10% of cases, there is an associated arterial aneurysm, while 1–2% of patients presenting with aneurysms have associated arteriovenous malformations. Clinical presentation may relate to hemorrhage from the malformation or an associated aneurysm or may relate to cerebral ischemia due to diversion of blood by the anomalous arteriovenous shunt or due to venous stagnation. Regional maldevelopment of the brain, compression or distortion of adjacent cerebral tissue by enlarged anomalous vessels, and progressive gliosis due to mechanical and ischemic factors may also be contributory. In addition, communicating or obstructive hydrocephalus may occur and lead to symptoms.

Clinical Findings

A. Symptoms and Signs:

1. Supratentorial lesions–Most cerebral arteriovenous malformations are supratentorial, usually lying in the territory of the middle cerebral artery. Initial symptoms consist of hemorrhage in 30–60% of cases, epilepsy in 20–40%, headache in 5–25%, and miscellaneous complaints (including focal deficits) in 10–15%. Up to 70% of arteriovenous malformations bleed at some point in their natural history, most commonly before the patient reaches the age of 40 years. This tendency to bleed is unrelated to the lesion site or to the patient's sex, but small arteriovenous malformations are more likely to bleed than large ones. Arteriovenous malformations that have bled once are more likely to bleed again. Hemorrhage is commonly intracerebral as well as into the subarachnoid space, and it has a fatal outcome in about 10% of cases. Focal or generalized seizures may accompany or follow hemorrhage, or they may be the initial presentation, especially with frontal or parietal arteriovenous malformations. Headaches are especially likely when the external carotid arteries are involved in the malformation. These sometimes simulate migraine but more commonly are nonspecific in character, with nothing about them to suggest an underlying structural lesion.

In patients presenting with subarachnoid hemorrhage, examination may reveal an abnormal mental status and signs of meningeal irritation. Additional findings may help to localize the lesion and sometimes indicate that intracranial pressure is increased. A cranial bruit always suggests the possibility of a cerebral arteriovenous malformation, but bruits may also be found with aneurysms, meningiomas, acquired arteriovenous fistulas, and arteriovenous malformations involving the scalp, calvarium, or orbit. Bruits are best heard over the ipsilateral eye or mastoid region and are of some help in lateralization but of no help in localization. Absence of a bruit in no way excludes the possibility of arteriovenous malformation.

2. Infratentorial lesions–Brainstem arteriovenous malformations are often clinically silent, but they may hemorrhage, cause obstructive hydrocephalus, or lead to progressive or relapsing brainstem deficits. Cerebellar arteriovenous malformations may also be clinically inconspicuous but sometimes lead to cerebellar hemorrhage.

B. Imaging: In patients presenting with suspected hemorrhage, CT scanning indicates whether subarachnoid or intracerebral bleeding has recently occurred, helps to localize its source, and may reveal the arteriovenous malformation. If the CT scan shows no evidence of bleeding but subarachnoid hemorrhage is diagnosed clinically, the cerebrospinal fluid should be examined.

When intracranial hemorrhage is confirmed but the source of hemorrhage is not evident on the CT scan, arteriography is necessary to exclude aneurysm or arteriovenous malformation. MR angiography is not sensitive enough for this purpose. Even if the findings on CT scan suggest arteriovenous malformation, arteriography is required to establish the nature of the lesion with certainty and to determine its anatomic features so that treatment can be planned. The examination must generally include bilateral opacification of the internal and external carotid arteries and the vertebral arteries. Arteriovenous malformations typically appear as a tangled vascular mass with distended tortuous afferent and efferent vessels, a rapid circulation time, and arteriovenous shunting. Findings on plain radiographs of the skull are often normal unless an intracerebral hematoma is present, in which case there may be changes suggestive of raised intracranial pressure and displacement of a calcified pineal gland.

In patients presenting without hemorrhage, CT scan or MRI usually reveals the underlying abnormality, and MRI frequently also shows evidence of old or recent hemorrhage that may have been asymptomatic. The nature and detailed anatomy of any focal lesion identified by these means is delineated by angiography, especially if operative treatment is under consideration.

C. Laboratory and Other Studies: Electroencephalography is usually indicated in patients presenting with seizures and may show consistently focal or lateralized abnormalities resulting from the underlying cerebral arteriovenous malformation. This should be followed by CT scanning.

Treatment

Surgical treatment to prevent further hemorrhage is justified in patients with arteriovenous malformations that have bled, provided that the lesion is accessible and the patient has a reasonable life expectancy. Surgical treatment is also appropriate if intracranial pressure is increased and to prevent further progression of a focal neurologic deficit. In patients presenting solely with seizures, anticonvulsant drug treatment is usually sufficient, and operative treatment is unnecessary unless there are further developments.

Definitive operative treatment consists of excision of the arteriovenous malformation if it is surgically accessible. Arteriovenous malformations that are inoperable because of their location are sometimes treated solely by embolization; although the risk of hemorrhage is not reduced, neurologic deficits may be stabilized or even reversed by this procedure. Two other new techniques for the treatment of intracerebral arteriovenous malformations are injection of a vascular occlusive polymer through a flow-guided microcatheter and permanent occlusion of feeding vessels by positioning detachable balloon catheters in the desired sites and then inflating them with quickly solidifying contrast material. Stereotactic radiosurgery with the gamma knife is also useful in the management of inoperable cerebral arteriovenous malformations.

7. INTRACRANIAL VENOUS THROMBOSIS

Intracranial venous thrombosis may occur in association with intracranial or maxillofacial infections, hypercoagulable states, polycythemia, sickle cell disease, and cyanotic congenital heart disease and in pregnancy or during the puerperium. It is characterized by headache, focal or generalized convulsions, drowsiness, confusion, increased intracranial pressure, and focal neurologic deficits—and sometimes by evidence of meningeal irritation. The diagnosis is confirmed by CT scanning and MRI, MR venography, or angiography.

Treatment includes anticonvulsant drugs if seizures have occurred and antiedema agents (eg, dexamethasone, 4 mg four times daily and continued as necessary) to reduce intracranial pressure. Anticoagulation with dose-adjusted intravenous heparin reduces morbidity and mortality of venous sinus thrombosis.

8. SPINAL CORD VASCULAR DISEASES

Infarction of the Spinal Cord

Infarction of the spinal cord is rare. It occurs only in the territory of the anterior spinal artery because this vessel, which supplies the anterior two-thirds of the cord, is itself supplied by only a limited number of feeders. Infarction usually results from interrupted flow in one or more of these feeders, eg, with aortic dissection, aortography, polyarteritis, or severe hypotension, or after surgical resection of the thoracic aorta. The paired posterior spinal arteries, by contrast, are supplied by numerous arteries at different levels of the cord.

Since the anterior spinal artery receives numerous feeders in the cervical region, infarcts almost always occur caudally. Clinical presentation is characterized by acute onset of flaccid, areflexive paraplegia that evolves after a few days or weeks into a spastic paraplegia with extensor plantar responses. There is an accompanying dissociated sensory loss, with impairment of appreciation of pain and temperature but preservation of sensations of vibration and position. Treatment is symptomatic.

Aminoff MJ: Spinal vascular disease. In: *Spinal Cord Disease.* Critchley E, Eisen A (editors). Springer, 1997.

Epidural or Subdural Hemorrhage

Epidural or subdural hemorrhage may lead to sudden severe back pain followed by an acute compressive myelopathy necessitating urgent myelography and surgical evacuation. It may occur in patients with bleeding disorders or those who are taking anticoagulant drugs, sometimes following trauma or lumbar puncture. Epidural hemorrhage may also be related to a vascular malformation or tumor deposit.

Arteriovenous Malformation of the Spinal Cord

Arteriovenous malformations of the cord are congenital lesions that present with spinal subarachnoid hemorrhage or myeloradiculopathy. Since most of these malformations are located in the thoracolumbar region, they lead to motor and sensory disturbances in the legs and to sphincter disorders. Pain in the legs or back is often severe. Examination reveals an upper, lower, or mixed motor deficit in the legs; sensory deficits are also present and are usually extensive, although occasionally they are confined to radicular distribution. Cervical arteriovenous malformations lead also to symptoms and signs in the arms. Spinal MRI may not detect the arteriovenous malformation, and negative findings do not exclude the diagnosis. In general, the diagnosis is suggested at myelography (performed with the patient prone and supine) when serpiginous filling defects due to enlarged vessels are found. Selective spinal arteriography confirms the diagnosis. Most lesions are extramedullary, are posterior to the cord (lying either intra- or extradurally), and can easily be treated by ligation of feeding vessels and excision of the fistulous anomaly or by embolization procedures. Delay in treatment may lead to increased and irreversible disability or to death from recurrent subarachnoid hemorrhage.

INTRACRANIAL & SPINAL SPACE-OCCUPYING LESIONS

1. PRIMARY INTRACRANIAL TUMORS

Essentials of Diagnosis

- Generalized or focal disturbance of cerebral function, or both.
- Increased intracranial pressure in some patients.
- Neuroradiologic evidence of space-occupying lesion.

General Considerations

Half of all primary intracranial neoplasms (Table 24–3) are gliomas and the remainder meningiomas, pituitary adenomas, neurofibromas, and other tumors. Certain tumors, especially neurofibromas, hemangioblastomas, and retinoblastomas, may have a familial basis, and congenital factors bear on the development of craniopharyngiomas. Tumors may occur at any age, but certain gliomas show particular age predilections (Table 24–3).

Clinical Findings

A. Symptoms and Signs: Intracranial tumors may lead to a generalized disturbance of cerebral function and to symptoms and signs of increased intracranial pressure. In consequence, there may be personality changes, intellectual decline, emotional lability, seizures, headaches, nausea, and malaise. If the pressure is increased in a particular cranial compartment, brain tissue may herniate into a compartment with lower pressure. The most familiar syndrome is herniation of the temporal lobe uncus through the tentorial hiatus, which causes compression of the third cranial nerve, midbrain, and posterior cerebral artery. The earliest sign of this is ipsilateral pupillary dilation, followed by stupor, coma, decerebrate posturing, and respiratory arrest. Another important herniation syndrome consists of displacement of the cerebellar tonsils through the foramen magnum, which causes medullary compression leading to apnea, circulatory collapse, and death. Other herniation syndromes are less common and of less clear clinical importance.

Intracranial tumors also lead to focal deficits depending on their location.

1. Frontal lobe lesions–Tumors of the frontal lobe often lead to progressive intellectual decline, slowing of mental activity, personality changes, and contralateral grasp reflexes. They may lead to expressive aphasia if the posterior part of the left inferior frontal gyrus is involved. Anosmia may also occur as a consequence of pressure on the olfactory nerve. Precentral lesions may cause focal motor seizures or contralateral pyramidal deficits.

2. Temporal lobe lesions–Tumors of the uncinate region may be manifested by seizures with olfactory or gustatory hallucinations, motor phenomena such as licking or smacking of the lips, and some impairment of external awareness without actual loss of consciousness. Temporal lobe lesions also lead to depersonalization, emotional changes, behavioral disturbances, sensations of déjà vu or jamais vu, micropsia or macropsia, visual field defects (crossed upper quadrantanopia), and auditory illusions or hallucinations. Left-sided lesions may lead to dysnomia and receptive aphasia, while right-sided involvement sometimes disturbs the perception of musical notes and melodies.

3. Parietal lobe lesions–Tumors in this location characteristically cause contralateral disturbances of sensation and may cause sensory seizures, sensory loss or inattention, or some combination of these symptoms. The sensory loss is cortical in type and involves postural sensibility and tactile discrimination, so that the appreciation of shape, size, weight, and texture is impaired. Objects placed in the hand may not be recognized (astereognosis). Extensive parietal lobe lesions may produce contralateral hyperpathia and spontaneous pain (thalamic syndrome). Involvement of the optic radiation leads to a contralateral homonymous field defect that sometimes consists solely of lower quadrantanopia. Lesions of the left angular gyrus cause Gerstmann's syndrome (a combination of alexia, agraphia, acalculia, right-left confusion, and finger agnosia), whereas involvement of the left submarginal gyrus causes ideational apraxia. Anosognosia (the denial, neglect, or rejection of a paralyzed limb) is seen in patients with lesions of the nondominant (right) hemisphere. Constructional apraxia and dressing apraxia may also occur with right-sided lesions.

4. Occipital lobe lesions–Tumors of the occipital lobe characteristically produce crossed homonymous hemianopia or a partial field defect. With left-sided or bilateral lesions, there may be visual agnosia both for objects and for colors, while irritative lesions on either side can cause unformed visual hallucinations. Bilateral occipital lobe involvement causes cortical blindness in which there is preservation of pupillary responses to light and lack of aware-

Table 24–3. Primary intracranial tumors.

Tumor	Clinical Features	Treatment and Prognosis
Glioblastoma multiforme	Presents commonly with nonspecific complaints and increased intracranial pressure. As it grows, focal deficits develop.	Course is rapidly progressive, with poor prognosis. Total surgical removal is usually not possible, and response to radiation therapy is poor.
Astrocytoma	Presentation similar to glioblastoma multiforme but course more protracted, often over several years. Cerebellar astrocytoma may have a more benign course.	Prognosis is variable. By the time of diagnosis, total excision is usually impossible; tumor often is not radiosensitive. In cerebellar astrocytoma, total surgical removal is often possible.
Medulloblastoma	Seen most frequently in children. Generally arises from roof of fourth ventricle and leads to increased intracranial pressure accompanied by brainstem and cerebellar signs. May seed subarachnoid space.	Treatment consists of surgery combined with radiation therapy and chemotherapy.
Ependymoma	Glioma arising from the ependyma of a ventricle, especially the fourth ventricle; leads early to signs of increased intracranial pressure. Arises also from central canal of cord.	Tumor is not radiosensitive and is best treated surgically if possible.
Oligodendroglioma	Slow-growing. Usually arises in cerebral hemisphere in adults. Calcification may be visible on skull x-ray.	Treatment is surgical and usually successful.
Brainstem glioma	Presents during childhood with cranial nerve palsies and then with long tract signs in the limbs. Signs of increased intracranial pressure occur late.	Tumor is inoperable; treatment is by irradiation and shunt for increased intracranial pressure.
Cerebellar hemangioblastoma	Presents with dysequilibrium, ataxia of trunk or limbs, and signs of increased intracranial pressure. Sometimes familial. May be associated with retinal and spinal vascular lesions, polycythemia, and renal cell carcinoma.	Treatment is surgical.
Pineal tumor	Presents with increased intracranial pressure, sometimes associated with impaired upward gaze (Parinaud's syndrome) and other deficits indicative of midbrain lesion.	Ventricular decompression by shunting is followed by surgical approach to tumor; irradiation is indicated if tumor is malignant. Prognosis depends on histopathologic findings and extent of tumor.
Craniopharyngioma	Originates from remnants of Rathke's pouch above the sella, depressing the optic chiasm. May present at any age but usually in childhood, with endocrine dysfunction and bitemporal field defects.	Treatment is surgical, but total removal may not be possible.
Acoustic neurinoma	Ipsilateral hearing loss is most common initial symptom. Subsequent symptoms may include tinnitus, headache, vertigo, facial weakness or numbness, and long tract signs. (May be familial and bilateral when related to neurofibromatosis.) Most sensitive screening tests are MRI and brainstem auditory evoked potential.	Treatment is excision by translabyrinthine surgery, craniectomy, or a combined approach. Outcome is usually good.
Meningioma	Originates from the dura mater or arachnoid; compresses rather than invades adjacent neural structures. Increasingly common with advancing age. Tumor size varies greatly. Symptoms vary with tumor site—eg, unilateral exophthalmos (sphenoidal ridge); anosmia and optic nerve compression (olfactory groove). Tumor is usually benign and readily detected by CT scanning; may lead to calcification and bone erosion visible on plain x-rays of skull.	Treatment is surgical. Tumor may recur if removal is incomplete.
Primary cerebral lymphoma	Associated with AIDS and other immunodeficient states. Presentation may be with focal deficits or with disturbances of cognition and consciousness. May be indistinguishable from cerebral toxoplasmosis.	Treatment is by whole brain irradiation; chemotherapy may have an adjunctive role. Prognosis depends upon CD4 count at diagnosis.

ness of the defect by the patient. There may also be loss of color perception, prosopagnosia (inability to identify a familiar face), simultagnosia (inability to integrate and interpret a composite scene as opposed to its individual elements), and Balint's syndrome (failure to turn the eyes to a particular point in space, despite preservation of spontaneous and reflex eye movements). The denial of blindness or a field defect constitutes Anton's syndrome.

5. Brainstem and cerebellar lesions–Brainstem lesions lead to cranial nerve palsies, ataxia, incoordination, nystagmus, and pyramidal and sensory deficits in the limbs on one or both sides. Intrinsic brainstem tumors, such as gliomas, tend to produce an increase in intracranial pressure only late in their course. Cerebellar tumors produce marked ataxia of the trunk if the vermis cerebelli is involved and ipsilateral appendicular deficits (ataxia, incoordination and hypotonia of the limbs) if the cerebellar hemispheres are affected.

6. False localizing signs–Tumors may lead to neurologic signs other than by direct compression or infiltration, thereby leading to errors of clinical localization. These false localizing signs include third or sixth nerve palsy and bilateral extensor plantar responses produced by herniation syndromes, and an extensor plantar response occurring ipsilateral to a hemispheric tumor as a result of compression of the opposite cerebral peduncle against the tentorium.

B. Imaging: CT scanning or MRI with gadolinium enhancement may detect the lesion and may also define its location, shape, and size; the extent to which normal anatomy is distorted; and the degree of any associated cerebral edema or mass effect. CT scanning is less helpful with tumors in the posterior fossa, but MRI is of particular value there. The characteristic appearance of meningiomas on CT scanning is virtually diagnostic; ie, a lesion in a typical site (parasagittal and sylvian regions, olfactory groove, sphenoidal ridge, tuberculum sellae) that appears as a homogeneous area of increased density in noncontrast CT scans and enhances uniformly with contrast.

Arteriography may show stretching or displacement of normal cerebral vessels by the tumor and the presence of tumor vascularity. The presence of an avascular mass is a nonspecific finding that could be due to tumor, hematoma, abscess, or any space-occupying lesion. In patients with normal hormone levels and an intrasellar mass, angiography is necessary to distinguish with confidence between a pituitary adenoma and an arterial aneurysm.

C. Laboratory and Other Studies: The electroencephalogram provides supporting information concerning cerebral function and may show either a focal disturbance due to the neoplasm or a more diffuse change reflecting altered mental status. Lumbar puncture is rarely necessary; the findings are seldom diagnostic, and the procedure carries the risk of causing a herniation syndrome.

Treatment

Treatment depends on the type and site of the tumor (Table 24–3) and the condition of the patient. Complete surgical removal may be possible if the tumor is extra-axial (eg, meningioma, acoustic neuroma) or is not in a critical or inaccessible region of the brain (eg, cerebellar hemangioblastoma). Surgery also permits the diagnosis to be verified and may be beneficial in reducing intracranial pressure and relieving symptoms even if the neoplasm cannot be completely removed. Clinical deficits are sometimes due in part to obstructive hydrocephalus, in which case simple surgical shunting procedures often produce dramatic benefit. In patients with malignant gliomas, radiation therapy increases median survival rates regardless of any preceding surgery, and its combination with chemotherapy provides additional benefit. Indications for irradiation in the treatment of patients with other primary intracranial neoplasms depend upon tumor type and accessibility and the feasibility of complete surgical removal. Corticosteroids help reduce cerebral edema and are usually started before surgery. Herniation is treated with intravenous dexamethasone (10–20 mg as a bolus, followed by 4 mg every 6 hours) and intravenous mannitol (20% solution given in a dose of 1.5 g/kg over about 30 minutes). Anticonvulsants are also commonly administered in standard doses (Table 24–2). For those patients whose disease deteriorates despite treatment, palliative care is important (Chapter 5).

Chamberlain MC et al: Practical guidelines for the treatment of malignant gliomas. West J Med 1998;168:114. [NLM Cit ID: 98160724]

DeAngelis LM et al: Malignant glioma: who benefits from adjuvant chemotherapy. Ann Neurol 1998;44:691. [NLM Cit ID: 98449720]

Leighton C et al: Supratentorial low-grade glioma in adults. J Clin Oncol 1997;15:1294. [NLM Cit ID: 97336573] (Prognostic factors and response to radiation.)

Nussbaum ES et al: Brain metastases. Histology, multiplicity, surgery, and survival: Cancer 1996;78:1781. [NLM Cit ID: 97012377]

Pech IV et al: Chemotherapy for brain tumors. Oncology 1998;12:537. [NLM Cit ID: 98236440]

2. METASTATIC INTRACRANIAL TUMORS

Cerebral Metastases

Metastatic brain tumors present in the same way as other cerebral neoplasms, ie, with increased intracranial pressure, with focal or diffuse disturbance of cerebral function, or with both of these manifestations. Indeed, in patients with a single cerebral lesion, the metastatic nature of the lesion may only become evident on histopathologic examination. In other patients, there is evidence of widespread metastatic disease, or an isolated cerebral metastasis develops during treatment of the primary neoplasm.

The most common source of intracranial metastasis is carcinoma of the lung; other primary sites are the breast, kidney, and gastrointestinal tract. Most cerebral metastases are located supratentorially. Laboratory and radiologic studies used to evaluate patients with metastases are those described for primary neoplasms. They include MRI and CT scanning performed both with and without contrast material. Lumbar puncture is necessary only in patients with suspected carcinomatous meningitis (see below). In patients with verified cerebral metastasis from an unknown primary, investigation is guided by symptoms and signs. In women, mammography is indicated; in men under 50, germ cell origin is sought since both have therapeutic implications.

In patients with only a single cerebral metastasis who are otherwise well, it may be possible to remove the lesion and then treat with irradiation; the latter may also be selected as the sole treatment. In patients with multiple metastases or widespread systemic disease, the prognosis is gloomy, and treatment is palliative only.

Leptomeningeal Metastases (Carcinomatous Meningitis)

The neoplasms metastasizing most commonly to the leptomeninges are carcinoma of the breast, lymphomas, and leukemia. Leptomeningeal metastases lead to multifocal neurologic deficits, which may be associated with infiltration of cranial and spinal nerve roots, direct invasion of the brain or spinal cord, obstructive hydrocephalus, or some combination of these factors.

The diagnosis is confirmed by examination of the cerebrospinal fluid. Findings may include elevated cerebrospinal fluid pressure, pleocytosis, increased protein concentration, and decreased glucose concentration. Cytologic studies may indicate that malignant cells are present; if not, spinal tap should be repeated at least twice to obtain further samples for analysis.

CT scans showing contrast enhancement in the basal cisterns or showing hydrocephalus without any evidence of a mass lesion support the diagnosis. Gadolinium-enhanced MRI frequently shows enhancing foci in the leptomeninges. Myelography may show deposits on multiple nerve roots.

Treatment is by irradiation to symptomatic areas, combined with intrathecal methotrexate. The long-term prognosis is poor—only about 10% of patients survive for 1 year—and palliative care is therefore important (Chapter 5).

3. INTRACRANIAL MASS LESIONS IN AIDS PATIENTS

AIDS patients may present with **primary cerebral lymphoma.** This leads to disturbances in cognition or consciousness, focal motor or sensory deficits, aphasia, seizures, and cranial neuropathies. Similar clinical disturbances may result from **cerebral toxoplasmosis,** which is also a common complication in patients with AIDS. Neither CT nor MRI findings distinguish these two disorders, and serologic tests for toxoplasmosis are unreliable in AIDS patients. Accordingly, for neurologically stable patients, a trial of treatment with sulfadiazine (100 mg/kg/d up to 8 g/d in four divided doses) and pyrimethamine (75 mg/d for 3 days, then 25 mg/d) is recommended for 3 weeks; the imaging studies are then repeated, and if any lesion has improved, the antitoxoplasmosis regimen is continued indefinitely. If any lesion does not improve, cerebral biopsy is necessary. Primary cerebral lymphoma is treated with whole-brain irradiation.

Cryptococcal meningitis is also a commonly opportunistic infection in AIDS patients. Clinically, it may resemble cerebral toxoplasmosis or lymphoma, but cranial CT scans are usually normal. The diagnosis is made on the basis of cerebrospinal fluid studies, with positive India ink staining in 75–80% and cryptococcal antigen tests in 95% of cases. Treatment is with amphotericin B, sometimes accompanied by flucytosine, as set forth in Table 36–1.

Berger JR: AIDS and the nervous system. In: *Neurology and General Medicine,* 2nd ed. Aminoff MJ (editor). Churchill Livingstone, 1995. (Clinical review.)

Evaluation and management of intracranial mass lesions in AIDS. Report of the Quality Standards Subcommittee of the American Academy of Neurology. Neurology 1998;50:21. [NLM Cit ID: 98103689]

4. PRIMARY & METASTATIC SPINAL TUMORS

Approximately 10% of spinal tumors are intramedullary. Ependymoma is the most common type of intramedullary tumor; the remainder are other types of glioma. Extramedullary tumors may be extradural or intradural in location. Among the primary extramedullary tumors, neurofibromas and meningiomas are relatively common, are benign, and may be intra- or extradural. Carcinomatous metastases, lymphomatous or leukemic deposits, and myeloma are usually extradural; in the case of metastases, the prostate, breast, lung, and kidney are common primary sites.

Tumors may lead to spinal cord dysfunction by direct compression, by ischemia secondary to arterial or venous obstruction, and, in the case of intramedullary lesions, by invasive infiltration.

Clinical Findings

A. Symptoms and Signs: Symptoms usually develop insidiously. Pain is often conspicuous with extradural lesions; is characteristically aggravated by coughing or straining; may be radicular, localized to the back, or felt diffusely in an extremity; and may be accompanied by motor deficits, paresthesias, or numbness, especially in the legs. When sphincter disturbances occur, they are usually particularly disabling. Pain, however, often precedes specific neurologic symptoms from epidural metastases.

Examination may reveal localized spinal tenderness. A segmental lower motor neuron deficit or dermatomal sensory changes (or both) are sometimes found at the level of the lesion, while an upper motor neuron deficit and sensory disturbance are found below it.

B. Imaging: Findings on plain radiography of the spine may be normal but are commonly abnormal when there are metastatic deposits. CT myelography or MRI may be necessary to identify and localize the site of cord compression. The combination of known tumor elsewhere in the body, back pain, and either abnormal plain films of the spine or neurologic signs of cord compression is an indication to perform these studies on an urgent basis. Some clinicians proceed to myelography based solely on new back pain in a cancer patient. If a complete block is present at lumbar myelography, a cisternal myelogram is performed to determine the upper level of the block and to investigate the possibility of block higher in the cord.

C. Laboratory Findings: The cerebrospinal fluid removed at myelography is often xanthochromic and contains a greatly increased protein concentration with normal cell content and glucose concentration.

Treatment

Intramedullary tumors are treated by decompression and surgical excision (when feasible) and by irradiation. The prognosis depends upon the cause and severity of cord compression before it is relieved.

Treatment of epidural spinal metastases consists of irradiation, irrespective of cell type. Dexamethasone is also given in a high dosage (eg, 25 mg four times daily for 3 days, followed by rapid tapering of the dosage, depending on response) to reduce cord swelling and relieve pain. Surgical decompression is reserved for patients with tumors that are unresponsive to irradiation or have previously been irradiated and for cases in which there is some uncertainty about the diagnosis. The long-term outlook is poor, but radiation treatment may at least delay the onset of major disability.

5. BRAIN ABSCESS

Cerebral abscess presents as an intracranial space-occupying lesion and arises as a sequela of disease of the ear or nose, may be a complication of infection elsewhere in the body, or may result from infection introduced intracranially by trauma or surgical procedures. The most common infective organisms are streptococci, staphylococci, and anaerobes; mixed infections are not uncommon. Headache, drowsiness, inattention, confusion, and seizures are early symptoms, followed by signs of increasing intracranial pressure and then a focal neurologic deficit. There may be little or no systemic evidence of infection.

A CT scan of the head characteristically shows an area of contrast enhancement surrounding a low-density core. Similar abnormalities may be found in patients with metastatic neoplasms. MRI findings often permit earlier recognition of focal cerebritis or an abscess. Arteriography indicates the presence of a space-occupying lesion, which appears as an avascular mass with displacement of normal cerebral vessels, but this procedure provides no clue to the nature of the lesion.

Treatment consists of intravenous antibiotics, combined with surgical drainage (aspiration or excision) if necessary to reduce the mass effect, or sometimes to establish the diagnosis. Abscesses smaller than 2 cm can often be cured medically. Broad-spectrum antibiotics are used if the infecting organism is unknown. A common regimen is penicillin G (2 million units every 2 hours intravenously) plus either chloramphenicol (1–2 g intravenously every 6 hours), metronidazole (750 mg intravenously every 6 hours), or both. Nafcillin is added if *Staphylococcus aureus* infection is suspected. Dexamethasone (4–25 mg four times daily, depending on severity, followed by tapering of dose, depending on response) may reduce any associated edema.

Pons V: Acute bacterial infections of the central nervous system. In: *Neurology and General Medicine,* 2nd ed. Aminoff MJ (editor). Churchill Livingstone, 1995.

NONMETASTATIC NEUROLOGIC COMPLICATIONS OF MALIGNANT DISEASE

A variety of nonmetastatic neurologic complications of malignant disease can be recognized:

(1) Metabolic encephalopathy due to electrolyte abnormalities, infections, drug overdose, or the failure of some vital organ may be reflected by drowsiness, lethargy, restlessness, insomnia, agitation, confusion, stupor, or coma. The mental changes are usually associated with tremor, asterixis, and multifocal myoclonus. The electroencephalogram is generally diffusely slowed. Laboratory studies are necessary to detect the cause of the encephalopathy, which must then be treated appropriately.

(2) Immune suppression resulting from either the malignant disease or its treatment (eg, by chemotherapy) predisposes patients to brain abscess, progressive multifocal leukoencephalopathy, meningitis, herpes zoster infection, and other opportunistic infectious diseases. Moreover, an overt or occult cerebrospinal fluid fistula, as occurs with some tumors, may also increase the risk of infection. CT scanning aids in the early recognition of a brain abscess, but metastatic brain tumors may have a similar appearance. Examination of the cerebrospinal fluid is essential in the evaluation of patients with meningitis but is of no help in the diagnosis of brain abscess. Treatment should be specific for the infective organism.

(3) Cerebrovascular disorders that cause neurologic complications in patients with systemic cancer include nonbacterial thrombotic endocarditis and septic embolization. Cerebral, subarachnoid, or subdural hemorrhages may occur in patients with myelogenous leukemia and may be found in association with

metastatic tumors, especially malignant melanoma. Spinal subdural hemorrhage sometimes occurs after lumbar puncture in patients with marked thrombocytopenia.

Disseminated intravascular coagulation occurs most commonly in patients with acute promyelocytic leukemia or with some adenocarcinomas and is characterized by a fluctuating encephalopathy, often with associated seizures, that frequently progresses to coma or death. There may be few accompanying neurologic signs.

Venous sinus thrombosis, which usually presents with convulsions and headaches, may also occur in patients with leukemia or lymphoma. Examination commonly reveals papilledema and focal or diffuse neurologic signs. Anticonvulsants, anticoagulants, and drugs to lower the intracranial pressure may be of value.

(4) Paraneoplastic cerebellar degeneration occurs most commonly in association with carcinoma of the lung. Symptoms may precede those due to the neoplasm itself, which may be undetected for several months or even longer. Typically, there is a pancerebellar syndrome causing dysarthria, nystagmus, and ataxia of the trunk and limbs. The disorder probably has an autoimmune basis. Treatment is of the underlying malignant disease.

(5) Encephalopathy, characterized by impaired recent memory, disturbed affect, hallucinations, and seizures, occurs in some patients with carcinomas. The cerebrospinal fluid is often abnormal. EEGs may show diffuse slow-wave activity, especially over the temporal regions. Pathologic changes are most marked in the inferomedian portions of the temporal lobes. There is no specific treatment.

(6) Malignant disease may be associated with sensorimotor polyneuropathy and less commonly with pure sensory neuropathy (ie, dorsal root ganglionitis) or autonomic neuropathy. A subacute motor neuronopathy may be associated with lymphomas.

(7) Dermatomyositis or a myasthenic syndrome may be seen in patients with underlying carcinoma (see Chapter 20). The myasthenic syndrome may have an autoimmune basis and differs clinically from myasthenia gravis.

Posner JB: Paraneoplastic syndromes involving the nervous system. In: *Neurology and General Medicine,* 2nd ed. Aminoff MJ (editor). Churchill Livingstone, 1995.

PSEUDOTUMOR CEREBRI (Benign Intracranial Hypertension)

Symptoms of pseudotumor cerebri consist of headache, diplopia, and other visual disturbances due to papilledema and abducens nerve dysfunction. Examination reveals the papilledema and some enlargement of the blind spots, but patients otherwise look well. Investigations reveal no evidence of a space-occupying lesion, and the CT scan shows small or normal ventricles. Lumbar puncture confirms the presence of intracranial hypertension, but the cerebrospinal fluid is normal.

There are many causes of pseudotumor cerebri. Thrombosis of the transverse venous sinus as a noninfectious complication of otitis media or chronic mastoiditis is one cause, and sagittal sinus thrombosis may lead to a clinically similar picture. MR venography is helpful in screening for these disorders. Other causes include chronic pulmonary disease, endocrine disturbances such as hypoparathyroidism or Addison's disease, vitamin A toxicity, and the use of tetracycline or oral contraceptives. Cases have also followed withdrawal of corticosteroids after long-term use. In many instances, however, no specific cause can be found, and the disorder remits spontaneously after several months.

Untreated pseudotumor cerebri leads to secondary optic atrophy and permanent visual loss. Repeated lumbar puncture to lower the intracranial pressure by removal of cerebrospinal fluid is effective, but pharmacologic approaches to treatment are now more satisfactory. Acetazolamide (250 mg orally three times daily) reduces formation of cerebrospinal fluid and can be used to start treatment. Oral corticosteroids (eg, prednisone, 60–80 mg daily) may also be necessary. Obese patients should be advised to lose weight. Treatment is monitored by checking visual acuity and visual fields, funduscopic appearance, and pressure of the cerebrospinal fluid.

If medical treatment fails to control the intracranial pressure, surgical placement of a lumboperitoneal or other shunt—or subtemporal decompression or optic nerve sheath fenestration—should be undertaken to preserve vision.

In addition to the above measures, any specific cause of pseudotumor cerebri requires appropriate treatment. Thus, hormone therapy should be initiated if there is an underlying endocrine disturbance. Discontinuing the use of tetracycline, oral contraceptives, or vitamin A will allow for resolution of pseudotumor cerebri due to these agents. If corticosteroid withdrawal is responsible, the medication should be reintroduced and then tapered more gradually.

Kessler LA et al: Surgical treatment of benign intracranial hypertension—subtemporal decompression revisited. Surg Neurol 1998;50:73. [NLM Cit ID: 98319601] (Clinical study.)

SELECTED NEUROCUTANEOUS DISEASES

Tuberous Sclerosis

Tuberous sclerosis may occur sporadically or on a familial basis with autosomal dominant inheritance.

The responsible gene is located on the long arm of chromosome 9 in at least some cases. Its pathogenesis is unknown. Neurologic presentation is with seizures and progressive psychomotor retardation beginning in early childhood. The cutaneous abnormality, adenoma sebaceum, becomes manifest usually between 5 and 10 years of age and typically consists of reddened nodules on the face (cheeks, nasolabial folds, sides of the nose, and chin) and sometimes on the forehead and neck. Other typical cutaneous lesions include subungual fibromas, shagreen patches (leathery plaques of subepidermal fibrosis, situated usually on the trunk), and leaf-shaped hypopigmented spots. Associated abnormalities include retinal lesions and tumors, benign rhabdomyomas of the heart, lung cysts, benign tumors in the viscera, and bone cysts.

The disease is slowly progressive and leads to increasing mental deterioration. There is no specific treatment, but anticonvulsant drugs may help in controlling seizures.

Neurofibromatosis

Neurofibromatosis may occur either sporadically or on a familial basis with autosomal dominant inheritance. Two distinct forms are recognized: Type 1 **(Recklinghausen's disease)** is characterized by multiple hyperpigmented macules and neurofibromas and type 2 by **eighth nerve tumors,** often accompanied by other intracranial or intraspinal tumors. Among familial cases, the gene for type 1 is located on chromosome 17 and that for type 2 on chromosome 22.

Neurologic presentation is usually with symptoms and signs of tumor. Multiple neurofibromas characteristically are present and may involve spinal or cranial nerves, especially the eighth nerve. Examination of the superficial cutaneous nerves usually reveals palpable mobile nodules. In some cases, there is an associated marked overgrowth of subcutaneous tissues (plexiform neuromas), sometimes with an underlying bony abnormality. Associated cutaneous lesions include axillary freckling and patches of cutaneous pigmentation (café au lait spots). Malignant degeneration of neurofibromas occasionally occurs and may lead to peripheral sarcomas. Meningiomas, gliomas (especially optic nerve gliomas), bone cysts, pheochromocytomas, scoliosis, and obstructive hydrocephalus may also occur.

It may be possible to correct disfigurement by plastic surgery. Intraspinal or intracranial tumors and tumors of peripheral nerves should be treated surgically if they are producing symptoms.

Gutmann DH et al: The diagnostic evaluation and multidisciplinary management of neurofibromatosis 1 and neurofibromatosis 2. JAMA 1997;278:51. [NLM Cit ID: 97350963]

Sturge-Weber Syndrome

Sturge-Weber syndrome consists of a congenital, usually unilateral, cutaneous capillary angioma involving the upper face, leptomeningeal angiomatosis, and, in many patients, choroidal angioma. It has no sex predilection and usually occurs sporadically. The cutaneous angioma sometimes has a more extensive distribution over the head and neck and is often quite disfiguring, especially if there is associated overgrowth of connective tissue. Focal or generalized seizures are the usual neurologic presentation and may commence at any age. There may be contralateral homonymous hemianopia, hemiparesis and hemisensory disturbance, ipsilateral glaucoma, and mental subnormality. Skull x-rays taken after the first 2 years of life usually reveal gyriform ("tramline") intracranial calcification, especially in the parieto-occipital region, due to mineral deposition in the cortex beneath the intracranial angioma.

Treatment is aimed at controlling seizures pharmacologically. Ophthalmologic advice should be sought concerning the management of choroidal angioma and of increased intraocular pressure.

MOVEMENT DISORDERS

1. BENIGN ESSENTIAL (FAMILIAL) TREMOR

The cause of benign essential tremor is uncertain, but it is sometimes inherited in an autosomal dominant manner. Tremor may begin at any age and is enhanced by emotional stress. The tremor usually involves one or both hands, the head, or the hands and head, while the legs tend to be spared. Examination reveals no other abnormalities. Ingestion of a small quantity of alcohol commonly provides remarkable but short-lived relief by an unknown mechanism.

Although the tremor may become more conspicuous with time, it generally leads to little disability, and treatment is often unnecessary. Occasionally, it interferes with manual skills and leads to impairment of handwriting. Speech may also be affected if the laryngeal muscles are involved. In such circumstances, propranolol may be helpful but will need to be continued indefinitely in daily doses of 60–240 mg. However, intermittent therapy is sometimes useful in patients whose tremor becomes exacerbated in specific predictable situations. Primidone may be helpful when propranolol is ineffective, but patients with essential tremor are often very sensitive to it. They are therefore started on 50 mg daily, and the daily dose is increased by 50 mg every 2 weeks depending on the response; a maintenance dose of 125 mg three times daily is commonly effective. Occasional patients fail to respond to these measures but are helped by alprazolam (up to 3 mg daily in divided doses), clozapine (30–50 mg twice daily), or mirtazapine (15 or 30 mg at night).

Disabling tremor unresponsive to medical treatment may be helped by contralateral thalamotomy.

Unilateral high-frequency thalamic stimulation is an alternative approach that is equally effective, is associated with only mild and transient side effects, and is therefore preferred. Bilateral thalamotomy has significant morbidity, whereas the risks of bilateral stimulation are appreciably lower.

Ceravolo R et al: Acute and chronic effects of clozapine in essential tremor. Mov Disord 1999;14:468. [NLM Cit ID: 99276227] (Double-blind clinical trial.)

Pact V et al: Mirtazapine treats resting tremor, essential tremor, and levodopa-induced dyskinesias. Neurology 1999;53:1154. [NLM Cit ID: 99424609] (Clinical report.)

2. PARKINSONISM

Essentials of Diagnosis

- Any combination of tremor, rigidity, bradykinesia, progressive postural instability.
- Seborrhea of skin quite common.
- Mild intellectual deterioration is often observed.

General Considerations

Parkinsonism is a relatively common disorder that occurs in all ethnic groups, with an approximately equal sex distribution. The most common variety, idiopathic Parkinson's disease (paralysis agitans), begins most often between 45 and 65 years of age.

Etiology

Parkinsonism may rarely occur on a familial basis, and the parkinsonian phenotype may result from mutations of several different genes. Postencephalitic parkinsonism is becoming increasingly rare. Exposure to certain toxins (eg, manganese dust, carbon disulfide) and severe carbon monoxide poisoning may lead to parkinsonism. Typical parkinsonism has occurred in individuals who have taken 1-methyl-4-phenyl-1,2,5,6-tetrahydropyridine (MPTP) for recreational purposes. This compound is converted in the body to a neurotoxin that selectively destroys dopaminergic neurons in the substantia nigra. Reversible parkinsonism may develop in patients receiving neuroleptic drugs (see Chapter 25), reserpine, or metoclopramide. Only rarely is hemiparkinsonism the presenting feature of a progressive space-occupying lesion.

In idiopathic parkinsonism, dopamine depletion due to degeneration of the dopaminergic nigrostriatal system leads to an imbalance of dopamine and acetylcholine, which are neurotransmitters normally present in the corpus striatum. Treatment is directed at redressing this imbalance by blocking the effect of acetylcholine with anticholinergic drugs or by the administration of levodopa, the precursor of dopamine.

Clinical Findings

Tremor, rigidity, bradykinesia, and postural instability are the cardinal features of parkinsonism and may be present in any combination. There may also be a mild decline in intellectual function. The tremor of about four to six cycles per second is most conspicuous at rest, is enhanced by emotional stress, and is often less severe during voluntary activity. Although it may ultimately be present in all limbs, the tremor is commonly confined to one limb or to the limbs on one side for months or years before it becomes more generalized. In some patients, tremor is absent.

Rigidity (an increase in resistance to passive movement) is responsible for the characteristically flexed posture seen in many patients, but the most disabling symptoms of parkinsonism are due to bradykinesia, manifested as a slowness of voluntary movement and a reduction in automatic movements such as swinging of the arms while walking. Curiously, however, effective voluntary activity may briefly be regained during an emergency (eg, the patient is able to leap aside to avoid an oncoming motor vehicle).

Clinical diagnosis of the well-developed syndrome is usually simple. The patient has a relatively immobile face with widened palpebral fissures, infrequent blinking, and a certain fixity of facial expression. Seborrhea of the scalp and face is common. There is often mild blepharoclonus, and a tremor may be present about the mouth and lips. Repetitive tapping (about twice per second) over the bridge of the nose produces a sustained blink response (Myerson's sign). Other findings may include saliva drooling from the mouth, perhaps due to impairment of swallowing; soft and poorly modulated voice; a variable rest tremor and rigidity in some or all of the limbs; slowness of voluntary movements; impairment of fine or rapidly alternating movements; and micrographia. There is typically no muscle weakness (provided that sufficient time is allowed for power to be developed) and no alteration in the tendon reflexes or plantar responses. It is difficult for the patient to arise from a sitting position and begin walking. The gait itself is characterized by small shuffling steps and a loss of the normal automatic arm swing; there may be unsteadiness on turning, difficulty in stopping, and a tendency to fall.

Differential Diagnosis

Diagnostic problems may occur in mild cases, especially if tremor is minimal or absent. For example, mild hypokinesia or slight tremor is commonly attributed to old age. Depression, with its associated expressionless face, poorly modulated voice, and reduction in voluntary activity, can be difficult to distinguish from mild parkinsonism, especially since the two disorders may coexist; in some cases, a trial of antidepressant drug therapy is necessary. The family history, the character of the tremor, and lack of other neurologic signs should distinguish essential tremor from parkinsonism. Wilson's disease can be distinguished by its early age at onset, the presence of other abnormal movements, Kayser-Fleischer rings, and chronic hepatitis, and by increased concentrations of copper in the tissues. Huntington's disease presenting with rigidity and bradykinesia may be mistaken for parkinsonism unless the family history and accompanying dementia are recognized. In Shy-Drager syndrome, the clinical features of parkinsonism are accompanied by autonomic insufficiency (leading to postural hypotension, anhidrosis, disturbances of sphincter control, impotence, etc) and more widespread neurologic deficits (pyramidal, lower motor neuron, or cerebellar signs). In progressive supranuclear palsy, bradykinesia and rigidity are accompanied by a supranuclear disorder of eye movements, pseudobulbar palsy, and axial dystonia. Creutzfeldt-Jakob disease may be accompanied by features of parkinsonism, but dementia is usual, myoclonic jerking is common, ataxia and pyramidal signs may be conspicuous, and the electroencephalographic findings are usually characteristic. In cortical-basal ganglionic degeneration, parkinsonism is accompanied by conspicuous signs of cortical dysfunction (eg, apraxia, sensory inattention, dementia, aphasia).

Treatment

A. Medical Measures: Drug treatment is not required early in the course of parkinsonism, but the nature of the disorder and the availability of medical treatment for use when necessary should be discussed with the patient.

1. Amantadine–Patients with mild symptoms but no disability may be helped by amantadine. This drug improves all of the clinical features of parkinsonism, but its mode of action is unclear. Side effects include restlessness, confusion, depression, skin rashes, edema, nausea, constipation, anorexia, postural hypotension, and disturbances of cardiac rhythm. However, these are relatively uncommon with the usual dose (100 mg twice daily).

2. Anticholinergic drugs–Anticholinergics are more helpful in alleviating tremor and rigidity than bradykinesia. Treatment is started with a small dose (Table 24–4) and gradually increased until benefit occurs or side effects limit further increments. If treatment is ineffective, the drug is gradually withdrawn and another preparation then tried.

Common side effects include dryness of the mouth, nausea, constipation, palpitations, cardiac arrhythmias, urinary retention, confusion, agitation, restlessness, drowsiness, mydriasis, increased intraocular pressure, and defective accommodation.

Anticholinergic drugs are contraindicated in patients with prostatic hypertrophy, narrow-angle glaucoma, or obstructive gastrointestinal disease and are often tolerated poorly by the elderly.

Table 24–4. Some anticholinergic antiparkinsonian drugs.[1]

Drug	Usual Daily Dose
Benztropine mesylate (Cogentin)	1–6 mg
Biperiden (Akineton)	2–12 mg
Chlorphenoxamine (Phenoxene)	150–400 mg
Cycrimine (Pagitane)	5–20 mg
Orphenadrine (Disipal, Norflex)	150–400 mg
Procyclidine (Kemadrin)	7.5–30 mg
Trihexyphenidy (Artane)	6–20 mg

[1]Modified, with permission, from Aminoff MJ. Pharmacologic management of parkinsonism and other movement disorders. In: *Basic & Clinical Pharmacology,* 6th ed. Katzung BG (editor). Appleton & Lange, 1994.

3. Levodopa–Levodopa, which is converted in the body to dopamine, improves all of the major features of parkinsonism, including bradykinesia, but does not stop progression of the disorder. The commonest early side effects of levodopa are nausea, vomiting, and hypotension, but cardiac arrhythmias may also occur. Dyskinesias, restlessness, confusion, and other behavioral changes tend to occur somewhat later and become more common with time. Levodopa-induced dyskinesias may take any conceivable form, including chorea, athetosis, dystonia, tremor, tics, and myoclonus. An even later complication is the "on-off phenomenon," in which abrupt but transient fluctuations in the severity of parkinsonism occur unpredictably but frequently during the day. The "off" period of marked bradykinesia has been shown to relate in some instances to falling plasma levels of levodopa. During the "on" phase, dyskinesias are often conspicuous but mobility is increased.

Carbidopa, which inhibits the enzyme responsible for the breakdown of levodopa to dopamine, does not cross the blood-brain barrier. When levodopa is given in combination with carbidopa, the extracerebral breakdown of levodopa is diminished. This reduces the amount of levodopa required daily for beneficial effects, and it lowers the incidence of nausea, vomiting, hypotension, and cardiac irregularities. Such a combination does not prevent the development of the "on-off phenomenon," and the incidence of other side effects (dyskinesias or psychiatric complications) may actually be increased.

Sinemet, a commercially available preparation that contains carbidopa and levodopa in a fixed ratio (1:10 or 1:4), is generally used. Treatment is started with a small dose—eg, one tablet of Sinemet 25/100 (containing 25 mg of carbidopa and 100 mg of levodopa) three times daily—and gradually increased depending on the response. Sinemet CR is a controlled-release formulation (containing 25 or 50 mg of carbidopa and 100 or 200 mg of levodopa). It is sometimes helpful in reducing fluctuations in clinical response to treatment and in reducing the frequency with which medication must be taken. Response fluctuations are also reduced by keeping the daily intake of protein at the recommended minimum and taking the main protein meal as the last meal of the day.

The dyskinesias and behavioral side effects of levodopa are dose-related, but reduction in dose may eliminate any therapeutic benefit.

Levodopa therapy is contraindicated in patients with psychotic illness or narrow-angle glaucoma. It should not be given to patients taking monoamine oxidase A inhibitors or within 2 weeks of their withdrawal, because hypertensive crises may result. Levodopa should be used with care in patients with suspected malignant melanomas or with active peptic ulcers because of concerns that it may exacerbate these disorders.

4. **Dopamine agonists**–Dopamine agonists act directly on dopamine receptors, and their use in parkinsonism is associated with a lower incidence of the response fluctuations and dyskinesias that occur with long-term levodopa therapy. They were previously reserved for patients who had either become refractory to levodopa or developed the "on-off phenomenon." However, they are now best given either before the introduction of levodopa or with a low dose of Sinemet-25/100 (carbidopa 25 mg and levodopa 100 mg), one tablet three times daily when dopaminergic therapy is first introduced; the dose of Sinemet is kept constant, while the dose of the agonist is gradually increased. Two widely used agonists are bromocriptine and pergolide, which are equally effective ergot derivatives. The initial dosage of bromocriptine is 1.25 mg twice daily; this is increased by 2.5 mg at 2-week intervals until benefit occurs or side effects limit further increments. The usual daily maintenance dose in patients with parkinsonism is between 10 and 30 mg. Pergolide is similarly started in a low dose (eg, 0.05 mg daily) and built up gradually depending on the response and tolerance.

Side effects include anorexia, nausea, vomiting, constipation, postural hypotension, digital vasospasm, cardiac arrhythmias, various dyskinesias and mental disturbances, headache, nasal congestion, erythromelalgia, and pulmonary infiltrates. Bromocriptine and pergolide are contraindicated in patients with a history of mental illness or recent myocardial infarction and are probably best avoided in those with peripheral vascular disease or peptic ulcers as bleeding from the latter has been reported.

Pramipexole and ropinirole are two newer dopamine agonists that are not ergot derivatives. It is not clear that they have any benefit over the older agents, except that ergot-related side effects are unlikely. They are effective in early Parkinson's disease as well as in advanced stages of the disease. In each case, the daily dose is built up gradually. Pramipexole is started at a dosage of 0.125 mg three times daily, and the dose is doubled after 1 week and again after another week; the daily dose is then increased by 0.75 mg at weekly intervals depending on response and tolerance. Most patients require between 0.5 and 1.5 mg three times daily. Ropinirole is begun in a dosage of 0.25 mg three times daily, and the total daily dose is increased at weekly intervals by 0.75 mg until the fourth week and by 1.5 mg thereafter. Most patients require between 2 and 8 mg three times daily for benefit. Adverse effects include fatigue, somnolence, nausea, peripheral edema, dyskinesias, confusion, and postural hypotension. Less commonly, an irresistible urge to sleep may occur, sometimes in appropriate and hazardous circumstances.

5. **Selegiline**–Selegiline is a monoamine oxidase B inhibitor that is sometimes used as adjunctive treatment for parkinsonism in patients receiving levodopa. By inhibiting the metabolic breakdown of dopamine, selegiline has been used to improve fluctuations or declining response to levodopa. In general, however, the response to treatment with it has been disappointing. The drug is taken in a standard dose of 5 mg with breakfast and 5 mg with lunch. It may increase any adverse effects of levodopa.

There are reasons to believe that selegiline may arrest the progression of Parkinson's disease. Studies have failed to establish this conclusively, but this remains an important consideration for patients who are young or have mild disease.

6. **Atypical antipsychotics**–Confusion and psychotic symptoms, which may be iatrogenic, often respond to atypical antipsychotic agents, which have few extrapyramidal side effects and do not block the effects of dopaminergic medication. Olanzapine and risperidone may be tried, but the most effective of these agents is clozapine, a dibenzodiazepine derivative. Clozapine may rarely cause marrow suppression, and weekly blood counts are therefore necessary for patients taking it. The patient is started on 6.25 mg at bedtime and the dosage increased to 25–100 mg/d as needed. In low doses, it may also improve iatrogenic dyskinesias.

7. **COMT inhibitors**–Catecholamine-*O*-methyltransferase inhibitors reduce the metabolism of levodopa to 3-*O*-methyldopa and thereby alter the plasma pharmacokinetics of levodopa, leading to more sustained plasma levels and more constant dopaminergic stimulation of the brain. Two such agents, tolcapone and entacapone, are currently available and may be used as an adjunct to levodopa-carbidopa in patients with response fluctuations or an otherwise inadequate response and who either have failed with other adjunctive therapies or are not candidates for such therapies. Treatment results in reduced response fluctuations, with a greater period of responsiveness to administered levodopa. Tolcapone is given in a dosage of 100 mg or

200 mg three times daily, and entacapone is given as 200 mg with each dose of Sinemet (levodopa-carbidopa). The dosage of Sinemet (levodopa/carbidopa) taken concurrently may have to be reduced by up to one-third to avoid side effects such as dyskinesias, confusion, hypotension, and syncope. Diarrhea is sometimes troublesome. Because rare cases of fulminant hepatic failure have followed its use, tolcapone should be avoided in patients with preexisting liver disease. Serial liver function tests should be performed at 2-week intervals for the first year and at longer intervals thereafter in patients receiving the drug—as recommended by the manufacturer. Hepatotoxicity has not been reported with entacapone, and serial liver function tests are not required.

B. General Measures: Physical therapy or speech therapy helps many patients. The quality of life can often be improved by the provision of simple aids to daily living, eg, rails or banisters placed strategically about the home, special table cutlery with large handles, nonslip rubber table mats, and devices to amplify the voice.

C. Surgical Measures: Thalamotomy or pallidotomy may be helpful for patients who become unresponsive to medical treatment or have intolerable side effects from antiparkinsonian agents, especially if they have no evidence of diffuse vascular disease or significant cognitive decline. Surgery should generally be confined to one side because the morbidity is considerably greater after bilateral procedures. Surgical implantation of adrenal medullary or fetal substantia nigra tissue into the caudate nucleus has recently been reported to benefit some patients, but other investigators have failed to substantiate such claims or have found only modest benefits, and the procedure is still being evaluated.

D. Brain Stimulation: High-frequency thalamic stimulation is effective in suppressing the rest tremor of Parkinson's disease, and investigational studies in small numbers of patients indicate that chronic bilateral stimulation of the subthalamic nuclei or globus pallidus internus may relieve all the major features of the disease. Electrical stimulation of the brain has the advantage of being reversible and of causing minimal or no damage to the brain, and its utility is being explored in several centers.

Adler CH et al: Ropinirole for the treatment of early Parkinson's disease. Neurology 1997;49:393. [NLM Cit ID: 97416617] (Clinical trial.)

Durif F et al: Low-dose clozapine improves dyskinesias in Parkinson's disease. Neurology 1997;48:658. [NLM Cit ID: 97217882]

Lang AE et al: Parkinson's disease. (Part 1.) N Engl J Med 1998;339:1044. [NLM Cit ID: 98425650]

Lang AE et al: Parkinson's disease. (Part 2.) N Engl J Med 1998;339:1130. [NLM Cit ID: 98432454]

Obeso JA et al: Surgery for Parkinson's disease. J Neurol Neurosurg Psychiatry 1997;62:2. [NLM Cit ID: 97163582] (Review of pathophysiologic basis and results of surgery.)

Olanow CW et al: An algorithm (decision tree) for the management of Parkinson's disease: Treatment guidelines. Neurology 1998;50(3 Suppl 3):S1. [NLM Cit ID: 98185240]

Starr PA et al: Deep brain stimulation for movement disorders. Neurosurg Clin North Am 1998;9:381. [NLM Cit ID: 98163479]

3. HUNTINGTON'S DISEASE

Essentials of Diagnosis

- Gradual onset and progression of chorea and dementia.
- Family history of the disorder.
- Responsible gene identified on chromosome 4.

General Considerations

Huntington's disease is characterized by chorea and dementia. It is inherited in an autosomal dominant manner and occurs throughout the world, in all ethnic groups, with a prevalence rate of about 5 per 100,000. The gene responsible for the disease has been located on the short arm of chromosome 4. At 4p16.3 there is an expanded and unstable CAG trinucleotide repeat.

Clinical Findings

Clinical onset is usually between 30 and 50 years of age. The disease is progressive and usually leads to a fatal outcome within 15–20 years. The initial symptoms may consist of either abnormal movements or intellectual changes, but ultimately both occur. The earliest mental changes are often behavioral, with irritability, moodiness, antisocial behavior, or a psychiatric disturbance, but a more obvious dementia subsequently develops. The dyskinesia may initially be no more than an apparent fidgetiness or restlessness, but eventually choreiform movements and some dystonic posturing occur. Progressive rigidity and akinesia (rather than chorea) sometimes occur in association with dementia, especially in cases with childhood onset. CT scanning usually demonstrates cerebral atrophy and atrophy of the caudate nucleus in established cases. MRI and positron emission tomography (PET) have shown reduced glucose utilization in an anatomically normal caudate nucleus.

Chorea developing with no family history of choreoathetosis should not be attributed to Huntington's disease, at least not until other causes of chorea have been excluded clinically and by appropriate laboratory studies. In younger patients, self-limiting Sydenham's chorea develops after group A streptococcal infections on rare occasions. If a patient presents solely with progressive intellectual failure, it may not be possible to distinguish Huntington's disease from other causes of dementia unless there is a characteristic family history or a dyskinesia develops.

Treatment

There is no cure for Huntington's disease, progression cannot be halted, and treatment is purely symptomatic. The reported biochemical changes suggest a relative underactivity of neurons containing gamma-aminobutyric acid (GABA) and acetylcholine or a relative overactivity of dopaminergic neurons. Treatment with drugs blocking dopamine receptors, such as phenothiazines or haloperidol, may control the dyskinesia and any behavioral disturbances. Haloperidol treatment is usually begun with a dose of 1 mg once or twice daily, which is then increased every 3 or 4 days depending on the response. Tetrabenazine, a drug that depletes central monoamines, is widely used in Europe to treat dyskinesia but is not available in the USA. Reserpine is similar in its actions to tetrabenazine and may be helpful; the daily dose is built up gradually to between 2 and 5 mg, depending on the response. Behavioral disturbances may respond to clozapine. Attempts to compensate for the relative GABA deficiency by enhancing central GABA activity or to compensate for the relative cholinergic underactivity by giving choline chloride have not been therapeutically helpful. High levels of somatostatin (a neuropeptide) have recently been reported in certain areas of the brain in patients with Huntington's disease, and the therapeutic response to cysteamine (a selective depleter of somatostatin in the brain) is currently under study.

Offspring should be offered genetic counseling. Genetic testing permits presymptomatic detection and definitive diagnosis of the disease.

Ross CA et al: Huntington disease and the related disorder, dentatorubral-pallidoluysian atrophy (DRPLA). Medicine 1997;76:305. [NLM Cit ID: 98014102]

4. IDIOPATHIC TORSION DYSTONIA

Essentials of Diagnosis

- Dystonic movements and postures.
- Normal birth and developmental history. No other neurologic signs.
- Investigations (including CT scan or MRI) reveal no cause of dystonia.

General Considerations

Idiopathic torsion dystonia may occur sporadically or on a hereditary basis, with autosomal dominant, autosomal recessive, and X-linked recessive modes of transmission. The responsible gene is located at 9q34 (and has been named *DYT1*) and involves a unique mutation consisting of a GAG deletion in the dominantly inherited disorder and to the long arm of the X chromosome in the X-linked recessive form; the responsible gene in the autosomal recessive disorder is unknown. Other autosomal dominant forms have also been recognized, with different or unidentified genetic loci. Symptoms may begin in childhood or later and persist throughout life.

Clinical Findings

The disorder is characterized by the onset of abnormal movements and postures in a patient with a normal birth and developmental history, no relevant past medical illness, and no other neurologic signs. Investigations (including CT scan) reveal no cause for the abnormal movements. Dystonic movements of the head and neck may take the form of torticollis, blepharospasm, facial grimacing, or forced opening or closing of the mouth. The limbs may also adopt abnormal but characteristic postures. The age at onset influences both the clinical findings and the prognosis. With onset in childhood, there is usually a family history of the disorder, symptoms commonly commence in the legs, and progression is likely until there is severe disability from generalized dystonia. In contrast, when onset is later, a positive family history is unlikely, initial symptoms are often in the arms or axial structures, and severe disability does not usually occur, although generalized dystonia may ultimately develop in some patients. If all cases are considered together, about one-third of patients eventually become so severely disabled that they are confined to chair or bed, while another one-third are affected only mildly.

Before a diagnosis of idiopathic torsion dystonia is made, it is imperative to exclude other causes of dystonia. For example, perinatal anoxia, birth trauma, and kernicterus are common causes of dystonia, but abnormal movements usually then develop before the age of 5, the early development of the patient is usually abnormal, and a history of seizures is not unusual. Moreover, examination may reveal signs of mental retardation or pyramidal deficit in addition to the movement disorder. Dystonic posturing may also occur in Wilson's disease, Huntington's disease, or parkinsonism; as a sequela of encephalitis lethargica or previous neuroleptic drug therapy; and in certain other disorders. In these cases, diagnosis is based on the history and accompanying clinical manifestations.

Treatment

Idiopathic torsion dystonia usually responds poorly to drugs. Levodopa, diazepam, baclofen, carbamazepine, amantadine, or anticholinergic medication (in high dosage) is occasionally helpful; if not, a trial of treatment with phenothiazines or haloperidol may be worthwhile. In each case, the dose has to be individualized, depending on response and tolerance. However, the doses of these latter drugs that are required for benefit lead usually to mild parkinsonism. Stereotactic thalamotomy is sometimes helpful in patients with predominantly unilateral dystonia, especially when this involves the limbs.

Bressman SB: Dystonia. Curr Opin Neurol 1998;11:363. [NLM Cit ID: 98392704] (Review of recent advances.)

Ozelius LJ et al: The early-onset torsion dystonia gene (*DYT1*) encodes an ATP-binding protein. Nat Genet 1997;17:40. [NLM Cit ID: 97434210] (Identification of gene.)

5. FOCAL TORSION DYSTONIA

A number of the dystonic manifestations that occur in idiopathic torsion dystonia may also occur as isolated phenomena. They are best regarded as focal dystonias that either occur as formes frustes of idiopathic torsion dystonia in patients with a positive family history or represent a focal manifestation of the adult-onset form of that disorder when there is no family history. Mapping of responsible genes to chromosome 8 *(DYT6)* and chromosome 18 *(DYT17)* has been reported in some instances of cervical or cranial dystonia. Medical treatment is generally unsatisfactory. A trial of the drugs used in idiopathic torsion dystonia is worthwhile, however, since a few patients do show some response. In addition, with restricted dystonias such as blepharospasm or torticollis, local injection of botulinum A toxin into the overactive muscles may produce worthwhile benefit for several weeks or months and can be repeated as needed.

Both blepharospasm and oromandibular dystonia may occur as an isolated focal dystonia. The former is characterized by spontaneous involuntary forced closure of the eyelids for a variable interval. Oromandibular dystonia is manifested by involuntary contraction of the muscles about the mouth causing, for example, involuntary opening or closing of the mouth, roving or protruding tongue movements, and retraction of the platysma.

Spasmodic torticollis, usually with onset between 25 and 50 years of age, is characterized by a tendency for the neck to twist to one side. This initially occurs episodically, but eventually the neck is held to the side. Spontaneous resolution may occur in the first year or so. The disorder is otherwise usually lifelong. Selective section of the spinal accessory nerve and the upper cervical nerve roots is sometimes helpful if medical treatment is unsuccessful. Local injection of botulinum A toxin provides benefit in most cases.

Writer's cramp is characterized by dystonic posturing of the hand and forearm when the hand is used for writing and sometimes when it is used for other tasks, eg, playing the piano, using a screwdriver or eating utensils. Drug treatment is usually unrewarding, and patients are often best advised to learn to use the other hand for activities requiring manual dexterity. Injections of botulinum A toxin are helpful in some instances.

6. MYOCLONUS

Occasional myoclonic jerks may occur in anyone, especially when drifting into sleep. General or multifocal myoclonus is common in patients with idiopathic epilepsy and is especially prominent in certain hereditary disorders characterized by seizures and progressive intellectual decline, such as the lipid storage diseases. It is also a feature of various rare degenerative disorders, notably Ramsay Hunt syndrome, and is common in subacute sclerosing panencephalitis and Creutzfeldt-Jakob disease. Generalized myoclonic jerking may accompany uremic and other metabolic encephalopathies, result from levodopa therapy, occur in alcohol or drug withdrawal states, or follow anoxic brain damage. It also occurs on a hereditary or sporadic basis as an isolated phenomenon in otherwise healthy subjects.

Segmental myoclonus is a rare manifestation of a focal spinal cord lesion. It may also be the clinical expression of **epilepsia partialis continua,** a disorder in which a repetitive focal epileptic discharge arises in the contralateral sensorimotor cortex, sometimes from an underlying structural lesion. An electroencephalogram is often helpful in clarifying the epileptic nature of the disorder, and CT or MRI scan may reveal the causal lesion.

Myoclonus may respond to certain anticonvulsant drugs, especially valproic acid, or to one of the benzodiazepines, particularly clonazepam (Table 24–2). It may also respond to piracetam (up to 16.8 g daily). Myoclonus following anoxic brain damage is often responsive to oxitriptan (5-hydroxytryptophan), an investigational agent that is the precursor of serotonin, and sometimes to clonazepam. Oxitriptan is given in gradually increasing doses up to 1–1.5 mg daily. In patients with segmental myoclonus, a localized lesion should be searched for and treated appropriately.

Caviness JN: Myoclonus. Mayo Clin Proc 1996;71:679. [NLM Cit ID: 96269448]

7. WILSON'S DISEASE

In this metabolic disorder, abnormal movement and posture may occur with or without coexisting signs of liver involvement. It is discussed in Chapter 15.

8. DRUG-INDUCED ABNORMAL MOVEMENTS

Phenothiazines and butyrophenones may produce a wide variety of abnormal movements, including parkinsonism, akathisia (ie, motor restlessness), acute dystonia, chorea, and tardive dyskinesia. These complications are discussed in Chapter 25. Chorea may also develop in patients receiving levodopa, bromocriptine, anticholinergic drugs, phenytoin, carbamazepine, lithium, amphetamines, or oral contraceptives, and it resolves with withdrawal of the offending substance. Similarly, dystonia may be produced by levodopa, bromocriptine, lithium, metoclopramide, or carbamazepine; and parkinsonism by reserpine, tetrabenazine, and metoclopramide. Postural tremor may occur with a variety of drugs, including epinephrine, isoproterenol, theophylline, caffeine, lithium, thyroid hormone, tricyclic antidepressants, and valproic acid.

9. GILLES DE LA TOURETTE'S SYNDROME

Essentials of Diagnosis

- Multiple motor and phonic tics.
- Symptoms begin before age 21 years.
- Tics occur frequently for at least 1 year.
- Tics vary in number, frequency, and nature over time.

Clinical Findings

Motor tics are the initial manifestation in 80% of cases and most commonly involve the face whereas in the remaining 20%, the initial symptoms are phonic tics; all patients ultimately develop a combination of different motor and phonic tics. These are noted first in childhood, generally between the ages of 2 and 15. Motor tics occur especially about the face, head, and shoulders (eg, sniffing, blinking, frowning, shoulder shrugging, head thrusting, etc). Phonic tics commonly consist of grunts, barks, hisses, throat-clearing, coughs, etc, but sometimes also of verbal utterances including coprolalia (obscene speech). There may also be echolalia (repetition of the speech of others), echopraxia (imitation of others' movements), and palilalia (repetition of words or phrases). Some tics may be self-mutilating in nature, such as nail-biting, hair-pulling, or biting of the lips or tongue. The disorder is chronic, but the course may be punctuated by relapses and remissions. Obsessive-compulsive behaviors are commonly associated and may be more disabling than the tics themselves.

Examination usually reveals no abnormalities other than the tics. In addition to obsessive-compulsive behavior disorders, psychiatric disturbances may occur because of the associated cosmetic and social embarrassment. Electroencephalography may show minor nonspecific abnormalities of no diagnostic relevance.

The diagnosis of the disorder is often delayed for years, the tics being interpreted as psychiatric illness or some other form of abnormal movement. Patients are thus often subjected to unnecessary treatment before the disorder is recognized. The tic-like character of the abnormal movements and the absence of other neurologic signs should differentiate this disorder from other movement disorders presenting in childhood. Wilson's disease, however, can simulate the condition and should be excluded.

Treatment

Treatment is symptomatic and may need to be continued indefinitely. Haloperidol is generally regarded as the drug of choice. It is started in a low daily dose (0.25 mg) that is gradually increased (by 0.25 mg every 4 or 5 days) until there is maximum benefit with a minimum of side effects or until side effects limit further increments. A total daily dose of between 2 and 8 mg is usually optimal, but higher doses are sometimes necessary. Treatment with clonazepam (in a dose that depends on response and tolerance) or clonidine (2–5 μg/kg/d) may also be helpful, and it seems sensible to begin with one of these drugs in order to avoid some of the long-term extrapyramidal side effects of haloperidol. Phenothiazines, such as fluphenazine (2–15 mg daily), have been used, but patients unresponsive to haloperidol are usually unresponsive to these as well.

Pimozide, an oral dopamine-blocking drug related to haloperidol, may be helpful in patients who cannot tolerate or have not responded to haloperidol. Treatment is started with 1 mg daily and the daily dose increased by 1–2 mg every 10 days; the average dose is between 7 and 16 mg daily.

Treatment with risperidone, calcium channel blockers, tetrabenazene, or clomipramine has yielded mixed results.

Robertson MM et al: The Gilles de la Tourette syndrome. Crit Rev Neurobiol 1997;11:1. [NLM Cit ID: 97247684] (General review of clinical features, epidemiology, genetics, and treatment.)

DEMENTIA

Dementia, the symptom complex of progressive global impairment of intellectual function, is a major medical, social, and economic problem that is worsening as the number of elderly people in the general population increases. It is discussed in Chapter 4, and the only point to be reiterated here is the importance of recognizing early any treatable or reversible causes of dementia, such as normal-pressure hydrocephalus, intracranial mass lesions, vascular disease, hypothyroidism, thiamin or vitamin B_{12} deficiency, Wilson's disease, hepatic or renal failure, neurosyphilis, and the chronic meningitides.

MULTIPLE SCLEROSIS

Essentials of Diagnosis

- Episodic neurologic symptoms.
- Patient usually under 55 years of age at onset.
- Single pathologic lesion cannot explain clinical findings.
- Multiple foci best visualized by MRI.

General Considerations

This common neurologic disorder, which probably has an autoimmune basis, has its greatest incidence in young adults. Epidemiologic studies indicate that multiple sclerosis is much more common in persons of western European lineage who live in temperate zones. No population with a high risk for multiple sclerosis exists between latitudes 40 °N and 40 °S. Genetic, dietary, and climatic factors cannot account for these differences. Nevertheless, a genetic susceptibility to the disease is likely, based on twin studies, familial cases, and an association with specific HLA antigens (HLA-DR2). Pathologically, focal—often perivenular—areas of demyelination with reactive gliosis are found scattered in the white matter of brain and spinal cord and in the optic nerves.

Clinical Findings

A. Symptoms and Signs: The common initial presentation is weakness, numbness, tingling, or unsteadiness in a limb; spastic paraparesis; retrobulbar neuritis; diplopia; disequilibrium; or a sphincter disturbance such as urinary urgency or hesitancy. Symptoms may disappear after a few days or weeks, although examination often reveals a residual deficit.

Several forms of the disease are recognized. In most patients, there is an interval of months or years after the initial episode before new symptoms develop or the original ones recur **(relapsing-remitting disease).** Eventually, however, relapses and usually incomplete remissions lead to increasing disability, with weakness, spasticity, and ataxia of the limbs, impaired vision, and urinary incontinence. The findings on examination at this stage commonly include optic atrophy, nystagmus, dysarthria, and pyramidal, sensory, or cerebellar deficits in some or all of the limbs. In some of these patients, the clinical course changes so that a steady deterioration occurs, unrelated to acute relapses **(secondary progressive disease).**

Less commonly, symptoms are steadily progressive from their onset, and disability develops at a relatively early stage **(primary progressive disease).** The diagnosis cannot be made with confidence unless the total clinical picture indicates involvement of different parts of the central nervous system at different times.

A number of factors (eg, infection, trauma) may precipitate or trigger exacerbations. Relapses are also more likely during the 2 or 3 months following pregnancy, possibly because of the increased demands and stresses that occur in the postpartum period.

B. Imaging: MRI of the brain or cervical cord is often helpful in demonstrating the presence of a multiplicity of lesions. CT scans are less helpful.

In patients presenting with myelopathy alone and in whom there is no clinical or laboratory evidence of more widespread disease, myelography or MRI may be necessary to exclude a congenital or acquired surgically treatable lesion. The foramen magnum region must be visualized to exclude the possibility of Arnold-Chiari malformation, in which part of the cerebellum and the lower brainstem are displaced into the cervical canal and produce mixed pyramidal and cerebellar deficits in the limbs.

C. Laboratory and Other Studies: A definitive diagnosis can never be based solely on the laboratory findings. If there is clinical evidence of only a single lesion in the central nervous system, multiple sclerosis cannot properly be diagnosed unless it can be shown that other regions are affected subclinically. The electrocerebral responses evoked by monocular visual stimulation with a checkerboard pattern stimulus, by monaural click stimulation, and by electrical stimulation of a sensory or mixed peripheral nerve have been used to detect subclinical involvement of the visual, brainstem auditory, and somatosensory pathways, respectively. Other disorders may also be characterized by multifocal electrophysiologic abnormalities.

There may be mild lymphocytosis or a slightly increased protein concentration in the cerebrospinal fluid, especially soon after an acute relapse. Elevated IgG in cerebrospinal fluid and discrete bands of IgG (oligoclonal bands) are present in many patients. The presence of such bands is not specific, however, since they have been found in a variety of inflammatory neurologic disorders and occasionally in patients with vascular or neoplastic disorders of the nervous system.

Treatment

At least partial recovery from acute exacerbations can reasonably be expected, but further relapses may occur without warning, and there is no means of preventing progression of the disorder. Some disability is likely to result eventually, but about half of all patients are without significant disability even 10 years after onset of symptoms.

Recovery from acute relapses may be hastened by treatment with corticosteroids, but the extent of recovery is unchanged. A high dose (eg, prednisone, 60 or 80 mg) is given daily for 1 week, after which medication is tapered over the following 2 or 3 weeks. Such a regimen is often preceded by methylprednisolone, 1 g intravenously for 3 days. Long-term treatment with steroids provides no benefit and does not prevent further relapses.

In patients with relapsing-remitting or secondary progressive disease, treatment with beta interferon or with daily subcutaneous administration of copolymer 1 (a mixture of random polymers simulating those of myelin basic protein) reduces the frequency of exacerbations. Several recent studies have suggested that intensive immunosuppressive therapy with cyclophosphamide or azathioprine may help to arrest the course of chronic progressive active multiple sclerosis. The evidence of benefit is incomplete, however, and further clinical trials are in progress. There is little evidence that plasmapheresis enhances any beneficial effects of immunosuppression in multiple sclerosis, and its role—and that of intravenous immune globulins—in the management of the various clinical forms of the disease is uncertain.

Treatment for spasticity (see below) and for neurogenic bladder may be needed in advanced cases. Excessive fatigue must be avoided, and patients should rest during periods of acute relapse.

Giovannoni G et al: Multiple sclerosis and its treatment. J R Coll Physicians Lond 1999;33:315. [NLM Cit ID: 99401238]

Placebo-controlled multicentre randomised trial of interferon beta-1b in treatment of secondary progressive multiple sclerosis. European Study Group on interferon beta-1b in secondary progressive MS. Lancet 1998;352:1491. [NLM Cit ID: 99036182] (Clinical trial.)

VITAMIN E DEFICIENCY

Vitamin E deficiency may produce a disorder somewhat similar to Friedreich's ataxia (see below). There is spinocerebellar degeneration involving particularly the posterior columns of the spinal cord and leading to limb ataxia, sensory loss, absent tendon reflexes, slurring of speech, and, in some cases, pigmentary retinal degeneration. The disorder may occur as a consequence of malabsorption or on a hereditary basis. Treatment is with alpha-tocopheryl acetate (eg, Aquasol E capsules or drops), as discussed in Chapter 29.

SPASTICITY

The term "spasticity" is commonly used for an upper motor neuron deficit, but it properly refers to a velocity-dependent increase in resistance to passive movement that affects different muscles to a different extent, is not uniform in degree throughout the range of a particular movement, and is commonly associated with other features of pyramidal deficit. It is often a major complication of stroke, cerebral or spinal injury, static perinatal encephalopathy, and multiple sclerosis.

Physical therapy with appropriate stretching programs is important during rehabilitation after the development of an upper motor neuron lesion and in subsequent management of the patient. The aim is to prevent joint and muscle contractures and perhaps to modulate spasticity.

Drug management is important also, but treatment may increase functional disability when increased extensor tone is providing additional support for patients with weak legs. Dantrolene weakens muscle contraction by interfering with the role of calcium. It is best avoided in patients with poor respiratory function or severe myocardial disease. Treatment is begun with 25 mg once daily, and the daily dose is built up by 25 mg increments every 3 days, depending on tolerance, to a maximum of 100 mg four times daily. Side effects include diarrhea, nausea, weakness, hepatic dysfunction (that may rarely be fatal, especially in women older than 35), drowsiness, light-headedness, and hallucinations.

Baclofen is an effective drug for treating spasticity of spinal origin and painful flexor (or extensor) spasms. The maximum recommended daily dose is 80 mg; treatment is started with a dose of 5 or 10 mg twice daily and then built up gradually. Side effects include gastrointestinal disturbances, lassitude, fatigue, sedation, unsteadiness, confusion, and hallucinations. Diazepam may modify spasticity by its action on spinal interneurons and perhaps also by influencing supraspinal centers, but effective doses often cause intolerable drowsiness and vary with different patients. Tizanidine, a centrally acting α_2-adrenergic agonist, is as effective as these other agents but is probably better tolerated. The daily dose is built up gradually, usually to 8 mg taken three times daily. Side effects include sedation, lassitude, hypotension, and dryness of the mouth.

Motor-point blocks by intramuscular phenol have been used to reduce spasticity selectively in one or a few important muscles and may permit return of function in patients with incomplete myelopathies. Intramuscular administration of botulinum toxin may also be helpful. Intrathecal injection of phenol or absolute alcohol may be helpful in more severe cases, but greater selectivity can be achieved by nerve root or peripheral nerve neurolysis. These procedures should not be undertaken until the spasticity syndrome is fully evolved, ie, only after about 1 year or so, and only if long-term drug treatment either has been unhelpful or carries a significant risk to the patient.

A number of surgical procedures, eg, adductor or heel cord tenotomy, may help in the management of spasticity. Neurectomy may also facilitate patient management. For example, obturator neurectomy is helpful in patients with marked adductor spasms that interfere with personal hygiene or cause gait disturbances. Posterior rhizotomy reduces spasticity, but its effect may be short-lived, whereas anterior rhizotomy produces permanent wasting and weakness in the muscles that are denervated.

Spasticity may be exacerbated by decubitus ulcers, urinary or other infections, and nociceptive stimuli.

Auff E et al: Clinical applications of botulinum toxin type A. Eur J Neurol 1999;6:Suppl 4. (Entire issue provides a review of clinical uses.)

Hesse S et al: Management of spasticity. Curr Opin Neurol 1997;10:498. [NLM Cit ID: 98086723]

MYELOPATHIES IN AIDS

Patients with AIDS may develop a subacute or chronic vacuolar myelopathy leading to paraparesis or quadriparesis, sphincter dysfunction, and sensory disturbances. Treatment is with drug combinations to suppress the underlying systemic infection. Myelitis or radiculomyelitis may occur also in AIDS patients as a result of opportunistic viral infections. When extradural lymphomatous deposits cause compressive myelopathy, pain and spinal tenderness are conspicuous, and MRI or myelography reveals the underlying lesion. Treatment is with corticosteroids, radiotherapy, and chemotherapy. Lymphomatous meningitis occurring in AIDS patients has the features described above.

MYELOPATHY OF HUMAN T CELL LEUKEMIA VIRUS

Human T cell leukemia virus (HTLV-1), a human retrovirus, is transmitted by breast feeding, sexual contact, blood transfusion, and contaminated needles. Most patients are asymptomatic, but after a variable latent period (may be as long as several years) a myelopathy develops in some instances. The MRI, electrophysiologic, and cerebrospinal fluid findings are similar to those of multiple sclerosis, but HTLV-1 antibodies are present in serum and spinal fluid. There is no specific treatment.

Engstrom JW: HTLV-I infection and the nervous system. In: *Neurology and General Medicine*, 2nd ed. Aminoff MJ (editor). Churchill Livingstone, 1995. (Clinical review.)

SUBACUTE COMBINED DEGENERATION OF THE SPINAL CORD

Subacute combined degeneration of the spinal cord is due to vitamin B_{12} deficiency, such as occurs in pernicious anemia. It is characterized by myelopathy with predominant pyramidal and posterior column deficits, sometimes in association with polyneuropathy, mental changes, or optic neuropathy. Megaloblastic anemia may also occur, but this does not parallel the neurologic disorder, and the former may be obscured if folic acid supplements have been taken. Treatment is with vitamin B_{12}. For pernicious anemia, a convenient therapeutic regimen is 100 mg cyanocobalamin intramuscularly daily for 1 week, then weekly for 1 month, and then monthly for the remainder of the patient's life.

Savage DG et al: Neurological complications of acquired cobalamin deficiency: Clinical aspects. Baillieres Clin Haematol 1995;8:657. [NLM Cit ID: 96119767]

WERNICKE'S ENCEPHALOPATHY

Wernicke's encephalopathy is characterized by confusion, ataxia, and nystagmus leading to ophthalmoplegia (lateral rectus muscle weakness, conjugate gaze palsies); peripheral neuropathy may also be present. It is due to thiamin deficiency and in the USA occurs most commonly in alcoholics. It may also occur in patients with AIDS. In suspected cases, thiamin (50 mg) is given intravenously immediately and then intramuscularly on a daily basis until a satisfactory diet can be ensured. Intravenous glucose given before thiamin may precipitate the syndrome or worsen the symptoms. The diagnosis is confirmed by the response to treatment, which must not be delayed while laboratory confirmation is obtained.

Messing RO, Greenberg DA: Alcohol and the nervous system. In: *Neurology and General Medicine*, 2nd ed. Aminoff MJ (editor). Churchill Livingstone, 1995. (Clinical review.)

STUPOR & COMA

The patient who is stuporous is unresponsive except when subjected to repeated vigorous stimuli, while the comatose patient is unarousable and unable to respond to external events or inner needs, although reflex movements and posturing may be present.

Coma is a major complication of serious central nervous system disorders. It can result from seizures, hypothermia, metabolic disturbances, or structural lesions causing bilateral cerebral hemispheric dysfunction or a disturbance of the brainstem reticular activating system. A mass lesion involving one cerebral hemisphere may cause coma by compression of the brainstem.

Assessment & Emergency Measures

The diagnostic workup of the comatose patient must proceed concomitantly with management. Supportive therapy for respiration or blood pressure is initiated; in hypothermia, all vital signs may be absent, all such patients should be rewarmed before the prognosis is assessed.

The patient can be positioned on one side with the neck partly extended, dentures removed, and secretions cleared by suction; if necessary, the patency of the airways is maintained with an oropharyngeal airway. Blood is drawn for serum glucose, electrolyte, and calcium levels; arterial blood gases; liver and renal function tests; and toxicologic studies as indicated. Dextrose 50% (25 g), naloxone (0.4–1.2 mg), and thiamine (50 mg) are given intravenously.

Further details are then obtained from attendants of the patient's medical history, the circumstances surrounding the onset of coma, and the time course of subsequent events. Abrupt onset of coma suggests subarachnoid hemorrhage, brainstem stroke, or intracerebral hemorrhage, whereas a slower onset and progression occur with other structural or mass lesions. A metabolic cause is likely with a preceding intoxicated state or agitated delirium. On examination, attention is paid to the behavioral response to painful stimuli, the pupils and their response to light, the position of the eyes and their movement in response to passive movement of the head and ice-water caloric stimulation, and the respiratory pattern.

A. Response to Painful Stimuli: Purposive limb withdrawal from painful stimuli implies that sensory pathways from and motor pathways to the stimulated limb are functionally intact. Unilateral absence of responses despite application of stimuli to both sides of the body in turn implies a corticospinal lesion; bilateral absence of responsiveness suggests brainstem involvement, bilateral pyramidal tract lesions, or psychogenic unresponsiveness. Inappropriate responses may also occur. Decorticate posturing may occur with lesions of the internal capsule and rostral cerebral peduncle, decerebrate posturing with dysfunction or destruction of the midbrain and rostral pons, and decerebrate posturing in the arms accompanied by flaccidity or slight flexor responses in the legs in patients with extensive brainstem damage extending down to the pons at the trigeminal level.

B. Ocular Findings:

1. Pupils–Hypothalamic disease processes may lead to unilateral Horner's syndrome, while bilateral diencephalic involvement or destructive pontine lesions may lead to small but reactive pupils. Ipsilateral pupillary dilation with no direct or consensual response to light occurs with compression of the third cranial nerve, eg, with uncal herniation. The pupils are slightly smaller than normal but responsive to light in many metabolic encephalopathies; however, they may be fixed and dilated following overdosage with atropine, scopolamine, or glutethimide, and pinpoint (but responsive) with opiates. Pupillary dilation for several hours following cardiopulmonary arrest implies a poor prognosis.

2. Eye movements–Conjugate deviation of the eyes to the side suggests the presence of an ipsilateral hemispheric lesion or a contralateral pontine lesion. A mesencephalic lesion leads to downward conjugate deviation. Dysconjugate ocular deviation in coma implies a structural brainstem lesion unless there was preexisting strabismus.

The oculomotor responses to passive head turning and to caloric stimulation relate to each other and provide complementary information. In response to brisk rotation of the head from side to side and to flexion and extension of the head, normally conscious patients with open eyes do not exhibit contraversive conjugate eye deviation (doll's-head eye response) unless there is voluntary visual fixation or bilateral frontal pathology. With cortical depression in lightly comatose patients, a brisk doll's-head eye response is seen. With brainstem lesions, this oculocephalic reflex becomes impaired or lost, depending on the site of the lesion.

The oculovestibular reflex is tested by caloric stimulation using irrigation with ice water. In normal subjects, jerk nystagmus is elicited for about 2 or 3 minutes, with the slow component toward the irrigated ear. In unconscious patients with an intact brainstem, the fast component of the nystagmus disappears, so that the eyes tonically deviate toward the irrigated side for 2–3 minutes before returning to their original position. With impairment of brainstem function, the response becomes perverted and finally disappears. In metabolic coma, oculocephalic and oculovestibular reflex responses are preserved, at least initially.

C. Respiratory Patterns: Diseases causing coma may lead to respiratory abnormalities. Cheyne-Stokes respiration may occur with bihemispheric or diencephalic disease or in metabolic disorders. Central neurogenic hyperventilation occurs with lesions of the brainstem tegmentum; apneustic breathing (in which there are prominent end-inspiratory pauses) suggests damage at the pontine level (eg, due to basilar artery occlusion); and atactic breathing (a completely irregular pattern of breathing with deep and shallow breaths occurring randomly) is associated with lesions of the lower pontine tegmentum and medulla.

1. STUPOR & COMA DUE TO STRUCTURAL LESIONS

Supratentorial mass lesions tend to affect brain function in an orderly way. There may initially be signs of hemispheric dysfunction, such as hemiparesis. As coma develops and deepens, cerebral function becomes progressively disturbed, producing a predictable progression of neurologic signs that suggest rostrocaudal deterioration.

Thus, as a supratentorial mass lesion begins to impair the diencephalon, the patient becomes drowsy, then stuporous, and finally comatose. There may be Cheyne-Stokes respiration; small but reactive pupils; doll's-head eye responses with side-to-side head movements but sometimes an impairment of reflex upward gaze with brisk flexion of the head; tonic ipsilateral deviation of the eyes in response to vestibular stimulation with cold water; and initially a positive response to pain but subsequently only decorticate posturing. With further progression, midbrain failure occurs. Motor dysfunction progresses from decorticate to bilateral decerebrate posturing in response to painful stimuli; Cheyne-Stokes respiration is gradually replaced by sustained central hyperventilation; the pupils become middle-sized and fixed; and the oculocephalic and oculovestibular reflex responses become impaired, perverted, or lost.

As the pons and then the medulla fail, the pupils remain unresponsive; oculovestibular responses are unobtainable; respiration is rapid and shallow; and painful stimuli may lead only to flexor responses in the legs. Finally, respiration becomes irregular and stops, the pupils often then dilating widely.

In contrast, a subtentorial (ie, brainstem) lesion may lead to an early, sometimes abrupt disturbance of consciousness without any orderly rostrocaudal progression of neurologic signs. Compressive lesions of the brainstem, especially cerebellar hemorrhage, may be clinically indistinguishable from intraparenchymal processes.

A structural lesion is suspected if the findings suggest focality. In such circumstances, a CT scan should be performed before, or instead of, a lumbar puncture in order to avoid any risk of cerebral herniation. Further management is of the causal lesion and is considered separately under the individual disorders.

2. STUPOR & COMA DUE TO METABOLIC DISTURBANCES

Patients with a metabolic cause of coma generally have signs of patchy, diffuse, and symmetric neurologic involvement that cannot be explained by loss of function at any single level or in a sequential manner, although focal or lateralized deficits may occur in hypoglycemia. Moreover, pupillary reactivity is usually preserved, while other brainstem functions are often grossly impaired. Comatose patients with meningitis, encephalitis, or subarachnoid hemorrhage may also exhibit little in the way of focal neurologic signs, however, and clinical evidence of meningeal irritation is sometimes very subtle in comatose patients. Examination of the cerebrospinal fluid in such patients is essential to establish the correct diagnosis.

In patients with coma due to cerebral ischemia and hypoxia, the absence of pupillary light reflexes at the time of initial examination indicates that there is little chance of regaining independence; by contrast, preserved pupillary light responses, the development of spontaneous eye movements (roving, conjugate, or better), and extensor, flexor, or withdrawal responses to pain at this early stage imply a relatively good prognosis.

Treatment of metabolic encephalopathy is of the underlying disturbance and is considered in other chapters. If the cause of the encephalopathy is obscure, all drugs except essential ones may have to be withdrawn in case they are responsible for the altered mental status.

Feske SK: Coma and confusional states: Emergency diagnosis and management. Neurol Clin North Am 1998;16:237. [NLM Cit ID: 98205043]

Young GB (editor): *Coma and Impaired Consciousness: A Clinical Perspective.* McGraw-Hill, 1998.

3. BRAIN DEATH

The definition of brain death is controversial, and diagnostic criteria have been published by many different professional organizations. In order to establish brain death, the irreversibly comatose patient must be shown to have lost all brainstem reflex responses, including the pupillary, corneal, oculovestibular, oculocephalic, oropharyngeal, and respiratory reflexes, and should have been in this condition for at least 6 hours. Spinal reflex movements do not exclude the diagnosis, but ongoing seizure activity or decerebrate or decorticate posturing is not consistent with brain death. The apnea test (presence or absence of spontaneous respiratory activity at a $PaCO_2$ of at least 60 mm Hg) serves to determine whether the patient is capable of respiratory activity.

Reversible coma simulating brain death may be seen with hypothermia (temperature < 32 °C) and overdosage with central nervous system depressant drugs, and these conditions must be excluded. Certain ancillary tests may assist the determination of brain death but are not essential. An isoelectric electroencephalogram, when the recording is made according to the recommendations of the American Electroencephalographic Society, is especially helpful in confirming the diagnosis. Alternatively, the demonstration of an absent cerebral circulation by intravenous radioisotope cerebral angiography or by four-vessel contrast cerebral angiography can be confirmatory.

Beresford HR: Brain death. Neurol Clin 1999;17:295. [NLM Cit ID: 99214411] (Review.)

4. PERSISTENT VEGETATIVE STATE

Patients with severe bilateral hemispheric disease may show some improvement from an initially comatose state, so that, after a variable interval, they appear to be awake but lie motionless and without evidence of awareness or higher mental activity. This persistent vegetative state has been variously referred to as akinetic mutism, apallic state, or coma vigil. Most patients in this persistent vegetative state will die in months or years, but partial recovery has occasionally occurred and in rare instances has been sufficient to permit communication or even independent living.

5. LOCKED-IN SYNDROME (De-efferented State)

Acute destructive lesions (eg, infarction, hemorrhage, demyelination, encephalitis) involving the ventral pons and sparing the tegmentum may lead to a mute, quadriparetic but conscious state in which the patient is capable of blinking and of voluntary eye movement in the vertical plane, with preserved pupillary responses to light. Such a patient can mistakenly be regarded as comatose. Physicians should recognize that "locked-in" individuals are fully aware of their surroundings. The prognosis is variable, but recovery has occasionally been reported—in some cases including resumption of independent daily life, though this may take up to 2 or 3 years.

HEAD INJURY

Trauma is the most common cause of death in young people, and head injury accounts for almost half of these trauma-related deaths. The prognosis following head injury depends upon the site and severity of brain damage. Some guide to prognosis is provided by the mental status, since loss of consciousness for more than 1 or 2 minutes implies a worse prognosis than otherwise. Similarly, the degree of retrograde and posttraumatic amnesia provides an indication of the severity of injury and thus of the prognosis. Absence of skull fracture does not exclude the possibility of severe head injury. During the physical examination, special attention should be given to the level of consciousness and extent of any brainstem dysfunction.

Note: Patients who have lost consciousness for 2 minutes or more following head injury should be admitted to the hospital for observation, as should patients with focal neurologic deficits, lethargy, or skull fractures. If admission is declined, responsible family members should be given clear instructions about the need for, and manner of, checking on them at regular (hourly) intervals and for obtaining additional medical help if necessary.

Skull radiographs or CT scans may provide evidence of fractures. Because injury to the spine may have accompanied head trauma, cervical spine radiographs (especially in the lateral projection) should always be obtained in comatose patients and in patients with severe neck pain or a deficit possibly related to cord compression. CT scanning has an important role in demonstrating intracranial hemorrhage and may also provide evidence of cerebral edema and displacement of midline structures.

Cerebral Injuries

These are summarized in Table 24–5 along with comments about treatment. Increased intracranial pressure may result from ventilatory obstruction, abnormal neck position, seizures, dilutional hyponatremia, or cerebral edema; an intracranial hematoma requiring surgical evacuation may also be responsible. Other measures that may be necessary to reduce intracranial pressure include induced hyperventilation, intravenous mannitol infusion, and intravenous furosemide; corticosteroids provide no benefit in this context.

Scalp Injuries & Skull Fractures

Scalp lacerations and depressed or compound depressed skull fractures should be treated surgically as appropriate. Simple skull fractures require no specific treatment.

The clinical signs of basilar skull fracture include bruising about the orbit (raccoon sign), blood in the external auditory meatus (Battle's sign), and leakage of cerebrospinal fluid (which can be identified by its glucose content) from the ear or nose. Cranial nerve palsies (involving especially the first, second, third,

Table 24–5. Acute cerebral sequelae of head injury.

Sequelae	Clinical Features	Pathology
Concussion	Transient loss of consciousness with bradycardia, hypotension, and respiratory arrest for a few seconds followed by retrograde and posttraumatic amnesia. Occasionally followed by transient neurologic deficit.	Bruising on side of impact (coup injury) or contralaterally (contrecoup injury).
Cerebral contusion or laceration	Loss of consciousness longer than with concussion. May lead to death or severe residual neurologic deficit.	Cerebral contusion, edema, hemorrhage, and necrosis. May have subarachnoid bleeding.
Acute epidural hemorrhage	Headache, confusion, somnolence, seizures, and focal deficits occur several hours after injury and lead to coma, respiratory depression, and death unless treated by surgical evacuation.	Tear in meningeal artery, vein, or dural sinus, leading to hematoma visible on CT scan.
Acute subdural hemorrhage	Similar to epidural hemorrhage, but interval before onset of symptoms is longer. Treatment is by surgical evacuation.	Hematoma from tear in veins from cortex to superior sagittal sinus or from cerebral laceration, visible on CT scan.
Cerebral hemorrhage	Generally develops immediately after injury. Clinically resembles hypertensive hemorrhage. Surgical evacuation is sometimes helpful.	Hematoma, visible on CT scan.

fourth, fifth, seventh, and eighth nerves in any combination) may also occur. If there is any leakage of cerebrospinal fluid, conservative treatment, with elevation of the head, restriction of fluids, and administration of acetazolamide (250 mg four times daily), is often helpful; but if the leak continues for more than a few days, lumbar subarachnoid drainage may be necessary. Antibiotics are given if infection occurs, based on culture and sensitivity studies. Only very occasional patients require intracranial repair of the dural defect because of persistence of the leak or recurrent meningitis.

Late Complications of Head Injury

The relationship of chronic subdural hemorrhage to head injury is not always clear. In many elderly persons there is no history of trauma, but in other cases a head injury, often trivial, precedes the onset of symptoms by several weeks. The clinical presentation is usually with mental changes such as slowness, drowsiness, headache, confusion, memory disturbances, personality change, or even dementia. Focal neurologic deficits such as hemiparesis or hemisensory disturbance may also occur but are less common. CT scan is an important means of detecting the hematoma, which is sometimes bilateral. Treatment is by surgical evacuation to prevent cerebral compression and tentorial herniation. There is no clear evidence that prophylactic anticonvulsant therapy reduces the incidence of posttraumatic seizures.

Normal-pressure hydrocephalus may follow head injury, subarachnoid hemorrhage, or meningoencephalitis.

Other late complications of head injury include posttraumatic seizure disorder and posttraumatic headache.

Attia J et al: Prognosis in anoxic and traumatic coma. Crit Care Clin 1998;14:497. [NLM Cit ID: 98365801] (Meta-analysis.)

Schierhout G et al: Prophylactic antiepileptic agents after head injury: A systematic review. J Neurol Neurosurg Psychiatry 1998;64:108. [NLM Cit ID: 98097238] (Meta-analysis.)

SPINAL TRAUMA

While spinal cord damage may result from whiplash injury, severe injury usually relates to fracture-dislocation causing compression or angular deformity of the cord either cervically or in the lower thoracic and upper lumbar regions. Extreme hypotension following injury may also lead to cord infarction.

Total cord transection results in immediate flaccid paralysis and loss of sensation below the level of the lesion. Reflex activity is lost for a variable period, and there is urinary and fecal retention. As reflex function returns over the following days and weeks, spastic paraplegia or quadriplegia develops, with hyperreflexia and extensor plantar responses, but a flaccid atrophic (lower motor neuron) paralysis may be found depending on the segments of the cord that are affected. The bladder and bowels also regain some reflex function, permitting urine and feces to be expelled at intervals. As spasticity increases, flexor or extensor spasms (or both) of the legs become troublesome, especially if the patient develops bed sores or a urinary tract infection. Paraplegia with the legs in flexion or extension may eventually result.

With lesser degrees of injury, patients may be left with mild limb weakness, distal sensory disturbance, or both. Sphincter function may also be impaired, urinary urgency and urgency incontinence being especially common. More particularly, a unilateral cord lesion leads to an ipsilateral motor disturbance with accompanying impairment of proprioception and contralateral loss of pain and temperature appreciation below the lesion (Brown-Séquard's syndrome). A central cord syndrome may lead to a lower motor neuron deficit and loss of pain and temperature appreciation, with sparing of posterior column functions. A radicular deficit may occur at the level of the injury—or, if the cauda equina is involved, there may be evidence of disturbed function in several lumbosacral roots.

Treatment of the injury consists of immobilization and—if there is cord compression—decompressive laminectomy and fusion. Early treatment with high doses of corticosteroids (eg, methylprednisolone, 30 mg/kg by intravenous bolus, followed by 5.4 mg/kg/h for 23 hours) has been shown to improve neurologic recovery if commenced within 8 hours after injury. Treatment with G_{M1} ganglioside for 3 or 4 weeks is an experimental approach that has also been helpful. Anatomic realignment of the spinal cord by traction and other orthopedic procedures is also important. Subsequent care of the residual neurologic deficit—paraplegia or quadriplegia—requires treatment of spasticity and care of the skin, bladder, and bowels.

Yu D: A crash course in spinal cord injury. Postgrad Med 1998;104:109. [NLM Cit ID: 98388554]

SYRINGOMYELIA

Destruction or degeneration of gray and white matter adjacent to the central canal of the cervical spinal cord leads to cavitation and accumulation of fluid within the spinal cord. The precise pathogenesis is unclear, but many cases are associated with Arnold-Chiari malformation, in which there is displacement of the cerebellar tonsils, medulla, and fourth ventricle into the spinal canal, sometimes with accompanying meningomyelocele. In such circumstances, the cord cavity connects with and may merely represent a dilated central canal. In other cases, the cause of cavitation is less clear. There is a characteristic clinical picture, with segmental atrophy and areflexia and loss of pain and temperature appreciation in a "cape" distribution owing to the destruction of fibers crossing in front of the central canal. Thoracic kyphoscoliosis is usually present. With progression, involvement of the long motor and sensory tracts occurs as well, so that a pyramidal and sensory deficit develops in the legs. Upward extension of the cavitation (syringobulbia) leads to dysfunction of the lower brainstem and thus to bulbar palsy, nystagmus, and sensory impairment over one or both sides of the face.

Syringomyelia, ie, cord cavitation, may also occur in association with an intramedullary tumor or following severe cord injury, and the cavity then does not communicate with the central canal.

In patients with Arnold-Chiari malformation, there are commonly skeletal abnormalities on plain x-rays of the skull and cervical spine. CT scans show caudal displacement of the fourth ventricle. MRI or positive contrast myelography may demonstrate the malformation itself. Focal cord enlargement is found at myelography or by MRI in patients with cavitation related to past injury or intramedullary neoplasms.

Treatment of Arnold-Chiari malformation with associated syringomyelia is by suboccipital craniectomy and upper cervical laminectomy, with the aim of decompressing the malformation at the foramen magnum. The cord cavity should be drained, and if necessary an outlet for the fourth ventricle can be made. In cavitation associated with intramedullary tumor, treatment is surgical, but radiation therapy may be necessary if complete removal is not possible. Posttraumatic syringomyelia is also treated surgically if it leads to increasing neurologic deficits or to intolerable pain.

Kramer KM et al: Posttraumatic syringomyelia: A review of 21 cases. Clin Orthop Rel Res 1997;334:190. [NLM Cit ID: 97158553] (Retrospective study.)

MOTOR NEURON DISEASES

This group of disorders is characterized clinically by weakness and variable wasting of affected muscles, without accompanying sensory changes.

Motor neuron disease in adults generally commences between 30 and 60 years of age. There is degeneration of the anterior horn cells in the spinal cord, the motor nuclei of the lower cranial nerves, and the corticospinal and corticobulbar pathways. The disorder is usually sporadic, but familial cases may occur.

Classification

Five varieties have been distinguished on clinical grounds.

A. Progressive Bulbar Palsy: Bulbar involvement predominates owing to disease processes affecting primarily the motor nuclei of the cranial nerves.

B. Pseudobulbar Palsy: Bulbar involvement predominates in this variety also, but it is due to bilateral corticobulbar disease and thus reflects upper motor neuron dysfunction.

C. Progressive Spinal Muscular Atrophy: This is characterized primarily by a lower motor neuron deficit in the limbs due to degeneration of the anterior horn cells in the spinal cord.

D. Primary Lateral Sclerosis: There is a purely upper motor neuron deficit in the limbs.

E. Amyotrophic Lateral Sclerosis: A mixed upper and lower motor neuron deficit is found in the limbs. This disorder is sometimes associated with dementia or parkinsonism.

Clinical Findings

A. Symptoms and Signs: Difficulty in swallowing, chewing, coughing, breathing, and talking (dysarthria) occur with bulbar involvement. In progressive bulbar palsy, there is drooping of the palate, a depressed gag reflex, pooling of saliva in the pharynx, a weak cough, and a wasted, fasciculating tongue. In pseudobulbar palsy, the tongue is contracted and spastic and cannot be moved rapidly from side to side. Limb involvement is characterized by motor disturbances (weakness, stiffness, wasting, fasciculations) reflecting lower or upper motor neuron dysfunction; there are no objective changes on sensory examination, though there may be vague sensory complaints. The sphincters are generally spared.

The disorder is progressive and usually fatal within 3–5 years; death usually results from pulmonary infections. Patients with bulbar involvement generally have the poorest prognosis.

B. Laboratory and Other Studies: Electromyography may show changes of chronic partial denervation, with abnormal spontaneous activity in the resting muscle and a reduction in the number of motor units under voluntary control. In patients with suspected spinal muscular atrophy or amyotrophic lateral sclerosis, the diagnosis should not be made with confidence unless such changes are found in at least three extremities. Motor conduction velocity is usually normal but may be slightly reduced, and sensory conduction studies are also normal. Biopsy of a wasted muscle shows the histologic changes of denervation. The serum creatine kinase may be slightly elevated but never reaches the extremely high values seen in some of the muscular dystrophies. The cerebrospinal fluid is normal.

A familial form of amyotrophic lateral sclerosis has been described with autosomal dominant inheritance, related to mutations in the copper-zinc superoxide dismutase gene on the long arm of chromosome 21. X-linked bulbospinal neuronopathy is associated with an expanded trinucleotide repeat sequence on the androgen receptor gene and carries a more benign prognosis than other forms of motor neuron disease. There have been recent reports of juvenile spinal muscular atrophy due to hexosaminidase deficiency, with abnormal findings on rectal biopsy and reduced hexosaminidase A in serum and leukocytes. Pure motor syndromes resembling motor neuron disease may also occur in association with monoclonal gammopathy or multifocal motor neuropathies with conduction block. A motor neuronopathy may also develop in Hodgkin's disease and has a relatively benign prognosis.

Treatment

Riluzole, which reduces the presynaptic release of glutamate, may slow progression of amyotrophic lateral sclerosis. There is otherwise no specific treatment except in patients with gammopathy, in whom plasmapheresis and immunosuppression may lead to improvement. Therapeutic trials of various neurotrophic factors to slow disease progression are, however, in progress. Symptomatic and supportive measures may include prescription of anticholinergic drugs (such as trihexyphenidyl, amitriptyline, or atropine) if drooling is troublesome, braces or a walker to improve mobility, and physical therapy to prevent contractures. Spasticity may be helped by baclofen or diazepam. A semiliquid diet or nasogastric tube feeding may be needed if dysphagia is severe. Gastrostomy or cricopharyngomyotomy is sometimes resorted to in extreme cases of predominant bulbar involvement, and tracheostomy may be necessary if respiratory muscles are severely affected; however, in the terminal stages of these disorders, the aim of treatment should be to keep patients as comfortable as possible.

Miller RG: New approaches to therapy of amyotrophic lateral sclerosis. West J Med 1998;168:262. [NLM Cit ID: 98245644]

Parton MJ et al: Motor neuron disease and its management. J R Coll Physicians Lond 1999;33:212. [NLM Cit ID: 99330977] (Review.)

PERIPHERAL NEUROPATHIES

Peripheral neuropathies can be categorized on the basis of the structure primarily affected. The predominant pathologic feature may be axonal degeneration (axonal or neuronal neuropathies) or paranodal or segmental demyelination. The distinction may be possible on the basis of neurophysiologic findings. Motor and sensory conduction velocity can be measured in accessible segments of peripheral nerves. In axonal neuropathies, conduction velocity is normal or reduced only mildly and needle electromyography provides evidence of denervation in affected muscles. In demyelinating neuropathies, conduction may be slowed considerably in affected fibers, and in more severe cases, conduction is blocked completely, without accompanying electromyographic signs of denervation.

Nerves may be injured or compressed by neighboring anatomic structures at any point along their course. Common **mononeuropathies** of this sort are considered below. They lead to a sensory, motor, or mixed deficit that is restricted to the territory of the affected nerve. A similar clinical disturbance is produced by peripheral nerve tumors, but these are rare except in patients with Recklinghausen's disease. Multiple mononeuropathies suggest a patchy multifocal disease process such as vasculopathy (eg, diabetes, arteritis), an infiltrative process (eg, leprosy, sarcoidosis), radiation damage, or an immunologic disorder (eg, brachial plexopathy). Diffuse **polyneuropathies** lead to a symmetric sensory, motor, or mixed deficit, often most marked distally. They include the hereditary, metabolic, and toxic disorders; idiopathic inflammatory polyneuropathy (Guillain-Barré syndrome); and the peripheral neuropathies that may occur as a nonmetastatic complication of malignant diseases. Involvement of motor fibers leads to flaccid weakness that is most marked distally; dysfunction of sensory fibers causes impaired sensory perception. Tendon reflexes are depressed or absent. Paresthesias, pain, and muscle tenderness may also occur.

1. POLYNEUROPATHIES & MONONEURITIS MULTIPLEX

The cause of polyneuropathy or mononeuritis multiplex is suggested by the history, mode of onset, and predominant clinical manifestations. Laboratory workup includes a complete blood count and sedimentation rate, serum protein electrophoresis, determination of plasma urea and electrolytes, liver and thyroid function tests, tests for rheumatoid factor and antinuclear antibody, HBsAg determination, a serologic test for syphilis, fasting blood glucose level, urinary heavy metal levels, cerebrospinal fluid examination, and chest radiography. These tests should be ordered selectively, as guided by symptoms and signs. Measurement of nerve conduction velocity is important in confirming the peripheral nerve origin of symptoms and providing a means of following clinical changes, as well as indicating the likely disease process (ie, axonal or demyelinating neuropathy). Cutaneous nerve biopsy may help establish a precise diagnosis (eg, polyarteritis, amyloidosis). In about half of cases, no specific cause can be established; of these, slightly less than half are subsequently found to be heredofamilial.

Treatment is of the underlying cause, when feasible, and is discussed below under the individual disorders. Physical therapy helps prevent contractures, and splints can maintain a weak extremity in a position of useful function. Anesthetic extremities must be protected from injury. To guard against burns, patients should check the temperature of water and hot surfaces with a portion of skin having normal sensation, measure water temperature with a thermometer, and use cold water for washing or lower the temperature setting of their hot-water heaters. Shoes should be examined frequently during the day for grit or foreign objects in order to prevent pressure lesions.

Patients with polyneuropathies or mononeuritis multiplex are subject to additional nerve injury at pressure points and should therefore avoid such behavior as leaning on elbows or sitting with crossed legs for lengthy periods.

Neuropathic pain is sometimes troublesome and may respond to simple analgesics such as aspirin. Narcotics or narcotic substitutes may be necessary for severe hyperpathia or pain induced by minimal stimuli, but their use should be avoided as far as possible. The use of a frame or cradle to reduce contact with bedclothes may be helpful. Many patients experience episodic stabbing pains, which may respond to phenytoin, carbamazepine, or tricyclic antidepressants.

Symptoms of autonomic dysfunction are occasionally troublesome. Postural hypotension is often helped by wearing waist-high elastic stockings and sleeping in a semierect position at night. Fludrocortisone reduces postural hypotension, but doses as high as 1 mg/d are sometimes necessary in diabetics and may lead to recumbent hypertension. Midodrine, an alpha agonist, is sometimes helpful. Impotence and diarrhea are difficult to treat; a flaccid neuropathic bladder may respond to parasympathomimetic drugs such as bethanechol chloride, 10–50 mg three or four times daily.

Inherited Neuropathies

A. Charcot-Marie-Tooth Disease: Several distinct varieties of Charcot-Marie-Tooth disease can be recognized. There is usually an autosomal dominant mode of inheritance, but occasional cases occur on a sporadic, recessive, or X-linked basis. The responsible gene is commonly located on the short arm of chromosome 17 and less often shows linkage to chromosome 1 or the X chromosome. Clinical presentation may be with foot deformities or gait disturbances in childhood or early adult life. Slow progression leads to the typical features of polyneuropathy, with distal weakness and wasting that begin in the legs, a variable amount of distal sensory loss, and depressed or absent tendon reflexes. Tremor is a conspicuous feature in some instances. Pathologic examination reveals segmental demyelination and remyelination of peripheral nerves, an increase in their transverse fascicular area, and hyperplasia of Schwann cells. Electrodiagnostic studies show a marked reduction in motor and sensory conduction velocity (hereditary motor and sensory neuropathy [HMSN] type I).

In other instances (HMSN type II), motor conduction velocity is normal or only slightly reduced, sensory nerve action potentials may be absent, and signs of chronic partial denervation are found in affected muscles electromyographically. The predominant pathologic change is axonal loss rather than segmental demyelination.

A similar disorder may occur in patients with progressive distal spinal muscular atrophy, but there is no sensory loss; electrophysiologic investigation reveals that motor conduction velocity is normal or only slightly reduced, and nerve action potentials are normal.

B. Dejerine-Sottas Disease (HMSN Type III): Most cases are sporadic or autosomal recessive. The recessive form has its onset in infancy or childhood and leads to a progressive motor and sensory polyneuropathy with weakness, ataxia, sensory loss, and depressed or absent tendon reflexes. The peripheral nerves may be palpably enlarged and are characterized pathologically by segmental demyelination, Schwann cell hyperplasia, and thin myelin sheaths. Electrophysiologically, there is slowing of conduction, and sensory action potentials may be unrecordable.

C. Friedreich's Ataxia: Patients generally present in childhood or early adult life with this autosomal recessive disorder, which has been related to an unstable mutation of the *X25* gene on chromosome 9q13–q21.1. The gait becomes atactic, the hands become clumsy, and other signs of cerebellar dysfunction develop accompanied by weakness of the legs and extensor plantar responses. Involvement of peripheral sensory fibers leads to sensory disturbances in the limbs and depressed tendon reflexes. There is bilateral pes cavus. Pathologically, there is a marked loss of cells in the posterior root ganglia and degeneration of peripheral sensory fibers. In the central nervous system, changes are conspicuous in the posterior and lateral columns of the cord. Electrophysiologically, conduction velocity in motor fibers is normal or only mildly reduced, but sensory action potentials are small or absent.

D. Refsum's Disease (HMSN Type IV): This autosomal recessive disorder is due to a disturbance in phytanic acid metabolism. Clinically, pigmentary retinal degeneration is accompanied by progressive sensorimotor polyneuropathy and cerebellar signs. Auditory dysfunction, cardiomyopathy, and cutaneous manifestations may also occur. Motor and sensory conduction velocity is reduced, often markedly, and there may be electromyographic evidence of denervation in affected muscles. Dietary restriction of phytanic acid and its precursors may be helpful therapeutically.

E. Porphyria: Peripheral nerve involvement may occur during acute attacks in both variegate porphyria and acute intermittent porphyria. Motor symptoms usually occur first, and weakness is often most marked proximally and in the upper limbs rather than the lower. Sensory symptoms and signs may be proximal or distal in distribution. Autonomic involvement is sometimes pronounced. The electrophysiologic findings are in keeping with the results of neuropathologic studies suggesting that the neuropathy is axonal in type. Hematin (4 mg/kg intravenously over 15 minutes once or twice daily) may lead to rapid improvement. A high-carbohydrate diet and, in severe cases, intravenous glucose or levulose may also be helpful. Propranolol (up to 100 mg every 4 hours) may control tachycardia and hypertension in acute attacks. Porphyria is discussed further in Chapter 40.

Neuropathies Associated With Systemic & Metabolic Disorders

A. Diabetes Mellitus: In this disorder, involvement of the peripheral nervous system may lead to symmetric sensory or mixed polyneuropathy, asymmetric motor neuropathy (diabetic amyotrophy), thoracoabdominal radiculopathy, autonomic neuropathy, or isolated lesions of individual nerves. These may occur singly or in any combination.

Sensory polyneuropathy, the most common manifestation, may lead to no more than depressed tendon reflexes and impaired appreciation of vibration in the legs. When symptomatic, there may be pain, paresthesias, or numbness in the legs, but in severe cases distal sensory loss occurs in all limbs. Diabetic amyotrophy is characterized by asymmetric weakness and wasting involving predominantly the proximal muscles of the legs, accompanied by local pain. Thoracoabdominal radiculopathy leads to pain over the trunk. In patients with autonomic neuropathy, postural hypotension, impaired thermoregulatory sweating, postgustatory hyperhidrosis, constipation, flatulence, diarrhea, impotence, urinary retention, and incontinence may occur, and there may be abnormal pupillary responses. Isolated lesions of individual peripheral nerves are common and in the limbs tend to occur at sites of compression or entrapment. Treatment is symptomatic. Entrapment neuropathies may be helped by surgical decompression. Treatment of neuropathic pain is discussed above.

B. Uremia: Uremia may lead to a symmetric sensorimotor polyneuropathy that tends to affect the lower limbs more than the upper limbs and is more marked distally than proximally. The diagnosis can be confirmed electrophysiologically, for motor and sensory conduction velocity is moderately reduced. The neuropathy improves both clinically and electrophysiologically with renal transplantation and to a lesser extent with chronic dialysis.

C. Alcoholism and Nutritional Deficiency: Many alcoholics have an axonal distal sensorimotor polyneuropathy that is frequently accompanied by painful cramps, muscle tenderness, and painful paresthesias and is often more marked in the legs than in the arms. Symptoms of autonomic dysfunction may also be conspicuous. Motor and sensory conduction velocity may be slightly reduced, even in subclinical cases, but gross slowing of conduction is uncommon. A similar distal sensorimotor polyneuropathy is a well-recognized feature of beriberi (thiamin deficiency). In vitamin B_{12} deficiency, distal sensory polyneuropathy may develop but is usually overshadowed by central nervous system manifestations (eg, myelopathy, optic neuropathy, or intellectual changes).

D. Paraproteinemias: A symmetric sensorimotor polyneuropathy that is gradual in onset, progressive in course, and often accompanied by pain and dysesthesias in the limbs may occur in patients (especially men) with multiple myeloma. The neuropathy is of the axonal type in classic lytic myeloma, but segmental demyelination (primary or secondary) and axonal loss may occur in sclerotic myeloma and lead to predominantly motor clinical manifestations. Both demyelinating and axonal neuropathies are also observed in patients with paraproteinemias without myeloma. A small fraction will develop myeloma if serially followed. The demyelinating neuropathy in these patients may be due to the monoclonal protein's reacting to a component of the nerve myelin. The neuropathy of classic multiple myeloma is poorly responsive to therapy. The polyneuropathy of benign monoclonal gammopathy may respond to immunosuppressant drugs and plasmapheresis.

Polyneuropathy may also occur in association with macroglobulinemia and cryoglobulinemia and sometimes responds to plasmapheresis. Entrapment neuropathy, such as carpal tunnel syndrome, is more common than polyneuropathy in patients with (nonhereditary) generalized amyloidosis. With polyneuropathy due to amyloidosis, sensory and autonomic symptoms are especially conspicuous, whereas distal wasting and weakness occur later; there is no specific treatment.

Neuropathies Associated With Infectious & Inflammatory Diseases

A. Leprosy: Leprosy is an important cause of peripheral neuropathy in certain parts of the world. Sensory disturbances are mainly due to involvement of intracutaneous nerves. In tuberculoid leprosy, they develop at the same time and in the same distribution as the skin lesion but may be more extensive if nerve trunks lying beneath the lesion are also involved. In lepromatous leprosy, there is more extensive sensory loss, and this develops earlier and to a greater extent in the coolest regions of the body, such as the dorsal surfaces of the hands and feet, where the bacilli proliferate most actively. Motor deficits result from involvement of superficial nerves where their temperature is lowest, eg, the ulnar nerve in the region proximal to the olecranon groove, the median nerve as it emerges from beneath the forearm flexor muscle to run toward the carpal tunnel, the peroneal nerve at the head of the fibula, and the posterior tibial nerve in the lower part of the leg; patchy facial muscular weakness may also occur owing to involvement of the superficial branches of the seventh cranial nerve.

Motor disturbances in leprosy are suggestive of multiple mononeuropathy, whereas sensory changes resemble those of distal polyneuropathy. Examination, however, relates the distribution of sensory deficits to the temperature of the tissues; in the legs, for example, sparing frequently occurs between the toes and in the popliteal fossae, where the temperature is higher. Treatment is with antileprotic agents (see Chapter 33).

B. AIDS: A variety of neuropathies occur in HIV-infected patients. Patients with AIDS may develop a chronic symmetric sensorimotor axonal **polyneuropathy** associated usually with no abnormal cerebrospinal fluid findings. Treatment is symptomatic. AIDS patients may also develop progressive **polyradiculopathy** or radiculomyelopathy that leads to leg weakness and urinary retention; sensory loss is less conspicuous than in polyneuropathy. The cerebrospinal fluid may show mononuclear pleocytosis and increased protein and low glucose concentrations. Cytomegalovirus is responsible in at least some cases. The prognosis is generally poor, but some patients respond to intravenous ganciclovir (2.5 mg/kg every 8 hours for 10 days, then 7.5 mg/kg daily 5 days per week).

An inflammatory **demyelinating polyradiculoneuropathy** sometimes occurs in HIV-seropositive patients without AIDS and may follow an acute, subacute, or chronic course. Weakness is usually more conspicuous distally than proximally and tends to overshadow sensory symptoms. Tendon reflexes are depressed or absent. The cerebrospinal fluid shows an increased cell count and protein concentration. Treatment with plasmapheresis has helped some patients. Spontaneous improvement may also occur. Seropositive patients without AIDS may also develop a **mononeuropathy multiplex** that sometimes responds to treatment with plasmapheresis.

C. Lyme Borreliosis: The neurologic manifestations of Lyme disease include meningitis, meningoencephalitis, polyradiculoneuropathy, mononeuropathy multiplex, and cranial neuropathy. Serologic tests establish the underlying disorder. Treatment is as described in Chapter 34.

D. Sarcoidosis: Cranial nerve palsies (especially facial palsy), multiple mononeuropathy, and, less commonly, symmetric polyneuropathy may all occur, the latter sometimes preferentially affecting either motor or sensory fibers. Improvement may occur with use of corticosteroids.

E. Polyarteritis: Involvement of the vasa nervorum by the vasculitic process may result in infarction of the nerve. Clinically, one encounters an asymmetric sensorimotor polyneuropathy (mononeuritis multiplex) that pursues a waxing and waning course. Steroids and cytotoxic agents—especially cyclophosphamide—may be of benefit in severe cases.

F. Rheumatoid Arthritis: Compressive or entrapment neuropathies, ischemic neuropathies, mild distal sensory polyneuropathy, and severe progressive sensorimotor polyneuropathy can occur in rheumatoid arthritis.

Neuropathy Associated With Critical Illness

Patients in intensive care units with sepsis and multiorgan failure sometimes develop polyneuropathies. This may be manifested initially by unexpected difficulty in weaning patients from a mechanical ventilator and in more advanced cases by wasting and weakness of the extremities and loss of tendon reflexes. Sensory abnormalities are relatively inconspicuous. The neuropathy is axonal in type. Its pathogenesis is obscure, and treatment is supportive. The prognosis is good provided patients recover from the underlying critical illness.

Toxic Neuropathies

Axonal polyneuropathy may follow exposure to industrial agents or pesticides such as acrylamide, organophosphorus compounds, hexacarbon solvents, methyl bromide, and carbon disulfide; metals such as arsenic, thallium, mercury, and lead; and drugs such as phenytoin, perhexiline, isoniazid, nitrofurantoin, vincristine, and pyridoxine in high doses. Detailed occupational, environmental, and medical histories and recognition of clusters of cases are important in suggesting the diagnosis. Treatment is by preventing further exposure to the causal agent. Isoniazid neuropathy is prevented by pyridoxine supplementation.

Diphtheritic neuropathy results from a neurotoxin released by the causative organism and is common in many areas. Palatal weakness may develop 2–4 weeks after infection of the throat, and infection of the skin may similarly be followed by focal weakness of neighboring muscles. Disturbances of accommodation may occur about 4–5 weeks after infection and distal sensorimotor demyelinating polyneuropathy after 1–3 months.

Neuropathies Associated With Malignant Diseases

Both a sensorimotor and a purely sensory polyneuropathy may occur as a nonmetastatic complication of malignant diseases. The sensorimotor polyneuropathy may be mild and occur in the course of known malignant disease; or it may have an acute or subacute onset, lead to severe disability, and occur before there is any clinical evidence of the cancer, occasionally following a remitting course.

Acute Idiopathic Polyneuropathy (Guillain-Barré Syndrome)

This acute or subacute polyradiculoneuropathy sometimes follows infective illness, inoculations, or surgical procedures. There is an association with preceding *Campylobacter jejuni* enteritis. The disorder probably has an immunologic basis, but the precise mechanism is unclear. The main complaint is of weakness that varies widely in severity in different patients and often has a proximal emphasis and symmetric distribution. It usually begins in the legs, spreading to a variable extent but frequently involving the arms and often one or both sides of the face. The muscles of respiration or deglutition may also be affected. Sensory symptoms are usually less conspicuous than motor ones, but distal paresthesias and dysesthesias are common, and neuropathic or radicular pain is present in many patients. Autonomic disturbances are also common, may be severe, and are sometimes life-threatening; they include tachycardia, cardiac irregularities, hypotension or hypertension, facial flushing, abnormalities of sweating, pulmonary dysfunction, and impaired sphincter control.

The cerebrospinal fluid characteristically contains a high protein concentration with a normal cell content, but these changes may take 2 or 3 weeks to develop. Electrophysiologic studies may reveal marked abnormalities, which do not necessarily parallel the clinical disorder in their temporal course. Pathologic examination has shown primary demyelination or, less commonly, axonal degeneration.

When the diagnosis is made, the history and appropriate laboratory studies should exclude the possibility of porphyric, diphtheritic, or toxic (heavy metal, hexacarbon, organophosphate) neuropathies. Poliomyelitis, botulism, and tick paralysis must also be considered. The presence of pyramidal signs, a markedly asymmetric motor deficit, a sharp sensory level, or early sphincter involvement should suggest a focal cord lesion.

Most patients eventually make a good recovery, but this may take many months, and 10–20% patients of are left with persisting disability. Treatment with prednisone is ineffective and may actually affect the outcome adversely by prolonging recovery time. Plasmapheresis is of value; it is best performed within the first few days of illness and is best reserved for clinically severe or rapidly progressive cases or those with ventilatory impairment. Intravenous immunoglobulin (400 mg/kg/d for 5 days) is also helpful and imposes less stress on the cardiovascular system than plasmapheresis. Patients should be admitted to intensive care units if their forced vital capacity is declining, and intubation is considered if the forced vital capacity reaches 15 mL/kg, dyspnea becomes evident, or the oxygen saturation declines. Respiratory toilet and chest physical therapy help prevent atelectasis. Marked hypotension may respond to volume replacement or pressor agents. Low-dose heparin to prevent pulmonary embolism should be considered.

Approximately 3% of patients with acute idiopathic polyneuropathy have one or more clinically similar relapses, sometimes several years after the initial illness. Plasma exchange therapy may produce improvement in chronic and relapsing inflammatory polyneuropathy.

Chronic Inflammatory Polyneuropathy

Chronic inflammatory demyelinating polyneuropathy, an acquired immunologically mediated disorder, is clinically similar to Guillain-Barré syndrome except that it has a relapsing or steadily progressive course over months or years. In the relapsing form, partial recovery may occur after some relapses, but in other instances there is no recovery between exacerbations. Although remission may occur spontaneously with time, the disorder frequently follows a progressive downhill course leading to severe functional disability.

Electrodiagnostic studies show marked slowing of motor and sensory conduction, and focal conduction block. Signs of partial denervation may also be present owing to secondary axonal degeneration. Nerve biopsy may show chronic perivascular inflammatory infiltrates in the endoneurium and epineurium, without accompanying evidence of vasculitis. However, a normal nerve biopsy result or the presence of nonspecific abnormalities does not exclude the diagnosis.

Corticosteroids may be effective in arresting or reversing the downhill course. Treatment is usually begun with prednisone, 60 mg daily, continued for 2–3 months or until a definite response has occurred. If no response has occurred despite 3 months of treatment, a higher dose may be tried. In responsive cases, the dose is gradually tapered, but most patients become corticosteroid-dependent, often requiring prednisone, 20 mg daily on alternate days, on a long-term basis. Patients unresponsive to corticosteroids may benefit instead from treatment with a cytotoxic drug such as azathioprine. There are increasing anecdotal reports of short-term benefit with plasmapheresis; high-dose intravenous immunoglobulin treatment (eg, 400 mg/kg/d) may produce clinical improvement lasting for weeks to months.

Aminoff MJ: *Electromyography in Clinical Practice: Clinical and Electrodiagnostic Aspects of Neuromuscular Disease*, 3rd ed. Churchill Livingstone, 1998.

Boulton AJ et al: Diabetic neuropathy. Med Clin North Am 1998;82:909. [NLM Cit ID: 98371383]

Hahn AF: Guillain-Barré syndrome: Lancet 1998;352:635. [NLM Cit ID: 98417122]

Ropper AH et al: Neuropathies associated with paraproteinemia. N Engl J Med 1998;338:1601. [NLM Cit ID: 98252468]

Thomas PK: Classification, differential diagnosis, and staging of diabetic peripheral neuropathy. Diabetes 1997; 46(Suppl 2) S54. [NLM Cit ID: 97429862]

2. MONONEUROPATHIES

An individual nerve may be injured along its course or may be compressed, angulated, or stretched by neighboring anatomic structures, especially at a point where it passes through a narrow space (entrapment neuropathy). The relative contributions of mechanical factors and ischemia to the local damage are not clear. With involvement of a sensory or mixed nerve, pain is commonly felt distal to the lesion. Symptoms never develop with some entrapment neuropathies, resolve rapidly and spontaneously in others, and become progressively more disabling and distressing in yet other cases. The precise neurologic deficit depends on the nerve involved. Percussion of the nerve at the site of the lesion may lead to paresthesias in its distal distribution.

Entrapment neuropathy may be the sole manifestation of subclinical polyneuropathy, and this must be borne in mind and excluded by nerve conduction studies. Such studies are also indispensable for the accurate localization of the focal lesion.

In patients with acute compression neuropathy such as Saturday night palsy, no treatment is necessary. Complete recovery generally occurs, usually within 2 months, presumably because the underlying pathology is demyelination. However, axonal degeneration can occur in severe cases, and recovery then takes longer and may never be complete.

In chronic compressive or entrapment neuropathies, avoidance of aggravating factors and correction of any underlying systemic conditions are important. Local infiltration of the region about the nerve with corticosteroids may be of value; in addition, surgical decompression may help if there is a progressively increasing neurologic deficit or if electrodiagnostic studies show evidence of partial denervation in weak muscles.

Peripheral nerve tumors are uncommon, except in Recklinghausen's disease, but also give rise to mononeuropathy. This may be distinguishable from entrapment neuropathy only by noting the presence of a mass along the course of the nerve and by demonstrating the precise site of the lesion with appropriate electrophysiologic studies. Treatment of symptomatic lesions is by surgical removal if possible.

Carpal Tunnel Syndrome

See Chapter 20.

Pronator Teres or Anterior Interosseous Syndrome

The median nerve gives off its motor branch, the anterior interosseous nerve, below the elbow as it descends between the two heads of the pronator teres muscle. A lesion of either nerve may occur in this region, sometimes after trauma or owing to compression from, for example, a fibrous band. With anterior interosseous nerve involvement, there is no sensory loss, and weakness is confined to the pronator quadratus, flexor pollicis longus, and the flexor digitorum profundus to the second and third digits. Weakness is more widespread and sensory changes occur in an appropriate distribution when the median nerve itself is affected. The prognosis is variable. If improvement does not occur spontaneously, decompressive surgery may be helpful.

Ulnar Nerve Lesions

Ulnar nerve lesions are likely to occur in the elbow region as the nerve runs behind the medial epicondyle and descends into the cubital tunnel. In the condylar groove, the ulnar nerve is exposed to pressure or trauma. Moreover, any increase in the carrying angle of the elbow, whether congenital, degenerative, or traumatic, may cause excessive stretching of the nerve when the elbow is flexed. Ulnar nerve lesions may also result from thickening or distortion of the anatomic structures forming the cubital tunnel, and the resulting symptoms may also be aggravated by flexion of the elbow, because the tunnel is then narrowed by tightening of its roof or inward bulging of its floor. A severe lesion at either site causes sensory changes in the medial 1½ digits and along the medial border of the hand. There is weakness of the ulnar-innervated muscles in the forearm and hand. With a cubital tunnel lesion, however, there may be relative sparing of the flexor carpi ulnaris muscle. Electrophysiologic evaluation using nerve stimulation techniques allows more precise localization of the lesion.

If conservative measures are unsuccessful in relieving symptoms and preventing further progression, surgical treatment may be necessary. This consists of nerve transposition if the lesion is in the condylar groove, or a release procedure if it is in the cubital tunnel.

Ulnar nerve lesions may also develop at the wrist or in the palm of the hand, usually owing to repetitive trauma or to compression from ganglia or benign tumors. They can be subdivided depending upon their presumed site. Compressive lesions are treated surgically. If repetitive mechanical trauma is responsible, this is avoided by occupational adjustment or job retraining.

Radial Nerve Lesions

The radial nerve is particularly liable to compression or injury in the axilla (eg, by crutches or by pressure when the arm hangs over the back of a chair). This leads to weakness or paralysis of all the muscles supplied by the nerve, including the triceps. Sensory changes may also occur but are often surprisingly inconspicuous, being marked only in a small area on the back of the hand between the thumb and index finger. Injuries to the radial nerve in the spiral groove occur characteristically during deep sleep, as in intoxicated individuals (Saturday night palsy), and there is then sparing of the triceps muscle, which is supplied more proximally. The nerve may also be injured at or above the elbow; its purely motor posterior interosseous branch, supplying the extensors of the wrist and fingers, may be involved immediately below the elbow, but then there is sparing of the extensor carpi radialis longus, so that the wrist can still be extended. The superficial radial nerve may be compressed by handcuffs or a tight watch strap.

Femoral Neuropathy

The clinical features of femoral nerve palsy consist of weakness and wasting of the quadriceps muscle, with sensory impairment over the anteromedian aspect of the thigh and sometimes also of the leg to the medial malleolus, and a depressed or absent knee jerk. Isolated femoral neuropathy may occur in diabetics or from compression by retroperitoneal neoplasms or hematomas (eg, expanding aortic aneurysm). Femoral neuropathy may also result from pressure from the inguinal ligament when the thighs are markedly flexed and abducted, as in the lithotomy position.

Meralgia Paresthetica

The lateral femoral cutaneous nerve, a sensory nerve arising from the L2 and L3 roots, may be compressed or stretched in obese or diabetic patients and during pregnancy. The nerve usually runs under the outer portion of the inguinal ligament to reach the thigh, but the ligament sometimes splits to enclose it. Hyperextension of the hip or increased lumbar lordosis—such as occurs during pregnancy—leads to nerve compression by the posterior fascicle of the ligament. However, entrapment of the nerve at any point along its course may cause similar symptoms, and several other anatomic variations predispose the nerve to damage when it is stretched. Pain, paresthesia, or numbness occurs about the outer aspect of the thigh, usually unilaterally, and is sometimes relieved by sitting. Examination shows no abnormalities except in severe cases when cutaneous sensation is impaired in the affected area. Symptoms are usually mild and commonly settle spontaneously. Hydrocortisone injections medial to the anterosuperior iliac spine often relieve symptoms temporarily, while nerve decompression by transposition may provide more lasting relief.

Sciatic & Common Peroneal Nerve Palsies

Misplaced deep intramuscular injections are probably still the most common cause of sciatic nerve palsy. Trauma to the buttock, hip, or thigh may also be responsible. The resulting clinical deficit depends on whether the whole nerve has been affected or only certain fibers. In general, the peroneal fibers of the sciatic nerve are more susceptible to damage than those destined for the tibial nerve. A sciatic nerve lesion may therefore be difficult to distinguish from peroneal neuropathy unless there is electromyographic evidence of involvement of the short head of the biceps femoris muscle. The common peroneal nerve itself may be compressed or injured in the region of the head and neck of the fibula, eg, by sitting with crossed legs or wearing high boots. There is weakness of dorsiflexion and eversion of the foot, accompanied by numbness or blunted sensation of the anterolateral aspect of the calf and dorsum of the foot.

Tarsal Tunnel Syndrome

The tibial nerve, the other branch of the sciatic, supplies several muscles in the lower extremity, gives origin to the sural nerve, and then continues as the posterior tibial nerve to supply the plantar flexors of the foot and toes. It passes through the tarsal tunnel behind and below the medial malleolus, giving off calcaneal branches and the medial and lateral plantar nerves that supply small muscles of the foot and the skin on the plantar aspect of the foot and toes. Compression of the posterior tibial nerve or its branches between the bony floor and ligamentous roof of the tarsal tunnel leads to pain, paresthesias, and numbness over the bottom of the foot, especially at night, with sparing of the heel. Muscle weakness may be hard to recognize clinically. Compressive lesions of the individual plantar nerves may also occur more distally, with similar clinical features to those of the tarsal tunnel syndrome. Treatment is surgical decompression.

Aminoff MJ: *Electromyography in Clinical Practice: Clinical and Electrodiagnostic Aspects of Neuromuscular Disease,* 3rd ed. Churchill Livingstone, 1998.

Facial Neuropathy

An isolated facial palsy may occur in patients with HIV seropositivity, sarcoidosis, or Lyme disease (Chapter 34), but most often it is idiopathic (Bell's palsy).

3. BELL'S PALSY

Bell's palsy is an idiopathic facial paresis of lower motor neuron type that has been attributed to an inflammatory reaction involving the facial nerve near the stylomastoid foramen or in the bony facial canal. A relationship of Bell's palsy to reactivation of herpes simplex virus has recently been suggested, but there is little evidence to support this.

The clinical features of Bell's palsy are characteristic. The facial paresis generally comes on abruptly, but it may worsen over the following day or so. Pain about the ear precedes or accompanies the weakness in many cases but usually lasts for only a few days. The face itself feels stiff and pulled to one side. There may be ipsilateral restriction of eye closure and difficulty with eating and fine facial movements. A disturbance of taste is common, owing

during the first few days after presentation. Patients with clinically complete palsy when first seen are less likely to make a full recovery than those with an incomplete one. A poor prognosis for recovery is also associated with advanced age, hyperacusis, and severe initial pain. Electromyography and nerve excitability or conduction studies provide a guide to prognosis but not early enough to aid in the selection of patients for treatment.

The only medical treatment that may influence the outcome is administration of corticosteroids with or without acyclovir, but studies supporting this concept have been criticized. Many physicians nevertheless routinely prescribe corticosteroids for patients with Bell's palsy seen within 5 days of onset. The author prescribes them only when the palsy is clinically complete or there is severe pain. Treatment with prednisone, 60 or 80 mg daily in divided doses for 4 or 5 days, followed by tapering of the dose over the next 7–10 days, is a satisfactory regimen. It is helpful to protect the eye with lubricating drops (or lubricating ointment at night) and a patch if eye closure is not possible. There is no evidence that surgical procedures to decompress the facial nerve are of benefit.

Adour KK et al: Bell's palsy treatment with acyclovir and prednisone compared with prednisone alone: A double-blind, randomized, controlled trial. Ann Otol Rhinol Laryngol 1996;105:371. [NLM Cit ID: 98432298] (Treatment with acyclovir-prednisone was statistically more effective in returning volitional muscle motion and in preventing partial nerve degeneration than placebo-prednisone treatment.)

DISCOGENIC NECK PAIN*

A variety of congenital abnormalities may involve the cervical spine and lead to neck pain; these include hemivertebrae, fused vertebrae, basilar impression, and instability of the atlantoaxial joint. Traumatic, degenerative, infective, and neoplastic disorders may also lead to pain in the neck. When rheumatoid arthritis involves the spine, it tends to affect especially the cervical region, leading to pain, stiffness, and reduced mobility; displacement of vertebrae or atlantoaxial subluxation may lead to cord compression that can be life-threatening if not treated by fixation. Further details are given in Chapter 20, and discussion here is restricted to disk disease.

Acute Cervical Disk Protrusion

Acute cervical disk protrusion leads to pain in the neck and radicular pain in the arm, exacerbated by head movement. With lateral herniation of the disk, motor, sensory, or reflex changes may be found in a radicular (usually C6 or C7) distribution on the affected side (Figure 24–1); with more centrally directed herniations, the spinal cord may also be involved, leading to spastic paraparesis and sensory disturbances in the legs, sometimes accompanied by impaired sphincter function. The diagnosis is confirmed by MRI or CT myelography. In mild cases, bed rest or intermittent neck traction may help, followed by immobilization of the neck in a collar for several weeks. If these measures are unsuccessful or the patient has a significant neurologic deficit, surgical removal of the protruding disk may be necessary.

Cervical Spondylosis

Cervical spondylosis results from chronic cervical disk degeneration, with herniation of disk material, secondary calcification, and associated osteophytic outgrowths. One or more of the cervical nerve roots may be compressed, stretched, or angulated; and myelopathy may also develop as a result of compression, vascular insufficiency, or recurrent minor trauma to the cord. Patients present with neck pain and restricted head movement, occipital headaches, radicular pain and other sensory disturbances in the arms, weakness of the arms or legs, or some combination of these symptoms. Examination generally reveals that lateral flexion and rotation of the neck are limited. A segmental pattern of weakness or dermatomal sensory loss (or both) may be found unilaterally or bilaterally in the upper limbs, and tendon reflexes mediated by the affected root or roots are depressed. The C5 and C6 nerve roots are most commonly involved, and examination frequently then reveals weakness of muscles supplied by these roots (eg, deltoids, supra- and infraspinatus, biceps, brachioradialis), pain or sensory loss about the shoulder and outer border of the arm and forearm, and depressed biceps and brachioradialis reflexes. Spastic paraparesis may also be present if there is an associated myelopathy, sometimes accompanied by posterior column or spinothalamic sensory deficits in the legs.

Plain radiographs of the cervical spine show osteophyte formation, narrowing of disk spaces, and encroachment on the intervertebral foramina, but such changes are common in middle-aged persons and may be unrelated to the presenting complaint. CT or MRI helps to confirm the diagnosis and exclude other structural causes of the myelopathy.

Restriction of neck movements by a cervical collar may relieve pain. Operative treatment may be necessary to prevent further progression if there is a significant neurologic deficit or if root pain is severe, persistent, and unresponsive to conservative measures.

BRACHIAL & LUMBAR PLEXUS LESIONS

Brachial Plexus Neuropathy

Brachial plexus neuropathy may be idiopathic, sometimes occurring in relationship to a number of

*Low back pain is discussed in Chapter 20.

different nonspecific illnesses or factors. In other instances, brachial plexus lesions follow trauma or result from congenital anomalies, neoplastic involvement, or injury by various physical agents. In rare instances, the disorder occurs on a familial basis.

Idiopathic brachial plexus neuropathy (neuralgic amyotrophy) characteristically begins with severe pain about the shoulder, followed within a few days by weakness, reflex changes, and sensory disturbances involving especially the C5 and C6 segments (Figure 24–1). Symptoms and signs are usually unilateral but may be bilateral. Wasting of affected muscles is sometimes profound. The disorder relates to disturbed function of cervical roots or part of the brachial plexus, but its precise cause is unknown. Recovery occurs over the ensuing months but may be incomplete. Treatment is purely symptomatic.

Cervical Rib Syndrome

Compression of the C8 and T1 roots or the lower trunk of the brachial plexus by a cervical rib or band arising from the seventh cervical vertebra leads to weakness and wasting of intrinsic hand muscles, especially those in the thenar eminence, accompanied by pain and numbness in the medial two fingers and the ulnar border of the hand and forearm. The subclavian artery may also be compressed, and this forms the basis of Adson's test for diagnosing the disorder; the radial pulse is diminished or obliterated on the affected side when the seated patient inhales deeply and turns the head to one side or the other. Electromyography, nerve conduction studies, and somatosensory evoked potential studies may help confirm the diagnosis. X-rays sometimes show the cervical rib or a large transverse process of the seventh cervical vertebra, but normal findings do not exclude the possibility of a cervical band. Treatment of the disorder is by surgical excision of the rib or band.

Lumbosacral Plexus Lesions

A lumbosacral plexus lesion may develop in association with diseases such as diabetes, cancer, or bleeding disorders or in relation to injury. It occasionally occurs as an isolated phenomenon similar to idiopathic brachial plexopathy, and pain and weakness then tend to be more conspicuous than sensory symptoms. The distribution of symptoms and signs depends on the level and pattern of neurologic involvement.

DISORDERS OF NEUROMUSCULAR TRANSMISSION

1. MYASTHENIA GRAVIS

Essentials of Diagnosis

- Fluctuating weakness of commonly used voluntary muscles, producing symptoms such as diplopia, ptosis, and difficulty in swallowing.
- Activity increases weakness of affected muscles.
- Short-acting anticholinesterases transiently improve the weakness.

General Considerations

Myasthenia gravis occurs at all ages, sometimes in association with a thymic tumor or thyrotoxicosis, as well as in rheumatoid arthritis and lupus erythematosus. It is commonest in young women with HLA-DR3; if thymoma is associated, older men are more commonly affected. Onset is usually insidious, but the disorder is sometimes unmasked by a coincidental infection that leads to exacerbation of symptoms. Exacerbations may also occur before the menstrual period and during or shortly after pregnancy. Symptoms are due to a variable degree of block of neuromuscular transmission caused by autoantibodies binding to acetylcholine receptors; these are found in most patients with the disease and have a primary role in reducing the number of functioning acetylcholine receptors. Additionally, cellular immune activity against the receptor is found. Clinically, this leads to weakness; initially powerful movements fatigue readily. The external ocular muscles and certain other cranial muscles, including the masticatory, facial, and pharyngeal muscles, are especially likely to be affected, and the respiratory and limb muscles may also be involved.

Clinical Findings

A. Symptoms and Signs: Patients present with ptosis, diplopia, difficulty in chewing or swallowing, respiratory difficulties, limb weakness, or some combination of these problems. Weakness may remain localized to a few muscle groups, especially the ocular muscles, or may become generalized. Symptoms often fluctuate in intensity during the day, and this diurnal variation is superimposed on a tendency to longer-term spontaneous relapses and remissions that may last for weeks. Nevertheless, the disorder follows a slowly progressive course and may have a fatal outcome owing to respiratory complications such as aspiration pneumonia.

Clinical examination confirms the weakness and fatigability of affected muscles. In most cases, the extraocular muscles are involved, and this leads to ocular palsies and ptosis, which are commonly asymmetric. Pupillary responses are normal. The bulbar and limb muscles are often weak, but the pattern of involvement is variable. Sustained activity of affected muscles increases the weakness, which improves after a brief rest. Sensation is normal, and there are usually no reflex changes.

The diagnosis can generally be confirmed by the response to a short-acting anticholinesterase. Edrophonium can be given intravenously in a dose of 10 mg (1 mL), 2 mg being given initially and the remaining 8 mg about 30 seconds later if the test dose is well tolerated; in myasthenic patients, there is an obvious improvement in strength of weak muscles lasting for about 5 minutes. Alternatively, 1.5 mg of neostigmine can be given intramuscularly, and the response then lasts for about 2 hours; atropine sulfate (0.6 mg) should be available to reverse muscarinic side effects.

B. Imaging: Lateral and anteroposterior x-rays of the chest and CT scans should be obtained to demonstrate a coexisting thymoma, but normal studies do not exclude this possibility.

C. Laboratory and Other Studies: Electrophysiologic demonstration of a decrementing muscle response to repetitive 2- or 3-Hz stimulation of motor nerves indicates a disturbance of neuromuscular transmission. Such an abnormality may even be detected in clinically strong muscles with certain provocative procedures. Needle electromyography of affected muscles shows a marked variation in configuration and size of individual motor unit potentials, and single-fiber electromyography reveals an increased jitter, or variability, in the time interval between two muscle fiber action potentials from the same motor unit.

Assay of serum for elevated levels of circulating acetylcholine receptor antibodies is another approach—increasingly used—to the laboratory diagnosis of myasthenia gravis and has a sensitivity of 80–90%.

Treatment

Medication such as aminoglycosides that may exacerbate myasthenia gravis should be avoided. Anticholinesterase drugs provide symptomatic benefit without influencing the course of the disease. Neostigmine, pyridostigmine, or both can be used, the dose being determined on an individual basis. The usual dose of neostigmine is 7.5–30 mg (average, 15 mg) taken four times daily; of pyridostigmine, 30–180 mg (average, 60 mg) four times daily. Overmedication may temporarily increase weakness, which is then unaffected or enhanced by intravenous edrophonium.

Thymectomy usually leads to symptomatic benefit or remission and should be considered in all patients younger than age 60, unless weakness is restricted to the extraocular muscles. If the disease is of recent onset and only slowly progressive, operation is sometimes delayed for a year or so, in the hope that spontaneous remission will occur.

Treatment with corticosteroids is indicated for patients who have responded poorly to anticholinesterase drugs and have already undergone thymectomy. It is introduced with the patient in the hospital, since weakness may initially be aggravated. Once weakness has stabilized after 2–3 weeks or any improvement is sustained, further management can be on an outpatient basis. Alternate-day treatment is usually well tolerated, but if weakness is enhanced on the nontreatment day it may be necessary for medication to be taken daily. The dose of corticosteroids is determined on an individual basis, but an initial high daily dose (eg, prednisone, 60–100 mg) can gradually be tapered to a relatively low maintenance level as improvement occurs; total withdrawal is difficult, however. Treatment with azathioprine may also be effective. The usual dose is 2–3 mg/kg orally daily after a lower initial dose.

In patients with major disability in whom conventional treatment is either unhelpful or contraindicated, plasmapheresis or intravenous immunoglobulin therapy may be beneficial. It may also be useful for stabilizing patients before thymectomy and for managing acute crisis.

Keesey J: Myasthenia gravis. Arch Neurol 1998;55:745. [NLM Cit ID: 98266774]

2. MYASTHENIC SYNDROME (Lambert-Eaton Syndrome)

Myasthenic syndrome may be associated with small-cell carcinoma, sometimes developing before the tumor is diagnosed, and occasionally occurs with certain autoimmune diseases. There is defective release of acetylcholine in response to a nerve impulse, and this leads to weakness especially of the proximal muscles of the limbs. As is not the case in myasthenia gravis, however, power steadily increases with sustained contraction. The diagnosis can be confirmed electrophysiologically, because the muscle response to stimulation of its motor nerve increases remarkably if the nerve is stimulated repetitively at high rates, even in muscles that are not clinically weak.

Treatment with plasmapheresis and immunosuppressive drug therapy (prednisone and azathioprine) may lead to clinical and electrophysiologic improvement, in addition to therapy aimed at tumor when present. Prednisone is usually initiated in a daily dose of 60–80 mg and azathioprine in a daily dose of 2 mg/kg. Guanidine hydrochloride (25–50 mg/kg/d in divided doses) is occasionally helpful in seriously disabled patients, but adverse effects of the drug include marrow suppression. The response to treatment with anticholinesterase drugs such as pyridostigmine or neostigmine, either alone or in combination with guanidine, is variable.

3. BOTULISM

The toxin of *Clostridium botulinum* prevents the release of acetylcholine at neuromuscular junctions and autonomic synapses. Botulism occurs most commonly following the ingestion of contaminated home-canned food and should be suggested by the development of sudden, fluctuating, severe weakness in a previously healthy person. Symptoms begin within 72 hours following ingestion of the toxin and may progress for several days. Typically, there is diplopia, ptosis, facial weakness, dysphagia, and nasal speech, followed by respiratory difficulty and finally by weakness that appears last in the limbs. Blurring of vision (with unreactive dilated pupils) is characteristic, and there may be dryness of the mouth, constipation (paralytic ileus), and postural hypotension. Sensation is preserved, and the tendon reflexes are not affected unless the involved muscles are very weak. If the diagnosis is suspected, the local health authority should be notified and a sample of serum and contaminated food (if available) sent to be assayed for toxin. Support for the diagnosis may be obtained by electrophysiologic studies; with repetitive stimulation of motor nerves at fast rates, the muscle response increases in size progressively.

Patients should be hospitalized in case respiratory assistance becomes necessary. Treatment is with trivalent antitoxin, once it is established that the patient is not allergic to horse serum. Guanidine hydrochloride (25–50 mg/kg/d in divided doses) to facilitate release of acetylcholine from nerve endings sometimes helps to increase muscle strength. Anticholinesterase drugs are of no value. Respiratory assistance and other supportive measures should be provided as necessary. Further details are provided in Chapter 33.

4. DISORDERS ASSOCIATED WITH USE OF AMINOGLYCOSIDES

Aminoglycoside antibiotics, eg, gentamicin, may produce a clinical disturbance similar to botulism by preventing the release of acetylcholine from nerve endings, but symptoms subside rapidly as the responsible drug is eliminated from the body. These antibiotics are particularly dangerous in patients with preexisting disturbances of neuromuscular transmission and are therefore best avoided in patients with myasthenia gravis.

MYOPATHIC DISORDERS

Muscular Dystrophies

These inherited myopathic disorders are characterized by progressive muscle weakness and wasting. They are subdivided by mode of inheritance, age at onset, and clinical features, as shown in Table 24–6. In the Duchenne type, pseudohypertrophy of muscles frequently occurs at some stage; intellectual retardation is common; and there may be skeletal deformities, muscle contractures, and cardiac involvement. The serum creatine kinase level is increased, especially in the Duchenne and Becker varieties, and mildly increased also in limb-girdle dystrophy. Electromyography may help to confirm that weakness is myopathic rather than neurogenic. Similarly, histopathologic examination of a muscle biopsy specimen may help to confirm that weakness is due to a primary disorder of muscle and to distinguish between various muscle diseases.

A genetic defect on the short arm of the X chromosome has been identified in Duchenne dystrophy. The affected gene codes for the protein dystrophin, which is markedly reduced or absent from the muscle of patients with the disease. Dystrophin levels are generally normal in the Becker variety, but the protein is qualitatively altered.

Duchenne muscular dystrophy can now be recognized early in pregnancy in about 95% of women by

Table 24–6. The muscular dystrophies.

Disorder	Inheritance	Age at Onset (years)	Distribution	Prognosis
Duchenne type	X-linked recessive	1–5	Pelvic, then shoulder girdle; later, limb and respiratory muscles	Rapid progression. Death within about 15 years after onset.
Becker's	X-linked recessive	5–25	Pelvic, then shoulder girdle	Slow progression. May have normal life span.
Limb-girdle (Erb's)	Autosomal recessive (may be sporadic or dominant)	10–30	Pelvic or shoulder girdle initially, with later spread to the other	Variable severity and rate of progression. Possible severe disability in middle life.
Facioscapulo-humeral	Autosomal dominant	Any age	Face and shoulder girdle initially; later pelvic girdle and legs	Slow progression. Minor disability. Usually normal life span.
Distal	Autosomal dominant (may be recessive)	40–60	Onset distally in extremities; proximal involvement later	Slow progression.
Ocular	Autosomal dominant (may be recessive)	Any age (usually 5–30)	External ocular muscles; may also be mild weakness of face, neck, and arms	
Oculopharyngeal	Autosomal dominant	Any age	As in the ocular form but with dysphagia	

genetic studies; in late pregnancy, DNA probes can be used on fetal tissue obtained for this purpose by amniocentesis. The gene causing facioscapulohumeral dystrophy has recently been localized to the long arm of chromosome 4. The genetic defect has been characterized, but the abnormal gene product is not yet known.

There is no specific treatment for the muscular dystrophies, but it is important to encourage patients to lead as normal lives as possible. Prolonged bed rest must be avoided, as inactivity often leads to worsening of the underlying muscle disease. Physical therapy and orthopedic procedures may help to counteract deformities or contractures.

Myotonic Dystrophy

Myotonic dystrophy, a slowly progressive, dominantly inherited disorder, usually manifests itself in the third or fourth decade but occasionally appears early in childhood. The genetic defect has been localized to the long arm of chromosome 19. Myotonia leads to complaints of muscle stiffness and is evidenced by the marked delay that occurs before affected muscles can relax after a contraction. This can often be demonstrated clinically by delayed relaxation of the hand after sustained grip or by percussion of the belly of a muscle. In addition, there is weakness and wasting of the facial, sternocleidomastoid, and distal limb muscles. Associated clinical features include cataracts, frontal baldness, testicular atrophy, diabetes mellitus, cardiac abnormalities, and intellectual changes. Electromyographic sampling of affected muscles reveals myotonic discharges in addition to changes suggestive of myopathy.

Myotonia can be treated with quinine sulfate (300–400 mg three times daily), procainamide (0.5–1 g four times daily), or phenytoin (100 mg three times daily). More recently, tocainide and mexiletine have been used. In myotonic dystrophy, phenytoin is preferred, since the other drugs may have undesirable effects on cardiac conduction. Neither the weakness nor the course of the disorder is influenced by treatment.

Myotonia Congenita

Myotonia congenita is commonly inherited as a dominant trait. The responsible gene may be on the long arm of chromosome 7. Generalized myotonia without weakness is usually present from birth, but symptoms may not appear until early childhood. Patients complain of muscle stiffness that is enhanced by cold and inactivity and relieved by exercise. Muscle hypertrophy, at times pronounced, is also a feature. A recessive form with later onset is associated with slight weakness and atrophy of distal muscles. Treatment with quinine sulfate, procainamide, tocainide, mexiletine, or phenytoin may help the myotonia, as in myotonic dystrophy.

Polymyositis & Dermatomyositis

See Chapter 20.

Inclusion Body Myositis

This disorder, of unknown cause, begins insidiously, usually after middle age, with progressive proximal weakness of first the lower and then the upper extremities. Distal weakness is usually mild. Serum creatine kinase levels may be normal or increased. The diagnosis is confirmed by muscle biopsy. In contrast to polymyositis, corticosteroid therapy is usually ineffective.

Amato AA et al: Idiopathic inflammatory myopathies. Neurol Clin 1997;15:615. [NLM Cit ID: 97372210]

Mitochondrial Myopathies

The mitochondrial myopathies are a clinically diverse group of disorders that on pathologic examination of skeletal muscle with the modified Gomori stain show characteristic "ragged red fibers" containing accumulations of abnormal mitochondria. Patients may present with progressive external ophthalmoplegia or with limb weakness that is exacerbated or induced by activity. Other patients present with central neurologic dysfunction, eg, myoclonic epilepsy (myoclonic epilepsy, ragged red fiber syndrome, or MERRF), or the combination of myopathy, encephalopathy, lactic acidosis, and stroke-like episodes (MELAS). These disorders result from separate abnormalities of mitochondrial DNA. (See also Chapter 19.)

Myopathies Associated With Other Disorders

Myopathy may occur in association with chronic hypokalemia, any endocrinopathy, and in patients taking corticosteroids, chloroquine, colchicine, clofibrate, emetine, aminocaproic acid, lovastatin, bretylium tosylate, or drugs causing potassium depletion. Weakness is mainly proximal, and serum creatine kinase is typically normal, except in hypothyroidism and some of the toxic myopathies. Treatment is of the underlying cause. Myopathy also occurs with chronic alcoholism, whereas acute reversible muscle necrosis may occur shortly after acute alcohol intoxication. Inflammatory myopathy may occur in patients taking penicillamine; myotonia may be induced by clofibrate; and preexisting myotonia may be exacerbated or unmasked by depolarizing muscle relaxants (eg, suxamethonium), beta-blockers (eg, propranolol), fenoterol, ritodrine, and, possibly, certain diuretics.

PERIODIC PARALYSIS SYNDROME

Periodic paralysis may have a familial (dominant inheritance) basis. Episodes of flaccid weakness or paralysis occur, sometimes in association with abnormalities of the plasma potassium level. Strength is normal between attacks. The **hypokalemic** variety is characterized by attacks that tend to occur on awakening, after exercise, or after a heavy meal and may last for several days. Patients should avoid excessive exertion. A low-carbohydrate and low-salt diet may help prevent attacks, as may acetazolamide, 250–750 mg/d. An ongoing attack may be aborted by potassium chloride given orally or by intravenous drip, provided the ECG can be monitored and renal function is satisfactory. In young Asian men, it is commonly associated with hyperthyroidism; treatment of the endocrine disorder then prevents recurrences. In **hyperkalemic** periodic paralysis, attacks also tend to occur after exercise but usually last for less than an hour. They may be terminated by intravenous calcium gluconate (1–2 g) or by intravenous diuretics (furosemide, 20–40 mg), glucose, or glucose and insulin; daily acetazolamide or chlorothiazide may prevent recurrences. Genetic linkage studies suggest that many families with this disorder have a defect in the sodium channel gene on the long arm of chromosome 17. **Normokalemic** periodic paralysis is similar clinically to the hyperkalemic variety, but the plasma potassium level remains normal during attacks; treatment is with acetazolamide.

Ptacek L: The familial periodic paralyses and nondystrophic myotonias. Am J Med 1998;104:58. [NLM Cit ID: 98351308]

RELEVANT WORLD WIDE WEB SITES

[Acute Cerebral Infarction]
http://www.brighamrad.harvard.edu/Cases/bwh/hcache/93/full.html

[Anaplastic Astrocytoma]
http://www.brighamrad.harvard.edu/Cases/bwh/hcache/49/full.html

[Brain Death]
http://www.brighamrad.harvard.edu/Cases/bwh/hcache/20/full.html

[Carotid Artery Stenosis]
http://www.brighamrad.harvard.edu/Cases/bwh/hcache/6/full.html

[CMTnet]
http://www.ultranet.com/~smith/CMTnet.html

[Epidural Hematoma]
http://www.brighamrad.harvard.edu/Cases/bwh/hcache/100/full.html

[Ganglioglioma]
http://www.brighamrad.harvard.edu/Cases/bwh/hcache/171/full.html

[Glioblastoma Multiforme Demonstration Case]
http://www.brighamrad.harvard.edu/Cases/bwh/hcache/125/full.html

[Johns Hopkins Center for Hearing and Balance—Vestibular Disorders]
http://www.bme.jhu.edu/labs/chb/disorders/disorder.html

[List of Clinical Trials for Brain Tumors]
http://www.virtualtrials.com

[Spongiform Encephalopathy Consistent With Creutzfeldt-Jakob Disease]
http://www.brighamrad.harvard.edu/Cases/bwh/hcache/156/full.html

[Subdural Hematoma]
http://www.brighamrad.harvard.edu/Cases/bwh/hcache/98/full.html

[The Whole Brain Atlas]
http://www.med.harvard.edu:80/AANLIB/home.html

[3-D Visualization of Brain Aneurysms]
http://everest.radiology.uiowa.edu/nlm/app/aneur/brain/aneur.html

25 Psychiatric Disorders

See http://www.current-med.com/ch25.html for updated addresses of Web sites referenced in this chapter.

Stuart J. Eisendrath, MD, & Jonathan E. Lichtmacher, MD

Psychiatric disorders are functional impairments that may result from disturbance of one or more of the following interrelated factors: (1) biologic function, (2) psychodynamic adaptation, (3) learned behavior, and (4) social and environmental conditions. Although the clinical situation at a given time determines which area of dysfunction will be emphasized, proper patient care requires an approach that adequately evaluates all factors.

Biologic Function

Psychiatric disorders of biologic origin may be secondary to identifiable physical illness or caused by biochemical disturbances of the brain. A wide variety of psychiatric disorders (eg, psychosis, depression, delirium, anxiety) as well as nonspecific symptoms are caused by organic brain disease or by derangement of cerebral metabolism resulting from illness, biochemical aberrations (usually neurotransmitter dysfunction), nutritional deficiencies, or toxic agents.

Neurotransmitter functions have been correlated with the major psychiatric disorders. Cholinergic deficiency is present in some dementias, and adrenergic imbalance is important in some psychoses. Serotonergic mechanisms are significantly involved in affective disorders, aggression, autism, and the anxiety disorders, particularly obsessive-compulsive disorders and panic disorder.

Psychodynamic Maladaptation

Psychodynamic maladaptation involves intrapsychic aberrations and is usually treated by a psychotherapeutic approach. There are many forms of psychotherapy: supportive, interpretive, cognitive, persuasive, educative, or some combination of these methods. Depth, duration, intensity, and frequency of sessions may vary.

Learned Behavior

Learned behavior is part of the pathogenetic mechanism in all psychiatric disorders. For example, in somatization disorder, the patient may have learned that being sick is the only way to get attention. Altering such positive reinforcement may be critical in producing a change in behavior. Personality disorders are examples of failure to learn to incorporate patterns of behavior acceptable in social surroundings.

Social & Environmental Conditions

Social and environmental factors have always been considered of vital importance in the mental balance of the individual. Without encounter with the environment, there can be no socially recognized illness: The exigencies of everyday life contribute both to the development of a stable personality and to the deviations from the norm. There is a constantly changing cultural mix of influences that determines which types of behavior will be tolerated or considered deviant. Cultural attitudes and fears play key roles in the perception of illness and acceptance of treatment.

Gabbard GO: Mind and brain in psychiatric treatment. In: *Synopsis of Treatment of Psychiatric Disorders,* 2nd ed. Gabbard SD, Atkinson SD (editors). American Psychiatric Press, 1996.

Olfson M et al: Mental disorders and disability among patients in a primary care group practice. Am J Psychiatry 1997;154:1734. [NLM Cit ID: 98059087] (Mental disorders in a population of primary care patients are significantly associated with a decline in work, family, and social functioning.)

Pincus HA et al: Prescribing trends in psychotropic medications: Primary care, psychiatry and other medical specialties. JAMA 1998;279:526. [NLM Cit ID: 98140732] (Primary care physicians tend to lag behind specialties in prescribing new psychotropics.)

PSYCHIATRIC ASSESSMENT

Psychiatric diagnosis rests upon the established principles of a thorough history and examination. All of the forces contributing to the individual's life situation must be identified, and this can be done only if the examination includes the history; mental status; medical conditions (including drugs); and pertinent social, cultural, and environmental factors impinging on the individual.

Interview

Every psychiatric history should cover the following points: (1) complaint, from the patient's viewpoint; (2) the present illness, or the evolution of the symptoms; (3) neurovegetative signs such as libido, appetite, and sleep; (4) previous disorders and the nature and extent of their treatment; (5) the family history—important for genetic aspects and family influences; (6) the personal history—childhood development, adolescent adjustment, level of education, and adult coping patterns; (7) current life functioning, with attention to vocational, social, educational, and avocational areas; and (8) present or past use of alcohol and other drugs.

It is often essential to obtain additional information from the family. Observing interactions of the patient with significant others in the context of a family interview may give important diagnostic information and may even underscore the nature of the problem and suggest a therapeutic approach.

The formal mental status examination should be particularly detailed when there is any evidence or high risk of cognitive dysfunction. The mental status examination includes the following: (1) Appearance: Note unusual modes of dress, use of makeup, etc. (2) Activity and behavior: Gait, gestures, coordination of bodily movements, etc. (3) Affect: Outward manifestation of emotions such as depression, anger, elation, fear, resentment, or lack of emotional response. (4) Mood: The patient's report of feelings and observable emotional manifestations. (5) Speech: Coherence, spontaneity, articulation, hesitancy in answering, and duration of response. (6) Content of thought: Associations, preoccupations, obsessions, depersonalization, delusions, hallucinations, paranoid ideation, anger, fear, or unusual experiences; suicidal and homicidal ideation. (7) Thought process: Loose associations, flight of ideas, thought blocking, tangentiality, circumstantiality, perseveration, racing thought. (8) Cognition: (a) orientation to person, place, time, and circumstances; (b) remote and recent memory and recall; (c) calculations, digit retention (six forward is normal), serial sevens or threes; (d) general fund of knowledge (presidents, states, distances, events); (e) abstracting ability, often tested with common proverbs or with analogies and differences (eg, "How are a lie and a mistake the same, and how are they different?"); (f) ability to identify by naming, reading, and writing specified test names and objects; (g) ideomotor function, which combines understanding and the ability to perform a task (eg, "Show me how to throw a ball"); (h) ability to reproduce geometric constructions (eg, parallelogram, intersecting squares); and (i) right-left differentiation. (9) Judgment regarding commonsense problems such as what to do when one runs out of medicine. (10) Insight into the nature and extent of the current difficulty and its ramifications in the patient's daily life.

Formal cognitive screens can quantify impairments and point to the need for further evaluation. The Mini-Mental State Examination produces a numerical score with up to 30 points given for correct answers to questions (likely organic < 27 points) (Figure 25–1). Specific cognitive assessment must be performed, since many patients are able to cover a deficit in routine conversation.

The examination of a psychiatric patient must include a complete medical history and physical examination (with emphasis on the neurologic examination) as well as all necessary laboratory and other special studies. Physical illness may frequently present as psychiatric disease, and vice versa.

Special Diagnostic Aids

Many tests and evaluation procedures are available that can be used to support and clarify initial diagnostic impressions.

A. Psychologic Testing: Testing by a psychologist may measure intelligence and cognitive functioning; provide information about personality, feelings, psychodynamics, and psychopathology; and differentiate psychic problems from organic ones. The place of such tests is similar to that of other tests in medicine—helpful in diagnostic problems but may be an unnecessary expense.

1. Objective tests–These tests provide quantitative evaluation compared to standard norms.

a. Intelligence tests–The test most frequently used is the Wechsler Adult Intelligence Scale–Revised (WAIS-R). Intelligence tests often reveal more than IQ. The results, given expert interpretation, can quantify intellectual deterioration that has occurred.

b. Minnesota Multiphasic Personality Inventory (MMPI)–The MMPI is an empirically based test of personality assessment. The patient's scores are interpreted in comparison with data about others with the same response pattern to assess psychopathologic changes.

c. Screening instruments–These tests include the Beck Depression Inventory, which quantifies degrees of dysphoria; and the Mental Health Screener (Prime MD), which is a broad measure of the patient's concerns and assists with differential diagnosis.

d. Neuropsychologic assessment–Such an assessment is made when an organic deficit is present but information on anatomic location and extent of dysfunction is required.

2. Projective tests–These tests are unstructured, so that the patient is forced to respond in ways that reflect fantasies and individual modes of adaptation. They are particularly useful in identifying psychotic disorders and unconscious motivations.

COMPLETE IF INDICATED CLINICALLY *(Ask general question and then ask specific questions to the right.)*		
Orientation	*(Score 1 for each correct. max = 10)*	
Where are you?	Name this place (building or hospital)	____
	What floor are you on now?	____
	What state are you in?	____
	What country are you in? (If not in a country, score correct if city is correct.)	____
	What city are you in (or near) now?	____
What is the date today?	What year is it?	____
	What season is it?	____
	What month is it?	____
	What is the day of the week?	____
	What is the date today?	____
Registration	*(Score 1 for each object correctly repeated. max = 3)*	
	Name three objects (ball, flag, and tree) and have patient repeat them. *(Say objects at about 1 word per second. If patient misses object, ask patient to repeat them after you until he/she learns them. Stop at 6 repeats.)*	____
Attention and calculation	*(Score 1 for each correct to 65. max = 5)*	
	Subtract 7s from 100 in a serial fashion to 65 *(Alternatively, ask serial 3s from 20 or spell WORLD backwards.)*	____
Recall	*(Score 1 for each object recalled. max = 3)*	
	Do you recall the names of the three objects?	____
Language	(max = 8)	
	Ask the patient to provide names of a watch and pen as you show them to him/her *(Score 1 for each object correct. max = 2)*	____
	Repeat "No ifs, ands, or buts." *(Only one trial. Score 1 if correct. max = 1)*	____
	Give the patient a piece of plain blank paper and say, "Take the paper in your right hand (1), fold it in half (2), and put it on the floor (3)." *(Score 1 for each part done correctly. max = 3)*	____
	Ask the patient to read and perform the following task written on paper: "Close your eyes." *(Score 1 if patient closes eyes. max = 1)*	____
	Ask the patient to write a sentence on a piece of paper. *(Score total of 1 if sentence has a subject, object and verb. max = 1)*	____
Construction		
	Ask patient to copy the design of the interlocking five-sided figures. *(Score total of 1, if all 10 angles are present and two angles intersect. Ignore tremor and rotation. max = 1)*	____
	Total Score *(Maximum = 30)*	____

Figure 25–1. MINI-MENTAL STATE EXAM (Optional). (Adapted from Folstein MF et al: Mini-mental state: A practical method for grading the cognitive state of patients for the clinician. J Psychiatr Res 1975;12:189.)

a. Rorschach Psychodiagnostics–This test utilizes ten inkblots to provide important information on psychodynamic themes and aberrations.

b. Thematic Apperception Test (TAT)–This test uses 20 pictures of people in different situations to assess areas of interpersonal conflicts.

B. Neurologic Evaluation: Consultation is often necessary and may include specialized tests. Brain imaging is useful for detecting structural abnormalities in the patient who presents with a nondefinitive history and examination (eg, dissociative episodes, unusual psychotic episodes not explained by drug abuse). MRI is particularly useful in delineating lesions and identifying demyelinating and degenerative diseases (eg, Huntington's disease). Electroencephalography is particularly useful for the diagnosis of seizure disorders and in differentiating delirium from depression or dementia. Typically, delirium is associated with generalized electroencephalographic slowing, while depression and dementia do not have this change. Single photon emission computed tomography (SPECT) is a gamma imaging technology like PET, and both provide tomographic images of brain activity. SPECT is cheaper but has the disadvantages of lower image resolution and lower quantification of regional brain activity.

Formulation of the Diagnosis

A psychiatric diagnosis must be based upon positive evidence accumulated by the above techniques. It must not be based simply on the exclusion of organic findings.

A thorough psychiatric evaluation has therapeutic as well as diagnostic value and should be expressed in ways best understood by the patient, family, and other physicians.

Crum RM et al: Population-based norms for the Mini-Mental State Examination by age and educational level. JAMA 1993;269:2386. [NLM Cit ID: 93240678] (Older or less well educated subjects may score somewhat lower but still may be normal.)

Reifler DR et al: Impact of screening for mental health concerns on health service utilization and functional status in primary care patients. Arch Intern Med 1996;156:2593. [NLM Cit ID: 97109023]

Spitzer RL et al: Validation and utility of a self-report version of Prime-MD: the PHQ primary care study. JAMA 1999;282:1737. [NLM Cit ID: 20033294] (This increasingly popular test is self-administered and is an excellent screen for common mental health problems.)

TREATMENT APPROACHES

The approaches to treatment of psychiatric patients are, in a broad sense, similar to those in other branches of medicine. For example, the internist treating a patient with heart disease uses not only **medical** measures such as drugs and pacemakers but also **psychologic** techniques to change attitudes and behaviors, **social** and **environmental** manipulation to mitigate deleterious influences, and **behavioral** techniques to change behavior patterns.

Regardless of the methods employed, treatment must be directed toward an objective, ie, it must be **goal-oriented.** This usually involves (1) obtaining active cooperation on the part of the patient; (2) establishing reasonable goals and modifying the goal if failure occurs; (3) emphasizing positive behavior (goals) instead of symptom behavior (problems); (4) delineating the method; and (5) setting a time frame (which can be modified later).

The physician must resist pressures for instantaneous results. In almost all cases, psychiatric treatment involves the active participation of the significant people in the patient's life. Time must be spent with the patient, but the frequency and duration of appointments are highly variable and should be adjusted to meet both the patient's psychologic needs and financial restrictions. Adherence (collaboration) is the end product of many factors, the most important being clear communication, attention to cost, and simple dosage regimens when drugs are prescribed. The physician can unwittingly promote chronic illness by prescribing medication inappropriately. The patient may come to believe that problems respond only to medication, and the more drugs prescribed, the stronger the misconception becomes.

Psychiatric Consultation

All clinicians are in an excellent position to meet their patients' emotional needs in an organized and competent way, referring to psychiatrists for consultation or for ongoing treatment of patients whose problems are considered beyond the expertise of the referring clinician. The most pressing problems involve evaluation of suicidal or assaultive potential and diagnostic differentiation in mood disorders and psychoses. Psychiatric problems associated with unusual psychopharmacologic therapy and with medications used in other branches of medicine may require pharmacologic consultation. When a psychiatric referral is made, it should be conducted like any other referral in an open manner, with full explanation of the problem to the patient.

Hospitalization

Hospital care may be indicated when patients are too sick to care for themselves or when they present serious threats to themselves or others; when observation and diagnostic procedures are necessary; or when specific kinds of treatment such as complex medication trials or a hospital environment ("milieu therapy") are required. Symptoms calling for hospitalization include self-neglect, violent or bizarre behavior, suicidal risk, paranoid ideation or delusions, marked intellectual impairment, and poor judgment. The trend over recent years has been to admit patients to hospitals, treat patients aggressively, and discharge them promptly to the next appropriate level of treatment—day hospital, halfway house, outpatient therapy, etc. Sixty percent of all psychiatric admissions are readmissions. The decision to propose involuntary hospitalization should be taken only after weighing the potential benefits to the patient and the community against the individual's loss of autonomy.

The disadvantages of psychiatric hospitalization include decreased self-confidence as a result of needing hospitalization; the stigma of being a "psychiatric

"habits"—persistent patterns of nonadaptive behavior acquired by learning. The "habits," being nonadaptive, are unsatisfactory ways of dealing with life's problems—hence the resultant anxiety. Help is sought only when the anxiety becomes too painful. Exogenous factors such as stimulants (eg, caffeine, cocaine) must be considered as a contributing factor.

Clinical Findings

A. Generalized Anxiety Disorder: This is the most common of the clinically significant anxiety disorders. Initial manifestations appear at age 20–35 years, and there is a slight predominance in women. The anxiety symptoms of apprehension, worry, irritability, difficulty in concentrating, insomnia, and somatic complaints are present more days than not for at least 6 months. Manifestations include cardiac (eg, tachycardia, increased blood pressure), gastrointestinal (eg, increased acidity, nausea, epigastric pain), and neurologic (eg, headache, near-syncope) systems. The focus of the anxiety may be a number of everyday activities.

B. Panic Disorder: This is characterized by short-lived, recurrent, unpredictable episodes of intense anxiety accompanied by marked physiologic manifestations. Agoraphobia may be present. Distressing symptoms and signs such as dyspnea, tachycardia, palpitations, headaches, dizziness, paresthesias, choking, smothering feelings, nausea, and bloating are associated with feelings of impending doom (alarm response). Recurrent sleep panic attacks (not nightmares) occur in about 30% of panic disorders. Anticipatory anxiety develops in all these patients and further constricts their daily lives. Panic disorder tends to be familial, with onset usually under age 25; it affects 3–5% of the population, and the female-to-male ratio is 2:1. The premenstrual period is one of heightened vulnerability. Patients frequently undergo emergency medical evaluations (eg, for "heart attacks" or "hypoglycemia") before the correct diagnosis is made. Gastrointestinal symptoms are especially common, occurring in about one-third of cases. Myocardial infarction, pheochromocytoma, hyperthyroidism, and various recreational drug reactions can mimic panic disorder. Mitral valve prolapse may be present but is not usually a significant factor. Patients with recurrent panic disorder often become **demoralized, hypochondriacal, agoraphobic,** and **depressed.** These individuals are at increased risk for major depression and the suicide attempts associated with that disorder. Alcohol abuse (about 20%) results from self-treatment and is not infrequently combined with dependence on sedatives. Some patients have atypical panic attacks associated with seizure-like symptoms that often include psychosensory phenomena (a history of stimulant abuse often emerges). About 25% of panic disorder patients also have obsessive-compulsive disorder.

C. Obsessive-Compulsive Disorder (OCD): In the obsessive-compulsive reaction, the irrational idea or the impulse persistently intrudes into awareness. Obsessions (constantly recurring thoughts such as fears of exposure to germs) and compulsions (repetitive actions such as washing the hands many times before peeling a potato) are recognized by the individual as absurd and are resisted, but anxiety is alleviated only by ritualistic performance of the action or by deliberate contemplation of the intruding idea or emotion. The primary underlying concern of the patient is not to lose control. Many patients do not mention the symptoms and must be asked about them. These patients are usually predictable, orderly, conscientious, and intelligent—traits that are seen in many compulsive behaviors such as food binging and purging and compulsive running. There is an overlapping of obsessive-compulsive disorder and other behaviors ("OCD spectrum"), including tics, trichotillomania (hair pulling), onychophagia (nail biting), hypochondriasis, Tourette's syndrome, and eating disorders (see Chapter 29). The 2–3% incidence of OCD in the general population is much higher than was previously recognized. In addition, there is a high comorbidity of OCD and major depression; two-thirds of OCD patients will develop major depression during their lifetime. Male:female ratios are similar, with the highest rates occurring in the young, divorced, separated, and unemployed (all high stress categories). Neurologic abnormalities of fine motor coordination and involuntary movements are common. Under extreme stress, these patients sometimes exhibit paranoid and delusional behaviors, often associated with depression, and can mimic schizophrenia.

D. Phobic Disorder: Phobic ideation can be considered a mechanism of "displacement" in which patients transfer feelings of anxiety from their true object to one that can be avoided. However, since phobias are ineffective defense mechanisms, there tends to be an increase in their scope, intensity, and number. Social phobias are global or specific; in the former, all social situations are poorly tolerated, while the latter group includes performance anxiety or well-delineated phobias. Agoraphobia (fear of open places and public areas) is frequently associated with severe panic attacks. Patients often develop the agoraphobia in early adult life, making a normal lifestyle difficult.

E. Dissociative Disorder: Fugue (the sudden, unexpected travel away from one's home with inability to recall one's past), amnesia, somnambulism, dissociative identity disorder (multiple personality disorder), and depersonalization are all dissociative states. The reaction is precipitated by emotional crisis. The symptom produces anxiety reduction and a temporary solution of the crisis. Mechanisms include repression and isolation as well as particularly limited concentration as seen in hypnotic states. Dissociative symptoms are similar in many ways to symptoms seen in patients with temporal lobe dysfunction.

Treatment

In all cases, underlying medical disorders must be ruled out (eg, cardiovascular, endocrine, respiratory, and neurologic disorders and substance-related syndromes, both intoxication and withdrawal states). These and other disorders can coexist with panic disorder.

A. Medical:

1. Generalized Anxiety–Benzodiazepines are the anxiolytics of choice in the acute management of generalized anxiety (Table 25–1). They are almost immediately effective. Antidepressants can be efficacious for the long-term treatment of generalized anxiety disorder, panic disorder, social phobia, and obsessive-compulsive disorder.

All of the benzodiazepines may be given orally, and several are available in parenteral formulations. Benzodiazepines such as lorazepam are absorbed rapidly when given intramuscularly. In psychiatric disorders, the benzodiazepines are usually given orally; in controlled medical environments (eg, the ICU), where the rapid onset of respiratory depression can be assessed, they are often given intravenously. Onset of action is a function of the rate of absorption (related to lipophilic property) and varies, with diazepam and clorazepate being the most rapidly absorbed. This characteristic, along with high lipid solubility, may explain the popularity of diazepam. In the average case of anxiety, diazepam, 5–10 mg orally every 6–8 hours as needed, is a reasonable starting regimen.

The duration of action of the benzodiazepines varies as a function of the active metabolites they produce. Benzodiazepines such as lorazepam do not produce active metabolites and have intermediate half-lives of 10–20 hours, characteristics useful in treating elderly patients. Ultra-short-acting agents such as triazolam have half lives of 1–3 hours and may lead to rebound withdrawal anxiety. Longer-acting benzodiazepines such as flurazepam and diazepam produce active metabolites, have half-lives of 20–120 hours, and should be avoided in the elderly. Since people vary widely in their response and since the drugs are long-lasting, one must individualize the dosage. Once this is established, an adequate dose early in the course of symptom development will obviate the need for "pill popping," which contributes to dependency problems. Panic disorder does not usually respond to benzodiazepines other than clonazepam and alprazolam. Those high-potency benzodiazepines and the antidepressants are most commonly used for panic disorder. Notably, alprazolam has a relatively short half-life and over time can lead to interdose rebound anxiety.

Table 25–1. Commonly used antianxiety and hypnotic agents.

	Usual Daily Oral Dose	Usual Daily Maximum Dose	Cost for 30 Days' Treatment Based on Maximum Dosage[1]
Benzodiazepines (used for anxiety)			
Alprazolam (Xanax)[2]	0.5 mg	4 mg	$92.40
Chlordiazepoxide (Librium)[3]	10–20 mg	100 mg	$27.60
Clonazepam (Klonopin)[3]	1–2 mg	10 mg	$169.50
Clorazepate (Tranxene)[3]	15–30 mg	60 mg	$236.40
Diazepam (Valium)[3]	5–15 mg	30 mg	$10.80
Lorazepam (Ativan)[2]	2–4 mg	4 mg	$76.80
Oxazepam (Serax)[2]	10–30 mg	60 mg	$86.40
Benzodiazepines (used for sleep)			
Estazolam (Prosom)[2]	1 mg	2 mg	$41.70
Flurazepam (Dalmane)[3]	15 mg	30 mg	$8.70
Midazolam (Versed IV)[4]	5 mg IV		$11.45/dose
Quazepam (Doral)[3]	7.5 mg	15 mg	$76.20
Temazepam (Restoril)[2]	15 mg	30 mg	$14.40
Triazolam (Halcion)[5]	0.125 mg	0.25 mg	$21.60
Miscellaneous (used for anxiety)			
Buspirone (Buspar)[2]	10–30 mg	60 mg	$134.40
Phenobarbital[3]	15–30 mg	90 mg	$1.26
Miscellaneous (used for sleep)			
Chloral hydrate (Noctec)[2]	500 mg	1000 mg	$12.00
Hydroxyzine (Vistaril)[2]	50 mg	100 mg	$25.20
Zolpidem (Ambien)[5]	5–10 mg	10 mg	$64.20
Zaleplon (Sonata)[6]	5–10 mg	10 mg	$63.60

[1]Cost to pharmacist (average wholesale price, generic when possible) for quantity listed. Source: *Drug Topics Red Book,* March 2000; Vol. 19, No. 3.
[2]Intermediate physical half-life (10–20 hours).
[3]Long physical half-life (> 20 hours).
[4]Intravenously for procedures.
[5]Short physical half-life (1–5 hours).
[6]Short physical half-life (about 1 hour)

Whether the indications for benzodiazepines are anxiety or insomnia, the drugs should be used judiciously. The longer-acting benzodiazepines are used for the treatment of alcohol withdrawal and anxiety symptoms; the intermediate drugs are useful as sedatives for insomnia (eg, lorazepam), while short-acting agents (eg, midazolam) are used for medical procedures such as endoscopy.

The side effects of all the benzodiazepine antianxiety agents are mainly behavioral and depend on patient reaction and dosage. As the dosage exceeds the levels necessary for sedation, the side effects include disinhibition, ataxia, dysarthria, nystagmus, and errors of commission. (The patient should be told not to operate machinery until he is well stabilized without side effects.)

Paradoxical agitation, anxiety, psychosis, confusion, mood lability, and anterograde amnesia have been reported, particularly with the shorter-acting benzodiazepines. These agents produce cumulative clinical effects with repeated dosage (especially if the patient has not had time to metabolize the previous dose); additive effects when given with other classes of sedatives or alcohol (many apparently "accidental" deaths are the result of concomitant use of sedatives and alcohol); and residual effects after termination of treatment (particularly in the case of drugs that undergo slow biotransformation).

Overdosage results in respiratory depression, hypotension, shock syndrome, coma, and death. Flumazenil, a benzodiazepine antagonist, is effective in overdosage. Overdosage (see Chapter 39) and withdrawal states are medical emergencies. Serious side effects of chronic excessive dosage are development of tolerance, resulting in increasing dose requirements, and physiologic dependence, resulting in withdrawal symptoms similar in appearance to alcohol and barbiturate withdrawal (withdrawal effects must be distinguished from reemergent anxiety). Abrupt withdrawal of sedative drugs may cause serious and even fatal convulsive seizures. Psychosis, delirium, and autonomic dysfunction have also been described. Both duration of action and duration of exposure are major factors. Common withdrawal symptoms after low to moderate daily use of benzodiazepines are classified as **somatic** (disturbed sleep, tremor, nausea, muscle aches), **psychologic** (anxiety, poor concentration, irritability, mild depression), or **perceptual** (poor coordination, mild paranoia, mild confusion). The presentation of symptoms will vary depending on the half-life of the drug. There are no significant side effects on organ systems other than the brain, and the drugs are safe in most medical conditions. Benzodiazepine interactions with other drugs are listed in Table 25–2.

Antidepressants are the first-line medications for sustained treatment of generalized anxiety, having the advantage of not causing serious physiologic dependency problems. At initiation of treatment, antidepressants can themselves be anxiogenic—thus, an initial dose, in conjunction with short-term treatment with a benzodiazepine, is often indicated. A sustained-release serotonin and norepinephrine reuptake inhibitor—venlafaxine (Effexor XR)—was approved by the FDA in 1999 for the treatment of generalized anxiety disorder in usual depression doses (75–225 mg). Similarly, buspirone, sometimes used as an augmenting agent in the treatment of agitated depression and compulsive behaviors, is also effective for generalized anxiety. Buspirone is usually given in a dosage of 15–60 mg/d in three divided doses. Higher doses tend to be counterproductive and produce gastrointestinal symptoms and dizziness. There is a 2- to 4-week delay before antidepressants and buspirone take effect, and patients require education regarding this lag. Sleep is sometimes negatively effected. Beta-blockers such as propranolol may help reduce peripheral somatic symptoms. Ethanol is the most frequently self-administered drug and should be interdicted. The highly addicting drugs with a narrow margin of safety such as glutethimide, ethchlorvynol, methprylon, meprobamate, and the barbiturates (with the exception of phenobarbital) should be avoided. Phenobarbital, in addition to its anticonvulsant properties, is a reasonably safe and very cheap sedative but has the disadvantage of causing hepatic microsomal enzyme stimulation (not the case with benzodiazepines), which markedly reduces its usefulness if any other relevant medications are being used by the patient.

Table 25–2. Benzodiazepine interactions with other drugs.

Drug	Effects
Antacids	Decreased absorption of benzodiazepines
Cimetidine	Increased half-life of diazepam and triazolam
Contraceptives	Increased levels of diazepam and triazolam
Digoxin	Alprazolam and diazepam raise digoxin level
Disulfiram	Increased duration of action of sedatives
Isoniazid	Increased plasma diazepam
Levodopa	Inhibition of antiparkinsonism effect
Propoxyphene	Impaired clearance of diazepam
Rifampin	Decreased plasma diazepam
Warfarin	Decreased prothrombin time

2. Panic attacks–Panic attacks may be treated in several ways. A sublingual dose of lorazepam (0.5–2 mg) or alprazolam (0.5–1 mg) is often effective for urgent treatment. For sustained treatment, serotonin-selective reuptake inhibitors (SSRIs) are the initial drugs of choice (adequate blood levels will require dosages similar to those used in the treatment of depression). For example, sertraline starting at 25 mg/d and increased after 1 week to 50 mg/d may be effective. As in depression, lithium may be used to augment the antidepressant drugs. Because of initial agitation in response to antidepressants, doses should start low and be very gradually increased. High-potency benzodiazepines may be used for symptomatic treatment as the antidepressant dose is titrated upward. Clonazepam (1–6 mg/d orally) and alprazolam (0.5–6 mg/d orally) are effective alternatives to antidepressants. Both drugs may produce marked withdrawal if stopped abruptly and should always be tapered. Because of chronicity of the disorders and the problem of dependency with benzodiazepine drugs, it is generally desirable to use antidepressant drugs as the principal pharmacologic approach. Antidepressants have been used in conjunction with beta-blockers in resistant cases. Propranolol (40–160 mg/d orally) can mute the peripheral symptoms of anxiety without significantly affecting motor performance. They block symptoms mediated by sympathetic stimulation (eg, palpitations, tremulousness) but not nonadrenergic symptoms (eg, diarrhea, muscle tension). Contrary to current belief, they usually do not cause depression as a side effect. Valproate has been found to be as effective in panic disorder as the antidepressants and is another useful alternative.

3. Phobic disorder–Phobic disorder may be part of the panic disorder and is treated within that framework. Global social phobias may be treated with SSRIs, such as paroxetine, sertraline, and fluvoxamine, or MAO inhibitors in the same dosage as used for depression. Gabapentin, an anticonvulsant with anxiolytic properties, may be an alternative to antidepressants in the treatment of social phobia in a dosage of 900–3600 mg/d. Specific phobias such as performance anxiety may respond to moderate doses of beta-blockers, such as propranolol, 20–40 mg 1 hour prior to exposure. A sustained effect is often not obtained with drugs alone; a combination of drugs, behavioral techniques, and cognitive psychotherapy is most effective. If there is any indication of seizure-like phenomena, carbamazepine or valproic acid should be considered.

4. Obsessive-compulsive disorders–Obsessive-compulsive disorders respond to serotonergic drugs in about 60% of cases. Clomipramine has proved effective in doses equivalent to those used for depression. Fluoxetine (an SSRI drug) has been widely used in this disorder but in doses higher than those used in depression (up to 60–80 mg/d). The other SSRI drugs such as sertraline, paroxetine, and fluvoxamine are being used with comparable efficacy, each with its own side effect profile. Buspirone in doses of 15–60 mg/d appears to be effective primarily as an antiobsessional augmenting agent for the aforementioned drugs. Psychosurgery has a limited place in selected cases of severe unremitting obsessive-compulsive disorder. The stereotactic techniques now being used, including modified cingulotomy, are great improvements over the crude methods of the past.

B. Behavioral: Behavioral approaches are widely used in various anxiety disorders, often in conjunction with medication. Any of the behavioral techniques (see above) can be used beneficially in altering the contingencies (precipitating factors or rewards) supporting any anxiety-provoking behavior. Relaxation techniques can sometimes be helpful in reducing anxiety. Desensitization, by exposing the patient to graded doses of a phobic object or situation, is an effective technique and one that the patient can practice outside the therapy session. Emotive imagery, wherein the patient imagines the anxiety-provoking situation while at the same time learning to relax, helps to decrease the anxiety when the patient faces the real-life situation. Physiologic symptoms in panic attacks respond well to relaxation training.

C. Psychologic: Cognitive approaches have been effective in treatment of panic disorders, phobias, and obsessive-compulsive disorder when erroneous beliefs need correction. The combination of medical and cognitive therapy is more effective than either alone. Group therapy is the treatment of choice when the anxiety is clearly a function of the patient's difficulties in dealing with others, and if these other people are part of the family it is appropriate to include them and initiate family or couples therapy.

D. Social: Peer support groups for panic disorder and agoraphobia have been particularly helpful. Social modification may require measures such as family counseling to aid acceptance of the patient's symptoms and avoid counterproductive behavior in behavioral training. Any help in maintaining the social structure is anxiety-alleviating, and work, school, and social activities should be maintained. School and vocational counseling may be provided by professionals, who often need help from the physician in defining the patient's limitations.

Prognosis

Anxiety disorders are usually of long standing and may be quite difficult to treat. All can be relieved to varying degrees with medications and behavioral techniques. The prognosis is much better if one can break the commonly observed anxiety-panic-phobia-depression cycle with a combination of the therapeutic interventions discussed above.

Barlow DH: Cognitive-behavioral therapy for panic disorder: Current status. J Clin Psychiatry 1997;58(Suppl 2):32. [NLM Cit ID: 97234124] (Efficacy of cognitive-behavioral therapy for panic disorder and current attempts to evaluate combined medication and psychologic interventions.)

Cowley DS et al: Determinants of pharmacologic treatment failure in panic disorder. J Clin Psychiatry 1997;58:555. [NLM Cit ID: 98110113] (Suggests that the most common reasons for treatment failure are medication side effects and inadequate dose and trial duration.)

Hohagen F: Cognitive-behavioral therapy and integrated approaches in the treatment of obsessive-compulsive disorder. CNS Spectrums 1999;5:35. (Cognitive-behavioral therapy and SSRIs can be used together or independently in the treatment of obsessive-compulsive disorder. Further research may refine their application in subtypes of the disorder.)

JAMA patient page: Obsessive-compulsive disorder. JAMA 1998;280:1806. [NLM Cit ID: 99057094]

Pande AC et al: Treatment of social phobia with gabapentin: a placebo controlled study. J Clin Psychopharmacol 1999;19:341. [NLM Cit ID: 99367074] (Gabapentin may have efficacy in the treatment of social phobia.)

Pohl RB et al: Sertraline in the treatment of panic disorder: A double-blind multicenter trial. Am J Psychiatry 1998;155:1189. [NLM Cit ID: 98403610] (Effective and well tolerated.)

Stein MB et al: Paroxetine treatment of generalized social phobia (social anxiety disorder). JAMA 1998;280:708. [NLM Cit ID: 98396814] (Symptoms and disability were substantially reduced.)

SOMATOFORM DISORDERS (Abnormal Illness Behaviors)

Essentials of Diagnosis

- Physical symptoms may involve one or more organ systems and are not intentional.
- Subjective complaints exceed objective findings.
- Correlations of symptom development and psychosocial stresses.
- Combination of biogenetic and developmental patterns.

General Considerations

A major source of diagnostic confusion in medicine has been to assume cause-and-effect relationships when parallel conditions exist. This problem is particularly vexing in situations where the individual exhibits psychosocial distress that could well be secondary to a chronic illness but has been assumed to be primary and causative. An example is the person with a chronic bowel disease who becomes querulous and demanding. Is this behavior a result of problems of coping with a chronic disease, or is it a personality pattern that causes the gastrointestinal problem?

Vulnerability in one or more organ systems and exposure to family members with somatization problems play a major role in the development of particular symptoms, and the "functional" versus "organic" dichotomy is a hindrance to good treatment. Physicians should suspect psychiatric disorders in a number of conditions. For example, 45% of patients complaining of palpitations had lifetime psychiatric diagnoses including generalized anxiety, depression, panic, and somatization disorders. Similarly, 33–44% of patients who undergo coronary angiography for chest pain but have negative results have been found to have panic disorder.

In any patient presenting with a condition judged to be somatoform, depression must be considered in the diagnosis.

Clinical Findings

A. Conversion Disorder: "Conversion" (formerly "hysterical conversion") of psychic conflict into physical symptoms in parts of the body innervated by the sensorimotor system (eg, paralysis, aphonia) is a disorder that is more common in individuals from lower socioeconomic classes and certain cultures. The defense mechanisms utilized in this condition are repression (a barring from consciousness) and isolation (a splitting of the affect from the idea). The somatic manifestation that takes the place of anxiety is typically paralysis, and in some instances the organ dysfunction may have symbolic meaning (eg, arm paralysis in marked anger). Pseudoepileptic ("hysterical") seizures are often difficult to differentiate from intoxication states or panic attacks. Retention of consciousness, random flailing with asynchronous movements of the right and left sides, and resistance to having the nose and mouth pinched closed during the attack all point toward a pseudoepileptic event. Electroencephalography, particularly in a video-EEG assessment unit, during the attack is the most helpful diagnostic aid in excluding genuine seizure states. Serum prolactin levels rise abruptly in the postictal state only in true epilepsy. La belle indifférence (a lack of affect) is not a significant characteristic, as commonly believed. Important criteria in diagnosis include a history of conversion or somatization disorder, modeling the symptom after someone else who had a similar presentation, a serious precipitating emotional event, associated psychopathology (eg, schizophrenia, personality disorders), a temporal correlation between the precipitating event and the symptom, and a temporary "solving of the problem" by the conversion. It is important to identify physical disorders with unusual presentations (eg, multiple sclerosis).

B. Somatization Disorder (Briquet's Syndrome, Hysteria): This is characterized by multiple physical complaints referable to several organ systems. Anxiety, panic disorder, and depression are often present, and **major depression** is an important consideration in the differential diagnosis. There is a significant relationship (20%) to a lifetime history of panic-agoraphobia-depression. It usually occurs before age 30 and is ten times more common in women. Polysurgery is often a feature of the history. Preoccupation with medical and surgical therapy becomes a lifestyle that excludes most other activities. The symptoms are a reflection of maladaptive coping techniques and reactivity of the particular organ system. There is often evidence of long-standing somatic symptoms (particularly dysmenorrhea, a lump in the throat, vomiting, shortness of breath, burning in the sex organs, painful extremities, and amnesia), often with a history of similar organ system involvement in other family members. Multiple symptoms that constantly change and inability of more than three doctors to make a diagnosis are strong clues to the problem.

C. Pain Disorder Associated With Psychologic Factors (Formerly Somatoform Pain Disorder): This involves a long history of complaints of severe pain not consonant with anatomic and clinical signs. This diagnosis must not be one of exclusion and should be made only after extended evaluation has established a clear correlation of psychogenic factors with exacerbations and remissions of complaints.

D. Hypochondriasis: This is a fear of disease and preoccupation with the body, with perceptual amplification and heightened responsiveness. A process of social learning is usually involved, frequently with a role model who was a member of the family and may be a part of the underlying psychodynamic causation. It is common in panic disorders.

E. Factitious Disorders: These disorders, in which symptom production is intentional, are not somatoform conditions in that symptoms are produced consciously, in contrast to the unconscious process of the above conditions. They are characterized by self-induced symptoms or false physical and laboratory findings for the purpose of deceiving physicians or other hospital personnel. The deceptions may involve self-mutilation, fever, hemorrhage, hypoglycemia, seizures, and an almost endless variety of manifestations—often presented in an exaggerated and dramatic fashion (Munchausen syndrome). "Munchausen by proxy" is the term used when a parent creates an illness in a child so the adult (usually the mother) can maintain a relationship with physicians. The duplicity may be either simple or extremely complex and difficult to recognize. The patients are frequently connected in some way with the health professions; they are often migratory; and there is no apparent external motivation other than achieving the patient role.

Complications

A poor doctor-patient relationship, with iatrogenic disorders and "doctor shopping," tends to exacerbate the problem. Sedative and analgesic dependency is the most common iatrogenic complication.

Treatment

A. Medical: Medical support with careful attention to building a therapeutic doctor-patient relationship is the mainstay of treatment. It must be accepted that the patient's distress is real. Every problem not found to have an organic basis is not necessarily a mental disease. Diligent attempts should be made to relate symptoms to adverse developments in the patient's life. It may be useful to have the patient keep a meticulous diary, paying particular attention to various pertinent factors evident in the history. Regular, frequent, short appointments that are not symptom-contingent may be helpful. Drugs (frequently abused) should not be prescribed to replace appointments. One doctor should be the primary physician, and consultants should be used mainly for evaluation. An empathic, realistic, optimistic approach must be maintained in the face of the expected ups and downs. Ongoing reevaluation is necessary, since somatization can coexist with a concurrent physical illness.

B. Psychologic: Psychologic approaches can be used by the primary physician when it is clear that the patient is ready to make some changes in lifestyle in order to achieve symptomatic relief. This is often best approached on a here-and-now basis and oriented toward pragmatic changes rather than an exploration of early experiences that the patient frequently fails to relate to current distress. Group therapy with other individuals who have similar problems is sometimes of value to improve coping, allow ventilation, and focus on interpersonal adjustment. Hypnosis or amobarbital interviews used early are helpful in resolving conversion disorders. If the primary physician has been working with the patient on psychologic problems related to the physical illness, the groundwork is often laid for successful psychiatric referral.

For patients who have been identified as having a factitious disorder, early psychiatric consultation is indicated. There are two main treatment strategies for these patients. One consists of a conjoint confrontation of the patient by both the primary physician and the psychiatrist. The patient's disorder is portrayed as a cry for help, and psychiatric treatment is recommended. The second approach avoids direct confrontation and attempts to provide a face-saving way to relinquish the symptom without overt disclosure of the disorder's origin. Techniques such as biofeedback and self-hypnosis may foster recovery using this strategy. Another face-saving approach is to utilize a double bind with the patient. For example, the patient is told there are two possible diagnoses: (1) an organic disease that should respond to the next medical intervention (usually modest and noninvasive), or (2) factitious disorder for which the patient will need psychiatric treatment. Given these options, many patients will choose to recover and not have to admit the origin of their problem

C. Behavioral: Behavioral therapy is probably best exemplified by biofeedback techniques. In biofeedback the particular abnormality (eg, increased peristalsis) must be recognized and monitored by the patient and therapist (eg, by an electronic stethoscope to amplify the sounds). This is immediate feedback, and after learning to recognize it the patient can then learn to identify any change thus produced (eg, a decrease in bowel sounds) and so become a conscious originator of the feedback instead of a passive recipient. Relief of the symptom operantly conditions the patient to utilize the maneuver that relieves symptoms (eg, relaxation causing a decrease in bowel sounds). With emphasis on this type of learning, the patient is able to identify symptoms early and initiate the countermaneuvers, thus decreasing the symptomatic problem. Migrainoid and tension headaches have been particularly responsive to biofeedback methods.

D. Social: Social endeavors include family, work, and other interpersonal activity. Family members should come for some appointments with the patient so they can learn how best to live with the patient. This is particularly important in treatment of somatization and pain disorders. Peer support groups provide a climate for encouraging the patient to accept and live with the problem. Ongoing communication with the employer may be necessary to encourage long-term continued interest in the employee. Employers can become just as discouraged as physicians in dealing with employees who have chronic problems.

Prognosis

The prognosis is much better if the primary physician is able to intervene early before the situation has deteriorated. After the problem has crystallized into chronicity, it is very difficult to effect change.

Eisendrath SJ: Factitious physical disorders. West J Med 1994;160:177. [NLM Cit ID: 94212678]

Eisendrath SJ et al: Somatization disorders: Effective management in primary care. J Musculoskel Med 1997;4:47. (The successful physician-patient relationship is the main "medicine" for this population.)

Noyes R et al: Fluvoxamine for somatoform disorders: an open trial. Gen Hosp Psychiatry 1998;20:339. [NLM Cit ID: 99077074] (Modest benefits in the treatment of patients with somatoform disorders may warrant further study.)

CHRONIC PAIN DISORDERS

Essentials of Diagnosis

- Chronic complaints of pain.
- Symptoms frequently exceed signs.
- Minimal relief with standard treatment.
- History of having seen many clinicians.
- Frequent use of several nonspecific medications.

General Considerations

A problem in the management of pain is the lack of distinction between acute and chronic pain syndromes. Most clinicians are adept at dealing with acute pain problems but have difficulty handling the patient with a chronic pain disorder. This type of patient frequently takes too many medications, stays in bed a great deal, has seen many clinicians, has lost skills, and experiences little joy in either work or play. All relationships suffer (including those with clinicians), and life becomes a constant search for succor. The search results in complex clinician-patient relationships that usually include many drug trials, particularly sedatives, with adverse consequences (eg, irritability, depressed mood) related to long-term use. Treatment failures provoke angry responses and depression from both the patient and the clinician, and the pain syndrome is exacerbated. When frustration becomes too great, a new clinician is found, and the cycle is repeated. The longer the existence of the pain disorder, the more important become the psychologic factors of anxiety and depression. As with all other conditions, it is counterproductive to speculate about whether the pain is "real." It is real to the patient, and acceptance of the problem must precede a mutual endeavor to alleviate the disturbance.

Clinical Findings

Components of the chronic pain syndrome consist of anatomic changes, chronic anxiety and depression, anger, and changed lifestyle. Usually, the anatomic problem is irreversible, since it has already been subjected to many interventions with increasingly unsatisfactory results. An algorithm for assessing chronic pain and differentiating from other psychiatric conditions is illustrated in Figure 25–2.

Chronic anxiety and depression produce heightened irritability and overreaction to stimuli. A marked decrease in pain threshold is apparent. This pattern develops into a hypochondriacal preoccupation with the body and a constant need for reassurance. The pressure on the doctor becomes wearing and often leads to covert rejection devices, such as not being available or making referrals to other physicians. This is perceived by the patient, who then intensifies the effort to find help, and the typical cycle is repeated. Anxiety and depression are seldom discussed, almost as if there is a tacit agreement not to deal with these issues.

Changes in lifestyle involve some of the so-called pain games. These usually take the form of a family script in which the patient accepts the role of being sick, and this role then becomes the focus of most family interactions and may become important in maintaining the family, so that neither the patient nor the family wants the patient's role to change. Demands for attention and efforts to control the behavior of others revolve around the central issue of control of other people (including physicians). Cultural factors frequently play a role in the behavior of the patient and how the significant people around the patient cope with the problem. Some cultures encourage demonstrative behavior, while others value the stoic role.

Another secondary gain that frequently maintains the patient in the sick role is financial compensation or other benefits ("green poultice"). Frequently, such systems are structured so that they reinforce the maintenance of sickness and discourage any attempts to give up the role. Physicians unwittingly reinforce this role because of the very nature of the practice of medicine, which is to respond to complaints of illness. Helpful suggestions from the physician are

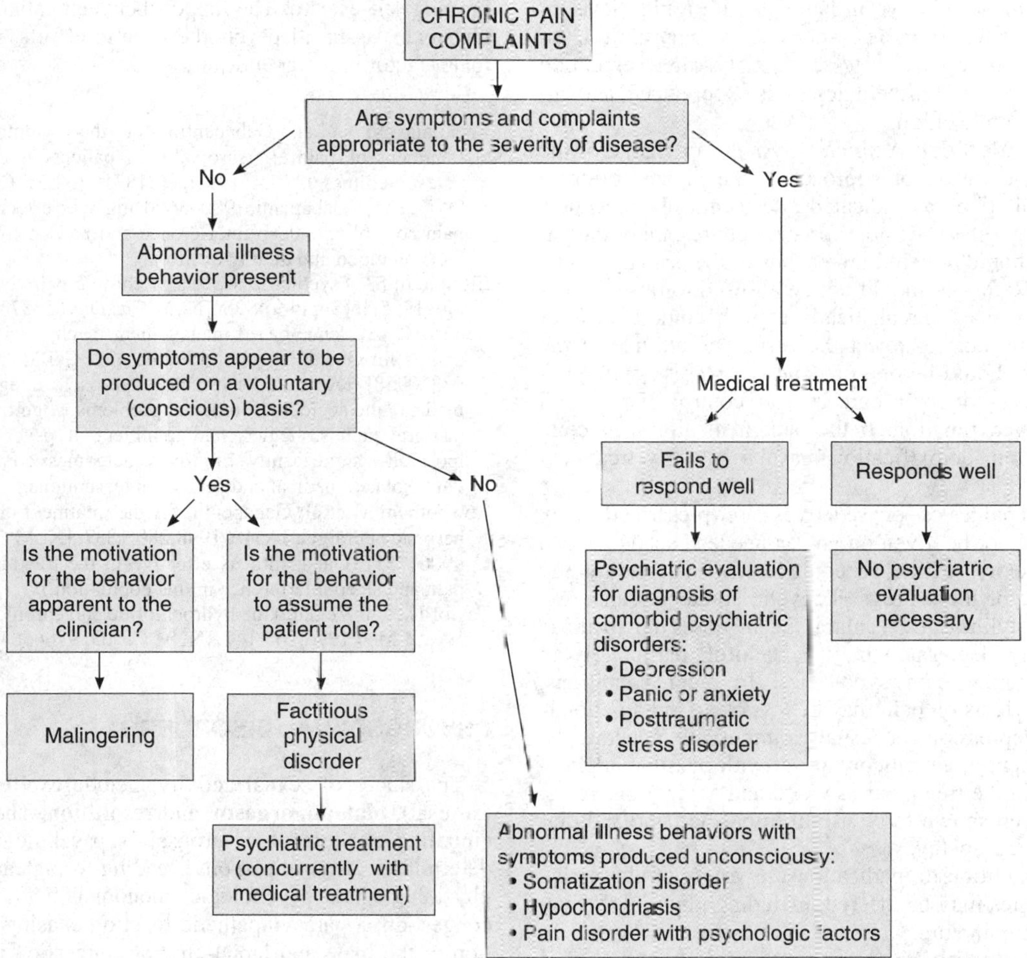

Figure 25–2. Algorithm for assessing psychiatric component of chronic pain. (Modified and reproduced, with permission, from Eisendrath SJ: Psychiatric aspects of chronic pain. Neurology 1995;45[Suppl 9]:S20.)

often met with responses like, "Yes, but. . . " Medications then become the principal approach, and drug dependency problems may develop.

Treatment

A. Behavioral: The cornerstone of a unified approach to chronic pain syndromes is a comprehensive behavioral program. This is necessary to identify and eliminate pain reinforcers, to decrease drug use, and to use effectively those positive reinforcers that shift the focus from the pain. It is critical that the patient be made a partner in the effort to alleviate pain. The physician must shift from the idea of biomedical cure to ongoing care of the patient. The patient should agree to discuss the pain only with the physician and not with family members; this tends to stabilize the patient's personal life, since the family is usually tired of the subject. At the beginning of treatment, the patient should be assigned self-help tasks graded up to maximal activity, as a means of positive reinforcement. The tasks should not exceed capability. The patient can also be asked to keep a self-rating chart to log accomplishments, so that progress can be measured and remembered. Instruct the patient to record degrees of pain on a self-rating scale in relation to various situations and mental attitudes so that similar circumstances can be avoided or modified.

Avoid positive reinforcers for pain such as marked sympathy and attention to pain. Emphasize a positive response to productive activities, which remove the focus of attention from the pain. Activity is also desensitizing, since the patient learns to tolerate increasing activity levels.

Biofeedback techniques (see Somatoform Disorders, above) and hypnosis have been successful in ameliorating some pain syndromes. Hypnosis tends to be most effective in patients with a high level of denial, who are more responsive to suggestion. Hypnosis can be used to lessen anxiety, alter perception of the length of time that pain is experienced, and encourage relaxation.

B. Medical: A *single physician* in charge of the multiple treatment approach is the highest priority. Consultations as indicated and technical procedures done by others are appropriate, but the care of the patient should remain in the hands of the primary physician. Referrals should not be allowed to raise the patient's hopes unrealistically or to become a way for the physician to reject the case. The attitude of the doctor should be one of honesty, interest, and hopefulness—not for a cure but for control of pain and improved function. If the patient manifests narcotic addiction, detoxification may be an early treatment goal.

If analgesics or sedatives are prescribed, they should not be given on an "as-needed" schedule (see Chapter 1). A fixed schedule lessens the conditioning effects of these drugs. Tricyclic antidepressants (eg, nortriptyline) and venlafaxine in doses up to those used in depression may be helpful, particularly in neuropathic pain syndromes. In other conditions, their effects on pain may be less clear, but ameliorating depression is usually important nonetheless. Gabapentin, an anticonvulsant with possible applications in the treatment of mood and anxiety disorders, has been shown to be useful in postherpetic and diabetic neuropathy.

In addition to medications, a variety of alternative strategies may be offered, including physical therapy and acupuncture.

C. Social: Involvement of family members and other significant persons in the patient's life should be an early priority. The best efforts of both patient and therapists can be unwittingly sabotaged by other persons who may feel that they are "helping" the patient. They frequently tend to reinforce the negative aspects of the chronic pain disorder. The patient becomes more dependent and less active, and the pain syndrome becomes an immutable way of life. The more destructive "pain games" described by many experts in chronic pain disorders are the results of well-meaning but misguided efforts of family members. Ongoing therapy with the family can be helpful in the early identification and elimination of these behavior patterns.

D. Psychologic: In addition to group therapy with family members and others, groups of patients can be helpful if properly led. The major goal, whether of individual or group therapy, is to gain patient involvement. A group can be a powerful instrument for achieving this goal, with the development of group loyalties and cooperation. People will frequently make efforts with group encouragement that they would never make alone. Individual therapy should be directed toward strengthening existing defenses and improving self-esteem. The rapport between patient and physician, as in all psychotherapeutic efforts, is the major factor in therapeutic success.

Backonja NI et al: Gabapentin for the symptomatic treatment of painful neuropathy in patients with diabetes mellitus. JAMA 1998;280:1831. [NLM Cit ID: 99061234] (Gabapentin 900–3600 mg was effective in pain control and sleep interference and had positive effects on mood and quality of life.)

Eisendrath SJ: Psychiatric aspects of chronic pain. Neurology 1995;45(Suppl 9):S26. [NLM Cit ID: 96133738]

Reiter RC: Evidence-based management of chronic pelvic pain. Clin Obstet Gynecol 1998;41:422. [NLM Cit ID: 98310958] (A multidisciplinary approach integrating medical and socioenvironmental problems, cognitive behavioral pain strategies, and treatment of psychologic morbidity significantly improves outcomes compared with isolated medical and surgical interventions.)

Rowbotham M et al: Gabapentin for the treatment of postherpetic neuralgia. JAMA 1998;280:1837. [NLM Cit ID: 99061235] (Gabapentin is effective in the treatment of pain and sleep interference in this population.)

Taylor K et al: Venlafaxine hydrochloride and chronic pain. West J Med 1996;165:147. [NLM Cit ID: 97065679]

PSYCHOSEXUAL DISORDERS

The stages of sexual activity include **excitement** (arousal), **plateau, orgasm,** and **resolution.** The precipitating excitement or arousal is psychologically determined. Arousal response leading to plateau is a physiologic and psychologic phenomenon of vasocongestion, a parasympathetic reaction causing erection in the male and labial-clitoral congestion in the female. The orgasmic response includes emission in the male and clonic contractions of the analogous striated perineal muscles of both male and female. Resolution is a gradual return to normal physiologic status.

While the arousal stimuli—vasocongestive and orgasmic responses—constitute a single response in a well-adjusted person, they can be considered as separate stages that can produce different syndromes responding to different treatment procedures.

Clinical Findings

There are three major groups of sexual disorders.

A. Paraphilias (Sexual Arousal Disorders): In these conditions, formerly called "deviations" or "variations," the excitement stage of sexual activity is associated with sexual objects or orientations different from those usually associated with adult sexual stimulation. The stimulus may be a woman's shoe, a child, animals, instruments of torture, or incidents of aggression. The pattern of sexual stimulation is usually one that has early psychologic roots. Poor experiences with sexual activity frequently reinforce this pattern over time.

Exhibitionism is the impulsive behavior of exposing the genitalia to unsuspecting strangers in order to achieve sexual excitation. It is a childhood sexual behavior carried into adult life.

Transvestism consists of recurrent cross-dressing behavior in a heterosexual male for the purpose of sexual excitation. Such fetishistic behavior can be part of masturbation foreplay. Transvestism in homosexuality and transsexualism is not for the purpose of sexual excitement but is a function of the homosexual preference or gender disorder.

Voyeurism involves the achievement of sexual arousal by watching the activities of an unsuspecting person, usually in various stages of undress or sexual activity. In both exhibitionism and voyeurism, excitation leads to masturbation as a replacement for sexual activity.

Pedophilia is the use of a child of either sex to achieve sexual arousal and, in many cases, gratification. Contact is frequently oral, with either participant being dominant, but pedophilia includes intercourse of any type. Adults of both sexes engage in this behavior, but because of social and cultural factors it is more commonly identified with males. The pedophile has difficulty in adult sexual relationships, and males who perform this act are frequently impotent.

Incest involves a sexual relationship with a person in the immediate family, most frequently a child. In many ways it is similar to pedophilia (intrafamilial pedophilia). Incestuous feelings are fairly common, but cultural mores are usually sufficiently strong to act as a barrier to the expression of sexual feelings.

Sexual sadism is the attainment of sexual arousal by inflicting pain upon the sexual object. Much sexual activity has aggressive components (eg, biting, scratching). However, forced sexual acquiescence (eg, rape) is considered to be primarily an act of aggression.

Sexual masochism is the achievement of erotic pleasure by being humiliated, enslaved, physically bound, and restrained. It is life-threatening, since neck binding or partial asphyxiation usually forms part of the ritual. It is estimated that bondage is responsible for about 1000 accidental deaths a year in males (the practice is much less common in females).

Necrophilia is sexual intercourse with a dead body or the use of parts of a dead body for sexual excitation, often with masturbation.

B. Gender Identity Disorder: Core gender identity reflects a biologic self-image—the conviction that "I am a male" or "I am a female" that is usually well developed by age 3 or 4. Gender dysphoria refers to the development of a sexual identity that is the opposite of the biologic one.

Transsexualism is an attempt to deny and reverse biologic sex by maintaining sexual identity with the opposite gender. Transsexuals do not alternate between gender roles; rather, they assume a fixed role of attitudes, feelings, fantasies, and choices consonant with those of the opposite sex, all of which clearly date back to early development. For example, male transsexuals in early childhood behave, talk, and fantasize as if they were girls. They do not grow out of feminine patterns; they do not work in professions traditionally considered to be masculine; and they have no interest in their own penises either as evidence of maleness or as organs for erotic behavior. The desire for sex change starts early and may culminate in assumption of a feminine lifestyle, hormonal treatment, and use of surgical procedures, eg, castration and vaginoplasty.

C. Psychosexual Dysfunction: This category includes a large group of vasocongestive and orgasmic disorders. Often, they involve problems of sexual adaptation, education, and technique that are often initially discussed with, diagnosed by, and treated by the primary care provider.

There are two conditions common in the male: erectile dysfunction and ejaculation disturbances.

Erectile dysfunction (impotence) is inability to achieve or maintain an erection firm enough for satisfactory intercourse; patients sometimes use the term to mean premature ejaculation. Careful questioning is necessary, since causes of this vasocongestive disorder can be psychologic, physiologic, or both. The majority are pathophysiologic and, to varying degrees, treatable. After onset of the problem, a history of occasional erections—especially nocturnal penile tumescence, which may be evaluated by a simple monitoring device, or a sleep study in the sleep laboratory—is usually evidence that the dysfunction is psychologic in origin, with the caveat that decreased nocturnal penile tumescence occurs in some depressed patients. **Psychologic erectile dysfunction** is caused by interpersonal or intrapsychic factors (eg, marital disharmony, depression). **Organic factors** are discussed in Chapter 23.

Ejaculation disturbances include premature ejaculation, inability to ejaculate, and retrograde ejaculation. (One may ejaculate even though impotent.) Ejaculation is usually connected with orgasm, and ejaculatory control is an acquired behavior that is minimal in adolescence and increases with experience. Pathogenic factors are those that interfere with learning control, most frequently sexual ignorance. Intrapsychic factors (anxiety, guilt, depression) and interpersonal maladaptation (marital problems, unresponsiveness of mate, power struggles) are also common. Organic causes include interference with sympathetic nerve distribution (often due to surgery or trauma) and the effects of pharmacologic agents (eg, SSRIs or sympatholytics).

In females, the two most common forms of sexual dysfunction are vaginismus and frigidity.

Vaginismus is a conditioned response in which a spasm of the perineal muscles occurs if there is any stimulation of the area. The desire is to avoid penetration. Sexual responsiveness and vasocongestion may be present, and orgasm can result from clitoral stimulation.

Frigidity is a complex condition in which there is a general lack of sexual responsiveness. The woman has difficulty in experiencing erotic sensation and does not have the vasocongestive response. Sexual activity varies from active avoidance of sex to an occasional orgasm. Orgasmic dysfunction—in which a woman has a vasocongestive response but varying degrees of difficulty in reaching orgasm—is sometimes differentiated from frigidity. Causes for the dysfunctions include poor sexual techniques, early traumatic sexual experiences, interpersonal disharmony (marital struggles, use of sex as a means of control), and intrapsychic problems (anxiety, fear, guilt). Organic causes include any conditions that might cause pain in intercourse, pelvic pathology, mechanical obstruction, and neurologic deficits.

Disorders of sexual desire consist of diminished or absent libido in either sex and may be a function of organic or psychologic difficulties (eg, anxiety, phobic avoidance). Any chronic illness can sap desire. Hormonal disorders, including hypogonadism or use of antiandrogen compounds such as cyproterone acetate, and chronic renal failure contribute to deterioration in sexual activity. Alcohol, sedatives, narcotics, marijuana, and some medications may affect sexual drive and performance.

Treatment

A. Paraphilias and Gender Identity Disorders:

1. Psychologic–Sexual arousal disorders involving variant sexual activity (paraphilia), particularly those of a more superficial nature (eg, voyeurism) and those of recent onset, are responsive to psychotherapy in a moderate percentage of cases. The prognosis is much better if the motivation comes from the individual rather than the legal system; unfortunately, however, judicial intervention is frequently the only stimulus to treatment, because the condition persists and is reinforced until conflict with the law occurs. Therapies frequently focus on barriers to normal arousal response; the expectation is that the variant behavior will decrease as normal behavior increases.

2. Behavioral–Aversive and operant conditioning techniques have been tried frequently in gender role disorders but have only occasionally been successful. In some cases, the sexual arousal disorders improve with modeling, role-playing, and conditioning procedures. Emotive imagery is occasionally helpful in lessening anxiety in fetish problems.

3. Social–Although they do not produce a change in sexual arousal patterns or gender role, self-help groups have facilitated adjustment to an often hostile society. Attention to the family is particularly important in helping persons in such groups to accept their situation and alleviate their guilt about the role they think they had in creating the problem.

4. Medical–Medroxyprogesterone acetate, a suppressor of libidinal drive, is used to mute disruptive sexual behavior in males of all ages. Onset of action is usually within 3 weeks, and the effects are generally reversible. Fluoxetine or other SSRIs may reduce some of the compulsive sexual behaviors including the paraphilias. Although some transsexuals are treated with genital reconstructive surgery, many others are screened out by trial periods of living as females prior to operation.

B. Psychosexual Dysfunction:

1. Medical–Identification of a contributory reversible cause is most important. Even if the condition is not reversible, identification of the specific cause helps the patient to accept the condition. Marital disharmony, with its exacerbating effects, may thus be avoided. Of all the sexual dysfunctions, erectile dysfunction is the condition most likely to have an organic basis. Sildenafil citrate is an effective oral agent for the treatment of penile erectile dysfunction in the recommended dose of 25–100 mg 1 hour prior to intercourse. Use of the medication in conjunction with any nitrates, particularly in individuals with coronary artery disease, can have significant hypotensive effects leading to death in some cases. The medication, which does not appear to impact sexual desire, should be used only once a day. Because of their common effect in delaying ejaculation, the SSRIs have been effective in premature ejaculation.

2. Behavioral–Syndromes resulting from conditioned responses have been treated by conditioning techniques, with excellent results. Vaginismus responds well to desensitization with graduated Hegar dilators along with relaxation techniques. Masters and Johnson have used behavioral approaches in all of the sexual dysfunctions, with concomitant supportive psychotherapy and with improvement of the communication patterns of the couple.

3. Psychologic–The use of psychotherapy by itself is best suited for those cases in which interpersonal difficulties or intrapsychic problems predominate. Anxiety and guilt about parental injunctions against sex may contribute to sexual dysfunction. Even in these cases, however, a combined behavioral-psychologic approach usually produces results most quickly.

4. Social–The proximity of other people (eg, a mother-in-law) in a household is frequently an inhibiting factor in sexual relationships. In such cases, some social engineering may alleviate the problem.

[NIH Consensus Statement: Erectile Dysfunction] http://odp.od.nih.gov/consensus/cons/091/091_intro.htm

Goldstein I et al: Oral sildenafil in the treatment of erectile dysfunction. N Engl J Med 1998;338:1397. [NLM Cit ID: 98234126]

JAMA patient page: Sexual abuse. JAMA 1998;280:1888. [NLM Cit ID: 99061247]

JAMA patient page: Sexual dysfunction. JAMA 1999; 281:584. [NLM Cit ID: 99144715]

Kravitz HM et al: Medroxyprogesterone and paraphiles: Do testosterone levels matter? Bull Am Acad Psychiatry Law 1996;24:73. [NLM Cit ID: 97046402] (Medroxyprogesterone can be effective in preventing relapse in sexual offenders.)

Speckens AE et al: Psychosexual functioning of partners of men with presumed nonorganic erectile dysfunction: Cause or consequence of the disorder? Arch Sex Behav 1995;24:157. [NLM Cit ID: 95314452] (Relationship problems, female psychosexual dysfunction, and the possible effect of relatively high levels of female sexual interest may contribute to the onset, exacerbation, and maintenance of erectile dysfunction.)

PERSONALITY DISORDERS

Essentials of Diagnosis

- Long history dating back to childhood.
- Recurrent maladaptive behavior.
- Low self-esteem and lack of confidence.
- Minimal introspective ability with a tendency to blame others for all problems.
- Major difficulties with interpersonal relationships or society.
- Depression with anxiety when maladaptive behavior fails.

General Considerations

Personality—a hypothetical construct—is the result of a genetic substrate and the prolonged interaction of an individual with personal drives and with outside influences (parent-child interactions, peer influences, random events). The sum of the effects produces the enduring and unique patterns of behavior that are adopted in order to cope with the environment and which characterize one as an individual. The personality structure, or character, is an integral part of self-image and is important to one's sense of personal identity.

The classification of subtypes depends upon the predominant symptoms and their severity. The most severe disorders—those that bring the patient into greatest conflict with society—tend to be classified as antisocial (psychopathic) or borderline.

Personality disorders can be considered a matrix for some of the more severe psychiatric problems (eg, schizotypal, relating to schizophrenia; avoidance types, relating to some anxiety disorders).

Classification & Clinical Findings

See Table 25–3.

Table 25–3. Personality disorders: Classification and clinical findings.

Personality Disorder	Clinical Findings
Paranoid	Defensive, oversensitive, secretive, suspicious, hyperalert, with limited emotional response.
Schizoid	Shy, introverted, withdrawn, avoids close relationships.
Obsessive-compulsive	Perfectionist, egocentric, indecisive, with rigid thought patterns and need for control.
Histrionic (hysterical)	Dependent, immature, seductive, egocentric, vain, emotionally labile.
Schizotypal	Superstitious, socially isolated, suspicious, with limited interpersonal ability and odd speech.
Narcissistic	Exhibitionist, grandiose, preoccupied with power, lacks interest in others, with excessive demands for attention.
Avoidant	Fears rejection, hyperreacts to rejection and failure, with poor social endeavors and low self-esteem.
Dependent	Passive, overaccepting, unable to make decisions, lacks confidence, with poor self-esteem.
Antisocial	Selfish, callous, promiscuous, impulsive, unable to learn from experience, has legal problems.
Borderline	Impulsive; has unstable and intense interpersonal relationships; is suffused with anger, fear, and guilt; lacks self-control and self-fulfillment; has identity problems and affective instability; is suicidal (a serious problem—up to 80% of hospitalized borderline patients make an attempt at some time during treatment, and the incidence of completed suicide is as high as 5%); aggressive behavior, feelings of emptiness, and occasional psychotic decompensation. This group has a high drug abuse rate, which plays a role in symptomatology. There is extensive overlap with other diagnostic categories, particularly mood disorders and posttraumatic stress disorder.

Differential Diagnosis

Patients with personality disorders tend to show anxiety and depression when pathologic coping mechanisms fail, and their symptoms can be similar to those occurring with anxiety disorders. Occasionally, the more severe cases may decompensate into psychosis under stress and mimic other psychotic disorders.

Treatment

A. Social: Social and therapeutic environments such as day hospitals, halfway houses, and self-help communities utilize peer pressures to modify the self-destructive behavior. The patient with a personality disorder often has failed to profit from experience, and difficulties with authority impair the learning experience. The use of peer relationships and the repetition possible in a structured setting of a helpful com-

disturbed interpersonal relationships and a reduced ability to experience pleasure. Dependency and a poor self-image are common. **Verbal utterances** are variable, the language being concrete yet symbolic, with unassociated rambling statements (at times interspersed with mutism) during an acute episode. Neologisms (made-up words or phrases), echolalia (repetition of words spoken by others), and verbigeration (repetition of senseless words or phrases) are occasionally present. **Affect** is usually flattened, with occasional inappropriateness. **Depression** is present in almost all cases but may be less apparent during the acute psychotic episode and more obvious during recovery. Depression is sometimes confused with akinetic side effects of antipsychotic drugs. It is also related to **boredom,** which increases symptoms and decreases the response to treatment. Work is generally unavailable and time hangs heavy, providing opportunities for counterproductive activities such as drug abuse, withdrawal, and increased psychotic symptoms.

Thought content may vary from a paucity of ideas to a rich complex of delusional fantasy with archaic thinking. One frequently notes after a period of conversation that little if any information has actually been conveyed. Incoming stimuli produce varied responses. In some cases a simple question may trigger explosive outbursts, whereas at other times there may be no overt response whatsoever (catatonia). When paranoid ideation is present, the patient is often irritable and less cooperative. **Delusions** (false beliefs) are characteristic of paranoid thinking, and they usually take the form of a preoccupation with the supposedly threatening behavior exhibited by other individuals. This ideation may cause the patient to adopt active countermeasures such as locking doors and windows, taking up weapons, covering the ceiling with aluminum foil to counteract radar waves, and other bizarre efforts. Somatic delusions revolve around issues of bodily decay or infestation. **Perceptual distortions** usually include auditory hallucinations—visual hallucinations are more commonly associated with organic mental states—and may include illusions (distortions of reality) such as figures changing in size or lights varying in intensity. Cenesthetic hallucinations (eg, a burning sensation in the brain, feeling blood flowing in blood vessels) occasionally occur. Lack of humor, feelings of dread, depersonalization (a feeling of being apart from the self), and fears of annihilation may be present. Any of the above symptoms generate higher anxiety levels, with heightened arousal and occasional panic and suicidal ideation, as the individual fails to cope.

Schizophrenic symptoms have been classified into positive and negative categories. Positive symptoms include hallucinations, delusions, and formal thought disorders. These symptoms appear to be related to increased (D_2) dopaminergic activity in the mesolimbic region. Negative symptoms include diminished sociability, restricted affect, and poverty of speech and appear to be related to decreased dopaminergic activity in the mesocortical system.

Ventricular enlargement and cortical atrophy, as seen on the CT scan, have been correlated with a chronic course, severe cognitive impairment, and nonresponsiveness to neuroleptic medications. Decreased frontal lobe activity on positron emission tomography has been associated with negative symptoms.

The development of the acute episode in schizophrenia frequently is the end product of a gradual decompensation. Frustration and anxiety appear early, followed by depression and alienation, along with decreased effectiveness in day-to-day coping. This often leads to feelings of panic and increasing disorganization, with loss of the ability to test and evaluate the reality of perceptions. The stage of so-called psychotic resolution includes delusions, autistic preoccupations, and psychotic insight, with acceptance of the decompensated state. The process is frequently complicated by the use of caffeine, alcohol, and other recreational drugs. Life expectancy of schizophrenics is as much as 20% shorter than that of cohorts in the general population (usually because of a higher mortality rate in younger people).

Polydipsia may produce water intoxication with hyponatremia—characterized by symptoms of confusion, lethargy, psychosis, seizures, and occasionally death—in any psychiatric disorder, but most commonly in schizophrenia. These problems exacerbate the schizophrenic symptoms. Possible pathogenetic factors include a hypothalamic defect, inappropriate ADH secretion, neuroleptic medications (anticholinergic effects, stimulation of hypothalamic thirst center, effect on ADH), smoking (nicotine and SIADH), psychotic thought processes (delusions), and other medications (eg, diuretics, antidepressants, lithium, alcohol). Other causes of polydipsia must be ruled out (eg, diabetes mellitus, diabetes insipidus, renal disease).

Differential Diagnosis

One should not hesitate to reconsider the diagnosis of schizophrenia in any person who has received that diagnosis in the past, particularly when the clinical course has been atypical. A number of these patients have been found to actually have atypical episodic affective disorders that have responded well to lithium. Manic episodes often mimic schizophrenia. Furthermore, many individuals have been diagnosed as schizophrenic because of inadequacies in psychiatric nomenclature. Thus, persons with brief reactive psychoses, obsessive-compulsive disorder, paranoid disorders, and schizophreniform disorders were often inappropriately diagnosed as having schizophrenia.

Psychotic depressions, psychotic organic mental states, and any illness with psychotic ideation tend to be confused with schizophrenia, partly because of the regrettable tendency to use the terms interchangeably. Adolescent phases of growth and counterculture behaviors constitute another area of diagnostic confusion. It is particularly important to avoid a misdiagnosis in these groups, because of the long-term implications arising from having such a serious diagnosis made in a formative stage of life.

Medical disorders such as thyroid dysfunction, adrenal and pituitary disorders, reactions to toxic materials (eg, mercury, PCBs), and almost all of the organic mental states in the early stages must be ruled out. Postpartum psychosis is discussed under Mood Disorders. **Complex partial seizures,** especially when psychosensory phenomena are present, are an important differential consideration. Toxic drug states arising from prescription, over-the-counter, and street drugs may mimic all of the psychotic disorders. The chronic use of amphetamines, cocaine, and other stimulants frequently produces a psychosis that is almost identical to the acute paranoid schizophrenic episode. The presence of formication and stereotypy suggests the possibility of stimulant abuse. Phencyclidine (see below) has become a very common street drug, and in many cases a reaction to it is difficult to distinguish from other psychotic disorders. Cerebellar signs, excessive salivation, dilated pupils, and increased deep tendon reflexes should alert the physician to the possibility of a toxic psychosis. Industrial chemical toxicity (both organic and metallic), degenerative disorders, and metabolic deficiencies must be considered in the differential diagnosis.

Catatonic syndrome, frequently assumed to exist solely as a component of schizophrenic disorders, is actually the end product of a number of illnesses, including various organic conditions. Neoplasms, viral and bacterial encephalopathies, central nervous system hemorrhage, metabolic derangements such as diabetic ketoacidosis, sedative withdrawal, and hepatic and renal malfunction have all been implicated. It is particularly important to realize that drug toxicity (eg, overdoses of antipsychotic medications such as fluphenazine or haloperidol) can cause catatonic syndrome, which may be misdiagnosed as a catatonic schizophrenic disorder and inappropriately treated with more antipsychotic medication.

Treatment

A. Medical: Hospitalization is often necessary, particularly when the patient's behavior shows gross disorganization. The presence of competent family members lessens the need for hospitalization, and each case should be judged individually. The major considerations are to prevent self-inflicted harm or harm to others and to provide the patient's basic needs. A full medical evaluation and CT scan or MRI should be considered in first episodes of schizophreniform disorder and other psychotic episodes of unknown cause.

Antipsychotic medications (see below) are the treatment of choice. They block the response to stimulation. The relapse rate can be reduced by 50% with proper maintenance neuroleptic therapy. Long-acting, injectable depot neuroleptics are used in noncompliant patients or nonresponders to oral medication. So-called **positive symptoms** such as hallucinations and delusions respond best, while **negative symptoms** such as withdrawal, psychomotor retardation, and poor interpersonal relationships may show little improvement. Atypical antipsychotics such as clozapine, risperidone, olanzapine, and quetiapine may reduce these negative symptoms. Antidepressant drugs may be used in conjunction with neuroleptics if significant depression is present. Resistant cases may require concomitant use of lithium, carbamazepine, or valproic acid. The addition of a benzodiazepine drug to the neuroleptic regimen may prove helpful in treating the agitated or catatonic psychotic patient who has not responded to neuroleptics alone—lorazepam, 1–2 mg orally, can produce a rapid resolution of catatonic symptoms; the benzodiazepine may allow maintenance with a lower neuroleptic dose. ECT has also been effective in treating catatonia.

Antipsychotic drugs include **phenothiazines, thioxanthenes** (both similar in structure), **butyrophenones, dihydroindolones, dibenzoxazepines,** and **benzisoxazoles** (Table 25–4). Generally, increasing milligram potency is associated with decreasing anticholinergic and adrenergic side effects and increasing extrapyramidal symptoms (Table 25–5). For example, chlorpromazine has lower potency and more severe anticholinergic and adrenergic side effects. The increased anticholinergic effect of chlorpromazine, however, lowers the risk of extrapyramidal symptoms.

The phenothiazines comprise the bulk of the currently used neuroleptic drugs. The only butyrophenone commonly used in psychiatry is haloperidol, which is totally different in structure but very similar in action and side effects to the piperazine phenothiazines such as fluphenazine, perphenazine, and trifluoperazine. These drugs and haloperidol (dopamine [D_2] receptor blockers) have high potency, a paucity of autonomic side effects, and act to markedly lower arousal levels. Molindone and loxapine, while less potent, are similar in action, side effects, and safety to the piperazine phenothiazines.

Clozapine, risperidone, olanzapine, and quetiapine are the first generation of "atypical" (novel) antipsychotic drugs. Clozapine, a dibenzodiazepine derivative, has dopamine (D_4) receptor blocking activity as well as central serotonergic, histaminergic, and alpha-noradrenergic receptor blocking activity. It is effective in the treatment of about 30% of psychoses resistant to other neuroleptic drugs. It has a 1% risk of agranulocytosis which requires weekly white blood cell count monitoring. Risperidone is an antipsychotic that blocks some serotonin receptors (5-HT_2) and dopamine receptors (D_2). Risperidone causes fewer extrapyramidal side effects than the typ-

Table 25–4. Commonly used antipsychotics.

	Chlorpromazine Ratio	Usual Daily Oral Dose	Usual Daily Maximum Dose[1]	Cost per Unit	Cost for 30 Days' Treatment Based on Maximum Dosage[2]
Phenothiazines					
Chlorpromazine (Thorazine; others)	1:1	100–400 mg	1 g	$0.95/200 mg	$142.50
Thioridazine (Mellaril)	1:1	100–400 mg	600 mg	$0.95/200 mg	$85.50
Mesoridazine (Serentil)	1:2	50–200 mg	400 mg	$1.24/100 mg	$148.80
Perphenazine (Trilafon)[3]	1:10	16–32 mg	64 mg	$1.08/16 mg	$129.60
Trifluoperazine (Stelazine)	1:20	5–15 mg	60 mg	$1.63/10 mg $1.15/10 mg	$293.40 $207.00
Fluphenazine (Permitil, Prolixin)[3]	1:50	2–10 mg	60 mg		
Thioxanthenes					
Thiothixene (Navane)[3]	1:20	5–10 mg	80 mg	$0.65/10 mg	$156.00
Dihydroindolone					
Molindone (Moban)	1:12	30–100 mg	225 mg	$3.00/50 mg	$405.00
Dibenzoxazepine					
Loxapine (Loxitane)	1:10	20–60 mg	200 mg	$1.80/50 mg	$216.00
Dibenzodiazepine					
Clozapine (Clozaril)	1:1	300–450 mg	900 mg	$3.33/100 mg	$899.10
Butyrophenone					
Haloperidol (Haldol)	1:50	2–5 mg	60 mg	$1.16/20 mg	$104.40
Benzisoxazole					
Risperidone[4] (Risperdal)	1:100	2–6 mg	10 mg	$4.22/2 mg	$633.00
Thienbenzodiazepine					
Olanzapine (Zyprexa)	1:50	5–10 mg	10 mg	$8.64/10 mg	$259.32
Dibenzothiazepine					
Quetiapine (Seroquel)	?	200–400 mg	800 mg	$4.68/200 mg	$561.60

[1]Can be higher in some cases.
[2]Cost to pharmacist (average wholesale price, generic when possible) for quantity listed. Source: *Drug Topics Red Book,* March 2000; Vol. 19, No. 3.
[3]Indicates piperazine structure.
[4]For risperidone, daily doses above 6 mg increase the risk of extrapyramidal syndrome. Risperidone 6 mg is approximately equivalent to haloperidol 20 mg.

ical antipsychotics at doses less than 6 mg. It appears to be as effective as haloperidol and possibly as effective as clozapine in treatment-resistant patients without requiring weekly white cell counts.

Olanzapine is a potent blocker of muscarinic, anticholinergic, 5-HT_2, and dopamine D_1, D_2, and D_4 receptors. High doses of olanzapine (12.5–17.5 mg daily) appear to be more effective than lower doses. The drug appears to be more effective than haloperidol in the treatment of negative symptoms. It has, however, been associated with more elevated serum alanine aminotransferase than those taking haloperidol. It is associated with a much lower incidence of dystonic reaction than haloperidol and is perhaps less likely to induce tardive dyskinesia. Its most common side effects include somnolence, agitation, nervousness, headache, insomnia, dizziness, weight gain, and dyspepsia. Its role in treatment-refractory patients remains to be explored.

Quetiapine is a neuroleptic with greater 5-HT_2 relative to D_2 receptor blockade as well as a relatively high affinity for α_1- and α_2-adrenergic receptors. It appears to be as efficacious as haloperidol in treating positive and negative symptoms of schizophrenia, with less extrapyramidal side effects even at high doses. More common side effects include somnolence, dizziness, and postural hypotension. Because of an association with lens changes seen in patients on long-term treatment, an eye examination to detect cataract formation is recommended at initiation of treatment and then at 6-month intervals during treatment.

None of the antipsychotics produce true physical dependency, and they have wide safety margins between therapeutic and toxic effects. All decrease adrenergic responses. Atypical neuroleptics are often considered preferable to traditional antipsychotics because of their perhaps reduced extrapyramidal symptoms and lesser risk of tardive dyskinesia.

Clinical Indications

The antipsychotics are used to treat all forms of the schizophrenias as well as psychotic ideation in or-

Table 25–5. Relative potency and side effects of antipsychotics.

	Chlorpromazine Potency Ratio	Anticholinergic Effects	Extrapyramidal Effects
Phenothiazines			
Chlorpromazine	1:1	4	1
Thioridazine	1:1	4	1
Mesoridazine	1:2	3	2
Perphenazine	1:10	2	3
Trifluoperazine	1:20	1	4
Fluphenazine	1:50	1	4
Thioxanthene			
Thiothixene	1:20	1	4
Dihydroindolone			
Molindone	1:7	2	3
Dibenzoxazepine			
Loxapine	1:10	2	3
Butyrophenone			
Haloperidol	1:50	1	4
Dibenzodiazepine			
Clozapine	1:1	4	—
Benzisoxazole			
Risperidone	1:50	1	1
Thienbenzodiazepine			
Olanzapine	1:20	1	1
Dibenzothiazepine			
Quetiapine	1:1	1	—

Key: 4 = strong effect; 1 = weak effect

ganic brain psychoses, delirium and dementia, drug-induced psychoses, psychotic depression, and mania. They are also effective in Tourette's disorder. They quickly lower the arousal (activity) level and, perhaps indirectly, gradually improve socialization and thinking. The improvement rate is about 80%. Patients whose behavioral symptoms worsen with use of antipsychotic drugs may have an undiagnosed organic condition such as anticholinergic toxicity.

Symptoms that are ameliorated by these drugs include hyperactivity, hostility, aggression, delusions, hallucinations, irritability, and poor sleep. Individuals with acute psychosis and good premorbid function respond quite well. The most common cause of failure in the treatment of acute psychosis is inadequate dosage, and the most common cause of relapse is noncompliance.

Dosage Forms & Patterns

The dosage range is quite broad. For example, haloperidol, 1 mg orally at bedtime, may be sufficient for the elderly person with mild dementia, whereas 60 mg/d may be used in a young patient with acute schizophrenia. A dosage of 10–20 mg/d is adequate initially for most patients. For quick response, one may start with haloperidol, 10 mg intramuscularly, which is absorbed rapidly and achieves an initial tenfold plasma level advantage over equal oral doses. Psychomotor agitation, racing thoughts, and general arousal are quickly reduced. The dose can be repeated every 3–4 hours; when the patient is less symptomatic, oral doses can replace parenteral administration in most cases.

Various factors play a role in the absorption of oral medications. Of particular importance are previous gastrointestinal surgery and concomitant administration of other drugs, eg, antacids (Table 25–6). There are racial differences in metabolizing the neuroleptic drugs—eg, many Asians require only about half the usual dosage. Bioavailability is influenced by other factors such as smoking or hepatic microsomal enzyme stimulation with alcohol or barbiturates and enzyme-altering drugs such as carbamazepine or methylphenidate. Plasma drug level determinations are not currently of major clinical assistance.

Divided daily doses are not necessary after a maintenance dose has been established, and most patients can then be maintained on a single daily dose, usually taken at bedtime. This is particularly appropriate in a case where the sedative effect of the drug is desired for nighttime sleep, and undesirable sedative effects can be avoided during the day. Risperidone is an ex-

Table 25–6. Antipsychotic drug interactions with other drugs.

Drug	Effects
Antacids	Decreased absorption of antipsychotic drugs
All anticholinergics	Increased anticholinergic effects
Barbiturates	Central nervous system depression and decreased antipsychotic drug levels
Carbamazepine	Decreased neuroleptic levels
Cimetidine	Increased chlorpromazine levels
Tricyclic antidepressants	Increased antidepressant blood levels
Guanethidine	Decreased hypotensive effect
Indomethacin	Severe drowsiness (with haloperidol)
Levodopa	Decreased antiparkinsonism effect
Methyldopa	Decreased hypotensive effect
Phenytoin	Increased phenytoin levels
Propranolol	Increased thioridazine levels
Thiazide diuretics	Increased hypotensive effect
Trihexyphenidyl	Decreased antipsychotic levels

ception, being given twice daily. First-episode patients especially should be tapered off medications after about 6 months of stability and carefully monitored; their rate of relapse is lower than that of multiple-episode patients.

Psychiatric patients—particularly paranoid individuals—often neglect to take their medication. In these cases and in nonresponders to oral medication, the enanthate and decanoate (the latter is slightly longer-lasting and has fewer extrapyramidal side effects) forms of fluphenazine or the decanoate form of haloperidol may be given by deep subcutaneous injection or intramuscularly to achieve an effect that will usually last 7–28 days. A patient who cannot be depended on to take oral medication (or who overdoses on minimal provocation) will generally agree to come to the physician's office for a "shot." The usual dose of the fluphenazine long-acting preparations is 25 mg every 2 weeks. Dosage and frequency of administration vary from about 100 mg weekly to 12.5 mg monthly. Use the smallest effective amount as infrequently as possible. A monthly injection of 25 mg of fluphenazine decanoate is equivalent to about 15–20 mg of oral fluphenazine daily. Concomitant use of a benzodiazepine (eg, lorazepam, 2 mg orally twice daily) may permit reduction of the required dosage of oral or parenteral antipsychotic drug.

Intravenous haloperidol, the neuroleptic most commonly used by this route, is often used in critical care units in the management of agitated, delirious patients. Intravenous haloperidol should be given no faster than 1 mg/min to reduce cardiovascular side effects and is associated with a lower risk of extrapyramidal side effects.

Side Effects

The side effects *decrease* as one goes from the sedating, lower milligram potency drugs such as chlorpromazine or thioridazine to those of higher milligram potency such as fluphenazine and haloperidol. However, the extrapyramidal effects *increase* as one goes down the list (consider chlorprothixene as similar to chlorpromazine).

The most common anticholinergic side effects include dry mouth (which can lead to ingestion of caloric liquids and weight gain or hyponatremia), blurred near vision, urinary retention (particularly in elderly men with enlarged prostates), delayed gastric emptying, esophageal reflux, ileus, delirium, and precipitation of acute glaucoma in patients with narrow anterior chamber angles. Other autonomic effects include orthostatic hypotension and sexual dysfunction—problems in achieving erection, ejaculation (including retrograde ejaculation), and orgasm in males (approximately 50% of cases) and females (approximately 30%). Delay in achieving orgasm is often a factor in medication noncompliance. Electrocardiographic changes occur frequently, but clinically significant arrhythmias are much less common. Elderly patients and those with preexisting cardiac disease are at greater risk. The most frequently seen electrocardiographic changes include diminution of the T wave amplitude, appearance of prominent U waves, depression of the ST segment, and prolongation of the QT interval. These electrocardiographic findings usually do not call for any change in treatment. In some critical care patients, however, torsade de pointes has been associated with the use of high-dose intravenous haloperidol (usually > 30 mg/24 h).

Metabolic and endocrine effects include weight gain, hyperglycemia, infrequent temperature irregularities (particularly in hot weather), and water intoxication that may be due to inappropriate antidiuretic hormone secretion. Lactation and menstrual irregularities are common (antipsychotic drugs should be avoided, if possible, in breast cancer patients because of potential trophic effects of elevated prolactin levels on the breast). Both antipsychotic and antidepressant drugs inhibit sperm motility. Bone marrow depression and cholestatic jaundice occur rarely; these are hypersensitivity reactions, and they usually appear in the first 2 months of treatment. They subside on discontinuance of the drug. There is cross-sensitivity among all of the phenothiazines, and a drug from a different group should be used when allergic reactions occur.

Clozapine is associated with a 1.6% risk of **agranulocytosis** (higher in persons of Ashkenazi Jewish ancestry), and its use must be strictly monitored with weekly blood counts. It also lowers the seizure threshold and has many side effects, including sedation, hypotension, increased liver enzyme levels, hypersalivation, respiratory arrest, weight gain, and changes in both ECG and EEG.

Photosensitivity, retinopathy, and hyperpigmentation are associated with use of fairly high dosages of chlorpromazine and thioridazine. The appearance of particulate melanin deposits in the lens of the eye is related to the total dose given, and patients on long-term medication should have periodic eye examinations. Teratogenicity has not been causally related to these drugs, but prudence is indicated particularly in the first trimester of pregnancy. The seizure threshold is lowered, but it is safe to use these medications in epileptics controlled by anticonvulsants.

The **neuroleptic malignant syndrome (NMS)** is a catatonia-like state manifested by extrapyramidal signs, blood pressure changes, altered consciousness, and hyperpyrexia; it is an uncommon but serious complication of neuroleptic treatment. Muscle rigidity, involuntary movements, confusion, dysarthria, and dysphagia are accompanied by pallor, cardiovascular instability, fever, pulmonary congestion, and diaphoresis and may result in stupor, coma, and death. The cause may be related to a number of factors, including poor dosage control of neuroleptic medication, affective illness, decreased serum iron, dehydration, and increased sensitivity of dopamine receptor sites. Lithium in combination with a neuroleptic drug may increase vulnerability, which is already increased in patients with an affective disorder. In most cases, the symptoms develop within the first 2 weeks of antipsychotic drug treatment. The syndrome may occur with small doses of the drugs. Intramuscular administration is a risk factor. Elevated creatine kinase and leukocytosis with a shift to the left are present early in about half of cases. Treatment includes controlling fever and providing fluid support. Dopamine agonists such as bromocriptine, 2.5–10 mg orally three times a day, and amantadine, 100–200 mg orally twice a day, have also been useful. Dantrolene, 50 mg intravenously as needed, is used to alleviate rigidity (do not exceed 10 mg/kg/d). There is ongoing controversy about the efficacy of these three agents as well as the use of calcium channel blockers and benzodiazepines. Electroconvulsive therapy has been used effectively in resistant cases. Clozapine has been used with relative safety and fair success as an antipsychotic drug for patients who have had NMS. The syndrome must be differentiated from acute lethal catatonia, malignant hyperthermia, neurotoxic syndromes (including AIDS), and a variety of other conditions such as viral encephalitis, Wilson's disease, central anticholinergic syndrome, and hypertonic states (eg, tetany, strychnine poisoning).

Akathisia is the most common (about 20%) so-called **extrapyramidal symptom.** It usually occurs early in treatment (but may persist after neuroleptics are discontinued) and is frequently mistaken for anxiety or exacerbation of psychosis. It is characterized by a subjective desire to be in constant motion followed by an inability to sit or stand still and consequent pacing. It may include suicidality or feelings of fright, rage, terror, or sexual torment. Insomnia is often present. In all cases, reevaluate the dosage requirement or the type of neuroleptic drug. One should inquire also about cigarette smoking, which in women has been associated with an increased incidence of akathisia. Antiparkinsonism drugs such as trihexyphenidyl, 2–5 mg orally three times daily, or benztropine mesylate, 1–2 mg twice daily, may be helpful. In resistant cases, symptoms may be alleviated by propranolol, 30–80 mg/d orally; diazepam, 5 mg three times daily; or amantadine, 100 mg orally three times daily.

Acute dystonias usually occur early, though a late (tardive) occurrence is reported in patients (mostly males after several years of therapy) who previously had early severe dystonic reactions and a mood disorder (see below). Younger patients are at higher risk for acute dystonias. The most common signs are bizarre muscle spasms of the head, neck, and tongue. Frequently present are torticollis, oculogyric crises, swallowing or chewing difficulties, and masseter spasms. Laryngospasm is particularly dangerous. Back, arm, or leg muscle spasms are occasionally reported. Diphenhydramine, 50 mg intramuscularly, is effective for the acute crisis; one should then give benztropine mesylate, 2 mg orally twice daily, for several weeks, and then discontinue gradually, since few of the extrapyramidal symptoms require long-term use of the antiparkinsonism drugs (all of which are about equally efficacious—though trihexyphenidyl tends to be mildly stimulating and benztropine mildly sedating).

Drug-induced parkinsonism is indistinguishable from idiopathic parkinsonism, but it is reversible, occurs later in treatment than the preceding extrapyramidal symptoms, and in some cases appears after neuroleptic withdrawal. The condition includes the typical signs of apathy and reduction of facial and arm movements (akinesia, which can mimic depression), festinating gait, rigidity, loss of postural reflexes, and pill-rolling tremor. AIDS patients seem particularly vulnerable to extrapyramidal side effects. High-potency neuroleptics often require antiparkinsonism drugs (Table 24–5). The neuroleptic dosage should be reduced, and immediate relief can be achieved with antiparkinsonism drugs in the same dosages as above. After 4–6 weeks, these antiparkinsonism drugs can often be discontinued with no recurrent symptoms. In any of the extrapyramidal symptoms, amantadine, 100–400 mg daily, may be used instead of the antiparkinsonism drugs. Neuroleptic-induced catatonia is similar to catatonic stupor with rigidity, drooling, urinary incontinence, and cogwheeling. It usually responds slowly to withdrawal of the offending medication and use of antiparkinsonism agents.

Tardive dyskinesia is a syndrome of abnormal involuntary stereotyped movements of the face, mouth, tongue, trunk, and limbs that may occur after months or (usually) years of treatment with neuroleptic agents. The syndrome affects 20–35% of patients who have undergone long-term neuroleptic therapy. Predisposing factors include older age, many years of treatment, cigarette smoking, and diabetes mellitus. Pineal calcification is higher in this condition by a margin of 3:1. There are no known differences among any of the antipsychotic drugs in the development of this syndrome.

Early manifestations include fine worm-like movements of the tongue at rest, difficulty in sticking out the tongue, facial tics, increased blink frequency, or jaw movements of recent onset. Later manifestations may include bucco-linguo-masticatory movements, lip smacking, chewing motions, mouth opening and closing, disturbed gag reflex, puffing of the cheeks, disrupted speech, respiratory distress, or choreoathetoid movements of the extremities (the last being more prevalent in younger patients). The symptoms do not necessarily worsen and in rare cases may lessen even though neuroleptic drugs are continued. The dyskinesias do not occur during sleep and can be voluntarily suppressed for short periods. Stress and movements in other parts of the body will often aggravate the condition.

Early signs of dyskinesia must be differentiated from those reversible signs produced by ill-fitting dentures or nonneuroleptic drugs such as levodopa, tricyclic antidepressants (TCAs), antiparkinsonism agents, anticonvulsants, and antihistamines. Other neurologic conditions such as Huntington's chorea can be differentiated by history and examination.

The emphasis should be on prevention. Use the least amount of neuroleptic drug necessary to mute the psychotic symptoms. Detect early manifestations of dyskinesias. When these occur, stop anticholinergic drugs and gradually discontinue neuroleptic drugs. Weight loss and cachexia sometimes appear on withdrawal of neuroleptics. In an indeterminate number of cases, the dyskinesias will remit. Keep the patient off the drugs until reemergent psychotic symptoms dictate their resumption, at which point they are restarted in low doses and gradually increased until there is clinical improvement. If neuroleptic drugs are restarted, clozapine and olanzapine appear to offer less risk of recurrence. The use of adjunctive agents such as benzodiazepines or lithium may help directly or indirectly by allowing control of psychotic symptoms with a low dosage of neuroleptics. If the dyskinesic syndrome recurs and it is necessary to continue neuroleptic drugs to control psychotic symptoms, informed consent should be obtained. Benzodiazepines, buspirone (in doses of 15–60 mg/d), phosphatidylcholine, clonidine, calcium channel blockers, vitamin E, and propranolol all have had limited usefulness in treating the dyskinetic side effects.

B. Social: Environmental considerations are most important in the individual with a chronic illness, who usually has a history of repeated hospitalizations, a continued low level of functioning, and symptoms that never completely remit. Family rejection and work failure are common. In these cases, board and care homes staffed by personnel experienced in caring for psychiatric patients are most important. There is frequently an inverse relationship between stability of the living situation and the amounts of required antipsychotic drugs, since the most salutary environment is one that reduces stimuli. Nonresidential self-help groups such as Recovery, Inc., should be utilized whenever possible. They provide a setting for sharing, learning, and mutual support and are frequently the only social involvement with which this type of patient is comfortable. Vocational rehabilitation and work agencies (eg, Goodwill Industries, Inc.) provide assessment, training, and job opportunities at a level commensurate with the person's clinical condition.

C. Psychologic: The need for psychotherapy varies markedly depending on the patient's current status and history. In a person with a single psychotic episode and a previously good level of adjustment, supportive psychotherapy may help the patient reintegrate the experience, gain some insight into antecedent problems, and become a more self-observant individual who can recognize early signs of stress. Insight-oriented psychotherapy is often counterproductive in this type of disorder. More importantly, family therapy should be given concomitantly to help alleviate the patient's stress and to assist relatives in coping with the patient.

D. Behavioral: Behavioral techniques (see above) are most frequently used in therapeutic settings such as day treatment centers, but there is no reason why they cannot be incorporated into family situations or any therapeutic setting. Many behavioral techniques are used unwittingly (eg, positive reinforcement—whether it be a word of praise or an approving nod—after some positive behavior), and with some careful thought this approach can be a powerful instrument for helping a person learn behaviors that will facilitate social acceptance. Music from portable cassette players with earphones is one of many ways to divert the patient's attention from auditory hallucinations.

Prognosis

In any psychosis in the large majority of patients, the prognosis is excellent for alleviation of positive symptoms such as hallucinations or delusions treated with medication. Negative symptoms such as diminished affect and sociability are much more difficult to treat and are the principal reason schizophrenic patients do not achieve optimal function. Unavailability of structured work situations and lack of family therapy are two other reasons why the prognosis is so guarded in such a large percentage of schizophrenic patients. Psychosis connected with a history of serious drug abuse has a guarded prognosis because of the central nervous system damage, usually from the drugs themselves and associated medical illnesses.

Andersson C et al: Emerging roles for novel antipsychotic medications in the treatment of schizophrenia. Psychiatr Clin North Am 1998;21:151. [NLM Cit ID: 98212859] (Superior efficacy and more benign side effect profile of atypical antipsychotics provide a rationale for their use as first-line treatment.)

Eisendrath SJ: Psychiatry in the critical care unit. In: *Current Critical Care Diagnosis and Treatment.* Bongard FS, Sue DY (editors). Appleton & Lange, 1994.

Kane JM: Schizophrenia. N Engl J Med 1996;334:34. [NLM Cit ID: 96105284] (Broad review of current approaches.)

Sharma ND et al: Torsades de pointes associated with intravenous haloperidol in ill patients. Am J Cardiol 1998;81:238. [NLM Cit ID: 98252610]

Tran PV et al: Extrapyramidal symptoms and tolerability of olanzapine versus haloperidol in the acute treatment of schizophrenia. J Clin Psychiatry 1997;58:205. [NLM Cit ID: 97328056]

MOOD DISORDERS (Depression & Mania)

Essentials of Diagnosis

Present in most depressions:

- Lowered mood, varying from mild sadness to intense feelings of guilt, worthlessness, and hopelessness.
- Difficulty in thinking, including inability to concentrate, ruminations, and lack of decisiveness.
- Loss of interest, with diminished involvement in work and recreation.
- Somatic complaints such as headache; disrupted, lessened, or excessive sleep; loss of energy; change in appetite; decreased sexual drive.
- Anxiety.

Present in some severe depressions:

- Psychomotor retardation or agitation.
- Delusions of a hypochondriacal or persecutory nature.
- Withdrawal from activities.
- Physical symptoms of major severity, eg, anorexia, insomnia, reduced sexual drive, weight loss, and various somatic complaints.
- Suicidal ideation.

Present in mania:

- Mood ranging from euphoria to irritability.
- Sleep disruption.
- Hyperactivity.
- Racing thoughts.
- Grandiosity.
- Variable psychotic symptoms.

General Considerations

Depression is extremely common, with up to 30% of primary care patients having depressive symptoms. Depression may be the final expression of (1) genetic factors (neurotransmitter dysfunction), (2) developmental problems (personality defects, childhood events), or (3) psychosocial stresses (divorce, unemployment). It frequently presents in the form of somatic complaints with negative medical workups. Although sadness and grief are normal responses to loss, depression is not. Patients experiencing normal grief tend to produce sympathy and sadness in the physician caregiver; depression often produces frustration and irritation in the physician. Grief is usually accompanied by intact self-esteem, whereas depression is marked by a sense of guilt and worthlessness.

Mania is often combined with depression and may occur alone, together with mania in a mixed episode, or in cyclic fashion with depression.

Clinical Findings

In general, there are four major types of depressions, with similar symptoms in each group.

A. Adjustment Disorder With Depressed Mood: Depression may occur in reaction to some identifiable stressor or adverse life situation, usually loss of a person by death (grief reaction), divorce, etc; financial reversal (crisis); or loss of an established role, such as being needed. Anger is frequently associated with the loss, and this in turn often produces a feeling of guilt. The disorder occurs within 3 months of the stressor and causes significant impairment in social or occupational functioning. The symptoms range from mild sadness, anxiety, irritability, worry, lack of concentration, discouragement, and somatic complaints to the more severe symptoms of the next group.

B. Depressive Disorders: The subclassifications include major depressive disorder and dysthymia.

1. A major depressive disorder (eg, "endogenous" unipolar disorder, melancholia) consists of at least one episode of serious mood depression that occurs at any time of life. Many consider a physiologic or metabolic aberration to be causative. Complaints vary widely but most frequently include a loss of interest and pleasure (anhedonia), withdrawal from activities, and feelings of guilt. Also included are inability to concentrate, some cognitive dysfunction, anxiety, chronic fatigue, feelings of worthlessness, somatic complaints (unidentifiable somatic complaints frequently indicate depression), loss of sexual drive, and thoughts of death. Diurnal variation with improvement as the day progresses is common. Vegetative signs that frequently occur are insomnia, anorexia with weight loss, and constipation. Occasionally, severe agitation and psychotic ideation (paranoid thinking, somatic delusions) are present. These symptoms are more common in postmenopausal depression (involutional melancholia). Paranoid symptoms may range from general suspiciousness to ideas of reference with delusions. The somatic delusions frequently revolve around feelings of impending annihilation or hypochondriacal beliefs (eg, that the body is rotting away with cancer). Hallucinations are uncommon.

Subcategories include **major depression with atypical features** characterized by hypersomnia, overeating, lethargy, and rejection sensitivity. **Major depression with a seasonal onset (seasonal affective disorder)** is a dysfunction of circadian rhythms that occurs more commonly in the winter months and is believed to be due to decreased exposure to full-spectrum light. Common symptoms include carbohydrate craving, lethargy, hyperphagia, and hypersomnia. **Major depression with postpartum onset** usually occurs 2 weeks to 6 months postpartum.

Most women (up to 80%) experience some mild letdown of mood in the postpartum period. For some of these (10–15%), the symptoms are more severe and similar to those usually seen in serious depression, with an increased emphasis on concerns related to the baby (obsessive thoughts about harming it or inability to care for it). When psychotic symptoms occur, there is frequently associated sleep deprivation, volatility of behavior, and manic-like symptoms. Postpartum psychosis is much less common (< 2%), often occurs within the first 2 weeks, and requires early and aggressive management. Biologic vulnerability with hormonal changes and psychosocial stressors all play a role. The chances of a second episode are about 25% and may be reduced with prophylactic treatment.

2. Dysthymia is a chronic depressive disturbance. Sadness, loss of interest, and withdrawal from activities over a period of 2 or more years with a relatively persistent course is necessary for this diagnosis. Generally, the symptoms are milder but longer-lasting than those in a major depressive episode.

3. Premenstrual dysphoric disorder usually has depressive symptoms during the late luteal phase of the menstrual cycles throughout the year.

C. Bipolar Disorders: Bipolar disorders (manic and depressive episodes) and individual manic episodes usually occur earlier (late teens or early adult life) than major depressive episodes.

1. A manic episode is a mood change characterized by elation with hyperactivity, overinvolvement in life activities, increased irritability, flight of ideas, easy distractibility, and little need for sleep. The overenthusiastic quality of the mood and the expansive behavior initially attract others, but the irritability, mood lability with swings into depression, aggressive behavior, and grandiosity usually lead to marked interpersonal difficulties. Activities may occur that are later regretted, eg, excessive spending, resignation from a job, a hasty marriage, sexual acting out, and exhibitionistic behavior, with alienation of friends and family. Atypical manic episodes can include gross delusions, paranoid ideation of severe proportions, and auditory hallucinations usually related to some grandiose perception. The episodes begin abruptly (sometimes precipitated by life stresses) and may last from several days to months. Spring and summer tend to be the peak periods. Generally, the manic episodes are of shorter duration than the depressive episodes. In almost all cases, the manic episode is part of a broader bipolar (manic-depressive) disorder. Patients with four or more discrete episodes of a mood disturbance in 1 year are called "rapid cyclers." (Substance abuse, particularly cocaine, can mimic rapid cycling.) These patients have a higher incidence of hypothyroidism. Manic patients differ from schizophrenics in that the former use more effective interpersonal maneuvers, are more sensitive to the social maneuvers of others, and are more able to utilize weakness and vulnerability in others to their own advantage. Creativity has been positively correlated with mood disorders, but the best work done is between episodes of mania and depression.

2. Cyclothymic disorders are chronic mood disturbances with episodes of depression and hypomania. The symptoms must have at least a 2-year duration and are milder than those that occur in depressive or manic episodes. Occasionally, the symptoms will escalate into a full-blown manic or depressive episode, in which case reclassification as bipolar disorder would be warranted.

D. Mood Disorders Secondary to Illness and Drugs: Any illness, severe or mild, can cause significant depression. Conditions such as rheumatoid arthritis, multiple sclerosis, and chronic heart disease are particularly likely to be associated with depression, as are other chronic illnesses. Hormonal variations clearly play a role in some depressions. Varying degrees of depression occur at various times in schizophrenic disorders, central nervous system disease, and organic mental states. **Alcohol dependency** frequently coexists with serious depression.

The classic model of drug-induced depression occurs with the use of reserpine, both in a clinical and a neurochemical sense. Corticosteroids and oral contraceptives are commonly associated with affective changes. Antihypertensive medications such as methyldopa, guanethidine, and clonidine have been associated with the development of depressive syndromes, as have digitalis and antiparkinsonism drugs (eg, levodopa). It is unusual for beta-blockers to produce depression when given for short periods, such as in the treatment of performance anxiety. Sustained use of beta-blockers for medical conditions such as hypertension may produce depression in some patients, though the literature is unclear on this subject. It is also unclear whether non-lipid-soluble beta-blockers are less likely to be associated with depression than lipid-soluble ones. Infrequently, disulfiram and anticholinesterase drugs may be associated with symptoms of depression. All stimulant use results in a depressive syndrome when the drug is withdrawn. Alcohol, sedatives, opiates, and most of the psychedelic drugs are depressants and, paradoxically, are often used in self-treatment of depression.

Differential Diagnosis

Since depression may be a part of any illness—either reactively or as a secondary symptom—careful attention must be given to personal life adjustment problems and the role of medications (eg, reserpine, corticosteroids, levodopa). Schizophrenia, partial complex seizures, organic brain syndromes, panic disorders, and anxiety disorders must be differentiated. Subtle thyroid dysfunction must be ruled out.

Complications

The longer the depression continues, the more crystallized it becomes—particularly when there is an element of secondary reinforcement. The most important complication is suicide, which often includes some elements of aggression. Suicide rates in the general population vary from 9 per 100,000 in Spain to 20 per 100,000 in the USA to 58 per 100,000 in Hungary. In individuals with depression, the lifetime risk rises to 10–15%. Males tend toward successful suicide, particularly in older age groups, whereas women make more attempts with lower mortality rates. An increased suicide rate is being observed in the younger population, ages 15–35. Patients with cancer, respiratory illnesses, AIDS, and those being maintained on hemodialysis have higher suicide rates. Alcohol is a significant factor in many suicide attempts.

There are four major groups of people who make suicide attempts:

(1) Those who are overwhelmed by problems in living (the despair of ordinary people). By far the greatest number fall into this category. There is often great ambivalence; they don't really want to die, but they don't want to go on as before either. These may be impulsive or aggressive acts not associated with significant depression.

(2) Those who are clearly attempting to control others. This is the blatant attempt in the vicinity of a significant other person in order to hurt or control that person.

(3) Those with severe depressions (high-risk group). This group includes both exogenous conditions (eg, AIDS, whose victims have a suicide rate over 30 times that of the general population) and endogenous conditions (eg, panic disorders). It also includes those who may not be diagnosed as having depression but who are overwhelmed by a serious stressful situation (eg, the man charged with child molestation who hangs himself in his cell). Anxiety, panic, and fear are major findings in suicidal behavior. A patient may seem to make a dramatic improvement, but the lifting of depression may be due to the patient's decision to commit suicide.

(4) Those with psychotic illness (high-risk group). These individuals tend not to verbalize their concerns, are unpredictable, and are often successful but comprise a small percentage of the total. (Suicide is ten times more prevalent in schizophrenics than in the general population, and jumping from bridges is more common. In one study of 100 jumpers, 47% were schizophrenic.)

The immediate goal of psychiatric evaluation is to assess the current suicidal risk and the need for hospitalization versus outpatient management. The intent is less likely to be truly suicidal, for example, if small amounts of poison or drugs were ingested or scratching of wrists was superficial; if the act was performed in the vicinity of others or with early notification of others; or if the attempt was arranged so that early detection would be anticipated. Alcohol, hopelessness, delusional thoughts, and complete or nearly complete loss of interest in life or ability to experience pleasure are all positively correlated with suicide attempts. Other risk factors are previous attempts, a family history of suicide, medical or psychiatric illness (eg, anxiety, depression, psychosis), male sex, older age, contemplation of violent methods, and drug use (including long-term sedative or alcohol use), which contributes to impulsiveness or mood swings. Successful treatment of the patient at risk for suicide cannot be achieved if the patient continues to abuse drugs.

The patient's current mood status is best evaluated by direct evaluation of plans and concerns about the future, personal reactions to the attempt, and thoughts about the reactions of others. The patient's immediate resources should be assessed—people who can be significantly involved (most important), family support, job situation, financial resources, etc.

If hospitalization is not indicated (eg, gestures, impulsive attempts; see above), the physician must formulate and institute a treatment plan or make an adequate referral. Medication should be dispensed in small amounts to at-risk patients. Although tricyclics and SSRIs are associated with an equal incidence of suicide attempts, the risk of successful suicide is higher with tricyclic overdose. Guns and drugs should be removed from the patient's household. Driving should be interdicted until the patient improves. The problem is often worsened by the long-term complications of the suicide attempt, eg, brain damage due to hypoxia; peripheral neuropathies caused by staying for long periods in one position, causing nerve compressions; and medical or surgical problems such as esophageal strictures and tendon dysfunctions.

The reasons for self-mutilation, most commonly wrist cutting (but also autocastration, autoamputation, and autoenucleation, which are associated with psychoses), may be very different from the reasons for a suicide attempt. The initial treatment plan, however, should presume suicidal ideation, and conservative treatment should be initiated.

Sleep disturbances in the depressions are discussed below.

Treatment of Depression

A. Medical: Depression associated with reactive disorders usually does not call for drug therapy and can be managed by psychotherapy and the passage of time. In severe cases—particularly when vegetative signs are significant and symptoms have persisted for more than a few weeks—antidepressant drug therapy is often effective. Drug therapy is also suggested by a family history of major depression in first-degree relatives or a past history of prior episodes.

The antidepressant drugs may be conveniently classified into three groups: (1) the newer antidepressants, including the serotonin-selective reuptake inhibitors (SSRIs) and bupropion, venlafaxine, nefazodone, and mirtazapine; (2) the tricyclic antidepressants (TCAs) and clinically similar drugs; and (3) the monoamine oxidase (MAO) inhibitors. These groups are described in greater detail below. Electroconvulsive therapy is effective in all types of depression (particularly involutional melancholia) and will also rapidly resolve a manic episode. It is also very effective for postpartum depression. Megavitamin treatment, acupuncture, and electrosleep are of unproved usefulness for any psychiatric condition.

Hospitalization is necessary if suicide is a major consideration or if complex treatment modalities are required.

Drug selection is influenced by the history of previous responses if that information is available. If a relative has responded to a particular drug, this suggests that the patient may respond similarly. If no background information is available, a drug such as desipramine, starting with 50 mg and gradually increasing to 150 mg daily, or sertraline, 50 mg daily, can be selected and a *full trial* instituted. The medication trial should be monitored every 1–2 weeks until week 6. If successful, the medication should be continued for 6–12 months at the full therapeutic dose before tapering is considered. Antidepressants should be continued indefinitely at full dosage in individuals with more than two episodes after age 40 or one episode after age 50. If the response is inadequate despite a diagnosis supported by review and adequate drug levels, a drug from a different group (eg, fluoxetine) is given a trial. If the second drug fails, augmentation with lithium (eg, 600–900 mg/d) or thyroid medication (eg, liothyronine, 25 μg/d) should be considered. Dysthymia is also treated in this way. The Agency for Health Care Policy and Research has produced clinical practice guidelines that outline one algorithm of treatment decisions (Figure 25–3).

Psychotic depression can be treated with a combination of an antipsychotic such as perphenazine (used initially) and an antidepressant such as an SSRI at their usual doses.

Major depression with atypical features or seasonal onset can be treated with an MAO inhibitor or an SSRI with good results.

Stimulants such as dextroamphetamine (5–30 mg/d) and methylphenidate (10–45 mg/d) have enjoyed a resurgence of interest for the short-term treatment of depression in medically ill and geriatric patients. Their 50–60% efficacy rate is slightly below that of other agents. The stimulants are notable for rapid onset of action (hours) and a paucity of side effects (tachycardia, agitation) in most patients. They are usually given in two divided doses early in the day (eg, 7 AM and noon) so as to avoid interfering with sleep. These agents may also be useful as adjunctive agents in refractory depression.

Caution: Depressed patients may have suicidal thoughts, and the amount of drug dispensed should be appropriately controlled. The older tricyclics have a narrow therapeutic index, and one advantage of the newer drugs is their wider margin of safety. In all cases of pharmacologic management of depressed states, caution is indicated until the risk of suicide is considered minimal.

1. SSRIs and atypical antidepressants–The chief advantages of these agents are that they do not cause significant cardiovascular or anticholinergic side effects or significant weight gain, as do the tricyclic agents. The serotonin-selective reuptake inhibitors (SSRIs) include fluoxetine, sertraline, paroxetine, fluvoxamine, and citalopram. The atypical antidepressants are bupropion, which appears to exert its effect through the dopamine neurotransmitter system; venlafaxine, which inhibits the reuptake of both serotonin and norepinephrine; nefazodone, which blocks the reuptake of serotonin but also inhibits the 5-HT_2 postsynaptic receptors; and mirtazapine, which selectively blocks presynaptic α_2-adrenergic receptors and enhances both noradrenergic and serotonergic transmission. All of these antidepressants are effective in the treatment of depression, both typical and atypical. The SSRI drugs have been effective in the treatment of panic attacks, bulimia, and obsessive-compulsive disorders, while bupropion may have some particular effectiveness in the treatment of rapid-cycling bipolar disorder. They do not seem to be as clearly effective in some pain syndromes as the tricyclics, though venlafaxine may have some efficacy in the treatment of neuropathic pain.

Most of the drugs in this group tend to be activating and are given in the morning so as not to interfere with sleep. Some patients, however, may have sedation, requiring that the drug be given at bedtime. This reaction occurs most commonly with paroxetine, fluvoxamine, and mirtazapine. The SSRIs can be given in once-daily dosage. Bupropion is usually given in three divided doses daily. Nefazodone and venlafaxine are usually given twice daily. Bupropion and venlafaxine are available in extended-release formulations. There is usually some delay in response; fluoxetine, for example, requires 2–6 weeks to act in depression, 4–8 weeks to be effective in panic disorder, and 6–12 weeks in treatment of obsessive-compulsive disorder. The starting dose (10–20 mg) is the usual daily dose for depression, while obsessive-compulsive disorder may require up to 80 mg daily. Some patients, particularly the elderly, may tolerate

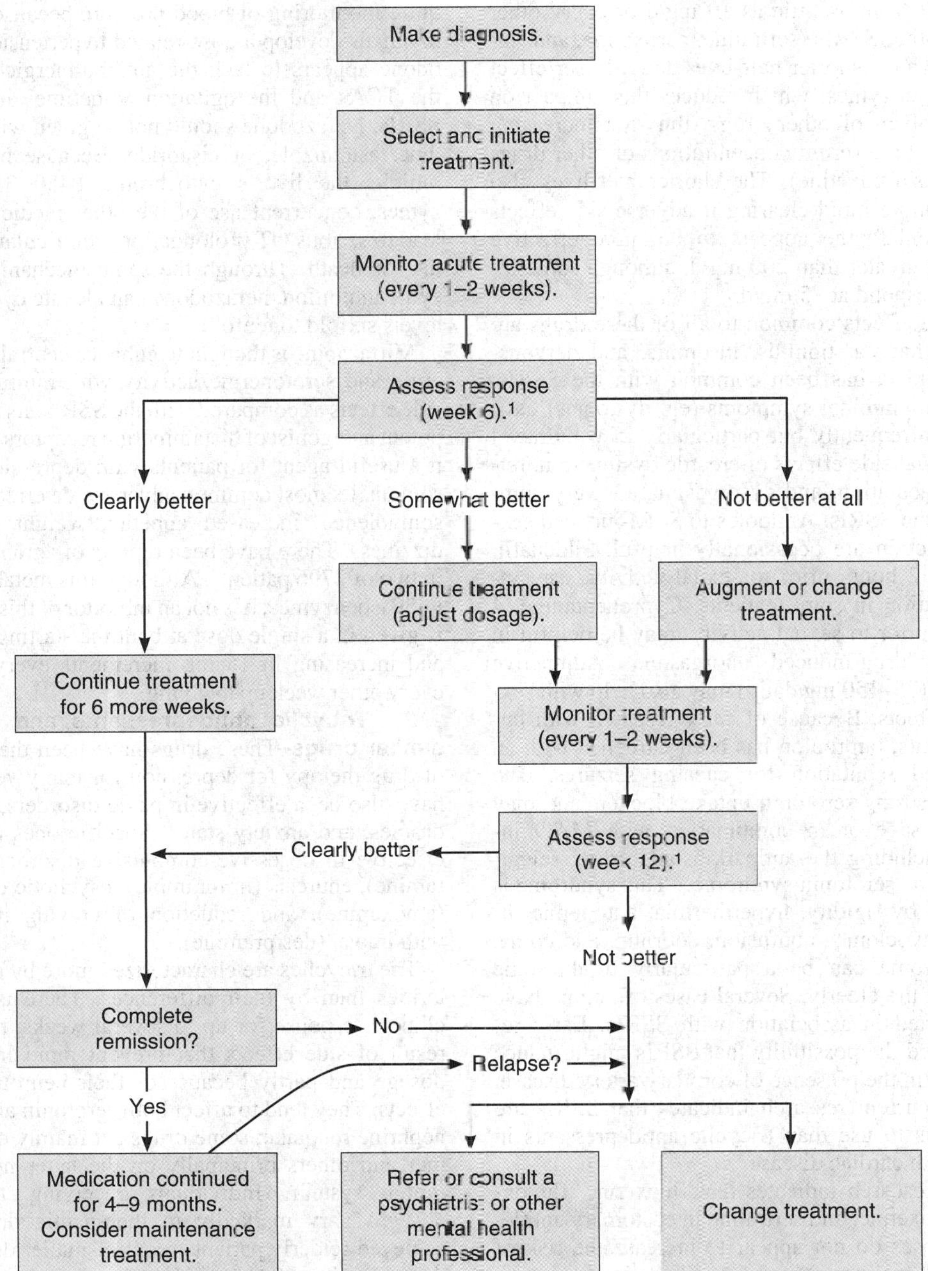

Figure 25–3. Overview of treatment for depression. (Reproduced, with permission, from Agency for Health Care Policy and Research: *Depression in Primary Care*. Vol. 2: *Treatment of Major Depression*. United States Department of Health and Human Services, 1993.)

and benefit from as little as 10 mg/d or every other day. The other SSRIs (sertraline, paroxetine, and fluvoxamine) have shorter half-lives and a lesser effect on hepatic enzymes, which reduces their impact on the metabolism of other drugs (thus not increasing significantly the serum concentrations of other drugs as much as fluoxetine). The shorter half-lives also allow for more rapid clearing if adverse side effects appear. Venlafaxine appears to be more effective with doses greater than 200 mg/d, although some individuals respond at 75 mg/d.

The side effects common to all of these drugs are headache, nausea, tinnitus, insomnia, and nervousness. Akathisia has been common with the SSRIs; other extrapyramidal symptoms (eg, dystonias) have occurred infrequently but particularly in withdrawal states. Sexual side effects of erectile dysfunction, retrograde ejaculation, and dysorgasmia are very common with the SSRIs. Antidotes to SSRI-induced sexual dysfunction are occasionally helpful. Sildenafil, 25–50 mg 2 hours prior to sexual activity, can improve function in some patients. Cyproheptadine, 4 mg orally prior to sexual activity, may be helpful in countering drug-induced anorgasmia. Adjunctive bupropion (75–150 mg daily) may also help with sexual side effects. Because of early research with bulimic patients, bupropion has been burdened with an unwarranted reputation for causing seizures. The SSRIs are strong serotonin uptake blockers and may in high dosage or in combination with MAO inhibitors, including the antiparkinsonian drug selegiline, cause a "serotonin syndrome." This syndrome is manifested by rigidity, hyperthermia, autonomic instability, myoclonus, confusion, delirium, and coma. This syndrome can be a particularly troublesome problem in the elderly. Several cases of angina have been reported in association with SSRIs. Early research raised the possibility that SSRIs might induce vasospasm in the presence of coronary artery disease. However, current research indicates that SSRIs are safer agents to use than tricyclic antidepressants in patients with cardiac disease.

Recent research indicates that fluoxetine, fluvoxamine, paroxetine, and sertraline in customary antidepressant doses do not appear to increase the risk of major fetal malformation when used in pregnancy. Postpartum developmental effects are thought to be minimal, but this question has not been well studied. Both TCAs and fluoxetine are associated with a higher risk of miscarriage, but this may be related to the underlying depressive disorder. The decision to use SSRIs and other psychotropic agents during pregnancy must be based on a risk-benefit analysis for each individual.

Venlafaxine is reported to be well tolerated without significant anticholinergic or cardiovascular side effects. Nausea, nervousness, and profuse sweating appear to be the major side effects. Venlafaxine appears to have few drug-drug interactions. It does require monitoring of blood pressure because some individuals develop a dose-related hypertension. Nefazodone appears to lack the anticholinergic effects of the TCAs and the agitation sometimes induced by SSRIs. Nefazodone should not be given with terfenadine, astemizole, or cisapride. Because nefazodone inhibits the liver's cytochrome P450 3A4 isoenzymes, concurrent use of the other medications can lead to serious QT prolongation, ventricular tachycardia, or death. Through the same mechanism of enzyme inhibition, nefazodone can elevate cyclosporine levels sixfold to tenfold.

Mirtazapine is thought to enhance central noradrenergic and serotonergic activity with minimal sexual side effects as compared with the SSRIs. Its action as a potent antagonist of histaminergic receptors may make it a useful agent for patients with depression and insomnia. Its most common adverse side effects include somnolence, increased appetite, weight gain, and dizziness. There have been reports of agranulocytosis in two of 2796 patients. Although it is metabolized by P450 isoenzymes, it is not an inhibitor of this system. It is given in a single dose at bedtime starting at 15 mg and increasing in 15 mg increments every week or every other week up to 45 mg.

2. Tricyclic antidepressants and clinically similar drugs–These drugs have been the mainstay of drug therapy for depression for many years. They have also been effective in panic disorders, pain syndromes, and anxiety states. Specific ones have been effective in obsessive-compulsive disorder (clomipramine), enuresis (imipramine), psychotic depression (amoxapine), and reduction of craving in cocaine withdrawal (desipramine).

The tricyclics are characterized more by their similarities than by their differences. There is a lag in clinical response for up to several weeks, partly as a result of side effects that prevent rapid increase in dosage and partly because of their neurotransmitter effects. They tend to affect both serotonin and norepinephrine reuptake; some drugs act mainly on the former and others principally on the latter neurotransmitter system. Individuals receiving the same dosages vary markedly in therapeutic drug levels achieved (elderly patients require smaller doses), and determination of plasma drug levels is helpful when clinical response has been disappointing. Nortriptyline is usually effective when plasma levels are between 50 and 150 ng/mL; imipramine at plasma levels of 200–250 ng/mL; and desipramine at plasma levels of 100–250 ng/mL. High blood levels are not more effective than moderate levels and may be counterproductive (eg, delirium, seizures). Patients with gastrointestinal side effects benefit from plasma level monitoring to assess absorption of the drug. Most of the tricyclics can be given in a single dose at bedtime, starting at fairly low doses (eg, nortriptyline 25 mg orally) and increasing by 25 mg every several days as tolerated until the therapeutic response is achieved (eg, nortriptyline, 100–150 mg) or to maximum dose if necessary (eg, nortriptyline, 150 mg). The most common cause of treatment failure is an inadequate trial. A full trial consists of giving maximum daily dosage for at least 2 and preferably 4 weeks. To reach maximum dosage, the trial encompasses a total of about 6 weeks. Because of marked anticholinergic and sedating side effects, clomipramine is started at a low dose (25 mg/d orally) and increased slowly in divided doses up to 100 mg/d, held at that level for several days, and then gradually increased as necessary up to 250 mg/d. Any of the TCA-like drugs should be started at very low doses (eg, 10–25 mg/d) and increased slowly in the treatment of panic disorder.

The tricyclic antidepressants have anticholinergic side effects to varying degrees (amitriptyline 100 mg is equivalent to atropine 5 mg). One must be particularly wary of the effect in elderly men with prostatic hyperplasia. The anticholinergic effects also predispose to other medical problems such as heat stroke or dental problems from xerostomia. Orthostatic hypotension is fairly common, may not remit with time, and is a major problem in elderly women with osteoporosis who may suffer a hip fracture after a fall. Cardiac effects of the TCAs are functions of the anticholinergic effect, direct myocardial depression (quinidine-like effect), and interference with adrenergic neurons. These factors may produce altered rate, rhythm, and contractility, particularly in patients with preexisting cardiac disease, such as bundle-branch or bifascicular block. Electrocardiographic changes range from benign ST segment and T wave changes and sinus tachycardia to a variety of complex and serious arrhythmias, the latter requiring a change in medication. Because TCAs have class I antiarrhythmic effects, they should be used with caution in patients with ischemic heart disease, arrhythmias, or conduction disturbances. SSRIs or the atypical antidepressants may be better initial choices for this population. TCAs lower the seizure threshold so this is of particular concern in patients with a propensity for seizures (eg, previous head injury, alcohol withdrawal). Loss of libido and erectile, ejaculatory, and orgasmic dysfunction are fairly common and can compromise compliance. Trazodone rarely causes priapism, which requires treatment within 12 hours (epinephrine 1:1000 injected into the corpus cavernosum). Delirium, agitation, and mania are infrequent complications. Sudden discontinuation of some of these drugs can produce "cholinergic rebound," manifested by headaches and nausea with abdominal cramps. Overdoses of the tricyclic compounds are often serious because of the narrow therapeutic index and quinidine-like effects (see Chapter 39).

3. Monoamine oxidase inhibitors–The MAO inhibitors are now generally used as third-line drugs for depression (after a failure of tricyclics, SSRIs, or the atypical antidepressants) because of the dietary and other restrictions required (see below and Table 25–7). They should be considered as drugs of first choice in atypical depression (with rejection sensitivity) or as useful agents for panic disorder or refractory depression.

MAO inhibitors are administered in gradual stepwise dosage and may be given in the morning or evening, depending upon their effect on sleep. They tend to take effect in a fairly low dosage range (Table 25–8). Blood levels are not congruent with therapeutic response.

The MAO inhibitors commonly cause symptoms of orthostatic hypotension (which may persist) and sympathomimetic effects of tachycardia, sweating, and tremor. Nausea, insomnia (often associated with intense afternoon drowsiness), and sexual dysfunction are common. Trazodone, 25–75 mg orally at bedtime, may ameliorate the MAO-induced insomnia. Central nervous system effects include agitation and toxic psychoses. Dietary limitations (Table 25–7) and abstinence from drug products containing phenylpropanolamine, phenylephrine, meperidine, dextromethorphan, and pseudoephedrine are mandatory for MAO-A type inhibitors (those marketed for treatment of depression), since the reduction of available monoamine oxidase leaves the patient vulnerable to exogenous amines (eg, tyramine in foodstuffs).

Treatment for a resultant hypertensive crisis has been the same as for pheochromocytoma (see Chapter 26), but there have been reports of success with nifedipine, 10 mg chewed and placed under the tongue, normalizing blood pressure in 1–5 minutes. The restrictions on the proscribed foodstuffs and sympathomimetic drugs are in effect during treatment and for 2–3 weeks after cessation of therapy. Termination of therapy with MAO inhibitors may be associated with anxiety, agitation, cognitive slowing, and headache. Very gradual withdrawal and short-term benzodiazepine therapy will ameliorate symptoms.

4. Switching and combination therapy–If the therapeutic response has been poor after an adequate trial with the chosen drug, one should reassess the diagnosis. Assuming that the trial has been adequate and the diagnosis is correct, a trial with a drug from another group is appropriate. In switching from one group to another, an adequate "washout time" must be allowed. This is critical in certain situations—eg, in switching from an MAO inhibitor to a

Table 25–7. Principal dietary restrictions in MAOI use.

1. Cheese, except cream cheese and cottage cheese and fresh yogurt
2. Fermented or aged meats such as bologna, salami
3. Broad bean pods such as Chinese bean pods
4. Liver of all types
5. Meat and yeast extracts
6. Red wine, sherry, vermouth, cognac, beer, ale
7. Soy sauce, shrimp paste, sauerkraut

Table 25–8. Commonly used antidepressants.

	Usual Daily Oral Dose (mg)	Usual Daily Maximum Dose (mg)	Sedative Effects[1]	Anticholinergic Effects[1]	Cost per Unit	Cost for 30 Days' Treatment Based on Maximum Dosage[2]
TRICYCLIC AND CLINICALLY SIMILAR COMPOUNDS						
Amitriptyline (Elavil)	150–250	300	4	4	$0.31/150 mg	$18.60
Amoxapine (Asendin)	150–200	400	2	2	$1.67/100 mg	$200.40
Clomipramine (Anafranil)	100	250	3	3	$1.33/75 mg	$119.70
Desipramine (Norpramin)	100–250	300	1	1	$1.07/100 mg	$96.30
Doxepin (Sinequan)	150–200	300	4	3	$1.00/100 mg	$90.00
Imipramine (Tofranil)	150–200	300	3	3	$0.69/50 mg	$24.20
Maprotiline (Ludiomil)	100–200	300	4	2	$0.89/75 mg	$106.80
Nortriptyline (Aventyl, Pamelor)	100–150	150	2	2	$1.55/50 mg	$139.50
Protriptyline (Vivactil)	15–40	60	1	3	$0.64/10 mg	$115.20
Trazodone (Desyrel)	100–300	400	4	< 1	$0.41/100 mg	$49.20
Trimipramine (Surmontil)	75–200	200	4	4	$1.87/100 mg	$112.20
Bupropion (Wellbutrin)	300[3]	450[3]		< 1	$1.07/100 mg	$144.45
Bupropion SR (Wellbutrin SR)	300	400[4]		< 1	$1.43/100 mg $1.53/150 mg	$85.80 $91.80
SSRIs AND OTHER NEW COMPOUNDS						
Fluoxetine (Prozac)	5–40	80	< 1	< 1	$2.64/20 mg	$316.80
Fluvoxamine (Luvox)	100–300	300	1	< 1	$2.82/100 mg	$253.80
Nefazodone (Serzone)	300–600	600	2	< 1	$1.24/200 mg	$111.60
Paroxetine (Paxil)	20–30	50	1	1	$2.43/20 mg	$182.25
Sertraline (Zoloft)	50–150	200	< 1	< 1	$2.41/100 mg	$144.60
Venlafaxine (Effexor)	150–225	375	1	< 1	$1.31/75 mg	$196.50
Venlafaxine XR (Effexor)	150–225	225	1	< 1	$2.32/75 mg	$208.80
Mirtazepine (Remeron)	15–45	45	4	2	$2.55/30 mg	$114.75
Citalopram (Celexa)	20	40	< 1	1	$2.10/40 mg	$63.00
MONOAMINE OXIDASE INHIBITORS						
Phenelzine (Nardil)	45–60	90	...	...	$0.46/15 mg	$82.80
Tranylcypromine (Parnate)	20–30	50	...	...	$0.55/10 mg	$82.50

[1]**Key:** 4 = strong effect; 1 = weak effect
[2]Cost to pharmacist (average wholesale price, generic when possible) for quantity listed. Source: *Drug Topics Red Book,* March 2000; Vol. 19, No. 3.
[3]No single dose should exceed 150 mg.
[4]200 mg twice daily.

tricyclic, allow 2–3 weeks between stopping one drug and starting another; in switching from an SSRI to an MAO inhibitor, allow 4–5 weeks. In switching within groups—eg, from one tricyclic to another (amitriptyline to desipramine, etc)—no washout time is needed, and one can rapidly decrease the dosage of one drug while increasing the other. Combining two antidepressants requires caution and is usually reserved for refractory patients after psychiatric consultation.

However, in any of the three groups, one can augment the antidepressant drug if the therapeutic response has been less than satisfactory. Lithium and thyroid hormone (eg, 25 μg daily of liothyronine) are the most commonly used augmenting agents. Lithium is an excellent augmentation agent for the 25–40% of depressed patients who fail to respond to an adequate trial of an antidepressant. One-half of these patients will respond to the addition of lithium

(600–900 mg/d) with an enhanced antidepressant effect.

5. Maintenance and tapering–When clinical relief of symptoms is obtained, medication is continued for 12 months in the effective maintenance dosage, which is the dosage required in the acute stage. The full dosage should be continued indefinitely when the individual has a first episode before age 20 or after age 50; is over age 40 with two episodes; or has had three episodes at any age. Major depression should often be considered as a chronic disease. If the medication is being tapered, it should be done gradually over several months, monitoring closely for relapse.

6. Drug interactions–Interactions with other drugs are listed in Table 25–9.

7. Electroconvulsive therapy (ECT)–ECT causes a generalized central nervous system seizure (peripheral convulsion is not necessary) by means of electric current. The key objective is to exceed the seizure threshold, which can be accomplished by a variety of means. Electrical stimulation is more reliable and simpler than the use of chemical convulsants. The mechanism of action is not known, but it is thought to involve major neurotransmitter responses at the cell membrane. Current insufficient to cause a seizure produces no therapeutic benefit.

Electroconvulsive therapy is the most effective (about 70–85%) treatment of severe depression, particularly the delusions and agitation commonly seen with depression in the involutional period. It is indicated when medical conditions preclude the use of antidepressants or in cases of nonresponsiveness to these medications. Comparative controlled studies of electroconvulsive therapy in severe depression show that it is more effective than chemotherapy. It is also effective in the manic disorders and psychoses during pregnancy (when drugs may be contraindicated). It has not been shown to be helpful in chronic schizophrenic disorders, and it is generally not used in acute schizophrenic episodes unless drugs are not effective and it is urgent that the psychosis be controlled (eg, a catatonic stupor complicating an acute medical condition).

The most common side effects are memory disturbance and headache. Memory loss or confusion is usually related to number and frequency of electroconvulsive therapy treatments and proper oxygenation during treatment. Some memory loss is occasionally permanent, but most memory faculties return to full capacity within several weeks. There have been reports that lithium administration concurrent with electroconvulsive therapy resulted in greater memory loss. Before anesthesia was used, spinal compression fractures and severe anticipatory anxiety were common.

Increased intracranial pressure is a serious contraindication. Other problems such as cardiac disorders, aortic aneurysms, bronchopulmonary disease, and venous thrombosis are relative contraindications and must be evaluated in light of the severity of the medical problem versus the need for electroconvulsive therapy. Serious complications arising from electroconvulsive therapy occur in less than one in 1000 cases. Most of these problems are cardiovascular or respiratory in nature (eg, aspiration of gastric contents). Poor patient understanding and lack of acceptance of the technique by the public are the biggest obstacles to the use of electroconvulsive therapy.

Table 25–9. Antidepressant drug interactions with other drugs.

Drug	Effects
Tricyclic and other non-MAOI antidepressants	
Antacids	Decreased absorption of antidepressants.
Anticoagulants	Increased hypoprothrombinemic effect.
Cimetidine	Increased antidepressant blood levels and psychosis.
Clonidine	Decreased antihypertensive effect.
Digitalis	Increased incidence of heart block.
Disulfiram	Increased antidepressant blood levels.
Guanethidine	Decreased antihypertensive effect.
Haloperidol	Increased clomipramine levels.
Insulin	Decreased blood sugar.
Lithium	Increased lithium levels with fluoxetine.
Methyldopa	Decreased antihypertensive effect.
Other anticholinergic drugs	Marked anticholinergic responses.
Phenytoin	Increased blood levels.
Procainamide	Decreased ventricular conduction.
Procarbazine	Hypertensive crisis.
Propranolol	Increased hypotension.
Quinidine	Decreased ventricular conduction.
Rauwolfia derivatives	Increased stimulation.
Sedatives	Increased sedation.
Sympathomimetic drugs	Increased pressor effect.
Terfenadine	Torsades de pointes
Monoamine oxidase inhibitors	
Antihistamines	Increased sedation.
Belladonna-like drugs	Increased blood pressure.
Dextromethorphan	Same as meperidine.
Guanethidine	Decreased blood pressure.
Insulin	Decreased blood sugar.
Levodopa	Increased blood pressure.
Meperidine	Increased agitation, seizures, coma, death.
Methyldopa	Decreased blood pressure.
Pseudoephedrine	Hypertensive crisis (increased blood pressure).
Reserpine	Increased blood pressure and temperature.
Succinylcholine	Increased neuromuscular blockade.
Sulfonylureas	Decreased blood sugar.
Sympathomimetic drugs	Increased blood pressure.

3. Phototherapy is used in major depression with seasonal onset. It consists of exposure (at a 3-foot distance) to a light source of 2500 lux for 2 hours daily. Light visors are an adaptation that provides greater mobility and an adjustable light intensity. The price of these full-spectrum light sources range between $300 and $400. The dosage varies, with some patients requiring morning and night exposure. One effect is alteration of biorhythm through melatonin mechanisms.

B. Psychologic: It is seldom possible to engage an individual in penetrating psychotherapeutic endeavors during the acute stage of a severe depression. While medications may be taking effect, a supportive approach to strengthen existing defenses and appropriate consideration of the patient's continuing need to function at work, to engage in recreational activities, etc, are necessary as the severity of the depression lessens. If the patient is not seriously depressed, it is often quite appropriate to initiate intensive psychotherapeutic efforts, since flux periods are a good time to effect change. A catharsis of repressed anger and guilt may be beneficial. Therapy during or just after the acute stage may focus on coping techniques, with some practice of alternative choices. When lack of self-confidence and identity problems are factors in the depression, individual psychotherapy can be oriented to ways of improving self-esteem, increasing assertiveness, and lessening dependency. Cognitive psychotherapy addresses patients' patterns of negative thoughts, called cognitive distortions, that lead to feelings of depression and anxiety. Treatment usually includes homework assignments such as keeping a journal of cognitive distortions and of positive responses to them. As previously noted, numerous studies have shown that the combination of drug therapy plus cognitive psychotherapy is more effective than either modality alone. It is usually helpful to involve the spouse or other significant family members early in treatment.

C. Social: Flexible use of appropriate social services can be of major importance in the treatment of depression. Since alcohol is often associated with depression, early involvement in alcohol treatment programs such as Alcoholics Anonymous can be important to future success (see Alcohol Dependency and Abuse, below). The structuring of daily activities during severe depression is often quite difficult for the patient, and loneliness is often a major factor. The help of family, employer, or friends is often necessary to mobilize the patient who experiences no joy in daily activities and tends to remain uninvolved and to deteriorate. Insistence on sharing activities will help involve the patient in simple but important daily functions. In some severe cases, the use of day treatment centers or support groups of a specific type (eg, mastectomy groups) is indicated. It is not unusual for a patient to have multiple legal, financial, and vocational problems requiring legal and vocational assistance.

D. Behavioral: When depression is a function of self-defeating coping techniques such as passivity, the role-playing approach can be useful. Behavioral techniques, including desensitization, may be used in problems such as phobias where depression is a by-product. When depression is a regularly used interpersonal style, behavioral counseling to family members or others can help in extinguishing the behavior in the patient.

Treatment of Mania

Acute manic or hypomanic symptoms will respond to lithium therapy after several days of treatment, but it is common to use neuroleptic drugs or high-potency benzodiazepines (eg, clonazepam) to immediately treat the excited or psychotic manic stage. Some schizoaffective disorders and some cases of so-called schizophrenia are probably atypical bipolar affective disorder, for which lithium treatment may be effective.

A. Neuroleptics: Acute manic symptoms of agitation and psychosis may be initially treated with haloperidol, 5–10 mg orally or intramuscularly every 2–3 hours until symptoms subside. The dosage of haloperidol is gradually reduced after lithium or another mood stabilizer is started (see below). Recent studies indicate that the atypical neuroleptic olanzapine (5–20 mg/d) is as efficacious as haloperidol in the treatment of acute mania.

B. Clonazepam: Clonazepam is an alternative to a neuroleptic such as haloperidol in controlling acute behavioral symptoms. Clonazepam has the advantage of causing no extrapyramidal side effects. Although 1–2 mg orally every 4–6 hours may be effective, up to 16 mg/d may be necessary.

C. Lithium: As a prophylactic drug for bipolar affective disorder, lithium significantly decreases the frequency and severity of both manic and depressive attacks in about 70% of patients. A positive response is more predictable if the patient has a low frequency of episodes (no more than two per year with intervals free of psychopathology). A positive response occurs more frequently in individuals who have blood relatives with a diagnosis of manic or hypomanic attacks. Patients who swing rapidly back and forth between manic and depressive attacks (at least four cycles per year) usually respond poorly to lithium prophylaxis initially, but some improve with continued long-term treatment. Carbamazepine (see below) has been used with success in this group.

In addition to its use in manic states, lithium is sometimes useful in the prophylaxis of recurrent unipolar depressions (perhaps undiagnosed bipolar disorder). Lithium may ameliorate nonspecific aggressive behaviors and dyscontrol syndromes. The dosages are the same as used in bipolar disorder. Most patients with bipolar disease can be managed long-term with lithium alone, though some will require continued or intermittent use of a neuroleptic, antidepressant, or carbamazepine. An excellent resource for information pertaining to lithium is the Lithium Information Center, Dean Foundation, 8000 Excelsior Drive, Suite 302, Madison, WI 53717-1914.

Before treatment, the clinical workup should include a medical history and physical examination; complete blood count; T_4, TSH, blood urea nitrogen, serum creatinine, and serum electrolyte determinations; urinalysis; and electrocardiography in patients over age 45 or with a history of cardiac disease.

1. Dosage–Lithium carbonate is generally prescribed in the 300 mg unit. In a small minority of patients, a slow release form or units of different dosage may be required. Lithium citrate is available as a syrup. The dosage is that required to maintain blood levels in the therapeutic range. For acute attacks, this ranges from 1 to 1.5 meq/L. Although there is controversy about the optimal chronic maintenance dose, many clinicians reduce the acute level to 0.6–1 meq/L in order to reduce side effects. The dose required to meet this need will vary in different individuals. For acute mania, doses of 1200–1800 mg/d are generally recommended. Augmentation of antidepressants is usually achieved with one-half of these doses. Once-a-day dosage is acceptable, but most patients have less nausea when they take the drug in divided doses with meals.

Lithium is readily absorbed, with peak serum levels occurring within 1–3 hours and complete absorption in 8 hours. Half of the total body lithium is excreted in 18–24 hours (95% in the urine). Blood for lithium levels should be drawn 12 hours after the last dose. Serum levels should be measured 5–7 days after initiation of treatment and changes in dose. For maintenance treatment, lithium levels should be monitored initially every 1–2 months but may be measured every 6–12 months in stable, long-term patients. Levels should be monitored more closely when there is any condition that causes volume depletion (eg, diarrhea; dehydration; use of diuretics).

2. Side effects–Mild gastrointestinal symptoms (take lithium with food), fine tremors (treat with propranolol, 20–60 mg/d orally, only if persistent), slight muscle weakness, and some degree of somnolence are early side effects that are usually transient. Moderate polyuria (reduced renal responsiveness to antidiuretic hormone) and polydipsia (associated with increased plasma renin concentration) are often present. Potassium administration can blunt this effect, as may once-daily dosing of lithium. Weight gain (often a result of calories in fluids taken for polydipsia) and leukocytosis not due to infection are fairly common.

Other side effects include goiter (3%; often euthyroid), hypothyroidism (10%; concomitant administration of lithium and iodide or lithium and carbamazepine enhances the hypothyroid and goitrogenic effect of either drug), changes in the glucose tolerance test toward a diabetes-like curve, nephrogenic diabetes insipidus (usually resolving about 8 weeks after cessation of lithium therapy), nephrotic syndrome, edema, folate deficiency, and pseudotumor cerebri (ophthalmoscopy is indicated if there are complaints of headache or blurred vision). A metallic taste, hair loss, and Raynaud's phenomenon have been reported in a few cases. Thyroid and kidney function should be checked at 3- to 4-month intervals. Most of these side effects subside when lithium is discontinued; when residual side effects exist, they are usually not serious. Most clinicians treat lithium-induced hypothyroidism (more common in women) with thyroid hormone while continuing lithium therapy. Hypercalcemia and elevated parathyroid hormone levels occur in some patients. Electrocardiographic abnormalities (principally T wave flattening or inversion) may occur during lithium administration but are not of major clinical significance. Sinoatrial block may occur, particularly in the elderly. It is important that other drugs which prolong intraventricular conduction, such as tricyclics, be used with caution in conjunction with lithium. Lithium impairs ventilatory function in patients with airway obstruction. Lithium alone does not have a significant effect on sexual function, but when combined with benzodiazepines (clonazepam in most symptomatic patients) it causes sexual dysfunction in about 50% of male patients. Lithium may precipitate or exacerbate psoriasis in some patients.

Patients receiving long-term lithium therapy may have cogwheel rigidity and, occasionally, other extrapyramidal signs. Lithium potentiates the parkinsonian effects of haloperidol. Long-term lithium therapy has also been associated with a relative lowering of the level of memory and perceptual processing (affecting compliance in some cases). Some impairment of attention and emotional reactivity has also been noted. Lithium-induced delirium with therapeutic lithium levels is an infrequent complication usually occurring in the elderly and may persist for several days after serum levels have become negligible. Encephalopathy has occurred in patients receiving combined lithium and neuroleptic therapy and in those who have cerebrovascular disease, thus requiring careful evaluation of patients who develop neurotoxic signs at subtoxic blood levels.

Some reports have suggested that the long-term use of lithium may have adverse effects on renal function (with interstitial fibrosis or tubular atrophy). A rise in serum creatinine levels is an indication for in-depth evaluation of renal function. Incontinence has been reported in women, apparently related to changes in bladder cholinergic-adrenergic balance.

Lithium exposure in early pregnancy increases the frequency of congenital anomalies, especially Ebstein's and other major cardiovascular anomalies. It is advisable for women using lithium either to avoid pregnancy or not to use lithium at all during a planned pregnancy, particularly during the first trimester. Recent prospective studies suggest that the risk imposed by lithium in pregnancy may be overemphasized. Indeed, the risk of untreated bipolar disorder carries its own risks for pregnancy. Formula feeding should be considered in mothers using lithium, since concentration in breast milk is one-third to one-half that in serum.

Frank toxicity usually occurs at blood lithium levels above 2 meq/L. Because sodium and lithium are reabsorbed at the same loci in the proximal renal tubules, any sodium loss (diarrhea, use of diuretics, or excessive perspiration) results in increased lithium levels. Symptoms and signs include vomiting and diarrhea, the latter exacerbating the problem since more sodium is lost and more lithium is absorbed. Other symptoms and signs, some of which may not be reversible, include tremors, marked muscle weakness, confusion, dysarthria, vertigo, choreoathetosis, ataxia, hyperreflexia, rigidity, lack of coordination, myoclonus, seizures, opisthotonos, and coma. Toxicity is more severe in the elderly, who should be maintained on slightly lower serum levels. Lithium overdosage may be accidental or intentional or may occur as a result of poor monitoring.

Patients with massive ingestions of lithium or blood lithium levels above 2.5 meq/L should be treated with induced emesis and gastric lavage. If renal function is normal, osmotic and saline diuresis increases renal lithium clearance. Urinary alkalinization is also helpful, since sodium bicarbonate decreases lithium reabsorption in the proximal tubule, as does acetazolamide as well. Aminophylline potentiates the diuretic effect by increasing the glomerular filtration rate of lithium. Drugs affecting the distal loop have no effect on lithium reabsorption. Blood lithium levels above 2.5 meq/L (confirmed by cerebrospinal fluid lithium levels) should be considered an indication for hemodialysis.

Compliance with lithium therapy is adversely affected by the loss of some hypomanic experiences valued by the patient. These include social extroversion and a sense of heightened enjoyment in many activities such as sex and business dealings, often with increased productivity in the latter.

3. Drug interactions–Patients receiving lithium should use diuretics with caution and only under close medical supervision. The thiazide diuretics cause increased lithium reabsorption from the proximal renal tubules, resulting in increased serum lithium levels (Table 25–10), and adjustment of lithium intake must be made to compensate for this. Reduce lithium dosage by 25–40% when the patient is receiving 50 mg of hydrochlorothiazide daily. Potassium-sparing diuretics (spironolactone, amiloride, triamterene) may also cause increased serum lithium levels and require careful monitoring of lithium levels. Loop diuretics (furosemide, ethacrynic acid, bumetanide) do not appear to alter serum lithium levels. Concurrent use of lithium and ACE inhibitors requires a 50–75% reduction in lithium intake to achieve therapeutic lithium levels.

Table 25–10. Lithium interactions with other drugs.

Drug	Effects
ACE inhibitors	↑ Lithium levels
Fluoxetine	↑ Lithium levels
Ibuprofen	↑ Lithium levels
Indomethacin	↑ Lithium levels
Methyldopa	Rigidity, mutism, fascicular twitching
Osmotic diuretics (urea, mannitol)	↑ Lithium excretion
Phenylbutazone	↑ Lithium levels
Potassium-sparing diuretics (spironolactone, amiloride, triamterene)	↑ Lithium levels
Sodium bicarbonate	↑ Lithium excretion
Succinylcholine	↑ Duration of action of succinylcholine
Theophylline, aminophylline	↑ Lithium excretion
Thiazide diuretics	↑ Lithium levels
Valproic acid	↓ Lithium levels

D. Valproic Acid: Valproic acid (divalproex) is an antiseizure drug whose activity is at least partially related to GABA neurotransmission. It is gaining favor as a first-line treatment for mania because it has a broader index of safety than lithium. This issue is particularly important in AIDS or other medically ill patients prone to dehydration or malabsorption with wide swings in serum lithium levels. Valproic acid has also been utilized effectively in panic disorder and migraine headache. Treatment is often started at a dose of 750 mg/d orally in divided doses, and dosage is then titrated to achieve therapeutic serum levels. Oral loading in acutely manic bipolar patients in an inpatient setting (initiated at a dosage of 20 mg/kg/d) can safely achieve serum therapeutic levels in 2–3 days. Concomitant use of aspirin, carbamazepine, warfarin, or phenytoin may affect serum levels. Gastrointestinal symptoms are the main side effects. Liver function tests and complete blood counts should be monitored, and teratogenic effects are a concern.

E. Carbamazepine: Carbamazepine, an antiseizure drug that stabilizes the activity of cell membranes, has been used with increasing frequency in the treatment of bipolar patients who cannot be satisfactorily treated with lithium (nonresponsive, excessive side effects, or rapid cycling). It is often effective at 800–1600 mg/d orally. It has also been used in the treatment of resistant depressions, alcohol withdrawal, and hallucinations (in conjunction with neuroleptics) and in patients with behavioral dyscontrol or panic attacks. It suppresses some phases of kindling (see Stimulants) and has been used to treat residual symptoms in previous stimulant abusers (eg, posttraumatic stress disorder with impulse control problems). Dose-related side effects include sedation and ataxia. Dosages start at 400–600 mg orally daily and are increased slowly to therapeutic levels. Skin rashes and a mild reduction in white count are common. SIADH occurs rarely. Nonsteroidal anti-inflammatory drugs (except aspirin); the antibiotics erythromycin, troleandomycin, and isoniazid; the calcium channel blockers verapamil and diltiazem (but not nifedipine); fluoxetine, propoxyphene, and cimetidine all increase carbamazepine levels. Carbamazepine can be effective in conjunction with lithium, though there have been reports of reversible neurotoxicity with the combination. Carbamazepine stimulates hepatic microsomal enzymes and so tends to decrease levels of haloperidol and oral contraceptives. It also lowers T_4, free T_4, and T_3 levels. Cases of fetal malformation (particularly spina bifida) have been reported along with growth deficiency and developmental delay. Liver tests and complete blood counts should be monitored in patients taking carbamazepine.

F. Calcium Channel Blockers: Calcium channel blockers (eg, verapamil) have been used in bipolar states that have failed to respond to lithium, carbamazepine, or valproic acid. This has come about with the realization that a number of drugs used in psychiatry (eg, lithium, antidepressants, neuroleptics, and carbamazepine) have calcium channel-blocking activity. There is also preliminary evidence that these drugs may be useful in the treatment of tardive dyskinesia and panic attacks. Verapamil may be safer than lithium or carbamazepine during pregnancy, though it decreases uterine contractility and must be discontinued before delivery.

G. Newer Anticonvulsants: Two newer additions to the family of anticonvulsants, both with a primary indication for adjunctive treatment of partial seizures, may have some efficacy in the treatment of refractory affective disorders. Lamotrigine is thought to inhibit neuronal sodium channels and the release of excitatory amino acids, glutamate and aspartate. Early case reports and open label studies suggest its efficacy in the treatment of depression and bipolar disorder, including rapid cycling type, both as adjunctive therapy and monotherapy. Its metabolism is inhibited by coadministration of valproic acid, doubling its half-life, and accelerated by hepatic enzyme-inducing agents such as carbamazepine. More frequent mild side effects include headache, dizziness, nausea, and diplopia. Rash occurring in 10% of patients is an indication for immediate cessation of dosing since lamotrigine has been associated with Stevens-Johnson syndrome (1:1000) and, rarely, toxic epidermal necrolysis. Dosing starts at 25–50 mg/d and is titrated upward slowly to decrease the likelihood of rash. Gabapentin, an anticonvulsant structurally related to γ-aminobutyric acid (GABA), does not interact with GABA or GABA receptors, and its mechanism of action is unknown. Case reports suggest its possible role as an adjunct in the treatment of refractory bipolar illness, though an association with increased rapid cycling and hypomania has been reported. An effective dose (900–1800 mg/d in three divided doses) can be achieved over a few days. Gabapentin is renally excreted, has little protein-binding and limited drug interactions. Most common side effects include fatigue, somnolence, and dizziness. Topiramate has been found useful in the treatment of bipolar disorder. Omega-3 fatty acids, which have been used as an alternative medicine approach to bipolar disease, are thought to work through the same mechanism.

Prognosis

Reactive depressions are usually time-limited, and the prognosis with treatment is good if a pathologic pattern of adjustment does not intervene. Major affective disorders frequently respond well to a full trial of drug treatment.

Mania and bipolar disorder have a good prognosis with adequate treatment.

[AHCPR: Depression in Primary Care—Diagnosis and Treatment]
http://text.nlm.nih.gov/ftrs/pick?dbName=dep1c&ftrsK=46227&cp=1&t=928429453&collect=ahcpr

Calabrese JR et al: A double-blind placebo-controlled study of lamotrigine monotherapy in outpatients with bipolar I depression. J Clin Psychiatry 1999;60:79. [NLM Cit ID: 99182124] (Lamotrigine monotherapy is effective treatment for bipolar disorder.)

Fatemi SH et al: Lamotrigine in rapid-cycling bipolar disorder. J Clin Psychiatry 1997;58:522. [NLM Cit ID: 98110104]

Fava GA et al: Six-year outcome for cognitive behavioral treatment of residual symptoms in major depression. Am J Psychiatry 1998;155:1443 [NLM Cit ID: 98438170] (Cognitive behavioral treatment improved the long-term outcome of major depression in terms of decreased number of recurrences.)

Glass RM: Treating depression as a recurrent or chronic disease. JAMA 1999;281:83 [NLM Cit ID: 99107474] (Current thinking regarding major depression requires a long-term view of the illness, just as with other chronic medical problems.)

JAMA patient page: Depression. JAMA 1998;279:1760. [NLM Cit ID: 98285514]

Kulin NA et al: Pregnancy outcome following maternal use of the new selective serotonin reuptake inhibitors: A prospective controlled multicenter study. JAMA 1998; 279:609. [NLM Cit ID: 98146161] (Prospective multicenter controlled study suggests that fluvoxamine, paroxetine, and sertraline at recommended doses do not increase teratogenic risk.)

Ohman R et al: Excretion of paroxetine in breast milk. J Clin Psychiatry 1999;60:519. [NLM Cit ID: 99413643] (Paroxetine levels in breast milk may be lower than those of citalopram and fluoxetine and higher than those of sertraline and fluvoxamine.)

Reimherr FW et al: Optimal length of continuation therapy in depression: A prospective assessment during long-term fluoxetine treatment. Am J Psychiatry 1998; 155:1247. [NLM Cit ID: 98403619] (For first episode patients who respond to fluoxetine, it should be continued for 9 months to minimize risk of relapse.)

Reynolds CF et al: Nortriptyline and interpersonal psychotherapy as maintenance therapies for recurrent major depression: A randomized controlled trial in patients older than 59 years. JAMA 1999;281:39. [NLM Cit ID: 99107467] (In geriatric patients, maintenance treatment with nortriptyline or interpersonal therapy is effective in preventing recurrence. Combining both treatments appears to be the optimal strategy.)

Roose SP et al: Comparison of paroxetine and nortriptyline in depressed patients with ischemic heart disease. JAMA 1998;279:287. [NLM Cit ID: 98111173] (Paroxetine had a significantly lower risk of adverse cardiac events.)

Solomon DA et al: Multiple recurrences of major depressive disorder. Am J Psychiatry 2000;2:229. [NLM Cit ID: 20137964] (The risk of recurrence of major depressive disorder increases with successive episodes and decreases with longer periods of recovery.)

Stoll AL et al: Omega 3 fatty acids in bipolar disorder. Arch Gen Psychiatry 1999;56:407. [NLM Cit ID: 99247254] (Omega-3 fatty acids are well tolerated and may have some efficacy as adjunctive treatment in bipolar disorder, though further research needs to be done.)

Young LT et al: Double-blind comparison of addition of second mood stabilizer versus an anti-depressant to an initial mood stabilizer for treatment of patients with bipolar depression. Am J Psychiatry 2000;157:124. [NLM Cit ID: 20084830] (Both treatments are effective, but paroxetine was better tolerated than the second mood-stabilizer.)

SLEEP DISORDERS

Sleep consists of two distinct states as shown by electroencephalographic studies: REM (rapid eye movement) sleep, also called dream sleep, D state sleep, paradoxic sleep; and NREM (non-REM) sleep, also called S stage sleep, which is divided into stages 1, 2, 3, and 4 recognizable by different electroencephalographic patterns. Stages 3 and 4 are "delta" sleep. Dreaming occurs mostly in REM and to a lesser extent in NREM sleep.

Sleep is a cyclic phenomenon, with four or five REM periods during the night accounting for about one-fourth of the total night's sleep (1½–2 hours). The first REM period occurs about 80–120 minutes after onset of sleep and lasts about 10 minutes. Later REM periods are longer (15–40 minutes) and occur mostly in the last several hours of sleep. Most stage 4 (deepest) sleep occurs in the first several hours.

Age-related changes in normal sleep include an unchanging percentage of REM sleep and a marked decrease in stage 3 and stage 4 sleep, with an increase in wakeful periods during the night. These normal changes, early bedtimes, and daytime naps play a role in the increased complaints of insomnia in older people. Variations in sleep patterns may be due to circumstances (eg, "jet lag") or to idiosyncratic patterns ("night owls") in persons who perhaps because of different "biologic rhythms" habitually go to bed late and sleep late in the morning. Creativity and rapidity of response to unfamiliar situations are impaired by loss of sleep. There are also rare individuals who have chronic difficulty in adapting to a 24-hour sleep-wake cycle (desynchronization sleep disorder), which can be resynchronized by altering exposure to light.

The three major sleep disorders are discussed below.

1. DYSSOMNIAS (Insomnia)

Classification & Clinical Findings

Patients may complain of difficulty getting to sleep or staying asleep, intermittent wakefulness during the night, early morning awakening, or combinations of any of these. Transient episodes are usually of little significance. Stress, caffeine, physical discomfort, daytime napping, and early bedtimes are common factors.

Psychiatric disorders are often associated with persistent insomnia. **Depression** is usually associated with fragmented sleep, decreased total sleep time, earlier onset of REM sleep, a shift of REM activity to the first half of the night, and a loss of slow wave sleep—all of which are nonspecific findings. In **manic disorders,** sleeplessness is a cardinal feature and an important early sign of impending mania in bipolar cases. Total sleep time is decreased, with shortened REM latency and increased REM activity. Sleep-related panic attacks occur in the transition from stage 2 to stage 3 sleep in some patients with a longer REM latency in the sleep pattern preceding the attacks.

Abuse of alcohol may cause or be secondary to the sleep disturbance. There is a tendency to use alcohol as a means of getting to sleep without realizing that it disrupts the normal sleep cycle. Acute alcohol intake produces a decreased sleep latency with reduced REM sleep during the first half of the night. REM sleep is increased in the second half of the night, with an increase in total amount of slow wave sleep (stages 3 and 4). Vivid dreams and frequent awakenings are common. Chronic alcohol abuse increases stage 1 and decreases REM sleep (most drugs delay or block REM sleep), with symptoms persisting for many months after the individual has stopped drinking. Acute alcohol or other sedative withdrawal causes delayed onset of sleep and REM rebound with intermittent awakening during the night.

Heavy smoking (more than a pack a day) causes difficulty falling asleep—apparently independently of the often associated increase in coffee drinking. Excess intake near bedtime of caffeine, cocaine, and other stimulants (eg, OTC cold remedies) causes decreased total sleep time—mostly NREM sleep—with some increased sleep latency.

Sedative-hypnotics—specifically, the benzodiazepines, which are the prescription drugs of choice to promote sleep—tend to increase total sleep time, decrease sleep latency, and decrease nocturnal awakening, with variable effects on NREM sleep. Withdrawal causes just the opposite effects and results in continued use of the drug for the purpose of preventing withdrawal symptoms. Antidepressants decrease REM sleep (with marked rebound on withdrawal in the form of nightmares) and have varying effects on NREM sleep. The effect on REM sleep correlates with reports that REM sleep deprivation produces improvement in some depressions.

Persistent insomnias are also related to a wide variety of medical conditions, particularly delirium, pain, respiratory distress syndromes, uremia, asthma, and hypothyroidism. Adequate analgesia and proper treatment of medical disorders will reduce symptoms and decrease the need for sedatives.

Treatment

In general, there are two broad classes of treatment for insomnia, and the two may be combined: psychologic (cognitive-behavioral) and pharmacologic. In situations of acute distress, such as a grief reaction, pharmacologic measures may be most appropriate. With primary insomnia, however, initial efforts should be psychologically based. This is particularly true in the elderly to avoid the potential adverse reactions of medications. The elderly population is at risk for complaints of insomnia because sleep becomes lighter and more easily disrupted with aging. Medical disorders that become more common with age may also predispose to insomnia.

A. Psychologic: Psychologic strategies should include educating the patient regarding good sleep hygiene: (1) Go to bed only when sleepy. (2) Use the bed and bedroom only for sleeping and sex. (3) If still awake after 20 minutes, leave the bedroom and only return when sleepy. (4) Get up at the same time every morning regardless of the amount of sleep during the night. (5) Discontinue caffeine and nicotine, at least in the evening if not completely. (6) Establish a daily exercise regimen. (7) Avoid alcohol as it may disrupt continuity of sleep. (8) Limit fluids in the evening. (9) Learn and practice relaxation techniques.

The physician should also discuss any myths or misconceptions about sleep that the patient may hold.

B. Medical: When the above measures are insufficient, medications may be useful. Pharmacologic measures currently rely primarily on safe hypnotic medications that are difficult to overdose with. Lorazepam (0.5 mg nightly), temazepam (7.5–15 mg nightly), and zolpidem (2.5–5 mg nightly) are often effective for the elderly population and can be given in larger doses (twice what is prescribed for the elderly) in younger populations. It is important to note that short-acting agents like triazolam or zolpidem may lead to amnestic episodes if used on a daily ongoing basis. Longer-acting agents such as flurazepam (half-life of > 48 hours) may accumulate in the elderly and lead to cognitive slowing, ataxia, falls, and somnolence. In general, it is appropriate to use medications for short courses of 1–2 weeks. The medications described above have largely replaced barbiturates as hypnotic agents because of their greater safety in overdose and their lesser hepatic enzyme induction effects. Antihistamines such as diphenhydramine (25 mg nightly) or hydroxyzine (25 mg nightly) may also be useful for sleep, as they produce no pharmacologic dependency; their anticholinergic effects may, however, produce confusion or urinary symptoms in the elderly. Trazodone, an atypical antidepressant, is a non-habit-forming, effective sleep medication in lower than antidepressant doses (25–150 mg at bedtime). Priapism is a rare side effect requiring emergent treatment.

Triazolam has achieved popularity as a hypnotic drug because of its very short duration of action. Because it has been associated with dependency, transient psychotic reactions, anterograde amnesia, and rebound anxiety, it has been removed from the market in several European countries. If used, it must be prescribed only for short periods of time.

2. HYPERSOMNIAS (Disorders of Excessive Sleepiness)

The hypersomnias are a more severe problem than insomnia.

Classification & Clinical Findings

A. Sleep Apnea: This disorder is characterized by cessation of breathing for at least 30 episodes (each lasting about 10 seconds) during the night. There are two types: obstructive and central. The obstructive type is discussed in Chapter 9. Central sleep apnea is due to failure during sleep of the respiratory drive mechanism. Obese middle-aged and older men with hypertension and associated congestive heart failure are most often affected. Both types may occur simultaneously. Symptoms include snoring, restless sleep, and excessive daytime sleepiness, which may be associated with headaches, memory impairment, and depression. Cardiac arrhythmias (particularly bradycardia) and blood gas abnormalities occur during episodes. The patients tend to have poor judgment and a history of work-related problems. Definitive diagnostic evaluation may include thyroid evaluation and otolaryngologic examination; polysomnography in the hospital to record sleep, heart rate, and respiratory movement; and oxygen saturation studies. Moderate alcohol intake at bedtime has produced sleep apnea episodes (10–12 nightly) in healthy men.

B. Narcolepsy: Narcolepsy consists of a tetrad of symptoms: (1) Sudden, brief (about 15 minutes) sleep attacks that may occur during any type of activity; (2) cataplexy—sudden loss of muscle tone involving specific small muscle groups or generalized muscle weakness that may cause the person to slump to the floor, unable to move, often associated with emotional reactions and sometimes confused with seizure disorder; (3) sleep paralysis—a generalized flaccidity of muscles with full consciousness in the transition zone between sleep and waking; and (4) hypnagogic hallucinations, visual or auditory, which may precede sleep or occur during the sleep attack. The attacks are characterized by an abrupt transition into REM sleep—a necessary criterion for diagnosis. The disorder begins in early adult life, affects both sexes equally, and usually levels off in severity at about 30 years of age.

REM sleep behavior disorder, characterized by motor dyscontrol and often violent dreams during REM sleep, may be related to narcolepsy.

C. Kleine-Levin Syndrome: This syndrome, which occurs mostly in young males, is characterized by hypersomnic attacks three or four times a year lasting up to 2 days, with hyperphagia, hypersexuality, irritability, and confusion on awakening. It has often been associated with antecedent neurologic insults. It usually remits after age 40.

D. Nocturnal Myoclonus: Periodic lower leg movements occur during sleep with subsequent daytime sleepiness, anxiety, depression, and cognitive impairment.

Treatment

Treatment of sleep apnea may include medical measures such as weight reduction and administration during sleep of air under continuous pressure through the nasopharynx. Surgical treatment is discussed in Chapter 9. Diaphragmatic pacing has also been helpful for central sleep apnea. Trials with protriptyline have improved daytime somnolence and nocturnal oxygenation, with no significant change, however, in the number of apneic episodes. Acetazolamide has shown some promise, probably by creating a metabolic acidosis and the resultant hypercapnic ventilatory response.

Narcolepsy is managed by daily administration of a stimulant such as dextroamphetamine sulfate, 10 mg in the morning, with increased dosage as necessary. Imipramine, 75–100 mg daily, has been effective in treatment of cataplexy but not narcolepsy.

Nocturnal myoclonus and REM sleep behavior disorder can be treated with clonazepam with variable results. There is no treatment for Kleine-Levin syndrome.

3. PARASOMNIAS (Abnormal Behaviors During Sleep)

These disorders are fairly common in children and less so in adults.

Classification & Clinical Findings

A. Sleep Terror: Sleep terror (pavor nocturnus) is an abrupt, terrifying arousal from sleep, usually in preadolescent boys though it may occur in adults as well. It is distinct from sleep panic attacks. Symptoms are fear, sweating, tachycardia, and confusion for several minutes, with amnesia for the event.

B. Nightmares: Nightmares occur during REM sleep; sleep terrors in stage 3 or stage 4 sleep.

C. Sleepwalking: Sleepwalking (somnambulism) includes ambulation or other intricate behaviors while still asleep, with amnesia for the event. It affects mostly children aged 6–12 years, and episodes occur during stage 3 or stage 4 sleep in the first third of the night and in REM sleep in the later sleep hours. Sleepwalking in elderly people may be a feature of dementia. Idiosyncratic reactions to drugs (eg, marijuana, alcohol) and medical conditions (eg, partial complex seizures) may be causative factors in adults.

D. Enuresis: Enuresis is involuntary micturition during sleep in a person who usually has voluntary control. Like other parasomnias, it is more common in children, usually in the 3–4 hours after bedtime, but is not limited to a specific stage of sleep. Confusion during the episode and amnesia for the event are common.

Treatment

Treatment for sleep terrors is with benzodiazepines (eg, diazepam, 5–20 mg at bedtime), since it will suppress stage 3 and stage 4 sleep. Somnambulism responds to the same treatment for the same reason, but simple safety measures should not be neglected. Enuresis may respond to imipramine, 50–100 mg at bedtime, though desmopressin nasal spray (an antidiuretic hormone preparation) has increasingly become the treatment of choice for nocturnal enuresis. Behavioral approaches (eg, bells that ring when the pad gets wet) have also been successful.

Farney RJ et al: Office management of common sleep-wake disorders. Med Clin North Am 1995;79:391. [NLM Cit ID: 95182698]

JAMA patient page: Insomnia. JAMA 1999;281:1056. [NLM Cit ID: 99184246]

Morin CM et al: Behavioral and pharmacological therapies for late-life insomnia; a randomized controlled trial. JAMA 1999;281:991. [NLM Cit ID: 98184237] (Behavioral treatment for late-life insomnia may have more sustained efficacy than pharmacotherapy, though both are effective.)

Simon GE et al: Prevalence, burden and treatment of insomnia in primary care. Am J Psychiatry 1997;154:1417. [NLM Cit ID: 97467616] (Insomnia among primary care patients is associated with broad functional impairment comparable to that found with other psychiatric and medical conditions.)

DISORDERS OF AGGRESSION

Acts performed with the deliberate intent of causing physical harm to persons or property have a wide variety of causative features. Aggression and violence are symptoms rather than diseases, and most frequently they are not associated with an underlying medical condition. Clinicians are unable to predict dangerous behavior with greater than chance accuracy. In terms of demographic characteristics, the perpetrator of an act of aggression is often a male under age 25, a member of a socioeconomically deprived group, and a resident of an inner city area. Depression, schizophrenia, personality disorders, mania, paranoia, temporal lobe dysfunction, and organic mental states may be associated. Anabolic steroid usage by athletes has been associated with increased tendencies toward violent behavior.

In the USA, a significant proportion of all violent deaths are alcohol-related. The ingestion of even small amounts of alcohol can result in pathologic intoxication that resembles an acute organic mental condition. Amphetamines, crack cocaine, and other stimulants are frequently associated with aggressive behavior. Phencyclidine is a drug commonly associated with violent behavior that is occasionally of a bizarre nature, partly due to lowering of the pain threshold. Impulse control disorders are characterized by physical abuse, usually of the aggressor's domestic partner or children, pathologic intoxication, impulsive sexual activities, and reckless driving.

Domestic violence and rape are much more widespread than heretofore recognized. Awareness of the problem is to some degree due to increasing recognition of the rights of women and the understanding by women that they do not have to accept abuse. Acceptance of this kind of aggression inevitably leads to more, with the ultimate aggression being murder—20–50% of murders in the USA occur within the family. Police are called in more domestic disputes than all other criminal incidents combined. Children living in such family situations frequently become victims of abuse.

Features of individuals who have been subjected to chronic physical or sexual abuse are as follows: trouble expressing anger, staying angry longer, general passivity in relationships, feeling "marked for life" with an accompanying feeling of deserving to be victimized, lack of trust, and dissociation of affect from experiences. They are prone to express their psychologic distress with somatization symptoms, often pain complaints. They may also have symptoms related to posttraumatic stress, as discussed above. The physician should be suspicious about the origin of any injuries not fully explained, particularly if such incidents recur.

Treatment

A. Psychologic: Management of any violent individual includes appropriate psychologic maneuvers. Move slowly, talk slowly with clarity and reassurance, and evaluate the situation. Strive to create a setting that is minimally disturbing and eliminate people or things threatening to the violent individual. Do not threaten or abuse and do not touch or crowd the person. Allow no weapons in the area (an increasing problem in hospital emergency rooms). Proximity to a door is comforting to both the patient and the examiner. Use a negotiator the violent person can relate to comfortably. Food and drink are helpful in defusing the situation (as are cigarettes for those who smoke). Honesty is important. Make no false promises, bolster the patient's self-esteem, and continue to engage the subject verbally until the situation is under control. This type of individual does better with strong external controls to replace the lack of inner controls over the long term. Close probationary supervision and judicially mandated restrictions can be most helpful. There should be a major effort to help the individual avoid drug use (eg, Alcoholics Anonymous). Victims of abuse are essentially treated as any victim of trauma and, not infrequently, have evidence of posttraumatic stress disorder.

B. Pharmacologic: Pharmacologic means are often necessary whether or not psychologic approaches have been successful. This is particularly true in the agitated or psychotic patient. The drug of choice in psychotic aggressive states is haloperidol, 5–10 mg intramuscularly every hour until symptoms are alleviated. Benzodiazepine sedatives (eg, diazepam, 5 mg orally or intravenously every several hours) can be used for mild to moderate agitation, but an antipsychotic drug is preferred for management of the seriously violent and psychotic patient. Chronic aggressive states, particularly in retardation and brain damage (rule out causative organic conditions and medications such as anticholinergic drugs in amounts sufficient to cause confusion), have been ameliorated with propranolol, 40–240 mg/d orally, or pindolol, 5 mg twice daily orally (pindolol causes less bradycardia and hypotension). Carbamazepine and valproic acid are effective in the treatment of aggression and explosive disorders, particularly when associated with known or suspected brain lesions. Lithium and SSRIs are also effective for some intermittent explosive outbursts. Buspirone (10–45 mg/d orally) is helpful for aggression, particularly in mentally retarded patients.

C. Physical: Physical management is necessary if psychologic and pharmacologic means are not sufficient. It requires the active and visible presence of an adequate number of personnel (five or six) to reinforce the idea that the situation is under control despite the patient's lack of inner controls. Such an approach often precludes the need for actual physical restraint. When adequate personnel are not available, however, two people shielded by a mattress (single-bed size) can usually corner and subdue the patient without injury to anyone. Seclusion rooms and restraints should be used only when necessary (ambulatory restraints are an alternative), and the patient must then be observed at frequent intervals. Design of corridors and seclusion rooms is important. Narrow corridors, small spaces, and crowded areas exacerbate the potential for violence in an anxious patient.

D. Other: The treatment of victims (eg, battered women) is challenging and often complicated by their reluctance to leave the situation. Reasons for staying vary, but common themes include the fear of more violence because of leaving; the hope that the situation may ameliorate (in spite of steady worsening); and the financial aspects of the situation, which are seldom to the woman's advantage. Concerns for the children often finally compel the woman to seek help. An early step is to get the woman into a therapeutic situation that provides the support of others in similar straits. Al-Anon is frequently a valuable asset and quite appropriate when alcohol is a factor. The group can support the victim while she gathers strength to consider alternatives without being paralyzed by fear. Many cities now offer temporary emergency centers and counseling. Use the available resources, attend to any medical or psychiatric problems, and maintain a compassionate interest. Some states now require physicians to report injuries caused by abuse to police authorities.

Abbott J et al: Domestic violence against women: Incidence and prevalence in an emergency department population. JAMA 1995;273:1763. [NLM Cit ID: 95287569] (The incidence of acute domestic violence among the 418 women with a current male partner was 11.7%.)

Rodriguez MA et al: Patient attitudes about mandatory reporting of domestic violence: Implications for health care professionals. West J Med 1998;169:337. [NLM Cit ID: 99083662] (Mandatory reporting may pose a threat to the safety of abused women.)

Swanston HY et al: Sexually abused children 5 years after presentation: A case-control study. Pediatrics 1997;100:600. [NLM Cit ID: 97456210] (Children who have been abused may experience four types of injury: traumatic sexualization, betrayal, powerlessness, and stigmatization.)

SUBSTANCE USE DISORDERS (Drug Dependency, Drug Abuse)

The term "drug dependency" is used in a broad sense here to include both addictions and habituations. It involves the triad of compulsive drug use referred to as drug addiction, which includes (1) a **psychologic** dependence or craving and the behavior included in the procurement of the drug; (2) **physiologic dependence,** with withdrawal symptoms on discontinuance of the drug; and (3) **tolerance,** ie, the need to increase the dose to obtain the desired effects. Drug dependency is a function of the amount of drug used and the duration of usage. The amount needed to produce dependency varies with the nature of the drug and the idiosyncratic nature of the user. The frequency of use is usually daily, and the duration is inevitably greater than 2–3 weeks. Polydrug abuse is very common. Transgenerational continuity of drug abuse is also common. A large percentage of drug abusers present themselves for something other than treatment (eg, avoiding legal sanctions, obtaining more drugs).

There is accumulating evidence that an impairment syndrome exists in many former (and current) drug users. It is believed that drug use produces damaged neurotransmitter receptor sites and that the consequent imbalance produces symptoms that may mimic other psychiatric illnesses. **"Kindling"**—repeated stimulation of the brain—renders the individual more susceptible to focal brain activity with minimal stimulation. Stimulants and depressants can produce kindling, leading to relatively spontaneous effects no longer dependent on the original stimulus. These effects may be manifested as mood swings, panic, psychosis, and occasionally overt seizure activity. The imbalance also results in personal nonproductivity: frequent job changes, marital problems, and generally erratic behavior. Patients with posttraumatic stress disorder frequently have treated themselves with a variety of drugs. Chronic abusers of a wide variety of drugs exhibit cerebral atrophy on CT scans, a finding that may relate to the above symptoms. Early recognition is important, mainly to establish realistic treatment programs that are chiefly symptom-directed.

The physician faces three problems with substance abuse: (1) the prescribing of substances such as sedatives, stimulants, or narcotics that might produce dependency; (2) the treatment of individuals who have already abused drugs, most commonly alcohol; and (3) the detection of illicit drug use in patients presenting with psychiatric symptoms. The usefulness of urinalysis for detection of drugs varies markedly with different drugs and under different circumstances (pharmacokinetics is a major factor). Water-soluble drugs (eg, alcohol, stimulants, opioids) are eliminated in a day or so. Lipophilic substances (eg, barbiturates, tetrahydrocannabinol) appear in the urine over longer periods of time: several days in most cases, 1–2 months in chronic marijuana users. Sedative drug determinations are quite variable, amount of drug and duration of use being important determinants. False-positives can be a problem related to ingestion of some legitimate drugs (eg, phenytoin for barbiturates, phenylpropanolamine for amphetamines, chlorpromazine for opioids) and some foods (eg, poppy seeds for opioids, coca leaf tea for cocaine). Manipulations can alter the legitimacy of the testing. Dilution, either in vivo or in vitro, can be detected by checking urine specific gravity. Addition of ammonia, vinegar, or salt may invalidate the test, but odor and pH determinations are simple. Hair analysis can determine drug use over longer periods, particularly sequential drug-taking patterns. The sensitivity and reliability of such tests are considered good, and the method may be complementary to urinalysis.

Botvin GJ et al: Long-term follow-up results of a randomized drug abuse prevention trial in a white middle-class population. JAMA 1995;273:1106. [NLM Cit ID: 95222827] (Drug abuse prevention programs conducted during junior high school can produce meaningful and durable reductions in tobacco, alcohol, and marijuana use.)

Gil-Rivas V et al: Sexual abuse, physical abuse, and post-traumatic stress disorder among women participating in outpatient drug abuse treatment. J Psychoactive Drugs 1996;28:95. [NLM Cit ID: 96282924] (Women are more likely to have suffered abuse but are also more willing to engage in treatment groups that mitigate substance abuse relapses.)

Parran T Jr: Prescription drug abuse: A question of balance. Med Clin North Am 1997;81:967. [NLM Cit ID: 97365436] (Short therapeutic courses and appropriate regard to patients' substance abuse histories leads to improved prescribing practice.)

Stewart SH: Alcohol abuse in individuals exposed to trauma: A critical review. Psychol Bull 1996;120:83. [NLM Cit ID: 96282437] (Strong relationship.)

ALCOHOL DEPENDENCY & ABUSE (Alcoholism)

Essentials of Diagnosis

Major criteria:

- Physiologic dependence as manifested by evidence of withdrawal when intake is interrupted.
- Tolerance to the effects of alcohol.
- Evidence of alcohol-associated illnesses, such as alcoholic liver disease, cerebellar degeneration.
- Continued drinking despite strong medical and social contraindications and life disruptions.
- Impairment in social and occupational functioning.
- Depression.
- Blackouts.

Other signs:

- Alcohol stigmas: alcohol odor on breath, alcoholic facies, flushed face, scleral injection, tremor, ecchymoses, peripheral neuropathy.
- Surreptitious drinking.
- Unexplained work absences.
- Frequent accidents, falls, or injuries of vague origin; in smokers, cigarette burns on hands or chest.
- Laboratory tests (elevated values of liver function tests, mean corpuscular volume, serum uric acid and triglycerides).

General Considerations

Alcoholism is a syndrome consisting of two phases: problem drinking and alcohol addiction. Problem drinking is the repetitive use of alcohol, often to alleviate anxiety or solve other emotional problems. Alcohol addiction is a true addiction similar to that which occurs following the repeated use of other sedative-hypnotics. There is a high incidence among homeless individuals. Alcohol and other drug abuse patients have a much higher prevalence of lifetime psychiatric disorders. While male-to-female ratios in alcoholic treatment agencies remain at 4:1, there is evidence that the rates are converging. Women delay seeking help, and when they do they tend to seek it in medical or mental health settings. Adoption and twin studies indicate some genetic influence. Ethnic distinctions are important—eg, 40% of Japanese have aldehyde dehydrogenase deficiency and are more susceptible to the effects of alcohol. Depression is often present and should be evaluated carefully. The majority of suicides and intrafamily homicides involve alcohol, and alcohol is a major factor in rapes and other assaults also.

There are several screening instruments that may help identify alcoholism. One of the most useful is the CAGE questionnaire (Table 1–9).

Clinical Findings

A. Acute Intoxication: The signs of alcoholic intoxication are the same as those of overdosage with any other central nervous system depressant: drowsiness, errors of commission, psychomotor dysfunction, disinhibition, dysarthria, ataxia, and nystagmus. For a 70-kg person, an ounce of whiskey, a glass of wine, or a 12-oz bottle of beer (roughly 15, 11, and 13 grams of alcohol, respectively) may raise the level of alcohol in the blood by 25 mg/dL. For a 50-kg person, the blood alcohol level would rise even higher (35 mg/dL) with the same consumption. Blood alcohol levels below 50 mg/dL rarely cause significant motor dysfunction. Intoxication as manifested by ataxia, dysarthria, and nausea and vomiting indicates a blood level above 150 mg/dL, and lethal blood levels range from 350 to 900 mg/dL. In severe cases, overdosage is marked by respiratory depression, stupor, seizures, shock syndrome, coma, and death. Serious overdoses are frequently due to a combination of alcohol with other sedatives.

B. Withdrawal: There is a wide spectrum of manifestations of alcoholic withdrawal, ranging from anxiety, decreased cognition, and tremulousness through increasing irritability and hyperreactivity to full-blown **delirium tremens.** Symptoms of mild withdrawal, including tremor, elevated vital signs, and anxiety, begin within about 8 hours after the last drink and usually have passed by day 3. Generalized seizures occur within the first 24–38 hours and are more prevalent in persons who have a history of withdrawal syndromes. Delirium tremens is an acute organic psychosis that is usually manifest within 24–72 hours after the last drink (but may occur up to 7–10 days later). It is characterized by mental confusion, tremor, sensory hyperacuity, visual hallucinations (often of snakes, bugs, etc), autonomic hyperactivity, diaphoresis, dehydration, electrolyte disturbances (hypokalemia, hypomagnesemia), seizures, and cardiovascular abnormalities. The acute withdrawal syndrome is often completely unexpected and occurs when the patient has been hospitalized for some unrelated problem and presents as a diagnostic problem. Suspect alcohol withdrawal in every unexplained delirium. The mortality rate from delirium tremens has steadily decreased with early diagnosis and improved treatment.

In addition to the immediate withdrawal symptoms, there is evidence of persistent longer-term ones, including sleep disturbances, anxiety, depression, excitability, fatigue, and emotional volatility. These symptoms may persist for 3–12 months, and in some cases they become chronic.

C. Alcoholic (Organic) Hallucinosis: This syndrome occurs either during heavy drinking or on withdrawal and is characterized by a paranoid psychosis without the tremulousness, confusion, and clouded sensorium seen in withdrawal syndromes. The patient appears normal except for the auditory hallucinations, which are frequently persecutory and may cause the patient to behave aggressively and in a paranoid fashion.

D. Chronic Alcoholic Brain Syndromes: These encephalopathies are characterized by increasing erratic behavior, memory and recall problems, and emotional instability—the usual signs of organic brain injury due to any cause. Wernicke-Korsakoff syndrome due to thiamin deficiency may develop with a series of episodes. Wernicke's encephalopathy consists of the triad of confusion, ataxia, and ophthalmoplegia (typically sixth nerve). Early recognition and treatment with thiamine can minimize damage. One of the possible sequelae is Korsakoff's psychosis, characterized by both anterograde and retrograde amnesia, with confabulation early in the course. Early recognition and treatment of the alcoholic with intravenous thiamine and B complex vitamins can minimize damage.

Differential Diagnosis

The differential diagnosis of problem drinking is essentially between primary alcoholism (when no other major psychiatric diagnosis exists) and secondary alcoholism, when alcohol is used as self-medication for major underlying psychiatric problems such as schizophrenia or affective disorder. The differentiation is important, since the latter group requires treatment for the specific psychiatric problem.

The differential diagnosis of alcohol withdrawal includes other sedative withdrawals and other causes of delirium. Acute alcoholic hallucinosis must be differentiated from other acute paranoid states such as amphetamine psychosis or paranoid schizophrenia. An accurate history is the most important differentiating factor. The history and laboratory test results (elevated liver function tests, increased mean corpuscular volume, increased serum uric acid and triglycerides, decreased serum potassium and magnesium) are the most important features in differentiating chronic organic brain syndromes due to alcohol from those due to other causes. The form of the brain syndrome is of little help—eg, chronic brain syndromes from lupus erythematosus may be associated with confabulation similar to that resulting from longstanding alcoholism.

Complications

The medical, economic, and psychosocial problems of alcoholism are staggering. The central and peripheral nervous system complications include chronic brain syndromes, cerebellar degeneration, cardiomyopathy, and peripheral neuropathies. Direct effects on the liver include cirrhosis, esophageal varices, and eventual hepatic failure. Indirect effects include protein abnormalities, coagulation defects, hormone deficiencies, and an increased incidence of liver neoplasms.

Fetal alcohol syndrome includes one or more of the following developmental defects in the offspring of alcoholic women: (1) low birth weight and small size with failure to catch up in size or weight; (2) mental retardation, with an average IQ in the 60s; and (3) a variety of birth defects, with a large percentage of facial and cardiac abnormalities. The fetuses are very quiet in utero, and there is an increased frequency of breech presentations. There is a higher incidence of delayed postnatal growth and behavior development. The risk is appreciably higher the more alcohol ingested by the mother each day. Cigarette and marijuana smoking as well as cocaine use can produce similar effects on the fetus.

Treatment of Problem Drinking

A. Psychologic: The most important consideration for the physician is to suspect the problem early and take a nonjudgmental attitude, though this does not mean a passive one. The problem of **denial** must be faced, preferably with significant family members at the first meeting. This means dealing from the beginning with any enabling behavior of the spouse or other significant people. Enabling behavior allows the alcoholic to avoid facing the consequences of his or her behavior.

There must be an emphasis on the things that can be done. This approach emphasizes the fact that the physician cares and strikes a positive and hopeful note early in treatment. Valuable time should not be wasted trying to find out why the patient drinks; come to grips early with the immediate problem of how to stop the drinking. Total abstinence (not "controlled drinking") should be the goal.

B. Social: Get the patient into Alcoholics Anonymous (AA) and the spouse into Al-Anon. Success is usually proportionate to the utilization of AA, religious counseling, and other resources. The patient should be seen frequently for short periods and charged an appropriate fee.

Do not underestimate the importance of religion, particularly since the alcoholic is often a dependent person who needs a great deal of support. Early enlistment of the help of a concerned religious adviser can often provide the turning point for a personal conversion to sobriety.

One of the most important considerations is the patient's job—fear of losing a job is one of the most powerful motivations for giving up drink. The business community has become painfully aware of the problem, with the result that about 70% of the Fortune 500 companies offer programs to their employees to help with the problem of alcoholism. In the latter case, some specific recommendations to employers can be offered: (1) Avoid placement in jobs where the alcoholic must be alone, eg, as a traveling buyer or sales executive. (2) Use supervision but not surveillance. (3) Keep competition with others to a minimum. (4) Avoid positions that require quick decision making on important matters (high stress situations).

C. Medical: Hospitalization is not usually necessary. It is sometimes used to dramatize a situation and force the patient to face the problem of alcoholism, but generally it should be used on medical indications.

Because of the many medical complications of alcoholism, a complete physical examination with appropriate laboratory tests is mandatory, with special attention to the liver and nervous system. Two tests that may provide clues to an alcohol problem are γ-glutamyl transpeptidase measurement (levels above 30 units/L are suggestive of heavy drinking) and mean corpuscular volume (> 95 fL in males and > 100 fL in females). If both are elevated, a serious drinking problem is likely. Use of other recreational drugs with alcohol skews and negates the significance of these tests. HDL cholesterol elevations combined with elevated γ-glutamyl transpeptidase concentrations also can help to identify heavy drinkers.

Use of sedatives as a replacement for alcohol is not desirable. The usual result is concomitant use of sedatives and alcohol and worsening of the problem. Lithium is not helpful in the treatment of alcoholism.

Disulfiram (250–500 mg/d orally) has been used for many years as an aversive drug to discourage alcohol use. Disulfiram inhibits alcohol dehydrogenase, causing toxic reactions when alcohol is consumed. The results have generally been of limited effectiveness and depend on the motivation of the individual to be compliant.

Naltrexone, an opiate antagonist, in a dosage of 50 mg daily, has been helpful in lowering relapse rates over the 3–6 months after cessation of drinking, apparently by lessening the pleasurable effects of alcohol. It has been approved by the FDA for maintenance therapy. Studies indicate that it reduces alcohol craving when used as part of a comprehensive treatment program.

D. Behavioral: Conditioning approaches have been used in some settings in the treatment of alcoholism, most commonly as a type of aversion therapy. For example, the patient is given a drink of whiskey and then a shot of apomorphine, and proceeds to vomit. In this way a strong association is built up between the vomiting and the drinking. Although this kind of treatment has been successful in some cases, many people do not sustain the learned aversive response.

Treatment of Hallucinosis & Withdrawal

A. Medical:

1. Alcoholic hallucinosis–Alcoholic hallucinosis, which can occur either during or on cessation of a prolonged drinking period, is not a typical withdrawal syndrome and is handled differently. Since the symptoms are primarily those of a psychosis in the presence of a clear sensorium, they are handled like any other psychosis: hospitalization (when indicated) and adequate amounts of antipsychotic drugs. Haloperidol, 5 mg orally twice a day for the first day or so, usually ameliorates symptoms quickly, and the drug can be decreased and discontinued over several days as the patient improves. It then becomes necessary to deal with the chronic alcohol abuse, which has been discussed.

2. Withdrawal symptoms–The onset of withdrawal symptoms is usually 8–12 hours and the peak intensity of symptoms is 48–72 hours after alcohol consumption is stopped. Providing adequate central nervous system depressants (eg, benzodiazepines) is important to counteract the excitability resulting from sudden cessation of alcohol intake. The choice of a specific sedative is less important than using adequate doses to bring the patient to a level of moderate sedation, and this will vary from person to person. Mild dependency requires "drying out." In some instances for outpatients, a short course of tapering benzodiazepines—eg, 20 mg of diazepam initially, decreasing by 5 mg daily—may be a useful adjunct. In moderate to severe withdrawal, hospitalize the patient and use diazepam orally in a dosage of 5–10 mg hourly depending on the clinical need as judged by withdrawal symptoms, including nausea, tremor, autonomic hyperactivity, agitation; tactile, visual, and auditory hallucinations; and disorientation. This type of symptom-driven medication regimen for withdrawal appears to reduce total benzodiazepine usage over fixed-dose schedules. Antipsychotic drugs should not be used. Monitoring of vital signs and fluid and electrolyte levels is essential for the severely ill patient.

In very severe withdrawal, intravenous administration is necessary. After stabilization, the amount of diazepam required to maintain a sedated state may be given orally every 8–12 hours. If restlessness, tremulousness, and other signs of withdrawal persist, the dosage is increased until moderate sedation occurs. The dosage is then gradually reduced by 20% every 24 hours until withdrawal is complete. This usually requires a week or so of treatment. Clonidine, 5 μg/kg orally every 2 hours, or the patch formulation of appropriate dosage strength, suppresses cardiovascular signs of withdrawal and has some anxiolytic effect. Carbamazepine, 400–800 mg daily orally, compares favorably with benzodiazepines for alcohol withdrawal.

Atenolol, as an adjunct to benzodiazepines, can reduce symptoms of alcohol withdrawal. The daily oral atenolol dose is 100 mg when the heart rate is above 80 beats per minute and 50 mg for a heart rate between 50 and 80 beats per minute. Atenolol should not be used when bradycardia is present.

Meticulous examination for other medical problems is necessary. Alcoholic hypoglycemia can occur with low blood alcohol levels (see Chapter 27). Alcoholics commonly have liver disease and associated clotting problems and are also prone to injury—and the combination all too frequently leads to undiagnosed subdural hematoma.

Phenytoin does not appear to be useful in managing alcohol withdrawal seizures per se. Sedating doses of benzodiazepines are effective in treating alcohol withdrawal seizures. Thus, other anticonvulsants are not usually needed unless there is a preexisting seizure disorder.

A general diet should be given, and vitamins in high doses: thiamine, 50 mg intravenously initially, then intramuscularly on a daily basis; pyridoxine, 100 mg/d; folic acid, 1 mg/d; and ascorbic acid, 100 mg twice a day. Intravenous glucose solutions should not be given prior to thiamine for fear of precipitation of Wernicke's syndrome. Thiamine is necessary as a ketolase enzyme cofactor. Concurrent administration is satisfactory, and hydration should be meticulously assessed on an ongoing basis.

Chronic brain syndromes secondary to a long history of alcohol intake are not clearly responsive to thiamine and vitamin replenishment. Attention to the social and environmental care of this type of patient is paramount.

B. Psychologic and Behavioral: The comments in the section on problem drinking apply here also; these methods of treatment become the primary consideration after successful treatment of withdrawal or alcoholic hallucinosis. Psychologic and social measures should be initiated in the hospital shortly before discharge. This increases the possibility of continued posthospitalization treatment.

Adams WL et al: Screening for problem drinking in older primary care patients. JAMA 1996;276:1964. [NLM Cit ID: 97126141] (The CAGE survey and other questions can identify alcohol abuse in elderly populations.)

Becker HC: Alcohol withdrawal: Neuroadaptation and sensitization. CNS Spectrums 1999;4:38. (Repeated episodes of withdrawal may lead to kindling-like effects that result in neurologic damage and efforts to control the kindling which in turn produce relapse episodes.)

Cornelius JR et al: Fluoxetine in depressed alcoholics. Arch Gen Psychiatry 1997;54:700. [NLM Cit ID: 97429154] (In patients with major depression and alcohol dependence, fluoxetine reduces symptoms and alcohol consumption.)

JAMA patient page: Alcohol. JAMA 1999;281:1352. [NLM Cit ID: 99222834]

Lieber CS: Medical disorders of alcoholism. N Engl J Med 1995;333:1058. [NLM Cit ID: 95405435]

O'Malley SS: Opioid antagonists in the treatment of alcohol dependence: Clinical efficacy and prevention of relapse. Alcohol Alcohol 1996;31:77. [NLM Cit ID: 96346233] (Naltrexone can help reduce craving and prevent relapse in some patients.)

Pages KP et al: Use of anticonvulsants in benzodiazepine withdrawal. Am J Addict 1998;7:198. [NLM Cit ID: 98367664] (Valproate and carbamazepine can be effective in treating withdrawal syndromes.)

Ragan PW et al: Brain injury associated with chronic alcoholism. CNS Spectrums 1999;4:38. (Release of neuroexcitatotoxins, thiamin deficiency, and magnesium wasting contribute to brain injury.)

See also Substance Abuse references in Chapter 1.

OTHER DRUG & SUBSTANCE DEPENDENCIES

Opioids

The terms "opioids" and "narcotics" are used interchangeably and include a group of drugs with actions that mimic those of morphine. The group includes natural derivatives of opium (opiates), synthetic surrogates (opioids), and a number of polypeptides, some of which have been discovered to be natural neurotransmitters. The principal narcotic of abuse is heroin (metabolized to morphine), which is not used as a legitimate medication. The other common narcotics are prescription drugs and differ in milligram potency, duration of action, and agonist and antagonist capabilities (see Chapter 1). All of the narcotic analgesics can be reversed by the narcotic antagonist naloxone.

The clinical symptoms and signs of mild narcotic intoxication include changes in mood, with feelings of euphoria; drowsiness; nausea with occasional emesis; needle tracks; and miosis. The incidence of snorting and inhaling heroin ("smoking") is increasing, particularly among cocaine users. This coincides with a decrease in the availability of methaqualone (no longer marketed) and other sedatives used to temper the cocaine "high" (see discussion of cocaine under Stimulants, below). Overdosage causes respiratory depression, peripheral vasodilation, pinpoint pupils, pulmonary edema, coma, and death.

Dependency is a major concern when continued use of narcotics occurs, though withdrawal causes only moderate morbidity (similar in severity to a bout of "flu"). Addicts sometimes consider themselves more addicted than they really are and may not require a withdrawal program. Grades of withdrawal are categorized from 0 to 4: grade 0 includes craving and anxiety; grade 1, yawning, lacrimation, rhinorrhea, and perspiration; grade 2, previous symptoms plus mydriasis, piloerection, anorexia, tremors, and hot and cold flashes with generalized aching; grades 3 and 4, increased intensity of previous symptoms and signs, with increased temperature, blood pressure, pulse, and respiratory rate and depth. In withdrawal from the most severe addiction, vomiting, diarrhea, weight loss, hemoconcentration, and spontaneous ejaculation or orgasm commonly occur. Complications of heroin administration include infections (eg, pneumonia, septic emboli, hepatitis, and HIV infection from using nonsterile needles), traumatic insults (eg, arterial spasm due to drug injection, gangrene), and pulmonary edema.

Treatment for overdosage (or suspected overdosage) is naloxone, 2 mg intravenously. If an overdose has been taken, the results are dramatic and occur within 2 minutes. Since the duration of action of naloxone is much shorter than that of the narcotics, the patient must be under close observation. Hospitalization, supportive care, repeated naloxone administration, and observation for withdrawal from other drugs should be maintained for as long as necessary.

Treatment for withdrawal begins if grade 2 signs develop. If a withdrawal program is necessary, use methadone, 10 mg orally (use parenteral administration if the patient is vomiting), and observe. If signs (piloerection, mydriasis, cardiovascular changes) persist for more than 4–6 hours, give another 10 mg; continue to administer methadone at 4- to 6-hour intervals until signs are not present (rarely more than 40 mg of methadone in 24 hours). Divide the total amount of drug required over the first 24-hour period by 2 and give that amount every 12 hours. Each day, reduce the total 24-hour dose by 5–10 mg. Thus, a moderately addicted patient initially requiring 30–40 mg of methadone could be withdrawn over a 4- to 8-day period. Clonidine, 0.1 mg several times daily over a 10- to 14-day period, is both an alternative and an adjunct to methadone detoxification; it is not necessary to taper the dose. Clonidine is helpful in alleviating cardiovascular symptoms but does not significantly relieve anxiety, insomnia, or generalized aching. There is a protracted abstinence syndrome of metabolic, respiratory, and blood pressure changes over a period of 3–6 months.

Alternative strategies for the treatment of opioid withdrawal include rapid and ultrarapid detoxification techniques. In rapid detoxification, withdrawal is precipitated by opioid antagonists followed by naltrexone maintenance. Ultrarapid detoxification precipitates withdrawal with opioid antagonists under general anesthesia in a hospital. The impact of rapid detoxification on relapse rates, compared to more traditional methods, is not known at this time.

Methadone maintenance programs are of some value in chronic recidivism. Under carefully controlled supervision, the narcotic addict is maintained on fairly high doses of methadone (40–120 mg/d) that satisfy craving and block the effects of heroin to a great degree.

Narcotic antagonists (eg, naltrexone) can also be used successfully for treatment of the patient who has been free of opioids for 7–10 days. Naltrexone blocks the narcotic "high" of heroin when 50 mg is given orally every 24 hours initially for several days and then 100 mg is given every 48–72 hours. Liver disorders are a major contraindication. Compliance tends to be poor, partly because of the dysphoria that can persist long after opioid discontinuance.

Sedatives (Anxiolytics)

See Anxiety Disorders, above.

Psychedelics

About 6000 species of plants have psychoactive properties. All of the common psychedelics (LSD, mescaline, psilocybin, dimethyltryptamine, and other derivatives of phenylalanine and tryptophan) can produce similar behavioral and physiologic effects. An initial feeling of tension is followed by emotional release such as crying or laughing (1–2 hours). Later, perceptual distortions occur, with visual illusions and hallucinations, and occasionally there is fear of ego disintegration (2–3 hours). Major changes in time sense and mood lability then occur (3–4 hours). A feeling of detachment and a sense of destiny and control occur (4–6 hours). Of course, reactions vary among individuals, and some of the drugs produce markedly different time frames. Occasionally, the acute episode is terrifying (a "bad trip") which may include panic, depression, confusion, or psychotic symptoms. Preexisting emotional problems, the attitude of the user, and the setting where the drug is used affect the experience

Treatment of the acute episode primarily involves protection of the individual from erratic behavior that may lead to injury or death. A structured environment is usually sufficient until the drug is metabolized. In severe cases, antipsychotic drugs with minimal side effects (eg, haloperidol, 5 mg intramuscularly) may be given every several hours until the individual has regained control. In cases where "flashbacks" occur (mental imagery from a "bad trip" that is later triggered by mild stimuli such as marijuana, alcohol, or psychic trauma), a short course of an antipsychotic drug (eg, trifluoperazine, 5 mg orally) for several days is usually sufficient. An occasional patient may have "flashbacks" for much longer periods and require small doses of neuroleptic drugs over the longer term.

Phencyclidine

Phencyclidine (PCP, angel dust, peace pill, hog), developed as an anesthetic agent, first appeared as a street drug deceptively sold as tetrahydrocannabinol (THC). Because it is simple to produce and mimics to some degree the traditional psychedelic drugs, PCP has become a common deceptive substitute for LSD, THC, and mescaline. It is available in crystals, capsules, and tablets to be inhaled, injected, swallowed, or smoked (it is commonly sprinkled on marijuana).

Absorption after smoking is rapid, with onset of symptoms in several minutes and peak symptoms in 15–30 minutes. Mild intoxication produces euphoria accompanied by a feeling of numbness. Moderate intoxication (5–10 mg) results in disorientation, detachment from surroundings, distortion of body image, combativeness, unusual feats of strength (partly due to its anesthetic activity), and loss of ability to integrate sensory input, especially touch and proprioception. Physical symptoms include dizziness, ataxia, dysarthria, nystagmus, retracted upper eyelid with blank stare, hyperreflexia, and tachycardia. There are increases in blood pressure, respiration, muscle tone, and urine production. Usage in the first trimester of pregnancy is associated with an increase in spontaneous abortion and congenital defects. Severe intoxication (20 mg or more) produces an increase in degree of moderate symptoms, with the addition of seizures, deepening coma, hypertensive crisis, and severe psychotic ideation. The drug is particularly long-lasting (several days to several weeks) owing to high lipid solubility, gastroenteric recycling, and the production of active metabolites. Overdosage may be fatal, with the major causes of death being hypertensive crisis, respiratory arrest, and convulsions. Acute rhabdomyolysis has been reported and can result in myoglobinuric renal failure.

Differential diagnosis involves the whole spectrum of street drugs, since in some ways phencyclidine mimics sedatives, psychedelics, and marijuana in its effects. Blood and urine testing can detect the acute problem.

Treatment is discussed in Chapter 39.

Marijuana

Cannabis sativa, a hemp plant, is the source of marijuana. The parts of the plant vary in potency. The resinous exudate of the flowering tops of the female plant (hashish, charas) is the most potent, followed by the dried leaves and flowering shoots of the female plant (bhang) and the resinous mass from small leaves of inflorescence (ganja). The least potent parts are the lower branches and the leaves of the female plant and all parts of the male plant. Mercury may be a contaminant in marijuana grown in volcanic soil. The drug is usually inhaled by smoking. Effects occur in 10–20 minutes and last 2–3 hours. "Joints" of good quality contain about 500 mg of marijuana (which contains approximately 5–15 mg of tetrahydrocannabinol with a half-life of 7 days). Marijuana soaked in formaldehyde and dried ("AMP") has produced unusual effects, including autonomic discharge and severe though transient cognitive impairment.

With moderate dosage, marijuana produces two phases: mild euphoria followed by sleepiness. In the acute state, the user has an altered time perception, less inhibited emotions, psychomotor problems, impaired immediate memory, and conjunctival injection. High doses produce transient psychotomimetic effects. No specific treatment is necessary except in the case of the occasional "bad trip," in which case the person is treated in the same way as for psychedelic usage. Marijuana frequently aggravates existing mental illness, adversely affects motor performance, and slows the learning process in children.

Studies of long-term effects have conclusively shown abnormalities in the pulmonary tree. Laryngitis and rhinitis are related to prolonged use, along with chronic obstructive pulmonary disease. Electrocardiographic abnormalities are common, but no long-term cardiac disease has been linked to marijuana use. Chronic usage has resulted in depression of plasma testosterone levels and reduced sperm counts. Abnormal menstruation and failure to ovulate have occurred in some female users. Cognitive impairments are probable, though studies are not conclusive. Health care utilization for a variety of health problems is increased in chronic marijuana smokers. Sudden withdrawal produces insomnia, nausea, myalgia, and irritability. Psychologic effects of chronic marijuana usage are still unclear. Urine testing is reliable if samples are carefully collected and tested. Detection periods span 4–6 days in acute users and 20–50 days in chronic users.

Stimulants: Amphetamines & Cocaine

Stimulant abuse is quite common, either alone or in combination with abuse of other drugs. The **amphetamines,** including Methedrine ("speed")—one variant is a smokable form called "ice," which gives an intense and fairly long-lasting high—methylphenidate, and phenmetrazine, are under prescription control, but street availability remains high. Moderate usage of any of the stimulants produces hyperactivity, a sense of enhanced physical and mental capacity, and sympathomimetic effects. The clinical picture of acute stimulant intoxication includes sweating, tachycardia, elevated blood pressure, mydriasis, hyperactivity, and an acute brain syndrome with confusion and disorientation. Tolerance develops quickly and, as the dosage is increased, hypervigilance, paranoid ideation (with delusions of parasitosis), stereotypy, bruxism, tactile hallucinations of insect infestation, and full-blown psychoses occur, often with persecutory ideation and aggressive responses. Stimulant withdrawal is characterized by depression with symptoms of hyperphagia and hypersomnia.

People who have used stimulants chronically (eg, anorexigenics) occasionally become sensitized **("kindling")** to future use of stimulants. In these individuals, even small amounts of mild stimulants such as caffeine can cause symptoms of paranoia and auditory hallucinations.

Cocaine is a stimulant. It is a product of the coca plant. The derivatives include seeds, leaves, coca paste, cocaine hydrochloride, and the free base of cocaine. Coca paste is a crude extract that contains 40–80% cocaine sulfate and other impurities. Cocaine hydrochloride is the salt and the most commonly used form. Free base, a purer (and stronger) derivative called "crack," is prepared by simple extraction from cocaine hydrochloride.

There are various modes of use. Coca leaf chewing involves toasting the leaves and chewing with alkaline material (eg, the ash of other burned leaves) to enhance buccal absorption. One achieves a mild high, with onset in 5–10 minutes and lasting for about an hour. Intranasal use is simply snorting cocaine through a straw. Absorption is slowed somewhat by vasoconstriction (which may eventually cause tissue necrosis and septal perforation); the onset of action is in 2–3 minutes, with a moderate high (euphoria, excitement, increased energy) lasting about 30 minutes. The purity of the cocaine is a major determinant of the high. Intravenous use of cocaine hydrochloride or "freebase" is effective in 30 seconds and produces a short-lasting, fairly intense high of about 15 minutes' duration. The combined use of cocaine and ethanol results in the metabolic production of cocaethylene by the liver. This substance produces more intense and long-lasting cocaine-like effects. Smoking freebase (volatilized cocaine because of the lower boiling point) acts in seconds and results in an intense high lasting several minutes. The intensity of the reaction is related to the marked lipid solubility of the freebase form and produces by far the most severe medical and psychiatric symptoms.

Cardiovascular collapse, arrhythmias, myocardial infarction, and transient ischemic attacks have been reported. Seizures, strokes, migraine symptoms, hyperthermia, and lung damage may occur, and there are several obstetric complications, including spontaneous abortion, abruptio placentae, teratogenic effects, delayed fetal growth, and prematurity. Cocaine can cause anxiety, mood swings, and delirium, and chronic use can cause the same problems as other stimulants (see above).

Physicians should be alert to cocaine use in patients presenting with unexplained nasal bleeding, headaches, fatigue, insomnia, anxiety, depression, and chronic hoarseness. Sudden withdrawal of the drug is not life-threatening but usually produces craving, sleep disturbances, hyperphagia, lassitude, and severe depression (sometimes with suicidal ideation) lasting days to weeks.

Treatment is imprecise and difficult. Since the high is related to blockage of dopamine reuptake, the dopamine agonist bromocriptine, 1.5 mg orally three times a day, alleviates some of the symptoms of craving associated with acute cocaine withdrawal. Other dopamine agonists such as apomorphine, levodopa, and amantadine are under study for this purpose. There is preliminary evidence that carbamazepine in the usual doses reduces craving in withdrawal (probably owing to its effect on kindling), and desipramine in moderate doses has been useful in helping maintain abstinence in the early stages of treatment. Treatment of psychosis is the same as that of any psychosis: antipsychotic drugs in dosages sufficient to alleviate the symptoms. Any medical symptoms (eg, hyperthermia, seizures, hypertension) are treated specifically. These approaches should be used in conjunction with a structured program, most often based on the AA model. Hospitalization may be required if self-harm or violence toward others is a perceived threat (usually indicated by paranoid delusions).

Caffeine

Caffeine, along with nicotine and alcohol, is one of the most commonly used drugs worldwide. About 10 billion pounds of coffee (the richest source of caffeine) are consumed yearly throughout the world. Tea, cocoa, and cola drinks also contribute to an intake of caffeine that is often astoundingly high in a large number of people. Low to moderate doses (30–200 mg/d) tend to improve some aspects of performance (eg, vigilance). The approximate content of caffeine in a (180 mL) cup of beverage is as follows: brewed coffee, 80–140 mg; instant coffee, 60–100 mg; decaffeinated coffee, 1–6 mg; black leaf tea, 30–80 mg; tea bags, 25–75 mg; instant tea, 30–60 mg; cocoa, 10–50 mg; and 12-oz cola drinks, 30–65 mg. A 2-oz chocolate candy bar has about 20 mg. Some herbal teas (eg, "morning thunder") contain caffeine. Caffeine-containing analgesics usually contain approximately 30 mg per unit. Symptoms of caffeinism (usually associated with ingestion of over 500 mg/d) include anxiety, agitation, restlessness, insomnia, a feeling of being "wired," and somatic symptoms referable to the heart and gastrointestinal tract. It is common for a case of caffeinism to present as an anxiety disorder. It is also common for caffeine and other stimulants to precipitate severe symptoms in compensated schizophrenic and manic-depressive patients. Chronically depressed patients often use caffeine drinks as self-medication. This diagnostic clue may help distinguish some major affective disorders. Withdrawal from caffeine (> 250 mg/d) can produce headaches, irritability, lethargy, and occasional nausea.

Miscellaneous Drugs, Solvents

The principal OTC drugs of concern are phenylpropanolamine and an assortment of antihistaminic agents. Frequently, these drugs are sold in combination with a mild analgesic as cold remedies (eg, Dristan, Triaminic). Most appetite suppressant drugs are combinations of phenylpropanolamine and caffeine; these drugs are also heavily marketed as "stay-awake" drugs. Practically all of the so-called sleep aids are now antihistamines. Scopolamine and bromides have generally been removed from OTC products.

The major problem in the use of all these drugs relates to phenylpropanolamine, which has all the side effects of any stimulant, including precipitation of anxiety states, increased pressor effect, auditory and visual hallucinations, paranoid ideation, and, occasionally, delirium. Aggressiveness and some loss of impulse control have been reported. Sleep disturbances are common even with reasonably small doses.

Antihistamines usually produce some central nervous system depression—thus their use as OTC sedatives. Drowsiness may be a problem. The mixture of antihistamines with alcohol usually exacerbates the central nervous system effects.

The abuse of laxatives sometimes can lead to electrolyte disturbances that may contribute to the manifestations of a delirium. The greatest use of laxatives tends to be in the elderly and in those with eating disorders, both of whom are the most vulnerable to physiologic changes.

Anabolic steroids are being abused by people who wish to increase muscle mass for cosmetic reasons or for greater strength. In addition to the medical problems, the practice is associated with significant mood swings, aggressiveness, and paranoid delusions. Alcohol and stimulant use is higher in these individuals. Withdrawal symptoms of steroid dependency include fatigue, depressed mood, restlessness, and insomnia.

Amyl nitrite, a drug useful in angina pectoris, has been used in recent years as an "orgasm expander." The changes in time perception, "rush," and mild euphoria caused by the drug prompted its nonmedical use, and popular lore concerning the effects of inhalation just prior to orgasm has led to increased use. Subjective effects last from 5 seconds to 15 minutes. Tolerance develops readily, but there are no known withdrawal symptoms. Abstinence for several days reestablishes the previous level of responsiveness. Long-term effects may include damage to the immune system and respiratory difficulties.

Sniffing of solvents and inhaling of gases (including aerosols) produce a form of inebriation similar to that of the volatile anesthetics. Agents include gasoline, toluene, petroleum ether, lighter fluids, cleaning fluids, paint thinners, and solvents that are present in many household products (eg, nail polish, typewriter correction fluid). Typical intoxication states include euphoria, slurred speech, hallucinations, and confusion, and with high doses, acute manifestations are unconsciousness and cardiorespiratory depression or failure; chronic exposure produces a variety of symptoms related to the liver, kidney, bone marrow, or heart. Lead encephalopathy can be associated with sniffing leaded gasoline. In addition, studies of workers chronically exposed to jet fuel showed significant increases in neurasthenic symptoms, including fatigue, anxiety, mood changes, memory difficulties, and somatic complaints. These same problems have been noted in long-term solvent abuse.

The so-called designer drugs are synthetic substitutes for commonly used recreational drugs and are produced in small, clandestine laboratories. The most common designer drugs have been methyl analogues of fentanyl and have been used as heroin substitutes. MDMA (methylenedioxymethamphetamine), an amphetamine derivative sometimes called "ecstasy," is also a designer drug with high abuse potential and neurotoxicity. Manufacture and use of these substances are a vexing problem for law enforcement, since the newest drugs have not yet achieved illegal status and there are no tests developed for detection. Furthermore, they present problems for physicians faced with symptoms from a totally unknown cause.

Harder S et al: Concentration-effect relationship of delta-9-tetrahydrocannabinol and prediction of psychotropic effects after smoking marijuana. Int J Clin Pharmacol Ther 1997;35:155. [NLM Cit ID: 97266342] (Smoking marijuana can lead to a plateau THC blood level that persists for 150 minutes after the last joint.)

National Consensus Development Panel on Effective Medical Treatment of Opiate Addiction: Effective medical treatment of opiate addiction. JAMA 1998;280:1936. [NLM Cit ID: 99066805] (Patients with opiate dependence should have access to methadone hydrochloride maintenance therapy.)

O'Brien CP: Recent developments in the pharmacotherapy of substance abuse. J Consult Clin Psychol 1996;64:677. [NLM Cit ID: 96396236]

O'Connor PG et al: Rapid and ultrarapid opioid detoxification techniques. JAMA 1998;279:229. [NLM Cit ID: 98099583]

DELIRIUM, DEMENTIA, & OTHER COGNITIVE DISORDERS (Formerly: Organic Brain Syndrome [OBS])

Essentials of Diagnosis

- Transient or permanent brain dysfunction.
- Cognitive impairment to varying degrees: may include impaired recall and recent memory, inability

to focus attention, random psychomotor activity such as stereotypy, and problems in perceptual processing, often with psychotic ideation.

- Emotional disorders frequently present: depression, anxiety, irritability.
- Behavioral disturbances may include problems of impulse control, sexual acting-out, attention deficits, aggression, and exhibitionism.

General Considerations

The organic problem may be a primary brain disease or a secondary manifestation of some general disorder. All of the cognitive disorders show some degree of impaired thinking depending on the site of involvement, the rate of onset and progression, and the duration of the underlying brain lesion. Emotional disturbances (eg, depression) are often present as significant comorbidities. The behavioral disturbances tend to be more common with chronicity, more directly related to the underlying personality or central nervous system vulnerability to drug side effects, and not necessarily correlated with cognitive dysfunction.

Etiology

A. Intoxication: Alcohol, sedatives, bromides, analgesics (eg, pentazocine), psychedelic drugs, stimulants, and household solvents.

B. Drug Withdrawal: Withdrawal from alcohol, sedative-hypnotics, corticosteroids.

C. Long-Term Effects of Alcohol: Wernicke-Korsakoff syndrome.

D. Infections: Septicemia; meningitis and encephalitis due to bacterial, viral, fungal, parasitic, or tuberculous organisms or to central nervous system syphilis; acute and chronic infections due to the entire range of microbiologic pathogens.

E. Endocrine Disorders: Thyrotoxicosis, hypothyroidism, adrenocortical dysfunction (including Addison's disease and Cushing's syndrome), pheochromocytoma, insulinoma, hypoglycemia, hyperparathyroidism, hypoparathyroidism, panhypopituitarism, diabetic ketoacidosis.

F. Respiratory Disorders: Hypoxia, hypercapnia.

G. Metabolic Disturbances: Fluid and electrolyte disturbances (especially hyponatremia, hypomagnesemia, and hypercalcemia), acid-base disorders, hepatic disease (hepatic encephalopathy), renal failure, porphyria.

H. Nutritional Deficiencies: Deficiency of vitamin B_1 (beriberi), vitamin B_{12} (pernicious anemia), folic acid, nicotinic acid (pellagra); protein-calorie malnutrition.

I. Trauma: Subdural hematoma, subarachnoid hemorrhage, intracerebral bleeding, concussion syndrome.

J. Cardiovascular Disorders: Myocardial infarctions, cardiac arrhythmias, cerebrovascular spasms, hypertensive encephalopathy, hemorrhages, embolisms, and occlusions indirectly cause decreased cognitive function.

K. Neoplasms: Primary or metastatic lesions of the central nervous system, cancer-induced hypercalcemia.

L. Seizure Disorders: Ictal, interictal, and postictal dysfunction.

M. Collagen and Immunologic Disorders: Autoimmune disorders, including systemic lupus erythematosus, Sjögren's syndrome, and AIDS.

N. Degenerative Diseases: Alzheimer's disease, Pick's disease, multiple sclerosis, parkinsonism, Huntington's chorea, normal pressure hydrocephalus.

O. Medications: Anticholinergic drugs, antidepressants, H_2-blocking agents, digoxin, salicylates (chronic use), and a wide variety of other OTC and prescribed drugs.

Clinical Findings

The manifestations are many and varied and include problems with orientation, short or fluctuating attention span, loss of recent memory and recall, impaired judgment, emotional lability, lack of initiative, impaired impulse control, inability to reason through problems, depression (worse in mild to moderate types), confabulation (not limited to alcohol organic brain syndrome), constriction of intellectual functions, visual and auditory hallucinations, and delusions. Physical findings will naturally vary according to the cause. The EEG usually shows generalized slowing in delirium.

A. Delirium: Delirium (acute confusional state) is a transient global disorder of attention, with clouding of consciousness, usually a result of systemic problems (eg, drugs, hypoxemia). Onset is usually rapid. The mental status fluctuates (impairment is usually least in the morning), with varying inability to concentrate, maintain attention, and sustain purposeful behavior. ("Sundowning"—mild to moderate delirium at night—is more common in patients with preexisting dementia and may be precipitated by hospitalization, drugs, and sensory deprivation.) There is a marked deficit of short-term memory and recall. Anxiety and irritability are common. Amnesia is retrograde (impaired recall of past memories) and anterograde (inability to recall events after the onset of the delirium). Orientation problems follow the inability to retain information. Perceptual disturbances (often visual hallucinations) and psychomotor restlessness with insomnia are common. Autonomic changes include tachycardia, dilated pupils, and sweating. The average duration is about 1 week, with full recovery in most cases. Delirium can coexist with dementia.

B. Dementia: (See also Chapter 3.) Dementia is characterized by chronicity and deterioration of selective mental functions. Onset is insidious over months to years in most cases. Dementia is usually progressive, more common in the elderly, and rarely reversible even if underlying disease can be corrected. Dementia can be classified as cortical or subcortical.

There are three types of cortical dementia: (1) primary degenerative dementia (eg, Alzheimer's), accounting for about 50–60% of cases; (2) atherosclerotic (multi-infarct) dementia, 15–20% of cases (this figure is probably low because of the tendency to overuse the diagnosis of Alzheimer's dementia); and (3) mixtures of the first two types or dementia due to miscellaneous causes, 15–20% of cases (see also Chapter 3). Examples of primary degenerative dementia are Alzheimer's dementia (most common) and Pick, Creutzfeldt-Jakob, and Huntington dementias (less common).

In all types, loss of impulse control (sexual and language) is common. The tenuous level of functioning makes the individual most susceptible to minor physical and psychologic stresses. The course depends on the underlying cause, and the general trend is steady deterioration.

HIV infection can produce a primary neurogenic disorder (partially due to neuronal loss) and secondary effects due to opportunistic infections, neoplasias, or the effects of drug therapy. At present there has been a reduction in dementia symptoms in both early and late stages, perhaps due to earlier use of zidovudine. The general trend is variable, and patients require ongoing monitoring of neuropsychiatric status.

Pseudodementia is a term applied to depressed patients who appear to be demented. These patients are often identifiable by their tendency to complain about memory problems vociferously rather than try to cover them up. They usually say they can't complete cognitive tasks but with encouragement can often do so.

C. Amnestic Syndrome: This is a memory disturbance without delirium or dementia. It is usually associated with thiamin deficiency and chronic alcohol use (eg, Korsakoff's syndrome). There is an impairment in the ability to learn new information or recall previously learned information.

D. Substance-Induced Hallucinosis: This condition is characterized by persistent or recurrent hallucinations (usually auditory) without the other symptoms usually found in delirium or dementia. Alcohol or hallucinogens are often the cause. There does not have to be any other mental disorder, and there may be complete spontaneous resolution.

E. Personality Changes Due to a General Medical Condition (Formerly Organic Personality Syndrome): This syndrome is characterized by emotional lability and loss of impulse control along with a general change in personality. Cognitive functions are preserved. Social inappropriateness is common. Loss of interest and lack of concern with the consequences of one's actions are often present. The course depends on the underlying cause (eg, frontal lobe contusion may resolve completely).

Differential Diagnosis

The differential diagnosis consists mainly of schizophrenia and the other psychoses, which are sometimes confused with cognitive disorders which are often accompanied by psychotic symptoms.

Complications

Chronicity may result from delayed correction of the defect, eg, subdural hematoma, low-pressure hydrocephalus. Accidents secondary to impulsive behavior and poor judgment are a major consideration. Secondary depression and impulsive behavior not infrequently lead to suicide attempts. Drugs—particularly sedatives—may worsen thinking abilities and contribute to the overall problems.

Treatment (See also Chapter 3.)

A. Medical: Delirium should be considered a syndrome of acute brain dysfunction analogous to acute renal failure. The first aim of treatment is to identify and correct the etiologic medical problem. Evaluation should consist of a comprehensive physical examination including a search for neurologic abnormalities, infection, or hypoxia. Routine laboratory tests may include serum electrolytes, serum glucose, BUN, serum creatinine, liver function tests, thyroid function tests, arterial blood gases, complete blood count, serum calcium, phosphorus, magnesium, vitamin B_{12}, folate, blood cultures, urinalysis, and cerebrospinal fluid analysis. Discontinue drugs that may be contributing to the problem (eg, analgesics, corticosteroids, cimetidine, lidocaine, anticholinergic drugs, central nervous system depressants, mefloquine). Do not overlook any possibility of reversible organic disease. Electroencephalography, CT, MRI, PET, and SPECT evaluations may be helpful in diagnosis. Ideally, the patient should be monitored without further medications while the evaluation is carried out. There are, however, two indications for medication in delirious states: behavioral control (eg, pulling out lines) and subjective distress (eg, pronounced fear due to hallucinations). If these indications are present, medications may be employed. If there is any hint of alcohol or substance withdrawal (the most common cause of delirium in the general hospital), a benzodiazepine such as lorazepam (1–2 mg every hour) can be given parenterally. If there is little likelihood of withdrawal syndrome, haloperidol is often used in doses of 1–10 mg every hour. Given intravenously, it appears to impose slight risk of extrapyramidal side effects. In addition to the medication, a pleasant, comfortable, nonthreatening, and physically safe environment with adequate nursing or attendant services should be provided. Once the underlying condition has been identified and treated, adjunctive medications can be tapered.

Treatment of dementia syndrome usually involves symptomatic management with one exception. Since there is a cholinergic deficiency in Alzheimer's disease, research has focused on drugs to increase cholinergic activity (eg, tacrine, phosphatidylcholine, and donepezil). Tacrine (tetrahydroaminoacridine, THA) is a reversible cholinesterase inhibitor for treatment of cognitive deficits associated with Alzheimer's disease. Studies suggest that tacrine (80–160 mg/d in four divided doses) may improve cognition in 25–42% of patients, with higher doses producing better effects. There was, however, no functional improvement in the subjects. Serum ALT levels increase in 50% of patients, with most returning to normal when the drug is discontinued. Many patients who discontinue tacrine due to elevated liver enzymes may be retried on it successfully with careful monitoring. Donepezil is a cholinesterase inhibitor found to enhance cognition and improve function in mild to moderate Alzheimer's disease. It has less benefit as the disease progresses. Unlike tacrine, it is dosed once a day, does not require hepatic monitoring, and is generally well tolerated. Common side effects are nausea, diarrhea, and vomiting. Neither tacrine nor donepezil is thought to slow disease progression.

Aggressiveness and rage states in central nervous system disease can be reduced with lipophilic beta-blockers (eg, propranolol, metoprolol) in moderate doses. Since the serotonergic system has been implicated in arousal conditions, drugs that affect serotonin have been found to be of some benefit in aggression and agitation. Included in this group are lithium, trazodone, buspirone, and clonazepam. Dopamine blockers (eg, the neuroleptic drugs such as haloperidol) have been used for many years to attenuate aggression. There are recent reports of reduced agitation in Alzheimer's disease from carbamazepine, 100–400 mg/d orally (with slow increase as needed). Emotional lability in some cases responds to small doses of imipramine (25 mg orally one to three times per day) or fluoxetine (5–20 mg/d orally); and depression, which often occurs early in the course of Alzheimer's dementia, responds to the usual doses of antidepressant drugs, preferably those with the least anticholinergic side effects (eg, SSRIs and MAO inhibitors).

Cerebral vasodilators were originally used on the assumption that cerebral arteriosclerosis and ischemia were the principal causes of the dementias. Although there is a slight reduction of blood flow in primary degenerative dementia (probably as a result of the basic disorder), there is no evidence that this is a major factor in this group of disorders or that vasodilators are of value. Ergotoxine alkaloids (ergoloid mesylates: Hydergine, others) have been studied with mixed results; improvement in ambulatory self-care and depressed mood has been noted, but there has been no improvement of cognitive functioning on any standardized tests. Hyperbaric oxygen treatment has not produced significant improvement. Stimulant drugs (eg, methylphenidate) do not change cognitive function but can improve affect and mood, which helps the caretakers cope with the problem.

Failing sensory functions should be supported as necessary, with hearing aids, cataract surgery, etc.

B. Social: Substitute home care, board and care, or convalescent home care may be most useful when the family is unable to care for the patient. The setting should include familiar people and objects, lights at night, and a simple schedule. Counseling may help the family to cope with problems and may help keep the patient at home as long as possible. Information about local groups can be obtained from the Alzheimer's Disease and Related Disorders Association, 70 East Lake Street, Suite 600, Chicago, IL 60601. Volunteer services, including homemakers, visiting nurses, and adult protective services, may be helpful in maintaining the patient at home.

C. Behavioral: Behavioral techniques include operant responses that can be used to induce positive behaviors, eg, paying attention to the patient who is trying to communicate appropriately, and extinction by ignoring inappropriate responses. Alzheimer's patients can learn skills and retain them but do not recall the circumstances in which they were learned.

D. Psychologic: Formal psychologic therapies are not usually helpful and may make things worse by taxing the patient's limited cognitive resources.

Prognosis

The prognosis is good for recovery of mental functioning in delirium when the underlying condition is reversible. For most dementia syndromes, the prognosis is for gradual deterioration, though new drug treatments may prove helpful.

Delagarza VW: New drugs for Alzheimer's disease. Am Fam Physician 1998;58:1175. [NLM Cit ID: 97266342]

Gruetzner H: *Alzheimer's: A Complete Guide for Families and Loved Ones.* Wiley, 1997. (An excellent guide for family caregivers.)

JAMA patient page: Alzheimer disease. JAMA 1998; 280:674. [NLM Cit ID: 98382165]

Rogers SL: Perspective in the management of disease: Clinical profile of donepezil. Dement Geriatr Cogn Disord 1998;9:29. [NLM Cit ID: 99070312]

GERIATRIC PSYCHIATRIC DISORDERS (See also Chapter 3.)

There are three basic factors in the process of aging: biologic, sociologic, and psychologic.

The complex **biologic** changes depend on inherited characteristics (the best chance of long life is to have long-lived parents), nutrition, declining sensory functions such as hearing or vision, disease, trauma, and lifestyle. A definite correlation between hearing loss and paranoid ideation exists in the elderly. (See Organic Brain Syndrome, above.) As a person ages, relatively minor disorders or combinations of disorders may cause deficits in cognition and affective response. Hypochondriasis is frequently a mechanism of compensating for decreased function (eg, preoccupation with bowel function).

The **sociologic** factors derive from stresses connected with occupation, family, and community. Any or all of these areas may be disrupted in a general phenomenon of "disengagement" and lack of intimacy that older people experience as friends die, the children move away, and the surroundings become less familiar. Retirement commonly precipitates a major disruption in a well-established life structure. This is particularly stressful in the person whose compulsive devotion to a job has inhibited the development of other interests, so that sudden loss of this outlet leaves a void that is not easily filled. New duties, such as caring for a spouse with dementia, may also lead to depression.

The **psychologic** withdrawal of the elderly person is frequently related to a loss of self-esteem, which is based on the economic insecurity of older age with its congruent loss of independence, the recognition of decreasing physical and mental ability, loneliness, and the fear of approaching death. The process of aging is often poorly accepted, and the real or imagined loss of physical attractiveness may have a traumatic impact that the plastic surgeon can only soften for a time. In a culture that stresses physical and sexual attractiveness, it is difficult for some people to accept the change.

Clinical Findings & Complications

The most common psychiatric syndrome in the elderly is dementia (organic brain syndrome) of varying degree. Psychotic ideation (usually paranoid) may coexist with dementia. Frequently, in milder cases, the individual is aware of the deficiency in cognition and becomes depressed about actual or threatened loss of function. Depression may then amplify the apparent cognitive decline.

Overt depression, often presenting as a somatic complaint, is often related to life changes (80% of people over age 65 have some kind of medical problem). Alcoholism is present in approximately 15% of older patients presenting with psychiatric symptoms. The incidence of suicide is higher in elderly people—loneliness, age, and medical problems being directly related. Deprivation of full-spectrum light may be a factor in some patients (eg, nursing home residents). Anxiety, often associated with organic illness, heightens preexisting confusion in the patient with cognitive dysfunction.

Abuse of the elderly—both physical neglect (passive) and physical injury (active)—demands early recognition. Bruises, welts, fractures, and debilitation should alert the physician. The battered elderly are probably just as numerous as battered children, but less reported, and require the same diligence in physician recognition.

Polypharmacy (with both prescription and OTC drugs) is a major cause of accidents (often with resultant hip fracture) and illness in the elderly. Cognitive impairment increases as the number of drugs used increases; sedatives and anticholinergic drugs are the major culprits (eg, overuse in sleep problems). The increased and varied complaints are often an attempt to compensate and divert attention from decreased mental function.

Treatment

A. Social: Socialization, a structured schedule of activities, familiar surroundings, continued achievement, and avoidance of loneliness (probably the most important factor) are some of the major considerations in prevention and amelioration of the psychiatric problems of old age. The patient can be supported in the primary environment by various agencies that can help avoid a premature change of habits. For patients with disabilities that make it difficult to cope with the problems of living alone, homemaker services can assist in continuing the day-to-day activities of the household; visiting nurses can administer medications and monitor the physical condition of the patient; and geriatric social groups can help maintain socialization and human contacts. In the hospital or nursing home, attention to the kinds of people placed in the same room is most important (mix active and inactive patients).

B. Medical: Treatment of any reversible components of a dementia syndrome is obviously the major medical consideration. One commonly overlooked factor is self-medication, frequently with nonprescription drugs that further impair the patient's already precarious functioning. Common culprits are antihistamines and anticholinergic drugs, sometimes mixed with ethanol abuse.

Any signs of psychosis, such as paranoid ideation, agitation, and delusions, respond very well to *small doses* of antipsychotics. Trifluoperazine, 2–5 mg orally once a day, or fluphenazine, 1–2 mg orally daily, will usually decrease psychotic ideation markedly.

Do not use drugs that cause significant orthostatic hypotension (resulting in dizziness, falls, fractures).

Antidepressants (in one-third to one-half the doses given to young adults) are used when indicated for depression. Occasionally, a stimulant in small doses (eg, methylphenidate, 5–30 mg orally usually given in two doses at 7 AM and noon) can be used to treat apathy. The stimulant may help increase the patient's energy for social involvement and help the patient to maintain life activities.

The appropriate use of wine and beer for mild sedative effects is quite rewarding in the hospital and other care facilities as well as at home.

C. Behavioral: The impaired cognitive abilities of the geriatric patient necessitate simple behavioral techniques. Positive responses to appropriate behavior encourage the patient to repeat desirable kinds of behavior, and frequent repetition offsets to some degree the defects in recent memory and recall. It also results in participation—a most important element, since there is a tendency in the older population to withdraw, thus increasing isolation and functional decline.

One must be careful not to reinforce and encourage obstreperous behavior by responding to it; in this way, extinction or at least gradual reduction of inappropriate behavior will occur. At the same time, the obstreperous behavior often represents a nondirective response to frustration and inability to function, and a structured program of activity is necessary.

D. Psychologic: Patients may require help in adjusting to changing roles and commitments and in finding new goals and viewpoints. The older person steadily loses an important commodity—the future—and may attempt to compensate by preoccupation with the past. Involvement with the present and psychotherapy on a here-and-now basis can help make the adjustment easier.

Grossman F: A review of anticonvulsants in treating agitated demented elderly patients. Pharmacotherapy 1998; 18:600. [NLM Cit ID: 98281420] (Divalproex sodium and carbamazepine are effective and well tolerated.)

Verma SD et al: Management of the agitated elderly patient in nursing homes: The role of the atypical antipsychotics. J Clin Psychiatry 1998;59(Suppl 19):50. [NLM Cit ID: 99061509] (Although behavioral interventions are often effective, the newer antipsychotics appear to impose a lesser risk of tardive dyskinesia and extrapyramidal side effects.)

PSYCHIATRIC PROBLEMS ASSOCIATED WITH HOSPITALIZATION & MEDICAL & SURGICAL DISORDERS

Diagnostic Categories

A. Acute Problems:

1. Delirium with psychotic features secondary to the medical or surgical problem, or compounded by effect of treatment.

2. Acute anxiety, often related to ignorance and fear of the immediate problem as well as uncertainty about the future.

3. Anxiety as an intrinsic aspect of the medical problem (eg, hyperthyroidism).

4. Denial of illness, which may present during acute or intermediate phases of illness.

B. Intermediate Problems:

1. Depression as a function of the illness or acceptance of the illness, often associated with realistic or fantasied hopelessness about the future.

2. Behavioral problems, often related to denial of illness and in extreme cases, causing the patient to leave the hospital against medical advice.

C. Recuperative Problems:

1. Decreasing cooperation as the patient sees improvement and compliance is not compelled.

2. Readjustment problems with family, job, and society.

General Considerations

A. Acute Problems:

1. "Intensive care unit psychosis" is a delirium. The stressful environment may contribute to the problem. Critical care unit factors include sleep deprivation, increased arousal, mechanical ventilation, and social isolation. Other causes include those common to delirium and require vigorous investigation (see Delirium, above).

2. Pre- and postsurgical anxiety states are common—and commonly ignored. Presurgical anxiety is very common and is principally a fear of death (many surgical patients make out their wills). Patients may be fearful of anesthesia (improved by the preoperative anesthesia interview), the mysterious operating room, and the disease processes that might be uncovered by the surgeon. Such fears frequently cause people to delay examinations that might result in earlier surgery and a greater chance of cure.

The opposite of this is **surgery proneness,** the quest for surgery to escape from overwhelming life stresses. Polysurgery patients are not easily categorized. Dynamic motivations include narcissism, societal pressures (eg, breast implants), unconscious guilt, a masochistic need to suffer, an attempt to deal with another family member's illness, and somatoform disorders and body dysmorphic disorder (an obsession that a body part is disfigured). More apparent reasons may include an attempt to get relief from pain and a lifestyle that has become almost exclusively medically oriented, with all of the risks entailed in such an endeavor.

Postsurgical anxiety states are usually related to pain, procedures, and loss of body image. Acute pain problems are quite different from chronic pain disorders (see Chronic Pain Disorders, above); the former are readily handled with adequate analgesic medication (see Chapter 1). Alterations in body image, as with amputations, ostomies, and mastectomies, often raise concerns about relationships with others.

3. Iatrogenic problems usually pertain to medications, complications of diagnostic and treatment procedures, and impersonal and unsympathetic staff behavior. Polypharmacy is often a factor. Patients with unsolved diagnostic problems are at higher risk. They are desirous of relief, and the quest engenders more diagnostic procedures with a higher incidence of complications. The upset patient and family may be very demanding. Excessive demands usually result from anxiety. Such behavior is best handled with calm and measured responses.

B. Intermediate Problems:

1. Prolonged hospitalization presents unique problems in certain hospital services, eg, burn units, orthopedic services, and tuberculosis wards. The acute problems of the severely burned patient are discussed in Chapter 38. The problems often are behavioral difficulties related to length of hospitalization and necessary procedures. For example, in burn units, pain is a major problem in addition to anxiety about procedures. Disputes with staff are common and often concern pain medication or ward privileges. Some patients regress to infantile behavior and dependency. Staff members must agree about their approach to the patient in order to ensure the smooth functioning of the unit.

Denial of illness may present in the patient with acute myocardial infarction. Intervention by an authority figure (eg, immediate work supervisor) may help the patient accept treatment and eventually abandon the defense of denial.

2. Depression frequently occurs during this period. Therapeutic drugs (eg, corticosteroids) may be a factor. Depression can contribute to irritability and overt anger. Severe depression can lead to anorexia, which further complicates healing and metabolic balance. It is during this period that the issue of disfigurement arises—relief at survival gives way to concern about future function and appearance.

C. Recuperative Problems:

1. Anxiety about return to the posthospital environment can cause regression to a dependent position. Complications increase, and staff forbearance again is tested. Anxiety occurring at this stage usually is handled more easily than previous behavior problems.

2. Posthospital adjustment is related to the severity of the deficits and the use of outpatient facilities (eg, physical therapy, rehabilitation programs, psychiatric outpatient treatment). Some patients may experience posttraumatic stress symptoms (eg, from traumatic injuries or even from necessary medical treatments). Lack of appropriate follow-up can contribute to depression in the patient, who may feel that he or she is making poor progress and may have thoughts of "giving up." Reintegration into work, educational, and social endeavors may be slow. Life is simply much more difficult when one is disfigured, disabled, or disfranchised.

Clinical Findings

The symptoms that occur in these patients are similar to those discussed in previous sections of this chapter, eg, organic brain syndrome, stress and adjustment disorders, anxiety, and depression. Behavior problems may include lack of cooperation, increased complaints, demands for medication, sexual approaches to nurses, threats to leave the hospital, and actual signing out against medical recommendations. The underlying personality structure of the individual is a major factor in coping styles (eg, the compulsive individual increases indecision, the hysterical individual increases dramatic behavior).

Differential Diagnosis

Delirium and dementia (including cases associated with HIV infection and drug abuse) must always be ruled out, since they often present with symptoms resembling anxiety, depression, or psychosis. Personality disorders existing prior to hospitalization often underlie the various behavior problems, but particularly the management problems.

Complications

Prolongation of hospitalization causes increased expense, deterioration of patient-staff relationships, and increased probabilities of iatrogenic and legal problems. The possibility of increasing posthospital treatment problems is enhanced.

Treatment

A. Medical: The most important consideration by far is to have one physician in charge, a physician whom the patient trusts and who is able to oversee multiple treatment approaches (see Somatoform Disorders, above). In acute problems, attention must be paid to metabolic imbalance, alcohol withdrawal, and previous drug use—prescribed, recreational, or OTC. Adequate sleep and analgesia are important in the prevention of delirium.

Most physicians are attuned to the early detection of the surgery-prone patient. Plastic and orthopedic surgeons are at particular risk. Appropriate consultations may help detect some problems and mitigate future ones.

Postsurgical anxiety states can be alleviated by personal attention from the surgeon. Anxiety is not so effectively lessened by ancillary medical personnel, whom the patient perceives as lesser authorities, until after the physician has reassured the patient. Inappropriate use of "as needed" analgesia places an unfair burden on the nurse. "Patient-controlled analgesia" can improve pain control, decrease anxiety, and minimize side effects (see Chapter 1).

Depression should be recognized early. If severe, it may be treated by antidepressant medications (see Antidepressant Drugs, above). High levels of anxiety can be lowered with judicious use of anxiolytic agents. Unnecessary medications tend to reinforce the patient's impression that there must be a serious illness or medication would not be required.

B. Psychologic: Prepare the patient and family for what is to come. This includes the types of units where the patient will be quartered, the procedures that will be performed, and any disfigurements that will result from surgery. Repetition improves understanding. The nursing staff can be helpful, since patients frequently confide a lack of understanding to a nurse but are reluctant to do so to the physician.

Denial of illness is frequently a block to acceptance of treatment. This too should be handled with family members present (to help the patient face the reality of the situation) in a series of short interviews (for reinforcement). Dependency problems resulting from long hospitalization are best handled by focusing on the changes to come as the patient makes the transition to the outside world. Key figures are teachers, vocational counselors, and physical therapists. Challenges should be realistic and practical and handled in small steps.

Depression is usually related to the loss of familiar hospital supports, and the outpatient therapists and counselors help to lessen the impact of the loss. Some of the impact can be alleviated by anticipating, with the patient and family, the signal features of the common depression to help prevent the patient from assuming a permanent sick role (invalidism).

Suicide is always a concern when a patient is faced with despair. An honest, compassionate, and supportive approach will help sustain the patient during this trying period.

C. Behavioral: Prior desensitization can significantly allay anxiety about medical procedures. A "dry run" can be done to reinforce the oral description. Cooperation during acute problem periods can be enhanced by the use of appropriate reinforcers such as a favorite nurse or helpful family member. People who are positive reinforcers are even more helpful during the intermediate phases when the patient becomes resistant to the seemingly endless procedures (eg, debridement of burned areas).

Specific situations (eg, psychologic dependency on the respirator) can be corrected by weaning with appropriate reinforcers (eg, watching a favorite movie on a videorecorder when disconnected from the ventilator). Behavioral approaches should be employed in a positive and optimistic way for maximal reinforcement.

Relaxation techniques and attentional distraction can be used to block side effects of a necessary treatment (eg, nausea in cancer chemotherapy).

D. Social: A change in environment requires adaptation. Because of the illness, admission and hospitalization may be more easily handled than discharge. Reintegration into society can be difficult. In some cases, the family is a negative influence. A predischarge evaluation must be made to determine whether the family will be able to cope with the physical or mental changes in the patient. Working with the family while the patient is in the acute stage may presage a successful transition later on.

Development of a new social life can be facilitated by various self-help organizations (eg, the stoma club). Sharing problems with others in similar circumstances eases the return to a social life which may be quite different from that prior to the illness.

Prognosis

The prognosis is good in all patients who have reversible medical and surgical conditions. It is guarded when there is serious functional loss that impairs vocational, educational, or societal possibilities—especially in the case of progressive and ultimately life-threatening illness.

Bone RC et al: Recognition, assessment, and treatment of anxiety in the critical care patient. Dis Mon 1995 May;41:293. [NLM Cit ID: 95254987] (Anxiety is ubiquitous in critical care units and can interfere with recovery if left untreated.)

Herrmann C et al: Diagnostic groups and depressed mood as predictors of 22-month mortality in medical inpatients. Psychosom Med 1998;60:570. [NLM Cit ID: 98444744] (Depressed mood was an independent risk factor associated with an odds ratio of 3.2 in predicting 22-month survival.)

Nemeroff CB et al: Depression and cardiac disease. Depress Anxiety 1998;(8 Suppl 1):71. [NLM Cit ID: 98444744] (Depression is a major risk factor for increased mortality of coronary artery disease but is often underdiagnosed and undertreated.)

RELEVANT WORLD WIDE WEB SITES

[American Hyperlexia Association—Hyperlexia]
http://www.hyperlexia.org/hyperlexia.html

[American Psychiatric Association—Let's Talk Facts About Series]
http://www.psych.org/public_info/talk_facts.html

[Autism]
http://www.autism.org/overview.html

[Children and Adults With Attention Deficit/Hyperactivity Disorder]
http://www.chadd.org

[Internet Mental Health]
http://www.mentalhealth.com/t30.html

[Mental Disorders Symptoms and Treatment Mental Health Net]
http://www.mhnet.org/sxlist.htm

[Psychopharmacology Tips]
http://uhs.bsd.uchicago.edu/~bhsiung/tips/tips.html

[Psychiatry On Line]
http://www.priory.com/psych.htm

26 Endocrinology

See http://www.current-med.com/ch26.html for updated addresses of Web sites referenced in this chapter.

Paul A. Fitzgerald, MD

Hormones exert their effects by interacting with receptors on the cell surface (catecholamines and peptide hormones) or inside the cell (thyroid and steroid hormones). Endocrine disorders result from an excess or deficiency of hormonal effects.

COMMON PRESENTATIONS IN ENDOCRINOLOGY

Obesity

Obesity is a common problem, but rarely is there an identifiable endocrine cause. Instead, obesity can usually be attributed to other factors. Most obese people underestimate their caloric intake. Physical inactivity can cause some weight gain. Aging also plays a role in obesity, since adults gain an average of 0.1 kg/m^2 yearly between ages 20 and 63 years. Genetics is the most important determinant for obesity. Studies of twins indicate that about 70% of obesity is due to genetic factors.

A gene regulating obesity (the *ob* gene) produces leptin, a cytokine secreted by fat cells in response to fat storage. With fatty weight gain, leptin acts upon the hypothalamus to promote satiety and increase the body's metabolic rate. Serum levels of leptin are an average of four times higher in most obese individuals than in their nonobese counterparts, indicating that most obesity is related to the brain's insensitivity to circulating leptin. A small percentage of cases of human obesity are due to a deficiency or detectable mutation in the gene for leptin or its receptor. Such patients have early-onset morbid obesity and hypogonadotropic hypogonadism.

Several endocrine disorders do cause obesity. Cushing's syndrome causes central obesity (due to intraperitoneal fat) with relatively thin extremities; such patients usually have plethoric, rounded (moon) facies along with prominent supraclavicular and dorsocervical fat pads (buffalo humps). Alcoholism causes hypercortisolism and a similar syndrome. Hypothyroidism occasionally causes mild weight gain due to edema and fat accumulation. Hyperthyroidism may cause mild weight gain due to hyperphagia. Pancreatic insulinomas secrete excessive amounts of insulin, causing hypoglycemia and compensatory overeating. Growth hormone deficiency usually causes mild obesity in both children and adults.

Estrogen replacement therapy and oral estrogen-containing contraceptives cause minimal weight gain. Insulin therapy for type II diabetes usually worsens obesity.

Obesity may be associated with other disorders as part of several recognized syndromes. Syndrome X (the cluster of obesity, diabetes, and hypertension) has a 50% hereditary component. Polycystic ovary syndrome refers to the combination of obesity with anovulation, amenorrhea, cystic ovaries, and hirsutism. Hypothalamic lesions can cause massive obesity and are often associated with headache, lethargy, depression, diabetes insipidus, and hypopituitarism. Congenital obesity may be due to various uncommon syndromes of hypothalamic obesity and hypogonadotropic hypogonadism.

Clement K et al: A mutation in the human leptin receptor gene causes obesity and pituitary dysfunction. Nature 1998;392:398. [NLM Cit ID: 98196670]

Overweight, obesity, and health risk. National Task Force on the Prevention and Treatment of Obesity. Arch Intern Med 2000;160:898. [NLM Cit ID: 20222590]

Pi-Sunyer FX et al: Therapeutic controversy: obesity—a modern epidemic. J Clin Endocrinol Metab 1999;84:3. [NLM Cit ID: 99116782]

Unintended Weight Loss

Uncontrolled diabetes mellitus may be associated with weight loss, polyphagia, polydipsia, and polyuria. Anorexia and nausea may be seen with diabetic ketoacidosis and with adrenal insufficiency (due either to pituitary ACTH deficiency or to Addison's disease). Patients with severe diabetes insipidus may also lose weight. Patients with hyperthyroidism typically lose weight despite increased appetite; some patients with hypothyroidism lose weight because of diminished appetite. About 15% of patients with pheochromocytoma lose over 10% of their basal weight. Some patients with Cushing's syndrome lose weight as a result of muscle wasting.

A great variety of nonendocrine conditions enter into the differential diagnosis of unintended weight loss (see Chapter 1). Anorexia is frequently a side effect of medications or radiation therapy and is also seen with azotemia, AIDS, and many gastrointestinal conditions. Malignancies typically produce diminished appetite and cachexia. Tuberculosis may cause weight loss even when occult. Chronic respiratory insufficiency is often associated with weight loss. Psychiatric illnesses producing diminished appetite include depressed or agitated affective disorder, catatonia, and anorexia nervosa.

Abnormal Skin Pigmentation

Increased skin pigmentation can be caused by excessive ACTH secretion in Addison's disease and can occur after bilateral adrenalectomy for Cushing's disease (Nelson's syndrome). Pigmentation can be generalized or may be localized to palmar creases, extensor joint surfaces, tongue, nails, belt or bra lines, freckles, or new scars.

Pigmentation of the upper lip, forehead, or malar eminences, known as **chloasma** can be caused by pregnancy ("mask of pregnancy"), oral contraceptives, or estrogen replacement therapy.

Acanthosis nigricans presents as velvety brown thickened skin of the neck and axillae. It may be associated with syndromes of severe insulin resistance type A (ovarian dysfunction and hirsutism) or type B (autoimmune). It may also be familial or associated with obesity, acromegaly, or thyroid disease. Acanthosis presenting after age 40 is often a sign of an underlying malignancy.

Pretibial areas of pigmentation are common in diabetes ("diabetic shin spots") as a result of minor trauma or following necrobiosis lipoidica diabeticorum.

Prominent lentigines can be a sign of Carney's complex, an autosomal dominant condition associated with atrial myxomas, schwannomas, and endocrine overactivity (eg, tumors of the thyroid, gonads, or pigmented adrenal nodular hyperplasia). Similar skin pigmentation is seen in Peutz-Jeghers syndrome with an increased risk of intestinal polyposis, adenocarcinoma, breast cancer, and tumors of the gonads and thyroid.

Diffuse hyperpigmentation is seen in POEMS syndrome (polyneuropathy, organomegaly, endocrinopathy, monoclonal gammopathy, skin changes); adrenal insufficiency, hypoparathyroidism, diabetes, osteosclerotic bone lesions, or thiamin deficiency may occur. Other causes of skin pigmentation include sprue, malnutrition, HIV infection, or drug effect (chlorpromazine, arsenic, minocycline, clofazimine, zidovudine, chloroquine, bleomycin, busulfan).

Gray-brown ("bronze") hyperpigmentation is caused by hemochromatosis, which can cause endocrine deficiencies such as diabetes mellitus. An orange skin discoloration is characteristic of jaundice and carotenodermia (caused by ingestion of large amounts of carotene in vegetables, seaweed, or vitamin preparations).

Patchy hypopigmentation can be due to vitiligo, a condition sometimes associated with Addison's disease and with other endocrine deficiencies as part of the polyglandular autoimmune syndrome. Hypopigmentation can also be a manifestation of cobalamin deficiency, trisomy 13, and various dermatologic conditions.

Stratakis CA et al: Carney complex, Peutz-Jeghers syndrome, Cowden disease, and Bannayan-Zonana syndrome share cutaneous and endocrine manifestations, but not genetic loci. J Clin Endocrinol Metab 1998; 83:2972. [NLM Cit ID: 98373752]

Gynecomastia

Gynecomastia is a glandular enlargement of the male breast that may be tender and is often asymmetric or unilateral. It must be distinguished from tumors and from the fatty breast enlargement of obesity.

Pubertal gynecomastia is common and is characterized by tender discoid enlargement of breast tissue 2–3 cm in diameter beneath the areola; the swelling usually subsides spontaneously within a year. Gynecomastia is also common among elderly men, particularly when there is associated weight gain. Gynecomastia can be the first sign of a serious disorder. Patients with Peutz-Jeghers syndrome are prone to development of gynecomastia caused by testicular tumors.

The causes of gynecomastia are multiple and diverse (Table 26–1).

The history and physical examination will often clarify the cause of gynecomastia. A careful drug history is important. An adolescent with slight gynecomastia or a man with prostatic carcinoma taking diethylstilbestrol needs no further study. Careful examination of the testes is mandatory to look for a testicular tumor. Small, firm testes are characteristic of Klinefelter's syndrome. Eunuchoid features, signs of liver disease, or the enlarged thyroid of Graves' disease are also helpful.

Laboratory investigation of unclear cases should include the following:

(1) A chest x-ray to search for metastatic or bronchogenic carcinoma.

(2) Measurements of plasma levels of prolactin (see Hyperprolactinemia) and the beta subunit of human chorionic gonadotropin (β-hCG). Detectable levels implicate a testicular tumor (germ cell or Sertoli cell) or other malignancy (usually lung or liver). Detectable low levels of serum β-hCG (< 5 mU/mL) may be reported in men with primary hypogonadism

Table 26–1. Causes of gynecomastia.

Idiopathic	**Drugs (partial list)**
	Alcohol
Physiologic causes	Alkylating agents
Neonatal period	Amiodarone
Puberty	Androgens
Aging	Busulfan
Obesity	Chorionic gonadotropin
	Cimetidine
Endocrine diseases	Clomiphene
Androgen resistance syndromes	Cyclophosphamide
	Diazepam
Hyperprolactinemia	Diethylstilbestrol
Hyperthyroidism	Digitalis preparations
Klinefelter's syndrome	Estrogens
Male hypogonadism	Ethionamide
Partial 17-ketosteroid reductase deficiency	Finasteride
	Flutamide
	Haloperidol
Systemic diseases	Hydroxyzine
Chronic liver disease	Isoniazid
Chronic renal disease	Ketoconazole
Refeeding after starvation	Marijuana
Spinal cord injury	Meprobamate
	Methadone
Neoplasms	Methyldopa
Adrenal tumors	Metoclopramide
Bronchogenic carcinoma	Narcotics
Carcinoma of the breast	Omeprazole
Testicular tumors	Penicillamine
Hepatocellular carcinoma (rare)	Phenothiazines
	Progestins
	Protease inhibitors
	Reserpine
	Spironolactone
	Testosterone
	Tricyclic antidepressants

and high serum LH levels if the assay for β-hCG cross-reacts with LH.

(3) Measurements of plasma testosterone and luteinizing hormone (LH) are valuable in the diagnosis of primary or secondary hypogonadism. A low testosterone and high LH are seen in primary hypogonadism. High testosterone levels *plus* high LH levels characterize partial androgen resistance.

(4) Other tests: Serum estradiol is determined but is usually normal; increased levels may result from testicular tumors, increased β-hCG, liver disease, obesity, adrenal tumors (rare), or true hermaphroditism (rare). Many estrogens and substances with estrogenic activity are not detected by estradiol assays. Serum TSH (sensitive) and free thyroxine levels are also determined. A karyotype (for Klinefelter's syndrome) is obtained in men with persistent gynecomastia without obvious cause.

(5) Needle biopsy with cytologic examination may be performed on suspicious areas of male breast enlargement (especially when unilateral or asymmetric) to distinguish gynecomastia from tumor.

The treatment of gynecomastia is that of the underlying condition. Idiopathic and pubertal gynecomastia usually resolve spontaneously within 1–2 years. Drug-induced gynecomastia resolves after the offending drug is removed. Painful gynecomastia may be treated with tamoxifen (an antiestrogen), 10 mg orally twice daily; discomfort improves, but breast size reduction occurs in only 50% and is usually minor. Surgical correction is reserved for persistent or severe gynecomastia, since results are often disappointing. Subcutaneous liposuction mastectomy by a surgeon experienced in the technique may produce acceptable results.

Chan WB et al: Gynaecomastia as a presenting feature of thyrotoxicosis. Postgrad Med J 1999;75:229. [NLM Cit ID: 20180655]

Evans NA: Gym and tonic: A profile of 100 male steroid users. Br J Sports Med 1997;31:54. [NLM Cit ID: 97227142] (Anabolic steroid use is common among athletes. Gynecomastia, acne, and striae occur along with muscle hypertrophy.)

Smyth CM et al: Klinefelter syndrome. Arch Intern Med 1998;158:1309. [NLM Cit ID: 98307756) (Klinefelter syndrome affects 1 in 500 male patients, with gynecomastia and other variable manifestations.)

Galactorrhea

Lactation that occurs in the absence of nursing is termed galactorrhea. A small amount of breast milk can be expressed from the nipple in many parous women and is not cause for concern. Normal breast milk may be various colors besides white. Galactorrhea requires evaluation when it occurs in significant amounts or in nulliparous women or when it is associated with amenorrhea, headache, visual field abnormalities, or other symptoms implying systemic illness.

Evaluation begins with serum prolactin measurement; a persistently elevated level should prompt further investigation to determine its cause (Table 26–4). MRI of the pituitary and hypothalamus is done for nonpregnant patients with serum prolactin levels over 200 mg/dL, those with headaches or visual field defects, and women with persistently elevated prolactin levels with no discernible cause. Treatment is directed at correcting the cause of the elevated prolactin. Galactorrhea due to antipsychotic drugs may resolve if the neuroleptic is changed to clozapine, an atypical antipsychotic. Galactorrhea may occur in the absence of elevated serum prolactin levels (idiopathic). Whatever the cause, galactorrhea can be reduced with bromocriptine or cabergoline administration.

Erectile Dysfunction & Diminished Libido in Men

Erectile dysfunction is a frequent problem. Psychogenic factors as well as endocrine, vascular, or neurologic abnormalities may be important. Hypogonadism of whatever origin (Table 26–14) is associated with lack of libido and erectile dysfunction. These can also be the first clinical manifestations of a hyperprolactinemic disorder (Table 26–4). Other endocrine causes include hyperthyroidism, Addison's disease, and acromegaly. Impotence in diabetes may be related to inadequate penile blood flow or autonomic neuropathy. Vascular disease is a frequent factor in impotence in elderly men. Vascular claudication of the legs along with related impotence is known as **Leriche's syndrome.**

Many pharmacologic agents are known to cause varying degrees of impotence (Table 26–2). Selective serotonin reuptake inhibitors (SSRIs, eg, fluoxetine) cause reduced libido. SSRIs and clomipramine cause delayed ejaculation.

Evaluation and treatment of erectile dysfunction are covered in Chapter 23.

Cryptorchism

One or both testes may be absent from the scrotum at birth in about 20% of premature males and in 3–6% at full term. Cryptorchism is found in 1–2% of males after 1 year of age but must be distinguished from retractile testes, which require no treatment. Cryptorchism should be corrected before age 18–24 months in an attempt to reduce the risk of infertility, which occurs in up to 75% of men with bilateral cryptorchism and in 50% with unilateral cryptorchism. It is not clear, however, whether early orchiopexy improves ultimate fertility. Many patients have underlying hypogonadism.

The ultimate incidence of significant testicular neoplasia is about 0.002% in normal males, 0.06% in cryptorchid males, and up to 5% in patients with intra-abdominal testes.

If the testes are not palpable, ultrasound or MRI can be used to locate them. Alternatively, human chorionic gonadotropin, 1500 units intramuscularly daily for 3 days, causes a significant rise in testosterone if the testes are present.

Orchiopexy decreases the risk of neoplasia when performed before 10 years of age. Orchiectomy after puberty is an option for intra-abdominal testes.

Rogers E et al: The role of orchiectomy in the management of postpubertal cryptorchidism. J Urol 1998;159:851. [NLM Cit ID: 98134442] (A review: 62% of undescended testes were palpable. Diminished spermatogenesis was related to age and the severity of the maldescent; only 2% had normal spermatogenesis. Carcinoma in situ was present in 4%, torsion of the undescended testis in 2%.)

Table 26–2. Drugs causing erectile dysfunction.

Alcohol	Marijuana
Amphetamines	Methadone
Antihistamines	Methyldopa
Barbiturates	Metoclopramide
Beta-blockers	Monoamine oxidase inhibitors
Butyrophenones	Opioids
Carbamazepine	Phenothiazines
Cimetidine	Sedatives
Clonidine	Spironolactone
Cocaine	Thiazides
Guanethidine	Tricyclic antidepressants
Ketoconazole	
Leuprolide	

Bone Pain & Pathologic Fractures

Onset of pathologic fractures at an early age is seen in osteogenesis imperfecta (blue scleras may be present). Painful bowing of the bones and pseudofractures suggest rickets or osteomalacia. Hyperparathyroidism or malignancy is suspected in patients with bone pain and hypercalcemia. Back pain or pathologic fractures in hypogonadal men and women implicate osteoporosis; such pain may be relieved with calcitonin. In cases of osteopenia of unknown cause, hyperthyroidism and Cushing's syndrome should also be considered. Bone pain may occur also as a result of primary or metastatic tumors, multiple myeloma, and Paget's disease; such pain may be relieved with bisphosphonates such as pamidronate or alendronate. Treatment is that of the underlying disorder.

Koeberle D et al: Pamidronate treatment in patients with malignant osteolytic bone disease and pain: a prospective randomized double-blind trial. Support Care Cancer 1999;7:21. [NLM Cit ID: 99124160] (Pamidronate 60 mg or 90 mg intravenously every 3 weeks for a maximum of six cycles led to a sustained reduction in pain intensity in approximately 60% of both groups.)

Muscle Cramps & Tetany

Muscle cramps are usually caused by sports or occupational muscle injury. Nocturnal leg cramps are commonly idiopathic but are seen in diabetes mellitus, Parkinson's disease, central nervous system or spinal cord lesions, a variety of neuromuscular conditions, peripheral neuropathy, hemodialysis, peripheral vascular disease, and—in those receiving cisplatin or vincristine—chemotherapy. Various other drugs can cause myalgias that patients describe as cramps (eg, cimetidine, cholestyramine). Alkalosis due to any cause (eg, severe vomiting or hyperventilation) may decrease ionized calcium and cause muscle cramping and paresthesias. Leg cramps during walking may be due to vascular insufficiency, hyperthyroidism, or hypothyroidism.

Diffuse, recurrent, or severe muscle cramping requires evaluation for hypocalcemia (Table 21–8). Treatment of hypocalcemia is discussed in Chapter 21. Magnesium deficiency must be considered in tetany unresponsive to calcium. Given the risk of potentially life-threatening arrhythmias, however rarely they may occur, quinine can no longer be recommended for leg cramps.

Recurrent cervicofacial and laryngeal dystonias, as well as hand cramps have been successfully treated with injections of botulinum toxin.

Haskell SG et al: Clinical epidemiology of nocturnal leg cramps in male veterans. Am J Med Sci 1997;313:210. [NLM Cit ID: 97253912]

Mental Changes

Disturbances of mentation may be important indications of underlying endocrine disorders. Nervousness and excitability are characteristic of the menopause and hyperthyroidism. Adult cretinism is the result of prolonged hypothyroidism in infancy. In adults, hypothyroidism is accompanied by mental slowness, depression, and lethargy. Occasionally it may be manifested by delusional psychosis ("myxedema madness"). Pheochromocytoma may cause anxiety, confusion, or psychosis. Prolonged hypocalcemia from untreated hypoparathyroidism may be associated with intellectual deterioration. Hypoglycemia of any origin may cause confusion, abnormal speech, and behavioral or personality changes as well as sudden loss of consciousness, somnolence and prolonged lethargy, or coma. Frank psychosis can occur but is rare. Mild hypercalcemia causes fatigue and emotional irritability. Severe hypercalcemia can cause confusion, psychosis, and coma. Confusion may occur in hypopituitarism or Addison's disease. Confusion, lethargy, and nausea may be the presenting symptoms of hyponatremia. Insomnia, mood changes, anxiety, and psychosis can be associated with Cushing's syndrome. Rapid changes in glucocorticoid status (either a sudden increase or a sudden decrease) may be associated with acute psychosis. Porphyria may cause affective and thought disorders, particularly during acute attacks.

Mental changes may result from vitamin deficiencies caused by malnutrition, malabsorption, and other conditions. Deficiency in vitamin B_1 (thiamin) is usually seen in alcoholism and can cause Korsakoff's syndrome with typical memory loss and confabulation. Deficiency in vitamin B_2 (riboflavin) may cause personality deterioration and occurs commonly with psychotropic and antimalarial drugs and with diabetes and other diseases. Vitamin B_3 (niacin) deficiency is seen with poor nutrition, alcoholism, mercaptopurine toxicity, and malignant carcinoid syndrome and can cause irritability, dementia, dermatitis, and diarrhea. Vitamin B_6 (pyridoxine) deficiency is frequently seen in alcoholics or during treatment with isoniazid or levodopa and can cause irritability, depression, and neuropathy. Deficiency of vitamin B_{12} (cobalamin) is caused by deficiency in gastric intrinsic factor and may be seen at any age; however, it is more common in the elderly, affecting about 10% of people over age 70 years. Vitamin B_{12} deficiency may cause depression, irritability, paranoia, confusion, and dementia. It is usually associated with other neurologic symptoms such as paresthesias and leg weakness. Mental changes may occur in the absence of megaloblastic anemia.

DISEASES OF THE HYPOTHALAMUS & PITUITARY GLAND

Anterior pituitary gland function is controlled by regulating hormones produced by the hypothalamus and by direct feedback inhibition. The **posterior pituitary** receives antidiuretic hormone and oxytocin from the hypothalamus, secreting them under central nervous system control (Table 26–3). Hypothalamic hormones generally stimulate the anterior pituitary except for dopamine, which inhibits the pituitary from spontaneously secreting prolactin.

HYPOPITUITARISM

Essentials of Diagnosis

- Sexual dysfunction; weakness; easy fatigability; lack of resistance to stress, cold, and fasting; axillary and pubic hair loss.
- Low blood pressure; pituitary tumors may cause visual field defects.
- Low free thyroxine; deficient cortisol response to cosyntropin.
- Low serum testosterone (men); amenorrhea; serum prolactin may be elevated; FSH and LH are low or low normal.
- MRI may reveal a pituitary or hypothalamic lesion.

General Considerations

Patients with hypopituitarism may have single or multiple hormonal deficiencies. When one hormonal deficiency is discovered, others must be sought.

Causes include mass lesions such as pituitary adenomas, brain tumors or aneurysms, apoplexy, metastatic carcinoma, granulomas, multifocal Langerhans cell granulomatosis, and pituitary abscess. Autoimmune hypophysitis, postpartum pituitary necrosis (Sheehan's syndrome), eclampsia-preeclampsia, sickle cell disease, and African trypanosomiasis are rare causes.

Table 26–3. Pituitary hormones.

Anterior pituitary
Growth hormone (GH)[1]
Prolactin (PRL)
Adrenocorticotropic hormone (ACTH)
Thyroid-stimulating hormone (TSH)
Luteinizing hormone (LH)[2]
Follicle-stimulating hormone (FSH)
Posterior pituitary
Arginine vasopressin (AVP)[3]
Oxytocin

[1]GH closely resembles human placental lactogen (hPL).
[2]LH closely resembles human chorionic gonadotropin (hCG).
[3]AVP is identical with antidiuretic hormone (ADH).

Hypopituitarism without mass lesions may be idiopathic or may be caused by trauma, radiation, surgery, encephalitis, hemochromatosis, autoimmunity, or stroke. It may also occur after coronary artery bypass grafting. Pituitary hormone deficiencies may be congenital and caused by a *PIT1* gene mutation.

A pituitary tumor may be part of the syndrome of multiple endocrine neoplasia (type 1), with tumors of the parathyroid glands and pancreatic islets.

Clinical Findings

Manifestations of hypopituitarism vary depending upon which specific hormones are lacking and whether their deficiency is partial or complete.

A. Symptoms and Signs: Gonadotropin deficiency includes loss of luteinizing hormone (LH) and follicle-stimulating hormone (FSH), which causes hypogonadism and infertility. Patients with isolated gonadotropin deficiency may present as delayed adolescence. (See also discussion of primary amenorrhea.) Congenital gonadotropin deficiency may be associated with micropenis, cryptorchism, or a decreased sense of smell (from hypoplasia of the olfactory bulbs) in Kallmann's syndrome. In acquired gonadotropin deficiency, both men and women lose axillary, pubic, and body hair gradually, particularly if they are also hypoadrenal. Men may note diminished beard growth. Libido is diminished. Women have amenorrhea; men note decreased erections. Most patients are infertile. (See section on secondary amenorrhea.)

Thyroid-stimulating hormone (TSH) deficiency causes hypothyroidism with manifestations such as fatigue, weakness, weight change, and hyperlipidemia. (See Hypothyroidism and Myxedema.)

Adrenocorticotropic hormone (ACTH) deficiency results in diminished cortisol secretion (see Adrenocortical Hypofunction). Symptoms include weakness, fatigue, weight loss, and hypotension. Adrenal mineralocorticoid secretion continues, so manifestations of adrenal insufficiency in hypopituitarism are usually less striking than in bilateral adrenal gland destruction (Addison's disease).

Growth hormone (GH) deficiency in adulthood tends to cause mild to moderate obesity, asthenia, and reduced cardiac output.

Panhypopituitarism is the absence of all anterior pituitary hormones. Besides the manifestations noted above, patients with long-standing hypopituitarism tend to have dry, pale, finely textured skin. The face has fine wrinkles and an apathetic countenance.

B. Laboratory Findings: The fasting blood glucose may be low. Hyponatremia is often present. Hyperkalemia usually does not occur, since aldosterone production is not affected.

The free T_4 level is low, and TSH is not elevated. Plasma levels of sex steroids (testosterone and estradiol) are low or low normal, as are the serum gonadotropins as well. Elevated prolactin levels are found in patients with prolactinomas, acromegaly, and hypothalamic disease.

In secondary hypoadrenalism, administration of cosyntropin (synthetic $ACTH_{1-24}$), 0.25 mg (intramuscularly or intravenously) usually causes serum cortisol to rise to less than 20 μg/dL by 30–60 minutes after the injection. A low-dose cosyntropin test (0.001 mg intravenously) is slightly more sensitive in detecting subtle ACTH-cortisol insufficiency. A baseline ACTH level is low or normal in secondary hypoadrenalism, distinguishing it from primary adrenal disease.

Patients with a normal cosyntropin test but with clinically suspected pituitary-adrenal insufficiency may have a metyrapone stimulation test: Metyrapone, 1.5 g orally, is administered at 11 PM; serum is collected at 8 AM for 11-deoxycortisol and cortisol determinations. Patients with hypoadrenalism usually have an 11-deoxycortisol concentration under 7 μg/dL in the presence of a cortisol suppressed to less than 5 μg/dL. The metyrapone test must be performed in the absence of replacement glucocorticoid. Side effects include frequent nausea and occasional vomiting.

The diagnosis of growth hormone (GH) deficiency is difficult because of the pulsatile nature of the hormone's secretion. GH deficiency is present in 90% of patients with multiple other pituitary hormone deficiencies. The insulin hypoglycemia test most accurately diagnoses GH deficiency but is dangerous for elderly or seizure-prone patients. IGF-I levels may be low in GH deficiency, but there is considerable overlap with normal. IGF-I may be low in patients with liver disease or malnutrition. Exercise-stimulated GH levels are usually under 5 ng/mL; however, by about age 40 years most normal adults have lost their GH response to exercise.

C. Imaging: MRI provides the best visualization of parasellar lesions. In hemochromatosis, MRI shows a very hypointense anterior lobe on T1-weighted images, which is surrounded by hyperintense cerebrospinal fluid on T2-weighted images. The posterior pituitary usually has a high-intensity signal on sagittal MRI that is lacking in central diabetes insipidus.

Differential Diagnosis

Reversible physiologic hypogonadotropic hypogonadism may occur during any serious illness and with malnutrition or anorexia nervosa. The clinical situation, presence of normal sex hair, and normal adrenal and thyroid function allow ready distinction from hypopituitarism.

Primary adrenal or thyroid insufficiency is easily differentiated from pituitary insufficiency, since serum ACTH and TSH are not elevated in hypopituitarism.

Severe illness causes functional suppression of TSH and thyroxine. Hyperthyroxinemia reversibly suppresses TSH. Glucocorticoids or megestrol treatment reversibly suppresses endogenous ACTH and cortisol secretion.

Complications

Patients with destructive lesions (eg, tumors) may develop complications related to them or to surgery or radiation therapy. Visual field impairment may occur. Hypothalamic damage may result in morbid obesity as well as cognitive and emotional problems. Conventional radiation therapy results in an increased incidence of small vessel ischemic strokes and second tumors.

Patients with untreated hypoadrenalism and a stressful illness may become febrile and die in shock and coma.

Adults with growth hormone deficiency have experienced an increased cardiovascular morbidity. Rarely, acute hemorrhage may occur in large pituitary tumors, manifested by rapid loss of vision, headache, and evidence of acute pituitary failure (pituitary apoplexy) requiring emergency decompression of the sella.

Treatment

Transsphenoidal removal of pituitary tumors will sometimes reverse hypopituitarism. Hypogonadism due to prolactin excess usually resolves during treatment with dopamine agonists. Endocrine substitution therapy must be used before, during, and often permanently after such procedures.

GH-secreting tumors may respond to octreotide (see section on acromegaly). Radiation therapy with x-ray, gamma knife, or heavy particles may be necessary but increases the likelihood of hypopituitarism.

The mainstay of substitution therapy for pituitary insufficiency remains lifetime hormone replacement.

A. Corticosteroids: Give hydrocortisone tablets, 15–25 mg/d orally in divided doses. Most patients do well with 15 mg in the morning and 5–10 mg in the late afternoon. Some patients feel better taking prednisone, 3–7.5 mg/d, or dexamethasone, 0.25 mg/d. A mineralocorticoid is rarely needed. Additional hydrocortisone must be given during states of stress, eg, during infection, trauma, or surgical procedures. For mild illness, corticosteroid doses are doubled or tripled. For trauma or surgical stress, hydrocortisone is given in doses of 50 mg intramuscularly or intravenously every 6 hours and then reduced to normal doses as the stress subsides.

Patients with secondary adrenal insufficiency due to treatment with glucocorticoids at supraphysiologic doses require their usual daily dose of glucocorticoid during surgery and acute illness; supplemental hydrocortisone is not usually required.

B. Thyroid: Levothyroxine is given to correct hypothyroidism only after the patient is assessed for cortisol deficiency or is already receiving glucocorticoids. (See Hypothyroidism.) The usual maintenance dose is 0.125 mg daily (range, 0.05–0.3 mg daily).

C. Sex Hormones:

1. Androgen replacement is discussed in the section on male hypogonadism.

2. Estrogen replacement is discussed in the section on female hypogonadism.

3. To improve spermatogenesis, chorionic gonadotropin (equivalent to luteinizing hormone) may be given at a dosage of 2000–3000 units intramuscularly three times weekly and testosterone replacement is discontinued. The dose of hCG is adjusted to normalize serum testosterone levels. After 6–12 months of hCG treatment, if the sperm count remains low, hCG injections are continued along with injections of FSH: follitropin beta (synthetic recombinant FSH) or urofollitropins (urine-derived FSH). An alternative for patients with an intact pituitary (eg, Kallmann's syndrome) is the use of leuprolide (GnRH analog) by intermittent subcutaneous infusion. With either treatment, testicular volumes double within 5–12 months, and spermatogenesis occurs in most cases. With the help of intracytoplasmic sperm injection for some cases, the total pregnancy success rate is about 70%. Clomiphene, 25–50 mg orally daily, can sometimes stimulate a man's own pituitary gonadotropins (when his pituitary is intact), thereby increasing testosterone and sperm production.

4. For fertility induction in females, ovulation may be induced with clomiphene, 50 mg daily for 5 days every 2 months. Follitropins and chorionic gonadotropin can induce multiple births and should be used only by those experienced with their administration. (See Chapter 17.)

D. Human Growth Hormone: hGH (somatotropin) is synthesized by recombinant DNA techniques. Symptomatic adults with severe growth hormone deficiency may be treated with subcutaneous somatotropin injection starting at a dosage of about 0.2 mg (0.6 IU) three times weekly or daily. The dosage is increased until side effects occur or a salutary response is achieved: every 2–4 weeks by 0.1 mg (0.3 IU) up to 0.7 mg (2.1 IU) daily. Women tend to require higher doses than men. The somatotropin dosage may be further increased by 0.1 mg (0.3 IU) at monthly intervals to a maximum of about 1 mg (3 IU) daily. If the desired effects (eg, improved energy, muscle strength) are not seen within about 3 months at maximum tolerated dosage, the somatotropin is discontinued.

Side effects of somatotropin therapy may include peripheral edema, hand stiffness, arthralgias, myalgias, headache, gynecomastia, carpal tunnel syndrome, tarsal tunnel syndrome, hypertension, and proliferative retinopathy. Such symptoms usually remit promptly after a sufficient reduction in dosage. Excessive doses of somatotropin could cause acromegaly; patients receiving chronic therapy require careful clinical monitoring.

GH levels normally decline with aging. GH deficiency and aging have similar manifestations regarding body composition and loss of strength. Elderly men treated with somatotropin for 6 months were found to have an increase in muscle mass and bone density and a 13% drop in fat mass, but functional abilities were unchanged. Available data do not support the use of hGH to reverse normal aging effects.

E. Other Drugs: Cabergoline, bromocriptine, or quinagolide may reverse the hypogonadism seen in hyperprolactinomas. (See Disorders of Prolactin Secretion.)

Prognosis

The prognosis depends on the primary cause. Hypopituitarism resulting from a pituitary tumor may be reversible with bromocriptine, cabergoline, or quinagolide or with careful selective resection of the tumor. Spontaneous recovery from hypopituitarism associated with pituitary stalk enlargement has been reported. Patients can also recover from functional hypopituitarism, eg, hypogonadism due to starvation or severe illness, suppression of ACTH by glucocorticoids, or suppression of TSH by hyperthyroidism.

Buchter D et al: Pulsatile GnRH or human chorionic gonadotropin/human menopausal gonadotropin as effective treatment for men with hypogonadotropic hypogonadism: a review of 42 cases. Eur J Endocrinol 1998; 139:298. [NLM Cit ID: 98429406]

Chico A et al: Reversible endocrine dysfunction and pituitary stalk enlargement. J Endocrinol Invest 1998; 21:122. [NLM Cit ID: 98244786]

Drake WM et al: Optimizing growth hormone replacement therapy by dose titration in hypopituitary adults. J Clin Endocrinol Metab 1998;83:3913. [NLM Cit ID: 99029605]

Schmidt DN et al: How to diagnose hypopituitarism. Learning the features of secondary hormonal deficiencies. Postgrad Med 1998;104:77. [NLM Cit ID: 98341356]

DIABETES INSIPIDUS

Essentials of Diagnosis

- Polyuria (2–20 L/d); polydipsia.
- Urine specific gravity usually < 1.006 during ad libitum fluid intake.
- Vasopressin reduces urine output (except in nephrogenic diabetes insipidus).

General Considerations

Diabetes insipidus is an uncommon disease characterized by an increase in thirst and the passage of large quantities of urine of low specific gravity. The urine is otherwise normal. It is caused by a deficiency of or resistance to vasopressin.

The causes may be classified as follows:

A. Deficiency of Vasopressin:

1. Primary diabetes insipidus (without an identifiable organic lesion noted on MRI of the pituitary and hypothalamus) may be familial, occurring as a dominant trait, or sporadic ("idiopathic").

2. Secondary diabetes insipidus is due to damage to the hypothalamus or pituitary stalk by tumor, anoxic encephalopathy, surgical or accidental trauma, infection (eg, encephalitis, tuberculosis, syphilis), sarcoidosis, or multifocal Langerhans cell (eosinophilic) granulomatosis ("histiocytosis X"). Metastases to the pituitary are more likely to cause diabetes insipidus (33%) than are pituitary adenomas (1%).

3. Vasopressinase-induced diabetes insipidus may be seen in the last trimester of pregnancy and in the puerperium; it is often associated with oligohydramnios, preeclampsia, or hepatic dysfunction. A circulating enzyme destroys native vasopressin; however, synthetic desmopressin is unaffected. The condition usually responds to desmopressin therapy (see below) and subsides spontaneously.

B. "Nephrogenic" Diabetes Insipidus: This disorder is due to a defect in the kidney tubules that interferes with water reabsorption. The polyuria is unresponsive to vasopressin. These patients have normal secretion of vasopressin. Congenital nephrogenic diabetes insipidus is present from birth and is due to defective expression of renal vasopressin V2 receptors or vasopressin-sensitive water channels. It occurs as a familial X-linked trait; adults often have hyperuricemia as well.

Acquired forms of vasopressin-resistant diabetes insipidus are usually less severe and are seen in pyelonephritis, renal amyloidosis, myeloma, potassium depletion, Sjögren's syndrome, sickle cell anemia, or chronic hypercalcemia. The disorder may occur also as a glucocorticoid effect or as an acute side effect of diuretics. Certain drugs (eg, demeclocycline, lithium, foscarnet, or methicillin) may induce nephrogenic diabetes insipidus. The recovery from acute tubular necrosis may also be associated with transient nephrogenic diabetes insipidus.

Clinical Findings

A. Symptoms and Signs: The symptoms of the disease are intense thirst, especially with a craving for ice water, and polyuria, the volume of ingested fluid varying from 2 L to 20 L daily, with correspondingly large urine volumes. Partial diabetes insipidus presents with less intense symptoms and should be suspected in patients with unremitting enuresis. Diabetes insipidus may present with hypernatremia and dehydration, especially after hypothalamic damage due to shock or anoxia.

B. Laboratory Findings: Evaluation for diabetes insipidus should include a 24-hour urine collection for volume, glucose, and creatinine and serum for glucose, urea nitrogen, calcium, uric acid, potassium, and sodium.

The diagnosis of diabetes insipidus as a cause of polyuria or hypernatremia requires mostly clinical judgment. There is no single diagnostic laboratory test. Hyperuricemia implicates central diabetes insipidus, since reduced stimulation of the renal V1 receptor causes reduced urate clearance.

If the clinical situation implicates central diabetes insipidus (and no other causes for polyuria are present; see Differential Diagnosis, below), a supervised "vasopressin challenge test" may be given: Desmopressin acetate is given in an initial dose of 0.05–0.1 mL (5–10 μg) intranasally (or 1 μg subcutaneously or intravenously), with measurement of urine volume for 12 hours prior to and 12 hours after administration. Serum sodium must be obtained immediately in the event of symptoms of hyponatremia. The dosage of desmopressin is doubled if the response is marginal. Patients with central diabetes insipidus notice a distinct reduction in thirst and polyuria; serum sodium stays normal except in some salt-losing conditions.

When nephrogenic diabetes insipidus is a diagnostic consideration, measurement of serum vasopressin is done during modest fluid restriction; typically, the vasopressin level is high.

In nonfamilial central diabetes insipidus, MRI of the pituitary and hypothalamus and of the skull is done to look for mass lesions. Absence of a posterior pituitary "bright spot" on T1-weighted MRI is suggestive of central diabetes insipidus.

Differential Diagnosis of Polyuria

Central diabetes insipidus must be distinguished from polyuria caused by Cushing's syndrome or glucocorticoid treatment, lithium, and the nocturnal polyuria of Parkinson's disease. It must also be distinguished from the excessive fluid intake seen in psychogenic polydipsia, central nervous system sarcoidosis, and intravenous fluid administration.

Central diabetes insipidus is distinguished from diabetes mellitus by checking the urine for glucose. It must also be distinguished from nephrogenic diabetes insipidus (see above).

Complications

If water is not readily available, the excessive output of urine will lead to severe dehydration. Patients with an impaired thirst mechanism are very prone to hypernatremia, particularly since they usually also have impaired mentation and forget to take their desmopressin. All the complications of the primary disease may eventually become evident. In patients who are receiving desmopressin acetate therapy, there is a danger of induced water intoxication.

Treatment

A. Desmopressin: Desmopressin acetate is the treatment of choice for central diabetes insipidus. It is also useful in diabetes insipidus associated with pregnancy or the puerperium, since desmopressin is resistant to degradation by the circulating vasopressinase. It is usually given intranasally (100 μg/mL solution) every 12–24 hours as needed for thirst and polyuria. It may be administered via metered-dose nasal inhaler containing 0.1 mL/spray or via a plastic calibrated tube. Patients are started with 0.05–0.1 mL every 12–24 hours, and the dose is then individualized according to response.

Desmopressin is also available as a parenteral preparation containing 4 μg/mL. For central diabetes insipidus, it is given intravenously, intramuscularly, or subcutaneously in doses of 1–4 μg every 12–24 hours as needed to treat thirst or hypernatremia.

Desmopressin is also available as an oral preparation (0.1 or 0.2 mg tablets) which are given in a starting dose of 0.1 mg daily and increased to a maximum of 0.2 mg every 8 hours, if required. Mild increases in hepatic enzymes are common, so the drug is not given to patients with liver disease. Gastrointestinal symptoms and asthenia may occur.

Adverse reactions to desmopressin have included nasal irritation, occasional agitation, and erythromelalgia. Hyponatremia is uncommon if minimum effective doses are used and the patient allows thirst to occur periodically.

B. Other Measures: Mild cases require no treatment other than adequate fluid intake. Reduction of aggravating factors (eg, glucocorticoids, which directly increase renal free water clearance) will improve polyuria. Both central and nephrogenic diabetes insipidus respond partially to hydrochlorothiazide, 50–100 mg/d (with potassium supplement or amiloride). Nephrogenic diabetes insipidus may respond to combined treatments of indomethacin-hydrochlorothiazide, indomethacin-desmopressin, or indomethacin-amiloride. Indomethacin, 50 mg every 8 hours, is effective acutely.

Psychotherapy is required for most patients with compulsive water drinking. Thioridazine and lithium are best avoided if drug therapy is needed, since they cause polyuria.

Prognosis

Central diabetes insipidus appearing after pituitary surgery usually remits after days to weeks but may be permanent if the upper pituitary stalk is cut.

Central diabetes insipidus is made transiently worse by glucocorticoids in the high doses frequently given perioperatively.

Chronic diabetes insipidus is more an inconvenience than a dire medical condition. Treatment with desmopressin allows normal sleep and activity. Hypernatremia can occur, especially when the thirst center is damaged, but diabetes insipidus itself does not reduce life expectancy, and the prognosis is that of the underlying disorder.

Bichet DG: Nephrogenic diabetes insipidus. Am J Med 1998;105:431. [NLM Cit ID: 99047323]

Singer I et al: The management of diabetes insipidus in adults. Arch Intern Med 1997;157:1293. [NLM Cit ID: 97344621]

ACROMEGALY & GIGANTISM

Essentials of Diagnosis

- Excessive growth of hands (increased glove and ring size), feet (increased shoe width), jaw (protrusion of lower jaw), and internal organs; or gigantism before closure of epiphyses.
- Coarsening facial features; deeper voice.
- Amenorrhea, headaches, visual field loss, sweating, weakness.
- Soft, doughy, sweaty handshake.
- Serum GH not suppressed following oral glucose.
- Elevated insulin-like growth factor I (IGF-I).
- Imaging: Terminal phalangeal "tufting" on radiographs. CT or MRI demonstration of pituitary tumor in 90%.

General Considerations

Growth hormone exerts much of its growth-promoting effects through the release of IGF-I produced in the liver and other tissues.

Acromegaly is nearly always caused by a pituitary adenoma. These tumors may be locally invasive, particularly into the cavernous sinus. Fewer than 1% are malignant. Most are macroadenomas (over 1 cm in diameter). Acromegaly is usually sporadic but may rarely be familial. The disease may be associated with endocrine tumors of the parathyroids or pancreas (multiple endocrine neoplasia type 1). Acromegaly may also be seen in McCune-Albright syndrome and as part of Carney's complex (atrial myxoma, acoustic neuroma, and spotty skin pigmentation). Acromegaly is rarely caused by ectopic GHRH or GH secreted by hypothalamic or bronchial carcinoid or pancreatic tumors. Rarely, the disease is transient and followed by partial pituitary insufficiency.

Clinical Findings

A. Symptoms and Signs: Excessive growth hormone causes tall stature and gigantism if it occurs before closure of epiphyses. Afterward, acromegaly develops. The term "acromegaly," meaning extremity enlargement, seriously understates the manifestations. The hands enlarge and a doughy, moist handshake is characteristic. The fingers widen, causing patients to enlarge their rings. Carpal tunnel syndrome is common. The feet also grow, particularly in width. Facial features coarsen since the bones and sinuses of the skull enlarge; hat size increases. The mandible becomes more prominent, causing prognathism and malocclusion. Tooth spacing widens.

Macroglossia occurs, as does hypertrophy of pharyngeal and laryngeal tissue; this causes a deep, coarse voice and sometimes makes intubation difficult. Obstructive sleep apnea may occur. A goiter may be noted. Hypertension (50%) and cardiomegaly are common; cardiovascular morbidity is increased. Weight gain is typical, particularly of muscle and bone. Insulin resistance is usually present and frequently causes diabetes mellitus (30%). Arthralgias and degenerative arthritis occur. Overgrowth of vertebral bone can cause spinal stenosis. Colon polyps are common, especially in patients with skin papillomas. The skin may also manifest hyperhidrosis, thickening, cystic acne, and areas of acanthosis nigricans.

GH-secreting pituitary tumors usually cause some degree of hypogonadism, either by cosecretion of prolactin or by direct pressure upon normal pituitary tissue. Decreased libido and impotence are common, as are irregular menses or amenorrhea. Secondary hypothyroidism sometimes occurs; hypoadrenalism is unusual. Headaches are frequent. Temporal hemianopia may occur as a result of the optic chiasm being impinged by a suprasellar growth of the tumor.

B. Laboratory Findings: After an overnight fast, a fasting serum specimen is obtained and assayed for prolactin (cosecreted by many GH-secreting tumors), IGF-I (increased to over five times normal in most acromegalics), glucose (diabetes is common in acromegaly), liver enzymes and BUN, serum inorganic phosphorus (frequently elevated), serum free thyroxine, and TSH (secondary hypothyroidism is common in acromegaly; primary hypothyroidism may increase prolactin).

Glucose syrup (100 g) is then administered orally, and serum GH is measured 60 minutes afterward. A GH level higher than 2 ng/mL (males) or 5 ng/mL (females) is evidence of acromegaly.

Misleadingly high serum GH levels can be caused by exercise or eating just prior to the test, acute illness or agitation, hepatic or renal failure, malnourishment, diabetes mellitus or concurrent treatment with estrogens, beta-blockers, or clonidine. Some patients with acromegaly have normal serum GH concentrations.

C. Imaging: MRI shows a pituitary tumor in 90% of acromegalics. MRI is generally superior to CT scanning especially in the postoperative setting. X-rays of the skull may show an enlarged sella and thickened skull. X-rays may also show tufting of the terminal phalanges of the fingers and toes. A lateral view of the foot shows increased thickness of the heel pad.

Differential Diagnosis

Active acromegaly must be distinguished from familial coarse features, large hands and feet, and isolated prognathism and from inactive ("burned-out") acromegaly in which there has been a spontaneous remission due to infarction of the pituitary adenoma. GH-induced gigantism must be differentiated from familial tall stature and from aromatase deficiency. (See Osteoporosis.) Acromegaly is differentiated from these conditions by testing (see above) and by ongoing enlargement in ring or shoe size and by progressive coarsening of facial features, which can be seen in serial photographs.

Complications

Complications include hypopituitarism, hypertension, glucose intolerance or frank diabetes mellitus, cardiac enlargement, and cardiac failure. Carpal tunnel syndrome may cause thumb weakness and thenar atrophy. Arthritis of hips, knees, and spine can be troublesome. Cord compression may be seen. Visual field defects may be severe and progressive. Acute loss of vision or cranial nerve palsy may occur if the tumor undergoes spontaneous hemorrhage and necrosis (pituitary apoplexy).

Treatment

Transsphenoidal pituitary microsurgery removes the adenoma while preserving anterior pituitary function in most patients. Growth hormone levels fall immediately; diaphoresis and carpal tunnel syndrome often improve within a day after surgery. Transsphenoidal surgery is usually well tolerated, but major complications can occur in about 10%, including infection, cerebrospinal fluid leak, and hypopituitarism. Hyponatremia can occur 4–13 days postoperatively and is manifested by nausea, vomiting, headache, malaise, or seizure.

Octreotide, a costly somatostatin analog, can be used to treat acromegaly that persists after transsphenoidal surgery and a trial of cabergoline or quinagolide. Treatment is begun with short-acting octreotide acetate in doses of 50 μg injected subcutaneously three times daily; the dosage is increased to 200 μg as tolerated. Patients who are deemed to be responders—as judged by serum GH levels and clinical response—and who tolerate the drug can be switched to octreotide acetate injectable suspension (Sandostatin LAR Depot) in doses of 20 mg intragluteally per month. The dosage may be adjusted—up to a maximum of 40 mg monthly—to maintain the serum GH between 1 ng and 2.5 ng/mL, keeping IGF-I levels normal. Gastrointestinal side effects are common, as is injection site discomfort. This treatment must be continued indefinitely or until radiation therapy has had its effect. It suppresses GH to < 5 ng/mL in 60% of treated patients within 3–6 months. Headache often improves, but tumor shrinkage is usually marginal. Octreotide may also be effective in ectopic acromegaly. Side effects are experienced by about one-third of patients and include injection site pain, loose acholic stools, abdominal discomfort, or cholelithiasis.

Dopamine agonists can occasionally be effective, particularly for tumors that cosecrete PRL with GH. About one-third of such tumors shrink by more than 50%. The optimal ergot-derived dopamine agonist is cabergoline in doses of 1–1.75 mg/wk orally. Side effects may include nausea, headache, and hypotension; these symptoms often remit with dosage reduction.

Pituitary irradiation is suggested for patients who are not cured by surgical and medical therapy.

Prognosis

Patients with untreated or persistent acromegaly tend to have premature cardiovascular disease and progressive acromegalic symptoms. Transsphenoidal pituitary surgery is successful in 90% of patients with tumors less than 2 cm in diameter and GH levels less than 50 ng/mL. Postoperatively, normal pituitary function is usually preserved. Soft tissue swelling regresses but bone enlargement is permanent. Hypertension frequently persists despite successful surgery. Conventional radiation therapy (alone) produces a remission in about 40% by 2 years and 75% by 5 years after treatment. Gamma knife radiation reduces GH levels an average of 77%, with 20% having a full remission after 12 months. Heavy particle pituitary radiation produces a remission in about 70% by 2 years and 80% by 5 years. Radiation therapy eventually produces some degree of hypopituitarism in most patients. Conventional radiation therapy may cause some degree of organic brain syndrome and predisposes to small strokes. Growth hormone levels over 5 ng/mL and rising usually indicate a recurrent tumor.

Abosch A et al: Transsphenoidal microsurgery for growth hormone-secreting pituitary adenomas: initial outcome and long-term results. J Clin Endocrinol Metab 1998; 83:3411. [NLM Cit ID: 98439576] (The surgical cure rate was 76%, with long-term recurrence rate of 7%.)

Colao A et al: Effect of different dopamine agents in the treatment of acromegaly. J Clin Endocrinol Metab 1997;82:518. [NLM Cit ID: 97176708] (Quinagolide normalized GH levels in 48% of acromegalics in this series.)

Davies PH et al: Long-term therapy with long-acting octreotide (Sandostatin–LAR) for the management of acromegaly. Clin Endocrinol 1998;48:311. [NLM Cit ID: 98239969] (Serum GH fell to < 5 ng/mL in 50% and IGF-I dropped to normal in 60% of acromegalics treated with long-acting octreotide after one year.)

HYPERPROLACTINEMIA

Essentials of Diagnosis

- Women: Menstrual cycle disturbances (oligomenorrhea, amenorrhea); galactorrhea; infertility.
- Men: Hypogonadism; decreased libido and erectile dysfunction; infertility.
- Elevated serum prolactin.
- CT scan or MRI often demonstrates pituitary adenoma.

Normal Physiology

Prolactin's main role is to induce lactation. Serum prolactin levels increase during pregnancy from a normal (follicular phase) level of less than 20 ng/mL to as high as 600 ng/mL by the time of delivery. Under the combined effect of prolactin, increased estrogen, and progesterone, breast development takes place, with eventual formation of milk in the acini. Estrogens inhibit the actual secretion of milk. After parturition, the sudden withdrawal of estrogen caused by expulsion of the placenta results in the onset of lactation. During the puerperal period, suckling constitutes a powerful stimulus for the continued production of prolactin as well as oxytocin. Lactation will cease if prolactin secretion is interrupted by prolactin-lowering drugs or by pituitary destruction. Prolactin is an unusual hormone in terms of control of secretion in that it is under mainly inhibitory control. Thus, section of the pituitary stalk will result in marked increases in prolactin secretion. Prolactin inhibitory factor (PIF) is dopamine.

Elevated serum prolactin can be caused by numerous conditions (Table 26–4).

General Considerations

Prolactin-secreting pituitary tumors are more common in women than in men and are usually sporadic but may rarely be familial as part of multiple endocrine neoplasia (MEN type 1). Most are microadenomas (< 1 cm in diameter) which do not grow even with pregnancy or oral contraceptives. However, some are quite large and can spread into the cavernous sinuses and suprasellar areas; rarely, they may erode the floor of the sella to invade the sinuses.

Clinical Findings

A. Symptoms and Signs: Hyperprolactinemia due to any cause may result in hypogonadotropic hypogonadism. Men usually have erectile dysfunction and diminished libido; gynecomastia sometimes occurs, but never with galactorrhea. Women may note oligomenorrhea or amenorrhea, though some women continue to menstruate normally; galactorrhea is common. Of women with secondary amenorrhea and galactorrhea, about 70% have hyperprolactinemia. Untreated hypogonadism ultimately increases the risk for developing osteoporosis.

Pituitary prolactinomas may cosecrete growth hormone and cause acromegaly (see above). Large tumors may cause headaches, visual symptoms, and pituitary insufficiency.

B. Laboratory Findings: Patients found to have hyperprolactinemia are evaluated for conditions known to cause it, particularly pregnancy (serum hCG), hypothyroidism (serum free thyroxine and TSH), renal failure (BUN and serum creatinine), and cirrhosis (clinical evaluation and serum bilirubin and liver enzymes). In the absence of renal failure or late pregnancy, serum prolactin levels greater than 250 ng/mL are virtually diagnostic of prolactinoma. Patients having pituitary macroadenomas (> 3 cm in diameter) should have prolactin measured on serial dilutions of serum, since certain assays may otherwise report falsely low titers. Women with amenorrhea are screened for estrogen deficiency (eg, vaginal hormonal cytology) and for concomitant primary hypogonadism (serum FSH, LH).

C. Imaging: When hyperprolactinemia persists without obvious cause, MRI of the pituitary and hypothalamus is indicated. Small prolactinomas may thus be demonstrated, but clear differentiation from normal variants is not always possible.

Differential Diagnosis

The differential diagnosis of prolactinoma should include acromegaly, since pituitary tumors often cosecrete prolactin and growth hormone. However, the most common causes of hyperprolactinemia are pregnancy and suckling. High prolactin levels are also commonly seen in conditions such as hypothyroidism, cirrhosis, renal failure, systemic lupus erythematosus, and hypothalamic disease. Chronic nipple stimulation, nipple piercing, augmentation mammoplasty, and mastectomy may stimulate prolactin secretion. Hyperprolactinemia may also be idiopathic or associated

Table 26–4. Causes of hyperprolactinemia.

Physiologic Causes	Pharmacologic Causes	Pathologic Causes
Exercise	Amoxapine	Acromegaly
Idiopathic (eg, "big" prolactin)	Amphetamines	Chronic chest wall stimulation (post-thoracotomy, postmastectomy, herpes zoster, breast problems, nipple rings, etc)
Pregnancy	Anesthetic agents	Cirrhosis
Puerperium	Butyrophenones	Hypothalamic disease
Sleep (REM phase)	Cimetidine	Hypothyroidism
Stress (trauma, surgery)	Estrogens	Multiple sclerosis
Suckling	Hydroxyzine	Optic neuromyelitis
	Methyldopa	Pituitary stalk section
	Metoclopramide	Prolactin-secreting tumors
	Narcotics	Pseudocyesis (false pregnancy)
	Nicotine	Renal failure (especially with zinc deficiency)
	Phenothiazines	Spinal cord lesions
	Progestins	Systemic lupus erythematosus
	Reserpine	
	Risperidone	
	Selective serotonin reuptake inhibitors	
	Tricyclic antidepressants	
	Verapamil	

with secretion of inactive "big" prolactin. Many drugs cause hyperprolactinemia, particularly psychotropic agents, cimetidine, tricyclic antidepressants, and oral contraceptives. (See Table 26–4.)

Treatment

Medications known to increase prolactin are stopped if possible. Hyperprolactinemia due to hypothyroidism is corrected by thyroxine. Patients with hyperprolactinemia not induced by drugs, hypothyroidism, or pregnancy should be examined by pituitary MRI. Women with microprolactinomas who have amenorrhea or are desirous of contraception may safely take oral contraceptives or estrogen replacement—there is minimal risk of stimulating enlargement of the adenoma. Since estrogens or testosterone treatment can stimulate the growth of macroprolactinomas, they should not be used by patients with large pituitary adenomas unless in full remission with dopamine agonist medication or surgery.

Dopamine Agonists: Dopamine agonists are the initial treatment of choice for patients with macroprolactinomas and those with hyperprolactinemia desiring restoration of normal sexual function and fertility. Of the ergot-derived dopamine agonists, cabergoline is usually the best tolerated and is prescribed beginning with a dosage of 0.25 mg orally once weekly for 1 week, then 0.25 mg twice weekly for the next week, then 0.5 mg twice weekly. Further dosage increases may be required monthly, based upon serum prolactin levels, up to a maximum of 1.5 mg twice weekly. Alternative drugs include bromocriptine (1.25–20 mg/d orally) and pergolide (0.125–2 mg/d orally). Women who experience nausea with oral preparations may find relief with deep vaginal insertion of cabergoline or bromocriptine tablets; vaginal irritation sometimes occurs. Quinagolide (Norprolac; not available in USA) is a non-ergot-derived dopamine agonist for patients intolerant or resistant to ergot-derived medications; the starting dosage is 0.075 mg/d orally, increasing as needed and tolerated to a maximum of 0.6 mg/d.

Dopamine agonists are given at bedtime to minimize side effects of fatigue, nausea, dizziness, and orthostatic hypotension. These symptoms usually improve with dosage reduction and continued use. Erythromelalgia is rare. A variety of psychiatric side effects may be seen which are not dose-related and may take weeks to resolve once the dopamine agonist is discontinued.

With dopamine agonist treatment, 90% of patients with prolactinomas experience a fall in serum prolactin to 10% or less of pretreatment levels; 67% of treated patients achieve a normal serum prolactin level. Shrinkage of a pituitary adenoma occurs early, but maximum effect may take up to a year. Nearly half—even massive tumors—shrink more than 50%. Discontinuing therapy after months or years usually results in reappearance of hyperprolactinemia and galactorrhea-amenorrhea, but a few patients with microadenomas remain in remission. Since fertility is usually promptly restored with dopamine agonists, many pregnancies have resulted, with no evidence of teratogenicity. Women with microadenomas may have treatment safely withdrawn during pregnancy. Macroadenomas may enlarge significantly during pregnancy; if therapy is withdrawn, patients must be followed clinically and with computer-assisted visual field perimetry.

B. Surgical Treatment: Transsphenoidal pituitary surgery may be urgently required for large tumors undergoing apoplexy or those severely compromising visual fields. It is also used electively for patients who do not tolerate or respond to dopamine agonists. Craniotomy is rarely indicated, since even large tumors can usually be decompressed via the transsphenoidal approach.

C. Radiation Therapy: Radiation therapy is reserved for patients with macroadenomas that are growing despite treatment with dopamine agonists. Conventional radiation therapy is most commonly used, but it must be given over 5 weeks and carries a high risk of eventual hypopituitarism. Other possible side effects include some degree of memory impairment and an increased long-term risk of second tumors and small vessel ischemic strokes. After radiation therapy, patients are advised to take low-dose aspirin to reduce their stroke risk. A single gamma knife treatment may be preferable for certain patients whose optic chiasm is clear of tumor, since it is generally safer and more convenient.

Barkan AL et al: Giant pituitary prolactinoma with falsely low serum prolactin: the pitfall of the "high-dose hook effect": case report. Neurosurgery 1998;42:913. [NLM Cit ID: 98233844]

Ferrari CI et al: Treatment of macroprolactinomas with cabergoline: A study of 85 patients. Clin Endocrinol 1997;46:409. [NLM Cit ID: 97340092] (Macroadenomas became smaller in 66%. Visual field abnormalities resolved in 50%, amenorrhea in 80%, erectile dysfunction in 87%. Twenty-five percent experienced adverse reactions, severe enough in 5% to require discontinuation of treatment.)

Orrego JJ et al: Pituitary disorders. Drug treatment options. Drugs 2000;59:93. [NLM Cit ID: 28181029]

DISEASES OF THE THYROID GLAND

An adult's thyroid gland normally weighs about 15–20 g. Embryologic defects may result in a rare lingual thyroid, retrosternal thyroid, or agenesis of one or both lobes.

Thyroid-stimulating hormone (TSH, thyrotropin) is secreted by the pituitary and stimulates several steps of thyroid hormone production: trapping of iodine, peroxidase linking of iodine to tyrosine, coupling of monoiodotyrosine or diiodotyrosine to form T_3 (triiodothyronine) or T_4 (thyroxine), and release of T_3 and T_4. The thyroid secretes mostly T_4 and very little T_3. About 90% of circulating T_3, the most active thyroid hormone, is derived from peripheral deiodination of T_4. Circulating thyroid hormones have a direct feedback inhibition effect upon the pituitary thyrotroph cells, desensitizing them from the stimulatory effect of hypothalamic thyrotropin-releasing hormone (TRH).

Over 99% of circulating thyroid hormones are bound to serum proteins, mostly thyroid-binding globulin (TBG). Only free hormone enters cells, binding to nuclear hormone receptors, which regulate DNA control of oxidative processes throughout the body.

The thyroid tests discussed in the following section are ordinarily very helpful in the evaluation of thyroid disorders. However, many conditions and drugs alter serum thyroxine levels without affecting clinical status (Table 26–5). Furthermore, a serum thyroxine determination is not sufficiently sensitive to detect mild degrees of hypo- or hyperthyroidism. Therefore, other tests may be used, but all are imperfect.

TESTS OF THYROID FUNCTION (Table 26–6)

The tests most widely used in clinical practice are serum immunoassays for TSH and "free" thyroxine (FT_4). Assays for FT_4 have largely supplanted measurements of total thyroxine (T_4), resin T_3 uptake (RT_3U), and free thyroxine index (FT_4I).

1. SERUM THYROID TESTS

Thyroid-Stimulating Hormone (TSH) Immunoassay

TSH levels as low as 0.01 mU/L can be detected by ultrasensitive "third-generation" assays. In order to diagnose hyperthyroidism, an assay sensitive to at least 0.1 mU/L (sensitive "second-generation" assay) should be employed. Owing to discrepancies between different TSH assay methods, it is prudent to recheck unexpected results with a different assay.

TSH levels are **decreased** in patients with primary hyperthyroidism (eg, Graves' disease, toxic multinodular goiter, toxic nodule, subacute thyroiditis, or release of stored hormone in Hashimoto's thyroiditis). TSH levels may also be suppressed in some clinically euthyroid individuals with autonomous thyroid secretion (eg, euthyroid Graves' ophthalmopathy). TSH can also be suppressed by thyroid hormone administration in either excessive or adequate replacement amounts. TSH is also frequently low during severe nonthyroidal illness; distinction from hypopituitarism can usually be made clinically.

Dopamine and dopamine agonists (levodopa, bromocriptine) can cause suppression of TSH and may

Table 26–5. Factors falsely altering serum thyroxine measurements without affecting clinical status.[1,2]

Factors Increasing T_4	Factors Decreasing T_4
Laboratory error	Laboratory error
Autoimmunity	Severe illness (eg chronic renal failure, major surgery, caloric deprivation)
Acute illness (eg, viral hepatitis, chronic active hepatitis; primary biliary cirrhosis; acute intermittent porphyria; AIDS)	Acute psychiatric problems
High-estrogen states (may also increase T_3)	Cirrhosis
Oral estrogen-containing contraceptives	Nephrotic syndrome
Pregnancy	Hereditary TBG deficiency
Estrogen replacement therapy	Drugs
Tamoxifen	Androgens
Acute psychiatric problems	Asparaginase
Hyperemesis gravidarum and morning sickness (may also increase T_3)	Carbamazepine
Familial thyroid-binding abnormalities	Chloral hydrate
Generalized resistance to thyroid hormone	Fenclofenac
Drugs	Fluorouracil
Amiodarone	Glucocorticoids
Amphetamines	Halofenate (lowers triglycerides and uric acid; not marketed in USA)
Clofibrate	Mitotane
Heparin (dialysis method)	Nicotinic acid
Heroin	Phenobarbital
Levothyroxine (T_4) replacement therapy	Phenylbutazone
Methadone (may also increase T_3)	Phenytoin (T_4 may be as low as 2 µg/dL)
Perphenazine	Salicylates (large doses)
	Sertraline
	Triiodothyronine (T_3) therapy

[1]Reproduced, with permission, from Fitzgerald PA: *Handbook of Clinical Endocrinology*, 2nd ed. Originally published by Appleton & Lange. Copyright © 1992 by The McGraw-Hill Companies, Inc.
[2]Symptomatic hyperthyroidism or hypothyroidism may also be present incidentally.

Table 26–6. Appropriate use of thyroid tests.

Purpose	Test	Comment
Screening	Serum TSH (sensitive assay)	Most sensitive test for primary hypothyroidism and hyperthyroidism
	Free T_4	Excellent test
For hypothyroidism	Serum TSH	High in primary and low in secondary hypothyroidism
	Antithyroglobulin and antithyroid peroxidase antibodies	Elevated in Hashimoto's thyroiditis
For hyperthyroidism	Serum TSH (sensitive assay)	Suppressed except in TSH-secreting pituitary tumor or hyperplasia (rare)
	T_3 (RIA)	Elevated
	^{123}I uptake and scan	Increased diffuse versus "hot" areas
	Antithyroglobulin and antimicrosomal antibodies	Elevated in Graves' disease
	TSH receptor antibody (TSH-R Ab [stim])	Usually positive in Graves' disease
For nodules	Fine-needle aspiration (FNA)	Best diagnostic method for thyroid cancer
	^{123}I uptake and scan	Cancer is usually "cold." Less reliable than FNA.
	^{99m}Tc scan	Vascular versus avascular
	Ultrasonography	Solid versus cystic. Pure cysts are usually not malignant.

cause true secondary hypothyroidism during prolonged administration. Other conditions associated with decreased TSH include pregnancy (especially with morning sickness), hCG-secreting trophoblastic tumors, acute psychiatric illness (1% incidence), and acute administration of glucocorticoids. Certain drugs cause mild suppression of TSH without clinical hyperthyroidism; these include nonsteroidal anti-inflammatory agents, amphetamine, octreotide, opioids, and certain calcium channel blockers (especially nifedipine; also verapamil, but not diltiazem).

In clinically euthyroid persons age 60 or older, the TSH is very low (≤ 0.1 mU/L) in 3% and mildly low (0.1–0.4 mU/L) in 9%. The chance of developing atrial fibrillation is higher with very low TSH (2.8% yearly) than with normal TSH (1.1% yearly). Asymptomatic patients with very low TSH are followed closely but not treated unless they develop atrial fibrillation or other manifestations of hyperthyroidism.

TSH levels are **elevated** in primary hypothyroidism, either clinical or subclinical. TSH may also be elevated or inappropriately normal in the very rare cases of hyperthyroidism due to pituitary neoplastic or nonneoplastic inappropriate secretion of thyrotropin. Autoimmune disease may also falsely elevate serum TSH levels by interfering with the assay. TSH may be transiently elevated during recovery from nonthyroidal illness and in about 14% of patients with acute psychiatric admissions; the TSH returns to normal in the great majority of these patients. TSH may be increased by dopamine antagonists (eg, metoclopramide), phenothiazines, and atypical antipsychotics). TSH may be mildly elevated in some individuals, especially elderly women (10% incidence). Such patients with normal T_4 levels must be carefully evaluated for subtle signs of hypothyroidism (eg, fatigue, depression, hyperlipidemia). About 18% later become definitely hypothyroid.

Free Thyroxine Immunoassay (FT_4)

FT_4 is a direct measurement of the serum concentration of free (unbound) thyroxine. FT_4 represents only about 0.025% of the serum concentration of the total T_4. It is the only metabolically active fraction of T_4 that freely enters cells to produce its effects.

When performed properly, this assay is superior to the total T_4 assay and free thyroxine index, since it is not affected by variations in protein binding. It is the procedure of choice for following the thyroid's changing secretion of T_4 during treatment for hyperthyroidism. Serum FT_4 levels may be suppressed in patients with severe nonthyroid illness. In patients receiving heparin, measured levels of FT_4 may be falsely high, particularly when a dialysis assay is used. Serum FT_4 levels rise transiently in acute nonthyroidal illness, when thyroid-binding protein frequently falls.

T_4 Immunoassay

This test measures the total serum concentration of thyroxine (bound and free). An increased serum T_4 confirms a clinical diagnosis of hyperthyroidism, while a decreased serum T_4 confirms a clinical diagnosis of hypothyroidism. It is affected by altered states of thyroxine binding (see Table 26–5). Therefore, this test is usually run with a resin T_3 uptake to provide a free thyroxine index (see below).

Resin T_3 (or T_4) Uptake

This is an indirect inverse test of serum thyroid-binding proteins (TBP)—ie, it is high when thyroid-binding proteins are low. The assay involves adding labeled T_3 or T_4 to the serum sample; it competes with the patient's thyroxine for binding to TBP. This mixture is then added to a thyroid hormone-binding resin. The resin is then assayed for its uptake of the label. A high resin uptake indicates that the patient's serum contains relatively low amounts of TBP or high levels of thyroxine.

This test corrects a total serum thyroxine measurement for the effect of increased or decreased binding, creating a free thyroxine index (see below). A low resin uptake (high TBP) is seen with estrogen therapy, pregnancy, acute hepatitis, genetic TBP increase, and hypothyroidism. A low resin uptake with low TBP may be seen in severe illness. A high resin uptake (low TBP) is seen with hyperthyroidism and with chronic liver disease, nephrotic syndrome, anabolic steroid administration, and high-dose glucocorticoid administration.

Free Thyroxine Index (FTI)

The product of T_4 and resin T_3 uptake ($T_4 \times T_3$ uptake) helps correct for abnormalities of thyroxine binding. A good free T_4 assay is more accurate.

The FTI, when calculated using the RT_3U, may be elevated in euthyroid patients with familial dysalbuminemic hyperthyroxinemia. This is a benign autosomal dominant trait in which an abnormal albumin molecule binds T_4 with much greater affinity than T_3. The RT_3U is not decreased (failing to compensate for the increased binding, as it would for TBG excess), because the T_3 used in the RT_3U assay is not significantly affected. Serum levels of free thyroxine and TSH are normal.

T_3

This test is of value in the diagnosis of thyrotoxicosis with normal T_4 values (T_3 thyrotoxicosis). It is not useful for the diagnosis of hypothyroidism.

Free T_3

This test measures the very tiny amount of T_3 that circulates unbound. It is sometimes useful in looking for hyperthyroidism in women taking oral estrogen and thyroxine replacement.

2. THYROID RADIOACTIVE IODINE UPTAKE & SCAN

Radioiodine (^{123}I or ^{131}I) Uptake of Thyroid Gland

A. Elevated: Graves' disease, dietary iodine deficiency, toxic nodular goiter, pregnancy, early Hashimoto's thyroiditis, some thyroid enzyme deficiencies, nephrotic syndrome, recovery from subacute thyroiditis, recovery from thyroid hormone suppression.

B. Low: Administration of iodides or iodine in any form (drugs, radiology contrast dyes, etc), antithyroid drugs, subacute thyroiditis, thyroid hormone administration, thyroid gland damage (from thyroiditis, surgery, or radioiodine), hypopituitarism, ectopic functioning thyroid tissue, azotemia, severe (high-turnover) Graves' disease, heart failure, and some thyroid enzyme abnormalities.

Radioiodine (RAI) Scans

A rectilinear scan over the neck may be obtained after radioiodine administration, thereby obtaining a life-sized picture of thyroid uptake. RAI scans are useful also for detecting metastatic thyroid cancer. (See Thyroid Cancer.) Following administration of a treatment dose of ^{131}I for thyroid cancer, a whole body scan is useful for detecting metastases.

3. OTHER THYROID TESTS

Thyroid Antibodies

Antibodies against several thyroid constituents (thyroglobulin and thyroperoxidase) are most commonly found in Hashimoto's thyroiditis and Graves' disease. Antithyroid antibodies are found in about 5–10% of normal subjects. There is an increasing incidence with age. About 20% of hospitalized patients have detectable antithyroid antibodies. In the latter, the titers tend to be low, and they increase with age. TSH receptor antibody (TSH-R Ab [stim]) titers are elevated in approximately 80% of patients with Graves' disease. These titers—and those of antithyroglobulin and antithyroperoxidase antibodies—often decrease during pregnancy and during treatment of Graves' disease with antithyroid drugs. TSH-R Ab [stim] titers have been used with variable results to predict the rate of relapse of Graves' disease after chronic thiourea therapy.

Serum Thyroglobulin

The level of serum thyroglobulin rises in autoimmune thyroid disease, thyroid injury or inflammation, and thyroid cancer. Levels are of little value in diagnosing or distinguishing among these conditions, but they provide a useful marker in thyroid cancer to indicate recurrence of disease and the need for further studies and therapy. Serum thyroglobulin is to be distinguished from serum thyroid binding globulin (see above).

Calcitonin Assay

This test is elevated in medullary thyroid carcinoma, azotemia, hypercalcemia, pernicious anemia, thyroiditis, and pregnancy. High levels are also seen in many other malignancies such as carcinomas of the lung (45%), pancreas, breast (38%), and colon (24%).

Ultrasound

Ultrasound may be used to guide fine-needle aspiration biopsy of clinically suspicious thyroid nodules and nodes. In patients with established thyroid malignancy, ultrasound of the neck is useful for surveillance, localization, and quantitation of residual or recurrent tumor. Small nonpalpable nodules are detected in half of "normal" thyroids and are rarely malignant.

Fine-Needle Thyroid Biopsy

Aspiration of thyroid tissue with a fine needle (25-gauge) is helpful in the diagnosis of thyroid disorders, especially nodular lesions. This technique has become the preferred approach to the diagnosis of thyroid masses. (See Nodular Thyroid.)

4. EFFECT OF NONTHYROIDAL ILLNESS & DRUGS UPON THYROID FUNCTION TESTS

Many factors affect thyroid function tests, causing misleading laboratory evidence of hypothyroidism or hyperthyroidism in patients who are clinically euthyroid. (See Table 26–5.)

Serum thyroxine is frequently low in patients with severe illness, caloric deprivation, or major surgery who have accelerated peripheral metabolism of serum T_4 to reverse T_3 (rT_3). Furthermore, in most patients who are critically ill, there is a circulating inhibitor of thyroid hormone binding to serum thyroid binding proteins. This causes the resin uptake of thyroid hormone (RT_3U) to be misleadingly low, causing the computed free thyroxine index to be very low. The presence of a very low serum T_4 in severe nonthyroidal illness indicates a poor prognosis. In one series of such patients with serum T_4 levels under 3 μg/dL, there was a mortality rate of 84%.

Direct assays of free thyroxine often show low levels of FT_4 in severe illness. Since studies of giving replacement thyroxine to such patients have shown no improvement in survival, they are considered "euthyroid." Serum TSH tends to be suppressed in severe nonthyroidal illness, making the diagnosis of concurrent primary hypothyroidism quite difficult, although the presence of a goiter suggests the diagnosis.

The clinician must decide whether such severely ill patients (with a low serum T_4 but nonelevated TSH) might have hypothyroidism due to pituitary insufficiency. Patients without symptoms of prior brain lesion or hypopituitarism are very unlikely to suddenly develop hypopituitarism during an unrelated illness. Patients with diabetes insipidus, hypopituitarism, or other signs of a central nervous system lesion may have thyroxine given empirically. Patients receiving prolonged dopamine infusions may develop true secondary hypothyroidism due to direct dopamine suppression of TSH-secreting cells.

DeGroot LJ: Dangerous dogmas in medicine: the nonthyroidal illness syndrome. J Clin Endocrinol Metab 1999;84:151. [NLM Cit ID: 99116804]

Despres N et al: Antibody interference in thyroid assays: a potential for clinical misinformation. Clin Chem 1998;44:440. [NLM Cit ID: 98171836]

Nordyke RA et al: Alternative sequences of thyrotropin and free thyroxine assays for routine thyroid function testing. Quality and cost. Arch Intern Med 1998;158:266. [NLM Cit ID: 98132792] (Sensitive TSH better detects subclinical thyroid dysfunction and monitors thyroxine treatment, while FT_4 better detects pituitary hypothyroidism and rapidly changing thyroid function.)

THE NODULAR THYROID

Essentials of Diagnosis

- Single or multiple thyroid nodules are commonly found with careful thyroid examinations.
- Thyroid function tests mandatory.
- Thyroid biopsy for single or dominant nodules or for a history of prior head-neck radiation.
- Ultrasound examination sometimes useful for biopsy and follow-up.
- Clinical follow-up required.

General Considerations

Enlargement of the thyroid (goiter) may be diffuse or irregular (nodular) and may often be discovered on physical examination. Nodular goiters are very common in regions of dietary iodine deficiency and may grow to large size (see Iodine Deficiency Disorders, below). Patients with a history of past head-neck radiation have about a 25% chance of developing thyroid disease years later, including a high rate of thyroid carcinoma. In others, a solitary nodule by palpation is most often a benign adenoma or colloid nodule. Thyroid adenomas may occasionally function enough to produce thyrotoxicosis. Other thyroid pathology may include cysts, thyroiditis, infections, and primary or metastatic neoplasms.

Clinical Evaluation (Table 26–7)

A. Symptoms and Signs: The thyroid is best examined in a well-lighted room. The seated patient is given water to drink and the anterior neck is observed during swallowing. The thyroid moves upward during swallowing and may be visible in a thin neck; enlargement or asymmetry of the thyroid may be noted. Palpation of the thyroid is best done from behind a seated patient using the second and third fingers of both hands. As the patient swallows water, thyroid nodules may be perceived moving beneath

Table 26–7. Clinical evaluation of thyroid nodules.[1]

Clinical Evidence	Low Index of Suspicion	High Index of Suspicion
History	Family history of goiter; residence in area of endemic goiter	Previous therapeutic radiation of head, neck, or chest; hoarseness
Physical characteristics	Older women; soft nodule; multinodular goiter	Young adults, men; solitary, firm nodule; vocal cord paralysis; enlarged lymph nodes; distant metastatic lesions
Serum factors	High titer of antithyroid antibody; hypothyroidism; hyperthyroidism	
Fine-needle aspiration biopsy	Colloid nodule or adenoma	Papillary carcinoma, follicular neoplasm, medullary or anaplastic carcinoma
Scanning techniques		
Uptake of ^{123}I	"Hot" nodule	"Cold" nodule
Ultrasonogram	Cystic lesion	Solid lesion
Roentgenogram	Shell-like calcification	Punctate calcification
Thyroxine therapy	Regression after 0.05–0.1 mg/d for 6 months or more	Increase in size

[1]Clinically suspicious nodules should be evaluated with fine-needle aspiration biopsy.

the fingers. The location of any nodules should be noted, along with their size, firmness, and tenderness. The neck should be examined for lymphadenopathy. Enlarged thyroids should be examined by auscultation for bruits.

Patients with thyroid enlargement should be questioned and examined for symptoms and signs of thyroid eye disease, hyperthyroidism, or hypothyroidism (see below).

Patients discovered to have thyroid enlargement are questioned further about any family history of thyroid disorders, prior medical history of thyroid problems, and prior radiation therapy to the head or neck or other exposure to radiation.

B. Laboratory Findings: Thyroid nodules are an indication for thyroid function testing. Serum determinations for TSH (sensitive assay) and free thyroxine (FT_4) are preferred. Tests for antithyroperoxidase antibodies and antithyroglobulin antibodies may also be helpful. Very high antibody levels are found in Hashimoto's thyroiditis. However, thyroiditis frequently coexists with malignancy, so a suspicious nodule should be biopsied.

Fine-needle aspiration (FNA) biopsy is the best way to assess a nodule for malignancy. A 25-gauge needle is used to biopsy suspicious nodules. The needle is attached to a syringe and special syringe holder. The biopsy is done without local anesthesia. The success rate of FNA biopsy is increased by ultrasound guidance. Care must be taken to avoid bloody dilution of the specimens. Material obtained is placed on a slide; a thin smear is obtained by laying a second slide over the material and then drawing the slides apart. One slide is air-dried while the other is preserved in 95% alcohol. Two or more biopsies may be obtained. Reading by an experienced cytopathologist is mandatory.

In one review of thyroid biopsies, about 70% were benign, 10% follicular neoplasm (suspicious), 5% malignant, and 15% nondiagnostic. Overall, about 20% of patients with "suspicious" cytology harbor a malignancy, but the risk is higher in young patients and those with nodules that are fixed or over 3 cm in diameter. Most such patients undergo thyroid surgery. However, a subgroup of elderly patients with "suspicious" cytology (nodules < 4 cm in diameter) have a malignancy rate of just 5%; such patients may elect to be followed every 6 months with palpation and ultrasound.

Cystic nodules yielding serous fluid are usually benign, but fluid should be submitted for cytology. Cystic nodules yielding bloody fluid have a higher chance of being malignant. Repeat FNA biopsy is done if the cytology is nondiagnostic (eg, diluted with blood or hypocellular) and the lesion remains palpable.

C. Imaging Studies: Since the advent of needle biopsy, radioactive iodine (RAI; ^{123}I or ^{131}I) scans are of less use in evaluating thyroid nodules because both hypofunctioning (cold) and hyperfunctioning (hot) nodules may sometimes be malignant. RAI scanning and uptake is helpful if a patient is found to have evidence of hyperthyroidism. (See Hyperthyroidism, below.) Ultrasound evaluation of thyroid nodules may be of benefit to determine whether a palpable nodule is really just one of many nodules, thus having less chance of being malignant. It may also be helpful in following thyroid nodules and in difficult biopsies. Ultrasound is generally preferred over CT and MRI because of its accuracy, ease of use, and lower cost.

Treatment

All thyroid nodules, including those with benign cytology, need to be followed by regular periodic palpation and rebiopsied if growth occurs. Patients with elevated levels of serum TSH are treated with thyroxine replacement. Otherwise, for small nodules, thyroxine is not required. For larger nodules (> 2 cm), if TSH levels are elevated or normal, "suppression" with levothyroxine sodium (0.05–0.1 mg daily) can be considered. Levothyroxine should not be administered if the baseline TSH is low, since that is an indication of autonomous thyroid secretion, such that levothyroxine treatment will be ineffective and liable to cause clinical thyrotoxicosis. Long-term levothyroxine suppression of TSH tends to keep nodules from enlarging, but only a few will actually shrink. Additional nodules develop in fewer treated patients. Suppressive levothyroxine therapy is most suitable for younger patients. All patients require regular careful clinical evaluation and thyroid palpation or ultrasound examinations. Levothyroxine suppression therapy should usually not be given to patients with certain cardiovascular problems since it may increase the risk for angina and arrhythmia. Levothyroxine suppression causes a small loss of bone density in many postmenopausal women not taking estrogen replacement; estrogen appears protective in this regard. Patients at risk for osteoporosis are advised to have periodic bone density testing.

A. Solitary Thyroid Nodules: Palpable solitary thyroid nodules call for fine-needle aspiration biopsy (see above). A solitary thyroid nodule in a patient with a remote history of radiation therapy to the head or neck (or exposure to nuclear fallout) is considered at high risk of malignancy and the nodule is resected. Cystic nodules can be managed by removal of fluid for cytologic examination, which may deflate the cyst. However, cysts tend to recur, requiring repeated aspirations. Solitary nodules in a patient with hyperthyroidism are an indication for radioactive iodine scan, which generally distinguishes toxic adenoma from Graves' disease. However, Graves' disease may occasionally be unilateral owing to agenesis of the contralateral lobe, so additional studies with antithyroid antibodies may be helpful. A "hot" nodule is usually benign but is resected to cure the hyperthyroidism.

B. Multinodular Goiters: A thyroid containing multiple nodules is likely to be a benign multinodular goiter. Nevertheless, fine-needle aspiration biopsy is performed on any nodule that is growing or is particularly dominant or hard. Large retrosternal goiters rarely harbor a malignancy but can be followed by CT scan or MRI. Continued growth or compressive symptoms are reasons for surgical excision. Patients found to be hyperthyroid may have a radioactive iodine scan and uptake for additional evaluation, especially if ^{131}I is a therapeutic consideration.

C. Nonpalpable Thyroid Nodules: Nonpalpable small thyroid nodules are detected in about 50% of scans of the neck (MRI, CT, ultrasound) done for other reasons. In one series, only 2% of such thyroids were found to have significant malignancy after surgical resection. Therefore, ultrasound-guided FNA biopsy is considered only for patients with nonpalpable nodules over 1.5 cm in diameter and for those with a history of head-neck irradiation.

Microscopic "micropapillary" carcinoma is a variant of normal, being found in 24% of thyroidectomies performed for benign thyroid disease when 2 mm sections were carefully examined. It thus appears that the overwhelming majority of these microscopic foci never become clinically significant. The surgical pathology report of such a tiny papillary carcinoma that is otherwise benign does not justify aggressive follow-up or treatment because a cancer diagnosis is unwarranted and harmful. All that may be required is yearly follow-up with palpation of the neck and mild TSH suppression by thyroxine.

Prognosis

The great majority of thyroid nodules are benign. Benign thyroid nodules tend to persist or grow slowly, but they may involute. Only about 1% of benign nodules increase in diameter with follow-up. Conversion to a malignant nodule is rare. The prognosis for patients with thyroid nodules that prove to be malignant is determined by the histologic type and other factors (see below). Overall, differentiated thyroid carcinoma has an excellent prognosis, but metastases do occur. Multinodular goiters tend to persist or grow slowly, even in iodine-deficient areas where iodine repletion usually does not shrink established goiters. Patients with small incidentally discovered nonpalpable thyroid nodules are at very low risk for malignancy, and even those that are malignant have a minor effect on morbidity and mortality.

Gharib H et al: Thyroxine suppressive therapy in patients with nodular thyroid disease. Ann Intern Med 1998; 128:386. [NLM Cit ID: 98138824] (Patients with cytologically benign nodules are best followed without thyroxine suppression. Nodules that increase in size should be rebiopsied or resected.)

Papini E et al: Long-term changes in nodular goiter: A 5-year prospective randomized trial of levothyroxine suppressive therapy for benign cold thyroid nodules. J Clin Endocrinol Metab 1998;83:780. [NLM Cit ID: 98165570] (Long-term thyroxine suppression can reduce the risk of nodular growth. But see Gharib reference, above; and see text.)

Schlinkert RT et al: Factors that predict malignant thyroid lesions when fine-needle aspiration is "suspicious for malignancy." Mayo Clin Proc 1997;72:913. [NLM Cit ID: 98018748]

THYROID CANCER (Table 26–8)

Essentials of Diagnosis

- Painless swelling in region of thyroid.
- Thyroid function tests usually normal.

Table 26–8. Some characteristics of thyroid cancer.

	Papillary	Follicular	Medullary	Anaplastic
Incidence	Most common	Common	Uncommon	Rare
Average age	42	50	50	57
Females	70%	72%	56%	56%
Deaths due to thyroid cancer	6%	24%	33%	98%
Invasion:				
Juxtanodal	++++	+	++++++	+++
Blood vessels	+	+++	+++	+++++
Distant sites	+	+++	++	++++
Resemblance to normal thyroid	+	+++	+	±
^{123}I uptake	+	++++	0	0
Degree of malignancy	+	++ to +++	+ to ++++	+++++++

- Past history of irradiation to head and neck region may be present.
- Positive thyroid needle aspiration.

General Considerations

The incidence of papillary and follicular (differentiated) thyroid carcinomas increases with age. The female:male ratio is 3:1. Clinically detectable thyroid carcinoma constitutes less than 1% of cancers, but in situ microcarcinomas can be found in up to 35% of thyroids in adult autopsy series. Most differentiated (papillary and follicular) thyroid carcinomas secrete thyroglobulin, which can be used as a serum tumor marker after total thyroidectomy.

Papillary carcinoma is the most common thyroid malignancy. Pure papillary or mixed papillary-follicular carcinoma represents about 76% of all thyroid cancers. It usually presents as a single nodule, but it can arise out of a multinodular goiter. Patients who have had external x-ray treatments to the neck or head during childhood have an increased lifelong risk. Similarly, childhood exposure to radioactive isotopes of iodine in nuclear fallout (eg, after the Chernobyl accident) carries a high risk for later development of papillary thyroid cancer. It may also be familial (3%) or associated with Cowden's disease (multiple hamartomas of the skin and mucous membranes with a high incidence of breast cancer) or adenomatous polyposis coli.

Generally speaking, papillary carcinoma is the least aggressive thyroid malignancy. However, the tumor spreads via lymphatics within the thyroid, becoming multifocal in 60% and involving both lobes in 30%. It frequently spreads to local and regional lymph nodes and sometimes to the lungs. Radioiodine thyroid scans usually depict papillary carcinomas as relatively "cold" nodules; however, most such carcinomas do concentrate some iodine, making possible diagnostic scanning and treatment with ^{131}I after total thyroidectomy. Certain papillary histopathologic features are associated with a higher risk of recurrence: tall cell, columnar cell, and diffuse sclerosing types. Chronic low-grade papillary carcinoma can sometimes undergo a late anaplastic transformation into an aggressive carcinoma.

Follicular carcinoma accounts for about 16% of thyroid malignancies and is generally more aggressive than papillary carcinoma. Rarely, some follicular carcinomas secrete enough thyroxine to cause thyrotoxicosis if the tumor load becomes significant. Metastases commonly are found in neck nodes, bone, and lungs. Most follicular thyroid carcinomas avidly absorb iodine, making possible diagnostic scanning and treatment with ^{131}I after total thyroidectomy. Certain follicular histopathologic features are associated with a high risk of metastasis and recurrence: poorly differentiated and Hürthle cell (oncocytic) variants. The latter variants rarely take up radioiodine.

Medullary thyroid carcinoma represents about 4% of thyroid cancers. About one-third are sporadic; one-third are familial; and one-third are associated with multiple endocrine neoplasia (MEN) type 2. Therefore, discovery of a medullary thyroid carcinoma makes family surveillance advisable. It arises from parafollicular thyroid cells that can secrete calcitonin, prostaglandins, serotonin, ACTH, corticotropin-releasing hormone (CRH), and other peptides. These peptides can cause symptoms and can be used as tumor markers. Early local metastases are usually present, usually to adjacent muscle and trachea as well as to local and mediastinal lymph nodes. Eventually, late metastases may appear in the bones, lungs, adrenals, or liver. This tumor does not concentrate iodine.

Anaplastic thyroid carcinoma represents about 1% of thyroid cancers. It usually presents in an older patient as a rapidly enlarging mass in a multinodular goiter. It is the most aggressive thyroid carcinoma and metastasizes early to surrounding nodes and distant sites. Local pressure symptoms include dysphagia or vocal cord paralysis. This tumor does not concentrate iodine.

Other thyroid malignancies together represent about 3% of thyroid cancers. Lymphoma of the thyroid is more common in women than in men. It usually presents as a rapidly enlarging, painful mass arising out of a multinodular or diffuse goiter affected by autoimmune thyroiditis, with which it may be confused microscopically. About 20% of cases have concomitant hypothyroidism. It may also be seen as part of systemic lymphoma. Thyroid lymphomas resolve with external radiation therapy; systemic lymphomas are also treated with chemotherapy. Thyroidectomy is rarely required. Metastatic cancers may sometimes involve the thyroid, particularly bronchogenic, breast, and renal carcinomas and malignant melanoma.

Clinical Findings

A. Symptoms and Signs: The principal sign of thyroid carcinoma is a palpable, firm and nontender nodule in the thyroid area. Anterior cervical lymph nodes may be enlarged. Metastatic functioning differentiated thyroid carcinoma can sometimes secrete enough thyroid hormone to produce thyrotoxicosis.

Medullary thyroid carcinoma frequently causes flushing and diarrhea (30%), fatigue, and other symptoms; about 5% develop Cushing's syndrome from secretion of ACTH or CRH. Signs of pressure or invasion of surrounding tissues are present in anaplastic or long-standing tumors with recurrent laryngeal nerve palsy or fixation of nodule to neighboring structures.

B. Laboratory Findings: (Fine-needle aspiration is discussed above in the section on nodular thyroid.) Thyroid function tests are generally normal unless there is concomitant thyroiditis. Follicular carcinoma may secrete enough thyroxine to suppress TSH and cause clinical hyperthyroidism.

Serum thyroglobulin is high in most metastatic papillary and follicular tumors, making this a useful marker for recurrent or metastatic disease. Caution must be exercised for the following reasons: (1) Circulating antithyroglobulin antibodies can cause erroneous thyroglobulin determinations. (2) Thyroglobulin levels may be misleadingly elevated in thyroiditis, which often coexists with carcinoma. (3) Certain thyroglobulin assays falsely report the continued presence of thyroglobulin after total thyroidectomy and tumor resection, causing undue concern about possible metastases. Therefore, unexpected thyroglobulin levels should prompt a repeat assay in another reference laboratory.

Serum calcitonin levels are frequently elevated in medullary thyroid carcinoma, making this a marker for metastatic disease. However, serum calcitonin may be elevated in many other conditions such as thyroiditis, pregnancy, azotemia, hypercalcemia, and other malignancies, including pheochromocytomas, carcinoid tumors, and carcinomas of the lung, pancreas, breast, and colon.

Serum carcinoembryonic antigen (CEA) levels are usually elevated with medullary carcinoma, making this a useful second marker; however, it is not specific for this carcinoma.

Serum determinations for calcitonin and CEA should be obtained before surgery for medullary carcinoma, then periodically in postoperative follow-up. Calcitonin levels remain elevated in patients with persistent tumor but also in some patients with apparent cure. Therefore, rising levels of calcitonin or CEA are the best indication for recurrence.

Since two-thirds of medullary carcinoma cases are familial or MEN type 2, siblings and children of patients with medullary carcinoma are advised to have genetic testing to detect *RET* proto-oncogene mutations (see MEN type 2a).

C. Imaging: Ultrasound of the neck is useful in determining the size and location of the malignancy as well as neck metastases. Bone and soft tissue metastases that take up radioiodine may be demonstrable on radioisotope scans. Chest x-ray or CT may demonstrate metastases. Medullary carcinoma in the thyroid, nodes, and liver may calcify, but lung metastases rarely do so; metastases may be detected with positron emission tomography (PET) scanning and MRI.

Differential Diagnosis

Lymphocytic thyroiditis, multinodular goiter, and colloid nodules can be distinguished from malignancies by FNA biopsy. However, FNA cannot distinguish benign follicular adenoma from follicular carcinoma. Overall, in such "suspicious" cases, the risk of malignancy is about 20%—higher in fixed lesions over 4 cm in diameter. The risk of malignancy is 5% for nodules in elderly patients with lesions under 4 cm in diameter having "suspicious" cytology.

Neuroendocrine carcinomas may metastasize to the thyroid and be confused with medullary thyroid carcinoma.

False-positive ^{131}I scans are common with normal residual thyroid tissue and have been reported with Zenker's diverticulum, ovary, pleuropericardial cyst, gastric pull-up, and ^{131}I-contaminated bodily secretions. False-negative ^{131}I scans are common in early metastatic differentiated thyroid carcinoma but occur also in more advanced disease, including 14% of bone metastases.

Complications

The complications vary with the type of carcinoma. Differentiated thyroid carcinomas may have local or distant metastases. One-third of medullary carcinomas may secrete serotonin and prostaglandins, producing flushing and diarrhea, and may be complicated by the coexistence of pheochromocytomas or hyperparathyroidism. The complications of radical neck surgery often include permanent hypoparathyroidism and, less commonly, vocal cord palsy; permanent hypothyroidism is expected and should always be treated adequately.

Treatment of Differentiated Thyroid Carcinoma

A. Surgical Treatment: Surgical removal is the treatment of choice for thyroid carcinomas. Neck ultrasound is useful both preoperatively and in follow-up. Highly skilled surgeons can perform near-total thyroidectomies with a less than 1% rate of serious complications (hypoparathyroidism or recurrent laryngeal nerve damage). Other series have reported up to an 11% incidence of permanent hypoparathyroidism after total thyroidectomy.

Following thyroidectomy, patients should be hospitalized as inpatients until it is determined that they have safely recovered from surgery. This requires at least an overnight hospital admission, since late bleeding, airway problems, and tetany can occur. Ambulatory thyroidectomy is potentially dangerous and should not be done.

The incidence of hypoparathyroidism may be reduced if accidentally resected parathyroids are immediately autotransplanted into the neck muscles. The advantage of near-total thyroidectomy for differentiated thyroid carcinoma is that multicentric foci of carcinoma are more apt to be resected and there is then less normal thyroid tissue to compete with cancer for ^{131}I administered later for scans or treatment. Subtotal thyroidectomy is acceptable for adults under age 45 who have a single small tumor ($\leq$ 1 cm in diameter). Neck muscle dissections are usually avoided for differentiated thyroid carcinoma. Thyroxine is prescribed in doses of 0.05–0.1 mg/d immediately postoperatively. The dosage is adjusted to keep the serum TSH slightly suppressed during long-term follow-up of differentiated thyroid carcinoma.

About 2–4 months after surgery, a whole-body ^{131}I scan is performed: Thyroxine is stopped for 6 weeks prior to the scan, thereby causing hypothyroidism; TSH then rises and stimulates iodide uptake and thyroglobulin release from residual tumor or normal thyroid. Iodine-containing foods and contrast media are avoided.

B. Medical Treatment: Thyrotropin alfa injections can stimulate uptake of ^{131}I by thyroid cancer or residual thyroid. The dosage is 0.9 mg intragluteally (not intravenously) every 24 hours for two doses or every 72 hours for three doses. Radioiodine is administered 24 hours after the final thyrotropin injection; 72 hours after the final injection, a whole-body scan is obtained and blood is drawn for serum thyroglobulin determination. Side effects of thyrotropin injections include nausea (11%) and headache (7%). Hyperthyroidism can occur in patients with significant metastases or residual normal thyroid. Thyrotropin has caused neurologic deterioration in 7% of patients with central nervous system metastases. The combination of thyrotropin-stimulated scan and thyroglobulin (Tg) level detects a thyroid remnant or cancer with a sensitivity of 94% (three injections) or 84% (two injections). The presence of anti-Tg antibodies renders the serum Tg determination uninterpretable. Thyrotropin injections do not stimulate radioiodine uptake sufficiently to allow ^{131}I ablative therapy of thyroid cancer.

Thyroid hormone withdrawal, with radioiodine imaging and serum Tg testing during hypothyroidism, remains the most sensitive means of determining the location and extent of differentiated thyroid cancer. Thyrotropin-stimulated scans and Tg may be useful for some patients who have no anti-Tg antibodies and a very low risk of metastatic thyroid cancer or who refuse thyroid hormone withdrawal because of the discomforts of hypothyroidism.

C. Radioiodine: Sodium iodide I 131, 30–50 mCi, is administered to patients with an original papillary or follicular carcinoma $\geq$ 1.5 cm in diameter and also to patients having persistent radioiodine uptake in the thyroid bed. Patients with extrathyroidal uptake from metastatic disease are given larger doses of 100–200 mCi in the hospital. Another whole-body scan several days after ^{131}I treatment will sometimes detect metastases not visible on pretreatment scans.

^{131}I ablation in doses over 100 mCi can cause sialadenitis, gastritis, and temporary oligospermia. Cumulative doses of ^{131}I over 500 mCi can cause infertility, pancytopenia (4%), and leukemia (0.3%).

D. External Radiation Therapy: External radiation may be delivered to bone metastases. Brain metastases do not usually respond to ^{131}I and are best resected or treated with gamma knife radiation therapy.

E. Surveillance: Patients with differentiated thyroid carcinoma are followed clinically with neck palpation, physical examination, and chest x-ray and observed for thyrotoxicosis that might indicate functioning metastases. About 6–12 months after their postoperative scan, patients usually receive another ^{131}I whole body scan and serum thyroglobulin measurement while hypothyroid; these have a combined sensitivity of 95% for metastases. Serum thyroglobulin in a patient receiving thyroxine has a lower sensitivity of 62%.

Thallium-201 (^{201}Tl) scans may be useful for detecting metastatic differentiated thyroid carcinoma when ^{131}I scan is normal but serum thyroglobulin is elevated. MRI or ultrasound is useful in distinguishing recurrent thyroid tumor from postoperative changes.

Patients with papillary carcinoma should have at least two consecutively negative scans before they are considered in remission. Further scans may be required for patients with more aggressive follicular carcinomas, prior metastases, rising serum thyroglobulin, or other evidence of metastases.

Treatment of Other Thyroid Malignancies

Patients with anaplastic thyroid carcinoma are treated with local resection and radiation. Thyroid lymphomas are best treated with external radiation therapy; chemotherapy is added for extensive lymphoma.

Medullary thyroid carcinoma is treated surgically; repeated neck dissections are often required over time. Patients found to have *RET* protooncogene mutations are advised to have a prophylactic total thyroidectomy, ideally at age 6 years. This cancer does not take up ^{131}I.

Anaplastic thyroid carcinoma is also treated surgically. It does not take up ^{131}I.

Prognosis

The prognosis for differentiated (papillary and follicular) thyroid carcinoma is generally excellent, particularly for adults under age 45 years. Staging and survival rates are presented in Table 26–9. Patients with follicular carcinoma have a cancer mortality rate that is 3.4 times higher than patients with papillary carcinoma. The Hürthle cell variant of follicular carcinoma is more aggressive. Patients with primary tumors over 1 cm in diameter who undergo limited thyroid surgery (subtotal thyroidectomy or lobectomy) have a 2.2-fold increased mortality over those having total or near-total thyroidectomies. Patients who have not received ^{131}I ablation have mortality rates that are increased twofold by 10 years and threefold by 25 years (over those who have received ablation). The risk of cancer recurrence is twofold higher in men than in women and 1.7-fold higher in multifocal than in unifocal tumors.

Medullary thyroid carcinoma has a variable prognosis. Patients with sporadic disease usually have lymph node involvement at the time of diagnosis, whereas distal metastases may not be noted for years; the 5-year survival is 82% and the 10-year survival rate is 69%. Familial cases or those associated with MEN 2a tend to be less aggressive; the 10-year survival rate is higher, in part due to earlier detection. Women with medullary thyroid carcinoma who are under age 40 also have a better prognosis. The mortality rate is increased 4.5-fold when primary or metastatic tumor tissue stains heavily for myelomonocytic antigen M-1. Conversely, tumors with heavy immunoperoxidase staining for calcitonin are associated with prolonged survival even in the presence of significant metastases.

Anaplastic thyroid carcinoma has a 1-year survival rate of about 10%, and a 5-year survival rate of about 5%. Patients with fully localized tumors on MRI have a better prognosis.

Thyroid non-Hodgkin lymphomas have an excellent prognosis when treated by radiation therapy and chemotherapy. Patients with localized lymphoma have nearly 100% 5-year survival. Those with disease outside the thyroid have a 63% 5-year survival. However, the prognosis is better for those with the mucosa-associated lymphoid tissue (MALT) type. Patients presenting with stridor, pain, laryngeal nerve palsy or mediastinal extension tend to fare worse.

Table 26–9. Pathologic tumor-node-metastasis (pTNM) staging and survival rates for adults with appropriately treated differentiated (papillary and follicular) thyroid carcinoma based upon patient age, primary tumor size and invasiveness (T), lymph node involvement (N), and distant metastases (M).[1]

	Description	Five-Year Survival	Ten-Year Survival
Stage 1	Under 45: Any T, any N, no M Over 45: T ≤1 cm, no N, no M	100%	98%
Stage 2	Under 45: Any T, any N, any M Over 45: T >1 cm limited to thyroid, no N, no M	99%	85%
Stage 3	Over 45: T beyond thyroid capsule, no N, no M; or any T, regional N, no M	95%	70%
Stage 4	Over 45: Any T, any N, any M	80%	61%

[1]From Loh KC et al: J Endocrinol Metab 1997;82:3553; and Hay ID: Endocrinol Metabol Clin North Am 1990;19:545.

Clark OH et al: Ambulatory thyroid surgery: Unnecessary and dangerous. J Clin Endocrinol Metab 1998;83:1100.

Dralle H et al: Prophylactic thyroidectomy in 75 children and adolescents with hereditary medullary thyroid carcinoma: German and Austrian experience. World J Surg 1998;22:744. [NLM Cit ID: 98270983] (Recommendation: prophylactic total thyroidectomy at age 6 years.)

Schlumberger MJ: Papillary and follicular thyroid carcinoma. N Engl J Med 1998;338:297. [NLM Cit ID: 98092076]

ENDEMIC & MULTINODULAR GOITER

Essentials of Diagnosis

- Common in regions of the world with low-iodine diets.
- High rate of congenital hypothyroidism and cretinism.
- Goiters may become multinodular and grow to great size.
- Most adults with endemic goiter are found to be euthyroid; however, some are hypothyroid or hyperthyroid.
- Impaired cognition and hearing may be subtle or severe in congenital hypothyroidism.

General Considerations

Approximately 5% of the world's population have goiters. Of these, about 75% are in persons dwelling in areas of iodine deficiency. Such areas are found in

115 countries, mostly in developing areas but also in Europe. In Pescopagano, Italy, 60% of adults have goiters. Hyperthyroidism (present or past) occurred in 2.9%; hypothyroidism was overt in 0.2% and subclinical in 3.8%. The incidence of thyroid cancer was less than 0.1%. Up to 0.5% of iodine-deficient populations have full-blown cretinism, with less severe manifestations of congenital hypothyroidism being even more common (eg, isolated deafness, short stature, or impaired mentation). Intelligence quotients in iodine-deficient adults are an average of 13 points lower than expected. Although iodine deficiency is the most common cause of endemic goiter, certain foods (eg, sorghum, millet, maize, cassava) and water pollutants can themselves cause goiter or aggravate a goiter proclivity caused by iodine deficiency. Some individuals are particularly susceptible to goiter owing to congenital partial defects in thyroid enzyme activity.

Clinical Findings

A. Symptoms and Signs: Endemic goiters may become multinodular and very large. Growth often occurs during pregnancy and may cause compressive symptoms.

Substernal goiters are usually asymptomatic but can cause tracheal compression, respiratory distress and failure, dysphagia, superior vena cava syndrome, gastrointestinal bleeding from esophageal varices, palsies of the phrenic or recurrent laryngeal nerves, or Horner's syndrome. Cerebral ischemia and stroke can result from arterial compression or thyrocervical steal syndrome. Substernal goiters can rarely cause pleural or pericardial effusions. The incidence of significant malignancy is less than 1%.

Some patients with endemic goiter may become hypothyroid. Others may become thyrotoxic as the goiter grows and becomes more autonomous, especially if iodine is added to the diet.

B. Laboratory Findings: The serum thyroxine is usually normal. Serum TSH is generally normal. TSH falls in the presence of hyperthyroidism if a multinodular goiter has become autonomous in the presence of sufficient amounts of iodine for thyroid hormone synthesis. TSH rises with hypothyroidism. Thyroid radioactive iodine uptake is usually elevated, but it may be normal if iodine intake has improved. Serum levels of antithyroid antibodies are usually either undetectable or in low titers. Serum thyroglobulin is often elevated.

Differential Diagnosis

Endemic goiter must be distinguished from all other forms of nodular goiter that may coexist in an endemic region (see above).

Prevention

Iodine supplementation was started in Switzerland in 1922, initially by adding 5 mg of potassium iodide per kilogram of salt, with later increases to the current level of 20 mg/kg salt. Iodized salt has greatly reduced the incidence of endemic goiter. Unfortunately, many iodine-deficient countries have inadequate programs for iodine supplementation. The minimum dietary requirement for iodine is about 50 μg daily, with optimal iodine intake being 150–300 μg daily. Iodine sufficiency is assessed by measurement of urinary iodide excretion, the target being more than 10 μg/dL.

Initiating iodine supplementation in a geographic area causes an increased frequency of hyperthyroidism in the first year, followed by greatly reduced rates of toxic nodular goiter and Graves' disease thereafter.

Treatment

The addition of potassium iodide to table salt greatly reduces the prevalence of endemic goiter and cretinism but is less effective in shrinking established goiter. Dietary iodine supplementation increases the risk of autoimmune thyroid dysfunction with hypothyroidism or thyrotoxicosis. Thyroxine supplementation can shrink goiters and reduce the risk of further goiter growth, but such treatment likewise carries a risk of inducing hyperthyroidism in individuals with autonomous multinodular goiters; therefore, thyroxine suppression should not be started in patients with suppressed TSH levels.

Adults with large multinodular goiter may require thyroidectomy for cosmesis, compressive symptoms, or thyrotoxicosis. Following partial thyroidectomy in iodine-deficient geographic areas, there is a high goiter recurrence rate, so total thyroidectomy is preferred when surgery is indicated. Certain patients at high surgical risk may be treated with ^{131}I for large compressive multinodular goiters. Such patients may rarely develop Graves' disease 3–10 months after treatment.

Aghini-Lombardi F et al: The spectrum of thyroid disorders in an iodine-deficient community: The Pescopagano survey. J Clin Endocrinol Metab 1999;84:561. [NLM Cit ID: 99145014]

Anders HJ: Compression syndromes caused by substernal goitres. Postgrad Med J 1998;74:327. [NLM Cit ID: 99016266]

Kahaly GJ et al: Iodide induces thyroid autoimmunity in patients with endemic goitre: a randomised, double-blind, placebo-controlled trial. Eur J Endocrinol 1998;139:290. [NLM Cit ID: 98429405] (In 62 patients with endemic goiter, thyroxine [0.125 mg/d] caused an average decrease in thyroid volume from 32 mL to 17 mL. Iodine [0.5 mg/d] caused an average decrease in thyroid volume from 33 mL to 21 mL, but was associated with the development of antithyroid antibodies in 19%; hypothyroidism developed in 13% and hyperthyroidism in 6%. Thyroid dysfunction remitted when iodine supplementation was withdrawn.)

caused by diarrhea of any cause or malabsorption due to sprue, regional enteritis, liver disease, or pancreatic exocrine insufficiency. Serum TSH may be elevated transiently in acute psychiatric illness and during recovery from nonthyroidal illness. Autoimmune disease can cause false elevations of TSH by interfering with the assay. A high TSH can also be caused by thyrotropin-secreting pituitary tumors.

Suppressed serum TSH levels < 0.1 mU/L (using a sensitive assay) may indicate overreplacement with levothyroxine; if such a patient has manifestations of hyperthyroidism, the dosage is reduced. However, patients with suppressed serum TSH levels may exhibit no symptoms of hyperthyroidism. For such patients, it is important to determine whether hypopituitarism or severe nonthyroidal illness is present, which can result in low serum TSH levels without hyperthyroidism. TSH can also be suppressed by certain medications, such as nonsteroidal anti-inflammatory agents, opioids, nifedipine, verapamil, and acute administration of glucocorticoids. Absent such conditions, a clinically euthyroid patient with a low serum TSH should be given a lower dosage of levothyroxine unless symptoms of hypothyroidism develop.

Some hypothyroid patients treated with levothyroxine complain of hypothyroid type symptoms despite having normal or suppressed levels of TSH and normal levels of free T_4. Such patients require careful assessment for other concurrent illnesses such as adrenal insufficiency, hypogonadism, anemia, or depression. If such conditions are ruled out or treated and hypothyroid type symptoms persist despite normal or low TSH levels, a serum T_3 level (free T_3 in women receiving oral estrogens) may help make the difficult decision about whether to increase the levothyroxine dose. If the T_3 level is low or low normal, such a patient may benefit from a careful increase in thyroxine dosage; if a definite clinical benefit is achieved, the higher dose is continued. However, long-term surveillance for atrial arrhythmias and for osteoporosis is recommended for such patients, though such complications are uncommon in those who are clinically euthyroid. The malaise felt by some hypothyroid patients despite apparent optimal replacement therapy with T_4 may be due to an abnormally low ratio of T_3/T_4 levels in certain tissues. In one recent small study, the addition of triiodothyronine, 12.5 μg daily, to the levothyroxine regimen caused an improvement in cognition, mood, and physical symptoms in some patients.

Prognosis

With early treatment, striking transformations take place both in appearance and mental function. Return to a normal state is usually the rule, but relapses will occur if treatment is interrupted. The patient may rarely die from the complications of myxedema coma. On the whole, response to thyroid treatment is most satisfactory. Hypothyroidism caused by interferon-alfa resolves within 17 months of stopping the drug in 50% of patients. Chronic maintenance therapy with unduly large doses of thyroid hormone may lead to subtle but important side effects (eg, bone demineralization) and is to be avoided.

Adlin V: Subclinical hypothyroidism: Deciding when to treat. Am Fam Physician 1998;57:776. [NLM Cit ID: 98151700] (Patients with definite and persistent TSH elevation should be considered for thyroid treatment even if their free thyroxine levels are normal.)

Bunevicius R et al: Effects of thyroxine as compared with thyroxine plus triiodothyronine in patients with hypothyroidism. N Engl J Med 1999;340:424. [NLM Cit ID: 99122622]

Dong BJ et al: Bioequivalence of generic and brand-name levothyroxine products in the treatment of hypothyroidism. JAMA 1997;277:1205. [NLM Cit ID: 97256503]

Harjai KJ et al: Effects of amiodarone on thyroid function. Ann Intern Med 1997;126:63. [NLM Cit ID: 971279530]

Helfand M et al: Clinical guideline, part 2. Screening for thyroid disease: an update. American College of Physicians. Ann Intern Med 1998;129:144. [NLM Cit ID: 98318198] (Screening with serum TSH can detect symptomatic but unsuspected overt thyroid dysfunction. The highest yield is among women over age 50, in whom one in 71 was found to have symptomatic hypothyroidism that could benefit from treatment.)

Hierholzer K et al: Myxedema. Kidney Int 1997;59 (Suppl):582. [NLM Cit ID: 97328573]

Loh LK et al: Interferon-alpha induced thyroid dysfunction: three clinical presentations and a review of the literature. Thyroid 1997;7:891. [NLM Cit ID: 98119721]

Mulder JE: Thyroid disease in women. Med Clin North Am 1998;82:103. [NLM Cit ID: 98118336]

HYPERTHYROIDISM (Thyrotoxicosis)

Essentials of Diagnosis

- Sweating, weight loss or gain, anxiety, loose stools, heat intolerance, irritability, fatigue, weakness, menstrual irregularity.
- Tachycardia; warm, moist skin; stare; tremor.
- In Graves' disease: goiter (often with bruit); ophthalmopathy.
- Suppressed TSH in primary hyperthyroidism; increased T_4, free T_4, and free T_4 index.

General Considerations

The term "thyrotoxicosis" refers to the clinical manifestations associated with serum levels of thyroxine or triiodothyronine that are excessive for the individual.

The various causes include the following:

(1) Graves' disease: By far the most common form of thyrotoxicosis is that associated with diffuse enlargement of the thyroid, hyperactivity of the gland, and the presence of antibodies against different fractions of the thyroid gland. This autoimmune thyroid disorder is called **Graves' disease** (Basedow's disease). It is much more common in women than in men (8:1), and its onset is usually between the ages of 20 and 40. It may be accompanied by infiltrative ophthalmopathy (Graves' exophthalmos) and, less commonly, by infiltrative dermopathy (pretibial myxedema). It may also be associated with other systemic autoimmune disorders such as pernicious anemia, myasthenia gravis, diabetes mellitus, etc. It has a familial tendency, and histocompatibility studies have shown an association with group HLA-B8 and HLA-DR3. The pathogenesis of the hyperthyroidism of Graves' disease involves the formation of autoantibodies that bind to the TSH receptor in thyroid cell membranes and stimulate the gland to hyperfunction. TSH receptor antibodies (TSH-R Ab [stim]) are demonstrable in the plasma of about 80% of patients with Graves' disease. Other antibodies such as ANA are generated in Graves' disease, with antimicrosomal or antithyroglobulin antibodies being increased in most patients.

(2) Autonomous toxic adenomas of the thyroid may be single (Plummer's disease) or multiple (toxic multinodular goiter). These adenomas are not accompanied by infiltrative ophthalmopathy or dermopathy. Antithyroid antibodies are usually not present in the plasma, and tests for TSH-R Ab [stim] are negative.

(3) Subacute thyroiditis (thought to be due to viral infection) is characterized by a moderately enlarged, tender thyroid. If the gland is nontender, the disorder is called "silent thyroiditis." Hyperthyroidism is followed by hypothyroidism. During thyrotoxicosis, thyroid RAIU is low. A similar problem is seen with interleukin-2 therapy and after neck surgery for hyperparathyroidism.

(4) Jodbasedow disease, or iodine-induced hyperthyroidism, may occur in patients with multinodular goiters after intake of large amounts of iodine in the diet or in the form of radiographic contrast materials or drugs, especially amiodarone.

(5) Thyrotoxicosis factitia is due to ingestion of excessive amounts of exogenous thyroid hormone. Isolated epidemics of thyrotoxicosis have been caused by consumption of ground beef contaminated with bovine thyroid gland.

(6) Struma ovarii–Thyroid tissue is contained in about 3% of ovarian dermoid tumors and teratomas. This thyroid tissue may autonomously secrete thyroid hormone due to a toxic nodule or in concert with the woman's thyroid gland in Graves' disease or toxic multinodular goiter.

(7) TSH hypersecretion by the pituitary may be caused by a tumor and is a rare cause of hyperthyroidism. Serum TSH is elevated or normal (determined by a sensitive TSH assay) in the presence of true thyrotoxicosis. No ophthalmopathy is present. Antithyroid antibodies and TSH-R Ab [stim] are usually normal. TSH hypersecretion may be caused by a pituitary adenoma, in which case it is known as "neoplastic inappropriate secretion of thyrotropin." The tumor may present as a mass lesion following treatment of hyperthyroidism. The pituitary adenoma is usually removed by transsphenoidal surgery; larger tumors may require radiation therapy. Tumors may sometimes respond to bromocriptine or octreotide. Hyperthyroidism is treated symptomatically with propranolol.

This condition may also be due to pituitary hyperplasia, in which case it is known as "nonneoplastic inappropriate secretion of thyrotropin." Pituitary hyperplasia may be detected on MRI scan as pituitary enlargement without a discrete adenoma being visible. This condition appears to be due to a diminished feedback effect of T_4 upon the pituitary. It may be familial, but it can also be caused by prolonged untreated hypothyroidism, especially in youth. Hyperthyroid symptoms are treated with propranolol. Definitive treatment is with radioactive iodine or thyroid surgery.

(8) Hashimoto's thyroiditis may cause transient hyperthyroidism during the initial destructive phase. It may occur transiently postpartum. This is also seen in some patients receiving interferon-alfa, interferon-beta, and interleukin-2.

(9) Pregnancy and trophoblastic tumors–Although hCG generally has a low affinity for the thyroid's TSH receptors, very high serum levels of hCG may cause sufficient receptor activation to cause thyrotoxicosis. Mild gestational hyperthyroidism may occur during the first 4 months of pregnancy, when hCG levels are very high. Pregnant women are more likely to have thyrotoxicosis and hyperemesis gravidarum if they have high serum levels of sialo-hCG, a subfraction of hCG with greater affinity for TSH receptors.

Thyrotoxicosis may also be caused by the high serum levels of hCG seen in molar pregnancy, choriocarcinoma, and testicular malignancies.

(10) Metastatic functioning thyroid carcinoma is a rare cause of thyrotoxicosis.

(11) Amiodarone, used for chronic treatment of cardiac arrhythmias, causes symptomatic hyperthyroidism in about 2.5% of patients. Since high levels of T_4 and free T_4 are normally seen in patients taking amiodarone, suppressed TSH (sensitive assay) must be present along with a greatly elevated T_4 (> 20 μg/dL) or T_3 (> 200 ng/dL). Treatment involves withdrawing the drug, if possible, but hyperthyroidism is slow to resolve. Patients in atrial fibrillation usually require anticoagulation with warfarin; close monitoring of the INR is required, since both methimazole and hyperthyroidism potentiate the hypoprothrombinemia of anticoagulants. Hyperthyroidism increases the catabolism of vitamin K-dependent clotting factors, and methimazole potentiates anti-vitamin K activity. Changing thyroid levels also modify the coagulation profile. Propranolol provides symptomatic relief. Methimazole, 40–60 mg/d initially, is given orally, and serum free T_4 and TSH levels are monitored regularly; the dosage is reduced to 10 mg/d once the free T_4 is normal or TSH is elevated. If TSH remains elevated, thyroxine is added carefully. Methimazole may require months to produce euthyroidism; therefore, after 2 days of methimazole, ipodate sodium or iopanoic acid, 500 mg/d orally, is added to block peripheral conversion of T_4 to T_3. Thyroidectomy is necessary in some patients. Radioactive iodine treatment is possible in some patients whose radioiodine uptake is adequate.

Clinical Findings

A. Symptoms and Signs: Thyrotoxicosis due to any cause produces many different manifestations of variable intensity among different individuals. Patients may complain of nervousness, restlessness, heat intolerance, increased sweating, fatigue, weakness, muscle cramps, frequent bowel movements, or weight change (usually loss). There may be palpitations or angina pectoris. Women frequently report menstrual irregularities.

Hypokalemic periodic paralysis occurs in about 15% of Asian or Native American men with thyrotoxicosis. It usually presents abruptly with paralysis (and few thyrotoxic symptoms), often after intravenous dextrose, oral carbohydrate, or vigorous exercise. Attacks last 7–72 hours.

Signs of thyrotoxicosis may include stare and lid lag, tachycardia or atrial fibrillation, fine resting finger tremors, moist warm skin, hyperreflexia, fine hair, onycholysis, and (rarely) heart failure. Chronic thyrotoxicosis may cause osteoporosis. At times there may be clubbing and swelling of the fingers (acropachy). Graves' disease usually presents with additional findings of goiter (often with a bruit).

Ophthalmopathy is clinically apparent in 20–40% of patients with Graves' disease and usually consists of chemosis, conjunctivitis, and mild proptosis. More severe lymphocytic infiltration of the eye muscles occurs in 5–10% and may produce exophthalmos and sometimes diplopia due to extraocular muscle entrapment. The optic nerve may be compressed in severe cases. Corneal drying may occur with inadequate lid closure. Eye changes may sometimes be asymmetric or unilateral. The severity of the eye disease is not closely correlated with the severity of the thyrotoxicosis. Some patients with Graves' ophthalmopathy are clinically euthyroid.

Diplopia can also be caused by coexistent ocular **myasthenia gravis,** which is more common in Graves' disease and is usually mild, often with selective eye involvement. Acetylcholinesterase receptor antibody (AchRAb) levels are elevated in only 36% of such patients, and a thymoma is present in 9%.

Skin "myxedema" occurs in about 3% of Graves' disease patients, usually in the pretibial region. Its texture resembles the skin of an orange.

B. Laboratory Diagnosis: Serum T_3, T_4, thyroid resin uptake, and free thyroxine are usually all increased. Sometimes the T_4 level may be normal but the serum T_3 is elevated. A reliable sensitive TSH assay is the best test for thyrotoxicosis; it is suppressed except in the very rare cases of pituitary inappropriate secretion of thyrotropin. Other laboratory abnormalities may include hypercalcemia, increased alkaline phosphatase, anemia, and decreased granulocytes.

TSH receptor antibody (TSH-R Ab [stim]) levels are usually high (80%), but TSH-R Ab [stim] measurement is not ordinarily required for diagnosis. Antithyroglobulin or antimicrosomal antibodies are usually elevated in Graves' disease. Serum ANA and anti-double-stranded DNA antibodies are also usually elevated without any evidence of lupus erythematosus or other collagen-vascular disease.

Patients with subacute thyroiditis often have an increased erythrocyte sedimentation rate.

Thyroid radioactive iodine uptake and scan is usually performed on patients with an established diagnosis of thyrotoxicosis. A high radioactive iodine uptake is seen in Graves' disease and toxic nodular goiter but can be seen in other conditions as well. A low radioactive iodine uptake is characteristic of subacute thyroiditis but can also be seen in other conditions. (For conditions affecting radioactive iodine uptake, see section on tests of thyroid function.)

C. Imaging: MRI of the orbits is the imaging method of choice to visualize Graves' ophthalmopathy affecting the extraocular muscles. CT scanning and ultrasound can also be used. Imaging is required only in severe cases or in euthyroid exophthalmos that must be distinguished from orbital tumors or other disorders.

Differential Diagnosis

True thyrotoxicosis must be distinguished from those conditions elevating serum thyroxine without affecting clinical status (Table 26–5).

Hyperthyroidism may be confused with anxiety neurosis or mania, but in the latter the thyroid is not enlarged and thyroid function tests are usually normal. Problems of diagnosis occur in patients with acute psychiatric disorders, about 30% of whom have hyperthyroxinemia without thyrotoxicosis. The TSH is not suppressed, distinguishing psychiatric disorder from true hyperthyroidism. T_4 levels return to normal gradually.

Exogenous thyroid administration will present the same laboratory features as thyroiditis. A rare pituitary tumor may produce the picture of thyrotoxicosis with high levels of TSH.

Some states of hypermetabolism without thyrotoxicosis—notably severe anemia, leukemia, polycythemia, and cancer—rarely cause confusion. Pheochromocytoma is often associated with hypermetabolism, tachycardia, weight loss, and profuse sweating. Acromegaly may also produce tachycardia, sweating, and thyroid enlargement. Appropriate laboratory tests will easily distinguish these entities.

Cardiac disease (eg, atrial fibrillation, angina) refractory to treatment suggests the possibility of underlying ("apathetic") hyperthyroidism. Other causes of ophthalmoplegia (eg, myasthenia gravis) and exophthalmos (eg, orbital tumor, pseudotumor) must be considered. Thyrotoxicosis must also be considered in the differential diagnosis of muscle weakness and osteoporosis. Diabetes mellitus and Addison's disease may coexist with thyrotoxicosis.

Complications

Cardiac complications of thyrotoxicosis include atrial fibrillation with a ventricular response that is difficult to control. Episodes of periodic paralysis induced by exercise or heavy carbohydrate ingestion and accompanied by hypokalemia may complicate thyrotoxicosis in Asian or Native American men. Hypercalcemia, osteoporosis, and nephrocalcinosis may occur. Decreased libido, impotence, decreased sperm count, and gynecomastia may be noted in men with hyperthyroidism.

Patients who have "subclinical hyperthyroidism" (suppressed TSH but normal free T_4 and clinically euthyroid) generally do well without treatment. No accelerated bone loss has been noted.

Treatment

The methods used to treat thyrotoxicosis will vary according to the cause and severity of the hyperthyroidism, the patient's age, the clinical situation, and the desires of the patient.

A. Graves' Disease: The treatment of Graves' disease involves a choice of methods rather than a method of choice:

1. Propranolol–Propranolol is generally used for symptomatic relief until the hyperthyroidism is resolved. It effectively relieves the tachycardia, tremor, diaphoresis, and anxiety that occur with hyperthyroidism due to any cause. It is the initial treatment of choice for thyroid storm. The periodic paralysis seen in association with thyrotoxicosis is also effectively treated with beta blockade. It has no effect on thyroid hormone secretion. Treatment is usually begun with 10 mg orally and increased progressively until an adequate response is achieved, usually 20 mg four times daily. Doses as high as 80 mg four times daily are occasionally required. Propranolol is available in a long-acting formulation that provides more consistent relief.

2. Thiourea drugs–Methimazole or propylthiouracil is generally used for young adults or patients with mild thyrotoxicosis, small goiters, or fear of isotopes. Aged patients usually respond particularly well. These drugs are also useful for preparing hyperthyroid patients for surgery and elderly patients for radioactive iodide treatment. The drugs do not permanently damage the thyroid and are associated with a lower chance of posttreatment hypothyroidism (compared with radioactive iodide or surgery). Unfortunately, there is a high rate of recurrent hyperthyroidism (about 50%) after a year or more of therapy. A greater likelihood of long-term remission is seen in patients with small goiters or mild hyperthyroidism. Patients whose thyroperoxidase and thyroglobulin antibodies remain high after 2 years of therapy have been reported to have only a 10% rate of relapse.

Agranulocytosis is an uncommon but serious complication of thiourea therapy, being reported in about 0.1% of patients taking methimazole and about 0.4% of patients taking propylthiouracil. Patients are warned that if they develop a sore throat or febrile illness, they should stop the drug while a white blood count is rechecked. The agranulocytosis is generally reversible and may be treated with filgrastim (G-CSF). Periodic surveillance of the white blood count during treatment has been advocated by some clinicians, but onset is generally abrupt.

Other side effects common to thiourea drugs include pruritus, allergic dermatitis, nausea, and dyspepsia. Antihistamines may control mild pruritus without discontinuation of the drug. Since the two thiourea drugs are similar patients who have had a major allergic reaction from one should not be given the other.

Primary hypothyroidism may occur. The patient may become clinically hypothyroid for 2 weeks or more before TSH levels rise, having been suppressed by the preceding hyperthyroidism. Therefore, the patient's changing thyroid status is best followed clinically and with serum levels of free thyroxine. Rapid growth of the goiter usually occurs if the patient is allowed to develop prolonged hypothyroidism; the goiter may sometimes become massive but usually regresses rapidly with thyroid hormone replacement.

a. Methimazole–Methimazole has the advantage of requiring less frequent dosing and fewer pills than propylthiouracil, making treatment more convenient. It is also associated with a lower incidence of acute hepatic necrosis. Rare complications peculiar to methimazole include serum sickness, cholestatic jaundice, loss of taste, alopecia, nephrotic syndrome, and hypoglycemia. Methimazole is given orally in initial doses of 30–60 mg once daily. The dosage is usually reduced as manifestations of hyperthyroidism resolve and as the free thyroxine level becomes normal.

b. Propylthiouracil–Propylthiouracil has been considered the drug of choice during breast feeding or pregnancy, possibly causing fewer problems in the newborn. It blocks the peripheral conversion of T_4 to T_3 and is of some theoretic advantage over methimazole in thyroid storm, but this effect has not been demonstrated to be clinically significant. Rare complications peculiar to propylthiouracil include arthritis, lupus erythematosus, aplastic anemia, thrombocytopenia, and hypoprothrombinemia. Acute hepatitis occurs rarely and is treated with prednisone but may progress to liver failure. Propylthiouracil is given orally in initial doses of 300–600 mg daily in four divided doses. The dosage and frequency of administration are generally reduced as symptoms of hyperthyroidism resolve and the free thyroxine level becomes normal. During pregnancy, the dose is kept below 200 mg/d in order to avoid goitrous hypothyroidism in the infant.

3. Iodinated contrast agents–These agents provide effective treatment for thyrotoxicosis of any cause. Iopanoic acid (Telepaque) or ipodate sodium (Bilivist, Oragrafin) is given orally in a dosage of 500 mg twice daily. Within 24 hours, serum T_3 levels fall an average of 62%. For patients with Graves' disease, methimazole is begun first in order to block iodine organification; the next day, ipodate sodium or iopanoic acid may be added. The iodinated contrast agents are particularly useful for patients who are very symptomatically thyrotoxic (see Thyroid Storm, below). They offer a therapeutic option for patients intolerant to thioureas and for newborns with thyrotoxicosis (due to maternal Graves' disease). Treatment periods of 8 months or more are possible, but efficacy tends to wane with time. Thyroid radioiodine uptake may be suppressed during treatment but returns to pretreatment uptake by 7 days after discontinuation of the drug, allowing ^{131}I treatment.

4. Radioactive iodine (^{131}I)–The administration of radioiodine is an excellent method of destroying overactive thyroid tissue (either diffuse or toxic nodular goiter). The radioiodine damages the cells that concentrate it. Patients have no apparent risk of subsequent thyroid cancer, leukemia, or other malignancies. Children born to parents previously treated with ^{131}I show normal rates of congenital abnormalities.

Since fetal radiation is harmful, *radioactive iodine should not be given to pregnant women.* It is prudent to obtain a sensitive pregnancy test (serum β-hCG) on all women of reproductive age prior to ^{131}I therapy.

Most patients may receive radioiodine while being symptomatically treated with just propranolol, which is then reduced in dosage as hyperthyroxinemia resolves. However, some patients (those with coronary diseases, the elderly, or those with severe hyperthyroidism) are usually rendered euthyroid with a thiouracil drug (see above) while the dosage of propranolol is reduced. Since pretreatment with propylthiouracil causes the risk of ^{131}I treatment failure to increase from 3% (without pretreatment) to 23%, the thiourea is stopped for 2 weeks (if possible) before ^{131}I treatment and a somewhat higher dose of ^{131}I is administered.

Following ^{131}I treatment for hyperthyroidism, Graves' ophthalmopathy appears or worsens in 15% and improves in none, whereas during treatment with methimazole, ophthalmopathy worsens in 3% and improves in 2%. Among patients receiving 3 months of prednisone following ^{131}I treatment, preexistent ophthalmopathy worsens in none and improves in 67%.

Smoking increases the risk of having a flare in ophthalmopathy following ^{131}I treatment and also reduces the effectiveness of prednisone treatment. Therefore, patients who smoke are strongly encouraged to quit prior to ^{131}I treatment.

Free T_4 levels may sometimes drop within 2 months after starting ^{131}I treatment but then rise again to thyrotoxic levels, at which time thyroid radioiodine uptake is low. This phenomenon is caused by a release of stored thyroid hormone from injured thyroid cells and does not indicate a treatment failure. In fact, serum free T_4 then falls abruptly to hypothyroid levels.

There is a high incidence of hypothyroidism several years after ^{131}I even when small doses are given. However, hypothyroidism also occurs quite frequently years after surgical or medical treatment of Graves' disease, and eventual hypothyroidism may be part of the natural history of this condition. Lifelong clinical follow-up is mandatory, with measurements of free T_4 and TSH when indicated.

5. Thyroid surgery–Thyroid surgery for Graves' disease and toxic nodular goiter has been performed less frequently as radioiodine treatment has become more widely accepted. Surgery is usually preferred for pregnant women whose thyrotoxicosis is not controlled with low doses of thioureas, for patients with particularly large goiters, and whenever there is a significant chance of malignancy.

Patients are ordinarily rendered euthyroid with a thiourea drug or ipodate preoperatively. Propranolol is given until the T_3 is normal preoperatively. Thyroid vascularity is reduced by preoperative treatment with either ipodate sodium or iopanoic acid (500 mg twice daily for 3 days) or iodine (eg, Lugol's solution, 2 or 3 drops orally daily for several days). If a patient undergoes surgery while thyrotoxic, larger doses of propranolol are given perioperatively to reduce the likelihood of thyroid crisis.

Morbidity includes possible damage to the recurrent laryngeal nerve that causes vocal cord paralysis. Hypoparathyroidism also occurs, which means that calcium levels must be checked postoperatively. These complications are unusual (< 1%) when the surgery is performed by a competent, experienced neck surgeon. Thyroid surgery should be performed as an inpatient, with at least an overnight observational period.

B. Toxic Solitary Thyroid Nodules: Hyperthyroidism caused by a single hyperfunctioning thyroid nodule may be treated symptomatically with propranolol as in Graves' disease. Definitive treatment is with surgery or radioactive iodine. For patients under age 40, surgery is usually recommended;

patients are made euthyroid with a thiourea preoperatively and given several days of iodine, ipodate sodium, or iopanoic acid before surgery as in Graves' disease (see above). Transient postoperative hypothyroidism resolves spontaneously. Permanent hypothyroidism occurs in about 14% of patients by 6 years after surgery. Patients over age 40 with a toxic solitary nodule are offered radioactive iodine. Permanent hypothyroidism occurs in about one-third of patients by 8 years after radioactive iodine. The nodule remains palpable in half and may grow in 10% of patients after radioactive iodine.

C. Toxic Multinodular Goiter: Hyperthyroidism caused by a toxic multinodular goiter may also be treated symptomatically with propranolol as in Graves' disease. This disorder usually affects older individuals, so radioactive iodine is ordinarily selected over surgery as definitive treatment. Thioureas do reverse hyperthyroidism, but there is a 95% recurrence rate after they are stopped. Older patients who are quite thyrotoxic are rendered nearly euthyroid with methimazole, which is stopped at least 3 days before radioactive iodine treatment. Meanwhile, the patient follows a low-iodine diet; this is done to enhance the thyroid gland's uptake of radioactive iodine, which may be relatively low in this condition (compared to Graves' disease). Relatively high doses of radioactive iodine are usually required; recurrent thyrotoxicosis and hypothyroidism are common, so patients must be followed closely. Surgery is generally reserved for pressure symptoms or cosmetic indications. Patients are prepared for surgery as in Graves' disease (see above).

D. Subacute Thyroiditis: Patients with hyperthyroidism due to subacute thyroiditis are treated symptomatically with propranolol. Ipodate sodium or iopanoic acid, 500 mg orally daily, promptly corrects elevated T_3 levels and is continued for 15–60 days until the serum FT_4 level normalizes. The condition subsides spontaneously within weeks to months. Thioureas are ineffective, since thyroid hormone production is actually low in this condition. Radioactive iodine is ineffective, since the thyroid's iodine uptake is low. Since periods of hypothyroidism may occur following the initial inflammatory episode, patients should have close clinical follow-up, with serum free thyroxine measurement when necessary. Prompt treatment of the transient hypothyroidism may reduce the incidence of recurrent thyroiditis. Pain can usually be managed with aspirin or other nonsteroidal anti-inflammatory agents.

E. Hashimoto's Thyroiditis: Rarely, patients develop hyperthyroidism as a result of release of stored thyroid hormone during severe Hashimoto's thyroiditis. The thyroperoxidase or thyroglobulin antibodies are usually high, but radioiodine uptake is low, thus distinguishing it from Graves' disease. This is especially common in postpartum women, in whom it may be transient. Treatment is with propranolol. Patients are followed carefully for the development of hypothyroidism and treated according to their thyroid status.

F. Treatment of Complications:

1. Graves' ophthalmopathy–The risk of having a "flare" of ophthalmopathy following ^{131}I treatment for hyperthyroidism is about 6% for nonsmokers and 23% for smokers. For progressive exophthalmos, prednisone must be given promptly in doses of 40–60 mg/d, with dosage reduction over several weeks. Higher initial prednisone doses of 80–120 mg/d are used when there is optic nerve compression. Prednisone alleviates eye symptoms in 64% of nonsmokers, but only 14% of smokers respond well. Another treatment is low-dose radiation therapy (cumulative dose 20 Gy to each orbit over 2 weeks) to the extraocular muscles, avoiding the cornea and lens. Intravenous immune globulin (IGIV) is reportedly comparable to prednisone in effectiveness in doses of 1 g/kg for 2 consecutive days and repeated every 3 weeks for 3–4 months. For severe cases, orbital decompression surgery may save vision, though diplopia often persists postoperatively. General eye protective measures include wearing glasses to protect the protruding eye and taping the lids shut during sleep if corneal drying is a problem. Methylcellulose drops and gels ("artificial tears") may also help. Tarsorrhaphy or canthoplasty can frequently help protect the cornea and provide improved appearance. Hypothyroidism and hyperthyroidism must be treated promptly.

2. Cardiac complications–

a. Sinus tachycardia or heart pounding is usually present in thyrotoxicosis. Treatment consists of treating the thyrotoxicosis. A beta-blocker (as described above) such as propranolol is used in the interim unless there is an associated cardiomyopathy.

b. Atrial fibrillation is commonly seen in thyrotoxicosis and may be the presenting manifestation. Electrical cardioversion is unlikely to convert atrial fibrillation to normal sinus rhythm while the patient is thyrotoxic. Spontaneous conversion to normal sinus rhythm tends to occur with achievement of euthyroidism, but that likelihood decreases with age. Hyperthyroidism must be treated (see above). Other drugs may be required:

(1) Digoxin is used to slow a fast ventricular response to thyrotoxic atrial fibrillation; it must be used in larger than normal doses because of increased clearance and an increased number of cardiac sodium transport units requiring inhibition. Digoxin doses are reduced as hyperthyroidism is corrected.

(2) Beta-blockers may also reduce the ventricular rate, but they must be used with caution—particularly in patients with cardiomegaly or signs of heart failure—since their negative inotropic effect may precipitate congestive heart failure. Therefore, an initial trial of a short-duration beta-blocker should be considered, such as esmolol intravenously. If a beta-blocker is used, doses of digoxin must be reduced.

(3) Anticoagulation is indicated to prevent arterial thromboembolism in thyrotoxicosis-induced atrial fibrillation in the following situations: left atrial enlargement on echocardiogram, global left ventricular dysfunction, recent congestive heart failure, hypertension, recurrent atrial fibrillation, or a history of previous thromboembolism. The doses of warfarin required in thyrotoxicosis are smaller than normal because of an accelerated plasma clearance of vitamin K-dependent clotting factors. Higher warfarin doses are usually required as hyperthyroidism subsides.

c. Heart failure due to thyrotoxicosis may be caused by extreme tachycardia, cardiomyopathy, or both. Very aggressive treatment of the hyperthyroidism is required in either case (see Thyroid Crisis, below). The tachycardia from atrial fibrillation is treated with digoxin as above. Intravenous furosemide is typically required. If tachycardia appears to be the main cause of the failure, beta-blockers are administered cautiously as described above.

Thyrotoxic dilated cardiomyopathy is caused by a direct toxic effect of prolonged excess thyroid hormone upon the heart and may occur at any age. Beta-blockers and calcium channel blockers are avoided. Emergency treatment may include afterload reduction, diuretics, digoxin, and other inotropic agents while the patient is being rendered euthyroid.

d. Apathetic hyperthyroidism may present with angina pectoris. Treatment is directed at reversing the hyperthyroidism as well as providing standard antianginal therapy. Coronary angioplasty or bypass grafting can often be avoided by prompt diagnosis and treatment.

3. Thyroid crisis or "storm"–This disorder, rarely seen today, is an extreme form of thyrotoxicosis that may occur with stressful illness, thyroid surgery, or radioactive iodine administration and is manifested by marked delirium, severe tachycardia, vomiting, diarrhea, dehydration, and, in many cases, very high fever. The mortality rate is high.

A thiourea drug is given (eg, propylthiouracil, 150–250 mg every 6 hours; or methimazole, 15–25 mg every 6 hours). Iodide is given 1 hour later as Lugol's solution (10 drops three times daily orally) or as sodium iodide (1 g intravenously slowly). Ipodate sodium (500 mg/d orally) can be helpful if begun 1 hour after the first dose of thiourea. Propranolol is given (cautiously in the presence of heart failure; see above) in a dosage of 0.5–2 mg intravenously every 4 hours or 20–120 mg orally every 6 hours. Hydrocortisone is usually given in doses of 50 mg every 6 hours, with rapid dosage reduction as the clinical situation improves. Aspirin is avoided since it displaces T_4 from thyroid-binding globulin, raising free T_4 serum levels. Definitive treatment with ^{131}I or surgery is delayed until the patient is euthyroid.

4. Hyperthyroidism and pregnancy–The prevalence of hyperthyroidism in pregnancy—most commonly due to Graves' disease—is about 0.2%. Struma ovarii is rare. Diagnosis may be difficult, since normal pregnancy may be accompanied by tachycardia, warm skin, heat intolerance, increased sweating, and a palpable thyroid. Laboratory tests are helpful: The free T_4 is clearly elevated, while the TSH is suppressed. However, apparent lack of full TSH suppression can be seen due to misidentification of hCG as TSH in certain assays. Although the total T_4 is elevated in most pregnant women, values over 20 μg/dL are encountered only in hyperthyroidism. The T_3 resin uptake, which is low in normal pregnancy because of high TBG concentration, is normal or high in thyrotoxic subjects. Pregnancy can have a beneficial effect upon the thyrotoxicosis of Graves' disease, with decreasing antibody titers and decreasing free T_4 levels as the pregnancy advances. However, there is an increased risk of thyroid storm, preeclampsia-eclampsia, congestive heart failure, premature delivery, and abruptio placentae. Newborns have an increased risk of intrauterine growth retardation, prematurity, and transient thyrotoxicosis from transplacental transfer of TSH-R Ab [stim]. Pregnant women with hyperthyroidism are treated with methimazole or propylthiouracil in the smallest dose possible, permitting mild hyperthyroidism to occur since it is usually well tolerated. The drug does cross the placenta and rarely may induce TSH hypersecretion and fetal goiter. Thyroid hormone administration to the mother does not prevent hypothyroidism in the fetus, since T_4 and T_3 do not freely cross the placenta. Fetal hypothyroidism is rare if the mother's hyperthyroidism is controlled with small daily doses of propylthiouracil (50–150 mg/d) or methimazole (5–15 mg/d). Thyroidectomy is reserved for women who are allergic or resistant to antithyroid drugs (usually due to noncompliance) or who have very large goiters.

Only minimal amounts of propylthiouracil are transferred to the maternal milk, so breast feeding is apt to be safe. This is less true for methimazole, which appears in higher concentrations in the milk.

5. Dermopathy–An uncommon complication of Graves' disease, dermopathy is an abnormal thickening of the skin due to deposition of glycosaminoglycans. It is known as "pretibial myxedema" since it usually occurs in the anterior lower leg, sometimes also including the dorsum of the foot. Treatment involves application of a topical glucocorticoid (eg, fluocinolone) with nocturnal plastic occlusive dressings.

Prognosis

Graves' disease may rarely subside spontaneously and may even result in spontaneous hypothyroidism. However, it usually progresses. The ocular, cardiac, and psychologic complications often are more serious than the chronic wasting of tissues and may become irreversible even after treatment. Permanent hypoparathyroidism and vocal cord palsy are risks of surgical thyroidectomy. Recurrences are common following thiourea therapy but also occur after low-dose ^{131}I therapy or subtotal thyroidectomy. With adequate treatment and long-term follow-up, the results are usually good. However, despite treatment for their hyperthyroidism, women experience an increased long-term risk of death from thyroid disease, cardiovascular disease, stroke, and fracture of the femur. Posttreatment hypothyroidism is common. It may occur within a few months or up to several years after radioactive iodine therapy or subtotal thyroidectomy. Malignant exophthalmos has a poor prognosis unless treated aggressively.

Bartalena L et al: Cigarette smoking and treatment outcomes in Graves ophthalmopathy. Ann Intern Med 1998;129:632. [NLM Cit ID: 98442933] (Smokers with thyroid-associated ophthalmopathy are more likely to have a flare in eye disease after ^{131}I treatment for hyperthyroidism and are less likely to respond to prednisone.)

Bauer DC et al: Low thyrotropin levels are not associated with bone loss in older women: A prospective study. J Clin Endocrinol Metab 1997;82:2931. [NLM Cit ID: 97430615]

Kannan CR et al: Thyrotoxicosis. Dis Mon 1997 Sep;43:601. [NLM Cit ID: 97447194]

Tomaske SM et al: Sodium ipodate (Cragrafin) in the preoperative preparation of Graves' hyperthyroidism. Laryngoscope 1997;107:1066. [NLM Cit ID: 97405966]

Turton DB et al: Time interval between the last dose of propylthiouracil and I-131 therapy influences cure rates in hyperthyroidism caused by Graves' disease. Clin Nucl Med 1998;23:810. [NLM Cit ID: 99074002]

THYROIDITIS

Essentials of Diagnosis

- Swelling of thyroid gland, often causing pressure symptoms in acute and subacute forms; painless enlargement in chronic form.
- Thyroid function tests variable.
- Serum antithyroid antibody tests often positive.

General Considerations

Thyroiditis may be classified as follows: (1) chronic lymphocytic ("Hashimoto's") thyroiditis due to autoimmunity, (2) subacute thyroiditis, (3) suppurative thyroiditis, and (4) Riedel's thyroiditis.

Clinical Findings

A. Symptoms and Signs:

1. Hashimoto's thyroiditis–Hashimoto's thyroiditis—also called chronic lymphocytic thyroiditis—is the most common form of thyroiditis and probably the most common thyroid disorder in the USA. It tends to be familial and is six times more common in women than in men. Its frequency is increased by dietary iodine supplementation. Certain drugs (amiodarone, alpha interferon, interleukin-2, granulocyte-colony stimulating factor) frequently induce thyroid autoantibodies.

The thyroid gland is usually diffusely enlarged, firm, and finely nodular. One thyroid lobe may be asymmetrically enlarged, raising concerns about neoplasm. Although patients may complain of neck tightness, pain and tenderness are not usually present. About 10% of cases are atrophic, the gland being fibrotic, particularly in elderly women.

Thyroiditis often progresses to hypothyroidism, which is usually permanent, remitting in fewer than 5% of cases. Uncommonly, thyroiditis causes acute destruction of thyroid tissue and release of stored thyroid hormone, causing thyrotoxicosis. Rarely, a hypofunctioning gland may become hyperfunctioning with the onset of coexistent Graves' disease.

Systemic manifestations of Hashimoto's thyroiditis are mostly related to ambient levels of thyroid hormone. However, depression and chronic fatigue are more common in such patients, even after correction of hypothyroidism. About one-third of patients with Hashimoto's thyroiditis have mild dry mouth (xerostomia) or dry eyes (keratoconjunctivitis sicca) of an autoimmune nature related to Sjögren's syndrome. It may be associated with myasthenia gravis, which is usually of mild severity, mainly affecting the extraocular muscles and having a relatively low incidence of detectable acetylcholinesterase receptor antibodies or thymic disease.

Hashimoto's thyroiditis is sometimes associated with adrenal insufficiency (Schmidt's syndrome) and other endocrine deficiencies as part of polyglandular autoimmunity. Thyroiditis is also more common in patients with other autoimmune conditions, such as inflammatory bowel disease, or celiac disease (10%). Women with gonadal dysgenesis (Turner's syndrome) have a 15% incidence of significant thyroid dysfunction by age 40 years. Thyroiditis is also commonly seen in patients with hepatitis C and during treatment with amiodarone or cytokines (eg, interferon-alfa, interferon-beta, interleukin-2).

Patients with clinically evident disease usually have increased circulating levels of antithyroid peroxidase (95%) or antithyroglobulin (60%) antibodies.

Subclinical thyroiditis is very common, and in autopsy series about 40% of women and 20% of men exhibit focal thyroiditis. Low serum titers of antithyroid antibodies are found in 13% of women and 3% of men. However, only 1% of the population has antibody titers greater than 1:6400.

Postpartum thyroiditis is a form of autoimmune thyroiditis occurring soon after parturition and accompanied by transient hyperthyroidism followed by hypothyroidism; recovery of normal function occurs in most cases.

2. Subacute thyroiditis–This fairly common disorder—also called de Quervain's thyroiditis, granulomatous thyroiditis, and giant cell thyroiditis—is an acute, usually painful enlargement of the thyroid gland, with dysphagia. The pain may radiate to the ears. If there is no pain, it is called "silent thyroiditis." The manifestations may persist for weeks or months and may be associated with signs of thyrotoxicosis and malaise. Young and middle-aged women are most commonly affected. Viral infection has been suggested as the cause. The erythrocyte sedimentation rate is markedly elevated, and antithyroid antibodies are low, which helps differentiate this form of thyroiditis from others. Radioactive iodine uptake is low, distinguishing this disorder from Graves' disease. Aspiration biopsy is usually not required but shows characteristic giant multinucleated cells.

3. Suppurative thyroiditis–Suppurative thyroiditis is a rare disorder causing severe pain, tenderness, redness, and fluctuation in the region of the thyroid gland. It is caused by pyogenic organisms, usually in the course of systemic infection.

4. Riedel's thyroiditis–Riedel's thyroiditis is also called invasive fibrous thyroiditis, Riedel's struma, woody thyroiditis, ligneous thyroiditis, and invasive thyroiditis. It usually causes hypothyroidism and may cause hypoparathyroidism as well. It is the rarest form of thyroiditis and is found most frequently in middle-aged or elderly women. Enlargement is often asymmetric; the gland is stony hard and adherent to the neck structures, causing signs of compression and invasion, including dysphagia, dyspnea, pain, and hoarseness. It is usually a manifestation of a multifocal systemic fibrosis syndrome, with anterior neck symptoms predominating. Related conditions include retroperitoneal fibrosis, fibrosing mediastinitis, sclerosing cervicitis, subretinal fibrosis, and biliary tract sclerosis. It responds to therapy with tamoxifen (see Treatment, below).

B. Laboratory Findings: The T_4 and T_3 resin uptake are usually markedly elevated in acute and subacute thyroiditis and normal or low in the chronic forms. Radioiodine uptake is characteristically very low in the initial, hyperthyroid phase of subacute thyroiditis; it may be high with an uneven scan in chronic thyroiditis, with enlargement of the gland, and low in Riedel's struma. Thyroid autoantibodies are most commonly demonstrable in Hashimoto's thyroiditis but are also found in the other types. The serum TSH level is elevated if thyroid hormone is not elaborated in adequate amounts by the thyroid gland.

Complications

In the suppurative forms of thyroiditis, any of the complications of infection may occur; the subacute and chronic forms of the disease are complicated by the effects of pressure on the neck structures: dyspnea and, in Riedel's struma, vocal cord palsy. Hashimoto's thyroiditis may lead to hypothyroidism or transient thyrotoxicosis. Graves' disease may sometimes develop. Carcinoma or lymphoma may be associated with chronic thyroiditis and must be considered in the diagnosis of uneven painless enlargements that continue in spite of treatment. Hashimoto's thyroiditis may be associated with Addison's disease, hypoparathyroidism, diabetes, pernicious anemia, biliary cirrhosis, vitiligo, and other autoimmune conditions.

Differential Diagnosis

Thyroiditis must be considered in the differential diagnosis of all types of goiters, especially if enlargement is rapid. The very low radioiodine uptake in subacute thyroiditis with elevated T_4 and T_3 are helpful. Chronic thyroiditis, especially if the enlargement is uneven and if there is pressure on surrounding structures, may resemble carcinoma, and both disorders may be present in the same gland. The subacute and suppurative forms of thyroiditis may resemble any infectious process in or near the neck structures. Thyroid autoantibody tests have been of help in the diagnosis of chronic lymphocytic (Hashimoto's) thyroiditis, but the tests are not specific and may also be positive in patients with goiters, carcinoma, and thyrotoxicosis—though the titers are usually higher in Hashimoto's thyroiditis. Biopsy may be required for diagnosis.

Treatment

A. Suppurative Thyroiditis: Treatment is with antibiotics and with surgical drainage when fluctuation is marked.

B. Subacute Thyroiditis: All treatment is empirical and must be continued for several weeks. Recurrence is common. The drug of choice is aspirin, which relieves pain and inflammation. Thyrotoxic symptoms are treated with propranolol, 10–40 mg every 6 hours. Transient hypothyroidism is treated with thyroxine (0.05–0.1 mg/d) if symptomatic.

C. Hashimoto's Thyroiditis: Levothyroxine should be given in the usual doses (0.05–0.2 mg daily) if hypothyroidism or large goiter is present. If the thyroid gland is only minimally enlarged and the patient is euthyroid (with normal TSH levels), regular observation is in order, since hypothyroidism may develop subsequently—often years later. (See Hypothyroidism section.)

D. Riedel's Struma: The treatment of choice for invasive fibrous thyroiditis, like that of its related conditions, is oral tamoxifen, which causes remarkable partial to complete remissions in most patients within 3–6 months. Tamoxifen treatment must be continued for years. Its mode of action appears to be unrelated to its antiestrogen activity. Short-term glucocorticoid treatment may be added for partial alleviation of pain and compression symptoms. Surgical decompression usually fails to permanently alleviate compression symptoms; such surgery is difficult due to dense fibrous adhesions, making surgical complications more likely.

Prognosis

The course of this group of diseases is quite variable. Spontaneous remissions and exacerbations are common in the subacute form, and therapy is nonspecific. The disease process may smolder for months. Hashimoto's thyroiditis is occasionally associated with other autoimmune disorders (diabetes mellitus, Addison's disease, pernicious anemia, etc). In general, however, patients with Hashimoto's thyroiditis have an excellent prognosis, since the condition either remains stable for years or progresses slowly to hypothyroidism, which is easily treated. Women with postpartum thyroiditis usually regain normal thyroid function.

Dayan CM et al: Chronic autoimmune thyroiditis. N Engl J Med 1996;335:99. [NLM Cit ID: 96266361]

Few J et al: Riedel's thyroiditis: treatment with tamoxifen. Surgery 1996;120:993. [NLM Cit ID: 97116397]

Mulder JE: Thyroid disease in women. Med Clin North Am 1998;82:103. [NLM Cit ID: 98118336]

Schuppert F et al: Patients treated with interferon-alpha, interferon-beta, and interleukin-2 have a different thyroid autoantibody pattern than patients suffering from endogenous autoimmune thyroid disease. Thyroid 1997;7:837. [NLM Cit ID: 98119713]

THE PARATHYROIDS

The main physiologic effects of parathyroid hormone are as follows: (1) It increases the osteoclastic activity in bone, with increased delivery of calcium and phosphorus to the circulation; (2) it increases the renal tubular reabsorption of calcium in the glomerular filtrate; (3) it inhibits the net absorption of phosphate and bicarbonate by the renal tubule; and (4) it stimulates the synthesis of 1,25-dihydroxycholecalciferol by the kidney. All of these steps result in a net increase in the amount of serum ionized calcium. Serum calcium is largely bound to albumin. Therefore, ionized calcium should be determined, or the serum calcium level should be corrected for serum albumin level as follows:

$$\text{"Corrected" serum } Ca^{2+} = \text{Serum } Ca^{2+} \text{ mg/dL} - (0.8 \times [4.0 - \text{Albumin g/dL}])$$

HYPOPARATHYROIDISM & PSEUDOHYPOPARATHYROIDISM

Essentials of Diagnosis

- Tetany, carpopedal spasms, tingling of lips and hands, muscle and abdominal cramps, psychologic changes.
- Positive Chvostek's sign and Trousseau's phenomenon; defective nails and teeth; cataracts.
- Serum calcium low; serum phosphate high; alkaline phosphatase normal; urine calcium excretion reduced.
- Serum magnesium may be low.

General Considerations

Hypoparathyroidism is most commonly seen following thyroidectomy, when it is usually transient but may be permanent. It may also occur after surgical removal of a parathyroid adenoma for primary hyperparathyroidism due to suppression of the remaining normal parathyroids and accelerated remineralization of the skeleton (hungry bone syndrome).

Hypoparathyroidism may be autoimmune (rarely) and occur sporadically or as part of polyglandular autoimmune syndrome (PGA type 1). This is also known as autoimmune polyendocrinopathy-candidiasis-ectodermal dystrophy (APECED). PGA type 1 presents in childhood with at least two of the following: candidiasis, hypoparathyroidism, or Addison's disease. Patients may also develop cataracts, uveitis, alopecia, vitiligo, or immune thyroid disease.

Parathyroid deficiency can also occur from dysembryogenesis (DiGeorge's syndrome) or as a result of damage from heavy metals (Wilson's disease, transfusion hemosiderosis, hemochromatosis), granulomas, metastatic tumors, or infection.

Functional hypoparathyroidism may also occur as a result of magnesium deficiency (malabsorption, chronic alcoholism), which prevents the secretion of PTH. Correction of hypomagnesemia results in rapid disappearance of the condition. Hypoparathyroidism may rarely occur after neck irradiation.

Pseudohypoparathyroidism is a group of diseases characterized by hypocalcemia due to renal resistance to parathyroid hormone. There are several subtypes caused by different mutations involving the parathyroid hormone receptor or its G protein or adenylyl cyclase. PTH levels are high and the PTH receptors in bone are typically not involved, such that bony changes of hyperparathyroidism may be evident. Various phenotypic abnormalities may be associated—classically, short stature, round face, obesity, short fourth metacarpals, ectopic bone formation, and mental retardation. Patients without hypocalcemia but sharing the phenotypic abnormalities are said to have "pseudopseudohypoparathyroidism."

Clinical Findings

A. Symptoms and Signs: Acute hypoparathyroidism causes tetany, with muscle cramps, irritability, carpopedal spasm, and convulsions; tingling of the circumoral area, hands, and feet is almost always present. Symptoms of the chronic disease are lethargy, personality changes, anxiety state, blurring of vision due to cataracts, and mental retardation.

Chvostek's sign (facial muscle contraction on tapping the facial nerve in front of the ear) is positive, and Trousseau's phenomenon (carpal spasm after application of a cuff) is present. Cataracts may occur; the nails may be thin and brittle; the skin is dry and scaly, at times with fungus infection (candidiasis), and there may be loss of hair (eyebrows); deep tendon reflexes may be hyperactive. Papilledema and elevated cerebrospinal fluid pressure are occasionally seen. Teeth may be defective if the onset of the disease occurs in childhood.

B. Laboratory Findings: Serum calcium is low, serum phosphate high, urinary calcium low, and alkaline phosphatase normal. Parathyroid hormone levels are low. Serum magnesium should be determined since hypomagnesemia frequently accompanies hypocalcemia and may exacerbate symptoms and decrease parathyroid function.

C. Imaging: Radiographs or CT scans of the skull may show basal ganglia calcifications; the bones may be denser than normal.

D. Other Examinations: Slitlamp examination may show early posterior lenticular cataract formation. The ECG shows prolonged QT intervals and T wave abnormalities.

Complications

Acute tetany with stridor, especially if associated with vocal cord palsy, may lead to respiratory obstruction requiring tracheostomy. The complications of chronic hypoparathyroidism depend largely upon the duration of the disease. There may be associated autoimmunity causing sprue syndrome, pernicious anemia, or Addison's disease. In long-standing cases, cataract formation and calcification of the basal ganglia are seen. Occasionally, parkinsonian symptoms or choreoathetosis develops. Ossification of the paravertebral ligaments may occur with nerve root compression; surgical decompression may be required. Seizures are common in untreated patients. Overtreatment with vitamin D and calcium may produce nephrocalcinosis and impairment of renal function.

Differential Diagnosis

The symptoms of hypocalcemic tetany may be confused with paresthesias, muscle cramps, or tetany due to respiratory alkalosis, in which the serum calcium is normal. In fact, hyperventilation tends to accentuate hypocalcemic symptoms. Chronic hypocalcemia can cause heart failure and be confused with myocardial infarction and ischemic cardiomyopathy.

At times hypoparathyroidism is misdiagnosed as idiopathic epilepsy, choreoathetosis, or brain tumor (on the basis of brain calcifications, convulsions, choked disks) or, more rarely, as "asthma" (on the basis of stridor and dyspnea). Hypocalcemia is frequently seen in patients with hypoalbuminemia; serum levels of ionized calcium are normal.

Hypocalcemia may also be due to malabsorption of calcium, magnesium, or vitamin D; patients do not always have diarrhea. It may also be caused by certain drugs such as loop diuretics, plicamycin, phenytoin, alendronate, and foscarnet. In addition, hypocalcemia may be seen in cases of rapid intravascular volume expansion or due to chelation from transfusions of large volumes of citrated blood. Hypocalcemia is also frequently seen following parathyroidectomy for hyperparathyroidism. It is also observed in patients with acute pancreatitis. Some patients with certain osteoblastic metastatic carcinomas (especially breast, prostate) may develop hypocalcemia instead of the expected hypercalcemia. Hypocalcemia with hyperphosphatemia (simulating hypoparathyroidism) is seen in azotemia but may also be caused by large doses of intravenous, oral, or rectal phosphate preparations and by chemotherapy of responsive lymphomas or leukemias.

Hypocalcemia with hypercalciuria may be due to a familial syndrome involving a mutation in the calcium-sensing receptor; such patients have levels of serum PTH that are in the normal range, distinguishing it from hypoparathyroidism. It is transmitted as an autosomal dominant. Such patients are hypercalciuric; treatment with calcium and vitamin D may cause nephrocalcinosis.

Treatment

A. Emergency Treatment for Acute Attack (Hypoparathyroid Tetany): This usually occurs after surgery and requires immediate treatment.

1. Be sure an adequate airway is present.

2. Intravenous calcium gluconate–Calcium gluconate, 10–20 mL of 10% solution intravenously, may be given *slowly* until tetany ceases. Ten to 50 mL of 10% calcium gluconate may be added to 1 L of 5% glucose in water or saline and administered by slow intravenous drip. The rate should be so adjusted that the serum calcium is maintained between 8 and 9 mg/dL.

3. Oral calcium–Calcium salts should be given orally as soon as possible to supply 1–2 g of calcium daily. Liquid calcium carbonate (Titralac Plus), 500 mg/5 mL, may be especially useful. The dosage is 1–3 g calcium daily. Calcium citrate contains 21% calcium, but a higher proportion is absorbed with less gastrointestinal intolerance.

4. Vitamin D preparations–(Table 26–10.) Therapy should be started as soon as oral calcium is begun. The treatment of choice for chronic hypoparathyroidism is vitamin D_2 (ergocalciferol). The usual dose ranges from 25,000 to 150,000 units/d. It is a slow-acting preparation, and if toxicity develops, hypercalcemia—treatable with hydration and prednisone—may persist for weeks after it is discontinued. Ergocalciferol usually gives a more stable serum calcium level than do the shorter-acting preparations.

The active metabolite of vitamin D, 1,25-dihydroxycholecalciferol (calcitriol), has a very rapid onset of action, and if toxicity develops it is not long-lasting. It is of great use in the treatment of acute hypocalcemia in doses ranging from 0.25 to 4 μg/d.

Table 26–10. Vitamin D preparations used in the treatment of hypoparathyroidism.[1]

	Potency	How Supplied	Daily Dose (Range)	Time Required for Hypercalcemia to Subside
Ergocalciferol (ergosterol, vitamin D_2)	40,000 USP units/mg	Capsules of 25,000 and 50,000 units; solution, 8000 units/mL	25,000–200,000 units	6–18 weeks
Dihydrotachysterol (Hytakerol)	120,000 USP units/mg	Tablets of 0.125, 0.2, and 0.4 mg	0.2–1 mg	1–3 weeks
Calcifediol (Calderol)	. . .	Capsules of 20 and 50 μg	20–200 μg	3–6 weeks
Calcitriol (Rocaltrol)	. . .	Capsules of 0.25 and 0.5 μg	0.25–4 μg	1/2–2 weeks

[1]Reproduced, with permission, from Greenspan FS, Baxter JD (editors): *Basic & Clinical Endocrinology,* 4th ed. Originally published by Appleton & Lange. Copyright © 1994 by The McGraw-Hill Companies, Inc.

Despite its high cost, calcitriol is being used with increasing frequency for the treatment of chronic hypocalcemia. Therapy is commenced at a dosage of 0.25 μg orally each morning with upward dosage titration to near-normocalcemia. Ultimately, doses of 0.5–2 μg/d are usually required.

Calcifediol (25-hydroxyvitamin D_3) is another option for treatment which has an intermediate onset and duration of action; the usual starting dose is 20 μg/d orally.

Dihydrotachysterol is faster in onset of action and is three times more potent than ergocalciferol. The usual daily maintenance dose is 0.125–1 mg/d. It is more expensive than vitamin D_2.

5. Magnesium–If hypomagnesemia is present (chronic alcoholism, malnutrition, renal loss, drugs such as cisplatin, etc), it must be corrected in order to treat the resulting hypocalcemia. Acutely, $MgSO_4$ is given intravenously, 1–2 g every 6 hours. Chronic magnesium replacement may be given as magnesium oxide tablets (600 mg), one or two per day, or as a combined magnesium and calcium preparation (Dolomite, others).

6. Transplantation of cryopreserved parathyroid tissue removed during prior surgery restores normocalcemia in about 23%.

B. Maintenance Treatment: The goal should be to maintain the serum calcium in a slightly low but asymptomatic range (8–8.6 mg/dL). This will minimize the hypercalciuria that would otherwise occur and provides a margin of safety against overdosage and hypercalcemia, which may produce permanent damage to renal function. Calcium supplementation (1–2 g/d) is continued, and a vitamin D preparation (see above) is given. Monitoring of serum calcium at regular intervals (at least every 3 months) is mandatory. One should also monitor urine calcium with "spot" urine determinations and keep the level below 30 mg/dL if possible. Hypercalciuria may respond to oral hydrochlorothiazide, usually given with a potassium supplement.

Caution: Phenothiazine drugs should be administered with caution to hypocalcemic patients, since they may precipitate extrapyramidal symptoms. Furosemide should be avoided, since it may worsen hypocalcemia.

Prognosis

The outlook is good if the diagnosis is made promptly and treatment instituted. Any dental changes, cataracts, and brain calcifications are permanent. Periodic blood chemical evaluation is required, since changes in calcium levels may call for modification of the treatment schedule. Hypercalcemia that develops in patients with seemingly stable, treated hypoparathyroidism may be a presenting sign of Addison's disease.

Caccitolo JA et al: The current role of parathyroid cryopreservation and autotransplantation in parathyroid surgery: An institutional experience. Surgery 1997;122:1062. [NLM Cit ID: 98037800]

Callies F et al: Management of hypoparathyroidism during pregnancy—report of twelve cases. Eur J Endocrinol 1998;139:284. [NLM Cit ID: 98429404] (Hypoparathyroid women were treated during pregnancy with calcitriol 0.25 μg/d up to 3.25 μg/d, with a requirement for the higher doses as the pregnancies progressed.)

Eubanks PJ et al: Osteitis fibrosa cystica with renal parathyroid resistance: a review of pseudohypoparathyroidism with insight into calcium homeostasis. Arch Surg 1998;133:673. [NLM Cit ID: 98299584]

Yamashita H et al: Postoperative tetany in Graves' disease: Important role of vitamin D metabolites. Ann Surg 1999;229:237. [NLM Cit ID: 99146711]

HYPERPARATHYROIDISM

Essentials of Diagnosis

- Patients frequently asymptomatic, detected by screening.
- Renal stones, polyuria, hypertension, constipation, fatigue, mental changes.

- Bone pain; rarely, cystic lesions and pathologic fractures.
- Serum and urine calcium elevated; urine phosphate high with low to normal serum phosphate; alkaline phosphatase normal to elevated.
- Elevated parathyroid hormone.

General Considerations

Primary hyperparathyroidism is an increasingly recognized disorder, present in up to 0.1% of adult patients examined. It can be seen at any age but is more frequent in persons over the age of 50 and is three times more common in women than in men.

The disease is caused by hypersecretion of parathyroid hormone, usually by a parathyroid adenoma, and less commonly by hyperplasia or carcinoma (rare). However, when hyperparathyroidism presents before age 30, there is a higher incidence of multiglandular disease (36%) and carcinoma (5%). The size of the parathyroid adenoma correlates with the serum parathyroid hormone level.

Parathyroid adenomas or hyperplasia can be familial (about 5%) and may be part of multiple endocrine neoplasia types 1, 2a, and 2b. (See Table 26–16.)

Hyperparathyroidism causes excessive excretion of calcium and phosphate by the kidneys. Parathyroid hormone stimulates renal tubular reabsorption of calcium; however, hyperparathyroidism causes hypercalcemia and an increase in calcium in the glomerular filtrate that overwhelms tubular reabsorption capacity, resulting in hypercalciuria. At least 5% of renal stones are associated with this disease. Diffuse parenchymal calcification (nephrocalcinosis) is seen less commonly. Chronic bone resorption induced by excessive PTH in the circulation may produce diffuse demineralization, pathologic fractures, or cystic bone lesions throughout the skeleton ("osteitis fibrosa cystica").

In chronic renal failure, hyperphosphatemia and decreased renal production of $1,25(OH)_2D_3$ initially produce a decrease in ionized calcium. The parathyroid glands are stimulated (secondary hyperparathyroidism) and may enlarge, becoming autonomous (tertiary hyperparathyroidism). The bone disease seen in this setting is known as "renal osteodystrophy." Diabetics seem somewhat less prone to develop this syndrome. Hypercalcemia often occurs after renal transplant but usually subsides spontaneously.

Parathyroid carcinoma is an unusual cause of hyperparathyroidism but is more common in patients with severe hypercalcemia.

Clinical Findings

A. Symptoms and Signs: Hypercalcemia is frequently discovered accidentally by routine chemistry panels. Most patients are asymptomatic. Parathyroid adenomas are usually so small and deeply located in the neck that they are almost never palpable; when a mass is palpated, it usually turns out to be an incidental thyroid nodule.

Although many patients with mild hypercalcemia offer no complaints, symptomatic patients are said to have problems with "bones, stones, abdominal groans, psychic moans, with fatigue overtones." The manifestations are more formally categorized as follows:

1. Skeletal manifestations–Hyperparathyroidism causes a loss of cortical bone and a gain of trabecular bone. Bone mineral concentration tends to be decreased in the distal radius and in the midshaft of the femur but not in the femoral neck. Similarly, bone mineral is decreased in vertebral posterior processes but increased in the vertebral bodies. Significant bone demineralization is uncommon in mild hyperparathyroidism, but osteitis fibrosa cystica may present as pathologic fractures or as "brown tumors" or cysts of the jaw. More commonly, patients have bone pain and arthralgias.

2. Urinary tract manifestations–Polyuria and polydipsia may be present and are due to hypercalcemia-induced nephrogenic diabetes insipidus. Calcium-containing kidney stones are reported in about 18% of those with newly discovered primary hyperparathyroidism. Nephrocalcinosis and renal failure can occur.

3. Manifestations of hypercalcemia–Mild hypercalcemia is often asymptomatic. In more severe cases, thirst, anorexia, nausea, and vomiting are present. Constipation, fatigue, anemia, weight loss, and hypertension are commonly found. Pancreatitis occurs in 3%. Some patients present primarily with neuromuscular disorders such as muscle weakness, easy fatigability, or paresthesias. Depression, intellectual weariness, and increased sleep requirement are common. Pruritus and psychosis or even coma may accompany severe hypercalcemia. Calcium may precipitate in the corneas ("band keratopathy") or soft tissue (calciphylaxis). Pancreatitis can occur.

B. Laboratory Findings: The hallmark of primary hyperparathyroidism is hypercalcemia (serum calcium > 10.5 mg/dL when corrected for serum albumin; see above). In hyperproteinemic states, the total serum calcium may be elevated but the ionized fraction is normal, whereas in primary hyperparathyroidism the ionized calcium is almost always elevated. The serum phosphate is often low (< 2.5 mg/dL). The urine calcium excretion may be high or normal (averaging 250 mg/g creatinine) but it is usually low for the degree of hypercalcemia. There is an excessive loss of phosphate in the urine in the presence of low (25% of cases) to low normal serum phosphate. (In secondary hyperparathyroidism due to renal failure, the serum phosphate is high.) The alkaline phosphatase is elevated only if bone disease is present. The plasma chloride and uric acid levels may be elevated. Elevated levels of parathyroid hormone confirm the diagnosis. The best immunoassay recognizes the intact molecule at two different sites—the amino terminal and the carboxyl terminal ends—with two different antibodies. This assay, known as immunoradiometric assay (IRMA), is specific and sensitive, making it easier to distinguish primary hyperparathyroidism from other causes of hypercalcemia.

C. Imaging: Unguided neck exploration by an experienced parathyroid surgeon is about equally successful at identifying a parathyroid adenoma as the best localization procedures. Localizing preoperative imaging may be reserved for patients with prior neck surgery. In such cases, performing two different types of studies reduces the chance of false positives. Since the gland or glands affected are rarely larger than 1.5 cm in diameter (and usually *much* smaller), preoperative imaging techniques are often unsuccessful. Imaging techniques include ultrasonography, CT, MRI, and Tc-99m MIBI studies. The accuracy of a given technique depends upon the available equipment and technical personnel. Tc-99m MIBI scintigraphy can detect about 90% of solitary parathyroid adenomas but only about 55% of abnormal glands in patients with multiglandular disease. Three-dimensional scintigraphic imaging techniques can help localize ectopic glands. Tc-99m MIBI specificity is over 95%, but false-positive scans can occur. Incidental small benign thyroid nodules are discovered incidentally in nearly half of patients with hyperparathyroidism who have imaging with ultrasound or MRI.

Bone x-rays are usually normal and not required to make the diagnosis of hyperparathyroidism. There may be demineralization, subperiosteal resorption of bone (especially in the radial aspects of the fingers), or loss of the lamina dura of the teeth. There may be cysts throughout the skeleton, mottling of the skull ("salt-and-pepper appearance"), or pathologic fractures. Articular cartilage calcification (chondrocalcinosis) is sometimes found.

Patients with renal osteodystrophy may have ectopic calcifications around joints or in soft tissue. Such patients may exhibit x-ray changes of osteopenia, osteitis fibrosa, or osteosclerosis, alone or in combination. Osteosclerosis of the vertebral bodies is known as "rugger jersey spine."

Complications

Pathologic fractures are more common, especially in women. Urinary tract infection due to stone and obstruction may lead to renal failure and uremia. If the serum calcium level rises rapidly, clouding of sensorium, renal failure, and rapid precipitation of calcium throughout the soft tissues may occur. Peptic ulcer and pancreatitis may be intractable before surgery. Insulinomas or gastrinomas may be associated, as well as pituitary tumors (multiple endocrine neoplasia type 1). Pseudogout may complicate hyperparathyroidism both before and after surgical removal of tumors. Hypercalcemia during gestation produces neonatal hypocalcemia.

In secondary hyperparathyroidism due to renal failure, high serum calcium and phosphate levels may cause disseminated calcification in the skin, soft tissues, and arteries (calciphylaxis); this can result in painful ischemic necrosis of skin and gangrene, cardiac arrhythmias, and respiratory failure. The actual serum levels of calcium and phosphate have not correlated well with calciphylaxis, but a calcium (mg/dL) × phosphate (mg/dL) product over 70 is usually present.

Differential Diagnosis

(1) Artifact: A report of hypercalcemia may be due to laboratory error or excess tourniquet time and should always be repeated. Hypercalcemia may be due to high serum protein concentrations; serum calcium should be corrected for albumin (see above). It may also be seen with dehydration.

(2) Hypercalcemia of malignancy: Many malignant tumors (breast, lung, pancreas, uterus, hypernephroma, etc) can produce hypercalcemia. In some cases (breast carcinoma especially), bony metastases are present. In others, no metastases to bone can be demonstrated. Most of these tumors secrete parathyroid hormone-related protein, which has tertiary structural homologies to PTH and causes bone resorption and hypercalcemia similar to those of parathyroid hormone. The clinical features of the hypercalcemia of cancer can closely simulate hyperparathyroidism. Serum phosphate is often low, but the plasma level of PTH by IRMA is *low*.

Multiple myeloma is a common cause of hypercalcemia in the older population. Many other hematologic cancers such as monocytic leukemia, T cell leukemia and lymphoma, Burkitt's lymphoma, etc, have also been associated with hypercalcemia. Multiple myeloma causes renal dysfunction; resultant increased levels of carboxyl terminal PTH may cause it to be confused with hyperparathyroidism if a carboxyl terminal PTH assay is used. Serum protein and urine electrophoresis and bone marrow biopsy establish the diagnosis.

(3) Sarcoidosis and other granulomatous disorders: Macrophages and perhaps other cells present in granulomatous tissue have the ability to synthesize 1,25-dihydroxycholecalciferol. Hypercalcemia has been reported in patients with tuberculosis, sarcoidosis, berylliosis, histoplasmosis, coccidioidomycosis, leprosy, and even foreign-body granuloma. Increased intestinal calcium absorption and hypercalciuria are more common than hypercalcemia. Serum levels of 1,25-dihydroxycholecalciferol are elevated.

(4) Calcium or vitamin D ingestion: Ingestion of large amounts of calcium (usually as an antacid) or vitamin D can cause hypercalcemia, which is reversible following its cessation. If it persists, the possibility of associated hyperparathyroidism should be strongly considered.

Table 26–11. Etiologic classification of osteoporosis.[1,2]

Hormone deficiency	**Genetic disorders**
Estrogen (women)	Aromatase deficiency
Androgen (men)	Type I collagen mutations
Hormone excess	Osteogenesis imperfecta
Cushing's syndrome or glucocorticoid administration	Idiopathic juvenile and adult osteoporosis
Thyrotoxicosis	Ehlers-Danlos syndrome
Hyperparathyroidism	Marfan's syndrome
Immobilization and microgravity	Homocystinuria
Tobacco	**Miscellaneous**
Alcoholism	Anorexia nervosa
Malignancy, especially multiple myeloma	Protein-calorie malnutrition
Medications	Vitamin C deficiency
Excessive vitamin D intake	Copper deficiency
Excessive vitamin A intake	Liver disease
Heparin therapy	Rheumatoid arthritis
	Uncontrolled diabetes mellitus
	Systemic mastocytosis

[1]Modified, with permission, from Fitzgerald PA: *Handbook of Clinical Endocrinology,* 2nd ed. Originally published by Appleton & Lange. Copyright © 1992 by The McGraw-Hill Companies, Inc.
[2]See Table 26–12 for causes of osteomalacia.

Clinical Findings

A. Symptoms and Signs: Osteoporosis is usually asymptomatic until fractures occur. It may present as backache of varying degrees of severity or as a spontaneous fracture or collapse of a vertebra. Loss of height is common.

B. Laboratory Findings: Serum calcium, phosphate, and PTH are normal. The alkaline phosphatase is usually normal but may be slightly elevated, especially following a fracture.

C. Imaging: The principal areas of demineralization are the spine and pelvis, especially in the femoral neck and head; demineralization is less marked in the skull and extremities. Compression of vertebrae is common. Bone densitometry permits screening for osteopenia in high-risk individuals and allows assessment of response to therapy. CT densitometry of vertebrae is highly accurate and reproducible. Dual energy x-ray absorptiometry (DEXA) can determine the density of any bone, is quite accurate, and delivers negligible radiation.

Differential Diagnosis

Osteoporosis has many causes (Table 26–11). Additionally, osteopenia and fractures can be caused by osteomalacia (see below) and bone marrow neoplasia such as myeloma or metastatic bone disease. These conditions coexist in many patients.

Treatment

A. Specific Measures: Several treatment options are available, so a regimen is tailored to each patient.

1. Sex hormones–Women with hypogonadism should be considered for replacement estrogen (see Hormone Replacement Therapy) or raloxifene (see below). Men with hypogonadism are treated with testosterone (see Male Hypogonadism).

2. Bisphosphonates–These agents work similarly, inhibiting osteoclast-induced bone resorption. To ensure intestinal absorption, bisphosphonates must be taken in the morning with at least 8 oz of plain water at least 30 minutes before consumption of anything else. The patient must remain upright after taking alendronate to reduce the risk of esophagitis.

Alendronate, 10 mg/d orally, has proved effective for increasing bone density and reducing fracture risk; esophagitis can occur, especially in patients with hiatal hernia. Gastritis, anorexia, and weight loss are common side effects. Alendronate 70 mg orally once weekly appears to be as effective as daily dosing and is more convenient and possibly better-tolerated. Hypocalcemia may occur and require treatment with vitamin D. Etidronate appears to be somewhat less effective but is less expensive and often better tolerated; it is given cyclically in a dose of 400 mg daily for 2 weeks every 3 months. Pamidronate is a parenteral bisphosphonate that can be given in doses of 60 mg by slow intravenous infusion in normal saline solution every 3 months for patients with osteoporosis who cannot tolerate the oral bisphosphonate preparations.

Bisphosphonates have been effective in preventing corticosteroid-induced osteoporosis.

3. Selective estrogen receptor modulators (SERMs)–Raloxifene, 60 mg/d orally, can be used by postmenopausal women in place of estrogen for prevention of osteoporosis. Bone density increases about 1% over 2 years in postmenopausal women versus 2% increases with estrogen replacement. Raloxifene produces a reduction in LDL cholesterol but not the rise in HDL cholesterol seen with estrogen. It has no direct effect on coronary plaque. Unlike estrogen, raloxifene does not reduce hot flushes; in fact, it often intensifies them. It does not relieve vaginal dryness. Unlike estrogen, raloxifene does not cause endometrial hyperplasia, uterine bleeding, or cancer, nor does it cause breast soreness or increase the risk of breast cancer. Since it is a potential teratogen, it is contraindicated in premenopausal women.

Raloxifene increases the risk for thromboembolism and should not be used by women with such a history. Leg cramps can also occur.

4. Calcitonin–A nasal spray of calcitonin-salmon (Miacalcin) is available that contains 2200 units/mL in 2 mL metered-dose bottles. The usual dose is one puff (0.09 mL, 200 IU) once daily, alternating nostrils. Nasal administration causes significantly less nausea and flushing than the parenteral route. However, nasal symptoms such as rhinitis and epistaxis occur commonly; other less common adverse reactions include flu-like symptoms, allergy, arthralgias, back pain, and headache. Five years of therapy increases bone 2–3% and reduces the number of new vertebral fractures. Both nasal and parenteral calcitonin have analgesic effects on bone pain; reduction of pain may be noted within 2–4 weeks after commencing therapy.

5. Calcium and vitamin D–Adequate oral intakes of calcium and vitamin D are required throughout life in order to maintain peak bone mass and reduce the risk of subsequent osteoporosis and osteomalacia. Supplements are recommended for patients at high risk for osteoporosis (see above) and for those with established osteoporosis. Other possible benefits are that the risk of breast cancer is reduced by vitamin D and that calcium supplements may reduce the risk of colon cancer. Calcium supplementation may be given as calcium citrate (0.4–0.6 g elemental calcium per day) or calcium carbonate (1–1.5 g elemental calcium per day). Vitamin D_2 is given in doses of 400–1000 IU daily.

Precautions: Patients who are taking glucocorticoids and thiazide diuretics may develop hypercalcemia when given oral calcium supplements. Calcium salts are given with meals in order to reduce the risk of calcium oxalate nephrolithiasis. Patients with renal failure who take calcium carbonate supplements experience a higher risk of calciphylaxis.

B. General Measures: For prevention and treatment of osteoporosis, the diet should be adequate in protein, total calories, calcium, and vitamin D. Pharmacologic glucocorticoid doses should be reduced or discontinued if possible. Thiazides may be useful if hypercalciuria is present. Regular exercise is recommended in the form of walking or running. Weight training is also helpful to increase muscle strength as well as bone density. Measures should be taken to avoid falls at home (eg, adequate lighting, handrails on stairs, handholds in bathrooms). Patients who have weakness or balance problems must use a cane or a walker; rolling walkers should have a brake mechanism. Balance exercises (eg, tai chi) can reduce the risk of falls. Patients should be kept active; bedridden patients should be given active or passive exercises. The spine may be adequately supported (though braces or corsets are usually not well tolerated), but rigid or excessive immobilization must be avoided. Alcohol and smoking should be avoided.

Prognosis

The prognosis is good for preventing postmenopausal osteoporosis if estrogen therapy or raloxifene is started early and maintained for years. Bisphosphonates can reverse osteoporosis and decrease fracture risk.

Bone HG et al: Dose-response relationships for alendronate treatment in osteoporotic elderly women. Alendronate Elderly Osteoporosis Study Centers. J Clin Endocrinol Metab 1997;82:265. [NLM Cit ID: 97143261]

Garland CF et al: Calcium and vitamin D. Their potential roles in colon and breast cancer prevention. Ann N Y Acad Sci 1999;889:107. [NLM Cit ID: 20133666]

Graham DY et al: Alendronate gastric ulcers. Aliment Pharmacol Ther 1999;13:515. [NLM Cit ID: 99234441] (Significant erosions of the gastric antrum and esophagus occurred after just 7–14 days of treatment.)

Homik JE et al: A metaanalysis on the use of bisphosphonates in corticosteroid induced osteoporosis. J Rheumatol 1999;26:1148. [NLM Cit ID: 99263777] (Bisphosphonates prevented prednisone-induced bone loss at the lumbar spine; a 24% reduction in spinal fractures did not reach statistical significance.)

Khovidhunkit W et al: Clinical effects of raloxifene hydrochloride in women. Ann Intern Med 1999;130:431. [NLM Cit ID: 99156327]

Layne JE, Nelson ME: The effects of progressive resistance training on bone density: a review. Med Sci Sports Exerc 1999;31:25. [NLM Cit ID: 99124196]

Mortensen L et al: Risedronate increases bone mass in an early postmenopausal population: Two years of treatment plus one year of follow-up. J Clin Endocrinol Metab 1998;83:396. [NLM Cit ID: 98128576]

Schnitzer T et al: Therapeutic equivalence of alendronate 70 mg once-weekly and alendronate 10 mg daily in the treatment of osteoporosis. Alendronate Once-Weekly Study Group. Aging 2000;12:1. [NLM Cit ID: 20208195] (Three different regimens for oral alendronate were equally effective in increasing lumbar bone mineral density: 10 mg/d, 35 mg twice weekly, or 70 mg/wk.)

OSTEOMALACIA

Essentials of Diagnosis

- Painful proximal muscle weakness (especially pelvic girdle); bone pain and tenderness.
- Decreased bone density from diminished mineralization of osteoid.
- Laboratory abnormalities may include increases in alkaline phosphatase, decreased 25-hydroxyvitamin D, or hypocalcemia, hypocalciuria, hypophosphatemia, secondary hyperparathyroidism.
- Classic radiologic features may be present.

General Considerations

Defective mineralization of the growing skeleton in childhood causes permanent bone deformities (rickets). Defective skeletal mineralization in adults is known as osteomalacia.

Osteomalacia is commonly caused by a deficiency in vitamin D, which is a hormone with a complex set of actions and mechanism of synthesis. Ergocalciferol (vitamin D_2) is derived from plants and is used in most pharmaceutical preparations of vitamin D. Cholecalciferol (vitamin D_3) is synthesized in the skin, under the influence of ultraviolet radiation, from 7-dehydrocholesterol. Both vitamin D_2 and vitamin D_3 are used to fortify foods and have equivalent potency. Two sequential hydroxylations are necessary for full biologic activity: The first one takes place in the liver—to 25-hydroxycholecalciferol (25[OH]D_3)—and the second one in the kidney, resulting in the formation of the most potent biologic metabolite of vitamin D, 1,25-dihydroxycholecalciferol (1,25[OH]$_2D_3$). The main action of vitamin D is to increase the absorption of calcium and phosphate from the intestine. However, vitamin D appears to have other systemic effects, since 1,25$(OH)_2$D receptors are also found in other tissues, including the parathyroids, bones, kidneys, skin, brain, pituitary, activated lymphocytes, and various tumors.

Etiology (Table 26–12)

Osteomalacia is a common disorder and is caused by any condition that results in inadequate calcium or phosphate mineralization of bone osteoid.

A. Vitamin D Deficiency and Resistance: Vitamin D deficiency impairs the intestinal absorption of calcium and is the most common cause of osteomalacia. Deficiency of vitamin D may arise from insufficient sun exposure, malnutrition, or malabsorption (due to pancreatic insufficiency, cholestatic liver disease, sprue, inflammatory bowel disease, jejunoileal bypass, Billroth type II gastrectomy, etc). Cholestyramine binds bile acids necessary for vitamin D absorption. Patients with severe nephrotic syndrome lose large amounts of vitamin D-binding protein in the urine and may also develop osteomalacia.

Vitamin D-dependent rickets type I is caused by a rare autosomal recessive defect in renal synthesis of 1,25$(OH)_2$D. It presents in childhood with rickets; adults develop osteomalacia unless treated with oral calcitriol in doses of 0.5–1 μg daily. Vitamin D-dependent rickets type II (now better known as hereditary 1,25$(OH)_2$D-resistant rickets) is caused by a genetic defect in the 1,25$(OH)_2$D receptor. It presents in childhood with rickets and alopecia. Adults respond variably to oral calcitriol in very large doses (2–6 μg daily).

Anticonvulsants (eg, phenytoin, carbamazepine, valproate, phenobarbital) inhibit the hepatic production of 25(OH)D and sometimes cause osteomalacia.

Table 26–12. Causes of osteomalacia.[1,2]

Vitamin disorders
Decreased availability of vitamin D
Insufficient sunlight exposure
Nutritional deficiency of vitamin D
Malabsorption
Nephrotic syndrome
Vitamin D-dependent rickets type I
Liver disease
Chronic renal failure
Phenytoin, carbamazepine, or barbiturate therapy
Dietary calcium deficiency
Phosphate deficiency
Decreased intestinal absorption
Nutritional deficiency of phosphorus
Malabsorption
Phosphate-binding antacid therapy
Increased renal loss
X-linked hypophosphatemic rickets
Tumoral hypophosphatemic osteomalacia
Association with other disorders, including paraproteinemias, glycogen storage diseases, neurofibromatosis, Wilson's disease, and Fanconi's syndrome
Disorders of bone matrix
Hypophosphatasia
Fibrogenesis imperfecta
Axial osteomalacia
Inhibitors of mineralization
Aluminum
Bisphosphonates

[1]Modified, with permission, from Fitzgerald PA: *Handbook of Clinical Endocrinology*, 2nd ed. Originally published by Appleton & Lange. Copyright © 1992 by The McGraw-Hill Companies, Inc.
[2]See Table 26–11 for causes of osteoporosis.

Phenytoin can also directly inhibit bone mineralization. Serum levels of 1,25$(OH)_2$D are usually normal.

B. Deficient Calcium Intake: Rickets and osteomalacia continue to be common problems in many tropical countries despite adequate exposure to sunlight. A nutritional deficiency of calcium can occur in any severely malnourished patient. Some degree of calcium deficiency is common in the elderly, since intestinal calcium absorption declines with age.

C. Phosphate Deficiency: Congenital phosphate deficiency is caused most commonly by *PHEX* gene mutations which result in a familial or sporadic X-linked renal tubular defect of phosphate resorption (vitamin D-resistant rickets). Acquired hypophosphatemia can be caused by poor nutrition, alcoholism, or chelation of phosphate in the gut by aluminum hydroxide antacids. Oncogenic hypophosphatemia is caused by a wide variety of soft tissue tumors (87% benign) which secrete 56 kDa and 58 kDa peptides that block the renal tubular reabsorption of phosphate and also block the renal production of 1,25$(OH)_2$D. Excessive renal phosphate losses are also seen in proximal renal tubular acidosis and Fanconi's syndrome. Some cases of hyperphosphaturia are idiopathic.

D. Aluminum Toxicity: Bone mineralization is

inhibited by aluminum. Osteomalacia may occur in patients receiving chronic renal hemodialysis with tap water dialysate or from aluminum-containing antacids used to reduce phosphate levels. Patients being maintained on long-term total parenteral nutrition may develop osteomalacia if the casein hydrolysate used for amino acids contains high levels of aluminum.

E. Hypophosphatasia: Osteomalacia results from an autosomal recessive deficiency of bone alkaline phosphatase, which usually inactivates pyrophosphate; pyrophosphate inhibits bone mineralization. It may present in childhood as rickets or in adulthood as a propensity to fracture—due to osteomalacia. Patients have low serum levels of alkaline phosphatase and high urinary excretion of phosphoethanolamine.

F. Fibrogenesis Imperfecta Ossium: This rare condition sporadically affects middle-aged patients, who present with progressive bone pain and pathologic fractures. Bones have a dense "fishnet" appearance on x-ray. MRI of unfractured bone shows low signal intensity on both T1- and T2-weighted imaging. Serum alkaline phosphatase levels are elevated. Some patients have a monoclonal gammopathy, indicating a possible plasma cell dyscrasia causing an impairment in osteoblast function and collagen disarray. Remission has been reported after repeated courses of melphalan, corticosteroids, and vitamin D analog over 3 years.

Clinical Findings

The clinical manifestations of defective bone mineralization depend on the age at onset and the severity. In adults, osteomalacia is typically asymptomatic at first. Eventually, bone pain occurs, along with muscle weakness due to calcium deficiency. Fractures may occur with little or no trauma.

Diagnostic Tests

Serum is obtained for calcium, albumin, phosphate, alkaline phosphatase, parathyroid hormone. and 25-hydroxyvitamin D (25[OH]D_3) determinations. Bone densitometry helps document the degree of osteopenia. X-rays may show diagnostic features.

In one series of biopsy-proved osteomalacia, alkaline phosphatase was elevated in 94%; the calcium or phosphorus was low in 47%; 25(OH)D_3 was low in 29%; pseudofractures were seen in 18%; and urinary calcium was low in 18%. 1,25$(OH)_2D_3$ may be low even when 25(OH)D_2 levels are normal.

Bone biopsy is not usually necessary but is diagnostic of osteomalacia if there is significant unmineralized osteoid.

Differential Diagnosis

Osteomalacia usually can be distinguished from osteoporosis by the relative absence of biochemical abnormalities in the latter. Phosphate deficiency must be distinguished from hypophosphatemia seen in hyperparathyroidism.

Prevention & Treatment

Prevention of vitamin D deficiency may be achieved with adequate sunlight exposure and vitamin D supplements. In the USA, the current recommended daily allowance (RDA) of vitamin D is at least 10 μg (400 IU) daily. However, in sunlight-deprived individuals (eg, veiled women, confined patients, or residents of higher latitudes during winter), the RDA should be 1000 IU daily. Patients receiving chronic phenytoin therapy may be treated prophylactically with vitamin D, 50,000 IU orally every 2–4 weeks.

Vitamin D deficiency is treated with ergocalciferol (D_2), 50,000 IU orally once or twice weekly for 6–12 months, followed by at least 1000 IU daily. Ergocalciferol has a long duration of action and may also be given orally every 2 months in doses of 50,000 IU. In patients with intestinal malabsorption, oral doses of 25,000–100,000 IU of vitamin D_2 daily may be required. Some patients with steatorrhea respond better to oral 25(OH)D (calcifediol), 50–100 μg daily. All patients receive supplemental oral calcium salts (eg, calcium citrate or calcium carbonate), which are given with meals. Recommended doses of calcium are as follows: calcium citrate (eg, Citracal), 0.4–0.6 g elemental calcium per day; or calcium carbonate (eg, OsCal, Tums), 1–1.5 g elemental calcium per day.

In hypophosphatemic osteomalacia, nutritional deficiencies are corrected, aluminum-containing antacids are discontinued, and patients with renal tubular acidosis are given bicarbonate therapy. In patients with sporadic adult-onset hypophosphatemia, hyperphosphaturia, and low serum 1,25$(OH)_2$D levels, a search is conducted for occult tumors that may be resected; whole-body MRI scanning may be required.

For those with X-linked or idiopathic hypophosphatemia and hyperphosphaturia, oral phosphate supplements must be given chronically; calcitriol, 0.25–0.5 μg/d, is given also to improve the impaired calcium absorption caused by the oral phosphate. Human recombinant growth hormone reduces phosphaturia and may be added to the above regimen if necessary, with appropriate precautions (see Growth Hormone).

Glerup H et al: Commonly recommended daily intake of vitamin D is not sufficient if sunlight exposure is limited. J Intern Med 2000;247:260. [NLM Cit ID: 20156565]

Heller HJ et al: Pharmacokinetics of calcium absorption from two commercial calcium supplements. J Clin Pharm 1999;39:1151. [NLM Cit ID: 20046107] (The gastrointestinal absorption of 500 mg of elemental calcium was 2.5 times higher for the calcium citrate preparation than for calcium carbonate.)

PAGET'S DISEASE OF BONE (Osteitis Deformans)

Essentials of Diagnosis

- Often asymptomatic.
- Bone pain may be the first symptom.
- Kyphosis, bowed tibias, large head, deafness, and frequent fractures that vary with location of process.
- Serum calcium and phosphate normal; alkaline phosphatase elevated; urinary hydroxyproline elevated.
- Dense, expanded bones on x-ray.

General Considerations

Paget's disease is a bone disease that may be related to a paramyxovirus (canine distemper) infection. It causes excessive bone destruction and repair—with associated deformities, since the repair takes place in an unorganized fashion. Up to 3% of persons over age 50 have isolated lesions, but clinically important disease is much less common. Familial Paget's disease is unusual but is generally more severe than sporadic cases. A rare form occurs in young people.

Clinical Findings

A. Symptoms and Signs: Paget's disease is usually diagnosed in patients over 40 years of age and often mild and asymptomatic. It can involve just one bone (monostotic) or multiple bones (polyostotic), particularly the skull, femur, tibia, pelvis, and humerus. Pain is the usual first symptom. The bones become soft, leading to bowed tibias, kyphosis, and frequent fractures with slight trauma. If the skull is involved, the patient may report headaches and an increased hat size. Deafness may occur. Increased vascularity over the involved bones causes increased warmth.

B. Laboratory Findings: Serum calcium and phosphorus are normal, but serum alkaline phosphatase is markedly elevated. Urinary hydroxyproline is also elevated in active disease. Serum calcium may be elevated, particularly if the patient is at bed rest.

C. Imaging: On radiographs the involved bones are expanded and denser than normal. Multiple fissure fractures may be seen in the long bones. The initial lesion may be destructive and radiolucent, especially in the skull ("osteoporosis circumscripta"). Technetium pyrophosphate bone scans are helpful in delineating activity of bone lesions even before any radiologic changes are apparent.

Differential Diagnosis

Paget's disease must be differentiated from primary bone lesions such as osteogenic sarcoma, multiple myeloma, and fibrous dysplasia and from secondary bone lesions such as metastatic carcinoma and osteitis fibrosa cystica. Fibrogenesis imperfecta ossium is a rare symmetric disorder that can mimic the features of Paget's disease; alkaline phosphate is likewise elevated. If serum calcium is elevated, hyperparathyroidism may be present in some patients as well.

Complications

Fractures are frequent and occur with minimal trauma. If immobilization takes place and there is an excessive calcium intake, hypercalcemia and kidney stones may develop. Vertebral collapse may lead to spinal cord compression. Osteosarcoma may develop in long-standing lesions. Sarcomatous change is suggested by marked increase in bone pain, sudden rise in alkaline phosphatase, and appearance of a new lytic lesion. The increased vascularity may give rise to high-output cardiac failure. Arthritis frequently develops in joints adjacent to involved bone.

Extensive skull involvement may cause cranial nerve palsies from impingement of the neural foramina. Ischemic neurologic events may occur as a result of a vascular "steal" phenomenon. Involvement of the auditory region frequently causes hearing loss (mixed sensorineural and conductive) and occasionally tinnitus or vertigo.

Treatment

Asymptomatic patients require no treatment except for those with extensive skull involvement, in whom prophylactic treatment may prevent deafness and stroke.

A. Bisphosphonates: Bisphosphonates have become the treatment of choice for Paget's disease. The oral compounds should all be taken with 8 oz of plain water only. Bisphosphonates are usually given cyclically. Therapy is given until a therapeutic response occurs, as evidenced by normalization of the serum alkaline phosphatase. Patients are then given a break from therapy for about 3 months or until the serum alkaline phosphatase becomes elevated again; another cycle is then commenced.

1. Tiludronate, 400 mg orally daily for 3 months, is very effective in reducing the activity of bone lesions. It should not be taken within 2 hours of meals, aspirin, indomethacin, calcium, magnesium, or aluminum-containing antacids. Esophagitis is uncommon, so recumbency after dosing is not restricted, and it may be taken in the evening as well as during the day. The most common side effects have been gastrointestinal, including abdominal pain in 13% and nausea in 9%.

2. Alendronate, 20–40 mg orally daily for 3-month cycles, is also effective. It must be taken in the morning, at least one-half to 1 hour before breakfast. Its main side effect is esophagitis, so recumbency after dosing is prohibited, and the drug is contraindicated in patients with a history of esophagitis, esophageal stricture, dysphagia, hiatal hernia, or achalasia.

3. Risedronate, 30 mg orally daily for 3-month cycles, has been effective in normalizing alkaline phosphatase and eliminating bone pain in the majority of patients. It has been generally well tolerated, but arthralgias and gastrointestinal side effects do occur.

4. Etidronate disodium is given in doses of 5 mg/kg orally daily for 90–180 days. In severe disease, 10 mg/kg daily may be used for 90 days, with a rest period before another course is given. Etidronate can aggravate bone pain, particularly in the femur. It is much less effective than the other bisphosphonates.

5. Pamidronate, 60–120 mg intravenously over 2–4 hours, may produce improvements lasting several months. Alkaline phosphatase may continue to drop for 6 months after treatment. (See Treatment of Hypercalcemia.)

B. Nasal Calcitonin-Salmon: Miacalcin, 200 IU/unit dose spray, is administered as one spray daily, alternating nostrils. It is just as effective as the parenteral preparation and is associated with fewer side effects. Nasal irritation may occur, as may occasional epistaxis. Calcitonin has been used for many years to treat Paget's disease. However, its use has declined dramatically with the introduction of more potent bisphosphonates.

Prognosis

The prognosis in general is good, but sarcomatous changes (in 1–3%) can alter the prognosis unfavorably. In general, the prognosis is worse the earlier in life the disease starts. Fractures usually heal well. In the severe forms, marked deformity, intractable pain, and cardiac failure are found. These complications should become rare with prompt bisphosphonate treatment.

Fraser WD et al: A double-blind, multi-centre, placebo-controlled study of tiludronate in Paget's disease of bone. Postgrad Med J 1997;73:496. [NLM Cit ID: 97452952] (Tiludronate, 400 mg orally once daily, reduced alkaline phosphatase by over half in 52% after 12 weeks and in 70% after 24 weeks, affording prolonged remissions. Gastrointestinal side effects occurred in 6%.)

Hosking DJ et al: Paget's disease of bone: Reduction in disease activity with oral risedronate. Bone 1998;22:51. [NLM Cit ID: 98100167] (Risedronate, 30 mg orally daily for 12 weeks, normalized alkaline phosphatase in most patients.)

Lombardi A: Treatment of Paget's disease of bone with alendronate. Bone 1999;24:59S. [NLM Cit ID: 99253848] (The majority of patients with Paget's disease, treated with oral alendronate 40 mg/d, normalize their serum alkaline phosphatase within 6 months. The majority of those patients are likely to maintain biochemical remission for several years.)

DISEASES OF THE ADRENAL CORTEX

ADRENAL CORTEX PHYSIOLOGY

Aldosterone is the major mineralocorticoid secreted by the zona glomerulosa, the outer layer of the adrenal cortex. It stimulates the renal tubule to reabsorb sodium and excrete potassium, thereby protecting against hypovolemia and hyperkalemia.

Aldosterone secretion is stimulated by hypovolemia in an indirect way. Hypovolemia causes the renal juxtaglomerular cells to secrete renin; renin stimulates the peripheral conversion of angiotensin I to angiotensin II; angiotensin II then causes aldosterone secretion. Hyperkalemia directly stimulates aldosterone secretion. Secretion is inhibited by atrial natriuretic factor and by dopamine.

Cortisol is the major glucocorticoid secreted by the middle zona fasciculata and the inner zona reticularis of the adrenal cortex.

Cortisol counters insulin effects, tending to cause hyperglycemia by inhibiting insulin secretion and by increasing hepatic gluconeogenesis, substrate being provided by the increased amino acids made available by cortisol's inhibition of protein synthesis in muscles.

Cortisol is secreted in a diurnal pattern, being highest upon awakening and lowest at bedtime. Cortisol production normally increases during exercise, making more glucose and fatty acids available for energy. Cortisol is also secreted in response to acute trauma, infection, and other stresses; it dampens defense mechanisms, helping prevent their dangerous overactivity. It inhibits the production or action of many mediators of inflammation and immunity such as interleukin-6 (IL-6), lymphokines, prostaglandins, and histamine. Cortisol is required for production of angiotensin II, thereby helping maintain adequate vascular tone.

Glucocorticoids increase renal free water clearance. They lower serum calcium by inhibiting calcium uptake by the renal tubule and gut and by redistributing calcium intracellularly.

Androgens are produced in the adrenal cortex, mostly by the inner zona fasciculata. The adrenal cortex's fetal zone atrophies after birth, but the adrenal continues to make large amounts of dehydroepiandrosterone sulfate (DHEAS) and dehydroepiandrosterone (DHEA), which have no known significance during adult life, having minimal androgenic activity; but they continue to be the adrenals' most abundantly secreted steroids. DHEAS secretion declines steadily with age. There are individual differences in secretion, and—for unknown reasons—

there is a positive correlation between DHEAS levels and longevity.

Testosterone and androstenedione are the major functional androgens secreted by the adrenal. Their secretion causes adrenarche, which precedes gonadal androgen secretion and stimulates the first sexual hair of puberty.

ADRENOCORTICAL INSUFFICIENCY (Addison's Disease)

1. ACUTE ADRENAL INSUFFICIENCY (Adrenal Crisis)

Essentials of Diagnosis

- Weakness, abdominal pain, fever, confusion, nausea, vomiting, and diarrhea.
- Low blood pressure, dehydration; skin pigmentation may be increased.
- Serum potassium high, sodium low, blood urea nitrogen high.
- Cosyntropin ($ACTH_{1-24}$) unable to stimulate a normal increase in serum cortisol.

General Considerations

Acute adrenal insufficiency is an emergency caused by insufficient cortisol. Crisis may occur in the course of chronic treated insufficiency, or it may be the presenting manifestation of adrenal insufficiency. Acute adrenal crisis is more commonly seen in primary adrenal insufficiency (Addison's disease) than in disorders of the pituitary gland causing secondary adrenocortical hypofunction.

Adrenal crisis may occur in the following situations: (1) Following stress, eg, trauma, surgery, infection, or prolonged fasting in a patient with latent insufficiency. (2) Following sudden withdrawal of adrenocortical hormone in a patient with chronic insufficiency or in a patient with temporary insufficiency due to suppression by exogenous glucocorticoids. (3) Following bilateral adrenalectomy or removal of a functioning adrenal tumor that had suppressed the other adrenal. (4) Following sudden destruction of the pituitary gland (pituitary necrosis), or when thyroid is given to a patient with hypoadrenalism. (5) Following injury to both adrenals by trauma, hemorrhage, anticoagulant therapy, thrombosis, infection, or, rarely, metastatic carcinoma.

Clinical Findings

A. Symptoms and Signs: The patient complains of headache, lassitude, nausea and vomiting, abdominal pain, and often diarrhea. Confusion or coma may be present. Fever may be 40.6 °C or more. The blood pressure is low. Other signs may include cyanosis, dehydration, skin hyperpigmentation, and sparse axillary hair (if hypogonadism is also present). Meningococcemia may be associated with purpura and adrenal insufficiency secondary to adrenal infarction (Waterhouse-Friderichsen syndrome).

B. Laboratory Findings: The eosinophil count may be high. Hyponatremia or hyperkalemia (or both) are usually present. Hypoglycemia is frequent. Hypercalcemia may be present. Blood, sputum, or urine culture may be positive if bacterial infection is the precipitating cause of the crisis.

The diagnosis is made by a simplified cosyntropin stimulation test, which is performed as follows: (1) Synthetic $ACTH_{1-24}$ (cosyntropin), 0.25 mg, is given parenterally. (2) Serum is obtained for cortisol between 30 and 60 minutes after cosyntropin is administered. Normally, serum cortisol rises to at least 20 μg/dL. For patients receiving glucocorticoid treatment, hydrocortisone must not be given for at least 8 hours before the test. Other glucocorticoids (eg, prednisone, dexamethasone) do not interfere with specific assays for cortisol.

Plasma ACTH is markedly elevated if the patient has primary adrenal disease (generally > 200 pg/mL).

Differential Diagnosis

Acute adrenal insufficiency must be distinguished from other causes of shock (eg, septic, hemorrhagic, cardiogenic). Hyperkalemia is also seen with gastrointestinal bleeding, rhabdomyolysis, hyperkalemic paralysis, and certain drugs (eg, ACE inhibitors, spironolactone). Hyponatremia is seen in many other conditions (eg, hypothyroidism, diuretic use, heart failure, cirrhosis, vomiting, diarrhea, severe illness, or major surgery). It must also be distinguished from an acute abdomen where neutrophilia is the rule, whereas eosinophilia and lymphocytosis are characteristic of adrenal insufficiency.

Treatment

A. Acute Phase: If the diagnosis is suspected, draw a blood sample for cortisol determination and treat with hydrocortisone, 100–300 mg intravenously, and saline *immediately*, without waiting for the results. Thereafter, give hydrocortisone phosphate or hydrocortisone sodium succinate, 100 mg intravenously immediately, and continue intravenous infusions of 50–100 mg every 6 hours for the first day. Give the same amount every 8 hours on the second day and then adjust the dosage in view of the clinical picture.

Since bacterial infection frequently precipitates acute adrenal crisis, broad-spectrum antibiotics should be administered empirically while waiting for the results of initial cultures. Hypoglycemia should be vigorously treated while serum electrolytes, blood urea nitrogen, and creatinine are monitored.

B. Convalescent Phase: When the patient is able to take food by mouth, give oral hydrocortisone, 10–20 mg every 6 hours, and reduce dosage to maintenance levels as needed. Most patients ultimately require hydrocortisone twice daily (AM, 10–20 mg; PM, 5–10 mg). Mineralocorticoid therapy is not needed when large amounts of hydrocortisone are being given, but as the dose is reduced it is usually necessary to add fludrocortisone acetate, 0.05–0.2 mg daily. Some patients never require fludrocortisone or become edematous at doses of more than 0.05 mg once or twice weekly. Once the crisis has passed, the patient must be investigated to assess the degree of permanent adrenal insufficiency and to establish the cause if possible.

Prognosis

Rapid treatment will usually be life-saving. However, acute adrenal insufficiency is frequently unrecognized and untreated since its manifestations mimic more common conditions; lack of treatment leads to shock that is unresponsive to volume replacement and vasopressors, resulting in death.

Aygen B et al: Adrenal function in patients with sepsis. Exp Clin Endocrinol Diabetes 1997;105:182. [NLM Cit ID: 97372276] (Of 49 patients with sepsis, 16% had adrenal insufficiency as determined by ACTH stimulation tests. There was a 43% mortality.)

Barquist E et al: Adrenal insufficiency in the surgical intensive care unit patient. J Trauma 1997;42:27. [NLM Cit ID: 97156873]

Oelkers W: Adrenal insufficiency. N Engl J Med 1996; 335:1206. [NLM Cit ID: 96399029]

2. CHRONIC ADRENOCORTICAL INSUFFICIENCY (Addison's Disease)

Essentials of Diagnosis

- Weakness, easy fatigability, anorexia, weight loss; nausea and vomiting, diarrhea; abdominal pain, muscle and joint pains; amenorrhea.
- Sparse axillary hair; increased skin pigmentation, especially of creases, pressure areas, and nipples.
- Hypotension, small heart.
- Serum sodium may be low; potassium, calcium, and urea nitrogen may be elevated; neutropenia, mild anemia, eosinophilia, and relative lymphocytosis may be present.
- Plasma cortisol levels are low or fail to rise after administration of corticotropin.
- Plasma ACTH level elevated.

General Considerations

Addison's disease is an uncommon disorder caused by destruction or dysfunction of the adrenal cortices. It is characterized by chronic deficiency of cortisol, aldosterone, and adrenal androgens and causes skin pigmentation that can be subtle or strikingly dark. Volume and sodium depletion and potassium excess eventually occur in primary adrenal failure. In contrast, if chronic adrenal insufficiency is secondary to pituitary failure (atrophy, necrosis, tumor), mineralocorticoid production (controlled by the renin-angiotensin system) persists and hyperkalemia is not present. Furthermore, if ACTH is not elevated, skin pigmentary changes are not encountered.

Etiology

(1) Autoimmune destruction of the adrenals is the most common cause of Addison's disease in the USA (accounting for about 80% of spontaneous cases). It may occur alone or as part of a polyglandular autoimmune (PGA) syndrome. Type 1 PGA is also known as autoimmune polyendocrinopathy-candidiasis-ectodermal dystrophy (APCED) syndrome and is caused by a defect in T cell-mediated immunity inherited as an autosomal recessive trait. It usually presents in early childhood with mucocutaneous candidiasis, followed by hypoparathyroidism and dystrophy of the teeth and nails; Addison's disease usually appears by age 15 years. Partial or late expression of the syndrome is common. A varied spectrum of associated diseases may be seen in adulthood, including hypogonadism, hypothyroidism, pernicious anemia, alopecia, vitiligo, hepatitis, malabsorption, and Sjögren's syndrome.

Type 2 PGA usually presents in adulthood with autoimmune adrenal insufficiency (no hypoparathyroidism) that is HLA-related. It is associated with autoimmune thyroid disease (usually hypothyroidism, sometimes hyperthyroidism), vitiligo, type 1 diabetes, alopecia areata, or celiac sprue. Autoimmune Addison's disease can also be associated with primary ovarian failure (40% of women before age 50), testicular failure (5%), and pernicious anemia (4%). The combination of Addison's disease and hypothyroidism is known as Schmidt's syndrome.

(2) Tuberculosis was formerly a leading cause of Addison's disease. The association is now relatively rare in the USA but common where tuberculosis is more prevalent.

(3) Bilateral adrenal hemorrhage may occur in patients taking anticoagulants, during open heart surgery, and during other major trauma. It may also occur about 1 week postoperatively, presenting with pain, fever, and shock. Some cases are associated with antiphospholipid antibody syndrome.

(4) Adrenoleukodystrophy is an X-linked peroxisomal disorder causing accumulation of very long chain fatty acids in the adrenal cortex, testes, brain, and spinal cord. It may present at any age and accounts for one-third of cases of Addison's disease in boys. Aldosterone deficiency occurs in 9%. Hypogonadism is common. Psychiatric symptoms often include mania, psychosis, or cognitive impairment. Neurologic deterioration may be severe or mild (particularly in heterozygote women), mimics symptoms of multiple sclerosis, and can occur years after the onset of adrenal insufficiency.

(5) Rare causes of adrenal insufficiency include lymphoma, metastatic carcinoma, coccidioidomycosis, histoplasmosis, cytomegalovirus infection (more frequent in patients with AIDS), syphilitic gummas, scleroderma, amyloid disease, and hemochromatosis.

Adults with hereditary cortisol deficiency due to adrenal insensitivity to ACTH may develop achalasia, alacrima, and neurologic disease (Allgrove's syndrome); cortisol deficiency usually presents in childhood but may not occur until the third decade. Adults with congenital adrenal hypoplasia may have hypogonadotropic hypogonadism, myopathy, and high-frequency hearing loss.

Patients with hereditary defects in adrenal enzymes for cortisol synthesis develop "congenital adrenal hyperplasia" due to ACTH stimulation. The most common enzyme defect is P450c21 (21-hydroxylase). Patients with severely defective P450c21 enzymes manifest deficiency of mineralocorticoids (salt wasting) in addition to deficient cortisol and excessive androgens. Women with milder enzyme defects have adequate cortisol but develop hirsutism in adolescence or adulthood and are said to have "late-onset" congenital adrenal hyperplasia. (See Hirsutism section.)

Clinical Findings

A. Symptoms and Signs: The symptoms may include weakness and fatigability, weight loss, myalgias, arthralgias, fever, anorexia, nausea and vomiting, anxiety, and mental irritability. Some of these symptoms may be due to high serum levels of IL-6. Pigmentary changes consist of diffuse tanning over nonexposed as well as exposed parts or multiple freckles; hyperpigmentation is especially prominent over the knuckles, elbows, knees, and posterior neck and in palmar creases and nail beds. Nipples and areolas tend to darken. The skin in pressure areas such as the belt or brassiere lines and the buttocks also darkens. New scars are pigmented. Some patients have associated vitiligo (10%). Emotional changes are common. Hypoglycemia, when present, may worsen the patient's weakness and mental functioning, rarely leading to coma. Manifestations of other autoimmune disease (see above) may be present. Patients tend to be hypotensive and orthostatic; about 90% have systolic blood pressures under 110 mm Hg; blood pressure over 130 mm Hg is rare. Other findings may include a small heart, hyperplasia of lymphoid tissues, and scant axillary and pubic hair (especially in women).

Patients with adult-onset adrenoleukodystrophy may present with neuropsychiatric symptoms, sometimes without adrenal insufficiency.

B. Laboratory Findings: The white count usually shows moderate neutropenia, lymphocytosis, and a total eosinophil count over 300/μL. Among patients with *chronic* Addison's disease, the serum sodium is usually low (90%) while the potassium is elevated (65%). Patients with diarrhea may not be hyperkalemic. Fasting blood glucose may be low. Hypercalcemia may be present. Young men with idiopathic Addison's disease are screened for adrenoleukodystrophy by determining plasma very long chain fatty acid levels; affected patients have high levels.

Low plasma cortisol (< 5 mg/dL) at 8 AM is diagnostic, especially if accompanied by simultaneous elevation of the plasma ACTH level (usually > 200 pg/mL). The cosyntropin stimulation test is performed as described above. Antiadrenal antibodies are found in the serum in about 50% of cases of autoimmune Addison's disease. Antibodies to thyroid (45%) and other tissues may be present.

C. Imaging: When Addison's disease is not clearly autoimmune, a chest x-ray is obtained to look for tuberculosis, fungal infection, or cancer as possible causes. CT scan of the abdomen will show small noncalcified adrenals in autoimmune Addison's disease. The adrenals are enlarged in about 85% of cases due to metastatic or granulomatous disease. Calcification is noted in about 50% of cases of tuberculous Addison's disease but is also seen with hemorrhage, fungal infection, pheochromocytoma, and melanoma.

Differential Diagnosis

Addison's disease should be considered in any patient with hypotension or hyperkalemia. Unexplained weight loss, weakness, and anorexia may be mistaken for occult cancer. Nausea, vomiting, diarrhea, and abdominal pain may be misdiagnosed as intrinsic gastrointestinal disease. The hyperpigmentation may be confused with that due to ethnic or racial factors. Weight loss may simulate anorexia nervosa. The neurologic manifestations of Allgrove's syndrome and adrenoleukodystrophy (especially in women) often mimic multiple sclerosis. Hemochromatosis also enters the differential diagnosis of skin hyperpigmentation, but it should be remembered that it may truly be a cause of Addison's disease as well as diabetes mellitus and hypoparathyroidism. Serum ferritin is increased in most cases of hemochromatosis and is a useful screening test. About 17% of patients with AIDS have symptoms of cortisol resistance. AIDS can also cause frank adrenal insufficiency.

Complications

Any of the complications of the underlying disease (eg, tuberculosis) are more likely to occur, and the patient is susceptible to intercurrent infections that may precipitate crisis. Associated autoimmune diseases are common (see above).

Treatment

A. Specific Therapy: Replacement therapy should include a combination of glucocorticoids and mineralocorticoids. In mild cases, hydrocortisone alone may be adequate.

1. **Hydrocortisone** is the drug of choice. Most addisonian patients are well maintained on 15–25 mg of hydrocortisone orally daily in two divided doses, two-thirds in the morning and one-third in the late afternoon or early evening. Some patients respond better to prednisone in a dosage of about 3 mg in the morning and 2 mg in the evening. Many patients, however, do not obtain sufficient salt-retaining effect and require fludrocortisone supplementation or extra dietary salt.

2. **Fludrocortisone acetate** has a potent sodium-retaining effect. The dosage is 0.05–0.3 mg orally daily or every other day. If postural hypotension, hyperkalemia, or weight loss occurs, raise the dose. If edema, hypokalemia, or hypertension ensues, lower the dose.

3. **Dehydroepiandrosterone (DHEA)** is given to some women with adrenal insufficiency. Women taking DHEA 50 mg orally each morning have experienced an improvement in their overall sense of well-being, mood, and sexuality. Since over-the-counter preparations of DHEA have variable potencies, it is best to have the pharmacy formulate this with pharmaceutical-grade DHEA.

B. General Measures: Treat all infections immediately and vigorously, and raise the dose of hydrocortisone appropriately. The dose of glucocorticoid should also be raised in case of trauma, surgery, stressful diagnostic procedures, or other forms of stress. The maximum hydrocortisone dose for severe stress is 50 mg intravenously or intramuscularly every 6 hours. Lower doses, oral or parenteral, are used for lesser stress. The dose is reduced back to normal as the stress subsides. Patients are advised to wear a medical alert bracelet or medal reading, "Adrenal insufficiency—takes hydrocortisone."

For patients with adrenoleukodystrophy, therapy with "Lorenzo's oil" normalizes serum very long-chain fatty acid concentrations but is ineffective clinically. Neurologic manifestations may improve following hematopoietic stem cell transplantation from normal donors.

Prognosis

With adequate replacement therapy, the life expectancy of patients with Addison's disease is markedly prolonged. Active tuberculosis responds to specific treatment. Withdrawal of treatment or increased demands due to infection, trauma, surgery, or other types of stress may precipitate crisis with a sudden fatal outcome unless large doses of parenteral corticosteroids are employed. With appropriate therapy, however, a fully active life is possible for most patients.

Arlt W et al: Dehydroepiandrosterone replacement in women with adrenal insufficiency. N Engl J Med 1999;341:1013. (See editorial on page 1073.) [NLM Cit ID: 99417078] (DHEA raised initially low serum concentrations of DHEA, androstenedione, and testosterone to normal, and serum concentrations of sex hormone-binding globulin, cholesterol, and HDL cholesterol decreased.)

Betterle C et al: Clinical review 93: Autoimmune polyglandular syndrome type 1. J Clin Endocrinol Metab 1998;83:1049. [NLM Cit ID: 98202115]

Flemming TG et al: Quality of self-care in patients on replacement therapy with hydrocortisone. J Intern Med 1999;246:497. [NLM Cit ID: 20050800] (Nearly half were insufficiently prepared to cope with physical stress, and 20% did not possess a "steroid warning card.")

Satta MA et al: Adrenal insufficiency as the first clinical manifestation of the primary antiphospholipid antibody syndrome. Clin Endocrinol 2000;52:123. [NLM Cit ID: 20191666]

CUSHING'S SYNDROME (Hypercortisolism)

Essentials of Diagnosis

- Central obesity, muscle wasting, thin skin, easy bruisability, psychologic changes, hirsutism, purple striae.
- Osteoporosis, hypertension, poor wound healing.
- Hyperglycemia, glycosuria, leukocytosis, lymphocytopenia, hypokalemia.
- Elevated serum cortisol and urinary free cortisol. Lack of normal suppression by dexamethasone.

General Considerations

The term Cushing's "syndrome" refers to the manifestations of excessive corticosteroids, commonly due to supraphysiologic doses of glucocorticoid drugs and rarely due to spontaneous production of excessive corticosteroids by the adrenal cortex. Adult cases of spontaneous Cushing's syndrome have several possible causes:

(1) About 70% are due to Cushing's "disease," which refers to the manifestations of hypercortisolism due to ACTH hypersecretion by the pituitary. It is usually caused by a benign pituitary adenoma that is typically very small (< 5 mm). It is at least five times more frequent in women than men.

(2) About 15% are due to nonpituitary neoplasms (eg, small-cell lung carcinoma), which produce excessive amounts of ectopic ACTH. Hypokalemia and hyperpigmentation are commonly found in this group.

(3) About 15% are unrelated to ACTH and are caused by excessive cortisol secretion by an adrenal tumor (adenoma or carcinoma) or rarely by bilateral adrenal nodular hyperplasia. Adrenal adenomas are generally small and produce mostly cortisol, whereas adrenal carcinomas are usually large when discovered and can also produce excessive amounts of androgens with resultant hirsutism and virilization.

Clinical Findings

A. Symptoms and Signs: Patients with Cushing's syndrome usually have central obesity with a plethoric "moon face," "buffalo hump," supraclavicular fat pads, protuberant abdomen, and thin extremi-

lite of dihydrotestosterone that is produced by skin in cosmetically unacceptable amounts.

(2) Polycystic ovary syndrome (hyperthecosis, Stein-Leventhal syndrome): This is a common functional disorder of the ovaries which accounts for at least half the cases of clinical hirsutism. Patients frequently have amenorrhea or oligomenorrhea with anovulation and obesity. The serum LH:FSH ratio is often greater than 2.0. Both adrenal and ovarian androgen hypersecretion are commonly present. Insulin resistance and obesity are common; fasting insulin levels are elevated in 70%. Diabetes mellitus is present in about 13%. Women frequently regain normal menstrual cycles with aging.

(3) Adrenal enzyme defects: Baby girls with "classic" 21-hydroxylase deficiency have ambiguous genitalia and may become virilized unless treated with corticosteroid replacement; about half of such patients have clinically evident mineralocorticoid deficiency (salt-wasting) as well.

About 2% of patients with adult-onset hirsutism have been found to have a partial defect in adrenal 21-hydroxylase, whose phenotypic expression is delayed until adolescence or adulthood; such patients do not have salt wasting.

Some rare patients with hyperandrogenism and hypertension have 11-hydroxylase deficiency. This is distinguished from cortisol resistance by high cortisol levels in the latter and by high 11-deoxycortisol levels in the former.

(4) Ovarian tumors are very uncommon causes of hirsutism (0.8%) and include arrhenoblastomas, Sertoli-Leydig cell tumors, dysgerminomas, and hilar cell tumors.

(5) Adrenal carcinoma is a rare cause of hyperandrogenism that can be quite virilizing.

(6) Other rare causes of hirsutism include ACTH-induced Cushing's syndrome and acromegaly. Maternal virilization during pregnancy may occur as a result of a luteoma of pregnancy, hyperreactio luteinalis, or polycystic ovaries. In postmenopausal women, diffuse stromal Leydig cell hyperplasia is a rare cause of hyperandrogenism. Pharmacologic causes include minoxidil, cyclosporine, phenytoin, anabolic steroids, diazoxide, and certain progestins.

Clinical Findings

A. Symptoms and Signs: Modest androgen excess from any source increases sexual hair (chin, upper lip, abdomen, and chest) and increases sebaceous gland activity, producing acne. Menstrual irregularities, anovulation, and amenorrhea are common. If androgen excess is pronounced, defeminization (decrease in breast size, loss of feminine adipose tissue) and virilization (frontal balding, muscularity, clitoromegaly, and deepening of the voice) occurs. Virilization implicates the presence of an androgen-producing neoplasm.

Hypertension may be seen in rare patients with Cushing's syndrome, adrenal 11-hydroxylase deficiency, or cortisol resistance syndrome.

A pelvic examination may disclose clitoromegaly or ovarian enlargement that may be cystic or neoplastic.

B. Laboratory Testing and Imaging: Serum androgen testing is mainly useful to screen for rare occult adrenal or ovarian neoplasms. Some general guidelines are presented here, though exceptions are common:

Serum is assayed for total testosterone and free testosterone. Certain assays for free testosterone are not reliable, including the free androgen index, the analog free testosterone assay, and the electrochemical luminescence assay. It is best to specify the assay desired, eg, free testosterone by equilibrium dialysis, calculated free testosterone, or non-sex hormone-bound testosterone assay.

A serum testosterone level greater than 200 ng/dL or free testosterone greater than 40 ng/dL indicates the need for pelvic examination and ultrasound. If that is negative, an adrenal CT scan is performed.

A serum androstenedione greater than 1000 ng/dL also implicates an ovarian or adrenal neoplasm.

Patients with milder elevations of serum testosterone or androstenedione usually are treated with an oral contraceptive.

Patients with very elevated serum DHEAS (> 700 μg/dL) have an adrenal source of androgen. This usually is due to adrenal hyperplasia and rarely to adrenal carcinoma. An adrenal CT scan is performed.

No firm guidelines exist as to which patients (if any) with hyperandrogenism should be screened for "late-onset" 21-hydroxylase deficiency. The evaluation requires levels of serum 17-hydroxyprogesterone to be drawn at baseline and at 30–60 minutes after the intramuscular injection of 0.25 mg of cosyntropin ($ACTH_{1-24}$). Patients with congenital adrenal hyperplasia will usually have a baseline 17-hydroxyprogesterone over 300 ng/dL or a stimulated level over 1000 ng/dL. The diagnosis, once made, is interesting academically but not helpful to the patient since glucocorticoid treatment is not particularly more effective in this condition than are other treatment modalities (see below).

Patients with any clinical signs of Cushing's syndrome should receive a screening test. (See Cushing's Syndrome.)

Serum levels of FSH and LH are elevated if amenorrhea is due to ovarian failure. An LH:FSH ratio greater than 2.0 is common in patients with polycystic ovary syndrome. On abdominal ultrasound, about 33% of normal young women have polycystic ovaries, so the appearance of ovarian cysts on ultrasound is not helpful diagnostically.

Treatment

Any underlying cause of hyperandrogenism must be detected and treated if possible. Postmenopausal women with severe hyperandrogenism should undergo laparoscopic bilateral oophorectomy (if CT scan of the adrenals and ovaries is normal), since small hilar cell tumors of the ovary may not be visible on scans. Any drugs causing hirsutism are stopped. Treatment options for other cases include the following:

(1) Spironolactone may be taken in doses of 50–100 mg twice daily on days 5–25 of the menstrual cycle or daily if used concomitantly with an oral contraceptive. Hyperkalemia or hyponatremia is uncommon.

(2) Cyproterone acetate is a potent antiandrogen with progestational activity. A dose of 2 mg is effective. An oral contraceptive is usually prescribed also. Cyproterone is not available in the USA. It is available elsewhere as the progestin element in an oral contraceptive (Diane-35: ethinyl estradiol 35 μg with cyproterone acetate 2 mg). Side effects may include fatigue, nausea, or depression.

(3) Finasteride inhibits 5α-reductase, the enzyme that converts testosterone to active dihydrotestosterone in the skin. Given as 5 mg doses orally daily, it provides modest reduction in hirsutism over 6 months—comparable to results achieved with spironolactone. Side effects are rare.

(4) Flutamide, 250–375 mg/d, inhibits androgen reception uptake and also suppresses serum androgen. Used with an oral contraceptive, it appears to be more effective than spironolactone in improving hirsutism, acne, and male pattern baldness. Hepatotoxicity has been reported but is rare.

(5) Oral contraceptives stimulate menses, if desired, but are less effective for hirsutism. Contraceptives with low-androgenic progestins (desogestrel, gestodene) may be tried.

(6) Metformin, 500–1000 mg twice daily, in women with polycystic ovary syndrome and amenorrhea tends to restore normal menses and reduce hirsutism. It is contraindicated in renal disease. Gastrointestinal side effects are usually tolerable. Metformin can be taken by nondiabetics without causing hypoglycemia.

(7) Local treatment by shaving or depilatories, waxing, electrolysis, or bleaching should be encouraged.

Note: Antiandrogen treatments must be given only to nonpregnant women. Women must be counseled to take oral contraceptives, when indicated, and avoid pregnancy, since use during pregnancy causes malformations and pseudohermaphroditism in male infants.

Elting MW et al: Women with polycystic ovaries gain regular menstrual cycles when aging. Hum Reprod 2000; 15:24. [NLM Cit ID: 20079187]

Glueck CJ et al: Metformin-induced resumption of normal menses in 19 of 23 (83%) previously amenorrheic women with polycystic ovary syndrome. J Invest Med 1998;46:208A.

Goldberg DJ: Unwanted hair: evaluation and treatment with lasers and light source technology. Adv Dermatol 1999;14:115. [NLM Cit ID: 20108109]

Michelmore KF et al: Polycystic ovaries and associated clinical and biochemical features in young women. Clin Endocrinol 1999;51:779. [NLM Cit ID: 20086804] (Women with polycystic ovaries were 20% more prone to irregular menses but did not have increases in acne, hirsutism, or body mass index when compared with those showing no ovarian cysts on ultrasound.)

Tartagni M et al: Comparison of Diane 35 and Diane 35 plus finasteride in the treatment of hirsutism. Fertil Steril 2000;73:718. [NLM Cit ID: 20198098] (Diane 35 is an oral contraceptive with 35 μg ethinyl estradiol and 2 mg cyproterone acetate, an anti-androgen progestin. Combining this treatment with finasteride 5 mg/d for 2 weeks monthly led to rapid improvement in hirsutism.)

PRIMARY HYPERALDOSTERONISM

Essentials of Diagnosis

- Hypertension, polyuria, polydipsia, muscular weakness.
- Hypokalemia, alkalosis.
- Elevated plasma and urine aldosterone levels and low plasma renin level.

General Considerations

Classic hyperaldosteronism (with hypokalemia) accounts for about 0.7% of cases of hypertension; milder hyperaldosteronism is more frequent. The disorder is more common in females. Primary hyperaldosteronism may be due to unilateral adrenocortical adenoma (Conn's syndrome, 73%) or bilateral cortical hyperplasia (27%), which may be glucocorticoid-suppressible due to an autosomal dominant genetic defect allowing ACTH stimulation of aldosterone production.

Clinical Findings

A. Symptoms and Signs: Hypertension, muscular weakness (at times with paralysis simulating periodic paralysis), paresthesias with frank tetany, headache, polyuria, and polydipsia are the main complaints. Hypertension is typically moderate. Some patients have only diastolic hypertension, without other symptoms and signs. Malignant hypertension is rare. Edema is rarely seen in primary hyperaldosteronism.

B. Laboratory Findings: For a patient to be properly tested for hyperaldosteronism, all antihypertensive medications must be discontinued. Calcium channel blockers can normalize aldosterone secretion, thus interfering with the diagnosis. The patient must have a high sodium intake (> 120 meq/d) during the entire evaluation period; serum potassium is low. A 24-hour urine collection is assayed for aldosterone, free cortisol, and creatinine. A low plasma renin activity (<5 μg/dL) with 24-hour urine aldosterone over 20 μg indicates hyperaldosteronism. A urine aldosterone of less than 20 μg/24 h is seen with rare adrenal or gonadal enzyme defects in the activity of 17α-hydroxylase (associated with ambiguous genitalia or primary amenorrhea) or 11β-hydroxylase (associated with virilization).

Once hyperaldosteronism is diagnosed, plasma is assayed for 18-hydroxycorticosterone; a level over 85 μg/dL is seen with adrenal neoplasms, whereas levels under 85 μg/dL are nondiagnostic. Additionally, plasma can be assayed for aldosterone at 8 AM while the patient is supine after overnight recumbency and again after 4 hours upright. Patients with an adrenal adenoma usually have a baseline plasma aldosterone greater than 20 μg/dL which does not rise. Patients with hyperplasia typically have a baseline plasma aldosterone less than 20 μg/dL which rises during upright posture. Exceptions occur.

C. Imaging: If biochemical testing implicates an adrenal aldosterone-secreting adenoma, a thin-section CT scan of the adrenals is obtained. A discrete adrenal adenoma (> 1 cm in diameter with normal contralateral adrenal) is found is 60–80% of such patients. However, about 20% of such "adenomas" are found to be hyperplasia at surgery. Therefore, it is prudent to supplement CT localization with either adrenal vein catheterization for aldosterone or a dexamethasone-suppressed adrenal scan using ^{131}I-labeled 6β-iodomethyl-19-norcholesterol.

Differential Diagnosis

The differential diagnosis of hyperaldosteronism includes other causes of hypokalemia (see Chapter 21) in patients with essential hypertension. For example, many hypertensive patients taking diuretics develop hypokalemia even while taking potassium-sparing diuretics or potassium supplements. Chronic depletion of intravascular volume stimulates renin secretion and secondary hyperaldosteronism. Thus, it is important to discontinue diuretics and ensure adequate hydration and sodium intake when assessing a patient for primary hyperaldosteronism (see above).

Excessive ingestion of real licorice (black and derived from anise) may produce hypertension and hypokalemia caused by a derivative of its glycyrrhizinic acid inhibiting 11β-hydroxysteroid dehydrogenase, thereby enhancing cortisol's mineralocorticoid effect. Oral contraceptives may increase aldosterone secretion in some patients. Renal vascular disease can cause severe hypertension with hypokalemia; plasma renin activity is high, distinguishing it from primary hyperaldosteronism.

Excessive adrenal secretion of other corticosteroids (besides aldosterone) may also cause hypertension with hypokalemia. This occurs with certain congenital adrenal enzyme disorders such as P450c11 deficiency (increased deoxycorticosterone with virilization and deficient cortisol) or P450c17 deficiency (increased deoxycorticosterone, corticosterone, and progesterone but deficient estradiol and testosterone). Primary cortisol resistance can cause hypertension and hypokalemia; renin and aldosterone are suppressed, while plasma levels of cortisol, ACTH, and deoxycorticosterone are high. Liddle's syndrome is an autosomal dominant cause of hypertension and hypokalemia resulting from excessive sodium absorption from the renal tubule; renin and aldosterone levels are low. Hyperaldosteronism may rarely be due to a malignant ovarian tumor.

Complications

All of the complications of chronic hypertension are encountered in primary hyperaldosteronism. Progressive renal damage is less reversible than hypertension.

Treatment

Conn's syndrome (unilateral adrenal adenoma secreting aldosterone) is treated by laparoscopic adrenalectomy, though lifelong spironolactone therapy is an option. Bilateral adrenal hyperplasia is best treated with spironolactone; bilateral adrenalectomy corrects the hypokalemia but not the hypertension and should *not* be performed. Antihypertensive agents may also be necessary. Hyperplasia sometimes responds well to dexamethasone suppression.

Prognosis

The hypertension is reversible in about two-thirds of cases but persists or returns in spite of surgery in the remainder. The prognosis is much improved by early diagnosis and treatment. Only 2% of aldosterone-secreting adrenal tumors are malignant.

The low renin levels found in this condition (and in about 25% of cases of essential hypertension) also confer a relatively good prognosis.

Brown MJ et al: Calcium-channel blockade can mask the diagnosis of Conn's syndrome. Postgrad Med J 1999;75:235. [NLM Cit ID: 20180658]

Ganguly A: Primary aldosteronism. N Engl J Med 1998; 339:1828. [NLM Cit ID: 99061028]

Harper R et al: Accuracy of CT scanning and adrenal vein sampling in the pre-operative localization of aldosterone-secreting adrenal adenomas. QJM 1999;92:643. [NLM Cit ID: 20113084]

Young WF Jr: Pheochromocytoma and primary aldosteronism: Diagnostic approaches. Endocrinol Metab Clin North Am 1997;26:801. [NLM Cit ID: 98091696]

DISEASES OF THE ADRENAL MEDULLA

PHEOCHROMOCYTOMA

Essentials of Diagnosis

- "Attacks" of headache, perspiration, palpitations.
- Hypertension, frequently sustained but often paroxysmal, especially during surgery or delivery.

- Attacks of nausea, abdominal pain, chest pain, weakness, dyspnea, tremor, visual disturbance.
- Anxiety, tremor, weight loss, or heat intolerance.
- Elevated urinary catecholamines or their metabolites. Normal serum T_4 and TSH.

General Considerations

Pheochromocytomas are rare, being found in less than 0.1% of hypertensive individuals. The incidence is higher in patients with moderate to severe hypertension. About two new cases per million population are discovered annually. The hypertension is caused by excessive plasma levels of norepinephrine or neuropeptide Y. Patients have disease characterized by paroxysmal or sustained hypertension due to a tumor located in either or both adrenals or anywhere along the sympathetic nervous chain, and rarely in such aberrant locations as the thorax, bladder, or brain. Primary extra-adrenal pheochromocytomas are known as "paragangliomas." Pheochromocytomas are characterized by a rough "rule of tens": About 10% of cases are not associated with hypertension; 10% are extra-adrenal, and of those about 10% are extra-abdominal; 10% occur in children; most tumors are sporadic, with only 10–15% familial; in about 10%, the tumor involves both adrenal glands (bilateral adrenal tumors tend to occur more frequently in familial cases); and about 10% have metastatic disease noted around the time of diagnosis. Initially occult metastases are later discovered in another 5%.

Familial pheochromocytoma may be associated with the following: calcitonin-secreting medullary thyroid carcinoma and hyperparathyroidism (multiple endocrine neoplasia type 2); medullary thyroid carcinoma and the syndrome of multiple mucosal neuromas (multiple endocrine neoplasia type 2b); neurofibromatosis (Recklinghausen's disease); and islet cell tumors (rare).

Pheochromocytomas develop in about 20% of patients with von Hippel-Lindau disease (hemangiomas of the retina, cerebellum, brainstem, and spinal cord; pancreatic cysts; renal cysts, adenomas and carcinomas); inheritance is autosomal dominant.

Clinical Findings

A. Symptoms and Signs: Pheochromocytoma typically causes attacks of severe headache (80%), perspiration (70%), and palpitations (60%); other symptoms may include anxiety (50%), a sense of impending doom, or tremor (40%). Vasomotor changes (including facial pallor) may occur, along with tachycardia, precordial or abdominal pain, vomiting, increasing nervousness and irritability, increased appetite, and loss of weight. Anginal attacks may occur. Physical findings usually include hypertension (90%), which may be sustained (20%), sustained with paroxysms (50%), or paroxysmal only (25%). There may be cardiac enlargement; postural tachycardia (change of more than 20 beats/min) and postural hypotension; and mild elevation of basal body temperature. Retinal hemorrhage or cerebrovascular hemorrhage occurs occasionally.

The manifestations of pheochromocytoma are quite varied. Besides the above symptoms, some patients can present with psychosis or confusion, seizures, hyperglycemia, bradycardia, hypotension, paresthesias, or Raynaud's phenomenon. Other patients may have pulmonary edema and heart failure due to cardiomyopathy. Epinephrine secretion may cause episodic hypotension or syncope. Other patients may be entirely asymptomatic despite high serum levels of catecholamines. Some patients present with abdominal discomfort due to a pheochromocytoma presenting as a large abdominal mass.

Besides catecholamines and their metabolites, pheochromocytomas secrete a wide range of other peptides that can sometimes cause Cushing's syndrome (ACTH), erythrocytosis (erythropoietin), or hypercalcemia (parathyroid-related peptide; PthRP). Serum chromogranin A is elevated in 90% and can serve as a tumor marker.

B. Laboratory Findings: Hypermetabolism is present; thyroid function tests are normal, including serum T_4, free T_4, T_3, and TSH. Hyperglycemia is present in about 35% but is usually mild. Leukocytosis is common The erythrocyte sedimentation rate is sometimes elevated.

C. Special Tests:

1. Assay of urinary catecholamines (total and fractionated), metanephrines, vanillylmandelic acid (VMA), and creatinine detects most pheochromocytomas, especially when samples are obtained during or immediately following an episodic attack. A 24-hour urine specimen is usually obtained, although an overnight or shorter collection may be used: patients with pheochromocytomas generally have more that 2.2 μg of metanephrine per milligram of creatinine, and more than 135 μg total catecholamines per gram creatinine.

Testing for catecholamines should be done using high-performance liquid chromatography with electrochemical detection (HPLC-ECD); this minimizes false test results. Nevertheless, some drugs and foods can interfere with certain assays, and stresses can also cause misleading elevations in catecholamine excretion (Table 26–13).

2. Direct assay of epinephrine and norepinephrine in blood and urine during or following an attack is the most sensitive test for pheochromocytoma associated with paroxysmal hypertension. High epinephrine levels favor tumor localization within the adrenal gland. Proper, quiet collection of plasma specimens is essential.

3. Imaging should not replace biochemical testing since incidental adrenal adenomas are common (2–4% of scans) and can be misleading. CT scanning of the adrenals will detect the pheochromocytoma in 90% of cases. If no adrenal tumor is found, the CT scan

Table 26–13. Factors potientially causing misleading catecholamine or metanephrine results: High pressure liquid chromatography with electrochemical detection (HPLC-ECD).

Drugs	Foods	Conditions
Acetaminophen[2]	Bananas[1]	Amyotrophic lateral sclerosis[1]
Aldomet[2]	Caffeine[1]	Brain lesions[1]
Amphetamines[1]	Coffee[2]	Carcinoid[1]
Bronchodilators[1]	Peppers[2]	Eclampsia[1]
Buspirone[2]		Emotion, severe[1]
Captopril[2]		Exercise, vigorous[1]
Cocaine[1]		Guillain-Barré syndrome[1]
Cimetidine[2]		Hypoglycemia[1]
Codeine[2]		Lead poisoning[1]
Decongestants[1]		Myocardial infarct, acute[1]
Ephedrine[1]		Pain, severe[1]
Fenfluramine[3]		Porphyria, acute[1]
Isoproterenol[1]		Psychosis, acute[1]
Levodopa[2]		Quadriplegia[1]
Labetalol[1,2]		Renal failure[3]
Mendelamine[2]		
Metoclopramide[2]		
Nitroglycerine[1]		
Vilozaxine[2]		

[1]Increases catecholamine excretion.
[2]May cause confounding peaks on HPLC chromatograms.
[3]Decreases catecholamine excretion.

is extended to include the entire abdomen, pelvis, and chest. A whole body ^{123}I MIBG scan can localize tumors with a sensitivity of 85% and a specificity of 99%. MRI can visualize suspected bone metastases.

4. Pharmacologic provocative and suppressive tests that evaluate the rise or fall in blood pressure are usually not required or recommended.

Differential Diagnosis

Tachycardia, tremor, palpitation, and hypermetabolism may give rise to confusion with thyrotoxicosis. Pheochromocytoma may also be misdiagnosed as essential hypertension, myocarditis, glomerulonephritis or other renal lesions, toxemia of pregnancy, eclampsia, and psychoneurosis (anxiety attack). It can sometimes be mistaken for an acute abdomen.

Other conditions that have manifestations similar to those of pheochromocytoma include acute intermittent porphyria, hypogonadal vascular instability (hot flushes), cocaine or amphetamine use, clonidine withdrawal, hypertensive crisis caused by foods containing tyramine (eg, cheeses) in patients taking MAO inhibitor antidepressants, labile hypertension, and unstable angina.

False-positive testing for catecholamines and metabolites occurs in about 10% of hypertensives, but levels are usually less than 50% above normal and typically normalize with repeat testing.

Complications

All of the complications of severe hypertension may be encountered. Hypertensive crises with sudden blindness or cerebrovascular accidents are not uncommon. These may be precipitated by sudden movement, by manipulation during or after pregnancy, by emotional stress or trauma, or during surgical removal of the tumor. Cardiomyopathy may develop. Occasionally, the initial manifestation of pheochromocytoma may be hypotension or even shock.

After removal of the tumor, a state of severe hypotension and shock (resistant to epinephrine and norepinephrine) may ensue with precipitation of renal failure or myocardial infarction. Hypotension and shock may occur from spontaneous infarction or hemorrhage of the tumor; emergency surgical removal of the tumor is necessary in these cases.

On rare occasions, a patient dies as a result of the complications of diagnostic tests or during surgery. No patient with suspected pheochromocytoma should be subjected either to an invasive diagnostic procedure or to surgery unless there has been adequate alpha blockade with phenoxybenzamine.

Treatment

Laparoscopic removal of the tumor or tumors is the treatment of choice. Very large and invasive tumors are treated with open laparotomy. Preoperative administration of α-adrenergic blocking drugs has made pheochromocytoma surgery a great deal safer in recent years. Give phenoxybenzamine, 10 mg orally every 12 hours, and increase the dose gradually—about every 3 days—until hypertension is controlled. The usual maintenance dose is 40–120 mg daily. Optimal alpha blockade is achieved when supine arterial pressure is below 160/90 mm Hg and standing arterial pressure is above 80/45 mm Hg. Calcium channel blockers can also be effective and are better-tolerated than alpha-blockers.

After appropriate antihypertensive therapy, the beta-blocker propranolol (10–40 mg four times daily) can be employed to control tachycardia and other arrhythmias. Maintain blood pressure control for a minimum of 4–7 days or until optimal cardiac status is established. Monitor the ECG until it becomes stable. (It may take a week or even months to correct electrocardiographic changes in patients with catecholamine myocarditis, and it is prudent to defer surgery until then in such cases.) Patients must be very closely monitored during surgery in order to promptly detect sudden changes in blood pressure or cardiac arrhythmias.

Hypertensive crisis can initially be managed with sublingual administration of nifedipine 10 mg (pierced capsule). Intraoperative severe hypertension is managed with continuous intravenous nicardipine (a short-acting calcium channel blocker), 2–6 μg/kg/min; or nitroprusside, 0.5–10 μg/kg/min. Tachyarrhythmia is treated with intravenous atenolol (1 mg boluses), esmolol, or lidocaine.

Autotransfusion of 1–2 units of blood at 12 hours preoperatively plus generous intraoperative volume replacement reduces the risk of postresection hypotension caused by desensitization of the vascular α_1 receptors. Shock may therefore occur following removal of the pheochromocytoma. It is treated with intravenous saline or colloid and high doses of intravenous norepinephrine. Intravenous 5% dextrose is infused postoperatively to prevent hypoglycemia.

Since there may be multiple or metastatic tumors, it is essential to recheck urinary catecholamine levels postoperatively (1–2 weeks after surgery). Thereafter, blood pressure and symptoms must be rechecked regularly; urinary catecholamines and metanephrines are rechecked postoperatively and if hypertension or symptoms recur or if metastases are evident.

For inoperable or metastatic tumors, metyrosine may be added to reduce catecholamine synthesis. Metyrosine is a competitive blocker in the synthesis of catecholamines that is also useful; the initial dosage is 250 mg four times daily, increased daily by increments of 250–500 mg to a maximum of 4 g/d. Metastatic pheochromocytomas may be treated with combination chemotherapy (eg, cyclophosphamide, vincristine, and dacarbazine) or with high doses of ^{131}I MIBG, which is available at some medical centers.

Prognosis

The prognosis depends upon how early the diagnosis is made. The malignancy of a pheochromocytoma cannot be determined by histologic examination. A tumor is considered malignant if metastases are present; this may take many years to become clinically evident. If the tumor is successfully removed before irreparable damage to the cardiovascular system has occurred, a complete cure is usually achieved. Complete cure (or improvement) may follow removal of a tumor that has been present for many years. In about 25%, hypertension persists or returns in spite of successful surgery. Although this may be essential hypertension, biochemical reevaluation is then required, looking for a second or metastatic pheochromocytoma.

Before the advent of blocking agents, the surgical mortality rate was as high as 30%, but this has rapidly decreased. The importance of a team approach—endocrinologist, anesthesiologist, and surgeon—cannot be overemphasized. With optimal management, the surgical mortality rate is less than 3%.

Patients with metastatic pheochromocytoma have a 50% 5-year survival rate; however, prolonged survivals do occur.

Colson P et al: Haemodynamic heterogeneity and treatment with the calcium channel blocker nicardipine during phaeochromocytoma surgery. Acta Anaesthesiol Scand 1998;42:1114. [NLM Cit ID: 99026627]

Januszewicz W et al: Alterations in plasma neuropeptide Y immunoreactivity and catecholamine levels during surgical removal of pheochromocytoma. J Hypertens 1998; 16:543. [NLM Cit ID: 99011225]

Loh KC et al: The treatment of malignant pheochromocytoma with iodine-131 metaiodobenzylguanidine (^{131}I-MIBG): A comprehensive review of 116 reported patients. J Endocrinol Invest 1997;20:648. [NLM Cit ID: 98151067]

Peaston RT et al: Overnight excretion of urinary catecholamines and metabolites in the detection of pheochromocytoma. J Clin Endocrinol Metab 1996;81:1378. [NLM Cit ID 96186135] (Compared with 24-hour results, overnight urinary norepinephrine levels provided a better diagnostic sensitivity [100%] and specificity [98%].)

PANCREATIC NEUROENDOCRINE TUMORS*

ISLET CELL TUMORS

Essentials of Diagnosis

- Half the tumors are nonsecretory, and patients present with weight loss, abdominal pain, or jaundice.
- Secretory tumors cause a variety of manifestations depending upon the hormones secreted.

General Considerations

The pancreatic islets are composed of several types of cells, each with distinct chemical and microscopic features: the A cells (20%) secrete glucagon, the B cells (70%) secrete insulin, and the D cells (5%) secrete somatostatin or gastrin. F cells secrete "pancreatic polypeptide." Each type of cell may give rise to benign or malignant neoplasms that may be multiple and usually present with a clinical syndrome related to hypersecretion of a native or ectopic hormonal product. The endocrine diagnosis of a particular pancreatic islet neoplasm depends upon first suspecting it from its clinical manifestations. Many tumors secrete two or more different hormones.

Insulinomas are usually (about 85%) benign and secrete excessive amounts of insulin (as well as proinsulin and C-peptide), which causes hypoglycemia. The tumors may be multiple, especially in familial cases of MEN type 1.

Gastrinomas are generally benign and secrete excessive gastrin (as well as "big" gastrin), which stimulates the stomach to hypersecrete acid, thereby causing peptic ulceration (Zollinger-Ellison syndrome). About 25% are ultimately found to have multiple endocrine neoplasia, with hyperparathyroidism occurring from

*Diabetes mellitus is discussed in Chapter 27.

testes must also be carefully palpated for masses, since Leydig cell tumors may secrete estrogen and present with hypogonadism. The testicles must be carefully examined for evidence of trauma, infiltrative lesions (eg, lymphoma), or ongoing infection (eg, leprosy, tuberculosis).

B. Laboratory Findings: The hemoglobin and hematocrit may be slightly below the male range due to hypogonadism.

To evaluate a man for hypogonadism, the morning serum total testosterone concentration is determined. Normal ranges for serum testosterone have been derived from nonfasting morning blood specimens, which tend to be the highest of the day. Later in the day, serum testosterone levels are 25–50% lower, especially in older men. Therefore, a serum testosterone drawn fasting or late in the day may be misleadingly below the "normal range." Serum testosterone levels in men are highest at age 20–30 years and slightly lower at age 30–40 years; testosterone falls gradually but progressively after age 40 years. Elderly men have higher levels of SHBG, with consequently lower levels of free testosterone. The electrochemical luminescence assay for measuring serum total testosterone suffers interference in hyperlipidemic patients.

Serum free testosterone levels are low in hypogonadism. Different assay methodologies for free testosterone are in use. Assays employing equilibrium dialysis, calculated free testosterone, and non SHBG-bound testosterone are reasonably accurate. However, the free androgen index and analog free testosterone assays are inaccurate.

In patients with low or borderline-low serum testosterone levels, serum LH and FSH should be measured. LH and FSH tend to be high in patients with hypergonadotropic hypogonadism but low or inappropriately normal in men with hypogonadotropic hypogonadism. Bone densitometry may be reduced in long-standing male hypogonadism.

1. Hypogonadotropic hypogonadism–Men with hypogonadotropic hypogonadism have low serum testosterone levels without a compensatory increase in gonadotropins. A serum prolactin determination is obtained but may be elevated for many reasons (Table 26–4). Men with gynecomastia may be screened for partial 17-ketosteroid reductase deficiency with serum determinations for androstenedione and estrone, which are elevated in this condition. The serum estradiol level may be elevated in patients with cirrhosis and in rare cases of estrogen-secreting tumors (testicular Leydig cell tumor or adrenal carcinoma). Men with no discernible definite cause for hypogonadotropic hypogonadism should have an MRI of the pituitary and hypothalamic region to look for a tumor or other lesion. (See Hypopituitarism.)

2. Hypergonadotropic hypogonadism–Men with hypergonadotropic hypogonadism have low serum testosterone levels with a compensatory increase in gonadotropins. Klinefelter's syndrome can be confirmed by karyotyping or by measurement of leukocyte X-inactive-specific transcriptase (XIST). Testicular biopsy is usually reserved for younger patients in whom the reason for primary hypogonadism is unclear.

Treatment

Before treating hypogonadism in men over 40 years of age, it is prudent to screen for prostate cancer. Hypogonadism is usually treated with parenteral testosterone (enanthate or cypionate). The usual dose is about 300 mg intramuscularly every 3 weeks or 200 mg every 2 weeks. The preparation is oil-based and is usually given in the gluteal area. The dose is adjusted according to the patient's response. Oral androgen preparations include methyltestosterone and fluoxymesterone. These oral preparations have rarely caused liver tumors or peliosis hepatis with long-term use. Cholestatic jaundice occurs in 1–2% but usually remits after the medication is discontinued. The oral androgens are not as effective as parenteral testosterone.

Testosterone transdermal systems (skin patches) are available in two formulations for application to nongenital skin. The testosterone may be mixed with the adhesive (eg, Testoderm II, 5 mg/d) with a new patch applied daily to a different site; this system leaves a sticky residue but causes little skin irritation. A different patch uses testosterone in a reservoir system applied to skin (eg, Androderm); this system adheres more tightly to the skin but may cause more skin irritation. Both produce reliable serum levels of testosterone which are somewhat lower that those achieved with injections.

Topical 1% testosterone gel is commercially available as Androgel (2.5 g and 5 g packets). The starting dose is 5 g (50 mg testosterone) applied once daily to clean, dry skin of the shoulders, upper arms, or abdomen. The gel should not be applied to the genitals. The entire contents of a packet are squeezed onto the palm and then immediately applied. The hands should be washed and the application site allowed to dry for 3–5 minutes before dressing. A shirt must be worn during contact with women or children to prevent transfer of testosterone to them. The serum testosterone level should be determined about 14 days after starting therapy; if the level remains below normal or the clinical response is inadequate, the dose may be increased to 7.5 g or 10 g.

Side effects of any testosterone therapy may include acne, gynecomastia, and reduced HDL levels.

Men with hypogonadism due to endocrine therapy for prostate cancer usually develop severe hot flushes. Symptomatic relief can be obtained with the progestational agent megestrol acetate, 20 mg orally twice daily. Megestrol has some glucocorticoid-like activity and tends to increase appetite and cause weight gain. Hyperglycemia and hypertriglyceridemia may occur, so the dosage should be kept minimal.

Men with hypogonadotropic hypogonadism must receive further evaluation and specific treatment (see Hypopituitarism).

Prognosis of Hypogonadism

If hypogonadism is due to a pituitary lesion, the prognosis is that of the primary disease (eg, tumor, necrosis). The prognosis for restoration of virility is good if testosterone is given.

Androgel. Med Lett Drugs Ther 2000;42:49. [NLM Cit ID: 20318866] (After application of 1% testosterone gel, the skin serves as a reservoir which slowly releases about 10% of the testosterone into the blood. During once-daily application of 10 g gel (100 mg testosterone), serum testosterone levels rise to normal within 2–4 hours and reach a steady state in 1–3 days. Side effects in men receiving the 10 g dose daily for 1 year included acne in 12% and prostate disorders (elevated PSA or enlarged glands; one new case of cancer) in 18%. Vigorous daily skin-to-skin contact for 15 minutes 2–12 hours after testosterone gel application leads to over two times the basal testosterone levels in female partners. Wearing a shirt over the application area prevents this, but the transferability to women and children is a concern. This preparation is significantly more expensive than testosterone patches.)

Katznelson L et al: Increase in bone density and lean body mass during testosterone administration in men with acquired hypogonadism. J Clin Endocrinol Metab 1996;81: 4358. [NLM Cit ID: 97112362] (The beneficial effects of androgen administration on body composition and bone density may provide additional indications for testosterone therapy in hypogonadal men.)

Morales A et al: Andropause: a misnomer for a true clinical entity. J Urol 2000;163:705. [NLM Cit ID: 20150669]

Smyth CM et al: Klinefelter syndrome. Arch Intern Med 1998;158:1309. [NLM Cit ID: 98307756]

Wang C et al: Pharmacokinetics of transdermal testosterone gel in hypogonadal men: application of gel at one site versus four sites: a general clinical research study. J Clin Endocrinol Metab 2000;85:964. [NLM Cit ID: 20182943] (Nine hypogonadal men applied 100 mg testosterone gel either all at one skin site or over a larger total skin area at four skin sites. Serum testosterone levels were only slightly higher following application to the larger skin area.)

TESTICULAR TUMORS IN ADULTS (See also Chapter 23.)

About 95% of testicular tumors are germ cell tumors (seminomas or nonseminomas). They may produce (as serum markers) hCG and alpha-fetoprotein. Seminomas do not produce alpha-fetoprotein, but about 5–10% produce some hCG; nonseminomas, on the other hand, produce increased serum levels of one or both of these markers in about 90% of cases. Men with liver disease may have misleadingly high levels of alpha-fetoprotein.

About 5% of testicular tumors are Leydig or Sertoli cell tumors. Leydig cell tumors tend to produce estrogen (75%) and cause gynecomastia and impotence on that basis; they may sometimes produce androgens that can cause pseudoprecocious puberty in boys. Sertoli cell tumors may also produce estrogen (30%) with feminization; gynecomastia may be due to hCG secretion (25%).

Some testicular tumors may be small and nonpalpable yet may secrete sufficient amounts of hCG or estrogen to cause gynecomastia or impotence. Testicular ultrasound may help reveal small tumors.

After unilateral orchiectomy for testicular cancer, an elevated FSH level prior to further treatment indicates a patient at higher risk for cancer in the remaining testis.

Horwich A et al: Markers and management of germ-cell tumors of the testes. Lancet 1998;352:1535. [NLM Cit ID: 99036204]

Nichols CR: Testicular cancer. Curr Probl Cancer 1998; 22:187. [NLM Cit ID: 98414020] (A comprehensive review.)

AMENORRHEA & MENOPAUSE (See also Chapter 17.)

PRIMARY AMENORRHEA

Menarche ordinarily occurs between ages 11 and 15 years (average in USA: 12.7 years). The failure of any menses to appear is termed primary amenorrhea, and evaluation is commenced (1) at age 14 if neither menarche nor breast development has occurred or if height is in the lowest 3%, or (2) at age 16 if menarche has not occurred.

Etiology

The causes of primary amenorrhea include the following:

A. Hypothalamic-Pituitary Causes (With Low-Normal FSH): A genetic deficiency of GnRH and gonadotropins may be isolated or associated with other pituitary deficiencies or diminished olfaction (Kallmann's syndrome). Hypothalamic lesions, particularly craniopharyngioma, may be present. Pituitary tumors may be nonsecreting or may secrete prolactin or growth hormone. Cushing's syndrome may be caused by glucocorticoid treatment, a cortisol-secreting adrenal tumor, or an ACTH-secreting pituitary tumor. Hypothyroidism can delay adolescence. Head trauma or encephalitis can cause gonadotropin deficiency. Primary amenorrhea may also be caused by constitutional delay of adolescence, organic illness, vigorous exercise (eg, ballet dancing, running), stressful life events, dieting, or anorexia nervosa; however, these conditions should not be assumed to account for amenorrhea without a full physical and endocrinologic evaluation. (See section on hypopituitarism.)

B. Hyperandrogenism (With Low-Normal FSH): Excess testosterone may be secreted by adrenal tumors or by adrenal hyperplasia caused by steroidogenic enzyme defects such as P450c21 deficiency (salt-wasting) or P450c11 deficiency (hypertension). Ovarian tumors or polycystic ovaries may also secrete excess testosterone. Androgenic steroids may also cause this syndrome.

C. Ovarian Causes (With High FSH): Gonadal dysgenesis (Turner's syndrome and variants; see below) is a frequent cause of primary amenorrhea. Ovarian failure due to autoimmunity is a common cause. Rare deficiencies in certain ovarian steroidogenic enzymes are causes of primary hypogonadism without virilization: 3β-hydroxysteroid dehydrogenase deficiency (adrenal insufficiency with low serum 17-hydroxyprogesterone) and P450c17 deficiency (hypertension and hypokalemia with high serum 17-hydroxyprogesterone). A whole-body deficiency in P450arom activity produces female hypogonadism associated with polycystic ovaries, tall stature, osteoporosis, and virilization.

D. Pseudohermaphroditism (With High LH): An enzymatic defect in testosterone synthesis may present as a sexually immature phenotypic girl with primary amenorrhea. Complete androgen resistance (testicular feminization) presents as a phenotypic young woman without sexual hair but with normal breast development and primary amenorrhea. In both cases, the uterus is absent and testes are intra-abdominal or cryptorchid. Intra-abdominal testes are surgically resected. Such patients are treated as normal but infertile, hypogonadal women.

E. Uterine Causes (With Normal FSH): Congenital absence or malformation of the uterus may be responsible for primary amenorrhea, as may an unresponsive or atrophic endometrium. An imperforate hymen is occasionally the reason for the absence of visible menses.

F. Pregnancy (With High hCG): Pregnancy may be the cause of primary amenorrhea even when the patient denies ever having had sexual intercourse.

Clinical Findings

A. Symptoms and Signs: Patients with primary amenorrhea require a thorough history and physical examination to look for signs of the conditions noted above. Headaches or visual field abnormalities implicate a hypothalamic or pituitary tumor. Signs of pregnancy may be present. Blood pressure abnormalities, acne, and hirsutism should be noted. Short stature may be seen with an associated growth hormone or thyroid hormone deficiency. Short stature with manifestations of gonadal dysgenesis indicates Turner's syndrome (see below). Olfaction testing screens for Kallmann's syndrome. Obesity and short stature may be signs of Cushing's syndrome. Tall stature may be due to eunuchoidism or gigantism. Hirsutism or virilization suggests excessive testosterone.

An external pelvic examination plus a rectal examination should be performed to assess hymenal patency and the presence of a uterus.

B. Laboratory Findings: The initial endocrine evaluation should include serum determinations of FSH, LH, PRL, testosterone, TSH, free T_4, and hCG (pregnancy test). Patients who are virilized or hypertensive require serum electrolyte determinations and further hormonal evaluation. Girls with low-normal FSH and LH—especially those with high PRL levels—are evaluated by MRI of the hypothalamus and pituitary. Girls who have a normal uterus and high FSH without the classic features of Turner's syndrome may require a karyotype to diagnose X chromosome mosaicism.

Treatment

Treatment of primary amenorrhea is directed at the underlying cause. Girls with permanent hypogonadism are treated with estrogen replacement therapy (see below).

SECONDARY AMENORRHEA

Secondary amenorrhea is defined as absence of menses for 3 consecutive months in women who have passed menarche.

Etiology

The causes of secondary amenorrhea include the following:

A. Pregnancy (High hCG): Pregnancy is the most common cause for secondary amenorrhea in women of childbearing age. The differential diagnosis includes rare ectopic secretion of hCG by a choriocarcinoma or bronchogenic carcinoma.

B. Hypothalamic-Pituitary Causes (With Low-Normal FSH): Prolactin elevation due to any cause (see section on hyperprolactinemia) may cause amenorrhea. Pituitary tumors or other lesions may cause hypopituitarism. Glucocorticoid excess of any cause suppresses gonadotropins. Patients with signs of adrenal insufficiency require a cosyntropin stimulation test (see section on adrenal insufficiency).

Secondary "hypothalamic" amenorrhea may be caused by stressful life events such as school examinations or leaving home. Such women usually have a history of normal sexual development and irregular menses since menarche. Amenorrhea may also be the result of strict dieting, vigorous exercise, organic illness, or anorexia nervosa. These conditions should not be assumed to account for amenorrhea without a full physical and endocrinologic evaluation. Young women in whom the results of evaluation and progestin withdrawal test are normal have noncyclic secretion of gonadotropins resulting in anovulation. Such women typically recover spontaneously but should have regular evaluations and a progestin withdrawal test about every 3 months to detect loss of estrogen effect.

C. Hyperandrogenism (With Low-Normal FSH): Elevated serum levels of testosterone can cause hirsutism, virilization, and amenorrhea. The cause is typically polycystic ovary syndrome or, less commonly, adrenal P450c21 deficiency. Rare causes include ovarian or adrenal malignancies, ectopic ACTH secretion by a malignancy, and Cushing's disease. Anabolic steroids also cause amenorrhea.

D. Uterine Causes (With Normal FSH): Infection of the uterus commonly occurs following delivery or D&C but may occur spontaneously. Endometritis due to tuberculosis or schistosomiasis should be suspected in endemic areas. Endometrial scarring may result, causing amenorrhea (Asherman's syndrome). Such women typically continue to have monthly premenstrual symptoms. The vaginal estrogen effect is normal. Diagnosis and treatment is best done by direct hysteroscopic inspection of the endometrium and lysis of adhesions. A small Foley catheter is left in the uterus for 1 week while antibiotics are given. The catheter is then replaced by an IUD for about 2 months. Cyclic estrogen and progestin is given to build up the endometrial lining. After such treatment, menses usually resume and fertility is possible, but spontaneous abortions and other pregnancy complications occur commonly.

E. Premature Ovarian Failure (High FSH): This refers to primary hypogonadism that occurs before age 40. This affects about 1% of women. About 30% of such cases are due to autoimmunity against the ovary. About 8% of cases are due to X chromosome mosaicism. Other causes include surgical bilateral oophorectomy, radiation therapy for pelvic malignancy, and chemotherapy. Women who have undergone hysterectomy are prone to premature ovarian failure even though the ovaries were left intact. Myotonic dystrophy, galactosemia, and mumps oophoritis are additional causes. Other cases may be familial or idiopathic. Ovarian failure is usually irreversible. Treatment consists of estrogen replacement therapy plus a progestin if the uterus is present.

F. Menopause (High FSH): "Climacteric" is defined as the period of natural physiologic decline in ovarian function, generally occurring over about 10 years. By about age 40, the remaining ovarian follicles are those that are the least sensitive to gonadotropins. Increasing titers of FSH are required to stimulate estradiol secretion. Estradiol levels may actually rise during early climacteric. Frequent anovulation tends to cause menometrorrhagia (dysfunctional uterine bleeding). Fertility declines progressively. Psychologic symptoms may include depression and irritability. Women may experience fatigue, insomnia, headache, diminished libido, or rheumatologic symptoms. Vasomotor instability (hot flushes) are experienced by 80% of women, lasting seconds to many minutes. Hot flushes may be most severe at night or may be triggered by emotional stress. Some women continue to menstruate for many months despite symptoms of estrogen deficiency. Estrogen supplementation provides symptomatic relief.

"Menopause" is defined as the terminal episode of naturally occurring menses. It is a retrospective diagnosis, usually made after 6 months of amenorrhea. The normal age for menopause in the USA ranges between 48 and 55 years, with an average of about 51.5 years. Serum estradiol levels fall and the remaining estrogen after menopause is estrone, derived mainly from peripheral aromatization of adrenal androstenedione. Such peripheral production of estrone is enhanced by obesity and liver disease. Individual differences in estrone levels partly explain why the symptoms noted above may be minimal in some women but severe in others. The acute symptoms of estrogen deficiency noted above tend to decline in severity within several years after menopause. However, about 35% of women have symptoms for more than 5 years. The late manifestations of estrogen deficiency include urogenital atrophy with vaginal dryness and dyspareunia; dysuria, frequency, and incontinence may occur. Increased bone osteoclastic activity increases the risk for osteoporosis and fractures. The skin becomes more wrinkled. Increases in the LDL:HDL cholesterol ratio cause an increased risk for arteriosclerosis.

Clinical Findings

A. Symptoms and Signs: All women with amenorrhea require a complete history and physical examination. Nausea and breast engorgement are typical signs of early pregnancy. Hot flushes are common in ovarian failure. Headache or visual field abnormalities are seen with pituitary or hypothalamic tumors. Complaints of thirst and polyuria require evaluation; diabetes insipidus implicates a hypothalamic lesion. Goiter may be due to hyperthyroidism. Weight loss, diarrhea, or skin darkening may indicate adrenal insufficiency. Weight loss with a distorted body image implicates anorexia nervosa. The breasts are examined carefully for galactorrhea, a common sign of hyperprolactinemia. Hirsutism or virilization may be a sign of hyperandrogenism. Manifestations of hypercortisolism (eg, weakness, psychiatric changes, hypertension, central obesity, hirsutism, thin skin, ecchymoses) may indicate alcoholism or Cushing's syndrome. Signs of acromegaly or gigantism may also indicate a pituitary tumor. Signs of systemic illness (eg, cirrhosis, renal failure) should be appreciated. Various drugs may elevate prolactin and cause amenorrhea (see section on hyperprolactinemia). Needle tracks may indicate heroin or amphetamine abuse.

A careful pelvic examination is always required to check for uterine or adnexal enlargement and to obtain a Papanicolaou smear and a vaginal smear for assessment of estrogen effect. Various life stresses, vigorous exercise, and "crash" dieting all predispose to amenorrhea; however, such factors should not be assumed to account for amenorrhea without a complete workup to screen for other causes.

B. Laboratory Findings: Since pregnancy is the most common cause of amenorrhea, women of childbearing age are immediately screened with a serum or urine hCG (pregnancy test). An elevated hCG overwhelmingly indicates pregnancy; false-positive testing may occur very rarely with ectopic hCG secretion (eg, choriocarcinoma or bronchogenic carcinoma). Women without an elevated hCG receive further laboratory evaluation including serum PRL, FSH, LH, TSH, and plasma potassium. Hyperprolactinemia or hypopituitarism (without obvious cause; see section on hypopituitarism) should prompt an MRI study of the pituitary region. Routine testing for renal and hepatic function (eg, BUN, serum creatinine, bilirubin, alkaline phosphatase, and ALT) is also performed. A serum testosterone level is obtained in hirsute or virilized women. Patients with manifestations of hypercortisolism receive a 1 mg overnight dexamethasone suppression test for initial screening (see section on Cushing's syndrome). Nonpregnant women without any laboratory abnormality may receive a 10-day course of a progestin (eg, medroxyprogesterone acetate, 10 mg/d); absence of withdrawal menses typically indicates a lack of estrogen or a uterine abnormality.

Treatment

Treatment of secondary amenorrhea is directed at the cause. Therapy of hypogonadism generally consists of estrogen replacement therapy (see below). The doses of estrogen required for symptomatic relief from vasomotor symptoms are sometimes higher than typical physiologic replacement doses. If estrogen replacement therapy is declined or contraindicated, partial symptomatic relief from hot flushes may sometimes be afforded by medroxyprogesterone acetate or clonidine. Tamoxifen, an antiestrogen used in breast cancer management, gives some bone protection but no relief from hot flushes. Treatment or prevention of postmenopausal osteoporosis with bisphosphonates such as alendronate (see section on osteoporosis) is another therapeutic option.

Estrogen Replacement Therapy

The goals of estrogen replacement therapy are several:

(1) Replace adequate estrogen to prevent osteoporosis.

(2) Restore menses when the patient wants this for psychologic reasons.

(3) Reduce manifestations of estrogen deficiency such as hot flushes, mood changes, vaginal dryness, urinary incontinence, and skin wrinkling.

(4) Improve serum lipid profile, reducing the risk of cardiovascular disease.

(5) May reduce the risks of Alzheimer's disease and of colon and lung cancer.

Estrogen replacement therapy should begin with the onset of hypogonadism. However, it is not necessary to treat all cases, especially temporary amenorrhea or irregular menses. Patients who have normal menses after a short course of medroxyprogesterone acetate (see above) may have menses induced every 1–3 months in this manner.

Oral estrogen preparations include conjugated equine estrogens (0.3, 0.625, 0.9, 1.25, and 2.5 mg), ethinyl estradiol (20 and 50 μg), estradiol (0.5, 1, and 2 mg), estropipate (0.75, 1.5, and 3 mg), and plant-derived estrogen (eg, Estratab, 0.3, 0.625, 1.25, and 2.5 mg).

Estradiol transdermal systems (skin patches): Estradiol can be delivered systemically with different transdermal systems:

(1) Transdermal systems with estradiol mixed with adhesive: These systems tend to cause minimal skin irritation. Available preparations include the following: Climara (0.05 mg/d or 0.1 mg/d), replaced weekly; Fempatch (0.025 mg/d), replaced weekly; Alora (0.05 mg/d, 0.075 mg/d, or 0.1 mg/d), replaced twice weekly; Vivelle (0.0375 mg/d, 0.05 mg/d, 0.075 mg/d, or 0.1 mg/d), replaced twice weekly.

(2) Transdermal systems with estradiol in a drug reservoir: These systems cause significant skin irritation in some women. Available preparations include Estraderm (0.05 mg/d, or 0.1 mg/d), replaced twice weekly.

(3) Transdermal systems with estradiol (E) and norethindrone acetate (NA) mixed with adhesive: Available preparations include Combipatch (0.05 mg/d E & 0.14 mg/d NA, or 0.05 mg/d E & 0.25 mg/d NA), replaced twice weekly.

Intramuscular estrogen preparations include estradiol cypionate in oil (5 mg/mL; 1–5 mL every 3–4 weeks) and estradiol valerate (10, 20, and 40 mg/mL; 10–20 mg every 3-4 weeks).

Women who have had a hysterectomy may receive estrogen alone on either a continuous or cyclic regimen. Women with an intact uterus may be treated with estrogen (as above) but must also receive a progestin in order to decrease the risk of estrogen-induced endometrial carcinoma. Women receiving unopposed estrogen (conjugated estrogens, 0.625 mg/d or more) have a risk of endometrial carcinoma that is ten times greater than the risk in untreated patients. However, daily conjugated estrogens, 0.3 mg/d, does not appear to cause such an increased risk. The lower estrogen doses also cause less mastalgia, so it is prudent to initiate estrogen at a low dose. The addition of a progestin reduces the risk below that of untreated women. The progestin of choice is medroxyprogesterone acetate. Medroxyprogesterone acetate (5–10 mg) is given on days 16–25 of the calendar month; estrogen is given daily on days 1–25 of the month. Alternatively, medroxyprogesterone may be given as 2.5–5 mg daily with the estrogen; this continuous regimen is initially associated with some breakthrough bleeding, but this declines over time. Another alternative is to give daily estrogen and add medroxyprogesterone, 5 mg/d, for 10 days monthly. Continued abnormal bleeding necessitates a pelvic examination; endometrial biopsy may be done using a Vibra aspiration technique. These regimens can be tailored to the individual's requirements and response.

Long-term estrogen replacement therapy is associated with a significant reduction in the overall mortality of postmenopausal women. This is mainly due to a reduction in cardiovascular deaths, probably caused by both a "healthy user" effect and an improvement in lipoprotein parameters in most women. Serum levels of atherogenic lipoprotein(a) are reduced by estrogen replacement, with or without daily or cycled medroxyprogesterone. Improvement in serum HDL cholesterol is greatest with unopposed estrogen but is also seen with the addition of a progestin. However, in the HERS study, postmenopausal women with established coronary disease who received conjugated estrogens plus progestin were not protected from further coronary events. In that study, women receiving hormone replacement actually had more coronary events in the first year of therapy and fewer events in the fourth and fifth years. Because of these findings, the presence of known coronary artery disease in women is not an indication for beginning hormone replacement therapy.

The effect of long-term estrogen replacement therapy upon the risk of breast cancer is controversial. The overall absolute risk of diagnosed breast cancer is probably increased by about 3% among women taking estrogen replacement therapy for 10 years or longer; however, no increased mortality from breast cancer has been noted. The Nurses' Health Study indicated an increased risk, but only for women who consumed alcohol. The Iowa Women's Health Study reported an increase in breast cancer with estrogen replacement only in women consuming more than 1 oz of alcohol weekly. No accelerated risk of breast cancer has been seen in users of estrogen replacement therapy who have benign breast disease or a family history of breast cancer.

Certain studies suggest that women receiving estrogen replacement therapy have a reduced incidence of Alzheimer's disease and a lower mortality rate from lung and colon cancers. Estrogen replacement also reduces bone loss and the risk of osteoporotic fractures.

Relative contraindications to estrogen replacement therapy include breast cancer, history of thromboembolic disease, seizure disorders, and large pituitary prolactinomas.

Side effects of estrogen replacement may include weight gain, edema, and breast tenderness. There is an increased risk of venous thrombosis with oral estrogen. Oral estrogen therapy may cause hypertriglyceridemia, particularly in patients with preexistent hyperlipidemia, which may rarely result in pancreatitis. Transdermal estrogen replacement appears less likely to worsen hypertriglyceridemia.

Hypogonadal women usually have diminished ovarian androgen secretion. This contributes to hot flushes, loss of libido and sexual hair, muscle atrophy, and osteoporosis. Selected women may be treated with low-dose methyltestosterone, which is available in combination with conjugated estrogens (eg, Estratest). Tablets contain either 1.25 mg conjugated estrogens with 2.5 mg methyltestosterone or 0.625 mg conjugated estrogens with 1.25 mg methyltestosterone. Estratest is usually started at the lowest strength every 2 days, alternating days with standard estrogen replacement (see above). It should be given cyclically at the lowest dose that controls symptoms. At such small doses, side effects are usually minimal but may include nausea, polycythemia, emotional changes, paresthesias, electrolyte disturbances, and potentiation of anticoagulant therapy. Reduction in HDL cholesterol may negate the beneficial effect on cardiovascular mortality conferred by estrogen replacement therapy. Cholestatic jaundice and elevation of liver enzymes occur rarely. Hepatocellular neoplasms and peliosis hepatis, rare complications of oral androgens at higher doses, have not been reported with lower doses. Side effects of excess androgen treatment include hirsutism and virilization. Androgens should not be given to women with liver disease or during pregnancy or breast feeding.

A high intake of soy has been reported to reduce the severity of hot flushes, lower LDL:HDL ratios, and improve bone density.

Selective estrogen receptor modulators (SERMs—eg, raloxifene; Evista) are an alternative to estrogen replacement for hypogonadal women at risk for osteoporosis who prefer not to take estrogens because of their contraindications (eg, breast or uterine cancer) or side effects. Raloxifene does not reduce hot flushes, vaginal dryness, skin wrinkling, or breast atrophy. However, in doses of 60 mg/d orally, it inhibits bone loss without stimulating effects upon the breasts or endometrium. Since raloxifene may slightly increase the risk of venous thromboembolism, it should not be used by women at prolonged bed rest or by those prone to thrombosis. In contrast with the use of estrogen replacement therapy, concomitant progesterone therapy is not needed, and raloxifene does not increase the risk of development of breast cancer.

Colditz GA: Relationship between estrogen levels, use of hormone replacement therapy, and breast cancer. J Natl Cancer Inst 1998;90:814. [NLM Cit ID: 98286833] (This review concludes that the magnitude of the increase in breast cancer risk per year of estrogen replacement is comparable to that associated with delaying menopause by a year.)

Ettinger B et al: Unexpected vaginal bleeding and associated gynecologic care in postmenopausal women using hormone replacement therapy: comparison of cyclic versus continuous combined schedules. Fertil Steril 1998; 69:865. [NLM Cit ID: 98252168] (Unexpected vaginal bleeding was common with initiation of hormone replacement, and after 2 years became less common in women on continuous replacement [22 events per 100 patient-years] but remained unchanged in women on cyclic replacement [38 events per 100 patient-years.])

Genant HK et al: Low-dose esterified estrogen therapy: Effects on bone, plasma estradiol concentrations, endometrium, and lipid levels. Arch Intern Med 1997; 157:2609. [NLM Cit ID: 98189716] (Esterified estrogens, 0.3 mg daily, improved bone density and lipids without causing endometrial hyperplasia.)

Grodstein F et al: Postmenopausal hormone use and risk for colorectal cancer and adenoma. Ann Intern Med 1998;128:705. [NLM Cit ID: 98213264] (A Nurses' Health Study with 59,002 participants determined that women currently receiving estrogen replacement have a reduced risk of colorectal cancer; relative risk = 0.65.)

Hulley S et al: Randomized trial of estrogen plus progestin for secondary prevention of coronary heart disease in postmenopausal women. Heart and Estrogen/Progestin Replacement Study (HERS) Research Group. JAMA 1998;280:605. [NLM Cit ID: 98382151] (A randomized prospective placebo-controlled study of 2763 postmenopausal women with coronary disease. With an average follow-up of 4.1 years, treatment with oral conjugated equine estrogen plus medroxyprogesterone acetate did not reduce the overall mortality or risk of coronary events. There were more coronary events during the first year but fewer during the fourth and fifth years. More women in the hormone group experienced thromboembolic events [34 versus 12] and gallbladder disease [84 versus 62].)

Inestrosa NC et al: Cellular and molecular basis for estrogen's neuroprotection. Potential relevance for Alzheimer's disease. Mol Neurobiol 1998;17:73. [NLM Cit ID: 99104394]

Khovidhunkit W, Shoback DM: Clinical effects of raloxifene hydrochloride in women. Ann Intern Med 1999;130:431. [NLM Cit ID: 99104394]

Sherwin BB: Can estrogen keep you smart? Evidence from clinical studies. J Psychiatry Neurosci 1999;24:315. [NLM Cit ID: 99445971] (A review of 16 prospective, placebo-controlled studies in humans concludes that estrogen maintains verbal memory in women and may delay the deterioration of memory that occurs with aging. Some evidence indicates that estrogen replacement may reduce the risk of Alzheimer's disease or retard its onset.)

Zumoff B: The critical role of alcohol consumption in determining the risk of breast cancer with postmenopausal estrogen administration. J Clin Endocrinol Metab 1997;82:1656. [NLM Cit ID: 97320506]

TURNER'S SYNDROME (Gonadal Dysgenesis)

Turner's syndrome is a chromosomal disorder associated with primary hypogonadism, short stature, and other phenotypic anomalies. It is a common cause of primary amenorrhea. Patients with the classic syndrome lack one of the two X chromosomes and have a 45,XO karyotype.

Typical Turner's Syndrome (45,XO Gonadal Dysgenesis)

Features of Turner's syndrome (Table 26–15) are variable and may be subtle in girls with mosaicism.

Table 26–15. Manifestations of Turner's syndrome.

Short stature
Distinctive facial features
  Ptosis
  Micrognathia
  Low-set ears
  Epicanthal folds
Sexual infantilism due to gonadal dysgenesis
Webbed neck (40%)
Low hairline
High-arched palate
Cubitus valgus
Short fourth metacarpals (50%)
Lymphedema of hands and feet (30%)
Hypoplastic widely spaced nipples
Hyperconvex nails
Pigmented nevi
Keloid formation
Recurrent otitis media
Renal abnormalities (60%)
  Horseshoe kidney
  Hydronephrosis
Hypertension (idiopathic or due to coarctation or renal disease)
Gastrointestinal bleeding from intestinal telangiectases (rare)
Impaired space-form recognition, direction sense, and mathematical reasoning
Cardiovasular anomalies
  Coarctation of the aorta (10–20%)
  Aortic stenosis
  Bicuspid aortic valve
  Aortic dissection due to coarctation and cystic medial necrosis of aorta (rare)
Associated conditions
  Obesity
  Diabetes mellitus (types 1 and 2)
  Dyslipidemia
  Hyperuricemia
  Hashimoto's thyroiditis
  Achlorhydria
  Cataracts, corneal opacities
  Neuroblastoma (1%)
  Rheumatoid arthritis
  Inflammatory bowel disease

Typical manifestations in adulthood include short stature, hypogonadism, webbed neck, high-arched palate, wide-spaced nipples, hypertension, and renal abnormalities. 45,XO zygotes account for about 0.8 of all conceptuses, making this the most common major chromosomal abnormality in humans. Less than 3% of these zygotes survive to term, with the incidence of Turner's syndrome being about 1:10,000 female newborns.

Girls with Turner's syndrome may be diagnosed at birth, since they tend to be small and may exhibit severe lymphedema. Evaluation for childhood short stature often leads to the diagnosis. Growth hormone and somatomedin levels are normal. Hypogonadism presents as "delayed adolescence"; FSH and LH are high, making a diagnosis of primary hypogonadism. A blood karyotype showing 45,XO (or X chromosome abnormalities or mosaicism) establishes the diagnosis.

Treatment of short stature with daily injections of growth hormone (0.1 unit/kg/d) plus an androgen (eg, oxandrolone) for at least 4 years before epiphysial fusion increases final height by a mean of about 10.3 cm over the mean predicted height of 144.2 cm. After age 12, estrogen therapy is begun with low doses of conjugated estrogens (0.3 mg) or ethinyl estradiol (5 μg) given on days 1–21 per month. When growth stops, 0.625–1.25 mg of conjugated estrogens or 10–20 μg of ethinyl estradiol is given on days 1–25 per month. Medroxyprogesterone acetate, 5 mg, is added on days 16–25 of the month to induce menses.

Women with Turner's syndrome have a reduced life expectancy due in part to their increased risk for diabetes mellitus (types 1 and 2), hypertension, dyslipidemia, and osteoporosis. Diagnostic vigilance and aggressive treatment of these conditions reduces the risk of ischemic heart disease, stroke, and fracture. Yearly ocular examinations and periodic thyroid evaluations are recommended.

Turner's Syndrome Variants

A. 46,X (Abnormal X) Karyotype: An abnormality or deletion of certain genes on the short arm of the X chromosome causes short stature and other signs of Turner's syndrome; some gonadal function and even fertility is possible. Transmission of Turner's syndrome from mother to daughter can occur. There may be an increased risk of trisomy 21 in the conceptuses of women with Turner's syndrome. Abnormalities or deletions of other genes located on both the long and short arms of the X chromosome can produce gonadal dysgenesis with few other somatic features.

B. 45,XO/46,XX Mosaicism: This karyotype results in a modified form of Turner's syndrome. Such girls tend to be taller and may have more gonadal function and fewer other manifestations of Turner's syndrome.

C. Other Variants: 45,XO/46,XY mosaicism can produce some manifestations of Turner's syndrome. Patients may have ambiguous genitalia or male infertility with an otherwise normal phenotype.

Blumenthal AL et al: Turner syndrome in a mother and daughter: r(x) and fertility. Clin Genet 1997;52:87. [NLM Cit ID: 98018322]

Gravholt C et al: Morbidity in Turner's syndrome. J Clin Epidemiol 1998;51:147. [NLM Cit ID: 98134350]

Nathwani NC et al: The influence of renal and cardiovascular abnormalities on blood pressure in Turner syndrome. Clin Endocrinol 2000;52:371. [NLM Cit ID: 20183559] (Patients with Turner's syndrome suffer a high rate of cardiovascular mortality. Over 30% were found to be mildly hypertensive without detectable renovascular causes.)

Rosenfeld RG et al: Growth hormone therapy for Turner's syndrome: Beneficial effect on adult height. J Pediatr 1998;132:319. [NLM Cit ID: 98165492]

MULTIPLE ENDOCRINE NEOPLASIA

Several syndromes with multiple gland involvement have been described (Table 26–16).

MEN 1 (Wermer's Syndrome)

The most common multiglandular syndrome is multiple endocrine neoplasia type 1 (MEN 1). Biochemical testing identifies affected individuals by age 14–18 years, but the syndrome usually becomes clinically manifest in the fourth decade. **Hyperparathyroidism** occurs in over 80% of patients; it presents with hypercalcemia and usually involves hyperplasia or adenomas of several parathyroid glands. **Pancreatic islet cell tumors** occur in about 75% of patients; gastrinomas are the most common tumor and can result in gastric hyperacidity (Zollinger-Ellison syndrome) with peptic ulcer disease or diarrhea. Islet cell tumors may also secrete insulin, somatostatin, or glucagon. **Pituitary adenomas** occur in about 60% and may secrete prolactin, growth hormone, or ACTH but are usually nonfunctional; such tumors may produce local pressure effects and hypopituitarism. About 37% of these patients have adrenal cortical adenomas or hyperplasia—bilateral in about half. They are generally benign and nonfunctional. In one series, one out of 12 such patients developed a feminizing adrenal carcinoma. These adrenal lesions are pituitary-independent.

Tumors of the pituitary gland, the parathyroid gland, and the pancreatic islets may occur in the same patient, though not necessarily at the same time. Some individuals in the same family express the abnormality as children, whereas in others the clinical manifestations may not appear until late in adult life.

Table 26–16. Multiple endocrine neoplasia (MEN) syndromes: Incidence of tumor types.[1]

Tumor Type	MEN 1 (Wermer's Syndrome)	MEN 2a (Sipple's Syndrome)	MEN 2b
Parathyroid	> 80%	50%	Rare
Pancreatic	75%		
Pituitary	60%		
Medullary thyroid carcinoma		> 50%	80%
Pheochromocytoma		20%	60%
Mucosal and gastrointestinal ganglioneuromas		Rare	> 90%
Lipoma	Occasional		
Adrenocortical adenoma	Occasional		
Carcinoid	Occasional		
Thyroid adenoma	Occasional		

[1]Modified from Fitzgerald PA (editor): *Handbook of Clinical Endocrinology*, 2nd ed. Originally published by Appleton & Lange. Copyright © 1992 by The McGraw-Hill Companies, Inc.

The clinical manifestations of MEN 1 are extremely variable, since the glandular tumors may secrete a variety of different hormones.

The kindreds expressing MEN 1 have been shown to harbor a gene mutation on the long arm of chromosome 11 (11q13), which causes phenotypic expression as a dominant trait. Genetic linkage analysis can be used to determine which other family members will express this syndrome, permitting informed genetic counseling and avoiding unnecessary testing for unaffected individuals.

The differential diagnosis of MEN 1 includes sporadic or familial tumors of the pituitary, parathyroids, or pancreatic islets. Hypercalcemia (from any cause) may cause gastrointestinal symptoms and increased gastrin levels, simulating a gastrinoma. Treatment of gastrointestinal symptoms with H_2 blockers or metoclopramide causes hyperprolactinemia, simulating a pituitary prolactinoma.

Surgical treatment of hyperparathyroidism in MEN 1 can induce prolonged remissions, but relapse is typical. Aggressive parathyroid resection can cause permanent hypoparathyroidism. Medical treatment of hyperparathyroidism with bisphosphonates (eg, alendronate) is thus an important option.

MEN 2a (Sipple's Syndrome)

A separate disorder of multiglandular hypersecretion of hormones is multiple endocrine neoplasia type 2a. It too is inherited as an autosomal dominant trait. In MEN 2a, patients may have **medullary thyroid carcinoma** (> 90%); hyperparathyroidism (20–50%), due to hyperplasia or multiple adenomas in over 70% of cases; **pheochromocytomas** (20–35%), which are often bilateral; or **Hirschsprung's disease.** The medullary thyroid carcinoma is of mild to moderate aggressiveness and generally occurs in the third or fourth decade in the familial syndrome and in the sixth decade in sporadic cases.

Siblings or children of patients with MEN 2a can have genetic testing to determine if they have a mutation of the *RET* proto-oncogene, which identifies about 98% of such individuals. There is incomplete penetrance and about 30% of those with such mutations never manifest endocrine tumors. Alternatively, patients may have periodic serum calcitonin measurements after pentagastrin stimulation to screen for early medullary thyroid carcinoma: pentagastrin, 0.5 μg/kg, is given intravenously over 15 seconds; serum samples for calcitonin are obtained at intervals of 1.5, 5, and 10 minutes; a peak level over 190 pg/mL in males or over 80 pg/mL in females implicates an occult medullary thyroid carcinoma. Alternatively, patients may be screened with a serum calcitonin drawn after 3 days of omeprazole, 20 mg orally twice daily; calcitonin levels rise in the presence of medullary thyroid carcinoma to levels seen with the pentagastrin test. Patients with *RET* mutations or abnormal stimulation testing are advised to have a total thyroidectomy after screening for latent pheochromocytoma.

MEN 2b

Patients with MEN 2b have a syndrome characterized by mucosal neuromas (> 90% with bumpy lips, enlarged tongue, Marfan-like habitus), pheochromocytomas (60%), and medullary thyroid carcinoma (80%), which can be quite aggressive. Patients also have intestinal abnormalities (75%), skeletal abnormalities (87%), and delayed puberty (43%). The medullary thyroid carcinoma is aggressive and tends to present in the third to fourth decades. Prophylactic thyroidectomy is advisable for patients with mucosal neuromas and family members with the syndrome or

RET proto-oncogene mutations after screening for pheochromocytoma.

Burgess JR et al: The outcome of subtotal parathyroidectomy for the treatment of hyperparathyroidism in multiple endocrine neoplasia type 1. Arch Surg 1998;133:126. [NLM Cit ID: 98143250]

Eng C: Seminars in medicine of the Beth Israel Hospital, Boston. The RET proto-oncogene in multiple endocrine neoplasia type 2 and Hirschsprung's disease. N Engl J Med 1996;335:943. [NLM Cit ID: 96365281]

Erdoǧan MF et al: Omeprazole:calcitonin stimulation test for the diagnosis, follow-up, and family screening in medullary thyroid carcinoma. J Clin Endocrinol Metab 1997;82:897. [NLM Cit ID: 97216246]

Ledger GA et al: Genetic testing in the diagnosis and management of multiple endocrine neoplasia type II. Ann Intern Med 1995;122:118. [NLM Cit ID: 95085156]

CLINICAL USE OF GLUCOCORTICOIDS

Mechanisms of Action

Cortisol is a steroid hormone that is normally secreted by the adrenal cortex in response to ACTH. It exerts its action by binding to nuclear receptors which then act upon chromatin to regulate gene expression, producing effects throughout the body.

Relative Potencies

Hydrocortisone and cortisone acetate, like cortisol, have mineralocorticoid effects that become excessive at higher doses. Other synthetic glucocorticoids such as prednisone, dexamethasone, and deflazacort (an oxazoline derivative of prednisolone) have minimal mineralocorticoid activity. The relative potencies relative to hydrocortisone are listed in Table 26–17. Anticonvulsant drugs (eg, phenytoin, carbamazepine, phenobarbital) accelerate the metabolism of glucocorticoids other than hydrocortisone, making them significantly less potent. Megestrol, a synthetic progestin, has slight glucocorticoid activity that becomes significant when administered in high doses for appetite stimulation.

Adverse Effects

Prolonged treatment with systemic glucocorticoids causes a variety of adverse effects that can be life-threatening. Patients should be thoroughly informed of the major possible side effects of treatment such as insomnia, personality change, weight gain, muscle weakness, polyuria, kidney stones, diabetes mellitus, sex hormone suppression, occasional amenorrhea in women, candidiasis and opportunistic infections, osteoporosis with fractures, or aseptic necrosis of bones, particularly of the hips, which may become manifest many months after even brief treatment (see section on Cushing's syndrome). Oral bisphosphonates can prevent osteoporosis. It is wise to follow an organized treatment plan such as the one outlined in Table 26–18.

Table 26–17. Systemic versus topical activity of corticosteroids. (Hydrocortisone = 1 in potency.)

	Systemic Activity	Topical Activity
Prednisone	4–5	1–2
Fluprednisolone	8–10	10
Triamcinolone	5	1
Triamcinolone acetonide	5	40
Dexamethasone	30–120	10
Betamethasone	30	5–10
Betamethasone valerate	. . .	50–150
Methylprednisolone	5	5
Fluocinolone acetonide	. . .	40–100
Flurandrenclone acetonide	. . .	20–50
Fluorometholone	1–2	40
Deflazocort	3–4	. . .

Adachi JD et al: Management of corticosteroid-induced osteoporosis. Semin Arthritis Rheum 2000;29:228. [NLM Cit ID: 20170264] (Bisphosphonates are the agents of choice for the prevention and treatment of corticosteroid osteoporosis.)

Gonnelli S et al: Prevention of corticosteroid-induced osteoporosis with alendronate in sarcoid patients. Calcif Tissue Int 1997;61:382. [NLM Cit ID: 98035139] (Alendronate, 5 mg/d orally, prevented bone loss in patients receiving prednisone over 12 months.)

Millard PS: Corticosteroid-induced bone loss. J Fam Pract 1996;42:347. [NLM Cit ID: 96196458]

Roux C et al: Randomized trial of effect of cyclical etidronate in the prevention of corticosteroid-induced bone loss. J Clin Endocrinol Metab 1998;83:1128. [NLM Cit ID: 98202129]

Steer KA et al: Megestrol-induced Cushing's syndrome. Clin Endocrinol 1995;42:91. [NLM Cit ID: 95196348]

RELEVANT WORLD WIDE WEB SITES

[A Clinical Evaluation of the Thyroid in Health and Disease]
http://www.meddean.luc.edu/lumen/MedEd/medicine/endo/thyroid.htm

[Adrenal Leukodystrophy Module]
http://www.vh.org/Providers/TeachingFiles/RCW/012696/012696.html

[Medullary Nephrocalcinosis Secondary to Parathyroid Adenoma]
http://www.brighamrad.harvard.edu/Cases/bwh/hcache/186/full.html

Table 26–18. Management of patients receiving systemic glucocorticoids.[1]

Do not administer glucocorticoids unless absolutely indicated or more conservative measures have failed.

Keep dosage and duration of administration to the minimum required for adequate treatment.

Screen for tuberculosis before treatment with a PPD test or chest x-ray.

Screen for diabetes mellitus before treatment and at each physician visit. Train the patient to test urine weekly for glucose.

Screen for hypertension before treatment and at each physician visit.

Screen for glaucoma and cataracts before treatment, 3 months into treatment, and then at least yearly.

Prepare the patient and family for possible adverse effects on mood, memory, and cognitive function. Inform them about other possible side effects, particularly weight gain, osteoporosis, and aseptic necrosis of bone.

Institute a vigorous physical exercise and isometric regimen tailored to each patient's disabilities.

Administer calcium (1 g elemental calcium) and vitamin D_3, 400–800 IU orally daily. Check spot morning urines, and alter dosage to keep urine calcium concentration below 30 mg/dL. If the patient is receiving thiazide diuretics, check for hypercalcemia, and administer only 500 mg elemental calcium daily. Consider a bisphosphonate such as alendronate (5–10 mg each morning) or etidronate (cycles of 400 mg/d for 2 weeks), then oral calcium for 6 weeks for prophylaxis against osteoporosis.

Avoid prolonged bed rest that will accelerate muscle weakness and bone mineral loss. Ambulate early after fractures.

Treat hypogonadism in women or men.

Avoid elective surgery, if possible. Vitamin A in a daily dose of 20,000 units orally for 1 week may improve wound healing, but it is not prescribed in pregnancy.

Avoid activities that could cause falls or other trauma.

Watch for fungal or yeast infections of skin, nails, mouth, vagina, and rectum, and treat appropriately.

Ulcer prophylaxis: Administer oral glucocorticoids with meals. If administered with nonsteroidals, consider prophylaxis with omeprazole, 20–40 mg/d. Glucocorticoids alone do not need prophylaxis with H_2 blockers or omeprazole. Avoid large doses of antacids containing aluminum hydroxide (many popular brands); aluminum hydroxide binds phosphate and may cause a hypophosphatemic osteomalacia that can compound glucocorticoid osteoporosis.

Treat infections aggressively. Consider unusual pathogens.

Weigh daily. Use dietary measures to avoid obesity and optimize nutrition.

Measure height frequently. This serves to document the degree of axial spine demineralization and compression.

Treat edema as indicated.

Monitor plasma potassium for hypokalemia. Treat as indicated.

Obtain bone densitometry before treatment and then periodically. Treat osteoporosis.

Avoid smoking and excessive ethanol consumption.

With dosage reduction, watch for signs of adrenal insufficiency or glucocorticoid withdrawal syndrome.

[1]Modified and reproduced, with permission, from Fitzgerald PA: *Handbook of Clinical Endocrinology*, 2nd ed. Originally published by Appleton & Lange. Copyright © 1992 by The McGraw-Hill Companies, Inc.

[McCune-Albright Syndrome With Fibrous Dysplasia]
http://www.brighamrad.harvard.edu/Cases/bwh/hcache/92/full.html

[Paget's Disease]
http://www.brighamrad.harvard.edu/Cases/bwh/hcache/12/full.html

[Paget's Disease With Tibial Fracture]
http://www.brighamrad.harvard.edu/Cases/bwh/hcache/120/full.html

[Parathyroid Adenoma]
http://www.brighamrad.harvard.edu/Cases/bwh/hcache/17/full.html

[Pheochromocytoma]
http://www.brighamrad.harvard.edu/Cases/bwh/hcache/169/full.html

[Renal Osteodystrophy Demonstration Case]
http://www.brighamrad.harvard.edu/Cases/bwh/hcache/21/full.html

Diabetes Mellitus & Hypoglycemia 27

See http://www.current-med.com/ch27.html for updated addresses of Web sites referenced in this chapter.

Umesh Masharani, MRCP(UK), & John H. Karam, MD

DIABETES MELLITUS

Essentials of Diagnosis

Type 1 diabetes:

- Polyuria, polydipsia, and rapid weight loss associated with random plasma glucose ≥ 200 mg/dL.
- Plasma glucose of 126 mg/dL or higher after an overnight fast, documented on more than one occasion.
- Ketonemia, ketonuria, or both.

Type 2 diabetes:

- Most patients are over 40 years of age and obese.
- Polyuria and polydipsia. Ketonuria and weight loss generally are uncommon at time of diagnosis. Candidal vaginitis in women may be an initial manifestation. Many patients have few or no symptoms.
- Plasma glucose of 126 mg/dL or higher after an overnight fast on more than one occasion. After 75 g oral glucose, diagnostic values are 200 mg/dL or more 2 hours after the oral glucose.
- Hypertension, dyslipidemia, and atherosclerosis are often associated.

Classification & Pathogenesis (Table 27–1)

Diabetes mellitus is a syndrome with disordered metabolism and inappropriate hyperglycemia due to either a deficiency of insulin secretion or to a combination of insulin resistance and inadequate insulin secretion to compensate. An international committee of experts in the field has recommended several changes in the classification of diabetes mellitus that include the following:

(1) The terms "insulin-dependent diabetes mellitus" and "non-insulin-dependent diabetes mellitus" and their acronyms (IDDM and NIDDM) were eliminated since they are based on pharmacologic rather than etiologic considerations.

(2) The terms "type 1 and type 2 diabetes" are retained, with arabic numerals being used rather than roman numerals, since the numeral II can be confused with the number 11. Type 1 diabetes is due to pancreatic islet B cell destruction predominantly by an autoimmune process, and these patients are prone to ketoacidosis. Type 2 diabetes is the more prevalent form and results from insulin resistance, mainly caused by visceral obesity, with a defect in compensatory insulin secretion.

A. Type 1 Diabetes Mellitus: This form of diabetes is immune-mediated in over 90% of cases and idiopathic in less than 10%. The rate of pancreatic B cell destruction is quite variable, being rapid in some individuals and slow in others. Type 1 diabetes is usually associated with ketosis in its untreated state. It occurs most commonly in juveniles but occasionally in adults, especially the nonobese and those who are elderly when hyperglycemia first appears. It is a catabolic disorder in which circulating insulin is virtually absent, plasma glucagon is elevated, and the pancreatic B cells fail to respond to all insulinogenic stimuli. Exogenous insulin is therefore required to reverse the catabolic state, prevent ketosis, reduce the hyperglucagonemia, and reduce blood glucose.

The highest prevalence of immune-mediated type 1 diabetes is in Scandinavia, where it comprises as many as 20% of the total number of patients with diabetes. This decreases in prevalence to 15% in southern Europe and 10% in the USA, while in Japan and China less than 1% of patients with diabetes have type 1.

Certain human leukocyte antigens (HLA) are strongly associated with the development of type 1 diabetes. About 95% of type 1 patients possess either HLA-DR3 or HLA-DR4, compared with 45–50% of Caucasian controls. HLA-DQ genes are even more specific markers of type 1 susceptibility, since a particular variety (HLA-DQw3.2) is found in the DR4 patients with type 1, while a "protective" gene (HLA-DQw3.1) is often present in the DR4 controls. In addition, circulating islet cell antibodies have been detected in as many as 85% of patients tested in the first few weeks of their diabetes, and when sensitive immunoassays are used, the majority of these patients also have detectable anti-insulin antibodies prior to

Table 27–1. Clinical classification of common diabetes mellitus syndromes.

Type	Ketosis	Islet Cell Antibodies	HLA Association	Treatment
Type 1 (a) Immune-mediated	Present	Present at onset	Positive	Eucaloric healthy diet and preprandial rapid-acting insulin, plus basal insulin replacement with intermediate-acting or long-acting insulin
(b) Idiopathic	Present	Absent	Absent	
Type 2 (a) Nonobese	Absent	Absent	Negative	(1) Eucaloric diet alone (2) Diet plus insulin or oral agents
(b) Obese	Absent	Absent	Negative	(1) Weight reduction (2) Hypocaloric diet, plus oral agents or insulin

receiving insulin therapy. Most islet cell antibodies are directed against glutamic acid decarboxylase, an enzyme localized within pancreatic B cells. Immunoassays for this marker of type 1 diabetes facilitate screening of siblings of affected children as well as adults with atypical features of type 2 for an autoimmune cause of their diabetes.

Certain unrecognized patients with a milder expression of type 1 diabetes initially retain enough B cell function to avoid ketosis but later in life develop increasing dependency on insulin therapy as their B cell mass diminishes. Islet cell antibody surveys indicate 15% of "type 2" patients may actually have this mild form of type 1 diabetes.

1. Immune-mediated type 1 diabetes mellitus–Immune-mediated type 1 diabetes is felt to result from an infectious or toxic insult to persons whose immune system is genetically predisposed to develop a vigorous autoimmune response either against altered pancreatic B cell antigens or against molecules of the B cell resembling the viral protein (molecular mimicry). Extrinsic factors that affect B cell function include damage caused by viruses such as mumps or coxsackie B4 virus, by toxic chemical agents, or by destructive cytotoxins and antibodies released from sensitized immunocytes. Specific HLA genes may increase susceptibility to a diabetogenic virus or be linked to certain immune response genes that predispose patients to a destructive autoimmune response against their own islet cells (autoaggression). Amelioration of hyperglycemia in patients given an immunosuppressive agent (eg, cyclosporine) shortly after onset of type 1 diabetes lends further support to the pathogenetic role of autoimmunity.

2. Idiopathic type 1 diabetes mellitus–Fewer than 10% of subjects have no evidence of pancreatic B cell autoimmunity to explain their insulinopenia and ketoacidosis. This subgroup has been classified as "idiopathic type 1 diabetes." Although only a minority of patients with type 1 diabetes fall into this group, most of these are of Asian or African origin.

B. Type 2 Diabetes: This represents a heterogeneous group comprising milder forms of diabetes that occur predominantly in adults but occasionally in juveniles. More than 90% of all diabetics in the USA are included under this classification. Circulating endogenous insulin is sufficient to prevent ketoacidosis but is inadequate to prevent hyperglycemia in the face of increased needs owing to tissue insensitivity. In most cases of this type of diabetes, the cause is unknown.

Tissue insensitivity to insulin has been noted in most type 2 patients irrespective of weight and has been attributed to several interrelated factors. These include a putative (and as yet undefined) genetic factor, which is aggravated in time by additional enhancers of insulin resistance such as aging, a sedentary lifestyle, and abdominal-visceral obesity. In addition, there is an accompanying deficiency in the response of pancreatic B cells to glucose. Both the tissue resistance to insulin and the impaired B cell response to glucose appear to be further aggravated by increased hyperglycemia, and both defects are ameliorated by treatment that reduces the hyperglycemia toward normal. Attempts to identify a genetic marker for type 2 have as yet been unsuccessful, though linkage to a site on chromosome 2 has been reported in one Mexican-American population. However, most epidemiologic data indicate strong genetic influences, since in monozygotic twins over 40 years of age, concordance develops in over 70% of cases within a year whenever one twin develops type 2 diabetes.

Two subgroups of patients are currently distinguished by the absence or presence of obesity. The degree and prevalence of obesity varies among different racial groups. While obesity is apparent in no more than 30% of Chinese and Japanese patients with type 2, it is found in 60–70% of North Americans, Europeans, or Africans with type 2 and approaches 100% of patients with type 2 among Pima Indians or Pacific Islanders from Nauru or Samoa.

1. Nonobese type 2 patients–These patients generally show an absent or blunted early phase of insulin release in response to glucose; however, it can be elicited in response to other insulinogenic stimuli such as acute intravenous administration of sulfonylureas, glucagon, or arginine.

Although insulin resistance may be detected with special tests, it does not seem to be clinically relevant to the treatment of most nonobese type 2 patients, who generally respond to appropriate therapeutic supplements of insulin in the absence of rare associated conditions such as lipoatrophy or acanthosis nigricans.

Among this heterogeneous subgroup of patients with nonobese type 2 diabetes, the majority are idiopathic. However, with increasing frequency, a variety of etiologic genetic abnormalities have been documented in a subset of these patients who have recently been reclassified within a group designated "other specific types." (See Table 27–2.)

C. Other Specific Types of Diabetes Mellitus:

1. Maturity-onset diabetes of the young (MODY)–This subgroup is a relatively rare monogenic disorder characterized by non-insulin-dependent diabetes with autosomal dominant inheritance and an age at onset of 25 years or younger. Patients are nonobese, and their hyperglycemia is due to impaired glucose-induced secretion of insulin. Five types of MODY have been described, with single gene defects localized to chromosomes 20, 7, 12, 13, and 17. Except for MODY 2, all types involve mutations of a nuclear transcription factor that regulates islet gene expression.

a. MODY 1 includes 74 members of a pedigree known as the R-W family, who are descendants of a German couple who immigrated to Michigan in 1861. Their extremely rare genetic defect was shown to be a nonsense mutation of a nuclear transcription factor found in liver as well as in pancreatic B cells. This gene has been termed hepatocyte nuclear factor-4α (HNF-4α) and is found on chromosome 20. How it reduces glucose-induced insulin secretion has not yet been clarified. Six families with mutations of this gene have been reported.

Table 27–2. Factors reducing response to insulin.

Prereceptor inhibitors:
Anti-insulin antibodies
Receptor inhibitors:
Insulin receptor antibodies
"Down-regulation" of receptors by hyperinsulinism:
- Primary hyperinsulinism (B cell adenoma)
- Hyperinsulinism secondary to a postreceptor defect (obesity, Cushing's syndrome, acromegaly, pregnancy) or prolonged glycemia (diabetes mellitus, post-glucose tolerance test)

Postreceptor influences:
- Poor responsiveness of principal target organs; obesity; hepatic disease; muscle inactivity; sustained hyperglycemia
- Hormonal excess: glucocorticoids, growth hormone, oral contraceptive agents, progesterone, human chorionic somatomammotropin, catecholamines, thyroxine

b. MODY 2 has been described in all parts of the world, and at least 26 different mutations of the glucokinase gene on chromosome 7 have been identified. Reduced sensitivity of pancreatic B cell glucokinase to plasma glucose causes impaired insulin secretion, resulting in fasting hyperglycemia and mild diabetes. Most of these patients have a benign course without long-term complications and respond well to diet or oral agents.

c. MODY 3 is caused by mutations of the hepatocyte nuclear factor-1α (HNF-1α), whose gene is located on chromosome 12. Approximately two-thirds of all known cases of MODY are due to MODY 3, with 41 different mutations reported in 61 families. This transcription factor is expressed in pancreatic B cells as well as in liver and is a weak transactivator of the insulin gene. This may explain how mutations of HNF-1α impair glucose-induced insulin secretion. Unlike most type 2 diabetes, there is no associated insulin resistance, but the clinical course of these two disorders is otherwise similar regarding prevalence of microangiopathy and failure to continue to respond to oral agents with time.

d. MODY 4 results from mutation of a pancreatic nuclear transcription factor known as insulin promoter factor-1 (IPF-1), whose gene is on chromosome 13. It mediates insulin gene transcription as well as regulates expression of other B cell-specific genes such as glucokinase and the glucose transporter-2. When both alleles of this gene are nonfunctioning, agenesis of the entire pancreas results; but in the presence of a heterozygous mutation of IPF-1, a mild form of MODY has been described in a family in whom affected individuals developed diabetes at a later age (mean onset at 35 years) than occurs with the other forms of MODY in which onset generally occurs before the age of 25 years.

e. MODY 5, the latest form of early-onset type 2 diabetes reported, is in a Japanese family with a mutation of HNF-1β, a hepatic nuclear transcription factor that acts with HNF-1α to regulate gene expression in pancreatic islets. This mutation caused a moderately severe form of MODY with progression to insulin treatment and severe diabetic complications in those affected. In addition, a nephropathy was seen in affected individuals prior to the onset of diabetes, suggesting that decreased levels of this transcription factor in the kidney, where it is also normally expressed in high levels, may contribute to renal dysfunction.

2. Diabetes due to mutant insulins–This is a very rare subtype of nonobese type 2 diabetes, with no more than ten families having been described. Since affected individuals were heterozygous and possessed one normal insulin gene, diabetes was mild, did not appear until middle age, and showed autosomal dominant genetic transmission. There is generally no evidence of clinical insulin resistance and these patients respond well to standard therapy.

3. Diabetes due to mutant insulin receptors–Defects in the insulin receptor gene have been found in more than 40 people with diabetes, but most have extreme insulin resistance associated with acanthosis nigricans.

4. Diabetes mellitus associated with a mutation of mitochondrial DNA–Since sperm do not contain mitochondria, only the mother transmits mitochondrial genes to her offspring. Diabetes due to a mutation of mitochondrial DNA that impairs the transfer of leucine into mitochondrial proteins has been described in Japanese families as well as in isolated case reports in Caucasians. Most patients have a mild form of diabetes that responds to oral hypoglycemic agents, some a nonimmune form of type 1 diabetes. Two-thirds of patients with this subtype of diabetes have a hearing loss, and a smaller proportion (15%) had a syndrome of myopathy, encephalopathy, lactic acidosis, and stroke-like episodes (MELAS). A lysine transfer defect has also recently been found in a family with maternally transmitted diabetes.

5. Obese type 2 patients–This form of diabetes is secondary to extrapancreatic factors that produce insensitivity to endogenous insulin. When an associated defect of insulin production prevents adequate compensation for this insulin resistance, nonketotic mild diabetes occurs. The primary problem is a "target organ" disorder resulting in ineffective insulin action (Table 27–2) that can secondarily influence pancreatic B cell function. Hyperplasia of pancreatic B cells is often present and probably accounts for the fasting hyperinsulinism and exaggerated insulin and proinsulin responses to glucose and other stimuli seen in the milder forms of this disorder. In more severe cases, especially after several years' duration of diabetes, failure of B cell secretion may result. Chronic deposition of amyloid in the islets may combine with inherited genetic defects to progressively impair B cell function. Obesity is generally associated with abdominal distribution of fat, producing an abnormally high waist-to-hip ratio. This "visceral" obesity, due to accumulation of fat in the omental and mesenteric regions, correlates with insulin resistance; subcutaneous abdominal fat has little if any association with insulin insensitivity. Visceral metabolites released into the portal circulation alter liver metabolism and increase hepatic glucose output more than peripheral fat mobilization into systemic veins. Exercise may affect the deposition of visceral fat as suggested by CT scans of Japanese wrestlers, whose extreme obesity is predominantly subcutaneous. Their daily vigorous exercise program prevents accumulation of visceral fat, and they have normal serum lipids and euglycemia despite daily intakes of 5000–7000 kcal and development of massive subcutaneous obesity.

A major cause of the observed resistance to insulin in target tissues of obese patients is believed to be a postreceptor defect in insulin action. This is associated with overdistended visceral fat depots, and there is a reduced ability to clear nutrients from the circulation after meals. The resulting hyperinsulinism can further enhance insulin resistance by down-regulation of insulin receptors. Moreover, when hyperglycemia develops, hexosamines accumulate in muscle and fat tissue to further inhibit glucose transport. This contributes to further defects in postreceptor insulin action, thereby aggravating hyperglycemia.

When exercise increases blood flow to muscle as well as increasing muscle mass, and when overfeeding is corrected so that storage depots become less saturated, the cycle is interrupted. There is improvement in insulin sensitivity, which is further restored toward normal by a reduction of both the hyperinsulinism and the hyperglycemia.

Epidemiologic Considerations

An estimated 16 million people in the USA are known to have diabetes, of which 1.4 million have type 1 diabetes and approximately 14.5 million have type 2 diabetes. The remainder, numbered only in the thousands, comprise a third group which was designated as "other specific types" by the American Diabetes Association (see above). These other types include disorders for which causes are known. Among these are the rare monogenic defects of either B cell function or of insulin action, primary diseases of the exocrine pancreas, endocrinopathies, and drug-induced diabetes.

Insulin resistance syndrome (syndrome X, CHAOS). In obese patients with type 2 diabetes, the association of **hyperglycemia, hyperinsulinemia, dyslipidemia,** and **hypertension,** which leads to coronary artery disease and stroke, may result from a genetic defect producing insulin resistance, exaggerated by obesity. This suggests that insulin resistance predisposes to hyperglycemia, which results in hyperinsulinemia, which may or may not be of sufficient magnitude to correct the hyperglycemia; and that this excessive insulin level then contributes to increased VLDL production in the liver, leading to hypertriglyceridemia and to increased sodium retention by renal tubules, thus inducing hypertension. Moreover, high insulin levels can stimulate endothelial proliferation—by virtue of insulin's action on growth factor receptors—to initiate atherosclerosis. In Australia, this association of disorders is called "CHAOS" (*c*oronary artery disease, *h*ypertension, *a*therosclerosis, *o*besity, and *s*troke). While these associations have been well known, the mechanism for their interrelationship remains speculative and an invitation to experimental investigation. Some question the role of hyperinsulinism in hypertension, since they often coexist in Caucasians but not in blacks or Pima Indians. Moreover, patients with hyperinsulinism due to insulinoma are not hypertensive, and there is no fall in blood pressure after surgical removal of the insulinoma restores normal insulin levels. The main value of grouping these disorders as a syndrome, however, is to remind physicians that the therapeutic goals are not only to correct hyperglycemia but also to manage the elevated blood pressure and dyslipidemia that result in increased cerebrovascular and cardiac morbidity and mortality in these patients. Physicians aware of this syndrome are more cautious in prescribing therapies that correct hypertension but may raise lipids (diuretics, beta-blockers) or that correct hyperlipidemia but increase insulin resistance, with aggravation of diabetes (niacin). Finally, the use of long-acting insulins and sulfonylureas that promote sustained hyperinsulinism may have to be moderated, with an insulin-sparing drug such as metformin being preferable, if the hypothesis behind the insulin-resistance syndrome is ever substantiated.

Plasminogen activator-inhibitor 1 (PAI-1), produced by omental and visceral adipocytes, is elevated in the plasma of these patients. This contributes to the reduced fibrinolysis and higher risk for atherothrombosis in this syndrome.

Clinical Findings

The principal clinical features of the two major types of diabetes mellitus are listed for comparison in Table 27–3.

Patients with type 1 diabetes present with a characteristic symptom complex. An absolute deficiency of insulin results in accumulation of circulating glucose and fatty acids, with consequent hyperosmolality and hyperketonemia.

Patients with type 2 diabetes may or may not present with characteristic features. The presence of obesity or a strongly positive family history for mild diabetes suggests a high risk for the development of type 2 diabetes.

A. Symptoms and Signs:

1. Type 1 diabetes–Increased urination is a consequence of osmotic diuresis secondary to sustained hyperglycemia. This results in a loss of glucose as well as free water and electrolytes in the urine. Thirst is a consequence of the hyperosmolar state, as is blurred vision, which often develops as the lenses and retinas are exposed to hyperosmolar fluids.

Table 27–3. Clinical features of diabetes at diagnosis.

	Type 1 Diabetes	Type 2 Diabetes
Polyuria and thirst	++	+
Weakness or fatigue	++	+
Polyphagia with weight loss	++	–
Recurrent blurred vision	+	++
Vulvovaginitis or pruritus	+	++
Peripheral neuropathy	+	++
Nocturnal enuresis	++	–
Often asymptomatic	–	++

Weight loss despite normal or increased appetite is a common feature of type 1 when it develops subacutely. The weight loss is initially due to depletion of water, glycogen, and triglycerides; thereafter, reduced muscle mass occurs as amino acids are diverted to form glucose and ketone bodies.

Lowered plasma volume produces symptoms of postural hypotension. Total body potassium loss and the general catabolism of muscle protein contribute to the weakness.

Paresthesias may be present at the time of diagnosis of type 1 diabetes, particularly when the onset is subacute. They reflect a temporary dysfunction of peripheral sensory nerves, which clears as insulin replacement restores glycemic levels closer to normal, suggesting neurotoxicity from sustained hyperglycemia.

When absolute insulin deficiency is of acute onset, the above symptoms develop abruptly. Ketoacidosis exacerbates the dehydration and hyperosmolality by producing anorexia and nausea and vomiting, interfering with oral fluid replacement.

The patient's level of consciousness can vary depending on the degree of hyperosmolality. When insulin deficiency develops relatively slowly and sufficient water intake is maintained, patients remain relatively alert and physical findings may be minimal. When vomiting occurs in response to worsening ketoacidosis, dehydration progresses and compensatory mechanisms become inadequate to keep serum osmolality below 320–330 mosm/L. Under these circumstances, stupor or even coma may occur. The fruity breath odor of acetone further suggests the diagnosis of diabetic ketoacidosis.

Hypotension in the recumbent position is a serious prognostic sign. Loss of subcutaneous fat and muscle wasting are features of more slowly developing insulin deficiency. In occasional patients with slow, insidious onset of insulin deficiency, subcutaneous fat may be considerably depleted. An enlarged liver, eruptive xanthomas on the flexor surface of the limbs and on the buttocks, and lipemia retinalis indicate that chronic insulin deficiency has resulted in chylomicronemia, with circulating triglycerides elevated usually to over 2000 mg/dL.

2. Type 2 diabetes–While many patients with type 2 diabetes present with increased urination and thirst, many others have an insidious onset of hyperglycemia and are asymptomatic initially. This is particularly true in obese patients, whose diabetes may be detected only after glycosuria or hyperglycemia is noted during routine laboratory studies. Occasionally, type 2 patients may present with evidence of neuropathic or cardiovascular complications because of occult disease present for some time prior to diagnosis. Chronic skin infections are common. Generalized pruritus and symptoms of vaginitis are frequently the initial complaints of women. Diabetes should be suspected in women with chronic candidal vulvovaginitis as well as in those who have delivered large babies (> 9 lb, or 4.1 kg) or have had polyhydramnios, preeclampsia, or unexplained fetal losses.

Obese diabetics may have any variety of fat distribution; however, diabetes seems to be more often associated in both men and women with localization of fat deposits on the upper segment of the body (particularly the abdomen, chest, neck, and face) and relatively less fat on the appendages, which may be quite muscular. Standardized tables of waist-to-hip ratio indicate that ratios of "greater than 0.9" in men and "greater than 0.8" in women are associated with an increased risk of diabetes in obese subjects. Mild hypertension is often present in obese diabetics.

B. Laboratory Findings:

1. Urinalysis–

a. Glucosuria–A specific and convenient method to detect glucosuria is the paper strip impregnated with glucose oxidase and a chromogen system (Clinistix, Diastix), which is sensitive to as little as 0.1% glucose in urine. Diastix can be directly applied to the urinary stream, and differing color responses of the indicator strip reflect glucose concentration.

A normal renal threshold for glucose as well as reliable bladder emptying is essential for interpretation.

b. Ketonuria–Qualitative detection of ketone bodies can be accomplished by nitroprusside tests (Acetest or Ketostix). Although these tests do not detect β-hydroxybutyric acid, which lacks a ketone group, the semiquantitative estimation of ketonuria thus obtained is nonetheless usually adequate for clinical purposes.

2. Blood testing procedures–

a. Glucose tolerance test–

(1) Methodology and normal fasting glucose–Plasma or serum from venous blood samples has the advantage over whole blood of providing values for glucose that are independent of hematocrit and that reflect the glucose concentration to which body tissues are exposed. For these reasons, and because plasma and serum are more readily measured on automated equipment, they are used in most laboratories. If serum is used, samples should be refrigerated and separated within 1 hour after collection.

(2) Criteria for laboratory confirmation of diabetes mellitus–If the fasting plasma glucose level is 126 mg/dL or higher on more than one occasion, further evaluation of the patient with a glucose challenge is unnecessary. However, when fasting plasma glucose is less than 126 mg/dL in suspected cases, a standardized oral glucose tolerance test may be done (Table 27–4).

For proper evaluation of the test, the subjects should be normally active and free from acute illness.

Table 27–4. The Diabetes Expert Committee criteria for evaluating the standard oral glucose tolerance test.[1]

	Normal Glucose Tolerance	Impaired Glucose Tolerance	Diabetes Mellitus[2]
Fasting plasma glucose (mg/dL)	< 110	110–125	≥ 126
Two hours after glucose load (mg/dL)	< 140	≥ 140 but < 200	≥ 200

[1]Give 75 g of glucose dissolved in 300 mL of water after an overnight fast in subjects who have been receiving at least 150–200 g of carbohydrate daily for 3 days before the test.
[2]A fasting plasma glucose ≥ 126 mg/dL is diagnostic of diabetes if confirmed on a subsequent day.

Medications that may impair glucose tolerance include diuretics, contraceptive drugs, glucocorticoids, niacin, and phenytoin.

Because of difficulties in interpreting oral glucose tolerance tests and the lack of standards related to aging, these tests are being replaced by documentation of fasting hyperglycemia.

Since fasting plasma glucose is known to increase with aging, physicians should be more tolerant of slight abnormalities of fasting glucose values in older people (over 70 years of age) and not deprive patients of occasional sugar-containing snacks when symptoms are not evident. However, an occasional elderly patient may benefit from the diagnosis of mild diabetes in that macular edema may be detected earlier and laser treatment initiated before vision deteriorates permanently.

b. Glycosylated hemoglobin (hemoglobin A_1) measurements–Glycosylated hemoglobin is abnormally high in diabetics with chronic hyperglycemia and reflects their metabolic control. It is produced by nonenzymatic condensation of glucose molecules with free amino groups on the globin component of hemoglobin. The higher the prevailing ambient levels of blood glucose, the higher will be the level of glycosylated hemoglobin. The major form of glycohemoglobin is termed hemoglobin A_{1c}, which normally comprises only 4–6% of the total hemoglobin. The remaining glycohemoglobins (2–4% of the total) consist of phosphorylated glucose or fructose and are termed hemoglobin A_{1a} and hemoglobin A_{1b}. Many laboratories measure the sum of these three glycohemoglobins and report it as hemoglobin A_1, but more laboratories are converting to the more intricate but highly specific HbA_{1c} assay.

Since glycohemoglobins circulate within red blood cells whose life span lasts up to 120 days, they generally reflect the state of glycemia over the preceding 8–12 weeks, thereby providing an improved method of assessing diabetic control. Glycohemoglobins are extremely useful in monitoring the progress of patients. Measurements should be made in patients with either type of diabetes mellitus at 3- to 4-month intervals so that adjustments in therapy can be made if glycohemoglobin is either subnormal or if it is more than 2% above the upper limits of normal for a particular laboratory. In patients monitoring their own blood glucose levels, glycohemoglobin values provide a valuable check on the accuracy of monitoring. In patients who do not monitor their own blood glucose levels, glycohemoglobin values are essential for adjusting therapy. Use of glycohemoglobin for screening is controversial. Sensitivity in detecting known diabetes cases by hemoglobin A_{1c} measurements is only 85%, indicating that diabetes cannot be excluded by a normal value. On the other hand, elevated hemoglobin A_{1c} assays are quite specific (91%) in identifying the presence of diabetes.

Occasionally, fluctuations in hemoglobin A_1 are due to an acutely generated, reversible, intermediary (aldimine-linked) product that can falsely elevate glycohemoglobins when measured with "short-cut" chromatographic methods. This can be eliminated by using specific HPLC methods that detect HbA_{1c} or by dialysis of the hemolysate before chromatography. When hemoglobin variants are present, such as negatively charged hemoglobin F, acetylated hemoglobin from high-dose aspirin therapy, or carbamoylated hemoglobin produced by the complexing of urea with hemoglobin in uremia, falsely high "hemoglobin A_1" values are obtained with commonly used chromatographic methods. In the presence of positively charged hemoglobin variants such as hemoglobin S or C, or when the life span of red blood cells is reduced by increased hemolysis or hemorrhage, falsely low values for "hemoglobin A_1" result.

Serum fructosamine is formed by nonenzymatic glycosylation of serum proteins (predominantly albumin). Since serum albumin has a much shorter half-life than hemoglobin, serum fructosamine generally reflects the state of glycemic control for only the preceding 2 weeks. When abnormal hemoglobins or hemolytic states affect the interpretation of glycohemoglobin or when a narrower time frame is required, such as for ascertaining glycemic control at the time of conception in a diabetic woman who has recently become pregnant, serum fructosamine assays offer some advantage. Normal values are 1.5–2.4 mmol/L when the serum albumin level is 5 g/dL.

c. Self-monitoring of blood glucose–Capillary blood glucose measurements performed by patients themselves, as outpatients, are extremely useful. In type 1 patients in whom "tight" metabolic control is attempted, they are indispensable. A portable battery-operated glucometer provides a digital readout of the intensity of color developed when glucose oxidase paper strips are exposed to a drop of capillary blood for up to 45 seconds. Second-generation glucometers—One Touch Basic (Lifescan, Inc), Glucometer Elite (Ames Co.), Precision Q&D (Medisense Co.), or ExacTech (Baxter Corp)—automatically time the reaction as soon as a drop of blood is applied to the previously inserted test strip. This relieves patients of the need to wipe off the strip after an exact interval of time and eliminates technical errors from improper blotting or timing. The timing for glucometer readouts varies from 12 to 45 seconds, with the most rapid result obtained from the Accu-Chek "Instant," which requires only 12 seconds. The memory in this device only holds nine entries, whereas other glucometers can retain memories of as many as 500 tests. As little as 2–5 μL of blood are needed for analysis by most meters, though the Accu-Chek "Instant" requires 12–50 μL. Various glucometers appeal to a particular consumer need and are relatively inexpensive, ranging from $50.00 to $100.00 each. The more expensive models compute blood glucose averages and can be attached to printers for data records and graph production. Test strips remain a major expense, costing 50–75 cents apiece. In self-monitoring of blood glucose, patients must prick their finger with a 28-gauge lancet (Monolet, Ames Co.), which can be facilitated by a small plastic trigger device such as an Autolet (Ames Co.), SoftClix (Boehringer-Mannheim), or Penlet (Lifescan, Inc.). When used for multiple patients, as in a clinic, physician's office, or hospital ward, disposable finger-rest platforms are required to avoid inadvertent transmission of blood-borne viral diseases.

The accuracy of data obtained by glucose monitoring requires education of the patient in sampling and measuring procedures as well as in proper calibration of the instruments. Bedside glucose monitoring in a hospital setting requires rigorous quality control programs and certification of personnel to avoid errors. When this is not feasible, glucose testing at the bedside is best done by technicians from the central laboratory.

Noninvasive glucose monitoring is a subject of intensive research interest, and a prototype, the GlucoWatch, was recently approved by the FDA. It utilizes reverse iontophoresis to measure interstitial glucose values with acceptable accuracy. Because of a lag period of 20 minutes, it records measurements only three times an hour, and sweating can result in skipped readings. Further experience is needed to evaluate its clinical value.

3. Lipoprotein abnormalities in diabetes–Circulating lipoproteins are just as dependent on insulin as is the plasma glucose. In type 1 diabetes, moderately deficient control of hyperglycemia is associated with only a slight elevation of LDL cholesterol and serum triglycerides and little if any change in HDL cholesterol. Once the hyperglycemia is corrected, lipoprotein levels are generally normal. However, in obese patients with type 2 diabetes, a distinct "diabetic dyslipidemia" is characteristic of the insulin resistance syndrome. Its features are a high serum triglyceride level (300–400 mg/dL), a low HDL-cholesterol (less than 30 mg/dL), and a qualitative change in LDL particles, producing a smaller dense LDL whose membrane carries supranormal amounts of free cholesterol. Since a low HDL-cholesterol is a major feature predisposing to macrovascular disease, the term "dyslipidemia" has preempted the term "hyperlipidemia," which mainly denoted the elevated triglycerides. Measures designed to correct the obesity and hyperglycemia, such as exercise, diet, and hypoglycemic therapy, are the treatment of choice for diabetic dyslipidemia, and in occasional patients in whom normal weight was achieved, all features of the lipoprotein abnormalities cleared. Since primary disorders of lipid metabolism may coexist with diabetes, persistence of lipid abnormalities after restoration of normal weight and blood glucose should prompt a diagnostic workup and possible pharmacotherapy of the lipid disorder. Chapter 28 discusses these matters in detail.

Differential Diagnosis

A. Hyperglycemia Secondary to Other Causes: (Table 27–5.) Secondary hyperglycemia has been associated with various disorders of insulin target tissues (liver, muscle, and adipose tissue).

Other secondary causes of carbohydrate intolerance include endocrine disorders—often specific endocrine tumors—associated with excess production of growth hormone, glucocorticoids, catecholamines, glucagon, or somatostatin. In the first four situations, peripheral responsiveness to insulin is impaired. With excess of glucocorticoids, catecholamines, or glucagon, increased hepatic output of glucose is a contributory factor; in the case of catecholamines, decreased insulin release is an additional factor in producing carbohydrate intolerance, and with excess somatostatin production it is the major factor.

A rare syndrome of extreme insulin resistance associated with acanthosis nigricans afflicts either young women with androgenic features as well as insulin receptor mutations or older people, mostly women, in whom a circulating immunoglobulin binds to insulin receptors and reduces their affinity to insulin.

Medications such as diuretics, phenytoin, niacin, and high-dose glucocorticoids can produce hyperglycemia that is reversible once the drugs are discontinued or when diuretic-induced hypokalemia is corrected. Chronic pancreatitis or subtotal pancreatectomy reduces the number of functioning B cells and can result in a metabolic derangement very similar to that of genetic type 1 diabetes except that a concomitant reduction in pancreatic A cells may reduce glucagon secretion so that relatively lower doses of insulin replacement are needed. Insulin-dependent diabetes is occasionally associated with Addison's disease and autoimmune thyroiditis (**Schmidt's syndrome,** or **polyglandular failure syndrome**). This occurs more commonly in women and represents an autoimmune disorder in which there are circulating antibodies to adrenocortical and thyroid tissue, thyroglobulin, and gastric parietal cells.

B. Nondiabetic Glycosuria: Nondiabetic glycosuria (renal glycosuria) is a benign, asymptomatic condition wherein glucose appears in the urine despite a normal amount of glucose in the blood, either basally or during a glucose tolerance test. Its cause may vary from an autosomally transmitted genetic disorder to one associated with dysfunction of the proximal renal tubule (Fanconi's syndrome, chronic renal failure), or it may merely be a consequence of the increased load of glucose presented to the tubules by the elevated glomerular filtration rate during pregnancy. As many as 50% of pregnant women normally have demonstrable sugar in the urine, especially during the third and fourth months. This sugar is practically always glucose except during the late weeks of pregnancy, when lactose may be present.

Table 27–5. Secondary causes of hyperglycemia.

Hyperglycemia due to tissue insensitivity to insulin
Hormonal tumors (acromegaly, Cushing's syndrome, glucagonoma, pheochromocytoma)
Pharmacologic agents (glucocorticoids, sympathomimetic drugs, niacin)
Liver disease (cirrhosis, hemochromatosis)
Muscle disorders (myotonic dystrophy)
Adipose tissue disorders (lipodystrophy, truncal obesity)
Insulin receptor disorders (acanthosis nigricans syndromes, leprechaunism)
Hyperglycemia due to reduced insulin secretion
Hormonal tumors (somatostatinoma, pheochromocytoma)
Pancreatic disorders (pancreatitis, hemosiderosis, hemochromatosis)
Pharmacologic agents (thiazide diuretics, phenytoin, pentamidine)

Treatment

A. Goals of Treatment of Diabetes: Diabetes mellitus requires ongoing medical care as well as patient and family education both to prevent acute illness and to reduce the risk of long-term complications. The Diabetes Control and Complications Trial of type 1 diabetes and the United Kingdom Prospective Diabetes Study of type 2 diabetes (see below) both indicate that the therapeutic objective is to restore known metabolic derangements toward normal in order to prevent and delay progression of diabetic complications.

B. Treatment Regimens:

1. Diet–A well-balanced, nutritious diet remains a fundamental element of therapy. However, in more than half of cases, diabetic patients fail to follow their diet. In prescribing a diet, it is important to relate dietary objectives to the type of diabetes. In obese patients with mild hyperglycemia, the major goal of diet therapy is weight reduction by caloric restriction. Thus, there is less need for exchange lists, emphasis on timing of meals, or periodic snacks, all of which are so essential in the treatment of insulin-requiring nonobese diabetics. This type of patient represents the most frequent challenge for the physician. Weight reduction is an elusive goal that can only be achieved by close supervision and education of the obese patient. See Chapter 29 for dietary management of obesity.

a. Revised ADA recommendations–Since 1994, the American Diabetes Association has released an annual position statement on medical nutrition therapy that replaced the calculated ADA diet formula of the past with suggestions for an individually tailored dietary prescription based on metabolic, nutritional, and life-style requirements. They contend that the concept of one diet for "diabetes" and the prescription of an "ADA diet" no longer can apply to both major types of diabetes. In their recommendations for persons with type 2 diabetes, the 55–60% carbohydrate content of previous diets has been reduced considerably because of the tendency of high carbohydrate intake to cause hyperglycemia, hypertriglyceridemia, and a lowered HDL-cholesterol. In obese type 2 patients, glucose and lipid goals join weight loss as the focus of therapy. These patients are advised to limit their carbohydrate content by substituting noncholesterologenic monounsaturated oils such as olive oil, rapeseed (canola) oil, or the oils in nuts and avocados. This maneuver is also indicated in type 1 patients on intensive insulin regimens in whom near-normoglycemic control is less achievable on higher carbohydrate diets. They should be taught "carbohydrate counting" so they can administer 1 unit of regular insulin or insulin lispro for each 10 or 15 g of carbohydrate eaten at a meal. In these patients, the ratio of carbohydrate to fat will vary among individuals in relation to their glycemic responses, insulin regimens, and exercise pattern.

The current recommendations for both types of diabetes continue to limit cholesterol to 300 mg daily and advise a daily protein intake of 10–20% of total calories. They suggest that saturated fat be no higher than 8–9% of total calories with a similar proportion of polyunsaturated fat and that the remainder of caloric needs be made up of an individualized ratio of monounsaturated fat and of carbohydrate containing 20–35 g of dietary fiber. Poultry, veal, and fish continue to be recommended as a substitute for red meats for keeping saturated fat content low. The present ADA position statement proffers no evidence that reducing protein intake below 10% of intake (about 0.8 g/kg/d) is of any benefit in patients with nephropathy and renal impairment, and doing so may be detrimental.

Exchange lists for meal planning can be obtained from the American Diabetes Association and its affiliate associations or from the American Dietetic Association, 216 W. Jackson Blvd., Chicago, IL 60606 (312-899-0040). Their Internet address is http://www.eatright.org.

b. Dietary fiber–Plant components such as cellulose, gum, and pectin are indigestible by humans and are termed dietary "fiber." Insoluble fibers such as cellulose or hemicellulose, as found in bran, tend to increase intestinal transit and may have beneficial effects on colonic function. In contrast, soluble fibers such as gums and pectins, as found in beans, oatmeal, or apple skin tend to retard nutrient absorption rates so that glucose absorption is slower and hyperglycemia may be slightly diminished. Although its recommendations do not include insoluble fiber supplements such as added bran, the ADA recommends food such as oatmeal, cereals, and beans with relatively high soluble fiber content as staple components of the diet in diabetics. High soluble fiber content in the diet may also have a favorable effect on blood cholesterol levels.

c. Artificial sweeteners–Aspartame (NutraSweet) has proved to be a popular sweetener for diabetic patients. It consists of two amino acids (aspartic acid and phenylalanine) that combine to produce a nutritive sweetener 180 times as sweet as sucrose. A major limitation is that it cannot be used in baking or cooking because of its lability to heat.

The nonnutritive sweetener saccharin continues to be available in certain foods and beverages despite warnings by the FDA about its potential long-term carcinogenicity to the bladder. The 1994 position statement of the ADA concludes that all nonnutritive sweeteners that have been approved by the FDA (such as aspartame and saccharin) are safe for consumption by all people with diabetes. Two other nonnutritive sweeteners have been approved by the FDA as safe for general use: sucralose (Splenda) and acesulfame potassium (Sunett, Sweet One, DiabetiSweet). These are both highly stable and, in contrast to aspartame, can be used in cooking and baking.

Nutritive sweeteners such as sorbitol and fructose have increased in popularity. Except for acute diarrhea induced by ingestion of large amounts of sorbitol-containing foods, their relative risk has yet to be established. Fructose represents a "natural" sugar substance that is a highly effective sweetener which induces only slight increases in plasma glucose levels. However, because of potential adverse effects of large amounts of fructose (up to 20% of total calories) on raising serum cholesterol and LDL-cholesterol, the ADA feels it may have no overall advantage as a sweetening agent in the diabetic diet. This does not preclude, however, ingestion of fructose-containing fruits and vegetables or fructose-sweetened foods in moderation.

2. Oral drugs for treating hyperglycemia–(Table 27–6.) The drugs for treating type 2 diabetes fall into three categories: (1) Drugs that primarily stimulate insulin secretion: Sulfonylureas remain the most widely prescribed drugs for treating hyperglycemia. The meglitinide analog repaglinide also binds the sulfonylurea receptor and stimulates insulin

Table 27–6. Oral antidiabetic drugs.

Drug	Tablet Size	Daily Dose	Duration of Action	Cost per Unit	Cost for 30 Days' Treatment Based on Maximum Dosage[1]
Sulfonylureas					
Tolbutamide (Orinase)	250 and 500 mg	0.5–2 g in 2 or 3 divided doses	6–12 hours	\$0.26/500 mg	\$31.20
Tolazamide (Tolinase)	100, 250, and 500 mg	0.1–1 g as single dose or in 2 divided doses	Up to 24 hours	\$0.25/250 mg	\$30.00
Acetohexamide (Dymelor)[2]	250 and 500 mg	0.25–1.5 g as single dose or in 2 divided doses	8–24 hours	\$0.37/500 mg	\$33.30
Chlorpropamide (Diabinese)[2]	100 and 250 mg	0.1–0.5 g as single dose	24–72 hours	\$0.67/250 mg	\$40.20
Glyburide (Diaβeta, Micronase)	1.25, 2.5, and 5 mg	1.25–20 mg as single dose or in 2 divided doses	Up to 24 hours	\$0.68/5 mg	\$81.60
(Glynase)	1.5, 3, and 6 mg	1.5–18 mg as single dose or in 2 divided doses	Up to 24 hours	\$1.02/6 mg	\$91.80
Glipizide (Glucotrol)	5 and 10 mg	2.5–40 mg as single dose or in 2 divided doses on an empty stomach.	6–12 hours	\$0.59/10 mg	\$70.80
(Glucotrol XL)	5 and 10 mg	Up to 20 or 30 mg daily as a single dose	Up to 24 hours	\$0.70/10 mg	\$63.00
Glimeperide (Amaryl)	1, 2, and 4 mg	1–4 mg as single dose	Up to 24 hours	\$0.78/4 mg	\$23.40
Meglitinide analogs					
Repaglinide (Prandin)	0.5, 1, and 2 mg	4 mg in two divided doses given 15 minutes before breakfast and dinner	3 hours	\$0.83/2 mg	\$49.80
Biguanides					
Metformin (Glucophage)	500 and 850 mg	1–2.5 g. One tablet with meals 2 or 3 times daily	7–12 hours	\$0.65/500 mg \$1.10/850 mg	\$99.00
Thiazolidinediones					
Rosiglitazone (Avandia)	2, 4, 8 mg	4–8 mg daily (can be divided)	Up to 24 hours	\$4.56/8 mg	\$136.90
Pioglitazone (Actos)	15, 30, 45 mg	15–45 mg daily	Up to 24 hours	\$4.56/30 mg	\$136.90
Alpha-glucosidase inhibitors					
Acarbose (Precose)	50 and 100 mg	75–300 mg in 3 divided doses with first bite of food	4 hours	\$0.67/100 mg	\$60.30
Miglitol (Glyset)	25, 50, and 100 mg	75–300 mg in 3 divided doses with first bite of food	4 hours	\$0.49/25 mg \$0.66/100 mg	\$59.40 (100 mg 3 times daily)

[1]Cost to pharmacist (average wholesale price, generic when possible) for maximum dosage listed. Source: *Drug Topics Red Book,* March 2000; Vol. 19, No. 3.
[2]There has been a decline in use of these formulations. In the case of chlorpropamide, the decline is due to its numerous side effects (see text).

secretion. Nateglinide, a D-phenylalanine derivative, is another insulin secretagogue and is being reviewed by the FDA for clinical use. (2) Drugs that alter insulin action: Metformin works primarily in the liver. The thiazolidinediones appear to have their main effect on skeletal muscle and adipose tissue. (3) Drugs that principally affect absorption of glucose: The α-glucosidase inhibitors acarbose and miglitol are such currently available drugs.

a. Sulfonylureas–The mechanism of action of the sulfonylureas when they are acutely administered is due to their insulinotropic effect on pancreatic B cells. Sulfonylureas specifically bind to a receptor that closes an ATP-sensitive potassium channel of the pancreatic B cell, thereby depolarizing the cell membrane. This results in an influx of extracellular calcium through voltage-gated calcium channels, which causes insulin granules to move toward the cell surface, facilitating exocytosis.

Sulfonylureas are presently not indicated in the juvenile type ketosis-prone insulin-dependent diabetic, since these drugs seem to depend on functioning pancreatic B cells. There is little, if any, potentiation of insulin effectiveness on long-term glycemic control when sulfonylureas are added in type 1 patients, which argues against any substantial extrapancreatic effect of sulfonylureas.

The sulfonylureas seem most appropriate for use in nonobese mild type 2 diabetic patients. In this group, acute administration of sulfonylureas improves the early phase of insulin release that is refractory to acute glucose stimulation. In obese mild diabetics and others with peripheral insensitivity to levels of circulating insulin, primary emphasis should be on weight reduction. When hyperglycemia in obese diabetics has been more severe, with consequent impairment of pancreatic B cell function, sulfonylureas may improve glycemic control until concurrent measures such as diet, exercise, and weight reduction can sustain the improvement without the need for oral drugs. Sulfonylureas are generally contraindicated in patients with hepatic or renal impairment. Idiosyncratic reactions are rare, with skin rashes or hematologic toxicity (leukopenia, thrombocytopenia) occurring in less than 0.1% of users.

(1) Tolbutamide is supplied as 500 mg tablets. It is rapidly oxidized in the liver to inactive metabolites, and its approximate duration of effect is relatively short (6–10 hours). Tolbutamide is probably best administered in divided doses (eg, 500 mg before each meal and at bedtime); however, some patients require only one or two tablets daily with a maximum dose of 3000 mg/d. Because of its short duration of action, which is independent of renal function, tolbutamide is probably the safest sulfonylurea to use if liver function is normal. Prolonged hypoglycemia has been reported rarely with tolbutamide, mostly in patients receiving certain antibacterial sulfonamides (sulfisoxazole), phenylbutazone for arthralgias, or the oral azole antifungal drugs to treat candidiasis. These drugs apparently compete with tolbutamide for oxidative enzyme systems in the liver, resulting in maintenance of high levels of unmetabolized, active sulfonylurea in the circulation.

(2) Tolazamide is supplied in tablets of 100, 250, and 500 mg. It has a longer duration of action than tolbutamide, lasting up to 20 hours, with maximal hypoglycemic effect occurring between the fourth and fourteenth hours. It is often effective, as are other longer-acting sulfonylureas also, when tolbutamide fails to correct prebreakfast hyperglycemia. Tolazamide is metabolized to several compounds that retain hypoglycemic effects. If more than 500 mg/d is required, the dose should be divided and given twice daily. Doses larger than 1000 mg daily do not improve the degree of glycemic control.

(3) Acetohexamide is supplied in tablets of 250 and 500 mg. Its duration of action is about 10–16 hours, being intermediate in action between tolbutamide and chlorpropamide. A dose of 0.25–1.5 g is given daily in one or two doses. Liver metabolism is rapid, but the metabolite produced remains active.

(4) Chlorpropamide is supplied in tablets of 100 and 250 mg. This drug, with a half-life of 32 hours, is slowly metabolized, with approximately 20–30% excreted unchanged in the urine. Since the metabolites retain hypoglycemic activity, elimination of the biologic effect is almost completely dependent on renal excretion. Its use is therefore contraindicated in patients with renal insufficiency because of its increased duration of action and prolonged half-life. The average maintenance dose is 250 mg daily, given as a single dose in the morning. Chlorpropamide is a potent agent, and prolonged hypoglycemic reactions are more common than with tolbutamide, particularly in elderly patients, in whom chlorpropamide therapy is contraindicated. A flush may occur when alcohol is ingested by patients taking chlorpropamide, appearing within 8 minutes of ingesting the alcohol and lasting for 10–12 minutes; it is believed to be dose-related and similar to a mild disulfiram reaction.

Chlorpropamide both stimulates vasopressin secretion and potentiates its action at the renal tubule, resulting in hyponatremia in some patients, especially those taking diuretics. Since second-generation sulfonylureas are available with comparable potency but without the disadvantage of causing water retention or alcohol-induced flushing, there is less need to prescribe chlorpropamide. In the UKPDS, subjects on chlorpropamide had, unlike the glibenclamide group, progression of retinopathy despite equivalent glycemic control. The reason for this is unclear, but the observation does make use of this drug even less desirable.

(5) Second-generation sulfonylureas (glyburide, glipizide, and glimeperide)–Glyburide, glipizide, and glimeperide are from 100 to 200 times more potent than tolbutamide. These drugs should be used with caution in patients with cardiovascular disease or in elderly patients, in whom prolonged hypoglycemia would be especially dangerous.

(a) Glyburide–Glyburide is available in 1.25, 2.5, and 5 mg tablets. The usual starting dose is 2.5 mg/d, and the average maintenance dose is 5–10 mg/d given as a single morning dose; maintenance doses higher than 20 mg/d are not recommended. Some reports suggest that 10 mg is a maximum daily therapeutic dose, with 15–20 mg having no additional benefit in poor responders and doses over 20 mg actually worsening hyperglycemia. Glyburide is metabolized in the liver into products with hypoglycemic activity, which probably explains why assays specific for the unmetabolized compound suggest a plasma half-life of only 1–2 hours, yet the biologic effects of glyburide are clearly persistent 24 hours after a single morning dose in diabetic patients. Glyburide is unique among sulfonylureas in that it not only binds to the pancreatic B cell membrane sulfonylurea receptor but also becomes sequestered within the B cell. This may also contribute to its prolonged biologic effect despite its relatively short circulating half-life. A recently marketed "Press Tab" formulation of "micronized" glyburide—easy to divide in half with slight pressure if necessary—is currently available in tablet sizes of 1.5 mg, 3 mg, and 6 mg.

Glyburide has few adverse effects other than its potential for causing hypoglycemia, which at times can be prolonged. Flushing has rarely been reported after ethanol ingestion. It does not cause water retention, as chlorpropamide does, but rather slightly enhances free water clearance. Glyburide is absolutely contraindicated in the presence of hepatic impairment and should not be used in patients with renal insufficiency, in elderly patients, or in those who would be put at serious risk from an episode of hypoglycemia.

(b) Glipizide–Glipizide is available in 5 and 10 mg tablets. For maximum effect in reducing postprandial hyperglycemia, this agent should be ingested 30 minutes before meals, since rapid absorption is delayed when the drug is taken with food. The recommended starting dose is 5 mg/d with up to 15 mg/d given as a single daily dose before breakfast. When higher daily doses are required, they should be divided and given before meals. The maximum dose recommended by the manufacturer is 40 mg/d, though doses above 10–15 mg probably provide little additional benefit in poor responders and may even be *less* effective than smaller doses.

At least 90% of glipizide is metabolized in the liver to inactive products, and 10% is excreted unchanged in the urine. Glipizide therapy is therefore contraindicated in patients with hepatic or renal impairment, who would be at high risk for hypoglycemia, but because of its lower potency and shorter duration of action it is preferable to glyburide in elderly patients. Glipizide has also been marketed as Glucotrol-XL in 5 mg and 10 mg tablets. It provides extended release during transit through the gastrointestinal tract with greater effectiveness in lowering prebreakfast hyperglycemia than the shorter-duration immediate-release standard glipizide tablets. However, this formulation appears to have sacrificed its lower propensity for severe hypoglycemia compared with longer-acting glyburide without showing any demonstrable therapeutic advantages over glyburide.

(c) Glimeperide–This sulfonylurea is given once daily as monotherapy or in combination with insulin to lower blood glucose in diabetes patients who cannot control their glucose level through diet and exercise. Glimeperide achieves blood glucose lowering with the lowest dose of any sulfonylurea compound and this tends to increase its cost-effectiveness. A single daily dose of 1 mg/d has been shown to be effective, and the maximal recommended dose is 8 mg. It has a long duration of action with a pharmacodynamic half-life of 5 hours, allowing once-daily administration, which improves compliance. It is completely metabolized by the liver to relatively inactive metabolic products.

b. Meglitinide analogs–Repaglinide is similar to glyburide but lacks the sulfonic acid-urea moiety. It acts by binding to the sulfonylurea receptor and closing the ATP-sensitive potassium channel. It is rapidly absorbed from the intestine and then undergoes complete metabolism in the liver to inactive biliary products, giving it a plasma half-life of less than 1 hour. The drug therefore causes a brief but rapid pulse of insulin. The starting dose is 0.5 mg three times a day 15 minutes before each meal. The dose can be titrated to a maximal daily dose of 16 mg. Like the sulfonylureas, repaglinide can be used in combination with metformin. Hypoglycemia is the main side effect. In clinical trials, when the drug was compared with a long-duration sulfonlyurea (glyburide), there was a trend toward less hypoglycemia. Like the sulfonylureas also, repaglinide causes weight gain. Metabolism is by cytochrome P450 3A4 isoenzyme, and other drugs that induce or inhibit this isoenzyme may increase or inhibit (respectively) the metabolism of repaglinide. The drug may be useful in patients with renal impairment or in the elderly. It remains to be shown that this drug has significant advantages over short-acting sulfonylureas.

c. Metformin and other biguanides–The biguanides were introduced in the 1950s for the management of type 2 diabetes mellitus. Phenformin was available in the USA until 1977, when it was discontinued because of its association with lactic acidosis. Only metformin is discussed here.

Metformin (1,1-dimethylbiguanide hydrochloride) was introduced in France in 1957 as an oral agent for therapy of type 2 diabetes, either alone or in conjunction with sulfonylureas. In 1995 it became available in the United States.

(1) Clinical pharmacology–The exact mechanism of action of metformin remains unclear. It reduces both the fasting level of blood glucose and the degree of postprandial hyperglycemia in patients with type 2 diabetes but has no effect on fasting blood glucose in normal subjects. Metformin is particularly effective in reducing hepatic gluconeogenesis by interfering with lactate oxidation and uptake by the liver. Other proposed mechanisms include a slowing down of gastrointestinal absorption of glucose and increased glucose uptake by skeletal muscle, which have been reported in some but not all clinical studies. Because of its very high concentration in intestinal cells after oral administration, metformin increases glucose to lactate turnover, which may account for a reduction in hyperglycemia.

Metformin has a half-life of 1½–3 hours, is not bound to plasma proteins, and is not metabolized in humans, being excreted unchanged by the kidneys.

(2) Indications and dosage–Metformin may be used as an adjunct to diet for the control of hyperglycemia and its associated symptomatology in patients with type 2 diabetes, particularly those who are obese or are not responding optimally to maximal doses of sulfonylureas. A side benefit of metformin therapy is its tendency to improve both fasting and postprandial hyperglycemia and hypertriglyceridemia in obese diabetics without the weight gain associated with insulin or sulfonylurea therapy. Metformin is not indicated for patients with type 1 diabetes and is contraindicated in diabetics with serum creatinine levels of 1.5 mg/dL or higher, hepatic insufficiency, alcoholism, or a propensity to develop tissue hypoxia.

Metformin is dispensed as 500 mg, 850 mg, and 1000 mg tablets. Although the maximal dosage is 2.55 g, little benefit is seen above a total dose of 2000 mg. It is important to begin with a low dose and increase the dosage very gradually in divided doses—taken with meals—to reduce minor gastrointestinal upsets. A common schedule would be one 500 mg tablet three times a day with meals or one 850 mg or 1000 mg tablet twice daily at breakfast and dinner.

(3) Adverse reactions–The most frequent side effects of metformin are gastrointestinal symptoms (anorexia, nausea, vomiting, abdominal discomfort, diarrhea), which occur in up to 20% of patients. These effects are dose-related, tend to occur at onset of therapy, and often are transient. However, in 3–5% of patients, therapy may have to be discontinued because of persistent diarrheal discomfort.

Hypoglycemia does not occur with therapeutic doses of metformin, which permits its description as a "euglycemic" or "antihyperglycemic" drug rather than an oral hypoglycemic agent. Dermatologic or hematologic toxicity is rare.

Lactic acidosis (see below) has been reported as a side effect but is uncommon with metformin in contrast to phenformin. While therapeutic doses of metformin reduce lactate uptake by the liver, serum lactate levels rise only minimally if at all, since other organs such as the kidney can remove the slight excess. However, if tissue hypoxia occurs, the metformin-treated patient is at higher risk for lactic acidosis due to compromised lactate removal. Similarly, when renal function deteriorates, affecting not only lactate removal by the kidney but also metformin excretion, plasma levels of metformin rise far above the therapeutic range and block hepatic uptake enough to provoke lactic acidosis without associated increases in lactic acid production. Almost all reported cases have involved subjects with associated risk factors that should have contraindicated its use (renal, hepatic, or cardiorespiratory insufficiency, alcoholism, advanced age). Acute renal failure can occur rarely in certain patients receiving radiocontrast agents. Metformin therapy should therefore be temporarily halted on the day of the test and for 2 days following injection of radiocontrast agents to avoid potential lactic acidosis if renal failure occurs.

d. Thiazolidinediones–Drugs of this new class of antihyperglycemic agents sensitize peripheral tissues to insulin. They bind a nuclear receptor called peroxisome proliferator-activated receptor gamma (PPAR-γ) and affect the expression of a number of genes. The exact mechanism by which these drugs improve tissue sensitivity to insulin is not known. Observed effects include increased glucose transporter expression (GLUT 1 and GLUT 4), decreased free fatty acid levels, decreased hepatic glucose output, and increased differentiation of preadipocytes into adipocytes. Like the biguanides, this class of drugs does not cause hypoglycemia.

Troglitazone was the first drug in this class to go into widespread clinical use. Unfortunately, about 1.9% of patients taking this drug developed elevations in liver enzymes greater than three times normal, which resolved when the drug was stopped. Liver failure, however, occurred if the drug was continued—at least 90 cases have been reported, and 63 of these patients have died. The drug has therefore been withdrawn from clinical use.

Two other drugs in the same class are available for clinical use: Rosiglitazone and pioglitazone. Both are effective as monotherapy and in combination with sulfonylureas, metformin, and insulin. When used as monotherapy, they lower HbA_{1c} by about 1 or 2 percentage points. When used in combination with insulin, they can result in a 30–50% reduction in insulin dosage, and some patients can come off insulin completely. The combination of a thiazolidinedione and metformin has the advantage of not causing hypoglycemia. Patients inadequately managed on sulfonylureas can do well on a combination of sulfonylurea and rosiglitazone or pioglitazone. About 25% of patients in clinical trials fail to respond to these drugs, presumably because they are significantly insulinopenic.

Rosiglitazone therapy is associated with increases in total cholesterol, LDL cholesterol (15%), and HDL cholesterol (10%). There is reduction in free fatty acids of about 8–15%. The changes in triglycerides were generally not different from placebo. The increase in the LDL cholesterol need not necessarily be detrimental—studies with troglitazone showed that there is a shift from the atherogenic small dense LDL particles to larger, less dense LDL particles. Pioglitazone in clinical trials lowered triglycerides (9%) and increased HDL cholesterol (15%) but did not cause a consistent change in total cholesterol and LDL cholesterol levels. There have not been any direct comparisons of rosiglitazone and pioglitazone, and the purported differences in the lipid profiles may simply reflect differences in the clinical study design rather than real differences in the drugs. Anemia occurs in 4% of patients treated with these drugs, but this effect may be due to a dilutional effect of increased plasma volume rather than a reduction in red cell mass. Weight gain occurs especially when the drug is combined with a sulfonylurea or insulin. A recent short-term study reported that over a 12-week period, troglitazone caused a decrease in intra-abdominal fat mass but did not affect total body fat or weight. This study suggests that this class of drugs may be of particular benefit in patients with syndrome X.

The dosage of rosiglitazone is 4–8 mg daily and of pioglitazone 15–45 mg daily, and the drugs do not have to be taken with food. Rosiglitazone is primarily metabolized by the CYP2C8 isoenzyme and unlike troglitazone does not appear to affect CYP3A4 isoenzyme and has no significant clinical effect on oral contraceptives. Pioglitazone is metabolized by CYP2C8 and CYP3A4. The pharmacokinetics of coadministration of pioglitazone and oral contraceptives has not been evaluated.

These two agents in the clinical trials (unlike troglitazone) did not show evidence of causing drug-induced hepatotoxicity. The FDA has, however, recommended that patients should not initiate drug therapy if the ALT is 2.5 times greater than the upper limit of normal. Obviously, caution should be used in initiation of therapy in patients with even mild ALT elevations. Liver function tests should be performed once every 2 months for the first year and periodically thereafter.

The thiazolidinediones have only recently become clinically available, and obviously it will take some time before their safety is established. Based on the clinical trial data and the limited clinical experience so far, it would be considered good practice to start patients on these drugs only if combinations of the other oral agents and insulin fail to achieve glycemic control.

e. Alpha-glucosidase inhibitors–This family of drugs competitively inhibits the alpha-glucosidase enzymes in the gut which digest dietary starch and sucrose. Two of these drugs—acarbose and miglitol—are available for clinical use. Both are potent inhibitors of glucoamylase, α-amylase, and sucrase but have less effect on isomaltase and hardly any on trehalase and lactase. A fundamental difference between acarbose and miglitol is in their absorption. Acarbose has the molecular mass and structural features of a tetrasaccharide, and very little (about 2%) crosses the microvillar membrane. Miglitol, however, has a structural similarity with glucose and is absorbable. Both drugs delay the absorption of carbohydrate and lower postprandial glycemic excursion.

(1) Acarbose–Acarbose binds 1000 times more avidly to the intestinal disaccharidases than do products of carbohydrate digestion or sucrose. In diabetic patients, acarbose reduces postprandial hyperglycemia by 30–50%, and its overall effect is to lower the HbA_{1c} by 0.5–1%. The principal adverse effect, seen in 20–30% of patients, is flatulence. This is caused by undigested carbohydrate reaching the lower bowel, where gases are produced by bacterial flora. In 3% of cases, troublesome diarrhea occurs. This gastrointestinal discomfort tends to discourage excessive carbohydrate consumption and promotes improved compliance of type 2 patients with their diet prescriptions. The recommended starting dose of acarbose is 25 mg once or twice daily. This can be titrated upward slowly over 1 or 2 months to a maximum dosage of 100 mg three times a day. The more slowly the dose is raised, the less the bowel discomfort. For maximal benefit on postprandial hyperglycemia, acarbose should be given with the first mouthful of food ingested. When acarbose is given alone, there is no risk of hypoglycemia. However if combined with insulin or sulfonylureas, it might increase the risk of hypoglycemia from these agents. A slight rise in hepatic aminotransferases has been noted in clinical trials with acarbose (5% versus 2% in placebo controls, and particularly with doses > 300 mg/d). The levels generally return to normal on stopping the drug.

In the UKPDS, approximately 2000 patients on diet, sulfonylurea, metformin, or insulin therapy were randomized to acarbose or placebo therapy. By 3 years, 60% of the patients had discontinued the drug, mostly because of gastrointestinal symptoms. If one looked only at the 40% who remained on the drug, they had an 0.5% lower HbA_{1c} compared with placebo.

(2) Miglitol–Miglitol is similar to acarbose in terms of its clinical effects. It is indicated for use in diet- or sulfonylurea-treated patients with type 2 diabetes. Therapy is initiated at the lowest effective dosage of 25 mg three times a day. The usual maintenance dose is 50 mg three times a day, though some patients may benefit from increasing the dose to 100 mg three times a day. Gastrointestinal side effects occur as with acarbose. The drug is not metabolized and is excreted unchanged by the kidney. Theoretically, absorbable α-glucosidase inhibitors could induce a deficiency of one or more of the α-glucosidases involved in cellular glycogen metabolism and biosynthesis of glycoproteins. This does not occur in practice because, unlike the intestinal mucosa, which sees a high concentration of the drug, the blood level is 200-fold to 1000-fold lower than the concentration needed to inhibit intracellular α-glucosidases. Miglitol should not be used in renal failure, when its clearance would be impaired.

f. Safety of the oral hypoglycemic agents–The University Group Diabetes Program (UGDP) reported that the number of deaths due to cardiovascular disease in diabetic patients treated with tolbutamide or the no longer used phenformin was excessive compared to either insulin-treated patients or those receiving placebos. However, the recently published United Kingdom Prospective Diabetes Study of type 2 diabetes (see below) has refuted these conclusions regarding sulfonylureas. It did not confirm any cardiovascular hazard among over 1500 patients treated intensively with sulfonylureas for over 10 years, compared with a comparable number who received either insulin or diet therapy. Analysis of a subgroup of obese patients receiving metformin also showed no hazard and even a slight reduction in cardiovascular deaths compared with conventional therapy. As yet there has not been a revision of the package insert rescinding the warning of potential cardiac deaths in patients receiving these oral drugs.

The safety of the thiazolidinediones (see above) as regards the frequency of life-threatening hepatic toxicity remains to be determined. Lactic acidosis from metformin (see above) is quite rare and probably not a major problem with its use in the absence of major risk factors such as impaired renal or hepatic disease or conditions predisposing to hypoxia.

3. Insulin–Insulin is indicated for type 1 diabetes as well as for type 2 diabetic patients with insulinopenia whose hyperglycemia does not respond to diet therapy either alone or combined with oral hypoglycemic drugs.

With the development of highly purified human insulin preparations, immunogenicity has been markedly reduced, thereby decreasing the incidence of therapeutic complications such as insulin allergy, immune insulin resistance, and localized lipoatrophy at the injection site. However, the problem of achieving optimal insulin delivery remains unsolved with the present state of technology. It has not been possible to reproduce the physiologic patterns of intraportal insulin secretion with subcutaneous injections of soluble or longer-acting insulin suspensions. Even so, with the help of appropriate modifications of diet and exercise and careful monitoring of capillary blood glucose levels at home, it has often been possible to achieve acceptable control of blood glucose by using various mixtures of short- and longer-acting insulins injected at least twice daily or portable insulin infusion pumps.

a. Characteristics of available insulin preparations–Commercial insulin preparations differ with respect to the animal species from which they are obtained, their purity and solubility, and the time of onset and duration of their biologic action. As many as 17 different formulations of insulin are available in the USA.

(1) Species of insulin–Human insulin is now produced by recombinant DNA techniques (biosynthetic human insulin). It has been introduced for clinical use as Humulin (Eli Lilly) and as Novolin (Novo Nordisk) and dispensed as either Regular (R), NPH (N), Lente (L), or Ultralente (U) formulations (see Table 27–7). A very rapidly-acting analog of human insulin with reversal of the 28 and 29 amino acids of the B chain is now available for human use (see Insulin Lispro, below). Because of declining costs for biosynthetic insulin production, the Eli Lilly Company in 1998 discontinued manufacturing its standard preparation of Iletin I, composed of 70% beef insulin and 30% pork insulin. However, a limited supply of their monospecies pork insulin (Iletin II) remains available for use in certain patients who may benefit from the slightly more prolonged and sustained effect of animal insulin, compared with human insulin. The cost of human insulin is slightly less than the cost of purified pork insulin.

(2) Purity of insulin–Improvements in purification techniques for insulins have reduced or eliminated contaminating insulin precursors which were capable of inducing anti-insulin antibodies. "Purified" insulin is defined by FDA regulations as the degree of purity wherein proinsulin contamination is less than 10 ppm, whether extracted from animal pancreas or produced from biosynthetic proinsulin. In 1998, Eli Lilly discontinued its "standard" formulations of beef-pork insulin, which contained between 10 ppm and 25 ppm of proinsulin. All human insulin and pork insulin products of Novo Nordisk and Eli Lilly presently available contain less than 10 ppm of proinsulin and are labeled as "purified." These purified insulins seem to preserve their potency quite well, so that refrigeration is recommended but not crucial. During travel, reserve supplies of insulin can thus be readily transported for weeks without losing potency if protected from extremes of heat or cold.

(3) Concentration of insulin–At present, insulins are available in a concentration of 100 units/mL (U100), and all are dispensed in 10 mL vials. With the popularity of "low-dose" (0.5 or 0.3 mL) disposable insulin syringes, U100 can be measured with acceptable accuracy in doses as low as 1–2 units. For use in rare cases of severe insulin resistance in which large quantities of insulin are required, U500 regular human insulin (Humulin R) is available from Eli Lilly.

b. Insulin preparations–(Table 27–7.) Four principal types of insulins are available: (1) ultrashort-acting, with very rapid onset and short duration; (2) short-acting, with rapid onset of action; (3) intermediate-acting; and (4) long-acting, with slow onset of action (Table 27–7 and Figure 27–1). Ultrashort-acting and short-acting insulins are dispensed

Table 27–7. Some insulin preparations available in the USA.[1,2]

Preparation	Species Source	Concentration	Cost[2]
Ultra-short-acting insulins			
Insulin lispro (Humalog, Lilly)	Human analog (recombinant)	U100	$33.08
Short-acting insulins			
"Purified"[3]			
Regular (Novo Nordisk)[4]	Human	U100	$22.94
Regular Humulin (Lilly)	Human	U100, U500	$22.94, $165.07
Regular Iletin II (Lilly)	Pork	U100	$46.13
Velosulin (Novo Nordisk)[5]	Human	U100	$31.40
Intermediate-acting insulins			
"Purified"[3]			
Lente Humulin (Lilly)	Human	U100	$22.94
Lente Iletin II (Lilly)	Pork	U100	$46.13
Lente (Novo Nordisk) Novolin	Human	U100	$22.94
NPH Humulin (Lilly)	Human	U100	$22.94
NPH Iletin II (Lilly)	Pork	U100	$46.13
NPH (Novo Nordisk) Novolin	Human	U100	$22.94
Premixed insulins (% NPH/% regular)			
Novolin 70/30 (Novo Nordisk)	Human	U100	$22.94
Humulin 70/30 and 50/50 (Lilly)	Human	U100	$22.94
% NPL/% insulin lispro			
Humalog Mix 75/25 (Lilly)	Human analog (recombinant)	U100 (insulin pen, prefilled syringes, 15 mL)	$87.64
Long-acting insulins			
"Purified"[3]			
Ultralente Humulin (Lilly)	Human	U100	$22.94

[1]Modified and reproduced, with permission, from Katzung BG (editor): *Basic and Clinical Pharmacology,* 7th ed. Appleton & Lange, 1997.
[2]All of these agents (except insulin lispro and U500) are available without a prescription. Cost to pharmacist (average wholesale price, generic when possible) for quantity listed. Source: *Drug Topics Red Book,* March 2000; Vol. 19, No. 3. Wholesale prices for all human preparations (except insulin lispro and U500) are similar.
[3]Less than 10 ppm proinsulin.
[4]Novo Nordisk human insulins are termed Novolin R, L, and N.
[5]Velosulin contains phosphate buffer, which favors its use to prevent insulin aggregation in pump tubing but precludes its being mixed with lente insulin. It is the only FDA-approved insulin for pump use.

as clear solutions at neutral pH and contain small amounts of zinc to improve their stability and shelf life. All other commercial insulins have been modified to provide prolonged action and are dispensed as turbid suspensions at neutral pH with either protamine in phosphate buffer (NPH insulin) or varying concentrations of zinc in acetate buffer (ultralente and lente insulins). These suspensions of insulin are designed for subcutaneous administration only, while the short-acting and ultra-short-acting insulins can also be given intravenously.

(1) Ultra-short-acting insulin–Insulin lispro (Humalog) is an insulin analog, produced by recombinant technology, wherein two amino acids near the carboxyl terminal of the B chain have been reversed in position: proline at position B28 has been moved to B29 and lysine has been moved from B29 to B28. Reversing these two amino acids results in a much lower propensity to form hexamers in contrast to human insulin. When injected subcutaneously, insulin lispro quickly dissociates into monomers and is absorbed very rapidly, reaching peak serum values in as early as 1 hour—in contrast to regular human insulin, whose hexamers require considerably more time to dissociate and become absorbed. Moreover, reversing these two amino acids does not interfere

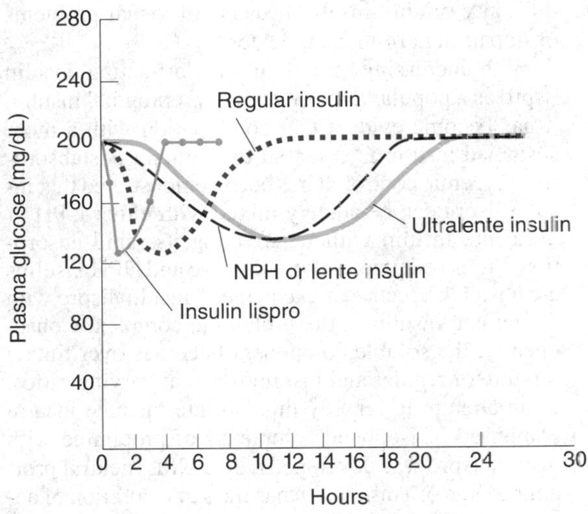

Figure 27–1. Extent and duration of action of various insulins (in a fasting diabetic). Duration is extended considerably when the dose of a given formulation increases above average therapeutic doses (except for insulin lispro).

with insulin lispro's binding to the insulin receptor, its circulating half-life, or its immunogenicity, which are all identical with that of human regular insulin.

Clinical trials have demonstrated that optimal time of preprandial subcutaneous injection of comparable doses of insulin lispro and of regular human insulin are 20 minutes and 60 minutes before the meal, respectively, in insulin-dependent diabetics requiring intensive insulin therapy. While this ultra-rapid onset of action of insulin lispro has been welcomed as a great convenience by diabetic patients who object to waiting as long as 60 minutes after injecting regular human insulin before they can begin their meal, patients must be taught to ingest adequate absorbable carbohydrate early in the meal to avoid hypoglycemia during the meal. Moreover, a property of insulin lispro which tends to reduce the frequency of late hypoglycemia following meals is that its duration of action, in contrast to regular human insulin, is not prolonged by increasing the dosage of the insulin. Regardless of the dose of insulin lispro injected subcutaneously, its duration is no more than 3–4 hours, whereas regular human insulin in moderate doses (15–40 units) lasts much longer, with its duration of action being proportionate to the dose. When the FDA approved insulin lispro, it indicated that—in contrast to other over-the-counter insulin formulations—insulin lispro will require a physician's prescription and medical supervision of its use until more experience with its novel pharmacokinetics is available.

(2) Short-acting insulin–Regular insulin is a short-acting soluble crystalline zinc insulin whose effect appears within 30 minutes after subcutaneous injection and lasts 5–7 hours when usual quantities are administered. Intravenous infusions of regular insulin are particularly useful in the treatment of diabetic ketoacidosis and during the perioperative management of insulin-requiring diabetics. When intravenous insulin is needed for hyperglycemic emergencies, insulin lispro has no advantage over regular human insulin, which is instantly converted to the monomeric form when given intravenously and which is 30–40% less costly than insulin lispro. Regular insulin is indicated when the subcutaneous insulin requirement is changing rapidly, such as after surgery or during acute infections, although insulin lispro may be preferable in these situations.

Aggregation of insulin solutions which cause clogging of tubing in insulin infusion pumps appears to be reduced by use of phosphate-buffered insulins. Novo Nordisk's Velosulin human insulin is the only buffered regular insulin approved by the FDA for pump users. Although infusion sets made of newer materials such as polyfin seem to reduce aggregation tendencies of unbuffered regular insulin, it remains advisable to recommend buffered Velosulin for use with insulin pumps. The FDA has approved insulin lispro for injection only and not yet for use in insulin pumps. Many patients are in fact using this insulin in their pumps. In a double-blind crossover study comparing insulin lispro with regular insulin in insulin pumps, subjects while using insulin lispro had lower HbA_{1c} values and improved postprandial glucose control with the same frequency of hypoglycemia. The concern remains that in the event of pump failure, insulin lispro would result in more rapid onset of hyperglycemia and ketosis.

(3) Intermediate- and long-acting insulins– Lente insulin is a mixture of 30% semilente (an amorphous precipitate of insulin with zinc ions) with 70% ultralente insulin (an insoluble crystal of zinc and insulin). Its onset of action is delayed for up to 2 hours (Figure 27–1), and because its duration of action often is less than 24 hours (with a range of 18–24 hours), most patients require at least two injections daily to maintain a sustained insulin effect. Lente insulin has its peak effect in most patients between 8 and 12 hours, but individual variations in peak response time must be considered when interpreting unusual or unexpected patterns of glycemic responses in individual patients. While lente insulin is the most widely used of the lente series, particularly in conjunction with regular insulin, there has recently been a resurgence of use of ultralente in combination with multiple injections of rapid-acting insulin (regular insulin or insulin lispro) as a means of attempting optimal control in type 1 patients. Manufacturers have discontinued production of beef ultralente insulin, and only the less sustained and much shorter-acting ultralente made from human insulin is currently available (Table 27–7). Because of its less sustained action compared with beef ultralente, it is generally recommended that the daily dose of Humulin Ultralente be split into two equal doses given every 12 hours.

NPH (neutral protamine Hagedorn or isophane) insulin is an intermediate-acting insulin whose onset of action is delayed by combining two parts soluble crystalline zinc insulin with 1 part protamine zinc insulin. This produces equivalent amounts of insulin and protamine, so that neither is present in an uncomplexed form ("isophane").

The onset and duration of action of NPH insulin are comparable to those of lente insulin (Figure 27–1); it is usually mixed with regular insulin and given at least twice daily for insulin replacement in type 1 patients. Occasional vials of NPH insulin have tended to show unusual clumping of their contents or "frosting" of the container, with considerable loss of bioactivity. This instability is rare and occurs less frequently if NPH human insulin is refrigerated when not in use and if bottles are discarded after 1 month of use.

(4) Mixtures of insulin–Since intermediate insulins require several hours to reach adequate therapeutic levels, their use in type 1 patients requires supplements of regular or lispro insulin preprandially. It is well established that insulin mixtures containing increased proportions of lente to regular insulins may retard the rapid action of admixed regular insulin. The excess zinc in lente insulin binds the soluble insulin and partially blunts its action, particularly when a relatively small proportion of regular insulin is mixed with lente (eg, 1 part regular to 1½ or more parts lente). NPH preparations do not contain excess protamine and so do not delay absorption of admixed regular insulin. They are therefore preferable to lente when mixtures of intermediate and regular insulins are prescribed. For convenience, regular and NPH insulin may be mixed together in the same syringe and injected subcutaneously in split dosage before breakfast and supper. It is recommended that the regular insulin be withdrawn first, then the NPH insulin. No attempt should be made to mix the insulins in the syringe, and the injection is preferably given immediately after loading the syringe. Stable premixed insulins (70% NPH and 30% regular or 50% of each) are available as a convenience to patients who have difficulty mixing insulin because of visual problems or impairment of manual dexterity.

With increasing use of ultra-short-acting insulin lispro as a popular and convenient preprandial insulin, it has become evident that combination with a more sustained insulin is essential to maintain postabsorptive glycemic control. It has been demonstrated that insulin lispro can be acutely mixed with either NPH or ultralente insulin without affecting its rapid absorption. Premixed preparations of lispro and NPH insulins are unstable because of exchange of insulin lispro with the human insulin in the protamine complex. Consequently, the soluble component becomes over time a mixture of regular and insulin lispro at varying ratios. In an attempt to remedy this, an intermediate insulin composed of isophane complexes of protamine with insulin lispro was developed called NPL (neutral protamine lispro). This insulin has the same duration of action as NPH insulin. Premixed combinations of NPL and insulin lispro (eg, 75:25, 50:50, and 25:75 of NPL:insulin lispro) have been tested. The 75% NPL:25% insulin lispro mixture (Humalog Mix 75/25) is available for clinical use. It is marketed only in the form of a disposable insulin pen, and vials are not available. This new mixture has a more rapid onset of glucose-lowering activity compared with the 70% NPH:30% regular human insulin mixture, and it can therefore be given within 15 minutes of starting a meal. It remains to be shown that this new mixture has any other clinical advantage over the usual 70% NPH:30% regular mixture.

Since insulin lispro resists hexamer formation at pharmacologic concentrations, it appears to resist precipitation by high concentrations of zinc and thus cannot be used to make a lente or ultralente formulation. However, this lack of precipitation by zinc allows it to be mixed with any of the lente series—in contrast to regular insulin, which tends to be precipitated by the excess zinc in the lente series when mixed prior to injection.

c. Methods of insulin administration–

(1) Insulin syringes and needles–Plastic disposable syringes with half-inch ultrafine needles attached are available in 1 mL, 0.5 mL, 0.3 mL, and 0.25 mL sizes. In cases where very low insulin doses are prescribed, the specially calibrated 0.3 mL and 0.25 mL disposable syringes facilitate accurate measurement of U100 insulin in doses up to 30 or 25 units, respectively. The "low-dose" syringes have become increasingly popular, because diabetics generally should not take more than 25–30 units of insulin in a single injection, except in rare instances of extreme insulin resistance. Two lengths of needles are available: short, 8 mm, and long, 12.7 mm. Long needles are preferable in obese patients to reduce variability of insulin absorption. Ultrafine needles as small as 30 gauge reduce the pain of injections. "Disposable" syringes may be reused until blunting of the needle occurs (usually after three to five injections).

Sterility adequate to avoid infection with reuse appears to be maintained by recapping syringes between uses. Cleansing the needle with alcohol may not be desirable since it can dissolve the silicon coating and can increase the pain of skin puncturing.

(2) Site of injection–Any part of the body covered by loose skin can be used, such as the abdomen, thighs, upper arms, flanks, and upper buttocks. Preparation with alcohol is no longer required prior to injection as long as the skin is clean. Rotation of sites continues to be recommended to avoid delayed absorption when fibrosis or lipohypertrophy occurs from repeated use of a single site. However, considerable variability of absorption rates from different sites, particularly with exercise, may contribute to the instability of glycemic control in certain type 1 patients if injection sites are rotated too frequently in different areas of the body. Consequently, it is best to limit injection sites to a single region of the body and rotate sites within that region. The abdomen is recommended for subcutaneous injections, since regular insulin has been shown to absorb more rapidly from there than from other subcutaneous sites.

(3) Insulin delivery systems–In the United States, both MiniMed and the Disetronic insulin infusion pumps are available for subcutaneous delivery of insulin. These pumps are small (about the size of a pager) and very easy to program. They have a large number of features, including the ability to set a number of different basal rates throughout the 24 hours and adjust the time over which bolus doses are given. They also are able to detect pressure build-up if the catheter is kinked. Improvements have also been made in the infusion sets. The catheter connecting the insulin reservoir to the subcutaneous cannula can be disconnected, allowing the patient to remove the pump temporarily (eg, for bathing). The great advantage of continuous subcutaneous insulin infusion (CSII) is that it allows for establishment of a basal profile tailored to the patient. The patient therefore is able to eat with less regard to timing because the basal insulin infusion should maintain constant blood glucose between meals.

CSII therapy is appropriate for patients who are motivated, mechanically inclined, educated about diabetes (diet, insulin action, treatment of hypo- and hyperglycemia), and willing to monitor their blood glucose four to six times a day. Known complications of CSII include ketoacidosis, which can occur when insulin delivery is interrupted, and skin infections. Another disadvantage is its cost and the time demanded of physicians and staff in initiating therapy.

Standard methods of insulin administration with multiple subcutaneous injections of soluble, rapid-acting insulin before meals and injections of long-acting insulin or intermediate-acting insulin to maintain basal levels are therefore widely used for intensive insulin therapy. These regimens usually provide acceptable glycemic control if frequent self-monitoring of blood glucose is practiced.

To facilitate these multiple injection regimens, portable pen-sized injectors have been introduced which contain cartridges of U100 regular human insulin and retractable needles (NovoPen, NovolinPen, Insuject). Cartridges of insulin lispro (Humalog) are available as well as dispcsable pens containing insulin lispro, NPH, 70/30 mixtures, and Humalog Mix 75/25. These injectors eliminate the need for carrying an insulin bottle and syringes during the day to provide multiple injections of insulin.

4. Insulin-like growth factor-1 (IGF-1) therapy–In patients with severe insulin resistance who respond poorly to insulin, the use of IGF-1 has been advocated. IGF-1 is a 70-amino-acid peptide which is homologous to human proinsulin. An intravenous bolus of 13 nmol produces hypoglycemia in humans similar to a bolus of 1 nmol of insulin. Several patients with severe insulin resistance due to insulin receptor mutations have responded to IGF-1 but not to insulin, suggesting that the hypoglycemic action of IGF-1 is via its own receptor and not by cross-reacting with the receptor for insulin. Although its use in some cases of severe insulin resistance has been advocated, IGF-1 may promote tumor growth, and there are serious questions about its safety in other than short-term use.

5. Aspirin therapy–A dose of 81–325 mg of enteric-coated aspirin given once daily has been shown to effectively inhibit thromboxane synthesis by platelets and reduce the risk of diabetic atherothrombosis without increasing risks of either vitreous or gastrointestinal hemorrhage. Since diabetic patients have up to a fourfold increase in risk of dying from cardiovascular disease, the use of low-dose enteric-coated aspirin is recommended in diabetic adults with evident macrovascular disease or in those with increased cardiovascular risk factors. Contraindications for aspirin therapy are patients with aspirin allergy, bleeding tendency, recent gastrointestinal bleeding, or active hepatic disease.

C. General Considerations in Treatment of Diabetes: Insulin-treated patients with diabetes can have a full and satisfying life. However, "free" diets and unrestricted activity are still not advised. Until new methods of insulin replacement are developed that provide more normal patterns of insulin delivery in response to metabolic demands, multiple feedings with carbohydrate counting will continue to be recommended, and certain occupations potentially hazardous to the patient or others will continue to be prohibited because of risks due to hypoglycemia. The American Diabetic Association can act as a patient advocate in case of employment questions.

Exercise increases the effectiveness of insulin, and moderate exercise is an excellent means of improving utilization of fat and carbohydrate in diabetic patients. A judicious balance of the size and frequency of meals with moderate regular exercise can often stabilize the insulin dosage in diabetics who tend to slip out of control easily. Strenuous exercise can precipitate hypoglycemia in an unprepared patient, and diabetics must therefore be taught to reduce their insulin dosage in anticipation of strenuous activity or to take supplemental carbohydrate. Injection of insulin into a site farthest away from the muscles most involved in exercise may help ameliorate exercise-induced hypoglycemia, since insulin injected in the proximity of exercising muscle may be more rapidly mobilized.

All diabetic patients must receive adequate instruction on personal hygiene, especially with regard to care of the feet (see below), skin, and teeth. All infections (especially pyogenic ones) provoke the release of high levels of insulin antagonists such as catecholamines or glucagon and thus bring about a marked increase in insulin requirements. Supplemental regular insulin is often required to correct hyperglycemia during infection.

D. The Diabetes Control and Complications Trial (DCCT): A long-term study involving 1441 type 1 patients reported that "near" normalization of blood glucose resulted in a delay in the onset and a major slowing of the progression of established microvascular and neuropathic complications of diabetes during an up to 10-year follow-up.

Multiple insulin injections (66%) or insulin pumps (34%) were used in the intensively treated group who were trained to modify their therapy depending on frequent glucose monitoring. The conventionally treated groups used no more than two insulin injections, and clinical well-being was the goal with no attempt to modify management based on HbA_{1c} or their glucose results.

In one-half of the subjects, a mean hemoglobin A_{1c} of 7.2% (normal: < 6%) and a mean blood glucose of 155 mg/dL was achieved using intensive therapy, while in the conventionally treated group, HbA_{1c} averaged 8.9% with an average blood glucose of 225 mg/dL. Over the study period, which averaged 7 years, there was an approximately 60% reduction in risk between the two groups in regard to diabetic retinopathy, nephropathy, and neuropathy.

Intensively treated patients had a threefold greater risk of serious hypoglycemia as well as a greater tendency toward weight gain. However, there were no deaths definitely attributable to hypoglycemia in any subjects in the DCCT study, and no evidence of posthypoglycemic cognitive damage was detected.

Reinterpretation of the published data from the DCCT trial suggests that "moderate" glycemic control (HbA_{1c} no higher than 2% above the upper limits of normal) rather than "tight" control was just as beneficial in reducing complications while producing fewer episodes of severe hypoglycemia. This implies that adjusting therapeutic glycemic goals a bit higher than those of the DCCT should retain the benefits of intensive insulin therapy at a somewhat lower risk.

The general consensus of the American Diabetes Association is that intensive insulin therapy associated with comprehensive self-management training should become standard therapy in type 1 patients after the age of puberty. Exceptions include those with advanced renal disease and the elderly, since, in these groups, the detrimental risks of hypoglycemia outweigh the benefits of tight glycemic control.

While patients with type 2 were not studied in the DCCT, there is no reason to believe that the effects of better control of blood glucose levels would not also apply to type 2. The eye, kidney, and nerve abnormalities are quite similar in both types of diabetes, and it is likely that similar underlying mechanisms apply. Several important differences, however, must be considered. Since these patients are generally from an older population with a high incidence of macrovascular disease, an episode of severe hypoglycemia entails much greater risk than it would in younger type 1 patients of the DCCT. Moreover, weight gain may be much greater in obese type 2 patients in whom intensive insulin therapy is attempted. These risks take on greater relevance in older type 2 patients who have a relatively lower prevalence of microangiopathy than type 1 patients and in whom prevention of microvascular disease over the long term is much less likely to influence morbidity and mortality because of the much more ominous consequences of their macrovascular disease.

To address these issues raised by the DCCT findings as well as a previous concern that sulfonylureas may *increase* cardiovascular deaths, as reported in 1970 by the University Group Diabetes Program, several randomized clinical therapeutic trials have been conducted, as summarized in the following paragraphs.

E. Clinical Trials in Type 2 Diabetes: These include the Kumamoto Study, the Veterans Affairs Cooperative Study, and the much more extensive United Kingdom Prospective Diabetes Study (UKPDS).

1. The Kumamoto Study involved a relatively small number of type 2 patients (N = 110) who were nonobese and only slightly insulin-resistant, requiring less than 30 units of insulin a day for intensive therapy. Over a 6-year period, it was shown that intensive insulin therapy, achieving a mean HbA_{1c} of 7.1%, significantly reduced microvascular end points compared with conventional insulin therapy, achieving a mean HbA_{1c} of 9.4%. Cardiovascular events were neither worsened nor improved by intensive therapy, and weight changes were not influenced by either form of treatment.

2. The Veterans Administration Cooperative Study involved 153 obese men who were moderately insulin-resistant and who were followed for only 27 months. Intensive insulin treatment resulted in mean HbA_{1c} differences from conventional insulin treatment (7.2% versus 9.5%) that were comparable to those reported from the Kumamoto Study. However, a difference in cardiovascular outcome in this study has prompted some concern. While conventional insulin therapy resulted in 26 total cardiovascular events, there were 35 total cardiovascular events in the inten-

INSTRUCTIONS IN THE CARE OF THE FEET FOR PERSONS WITH DIABETES MELLITUS OR VASCULAR DISTURBANCES

Hygiene of the Feet

(1) Wash feet daily with mild soap and lukewarm water. Dry thoroughly between the toes by pressure. Do not rub vigorously, as this is apt to break the delicate skin.

(2) When feet are thoroughly dry, rub well with vegetable oil to keep them soft, prevent excess friction, remove scales, and prevent dryness. Care must be taken to prevent foot tenderness.

(3) If the feet become too soft and tender, rub them with alcohol about once a week.

(4) When rubbing the feet, always rub upward from the tips of the toes. If varicose veins are present, massage the feet very gently; never massage the legs.

(5) If the toenails are brittle and dry, soften them by soaking for one-half hour each night in lukewarm water containing 1 tbsp of powdered sodium borate (borax) per quart. Follow this by rubbing around the nails with vegetable oil. Clean around the nails with an orangewood stick. If the nails become too long, file them with an emery board. File them straight across and no shorter than the underlying soft tissues of the toe. Never cut the corners of the nails. (The podiatrist should be informed if a patient has diabetes.)

(6) Wear low-heeled shoes of soft leather that fit the shape of the feet correctly. The shoes should have wide toes that will cause no pressure, fit close in the arch, and grip the heels snugly. Wear new shoes one-half hour only on the first day and increase by 1 hour each day following. Wear thick, warm, loose stockings.

Treatment of Corns & Calluses

(1) Corns and calluses are due to friction and pressure, most often from improperly fitted shoes and stockings. Wear shoes that fit properly and cause no friction or pressure.

(2) To remove excess calluses or corns, soak the feet in lukewarm (not hot) water, using a mild soap, for about 10 minutes and then rub off the excess tissue with a towel or file. Do not tear it off. Under no circumstances must the skin become irritated.

(3) Do not cut corns or calluses. If they need attention it is safer to see a podiatrist.

(4) Prevent callus formation under the ball of the foot (a) by exercise, such as curling and stretching the toes several times a day; (b) by finishing each step on the toes and not on the ball of the foot; and (c) by wearing shoes that are not too short and that do not have high heels.

Aids in Treatment of Impaired Circulation (Cold Feet)

(1) Never use tobacco in any form. Tobacco contracts blood vessels and so reduces circulation.

(2) Keep warm. Wear warm stockings and other clothing. Cold contracts blood vessels and reduces circulation.

(3) Do not wear circular garters, which compress blood vessels and reduce blood flow.

(4) Do not sit with the legs crossed. This may compress the leg arteries and shut off the blood supply to the feet.

(5) If the weight of the bedclothes is uncomfortable, place a pillow under the covers at the foot of the bed.

(6) Do not apply any medication to the feet without directions from a physician. Some medicines are too strong for feet with poor circulation.

(7) Do not apply heat in the form of hot water, hot water bottles, or heating pads without a physician's consent. Even moderate heat can injure the skin if circulation is poor.

(8) If the feet are moist or the patient has a tendency to develop athlete's foot, a prophylactic dusting powder should be used on the feet and in shoes and stockings daily. Change shoes and stockings at least daily or oftener.

Treatment of Abrasions of the Skin

(1) Proper first-aid treatment is of the utmost importance even in apparently minor injuries. Consult a physician immediately for any redness, blistering, pain, or swelling. Any break in the skin may become ulcerous or gangrenous unless properly treated by a physician.

(2) Dermatophytosis (athlete's foot), which begins with peeling and itching between the toes or discoloration or thickening of the toenails, should be treated immediately by a physician or podiatrist.

(3) Avoid strong irritating antiseptics such as tincture of iodine.

(4) As soon as possible after any injury, cover the area with sterile gauze, which may be purchased at drugstores. Only fine paper tape or cellulose tape should be used on the skin if adhesive retention of the gauze is required.

(5) Elevate and, as much as possible until recovery, avoid using the foot.

sively treated group. This difference in the relatively small population was not statistically significant, but when the total events were broken down to *major* events (myocardial infarction, stroke, cardiovascular death, congestive heart failure, or amputation), the 18 major events in the group treated intensively with insulin was reported to be statistically greater ($p = .04$) than the ten major events occurring with conventional treatment. While this difference may be a chance consequence of studying too few patients for too short a time, it raises the possibility that insulin-resistant patients with visceral obesity and long-standing type 2 diabetes may develop a greater risk of serious cardiovascular mishap when intensively treated with high doses of insulin. At the end of the study, 64% of the intensively treated group were either receiving (1) an average of 113 units of insulin per day when only two injections per day were used or (2) a mean dosage of 133 units per day when multiple injections were used. Unfortunately, the UKPDS (see below), which did not discern any effect of intensive therapy on cardiovascular outcomes, does not resolve the concern generated by the Veterans Administration Study since their patient population consisted of newly diagnosed diabetic patients in whom the obese subgroup seemed to be less insulin-resistant, requiring a median insulin dose for intensive therapy of only 60 units per day by the 12th year of the study.

3. The United Kingdom Prospective Diabetes Study (UKPDS) began in 1977 as a multicenter clinical trial designed to establish, in type 2 diabetic patients, whether the risk of macrovascular or microvascular complications could be reduced by intensive blood glucose control with oral hypoglycemic agents or insulin and whether any particular therapy was of advantage. Newly diagnosed type 2 diabetic patients aged 25–65 years were recruited between 1977 and 1991, and a total of 3867 were studied over 10 years. The median age at baseline was 54 years; 44% were overweight (> 120% over ideal weight); and baseline HbA_{1c} was 9.1%. Therapies were randomized to include a control group on diet alone and separate groups intensively treated with either insulin, chlorpropamide, glyburide, or glipizide. Metformin was included as a randomization option in a subgroup of 342 overweight patients, and much later in the study an additional subgroup of both normal weight and overweight patients who were responding unsatisfactorily to sulfonylurea therapy were randomized to either continue on their sulfonylurea therapy alone or to have metformin combined with it.

In 1987, an additional modification was made to evaluate whether tight control of blood pressure with stepwise antihypertensive therapy would prevent macrovascular and microvascular complications in 758 hypertensive patients among this UKPDS population compared with 390 of them whose blood pressure was treated less intensively. The tight control group was randomly assigned to treatment with either an angiotensin-converting enzyme (ACE) inhibitor (captopril) or a beta-blocker (atenolol). Both drugs were stepped up to maximum dosages of 100 mg/d and then, if blood pressure remained higher than the target level of < 150/85 mm Hg, more drugs were added in the following stepwise sequence: a diuretic, slow-release nifedipine, methyldopa, and prazosin—until the target level of tight control was achieved. In the control group, hypertension was conventionally treated to achieve target levels < 180/105 mm Hg, but these patients were not prescribed either ACE inhibitors or beta-blockers.

a. Intensive glycemic therapy in the entire group of 3897 newly diagnosed type 2 diabetic patients followed over 10 years showed the following: Intensive treatment with either sulfonylureas, metformin, combinations of those two, or insulin achieved mean HbA_{1c} levels of 7%. This level of glycemic control decreases the risk of microvascular complications in comparison with conventional therapy (mostly diet alone), which achieved mean levels of HbA_{1c} of 7.9%. Weight gain occurred in intensively treated patients except when metformin was used as monotherapy. No cardiovascular benefit and no adverse cardiovascular outcomes were noted regardless of the therapeutic agent. Hypoglycemic reactions occurred in the intensive treatment groups, but only one death from hypoglycemia was documented during 27,000 patient-years of intensive therapy.

When therapeutic subgroups were analyzed, some unexpected and paradoxical results were noted. Among the obese patients, intensive treatment with insulin or sulfonylureas did not reduce microvascular complications compared with diet therapy alone. This was in contrast to the significant benefit of intensive therapy with these drugs in the total group. Furthermore, intensive therapy with metformin was more beneficial in obese persons than diet alone as regards less myocardial infarctions, strokes, and diabetes-related deaths, but there was no significant reduction by metformin of diabetic microvascular complications as compared with the diet group. Moreover, in the subgroup of obese and nonobese patients in whom metformin was added to sulfonylurea failures, rather than showing a benefit, there was a 96% *increase* in diabetes-related deaths compared with the matched cohort of patients with unsatisfactory glycemic control on sulfonylureas who remained on their sulfonylurea therapy. Chlorpropamide also came out poorly on subgroup analysis in that those receiving it as intensive therapy did less well as regards progression to retinopathy than those conventionally treated with diet.

b. Intensive antihypertensive therapy to a mean of 144/82 mm Hg had beneficial effects on microvascular disease as well as on all diabetes-related end points, including virtually all cardiovascular outcomes, in comparison with looser control at a mean of 154/87 mm Hg. In fact, the advantage of reducing hypertension by this amount was substantially more impressive than the benefit accrued by improving the degree of glycemic control from a mean HbA_{1c} of 7.9% to 7%. More than half of the patients needed two or more drugs for adequate therapy of their hypertension, and there was no demonstrable advantage of ACE-inhibitor therapy over therapy with beta-blockers as regards diabetes end points. Use of a calcium channel blocker added to both treatment groups appeared to be safe over the long term in this diabetic population despite some controversy in the recent literature about its safety in diabetics.

Implications of the UKPDS

It appears that glycemic control to levels of HbA_{1c} to 7% shows benefit in reducing total diabetes end points, including a 25% reduction in microvascular disease as compared with HbA_{1c} levels of 7.9%. This reassures those who have questioned whether the value of intensive therapy, so convincingly shown by the DCCT in type 1 diabetes, can safely be extrapolated to older patients with type 2 diabetes. It also argues against the concept of a "threshold" of glycemic control since in this group there was a benefit from this modest reduction of HbA_{1c} below 7.9% whereas in the DCCT a threshold was suggested in that further benefit was less apparent at HbA_{1c} levels below 8%.

Because of the complexity of the overall design in which many of the original therapy groups received additional medications to achieve glycemic goals but remained assigned to the group, statistical analysis may have been compromised by these multiple crossovers. For instance, in the diet group that was used as a control for all the drug treatment groups, only 58% of their total "patient-years" were actually drug-free while the remainder consisted of nonintensive therapy with various hypoglycemic drug regimens to avoid unacceptable hyperglycemia. This probably partly explains why the mean HbA_{1c} for this group was only 7.9% on "diet alone" therapy for over 10 years. In view of these crossovers within treatment groups, caution is suggested regarding several subgroup analyses that are controversial. These include the implication that metformin was superior to insulin or sulfonylureas in reducing diabetes-related end points in obese patients compared with diet therapy even though all three treatment groups achieved the same degree of glycemic control. Conversely, the finding of excess mortality in the subgroup of patients receiving combination therapy with metformin and sulfonylureas need not necessarily preclude this combination in patients doing poorly on sulfonylureas alone, though it certainly indicates a need for clarification of this important question.

Probably the most striking implication of the UKPDS is the benefit to the *hypertensive* type 2 diabetic patient of intensive control of blood pressure. Of interest was the observation that there was no demonstrable advantage of ACE inhibitor therapy on outcome despite a number of short-term reports in smaller populations implying that these drugs have special efficacy in reducing glomerular pressure beyond their general antihypertensive effects. Moreover, slow-release nifedipine showed no evidence of cardiac toxicity in this study despite some previous reports claiming that calcium channel blockers may be hazardous in patients with diabetes. Finally, the greater benefit in diabetes end points from antihypertensive than from antihyperglycemic treatments may be that the difference between the mean blood pressures achieved (144/82 mm Hg versus 154/87 mm Hg) is therapeutically more influential than the slight difference in HbA_{1c} (7% versus 7.9%). Greater hyperglycemia in the control group would most likely have rectified this discrepancy in outcomes. At present, the American Diabetes Association recommends vigorous treatment of both hyperglycemia and hypertension when they occur with an expectation that reductions in microvascular and cardiovascular outcomes will be additive.

Steps in the Management of the Diabetic Patient

A. Diagnostic Examination: Any features of the clinical picture that suggest end-organ insensitivity to insulin, such as visceral obesity, must be identified. The family history should document not only the incidence of diabetes in other members of the family but also the age at onset, whether it was associated with obesity, and whether insulin was required. Other factors that increase cardiac risk, such as smoking history, presence of hypertension or hyperlipidemia, or oral contraceptive pill use, should be recorded.

Laboratory diagnosis should document fasting plasma glucose levels above 126 mg/dL or postprandial values consistently above 200 mg/dL and whether ketonuria accompanies the glycosuria. A glycohemoglobin measurement is useful for assessing the effectiveness of future therapy. Some flexibility of clinical judgment is appropriate when diagnosing diabetes mellitus in the elderly patient with borderline hyperglycemia.

Baseline values include fasting plasma triglycerides, total cholesterol and HDL cholesterol, electrocardiography, renal function studies, peripheral pulses, and neurologic, podiatric, and ophthalmologic examinations to help guide future assessments.

B. Patient Education (Self-Management Training): Since diabetes is a lifelong disorder, education of the patient and the family is probably the most important obligation of the physician who provides initial care. The best persons to manage a disease that is affected so markedly by daily fluctuations in environmental stress, exercise, diet, and infections are the patients themselves and their families. The "teaching curriculum" should include explanations by the physician or nurse of the nature of diabetes and its potential acute and chronic hazards and how they can be recognized early and prevented or treated. The importance of regular tests for glucose on capillary blood specimens should be stressed and instructions on proper testing and recording of data provided. Moreover, patients should be provided with algorithms they can use to adjust the timing and quantity of their insulin dose, food, and exercise in response to recorded blood glucose values for optimal blood glucose control. The targets for blood glucose control should be elevated appropriately in elderly patients since they have the greatest risk if subjected to hypoglycemia and the least long-term benefit from more rigid glycemic control. Advice on personal hygiene, including detailed instructions on foot care, as well as individual instruction on diet and specific hypoglycemic therapy, should be provided. Patients should be told about community agencies, such as Diabetes Association chapters, that can serve as a continuing source of instruction. Finally, vigorous efforts should be made to persuade new diabetics who smoke to give up the habit, since large vessel peripheral vascular disease and debilitating retinopathy are less common in nonsmoking diabetic patients.

C. Self-Monitoring of Blood Glucose: Monitoring of blood glucose by patients has allowed greater flexibility in management while achieving improved glycemic control.

Self-monitoring of blood glucose is particularly useful in brittle diabetics, those attempting "ideal" glycemic control such as during pregnancy, patients who have little or no early warning of hypoglycemic attacks, and those with impaired gastric emptying from diabetic neuropathy or altered renal thresholds for glucose. Self-monitoring of blood glucose is recommended for all insulin-treated diabetic patients. The expert consensus on self-monitoring is that its proper use is to develop a database as an aid in making day-to-day informal decisions about therapy as well as to determine when emergency situations arise. It is particularly valuable as an educational and training tool to enhance understanding of diabetes by patients and their families. The usefulness of self-monitoring depends on the accuracy of the results obtained. Patients must be taught proper techniques, cautioned to calibrate instruments properly despite the expense of strips, to keep proper records, and, particularly, *how to respond to unacceptably high or low blood glucose levels with appropriate therapeutic maneuvers.* Self-monitoring has proved to be an effective and safe clinical tool that can improve glycemic control in compliant patients.

D. Initial Therapy: Treatment must be individualized on the basis of the type of diabetes and specific needs of each patient. However, certain general principles of management can be outlined for hyperglycemic states of different types.

1. The obese type 2 patient–The most common type of diabetic patient is obese, is non-insulin-dependent, and has hyperglycemia because of insensitivity to normal or elevated circulating levels of insulin.

a. Weight reduction–Treatment is directed toward achieving weight reduction, and prescribing a diet is only one means to this end. Behavior modification to achieve adherence to the diet, as well as increased physical activity to expend energy, is also required. Cure can be achieved by reducing adipose stores, with consequent restoration of tissue sensitivity to insulin, but weight reduction is hard to achieve and even more difficult to maintain with our current therapies. The presence of diabetes with its added risk factors may motivate the obese diabetic to greater efforts to lose weight. (See also Chapter 29.)

b. Hypoglycemic agents–Neither insulin nor sulfonylureas are indicated for long-term use in the obese patient with mild diabetes. The weight reduction program can be upset by real or imagined hypoglycemic reactions when insulin therapy or sulfonylureas are used and weight gain is a frequent complication. Monotherapy with alpha-glucosidase inhibitors or metformin may be useful in the obese patient with mild diabetes if pharmacotherapy is required since they are not associated with weight gain or drug-induced hypoglycemia.

If metformin therapy (combined with a weight reduction regimen) is inadequate to control symptoms of hyperglycemia (eg, nocturia, blurred vision, or candidal vulvovaginitis), a sulfonylurea should be added. If this combination of metformin and sulfonylurea is ineffective in achieving appropriate glycemic control, addition of a thiazolidinedione should be considered. Insulin therapy should be instituted if the combination of these three drugs fails to restore euglycemia. Generally, the sulfonylurea is discontinued when insulin therapy is instituted but the patient can stay on the metformin and the thiazolidinedione. Weight-reducing interventions should continue and may allow for simplification of this regimen in the future.

2. The nonobese patient–In the nonobese diabetic, mild to severe hyperglycemia is usually due to refractoriness of B cells to glucose stimulation. Treatment depends on whether insulinopenia is mild (type 2 or mild type 1 in partial remission) or severe, with ketoacidosis.

a. Diet therapy–If hyperglycemia is mild, normal metabolic control can occasionally be restored by means of multiple feedings of a diet limited in simple sugars and with a caloric content sufficient to maintain ideal weight. Restriction of saturated fats and cholesterol is also strongly advised.

b. Oral hypoglycemic agents–When diet therapy in nonketotic type 2 pateints is not sufficient to correct hyperglycemia, a trial of sulfonylureas is often successful in reducing the glycohemoglobin concentration below 9.5%. Once the dosage of one of the more potent sulfonylureas reaches the upper recommended limit in a compliant patient without maintaining fasting blood glucose below 140 mg/dL during the day, combination therapy with metformin (up to 850 mg two or three times daily) and sulfonylureas should be tried. This has been effective in up to 50% of sulfonylurea failures. If the sulfonylurea and metformin combination fails to keep the fasting blood glucose below 140 mg/dL, a thiazolidinedione can be added. When the patient fails the combination of these three drugs, insulin therapy is indicated.

c. Treatment of type 1 with insulin–(Table 27–8.) The patient requiring insulin therapy should be initially regulated under conditions of optimal diet and normal daily activities. Traditional once- or twice-daily insulin regimens are usually ineffective in type 1 patients without residual endogenous insulin despite their widespread use. In these patients, information and counseling based on the findings of the DCCT (see above) should be provided about the advantages of taking multiple injections of insulin in conjunction with self blood glucose monitoring. If near-normalization of blood glucose is attempted, urine glucose measurements are not sufficient, and at least three measurements of capillary blood glucose are required daily to avoid frequent hypoglycemic reactions. Table 27–8 sets forth the advantages and disadvantages of various insulin regimens in this type of diabetes.

(1) Conventional split-dose insulin mixtures–A typical initial dose schedule in a 70-kg patient taking 2200 kcal divided into six or seven feedings might be 10 units of regular and 15 units of NPH insulin in the morning and 5 units of regular and 5 units of NPH insulin in the evening. The morning capillary blood glucose gives a measure of the effectiveness of NPH insulin administered the previous evening; the noon blood glucose reflects the effects of the morning regular insulin; and the 5:00 PM and 9:00 PM sugars represent the effects of the morning NPH and evening regular insulins, respectively. A properly educated patient should be taught to adjust insulin dosage by observing the pattern of glycemia and correlating it with the approximate duration of action and the time of peak effect after injection of the various insulin preparations (Figure 27–1). Adjustments to correct patterns of hyperglycemia should include the following options, either alone or in combination: modification of diet and exercise programs and changes in the insulin dose or its preprandial timing.

(2) Intensive insulin therapy–In most type 1 diabetes cases, conventional split doses of insulin mixtures cannot maintain near normalization of blood glucose without hypoglycemia, particularly at night, and multiple injections of insulin are usually required. An increasingly popular regimen consists of reducing or omitting the evening dose of intermediate insulin and adding a portion of it at bedtime. For example, 10 units of regular insulin mixed with 10 units of NPH insulin in the morning, 8–10 units of regular insulin before the evening meal, and 6 units of NPH insulin at bedtime is often more efficacious than the conventional split-dose regimen mentioned above. The dose of regular insulin prior to a meal should be selected so that each 10–15 g of carbohydrate is covered by 1 unit of regular insulin. With current availability of nutritional labeling, the counting of nutrient carbohydrates should be taught to all patients receiving intensive insulin therapy.

In cases where hypoglycemia occurs unexpectedly day or night, variable or delayed insulin absorption from large subcutaneous depots containing both regular and NPH insulin may be a contributing factor. Reducing the size and changing the character of the depots by administering small doses of regular insulin

Table 27–8. Advantages and disadvantages of various insulin regimens in treatment of type 1 diabetes.

Two Injections (Conventional Split Doses of Regular and NPH Insulin Twice Daily)	Three Injections (Mixtures of Regular and NPH in AM; Regular at Dinner; NPH at Bedtime)	Four Injections (Regular or Insulin Lispro Before Meals and Long-Acting Insulin to Maintain Basal Insulin Levels)
	ADVANTAGES	
Relatively convenient. Controls postprandial glycemia at breakfast and dinner.	Controls postprandial glycemia at breakfast and dinner. Can prevent prebreakfast hyperglycemia with less risk of nocturnal hypoglycemia. Less variability of absorption of NPH, since lower doses are injected to last overnight.	Controls postprandial glycemia. Allows flexibility of meal schedules and quantity. Less variability of absorption of small doses of insulins given more frequently. Tight glycemic control is possible with least risk of hypoglycemia.
	DISADVANTAGES	
Prebreakfast hyperglycemia is common. Increased risk of nocturnal hypoglycemia in attempt to control prebreakfast hyperglycemia. Variability of absorption due to relatively large NPH doses to last overnight.	Less convenient. Lunch schedule is relatively inflexible as to time and quantity to avoid hypoglycemia from morning NPH. Dinner schedule cannot be delayed without extra feedings.	Relatively inconvenient. Pumps are expensive and are generally less convenient than multiple injections and add risk of skin infections and pump failures.

more frequently (eg, three times a day before meals), with one injection of a long-acting insulin (eg, ultralente insulin) at bedtime has often been most helpful in reducing the frequency and severity of hypoglycemia in patients attempting near normalization of blood glucose. This regimen has become more convenient with the advent of pen-injectors and gives greater flexibility regarding meal patterns and diet than conventional therapy with split-dose insulin mixtures.

Insulin lispro has been advocated as a safer and much more convenient alternative to regular human insulin for preprandial use in regimens of intensive insulin therapy. In a study comparing regular insulin with insulin lispro, daily insulin doses and hemoglobin A_{1c} levels were similar, but insulin lispro improved postprandial control, reduced hypoglycemic episodes, and improved patient convenience compared with regular insulin. However, because of its relatively short duration (no more than 3–4 hours), it requires two injections of ultralente insulin at 12-hour intervals or concomitant small doses of intermediate-acting insulin with each preprandial injection to provide basal insulin and thus avoid hyperglycemia prior to the subsequent meal or bedtime snack. In addition to carbohydrate content of the meal, the effect of simultaneous fat ingestion must also be considered a factor in determining the insulin lispro dosage required to control the glycemic increment during and just after the meal. With low-carbohydrate content and high-fat intake there is an increased risk of hypoglycemia from insulin lispro within 2 hours after the meal. In a 65 kg person with type 1 diabetes eating meals of standard carbohydrate content and a moderate to low fat content, a possible regimen of insulin lispro might be started, with the following doses injected only 5–20 minutes before meals and adjusted depending on target blood glucose levels (see Table 27–9).

Since insulin lispro reaches a peak serum level so quickly after subcutaneous administration, smaller doses are generally required compared with regular human insulin. Multiple injections of NPH insulin (or twice-daily ultralente insulin) can be mixed in the same syringe as the insulin lispro.

Occasional patients do not accept multiple injections of insulin and prefer continuous subcutaneous infusions with portable open-loop insulin pumps, which require subcutaneous needle insertion only every 48 hours.

(3) Management of early morning hyperglycemia in type 1–(Table 27–10.) One of the more difficult therapeutic problems in managing patients with type 1 is determining the proper adjustment of insulin dose when the prebreakfast blood glucose level is high.

(a) Somogyi effect–Patients with type 1 may develop nocturnal hypoglycemia, which may in turn stimulate a surge of counterregulatory hormones (Somogyi effect) to produce high blood glucose levels by 7:00 AM. Reducing inappropriately high doses of administered insulin improves morning hyperglycemia.

(b) Dawn phenomenon–The dawn phenomenon is present in as many as 75% of type 1 patients and occurs in most type 2 and normal subjects as well. It is characterized by reduced tissue sensitivity to insulin developing between 5:00 AM and 8:00 AM. This phenomenon may be evoked by spikes of growth hormone released hours before, at the onset of sleep. When the dawn phenomenon occurs alone, it may produce only mild hyperglycemia in the early morning, but when it is associated with the Somogyi effect or the waning phenomenon (or both), the hyperglycemia may be more severe.

(c) Waning of circulating insulin levels–The most common cause of prebreakfast hyperglycemia is probably the waning of circulating insulin levels. This would suggest that more rather than less intermediate-acting insulin should be given in the evening.

Table 27–10 shows that diagnosis of the cause of prebreakfast hyperglycemia can be facilitated by self-monitoring of blood glucose at 3:00 AM in addition to the usual bedtime and 7:00 AM measurements. This is required for only a few nights until the diagnosis is established and appropriate adjustment of bedtime insulin dose or nighttime feeding is achieved.

(d) Therapy of prebreakfast hyperglycemia– When a particular pattern emerges from monitoring

Table 27–9. Two examples of intensive insulin regimens using insulin lispro and either ultralente or NPH insulin in a 70 kg man with type 1 diabetes.[1]

	Pre-Breakfast	Pre-Lunch	Pre-Dinner	At Bedtime
Insulin lispro	5 units	4 units	6 units	—
Ultralente insulin	12 units	—	12 units	—
		OR		
Insulin lispro	5 units	4 units	8 units	—
NPH insulin	3 units	3 units	2 units	8–14 units

[1]The dose of insulin lispro can be raised by 1 or 2 units if extra carbohydrate (15–30 g) is ingested or if premeal blood glucose is > 170 mg/dL. Insulin lispro can be mixed in the same syringe with ultralente or NPH insulin.

Table 27–10. Prebreakfast hyperglycemia: Classification by blood glucose and insulin levels.

	Blood Glucose (mg/dL)			Free Immunoreactive Insulin (μU/mL)		
	10:00 PM	3:00 AM	7:00 AM	10:00 PM	3:00 AM	7:00 AM
Somogyi effect	90	40	200	High	Slightly high	Normal
Dawn phenomenon	110	110	150	Normal	Normal	Normal
Waning of insulin dose plus dawn phenomenon	110	190	220	Normal	Low	Low
Waning of insulin dose plus dawn phenomenon plus Somogyi effect	110	40	380	High	Normal	Low

blood glucose levels overnight, appropriate therapeutic measures can be taken. The Somogyi effect can be treated by eliminating the dose of intermediate insulin at dinnertime and giving it at a lower dosage at bedtime or by supplying more food at bedtime. When the dawn phenomenon alone is present, the dosage of intermediate insulin can be divided between dinnertime and bedtime, or when insulin pumps are used, the basal infusion rate can be increased (eg, from 0.8 unit/h to 1 unit/h from 6:00 AM until breakfast). With waning insulin levels, either increasing the evening dose or shifting it from dinnertime to bedtime, or both, can be effective. A bedtime dose of NPH made from pork insulin provides more sustained overnight insulin levels than human NPH or human ultralente insulin and may be effective in managing refractory prebreakfast hyperglycemia. If this fails, insulin pump therapy may be required.

d. Treatment of type 2 with insulin–When the combination of metformin, sulfonylurea, and a thiazolidinedione fail and type 2 patients require insulin, various insulin regimens may be effective. Although a single morning injection of insulin is not recommended in type 1 diabetes, in some patients with type 2 diabetes enough residual insulin secretion persists to allow a single morning injection of 25–30 units of NPH or lente insulin to replace their deficient insulin secretion. If prebreakfast hyperglycemia persists on this regimen or if hypoglycemia occurs before dinner, a number of alternatives are available. A convenient regimen includes split doses of a fixed 70:30 mixture of NPH:regular insulin, which can be started as 20 units before breakfast and 15 units before dinner and increased appropriately depending on target blood glucoses at 7:00 AM and 5:00 PM. When more than 50 units a day are required without achieving proper control, these patients may benefit from three or four injection regimens as described for type 1 in Table 27–9.

e. Acceptable levels of glycemic control: See above for a discussion of the Diabetes Control and Complications Trial (DCCT) and the United Kingdom Prospective Diabetes Study (UKPDS) and their implications for diabetes therapy. A reasonable aim of therapy is to approach normal glycemic excursions without provoking severe or frequent hypoglycemia. What has been considered "acceptable" control includes blood glucose levels of 90–130 mg/dL before meals and after an overnight fast, and levels no higher than 180 mg/dL 1 hour after meals and 150 mg/dL 2 hours after meals. Glycohemoglobin levels should be no higher than 2% above the upper limit of the normal range for any particular laboratory. It should be emphasized that the value of blood pressure control was as great as or greater than glycemic control in type 2 patients as regards microvascular as well as macrovascular complications.

Complications of Insulin Therapy

A. Hypoglycemia: Hypoglycemic reactions, the most common complication of insulin therapy, may result from delay in taking a meal or unusual physical exertion. With more type 1 patients attempting "tight" control, this complication has become even more frequent. In older diabetics, in those taking only longer-acting insulins, and often in those attempting to maintain euglycemia on infusion pumps, autonomic counterregulatory responses are less readily elicited during hypoglycemia, and central nervous system dysfunction may occur, ie, mental confusion, bizarre behavior, and ultimately coma. Even focal neurologic deficits mimicking stroke may be observed. More rapid development of hypoglycemia from the effects of regular insulin causes signs of autonomic hyperactivity, both sympathetic (tachycardia, palpitations, sweating, tremulousness) and parasympathetic (nausea, hunger), that may progress to coma and convulsions. Except for sweating, most of the sympathetic symptoms of hypoglycemia are blunted in patients receiving beta-blocking agents for angina or hypertension. Though not absolutely contraindicated, these drugs must be used with caution in insulin-requiring diabetics, and, β_1-selective blocking agents are preferred.

1. Altered awareness of hypoglycemia–Since autonomic responses correlate strongly with "awareness" of hypoglycemia, many poorly controlled diabetics—whose nervous systems have adapted to chronic hyperglycemia—may trigger adrenergic alarms at levels of blood glucose above the usual hypoglycemic range. Conversely, type 1 patients overtreated with insulin may be unaware of critically low levels of blood glucose because of an adaptive blunting of their alarm systems owing to repeated episodes of hypoglycemia. This has been shown to be reversible if higher average blood glucose levels are maintained in these patients to avoid recurrent hypoglycemia over a period of several weeks.

As evidenced by results of the DCCT, the risk of frequent severe hypoglycemic episodes is greatly increased when "normalization" of the blood glucose is attempted with presently available methods of insulin delivery, and this is independent of the species of insulin used. "Near normalization" is therefore a safer target for therapy to avoid hypoglycemic unawareness.

2. Lack of glucagon response in type 1–For unexplained reasons, patients with type 1 lose their glucagon responses to hypoglycemia (but not to amino acids in protein-containing meals) within a year or so after developing diabetes. These patients then rely predominantly on the sympathetic nervous system to counterregulate hypoglycemia and are at special risk in later years when aging, autonomic neuropathy, or frequent hypoglycemic episodes blunt their sympathetic responses.

3. Prevention and treatment of hypoglycemia–Because of the potential danger of insulin-induced reactions, the diabetic patient should carry packets of table sugar or a candy roll at all times for use at the onset of hypoglycemic symptoms. Tablets containing 3 g of glucose are available (dextrosol). The educated patient soon learns to take the amount of glucose needed and avoids the excess that may occur with eating candy or drinking orange juice, causing very high hyperglycemia. An ampule of glucagon (1 mg) should be provided to every diabetic receiving insulin therapy, and family or friends should be instructed how to inject it intramuscularly in the event that the patient is unconscious or refuses food. An identification MedicAlert bracelet, necklace, or card in the wallet or purse should be carried by every diabetic receiving hypoglycemic drug therapy. The telephone number for the MedicAlert Foundation International in Turlock, California, is 800-ID-ALERT.

All of the manifestations of hypoglycemia are rapidly relieved by glucose administration. If more severe hypoglycemia has produced unconsciousness or stupor, the treatment is 50 mL of 50% glucose solution by rapid intravenous infusion. If intravenous therapy is not available, 1 mg of glucagon injected intramuscularly will usually restore the patient to consciousness within 15 minutes to permit ingestion of sugar. If the patient is stuporous and glucagon is not available, small amounts of honey or syrup can be inserted within the buccal pouch, but, in general, oral feeding is contraindicated in unconscious patients. Rectal administration of syrup or honey (30 mL per 500 mL of warm water) has been effective.

B. Immunopathology of Insulin Therapy: At least five molecular classes of insulin antibodies are produced during the course of insulin therapy in diabetes, including IgA, IgD, IgE, IgG, and IgM. With the increased therapeutic use of purified pork and especially human insulin, the various immunopathologic syndromes such as insulin allergy, immune insulin resistance, and lipoatrophy have become quite rare since the titers and avidity of these induced antibodies are generally quite low. However, in parts of the world where less purified forms of beef insulin are still used, these disorders remain a clinical concern among some insulin-treated patients.

1. Insulin allergy–Insulin allergy, or immediate-type hypersensitivity, is a rare condition in which local or systemic urticaria is due to histamine release from tissue mast cells sensitized by adherence of anti-insulin IgE antibodies. In severe cases, anaphylaxis results. When only human insulin has been used from the onset of insulin therapy, insulin allergy is exceedingly rare. Antihistamines, corticosteroids, and even desensitization may be required, especially for systemic hypersensitivity. There have been case reports of successful use of insulin lispro in those rare patients who have a generalized allergy to human insulin or insulin resistance due to a high titer of insulin antibodies.

2. Immune insulin resistance–Most insulin-treated patients develop a low titer of circulating IgG anti-insulin antibodies that neutralize to a small extent the action of insulin. However, under rare circumstances, in some type 2 diabetic patients, principally those with some degree of tissue insensitivity to insulin (such as in the obese) and with a history of interrupted exposure to therapy with beef insulin, a high titer of circulating IgG anti-insulin antibodies may develop. This results in extremely high insulin requirements—often more than 200 units daily. This is often a self-limited condition and may clear spontaneously after several months. However, with advances in insulin purification and the use of human insulins, this syndrome has essentially disappeared in all industrialized countries.

C. Lipodystrophy at Injection Sites: Atrophy of subcutaneous fatty tissue leading to disfiguring excavations and depressed areas may rarely occur at the site of injection. This complication results from an immune reaction, and it has become rarer with the development of pure insulin preparations. Injection of these preparations directly into the atrophic area often results in restoration of normal contours. Lipohypertrophy, on the other hand, is a consequence of the pharmacologic effects of insulin being deposited in the same location repeatedly. It can occur with purified insulins and is best treated with localized liposuction of the hypertrophic areas by an experienced plastic surgeon. Rotation of injection sites will prevent lipohypertrophy. There is a case report of a patient who had intractable lipohypertrophy with human insulin but no longer had the problem when he switched to insulin lispro.

Chronic Complications of Diabetes

Late clinical manifestations of diabetes mellitus include a number of pathologic changes that involve small and large blood vessels, cranial and peripheral nerves, the skin, and the lens of the eye. These lesions lead to hypertension, renal failure, blindness, autonomic and peripheral neuropathy, amputations of the lower extremities, myocardial infarction, and cerebrovascular accidents. These late manifestations correlate with the duration of the diabetic state subsequent to the onset of puberty. In type 1 diabetes, up to 40% of patients develop end-stage renal disease, compared with less than 20% of patients with type 2 diabetes. As regards proliferative retinopathy, it ultimately develops in both types of diabetes but has a slightly higher prevalence in type 1 patients (25% after 15 years' duration). In patients with type 1 diabetes, complications from end-stage renal disease are a major cause of death, whereas patients with type 2 diabetes are more likely to have macrovascular diseases leading to myocardial infarction and stroke as the main causes of death.

A. Ocular Complications:

1. Diabetic cataracts–Premature cataracts occur in diabetic patients and seem to correlate with both the duration of diabetes and the severity of chronic hyperglycemia. Nonenzymatic glycosylation of lens protein is twice as high in diabetic patients as in age-matched nondiabetic persons and may contribute to the premature occurrence of cataracts.

2. Diabetic retinopathy–Three main categories exist: background, or "simple," retinopathy, consisting of microaneurysms, hemorrhages, exudates, and retinal edema; preproliferative retinopathy with arteriolar ischemia manifested as cotton-wool spots (small infarcted areas of retina); and proliferative, or "malignant," retinopathy, consisting of newly formed vessels. Proliferative retinopathy is a leading cause of blindness in the USA, particularly since it increases the risk of retinal detachment. Vision-threatening retinopathy virtually never appears in type 1 patients in the first 3–5 years of diabetes or before puberty. Up to 20% of patients with type 2 diabetes have retinopathy at the time of diagnosis. Annual consultation with an ophthalmologist should be arranged for patients who have had type 1 diabetes for more than 3–5 years and for all patients with type 2 diabetes, because many were probably diabetic for an extensive period of time before diagnosis. Patients with any macular edema, severe nonproliferative retinopathy, or any proliferative retinopathy require the care of an ophthalmologist. Extensive "scatter" xenon or argon photocoagulation and focal treatment of new vessels reduce severe visual loss in those cases in which proliferative retinopathy is associated with recent vitreous hemorrhages or in which extensive new vessels are located on or near the optic disk. Macular edema, which is more common than proliferative retinopathy in patients with type 2 diabetes (up to 20% prevalence), has a guarded prognosis, but it has also responded to scatter therapy with improvement in visual acuity if detected early. Avoiding tobacco use and correction of associated hypertension are important therapeutic measures in the management of diabetic retinopathy.

3. Glaucoma–Glaucoma occurs in approximately 6% of persons with diabetes. It is responsive to the usual therapy for open-angle disease. Neovascularization of the iris in diabetics can predispose to closed-angle glaucoma, but this is relatively uncommon except after cataract extraction, when growth of new vessels has been known to progress rapidly, involving the angle of the iris and obstructing outflow.

B. Diabetic Nephropathy: As many as 4000 cases of end-stage renal disease occur each year among diabetic people in the United States. This is about one-third of all patients being treated for end-stage renal disease and represents a considerable national health expense.

The cumulative incidence of nephropathy differs between the two major types of diabetes. Patients with type 1 diabetes have a 30–40% chance of having nephropathy after 20 years—in contrast to the much lower frequency in type 2 diabetes patients, in whom only about 15–20% develop clinical renal disease. However, since there are many more individuals affected with type 2 diabetes, end-stage renal disease is much more prevalent in type 2 than in type 1 diabetes in the United States and especially throughout the rest of the world. Improved glycemic control and more effective therapeutic measures to correct hypertension—and with the beneficial effects of angiotensin-converting enzyme inhibitors—can reduce the development of end-stage renal disease among diabetics.

Diabetic nephropathy is initially manifested by proteinuria; subsequently, as kidney function declines, urea and creatinine accumulate in the blood.

1. Microalbuminuria–Sensitive radioimmunoassay methods of detecting small amounts of urinary albumin have permitted detection of microgram concentrations—in contrast to the less sensitive dipstick strips, whose minimal detection limit is 0.3–0.5%. Conventional 24-hour urine collections, in addition to being inconvenient for patients, also show wide variability of albumin excretion, since several factors such as sustained erect posture, dietary protein, and exercise tend to increase albumin excretion rates. For these reasons, most laboratories prefer to measure a timed overnight urine collection beginning at bedtime, when the urine is discarded and the time noted. Normal subjects excrete less than 15 μg/min during overnight urine collections; values of 20 μg/min or higher are considered to represent abnormal microalbuminuria. A convenient screening method involves analysis of the albumin-creatinine ratio in an early morning spot urine collected upon awakening and brought in by the patient. A ratio of albumin (μg/L) to creatinine (mg/L) of < 30 μg/mg creatinine is normal, and a ratio of 30–300 μg/mg creatinine suggests abnormal microalbuminuria. At least two of three timed overnight urine collections over a 3- to 6-month period should be abnormal before a diagnosis of microalbuminuria is justified.

Subsequent renal failure can be predicted by persistent urinary albumin excretion rates exceeding 30 μg/min. Increased microalbuminuria correlates with increased levels of blood pressure and increased LDL cholesterol, and this may explain why increased proteinuria in diabetic patients is associated with an increase in cardiovascular deaths even in the absence of renal failure. Glycemic control as well as a low-protein diet (0.8 g/kg/d) may reduce both the hyperfiltration and the elevated microalbuminuria in patients in the early stages of diabetes and those with incipient diabetic nephropathy. Antihypertensive therapy also decreases microalbuminuria. Evidence from some studies—but not the UKPDS—supports a specific role for ACE inhibitors in reducing intraglomerular pressure in addition to their lowering of systemic hypertension. An ACE inhibitor (captopril, 50 mg twice daily) in normotensive diabetics impedes progression to proteinuria and prevents the increase in albumin excretion rate. Since microalbuminuria has been shown to correlate with elevated *nocturnal* systolic blood pressure, it is possible that "normotensive" diabetic patients with microalbuminuria have slightly elevated systolic blood pressure during sleep which is lowered during antihypertensive therapy. This action may contribute to the reported efficacy of ACE inhibitor drugs in reducing microalbuminuria in "normotensive" patients.

2. Progressive diabetic nephropathy–Progressive diabetic nephropathy consists of proteinuria of varying severity occasionally leading to nephrotic syndrome with hypoalbuminemia, edema, and an increase in circulating betalipoproteins as well as progressive azotemia. In contrast to all other renal disorders, the proteinuria associated with diabetic nephropathy does not diminish with progressive renal failure (patients continue to excrete 10–11 g daily as creatinine clearance diminishes). As renal failure progresses, there is an elevation in the renal threshold at which glycosuria appears.

Hypertension develops with progressive renal involvement, and coronary and cerebral atherosclerosis seems to be accelerated. Approximately two-thirds of adult patients with diabetes have hypertension. Once diabetic nephropathy has progressed to the stage of hypertension, proteinuria, or early renal failure, glycemic control is not beneficial in influencing its course. In this circumstance, antihypertensive medications, including ACE inhibitors, and restriction of dietary protein to 0.8 g/kg body weight per day are recommended. ACE inhibitors have been shown to protect against deterioration in renal function in type 1 diabetic patients with clinical nephropathy. This beneficial effect appears to be due to improved glomerular hemodynamics that cannot be explained only by the antihypertensive action of these drugs. Captopril (25 mg three times daily) has shown a 50% reduction in the risk of the combined end points of death, dialysis and transplantation in type 1 subjects with diabetic nephropathy and clinical proteinuria. During initiation of ACE-inhibitor therapy, an increment in serum creatinine greater than 2 mg/dL due to a rapid fall in intraglomerular pressure—or the occurrence of persistent hyperkalemia (above 6 meq/L) due to hyporeninemic hypoaldosteronism—is an indication to stop this medication.

Dialysis has been of limited value in the long-term treatment of renal failure due to diabetic nephropathy. At present, experience in renal transplantation—especially from related donors—is more promising and is the treatment of choice in cases where there are no contraindications such as severe cardiovascular disease.

C. Gangrene of the Feet: The incidence of gangrene of the feet in diabetics is 20 times the incidence in matched controls. The factors responsible for its development are ischemia, peripheral neuropathy, and secondary infection. Occlusive vascular disease involves both microangiopathy and atherosclerosis of large and medium-sized arteries. Cigarette smoking should be avoided, and prevention of foot disease should be emphasized, since treatment is difficult once ulceration and gangrene have developed. Patients should be examined with a 10-g Semmes-Weinstein monofilament to ensure that protective sensation is intact. If it is not, cushioned socks, athletic shoes, and special foot care are needed since insensitive feet are at high risk for development of neuropathic ulcers. Patients should be instructed to inspect their feet daily for reddened areas, blisters, abrasions, or lacerations (see Instructions in the Care of the Feet). Physicians should inspect the feet at each visit and instruct patients as necessary on filing calluses with an emery board, cutting toenails straight across, not walking barefoot, and avoiding tight shoes. When an uncomplicated neuropathic ulcer is present and blood flow is not impaired, consultation with a podiatrist or orthopedist is recommended. Cholesterol-lowering agents are useful as adjunctive therapy when early ischemic signs are detected. If blood supply is diminished or absent, patients with foot ulcers should be referred to an appropriate specialist (vascular or orthopedic surgeon). When chronic foot ulcers are refractory to standard debridement and antibiotics, platelet-derived growth factor should be considered for local application. Regranex has been safe and effective. Special custom-built shoes are usually required to redistribute weight evenly over an insensitive foot when it has been deformed by surgery or asymptomatic fractures (Charcot's joint). Amputation of the lower extremities is sometimes required, but appropriate prophylactic foot care has greatly reduced its frequency.

Nonselective beta-blockers are relatively contraindicated in patients with ischemic foot ulcers, because these drugs may potentially reduce peripheral blood flow.

D. Diabetic Neuropathy: Peripheral and autonomic neuropathy, the two most common chronic complications of diabetes, are poorly understood.

1. Peripheral neuropathy–

a. Distal symmetric polyneuropathy–This is the most common form of diabetic peripheral neuropathy where loss of function appears in a stocking-glove pattern and is due to an axonal neuropathic process. Sensory involvement usually occurs first and is generally bilateral, symmetric, and associated with dulled perception of vibration, pain, and temperature, particularly in the lower extremities. At times, discomfort of the lower extremities can be incapacitating. Both motor and sensory nerve conduction are delayed in peripheral nerves, and ankle jerks may be absent. In most cases, motor weakness is mild and confined to the most distal intrinsic muscles of the hands and feet. Long-term complications of diabetic polyneuropathy include insensitivity of the feet, leading to repeated "silent" trauma that predisposes to neuropathic plantar ulcers or deformities of the feet secondary to multiple "silent" fractures (Charcot's joint).

b. Isolated peripheral neuropathy–Involvement of the distribution of only one nerve ("mononeuropathy"), or of several nerves ("mononeuropathy multiplex") is characterized by sudden onset with subsequent recovery of all or most of the function. This neuropathology has been attributed to vascular ischemia or traumatic damage. Femoral and cranial nerves are commonly involved, and motor abnormalities predominate. These can result in sudden onset of diplopia due to ophthalmoplegia or in acute pain and weakness of thigh muscles (diabetic amyotrophy). Spontaneous resolution of these ischemic neuropathies generally occurs in 6–12 weeks. In more severe cases with extensive atrophy of limb musculature, this disorder has been termed "malignant cachexia" and mimics the end stages of advanced neoplasia, particularly when depression produces anorexia and weight loss. With this more severe manifestation of diabetic amyotrophy, recovery of muscle function may only be partial.

c. Painful diabetic neuropathy–Hypersensitivity to light touch and occasionally severe "burning" pain, particularly at night, can become physically and emotionally disabling. Amitriptyline, 25–75 mg at bedtime, has been recommended for pain associated with diabetic neuropathy. Dramatic relief has often resulted within 48–72 hours. This rapid response is in contrast to the 2 or 3 weeks required for an antidepressive effect. Patients often attribute benefit to their having a full night's sleep after amitriptyline compared to many previously sleepless nights occasioned by neuropathic pain. Mild to moderate morning drowsiness is a side effect that generally improves with time or can be lessened by giving the medication several hours before bedtime. This drug should not be continued if improvement has not occurred after 5 days of therapy. Desipramine in doses of 25–150 mg/d seems to have the same efficacy as amitriptyline. Gabapentin (900–1800 mg/d in three divided doses) has also been shown to be effective in the treatment of painful neuropathy and should be tried if the tricyclic drugs prove ineffective. There has also been interest in use of the antiarrhythmic drug mexiletine for this purpose in doses of up to 10 mg/kg/d. Capsaicin, a topical irritant, has been found to be effective in reducing local nerve pain; it is dispensed as a cream (Zostrix 0.025%, Zostrix-HP 0.075%) to be rubbed into the skin over the painful region two to four times daily. Gloves should be used for application since hand contamination could result in discomfort if the cream comes in contact with eyes or sensitive areas such as the genitalia.

2. Autonomic neuropathy–With autonomic neuropathy, there is evidence of postural hypotension, decreased cardiovascular response to Valsalva's maneuver, gastroparesis, alternating bouts of diarrhea (particularly nocturnal) and constipation, inability to empty the bladder, and impotence. Gastroparesis should be considered in insulin-dependent diabetic patients who develop unexpected fluctuations and variability in their blood glucose levels after meals. Impotence due to neuropathy differs from psychogenic impotence in that the latter may be intermittent (erections occur under special circumstances), whereas diabetic impotence is usually persistent; aortoiliac occlusive disease may contribute to this problem.

a. Management of autonomic neuropathy– There is no consistently effective treatment for diabetic autonomic neuropathy. Metoclopramide has been of some help in treating diabetic gastroparesis over the short term, but its effectiveness seems to diminish over time. It is a dopamine antagonist that has central antiemetic effects as well as a cholinergic action to facilitate gastric emptying. It can be given intravenously (10 mg three or four times a day, 30 minutes before meals and at bedtime) or orally (20 mg of liquid metoclopramide) before breakfast and dinner. Drowsiness, restlessness, fatigue, and lassitude are common adverse effects. Tardive dyskinesia and extrapyramidal effects also occur. Cisapride (10 mg three or four times daily) can improve the rate of gastric emptying of both liquids and solids by virtue of its cholinergic and antiserotonergic actions. It appears to be better tolerated and to cause fewer central nervous system side effects than metoclopramide, but it may cause troublesome increased stool frequency in some patients. Cisapride can cause life-threatening cardiac arrhythmias, including ventricular tachycardia, ventricular fibrillation, torsade de pointes, and QT prolongation. Many of the patients in whom this occurred were also taking drugs that inhibit cytochrome P450 3A4 isoenzyme and increase cisapride blood levels (eg, macrolides, azole antifungals). Eighty deaths have been reported, and Janssen Pharmaceutical has therefore withdrawn the drug from the United States. The company will, however, make the drug available to patients in whom the benefits far outweigh the risks (contact 1-800-526-7736). Erythromycin appears to bind to motilin receptors in the stomach and has been found to improve gastric emptying in doses of 250 mg three times daily. Diarrhea associated with autonomic neuropathy has occasionally responded to broad-spectrum antibiotic therapy, though it often undergoes spontaneous remission. Refractory diabetic diarrhea is often associated with impaired sphincter control and fecal incontinence. Therapy with loperamide, 4–8 mg daily, or diphenoxylate with atropine, two tablets up to four times a day, may provide relief. In more severe cases, tincture of paregoric or codeine (60 mg tablets) may be required to reduce the frequency of diarrhea and improve the consistency of the stools. Clonidine has been reported to lessen diabetic diarrhea, but its tendency to lower blood pressure in these patients who already have autonomic neuropathy and some orthostatic hypotension often limits its usefulness. Bethanechol in doses of 10–50 mg three times a day has occasionally improved emptying of the atonic urinary bladder. Catheter decompression of the distended bladder has been reported to improve its function, and considerable benefit has been reported after surgical severing of the internal vesicle sphincter. Mineralocorticoid therapy with fludrocortisone, 0.2–0.3 mg/d, and elastic stockings or pressure suits have reportedly been of some help in patients with orthostatic hypotension occurring as a result of loss of postural reflexes.

b. Management of erectile dysfunction– There are medical, mechanical, and surgical treatments available for treatment of erectile dysfunction. Penile erection depends on relaxation of the smooth muscle in the arteries of the corpus cavernosum, and this is mediated by nitric oxide-induced cyclic 3′,5′-guanosine monophosphate (cGMP) formation. Sildenafil (Viagra) is a selective inhibitor of cGMP-specific phosphodiesterase type 5. In response to sexual stimulation, there is local release of nitric oxide and cGMP production, and sildenafil, by inhibiting the breakdown of cGMP, improves the ability to attain and maintain an erection. The recommended dose for most patients is one 50 mg tablet taken approximately 1 hour before sexual activity. The peak effect is at 1.5–2 hours, with some effect persisting for 4 hours. Patients with diabetes mellitus using sildenafil reported 50–60% improvement in erectile function. The maximum recommended dose is 100 mg. In clinical trials, only a few adverse effects have been reported—transient mild headache, flushing, dyspepsia, and some altered color vision, particularly with the 100 mg dose. There was no priapism or increase in libido. Because of sildenafil's potentiation of the hypotensive effects of nitrates, its use is contraindicated in patients who are concurrently using organic nitrates in any form. Following its approval and release, a number of deaths have resulted from its use in men with active cardiovascular disease. The FDA has mandated a warning label change in the package insert, advising caution for men who have suffered a heart attack, stroke, or life-threatening arrhythmia within the previous 6 months; men who have resting hypotension or hypertension; and men who have a history of cardiac failure or have unstable angina.

Intracorporeal injection of vasoactive drugs causes penile engorgement and erection. Drugs most commonly used include papaverine alone, papaverine with phentolamine, and alprostadil (prostaglandin E_1). Alprostadil injections are relatively painless, but careful instruction is essential to prevent local trauma, priapism, and fibrosis. Intraurethral pellets of alprostadil avoid the problem of injection of the drug.

External vacuum therapy (Erec-Aid System) is a nonsurgical treatment consisting of a suction chamber operated by a hand pump that creates a vacuum around the penis. This draws blood into the penis to produce an erection which is maintained by a specially designed tension ring inserted around the base of the penis and which can be kept in place for up to 20–30 minutes. While this method is generally effective, its cumbersome nature limits its appeal.

In view of the recent development of nonsurgical approaches to therapy of erectile dysfunction, resort to surgical implants of penile prostheses is becoming less common.

E. Skin and Mucous Membrane Complications: Chronic pyogenic infections of the skin may occur, especially in poorly controlled diabetic patients. Eruptive xanthomas can result from hypertriglyceridemia, associated with poor glycemic control. An unusual lesion termed **necrobiosis lipoidica diabeticorum** is usually located over the anterior surfaces of the legs or the dorsal surfaces of the ankles. They are oval or irregularly shaped plaques with demarcated borders and a glistening yellow surface and occur in women two to four times more frequently than in men.

"Shin spots" are not uncommon in adult diabetics. They are brownish, rounded, painless atrophic lesions of the skin in the pretibial area. Candidal infection can produce erythema and edema of intertriginous areas below the breasts, in the axillas, and between the fingers. It causes vulvovaginitis in most chronically uncontrolled diabetic women with persistent glucosuria and is a frequent cause of pruritus.

While antifungal creams containing miconazole or

clotrimazole offer immediate relief of vulvovaginitis, recurrence is frequent unless glucosuria is reduced.

F. Special Situations:

1. Insulin replacement during surgery–It is likely that target glucose levels between 100 and 250 mg/dL are adequate in most patients to avoid postoperative infections or wound dehiscence, though this view is based on clinical observations rather than conclusive evidence. All diabetic patients should have serum electrolytes measured preoperatively so that abnormalities can be corrected prior to surgery. During major surgery and in the immediate recovery period in patients with type 1 diabetes, 5% dextrose in physiologic saline containing 20 meq of potassium chloride should be infused intravenously at a rate of 100–200 mL/h with regular human insulin (25 units/250 mL 0.9% saline) infused into the intravenous tubing at a rate of 1–3 units/h. The patient's blood glucose should be monitored every hour initially and the rates of insulin or dextrose adjusted to maintain blood glucose values between 120 and 190 mg/dL (although levels up to 250 mg/dL may be acceptable).

Most patients with type 2 diabetes, whether or not they are receiving insulin therapy, should be treated with insulin during major surgery. In these patients, 10 units of regular human insulin added to 1000 mL of a D_5W solution containing 20 meq of potassium chloride and infused at a rate of 100 mL/h (1 unit/h) is generally adequate to regulate glycemia during surgery. The patient's glucose should be monitored hourly to prevent extremes of hyper- or hypoglycemia. If blood glucose values remain above 250 mg/dL at 1–2 hours, an infusion concentration of 15 units/L can be substituted.

Type 2 patients facing minor surgical procedures not requiring general anesthesia who have previously been controlled on oral agents or diet alone do not generally require insulin infusions. Glucose-containing solutions should be avoided during surgery in these patients, and blood glucose levels should be monitored every 4 hours. Regular human insulin or insulin lispro should be administered subcutaneously if needed to maintain blood glucose below 250 mg/dL (see Chapter 2).

2. Pregnancy and the diabetic patient–Several features distinguish the management of diabetics during pregnancy from the general therapy of diabetes These include the following: (1) Oral hypoglycemic agents are contraindicated. (2) Weight reduction is not advised, since fetal nutrition can be adversely affected (3) Intensive insulin therapy with frequent self-monitoring of blood glucose is generally recommended to improve the likelihood of having healthy normal babies. Every effort should be made, utilizing multiple injections of insulin or a continuous infusion of insulin by pump, to maintain near-normalization of fasting and preprandial blood glucose values while avoiding hypoglycemia. Glycohemoglobin should be maintained in the normal range.

Since many diabetic pregnancies persist beyond the expected term—or because the infants are usually large and hydramnios may be present—it has been suggested that pregnancy be terminated early (at 37–38 weeks), especially if glycemic control during pregnancy has been inadequate (eg, glycohemoglobin > 10%). There is a present trend away from elective cesarean section and toward induction of labor.

See Chapter 18 for further details.

Prognosis

The Diabetes Control and Complications Trial (DCCT) showed that the previously poor prognosis for as many as 40% of patients with type 1 diabetes is markedly improved by optimal care. DCCT participants were generally young and highly motivated and were cared for in academic centers by skilled diabetes educators and endocrinologists who were able to provide more attention and services than are usually available. Improved training of primary care providers may be beneficial.

For type 2 diabetes, the UKPDS documented a reduction in microvascular disease with glycemic control, though this was not apparent in the obese subgroup. Cardiovascular outcomes were not improved by glycemic control, though among hypertensive patients antihypertensive therapy showed benefit in reducing the number of adverse cardiovascular complications as well as in reducing the occurrence of microvascular disease. In those with visceral obesity, its successful management remains a major challenge in the attempt to achieve appropriate control of hyperglycemia, hypertension, and dyslipidemia. Once safe and effective methods are devised to prevent or manage obesity, the prognosis of type 2 diabetes with its high cardiovascular risks should improve considerably.

In addition to poorly understood genetic factors relating to differences in individual susceptibility to development of long-term complications of hyperglycemia, it is clear that in both types of diabetes, the diabetic patient's intelligence, motivation, and awareness of the potential complications of the disease contribute significantly to the ultimate outcome.

Internet Addresses

[American Association of Diabetes Educators]
http://www.aadenet.org/

[American Diabetes Association]
http://www.diabetesnet.com/ada.html

[American Dietetic Association]
http://www.eatright.org

[Juvenile Diabetes Foundation]
http://www.jdf.org/index.html

Classification, Pathophysiology, & Diagnosis of Diabetes Mellitus

Ferrannini E: Insulin resistance versus insulin deficiency in non-insulin-dependent diabetes mellitus: Problems and prospects. Endocr Rev 1998;19:477. [NLM Cit ID:

98381165] (This comprehensive review of the pathophysiology of type 2 diabetes emphasizes the presence of both insulin resistance and a defect in insulin secretion in most patients with this syndrome. While genetic factors could explain either or both of these abnormalities, the author indicates how acquired causes contribute to both defects and might even be primarily responsible. Until specific genes are identified, the relative influence of inheritance and environment on the etiology of type 2 diabetes remains to be clarified.)

Gottlieb PA et al: Diagnosis and treatment of pre-insulin dependent diabetes. Annu Rev Med 1998;49:391. [NLM Cit ID: 98170009] (The identification of certain genetic and serological markers allows identification of subjects at high risk for the development of autoimmune type 1 diabetes. This review discusses current clinical approaches to preventing full expression of clinical diabetes in these individuals and updates current concepts of the etiology of type 1 diabetes.)

Hunter SJ et al: Insulin action and insulin resistance: Diseases involving defects in insulin receptors, signal transduction, and the glucose transport effector system. Am J Med 1998;105:331. [NLM Cit ID: 99025567] (A current review of the molecular basis of insulin resistance in various human diseases, including cases of insulin receptor mutations, polycystic ovary syndrome, and type 2 diabetes.)

JAMA patient page: Diabetes. JAMA 1998;280:202. [NLM Cit ID: 98332462]

Report of the expert committee on the diagnosis and classification of diabetes mellitus. Diabetes Care 2000;23 (Suppl 1):S4. (This revision of the previous 1997 therapeutic classification drops the terms "insulin-dependent" and "non-insulin dependent diabetes mellitus" and the acronyms IDDM and NIDDM. It provides an etiologic classification for a number of disorders of carbohydrate metabolism, including those whose genetic mechanisms are known, such as the forms of maturity-onset diabetes of the young, mitochondrial mutations of the pancreatic B cells, mutations of the insulin receptor, and other specific types of diabetes.)

Winter WE et al: Monogenic diabetes mellitus in youth. The MODY syndromes. Endocrinol Metab Clin North Am 1999;28:765. [NLM Cit ID: 20077119] (A current review of the genetic mutations responsible for the various clinical forms of MODY, with a discussion of the difficulties in distinguishing between MODY and idiopathic type 1 diabetes among blacks.)

Yamashita S et al: Insulin resistance and body fat distribution: Contribution of visceral fat accumulation to the development of insulin resistance and atherosclerosis. Diabetes Care 1996;19:287. [NLM Cit ID: 96341969] (Using CT scans, the ratio of visceral fat area to subcutaneous fat area [V/S ratio] was used to define certain obese patients with the "visceral fat syndrome." This highly atherogenic state includes visceral fat accumulation, glucose intolerance [insulin resistance], hyperlipidemia, and hypertension.)

Therapy of Diabetes Mellitus

American Diabetes Association: Clinical practice recommendations 1999. Diabetes Care 2000;23(Suppl 1):S1. (A detailed compendium of all the current position statements of the ADA regarding screening, diagnostic procedures, and standards of medical care for treating the acute and chronic complications of type 1 and type 2 diabetes.)

American Diabetes Association: Diabetes mellitus and exercise. (Position statement) Diabetes Care 2000;23 (Suppl 1):S50. (Discussion on how to evaluate a patient with diabetes who wants to start an exercise program. There is also a discussion on the effects of exercise on metabolic control in both type 1 and type 2 diabetes.)

American Diabetes Association: Nutrition recommendations and principles for people with diabetes mellitus. (Position statement.) Diabetes Care 2000;23(Suppl 1):S43. (Major changes in nutritional therapy of diabetes include the elimination of "ADA diet prescriptions," allowing freer substitution of sucrose in the meals and recommending tailored prescriptions for each diabetic patient based on individual goals.)

Colwell JA: The feasibility of intensive insulin management in non-insulin-dependent diabetes mellitus: Implications of the Veterans Affairs Cooperative Study on Glycemic Control and Complications in NIDDM. Ann Intern Med 1996;124(1 Part 2):131. [NLM Cit ID: 96147231] (This preliminary study at five VAMCs in 153 men with type 2 diabetes in whom standard pharmacologic therapy had failed raised concern that intensive insulin therapy over 27 months was accompanied by more major cardiovascular events than did standard insulin therapy. Because of the small sample size and the relatively short duration of the study, the authors feel that a longer expanded trial is needed before this unexpected conclusion can be accepted.)

Cusi K, DeFronzo RA: Metformin: A review of its metabolic effects. Diabetes Rev 1998;6:89. (A very comprehensive review that includes 471 references related to the pharmacology of metformin and its clinical efficacy when given alone or with other hypoglycemic drugs. The authors, who have extensive experience with this drug, conclude that metformin is an effective therapeutic agent in type 2 diabetes and relatively safe in the absence of impaired renal function or conditions predisposing to hypotension or hypoxia.)

Day C: Thiazolidinediones: a new class of antidiabetic drugs. Diabet Med 1999;16:179. [NLM Cit ID: 99242101] (A review of the pharmacology of the thiazolidinediones and summary of the clinical studies using troglitazone.)

DCCT Research Group: Hypoglycemia in the Diabetes Control and Complications Trial. Diabetes 1997;46:271. [NLM Cit ID: 97153415] (This report emphasizes the threefold higher risk of severe hypoglycemia among type 1 diabetic patients receiving intensive insulin therapy and analyzes the factors that were the strongest predictors of the risk of future episodes of hypoglycemia in these patients.)

Holleman F et al: Insulin lispro. N Engl J Med 1997; 337:176. [NLM Cit ID: 97347219] (Lists the documented advantages of insulin lispro, including its superiority over regular insulin regarding reduced postprandial blood glucose, its reduced frequency of hypoglycemia in type 1 patients, and its much greater convenience by avoiding the need for a long interval before preprandial injections.)

Lebovitz HE: Alpha-glucosidase inhibitors as agents in the treatment of diabetes. Diabetes Rev 1998;6:132. (An update of the clinical experience with drugs such as acarbose and miglitol that delay digestion of complex carbohydrates by competitively inhibiting intestinal alpha-glucosidase enzymes. Clinical studies show that acarbose reduces the rise of postprandial glucose by a mean of 54 mg/dL in type 2 patients and reduces HbA_{1c} by a mean of 0.9%.)

Lebovitz HE: Insulin secretagogues: old and new. Diabetes Rev 1999;7:139. (A review of the mechanism of action and clinical effects of the three classes of insulin secretagogues: sulfonylureas, meglitinides, and D-phenylalanine derivatives.)

United Kingdom Prospective Diabetes Study (UKPDS) Group: (1) Intensive blood-glucose control with sulphonylureas or insulin compared with conventional treatment and risk of complications in patients with type 2 diabetes (UKPDS 33). Lancet 1998;352:837. [NLM Cit ID: 98413908] (Intensive glycemic control over a 10-year period in 3867 newly diagnosed type 2 patients with either sulfonylureas or insulin decreased the risk of microvascular complications but not macrovascular disease. All intensive treatment with these drugs increased the risk of hypoglycemia and weight gain. There were no adverse effects on cardiovascular outcomes.)

United Kingdom Prospective Diabetes Study (UKPDS) Group: (2) Effect of intensive blood-glucose control with metformin on complications in overweight patients with type 2 diabetes (UKPDS 34). Lancet 1998;352:854. [NLM Cit ID: 98413909] (Seven hundred and fifty-three obese newly diagnosed type 2 patients were randomized into groups receiving intensive therapy with metformin [n = 342], chlorpropamide [n = 265], glibenclamide [n = 277], or insulin [n = 409], and compared over a median duration of 10.7 years to a group receiving conventional therapy primarily with diet alone [n = 411]. In contrast to the results in the overall study population [see UKPDS 33 above], intensive therapy in these subgroups of obese patients did not reduce microvascular complications no matter what drug was used, as compared with conventional treatment with diet. A paradoxical finding was that metformin monotherapy reduced the risk for diabetes-related death and all-cause mortality compared with diet alone, but in a subgroup of 537 nonobese and obese patients responding poorly to sulfonylurea drugs alone, addition of metformin in half the group showed an increased risk of diabetes-related death compared with those staying on sulfonylureas alone. Since weight gain was less when type 2 obese patients received monotherapy with metformin and since hypoglycemia was uncommon, metformin was recommended as the first choice for drug therapy in obese type 2 patients.)

United Kingdom Prospective Diabetes Study (UKPDS) Group: (3) Tight blood pressure control and risk of macrovascular and microvascular complications in type 2 diabetes: UKPDS 38. BMJ 1998;317:703. [NLM Cit ID: 98404064] (In this long-term study of 1148 hypertensive type 2 diabetic patients studied for a mean of 8.4 years, tight blood pressure control [mean of 144/82 mm Hg] reduced the risk of deaths related to diabetes as well as reducing microvascular complications related to diabetes such as progression of diabetic retinopathy and deterioration in visual acuity compared with less tight control with a mean blood pressure of 154/87 mm Hg. Intensive antihypertensive therapy was initially done with either atenolol or captopril, but stepwise addition of diuretics, long-acting nifedipine, and other drugs was needed to achieve target levels. At least 29% of the patients required three drugs to achieve tight control of blood pressure.)

United Kingdom Prospective Diabetes Study (UKPDS) Group: (4) Efficacy of atenolol and captopril in reducing risk of macrovascular and microvascular complications in type 2 diabetes: UKPDS 39. BMJ 1998;317:713. [NLM Cit ID: 98404065] (This analysis indicates that atenolol was just as effective as the ACE inhibitor captopril in reducing macrovascular and microvascular end points in hypertensive type 2 diabetes. Captopril had no specific beneficial effect regarding diabetic renal complications, suggesting that blood pressure reduction in itself may be more important than the medication used.)

Chronic Complications of Diabetes Mellitus

Aiello LP et al: Diabetic retinopathy. Diabetes Care 1998;21:143. [NLM Cit ID: 98199813] (Screening strategies for comprehensive eye examinations in diabetic patients, lists outcomes of specific clinical therapies for retinopathy, and gives recommendations for treatment of the various stages of diabetic retinopathy. The American Diabetes Association based its 1998 statement upon evidence reviewed in this publication.)

American Diabetes Association Position Statement: Diabetes nephropathy. Diabetes Care 2000;23(Suppl 1):S69. (Reviews the natural history of diabetic nephropathy, discusses techniques to screen for microalbuminuria, and outlines therapy, including improved glycemic control, and aggressive antihypertensive treatment.)

American Diabetes Association Position Statement: Preventive foot care in people with diabetes. Diabetes Care 2000;23(Suppl 1):S55. (An update on the foot examination in patients with diabetes and recommendations regarding prevention and management of high-risk foot problems.)

Dejgaard A: Pathophysiology and treatment of diabetic neuropathy. Diabetic Med 1998;15:97. [NLM Cit ID: 98167327] (A comprehensive overview of pathogenesis and management of the wide range of subclinical and clinical syndromes comprising diabetic neuropathy. It reflects clinical experience as well as a careful review of numerous clinical trials regarding outcome of various pharmacotherapies with special attention to the use of local anesthetic agents in treating painful diabetic neuropathy.)

Lipshultz LI et al: Treatment of erectile dysfunction in men with diabetes. JAMA 1999;281:465. [NLM Cit ID: 91135681] (All available therapeutic options are discussed, including a useful critical commentary reviewing the promising results of clinical trials with sildenafil [Viagra] while emphasizing the selection criteria needed to minimize cardiovascular complications.)

DIABETIC COMA

Coma may be due to a variety of causes not directly related to diabetes. Certain causes directly related to diabetes require differentiation: (1) Hypoglycemic coma resulting from excessive doses of insulin or oral hypoglycemic agents. (2) Hyperglycemic coma associated with either severe insulin deficiency (diabetic ketoacidosis) or mild to moderate insulin deficiency (hyperglycemic nonketotic hyperosmolar coma). (3) Lactic acidosis associated with diabetes, particularly in diabetics stricken with severe infections or with cardiovascular collapse.

DIABETIC KETOACIDOSIS

Essentials of Diagnosis

- Hyperglycemia > 250 mg/dL.
- Acidosis with blood pH < 7.3.
- Serum bicarbonate < 15 meq/L.
- Serum positive for ketones.

General Considerations

Diabetic ketoacidosis may be the initial manifestation of type 1 diabetes or may result from increased insulin requirements in type 1 diabetes patients during the course of infection, trauma, myocardial infarction, or surgery. It is a life-threatening medical emergency with a mortality rate just under 5%. Type 2 diabetics may develop ketoacidosis under severe stress such as sepsis or trauma. Recently, diabetic ketoacidosis has been found to be one of the more common serious complications of insulin pump therapy, occurring in approximately one per 80 patient-months of treatment. Many patients who monitor capillary blood glucose regularly ignore urine ketone measurements, which would signal the possibility of insulin leakage or pump failure before serious illness develops. Poor compliance is one of the most common causes of diabetic ketoacidosis, particularly when episodes are recurrent.

Clinical Findings

A. Symptoms and Signs: The appearance of diabetic ketoacidotic coma is usually preceded by a day or more of polyuria and polydipsia associated with marked fatigue, nausea and vomiting, and, finally, mental stupor that can progress to coma. On physical examination, evidence of dehydration in a stuporous patient with rapid deep breathing and a "fruity" breath odor of acetone would strongly suggest the diagnosis. Hypotension with tachycardia indicates profound fluid and electrolyte depletion, and mild hypothermia is usually present. Abdominal pain and even tenderness may be present in the absence of abdominal disease. Conversely, cholecystitis or pancreatitis may occur with minimal symptoms and signs.

B. Laboratory Findings: (Table 27–11.) Glycosuria of 4+ and strong ketonuria with hyperglycemia, ketonemia, low arterial blood pH, and low plasma bicarbonate are typical of diabetic ketoacidosis. Serum potassium is often elevated despite total body potassium depletion resulting from protracted polyuria or vomiting. Elevation of serum amylase is common but often represents salivary as well as pancreatic amylase. Thus, in this setting, an elevated serum amylase is not specific for acute pancreatitis. Azotemia may be a better indicator of renal status than serum creatinine, since multichannel chemical analysis of serum creatinine (SMA-6) is falsely elevated by nonspecific chromogenicity of keto acids and glucose. Most laboratories, however, now routinely eliminate this interference. Leukocytosis as high as 25,000/μL with a left shift may occur with or without associated infection. The presence of an elevated or even a normal temperature would suggest the presence of an infection, since patients with diabetic ketoacidosis are generally hypothermic if uninfected.

Complications

The two major metabolic aberrations of diabetic ketoacidosis are hyperglycemia and ketoacidemia, both due to insulin lack associated with hyperglucagonemia.

A. Hyperglycemia: Hyperglycemia results from increased hepatic production of glucose as well as diminished glucose uptake by peripheral tissues. He-

Table 27–11. Laboratory diagnosis of coma in diabetic patients.

	Urine		Plasma		
	Glucose	Acetone	Glucose	Bicarbonate	Acetone
Related to diabetes					
Hypoglycemia	0[1]	0 or +	Low	Normal	0
Diabetic ketoacidosis	++++	++++	High	Low	++++
Nonketotic hyperglycemic coma	++++	0	High	Normal or slightly low	0
Lactic acidosis	0 or +	0 or +	Normal or low or high	Low	0 or +
Unrelated to diabetes					
Alcohol or other toxic drugs	0 or +	0 or +	May be low	Normal or low[2]	0 or +
Cerebrovascular accident or head trauma	+ or 0	0	Often high	Normal	0
Uremia	0 or +	0	High or normal	Low	0 or +

[1]Leftover urine in bladder might still contain glucose from earlier hyperglycemia.
[2]Alcohol can elevate plasma lactate as well as keto acids to reduce pH.

patic glucose output is a consequence of increased gluconeogenesis resulting from insulinopenia as well as from an associated hyperglucagonemia. When serum hyperosmolality exceeds 320–330 mosm/L, central nervous system depression or coma may ensue. Coma in a diabetic patient with a lower osmolality should prompt a search for cause of coma other than hyperosmolality.

B. Ketoacidemia: Ketoacidemia represents the effect of insulin lack at multiple enzyme loci. Insulin lack associated with elevated levels of growth hormone and glucagon contributes to an increase in lipolysis from adipose tissue and in hepatic ketogenesis. In addition, there is evidence that reduced ketolysis by insulin-deficient peripheral tissues contributes to the ketoacidemia. The only true "keto" acid present is acetoacetic acid, which, along with its by-product acetone, is measured by nitroprusside reagents (Acetest and Ketostix). The sensitivity for acetone, however, is poor, requiring over 10 mmol, which is seldom reached in the plasma of ketoacidotic subjects—although this detectable concentration is readily achieved in urine. Thus, in the plasma of ketotic patients, only acetoacetate is measured by these reagents. The more prevalent β-hydroxybutyric acid has no ketone group and is therefore not detected by conventional nitroprusside tests. This takes on special importance in the presence of circulatory collapse during diabetic ketoacidosis, wherein an increase in lactic acid can shift the redox state to increase β-hydroxybutyric acid at the expense of the readily detectable acetoacetic acid. Bedside diagnostic reagents would then be unreliable, suggesting no ketonemia in cases where β-hydroxybutyric acid is a major factor in producing the acidosis.

Treatment

A. Prevention: Education of diabetic patients to recognize the early symptoms and signs of ketoacidosis has done a great deal to prevent severe acidosis. Urine ketones should be measured in patients with signs of infection or in insulin pump-treated patients when capillary blood glucose is unexpectedly and persistently high. When heavy ketonuria and glycosuria persist on several successive examinations, supplemental regular insulin should be administered and liquid foods such as lightly salted tomato juice and broth should be ingested to replenish fluids and electrolytes. The patient should be instructed to contact the physician if ketonuria persists, and especially if vomiting develops or if appropriate adjustment of the infusion rate on an insulin pump does not correct the hyperglycemia and ketonuria. In juvenile-onset diabetics, particularly in the teen years, recurrent episodes of severe ketoacidosis often indicate poor compliance with the insulin regimen, and these patients will require intensive family counseling.

B. Emergency Measures: If ketosis is severe, the patient should be placed in the hospital for correction of the hyperosmolality as well as the ketoacidemia. An intensive care unit or, at the least, a step-down unit is preferable for more severe cases.

1. Therapeutic flow sheet–One of the most important steps in initiating therapy is to start a flow sheet listing vital signs and the time sequence of diagnostic laboratory values in relation to therapeutic maneuvers. Indices of the metabolic defects include urine glucose and ketones as well as arterial pH, plasma glucose, acetone, bicarbonate, serum urea nitrogen, and electrolytes. Serum osmolality should be measured or estimated and tabulated during the course of therapy.

A convenient method of estimating effective serum osmolality is as follows (normal values in humans are 280–300 mosm/kg):

$$\textbf{mosm/kg} = \textbf{2[Na}^{+}\textbf{]} + \frac{\textbf{Glucose (mg/dL)}}{\textbf{18}}$$

These calculated estimates are usually 10–20 mosm/kg lower than values measured by standard cryoscopic techniques in patients with diabetic coma. While urea exerts an effect on freezing point depression as measured in the laboratory, it is freely permeable across cell membranes and therefore not included in calculations of effective serum osmolality. One physician should be responsible for maintaining this therapeutic flow sheet and prescribing therapy. An indwelling urinary catheter is required in all comatose patients but should be avoided if possible in a fully cooperative diabetic because of the risk of introducing bladder infection. Fluid intake and output should be recorded. Gastric intubation is recommended in the comatose patient to correct the commonly associated gastric dilatation that may lead to vomiting and aspiration. The patient should not receive sedatives or narcotics.

2. Insulin replacement–Only regular insulin should be used initially in all cases of severe ketoacidosis, and it should be given immediately after the diagnosis is established. Regular insulin can be given in a loading dose of 0.1 unit/kg as an intravenous bolus followed by 0.1 unit/kg/h, continuously infused or given hourly as an intramuscular injection; this is sufficient to replace the insulin deficit in most patients. Replacement of insulin deficiency helps correct the acidosis by reducing the flux of fatty acids to the liver, reducing ketone production by the liver, and also improving removal of ketones from the blood. Insulin treatment reduces the hyperosmolality by reducing the hyperglycemia. It accomplishes this by increasing removal of glucose through peripheral utilization as well as by decreasing production of glucose by the liver. This latter effect is accomplished by direct inhibition of gluconeogenesis and glycogenolysis, as well as by lowered amino acid flux from muscle to liver and reduced hyperglucagonemia.

The insulin dose should be "piggy-backed" into the fluid line so the rate of fluid replacement can be changed without altering the insulin delivery rate. For optimal effects, continuous low-dose insulin infusions should always be preceded by a rapid intravenous loading dose of regular insulin, 0.1 unit/kg, to prime the tissue insulin receptors. If the plasma glucose level fails to fall at least 10% in the first hour, a repeat loading dose is recommended. The availability of bedside glucometers and of laboratory instruments for rapid and accurate glucose analysis (Beckman or Yellow Springs glucose analyzer) has contributed much to achieving optimal insulin replacement. Rarely, a patient with immune insulin resistance is encountered, and this requires doubling the insulin dose every 2–4 hours if hyperglycemia does not improve after the first two doses of insulin.

3. Fluid and electrolyte replacement–In most patients, the fluid deficit is 4–5 L. Initially, 0.9% saline solution is the solution of choice to help reexpand the contracted vascular volume and should be started in the emergency room as soon as the diagnosis is established. The use of sodium bicarbonate has been questioned since clinical benefit was not demonstrated in one prospective randomized trial and because of the following potentially harmful consequences: (1) hypokalemia from rapid potassium shifts into cells; (2) tissue hypoxia from reduced dissociation of oxygen from hemoglobin when acidosis is rapidly reversed; (3) cerebral acidosis resulting from a reduction of cerebrospinal fluid pH; and (4) a worsening of hyperosmolality. However, these concerns are relatively less important in certain clinical settings, and 1–2 ampules of sodium bicarbonate (44 meq per 50 mL ampule) added to a bottle of hypotonic saline solution may be administered whenever the blood pH is 7.0 or less or blood bicarbonate is below 9 meq/L. *Once the pH reaches 7.1, no further bicarbonate should be given, since it aggravates rebound metabolic alkalosis as ketones are metabolized.* Alkalosis causes potassium shifts that increase the risk of cardiac arrhythmias. In the first hour, at least 1 L of 0.9% saline should be infused, and fluid should be given thereafter at a rate of 300–500 mL/h with careful monitoring of serum potassium. Failure to give enough volume replacement (at least 3–4 L in 8 hours) to restore normal perfusion is one of the most serious therapeutic shortcomings affecting satisfactory recovery. Likewise, excessive fluid replacement (more than 5 L in 8 hours) may contribute to acute respiratory distress syndrome or cerebral edema. When blood glucose falls to 250 mg/dL or less, 5% glucose solutions should be used to maintain blood glucose between 200 and 300 mg/dL while insulin therapy is continued in order to clear the ketonemia. Glucose administration has the dual advantage of preventing hypoglycemia and furthermore of reducing the likelihood of cerebral edema, which could result from too rapid a decline in hyperglycemia.

During therapy, **hyperchloremic acidosis** develops because of the considerable loss of keto acids in the urine during the initial phase of treatment. A portion of the bicarbonate deficit is replaced with chloride ions infused in large amounts as saline to correct the dehydration. Thus, in most patients, as the ketoacidosis clears during insulin replacement, they show a hyperchloremic, low bicarbonate pattern with a normal anion gap. This is a relatively benign condition that reverses itself over the subsequent 12–24 hours once intravenous saline is no longer being administered.

4. Potassium and phosphate replacement– Total body potassium loss from polyuria as well as from vomiting may be as high as several hundred milliequivalents. However, because of shifts from cells due to the acidosis, serum potassium is usually normal or high until after the first few hours of treatment, when acidosis improves and serum potassium returns into cells. Potassium in doses of 20–30 meq/h should be infused within 2–3 hours after beginning therapy, or sooner if initial serum potassium is inappropriately low. Potassium replacement should be deferred if serum potassium fails to respond to initial therapy and remains above 5 meq/L, as in cases of renal insufficiency.

Foods high in potassium content can be prescribed when the patient has recovered sufficiently to take food orally. (Tomato juice and grapefruit juice contain 14 meq of potassium per 240 mL and a medium-sized banana 10 meq.) See Chapter 21 for potassium content of foods.

Phosphate replacement is seldom required in treating diabetic ketoacidosis. A significant therapeutic benefit of routine phosphate replacement has not been documented in several randomized trials. However, if severe hypophosphatemia of less than 0.35 mmol/L (< 1 mg/dL) develops during insulin therapy, a small amount of phosphate can be replaced as the potassium salt. Hypophosphatemia of this severity is detrimental to membranes of skeletal muscle and may lyse red blood cells. The potassium need is several times that of phosphate and should be replaced separately, since replacing phosphorus ions too rapidly (while meeting potassium requirements) can precipitate serum calcium in the tissues and induce tetany.

However, certain potential advantages have been suggested. Treatment of hypophosphatemia helps to restore the buffering capacity of the plasma, thereby facilitating renal excretion of hydrogen; and it corrects the impaired oxygen dissociation from hemoglobin by regenerating 2,3-diphosphoglycerate. To minimize the risk of inducing tetany from an overload of phosphate replacement, an average deficit of 40–50 mmol phosphate in adults with diabetic ketoacidosis should be replaced by intravenous infusion at a rate not to exceed 3 mmol/h.

A stock solution available from Abbott Laboratories provides a mixture of 1.12 g KH_2PO_4 and 1.18 g

K_2HPO_4 in a 5 mL single-dose vial representing 22 meq potassium and 15 mmol phosphate (27 meq). Five milliliters of this stock solution in 2 L of either 0.45% saline or 5% dextrose in water, infused at 400 mL/h, will replace the phosphate at the optimal rate of 3 mmol/h and will provide 4.4 meq of potassium per hour. If serum phosphate remains below 0.35 mmol/L (1 mg/dL), a repeat 5-hour infusion of potassium phosphate at a rate of 3 mmol/h would be reasonable.

5. Treatment of associated infection–Antibiotics are prescribed as indicated. Cholecystitis and pyelonephritis may be particularly severe in these patients.

Prognosis

The frequency of deaths due to diabetic ketoacidosis has been dramatically reduced by improved therapy of young diabetics, but this complication remains a significant risk in the aged and in patients in profound coma in whom treatment has been delayed. Acute myocardial infarction and infarction of the bowel following prolonged hypotension worsen the outlook. A serious prognostic sign is renal failure, and prior kidney dysfunction worsens the prognosis considerably because the kidney plays a key role in compensating for massive pH and electrolyte abnormalities. Cerebral edema has been reported to occur rarely as metabolic deficits return to normal. This is best prevented by avoiding sudden reversal of marked hyperglycemia. Maintaining glycemic levels of 200–300 mg/dL for the initial 24 hours after correction of severe hyperglycemia reduces this risk.

Kitabchi AE, Wall BM: Management of diabetic ketoacidosis. Am Fam Physicians 1999;60:455. [NLM Cit ID: 99392890] (This update reviews the clinical features and current therapeutic recommendations for this critical emergency and reflects the extensive clinical experience of the authors.)

Wagner A et al: Therapy of severe diabetic ketoacidosis. Zero mortality under very-low-dose insulin application. Diabetes Care 1999;22:674. [NLM Cit ID: 99265068] (A prospective study of 65 patients admitted with severe diabetic ketoacidosis from 1994 to 1997 were all treated successfully in an intensive care unit without routine administration of sodium bicarbonate and with relatively low doses of insulin [average bolus of 6.2 units and infusions at doses no higher than 4 units per hour].)

NONKETOTIC HYPERGLYCEMIC HYPEROSMOLAR COMA

Essentials of Diagnosis

- Hyperglycemia > 600 mg/dL.
- Serum osmolality > 310 mosm/kg.
- No acidosis; blood pH above 7.3.
- Serum bicarbonate > 15 meq/L.
- Normal anion gap (< 14 meq/L).

General Considerations

This second most common form of hyperglycemic coma is characterized by severe hyperglycemia in the absence of significant ketosis, with hyperosmolality and dehydration. It occurs in patients with mild or occult diabetes, and most patients are at least middle-aged to elderly. Lethargy and confusion develop as serum osmolality exceeds 310 mosm/kg, and coma can occur if osmolality exceeds 320–330 mosm/kg. Underlying renal insufficiency or congestive heart failure is common, and the presence of either worsens the prognosis. A precipitating event such as infection, myocardial infarction, stroke, or recent operation is often present. Certain drugs such as phenytoin, diazoxide, glucocorticoids, and diuretics have been implicated in its pathogenesis, as have procedures associated with glucose loading such as peritoneal dialysis.

Pathogenesis

A partial or relative insulin deficiency may initiate the syndrome by reducing glucose utilization of muscle, fat, and liver while inducing hyperglucagonemia and increasing hepatic glucose output. With massive glycosuria, obligatory water loss ensues. If a patient is unable to maintain adequate fluid intake because of an associated acute or chronic illness or has suffered excessive fluid loss, marked dehydration results. As plasma volume contracts, renal insufficiency develops, and the resultant limitation of renal glucose loss leads to increasingly higher blood glucose concentrations. Severe hyperosmolality develops that causes mental confusion and finally coma. It is not clear why ketosis is virtually absent under these conditions of insulin insufficiency, although reduced levels of growth hormone may be a factor, along with portal vein insulin concentrations sufficient to restrain ketogenesis.

Clinical Findings

A. Symptoms and Signs: Onset may be insidious over a period of days or weeks, with weakness, polyuria, and polydipsia. The lack of features of ketoacidosis may retard recognition of the syndrome and delay therapy until dehydration becomes more profound than in ketoacidosis. Reduced intake of fluid is not an uncommon historical feature, due to either inappropriate lack of thirst, nausea, or inaccessibility of fluids to elderly, bedridden patients. Lethargy and confusion develop, progressing to convulsions and deep coma. Physical examination confirms the presence of profound dehydration in a lethargic or comatose patient without Kussmaul respirations.

B. Laboratory Findings: Severe hyperglycemia is present, with blood glucose values ranging from 600 to 2400 mg/dL. In mild cases, where dehydration is less severe, dilutional hyponatremia as well as urinary sodium losses may reduce serum sodium to 120–125 meq/L, which protects to some extent against extreme hyperosmolality. However, as dehydration progresses, serum sodium can exceed 140 meq/L, producing serum osmolality readings of 330–440 mosm/kg. Ketosis and acidosis are usually absent or mild. Prerenal azotemia is the rule, with serum urea nitrogen elevations over 100 mg/dL being typical.

Treatment

A. Saline: Fluid replacement is of paramount importance in treating nonketotic hyperglycemic coma. The onset of hyperosmolarity is more insidious in elderly people without ketosis than in younger individuals with high serum ketone levels, which provide earlier indicators of severe illness (vomiting, rapid deep breathing, acetone odor, etc). Consequently, diagnosis and treatment are often delayed until fluid deficit has reached levels of 6–10 L.

If hypovolemia is present as evidenced by hypotension and oliguria, fluid therapy should be initiated with isotonic saline. In all other cases, hypotonic (0.45%) saline appears to be preferable as the initial replacement solution because the body fluids of these patients are markedly hyperosmolar. As much as 4–6 L of fluid may be required in the first 8–10 hours. Careful monitoring of the patient is required for proper sodium and water replacement. Once blood glucose reaches 250 mg/dL, fluid replacement should include 5% dextrose in either water, 0.45% saline solution, or 0.9% saline solution. The rate of dextrose infusion should be adjusted to maintain glycemic levels of 250–300 mg/dL in order to reduce the risk of cerebral edema. An important end point of fluid therapy is to restore urine output to 50 mL/h or more.

B. Insulin: Less insulin may be required to reduce the hyperglycemia in nonketotic patients as compared to those with diabetic ketoacidotic coma. In fact, fluid replacement alone can reduce hyperglycemia considerably by correcting the hypovolemia, which then increases both glomerular filtration and renal excretion of glucose. An initial dose of only 15 units intravenously and 15 units subcutaneously of regular insulin is usually quite effective, and in most cases subsequent doses need not be greater than 10–20 units subcutaneously every 4 hours.

C. Potassium: With the absence of acidosis, there may be no initial hyperkalemia unless associated renal failure is present. This results in less severe total potassium depletion than in diabetic ketoacidosis, and less potassium replacement is therefore needed. However, because initial serum potassium is usually not elevated and because it declines rapidly as a result of insulin's effect on driving potassium intracellularly, it has been recommended that potassium replacement be initiated earlier than in ketotic patients, assuming that no renal insufficiency or oliguria is present. Potassium chloride (10 meq/L) can be added to the initial bottle of fluids administered if the patient's serum potassium is not elevated.

D. Phosphate: If severe hypophosphatemia (serum phosphate < 1 mg/dL [< 0.35 mmol/L]) develops during insulin therapy, phosphate replacement can be given as described for ketoacidotic patients (at 3 mmol/h).

Prognosis

The overall mortality rate of hyperglycemic, hyperosmolar, nonketotic coma is more than ten times that of diabetic ketoacidosis, chiefly because of its higher incidence in older patients, who may have compromised cardiovascular systems or associated major illnesses and whose dehydration is often excessive because of delays in recognition and treatment. (When patients are matched for age, the prognoses of these two hyperglycemic emergencies are reasonably comparable.) When prompt therapy is instituted, the mortality rate can be reduced from nearly 50% to that related to the severity of coexistent disorders.

Matz R: Management of the hyperosmolar, hyperglycemic syndrome. Am Fam Physician 1999;60:1468. [NLM Cit ID: 99452122] (A comprehensive review of the prevalence, pathogenesis, and diagnosis of this diabetic emergency as well as a detailed outline of treatment, emphasizing the need for fluid replacement and insulin administration.)

LACTIC ACIDOSIS (See also Metformin & Other Biguanides.)

Essentials of Diagnosis

- Severe acidosis with hyperventilation.
- Blood pH below 7.30.
- Serum bicarbonate < 15 meq/L.
- Anion gap > 15 meq/L.
- Absent serum ketones.
- Serum lactate > 5 mmol/L.

General Considerations

Lactic acidosis is characterized by accumulation of excess lactic acid in the blood. Normally, the principal sources of this acid are the erythrocytes (which lack enzymes for aerobic oxidation), skeletal muscle, skin, and brain. Conversion of lactic acid to glucose and its oxidation principally by the liver but also by the kidneys represent the chief pathways for its removal. Overproduction of lactic acid (tissue hypoxia), deficient removal (hepatic failure), or both (circulatory collapse) can cause accumulation. Lactic acidosis is not uncommon in any severely ill patient suffering from cardiac decompensation, respiratory or hepatic failure, septicemia, or infarction of bowel or extremities. With the discontinuance of phenformin therapy in the USA, lactic acidosis in patients with diabetes mellitus has become uncommon but occasionally occurs in metformin-treated patients (see above) and it still must be considered in the acidotic diabetic, especially if the patient is seriously ill.

Clinical Findings

A. Symptoms and Signs: The main clinical feature of lactic acidosis is marked hyperventilation. When lactic acidosis is secondary to tissue hypoxia or vascular collapse, the clinical presentation is variable, being that of the prevailing catastrophic illness. However, in the idiopathic, or spontaneous, variety, the onset is rapid (usually over a few hours), blood pressure is normal, peripheral circulation is good, and there is no cyanosis.

B. Laboratory Findings: Plasma bicarbonate and blood pH are quite low, indicating the presence of severe metabolic acidosis. Ketones are usually absent from plasma and urine or at least not prominent. The first clue may be a high anion gap (serum sodium minus the sum of chloride and bicarbonate anions [in meq/L] should be no greater than 15). A higher value indicates the existence of an abnormal compartment of anions. If this cannot be clinically explained by an excess of keto acids (diabetes), inorganic acids (uremia), or anions from drug overdosage (salicylates, methyl alcohol, ethylene glycol), then lactic acidosis is probably the correct diagnosis. (See Chapter 21 also.) In the absence of azotemia, hyperphosphatemia may be a clue to the presence of lactic acidosis for reasons that are not clear. The diagnosis is confirmed by demonstrating, in a sample of blood that is promptly chilled and separated, a plasma lactic acid concentration of 5 mmol/L or higher (values as high as 30 mmol/L have been reported). Normal plasma values average 1 mmol/L, with a normal lactate/pyruvate ratio of 10:1. This ratio is greatly exceeded in lactic acidosis.*

Treatment

Aggressive treatment of the precipitating cause of lactic acidosis is the main component of therapy, such as ensuring adequate oxygenation and vascular perfusion of tissues. Empirical antibiotic coverage for sepsis should be given after culture samples are obtained in any patient in whom the cause of the lactic acidosis is not apparent.

Alkalinization with intravenous sodium bicarbonate to keep the pH above 7.2 has been recommended by some in the emergency treatment of lactic acidosis; as much as 2000 meq in 24 hours has been used. However, there is no evidence that the mortality rate is favorably affected by administering bicarbonate. Hemodialysis may be useful in cases where large sodium loads are poorly tolerated.

Prognosis

The mortality rate of spontaneous lactic acidosis is high. The prognosis in most cases is that of the primary disorder that produced the lactic acidosis.

Chan NN et al: Metformin-associated lactic acidosis: a rare or very rare clinical entity? Diabet Med 1999;16:273. [NLM Cit ID: 99235606] (Analysis of over 170 reported cases of metformin-associated lactic acidosis found it to be 20 times less common than that associated with phenformin. They concluded that if recommended therapeutic guidelines are adhered to, metformin use appears to be safe and the case fatality rate is no higher than that seen in sulfonylurea-induced hypoglycemia.)

Forsythe SM, Schmidt GA: Sodium bicarbonate for the treatment of lactic acidosis. Chest 2000;117:260. [NLM Cit ID: 20098447] (This perspective focuses on the treatment of lactic acidosis and presents evidence from an extensive literature search—as well as from the authors' extensive experience—that the use of sodium bicarbonate cannot be condoned for treating patients with lactic acidosis.)

THE HYPOGLYCEMIC STATES

Spontaneous hypoglycemia in adults is of two principal types: fasting and postprandial. Symptoms begin at plasma glucose levels in the range of 60 mg/dL and impairment of brain function at approximately 50 mg/dL. Fasting hypoglycemia is often subacute or chronic and usually presents with neuroglycopenia as its principal manifestation; postprandial hypoglycemia is relatively acute and is often heralded by symptoms of neurogenic autonomic discharge (sweating, palpitations, anxiety, tremulousness).

Differential Diagnosis (Table 27–12)

Fasting hypoglycemia may occur in certain endocrine disorders, such as hypopituitarism, Addison's disease, or myxedema; in disorders related to liver malfunction, such as acute alcoholism or liver failure; and in instances of renal failure, particularly in patients requiring dialysis. These conditions are usually obvious, with hypoglycemia being only a secondary feature. When fasting hypoglycemia is a primary manifestation developing in adults without apparent endocrine disorders or inborn metabolic diseases from childhood, the principal diagnostic possibilities include (1) hyperinsulinism, due to either pancreatic B cell tumors or surreptitious administration of insulin (or sulfonylureas); and (2) hypoglycemia due to non-insulin-producing extrapancreatic tumors.

Postprandial (reactive) hypoglycemia may be classified as early (within 2–3 hours after a meal) or late (3–5 hours after eating). Early, or alimentary, hypoglycemia occurs when there is a rapid discharge of ingested carbohydrate into the small bowel followed by rapid glucose absorption and hyperinsulinism. It

*In collecting samples, it is essential to rapidly chill and separate the blood in order to remove red cells, whose continued glycolysis at room temperature is a common source of error in reports of high plasma lactate. Frozen plasma remains stable for subsequent assay.

Table 27–12. Common causes of hypoglycemia in adults.[1]

Fasting hypoglycemia
Hyperinsulinism
Pancreatic B cell tumor
Surreptitious administration of insulin or sulfonylureas
Extrapancreatic tumors
Postprandial (reactive) hypoglycemia
Early hypoglycemia (alimentary)
Postgastrectomy
Functional (increased vagal tone)
Late hypoglycemia (occult diabetes)
Delayed insulin release due to B cell dysfunction
Counterregulatory deficiency
Idiopathic
Alcohol-related hypoglycemia
Immunopathologic hypoglycemia
Idiopathic anti-insulin antibodies (which release their bound insulin)
Antibodies to insulin receptors (which act as agonists)
Pentamidine-induced hypoglycemia

[1]In the absence of clinically obvious endocrine, renal, or hepatic disorders and exclusive of diabetes treated with hypoglycemic agents.

may be seen after gastrointestinal surgery and is particularly associated with the dumping syndrome after gastrectomy. In some cases, it is functional and may represent overactivity of the parasympathetic nervous system mediated via the vagus nerve. Rarely, it results from defective counterregulatory responses such as deficiencies of growth hormone, glucagon, cortisol, or autonomic responses.

Alcohol-related hypoglycemia is due to hepatic glycogen depletion combined with alcohol-mediated inhibition of gluconeogenesis. It is most common in malnourished alcohol abusers but can occur in anyone who is unable to ingest food after an acute alcoholic episode followed by gastritis and vomiting.

Immunopathologic hypoglycemia is an extremely rare condition in which anti-insulin antibodies or antibodies to insulin receptors develop spontaneously. In the former case, the mechanism appears to relate to increasing dissociation of insulin from circulating pools of bound insulin. When antibodies to insulin receptors are found, most patients do not have hypoglycemia but rather severe insulin-resistant diabetes and acanthosis nigricans. However, during the course of the disease in these patients, certain anti-insulin receptor antibodies with agonist activity mimicking insulin action may develop, producing severe hypoglycemia.

Factitious hypoglycemia is self-induced hypoglycemia due to surreptitious administration of insulin or sulfonylureas.

HYPOGLYCEMIA DUE TO PANCREATIC B CELL TUMORS

Fasting hypoglycemia in an otherwise healthy, well-nourished adult is rare, and is most commonly due to an adenoma of the islets of Langerhans. Ninety percent of such tumors are single and benign, but multiple adenomas can occur as well as malignant tumors with functional metastases. B cell hyperplasia as a cause of fasting hypoglycemia is rare but has been documented in adults. Adenomas may be familial, and multiple adenomas have been found in conjunction with tumors of the parathyroids and pituitary (multiple endocrine neoplasia type 1 [MEN 1]).

Clinical Findings

A. Symptoms and Signs: The most important prerequisite to diagnosing an insulinoma is simply to consider it, particularly in relatively healthy-appearing persons who have fasting hypoglycemia associated with some degree of central nervous system dysfunction such as confusion or abnormal behavior. A delay in diagnosis can result in unnecessary treatment for psychomotor epilepsy or psychiatric disorders and may cause irreversible brain damage. In long-standing cases, obesity can result as a consequence of overeating to relieve symptoms.

Whipple's triad is characteristic of hypoglycemia regardless of the cause. It consists of (1) a history of hypoglycemic symptoms, (2) an associated fasting blood glucose of 40 mg/dL or less, and (3) immediate recovery upon administration of glucose. The hypoglycemic symptoms in insulinoma often develop in the early morning or after missing a meal. Occasionally, they occur after exercise. They typically begin with evidence of central nervous system glucose lack and can include blurred vision or diplopia, headache, feelings of detachment, slurred speech, and weakness. Personality and mental changes vary from anxiety to psychotic behavior, and neurologic deterioration can result in convulsions or coma. Sweating and palpitations may not occur.

Hypoglycemic unawareness is very common in patients with insulinoma. They adapt to chronic hypoglycemia by increasing their efficiency in transporting glucose across the blood-brain barrier, which masks awareness that their blood glucose is approaching critically low levels. Counterregulatory hormonal responses as well as neurogenic symptoms such as tremor, sweating, and palpitations are therefore blunted during hypoglycemia. If lack of these warning symptoms prevents recognition of the need to eat to correct the problem, patients can lapse into severe hypoglycemic coma. However, symptoms and normal hormone responses during experimental insulin-induced hypoglycemia have been shown to be restored after successful surgical removal of the insulinoma. Presumably with return of euglycemia, adaptive effects on glucose transport into the brain are corrected and thresholds of counterregulatory responses and neurogenic autonomic symptoms are therefore restored to normal.

B. Laboratory Findings: B cell adenomas do not reduce secretion in the presence of hypoglycemia, and the critical diagnostic test is to demonstrate inappropriately elevated serum insulin levels at a time when hypoglycemia is present. A reliable serum insulin level of 6 μU/mL or more in the presence of blood glucose values below 40 mg/dL is diagnostic of inappropriate hyperinsulinism. Other causes of hyperinsulinemic hypoglycemia must be considered, including factitious administration of insulin or sulfonylureas. An elevated circulating proinsulin level is characteristic of most B cell adenomas and does not occur in factitious hyperinsulinism.

In patients with epigastric distress, a history of renal stones, or menstrual or erectile dysfunction, a serum calcium, gastrin, or prolactin level may be useful in screening for MEN-1 associated with insulinoma.

C. Diagnostic Tests:

1. Prolonged fasting under hospital supervision until hypoglycemia is documented is probably the most dependable means of establishing the diagnosis, especially in men. In 30% of patients with insulinoma, the blood glucose levels often drop below 40 mg/dL after an overnight fast, but some patients require up to 72 hours to develop symptomatic hypoglycemia. However, the term "72-hour fast" is actually a misnomer in most cases since the fast should be immediately terminated as soon as symptoms appear and laboratory confirmation of hypoglycemia is available. In normal male subjects, the blood glucose does not fall below 55–60 mg/dL during a 3-day fast. In contrast, in premenopausal women who have fasted for only 24 hours, the plasma glucose may fall normally to such an extent that it can reach values as low as 35 mg/dL. In these cases, however, the women are not symptomatic, presumably owing to the development of sufficient ketonemia to supply energy needs to the brain. Insulinoma patients, on the other hand, become symptomatic when plasma glucose drops to subnormal levels, since inappropriate insulin secretion restricts ketone formation. Moreover, the demonstration of a nonsuppressed insulin level (≥ 6 μU/mL) in the presence of hypoglycemia suggests the diagnosis of insulinoma. If hypoglycemia does not develop in a male patient after fasting for up to 72 hours—and particularly when this prolonged fast is terminated with a period of moderate exercise—insulinoma must be considered an unlikely diagnosis.

2. Proinsulin determinations–In contrast to normal subjects, whose proinsulin concentration is less than 20% of the total immunoreactive insulin, patients with insulinoma have elevated levels of proinsulin representing 30–90% of total immunoreactive insulin. However, this assay is seldom required in the routine diagnosis of insulinoma.

3. Stimulation tests with pancreatic B cell secretagogues such as tolbutamide, glucagon, or leucine are generally not needed in most cases if basal insulin is found to be nonsuppressible and therefore inappropriately elevated during fasting hypoglycemia.

Intravenous glucagon (1 mg over 1 minute) can be useful in patients with "borderline" fasting inappropriate hyperinsulinism. A serum insulin rise above baseline of 200 μU/mL or more at 5 and 10 minutes strongly suggests insulinoma, although poorly differentiated tumors may not respond. Glucagon has the advantage over tolbutamide of correcting rather than provoking hypoglycemia during stimulation testing and is diagnostic in 60–70% of patients with insulinoma. False-negative results can occur if the tumor is poorly differentiated and agranular.

D. Preoperative Localization of B Cell Tumors: Radiographic and arteriographic techniques are seldom helpful in localizing insulinomas preoperatively owing to the small size of most of these tumors (averaging 1.5 cm in diameter in one large series). These methods are often positive only when the tumor is large enough to be easily visualized or palpated intraoperatively.

Currently, there is a growing consensus among experts in this field that present techniques for preoperative localization are of limited usefulness and should be replaced by careful intraoperative ultrasonography and palpation by a surgeon experienced in insulinoma surgery. This approach has a success rate of over 90% in recent surveys and is the sole localizing approach relied upon by many centers, though a CT scan or MRI can be useful to screen for hepatic metastases from a malignant islet cell tumor.

When the insulinoma is not found at the initial surgery, three localization methods are available prior to reoperation. (1) The least invasive is a kinetic MRI with multiple imaging during gadolinium injection, but its accuracy for small tumors is no better than 40%. (2) Percutaneous transhepatic pancreatic vein catheterization with insulin assay can also be useful for localizing small insulinomas with about 70% reliability. However, this technique is not widely available, is invasive and expensive, and is associated with considerable discomfort and some risk to the patient. (3) A promising modification correlates imaging from selective arteriography of segments of the pancreas with simultaneous hepatic vein sampling for insulin during a bolus of intra-arterial calcium delivered selectively to these same pancreatic segments. Calcium has been found to be a secretagogue only for insulinomas and not for normal islet tissue, so that a rise in hepatic insulin concentration indicates segmental localization of an insulinoma. Furthermore, this technique may provide data which are particularly helpful when multiple insulinomas are suspected as in patients with coexisting pituitary or parathyroid adenomas or in rare instances of pancreatic hyperplasia due to nesidioblastosis.

Treatment

A. Surgical Measures: It is imperative that the surgeon be convinced that the diagnosis of insulinoma has been unequivocally made by clinical and laboratory findings. Only then should surgery be considered, as there is no justification for exploratory operation—just as there is none for the use of current localization techniques as a preoperative diagnostic tool. Resection by a surgeon with previous experience in removing pancreatic B cell tumors is the treatment of choice. In patients with a single benign adenoma 90–95% have a successful cure at the first surgical attempt when intraoperative ultrasound is used by a skilled surgeon. Diazoxide, 300–400 mg/d orally, inhibits insulin release from most tumors and is useful in the interval prior to surgery for prevention of hypoglycemic episodes. Hydrochlorothiazide, 25–50 mg daily, should also be prescribed to counteract the edema and hyperkalemia secondary to diazoxide therapy as well as to potentiate its hyperglycemic effect. However, because effective doses are tolerated poorly over the long term—particularly because of its tendency to produce hirsutism in women—diazoxide is not considered a desirable alternative to surgical excision. Blood glucose should be monitored throughout surgery, and 10% dextrose in water should be infused at a rate of 100 mL/h or faster. In cases where the diagnosis has been established but no adenoma is located after careful palpation and use of intraoperative ultrasound, it is no longer advisable to blindly resect the body and tail of the pancreas, since a nonpalpable tumor missed by ultrasound is most likely embedded within the fleshy head of the pancreas that is left behind with subtotal resections. Most surgeons prefer to close the incision and schedule a selective arterial calcium stimulation with hepatic venous sampling to locate the tumor site prior to a repeat operation. Total pancreatectomy is seldom required now in view of the efficacy of long-term medical therapy with diazoxide in most patients with insulinomas that are not surgically correctable.

B. Diet and Medical Therapy: In patients with inoperable functioning islet cell carcinoma and in approximately 5–10% of MEN-1 cases when subtotal removal of the pancreas has failed to produce cure, reliance on frequent feedings is necessary. Since most tumors are not responsive to glucose, carbohydrate feedings every 2–3 hours are usually effective in preventing hypoglycemia, although obesity may become a problem. Glucagon should be available for emergency use as indicated in the discussion of treatment of diabetes, but its beneficial effect may be diminished by a concomitant stimulation of insulin release from the tumor. Diazoxide, 300–600 mg daily orally, has been useful with thiazide diuretic therapy to control sodium retention. When patients are unable to tolerate diazoxide because of gastrointestinal upset, hirsutism, or edema, the calcium channel blocker verapamil may be beneficial in view of its inhibitory effect on insulin release from insulinoma cells. Octreotide, a potent long-acting synthetic octapeptide analog of somatostatin, has been used to inhibit release of hormones from a number of endocrine tumors. A dose of 50 μg of octreotide injected subcutaneously twice daily has been tried in cases where surgery failed to remove the source of hyperinsulinism. However, its effectiveness is limited since its affinity for somatostatin receptors of the pancreatic B cell is very much less than for those of the anterior pituitary somatotrophs for which it was originally designed as treatment for acromegaly. When hypoglycemia persists after attempted surgical removal of the insulinoma and if diazoxide or verapamil is poorly tolerated or ineffective, multiple small feedings may be the only recourse until more selective somatostatin receptor agonists are available. Streptozocin can decrease insulin secretion in islet cell carcinomas, and effective doses have been delivered via selective arterial catheter so that the undue renal toxicity that characterized early experience is less of a problem.

Prognosis

When insulinoma is diagnosed early and cured surgically, complete recovery is likely, although brain damage following prolonged severe hypoglycemia is not reversible. A significant increase in survival rate has been shown in streptozocin-treated patients with islet cell carcinoma, with reduction in tumor mass as well as decreased hyperinsulinism.

Boukhman MP et al: Localization of insulinomas. Arch Surg 1999;134:818. [NLM Cit ID: 99371403] (Surgical treatment of 58 insulinoma patients showed that extensive preoperative radiologic localization did not generally improve surgical outcome and that it was not cost-effective. Careful palpation with intraoperative ultrasonography was superior for tumor localization and led to successful operations for single benign tumors in 96% of patients.)

Grant CS: Surgical aspects of hyperinsulinemic hypoglycermia. Endocrinol Metab Clin North Am 1999;28:533. [NLM Cit ID: 99430717] (A comprehensive review of the Mayo Clinic experience in 132 consecutive patients in whom 88% had a single tumor with an average size of 1.5 cm and in whom intraoperative ultrasound surpassed all other techniques for tumor localization, with a sensitivity of 96%.)

HYPOGLYCEMIA DUE TO EXTRAPANCREATIC TUMORS

These rare causes of hypoglycemia include mesenchymal tumors such as retroperitoneal sarcomas, hepatocellular carcinomas, adrenocortical carcinomas, and miscellaneous epithelial type tumors. The tumors are frequently large and readily palpated or visualized on CT scans or MRI.

The mechanism of these tumors' hypoglycemic effects has only recently been elucidated. The expression and release of an incompletely processed insulin-like growth factor-2 (IGF-2) has provided the best explanation for the clinical manifestations of hypoglycemia in these cases. A larger immature form of the IGF-2 molecule is released which binds to a carrier protein but not to an acid-labile component of serum which inactivates normal IGF-2. This immature IGF-2 complex therefore remains active and binds to insulin receptors in muscle to promote glucose transport and to insulin receptors in liver and kidney to reduce glucose output. It also binds to receptors for IGF-1 in the pancreatic B cell to inhibit insulin secretion. Serum levels of IGF-2 may be increased but often are "normal" in quantity, despite the presence of the immature, higher-molecular-weight form of IGF-2, which can only be detected by special laboratory techniques. Laboratory diagnosis depends upon documenting fasting hypoglycemia associated with undetectable serum insulin levels.

The prognosis for these tumors is generally poor, and surgical removal should be attempted when feasible. Dietary management of the hypoglycemia is the mainstay of medical treatment, since diazoxide is usually ineffective.

Le Roith D: Tumor-induced hypoglycemia. N Engl J Med 1999;341:757. [NLM Cit ID: 99383629] (An abnormal incompletely processed insulin-like growth factor-2 [IGF-2], with a high molecular weight, appears to explain many, but not all, cases of hypoglycemia secondary to extrapancreatic tumors.)

POSTPRANDIAL HYPOGLYCEMIA (Reactive Hypoglycemia)

Postgastrectomy Alimentary Hypoglycemia

Reactive hypoglycemia following gastrectomy is a consequence of hyperinsulinism resulting from rapid gastric emptying of ingested food. Symptoms result from adrenergic hyperactivity in response to the hypoglycemia. Treatment consists of more frequent feedings with smaller portions of less rapidly assimilated carbohydrate and more slowly absorbed fat and protein.

Functional Alimentary Hypoglycemia

This syndrome is classified as functional when no postsurgical explanation exists for the presence of early alimentary type reactive hypoglycemia. It is most often associated with chronic fatigue, anxiety, irritability, weakness, poor concentration, decreased libido, headaches, hunger after meals, and tremulousness. However, most patients with these symptoms do not have hypoglycemia. (See Chronic Fatigue Syndrome in Chapter 1.)

Indiscriminate use and overinterpretation of glucose tolerance tests have led to an unfortunate tendency to overdiagnose functional hypoglycemia. As many as one-third or more of normal subjects have hypoglycemia reaching nadirs as low as 40–50 mg/dL with or without symptoms during a 4-hour glucose tolerance test. Accordingly, to increase diagnostic reliability, hypoglycemia should preferably be documented during a spontaneous symptomatic episode accompanying routine daily activity, with clinical improvement following feeding. Oral glucose tolerance tests are overly sensitive and mixed meals are relatively insensitive in detecting postprandial reactive hypoglycemia. It has been shown that a high-carbohydrate breakfast has proved useful in differentiating persons with postprandial reactive hypoglycemia from normal controls. The test resulted in reactive hypoglycemia to levels below 59 mg/dL in 47% of 38 subjects, in contrast to only 2.2% of the 43 controls. This test was found to be much more sensitive than a standard mixed meal, which was also given to these two groups.

In patients with documented postprandial hypoglycemia on a functional basis, there is no harm and occasional benefit in reducing the proportion of carbohydrate in the diet while increasing the frequency and reducing the size of meals. Support and mild sedation should be the mainstays of therapy, with dietary manipulation only an adjunct.

Late Hypoglycemia (Occult Diabetes)

This condition is characterized by a delay in early insulin release from pancreatic B cells, resulting in initial exaggeration of hyperglycemia during a glucose tolerance test. In response to this hyperglycemia, an exaggerated insulin release produces a late hypoglycemia 4–5 hours after ingestion of glucose. These patients are usually quite different from those with early hypoglycemia occurring 2–3 hours after glucose ingestion, often being obese and frequently having a family history of diabetes mellitus.

In obese patients, treatment is directed at weight reduction to achieve ideal weight. Like all patients with postprandial hypoglycemia, regardless of cause, these patients often respond to reduced carbohydrate intake with multiple, spaced, small feedings high in protein. They should be considered potential diabetics and advised to have periodic medical evaluations.

Brun JF et al: Evaluation of a standardized hyperglucidic breakfast test in postprandial reactive hypoglycaemia. Diabetologia 1995;38:494. [NLM Cit ID: 95317510] (A high-carbohydrate breakfast was found to differentiate patients referred for symptomatic postprandial hypoglycemia [n = 38] from a control population [n = 43] much better than did a standard mixed meal. Blood glucose levels less than 59 mg/dL were found in 47% of the referred subjects after the hyperglucidic breakfast but in only 2.2% of the controls, implying that this may be a useful test in identifying postprandial reactive hypoglycemia.)

ALCOHOL-RELATED HYPOGLYCEMIA

Fasting Hypoglycemia After Ethanol

During the postabsorptive state, normal plasma glucose is maintained by hepatic glucose output derived from both glycogenolysis and gluconeogenesis. With prolonged starvation, glycogen reserves become depleted within 18–24 hours and hepatic glucose output becomes totally dependent on gluconeogenesis. Under these circumstances, a blood concentration of ethanol as low as 45 mg/dL can induce profound hypoglycemia by blocking gluconeogenesis. Neuroglycopenia in a patient whose breath smells of alcohol may be mistaken for alcoholic stupor. Prevention consists of adequate food intake during ethanol ingestion. Therapy consists of glucose administration to replenish glycogen stores until gluconeogenesis resumes.

Postethanol Reactive Hypoglycemia

When sugar-containing soft drinks are used as mixers to dilute alcohol in beverages (gin and tonic, rum and cola), there seems to be a greater insulin release than when the soft drink alone is ingested and a tendency for more of a late hypoglycemic overswing to occur 3–4 hours later. Prevention would consist of avoiding sugar mixers while ingesting alcohol and ensuring supplementary food intake to provide sustained absorption.

FACTITIOUS HYPOGLYCEMIA

Factitious hypoglycemia may be difficult to document. A suspicion of self-induced hypoglycemia is supported when the patient is associated with the health professions or has access to insulin or sulfonylurea drugs taken by a diabetic member of the family. The triad of hypoglycemia, high immunoreactive insulin, and suppressed plasma C peptide immunoreactivity is pathognomonic of exogenous insulin administration. Demonstration of circulating insulin antibodies supports this diagnosis in suspected cases. When sulfonylureas are suspected as a cause of factitious hypoglycemia, a chemical test of the plasma to detect the presence of these drugs may be required to distinguish laboratory findings from those of insulinoma.

IMMUNOPATHOLOGIC HYPOGLYCEMIA

This rare cause of hypoglycemia, documented in isolated case reports, may occur as two distinct disorders: one associated with spontaneous development of circulating anti-insulin antibodies and another associated with antibodies to insulin receptors, in which the antibodies apparently have agonist capabilities. This latter disorder is extremely rare, having been documented in no more than five cases. However, development of anti-insulin antibodies has been reported in over 200 patients most of whom were being treated with methimazole for thyrotoxicosis. In western countries, 23 cases have been reported and include patients with a lupus-like syndrome or with various paraproteinemias. The hypoglycemia occurs 3–4 hours after meals following an initial postprandial hyperglycemic phase that is due to the antibodies interfering with the exit of insulin from the plasma to reach its target tissues. Later, after most of the meal is absorbed, inappropriate high levels of insulin dissociate from this antibody-bound compartment, resulting in hypoglycemia.

Redmon JB et al: Autoimmune hypoglycemia. Endocrinol Metab Clin North Am 1999;28:603. [NLM Cit ID: 99430720] (A comprehensive review of this rare syndrome of hypoglycemia caused by the interaction of endogenous antibodies with insulin or the insulin receptor. Clinical manifestations, diagnosis, and therapy are discussed.)

PENTAMIDINE-INDUCED HYPOGLYCEMIA

With the increased prevalence of pulmonary infection by *Pneumocystis carinii* in patients with acquired immune deficiency syndrome, pentamidine given intravenously or by aerosol is being used more frequently and in 10–20% of patients produces symptomatic hypoglycemia, particularly when administered intravenously. This apparently is due to lytic destruction of pancreatic B cells, causing acute hyperinsulinemia and hypoglycemia, followed later by insulinopenia and hyperglycemia which occasionally is persistent. Intravenous glucose should be administered during intravenous pentamidine administration and for the period immediately following to prevent or ameliorate hypoglycemic symptoms. Following a complete course of therapy with pentamidine, fasting blood glucose or a subsequent glycohemoglobin should be monitored to assess the extent of pancreatic B cell recovery or residual damage.

Assan R et al: Pentamidine-induced derangements of glucose homeostasis: Determinant roles of renal failure and drug accumulation—a study of 128 patients. Diabetes Care 1995;18:47. [NLM Cit ID: 95212191] (Hypoglycemia associated with elevated insulin levels in plasma occurred in 25 of 128 pentamidine-treated patients due to pancreatic B cell toxicity. Drug accumulation due to excessive doses or renal impairment is the determining risk factor.)

Service FJ: Diagnostic approach to adults with hypoglycemic disorders. Endocrinol Metab Clin North Am 1999;28:519. [NLM Cit ID: 99430716] (Reviews hypoglycemia—its clinical presentation and the diagnostic steps needed to confirm its etiology.)

RELEVANT WORLD WIDE WEB SITES

[Managing Your Diabetes]
http://diabetes.lilly.com/

[American Diabetes Association]
http://www.diabetes.org/default.htm

[American Association of Diabetes Educators]
http://www.aadenet.org/

[American Dietetic Assocation]
http://www.eatright.org

[Juvenile Diabetes Foundation]
http://www.jdf.org/index.html

28 Lipid Abnormalities

See http://www.current-med.com/ch28.html for updated addresses of Web sites referenced in this chapter.

Robert B. Baron, MD, MS

Lowering high blood cholesterol reduces the incidence of coronary heart disease and has given impetus to nationwide campaigns to reduce serum cholesterol levels. For patients with known cardiovascular disease (secondary prevention), benefits from cholesterol lowering include a reduction in total mortality in both men and women and in both middle-aged patients and older patients. Among patients without cardiovascular disease (primary prevention), however, the data are less conclusive. One study showed a beneficial effect on heart disease mortality and all-cause mortality in middle-aged men. Other studies have demonstrated reduction in coronary artery events but not reduction in mortality. The effects of cholesterol lowering on total mortality in women, young men, and the elderly have not been effectively studied. Nonetheless, treatment algorithms have been designed to assist clinicians in selecting patients for cholesterol-lowering therapy based on their lipid levels and their overall risk of developing cardiovascular disease.

LIPIDS & LIPOPROTEINS

The two main lipids in blood are cholesterol and triglyceride. They are carried in lipoproteins, which are globular packages that also contain proteins known as apoproteins. Cholesterol is an essential element of all animal cell membranes and forms the backbone of steroid hormones and bile acids; triglycerides are important in transferring energy from food into cells. Why lipids are deposited into the walls of large and medium-sized arteries—an event with potentially lethal consequences—is not known.

Lipoproteins are usually classified on the basis of how dense they are. Density is determined by the amounts of triglyceride (which makes them less dense) and apoproteins (which have the opposite effect). The least dense particles, known as chylomicrons, are normally found in the blood only after fat-containing foods have been eaten. Chylomicrons rise as a creamy layer when nonfasting serum is allowed to stand. The other lipoproteins are suspended in serum and must be separated using a centrifuge. The densest (and smallest) family of particles consists mainly of apoproteins and cholesterol and are called high-density lipoproteins (HDL). Somewhat less dense are the low-density lipoproteins (LDL). Least dense are the large, very-low-density lipoproteins (VLDL), consisting mainly of triglyceride. In fasting serum, most of the cholesterol is carried on LDL particles and is therefore referred to as LDL cholesterol; most of the triglyceride is found in VLDL particles. Specific apoproteins are associated with each lipoprotein class.

Chylomicrons are made in the gut and travel via the portal vein into the liver and via the thoracic duct into the circulation. They are normally completely metabolized, transferring energy from food into muscle and fat cells. The liver manufactures VLDL particles from its own stores of fat and carbohydrate. VLDL particles transfer triglyceride to cells; after losing enough, they eventually become LDL particles, which provide cholesterol for cellular needs. Excess LDL particles are taken up by the liver, and the cholesterol they contain is then excreted into the bile. HDL particles are made in the liver and intestine and appear to facilitate the transfer of apoproteins among lipoproteins. They also participate in reverse cholesterol transport, either by transferring cholesterol into other lipoproteins or directly into the liver.

LIPOPROTEINS & ATHEROGENESIS

The plaques found in the arterial walls of patients with atherosclerosis contain large amounts of cholesterol, providing an early clue that serum cholesterol might be an important factor in their development. The higher the level of LDL cholesterol, the greater the risk of atherosclerotic heart disease; conversely, the higher the level of HDL cholesterol, the lower the risk of coronary heart disease. This is true in men and women, in different racial and ethnic groups, and at all adult ages. Because most cholesterol in serum is LDL, high total cholesterol levels are also associated with an increased risk of coronary heart disease. Middle-aged men whose serum cholesterol levels are in the highest quintile for age (above about 230 mg/dL) have a risk of coronary death before age 65 of about 11%; men in the lowest quintile (below about 170 mg/dL) have a 3% risk. Death from coronary heart disease before age 65 is less common in women, with equivalent risks about one-third those of men. As a general approximation in men, each 10 mg/dL increase in cholesterol (or LDL cholesterol) increases the risk of coronary heart disease by about 10%; each 5 mg/dL increase in HDL reduces the risk by about 10%. The effect of HDL cholesterol is greater in women, whereas the effects of total and LDL cholesterol are smaller. All of these relationships tend to diminish with age.

The exact mechanism by which LDL particles result in the formation of atherosclerotic plaques—or the means whereby HDL particles protect against their formation—is not known. The simple model of LDL carrying cholesterol into the walls of arteries, with HDL removing it, is more useful as a mnemonic than as a representation of what is known. LDL particles which have become oxidized (a process that occurs naturally) may be particularly atherogenic. Receptors on the surface of macrophages within atherosclerotic plaques bind and accumulate oxidized LDL. The formation of antibodies to oxidized LDL may also be important in plaque formation. Thus, there is growing interest in the role of antioxidants in the prevention and treatment of atherosclerotic disease. The size of the LDL molecule itself may also influence its atherogenesis; at the same LDL concentrations, those persons with large numbers of smaller particles appear to be at higher risk for coronary heart disease.

The relationship of VLDL cholesterol to atherogenesis is less certain. Perhaps the number, or size, or subtype of VLDL particles—rather than the total amount in serum—is important. In addition, HDL and VLDL levels are inversely related. Patients with a high VLDL level are likely to have a low HDL level and thus be at increased risk for coronary heart disease for that reason alone.

There are several genetic disorders that provide insight into the pathogenesis of lipid-related diseases. Most important—but rare in the homozygous state (about one per million)—is a condition in which the cell-surface receptors for the LDL molecule are absent or defective, **familial hypercholesterolemia.** These patients have reduced ability to metabolize LDL particles, resulting in high LDL levels and premature atherosclerosis. Patients with two abnormal genes (homozygotes) have extremely high LDL levels—up to eight times normal—and may present with atherosclerotic disease in childhood. Homozygotes may require liver transplantation to correct their severe lipid abnormalities. Those with one defective gene (heterozygotes) have LDL concentrations that are approximately twice normal; persons with this condition often present with coronary heart disease in their 30s or 40s.

Another rare condition is characterized by an abnormality of lipoprotein lipase, the enzyme that enables peripheral tissues to take up triglyceride from chylomicrons and VLDL particles. Patients with this condition, one cause of **familial hyperchylomicronemia,** have marked hypertriglyceridemia and usually present with recurrent pancreatitis and hepatosplenomegaly in childhood.

There are numerous other genetic abnormalities of lipid metabolism. These may be named for the abnormality that appears when serum is electrophoresed (eg, **dysbetalipoproteinemia**) or from the particular combinations of lipid abnormalities that appear in families (eg, **familial combined hyperlipidemia**). These entities are important to the clinician because of the need to screen family members of patients with severe lipid disorders. Other patients have abnormalities in the production of various apoproteins, such as increased levels of apoprotein B and its affiliated lipoproteins, LDL and VLDL, or reduced production of apoprotein AII and its affiliated particle, or excess levels of lipoprotein(a). Mutations of many other proteins and enzymes involved in lipid metabolism may also be clinically important. Examples include mutations in lipoprotein lipase and mutations in the gene encoding for a newly described protein, cholesterol efflux regulatory protein.

Castelli WP: The new pathophysiology of coronary artery disease. Am J Cardiol 1998;82(10B):60T. [NLM Cit ID: 99075721] (Unstable, soft plaque that cannot be seen angiographically is prone to rupture and results in infarction.)

Marcil M et al: Mutations in the *ABC1* gene in familial HDL deficiency with defective cholesterol efflux. Lancet 1999;354:1341. [NLM Cit ID: 20001430] (Mutations in the gene that regulates the cholesterol efflux protein are a major cause of familial HDL deficiency.)

Miwa K et al: Lipoprotein(a) is a risk factor for occurrence of acute myocardial infarction in patients with coronary vasospasm. J Am Coll Cardiol 2000;35:1200. [NLM Cit ID: 20220711] (Elevated serum Lp[a] is associated with a history of prior myocardial infarction in patients with coronary spasm. This suggests that Lp[a] may play an important role in the genesis of thrombotic coronary occlusion and the occurrence of acute myocardial infarction subsequent to coronary spasm.)

Saku K et al: Hyperinsulinemic hypoalphalipoproteinemia as a new indicator for coronary heart disease. J Am Coll Cardiol 1999;34:1443. [NLM Cit ID: 20017853] (Hyperinsulinemic hypoalphalipoproteinemia is a more potent indicator for coronary heart disease than either insulin resistance or low serum HDL-C levels alone. The adverse effects of hyperinsulinemia seem to be ameliorated by high HDL-C levels.)

Shlipak MG et al: Estrogen and progestin, lipoprotein(a), and the risk of recurrent coronary heart disease events after menopause. JAMA 2000;283:1845. [NLM Cit ID: 20230915] (Lp[a] is an independent risk factor for recurrent coronary heart disease in postmenopausal women, and treatment with estrogen and progestin lowers Lp[a] levels.)

Sloop GD: A critical analysis of the role of cholesterol in atherogenesis. Atherosclerosis 1999;142:265. [NLM Cit ID: 99153447] (Presents evidence that serum hypercholesterolemia accelerates atherogenesis by increasing blood viscosity and the mechanical fragility of plaques, making them vulnerable to rupture and thrombosis.)

Stein JH et al: Lipoprotein Lp(a) excess and coronary heart disease. Arch Intern Med 1997;157:1170. [NLM Cit ID: 97326406] (Lipoprotein Lp(a) is a potent predictor of premature atherosclerotic disease.)

Steinberg D et al: Oxidative modification of LDL and atherogenesis. Circulation 1997;95:1062. [NLM Cit ID: 97207478] (Excellent review of the pathogenesis of atherosclerosis.)

Vogel RA et al: Cholesterol, cholesterol lowering, and endothelial function. Prog Cardiovasc Dis 1998;41:117. [NLM Cit ID: 99005073] (Atherosclerosis at least in part is caused by endothelial dysfunction that favors cellular proliferation, explaining the early and substantial reductions in major cardiovascular events associated with cholesterol lowering.)

Wittrup HH et al: Lipoprotein lipase mutations, plasma lipids and lipoproteins, and risk of ischemic heart disease. A meta-analysis. Circulation 1999;99:2901. [NLM Cit ID: 99289694] (Carriers of certain lipoprotein lipase mutations have an increased risk of ischemic heart disease. Other mutations are associated with reduced risk.)

LIPID FRACTIONS & THE RISK OF CORONARY HEART DISEASE

In fasting serum, cholesterol is carried primarily on three different lipoproteins—the VLDL, LDL, and HDL molecules. Total cholesterol equals the sum of these three components:

$$\text{Total cholesterol} = \text{HDL cholesterol} + \text{VLDL cholesterol} + \text{LDL cholesterol}$$

Most clinical laboratories measure the total cholesterol, the total triglycerides, and the amount of cholesterol found in the HDL fraction, which is easily precipitated from serum. The vast majority of triglyceride is found in VLDL particles, which contain about five times as much triglyceride by weight as cholesterol. Thus, the amount of cholesterol found in the VLDL fraction can be estimated by dividing the triglyceride by 5:

$$\text{VLDL cholesterol} = \frac{\text{Triglycerides}}{5}$$

Because the triglyceride level is used as a proxy for the amount of VLDL, this formula only works in fasting samples. Furthermore, it only works when the triglyceride level is less than 400–500 mg/dL. At higher triglyceride levels (as is the case when serum appears lipemic), LDL and VLDL cholesterol levels can be determined after ultracentrifugation.

The total cholesterol is reasonably stable over time; however, measurements of HDL and especially triglycerides may vary considerably because of analytic error in the laboratory and because of biologic variation in a patient's lipid level. Thus, the LDL should always be estimated as the mean of at least two determinations; if those two estimates differ by more than 10%, a third lipid profile should be obtained. It is estimated as follows:

$$\text{LDL cholesterol} = \text{Total cholesterol} - \text{HDL cholesterol} - \frac{\text{Triglycerides}}{5}$$

When using SI units (which measure lipids by moles rather than weight), the formula becomes:

$$\text{LDL cholesterol} = \frac{\text{Total cholesterol}}{\text{(mmol/L)}} - \frac{\text{HDLcholesterol}}{\text{(mmol/L)}} - \frac{\text{Triglycerides (mmol/L)}}{2.2}$$

Understanding the relationships of the different lipid fractions leads to a more sophisticated and clinically accurate understanding of a patient's lipid-related coronary risk than simply knowing the total cholesterol level. Two persons with the same total cholesterol of 275 mg/dL may have very different lipid profiles. One may have an HDL cholesterol of 110 mg/dL with a triglyceride of 150 mg/dL, giving an estimated LDL cholesterol of 135 mg/dL; the other may have an HDL cholesterol of 25 mg/dL with a triglyceride of 200 mg/dL and an LDL cholesterol of 210 mg/dL. All other risk factors being equal, the second patient would have more than a tenfold higher coronary heart disease risk than the first. Because high HDL cholesterol levels are common in women, many women with apparently high total cholesterol levels actually have favorable lipid profiles. Thus, evaluation of the lipid fractions is essential before therapy for high blood cholesterol in individual patients is initiated.

Some authorities use the ratio of the total cholesterol to HDL cholesterol as an indicator of lipid-related coronary risk: the lower this ratio is, the better. (In the example from the previous paragraph, the first person would have a ratio of 275 ÷ 110 = 2.5, while the second would have a much less favorable ratio of 275 ÷ 25 = 11.) While intuitively convenient, the ratio may obscure important information (a total cholesterol of 300 mg/dL and an HDL of 60 mg/dL results in the same ratio of 5 as a total cholesterol of 150 mg/dL with an HDL of 30 mg/dL). Moreover, errors in the measurement of HDL cholesterol are common in many laboratories, and the total cholesterol-to-HDL cholesterol ratio magnifies their importance.

There is no "normal" range for serum lipids. In Western populations, cholesterol values are about

20% higher than in Asian populations and exceed 300 mg/dL in nearly 5% of adults. About 10% of adults have LDL cholesterol levels above 200 mg/dL. In general, total and LDL cholesterol levels rise with age.

Declines in cholesterol levels are seen when a patient is acutely ill. Thus, it is rarely appropriate to measure lipid levels in an ill or hospitalized patient, with the notable exception of the serum triglyceride level in a patient with pancreatitis. Cholesterol levels (even when expressed as an age-matched percentile rank, such as the highest 20%) do not remain constant over time, especially from childhood through adolescence and young adulthood. Thus, children and young adults with relatively high cholesterol levels may have lower levels later in life, whereas those with low cholesterol levels may later have higher levels.

THERAPEUTIC EFFECTS OF LOWERING CHOLESTEROL

Most studies of the effect of cholesterol lowering have distinguished between primary prevention (treating high blood cholesterol in persons free of coronary heart disease) and secondary prevention (treating persons with manifest coronary heart disease). The important distinction is that primary prevention trials enroll healthy subjects who have relatively low rates of coronary disease but in whom other causes of morbidity and mortality are proportionately more common. Secondary prevention trials, on the other hand, follow patients who have a high rate of subsequent coronary disease; other causes of mortality are relatively less important.

Reducing cholesterol levels in healthy middle-aged men without coronary heart disease (primary prevention) reduces their risk, and the reduction in risk is proportionate to the reduction in LDL cholesterol and the increase in HDL cholesterol. Patients in the treatment groups have had statistically significant and clinically important reductions in the rates of myocardial infarctions, new cases of angina, and need for coronary artery bypass procedures. The West of Scotland Study, for example, showed a 31% decrease in myocardial infarctions in middle-aged men treated with pravastatin compared with placebo. The recent AFCAPS/TexCAPS study of middle-aged men and women with average LDL cholesterol and below-average HDL cholesterol and no evidence of coronary artery disease also showed substantial reductions (37%) in the incidence of first major coronary events when treated with lovastatin. As with most primary prevention interventions, however, large numbers of healthy patients need to be treated to prevent a single event.

Primary prevention studies have found a less consistent effect on total mortality. Although the West of Scotland Study found a 22% decrease in total mortality that was almost statistically significant ($p = .051$), the AFCAPS/TexCAPS study resulted in no change in mortality. Seventy-seven patients treated with placebo died during the study compared with 80 treated with lovastatin.

In patients who already have coronary heart disease, the net benefits of cholesterol lowering are clearer, with reductions in the progression of coronary atherosclerosis, fewer subsequent coronary events, less mortality from coronary heart disease, and a reduction in mortality from all causes. Three major randomized clinical trials with statins have shown significant reductions in cardiovascular events, cardiovascular deaths, and all-cause mortality in men and women with coronary artery disease. Studies with statins have also shown that aggressive cholesterol lowering causes regression of atherosclerotic plaques in some patients, reduces the progression of atherosclerosis in saphenous vein grafts, and can slow or reverse carotid artery atherosclerosis. A recent meta-analysis suggests that this latter effect results in a significant decrease in strokes in patients treated with statins. The results with other classes of medications have been less consistent. A recent study compared gemfibrozil and placebo in patients with coronary artery disease who had a low HDL-cholesterol. Gemfibrozil-treated subjects had fewer cardiovascular events, but there was no benefit reflected in all-cause mortality.

The apparent disparities in results between primary and secondary prevention studies highlight several important points. The benefits and adverse effects of cholesterol lowering appear to be specific to each type of drug; the clinician cannot assume that the effects will generalize to other classes of medication. Second, the net benefits from cholesterol lowering depend upon the underlying risk of coronary heart disease and of other disease. In patients with manifest atherosclerosis, morbidity and mortality rates associated with coronary heart disease are high, and measures that reduce coronary heart disease are more likely to be beneficial even if they have no effect—or even slightly harmful effects—on other diseases. Third, the full effects of cholesterol lowering in women and in older and younger men are uncertain.

Bucher HC et al: Effect of HMG-CoA reductase inhibitors on stroke: a meta-analysis of randomized controlled trials. Ann Intern Med 1998;128:89. [NLM Cit ID: 98085833] (Meta-analysis of randomized, controlled trials suggests that in hyperlipidemic patients who have not previously had stroke, HMG-CoA reductase inhibitors reduce the incidence of stroke. Other antilipidemic drugs and dietary interventions are not efficacious for stroke prevention.)

Downs JR et al: Primary prevention of acute coronary events with lovastatin in men and women with average cholesterol levels: Results of AFCAPS/TexCAPS. JAMA 1998;279:1615. [NLM Cit ID: 98273991]

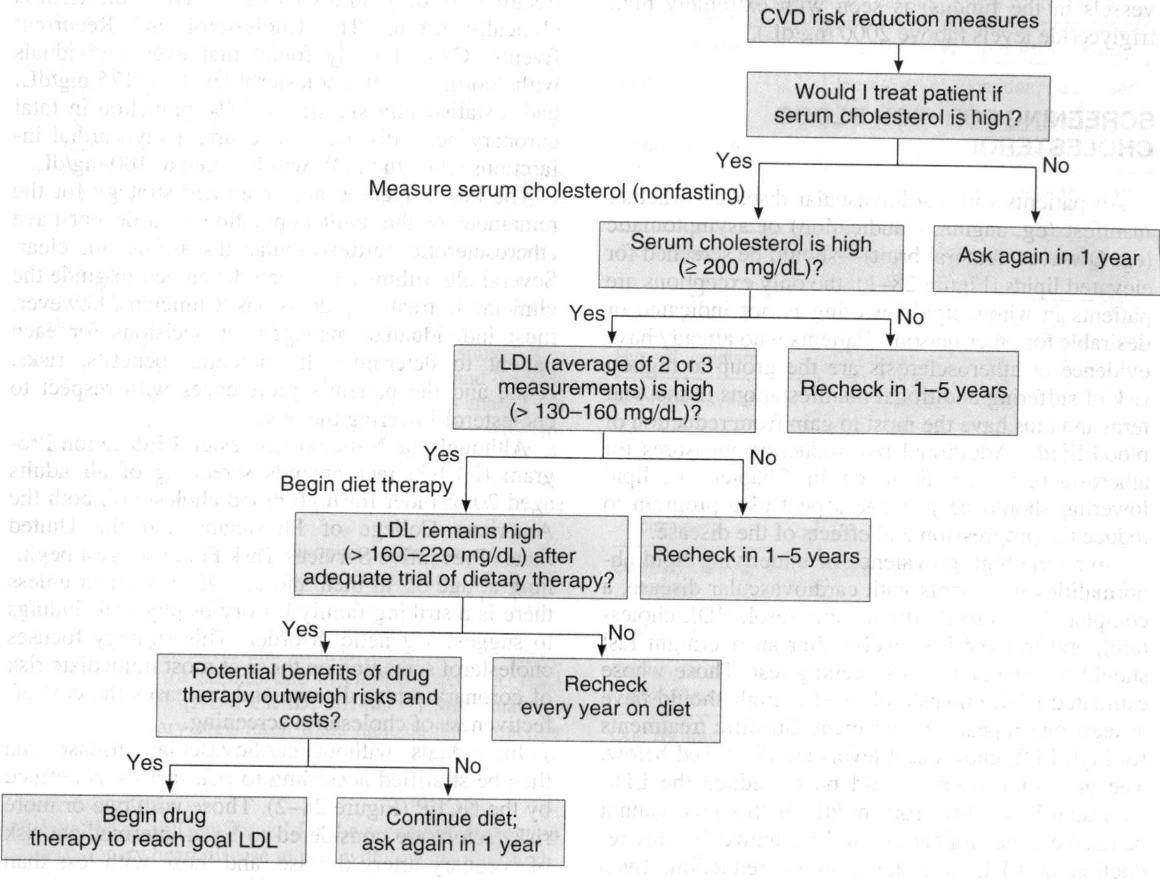

Figure 28–2. Algorithm for screening and management of patients free of cardiovascular disease. Treatment cutpoints, goals, and variations are discussed in the text.

two are at low risk. Risk factors include age and gender (men aged 45 or older, women aged 55 or older); a family history of premature coronary heart disease (myocardial infarction or sudden cardiac death before age 55 in a first-degree male relative or before age 65 in a first-degree female relative); hypertension (whether treated or not); current cigarette smoking (ten or more cigarettes per day); diabetes mellitus (whether treated or not); and low HDL cholesterol (< 35 mg/dL). Because HDL cholesterol is protective against coronary heart disease, a risk factor is subtracted if the level is greater than 60 mg/dL. Newer algorithms have been proposed to further improve risk stratification. Placing additional emphasis on age can improve discrimination between high- and low-risk adults.

Several strategies for obtaining the initial cholesterol measurement have been proposed, including (1) measuring total cholesterol alone, (2) measuring total cholesterol and HDL cholesterol, or (3) measuring only LDL and HDL cholesterol. Each is acceptable as long as all treatment decisions are based on the LDL and HDL cholesterol levels. Measurement of the total cholesterol alone is the least expensive strategy and is adequate for low-risk individuals; those with total cholesterol greater than 200 mg/dL should then be reevaluated with a fasting LDL and HDL cholesterol measurement. Measurement of the total cholesterol and HDL cholesterol allows for better characterization of the risk factor profile but also requires reevaluation if the total cholesterol is greater than 200 mg/dL. Initial measurement of the LDL and HDL cholesterol is least likely to lead to patient misinformation and misclassification and is the strategy preferred by many clinicians.

Treatment decisions are based upon the LDL cholesterol and the patient's risk factor profile (including the HDL cholesterol level). Patients in the intermediate risk group (two or more risk factors) are selected for diet therapy if LDL cholesterol is greater than 130 mg/dL and for drug therapy if it is greater than 160 mg/dL. Low-risk individuals are selected for diet therapy if LDL cholesterol is greater than 160 mg/dL and for drug therapy if it is greater than 190 mg/dL. Young individuals (men under age 35 and women under age 45) require an LDL cholesterol of 220 mg/dL or more before drug therapy is warranted.

Screening in Women

The foregoing screening and treatment guidelines, based largely on LDL cholesterol levels, are designed for both male and female patients. Yet observational studies suggest that a low HDL cholesterol is a more important risk factor for coronary heart disease in women than a high LDL cholesterol. Meta-analysis of clinical trials that have included women with known heart disease, however, has found that medications which primarily lower LDL cholesterol do prevent recurrent myocardial infarctions in women. There is insufficient evidence to be certain of a similar effect from LDL-lowering therapy in women without evidence of coronary heart disease. Although most experts recommend application of the same primary prevention guidelines for women as for men, clinicians should be aware of the uncertainty in this area.

Screening in Older Patients

Meta-analysis of observational evidence relating cholesterol to coronary heart disease in the elderly suggests that cholesterol is not a risk factor for coronary heart disease for persons over age 75. Clinical trials have rarely included such individuals. Although the NCEP recommends continuing treatment in the elderly, many clinicians will prefer to stop screening and treatment in patients age 75 or older who do not have coronary heart disease. In patients age 75 or older who have coronary heart disease, LDL-lowering therapy can be continued as recommended for younger patients with the disease. Decisions to discontinue therapy should be based on overall functional status and life expectancy, comorbidities, and patient preference and should be made in context with overall therapeutic goals and end-of-life decisions.

Ansell BJ et al: An evidence-based assessment of the NCEP Adult Treatment Panel II guidelines. National Cholesterol Education Program. JAMA 1999;282:2051. [NLM Cit ID: 20057345] (Lipid-lowering therapy should be more aggressively applied to patients with diabetes or coronary heart disease. Statins are preferred to estrogen replacement use in secondary coronary heart disease prevention in postmenopausal women. Further studies are needed to address the effects of lipid modification in primary prevention of coronary heart disease in populations other than middle-aged men and to study markers of lipid metabolism other than LDL-C.)

Avins AL et al: Improving the prediction of coronary heart disease to aid in the management of high cholesterol levels. What a difference a decade makes. JAMA 1998;279:445. [NLM Cit ID: 98126113] (Placing greater emphasis on age as a risk factor for coronary heart disease improves the ability to discriminate between higher and lower risks.)

Carlsson CM et al: Managing dyslipidemia in older adults. J Am Geriatr Soc 1999;47:1458. [NLM Cit ID: 20057200] (Improving lipid levels in older adults with coronary heart disease decreases the risk of future coronary events by up to 45%, with effects seen within 2 years after initiation of therapy.)

Cleeman JI: Adults aged 20 and older should have their cholesterol measured. Am J Med 1997;102:31. [NLM Cit ID: 97360620] (An argument in defense of the NCEP recommendations to screen young adults.)

Corti MC et al: Clarifying the direct relation between total cholesterol levels and death from coronary heart disease in older persons. Ann Intern Med 1997;126:753. [NLM Cit ID: 97282912] (A recent longitudinal study that contradicts earlier studies of the impact of cholesterol in the elderly.)

Goldman L et al: The relative influence of secondary versus primary prevention using the National Cholesterol Education Program Adult Treatment Panel II guidelines. J Am Coll Cardiol 1999;34:768. [NLM Cit ID: 99411760] (The NCEP guidelines for targeted primary prevention can be a useful component of a rational public health strategy but only as a complement to the more appealing strategies of secondary prevention and "across-the-board" programs to lower all cholesterol levels.)

Grundy SM: The role of cholesterol management in coronary disease risk reduction in elderly patients. Endocrinol Metab Clin North Am 1998;27:655. [NLM Cit ID: 99001238] (Factors taken into account when making decisions about particular therapies for the management of high serum cholesterol in older persons.)

Newman TB et al: Cholesterol screening in children and adolescents. Pediatrics 2000;105:637. [NLM Cit ID: 20164980] (The evidence does not support routine screening for lipid abnormalities in children and adolescents.)

TREATMENT OF HIGH LDL CHOLESTEROL

Reduction of LDL cholesterol is just one part of a program to reduce the risk of cardiovascular disease. Other measures—including smoking cessation, hypertension control, and aspirin—are also of central importance. Less well studied but potentially of great value is raising the HDL cholesterol level. Several "healthy habits" have more than one benefit. Quitting smoking, for example, reduces the effect of other cardiovascular risk factors (such as a high cholesterol level); it may also increase the HDL cholesterol level. Exercise (and weight loss) may reduce the LDL cholesterol level and increase the HDL cholesterol level. Modest alcohol use (1–2 ounces a day) also raises HDL levels and appears to have a salutary effect on coronary heart disease rates. While the clinician may not wish to recommend alcohol use to patients, its use in moderation need not be discouraged.

Diet Therapy

Most treatment algorithms recommend diet therapy as the initial step for all patients with high blood cholesterol. Unfortunately, studies of nonhospitalized adults have reported only modest cholesterol-lowering benefits from such therapy, typically in the range of a 5–10% decrease in LDL cholesterol. The results of studies with longer periods of follow-up suggest that the long-term impact of diet therapy is even less. The effect of diet therapy, however, varies considerably among individuals. Although most patients will have a quite modest effect with dietary changes, some patients will have striking reductions in LDL cholesterol—up to a 25–30% decrease—while others will have clinically important increases. Thus, the results of diet therapy should be carefully monitored, typically about 4 weeks after initiation.

Cholesterol-lowering diets may also have a variable effect on lipid fractions. For example, diets that are very low in total fat or very low in saturated fat may lower HDL cholesterol as much as LDL cholesterol. It is not known how these diet-induced changes affect coronary risk.

Several nutritional approaches to diet therapy are available (Table 28–2). Most Americans currently eat 35–40% of calories as fat. Approximately 15% is saturated fat. Dietary cholesterol intake averages 400 mg/d. A standard "Step 1" cholesterol-lowering diet recommends reducing total fat to 30% and saturated fat to 10% of calories. Dietary cholesterol is limited to 300 mg/d. The "Step 2" diet further restricts saturated fat to 7% of calories and dietary cholesterol to 200 mg/d. These diets replace fat, particularly saturated fat, with carbohydrate. In most instances, this approach will also result in fewer total calories consumed and will facilitate weight loss in overweight patients. Other diet plans, including the Dean Ornish Diet, the Pritikin Diet, and most vegetarian diets, restrict fat even further. Low-fat, high-carbohydrate diets may, however, result in reductions in HDL cholesterol.

An alternative strategy is the "Mediterranean diet," which maintains total fat at approximately 35–40% of total calories but replaces saturated fat with monounsaturated fat such as that found in canola oil and in olives, peanuts, avocados, and their oils. This diet is equally effective at lowering LDL cholesterol but is less likely to lead to reductions in HDL cholesterol. Because of the substantial intake of dietary fat, this diet is less likely to lead to weight loss. Thus, a traditional low-fat approach is still preferred for patients with lipid disorders who are overweight. In thin patients, however, a Mediterranean diet can be considered.

Other dietary changes may also result in beneficial changes in blood lipids. Soluble fiber, such as that found in oat bran or psyllium, may reduce LDL cholesterol by 5–10%. Garlic, soy protein, vitamin C, and certain plant sterols may also result in reduction of LDL cholesterol. Because of current interest in oxidation of LDL cholesterol as an initiating event in atherogenesis, diets should also be rich in antioxidant vitamins, found primarily in fruits and vegetables (see Chapter 29).

Anderson JW et al: Cholesterol-lowering effects of psyllium intake adjunctive to diet therapy in men and women with hypercholesterolemia: meta-analysis of 8 controlled trials. Am J Clin Nutr 2000;71:472. [NLM Cit ID: 20123714] (Psyllium lowers total and LDL-cholesterol concentrations in subjects consuming a low-fat diet.)

Berglund L et al: HDL-subpopulation patterns in response to reductions in dietary total and saturated fat intakes in healthy subjects. Am J Clin Nutr 1999;70:992. [NLM Cit ID: 20051092] (A reduction in dietary total and saturated fat decreased both large (HDL[2] and HDL[2b]) and small, dense HDL subpopulations.)

Brown L et al: Cholesterol-lowering effects of dietary fiber: a meta-analysis. Am J Clin Nutr 1999;69:30. [NLM Cit ID: 99122508] (Various soluble fibers reduce total and LDL cholesterol by similar amounts, but the effect is small within the practical range of intake.)

Knopp RH et al: Long-term cholesterol-lowering effects of 4 fat-restricted diets in hypercholesterolemic and combined hyperlipidemic men. The Dietary Alternatives Study. JAMA 1997;278:1509. [NLM Cit ID: 98028601] (Severe restriction of dietary fat to less than 30% of total calories resulted in no further decrease in LDL cholesterol when compared with diets containing 30% of calories as fat. In some patients, lower-fat diets resulted in significant reductions in HDL cholesterol.)

Table 28–2. Macronutrient composition of three lipid-modifying diets.

	Recommended Intake		
Nutrient	**Step 1 Diet**	**Step 2 Diet**	**Mediterranean Diet**
Total fat	< 30% of calories	< 30% of calories	< 40% of calories
Saturated fat	< 10% of calories	< 7% of calories	< 10% of calories
Polyunsaturated fat	< 10% of calories	< 10% of calories	< 10% of calories
Monounsaturated fat	< 10% of calories	< 10% of calories	< 20% of calories
Carbohydrate	50–60% of calories	50–60% of calories	40–50% of calories
Protein	10–20% of calories	10–20% of calories	10–20% of calories
Cholesterol	< 300 mg/d	< 200 mg/d	< 300 mg/d
Total calories	For desirable weight	For desirable weight	For desirable weight

LaRosa JC: The role of diet and exercise in the statin era. Prog Cardiovasc Dis 1998;41:137. [NLM Cit ID: 99005074] (Diet, exercise, and other nonpharmacologic interventions have a role in the age of statins, not only to augment the effects of these drugs in high-risk patients but also, by preventing atherogenesis in the first place, to reduce the number of at-risk patients.)

Lichtenstein AH: Soy protein, isoflavones and cardiovascular disease risk. J Nutr 1998;128:1589. [NLM Cit ID: 98445483] (Nutritional components in soy lower cholesterol; consumption of products containing soy protein may displace foods relatively high in saturated fat and cholesterol from the diet and hence have an indirect blood cholesterol-lowering effect.)

Lorgeril M et al: Mediterranean diet, traditional risk factors and the rate of cardiovascular complications after myocardial infarction: Final report of the Lyon Diet Heart Study. Circulation 1999;99:779. [NLM Cit ID: 99145700] (The protective effect of the Mediterranean diet was maintained up to 4 years.)

Morgan WA et al: Pecans lower low-density lipoprotein cholesterol in people with normal lipid levels. J Am Diet Assoc 2000;100:312. [NLM Cit ID: 20184318] (LDL-C was significantly lowered in the pecan treatment group.)

Sikand G et al: Medical nutrition therapy lowers serum cholesterol and saves medication costs in men with hypercholesterolemia. J Am Diet Assoc 1998;98:889. [NLM Cit ID: 98376518] (Diet therapy in men with hypercholesterolemia leads to reduction in total cholesterol levels and LDL-C, reduces the number of patients needing drug therapy, and results in substantial cost savings.)

Superko HR et al: Garlic powder, effect on plasma lipids, postprandial lipemia, low-density lipoprotein particle size, high-density lipoprotein subclass distribution and lipoprotein(a). J Am Coll Cardiol 2000;35:321. [NLM Cit ID: 20139846] (Garlic therapy has no effect on major plasma lipoproteins or on HDL subclasses, Lp[a], apolipoprotein B, postprandial triglycerides, or LDL subclass distribution.)

Tang JL et al: Systematic review of dietary intervention trials to lower blood total cholesterol in free-living subjects. BMJ 1998;316:1213. [NLM Cit ID: 98221047] (Dietary advice to free-living subjects can be expected to reduce blood total cholesterol by only 3–6%. More intensive diets—such as the step 1 and step 2 diets of the American Heart Association—achieve a greater reduction in serum cholesterol concentration.)

Pharmacologic Therapy (Table 28–3)

All patients whose risk from coronary heart disease is considered high enough to warrant pharmacologic therapy of an elevated LDL cholesterol should be given aspirin prophylaxis at a dose of 81–325 mg/d unless there are contraindications such as aspirin sensitivity, bleeding diatheses, or active peptic

Table 28–3. Effects of selected lipid-modifying drugs.

Drug	Lipid-Modifying Effects			Initial Daily Dose	Maximum Daily Dose	Cost for 30 Days' Treatment With Dose Listed[1]
	LDL	HDL	Triglyceride			
Atorvastatin (Lipitor)	–25 to –40%	+5 to –10%	↓↓	10 mg once	80 mg once	$87.14 (20 mg once)
Cerivastatin (Baycol)	–30%	+5 to –10%	↓	0.3 mg once	0.3 mg once	$42.60 (0.3 mg once)
Cholestyramine (Questran, others)	–15 to –25%	+5%	±	4 g bid	24 g divided	$110.71 (8 g divided)
Colestipol (Colestid)	–15 to –25%	+5%	±	5 g bid	30 g divided	$99.78 (10 g divided)
Fluvastatin (Lescol)	–20 to –30%	+5 to –10%	↓	20 mg once	40 mg once	$39.90 (20 mg once)
Gemfibrozil (Lopid)	–10 to –15%	+15 to –20%	↓↓	600 mg once	1200 mg divided	$64.69 (600 mg bid)
Lovastatin (Mevacor)	–25 to –40%	+5 to –10%	↓	10 mg once	80 mg divided	$72.50 (20 mg once)
Niacin	–15 to –25%	+25 to –35%	↓↓	100 mg once	3–4.5 g divided	$7.20 (1.5 g bid)
Pravastatin (Pravachol)	–25 to –40%	+5 to –10%	↓	20 mg once	40 mg once	$72.90 (20 mg once)
Simvastatin (Zocor)	–25 to –40%	+5 to –10%	↓↓	5 mg once	80 mg once	$65.45 (10 mg once)

[1]Cost to pharmacist (average wholesale price, generic when possible) for quantity listed. Source: *Drug Topics Red Book,* March 2000; Vol. 19, No. 3.

± = variable, if any.

ulcer disease. Current data suggest that the effect of aspirin in reducing the risk of coronary heart disease is equivalent to that of cholesterol lowering. Other coronary heart disease risk factors, such as hypertension and smoking, should also be controlled.

If the decision to treat a patient with an LDL-lowering drug is made, the clinician must select an appropriate agent based on the safety, efficacy, cost, and effects on lipid levels (Tables 28–3 and 28–4) and set a goal for treatment. As with all therapies for chronic conditions, the therapeutic goal is best approached slowly and steadily, watching carefully for side effects and encouraging continued compliance with nonpharmacologic measures. Combinations of drugs may be necessary. Once the goal is reached, the lipid profile should be monitored periodically (every 6–12 months), with consideration given to periodic reductions in drug dose. With the exception of niacin (available generically for a few dollars per month), lipid-lowering agents are expensive and may need to be given for decades. Thus, their cost-effectiveness is generally low, especially in primary prevention. Balancing the risks and benefits of any therapy, especially one that may be lifelong, is essential.

A. Niacin (Nicotinic Acid): Niacin was the first lipid-lowering agent that was associated with a reduction in total mortality. Long-term follow-up of a secondary prevention trial of middle-aged men with previous myocardial infarction disclosed that about 52% of those who had been previously treated with niacin had died, compared with 58% in the placebo group. This favorable effect on mortality was not seen during the trial itself, though there was a reduction in the incidence of coronary heart disease.

Niacin reduces the production of VLDL particles, with secondary reduction in LDL and increases in HDL cholesterol levels. The average effect of full-dose niacin therapy, 3–4.5 g/d, is a 15–25% reduction in LDL cholesterol and a 25–35% increase in HDL cholesterol. Full doses of niacin are required to obtain the LDL effect, but the HDL effect is observed at lower doses, eg, 1 g/d. Niacin will also reduce triglycerides by half and will lower lipoprotein(a) (Lp[a]) levels. Thus, its effect on blood lipids is nearly optimal. Unfortunately, intolerance to niacin is common; only 50–60% of subjects in clinical trials tolerate full doses. Niacin causes a prostaglandin-mediated flushing that patients may describe as hot flashes or pruritus. This problem can be decreased by pretreatment with aspirin (81–325 mg/d) or other nonsteroidal anti-inflammatory agents. Flushing may also be decreased by initiating niacin therapy with a very small dose, eg, 50–100 mg with the evening meal. The dose can be doubled each week until 1.5 g/d is tolerated. After rechecking blood lipids, the dose is divided and increased until the goal of 3–4.5 g/d is reached. Only immediate-release niacin is recommended for lipid modification. Sustained-release preparations are more expensive and have less effect on raising HDL cholesterol. Both immediate-release and sustained-release niacin are associated with hepatitis, but the most severe cases have been reported with the sustained-release preparations. It is not known whether routine monitoring of liver enzymes results in early detection and thus reduced severity of this side effect. Niacin can also exacerbate gout and peptic ulcer disease and may worsen hyperglycemia in patients with diabetes mellitus.

Table 28–4. Selection of lipid-modifying medications.

Primary prevention
- Premenopausal women (rare):
  - Statins, niacin, resins
- Men (35–75 years):
  - Statins, niacin, resins
- Postmenopausal women (< 75 years):
  - Statins, niacin

Secondary prevention
- Men:
  - Statins, niacin, combinations
- Women:
  - Statins, niacin, combinations

B. Bile Acid-Binding Resins (Cholestyramine, Colestipol): Treatment with these agents has been shown to reduce the incidence of coronary events (such as myocardial infarction) in middle-aged men by about 20%, with no significant effect on total mortality. The resins work by binding bile acids in the intestine. The resultant reduction in the enterohepatic circulation causes the liver to increase its production of bile acids, using hepatic cholesterol to do so. Thus, hepatic LDL receptor activity increases, with a decline in plasma LDL levels. The triglyceride level tends to increase slightly in some patients treated with bile acid-binding resins; they should be used with caution in those with elevated triglycerides and probably not at all in patients who have triglyceride levels above about 500 mg/dL. The clinician can anticipate a reduction of 15–25% in the LDL cholesterol level, with minor (if any) increases in the HDL level.

The usual dose of cholestyramine is 12–36 g of resin per day in divided doses with meals, mixed in water or, more palatably, juice. The prepackaged 4 g doses are more expensive than the bulk form; the "candy bars" are even more expensive. Doses of colestipol are 20% higher (the packets each contain 5 g of resin).

These agents often cause gastrointestinal symptoms, such as constipation and gas. They may interfere with the absorption of fat-soluble vitamins (thereby complicating the management of patients receiving warfarin) and may bind other drugs in the intestine. Concurrent use of psyllium may ameliorate the gastrointestinal side effects.

C. HMG-CoA Reductase Inhibitors (Lovastatin, Pravastatin, Simvastatin, Fluvastatin, Atorvastatin, Cerivastatin): These agents work by inhibiting the rate-limiting enzyme in the formation of cholesterol. They have been shown to reduce coronary heart disease and total mortality in secondary prevention settings, as well as in middle-aged men free of coronary heart disease. A recent meta-analysis also demonstrates significant reduction in risk of stroke. Cholesterol synthesis in the liver is reduced, with a compensatory increase in hepatic LDL receptors (presumably so that the liver can take more of the cholesterol that it needs from the blood), and a reduction in the circulating LDL cholesterol level by up to 35%. There are also modest increases in HDL levels and decreases in triglyceride levels.

Doses are as follows: lovastatin, 10–80 mg/d; pravastatin, 10–40 mg/d; simvastatin, 5–40 mg/d; fluvastatin, 20–40 mg/d; atorvastatin, 10–80 mg/d; and cerivastatin, 0.3 mg/d. These agents are usually given once a day in the evening (most cholesterol synthesis takes place overnight); at the high end of the dose ranges, twice-a-day dosing may be used. Side effects include myositis, whose incidence may be higher in patients concurrently taking fibrates or niacin. Manufacturers recommend monitoring liver and muscle enzymes. Several agents (notably erythromycin, cyclosporine, and azole antifungals) reduce the metabolism of these agents.

D. Fibric Acid Derivatives (Gemfibrozil, Clofibrate, Fenofibrate): In the largest clinical trial that used clofibrate, there were significantly more deaths—especially due to cancer—in the treatment group than in the control group. Although still available, clofibrate is rarely used. Gemfibrozil reduced coronary heart disease rates in hypercholesterolemic middle-aged men free of coronary disease in the Helsinki Heart Study. The effect was only observed among those who also had lower HDL cholesterol levels and high triglyceride levels. Among men with previous myocardial infarction, however, gemfibrozil increased overall mortality as well as that due to coronary heart disease. Clinicians should also be aware of the trend toward increased numbers of cancer deaths among subjects treated with gemfibrozil in the Helsinki Heart Study.

The fibrates reduce the synthesis and increase the breakdown of VLDL particles, with secondary effects on LDL and HDL levels. They reduce LDL levels by about 10–15% and triglyceride levels by about 40% and raise HDL levels by about 15–20%. The usual dose of gemfibrozil is 600 mg once or twice a day. Side effects include cholelithiasis, hepatitis, and myositis. The incidence of the latter two conditions may be higher among patients also taking other lipid-lowering agents. Given that clofibrate caused a statistically significant increase in cancer mortality, it should not be used.

E. Probucol: The effects of probucol on coronary heart disease—and its long-term safety—are not known. It does reduce the deposition of LDL into xanthomas in humans (and into atherosclerotic plaques in rabbits). The mechanism of action of probucol is not clear. It apparently reduces the amount of oxidized LDL (it was originally used as an industrial antioxidant). Probucol reduces LDL levels by 10–15% but has the potentially important adverse effect of lowering HDL levels by up to 10%. Probucol, if used at all, should be reserved for patients with a clear genetic disorder who have failed other therapies.

Initial Selection of Medication

At present there are no absolute guidelines for selection of available lipid-modifying medications in particular patients. Nonetheless, the results of clinical trials can provide some guidance (Table 28–4). For men with known coronary heart disease who require a lipid-modifying medication, an HMG-CoA reductase inhibitor is preferred. Although niacin will also have beneficial effects on lipids in both men and women with coronary heart disease, there is less evidence from clinical trials demonstrating the desired effects on coronary heart disease and all-cause mortality. Although estrogen also has beneficial effects on lipids in postmenopausal women, the recent Heart and Estrogen/Progestin Replacement Study (HERS) suggests that estrogen should not be used to treat lipid disorders in women with coronary heart disease (see Chapter 26).

For patients without known coronary heart disease, the choice of medications (and proof of a beneficial effect) is less clear. For men 45–64 years of age, an HMG-CoA reductase inhibitor is preferred. For men aged 35–44 and for men aged 65–75, either an HMG-CoA reductase inhibitor or niacin can be equally considered. For postmenopausal women up to age 75, an HMG-CoA reductase inhibitor or niacin can also be used. Hormone therapy (estrogen and progestin) will improve lipids as well, but the effect on heart disease outcomes is still unknown Premenopausal women rarely require lipid-modifying therapy. Resins are the only lipid-modifying medication considered safe in pregnancy. If pregnancy is not a concern, an HMG-CoA reductase inhibitor or niacin can be considered.

Combinations of lipid-modifying medications can also be used. Combinations may be more cost-effective than high doses of a single medication (usually an HMG-CoA reductase inhibitor) and may have beneficial effects on lipids. Low-dose niacin (0.5–1 g/d), for example, will substantially increase the HDL cholesterol when added to an HMG-CoA reductase inhibitor. Combinations, however, may increase the risk of severe complications of drug therapy. The combination of gemfibrozil and HMG-CoA reductase inhibitors increases the risk of myopathy more than either drug alone.

Bucher HC et al: Systematic review on the risk and benefit of different cholesterol-lowering interventions. Arterioscler Thromb Vasc Biol 1999;19:187. [NLM Cit ID: 99141278] (Statins have the largest effect on the reduction of cardiovascular and all-cause mortality, and this result recommends their use in preference to other antilipidemic agents.)

Choice of lipid-lowering drugs. Med Lett Drugs Ther 1998;40:117. [NLM Cit ID: 99100410]

Garg R et al: Niacin treatment increases plasma homocyst(e)ine levels. Am Heart J 1999;138:1082. [NLM Cit ID: 20044326] (Niacin substantially increases plasma homocyst[e]ine levels).

Guyton JR et al: Treatment of hyperlipidemia with combined niacin-statin regimens. Am J Cardiol 1998; 82:82U; discussion 85U. [NLM Cit ID: 99112873] (This combination therapy can be used safely as long as careful attention is given to niacin formulation and dosing, liver function is monitored, and patients are educated to recognize symptoms of myopathy.)

Guyton JR: Effect of niacin on atherosclerotic cardiovascular disease. Am J Cardiol 1998;82:18U; discussion 39U. [NLM Cit ID: 99112864] (The use of niacin to prevent or treat atherosclerotic cardiovascular disease is based on strong and consistent evidence from clinical trials.)

Hilleman DE et al: A population-based treat-to-target pharmacoeconomic analysis of HMG-CoA reductase inhibitors in hypercholesterolemia. Clin Ther 1999;21:536. [NLM Cit ID: 99253339] (Atorvastatin was the most cost-effective drug for high-risk patients, whereas fluvastatin was the most cost-effective agent for low-risk and moderate-risk patients. If one drug is chosen to treat all patients—in cases of formulary restriction—atorvastatin would be the most cost-effective agent.)

Hulley SB et al: Randomized trial of estrogen plus progestin for secondary prevention of coronary heart disease in postmenopausal women. JAMA 1998;280:605. [NLM Cit ID: 98382151] (Treatment with oral conjugated equine estrogen plus medroxyprogesterone acetate did not reduce the overall rate of coronary heart disease events in postmenopausal women with established coronary disease.)

Hunninghake D et al: Treating to meet NCEP-recommended LDL-cholesterol concentrations with atorvastatin, fluvastatin, lovastatin or simvastatin in patients with risk factors for coronary heart disease. J Fam Pract 1998;47:349. [NLM Cit ID: 99051834] (A greater percentage of patients reached their target LDL with atorvastatin than with other statins.)

Knopp RH: Clinical profiles of plain versus sustained-release niacin (Niaspan) and the physiologic rationale for nighttime dosing. Am J Cardiol 1998;82:24. [NLM Cit ID: 99112865] (Bedtime administration of 1.5 g extended-release niacin was shown to have the same beneficial effects as 1.5 g plain niacin in three divided doses and to be well tolerated.)

Zema MJ: Gemfibrozil, nicotinic acid and combination therapy in patients with isolated hypoalphalipoproteinemia: a randomized, open-label, crossover study. J Am Coll Cardiol 2000;35:640. [NLM Cit ID: 20179210] (In patients with clinical atherosclerotic disease and isolated hypoalphalipoproteinemia, pharmacologic therapy with gemfibrozil and niacin, alone or in combination, will raise HDL-C.)

HIGH BLOOD TRIGLYCERIDES

Patients with very high levels of serum triglycerides are at risk of pancreatitis. The pathophysiology is not certain, since there are some patients with very high triglyceride levels who never develop pancreatitis. Most patients with congenital abnormalities in triglyceride metabolism present in childhood; hypertriglyceridemia-induced pancreatitis that first presents in adults is more commonly due to an acquired problem in lipid metabolism.

Although there are no clear triglyceride levels that always result in pancreatitis, most clinicians are uncomfortable with levels above 1000 mg/dL. The risk of pancreatitis may be more related to the triglyceride level following consumption of a fatty meal. Because postcibal increases in triglyceride are inevitable if fat-containing foods are eaten, fasting triglyceride levels in persons prone to pancreatitis should be kept well below that level.

The primary therapy for high triglyceride levels is dietary, avoiding alcohol and fatty foods and restricting calories. Control of secondary causes of high triglyceride levels (see Table 28–1) may also be helpful. In patients with persistent elevations in the pancreatitis range despite adequate dietary compliance—and certainly in those with a previous episode of pancreatitis—therapy with a triglyceride-lowering drug (eg, niacin, in doses as described above) is indicated.

Whether patients with elevated triglycerides (> 250 mg/dL) and no other lipoprotein abnormalities are at increased risk of atherosclerotic disease is not known. Some of these patients may belong to families with a genetic disorder known as **familial combined hyperlipidemia.** This disorder is characterized by a variety of lipid abnormalities in different family members: Some have high cholesterol levels, some high triglyceride levels, and some both. It now appears that the common link is an abnormality in one of the LDL-associated apoproteins (B-100), and that this may be a coronary risk factor. However, the effect on coronary heart disease risk of treating an isolated high triglyceride level in these patients is not known.

Current indications for treatment of high blood triglycerides to prevent coronary heart disease are controversial. In patients with known coronary heart disease, it is reasonable to treat isolated increases in triglycerides to 400 mg/dL or greater with an HMG-CoA reductase inhibitor. Most of these patients will have elevated LDL cholesterol (≥ 130 mg/dL) and will benefit from drug therapy even though estimation of the LDL cholesterol level will not be possible until the triglyceride is below 400 mg/dL. In patients without known coronary heart disease, the optimal strategy is not known. Triglyceride levels above 400 mg/dL can be treated first with nonpharmacologic approaches, including weight loss, low-fat diet, avoidance of excess alcohol, and regular aerobic exercise. If serum triglyceride levels remain greater than 400 mg/dL (but < 1000 mg/dL), LDL cholesterol can be measured directly by ultracentrifugation. Treatment decisions can then be based on the LDL cholesterol level.

Gotto AM Jr: Triglyceride as a risk factor for coronary artery disease. Am J Cardiol 1998;82:22Q. [NLM Cit ID: 99034409] (The data for an independent association between triglyceride concentrations and risk for coronary artery disease are equivocal, unlike the data for LDL and HDL cholesterol, which show strong, consistent, and opposing correlations with coronary artery disease risk.)

Kesaniemi YA: Serum triglycerides and clinical benefit in lipid-lowering trials. Am J Cardiol 1998;81:70B. [NLM Cit ID: 98186013] (The role of serum triglyceride reduction in achieving clinical benefit is unclear and poorly documented. On the other hand, no specific trials have studied the importance of triglyceride lowering among patients with marked hypertriglyceridemia. One of the problems in assessing patients with high serum triglyceride levels may be the heterogeneous background of the molecular mechanisms that result in hypertriglyceridemia.)

Sattar N et al: The end of triglycerides in cardiovascular risk assessment? Rumours of death are greatly exaggerated. BMJ 1998;317:553. [NLM Cit ID: 98387791]

Stein EA et al: Comparison of statins in hypertriglyceridemia. Am J Cardiol 1998;81:66B. [NLM Cit ID: 98186012] (All statins are effective in decreasing triglyceride levels, but only in hypertriglyceridemic patients. Owing to the relatively constant triglyceride:LDL cholesterol ratio, our analysis indicates that the more effective the statin is in decreasing LDL cholesterol, the more effective it will also be in decreasing triglyceride levels.)

RELEVANT WORLD WIDE WEB SITES

[CIC Food and Nutrition]
http://www.gsa.gov/staff/pa/cic/food.htm

[Elevated Cholesterol—Doctor's Guide to the Internet]
http://www.pslgroup.com/ELEVCHOL.HTM

[NHLBI—National Cholesterol Education Program]
http://rover.nhlbi.nih.gov/chd/
http://www.nhlbi.nih.gov/about/ncep/index.htm

[NHLBI—Recommendations Regarding Public Screening for Measuring Blood Cholesterol]
http://www.nhlbi.nih.gov/guidelines/cholesterol/chol_scr.htm

[NHBLI—Second Report of the Expert Panel on Detection, Evaluation, and Treatment of High Blood Cholesterol in Adults (ATP II)]
http://www.nhlbi.nih.gov/guidelines/cholesterol/atp_ii.htm

[NIH Consensus Development Program—Triglyceride, High Density Lipoprotein, and Coronary Heart Disease]
http://www.odp.od.nih.gov/consensus/cons/089/089_intro.htm

[The Nutritionist's Tool Box]
http://fscn.che.umn.edu/tools.htm

29 Nutrition

See http://www.current-med.com/ch29.html for updated addresses of Web sites referenced in this chapter.

Robert B. Baron, MD, MS

NUTRITIONAL REQUIREMENTS

Approximately 40 nutrients are required by the human body. Nutrients are essential if they cannot be synthesized by the body and if a deficiency causes recognizable abnormalities that disappear when the deficit is corrected. Required nutrients include the essential amino acids, water-soluble vitamins, fat-soluble vitamins, minerals, and the essential fatty acids. The body also requires an adequate energy substrate, a small amount of metabolizable carbohydrate, indigestible carbohydrate (fiber), additional nitrogen, and water.

Nutritional requirements have been most commonly expressed by recommended dietary allowances (RDAs). Published and periodically reviewed by the Food and Nutrition Board of the National Academy of Sciences, the RDAs were initially designed to meet the known nutritional needs of practically all healthy persons. RDAs have been established for energy and protein; the water-soluble vitamins thiamin, riboflavin, niacin, vitamin B_6, folic acid, vitamin B_{12}, and vitamin C; the fat soluble vitamins A, D, and K; and the minerals calcium, phosphorus, magnesium, iron, zinc, iodine, and selenium (Table 29–1).

Recently, the Food and Nutrition Board has developed a new approach to defining nutritional adequacy. Known as dietary reference intakes (DRIs), these new guidelines go beyond the prevention of classic nutritional deficiency diseases and address the role of nutrients and other food components in long-term health and the reduction of risk of chronic diseases. The DRIs consist of four reference intakes: the RDA, the estimated average requirement (EAR), the tolerable upper intake level (UL), and the adequate intake (AI). The RDA remains the dietary intake that is sufficient to meet the nutritional requirements of nearly all individuals in an age- and gender-specific group. RDAs are intended as goals for individuals. The EAR is the intake value that is estimated to meet the requirements of 50% of individuals in an age- and gender-specific group. The UL is the maximum level of daily nutrient intake that is unlikely to pose risks of adverse health to almost all individuals. The AI is given when insufficient data are available to establish the EAR and RDA for a given nutrient. It is based on fewer data and more expert opinion but is also intended as goals for individuals. DRIs are divided into seven nutrient groups: (1) calcium, vitamin D, phosphorus, magnesium and fluoride; (2) folate and other B vitamins; (3) antioxidants (eg, vitamins C and E and selenium); (4) macronutrients (eg, protein, fat, carbohydrates); (5) trace elements (eg, iron and zinc); (6) electrolytes and water; and (7) other food components (eg, fiber, phytoestrogens). Reports have been issued establishing DRIs for the first three groups.

ENERGY

The body requires energy to support normal functions and physical activity, growth, and repair of damaged tissues. Energy is provided by oxidation of dietary protein, fat, carbohydrate, and alcohol. Oxidation of 1 g of each provides 4 kcal of energy from protein and carbohydrate, 9 kcal from fat, and 7 kcal from alcohol.

In healthy adults, energy expenditure is primarily determined by three factors: basal energy expenditure (BEE), thermic effect of food (TEF), and physical activity.

The BEE is the amount of energy required to maintain basic physiologic functions. It is measured while the subject is resting in a warm room, not having eaten for 12 hours. In healthy persons, the BEE (in kcal/24 h) can be estimated by the Harris-Benedict equation, which will correctly predict measured BEE in 90% ± 10% of healthy subjects (see Nutritional Requirement, below). In clinical practice, patients rarely meet the strict criteria for basal measurement. Energy expenditure measured in individuals at rest without food for 2 hours is the resting energy expenditure (REE) and is about 10% greater than BEE.

Table 29–1. Recommended daily dietary allowances for adults (revised 1989).[1]

Category	Age (years) or Condition	Weight (kg)	Weight (lb)	Height (cm)	Height (in)	Protein (g)	Fat-Soluble Vitamins: Vitamin A (mg RE)	Vitamin D (mg)	Vitamin E (mg α-TE)	Vitamin K (mg)	Water-Soluble Vitamins: Vitamin C (mg)	Thiamine (mg)	Riboflavin (mg)	Niacin (mg)	Vitamin B_6 (mg)	Folate (μg)	Vitamin B_{12} (μg)	Minerals: Calcium (mg)	Phosphorus (mg)	Magnesium (mg)	Iron (mg)	Zinc (mg)	Iodine (μg)	Selenium (μg)
Males	15–18	66	145	176	69	59	1000	10	10	65	60	1.5	1.8	20	2.0	200	2.0	1200	1200	400	12	15	150	50
	19–24	72	160	177	70	58	1000	10	10	70	60	1.5	1.7	19	2.0	200	2.0	1200	1200	350	10	15	150	70
	25–50	79	174	176	70	63	1000	5	10	80	60	1.5	1.7	19	2.0	200	2.0	800	800	350	10	15	150	70
	51+	77	170	173	68	63	1000	5	10	80	60	1.2	1.4	15	2.0	200	2.0	800	800	350	10	15	150	70
Females	15–18	55	120	163	64	44	800	10	8	55	60	1.1	1.3	15	1.5	160	2.0	1200	1200	300	15	12	150	50
	19–24	58	128	164	65	46	800	10	8	60	60	1.1	1.3	15	1.6	180	2.0	1200	1200	280	15	12	150	55
	25–50	63	138	163	64	50	800	5	8	65	60	1.1	1.3	15	1.6	180	2.0	800	800	280	15	12	150	55
	51+	65	143	160	63	50	800	5	8	65	60	1.0	1.2	13	1.6	180	2.0	800	800	280	10	12	150	55
Pregnant						60	800	10	10	65	70	1.5	1.6	17	2.2	400	2.2	1200	1200	320	30	15	175	65
Lactating	1st 6 months					65	1300	10	12	65	95	1.6	1.8	20	2.1	280	2.6	1200	1200	355	15	19	200	75
	2nd 6 months					62	1300	10	11	65	95	1.6	1.7	20	2.1	260	2.6	1200	1200	340	15	19	200	75

[1]From: National Research Council: *Recommended Dietary Allowances,* 10th ed. National Academy of Sciences, 1989.

Table 29–4. Essential macrominerals: Summary of major characteristics.[1]

Elements	Functions	Deficiency Disease or Symptoms	Toxicity Disease or Symptoms[2]
Calcium	Constituent of bones, teeth; regulation of nerve, muscle function.	Children: rickets. Adults: osteomalacia. May contribute to osteoporosis.	Occurs with excess absorption due to hypervitaminosis D or hypercalcemia due to hyperparathyroidism or other causes of hypercalcemia.
Phosphorus	Constituent of bones, teeth, ATP, phosphorylated metabolic intermediates. Nucleic acids.	Children: rickets. Adults: osteomalacia.	Low serum Ca^{2+}:P_i ratio stimulates secondary hyperparathyroidism; may lead to bone loss.
Sodium	Principal cation in extracellular fluid. Regulates plasma volume, acid-base balance, nerve and muscle function, Na^+-K^+ ATPase.	Unknown on normal diet, secondary to injury or illness.	Hypertension (in susceptible individuals).
Potassium	Principal cation in intracellular fluid; nerve and muscle function, Na^+-K^+ ATPase.	Occurs secondary to illness, injury, or diuretic therapy; muscular weakness, paralysis, mental confusion.	Cardiac arrest, small bowel ulcers.
Chloride	Fluid and electrolyte balance; gastric fluid.	Infants fed salt-free formula. Secondary to vomiting, diuretic therapy, renal disease.	Cardiac arrest, small bowel ulcers.
Magnesium	Constituent of bones, teeth; enzyme cofactor (kinases, etc).	Secondary to malabsorption or diarrhea, alcoholism.	Depressed deep tendon reflexes and respiration.

[1]Modified from Murray RK et al: *Harper's Biochemistry,* 25th ed. Appleton & Lange, 1998.
[2]Excess mineral intake produces toxic symptoms. Unless otherwise specified, symptoms include nonspecific nausea, diarrhea, and irritability.

In the last 2 decades, numerous authorities have published dietary recommendations that address these issues. Although attention has been directed to the differences between these reports, most agree on the basic principles of eating a wide variety of foods; increasing the consumption of foods containing complex carbohydrates; reducing the intake of sugar, fat (particularly saturated fat), cholesterol, salt, and alcohol; and maintaining an ideal body weight.

A nutrition education guide, the "Food Guide Pyramid" (Figure 29–1), has been published by the USDA. The Pyramid emphasizes consumption of bread, cereal, rice, and pasta (six to eleven servings); vegetables (three to five servings); and fruit (two to four servings); lesser emphasis on milk, yogurt, and cheese (two or three servings) and meat, poultry, fish, dry beans, eggs, and nuts (two or three servings); and recommends that fats, oils, and sweets be used sparingly.

"Food guide pyramids" have also been developed recently for use with older individuals and with children.

[American Dietetic Association: Position of the American Dietetic Association: The Role of Nutrition in Health Promotion and Disease Prevention Programs] http://www.eatright.org. (Optimal nutrition and physical activity can promote health and reduce the risk of chronic disease.)

Bryant RJ et al: The new dietary reference intakes for calcium: implications for osteoporosis. J Am Coll Nutr 1999;18(5 Suppl):406S. [NLM Cit ID: 99439339] (The new Dietary Reference Intakes [DRI] recommend calcium intakes for adults of 1000–1200 mg/d. Most people do not consume these amounts of calcium.)

Liu S et al: Whole-grain consumption and risk of coronary heart disease: results from the Nurses' Health Study. Am J Clin Nutr 1999;70:412. [NLM Cit ID: 99409013] (Increased intake of whole grains may protect against coronary heart disease.)

Millward DJ: Optimal intakes of protein in the human diet. Proc Nutr Soc 1999;58:403. [NLM Cit ID: 99395678] (Risks of high intakes of protein in adults may be overestimated. There is evidence to support raising the safe upper limit to more than the current value of 1.5 g/kg/d.)

Rock CL: Dietary Reference Intakes, antioxidants, and beta-carotene. J Am Diet Assoc 1998;98:1410. [NLM Cit ID: 99065359] (Nutrient recommendations for antioxidants.)

Suitor CW et al: Dietary folate equivalents: interpretation and application. J Am Diet Assoc 2000;100:88. [NLM Cit ID: 20111479] (Dietary requirements for folate are expressed in dietary folate equivalents [DFEs]. DFEs account for the differences in absorption of naturally occurring food folate and the more bioavailable synthetic folic acid.)

Yates AA et al: Dietary Reference Intakes: The new basis for recommendations for calcium and related nutrients, B vitamins, and choline. J Am Diet Assoc 1998;98:699. [NLM Cit ID: 98291100] (DRIs are a new comprehensive approach to define nutrient intakes.)

ASSESSMENT OF NUTRITIONAL STATUS

No single biochemical test or clinical technique is sufficiently accurate to serve as a reliable test for malnutrition. Techniques of nutritional assessment

Table 29–5. Effect of drugs on nutrient absorption and metabolism.

Drug	Effect
Analgesics and anti-inflammatories	
Salicylates	Decrease serum ascorbic acid; increase urinary loss of ascorbic acid, potassium, and amino acids.
Sulfasalazine	Impairs folate absorption and antagonizes folate supplementation.
Antacids	
Aluminum antacids	Decrease absorption of phosphate and vitamin A.
H_2 blockers	Decrease iron and vitamin B_{12} absorption.
Octreotide acetate	Hypo- and hyperglycemia; decreases fat and carotene absorption.
Anticonvulsants	
Phenobarbital	Decreases serum folate; increases vitamin D and vitamin K turnover and may cause deficiency.
Phenytoin	Decreases serum folate; increases vitamin D and vitamin K turnover and may cause deficiency.
Primidone	Decreases serum folate and vitamins B_6 and B_{12}; decreases calcium absorption; increases vitamin D and vitamin K turnover and may cause anxiety.
Antimicrobials	
Neomycin	Binds bile acids. Decreases absorption of fat and carotene; of vitamins A, D, K, and B_{12}; and of potassium, sodium, calcium, and nitrogen.
Amphotericin B	Decreases serum magnesium and potassium.
Aminosalicylic acid	Increases absorption of folate, vitamin B_{12}, iron, cholesterol, and fat.
Chloramphenicol	Increases need for vitamins B_2, B_6, B_{12}; increases serum iron.
Penicillin	Hypokalemia; renal potassium wasting.
Tetracycline	Calcium, iron, magnesium inhibit drug absorption; decreases vitamin K synthesis.
Cycloserine	May decrease absorption of calcium, magnesium; may decrease serum folate and vitamins B_6 and B_{12}; decreases protein synthesis.
Isoniazid	Vitamin B_6 antagonist; may cause deficiency.
Sulfonamide	Decreases absorption of folate; decreases serum folate, iron.
Nitrofurantoin	Decreases serum folate.
Pyrimethamine	Decreases serum B_{12} and folate.
Antimitotics	
Methotrexate	Decreases activation of folate.
Colchicine	Decreases absorption of vitamin B_{12}, carotene, fat, sodium, potassium, cholesterol, lactose, nitrogen.
Cathartics	
Phenolphthalein	Malabsorption, hypokalemia; deficiency of vitamin D, calcium.
Mineral oil	Malabsorption; decreased absorption of vitamins A, D, K.
Diuretics	Some cause hypokalemia, hypomagnesemia; may increase urinary excretion of vitamins B_1 and B_6; calcium, magnesium, potassium.
Hypocholesterolemics	
Cholestyramine	Binds bile acids; decreases absorption of fat, carotene; vitamins A, D, K, and B_{12}; folate, iron.
Clofibrate	Decreases absorption of carotene, vitamin B_{12}, iron, glucose.
Hypotensives	
Hydralazine	Vitamin B_6 deficiency.
Captopril	May cause hyponatremia, hyperkalemia; decreases taste acuity.
Oral contraceptives	Vitamin B_6, folate deficiency; may increase the need for other nutrients.

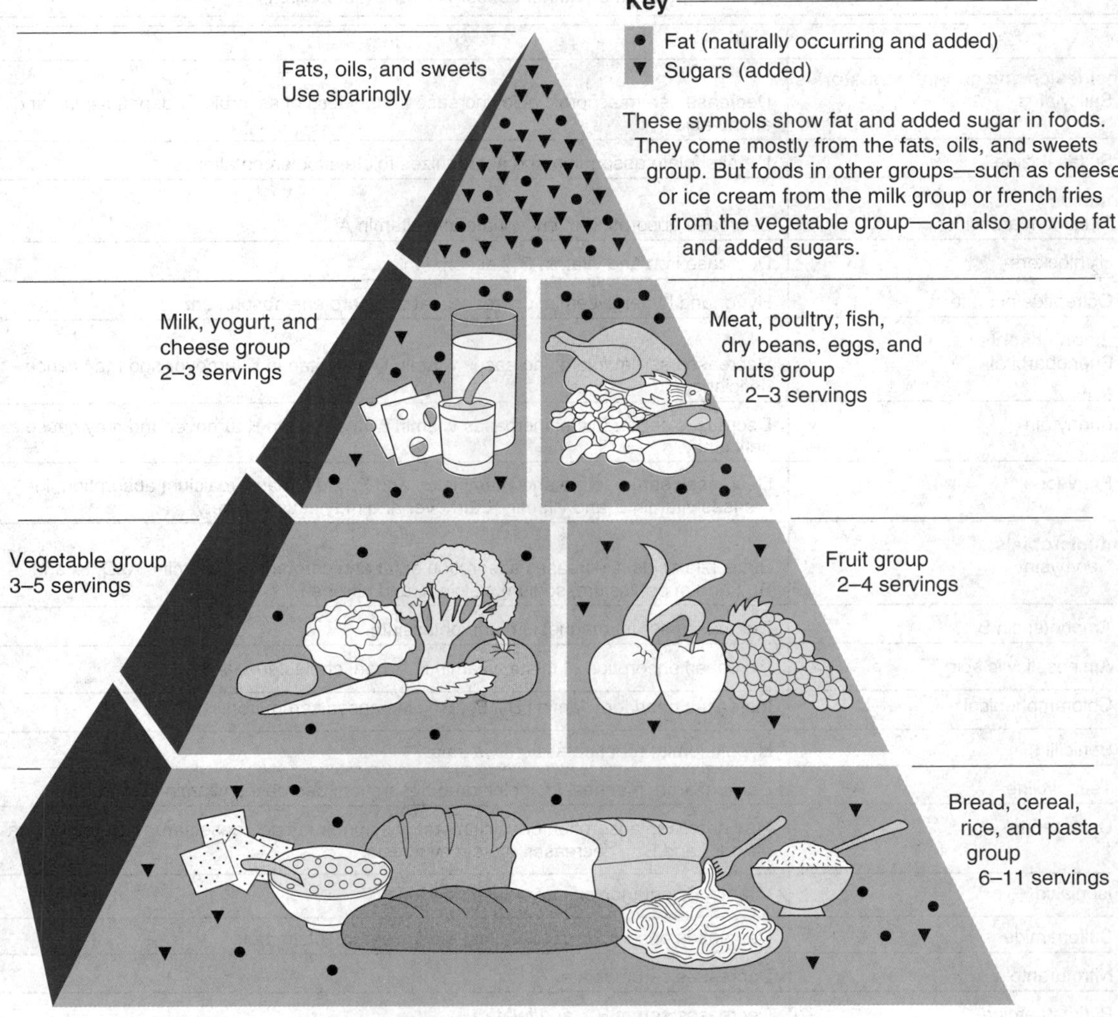

Key
Fat (naturally occurring and added)
Sugars (added)
These symbols show fat and added sugar in foods. They come mostly from the fats, oils, and sweets group. But foods in other groups—such as cheese or ice cream from the milk group or french fries from the vegetable group—can also provide fat and added sugars.
Fats, oils, and sweets
Use sparingly
Milk, yogurt, and cheese group
2–3 servings
Meat, poultry, fish, dry beans, eggs, and nuts group
2–3 servings
Vegetable group
3–5 servings
Fruit group
2–4 servings
Bread, cereal, rice, and pasta group
6–11 servings
Looking at the Pieces of the Pyramid
The Food Guide Pyramid emphasizes foods from the five major food groups shown in the three lower sections of the Pyramid. Each of these food groups provides some, but not all, of the nutrients you need. Foods in one group can't replace those in another. No one of these major food groups is more important than another—for good health, you need them all.

Figure 29–1. The Food Guide Pyramid. A guide to daily food choices.

utilize a combination of methods, including evaluation of dietary intake, anthropometric measurements, clinical examination, and laboratory tests.

DIETARY HISTORY

Patients undergoing a history and physical examination should be asked questions to help identify those high-risk patients who require further evaluation for malnutrition. Of particular importance are the regularity and availability of meals; who does the shopping and food preparation; recent changes in appetite, intake, or body weight; use of special diets or dietary supplements; use of alcohol, drugs, or medications; food preferences and food allergies; and the presence of illnesses affecting nutritional intakes, losses, or requirements. Elderly and adolescent patients, pregnant or lactating women, and the poor and socially isolated are at particular risk for nutritional problems.

Further quantification of dietary intake can be performed using a variety of techniques. **Twenty-four-hour diet recalls** provide rough estimates of nutrient intakes. Patients are asked to describe their dietary in-

What Counts as One Serving?

The amount of food that counts as one serving is listed below. If you eat a larger portion, count it as more than one serving. For example, a dinner portion of spaghetti would count as two or three servings of pasta.

Be sure to eat at least the lowest number of servings from the five major food groups listed below. You need them for the vitamins, minerals, carbohydrates, and protein they provide. Just try to pick the lowest fat choices from the food groups. No specific serving size is given for the fats, oils, and sweets group because the message is USE SPARINGLY.

Food groups

Milk, yogurt, and cheese

1 cup of milk or yogurt	1½ ounces of natural cheese	2 ounces of processed cheese

Meat, poultry, fish, dry beans, eggs, and nuts

2–3 ounces of cooked lean meat, poultry, or fish	½ cup of cooked dry beans, 1 egg, or 2 tablespoons of peanut butter count as 1 ounce of lean meat

Vegetable

1 cup of raw leafy vegetables	½ cup of other vegetables, cooked or chopped raw	¾ cup of vegetable juice

Fruit

1 medium apple, banana, orange	½ cup of chopped, cooked, or canned fruit	¾ cup of fruit juice

Bread, cereal, rice, and pasta

1 slice of bread	1 ounce of ready-to-eat cereal	½ cup of cooked cereal, rice, or pasta

How many servings do you need each day?

	Many women, older adults	Children, teenage girls, active women, most men	Teen-age boys, active men
Calorie level[1]	About 1600	About 2200	About 2800
Bread group servings	6	9	11
Vegetable group servings	3	4	5
Fruit group servings	2	3	4
Milk group servings	2–3[2]	2–3[2]	2–3[2]
Meat group servings	2, for a total of 5 ounces	2, for a total of 6 ounces	3, for a total of 7 ounces
Total fat (grams)	53	73	93

[1] These are the calorie levels if you choose low-fat, lean foods from the five major groups and use foods from the fats, oils, and sweets group sparingly.

[2] Women who are pregnant or breast feeding, teenagers, and young adults to age 24 need three servings.

Figure 29–1. (*continued*)

take over the preceding day, including snacks, beverages, and alcohol. Problems with this technique include inaccurate reporting, difficulties in estimating serving sizes, and the problem of generalizing from a single day's intake. More accurate information can be obtained by asking patients to complete a **3- to 5-day diet record.** Nutrient composition can then be analyzed with the aid of standard handbooks or computer software. Although prospective and less likely to be invalidated by memory lapses, omissions are still common as well as the usual difficulties in estimating serving sizes.

CLINICAL EXAMINATION

A nutritionally focused physical examination should be performed on each patient at risk for nutritional problems. The examination emphasizes muscle wasting, fat stores, volume status, and signs of micronutrient deficiencies (Table 29–6).

Evaluation of body weight is particularly useful. Body weight in relation to height can be assessed as the **relative weight,** the current weight/desirable weight (Table 29–7) × 100, or as the **body mass index weight** (in kilograms)/height (in meters)^2. In

Table 29–6. Clinical signs that may be due to nutrient deficiency.

Clinical Sign	Nutrient Deficiency	Clinical Sign	Nutrient Deficiency
Hair		**Neck**	
Transverse depigmentation	Protein, copper	Goiter	Iodine
Easily pluckable	Protein	**Chest**	
Sparse and thin	Protein, zinc, biotin	Thoracic rosary	Vitamin D
Skin		**Heart**	
Dry, scaling	Zinc, vitamin A, essential fatty acids	High-output failure	Thiamin
		Decreased output	Protein-calorie
Flaky paint dermatitis	Protein, niacin, riboflavin	**Abdomen**	
Follicular hyperkeratosis	Vitamins A and C	Hepatosplenomegaly	Protein-calorie
Perifollicular petechiae	Vitamin C	Distention	Protein-calorie
Petechiae, purpura	Vitamins C and K	Diarrhea	Niacin, folate, vitamin B_{12}
Pigmentation, desquamation	Niacin	**Extremities**	
		Muscle tenderness, pain	Thiamin, vitamin C
Nasolabial seborrhea	Niacin, riboflavin, pyridoxine	Muscle wasting	Protein-calorie
Pallor	Iron, folate, vitamin B_{12}, copper	Edema	Protein, thiamin
		Bone tenderness	Vitamin C, vitamin D, calcium, phosphorus
Scrotal/vulvar dermatoses	Riboflavin		
Subcutaneous fat loss	Calories	**Neurologic**	
Nails		Hyporeflexia	Thiamin
Spooning	Iron	Decreased position and vibratory sense	Vitamin B_{12}, thiamin
Transverse lines, ridging	Protein-calorie		
Head		Paresthesias	Vitamin B_{12}, thiamin, niacin
Temporal muscle wasting	Protein-calorie	Confabulation, disorientation	Thiamin
Parotid enlargement	Protein		
Eyes		Dementia	Niacin
Night blindness	Vitamin A, zinc	Ophthalmoplegia	Thiamin, phosphorus
Corneal vascularization	Riboflavin	Tetany	Calcium, magnesium
Xerosis, Bitot's spots, keratomalacia	Vitamin A	**Other**	
		Delayed wound healing	Zinc, protein-calorie, vitamin C
Conjunctival inflammation	Riboflavin		
Mouth			
Glossitis (scarlet, raw)	Niacin, pyridoxine, riboflavin, vitamin B_{12}, folate		
Bleeding gums	Vitamin C, riboflavin		
Cheilosis, angular stomatitis	Riboflavin		
Atrophic lingual papillae	Niacin, iron, riboflavin, folate, vitamin B_{12}		
Hypogeusia	Zinc, vitamin A		
Tongue fissuring	Niacin		

adult patients, however, a recent change in body weight is usually a better index of undernutrition than a low relative weight or a low body mass index. Changes in body weight are best expressed as a percentage of usual weight lost per unit of time. A loss of 10% or more of usual weight within a period of 1–2 months is generally considered to be predictive of a poor clinical outcome.

Evaluation of body composition—particularly fat stores and skeletal muscle—can be performed by visual inspection or, more quantitatively, by using **anthropometric measurements.** The most commonly used are the triceps skin fold, and mid arm muscle circumference. Because of individual variations and technical variations in measurement, it has limited clinical utility.

A number of more sophisticated techniques are available for assessment of body composition. Most have little role in patient care. These include bioelectrical impedance, dual energy x-ray absorptiometry, air-displacement plethysmography, hydrodensitometry, spectroscopy and mass spectrometry, neutron activation analysis, and MRI and body line scanners.

LABORATORY TESTS

Serum albumin is the most important laboratory test for the diagnosis of protein-calorie undernutrition. Most patients with severe protein depletion will have low serum albumin levels. Many nonnutritional conditions can also reduce serum albumin—particularly liver disease and severe illness in general. Other serum proteins with shorter half-lives (transferrin, transthyretin, etc) may reflect short-term changes in nutritional status but suffer from similar shortcomings.

Qualitative and quantitative tests of cellular immunity are also abnormal in many patients with protein-calorie undernutrition. Measurements of the **total**

Table 29–7. Body mass index chart.

	BODY MASS INDEX (kg/m²)																
	19	**20**	**21**	**22**	**23**	**24**	**25**	**26**	**27**	**28**	**29**	**30**	**31**	**32**	**33**	**34**	**35**
Height (inches)	**Body weight (pounds)**																
58	91	96	100	105	110	115	119	124	129	134	138	143	148	153	158	162	167
59	94	99	104	109	114	119	124	128	133	138	143	148	153	158	163	168	173
60	97	102	107	112	118	123	128	133	138	143	148	153	158	163	168	174	179
61	100	106	111	116	122	127	132	137	143	148	153	158	164	169	174	180	185
62	104	109	115	120	126	131	136	142	147	153	158	164	169	175	180	186	191
63	107	113	118	124	130	135	141	146	152	158	163	169	175	180	186	191	197
64	110	116	122	128	134	140	145	151	157	163	169	174	180	186	192	197	204
65	114	120	126	132	138	144	150	156	162	168	174	180	186	192	198	204	210
66	118	124	130	136	142	148	155	161	167	173	179	186	192	198	204	210	216
67	121	127	134	140	146	153	159	166	172	178	185	191	198	204	211	217	223
68	125	131	138	144	151	158	164	171	177	184	190	197	203	210	216	223	230
69	128	135	142	149	155	162	169	176	182	189	196	203	209	216	223	230	236
70	132	149	146	153	160	167	174	181	188	195	202	209	216	222	229	236	243
71	136	143	150	157	165	172	179	186	193	200	208	215	222	229	236	243	250
72	140	157	154	162	169	177	184	191	199	206	213	221	228	235	242	250	258
73	144	151	159	166	174	182	189	197	204	212	219	227	235	242	250	257	265
74	148	155	163	171	179	186	194	202	210	218	225	233	241	249	256	264	272
75	152	160	168	176	184	192	200	208	216	224	232	240	248	256	264	272	279
76	156	164	172	180	189	197	205	213	221	230	238	246	254	263	271	279	287

To use this table, find the appropriate height in the left-hand column. Move across to a given weight. The number at the top of the column is the BMI (in kg/m²) at that height and weight. Pounds have been rounded off. A normal BMI is 18.5–24.9 kg/m². Overweight is defined as a BMI of 25–29.9 kg/m². Class I obesity is 30–34.9 kg/m²; class II obesity is a BMI of 35–39.9 kg/m²; and class III (extreme) obesity is a BMI of > 40 kg/m².

lymphocyte count and **delayed hypersensitivity reactions** to common skin test antigens are nonspecific; abnormalities may be due to nonnutritional factors.

Despite their uncertain diagnostic utility, these tests are useful prognostically. Patients with abnormal nutritional assessment parameters have a markedly increased risk of poor clinical outcomes.

Despite the use of a nutritionally focused history, physical examination, and laboratory tests, it is often difficult to confirm a diagnosis of malnutrition. Monitoring dietary intakes during hospitalization is helpful. **Calorie counts** estimate energy and protein intakes for comparison with requirements.

Ahmad A et al: An evaluation of resting energy expenditure in hospitalized, severely underweight patients. Nutrition 1999;15:384. [NLM Cit ID: 99281983] (Commonly employed formulas routinely underestimate the energy needs of severely underweight [< 50 kg] patients. An empirical calculation using 30–32 kcal/kg can be used when direct measurements are unavailable.)

Baxter JP: Problems of nutritional assessment in the acute setting. Proc Nutr Soc 1999;58:39. [NLM Cit ID: 99274806] (Twenty to 50 percent of hospitalized patients suffer from nutritional depletion, and there is failure to recognize its existence and significance. More emphasis must be placed in clinical medicine on identifying subjects who are at high risk of developing disease-related malnutrition.)

Beck AM et al: At which body mass index and degree of weight loss should hospitalized elderly patients be considered at nutritional risk? Clin Nutr 1998;17:195. [NLM Cit ID: 99223689] (BMI less than 24 kg/m² or any degree of weight loss should be used to identify elderly patients who may benefit from nutrition support.)

Edington J: Problems of nutritional assessment in the community. Proc Nutr Soc 1999;58:47. [NLM Cit ID: 99274807] (Nutritional screening tools have been developed for community use. Most are aimed at the elderly population, but others are available to assess nutritional risk in children with developmental disabilities and in the general population.)

Elia M et al: New techniques in nutritional assessment: body composition methods. Proc Nutr Soc 1999;58:33. [NLM Cit ID: 99274805] (Several new techniques are improving the reproducibility and validity of body composition measurements.)

Jeejeebhoy KN: Nutritional assessment. Gastroenterol Clin North Am 1998;27:347. [NLM Cit ID: 98313707] (Nutritional assessment should be used to predict clinical outcomes.)

Niyongabo T et al: Comparison of methods for assessing nutritional status in HIV-infected adults. Nutrition 1999; 15:740. [NLM Cit ID: 99429393] (Subjective global assessment of nutritional status can serve as a basis for prescribing artificial nutrition, but assessment of body weight loss detects malnutrition at an earlier stage.)

Omran ML et al: Assessment of protein energy malnutrition in older persons, Part I: History, examination, body composition, and screening tools. Nutrition 2000;16:50.

[NLM Cit ID: 2013919] (The goal of nutrition assessment is to promote disease-free, active, and successful aging.)

Omran ML et al: Assessment of protein energy malnutrition in older persons, Part II: Laboratory evaluation. Nutrition 2000;16:131. [NLM Cit ID: 20161628] (Biochemical measurements are a useful part of nutritional assessment in the elderly.)

NUTRITIONAL DISORDERS

PROTEIN-ENERGY MALNUTRITION

Essentials of Diagnosis

- History of decreased intake of energy or protein, increased nutrient losses, or increased nutrient requirements.
- Manifestations range from weight loss and growth failure to distinct syndromes, kwashiorkor, and marasmus.
- In severe cases, virtually all organ systems affected.

General Considerations

Protein-energy malnutrition occurs as a result of a relative or absolute deficiency of energy and protein. It may be primary, due to inadequate food intake, or secondary, as a result of other illness. For most developing nations, primary protein-energy malnutrition remains among the most significant health problems. Protein-energy malnutrition has been described as two distinct syndromes. **Kwashiorkor,** caused by a deficiency of protein in the presence of adequate energy, is typically seen in weaning infants at the birth of a sibling in areas where foods containing protein are insufficiently abundant. **Marasmus,** caused by combined protein and energy deficiency, is most commonly seen where adequate quantities of food are not available.

In industrialized societies, protein-energy malnutrition is most often secondary to other diseases. **Kwashiorkor-like secondary protein-energy malnutrition** occurs primarily in association with hypermetabolic acute illnesses such as trauma, burns, and sepsis. **Marasmus-like secondary protein-energy malnutrition** typically results from chronic diseases such as COPD, congestive heart failure, cancer, or AIDS. These syndromes have been estimated to be present in at least 20% of hospitalized patients. A substantially greater number of patients have risk factors that could result in these syndromes but remain unrecognized and are not prevented. In both syndromes, protein-energy malnutrition is caused either by decreased intake of energy and protein, increased nutrient losses, or increased nutrient requirements dictated by the underlying illness. For example, diminished oral intake may result from poor dentition or various gastrointestinal disorders. Loss of nutrients results from malabsorption and diarrhea as well as from glycosuria. Requirements are increased by fever, surgery, neoplasia, and burns.

Pathophysiology

Protein-energy malnutrition results in pathophysiologic changes affecting every organ system. The most obvious results are loss of body weight, adipose stores, and skeletal muscle mass. Weight losses of 5–10% are usually tolerated without loss of physiologic function; losses of 35–40% of body weight usually result in death. Loss of protein from skeletal muscle and internal organs is usually proportionate to weight loss. Protein mass is lost from the liver, gastrointestinal tract, kidneys, and heart.

As protein-energy malnutrition progresses, organ dysfunction develops. Hepatic synthesis of serum proteins decreases, and depressed levels of circulating proteins are observed. Cardiac output and contractility are decreased, and the ECG may show decreased voltage and a rightward axis shift. Autopsies of patients who die with severe undernutrition show myofibrillar atrophy and interstitial edema of the heart.

The lungs are affected primarily by weakness and atrophy of the muscles of respiration. Vital capacity and tidal volume are depressed, and mucociliary clearance is abnormal. The gastrointestinal tract is most importantly affected by mucosal atrophy and loss of villi of small intestine, resulting in malabsorption. Intestinal disaccharidase deficiency and mild pancreatic insufficiency also contribute.

Changes in immunologic function are among the most important changes seen in protein-calorie undernutrition. T lymphocyte number and function are depressed. Changes in B cell function are more variable. Impaired complement activity, granulocyte function, and anatomic barriers to infection are noted, and wound healing is poor.

Clinical Findings

The clinical manifestations of protein-energy malnutrition range from mild growth failure and weight loss to a number of distinct clinical syndromes. Children in the developing world manifest marasmus and kwashiorkor. In secondary protein-energy malnutrition as seen in industrialized nations, clinical manifestations are affected by the degree of protein and energy deficiency, the underlying illness that resulted in the deficiency, and the patient's nutritional status prior to illness.

In marasmus-like secondary protein-energy malnutrition, most patients typically develop progressive wasting that begins with weight loss and proceeds to more severe cachexia. In the most severe form of this disorder, virtually all body fat stores disappear and muscle mass decreases, most noticeably in the temporalis and interosseus muscles. Laboratory studies may be unremarkable—serum albumin, for example, may be normal or slightly decreased, rarely decreasing to < 2.8 g/dL. In contrast, owing to its rapidity of onset, kwashiorkor-like secondary protein-energy malnutrition may develop in patients with normal subcutaneous fat and muscle mass or, if the patient is obese, in patients with excess fat and muscle. The serum protein level, however, typically declines and the serum albumin is often < 2.8 g/dL. Dependent edema, ascites, or anasarca may develop. As with primary protein-energy malnutrition, combinations of the marasmus-like and kwashiorkor-like syndromes can occur simultaneously, typically in patients with progressive chronic disease who develop a superimposed acute illness.

Treatment

The treatment of severe protein-energy malnutrition is a slow process requiring great care. Initial efforts should be directed at correcting fluid and electrolyte abnormalities and infections. Of particular concern is depletion of potassium, magnesium, and calcium in addition to acid-base abnormalities. The second phase of treatment is directed at repletion of protein, energy, and micronutrients. Treatment is started with modest quantities of protein and calories calculated according to the patient's actual body weight. Adult patients are given 1 g of protein and 30 kcal per kilogram. Concomitant administration of vitamins and minerals is obligatory. Either the enteral or parenteral route can be used, although the former is preferable. Enteral fat and lactose are withheld initially. Patients with less severe protein-calorie undernutrition can be given calories and protein simultaneously with the correction of fluid and electrolyte abnormalities. Similar quantities of protein and calories are recommended for initial treatment.

Patients treated for protein-energy malnutrition require close follow-up. Both calories and protein are advanced as tolerated, adults to 1.5 g/kg/d of protein and 40 kcal/kg/d of calories.

Patients who are refed too rapidly develop a number of untoward clinical sequelae. During refeeding, circulating potassium, magnesium, phosphorus, and glucose move intracellularly and can result in low serum levels of each. The administration of water and sodium with carbohydrate refeeding overloads hearts with depressed cardiac function and results in congestive heart failure. Enteral refeeding leads to malabsorption and diarrhea due to abnormalities in the gastrointestinal tract.

Refeeding edema is a benign condition to be differentiated from congestive heart failure. Changes in renal sodium reabsorption and poor skin and blood vessel integrity result in the development of dependent edema without other signs of heart disease. Treatment includes reassurance, elevation of the dependent area, and modest sodium restriction. Diuretics are usually ineffective, may aggravate electrolyte deficiencies, and should not be used.

The prevention and early detection of protein-energy malnutrition in hospitalized patients require awareness of the possibility by caregivers. Patients at risk require formal assessment of nutritional status and close observation of dietary intake, body weight, and nutritional requirements during the hospital stay.

Chandra RK: Nutrition and immunology: from the clinic to cellular biology and back again. Proc Nutr Soc 1999;58:681. [NLM Cit ID: 20071870] (The interactions between nutrition and the immune system are of clinical, practical, and public health importance.)

Herselman M et al: Protein-energy malnutrition as a risk factor for increased morbidity in long-term hemodialysis patients. J Ren Nutr 2000;10:7. [NLM Cit ID: 20138715] (Protein-energy malnutrition contributes to morbidity in hemodialysis patients, possibly via an effect on the immune system and infection.)

Koretz RL: Does nutritional intervention in protein-energy malnutrition improve morbidity or mortality? J Ren Nutr 1999;9:119. [NLM Cit ID: 99362929] (There is still need for large randomized controlled trials to establish or refute the efficacy of nutritional support in renal disease.)

Sullivan DH et al: Protein-energy undernutrition among elderly hospitalized patients: a prospective study. JAMA 1999;281:2013. [NLM Cit ID: 99285923] (Many hospitalized elderly patients were maintained on nutrient intakes far less than their estimated maintenance energy requirements, which may contribute to an increased risk of mortality.)

OBESITY

Essentials of Diagnosis

- Excess adipose tissue, resulting in body mass index > 30 kg/m^2.
- Upper body obesity (abdomen and flank) of greater health consequence than lower body obesity (buttocks and thighs).
- Associated with multiple metabolic and structural disorders.

General Considerations

Obesity is one of the most common disorders in medical practice and among the most frustrating and difficult to manage. Little progress has been made in treatment, yet major changes have occurred in our understanding of its causes and its implications for health.

Definition & Measurement

Obesity is defined as an excess of adipose tissue. Accurate quantification of body fat requires sophisticated techniques not usually available in clinical practice. Physical examination is usually sufficient to detect excess body fat. Two methods commonly used

Several medications remain available for treatment of obesity. Older catecholaminergic medications (eg, phentermine, diethyproprion, mazindol) are approved for short-term use only and have limited utility. **Sibutramine,** typically at doses of 10 mg/d, results in average weight losses of 5–10 kg in 6-month studies. Sibutramine also appears to improve 1-year outcomes in patients on very low-calorie diets. Side effects include dry mouth, anorexia, constipation, insomnia, and dizziness. In some patients (< 5%), sibutramine may substantially increase blood pressure.

Orlistat is the first approved medication for obesity that works in the gastrointestinal tract rather than the central nervous system. By inhibiting intestinal lipase, orlistat reduces fat absorption. As expected, orlistat may result in diarrhea, gas, and cramping and perhaps also reduced absorption of fat-soluble vitamins. In randomized trials with up to 2 years of follow-up, orlistat has resulted in 2–4 kg greater weight loss than placebo. The recommended dose of orlistat is 120 mg three times daily with meals.

No studies have been published using combinations of sibutramine and orlistat, but their distinct mechanisms of action make such combinations theoretically feasible.

Despite FDA approval of sibutramine and orlistat and NIH guidelines supporting their use, long-term clinical benefits have not been demonstrated. Although these medications result in some additional weight loss at the end of 1- and 2-year clinical trials and, in some studies, improved obesity-related metabolic parameters, the impact of these medications on obesity-related clinical outcomes is unknown.

Although surgery is the last resort for treatment of obesity, large numbers of patients have had bariatric surgery. In the United States, gastric operations are considered the procedures of choice. Most popular are the vertical banded gastroplasty (VBG) and roux-en-Y gastric bypass (GBP). In some centers, these procedures can be done laparoscopically. Both operations lead to substantial amounts of weight loss—close to 50% of initial body weight in some studies. Direct comparisons of the two operations suggest that GBP is the more effective procedure. Complications occur in up to 50% of subjects undergoing both operations and include peritonitis due to anastomotic leak, abdominal wall hernias, staple line disruption, gallstones, neuropathy, marginal ulcers, stomal stenosis, wound infections, thromboembolic disease, and various nutritional deficiencies and gastrointestinal symptoms. Within 30-day operative mortality rates are nil to 1%. NIH consensus panel recommendations are to limit obesity surgery to patients with BMIs over 40, or over 35 if obesity-related comorbidities are present. Many third-party payers now cover obesity surgery.

Apfelbaum M et al: Long-term maintenance of weight loss after a very-low-calorie diet: a randomized blinded trial of the efficacy and tolerability of sibutramine. Am J Med 1999;106:179. [NLM Cit ID: 99245778] (Seventy-five percent of subjects treated with sibutramine maintained at least 100% of the weight loss achieved with a very-low-calorie diet, compared with 42% in the placebo group.)

Bach DS et al: Absence of cardiac valve dysfunction in obese patients treated with sibutramine. Obes Res 1999;7:363. [NLM Cit ID: 99367204] (In a controlled study of 210 patients, there was no increase in cardiac valve dysfunction with sibutramine.)

Comuzzie AG et al: The search for human obesity genes. Science 1998;280:1374. [NLM Cit ID: 98267295] (Numerous candidate genes for human obesity have been identified, but only a very small number of humans have been found with single-gene mutations. Obesity develops from the interactions of multiple genes, environmental factors, and behavior.)

Davidson MH et al: Weight control and risk factor reduction in obese subjects treated for 2 years with orlistat: A randomized controlled trial. JAMA 1999;281:235. [NLM Cit ID: 99115037] (After 2 years of treatment, orlistat 120 mg three times per day resulted in modest weight loss compared with placebo.)

Devereux RB: Appetite suppressants and valvular heart disease. N Engl J Med 1998;339:765. [NLM Cit ID: 98391453] (Although appetite suppressant medications are clearly associated with valvular heart disease, the risk is less than initially feared.)

Executive summary of the clinical guidelines on the identification, evaluation, and treatment of overweight and obesity in adults. Arch Intern Med 1998;158:1855. [NLM Cit ID: 98430481] (Comprehensive evidence-based review of diagnosis and treatment of obesity from the NIH.)

Hansen DL et al: The effect of sibutramine on energy expenditure and appetite during chronic treatment without dietary restriction. Int J Obes Relat Metab Disord 1999;23:1016. [NLM Cit ID: 20025770] (The weight-reducing effect of sibutramine in humans is caused by a dual mechanism: reduction of energy intake by increasing satiety and decreasing hunger, and prevention of the decline in energy expenditure that follows weight loss.)

Hauptman J et al: Orlistat in the long-term treatment of obesity in primary care settings. Arch Fam Med 2000;9:160. [NLM Cit ID: 20155401] (Orlistat was associated with a 4-kg greater weight loss than placebo.)

Heymsfield SB et al: Recombinant leptin for weight loss in obese and lean adults: a randomized, controlled, dose-escalation trial. JAMA 1999;282:1568. [NLM Cit ID: 20012188] (Leptin injections induced weight loss in some obese subjects with elevated endogenous serum leptin concentrations.)

Jakicic JM et al: Effects of intermittent exercise and use of home exercise equipment on adherence, weight loss, and fitness in overweight women: a randomized trial. JAMA 1999;282:1554. [NLM Cit ID: 20012186] (A dose-response relationship exists between amount of exercise and long-term weight loss in overweight adult women.)

JAMA patient page: Weight management. JAMA 1999; 281:296. [NLM Cit ID: 99115047]

Nguyen NT et al: Laparoscopic roux-en-Y gastric bypass for super/super obesity. Obes Surg 1999;9:403. [NLM Cit ID: 99412132] (Roux-en-Y gastric bypass is increasingly done using a laparoscopic technique.)

Rossner S et al: Weight loss, weight maintenance, and improved cardiovascular risk factors after 2 years treatment with orlistat for obesity. European Orlistat Study Group. Obes Res 2000;8:49. [NLM Cit ID: 20141727] (Orlistat-treated patients lost more weight than placebo-treated patients [6.6% versus 9.7% of initial weight] and regained less weight at 2-year follow-up.)

Sharma L et al: The mechanism of the effect of obesity in knee osteoarthritis: the mediating role of malalignment. Arthritis Rheum 2000;43:568. [NLM Cit ID: 20191094] (Obesity was related to osteoarthritis severity in those with varus knee deformities but not in those with valgus knee deformities.)

Shively BK et al: Prevalence and determinants of valvulopathy in patients treated with dexfenfluramine. Circulation 1999;100:2161. [NLM Cit ID: 20040181] (The prevalence of valvular dysfunction with dexfenfluramine is less than initial estimates. Valvulopathy may regress after discontinuation of the drug.)

Stevens J et al: The effect of age on the association between body-mass index and mortality. N Engl J Med 1998; 338:1. [NLM Cit ID: 98069938] (Analysis of body weight and mortality. Although excess body weight increases the risk of death in adults, the risk is less than previously estimated and is no longer a factor in adults after age 75.)

Wei M et al: Relationship between low cardiorespiratory fitness and mortality in normal-weight, overweight, and obese men. JAMA 1999;282:1547. [NLM Cit ID: 20012185] (Fitness was an independent predictor of outcomes in obese subjects.)

EATING DISORDERS

ANOREXIA NERVOSA

Essentials of Diagnosis

- Disturbance of body image and intense fear of becoming fat.
- Weight loss leading to body weight 15% below expected.
- In females, absence of three consecutive menstrual cycles.

General Considerations

Anorexia nervosa begins in the years between adolescence and young adulthood. Ninety percent of patients are females, most from the middle and upper socioeconomic strata. The diagnosis is based on weight loss leading to body weight 15% below expected, a distorted body image, fear of weight gain or of loss of control over food intake, and, in females, the absence of at least three consecutive menstrual cycles. Other medical or psychiatric illnesses that can account for anorexia and weight loss must be excluded.

The prevalence of anorexia nervosa is greater than previously suggested. In Rochester, Minnesota, for example, the prevalence per 100,000 population is estimated to be 270 for females and 22 for males. Many other adolescent girls have features of the disorder without the severe weight loss.

The cause of anorexia nervosa is not known. Although multiple endocrinologic abnormalities exist in these patients, most authorities believe they are secondary to malnutrition and not primary disorders. Most authors favor a primary psychiatric origin, but no hypothesis explains all cases. The patient characteristically comes from a family whose members are highly goal- and achievement-oriented. Interpersonal relationships may be inadequate or destructive. The parents are usually overly directive and concerned with slimness and physical fitness, and much of the family conversation centers around dietary matters. One theory holds that the patient's refusal to eat is an attempt to regain control of her body in defiance of parental control. The patient's unwillingness to inhabit an "adult body" may also represent a rejection of adult responsibilities and the implications of adult interpersonal relationships. Patients are commonly perfectionistic in behavior and exhibit obsessional personality characteristics. Marked depression or anxiety may be present.

Clinical Findings

A. Symptoms and Signs: Clinically, patients with anorexia nervosa may exhibit severe emaciation and may complain of cold intolerance or constipation. Amenorrhea is almost always present. Bradycardia, hypotension, and hypothermia may be present in severe cases. Examination demonstrates loss of body fat, dry and scaly skin, and increased lanugo body hair. Parotid enlargement and edema may also be present.

B. Laboratory Findings: Laboratory findings are variable but may include anemia, leukopenia, electrolyte abnormalities, and elevations of BUN and serum creatinine. Serum cholesterol levels are often increased. Endocrine abnormalities include depressed levels of luteinizing and follicle-stimulating hormones and impaired response of LH to luteinizing hormone-releasing hormone.

Diagnosis & Differential Diagnosis

The diagnosis can be difficult, since many common social and cultural factors promote and maintain anorexic behavior. It depends upon identification of the common behavioral features and exclusion of medical disorders that would account for weight loss.

Behavioral features required for the diagnosis include intense fear of becoming obese, disturbance of body image, weight loss of at least 25%, and refusal to exceed a minimal normal weight.

The differential diagnosis includes endocrine and metabolic disorders such as panhypopituitarism, Addison's disease, hyperthyroidism, and diabetes mellitus; gastrointestinal disorders such as Crohn's disease and celiac sprue; chronic infections and cancers such as tuberculosis and lymphoma; and rare central nervous system disorders such as hypothalamic tumors.

Treatment

The goal of treatment is restoration of normal body weight and resolution of psychologic difficulties. Hospitalization may be necessary. Treatment programs conducted by experienced teams are successful in about two-thirds of cases, restoring normal weight and menstruation. One-half continue to experience difficulties with eating behavior and psychiatric problems. Occasional patients with anorexia develop obesity after treatment. Two to 6% of patients die from the complications of the disorder or commit suicide.

Various treatment methods have been used without clear evidence of superiority of one over another. Supportive care by physicians and nurses is probably the most important feature of therapy. Structured behavioral therapy, intensive psychotherapy, and family therapy may be tried. A variety of medications including tricyclic antidepressants, selective serotonin reuptake inhibitors, and lithium carbonate are effective in some cases. Patients with severe malnutrition must be hemodynamically stabilized and may require enteral or parenteral feeding. Forced feedings should be reserved for life-threatening situations, since the goal of treatment is to reestablish normal eating behavior.

[American Dietetic Association: Position of the American Dietetic Association: Nutrition intervention in the treatment of anorexia nervosa, bulimia nervosa, and binge eating]

http://www.eatright.org/aanorexiainter.html (Nutrition education and interventions should be integrated into the team treatment of patients with anorexia nervosa and other eating disorders.)

Becker AE et al: Eating disorders. N Engl J Med 1999;340:1092. [NLM Cit ID: 99192007] (Patients with eating disorders should be evaluated and treated for medical complications of the disease at the same time that psychotherapy and nutritional counseling are undertaken. Pharmacologic agents are often useful as adjuncts to psychotherapy for bulimia nervosa or binge-eating disorder; in anorexia nervosa, medication is generally reserved for patients with concurrent psychiatric illness.)

Kaye WH: Anorexia nervosa, obsessional behavior, and serotonin. Psychopharmacol Bull 1997;33:335. [NLM Cit ID: 98212233] (Recent data suggest that SSRI-type medication improves outcomes and prevents relapse in patients with anorexia nervosa.)

Kreipe RE et al: Eating disorders in adolescents and young adults. Obstet Gynecol Clin North Am 2000;27:101. [NLM Cit ID: 20157574] (Eating disorders frequently result in gynecologic disorders.)

Pike KM: Long-term course of anorexia nervosa: response, relapse, remission, and recovery. Clin Psych Rev 1998;18:447. [NLM Cit ID: 98302213] (Review of long term outcomes of anorexia and current treatment options.)

Practice guideline for the treatment of patients with eating disorders (revision). American Psychiatric Association Work Group on Eating Disorders. Am J Psychiatry 2000;157(Suppl 1):1. [NLM Cit ID: 20107394]

BULIMIA NERVOSA

Essentials of Diagnosis

- Uncontrolled episodes of binge eating.
- Recurrent inappropriate compensation to prevent weight gain such as self-induced vomiting, laxatives, diuretics, fasting, or excessive exercise.
- A minimum average of two binge eating episodes a week for at least 3 months.
- Overconcern with weight and body shape.

General Considerations

Bulimia nervosa is the episodic uncontrolled ingestion of large quantities of food followed by recurrent inappropriate compensatory behavior in order to prevent weight gain such as self-induced vomiting, diuretics or cathartics, or strict dieting or vigorous exercise.

Like anorexia nervosa, bulimia nervosa is predominantly a disorder of young, white middle- and upper-class women. It is more difficult to detect than anorexia, and some studies have estimated that the prevalence may be as high as 19% in college-age women.

Patients with bulimia nervosa typically consume large quantities of easily ingested high-calorie foods, usually in secrecy. Some patients may have several such episodes a day for a few days; others report regular and persistent patterns of binge eating. Binging is usually followed by vomiting, cathartics, or diuretics and is usually accompanied by feelings of guilt or depression. Periods of binging may be followed by intervals of self-imposed starvation. Body weights may fluctuate but generally are within 20% of desirable weights.

Some patients with bulimia nervosa also have a cryptic form of anorexia nervosa with significant weight loss and amenorrhea. Family and psychologic issues are generally similar to those encountered among patients with anorexia nervosa. Bulimics, however, have a higher incidence of premorbid obesity, greater use of cathartics and diuretics, and more impulsive or antisocial behavior. Menstruation is usually preserved.

Medical complications are numerous. Gastric dilatation and pancreatitis have been reported after binges. Vomiting can result in poor dentition, pharyngitis, esophagitis, aspiration, and electrolyte abnormalities. Cathartic and diuretic abuse also cause electrolyte abnormalities or dehydration. Constipation and hemorrhoids are common.

Treatment of bulimia and bulimarexia requires supportive care and psychotherapy. Individual, group, family, and behavioral therapy have all been utilized. Antidepressants may be helpful. The best results have been with fluoxetine hydrochloride and other selective serotonin reuptake inhibitors. Although death from bulimia is rare, the long-term psychiatric prognosis in severe bulimia is worse than that in anorexia nervosa.

Bulik CM et al: Predictors of 1-year treatment outcome in bulimia nervosa. Compr Psychiatry 1998;39:206. [NLM Cit ID: 98340105] (A history of obesity, the presence of depression, and several personality factors were predictive of poor treatment outcomes.)

Fitzgibbon ML et al: Binge eating disorder and bulimia nervosa: differences in the quality and quantity of binge eating episodes. Int J Eat Disord 2000;27:238. [NLM Cit ID: 2012578] (Patients with binge eating disorder have as many binges as patients with bulimia nervosa, but patients with binge eating disorder do not purge and are more likely to be obese.)

Mcgilley BM et al: Assessment and treatment of bulimia nervosa. Am Fam Physician 1998;57:2743. [NLM Cit ID: 98299966]

Sullivan PF et al: The epidemiology and classification of bulimia nervosa. Psychol Med 1998;28:599. [NLM Cit ID: 98290018] (*DSM-IV* criteria may underestimate the spectrum of bulimic behaviors in the population.)

DISORDERS OF VITAMIN METABOLISM

Deficiencies of single vitamins are less often encountered than those of multiple vitamins along with protein-calorie undernutrition. Although any cause of protein-calorie undernutrition can result in concurrent vitamin deficiency, most such instances are associated with malabsorption, alcoholism, medications hemodialysis, total parenteral nutrition, food faddism, or inborn errors of metabolism.

Vitamin deficiency syndromes develop gradually Symptoms are commonly nonspecific, and the physical examination is rarely helpful in early diagnosis Most characteristic physical findings are seen late in the course of the syndrome. Other characteristic physical findings, such as glossitis and cheilosis, are seen with deficiencies of many B vitamins. Such abnormalities suggest the presence of a nutritional deficiency but do not indicate which nutrient is deficient.

Despite the relative ease of meeting the recommended daily allowances with a mixed diet, many adults in the USA take vitamin supplements. In fact, syndromes of vitamin excess may be more common than deficiency syndromes, particularly those due to excess of vitamins A, D, and B_6. Most claims for significant health benefits of such supplements, particularly those taken in megadoses, remain unsubstantiated.

Some vitamins can be used efficaciously as drugs. Derivatives of vitamin A are used to treat cystic acne and, more recently, skin wrinkles. Niacin is an effective medication for hyperlipidemia. Vitamin-responsive inborn errors of metabolism also commonly require pharmacologic doses of vitamins.

WATER-SOLUBLE VITAMINS

1. THIAMIN (B_1)

The primary role of thiamin is as precursor of thiamin pyrophosphate, a coenzyme required for several important biochemical reactions necessary for carbohydrate oxidation. Thiamin is also thought to have an independent role in nerve conduction in peripheral nerves. The recommended daily allowances of thiamin are listed in Table 29–1.

Thiamin Deficiency

A. Clinical Findings: Most thiamin deficiency in the USA is due to alcoholism. Chronic alcoholics may have poor dietary intakes of thiamin and impaired thiamin absorption, metabolism, and storage. Thiamin deficiency is also associated with malabsorption, dialysis, and other causes of chronic protein-calorie undernutrition. Thiamin deficiency can be precipitated in patients with marginal thiamin status with intravenous dextrose solutions.

Early manifestations of thiamin deficiency include anorexia, muscle cramps, paresthesias, and irritability. Advanced deficiency affects chiefly the cardiovascular system ("wet beriberi") or the nervous system ("dry beriberi"). Wet beriberi occurs if severe physical exertion and high carbohydrate intakes accompany thiamin deficiency, whereas dry beriberi is seen with inactivity and low-calorie intake.

Beriberi heart disease is characterized by marked peripheral vasodilation resulting in high-output heart failure with dyspnea, tachycardia, cardiomegaly, and pulmonary and peripheral edema, with warm extremities mimicking cellulitis.

Neurologic manifestations include both the peripheral and the central nervous systems. Peripheral nerve involvement is typically a symmetric motor and sensory neuropathy with pain, paresthesias, and loss of reflexes. The legs are affected more than the arms. Central nervous system involvement results in Wernicke-Korsakoff syndrome. Wernicke's encephalopathy consists of nystagmus progressing to ophthalmoplegia, truncal ataxia, and confusion. Korsakoff's syndrome includes amnesia, confabulation, and impaired learning.

6. VITAMIN C (Ascorbic Acid)

Vitamin C is a potent antioxidant involved in many oxidation-reduction reactions and is also required for the synthesis of collagen. It increases the absorption of nonheme iron and is involved in tyrosine metabolism, wound healing, and drug metabolism. With the exception of collagen synthesis, the mechanism of action for these functions is poorly understood. The recommended daily allowances of vitamin C are listed in Table 29–1; major food sources are fresh fruits and vegetables.

Vitamin C Deficiency

A. Clinical Findings: Most cases of vitamin C deficiency seen in the USA are due to dietary inadequacy in the urban poor, the elderly, and chronic alcoholics. Patients with chronic illnesses such as cancer and chronic renal failure and individuals who smoke cigarettes are also at risk.

Early manifestations of vitamin C deficiency are nonspecific and include malaise and weakness. In more advanced stages, the typical features of scurvy develop. Manifestations include perifollicular hemorrhages, perifollicular hyperkeratotic papules, petechiae and purpura, splinter hemorrhages, bleeding gums, hemarthroses, and subperiosteal hemorrhages. Periodontal signs do not occur in edentulous patients. Anemia is common, and wound healing is impaired. The late stages of scurvy are characterized by edema, oliguria, neuropathy, intracerebral hemorrhage, and death.

B. Diagnosis: The diagnosis of advanced scurvy can be made clinically on the basis of the skin lesions in the proper clinical situation. Atraumatic hemarthrosis is also highly suggestive. The diagnosis can be confirmed with decreased plasma ascorbic acid levels, typically below 0.1 mg/dL.

C. Treatment: Adult scurvy can be treated with 300–1000 mg of ascorbic acid per day. Improvement typically occurs within days. Some studies have suggested that high intakes of vitamin C are associated with a decreased risk of cancer. Vitamin C may also protect against coronary heart disease by modifying blood cholesterol levels and preventing LDL-cholesterol from oxidation. A decrease in all-cause and coronary heart disease mortality in individuals with high intakes (approximately 300–400 mg/d) has been reported.

Vitamin C Toxicity

Very large doses of vitamin C can have side effects. Most common are gastric irritation, flatulence, or diarrhea. Oxalate kidney stones are of theoretic concern because ascorbic acid is metabolized to oxalate, but stone formation has not been frequently reported. Vitamin C can also confound common diagnostic tests by causing false-negative tests for fecal occult blood and both false-negative and false-positive tests for urine glucose.

JAMA patient page: Vitamin C. JAMA 1999;281:1460. [NLM Cit ID: 99231414]

Johnston CS et al: People with marginal vitamin C status are at high risk of developing vitamin C deficiency. J Am Diet Assoc 1999;99:854. [NLM Cit ID: 99334158]

Levine M et al: Criteria and recommendations for vitamin C intake. JAMA 1999;281:1415. [NLM Cit ID: 99231410] (New evidence suggests the RDA for vitamin C, currently 60 mg/d, should be raised to 120 mg/d.)

Rimm EB et al: Antioxidants for vascular disease. Med Clin North Am 2000;84:239. [NLM Cit ID: 20149398] (The epidemiologic data do not support a role for vitamin C in reducing risk of coronary disease.)

FAT-SOLUBLE VITAMINS

1. VITAMIN A

Vitamin A (retinol) is a high-molecular-weight alcohol either ingested preformed or synthesized from plant carotenoids, particularly β-carotene. Isomers and derivatives of retinol are commonly called retinoids. Vitamin A is essential for normal retinal function and plays an important but still not fully understood role in cell growth and differentiation, particularly of epithelial cells. Vitamin A is also necessary for normal wound healing. The recommended daily allowances of vitamin A are listed in Table 29–1; the principal food sources are highly pigmented vegetables.

Because of its role in cell differentiation, vitamin A has been postulated to have a role in cancer prevention. The role of retinoids for chemoprevention of cancer is under intense investigation. The provitamin β-carotene may play an even more important role in prevention of cancer and heart disease by virtue of its antioxidant activity.

Vitamin A Deficiency

A. Clinical Findings: Vitamin A deficiency is one of the most common vitamin deficiency syndromes, particularly in developing countries. In many such regions, it is the most common cause of blindness. In the USA, vitamin A deficiency is usually due to fat malabsorption syndromes or mineral oil laxative abuse and occurs most commonly in the elderly and urban poor.

Night blindness is the earliest symptom. Dryness of the conjunctiva (xerosis) and the development of small white patches on the conjunctiva (Bitot's spots) are early signs. Ulceration and necrosis of the cornea (keratomalacia), perforation, endophthalmitis, and blindness are late manifestations. Xerosis and hyperkeratinization of the skin and loss of taste may also occur.

B. Diagnosis: Abnormalities of dark adaptation are strongly suggestive of vitamin A deficiency. Serum levels below the normal range of 30–65 mg/dL are commonly seen in advanced deficiency.

C. Treatment: Night blindness, poor wound healing, and other signs of early deficiency can be effectively treated with 30,000 IU of vitamin A daily for 1 week. Advanced deficiency with corneal damage calls for administration of 20,000 units/kg for at least 5 days. The potential antioxidant effects of β-carotene can be achieved with supplements of 25,000–50,000 IU of β-carotene.

Vitamin A Toxicity

Excess intake of β-carotenes (hypercarotenosis) results in staining of the skin a yellow-orange color but is otherwise benign. Skin changes are most marked on the palms and soles, while the scleras remain white, clearly distinguishing hypercarotenosis from jaundice. Large doses of β-carotene are otherwise safe.

Excessive vitamin A (hypervitaminosis A), on the other hand, can be quite toxic. Chronic toxicity usually occurs after ingestion of daily doses of over 50,000 units/d for more than 3 months. Early manifestations include dry, scaly skin, hair loss, mouth sores, painful hyperostoses, anorexia, and vomiting. Hypercalcemia may be noted. More serious findings include increased intracranial pressure, with papilledema, headaches, and decreased cognition; and hepatomegaly, occasionally progressing to cirrhosis. Acute toxicity can result from ingestion of massive doses of vitamin A, such as in drug overdoses or consumption of polar bear liver. Manifestations include nausea, vomiting, abdominal pain, headache, papilledema, and lethargy.

The diagnosis can be confirmed by elevations of serum vitamin A levels. The only treatment is withdrawal of vitamin A from the diet. Most symptoms and signs improve rapidly.

Dawson MI: The importance of vitamin A in nutrition. Curr Pharm Des 2000;6:311. [NLM Cit ID: 20105754] (Observational studies on vitamin A use and cancer prevention have produced mixed results.)

McLaren DS: Vitamin A deficiency disorders. J Indian Med Assoc 1999;97:320. [NLM Cit ID: 20107796]

2. VITAMIN D

Vitamin D is discussed in Chapter 26. The recommended daily allowances of vitamin D are listed in Table 29–1; a major food source is fortified milk, but sunlight on the skin is a prime resource as well.

LeBoff MS et al: Occult vitamin D deficiency in postmenopausal US women with acute hip fracture. JAMA 1999;281:1505. [NLM Cit ID: 99241859] (Postmenopausal community-living women who presented with hip fracture showed occult vitamin D deficiency.)

3. VITAMIN E

Vitamin E activity is derived from at least eight naturally occurring tocopherols, the most potent of which is α-tocopherol. Although the exact function and mechanism of action of vitamin E in humans are unclear, it is commonly thought to function as an antioxidant, protecting membranes and other cellular structures from attack by free radicals. Dietary selenium and other antioxidants work in conjunction with vitamin E and may partially spare its requirement and reverse signs of vitamin E deficiency in animals. The recommended daily allowances of vitamin E are listed in Table 29–1; the major food source is vegetable seed oil.

Vitamin E, like β-carotene and vitamin C, may also play a role in protection against cancer, coronary heart disease, and cataracts through its antioxidant function.

Vitamin E Deficiency

A. Clinical Findings: Clinical deficiency of vitamin E is most commonly due to severe malabsorption, the genetic disorder abetalipoproteinemia, or, in children with chronic cholestatic liver disease, biliary atresia or cystic fibrosis. Manifestations of deficiency include areflexia, disturbances of gait, decreased proprioception and vibration, and ophthalmoplegia.

B. Diagnosis: Plasma vitamin E levels can be measured; normal levels are 0.5–0.7 mg/dL or higher. Since vitamin E is normally transported in lipoproteins, the serum level should be interpreted in relation to circulating lipids.

C. Treatment: The optimum therapeutic dose of vitamin E has not been clearly defined. Large doses, often administered parenterally, can be used to improve the neurologic complications seen in abetalipoproteinemia and cholestatic liver disease. The potential antioxidant benefits of vitamin E can be achieved with supplements of 100–400 units/d.

Vitamin E Toxicity

Vitamin E is the least toxic of the fat-soluble vitamins. Large doses, 20–80 times the recommended daily requirement, have been taken for extended periods of time without apparent harm, although nausea, flatulence, and diarrhea have been reported. Large doses of vitamin E can increase the vitamin K requirement and can result in bleeding in patients taking oral anticoagulants.

Christen WG et al: Design of Physicians' Health Study II—a randomized trial of beta-carotene, vitamins E and C, and multivitamins, in prevention of cancer, cardiovascular disease, and eye disease, and review of results of completed trials. Ann Epidemiol 2000;10:125. [NLM Cit ID: 20152925] (A large clinical trial is under way to assess the balance of benefits and risks of vitamin E on cancer and cardiovascular disease.)

Grundman M: Vitamin E and Alzheimer disease: the basis for additional clinical trials. Am J Clin Nutr 2000;71:630S. [NLM Cit ID: 20142740] (A placebo-controlled clinical trial indicated that vitamin E may slow functional deterioration leading to nursing home placement. A new trial is planned to see if vitamin E can delay or prevent a clinical diagnosis of Alzheimer disease in elderly persons with mild cognitive impairment.)

Rimm EB et al: Antioxidants for vascular disease. Med Clin North Am 2000;84:239. [NLM Cit ID: 20149398] (Observational and experimental evidence consistently support an effect for vitamin E in reducing risk of coronary disease.)

4. VITAMIN K

Vitamin K is discussed in Chapter 13. The recommended daily allowances of vitamin K are listed in Table 29–1. It is synthesized by intestinal bacteria.

Booth SL et al: Vitamin K: a practical guide to the dietary management of patients on warfarin. Nutr Rev 1999; 57(9 Part 1):288. [NLM Cit ID: 20034336] (A constant dietary intake of vitamin K that meets current dietary recommendations of 65–80 μg/day is the most acceptable practice for patients on warfarin therapy.)

Rashid M et al: Prevalence of vitamin K deficiency in cystic fibrosis. Am J Clin Nutr 1999;70:378. [NLM Cit ID: 99409009] (Vitamin K deficiency is common in unsupplemented patients with cystic fibrosis and pancreatic insufficiency. Routine supplementation should be considered in all of these patients.)

Vatassery GT: Vitamin E and other endogenous antioxidants in the central nervous system. Geriatrics 1998; 53(Suppl 1):S25. [NLM Cit ID: 98418154] (Among the antioxidants, vitamin E has shown some promise in the treatment of Alzheimer's disease and cardiovascular disease.)

Yates AA et al: Dietary Reference Intakes: the new basis for recommendations for calcium and related nutrients, B vitamins, and choline. J Am Diet Assoc 1998;98:699. [NLM Cit ID: 98291100] (Dietary reference intakes [DRIs] represent the new approach adopted by the Food and Nutrition Board to providing quantitative estimates of nutrient intakes.)

DIET THERAPY

Specific therapeutic diets can be designed to facilitate the medical management of most common illnesses. In most cases, consultation with a registered dietitian is necessary in order to design and implement major dietary changes. Physicians should be familiar with the indications for special diets and their basic composition to facilitate patient referrals and to maximize patient compliance. Diet therapy is a difficult process, and not all patients are able to cooperate fully. Requesting the patient to record dietary intake for 3–5 days may provide useful insight into the patient's motivation.

Therapeutic diets can be divided into three groups: (1) diets that alter the consistency of food; (2) diets that restrict or otherwise modify dietary components; and (3) diets that supplement dietary components.

DIETS THAT ALTER CONSISTENCY

Clear Liquid Diet

This diet provides adequate water, 500–1000 kcal as simple sugar, and some electrolytes. It is fiber-free and requires minimal digestion or intestinal motility.

A clear liquid diet is useful for patients with resolving postoperative ileus, acute gastroenteritis, partial intestinal obstruction, and as preparation for diagnostic gastrointestinal procedures. It is commonly used as the first diet for patients who have been taking nothing by mouth for long periods. Because of the low calorie and minimal protein content of the clear liquid diet, it is used only for short periods.

Full Liquid Diet

The full liquid diet provides adequate water and can be designed to provide adequate calories and protein. Vitamins and minerals—especially folic acid, iron, and vitamin B_6—may be inadequate and should be provided in the form of supplements. Dairy products, soups, eggs, and soft cereals are used to supplement clear liquids. Commercial oral supplements can also be incorporated into the diet or used alone.

This diet is low in residue and can be used in many instances instead of the clear liquid diet described above—especially in patients with difficulty in chewing or swallowing, with partial obstructions, or in preparation for some diagnostic procedures. Full liquid diets are commonly used following clear liquid diets to advance diets in patients who have been taking nothing by mouth for long periods.

Soft Diets

Soft diets are designed for patients unable to chew or swallow hard or coarse food. Tender foods are used, and most raw fruits and vegetables and coarse breads and cereals are eliminated. Soft diets are commonly used to assist in progression from full liquid diets to regular diets in postoperative patients and patients who are too weak or those whose dentition is too poor to handle a general diet.

Mechanical soft diets include chopped, ground, and pureed foods as well as any foods patients are able to masticate. These diets are used for head and neck surgical patients, those with dental problems and esophageal strictures, and other patients who have difficulty with chewing or swallowing.

The soft diet can be designed to meet all nutritional requirements.

DIETS THAT RESTRICT NUTRIENTS

Diets can be designed to restrict (or eliminate) virtually any nutrient or food component. The most commonly used restricted diets are those that limit sodium, fat, and protein. Other restrictive diets include gluten restriction in sprue, potassium and phosphate reduction in renal insufficiency, and various elimination diets for food allergies.

Sodium-Restricted Diets

Low-sodium diets are useful in the management of hypertension and in conditions in which sodium retention and edema are prominent features, particularly congestive heart failure, chronic liver disease, and chronic renal failure. Sodium restriction is beneficial with or without diuretic therapy. When used in conjunction with diuretics, sodium restriction allows lower dosage of the diuretic medication and may prevent side effects. Potassium excretion, in particular, is directly related to distal renal tubule sodium delivery, and sodium restriction will decrease diuretic-related potassium losses.

Typical American diets contain a minimum of 4–6 g (175–260 meq) of sodium per day. A no-added-salt diet contains approximately 3 g of sodium (132 meq) per day. Further restriction can be achieved with sodium diets 2 g or 1 g per day. Diets with more severe restriction are poorly accepted by patients and are rarely used.

Dietary sodium includes sodium naturally occurring in foods, sodium added during food processing, and sodium added by the consumer during cooking and at the table. About a third of current dietary intake is derived from each. Diets that allow 2000 mg of sodium daily are easiest to design and implement. Such diets generally eliminate added salt, most processed foods, and selected foods with particularly high sodium content. Patients who follow such diets for 2–3 months lose their craving for salty foods and can often continue to restrict their sodium intake indefinitely. Many patients with mild hypertension will achieve significant reductions in blood pressure (approximately 5 mm Hg diastolic) with this degree of sodium restriction. Other patients require more severe sodium restriction (approximately 1000 mg of sodium per day) for reduction in blood pressure.

Diets allowing 1000 mg of sodium require further restriction of commonly eaten foods. Special "low-sodium" products are now available to facilitate such diets. These diets are difficult for most people to follow and are generally reserved for hospitalized patients and highly motivated outpatients—most commonly those with severe liver disease and ascites.

Fat-Restricted Diets

Traditional fat-restricted diets are useful in the treatment of fat malabsorption syndromes. Such diets will improve the symptoms of diarrhea with steatorrhea independently of the primary physiologic abnormality by limiting the quantity of fatty acids that reach the colon. The degree of fat restriction necessary to control symptoms must be individualized. Patients with severe malabsorption can be limited to 40–60 g of fat per day. Diets containing 60–80 g of fat per day can be designed for patients with less severe abnormalities.

In general, fat-restricted diets require broiling, baking, or boiling meat and fish; discarding the skin of poultry and fish and using those foods as the main protein source; using nonfat dairy products; and avoiding desserts, sauces, and gravies.

Low-Cholesterol, Low-Saturated-Fat Diets

Fat-restricted diets that specifically restrict saturated fats and dietary cholesterol are the mainstay of dietary treatment of hyperlipidemia (see Chapter 28). Similar diets are recommended also for diabetes (Chapter 27) and for the prevention of coronary artery disease (Chapter 10). Current recommendations for the prevention of cancer by dietary modification also include fat restriction.

The aim of these diets is to restrict total fat to 30% of calories and to achieve a normal body weight by caloric restriction. Saturated fat is restricted to 10% of calories and dietary cholesterol to 300 mg/d. Saturated fat can be replaced either with complex carbohydrates or, if energy balance permits, with monounsaturated fats. Saturated fat, total fat, and dietary cholesterol can be restricted further, but studies suggest that more extreme restriction offers little further advantage in overall modification of serum lipids.

Protein-Restricted Diets

Protein-restricted diets are most commonly used in patients with hepatic encephalopathy due to chronic liver disease and in patients with renal failure to ameliorate the progression of early disease and to decrease symptoms of uremia in more severe disease. Patients with selected inborn errors of amino acid metabolism and other abnormalities resulting in hyperammonemia also require restriction of protein or of specific amino acids.

Protein restriction is intended to limit the production of nitrogenous waste products. Energy intake must be adequate to facilitate the efficient use of dietary protein. Proteins must be of high biologic value and be provided in sufficient quantity to meet minimal requirements. For most patients, the diet should contain at least 0.6 g/kg/d of protein. Patients with encephalopathy who fail to respond to this degree of restriction are unlikely to respond to more severe restriction.

DIETS THAT SUPPLEMENT NUTRIENTS

High-Fiber Diet

Dietary fiber is a diverse group of plant constituents that are resistant to digestion by the human digestive tract. Typical American diets contain about 5–10 g of dietary fiber per day. Epidemiologic evidence has suggested that populations consuming greater quantities of fiber have a lower incidence of certain gastrointestinal disorders, including diverticulitis and colon cancer. Most authorities currently recommend higher intakes of dietary fiber for health maintenance.

Diets high in dietary fiber (20–35 g/d) are also commonly used in management of a variety of gastrointestinal disorders, particularly irritable bowel syndrome and recurrent diverticulitis. Diets high in fiber may also be useful to reduce blood sugar in patients with diabetes and to reduce cholesterol levels in patients with hypercholesterolemia. Such diets include greater intakes of fresh fruits and vegetables, whole grains, legumes and seeds, and bran products. For some patients, the addition of psyllium seed (2 tsp per day) or natural bran (½ cup per day) may be preferable.

High-Potassium Diets

Potassium-supplemented diets are used most commonly to compensate for potassium losses caused by diuretics. Although potassium losses can be partially prevented by using lower doses of diuretics, concurrent sodium restriction, and potassium-sparing diuretics, some patients require additional potassium to prevent hypokalemia. High-potassium diets may also have a direct antihypertensive effect. Typical American diets contain about 3 g (80 meq) of potassium per day. High-potassium diets commonly contain 4.5–7 g (120–180 meq) of potassium per day.

Most fruits, vegetables, and their juices contain high concentrations of potassium (see Chapter 21). Supplemental potassium can also be provided with potassium-containing salt substitutes (up to 20 meq in ¼ tsp) or as potassium chloride in solution or capsules, but this is rarely necessary if the above measures are followed to prevent potassium losses and supplement dietary potassium.

High-Calcium Diets

Additional intakes of dietary calcium have recently been recommended for the prevention of postmenopausal osteoporosis, the prevention and treatment of hypertension, and the prevention of colon cancer. Although the evidence in each case is preliminary, authorities recommend intakes of 1 g of calcium per day for most adults and 1.5 g/d for postmenopausal women. Current USA intakes are approximately 700 mg/d.

Low-fat and nonfat dairy products are the mainstay of supplemental calcium intakes. Patients with lactose intolerance who cannot tolerate liquid dairy products may be able to tolerate nonliquid products such as cheese and yogurt. Leafy green vegetables and canned fish with bones also contain high concentrations of calcium, although the latter is also very high in sodium.

[American Dietetic Association Web Page.] http://www.eatright.org. (Position papers on medical nutrition therapy.)

Position of the American Dietetic Association: Medical nutrition therapy and pharmacotherapy. J Am Diet Assoc 1999;99:227. [NLM Cit ID: 99138142] (Medical nutrition therapy and lifestyle counseling are integral components of the medical treatment of many conditions for which medications are also required.)

Appel LJ et al: A clinical trial of the effects of dietary patterns on blood pressure. N Engl J Med 1997;336:1117. [NLM Cit ID: 97238752] (A diet rich in fruits and vegetables and reduced saturated fats resulted in substantial reductions of systolic and diastolic blood pressure.)

Gillespie SJ et al: Using carbohydrate counting in diabetes clinical practice. J Am Diet Assoc 1998;98:897. [NLM Cit ID: 98376519] (Carbohydrate counting is a meal planning approach used with clients who have diabetes that focuses on carbohydrate as the primary nutrient affecting postprandial glycemic response.)

Haynes RB et al: Nutritionally complete prepared meal plan to reduce cardiovascular risk factors: a randomized clinical trial. J Am Diet Assoc 1999;99:1077. [NLM Cit ID: 99420505] (A nutritionally complete prepackaged meal plan offers greater improvements in lipids, blood sugars, homocysteine, and weight loss than usual care diet therapy.)

Kasiske BL et al: A meta-analysis of the effects of dietary protein restriction on the rate of decline in renal function. Am J Kidney Dis 1998;31:954. [NLM Cit ID: 98293600] (Meta-analysis of 13 trials demonstrates that protein restriction retards only somewhat the rate of renal function decline.)

Knopp RH et al: Long-term cholesterol-lowering effects of 4 fat restricted diets in hypercholesterolemic men and combined hyperlipidemic men. JAMA 1997;278:1509. [NLM Cit ID: 98028601] (Restriction of dietary fat beyond 30% of calories did not result in additional benefit and may have undesirable effects on blood lipids.)

Lipkin E: New strategies for the treatment of type 2 diabetes. J Am Diet Assoc 1999;99:329. [NLM Cit ID: 9917588] (Nutrition therapy is still considered the first-line therapy for type 2 diabetes.)

Nuttall FQ et al: Nutrition and the management of type 2 diabetes. J Fam Pract 1998;47(5 Suppl):S45. [NLM Cit ID: 99051820] (Six general principles for the nutritional management of type 2 diabetes mellitus.)

Sheils JF et al: The estimated costs and savings of medical nutrition therapy: the Medicare population. J Am Diet Assoc 1999;99:428. [NLM Cit ID: 99223801] (After an initial period of implementation, coverage for medical nutrition therapy can result in a net reduction in health services utilization and costs for at least some populations. In the case of persons aged 55 years and older, the savings in utilization of hospital and other services will exceed the cost of providing the medical nutrition therapy benefit.)

Windhauser MM et al: Translating the Dietary Approaches to Stop Hypertension diet from research to practice: dietary and behavior change techniques. DASH Collaborative Research Group. J Am Diet Assoc 1999;99(8 Suppl):S90. [NLM Cit ID: 99378794] (Dietary advice and counseling suggestions for tailoring interventions to match patients' readiness for adopting the DASH diet.)

Young JS: HIV and medical nutrition therapy. J Am Diet Assoc 1997;97(10 Suppl 2):S161. [NLM Cit ID: 97477578] (In those who are infected with HIV, malnutrition may be prevented or reversed by medical nutrition therapy that includes nutrition assessment, planning, and implementation.)

NUTRITIONAL SUPPORT

Nutritional support is the provision of nutrients to patients who cannot meet their nutritional requirements by eating standard diets. Nutrients may be delivered enterally, using oral nutritional supplements, nasogastric and nasoduodenal feeding tubes, and tube enterostomies; or parenterally, using lines or catheters placed in peripheral or central veins, respectively. Current nutritional support techniques permit adequate nutrient delivery to virtually any patient. Nutrition support should only be utilized, however, if it is likely to improve the patient's clinical outcome. The financial costs and risks of side effects must be balanced against the potential advantages of improved nutritional status in each clinical situation.

INDICATIONS FOR NUTRITIONAL SUPPORT

The precise indications for nutritional support remain controversial. Most authorities agree that nutritional support is indicated for at least four groups of adult patients: (1) those with inadequate bowel syndromes; (2) those with severe prolonged hypercatabolic states (eg, due to extensive burns, multiple trauma, mechanical ventilation); (3) those requiring prolonged therapeutic bowel rest; and (4) those with severe protein-calorie undernutrition with a treatable disease who have sustained a loss of over 25% of body weight.

It has been difficult to prove the efficacy of nutritional support in the treatment of most other conditions. In most cases it has not been possible to show a clear advantage of treatment by means of nutritional support over treatment without such support.

The American Society for Parenteral and Enteral Nutrition (ASPEN) has published recommendations for the rational use of nutritional support. The recommendations emphasize the need to individualize the decision to begin nutritional support, weighing the risks and costs against the benefit to each patient. They also demonstrate the need to identify high-risk malnourished patients by nutritional assessment.

NUTRITIONAL SUPPORT METHODS

Selection of the most appropriate nutritional support method involves consideration of gastrointestinal function, the anticipated duration of nutritional support, and the ability of each method to meet the patient's nutritional requirements. The method chosen should meet the patient's nutritional needs with the lowest risk and lowest cost possible. For most patients, enteral feeding is safer and cheaper and offers significant physiologic advantages. An algorithm for selection of the most appropriate nutritional support method is presented in Figure 29–2.

Prior to initiating specialized enteral nutritional support, efforts should be made to supplement food intake. Attention to patient preferences, timing of meals, diagnostic procedures and use of medications, and the use of foods brought to the hospital by family and friends can often increase oral intake. Patients unable to eat enough at regular mealtimes to meet nutritional requirements can be given **oral supplements** as snacks or to replace low-calorie beverages. Supplements of differing nutritional composition are available for the purpose of individualizing the diet in accordance with specific clinical requirements. Fiber and lactose content, caloric density, protein level, and amino acid profiles can all be modified as necessary.

Patients unable to take adequate oral nutrients who have functioning gastrointestinal tracts and who meet the criteria for nutritional support are candidates for **tube feedings.** Small-bore feeding tubes are placed via the nose into the stomach or duodenum. Patients able to sit up in bed who can protect their airways can be fed into the stomach. Because of the increased risk of aspiration, patients who cannot adequately protect their airways should be fed nasoduodenally. Feeding tubes can be passed into the duodenum by leaving an extra length of tubing and placing the patient in the right decubitus position. Metoclopramide, 10 mg intravenously, can be given 20 minutes prior to insertion and continued every 6 hours thereafter to facilitate passage through the pylorus. Occasionally patients will require fluoroscopy or endoscopic guidance to insert the tube distal to the pylorus. Placement of nasogastric and, particularly, nasoduodenal

Table 29–8. Enteral solutions.

Complete
Blenderized (eg, Compleat Regular, Compleat Modified,[1] Vitaneed[1])
Whole protein, lactose-containing (eg, Mentene, Carnation and Delmark Instant Breakfast, Forta Shake)
Whole protein, lactose-free, low-residue:
1 kcal/mL (eg, Ensure, Isocal, Osmolite, Nutren 1.0,[1] Nutrilan, Isolan,[1] Sustacal, Resource)
1.5 kcal/mL (eg, Ensure Plus, Sustacal HC, Comply, Nutren 1.5, Resource Plus)
2 kcal/mL (eg, Isocal HCN, Magnacal, TwoCal HN)
High-nitrogen: > 15% total calories from protein (eg, Ensure HN, Attain,[1] Osmolite HN,[1] Replete, Entrition HN,[1] Isolan,[1] Isocal HN,[1] Sustacal HC, Isosource HN,[1] Ultralan)
Whole protein, lactose-free, high-residue:
1 kcal/mL (eg, Jevity,[1] Profiber,[1] Nutren 1.0 with fiber,[1] Fiberian,[1] Sustacal with fiber, Ultracal,[1] Ensure with fiber, Fibersource)
Chemically defined peptide- or amino acid-based (eg, Accupep HPF, Criticare HN, Peptamen,[1] Reabfin, Vital HN, AlitraQ, Tolerex, Vivonex TEN)
"Disease-specific" formulas
Renal failure: with essential amino acids (eg, Amin-Aid, Travasorb Renal, Aminess)
Malabsorption: with medium-chain triglycerides (eg, Portagen,[1] Travasorb MCT)
Respiratory failure: with > 50% calories from fat (eg, Pulmocare, NutriVent)
Hepatic encephalopathy: with high amounts of branched-chain amino acids (eg, Hepatic-Acid II, Travasorb Hepatic)
Incomplete (modular)
Protein (eg, Nutrisource Protein, Promed, Propac)
Carbohydrate (eg, Nutrisource Carbohydrate, Polycose, Sumacal)
Fat (eg, MCT Oil, Microlipid, Nutrisource Lipid)
Vitamins (eg, Nutrisource Vitamins)
Minerals (eg, Nutrisource Minerals)

[1]Isotonic.

isotonic solutions contain 1000 kcal and about 37–45 g of protein per liter.

Solutions containing hydrolyzed proteins or crystalline amino acids and with no significant fat content are called elemental solutions, since macronutrients are provided in their most "elemental" form. These solutions have been designed for patients with malabsorption, particularly pancreatic insufficiency and limited fat absorption. Elemental diets are extremely hypertonic and often result in more severe diarrhea. Their use should be limited to patients who cannot tolerate isotonic solutions.

Although formulas have been designed for specific clinical situations—solutions containing primarily essential amino acids (for renal failure), medium-chain triglycerides (for fat malabsorption), more fat (for respiratory failure and CO_2 retention), and more branched-chain amino acids (for hepatic encephalopathy and severe trauma)—they have not been shown to be superior to standard formulas for most patients.

Enteral solutions should be administered via continuous infusion, preferably with an infusion pump. Isotonic feedings should be started at full strength at about 25–33% of the estimated final infusion rate. Feedings can be advanced by similar amounts every 12 hours as tolerated. Hypertonic feedings should be started at half strength. The strength and the rate can then be advanced every 6 hours as tolerated.

COMPLICATIONS OF ENTERAL NUTRITIONAL SUPPORT

Minor complications of tube feedings occur in 10–15% of patients. Gastrointestinal complications include diarrhea (most common), inadequate gastric emptying, emesis, esophagitis, and occasionally gastrointestinal bleeding. Diarrhea associated with tube feeding may be due to intolerance to the osmotic load or to one of the macronutrients (eg, fat, lactose) in the solution. Patients being fed in this way may also have diarrhea from other causes (as side effect of antibiotics or other drugs; associated with infection, etc), and these possibilities should always be investigated in appropriate circumstances.

Mechanical complications of tube feedings are potentially the most serious. Of particular importance is aspiration. All patients receiving nasogastric tube feedings are at risk for this life-threatening complication. Limiting nasogastric feedings to those patients who can adequately protect their airway and careful monitoring of patients being fed by tube should limit these serious complications to 1–2% of cases. Minor mechanical complications are common and include tube obstruction and dislodgment.

Metabolic complications during enteral nutritional support are common but in most cases easily managed. The most important problem is hypernatremic dehydration, most commonly seen in elderly patients given excessive protein intake who are unable to respond to thirst. Abnormalities of potassium, glucose, and acid-base balance may also occur.

PARENTERAL NUTRITIONAL SUPPORT SOLUTIONS

Parenteral nutritional support solutions can be designed to deliver adequate nutrients to virtually any patient. The basic parenteral solution is composed of dextrose, amino acids, and water. Electrolytes, minerals, trace elements, vitamins, and medications can also be added. Most commercial solutions contain the monohydrate form of dextrose that provides 3.4 kcal/g. Crystalline amino acids are available in a variety of concentrations, so that a broad range of solutions can be made up that will contain specific amounts of dextrose and amino acids as required.

Typical solutions for central vein nutritional support contain 25–35% dextrose and 2.75–6% amino acids depending upon the patient's estimated nutrient and water requirements. These solutions typically have osmolalities in excess of 1800 mosm/L and require infusion into a central vein. A typical formula for patients without organ failure is shown in Table 29–9.

Solutions with lower osmolalities can also be designed for infusion into peripheral veins. Typical solutions for peripheral infusion contain 5–10% dextrose and 2.75–4.25% amino acids. These solutions have osmolalities between 800 and 1200 mosm/L and result in a high incidence of thrombophlebitis and line infiltration. These solutions will provide adequate protein for most patients but inadequate energy. Additional energy must be provided in the form of emulsified soybean or safflower oil. Such intravenous fat solutions are currently available in 10% and 25% solutions providing 1.1 and 2.2 kcal/mL, respectively. Intravenous fat solutions are isosmotic and well tolerated by peripheral veins. Typical patients are given 200–500 mL of a 20% solution each day. As much as 60% of total calories can be administered in this manner.

Intravenous fat can also be provided to patients receiving central vein nutritional support. In this instance, dextrose concentrations should be decreased to provide a fixed concentration of energy. Intravenous fat has been shown to be equivalent to intravenous dextrose in providing energy to spare protein. Intravenous fat is associated with less glucose intolerance, less production of carbon dioxide, and less fatty infiltration of the liver and has been increasingly utilized in patients with hyperglycemia, respiratory failure, and liver disease. Intravenous fat has also been increasingly used in patients with large estimated energy requirements. Recent studies suggest that the maximum glucose utilization rate is approximately 5–7 mg/min/kg. Patients who require additional calories can be given them as fat to prevent excess administration of dextrose. Intravenous fat can also be used to prevent essential fatty acid deficiency. The optimal ratio of carbohydrate and fat in parenteral nutritional support has not been determined.

Infusion of parenteral solutions should be started slowly to prevent hyperglycemia and other metabolic complications. Typical solutions are given initially at a rate of 50 mL/h and advanced by about the same amount every 24 hours until the desired final rate is reached.

Table 29–9. Typical solution (for stable patients without organ failure).

Dextrose (3.4 kcal/g)	25%	
Amino acids (4 kcal/g)	6%	
Na^+	50 meq/L	
K^+	40 meq/L	
Ca^{2+}	5 meq/L	
Mg^{2+}	8 meq/L	
Cl^-	60 meq/L	
P	12 meg/L	
Acetate	Balance	
MVI-12 (vitamins)	10 mL/d	
MTE (trace elements)	5 mL/d	
Fat emulsion 20%	250 mL 5 times a week	
Typical rate	Day 1: 30 mL/h Day 2: 60 mL/h	
By day 2, solution provides:	Calories:	1925 kcal total
	Protein:	86 g
	Fat:	19% of total kcal
	Fluid:	1690 mL

COMPLICATIONS OF PARENTERAL NUTRITIONAL SUPPORT

Complications of central vein nutritional support occur in up to 50% of patients. Although most are minor and easily managed, about 5% of patients will develop significant complications. Complications of central vein nutritional support can be divided into catheter-related complications and metabolic complications.

Catheter-related complications can occur during insertion or while the catheter is in place. Pneumothorax, hemothorax, arterial laceration, air emboli, and brachial plexus injury can occur during catheter placement. The incidence of these complications is inversely related to the experience of the physician performing the procedure but will occur in at least 1–2% of cases even in major medical centers. Each catheter placement should be documented by chest radiograph prior to initiation of nutritional support.

Catheter thrombosis and catheter-related sepsis are the most important complications of indwelling catheters. Patients with indwelling central vein catheters who develop fever without an apparent source should have their lines removed immediately, the tip cultured, and antibiotics begun empirically. Blood cultures should also be obtained from a separate site, as duration of antibiotic therapy is determined by their positivity and by the number of colonies on the line tip. Catheter-related sepsis occurs in 2–3% of patients even if maximal efforts are made to prevent infection.

Metabolic complications of central vein nutritional support occur in over 50% of patients (Table 29–10). Most are minor and easily managed, and termination of support is seldom necessary.

PATIENT MONITORING DURING NUTRITIONAL SUPPORT

Every patient receiving enteral or parenteral nutritional support should be followed closely. Formal nutritional support teams composed of a physician, a

Table 29–10. Metabolic complications of parenteral nutritional support.

Complication	Common Causes	Possible Solutions
Hyperglycemia	Too rapid infusion of dextrose, "stress," glucocorticoids	Decrease glucose infusion. Insulin. Replacement of dextrose with fat.
Hyperosmolar nonketotic dehydration	Severe, undetected hyperglycemia	Insulin, hydration, potassium
Hyperchloremic metabolic acidosis	High chloride administration	Decrease chloride
Azotemia	Excessive protein administration	Decrease amino acid concentration
Hyperphosphatemia, hypokalemia, hypomagnesemia	Extracellular to intracellular shifting with refeeding	Increase solution concentration
Liver enzyme abnormalities	Lipid trapping in hepatocytes, fatty liver	Decrease dextrose
Acalculous cholecystitis	Biliary stasis	Oral fat
Zinc deficiency	Diarrhea, small bowel fistulas	Increase concentration
Copper deficiency	Biliary fistulas	Increase concentration

nurse, a dietitian, and a pharmacist have been shown to decrease the rate of complications.

Patients should be monitored both for the adequacy of treatment and to prevent complications or detect them early when they occur. Because estimates of nutritional requirements are imprecise, frequent reassessment is necessary. Daily intakes should be recorded and compared with estimated requirements. Body weight, hydration status, and overall clinical status should be followed. Patients who do not appear to be responding as anticipated can be evaluated for nitrogen balance by means of the following equation:

$$\text{Nitrogen balance} = \frac{\text{24-hour protein intake (g)}}{6.25} - \left(\text{25-hour urinary nitrogen (g)} + 4\right)$$

Patients with positive nitrogen balances can be continued on their current regimens; patients with negative balances should receive moderate increases in calorie and protein intake and then be reassessed.

Monitoring for metabolic complications includes urine glucose determination every 6 hours; daily measurements of electrolytes; serum glucose, phosphorus, magnesium, calcium, and creatinine; and BUN until the patient is stabilized. Once the patient is stabilized, electrolytes, phosphorus, calcium, magnesium, and glucose should be obtained at least twice weekly. Red blood cell folate, zinc, and copper should be checked at least once a month.

Deitch EA et al: Prevention of multiple organ failure. Surg Clin North Am 1999;79:1471. [NLM Cit ID: 20091434] (Despite lack of clinical trial evidence, early nutritional support may be useful in preventing multiple organ failure in high risk patients.)

Ferreira IM et al: Nutritional support for individuals with COPD: a meta-analysis. Chest 2000;117:672. [NLM Cit ID: 20179545] (Nutritional support had no effect on improving anthropometric measures, lung function, or functional exercise capacity among patients with stable COPD.)

Finck C: How to provide nutritional support. Nutrition 2000;16:155. [NLM Cit ID: 20161636]

Hasselgren PO: Burns and metabolism. J Am Coll Surg 1999;188:98. [NLM Cit ID: 99146755]

Heyland DK: Nutritional support in the critically ill patient. A critical review of the evidence. Crit Care Clin 1998;14:423. [NLM Cit ID: 98365797]

Jensen GL: Hypoenergetic nutrition support in hospitalized obese patients: A simplified method for clinical application. J Parenter Enteral Nutr 1997;21:366. [NLM Cit ID: 98069211] (Hypocaloric feedings can be used in obese patients who require nutritional support.)

Klein GL: Metabolic bone disease of total parenteral nutrition. Nutrition 1998;14:149. [NLM Cit ID: 98100355] (The true incidence of parenteral nutrition-related metabolic bone disease remains unknown.)

Klein S et al: Nutrition support in clinical practice: A review of published data and recommendations for future research directions. National Institute of Health, American Society for Parenteral and Enteral Nutrition, and the American Society for Clinical Nutrition. J Parenter Enteral Nutr 1997;21:133. [NLM Cit ID: 97424272] (Extensive panel report on nutrition assessment, nutrition support in gastrointestinal diseases, nutrition support in wasting diseases, nutrition support in critically ill patients, and perioperative nutrition support.)

Mahesh C et al: Extended indications for enteral nutritional support. Nutrition 2000;16:129. [NLM Cit ID: 20161627] (Enteral nutrition can be given to many patients who otherwise would have received parenteral nutrition.)

Mathus-Vliegen LM et al: Percutaneous endoscopic gastrostomy and gastrojejunostomy: a critical reappraisal of patient selection, tube function and the feasibility of nutritional support during extended follow-up. Gastrointest Endosc 1999;50:746. [NLM Cit ID: 20040221] (Clinical outcomes in 286 patients referred for percutaneous endoscopic gastrostomy)

Phinney SD et al: Is there a role for parenteral feeding in clinical medicine? West J Med 1996;164:130. [NLM Cit ID: 96371903] (Critical review of the effectiveness of parenteral nutrition.)

Rabenek L et al: Long-term outcomes of patients receiving percutaneous endoscopic gastrostomy tubes. J Gen Intern Med 1996;11:287. [NLM Cit ID: 96338659] (Tube placement is common, often in the terminal phase of illness.)

Souba WW: Drug therapy: nutritional support. N Engl J Med 1997;336:41. [NLM Cit ID: 97122461]

Wilmore DW: Nutrition and metabolic support in the 21st century. JPEN J Parenter Enteral Nutr 2000;24:1. [NLM Cit ID: 20102002] (Recommends greater use of the enteral route for nutrient delivery, reductions in exogenous calories, utilization of nutrients for their pharmacologic effects, use of growth factors to enhance nutrient efficacy, and institution of nutritional supplementation before elective surgery.)

Zaloga GP: Early enteral nutritional support improves outcome: hypothesis or fact? Crit Care Med 1999;27:259. [NLM Cit ID: 99173339]

RELEVANT WORLD WIDE WEB SITES

[Food and Drug Administration]
http://www.fda.gov/

[Center for Food Safety and Applied Nutrition]
http://vm.cfsan.fda.gov/

[CIC Food and Nutrition]
http://www.gsa.gov/staff/pa/cic/food.htm

[American Society for Clinical Nutrition]
http://www.faseb.org/ascn/

[Food and Nutrition Information Center]
http://www.nal.usda.gov/fnic/

[American Dietetic Association]
http://www.eatright.org/

[Nutrition Analysis Tool]
http://www.ag.uiuc.edu/~food-lab/nat/

[The Nutritionist's Tool Box]
http://fscn.che.umn.edu/tools.htm

[Federal Consumer Information Catalog—Food]
http://www.pueblo.gsa.gov/food.htm

[Mayo Health—Nutrition Center]
http://www.mayohealth.org/mayo/common/htm/dietpage.htm

[Arbor Nutrition Guide]
http://www.arborcom.com/

[Nutrition Navigator]
http://navigator.tufts.edu/

[Veggie Heaven]
http://www.veggieheaven.com

[Vitamin Update]
http://bookman.com.au/vitamins

30 General Problems in Infectious Diseases

See http://www.current-med.com/ch30.html for updated addresses of Web sites referenced in this chapter.

Richard A. Jacobs, MD, PhD

Most infections are confined to specific organ systems. In a book such as this—arranged principally by organ system—many of the important infectious disease entities are discussed in chapters dealing with specific anatomic areas. In this chapter are discussed some important general problems related to infectious diseases that are not covered elsewhere.

FEVER OF UNKNOWN ORIGIN (FUO)

To fulfill the original criteria for FUO as set forth in 1961, a patient must have an illness of at least 3 weeks' duration, fever over 38.3 °C on several occasions, and must remain undiagnosed after 1 week of study in the hospital. The intervals specified are arbitrary ones intended to exclude patients with protracted but self-limited viral illnesses and to allow time for the usual radiographic, serologic, and cultural studies to be performed. Because of concerns over costs of hospitalization and the availability of most screening tests on an outpatient basis, the criterion requiring 1 week of hospitalization has been modified to accept patients who remain undiagnosed after three outpatient visits or 3 days of hospitalization.

Over the ensuing decades, several additional categories of FUO have been added: (1) Nosocomial FUO refers to the hospitalized patient with fever of 38.3 °C or higher on several occasions, due to a process not present or incubating at the time of admission, in whom initial cultures are negative and the diagnosis remains unknown after 3 days of investigation (see Nosocomial Infections, below). (2) Neutropenic FUO includes patients with fever of 38.3 °C or higher on several occasions with less than 500 neutrophils per milliliter in whom initial cultures are negative and the diagnosis remains uncertain after 3 days (see Chapter 4 and Infections in the Immunocompromised Patient, below). (3) HIV-associated FUO refers to HIV-positive patients with fever of 38.3 °C or higher who have been febrile for 4 weeks or more as an outpatient or 3 days as an inpatient, in whom the diagnosis remains uncertain after 3 days of investigation with at least 2 days for cultures to incubate (see Chapter 31). Although not usually considered a separate group, FUO in solid organ transplant recipients is a common scenario with a unique differential diagnosis and is discussed below.

For a general discussion of fever, see the section on fever and hyperthermia in Chapter 1.

Etiologic Considerations

Certain general principles about FUO should be kept in mind in the diagnostic approach to these patients.

A. Common Causes: Most cases represent unusual manifestations of common diseases and not rare or exotic diseases—ie, tuberculosis, endocarditis, gallbladder disease, and HIV (primary infection or opportunistic infection) are more common causes of FUO than Whipple's disease or familial Mediterranean fever.

B. Age of Patient: In adults, infections (25–40% of cases) and cancer (25–40% of cases) account for the majority of FUOs. In children, infections are the most common cause of FUO (30–50% of cases) and cancer a rare cause (5–10% of cases). Autoimmune disorders occur with equal frequency in adults and children (10–20% of cases), but the diseases differ. Juvenile rheumatoid arthritis is particularly common in children, whereas systemic lupus erythematosus, Wegener's granulomatosis, and polyarteritis nodosa are more common in adults. Adult Still's disease, giant cell arteritis, and polymyalgia rheumatica occur exclusively in adults.

C. Duration of Fever: The cause of FUO changes dramatically in patients who have been febrile for a prolonged period of time—ie, 6 months or longer. Infection, cancer, and autoimmune disorders combined account for only 20% of FUOs in these patients. Instead, other entities such as granulomatous diseases (granulomatous hepatitis, Crohn's disease, ulcerative colitis) and factitious fever become important causes. Up to 27% of patients who say they have been febrile for 6 months or longer actually have no true fever or underlying disease. Instead, the usual normal circadian variation in temperature (temperature 1–2 °C higher in the afternoon than in the morning) is interpreted as abnormal. Patients with episodic or recurrent fever (ie, those who meet the classic criteria for FUO but have fever-free periods of 2 weeks or longer) are similar to patients with prolonged fever. Infection, malignancy, and autoimmune disorders account for only 20–25% of such fevers, whereas various miscellaneous diseases (Crohn's disease, familial Mediterranean fever, allergic alveolitis) account for another 25%. Approximately 50% remain undiagnosed but have a benign course with eventual resolution of symptoms.

D. Immunologic Status: In the neutropenic patient, fungal infections and occult bacterial infection are important and common causes of FUO. In the patient taking immunosuppressive medications (particularly organ transplant patients), cytomegalovirus infections are a frequent cause of fever, as are fungal infections, nocardiosis, *Pneumocystis carinii* pneumonia, and mycobacterial infections.

E. Classification of Causes of FUO: Most patients with FUO will fit into one of five categories.

1. Infection–Both systemic and localized infections can cause FUO. Tuberculosis and endocarditis are the most common systemic infections, but mycoses, viral diseases (particularly infection with Epstein-Barr virus and cytomegalovirus), toxoplasmosis, brucellosis, Q fever, cat-scratch disease, salmonellosis, malaria, and many other less common infections have been implicated. Primary infection with human immunodeficiency virus (HIV) or opportunistic infections associated with the acquired immunodeficiency syndrome (AIDS)—particularly mycobacterial infections—can also present as FUO. The most common form of localized infection causing FUO is an occult abscess. Liver, spleen, kidney, brain, and bone are organs in which abscess may be difficult to find. A collection of pus may form in the peritoneal cavity or in the subdiaphragmatic, subhepatic, paracolic, or other areas. Cholangitis, osteomyelitis, urinary tract infection, dental abscess, or a collection of pus in a paranasal sinus may cause prolonged fever.

2. Neoplasms–Many cancers can present as FUO. The most common are lymphoma (both Hodgkin's and non-Hodgkin's) and leukemia. Other diseases of lymph nodes, such as angioimmunoblastic lymphoma and Castleman's disease, can also cause FUO. Primary and metastatic tumors of the liver also are frequently associated with fever, as are renal cell carcinomas. Atrial myxoma is an often forgotten neoplasm that can result in fever. Chronic lymphocytic leukemia and multiple myeloma are rarely associated with fever, and the presence of fever in patients with these diseases should prompt a careful search for infection.

3. Autoimmune disorders–Still's disease, systemic lupus erythematosus, cryoglobulinemia, and polyarteritis nodosa are the most common autoimmune causes of FUO. Giant cell arteritis and polymyalgia rheumatica are seen almost exclusively in patients over 50 years of age and are nearly always associated with an elevated erythrocyte sedimentation rate (> 40 mm/h).

4. Miscellaneous causes–Many other diseases have been associated with FUO but less commonly than the foregoing types of illness. Examples include hyperthyroidism, thyroiditis, sarcoidosis, Whipple's disease, familial Mediterranean fever, recurrent pulmonary emboli, alcoholic hepatitis, drug fever, factitious fever, and others.

5. Undiagnosed FUO–Despite extensive evaluation, in 10–15% of patients the diagnosis remains elusive. In about three-fourths of these patients, the fever abates spontaneously and the clinician never knows the cause; in the remainder, more classic manifestations of the underlying disease appear over time, and the diagnosis then becomes obvious.

Approach to Diagnosis of FUO

Because the evaluation of a patient with FUO is so costly and time-consuming, it is imperative to document the presence of fever. This is done most reliably by observing the patient while the temperature is being taken to make certain that fever is not factitious (self-induced). Associated findings that usually accompany fever include tachycardia, chills, and piloerection. A thorough history—including family, occupational, social (sexual practices, use of intravenous drugs), dietary (unpasteurized products, raw meat), exposures (animals, chemicals), and travel histories—may give clues to the underlying diagnosis. Detailed and repeated physical examination may reveal subtle, evanescent clinical findings that are the key to diagnosis.

In addition to routine laboratory studies, blood cultures should always be obtained, preferably when the patient has been off antibiotics for several days, and should be held by the laboratory for 2 weeks to detect slow-growing organisms. Cultures on special media should be requested if legionella, bartonella, or nutritionally deficient streptococci are considered possible pathogens. "Screening tests" with immunologic or microbiologic serologies ("febrile agglutinins") are of low yield and should not be done. Specific serologic tests are helpful if the history or physical examination suggests a specific diagnosis. A single elevated titer rarely allows one to make a diagnosis of infection; instead, one must demonstrate a fourfold rise or fall in titer to confirm a specific infectious cause. Because infection is the most common cause of FUO, other body fluids are usually cultured, ie, urine, sputum, stool, cerebrospinal fluid, and morning gastric aspirates (if one suspects tuberculosis). Direct examination of blood smears may establish a diagnosis of malaria or relapsing fever (borrelia).

All patients with FUO should have a chest radiograph. Other studies such as sinus films, upper gas-

eg, induced sputum yields a diagnosis of pneumocystis pneumonia in 50–80% of AIDS patients with this infection. In other situations, more invasive procedures may be required (bronchoalveolar lavage, transbronchial biopsy, or even open lung biopsy). Other procedures such as skin, liver, or bone marrow biopsy may be helpful in establishing a diagnosis.

(5) In patients who have undergone solid organ transplants, immediate postoperative infections often involve the transplanted organ. Following lung transplantation, pneumonia and mediastinitis are particularly common; following liver transplantation, intra-abdominal abscess, cholangitis, and peritonitis are common; following renal transplantation, urinary tract infections, perinephric abscesses, and infected lymphoceles can occur. In contrast to solid organ transplants, in bone marrow transplant patients the source of fever cannot be found in 60–70% of patients.

(6) The time of occurrence of infection, particularly following solid organ transplantation, can be helpful in determining the infectious origin. Most infections that occur in the first 2–4 weeks posttransplant are related to the operative procedure and to hospitalization itself (wound infection, intravenous catheter infection, urinary tract infection from a Foley catheter) or are related to the transplanted organ (see paragraph [5], above). Infections that occur between the first and sixth months are often related to immunosuppression. During this period, reactivation of viruses occurs, and herpes simplex, varicella-zoster, and CMV infections are quite common. Opportunistic infections with fungi (candida, aspergillus, cryptococcus, pneumocystis, and others), *Listeria monocytogenes,* nocardia, and toxoplasma are also common. After 6 months, when immunosuppression has been reduced to maintenance levels, common infections that are found in any population occur.

Prevention of Infection

There is great interest in preventing infection with prophylactic antimicrobial regimens, but there is no uniformity of opinion about what the optimal drugs or dosage regimens should be.

Trimethoprim-sulfamethoxazole, one double-strength tablet three times a week, one double-strength tablet twice daily on weekends, or one single-strength tablet daily for 3–6 months, is frequently used to prevent pneumocystis infections in transplant patients. It may also decrease the incidence of bacterial pneumonia, urinary tract infections, nocardia infections, and toxoplasmosis.

In patients allergic to trimethoprim-sulfamethoxazole, aerosolized pentamidine is used in a dosage of 300 mg once a month. Dapsone, 50 mg daily or 100 mg three times weekly, can also be used. (G6PD levels should be determined before therapy is instituted.) Acyclovir has been shown to be effective in preventing herpes simplex and varicella infections in transplant recipients.

Prevention of CMV is more difficult, and no uniformly accepted approach has been adopted. Prevention strategies often depend on the serologic status of the donor and recipient and the organ transplanted, which determines the level of immunosuppression after transplant. In solid organ transplants (liver, kidney, heart, lung), the greatest risk of developing CMV disease is in seronegative patients who receive organs from seropositive donors. These high-risk patients usually receive ganciclovir, 2.5–5 mg/kg intravenously twice daily, during hospitalization (usually about 10 days) and then are placed on a regimen of oral ganciclovir, 1 g three times daily, for 3 months. Other solid organ transplant recipients are at lower risk for developing CMV disease and usually receive intravenous ganciclovir while in the hospital followed by high-dose oral acyclovir at a dosage of 800 mg four times daily for 3 months. Both ganciclovir and acyclovir prevent herpesvirus reactivation. Because immunosuppression is increased during periods of rejection, patients treated for rejection usually receive intravenous ganciclovir during rejection therapy.

Recipients of bone marrow transplants are more severely immunosuppressed than recipients of solid organ transplants, are at greater risk for developing serious CMV infection, and thus usually receive more aggressive prophylaxis. Two approaches have been used: universal prophylaxis or preemptive therapy. In the former, all CMV-seropositive patients receive 7.5–10 mg/kg/d of ganciclovir for 1 week prior to transplantation and a lower dose of 5 mg/kg/d up to the time of engraftment (which usually occurs on about day 30). Thereafter, therapy is continued 3 days per week to day 90 posttransplant. Although effective in preventing infection and disease, this method is costly and associated with significant toxicity and is therefore being used less frequently. Alternatively, patients can be followed without specific therapy and have blood sampled weekly for the presence of CMV. If CMV is detected by an antigenemia assay, preemptive therapy with ganciclovir is given (5 mg/kg intravenously twice daily for 7 days, followed by 5 mg/kg daily for the first 100–120 days after transplantation). This approach is also effective but does miss a small number of patients who subsequently develop CMV disease. In allogeneic marrow transplant patients, intravenous immune globulin, 500–1000 mg/kg, is given every 1–2 weeks for the first 3 months after transplantation as CMV prophylaxis. Following autologous bone marrow transplantation, immune globulin is not recommended and may be associated with increased toxicity. Bone marrow transplant patients who are seronegative for CMV usually receive intravenous acyclovir (for prevention of other herpesvirus infections) at a dosage of 5 mg/kg/d in two divided doses until mucositis has resolved, followed by oral acyclovir, 200 mg three times daily, for the first year posttransplant.

In the neutropenic patient, the gastrointestinal tract is the source of many infections. Oral nonabsorbable antibiotics and quinolones have been used for gastrointestinal decontamination in an attempt to decrease bacteremia from this site. Because of poor compliance with nonabsorbable agents and concern about selection of resistant organisms with quinolones, neither approach has gained widespread acceptance. Small bowel decontamination with polymyxin E, gentamicin, and nystatin when given at least 3 days prior to liver transplantation is effective in reducing the incidence of postoperative infections. The role of prophylactic antifungal agents in neutropenic patients remains controversial. Fluconazole has been shown to decrease the incidence of superficial and invasive fungal infections due to *Candida albicans* but has been associated with selection of resistant organisms *(Candida krusei)* and an increase in infections with molds (aspergillus, mucor, and others). Itraconazole, like fluconazole, decreases infection with candida species, but it has had no effect on infection with aspergillus. Preliminary data on low-dose amphotericin B (0.1 mg/kg/d) for prophylaxis suggest efficacy in preventing invasive disease, but further data are required. Prophylaxis in HIV-positive patients is summarized in Chapter 31.

Handwashing is the simplest and most effective means of decreasing nosocomial infections in *all* patients, especially the compromised host. Invasive devices such as central and peripheral lines and Foley catheters are a potential source of infection. The need for these devices should be continually assessed and their use discontinued at the earliest possible time.

Approach to Treatment

In addition to providing antimicrobial therapy, it is important to improve host defenses whenever possible, correct electrolyte imbalances, and maintain adequate nutrition. Because immunosuppression is often the reason for infection, it is important to decrease immunosuppressive medications even in organ transplant patients. Reduction or discontinuation of immunosuppressive medication may jeopardize the viability of the transplanted organ, but in life-threatening infections it is necessary as an adjunct to effective antimicrobial therapy. Hematopoietic growth factors (granulocyte and granulocyte-macrophage colony-stimulating factors) stimulate proliferation of bone marrow stem cells, resulting in an increase in peripheral leukocytes. These agents shorten the period of neutropenia and have been associated with fewer infections. Use of growth factors in patients with prolonged neutropenia (> 7 days) is an effective means of reversing immunosuppression.

Antimicrobial drug therapy should be rationally based on culture results (see Chapter 37). Therapy should be specific for isolated pathogens, and bactericidal agents should be used. Combinations of antimicrobials are often required to provide synergy, to prevent resistance, or to serve as broad-spectrum coverage of multiple pathogens (since infections in these patients are often polymicrobial).

Empirical therapy is often instituted at the earliest sign of infection in the immunosuppressed patient because prompt therapy favorably affects outcome. The antibiotic or combination of antibiotics used depends on the type of immunocompromise and the site of infection. For example, in the febrile neutropenic patient, one is concerned primarily about bacterial and fungal infections. Often in this patient population an algorithmic approach to therapy is used, with initial treatment directed at gram-positive and gram-negative organisms. If the patient fails to respond, broader-spectrum antibiotics and antifungal drugs are added. Although a number of different agents can be used, choices should be based on local microbiologic trends. One example would be to initiate therapy with levofloxacin, 500 mg orally or intravenously daily, when the absolute neutrophil count falls below 500/μL. If fever develops, cultures should be obtained; vancomycin, 10–15 mg/kg every 12 hours, is given (to cover methicillin-resistant *S aureus, S epidermidis,* and enterococcus), and amphotericin B, 0.3 mg/kg/d, is added. If after 48–72 hours fever continues, broader-spectrum antibiotics can be added sequentially—eg, to better cover acinetobacter, citrobacter, and pseudomonas. levofloxacin may be switched to cefipime, 2 g every 8 hours intravenously; with continued fever, imipenem, 500 mg every 6 hours with or without tobramycin, 1.8 mg/kg every 8 hours, may be used in place of cefipime, and amphotericin B may be increased to 0.6–1 mg/kg/d. Regardless of whether the patient becomes afebrile, therapy is continued until resolution of neutropenia. Failure to continue antibiotics through the period of neutropenia is associated with a high incidence of relapse that can be associated with septic shock. Patients with fever and neutropenia who are at low risk for developing complications (neutropenia expected to persist for less than 10 days, no comorbid complications requiring hospitalization, and cancer adequately treated) can be treated with oral antibiotic regimens (ciprofloxacin, 750 mg every 12 hours, plus amoxicillin-clavulanic acid, 500 mg every 8 hours). In the organ transplant patient with interstitial infiltrates, one is concerned mainly about pneumocystis or legionella species, so that empirical treatment with intravenous erythromycin and trimethoprim-sulfamethoxazole would be reasonable. If the patient fails to respond to empirical treatment, one must often decide between empirical addition of more antimicrobial agents or undertaking invasive procedures (see above) to make a specific diagnosis. By making a specific diagnosis, therapy can be specific and polypharmacy with multiple potentially toxic agents avoided.

Alexander SW et al: Current considerations in the management of fever and neutropenia. Curr Clin Top Infect Dis 1999;19:160. [NLM Cit ID: 99401705]

Greene JN et al (editors): Infectious complications of cancer therapy. Infect Dis Clin North Am 1996;10(2). [NLM Cit ID: 96396501] (Entire issue contains articles on infections associated with antitumor chemotherapy.)

Hughes WT et al: 1997 guidelines for the use of antimicrobial agents in neutropenic patients with unexplained fever. Clin Infect Dis 1997;25:551. [NLM Cit ID: 97458113] (Current recommendation for prophylaxis and therapy by the Infectious Disease Society of America.)

Pizzo PA: Fever in immunocompromised patients. N Engl J Med 1999;341:893. [NLM Cit ID: 99404889] (Review of etiology diagnosis and therapy in immunocompromised patients.)

Stoupis A et al: Approach to fever in the neutropenic host. Cancer Treatment and Research 1998;96:77. [NLM Cit ID: 98377255] (Principles and sample algorithms for the febrile neutropenic host.)

NOSOCOMIAL INFECTIONS

Nosocomial infections are by definition those acquired during the course of hospitalization. In the USA, approximately 5% of patients who enter the hospital free of infection acquire a nosocomial infection resulting in prolongation of the hospital stay, increase in cost of care, significant morbidity, and a 5% mortality rate. Although most fevers that develop during the course of hospitalization are due to infections, about 25% of patients will have fever of noninfectious origin. Causes include drug fever, nonspecific postoperative fevers (atelectasis, tissue damage or necrosis), hematoma, pancreatitis, pulmonary embolus, myocardial infarction, and ischemic bowel disease. The most common infections are urinary tract infections, usually associated with Foley catheters or urologic procedures; bloodstream infections, most commonly from indwelling catheters but also from secondary sites such as surgical wounds, abscesses, pneumonia, the genitourinary tract, and the gastrointestinal tract; pneumonia in intubated patients or those with altered levels of consciousness; surgical wound infections; and *C difficile* colitis.

Some general principles are helpful in preventing, diagnosing, and treating nosocomial infections:

(1) Many infections are a direct result of the use of invasive devices for monitoring or therapy such as intravenous catheters (for hyperalimentation, fluids and electrolytes, medication, dialysis, hemodynamic monitoring, etc), Foley catheters, shunts, surgical drains, catheters placed by interventional radiology for drainage, nasogastric tubes and orotracheal or nasotracheal tubes for ventilatory support. To prevent infections associated with these devices, they should be removed as soon as is medically possible.

(2) Patients who develop nosocomial infections are often critically ill (in the intensive care unit), have been hospitalized for extended periods, and have received several courses of antibiotic therapy with agents that have a broad spectrum of activity. As a result, nosocomial infections are often caused by organisms that are multidrug-resistant and are different from those encountered in community-acquired infections. Examples of nosocomial pathogens are *S aureus* and *S epidermidis* (a frequent cause of prosthetic device infection) that may be resistant to nafcillin and cephalosporins and require vancomycin for therapy; *Enterococcus faecium* that is resistant to ampicillin and vancomycin (vancomycin-resistant enterococcus, or VRE); gram-negative infections caused by pseudomonas, citrobacter, enterobacter, acinetobacter, and stenotrophomonas, which may be sensitive only to fluoroquinolones, carbapenems, aminoglycosides, or trimethoprim-sulfamethoxazole. When choosing antibiotics to treat the seriously ill patient with a nosocomial infection, one must consider the previous antimicrobial the patient has received as well as the "local ecology" (ie, nosocomial pathogens for a given institution). It is often necessary to institute therapy with drugs such as vancomycin and a carbapenem (or aminoglycoside or a fluoroquinolone) until a specific agent is isolated and sensitivities are known, at which time the least toxic and most cost-effective drug can be used.

(3) Because widespread use of antimicrobial drugs contributes to the selection of drug-resistant organisms that cause nosocomial infections, every effort should be made to limit the use of antibiotics to treat documented infections. All too often, unreliable or uninterpretable specimens are obtained for culture that result in unnecessary use of antibiotics. The best example of this principle is the diagnosis of line-related or bloodstream infection in the febrile patient in the intensive care unit. Blood cultures from unidentified sites, a single blood culture from any site, or a blood culture through an existing line will often be positive for *S epidermidis* and will result in therapy with vancomycin. The likelihood that such a culture represents a true bacteremia is 10–20%. Unless two separate venipuncture cultures are obtained (*do not* sample through catheters), interpretation of results is impossible and unnecessary therapy is given. It has been estimated that every such "pseudobacteremia" increases laboratory costs, antibiotic use, and length of stay and increases costs of hospitalization by about $4500. To avoid unnecessary use of antibiotics, thoughtful consideration of culture results is mandatory. A positive wound culture without signs of inflammation or infection, a positive sputum culture without pulmonary infiltrates on chest x-ray, or a positive urine culture in a catheterized patient without signs or symptoms of pyelonephritis are all likely to represent colonization, not infection, and would not require antimicrobial therapy.

Prevention is of paramount importance in controlling nosocomial infections. The concept of universal precautions emphasizes that all patients should be treated as though they have a potential blood-borne transmissible disease, and thus all body secretions should be handled with care to prevent spread of disease. Almost all hospitals have implemented body substance isolation, which requires use of gloves whenever a health care worker anticipates contact with blood or other body secretions. The use of gloves is intended to prevent contamination of the hands of health care workers with infected secretions and subsequent spread of infection to other patients by direct contact. Hand washing is the easiest and most effective means of preventing nosocomial infections and should be done routinely even when gloves are utilized. Foley catheters, intravenous lines, hemodynamic monitoring devices, hyperalimentation lines, and similar invasive devices should be used only when critical to patient care and, when used, should be discontinued at the earliest possible time. Peripheral intravenous lines should be replaced every 3 days and arterial lines every 4 days. Lines in the central venous circulation (including those placed peripherally) can be left in indefinitely and are changed or removed when they are clinically suspected of being infected, when they are nonfunctional, or when they are no longer needed. Silver alloy-impregnated Foley catheters reduce the incidence of catheter-associated bacteriuria, and antibiotic-impregnated (minocycline plus rifampin) venous catheters reduce line infections and bacteremia. Whether the increased cost of these devices justifies their routine use is yet to be determined. Selective decontamination of the digestive tract with nonabsorbable antibiotics to prevent nosocomial pneumonia is widely used in Europe, but the therapeutic efficacy of this expensive intervention is controversial. Attentive nursing care (positioning to prevent decubitus ulcers, wound care, elevating the head during tube feedings to prevent aspiration) is critical in preventing nosocomial infections. In addition, careful monitoring of high-risk areas (intensive care units, neonatal units, surgical floors, hemodialysis and transplant units, etc) by skilled personnel—hospital epidemiologists—to detect increases in infection rates early is a key factor in prevention of these types of infections.

Several highly efficacious vaccines have been approved by the FDA that add to our armamentarium for prevention of certain nosocomial infections. Hepatitis A, hepatitis B, and the varicella vaccine should be considered in the appropriate setting. (See section below on Immunization Against Infectious Diseases.)

Gerberding JL et al: Emerging nosocomial infections and antimicrobial resistance. Curr Clin Top Infect Dis 1999;19:83. [NLM Cit ID: 99401701]

Ratula WA et al: (editors) Nosocomial infections. Infect Dis Clin North Am 1997;11(2). (A variety of issues are discussed, including drug-resistant organisms, nosocomial pneumonias, molecular epidemiology, and prevention.)

INFECTIONS OF THE CENTRAL NERVOUS SYSTEM

Infections of the central nervous system can be caused by almost any infectious agent, including bacteria, mycobacteria, fungi, spirochetes, protozoa, helminths, and viruses. Certain symptoms and signs are common to all types of central nervous system infection: headache, fever, sensorial disturbances, neck and back stiffness, positive Kernig and Brudzinski signs, and cerebrospinal fluid abnormalities. Although it is rare for all of these manifestations to be present in any one individual, the presence of even one of them should suggest the possibility of a central nervous system infection.

Central nervous system infection constitutes a *medical emergency*. Immediate diagnostic steps must be instituted to establish the specific cause. Normally, these include the history, physical examination, blood count, blood culture, lumbar puncture followed by careful study and culture of the cerebrospinal fluid, and a chest film. The fluid must be examined for cell count, glucose, and protein, and a smear must be stained for bacteria (and acid-fast organisms when appropriate) and cultured for pyogenic organisms and for mycobacteria and fungi when indicated. Latex agglutination tests can detect antigens of encapsulated organisms (*S pneumoniae, H influenzae, N meningitidis,* and *Cryptococcus neoformans*) but are rarely used except for detection of cryptococcus. Polymerase chain reaction (PCR) testing of cerebrospinal fluid has been employed to detect bacteria (*S pneumoniae, H influenzae, N meningitidis, Mycobacterium tuberculosis, Borrelia burgdorferi,* and *Tropheryma whippelii*) and viruses (herpes simplex, varicella-zoster, cytomegalovirus, Epstein-Barr virus, and enteroviruses) in patients with meningitis. The greatest experience is with PCR for herpes simplex, and the test is very sensitive (greater than 95%) and specific. Tests to detect the other organisms are generally more sensitive than culture, but the real value is the rapidity with which results are available, ie, hours compared with days or weeks. At present, with the exception of PCR for herpes simplex, these tests are performed only in reference laboratories. Although it is difficult to prove with existing clinical data that early antibiotic therapy improves outcome in bacterial meningitis, prompt therapy is still recommended.

Since performing a lumbar puncture in the presence of a space-occupying lesion (brain abscess, subdural hematoma, subdural abscess) can result in brain stem herniation and death, a CT scan is performed prior to lumbar puncture if a space-occupying lesion is suspected on the basis of papilledema, coma, seizures, or focal neurologic findings. If delays are encountered in obtaining a CT scan and bacterial meningitis is suspected, blood cultures should be drawn and antibiotics should be administered even before cerebrospinal fluid is obtained for culture to avoid unnecessary delays in treatment (Table 30–1). Animal studies suggest that antibiotics given within 4 hours before obtaining cerebrospinal fluid will not affect culture results.

Etiologic Classification

Central nervous system infections can be divided into several categories that usually can be readily distinguished from each other by cerebrospinal fluid examination as the first step toward etiologic diagnosis (Table 30–2).

A. Purulent Meningitis: Patients with bacterial meningitis usually present acutely within hours or 1–2 days after onset of symptoms. The organisms responsible depend primarily on the age of the patient as summarized in Table 30–1. The diagnosis is usually based on the Gram-stained smear (positive in 60–80%) or culture (positive in over 90%).

B. Chronic Meningitis: Patients with chronic meningitis present less acutely with a history of symptoms lasting weeks to months. The most common pathogens are *Mycobacterium tuberculosis,* atypical mycobacteria, fungi (cryptococcus, coccidioides, histoplasma), and spirochetes (*Treponema pallidum,* the agent of meningovascular syphilis; and *Borrelia burgdorferi,* the agent of Lyme disease). The diagnosis is made by culture or in some cases by serologic tests (cryptococcosis, coccidioidomycosis, syphilis, Lyme disease).

C. Aseptic Meningitis: Aseptic meningitis—a much more benign and self-limited syndrome than purulent meningitis—is caused principally by viruses, especially mumps virus and the enterovirus group (including coxsackieviruses and echoviruses). Infectious mononucleosis may be accompanied by aseptic meningitis. Leptospiral infection is usually placed in the aseptic group because of the lymphocytic cellular response and its relatively benign course. This type of meningitis also occurs during secondary syphilis and stage 2 Lyme disease.

D. Encephalitis: Encephalitis (due to herpesviruses, arboviruses, rabies virus, and many other viruses) produces disturbances of the sensorium, seizures, and many other manifestations. Patients present more acutely and are more ill than patients with aseptic meningitis. Cerebrospinal fluid may be entirely normal or may show some lymphocytes.

E. Partially Treated Bacterial Meningitis: Previous effective antibiotic therapy given for 12–24 hours will decrease the rate of positive Gram stain results by 20% and culture by 30–40% but will have little effect on cell count, protein, or glucose. Occasionally, previous antibiotic therapy will change a predominantly polymorphonuclear response to a lymphocytic pleocytosis, and some of the cerebrospinal fluid findings may be similar to those seen in aseptic meningitis.

F. Neighborhood Reaction: As noted in Table 30–2, this term denotes a purulent infectious process in close proximity to the central nervous system that spills some of the products of the inflammatory process—white blood cells or protein—into the cerebrospinal fluid. Such an infection might be a brain abscess, osteomyelitis of the vertebrae, epidural abscess, subdural empyema, or bacterial sinusitis or mastoiditis.

G. Noninfectious Meningeal Irritation: Meningismus, presenting with the classic signs of meningeal irritation with totally normal cerebrospinal fluid findings, may occur in the presence of other infections such as pneumonia and shigellosis. Carcinomatous meningitis, sarcoidosis, systemic lupus erythematosus, chemical meningitis, and certain drugs—NSAIDs, muromonab-CD3 (OKT3), trimethoprim-sulfamethoxazole, and others—can also produce symptoms and signs of meningeal irritation with associated cerebrospinal fluid pleocytosis, increased protein, and low or normal glucose.

Table 30–1. Initial antimicrobial therapy for purulent meningitis of unknown cause.

Age Group	Common Microorganisms	Standard Therapy
18–50 years	*S pneumoniae,*[1] *N meningitidis*	Cefotaxime or ceftriaxone[2]
Over 50 years	*S pneumoniae,*[1] *N meningitidis, L monocytogenes,* gram-negative bacilli	Ampicillin,[3] cefotaxime, or ceftriaxone[2]
Impaired cellular immunity	*L monocytogenes,* gram-negative bacilli, *S pneumoniae*	Ampicillin[3] plus ceftazidime[4]
Postsurgical or posttraumatic	*S aureus, S pneumoniae,*[1] gram-negative bacilli	Vancomycin[5] plus ceftazidime[4]

[1]In areas where penicillin-resistant pneumococcus is prevalent, vancomycin, 15 mg/kg every 8 hours, should be included in the regimen.
[2]The usual dose of cefotaxime is 2 g every 6 hours and that of ceftriaxone is 2 g every 12 hours. If the organism is sensitive to penicillin, 3–4 million units IV every 4 hours is given.
[3]The dose of ampicillin is usually 2 g IV every 4 hours.
[4]Ceftazidime is given in a dose of 50–100 mg/kg every 8 hours up to 2 g every 8 hours.
[5]The dose of vancomycin is 15 mg/kg every 8 hours.

Table 30–2. Typical cerebrospinal fluid findings in various central nervous system diseases.

Diagnosis	Cells/μL	Glucose (mg/dL)	Protein (mg/dL)	Opening Pressure
Normal	0–5 lymphocytes	45–85[1]	15–45	70–180 mm H_2O
Purulent meningitis (bacterial)[2] community-acquired	200–20,000 polymorphonuclear neutrophils	Low (< 45)	High (> 50)	Markedly elevated
Granulomatous meningitis (mycobacterial, fungal)[3]	100–1000, mostly lymphocytes[3]	Low (< 45)	High (> 50)	Moderately elevated
Spirochetal meningitis	100–1000, mostly lymphocytes[3]	Normal	Moderately high (> 50)	Normal to slightly elevated
Aseptic meningitis, viral or meningoencephalitis[4]	25–2000, mostly lymphocytes[3]	Normal or low	High (> 50)	Slightly elevated
"Neighborhood reaction"[5]	Variably increased	Normal	Normal or high	Variable

[1]Cerebrospinal fluid glucose must be considered in relation to blood glucose level. Normally, cerebrospinal fluid glucose is 20–30 mg/dL lower than blood glucose, or 50–70% of the normal value of blood glucose.
[2]Organisms in smear or culture of cerebrospinal fluid; counterimmunoelectrophoresis or latex agglutination may be diagnostic.
[3]Polymorphonuclear neutrophils may predominate early.
[4]Viral isolation from cerebrospinal fluid early; antibody titer rise in paired specimens of serum; PCR for herpesvirus.
[5]May occur in mastoiditis, brain abscess, epidural abscess, sinusitis, septic thrombus, brain tumor. Cerebrospinal fluid culture results usually negative.

H. Brain Abscess: Brain abscess presents as a space-occupying lesion; symptoms may include vomiting, fever, change of mental status, or focal neurologic manifestations. If brain abscess is suspected, a CT scan should precede lumbar puncture. The bacteriology of brain abscess is usually polymicrobial and includes *S aureus,* gram-negative bacilli, streptococci, and anaerobes (including anaerobic streptococci and prevotella species).

I. Amebic Meningoencephalitis: These infections are caused by free-living amebas and present as two distinct syndromes. The diagnosis is confirmed by culture or identification of the organism in cerebrospinal fluid or on biopsy specimens. No effective therapy is available.

1. Primary amebic meningoencephalitis is caused by *Naegleria fowleri* and is an acute fulminant disease characterized by signs of meningeal irritation that rapidly progresses to encephalitis and death. Anecdotal reports of cure of primary amebic meningoencephalitis have been reported with intravenous and intraventricular administration of amphotericin B.

2. Granulomatous amebic encephalitis is caused by acanthamoeba species. It is an indolent disease characterized by headache, nausea, vomiting, cranial neuropathies, seizures, and hemiparesis.

Treatment

Treatment consists of supportive care and specific antimicrobial therapy directed at the causative organism. Increased intracranial pressure due to brain edema often requires therapeutic attention. Hyperventilation, mannitol (25–50 g as a bolus intravenous infusion), and even drainage of cerebrospinal fluid by repeated lumbar punctures or by placement of ventricular catheters have been employed to control cerebral edema and increased intracranial pressure. Dexamethasone (4 mg every 4–6 hours) may also decrease cerebral edema. In the case of purulent meningitis, proper antimicrobial treatment is imperative. Since the identity of the causative microorganism may remain unknown or doubtful for a few days, initial antibiotic treatment as set forth in Table 30–1 should be directed against the microorganisms most common for each age group.

The duration of therapy for bacterial meningitis varies depending upon the etiologic agent: *H influenzae* 7 days; *N meningitidis* 7 days; *S pneumoniae* 10–14 days; *L monocytogenes* 14–21 days; gram-negative bacilli 21 days.

Although dexamethasone therapy is standard in infants and children with meningitis, prospective controlled studies have not been performed in adults. Nonetheless, because adverse effects are minimal and some benefit may occur, some clinicians have recommended dexamethasone, 0.15 mg/kg intravenously every 6 hours for 2–4 days, especially in patients with high bacterial loads (ie, positive Gram stain), increased intracranial pressure, or altered mental status.

Therapy of brain abscess consists of drainage (excision or aspiration) in addition to 3–4 weeks of systemic antibiotics directed against organisms isolated. A regimen often used includes metronidazole, 500 mg intravenously or orally every 8 hours, plus ceftizoxime, 2 g intravenously every 8 hours, or ceftriaxone, 2 g every 12 hours. In cases where abscesses are less than 2 cm in size, there are multiple abscesses that cannot be drained, or if an abscess is located in an area where significant neurologic sequelae would result from drainage, antibiotics for 6–8 weeks without drainage can be employed.

Therapy of other types of meningitis is discussed elsewhere in this book (fungal meningitis, Chapter 36; syphilis and Lyme borreliosis, Chapter 33; tuberculous meningitis, Chapter 34; herpes encephalitis, Chapter 32).

Johnson RT: Acute encephalitis. Clin Infect Dis 1996; 23:219. [NLM Cit ID: 96439942] (Comprehensive review.)

Quagliarello VJ et al: Treatment of bacterial meningitis. N Engl J Med 1997;336:708. [NLM Cit ID: 97177211] (Review of etiology and therapy, including use of corticosteroids and treatment of infection with penicillin-resistant pneumococci.)

Schaad UB (editor): Bacterial meningitis. Infect Dis Clin North Am 1997;13. (Entire issue.) (Several articles covering a variety of issues such as diagnosis, antibiotic therapy, drug resistance, anti-inflammatory therapy, and prophylaxis.)

Schuchat A et al: Bacterial meningitis in the United States in 1995. N Engl J Med 1997;337:970. [NLM Cit ID: 97441019] (Reviews 248 cases for recent trends in etiology by age.)

ANIMAL & HUMAN BITE WOUNDS

It is estimated that about 900 new dog bite injuries require emergency department attention each day and that about 1% of emergency room visits in urban areas are for treatment of animal and human bites. Dog bites occur most commonly in the summer months. Biting animals are usually known by their victims, and most biting incidents are provoked (ie, bites occur while playing with the animal or after surprising the animal or waking it abruptly from sleep). Failure to elicit a history of provocation is important, because an unprovoked attack raises the possibility that the animal is rabid. Human bites are usually inflicted by children while playing or fighting; in adults, bites are associated with alcohol use and closed-fist injuries that occur during fights.

The animal inflicting the bite, the location of the bite, and the type of injury inflicted are all important determinants of whether these injuries become infected. Cat bites are more likely to become infected than human bites—between 30% and 50% of all cat bites subsequently become infected. Infections following human bites are variable: Those inflicted by children rarely become infected, because they are superficial; and bites by adults become infected in 15–30% of cases, with a particularly high rate of infection in closed-fist injuries. Dog bites, for unclear reasons, become infected only 5% of the time. Bites of the head, face, and neck are less likely to become infected than bites on the extremities. Puncture wounds become infected more frequently than lacerations, probably because the latter are easier to irrigate and debride.

The bacteriology of bite infections depends upon the biting animal and when the infection occurs after the biting incident. Early infections (within 24 hours after the bite) following dog and cat bites are most frequently caused by *Pasteurella multocida.* These infections are characterized by rapid onset and progression, fevers, chills, cellulitis, and local adenopathy. Early infections following human bites are usually caused by mixed aerobic and anaerobic mouth flora and can produce a rapidly progressive necrotizing infection. Late infections (longer than 24 hours after the bite) are caused mainly by staphylococci, streptococci, and anaerobes (fusobacterium, bacteroides, prevotella), but innumerable organisms have been implicated in these infections. *Capnocytophaga canimorsus* (formerly called a DF2 organism), a gram-negative organism that is part of canine oral flora; *Eikenella corrodens,* another gram-negative organism that can be part of human mouth flora; haemophilus species, pseudomonas species, and other gram-negative organisms—all have been implicated in bite infections.

There have been no documented cases of HIV transmission by human bites.

Treatment

A. Local Care: Vigorous cleansing and irrigation of the wound as well as debridement of necrotic material are the most important factors in decreasing the incidence of infections. X-rays should be obtained to look for fractures and the presence of foreign bodies. Careful examination to assess the extent of the injury (tendon laceration, joint space penetration) is critical to appropriate care.

B. Suturing: If wounds require closure for cosmetic or mechanical reasons, suturing can be done. However, one should never suture a wound that is already infected, and wounds of the hand should generally not be sutured since a closed-space infection of the hand can result in loss of function.

C. Prophylactic Antibiotics: Prophylaxis is indicated in high-risk bites, eg, cat bites in any location (dicloxacillin, 0.5 g orally four times a day for 3–5 days) and hand bites by any animal or by humans (penicillin V, 0.5 g orally four times a day for 3–5 days). Although dicloxacillin and penicillin have been most extensively studied for prophylaxis, there is concern about their use because of their narrow spectrum of activity. Based on the microbiology of bite wounds noted above, other agents that have not been adequately studied but that have broader spectrums of activity may be even more effective as prophylactic agents. Examples include cefuroxime, amoxicillin-clavulanic acid, and, in the penicillin-allergic patient, clindamycin plus a fluoroquinolone. Immunocompromised patients and especially individuals without functional spleens are at risk for developing overwhelming bacteremia and sepsis following animal bites and should also receive prophylaxis.

D. Antibiotics: For wounds that are infected, antibiotics are clearly indicated. How they are given (orally or intravenously) and the need for hospitalization are individualized clinical decisions. In general, *P multocida* is best treated with penicillin or a tetracycline. Other active agents include second- and third-generation cephalosporins, fluoroquinolones, or azithromycin and clarithromycin. Response to therapy is slow, and therapy should be continued for at least 2–3 weeks. Human bites frequently require admission to the hospital and intravenous therapy with a β-lactam plus a β-lactamase inhibitor combination (Unasyn, Timentin, Zosyn), a second-generation cephalosporin with anaerobic activity (cefoxitin, cefotetan, cefmetazole), or, in the penicillin-allergic patient, clindamycin plus a fluoroquinolone. Because the bacteriology of these infections is so variable, one should always culture infected wounds and adjust therapy appropriately, especially if the patient is not responding to initial empirical treatment.

E. Tetanus and Rabies: All patients must be evaluated for the need for tetanus (see Chapter 33) and rabies (see Chapter 32) prophylaxis.

Goldstein EJ: Current concepts on animal bites: bacteriology and therapy. Curr Clin Top Infect Dis 1999;19:99. [NLM Cit ID: 99401702]

Talan DA et al: Bacteriologic analysis of infected dog and cat bites. N Engl J Med 1999;340:85. [NLM Cit ID: 99091092] (Prospective analysis of bacteriology with discussion of therapy.)

SEXUALLY TRANSMITTED DISEASES

Some infectious diseases are transmitted most commonly—or most efficiently—by sexual contact. Most of the infectious agents that cause sexually transmitted diseases are fairly easily inactivated when exposed to a harsh environment. They are thus particularly suited to transmission by contact with mucous membranes. They may be bacteria (eg, gonococci), spirochetes (syphilis), chlamydiae (nongonococcal urethritis, cervicitis), viruses (eg, herpes simplex, hepatitis B virus, cytomegalovirus, HIV), or protozoa (eg, trichomonas). In most infections caused by these agents, early lesions occur on genitalia or other sexually exposed mucous membranes; however, wide dissemination may occur, and involvement of nongenital tissues and organs may mimic many noninfectious disorders. All sexually transmitted diseases have subclinical or latent phases that play an important role in long-term persistence of the infection or in its transmission from infected (but largely asymptomatic) persons to other contacts. Laboratory examinations are of particular importance in the diagnosis of such asymptomatic patients. Simultaneous infection by several different agents is common, and any person with a sexually transmitted disease should be tested for syphilis. If the test is negative, a repeat study should be done in 3 months, since seroconversion can be delayed.

For each patient, there are one or more sexual contacts who require diagnosis and treatment. As a rule, sexual partners should be treated simultaneously to avoid prompt reinfection. The commonest sexually transmitted diseases are gonorrhea,* syphilis,* condyloma acuminatum, chlamydial genital infections, herpesvirus genital infections, *Trichomonas* vaginitis, chancroid,* granuloma inguinale,* scabies, louse infestation, and bacterial vaginosis (among lesbians). However, shigellosis,* hepatitis A, B, and C,* amebiasis,* giardiasis, cryptosporidiasis, salmonellosis,* and campylobacteriosis may also be transmitted by sexual (oral-anal) contact, especially in homosexual males. Homosexual contact is the most prevalent method of transmission of HIV and AIDS,* though bidirectional heterosexual transmission can also occur (see Chapter 31).

The risk of developing a sexually transmitted disease following a sexual assault has not been extensively studied. Victims of assault have a high baseline rate of infection (*N gonorrhoeae* 6%, *C trachomatis* 10%, *T vaginalis* 15%, and bacterial vaginosis 34%), and the risk of acquiring infection as a result of the assault is significant but is lower than the preexisting rate (*N gonorrhoeae* 6–12%, *C trachomatis* 4–17%, *T vaginalis* 12%, syphilis 0.5–3%, and bacterial vaginosis 19%). Victims should be evaluated within 24 hours after the assault, and cultures for *N gonorrhoeae, C trachomatis* (if culture is not available, nonculture tests, such as nucleic acid amplification tests, are acceptable), and herpes simplex virus should be obtained and vaginal secretions examined for trichomonas and bacterial vaginosis. In addition, a blood sample should be obtained for immediate serologic testing for syphilis, hepatitis B, and HIV. Follow-up examination for sexually transmitted disease should be repeated at 2 weeks, since concentrations of infecting organisms may not have been sufficient to produce a positive culture at the time of initial examination. Follow-up serologic testing for syphilis should be performed in 6, 12, and 24 weeks if the initial tests are negative. RNA testing for HIV should be done at 2 and 4 weeks if initial serologic tests are negative. Prophylactic antibiotics should be given if the assailant is known to be infected. The usefulness of presumptive therapy is controversial, some feeling that all patients should receive it and others that it should be limited to those in whom follow-up cannot be ensured or that it should be given

*Reportable to public health authorities.

only to those who request it. If therapy is given, a reasonable regimen would be hepatitis B vaccination (without hepatitis B immune globulin, the first dose given at the initial evaluation and follow-up doses at 1–2 months and 4–6 months) and one dose of ceftriaxone, 125 mg intramuscularly, plus metronidazole, 2 g orally as a single dose, plus doxycycline, 100 mg orally twice daily for 7 days, or azithromycin, 1 g orally as a single dose. If the patient is pregnant, azithromycin should be used instead of doxycycline, and metronidazole should be given only after the first trimester.

Although seroconversion to HIV has been reported following sexual assault when this was the only known risk, the risk of acquiring HIV is felt to be low. The likelihood of HIV transmission from anal or vaginal receptive intercourse when the source is known to be HIV positive is 1–3 per 1000. Because prophylactic antiretroviral therapy has not been studied in this setting, firm recommendations cannot be made and the decision to institute therapy should be individualized. Because of the time-dependent nature of postexposure prophylaxis, if therapy is given it should be as soon as possible after the assault and certainly within 72 hours.

Bamberger JD et al: Post-exposure prophylaxis for human immunodeficiency virus (HIV) infection following sexual assault. Am J Med 1999;106:323. [NLM Cit ID: 99204657] (Discussion of risk of infection and the risks and benefits of therapy with specific regimens.)

Hampton HL: Care of the woman who has been raped. N Engl J Med 1995;332:234. [NLM Cit ID: 95107364] (Review of medical, forensic, and psychologic issues associated with assault.)

1998 guidelines for treatment of sexually transmitted diseases. MMWR Morb Mortal Wkly Rep 1998;47(RR-1):1. [NLM Cit ID: 98120951]

INFECTIONS IN DRUG USERS

The abuse of parenterally administered narcotic drugs has increased enormously in recent years. There are now an estimated 300,000 or more intravenous drug users in the USA, mostly in or near large urban centers. Consequently, physicians and hospitals serving such urban and suburban populations must deal with many problems—including infections—related to drug abuse.

Common Infections That Occur With Greater Frequency in Drug Users

(1) **Skin infections** are associated with poor hygiene and use of nonsterile technique when injecting drugs. *S aureus* is the most common organism involved, but streptococci, enteric gram-negative organisms, and anaerobes can also cause skin infections. Cellulitis and subcutaneous abscesses occur most commonly. Myositis and necrotizing fasciitis occur infrequently but are life-threatening. Wound botulism in association with brown heroin use has also been reported.

(2) **Hepatitis** is very common among habitual drug users and is transmissible both by the parenteral (hepatitis B, C, and D virus) and by the fecal-oral route (hepatitis A). Multiple episodes of hepatitis with different agents can occur.

(3) **Aspiration pneumonia** and its complications (lung abscess, empyema, brain abscess) result from altered consciousness associated with drug abuse. Mixed aerobic and anaerobic mouth flora are usually involved.

(4) **Tuberculosis** also occurs in drug users, and infection with HIV has fostered the spread of tuberculosis in this population. Morbidity and mortality rates are increased in HIV-infected individuals with tuberculosis. Tuberculosis should be suspected in those who have classic radiographic findings and in those with infiltrates who do not respond to antibiotics.

(5) **Pulmonary septic emboli** may originate from venous thrombi or right-sided endocarditis.

(6) **Sexually transmitted diseases** are not directly related to drug abuse, but the practice of exchanging sex for drugs has resulted in an increased frequency of sexually transmitted diseases. Syphilis, gonorrhea, and chancroid are the most common.

(7) **AIDS** has a high incidence among intravenous drug users and their sexual contacts and the offspring of infected women (see Chapter 31).

(8) **Infective endocarditis** (see below). A number of complications of endocarditis can occur, including splenic abscesses, central nervous system infections (meningitis, brain abscess, subdural empyema, epidural abscess), and endophthalmitis.

(9) **Other vascular infections** include septic thrombophlebitis and mycotic aneurysms. Mycotic aneurysms resulting from direct trauma to a vessel with secondary infection most commonly occur in femoral arteries and less commonly in arteries of the neck. Aneurysms resulting from hematogenous spread of organisms frequently involve intracerebral vessels and are seen in association with endocarditis.

Infections Rare in USA

A. Tetanus: In the 1950s and 1960s, tetanus was commonly seen in drug users, especially in unimmunized women who injected drugs subcutaneously ("skin-popping"). Increased tetanus immunization among drug users has resulted in a decline in this disease, though cases are still reported.

B. Malaria: Needle transmission occurs from intravenous drug users who acquired the infection in malaria-endemic areas outside the USA.

C. Melioidosis: This chronic pulmonary infection caused by *Pseudomonas pseudomallei* is occasionally seen in debilitated drug users.

Osteomyelitis & Septic Arthritis

Osteomyelitis involving vertebral bodies, sternoclavicular joints, the pubic symphysis, the sacroiliac joints, and other sites usually results from hematogenous distribution of injected organisms or septic venous thrombi. Pain and fever precede radiographic changes, sometimes by several weeks. While staphylococci—often methicillin-resistant—are common organisms, serratia, pseudomonas, candida, and other pathogens rarely encountered in spontaneous bone or joint disease are found in intravenous drug users.

Infective Endocarditis

The organisms that cause infective endocarditis in those who use drugs intravenously are most commonly *S aureus,* candida (especially *Candida parapsilosis*), *Enterococcus faecalis,* other streptococci, and gram-negative bacteria (especially pseudomonas and *Serratia marcescens*).

Involvement of the right side of the heart is somewhat more frequent than involvement of the left side, and infection of more than one valve is not infrequent. Right-sided involvement, especially in the absence of murmurs, is often suggested by the presence of septic pulmonary emboli. The diagnosis must be established by blood culture. Therapy, including empirical treatment, is discussed in Chapter 33.

Approach to the Patient

A common and difficult clinical problem is management of the parenteral drug user who presents with fever. In general, after obtaining appropriate cultures (blood, urine, and sputum if the chest x-ray is abnormal), empirical therapy is begun. If the chest x-ray is suggestive of a community-acquired pneumonia (consolidation), therapy for outpatient pneumonia is begun with a second- or third-generation cephalosporin (many would add erythromycin to this regimen). If the chest x-ray is suggestive of septic emboli (nodular infiltrates), therapy for presumed endocarditis is initiated, usually with a combination of nafcillin and gentamicin. Ampicillin should be added if enterococci are a consideration. If the chest x-ray is normal and no focal site of infection can be found, endocarditis is presumed. While awaiting the results of blood cultures, empirical treatment with nafcillin and gentamicin (with or without ampicillin) is started. If blood cultures are positive for organisms that frequently cause endocarditis in drug users (see above), endocarditis is presumed to be present and treated accordingly. If blood cultures are positive for an organism that is an unusual cause of endocarditis, evaluation for an occult source of infection should go forward. In this setting, a transesophageal echocardiogram may be quite helpful since it is 90% sensitive in detecting vegetations and a negative study is strong evidence against endocarditis. If blood cultures are negative and the patient responds to antibiotics, therapy should be continued for 7–14 days (oral therapy can be given once an initial response has occurred). In every patient, careful examination for an occult source of infection (genitourinary, dental, sinus, gallbladder, etc) should be done.

Levine DP, Brown PD: Infections in injection drug users. In: *Principles and Practice of Infectious Diseases,* 5th ed. Mandell GL, Bennett JR, Dolin R (editors). Churchill Livingstone, 2000.

ACUTE INFECTIOUS DIARRHEA

Diarrheal syndromes are arbitrarily divided into acute (those lasting less than 2 weeks) and chronic diseases and are said to be mild if there are three or fewer stools per day, moderate if there are four or more stools in association with local symptoms (abdominal cramps, nausea, tenesmus), and severe if there are four or more stools per day with systemic symptoms (fevers, chills, dehydration). Acute diarrhea can be caused by a number of different factors, including emotional stress, food intolerance, inorganic agents (eg, sodium nitrite), organic substances (eg, mushrooms, shellfish), drugs, and infectious agents (including viruses, bacteria, and protozoa). From a diagnostic and therapeutic standpoint, it is helpful to classify infectious diarrhea into syndromes that produce inflammatory or bloody diarrhea and those that are noninflammatory, nonbloody, or watery. In general, the term "inflammatory diarrhea" suggests colonic involvement by invasive bacteria or parasites or toxin production that affects the large bowel. Clinically, patients present with frequent bloody, small-volume stools, often associated with fever, abdominal cramps, tenesmus, and fecal urgency. Common causes of this syndrome include shigella, salmonella, campylobacter, yersinia, invasive strains of *E coli, E coli* O157:H7, *Entamoeba histolytica,* and *Clostridium difficile.* Tests for fecal leukocytes are frequently positive, and definitive etiologic diagnosis requires stool culture. Noninflammatory diarrhea is generally a milder disease and is caused by viruses or toxins that affect the small intestine and interfere with salt and water balance, resulting in large-volume watery diarrhea, often with nausea, vomiting, and cramps. Common causes of this syndrome include viruses (eg, rotavirus, Norwalk virus, enteric adenoviruses, astrovirus, coronavirus), vibrios *(V cholerae, V parahaemolyticus, V vulnificus),* enterotoxin-producing *E coli, Giardia lamblia,* cryptosporidia, and agents that can cause food-borne gastroenteritis.

The term "food poisoning" denotes diseases caused by toxins present in consumed foods. When the incubation period is short (1–6 hours after consumption), the toxin is usually preformed and present in the contaminated food. Vomiting is usually a major complaint, and fever is usually absent. Examples include intoxication from *S aureus* or *Bacillus cereus,* and toxin can be detected in the food. When the incubation period is longer—between 8 and 16 hours—the organism is present in the food and produces toxin after being ingested. Vomiting is less prominent, abdominal cramps are frequent, and fever is often absent. The best example of this disease is that due to *Clostridium perfringens.* Toxin can be detected in food or stool specimens.

The inflammatory and noninflammatory diarrheas discussed above can also be transmitted by food and water and usually have incubation periods between 12 and 72 hours. Cyclospora, cryptosporidia, and isospora are protozoans capable of causing disease in both immunocompetent and immunocompromised patients. Characteristics of disease include profuse watery diarrhea that is prolonged but usually self-limited (1–2 weeks) in the immunocompetent patient but can be chronic in the compromised host. Epidemiologic features may be helpful in determining etiology. Recent hospitalization or antibiotic use suggests *C difficile;* recent foreign travel suggests salmonella, shigella, campylobacter, *E coli,* or *V cholerae;* undercooked hamburger suggests *E coli,* especially O157:H7; fried rice consumption is associated with *B cereus* toxin. Prominent features of some of these causes of diarrhea are listed in Table 30–3.

Treatment usually consists of replacement of fluids and electrolytes and, very rarely, management of hypovolemic shock and respiratory compromise. In general, most cases of acute gastroenteritis are self-limited and do not require therapy other than supportive measures. When symptoms persist beyond 3–4 days, initial presentation is accompanied by fever or bloody diarrhea, or the patient is immunocompromised, cultures of stool are usually obtained. Symptoms have often resolved by the time cultures are completed. In this case, even if a pathogen is isolated, therapy is not needed (except for shigella, since the infecting dose is so small that therapy to eradicate organisms from the stool is indicated for epidemiologic reasons). If symptoms persist and a pathogen is isolated, it is reasonable to institute specific treatment even though therapy has not been conclusively shown to alter the natural history of disease for most pathogens. Exceptions include gastroenteritis due to salmonella (where therapy may prolong the carrier state and increase the relapse rate) and campylobacter (early therapy shortens the course of disease). Several studies examining the effect of antibiotic therapy on domestically acquired diarrhea have suggested that ciprofloxacin, 500 mg every 12 hours for 5 days, is effective in shortening the course of illness compared with placebo. Because of concerns about selecting for resistant organisms coupled with the fact that most infectious diarrhea is self-limited, routine use of antibiotics for all patients with diarrhea is not recommended. Antibiotics should be considered in patients with evidence of invasive disease (white cells in stool, dysentery), with symptoms 3–4 days or more in duration, with multiple stools (eight to ten or more per day) and in those with impaired immune responses. Antimotility drugs may relieve cramping and decrease diarrhea in mild cases. Their use should be limited to patients without fever and without dysentery (bloody stools), and they should be used in low doses.

Therapeutic recommendations for specific agents can be found elsewhere in this book.

Aranda-Michel J et al: Acute diarrhea: a practical review. Am J Med 1999;106:670. [NLM Cit ID: 99304971] (Review of causes with discussion of who should receive cultures and be treated.)

TRAVELER'S DIARRHEA

Whenever a person travels from one country to another—particularly if the change involves a marked difference in climate, social conditions, or sanitation standards and facilities—diarrhea is likely to develop within 2–10 days. There may be up to ten or even more loose stools per day, often accompanied by abdominal cramps, nausea, occasionally vomiting, and rarely fever. The stools do not usually contain mucus or blood, and aside from weakness and dehydration there are no systemic manifestations of infection. The illness usually subsides spontaneously within 1–5 days, although 10% remain symptomatic for a week or longer, and in 2% symptoms persist for longer than a month.

Bacteria cause 80% of cases of traveler's diarrhea, with enterotoxigenic *E coli,* shigella species, and *Campylobacter jejuni* being the most common pathogens. Less common causative agents include aeromonas, salmonella, noncholera vibrios, *Entamoeba histolytica,* and *Giardia lamblia.* Contributory causes may at times include unusual food and drink, change in living habits, occasional viral infections (adenoviruses or rotaviruses), and change in bowel flora. In patients with fever and bloody diarrhea, stool culture may be indicated, but in most cases cultures are reserved for those who do not respond to antibiotics. Chronic watery diarrhea may be due to amebiasis or giardiasis or, rarely, tropical sprue.

For most individuals, the affliction is short-lived, and symptomatic therapy with opioids or loperamide is all that is required provided the patient is not systemically ill (fever ≥ 39 °C) and does not have dysentery (bloody stools), in which case antimotility agents should be avoided. Packages of oral rehydration salts to treat dehydration are available over the counter in the USA (Infalyte, Pedialyte, others) and in many foreign countries. Avoidance of fresh foods and water sources that are likely to be contaminated is recommended for travelers to developing countries, where infectious diarrheal illnesses are endemic. Prophylaxis is recommended for those with significant underlying disease (inflammatory bowel disease, AIDS, diabetes, heart disease in the elderly, conditions requiring immunosuppressive medications) and for those whose

Table 30–3. Acute bacterial diarrheas and "food poisoning."

Organism	Incubation Period (hours)	Vomiting	Diarrhea	Fever	Microbiology	Pathogenesis	Clinical Features and Treatment
Staphylococcus	1–8, rarely up to 18	+++	+	–	Staphylococci grow in meats and in dairy and bakery products and produce enterotoxin.	Enterotoxin acts on receptors in gut that transmit impulses to medullary centers.	Abrupt onset, intense vomiting for up to 24 hours, regular recovery in 24–48 hours. Occurs in persons eating the same food. No treatment usually necessary except to restore fluids and electrolytes.
Bacillus cereus	1–8, rarely up to 18	+++	+	–	Reheated fried rice causes vomiting or diarrhea.	Enterotoxins formed in food or in gut from growth of *B cereus*.	After 1–6 hours, mainly vomiting. After 8–16 hours, mainly diarrhea. Both self-limited to less than 1 day.
Clostridium perfringens	8–16	±	+++	–	Clostridia grow in rewarmed meat dishes and produce an enterotoxin.	Enterotoxin produced in food and in gut causes hypersecretion in small intestine.	Abrupt onset of profuse diarrhea; vomiting occasionally. Recovery usual without treatment in 1–4 days. Many clostridia in cultures of food and feces of patients.
Clostridium botulinum	24–96	±	Rare	–	Clostridia grow in anaerobic foods and produce toxin.	Toxin absorbed from gut blocks acetylcholine at neuromuscular junction.	Diplopia, dysphagia, dysphonia, respiratory embarrassment. Treatment requires clear airway, ventilation, and intravenous polyvalent antitoxin (see text). Toxin present in food and serum. Mortality rate high
Clostridium difficile	?	–	+++	+	Associated with antimicrobial drugs, eg, clindamycin.	Enterotoxin causes epithelial necrosis in colon; pseudomembranous colitis.	Especially after abdominal surgery, abrupt bloody diarrhea and fever. Toxin in stool. Oral vancomycin or metronidazole useful in therapy.
Escherichia coli (some strains)	24–72	±	+	–	Organisms grow in gut and produce toxin. May also invade superficial epithelium.	Enterotoxin causes hypersecretion in small intestine.	Usually abrupt onset of diarrhea; vomiting rare. A serious infection in neonates. In adults, "traveler's diarrhea" is usually self-limited to 1–3 days and does respond to a fluoroquinolone.

(*continued*)

Table 30–3. Acute bacterial diarrheas and "food poisoning." (continued)

Organism	Incubation Period (hours)	Vomiting	Diarrhea	Fever	Microbiology	Pathogenesis	Clinical Features and Treatment
Vibrio parahaemolyticus	6–96	+	+	±	Organisms grow in seafood and in gut and produce toxin or invade.	Hypersecretion in small intestine; stools may be bloody.	Abrupt onset of diarrhea in groups consuming the same food, especially crabs and other seafood. Recovery is usually complete in 1–3 days. Food and stool cultures are positive.
Vibrio cholerae (mild cases)	24–72	+	+++	–	Organisms grow in gut and produce toxin.	Enterotoxin causes hypersecretion in small intestine. Infective dose: 10^7–10^9 organisms.	Abrupt onset of liquid diarrhea in endemic area. Needs prompt replacement of fluids and electrolytes intravenously or orally. Tetracyclines shorten excretion of vibrios. Stool cultures positive.
Campylobacter jejuni	2–10 days	–	+++	+	Organisms grow in jejunum and ileum.	Invasion and enterotoxin production uncertain.	Fever, diarrhea; PMNs and fresh blood in stool, especially in children. Usually self-limited. Special media needed for culture at 43 °C. Give a fluoroquinolone in severe cases with invasion. Recovery in 5–8 days is usual.
Shigella species (mild cases)	24–72	±	+	+	Organisms grow in superficial gut epithelium and gut lumen and produce toxin.	Organisms invade epithelial cells; blood, mucus, and PMNs in stools. Infective dose: 10^2–10^3 organisms.	Abrupt onset of diarrhea, often with blood and pus in stools, cramps, tenesmus, and lethargy. Stool cultures are positive. Therapy depends on sensitivity testing, but the fluoroquinolones are most effective. Do not give opioids. Often mild and self-limited.
Salmonella species	8–48	±	+	+	Organisms grow in gut. Do not produce toxin.	Superficial infection of gut, little invasion. Infective dose: 10^5 organisms.	Gradual or abrupt onset of diarrhea and low-grade fever. No antimicrobials unless systemic dissemination is suspected, in which case give a fluoroquinolone. Stool cultures are positive. Prolonged carriage is common.
Yersinia enterocolitica	?	±	+	+	Fecal-oral transmission (occasionally). Food-borne. In pets.	Gastroenteritis or mesenteric adenitis. Occasional bacteremia. Enterotoxin produced.	Severe abdominal pain, diarrhea, fever. PMNs and blood in stool; polyarthritis, erythema nodosum in children. If severe, give tetracycline or gentamicin. Keep stool at 4 °C before culture.

full activity status during the trip is so essential that even short periods of diarrhea would be unacceptable. Prophylaxis is started upon entry into the destination country and is continued for 1 or 2 days after leaving. For stays of more than 3 weeks, prophylaxis is not recommended because of the cost and increased toxicity. For prophylaxis, bismuth subsalicylate is effective but turns the tongue and the stools black and can interfere with doxycycline absorption, which may be needed for malaria prophylaxis. Numerous antimicrobial regimens for once-daily prophylaxis also are effective, such as norfloxacin 400 mg, ciprofloxacin 500 mg, ofloxacin 300 mg, or trimethoprim-sulfamethoxazole 160/800 mg. Because not all travelers will have diarrhea and because most episodes are brief and self-limited, an alternative approach that is currently recommended is to provide the traveler with a supply of antimicrobials to be taken if significant diarrhea occurs during the trip. Loperamide (4 mg loading dose, then 2 mg after each loose stool to a maximum of 16 mg/d) with a single dose of ciprofloxacin (750 mg), levofloxacin (500 mg), or ofloxacin (300 mg) cures most cases of traveler's diarrhea. If diarrhea is severe, associated with fever or bloody stools, or persists despite single-dose ciprofloxacin treatment, then 3–5 days of ciprofloxacin 500 mg twice daily, levofloxacin 500 mg once daily, norfloxacin 400 mg twice daily, or ofloxacin 300 mg twice daily can be given. Trimethoprim-sulfamethoxazole 160/800 mg twice daily can be used as an alternative, but resistance is common in many areas.

Ansdell VE et al: Prevention and empiric treatment of traveler's diarrhea. Med Clin North Am 1999;83:945. [NLM Cit ID: 99382630] (Comprehensive review of epidemiology, prevention and therapy.)

DuPont HL et al: Persistent diarrhea in travelers. Clin Infect Dis 1996;22:124. [NLM Cit ID: 96422358] (Etiology, diagnosis, and therapy.)

Passaro DJ et al: Advances in prevention and management of traveler's diarrhea. Curr Clin Top Infect Dis 1998;18:217. [NLM Cit ID: 98452393] (Review of causes, prevention, and therapy.)

ACTIVE IMMUNIZATION AGAINST INFECTIOUS DISEASES

RECOMMENDED IMMUNIZATION OF INFANTS, CHILDREN, & ADOLESCENTS

Every individual—child or adult—should maintain an adequate defense against infectious disease by immunization. The recommended schedules and dosages change often, so that one should always consult the manufacturer's package inserts.

The schedule for active immunizations in children is presented in Table 30–4 Of note is the recommendation that all adolescents should see a health care provider at age 11–12. The objective is to ensure vaccination of those who have not received varicella or hepatitis B vaccine; to make certain that a second dose of measles-mumps-rubella (MMR) has been given as well as a booster for tetanus and diphtheria (Td); and to provide immunizations (influenza and pneumococcal vaccines) that may be indicated for certain high-risk individuals.

RECOMMENDED IMMUNIZATION OF ADULTS

Several vaccines are recommended for adults depending upon the individual's previous vaccination status and the risks of exposure to certain diseases.

Tetanus-Diphtheria Toxoid

Everyone should receive a primary series of immunizations against tetanus and diphtheria once (Table 30–4). Adults who have not previously been immunized should receive two doses of Td 1–2 months apart, followed by a booster dose 6–12 months later. Adults partially immunized in childhood with DTP need only a total of three doses of tetanus and diphtheria toxoid (ie, if one dose was given in childhood, give two doses of Td; if two doses were given, only one dose of Td is needed to complete primary immunization). The traditional recommendation has been to give booster doses of Td every 10 years throughout life. An alternative approach emphasizes ensuring that all adults receive primary immunization and recommending a single midlife (age 50 years) booster dose of Td to those who have received the full pediatric immunization, including the booster in the teenage years. If booster doses are given too frequently, an Arthus reaction as well as severe local pain and swelling can occur. An acellular pertussis vaccine, which is highly immunogenic but associated with far fewer adverse effects than the whole cell vaccine, is now included with tetanus-diphtheria toxoid for use in childhood immunization (DTaP). Preliminary data suggest that the acellular vaccine is well tolerated in adolescents and adults, but large-scale trials have not been performed. Even though adolescents and adults with waning immunity may be reservoirs for *B pertussis*—making immunization attractive—because of lack of data, routine immunization of this population with the acellular vaccine is not presently recommended.

For tetanus prophylaxis in wound management see Chapter 33.

Measles

Adults born before 1957 are considered immune to measles. Adults born in 1957 or later who lack docu-

Table 30–4. Recommended childhood immunization schedule[1] United States, January-December, 2000.

<table>
<tr><th rowspan="2">Vaccine</th><th colspan="12">Age</th></tr>
<tr><th>Birth</th><th>1 mo</th><th>2 mos</th><th>4 mos</th><th>6 mos</th><th>12 mos</th><th>15 mos</th><th>18 mos</th><th>24 mos</th><th>4–6 yrs</th><th>11–12 yrs</th><th>14–16 yrs</th></tr>
<tr><td rowspan="2">Hepatitis B[2]</td><td colspan="3">Hep B</td><td></td><td></td><td></td><td></td><td></td><td></td><td></td><td></td><td></td></tr>
<tr><td></td><td colspan="3">Hep B</td><td colspan="4">Hep B</td><td></td><td></td><td>Hep B</td><td></td></tr>
<tr><td>Diphtheria and tetanus toxoids and pertussis[3]</td><td></td><td></td><td>DTaP</td><td>DTaP</td><td>DTaP</td><td></td><td colspan="2">DTaP</td><td></td><td>DTaP</td><td colspan="2">Td</td></tr>
<tr><td>H influenzae type b[4]</td><td></td><td></td><td>Hib</td><td>Hib</td><td>Hib</td><td colspan="2">Hib</td><td></td><td></td><td></td><td></td><td></td></tr>
<tr><td>Polio[5]</td><td></td><td></td><td>IPV</td><td>IPV</td><td colspan="4">IPV</td><td></td><td>IPV</td><td></td><td></td></tr>
<tr><td>Measles-mumps-rubella[6]</td><td></td><td></td><td></td><td></td><td></td><td colspan="2">MMR</td><td></td><td></td><td>MMR</td><td>MMR</td><td></td></tr>
<tr><td>Varicella[7]</td><td></td><td></td><td></td><td></td><td></td><td colspan="3">Var</td><td></td><td></td><td>Var</td><td></td></tr>
<tr><td>Hepatitis A[8]</td><td></td><td></td><td></td><td></td><td></td><td></td><td></td><td colspan="3">Hep A in selected areas</td><td></td><td></td></tr>
</table>

Range of recommended ages for vaccination

Vaccines to be given if previously recommended doses were missed or were given earlier than the recommended minimum age.

Recommended in selected states and/or regions.

On October 22, 1999, the Advisory Committee on Immunization Practices (ACIP) recommended that Rotashield® (rhesus rotavirus vaccine-tetravalent [RRV-TV]), the only U.S.-licensed rotavirus vaccine, no longer be used in the United States (*MMWR,* Vol. 48, No. 43, November 5, 1999). Parents should be reassured that children who received rotavirus vaccine before July 1999 are not now at increased risk for intussusception.

[1]This schedule indicates the recommended ages for routine administration of licensed childhood vaccines as of November 1, 1999. Any dose not given at the recommended age should be given as a "catch-up" vaccination at any subsequent visit when indicated and feasible. Additional vaccines may be licensed and recommended during the year. Licensed combination vaccines may be used whenever any components of the combination are indicated and the vaccine's other components are not contraindicated. Providers should consult the manufacturers' package inserts for detailed recommendations.

[2]**Infants born to hepatitis B surface antigen (HBsAg)-negative mothers** should receive the first dose of hepatitis B vaccine (Hep B) by age 2 months. The second dose should be administered at least 1 month after the first dose. The third dose should be administered at least 4 months after the first dose and at least 2 months after the second dose, but not before age 6 months. **Infants born to HBsAg-positive mothers** should receive Hep B and 0.5 mL hepatitis B immune globulin (HBIG) within 12 hours of birth at separate sites. The second dose is recommended at age 1–2 months and the third dose at age 6 months. **Infants born to mothers whose HBsAg status is unknown** should receive Hep B within 12 hours of birth. Maternal blood should be drawn at delivery to determine the mother's HBsAg status; if the HBsAg test is positive, the infant should receive HBIG as soon as possible (no later than age 1 week). **All children and adolescents (through age 18 years)** who have not been vaccinated against hepatitis B may begin the series during any visit. Providers should make special efforts to vaccinate children who were born in or whose parents were born in areas of the world where hepatitis B virus infection is moderately or highly endemic.

[3]The fourth dose of diphtheria and tetanus toxoids and acellular pertussis vaccine (DTaP) can be administered as early as age 12 months, provided 6 months have elapsed since the third dose and the child is unlikely to return at age 15–18 months. Tetanus and diphtheria toxoids (Td) is recommended at age 11–12 years if at least 5 years have elapsed since the last dose of diphtheria and tetanus toxoids and pertussis vaccine (DTP), DTaP, or diphtheria and tetanus toxoids (DT). Subsequent routine Td boosters are recommended every 10 years.

[4]Three *Haemophilus influenzae* type b (Hib) conjugate vaccines are licensed for infant use. If Hib conjugate vaccine (PRP-OMP) (PedvaxHIB® or ComVax® [Merck]) is administered at ages 2 months and 4 months, a dose at age 6 months is not required. Because clinical studies in infants have demonstrated that using some combination products may induce a lower immune response to the Hib vaccine component, DTaP/Hib combination products should not be used for primary vaccination in infants at ages 2, 4, or 6 months unless approved by the Food and Drug Administration for these ages.

[5]To eliminate the risk for vaccine-associated paralytic poliomyelitis (VAPP), an all-inactivated poliovirus vaccine (IPV) schedule is now recommended for routine childhood polio vaccination in the United States. All children should receive four doses of IPV: at age 2 months, age 4 months, between ages 6 and 18 months, and between ages 4 and 6 years. Oral poliovirus vaccine (OPV) (if available) may be used only for the following special circumstances: 1) mass vaccination campaigns to control outbreaks of paralytic polio; 2) unvaccinated children who will be traveling in < 4 weeks to areas where polio is endemic or epidemic; and 3) children of parents who do not accept the recommended number of vaccine injections. Children of parents who do not accept the recommended number of vaccine injections may receive OPV only for the third or fourth dose or both; in this situation, health-care providers should administer OPV only after discussing the risk for VAPP with parents or caregivers. During the transition to an all-IPV schedule, recommendations for the use of remaining OPV supplies in physicians' offices and clinics have been issued by the American Academy of Pediatrics (*Pediatrics,* Vol. 104, No. 6, December 1999).

[6]The second dose of measles, mumps, and rubella vaccine (MMR) is recommended routinely at age 4–6 years and may be administered during any visit, provided at least 4 weeks have elapsed since receipt of the first dose and that both doses are administered beginning at or after age 12 months. Those who previously have not received the second dose should complete the schedule no later than the routine visit to a health-care provider at age 11–12 years.

[7]Varicella (Var) vaccine is recommended at any visit on or after the first birthday for susceptible children, ie, those who lack a reliable history of chickenpox (as judged by a health-care provider) and who have not been vaccinated. Susceptible persons aged ≥ 13 years should receive two doses given at least 4 weeks apart.

[8]Hepatitis A vaccine (Hep A) is recommended for use in selected states and regions. Information is available from local public authorities and *MMWR,* Vol. 48, No. RR-12, October 1, 1999.

Use of trade names and commercial sources is for identification only and does not constitute or imply endorsement by CDC or the U.S. Department of Health and Human Services.

Source: Advisory Committee on Immunization Practices (ACIP), American Academy of Family Physicians (AAFP), and American Academy of Pediatrics (AAP).

mentation of immunization after age 1 or who do not have a physician-documented history or laboratory evidence of previous infection should receive at least one dose of vaccine. Persons born between 1963 and 1967—a period when inactivated measles vaccine was the only product available—should also receive one dose of live attenuated vaccine. Persons vaccinated before their first birthday should also receive a single dose of vaccine. Because most adults do not have detailed information about childhood immunization or illnesses, a practical approach is to administer a single dose of MMR to all healthy adults born after 1956. Because outbreaks of measles have occurred in young adults who have received a single dose of measles vaccine, revaccination is recommended, particularly before going to college, entering a health care profession, or embarking on foreign travel to areas where measles is endemic. Even though birth before 1957 implies immunity, unvaccinated health care workers (especially women of childbearing age) who do not have a history of measles or laboratory evidence of immunity should be vaccinated. Entrants to colleges and universities and employees of health care institutions who have not previously been vaccinated should receive two doses of vaccine at least 1 month apart. Revaccination of an immune person is not associated with adverse effects—if the vaccination status is unknown and an indication for vaccination exists, it can be safely done. Vaccination of susceptible adults within 72 hours after exposure to an active case of measles is protective.

About 5–15% of unimmunized individuals will develop fever and about 5% a mild rash 5–12 days after vaccination. Fever and rash are self-limiting, lasting only 2–3 days. Local swelling and induration are particularly common in individuals previously vaccinated with inactivated vaccine. Pregnant women and immunosuppressed persons should not be vaccinated (with the exception of asymptomatic HIV-infected individuals who are not severely immunosuppressed [CD4 count < 200/μL], who should be vaccinated if susceptible). Recent data suggest that MMR vaccine can be safely given to patients with a history of egg allergy even when severe. A single 0.5 mL dose can be given without prior skin testing or desensitization as long as postvaccination observation for 90 minutes is possible.

Rubella

The major purpose of rubella vaccination is to prevent transmission to the fetus. Immunization is recommended for all adults but particularly for women of childbearing age who have not previously been immunized. Although persons born before 1957 are considered immune, this is not an acceptable criterion of immunity for women who could become pregnant. Thus, premenopausal women born before 1957 who might become pregnant should be vaccinated. In addition, both male and female hospital workers who may be exposed to patients with rubella or who might have contact with pregnant patients should be immunized. A single immunization is given. MMR trivalent vaccine is recommended, but if immunity to one or more of the components can be demonstrated, monovalent or bivalent vaccines can be used. Because of the expense of serologic testing to identify susceptible individuals and because revaccination of immune individuals is not associated with adverse effects, routine serologic testing is not required prior to vaccination.

Adverse effects are usually mild. Up to 40% of unvaccinated adults (usually women) experience joint pain. Joint symptoms begin 1–3 weeks after vaccination and are self-limited, lasting 3–10 days. Frank arthritis is rare. Although vaccination of pregnant women is *not* recommended, available data suggest that with the RA27/3 vaccine strain (the one presently available), the congenital rubella syndrome does not occur in the offspring of those inadvertently vaccinated during pregnancy or within 3 months before conception. Persons immunosuppressed by virtue of disease or medication should not receive vaccine. HIV infection is an exception—vaccine should be given to asymptomatic individuals who do not have evidence of severe immunosuppression (CD5 count < 200/μL) and may be considered in symptomatic patients. Since the vaccine contains trace amounts of neomycin, a history of anaphylaxis to this agent is a contraindication to vaccine use.

Mumps

Mumps vaccine is recommended for all adults thought to be susceptible. Persons born before 1957 are considered to be naturally immune and do not require vaccination. Those born in 1957 or later should be considered susceptible unless they can document infection, prove vaccination, or have laboratory evidence of immunity. Vaccination in those already immune is not associated with an increased incidence of adverse effects.

Mumps vaccine is generally safe. It should not be given to those who are immunosuppressed (except HIV-infected individuals) or who have a history of anaphylaxis to neomycin.

Influenza

Influenza vaccination is recommended yearly. Those at greatest risk for severe complications of influenza should have priority in vaccination programs: (1) Adults and children with chronic cardiopulmonary disease, including children with asthma. (2) Residents of nursing homes and other chronic care facilities. (3) Healthy adults 65 years of age or older. (4) Adults and children who have required either regular medical follow-up or hospitalization in the last year for chronic metabolic disorders (including diabetes) or renal disease, those with hemoglobinopathies, and those receiving immunosuppressive drugs. (5) Children and teenagers (age 6 months to 18 years) who are on long-term aspirin therapy and would be at increased risk for developing Reye's syndrome following influenza. (6) Women who will be in the second or third trimester of pregnancy during the influenza season. Certain high-risk groups of patients (the elderly, persons with AIDS, transplant patients) may have a poor antibody response to vaccine, but there is no reason not to vaccinate them. Recent studies have suggested that following vaccination of HIV-positive patients there is a brief (2- to 4-week) period of increased HIV viremia and viral replication. The clinical significance of this is not known, and progression of disease after vaccination has not been observed. Thus, the potential benefit of vaccination of HIV-positive individuals outweighs any theoretic risks. In an attempt to prevent disease in high-risk patients, vaccination is advised for household members and health care providers who have contact with these high-risk patients. Vaccination is recommended also for otherwise healthy adults who provide essential community services and for any individual who wants to decrease the risk of becoming ill with influenza.

Local reactions (erythema and tenderness) at the site of injection are common, but fevers, chills, and malaise (which last in any case only 2–3 days) are rare. Like measles, mumps, and yellow fever vaccines, influenza vaccine is prepared using embryonated chicken eggs, and persons with a history of anaphylaxis to eggs should not be vaccinated. The risk of Guillain-Barré syndrome is not increased following vaccination. Influenza vaccination may be associated with multiple false-positive serologic tests to HIV, HTLV-1, and hepatitis C. Seropositivity is self-limited, lasting 2–5 months.

Preliminary data suggest that a trivalent live attenuated influenza vaccine administered as a single-dose intranasal spray is effective in preventing disease. The product may be available for the next influenza season. Two neuraminidase inhibitors (zanamivir and oseltamivir) are approved for therapy of influenza but not prophylaxis.

Pneumococcal Pneumonia

Pneumococcal vaccine contains purified polysaccharide from 23 of the most common strains of *S pneumoniae,* which cause 90% of bacteremic episodes in the USA. Antibody response following vaccination is dependent upon the patient's immune status and the presence of concomitant disease. Healthy adults have an excellent antibody response, as do patients who are postsplenectomy and those with sickle cell disease. Elderly individuals and those with chronic diseases (diabetes mellitus, alcoholic cirrhosis, chronic obstructive pulmonary disease) have increased antibody levels following vaccination but to a lesser extent than young healthy adults. Patients with Hodgkin's disease respond to vaccination if it is given before splenectomy, radiation, or chemotherapy, whereas patients with leukemia, lymphoma, and HIV infection respond poorly.

Although the efficacy of pneumococcal vaccine has been questioned, most postlicensure studies indicate that vaccination is about 60–70% effective in preventing bacteremic disease in immunocompetent persons. It is 50% effective in patients with underlying diseases (not severely immunocompromised) and even less effective in immunocompromised patients (only 10% effective) largely because of inability to mount an antibody response in this population of patients. It is presently recommended for patients at increased risk for developing severe pneumococcal disease, especially asplenic patients and those with sickle cell disease. It is also recommended for adults who are at increased risk of developing pneumococcal disease, including those with chronic illnesses (eg, cardiopulmonary disease, alcoholism, cirrhosis, cerebrospinal fluid leaks), those who are immunocompromised (eg, patients with Hodgkin's disease, lymphoma, chronic lymphocytic leukemia, multiple myeloma, chronic renal failure, nephrotic syndrome, organ transplant recipients receiving immunosuppressive therapy, including long-term systemic steroids, and asymptomatic or symptomatic HIV infection), and those taking immunosuppressive medications. In addition, it is recommended for all individuals over 65 years of age. Whether 65 is the appropriate age to vaccinate healthy adults is unclear. Antibody response declines with age, and some have suggested routine immunization at age 50 similar to the recommendation for tetanus (see above). A single dose of vaccine usually confers lifelong immunity. Revaccination every 5 years should be considered only in those at highest risk of fatal pneumococcal infection (eg, functionally or anatomically asplenic patients), those known to have a rapid decline in antibody titers (eg, those with nephrotic syndrome or renal failure, HIV infection, leukemia, lymphoma, multiple myeloma, those taking immunosuppressive medications, transplant patients), and those 65 years of age if they received the vaccine 5 years or more previously and were under age 65 at the time of primary vaccination. Elderly individuals with unknown vaccination status should be immunized once. Individuals vaccinated at age 65 or older do not need revaccination. Revaccination should also be considered for high-risk individuals previously immunized with the older 14-valent vaccine. Since immunocompetent patients respond best to the vaccine, it should be given 2 weeks before splenectomy or before starting chemotherapy if that can be anticipated.

Mild reactions (erythema and tenderness) occur in up to 50% of recipients, but systemic reactions are uncommon. Similarly, revaccination at least 5 years after initial vaccination is associated with mild self-limited local reactions but not systemic reactions.

Hepatitis B

Recombinant hepatitis B vaccine is given intramuscularly in the deltoid (gluteal injection often results in deposition of vaccine in fat rather than muscle, with fewer serologic conversions) on three separate occasions: the first two doses 1 month apart and the last dose 5 months after the second one. It is recommended for all individuals at increased risk of developing hepatitis B for social reasons (intravenous drug users, male homosexuals), family reasons (household and sexual contacts of hepatitis B carriers), or occupational reasons (those with frequent exposure to blood and blood products, hemodialysis patients and staff, house officers, medical students, morticians). For immunosuppressed patients, those being maintained on hemodialysis, and chronic alcoholics, seroresponse to standard doses of vaccine is low, and for that reason preparations delivering a higher vaccine dose (40 μg/mL) have become available. In addition to higher vaccine doses, these patients may require more frequent immunizations, and some experts have recommended annual screening to determine whether booster doses are needed. Although most often used for preexposure prophylaxis, the vaccine is also given as postexposure prophylaxis along with hepatitis B immunoglobulin following needle stick injury or mucous membrane exposure to blood from an individual who is HBsAg-positive. It is also given along with hepatitis B immunoglobulin to infants of mothers who are HBsAg-positive (Table 30–4). Immunity wanes with time, but periodic serologic monitoring is not recommended, and routine administration of booster doses is not necessary. Adverse reactions are minor and limited to local soreness.

Following vaccination, 90–95% of healthy young individuals develop protective antibodies. A number of factors decrease serologic response, including increasing age over 30, renal failure, HIV infection, diabetes, chronic liver disease, obesity, and smoking. Postvaccination serologic testing is not routinely done. It is reserved for those whose clinical management would be influenced by their immune status (eg, health care workers, infants born to HBsAg-positive mothers, dialysis patients), and those who may have an impaired response. Those who do not respond should receive a second three-dose vaccine series with serologic testing 1–2 months after completion. Those who fail to respond should be considered susceptible, and if exposed they should receive hepatitis B immune globulin.

Varicella

A live attenuated varicella virus vaccine is currently recommended as part of routine childhood immunization (Table 30–4). Although only 10% of adults remain susceptible, varicella in adolescents and adults is a more severe disease. Only about 2% of all cases of varicella occur in adults, but almost 50% of all deaths are in the adult population. Thus, susceptible adolescents and adults should be immunized, with special emphasis on certain high-risk groups, ie, health care workers; susceptible household contacts of immunosuppressed individuals; persons who live or work in environments where transmission can occur, eg, teachers in day care centers or elementary schools, residents and workers in institutional settings such as the military and correctional institutions, college students; nonpregnant women of childbearing age; and international travelers. The role of the present vaccine in postexposure prophylaxis has not been widely studied, but several reports from Japan and the United States suggest that it is 90% effective in preventing varicella in an outbreak situation, particularly when given within 3–5 days after exposure. The Advisory Committee on Immunization Practices (ACIP) now recommends vaccination in susceptible persons following exposure. The vaccine is very immunogenic. Seroconversion occurs in 95% of children after a single dose. In adolescents (older than 12 years of age) and adults, seroconversion is seen in 78% after one dose and 99% after two doses. For this reason, two doses given 4–8 weeks apart are recommended in persons 12 years of age and older. The duration of immunity is not known but is probably 10 years. Although the vaccine is very effective in preventing disease, breakthrough infections do occur—but are much milder than in unvaccinated individuals (usually less than 50 lesions, with milder systemic symptoms). Although the vaccine is very safe, adverse reactions can occur as late as 4–6 weeks after vaccination. Tenderness and erythema at the injection site are seen in 25%, fever in 10–15%, a localized maculopapular or vesicular rash in 5%, and a smaller percentage develop a diffuse rash, usually with five or fewer vesicular lesions. Spread of virus from vaccinees to susceptible individuals is possible, but the risk of such transmission even to immunocompromised patients is small and disease, when it develops, is mild and treatable with acyclovir. Nonetheless, the vaccine, being a live attenuated virus, should not be given to immunocompromised individuals, including HIV-positive children and adults, or pregnant women. The vaccine is contraindicated in persons allergic to neomycin. For theoretic reasons, it is recommended that following vaccination salicylates should be avoided for 6 weeks (to prevent Reye's syndrome). Several unresolved issues remain, including the need for booster doses, whether universal childhood vaccination will shift the incidence of disease to adolescence or adulthood with the possibility of more severe disease, and whether vaccination might prevent development of herpes zoster.

Hepatitis A

Two inactivated hepatitis A vaccines (Havrix, VAQTA) are approved for use in the USA. They are indicated for individuals 2 years of age or older who

quires registration of the manufacturer and the batch number of the vaccine. Vaccination is available in the USA only at approved centers. (Contact the local health department for available resources.) Reimmunization is recommended at 10-year intervals if continued risk exists.

Because it is a live attenuated vaccine prepared in embryonated eggs, the yellow fever vaccine should not be given to immunosuppressed individuals or those with a history of anaphylaxis to eggs. Pregnancy is a relative contraindication to vaccination.

Japanese B Encephalitis

This is a mosquito-borne viral encephalitis that affects primarily children and older adults (65 years and older) and usually occurs from May to September. It is the leading cause of encephalitis in Asia. Because the risk of infection is low and because adverse effects of the vaccine can be serious, not all travelers to Asia should be vaccinated. Vaccine should be given to travelers to endemic areas who will be staying at least 30 days and who are traveling during the transmission season, particularly if they are visiting rural areas. Travelers who spend less than 30 days in the region should be considered for vaccination if they intend to visit areas of epidemic transmission or if extensive outdoor activities are planned in rural rice-growing areas. The recommended primary immunization schedule is 1 mL of vaccine administered subcutaneously on days 0, 7, and 30. If time constraints are compelling, the last dose can be given on day 14. The last dose should be given at least 10 days before embarkation because adverse effects in the form of urticaria and angioedema have been described, occurring from minutes up to 10 days after vaccination. Following vaccination, patients should be observed for 30 minutes and advised of the possibility of delayed reactions of angioedema and urticaria. In addition, local reactions have been reported in 20% of vaccinees and systemic reactions (fever, chills, malaise, headache) in 10%.

[The National Immunization Program] http://www.cdc.gov/nip/

Advice for travelers. Med Lett Drugs Ther 1998;40:47. [NLM Cit ID: 98253207] (Concise recommendations.)

Jong EC: Travel immunizations. Med Clin North Am 1999;83:903. [NLM Cit ID: 99382628] (Review of routine, required, and recommended vaccinations for travel.)

Reid KC et al: Immunizations: Recommendations for practice. Mayo Clin Proc 1999;74:377. [NLM Cit ID: 99236657] (Summary of indications for common adult immunizations.)

Thompson RF et al: Travel vaccines. Infect Dis Clin North Am 1999;13:149. [NLM Cit ID: 99215010] (Review of indications and preparations available for common vaccines.)

Vaccine side effects, adverse reactions, contraindications, and precautions: Recommendations of the Advisory Committee on Immunization Practices (ACIP). MMWR Morb Mortal Wkly Rep 1996;45(RR-12):1. [NLM Cit ID: 96379651] (Comprehensive review of adverse effects, with recommendations for vaccine use.)

HYPERSENSITIVITY TESTS & DESENSITIZATION

One should test for hypersensitivity before injecting antitoxin, materials derived from animal sources, or drugs (eg, penicillin) to which a patient has had a severe reaction in the past. If the test described below is negative, desensitization is not necessary, and a full dose of the material may be given. If the test is positive, alternative drugs should be strongly considered. If that is not feasible, desensitization is necessary.

Intradermal Test for Hypersensitivity

Penicillin is the drug that most frequently serves as an indication for sensitivity testing and desensitization. Skin testing requires two preparations: PPL (penicilloyl-polylysine) and a minor determinant mixture. Several points should be emphasized in performing and interpreting these tests. Whenever possible, both PPL and a minor determinant should be used, since 85% of skin test reactors are positive to PPL but 15% react only to the minor determinant mixture. In addition, if penicillin G is used instead of the minor determinant mixture, some allergic patients will be missed. About 25% of individuals who react to minor determinant mixture may not react to penicillin G, and such patients may still have an anaphylactic or accelerated reaction to penicillin. A pinprick test is performed with each solution at different sites by placing a small drop of solution on the skin and making small indentations of the skin with a needle. If there is no reaction within 10 minutes, 0.01–0.02 mL is injected intradermally, raising a small bleb. Development of a wheal greater than 5 mm in diameter is considered a positive test and an indication for desensitization. Even if the test is negative, about 1% of patients will have an immediate or accelerated reaction. Thus, if the test is negative, the drug can be administered with relative safety, but the precautions below should be followed.

Desensitization

A. Precautions:

1. The desensitization procedure is not innocuous—deaths from anaphylaxis have been reported. If extreme hypersensitivity is suspected, it is advisable to use an alternative structurally unrelated drug and to reserve desensitization for situations when treatment cannot be withheld and no alternative drug is available.

2. An antihistaminic drug (25–50 mg of hydroxyzine or diphenhydramine intramuscularly or orally) should be administered before desensitization is begun in order to lessen any reaction that occurs.

3. Desensitization should be conducted in an intensive care unit where cardiac monitoring and emergency endotracheal intubation can be performed.

4. Epinephrine, 1 mL of 1:1000 solution, must be ready for immediate administration.

B. Desensitization Method: Several methods of desensitization have been described for penicillin, including use of both oral and intravenous preparations. All methods start with very small doses of drug and gradually increase the dose until therapeutic doses are achieved. For penicillin, 1 unit of drug is given intravenously and the patient observed for 15–30 minutes. If there is no reaction, some recommend doubling the dose while others recommend increasing it tenfold every 15–30 minutes until a dosage of 2 million units is reached; then give the remainder of the desired dose.

For recommendations on skin testing and desensitization for other preparations (botulism antitoxin, diphtheria antitoxin, etc), one should consult the manufacturer's package inserts.

Treatment of Reactions

A. Mild Reactions: If a mild reaction occurs, drop back to the next lower dose and continue with desensitization. If a severe reaction occurs, administer epinephrine (see below) and discontinue the drug unless treatment is urgently needed. If desensitization is imperative, continue slowly, increasing the dosage of the drug more gradually.

B. Severe Reactions: If bronchospasm occurs, epinephrine, 0.3–0.5 mL of 1:1000 dilution, should be given subcutaneously every 10–20 minutes. The following can also be given if symptoms persist: inhaled metaproterenol (0.3 mL of a 5% solution in 2.5 mL of saline), intravenous aminophylline (0.3–0.9 mL/kg/h maintenance after a 6 mg/kg loading dose over 30 minutes), or corticosteroids (250 mg of hydrocortisone or 50 mg of methylprednisolone intravenously every 6 hours for two to four doses). Hypotension should be treated with intravenous fluids (saline or colloid), epinephrine (1 mL of 1:1000 dilution in 500 mL of D_5W intravenously at a rate of 0.5–5 μg/min), and antihistamines (25–50 mg of hydroxyzine or diphenhydramine intramuscularly or orally every 6–8 hours as needed). Cutaneous reactions, manifested as urticaria or angioedema, respond to epinephrine subcutaneously and antihistamines in the doses set forth above.

1998 guidelines for treatment of sexually transmitted diseases: MMWR Morb Mortal Wkly Rep 1998;47(RR-1):46. [NLM Cit ID: 98120951] (Section on oral or intravenous desensitization to penicillin in patients with positive skin tests.)

RELEVANT WORLD WIDE WEB SITES

[Centers for Disease Control and Prevention (CDC)]
http://www.cdc.gov
[CDC—Emerging Infectious Diseases]
http://www.cdc.gov/ncidod/eid/index.htm
[CDC—Morbidity and Mortality Weekly Report]
http://www.cdc.gov/epo/mmwr/mmwr.html
[CDC—National Center for Infectious Diseases]
http://www.cdc.gov/ncidod/index.htm
[CDC Travel Information]
http://www.cdc.gov/travel
[The Childhood Immunization Informatics Collaboratory]
http://paella.med.yale.edu/immserve/immshome.html
[Infectious Diseases of the Central Nervous System]
http://www.vh.org/Providers/TeachingFiles/CNSInfDisR2/ IDCNSHomePg.html
[Outbreak]
http://www.outbreak.org/cgi-unreg/dynaserve.exe/index.html
[Sexually Transmitted Diseases Tutorial]
http://edcenter.med.cornell.edu/Pathophysiology_Cases/STDs/STD_TOC.html
[Travel Health Information]
http://healthlink.mcw.edu/travel-links.html

31 HIV Infection

See http://www.current-med/ch31.html for updated addresses of Web sites referenced in this chapter.

Harry Hollander, MD, & Mitchell H. Katz, MD

Essentials of Diagnosis

- Risk factors: sexual contact with an infected person, parenteral exposure to infected blood by transfusion or needle sharing, perinatal exposure.
- Prominent systemic complaints such as sweats, diarrhea, weight loss, and wasting.
- Opportunistic infections due to diminished cellular immunity—often life-threatening.
- Aggressive cancers, particularly Kaposi's sarcoma and extranodal lymphoma.
- Neurologic manifestations, including dementia, aseptic meningitis, and neuropathy.

General Considerations

When AIDS was first recognized in the USA in 1981, cases were identified by finding severe opportunistic infections such as pneumocystis pneumonia that indicated profound defects in cellular immunity in the absence of other causes of immunodeficiency. When the syndrome was found to be caused by the human immunodeficiency virus (HIV), it became obvious that severe opportunistic infections and unusual neoplasms were at one end of a spectrum of disease, while healthy seropositive individuals were at the other end.

In 1993, the Centers for Disease Control and Prevention expanded the AIDS definition (Table 31–1). The 1993 definition includes all 23 opportunistic infections (eg, pneumocystis pneumonia) and neoplasms (eg, Kaposi's sarcoma) that were included in the 1987 definition. As with the 1987 definition, it also includes as AIDS cases persons with documented weight loss, diarrhea, or dementia and a positive HIV serology. There remain criteria for both definitive and presumptive diagnoses. The expansion is that persons with a positive HIV serology and who have ever had a CD4 lymphocyte count below 200 cells/μL or a CD4 lymphocyte percentage below 14% are considered to have AIDS. Inclusion of persons with low CD4 counts as AIDS cases reflects the recognition that immunodeficiency is the defining characteristic of AIDS. The choice of a cutoff point at 200 cells/μL is supported by several cohort studies showing that over 80% of persons with counts below this level will develop AIDS within 3 years in the absence of effective antiretroviral therapy. The 1993 definition was also expanded to include persons with positive HIV serology and pulmonary tuberculosis, recurrent pneumonia, and invasive cervical cancer. One consequence of the expanded definition has been that HIV-infected persons are diagnosed with AIDS an average of 1.6 years earlier in the course of the disease. The definition doubled to tripled the number of new cases of AIDS in 1993. However, the impact of the new definition on the number of new cases has been less since then.

The goal of the current definition is to enhance efforts at surveillance of HIV disease. It does not affect eligibility for most social services benefits, since the Social Security Administration has decided not to use the CDC definition as presumptive eligibility of disability. Instead, SSA has developed a functional assessment for determining eligibility for benefits for HIV-infected persons. In the past, the term "AIDS-related complex" (ARC) was used to denote those HIV-infected patients who were symptomatic but did not fit the CDC definition of AIDS. This group of patients is heterogeneous, with varying clinical problems and prognoses. Therefore, the use of the term "ARC" should be avoided.

Dramatic increases in the efficacy of antiretroviral treatments—especially those regimens that include protease inhibitors—have improved the prognosis of persons with HIV/AIDS. As antiretroviral and prophylactic regimens have become more complicated there has been greater attention paid to the experience of clinicians caring for persons with HIV and AIDS. Several studies have documented that persons cared for by clinicians experienced in this field have a better prognosis and receive more cost-effective care than patients of less experienced clinicians. While experience in dealing with the medical problems of infected persons is clearly important, subspecialty training per se has not been found to be related to quality of care.

Given that there are approximately 700,000 HIV-infected persons in the United States and that a substantial number of these cases occur in rural areas where there may be few HIV specialists, it is unreal-

Table 31–1. CDC AIDS case definition for surveillance of adults and adolescents.

Definitive AIDS diagnoses (with or without laboratory evidence of HIV infection)

1. Candidiasis of the esophagus, trachea, bronchi, or lungs.
2. Cryptococcosis, extrapulmonary.
3. Cryptosporidiosis with diarrhea persisting > 1 month.
4. Cytomegalovirus disease of an organ other than liver, spleen, or lymph nodes.
5. Herpes simplex virus infection causing a mucocutaneous ulcer that persists longer than 1 month; or bronchitis, pneumonitis, or esophagitis of any duration.
6. Kaposi's sarcoma in a patient < 60 years of age.
7. Lymphoma of the brain (primary) in a patient < 60 years of age.
8. *Mycobacterium avium* complex or *Mycobacterium kansasii* disease, disseminated (at a site other than or in addition to lungs, skin, or cervical or hilar lymph nodes).
9. *Pneumocystis carinii* pneumonia.
10. Progressive multifocal leukoencephalopathy.
11. Toxoplasmosis of the brain.

Definitive AIDS diagnoses (with laboratory evidence of HIV infection)

1. Coccidioidomycosis, disseminated (at a site other than or in addition to lungs or cervical or hilar lymph nodes).
2. HIV encephalopathy.
3. Histoplasmosis, disseminated (at a site other than or in addition to lungs or cervical or hilar lymph nodes).
4. Isosporiasis with diarrhea persisting > 1 month.
5. Kaposi's sarcoma at any age.
6. Lymphoma of the brain (primary) at any age.
7. Other non-Hodgkin's lymphoma of B cell or unknown immunologic phenotype.
8. Any mycobacterial disease caused by mycobacteria other than *Mycobacterium tuberculosis*, disseminated (at a site other than or in addition to lungs, skin, or cervical or hilar lymph nodes).
9. Disease caused by extrapulmonary *M tuberculosis*.
10. Salmonella (nontyphoid) septicemia, recurrent.
11. HIV wasting syndrome.
12. CD4 lymphocyte count below 200 cells/μL or a CD4 lymphocyte percentage below 14%.
13. Pulmonary tuberculosis.
14. Recurrent pneumonia.
15. Invasive cervical cancer.

Presumptive AIDS diagnoses (with laboratory evidence of HIV infection)

1. Candidiasis of esophagus: (a) recent onset of retrosternal pain on swallowing; and (b) oral candidiasis.
2. Cytomegalovirus retinitis. A characteristic appearance on serial ophthalmoscopic examinations.
3. Mycobacteriosis. Specimen from stool or normally sterile body fluids or tissue from a site other than lungs, skin, or cervical or hilar lymph nodes, showing acid-fast bacilli of a species not identified by culture.
4. Kaposi's sarcoma. Erythematous or violaceous plaque-like lesion on skin or mucous membrane.
5. *Pneumocystis carinii* pneumonia: (a) a history of dyspnea on exertion or nonproductive cough of recent onset (within the past 3 months); and (b) chest x-ray evidence of diffuse bilateral interstitial infiltrates or gallium scan evidence of diffuse bilateral pulmonary disease; and (c) arterial blood gas analysis showing an arterial oxygen partial pressure of < 70 mm Hg or a low respiratory diffusing capacity of < 80% of predicted values or an increase in the alveolar-arterial oxygen tension gradient; and (d) no evidence of a bacterial pneumonia.
6. Toxoplasmosis of the brain: (a) recent onset of a focal neurologic abnormality consistent with intracranial disease or a reduced level of consciousness; and (b) brain imaging evidence of a lesion having a mass effect or the radiographic appearance of which is enhanced by injection of contrast medium; and (c) serum antibody to toxoplasmosis or successful response to therapy for toxoplasmosis.
7. Recurrent pneumonia: (a) more than one episode in a 1-year period; and (b) acute pneumonia (new symptoms, signs, or radiologic evidence not present earlier) diagnosed on clinical or radiologic grounds by the patient's physician.
8. Pulmonary tuberculosis: (a) apical or miliary infiltrates and (b) radiographic and clinical response to antituberculous therapy.

istic to expect that all patients will be cared for by experienced clinicians. On the other hand, these findings emphasize the need for clinicians with limited experience in this area to educate themselves about disease manifestations and treatment. Resources are available to help clinicians care for HIV-infected persons. Clinicians should call their state medical associations for a list of local resources.

Specialists should be consulted for patients failing their current regimens, intolerant of standard antiviral drugs, those in need of systemic chemotherapy, and those with complicated opportunistic infections, particularly when invasive procedures or experimental therapies are needed. In many cases, a single consultation with follow-up to the primary care clinician will provide the needed expertise while ensuring continuity in care.

Epidemiology

The modes of transmission of HIV are similar to those of hepatitis B, in particular with respect to sexual, parenteral, and vertical transmission. The risk of sexual transmission varies with particular sexual practices; receptive anal intercourse is the riskiest. The risk of sustaining HIV infection from a needle stick with infected blood is approximately 1:300 in the absence of retroviral treatment. Between 13% and 40% of children born to HIV-infected mothers contract HIV infection. This risk can be decreased with the use of antiretroviral treatment during pregnancy. A multicenter trial showed that when zidovudine is administered to women during pregnancy, labor, and delivery and to their newborns, the rate of HIV transmission is decreased by two-thirds. An observational trial demonstrated that zidovudine treatment is almost as effective when begun during labor or when administered only to the infant, as long as treatment is begun within 48 hours after birth. Nonetheless, treatment begun by at least the second trimester is still recommended. Many women are currently being offered combination antiretroviral treatment to further lower the risk of transmission. The availability of treatment makes it essential that all women who are pregnant or considering pregnancy be offered HIV counseling and testing. The HIV has not been shown to be transmitted by respiratory droplet spread, by vectors such as mosquitoes, or by casual nonsexual contact.

Current estimates are that about 700,000 Americans are infected with HIV. Estimates of the number of people who have developed AIDS in the 1990s have been scaled down from prior estimates, based on recent AIDS incidence data. In 1999, there were 288,000 persons in the USA living with AIDS. Fifty-two percent of those cases are in gay or bisexual men; 28% are in heterosexual injection drug users; and 16% are in heterosexual noninjection drug users. Women account for 20% of cases. Among risk groups, the most rapid percentage increases are among young gay and bisexual men and heterosexual men and women, especially blacks and Hispanics.

The rapid increase of AIDS cases among women is of great concern. In 1985, women represented only 7% of new AIDS cases; in 1996, women represented 25% of new cases. Intravenous drug use and heterosexual contact with an infected partner are the two major risk factors for women. With the rapid increase of HIV infection among women, there has been a corresponding rise in the number of perinatally infected children.

The natural history of HIV infection is different in men than in women, though it has been difficult to determine whether the differences are due to biologic or to social factors. In general, women appear later for medical care than men. Therefore, those studies which compared men with women with reference to rates of progression to AIDS found that women progressed more rapidly. Most studies that have adequately adjusted for disease stage have reported no differences in rates of progression. However, one large study reported that women have shorter survival times than men and that many have died without an AIDS diagnosis. Violence toward women, drugs, pregnancy, and poverty may all play a role in this higher rate of death. In addition, women are at risk for gynecologic complications of HIV infection, including recurrent candidal vaginitis, pelvic inflammatory disease, and cervical dysplasia and cancer.

HIV infection will continue to spread outward from major metropolitan areas to suburban and rural parts of the country. Because blood donor screening using the HIV-enzyme-linked immunosorbent assay (ELISA) is universally practiced in the USA, the number of new AIDS cases due to transfusion has already peaked and is expected to decline further. The current risk of contracting HIV from a screened unit of blood is 1:100,000. Although "safer sex" campaigns dramatically decreased the rates of seroconversions among gay men living in metropolitan areas in the United States by the mid 1980s, there is concern that relapse to unsafe sexual practices will result in an increase in the number of new seroconversions. In particular, recent improvements in the efficacy of treatment may allay fear of contracting infection among persons at risk. A CDC study found that the number and proportion of gonorrhea cases in gay men between 1993 and 1996 increased in several large cities in the United States.

There are an estimated 10 million persons infected worldwide. In Central and East Africa in some urban areas, as many as one-third of sexually active adults are infected. HIV infection began to spread in Asia in the late 1980s, and new infections in Asia exceeded new infections in Africa by the late 1990s. The most common mode of transmission is bidirectional heterosexual spread. The reason for the greater risk for transmission with heterosexual intercourse in Africa and Asia than in the United States may relate to cofactors such as general health status, the presence of genital ulcers, and the number of sexual partners.

Gonorrhea among men who have sex with men—Selected sexually transmitted diseases clinics, 1993–1996. MMWR Morb Mortal Wkly Rep 1997;46:889. [NLM Cit ID: 97459819] (Study found increases in the proportion of gonorrhea cases occurring in gay men.)

Holmberg SD: The estimated prevalence and incidence of HIV in 96 large US metropolitan areas. Am J Public Health 1996;86:642. [NLM Cit ID: 96212357] (Synthesis of existing data provides estimates of prevalence and incidence by population within major metropolitan areas.)

Kitahata MM et al: Physicians' experience with the acquired immunodeficiency syndrome as a factor in patients' survival. N Engl J Med 1996;334:701. [NLM Cit ID: 96175166] (Risk of death was significantly lower for AIDS patients who had physicians who were more experienced in HIV and AIDS care.)

Wade NA et al: Abbreviated regimens of zidovudine prophylaxis and perinatal transmission of the human immunodeficiency virus. N Engl J Med 1998;339:1409. [NLM Cit ID: 99015390] (Zidovudine prophylaxis decreased the rate of perinatal transmission of HIV even if begun intrapartum or in the first 48 hours of life of the infant.)

Etiology

The syndromes described below are due to infection with human retroviruses known as human immunodeficiency viruses (HIV or HIV-1, formerly HTLV-III or LAV). Retroviruses depend upon a unique enzyme, reverse transcriptase (RNA-directed DNA-polymerase), to replicate within host cells. The other major pathogenic human retrovirus, HTLV-I, is associated with lymphoma, while HIV is not directly oncogenic. The HIV genomes contain genes for three basic structural proteins and at least five other regulatory proteins; *gag* codes for group antigen proteins, *pol* codes for polymerase, and *env* codes for the external envelope protein. The greatest variability in strains of HIV occurs in the viral envelope. Since neutralizing activity is found in antibodies directed against the envelope, this variability presents problems for vaccine development.

In addition to the classic AIDS virus (HIV-1), a group of related viruses, HIV-2, have been isolated in West African patients. HIV-2 has the same genetic organization as HIV-1, but there are significant differences in the envelope glycoproteins. Some infected individuals exhibit AIDS-like illnesses, but most West Africans infected with HIV-2 are currently asymptomatic. HIV-2 has been found in several people in the USA. Thus, this variant may be less pathogenic or have a longer period of latency preceding disease. Cases have been documented in which AIDS-like illnesses have occurred in the absence of HIV infection. The syndrome of idiopathic CD4 lymphocytopenia appears to represent a heterogeneous form of immunodeficiency. No convincing infectious or other cause has been identified.

Pathogenesis

The hallmark of symptomatic HIV infection is immunodeficiency caused by continuing viral replication. The virus can infect all cells expressing the T4 (CD4) antigen, which serves as a receptor for HIV. Once it enters a cell, HIV can replicate and cause cell fusion or death by unknown mechanisms. In many cases, a latent state is established, with integration of the HIV genome into the cell's genome. The cell principally infected is the CD4 (helper-inducer) lymphocyte, which directs many other cells in the immune network. With increasing duration of infection, the number of CD4 lymphocytes falls. Some of the immunologic defects, however, are explained not by *quantitative* abnormalities of lymphocyte subsets but by *qualitative* defects in CD4 responsiveness induced by HIV.

Other cells in the immune network that are infected by HIV include B lymphocytes and macrophages. The defect in B cells is mainly due to disordered CD4 lymphocyte function. These direct and indirect effects can lead to generalized hypergammaglobulinemia and can also depress B cell responses to new antigen challenges. Because of these defects, the immunodeficiency of HIV is mixed. Elements of humoral and cellular immunodeficiency are present, especially in children. Macrophages act as a reservoir for HIV and serve to disseminate it to other organ systems (eg, the central nervous system).

Apart from the immunologic effects of HIV, the virus can also directly cause a variety of neurologic effects. Rare glial cells and oligodendrocytes express CD4 antigen and thus may be permissive of infection by HIV. However, these cells are rarely infected, whereas multinucleated giant cells of macrophage origin are more commonly seen in brain specimens of infected individuals. Neuropathology largely results from the release of cytokines and other neurotoxins by infected macrophages. Other factors such as coexistent CMV infection may also be important. Perturbations of excitatory neurotransmitters and calcium flux may contribute to neurologic dysfunction.

Pathophysiology

Clinically, the syndromes caused by HIV infection are usually explicable by one of three known mechanisms. Some HIV-associated manifestations such as idiopathic diarrhea, however, are not explained by any of these proposed mechanisms.

A. Immunodeficiency: Immunodeficiency is a direct result of the effects of HIV upon immune cells. A spectrum of infections and neoplasms is seen, as in other congenital or acquired immunodeficiency states. Two remarkable features of HIV immunodeficiency are the low incidence of certain infections such as listeriosis and aspergillosis and the frequent occurrence of certain neoplasms such as lymphoma or Kaposi's sarcoma. This latter complication has been seen primarily in gay or bisexual men, and its incidence has steadily declined through the first 10 years of the epidemic. Evidence now strongly suggests that a herpesvirus (KSHV or HHV-8) is the cause of Kaposi's sarcoma.

B. Autoimmunity: Autoimmunity can occur as a result of disordered cellular immune function or B lymphocyte dysfunction. Examples of both lymphocytic infiltration of organs (eg, lymphocytic interstitial pneumonitis) and autoantibody production (eg, immunologic thrombocytopenia) occur. These phenomena may be the only clinically apparent disease or may coexist with obvious immunodeficiency.

C. Neurologic Dysfunction: See discussion in Pathogenesis, above.

Clinical Findings

The complications of HIV-related infections and neoplasms affect virtually every organ. The general approach to the HIV-infected person with symptoms is to evaluate the organ systems involved, aiming to diagnose treatable conditions rapidly. As can be seen in Figure 31–1, the CD4 lymphocyte count provides very important prognostic information. Certain infections may occur at any CD4 count, while others rarely occur unless the CD4 lymphocyte count has dropped below a certain level. For example, a patient

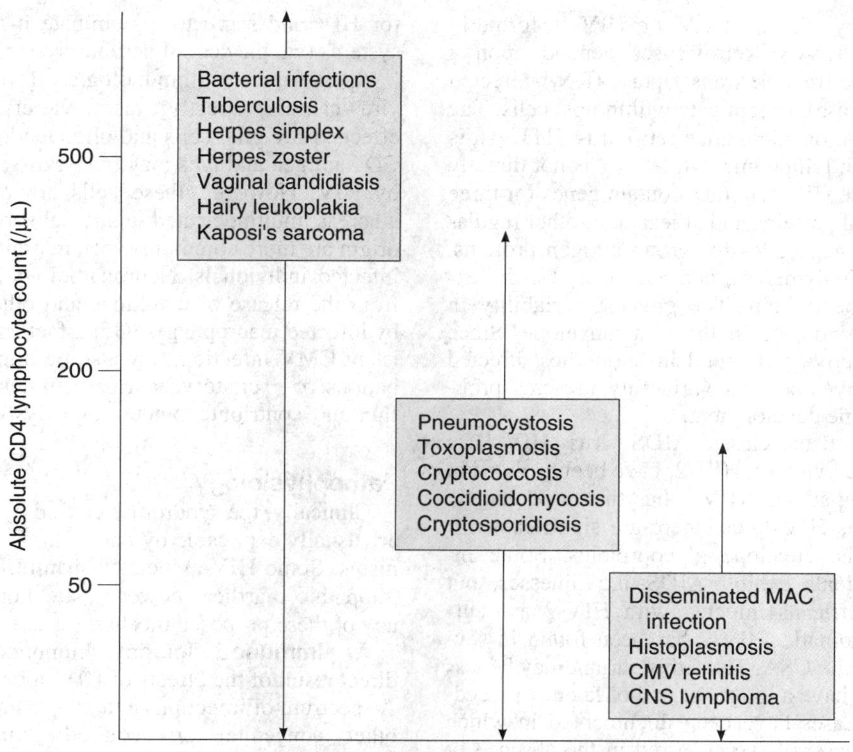

Figure 31–1. Relationship of CD4 count to development of opportunistic infections.

with a CD4 count of 600 cells/µL, cough, and fever may have a bacterial pneumonia but would be very unlikely to have pneumocystis pneumonia.

A. Symptoms and Signs: Many individuals with HIV infection remain asymptomatic for years even without antiretroviral therapy, with a mean time of approximately 10 years between exposure and development of AIDS. When symptoms occur, they may be remarkably protean and nonspecific. Since virtually all the findings may be seen with other diseases, a combination of complaints is more suggestive of HIV infection than any one symptom.

Physical examination may be entirely normal. Abnormal findings range from completely nonspecific to highly specific for HIV infection. Those that are predictive of HIV infection include hairy leukoplakia of the tongue, disseminated Kaposi's sarcoma, and cutaneous bacillary angiomatosis.

1. Systemic complaints–Fever, night sweats, and weight loss are common symptoms in HIV-infected patients and may occur without a complicating opportunistic infection. Patients with persistent **fever** and no localizing symptoms should nonetheless be carefully examined, and evaluated with a chest radiograph (pneumocystis pneumonia can present without respiratory symptoms), bacterial blood cultures if the fever is greater than 38.5 °C, serum cryptococcal antigen, and mycobacterial cultures of the blood. Sinus radiographs or sinus CT scans should be considered to evaluate occult sinusitis. If these studies are normal, patients should be observed closely. Antipyretics are useful because HIV-infected patients have a propensity for high fevers and subsequent dehydration. Generally, nonsteroidal anti-inflammatory agents are more effective than aspirin or acetaminophen in the relief of fever.

Weight loss is a particularly distressing complication of long-standing HIV infection. Patients typically have disproportionate loss of muscle mass, with maintenance or less substantial loss of fat stores. The mechanism of HIV-related weight loss is not completely understood but appears to be multifactorial.

Tumor necrosis factor (TNF; cachectin) is known to be elevated in AIDS patients with secondary infections such as pneumocystis pneumonia. TNF decreases lipoprotein lipase activity, decreases the synthesis of fatty acids, and promotes the breakdown of fat. AIDS patients also have high alpha interferon levels, which may result in decreased clearance of triglycerides. However, the exact roles of tumor necrosis factor, alpha interferon, and other cytokines, as well as their combined effect on weight loss, are still unknown.

AIDS patients frequently suffer from anorexia, nausea, and vomiting, all of which contribute to weight loss by decreasing caloric intake. In some cases, these symptoms are secondary to a specific infection, such as viral hepatitis. In other cases, however, evaluation of the symptoms yields no specific pathogen, and it is assumed to be due to a primary effect of HIV. Malabsorption also plays a role in decreased caloric intake. Patients may suffer diarrhea from infections with bacterial, viral, or parasitic agents.

Exacerbating the decrease in caloric intake, many AIDS patients have an increased metabolic rate. This increased rate has been shown to exist even among asymptomatic HIV-infected persons, but it accelerates with disease progression and secondary infection. AIDS patients with secondary infections also have decreased protein synthesis, which makes maintaining muscle mass difficult.

Several strategies have been developed to slow AIDS wasting. Patients should be counseled to maintain high caloric diets. Food supplementation with high-calorie drinks may enable patients with not much appetite to maintain their intake. Selected patients with otherwise good functional status and weight loss due to unrelenting nausea, vomiting, or diarrhea may benefit from total parenteral nutrition. It should be noted, however, that TPN is more likely to increase fat stores than to reverse the muscle wasting process.

Two pharmacologic approaches for increasing appetite and weight gain are the progestational agent megestrol acetate (80 mg four times a day) and the antiemetic agent dronabinol (2.5–5 mg three times a day). Side effects from megestrol acetate are rare. Thromboembolic phenomena, edema, nausea, vomiting, and rash have been reported. Euphoria, dizziness, paranoia, and somnolence and even nausea and vomiting have been reported in 3–10% of patients using dronabinol. Unfortunately, neither megestrol acetate or dronabinol increases lean body mass. Two regimens that have resulted in increases in lean body mass are growth hormone and anabolic steroids.

Growth hormone at a dose of 0.1 mg/kg/d subcutaneously for 12 weeks has resulted in modest increases in lean body mass; its cost is approximately $150 per day. Anabolic steroids also increase lean body mass among HIV-infected patients. They seem to work best for patients who are able to do weight training. The most commonly used regimens are testosterone enanthate or testosterone cypionate (100–200 mg intramuscularly every 2–4 weeks). Testosterone patches (4–6 mg/d) applied to the shaved scrotum can also be used. A transdermal delivery system (2.5 mg/d) is also available that can be applied to nonhairy parts of the body. The anabolic steroid oxandrolone (15–20 mg orally in two to four divided doses) has also been found to increase lean body mass.

Nausea leading to weight loss is sometimes due to esophageal candidiasis. Patients with oral candidiasis and nausea should be empirically treated with an oral antifungal agent. Patients with weight loss due to nausea of unclear origin may benefit from use of antiemetics prior to meals (prochlorperazine, 10 mg three times daily; metoclopramide, 10 mg three times daily; or ondansetron, 8 mg three times daily). Effective fever control decreases the metabolic rate and may slow the pace of weight loss. Dronabinol (5 mg three times daily) can also be used to increase appetite. Depression and adrenal insufficiency are two potentially treatable causes of weight loss.

2. Sinopulmonary disease–

a. Pneumocystis pneumonia–(See also discussions in Chapter 36.) The lungs are a frequently involved site of disease. Pneumocystis pneumonia is the most common opportunistic infection, affecting 75% of patients. Pneumocystis pneumonia may be difficult to diagnose because the symptoms—fever, cough, and shortness of breath—are nonspecific. Furthermore, the severity of symptoms ranges from fever and no respiratory symptoms through mild cough or dyspnea to frank respiratory distress.

Hypoxemia may be severe, with a Po_2 less than 60 mm Hg. The cornerstone of diagnosis is the chest radiograph. Diffuse or perihilar infiltrates are most characteristic, but only two-thirds of patients with pneumocystis pneumonia have this finding. Normal chest radiographs are seen in 5–10% of patients with pneumocystis pneumonia, while the remainder have atypical infiltrates. Apical infiltrates are commonly seen among patients with pneumocystis pneumonia who have been receiving aerosolized pentamidine prophylaxis. Large pleural effusions are uncommon with pneumocystis pneumonia; their presence suggests bacterial pneumonia, other infections such as tuberculosis, or pleural Kaposi's sarcoma.

Definitive diagnosis can be obtained by Wright-Giemsa stain of induced sputum in 50–80% of cases. Sputum induction is performed by having patients inhale an aerosolized solution of 3% saline produced by an ultrasonic nebulizer. Patients should not eat for at least 8 hours and should not use toothpaste or mouthwash prior to the procedure since they can interfere with test interpretation. The next step for patients with negative sputum examinations still suspected of having pneumocystis pneumonia should be bronchoalveolar lavage. This technique establishes the diagnosis in over 95% of cases.

In patients with symptoms suggestive of pneumocystis pneumonia but with negative or atypical chest radiographs and negative sputum examinations, other diagnostic tests may provide additional information in deciding whether to proceed to bronchoalveolar lavage. Elevation of serum lactate dehydrogenase occurs in 95% of cases of pneumocystis pneumonia, but the specificity of this finding is at best 75%. Elevation of serum LDH can also be seen with lymphoma, disseminated histoplasmosis, and long-term treatment with zidovudine. Patients with serum lactate dehydrogenase levels of 220 units/L or less and erythrocyte sedimentation rates less than 50 mm/h are unlikely to have pneumocystis pneumonia and may be clinically followed. In addition, a CD4 count above 250 cells/μL within 2 months prior to evaluation of respiratory symptoms makes a diagnosis of pneumocystis pneumonia unlikely; only 1–5% of cases occur at this CD4 count level (Figure 31–1).

Pneumothoraces are common in HIV-infected patients with a history of pneumocystis pneumonia, especially if they have received aerosolized pentamidine treatment. Because patients may have a pneumothorax as their presenting symptom of recurrent pneumocystis pneumonia, such patients who have not had therapy for pneumocystis pneumonia in the preceding 3 months may need evaluation for pneumocystis. Pneumothoraces in HIV-infected individuals should be treated initially in the same fashion as in other patients. Unfortunately, they frequently recur with clamping or removal of the chest tube. Sclerosis with bleomycin or talc is the treatment of choice for recurrent pneumothoraces, but it is not uniformly successful even when multiple treatments are performed. If sclerosis fails, thoracoscopic stapling or thoracotomy may be required.

b. Other infectious pulmonary diseases– Other infectious causes of pulmonary disease in AIDS patients include bacterial, mycobacterial, and viral pneumonias. An increased incidence of pneumococcal pneumonia with septicemia and *Haemophilus influenzae* pneumonia has been reported. *Pseudomonas aeruginosa* is an important respiratory pathogen in advanced disease. The incidence of infection with *Mycobacterium tuberculosis* has markedly increased in metropolitan areas because of HIV infection as well as homelessness. Tuberculosis occurs in an estimated 4% of persons who have AIDS. It is thought to result mainly from reactivation of prior infection; atypical infiltrates and disseminated disease occur more commonly than among immunocompetent hosts. Multidrug-resistant tuberculosis is a major problem in several metropolitan areas. Noncompliance with prescribed antituberculous drugs is a major risk factor. Several of the reported outbreaks appear to implicate nosocomial spread. The emergence of drug resistance makes it essential that antibiotic sensitivities be performed on all positive cultures. Drug therapy should be individualized. Patients with multidrug-resistant *M tuberculosis* infection should receive at least three drugs to which their organism is sensitive. Atypical mycobacteria can cause pulmonary disease in AIDS patients with or without preexisting lung disease and responds variably to treatment. Making a distinction between *M tuberculosis* and atypical mycobacteria requires culture of sputum specimens. If culture of the sputum produces acid-fast bacilli, definitive identification may take several weeks. DNA probes allow for presumptive identification usually within days of a positive culture. While awaiting definitive diagnosis, clinicians should err on the side of treating patients as if they have *M tuberculosis* infection. In cases where the risk of atypical mycobacteria is very high (eg, a person without risk for tuberculosis exposure with a CD4 count under 50 cells/μL—see Figure 31–1), clinicians may wait for definitive diagnosis if the person is smear-negative for acid-fast bacilli and not living in a communal setting. Isolation of cytomegalovirus from bronchoalveolar lavage fluid occurs commonly in AIDS patients but does not establish a definitive diagnosis. Diagnosis of cytomegalovirus pneumonia requires biopsy; response to treatment is poor.

c. Noninfectious pulmonary diseases–Noninfectious causes of lung disease include Kaposi's sarcoma, non-Hodgkin's lymphoma, and interstitial pneumonitis. In patients with known Kaposi's sarcoma, pulmonary involvement complicates the course in approximately one-third of cases. Non-Hodgkin's lymphoma may involve the lung as the sole site of disease but more commonly involves other organs as well, especially the brain, liver, and gastrointestinal tract. Both of these processes may show nodular or diffuse parenchymal involvement, pleural effusions, and mediastinal adenopathy on chest radiographs.

Nonspecific interstitial pneumonitis may mimic pneumocystis pneumonia. Pulmonary involvement by HIV may result in a lymphocytic interstitial pneumonitis seen in lung biopsies. Whether this pathologic pattern represents direct HIV infection or is an autoimmune response to infection is unclear. It has a variable clinical course. Typically, these patients present with several months of mild cough and dyspnea; chest radiographs show interstitial infiltrates. Many patients with this entity undergo transbronchial biopsies in an attempt to diagnose pneumocystis pneumonia. Instead, the tissue shows interstitial inflammation ranging from an intense lymphocytic infiltration (consistent with lymphoid interstitial pneumonitis) to a mild mononuclear inflammation. Corticosteroids may be helpful in some cases.

d. Sinusitis–Chronic sinusitis can be a frustrating problem for HIV-infected patients. Symptoms include sinus congestion and discharge, headache, and fever. Some patients may have radiographic evidence on sinus x-ray or sinus CT scan of sinus disease in the absence of significant symptoms. Nonsmoking patients with purulent drainage should be treated with amoxicillin (500 mg orally three times a day). Patients who smoke should be treated with amoxicillin-potassium clavulanate (500 mg orally three times a day) to cover *H influenzae.* Prolonged treatment (3–6 weeks) with an antibiotic and guaifenesin (600 mg orally twice daily) to decrease sinus congestion may be required. For patients not responding to amoxicillin-potassium clavulanate, ciprofloxacin should be tried (500 mg orally twice a day). Some patients may require referral to an otolaryngologist for sinus drainage.

3. Central nervous system disease–Central nervous system disease in HIV-infected patients can be divided into intracerebral space-occupying lesions, encephalopathy, meningitis, and spinal cord processes.

a. Toxoplasmosis–Toxoplasmosis is the most common space-occupying lesion in HIV-infected patients. Patients may present with headache, focal neurologic deficits, seizures, or altered mental status. The diagnosis is usually made presumptively based on the characteristic appearance of cerebral imaging studies. Typically, toxoplasmosis appears as multiple lesions, contrast-enhancing on CT scan, with a predilection for the basal ganglia.

Single lesions are atypical of toxoplasmosis. When a single lesion has been detected by CT scanning, MRI scanning—because of its greater sensitivity—may reveal multiple lesions. If a patient has a single lesion on MRI and is neurologically stable, clinicians may pursue a 2-week empirical trial of toxoplasmosis therapy. A repeat scan should be performed at 2 weeks. If the lesion has not diminished in size, biopsy of the lesion should be performed. Since many HIV-infected patients will have detectable titers, a positive toxoplasma serologic test does not confirm the diagnosis. Conversely, as many as 15% of patients with toxoplasmosis have negative titers by enzyme immunoassay or immunofluorescence assays. Polymerase chain reaction assays of cerebrospinal fluid are useful adjunctive tests.

b. Central nervous system lymphoma–Primary non-Hodgkin's lymphoma is the second most common space-occupying lesion in HIV-infected patients. Symptoms are similar to those with toxoplasmosis. While imaging techniques cannot distinguish these two diseases with certainty, lymphoma more often is solitary. Other less common lesions should be suspected if there is preceding bacteremia, positive tuberculin test, fungemia, or intravenous drug use. These include bacterial abscesses, cryptococcomas, tuberculomas, and nocardia lesions.

Because techniques for stereotactic brain biopsy have improved, this procedure plays an increasing role in diagnosing cerebral lesions. Biopsy should be strongly considered if lesions are solitary or do not respond to toxoplasmosis treatment, especially if they are easily accessible. Diagnosis of lymphoma is important because patients who have not had a prior opportunistic infection are likely to benefit from treatment (radiation therapy). In the future, it may be possible to avoid brain biopsy by utilizing PCR assay of cerebrospinal fluid for Epstein-Barr virus DNA, which is present in 90% of cases.

c. AIDS dementia complex–AIDS dementia complex (HIV-associated cognitive/motor complex) is the most common cause of mental status changes in HIV-infected patients. The diagnosis is one of exclusion based on a brain imaging study and spinal fluid analysis that exclude other pathogens. Neuropsychiatric testing is helpful in distinguishing patients with dementia from those with depression. Patients with AIDS dementia complex typically have difficulty with cognitive tasks and exhibit diminished motor speed. Patients may first notice a deterioration in their handwriting. The manifestations of dementia may wax and wane, with persons exhibiting periods of lucidity and confusion over the course of a day. Although the mechanism by which HIV causes neurologic dysfunction is not completely understood, many patients improve with effective antiretroviral treatment. The calcium channel blocker nimodipine has been shown to be well tolerated but is of uncertain efficacy. Metabolic abnormalities may also cause changes in mental status: hypoglycemia, hyponatremia, hypoxia, and drug overdose are important considerations in this population. Other less common infectious causes of encephalopathy include progressive multifocal leukoencephalopathy, cytomegalovirus, syphilis, and herpes simplex encephalitis.

d. Cryptococcal meningitis–Cryptococcal meningitis typically presents with fever and headache. Less than 20% of patients have meningismus. Diagnosis is based on a positive latex agglutination test (CRAG) or positive culture of spinal fluid for cryptococcus. Seventy to ninety percent of patients with cryptococcal meningitis have a positive serum CRAG. Thus, a negative serum CRAG test makes a diagnosis of cryptococcal meningitis unlikely and can be useful in the initial evaluation of a patient with headache, fever, and normal mental status. HIV meningitis, characterized by lymphocytic pleocytosis of the spinal fluid with negative culture, is common early in HIV infection and may mimic cryptococcal meningitis in its clinical presentation.

e. HIV myelopathy–Spinal cord function may also be impaired in HIV-infected individuals. HIV myelopathy presents with leg weakness and incontinence. Spastic paraparesis and sensory ataxia are seen on neurologic examination. Myelopathy is usually a late manifestation of HIV disease, and most patients will have concomitant HIV encephalopathy. Pathologic evaluation of the spinal cord reveals vacuolation of white matter. Because HIV myelopathy is a diagnosis of exclusion, symptoms suggestive of myelopathy should be evaluated by lumbar puncture to rule out cytomegalovirus polyradiculopathy (described below) and an MRI or CT scan to exclude epidural lymphoma.

f. Progressive multifocal leukoencephalopathy (PML)–PML is an untreatable viral infection of the white matter of the brain seen in patients with very advanced HIV infection. It typically results in focal neurologic deficits such as aphasia, hemiparesis, and cortical blindness. Imaging studies are strongly suggestive of the diagnosis if they show nonenhancing white matter lesions without mass effect. Extensive lesions may be difficult to differentiate from the changes caused by HIV. Several patients have stabilized or improved after the institution of combination antiretroviral therapy.

4. Peripheral nervous system–Peripheral nervous system syndromes include inflammatory polyneuropathies, sensory neuropathies, and mononeuropathies.

An inflammatory demyelinating polyneuropathy similar to Guillain-Barré syndrome occurs in HIV-infected patients, usually prior to frank immunodeficiency. The syndrome in many cases improves with plasmapheresis, supporting an autoimmune basis of the disease. Cytomegalovirus can cause an ascending polyradiculopathy characterized by lower extremity weakness and a neutrophilic pleocytosis on spinal fluid analysis with a negative bacterial culture. Transverse myelitis can be seen with herpes zoster or cytomegalovirus.

About 30% of patients with advanced HIV disease develop sensory neuropathies. Affected patients typically complain of numbness, tingling, and pain in their lower extremities. Symptoms are disproportionate to findings on gross sensory and motor evaluation. In contrast to inflammatory demyelinating polyneuropathy, sensory neuropathies occur late in HIV-disease progression and are due to axonal loss. Evaluation should rule out other causes of sensory neuropathy such as alcoholism, thyroid disease, vitamin B_{12} deficiency, and syphilis. Severe sensory neuropathy is a contraindication to initiation of three antiretroviral drugs, the dideoxynucleosides didanosine (ddI), zalcitabine (ddC), and stavudine (d4T), because they all can cause peripheral neuropathy. Occasionally, sensory neuropathies improve with zidovudine therapy, but more commonly treatment is symptomatic with amitriptyline. Gabapentin, at a starting dose of 300 mg orally three times a day, has also been anecdotally reported to improve symptoms in some patients. A randomized study of recombinant nerve growth factor administered subcutaneously has shown that individuals with moderate to severe neuropathy tended to experience some reduction of pain. However, this therapy is currently unavailable.

5. Rheumatologic manifestations–Arthritis, involving single or multiple joints, with or without effusion, has been commonly noted in HIV-infected patients. Involvement of large joints is most common. While the cause of HIV-related arthritis is unknown, most patients will respond to nonsteroidal anti-inflammatory agents. Patients with a sizable effusion, especially if the joint is warm or erythematous, should have the joint tapped, followed by culture of the fluid to rule out suppurative arthritis as well as fungal and mycobacterial disease.

Several rheumatologic syndromes, including Reiter's syndrome, psoriatic arthritis, sicca syndrome, and systemic lupus erythematosus, have been reported in HIV-infected patients (Chapter 19). However, it is unclear if the prevalence is greater than in the general population.

6. Myopathy–Myopathies are increasingly noted in HIV-infected patients. Proximal muscle weakness is typical, and patients may have varying degrees of muscle tenderness. The most important clinical distinction is between myopathy due to the primary effect of HIV and that due to zidovudine. Patients with symptomatic myopathy, especially with creatine kinase levels greater than 1000 units/L, should have their dose of zidovudine decreased or stopped and be considered for alternative antiviral therapy (didanosine or zalcitabine). A muscle biopsy can distinguish HIV myopathy from zidovudine myopathy and should be considered in patients for whom continuation of zidovudine is essential.

7. Retinitis–Complaints of visual changes must be evaluated immediately in HIV-infected patients. Cytomegalovirus retinitis, characterized by perivascular hemorrhages and fluffy exudates, is the most common retinal infection in AIDS patients and can be rapidly progressive. In contrast, cotton wool spots, which are also common in HIV-infected people, are benign, remit spontaneously, and appear as small indistinct white spots without exudation or hemorrhage. This distinction may be difficult at times for the nonspecialist, and patients with visual changes should be seen by an ophthalmologist. Other rare retinal processes include other herpesvirus infections or toxoplasmosis.

8. Oral lesions–The findings of oral candidiasis and hairy leukoplakia are significant for several reasons. First, these lesions are highly suggestive of HIV infection. Second, several studies have indicated that patients with these lesions have a high rate of progression to AIDS, though it is not known whether this increased risk within 3 years is independent of other parameters of immune function, such as the CD4 count.

Hairy leukoplakia is caused by the Epstein-Barr virus. The lesion is not usually troubling to patients and sometimes regresses spontaneously. Hairy leukoplakia is commonly seen as a white lesion on the lateral aspect of the tongue. It may be flat or slightly raised, is usually corrugated, and has vertical parallel lines with fine or thick ("hairy") projections. Patients who are bothered by hairy leukoplakia can be treated with acyclovir, 800 mg orally four times a day, until it resolves. It may, however, return once therapy is discontinued. Oral candidiasis can be bothersome to patients, many of whom report an unpleasant taste or mouth dryness. There are two types of oral candidiasis: pseudomembranous (removable white plaques) and erythematous (red friable plaques). Treatment is with topical agents such as clotrimazole 10 mg troches (one four or five times a day). Patients with candidiasis that does not respond to topical antifungals can be treated with fluconazole (50–100 mg orally once a day for 3–7 days). Chronic suppression of oral candidiasis with fluconazole has been associated with development of candidiasis resistant to all available azoles and thus should be avoided except in frequently recurring cases.

Angular cheilitis—fissures at the sides of the mouth—is usually due to candida as well and can be treated topically with ketoconazole cream (2%) twice a day.

Gingival disease is common in HIV-infected patients and is thought to be due to an overgrowth of microorganisms. It usually responds to professional dental cleaning and chlorhexidine rinses. Some HIV-infected patients will develop a particularly aggressive gingivitis or periodontitis; these patients should be started on antibiotics that cover anaerobic oral flora (eg, metronidazole, 250 mg four times a day for 4 or 5 days) and referred to oral surgeons with experience with these entities.

Aphthous ulcers are painful and may interfere with eating. They can be treated with fluocinonide (0.05% ointment mixed 1:1 with plain Orabase and applied six times a day to the ulcer). For lesions that are difficult to reach, patients should use dexamethasone swishes (0.5 mg in 5 mL elixir three times a day). The pain of the ulcers can be relieved with use of an anesthetic spray (10% lidocaine). For patients with refractory ulcers, thalidomide, 100–200 mg orally daily, has proved useful and may be obtained through a compassionate use protocol. Other lesions seen in the mouths of HIV-infected patients include Kaposi's sarcoma (usually on the hard palate), and warts.

9. Gastrointestinal manifestations–

a. Candidal esophagitis–(See also discussion in Chapter 14.) Esophageal candidiasis is a common AIDS infection. In a patient with characteristic symptoms, empirical antifungal treatment is begun with fluconazole (200 mg daily for 10–14 days). Further evaluation to identify other causes of esophagitis (herpes simplex, cytomegalovirus) is reserved for patients who do not improve with treatment.

b. Hepatic disease–Autopsy studies have demonstrated that the liver is a frequent site of infections and neoplasms in HIV-infected patients. However, many of these infections are not clinically symptomatic. Clinicians may note elevations of alkaline phosphatase and aminotransferases on routine chemistry panels. Mycobacterial disease, cytomegalovirus, hepatitis B virus, hepatitis C virus, and lymphoma cause liver disease and can present with varying degrees of nausea, vomiting, and right upper quadrant abdominal pain. Sulfonamides, imidazole drugs, antituberculous medications, pentamidine, clarithromycin, and didanosine (ddI) have also been associated with hepatitis. HIV-infected patients with chronic active hepatitis may have less severe bouts of hepatitis because of the concomitant immunodeficiency. Percutaneous liver biopsy may be helpful in diagnosing liver disease, but frequently the cause can be determined by other tests (eg, blood culture, biopsy of a more accessible site). Moreover, because the majority of hepatic infections do not respond well to treatment (eg, *M avium* complex), liver biopsy should be reserved for people with persistent symptoms and laboratory abnormalities in whom no other cause for illness can be determined.

c. Biliary disease–Biliary disease is common in AIDS patients. Cholecystitis presents with similar manifestations as seen in immunocompetent hosts but is more likely to be acalculous. Sclerosing cholangitis and papillary stenosis have also been increasingly reported in HIV-infected patients. Typically, the syndrome presents with severe nausea, vomiting, and right upper quadrant pain. Liver function tests generally show alkaline phosphatase elevations disproportionate to elevation of the aminotransferases. Although dilated ducts can be seen on ultrasound, the diagnosis is made by endoscopic retrograde cholangiopancreatography, which reveals intraluminal irregularities of the proximal intrahepatic ducts with "pruning" of the terminal ductal branches. Stenosis of the distal common bile duct at the papilla is commonly seen with this syndrome. Cytomegalovirus, cryptosporidium, and microsporidia are thought to play inciting roles in this syndrome. Initial reports of symptomatic improvement with performance of sphincterotomies were encouraging, but many patients had recurrence of symptoms.

d. Enterocolitis–Enterocolitis is a common problem in HIV-infected individuals. Organisms known to cause enterocolitis include bacteria (campylobacter, salmonella, shigella), viruses (cytomegalovirus, adenovirus), and protozoans (cryptosporidium, *Entamoeba histolytica,* giardia, isospora, microsporida). HIV itself may cause enterocolitis. Several of the organisms causing enterocolitis in HIV-infected individuals also cause diarrhea in immunocompetent hosts. However, HIV-infected patients tend to have more severe and more chronic symptoms, including high fevers and severe abdominal pain that can mimic acute abdominal catastrophes. Bacteremia and concomitant biliary involvement are also more common with enterocolitis in HIV-infected patients. Relapses of enterocolitis following adequate therapy have been reported with both salmonella and shigella infections.

Because of the wide range of agents known to cause enterocolitis, a stool culture and multiple stool examinations for ova and parasites (including modified acid-fast staining for cryptosporidium) should be performed. Those patients who have cryptosporidium in one stool with improvement in symptoms in less than 1 month should not be considered to have AIDS, as cryptosporidium is a cause of self-limited diarrhea in HIV-negative hosts. More commonly, HIV-infected patients with cryptosporidium have persistent enterocolitis with profuse watery diarrhea.

To date, no consistently effective treatments have been developed for cryptosporidium infection. There are anecdotal reports of good responses to paromomycin (500 mg orally four times daily for 2 weeks). Patients with high CD4 counts are more likely to respond to this regimen. Patients who respond may be given chronic suppression (500 mg twice daily). Patients who do not respond may be given a trial of paromomycin with azithromycin (500 mg daily) for 21 days. Nitazoxanide (NTZ) at a dosage of 1000 mg daily is not FDA-approved but is available through a compassionate use protocol (Romark Laboratories: 813-282-8544). Immune bovine colostrum, the newer macrolide antibiotics, and diclazuril are being evaluated as oral therapy. Patients should be given diphenoxylate with atropine (one or two tablets orally three or four times a day). Those who do not respond may be given paregoric with bismuth (5–10 mL orally three or four times a day). Octreotide in escalating doses (starting at 0.05 mg subcutaneously every 8 hours for 48 hours) has been found to ameliorate symptoms in approximately 40% of patients with cryptosporidial or idiopathic HIV-associated diarrhea.

Patients with a negative stool examination and persistent symptoms should be evaluated with colonoscopy and biopsy. Patients whose symptoms last longer than 1 month with no identified cause of diarrhea are considered to have a presumptive diagnosis of AIDS enteropathy. A primary effect of the HIV on the colonic epithelium may be the cause. Patients may respond to institution of effective antiretroviral treatment. Upper endoscopy with small bowel biopsy is not recommended as a routine part of the evaluation. Many patients who undergo upper endoscopy have nonspecific abnormalities, but these rarely reflect treatable diseases.

e. Other disorders–Two other important gastrointestinal abnormalities in HIV-infected patients are gastropathy and malabsorption. It has been documented that some HIV-infected patients do not produce normal levels of stomach acid and therefore are unable to absorb drugs such as itraconazole that require an acid medium. This decreased acid production may explain, in part, the susceptibility of HIV-infected patients to campylobacter, salmonella, and shigella, all of which are sensitive to acid concentration. There is no evidence that *Helicobacter pylori* is more common in HIV-infected persons.

A malabsorption syndrome occurs commonly in HIV-infected patients. It can be due to infection of the small bowel with *M avium* complex, cryptosporidium, or microsporidia. In other cases, biopsy of the small bowel reveals no pathogens but histologic changes consistent with Whipple's disease.

10. Endocrinologic manifestations–The adrenal gland is the most commonly afflicted endocrine gland in patients with AIDS. Abnormalities demonstrated on autopsy include infection (especially with cytomegalovirus and *M avium* complex), infiltration with Kaposi's sarcoma, and injury from hemorrhage and presumed autoimmunity. The prevalence of clinically significant adrenal insufficiency is low. Patients with suggestive symptoms should undergo a cosyntropin stimulation test.

While frank deficiency of cortisol is rare, an isolated defect in mineralocorticoid metabolism may lead to salt wasting and hyperkalemia. Such patients should be treated with fludrocortisone (0.1–0.2 mg daily).

AIDS patients appear to have abnormalities of thyroid function tests different from those of patients with other chronic diseases. AIDS patients have been shown to have high levels of triiodothyronine (T_3), thyroxine (T_4), and thyroid-binding globulin and low levels of reverse triiodothyronine (rT_3). The causes and clinical significance of these abnormalities are unknown.

11. Skin manifestations–HIV-infected patients commonly develop skin manifestations that can be grouped into viral, bacterial, fungal, neoplastic, and nonspecific dermatitides.

Herpes simplex infections occur more frequently, tend to be more severe, and are more likely to disseminate in AIDS patients than in immunocompetent hosts. Because of the risk of progressive local disease, all herpes simplex attacks should be treated with acyclovir (200 mg orally five times a day), or famciclovir (500 mg orally three times a day) for 7 days. To avoid the complications of attacks, many clinicians recommend chronic acyclovir administration (400 mg orally twice a day) for HIV-infected patients with a history of recurrent herpes. However, the finding of acyclovir resistance among some herpes strains cultured from HIV-infected patients raises concern about this practice.

Herpes zoster is a common manifestation of HIV infection. As with herpes simplex infections, patients with zoster should be treated with acyclovir to prevent dissemination (800 mg orally four or five times per day for 7 days). Vesicular lesions should be cultured if there is any question about their origin, since herpes simplex responds to much lower doses of acyclovir. Disseminated zoster and cases with ocular involvement should be treated with intravenous (10 mg/kg every 8 hours for 7–10 days) rather than oral acyclovir.

Molluscum contagiosum is seen in HIV-infected patients, as in other immunocompromised patients. Lesions have a propensity for spreading widely over the patient's skin and should be treated with topical liquid nitrogen.

Staphylococcus is the most common bacterial cause of skin disease in HIV-infected patients; it usually presents as folliculitis, superficial abscesses (furuncles), or bullous impetigo. Because dissemination with sepsis has been reported, attempts should be made to treat these lesions aggressively. Folliculitis is initially treated with topical clindamycin or mupirocin, and patients may benefit from regular washing with an antibacterial soap such as chlorhexidine. Intranasal mupirocin has been used successfully for staphylococcal decolonization in other settings. In HIV-infected patients with recurrent staphylococcal infections, weekly intranasal mupirocin should be considered in addition to topical care and systemic antibiotics. Abscesses often require incision and drainage. Patients may need antistaphylococcal antibiotics such as dicloxacillin, 250–500 mg orally four times daily, or erythromycin, 250 mg orally four times daily (with rifampin, 600 mg orally daily for 10 days for nasal staphylococcal decolonization), for severe folliculitis.

Bacillary angiomatosis is a well-described entity in HIV-infected patients. It is caused by two closely related organisms: *Bartonella henselae* and *Bartonella quintana.* The epidemiology of *B henselae* infection suggests zoonotic transmission from young cats. *B quintana* may be harbored by fleas. The most common manifestation is raised, reddish, highly vascular skin lesions that can mimic the lesions of Kaposi's sarcoma. Fever is a common manifestation of this infection; involvement of bone, lymph nodes, and liver has also been reported. Responses to doxycycline, 100 mg orally twice daily, and erythromycin, 250 mg orally four times daily, have been reported. Therapy is continued for at least 14 days, and patients who are seriously ill with visceral involvement may require months of therapy.

The majority of fungal rashes afflicting AIDS patients are due to dermatophytes and candida. These are particularly common in the inguinal region but may occur anywhere on the body. Fungal rashes generally respond well to topical clotrimazole (1% twice a day) or ketoconazole (2% twice a day).

Kaposi's sarcoma lesions are red or purple, flat or raised papules that generally do not blanch. Since they may be confused with lesions of bacillary angiomatosis, biopsy for definitive diagnosis should be performed. Cutaneous lesions can be treated with radiation or with intralesional injection of vinblastine, 0.01–0.02 mg in 0.1 mL of saline. Other dermatologic malignancies seen disproportionately among HIV-infected persons include basal cell and squamous cell carcinomas.

Seborrheic dermatitis is more common in HIV-infected patients. Scrapings of seborrhea have revealed *Malassezia furfur (Pityrosporum ovale),* implying that the seborrhea is caused by this fungus. Consistent with the isolation of this fungus is the clinical finding that seborrhea responds well to topical clotrimazole (1% cream) as well as hydrocortisone (1% cream).

Xerosis presents in HIV-infected patients with severe pruritus. The patient may have no rash, or nonspecific excoriations from scratching. Treatment is with emollients (eg, absorption base cream) and antipruritic lotions (eg, camphor 9.5% and menthol 0.5%).

Psoriasis can be very severe in HIV-infected patients. Phototherapy and etretinate (0.25–9.75 mg/kg/d orally in divided doses) may be used for recalcitrant cases in consultation with a dermatologist. Because of the underlying immunodeficiency, methotrexate should be avoided.

12. HIV-related malignancies–Four cancers are currently included in the CDC classification of AIDS: Kaposi's sarcoma, non-Hodgkin's lymphoma, primary lymphoma of the brain, and invasive cervical carcinoma. Epidemiologic studies have shown that between 1973 and 1987 among single men in San Francisco, the risk of Kaposi's sarcoma increased more than 5000-fold and the risk of non-Hodgkin's lymphoma more than tenfold. The increase in incidence of malignancies is probably a function of impaired cell-mediated immunity.

Kaposi's sarcoma is still the most common HIV-related malignancy. Kaposi's lesions may appear anywhere; careful examination of the eyelids, conjunctiva, pinnae, palate, and toe webs is mandatory to locate potentially occult lesions. In light-skinned individuals, Kaposi's lesions usually appear as purplish, nonblanching lesions that can be papular or nodular. In dark-skinned individuals, the lesions may appear more brown. In the mouth, lesions are most often palatal papules, though exophytic lesions of the tongue and gingivae may also be seen. Kaposi's lesions may be confused with other vascular lesions such as angiomas and pyogenic granulomas. About 40% of patients with dermatologic Kaposi's sarcoma will develop visceral disease (eg, gastrointestinal, pulmonary). Rapidly progressive dermatologic or visceral disease is best treated with systemic chemotherapy. Commonly used regimens include alternating weekly vincristine and vinblastine or combination doxorubicin, bleomycin, and vincristine. Alpha interferon has activity against Kaposi's sarcoma and may result in remission of lesions in minimally symptomatic patients with high CD4 counts and no history of opportunistic infection. However, even in this subgroup, subjective symptoms (eg, malaise, anorexia) limit the utility of this therapy. Bulky lesions of the lower extremities accompanied by lymphedema are a common presentation of Kaposi's sarcoma. Radiation and conservative measures (eg, leg elevation, elastic stockings) may be helpful.

Non-Hodgkin's lymphoma in HIV-infected persons tends to be very aggressive. The malignancies are usually of B cell origin and characterized as diffuse large-cell tumors. Over 70% of the malignancies are extranodal.

Patients with primary central nervous system disease are treated with radiation therapy. Systemic disease is treated with chemotherapy. Common regimens are CHOP (cyclophosphamide, doxorubicin, vincristine, and prednisone) and modified M-BACOD (methotrexate, bleomycin, doxorubicin, cyclophosphamide, vincristine, and dexamethasone).

Intrathecal chemotherapy is administered to prevent or treat meningeal involvement. Granulocyte colony-stimulating factor (G-CSF; filgrastim) is used to maintain white blood counts with this latter regimen.

Although Hodgkin's disease is not included as part of the CDC definition of AIDS, studies have found that HIV infection is associated with a fivefold increase in the incidence of Hodgkin's disease. HIV-infected persons with Hodgkin's disease are more likely to have mixed cellularity and lymphocyte depletion subtypes of Hodgkin's disease and to present at an advanced stage of disease.

Anal dysplasia and squamous cell carcinoma have been noted in HIV-infected homosexual men. These lesions have been strongly correlated with previous infection by human papillomavirus (HPV). While many of the infected men report a history of anal warts or have visible warts, a significant percentage have silent papillomavirus infection. Cytologic (using Papanicolaou smears) and papillomavirus DNA studies can easily be performed on specimens obtained by anal swab. Although many questions remain unanswered, the growing frequency of these problems and the risk of progression from dysplasia to cancer in immunocompromised patients suggest that annual anal swabs for cytologic examination should be done in all HIV-infected persons who have engaged in anal intercourse.

HPV also appears to play a causative role in cervical dysplasia and neoplasia. The incidence and clinical course of cervical disease in HIV-infected women are discussed below.

13. Gynecologic manifestations–Vaginal candidiasis, cervical dysplasia and neoplasia, and pelvic inflammatory disease are more common in HIV-infected women than in uninfected women. These manifestations also tend to be more severe when they occur in association with HIV infection. Therefore, HIV-infected women need frequent gynecologic care. Vaginal candidiasis may be treated with topical agents (see Chapter 36). However, HIV-infected women with recurrent or severe vaginal candidiasis may need systemic therapy.

The incidence of cervical dysplasia in HIV-infected women is 40%. Because of this finding, HIV-infected women should have Papanicolaou smears every 6 months (as opposed to the AHCPR Guideline recommendation for every 12 months). Some clinicians recommend routine colposcopy or cervicography because cervical intraepithelial neoplasia has occurred in women with negative Papanicolaou smears. Cone biopsy is indicated in cases of serious cervical dysplasia.

Cervical neoplasia appears to be more aggressive among HIV-infected women. Most HIV-infected women with cervical cancer die of that disease rather than of AIDS. Because of its frequency and severity, cervical neoplasia was added to the CDC definition of AIDS in 1993.

While pelvic inflammatory disease appears to be more common in HIV-infected women, the bacteriology of this condition appears to be the same as among HIV-uninfected women. At present, HIV-infected women with pelvic inflammatory disease should be treated with the same regimens as uninfected women (see Chapter 17). However, inpatient therapy is generally recommended.

B. Laboratory Findings: Specific tests for HIV include antibody and antigen detection (Table 31–2). Screening serology is done by enzyme-linked immunosorbent assay (ELISA). Positive specimens are then confirmed by a different method (eg, Western blot). The sensitivity of screening serologic tests is greater than 99.5%. The specificity of positive results by two different techniques approaches 100% even in low-risk populations. False-positive screening tests may occur as normal biologic variants or in association with recent influenza vaccination or other disease

Table 31–2. Laboratory findings with HIV infection.

Test	Significance
HIV enzyme-linked immunosorbent assay (ELISA)	Screening test for HIV infection. Sensitivity > 99.9%; to avoid false-positive results, repeatedly reactive results must be confirmed with Western blot.
Western blot	Confirmatory test for HIV. Specificity when combined with ELISA > 99.99%. Indeterminate results with early HIV infection, HIV-2 infection, autoimmune disease, pregnancy, and recent tetanus toxoid administration.
CBC	Anemia, neutropenia, and thrombocytopenia common with advanced HIV infection.
Absolute CD4 lymphocyte count	Most widely used predictor of HIV progression. Risk of progression to an AIDS opportunistic infection or malignancy is high with CD4 < 200 cells/μL.
CD4 lymphocyte percentage	Percentage may be more reliable than the CD4 count. Risk of progression to an AIDS opportunistic infection or malignancy is high with percentage < 20%.
HIV viral load tests	These tests measure the amount of actively replicating HIV virus. Correlates with disease progression and response to antiretroviral drugs. Levels > 5000–10,000 copies/mL indicate the need for treatment.
β_2-Microglobulin	Cell surface protein indicative of macrophage-monocyte stimulation. Levels > 3.5 mg/dL associated with rapid progression of disease. Not useful with intravenous drug users.

states, such as connective tissue disease. These are usually detected by negative confirmatory tests. Molecular biology techniques (polymerase chain reaction) show a small incidence of individuals (< 1%) who are infected with HIV for up to 36 months without generating an antibody response. However, the vast majority will develop antibodies detectable by screening serologic tests within several months of infection.

Nonspecific laboratory findings with HIV infection may include anemia, leukopenia (particularly lymphopenia) and thrombocytopenia in any combination, polyclonal hypergammaglobulinemia, and hypocholesterolemia. Cutaneous anergy is common.

Several laboratory markers are available to provide prognostic information and guide therapy decisions (Table 31–2). The most widely used marker is the absolute CD4 lymphocyte count. As counts decrease, the risk of serious opportunistic infection over the subsequent 3–5 years increases (Figure 31–1).

The limitations of the CD4 count have become more apparent. There is substantial diurnal variation (counts are generally lower in the morning), and counts may be depressed by any intercurrent illness. Therefore, the trend in counts is more important than any single value. Because of laboratory variation, serial counts should be performed in the same laboratory. The frequency of performance of counts depends on the patient's health status. Patients whose CD4 counts are substantially above the threshold for initiation of antiviral therapy (500 cells/μL) should have counts performed every 6 months. Those who have counts near or below 500 cells/μL should have counts performed every 3 months. This is necessary for evaluating the efficacy of antiviral therapy and for initiating *P carinii* prophylactic therapy when the CD4 count drops below 200 cells/μL. Some studies suggest that the percentage of CD4 lymphocytes is a more reliable indicator of prognosis than the absolute counts because the percentage does not depend on calculating a manual differential. While the CD4 count measures immune dysfunction, it does not provide a measure of how actively HIV is replicating in the body. This large gap in our ability to assess HIV replication has been filled by viral load tests. See further discussion of these tests in the section on antiretroviral treatment.

Koehler JE et al: Molecular epidemiology of *Bartonella* infections in patients with bacillary angiomatosis-peliosis. N Engl J Med 1997;337:1876. [NLM Cit ID: 98057268] (Emphasizes different transmission and clinical manifestations of the two species.)

McArthur JC: NeuroAIDS: Diagnosis and management. Hosp Pract (Off Ed) 1997 Aug;32:73. [NLM Cit ID: 99421845]

Mellors JW et al: Plasma viral load and CD4+ lymphocytes as prognostic markers of HIV-1 infection. Ann Intern Med 1997;126:946. [NLM Cit ID: 97315712] (Very useful stratification of risk of progression stratified by CD4 and HIV RNA subsets.)

Report of the NIH Panel to Define Principles of Therapy of HIV Infection. MMWR Morb Mortal Wkly Rep 1998; 47(RR-5):1. [NLM Cit ID: 98231829] (Guidelines for using antiretroviral treatment in a variety of settings.)

Schambelan M et al: Recombinant human growth hormone in patients with HIV-associated wasting: A randomized, placebo-controlled trial. Ann Intern Med 1996;125:873. [NLM Cit ID: 97067808] (Treatment with growth hormone increased body weight, lean body mass, and exercise tolerance.)

Differential Diagnosis

HIV infection may mimic a variety of other medical illnesses. Specific differential diagnosis depends upon the mode of presentation. In patients presenting with constitutional symptoms such as weight loss and fevers, differential considerations include cancer, chronic infections such as tuberculosis and endocarditis, and endocrinologic diseases such as hyperthyroidism. When pulmonary processes dominate the presentation, acute and chronic lung infections must be considered as well as other causes of diffuse interstitial pulmonary infiltrates. When neurologic disease is the mode of presentation, conditions that cause mental status changes or neuropathy—eg, alcoholism, liver disease, renal dysfunction, thyroid disease, and vitamin deficiency—should be considered. If a patient presents with headache and a cerebrospinal fluid pleocytosis, other causes of chronic meningitis enter the differential. When diarrhea is a prominent complaint, infectious enterocolitis, antibiotic-associated colitis, inflammatory bowel disease, and malabsorptive symptoms must be considered.

Prevention

A. Primary Prevention: Until vaccination is a reality, prevention of HIV infection will depend upon effective precautions regarding sexual practices and intravenous drug use, screening of blood products, and infection control practices in the health care setting. Primary care clinicians should routinely obtain a sexual history and provide risk factor assessment of their patients and, when appropriate, screening for HIV infection with pre- and posttest counseling. Pretest counseling should include review of risk factors for HIV infection, discussion of safe sex, and the meaning of a positive test. Posttest counseling should include a review of the importance of safe sex practices. For persons who test positive, information on available medical and mental health services should be provided as well as guidance for contacting sexual or needle-sharing partners. It is the duty of clinicians to counsel HIV-negative patients on how to avoid exposure to HIV. Patients should be counseled not to exchange bodily fluids unless they are in a long-term mutually monogamous relationship with someone who has tested HIV antibody-negative and has not engaged in unsafe sex for at least 6 months prior to or at any time since the negative test.

Only latex condoms should be used, along with a water-soluble lubricant. Although nonoxynol-9, a spermicide, kills HIV, it cannot be enthusiastically recommended as an ingredient in lubricants because of the possibility that it may cause genital ulcers which could facilitate HIV transmission. Patients should be counseled that condoms are not 100% effective. They should be made familiar with the use of condoms, including, specifically, the advice that condoms must be used every time; that space should be left at the tip of the condom as a receptacle for semen; that intercourse with a condom should not be attempted if the penis is only partially erect; that men should hold on to the base of the condom when withdrawing the penis to prevent slippage; and that condoms should not be reused. Although anal intercourse remains the sexual practice at highest risk of transmitting HIV, seroconversions have been documented with vaginal and oral intercourse as well. Therefore, condoms should be used when engaging in these activities. Women as well as men should understand how to use condoms so as to be sure that their partners are using them correctly.

Persons using intravenous drugs should be cautioned never to exchange needles or other drug paraphernalia. When sterile needles are not available, bleach does appear to inactivate HIV and should be used to clean needles.

Current efforts to screen blood and blood products have lowered the risk of HIV transmission with transfusion to 1:100,000.

In the hospital, concerns about nosocomial infection have led to the recommendation for universal body fluid precautions. This involves the rigorous use of gloves when handling any body fluid and the addition of gown, mask, and goggles for procedures that may result in splash or droplet spread. Reports of transmission of drug-resistant tuberculosis in health care settings also have had infection control implications. All patients with cough in outpatient settings should be encouraged to wear masks. Hospitalized HIV-infected patients with cough should be placed in respiratory isolation until tuberculosis can be excluded by chest x-ray and sputum smear examination. Primate model data have suggested that development of a protective vaccine may be possible, but clinical trials in humans using gp120 or its precursor gp160 have shown development of neutralizing antibodies to laboratory but not field isolates of HIV and may not be protective of infection.

B. Secondary Prevention: In the era prior to the development of highly effective antiretroviral treatment, cohort studies of individuals with documented dates of seroconversion demonstrate that approximately 50% of untreated seropositive persons develop AIDS within 10 years. Recent improvements in treatment would be expected to substantially improve this prognosis. Too few persons have been treated with these regimens prior to the development of AIDS to provide good data on progression of disease with these new regimens. Nevertheless, decreases in the incidence of AIDS reflecting successful treatment of HIV and successful HIV prevention efforts have been reported in the United States.

There is substantial evidence that medical intervention with antiretroviral and prophylactic regimens can prevent opportunistic infections and improve survival. Treatment prevents several infectious diseases, including tuberculosis and syphilis, which are transmissible to others. Recommendations are listed in Table 31–3.

Because of the increased occurrence of tuberculosis among HIV-infected patients, all such individuals should undergo PPD testing. Although anergy is common among AIDS patients, the likelihood of a false-negative result is much lower when the test is done early in infection. Those with positive tests (defined for HIV-infected patients as > 5 mm of induration) need a chest x-ray. Patients with an infiltrate in any location, especially if accompanied by mediastinal adenopathy, should have sputum sent for acid-fast staining. Patients with a positive PPD but negative evaluations for active disease should receive isoniazid (300 mg daily) with pyridoxine (50 mg daily)—or rifampin (600 mg daily) with pyrazinamide (20 mg/kg daily)—for 9 months to a year regardless of their age. Recent analysis suggests also that HIV-infected individuals at high risk for tuberculosis should receive a course of isoniazid prophylaxis regardless of PPD status. This may include homeless individuals and injection drug users.

HIV-infected patients are at increased risk of reactivation of syphilis and progression to tertiary syphilis despite standard treatment. Because the only

Table 31–3. Health care maintenance of HIV-infected individuals.

For all HIV-infected individuals
CD4 counts every 3–6 months
Viral load tests every 3–6 months and 1 month following a change in therapy
PPD with anergy controls
INH for those with positive PPD and normal chest x-ray
RPR or VDRL
Toxoplasma IgG serology
Cytomegalovirus IgG serology
Pneumococcal vaccine
Influenza vaccine in season
Hepatitis vaccine for those who are HBsAb-negative
Haemophilus influenzae b vaccination
Papanicolaou smears every 6 months for women
Consider anal swabs for cytologic evaluation yearly for men with history of receptive anal intercourse
For HIV-infected individuals with CD4 < 500 cells/μL
Antiretroviral therapy (see Figure 31–2)
For HIV-infected individuals with CD4 < 200 cells/μL
P carinii prophylaxis (see Table 31–6)
For HIV-infected individuals with CD4 < 100 cells/μL
M avium complex prophylaxis
Consider CMV prophylaxis

widely available tests for syphilis are serologic and because HIV-infected individuals are known to have disordered antibody production, there is concern about the interpretation of these titers. This concern has been fueled by a report of an HIV-infected patient with secondary syphilis and negative syphilis serologic testing. Furthermore, HIV-infected individuals may lose FTA-ABS reactivity after treatment for syphilis, particularly if they have low CD4 counts. Thus, in this population, a nonreactive treponemal test does not rule out a past history of syphilis. In addition, persistence of treponemes in the spinal fluid after one dose of benzathine penicillin has been demonstrated in HIV-infected patients with primary and secondary syphilis. Therefore, the CDC has recommended an aggressive diagnostic approach to HIV-infected patients with reactive RPR or VDRL tests of greater than 1 year or unknown duration. All such patients should have a lumbar puncture with cerebrospinal fluid cell count and CSF-VDRL. Those with a normal cerebrospinal fluid evaluation are treated as having late latent syphilis (benzathine penicillin G, 2.4 million units intramuscularly weekly for 3 weeks) with follow-up titers. Those with a pleocytosis or a positive CSF-VDRL test are treated as having neurosyphilis (aqueous penicillin G, 2–4 million units intravenously every 4 hours; or procaine penicillin G, 2.4 million units intramuscularly daily, with probenecid, 500 mg four times daily, for 10 days). Some clinicians take a less aggressive approach to patients who have low titers (less than 1:8), a history of having been treated for syphilis, and a normal neurologic examination. Close follow-up of titers is mandatory if such a course is taken. For a more detailed discussion of this topic, see Chapter 34.

The efficacy of pneumococcal vaccine is debated, but since it is safe, HIV-infected individuals should receive it. Patients without evidence of hepatitis B antigen or surface antibody should receive hepatitis B vaccination. Live vaccines, such as yellow fever vaccine, should be avoided. Measles vaccination, while a live virus vaccine, appears relatively safe when administered to HIV-infected individuals and should be given if the patient has never had measles or been adequately vaccinated.

HIV-infected individuals should be counseled with regard to safe sex. Because of the risk of transmission, they should be warned to use condoms with sexual intercourse, including oral intercourse. HIV-infected women should use latex barriers such as dental dams (available at dental supply stores) to prevent their partners from having direct oral contact with vaginal secretions. Substance abuse treatment should be recommended for persons who are using recreational drugs. They should be warned to avoid consuming raw meat or eggs to avoid infections with toxoplasma, campylobacter, and salmonella. Because of the emotional impact of HIV infection and subsequent illness, many patients will benefit from supportive counseling.

C. HIV Risk for Health Care Professionals: Epidemiologic studies show that needle sticks occur commonly among health care professionals, especially among surgeons performing invasive procedures, inexperienced hospital house staff, and medical students. Efforts to reduce needle sticks should focus on avoiding recapping needles and, whenever possible, doing invasive procedures under controlled circumstances. The risk of HIV transmission from a needle stick with blood from an HIV-infected patient is about 1:300. The risk from mucous membrane contact is too low to quantitate.

Health care professionals who sustain needle sticks should be counseled and offered HIV testing as soon as possible. HIV testing is done to establish a negative baseline for worker's compensation claims in case there is a subsequent conversion. Follow-up testing is usually performed at 6 weeks, 3 months, and 6 months.

A case-control study by the Centers for Disease Control and Prevention indicates that administration of zidovudine following a needle stick decreases the rate of HIV seroconversion by 79%. Furthermore, data from animal models suggest potential efficacy of zidovudine when given soon after exposure. Therefore, providers should be offered therapy with zidovudine (200 mg orally three times daily) and lamivudine (150 mg orally twice daily). Providers who have high-risk exposures (eg, deep punctures), exposures to source patients with advanced disease or with high viral loads (eg, > 50,000 copies per milliliter), or exposures to source patients who may have virus resistant to standard antiretroviral therapy should be offered a protease inhibitor in addition to the above regimen (eg, indinavir, 800 mg orally three times daily). Therapy should be started as soon as possible after exposure and continued for 4 weeks. Unfortunately, there have been documented cases of seroconversion following parenteral exposure to HIV despite prompt use of zidovudine prophylaxis. Counseling of the provider should include "safe sex" guidelines.

D. Postexposure Prophylaxis for Sexual and Drug Use Exposures to HIV: Following publication of a case-control study indicating that antiretroviral therapy decreased the odds of seroconversion among health care workers who had occupational exposure, some experts have recommended offering antiretroviral therapy following exposure to HIV through sexual or drug use exposures. While there are no efficacy data to support this practice, there are similarities between the immune response following transcutaneous and transmucosal exposures. The goal of postexposure prophylaxis is to reduce or prevent local viral replication prior to dissemination such that the infection can be aborted.

The choice of antiretroviral agents and the duration of treatment is the same as that for exposures that occur through the occupational route (see above).

In contrast to those with occupational exposures, some individuals may present very late after exposure. Because the likelihood of success declines with length of time from HIV exposure, it is not recommended that treatment be offered after 72 hours. In addition, because the psychosocial issues involved with postexposure prophylaxis for sexual and drug use exposures are complex, it should be offered only in the context of prevention counseling. Counseling should focus on how to prevent future exposures.

E. Preventing Perinatal Transmission of HIV: A multicenter trial showed that when zidovudine is administered to women during pregnancy, labor, and delivery and then to their newborns, the rate of transmission of HIV is decreased by two-thirds. For this reason, all women who are pregnant or considering pregnancy should be offered an HIV antibody test. At a minimum, pregnant HIV-infected women should be started on zidovudine during the second trimester. Many obstetricians recommend combination antiretroviral treatment, especially if zidovudine resistance is suspected. HIV-infected women receiving antiretroviral therapy in whom pregnancy is recognized during the first trimester should be counseled about the benefits and potential risks to the fetus of treatment during the first trimester. Since healthy mothers make healthy babies, continuation of therapy should be strongly considered. Because about half of fetal infections in non-breast-feeding women occur shortly before or during the birth process, antiretroviral therapy should be administered whenever a woman initiates perinatal care even if she did not begin therapy in the second trimester. Breast feeding is thought to increase the rate of transmission by 10–20% and should be avoided.

Cardo DM et al: A case-control study of HIV seroconversion in health care workers after percutaneous exposure. N Engl J Med 1997;337:1485. [NLM Cit ID: 98026764] (Zidovudine reduces the risk of seroconversion after percutaneous exposure by approximately 81%.)

Gordin F et al: Rifampin and pyrazinamide vs isoniazid for prevention of tuberculosis in HIV-infected persons: an international randomized trial. JAMA 2000;283:1445. [NLM Cit ID: 20195072] (A 2-month regimen of rifampin and pyrazinamide was equally efficacious as a year of isoniazid.)

Graham BS et al: Safety and immunogenicity of a candidate HIV-1 vaccine in healthy adults: Recombinant glycoprotein (rgp) 120. A randomized double-blind trial. Ann Intern Med 1996;125:270. [NLM Cit ID: 96301139]

Katz MH et al: The care of persons with recent sexual exposure to HIV. Ann Intern Med 1998;128:306. [NLM Cit ID: 98121792] (Information on the data supporting postexposure treatment, the indications for its use, the treatment regimen, and counseling recommendations.)

Management of possible sexual, injecting-drug-use, or other nonoccupational exposure to HIV, including considerations related to antiretroviral therapy. MMWR Morb Mortal Wkly Rep 1998;47(RR-17):1. [NLM Cit ID: 98434071] (Recommendations for treatment of nonoccupational exposure to HIV.)

Osborn EH et al: Occupational exposures to body fluids among medical students: A seven-year longitudinal study. Ann Intern Med 1999;130:45. [NLM Cit ID: 99087461]

Public Health Service guidelines for the management of health-care worker exposures to HIV and recommendations for postexposure prophylaxis. MMWR Morb Mortal Wkly Rep 1998;47(RR-7):1. [NLM Cit ID: 98264793] (Recommendations for treatment of occupational exposure to HIV.)

Public Health Service Task Force recommendations for the use of antiretroviral drugs in pregnant women infected with HIV-1 for maternal health and for reducing perinatal HIV-1 transmission in the United States. MMWR Morb Mortal Wkly Rep 1998;48(RR-2):1. [NLM Cit ID: 98120942] (Preclinical and clinical data regarding the use of a variety of antiretroviral regimens during pregnancy.)

Treatment

Treatment for HIV infection can be divided into four categories: therapy for opportunistic infections and malignancies, antiretroviral treatment, hematopoietic stimulating factors, and prophylaxis of opportunistic infections.

Experimental treatment regimens for HIV infection are constantly changing. Clinicians may obtain up-to-date information on experimental treatments by calling the AIDS Clinical Trials Information Service (ACTIS), 800-TRIALS-A (English and Spanish); the National AIDS Hot Line, 800-342-AIDS (English), 800-344-SIDA (Spanish), and 800-AIDS-TTY (hearing impaired).

A. Therapy for Opportunistic Infections and Malignancies: Treatment of common HIV infections and malignancies is detailed in Table 31–4. In general, AIDS patients require protracted therapy, including lifelong therapy for toxoplasmosis, cryptococcosis, and cytomegalovirus retinitis. It may be possible to discontinue therapy in some individuals who have had substantial immunologic improvement on highly active antiretroviral therapy (HAART). For example, maintenance therapy for CMV retinitis has been safely stopped in patients receiving HAART whose CD4 counts rose to at least 150 cells/μL. The emergence of resistance is more common for some infections of HIV-infected people (eg, acyclovir-resistant herpes simplex) than among immunocompetent individuals. In addition, HIV-infected patients have an increased incidence of side effects to standard drugs such as trimethoprim-sulfamethoxazole.

Treating patients with repeated episodes of the same opportunistic infection can pose difficult therapeutic challenges. For example, patients with second or third episodes of pneumocystis pneumonia may have developed allergic reactions to standard treatments with a prior episode. Fortunately, there are several alternatives available for the treatment of pneumocystis infection. Trimethoprim with dap-

Table 31–4. Treatment of AIDS-related opportunistic infections and malignancies.[1]

Infection or Malignancy	Treatment	Complications
P carinii infection[2]	Trimethoprim-sulfamethoxazole, 15 mg/kg/d (based on trimethoprim component) orally or IV for 14–21 days.	Nausea, neutropenia, anemia, hepatitis, drug rash. Stevens-Johnson syndrome.
	Pentamidine, 3–4 mg/kg/d IV for 14–21 days.	Hypotension, hypoglycemia, anemia, neutropenia, pancreatitis, hepatitis.
	Trimethoprim, 15 mg/kg/d orally, with dapsone, 100 mg/d orally, for 14–21 days.[3]	Nausea, rash, hemolytic anemia in G6PD-deficient patients. Methemoglobinemia (weekly levels should be < 10% of total hemoglobin).
	Primaquine, 15–30 mg/d orally, and clindamycin, 600 mg every 8 hours orally, for 14–21 days.	Hemolytic anemia in G6PD-deficient patients. Methemoglobinemia, neutropenia, colitis.
	Atovaquone, 750 mg orally 3 times daily for 14–21 days.	Rash, elevated aminotransferases, anemia, neutropenia.
	Trimetrexate, 45 mg/m^2 IV for 21 days (given with leucovorin calcium) if intolerant of all other regimens.	Leukopenia, rash, mucositis.
M avium complex infection	Clarithromycin, 500 mg orally twice daily with ethambutol, 15 mg/kg/d orally (maximum, 1 g). May also add:	Clarithromycin: hepatitis, nausea, diarrhea; ethambutol: hepatitis, optic neuritis.
	Rifabutin, 300 mg orally daily.	Rash, hepatitis, uveitis.
Toxoplasmosis	Pyrimethamine, 100–200 mg orally as loading dose, followed by 50–75 mg/d, combined with sulfadiazine, 4–6 g orally daily in 4 divided doses, and folinic acid, 10 mg daily for 4–8 weeks; then pyrimethamine, 25–50 mg/d, with clindamycin, 2 g/d, and folinic acid, 5 mg/d, until clinical and radiographic resolution is achieved.	Leukopenia, rash.
Lymphoma	Combination chemotherapy (eg, modified CHOP, M-BACOD,[4] with or without G-CSF or GM-CSF).[5] Central nervous system disease: radiation treatment with dexamethasone for edema.	Nausea, vomiting, anemia, leukopenia, cardiac toxicity (with doxorubicin).
Cryptococcal meningitis	Amphotericin B, 0.6 mg/kg/d IV, with or without flucytosine, 100 mg/kg/d orally in 4 divided doses for 2 weeks, followed by:	Fever, anemia, hypokalemia, and azotemia.
	Fluconazole, 400 mg orally daily for 6 weeks, then 200 mg orally daily.	Hepatitis.
Cytomegalovirus infection	Ganciclovir, 10 mg/kg/d IV in 2 divided doses for 10 days, followed by 6 mg/kg 5 days a week indefinitely. (Decrease dose for renal impairment.) May use ganciclovir as maintenance therapy (1 g orally with fatty foods 3 times a day).	Neutropenia (especially when used concurrently with zidovudine).
	Foscarnet, 60 mg/kg IV every 8 hours for 10–14 days (induction), followed by 90 mg/kg once daily. (Adjust for changes in renal function.)	Nausea, hypokalemia, hypocalcemia, hyperphosphatemia, azotemia.
Esophageal candidiasis or recurrent vaginal candidiasis	Fluconazole, 100–200 mg daily for 10–14 days.	Hepatitis, development of imidazole resistance.
	Ketoconazole, 200 mg orally twice daily for 10–14 days.	Hepatitis, adrenal insufficiency, ventricular tachycardia when given with terfenadine or astemizole.
Herpes simplex infection	Acyclovir, 200 mg 5 times daily for 7–10 days; or acyclovir, 5 mg/kg IV every 8 hours for severe cases.	Resistant herpes simplex with chronic therapy.
	Foscarnet, 40 mg/kg IV every 8 hours, for acyclovir-resistant cases. (Adjust for changes in renal function.)	See above.

(*continued*)

Table 31–4. Treatment of AIDS-related opportunistic infections and malignancies.[1] (continued)

Infection or Malignancy	Treatment	Complications
Herpes zoster	Acyclovir, 800 mg orally 4 or 5 times daily for 7–10 days. Intravenous therapy at 10 mg/kg every 8 hours for ocular involvement, disseminated disease.	See above.
	Famciclovir, 50 mg orally 3 times daily.	Headache, nausea.
	Foscarnet, 40 mg/kg IV every 8 hours for acyclovir-resistant cases. (Adjust for changes in renal function.)	See above.
Kaposi's sarcoma Limited cutaneous disease	Observation, intralesional vinblastine.	Inflammation, pain at site of injection.
Extensive or aggressive cutaneous disease	Systemic chemotherapy (eg, alternating weekly vinca alkaloids). Alpha interferon (for patients with CD4 > 200 cells/μL and no constitutional symptoms). Radiation (amelioration of edema).	Bone marrow suppression, peripheral neuritis, flu-like syndrome.
Visceral disease (eg, pulmonary)	Combination chemotherapy (eg, daunorubicin, bleomycin, vinblastine).	Bone marrow suppression, cardiac toxicity, fever.

[1]For treatment of *Mycobacterium tuberculosis* infection, see Chapter 9.
[2]For moderate to severe *P carinii* infection (oxygen saturation < 90%), corticosteroids should be given with specific treatment. The dose of prednisone is 40 mg twice daily for 5 days, then 40 mg daily for 5 days, and then 20 mg daily until therapy is complete.
[3]When considering use of dapsone, check G6PD level in African-American patients and those of Mediterranean origin.
[4]CHOP = cyclophosphamide, doxorubicin, vincristine (Oncovin), and prednisone. Modified M-BACOD = methotrexate, bleomycin, doxorubicin, cyclophosphamide, vincristine (Oncovin), and dexamethasone.
[5]G-CSF = granulocyte colony stimulating factor (filgrastim); GM-CSF = granulocyte-macrophage colony stimulating factor (sargramostim).

sone—and primaquine and clindamycin—are two combinations that often are tolerated in patients with a prior allergic reaction to trimethoprim-sulfamethoxazole and intravenous pentamidine. On the positive side, patients who develop second episodes of pneumocystis pneumonia while taking prophylaxis tend to have milder courses.

Well-established alternative regimens now also exist for most AIDS-related opportunistic infections: amphotericin B or fluconazole for cryptococcal meningitis; ganciclovir or foscarnet for cytomegalovirus infection; and sulfadiazine or clindamycin with pyrimethamine for toxoplasmosis.

Corticosteroids. Although conceptually it would seem that corticosteroid therapy should be avoided in HIV-infected patients, steroid use has been shown to improve the course of patients with moderate to severe pneumocystosis (oxygen saturation < 90%, Po_2 < 65 mm Hg) when administered within 72 hours after diagnosis. The mechanism of action is presumed to be a decrease in alveolar inflammation.

B. Antiretroviral Therapy: The availability of agents that alone and in combination suppress HIV replication (Table 31–5) has had a profound impact on the natural history of HIV infection. Patients who achieve excellent suppression of HIV generally have stabilization or improvement of their clinical course which results from partial immunologic reconstitution and a subsequent decrease in complications of immunosuppression. Concepts about the timing of such therapy have changed considerably. The recognition of continuous viral replication during early HIV infection and the considerable risk of disease progression in individuals with even low levels of circulating HIV RNA has given impetus to the concept of treating the majority of infected individuals with antiretroviral therapy even if the CD4 lymphocyte count is preserved. Although the long-term benefit of this strategy has not been proved, it is reasonable to offer immediate antiretroviral therapy to all patients except those at the very lowest risk for disease progression (ie, normal CD4 cell count and undetectable HIV viral load). The goal of reaching undetectable viral loads has been made harder to reach by the advent of highly sensitive viral load tests capable of detecting HIV viral loads as low as 50 copies. Early evidence suggests that patients with viral loads below 20–50 have a better prognosis than patients with viral loads between 20–50 and 400–500 copies (the cutoff of the older generation of tests).

Once a decision to initiate therapy has been made, several important principles should guide therapy. First, since HIV rapidly develops drug resistance to most of the antiretroviral agents, a major goal of therapy should be total suppression of viral replication as measured by the serum viral load, which has been shown to correlate with antiviral effect in other compartments. To achieve this and maintain virologic control over time, aggressive combination therapy is essential, and partially suppressive combinations

Table 31–5. Antiretroviral therapy.

Drug	Dose	Common Side Effects	Monitoring	Cost[1]	Cost/Month
Nucleoside analogs					
Zidovudine (AZT) (Retrovir)	500–600 mg orally daily in three divided doses	Anemia, neutropenia, nausea, malaise, headache, insomnia, myopathy	Complete blood count and differential (every 3 months once stable)	$1.77/100 mg	$318.60
Didanosine (ddI) (Videx)	125–200 mg orally twice daily (for pill formulation)	Peripheral neuropathy, pancreatitis, dry mouth, hepatitis	CBC and differential, aminotransferases, K^+, amylase, triglycerides, bimonthly neurologic questionnaire for neuropathy	$2.84/150 mg $4.74/250 mg powder	$170.40 $284.40
Zalcitabine (ddC) (Hivid)	0.375–0.75 mg orally 3 times daily	Peripheral neuropathy, aphthous ulcers, hepatitis	Monthly neurologic questionnaire for neuropathy, aminotransferases	$2.43/0.75 mg	$218.70
Stavudine (d4T) (Zerit)	40 mg orally twice daily	Peripheral neuropathy, hepatitis, pancreatitis	Monthly neurologic questionnaire for neuropathy, aminotransferases, amylase	$4.77/40 mg	$286.02
Lamivudine (3TC) (Epivir)	150 mg orally twice daily	Rash, peripheral neuropathy	No additional monitoring	$4.54/150 mg	$272.59
Protease inhibitors					
Saquinavir soft gel (Invirase)	600 mg orally three times daily	Gastrointestinal distress, headache	Bimonthly aminotransferases, cholesterol, triglycerides	$2.24/200 mg	$603.05
(Fortovase)	1200 mg three times daily			$1.15/200 mg	$623.13
Ritonavir (Norvir)	600 mg orally twice daily or 400 mg orally twice daily in combination with other protease inhibitors	Gastrointestinal distress, peripheral paresthesias	Bimonthly aminotransferases, CK, uric acid, triglycerides	$1.93/100 mg	$693.84
Indinavir (Crixivan)	800 mg orally three times daily	Kidney stones	Bimonthly aminotransferases, bilirubin level, cholesterol, triglycerides	$2.58/400 mg	$463.50
Nelfinavir (Viracept)	750 mg orally three times daily	Diarrhea	Cholesterol, triglycerides	$2.26/250 mg	$609.12
Nonnucleoside reverse transcriptase inhibitors (NNRTIs)					
Nevirapine (Viramune)	200 mg orally daily for 2 weeks, then 200 mg orally twice daily	Rash	No additional monitoring	$4.64/200 mg	$278.40
Delavirdine (Rescriptor)	400 mg orally three times daily	Rash	No additional monitoring	$0.79/100 mg	$282.96
Efavirenz (Sustiva)	600 mg orally daily	Neurologic disturbances	No additional monitoring	$1.10/50 mg, $2.19/100 mg, $4.38/200 mg	$394.20

[1]Cost to pharmacist (average wholesale price, generic when possible) for quantity listed. Source: *Drug Topics Red Book,* March 2000; Vol. 19, No. 3.

such as dual nucleoside therapy should be avoided. Similarly, if toxicity develops, it is preferable to interrupt the entire regimen rather than reduce individual doses. The current standard is to use at least three agents simultaneously. Since the number of drugs and potential combinations is finite and the development of drug resistance may severely compromise the efficacy of treatment, patients must be willing to endure the complexities, expense, and potential toxicities of such a regimen and must be rigorously counseled about the importance of adherence to the regimen.

Monitoring of antiretroviral therapy has two goals. Laboratory evaluation for toxicity depends upon the specific drugs in the combination but generally should be done approximately every 2–3 months once a patient is on a stable regimen. The second aspect of monitoring is to regularly measure objective markers of efficacy. The CD4 cell count and HIV viral load should be repeated 2–3 months after the initiation or change of antiretroviral regimen and every 3–4 months thereafter in clinically stable patients. Reasons for changing antiretroviral regimens include intolerable adverse reactions, clinical progression of disease, and continued immunologic deterioration as reflected by a declining CD4 cell count. Although a rebound in HIV viral load is cited as an indication to change therapy, exact parameters have not yet been established, and many patients appear to have continued clinical benefit in the face of rising viral load measurements. When therapy is modified, clinicians should attempt to start at least two agents to which an individual has not been exposed.

Although the ideal combination of drugs has not yet been defined, possible choices can be better understood after a review of the available agents. These drugs can be grouped into three major categories: nucleoside and nucleotide reverse transcriptase inhibitors, nonnucleoside reverse transcriptase inhibitors, and protease inhibitors.

1. Nucleoside and nucleotide analogs-

a. Zidovudine–Zidovudine (azidothymidine; AZT) was the first approved antiviral drug for HIV infection and remains an important agent. It is administered at a dose of 300 mg orally twice daily. A combination of zidovudine 300 mg and lamivudine 150 mg (Combivir) allows more convenient dosing of medication for individuals taking both of these agents. The cost of zidovudine (at a dose of 600 mg/d) is approximately $270 a month. Higher doses of zidovudine (1000–2000 mg/d) have been shown to be of possible benefit in individuals with HIV-associated dementia. Side effects seen with zidovudine are listed in Table 31–5. Approximately 40% of patients experience subjective side effects which usually remit within 6 weeks. The common dose-limiting side effects are anemia and neutropenia, which can be exacerbated by other drugs such as ganciclovir that cause bone marrow suppression. Anemia is usually mild, indolent in course, and characterized by macrocytosis. It is unresponsive to vitamin B_{12} or folate supplementation. A minority of patients have the more rapid onset of red cell aplasia. Bone marrow toxicity is generally reversible with cessation of the drug. Erythropoietin (epoetin alfa), at a starting dose of 8000 units subcutaneously three times a week, and G-CSF (filgrastim), at a dose of 300 μg subcutaneously one to three times a week, can ameliorate these side effects in situations where alternatives to zidovudine therapy are limited. Long-term zidovudine administration may also be complicated by myopathy, with wasting and weakness usually most prominent in the gluteus and quadriceps muscles.

In monitoring patients receiving zidovudine, complete blood counts—with platelet and differential counts—should be done monthly for the first 2 months of therapy and then every 3 months. Creatine phosphokinase levels should be checked every 6 months. Zidovudine can be taken concomitantly with other medicines except probenecid, which prolongs the serum half-life of zidovudine. Long-term administration of zidovudine with ganciclovir can pose a difficult problem. Only 15% of patients tolerate this combination without significant hematologic toxicity. One approach to neutropenia is to add G-CSF (filgrastim) to the regimen; another is to substitute another agent for zidovudine.

b. Didanosine–This agent also proved to have significant antiviral activity in early monotherapy trials and now is incorporated into combination regimens.

Administration of didanosine is inconvenient. Because the drug is degraded by stomach acid, patients must take the medication on an empty stomach (1 hour before or 2–3 hours after meals). It is supplied in two forms: pills and packets of powder. To receive adequate buffering agent, the pills should be taken two at a time and thoroughly chewed or dissolved in water. Diarrhea (due to the buffering agent used) is more common with the powder.

Dosing of these two formulations is by weight. For adults weighing < 60 kg, dosing is 125 mg (tablets) or 167 mg (powder) twice a day; for adults weighing ≥ 60 kg, 200 mg (tablets) or 250 mg (powder) twice a day. Didanosine may also be taken once daily. For adults over 60 kg, the dosage would be 400 mg (tablets). Unlike zidovudine, didanosine does not cause anemia but may cause neutropenia. It has also been associated with pancreatitis. The incidence of pancreatitis with didanosine is 5–10%—of fatal pancreatitis, less than 0.4%. Patients with a history of pancreatitis, as well as those taking other medications associated with pancreatitis (including trimethoprim-sulfamethoxazole and intravenous pentamidine) are at higher risk of this complication. Patients should be warned to use alcohol judiciously while taking didanosine. Clinicians should also teach patients to watch for the symptoms of pancreatitis and to stop treatment if they develop abdominal pain, nausea, or vomiting while taking didanosine until it can be determined if they have pancreatitis. Other common side effects with didanosine include a dose-related, reversible, painful peripheral neuropathy which occurs in about 15% of patients, and dry mouth. Fulminant hepatic failure and electrolyte abnormalities, including hypokalemia, hypocalcemia, and hypomagnesemia, have been reported in patients taking didanosine.

c. Zalcitabine–Zalcitabine is thought to be one of the least effective antiretroviral agents and is therefore uncommonly used. Its advantages are that it has several advantages as a potential antiviral agent. It is inexpensive, easy to administer, and has no known hematologic side effects. The usual dosage of zalcitabine is approximately 0.005–0.01 mg/kg orally every 8 hours. This drug is formulated in 0.375 mg and 0.75 mg tablets.

Zalcitabine, like didanosine, may cause peripheral neuropathy. It is also associated with aphthous ulcers, rash, and rare cases of pancreatitis.

d. Stavudine–Stavudine (d4T) has shown good activity as an antiretroviral drug. Side effects noted are peripheral neuropathy and, rarely, hepatitis. Pancreatitis has been reported in patients taking stavudine, but it is unclear if the drug was the cause of the pancreatitis. The dose is 40 mg orally twice daily for individuals weighing more than 70 kg.

e. Lamivudine–Lamivudine (3TC) is a safe and well-tolerated agent that has shown great promise when used in combination with zidovudine or stavudine. This combination results in more sustained suppression of viral replication and increase in CD4 cell counts than other combinations of nucleoside drugs studied to date. Zidovudine and lamivudine have a unique interaction whereby lamivudine suppresses the development and effect of zidovudine resistance mutations. The dose of lamivudine is 150 mg orally twice daily.

f. Abacavir–This is a highly active agent that was licensed in 1999. A daily dose of 600 mg results in potent antiretroviral activity, and the drug has pharmacokinetic features that allow twice-daily dosing. Abacavir retains activity against some HIV strains that have become resistant to other nucleoside drugs. The main toxicity is a hypersensitivity syndrome in about 5% of patients, characterized by rash and fever; individuals who develop this syndrome *should not* be rechallenged with this agent.

g. Adefovir–Adefovir was the first nucleotide agent considered for licensure as an antiretroviral agent. It showed moderate activity in phase I and phase II clinical trials but was associated with renal toxicity that precluded its licensure.

2. Protease inhibitors–Five protease inhibitors—indinavir, nelfinavir, ritonavir, amprenavir, and saquinavir—have been approved for use. Protease inhibitors have been shown to potently suppress HIV replication in vitro and in vivo and are always administered as part of a combination regimen, using either one or two agents from this class. If only one protease inhibitor is chosen as part of a regimen, possible choices include indinavir, ritonavir, or nelfinavir.

a. Indinavir–The standard dose of indinavir is 800 mg orally three times a day. Twice-daily dosing of indinavir is less effective and should not be used. It is recommended that indinavir be taken without food but with water 1 hour before or 2 hours after a meal. Nausea and headache are common complaints with this drug. Indinavir crystals are present in the urine in approximately 40% of patients; this results in clinically apparent nephrolithiasis in about 15% of patients receiving indinavir. Lower urinary tract symptoms and acute renal failure have been rarely reported. Patients taking this drug should be instructed to drink at least 48 ounces of fluid a day to ensure adequate hydration in an attempt to avoid these complications, but if stones occur repeatedly, an alternative protease inhibitor may be needed. Mild indirect hyperbilirubinemia is also commonly observed in patients taking indinavir, but this does not portend more serious hepatotoxicity and is not an indication to discontinue the drug.

b. Nelfinavir–This agent appears to have slightly less potent antiviral activity than either indinavir or ritonavir but has shown short-term benefit in combination regimens. This agent is also attractive in that it does not share all of the major drug resistance mutations required for development of high-level resistance to indinavir or ritonavir, though the clinical significance of this is not yet clear. The dose of nelfinavir is 750 mg orally three times daily. Preliminary results of twice-daily rather than three times daily (1250 mg orally) dosing have been promising. Diarrhea is a side effect in 25% of patients taking nelfinavir, and this symptom may be controlled in the majority of patients with over-the-counter antidiarrheal agents.

c. Ritonavir–Use of this potent protease inhibitor has been limited by its inhibition of the cytochrome P450 pathway causing a large number of drug-drug interactions and by its frequent side effects of fatigue, nausea, and paresthesias when the full dose of 600 mg orally twice daily is given. Ritonavir capsules require refrigeration. Difficulties in formulating the capsule version of ritonavir. have resulted in availability of only the liquid version. Because the liquid has a very bad taste, patients may find it easier to mix with chocolate milk or other thick liquids, such as nutritional supplements. The liquid does not require refrigeration if it is used within 30 days and kept at room temperature.

d. Saquinavir–As a single agent, in its original capsule formulation, saquinavir had limited bioavailability, which greatly curtailed its antiviral activity. A new soft-gel capsule formulation of saquinavir with greater bioavailability (Fortovase) is available. The dose of the soft gel formulation is 1200 mg three times a day with food. The most common side effects with saquinavir are diarrhea, nausea, dyspepsia, and abdominal pain. Soft-gel capsules of saquinavir do not require refrigeration if the capsules are kept at room temperature and used within 30 days.

a. Amprenavir–The fifth drug in this class, amprenavir, does not appear to have unique pharmacologic properties or resistance patterns that will differentiate it from the older protease inhibitor drugs.

Since all the protease inhibitors—to differing degrees—are metabolized by the cytochrome P450 system and since each can inhibit and induce various P450 isoenzymes, drug interactions are common and difficult to predict. Clinicians should consult the product inserts before prescribing protease inhibitors with other medications. Drugs that are known to induce the P450 system, such as rifabutin, should be avoided.

The fact that the protease inhibitors are dependent on metabolism through the cytochrome P450 system has led to some innovative dosing strategies. In particular, ritonavir dramatically increases the hepatic clearance of saquinavir, thereby enhancing its antiviral effect; the combination has demonstrated potent suppression of HIV. When the drugs are used together, the doses are reduced to 400 mg of ritonavir twice daily and 400–600 mg of saquinavir (soft gel) twice daily. The only additional toxicity observed with this combination has been elevation of hepatic aminotransferases. Thus, liver enzymes should be regularly monitored, especially in patients who have underlying liver disease.

When any protease inhibitor is used incorrectly, drug resistance develops rapidly. For this reason, it is important to stress to patients the importance of complying with the prescribed treatment regimen. Patients should be counseled that if they feel they will miss doses or days of treatment, it would be better for them to not take a protease inhibitor. Protease inhibitors should not be used alone. In general, they should not be dose-escalated. The one exception is ritonavir, which should be initiated with a dose escalation schedule. The reason is that the body metabolizes the drug more slowly at the start of therapy, so that full dosing results in overdosing in the initial period. The manufacturer recommends a schedule of 300 mg twice daily for 1 day, 400 mg twice daily for 2 days, 500 mg twice daily for 1 day, and then 600 mg twice daily thereafter. Some clinicians have slowed this dose escalation even further over a period of 10 days to 3 weeks, starting with doses of 200 mg orally twice daily for 2 days. Protease inhibitors have been linked to a constellation of metabolic abnormalities. These abnormalities include elevated cholesterol levels, elevated triglyceride levels, insulin resistance, diabetes mellitus, and changes in body fat composition (eg, abdominal obesity, skeletal wasting). The lipid abnormalities and body habitus changes are referred to as lipodystrophy. Much remains to be learned about this syndrome. Its prevalence is known to be increased among persons treated with protease inhibitors, but it has been seen also in HIV-infected persons who have never been treated with these agents.

3. Nonnucleoside reverse transcriptase inhibitors–These agents inhibit reverse transcriptase at a different site than the nucleoside and nucleotide agents described above. While they have significant antiviral activity, drug resistance develops rapidly, making it crucial to use them as a component of a completely suppressive regimen. Resistance to one drug uniformly predicts resistance to all other drugs in the class, which limits the possibilities for "salvage" regimens in patients previously exposed to any of these agents.

There are three available agents, **nevirapine, delavirdine,** and **efavirenz**. All three have shown antiviral activity as measured by HIV viral load and CD4 responses; clinical trials data demonstrate a clinical benefit when nevirapine is added to a dual nucleoside regimen. The target dose of nevirapine is 200 mg orally twice daily, but it is initiated at a dose of 200 mg once a day to decrease the incidence of rash, which is as high as 40% when full doses are begun immediately. Delavirdine is dosed at 400 mg orally three times a day. Rash is its most common side effect also, but the incidence is much lower than with nevirapine. With either agent, it is usually possible to treat through the rash. Diphenhydramine (25–50 mg orally three or four times daily) may provide symptomatic relief. These agents may cause alterations in the clearance of protease inhibitors, which may require dose modification if these two classes of drugs are administered concomitantly.

Efavirenz, the newest agent in this class, has the advantage that it can be given once daily as a single dose (600 mg orally). The major side effects are neurologic, with patients reporting symptoms ranging from lack of concentration and strange dreams to delusions and mania.

4. Novel agents–

a. Hydroxyurea–This drug has no direct activity against HIV but potentiates the effect of several dideoxynucleosides, particularly didanosine, by decreasing clearance of the active compound. When hydroxyurea (at a dosage of 500 mg orally twice a day) is combined with didanosine, it can result in a short-term decrease of HIV viral load by greater than 1.5 log, an effect comparable to that seen with dual nucleoside regimens. Because of its cytotoxic effect, patients treated with hydroxyurea tend to have less of a CD4 response to therapy than with other regimens; the clinical importance of this observation is unknown. The major toxicities of hydroxyurea are hematologic, with neutropenia being a dose-limiting toxicity about 8% of the time, and drug-induced hepatitis.

b. Peptide T20–Peptide T20 is the first drug in the new class of fusion inhibitors, which block the entry of HIV into cells. These drugs have antiviral activity even in heavily pretreated individuals.

5. Combination therapy–There is now little debate about the necessity for combining drugs from all of the available classes in order to achieve long-term suppression of HIV and its associated clinical benefit. Only combinations of drugs have been able to decrease HIV viral load by 2–3 logs and allow suppression of HIV RNA to below the threshold of detection for longer than 2 years in some individuals. Data from clinical trials have demonstrated the superiority of regimens that contain either nonnucleoside or protease inhibitor agents in addition to nucleoside agents alone. There is consensus about the desirability of treating aggressively once the decision to start antiretroviral therapy has been made rather than adding drugs sequentially over months or years. However, the ideal regimens for initial and second-line therapy have not yet been defined, so clinicians and their patients face difficult decisions in selecting therapy.

Several general principles should guide the choice of combinations. First, it is desirable to prescribe combinations that have demonstrated clinical benefit: since these data do not exist for many combinations, it is reassuring to know that the combination under consideration has shown beneficial effects upon HIV viral load levels in short-term studies. Second, to the extent possible, agents to which the patient has not been exposed are preferable to drugs for which resistance mutations may have already occurred. Third, toxicities should ideally be nonoverlapping. Fourth, an individual's relative contraindications to a given drug or drugs should be considered. Fifth, the regimen should not include agents that are either virologically antagonistic or incompatible in terms of drug-drug interactions. And finally, highly complex therapeutic regimens should be reserved for individuals who are capable of adhering to the rigorous demands of taking multiple medications and having this therapy closely monitored.

Possible ways of incorporating nonnucleoside agents and protease inhibitors into combinations are displayed in Figure 31–2. A number of points about the "nucleoside backbone" of regimens have become clearer. First, the dual nucleoside combinations with most activity probably include zidovudine plus lamivudine, zidovudine plus didanosine, stavudine plus lamivudine, and stavudine plus didanosine. In these pairings, both agents are given in full doses. The latter combination does not seem to lead to synergistic development of neuropathy despite both drugs' predilection to cause this side effect. Also notable is the fact that the addition of lamivudine to didanosine does not appear to result in the same level of viral suppression as when lamivudine is combined with zidovudine or stavudine. Finally, the nucleoside pair of zidovudine and stavudine are antagonistic and should never be used together. This results from stavudine inhibiting the phosphorylation of zidovudine to its active metabolite.

In choosing which third agent to include in an initial antiretroviral regimen, ease of administration, minimization of side effects, and future treatment options should all be considered. For example, for patients for whom it is important to minimize the number of pills, a regimen of lamivudine/zidovidine (Combivir) and nevirapine offers the simplest three drug regimen (two pills twice a day). Although protease inhibitors may be more potent than nonnucleoside reverse transcriptase inhibitors, some clinicians favor using the nonnucleoside reverse transcriptase inhibitors initially, thus sparing protease inhibitors for future use. Some persons who develop resistance to nelfinavir may still have sensitivity to indinavir and ritonavir. For this reason, many clinicians favor the use of nelfinavir as the initial protease inhibitor. Some clinicians advocate using two protease inhibitors simultaneously, particularly for patients with high viral loads (> 100,000/mL). The concern is that patients with particularly high viral loads are more likely to develop resistant virus on more conventional regimens. In addition to ritonavir-saquinavir, other combinations tried have included ritonavir-indinavir and indinavir-nelfinavir, with dosing of each agent reduced by roughly 50% of the usual recommended dose.

For some patients who have been heavily treated with antiretroviral agents it may be difficult to design second-line regimens when they are showing evidence of progression of disease on their existing regimen. In designing second-line regimens (sometimes called salvage regimens—a term that some patients may find offensive), the goal is to identify agents to which the patient is not resistant. This can be quite complicated because of cross resistance within types of agents. For example, the resistance patterns of ritonavir and indinavir are overlapping, and patients with virus resistant to these agents are unlikely to respond to nelfinavir or saquinavir even though they have never received treatment with these agents. Similarly, the resistance patterns of nevirapine and delavirdine are overlapping.

In addition to taking a careful history of what antiretroviral agents a patient has taken and for how long, genotypic and phenotypic resistance testing can provide useful information in designing second-line regimens. Of the two methods, genotypic testing is more easily performed and less expensive. The presence of certain genetic mutations confers resistance to particular agents. Although phenotypic testing would appear to be more relevant than genetic testing since it offers the promise of determining how a patient's virus actually responds to different agents, it is not well standardized and is expensive.

Some clinicians have advocated the use of mega-dose highly active antiretroviral (HAART) regi-

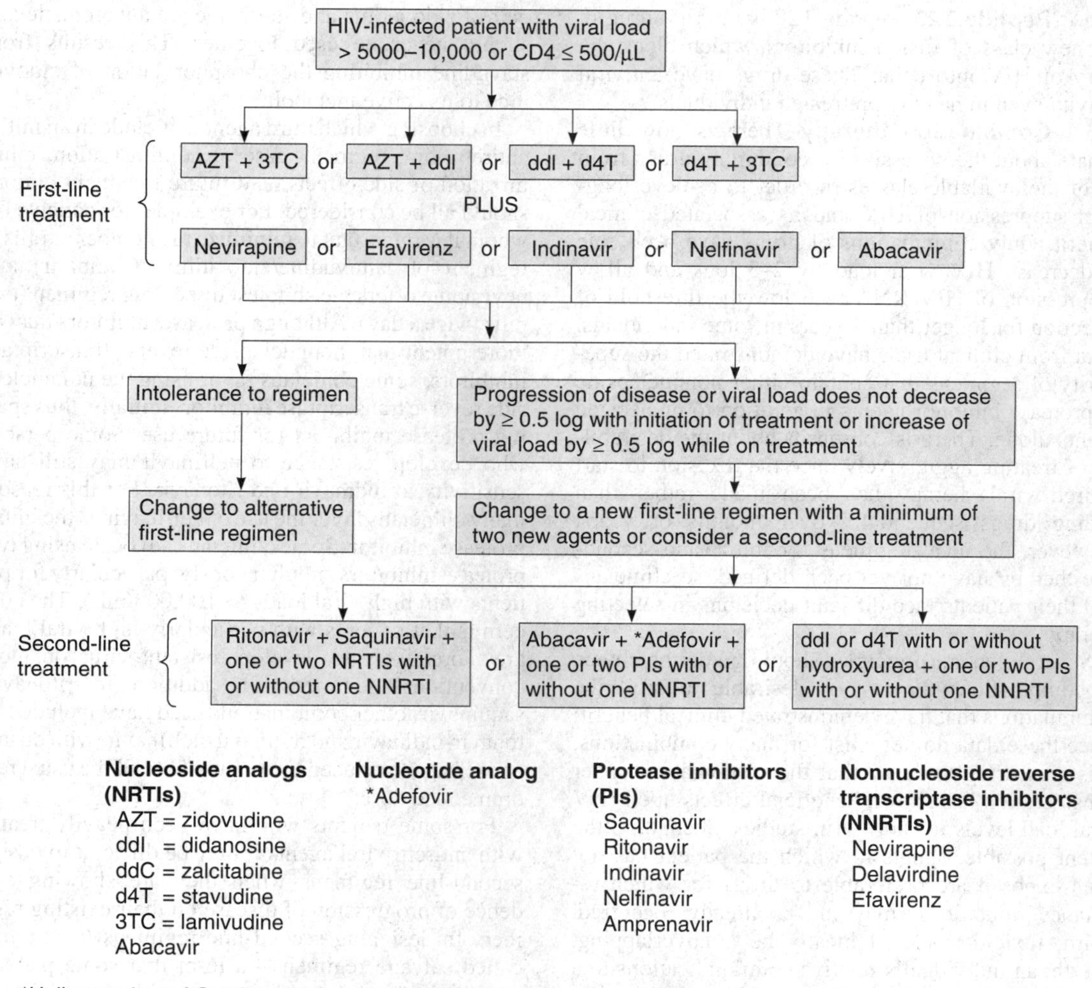

Figure 31–2. Approach to antiretroviral therapy.

mens—regimens with six or more agents—for patients who have progressed on standard regimens. Although their use in some patients has resulted in virologic improvement, these regimens are difficult to adhere to, side effects are common, and they are expensive. Whatever regimen is chosen, patients should be coached in ways to improve adherence. This should include taking medicines on an established schedule (eg, first thing in the morning), keeping a medication diary, and keeping medications in a variety of places the patient is likely to be (eg, car, workplace). For certain populations (eg, of unstably housed individuals), specially tailored programs that include drug dispensing are needed.

For some patients, it is impossible to construct a tolerable regimen that fully suppresses HIV. In such cases, clinicians and patients should consider their goals. Patients maintained on effective antiretroviral agents often benefit from these regimens (eg, higher CD4 counts, fewer opportunistic infections) even if their virus is detectable. In some cases, patients appear to benefit from a drug holiday during which patients are taken off all medications. Patients often immediately feel better because of the absence of drug side effects. After a period of time off medications, some patients may become more sensitive to existing medications, or new medications may become available. There are in development nonnucleoside reverse transcriptase inhibitors as well as one protease inhibitor (ABT 378) that appear to have less cross resistance with currently available medications. ABT 378 is combined with low-dose ritonavir to maximize its bioavailability. Patients should be monitored very closely during drug holidays.

C. Hematopoietic Stimulating Factors: Epoetin alfa (erythropoietin) is approved for use in HIV-infected patients with anemia, including those with anemia secondary to zidovudine use. It has been shown to decrease the need for blood transfusions. The drug is expensive, and a low endogenous erythropoietin level (less than 500 mU/mL) should be demonstrated before starting therapy. The starting dose is 8000 units subcutaneously three times a week. The target hematocrit is 35–40%. The dose may be increased by 12,000 units every 4–6 weeks as needed to a maximum dose of 48,000 units per week. Hypertension is the most common side effect.

Human granulocyte colony-stimulating factor (G-CSF [filgrastim]) and granulocyte-macrophage colony-stimulating factor (GM-CSF [sargramostim]) have been shown to increase the neutrophil counts of HIV-infected patients. G-CSF is preferred because of the theoretical concern of GM-CSF-stimulating HIV replication in infected monocytes. In patients receiving cytotoxic chemotherapy for lymphoma or Kaposi's sarcoma, daily subcutaneous doses of G-CSF at approximately 5 μg/kg (a 300 μg or 480 μg vial, depending upon weight) are given beginning 5–7 days after chemotherapy until the neutrophil count has rebounded to above 1000/μL. G-CSF may also have a role in ameliorating neutropenia caused by other drugs such as zidovudine or ganciclovir, when other therapeutic alternatives are not possible. Since the cost of this therapy is approximately $150 per vial, dosage should be closely monitored and minimized, aiming for a neutrophil count of 1000/μL. When the drug is used for indications other than cytotoxic chemotherapy, one or two doses at 5 μg/kg per week is usually sufficient.

D. Prophylaxis of Opportunistic Infections: Patients with a history of pneumocystis pneumonia should receive secondary prophylaxis for that disease. Primary prophylaxis should be offered to patients with CD4 counts below 200 cells/μL, or less than 14% CD4 lymphocyte counts, or weight loss or oral candidiasis.

Three regimens for prophylaxis are trimethoprim-sulfamethoxazole, aerosolized pentamidine, and dapsone (see Table 31–6). Trimethoprim-sulfamethoxazole is inexpensive and widely available. In two studies comparing once-daily double-strength trimethoprim-sulfamethoxazole with aerosolized pentamidine for primary and secondary prophylaxis of pneumocystis pneumonia, patients randomized to trimethoprim-sulfamethoxazole were significantly less likely to develop pneumocystis pneumonia. In the study of secondary prophylaxis, there was a threefold decrease in the risk of recurrence with trimethoprim-sulfamethoxazole. This study also found that patients randomized to trimethoprim-sulfamethoxazole were less likely to develop bacterial infections (eg, pneumonia, sinusitis) than persons in the aerosolized pentamidine group—another reason to use trimethoprim-sulfamethoxazole instead of aerosolized pentamidine. There is a higher incidence of side effects with trimethoprim-sulfamethoxazole (primarily fever, rash, and nausea and vomiting) than with aerosolized pentamidine. Nonetheless, trimethoprim-sulfamethoxazole (one double-strength tablet three times a week to once daily) should be considered the prophylactic agent of choice if tolerated. Patients who develop mild rashes on this regimen may be treated with diphenhydramine (25–50 mg every 4 hours). However, clinicians and patients must watch carefully for signs of Stevens-Johnson syndrome. Some clinicians are also using desensitization regimens to overcome allergic reactions. Reports suggest that desensitization may be successful in 40% of cases.

Aerosolized pentamidine has the advantage of minimal systemic side effects. Its disadvantages are expense (approximately $160 per monthly treatment) and decreased effectiveness in the apical and peripheral areas of the lung. Cases of extrapulmonary pneumocystis infections in patients receiving aerosolized pentamidine have also been reported

Aerosolized pentamidine may also increase the incidence of pneumothorax in patients with a history of pneumocystis infection.

Although dapsone has not been widely studied, it appears to be an effective prophylactic agent with minimal side effects. As with trimethoprim-sulfamethoxazole, it is inexpensive and widely available and may be used in patients with an allergic reaction to trimethoprim-sulfamethoxazole. Before prescribing dapsone, clinicians should document that the patient is not G6PD-deficient. Such patients are at high risk of developing hemolytic anemia with dapsone

Table 31–6. *Pneumocystis carinii* prophylaxis.

Drug	Dose	Side Effects	Limitations
Trimethoprim-sulfamethoxazole	One double-strength tablet 3 times a week to one tablet daily	Rash, neutropenia, hepatitis, Stevens-Johnson syndrome	Hypersensitivity reaction is common but, if mild, it may be possible to treat through.
Dapsone	50–100 mg daily or 100 mg 2 or 3 times per week	Anemia, nausea, methemoglobinemia, hemolytic anemia	Efficacy not established. G6PD level should be checked prior to therapy. Check methemoglobin level at 1 month.
Aerosolized pentamidine	300 mg monthly	Bronchospasm (pretreat with bronchodilators) rare reports of pancreatitis	Apical *P carinii* pneumonia, extrapulmonary *P carinii* infections, pneumothorax.

therapy. Patients taking dapsone concomitantly with didanosine should take the dapsone at least 2 hours prior to the didanosine. Dapsone is not absorbed well in the neutral pH stomach environment created by the didanosine buffering agent. Finally, atovaquone may be an option for individuals intolerant of other systemic therapies.

Patients who develop pneumocystis infection on a particular prophylactic regimen should be switched to a different one or should receive a combination regimen (eg, aerosolized pentamidine plus trimethoprim-sulfamethoxazole).

M avium complex infection occurs in at least one-third of AIDS patients. Once the CD4 count falls below 75–100 cells/μL, prophylaxis should be started with a macrolide agent. Clarithromycin (500 mg orally twice daily) and azithromycin (1200 mg orally weekly) have both been shown to decrease the incidence of disseminated disease by approximately 75%, with a low rate of breakthrough of resistant disease. The latter regimen is generally preferred on the basis of ease of compliance and cost. Adding rifabutin increases the toxicity of the regimen but does not significantly increase its efficacy and is therefore not recommended. As sole therapy, rifabutin (300 mg orally daily) is less effective and more toxic than clarithromycin or azithromycin. Clinicians should make certain that patients do not have active *M tuberculosis* infection by examination of a chest radiograph prior to starting rifabutin because of concern about the development of resistance to rifabutin with cross-resistance to rifampin. Similarly, clinicians should establish with a blood culture that the patient does not have disseminated *M avium* complex infection. Common side effects of both azithromycin and clarithromycin are nausea and diarrhea. Two common side effects with rifabutin are rash and hepatic dysfunction. Rifabutin may induce hepatic enzymes, thereby decreasing the activity of some drugs metabolized by the liver.

Prophylaxis for *M tuberculosis*—isoniazid, 300 mg daily for 9 months to a year—should be given to all HIV-infected patients with positive PPD reactions (defined for HIV-infected patients as > 5 mm of induration).

Toxoplasmosis prophylaxis is desirable in patients with positive IgG toxoplasma serology. Trimethoprim-sulfamethoxazole (one double-strength tablet daily) offers good protection against toxoplasmosis, as does a combination of pyrimethamine, 25 mg orally once a week, plus dapsone, 100 mg orally daily.

Cytomegalovirus infection is also common in late HIV disease. Oral ganciclovir has been approved for CMV prophylaxis among HIV-infected persons with CD4 counts below 50 cells/μL. However, because the drug causes neutropenia, it is not widely used. Clinicians should consider performing serum CMV IgG antibody testing. Persons who are CMV IgG-negative are not at risk for development of CMV disease. Importantly, patients who are CMV IgG-negative should receive CMV-negative blood if they require a transfusion. Because over 99% of gay men are positive for CMV IgG, it is appropriate to reserve testing for heterosexuals with HIV.

Cryptococcosis, candidiasis, and endemic fungal diseases are also candidates for prophylaxis. One prophylactic trial showed a decreased incidence of cryptococcal disease with the use of fluconazole, 200 mg orally daily, but the treated group had no benefit in terms of mortality. Fluconazole (200 mg orally once a week) was found to prevent oral and vaginal candidiasis in women with CD4 counts below 300 cells/μL. In areas of the world where histoplasmosis and coccidioidomycosis are endemic and are frequent complications of HIV infection, prophylactic use of fluconazole or itraconazole may prove to be useful prophylactic strategies. However, the problem of identifying individuals at highest risk makes the targeting of prophylaxis difficult.

Since individuals with advanced HIV infection are susceptible to a number of opportunistic pathogens, the use of agents with activity against more than one pathogen is envisioned. It has been shown, for example, that trimethoprim-sulfamethoxazole confers some protection against toxoplasmosis in individuals receiving this drug for pneumocystis prophylaxis. Similarly, clarithromycin and rifabutin may offer protection against development of cryptosporidiosis.

Discontinuation of Prophylaxis for Opportunistic Infections

Many patients experience significant increases in their CD4 counts following the initiation of HAART. This raises the question of whether prophylaxis can be safely discontinued. Based on limited experience, patients whose counts are above a CD4 count threshold of 300 cells/μL for at least 3–6 months and who have sustained reductions in their viral load can safely discontinue prophylaxis.

Course & Prognosis

The rate of progression to symptomatic disease is reviewed above. Once clinical findings develop, outcome varies. With improvements in therapy, some cohorts of patients are living longer after the diagnosis of AIDS. This has resulted in dramatic decreases in AIDS deaths nationally. In 1998 in the USA there were 17,171 deaths due to AIDS, compared with 49,895 deaths in 1995. It remains to be seen whether the decreases in number of deaths can be sustained over the long term. Maintaining access to quality care and treatment is one key element. Unfortunately, studies continue to show less access to treatment for some disfranchised groups, especially injecting drug users. Another key element in sustaining lower mortality is developing new treatments for patients who have been heavily treated with existing agents. Despite new therapeutic options, people continue to die from HIV infection. For patients whose disease progresses even though they are receiving appropriate treatment, meticulous palliative care must be provided (see Chapter 5).

[HIV/AIDS Information Outreach Program]
http://www.aidsnyc.org/

[HIV/AIDS National Treatment Information Service]
http://www.hivatis.org/

[HIV InSight—University of California, San Francisco]
http://hivinsite.ucsf.edu/

Carpenter CC et al: Antiretroviral therapy in adults: updated recommendations of the International AIDS Society–USA Panel. JAMA 2000;283:381. [NLM Cit ID: 20112328]

Chaisson RE et al: Prevention of opportunistic infections in the era of improved antiretroviral therapy. J Acquir Immune Defic Syndr Hum Retrovirol 1997;16(Suppl 1):S14. [NLM Cit ID: 98049179] (Review of epidemiology of opportunistic infections, impact of treatment on survival, drug resistance, drug toxicity, and recommendations for treatment.)

Deeks SG et al: HIV-1 protease inhibitors: A review for clinicians. JAMA 1997;277:145. [NLM Cit ID: 97144574] (Reviews available data on the use of protease inhibitors.)

Freedberg KA et al: The cost-effectiveness of prevention of AIDS-related opportunistic infections. JAMA 1998;279:130. [NLM Cit ID: 98101613] (Prophylaxis against pneumocystis pneumonia, toxoplasmosis, and MAC infection were the most cost-effective, while prophylaxis against CMV infection was the least.)

Gulick RM et al: Simultaneous versus sequential initiation of therapy with indinavir, zidovudine, and lamivudine for HIV-1 infection: 100-week follow-up. JAMA 1998;280:35. [NLM Cit ID: 98321798] (Sustained viral suppression for 2 years in the majority of people who adhered to this regimen.)

Hammer SM et al: A controlled trial of two nucleoside analogues plus indinavir in persons with human immunodeficiency virus infection and CD4 cell counts of 200 per cubic millimeter or less. AIDS Clinical Trials Group 320 Study Team. N Engl J Med 1997;337:725. [NLM Cit ID: 97413573] (First study to demonstrate survival benefit of triple therapy, even when the protease inhibitor is added to existing nucleoside therapy.)

Havlir DV et al: Prophylaxis against disseminated *Mycobacterium avium* complex with weekly azithromycin, daily rifabutin, or both. N Engl J Med 1996;335:392. [NLM Cit ID: 96293369] (As monotherapy, azithromycin is superior to rifabutin. Adding rifabutin increases side effects without significantly increasing efficacy.)

Jacobson MA et al: Altered natural history of AIDS-related opportunistic infections in the era of potent combination antiretroviral therapy. AIDS 1998;12(Suppl A):S157. [NLM Cit ID: 98296654] (Interesting review of newer manifestations of CMV, tuberculosis and other infections.)

JAMA patient page: HIV/AIDS. JAMA 1998;280:106. [NLM Cit ID: 98321810]

Ledergerber B et al. AIDS-related opportunistic illnesses occurring after initiation of potent antiretroviral therapy: the Swiss HIV Cohort Study. JAMA 1999;282:2220. [NLM Cit ID: 20071989] (Low rates of opportunistic infections among persons with undetectable viral loads after 5 months of HAART)

1999 USPHS/IDSA guidelines for the prevention of opportunistic infections in persons infected with human immunodeficiency virus. MMWR Morb Mortal Wkly Rep 1999;48(RR-10):1. [NLM Cit ID: 99428016]

Schuman P et al: Weekly fluconazole for the prevention of mucosal candidiasis in women with HIV infection. A randomized, double-blind, placebo-controlled trial. Ann Intern Med 1997;126:689. [NLM Cit ID: 97267478] (Low-dose fluconazole decreased the risk of candidiasis by 44% compared with placebo in women with CD4 counts less than 300 cells/µL.)

Staszewski S et al: Efavirenz plus zidovudine and lamivudine, efavirenz plus indinavir, and indinavir plus zidovudine and lamivudine in the treatment of HIV-1 infection in adults. N Engl J Med 1999;341:1865. [NLM Cit ID: 20046565] (The combination of efavirenz, zidovudine, and lamivudine had greater antiviral activity and was better tolerated than the combination of indinavir, zidovudine, and lamivudine.)

Whitcup SM et al: Discontinuation of anticytomegalovirus therapy in patients with HIV infection and cytomegalovirus retinitis. JAMA 1999;282:1633. [NLM Cit ID 20019217] (Maintenance therapy for CMV retinitis was safely stopped for patients with CD4 counts greater than 150 cells/µL who were being treated with HAART.)

RELEVANT WORLD WIDE WEB SITES

[AEGIS: AIDS Education Global Information System]
http://www.aegis.com

[American Academy of Family Physicians]
http://www.aafp.org/patientinfo/common11.html

[The Body]
http://www.thebody.com

[Center for AIDS Prevention Studies]
http://www.caps.ucsf.edu/capsweb/AIDSlist.html

[Centers for Disease Control and Prevention]
http://www.cdc.gov

[HIV/AIDS Prevention]
http://www.cdc.gov/hiv/dhap.htm

[HIV/AIDS Treatment Information Services]
http://www.hivatis.org

[The HIV InfoWeb]
http://www.infoweb.org

[HIV InSite]
http://HIVInsite.ucsf.edu/

[JAMA HIV/AIDS Information Center]
http://www.ama-assn.org/special/hiv/hivhome.htm

[Johns Hopkins University AIDS Service]
http://www.hopkins-aids.edu

[Merck, Inc.: Welcome to Crixivan]
http://www.crixivan.com/

[Project Inform]
http://www.projinf.org/

Table 32–1. Agents for viral infections.

Drug	Dosing	Spectrum	Renal Clearance? /Hemodialysis	CNS/CSF Penetration	Toxicities
Acyclovir	200–800 mg orally five times daily; 250–500 mg/m^2 IV every 8 hours for 7 days	HSV	Yes/Yes	Yes	Neurotoxic reactions, reversible renal dysfunction, local reactions
Amantadine	100 mg orally twice daily (100 mg/d in elderly) for 10 days	Influenza A	Yes/No	Yes	Confusion, gastrointestinal symptoms
Cidofovir	5 mg/kg IV weekly for 2 weeks, then every other week	CMV	Yes/NA	NA	Neutropenia, renal failure, ocular hypotonia
Famciclovir	500 mg orally 3 times daily	VZV, ?HSV	Yes/NA	NA	NA
Foscarnet	20 mg/kg IV bolus, then 120 mg/kg IV every 8 hours for 2 weeks; maintain with 60 mg/kg/d IV for 5 days each week	CMV, HSV resistant to acyclovir, VZV, HIV-1	Yes/Yes	Variable	Nephrotoxicity, genital ulcerations, calcium disturbances
Ganciclovir	5 mg/kg IV bolus every 12 hours for 14–21 days; maintain with 3.75 mg/kg/d IV for 5 days each week	CMV	Yes/Yes	Yes	Neutropenia, thrombocytopenia, CNS side effects
Idoxuridine	Topical, 0.1% every 1–2 hours for 3–5 days	HSV keratitis	—	—	Local reactions
Interferon alfa-2b	3–5 million IU SC 3 times weekly to daily Intralesionally: 1 million IU per 0.1 mL in up to 5 warts 3 times weekly for 3 weeks	HBV, HCV, papillomavirus	Yes/Yes		Influenza-like syndrome, myelosuppression, neurotoxicity
Interferon alfa-n3	0.05 mL/wart biweekly up to 8 weeks	HPV	NA/NA	NA	Local reactions
	3 mU IV 3 times per week	?HCV	NA/NA	NA	Influenza-like syndrome, myelosuppression, neurotoxicity
Lamivudine (3TC)	12 mg/kg/d	HIV-1, ?HIV-2, HBV	Yes/NA	Yes	Skin rash, headache, insomnia
Oseltamivir	75 mg twice daily for 5 days beginning 48 hours after onset of symptoms	Influenza A and B	Yes/NA	NA	Few
Ribavirin	Aerosol: 1.1 g/d as 20 mg/mL dilution over 12–18 hours for 3–7 days (See text for Lassa fever doses.)	RSV, severe influenza A or B, Lassa fever	Yes/No	Yes	Wheezing
Rimantadine	100 mg orally twice daily	Influenza A	Yes/No	Yes	Same as amantadine, but less severe
Stavudine (d4T)	40 mg twice daily	HIV-1, ?HIV-2	Yes (moderate)/ NA	Yes	Neuropathy, increased liver function tests, pancreatitis
Trifluridine	Topical, 1% drops every 2 hours to 9 drops/d	HSV keratitis	—	—	Local reactions

(continued)

pears to also be associated with EBV by serologic and virologic data.)

Syrjanen S et al: Oral ulcers in AIDS patients frequently associated with CMV and EBV infections. J Oral Pathol Med 1999;28:204. [NLM Cit ID: 99243529]

5. CYTOMEGALOVIRUS DISEASE

Most cytomegalovirus (CMV) infections are asymptomatic, with the virus remaining latent. The virus can be isolated from a variety of tissues under nonpathogenic conditions including up to 25% of salivary glands and 10% of uterine crevices. Nevertheless, the cells of latency are unknown. Seroprevalence increases with age and with the number of sexual partners. Detectable antibody is present in the serum of most homosexual men. Transmission is sexual, congenital, through blood products or transplantation, and person-to-person (eg, day care centers). Severe disease occurs primarily in the immunocompromised, especially AIDS and transplant patients.

Clinical Findings

A. Classification: There are three recognizable clinical syndromes.

1. Perinatal disease and CMV inclusion disease–This is a neonatal syndrome acquired in utero and seen in 10% of newborns born to mothers with primary CMV infection during pregnancy. It is characterized by jaundice, hepatosplenomegaly, thrombocytopenia, periventricular central nervous system calcifications, mental retardation, motor disability, and purpura. Neonatally acquired disease is often asymptomatic, but neurologic deficits may ensue later in life.

2. Acute acquired CMV infection–This syndrome, akin to EBV-associated infectious mononucleosis, is characterized by fever, malaise, myalgias and arthralgias (but not pharyngitis or respiratory symptoms), splenomegaly, atypical lymphocytes, and abnormal liver function tests. Leukopenia is more often observed than leukocytosis. Heterophil antibody is absent. Transmission occurs by sexual contact, in breast milk, via respiratory droplets among nursery or day care center attendants, and by transfusions of blood.

3. Disease in immunocompromised hosts–Tissue and bone marrow transplant patients are mainly at risk in the first 100 days after allograft transplantation. HIV-infected patients may have numerous manifestations. CMV is itself immunosuppressive and may worsen pneumocystis pneumonia.

a. CMV retinitis–Retinitis occurs primarily in AIDS patients with significant immunosuppression (CD4 count less than 50 cells/μL). Ophthalmologic documentation of neovascular, proliferative lesions ("pizza-pie" retinopathy) is required for diagnosis. With HAART, the frequency of retinitis is reduced, CD4 counts are less predictive, and active disease may be reversible.

b. Gastrointestinal and hepatobiliary CMV–Serious gastrointestinal CMV disease occurs in AIDS and after organ transplantation, cancer chemotherapy, or steroid therapy. Esophagitis presents with odynophagia; small bowel disease may mimic inflammatory bowel disease or may present as ulceration or perforation. Colonic CMV disease causes diarrhea, hematochezia, abdominal pain, fever, and weight loss. CMV has been identified, often with other pathogens, in up to 15% of patients with AIDS cholangiopathy. Diagnosis is by mucosal biopsy showing characteristic CMV histopathologic findings of intranuclear ("owl's eye") and intracytoplasmic inclusions.

c. Pulmonary CMV–Pulmonary CMV infection occurs in about 15% of bone marrow transplant recipients, in whom the mortality rate is 80–90% and in severely immunosuppressed AIDS patients, in whom the significant morbidity and high mortality in the developed world appear to be diminished by the use of highly active antiretroviral therapy (HAART). CMV seronegative blood products should be used in seronegative recipients of seronegative transplants. High-titer CMV immunoglobulins may be effective in preventing CMV pneumonia in seronegative recipients.

d. Neurologic CMV–The variety of neurologic syndromes associated with CMV include polyradiculopathy, transverse myelitis, and encephalitis. The encephalitis has a subacute onset in patients with advanced AIDS and is usually associated with disseminated CMV infection.

CMV can be isolated in the cerebrospinal fluid in cases of transverse myelitis or disseminated disease. Prolonged anti-CMV antivirals are indicated in therapy, given in combination with HAART for HIV-positive patients.

B. Laboratory Findings: Virus isolation is most useful when combined with the pathologic findings. Cultures alone are of little use in diagnosing AIDS-related CMV infections, but when positive have been associated with a risk of progressive retinitis. The acute mononucleosis-like syndrome is associated with lymphocytosis, often 2 weeks after the fever, but absolute leukopenia may also be noted. Serologic tests are useful primarily in seroepidemiologic studies and occasionally in confirming acute infection (with IgM) in nonimmunosuppressed patients. Antigen detection by virus technology (including the PCR technique) must be interpreted in the context of clinical and pathologic findings but appears to be highly predictive of CMV disease in immunocompromised patients.

Prevention

No vaccine is currently available. CMV hyperimmune globulin given to seronegative bone marrow transplant recipients is not clearly effective. Limiting transfusions, using products filtered to remove leukocytes, and selecting CMV-seronegative donors are all important in reducing the rate of CMV transmission. Ganciclovir at a dosage of 5 mg/kg intravenously twice daily for 5 days, beginning when the absolute neutrophil count is 750 cells/μL, then daily until day 100 posttransplant, reduces CMV infection and disease, leaving mortality unchanged. HAART is effective in preventing CMV infections in HIV-infected patients.

Treatment

Three antiviral agents with efficacy against CMV infections are ganciclovir, 5 mg/kg intravenously every 12 hours for 14–21 days; foscarnet, loading with 20 mg/kg intravenously, followed by 60 mg/kg every 8 hours over weeks; and cidofovir, 5 mg/kg, intravenously, every week for 2 weeks. A daily maintenance regimen using both ganciclovir (3.75 mg/kg intravenously) and foscarnet (60 mg/kg intravenously), each over 1 hour, has been shown to be safe and effective in inhibiting CMV replication. Cidofovir is given only every 2 weeks, 375 mg intravenously, for maintenance. Oral ganciclovir (1 g three times daily) is an expensive alternative for maintenance. Dosage adjustments of all three medications are needed for renal impairment. In addition, a sustained-release ganciclovir implant has been shown to control disease in the implanted eye (but not elsewhere) more effectively than intravenous ganciclovir. Again, the role of HAART in reducing the need for CMV antivirals is essential.

Abecassis MM et al: The role of PCR in the diagnosis and management of CMV in solid organ recipients: What is the predictive value for the development of disease and should PCR be used to guide antiviral therapy? Transplantation 1997;63:275. [NLM Cit ID: 97172246] (PCR had greatest predictive value among CMV seronegative recipients.)

Deayton J et al: Loss of CMV viraemia following HAART in the absence of specific anti-CMV therapy. AIDS 1999;13:1203. [NLM Cit ID: 99342912] (HAART can fully suppress CMV viremia and helps explain why the natural history of CMV is changed in AIDS.)

Lesprit P et al: Use of the CMV antigenemia assay for the rapid diagnosis of primary CMV infection in hospitalized adults. Clin Infect Dis 1998;26:646. [NLM Cit ID: 98185526]

Musch DC et al: Treatment of CMV retinitis with a sustained-release ganciclovir implant. The Ganciclovir Implant Study Group. N Engl J Med 1997;337:83. [NLM Cit ID: 97337875]

Whitley RJ et al: Guidelines for the treatment of CMV diseases in patients with AIDS in the era of potent antiretroviral therapy. Arch Intern Med 1998;158:957. [NLM Cit ID: 98247843]

6. HUMAN HERPESVIRUSES 6, 7, 8

Human herpesvirus 6 (HHV-6) is a B cell lymphotropic virus that is the principal cause of exanthema subitum (roseola infantum, sixth disease). Primary HHV-6 infection occurs most commonly in children under 2 years of age and is the most common cause of infantile febrile seizures. HHV-6 in adults is associated with immunocompromised states such as HIV and lymphoma. It has been associated with graft rejection and bone marrow suppression in transplant patients, with encephalitis and pneumonitis in AIDS, and has recently been mentioned as a factor in the etiology of multiple sclerosis.

Two variants (A and B) of HHV-6 have been identified. The latter is sensitive to ganciclovir, and both are sensitive to foscarnet. HHV-6 has been isolated from blood in lymphoma patients and appears to be involved in the pathogenesis of angioimmunoblastic lymphadenopathy with dysproteinemia.

HHV-7 is a T cell lymphotropic virus that has also been serologically associated with roseola. The membrane glycoprotein CD4 is involved in HHV-7 recognition, and an antagonistic interaction between HHV-7 and HIV has been shown.

HHV-8 is associated with Kaposi's sarcoma in AIDS patients. It has also been implicated in Castleman's disease and body-cavity lymphomas. See Chapter 31 for pathogenesis and management.

Dockrell DH et al: Human herpesvirus 6. Mayo Clin Proc 1999;74:163. [NLM Cit ID: 99166886]

Levy JA: Three new human herpesviruses (HHV6, 7, and 8). Lancet 1997;349:558. [NLM Cit ID: 97200974]

MAJOR VACCINE-PREVENTABLE VIRAL INFECTIONS

1. MEASLES

Essentials of Diagnosis

- Exposure 10–14 days before onset in an unvaccinated patient.
- Prodrome of fever, coryza, cough, conjunctivitis, malaise, irritability, photophobia, Koplik's spots.
- Rash: brick-red, irregular, maculopapular; onset 3–4 days after onset of prodrome; begins on the face and proceeds "downward and outward," affecting the palms and soles last.
- Leukopenia.

General Considerations

Measles is an acute systemic viral (paramyxovirus) infection transmitted by inhalation of infective droplets. This monocyte-tropic virus is a major worldwide cause of pediatric morbidity and mortality, with an estimated 1 million deaths annually. Illness confers permanent immunity. Communicability is greatest during the preeruptive and catarrhal stages but continues as long as the rash remains. Sporadic recent outbreaks of the disease in adults, adolescents, and unvaccinated preschool children in dense urban areas have led to changes in recommendations concerning prevention (see below).

Clinical Findings

A. Symptoms and Signs: (Table 32–2.) Fever is often as high as 40–40.6 °C. It persists through the prodrome and early rash (about 5–7 days). Malaise may be marked. Coryza (nasal obstruction, sneezing, and sore throat) resembles that seen with upper respiratory infections. Cough is persistent and nonproductive. Conjunctivitis manifests as redness, swelling, photophobia, and discharge.

Koplik's spots are pathognomonic of measles. They appear about 2 days before the rash and last 1–4 days as tiny "table salt crystals" on the dull red mucous membranes of the cheeks and often on inner conjunctival folds and vaginal mucous membranes. Other findings include pharyngeal erythema, a yellowish exudate on the tonsils, coating of the tongue in the center with a red tip and margins, moderate generalized lymphadenopathy, and, in occasional cases, splenomegaly.

The rash usually appears first on the face and behind the ears 4 days after the onset of symptoms. The initial lesions are pinhead-sized papules which coalesce to form a brick-red, irregular, blotchy maculopapular rash. In severe cases, the rash may coalesce to form a nearly uniform erythema on some body areas. The rash next appears on the trunk, followed by the extremities, including the palms and soles. It fades in order of appearance. Hyperpigmentation remains in fair-skinned individuals and severe cases. Slight desquamation may follow.

Atypical measles is a syndrome occurring in adults who received inactivated measles vaccine (available 1963–1967) or who received live measles vaccine before age 12 months and as a result developed hypersensitivity rather than protective immunity. When infected later with wild measles virus, such individuals may develop a potentially fatal illness with high fever, unusual rashes (papular, hemorrhagic) without Koplik's spots, headache, arthralgias, hepatitis, and interstitial or nodular infiltrates, occasionally with pleural effusions.

Measles may occur in HIV-infected individuals in an uncharacteristic fashion, with higher rates of pneumonitis and higher mortality. Vaccine failure rates, both primary and secondary, are higher in HIV-infected children. The frequent difficulty in establishing a diagnosis suggests that measles may be more readily transmitted in HIV-infected persons.

B. Laboratory Findings: Leukopenia is usually present unless secondary bacterial complications exist. A lymphocyte count under 2000/μL is a poor prognostic sign. Proteinuria is often observed. Although technically difficult, virus can be cultured from nasopharyngeal washings and from blood. A fourfold rise in serum hemagglutination inhibition antibody supports the diagnosis. Fluorescent antibody staining of respiratory or urinary epithelial cells can also confirm the diagnosis.

Differential Diagnosis

Measles is easily recognizable from the clinical picture but could be mistaken for other viral infections, including exanthems.

Complications

A. Central Nervous System Complications: Encephalitis occurs in approximately 0.05–0.1% of cases. Its onset is usually 3–7 days after the rash. Vomiting, convulsions, coma, and a variety of severe neurologic signs and symptoms develop. Treatment is symptomatic and supportive. Virus is usually not found in the central nervous system, though demyelination is prominent. There is an appreciable mortality rate (10–20%), and many patients are left with neurologic morbidity.

A similar form ("inclusion body encephalitis") is also reported to occur after measles vaccination but is associated with isolation of the measles virus.

Subacute sclerosing panencephalitis (SSPE) is a very late central nervous system complication, the measles virus acting as a "slow virus" to produce degenerative central nervous system disease years after the initial infection. SSPE is rare (1:100,000 cases of measles) and occurs more often when measles develops early in life, among males, and in persons living in rural environments.

An acute progressive encephalitis (subacute measles encephalitis), characterized by seizures, neurologic deficits, and often progressive stupor and death, can occur among immunosuppressed patients; measles virus opportunistically invades the central nervous system. Treatment is supportive, withholding immunosuppressive chemotherapy when feasible. Interferon and ribavirin have been variably successful.

B. Respiratory Tract Disease: Early in the course of the disease, bronchopneumonia or bronchiolitis due to the measles virus may occur in up to 5% and result in serious respiratory difficulties. Pneumonia occurring with or without an evanescent rash is seen in atypical measles.

C. Secondary Bacterial Infections: Immediately following measles, secondary bacterial infection, particularly cervical adenitis, otitis media, and pneumonia, occurs in about 15% of patients.

D. Tuberculosis: Measles produces temporary anergy to the tuberculin skin test.

E. Gastroenteritis: Diarrhea and protein-losing enteropathy (prodromal rectal Koplik spots may be seen) are significant complications when measles affects malnourished children.

Prevention

In the United States, it is recommended that children receive their first vaccine dose at 12–15 months and a second at age 4–6 years prior to entry into school (see Table 30–4). A recent outbreak in Alaska secondary to an imported case emphasizes the importance of the second dose of measles immunization.

Students beyond high school and medical staff starting employment must have the above vaccination schedule documented or must have serologic evidence of immunity if they were born after 1956. For individuals born before 1957, herd immunity can be assumed. Health care workers should be screened and vaccinated if necessary regardless of date of birth.

Outbreak control in the USA is similar. If outbreaks are occurring in preschool children under 1 year of age, initial vaccination may be given at 6 months, with repeat at 15 months. When outbreaks take place in day care centers, K–12 institutions, or colleges and universities, revaccination is probably indicated for all, in particular for students and their siblings born after 1956 who do not have documentation of immunity as defined above. Susceptible personnel who have been exposed should be isolated from patient contact from the fifth to the 21st day after exposure irrespective of whether they have been vaccinated or have received immune globulin. If they develop measles, they should be isolated from patient contact until 7 days after the rash develops.

Ancillary control measures used in the developing world include "catch-up days"—when all children regardless of immunization history are vaccinated—surveillance of acute cases, and confirmation of whether isolates from cases are imported or outbreak-associated.

When susceptible individuals are exposed to measles, the live virus vaccine can prevent disease if given within 5 days of exposure. This is rarely feasible in a household. Later, immune globulin (0.25 mL/kg [0.11 mL/lb] body weight) can be injected intramuscularly for prevention or modification of clinical illness if given within 6 days after exposure. This must be followed by active immunization with live measles vaccine 3 months later. Vaccination of all immunocompetent persons born after 1956 who travel to the developing world is essential.

Pregnant women and the immunosuppressed should *not* receive this vaccine. There are two exceptions: asymptomatic HIV-infected patients, who have not shown adverse effects from measles vaccination; and HIV-infected children, in whom exposure to vaccines improves survival after measles. In the developing world, the use of "high-titer" vaccine is associated with a higher delayed mortality rate. Immune globulin should be considered for postexposure prophylaxis in any HIV-infected person exposed to measles.

Treatment

A. General Measures: The patient should be isolated for the week following onset of rash and kept at bed rest until afebrile. Treatment is symptomatic as needed. Vitamin A, 400,000 units/d orally (the beneficial effects of which include maintenance of gastrointestinal and respiratory epithelial mucosa and perhaps immune enhancement), reduces pediatric morbidity and mortality rates.

B. Treatment of Complications: Secondary bacterial infections are treated with appropriate antimicrobial drugs. Postmeasles encephalitis, including SSPE, can only be treated symptomatically.

Prognosis

The mortality rate of measles in infants was 0.6% in a recent outbreak in California; the mortality rate may be as high as 10% in developing nations. Deaths in the USA are due principally to encephalitis (15% mortality rate) and secondary bacterial pneumonia. Deaths in the developing world are mainly related to diarrhea and protein-losing enteropathy.

Bitnun A et al: Measles inclusion-body encephalitis caused by the vaccine strain measles virus. Clin Infect Dis 1999;29:855. [NLM Cit ID: 20055848]

deQuadros CA et al: Measles eradication in the Americas. Bull WHO 1998;72(Suppl 2):47. (Record low rates in the last several years except 1997, when an outbreak occurred in Sao Paulo, Brazil.)

Global measles control and regional elimination, 1998–1999. MMWR Morb Mort Wkly Rep 1999;48:1124. [NLM Cit ID: 20097813]

Moss WJ et al: Implications of the HIV epidemic for control and eradication of measles. Clin Infect Dis 1999;29:106. [NLM Cit ID: 99360954]

Paunio M et al: Measles history and atopic diseases: a population-based cross-sectional study. JAMA 2000;283: 343. [NLM Cit ID: 20112322] (Despite theories that communicable diseases in childhood protect against atopic disease, this study shows an increased rate of atopy among Finnish children with a history of measles.)

2. MUMPS

Essentials of Diagnosis

- Exposure 14–21 days before onset.
- Painful, swollen salivary glands, usually parotid.
- Frequent involvement of other tissues, including testes, pancreas, and meninges, in unvaccinated individuals.

General Considerations

Mumps is a viral (paramyxovirus) disease spread by respiratory droplets that usually produces inflammation of the salivary glands and, less commonly, orchitis, aseptic meningitis, pancreatitis, and oophoritis. Most patients are children, and the incidence is highest in spring. The incubation period is 14–21 days (average, 18 days). Infectivity occurs via saliva and urine and precedes the symptoms by about 1 day and is maximal for 3 days but may last a week.

Clinical Findings

A. Symptoms and Signs: Parotid tenderness and overlying facial edema are the most common physical findings. Occasionally, swelling in one gland subsides completely before the other parotid or salivary glands become involved. Swelling and tenderness of the submaxillary and sublingual glands are variable. The orifice of Stensen's duct may be red and swollen.

Fever and malaise are variable and are often minimal in young children. High fever usually accompanies meningitis or orchitis. Neck stiffness, headache, and lethargy suggest meningitis. Testicular swelling and tenderness (unilateral in 75%) denote orchitis. Orchitis, which develops typically 7–10 days after the onset of parotitis, occurs in about 25–40% of postpubertal men, but sterility is rare. Upper abdominal pain, nausea, and vomiting suggest pancreatitis. Mumps is the leading cause of pancreatitis in children. Lower abdominal pain and ovarian enlargement suggest oophoritis, but the diagnosis may be difficult. Pain and swelling of one or both (75%) of the parotid or other salivary glands occur, usually in succession 1–3 days apart. Occasionally, one gland subsides completely (usually in 7 days or less) before others become involved.

B. Laboratory Findings: Relative lymphocytosis may be present. Serum amylase is commonly elevated with or without pancreatitis because of salivary gland involvement. Lymphocytic pleocytosis (and normal to low glucose) of the cerebrospinal fluid is present in meningitis, which may be asymptomatic. The diagnosis is confirmed by isolating mumps virus from saliva or cerebrospinal fluid or demonstrating a fourfold rise in complement-fixing antibodies in paired sera.

Differential Diagnosis

Swelling of the parotid gland may be due to calculi in the parotid ducts or to a reaction to iodides. Other causes include starch ingestion, sarcoidosis, cirrhosis, diabetes, bulimia, and Sjögren's syndrome. Parotitis may also be produced by pyogenic organisms (eg, *Staphylococcus aureus*), particularly in debilitated individuals, drug reaction (phenothiazines, propylthiouracil), and other viruses (influenza A, parainfluenza, EBV infection, coxsackieviruses). Swelling of the parotid gland must be differentiated from inflammation of the lymph nodes located more posteriorly and inferiorly than the parotid gland.

Complications

Other manifestations of the disease are less common than inflammation of the salivary glands. These usually follow the parotitis but may precede it or occur without salivary gland involvement: meningitis (30%), orchitis (on rare occasion leads to priapism or testicular infarction), pancreatitis, oophoritis, thyroiditis, neuritis, hepatitis, myocarditis, thrombocytopenia, migratory arthralgias, and nephritis.

Aseptic meningitis may occur without salivary gland involvement and low cerebrospinal fluid glucose occurs in some cases. Rare neurologic complications include encephalitis, Guillain-Barré syndrome, cerebellar ataxia, and transverse myelitis. Encephalitis is associated with cerebral edema, serious neurologic manifestations, and sometimes death. Deafness develops rarely from eighth nerve neuritis. Mumps has also been associated with cases of endocardial fibroelastosis.

Prevention

Mumps live virus vaccine is safe and highly effective. It is recommended for routine immunization for children over age 1 year, either alone or in combination with other virus vaccines (eg, with measles and rubella—in MMR vaccine). Reactions are reviewed in the measles section. It should not be given to pregnant women or to immunocompromised individuals, though the vaccine has been given to asymptomatic HIV-infected individuals without adverse sequelae. Its use has markedly decreased the incidence of mumps in the United States. The mumps skin test is less reliable in determining immunity than are serum neutralization titers.

Treatment

A. General Measures: The patient should be isolated until swelling subsides and kept at bed rest during the febrile period. Treatment is symptomatic as needed.

B. Management of Complications:

1. Meningitis–The treatment of aseptic meningitis is purely symptomatic. The management of encephalitis requires attention to cerebral edema, the airway, and vital functions.

2. Orchitis–The scrotum should be suspended in a suspensory or toweling "bridge" and ice bags applied. Incision of the tunica may be necessary in severe cases. Codeine or meperidine may be given as necessary for pain. Pain can also be relieved by injection of the spermatic cord at the external inguinal ring with 10–20 mL of 1% procaine solution. Hydrocortisone sodium succinate (100 mg intravenously, followed by 20 mg orally every 6 hours for 2 or 3 days) to reduce the inflammatory reaction is of questionable benefit.

3. Pancreatitis–Symptomatic treatment should be provided and parenteral fluids if necessary.

Prognosis

The entire course of mumps rarely exceeds 2 weeks. Fatalities (from encephalitis) are rare.

Galazka AM et al: Mumps and mumps vaccine: a global review. Bull WHO 1999;77:3. [NLM Cit ID: 99163142]

Lindberg B et al: Previous exposure to measles, mumps, and rubella—but not vaccination during adolescence—

correlates to the prevalence of pancreatic and thyroid autoantibodies. Pediatrics 1999;104:312. [NLM Cit ID: 99319082] (Measles and mumps antibody inhibit the development of thyroid antibodies, while exposure to rubella is associated with increased levels of pancreas islet cell antibodies.)

Measles, mumps, and rubella—vaccine use and strategies for elimination of measles, rubella, and congenital rubella syndrome and control of mumps. MMWR Morb Mortal Wkly Rep 1998;47(RR-8):1. [NLM Cit ID: 98301240]

Ni J et al: Viral infection of the myocardium in endocardial fibroelastosis. Molecular evidence for the role of mumps virus as an etiologic agent. Circulation 1997;95:133. [NLM Cit ID: 97147656]

3. POLIOMYELITIS

Essentials of Diagnosis

- Muscle weakness, headache, stiff neck, fever, nausea and vomiting, sore throat.
- Lower motor neuron lesion (flaccid paralysis) with decreased deep tendon reflexes and muscle wasting.
- Cerebrospinal fluid shows excess leukocytes, with lymphocytic predominance; count is rarely more than 500/μL.

General Considerations

Poliomyelitis virus, an enterovirus, is present in throat washings and stools. Infection is most commonly acquired by the fecal-oral route. Since the introduction of an effective vaccine, poliomyelitis has become a rare disease in developed areas of the world, and globally, between 1988 and 2000, the number of cases decreased 85%. Among 133 cases reported in the United States between 1980 and 1994, six were imported and 125 (94%) were vaccine-associated (two were indeterminate). Wild poliovirus disease has been eradicated from the Western hemisphere, and the Pacific Rim, Europe, and Central Asia appear to be polio-free. Polio remains endemic in Pakistan, India, and Southeast Asia, part of the Middle East (in particular Iraq), and Central and Western Africa. Three antigenically distinct types of poliomyelitis virus are recognized, with no cross-immunity between them. The incubation period is 5–35 days (usually 7–14 days). Disease with type 2 in particular is on the verge of extinction. Infectivity is maximal during the first week, but virus is excreted in stools for several weeks.

Clinical Findings

A. Symptoms and Signs: At least 95% of infections are asymptomatic, but in those who become ill the following manifestations are seen.

1. Minor illness (abortive poliomyelitis)–The symptoms are fever, headache, vomiting, diarrhea, constipation, and sore throat.

2. Nonparalytic poliomyelitis–In addition to the above symptoms, signs of meningeal irritation and muscle spasm occur.

3. Paralytic poliomyelitis–Paralytic poliomyelitis represents 0.1% of all poliomyelitis cases (the incidence is higher when infections are acquired later in life). Paralysis may occur at any time during the febrile period. Tremors, muscle weakness, constipation, and ileus may appear. Paralytic poliomyelitis may be divided into two forms, which may coexist: **(1) spinal poliomyelitis,** with involvement of the muscles supplied by the spinal nerves; and **(2) bulbar poliomyelitis,** with weakness of the muscles supplied by the cranial nerves (especially nerves IX and X) and of the respiratory and vasomotor centers.

In spinal poliomyelitis, paralysis of the shoulder girdle often precedes intercostal and diaphragmatic paralysis, which leads to diminished chest expansion and decreased vital capacity.

In bulbar poliomyelitis, symptoms include diplopia (uncommonly), facial weakness, dysphagia, dysphonia, nasal voice, weakness of the sternocleidomastoid and trapezius muscles, difficulty in chewing, inability to swallow or expel saliva, and regurgitation of fluids through the nose. The most life-threatening aspect of bulbar poliomyelitis is respiratory paralysis. Lethargy or coma may be due to hypoxia, most often from hypoventilation. Hypertension, hypotension, and tachycardia may occur. Convulsions are rare.

B. Laboratory Findings: The peripheral white blood cell count may be normal or mildly elevated. Cerebrospinal fluid pressure and protein are normal or slightly increased. Glucose is not decreased. White blood cells usually number fewer than 500/μL and are principally lymphocytes after the first 24 hours. Cerebrospinal fluid is normal in 5% of patients. The virus may be recovered from throat washings (early) and stools (early and late). Neutralizing and complement-fixing antibodies appear during the first or second week of illness.

Differential Diagnosis

Nonparalytic poliomyelitis is similar to other forms of enteroviral meningitis; the distinction is made serologically. Acute infectious polyneuritis (Guillain-Barré) and tick paralysis may initially resemble poliomyelitis. In Guillain-Barré syndrome (see Chapter 24), the weakness is more symmetric and ascending in most cases, but the Miller-Fisher variant is quite similar to bulbar polio. Cerebrospinal fluid usually has a high protein content but normal cell count.

Complications

Urinary tract infection, atelectasis, pneumonia, myocarditis, and pulmonary edema may occur. Respiratory failure may be a result of paralysis of respiratory muscles, airway obstruction from involvement of cranial nerve nuclei, or lesions of the respiratory center.

Prevention

Recommendations for prevention of poliomyelitis have been modified as a result of changing epidemiology, eradication of polio in the Western Hemisphere, and continued concern about vaccine-associated disease with the oral live vaccine. Current recommendations in the USA are to provide the inactive (Salk) parenteral vaccination for all four doses (at ages 2, 4, and 6–18 months and 4–6 years). Oral vaccination should be considered in special circumstances such as outbreak control, travel to endemic areas within the ensuing month, and in protection of children whose parents do not accept the recommended number of immunizations. The limited advantages of oral vaccination are the ease of administration, the effective local gastrointestinal and circulating immunity, and herd immunity, but it is not favored for public health use in the developed world because of occasional vaccine-associated disease both in vaccine recipients and in contacts.

Routine immunization of adults in the United States is not recommended because of the low incidence of the disease. However, adults who are exposed to poliomyelitis or plan to travel to endemic areas and who have not received polio immunization within the past decade should be given inactivated poliomyelitis vaccine (Salk). This vaccine should also be given when immunization of immunodeficient or immunosuppressed individuals and members of their households is required.

In the developing world, the interval between OPV doses should probably be longer than 1 month (because of interference from enteric pathogens). Intramuscular injections should be routinely avoided during the month following oral poliomyelitis vaccination to prevent provocation paralysis. Ancillary useful control measures in polio-endemic countries include national immunization days (mass campaigns in which all children are vaccinated twice, 4–6 weeks apart, regardless of vaccine history); cross-border vaccination activities; surveillance for acute flaccid paralysis, which serves as an indicator for poliomyelitis; and aggressive outbreak responses.

Treatment

Strict bed rest in the first few days of illness reduces the rate of paralysis. Cranial nerve involvement must be vigilantly sought. Comfortable but rotating positions should be maintained in a "polio bed": (firm mattress, footboard, sponge rubber pads or rolls, sandbags, and light splints). Fecal impaction and urinary retention (especially with paraplegia) are managed appropriately. In cases of respiratory weakness or paralysis, intensive care is needed.

Prognosis

During the febrile period, paralysis may develop or progress. Mild weakness of small muscles is more likely to regress than is severe weakness of large muscles. Bulbar poliomyelitis carries a mortality rate of up to 50%. New muscle weakness may develop and progress slowly years after recovery from acute paralytic poliomyelitis. This entity, postpoliomyelitis syndrome, presents with signs of chronic and new denervation, is not infectious in origin, and is associated with increasing dysfunction of surviving motor neurons.

Progress toward the global interruption of wild poliovirus type 2 transmission, 1999. MMWR Morb Mort Wkly Rep 1999;48:736. [NLM Cit ID: 99430900] (A map shows the distribution and dates of last type 2 isolates.)

Recommendations of the advisory committee on immunization practices: revised recommendations for routine poliomyelitis vaccination. MMWR Morb Mort Wkly Rep 1999;48:590. [NLM Cit ID: 99355052]

4. RUBELLA

Essentials of Diagnosis

- Exposure 14–21 days before onset.
- Arthralgia, particularly in young women.
- No prodrome in children (mild in adults); mild symptoms (fever, malaise, coryza) coinciding with eruption.
- Posterior cervical and postauricular lymphadenopathy 5–10 days before rash.
- Fine maculopapular rash of 3 days' duration; face to trunk to extremities.
- Leukopenia, thrombocytopenia.

General Considerations

Rubella is a systemic disease caused by a togavirus transmitted by inhalation of infective droplets. It is only moderately communicable. One attack usually confers permanent immunity. The incubation period is 14–21 days (average, 16 days). The disease is transmissible from 1 week before the rash appears until 15 days afterward.

The clinical picture of rubella is difficult to distinguish from other viral illnesses such as infectious mononucleosis, echovirus infections, and coxsackievirus infections, though arthritis is more prominent in rubella. Definitive diagnosis can be made only by isolating the virus or serologically.

The principal importance of rubella lies in its devastating effects on the fetus in utero, producing teratogenic effects and a continuing congenital infection. Congenital rubella syndrome continues to occur in parts of the developing world at rates equivalent to those reported from the industrialized world during the prevaccine era. Modeling estimates from 1996 suggest there are 110,000 cases annually in the developing world.

Clinical Findings

A. Symptoms and Signs: (Table 32–2.) Fever and malaise, usually mild, accompanied by tender suboccipital adenitis, may precede the eruption by 1 week. Mild coryza may be present. Polyarthritis occurs in about 25% of adult cases. These symptoms usually subside within 7 days but may persist for weeks.

Posterior cervical and postauricular lymphadenopathy is very common. Erythema of the palate and throat, sometimes patchy, may be noted. A fine, pink maculopapular rash appears on the face, trunk, and extremities in rapid progression (2–3 days) and fades quickly, usually lasting 1 day in each area. Rubella without rash may be at least as common as the exanthematous disease. Diagnosis can be suspected when there is epidemiologic evidence of the disease in the community but requires laboratory confirmation.

B. Laboratory Findings: Leukopenia may be present early and may be followed by an increase in plasma cells. Virus isolation and serologic tests of immunity (rubella virus hemagglutination inhibition and fluorescent antibody tests) are available. Definitive diagnosis is based on a fourfold rise in the antibody titer.

Complications

A. Exposure During Pregnancy: Rubella antibodies are sought for at the beginning of pregnancy, since fetal infection during the first trimester leads to congenital rubella in at least 80% of fetuses.

When a pregnant woman is exposed to a possible case of rubella, an immediate hemagglutination-inhibiting rubella antibody level should be obtained; there is no reason for concern in positive tests. If no antibodies are found, clinical and serologic follow-up is essential. Confirmation of rubella in the expectant mother raises the question of therapeutic abortion, an alternative to be considered in the light of personal, religious, legal, and other factors. The risk to the fetus is highest for maternal infection in the first trimester but continues into the second trimester.

B. Congenital Rubella: An infant acquiring the infection in utero may be normal at birth but more likely will have a wide variety of manifestations, including early-onset cataracts, microphthalmia, and glaucoma, hearing deficits, psychomotor retardation, congenital heart defects, organomegaly, and maculopapular rash. Viral excretion in the throat and urine persists for many months despite high antibody levels. The diagnosis is confirmed by isolation of the virus. A specific test for IgM rubella antibody is useful for diagnosis in the newborn. Treatment is directed to the many anomalies.

C. Postinfectious Encephalopathy: In 1:6000 cases, postinfectious encephalopathy develops 1–6 days after the rash; the virus cannot always be isolated. The mortality rate is 20%, but residual deficits are rare among the recovered. The mechanism is unknown.

Prevention

Live attenuated rubella virus vaccine should be given to all infants and to susceptible girls before the menarche. When women are immunized, they should not be pregnant, and the absence of antibodies should be established. (In the USA, about 80% of 20-year-old women are immune to rubella.) Birth control should be practiced for at least 3 months after vaccine administration, though there are no reports of congenital rubella syndrome after rubella immunization and inadvertent immunization of a pregnant woman is not considered an indication for therapeutic abortion. Arthritis is more marked after rubella vaccination than native disease and appears to be immunologically mediated. The association between chronic arthropathies and rubella vaccination is controversial. MMR may be given in conjunction with DPT boosters; adequate serologic response has been shown.

Treatment

Acetaminophen provides symptomatic relief. Encephalitis and non-life-threatening thrombocytopenia should be treated symptomatically.

Prognosis

Rubella is a mild illness and rarely lasts more than 3–4 days. Congenital rubella, on the other hand, has a high mortality rate, and the associated congenital defects are largely permanent.

Cutts FT et al: Modeling the incidence of congenital rubella syndrome in developing countries. Int J Epidemiol 1999;28:1176. [NLM Cit ID: 20125308]

Measles, mumps, and rubella—vaccine use and strategies for elimination of measles, rubella, and congenital rubella syndrome and control of mumps. MMWR Morb Mortal Wkly Rep 1998;47(RR-8):1. [NLM Cit ID: 98301240]

O'Neill JF: The ocular manifestations of congenital infection: a study of the early effect and long-term outcome of maternally transmitted rubella and toxoplasmosis. Trans Am Ophthalmol Soc 1998;96:813. [NLM Cit ID: 99288589]

OTHER NEUROTROPIC VIRUSES

1. RABIES

Essentials of Diagnosis

- History of animal bite.
- Paresthesia, hydrophobia, rage alternating with calm.
- Convulsions, paralysis, thick tenacious saliva.

General Considerations

Rabies is a viral (rhabdovirus) encephalitis transmitted by infected saliva that gains entry into the body by an animal bite or an open wound. Cases in the United States are rare but probably underreported.

Bats, skunks, foxes, and raccoons are widely infected. Biting species that cause rabies in the United States tend to be geographically determined: raccoons in the East and New England; skunks in the Midwest, Southwest, and California; coyotes in Texas; and foxes in the Southwest, New England, and Alaska. Dogs and cats are infected in developing countries (including the Mexican border), and 10 of 20 Americans with rabies acquired the disease abroad during the 1980s. Rodents and lagomorphs (eg, rabbits) are unlikely to have rabies. The virus gains entry into the salivary glands of dogs 5–7 days before their death from rabies, thus limiting their period of infectivity.

The incubation period may range from 10 days to many years but is usually 3–7 weeks. The interval is dependent in part on distance of the wound from the central nervous system. The virus travels in the nerves to the brain, multiplies there, and then migrates along the efferent nerves to the salivary glands.

Rabies is almost uniformly fatal, with surviving cases likely due to rabies-related viruses. The most common clinical problem confronting the physician is the management of a patient bitten by an animal (see Prevention).

Clinical Findings

A. Symptoms and Signs: There is usually a history of animal bite. Patients with scratches from rabid animals are about 50 times less likely than those with bites to develop rabies. Pain appears at the site of the bite, followed by paresthesias. The skin is quite sensitive to changes of temperature, especially air currents. Attempts at drinking cause extremely painful laryngeal spasm (hydrophobia). Restlessness, muscle spasm, extreme excitability and bizarre behavior, convulsions, and paralysis occur. Large amounts of thick tenacious saliva are present.

B. Laboratory Findings: Biting animals who are apparently well should be kept under observation for 7–10 days. Sick or dead animals should be examined for rabies. A wild animal, if captured, should be sacrificed and the head shipped on ice to the nearest laboratory qualified to examine the brain for evidence of rabies virus; the diagnosis is made by the fluorescent antibody technique. When the animal cannot be examined, skunks, bats, coyotes, foxes, and raccoons should be presumed to be rabid.

Fluorescent antibody testing of skin biopsy material from the posterior neck (where hair follicles are highly innervated) or a corneal impression may be positive early in the disease. The test may become negative after antibodies develop. PCR and genetic probes are available but are far more expensive and may not be sensitive early in the course of disease.

Prevention

Since rabies is almost always fatal, prevention is the only reasonable approach, and all exposures must be evaluated individually. Immunization of household dogs and cats and active immunization of persons with significant animal exposure (eg, veterinarians) are important. However, the most important common decisions concern animal bites.

A. Local Treatment of Animal Bites and Scratches: Thorough cleansing, debridement, and repeated flushing of wounds with soap and water are important. If rabies immune globulin or antiserum is to be used, a portion should be infiltrated locally around the wound (see below) and the remainder given intramuscularly. Wounds caused by animal bites should not be sutured.

B. Postexposure Immunization: Therapy is indicated when the disease is seriously under consideration. Medical decisions should be based on recommendations of the USPHS Advisory Committee but also be on circumstances of the bite, including the extent and location of the wound, the biting animal, history of prior vaccination, and the local endemicity of rabies. Consultation is available from state and local health departments. Postexposure treatment includes both passive antibody and vaccination.

The optimal form of passive immunization is rabies immune globulin (20 units/kg). Up to 50% of the globulin is infiltrated around the wound; the rest is administered intramuscularly. If immune globulin (human) is not available, equine rabies antiserum (20 units/kg) can be used after appropriate tests for horse serum sensitivity. An inactivated human diploid cell rabies vaccine (HDCV) is given as five injections of 1 mL intramuscularly (in the deltoid rather than the gluteal muscle) on days 0, 3, 7, 14, and 28 after exposure.

Several cell culture vaccines are available and are preferable to embryonated tissue vaccine (eg, duck embryo vaccine; DEV) because of better antigenic response and fewer systemic reactions. HDCV availability and cost limit its use in the developing world.

Rabies immune globulin and rabies vaccine (human diploid cell vaccine) should never be given in the same syringe or at the same site. Allergic reactions to the vaccine are rare, though local reactions (pruritus, erythema, tenderness) occur in about 25% and mild systemic reactions (headaches, myalgias, nausea) in about 20% of recipients. The vaccine is commercially available or can be obtained through health departments. For patients who previously received pre- or postexposure vaccine, rabies immune globulin should not be given; vaccine, 1 mL in the deltoid, should be given twice (on days 0 and 3).

In other countries, inactivated duck embryo vaccine or mouse brain vaccine may be available, but the method of administration is more complex, the rate of allergic reactions—including particularly ascending paralysis—is higher, and the efficacy is less.

C. Preexposure Immunization: Preexposure prophylaxis with three injections of diploid cell vaccine is recommended for persons at high risk of exposure: veterinarians (who should have rabies antibody titers checked every 2 years), animal handlers, Peace corps workers, and travelers to remote areas. An intradermal route is available for preexposure prophylaxis only. Immunosuppressive illness and agents including corticosteroids as well as antimalarials—in particular chloroquine—may diminish the antibody response.

Treatment

This very severe illness with an almost universally fatal outcome requires skillful intensive care with attention to the airway, maintenance of oxygenation, and control of seizures. Universal blood and body fluid precautions are essential.

Prognosis

Once the symptoms have appeared, death almost inevitably occurs after 7 days, usually from respiratory failure.

Dressen DW: A global review of rabies vaccines for human use. Vaccine 1997;15:S2. [NLM Cit ID: 97361389] (The regional differences in incidence and in availability of cell culture vaccine are considerable).

Human rabies prevention—United States, 1999. MMWR Morb Mortal Wkly Rep 1999;48(RR-1):1. [NLM Cit ID: 99175029]

Plotkin SA: Rabies. Clin Infect Dis 2000;30:4. [NLM Cit ID: 20086528] (Review and discussion of bat-related issues and detailed discussion of prophylaxis recommendations.)

2. ARBOVIRUS ENCEPHALITIDES

Essentials of Diagnosis

- Fever, malaise, stiff neck, sore throat, and nausea and vomiting, progressing to stupor, coma, and convulsions.
- Signs of an upper motor neuron lesion (exaggerated deep tendon reflexes, absent superficial reflexes, pathologic reflexes, spastic paralysis).
- Cerebrospinal fluid protein and opening pressure often increased, with lymphocytic pleocytosis.

General Considerations

The arboviruses are arthropod-borne agents that produce clinical manifestations in humans. They include three alphaviruses (causing Western, Eastern, and Venezuelan equine encephalitis), five flaviviruses (causing St. Louis and Japanese B encephalitis, dengue, yellow fever, and the West Nile agent [see below]), and bunyaviruses (the California serogroup of viruses [in particular California encephalitis caused by the Lacrosse agent] and a series of viral hemorrhagic fevers [Rift Valley fever; hemorrhagic fever with renal syndrome from the Hantaan agent]). The tick-borne causes of encephalitis include agents reviewed under hemorrhagic fevers, the flavivirus Powassan (northeastern United States and Canada), and tick-borne encephalitides of Europe. Only those agents causing primarily encephalitis in the United States will be discussed.

A new arboviral encephalitis in the USA was identified in 1999—West Nile encephalitis, with cases largely in the United States area and presenting similarly to St. Louis encephalitis. Bird infections in the New York area are now documented. The disease caused outbreaks in France in the early 1960s and in Romania in 1996, with occasional fatalities.

The leading causes of arbovirus encephalitis in the USA are St. Louis and California encephalitis. Agent-specific reservoirs (typically small mammals or birds) are responsible for maintaining the encephalitis-producing viruses in nature; horses serve as sentinels for infection with the equine agents, though birds maintain the life cycle. Eleven North Americans died of Japanese B encephalitis between 1981 and 1992—most of them military personnel stationed in Asia.

Clinical Findings

A. Symptoms and Signs: The symptoms are fever, malaise, sore throat, nausea and vomiting, lethargy, stupor, coma, and convulsions. Signs include stiff neck, meningeal irritation, tremors, convulsions, cranial nerve palsies, paralysis of extremities, exaggerated deep tendon reflexes, absent superficial reflexes, and pathologic reflexes.

While asymptomatic seroconversion is common, when frank encephalitis develops the outcome is age-dependent. St. Louis encephalitis occurs largely in adults, with residual damage principally in older patients. The other encephalitis-causing agents cause morbidity chiefly among children.

B. Laboratory Findings: The white blood cell count is variable. Cerebrospinal fluid pressure and protein content are often increased; glucose is normal; lymphocytic pleocytosis may be present (polymorphonuclear cells may predominate early). The virus may sometimes be isolated from blood or, rarely, from cerebrospinal fluid. PCR assays are available to assist with diagnosis. Serologic tests of blood or cerebrospinal fluid may be diagnostic in specific types of encephalitis (by demonstrating virus-specific IgM or a fourfold change in complement-fixing or neutralizing antibodies). CT or MRI of the brain showing basal ganglial or thalamic involvement may be useful in excluding the temporal lobe lesions of herpesvirus or other space-occupying processes.

Differential Diagnosis

Mild forms of encephalitis must be differentiated from aseptic meningitis, lymphocytic choriomeningitis, and nonparalytic poliomyelitis; severe forms of cerebrovascular accidents, brain tumors, brain abscess, and intoxications.

Arbovirus encephalitides are to be differentiated from other causes of viral encephalitis (herpes simplex virus, mumps virus, poliovirus or other enteroviruses, HIV), encephalitis accompanying exanthematous diseases of childhood (measles, varicella, infectious mononucleosis, rubella), encephalitis following vaccination (a demyelinating type following rabies, measles, pertussis), toxic encephalitis (from drugs, poisons, or bacterial toxins such as *Shigella dysenteriae* type 1), and Reye's syndrome.

Complications

Bronchial pneumonia, urinary retention and infection, and decubitus ulcers may occur. Late sequelae are mental deterioration, parkinsonism, and epilepsy.

Prevention

Effective measures include mosquito control (repellents, protective clothing, insecticides). A vaccine against Japanese B encephalitis is recommended for summer travelers to rural areas of East Asia.

Treatment

Although specific antiviral therapy is not available for most causative entities, vigorous supportive measures can be helpful. Such measures include reduction of intracranial pressure (mannitol) and monitoring of intraventricular pressure. The efficacy of corticosteroids in these infections is not established.

Prognosis

The prognosis is always guarded, especially in younger children. Sequelae may become apparent late in the course of what appears to be a successful recovery. The prognosis is generally better for Western equine than for Eastern equine or St. Louis encephalitis.

Balkhy HH et al: Severe La Crosse encephalitis with significant neurologic sequelae. Ped Infect Dis J 2000;19:77. [NLM Cit ID: 20106650] (A description of 6 cases with severe disease, requiring ICU care and causing neurologic sequelae.)

Cunha BA: West Nile encephalitis. Infectious Disease Practice for Clinicians 1999;23:85.

Deresiewicz RL et al: Clinical and neuroradiographic manifestations of eastern equine encephalitis. N Engl J Med 1997;336:1867. [NLM Cit ID: 97324063] (A mortality rate of 31% and a significant morbidity rate of 35% were reported in a series of 36 patients.)

Lanciotti RAS et al: Origin of the West Nile virus responsible for an outbreak of encephalitis in the northeastern United States. Science 1999;286:2333. [NLM Cit ID: 20070288] (The agent was isolated from fatal human cases from NYC, crows, exotic birds including a Chilean flamingo, and mosquitoes [all in the NYC area], and appears related to a virus isolated from a dead goose in Israel in 1998.)

Lowry PW: Arbovirus encephalitis in the United States and Asia. J Lab Clin Med 1997;129:405. [NLM Cit ID: 97258712] (Review article.)

Lundstrom JO: Mosquito-borne viruses in western Europe: a review. J Vector Ecol 1999;24:1. [NLM Cit ID: 99365929] (Of special concern are, again, West Nile encephalitis, and also the alphavirus Sindbis virus [a cause of fever, rash, and arthralgias in northern Europe], and the bunyavirus Tahyna [a cause of respiratory and CNS disease in central and eastern Europe].)

Outbreak of West Nile-like viral encephalitis—New York, 1999. MMWR Morb Mortal Wkly Rep 1999;48:845 and 890. [NLM Cit ID: 20025045] (Initial report and update with mention of five deaths among residents in NYC in late August.)

Wasay MN et al: St Louis encephalitis: a review of 11 cases in a 1995 Dallas, Texas, epidemic. Arch Neurol 2000;57:114. [NLM Cit ID: 20097923] (The authors suggest that substantia nigra involvement may be more common with St. Louis encephalitis and propose that HIV may be a risk factor, although only 2 cases independently fulfilled each of these characteristics.)

3. LYMPHOCYTIC CHORIOMENINGITIS

Essentials of Diagnosis

- "Influenza-like" prodrome of fever, chills, malaise, and cough, followed by meningitis with associated stiff neck.
- Aseptic meningitis with positive Kernig's sign, headache, nausea, vomiting, and lethargy.
- Cerebrospinal fluid: slight increase of protein, lymphocytic pleocytosis (500–3000/μL); low glucose in 25% of patients.
- Complement-fixing antibodies within 2 weeks.

General Considerations

Lymphocytic choriomeningitis is a viral (arenavirus) infection of the central nervous system. The reservoir of infection is the infected house mouse, although naturally infected guinea pigs, monkeys, dogs, and swine have been observed. Pet hamsters may be a source of infection. The virus is shed by the infected animal via oronasal secretions, urine, and feces, with transmission to humans probably through exposure to animal droppings via contaminated food and dust. The virus is not spread from person to person, though there appears to be vertical transmission, and lymphocytic choriomeningitis is considered a fetal teratogen. The incubation period is 8–13 days to the appearance of systemic manifestations and 15–21 days to the appearance of meningeal symptoms. CD4 cells may be involved in pathogenesis. Lymphocytic choriomeningitis is considered a model of cell-mediated immunity in vaccine development.

Outbreaks have occurred among persons with rodent exposure. Complications of clinical disease are rare.

This disease is principally confined to the eastern seaboard and northeastern states of the USA, and serologic evidence of infection is increased among women, the elderly, and members of lower socioeconomic groups.

Clinical Findings

A. Symptoms and Signs: Symptoms are biphasic. The prodromal illness is characterized by fever, chills, headache, myalgia, cough, and vomiting, the meningeal phase by headache, nausea and vomiting, and lethargy. Signs of pneumonia are occasionally present during the prodromal phase. During the meningeal phase there may be neck and back stiffness with a positive Kernig sign. Obstructive hydrocephalus is a rare complication. Arthralgias can develop late.

The prodrome may terminate in complete recovery, or meningeal symptoms may appear after a few days of remission.

B. Laboratory Findings: Leukocytosis or leukopenia and thrombocytopenia may be present. Cerebrospinal fluid lymphocytic pleocytosis (total count is often 500–3000/μL) may occur, with slight increase in protein and normal to low glucose in at least 25%. Complement-fixing antibodies appear during or after the second week. The virus may be recovered from the blood and cerebrospinal fluid by mouse inoculation. A PCR technique for the detection of lymphocytic choriomeningitis virus in the cerebrospinal fluid has been described.

Differential Diagnosis

The influenza-like prodrome and latent period help distinguish this from other aseptic meningitides, and bacterial and granulomatous meningitis. A history of exposure to mice or other potential vector is an important diagnostic clue.

Treatment

Treatment is supportive as for encephalitis or aseptic meningitis. A membrane protein called alpha-dystroglycan interacts with lymphocytic choriomeningitis and Lassa fever virus (both arenaviruses) may provide an avenue for future interventions.

Prognosis

Fatalities are rare. The illness usually lasts 1–2 weeks, although convalescence may be prolonged.

Barton LL et al: Lymphocytic choriomeningitis: pediatric pathogen and fetal teratogen. Pediatr Infect Dis J 1999; 18:540. [NLM Cit ID: 99318070]

Cao W et al: Identification of alpha-dystroglycan as a receptor for LCM and Lassa fever virus. Science 1998;282:2079. [NLM Cit ID: 99069625]

Klenerman P et al: What can we learn about HIV infection from a study of lymphocytic choriomeningitis virus? Immunol Rev 1997;159:5. [NLM Cit ID: 98078459] (A comparison is made between these two infections in light of the known and established scientific studies of lymphocytic choriomeningitis.)

4. PRION DISEASE

Several neurologic diseases are caused by communicable agents with slow replication and long latent intervals in the host. Such agents have been called *pro*teinaceous *in*fectious particles resistant to most procedures that modify nucleic acid and are increasingly being referred to as "prions." The transmissible agents require conversion of a brain protein to an abnormal isoform, a process that appears to be both genetically determined and in need of the infectious agent. The accumulated abnormal isoform proteins are associated with disease, although the method by which modes of pathogenesis result in the spongiform pathology and the accumulation in some cases of amyloid plaque remains to be determined. A variety of animal diseases exhibit these properties, including visna and scrapie in sheep and goats, chronic wasting disease of mule deer, and transmissible encephalopathy of mink. The agents or related agents that cause human disease are discussed here.

Kuru and **Creutzfeldt-Jakob disease** are transmissible in brain or eye tissue to primates, including humans. On reactivation from the latent state after months to years, diseases ensue that are characterized by an inexorably progressive downhill course. Kuru—once prevalent in central New Guinea but no longer seen since the abandonment of cannibalism—was characterized by cerebellar ataxia, tremors, dysarthria, and emotional lability.

Creutzfeldt-Jakob disease presents usually in late middle age with rapidly progressive dementia, myoclonic fasciculations, ataxia, and somnolence and has an electroencephalographic pattern characterized by paroxysms with high voltages and slow waves. The four forms of Creutzfeld-Jakob disease are sporadic (80–85%), familial (15%), iatrogenic (< 1%), and a new variant (also rare) described below. There is a rapid decline to akinetic mutism. There are no definitive risk factors for Creutzfeldt-Jakob disease. MRI typically shows bilateral areas of increased signal intensity, predominantly in the caudate and putamen.

There is no specific treatment, and the only known means of prevention is avoidance of contamination by affected brain tissue, electrodes, or neurosurgical tools or by transplants of cornea, dura, or cadaveric growth hormone from infected donors. Disinfection of equipment requires autoclaving at 15 psi for 1 hour, and disinfection of contaminated surfaces requires 5% hypochlorite or 0.1 N sodium hydroxide solution.

A variant of Creutzfeldt-Jakob disease has been described in a small outbreak from Britain. The patients were younger adults, the duration of disease was longer, the clinical symptomatology was unique (psychiatric symptoms and cerebellar signs were more common), and the electroencephalographic findings were not typical of classic Creutzfeldt-Jakob disease. The disease is believed to result from ingestion of beefsteak from livestock infected with **bovine spongiform encephalopathy (BSE)** ("mad cow disease").

Other prion diseases include fatal familial insomnia (rarely sporadic) and Gerstmann-Straussler-Scheinker disease (with dementia and spastic paraparesis).

Hedge RS et al: Transmissible and genetic prion diseases share a common pathway of neurodegeneration. Nature 1999;402:822. [NLM Cit ID: 20083494]

Johnson RT et al: Medical progress: Creutzfeldt-Jakob disease and related transmissible spongiform encephalopathies. N Engl J Med 1998;339:1994. [NLM Cit ID: 99077403] (An excellent review by leading investigators, outlining the differences between sporadic and familial Creutzfeldt-Jakob disease and between that disease and bovine spongiform encephalopathy.)

Prusiner SB: Prion diseases and the BSE crisis. Science 1997;278:245. [NLM Cit ID: 97465970] (The link between BSE and CJD and how faulty animal husbandry resulted in prion-contaminated feed for cattle.)

Tyler KL: Prions and prion diseases of the central nervous system. Curr Clin Top Infect Dis 1999;19:226. [NLM Cit ID: 99401709]

Will RG: Descriptive epidemiology of Creutzfeldt-Jakob disease in six European countries, 1993–1995. EU Collaborative Study Group for CJD. Ann Neurol 1998;43:763. [NLM Cit ID: 98291798] (A reminder that the link between BSE and Creutzfeld-Jakob disease to date is not firmly substantiated.)

5. PROGRESSIVE MULTIFOCAL LEUKOENCEPHALOPATHY

Progressive multifocal leukoencephalopathy is another progressive demyelinating central nervous system disorder with a propensity for immunosuppressed adults, including AIDS patients. The cause is JC virus (JCV), a papovavirus whose main central nervous system target is myelinating oligodendrocytes. JCV has also been cultured and identified by PCR—though not necessarily associated with disease—in central nervous system tissue from HIV-infected and other individuals. Highly active antiretroviral therapy (HAART) for HIV infection is effective in improving survival as well as the clinical and radiographic features associated with this disease.

Sadler M: Progressive multifocal leukoencephalopathy in HIV. Int J STD AIDS 1997;8:351. [NLM Cit ID: 97323154]

6. HUMAN T CELL LYMPHOTROPIC VIRUS (HTLV)

Retroviruses include both the lympholytic HIV agents and the lymphotropic oncoviruses, human T cell leukemia viruses types 1 and 2 (HTLV-1 and -2). The isolation of HTLV-1 from a young male with T cell lymphoma established an association of the virus with adult T cell lymphoma/leukemia (ATL) that has been confirmed from highly endemic areas (the Caribbean, southern Japan, sub-Saharan Africa—where over 10% of the population of Gabon and Cameroon are seropositive—and among intravenous drug users in the southeastern United States).

The lifetime risk of developing ATL among the seropositive is estimated to be 3% among females and 7% among males, with an incubation period of at least 15 years. HTLV-1 is oncogenic primarily through the simultaneous induction of both interleukin-2 and interleukin-2 receptor.

Common clinical features of ATL include diffuse lymphadenopathy, maculopapular skin lesions that may evolve into an erythroderma, organomegaly, lytic bone lesions, and sometimes hypercalcemia.

There is a predisposition to dermatophytoses, strongyloidiasis, and the usual AIDS-associated opportunistic infections (pneumocystis pneumonia, CMV infection, cryptococcosis). Diagnosis requires identification of HTLV antibodies. Confirmatory demonstration of monoclonal proviral DNA integration in tumor cells is helpful.

HTLV-1 also causes HTLV-associated myelopathy (HAM; tropical spastic paraparesis). It is characterized by progressive motor weakness with spastic paraparesis or paraplegia with hyperreflexia. Sensory disturbances and urinary incontinence are also seen. The disease may resemble multiple sclerosis but does not remit. Cranial nerve abnormalities are rare, and cognitive function is usually preserved. HAM develops in less than 1% of HTLV-1 seropositive individuals.

HTLV-2 was initially implicated in hairy cell leukemia, but this association has not been confirmed. HTLV-2 seropositivity is common in some Native American populations. It infects primarily CD8 cells, HTLV-1 primarily CD4 cells. The role of HTLV-2 in disease is under investigation.

Management of ATL is similar to that for non-Hodgkin's lymphoma and includes combination chemotherapy and radiation of particular sites (weight-bearing bony lesions, paraspinal masses, intracerebral lesions). HTLV-associated myelopathy has been treated successfully with corticosteroids. Antiretrovirals have not shown clear benefit for ATL or HTLV-associated myelopathy.

Screening of the blood supply for HTLV-1 is required in the United States, since transfusion is a recognized mode of transmission. Intravenous drug use is a common mode of transmission; less common routes are sexual activity, vertical transmission, and perhaps others since vertical transmission increases with age. Ten to 40 percent of HTLV-2 carriers are not cross-reactive to HTLV-1 screening assays, and new methods for improving blood screening are under development.

Ferreira OC Jr et al: HTLV: Epidemiology, biology, and pathogenesis. Blood Rev 1997;11:91. [NLM Cit ID: 97386929]

Vassilopoulos D et al: Rheumatologic manifestations of HIV-1 and HTLV-1 infections. Cleve Clin J Med 1998;65:436. [NLM Cit ID: 98441701] (There is considerable clinical mimicry between the two.)

OTHER SYSTEMIC VIRAL DISEASES

1. DENGUE

Essentials of Diagnosis

- Exposure 7–10 days before onset.
- Sudden onset of high fever, chills, severe aching, headache, sore throat, prostration, and depression.
- Biphasic fever curve: initial phase, 3–7 days; remission, few hours to 2 days; second phase, 1–2 days.
- The rash is biphasic: first evanescent, followed by maculopapular, scarlatiniform, morbilliform, or petechial changes from extremities to torso.
- Leukopenia and thrombocytopenia in the hemorrhagic form.

General Considerations

Dengue is a viral (togavirus, flavivirus) disease transmitted by the bite of the *Aedes* mosquito. It may be caused by one of several serotypes widely distributed between latitudes 25 °N and 25 °S (eg, Thailand, India, Philippines; Caribbean, including Puerto Rico and Cuba; Central America; Africa). It occurs only in the active mosquito season (warm weather). The incubation period is 3–15 days (usually 7–10 days). Transmission has occurred in the USA in southern Texas and nearby Mexican border towns in 1986 and 1999. A high level of suspicion for dengue is warranted in the southern United States since a new vector, the Asian tiger mosquito, *Aedes albopictus,* was admitted through imported tires in Texas in the 1980s.

Clinical Findings

A. Symptoms and Signs: Dengue is usually a nonspecific, self-limited, febrile illness, but its presentation may range from asymptomatic infection to severe hemorrhage **(dengue hemorrhagic fever)** and sudden fatal shock **(dengue shock syndrome).** Severe dengue begins with a sudden onset of high fever, chilliness, and severe aching ("breakbone") of the head, back, and extremities, accompanied by sore throat, prostration, and depression. There may be conjunctival redness and flushing or blotching of the skin. The initial febrile phase lasts 3–7 days, typically but not inevitably followed by a remission of a few hours to 2 days.

The rash appears in 80% of cases during the remission or during the second febrile phase, which lasts 1–2 days and is accompanied by similar but usually milder symptoms than in the first phase. The rash may be scarlatiniform, morbilliform, maculopapular, or petechial. It appears first on the dorsum of the hands and feet and spreads to the arms, legs, trunk, and neck but rarely to the face. The rash lasts 2 hours to several days and may be followed by desquamation.

Petechial rashes and gastrointestinal hemorrhages occur with dengue hemorrhagic fever, caused by strains of many subtypes in Asia and increasingly in the Caribbean, Mexico, and Central America, typically as an anamnestic response, most often to serotype 2, and less often to serotypes 3, 4, and 1 (in decreasing order of frequency). Some dengue virus envelope glycoproteins are homologous with segments of clotting factors, including plasminogen, and thus the hemorrhagic fever may represent an autoimmune reaction. A subset of patients progress to dengue shock syndrome, in which a capillary leak process is prominent.

Before the rash of dengue appears, it is difficult to distinguish from malaria, yellow fever, or influenza; the rash makes dengue far more likely. A positive tourniquet test should alert one to the possible development of hemorrhagic fever.

B. Laboratory Findings: Leukopenia is characteristic. Thrombocytopenia occurs in the hemorrhagic form of the disease and appears to correlate with early CD69 expression on peripheral lymphocytes. Virus may be recovered from the blood during the acute phase.

Complications

Depression, pneumonia, bone marrow failure, iritis, orchitis, and oophoritis are unusual complications. Dengue shock syndrome occurs among a small subset of patients with severe dengue hemorrhagic fever, and children appear to be at particular risk.

Prevention

Available prophylactic measures include control of mosquitoes by screening and insect repellents, particularly during early morning and late afternoon exposures. An effective vaccine has been developed but has not been produced commercially.

Treatment

Treatment entails the appropriate use of volume and pressors, acetaminophen rather than aspirin for analgesia, and the gradual restoration of activity during prolonged convalescence. Monitoring patients with platelet counts is useful in anticipating the complications of dengue hemorrhagic fever or shock syndrome.

Prognosis

Fatalities are rare, though convalescence tends to be slow.

Green S et al: Early CD69 expression on peripheral blood lymphocytes from children with dengue hemorrhagic fever. J Infect Dis 1999;180:1429. [NLM Cit ID: 99445606] (The expression of the CD69 antigen may be an important correlate with disease severity.)

Gubler DJ et al: Impact of dengue/dengue hemorrhagic fever on the developing world. Adv Virus Res 1999;35:53. [NLM Cit ID: 20048807]

Halstead SB et al: Resuscitation of patients with dengue hemorrhagic fever/dengue shock syndrome. (Editorial) Clin Infect Dis 1999;29:795. [NLM Cit ID: 20055835]

Rigau-Pérez JG et al: Dengue and dengue haemorrhagic fever. Lancet 1998;352:971. [NLM Cit ID: 98423756]

2. COLORADO TICK FEVER

Essentials of Diagnosis

- Onset 1–19 days (average, 4 days) following tick bite.
- Fever, chills, myalgia, headache, prostration.
- Leukopenia.
- Second attack of fever after remission lasting 2–3 days.

General Considerations

Colorado tick fever is an acute coltivirus infection transmitted by *Dermacentor andersoni* bites. The disease is limited to the western USA and Canada and is most prevalent during the tick season (March to November). The incubation period is 3–6 days.

Clinical Findings

A. Symptoms and Signs: The onset of fever (to 38.9–40.6 °C) is abrupt, sometimes with chills. Severe myalgia, headache, photophobia, anorexia, nausea and vomiting, and generalized weakness are prominent symptoms. Physical findings are limited to an occasional faint rash. Fever continues for 3 days, followed by a remission of 1–3 days and then by a full recrudescence lasting 2–4 days. In an occasional case there may be three bouts of fever.

The differential diagnosis includes influenza, Rocky Mountain spotted fever, and numerous other viral infections.

B. Laboratory Findings: Leukopenia (2000–3000/μL) with a shift to the left occurs. Viremia may be demonstrated by inoculation of blood into mice or by fluorescent antibody staining of the patient's red cells (with adsorbed virus). Complement-fixing antibodies appear during the third week of disease. A reverse transcriptase PCR technique has been developed for detection of the virus in serum.

Complications

Aseptic meningitis, encephalitis, and hemorrhagic fever occur rarely. Malaise may ensue, but fatalities are very rare.

Treatment

No specific treatment is available. Aspirin or another nonsteroidal anti-inflammatory agent—or codeine or hydrocodone—may be given for pain.

Prognosis

The disease is usually self-limited and benign.

Attoui H et al: Serologic and molecular diagnosis of Colorado tick fever viral infections. Am J Trop Med Hyg 1998;59:763. [NLM Cit ID: 99054329]

3. HEMORRHAGIC FEVERS

This is a diverse group of illnesses resulting from viral infections and immunologic responses to them. The common clinical features include high fever, leukopenia, altered mental status, and a hemorrhagic diathesis. Marked toxicity and death may occur. The viruses may be tick-borne (eg, Omsk hemorrhagic fever, Russia; Kyasanur Forest hemorrhagic fever, India); mosquito-borne (eg, Chikungunya hemorrhagic fever, yellow fever, dengue, and o'nyong-nyong fever); or zoonotic (often derived from rodents, eg, hemorrhagic fever with renal failure secondary to Hantaan virus infection [discussed below], Junin hemorrhagic fever, Argentina; Machupo hemorrhagic fever, Bolivia; Lassa hemorrhagic fever, West Africa; the Puumala virus, Scandinavia; Belgrade virus, Yugoslavia; Dobrava virus, the Balkans; Nipah virus, Malaysia and related to pig contact). The zoonotic group also includes Marburg hemorrhagic fever and possibly Ebola hemorrhagic fever in central Africa. Lassa fever has been associated with rodent consumption.

Persons who present with symptoms compatible with those of hemorrhagic fever and who have traveled from a possible endemic area should be isolated for diagnosis and symptomatic treatment. Diagnosis may be made by growing the virus from blood obtained early in the disease or by showing a significant specific antibody titer rise. Isolation is particularly important, because some of these infections are highly transmissible and carry a mortality rate of 50–90%.

For most of these entities, no specific treatment is available. Lassa fever and hemorrhagic fever with renal failure can be effectively treated with intravenous ribavirin if started promptly: 33 mg/kg as loading dose, followed by 16 mg/kg every 6 hours for

4 days and then 8 mg/kg every 8 hours for 3 days (see Chapter 37). It is important to differentiate hemorrhagic fever from differently treated entities such as meningococcemia or other septicemias, Rocky Mountain spotted fever, dengue, and malaria. The likelihood of hemorrhagic fevers among travelers is sufficiently low that febrile travelers should be evaluated in the context of a broad differential diagnosis.

Harrison LH et al: Clinical case definitions for Argentine hemorrhagic fever. Clin Infect Dis 1999;28:1091. [NLM Cit ID: 99379709] (Thrombocytopenia < 100,000/μL and leukopenia < 4000/μL appear to be highly sensitive screens for this disease in developing world settings.)

Pateon NI et al: Outbreak of Nipah-virus infection among abattoir workers with dyspnea. Lancet 1999;354:1253. [NLM Cit ID: 99448944] (Nipah virus is a highly fatal zoonotic infection related to hendraviruses of Australia. Pigs are the animal source, requiring slaughter for containment.)

Sodhi A: Ebola virus disease: Recognizing the face of a rare killer. Postgrad Med 1996;99:75. [NLM Cit ID: 96219037]

4. HANTAVIRUSES

Hantaviruses are rodent-borne RNA viruses with several distinct serotypes. These differ in rodent hosts, geographic distribution, and degree of pathogenicity for humans. They cause two major clinical syndromes: hemorrhagic fever (discussed above) and the **hantavirus pulmonary syndrome.** The ubiquitousness of hantaviruses is becoming recognized, with descriptions of infections from Paraguay and Argentina and serotypes reported from the Balkans. The Hantaan serotype viruses cause severe hemorrhagic fever with renal syndrome and are found primarily in Korea, China, and eastern Russia. The Seoul viruses produce a less severe form and are found primarily in Korea and China. The Puumala viruses are found in Scandinavia and Europe and are associated with a relatively mild form of the syndrome.

The recently discovered Sin Nombre (Muerto Canyon, Four Corners) virus is responsible for the **hantavirus pulmonary syndrome,** most cases of which have been seen in the southwestern United States, though South American cases have been observed and an outbreak was reported from Panama in early 2000. Two other hantaviruses associated with the syndrome in the United States are the Black Creek virus (in Florida) and Bayou virus (in Louisiana). It begins as a nonspecific febrile illness followed by rapid progression to a shock-like state, associated with increased pulmonary vascular permeability and ARDS. Hematologic features include thrombocytopenia, hemoconcentration, and leukocytosis.

Diagnosis can be made serologically, by immunohistochemical staining, or by PCR amplification of viral tissue DNA.

Since infection is thought to occur by inhalation of rodent wastes, prevention is aimed toward eradication of rodents in houses and avoidance of exposure to rodent excreta in rural settings. Person-to-person transmission, while documented, is rare.

No treatment has been established as definitely effective. Intravenous ribavirin has been used, since it is effective in treating severe cases of Hantaan virus infection.

Doyle TJ et al: Viral hemorrhagic fevers and hantavirus infections in the Americas. Infect Dis Clin North Am 1998;12:95. [NLM Cit ID: 98155936]

Schmaljohn C et al: Hantaviruses: A global disease problem. Emerg Infect Dis 1997;3:95. [NLM Cit ID: 97348239] (Entire issue on the ecology and epidemiology of this ubiquitous group of viruses.)

Update: Hantavirus pulmonary syndrome—United States, 1999. MMWR Morb Mort Wkly Rep 1999;38:521. [NLM Cit ID: 99328337].

Young JC et al: New World hantaviruses. Br Med Bull 1998;54:659. [NLM Cit ID: 99258142].

5. YELLOW FEVER

Essentials of Diagnosis

- Endemic area exposure (tropical South and Central America, Africa, but not Asia).
- Sudden onset of severe headache, aching in legs, and tachycardia.
- Brief (1 day) remission, followed by bradycardia, hypotension, jaundice, hemorrhagic tendency.
- Proteinuria, leukopenia, bilirubinemia, bilirubinuria.

General Considerations

Yellow fever is a zoonotic viral (group B arbovirus, togavirus) infection transmitted by the *Aedes* and jungle mosquitoes. It is endemic only in Africa and South America (tropical or subtropical), but epidemics have extended far into the temperate zone during warm seasons. Its role in thwarting economic development in tropical areas has been devastating.

The mosquito transmits the infection by first biting an individual having the disease and then biting a susceptible individual after the virus has multiplied within the mosquito's body. The incubation period in humans is 3–6 days. Adults and children are equally susceptible, though attack rates are highest among adult males because of their work habits.

Clinical Findings

A. Symptoms and Signs:

1. Mild form–Symptoms are malaise, headache, fever, retro-orbital pain, nausea, vomiting, and photophobia. Bradycardia may be present.

2. Severe form–About 15% of those infected with yellow fever develop severe illness. Initial symptoms are similar to the mild form, but a brief remission after about 3 days of acute illness is followed by a toxic phase manifested by fever and bradycardia (Faget's sign), hypotension, jaundice, hemorrhage (gastrointestinal, nasal, oral), and delirium that may progress to coma.

B. Laboratory Findings: Leukopenia occurs, although it may not be present at the onset. Proteinuria is present, sometimes as high as 5–6 g/L, and disappears completely with recovery. Abnormal liver function tests are seen, and prothrombin time may be elevated. Serologic diagnosis may be established by showing fourfold or greater increases in hemagglutination inhibition, complement fixation, or neutralizing antibodies. An IgM capture enzyme immunoassay (EIA) is a rapid, specific diagnostic aid.

Differential Diagnosis

It may be difficult to distinguish yellow fever from hepatitis, malaria, leptospirosis, dengue, and other hemorrhagic fevers on clinical evidence alone. Laboratory confirmation is often needed.

Prevention

Transmission is prevented through mosquito control. Live virus vaccine is highly effective, safe, and should be provided for immunocompetent adults living in or traveling to endemic areas. Pregnant women should not be immunized and should defer travel to endemic areas (see Chapter 30). Eradication is difficult because of the sylvatic cycle, with forest rodents serving as a reservoir. (See Chapter 30.)

Treatment

No specific antiviral therapy is available. Treatment is directed toward symptomatic relief and management of complications.

Prognosis

The mortality rate is high in the severe form, with death occurring most commonly between the sixth and the tenth days. In survivors, the temperature returns to normal by the seventh or eighth day. The prognosis in any individual case is guarded at the onset, since sudden changes for the worse are common. Intractable hiccups, copious black vomitus, melena, and anuria are unfavorable signs. Convalescence is prolonged, including 1–2 weeks of asthenia.

Arya SC: Yellow fever vaccine. Emerg Infect Dis 1999;5:487. [NLM Cit ID: 99276715]

Robertson SE et al: Yellow fever: A decade of reemergence. JAMA 1996;276:1157. [NLM Cit ID: 96425579]

Tomori O: Impact of yellow fever on the developing world. Adv Virus Res 1999;53:5. [NLM Cit ID: 20048806]

Tsai TF: Yellow fever. Bull WHO 1998;72(Suppl 2):158. [NLM Cit ID: 99163191]

COMMON VIRAL RESPIRATORY INFECTIONS

Infections of the respiratory tract are perhaps the most common human ailments. Specific associations of certain groups of viruses with certain disease syndromes have been established. In young infants and in the elderly, or in persons with impaired respiratory tract reserve bacterial superinfection increases morbidity and mortality.

Croup, epiglottitis, and the common cold are discussed in Chapter 8.

Glezen WP et al: Impact of respiratory virus infections on persons with chronic underlying conditions. JAMA 2000;283:499. [NLM Cit ID: 20123272] (Underlying respiratory conditions are a major risk factor for hospitalization when acute respiratory infections develop.)

Wang E et al: Antibiotic overprescribing for Canadian preschool children; evidence of overprescribing for viral respiratory infections. Clin Infect Dis 1999;29:155. [NLM Cit ID 99360961]: (An estimated 49% of costs were associated with overprescribing.)

1. RESPIRATORY SYNCYTIAL VIRUS

Respiratory syncytial virus (RSV) causes annual outbreaks of pneumonia, bronchiolitis, and tracheobronchitis in the very young. Reinfection is common and manifests itself typically as a mild upper respiratory tract infection and tracheobronchitis in older children or adults. Serious pulmonary RSV infections have been described in elderly and immunocompromised adults. Outbreaks with a high mortality rate in bone marrow transplant and pediatric liver transplant patients are reported. Infants with congenital heart disease are also at high risk.

Annual epidemics occur in winter and spring. The average incubation period is 5 days. Inoculation may occur through the nose or the eyes.

In bronchiolitis, proliferation and necrosis of bronchiolar epithelium develop, producing obstruction from sloughed epithelium and increased mucus secretion. Signs include low-grade fever, tachypnea, and wheezes. Hyperinflated lungs, decreased gas exchange, and increased work of breathing are present. Otitis media is a frequent complication.

RSV is the only respiratory pathogen that produces its most serious illness at a time when specific maternal antibody is invariably present, though high titers can modify or prevent infection.

Rapid diagnosis may be made by viral antigen identification of nasal washings using an ELISA or immunofluorescent assay. Culture of nasopharyngeal secretions remains the standard of diagnosis.

Treatment consists of hydration, humidification of inspired air and ventilatory support as needed. In infants with underlying cardiopulmonary disease, aerosolized ribavirin may help (1.1 g/d, diluted to 20 mg/mL, delivered as a particulate with oxygen over 12–18 hours per day for 3–7 days—although high-dose, short-duration therapy may be as effective). Pregnant women should avoid ribavirin exposure—and indeed, patients with upper respiratory RSV infections probably do not need ribavirin. Hyperimmune RSV immunoglobulin G (1500 mg/kg) is effective in combination with ribavirin in the management of RSV infections among immunocompromised adults; its role in the treatment of children with lower respiratory tract infections remains under study. Intravenous RSV immunoglobulin (RSV-IVIG), given as 750 mg/kg every 30 days, is, however, safe and effective in preventing lower respiratory tract infection in infants and young children, though immunoglobulin has been supplanted by palivizumab. This is a monoclonal antibody, used especially if the infants are premature or suffer from bronchopulmonary disease, especially bronchopulmonary dysplasia. They are at particular risk if there is prematurity or cardiopulmonary disease, especially with bronchopulmonary dysplasia. A subunit vaccine given to pregnant women may provide passive protection against RSV in neonates and in the institutionalized elderly. Because nosocomial RSV infections disseminate rapidly, prevention in hospitals entails rapid diagnosis, handwashing, and perhaps passive immunization.

Englund JA et al: Diagnosis of respiratory viruses in cancer and transplant patients. Curr Clin Top Infect Dis 1999;190:30. [NLM Cit ID: 99401699]

Garcia R et al: Nosocomial RSV infections: Prevention and control in bone marrow transplant patients. Infect Control Hosp Epidemiol 1997;18:412. [NLM Cit ID: 97325344]

Heikkinen T et al: Prevalence of various respiratory viruses in the middle ear during acute otitis media. N Engl J Med 1999;340:260. [NLM Cit ID: 99110541] (RSV was the principal cause of invasive acute otitis media, followed by parainfluenza and influenza viruses.)

Scott LJ: Palivizumab. Drugs 1999;58:305. [NLM Cit ID: 99400001] (Shown to be effective in children at high risk with cardiopulmonary conditions.)

Simoes EA: RSV infection. Lancet 1999;354:847. [NLM Cit ID: 99413751]

Update: RSV activity—United States, 1998–1999 season. MMWR Morb Mortal Wkly Rep 1999;48:1104. [NLM Cit ID: 20096160]

Walsh EE et al: Respiratory syncytial and other virus infection in persons with chronic cardiopulmonary disease. Am J Respir Crit Care Med 1999;160:791. [NLM Cit ID: 99403216] (Aggravates pulmonary status during the winter among patients with cardiopulmonary disease.)

2. INFLUENZA

Essentials of Diagnosis

- Cases usually in epidemic pattern, not sporadic.
- Abrupt onset with fever, chills, malaise, cough, coryza, and muscle aches.
- Aching, fever, and prostration out of proportion to catarrhal symptoms.
- Leukopenia.

General Considerations

Influenza (an orthomyxovirus) is transmitted by the respiratory route. In contrast to RSV and rhinoviruses, transmission occurs by droplet nuclei rather than fomites or large particle aerosols. Although sporadic cases occur, epidemics and pandemics appear at varying intervals, usually in the fall or winter. Antigenic types A and B produce clinically indistinguishable infections, whereas type C is usually a minor illness. New epidemic strains may evolve from reassortment, through pig vectors, between avian and human strains. Pandemics—associated with higher mortality—typically are associated with type A infections in which significant genetic recombination of the virus (antigenic shift) has taken place. The incubation period is 1–4 days.

A small number of human cases of a new strain of avian influenza A (H5N1) were reported from Hong Kong in December 1997. Surveillance suggested that the highest risk for disease occurred among those with poultry exposure, though person-to-person transmission was not fully excluded. A massive poultry slaughter ensued based on these findings. The continued surveillance for future potentially pandemic strains is an important aspect of influenza control.

It is difficult to diagnose influenza in the absence of an epidemic. The disease resembles many other mild febrile illnesses but is almost always accompanied by a cough. Influenza A (H3N2) has been the dominating strain for the last three seasons (1997–1999).

Clinical Findings

A. Symptoms and Signs: The onset is usually abrupt, with fever, chills, malaise, muscular aching, substernal soreness, headache, nasal stuffiness, and occasionally nausea. Fever lasts 1–7 days (usually 3–5). Coryza, nonproductive cough, and sore throat are present. Signs include mild pharyngeal injection, flushed face, and conjunctival redness.

B. Laboratory Findings: Leukopenia is common. Proteinuria may be present. The virus may be isolated from the throat washings by inoculation of embryonated eggs or cell cultures. Complement-fixing and hemagglutination-inhibiting antibodies appear during the second week.

Complications

Influenza causes necrosis of the respiratory epithelium, which predisposes to secondary bacterial infections. The interactions between bacteria and influenza are bidirectional, with bacterial enzymes (eg, proteases, trypsin-like compounds, streptokinase, plasminogen) activating influenza viruses. Frequent complications are acute sinusitis, otitis media, purulent bronchitis, and pneumonia; the elderly and the chronically ill are at high risk for complications.

Pneumonia is commonly due to bacterial infection with pneumococci or, less often, staphylococci or haemophilus or, on occasion, the influenza virus itself. Pericarditis, myocarditis, and thrombophlebitis sometimes occur.

Reye's syndrome is a rare and severe complication of influenza and other viral diseases (eg, varicella), particularly in young children. It consists of rapidly progressive hepatic failure and encephalopathy, and there is a 30% fatality rate. The pathogenesis is unknown, but the syndrome is associated with aspirin use in such viral infections. Hypoglycemia, elevation of serum aminotransferases and blood ammonia, prolonged prothrombin time, and change in mental status all occur within 2–3 weeks after onset of the virus infection. Histologically, the periphery of liver lobules shows striking fatty infiltration and glycogen depletion. Treatment is supportive and directed to the management of cerebral edema.

Prevention

Trivalent influenza virus vaccine provides partial immunity (about 85% efficacy) for a few months to 1 year. The vaccine's antigenic configuration changes yearly and is based on prevalent strains of the preceding year. Vaccination in October or November each year is recommended for persons over 65, children and teenagers receiving chronic aspirin therapy, nursing home residents, those with chronic lung or heart disease or other debilitating illnesses, and health care workers. The vaccine is contraindicated in persons with hypersensitivity to chicken eggs or other components of the vaccine, persons with an acute febrile illness, or thrombocytopenia. Concomitant warfarin or steroid therapy is not a contraindication. Side effects are infrequent and include tenderness, redness, or induration at the site of the injection and, rarely, myalgias or fever.

Adequate immunity is achieved about 2 weeks after vaccination. In healthy subjects, the antibody level remains sufficiently high throughout the season. Levels wane quickly, however, in elderly nursing home patients. Therefore, the vaccine should not be administered too early in the influenza season. The vaccination effectively reduces both morbidity (preventing 35–60% of hospital admissions in the elderly) and mortality (preventing 35–80% of hospital deaths). A live attenuated vaccine has been widely used among Russian adults.

HIV-infected persons can be safely vaccinated, and concerns about activating replication of the HIV virus by the immunogen appear to be exaggerated and may be less severe than the increase in HIV viral load associated with a full influenza infection. Vaccination is less effective when CD4 counts are less than 100/μL. False-positive assays with HIV, HTLV-1, and HCV have been reported in the wake of influenza vaccination.

Chemoprophylaxis for epidemiologically or virologically confirmed influenza A with amantadine hydrochloride, 200 mg/d orally in two divided doses (100 mg/d in the elderly, who may develop central nervous system side effects), or rimantadine (200 mg/d in two divided doses) will markedly reduce the attack rate among exposed unvaccinated individuals if begun immediately and continued for 10 days. Amantadine or rimantadine may also be used during an outbreak while waiting for immunity to develop following vaccination.

Treatment

Many patients with influenza prefer to rest in bed. Analgesics and a cough mixture may be used. Amantadine or rimantadine, in the same doses as are used for prophylaxis appreciably decrease the duration of signs and symptoms. Rimantadine is preferred in patients with renal failure. The clinical significance of resistance to antiviral agents is controversial. Ribavirin (1.1 g/d, diluted to 20 mg/mL and delivered as particulate aerosol with oxygen over 12–18 hours a day for 3–7 days [Table 32–1]) has helped severely ill patients with influenza A or B. Newer agents such as inhaled zanamivir and oral oseltamivir, neuraminidase inhibitors, are equally helpful in the prophylaxis and treatment of influenza but more costly. The latter agents are given only to patients over age 12 whose symptoms have not been present more than 48 hours.

Antibacterial antibiotics should be reserved for treatment of bacterial complications. Acetaminophen rather than aspirin should be used for fever in children.

Prognosis

The duration of the uncomplicated illness is 1–7 days, and the prognosis is excellent. Purulent bronchitis and bronchiectasis may result in chronic pulmonary disease and fibrosis that persist throughout life. Most fatalities are due to bacterial pneumonia. Influenzal pneumonia has a high mortality rate among pregnant women and persons with a history of rheumatic heart disease. In recent epidemics, the mortality rate has been low except in debilitated individuals.

If the fever persists for more than 4 days with productive cough and white cell count over 10,000/μL, secondary bacterial infection should be suspected. Pneumococcal pneumonia is most common and staphylococcal pneumonia most serious.

Bardsley-Elliot A et al: Oseltamivir. Drugs 1999;58:851. [NLM Cit ID: 20061314]

Couch RB et al: Improvement of inactivated influenza virus vaccines. J Infect Dis 1997;176:S38. [NLM Cit ID: 97382689]

Cox NH: New options for the prevention of influenza. N Engl J Med 1999;341:1387. [NLM Cit ID: 99450919]

Hayden FT et al: Use of the selective oral neuraminidase inhibitor oseltamivir to prevent influenza. N Engl J Med 1999;341:1336. [NLM Cit ID: 99450912] (May produce bronchospasm in asthmatics; comparison of its efficacy with zanamivir yet to be published.)

JAMA patient page: Flu. JAMA 1999;281:962. [NLM Cit ID: 99176382]

Mossad SB. Underused options for preventing and treating influenza. Cleve Clin J Med 1999;66:19. [NLM Cit ID: 99125543] (Influenza vaccine is the most effective preventive measure but is greatly underused.)

Neuraminidase inhibitors for treatment of influenza A and B infections. MMWR Morb Mortal Wkly Rep 1999;48(RR-14):1. [NLM Cit ID: 20096304] (Published erratum in MMWR Morb Mortal Wkly Rep 1999;48[49]:1139.)

Potter J et al: Influenza vaccination of health care workers in long-term-care hospitals reduces the mortality of elderly patients. J Infect Dis 1997;175:1. [NLM Cit ID: 97138163] (Vaccination of the staff caused a greater reduction in influenza mortality than did vaccination of the residents.)

Update: influenza activity—United States and worldwide, 1998–1999 season, and composition of the 1999–2000 vaccine. MMWR Morb Mortal Wkly Rep 1999;48:374. [NLM Cit ID: 99296269]

ADENOVIRUS INFECTIONS

Adenoviruses (there are more than 40 antigenic types) produce a variety of clinical syndromes. These infections are self-limited or clinically inapparent and most common among infants, young children, and military recruits. Outbreaks in liver, bone marrow, and renal transplant recipients have been reported, and dissemination may occur. The incubation period is 4–9 days.

Clinical syndromes of adenovirus infection, often overlapping, include the following: (1) The **common cold** (see Chapter 8) is characterized by rhinitis, pharyngitis, and mild malaise without fever. (2) **Nonstreptococcal exudative pharyngitis** is characterized by fever lasting 2–12 days and accompanied by malaise and myalgia. Sore throat is often manifested by diffuse injection, a patchy exudate, and cervical lymphadenopathy. Cough is sometimes accompanied by rales and x-ray evidence of pneumonitis. Conjunctivitis is often present. (3) Lower respiratory tract involvement may occur, including bronchiolitis, suggested by cough and rales, or pneumonia (type 7 commonly causes acute respiratory disease and pneumonia). (4) **Pharyngoconjunctival fever** is manifested by fever and malaise, conjunctivitis (often unilateral), and mild pharyngitis. (5) **Epidemic keratoconjunctivitis** (transmissible person-to-person) occurs in adults and is manifested by unilateral conjunctival redness, pain, tearing, and an enlarged preauricular lymph node. Keratitis leads to subepithelial opacities (especially with types 8, 19, or 37). (6) **Acute hemorrhagic cystitis** is a disorder of children often associated with adenovirus type 11. (7) Sexually transmitted **genitourinary ulcers** and **urethritis** may be caused by types 2, 8, and 37 in particular. (8) Adenoviruses also cause acute **gastroenteritis** (types 40, 41) and **intussusception** and have been rarely associated with **encephalitis** and **pericarditis.**

Infected liver transplant recipients tend to develop hepatitis (type 5 adenovirus), whereas bone marrow and renal transplant recipients tend to develop pneumonia or hemorrhagic cystitis. Ribavirin has been used to treat adenovirus infections among HIV-infected individuals.

Vaccines are not available for general use. Live oral vaccines containing attenuated type 4 and type 7 have been used in military personnel.

Treatment is symptomatic.

Grumbach IM et al: Adenoviruses and enteroviruses as pathogens in myocarditis and dilated cardiomyopathy. Acta Cardiol 1999;54:82. [NLM Cit ID: 99305782] (For myocarditis, enteroviruses are more commonly associated with disease than are adenoviruses).

Wilson JM et al: Adenoviruses as gene delivery vehicles. N Engl J Med 1996;334:1185. [NLM Cit ID: 96185738] (Adenoviruses, although a common cause of human disease, have received particular recognition through their role in gene therapy.)

OTHER EXANTHEMATOUS VIRAL INFECTIONS

1. PARVOVIRUS INFECTIONS

Parvovirus B19 causes several syndromes. In children, an exanthematous illness ("fifth disease," erythema infectiosum) is characterized by fiery red "slapped cheek," circumoral pallor, and a subsequent lacy, maculopapular, evanescent truncal rash. Malaise, headache, and pruritus occur, but little fever. In immunosuppressed patients, including those with HIV infection and hematologic conditions such as sickle cell disease, anemia due to red cell hypoplasia occurs as a consequence of binding to erythrocyte P antigen (globoside). Middle-aged persons (especially women) develop a symmetric polyarthritis that mimics lupus erythematosus and rheumatoid arthritis, preferentially involving the proximal interphalangeal joints of the hands and the wrists and knees. Arthralgias are uncommon in children. Rashes, especially facial, are uncommon in adults. Hepatitis may occur. In pregnancy, fetal loss and hydrops fetalis have been reported. An association with Henoch-Schönlein purpura has also been noted.

The diagnosis is clinical (Table 32–2) but may be confirmed by an elevated titer of IgM anti-parvovirus antibodies in serum. Scarlet fever is the most similar disorder. Besides arthritis with hypocomplementemia, which is common in some outbreaks, encephalitis, chronic hemolytic anemia, and hepatitis are rare complications.

Treatment in healthy persons is symptomatic. NSAIDs can be used to treat arthralgias and transfusions to treat transient aplastic crises. In immunosuppressed patients, intravenous immunoglobulin aids in treatment.

Screening of donated blood could potentially prevent transfusion-related infection. Several nosocomial outbreaks have been documented, and hospital infection control personnel should administer standard containment guidelines (handwashing after patient exposure, avoiding contact with pregnant women).

The prognosis is generally excellent in immunocompetent individuals. In immunosuppressed patients, persistent anemia may require continued transfusions and periodic evaluations.

Gabriel SE et al: The role of parvovirus B19 in the pathogenesis of giant cell arteritis: a preliminary evaluation. Arthritis Rheum 1999;42:1255. [NLM Cit ID: 99292241] (The authors documented a significant correlation between histologic evidence of giant cell arteritis and the presence of B19 DNA in temporal artery biopsy tissue.)

Scapellato PG et al: Improvement of anemia induced by parvovirus B19 in a patient with AIDS after combined antiretroviral therapy. Mayo Clin Proc 2000;75:215. [NLM Cit ID: 20147288]

Valeur-Jensen AK et al: Risk factors for parvovirus B19 infection in pregnancy. JAMA 1999;281:1099. [NLM Cit ID: 99202543] (Although nearly two-thirds of women were seropositive, during an outbreak period there was a 13% annual seroconversion rate and the risk of infections was highest among women who had contact with children.)

2. POXVIRUS INFECTIONS

Among the nine poxviruses causing disease in humans, the following are clinically important.

(1) **Variola:** Smallpox was a highly contagious disease characterized by severe headache, fever, and prostration and accompanied by a centrifugal rash developing in order of progression from macules to papules to vesicles to pustules. An international consensus among the scientific community resulted in a decision to consider destroying the virus since elimination of the disease had been achieved.

(2) **Molluscum contagiosum** may be transmitted sexually or by other close contact. It is manifested by pearly, raised, umbilicated skin nodules sparing the palms and soles. Marked and persistent lesions in AIDS patients appear to respond readily to combination antiretroviral therapy. The many anecdotal agents reported to hasten resolution include cimetidine and CO_2 laser therapy combined with natural interferon-beta gel. One percent imiquimod cream appeared to be effective in curing molluscum lesions. The disorder may be marked and persistent in AIDS patients.

(3) **Vaccinia:** Vaccination with vaccinia was responsible in part for smallpox eradication. Civilian vaccination is indicated only for laboratory workers who must handle virus. Vaccination is still practiced among some military forces but is not required for any international travel; it is effective in prevention of monkeypox (see below). Any form of immunosuppression is an absolute contraindication to smallpox vaccination. Eczema (or a history of it) in a patient or family member, other forms of dermatitis, and burns also contraindicate vaccination. There is no indication for therapeutic use of smallpox vaccine.

(4) **Orf** (contagious pustular dermatitis or ecthyma contagiosa) and **paravaccinia** (milkers' nodules) are occupational diseases acquired by contact with sheep and cattle, respectively.

(5) **Monkeypox,** first identified in 1970, is enzootic in the rain forests of equatorial Africa and presents in humans with a syndrome similar to smallpox; case fatalities are about 3% (to 11% among the unvaccinated), and secondary attack rates, which are hard to determine because of diagnostic confusion with varicella in older series, appear to be about 10%. Primary prevention entails the use of vaccinia immunization, a procedure accompanied by a risk of dissemination in HIV-infected persons—a real concern considering the coincident areas of endemicity of HIV-1 and monkeypox.

Breman JG et al: Poxvirus dilemmas—monkeypox, smallpox, and biologic terrorism. N Engl J Med 1998;339: 556. (Monkeypox threat unsubstantiated.)

Barquet N et al: Smallpox: The triumph over the most terrible of the ministers of death. Ann Intern Med 1997; 127:635. [NLM Cit ID: 97460344]

Heymann DL et al: Re-emergence of monkeypox in Africa: a review of the past six years. Br Med Bull 1998;54:693. [NLM Cit ID: 99258144] (The authors postulate that the termination of vaccinia vaccination after smallpox elimination may have increased the number of susceptibles and allowed this outbreak to emerge.)

Meadows KP et al: Resolution of recalcitrant molluscum contagiosum virus lesions in HIV-infected patients treated with cidofovir. Arch Dermatol 1997;133:1039. [NLM Cit ID: 97412593] (Cidofovir, used as a 3% cream or intravenously for concomitant CMV retinitis, was effective in clearing molluscum lesions.)

VIRUSES & GASTROENTERITIS

Viruses are responsible for probably 30–40% of cases of infectious diarrhea in the USA, and rotaviruses are a leading worldwide cause of dehydrating gastroenteritis in young children. The agents that can cause disease include group B rotaviruses, Norwalk agent (which causes epidemics of vomiting and diarrhea and is often transmitted by food—especially shellfish—and water), astroviruses, and enteric adenoviruses.

Rotaviruses (four major serotypes) are a major cause of diarrheal morbidity worldwide (due to dehydration) and can also cause infections in adults exposed to infected infants and are ubiquitous in the environment of an outbreak. (Secondary rates are between 16% and 30%.) The disease is usually mild, and cases have also occurred among travelers, in epidemic fashion, and after waterborne exposure. Sensitive and specific immunoassays to detect viral RNA in fecal specimens are available. Treatment is symptomatic, with fluid and electrolyte replacement. A tetravalent oral vaccine (RotaShield) was developed but is not available in the United States because of a possible association with small bowel intussusception.

The **Norwalk agent** and **Norwalk-like agents** are responsible for about 40% of cases of group-related or institutional diarrhea, transmission usually being by the fecal-oral route, though airborne transmission may also occur. Nausea and vomiting are especially common with Norwalk agent. An ELISA can detect the agent in stool samples, and a PCR assay is under development. Treatment again is symptomatic.

[CDC Advisory regarding rotavirus vaccine] http://www.cdc.gov/od/oc/media/pressrel/r990715.htm

Lundgren O et al: Role of the enteric nervous system in the fluid and electrolyte secretion of rotavirus diarrhea. Science 2000;287:491. [NLM Cit ID: 20111400]

Noel JS et al: Identification of a distinct common strain of "Norwalk-like viruses" having a global distribution. J Infect Dis 1999;179:1334. [NLM Cit ID: 99246332] (A particular isolate was responsible for over 60 outbreaks throughout the world.)

Withdrawal of rotavirus vaccine recommendation. MMWR Morb Mortal Wkly Rep 1999;48:1007. [NLM Cit ID: 20043427]

VIRUSES THAT PRODUCE SEVERAL SYNDROMES

1. COXSACKIEVIRUS INFECTIONS

Coxsackievirus infections cause several clinical syndromes. As with other enteroviruses, infections are most common during the summer. Two groups, A and B, are defined either serologically or by mouse bioassay. There are more than 50 serotypes.

Clinical Findings

A. Symptoms and Signs: The clinical syndromes associated with coxsackievirus infection may be described briefly as follows:

1. Summer grippe (A and B)–A febrile illness, principally of children, lasting 1–4 days. Minor symptoms and respiratory tract infection are often present.

2. Herpangina (A2–6, 10)–Sudden onset of fever, which may be as high as 40.6 °C, sometimes with febrile convulsions; headache, myalgia, vomiting; and sore throat, characterized early by petechiae or papules on the soft palate that become shallow ulcers in about 3 days and then heal.

3. Epidemic pleurodynia (Bornholm disease) (B1–5)–Pleuritic pain is prominent, and tenderness, hyperesthesia, and muscle swelling are present over the area of diaphragmatic attachment. Other findings include headache, sore throat, malaise, and nausea. Orchitis and aseptic meningitis are uncommon manifestations.

4. Aseptic meningitis (A and B)–Fever, headache, nausea, vomiting, stiff neck, drowsiness, and cerebrospinal fluid lymphocytosis without chemical abnormalities may occur, and pediatric clusters of group B meningitis are reported. A focal encephalitis and a transverse myelitis are reported with coxsackievirus group A and a disseminated encephalitis after group B infection.

5. Acute nonspecific pericarditis (B types)–Sudden onset of anterior chest pain, often worse with inspiration and in the supine position. Fever, myalgia, headache, and pericardial friction rub appear early. Examination may reveal signs of pericardial effusion with paradoxic pulse, increased venous pressure, and increased heart size. Electrocardiographic evidence of pericarditis is often present. Relapses may occur.

6. Myocarditis (B1–5)–Heart failure in the neonatal period secondary to in utero myocarditis and over 20% of adult cases of myocarditis and dilated cardiomyopathy are allegedly associated with group B infections. Among middle-aged men, a serologic association with myocardial infarction was recently noted.

7. Hand, foot, and mouth disease (A5, 10, 16)–Sometimes epidemic and characterized by stomatitis and a vesicular rash on hands and feet. Enterovirus 71 is also a causative agent.

8. Hepatitis (B1)–Fulminant neonatal hepatitis with thrombocytopenia and coagulopathy occur rarely.

9. Insulin-dependent diabetes mellitus (B types)–An association purportedly exists between coxsackievirus B infections and subsequent development of type 1 diabetes mellitus.

10. Glomerulopathy and tubular injury were recently reported with several group B infections.

B. Laboratory Findings: Routine laboratory studies show no characteristic abnormalities. Neutralizing antibodies appear during convalescence. The virus may be isolated from throat washings or stools inoculated into suckling mice.

Treatment & Prognosis

Treatment is symptomatic. With the exception of myocarditis, pericarditis, perhaps diabetes, and rare illnesses such as pancreatitis or polio-like syndrome, the syndromes caused by coxsackieviruses are benign and self-limited. There are anecdotal reports of success with immunoglobulin in severe disease.

Crowell RL: A short history and introductory background on the coxsackieviruses of group B. Curr Top Microbiol Immunol 1997;223:1. [NLM Cit ID: 97440719]

Gebhard JR et al: Coxsackievirus B3-induced myocarditis: Perforin exacerbates disease, but plays no detectable role in virus clearance. Am J Pathol 1998;153:417. [NLM Cit ID: 98372533] (CD8 T lymphocytes induce damage through the cytolytic protein perforin.)

Roivainen M et al: Enterovirus infections as a possible risk factor for myocardial infarction. Circulation 1998; 98:2534. [NLM Cit ID: 99060162]

Wang SM et al: Fatal coxsackievirus B infection in early infancy characterized by fulminant hepatitis. J Infect Dis 1998;37:270. [NLM Cit ID: 99107549]

2. ECHOVIRUS INFECTIONS

Echoviruses are enteroviruses that produce several clinical syndromes, particularly in children. Infection is most common during summer.

Over 30 serotypes have been demonstrated. Most cause aseptic meningitis, which may be associated with a rubelliform rash. Recent outbreaks of aseptic meningitis with type 30 were reported from Japan, France, Germany, and Canada (Saskatchewan). Type 16 causes Boston exanthem, characterized by sudden onset of fever, nausea, and sore throat and a roseola-like rash over the face and trunk that persists 1–10 days. Diseases associated with echoviruses range from common respiratory diseases and epidemic diarrhea (including type 22) to myocarditis, a hemorrhagic obstetric syndrome, keratoconjunctivitis, leukocytoclastic vasculitis, and neonatal as well as adult cases of encephalitis and sepsis to myocarditis, encephalitis, and septic shock.

As with other enterovirus infections, diagnosis is best established by correlation of clinical, epidemiologic, and laboratory evidence. Cytopathic effects are produced in tissue culture after recovery of virus from throat washings, blood, or cerebrospinal fluid. Fourfold or greater rises in antibody titer signify systemic infection.

Treatment is symptomatic. The prognosis is excellent, though there are reports of mild paralysis after central nervous system infection. Handwashing is an effective control measure in outbreaks of aseptic meningitis.

Chambon M et al: An outbreak due to echovirus type 30 in a neonatal unit in France in 1997: usefulness of PCR diagnosis. J Hosp Infect 1999;43:63. [NLM Cit ID: 99393583]

Mohle-Boetani JC et al: Viral meningitis in child care center staff and parents: an outbreak of echovirus 30 infections. Public Health Rep 1999;114:249. [NLM Cit ID: 99404644] (Emphasizes the importance of handwashing in preventing disease among contacts.)

II. RICKETTSIAL DISEASES

The rickettsioses are febrile exanthematous diseases caused by rickettsiae, small gram-negative obligate intracellular bacteria. In arthropods, rickettsiae grow in the gut lining, often without harming the host. Human infection results from either an arthropod bite or contamination with its feces. In humans, rickettsiae grow principally in endothelial cells of small blood vessels, producing vasculitis, cell necrosis, thrombosis of vessels, skin rashes, and organ dysfunctions.

Different rickettsiae and their vectors are endemic in different parts of the world, but two or more types may coexist in the same geographic area. New organisms are identified regularly. A summary of epidemiologic features is given in Table 32–3. The clinical picture is variable but usually includes a prodromal stage followed by fever, rash, and prostration. Isolation of rickettsiae from the patient is difficult. A promising new means of isolation is the centrifugation shell-vial technique. Diagnosis is usually based on clinical examination and epidemiologic evidence. Laboratory diagnosis relies on the development of specific antibodies detected by complement fixation (for diagnosis), immunofluorescence, or hemagglutination (for species identification) tests. PCR techniques are available for identification of some rickettsial organisms.

Prevention & Treatment

Preventive measures are directed at control of the vector, and avoidance of exposure by use of repellents and protective clothing. A search of body surfaces should be conducted after potential exposure and the vector (louse, tick, or mite) gently removed. Many patients do not recall exposure to a vector.

Rickettsiae can be inhibited by tetracyclines or chloramphenicol. All early infections respond to treatment with these drugs. Dosage schedules are listed below.

Hackstadt T: The biology of rickettsiae. Infect Agents Dis 1996;5:127. [NLM Cit ID: 96398226] (Discussion of the different pathogenesis of typhus and spotted fever group of rickettsiae.)

Russell RC: Vectors vs. humans in Australia—who is on top down under? An update on vector-borne disease and research on vectors in Australia. J Vector Ecol 1998 23:1. [NLM Cit ID: 98338716] (Description of vectors and associated diseases, including rickettsiae in Australia.)

Rydkina E et al: New rickettsiae in ticks collected in territories of the former Soviet Union. Emerg Infect Dis 1999;5:811. [NLM Cit ID: 20070438] (Siberian ticks

Table 32–3. Rickettsial diseases.

Disease	Rickettsial Pathogen	Geographic Areas of Prevalence	Insect Vector	Mammalian Reservoir
Typhus group				
Epidemic (louse-borne) typhus	*Rickettsia prowazekii*	South America, Africa, Asia, North America	Louse	Humans, flying squirrels
California flea rickettsiosis	*Rickettsia felis*	Southern California, Texas	Flea	Cats, opossums
Endemic (murine) typhus	*Rickettsia typhi*	Worldwide; small foci (USA: southeastern Gulf Coast)	Flea	Rodents
Scrub typhus	*Orientia tsutsugamushi*	Southeast Asia, Japan, Australia	Mite[1]	Rodents
Spotted fever group				
Rocky Mountain spotted fever	*Rickettsia rickettsii*	Western Hemisphere; USA (especially mid-Atlantic coast region)	Tick[1]	Rodents, dogs
Boutonneuse fever, Kenya tick typhus, South African tick fever, Indian tick typhus	*Rickettsia conorii*	Africa, India, Mediterranean regions	Tick[1]	Rodents, dogs
Queensland tick typhus	*Rickettsia australis*	Australia	Tick[1]	Rodents, marsupials
North Asian tick typhus	*Rickettsia sibirica*	Siberia, Mongolia	Tick[1]	Rodents
Rickettsialpox	*Rickettsia akari*	USA, Korea, former USSR	Mite[1]	Mice
RMSF-like	*Rickettsia canada*	North America	Tick[1]	Rodents
Other				
Ehrlichiosis	*Ehrlichia chaffeensis, E equi, E phagocytophilia, E sennetsu*	Southeastern North America	Tick[1]	Dogs
Q fever	*Coxiella burnetii*	Worldwide	None[2]	Cattle, sheep, goats

[1]Also serve as arthropod reservoir by maintaining rickettsiae through transovarian transmission.
[2]Human infection results from inhalation of dust.

were found to be infected with *R sibirica* [12%], *R conorii* [8%], and three new rickettsiae.)

Zavala-Velasquez JE et al: Serologic study of the prevalence of rickettsiosis in Yucatan: evidence for a prevalent spotted fever group rickettsiosis. Am J Trop Med Hyg 1999;61:405. [NLM Cit ID 99426268] (A rickettsiosis with symptoms similar to dengue fever has been discovered in Yucatan, Mexico; this appears to be most likely a close relative of *R akari.*)

TYPHUS GROUP

1. EPIDEMIC LOUSE-BORNE TYPHUS

Essentials of Diagnosis

- Prodrome of headache, then chills and fever.
- Severe, intractable headaches, prostration, persisting high fever.
- Macular rash appearing on the fourth to seventh days on the trunk and in the axillae, spreading to the rest of the body but sparing the face, palms, and soles.
- Diagnosis confirmed by specific antibodies using complement fixation, microagglutination, or immunofluorescence.

General Considerations

Epidemic louse-borne typhus is due to infection with *Rickettsia prowazekii,* a parasite of the body louse that ultimately kills the louse. Transmission is favored by crowded living conditions, famine, war, or any circumstances that predispose to heavy infestation with lice. When the louse sucks the blood of a person infected with *R prowazekii,* the organism becomes established in the gut of the louse and grows there. When the louse is transmitted to another person (through contact or clothing) and has a blood meal, it defecates simultaneously, and the infected feces are rubbed into the itching bite wound. Dry, infectious louse feces may also enter the respiratory tract.

In a person who recovers from clinical or subclinical typhus infection, *R prowazekii* may survive in lymphoid tissues. Years later, there may be a recrudescence of disease (Brill's disease) without exposure to infected lice.

Mild and atypical cases of *R prowazekii* have rarely occurred in the USA after contact with flying squirrels or their ectoparasites or decades following exposure (eg, among concentration camp victims of World War II). Cases can be acquired by travel to pockets of infection (eg, central and northeastern Africa).

Clinical Findings

A. Symptoms and Signs: (Table 32–3.) Prodromal malaise, cough, headache, backache, arthralgia, and chest pain begin after an incubation period of 10–14 days, followed by an abrupt onset of chills, high fever, and prostration, with flu-like symptoms progressing to delirium and stupor. The headache is severe, the fever prolonged.

Other findings consist of conjunctivitis, hearing loss from neuropathy of the eighth cranial nerve, flushed facies, rales at the lung bases, and often splenomegaly. A macular rash (that may become confluent) appears first in the axillas and then over the trunk, spreading to the extremities but rarely involving the face, palms, or soles. In severely ill patients, the rash becomes hemorrhagic, and hypotension becomes marked. There may be renal insufficiency, stupor, and delirium. In spontaneous recovery, improvement begins 13–16 days after onset with rapid drop of fever.

B. Laboratory Findings: The white blood cell count is variable. Proteinuria and hematuria commonly occur. Serum obtained 5–12 days after onset of symptoms usually shows specific antibodies for *R prowazekii* antigens as demonstrated by complement fixation, microagglutination, or immunofluorescence. In primary rickettsial infection, early antibodies are IgM; in recrudescence (Brill's disease), early antibodies are predominantly IgG.

C. Imaging: Radiographs of the chest may show patchy consolidation.

Differential Diagnosis

The prodromal symptoms and the early febrile stage are not specific enough to permit diagnosis in nonepidemic situations. The rash is usually sufficiently distinctive for diagnosis, but it may be absent in up to 10% of cases or may be difficult to observe in dark-skinned persons. A variety of other acute febrile diseases may have to be considered.

Brill's disease (recrudescent epidemic typhus) has a more gradual onset than primary *R prowazekii* infection, fever and rash are of shorter duration, and the disease is milder and rarely fatal.

Complications

Pneumonia, thromboses, vasculitis with major vessel obstruction and gangrene, circulatory collapse, myocarditis, and uremia may occur.

Prevention

Prevention consists of louse control with insecticides, particularly by applying chemicals to clothing or treating it with heat, and frequent bathing. A deloused and bathed typhus patient is not infectious. The disease is not transmitted from person to person. Patients are infective for the lice during the febrile period and perhaps 2–3 days after the fever returns to normal. Infected lice pass rickettsiae in their feces within 2–6 days after the blood meal and can be infective earlier if crushed. Rickettsiae remain viable in a dead louse for weeks.

Immunization with vaccines consisting of inactivated egg-grown *R prowazekii* gives some protection to laboratory personnel, physicians, or field workers who are exposed to the parasite. This vaccine is not currently commercially available in the USA or Canada. An improved cell culture vaccine is being developed.

Treatment

Treatment consists of either tetracycline (25 mg/kg/d in four divided doses) or chloramphenicol (50–100 mg/kg/d in four divided doses) for 4–10 days.

Prognosis

The prognosis depends greatly upon age and immunization status. In children under age 10, the disease is usually mild. The mortality rate is 10% in the second and third decades but in the past reached 60% in the sixth decade. Effective vaccination can convert a potentially serious disease into a mild one.

Andersson SG et al: Molecular phylogeny and rearrangement of rRNA genes in *Rickettsia* species. Mol Biol Evol 1999;16:987. [NLM Cit ID: 99334618] (The unique organization of the 23S rRNA genes provides a simple diagnostic tool for identification of rickettsiae.)

Raoult D et al: The body louse as a vector of reemerging human diseases. Clin Infect Dis 1998;352:353. [NLM Cit ID: 20055853] (A description of pathogens and epidemics associated with the body louse, *Pediculus humanus humanus*.)

Raoult D et al: Outbreak of epidemic typhus associated with trench fever in Burundi. Lancet 1998;353. [NLM Cit ID: 98382022] (A massive outbreak occurred at high altitudes in refugee camps of east Africa.)

2. ENDEMIC FLEA-BORNE TYPHUS (Murine Typhus)

Rickettsia typhi, a ubiquitous pathogen, is transmitted from rat to rat through the rat flea. Humans acquire the infection when bitten by an infected flea, which releases infected feces while sucking blood. Rare cases in the developed world follow travel, usually to Southeast Asia. A second causative agent, *R felis,* has been linked to the cat flea and opossum exposures. Most cases in the USA are reported from southern Texas and California.

Endemic typhus resembles recrudescent epidemic typhus in that it has a gradual onset and the fever and rash are of shorter duration (6–13 days). The symptoms are less severe than in epidemic typhus and may mimic measles, rubella, or roseola. The rash is maculopapular and concentrated on the trunk and fades fairly rapidly. Fatalities are rare (less than 1%) and limited to the elderly.

Clinical differentiation from Rocky Mountain spotted fever is established by the earlier seasonal onset of Rocky Mountain spotted fever and the character of the rash. Complement-fixing or immunofluorescent antibodies can be detected in the patient's serum with specific *R typhi* antigens.

Preventive measures are directed at control of rats and ectoparasites (rat fleas) with insecticides, rat poisons, and rat-proofing of buildings. Antibiotic treatment with tetracycline (25–50 mg/kg/d in four divided doses) or chloramphenicol (50–75 mg/kg/d in four divided doses) is indicated through 3 full days of defervescence.

Hudson HL et al: Retinal manifestations of acute murine typhus. Int Ophthalmol 1997;21:121. [NLM Cit ID: 98249408] (Rickettsial disease should be included in the differential diagnosis of fever and retinitis or neuroretinitis in healthy individuals.)

Reporter R et al: Murine typhus still exists in the United States. Clin Infect Dis 1995;21:859. [NLM Cit ID: 96412924]

3. SCRUB TYPHUS (Tsutsugamushi Fever)

Essentials of Diagnosis

- Exposure to mites in endemic area of Southeast Asia, the western Pacific (including Korea), and Australia.
- Black eschar at site of bite, with regional and generalized lymphadenopathy.
- Conjunctivitis and a short-lived macular rash.
- Frequent pneumonitis, encephalitis, and cardiac failure.
- Laboratory confirmation with agglutinins to proteus OXK and specific antibodies by immunofluorescence.

General Considerations

Scrub typhus is caused by *Orientia tsutsugamushi,* which is principally a parasite of rodents transmitted by mites in the endemic areas listed above. The mites live on vegetation but complete their maturation cycle by biting humans who come in contact with infested vegetation. Vertical transmission occurs, and blood transfusions may transmit the pathogen. Serosurveys from Bangkok show prevalences over 20% for blood donors and nearly 60% for febrile malaria clinic patients.

Clinical Findings

A. Symptoms and Signs: After a 1- to 3-week incubation period, malaise, chills, severe headache, and backache develop. At the site of the bite, a papule evolves into a flat black eschar. The regional lymph nodes are enlarged and tender, and there may be generalized adenopathy. Fever rises gradually, and a macular rash appears primarily on the trunk after a week of fever and may be fleeting or may last a week. The patient may become obtunded. During the second or third week, pneumonitis, myocarditis and cardiac failure, and encephalitis or meningitis, acute abdominal pain, granulomatous hepatitis, or acute renal failure may develop. An attack confers prolonged immunity against homologous strains and transient immunity against heterologous strains. Heterologous strains produce mild disease but when a year after the first episode the illness is clinically typical in manifestations.

B. Laboratory Findings: Blood obtained during the first few days of illness may permit isolation of the rickettsial organism by mouse inoculation. Fluorescein-labeled antirickettsial assays or commercial dot-blot ELISA dipstick assays are convenient means of establishing the diagnosis, though PCR may be the most sensitive test.

Differential Diagnosis

Leptospirosis, typhoid, dengue, malaria, and other rickettsial infections should be considered. Scrub typhus is a recognized cause of obscure tropical fevers, especially in children. When the rash is fleeting and the eschar not evident, laboratory results are required for diagnosis.

Prevention

Repeated application of long-acting miticides can make endemic areas safe. Insect repellents on clothing and skin provide some protection. For short exposure, chemoprophylaxis with doxycycline (200 mg weekly) can prevent the disease but permits infection. No effective vaccines are available.

Treatment & Prognosis

Without treatment, fever subsides spontaneously after 2 weeks, but the mortality rate may be 10–30%. Treatment for 3 days with doxycycline, 100 mg twice daily, or for 7 days with chloramphenicol, 25 mg/kg/d in four divided doses, virtually eliminates deaths and relapses, though chloramphenicol- and tetracycline-resistant strains have been reported from Southeast Asia, and azithromycin may become the drug of choice for children, pregnant women, and patients with refractory disease. HIV infection does not appear to influence the severity of scrub typhus.

Graves S et al: Rickettsia serosurvey in Kimberley, Western Australia. Am J Trop Med Hyg 1999;60:786. [NLM Cit ID: 99274450] (Of 920 serum samples nonrandomly examined, 5.6% showed antirickettsial antibodies, mostly against *Orientia tsutsugamushi.*)

Watt G et al: Azithromycin activities against *Orientia tsutsugamushi* strains isolated in cases of scrub typhus in Northern Thailand. Antimicrob Agents Chemother 1999;43:2817. [NLM Cit ID 20011200] (Azithromycin and doxycycline yielded comparable animal data, with success in pregnant women.)

SPOTTED FEVERS

1. ROCKY MOUNTAIN SPOTTED FEVER

Essentials of Diagnosis

- Exposure to tick bite in endemic area.
- An influenza-like prodrome followed by chills, fever, severe headache, myalgias, restlessness, and prostration; occasionally, delirium and coma.
- Red macular rash appears between the second and sixth days of fever, first on the wrists and ankles and then spreading centrally; it may become petechial.
- Laboratory confirmation by agglutination of proteus OX19 and OX2 and by specific antibodies with complement fixation and immunofluorescence.

General Considerations

Despite its name, most cases occur elsewhere than in the Rocky Mountains. The causative agent, *R rickettsii,* is transmitted to humans by the bite of ticks, including the wood tick, *Dermacentor andersoni,* in the western USA and by the bite of the dog tick, *Dermacentor variabilis,* in the eastern USA. Other hard ticks transmit the organism in the southern USA and in Central and South America and are responsible for transmitting it among rodents, dogs, porcupines, and other animals. Most human cases occur in late spring and summer. In the USA, most cases occur in the eastern third of the country, with about 1000 reported per year, primarily from April through September, and with a higher incidence among children and men.

Clinical Findings

A. Symptoms and Signs: Two to 14 days (mean, 7 days) after the bite of an infectious tick, symptoms begin with fever, chills, headache, nausea and vomiting, myalgias, restlessness, insomnia, and irritability. Cough and pneumonitis may develop. Delirium, lethargy, seizures, stupor, and coma may appear. The face is flushed and the conjunctiva injected. The rash (faint macules that progress to maculopapules and then petechiae) appears between days 2 and 6 of fever, first on the wrists and ankles, spreading centrally to the arms, legs, and trunk for 2–3 days; involvement of the palms and soles is characteristic. About 10% of cases occur without rash or with minimal rash. In some cases there is splenomegaly, hepatomegaly, jaundice, myocarditis, or uremia; acute respiratory distress syndrome (ARDS) is of greatest concern. About 3–5 % of reported cases in the USA during recent years have been fatal.

B. Laboratory Findings: Leukocytosis, thrombocytopenia, hyponatremia, proteinuria, and hematuria are common. Cerebrospinal fluid may show hypoglycorrhachia and mild pleocytosis. Intravascular dissemination is typical. Diagnosis during the acute phase of the illness can be made by immunohistologic demonstration of *R rickettsiae* in skin biopsy specimens, but this must be performed as soon as skin lesions become apparent to achieve maximum sensitivity. Isolation of the organism using the shell vial technique is available in some laboratories. A rise in antibody titer during the second week of illness can be detected by specific complement fixation, immunofluorescence, and microagglutination tests. Laboratory confirmation is established by immunofluorescent antibody (IFA), latex agglutination, or complement fixation.

Differential Diagnosis

The early signs and symptoms of Rocky Mountain spotted fever resemble those of many other infections. The rash may be confused with that of measles, typhoid, and ehrlichiosis, or—most importantly—meningococcemia. Blood cultures and cerebrospinal fluid examination establish the latter.

Prevention

Protective clothing, tick-repellent chemicals, and the removal of ticks at frequent intervals are helpful measures.

Treatment & Prognosis

In mild, untreated cases, fever subsides at the end of the second week. The response to chloramphenicol (25–50 mg/kg/d orally or intravenously in four divided doses) or doxycycline (200 mg daily intravenously or orally) is prompt if the drugs are started early. Treatment is given for 7 days or through the third day of defervescence.

The mortality rate for Rocky Mountain spotted fever varies strikingly with age. In the untreated elderly, it may be 70%, but it is usually less than 20% in children. Other risk factors for a fatal outcome include advanced age, atypical clinical features (absence of headache, no history of tick attachment, gastrointestinal symptoms), and a delay in treatment. The usual cause of death is pneumonitis with respiratory or cardiac failure. Sequelae, more common than formerly recognized, may include seizures, encephalopathy, peripheral neuropathy, paraparesis, bowel and bladder incontinence, cerebellar and vestibular dysfunction, hearing loss, and motor deficits.

Paddock CD et al: Hidden mortality attributable to Rocky Mountain spotted fever; immunohistochemical detection of fatal, serologically unconfirmed disease. J Infect Dis 1999;179:1469. [NLM Cit ID: 99246349] (Fatal cases with undetectable or low antibody levels but confirmed by immunohistochemical staining show that serologic assays underestimate the incidence and mortality.)

Quintal D: Rocky Mountain spotted fever. Clin Dermatol 1996;14:3. [NLM Cit ID: 96330674] (Entire issue devoted to rickettsial diseases.)

Thorner AR et al: Rocky Mountain spotted fever. Clin Infect Dis 1998;27:1353. [NLM Cit ID: 99085531]

2. RICKETTSIALPOX

Rickettsia akari is a parasite of mice, transmitted by mites *(Allodermanyssus sanguineus)*. Rickettsialpox occurs in humans where crowded conditions and mouse-infested housing allow transmission of the pathogen to humans. Pathologic findings include dermal edema, subepidermal vesicles, and at times a lymphocytic vasculitis. The incubation period is 7–12 days. Onset is sudden, with chills, fever, headache, photophobia, and disseminated aches and pains. The primary lesion is a painless red papule that vesicates and forms a black eschar. Two to 4 days after onset of symptoms, a widespread papular eruption appears that becomes vesicular and forms crusts that are shed in about 10 days. Early lesions may resemble those of chickenpox (typically vesicular versus papulovesicular in rickettsialpox).

Leukopenia and a rise in antibody titer to rickettsial antigen with complement fixation or indirect fluorescent assays using a conjugated antirickettsial globulin can identify antigen in punch biopsies of skin lesions.

Treatment includes tetracycline, 15 mg/kg/d orally in four divided doses for 3–5 days.

Even without treatment, the disease is fairly mild and self-limited, treatment only hastening resolution. Control requires the elimination of mice from human habitations after insecticide has been applied to suppress the mite vectors.

Boyd AS: Rickettsialpox. Dermatol Clin 1997;15:313. [NLM Cit ID: 97253197] (Review article.)

Comer JA et al: Serologic evidence of rickettsialpox infection among intravenous drug users in inner-city Baltimore, Maryland. Am J Trop Med Hyg 1999;60:894. [NLM Cit ID: 99330110] (Many showed a positive IFA against *R akari;* when present, antibodies against *R rickettsii* or HIV were less likely.)

3. TICK TYPHUS

The term "tick typhus" denotes a variety of spotted rickettsial fevers. They are often named by geography, eg, Israel tick fever, Kenya tick fever, Mediterranean spotted fever, Queensland tick typhus, Flinders Island spotted fever; or morphology, eg, boutonneuse fever. These illnesses are transmitted by tick vectors of the rickettsial agents *R conorii, R australis, R japonica, R africae,* and *R sibirica.* Dogs and wild animals may serve as reservoirs. The pathogens usually produce a black spot (tâche noire) at the site of the tick bite that may be useful in diagnosis, though spotless boutonneuse fever occurs. Rarely, papulovesicular lesions may resemble rickettsialpox. Endothelial injury produces perivascular edema and dermal necrosis; regional adenopathy, disseminated lesions, and focal hepatic necrosis may occur. The disease has occurred among travelers, with occasional cases recorded among returnees from Africa in particular. Diagnosis is clinical, with serologic or PCR confirmation. Prevention entails protective clothing, repellents, and inspection for and removal of ticks. Treatment is with the following drugs given for 7–10 days: tetracycline (25–50 mg/kg/d in four divided doses), chloramphenicol (50–75 mg/kg/d in four divided doses), or ciprofloxacin (500 mg twice daily).

Okabayashi T et al: Short report: prevalence of antibodies against spotted fever, murine typhus, and Q fever rickettsiae in humans living in Zambia. Am J Trop Med Hyg 1999;61:70. [NLM Cit ID: 99359006] (Seventeen percent showed antibodies against *R conorii,* 8% *C burnetii,* and 5% *R typhi.* Cattle breeding areas coincided with foci of *R conorii* and *C burnetii* infections.)

OTHER RICKETTSIAL & RICKETTSIAL-LIKE DISEASES

1. EHRLICHIOSIS

Ehrlichiosis presents two clinical entities: human monocytic ehrlichiosis and human granulocytic ehrlichiosis. The syndromes are caused by *Ehrlichia chaffeensis* and by closely related agents, *E equi* and *E phagocytophilia.* Human monocytic ehrlichiosis is caused by *Ehrlichia chaffeensis* and by the closely related agents *E equi* and *E canis.* Human granulocytic ehrlichiosis is caused by *E phagocytophilia. E sennetsu* is the etiologic agent of sennetsu fever, which appears to be confined to western Japan.

Ehrlichiae are small tick-borne gram-negative obligate intracellular bacteria. The major nonhuman hosts have not been definitively determined but include dogs. Ehrlichiae grow as microcolonies in phagosomes and form characteristic inclusions seen with Giemsa's stain. Human monocytic ehrlichiosis is seen primarily in the Southeast, mid-Atlantic, and South Central states of the USA, though serologic evidence now documents a much more global endemicity (Israel, Japan, Mexico). Its major vector is the Lone Star tick *(Amblyomma americanus).* Clinical disease ranges from mild to life-threatening. Typically, after about a 9-day incubation period and a prodrome consisting of malaise, rigors, and nausea, patients develop worsening fever and headache; a pleomorphic rash may occur. Leukopenia and absolute lymphopenia as well as thrombocytopenia occur often. Serious sequelae include acute respiratory failure and ARDS, encephalopathy, and acute renal failure, which may mimic thrombotic thrombocytopenic purpura. An indirect fluorescent antibody assay is available through CDC and requires acute and convalescent sera. A PCR assay applied to whole blood samples is a rapid diagnostic tool.

Human granulocytic ehrlichiosis is more recently described. It has a geographic area of distribution similar to that for Lyme disease, though the geographic boundaries are as yet not fully determined and seroconversion with clinically consistent cases are now reported from Israel and Europe also. The vectors are ticks of the *Ixodes* genus, and deer and possibly horses appear to be major nonhuman reservoirs. The incidence peaks in summer, but cases are seen year-round in warmer areas where ticks remain viable. The symptoms are similar to those seen with human monocytic ehrlichiosis. Coinfection with Lyme disease may occur, though patients with granulocytic ehrlichiosis appear to be older and sicker than those with acute Lyme disease.

Diagnosis is made by the history of tick exposure followed by a clinical illness with the characteristic signs and symptoms. Further laboratory evaluation is similar to that described for human monocytic ehrlichiosis.

Treatment for both forms of ehrlichiosis is with doxycycline, 200 mg orally or intravenously for at least 7 days or until 3 days of defervescence.

Buller RS et al: *Ehrlichia ewingii,* a newly recognized agent of human ehrlichiosis. N Engl J Med 1999;15:148. [NLM Cit ID: 99316833] (Reporting four patients from Missouri between 1996 and 1998, all with tick exposure, all of whom responded to doxycycline.)

Horowitz HW et al: Perinatal transmission of the agent of human granulocytic ehrlichiosis. N Engl J Med 1998;339:375. [NLM Cit ID: 98346820]

Martin GS et al: Rapidly fatal infection with *Ehrlichia chaffeensis.* N Engl J Med 1999;341:763. [NLM Cit ID: 99383633]

McQuiston JH et al: The human ehrlichiosis in the United States. Emerg Infect Dis 1999;5:635. [NLM Cit ID: 99442454] (An overview of ehrlichiosis in the United States.)

2. Q FEVER

Essentials of Diagnosis

- Exposure to sheep, goats, cattle, or their products is common; some infections are laboratory-acquired.
- An acute or chronic febrile illness with severe headache, cough, prostration, and abdominal pain.
- Extensive pneumonitis, hepatitis, or encephalopathy; rarely endocarditis.

General Considerations

Coxiella burnetii is unique among rickettsiae in that it is usually transmitted to humans not by arthropods but by inhalation or ingestion. It is distributed worldwide with few exceptions (New Zealand). Coxiella infections occur mostly in cattle, sheep, and goats, in which they cause mild or subclinical disease. Transmission by cows and goats is principally through the milk and placenta and by sheep through feces, placenta, and milk. Dry feces and milk, dust contaminated with them, and the tissues of these animals contain large numbers of infectious organisms that are spread by the airborne route. Inhalation of contaminated dust and of droplets from infected animal tissues is the main source of human infection. Outbreaks have been described in association with parturient cats. There is an occupational risk for animal handlers, slaughterhouse workers, veterinarians, and laboratory workers.

The route of acquisition appears to determine the main clinical syndrome. Endocarditis is an uncommon but serious form of coxiella infection and has been linked with immunocompromising conditions, urban residence, and raw milk ingestion. Coxiella is resistant to heat and drying, perhaps because the organism forms endospore-like structures. Thus, it survives in dust, on the fleece of infected animals, or in inadequately pasteurized milk. Spread from one human to another does not seem to occur even in the presence of florid pneumonitis, but maternal-fetal infection can occur.

Clinical Findings

A. Symptoms and Signs: After an incubation period of 1–3 weeks, a febrile illness develops with headache, prostration, and muscle pains, occasionally with a nonproductive cough. Physical signs of pneumonitis may occur. Granulomatous hepatitis is often present. Granulomatous hepatitis is often present during the acute phase. A rare but severe chronic manifestation of coxiella infections is endocarditis, usually of the aortic valve and found mainly in the setting of preexisting valve disease or immunosuppression. Other uncommon manifestations include encephalitis, hemolytic anemia, orchitis, acute renal failure, and mediastinal lymphadenopathy. The clinical course may be acute or chronic and relapsing.

B. Laboratory Findings: Laboratory examination during the acute phase shows elevated liver function tests, occasionally leukocytosis, and a diagnostic rise in complement-fixing antibodies. Antibodies to phospholipids and antibody against phase 2 antigens have been reported.

In Q fever endocarditis, there is an IgG titer of 1:200 or more by complement fixation or indirect immunofluorescence with IgA or IgG antibodies against phase 1 antigen of *C burnetii*. Isolation of *C burnetii* is possible using the shell-vial technique. A serum ELISA is also available.

C. Imaging: Radiographs of the chest show patchy pulmonary infiltrates, often more prominent than the physical signs.

Differential Diagnosis

Viral, mycoplasmal, and bacterial pneumonias; viral hepatitis; brucellosis; tuberculosis; psittacosis; and other animal-borne diseases must be considered. The history of exposure to animals or animal dusts or tissues (eg, in slaughterhouses) should lead to appropriate specific serologic tests. Unexplained fevers with negative blood cultures in association with embolic or cardiac disease should make one consider Q fever, especially in immunocompromised patients.

Prevention

Prevention is based on detection of the infection in livestock, reduction of contact with infected animals or dusts contaminated by them, special care when working with animal tissues, and effective pasteurization of milk. A vaccine of formalin-inactivated phase 1 coxiella is being developed for persons at high risk of infection and appears to be protective. A vaccine is available in some countries for persons with high-risk exposures.

Treatment & Prognosis

Treatment with tetracycline (25 mg/kg/d in four divided doses) or doxycycline (100 mg twice daily) can suppress symptoms and shorten the clinical course but does not always eradicate the infection. Treatment should continue through 3 full days of defervescence. Even in untreated patients, the mortality rate is usually low, except with endocarditis.

Treatment of endocarditis consists of protracted—often for years—antibiotic therapy with doxycycline (200 mg/d) and one of several alternatives, including trimethoprim-sulfamethoxazole (320/1600 mg/d), rifampin (900 mg/d), fluoroquinolones, or hydroxychloroquine. Potential interactions of antibiotics (rifampin, quinolones) with warfarin anticoagulation need be considered. Heart valves often need replacement, since the mainstays of antibiotic therapy (chloramphenicol, tetracycline) for rickettsial organisms are bacteriostatic. The combination of hydroxychloroquine and doxycycline is bactericidal in vitro, and human studies are under way using this regimen.

Caron F et al: Acute Q fever pneumonia: A review of 80 hospitalized patients. Chest 1998;114:808. [NLM Cit ID: 98414103] (When pneumonia occurs, it tends to be lobar or segmental and to involve the lower lobes.)

Domingo P et al: Acute Q fever in adult patients: report on 63 sporadic cases in an urban area. Clin Infect Dis 1999;29:874. [NLM Cit ID: 20055851] (Doxycycline was preferred agent in this outbreak from Barcelona.)

Fournier PE et al: Modification of the diagnostic criteria proposed by the Duke Endocarditis Service to permit improved diagnosis of Q fever endocarditis. Am J Med 1996;100:629. [NLM Cit ID: 96291119] (The sensitivity of the criteria were significantly increased by including serologic results and single blood culture as major diagnostic criteria.)

Raoult D et al: Treatment of Q fever endocarditis: Comparison of two regimens containing doxycycline and ofloxacin or hydroxychloroquine. Arch Intern Med 1999;159:167. [NLM Cit ID: 99124290]

Serbezov VS et al: Q fever in Bulgaria and Serbia. Emerg Infect Dis 1999;5:388. [NLM Cit ID: 99276691] (Tripling of the goat population is deemed responsible.)

Siegman-Igra Y et al: Q fever endocarditis in Israel and a worldwide review. Scand J Infect Dis 1997;29:41. [NLM Cit ID: 97266541] (The authors emphasize the importance of prompt initiation of combination chemotherapy for at least 3 years with long-term follow-up.)

Stein A et al: Pigeon pneumonia in Provence: a bird-borne Q fever outbreak. Clin Infect Dis 1999;20:617. [NLM Cit ID: 99458040]

Stein A et al: Q fever during pregnancy: A public health problem in southern France. Clin Infect Dis 1998; 27:592. [NLM Cit ID: 98442297]

KAWASAKI SYNDROME

Kawasaki syndrome is a worldwide multisystemic disease also known as mucocutaneous lymph node syndrome. It occurs mainly in children under 10 but occasionally in adults, at times in epidemic fashion. Asian children are at higher risk. The epidemiology suggests an infectious origin, though no agent has been identified. Disease is probably not mediated by a bacterial toxin, though a staphylococcal toxin may serve as a "superantigen" that interacts with T cells. The disease is characterized by fever and four of the following for at least 5 days: bilateral nonexudative conjunctivitis, mucous membrane changes of at least one type (injected pharynx, cracked lips, strawberry tongue); extremity changes of at least one type (edema, desquamation, erythema); a polymorphous rash; and cervical lymphadenopathy greater than 1.5 cm.

A major complication is arteritis of the coronary vessels, occurring in about 25% of untreated cases and on occasion causing myocardial infarction. Factors associated with the development of coronary artery aneurysms are leukocytosis and elevated C-reactive protein. Arteritis of extremity vessels and peripheral gangrene are reported also. Cerebrospinal fluid pleocytosis is reported in one-third of cases. The cause of these complications is likewise unknown.

Management is with aspirin (80–100 mg/kg/d in divided doses with subsequent tapering) and intravenous immune globulin in high doses. Plasmapheresis may be useful in cases unresponsive to immune globulin. Corticosteroids are used by some in refractory disease, though early Japanese reports suggest they may increase the likelihood of development of coronary aneurysms. Warfarin is indicated for the management of coronary artery aneurysms larger than 6.5 mm in diameter. Regular follow up by a cardiologist is recommended for patients with coronary artery disease or aneurysms.

Hall M et al: Kawasaki syndrome-like illness associated with infection caused by enterotoxin B-secreting *Staphylococcus aureus.* Clin Infect Dis 1999;29:586. [NLM Cit ID: 99458035] (Two cases that coincided with *S aureus* bacteremia.)

Leung DY et al: The immunopathogenesis and management of Kawasaki syndrome. Arthritis Rheum 1998;41:1538. [NLM Cit ID: 98421705]

Mason WH et al: Kawasaki syndrome. Clin Infect Dis 1999;28:169. [NLM Cit ID: 99161985] (An excellent review including guidelines for management of coronary artery complications.)

Newberger JW et al: Treatment of Kawasaki syndrome; corticosteroids revisited. J Pediatr 1999;135:411. [NLM Cit ID: 99447777] (Steroids may actually improve the course of disease according to these authors, and they refute the theory that steroids provoke coronary aneurysms.)

RELEVANT WORLD WIDE WEB SITES

[CMV Retinitis and Treatment]
http://hiv.medscape.com/Home/Topics/AIDS/AIDS.html

[The Hepatitis Information Network]
http://www.hepnet.com/

[HerpesZone]
http://www.herpeszone.com/MainMenu.htm

[Infectious Mononucleosis Case Study]
http://path.upmc.edu:80/cases/case37.html

[Influenza Treatment]
http://www2.cdc.gov/mmwr/

33 Infectious Diseases: Bacterial & Chlamydial

See http://www.current-med.com/ch33.html for updated addresses of Web sites referenced in this chapter.

Henry F. Chambers, MD

INFECTIONS CAUSED BY GRAM-POSITIVE BACTERIA

STREPTOCOCCAL INFECTIONS

1. PHARYNGITIS

Essentials of Diagnosis

- Abrupt onset of sore throat, fever, malaise, nausea, and headache.
- Throat red and edematous, with or without exudate; cervical nodes tender.
- Diagnosis confirmed by culture of throat.

General Considerations

Beta-hemolytic streptococci, classically group A, are the most common bacterial cause of exudative pharyngitis. Transmission is by droplets of infected secretions. Group A streptococci producing erythrogenic toxin may cause scarlet fever rashes in susceptible persons.

Clinical Findings

A. Symptoms and Signs: "Strep throat" is characterized by a sudden onset of fever, sore throat, pain on swallowing, tender cervical adenopathy, malaise, and nausea. The pharynx, soft palate, and tonsils are red and edematous. There may be a purulent exudate. The rash of scarlet fever is diffusely erythematous, resembling a sunburn, with superimposed fine red papules, and is most intense in the groin and axillas. It blanches on pressure, may become petechial, and fades in 2–5 days, leaving a fine desquamation. In scarlet fever, the face is flushed, with circumoral pallor; and the tongue is coated, with enlarged red papillae (strawberry tongue).

B. Laboratory Findings: Leukocytosis with neutrophil predominance is common. Throat culture onto a single blood agar plate has a sensitivity of 80–90%. Currently available rapid diagnostic tests, which are based on detection of streptococcal antigen, are slightly less sensitive than culture.

Complications

The suppurative complications of streptococcal sore throat include sinusitis, otitis media, mastoiditis, peritonsillar abscess, and suppuration of cervical lymph nodes, among others.

Nonsuppurative complications are rheumatic fever and glomerulonephritis. Rheumatic fever may follow recurrent episodes of pharyngitis beginning 1–4 weeks after the onset of symptoms. Glomerulonephritis follows a single infection with a nephritogenic strain of *Streptococcus* group A (eg, types 4, 12, 2, 49, and 60), more commonly on the skin than in the throat, and begins 1–3 weeks after the onset of the infection.

Differential Diagnosis

Streptococcal sore throat resembles (and cannot be reliably distinguished clinically from) pharyngitis caused by adenoviruses, Epstein-Barr virus, and other agents. Pharyngitis and lymphadenopathy are common findings in primary HIV infection. Generalized lymphadenopathy, splenomegaly, atypical lymphocytosis, and a positive serologic test (eg, Monospot) distinguish mononucleosis from streptococcal pharyngitis. Diphtheria is characterized by a pseudomembrane; candidiasis shows white patches of exudate and less erythema; and necrotizing ulcerative gingivostomatitis (Vincent's fusospirochetal disease) presents with shallow ulcers in the mouth. Retropharyngeal abscess or bacterial epiglottitis should be considered when odynophagia and difficulty in handling secretions are present and when the severity of symptoms is disproportionate to findings on examination of the pharynx.

Treatment

Antimicrobial therapy has a minimal effect on resolution of symptoms. Because its main purpose is prevention of complications, therapy may be withheld pending results of culture. Because throat culture (especially if a single plate is used) and rapid detection methods may be falsely negative in 30% or more of cases, when clinical suspicion is high (eg, presence of exudative pharyngitis, tender adenopathy, high fever, and absence of cough and rhinorrhea) and the risk of therapy is low (eg, no drug allergy), antimicrobial therapy may be given without laboratory evaluation.

A. Benzathine penicillin G, 1.2 million units intramuscularly as a single dose, is optimal therapy.

B. Penicillin VK, 500 mg orally four times a day (or amoxicillin, 750 mg orally twice daily), is effective, but compliance may be poor after the patient becomes asymptomatic in 2–4 days.

C. Macrolides—erythromycin, 500 mg orally four times a day, or azithromycin, 500 mg once daily for 3 days—are alternatives for the penicillin-allergic patient. Macrolides are less effective than penicillins. The prevalence of macrolide resistance among strains of group A streptococci is on the order of 25–40%. Therefore, macrolides are considered second-line agents because of the risk of treatment failure. The vast majority of macrolide-resistant strains are susceptible to clindamycin, which is an alternative for serious infections. A 10-day course of 300 mg three times a day orally should be effective.

Prevention of Recurrent Rheumatic Fever

Effectively controlling rheumatic fever depends upon identification and treatment of primary streptococcal infection and secondary prevention of recurrences. Patients who have had rheumatic fever should be treated with a continuous course of antimicrobial prophylaxis for at least 5 years. Effective regimens are erythromycin, 250 mg orally twice daily, or penicillin G, 500 mg orally daily.

Bronze MS et al: The reemergence of serious group A streptococcal infections and acute rheumatic fever. Am J Med Sci 1996;311:41. [NLM Cit ID: 96164691]

Carroll K et al: Microbiology and laboratory diagnosis of upper respiratory tract infections. Clin Infect Dis 1996;23:442. [NLM Cit ID: 97034105] (Microbial causes of pharyngitis and accuracy of various diagnostic tests.)

Kuhn S et al: Evaluation of the Strep A OIA assay versus culture methods: ability to detect different quantities of group A Streptococcus. Diagn Microbiol Infect Dis 1999;34:275. [NLM Cit ID: 99388769]

Kurtz B et al: Importance of inoculum size and sampling effect in rapid antigen detection for diagnosis of *Streptococcus pyogenes* pharyngitis. J Clin Microbiol 2000; 38:279. [NLM Cit ID: 20085147] (Evaluation of effect of inoculum on sensitivity and specificity of antigen detection versus culture for diagnosis of group A streptococcal pharyngitis.)

2. STREPTOCOCCAL SKIN INFECTIONS

Streptococci are not normal skin flora. Streptococcal skin infections usually result from colonization of normal skin by contact with other infected individuals or by preceding streptococcal respiratory infection.

Clinical Findings

A. Symptoms and Signs: Impetigo is a focal, vesicular, pustular lesion with a thick, amber-colored crust that has a "stuck-on" appearance.

Erysipelas is a painful superficial cellulitis that frequently involves the face. It is well demarcated from the surrounding normal skin. Erysipelas also affects skin with impaired lymphatic drainage, such as edematous lower extremities or wounds.

B. Laboratory Findings: Cultures obtained from a wound or pustule are likely to grow group A streptococci. Other cultures of the skin may be positive if the specimen is obtained from the leading edge of the cellulitis. Blood cultures are occasionally positive.

Treatment

Parenteral antibiotics are indicated for patients with facial erysipelas or evidence of systemic infection. Penicillin, 2 million units intravenously every 4 hours, is the drug of choice.

Cutaneous infections caused by staphylococci may at times be difficult to differentiate from streptococcal infections. Coinfection with staphylococci also occurs. Therefore, initial therapy for severely ill patients or those who have risk factors for staphylococcal infection (eg, intravenous drug use, wound infection, diabetes) should include an agent—such as nafcillin, 1.5 g intravenously every 6 hours—that also is active against *Staphylococcus aureus.* In the patient with minor penicillin allergy, cefazolin, 500 mg intravenously or intramuscularly every 8 hours, may be used. In the patient with a serious penicillin allergy (ie, anaphylaxis), vancomycin, 1000 mg intravenously every 12 hours, should be used.

Patients who do not require parenteral therapy may be treated with amoxicillin, 750 mg twice daily for 7–10 days. As mentioned for treatment of pharyngitis, a 25–40% prevalence of resistance among strains makes macrolides a less attractive alternative for penicillin-allergic patients. A first-generation oral cephalosporin, eg, cephalexin, 500 mg four times daily, or clindamycin, 300 mg orally three times daily, is an alternative to amoxicillin.

Bisno AL et al: Streptococcal infections of skin and soft tissue. N Engl J Med 1996;334:240. [NLM Cit ID: 96132561]

3. OTHER GROUP A STREPTOCOCCAL INFECTIONS

Arthritis, pneumonia, empyema, endocarditis, and necrotizing fasciitis are relatively uncommon infections that may be caused by group A streptococci. A toxic shock-like syndrome also occurs.

Arthritis generally occurs in association with cellulitis. In addition to intravenous therapy with penicillin G, 2 million units every 4 hours (or cefazolin or vancomycin in doses recommended above for penicillin-allergic patients), frequent percutaneous needle aspiration should be performed to remove joint effusions. Open surgical drainage may be necessary when percutaneous drainage is difficult to achieve—eg, when the hip or shoulder joint is infected.

Pneumonia and **empyema** often are characterized by extensive tissue destruction and an aggressive, rapidly progressive clinical course associated with significant morbidity and mortality rates. High-dose penicillin and chest tube drainage are indicated for treatment of empyema. Vancomycin is an acceptable substitute in penicillin-allergic patients.

Group A streptococci can cause **endocarditis.** This complication should be suspected when bacteremia accompanies pneumonia, particularly if the patient abuses parenteral drugs. The tricuspid valve is most commonly involved. A patient with suspected endocarditis should be treated with 4 million units of penicillin G every 4 hours for 4 weeks. Vancomycin, 1000 mg every 12 hours, is recommended for persons allergic to penicillin.

Necrotizing fasciitis is a rapidly spreading infection involving the fascia of deep muscle. The clinical findings at presentation may be those of severe cellulitis, but the presence of systemic toxicity and severe pain, which may be followed by anesthesia of the involved area due to destruction of nerves as infection advances through the fascial planes, are important clues to the diagnosis. Surgical exploration is mandatory when the diagnosis is suspected. Early and extensive debridement is essential for survival.

Any streptococcal infection—and necrotizing fasciitis in particular—can be associated with **streptococcal toxic shock-like syndrome,** characterized by invasion of skin or soft tissues, acute respiratory distress syndrome, and renal failure. The very young, the elderly, and those with underlying medical conditions are at particularly high risk for invasive disease. Bacteremia, which is uncommon in staphylococcal toxic shock syndrome, occurs in the majority of cases. Skin rash and desquamation may not be present. Mortality rates up to 80% have been reported for patients with the full-blown syndrome. The syndrome is due to elaboration of pyrogenic erythrotoxin (which also causes **scarlet fever**), a superantigen that stimulates massive release of inflammatory cytokines felt to mediate the shock. Clindamycin—but not penicillin—inhibits toxin production.

Penicillin remains the drug of choice for treatment of serious streptococcal infections, but some authorities recommend adding clindamycin (600 mg every 8 hours intravenously) to the regimen. Outbreaks of invasive disease have been associated with colonization by invasive clones that can be transmitted to close contacts who, though asymptomatic, may be a reservoir for disease. Tracing contacts of patients with invasive disease is controversial.

Bernaldo de Quirâos JC et al: Group A streptococcal bacteremia: A 10-year prospective study. Medicine 1997;76:238. [NLM Cit ID: 97425280]

Davies HD et al: Invasive group A streptococcal infections in Ontario, Canada. Ontario Group A Streptococcal Study Group. N Engl J Med 1996;335:547. [NLM Cit ID: 96310761] (Risk factors, including risk to household contacts of cases, and mortality rates for toxic shock-like syndrome and other invasive streptococcal infections are reported.)

Haywood CT et al: Clinical experience with 20 cases of group A streptococcus necrotizing fasciitis and myonecrosis: 1995 to 1997. Plast Reconstr Surg 1999; 103:1567. [NLM Cit ID: 99255289]

Sommer R et al: Group A beta-hemolytic streptococcus meningitis: clinical and microbiological features of nine cases. Clin Infect Dis 1999;29:929. [NLM Cit ID: 20055858]

4. NON-GROUP A STREPTOCOCCAL INFECTIONS

Non-group A streptococci produce a spectrum of disease similar to that of group A streptococci. Some non-group A streptococci are β-hemolytic (eg, groups B, C, and G). The treatment of infections caused by these strains is the same as for group A streptococci.

Group B streptococci are an important cause of sepsis, bacteremia, and meningitis in the neonate. This organism, which is part of the normal vaginal flora, may cause septic abortion, endometritis, or peripartum infections and, less commonly, cellulitis, bacteremia, and endocarditis in adults. Treatment of infections caused by group B streptococci is with either penicillin or vancomycin in doses recommended for group A streptococci. Because of in vitro synergism, some authorities recommend the addition of low-dose gentamicin, 1 mg/kg every 8 hours.

Viridans streptococci, which are nonhemolytic or α-hemolytic (ie, producing a green zone of hemolysis on blood agar), are part of the normal oral flora. Although these strains may produce focal pyogenic infection, they are most notable as the leading cause of native valve endocarditis (see below).

Group D streptococci include *Streptococcus bovis* and the enterococci. *S bovis* is a cause of endocarditis in association with bowel neoplasia or cirrhosis. Endocarditis caused by *S bovis* is treated like viridans streptococci.

Cabellos C et al: Streptococcal meningitis in adult patients: current epidemiology and clinical spectrum. Clin Infect Dis 1999;28:1104. [NLM Cit ID: 99379712]

Perovic O et al: Invasive group B streptococcal disease in nonpregnant adults. Eur J Clin Microbiol Infect Dis 1999;18:362. [NLM Cit ID: 99347394]

ENTEROCOCCAL INFECTIONS

Enterococci have been classified into a genus separate from other streptococci. Two species, *Enterococcus faecalis* and *Enterococcus faecium,* are responsible for most human enterococcal infections. Enterococci cause wound infections, urinary tract infections, and endocarditis. Except for serious infections such as meningitis, endocarditis, bacteremia in the immunocompromised host, and osteomyelitis, most enterococcal infections can still be treated with penicillin, 3 million units every 4 hours; ampicillin (which is slightly more active than penicillin in vitro), 2 g every 6 hours; or vancomycin, 1 g every 12 hours. Because these antibiotics are not bactericidal for enterococci, gentamicin in a dose of 1 mg/kg every 8 hours is added for treatment of endocarditis or other serious infection.

Enterococci, which are intrinsically resistant to multiple antibiotics, have until recently been susceptible to penicillin, vancomycin, and gentamicin. Strains that are resistant to all known antibiotics are now being encountered, and nosocomial outbreaks of infection caused by strains resistant to gentamicin or vancomycin are increasingly common. It is essential to determine antimicrobial susceptibility of clinical isolates in order to detect these resistant organisms. Infection control measures that may be indicated to limit their spread include isolation, strict adherence to barrier precautions, and avoidance of overuse of vancomycin and gentamicin. Optimal therapy for infection caused by vancomycin- and gentamicin-resistant strains is not known. Two agents have recently been approved by the FDA for treatment of infections caused by vancomycin-resistant enterococci: the streptogramin fixed combination of quinupristin/dalfopristin and linezolid. Quinupristin/dalfopristin is not active against strains of *Enterococcus faecalis* and should be used only for infections caused by *E faecium.* The dose is 7.5 mg/kg intravenously every 8–12 hours. Infusion-related events, including phlebitis and irritation at the infusion site (often requiring infusion via a central line), and an arthralgia-myalgia syndrome are relatively common side effects. Quinupristin/dalfopristin has important drug interactions with midazolam, nifedipine, and cyclosporine because it is an inhibitor of cytochrome P450 enzyme 3A4, which metabolizes these drugs. In open-label noncomparative trials, the reported microbiologic success rate was approximately 70% overall. Linezolid, an oxazolidinone, is active against both *E faecalis* and *E faecium.* The dose is 600 mg twice daily, and both intravenous and oral preparations are available. The overall microbiologic cure rate in open-label noncomparative trials is approximately 85%. The drug is well tolerated, with hematologic abnormalities as the principal toxicity.

Chien JW et al: Use of linezolid, an oxazolidinone, in the treatment of multidrug-resistant gram-positive bacterial infections. Clin Infect Dis 2000;30:146. [NLM Cit ID: 20086546]

Diekema DJ et al: Oxazolidinones: a review. Drugs 2000;59:7. [NLM Cit ID: 20181025]

Murray BE: Vancomycin-resistant enterococcal infections. N Engl J Med 2000;342:710. [NLM Cit ID: 20155741]

PNEUMOCOCCAL INFECTIONS

1. PNEUMOCOCCAL PNEUMONIA

Essentials of Diagnosis

- Productive cough, fever, rigors, dyspnea, early pleuritic chest pain
- Consolidating lobar pneumonia on chest x-ray.
- Lancet-shaped gram-positive diplococci on Gram stain of sputum.

General Considerations

The pneumococcus is the most common cause of community-acquired pyogenic bacterial pneumonia. Alcoholism, infection by HIV, sickle cell disease, splenectomy, and hematologic disorders are predisposing factors. The mortality rate remains high in the setting of advanced age, multilobar disease, severe hypoxemia, extrapulmonary complications, and bacteremia.

Clinical Findings

A. Symptoms and Signs: The illness typically evolves over a period of a few days. The patient presents with high fever, productive cough, occasionally hemoptysis, and pleuritic chest pain, features that distinguish it from mycoplasmal or pneumocystis pneumonia. Rigors occur within the first few hours of infection but are uncommon thereafter. Bronchial breath sounds are an early sign.

B. Laboratory Findings: Classically, pneumococcal pneumonia is a lobar pneumonia with radiographic signs of consolidation and occasionally effusion. Infiltrates may also be patchy.

Gram's stain of sputum always should be examined. Adequately collected samples (with < 10 epithelial cells and > 25 polymorphonuclear leukocytes per high-power field) show gram-positive diplococci 80–90% of the time. Sputum culture alone is less sensitive than Gram's stain, and false positives are common as well. Blood cultures are positive in up to 25% of selected cases and much more commonly so in HIV-positive patients.

Complications

Parapneumonic (sympathetic) effusion is common and may cause recurrence or persistence of fever. These sterile fluid accumulations need no specific therapy. Empyema occurs in 5% or less of cases and is differentiated from sympathetic effusion by the presence of organisms on Gram-stained fluid or positive pleural fluid cultures.

Pneumococcal pericarditis is a rare complication that can cause tamponade. Pneumococcal arthritis also is uncommon. Pneumococcal endocarditis usually involves the aortic valve and often occurs in association with meningitis and pneumonia. Early heart failure and multiple embolic events are typical.

Treatment

A. Specific Measures: Uncomplicated pneumococcal pneumonia (ie, arterial Po_2 > 60 mm Hg, no coexisting medical problems, and single-lobe disease without signs of extrapulmonary infection) may be treated on an outpatient basis with penicillin V potassium, 500 mg orally four times a day for 7–10 days. For penicillin-allergic patients, erythromycin, 500 mg orally four times a day, or azithromycin, one 500 mg dose on the first day and 250 mg once a day for the next 4 days, is an alternative. Patients should be followed for clinical response (eg, less cough, defervescence within 2–3 days) because pneumococci may be resistant to penicillin or any of the second-line agents. Lack of clinical response may indicate infection with a resistant strain, and hospitalization should be considered.

More seriously ill patients or those with other medical problems should be admitted and treated parenterally with aqueous penicillin G, 2 million units intravenously every 4 hours. A low-dose regimen of procaine penicillin, 600,000 units intramuscularly every 12 hours, is effective for pneumonia caused by penicillin-susceptible strains; however, because 10% or more of pneumococcal isolates are of intermediate or high-level resistance, higher doses of penicillin are recommended until susceptibility of the isolate is known. For penicillin-allergic patients without anaphylaxis or other serious reactions, cefazolin, 500 mg either intravenously or intramuscularly every 8 hours, is effective. For serious penicillin or cephalosporin allergy or infection caused by a highly penicillin-resistant strain (MIC > 1 μg/mL), vancomycin, 30 mg/kg/d, up to 2000 mg total, in two divided doses, can be used.

B. Treatment of Complications: Pleural effusions developing after initiation of antimicrobial therapy usually are sterile, and thoracentesis need not be performed if the patient is otherwise improving. Thoracentesis is indicated for an effusion that is present prior to initiation of therapy and in the patient who has significant fever or who otherwise has not responded to antibiotics after 3–4 days. Chest tube drainage may be required if pneumococci are identified by culture or Gram stain.

Echocardiography should be done if pericardial effusion is suspected. Patients with pericardial effusion who are responding to therapy and have no signs of tamponade may be followed and treated with indomethacin, 50 mg three times daily, for pain. In patients with increasing effusion, unsatisfactory clinical response, or evidence of tamponade, pericardiocentesis will determine if the pericardial space is infected. Infected fluid must be drained either percutaneously (by tube placement or needle aspiration), by placement of a pericardial window, or by pericardiectomy. Pericardiectomy eventually may be required to prevent or treat constrictive pericarditis, a common sequela of bacterial pericarditis.

Endocarditis should be treated with 24 million units of penicillin G intravenously (or vancomycin, 30 mg/kg/d, for penicillin-allergic patients or for infections caused by penicillin-resistant strains) daily for 3–4 weeks. Mild heart failure may respond to medical therapy alone, such as digoxin and diuretics, but moderate to severe heart failure is an indication for prosthetic valve implantation, as are systemic emboli or large friable vegetations as determined by echocardiography.

C. Penicillin-Resistant Pneumococci: The prevalence of penicillin-resistant pneumococci (MIC > 0.1 μg/mL) in the United States is increasing, accounting for 10–15% of bloodstream isolates in some regions. All blood and cerebrospinal fluid isolates should be tested for resistance to penicillin. The 1 μg oxacillin disk diffusion assay is an easily performed, reliable screen for resistance. Pneumonia caused by intermediately resistant strains (penicillin MIC > 0.1 μg/mL but ≤ 1 μg/mL) generally will respond to high-dose penicillin therapy. High-dose penicillin also may be effective for infections other than meningitis caused by highly penicillin-resistant strains (MIC > 1 μg/mL). However, some authorities recommend that ceftriaxone, 2 g once daily, cefotaxime 3 g every 6 hours, or vancomycin, 1 g every 12 hours be used instead, especially for immunocompromised patients, because of superior in vitro activity and a more favorable ratio between serum drug concentration and MIC. Fluoroquinolones with enhanced gram-positive activity (eg, levofloxacin 500 mg once daily, moxifloxacin 400 mg once daily, or gatifloxacin 400 mg once daily) are effective oral alternatives. Penicillin-resistant strains of pneumococci may be resistant to multiple antibiotics, including macrolides, trimethoprim-sulfamethoxazole, and chloramphenicol, and susceptibility to these agents must be documented prior to their use.

Lieu TA et al: Projected cost-effectiveness of pneumococcal conjugate vaccination of healthy infants and young children. JAMA 2000;283:1460. [NLM Cit ID: 20195074]

Pallares R: Treatment of pneumococcal pneumonia. Semin Respir Infect 1999;14:276. [NLM Cit ID: 99429423]

Schneider RF et al: Pneumococcal infections in HIV-infected adults. Semin Respir Infect 1999;14:237. [NLM Cit ID: 99429419] (This entire issue is devoted to pneumococcal infections. Four of the best articles address epidemiology, vaccination, clinical pathogenesis, and pathophysiology of the disease.)

2. PNEUMOCOCCAL MENINGITIS

Essentials of Diagnosis

- Fever, headache, altered mental status.
- Meningismus.
- Gram-positive diplococci on Gram stain of cerebrospinal fluid; counterimmunoelectrophoresis may be positive in partially treated cases.

General Considerations

Streptococcus pneumoniae is the most common cause of meningitis in adults and the second most common cause of meningitis in children over the age of 6 years. Head trauma, cerebrospinal fluid leaks, and sinusitis may precede pneumococcal meningitis.

Clinical Findings

A. Symptoms and Signs: The onset is rapid, with fever, headache, and altered mentation. Pneumonia may be present. Compared with meningitis caused by the meningococcus, pneumococcal meningitis lacks a rash, and focal neurologic deficits, cranial nerve palsies, and obtundation are more prominent features.

B. Laboratory Findings: The cerebrospinal fluid typically has more than 1000 white blood cells per microliter, over 60% of which are polymorphonuclear leukocytes; the glucose concentration is less than 40 mg/dL, or less than 50% of the simultaneous serum concentration; the protein usually exceeds 150 mg/dL. Not all cases of meningitis will have these typical findings, and alterations in cerebrospinal fluid cell counts and chemistries may be surprisingly minimal, overlapping with those of aseptic meningitis.

Gram stain of cerebrospinal fluid shows gram-positive cocci in 80–90% of cases, and in untreated cases blood or cerebrospinal fluid cultures are almost always positive. Tests such as counterimmunoelectrophoresis or latex agglutination to detect pneumococcal antigens in cerebrospinal fluid are less sensitive than culture and Gram stain. Antigen detection tests may occasionally be helpful in establishing the diagnosis in the patient who has been partially treated and in whom cultures and stains are negative.

Treatment

Antibiotics should be given as soon as the diagnosis of meningitis is suspected. If lumbar puncture must be delayed (eg, while awaiting results of an imaging study to exclude a mass lesion), ceftriaxone, 4 g, is given intravenously after blood cultures (positive in 50% of cases) have been obtained. If gram-positive diplococci are present on the Gram stain, then vancomycin, 45 mg/kg/d intravenously in three divided doses, should be administered in addition to ceftriaxone until the isolate is confirmed not to be penicillin-resistant. In the penicillin-allergic patient, chloramphenicol, 1.5 g every 6 hours, may be used, but some penicillin-resistant strains are also resistant to this antibiotic. Once susceptibility has been confirmed, penicillin, 24 million units daily in six divided doses, ceftriaxone, 4 g/d, or chloramphenicol, 6 g/d in four divided doses, is continued for 10–14 days in documented cases.

The best therapy for penicillin-resistant strains is not known. Penicillin-resistant strains often are cross-resistant to the third-generation cephalosporins as well as other antibiotics. Susceptibility testing is essential to proper management of this infection. Treatment failures have been reported with ceftriaxone or cefotaxime for meningitis caused by strains with penicillin MICs ≥ 2 μg/mL. If the MIC of ceftriaxone or cefotaxime is ≤ 0.5 μg/mL, single-drug therapy with either of these cephalosporins is likely to be effective. If the MIC is ≥ 1 μg/mL, treatment with a combination of ceftriaxone, 2 g every 12 hours, plus vancomycin, 45 mg/kg/d (up to 2 g/d) in three divided doses, is recommended. If a patient with a penicillin-resistant organism has not responded clinically to therapy with a third-generation cephalosporin, repeat lumbar puncture is indicated to assess the bacteriologic response.

The role of steroids in adjunctive therapy of meningitis in the adult remains controversial. Dexamethasone, 0.15 mg/kg intravenously every 6 hours, may be given when coma, focal deficits, or other signs of increased intracranial pressure are present.

Peltola H: Prophylaxis of bacterial meningitis. Infect Dis Clin North Am 1999;13:685. [NLM Cit ID: 99399583]

Quagliarello VJ et al: Treatment of bacterial meningitis. N Engl J Med 1997;336:708. [NLM Cit ID: 97177211]

Saez-Llorens X et al: Antimicrobial and anti-inflammatory treatment of bacterial meningitis. Infect Dis Clin North Am 1999;13:619. [NLM Cit ID: 99399579]

STAPHYLOCOCCUS AUREUS INFECTIONS

1. SKIN & SOFT TISSUE INFECTIONS

Essentials of Diagnosis

- Localized erythema with induration.
- Tendency toward abscess formation.
- Folliculitis commonly observed.

- Gram stain of pus with gram-positive cocci in clusters; cultures usually positive.

General Considerations

Most staphylococci found on cultures of normal skin belong to the *Staphylococcus epidermidis* group. *Staphylococcus aureus* is not normal skin flora. *S aureus* tends to cause more localized skin infections than streptococci, and abscess formation is common.

Clinical Findings

A. Symptoms and Signs: *S aureus* skin infections may begin around one or more hair follicles, causing folliculitis. These infections may localize to form boils (or furuncles) or spread to adjacent skin and deeper subcutaneous tissue (ie, a carbuncle). Myositis or fasciitis may occur, often in association with a deep wound or other inoculation or injection.

B. Laboratory Findings: Cultures of the wound or abscess material will almost always yield the organism. In patients with other systemic signs of infection, blood cultures should be obtained because of potential endocarditis, osteomyelitis, or metastatic seeding of other sites.

Treatment

Proper drainage of abscess fluid or other focal infections is the mainstay of therapy. Drainage may be all that is needed for cutaneous abscess. Antibiotic therapy alone is unlikely to be effective if collections of infected material are undrained.

For uncomplicated skin infections, oral therapy is satisfactory. An oral penicillinase-resistant penicillin or cephalosporin, such as dicloxacillin or cephalexin, 500 mg four times a day for 7–10 days, is the drug of choice. Erythromycin, 500 mg four times a day, may be used in the penicillin-allergic patient, although the prevalence of erythromycin-resistant strains (40–60%) makes this regimen less attractive empirically.

For more complicated infections with extensive cutaneous or deep tissue involvement or fever, parenteral therapy is indicated initially. A penicillinase-resistant penicillin such as nafcillin or oxacillin in a dosage of 1.5 g every 6 hours intravenously is the drug of choice. In allergic patients without a serious reaction, cefazolin, 0.5–1 g intravenously or intramuscularly every 8 hours, can be used. In patients with a serious allergy to β-lactam antibiotics or if the strain is methicillin-resistant, vancomycin, 1000 mg intravenously every 12 hours, is the drug of choice.

2. OSTEOMYELITIS

S aureus is the cause of approximately 60% of all cases of osteomyelitis. Osteomyelitis may be caused by direct inoculation, eg, from an open fracture or as a result of surgery; by extension from a contiguous focus of infection or open wound; or, more commonly, by hematogenous spread. Long bones and vertebrae are the usual sites. Epidural abscess with or without bone involvement is a common complication of vertebral osteomyelitis and should be suspected if fever and back pain are accompanied by radicular pain or neurologic symptoms or signs indicative of spinal cord compression (eg, incontinence).

Clinical Findings

A. Symptoms and Signs: The infection may be acute, with abrupt development of local symptoms and systemic toxicity; or indolent, with insidious onset of vague pain over the site of infection, progressing to local tenderness. Fever is absent in one-third or more of cases. Abscess formation is a late and unusual manifestation. Draining sinus tracts occur in chronic infections or infections of foreign body implants.

B. Laboratory Findings: The diagnosis is established by isolation of *S aureus* from the blood, bone, or a contiguous focus of a patient with signs and symptoms of focal bone infection. Blood culture will be positive in approximately 60% of untreated cases of staphylococcal osteomyelitis. Bone biopsy and culture should be considered if blood cultures are sterile.

C. Imaging: Bone scan and gallium scan, each with a sensitivity of approximately 95% and a specificity of 60–70%, are useful in identifying or confirming the site of bone infection. Plain bone films early in the course of infection are often normal but will become abnormal in most cases even with effective therapy. Spinal infection (unlike malignancy) traverses the disk space to involve the contiguous vertebral body. CT is more sensitive than plain films and can be useful in localizing associated abscesses. MRI is somewhat less sensitive than bone scan but has a specificity of 90%. MRI is indicated when epidural abscess is suspected in association with vertebral osteomyelitis.

Treatment

Prolonged therapy is required to cure staphylococcal osteomyelitis. Durations of 4–6 weeks or longer are recommended. Although oral regimens can be effective, parenteral regimens are advised during the acute phase of the infection for patients with systemic toxicity. Nafcillin or oxacillin, 9–12 g/d in six divided doses, is the drug of choice. Cefazolin, 1 g every 8 hours, also is effective. Vancomycin, 1 g every 12 hours, may be used for the penicillin-allergic patient.

Oral regimens are dicloxacillin or cephalexin, 1 g every 6 hours. Addition to the regimen of rifampin 300 mg twice daily probably prevents late relapse and should be strongly considered. For example, an oral regimen of ciprofloxacin 750 mg plus rifampin 300 mg twice daily improved outcome in implant-related staphylococcal infections, which are very prone to relapse.

Herwaldt LA: Control of methicillin-resistant *Staphylococcus aureus* in the hospital setting. Am J Med 1999; 106(Suppl 5A):11S. [NLM Cit ID: 99275815]

Zimmerli W et al: Role of rifampin for treatment of orthopedic implant-related staphylococcal infections: A randomized controlled trial. Foreign-Body Infection Study Group. JAMA 1998;279:1537. [NLM Cit ID: 98266934]

3. STAPHYLOCOCCAL BACTEREMIA

S aureus readily invades the bloodstream and infects sites distant from the primary site of infection, which may be relatively minor or even inapparent. Though commonly arising from skin lesions or intravenous lines, whenever *S aureus* is recovered from blood cultures, the possibility of endocarditis, osteomyelitis, or other metastatic deep infection must be considered. The appropriate duration of therapy for uncomplicated bacteremia arising from a removable source (eg, intravenous device) or drainable focus (eg, skin abscess) has not been well defined, but at least 10–14 days of parenteral therapy appear to be the minimum. However, approximately 5% or more of patients still relapse, usually with endocarditis or osteomyelitis, even if treated for 2 weeks.

Because of this tendency—and based on the impression that longer courses of therapy reduce the relapse rate—10–14 days of nafcillin or oxacillin, 1.5 g intravenously every four to six hours, cefazolin, 500–1000 mg every 8 hours, or vancomycin, 1000 mg every 12 hours, is recommended for uncomplicated staphylococcal bacteremia. Vancomycin should be reserved for patients with serious penicillin allergy or with infections caused by methicillin-resistant strains because of data suggesting that it is less active than β-lactam antibiotics. Longer courses of either parenteral or oral therapy may be considered for patients (eg, those with diabetes, immunocompromised persons) at risk for late complications from bacteremia and for those in whom endocarditis is suspected. Transesophageal echocardiography (TEE) is a sensitive and cost-effective method for excluding underlying endocarditis. It should be performed in all patients for whom the pretest probability of endocarditis is 5% or higher—and perhaps in all patients with *S aureus* bacteremia.

Treatment failures have been reported with the isolation of intermediate-resistant strains in foreign body infections, in association with prolonged or repeated courses of vancomycin therapy, and in patients with chronic renal failure. These strains have also been resistant to methicillin and numerous other antibiotics, severely limiting therapeutic options. However, limited data suggest that an antistaphylococcal penicillin in combination with vancomycin may be synergistic in vitro against vancomycin-resistant strains and is an option for infections that do not respond to vancomycin alone. Cases of vancomycin treatment failures in which the staphylococcal isolate exhibits a vancomycin MIC ≥ 4 μg/mL should be reported to CDC, as this information is critical for tracking this potentially serious and emerging problem.

Gopal AK et al: Prospective analysis of *Staphylococcus aureus* bacteremia in nonneutropenic adults with malignancy. J Clin Oncol 2000;18:1110. [NLM Cit ID: 20160758]

Rosen AB et al: Cost-effectiveness of transesophageal echocardiography to determine the duration of therapy for intravascular catheter-associated *Staphylococcus aureus* bacteremia. Ann Intern Med 1999;130:810. [NLM Cit ID: 99242203]

Smith TL et al: Emergence of vancomycin resistance in *Staphylococcus aureus*. N Engl J Med 1999;340:493. [NLM Cit ID: 99134018]

4. TOXIC SHOCK SYNDROME

Some strains of staphylococci elaborate toxins that can cause three important entities: "scalded skin syndrome" in children, toxic shock syndrome in adults, and enterotoxin food poisoning. Toxic shock syndrome is characterized by abrupt onset of high fever, vomiting, and watery diarrhea. Sore throat, myalgias, and headache are common. Hypotension with renal and cardiac failure is an ominous manifestation in severe cases. A diffuse macular erythematous rash and nonpurulent conjunctivitis are common, and desquamation, especially of palms and soles, is typical during recovery. Fatality rates may be as high as 15%. Although toxic shock syndrome has occurred in children and in males, most cases (90% or more) have been reported in women of childbearing age. Of these, symptoms begin in nearly all patients within 5 days of the onset of a menstrual period in women who have used tampons. The syndrome is possible in any patient with a focus of toxin-producing *S aureus*. Nonmenstrual cases of toxic shock syndrome are now about as common as menstrual cases. Organisms from various sites, including the nasopharynx, vagina, or rectum or from wounds, have all been associated with the illness. Toxic shock syndrome is most often caused by toxic shock syndrome toxin-1 (TSST-1). Nonmenstrual cases of toxic shock syndrome are frequently caused by strains that do not produce TSST-1. Blood cultures are negative, because symptoms are due to the effects of the toxin and not to the invasive properties of the organism.

Important aspects of treatment include rapid rehydration, antistaphylococcal drugs, management of renal or cardiac insufficiency, and removal of sources of toxin, eg, removal of tampon, drainage of abscess.

5. INFECTIONS CAUSED BY COAGULASE-NEGATIVE STAPHYLOCOCCI

Coagulase-negative staphylococci are an important cause of infections of intravascular and prosthetic devices and of wound infection following cardiothoracic surgery. Rarely, these organisms cause infections such as osteomyelitis and endocarditis in the absence of a prosthesis. More than 20 species have been identified, but most human infections are caused by *Staphylococcus epidermidis, S haemolyticus, S hominis, S warnerii, S saprophyticus, S saccharolyticus,* and *S cohnii.* These common nosocomial pathogens are less virulent than *S aureus,* and infections caused by them tend to be more indolent.

Because coagulase-negative staphylococci are normal inhabitants of human skin, it can be difficult to determine whether their isolation is caused by infection or contamination, the latter perhaps accounting for three-fourths of blood culture isolates. Infection is more likely if the patient has a foreign body (eg, sternal wires, prosthetic joint, prosthetic cardiac valve, intracranial pressure monitor, cerebrospinal fluid shunt, peritoneal dialysis catheter) or an intravascular device in place. Purulent or serosanguineous drainage, erythema, pain, or tenderness at the site of the foreign body or device suggests infection. Instability and pain are signs of prosthetic joint infection. Fever, a new murmur, instability of the prosthesis, or signs of systemic embolization are evidence of prosthetic valve infection. Immunosuppression and recent antimicrobial therapy also are risk factors for infection.

Infection is also more likely if the same strain is consistently isolated from two or more blood cultures (particularly if samples were obtained at different times) and from the foreign body site. Contamination rather than infection is favored by a single positive blood culture or if more than one strain is isolated from blood cultures. The antimicrobial susceptibility pattern and speciation is commonly used to determine whether one or more strains have been isolated. More sophisticated typing methods, eg, pulse-field gel electrophoresis of restriction enzyme digested chromosomal DNA, may be required to identify distinct strains.

Whenever possible, the intravascular device or foreign body suspected of being infected by coagulase-negative staphylococci should be removed. However, removal and replacement of some devices (eg, prosthetic joint, prosthetic valve, cerebrospinal fluid shunt) can be a difficult or risky procedure, and it may sometimes be preferable to treat with antibiotics alone with the understanding that the probability of cure is reduced and that surgical management may eventually be necessary.

Coagulase-negative staphylococci are commonly resistant to methicillin and multiple other antibiotics. For patients with normal renal function, vancomycin, 1 g intravenously every 12 hours, is the treatment of choice for suspected or confirmed infection caused by these organisms until susceptibility to penicillinase-resistant penicillins or other agents has been confirmed. Duration of therapy has not been established for relatively uncomplicated infections, such as those secondary to intravenous devices, which may be eliminated by simply removing the infected device. Infection involving bone or a prosthetic valve should be treated for 6 weeks. A combination regimen of vancomycin plus rifampin, 300 mg orally twice daily, and gentamicin, 1 mg/kg intravenously every 8 hours, is recommended for treatment of prosthetic valve endocarditis caused by methicillin-resistant strains.

Herwaldt LA et al: The positive predictive value of isolating coagulase-negative staphylococci from blood cultures. Clin Infect Dis 1996;22:14. [NLM Cit ID: 96422342] (Twenty-six percent of 227 episodes of blood cultures growing coagulase-negative staphylococci represented true bacteremia. Risk factors associated with true infection are discussed.)

CLOSTRIDIAL DISEASES

1. CLOSTRIDIAL MYONECROSIS (Gas Gangrene)

Essentials of Diagnosis

- Sudden onset of pain and edema in an area of wound contamination.
- Prostration and systemic toxicity.
- Brown to blood-tinged watery exudate, with skin discoloration of surrounding area.
- Gas in the tissue by palpation or x-ray.
- Gram-positive rods in culture or smear of exudate.

General Considerations

Gas gangrene or clostridial myonecrosis is produced by entry of one of several clostridia (*Clostridium perfringens, Clostridium ramosum, Clostridium bifermentans, Clostridium histolyticum, Clostridium novyi,* etc) into devitalized tissues. Toxins produced under anaerobic conditions result in shock, hemolysis, and myonecrosis.

Clinical Findings

A. Symptoms and Signs: The onset of gas gangrene is usually sudden, with rapidly increasing pain in the affected area, fall in blood pressure, and tachycardia. Fever is present but is not proportionate to the severity of the infection. In the last stages of the disease, severe prostration, stupor, delirium, and coma occur.

The wound becomes swollen, and the surrounding skin is pale. There is a foul-smelling brown, blood-tinged serous discharge. As the disease advances, the surrounding tissue changes from pale to dusky and finally becomes deeply discolored, with coalescent, red, fluid-filled vesicles. Gas may be palpable in the tissues.

B. Laboratory Findings: Gas gangrene is a clinical diagnosis, and empirical therapy is indicated whenever the diagnosis is suspected. Radiographic studies may show gas within the soft tissues, but this finding is not specific because other organisms may produce gas. The smear typically shows a remarkable absence of neutrophils and the presence of gram-positive rods. Anaerobic culture confirms the diagnosis.

Differential Diagnosis

Other types of infection can cause gas formation in the tissue, eg, enterobacter, escherichia, and mixed anaerobic infections including bacteroides and peptostreptococci. Clostridia may produce serious puerperal infection with hemolysis.

Treatment

Penicillin, 2 million units every 3 hours intravenously, is effective. Other agents (eg, tetracycline, clindamycin, metronidazole, chloramphenicol, cefoxitin) are active against clostridium species in vitro and probably in vivo as well. Adequate surgical debridement and exposure of infected areas is essential, with radical surgical excision often necessary. Hyperbaric oxygen therapy has been used, but clinical data supporting its efficacy consist only of retrospective case series and anecdotal reports. If hyperbaric oxygen therapy is used, it must be in conjunction with administration of an appropriate antibiotic and surgical debridement.

Petit L et al: *Clostridium perfringens:* toxinotype and genotype. Trends Microbiol 1999;7:104. [NLM Cit ID: 99226295]

TETANUS

Essentials of Diagnosis

- History of wound and possible contamination.
- Jaw stiffness followed by spasms of jaw muscles (trismus).
- Stiffness of the neck and other muscles, dysphagia, irritability, hyperreflexia.
- Finally, painful convulsions precipitated by minimal stimuli.

General Considerations

Tetanus is caused by the neurotoxin tetanospasmin, elaborated by *Clostridium tetani.* Spores of this organism are ubiquitous in soil. When introduced into a wound, spores may germinate. The vegetative bacteria produce the toxin, which is a zinc metalloprotease that cleaves synaptobrevin, a protein essential for neurotransmitter release. Tetanospasmin interferes with neurotransmission at spinal synapses of inhibitory neurons. As a result, minor stimuli result in uncontrolled spasms, and reflexes are exaggerated. The incubation period is 5 days to 15 weeks, with the average being 8–12 days.

In the United States, most cases occur in unvaccinated individuals. Persons at risk are the elderly, migrant workers, newborns, and injection drug users, who may acquire the disease through subcutaneous injections. While puncture wounds are recognized as particularly prone to causing tetanus, any wound, including decubiti, where dead tissue and anaerobic conditions are present may become colonized and infected by *C tetani.*

Clinical Findings

A. Symptoms and Signs: The first symptom may be pain and tingling at the site of inoculation, followed by spasticity of the muscles nearby. More frequently, however, the presenting symptoms are stiffness of the jaw, neck stiffness, dysphagia, and irritability. Hyperreflexia develops later, with spasms of the jaw muscles (trismus) or facial muscles and rigidity and spasm of the muscles of the abdomen, neck, and back. Painful tonic convulsions precipitated by minor stimuli are common. Spasms of the glottis and respiratory muscles may cause acute asphyxia. The patient is awake and alert throughout the illness. The sensory examination is normal. The temperature is normal or only slightly elevated.

B. Laboratory Findings: The diagnosis of tetanus is made clinically.

Differential Diagnosis

Tetanus must be differentiated from various acute central nervous system infections. Trismus may occasionally develop with the use of phenothiazines. Strychnine poisoning should also be considered.

Complications

Airway obstruction is common. Urinary retention and constipation may result from spasm of the sphincters. Respiratory arrest and cardiac failure are late, life-threatening events.

Prevention

Tetanus is completely preventable by active immunization. Immunizations for children include tetanus toxoid, usually as DTP (see Table 30–4 for schedule). For primary immunization of adults, tetanus toxoid is administered as two doses 4–6 weeks apart, with a third dose 6–12 months later. Booster doses are given every 10 years or at the time of major injury if it occurs more than 5 years after a dose.

Passive immunization should be used in nonimmunized individuals and those whose immunization status is uncertain whenever a wound is contaminated or likely to have devitalized tissue. Tetanus immune globulin, 250 units, is given intramuscularly. Active immunization with tetanus toxoid should be started concurrently. Table 33–1 provides a guide to prophylactic management.

Table 33–1. Guide to tetanus prophylaxis in wound management.[1]

History of Absorbed Tetanus Toxoid	Clean, Minor Wounds		All Other Wounds[2]	
	Td[3]	TIG[4]	Td[3]	TIG[4]
Unknown or < 3 doses	Yes	No	Yes	Yes
3 or more doses	No[5]	No	No[6]	No

[1]From the Centers for Disease Control and Prevention. Recommended childhood immunization schedule—United States, 2000. JAMA 2000;283:876. [NLM Cit ID: 20148136]
[2]Such as, but not limited to, wounds contaminated with dirt, feces, soil, saliva, etc; puncture wounds; avulsions; and wounds resulting from missiles, crushing, burns, and frostbite.
[3]Tetanus toxoid and diphtheria toxoid, adult form. Use only this preparation (Td-adult) in children older than 6 years.
[4]Tetanus immune globulin.
[5]Yes if more than 10 years have elapsed since last dose.
[6]Yes if more than 5 years have elapsed since last dose. (More frequent boosters are not needed and can enhance side effects.)

Treatment

A. Specific Measures: Give tetanus immune globulin, 5000 units intramuscularly. Tetanus does not produce natural immunity, and a full course of immunization with tetanus toxoid should be administered once the patient has recovered.

B. General Measures: Minimal stimuli can provoke spasms, so the patient should be placed at bed rest and monitored under the quietest conditions possible. Sedation, paralysis with curare-like agents, and mechanical ventilation are often necessary to control tetanic spasms. Penicillin, 20 million units daily, is administered to all patients—even those with mild illness—to eradicate toxin-producing organisms.

Prognosis

High mortality rates are associated with a short incubation period, early onset of convulsions, and delay in treatment. Contaminated lesions about the head and face are more dangerous than wounds on other parts of the body. The overall mortality rate historically is about 40%, but this can be considerably reduced with ventilator management as described.

Pellizzari R et al: Tetanus and botulinum neurotoxins: mechanism of action and therapeutic uses. Philos Trans R Soc London B Biol Sci 1999;354:259. [NLM Cit ID: 99228944]

BOTULISM

Essentials of Diagnosis

- History of recent ingestion of home-canned or smoked foods or of injection drug use and demonstration of toxin in serum or food.
- Sudden onset of diplopia, dry mouth, dysphagia, dysphonia, and muscle weakness progressing to respiratory paralysis.
- Pupils are fixed and dilated.

General Considerations

Botulism is food poisoning usually caused by ingestion of preformed toxin (usually type A, B, or E) of *Clostridium botulinum,* a ubiquitous, strictly anaerobic, spore-forming bacillus found in soil. Canned, smoked, or vacuum-packed anaerobic foods are involved—particularly home-canned vegetables, smoked meats, and vacuum-packed fish—but commercial foods have also been associated with outbreaks of botulism. Infant botulism and wound botulism, which occurs in injection drug users, differ in that organisms present in the gut or wound, respectively, elaborate toxin in vivo. Botulinum toxins, like tetanus toxin, are zinc metalloproteases that cleave specific components of the synaptic vesicle membrane docking and fusion complex. Botulinum toxin inhibits release of acetylcholine at the neuromuscular junction. Clinically, early nervous system involvement leads to respiratory paralysis. The mortality rate in untreated cases is high.

Clinical Findings

A. Symptoms and Signs: Twelve to 36 hours after ingestion of the toxin, visual disturbances appear, particularly diplopia and loss of accommodation. Ptosis, cranial nerve palsies with impairment of extraocular muscles, and fixed dilated pupils are characteristic signs. The sensory examination is normal. Other symptoms are dry mouth, dysphagia, and dysphonia. Nausea and vomiting may be present, particularly with type E toxin. The sensorium remains clear and the temperature normal. Respiratory paralysis may lead to death unless mechanical assistance is provided.

B. Laboratory Findings: Toxin in patients' serum and in suspected foods may be shown by mouse inoculation and identified with specific antiserum.

Differential Diagnosis

Cranial nerve involvement suggests vertebrobasilar insufficiency, the C. Miller Fisher variant of Guillain-Barré syndrome, myasthenia gravis, or any basilar meningitis, infectious or carcinomatous. Intestinal obstruction or other types of food poisoning are considered when nausea and vomiting are present.

Treatment

If botulism is suspected, the physician should contact the state health authorities or the Centers for Disease Control and Prevention for advice and help with procurement of botulinus antitoxin and for assistance in obtaining assays for toxin in serum, stool, or food. During off hours, the CDC provides assistance via a recorded message at 404-639-2206.

Respiratory failure is managed with intubation and

mechanical ventilation. Parenteral fluids or alimentation should be given while swallowing difficulty persists.

The removal of unabsorbed toxin from the gut may be attempted. Any remnants of suspected foods should be assayed for toxin. Persons who might have eaten the suspected food must be located and observed.

Pellizzari R et al: Tetanus and botulinum neurotoxins: mechanism of action and therapeutic uses. Philos Trans R Soc London B Biol Sci 1999;354:259. [NLM Cit ID: 99228944]

Shapiro RL et al: Botulism in the United States: A clinical and epidemiologic review. Ann Intern Med 1998;129: 221. [NLM Cit ID: 98348297]

ANTHRAX

Anthrax is a disease of sheep, cattle, horses, goats, and swine caused by *Bacillus anthracis,* a gram-positive spore-forming aerobic rod. The organism is transmitted to humans by inoculation of broken skin or mucous membranes or by inhalation, causing either cutaneous or pulmonary infection. Anthrax is a rare occupational disease of farmers, veterinarians, and tannery and wool workers; prospective military use of the organism may result in future cases.

In cutaneous anthrax, an erythematous papule appears on an exposed area of skin and becomes vesicular, with a purple to black center. The surrounding area is edematous and vesicular. The center of the lesion finally forms a necrotic eschar and sloughs. Regional adenopathy, fever, malaise, headache, and nausea and vomiting may be present. After the eschar sloughs, hematogenous spread and sepsis may occur, resulting in shock, cyanosis, sweating, and collapse. Hemorrhagic meningitis may also occur.

Pulmonary anthrax follows inhalation of spores from hides, bristles, or wool. It is characterized by fever, malaise, headache, dyspnea, and cough; congestion of the nose, throat, and larynx; and evidence of pneumonia or mediastinitis.

Culture of sputum, blood, or a skin lesion may be positive for *B anthracis.* Smears of skin lesions show gram-positive encapsulated rods.

The mortality rate is high despite proper therapy, especially in pulmonary disease. Penicillin G, 2 million units intravenously every 4 hours, is the therapy of choice. Tetracycline, 500 mg orally every 6 hours, may be used for mild, localized cutaneous infection.

Dixon TC et al: Anthrax. N Engl J Med 1999;341:815. [NLM Cit ID: 99393048]

Franz DR et al: Clinical recognition and management of patients exposed to biological warfare agents. JAMA 1997;278:399. [NLM Cit ID: 97386483]

Shafazand S et al: Inhalational anthrax: epidemiology, diagnosis, and management. Chest 1999;116:1369. [NLM Cit ID: 20025853]

DIPHTHERIA

Essentials of Diagnosis

- Tenacious gray membrane at portal of entry in pharynx.
- Sore throat, nasal discharge, hoarseness, malaise, fever.
- Myocarditis, neuropathy.
- Culture confirms the diagnosis.

General Considerations

Diphtheria is an acute infection, caused by *Corynebacterium diphtheriae,* that usually attacks the respiratory tract but may involve any mucous membrane or skin wound. The organism is spread chiefly by respiratory secretions. Exotoxin produced by the organism is responsible for myocarditis and neuropathy. This exotoxin inhibits elongation factor, which is required for protein synthesis.

Clinical Findings

A. Symptoms and Signs: Nasal, laryngeal, pharyngeal, and cutaneous forms of diphtheria occur. Nasal infection produces few symptoms other than a nasal discharge. Laryngeal infection may lead to upper airway and bronchial obstruction. In pharyngeal diphtheria, the most common form, a tenacious gray membrane covers the tonsils and pharynx. Mild sore throat, fever, and malaise are followed by toxemia and prostration.

Myocarditis and neuropathy are the most common and most serious complications. Myocarditis causes cardiac arrhythmias, heart block, and heart failure. The neuropathy usually involves the cranial nerves first, producing diplopia, slurred speech, and difficulty in swallowing.

B. Laboratory Findings: The diagnosis is made clinically but can be confirmed by culture of the organism.

Differential Diagnosis

Diphtheria must be differentiated from streptococcal pharyngitis, infectious mononucleosis, adenovirus or herpes simplex infection, Vincent's angina, and candidiasis. A presumptive diagnosis of diphtheria must be made on clinical grounds without waiting for laboratory verification, since emergency treatment is needed.

Prevention

Active immunization with diphtheria toxoid is part of routine childhood immunization (usually as DTP) with appropriate booster injections. The immunization schedule for adults is the same as for tetanus. In order to avoid major allergic reactions, only the "adult type" toxoid (Td) should be used.

Susceptible persons exposed to diphtheria should receive a booster dose of diphtheria toxoid plus active immunization if not previously immunized, as well as a course of penicillin or erythromycin.

Treatment

Antitoxin, which is prepared from horse serum, must be given in all cases when diphtheria is suspected. For mild early pharyngeal or laryngeal disease, the dose is 20,000–40,000 units; for moderate nasopharyngeal disease, 40,000–60,000 units; for severe, extensive, or late (3 days or more) disease, 80,000–100,000 units. Diphtheria equine antitoxin can be obtained from the Centers for Disease Control and Prevention.

Removal of membrane by direct laryngoscopy or bronchoscopy may be necessary to prevent or alleviate airway obstruction.

Either penicillin, 250 mg orally four times daily, or erythromycin, 500 mg orally four times daily, for 14 days is effective therapy, though erythromycin is slightly more effective in eliminating the carrier state. The patient should be isolated until three consecutive cultures at the completion of therapy have documented elimination of the organism from the oropharynx. Contacts to a case should receive erythromycin, 500 mg four times daily for 7 days, to eradicate carriage.

LISTERIOSIS

Listeria monocytogenes is a motile, gram-positive rod that is a facultative intracellular organism capable of invading several cell types. Most cases of infection caused by *L monocytogenes* are sporadic, but outbreaks have been traced to eating contaminated food, especially unpasteurized dairy products. Five types of infection are recognized:

(1) Infection during pregnancy, usually in the last trimester, is a mild febrile illness without an apparent primary focus. This is a relatively benign disease for both mother and fetus that may resolve without specific therapy.

(2) Granulomatosis infantisepticum is a neonatal infection acquired in utero and characterized by disseminated abscesses and granulomas and by a high mortality rate.

(3) Bacteremia with or without sepsis syndrome is an infection of neonates or immunocompromised adults. The presentation is that of a febrile illness without a recognized source.

(4) Meningitis caused by *L monocytogenes* affects infants under 2 months of age and adults, ranking third and fourth, respectively, among the common causes of bacterial meningitis. Adults with meningitis are usually immunocompromised, and cases have been associated with HIV infection. Cerebrospinal fluid shows a *neutrophilic* pleocytosis.

(5) Finally, focal infections, including adenitis, brain abscess, endocarditis, osteomyelitis, and arthritis, occur rarely.

Therapy of infections caused by listeria is controversial with respect both to the most effective agent and the duration of treatment. The drug of choice is probably ampicillin, 8–12 g/d intravenously in four to six divided doses (the higher dose being recommended in cases of meningitis). It has relatively good penetration into cerebrospinal fluid, and, although there are few data, the response to ampicillin seems to be better than that to penicillin, erythromycin, or chloramphenicol. Gentamicin is synergistic with ampicillin against listeria in vitro and in animal models, and the use of combination therapy may for that reason be considered during the first few days of treatment to enhance eradication of organisms. Mortality and morbidity rates still are high, and relapse does occur, perhaps related to poor penetration of ampicillin into cells where organisms reside. Anecdotal clinical data indicating efficacy of trimethoprim-sulfamethoxazole and its excellent penetration into cells and into the cerebrospinal fluid support its use for therapy of listeriosis. The dose is 10–20 mg/kg/d of the trimethoprim component. Therapy should be administered for at least 2–3 weeks. Longer durations—between 3 and 6 weeks—have been recommended for treatment of meningitis, especially in severely immunocompromised patients.

Charpentier E et al: Antibiotic resistance in *Listeria* spp. Antimicrob Agents Chemother 1999;43:2103. [NLM Cit ID: 99402661]

Silver HM: Listeriosis during pregnancy. Obstet Gynecol Surv 1998;53:737. [NLM Cit ID: 99087059]

INFECTIVE ENDOCARDITIS

Essentials of Diagnosis

- Preexisting organic heart lesion.
- Fever.
- New or changing heart murmur.
- Evidence of systemic emboli.
- Positive blood culture.
- Evidence of vegetation on echocardiography.

General Considerations

Important factors that determine the clinical presentation are (1) the nature of the infecting organism; (2) which valve or valves are infected; and (3) the route of infection, since endocarditis in intravenous drug users and infections acquired during open heart surgery have special features.

More virulent organisms—*Staphylococcus aureus* in particular—tend to produce a more rapidly progressive and destructive infection. Patients are more likely to present with acute febrile illnesses, early embolization, and acute valvular regurgitation and myocardial abscess formation. Still, these organisms can produce a more gradual illness, and more indolent organisms can occasionally cause the acute presentation. Viridans strains of streptococci, enterococci, and a variety of other gram-positive and gram-negative bacilli, yeasts, and fungi tend to cause a more subacute picture. Systemic and peripheral manifestations may predominate. Acute deterioration due to valve perforations or large emboli may supervene at any time.

Most patients who develop infective endocarditis have underlying cardiac disease, though this is not the case with intravenous drug users and hospital-acquired infections. Abnormal valves or endocardial changes due to jet flow effects in congenital lesions (most commonly ventricular septal defect, tetralogy of Fallot, coarctation of the aorta, or patent ductus arteriosus) provide a nidus for infection during bacteremic episodes. Predisposing valvular abnormalities include rheumatic involvement of any valve, bicuspid aortic valves, calcific or sclerotic aortic valves (which are very common in elderly hypertensives), hypertrophic subaortic stenosis, and mitral valve prolapse. In the past, rheumatic disease was the commonest predisposing condition; this is no longer the case in developed countries.

The initiating event in infective endocarditis is colonization of the valve by bacteria during a transient or persistent bacteremia. Transient bacteremia is common during dental, upper respiratory, urologic, and lower gastrointestinal diagnostic and surgical procedures. It is less common during upper gastrointestinal and gynecologic procedures, though a high incidence has been reported during suction abortion.

Approximately 90% of cases of native valve endocarditis are due to viridans streptococci (60%), *S aureus* (20%), and enterococci (5–10%). Gram-negative organisms and fungi account for a small percentage.

The microbiology of native valve endocarditis in intravenous drug users differs from that of other patients. *S aureus* accounts for 60% or more of all cases and for 80–90% of cases in which the tricuspid valve is infected. Enterococci and streptococci comprise the balance in about equal proportions. Gram-negative aerobic bacilli, fungi, and unusual organisms that rarely infect others may cause endocarditis in intravenous drug users.

The microbiology of prosthetic valve endocarditis also is distinctive. Early infections (ie, those occurring within 2 months after valve implantation) are commonly caused by staphylococci—both coagulase-positive and coagulase-negative—gram-negative organisms, and fungi. Late prosthetic valve endocarditis resembles native valve endocarditis, with the majority of infections caused by streptococci, though coagulase-negative staphylococci still cause a significant proportion of cases.

Clinical Findings

A. Symptoms and Signs: Most patients present with a febrile illness that has lasted several days to 2 weeks. Nonspecific symptoms are common. Cough, dyspnea, arthralgias or arthritis, diarrhea, and abdominal or flank pain may occur as a result of embolization or immunologically mediated phenomena. The initial symptoms or signs of endocarditis may be caused by arterial emboli or cardiac damage.

Most patients have readily documented fever, though fever may be absent in older individuals. Ninety percent have heart murmurs, but murmurs may be absent in patients with right-sided infections. The characteristic peripheral lesions—petechiae (on the palate or conjunctiva or beneath the fingernails); subungual ("splinter") hemorrhages; Osler nodes (painful, violaceous raised lesions of the fingers, toes, or feet); Janeway lesions (painless erythematous lesions of the palms or soles); and Roth spots (exudative lesions in the retina)—occur in 20–25% of patients. Pallor and splenomegaly are other helpful signs.

In acute endocarditis, leukocytosis is common; in subacute cases, anemia of chronic disease and a normal white count are the rule. Hematuria and proteinuria as well as renal dysfunction may result from emboli or immunologically mediated glomerulonephritis.

B. Diagnostic Studies: Blood culture is the single most important procedure for diagnosis of endocarditis. The current recommendation for maximizing the yield of blood cultures is to obtain three sets of blood cultures at least 1 hour apart before starting antibiotics. Even when this is done, a small but significant number of infected patients (up to 5% of cases) will be culture-negative, which is usually attributable to administration of antimicrobials prior to obtaining cultures. If antimicrobial therapy has been administered prior to cultures and the patient is clinically stable, it is reasonable to withhold further antimicrobial therapy for 2–3 days so that appropriate cultures can be obtained. These cases may also be due to a fungus (50% of patients with fungal endocarditis have negative blood cultures), organisms that require special media for growth (eg, legionella species, bartonella species, nutritionally deficient streptococci), organisms that do not grow on artificial media (agents of Q fever, psittacosis), or organisms that are slow-growing and may require several weeks to grow (eg, brucella, anaerobes, certain haemophilus species, *Actinobacillus actinomycetemcomitans, Cardiobacterium hominis, Eikenella corrodens,* and kingella species).

The chest x-ray may show evidence for the underlying cardiac abnormality and, in right-sided endocarditis, pulmonary infiltrates. The ECG is nondiagnostic. Changing conduction abnormalities suggest myocardial abscess formation.

Echocardiography is useful in diagnosis and may provide adjunctive information about the specific valve or valves that are infected. The sensitivity of transthoracic echocardiography is between 55% and 65%; therefore, it cannot reliably rule out endocarditis but may confirm a clinical suspicion. Transesophageal echocardiography is 90% sensitive in detecting vegetations and is particularly useful for identifying valve ring abscesses as well as pulmonary and prosthetic valve endocarditis.

Clinical criteria (commonly referred to as the Duke criteria) for the diagnosis of endocarditis have been proposed. Major criteria include (1) a positive blood culture for a microorganism that typically causes infective endocarditis from two separate blood cultures; and (2) evidence of endocardial involvement documented by echocardiography (definite vegetation, myocardial abscess, or new partial dehiscence of a prosthetic valve) or development of a new regurgitant murmur. Minor criteria include (1) the presence of a predisposing condition; (2) fever ≥ 38 °C; (3) embolic disease; (4) immunologic phenomena (glomerulonephritis, Osler nodes, Roth spots, rheumatoid factor); (5) positive blood cultures but not meeting the major criteria; and (6) a positive echocardiogram but not meeting the major criteria. A definite diagnosis can be made with 80% accuracy if two major criteria, one major criterion and three minor criteria, or five minor criteria are fulfilled. If none of these criteria are met and either an alternative explanation for illness is identified or the patient has defervesced within 4 days, endocarditis is highly unlikely.

Complications

The clinical course of infective endocarditis is determined by the degree of damage to the heart, by the site of infection (right- versus left-sided, aortic versus mitral valve), by whether embolization from the site of infection occurs, and by immunologically mediated processes. Destruction of infected heart valves is especially common and precipitous with *S aureus* and often enterococci but can occur with any organism. The resulting regurgitation can be mild or severe and can progress even after bacteriologic cure. The infection can also extend into the myocardium, resulting in abscesses leading to conduction disturbances, and can also involve the wall of the aorta, creating sinus of Valsalva aneurysms.

Peripheral embolization can occur with any organism. The most catastrophic are cerebral and myocardial embolizations, with resulting infarctions. The spleen and kidneys are also common sites. Peripheral emboli may initiate metastatic infections or may become established in vessel walls, leading to mycotic aneurysms. Right-sided endocarditis, which usually involves the tricuspid valve, often leads to septic pulmonary emboli, causing infarction and lung abscesses.

Prevention

Some cases of endocarditis occur after dental procedures or operations involving the upper respiratory, genitourinary, or intestinal tract. Prophylactic antibiotics should be given to patients with predisposing congenital or valvular anomalies who are to have any of these procedures (Tables 33–2 and 33–3). Current recommendations are given in Table 33–4.

Treatment

Empirical regimens for endocarditis while culture results are pending should include agents active against staphylococci, streptococci, and enterococci. Nafcillin or oxacillin, 1.5 g every 4 hours, plus penicillin, 2–3 million units every 4 hours (or ampicillin, 1.5 g every 4 hours), plus gentamicin, 1 mg/kg every 8 hours, is such a regimen. Vancomycin, 15 mg/kg every 12 hours, may be used instead of the penicillins in the penicillin-allergic patient.

Table 33–2. Cardiac lesions for which bacterial endocarditis prophylaxis is or is not recommended.[1,2]

Endocarditis prophylaxis recommended

1. High-risk category
   - Prosthetic cardiac valves, including bioprosthetic and homograft valves
   - Previous bacterial endocarditis, even in the absence of heart disease
   - Complex cyanotic congenital heart disease (eg, single ventricle states, transposition of the great arteries, tetralogy of Fallot)
   - Surgically constructed systemic pulmonary shunts or conduits
2. Moderate-risk category
   - Most congenital cardiac malformations (other than those listed above and below)
   - Rheumatic and other acquired valvular dysfunction, even after valvular surgery
   - Hypertrophic cardiomyopathy
   - Mitral valve prolapse with valvular regurgitation[3,4]

Endocarditis prophylaxis not recommended[5]

- Isolated secundum septal defect
- Surgical repair of atrial septal defect, ventricular septal defect, or patent ductus arteriosus (without residua beyond 6 months)
- Previous coronary artery bypass graft surgery
- Mitral valve prolapse without valvular regurgitation[6]
- Physiologic, functional, or innocent heart murmurs
- Previous Kawasaki disease without valvular dysfunction
- Previous rheumatic fever without valvular dysfunction
- Cardiac pacemakers (intravascular and epicardial) and implanted defibrillators

[1]Modified and reproduced, with permission, from Dajani AS et al: Prevention of bacterial endocarditis. Recommendations by the American Heart Association. JAMA 1997;277:1794. Copyright © 1997 by American Medical Association.
[2]This table lists selected conditions and is not meant to be all-inclusive.
[3]Mitral regurgitation determined by the presence of a murmur or by echo-Doppler.
[4]Men older than 45 without a consistent systolic murmur may warrant prophylaxis even in the absence of resting regurgitation.
[5]Negligible risk category—no greater than in the general population.
[6]Individuals who have a mitral valve prolapse associated with thickening or redundancy of the valve leaflets may be at increased risk for bacterial endocarditis.

Table 33–3. Procedures for which bacterial endocarditis prophylaxis is or is not recommended.[1,2]

Endocarditis prophylaxis recommended[3]

1. Dental
   - Dental extractions
   - Periodontal procedures
   - Dental implant placement or reimplantation
   - Endodontic (root canal) instrumentation or surgery only beyond the apex
   - Subgingival placement of antibiotic fibers or strips
   - Initial placement of orthodontic bands but not brackets
   - Intraligamentary local anesthetic injections
   - Prophylactic cleaning of teeth or implants where bleeding is anticipated
2. Respiratory tract
   - Tonsillectomy, adenoidectomy
   - Surgical operations that involve intestinal or respiratory mucosa
   - Bronchoscopy with a rigid bronchoscope
3. Gastrointestinal tract[4]
   - Sclerotherapy for esophageal varices
   - Esophageal stricture dilation
   - Endoscopic retrograde cholangiography with biliary obstruction
   - Biliary tract surgery
   - Surgical operations that involve intestinal mucosa
4. Genitourinary tract
   - Prostatic surgery
   - Cystoscopy
   - Urethral dilation

Endocarditis prophylaxis not recommended

1. Dental
   - Restorative dentistry (filling cavities, operative and prosthodontic) with or without retraction cord[5]
   - Local anesthetic injections (nonintraligamentary)
   - Intracanal endodontic treatment; post placement and buildup
   - Placement of rubber dams, removable prosthodontic, or orthodontic appliances
   - Postoperative suture removal
   - Taking of oral impression
   - Fluoride treatments
   - Orthodontic appliance adjustment
2. Respiratory
   - Endotracheal intubation
   - Bronchoscopy with a flexible bronchoscope, with or without biopsy[6]
   - Tympanostomy (insertion)
3. Gastrointestinal
   - Transesophageal echocardiography[6]
   - Endoscopy with or without gastrointestinal biopsy[6]
4. Genitourinary tract
   - Vaginal hysterectomy[6]
   - Vaginal delivery[6]
   - Cesarean section
   - In the absence of infection:
     - Urethral catheterization
     - Uterine dilation and curettage
     - Therapeutic abortion
     - Sterilization procedures
     - Insertion or removal of intrauterine devices
5. Other
   - Cardiac catheterization, including balloon angioplasty
   - Implanting cardiac pacemakers or defibrillators and coronary stents
   - Incision or biopsy of surgically scrubbed skin
   - Circumcision

[1]Reproduced, with permission, from Dajani AS et al: Prevention of bacterial endocarditis. Recommendation by the American Heart Association. JAMA 1997;277:1794. Copyright © 1997 by American Medical Association.
[2]This table lists selected procedures but is not meant to be all-inclusive.
[3]Recommended for individuals with high- and moderate-risk cardiac conditions (Table 33–2).
[4]Prophylaxis is recommended for high-risk patients, optional for moderate-risk patients.
[5]Clinical judgment may indicate antibiotic use in selected circumstances that may create significant bleeding.
[6]Prophylaxis is optional for high-risk patients.

A. Viridans Streptococci: For penicillin-susceptible viridans streptococcal endocarditis (ie, MIC ≤ 0.1 μg/mL), penicillin G, 2–3 million units intravenously every 4 hours for 4 weeks, is recommended. The duration of therapy can be shortened to 2 weeks if gentamicin, 1 mg/kg every 8 hours, is used with penicillin. Ceftriaxone, 2 g once daily intravenously or intramuscularly for 4 weeks, is also effective therapy for penicillin-susceptible strains and is a convenient regimen for home therapy. For the penicillin-allergic patient, vancomycin, 15 mg/kg every 12 hours for 4 weeks should be used. Two-week regimens with aminoglycosides have not been studied with any agent other than penicillin. Thus, if ceftriaxone or vancomycin is used to treat susceptible strains, a 4-week course is needed. The 2-week regimen is not recommended for patients with symptoms of more than 3 months' duration or patients with complications such as myocardial abscess or extracardiac infection. Prosthetic valve endocarditis should be treated with a 6-week course of penicillin with at least 2 weeks of gentamicin.

Viridans streptococci that are relatively resistant to penicillin (ie, MIC > 0.1 μg/mL but ≤ 0.5 μg/mL) should be treated for 4 weeks. Penicillin G, 3 million units intravenously every 4 hours is combined with gentamicin, 1 mL/kg every 8 hours for the first 2 weeks. In the patient with IgE-mediated allergy to penicillin, vancomycin alone, 15 mg/kg every 12 hours for 4 weeks, should be administered.

Viridans streptococci with an MIC > 0.5 μg/mL and nutritionally deficient streptococci should be treated like enterococci (see below).

B. Other Streptococci: Endocarditis caused by *Streptococcus pneumoniae, Streptococcus pyogenes* (group A streptococcus), and groups B, C, and G streptococci are unusual causes of endocarditis, and large studies to determine efficacy of antibiotic regimens have not been published. *S pneumoniae* sensitive to penicillin (MIC < 0.1 μg/mL) can be treated with penicillin alone, 2–3 million units every 4 hours for 4–6 weeks. Strains resistant to penicillin (MIC > 0.1 μg/mL) are being reported with increasing frequency, and optimal therapy is not known, though

Table 33–4. Endocarditis prophylaxis.[1,2]

	DENTAL, RESPIRATORY, OR ESOPHAGEAL PROCEDURES	
Oral	Amoxicillin	2 g 1 hour before procedure
Penicillin allergy	Clindamycin	600 mg 1 hour before procedure
	or	
	Cephalexin or cefadroxil[3]	2 g 1 hour before procedure
	or	
	Azithromycin or clarithromycin	500 mg 1 hour before procedure
Parenteral	Ampicillin	2 g IM or IV 30 minutes before procedure
Penicillin allergy	Clindamycin	600 mg IV 1 hour before procedure
	or	
	Cefazolin[3]	1 g IM or IV 30 minutes before procedure
	GASTROINTESTINAL (EXCEPT ESOPHAGEAL) OR GENITOURINARY PROCEDURES	
High-risk patient (Table 33–1)	Ampicillin plus gentamicin	Ampicillin, 2 g IM or IV, plus gentamicin, 1.5 mg/kg (not to exceed 120 mg) 30 minutes before procedure; 6 hours later, ampicillin, 1 g IM or IV, or amoxicillin, 1 g orally
Penicillin allergy	Vancomycin plus gentamicin	Vancomycin, 1 g IV over 1–2 hours, plus gentamicin, 1.5 mg/kg (not to exceed 120 mg) IV or IM; complete infusion or injection 30 minutes before procedure
Moderate-risk patient	Amoxicillin or ampicillin	Amoxicillin, 2 g orally 1 hour before procedure, or ampicillin, 2 g IM or IV 30 minutes before starting procedure
Penicillin allergy	Vancomycin	Vancomycin, 1 g IV over 1–2 hours; complete infusion 30 minutes before procedure

[1]Modified and reproduced, with permission, from Dajani AS et al: Prevention of bacterial endocarditis. Recommendations by the American Heart Association. JAMA 1997;277:1794. Copyright © 1997 by American Medical Association.
[2]Viridans streptococci are the most common cause of endocarditis occurring after dental or upper respiratory procedures; enterococci are the most common cause after gastrointestinal or genitourinary procedures.
[3]Cephalosporins should not be used in individuals with immediate type hypersensitivity reactions to penicillin.

vancomycin should be effective based on in vitro data. Group A streptococcal infection can be treated with penicillin, ceftriaxone, or vancomycin for 4–6 weeks. Groups B, C, and G streptococci tend to be more resistant to penicillin than group A streptococci, and some have recommended adding gentamicin, 1 mg/kg every 8 hours, to penicillin for the first 2 weeks of a 4- to 6-week course.

C. Enterococci: For enterococcal endocarditis, the relapse rate is unacceptably high when penicillin is used alone; either streptomycin or gentamicin must be included in the regimen. Because aminoglycoside resistance occurs in enterococci, susceptibility to it should be documented. Gentamicin is the aminoglycoside of choice, because streptomycin resistance is more common than gentamicin resistance and the nephrotoxicity of gentamicin is generally more easily managed than the vestibular toxicity of streptomycin. Ampicillin, 2 g intravenously every 4 hours, or penicillin G, 3–4 million units every 4 hours (or, in the penicillin-allergic patient, vancomycin, 15 mg/kg every 12 hours), plus gentamicin, 1 mg/kg every 8 hours, is recommended. Standard practice is to continue this regimen for at least 4 weeks, and patients at high risk for relapse (those with symptoms of more than 3 months' duration or those with prosthetic valve endocarditis) should be treated for 6 weeks. Experience is more extensive with penicillin and ampicillin than with vancomycin for therapy of enterococcal endocarditis, and penicillin and ampicillin are superior to vancomycin in in vitro studies. Thus, whenever possible, either ampicillin or penicillin should be used. If endocarditis is caused by an organism that demonstrates high-level resistance to aminoglycosides (ie, not inhibited by 500 μg/mL of gentamicin), then the addition of an aminoglycoside will not be beneficial. Therapy with high doses of penicillin (eg, 6 g/d) administered as a continuous infusion, is recommended for 8–12 weeks, but the relapse rate may be as high as 50%. Surgery may be the only option in such situations.

D. Staphylococci: For methicillin-susceptible *S aureus,* nafcillin or oxacillin, 1.5 g every 4 hours for 4–6 weeks, is the preferred therapy. For penicillin-allergic patients, cefazolin, 2 g intravenously every 8 hours, or vancomycin, 15 mg/kg every 12 hours, may be used. For methicillin-resistant strains, vancomycin is the only agent of proved effectiveness. Aminoglycoside combination regimens may be useful in shortening the duration of bacteremia. Their maximum benefit is achieved at low doses (1 mg/kg every 8 hours) and in the first 3–5 days of therapy, and they should not be continued beyond the early phase of therapy. For treatment of tricuspid valve endocarditis (with or without pulmonary involvement) in the injection drug user who does not have serious extrapulmonary sites of infection, the total duration of therapy can be shortened from 4 weeks to 2 weeks if an aminoglycoside is added to an antistaphylococcal drug for the entire 2 weeks of therapy. The effect of rifampin with antistaphylococcal drugs is variable, and its routine use is not recommended.

Because coagulase-negative staphylococci—a common cause of prosthetic valve endocarditis—are routinely resistant to methicillin, β-lactam antibiotics should not be used for this infection until the isolate is known to be susceptible. A combination of vancomycin for 6 weeks, rifampin, 300 mg every 8 hours for 6 weeks, and gentamicin, 1 mg/kg every 8 hours for the first 2 weeks, is the regimen of choice. If the organism is sensitive to methicillin, either nafcillin or oxacillin or cefazolin can be used in combination with rifampin and gentamicin. Combination therapy with nafcillin or oxacillin (vancomycin for methicillin-resistant strains or patients allergic to β-lactams), rifampin, and gentamicin is also recommended for treatment of *S aureus* prosthetic valve infection.

E. HACEK Organisms: HACEK organisms *(Haemophilus aphrophilus, Haemophilus parainfluenzae, Actinobacillus actinomycetemcomitans, Cardiobacterium hominis, Eikenella corrodens,* and *Kingella kingae)* are slow-growing, fastidious gram-negative coccobacilli or bacilli that are normal oral flora and cause about 5–10% of all cases of endocarditis. These organisms can produce β-lactamase, and thus the treatment of choice is ceftriaxone (or some other third-generation cephalosporin), 2 g once daily for 4 weeks. Prosthetic valve endocarditis should be treated for 6 weeks. In the penicillin-allergic patient, experience is limited, but trimethoprim-sulfamethoxazole, quinolones, and aztreonam have in vitro activity and should be considered.

F. Role of Surgery: While most cases can be successfully treated medically, operative management is sometimes required. Valvular regurgitation resulting in acute heart failure that does not resolve promptly after institution of medical therapy is an indication for valve replacement even if active infection is present, especially if the aortic valve is involved. Infections that do not respond to appropriate antimicrobial therapy after 7–10 days (ie, persistent fevers, positive blood cultures despite therapy) are more likely to be eradicated if the valve is replaced. Surgery is nearly always required for fungal endocarditis and is more often necessary with gram-negative bacilli. Surgery is also indicated when the infection involves the sinus of Valsalva or produces septal abscesses. Recurrent infection with the same organism often indicates that surgery is necessary, especially with infected prosthetic valves. Continuing embolization presents a difficult problem when the infection is otherwise responding but may be an indication for surgery. Embolization after bacteriologic cure, however, does not necessarily imply recurrence of endocarditis.

G. Role of Anticoagulation: Anticoagulation is contraindicated in native valve endocarditis because it imposes a greatly increased risk of intracerebral hemorrhage. The role of anticoagulant therapy during active prosthetic valve endocarditis is more controversial. Reversal of anticoagulation may result in thrombosis of the mechanical prosthesis, particularly in the mitral position. On the other hand, anticoagulation during active prosthetic valve endocarditis caused by *S aureus* has been associated with fatal intracerebral hemorrhage. Therefore, anticoagulation probably should be stopped during the septic phase of *S aureus* prosthetic valve endocarditis or if intracerebral hemorrhage has occurred as a complication of endocarditis due to any cause. Indications for anticoagulation following prosthetic valve implantation for endocarditis are the same as for patients with prosthetic valves without endocarditis (eg, nonporcine mechanical valves and valves in the mitral position).

Response to Therapy

If infection is caused by viridans streptococci, enterococci, or coagulase-negative staphylococci, defervescence occurs in 3–4 days on average, whereas if infection is caused by *Staphylococcus aureus* or *Pseudomonas aeruginosa,* patients may remain febrile for 9–12 days. If fevers persist, blood cultures should be obtained to ensure adequacy of therapy. Other causes of persistent fever are myocardial or metastatic abscess, sterile embolization, superimposed nosocomial infection, and drug reaction. Careful posttreatment monitoring is critical. Most relapses occur within 1–2 months after completion of therapy. Obtaining one or two blood cultures during this period allows for early detection of recurrent infection.

Bayer AS et al: Diagnosis and management of infective endocarditis and its complications. Circulation 1998;98:2936. [NLM Cit ID: 99077741]

Dajani AS et al: Prevention of bacterial endocarditis: Recommendations by the American Heart Association. JAMA 1997;277:1794. [NLM Cit ID: 97322139]

Röder BL et al: Clinical features of *Staphylococcus aureus* endocarditis: A 10-year experience in Denmark. Arch Intern Med 1999;159:462. [NLM Cit ID: 99173249]

Segreti J: Is antibiotic prophylaxis necessary for preventing prosthetic device infection? Infect Dis Clin North Am 1999;13:871. [NLM Cit ID: 20046075] (This article addresses the paucity of evidence for antibiotic prophylaxis.)

Strom BL et al: Dental and cardiac risk factors for infective endocarditis. A population-based, case-control study. Ann Intern Med 1998;129:761. [NLM Cit ID: 99015312]

Tornos P et al: Infective endocarditis due to *Staphylococcus aureus:* Deleterious effect of anticoagulant therapy. 1999. Intern Med 1999;159:473. [NLM Cit ID: 99173250]

Wilson WR et al: Antibiotic treatment of adults with infective endocarditis due to streptococci, enterococci, staphylococci, and HACEK microorganisms. JAMA 1995;274:1706. [NLM Cit ID: 96088939]

INFECTIONS CAUSED BY GRAM-NEGATIVE BACTERIA

BORDETELLA PERTUSSIS INFECTION (Whooping Cough)

Essentials of Diagnosis

- Predominantly in infants under age 2 years. Adults are an important reservoir of infection.
- Two-week prodromal catarrhal stage of malaise, cough, coryza, and anorexia.
- Paroxysmal cough ending in a high-pitched inspiratory "whoop."
- Absolute lymphocytosis, often striking; culture confirms diagnosis.

General Considerations

Pertussis is an acute infection of the respiratory tract caused by *Bordetella pertussis* that is transmitted by respiratory droplets. The incubation period is 7–17 days. Half of all cases occur before age 2 years. Neither immunization nor disease confers lasting immunity to pertussis. Consequently, adults are an important reservoir of the disease.

Clinical Findings

The symptoms of classic pertussis last about 6 weeks and are divided into three consecutive stages. The catarrhal stage is characterized by its insidious onset, with lacrimation, sneezing, and coryza, anorexia and malaise, and a hacking night cough that tends to become diurnal. The paroxysmal stage is characterized by bursts of rapid, consecutive coughs followed by a deep, high-pitched inspiration (whoop). The convalescent stage usually begins 4 weeks after onset of the illness with a decrease in the frequency and severity of paroxysms of cough. The diagnosis often is not considered in adults, who may not have a typical presentation. Cough persisting more than 2 weeks is suggestive of pertussis. Infection may also be asymptomatic.

The white blood cell count is usually 15,000–20,000/μL (rarely, as high as 50,000/μL or more), 60–80% of which are lymphocytes. The diagnosis is established by isolating the organism from nasopharyngeal culture. A special medium (eg, Bordet-Gengou agar) must be requested.

Prevention

Active immunization with pertussis vaccine is recommended for all infants, usually combined with diphtheria and tetanus toxoids (DTP). Infants and susceptible adults with significant exposure to pertussis should receive prophylaxis with erythromycin (40 mg/kg/d, up to 2 g/d, for 10 days). Booster doses of pertussis vaccine have not been recommended after age 6 except to control outbreaks. Recognition of adults as an important reservoir of infection and development of an effective acellular vaccine with fewer side effects than the whole cell vaccine undoubtedly will prompt a reevaluation of the current recommendations for vaccination of adults.

Treatment

Erythromycin, 500 mg four times a day orally for 10 days, shortens the duration of carriage. It also may diminish the severity of coughing paroxysms.

Cherry JD: Epidemiological, clinical, and laboratory aspects of pertussis in adults. Clin Infect Dis 1999;28 (Suppl 2):S112. [NLM Cit ID: 99374694] (Illustrates the atypical presentation in adults and emphasizes that pertussis is not exclusively a childhood disease.)

Hewlett EL: A commentary on the pathogenesis of pertussis. Clin Infect Dis 1999;28(Suppl 2):S94. [NLM Cit ID: 99374691]

MENINGOCOCCAL MENINGITIS

Essentials of Diagnosis

- Fever, headache, vomiting, confusion, delirium, convulsions.
- Petechial rash of skin and mucous membranes in many.
- Neck and back stiffness with positive Kernig and Brudzinski signs is characteristic.
- Purulent spinal fluid with gram-negative intracellular and extracellular diplococci.
- Culture of cerebrospinal fluid, blood, or petechial aspiration confirms the diagnosis.

General Considerations

Meningococcal meningitis is caused by *Neisseria meningitidis* of groups A, B, C, Y, W-135, and others. Meningitis due to serogroup A is uncommon in the United States. Serogroup B generally causes sporadic cases. The frequency of outbreaks of meningitis caused by group C meningococcus has increased in recent years, and this serotype is the most common cause of epidemic disease in the United States. Up to 40% of persons are nasopharyngeal carriers of meningococci, but relatively few develop disease. Infection is transmitted by droplets. The clinical illness may take the form of meningococcemia (a fulminant form of septicemia without meningitis), meningococcemia with meningitis, or predominantly meningitis. Chronic recurrent meningococcemia with fever, rash, and arthritis can occur, particular in those with terminal complement deficiencies (C7–C9).

Clinical Findings

A. Symptoms and Signs: High fever, chills, and headache; back, abdominal, and extremity pains; and nausea and vomiting are present. In severe cases, rapidly developing confusion, delirium, seizures, and coma occur.

On examination, nuchal and back rigidity are typical, with positive Kernig and Brudzinski signs. (Kernig's sign is pain in the hamstrings upon extension of the knee with the hip at 90-degree flexion; Brudzinski's sign is flexion of the knee in response to flexion of the neck.) A petechial rash often first appearing in the lower extremities and at pressure points is found in most cases. Petechiae may vary from pinhead-sized to large ecchymoses or even areas of skin gangrene that may later slough if the patient survives.

B. Laboratory Findings: Lumbar puncture typically reveals a cloudy or purulent cerebrospinal fluid, with elevated pressure, increased protein, and decreased glucose content. The fluid usually contains more than 1000 cells/μL, with polymorphonuclear cells predominating and containing gram-negative intracellular diplococci. The absence of organisms in a Gram-stained smear of the cerebrospinal fluid sediment does not rule out the diagnosis. The capsular polysaccharide can often be demonstrated in cerebrospinal fluid or urine by latex agglutination; this is especially useful in partially treated patients, though sensitivity is only 60–80%. The organism is usually demonstrated by smear or culture of the cerebrospinal fluid, oropharynx, blood, or aspirated petechiae.

Disseminated intravascular coagulation is an important complication of meningococcal infection. Prothrombin time and partial thromboplastin time are prolonged, fibrin dimers are elevated, fibrinogen is low, and the platelet count is depressed.

Differential Diagnosis

Meningococcal meningitis must be differentiated from other bacterial and viral meningitides. In small infants and in the elderly, the presentation may be atypical, without fever or stiff neck.

Rickettsial or echovirus infection and, rarely, other bacterial infections (eg, staphylococcal infections, scarlet fever) may also produce a petechial rash.

Prevention

Effective polysaccharide vaccines for groups A, C, Y, and W-135 are available. A and C vaccine has reduced the incidence of infections with these meningococcus groups in military recruits. The vaccines are effective for control of epidemics in civilian populations. The Advisory Committee on Immunization Practices now recommends immunization with a single dose of polyvalent vaccine (active against meningococcal groups A, C, Y, and W-135) for college freshmen—particularly those living in dormitories, who have been shown to have a modestly increased risk of invasive meningococcal disease.

Outbreaks in closed populations are best controlled by eliminating nasopharyngeal carriage of meningococci. Rifampin is the drug of choice; give 600 mg twice a day for 2 days. A single 500 mg oral dose of ciprofloxacin or one intramuscular 250 mg dose of ceftriaxone in adults is also effective.

Household members exposed to a person with meningococcal meningitis are at increased risk and should be given rifampin prophylaxis as outlined above. Day care center contacts are treated in the same manner. School and work contacts need not be treated. Hospital contacts need not be treated unless intense exposure has occurred (eg, mouth-to-mouth resuscitation).

Accidentally discovered carriers without known close contact with meningococcal disease do not require prophylactic antimicrobials.

Treatment

Blood cultures must be obtained and intravenous antimicrobial therapy started immediately. This may be done prior to lumbar puncture in patients in whom the diagnosis is not straightforward and who therefore require CT scanning to exclude mass lesions. Aqueous penicillin G is the antibiotic of choice (24 million units/24 h) in divided doses every 4 hours. In penicillin-allergic patients or those in whom *Haemophilus influenzae* or gram-negative meningitis is a consideration, ceftriaxone, 4 g intravenously once a day, should be used. Chloramphenicol, 1 g every 6 hours, is an alternative in the severely penicillin- or cephalosporin-allergic patient.

Treatment should be continued in full doses by the intravenous route until the patient is afebrile for 5 days. In the past, the recommended duration of therapy has been 7–10 days. More recent studies suggest that shorter courses—as few as 4 days if ceftriaxone is used—are also effective.

Obtundation or deterioration in mental status may result from cerebral edema and increased intracranial pressure. In critically ill patients with evidence of increased intracranial pressure, administration of dexamethasone (0.6 mg/kg/d in four divided doses) should be considered.

Heparinization is of theoretic value in disseminated intravascular coagulation and bleeding, but it does not influence prognosis.

Harrison LH et al: Risk of meningococcal infection in college students. JAMA 1999;281:1906. [NLM Cit ID: 99277397]

Peltola H: Prophylaxis of bacterial meningitis. Infect Dis Clin North Am 1999;13:685. [NLM Cit ID: 99399583]

Schuchat A et al: Bacterial meningitis in the United States in 1995. Active Surveillance Team. N Engl J Med

1997;337:970. [NLM Cit ID: 97441019] (Incidence of *H influenzae* meningitis in adults is falling because of vaccination of children.)

INFECTIONS CAUSED BY HAEMOPHILUS SPECIES

Haemophilus influenzae and other haemophilus species may cause sinusitis, otitis, bronchitis, epiglottitis, pneumonitis, cellulitis, arthritis, meningitis, and endocarditis. **Pneumonia** is one of the more common infections of adults caused by *H influenzae* type b, though nontypable strains actually are more common in HIV-infected patients. The presentation is that of a typical bacterial pneumonia, with purulent sputum containing a predominance of gram-negative, pleomorphic rods. Alcoholism, smoking, chronic lung disease, advanced age, and HIV infection are important risk factors. Haemophilus species frequently colonize the upper respiratory tract. Consequently, in the absence of positive pleural fluid or blood cultures, distinguishing pneumonia from colonization is difficult. Pneumonia from haemophilus species probably is overdiagnosed for this reason.

Beta-lactamase-producing strains are less common in adults than in children. For most adult patients with sinusitis, otitis, or respiratory tract infection, oral amoxicillin, 750 mg twice daily for 10–14 days, is adequate. For the penicillin-allergic patient, trimethoprim-sulfamethoxazole, 800 mg/160 mg, orally twice daily for 10–14 days, or azithromycin, 500 mg orally as a first dose and then 250 mg once a day for four days, is also effective.

In the more seriously ill patient (eg, the toxic patient with multilobar pneumonia), use of a second- or third-generation cephalosporin—cefuroxime, 750 mg every 8 hours, or ceftriaxone, 1 g/d—is advisable pending determination of whether the infecting strain is a β-lactamase producer. Trimethoprim-sulfamethoxazole, administered based on a dose of 10 mg/kg/d of trimethoprim, can be used for the penicillin-allergic patient. A 10- to 14-day course of therapy is adequate for most cases.

Epiglottitis, which occasionally occurs in adults, is characterized by an abrupt onset of high fever, drooling, and inability to handle secretions. Stridor and respiratory distress result from laryngeal obstruction. Early, elective intubation is recommended because airway obstruction may progress unpredictably and rapidly. The diagnosis is best made by direct visualization of the cherry-red, swollen epiglottis at laryngoscopy. Because laryngoscopy may provoke laryngospasm and obstruction, it should be performed in an intensive care unit or similar setting, and only at the time of intubation. Cefuroxime, 1.5 g every 8 hours for 7–10 days, or ceftriaxone, 1 g every 24 hours for 7–10 days, is the drug of choice. Trimethoprim-sulfamethoxazole (see above for dosage) or chloramphenicol, 4 g/d, may be used in the patient with serious penicillin allergy.

Meningitis, rare in adults, becomes a consideration in the patient who has meningitis associated with sinusitis or otitis. Initial therapy of suspected *H influenzae* meningitis should be with ceftriaxone, 4 g/d in one or two divided doses, until the strain is proved not to produce β-lactamase. Chloramphenicol, 100 mg/kg/d in four divided doses, can be used if the patient has a serious, life-threatening allergy to β-lactam antibiotics. Traditionally, meningitis has been treated for 10–14 days. Dexamethasone, 0.15 mg/kg intravenously every 6 hours, has been shown to be a valuable adjunctive agent in treatment of meningitis in infants and children, resulting in reduction in long-term sequelae, principally hearing loss. The role of steroids in adult meningitis is controversial.

INFECTIONS CAUSED BY *MORAXELLA CATARRHALIS*

Moraxella catarrhalis is a gram-negative aerobic coccus that is morphologically and biochemically similar to neisseria. This organism causes sinusitis, bronchitis, and pneumonia. Bacteremia and meningitis have also been reported in immunocompromised patients. The organism frequently colonizes the respiratory tract, and differentiation of colonization from infection can be difficult. If *M catarrhalis* is the predominant isolate, therapy should be directed against it. *M catarrhalis* typically produces β-lactamase and therefore is usually resistant to ampicillin and amoxicillin. It is susceptible to amoxicillin-clavulanate, ampicillin-sulbactam, trimethoprim-sulfamethoxazole, ciprofloxacin, and second- and third-generation cephalosporins. Treatment is similar to that for haemophilus infections.

McGregor K et al: *Moraxella catarrhalis:* clinical significance, antimicrobial susceptibility and BRO beta-lactamases. Eur J Clin Microbiol Infect Dis 1998;17:219. [NLM Cit ID: 98370801]

Niroumand M et al: Airway infection. Infect Dis Clin North Am 1998;12:671. [NLM Cit ID: 98452420] (Reviews common causes of upper airway infection in adults, including moraxella.)

LEGIONNAIRE'S DISEASE

Essentials of Diagnosis

- Patients are often immunocompromised, smokers, or have chronic lung disease.
- Scant sputum production, pleuritic chest pain, toxic appearance.
- Chest x-ray shows focal patchy infiltrates or consolidation.
- Gram's stain of sputum shows polymorphonuclear leukocytes and no organisms.

General Considerations

Legionella infection ranks among the three or four most common causes of community-acquired pneumonia. The diagnosis must be considered whenever the etiology of a pneumonia is in question. Legionnaire's disease is more common in immunocompromised persons, in smokers, and in those with chronic lung disease. Outbreaks of legionellosis have been associated with contaminated water sources, such as shower heads and faucets in patient rooms and air conditioning cooling towers.

Clinical Findings

A. Symptoms and Signs: Legionnaire's disease is one of the atypical pneumonias, so called because a Gram-stained smear of sputum does not show organisms. However, many features of Legionnaire's disease are more like typical pneumonia, with high fevers, a "toxic" appearance of the patient, pleurisy, and purulent sputum (without predominant or identifiable organisms). Classically, this pneumonia is caused by *Legionella pneumophila,* though other species can cause disease that is clinically indistinguishable.

B. Laboratory Findings: Culture onto charcoal-yeast extract agar or similar enriched medium is the most sensitive method (80–90% sensitivity) for diagnosis of legionellosis and permits identification of infections caused by species and serotypes other than *L pneumophila* serotype 1. Dieterle's silver staining of tissue, pleural fluid, or other infected material is also a reliable method for detecting legionella species. Direct fluorescent antibody stains and serologic testing are less sensitive because these will detect only infection caused by *L pneumophila* serotype 1.

Treatment

Erythromycin, 1 g every 6 hours intravenously, followed by 500 mg orally four times daily for 14–21 days, has been the preferred regimen for treatment of legionellosis. Alternative agents with excellent in vitro activity against legionella that are more easily administered and better tolerated than erythromycin are levofloxacin (500 mg once daily orally or intravenously), azithromycin (500 mg then 250 mg once daily, orally or intravenously), and clarithromycin (500 mg orally twice daily)—all administered for 10–14 days. Retrospective data indicate that azithromycin may be effective as a 5-day regimen. All indications are that these agents are just as effective as erythromycin and perhaps in some cases more effective. A 21-day course of treatment and combination therapy (eg, addition of rifampin 300 mg twice daily or macrolide-fluoroquinolone) have been recommended for legionellosis in the immunocompromised patient, but data supporting improved outcomes for combination regimens are lacking. Tetracyclines and trimethoprim-sulfamethoxazole also appear to be effective. Their use for documented infection has been limited, however, and they are best reserved for the patient who cannot be treated with either a macrolide or a fluoroquinolone.

File TM Jr et al: The role of atypical pathogens: *Mycoplasma pneumoniae, Chlamydia pneumoniae,* and *Legionella pneumophila* in respiratory infection. Infect Dis Clin North Am 1998;12:569. [NLM Cit ID: 98452415]

Stout JE et al: Legionellosis. N Engl J Med 1997;337:682. [NLM Cit ID: 97407846] (Epidemiology, pathogenesis, diagnosis, and treatment.)

GRAM-NEGATIVE BACTEREMIA & SEPSIS

There are several hundred thousand episodes of gram-negative sepsis annually. Patients with rapidly fatal underlying diseases (neutropenic patients or those immunosuppressed by virtue of an underlying disease or medication) have a mortality rate of 40–60%; patients with ultimately fatal underlying diseases (diseases likely to be fatal in 5 years, such as solid tumors, severe liver disease, and aplastic anemia) have a mortality rate of 15–20%; and patients with no underlying disease have a low mortality rate—5% or less. Gram-negative bacteremia can originate in a number of sites, the most common being the genitourinary system, hepatobiliary tract, gastrointestinal tract, and lungs. Less common sources include intravenous lines, infusion fluids, surgical wounds, surgical drains, and decubitus ulcers.

Clinical Findings

A. Symptoms and Signs: Most patients have fevers and chills, often with an abrupt onset. However, 15% of patients are hypothermic (temperature ≤ 36.4 °C) at the onset of sepsis, and 5% of patients never develop a temperature above 37.5 °C. Hyperventilation with respiratory alkalosis and changes in mental status are important early manifestations. Hypotension and shock, which occur in 20–50% of patients, are unfavorable prognostic signs.

B. Laboratory Findings: Neutropenia or neutrophilia, often with increased numbers of immature forms of polymorphonuclear leukocytes, is the most common laboratory abnormality in septic patients. Thrombocytopenia occurs in 50% of patients, laboratory evidence of coagulation abnormalities in 10%, and frank DIC in 2–3%. Both clinical manifestations and the laboratory abnormalities are nonspecific and insensitive, which accounts for the relatively low rate of blood culture positivity (approximately 20–40%) in patients with suspected gram-negative sepsis. If possible, three blood cultures from separate sites should be obtained in rapid succession before starting antimicrobial therapy. The chance of recovering the organism from the blood of the septic patient with bacteremia in at least one of the three blood cultures is greater than 95%. The false-negative rate for a single culture of 5–10 mL of blood is 30%. This may be reduced to a 5–10% false-negative rate (albeit with a slight false-positive rate due to isolation of contaminants) if a single volume of 30 mL is inoculated into several blood culture bottles. Because blood cultures may be falsely negative, if the patient with presumed septic shock, negative blood cultures, and no other good explanation for the clinical course responds to antimicrobials, therapy should be continued for 10–14 days.

Treatment

Several factors are important in the management of patients with sepsis.

A. Removal of Predisposing Factors: This usually means decreasing or stopping immunosuppressive medications and in certain circumstances (eg, documented positive blood cultures) giving granulocyte colony-stimulating factor (filgrastim; G-CSF) to the neutropenic patient.

B. Identifying the Source of Bacteremia: A search for the source of bacteremia should be made. By simply finding the source and either removing it (intravenous line) or draining it (abscess), it is possible to transform what might be a fatal disease into one that is easily treatable.

C. Supportive Measures: The use of fluids and pressors for maintaining blood pressure is discussed in Chapter 11; management of disseminated intravascular coagulation is discussed in Chapter 13.

D. Antibiotics: Antibiotics should be given as soon as the diagnosis of sepsis is seriously considered, since delays in therapy have been associated with increased mortality rates. In general, bactericidal antibiotics should be used and should be given intravenously to ensure therapeutic serum levels. Penetration of antibiotics into the site of primary infection is critical for successful therapy—ie, if the infection originates in the central nervous system, antibiotics that penetrate the blood-brain barrier should be used—eg, penicillin, ampicillin, chloramphenicol, and third-generation cephalosporins—but not first-generation cephalosporins or aminoglycosides, which penetrate poorly. Sepsis caused by gram-positive organisms cannot be differentiated on clinical grounds from that due to gram-negative bacteria. Therefore, initial therapy should include antibiotics active against both types of organisms.

The number of antibiotics necessary to treat sepsis remains controversial and depends upon the underlying disease. Table 37–2 provides a guide for empirical therapy. Most authorities believe that for patients with rapidly fatal underlying diseases, a synergistic combination of antibiotics, including an aminoglycoside, should be used. For patients with nonfatal and ultimately fatal underlying diseases and who are not in shock, a single-drug regimen with any of several broad-spectrum antibiotics (eg, a third-generation cephalosporin, ticarcillin-clavulanate, imipenem) is adequate. Therapy can be altered once results of culture and sensitivity are known.

E. Corticosteroids: There is no role for corticosteroids in the therapy of sepsis or septic shock.

F. Adjunctive Therapy: Expanded knowledge of the pathophysiology of sepsis and septic shock and recognition that cytokines play a critical role have led to novel approaches to reduce morbidity and mortality associated with sepsis. Strategies include blocking the effects of endotoxin with anti-endotoxin monoclonal antibodies; blockade of TNFα, a potent cytokine mediator of septic shock, with anti-TNF monoclonal antibody or soluble TNF receptor; and use of IL-1 receptor antagonists to inhibit the proinflammatory effects of IL-1 binding to its receptor. Results of clinical trials with these agents so far have been largely disappointing, with no significant improvement in overall survival. The ultimate role and long-term benefits of adjunctive therapy have yet to be defined.

Lazaron V et al: Gram-negative bacterial sepsis and the sepsis syndrome. Urol Clin North Am 1999;26:687. [NLM Cit ID: 20052006]

Opal SM et al: Clinical gram-positive sepsis: does it fundamentally differ from gram-negative bacterial sepsis? Crit Care Med 1999;27:1608. [NLM Cit ID: 99397374]

Sriskandan S et al: Gram-positive sepsis. Mechanisms and differences from gram-negative sepsis. Infect Dis Clin North Am 1999;13:397. [NLM Cit ID: 99271533] (The articles by Lazaron, Opal, and Sriskandan examine the similarities and differences of sepsis from different bacterial agents.)

Wheeler AW et al: Current concepts: Treating patients with severe sepsis. N Engl J Med 1999;340:207. [NLM Cit ID: 99101868]

SALMONELLOSIS

Salmonellosis includes infection by any of approximately 2000 serotypes of salmonellae. The taxonomy of salmonella species has been confusing. All salmonella serotypes are considered members of a single species, *S enterica.* Human infections are caused almost exclusively by *S enterica* subsp *enterica,* of which three serotypes—typhi, typhimurium, and choleraesuis—are predominantly isolated. Three clinical patterns of infection are recognized: (1) enteric fever, the best example of which is typhoid fever, due to serotype typhi; (2) acute enterocolitis, caused by serotype typhimurium, among others; and (3) the "septicemic" type, characterized by bacteremia and focal lesions, exemplified by infection with serotype choleraesuis. All types are transmitted by ingestion of the organism, usually from contaminated food or drink.

1. ENTERIC FEVER (Typhoid Fever)

Essentials of Diagnosis

- Gradual onset of malaise, headache, sore throat, cough, and either diarrhea or constipation.
- Rose spots, relative bradycardia, splenomegaly, and abdominal distention and tenderness.
- Slow (stepladder) rise of fever to maximum and then slow return to normal.
- Leukopenia; blood, stool, and urine culture positive for *S enterica* serotype typhi.

General Considerations

Enteric fever is a clinical syndrome characterized by constitutional and gastrointestinal symptoms and by headache. It can be caused by any salmonella species. The term "typhoid fever" applies when serotype typhi is the cause of enteric fever accompanied by bacteremia. Infection is transmitted by consumption of contaminated food or drink. The incubation period is 5–14 days. Salmonella is an intracellular pathogen. Infection begins when organisms breach the mucosal epithelium of the intestines by transcytosis, an organism-mediated transport process through the cell via an endocytic vesicle. Having crossed the epithelial barrier, organisms invade and replicate in macrophages in Peyer's patches, mesenteric lymph nodes, and the spleen. Serotypes other than typhi usually do not cause invasive disease, presumably because they lack the necessary human-specific virulence factors. Bacteremia occurs, and the infection then localizes principally in the lymphoid tissue of the small intestine (particularly within 60 cm of the ileocecal valve). Peyer's patches become inflamed and may ulcerate, with involvement greatest during the third week of disease. The organism may disseminate to the lungs, gallbladder, kidneys, or central nervous system.

Clinical Findings

A. Symptoms and Signs: The onset is usually insidious but in children may be abrupt, with chills and high fever. During the prodromal stage, there is increasing malaise, headache, cough, and sore throat, often with abdominal pain and constipation, while the fever ascends in a stepwise fashion. After about 7–10 days, the fever reaches a plateau and the patient is much more ill, appearing exhausted and often prostrated. There may be marked constipation, or "pea soup" diarrhea; marked abdominal distention occurs as well. If there are no complications, the patient's condition will gradually improve over 7–10 days. However, relapse may occur for up to 2 weeks after defervescence.

During the early prodrome, physical findings are few. Later, splenomegaly, abdominal distention and tenderness, relative bradycardia, dicrotic pulse, and occasionally meningismus appear. The rash (rose spots) commonly appears during the second week of disease. The individual spot, found principally on the trunk, is a pink papule 2–3 mm in diameter that fades on pressure. It disappears in 3–4 days.

B. Laboratory Findings: Typhoid fever is best diagnosed by isolation of the organism from blood culture, which is positive in the first week of illness in 80% of patients who have not taken antimicrobials. The rate of blood culture positivity declines thereafter, but one-fourth or more of patients still have positive blood cultures in the third week. Cultures of bone marrow occasionally are positive when blood cultures are not. Stool culture is not reliable because it may be positive in gastroenteritis without typhoid fever.

Differential Diagnosis

Enteric fever must be distinguished from other gastrointestinal illnesses and from other infections that have few localizing findings. Examples include tuberculosis, infective endocarditis, brucellosis, lymphoma, and Q fever. Often there is a history of recent travel to endemic areas, and viral hepatitis, malaria, or amebiasis may be in the differential diagnosis as well.

Complications

Complications occur in about 30% of untreated cases and account for 75% of all deaths. Intestinal hemorrhage, manifested by a sudden drop in temperature and signs of shock followed by dark or fresh blood in the stool, or intestinal perforation, accompanied by abdominal pain and tenderness, is most likely to occur during the third week. Less frequent complications are urinary retention, pneumonia, thrombophlebitis, myocarditis, psychosis, cholecystitis, nephritis, osteomyelitis, and meningitis.

Prevention

Immunization is not always effective but should be provided for household contacts of a typhoid carrier, for travelers to endemic areas, and during epidemic outbreaks. A multiple-dose oral vaccine and a single-dose parenteral vaccine are available. Their efficacies are similar, but oral vaccine causes fewer side effects. Boosters, when indicated, should be given every 5 years and 2 years for oral and parenteral preparations, respectively.

Adequate waste disposal and protection of food and water supplies from contamination are important public health measures to prevent salmonellosis. Carriers must not be permitted to work as food handlers.

Treatment

A. Specific Measures: Ampicillin, chloramphenicol, and trimethoprim-sulfamethoxazole may be effective. All can be given orally or intravenously depending on the patient's condition. Because resistance to ampicillin and chloramphenicol is common, trimethoprim-sulfamethoxazole, administered as 10 mg/kg/d of trimethoprim, is probably the first choice. Ceftriaxone, 2 g once a day, also is effective. Fluoroquinolones such as ciprofloxacin, 750 mg twice a day, also are effective, but their use is contraindicated in children and pregnant women. The recommended duration of therapy is 2 weeks, though limited data suggest that shorter courses are also effective.

B. Treatment of Carriers: Chemotherapy often is unsuccessful in eradicating the carrier state. While treatment of carriage with ampicillin, trimethoprim-sulfamethoxazole, or chloramphenicol may be successful, one recent study suggests that ciprofloxacin, 750 mg twice a day for 4 weeks, is highly effective. Cholecystectomy may also achieve this goal.

Prognosis

The mortality rate of typhoid fever is about 2% in treated cases. Elderly or debilitated persons are likely to do poorly. The course is milder in children.

With complications, the prognosis is poor. Relapses occur in up to 15% of cases. A residual carrier state frequently persists in spite of chemotherapy.

Akalin HE: Quinolones in the treatment of typhoid fever. Drugs 1999;58(Suppl 2):52. [NLM Cit ID: 20019134] (The strengths and weaknesses of quinolones as therapy for infectious diarrhea.)

Mermin JH et al: Typhoid fever in the United States, 1985–1994: Changing risks of international travel and increasing antimicrobial resistance. Arch Intern Med 1998;158:633. [NLM Cit ID: 98180524]

Rowe B et al: Multidrug-resistant *Salmonella typhi:* a worldwide epidemic. Clin Infect Dis 1997;24(Suppl 1):S106. [NLM Cit ID: 97148157]

2. SALMONELLA GASTROENTERITIS

By far the most common form of salmonellosis is acute enterocolitis. Numerous salmonella serotypes may cause enterocolitis. The incubation period is 8–48 hours after ingestion of contaminated food or liquid.

Symptoms and signs consist of fever (often with chills), nausea and vomiting, cramping abdominal pain, and diarrhea, which may be grossly bloody, lasting 3–5 days. Differentiation must be made from viral gastroenteritis, food poisoning, shigellosis, amebic dysentery, acute ulcerative colitis, and acute surgical abdominal conditions. The diagnosis is made by culturing the organism from the stool.

The disease is usually self-limited, but bacteremia with localization in joints or bones may occur, especially in patients with sickle cell disease.

Treatment of uncomplicated enterocolitis is symptomatic only. Malnourished or severely ill patients, those with sickle cell disease, and those with suspected bacteremia should be treated for 3–5 days with trimethoprim-sulfamethoxazole (one double-strength tablet twice a day), ampicillin (100 mg/kg intravenously or orally), or ciprofloxacin (750 mg twice a day).

3. SALMONELLA BACTEREMIA

Salmonella infection may be manifested by prolonged or recurrent fevers accompanied by bacteremia and local infection in bone, joints, pleura, pericardium, lungs, or other sites. Mycotic abdominal aortic aneurysms may also cause this problem. Serotypes other than typhi usually are isolated. This complication tends to occur in immunocompromised persons and is seen in HIV-infected individuals, who typically have bacteremia without an obvious source. Treatment is the same as for typhoid fever, plus drainage of any abscesses. In HIV-infected patients, relapse is common, and lifelong suppressive therapy may be needed. Ciprofloxacin, 750 mg twice a day, is effective both for therapy of acute infection and for suppression of recurrence.

SHIGELLOSIS

Essentials of Diagnosis

- Diarrhea, often with blood and mucus.
- Crampy abdominal pain and systemic toxicity.
- White blood cells in stools; organism isolated on stool culture.

General Considerations

Shigella dysentery is a common disease, often self-limited and mild but occasionally serious. *Shigella sonnei* is the leading cause in the USA, followed by *Shigella flexneri. Shigella dysenteriae* causes the most serious form of the illness. Shigellae are invasive organisms: The infective dose is 10^2–10^3 organisms. Recently, there has been a rise in strains resistant to multiple antibiotics.

Clinical Findings

A. Symptoms and Signs: The illness usually starts abruptly, with diarrhea, lower abdominal cramps, and tenesmus. The diarrheal stool often is mixed with blood and mucus. Systemic symptoms are fever, chills, anorexia and malaise, and headache. The patient becomes progressively weaker and more dehydrated. The abdomen is tender. Sigmoidoscopic examination reveals an inflamed, engorged mucosa with punctate, sometimes large areas of ulceration.

B. Laboratory Findings: The stool shows many leukocytes and red cells. Stool culture is positive for shigellae in most cases, but blood cultures grow the organism in less than 5% of cases.

Differential Diagnosis

Bacillary dysentery must be distinguished from salmonella enterocolitis and from disease due to enterotoxigenic *E coli,* campylobacter, and *Y enterocolitica.* Amebic dysentery may be similar clinically and is diagnosed by finding amebas in the fresh stool specimen. Ulcerative colitis in the adolescent and adult is an important cause of bloody diarrhea.

Complications

Temporary disaccharidase deficiency may follow the diarrhea. Reiter's syndrome is an uncommon complication, usually occurring in HLA-B27 individuals infected by shigella.

Treatment

Treatment of dehydration and hypotension is lifesaving in severe cases. The current antimicrobial treatment of choice is trimethoprim-sulfamethoxazole, one double-strength tablet twice a day for 7–10 days, or ciprofloxacin (contraindicated in pregnancy), 750 mg twice daily for 7–10 days, a fluoroquinolone (ciprofloxacin, 750 mg twice daily, or levofloxacin, 500 mg once daily) for 3 days. Fluoroquinolones are contraindicated in pregnancy. Shigellae resistant to ampicillin are common, but if the isolate is susceptible, a dose of 500 mg four times a day is also effective. Amoxicillin, which is less effective, should not be used.

GASTROENTERITIS CAUSED BY *ESCHERICHIA COLI*

Escherichia coli causes gastroenteritis by a variety of mechanisms. Enterotoxigenic *E coli* (ETEC) elaborates either a heat-stable or heat-labile toxin that mediates the disease. ETEC is an important cause of traveler's diarrhea. Enteroinvasive *E coli* (EIEC) differs from other *E coli* bowel pathogens in that these strains invade cells, causing bloody diarrhea and dysentery similar to infection with shigella species. EIEC is uncommon in the United States. Neither ETEC nor EIEC strains are routinely isolated and identified from stool cultures because there is no selective medium. Antimicrobial therapy directed against salmonella and shigella shortens the clinical course, but the disease is self-limited. Enterohemorrhagic *E coli* (EHEC) produces two shiga-like toxins that mediate the clinical manifestations, which include an asymptomatic carriage stage, nonbloody diarrhea, hemorrhagic colitis, hemolytic-uremic syndrome, and thrombotic thrombocytopenic purpura. Although there are several serotypes of EHEC, serotype O157:H7 is responsible for most cases in the United States. *E coli* O157:H7 has been responsible for several outbreaks of diarrhea and hemolytic-uremic syndrome related to consumption of undercooked hamburger and unpasteurized apple juice. Elderly individuals and young children are most severely affected, with hemolytic-uremic syndrome being a common and often fatal complication in the latter group. *E coli* O157:H7 is not identified by routine stool cultures. Isolation requires identification of sorbitol-negative colonies of *E coli* on sorbitol-MacConkey agar followed by serologic testing to confirm the serotype. Antimicrobial therapy does not alter the course of the disease, and treatment is primarily supportive. Hemolytic-uremic syndrome or thrombotic thrombocytopenic purpura occurring in association with a diarrheal illness suggests the diagnosis and should prompt evaluation for EHEC. Confirmed infections should be reported immediately to public health officials.

Besser RE et al: *Escherichia coli* O157:H7 gastroenteritis and the hemolytic uremic syndrome: an emerging infectious disease. Annu Rev Med 1999;50:355. [NLM Cit ID: 99172938]

Karch H et al: Epidemiology and diagnosis of Shiga toxin-producing *Escherichia coli* infections. Diagnostic Microbiol Infect Dis 1999;34:229. [NLM Cit ID: 99331535]

CHOLERA

Essentials of Diagnosis

- Voluminous diarrhea.
- Stool is liquid, gray, turbid, and without fecal odor, blood, or pus ("rice water stool").
- Rapid development of marked dehydration.
- History of travel in endemic area or contact with infected person.
- Positive stool cultures and agglutination of vibrios with specific sera.

General Considerations

Cholera is an acute diarrheal illness caused by certain serotypes of *Vibrio cholerae.* The disease is toxin-mediated, and fever is unusual. The toxin activates adenylyl cyclase in intestinal epithelial cells of the small intestines, producing hypersecretion of water and chloride ion and a massive diarrhea of up to 15 L per day. Death results from profound hypovolemia.

Cholera occurs in epidemics under conditions of crowding, war, and famine (eg, in refugee camps) and where sanitation is inadequate. Infection is acquired by ingestion of contaminated food or water. Cholera was rarely seen in the United States until 1991, when epidemic cholera returned to the Western Hemisphere, originating as an outbreak in coastal cities of Peru. The epidemic spread to involve several countries in South and Central America as well as Mexico, and cases have been imported into the United States. Cholera should be considered in the differential diagnosis of severe watery diarrhea, especially in those who have traveled to affected countries.

Clinical Findings

Cholera is characterized by a sudden onset of severe, frequent watery diarrhea (up to 1 L per hour).

The liquid stool is gray, turbid, and without fecal odor, blood, or pus ("rice water stool"). Dehydration and hypotension develop rapidly. Stool cultures are positive, and agglutination of vibrios with specific sera can be demonstrated.

Prevention

A vaccine is available that confers short-lived, limited protection and may be required for entry into or reentry after travel to some countries. It is administered in two doses 1–4 weeks apart. A booster dose every 6 months is recommended for persons remaining in areas where cholera is a hazard.

Vaccination programs are expensive and not particularly effective in managing outbreaks of cholera. When outbreaks occur, efforts should be directed toward establishing clean water and food sources and proper waste disposal.

Treatment

Treatment is by replacement of fluids. In mild or moderate illness, oral rehydration usually is adequate. A simple oral replacement fluid can be made from 1 teaspoon of table salt and 4 heaping teaspoons of sugar added to 1 L of water. Intravenous fluids are indicated for persons in shock or those with other signs of severe hypovolemia and those who cannot take adequate fluids orally. Lactated Ringer's infusion is satisfactory.

Antimicrobial therapy will shorten the course of illness. Several antimicrobials are active against *V cholerae,* including tetracycline, ampicillin, chloramphenicol, trimethoprim-sulfamethoxazole, and fluoroquinolones. Multiple antibiotic resistance does occur, so susceptibility testing, if available, is advisable.

Guerrant RL et al: How intestinal bacteria cause disease. J Infect Dis 1999;179(Suppl 2):S331. [NLM Cit ID: 99181345]

Sanchez JL et al: Cholera. Lancet 1997;349:1825. [NLM Cit ID: 97414534]

Seas C et al: Practical guidelines for the treatment of cholera. Drugs 1996;51:966. [NLM Cit ID: 96338539]

INFECTIONS CAUSED BY OTHER VIBRIO SPECIES

Vibrios other than *Vibrio cholerae* that cause human disease are *Vibrio parahaemolyticus, Vibrio vulnificus,* and *Vibrio alginolyticus.* All are halophilic marine organisms. Infection is acquired by exposure to organisms in contaminated, undercooked, or raw crustaceans or shellfish and warm (> 20 °C) ocean waters and estuaries. Infections are more common during the summer months from regions along the Atlantic coast and the Gulf of Mexico in the United States and from tropical waters around the world. Oysters are implicated in up to 90% of food-related cases. *V parahaemolyticus* causes an acute watery diarrhea with crampy abdominal pain and fever, typically occurring within 24 hours after ingestion of contaminated shellfish. The disease is self-limited, and antimicrobial therapy is usually not necessary. *V parahaemolyticus* may also cause cellulitis and sepsis, though these findings are more characteristic of *V vulnificus* infection.

V vulnificus and *V alginolyticus*—neither of which is associated with diarrheal illness—are important causes of cellulitis and primary bacteremia, which may follow ingestion of contaminated shellfish or exposure to sea water. Cellulitis with or without sepsis may be accompanied by bulla formation and necrosis with extensive soft tissue destruction, at times requiring debridement and amputation. The infection can be rapidly progressive and is particularly severe in immunocompromised individuals—especially those with cirrhosis—with death rates as high as 50%. Patients with chronic liver disease and those who are immunocompromised should be cautioned to avoid eating raw oysters.

Tetracycline at a dose of 500 mg four times a day for 7–10 days is the drug of choice for treatment of suspected or documented primary bacteremia or cellulitis caused by vibrio species. *V vulnificus* is susceptible in vitro to penicillin, ampicillin, cephalosporins, chloramphenicol, aminoglycosides, and fluoroquinolones, and these agents may also be effective. *V parahaemolyticus* and *V alginolyticus* produce β-lactamase and therefore are resistant to penicillin and ampicillin, but susceptibilities otherwise are similar to those listed for *V vulnificus.*

INFECTIONS CAUSED BY CAMPYLOBACTER SPECIES

Campylobacters are microaerophilic, motile, gram-negative rods. Two species infect humans: *Campylobacter jejuni,* an important cause of diarrheal disease; and *Campylobacter fetus* subsp *fetus,* which typically causes systemic infection and not diarrhea. Dairy cattle and poultry are an important reservoir for campylobacters. Outbreaks of enteritis have been associated with consumption of raw milk. Campylobacter gastroenteritis is associated with fever, abdominal pain, and diarrhea characterized by loose, watery, or bloody stools. The differential diagnosis includes shigellosis, salmonella gastroenteritis, and enteritis caused by *Yersinia enterocolitica* or invasive *Escherichia coli.* The disease is self-limited, but its duration can be shortened with antimicrobial therapy. Both erythromycin, 250–500 mg four times daily for 5–7 days, and ciprofloxacin, 500 mg twice daily for 3–5 days, are effective regimens. Pending identification of the causative agent of suspected bacterial gastroenteritis, ciprofloxacin is a rational choice for empirical therapy because all of the common bacterial pathogens are susceptible.

C fetus causes systemic infections that can be fatal, including primary bacteremia, endocarditis, meningitis, and focal abscesses. It infrequently causes gastroenteritis. Patients infected with *C fetus* are often elderly, debilitated, or immunocompromised. Closely related species, collectively termed campylobacter-like organisms, cause bacteremia in HIV-infected individuals. Systemic infections respond to therapy with gentamicin, chloramphenicol, ceftriaxone, or ciprofloxacin. Ceftriaxone or chloramphenicol should be used to treat infections of the central nervous system because of their ability to penetrate the blood-brain barrier.

BRUCELLOSIS

Essentials of Diagnosis

- Insidious onset: easy fatigability, headache, arthralgia, anorexia, sweating, irritability.
- Intermittent fever, especially at night, which may become chronic and undulant.
- Cervical and axillary lymphadenopathy; hepatosplenomegaly.
- Lymphocytosis, positive blood culture, elevated agglutination titer.

General Considerations

The infection is transmitted from animals to humans. *Brucella abortus* (cattle), *Brucella suis* (hogs), and *Brucella melitensis* (goats) are the main agents. Transmission to humans occurs by contact with infected meat (slaughterhouse workers), placentae of infected animals (farmers, veterinarians), or ingestion of infected unpasteurized milk or cheese. The incubation period varies from a few days to several weeks. The disorder may become chronic. In the USA, brucellosis is very rare except in the midwestern states (from *B suis*) and in visitors or immigrants from countries where brucellosis is endemic (eg, Mexico, Spain, South American countries).

Clinical Findings

A. Symptoms and Signs: The onset may be acute, with fever, chills, and sweats, but typically is insidious. It may be weeks before the patient seeks medical care for weakness, weight loss, low-grade fevers, sweats, and exhaustion upon minimal activity. Symptoms also include headache, abdominal or back pains with anorexia and constipation, and arthralgia. Epididymitis occurs in 10% of cases in men. The chronic form may assume an undulant nature, with periods of normal temperature between acute attacks; symptoms may persist for years, either continuously or intermittently.

Physical findings are minimal. Half of cases have peripheral lymph node enlargement and splenomegaly; hepatomegaly is less common.

B. Laboratory Findings: Early in the course of infection, the organism can be recovered from the blood, cerebrospinal fluid, urine, and bone marrow. Because the organism is slow-growing, cultures should be incubated for 21 days before being read as negative. Cultures are more likely to be negative in chronic cases. The diagnosis often is made by serologic testing. Rising serologic titers or an absolute agglutination titer of greater than 1:100 supports the diagnosis.

Differential Diagnosis

Brucellosis must be differentiated from any other acute febrile disease, especially influenza, tularemia, Q fever, mononucleosis, and enteric fever. In its chronic form it resembles Hodgkin's disease, tuberculosis, HIV infection, malaria, and disseminated fungal infections such as histoplasmosis and coccidioidomycosis.

Complications

The most frequent complications are bone and joint lesions such as spondylitis and suppurative arthritis (usually of a single joint), endocarditis, and meningoencephalitis. Less common complications are pneumonitis with pleural effusion, hepatitis, and cholecystitis.

Treatment

Single-drug regimens are not recommended because the relapse rate may be as high as 50%. Combination regimens of two or three drugs are more effective. Either (1) doxycycline plus rifampin or streptomycin (or both) *or* (2) trimethoprim-sulfamethoxazole plus rifampin or streptomycin (or both) is effective in doses as follows for 21 days: doxycycline, 100–200 mg/d in divided doses; trimethoprim 320 mg/d plus sulfamethoxazole 1600 mg/d in divided doses; rifampin, 600–1200 mg/d; and streptomycin, 500 mg intramuscularly twice a day. Longer courses of therapy (eg, several months) may be required to cure relapses, osteomyelitis, or meningitis.

Corbel MJ: Brucellosis: an overview. Emerg Infect Dis 1997;3:213. [NLM Cit ID: 97348256]

Solera J et al: Recognition and optimum treatment of brucellosis. Drugs 1997;53:245. [NLM Cit ID: 97180568]

Yagupsky P: Detection of brucellae in blood cultures. J Clin Microbiol 1999;37:3437. [NLM Cit ID: 99454824]

TULAREMIA

Essentials of Diagnosis

- Fever, headache, nausea, and prostration.
- Papule progressing to ulcer at site of inoculation.
- Enlarged regional lymph nodes.
- History of contact with rabbits, other rodents, and

biting arthropods (eg, ticks in summer) in endemic area.
- Serologic tests or culture of ulcer, lymph node aspirate, or blood confirm the diagnosis.

General Considerations

Tularemia is an infection of wild rodents—particularly rabbits and muskrats—with *Francisella (Pasteurella) tularensis.* Humans usually acquire the infection by contact with animal tissues (eg, trapping muskrats, skinning rabbits) or from ticks. Infection in humans often produces a local lesion and widespread organ involvement but may be entirely asymptomatic. The incubation period is 2–10 days.

Clinical Findings

A. Symptoms and Signs: Fever, headache, and nausea begin suddenly, and a local lesion—a papule at the site of inoculation—develops and soon ulcerates. Regional lymph nodes may become enlarged and tender and may suppurate. The local lesion may be on the skin of an extremity or in the eye. Pneumonia may develop from hematogenous spread of the organism or may be primary after inhalation of infected aerosols, which are responsible for human-to-human transmission. Following ingestion of infected meat or water, an enteric form may be manifested by gastrointestinal symptoms, stupor, and delirium. In any type of involvement, the spleen may be enlarged and tender and there may be nonspecific rashes, myalgias, and prostration.

B. Laboratory Findings: Culturing the organism from blood or infected tissue requires special media. For this reason and because cultures of *F tularensis* may be hazardous to laboratory personnel, the diagnosis is usually made serologically. A positive agglutination test (> 1:80) develops in the second week after infection and may persist for several years.

Differential Diagnosis

Tularemia must be differentiated from rickettsial and meningococcal infections, cat-scratch disease, infectious mononucleosis, and various bacterial and fungal diseases.

Complications

Hematogenous spread may produce meningitis, perisplenitis, pericarditis, pneumonia, and osteomyelitis.

Treatment

Streptomycin, 0.5 g intramuscularly every 6–8 hours, together with tetracycline 0.5 g orally every 6 hours, is administered until 4–5 days after the patient becomes afebrile. Chloramphenicol may be substituted for tetracycline in the same dosage.

Gill V et al: Tularemia pneumonia. Semin Respir Infect 1997;12:61. [NLM Cit ID: 97251707]

PLAGUE

Essentials of Diagnosis

- History of exposure to rodents in endemic area.
- Sudden onset of high fever, malaise, muscular pains, and prostration.
- Axillary or inguinal lymphadenitis (bubo).
- Bacteremia, sepsis, and pneumonitis may occur.
- Positive smear and culture from bubo and positive blood culture.

General Considerations

Plague is an infection of wild rodents with *Yersinia pestis,* a small bipolar-staining gram-negative rod. Plague is endemic in California, Arizona, Nevada, and New Mexico. It is transmitted among rodents and to humans by the bites of fleas or from contact with infected animals. If a plague victim develops pneumonia, the infection can be transmitted by droplets to other individuals. The incubation period is 2–10 days.

Following the flea bite, the organisms spread through the lymphatics to the lymph nodes, which become greatly enlarged (bubo). They may then reach the bloodstream to involve all organs. When pneumonia or meningitis develops, the outcome is often fatal.

Clinical Findings

A. Symptoms and Signs: The onset is sudden, with high fever, malaise, tachycardia, intense headache, and severe myalgias. The patient appears profoundly ill. Delirium may ensue. If pneumonia develops, tachypnea, productive cough, blood-tinged sputum, and cyanosis also occur. Signs of meningitis may develop. A pustule or ulcer at the site of inoculation and signs of lymphangitis may be observed. Axillary, inguinal, or cervical lymph nodes become enlarged and tender and may eventually suppurate and drain. With hematogenous spread, the patient may rapidly become toxic and comatose, with purpuric spots (black plague) appearing on the skin.

Primary plague pneumonia is a fulminant pneumonitis with bloody, frothy sputum and sepsis. It is usually fatal unless treatment is started within a few hours after onset.

B. Laboratory Findings: The plague bacillus may be found in smears from aspirates of buboes examined with Gram's stain. Cultures from bubo aspirate or pus and blood are positive but may grow slowly. In convalescing patients, an antibody titer rise may be demonstrated by agglutination tests.

Differential Diagnosis

The lymphadenitis of plague is most commonly mistaken for the lymphadenitis accompanying staphylococcal or streptococcal infections of an extremity, sexually transmitted diseases such as lymphogranuloma venereum or syphilis, and tularemia.

The systemic manifestations resemble those of enteric or rickettsial fevers, malaria, or influenza. The pneumonia resembles other bacterial pneumonias, and the meningitis is similar to those caused by other bacteria.

Prevention

Drug prophylaxis may provide temporary protection for persons exposed to the risk of plague infection, particularly by the respiratory route. Tetracycline hydrochloride, 500 mg orally once or twice daily for 5 days, is effective.

Plague vaccines—both live and killed—have been used for many years, but their efficacy is not clearly established.

Treatment

Therapy must be started promptly when plague is suspected. Streptomycin, 1 g intramuscularly, is administered immediately, and 0.5 g intramuscularly is then given every 6–8 hours. Tetracycline, 2 g daily orally (or parenterally if necessary), is given at the same time. Patients with plague pneumonia should be strictly isolated.

Cleri DJ et al: Plague pneumonia disease caused by *Yersinia pestis.* Semin Respir Infect 1997;12:12. [NLM Cit ID: 97251698]

Galimand M: Brief report: Multidrug resistance in *Yersinia pestis* mediated by a transferable plasmid. N Engl J Med 1999;340:677. [NLM Cit ID: 97407844]

Koornhof HJ et al: Yersiniosis. II: The pathogenesis of Yersinia infections. Eur J Clin Microbiol Infect Dis 1999;18:87. [NLM Cit ID: 99236314]

GONOCOCCAL INFECTIONS

Essentials of Diagnosis

- Purulent and profuse urethral discharge, especially in men, with dysuria, yielding positive smear.
- Epididymitis, prostatitis, periurethral inflammation, proctitis in men.
- Cervicitis in women with purulent discharge, or asymptomatic, yielding positive culture; vaginitis, salpingitis, proctitis also occur.
- Fever, rash, tenosynovitis, and arthritis with disseminated disease.
- Gram-negative intracellular diplococci seen in a smear or cultured from any site, particularly the urethra, cervix, pharynx, and rectum.

General Considerations

Gonorrhea is caused by *Neisseria gonorrhoeae,* a gram-negative diplococcus typically found inside polymorphonuclear cells. It is most commonly transmitted during sexual activity and has its greatest incidence in the 15- to 29-year-old age group. The incubation period is usually 2–8 days.

Anatomic Classification

A. Urethritis and Cervicitis: In men, there is initially burning on urination and a serous or milky discharge. One to 3 days later, the urethral pain is more pronounced and the discharge becomes yellow, creamy, and profuse, sometimes blood-tinged. The disorder may regress and become chronic or progress to involve the prostate, epididymis, and periurethral glands with acute, painful inflammation. Chronic infection leads to prostatitis and urethral strictures. Rectal infection is common in homosexual men. Atypical sites of primary infection (eg, the pharynx) must always be considered. Asymptomatic infection is common and occurs in both sexes.

Gonococcal infection in women often becomes symptomatic during menses. Women may have dysuria, urinary frequency, and urgency, with a purulent urethral discharge. Vaginitis and cervicitis with inflammation of Bartholin's glands are common. Infection may be asymptomatic, with only slightly increased vaginal discharge and moderate cervicitis on examination. Infection may remain as a chronic cervicitis—an important reservoir of gonococci. It may progress to involve the uterus and tubes with acute and chronic salpingitis and with ultimate scarring of tubes and sterility. In pelvic inflammatory disease, anaerobes and chlamydiae often accompany gonococci. Rectal infection may result from spread of the organism from the genital tract or from anal coitus.

Gram stain of urethral discharge in men, especially during the first week after onset, typically shows gram-negative diplococci in polymorphonuclear leukocytes. Gram stain is less often positive in women. Culture has been the gold standard for diagnosis, particularly when the Gram stain is negative. A ligase chain reaction (LCR) assay that detects both *N gonorrhoeae* and *Chlamydia trachomatis* in cervical and urethral swab specimens and urine permits more rapid diagnosis of gonococcal infection. LCR also has improved sensitivity (approximately 90–95% for urine and > 95% for swab) and high specificity (≥ 99%) compared with culture of swab specimens (overall sensitivity of approximately 80%). This test is likely to replace culture, particularly for screening, because of the convenience of obtaining a urine sample compared with swab and because it detects *C trachomatis* coinfection. Identification of *N gonorrhoeae* from rectal or pharyngeal sites and in joint fluid still requires culture.

B. Disseminated Disease: Systemic complications follow the dissemination of gonococci from the primary site via the bloodstream. Gonococcal bacteremia is associated with intermittent fever, arthralgia, and skin lesions ranging from maculopapular to pustular or hemorrhagic, which tend to be few in number and peripherally located. Rarely, gonococcal endocarditis or meningitis develops. Arthritis and tenosynovitis are common complications, particularly involving the knees, ankles, and wrists. One or occasionally a few joints usually are involved. Gonococci can be isolated from less than half of patients with gonococcal arthritis.

C. Conjunctivitis: The most common form of eye involvement is direct inoculation of gonococci into the conjunctival sac. In adults, this occurs by autoinoculation of a person with genital infection. The purulent conjunctivitis may rapidly progress to panophthalmitis and loss of the eye unless treated promptly. A single 1-g dose of ceftriaxone is effective.

Differential Diagnosis

Gonococcal urethritis or cervicitis must be differentiated from nongonococcal urethritis; cervicitis or vaginitis due to *Chlamydia trachomatis, Gardnerella vaginalis,* trichomonas, candida, and many other agents associated with sexually transmitted diseases; pelvic inflammatory disease, arthritis, proctitis, and skin lesions. Often, several such agents coexist in a patient. Reiter's disease (urethritis, conjunctivitis, arthritis) may mimic gonorrhea or coexist with it.

Prevention

Prevention is based on education, mechanical or chemical prophylaxis, and early diagnosis and treatment. The condom, if properly used, can reduce the risk of infection. Effective drugs taken in therapeutic doses within 24 hours of exposure can abort an infection.

Treatment

Therapy typically is administered before antimicrobial susceptibilities are known. The choice of which regimen to use should be based on the prevalence of penicillin-resistant organisms. Recent data indicate a nationwide distribution of penicillin- and tetracycline-resistant gonococci. Consequently, penicillin should no longer be considered first-line therapy. All sexual partners should be treated.

A. Uncomplicated Gonorrhea: For urethritis or cervicitis, either ceftriaxone, 125 mg intramuscularly, or cefixime, 400 mg orally, is the treatment of choice. A single oral dose of ciprofloxacin 500 mg, ofloxacin 400 mg, or levofloxacin 250 mg is also effective. Spectinomycin, 1 g intramuscularly once, may be used for the penicillin-allergic patient. Amoxicillin is no longer recommended owing to the prevalence of penicillin-resistant strains of gonococci. Anal gonorrhea in women responds to the same drugs, but in males ceftriaxone is most effective. Pharyngeal gonorrhea responds to ceftriaxone in the same dosage or to trimethoprim-sulfamethoxazole, nine regular-strength tablets orally daily for 5 days. Since coexistent chlamydial infection is common, one should give doxycycline, 100 mg twice daily orally for 7 days, or a single 1 g oral dose of azithromycin, concurrently.

B. Treatment of Other Infections: Salpingitis, prostatitis, bacteremia, arthritis, and other complications due to susceptible strains in adults should be treated with penicillin G, 10 million units intravenously daily, for 5 days. Ceftriaxone, 1 g intravenously daily for 5 days, or an oral fluoroquinolone (ciprofloxacin, 500 mg twice daily, or levofloxacin, 500 mg once daily) for 5 days also are effective. Endocarditis should be treated with ceftriaxone, 1 g every 12 hours intravenously, for at least 3 weeks. Postgonococcal urethritis and cervicitis, which is usually caused by chlamydia, is treated with a regimen of erythromycin, doxycycline, or azithromycin as described above. Serologic tests for syphilis should also be obtained.

Pelvic inflammatory disease requires cefoxitin, 2 g parenterally every 6 hours, or cefotetan, 2 g intravenously every 12 hours. Clindamycin, 900 mg intravenously every 8 hours, plus gentamicin, administered as a 2 mg/kg loading dose followed by 1.5 mg/kg every 8 hours, is also effective. Cefoxitin, 2 g intramuscularly, plus probenecid, 1 g orally as a single dose, followed by a 14-day oral regimen of doxycycline, 100 mg twice a day, is an effective outpatient regimen. Concurrent treatment for chlamydial infection also is indicated. Alternative drug choices exist.

Woodward C et al: Drug treatment of common STDs: Part I. Herpes, syphilis, urethritis, chlamydia and gonorrhea. Am Fam Physician 1999;60:1387. [NLM Cit ID: 200005778]

CHANCROID

Chancroid is a sexually transmitted disease caused by the short gram-negative bacillus *Haemophilus ducreyi.* The incubation period is 3–5 days. The initial lesion at the site of inoculation is a vesicopustule that breaks down to form a painful, soft ulcer with a necrotic base, surrounding erythema, and undermined edges. Multiple lesions—started by autoinoculation—and inguinal adenitis often develop. The adenitis is usually unilateral and consists of tender, matted nodes of moderate size with overlying erythema. These may become fluctuant and rupture spontaneously. With lymph node involvement, fever, chills, and malaise may develop. Balanitis and phimosis are frequent complications in men. Women may have no external signs of infection.

Swabs from lesions are best cultured on chocolate agar with 1% Isovitalex and vancomycin, 3 mg/mL, to yield *H ducreyi.* Mixed sexually transmitted disease is very common (including syphilis, herpes simplex, and HIV infection), as is infection of the ulcer with fusiforms, spirochetes, and other organisms.

Chancroid must be differentiated from other genital ulcers. The chancre of syphilis, by contrast, is clean and painless, with a hard base.

A single dose of either azithromycin, 1 g orally, or ceftriaxone, 250 mg intramuscularly, is effective treatment. Effective multiple-dose regimens are amoxicillin-potassium clavulanate (500/125) three times a day orally for 7 days; erythromycin, 500 mg orally four times a day for 7 days; or ciprofloxacin, 500 mg orally twice a day for 3 days.

Schmid GP: Treatment of chancroid, 1997. Clin Infect Dis 1999;28(Suppl 1):S14. [NLM Cit ID: 99152432]

GRANULOMA INGUINALE

Granuloma inguinale is a chronic, relapsing granulomatous anogenital infection due to *Calymmatobacterium (Donovania) granulomatis.* The pathognomonic cell, found in tissue scrapings or secretions, is large (25–90 μm) and contains intracytoplasmic cysts filled with bodies (Donovan bodies) that stain deeply with Wright's stain.

The incubation period is 8 days to 12 weeks. The onset is insidious. The lesions occur on the skin or mucous membranes of the genitalia or perineal area. They are relatively painless infiltrated nodules that soon slough. A shallow, sharply demarcated ulcer forms, with a beefy-red friable base of granulation tissue. The lesion spreads by contiguity. The advancing border has a characteristic rolled edge of granulation tissue. Large ulcerations may advance onto the lower abdomen and thighs. Scar formation and healing may occur along one border while the opposite border advances.

Superinfection with spirochete-fusiform organisms is common. The ulcer then becomes purulent, painful, foul-smelling, and extremely difficult to treat.

Several therapies are available. Because of the indolent nature of the disease, duration of therapy tends to be relatively long. Erythromycin or tetracycline, 500 mg four times a day for 21 days, is effective. Ampicillin, 500 mg four times a day, also is effective, but up to 12 weeks of therapy may be necessary.

Since other sexually transmitted diseases frequently coexist, cultures for these and a serologic test for syphilis must be performed.

Hart G: Donovanosis. Clin Infect Dis 1997;25:24. [NLM Cit ID: 97386965]

National guideline for the management of donovanosis (granuloma inguinale). Clinical Effectiveness Group (Association of Genitourinary Medicine and the Medical Society for the Study of Venereal Diseases). Sex Transm Infect 1999;75(Suppl 1):S38. [NLM Cit ID: 20083754]

BARTONELLA SPECIES

A revised classification of the α_2 subdivision of proteobacteria has grouped the species previously known as rochalimaea as members of the Bartonella based on ribosomal RNA. These organisms (which include *B quintana, B henselae, B vinsonii,* and *B elizabethae*) are responsible for a wide variety of clinical syndromes. **Bacillary angiomatosis,** an important manifestation of bartonellosis, is discussed in Chapter 31.

Trench fever is a self-limited, louse-borne relapsing febrile disease caused by *B quintana.* The disease has occurred epidemically in louse-infested troops and civilians during wars and endemically in residents of scattered geographic areas (eg, Central America). An urban equivalent of trench fever has been described among the homeless. Humans acquire infection when infected lice feces enter sites of skin breakdown. Onset of symptoms is abrupt and fever lasts 3–5 days, with relapses. The patient complains of weakness and severe pain behind the eyes and typically in the back and legs. Lymphadenopathy, splenomegaly, and a transient maculopapular rash may appear. Subclinical infection is frequent, and a carrier state is recognized. The differential diagnosis includes other febrile, self-limited states such as dengue, leptospirosis, malaria, relapsing fever, and typhus. Recovery occurs regularly even in the absence of treatment.

Brouqui P et al: Chronic *Bartonella quintana* bacteremia in homeless patients. N Engl J Med 1999;340:184. [NLM Cit ID: 99101864]

Raoult D et al: The body louse as a vector of reemerging human diseases. Clin Infect Dis 1999;29:888. [NLM Cit ID: 20055853]

CAT-SCRATCH DISEASE

This is an acute infection of children and young adults caused by *Bartonella henselae.* It is transmitted from cats to humans as the result of a scratch or bite. Within a few days, one-third of patients will develop a papule or ulcer at the inoculation site. One to 3 weeks later, fever, headache, and malaise occur. The regional lymph nodes become enlarged, often tender, and may suppurate. Lymphadenopathy from cat scratches must be differentiated from that due to neoplasm, tuberculosis, lymphogranuloma venereum, and bacterial lymphadenitis. The diagnosis is usually made clinically. Special cultures for bartonella or excisional biopsy, though rarely necessary, confirm the diagnosis. Cat-scratch disease is usually self-limited, requiring no specific therapy. Encephalitis occurs rarely.

Disseminated forms of the disease—bacillary angiomatosis and peliosis hepatis—occur in HIV-infected persons. Clinically, the lesions are vasculoproliferative and histopathologically distinct from those of cat-scratch disease. *Bartonella quintana,* the agent of trench fever, can also cause bacillary angiomatosis as well as culture-negative endocarditis. Bacillary angiomatosis and endocarditis respond to treatment with a macrolide or tetracycline administered in standard doses for 4–8 weeks. Relapse may occur.

Koehler JE et al: Molecular epidemiology of bartonella infections in patients with bacillary angiomatosis-peliosis. N Engl J Med 1997;337:1876. [NLM Cit ID: 98057268] (*Bartonella henselae* associated with peliosis hepatis and cat and flea exposure, *B quintana* associated with homelessness and lice.)

Robson JM et al: Cat-scratch disease with paravertebral mass and osteomyelitis. Clin Infect Dis 1999;28:274. [NLM Cit ID: 99162006]

ANAEROBIC INFECTIONS

Anaerobic bacteria make up the majority of normal human flora. Prominent members of the normal microbial flora of the mouth (anaerobic spirochetes, prevotella, fusobacteria), the skin (anaerobic diphtheroids), the large bowel (bacteroides, anaerobic streptococci, clostridia), and the female tract (bacteroides, anaerobic streptococci, fusobacteria) may produce disease when displaced from their normal sites into tissues or closed body spaces.

Certain characteristics are suggestive of anaerobic infections: (1) They are polymicrobial. (2) Abscess formation is the rule. (3) Pus and infected tissue often are malodorous. (4) Septic thrombophlebitis and metastatic infection are frequent and may require incision and drainage. Most of the important anaerobes except *Bacteroides fragilis* are highly sensitive to penicillin G. Diminished blood supply that favors proliferation of anaerobes because of reduced tissue oxygenation interferes with the delivery of antimicrobials to the site of anaerobic infection. (5) Bacteriologic examination may yield negative results or only inconsequential aerobes unless rigorous culture conditions are used.

Important types of infections that are most commonly caused by anaerobic organisms are listed below. Treatment of all these infections consists of surgical exploration and judicious excision in conjunction with administration of antimicrobial drugs.

Upper Respiratory Tract

Prevotella melaninogenica (formerly *Bacteroides melaninogenicus*) and anaerobic spirochetes are commonly involved in periodontal infections. These organisms, fusobacteria, and peptostreptococci may cause chronic sinusitis, peritonsillar abscess, chronic otitis media, and mastoiditis. Hygiene, drainage, and surgical debridement are as important in treatment as antimicrobials. Oral anaerobic organisms have been uniformly susceptible to penicillin, but there has been a recent trend of increasing penicillin resistance, usually due to β-lactamase production. Penicillin, 1–2 million units intravenously every 4 hours (if parenteral therapy is required) or 0.5 g orally four times daily for less severe infections or clindamycin can be used (600 mg intravenously every 8 hours or 300 mg orally every 6 hours). Duration of therapy depends upon clinical response; antimicrobial treatment is continued for a few days after signs and symptoms of infection have resolved. Indolent, established infections (eg, mastoiditis or osteomyelitis) may require prolonged courses of therapy, eg, 4–6 weeks or longer.

Chest Infections

Usually in the setting of poor oral hygiene and periodontal disease, aspiration of saliva (which contains 10^8 anaerobic organisms per milliliter in addition to aerobes) may lead to necrotizing pneumonia, lung abscess, and empyema. While polymicrobial infection is the rule, anaerobes—particularly *P melaninogenica,* fusobacteria, and peptostreptococci—are common etiologic agents. Most pulmonary infections respond to antimicrobial therapy alone. Percutaneous chest tube or surgical drainage is indicated for empyema.

Penicillin has long been considered the drug of choice for treatment of anaerobic lung infections, but penicillin-resistant *B fragilis* and *P melaninogenica* are isolated in up to 25% of cases and have been associated with clinical failures. Clindamycin, 600 mg intravenously once, followed by 300 mg orally every 6–8 hours, is the treatment of choice for these infections. Penicillin, 2 million units intravenously every 4 hours, followed by amoxicillin, 500 mg every 8 hours orally, is a reasonable alternative. These infections respond slowly. A duration of 3–4 weeks or more of antimicrobial therapy is typical. The second-generation cephalosporins cefoxitin, cefotetan, and cefmetazole are active in vitro against anaerobes, including those that are penicillin-resistant. Chloramphenicol is also effective, but it is used uncommonly given the numerous alternatives.

Central Nervous System

Anaerobes are a common cause of brain abscess, subdural empyema, or septic central nervous system thrombophlebitis. The organisms reach the central nervous system by direct extension from sinusitis, otitis, or mastoiditis or by hematogenous spread from chronic lung infections. Antimicrobial therapy—eg, penicillin, 20 million units intravenously, in combination with metronidazole, 750 mg intravenously, every 8 hours—is an important adjunct to surgical drainage. Duration of therapy is 6–8 weeks. Some small multiple brain abscesses can be treated with antibiotics alone without surgical drainage.

Intra-abdominal Infections

In the colon there are up to 10^{11} anaerobes per gram of content—predominantly *B fragilis,* clostridia, and peptostreptococci. These organisms play a central role in most intra-abdominal abscesses following trauma to the colon, diverticulitis, appendicitis, or perirectal abscess and may also participate in hepatic abscess and cholecystitis, often in association with aerobic coliform bacteria. The gallbladder wall may be infected with clostridia as well. The bacteriology includes anaerobes as well as enteric gram-negative rods and on occasion enterococci. Therapy should be directed both against anaerobes and gram-negative aerobes. Multiple antibiotics may be required. Antibiotics reliably active against *B fragilis* include metronidazole, chloramphenicol, imipenem, ampicillin-sulbactam, and ticarcillin-clavulanic acid. Cefoxitin, cefotetan, and clindamycin are active against 80–90% of strains, but most third-generation cephalosporins have poor activity, inhibiting only 50% of isolates. Non-fragilis species of bacteroides may be less susceptible to the cephalosporins.

Table 33–5 summarizes the antibiotic regimens for management of moderate to moderately severe infections (eg, patient hemodynamically stable, good surgical drainage possible or established, low APACHE score, no multiple organ failure) and severe infections (eg, major peritoneal soilage, large or multiple abscesses, patient hemodynamically unstable), particularly if drug-resistant organisms are suspected. An effective oral regimen for patients able to take oral medications is presented also.

Table 33–5. Treatment of anaerobic intra-abdominal infections.

Oral therapy
Ciprofloxacin, 750 mg twice daily, plus metronidazole, 500 mg three times daily
Intravenous therapy
Moderate to moderately severe infections:
Ticarcillin/clavulanate, 3 g/0.1 g every 6 hours
or—
Cefotetan, 2 g every 12 hours
or—
Clindamycin, 600 mg every 8 hours, or metronidazole, 500 mg every 8 hours, plus gentamicin, 5 mg/kg/d
Severe infections:
Imipenem, 0.5 g every 6–8 hours, or ceftriaxone, 1 g every 24 hours, plus either clindamycin, 600 mg every 8 hours, or metronidazole, 500 mg every 8 hours

Female Genital Tract & Pelvic Infections

The normal flora of the vagina and cervix includes several species of bacteroides, peptostreptococci, group B streptococci, lactobacilli, coliform bacteria, and, occasionally, spirochetes and clostridia. These organisms commonly cause genital tract infections and may disseminate from there.

While salpingitis is commonly caused by gonococci and chlamydiae, tubo-ovarian and pelvic abscesses are associated with anaerobes in a majority of cases. Postpartum infections may be caused by aerobic streptococci or staphylococci, but anaerobes are often found, and the most severe cases of postpartum or postabortion sepsis are associated with clostridia and bacteroides. These have a high mortality rate, and treatment requires both antimicrobials directed against anaerobes and coliforms (see above) and abscess drainage or early hysterectomy.

Bacteremia & Endocarditis

Anaerobic bacteremia usually originates from the gastrointestinal tract, the oropharynx, decubitus ulcers, or the female genital tract. Endocarditis due to anaerobic and microaerophilic streptococci and bacteroides originates from the same sites. Most cases of anaerobic or microaerophilic streptococcal endocarditis can be effectively treated with 12–20 million units of penicillin G daily for 4–6 weeks, but optimal therapy of other types of anaerobic bacterial endocarditis must rely on laboratory guidance. Anaerobic corynebacteria (propionibacterium), clostridia, and bacteroides occasionally cause endocarditis.

Skin & Soft Tissue Infections

Anaerobic infections in the skin and soft tissue usually follow trauma, inadequate blood supply, or surgery and are commonest in areas that are contaminated by oral or fecal flora. There may be progressive tissue necrosis and a putrid odor.

Several terms, such as bacterial synergistic gangrene, synergistic necrotizing cellulitis, necrotizing fasciitis, and nonclostridial crepitant cellulitis, have been used to classify these infections. Although there are some differences in microbiology among them, their differentiation on clinical grounds alone is difficult. All are mixed infections caused by aerobic and anaerobic organisms and require aggressive surgical debridement of necrotic tissue for cure. Surgical consultation is obligatory to assist in diagnosis and treatment.

Broad-spectrum antibiotics active against both anaerobes and gram-positive and gram-negative aerobes (eg, vancomycin plus metronidazole plus gentamicin or tobramycin) should be instituted empirically and modified by culture results (Table 37–2). They are given for about a week after progressive tissue destruction has been controlled and the margins of the wound remain free of inflammation.

Olsen I et al: A primer on anaerobic bacteria and anaerobic infections for the uninitiated. Infection 1999;27:159. [NLM Cit ID: 99305888]

ACTINOMYCOSIS

Essentials of Diagnosis

- History of recent dental infection or abdominal trauma.
- Chronic pneumonia or indolent intra-abdominal or cervicofacial abscess.
- Sinus tract formation.

General Considerations

Actinomyces israelii and other species of actinomyces occur in the normal flora of the mouth and tonsillar crypts. They are anaerobic, gram-positive, branching filamentous bacteria (1 μm in diameter) that may fragment into bacillary forms. When introduced into traumatized tissue and associated with other anaerobic bacteria, these actinomycetes become pathogens.

The most common site of infection is the cervicofacial area (about 60% of cases). Infection typically follows extraction of a tooth or other trauma. Lesions may develop in the gastrointestinal tract or lungs following ingestion or aspiration of the organism from its endogenous source in the mouth.

Clinical Findings

A. Symptoms and Signs:

1. Cervicofacial actinomycosis–Cervicofacial actinomycosis develops slowly. The area becomes markedly indurated, and the overlying skin becomes reddish or cyanotic. Abscesses eventually draining to the surface persist for long periods. Sulfur granules—masses of filamentous organisms—may be found in the pus. There is usually little pain unless there is secondary infection. Trismus indicates that the muscles of mastication are involved. Radiography may reveal bony involvement.

2. Thoracic actinomycosis–Thoracic involvement begins with fever, cough, and sputum production with night sweats and weight loss. Pleuritic pain may be present. Multiple sinuses may extend through the chest wall, to the heart, or into the abdominal cavity. Ribs may be involved. Radiography shows areas of consolidation and in many cases pleural effusion. Cervicofacial or thoracic disease may occasionally result in central nervous system complications, most commonly brain abscess or meningitis.

3. Abdominal actinomycosis–Abdominal actinomycosis usually causes pain in the ileocecal region, spiking fever and chills, vomiting, and weight loss and may be confused with Crohn's disease. Irregular abdominal masses may be palpated. Pelvic inflammatory disease caused by actinomycetes has been associated with prolonged use of an intrauterine contraceptive device. Sinuses draining to the exterior may develop. CT scanning reveals an inflammatory mass that may extend to involve bone.

B. Laboratory Findings: The anaerobic, gram-positive organism may be demonstrated as a granule or as scattered branching gram-positive filaments in the pus. Anaerobic culture is necessary to distinguish actinomyces from nocardia because specific therapy differs for the two infections.

Treatment

Penicillin G is the drug of choice. Ten to 20 million units are given via a parenteral route for 2–4 weeks, followed by oral penicillin V, 500 mg four times daily.

Sulfonamides such as sulfamethoxazole may be an alternative regimen at a total daily dosage of 2–4 g. Response to therapy is slow. Therapy should be continued for weeks to months after clinical manifestations have disappeared in order to ensure cure. Surgical procedures such as drainage and resection may be beneficial.

With penicillin and surgery, the prognosis is good. The difficulties of diagnosis, however, may permit extensive destruction of tissue before the diagnosis is identified and therapy is started.

Lippes J: Pelvic actinomycosis: a review and preliminary look at prevalence. Am J Obstet Gynecol 1999;180(2 Part 1):265. [NLM Cit ID: 99143014]

Zitsch RP 3rd et al: Actinomycosis: a potential complication of head and neck surgery. Am J Otolaryngol 1999;20:260. [NLM Cit ID: 99369391]

NOCARDIOSIS

Nocardia asteroides and *Nocardia brasiliensis,* aerobic filamentous soil bacteria, cause pulmonary and systemic nocardiosis. Bronchopulmonary abnormalities (eg, alveolar proteinosis) predispose to colonization, but infection is unusual unless the patient is also receiving systemic corticosteroids or is otherwise immunosuppressed.

Pulmonary involvement usually begins with malaise, loss of weight, fever, and night sweats. Cough and production of purulent sputum are the chief complaints. Radiography may show infiltrates accompanied by pleural effusion. The lesions may penetrate to the exterior through the chest wall, invading the ribs.

Dissemination may involve any organ. Brain abscesses and subcutaneous nodules are most frequent. Dissemination is seen exclusively in immunocompromised patients.

N asteroides is usually found as delicate, branching, gram-positive filaments. It may be weakly acid-fast, occasionally causing diagnostic confusion with tuberculosis. Identification is made by culture.

Therapy is initiated with intravenous trimethoprim-sulfamethoxazole administered at a dosage of 5–10 mg/kg/d (trimethoprim) and continued with oral trimethoprim-sulfamethoxazole, one double-strength tablet twice a day. Surgical procedures such as drainage and resection may be needed as adjunctive therapy.

Response may be slow, and therapy must be continued for at least 6 months. The prognosis in systemic nocardiosis is poor when diagnosis and therapy are delayed.

Case records of the Massachusetts General Hospital. Weekly clinicopathological exercises. Case 11-1999. A 60-year-old woman with epidural and paraspinal masses. N Engl J Med 1999;340:1188. [NLM Cit ID: 99200751]

INFECTIONS CAUSED BY MYCOBACTERIA

NONTUBERCULOUS ATYPICAL MYCOBACTERIAL DISEASES

About 10% of mycobacterial infections seen in clinical practice are caused not by *Mycobacterium tuberculosis* but by atypical mycobacteria. Atypical mycobacterial infections are among the most common opportunistic infections in advanced HIV disease. These organisms have distinctive laboratory characteristics, occur ubiquitously in the environment, are not communicable from person to person, and are often strikingly resistant to antituberculous drugs.

Disseminated *Mycobacterium avium* Infection

Mycobacterium avium complex (MAC) produces asymptomatic colonization or a wide spectrum of diseases, including coin lesions, bronchitis in patients with chronic lung disease, and invasive pulmonary disease that is often cavitary and occurs in patients with underlying lung disease. MAC is a common cause of disseminated disease in the late stages of HIV infection, when the CD4 cell count is less than 50–100/μL. Persistent fever and weight loss are the most common symptoms. The organism can usually be cultured from multiple sites, including blood, liver, lymph node, or bone marrow. Blood culture is the preferred means of establishing the diagnosis and has a sensitivity of 98%.

Agents with proved activity against MAC in humans are rifabutin, azithromycin, clarithromycin, and ethambutol. Amikacin and ciprofloxacin have activity in vitro, but clinical data are lacking. Single-agent therapy should not be used because of rapid emergence of secondary resistance. Clarithromycin, 500 mg orally twice daily, plus ethambutol, 15 mg/kg/d as a single dose, with or without rifabutin, 300 mg/d, is the treatment of choice. Azithromycin, 500 mg once daily, may be used instead of clarithromycin. Too few data are available to permit specific recommendations about second-line regimens for patients intolerant of macrolides or those who have disease caused by macrolide-resistant organisms. However, a combination of two or more active agents should be used. The recommendation has been lifelong therapy for disseminated infection for patients with AIDS. It is not known whether immune reconstitution in patients receiving highly active antiretroviral therapy (HAART) whose CD4 counts exceed 100–200/μL is sufficient to permit discontinuation of therapy without relapse. This decision should be made on an individual basis.

Several clinical trials have now shown that antimicrobial prophylaxis of MAC prevents disseminated disease and prolongs survival. It is the standard of care to offer prophylaxis against MAC to all HIV-infected patients with CD4 counts ≤ 50/μL. Duration of therapy is usually for life. Although firm data are lacking, it may be possible to discontinue MAC prophylaxis in patients who have responded to HIV protease inhibitor antiretroviral combination therapy with elevation of CD4 counts consistently above 50–100 cells/μL. Single-drug regimens of clarithromycin, 500 mg twice daily, azithromycin, 1200 mg once weekly, or rifabutin, 300 mg once daily, have been shown to be effective. Clarithromycin and azithromycin are more effective and better tolerated than rifabutin, and for that reason a macrolide is preferred over rifabutin. Patients who develop disseminated disease while receiving macrolide prophylaxis may have macrolide-resistant organisms, a factor to consider when pondering treatment options. Which regimen to use is not established, but most authorities recommend addition of rifabutin and ethambutol. Whether to continue the macrolide if the isolate is resistant in vitro is controversial.

Pulmonary Infections

MAC causes a chronic, slowly progressive pulmonary infection resembling tuberculosis in immunocompetent patients, who typically have underlying pulmonary disease.

Treatment of immunocompetent patients with pulmonary infection is almost completely empirical and based almost entirely on anecdotal data. A combination of agents should be used. Rifampin, 600 mg once daily, plus ethambutol, 15–25 mg/kg/d, plus streptomycin, 1 g intramuscularly three to five times a week for the first 4–6 months, have been used. The role of rifabutin, fluoroquinolones, and the macrolides is not known, but based upon their excellent efficacy in immunocompromised AIDS patients, they may actually be more effective than the relatively weak agents traditionally used in immunocompetent patients. Clarithromycin is a very potent drug in the treatment of MAC in AIDS patients. Based on this, inclusion of clarithromycin in the initial treatment regimen of immunocompetent patients should be strongly considered. Therapy is continued for a total of 18–24 months.

Mycobacterium kansasii can produce clinical disease resembling tuberculosis, but the illness progresses more slowly. Most such infections occur in patients with preexisting lung disease, though 40% of patients have no known pulmonary disease. Microbiologically, *M kansasii* is similar to *M tuberculosis* and is sensitive to the same drugs. Therapy with isoniazid, ethambutol, and rifampin for 2 years (or 1 year after sputum conversion) has been highly successful.

Less common causes of pulmonary disease include *Mycobacterium xenopi, Mycobacterium szulgai,* and *Mycobacterium gordonae.* These organisms have variable sensitivities, and treatment is based on results of sensitivity tests. *Mycobacterium fortuitum* and *Mycobacterium chelonei* also can cause pneumonia.

Lymphadenitis

Most cases of lymphadenitis (scrofula) in adults are caused by *Mycobacterium tuberculosis* and can be a manifestation of disseminated disease. In children, the majority of cases are due to nontuberculous mycobacterial species, with *Mycobacterium scrofulaceum* and MAC being the most common. *Mycobacterium kansasii, Mycobacterium bovis, Mycobacterium chelonei,* and *Mycobacterium fortuitum* are less commonly observed. Unlike disease caused by *M tuberculosis,* which requires systemic therapy for 6 months, infection with nontuberculous mycobacteria can be successfully treated by surgical excision without antituberculous therapy.

Skin & Soft Tissue Infections

Skin and soft tissue infections such as abscesses, septic arthritis, and osteomyelitis can result from direct inoculation or hematogenous dissemination or may occur as a complication of surgery.

M chelonei and *M fortuitum* are frequent causes of this type of infection. Most cases occur in the extremities and initially present as nodules. Ulceration with abscess formation often follows. The organisms are resistant to the usual antituberculous drugs but may be sensitive to a variety of antibiotics, including erythromycin, doxycycline, amikacin, cefoxitin, sulfonamides, imipenem, and ciprofloxacin. Therapy includes surgical debridement along with drug therapy. Initially, parenteral drugs are given for several weeks, and this is followed by an oral regimen to which the organism is sensitive. The duration of therapy is variable but usually continues for several months after the soft tissue lesions have healed.

Mycobacterium marinum infection ("swimming pool granuloma") presents as a nodular skin lesion following exposure to nonchlorinated water. The lesions respond to therapy with doxycycline, minocycline, or trimethoprim-sulfamethoxazole.

Mycobacterium ulcerans infection (Buruli ulcer) is seen mainly in Africa and Australia and produces a large ulcerative lesion. Therapy consists of surgical excision and skin grafting.

Diagnosis and treatment of disease caused by nontuberculous mycobacteria. Medical Section of the American Lung Association. Am J Respir Crit Care Med 1997;156(2 Part 2):S1. [NLM Cit ID: 97425234]

French AL et al: Nontuberculous mycobacterial infections. Med Clin North Am 1997;81:361. [NLM Cit ID: 97247099]

Horsburgh Jr CR: The pathophysiology of disseminated *Mycobacterium avium* complex disease in AIDS. J Infect Dis 1999;179(Suppl 3):S461. [NLM Cit ID: 99201459]

MYCOBACTERIUM TUBERCULOSIS INFECTIONS

The case rate of tuberculosis in the United States has been increasing since 1986, largely due to a dramatic increase in cases among HIV-infected individuals. Compared to a lifetime risk of developing active tuberculosis of approximately 10% in an infected immunocompetent person, the risk is up to 7% per year for the HIV-infected individual who is also infected with *M tuberculosis.* This greatly increased risk of developing active disease—as well as the recent occurrence in HIV-infected individuals of outbreaks of tuberculosis caused by strains of *M tuberculosis* resistant to multiple drugs—underscore the importance of early case identification and administration of effective antituberculous therapy. A complete discussion of initial and definitive therapy of tuberculosis is beyond the scope of this chapter. General principles and some specific recommendations for therapy are provided. More complete information and expert consultation can be obtained from the Francis J. Curry National Tuberculosis Center at the Web site http://www.nationaltbcenter.edu or, by phone, 415-502-4600, or fax, 415-502-4620. See also Chapter 9 of this book.

Treatment Considerations

A. Initial Therapy: Patients with suspected or documented active tuberculosis should be treated with at least two drugs to which the strain is susceptible. Single-drug regimens are notoriously ineffective, with failure rates of 70% or more due to emergence of resistant mutants, which occurs at a frequency of one bacillus in 10^6. Because 10^7 to 10^9 acid-fast bacilli typically are present at the site of active infection, resistant mutants are invariably present when therapy is initiated. Therapy with two drugs, each possessing a different mechanism of action, is effective because the odds that a bacillus is resistant to both are $10^{-6} \times 10^{-6}$, or one in 10^{12}, which is at least three orders of magnitude less than the number of infecting organisms.

The results of susceptibility tests usually are not known when therapy is initiated. Therefore, drugs are chosen based on their relative potency and on prior susceptibility data obtained from within the community or within the relevant patient population. Isoniazid and rifampin are the two most potent antituberculous agents, and because clinical isolates from newly diagnosed cases were predictably susceptible to both (98% or more of strains), initial therapy with these two drugs was until recently considered appropriate for most cases. Three or four drug regimens were reserved for patients who had one or more risk factors for drug-resistant tuberculosis. Patients at risk for infection with resistant strains were those who had been previously treated for tuberculosis; those who failed to complete a prescribed course of therapy or were otherwise noncompliant; and patients or their close contacts who were from regions (eg, the Philippines, China, Southeast Asia, and Haiti) where the prevalence of primary drug-resistant strains is above 5%.

Initial therapy with an oral four-drug regimen consisting of isoniazid (INH), 300 mg, rifampin, 600 mg, pyrazinamide, 25 mg/kg, and ethambutol, 15 mg/kg, each administered as a single daily dose, is recommended pending results of culture and susceptibility tests unless the patient has HIV infection and is receiving or will receive a protease inhibitor. In this case, rifabutin 150 mg once daily is used instead of rifampin. Ritonavir and hard-gel saquinavir are contraindicated because of unfavorable drug interactions. For indinavir, the dose should be increased from 800 mg to 1200 mg every 8 hours, and for nelfinavir the dose should be increased from 750 to 1250 mg three times daily. CDC has published recommendations for treatment of tuberculosis in the HIV-infected patient. This document can be obtained by calling 404-639-8094 or can be downloaded from the Division of TB Elimination Web site at http://www2.cdc.gov/mmwr/mmwr_rr.html. It may be reasonable to add or substitute other drugs (Table 33–6) depending on the epidemiologic data. For example, if a patient has had a relapse or has not responded to a particular regimen, two other drugs not used previously should be included in the regimen. If a strain is known to be resistant to a particular drug, another drug to which the strain is likely to be susceptible should be substituted. As a rule of thumb, at least two new drugs are added to a failing regimen. Which drug or drugs eventually are selected will also depend upon their toxicities and the ability of the patient to tolerate them.

B. Definitive Therapy: Assuming that the four-drug regimen recommended above is used and that the strain is susceptible, ethambutol can be discontinued and the three-drug regimen of isoniazid, rifampin, and pyrazinamide administered for a total of 2 months. The pyrazinamide is then stopped, and isoniazid and rifampin are administered for at least four more months (total of 6 months). If pyrazinamide is not used during the first 2 months of therapy, isoniazid and rifampin should be administered for a minimum of 9 months. If other drug combinations must be used because of toxicity or drug resistance, longer durations of therapy are required (Table 33–7).

The regimens used for treatment of active pulmonary tuberculosis are effective also against extrapulmonary disease. However, some authorities recommend longer durations (eg, 12 months of isoniazid plus rifampin instead of 6–9 months) for extrapulmonary disease such as meningitis or bone and joint infections, where drug penetration is an issue, and for disseminated infection. The relapse rate in HIV-infected patients treated with a 6-month regimen of isoniazid-rifampin-pyrazinamide is higher than in HIV-seronegative patients. Relapse has been associated with low CD4 counts (eg, < 50 cells/μL). Because extending therapy does not improve survival, current recommendations for treatment of active tuberculosis in HIV-infected patients are the same as for other patients.

Table 33–6. Antituberculous agents, ranked in order of preference, and usual daily doses.

Drug	Daily Dose and Route
First-line agents	
Isoniazid	300 mg orally or IM
Rifampin	600 mg orally or IV
Ethambutol	15–25 mg/kg orally
Pyrazinamide	25 mg/kg orally
Streptomycin	15 mg/kg IM
Second-line agents	
Amikacin	15 mg/kg IM
Capreomycin	15 mg/kg IM
Ethionamide	0.5–1 g orally
Cycloserine	0.5–1 g orally
Levofloxacin	500 mg orally once daily

Prognosis & Follow-Up

Response to therapy is monitored clinically and, if possible, bacteriologically. A qualitative decrease in numbers of acid-fast bacilli seen on sputum smears over the course of therapy is a reliable indicator of response. Most patients who are treated with the recommended four-drug regimen are culture-negative by 3 months. If sputum smears remain persistently positive, noncompliance should be suspected and institution of supervised daily therapy strongly considered. If noncompliance is unlikely, the possibility of drug

Table 33–7. Minimum recommended duration of antituberculous therapy.

Regimen	Duration (mo)
Isoniazid + rifampin + pyrazinamide[1]	6
Isoniazid + rifampin	9
Rifampin + pyrazinamide[1] + ethambutol	6–9
Rifampin + ethambutol	12
Isoniazid + ethambutol	18–24

[1]Pyrazinamide for the first 2 months only.

resistance should be entertained and the regimen altered accordingly.

The period of infectivity after initiation of chemotherapy is poorly defined. Three consecutive sputum smears negative for acid-fast bacilli using samples obtained on separate days are a reliable indication that the patient is no longer infectious to others.

Preventive Therapy

Administration of isoniazid, 300 mg once daily for 6–12 months, is approximately 80% effective in preventing active disease in persons with a positive tuberculin (PPD) skin test. A regimen of 900 mg twice weekly (directly observed) is also effective. The test is considered positive when there is ≥ 10 mm of induration at 48–72 hours after intradermal injection of 0.1 mL of tuberculin antigen (Table 9–12). The cutoff is ≥ 5 mm for HIV-infected individuals and close contacts of active cases of pulmonary tuberculosis. Isoniazid prophylaxis is recommended for tuberculin skin test-positive individuals aged 35 or younger and for all close contacts of active cases, HIV-infected or otherwise immunocompromised individuals, and the skin test converters (defined as individuals with a prior documented negative test within 2 years of a newly positive one) regardless of age. For patients unable to take isoniazid, an alternative is rifampin, 600 mg daily or twice weekly (or rifabutin 300 mg unless the patient is receiving a protease inhibitor, in which case the dose is 150 mg daily or 300 mg twice weekly).

A 3-month regimen of isoniazid plus rifampin 600 mg daily or twice weekly—or rifampin 600 mg plus pyrazinamide 20 mg/kg with daily dosing and 50 mg/kg for twice-weekly dosing—is also effective. Rifabutin at the doses given above should be used instead of rifampin in HIV-infected patients receiving a protease inhibitor.

Catanzaro AS et al: The role of clinical suspicion in evaluating a new diagnostic test for active tuberculosis: results of a multicenter prospective trial. JAMA 2000;283:639. [NLM Cit ID: 20127470]

Gordin F et al: Rifampin and pyrazinamide vs isoniazid for prevention of tuberculosis in HIV-infected persons: an international randomized trial. Terry Beirn Community Programs for Clinical Research on AIDS, the Adult AIDS Clinical Trials Group, the Pan American Health Organization, and the Centers for Disease Control and Prevention Study Group. JAMA 2000;283:1445. [NLM Cit ID: 20195072]

Jacobs MR: Activity of quinolones against mycobacteria. Drugs 1999;58(Suppl 2):19. [NLM Cit ID: 20019128]

JAMA patient page: Tuberculosis. JAMA 1998;280:1724. [NLM Cit ID: 99048848]

Prevention and treatment of tuberculosis among patients infected with human immunodeficiency virus: Principles of therapy and revised recommendations. MMWR Morb Mortal Wkly Rep 1998;47(RR-20):1. [NLM Cit ID: 99025615]

Pulido F et al: Relapse of tuberculosis after treatment in human immunodeficiency virus-infected patients. Arch Intern Med 1997;157:227. [NLM Cit ID: 97163147] (Shorter duration of treatment and a low CD4 cell count were associated with a greater probability of relapse, which occurred in 10 [24%] of 41 patients who were treated for less than 9 months.)

TUBERCULOUS MENINGITIS

Essentials of Diagnosis

- Gradual onset of listlessness, irritability, and anorexia.
- Headache, vomiting, and seizures common.
- Cranial nerve abnormalities typical.
- Tuberculosis focus may be evident elsewhere.
- Cerebrospinal fluid shows several hundred lymphocytes, low glucose, and high protein.

General Considerations

Tuberculous meningitis is caused by rupture of a meningeal tuberculoma resulting from earlier hematogenous seeding of tubercle bacillus from a pulmonary focus, or it may be a consequence of miliary spread.

Clinical Findings

A. Symptoms and Signs: The onset is usually gradual, with listlessness, irritability, anorexia, and fever, followed by headache, vomiting, convulsions, and coma. In older patients, headache and behavioral changes are prominent early symptoms. Nuchal rigidity and cranial nerve palsies occur as the meningitis progresses. Evidence of active tuberculosis elsewhere or a history of prior tuberculosis is present in up to 75% of patients.

B. Laboratory Findings: The spinal fluid is frequently yellowish, with increased pressure, 100–500 cells/μL (predominantly lymphocytes, though neutrophils may be present early during infection), increased protein, and decreased glucose. Acid-fast stains of cerebrospinal fluid usually are negative, and cultures also may be negative in 15–25% of cases. Chest x-ray often reveals abnormalities compatible with tuberculosis but may be normal.

Differential Diagnosis

Tuberculous meningitis may be confused with any other type of meningitis, but the gradual onset, the predominantly lymphocytic pleocytosis of the spinal fluid, and evidence of tuberculosis elsewhere often point to the diagnosis. The tuberculin skin test is usually positive, though in a significant proportion of patients it is negative.

Fungal and other granulomatous meningitides, syphilis, and carcinomatous meningitis are in the differential diagnosis.

Complications

Complications of tuberculous meningitis include chronic brain syndrome, seizure disorders, cranial nerve palsies, stroke, and obstructive hydrocephalus. These result from inflammatory exudate primarily involving the basilar meninges and arteries.

Treatment

Presumptive diagnosis followed by early, empirical antituberculous therapy is essential for survival and to minimize sequelae. Even if cultures are not positive, a full course of therapy is warranted if the clinical setting is suggestive of tuberculous meningitis.

Regimens that are effective for pulmonary tuberculosis are effective also for tuberculous meningitis (Table 33–6). Rifampin, isoniazid, and pyrazinamide all penetrate into cerebrospinal fluid well. The penetration of ethambutol is more variable, but therapeutic concentrations can be achieved, and the drug has been successfully used for meningitis. Aminoglycosides penetrate less well. Regimens that do not include both isoniazid and rifampin may be effective but are less reliable and generally must be given for longer periods. Other regimens may also be effective, but they are less reliable and generally must be given for longer periods.

Some authorities recommend the addition of corticosteroids for patients with focal deficits or altered mental status. Dexamethasone, 0.15 mg/kg four times daily for 1–2 weeks, then discontinued in a tapering regimen over 4 weeks, may be used.

LEPROSY

Essentials of Diagnosis

- Pale, anesthetic macular—or nodular and erythematous—skin lesions.
- Superficial nerve thickening with associated anesthesia.
- History of residence in endemic area in childhood.
- Acid-fast bacilli in skin lesions or nasal scrapings, or characteristic histologic nerve changes.

General Considerations

Leprosy is a chronic infectious disease caused by the acid-fast rod *Mycobacterium leprae.* The mode of transmission probably is respiratory and involves prolonged exposure in childhood. The disease is endemic in tropical and subtropical Asia, Africa, Central and South America and the Pacific regions, and southern USA.

Clinical Findings

A. Symptoms and Signs: The onset is insidious. The lesions involve the cooler body tissues: skin, superficial nerves, nose, pharynx, larynx, eyes, and testicles. Skin lesions may occur as pale, anesthetic macular lesions 1–10 cm in diameter; discrete erythematous, infiltrated nodules 1–5 cm in diameter; or a diffuse skin infiltration. Neurologic disturbances are manifested by nerve infiltration and thickening, with resultant anesthesia, neuritis, and paresthesia. Bilateral ulnar neuropathy is highly suggestive. In untreated cases, disfigurement due to the skin infiltration and nerve involvement may be extreme, leading to trophic ulcers, bone resorption, and loss of digits.

The disease is divided clinically and by laboratory tests into two distinct types: lepromatous and tuberculoid. The lepromatous type occurs in persons with defective cellular immunity. The course is progressive and malignant, with nodular skin lesions, slow, symmetric nerve involvement; abundant acid-fast bacilli in the skin lesions; and a negative lepromin skin test. In the tuberculoid type, cellular immunity is intact and the course is more benign and less progressive, with macular skin lesions, severe asymmetric nerve involvement of sudden onset with few bacilli present in the lesions, and a positive lepromin skin test. Intermediate ("borderline") cases are frequent. Eye involvement (keratitis and iridocyclitis), nasal ulcers, epistaxis, anemia, and lymphadenopathy may occur.

B. Laboratory Findings: Laboratory confirmation of leprosy requires the demonstration of acid-fast bacilli in a skin biopsy. Biopsy of skin or of a thickened involved nerve also gives a typical histologic picture. *M leprae* does not grow in artificial media.

Differential Diagnosis

The skin lesions of leprosy often resemble those of lupus erythematosus, sarcoidosis, syphilis, erythema nodosum, erythema multiforme, cutaneous tuberculosis, and vitiligo.

Complications

Renal failure and hepatomegaly from secondary amyloidosis may occur with long-standing disease.

Treatment

Combination therapy is recommended for treatment of all types of leprosy. Single-drug treatment is accompanied by emergence of resistance, and primary resistance to dapsone also occurs. For borderline and lepromatous cases, a three-drug regimen such as dapsone, 50–100 mg/d, clofazimine, 50 mg/d, and rifampin, 10 mg/kg/d (up to 600 mg/d), all given orally, should be used. The triple-drug combination should be administered for a minimum of 2–3 years and, ideally, until all biopsies are negative for acid-fast bacilli. For indeterminate and tuberculoid leprosy, the dapsone-rifampin combination is recommended for 6–12 months, often followed by a course of dapsone alone for 2 or more years.

Two reactional states—erythema nodosum leprosum and reversal reactions—may occur as a consequence of therapy. The reversal reaction, typical of borderline lepromatous leprosy, probably results from enhanced host immunity. Skin lesions and nerves become swollen and tender, but systemic manifestations are not seen. Erythema nodosum leprosum, typical of lepromatous leprosy, is a consequence of immune injury from antigen-antibody complex deposition in skin and other tissues; in addition to skin and nerve manifestations, fever and systemic involvement may be seen. Prednisone, 60 mg/d, or thalidomide, 300 mg/d (in the nonpregnant patient only), is effective for erythema nodosum leprosum. Improvement is expected within a few days after initiating prednisone, and thereafter the dose may be tapered over several weeks to avoid recurrence. Thalidomide is also tapered over several weeks to a 100 mg bedtime dose. Erythema nodosum leprosum is usually confined to the first year of therapy, and prednisone or thalidomide can be discontinued. Thalidomide is ineffective for reversal reactions, and prednisone, 60 mg/d, is indicated. Reversal reactions tend to recur, and the dose of prednisone should be slowly tapered over weeks to months. Therapy for leprosy should not be discontinued during treatment of reactional states.

Jacobson RR et al: Leprosy. Lancet 1999;353:655. [NLM Cit ID: 99153417]

INFECTIONS CAUSED BY CHLAMYDIAE

Chlamydiae are a large group of obligate intracellular parasites closely related to gram-negative bacteria. They are assigned to three species—*Chlamydia trachomatis, Chlamydia psittaci,* and *Chlamydia pneumoniae*—on the basis of intracellular inclusions, sulfonamide susceptibility, antigenic composition, and disease production. *C trachomatis* causes many different human infections involving the eye (trachoma, inclusion conjunctivitis), the genital tract (lymphogranuloma venereum, nongonococcal urethritis, cervicitis, salpingitis), or the respiratory tract (pneumonitis). *C psittaci* causes psittacosis in humans and many animal diseases. *Chlamydia pneumoniae* has recently been recognized as a cause of respiratory tract infections.

CHLAMYDIA TRACHOMATIS INFECTIONS

1. LYMPHOGRANULOMA VENEREUM

Essentials of Diagnosis

- Evanescent primary genital lesion.
- Lymph node enlargement, softening, and suppuration, with draining sinuses.
- Proctitis and rectal stricture in women or homosexual men.
- Positive complement fixation test.

General Considerations

Lymphogranuloma venereum is an acute and chronic sexually transmitted disease caused by *Chlamydia trachomatis* types L1–L3. After the genital lesion disappears, the infection spreads to lymph channels and lymph nodes of the genital and rectal areas. The disease is acquired during intercourse or through contact with contaminated exudate from active lesions. The incubation period is 5–21 days. Inapparent infections and latent disease are not uncommon.

Clinical Findings

A. Symptoms and Signs: In men, the initial vesicular or ulcerative lesion (on the external genitalia) is evanescent and often goes unnoticed. Inguinal buboes appear 1–4 weeks after exposure, are often bilateral, and have a tendency to fuse, soften, and break down to form multiple draining sinuses, with extensive scarring. In women, the genital lymph drainage is to the perirectal glands. Early anorectal manifestations are proctitis with tenesmus and bloody purulent discharge; late manifestations are chronic cicatrizing inflammation of the rectal and perirectal tissue. These changes lead to obstipation and rectal stricture and, occasionally, rectovaginal and perianal fistulas. They are also seen in homosexual men.

B. Laboratory Findings: The complement fixation test may be positive, but cross-reaction with other chlamydiae occurs. Although a positive reaction may reflect remote infection, high titers usually indicate active disease. Specific immunofluorescence tests for IgM are more specific for acute infection.

Differential Diagnosis

The early lesion of lymphogranuloma venereum must be differentiated from the lesions of syphilis, genital herpes, and chancroid; lymph node involvement must be distinguished from that due to tularemia, tuberculosis, plague, neoplasm, or pyogenic infection; rectal stricture must be distinguished from that due to neoplasm and ulcerative colitis.

Treatment

The antibiotic of choice is tetracycline (contraindicated in pregnancy), 0.25–0.5 g orally four times daily, or doxycycline, 0.1 g twice daily for 21 days. Erythromycin, 500 mg four times a day, or trimethoprim-sulfamethoxazole, 160/800 mg twice a day for 21 days, also is effective.

2. CHLAMYDIAL URETHRITIS & CERVICITIS

Chlamydia trachomatis immunotypes D–K are isolated in about 50% of cases of nongonococcal urethritis and cervicitis by appropriate techniques. In other cases, *Ureaplasma urealyticum* can be grown as a possible etiologic agent. *C trachomatis* is an important cause of postgonococcal urethritis. Co-infection with gonococci and chlamydiae is common, and postgonococcal (ie, chlamydial) urethritis may persist after successful treatment of the gonococcal component. Occasionally, epididymitis, prostatitis, or proctitis is caused by chlamydial infection.

Females infected with chlamydia may be asymptomatic or may have signs and symptoms of cervicitis, salpingitis, or pelvic inflammatory disease. Chlamydia is probably the leading cause of infertility in females in the United States.

The diagnosis of chlamydial infection has been clinical because *C trachomatis* is difficult and expensive to culture. The urethral or cervical discharge tends to be less painful, less purulent, and watery in chlamydial versus gonococcal infection. A patient with urethritis or cervicitis and absence of gram-negative diplococci on Gram stain and of *N gonorrhoeae* on culture is assumed to have chlamydial infection. Direct immunofluorescence assay, enzyme-linked immunoassay, and a DNA probe test, although less sensitive than culture, are sometimes used to confirm the diagnosis and for screening. The ligase chain reaction (LCR) test for *C trachomatis* has superior sensitivity compared with all other methods (eg, sensitivity of 60–70% for DNA probe versus 90–95% for LCR). LCR also has excellent specificity, approaching 100%, and it can be performed on urine. For these reasons, LCR will likely replace all other methods for diagnosis of chlamydial urethritis and cervicitis.

Therapy often must be given presumptively. Sexual partners of infected patients should also be treated. Effective treatment regimens are tetracycline or erythromycin, 500 mg four times a day, or doxycycline, 100 mg twice daily, for 7 days. Trimethoprim-sulfamethoxazole, 160/800 mg twice a day, is acceptable but may be less effective than tetracyclines or erythromycin. Erythromycin is the drug of choice in the pregnant patient. A single 1 g dose of azithromycin is effective for uncomplicated urethritis and cervicitis and has the advantage of improved patient compliance and minimal toxicity.

Cohen CR et al: Pathogenesis of chlamydia induced pelvic inflammatory disease. Sex Transm Infect 1999;75:21. [NLM Cit ID: 99377446]

CHLAMYDIA PSITTACI & PSITTACOSIS (Ornithosis)

Essentials of Diagnosis

- Fever, chills, and cough; headache common.
- Atypical pneumonia with slightly delayed appearance of signs of pneumonitis.
- Contact with infected bird (psittacine, pigeons, many others) 7–15 days previously.
- Isolation of chlamydiae or rising titer of complement-fixing antibodies.

General Considerations

Psittacosis is acquired from contact with birds (parrots, parakeets, pigeons, chickens, ducks, and many others), which may or may not be ill. The history may be difficult to obtain if the patient acquired infection from an illegally imported bird.

Clinical Findings

The onset is usually rapid, with fever, chills, myalgia, dry cough, and headache. Signs include temperature-pulse dissociation, dullness to percussion, and rales. Pulmonary findings may be absent early. Dyspnea and cyanosis may occur later. Endocarditis, which is culture-negative, may occur. The radiographic findings in typical psittacosis are those of atypical pneumonia, which tends to be interstitial and diffuse in appearance, though consolidation can occur. Psittacosis is indistinguishable from other bacterial or viral pneumonias by radiography.

The organism is rarely isolated from cultures. The diagnosis is usually made serologically; antibodies appear during the second week and can be demonstrated by complement fixation or immunofluorescence. Antibody response may be suppressed by early chemotherapy.

Differential Diagnosis

The illness is indistinguishable from viral, mycoplasmal, or other atypical pneumonias except for the history of contact with birds. Psittacosis is in the differential diagnosis of culture-negative endocarditis.

Treatment

Treatment consists of giving tetracycline, 0.5 g orally every 6 hours or 0.5 g intravenously every 12 hours, for 14–21 days. Erythromycin may be effective as well.

CHLAMYDIA PNEUMONIAE

Chlamydia pneumoniae causes pneumonia and bronchitis and has been associated seroepidemiologically with coronary artery disease. The clinical presentation of pneumonia is that of an atypical pneumonia. The organism accounts for approximately 10% of community-acquired pneumonias, ranking second to mycoplasma as an agent of atypical pneumonia. Its role in coronary artery disease remains to be defined, but *C pneumoniae* has been detected in up to 50% of coronary atheromatous lesions.

Like *C psittaci*, strains of *C pneumoniae* are resistant to sulfonamides. Erythromycin or tetracycline, 500 mg four times a day for 10–14 days, appears to be effective therapy. Some of the newer fluoroquinolones, such as levofloxacin or trovafloxacin, are active in vitro against *C pneumoniae* and probably are effective clinically. The oral dose is 500 mg (levofloxacin) or 200 mg once daily (trovafloxacin).

Campbell LA et al: Detection of *Chlamydia pneumoniae* TWAR in human coronary atherotomy tissue. J Infect Dis 1995;172:585. [NLM Cit ID: 95348569]

Gurfinkel EP et al: Emerging role of antibiotics in atherosclerosis. Am Heart J 1999;138(5 Part 2):S537. [NLM Cit ID: 20007596]

Marrie TJ et al: Ambulatory patients with community-acquired pneumonia: Frequency of atypical agents and clinical course. Am J Med 1996;101:508. [NLM Cit ID: 97104108]

Mattila KJ et al: Role of infection as a risk factor for atherosclerosis, myocardial infarction, and stroke. Clin Infect Dis 1998;26:719. [NLM Cit ID: 98185539] (Infections are being linked to atherosclerosis and thrombosis. *Chlamydia pneumoniae* is associated with coronary heart disease.)

Shor A et al: *Chlamydia pneumoniae* and atherosclerosis. JAMA 1999;282:2071. [NLM Cit ID: 20057348]

Stamm WE: *Chlamydia trachomatis* infections: progress and problems. J Infect Dis 1999;179(Suppl 2):S380. [NLM Cit ID: 99181352]

RELEVANT WORLD WIDE WEB SITES

[Hepatic Tuberculosis Case Study]
http://path.upmc.edu/cases/case30.html

[MedMicro Profiles]
http://endeavor.med.nyu.edu/courses/microbiology2/courseware/infect-disease

[Meningococcemia Case Study]
http://path.upmc.edu:80/cases/case53.html

[Pathology of Tuberculosis]
http://www-medlib.med.utah.edu/WebPath/TUTORIAL/MTB/MTB.html

[Centers for Disease Control and Prevention]
http://www.cdc.gov

Infectious Diseases: Spirochetal

34

See http://www.current-med.com/ch34.html for updated addresses of Web sites referenced in this chapter.

Richard A. Jacobs, MD, PhD

SYPHILIS

NATURAL HISTORY & PRINCIPLES OF DIAGNOSIS & TREATMENT

Syphilis is a complex infectious disease caused by *Treponema pallidum,* a spirochete capable of infecting almost any organ or tissue in the body and causing protean clinical manifestations (Table 34–1). Transmission occurs most frequently during sexual contact, through minor skin or mucosal lesions; sites of inoculation are usually genital but may be extragenital. The risk of developing syphilis after unprotected sex with an individual with early syphilis is approximately 30–50%. The organism is extremely sensitive to heat and drying but can survive for days in fluids; therefore, it can be transmitted in blood from infected persons. Syphilis can be transferred via the placenta from mother to fetus after the tenth week of pregnancy (congenital syphilis).

The immunologic response to infection is complex, but it provides the basis for most clinical diagnoses. The infection induces the synthesis of a number of antibodies, some of which react specifically with pathogenic treponemes and some with components of normal tissues (see below). If the disease is untreated, sufficient defenses develop to produce a relative resistance to reinfection; however, in most cases these immune reactions fail to eradicate existing infection and may contribute to tissue destruction in the late stages. Patients treated early in the disease are fully susceptible to reinfection.

The natural history of acquired syphilis is generally divided into two major clinical stages: early (infectious) syphilis and late syphilis. The two stages are separated by a symptom-free latent phase during the first part of which (early latency) the infectious stage is liable to recur. Infectious syphilis includes the primary lesions (chancre and regional lymphadenopathy); the secondary lesions (commonly involving skin and mucous membranes, occasionally bone, central nervous system, or liver); relapsing lesions during early latency; and congenital lesions. The hallmark of these lesions is an abundance of spirochetes; tissue reaction is usually minimal. Late syphilis consists of so-called benign (gummatous) lesions involving skin, bones, and viscera; cardiovascular disease (principally aortitis); and a variety of central nervous system and ocular syndromes. These forms of syphilis are not contagious. The lesions contain few demonstrable spirochetes, but tissue reactivity (vasculitis, necrosis) is severe and suggestive of hypersensitivity phenomena.

As a result of intensive public health efforts during and after World War II, there was a reduction in the incidence of infectious syphilis. With the marked increase in all sexually transmitted diseases since the 1970s, there has been a rise in the number of reported cases of syphilis. In the early 1980s, the incidence of infectious syphilis increased, with a particularly high rate among homosexual men. In the mid 1980s, there was a slight decrease in the incidence of syphilis, chiefly as a result of changes in sexual practices in response to the AIDS epidemic. Between 1985 and 1990, there was again a dramatic increase in infectious syphilis, with 50,223 cases of primary and secondary syphilis reported in 1990. This increase was broad-based, affecting both men and women in inner city urban and rural areas, particularly in the southern regions of the United States. Although adolescent and young adult blacks were primarily affected, increases were seen in other ethnic groups also, as well as adults over 60. Limited access to health care, decreases in health department clinical services, increased use of illicit drugs (especially "crack cocaine"), the exchange of sex for drugs or money to buy drugs, and the difficulty of contact tracing when multiple sexual partners are involved all contributed to the dramatic increase. Concomitantly with the increase in acquired syphilis, there has also been an increase in congenital syphilis, particularly in urban areas. In response to this increase in infectious syphilis, intensive syphilis control programs targeting high-risk populations—women of childbearing age, sexually active teens, drug users, inmates of penal institutions, persons with multiple sexual partners or those who have sex with

Table 34–1. Stages of syphilis and common clinical manifestations.

Primary syphilis
- Genital ulcer: painless ulcer with clean base and firm indurated borders
- Regional lymphadenopathy

Secondary syphilis
- Skin and mucous membranes
  - Rash: diffuse (including palms and soles), macular, papular, pustular, and combinations
  - Condylomata lata
  - Mucous patches: painless, silvery ulcerations of mucous membrane with surrounding erythema
- Generalized lymphadenopathy
- Constitutional symptoms
  - Fever, usually low-grade
  - Malaise
  - Anorexia
  - Arthralgias and myalgias
- Central nervous system
  - Asymptomatic
  - Symptomatic
  - Headache
  - Meningitis
  - Cranial neuropathies (II–VIII)
- Ocular
  - Iritis
  - Iridocyclitis
- Other
  - Renal: glomerulonephritis, nephrotic syndrome
  - Liver: hepatitis
  - Bone and joint: arthritis, periostitis

Late syphilis
- Late benign (gummatous): granulomatous lesion usually involving skin, mucous membranes and bones, but any organ can be involved
- Cardiovascular
  - Aortic insufficiency
  - Coronary ostial stenosis
  - Aortic aneurysm
- Neurosyphilis
  - Asymptomatic
  - Meningovascular
    - Seizures
    - Hemiparesis or hemiplegia
  - Tabes dorsalis
    - Impaired proprioception and vibratory sensation
    - Argyll Robertson pupil
    - Shooting pains
    - Ataxia
    - Romberg's sign
    - Urinary and fecal incontinence
    - Charcot joint
    - Cranial nerve involvement (II–VIII)
  - General paresis
    - Personality changes
    - Hyperactive reflexes
    - Argyll Robertson pupil
    - Decreased memory
    - Slurred speech
    - Optic atrophy

prostitutes—and emphasizing screening, early treatment, contact tracing, and condom use were instituted and have been successful in limiting the spread of this disease—as evidenced by the decrease in reported cases of primary and secondary syphilis to 6993 in 1998.

Laboratory Diagnosis

Since the infectious agent of syphilis cannot be cultured in vitro, diagnostic measures must rely mainly on serologic testing, microscopic detection of *T pallidum* in lesions, and other examinations (biopsies, lumbar puncture, x-rays) for evidence of tissue damage.

A. Serologic Tests for Syphilis: (Table 34–2.) There are two general categories of serologic tests for syphilis: (1) Nontreponemal tests detect antibodies to lipoidal antigens present in either the host or *T pallidum.* The original antigens used to measure these nonspecific antibodies (reagin) were crude extracts of beef heart or liver and resulted in significant false-positive reactions. The cardiolipin-cholesterol-lecithin preparation presently used is much purer and gives fewer false-positive reactions. (2) Treponemal tests employ live or killed *T pallidum* as antigen to detect antibodies specific for pathogenic treponemes.

1. Nontreponemal antigen tests–The most commonly used nontreponemal antigen tests are the VDRL and RPR, which measure the ability of heated serum to flocculate a suspension of cardiolipin-cholesterol-lecithin. The flocculation tests are easy, rapid, and inexpensive to perform and are therefore used primarily for routine (often automated) screening for syphilis. Quantitative expression of the reactivity of the serum, based upon titration of dilutions of serum, is valuable in establishing the diagnosis and in evaluating the efficacy of treatment.

The VDRL test (the nontreponemal test in widest use) generally becomes positive 4–6 weeks after infection, or 1–3 weeks after the appearance of a primary lesion; it is almost invariably positive in the secondary stage. The VDRL titer is usually high (> 1:32) in secondary syphilis and tends to be lower (< 1:4) or even negative in late forms of syphilis. These serologic tests are not highly specific and must be closely correlated with other clinical and laboratory findings. The tests are positive in patients with nonsexually transmitted treponematoses (see below). More importantly, "false-positive" serologic reactions are frequently encountered in a wide variety of nontreponemal states, including connective tissue diseases, infectious mononucleosis, malaria, febrile diseases, leprosy, intravenous drug use, infective endocarditis, old age, hepatitis C viral infection, and

Table 34–2. Percentage of patients with positive serologic tests for syphilis.[1]

Test	Stage		
	Primary	Secondary	Tertiary
VDRL[2]	70–75%	99%	75%
FTA-ABS[3]	85–95%	100%	98%

[1]Based on untreated cases.
[2]VDRL = Venereal Disease Research Laboratory test.
[3]FTA-ABS = Fluorescent treponemal antibody absorption test.

pregnancy. False-positive tests also occur more commonly in HIV-seropositive patients (4%) than in HIV-seronegative patients (0.8%). False-positive reactions are usually of low titer and transient and may be distinguished from true positives by specific treponemal antibody tests. False-negative results can be seen when very high antibody titers are present (the prozone phenomenon). If syphilis is strongly suspected and the nontreponemal test is negative, the laboratory should be instructed to dilute the specimen to detect a positive reaction. The rapid plasma reagin (RPR) test is a simple, rapid, and reliable substitute for the traditional VDRL test. RPR titers are often higher than VDRL titers and thus are not comparable. The RPR test is suitable for automated screening.

Nontreponemal antibody titers are used to assess adequacy of therapy. The time required for the VDRL or RPR to become negative depends on the stage of the disease, the height of the initial titer, and whether the infection is an initial or repeat episode. In general, individuals with repeat infections, higher initial titers, and more advanced stages of disease at the time of treatment have a slower seroconversion rate and are more likely to remain serofast (ie, titers do not become negative). Older data derived from more intensive treatment regimens than are presently used indicate that in primary and secondary syphilis, the VDRL usually decreases fourfold by 3 months and eightfold by 6 months. Furthermore, seronegativity was seen in 97% of those with primary syphilis and 76% of those with secondary syphilis at 2 years. More recent data based on currently recommended treatment regimens (see below) suggest that decreases in titer may be slower, ie, in primary and secondary syphilis it may take 6 months to see a fourfold decrease in titer and 12 months to see an eightfold drop. In patients with early latent syphilis, response is even slower, with a fourfold drop in titer taking 12–24 months. Seronegativity was seen in 72% of patients with primary syphilis and only 56% of those with secondary syphilis after 3 years. Additional studies support a slower decline in titers with currently recommended treatment regimens.

2. Treponemal antibody tests–The fluorescent treponemal antibody absorption (FTA-ABS) test is the most widely employed treponemal test. It measures antibodies capable of reacting with killed *T pallidum* after absorption of the patient's serum with extracts of nonpathogenic treponemes. The FTA-ABS test is of value principally in determining whether a positive nontreponemal antigen test is "false-positive" or is indicative of syphilis. Because of its great sensitivity, particularly in the late stages of the disease, the FTA-ABS test is also of value when there is clinical evidence of syphilis but the nontreponemal serologic test for syphilis is negative. The test is positive in most patients with primary syphilis and in virtually all with secondary syphilis. Like nontreponemal antigen tests, the specific treponemal antibody test may revert to negative with adequate therapy. This is seen almost exclusively in initial infections in individuals with primary syphilis. In one study, 11% of individuals with a first episode of primary syphilis were seronegative by the FTA-ABS test at 1 year posttreatment, and 24% were negative by 3 years. Immunologic status may also affect antibody titers. Seven percent of asymptomatic HIV-infected patients became seronegative after treatment, as opposed to 38% of symptomatic HIV-infected individuals. The long-held belief that a positive FTA-ABS persists indefinitely is clearly not valid, and this test therefore cannot be used as a reliable marker of previous infection. False-positive FTA-ABS tests occur rarely in systemic lupus erythematosus and in other disorders associated with increased levels of gamma globulins. It is noteworthy that Lyme disease may cause a false-positive FTA-ABS test but rarely causes a false-positive reaginic test. A *T pallidum* hemagglutination (TPHA) test and micrchemagglutination test for antibody to *T pallidum* (MHA-TP) are comparable in specificity and sensitivity to the FTA-ABS test but may become positive somewhat later in infection.

Investigational tests such as direct antigen detection, Western immunoblot, ELISA (CAPTIA Syph G, CAPTIA Syph M), and PCR are under study as diagnostic tools. They have shown promise in clinical trials, especially for diseases difficult to diagnose such as neurosyphilis and congenital syphilis. The increased sensitivity (ELISA) and specificity (Western blot) of these tests make them attractive, but because of lack of clinical evaluation in field trials they have not yet supplanted the more traditional methods of diagnosis.

Final decisions about the significance of the results of serologic tests for syphilis must be based upon a total clinical appraisal.

B. Microscopic Examination: In infectious syphilis, *T pallidum* may be shown by darkfield microscopic examination of fresh exudate from lesions or material aspirated from regional lymph nodes. The darkfield examination requires considerable experience and care in the proper collection of specimens and in the identification of pathogenic spirochetes by observing characteristic features of morphology and motility. Repeated examinations may be necessary. Spirochetes usually are not found in late syphilitic lesions by this technique.

An immunofluorescent staining technique for demonstrating *T pallidum* in dried smears of fluid taken from early syphilitic lesions is available. Slides are fixed and treated with fluorescein-labeled antitreponemal antibody that has been preabsorbed with nonpathogenic treponemes. The slides are then examined for fluorescing spirochetes in an ultraviolet microscope. Because of its simplicity and convenience to physicians (slides can be mailed), this technique has replaced darkfield microscopy in most health departments and medical center laboratories.

C. Spinal Fluid Examination: Cerebrospinal fluid findings in neurosyphilis are variable. In "classic" cases there is an elevation of total protein, lymphocytic pleocytosis, and a positive cerebrospinal fluid reagin test (VDRL). However, cerebrospinal fluid may be completely normal in neurosyphilis, and the VDRL may be negative. In one study, 25% of patients with primary or secondary syphilis in whom *T pallidum* was isolated from cerebrospinal fluid had a normal cerebrospinal fluid examination. In later stages of syphilis, normal cerebrospinal fluid analysis in the presence of infection can occur, but it is unusual. Because false-positive reagin tests rarely occur in the cerebrospinal fluid, a positive test confirms the presence of neurosyphilis. Because the cerebrospinal fluid VDRL may be negative in 30–70% of cases of neurosyphilis, *a negative test does not exclude neurosyphilis.* The use of cerebrospinal fluid FTA-ABS in the diagnosis of neurosyphilis is controversial. Some feel that it is more sensitive than the VDRL, but this is not accepted uniformly, and a high serum titer of FTA-ABS may result in a positive cerebrospinal fluid titer in the absence of neurosyphilis. However, the test is believed to be highly sensitive, and a negative cerebrospinal fluid FTA-ABS is strong evidence against the diagnosis of neurosyphilis. Other treponemal antibody tests, such as the MHA-TP and the TPHA index, likewise are not reliable in making the diagnosis of neurosyphilis, although a negative test is helpful in excluding the diagnosis.

Cerebrospinal fluid examination is recommended depending on clinical manifestations and stage of disease, as discussed below. Asymptomatic neurosyphilis (ie, positive cerebrospinal fluid findings without symptoms) requires prolonged penicillin treatment as given for symptomatic neurosyphilis. Adequate treatment is indicated by gradual decrease in cerebrospinal fluid cell count, protein concentration, and VDRL titer. Rarely, serologic tests of cerebrospinal fluid may remain positive for years after adequate treatment of neurosyphilis even though all other parameters have returned to normal.

Treatment

A. Specific Measures:

1. Penicillin, as benzathine penicillin G or aqueous procaine penicillin G, is the drug of choice for all forms of syphilis and other spirochetal infections. Effective tissue levels must be maintained for several days or weeks because of the spirochete's long generation time (about 30 hours). Penicillin is highly effective in early infections and variably effective in the late stages. The principal contraindication is hypersensitivity to the penicillins. The recommended treatment schedules are included below in the discussion of the various forms of syphilis.

2. Other antibiotic therapy–Oral tetracyclines are effective in the treatment of syphilis for patients who are sensitive to penicillin. Tetracycline, 500 mg orally four times daily for 14 days, or doxycycline, 100 mg orally twice daily for 14 days, is given for infectious syphilis. In syphilis of more than 1 year's duration or of unknown duration, treatment is continued for 28 days in the same doses.

Although azithromycin, 500 mg daily for 10 days (total dose 5 g) or 500 mg on alternate days for 11 days (total dose 3 g), has been shown in one study to be effective for infectious syphilis, large numbers of patients have not been treated, and long-term follow-up data to identify failures are lacking. Thus, although this therapy may be effective, it is not currently recommended.

Human clinical trials using ceftriaxone for infectious syphilis are limited, and this agent is therefore not officially recommended at present. However, based on animal data and pharmacologic predictions, some have suggested that ceftriaxone in multiple-dose regimens (1 g intravenously or intramuscularly once a day for 7–14 days) may be efficacious against infectious syphilis. Single-dose ceftriaxone therapy is not effective for established syphilis.

B. Local Measures (Mucocutaneous Lesions): Local treatment is usually not necessary. No local antiseptics or other chemicals should be applied to a suspected syphilitic lesion until specimens for microscopy have been obtained.

C. Public Health Measures: Patients with infectious syphilis must abstain from sexual activity until rendered noninfectious by antibiotic therapy. All cases of syphilis must be reported to the appropriate public health agency for assistance in identifying and treating contacts. In addition, all patients with syphilis should have an HIV test at the time of diagnosis. In areas of high HIV prevalence, a repeat HIV test should be performed in 3 months if the initial test was negative.

D. Empirical Postexposure Treatment: Patients who have been exposed to infectious syphilis within the preceding 3 months may be infected but seronegative and thus should be treated as for early syphilis. Persons exposed more than 90 days previously should be treated based on serologic results. If their partners are unavailable for testing or unreliable for follow-up, empirical therapy is indicated. Others at high risk either for infection (ie, those with other sexually transmitted diseases and those infected with HIV) or its consequences (ie, pregnant women) should undergo serologic tests for syphilis. The present recommended therapy for gonorrhea (ceftriaxone or quinolones) may not be effective in treating incubating syphilis. Therefore, patients with gonorrhea and a known exposure to syphilis should be treated with separate regimens effective against both diseases.

Complications of Specific Therapy

The Jarisch-Herxheimer reaction is ascribed to the sudden massive destruction of spirochetes by drugs and release of toxic products and is manifested by fever and aggravation of the existing clinical picture. It is most likely to occur in early syphilis. Treatment should not be discontinued unless the symptoms become severe or threaten to be fatal or unless syphilitic laryngitis, auditory neuritis, or labyrinthitis is present, where the reaction may cause irreversible damage.

The reaction may be prevented or modified by simultaneous administration of antipyretics or corticosteroids, though no proved method of prevention exists. It usually begins within the first 24 hours and subsides spontaneously within the next 24 hours of penicillin treatment.

Follow-Up Care

Because treatment failures can occur and reinfection is always a possibility, patients treated for syphilis should be followed clinically and serologically. Response to therapy is difficult to assess, and no definite criteria exist for cure in patients with primary or secondary syphilis. In primary and secondary syphilis, failure of nontreponemal antibody titers to decrease fourfold by 6 months may identify a group at high risk of treatment failure. Optimal management of these patients is unclear, but close clinical and serologic follow-up is indicated. If titers fail to decrease fourfold by 6 months, an HIV test should be repeated (all patients with syphilis should have an HIV test at the time of diagnosis), a lumbar puncture should be considered, and, if careful follow-up cannot be ensured (3-month intervals for HIV-positive individuals and 6-month intervals for HIV-negative patients), re-treatment should be given. When re-treatment is given, 2.4 million units of benzathine penicillin intramuscularly weekly for 3 weeks is administered. If symptoms or signs persist or recur after initial therapy or there is a fourfold or greater increase in nontreponemal titers, either the patient has failed therapy or has been reinfected. In those individuals, an HIV test should be performed, a lumbar puncture done (unless reinfection is a certainty) and re-treatment given as indicated above. In patients with latent syphilis, nontreponemal serologic tests should be repeated at 6, 12, and 24 months. If titers increase fourfold or initially high titers (≥ 1:32) fail to decrease fourfold by 12–24 months, or if symptoms or signs consistent with syphilis develop, an HIV test and lumbar puncture should be performed and re-treatment given according to the stage of the disease.

Prevention

Avoidance of sexual contact is the only completely reliable method of prophylaxis but is an impractical public health measure for obvious reasons.

A. Mechanical: The standard latex condom is effective but protects covered parts only. The exposed parts should be washed with soap and water as soon after contact as possible. This applies to both sexes.

B. Antibiotic: If there is known exposure to infectious syphilis, abortive penicillin therapy may be used. Give 2.4 million units of procaine penicillin G intramuscularly. Treatment of gonococcal (and chlamydial) infection with tetracyclines, and ceftriaxone is probably effective against incubating syphilis in most cases. However, other antimicrobial agents (eg, spectinomycin, quinolones) may be ineffective in aborting preclinical syphilis. Azithromycin administered as a single 1 g dose is also effective as preventive therapy in individuals exposed to infected partners. Because of concerns about treating incubating syphilis with nonpenicillin regimens, patients treated for gonorrhea should have a serologic test for syphilis 3–6 months after treatment.

Course & Prognosis (See Table 34–3.)

The lesions associated with primary and secondary syphilis are self-limiting and resolve with few or no residua. Late syphilis may be highly destructive and

Table 34–3. Natural course of untreated syphilis.

Stage of Disease	Likelihood of Developing Clinical Manifestations	Comment
Latent	24%	90% of relapses occur in first year after infection
Late		
Benign (gummatous)	15%	Many patients have more than one late manifestation.
Cardiovascular	10%	Seen only in those who develop syphilis after 15 years of age. Pathologic findings more common, ie, 50–80%.
Neurosyphilis	6.5%	Asymptomatic neurosyphilis has been reported in 8–40%.

permanently disabling and may lead to death. In broad terms, if no treatment is given, about one-third of people infected with syphilis will undergo spontaneous cure, about one-third will remain in the latent phase throughout life, and about one-third will develop serious late lesions.

CLINICAL STAGES OF SYPHILIS

1. PRIMARY SYPHILIS

Essentials of Diagnosis

- History of sexual contact (often unreliable).
- Painless ulcer on genitalia, perianal area, rectum, pharynx, tongue, lip, or elsewhere 2–6 weeks after exposure.
- Nontender enlargement of regional lymph nodes.
- Fluid expressed from lesion contains *T pallidum* by immunofluorescence or darkfield microscopy.
- Serologic test for syphilis often positive.

General Considerations

This is the stage of invasion and may pass unrecognized. The typical lesion is the chancre at the site or sites of inoculation, most frequently located on the penis, labia, cervix, or anorectal region. Anorectal lesions are especially common among men who have sex with men. The primary lesion occurs occasionally in the oropharynx (lip, tongue, or tonsil) and rarely on the breast or finger. The chancre starts as a small erosion 10–90 days (average, 3–4 weeks) after inoculation that rapidly develops into a painless superficial ulcer with a clean base and firm, indurated margins, associated with enlargement of regional lymph nodes, which are rubbery, discrete, and nontender. Bacterial infection of the chancre may occur and may lead to pain. Healing occurs without treatment, but a scar may form, especially with secondary bacterial infection.

Laboratory Findings

The serologic test for syphilis is usually positive 1–2 weeks after the primary lesion is noted; rising titers are especially significant when there is a history of previous infection. Immunofluorescence or darkfield microscopy shows treponemes in at least 95% of chancres. Cerebrospinal fluid pleocytosis has been reported in 10–20% of patients with primary syphilis.

Differential Diagnosis

The syphilitic chancre may be confused with chancroid, lymphogranuloma venereum, genital herpes, or neoplasm. Any lesion on the genitalia should be considered a possible primary syphilitic lesion.

Treatment

Benzathine penicillin G, 2.4 million units intramuscularly in the gluteal area, is given once. For the penicillin-allergic patient (who is not pregnant), doxycycline, 100 mg orally twice daily for 2 weeks, or tetracycline, 500 mg orally four times a day for 2 weeks, can be used. There is more clinical experience with tetracycline, but compliance is probably better with doxycycline. Erythromycin, 500 mg orally four times a day for 2 weeks, can be used, but this regimen is generally considered less effective than others, and careful follow-up is mandatory in individuals treated with erythromycin.

2. SECONDARY SYPHILIS

Essentials of Diagnosis

- Generalized maculopapular skin rash.
- Mucous membrane lesions, including patches and ulcers.
- Weeping papules (condylomas) in moist skin areas.
- Generalized nontender lymphadenopathy.
- Fever.
- Meningitis, hepatitis, osteitis, arthritis, iritis.
- Many treponemes in scrapings of mucous membrane or skin lesions by immunofluorescence or darkfield microscopy.
- Serologic tests for syphilis always positive.

General Considerations & Treatment

The secondary stage of syphilis usually appears a few weeks (or up to 6 months) after development of the chancre, when sufficient dissemination of *T pallidum* has occurred to produce systemic signs (fever, lymphadenopathy) or infectious lesions at sites distant from the site of inoculation. The most common manifestations are skin and mucosal lesions. The skin lesions are nonpruritic, macular, papular, pustular, or follicular (or combinations of any of these types), though the maculopapular rash is the most common. The skin lesions usually are generalized; involvement of the palms and soles is especially suspicious. Annular lesions simulating ringworm are observed in blacks. Mucous membrane lesions range from ulcers and papules of the lips, mouth, throat, genitalia, and anus ("mucous patches") to a diffuse redness of the pharynx. Both skin and mucous membrane lesions are highly infectious at this stage. Specific lesions—**condylomata lata**—are fused, weeping papules on the moist areas of the skin and mucous membranes.

Meningeal (aseptic meningitis or acute basilar meningitis), hepatic, renal, bone, and joint invasion may occur, with resulting cranial nerve palsies, jaundice, nephrotic syndrome, and periostitis. Alopecia (moth-eaten appearance) and uveitis may also occur.

All serologic tests for syphilis are positive in almost all cases. The cutaneous and mucous membrane lesions often show *T pallidum* on darkfield microscopic examination. A transient cerebrospinal fluid pleocytosis is seen in 30–70% of patients with secondary syphilis, though only 5% have positive serologic cerebrospinal fluid reactions. There may be evidence of hepatitis or nephritis (immune complex type). Circulating immune complexes exist in the blood and are deposited in blood vessel walls.

Skin lesions may be confused with the infectious exanthems, pityriasis rosea, and drug eruptions. Visceral lesions may suggest nephritis or hepatitis due to other causes. The diffusely red throat may mimic other forms of pharyngitis.

Treatment is as for primary syphilis unless central nervous system or ocular disease is present, in which case treatment is as for neurosyphilis (see below). Isolation of the patient is important.

3. RELAPSING SYPHILIS (Early Latent Syphilis)

The essentials of diagnosis are the same as in secondary syphilis.

The lesions of secondary syphilis heal spontaneously, but secondary syphilis may relapse if undiagnosed or inadequately treated. These relapses may include any of the findings noted under secondary syphilis: skin and mucous membrane, neurologic, ocular, bone, or visceral. Unlike the usual asymptomatic neurologic involvement of secondary syphilis, neurologic relapses may be fulminating, leading to death. Relapse is almost always accompanied by a rising titer in quantitative serologic tests; indeed, a rising titer may be the first or only evidence of relapse. About 90% of relapses occur during the first year after infection.

Treatment is as for primary syphilis unless central nervous system disease is present.

4. LATE LATENT ("HIDDEN") SYPHILIS

Essentials of Diagnosis

- No physical signs.
- History of syphilis with inadequate treatment.
- Positive serologic tests for syphilis.

General Considerations & Treatment

Latent syphilis is the clinically quiescent phase during the interval after disappearance of secondary lesions and before the appearance of tertiary symptoms. Early latency is defined as the first year after infection, during which time most infectious lesions recur ("relapsing syphilis"); after the first year, the patient is said to be in the late latent phase. Transmission to the fetus, however, can probably occur in any phase. There are (by definition) no clinical manifestations during the latent phase, and the only significant laboratory findings are positive serologic tests. A diagnosis of latent syphilis is justified only when the cerebrospinal fluid is entirely negative, x-ray and physical examination shows no evidence of cardiovascular involvement, and false-positive tests for syphilis have been ruled out. The latent phase may last from months to a lifetime.

It is important to differentiate latent syphilis from a false-positive serologic test for syphilis, which can be due to the many causes listed above.

Treatment is with benzathine penicillin G, 2.4 million units three times at 7-day intervals (total dose, 7.2 million units). In the penicillin-allergic patient, give tetracycline, 0.5 g orally four times a day for 28 days, or doxycycline, 100 mg orally twice daily for 28 days. If there is evidence of cerebrospinal fluid involvement, treat as for neurosyphilis. Only a small percentage of serologic tests will be appreciably altered by treatment with penicillin. The treatment of this stage of the disease is intended to prevent the late sequelae.

5. LATE (TERTIARY) SYPHILIS

Essentials of Diagnosis

- Infiltrative tumors of skin, bones, liver (gummas).
- Aortitis, aneurysms, aortic regurgitation.
- Central nervous system disorders, including meningovascular and degenerative changes, paresthesias, shooting pains, abnormal reflexes, dementia, or psychosis.

General Considerations

This stage may occur at any time after secondary syphilis, even after years of latency, and is seen in about one-third of untreated patients (Table 34–3). Late lesions probably represent, at least in part, a delayed hypersensitivity reaction of the tissue to the organism and are usually divided into two types: (1) a localized gummatous reaction, with a relatively rapid onset and generally prompt response to therapy ("benign late syphilis"); and (2) diffuse inflammation of a more insidious onset that characteristically involves the central nervous system and large arteries, is often fatal if untreated, and is at best arrested by treatment. Gummas may involve any area or organ of the body but most often the skin or long bones. Cardiovascular disease is usually manifested by aortic aneurysm, aortic regurgitation, or aortitis. Various forms of diffuse or localized central nervous system involvement may occur.

Late syphilis must be differentiated from neoplasms of the skin, liver, lung, stomach, or brain; other forms of meningitis; and primary neurologic lesions.

Although almost any tissue and organ may be involved in late syphilis, the following are the most common types of involvement.

Skin

Cutaneous lesions of late syphilis are of two varieties: (1) multiple nodular lesions that eventually ulcerate (lues maligna) or resolve by forming atrophic, pigmented scars; and (2) solitary gummas that start as painless subcutaneous nodules, then enlarge, attach to the overlying skin, and eventually ulcerate.

Mucous Membranes

Late lesions of the mucous membranes are nodular gummas or leukoplakia, highly destructive to the involved tissue.

Skeletal

Bone lesions are destructive, causing periostitis, osteitis, and arthritis with little or no associated redness or swelling but often marked myalgia and myositis of the neighboring muscles. The pain is especially severe at night.

Eyes

Late ocular lesions are gummatous iritis, chorioretinitis, optic atrophy, and cranial nerve palsies, in addition to the lesions of central nervous system syphilis.

Respiratory System

Respiratory involvement by late syphilis is caused by gummatous infiltrates into the larynx, trachea, and pulmonary parenchyma, producing discrete pulmonary densities. There may be hoarseness, respiratory distress, and wheezing secondary to the gummatous lesion itself or to subsequent stenosis occurring with healing.

Gastrointestinal System

Gummas involving the liver produce the usually benign, asymptomatic hepar lobatum. Occasionally a picture resembling Laennec's cirrhosis is produced by liver involvement. Gastric involvement can consist of diffuse infiltration into the stomach wall or focal lesions that endoscopically and microscopically can be confused with lymphoma or carcinoma. Epigastric pain, early satiety, regurgitation, belching, and weight loss are common symptoms.

Cardiovascular System

Cardiovascular lesions (10–15% of late syphilitic lesions) are often progressive, disabling, and life-threatening. Central nervous system lesions are often present also. Involvement usually starts as an arteritis in the supracardiac portion of the aorta and progresses to cause one or more of the following: (1) Narrowing of the coronary ostia with resulting decreased coronary circulation, angina, and acute myocardial infarction. (2) Scarring of the aortic valves, producing aortic regurgitation with its water-hammer pulse, aortic diastolic murmur, frequent aortic systolic murmur, cardiac hypertrophy, and eventually congestive heart failure. (3) Weakness of the wall of the aorta, with saccular aneurysm formation and associated pressure symptoms of dysphagia, hoarseness, brassy cough, back pain (vertebral erosion), and occasionally rupture of the aneurysm. Recurrent respiratory infections are common as a result of pressure on the trachea and bronchi.

Treatment of tertiary syphilis (excluding neurosyphilis; see below) is as for latent syphilis. Reversal of positive serologic tests does not usually occur. A second course of penicillin therapy may be given if necessary. There is no known method for reliable eradication of the treponeme from humans in the late stages of syphilis. Viable spirochetes are occasionally found in the eyes, in cerebrospinal fluid, and elsewhere in patients with "adequately" treated syphilis, but claims for their capacity to cause progressive disease are speculative.

Neurosyphilis

Neurosyphilis (15–20% of late syphilitic lesions; often present with cardiovascular syphilis) is also a progressive, disabling, and life-threatening complication. It develops more commonly in men than in women and in whites than in blacks.

A. Classification: There are four clinical types.

1. Asymptomatic neurosyphilis–This form is characterized by spinal fluid abnormalities (positive spinal fluid serology, increased cell count, occasionally increased protein) without symptoms or signs of neurologic involvement.

2. Meningovascular syphilis–This form is characterized by meningeal involvement or changes in the vascular structures of the brain (or both), producing symptoms of chronic meningitis (headache, irritability); cranial nerve palsies (basilar meningitis); unequal reflexes; irregular pupils with poor light and accommodation reflexes; and, when large vessels are involved, cerebrovascular accidents. The cerebrospinal fluid shows increased cells (100–1000/μL), elevated protein, and usually a positive serologic test for syphilis. The symptoms of acute meningitis are rare in late syphilis.

3. Tabes dorsalis–This form is a chronic progressive degeneration of the parenchyma of the posterior columns of the spinal cord and of the posterior sensory ganglia and nerve roots. The symptoms and signs are impairment of proprioception and vibration sense, Argyll Robertson pupils (which react poorly to light but well to accommodation), and muscular hypotonia and hyporeflexia. Impairment of proprioception results in a wide-based gait and inability to walk in the dark. Paresthesias, analgesia, or sharp recurrent pains in the muscles of the leg ("shooting" or "lightning" pains) may occur. Crises are also common in tabes: gastric crises, consisting of sharp abdominal pains with nausea and vomiting (simulating an acute abdomen); laryngeal crises, with paroxysmal cough and dyspnea; urethral crises, with painful bladder spasms; and rectal and anal crises. Crises may begin suddenly, last for hours to days, and cease abruptly. Neurogenic bladder with overflow incontinence is also seen. Painless trophic ulcers may develop over pressure points on the feet. Joint damage may occur as a result of lack of sensory innervation (Charcot joint). The cerebrospinal fluid may have a normal or increased cell count (3–200/μL), elevated protein, and variable results of serologic tests.

4. General paresis–This is generalized involvement of the cerebral cortex with insidious onset of symptoms. There is usually a decrease in concentrating power, memory loss, dysarthria, tremor of the fingers and lips, irritability, and mild headaches. Most striking is the change of personality; the patient becomes slovenly, irresponsible, confused, and psychotic. The cerebrospinal fluid findings resemble those of tabes dorsalis. Combinations of the various forms of neurosyphilis (especially tabes and paresis) are not uncommon.

B. Special Considerations in Treatment of Neurosyphilis: It is most important to prevent neurosyphilis by prompt diagnosis, adequate treatment, and follow-up of early syphilis. Indications for lumbar puncture vary depending upon the stage of the disease and the host's immune status. In early syphilis (primary and secondary syphilis and early latent syphilis of less than 1 year's duration), invasion of the central nervous system by *T pallidum* with cerebrospinal fluid abnormalities occur commonly, but neurosyphilis rarely develops in patients who have received the standard therapy outlined above. Thus, unless clinical symptoms and signs of neurosyphilis or ophthalmologic involvement (uveitis, neuroretinitis, optic neuritis, iritis) are present, a lumbar puncture in early syphilis is not recommended as part of the routine evaluation. In latent syphilis, the decision to perform a lumbar puncture should be individualized. Routine lumbar puncture for all patients is not indicated since the yield is low and findings rarely influence therapeutic decisions. Cerebrospinal fluid evaluation is recommended, however, in the later stages of syphilis if neurologic or ophthalmologic symptoms and signs are present; if therapy other than with penicillin is to be given; if the patient is HIV-positive (see next section); if there is evidence of treatment failure (see discussion above); if there is evidence of active tertiary syphilis (aortitis, iritis, optic atrophy, the presence of a gumma, etc); or if the serum nontreponemal antibody titer is ≥ 1:32. In the presence of definite cerebrospinal fluid or neurologic abnormalities, treat for neurosyphilis. The pretreatment clinical and laboratory evaluation should include neurologic, ocular, cardiovascular, psychiatric, and cerebrospinal fluid examinations.

The regimen of 2.4 million units of benzathine penicillin intramuscularly weekly for three consecutive weeks results in low to undetectable cerebrospinal fluid levels of penicillin, and treatment failures have been described when this regimen has been used to treat neurosyphilis. For these reasons, present recommendations for the therapy of neurosyphilis employ higher doses of short-acting penicillin in order to achieve better penetration and higher levels of drug in the cerebrospinal fluid. Recommended regimens include 3–4 million units of aqueous crystalline penicillin G intravenously every 4 hours for 10–14 days. Alternatively, 2.4 million units of procaine penicillin can be given intramuscularly once daily along with 500 mg of probenecid orally four times daily, both for 10–14 days. Because of concerns about slowly dividing organisms that may persist, many experts recommend subsequent administration of 2.4 million units of benzathine penicillin intramuscularly once weekly for 3 weeks as additional therapy. Alternative therapy to penicillin has not been established for treatment of neurosyphilis. Chloramphenicol (2 g daily for 30 days), doxycycline (200 mg twice daily for 21 days), and ceftriaxone (1 g daily for 14 days) have all been shown to achieve treponemicidal levels in the cerebrospinal fluid, but clinical experience is limited, and failures have been reported. Thus, patients with a history of penicillin allergy should be skin-tested, desensitized, and treated with penicillin.

All patients should have spinal fluid examinations at 6-month intervals until the cell count is normal. Response may be gauged by clinical improvement and reversal of cerebrospinal fluid changes. A second course of penicillin therapy may be given if the cell count has not decreased at 6 months or is not normal at 2 years. Not infrequently, there is progression of neurologic symptoms and signs despite high and prolonged doses of penicillin. It has been postulated that these treatment failures are related to the unexplained persistence of viable *T pallidum* in central nervous system or ocular lesions in at least some cases.

6. SYPHILIS IN HIV-INFECTED PATIENTS

Because syphilis has variable clinical manifestations and an unpredictable course, evaluation of case reports of unusual clinical or laboratory manifestations of syphilis in HIV-infected patients is difficult. Although unusual serologic responses have been reported in HIV-positive patients, including high titers of nontreponemal tests, delayed appearance of positive titers, and false-negative tests, most HIV-positive patients respond serologically in a way similar to noninfected patients. Thus, interpretation of serologic tests should be the same for HIV-positive and HIV-negative individuals. Because of concerns about false-negative serologic tests or a delayed immunologic response, if the diagnosis of syphilis is suggested on clinical grounds but reagin tests are negative, alternative tests should be performed. These tests include darkfield examination of lesions and direct fluorescent antibody staining for *T pallidum* of lesion exudate or biopsy specimens.

The diagnosis of neurosyphilis in HIV-infected patients is complicated by the fact that cerebrospinal fluid abnormalities are frequently seen and may be due to neurosyphilis or HIV infection itself. The significance of these abnormalities is unknown, and similar abnormalities are frequently seen in non-HIV-infected patients with primary or secondary syphilis. Despite occasional reports of HIV-infected patients who progress to develop neurosyphilis despite appropriate therapy for early disease, the vast majority of HIV-infected patients with primary or secondary syphilis respond appropriately to currently recommended regimens. Thus, although some recommend a cerebrospinal fluid examination for all HIV-positive patients with syphilis, it is probably not needed in those with early disease. In contrast, a lumbar puncture should be performed in HIV-positive patients if they have late latent syphilis or syphilis of unknown duration; if neurologic signs are present; or if they have failed therapy (as discussed above—the same criteria for failure apply to HIV-positive and HIV-negative patients, and re-treatment regimens are the same).

Treatment of HIV-positive patients with primary and secondary syphilis is the same as for HIV-negative patients. Because of concerns about the adequacy of this therapy, a large multicenter trial of therapy of early syphilis in HIV-positive and HIV-negative patients was undertaken to compare standard therapy with enhanced therapy (2.4 million units of benzathine penicillin followed by 2 g of amoxicillin plus 500 mg of probenecid taken orally three times a day for 10 days). In the 1 year of follow-up, no cases of neurosyphilis were observed, suggesting that current recommendations are adequate. Because of ongoing concerns about adequacy of therapy, careful clinical and serologic follow-up should be done at 3, 6, 9, 12, and 24 months.

HIV-infected patients with late latent syphilis, syphilis of unknown duration, and neurosyphilis should be treated like HIV-negative individuals, with follow-up at 6, 12, 18, and 24 months.

Because clinical experience treating HIV-infected patients with syphilis is based on penicillin regimens, all stages of syphilis should be treated with this drug. If severe allergy exists, the patient should be desensitized to penicillin.

7. SYPHILIS IN PREGNANCY

All pregnant women should have a nontreponemal serologic test for syphilis at the time of the first prenatal visit. In women suspected of being at increased risk for syphilis or for populations in which there is a high prevalence of syphilis, another nontreponemal test should be performed during the third trimester at 28 weeks and again at delivery. The serologic status of all women who have delivered should be known before discharge from the hospital. Seropositive women should be considered infected and should be treated unless prior treatment with fall in antibody titer is medically documented.

The preferred treatment is with penicillin in dosage schedules appropriate for the stage of syphilis (see above). Penicillin prevents congenital syphilis in 90% of cases, even when treatment is given late in pregnancy. Tetracycline and doxycycline are contraindicated in pregnancy, and erythromycin is associated with a high risk of failure in the fetus. Women with a history of penicillin allergy should be skin-tested and desensitized if necessary.

The infant should be evaluated immediately, as noted below, and at 6–8 weeks of age.

8. CONGENITAL SYPHILIS

Congenital syphilis is a transplacentally transmitted infection that occurs in infants of untreated or inadequately treated mothers. The physical findings at birth are quite variable: The infant may have many or only minimal signs or even no signs until 6–8 weeks of life (delayed form). The most common findings are on the mucous membranes and skin—maculopapular rash, condylomas, mucous membrane patches, and serous nasal discharge (snuffles). These lesions are infectious; *T pallidum* can easily be found microscopically, and the infant must be isolated. Other common findings are hepatosplenomegaly, anemia, or osteochondritis. These early active lesions subsequently heal, and if the disease is left untreated it produces the characteristic stigmas of syphilis—interstitial keratitis, Hutchinson's teeth, saddle nose, saber shins, deafness, and central nervous system involvement.

The presence of negative serologic tests at birth in both the mother and the infant usually means that the newborn is free of infection. However, recent infection near the time of delivery may result in negative tests because there has been insufficient time to develop a serologic response. Thus, one must maintain a high index of suspicion in infants who present with delayed onset of symptoms despite negative serologic tests at birth, especially in infants born to high-risk mothers (HIV-positive, illicit drug users).

Augenbraun MH et al: Treatment of syphilis, 1998: nonpregnant adults. Clin Infect Dis 1999;28(Suppl 1):S21. [NLM Cit ID: 99152433] (Recommended therapies with review of supporting evidence.)

1998 guidelines for treatment of sexually transmitted diseases. MMWR Morb Mortal Wkly Rep 1998;47(RR-1):1. [NLM Cit ID: 98120951] (Comprehensive summary of recommendations.)

Rolfs RT et al: A randomized trial of enhanced therapy for early syphilis in patients with and without human immunodeficiency virus infection. N Engl J Med 1997;337:307. [NLM Cit ID: 97365040] (A large trial concluding that present treatment regimens are adequate in both HIV-positive and HIV-negative patients.)

NON-SEXUALLY TRANSMITTED TREPONEMATOSES

A variety of treponemal diseases other than syphilis occur endemically in many tropical areas of the world. They are distinguished from disease caused by *T pallidum* by their nonsexual transmission, their relatively high incidence in certain geographic areas and among children, and their tendency to produce less severe visceral manifestations. As in syphilis, organisms can be demonstrated in infectious lesions with darkfield microscopy or immunofluorescence but cannot be cultured in artificial media; the serologic tests for syphilis are positive, including the newer tests such as CAPTIA Syph G; the diseases have primary, secondary, and sometimes tertiary stages; and penicillin is the drug of choice. There is evidence that infection with these agents may provide partial resistance to syphilis and vice versa. Treatment with penicillin in doses appropriate to primary syphilis (eg, 2.4 million units of benzathine penicillin G intramuscularly) is generally curative in any stage of the non-sexually transmitted treponematoses. In cases of penicillin hypersensitivity, tetracycline, 500 mg four times a day for 10–14 days, is usually the recommended alternative.

YAWS
(Frambesia)

Yaws is a contagious disease largely limited to tropical regions that is caused by *T pallidum* subsp *pertenue*. It is characterized by granulomatous lesions of the skin, mucous membranes, and bone. Yaws is rarely fatal, though if untreated it may lead to chronic disability and disfigurement. Yaws is acquired by direct nonsexual contact, usually in childhood, although it may occur at any age. The "mother yaw," a painless papule that later ulcerates, appears 3–4 weeks after exposure. There is usually associated regional lymphadenopathy. Six to 12 weeks later, similar secondary lesions appear and last for several months or years. Painful ulcerated lesions on the soles are frequent and are called "crab yaws." Late gummatous lesions may occur, with associated tissue destruction involving large areas of skin and subcutaneous tissues. The late effects of yaws, with bone change, shortening of digits, and contractions, may be confused with similar changes occurring in leprosy. Central nervous system, cardiac, or other visceral involvement is rare. See above for therapy.

PINTA

Pinta is a non-sexually transmitted spirochetal infection caused by *Treponema carateum*. It occurs endemically in rural areas of Latin America, especially in Mexico, Colombia, and Cuba, and in some areas of the Pacific. A nonulcerative, erythematous primary papule spreads slowly into a papulosquamous plaque showing a variety of color changes (slate, lilac, black). Secondary lesions resemble the primary one and appear within a year after it. These appear successively, new lesions together with older ones; are commonest on the extremities; and later show atrophy and depigmentation. Some cases show pigmentary changes and atrophic patches on the soles and palms, with or without hyperkeratosis, that are indistinguishable from "crab yaws." Very rarely, central nervous system or cardiovascular disease is observed late in the course of infection. See above for therapy.

ENDEMIC SYPHILIS

Endemic syphilis is an acute or chronic infection caused by an organism indistinguishable from *T pallidum* subsp *endemicum*. It has been reported in a number of countries, particularly in the eastern Mediterranean area, often with local names: bejel in Syria, Saudi Arabia, and Iraq; and dichuchwa, njovera, and siti in Africa. It also occurs in Southeast Asia. The local forms have distinctive features. Moist ulcerated lesions of the skin or oral or nasopharyngeal mucosa are the most common manifestations. Generalized lymphadenopathy and secondary and tertiary bone and skin lesions are also common. Deep leg pain points to periostitis or osteomyelitis. Cardiovascular and central nervous system involvement is rare. See above for therapy.

Chulay JD: *Treponema* species (yaws, pinta, bejel). In: *Principles and Practice of Infectious Diseases,* 5th ed. Mandell GL, Bennett JE, Dolin R (editors). Churchill Livingstone, 2000. (A textbook review of non-sexually transmitted treponemal diseases.)

MISCELLANEOUS SPIROCHETAL DISEASES

RELAPSING FEVER

Relapsing fever is endemic in many parts of the world. The main reservoir is rodents, which serve as the source of infection for ticks (eg, *Ornithodoros*).

The distribution and seasonal incidence of the disease are determined by the ecology of the ticks in different areas. In the USA, infected ticks are found throughout the West, especially in mountainous areas, but clinical cases are uncommon in humans.

The infectious organism is a spirochete, *Borrelia recurrentis,* though other poorly characterized borrelia-like organisms can cause similar disease. It may be transmitted transovarially from one generation of ticks to the next. The spirochetes occur in all tissues of the tick, and humans can be infected by tick bites or by rubbing crushed tick tissues or feces into the bite wound. Tick-borne relapsing fever is endemic but is not transmitted from person to person. Different species (or strain) names have been given to borrelia in different parts of the world where the organisms are transmitted by different ticks.

When an infected person harbors lice, the lice become infected with borrelia by sucking blood. A few days later, the lice serve as a source of infection for other persons. Large epidemics may occur in louse-infested populations, and transmission is favored by crowding, malnutrition, and cold climate.

Clinical Findings

A. Symptoms and Signs: There is an abrupt onset of fever, chills, tachycardia, nausea and vomiting, arthralgia, and severe headache. Hepatomegaly and splenomegaly may develop, as well as various types of rashes. Delirium occurs with high fever, and there may be various neurologic and psychic abnormalities. The attack terminates, usually abruptly, after 3–10 days. After an interval of 1–2 weeks, relapse occurs, but often it is somewhat milder. Three to ten relapses may occur before recovery.

B. Laboratory Findings: During episodes of fever, large spirochetes are seen in blood smears stained with Wright's or Giemsa's stain. The organisms can be cultured in special media but rapidly lose pathogenicity. The spirochetes can multiply in injected rats or mice and can be seen in their blood.

A variety of anti-borrelia antibodies develop during the illness; sometimes the Weil-Felix test for rickettsioses and nontreponemal serologic tests for syphilis may also be falsely positive. Infection with *Borrelia recurrentis* can cause false-positive indirect fluorescent antibody and Western blot tests for *Borrelia burgdorferi,* and some cases may be misdiagnosed as Lyme disease. Cerebrospinal fluid abnormalities occur in patients with meningeal involvement. Mild anemia and thrombocytopenia are common, but the white blood cell count tends to be normal.

Differential Diagnosis

The manifestations of relapsing fever may be confused with malaria, leptospirosis, meningococcemia, yellow fever, typhus, or rat-bite fever.

Prevention

Prevention of tick bites (as described for rickettsial diseases) and delousing procedures applicable to large groups can prevent illness. Arthropod vectors should be controlled if possible.

An effective means of chemoprophylaxis has not been developed.

Treatment

A single dose of tetracycline or erythromycin, 0.5 g orally, or a single dose of procaine penicillin G, 400,000–600,000 units intramuscularly, probably constitutes adequate treatment for louse-borne relapsing fevers. Because of higher relapse rates, tick-borne disease is treated with 0.5 g of tetracycline or erythromycin given four times daily for 5–10 days. Jarisch-Herxheimer reactions occur commonly following treatment and may be life-threatening. Treatment with aspirin—but not hydrocortisone—may ameliorate this reaction. The Jarisch-Herxheimer reaction is mediated in part by tumor necrosis factor, and administration of antibody to this cytokine prior to antibiotic therapy is effective in preventing the reaction.

Prognosis

The overall mortality rate is usually about 5%. Fatalities are most common in old, debilitated, or very young patients. With treatment, the initial attack is shortened and relapses are largely prevented.

Dworkin MS et al: Tick-borne relapsing fever in the northwestern United States and southwestern Canada. Clin Infect Dis 1998;26:122. [NLM Cit ID: 98116698] (Review of 182 cases.)

Johnson WD Jr, Golightly LM: *Borrelia* species: Relapsing fever. In: *Principles and Practice of Infectious Diseases,* 5th ed. Mandell GL, Bennett JE, Dolin R (editors). Churchill Livingstone, 2000.

RAT-BITE FEVER
(Spirillary Rat-Bite Fever, Sodoku)

Rat-bite fever is an uncommon acute infectious disease caused by *Spirillum minus.* It is transmitted to humans by the bite of a rat. Inhabitants of rat-infested slum dwellings and laboratory workers are at greatest risk.

Clinical Findings

A. Symptoms and Signs: The original rat bite, unless secondarily infected, heals promptly, but 1 to several weeks later the site becomes swollen, indurated, and painful; assumes a dusky purplish hue; and may ulcerate. Regional lymphangitis and lymphadenitis, fever, chills, malaise, myalgia, arthralgia, and headache are present. Splenomegaly may occur. A sparse, dusky-red maculopapular rash appears on the trunk and extremities in many cases, and there may be frank arthritis.

After a few days, both the local and systemic symptoms subside, only to reappear again in a few more days. This relapsing pattern of fever for 3–4 days alternating with afebrile periods lasting 3–9 days may persist for weeks. The other features, however, usually recur only during the first few relapses.

B. Laboratory Findings: Leukocytosis is often present, and the nontreponemal test for syphilis is often falsely positive. The organism may be identified in darkfield examination of the ulcer exudate or aspirated lymph node material; more commonly, it is observed after inoculation of a laboratory animal with the patient's exudate or blood. It has not been cultured in artificial media.

Differential Diagnosis

Rat-bite fever must be distinguished from the rat bite-induced lymphadenitis and rash of streptobacillary fever. Clinically, the severe arthritis and myalgias seen in streptobacillary disease is rarely seen in disease caused by *S minus*. Reliable differentiation requires an increasing titer of agglutinins against *Streptobacillus moniliformis* or identification of the causative organism. Rat-bite fever must also be distinguished from tularemia, rickettsial disease, *Pasteurella multocida* infections, and relapsing fever by identification of the causative organism.

Treatment

Treat with procaine penicillin G, 600,000 units intramuscularly every 12 hours; or tetracycline hydrochloride, 0.5 g every 6 hours for 10–14 days. Give supportive and symptomatic measures as indicated.

Prognosis

The reported mortality rate of about 10% should be markedly reduced by prompt diagnosis and antimicrobial treatment.

Washburn RG: *Spirillum minus* (rat-bite fever). In: *Principles and Practice of Infectious Diseases,* 5th ed. Mandell GL, Bennett JE, Dolin R (editors). Churchill Livingstone, 2000.

LEPTOSPIROSIS

Leptospirosis is an acute and often severe infection that frequently affects the liver or other organs and is caused by *Leptospira interrogans,* which is a diverse organism consisting of 23 serogroups and over 200 serovars. The three most common serovars of infection are *Leptospira icterohaemorrhagiae* of rats, *Leptospira canicola* of dogs, and *Leptospira pomona* of cattle and swine. Several other varieties can also cause the disease, but *L icterohaemorrhagiae* causes the most severe illness. The disease is worldwide in distribution, and the incidence is higher than usually supposed. The leptospires are often transmitted to humans by the ingestion of food and drink contaminated by the urine of the reservoir animal. The organism may also enter through minor skin lesions and probably via the conjunctiva. Recreational cases have followed swimming or rafting in contaminated water, and occupational cases occur among sewer workers, rice planters, abattoir workers, and farmers. Sporadic urban cases have been seen in the homeless exposed to rat urine. The incubation period is 2–20 days.

Clinical Findings

A. Symptoms and Signs: Anicteric leptospirosis is the more common and milder form of the disease and is often biphasic. The initial or "septicemic" phase begins with abrupt fever to 39–40 °C, chills, abdominal pain, severe headache, and myalgias, especially of the calf muscles. There is marked conjunctival suffusion. Leptospires can be isolated from blood, cerebrospinal fluid, and tissues. Following a 1- to 3-day period of improvement in symptoms and absence of fever, the second or "immune" phase begins. Leptospires are absent from blood and cerebrospinal fluid but are still present in the kidney, and specific antibodies appear. A recurrence of symptoms is seen as in the first phase of disease with the onset of meningitis. Uveitis (which can be unilateral or bilateral and usually involves the entire uveal tract), rash, and adenopathy may occur. The illness is usually self-limited, lasting 4–30 days, and complete recovery is the rule.

Icteric leptospirosis (Weil's syndrome) (usually caused by *L icterohaemorrhagiae*) is the most severe form of the disease, characterized by impaired renal and hepatic function, abnormal mental status, hypotension, and a 5–10% mortality rate. Symptoms and signs are continuous and not biphasic.

Pretibial fever, a mild form of leptospirosis caused by *Leptospira autumnalis,* occurred during World War II at Fort Bragg, USA. In pretibial fever, there is patchy erythema on the skin of the lower legs or generalized rash occurring with fever.

Leptospirosis with jaundice must be distinguished from hepatitis, yellow fever, and relapsing fever.

B. Laboratory Findings: The leukocyte count may be normal or as high as 50,000/μL, with neutrophils predominating. The urine may contain bile, protein, casts, and red cells. Oliguria is not uncommon, and in severe cases uremia may occur. In cases with meningeal involvement, organisms may be found in the cerebrospinal fluid during the first 10 days of illness. Early in the disease, the organism may be identified by darkfield examination of the patient's blood or by culture on a semisolid medium (eg, Fletcher's EMJH). Cultures take 1–6 weeks to become positive. The organism may also be grown from the urine from the tenth day to the sixth week. Diagnosis is usually made by means of serologic tests, of which several are available. Agglutination tests (microscopic, using live organisms; and macroscopic, using killed antigen) become positive after 7–10 days of illness, peak at 3–4 weeks, and may persist at high levels for many years. Thus, to make a diagnosis, a fourfold or greater rise in titer must be documented. The agglutination tests are cumbersome to perform and require trained personnel. Indirect hemagglutination, immunofluorescent antibody, and ELISA tests are also available. The IgM ELISA is particularly useful in making an early diagnosis, as it is positive as early as 2 days into illness, a time when the clinical manifestations may be nonspecific, and it is extremely sensitive and specific (93%). PCR methods (presently investigational) appear to be sensitive, specific, positive early in disease, and able to detect leptospiral DNA in blood, urine, cerebrospinal fluid, and aqueous humor. Serum CK is usually elevated in leptospirosis patients and normal in hepatitis patients.

Complications

Myocarditis, aseptic meningitis, renal failure, and pulmonary infiltrates with hemorrhage are not common but are the usual causes of death. Iridocyclitis may occur.

Treatment

Various antimicrobial drugs, including penicillin and tetracyclines, show antileptospiral activity. Penicillin (eg, 6 million units daily intravenously) is said to be beneficial in severe leptospirosis, especially if started within the first 4 days of illness. Jarisch-Herxheimer reactions may occur. Observe for evidence of renal failure, and treat as necessary. Effective prophylaxis consists of doxycycline, 200 mg orally once weekly during the risk of exposure. Doxycycline, 100 mg twice daily for 7 days, can also reduce the severity and duration of symptoms if given within 3 days after onset of disease.

Prognosis

Without jaundice, the disease is almost never fatal. With jaundice, the mortality rate is 5% for those under age 30 and 30% for those over age 60.

Farr RW: Leptospirosis. Clin Infect Dis 1995;21:1. [NLM Cit ID: 96065607] (Clinical review.)

Vinetz JM et al: Sporadic urban leptospirosis. Ann Intern Med 1996;125:794. [NLM Cit ID: 97037752] (Epidemiology of an urban outbreak.)

LYME DISEASE (Lyme Borreliosis)

Essentials of Diagnosis

- Erythema migrans, a flat or slightly raised red lesion that expands with central clearing.
- Headache or stiff neck.
- Arthralgias, arthritis, and myalgias; arthritis is often chronic and recurrent.
- Wide geographic distribution, with most United States cases in the Northeast, mid-Atlantic, Upper Midwest, and Pacific coastal regions.

General Considerations

This illness, named after the town of Old Lyme, Connecticut, is caused by the spirochete *Borrelia burgdorferi* and is transmitted to humans by ixodid ticks that are part of the *Ixodes ricinus* complex. Four genomic groups of the *B burgdorferi sensu lato* group have been identified: *B burgdorferi sensu stricto,* which causes disease in North America and less commonly in Europe and Asia; *B garinii,* and *B afzelii,* which are the predominant etiologic agents of Lyme disease in Europe and Asia; and the newly named *B bissettii* sp *nov* found in California. Lyme disease is the most common vector-borne disease in the United States and is being reported with increasing frequency, but the true incidence is not known, and overreporting remains a problem. In 1998 there were 16,801 cases reported from 46 states and the District of Columbia. Most cases (over 90%) were reported from the mid-Atlantic, northeastern, and North Central regions of the country. As in years past, cases were reported from states without known enzootic cycles of *B burgdorferi,* raising questions about the accuracy of diagnosis. Overdiagnosis of Lyme disease continues to be a problem. In a Lyme disease clinic at a major teaching hospital in an endemic area, 788 patients were referred over a 4.5-year period. Only 23% were found to have active disease. The remaining patients had adequately treated disease in the past and another concurrent illness (20%) or did not have Lyme disease at all (57%). The consequences of overdiagnosis and overtreatment of Lyme disease are substantial. Individuals with previously treated Lyme disease and another concurrent illness and those without Lyme disease were avid users of the health care system, with multiple office visits to several different physicians resulting in numerous prescriptions for unnecessary antibiotics (approximately 30% of patients received over 100 days of antibiotic therapy) that often caused adverse drug events. In addition, this group of patients seeking a diagnosis of Lyme disease had a significant number of days in which they were unable to perform normal activities and had a high incidence of depression and stress (40–50%). The overreporting and overdiagnosis of Lyme disease is in part explained by the recent discovery of a nonculturable spirochete in the Lone Star tick *(Amblyomma americanum).* This organism produces a Lyme disease-like illness with a skin lesion very similar to that of erythema migrans. As the lone star tick is found in the Midwest and Southern areas where enzootic cycles for *B burgdorferi* have not been reported, cases of Lyme disease reported from these areas are probably due to this newly discovered organism. The vector of Lyme disease varies geographically and is *Ixodes scapularis* (also known as *I dammini*) in the northeastern, North Central, and mid-Atlantic regions of the United States; *Ixodes pacificus* on the West Coast; *Ixodes ricinus* in Europe; and *Ixodes persulcatus* in Asia. The disease also occurs in Australia. Mice and deer make up the major animal reservoir of *B burgdorferi,* but other rodents and birds may also be infected. Domestic animals such as dogs, cattle, and horses can also develop clinical illness, usually manifested as arthritis.

Ticks feed once during each of their three stages of life. Larval ticks feed in late summer, nymphs in the following spring and early summer, and adults during the fall. In the northeastern United States and the mid-Atlantic states, the preferred host for the nymphs and larvae is the white-footed mouse (the black-striped mouse in Europe). This animal is tolerant of infection—a fact that is critical in maintaining infection, since the mouse can remain spirochetemic and transmit the agent to the larvae the following spring after being infected by the nymphal form in early summer. Adult ticks prefer the white-tailed deer as host. Although only 20–25% of nymphs harbor spirochetes compared with 50–65% of adults, most infections occur in the spring and summer (when nymphs are active), and fewer cases occur in the cooler months (October to April), when adults feed. This is probably due to the greater abundance of nymphs; greater human outdoor activity in spring and summer, when nymphs feed; and the fact that adult ticks are larger, easier to detect by the human host, and thus can be removed before disease is transmitted. Less than 1% of larvae are infected with spirochetes, and transmission of the disease through contact with larvae is unlikely. In the Western United States, the *Ixodes pacificus* nymph prefers to feed on lizards, which are not susceptible to infection. It is only the few nymph and larval ticks that feed on wood rats, which can be infected, that are capable of transmitting disease.

The increased incidence of Lyme disease is due in part to the resurgence of the once-decimated deer population, the spread of tick vectors to new areas (infected *Ixodes* ticks have been isolated from migratory birds), and the encroachment of suburbs on once rural areas, bringing humans and ticks into closer proximity. Factors contributing to increased reporting include enhanced provider awareness and better laboratory surveillance.

Under experimental conditions, ticks must feed for 24 hours or longer to transmit infections. Human epidemiologic studies have indicated that the incidence of disease is significantly higher when tick attachment is for longer than 72 hours than if it is less than 72 hours, though rare cases have been documented with attachment of less than 24 hours. In addition, the percentage of ticks infected varies on a regional basis. In the Northeast and Midwest, 15–65% of *I scapularis* ticks are infected with the spirochete; in the Western United States, only 2% of *I pacificus* are infected. These are important epidemiologic features in assessing the likelihood that tick exposure will result in disease. Exposure to *I pacificus* is unlikely to result in disease, since so few ticks are infected, but this is not true of exposure to *I scapularis.* Eliciting a history of brushing a tick off the skin (ie, the tick was not feeding) or removing a tick on the same day as exposure (ie, the tick did not feed long enough) decreases the likelihood that infection will develop, since the vast majority of cases occur when ticks feed for at least 24 hours.

Ixodes ticks are smaller than the more common dog ticks *(Dermacentor variabilis).* Larvae are less than 1 mm in size, and the adult female is 2–3 mm in size, with a red body and black legs. After a blood meal, ticks can reach two to three times their unengorged size. Because the tick is so small, the bite is usually painless and goes unnoticed. After feeding, the tick drops off in 2–4 days. If a tick is found, it should be removed immediately. The best way to accomplish this is to grab the mouth part—not the body—where it enters the skin with a fine-tipped tweezers and pull firmly and repeatedly until the tick releases its hold. Saving the tick in a bottle of alcohol for future identification may be useful, especially if symptoms develop.

Congenital infection has been documented, but the exact frequency and manifestations have not been clearly defined. Similarly, because the organism can be latent, it is not known if women infected prior to becoming pregnant can activate the disease and transmit infection to the fetus. In one retrospective study, 5 of 19 pregnancies complicated by Lyme disease resulted in an adverse outcome, but all of the outcomes were different and could not be conclusively linked to infection. Several serosurveys involving over 2000 pregnant women in endemic areas have not found any association between seropositivity in prospective mothers and the prevalence of congenital malformations, fetal death, and prematurity. Thus, if *B burgdorferi* causes a congenital syndrome like some other spirochetal illnesses, it must be extremely uncommon.

Clinical Findings

The typical clinical description of Lyme disease divides the illness into three stages: stage 1, flu-like symptoms and a typical skin rash **(erythema migrans)**; stage 2, weeks to months later, Bell's palsy or meningitis; and stage 3, months to years later, arthritis. The problem with this simplified scheme is that there is a great deal of overlap, and the skin, central nervous system, and musculoskeletal system can be involved early or late. A more accurate classification divides disease into early and late manifestations and specifies whether disease is localized or disseminated.

A. Symptoms and Signs:

1. Stage 1, early localized infection–Stage 1 infection is characterized by erythema migrans. About 1 week after the tick bite (range, 3–30 days; median 7–10 days), a flat or slightly raised red lesion appears at the site, which is commonly seen in areas of tight clothing such as the groin, thigh, or axilla. This lesion expands over several days, with central clearing. About 20% of patients either do not have typical skin lesions or the lesions go unnoticed. A flu-like illness with fever, chills, and myalgia occurs in about half of patients. Even without treatment, the symptoms and signs of erythema migrans resolve in 3–4 weeks. Although the classic lesion of erythema migrans is not difficult to recognize, atypical forms can occur that may lead to misdiagnosis. Vesicular, urticarial, and evanescent erythema migrans have been reported, as have lesions that develop central intensification instead of clearing. Similarly, chemical reactions to tick and spider bites, drug eruptions, urticaria, and staphylococcal and streptococcal cellulitis have been mistaken for erythema migrans.

2. Stage 2, early disseminated infection–In stage 2, the spirochete may spread in the patient's blood or lymph to cause a wide variety of symptoms and signs. This usually occurs within days to weeks after inoculation of the organism. The most common manifestations involve the skin, central nervous system, and musculoskeletal system. In about half of patients, secondary lesions develop that are not associated with a tick bite. These lesions are similar in appearance to the primary lesion but are usually smaller. A rare skin lesion (1% of patients) seen primarily in Europe is borrelia lymphocytoma. This presents as a small reddish nodule or plaque on the ear in children and on the nipple in adults. Headache and stiff neck can occur, as well as migratory pains in joints, muscles, and tendons. Fatigue and malaise are common. Generally, the neurologic and musculoskeletal symptoms are intermittent and last only hours to a few days, whereas fatigue is persistent. After hematogenous spread, the organism sequesters itself in certain areas and produces focal symptoms. Some patients experience cardiac (4–10% of patients) or neurologic (10–20% of patients) manifestations. Involvement of the heart includes myopericarditis, with atrial or ventricular arrhythmias and heart block. Neurologic disease is most commonly manifested as aseptic meningitis with mild headache and neck stiffness, Bell's palsy, or encephalitis with irritability, personality change, and forgetfulness that can wax and wane. Even in the absence of symptoms, seeding of the central nervous system can occur. Peripheral neuropathy (sensory or motor), transverse myelitis, and mononeuritis multiplex have also been described. Conjunctivitis, keratitis, and, rarely, panophthalmitis can occur.

3. Stage 3, late persistent infection–Stage 3 infection occurs months to years after the initial infection and again primarily manifests itself as musculoskeletal, neurologic, and skin disease. Up to 60% of patients develop musculoskeletal complaints. Clinical manifestations are quite variable and include (1) joint and periarticular pain without objective findings (perhaps a manifestation of fibromyalgia that may be triggered by Lyme disease); (2) frank arthritis, mainly of large joints, that is chronic or recurrent over years (recurrences become less severe, less frequent, and shorter with time); and (3) chronic synovitis, which may result in permanent disability. The pathogenesis of chronic Lyme arthritis may be an immunologic phenomenon rather than persistence of infection. The observations that individuals with chronic arthritis have an increased frequency of HLA-DR4 gene expression, antibodies to OspA and OspB protein in joint fluid (major outer surface proteins of *B burgdorferi*), lack *B burgdorferi* DNA in synovial fluid as detected by polymerase chain reaction (PCR), and often fail to respond to antibiotics—all support the inference of an immunologic mechanism.

Both the central and the peripheral nervous systems may be involved. Subacute encephalopathy, characterized by memory loss, mood changes, and sleep disturbance, is the most common chronic neurologic manifestation. An axonal polyneuropathy, manifested as distal sensory paresthesias or radicular pain, can occur either alone or, more commonly, in association with encephalopathy. Most of these patients have objective signs of disease when tested by electromyography. A rare form of chronic neurologic dysfunction—leukoencephalitis—presents with cognitive dysfunction, spastic paraparesis, ataxia, and bladder dysfunction. This form of the disease is seen more commonly in Europe than in the United States.

The cutaneous manifestation of late infection, which can occur up to 10 years after infection, is **acrodermatitis chronicum atrophicans.** It has been described mainly in Europe and is due to infection with *Borrelia afzelii,* a species that commonly causes disease in Europe but not the United States. There is usually bluish-red discoloration of a distal extremity with associated swelling. These lesions become atrophic and sclerotic with time and eventually resemble localized scleroderma. At least two cases of diffuse fasciitis with eosinophilia, a rare entity that resembles scleroderma, have been associated with infection with *B burgdorferi.*

B. Laboratory Findings: The diagnosis of Lyme disease is based on both clinical manifestations and laboratory findings. The National Surveillance Case Definition specifies a person with exposure to a potential tick habitat (within the 30 days just prior to developing erythema migrans) with (1) erythema migrans diagnosed by a physician or (2) at least one late manifestation of the disease and (3) laboratory confirmation as fulfilling the criteria for Lyme disease. Laboratory confirmation requires detection of specific antibodies to *B burgdorferi* in serum, either by indirect immunofluorescence assay (IFA) or enzyme-linked immunosorbent assay (ELISA); the latter is now preferred, because it is more sensitive and specific. A Western blot assay that can detect both IgM and IgG antibodies is used as a confirmatory test. IgM antibody appears first 2–4 weeks after onset of erythema migrans, peaks at 6–8 weeks, and then declines to low levels after 4–6 months of illness. The presence of IgM antibody in patients with prolonged symptoms persisting for several months is likely to be a false-positive result. IgG occurs later (6–8 weeks after onset of disease), peaks at 4–6 months, and may remain elevated at low levels indefinitely despite appropriate therapy and resolution of symptoms. A two-test approach is now recommended for the diagnosis of active Lyme disease. All specimens positive or equivocal by ELISA or IFA should be tested by Western immunoblot. When Western immunoblot is done during the first 4 weeks of illness, both IgM and IgG should be tested. If a patient with suspected early Lyme disease has negative serologic studies, acute and convalescent titers should be obtained since up to 50% of patients with early disease can be antibody-negative in the first several weeks of illness. A fourfold rise (or fall) in antibody titer would be diagnostic of recent infection. In patients with later stages of disease, almost all are antibody-positive. False-positive reactions in the ELISA and IFA have been reported in juvenile rheumatoid arthritis, rheumatoid arthritis, systemic lupus erythematosus, infectious mononucleosis, subacute infective endocarditis, syphilis, relapsing fever, leptospirosis, enteroviral and other viral illnesses, and patients with gingival disease (presumably because of cross-reactivity with oral treponemes). False-negative serologic reactions occur early in illness, and antibiotic therapy early in disease can abort subsequent seroconversion. Other investigational tests include an antibody-capture ELISA, which appears to be more specific and sensitive than the routine ELISA or IFA, especially in early disease. It is positive in up to 90% of patients with stage 1 disease. It is difficult to perform and is presently available only in reference and research laboratories. Use of flagellar antigen, which produces an early immune response, to detect antibodies by both ELISA and immunoblotting may improve the ability to detect early disease and is under investigation. Detection of immune complexes (specific antibody directed against *B burgdorferi* antigens) may be useful in diagnosing early disease and determining whether positive IgG serology is due to previous infection or active disease.

Caution should be exercised in basing the diagnosis of Lyme disease on serologic testing. In addition to the lack of sensitivity of the available tests as noted above, interlaboratory variation in test results is a major problem. In one study, aliquots of serum were sent to different laboratories, and there was a marked difference in reported test results, with known positive serum being identified in less than half of cases. When a second specimen of the same serum was sent 2 weeks later, 8 of 18 laboratories reported a fourfold difference in titers. These data demonstrate the difficulty in making the diagnosis of Lyme disease by serologic testing and emphasize the need for national standards. Lack of specificity is also a problem and several diseases can cause false-positive reactions as noted above.

Despite problems with the sensitivity and specificity of serologic tests, the lack of national standards, and the inter- and intralaboratory reproducibility of results, requests for laboratory tests for Lyme disease have increased rapidly, with several million tests done yearly. Testing is often done in patients with nonspecific symptoms such as headache, arthralgia, myalgia, fatigue, and palpitations. Even in endemic areas, the pretest probability of having Lyme disease is low in these patients, and the probability of a false-positive test result is greater than that of a true-positive. For these reasons, the American College of Physicians has established guidelines for laboratory evaluation of patients with suspected Lyme disease:

(1) The diagnosis of early Lyme disease is clinical (ie, exposure in an endemic area, with physician-documented erythema migrans), and does *not* require laboratory confirmation. (Tests are often negative at this stage.)

(2) Late disease requires objective evidence of clinical manifestations (recurrent brief attacks of mono- or oligoarticular arthritis of large joints; lymphocytic meningitis, cranial neuritis [Bell's palsy], peripheral neuropathy, or, rarely, encephalomyelitis—but *not* headache, fatigue, paresthesias, or stiff neck alone; atrioventricular conduction defects with or without myocarditis; and laboratory evidence of disease (two-stage testing with ELISA and Western blot, as described above).

(3) Patients with nonspecific symptoms without objective signs of Lyme disease should *not* have serologic testing done. It is in this setting that false-positive tests occur more commonly than true-positives.

(4) The role of serologic testing in neuroborreliosis is unclear, as sensitivity and specificity of cerebrospinal fluid serologic tests have not been determined. However, it is rare for a patient with neuroborreliosis to have positive serologic tests on cerebrospinal fluid without positive tests on serum (see below).

(5) Other tests such as the T cell proliferative assay, PCR testing, and urinary antigen detection have not yet been studied well enough to be routinely used (see discussion below).

B burgdorferi has rarely been cultured from blood or cerebrospinal fluid. Aspiration of erythema migrans lesions has yielded positive cultures in up to

29% of cases, and cultures of biopsy specimens (either central or peripheral aspects of the lesions) have been reported positive in 60–70%. The ability to culture organisms from skin lesions is greatly influenced by antibiotic therapy. Even a brief course of several days will result in negative cultures. Special silver staining of chronically inflamed synovial tissue demonstrates spirochetes in one-third of patients.

Detection of bacterial DNA by PCR may become a useful diagnostic tool in view of difficulties in culturing the organism and interpreting serologic tests. Although quite specific, the sensitivity of the test varies and depends upon which body fluid is tested and the stage of disease. In patients with arthritis, 85% of synovial fluid samples are positive for *B burgdorferi* DNA by PCR. Sensitivity in blood and cerebrospinal fluid is not as good. PCR is more sensitive than culture for detecting spirochetemia in early disease (18% versus 5%), but serology (IgG or IgM) detects over 50% of cases. Similarly, PCR can detect *B burgdorferi* DNA in cerebrospinal fluid of 25% of chronic cases of neuroborreliosis and 38% of acute cases, but sensitivity is obviously a limiting factor. The significance of a positive reaction is unclear. Whether a positive PCR indicates persistence of viable organisms that will respond to further treatment or is a marker for residual DNA (not active infection) has not been clarified and depends on the clinical specimen and the stage of disease. In chronic Lyme arthritis, some have suggested that a positive PCR indicates active infection that requires further therapy, while others have found a positive reaction despite months of therapy. At present, this test remains investigational.

The diagnosis of neuroborreliosis is often difficult since clinical manifestations, such as memory impairment, may be difficult to document. Most patients with neuroborreliosis have a history of previous mono- or polyarticular arthritis, and the vast majority have antibody present in serum. When cerebrospinal fluid is sampled, there is usually a pleocytosis or elevated protein (or both) and evidence of localized antibody production, ie, a ratio of cerebrospinal fluid to serum antibody of > 1.0. The role of other tests such as PCR in detection of DNA or ELISA in detecting the presence of OspA antigen is unclear, but in difficult cases these tests can be performed and, if positive, help establish the diagnosis. In addition, many patients with neuroborreliosis will have a peripheral neuropathy that may be detected by electromyography. In the absence of any of the above findings, it is difficult to make the diagnosis of central nervous system borrelia infection.

Nonspecific laboratory abnormalities can be seen, particularly in early disease. The most common are an elevated sedimentation rate of > 20 mm/h seen in 50% of cases and mildly abnormal liver function tests present in 30%. The abnormal liver function tests are transient and return to normal within a few weeks of treatment. A mild anemia, leukocytosis (11,000–18,000/μL), and microscopic hematuria have been reported in 10% or less of patients.

Prevention

Simple preventive measures such as avoiding tick-infested areas, covering exposed skin with long-sleeved shirts and wearing long trousers tucked into socks, using repellents, and inspecting for ticks after exposure will greatly reduce the number of tick bites. Environmental controls directed at limiting ticks on residential property would be helpful, but trying to limit the deer, tick, or white-footed mouse populations over large areas is not feasible.

The role of prophylactic antibiotics following tick bites is controversial. Analysis of the cost-effectiveness of prophylactic therapy suggests that antibiotics administered for 2 weeks would be beneficial in preventing illness in endemic areas, where the risk of acquiring disease following a tick bite is 3.6% or greater. However, studies designed to examine the effect of prophylaxis have not shown any significant benefit. In one study of almost 400 patients in a highly endemic area, amoxicillin, 250 mg three times daily for 10 days, was no better than placebo in preventing disease in patients who had been bitten by a deer tick within the previous 72 hours. Since most patients who develop Lyme disease are symptomatic and since treatment of early disease prevents late sequelae, it is reasonable to reserve treatment for patients who develop symptoms rather than to routinely administer prophylactic antibiotics. Exceptions might include situations where the follow-up is uncertain, the patient is extremely anxious, the patient is a pregnant woman, or the tick was engorged when removed.

A recombinant vaccine using a highly conserved region of *Borrelia burgdorferi* known as outer surface protein A (OspA) has recently been licensed by the FDA (LYMErix, SmithKline Beecham Pharmaceuticals). In a field study that excluded pregnant women, immunocompromised people, and those with chronic arthritis, almost 11,000 individuals between the ages of 15 and 70 years were immunized with three intramuscular injections at 0, 1, and 12 months. Efficacy was approximately 50% in those receiving two doses and 75% in those receiving all three. Adverse events were minor and included soreness at the site of injection (about 25%) and a flu-like illness with fevers and chills (about 4%). Reactions usually occurred within 48 hours after immunization and only lasted 3–4 days.

Several aspects of the vaccine and its use deserve emphasis. Antibodies decrease rapidly following immunization, and it is likely that boosters will be needed on a regular basis—but the exact frequency has not been determined. Although children are at highest risk for Lyme disease, the vaccine was not studied in this group, and safety and efficacy are unknown. Similarly, without data, the vaccine should not be used in pregnancy, in those older than 70, and in those with chronic arthritis. Few or no data are available for vaccine use in immunocompromised individuals, in those with chronic musculoskeletal disease, and in individuals with chronic joint, neurologic, or cardiac disease related to previous Lyme disease. As with any new product, long-term adverse effects are unknown. With this particular product, there are some concerns about causing chronic arthritis since patients with natural infection who have chronic arthritis have high antibody titers to OspA. Finally, immunization will affect the way a serologic diagnosis of Lyme disease is made because antibodies to OspA will cause a false-positive ELISA test. Thus, to make a diagnosis of Lyme disease in a vaccinated individual, the more expensive Western blot assay will be required.

Recommendations for use of the Lyme disease vaccine depend upon two epidemiologic factors—the entomologic risk (the density of ticks in a given area that are infected with *B burgdorferi*) and the human exposure risk (how likely an individual is to come into contact with infected ticks). The Centers for Disease Control and Prevention has stratified the United States into areas of high, moderate, low, and minimal or no risk of infection based on the density of infected ticks in the area. High and moderate risk areas include the northeastern, mid-Atlantic and North Central United States as well as one area on the Western slopes of the Sierra Nevada mountains in Northern California. All other areas are deemed to have low or minimal to no risk. Current recommendations, although somewhat vague and open to interpretation, state that vaccination should be considered for persons who live, work, or spend recreational time in areas of high or moderate risk and whose exposure to tick-infested areas is frequent or prolonged. Vaccination is not recommended for individuals who live or work in high or moderate risk areas if they have minimal or no tick exposure, and it is not recommended for individuals who live in low or minimal risk areas. Immunization should be considered in two additional groups: those who plan to travel to areas of high or moderate risk and who will have frequent or prolonged exposure to tick-infested areas, and individuals with previous uncomplicated Lyme disease who continue to be at risk.

Treatment

Antibiotic sensitivity of *B burgdorferi* has been established in vitro. Tetracycline is effective against the spirochete, but penicillin is only moderately so. Erythromycin is effective in vitro but has been disappointing in clinical trials. Ampicillin, ceftriaxone, azithromycin, cefuroxime, and imipenem are also effective in vitro, but aminoglycosides, ciprofloxacin, and rifampin are not.

Present recommendations for therapy are outlined in Table 34–4. In general, infection confined to skin is treated for 3–4 weeks. For central nervous system disease (with the exception of Bell's palsy), systemic therapy is used. Other organ system involvement usually responds to oral medication. For early disease, oral antibiotic therapy shortens the duration of rash and usually prevents late sequelae. Doxycycline, 100 mg twice daily, is most commonly used and has the advantage of being active against ehrlichia. Amoxicillin is also effective and is recommended for pregnant or lactating women and for those who cannot tolerate doxycycline. Cefuroxime axetil, 500 mg twice daily for 20 days, is as effective as doxycycline, 100 mg twice daily for 20 days. Erythromycin is less effective. Azithromycin, 500 mg/d for 7 days, was not as effective as amoxicillin, 500 mg three times a day for 20 days, for erythema migrans. Complete resolution of symptoms was less common in the azithromycin group, and relapses occurred more commonly. For acute disseminated disease (multiple erythema migrans lesions, carditis manifested as heart block, neurologic disease including Bell's palsy or radiculitis, and acute large joint arthritis), doxycy-

Table 34–4. Treatment of Lyme disease.

Manifestation	Drug and Dosage
Erythema migrans	Doxycycline, 100 mg twice daily for 3–4 weeks; or amoxicillin, 500 mg three times daily for 3–4 weeks; or cefuroxime axetil, 500 mg twice daily for 3–4 weeks
Neurologic disease	
Bell's palsy	Doxycycline, or amoxicillin as above for 3–4 weeks
Other central nervous system disease	Ceftriaxone, 2 g IV once daily for 2–4 weeks; or penicillin G, 20 million units daily IV in 6 divided doses for 2–4 weeks; or cefotaxime, 2 g IV every 8 hours for 2–4 weeks
Cardiac disease	
First-degree block (PR < 0.3 s)	Doxycycline or amoxicillin as above for 3–4 weeks
High-degree atrioventricular block	Ceftriaxone or penicillin G as above for 2–4 weeks
Arthritis	
Oral dosage	Doxycycline, or amoxicillin as above for 4 weeks
Parenteral dosage	Ceftriaxone or penicillin G as above for 2–4 weeks
Acrodermatitis chronicum atrophicans	Doxycycline or amoxicillin as above for 4 weeks

cline, 100 mg twice daily for 14 days, was as effective as ceftriaxone 2 g daily for 14 days, although most would treat for longer periods than 14 days. If other central nervous system manifestations are present (meningitis), ceftriaxone is given intravenously. Intravenous penicillin is also effective for central nervous system disease, but ceftriaxone penetrates into the cerebrospinal fluid better and can be given once daily. Mild cardiac disease (PR < 0.3 s) can be treated with oral agents, but high-degree atrioventricular block should be treated with either intravenous ceftriaxone or penicillin. Therapy of arthritis is difficult because some patients fail to respond to any therapy and others who do respond do so slowly. Initial studies suggested that intravenous penicillin was superior to benzathine penicillin. In one small study, ceftriaxone appeared to be superior to intravenous penicillin. In a recent study, however, oral agents (doxycycline or amoxicillin) were just as effective as intravenous regimens (penicillin or ceftriaxone). A reasonable approach to the patient with Lyme arthritis is to start with oral therapy and if this fails (no improvement in 1–2 months) treat for a longer period with oral medication (2 months) or switch to an intravenous agent. Data for treatment in pregnancy are limited. Tetracycline and doxycycline should not be used in pregnancy (because of subsequent tooth staining of infant). Because of the failure of oral agents to prevent fetal infection in one case, some have recommended parenteral therapy. In one study, 53 women in various trimesters with erythema migrans were treated with ceftriaxone for 2 weeks. The drug was tolerated well, no clinical disease developed in infants, and preterm births and congenital anomalies occurred no more frequently than in the general population.

Physicians are often confronted with patients with nonspecific symptoms (such as fatigue and myalgias) and positive serologic tests for Lyme disease who request (or demand) therapy for their illness. It is important in managing these patients to remember (1) that the diagnosis of Lyme disease is primarily a clinical one, and nonspecific symptoms alone are not diagnostic; (2) that serologic tests are fraught with difficulty (as noted above), and in areas where disease prevalence is low, false-positive serologic tests are much more common than true-positive tests; and (3) that parenteral therapy with ceftriaxone for 2–4 weeks is costly (approximately $5000) and has been associated with significant adverse effects (cholelithiasis). Parenteral therapy should be reserved for those most likely to benefit, ie, those with cutaneous, neurologic, cardiac, or rheumatic manifestations that are characteristic of Lyme disease. In addition, coinfection may present with an atypical clinical picture, eg, a patient with Lyme disease and ehrlichiosis may present with fever and rash but without the hematologic abnormalities characteristic of ehrlichiosis.

Prognosis

Most patients respond to appropriate therapy with prompt resolution of symptoms within 4 weeks. With adequate therapy, only a small percentage of patients will fail to respond or will develop a late relapse. True treatment failures are thus uncommon, and in most cases re-treatment or prolonged treatment of Lyme disease is instituted because of misdiagnosis or misinterpretation of serologic results rather than inadequate therapy. It is important to remember that most areas endemic for Lyme disease are also endemic for babesiosis and ehrlichiosis. Coinfection with the etiologic agents of these diseases may be associated with more severe symptoms than infection with either agent alone and is another possible explanation for failure to respond to therapy directed at Lyme disease.

The long-term outcome of adult patients with Lyme disease is not clear. Joint pain, memory impairment, and poor functional status secondary to pain are common subjective complaints in patients with Lyme disease, but physical examination and neurocognitive testing fail to document the presence of these symptoms as objective sequelae. Similarly, in highly endemic areas, patients with a diagnosis of Lyme disease commonly complain of pain, fatigue, and inability to perform certain physical activities when followed for several years. However, these complaints occur equally as commonly in age-matched controls without a history of Lyme disease. Attempts to document chronic cardiac disease in patients treated for Lyme disease also have been unsuccessful. It appears that long-term sequelae of adequately treated disease are uncommon.

Brown SL et al: Role of serology in the diagnosis of Lyme disease. JAMA 1999;282:62. [NLM Cit ID: 99331799] (Difficulties of making a serologic diagnosis.)

Guidelines for laboratory evaluation in the diagnosis of Lyme disease. (Two parts.) Ann Intern Med 1997; 127:1106, 1109. [NLM Cit ID: 98049721] (A summary followed by a detailed analysis of rationale for test utilization.)

Halperin JJ et al: Practice parameters for the diagnosis of patients with nervous system Lyme borreliosis (Lyme disease). Neurology 1996;46:619. [NLM Cit ID: 96173665] (Superb review of manifestations of neurologic disease, diagnostic criteria, and therapy.)

Nichol G et al: Test-treatment strategies for patients suspected of having Lyme disease: A cost-effectiveness analysis. Ann Intern Med 1998;128:37. [NLM Cit ID: 98069619] (Analyses of common clinical presentations and need to test or treat empirically.)

Recommendations for the use of Lyme disease vaccine. MMWR Morb Mortal Wkly Rep 1999;48(RR-7):1, 21. [NLM Cit ID: 99297664] (Official recommendations of an Advisory Committee on Immunization Procedures.)

Seltzer EG et al: Long-term outcomes of persons with Lyme disease. JAMA 2000;283:609. [NLM Cit ID: 20127466] (Cohort study comparing long-term sequelae in patients with and without a diagnosis of Lyme disease.)

Sigal LH et al: A vaccine consisting of recombinant *Borrelia burgdorferi* outer-surface protein A to prevent Lyme disease. N Engl J Med 1998;339:216. [NLM Cit ID: 98328628] (Safety, efficacy, and adverse events of the Connaught product.)

Steere AC et al: Vaccination against Lyme disease with recombinant *Borrelia burgdorferi* outer-surface lipoprotein A with adjuvant. N Engl J Med 1998;339:209. [NLM Cit ID: 98328627] (Full trial describing safety, efficacy, and adverse effects of LYMErix vaccine.)

RELEVANT WORLD WIDE WEB SITES

[CNS Lyme Disease Case Study]
http://path.upmc.edu:80/cases/case59.html

[Lyme Disease Information Resource]
http://www.x-l.net/Lyme/index.html

[Lyme Encephalopathy Case Study]
http://www.med.harvard.edu/AANLIB/cases/case19/mr1-tc1/020.html

35 Infectious Diseases: Protozoal & Helminthic

See http://www.current-med.com/ch35.html for updated addresses of Web sites referenced in this chapter.

Robert S. Goldsmith, MD, MPH, DTM&H

I. PROTOZOAL INFECTIONS

AFRICAN TRYPANOSOMIASIS (Sleeping Sickness)

Essentials of Diagnosis

- History of exposure to tsetse flies. Bite lesion.

Hemolymphatic stage (usually absent or unnoticed in *T b gambiense* infections):

- Irregular fevers, headaches, joint pains, malaise, pruritus, papular skin rash, edemas.
- Posterior cervical or generalized lymphadenopathy; hepatosplenomegaly.
- Anemia, weight loss.
- Trypanosomes in blood or lymph node aspirates; positive serology.

Meningoencephalitic stage:

- Insomnia, motor and sensory disorders, abnormal reflexes, somnolence to coma.
- Trypanosomes and increased white cells and protein in cerebrospinal fluid.

General Considerations

African trypanosomiasis is caused by *Trypanosoma brucei rhodesiense* and *Trypanosoma brucei gambiense,* both hemoflagellates. The organisms are transmitted by bites of tsetse flies (*Glossina* species), which inhabit shaded areas along streams and rivers. Trypanosomes ingested in a blood meal undergo a developmental period of 18–35 days in the fly; when the fly feeds again on a new mammalian host, the infective stage is injected. Human disease occurs locally throughout tropical Africa from south of the Sahara to about 20° south latitude. *T b gambiense* infections are in the moist sub-Saharan savannah and riverine forests of west and central Africa up to the eastern Rift Valley. *T b rhodesiense* occurs to the east of the Rift Valley in the savannah of east and southeast Africa and along the shores of Lake Victoria. Up to 50,000 deaths yearly are estimated to occur. The disease has been especially prevalent where fighting interfered with control programs, as in the Congo and southern Sudan.

T b rhodesiense infection is primarily a zoonosis of game animals; humans are infected sporadically. Humans are the principal mammalian host for *T b gambiense;* although domestic animals can be infected with this parasite, it is undetermined whether there is an animal reservoir. A third trypanosome, *T brucei brucei,* is morphologically identical to the human parasites but infects only wild and domestic animals.

Clinical Findings

A. Symptoms and Signs: *T b rhodesiense* infections go through the following three stages, are much more virulent, and untreated patients die within weeks to a year. In *T b gambiense* infections, however, chancres do not appear and the hemolymphatic stage is usually absent or goes unnoticed; when symptoms do become manifest after weeks to years, they are initially so mild that they are often ignored by the patient.

1. The trypanosomal chancre–This is a local pruritic, painful inflammatory reaction (3–10 cm) with regional lymphadenopathy that appears about 48 hours after the tsetse fly bite and lasts 2–4 weeks.

2. The hemolymphatic (early) stage–This stage usually begins 3–10 days later with invasion of the bloodstream and reticuloendothelial system. High fever, severe headache, joint pains, and malaise recur at irregular intervals corresponding to waves of parasitemia. Between febrile episodes there are symptom-free periods that last up to 2 weeks. Transient rashes may appear, often pruritic and papular or circinate. Examination reveals mild enlargement of the liver and spleen, and edema (peripheral, pleural, ascites, etc). Enlarged, rubbery, and painless lymph nodes occur in 75% of patients. In *T b gambiense,* only the posterior cervical group (Winterbottom's sign) may be enlarged. With progression of the disease, there is increasing weight loss and debilitation. Signs of myocardial involvement may appear early in Rhodesian infection, and the patient may succumb to myocarditis before signs of central nervous system invasion appear.

3. The meningoencephalitic (late) stage– This stage appears within a few weeks or months of onset of Rhodesian infection but in Gambian sleeping sickness develops more insidiously, starting 6 months to several years after onset. Insomnia, anorexia, personality changes, apathy, and headaches are among the early findings. A variety of motor or tonus disorders may develop, including tremors and disturbances of speech, gait, and reflexes; somnolence appears late. The patient becomes severely emaciated and, finally, comatose. Death often results from secondary infection.

B. Laboratory Findings: Definitive diagnosis requires identifying motile organisms in wet films and after Giemsa staining in specimens from the bite lesion aspirates (rare), lymph node aspirates, bone marrow, or cerebrospinal fluid. Because the number of trypanosomes in blood fluctuates and often is undetectable 3 out of 5 days, specimens should be examined daily for about 15 days, including after concentration by microhematocrit centrifugation of 10–15 mL of heparinized blood (trypanosomes are concentrated in the buffy coat). Other diagnostic tests with blood are the quantitative buffy coat technique, intraperitoneal inoculation into laboratory rodents (most sensitive approach, but only effective for *T b rhodesiense*), culture, Millipore filtration, and DEAE-cellulose anion exchange centrifugation. Only soft lymph nodes (not fibrosed) should be selected for aspiration (25-gauge needle); after the node is gently kneaded, the aspirate should be examined immediately for motile organisms. Cerebrospinal fluid shows an increase in lymphocytes and protein; centrifugation to detect the parasite should be done both rapidly and twice (at least twice as sensitive as single centrifugation). The fluid should also be inoculated into an experimental animal and culture medium. With progression of the disease, organisms are more likely to be found in cerebrospinal fluid than in blood or lymph nodes.

Serologic tests are available for IgM and IgG antibody. Circulating IgM levels become positive about 12 days after onset of infection and may reach 10–20 times normal. Normal or low levels, however, do not rule out the infection, for titers may fluctuate when brief periods of excess antigens may depress the titers, even to below detectable levels. In late central nervous system disease, though both circulating antibody and parasitemia may fall below detectable levels, serologic tests of the cerebrospinal fluid may yet prove useful. At any stage of the disease, an elevated IgM in the cerebrospinal fluid is pathognomonic for central nervous system infection except that false-negative results have been reported. Additional immunologic tests include ELISA, immunofluorescent assays, and a field-adapted card agglutination test; under evaluation are tests for circulating antigen.

Other findings include anemia, increased sedimentation rate, thrombocytopenia, reduced total serum protein, and increased serum globulin. Eosinophilia is not seen.

Differential Diagnosis

Trypanosomiasis may be mistaken for a variety of other diseases, including malaria, influenza, pneumonia, infectious mononucleosis, leukemia, lymphoma, the arbovirus encephalitides, cerebral tumor, and various psychoses. Serologic tests for syphilis may be falsely positive in trypanosomiasis.

Treatment

Because all of the drugs used (except eflornithine) are highly toxic (mortality during drug treatment can reach 5–10%), immunoassays are insufficient to make the diagnosis; detection of the organism is required. See references for details on treatments and adverse reactions.)

A. Early Disease, the Hemolymphatic Stage: Drugs of choice for both parasites are intravenous suramin (100–200 mg [test dose], then 1 g on days 1, 3, 7, 14, 21). Alternative drugs of choice only for *T b gambiense* are intravenous eflornithine (400 mg/kg/d in four divided doses for 14 days, followed by 300 mg/kg/d orally for 3–4 weeks), and pentamidine (4 mg/kg/d intramuscularly for 10 days).

B. Late Disease With Central Nervous System Involvement: Drugs of choice for both parasites are intravenous melarsoprol, 2–3.6 mg/k/d for 3 days; after 1 week, 3.6 mg/kg for 3 days; repeat after 10–21 days. Alternative treatments only against *T b gambiense* are eflornithine (as above) or intravenous tryparsamide, 30 mg/kg (maximum: 2 g) every 5 days for 12 injections, plus intravenous suramin, 100–200 mg (test dose), followed by 10 mg/kg every 5 days for 12 injections; the treatment may be repeated in 1 month.

Suramin, which does not pass the blood-brain barrier, cannot be used when the central nervous system is involved. Melarsoprol causes a reactive encephalopathy in up to 18% of patients; corticosteroids are used to prevent this. Eflornithine, approved for use in the USA but available only from WHO, is highly effective and associated with only mild toxicity in early and late *T b gambiense* infections, but it should not be used for *T b rhodesiense* infection, as its efficacy for this parasite is inconsistent. In the USA, suramin and melarsoprol are available only from the CDC Drug Service, Centers for Disease Control and Prevention, Atlanta, GA 30333. Telephone: 404-639-3670; 404-639-2888 evenings, weekends, and holidays.

Proper follow-up to ensure detection of the encephalitic stage requires initial cerebrospinal fluid examination, repeat studies at intervals during treatment, 3 months after treatment, and then at 6-month intervals for 2 years.

Prevention

Individual prevention in endemic areas should include wearing long sleeves and trousers, avoiding dark-colored clothing, and using mosquito nets while sleeping. Repellents have no effect. Pentamidine is used in chemoprophylaxis (controversial) only against the Gambian type. In *T b rhodesiense* infection, pentamidine may suppress early symptoms, resulting in recognition of the disease too late in its course for effective treatment. Excretion of pentamidine is slow; therefore, one intramuscular injection (4 mg/kg, maximum 300 mg) protects for 3–6 months. The drug is potentially toxic and should only be used for persons at high risk (ie, those with constant, heavy exposure to tsetse flies in areas with known transmission of Gambian disease). Performing serologic tests every 6 months during exposure and for 3 years afterward is the safest method for detecting the disease at an early stage.

Prognosis

Most patients—even those with advanced disease—recover following treatment. Relapses are uncommon (about 2%). When therapy is started late, irreversible brain damage or death is common. Most persons with African trypanosomiasis will die if untreated.

Atouguia J et al: Therapy of African trypanosomiasis: current situation. Memorias Instituto Oswaldo Cruz 1999; 94:221. [NLM Cit ID: 99242667]

Chimelli L et al: Trypanosomiasis. Brain Pathol 1997;7: 599. [NLM Cit ID: 97187115]

Doua F et al: The efficacy of pentamidine in the treatment of early-late stage *Trypanosoma brucei gambiense* trypanosomiasis. Am J Trop Med Hyg 1996;55:586. [NLM Cit ID: 97178260]

Drugs for parasitic infections: Med Lett Drugs Ther 1998;40:1. [NLM Cit ID: 98104976] (Important resource for dosages.)

Pepin J et al: Risk factors for encephalopathy and mortality during melarsoprol therapy of *Trypanosoma brucei gambiense* sleeping sickness. Trans R Soc Trop Med Hyg 1995;89:92. [NLM Cit ID: 95266138]

Pepin J et al: The treatment of human trypanosomiasis. Adv Parasitol 1994;33:1. [NLM Cit ID: 94168091]

Sinha A et al: African trypanosomiasis in two travelers from the United States. Clin Infect Dis 1999;29:840. [NLM Cit ID: 20055845]

AMERICAN TRYPANOSOMIASIS (Chagas' Disease)

Essentials of Diagnosis

Acute stage:

- Inflammatory lesion at site of inoculation; prolonged fever, tachycardia, hepatosplenomegaly, lymphadenopathy, signs of myocarditis.
- Parasites in peripheral blood, positive serologic tests.

Chronic stage:

- Heart failure with cardiac arrhythmias; decreased intensity of heart sounds; episodes of thromboembolism.
- In some geographic regions, dysphagia, severe constipation, and radiologic evidence of megaesophagus or megacolon.
- Positive xenodiagnosis or hemoculture, positive serologic tests; abnormal ECG.

General Considerations

Chagas' disease is caused by *Trypanosoma cruzi,* a protozoan parasite of humans and wild and domestic animals. *T cruzi* occurs only in the Americas; it is found in wild animals and to a lesser extent in humans from southern South America to southern USA. An estimated 16 million people are infected, mostly in rural areas, resulting in about 45,000 deaths yearly. In many countries of South America, Chagas' disease is the most important cause of heart disease. In southern USA, although the organism has been found in triatomine bugs and wild and domestic animals, only four confirmed indigenous cases have been reported. However, a large number of immigrants from Latin America (particularly Central America) are infected (estimated to be more than 50,000).

T cruzi is transmitted by many species of triatomine (reduviid) bugs that become infected by ingesting blood from infected animals or humans who have circulating trypanosomes. Multiplication occurs in the digestive tract of the bug; infective forms are eliminated in feces. Infection in humans is through "contamination" with bug feces; the parasite penetrates the skin (generally through the bite wound), mucus membranes, or the conjunctiva. Transmission can also occur by blood transfusion or in utero.

The trypanosomes first multiply close to the point of entry. They then enter the bloodstream as trypanosomes and later invade the heart and other tissues, where they assume a leishmanial form. Multiplication causes cellular destruction, inflammation, and fibrosis.

Clinical Findings

A. Symptoms and Signs: Although infection continues for many years—probably for life—as many as 70% of persons remain asymptomatic. The **acute stage,** seen principally in children, lasts 2–4 months and leads to death in up to 10% of cases. The earliest findings are at the site of inoculation either in the eye—Romaña's sign (unilateral bipalpebral edema, conjunctivitis, local lymphadenopathy)—or in the skin—a chagoma (furuncle-like lesion with local lymphadenopathy). Subsequent findings include fever, malaise, headache, hepatomegaly, mild splenomegaly, and generalized lymphadenopathy. Acute myocarditis may lead to biventricular failure, but arrhythmias are rare. Meningoencephalitis is limited to young children and is often fatal.

A **latent period** (indeterminate phase) may last from 10 to 30 years in which the patient is asymptomatic but in which serologic tests and sometimes parasitologic examination confirm the presence of the infection. Reactivation of Chagas' disease in AIDS has been reported.

The **chronic stage** is usually manifested by cardiac disease in the third and fourth decades of life, characterized by arrhythmias, congestive heart failure (often with prominent right-sided findings), and systemic or pulmonary embolization originating from mural thrombi. Sudden cardiac arrest in young persons may occur and is attributed to ventricular fibrillation. Megacolon and megaesophagus, caused by damage to nerve plexuses in the bowel or esophageal wall, occur in some areas of Chile, Argentina, and Brazil; findings include dysphagia, regurgitation, constipation, sigmoid volvulus, and parotid gland hypertrophy.

In immunosuppressed persons, latent Chagas' disease may reactivate. In HIV infection, a common finding is brain lesions indistinguishable from cerebral toxoplasmosis; cardiopathy also appears.

B. Laboratory Findings: Appropriate selection of tests allows a definitive parasitologic diagnosis in most acute cases and in up to 40% of chronic ones. In the acute stage, trypanosomes should be looked for (1) by examination of anticoagulated fresh blood or the buffy coat for motile organisms and (2) by examination of the following Giemsa-stained preparations: thick blood films, buffy coat, and the sediment after centrifuging (600 Hz) the supernatant of clotted blood. In the chronic stage, the parasite can only be detected by culture or xenodiagnosis. The latter consists of permitting uninfected laboratory-reared bugs of the local major vector to feed on the patients and then examining their intestinal contents for trypanosomes. In both acute and chronic infection, blood should also be cultured using Nicolle-Novy-MacNeal medium and inoculated into laboratory mice or rats 3–10 days old. *Trypanosoma rangeli,* a nonpathogenic blood trypanosome also found in humans in Central America and northern South America, must not be mistaken for *T cruzi.* Several highly sensitive serologic tests (hemagglutination inhibition, complement fixation, ELISA, immunofluorescence, others) are routinely used and are of presumptive value when positive. However, two or three tests should be done because false-positive tests are common, particularly with other infections—including leishmaniasis, malaria, syphilis, and *T rangeli* infection—and with autoimmune diseases. Antibodies of the IgM class are usually elevated early in the acute stage but are replaced by IgG antibodies as the disease progresses. Maximum titers are reached in 3–4 months; thereafter, titers can remain positive at a low level for life. In chronic infections, when circulating organisms are difficult to find, the polymerase chain reaction procedure shows promise as a sensitive detection method. Serologic tests generally fail to assess the effectiveness of chemotherapy. The most important electrocardiographic abnormalities are right bundle branch block, other conduction defects, and arrhythmias. In certain regions of South America, radiologic examination may show megaesophagus, megacolon, or cardiac enlargement with characteristic apical aneurysms.

Treatment

Therapy is unsatisfactory. Treatment is indicated in acute but not latent infection and is controversial in the chronic stage. Two drugs are used: nifurtimox and benznidazole—both must be used for long periods and are potentially toxic. In acute disease and congenital infections, the drugs are effective in reducing the duration and severity of infection, but cure is achieved in only about 50% of patients. In the chronic phase, although parasitemia and xenodiagnosis may become negative in up to 50% of patients, treatment does not alter the serologic reaction, cardiac function, or progression of the disease. Some evidence indicates that pathogenesis may have an autoimmune basis not dependent on persistence of infection. Some workers, therefore, treat only acute and latent stage infections but not chronic infections. Allopurinol and itraconazole continue under evaluation.

Nifurtimox is given orally in daily doses of 10 mg/kg in four divided doses after meals for 90–120 days. It generally produces anorexia, weight loss, tremors, and peripheral neuropathy. Hallucinations, pulmonary infiltrates, and convulsions are rare. In the USA, nifurtimox is available only from the Parasitic Disease Drug Service, Centers for Disease Control, Atlanta, GA 30333 (call 404-639-3670) Benznidazole, where available (not in the USA), is the alternative drug of choice at a dosage of 5 mg/kg/d for 60 days. Its side effects include granulocytopenia, rash, and peripheral neuropathy. The drug is better tolerated by children under 12 years of age.

In the chronic stage, diuretics are usually effective in cardiac failure, but digoxin is commonly not well tolerated. The most effective antiarrhythmic drug is amiodarone, but pulmonary and cardiac toxicity can be problems with its use. Arrhythmias are treated in the usual way; cardiac pacemakers are used for atrioventricular blocks. In endemic areas, blood should not be used for transfusion unless at least two serologic tests are negative; otherwise, blood can be treated with gentian violet to kill the parasites.

Control of Chagas' disease is continuing in large areas of South America through improvement of housing conditions, insecticidal spraying of infected houses, and discarding of infected blood donations. Immigrants from endemic areas to developed countries should be tested for antibodies.

Prognosis

Acute infections in infants and young children are often fatal, particularly when the central nervous system is involved. Adults with chronic cardiac disease also may ultimately succumb to the disease.

Antas PR et al: Early, intermediate, and late acute stages in Chagas' disease: a study combining anti-galactose IgG, specific serodiagnosis, and polymerase chain reaction analysis. Am J Trop Med Hyg 1999;61:308. [NLM Cit ID: 99391326] (By associating anti-Gal IgG with specific serology, early *T cruzi* infection can be detected with greater precision.)

Apt W et al: Treatment of chronic Chagas' disease with itraconazole and allopurinol. Am J Trop Med Hyg 1998;59:133. [NLM Cit ID: 98347783]

Ben BC: Chagas disease or American trypanosomiasis. Bull WHO 1998;76 Suppl 2:144. [NLM Cit ID: 99163184]

Marin Neto JA et al: Chagas' heart disease. Arq Bras Cardiol 1999;72:247. [NLM Cit ID: 99442530]

Pagano MA et al: Cerebral tumor-like American trypanosomiasis in acquired immunodeficiency syndrome. Ann Neurol 1999;45:403. [NLM Cit ID: 99170275]

AMEBIASIS

Essentials of Diagnosis

- Mild to moderate colitis: recurrent diarrhea and abdominal cramps, sometimes alternating with constipation; mucus may be present; blood is usually absent.
- Severe colitis: semiformed to liquid stools streaked with blood and mucus, fever, colic, prostration. In fulminant cases, ileus, perforation, peritonitis, and hemorrhage occur.
- Hepatic amebiasis: fever, hepatomegaly, pain, localized tenderness.
- Laboratory findings: amebas in stools or in abscess aspirate; serologic tests positive with severe colitis or hepatic abscess, which is readily imaged by ultrasonography or CT scan.

General Considerations

Amebiasis is infection of the large colon, liver, and other tissues by the protozoan parasite *Entamoeba histolytica.* Formerly considered one organism with varying virulence, it is now recognized that the entamoeba complex contains two morphologically identical species: (1) *E dispar* (about 90% of the complex), which remains in the colon as a stable commensal that is avirulent and produces an asymptomatic carrier state; and (2) *E histolytica*, which shows varying degrees of virulence ranging from a commensal state in the colon—in which it does not cause disease, yet is potentially invasive—to being invasive of the intestinal wall and resulting in acute diarrhea or dysentery or chronic diarrhea. *E histolytica* may also be carried by the blood to the liver, where they may produce hepatic abscesses. Rarely, they are carried to the lungs, brain, or other organs or invade the perianal skin.

Both *E histolytica* and *E dispar* exist as two forms in the lumen and mucosal crypts of the large bowel: identical-appearing cysts (10–14 μm) and motile trophozoites (12–50 μm). In the absence of diarrhea, trophozoites encyst in the large bowel. Trophozoites passed into the environment die rapidly, but cysts remain viable in soil and water for several weeks to months at appropriate temperature and humidity.

The infections are present worldwide but are most prevalent and severe in subtropical and tropical areas under conditions of crowding, poor sanitation, and poor nutrition. Using the new taxonomy, prevalence estimates have changed. Of perhaps 500 million persons worldwide infected with entamoeba, 90% are *E dispar* and 10% (50 million) *E histolytica.* Invasive *E histolytica* may constitute 5 million cases, with mortality in the range of 100,000 per year.

Humans are the only established host and are universally susceptible. Only cysts are infectious, since after ingestion they survive gastric acidity whereas trophozoites are destroyed. Transmission generally occurs through ingestion of cysts from fecally contaminated food or water. Flies and other arthropods also serve as mechanical vectors; to an undetermined degree, transmission results from contamination of food by the hands of food handlers. Where human excrement is used as fertilizer, it is often a source of food and water contamination. Person-to-person contact is also important in transmission; therefore, all household members as well as an infected person's sexual partner should have their stools examined. Sexual transmission of *E histolytica* among male homosexuals in some temperate urban areas is predominantly the nonpathogenic *E dispar.* In communal settings such as mental hospitals (but not child day care centers), prevalence rates as high as 50% have been reported. Amebiasis is rarely epidemic, but urban outbreaks have occurred because of common-source water contamination. Although entamoeba infections occur frequently among homosexuals, in the developed countries (except Japan) these infections are usually due to the *E dispar* and do not require treatment. In AIDS, *E histolytica* infection does not become an opportunistic infection.

Malnutrition and alcoholism probably predispose to enhanced virulence. Fulminant infections may occur in pregnancy and in young children. Corticosteroids and other immunosuppressive drugs often convert a commensal infection to an invasive one.

The characteristic intestinal lesion is the amebic ulcer, which can occur anywhere in the large bowel (including the appendix) and sometimes in the terminal ileum but predominates in the cecum, descending colon, and the rectosigmoid colon—areas of greatest fecal stasis. Trophozoites invade the colonic mucosa by means of their ameboid movement and proteolytic secretions and induce necrosis to form the characteristic flask-shaped ulcers. Ulcers are usually limited to the muscularis, but if penetration to the serous layer occurs, bowel perforation, local abscess, or generalized peritonitis may result. In fulminating cases, ulceration may be extensive, and the bowel becomes thin and friable. Hepatic abscesses range from a few millimeters to 15 cm or larger, usually are single, occur more often in the right lobe (particularly the upper portion), and are more common in men.

Clinical Findings

A. Symptoms and Signs: Amebiasis can be classified into intestinal and extraintestinal disease and further subdivided into the clinical syndromes described below. Some patients have an acute onset of severe diarrhea as early as 8 days (commonly 2–4 weeks) after infection. Others may have an asymptomatic or mild intestinal infection for months to several years before either intestinal symptoms or liver abscess appears. Transition may occur from one type of intestinal infection to another, and each may give rise to hepatic abscess, or the intestinal infection may clear spontaneously.

1. Intestinal amebiasis–

a. Asymptomatic infection–In most infected persons, the organism lives as a commensal, and the patient is without symptoms.

b. Mild to moderate colitis (nondysenteric colitis)–A few stools a day are passed that are semiformed and have mucus but no blood. There may be abdominal cramps, flatulence, fatigue, and weight loss; fever is uncommon. Periods of remission and recurrence may last days to weeks or longer; during remissions, the patient may have constipation. Abdominal examination may show distention, hyperperistalsis, and tenderness. In some patients with chronic infection, the colon is thick and palpable, particularly over the cecum and descending colon. Toxic products released as a result of the bowel infection may induce periportal inflammation, mild hepatomegaly, and low-grade liver enzyme abnormalities, but without demonstrable trophozoites in the liver.

c. Severe colitis (dysenteric colitis)–As the severity of intestinal infection increases, the number of stools increases, and they change from semiformed to liquid with streaks of blood beginning to appear. With larger numbers of stools, 10–20 or more, little fecal material is present, but blood (fresh or dark) and bits of necrotic tissue become increasingly evident. With increasing severity, the patient may become prostrate and toxic, with fever up to 40.5 °C, and have colic, tenesmus, vomiting, generalized abdominal tenderness, and nonspecific hepatic enlargement and tenderness. Rare complications include appendicitis, bowel perforation, fulminating colitis, massive mucosal sloughing, and hemorrhage. Death may follow.

d. Localized ulcerative lesions of the colon–Bowel ulcerations limited to the rectal area may result in passage of formed stools with bloody exudate. Ulcerations limited to the cecum may induce mild diarrhea and simulate acute appendicitis. Amebic appendicitis, in which the appendix is extensively involved but not the remainder of the large bowel, is rare.

e. Localized granulomatous lesions of the colon (ameboma)–This occurs as a result of excessive production of granulation tissue in response to amebic infection, either in the course of dysentery or slowly in chronic intestinal infection. These masses may present as an irregular tumor (single or multiple) that projects into the bowel or as an annular constricting mass up to several centimeters in length. Clinical findings (pain, obstructive symptoms, and hemorrhage) and x-ray findings may simulate bowel carcinoma, inflammatory bowel disease, tuberculosis, or lymphogranuloma venereum. At endoscopy, the mass is deep red and bleeds easily, and biopsy specimens show granulation tissue and *E histolytica,* though the number of organisms may be relatively few. Antiamebic drugs are usually adequate in treatment; surgical removal of the lesion without prior or immediate postoperative drug therapy is likely to result in death from disseminated disease.

2. Extraintestinal amebiasis–

a. Hepatic amebiasis–Amebic liver abscess, although a relatively infrequent consequence of intestinal amebiasis, is not uncommon given the large number of intestinal infections. A large proportion of patients with liver abscess do not have concurrent intestinal symptoms, nor can they recall having had chronic intestinal symptoms. The onset of symptoms can be sudden or gradual, ranging from a few days to many months. Cardinal manifestations are fever (often high), pain (continuous, stabbing, or pleuritic, and sometimes severe), and an enlarged and tender liver. Patients may also experience malaise or prostration, sweating, chills, anorexia, and weight loss. The liver enlargement may present subcostally, in the epigastrium, as a localized bulging of the rib cage, or, as a result of enlargement against the dome of the diaphragm, it may produce coughing and findings at the right lung base (dullness to percussion, rales, and diminished breath sounds). Intercostal tenderness is common. Localizing signs on the skin may be an area of edema or a point of maximum tenderness. Without prompt treatment, the hepatic abscess may rupture into the pleural, peritoneal, or pericardial space or other contiguous organs, and death may follow.

b. Other extraintestinal infections–Skin infections may develop in the perianal area. Metastatic infection may rarely occur throughout the body, particularly the lungs, brain, and genitalia.

B. Laboratory Findings:

1. Intestinal amebiasis–Diagnosis of intestinal amebiasis is by finding the antigen or the organism in stool. Serologic testing by the indirect hemagglutination test, though useful, may not be definitive as the test lacks sensitivity in early infections and does not distinguish recent from past infection.

Antigen detection in stools. Finding antigen is more sensitive and specific than microscopy. Unlike morphology, which does not distinguish *E histolytica* from nonpathogenic *E dispar,* antigen detection does differentiate them from each other and from the other pathogenic and nonpathogenic intestinal protozoa. Therefore, where possible, testing of stools for amebic antigen by the commercially-available TechLab test should replace microscopy.

Microscopic examination of stools. Standard microscopy of stool specimens is insensitive and permits false-positive findings. Testing three specimens obtained under optimal conditions will generally detect only 80% of entamoeba complex infections; three additional tests will raise the diagnostic rate to about 90%. Trophozoites predominate in liquid stools, cysts in formed stools. A standard procedure is to collect three specimens at 2-day intervals or longer, with one of the three obtained after a laxative such as (1) sodium sulfate or phosphate (Fleet's Phospho-Soda), 30–60 g in a glass of water; or (2) bisacodyl 5–15 mL. Oil laxatives such as mineral oil should not be used. Specimens should be collected in a clean container. Because trophozoites rapidly autolyze, specimens should be examined within about 30 minutes or should immediately be mixed with a preservative. If the patient has received specific therapy, antibiotics, antimalarials, antidiarrheal preparations (containing bismuth, kaolin, or magnesium hydroxide), barium, or mineral oil, specimen collection should be delayed

On sigmoidoscopic examination, no findings are typical in mild intestinal disease; in severe disease, ulcers may be found that are 1 mm to 2 cm across, with intact intervening mucosa. If present, exudate should be collected with a glass pipette (not with cotton, to which trophozoites may adhere) or by scraping with a metal curette and examined immediately. The colon should not be cleansed before sigmoidoscopy, since this washes exudate from ulcers and destroys trophozoites. In some centers, rectal biopsy has enhanced diagnosis; the specimens are best examined by immunofluorescence methods.

Serology. The standard serologic test—the indirect hemagglutination test—detects *E histolytica* infections but remains negative in *E dispar* infections. Because the test remains positive for as long as 10 years after successful treatment, a positive test does not distinguish between past and new infections. In commensal colon infections with *E histolytica,* the test is rarely positive. With invasive disease, the test can become positive within a week; with mild colitis, seropositivity may be less than 50%, whereas in dysentery it reaches 85% levels. The agar gel test, though less sensitive, is rapidly conducted and may detect current infection because it becomes negative 3–6 months after eradication of the organism. Other tests for serum antibody include the ELISA and immunofluorescent tests.

Other tests. Many patients with amebic colitis test positive for occult blood, whereas findings for fecal leukocytes are noncontributory. Detection of trophozoites that contain ingested red blood cells is nearly diagnostic for invasive *E histolytica* but may be confused with the occasional *E dispar* or macrophage that also contains the red blood cells. The white blood cell count can reach 20,000/μL or higher in amebic dysentery but is not elevated in mild colitis. A low-grade eosinophilia is occasionally present.

For research purposes, the diagnosis can also be made by isolating the two entamoeba species in culture (this requires specialized techniques) and then differentiating them by isoenzyme analysis, typing with monoclonal antibodies to surface antigens, polymerase chain reaction, or DNA probes.

2. Hepatic abscess–Elevation of the right dome of the diaphragm and the size and location of the abscess can be determined by ultrasonography (usually round or oval nonhomogeneous lesions, abrupt transition from normal liver to the lesion, hypoechoic center with diffuse echoes throughout the abscess), CT (well-defined, round, low-density lesions with an internal, nonhomogeneous structure), MRI, and radioisotope scanning. After intravenous injection of contrast material, CT may show a hyperdense halo around the periphery of the abscess. Gallium scans, only infrequently useful, show a cold spot (sometimes with a bright rim) as opposed to the increased gallium uptake in the center of pyogenic abscesses. Serologic tests are almost always positive (except early in the infection); however, a positive test does not distinguish recent from past infection. Examination of stools for antigen and the organism is frequently negative. The white count ranges from 15,000 to 25,000/μL. Eosinophilia is not present. Liver function test abnormalities, when present, are usually minimal. Indications and risks of percutaneous aspiration of abscesses when used in diagnosis and treatment are described below. Antigen detection in aspirate appears to be very sensitive.

Differential Diagnosis

Amebiasis should be considered in patients with acute or chronic diarrhea (including cases associated with only mild changes in bowel habits; in patients who have an exposure history, including travel or household or sexual exposure); liver abscess; and annular lesions of the colon. All patients with presumed inflammatory bowel disease should be tested for antibodies, by multiple stool examinations for antigen and the organism, and by colonoscopy with biopsy because of the risk of overwhelming amebic disease if corticosteroid therapy were to be given in the presence of amebiasis. The differential diagnosis of amebic liver abscess includes pyogenic abscess, echinococcal cyst, benign cyst, and hepatocellular carcinoma.

Treatment

E dispar is the more common cause of asymptomatic amebic infection and should not be treated. The decision to treat is based on finding *E histolytica* antigen or parasites in stool or in liver abscess aspirates. Occasionally, a positive serologic titer to *E histolytica* (*E dispar* does not induce seropositivity) plus appropriate clinical findings will be highly suggestive of present rather than past infection. The choice of drug depends on the type of clinical presentation and the site of drug action. Treatment may require the concurrent or sequential use of several drugs. Table 35–1 outlines a preferred and an alternative method of treatment for each clinical type of amebiasis.

The **tissue amebicides** dehydroemetine and emetine act on organisms in the bowel wall and in other tissues but not on amebas in the bowel lumen. Chloroquine is active principally against amebas in the liver. The **luminal amebicides** diloxanide furoate (not available in the USA), iodoquinol, and paromomycin act on organisms in the bowel lumen but are ineffective against amebas in the bowel wall or other tissues. Oral tetracycline inhibits the bacterial associates of *E histolytica* and thus has an indirect effect on amebas in the bowel lumen and bowel wall but not in other tissues. Given parenterally, antibiotics have little antiamebic activity at any site. Metronidazole (or tinidazole, which is not available in the USA) is unique in that it is effective both in the bowel lumen and in the bowel wall and other tissues, including the central nervous system. However, metronidazole when used alone for bowel infections is not sufficient as a luminal amebicide, for it fails to cure up to 50% of infections.

A. Asymptomatic Intestinal Infection: Cure rates with a single course of diloxanide furoate or iodoquinol are 80–85%. Alternatives for treatment or re-treatment are paromomycin or metronidazole plus iodoquinol or diloxanide furoate. Within endemic areas, asymptomatic carriers generally are not treated because of the frequency of reinfection.

B. Mild to Moderate Intestinal Infection: Metronidazole plus a luminal amebicide is the treatment of choice. Alternative treatments are set forth in Table 35–1. The minimum dose of chloroquine needed to destroy trophozoites carried to the liver or to eradicate an undetected early-stage liver abscess is not established.

C. Severe Intestinal Infection: Fluid and electrolyte therapy and opiates to control bowel motility are necessary adjuncts to specific therapy. Though opiates relieve symptoms, they should be used cautiously because of the potential risk of toxic megacolon.

D. Hepatic Abscess: Hospitalization and bed rest are necessary. Opinions differ on whether a course of chloroquine should follow metronidazole to avoid rare long-term failures. Regarding rare short-term metronidazole failures, if during the course of metronidazole treatment a satisfactory clinical response does not occur in about 3 days, the abscess should be drained for therapeutic purposes and to evaluate for pyogenic abscess. Continued failure to achieve an adequate clinical response of a suspected amebic abscess requires changing to the potentially toxic alternative drug dehydroemetine (or emetine) plus chloroquine. Treatment also requires a luminal amebicide (diloxanide furoate or iodoquinol), whether or not the organism is found in the stool. Antibiotics are added only when there is concomitant bacterial liver abscess, which is rare. However, metronidazole itself is highly effective against anaerobic bacteria, a major cause of bacterial liver abscesses. After successful treatment, imaging defects in the liver disappear slowly (range: 3–13 months); some calcify.

Most patients treated with metronidazole for an amebic liver abscess do not require percutaneous aspiration for diagnostic or therapeutic purposes. The indications for aspiration are (1) a large abscess, threatening rupture; (2) a left lobe abscess, which is associated with a higher rate of severe complications; (3) lack of medical response after about 3 days of metronidazole; and (4) a need to evaluate for pyogenic abscess. The risks of aspiration are bacterial superinfection, bleeding, peritoneal spillage, and inadvertent puncture of an infected hydatid cyst. The aspirate is divided into serial 30- to 50-mL aliquots, but only the last sample is examined, as organisms are found only at the edge of the abscess.

E. Adverse Drug Reactions: Metronidazole often induces transient nausea, vomiting, headache, or a metallic taste in the mouth; if alcohol is taken during or shortly after treatment, a disulfiram-like reaction may occur. See manufacturer's recommendations regarding drug interactions with some commonly used drugs (cimetidine, some anticoagulants, phenytoin, phenobarbital, lithium). Metronidazole increases the rate of naturally occurring tumors in mice but not in nonrodent species. Although some authorities consider the drug to be essentially free of cancer risk in humans, prudence requires that metronidazole be given to pregnant or nursing mothers only if other drugs cannot be used.

Dehydroemetine and emetine cause nausea, vomiting, and pain at the injection site. They are general protoplasmic poisons that have adverse effects on many tissues (particularly the heart) and a narrow range between therapeutic and toxic effects; dehydroemetine may be the safer of the two drugs. The tetracyclines should not be used for pregnant women; use erythromycin stearate or paromomycin instead. Paromomycin may cause mild gastrointestinal symptoms, infrequently intense diarrhea, and rarely overgrowth of nonsusceptible organisms. Paromomycin

Table 35–1. Treatment of amebiasis.

	Drug(s) of Choice	Alternative Drug(s)
Asymptomatic intestinal infection	Diloxanide furoate[1,2]	Iodoquinol (diiodohydroxyquin)[3] or paromomycin[4]
Mild to moderate intestinal infection (nondysenteric colitis)	(1) Metronidazole[5] or tinidazole[1,5] **plus** (2) Diloxanide furoate,[1,2] iodoquinol,[3] or paromomycin[4]	(1) Diloxanide furoate[2] or iodoquinol[3] **plus** (2) A tetracycline[6] **followed by** (3) Chloroquine[7] **or** (1) Paromomycin[4] **followed by** (2) Chloroquine[7]
Severe intestinal infection (dysentery)	(1) Metronidazole[5] or tinidazole[1,5] **plus** (2) Diloxanide furoate[1,2] or iodoquinol[3] **or, if parenteral therapy is needed initially:** (1) Intravenous metronidazole[8] until oral therapy can be started; (2) Then give oral metronidazole[5] plus diloxanide furoate[1,2] or iodoquinol[3]	(1) A tetracycline[6] **plus** (2) Diloxanide furoate[1,2] or iodoquinol[3] **followed by** (3) Chloroquine[9] **or, if parenteral therapy is needed initially:** (1) Dehydroemetine[10] or emetine[1,10] **followed by** (2) A tetracycline[6] plus diloxanide furoate[1,2] or iodoquinol[3] **followed by** (3) Chloroquine[9]
Hepatic abscess	(1) Metronidazole[5,8] or tinidazole[1,5] **plus** (2) Diloxanide furoate[1,2] or iodoquinol[3] **followed by** (3) Chloroquine[9]	(1) Dehydroemetine[10] or emetine[1,11] **followed by** (2) Chloroquine[12] **plus** (3) Diloxanide furoate[1,2] or iodoquinol[3]
Ameboma or extraintestinal infection	As for hepatic abscess, but not including chloroquine	As for hepatic abscess, but not including chloroquine

[1]Not available in the USA.
[2]Diloxanide furoate, 500 mg three times daily with meals for 10 days.
[3]Iodoquinol (diiodohydroxyquin), 650 mg three times daily for 21 days.
[4]Paromomycin, 25–30 mg/kg (base) (maximum 3 g) in three divided doses after meals daily for 7 days.
[5]Metronidazole, 750 mg three times daily for 10 days. In countries where it is available (not in the USA), tinidazole is preferred over metronidazole as the nitroimidazole component in treatment; although the two drugs are equally effective, tinidazole is given in a shorter course of treatment and is better tolerated. The tinidazole dosage is 800 mg three times daily for 3 days; in severe intestinal disease and hepatic abscess, continue for 5 days.
[6]Tetracycline, 250 mg four times daily for 10 days; in severe dysentery, give 500 mg four times daily for the first 5 days, then 250 mg four times daily for 5 days. Tetracycline should not be used during pregnancy.
[7]Chloroquine, 500 mg (salt) daily for 7 days.
[8]An intravenous metronidazole formulation is available; change to oral medication as soon as possible. See manufacturer's recommendation for dosage and cautions.
[9]Chloroquine, 500 mg (salt) daily for 14 days.
[10]Dehydroemetine or emetine, 1 mg/kg subcutaneously (preferred) or intramuscularly daily for the least number of days necessary to control severe symptoms (usually 3–5 days) (maximum daily dose for dehydroemetine is 90 mg; for emetine, 65 mg).
[11]Use dosage recommended in footnote 11 for 8–10 days.
[12]Chloroquine, 500 mg (salt) orally twice daily for 2 days and then 500 mg orally daily for 19 days.

should be used with caution in patients with ulcerative bowel conditions and should not be used in the presence of significant renal disease. Iodoquinol may cause mild, transient diarrhea. It should be taken with meals; used with caution in patients with optic neuropathy, renal, or thyroid disease; and discontinued in the event of iodine toxicity (dermatitis, fever). The neurotoxicity seen with extended treatment does not occur at the standard 3-week dosage. Diloxanide usage commonly results in flatulence.

Follow-Up Care

In follow-up, examine at least three stools at 2- to 3-day intervals, starting 2–4 weeks after the end of treatment. For some patients, colonoscopy and reexamination of stools within 3 months may be indicated.

Postdysenteric colitis is an uncommon sequela of severe amebic colitis. Following adequate treatment, diarrhea continues and the mucosa may be reddened and edematous, but no ulcers or organisms are found. Most such cases are self-limited, with permanent remission in weeks to months. Uncommonly, the diarrhea may be profound and unremitting and in some instances probably represents ulcerative colitis triggered by the amebic infection.

Prevention & Control

Prevention requires safe water supplies, sanitary disposal of human feces, adequate cooking of foods, protection of foods from fly contamination, washing hands after defecation and before preparing or eating foods, and, in endemic areas, avoidance of foods that cannot be cooked or peeled. Water supplies can be boiled (briefly) or treated with iodine (0.5 mL tincture of iodine per liter for 20 minutes, or longer if the water is cold). Filters are also available to purify drinking water. Disinfection dips for fruits and vegetables are not advised, and no drug is safe or effective in prophylaxis.

Prognosis

The mortality rate from untreated amebic dysentery, hepatic abscess, or ameboma may be high. With chemotherapy instituted early in the course of the disease, the prognosis is good.

Anand AC et al: Amoebiasis revisited: pathogenesis, diagnosis and management. Trop Gastroenterol 1999;20:2. [NLM Cit ID: 99393695]

Clark CG: Amoebic disease. *Entamoeba dispar,* an organism reborn. Trans R Soc Trop Med Hyg 1998;92:361. [NLM Cit ID: 99067368]

Freeman CD et al: Metronidazole: a therapeutic review and update. Drugs 1997;54:679. [NLM Cit ID: 98024358]

Haque R et al: Comparison of PCR, isoenzyme analysis, and antigen detection for diagnosis of *Entamoeba histolytica* infection. J Clin Microbiology 1998;36:449. [NLM Cit ID: 98126232] (Comparison of a convenient stool ELISA test with research tests to distinguish *E histolytica* from *E dispar.*)

Leber AL: Intestinal amebae. Clin Lab Med 1999;19:601. [NLM Cit ID: 20017194] (Epidemiology, control, and laboratory diagnosis of *E histolytica* and *B hominis* infection.)

Petri WA et al: Diagnosis and management of amebiasis. Clin Infect Dis 1999;29:1117. [NLM Cit ID: 99454644]

INFECTIONS WITH PATHOGENIC FREE-LIVING AMEBAS

Primary Amebic Meningoencephalitis

Primary amebic meningoencephalitis is a fulminating, hemorrhagic, necrotizing meningoencephalitis with a limited purulent exudate. It occurs in healthy children and young adults and is rapidly fatal. It is caused by free-living amebas, most commonly by the ameboflagellate *Naegleria fowleri.* Other causes are *Balamuthia mandrillaris* and the acanthamoeba species (see below), both of which may have a predilection for immunocompromised patients, including those with AIDS.

N fowleri is a thermophilic organism found in fresh and polluted warm lake water, domestic water supplies, swimming pools, thermal water, and sewers. Most patients give a history of exposure to fresh water; dust is also a possible source of infection. Nasal and throat swabs have shown a human carrier state, and serologic surveys suggest that inapparent infections occur.

The organism apparently invades the central nervous system through the cribriform plate. The incubation period varies from 2 to 15 days. Early symptoms include headache, fever, and lethargy, often associated with rhinitis and pharyngitis. Vomiting, disorientation, and other signs of meningoencephalitis develop within 1 or 2 days, followed by coma and then death on the fifth or sixth day. No distinctive clinical features distinguish the infection from acute bacterial meningoencephalitis. At autopsy, some victims have a nonspecific myocarditis.

Lumbar or ventricular cerebrospinal fluid contains several hundred to 25,000 leukocytes/μL (50–100% neutrophils) and erythrocytes (up to several thousand/μL). Protein is usually somewhat elevated, and glucose is normal or moderately reduced. If conventional examinations for bacteria and fungi are negative, the fluid must then be examined for free-living amebas to make the specific diagnosis. A wet mount examined by an ordinary optical microscope with the aperture restricted or condenser down will enhance contrast and refractility; a warm stage is not needed. The fluid should not be centrifuged or refrigerated, as this tends to immobilize the amebas (7–14 μm). Their brisk motility distinguishes them from leukocytes of various types, which they closely resemble. Staining, culture, and mouse inoculation should be performed. Serologic testing is only useful for surveys; patients die before antibodies are detectable.

Precise species identification is based on morphology, demonstration of flagellate transformation (naegleria only), and various immunologic methods.

Only four well-documented survivors of *N fowleri* infection have been reported. One was treated with intravenous and intrathecal amphotericin B and another with a combination of amphotericin B, miconazole, and oral rifampin. Experimental studies have shown a marked synergistic effect between amphotericin B and either tetracycline or rifampin. No treatment is available for *B mandrillaris* infection.

Acanthamoeba Infections

Free-living amebas of the genus acanthamoeba are found in soil and in fresh, brackish, and thermal water as trophozoites (15–45 μm) or cysts (10–25 μm). Several species are recognized as human pathogens that cause a number of poorly defined syndromes: (1) a subacute and chronic multifocal granulomatous necrotizing encephalitis that invariably has led to death in weeks to months, (2) skin lesions that resemble deep fungal infections, (3) granulomatous dissemination to many tissues, and (4) uveitis or chronic keratitis that may lead to blindness. Portals of entry may include the skin, eyes, or respiratory tract. A commensal nasal carrier state is established.

In the encephalitis syndrome, the clinical course is protracted (averaging 1 month), showing mental status abnormalities, stiff neck, and features of a space occupying lesion. Focal consolidation may be seen on chest films. Cerebrospinal fluid lymphocytosis has been described. Antemortem diagnosis has been made via biopsy specimens. Specific identification is based on morphology and immunologic methods. No treatment has been effective, but ketoconazole, miconazole, itraconazole, sulfonamides, clotrimazole, pentamidine, paromomycin, propamidine, neomycin, amphotericin B, or flucytosine can be tried.

Hundreds of cases of acanthamoeba keratitis have been documented, most associated with wearing contact lenses; some infections are due to penetrating corneal trauma or exposure to contaminated water. The clinical features suggestive of acanthamoeba keratitis are (1) a waxing and waning clinical course over several months with severe ocular pain, photophobia, tearing, blurred vision, and conjunctival injection; (2) partial or 360-degree paracentral stromal ring infiltrate on ophthalmologic examination; (3) recurrent corneal epithelial breakdown; and (4) a corneal lesion refractory to the usual medications. Typically, the keratitis progresses slowly over months. The diagnosis can be confirmed by vigorously scraping the cornea with a swab or platinum-tipped scapula. The material is microscopically examined (1) as a wet preparation for cysts and motile trophozoites, (2) after staining, (3) by use of immunofluorescent techniques, and (4) after being cultured on nonnutrient agar seeded with *E coli.* Isolates can be identified by isoenzyme analysis and DNA profiles and tested for drug sensitivity.

A large proportion of patients can expect a good visual result and cure with treatment that follows early medical diagnosis. Topical chlorhexidine digluconate 0.02% with propamidine isethionate (0.1%) is more effective than polyhexamethylene biguanide plus propamidine. Topical miconazole has also been used. Oral itraconazole or ketoconazole can be added for deep keratitis. Use of corticosteroid therapy is controversial. In spite of medical treatment, penetrating keratoplasty is often necessary to excise diseased tissue; corneal grafting can be done after the amebic infection has been eradicated.

Prevention requires immersion of contact lenses in disinfectant solutions or by heat sterilization. The lens should not be cleaned in homemade saline solutions nor be worn while swimming.

Duguid IG et al: Outcome of acanthamoeba keratitis treated with polyhexamethyl biguanide and propamidine. Ophthalmology 1997;104:1587. [NLM Cit ID: 97470735]

Huang ZH et al: Serum antibodies to *Balamuthia mandrillaris,* a free-living amoeba recently demonstrated to cause granulomatous amoebic encephalitis. J Infect Dis 1999;179:1305. [NLM Cit ID: 99208721] (Diagnosis and clinical presentation.)

Illingworth CD et al: *Acanthamoeba* keratitis. Surv Ophthalmol 1998;42:493. [NLM Cit ID: 98297823]

Kidney DD et al: CNS infections with free-living amebas: neuroimaging findings. AJR Am J Roentgenol 1998; 171:809. [NLM Cit ID: 98391137]

Martinez AJ et al: Free-living, amphizoic and opportunistic amebas. Brain Pathol 1997;7:583. [NLM Cit ID: 97187114]

Sell JJ et al: Granulomatous amebic encephalitis caused by acanthamoeba. Neuroradiology 1997;39:434. [NLM Cit ID: 97368711]

Szénási Z et al: Isolation, identification and increasing importance of "free-living" amoeba causing human disease. J Med Microbiol 1998;47:5. [NLM Cit ID: 98111598]

BABESIOSIS (Piroplasmosis)

Babesiae are tick-borne protozoal parasites of wild and domestic animals worldwide. Babesiosis in humans is a rare intraerythrocytic infection caused by two babesia species. Heretofore, the infection has been recognized only in Europe *(Babesia divergens)* (rare) and North America *(Babesia microti).* Serosurveys and limited confirmations of isolates suggest that the infection occurs in other parts of the world including Taiwan, China, Egypt, South Africa, and Mexico. In the USA, several hundred *B microti* infections have been reported from coastal and island areas of northeastern and mid-Atlantic states as well as from Wisconsin, Minnesota, Missouri, Washington, and California. A new *Babesia* species (WA1) has been described in humans in California (serosurvey prevalence in rural areas was 3–20%), Washington, and Georgia. Natural hosts for *B microti* are various wild and domestic animals, particularly the white-footed mouse and white-tailed deer. With extension of the deer's habitat, the range of human infection appears to be increasing as well.

Humans are infected as a result of *Ixodes scapularis* tick bites (mainly nymphal) but also by blood transfusion and perinatally. Coinfections with Lyme disease occur and probably also with ehrlichiosis. Without passing through an exoerythrocytic stage, *B microti* enters the red blood cell and multiplies, resulting in cell rupture followed by infection of other cells.

Surveys have shown an antibody prevalence of up to 2% in humans, which indicates a high level of subclinical infections. The incubation period is 1 week to several months, but patients usually do not recall the tick bite. The illness is characterized by irregular fever, chills, headache, diaphoresis, myalgia, and fatigue but is without malaria-like periodicity of symptoms. Other symptoms may occur including nausea, vomiting, jaundice, arthralgia, and emotional lability. Most patients have a moderate hemolytic anemia, and some have hemoglobinuria, hepatosplenomegaly, or thrombocytopenia. Although parasitemia may continue for months, with or without symptoms, the disease is self-limited and, after several weeks or months, most patients recover without sequelae. Splenectomized, elderly, or immunosuppressed persons are the most likely to have severe manifestations.

About 25 *B divergens* infections have been reported, all in splenectomized patients. These infections progress rapidly with high fever, severe hemolytic anemia, jaundice, hemoglobinuria, and renal failure; death usually follows.

Diagnosis is by identification of the intraerythrocytic parasite (2–3 μm) on Wright- or Giemsa-stained thick or thin blood smears; no gametocytes and no intracellular pigment are seen. A single red cell may contain different stages of the parasite, and parasitemia can exceed 10%. Repeated smears may be necessary; parasitemia is usually evident in 2–4 weeks. The organism must be differentiated from malarial parasites, particularly *Plasmodium falciparum.* Isolation can be attempted by inoculating patient blood into hamsters or gerbils. Antibody is detectable within 1–4 weeks after onset of symptoms and persists for 6–12 months. Testing with specific antigens in the immunofluorescent test is relatively species-specific; antibody titers against plasmodium are generally low or absent. Detection of specific IgM antibody confirms the diagnosis. The polymerase chain reaction method, where available, is more sensitive for low parasitemias but of equal specificity. The leukocyte count and the serum alkaline phosphatase concentration may be elevated.

No drug treatment is satisfactory. Since *B microti* infections in patients with an intact spleen are usually self-limiting, a common approach has been to treat most infections symptomatically. However, preliminary data suggests that even mildly ill patients may benefit from the standard 7-day course of treatment: quinine (650 mg three times a day) plus clindamycin (1.2 g twice daily intravenously or 650 mg three times a day). Exchange transfusion has been successful in several ill patients with parasitemia greater than 10%. New reports suggest effectiveness for azithromycin (500 mg twice daily for 3 days followed by 500 mg daily for 7 days) plus either atovaquone suspension (750 mg twice daily for 7–10 days) or quinine (see above). Management of *B divergens* infection can be attempted with exchange transfusion and clindamycin-quinine therapy.

Denes E et al: Management of *Babesia divergens* babesiosis without a complete course of quinine treatment. Eur J Clin Microbiol Infect Dis 1999;18:672. [NLM Cit ID: 20001761]

Dobroszycki J et al: A cluster of transfusion-associated babesiosis cases traced to a single asymptomatic donor. JAMA 1999;281:927. [NLM Cit ID: 99176376]

Gelfand JA et al: Babesiosis. Curr Top Infect Dis 1998;18:201. [NLM Cit ID: 98452392]

White DJ et al: Human babesiosis in New York State: Review of 139 hospitalized cases and analysis of prognostic factors. Arch Intern Med 1998;158:2149. [NLM Cit ID: 99015802]

BALANTIDIASIS

Balantidium coli is a large ciliated intestinal protozoan found worldwide, but particularly in the tropics. Pigs are considered the reservoir host, but the agent has been found in other animals and in insects. The disease is rare in humans, occurring as an acute infection (sporadic or in outbreaks) or as a chronic infection. Infection results from ingestion of cysts passed in stools of humans or swine. In the new host, the cyst wall dissolves and the trophozoite may invade the mucosa and submucosa of the terminal ileum, appendix, and large bowel, causing abscesses and irregularly rounded ulcerations. Many infections are asymptomatic and probably need not be treated. Chronic recurrent diarrhea, alternating with constipation, is most common, but mild to moderate diarrhea to severe dysentery with bloody mucoid stools, tenesmus, and colic may occur. Rare instances of infection in the lung, liver, and vagina have been reported.

Diagnosis is established by finding trophozoites in liquid stools, cysts in formed stools, or the trophozoite in scrapings or biopsy of ulcers of the large bowel. Specimens must be examined rapidly or placed in preservative.

The treatment of choice is tetracycline hydrochloride, 500 mg four times daily for 10 days. The alternative drug is iodoquinol (diiodohydroxyquin), 650 mg three times daily for 21 days. Occasional success has also been reported with metronidazole (750 mg three times daily for 5 days) or paromomycin (25–30 mg/kg [base] in three divided doses for 5–10 days).

In properly treated mild to moderate symptomatic cases, the prognosis is good, but in spite of treatment, fatalities have occurred in severe infections as a result of intestinal perforation or hemorrhage.

Esteban JH et al: Balantidiasis in Aymara children from the Northern Bolivian Altiplano. Am J Trop Med Hyg 1998; 59:922. [NLM Cit ID: 99101292]

Garcia LS: Flagellates and ciliates. Clin Lab Med 1999; 19:621. [NLM Cit ID: 20017195] (Review of *Giardia lamblia* and *Balantidium coli.*)

COCCIDIAL & MICROSPORIDIAL INFECTIONS: CRYPTOSPORIDIOSIS, ISOSPORIASIS, CYCLOSPORIASIS, & SARCOCYSTOSIS

Coccidiosis and microsporidiosis are intracellular infections of intestinal epithelial cells by spore-forming protozoa. Various species are the etiologic agents for microsporidiosis (see below). The causes of coccidiosis are *Cryptosporidium parvum, Isospora belli, Cyclospora cayetanensis,* and *Sarcocystis bovihominis* and *S suihominis;* all but the sarcocystis species complete their life cycle in a single host. Although once considered rare, many of these infections are now known to occur commonly worldwide, but particularly in the tropics and in regions where hygiene is poor. They are causes of traveler's diarrhea; endemic childhood gastroenteritis (particularly in malnourished children in developing countries); institutional and community outbreaks of diarrhea; and acute and chronic diarrhea in immunosuppressed patients, including those with AIDS, in whom infection can be life-threatening. Clustering occurs in households, day care centers, and among sexual partners. Diarrhea in non-AIDS patients—sporadic, epidemic, and traveler's—is more likely to be due to crypotosporidia and less often to cyclospora or microsporidia. Diarrhea in AIDS is more commonly due to the microsporidia, *Enterocytozoon bieneusi,* and *Encephalitozoon* (formerly *Septata*) *intestinalis,* but cryptosporidium, isospora, and cyclospora are also important causes.

The infectious agents are oocysts (spores) transmitted directly from person to person or by contaminated water or food. Ingested oocysts release sporozoites that invade and multiply in enterocytes, primarily in the small bowel. Liberated merozoites reinvade other cells in the process of asexual intracellular multiplication. Eventually, sexual stages are released; following fertilization, immature oocysts form which are then shed in feces. The oocysts mature on exposure to air and can remain viable in a moist environment for months to years.

The isospora and cyclospora species found in humans appear to be distinct to humans only. Cryptosporidiosis is a zoonosis in which infections in farm animals (cattle, goats, turkeys, and others) can be transmitted to humans; however, most human infections seem to be acquired from humans.

Although the small bowel is the usual location of infection, other sites can be involved. Colon infection is common in cryptosporidiasis and has been reported with microsporidiosis. Biliary tract infection, which occurs in cryptosporidiosis, microsporidiosis and isosporiasis, may result in either a sclerosing, cholangitis-like syndrome or an acalculous cholecystitis. Disseminated disease and corneal infections occur with several microsporidial species.

The pathogenesis of these diarrheas is not well understood. No enterotoxin has been identified. Voluminous secretory or malabsorption diarrhea (including vitamin B_{12}, D-xylose, and fat absorption dysfunction) can result. Although histologic examination of the small bowel can be normal, with intense infection there may be dense inflammatory infiltration accompanied by blunting to atrophy of the villi and crypt hyperplasia. The infections are nonulcerative and noninvasive except for *E intestinalis,* which can be invasive.

Clinical Findings

A. Symptoms and Signs: Generally, the forms of diarrhea caused by the coccidial and microsporidial agents are clinically indistinguishable from each other.

1. In immunocompetent persons, infection varies from no symptoms, to a mild diarrhea with flatulence and bloating, to severe and frequent watery diarrhea in which the onset may be explosive. Mucus may be present in stools, but no microscopic or gross blood. Other findings may include low-grade fever, malaise, anorexia, abdominal cramps, vomiting, and myalgia. These symptoms are generally self-limited, lasting a few days to several weeks (sometimes longer for isosporiasis). Weight loss can be marked. Parasitologic clearance, however, may take several months.

2. In immunologically deficient patients, the diarrhea can be profuse (up to 15 L daily has been reported), with cholera-like watery movements, accompanied by severe malabsorption, electrolyte imbalance, and marked weight loss; fever is uncommon. Mucus is seen in the stools, but blood and leukocytes are seldom present. The diarrhea may recur or persist, and passage of organisms continues for months to indefinitely.

B. Laboratory Findings: In diagnosis, three stool specimens should be obtained fresh and in preservative over 5–7 days and processed by a variety of flotation or concentration methods to detect the distinctive oocysts (differences are based on size and intracellular location). A modified acid-fast stain is used to stain for cryptosporidia, cyclospora, and isospora; in microsporidiosis, a modified trichrome or Weber stain is used. The four organisms can also be detected by duodenal aspiration or biopsy and seen by light microscopy. When examining stool specimens, some laboratories need to be notified in advance of concern for these infections to ensure that appropriate specialized techniques will be used.

Specific Diseases

A. Cryptosporidiosis: The organism is highly infectious (relatively few parasites can induce infection) and readily transmitted in health and day care settings and in households. The incubation period appears to be 5–21 days. Oocysts passed in stools are fully sporulated and infectious; therefore, hospitalized patients should be isolated and stool precautions strictly observed. The prevalence of asymptomatic human carriers in the USA is estimated to be about 1.5%. Outbreaks are of particular concern, as exemplified by the 1993 epidemic in Milwaukee in which 400,000 persons became ill. Since chlorine disinfection of water is not effective, adequate filtration is required. However, because of the oocysts' small size (2–5 μm), filtration is difficult and unreliable (the < 1 μm filters required frequently become clogged or fail).

In AIDS, infection may involve any part of the gastrointestinal tract, including the biliary tract (sclerosing cholangitis has been described); respiratory tract infection, hepatitis, pancreatitis, lymphadenopathy, and hepatosplenomegaly may occur, as well as multisystem involvement.

In diagnosis, fluorescent microscopy using auramine staining or a monoclonal antibody increases sensitivity and may be as specific as acid-fast staining. Commercially available ELISA tests that detect cryptosporidial antigen in feces appear to have high sensitivity and specificity and provide for ease of use. Stools rarely show white or red blood cells. Blood leukocytosis and eosinophilia are uncommon. Serodiagnostic tests have been developed, including ELISA and immunofluorescent tests that detect IgG and IgM antibody, but they are not yet useful in diagnosing acute disease. Radiologic changes have been reported in the stomach, intestines, and bile ducts in severe disease. In AIDS patients with unexplained diarrhea, the organism should also be looked for in sputum and bronchoalveolar lavage fluid; specimens obtained from lung tissue have sometimes been positive in patients with negative stool specimens.

B. Isosporiasis: *I belli* oocysts in feces are 20–30 × 10–20 μm. Opinion differs about whether the oocyst can be transmitted directly from person to person by anal-oral sexual contact or if it must pass into the environment and mature to its infectious stage. Outbreaks have occurred in day care centers and mental institutions. The incubation period is 7–11 days. A hemorrhagic ulcerative colitis has been described.

Diagnosis by stool examination is often difficult, for the organisms may be scanty even in the presence of significant symptoms. Because of their buoyancy, oocysts must be looked for just beneath the coverslip of the preparation. Frequently, diagnosis can be made only after duodenal biopsy and search of multiple serial sections. Serologic tests are not available.

C. Cyclosporiasis: *C cayetanensis* oocysts (8–10 μm) must undergo a period of sporulation in the environment before they become infectious. The incubation period appears to be 2–11 days. Transmission is presumed to be fecal-oral; the host range is unknown. The infection has been reported in many parts of the world, in travelers, and as the cause of water and food-borne outbreaks; raspberries and other foods have been implicated in outbreaks. Oocysts can be identified in stool by examination of wet mounts under phase microscopy, by use of modified acid-fast stains (oocysts are variably acid-fast), microwave-heated safranine staining, or by autofluorescence with ultraviolet epifluorescence microscopy. Antibodies have been detected, and titers increase during convalescence.

D. Sarcocystosis: Sarcocystis is a two-host coccidian. Human disease occurs as two syndromes, both rare: (1) an enteric infection in which humans are the definitive host and (2) a muscle infection in which humans are an intermediate host. In the enteric form, sporocysts passed in human feces are not infective for humans but must be ingested by cattle or pigs. Humans become infected by eating poorly cooked beef or pork containing oocysts of *Sarcocystis bovihominis* or *Sarcocystis suihominis,* respectively. Organisms enter intestinal epithelial cells and are transformed into oocysts that release sporocysts into the feces. Clinically, the intestinal infection is often asymptomatic or causes mild but protracted diarrhea; an eosinophilic necrotizing enteritis has been reported. Diagnosis is by stool examination using a flotation method.

The muscle form of sarcocystosis results when humans ingest sporocysts in feces from an infected carnivore that has eaten prey which harbored sarcocysts. The sporocysts liberate sporozoites that invade the intestinal wall and are disseminated to skeletal muscle. This results in subcutaneous and muscular inflammation lasting several days to 2 weeks and the finding of swellings at these sites, sometimes associated with local erythema, tenderness and myalgia, fever, and eosinophilia. Sarcocysts are often asymptomatic, however, such as those found incidentally at autopsy in cardiac muscle.

E. Microsporidiosis: Microsporidia are obligate intracellular protozoans that are pathogens of arthropods, fish, and vertebrates. In humans, the infections are seen mainly in immunoincompetent persons, particular those with AIDS. In chronic wasting AIDS diarrhea, the two most common intestinal parasites (up to 50% of diarrheal cases) are *Enterocytozoon bieneusi* and *Encephalitozoon intestinalis*. These parasites can also cause biliary infection (cholangitis, cholecystitis). In immunocompetent persons, the diarrhea due to these parasites (including traveler's diarrhea) is self-limited. *E intestinalis, E cuniculi, E helleum,* and *Nosema connori* can disseminate to many tissues, including the sinuses, lungs, liver, urinary tract, and brain. In *E cuniculi* infection, magnetic resonance imaging has shown contrast-enhancing brain lesions. Most of the above parasites and others can cause keratoconjunctivitis. Pleistophora species and *Trachipleistophora hominis* cause a myositis associated with high elevations of creatine phosphokinase, lactate dehydrogenase, and myoglobin. Thus, microsporidia should be considered in infections in immunoincompetent persons in whom no other infectious agent can be found.

Microsporidia are detected in feces, body fluids, and tissue biopsies (intestinal epithelium, cornea, conjunctiva, bronchi, and others) by light microscopy using various staining methods, particularly trichrome and Weber's chromatrope-based stains, followed by confirmatory fluorescence staining.

Treatment

Most acute infections in immunocompetent persons are self-limited and do not require treatment. Supportive treatment for severe or chronic diarrhea includes fluid and electrolyte replacement and, in chronic cases, parenteral nutrition.

In **isosporiasis,** effective treatment has been described using (1) trimethoprim (160 mg) and sulfamethoxazole (800 mg) (TMP-SMZ) four times daily for 10 days and then twice daily for 3 weeks; or (2) sulfadiazine, 4 g, and pyrimethamine, 35–75 mg, in four divided doses daily, plus leucovorin calcium, 10–25 mg daily, for 3–7 weeks. In immunocompromised patients, it may be necessary to continue a maintenance dose indefinitely with TMP-SMZ three times weekly or Fansidar once weekly. Efficacy in primary infection has also been reported for furazolidone (400 mg/d for 10 days), roxithromycin, nitrofurantoin, metronidazole, quinacrine, pyrimethamine, albendazole with ornidazole, and diclazuril.

In the treatment of **cyclosporiasis,** TMP (160 mg)-SMZ (800 mg) twice daily for 7 days is effective; in HIV infections, higher doses (four times daily for 10 days) and long-term maintenance (three times weekly) are needed. In **microsporidiosis,** the encephalitozoon species often respond to albendazole (400 mg two or three times daily for several weeks up to 3 months). In *E bieneusi* infection and in the various causes of disseminated disease, albendazole can be tried; although it has not had good success, amelioration may result. For ocular lesions, some infections have responded to oral albendazole plus fumagillin eyedrops.

No treatment has been successful for **sarcocystosis** or **cryptosporidiosis.** In cryptosporidiosis, the following have been useful in isolated cases: roxithromycin (300 mg twice daily for 4 weeks), spiramycin (1 g three times daily for 2 weeks or longer), paromomycin (25–35 mg/kg/d in three or four divided doses; duration uncertain), zidovudine (AZT), azithromycin, octreotide, eflornithine, letrazuril, and hyperimmune bovine colostrum.

Prevention

Measures to reduce exposure to these organisms are recommended for immunocompromised patients. These include reduced exposure to swimming in fresh water and boiling of drinking water (1 minute) or use of a filter that removes particles over 1 μm in size.

Ackers JP: Gut coccidia—*Isospora, Cryptosporidium, Cyclospora* and *Sarcocystis*. Semin Gastrointest Dis 1997;8:33. [NLM Cit ID: 97153210]

Clark DP: New insights into human cryptosporidiosis. Clin Microbiol Rev 1999;12:554. [NLM Cit ID: 99445442]

Connor BA et al: Cyclosporiasis: clinical and histopathologic correlates. Clin Infect Dis 1999;28:1216. [NLM Cit ID: 99378365]

Croft SL et al: Intestinal microsporidiosis. Semin Gastrointest Dis 1997;8:45. [NLM Cit ID: 97153211]

Dascomb K et al: Natural history of intestinal microsporidiosis among patients infected with human immunodeficiency virus. J Clin Microbiol 1999;37:3421. [NLM Cit ID: 99419187]

Didier ES: Microsporidiosis. Clin Infect Dis 1998;27:1. [NLM Cit ID: 98340042]

Fayer R: *Cryptosporidium and Cryptosporidiosis.* CRC Press, 1997.

Franzen C et al: Cryptosporidia and microsporidia–waterborne diseases in the immunocompromised host. Diagn Microbiol Infect Dis 1999;34:245. [NLM Cit ID: 99331536]

Soave R et al: Cyclospora. Infect Dis Clin North Am 1998;12:1. [NLM Cit ID: 98155929]

GIARDIASIS

Essentials of Diagnosis

- Most infections are asymptomatic.
- In some cases, acute or chronic diarrhea, mild to severe, with bulky, greasy, frothy, malodorous stools, free of blood and pus.
- Upper abdominal discomfort, cramps, distention, excessive flatus, and lassitude.
- Cysts and occasionally trophozoites in stools.
- Trophozoites in duodenal fluid.

General Considerations

Giardiasis is a protozoal infection of the upper small intestine caused by the flagellate *Giardia lam-*

blia (also called *G intestinalis* and *G duodenalis*). The parasite occurs worldwide, most abundantly in areas with poor sanitation. In the USA and Europe, the infection is considered the most common intestinal protozoal pathogen. Persons of all ages are affected, but occurrence is particularly high among children. In children in developing countries, prevalence rates can reach 20% and higher.

The organism occurs in feces as a symmetric, heart-shaped flagellated trophozoite measuring 10–25 × 6–12 μm and as a cyst measuring 11–14 × 7–10 μm. Only the cyst form is infectious by the oral route; trophozoites are destroyed by gastric acidity. Humans are a reservoir for the infection; animals, including dogs, cats, beavers, and other mammals have been implicated but not confirmed as reservoirs or zoonotic sources of infection. Under suitable moist, cool conditions, cysts can survive in the environment for weeks to months.

Cysts are transmitted as a result of fecal contamination of water or food, by person-to-person contact, or by anal-oral sexual contact. Multiple cases are common in households, children's day care centers (often the nidus for spread of organisms to the community), and mental institutions. Outbreaks occur as a result of contamination of water supplies. Giardiasis is a well-recognized problem in special groups including travelers abroad, campers who drink water from USA streams, male homosexuals, and persons with impaired immune states. Giardiasis has not been, however, an opportunistic infection in AIDS.

After the cysts are ingested, trophozoites emerge in the duodenum and jejunum. They can cause epithelial damage, atrophy of villi, hypertrophic crypts, and extensive cellular infiltration of the lamina propria; mucosal invasion is rare. It is likely that hypogammaglobulinemia, low secretory IgA levels in the gut, achlorhydria, and malnutrition favor the development of infection. Giardia has been detected in the stomach; to be determined is whether this represents reflux from the duodenum or localized infection.

Clinical Findings

A. Symptoms and Signs: A large proportion of infected persons (especially children) remain asymptomatic cyst carriers, and their infection clears spontaneously. Giardia should be considered in most cases of diarrhea, especially where there is prolonged diarrhea and marked weight loss. The clinical forms of giardiasis are (1) acute diarrhea, (2) chronic diarrhea, and (3) malabsorption syndrome. The incubation period is usually 1–3 weeks but may be longer. The illness may begin gradually or suddenly. The acute phase may last days or weeks, but it is usually self-limited, although cyst excretion may be prolonged. In a few patients, the disorder may become chronic and last for years, but it does not appear to last indefinitely.

In both the acute and chronic forms, diarrhea ranges from mild to severe; most often it is mild. There may be no complaints other than of one bulky, loose bowel movement a day, often after breakfast. With larger numbers of movements, the stools become increasingly watery and may contain mucus but are usually free of blood and pus; they are copious, frothy, malodorous, and greasy. The diarrhea may be daily or recurrent; if recurrent, stools may be normal to mushy during intervening days, or the patient may be constipated. Weight loss is frequent; weakness may occur. Infants and young children may show impaired growth and development. Less common are anorexia, nausea and vomiting, midepigastric discomfort and cramps (often after meals), belching, flatulence, borborygmi, and abdominal distention. Low-grade fever is infrequent; sometimes attributed to giardiasis but not confirmed are headache, urticaria, myalgia, arthralgia, synovitis, and "salt and pepper" retinal changes.

A malabsorption syndrome occasionally develops in the acute or chronic stage that may result in marked weight loss and debility. Findings may include fat- and protein-losing enteropathy and vitamin A, vitamin B_{12}, and disaccharidase deficiencies. The latter may persist for a long time in persons apparently cured after specific treatment.

B. Laboratory Tests: Diagnosis is by identifying cysts or trophozoites in feces or duodenal fluid or antigen in feces. Using commercial kits, coproantigen detection by ELISA and IFA tests is now the preferred diagnostic test because of its high sensitivity (91–98%)—which is greater than finding the organism in feces—and high specificity (nearly 100%). Antigen detection, however, should be reserved for situations when there is no need to examine feces for other parasitic causes of diarrhea, as among day care children.

Detection of the parasites in feces can be difficult because the number of organisms passed varies considerably from day to day. At the onset of infection, patients may have symptoms for about a week before organisms can be detected; in chronic diarrhea, stool examinations can be persistently negative. Three stool specimens collected at intervals of 2 days or longer should be examined following concentration methods. One specimen will detect 50–75% of cases and three specimens about 90%. Unless the specimens can be submitted within an hour, they should be preserved immediately in a fixative. Purges do not increase the likelihood of finding the organism. Use of barium, antibiotics, antacids, kaolin products, or oily laxatives may temporarily (about 10 days) reduce the number of parasites or interfere with detection. In the presence of a presumptive diagnosis but negative stool specimens, an empirical course of treatment is sometimes indicated or selected other diagnostic procedures may be warranted: (1) the duodenal string test (Entero-Test), (2) duodenal aspiration (followed by concentration [500 Hz for 5 minutes]), (3) endoscopic brush cytology, or (4) duodenal biopsy (a mucosal imprint for staining should be made before sectioning).

Serum antibody tests are generally not useful in diagnosis. A serum ELISA for IgG antibody test does not distinguish present from past infection; however, an IgM test appears to do so. Approximately one-third of infections show a short-lived IgA response. Radiologic examination is of little use; the small bowel is usually normal in mildly ill persons but may show nonspecific findings of increased transit time, altered motility, thickened mucosal folds, and barium column segmentation in patients with marked symptoms.

Treatment

Symptomatic patients should be treated. Although controversial, treatment of asymptomatic patients should be considered since they can transmit the infection to others and may occasionally become symptomatic themselves. In selected instances of asymptomatic infection, it may be best to wait a few weeks before starting treatment, as some infections will clear spontaneously in the absence of treatment.

Treatment is effective with tinidazole, metronidazole, quinacrine, or furazolidone. However, rare drug resistance (failure has also been induced experimentally) has resulted occasionally in treatment failures that require re-treatment with an alternative drug. Single-dose tinidazole (not available in the USA) is the drug of choice because it is as effective as a course of the other drugs. In follow-up, wait about 2 weeks before rechecking two or more stools at weekly intervals.

All of these drugs occasionally have unpleasant side effects. The potential carcinogenicity of furazolidone, metronidazole, and tinidazole appears to be negligible based on over 2 decades of use. None of the agents cure more than about 90% of cases (80% for furazolidone). Because of its rare potential for severe toxicity, quinacrine should be used only when no other drug is available.

A. Tinidazole: (Not available in the USA.) A dose of 2 g given once has had reported cure rates of 90–100%. Adverse reactions consist of mild gastrointestinal side effects in about 10% of patients; headache and vertigo are less common.

B. Metronidazole: The dose is 250 mg three times daily for 5 days. Metronidazole may cause gastrointestinal symptoms, headache, dizziness, a metallic taste, and candidal overgrowth. Patients must be warned that alcohol may cause a disulfiram-like reaction. In the USA, metronidazole for giardiasis treatment is only available for off-label use.

C. Furazolidone: The dose is 100 mg (in suspension) four times daily for 7–10 days. Gastrointestinal symptoms, fever, headache, rash, and a disulfiram-like reaction with alcohol occur. Furazolidone can cause mild hemolysis in glucose-6-phosphate dehydrogenase-deficient persons and rarely causes hypersensitivity reactions.

D. Quinacrine (Mepacrine): (Not available in the USA.) The dose is 100 mg three times daily after meals for 5–7 days. The drug has a bitter taste. Gastrointestinal symptoms, headache, and dizziness are common; harmless yellowing of the skin is infrequent. Toxic psychosis and exfoliative dermatitis, which are rare, may be severe and long-lasting. Quinacrine is contraindicated in psoriasis or in persons with a history of psychosis.

E. Others: Albendazole (400 mg daily for 5 days) has shown cure rates that range from 10% to 95%. Reports with **paromomycin** (25–35 mg/kg/d in three divided doses for 7 days) have been mixed; because the drug is not absorbed, it has been proposed for use in pregnancy.

Prevention

There is no effective chemoprophylaxis for giardiasis. Since community chlorination (0.4 mg/L) of water is relatively ineffective for inactivating cysts, filtration is required. For hikers, bringing water to a boil is adequate; halogenation with iodine or filtration with a pore size less than 1 μm can also be used. In day care centers, appropriate disposal of diapers and frequent hand washing are essential.

Prognosis

With treatment and successful eradication of the infection, there are no sequelae. Without treatment, severe malabsorption may rarely contribute to death from other causes.

Farthing MJ: Giardiasis. Gastroenterol Clin North Am 1996;25:493. [NLM Cit ID: 97016402]

Ortega YR et al: Giardia: Overview and update. Clin Infect Dis 1997;25:545. [NLM Cit ID: 97458112]

Vesy CJ et al: Review article: the management of giardiasis. Aliment Pharmacol Therap 1999;13:843. [NLM Cit ID: 99315240]

Zaat JO et al: A systematic review on the treatment of giardiasis. Trop Med Int Health 1997;2:63. [NLM Cit ID: 97171031]

LEISHMANIASIS

Leishmaniasis is infection by species of the genus leishmania. The disease is a zoonosis transmitted by bites of sand flies (*Phlebotomus* [Old World leishmaniasis] and *Lutzomyia* [New World leishmaniasis] species) from the wild animal reservoir (eg, rodents, Canidae, sloths, marsupials) and domestic dogs (they can die from *L infantum* infections) to humans; however, kala azar is transmitted directly from humans to humans. Leishmaniae have two distinct forms in their life cycle: (1) In mammalian hosts, the parasite is found in its amastigote form (Leishman-Donovan bodies, 2 × 5 μm) within mononuclear phagocytes. When sand flies feed on an infected host, the parasitized cells are ingested with a blood meal. (2) In the sand fly vector, the parasite converts to, multiplies, and is then transmitted during feeding as a flagellated extracellular promastigote (10–15 μm).

Four clinical syndromes occur, with overlap between them. The speciation of leishmaniasis is complex (about 20 species are known to infect humans) and unsettled, and some species, not all of which are noted below, can cause more than one syndrome.

(1) **Visceral leishmaniasis** (kala azar), characterized by hepatosplenomegaly and anemia, is caused mainly by the *L donovani* group of agents: *L donovani, L infantum,* and *L chagasi.*

(2) **Old World cutaneous leishmaniasis**—moist or dry cutaneous leishmaniasis—is caused mainly by *L tropica, L major,* and *L aethiopica.* **New World cutaneous leishmaniasis** is caused by the *L mexicana* complex.

(3) **Mucocutaneous leishmaniasis** (espundia), characterized by an initial cutaneous ulcer that is followed in months to years by destructive nasopharyngeal lesions, is caused by the leishmania (viannia) group of agents, principally by *L (V) braziliensis* and rarely by *L (V) panamensis.*

(4) **Diffuse cutaneous leishmaniasis** is a state of deficient cell-mediated immunity, in which the widespread, leprosy-like skin lesions are generally progressive and refractory to treatment. The causative organisms are the *L mexicana* complex in the New World and *L aethiopica* in the Old World.

In tropical and temperate zones, an estimated 12 million persons are infected; 1.5–2 million new cases occur yearly, of which more than 1 million are cutaneous and 500,000 visceral disease. Severity of infection ranges from subclinical or minimally pathologic (self-curing or easily treated cutaneous lesions) to persistent, disfiguring cutaneous and mucocutaneous lesions to potentially fatal visceral disease (about 5000 yearly). Large outbreaks of infection with some agents have occurred.

Leishmaniae are capable of latent infection and can become opportunistic pathogens in immunoincompetent persons; more than 1000 coinfections with HIV-visceral leishmaniasis have been reported from 25 countries, but the problem is worse in southern Europe (France, Italy, Spain, Portugal), where up to 17% of people with AIDS have coinfections. Coinfections are being increasingly reported with other leishmania species elsewhere in the world. In AIDS coinfection, both diagnosis and treatment may be difficult. Antibodies are often undetectable; in visceral leishmaniasis, splenomegaly may not be present.

Diagnosis

Definitive diagnosis is by finding (1) the intracellular nonflagellated amastigote in Giemsa-stained impression smears or sectioned tissue biopsies from skin or mucosal lesions or from visceral tissue (spleen, liver, bone marrow), or (2) the flagellated promastigote stage in culture of these tissues. Hamster or Balb/c mouse inoculation of the nose, footpad, or tail base may also be useful (requires 2–12 weeks). Culture requires up to 28 days, using specialized media held at 22–28 °C. Other tests that may facilitate diagnosis and increase sensitivity are serologic tests (ELISA, direct agglutination, others; none are sufficiently sensitive or specific to be used alone in diagnosis), skin tests (leishmanin—none approved for use in the USA), polymerase chain reaction, and monoclonal antibody staining of tissue smears. The serologic and skin tests do not reliably distinguish present from past infection. After culture isolation, organisms can be identified to species, usually by isoenzyme patterns, monoclonal antibodies, or polymerase chain reaction. Specimens from the skin lesions should be obtained at a raised ulcer margin through an area of intact skin cleansed with 70% alcohol. For scrapings, press the site with the fingers (to obtain tissue fluid, not blood) and incise a 3-mm slit. For needle aspiration, sterile preservative-free saline is inserted with a 23- to 27-gauge needle; the aspirate is then cytospun at 800 *g* for 5 minutes.

Treatment

Treatment is less than adequate because of drug toxicity, long courses required, and frequent need for hospitalization. The drug of choice is sodium stibogluconate; however, resistance to the agent is increasing in frequency in many countries. Second line drugs used in cases unresponsive to the antimonials—but potentially more toxic—are amphotericin B and pentamidine. In antimony-resistant infections, three new lipid-formulated amphotericins permit a shorter course of treatment with less toxicity and high effectiveness. AmBisome, recently approved for use in the USA, is considered by some workers to be the drug of choice for the treatment of visceral leishmaniasis. See specialized sources for additional details on toxicity and mode of treatment with these drugs.

A. Sodium Stibogluconate: Sodium stibogluconate is provided as a solution that contains 100 mg of antimony (Sb) per milliliter; only fresh solutions should be used. Treatment is started with a 200-mg Sb test dose followed by 20 mg Sb/kg/d, but there is no upper limit on the maximum daily dose. Although the drug can be administered as a 5% solution intramuscularly (may be locally painful), intravenous administration is preferred (cough may occur) when the volume is high, as is the case for most adults. Meglumine antimoniate (85 mg Sb/mL) is equal in efficacy and toxicity when used in equivalent Sb doses (20 mg Sb/kg/d). The appropriate volume of drug is mixed with 50 mL of 5% dextrose in water and infused over at least a 10-minute interval. The selected drug is given on consecutive days: 28 days for visceral and mucocutaneous leishmaniasis and 20 days for cutaneous leishmaniasis. In certain regions of the world, because of resistance, longer courses are indicated. Although few side effects occur initially, they are more likely to appear with cumulative doses. Most common are gastrointestinal symptoms, fever, myalgia, arthralgia, phlebitis, and rash; hemolytic anemia, hepatitis, renal and heart damage, and pancreatitis are rare. Patients should be monitored weekly for the first 3 weeks and twice weekly thereafter by serum chemistries, complete blood counts, and electrocardiography. Discontinue therapy if the following occur: aminotransferases three to four times normal levels or significant arrhythmias, corrected QT intervals greater than 0.50 s, or concave ST segments. Relapses should be treated at the same dosage level for at least twice the previous duration. In the USA, the only drug available is stibogluconate, obtainable from the Parasitic Drug Service, Centers for Disease Control and Prevention, Atlanta, GA 30333 (404-639-3670).

B. Amphotericin B: For the treatment of visceral leishmaniasis, the parenteral dosage of AmBisome (a liposomal formulation) is 3 mg/kg/d on days 1–5, 14, and 21; the dosage for immunoincompetent persons is 4 mg/kg/d on days 1–5, 10, 17, 24, 31, and 38. Infusion-related side effects (hypertension, hypotension, dyspnea, fever) and renal toxicity occur occasionally. The dosage for cutaneous and mucosal leishmaniasis has not been established. Conventional amphotericin B deoxycholate, as given in India, is slow infusion (4–6 hours) of 1 mg/kg daily for 20 days; this dosage achieved 99% cure rates and was well tolerated.

C. Pentamidine Isethionate: Pentamidine isethionate, 2–4 mg/kg intramuscularly (preferable) or intravenously, is given daily or on alternate days (fifteen doses for visceral and four doses for cutaneous leishmaniasis). For some forms of visceral leishmaniasis, it may be necessary to repeat treatment, but resistance may persist.

D. Paromomycin (Aminosidine): Success was limited in cutaneous leishmaniasis when the drug was applied topically (15% paromomycin, 12% methylbenzethonium chloride in soft white paraffin) twice daily for 15 days. The drug is showing promise in parenteral treatment (potentially severely toxic) of refractory visceral leishmaniasis in India and cutaneous disease in Central America.

Prevention & Control

Infection occurs when humans encroach on sand fly habitats—warm, humid microclimates, including rodent burrows, rock piles, or tree holes; these are often in sylvatic areas near forests or semiarid ecosystems. Biting is generally at twilight or at night but may occur in shaded areas during the day. Personal protection may fail but is partially accomplished by clothing (pants, long sleeves) that covers exposed skin, deet repellent (see under Malaria), avoidance of endemic areas (especially at night), use of mosquito coils, and use of fine-mesh sand fly netting for sleeping (may be too warm in tropical areas). Although sand flies can traverse the mesh of standard mosquito nets, insecticide-impregnated nets may prevent this. Often useful in control are destruction of animal reservoir hosts, mass treatment of humans in kala azar-prevalent areas, residual insecticide spraying in domestic and peridomestic areas, and keeping dogs and other domesticated animals out of the house, particularly at night.

Balana-Fouce R et al: The pharmacology of leishmaniasis. Gen Pharmacol 1998;30:435. [NLM Cit ID: 98182626]

Berman JD: Human leishmaniasis: Clinical, diagnostic, and chemotherapeutic developments in the last 10 years. Clin Infect Dis 1997;24:684. [NLM Cit ID: 97291130]

Desjeux P: Global control and *Leishmania* HIV coinfection. Clin Dermatol 1999;17:317. [NLM Cit ID: 99312865]

Herwaldt BL: Leishmaniasis. Lancet 1999;354:1191. [NLM Cit ID: 99441884]

Pearson RD et al: Clinical spectrum of leishmaniasis. Clin Infect Dis 1996;22:1. [NLM Cit ID: 96422341]

1. VISCERAL LEISHMANIASIS (Kala Azar)

Visceral leishmaniasis is infection of the reticuloendothelial system, resulting in fever, hepatosplenomegaly, and pancytopenia. More than 500,000 cases occur yearly, most of them fatal unless treated. The disease is caused mainly by the *Leishmania donovani* complex: (1) *L d donovani* (eastern India, Bangladesh, Southeast Asia, Sudan, Ethiopia, Kenya, scattered foci in sub-Saharan Africa, the central Asian part of Russia, and northern and eastern China); (2) *L infantum* (Mediterranean littoral, Middle East, China, central and southwestern Asia, Ethiopia, Sudan, Afghanistan, Pakistan); and (3) *L chagasi* (South America, Central America, Mexico). The number of cases is increasing, particularly in Sudan, Bangladesh, Brazil, and Nepal. In each locale, the disease has its own peculiar clinical and epidemiologic features. Two other species—*L tropica* in the Middle East, the Mediterranean littoral, Kenya, India, and western Asia and *L amazonensis* in the Amazon Basin—cause visceral leishmaniasis in a few patients, generally in a milder form. Although humans are the major reservoir, animal reservoirs such as the dog, other canids, and rodents are important. The incubation period is usually 4–6 months (range: 10 days to 24 months).

A local nonulcerating nodule at the site of the bite may precede systemic manifestations but usually is inapparent. The onset may be acute (as early as 2 weeks after infection) or insidious. Fever often peaks twice daily, with chills and sweats, weakness, weight loss, cough, and diarrhea. The spleen progressively becomes huge, hard, and nontender. The liver is somewhat enlarged, and generalized lymphadenopathy is common. Hyperpigmentation of skin, especially on the hands, feet, abdomen, and forehead, is marked in light-skinned patients. In blacks, there may be warty eruptions or skin ulcers. Petechiae, bleeding from the nose and gums, jaundice, edema, and ascites may occur. Wasting is progressive; death, often due to intercurrent infection, occurs within months to 1–2 years. In some regions, oral and nasopharyngeal or cutaneous manifestations occur with or without visceral involvement.

In HIV-infected persons—with or without AIDS—visceral leishmaniasis can be an opportunistic infection. Numerous cases have been reported from the Mediterranean area and some from South America. These patients may have a shorter duration of symptoms, no fever or splenomegaly, and a poor response to treatment.

The diagnosis is made by demonstrating the organism in buffy coat preparations of blood either directly or after culture; on stained smears of aspirates of sternal marrow or iliac crest, liver, enlarged lymph nodes, or spleen; nasopharyngeal swabs; and by culture. Although splenic aspiration is the most sensitive test, because of its hazard it should be reserved for last and be performed only by experienced persons; contraindications are a soft spleen in the acute phase, a prolonged prothrombin time, and platelet counts under 40,000/μL. Serologic tests are highly sensitive (> 90%), but false positives may occur. The direct agglutination IgM test and ELISAs are positive early; in most patients the immunofluorescent IgG test is positive at titers of 1:256 or higher. The leishmanin skin test is always negative during active disease and becomes positive months to years after recovery. Other characteristic findings are progressive leukopenia (seldom over 3000/μL after the first 1–2 months), with lymphocytosis and monocytosis, normochromic anemia, and thrombocytopenia. There is a marked increase in total protein up to or greater than 10 g/dL owing to an elevated IgG fraction; serum albumin is 3 g/dL or less. Liver function tests show hepatocellular damage. Proteinuria may be present.

The differential diagnosis includes leukemia, lymphoma, tuberculosis, histoplasmosis, infectious mononucleosis, brucellosis, malaria, typhoid, schistosomiasis, African trypanosomiasis, infective endocarditis, and cirrhosis.

Sodium stibogluconate (20 mg/kg/d for 30 days) is the drug of choice; however, some workers now use the liposomal amphotericin B formulations as the preferred treatment. Whereas Mediterranean kala-azar responds to 10–15 daily doses of stibogluconate, the disease in Kenya, Sudan, and India requires at least 30 days of treatment. With incomplete response or relapse, the treatment should be repeated for up to 60 days. Failure of stibogluconate or liposomal amphotericin B should lead to use of pentamidine. Other drugs under evaluation individually or in combination with antimony, pentamidine, or amphotericin B are allopurinol, human gamma interferon, atovaquone, multifosin, and parenteral paromomycin (aminosidine). In Bihar, India, where the infection is becoming increasingly unresponsive to antimonials (currently 40%), liposomal amphotericin B is usually effective. Miltefosine, a new oral treatment under evaluation, shows high cure rates and less toxicity than other treatments but does have potential fetal toxicity.

Without treatment, the case-fatality rate can reach 90%. Early diagnosis and treatment reduces the mortality rate to 2–5%. Relapses (up to 10% in India and 30% in Kenya) are most likely to occur within 6 months after completion of treatment.

Post kala azar dermal leishmaniasis may appear after apparent cure in the Indian subcontinent and east Africa. It may simulate leprosy, as multiple hypopigmented macules or nodules develop on preexisting lesions. Erythematous patches may appear on the face. Leishmaniae are present in the skin. Antimony treatment should be tried but is often ineffective.

Berman J et al: Treatment of visceral leishmaniasis with amphotericin B colloidal dispersion. Chemotherapy 1999;45(Suppl 1):54. [NLM Cit ID: 99323845]

Davidson RN: Visceral leishmaniasis in clinical practice. J Infect 1999;39:112. [NLM Cit ID: 20075618]

Jha TK et al: Randomized controlled trial of aminosidine (paromomycin) sodium stibogluconate for treating visceral leishmaniasis in North Bihar, India. BMJ 1998; 316:1200. [NLM Cit ID: 98245966]

Meyerhoff A: U.S. Food and Drug Administration approval of AmBisome (liposomal amphotericin B) for treatment of visceral leishmaniasis. Clin Infect Dis 1999;28:42. [NLM Cit ID: 99152395]

Sundar S et al: Trial of oral miltefosine for visceral leishmaniasis. Lancet 1998;352:1821. [NLM Cit ID: 99066708]

Thakur CP et al: Amphotericin B deoxycholate treatment of visceral leishmaniasis with new modes of administration and precautions: a study of 939 cases. Trans R Soc Trop Med Hyg 1999;93:319. [NLM Cit ID: 99422438]

2. CUTANEOUS LEISHMANIASIS

Cutaneous swellings appear 2 weeks to several months after sand fly bites and can be single or multiple. Depending on the leishmanial species and host immune response, lesions begin as small papules and develop into nonulcerated dry plaques or large encrusted ulcers with well-demarcated raised and indurated margins. Satellite lesions may be present. The lesions are painless unless secondarily infected. Local lymph nodes may be enlarged. Systemic symptoms are rare, but a low-grade fever of short duration may be present at the onset. For most species, healing usually occurs spontaneously in months to 1–3 years, starting with central granulation tissue that spreads peripherally. Pyogenic complications may be followed by lymphangitis or erysipelas. Contraction of scars can cause deformities and disfigurement, especially if lesions are on the face.

The differential diagnosis includes tuberculosis, leprosy, fungal infections, yaws, syphilis, neoplasms, and sarcoidosis.

Diffuse cutaneous leishmaniasis is caused by the *L mexicana* complex and *L aethiopica*. Nonulcerating lesions (that resemble lepromatous leprosy) occur over the entire body. The condition is associated with anergy, in which the skin test is negative but amastigotes are abundant. In spite of repeated doses of antimony, pentamidine, or amphotericin, cures are rare.

Definitive diagnosis is by identification of the organisms (see above). Microscopic examination of skin scrapings has limited sensitivity, particularly in chronic infections. Where available, species identification should be done by molecular methods. The serologic and leishmanin skin tests become positive in 4–6 weeks but are unreliable; most assays cannot distinguish between leishmaniasis and *Trypanosoma cruzi* infections and may cross-react at low titers in malaria, toxoplasmosis, and amebiasis. A PCR technique that used boiled dermal scrapings yielded a sensitivity and specificity of 100% in New World cutaneous leishmaniasis.

Old World Cutaneous Leishmaniasis

Agents of Old World cutaneous leishmaniasis are as follows:

(1) *L tropica* is the agent responsible for an urban infection of dogs and humans. It is found in the Middle East, northwestern India, East Africa, central Asian area of the former Soviet Union, Afghanistan, Pakistan, Turkey, Armenia, Greece, and southern France and Italy. The incubation period is 2 months or longer, and healing is complete in 1–2 years. The lesions of *L tropica* infection tend to be single and dry, to ulcerate slowly or not at all, and to persist for a year or longer. **Leishmaniasis recidivans** is a relapsing form of *L tropica* infection in which the primary lesion nearly heals, lateral spread follows, and scarring can be extensive; it is associated with hypersensitivity and a strongly positive skin test but scarce amastigotes. Visceral involvement by *L tropica* has been reported rarely (including after troop exposure in Operation Desert Storm) and is relatively resistant to antimony treatment.

(2) *L major* infection causes lesions in dry or desert rural areas and is primarily a disease of desert rodents. Human disease occurs in the Middle East, central Asian area of the former Soviet Union, Arabian peninsula, Afghanistan, and Africa (North, East, and sub-Saharan Africa from Senegal to Sudan and Kenya). The lesions are characterized by multiple, wet, rapidly ulcerating sores with crusting. Spontaneous healing is generally complete in 6–12 months.

(3) *L aethiopica* infection occurs in the Ethiopian and Kenyan highlands. Ulceration is rare; spontaneous healing is slow over several years. An uncommon complication is diffuse cutaneous leishmaniasis.

(4) *L donovani* sometimes causes cutaneous disease with visceral manifestations.

Old World leishmaniasis, especially in the Middle East, is generally self-healing in about 6 months and does not metastasize to the mucosa. Thus, it may be justified to withhold treatment if the lesions are small, in an unobtrusive place, and appear to be healing. Pentavalent antimony (20 days) should be used to treat patients with large or multiple lesions or if the lesions are on cosmetically or functionally important areas (eg, the wrist). Complete healing may not be evident until weeks after the course of treatment has been completed. Pentamidine or amphotericin B is used for failures. Other treatments for less severe disease are physical measures (local cryotherapy or heat therapy, electrocoagulation, surgical removal) and intralesional injection of sodium stibogluconate. Paromomycin ointment may also be effective. Lesions should be kept clean and antibiotics used if secondary infection occurs.

New World Cutaneous Leishmaniasis

Agents of New World cutaneous leishmaniasis are as follows:

(1) The *L mexicana* complex: *L mexicana* (Texas, Oklahoma, Arizona, Mexico, Central America); *L amazonensis* (Amazonian basin, Venezuela, Panama, Trinidad); *L chagasi* (Central and South America); other species (Venezuela and Dominican Republic).

(2) The leishmania (viannia) group: *L braziliensis* (Central and South America); *L panamensis* (Central America and northeastern South America); and *L guyanensis* (South America).

L mexicana and *L braziliensis* infections generally result from forest-related activities or from residence in dwellings situated near forests. *P panamensis* is also found in drier habitats. In parts of South America, several leishmania species are now transmitted in domestic environments.

Most New World cutaneous lesions are ulcers, but vegetative, verrucous, or nodular lesions may occur also. *L mexicana* ("chiclero's ulcer") in the Yucatan and Central America produces destructive lesions on the ear cartilage. Up to 80% of *L braziliensis* cutaneous lesions progress to espundia (see below); some *L braziliensis* complex strains also show a chain of palpable local lymph nodes, and some *L mexicana* and South American strains can cause diffuse cutaneous leishmaniasis.

In New World *L mexicana* infections from Mexico and Central America, solitary nodules or ulcers in inconspicuous sites generally will heal spontaneously, but metronidazole, 750 mg three times daily for 10 days, can be tried. Lesions on the ear, face, or hands should be treated with sodium antimony gluconate but usually require only a 12- to 14-day course. Under evaluation are ketoconazole, itraconazole, liposome-encapsulated compounds, combined sodium stibogluconate and allopurinol, and topically applied paromomycin. Cutaneous lesions acquired in regions of mucocutaneous leishmaniasis may be due to *L braziliensis* or *L panamensis* and should be treated with a full course of sodium stibogluconate.

Ashford RW: Cutaneous leishmaniasis: strategies for prevention. Clin Dermatol 1999;17:327. [NLM Cit ID: 99312866]

Belli A et al: Simplified polymerase chain reaction detection of New World *Leishmania* in clinical specimens of cutaneous leishmaniasis. Am J Trop Med Hyg 1998;58: 102. [NLM Cit ID: 98112679]

Salman SM et al: Cutaneous leishmaniasis: clinical features and diagnosis. Clin Dermatol 1999;17:291. [NLM Cit ID: 99312862] (Entire issue devoted to leishmaniasis.)

Samady JA et al: Old World cutaneous leishmaniasis. Int J Dermatol 1997;36:161. [NLM Cit ID: 97302747]

Vargas-Gonzales A et al: Response of cutaneous leishmaniasis (Chiclero's ulcer) to treatment with meglumine antimoniate in southeast Mexico. Am J Trop Med Hyg 1999;61:960. [NLM Cit ID: 20137143]

3. MUCOCUTANEOUS LEISHMANIASIS (Espundia)

Mucocutaneous leishmaniasis occurs in lowland forest areas and is caused by the leishmania (viannia) group of organisms, usually by *L (V) braziliensis* (Central and South America; most cases are in Brazil, Bolivia, and Peru) and rarely by *L (V) panamensis* (Central and northeastern South America) or *L (V) peruviana* (Peru). The initial lesion, single or multiple, is on exposed skin; at first it is papular (can be pruriginous or painful), then nodular, and later may ulcerate or become wart-like or papillomatous. Local healing follows, with scarring within several months to a year. Subsequent naso-oral involvement occurs in a small proportion of patients either by direct extension or, more often, metastatically to the mucosa. It may appear concurrently with the initial lesion, shortly after healing, or after many years. The mucosa of the anterior part of the nasal septum is generally the first area to be involved. Extensive destruction of the soft tissues and cartilage of the nose, oral cavity, and lips may follow and may extend to the larynx and pharynx. Gross and hideous destruction and marked suffering can result. Secondary bacterial infection is common. Regional lymphangitis, lymphadenitis, fever, weight loss, keratitis, and anemia may be present.

Diagnosis is by finding amastigotes in scrapings, biopsy impressions or histologic sections, or aspirated tissue fluid. The organism grows with difficulty in culture or after inoculation of hamsters; if positive, speciation should be attempted. The leishmanin skin test is useful if it produces a fully developed papule in 2–3 days that disappears after a week. The direct agglutination test for IgM antibodies becomes positive in 4–6 weeks. IgG antibodies are detectable in most cases and disappear with cure. The main considerations in the differential diagnosis are paracoccidioidomycosis and other fungal infections, polymorphic reticulosis, Wegener's granulomatosis, lymphoma, and nasopharyngeal carcinoma, yaws, syphilis, and sarcoidosis.

Treatment of this condition is difficult; failure rates are high in severe disease even when a full course (28 days) of sodium stibogluconate treatment is used (see above). If repeated and extended antimony treatment fails, amphotericin B is used. Under evaluation are the liposomal formulations of amphotericin B and combined antimony and gamma interferon treatment. Corticosteroids may be needed to control local inflammation due to release of antigens. Antibiotics are usually needed to treat associated bacterial or fungal infection.

Amato VS et al: An evaluation of clinical, serologic, anatomopathologic and immunohistological findings for fifteen patients with mucosal leishmaniasis before and after treatment. Rev Inst Med Trop Sao Paulo 1998;40:23. [NLM Cit ID: 98378756]

Berman JD: Treatment of New World cutaneous and mucosal leishmaniases. Clin Dermatol 1996;14:519. [NLM Cit ID: 97044259]

Llanos-Cuentas A et al: Efficacy of sodium stibogluconate alone and in combination with allopurinol for treatment of mucocutaneous leishmaniasis. Clin Infect Dis 1997;25:677. [NLM Cit ID: 97458132]

MALARIA

Essentials of Diagnosis

- History of exposure in a malaria-endemic area.
- Periodic attacks of sequential chills, fever, and sweating.
- Headache, myalgia, splenomegaly; anemia, leukopenia.
- Characteristic parasites in erythrocytes, identified in thick or thin blood films.
- Complications of falciparum malaria: Cerebral findings (mental disturbances, neurologic signs, convulsions), hemolytic anemia, hyperpyrexia, dysenteric or cholera-like stools, dark urine, anuria.

General Considerations

Four species of the genus plasmodium are responsible for human malaria: *P vivax, P malariae, P ovale,* and *P falciparum.* Although the disease has been eradicated from most temperate zone countries, it continues to be endemic in many parts of the tropics and subtropics, and imported cases occur in the USA and other countries free of transmission. Malaria is present in parts of Mexico, Haiti, Dominican Republic, Central and South America, Africa, the Middle East, the Indian subcontinent, Southeast Asia, China, and Oceania. *P vivax* and *P falciparum* are responsible for most infections and are found throughout the malarious regions; *P falciparum* is the predominant species in Africa and the only plasmodium in Haiti and the Dominican Republic. *P malariae* is also widely distributed but is less common. *P ovale,* although generally rare, seems to replace *P vivax* in West Africa. *P vivax* infection is uncommon among blacks because their red blood cells do not have the Duffy factor surface antigen. Annually worldwide, malaria causes clinical illness in 300–500 million people and results in 1.5–2.7 million deaths; its greatest impact is on young children, particularly in sub-Saharan Africa. The USA experiences each year an average of 1000 imported infections with different species; a few cases of locally acquired, mosquito-transmitted infection from an imported case; and an average of four deaths from falciparum malaria. Most of the imported infections are acquired in tropical Africa.

Malaria is transmitted from human to human by the bite of infected female *Anopheles* mosquitoes. **Induced malaria**—congenital transmission and transmission by blood transfusion—also occurs. Other than the mosquito, there are no animal reservoirs for human malaria.

The mosquito becomes infected by ingesting blood containing the sexual forms of the parasite (micro- and macrogametocytes). After a developmental phase in the mosquito, sporozoites in the salivary glands are inoculated into humans when the mosquito next feeds. The first stage of development in humans, the exoerythrocytic stage, takes place in the liver. In all four infections, the sporozoites invade hepatocytes to mature as tissue schizonts. However, in *P vivax* and *P ovale* infections only—but not in induced infections with these parasites—some sporozoites enter hepatocytes to become dormant hypnozoites; activation of the hypnozoites 6–8 months later results in a primary infection or in relapse. When liver schizonts escape from the liver into the bloodstream, they invade red blood cells, multiply, and 48 hours later (or 72 with *P malariae*) cause the red cells to rupture, releasing a new crop of parasites (merozoites). Within the bloodstream, this cycle of invasion, multiplication, and red cell rupture may be repeated many times.

In *P falciparum* and *P malariae* malaria, the liver infection ceases spontaneously in less than 4 weeks; thereafter, multiplication is confined to the red cells. Thus, 4 weeks after departure from an endemic area, treatment that eliminates these species from the red cells will cure the infection. Cure of *P vivax* and *P ovale* malaria, however, requires treatment to eradicate infection from both red cells and liver hypnozoites.

The incubation period after exposure or after stopping chemoprophylaxis is, for *P falciparum,* approximately 12 days (range: 9–60 days); for *P vivax* and *P ovale,* 14 days (range: 8–27 days [initial attacks for some temperate strains may not occur for up to 8 months]); and for *P malariae,* 30 days (range: 16–60 days). If untreated, *P falciparum* infections usually terminate spontaneously in 6–8 months but can persist for up to 1.5 years; *P vivax* and *P ovale* infections can persist without treatment for as long as 5 years; and *P malariae* infections have lasted for as long as 50 years. Protective immunity results from infection but decays after several years if reinfection does not occur.

Clinical Findings

A. Symptoms and Signs: Typical malarial attacks show sequentially, over 4–6 hours, shaking chills (the cold stage); fever (the hot stage) to 41 °C or higher; and marked diaphoresis (the sweating stage). Associated symptoms may include fatigue, headache, dizziness, gastrointestinal symptoms (anorexia, nausea, slight diarrhea, vomiting, abdominal cramps), myalgia, arthralgia, backache, and dry cough. These symptoms appear to be due in large part to release of tissue necrosis factor and other cytokines during schizogony.

Either from the onset or with progression of the disease, the attacks may show an every-other-day (tertian) periodicity in vivax, ovale, or falciparum malaria or an every-third-day (quartan) periodicity in malariae malaria. Splenomegaly usually appears when acute symptoms have continued for 4 or more days; the liver is frequently mildly enlarged. The patient may be tired between attacks but otherwise feels well. After this primary episode, recurrences are common, each separated by a latent period.

Because of its frequent and severe complications, *P falciparum* is the more serious infection and causes the most deaths, sometimes within 24 hours. In severe falciparum infections, red blood cell parasitemia is higher than 3–5%. Severe disease results in part from intense sequestration and cytoadherence of parasitized red cells in capillaries and postcapillary venules. Complications include (1) cerebral malaria with edema (headache, mental disturbances, neurologic signs, retinal hemorrhages, convulsions, delirium, coma); (2) hyperpyrexia; (3) hemolytic anemia; (4) noncardiogenic pulmonary edema; (5) acute tubular necrosis and renal failure—rarely, this is associated with blackwater fever (dark urine), which most commonly is due to severe hemolysis following quinine treatment; (6) acute hepatopathy, with centrilobular necrosis and marked jaundice but no liver failure; (7) hypoglycemia; (8) an adrenal insufficiency-like syndrome; (9) cardiac dysrhythmias; (10) gastrointestinal syndromes (including secretory diarrhea and dysentery); (11) lactic acidosis and hypoglycemia; (12) coexisting pneumonia; and (13) water and electrolyte imbalance. The prognosis is bad when there are multiple complications or if more than 20% of infected red cells contain mature parasites or more than 5% of neutrophils contain pigment. Gram-negative bacteremia may contribute to death.

Immunologic disorders resulting from chronic infection are tropical splenomegaly and nephrotic syndrome (the latter due to *P malariae* only). Malaria infections do not appear to act as an opportunistic infection in AIDS patients, with the possible exception of malaria infection in pregnancy.

B. Laboratory Findings: The thick and thin blood film, dehemoglobinized and Giemsa-stained or Wright-stained, is the mainstay of diagnosis. The much less sensitive thin film is used primarily for species differentiation after the presence of an infection is detected on a thick film. Because the level of parasitemia varies from hour to hour—especially for *P falciparum* infections, in which parasites may be difficult to find—blood should be examined at 8-hour intervals for 3 days, during and between febrile spikes. The newly described quantitative buffy coat method to detect parasitemia is slightly more sensitive than thick smears, but it is expensive and requires fluorescent microscopy.

The number of red cells infected seldom exceeds 2% of the total cells. During paroxysms, there may be transient leukocytosis; leukopenia develops subsequently, with a relative increase in large mononuclear cells. In severe falciparum malaria, parasitemia may reach 30% or higher; mature asexual forms disappear (sequestered in the microcirculation); hepatic function tests often become abnormal; and hemolytic jaundice, thrombocytopenia, and marked anemia with reticulocytosis may develop.

Serologic tests (ELISA and others) are not commonly used in the diagnosis of acute attacks. Antibody becomes detectable only 8–10 days after onset of symptoms—too late to be of use; also, because antibody persists for 10 or more years, it does not distinguish between current and past infection. In rare instances, however, serology may be useful in the differential diagnosis of chronic fevers. Available for field diagnosis for falciparum malaria only is a rapid and simply accomplished dipstick antigen capture assay; sensitivity and specificity range between 75% and 95%. Two fluorescent microscopy methods have high sensitivity, but they do not distinguish between parasitic species. A polymerase chain reaction method is highly specific and sensitive but requires specialized laboratory methods.

Differential Diagnosis

Uncomplicated malaria must be distinguished from a variety of other causes of fever, splenomegaly, anemia, or hepatomegaly. Often considered are influenza, urinary tract infections, typhoid fever, infectious hepatitis, dengue, kala azar, amebic liver abscess, leptospirosis, and relapsing fever. Malaria complications can mimic many diseases.

Prevention

Prevention is based on evaluating the risk of exposure to infection, preventing mosquito bites, and chemoprophylaxis. Advice should also be given regarding medical care if malaria-like symptoms occur while traveling. All persons who will be exposed should receive chemoprophylaxis; however, because of rare but potentially serious side effects, chemoprophylaxis should not be prescribed in the absence of malaria risk Travelers should be advised that in spite of all precautions, no prophylactic regimen gives complete protection. Fever or other symptoms can develop in malaria as early as 8 days (range: 8–60 days) after exposure or stopping prophylaxis; for *P vivax* infections, the delay may be up to 8–12 months.

A. Consultative Resources Regarding Risks, Chemoprophylaxis, and Treatment: Consultation with a center working on malaria may be necessary to obtain up-to-date information on malaria treatment, and risk and prophylaxis by country. A source of information and advice in the USA is the Malarial Branch, Centers for Disease Control and Prevention (CDC), Atlanta, Georgia. For recorded information on prophylaxis: fax response, 888-232-3299; Internet, http://www.cdc.gov (choose the Travelers' Health category). For additional information on prophylaxis or for management of acute attacks, phone 770-488-7788. See also CDC and WHO references, below.

B. Risk of Exposure: The risk of exposure to mosquitoes may be difficult to estimate since it varies by climate rainy season, altitude, degree of mosquito control in urban versus rural areas, and according to whether exposure will occur during the time malaria mosquitoes are biting (chiefly between dusk and dawn). Travel to urban areas of Central and South America and Southeast Asia entails minimal risk.

C. Preventing Mosquito Bites: When out of doors between dusk and dawn (the primary feeding time for *Anopheles* mosquitoes), protective measures should be used: Clothing should cover most of the body, and deet (N,N-diethyl-3-methylbenzamide) mosquito repellent should be applied to exposed areas every 3–4 hours. To minimize the slight risk of toxic encephalopathy from deet, it should be applied sparingly and only to exposed skin and outer clothing; avoid high concentrations (over 30%) of the repellent; avoid inhalation and contamination of eyes, mouth, wounds, or irritated skin; and wash skin after coming indoors. The Ultrathon formulation provides a reduced concentration of deet (33%) with extended protection (12 hours). Living quarters should preferably be air-conditioned or be well screened; if screening is not available, mosquito bed nets should be used at night, preferably ones impregnated every 6 months with permethrin (0.2 g/m^2) (Permonone). To kill

Table 35–2. Prevention of malaria in travelers.[1]

TO PREVENT ATTACKS OF ALL FORMS OF MALARIA AND TO ERADICATE *P FALCIPARUM* AND *P MALARIAE* INFECTIONS[2,3,4]

REGIONS WITH CHLOROQUINE-SENSITIVE *P FALCIPARUM* MALARIA: Central America west of the Panama Canal, the Caribbean, North Africa, and parts of the Middle East

Chloroquine[5]

Dose: Chloroquine phosphate, 500 mg salt (300 mg base) weekly. Give a single dose of chloroquine weekly starting 1 week before entering the endemic area, while there, and for 4 weeks after leaving.

REGIONS WITH CHLOROQUINE-RESISTANT *P FALCIPARUM* MALARIA: All other regions of the world; the frequency and intensity of resistance vary by region.

Mefloquine (preferred method)[6]

Dose: one 250-mg tablet salt (228 mg base) weekly. Give a single dose of mefloquine weekly starting 3 weeks before entering the endemic area, while there, and for 4 weeks after leaving.

Doxycycline (alternative method)[7]

Dose: 100 mg daily. Give the daily dose for 2 days before entering the endemic area, while there, and for 4 weeks after leaving.

Malarone (atovaquone [250 mg] combined with proguanil [100 mg] (second alternative method)

Dose: One tablet daily. Give one tablet the day before entering the endemic area, daily while there, and daily for 1 week after leaving.

Chloroquine[5] **combined with proguanil**[5,8] **(third alternative method)**

Dose:

Chloroquine, weekly at the above schedule.

Proguanil, 200 mg daily while in the endemic area and daily for 4 weeks after leaving.

TO ERADICATE *P VIVAX* AND *P OVALE* INFECTIONS[2]

Primaquine[9]

Start primaquine only after returning home, during the last 2 weeks of chemoprophylaxis. Dose: 26.3 mg salt (15 mg base) daily for 14 days. An alternative regimen in regions where chloroquine is effective in prophylaxis is chloroquine phosphate, 500 mg (salt), plus primaquine phosphate 78.9 mg (salt), weekly for 8 weeks.

[1]See text for additional information on drug cautions, contraindications, and side effects. For additional information on prophylaxis for specific countries, see the references or call the Centers for Disease Control and Prevention, Atlanta, GA at 770-488-7788 (for fax response: 888-232-3299). The information is also available on the Internet at http://www.cdc.gov (choose the Traveler's Health category).

[2]The blood schizonticides (chloroquine, mefloquine, Malarone, and doxycycline), when taken for 4 weeks after leaving the endemic area, are curative for sensitive *P falciparum* and *P malariae* infections; primaquine, however, is needed to eradicate the persistent liver stages of *P vivax* and *P ovale.* Give primaquine with meals.

[3]A test dose of the selected prophylactic drug should be given before departure to allow for changing to an alternative drug in the event of significant side effects: chloroquine (weekly for 2 weeks), atovaquone/proguanil (daily for 2 days), doxycycline (daily for 2 days), mefloquine (weekly for 3 weeks). Side effects from mefloquine sometimes do not appear until after the third or later doses.

[4]See text for standby drugs for emergency self-treatment of presumptive malaria; such drugs should be used only when a physician is not immediately available. It is imperative, however, that medical follow-up be sought promptly.

[5]Chloroquine and proguanil can be used by pregnant women.

[6]Because of the high frequency of resistance, mefloquine should not be used in Thailand or adjacent countries; it is now the preferred drug for sub-Saharan Africa. Mefloquine is not recommended in the first trimester of pregnancy or under some other conditions (see text).

[7]Doxycycline is used in Thailand and adjacent countries and in other regions by persons who cannot tolerate mefloquine. It is contraindicated in pregnant women. Take with evening meals. See text for side effects.

[8]The combination can be used in countries with a low frequency of chloroquine-resistant falciparum malaria such as southern Asia (not Bangladesh) and parts of the Middle East. Proguanil is not available in the USA but can be purchased in other countries.

[9]Primaquine is indicated only for persons who have had a high probability of exposure to *P vivax* or *P ovale* (see text), and who have not taken the drug for daily prophylaxis. The drug should be taken with food and is contraindicated in pregnancy. Before use, patients must be screened for glucose-6-phosphate dehydrogenase deficiency.

mosquitoes in living quarters, use an antimosquito pyrethrum-containing spray or a powdered insecticide dispenser of pyrethroid tablets or burn pyrethroid mosquito coils. Garments can also be impregnated (sprayed or soaked) with permethrin, which repels for several weeks.

D. Advice Regarding Treatment if Malaria-Like Febrile Symptoms Occur While Traveling: Medical care should be sought immediately. The traveler should insist that blood smears be done and, if negative, repeated at intervals. If malaria is suspected but blood smears cannot be done, malaria treatment should be started.

Emergency self-treatment (standby treatment): Individuals who may be exposed to malaria and for whom medical attention will not be readily available are advised to carry medication for self-treatment if they develop fever or flu-like symptoms. However, *it is imperative that medical follow-up be sought promptly.* Patients should be given written instructions. The choice among available drugs depends on the anticipated type of exposure to drug-resistant *P falciparum* (see above for areas of resistance and Table 35–3 for dosages): (1) in chloroquine-sensitive areas, for persons who have taken no prophylaxis, use the chloroquine 2-day course of treatment; (2) in chloroquine-resistant areas without Fansidar resistance, use Fansidar (three tablets once only); (3) in areas with Fansidar resistance, use atovaquone/proguanil (500 mg/200 mg) daily for 3 days, atovaquone/doxycycline (500 mg/100 mg) daily for 3 days, or use quinine for 3–7 days plus tetracycline for 7 days (7 days of quinine is toxic for some patients). Mefloquine and halofantrine are not recommended because of their potential for severe toxicity.

Drugs Used in Chemoprophylaxis & Treatment (Tables 35–2 and 35–3)

A. Drug Classification: By chemical groups, some of the major antimalarial drugs are as follows: **4-aminoquinolines**—chloroquine, hydroxychloroquine, amodiaquine;* **diaminopyrimidines**—pyrimethamine, trimethoprim; **biguanides**—proguanil* (chlorguanide,* chlorproguanil*); **8-aminoquinolines**—primaquine; **cinchona alkaloids**—quinine, quinidine; **sulfonamides**—sulfadoxine, sulfadiazine, sulfamethoxazole; **sulfones**—dapsone; **4-quinoline-carbinolamines**—mefloquine; and **antibiotics**—tetracycline, doxycycline, clindamycin; and **others**—halofantrine,* artemisinin (qinghaosu)* and its derivatives, and atovaquone.† Pyrimethamine and proguanil are known as **antifolates,** since they inhibit dihydrofolate reductase of plasmodia. Drug combinations used to treat *P falciparum* malaria resistant to chloroquine include Fansidar (pyrimethamine plus sulfadoxine), Maloprim (pyrimethamine plus dapsone), and Malarone (atovaquone plus proguanil).

The effectiveness of antimalarial drugs differs with different species of the parasite and with different stages of the life cycle. Drugs that act in the liver to eliminate developing exoerythrocytic schizonts or latent hypnozoites are called **tissue schizonticides** (primaquine). Those that act on blood schizonts are **blood schizonticides** or **suppressive agents** (eg, chloroquine, amodiaquine, proguanil, pyrimethamine, mefloquine, quinine, quinidine, halofantrine, artemisinin and its derivatives) and atovaquone. **Gametocides** are drugs that prevent infection of mosquitoes by destroying gametocytes in the blood (eg, primaquine for *P falciparum* and chloroquine for *P vivax, P malariae,* and *P ovale*). **Sporonticidal** agents are drugs that render gametocytes noninfective in the mosquito (eg, pyrimethamine, proguanil).

None of the drugs prevent infection (ie, are true **causal prophylactic drugs**). However, proguanil and chlorproguanil—and to some extent the antibiotics and primaquine—prevent maturation of the early *P falciparum* and *P vivax* hepatic schizonts. Blood schizonticides destroy circulating plasmodia and thus prevent malarial attacks **(suppressive prophylaxis)** and, when given weekly for 4 weeks after departure from the endemic area, result in cure of *P falciparum* and *P malariae* infections. Only primaquine destroys the hypnozoites of *P vivax* and *P ovale* and, when given with a blood schizonticide, prevents relapse from infection with these parasites and thus effects **radical cure (terminal prophylaxis).**

B. Parasite Resistance to Drugs:

1. *P falciparum* resistance—

a. Chloroquine-resistant strains of *P falciparum* have been confirmed or are probably present in all malarious areas except Haiti, the Dominican Republic, rural areas of Mexico, Central America north and west of the Panama Canal, North Africa, and most of the Middle East (resistance is present, however, in Oman, Yemen, and Iran). In regions of resistance, some strains of *P falciparum* are only partially resistant to the drug, as manifested by temporary subsidence of symptoms and transient decrease or disappearance in asexual parasitemia, followed by return of both after several days to weeks.

b. Resistance to pyrimethamine-sulfadoxine (Fansidar) is present at high levels in Southeast Asia. It is also reported in parts of the Indian subcontinent, the Amazon basin, sub-Saharan Africa, and Oceania. Fansidar shows no cross-resistance with other antimalarial drugs.

c. Resistance to pyrimethamine or proguanil when used alone is common in most endemic areas, but the degree and distribution are not accurately known.

d. Mefloquine—Sporadic or low levels of mefloquine resistance have been reported from Southeast and southern Asia and parts of Africa, South America, the Middle East, and Oceania. Along the Thai-Burmese and Thai-Cambodian borders, however, the frequency reaches 30–60%.

e. Quinine and quinidine—Variable degrees of decreased responsiveness have been reported rarely in Southeast Asia (particularly in the border regions of Thailand) and Oceania and apparently in sub-Saharan Africa and Brazil.

f. Halofantrine—A high degree of resistance has been reported in eastern Thailand. Strains resistant to halofantrine are sometimes resistant to mefloquine as well.

2. *P vivax* resistance—

a. Antifolates—Resistance of *P vivax* blood schizonts to pyrimethamine and proguanil, including the pyrimethamine-containing drugs Fansidar and

*Not available in the USA but available in some countries.
†Available in the USA but not approved for antimalarial use.

Maloprim, has been reported in many areas of the world, particularly Southeast Asia.

b. Primaquine–Partial resistance of some strains of *P vivax* hepatic schizonts to primaquine has been reported in areas of Southeast Asia, (17% failure rate in Thailand), Papua New Guinea (30%), the Amazon Basin, Central America, and Somalia (43% in American military personnel). Treatment is usually successful with a higher dose (30 mg of base daily for 14 days) or a longer course (15 mg of base daily for 28 days).

c. Chloroquine–There are reports from Indonesia and Papua New Guinea of *P vivax* blood schizonts resistant to chloroquine. Decreased susceptibility is also appearing in the Solomon Islands, Myanmar, India, Thailand, Guyana, Brazil, and Peru. Mefloquine, halofantrine, or quinine plus doxycycline appear to be effective in treatment.

3. *P ovale* and *P malariae*–These forms have not shown resistance.

C. Selected Drugs: Indications, Limitations, and Adverse Side Effects:

1. Chloroquine phosphate–Chloroquine is the drug of choice in chemoprophylaxis and in treatment for all forms of malaria except for infections due to resistant strains of *P falciparum* and *P vivax* (see above). However, in *P vivax* and *P ovale* infections, primaquine is needed to eradicate the persistent liver phases and thus prevent relapse.

Oral chloroquine is usually well tolerated when used for malaria prophylaxis or treatment and is safe to use in pregnancy. Gastrointestinal symptoms, mild headache, pruritus (especially in blacks), dizziness, blurred vision, anorexia, malaise, and urticaria may occur; taking the drug after meals or in divided twice-weekly doses may reduce these side effects.

In parenteral treatment of severely ill patients, quinine, quinidine, or the parenteral artemisinin derivatives are the preferred drugs. If none are available, chloroquine can be given intramuscularly or intravenously. However, parenteral chloroquine can be severely toxic unless it is given in small amounts (3.5 mg [base]/kg) intramuscularly every 6 hours or by slow intravenous infusion.

Rare reactions from oral chloroquine include impaired hearing, psychosis, convulsions, blood dyscrasias, skin reactions, hypotension, and hemolysis in G6PD-deficient persons. When given in large doses for prolonged periods as an anti-inflammatory agent in autoimmune diseases, chloroquine has caused ocu-

Table 35–3. Treatment of malaria in nonimmune adult populations.

Treatment[1] of Infection With All Species (Except Chloroquine-Resistant *P falciparum*)	Treatment[1] of Infection With Chloroquine-Resistant *P falciparum* Strains
Oral treatment of *P falciparum*[2] or *P malariae* infection Chloroquine phosphate, 1 g (salt)[3,4] as initial dose, then 0.5 g at 6, 24, and 48 hours. **Oral treatment of *P vivax*[5] or *P ovale* infection** Chloroquine[3,4] as above followed by 0.5 g on days 10 and 17 plus primaquine phosphate, 26.3 mg (salt)[3,4] daily for 14 days starting about day 4. **Parenteral treatment of severe attacks** Quinine dihydrochloride[6] or quinidine gluconate.[7] Start oral chloroquine therapy as soon as possible; follow with primaquine if the infection is due to *P vivax* or *P ovale.* **or** Artemether[13] (preferable), 3.2 mg/kg IM, followed by 1.6 mg/kg daily; or chloroquine hydrochloride IM;[14] repeat every 6 hours. For both regimens, start oral chloroquine as soon as possible; follow with primaquine if infection is due to *P vivax* or *P ovale.*	**Oral treatment** Quinine sulfate, 10 mg/kg 3 times daily for 3–7 days,[8] plus one of the following: (1) doxycycline,[9] 100 mg twice daily for 7 days; (2) clindamycin,[9] 900 mg 3 times daily for 5 days; (3) pyrimethamine, 25 mg twice daily for 3 days, and sulfadiazine, 500 mg 4 times daily for 5 days; (4) tetracycline,[9] 250–500 mg 4 times daily for 7 days; (5) once only, pyrimethamine, 75 mg, and sulfadoxine, 1500 mg (= 3 tablets of Fansidar[10]). **or** Mefloquine,[11] 1250 mg (salt) once or 750 mg followed after 6–8 hours by 500 mg. **or** Halofantrine[12,13] **or** Atovaquone/proguanil,[13] 500 mg/200 mg, twice daily for 3 days **or** Atovaquone/doxycycline, 500 mg/100 mg, twice daily for 3 days **or** Artesunate,[13] 4 mg/kg/d for 3 days followed by mefloquine,[11] 1250 mg (salt) once

(continued)

Table 35–3. Treatment of malaria in nonimmune adult populations (continued).

Treatment[1] of Infection With All Species (Except Chloroquine-Resistant *P falciparum*)	Treatment[1] of Infection With Chloroquine-Resistant *P falciparum* Strains
	Parenteral treatment of severe attacks Quinine dihydrochloride[6] or quinidine gluconate[7] plus intravenous doxycycline or clindamycin. Start oral therapy with quinine sulfate plus the second drug as soon as possible to complete 7 days of treatment. **or** Artemether,[13] 3.2 mg/kg IM initially, followed by 1.6 mg/kg daily; followed by mefloquine,[11] 1250 mg (salt) once

[1]See text for cautions, contraindications, and side effects of each drug. For advice on management, call the Centers for Disease Control and Prevention (CDC), Atlanta, GA (770-488-7760).
[2]In falciparum malaria, if the patient has not shown a clinical response to chloroquine (48–72 hours for mild infections, 24 hours for severe ones), parasitic resistance to chloroquine should be considered. Chloroquine should be stopped and treatment started with oral quinine plus doxycycline, or mefloquine, or halofantrine.
[3]500 mg chloroquine phosphate = 300 mg base; 26.3 mg of primaquine = 15 mg base.
[4]Chloroquine alone is curative for infection with sensitive strains of *P falciparum* and for *P malariae,* but primaquine is needed to eradicate the persistent liver stages of *P vivax* and *P ovale.* Start primaquine after the patient has recovered from the acute illness; continue chloroquine weekly during primaquine therapy. Patients should be screened for glucose-6-phosphate dehydrogenase deficiency before use of primaquine. An alternative mode for primaquine therapy is combined primaquine, 78.9 mg (salt), and chloroquine, 0.5 g (salt), weekly for 8 weeks.
[5]Strains of *P vivax* resistant to chloroquine have appeared in some regions (see text). For their treatment, give quinine (plus doxycycline or Fansidar), mefloquine, or halofantrine as used to treat *P falciparum* resistant to chloroquine.
[6]Quinine dihydrochloride. Give 10 mg/kg (salt) in 500 mL of 5% glucose solution IV slowly over 4 hours; repeat every 8 hours until oral therapy is possible (maximum, 1800 mg/d). Blood pressure and ECG should be monitored constantly to detect arrhythmias or hypotension. As severe hypoglycemia may occur, blood glucose levels should be monitored. A higher initial loading dose of quinine is given (20 mg/kg) to patients who acquired infections in Southeast Asia if it is known with certainty that they have not already taken the medication. Extreme caution is required in treating patients with quinine who previously have been taking mefloquine in prophylaxis. In the USA, quinine dihydrochloride is no longer available.
[7]When parenteral quinine is unavailable (as in the USA), quinidine gluconate can be used, administered as a continuous infusion. A loading dose of 10 mg/kg (salt) (maximum, 600 mg) is diluted in 300 mL of normal saline and administered over 1–2 hours, followed by 0.02 mg/kg/min (maximum, 10 mg/kg every 8 hours) by continuous infusion until oral quinine therapy is possible. If more than 48 hours of parenteral treament is required, some authorities reduce the quinidine dose by one-third to one-half. Fluid status, glucose, blood pressure, and ECG should be closely monitored; widening of the QRS interval or lengthening of the QT interval requires discontinuation.
[8]Although quinine sulfate is usually given for 3 days, it should be continued for 7 days in patients who acquired infections in Southeast Asia and South America, where diminished responsiveness to quinine has been noted.
[9]Contraindicated in pregnant women.
[10]Fansidar should not be used for infections acquired in Southeast Asia, the Amazon Basin, Bangladesh, or Oceania.
[11]Serious side effects are rare. See text for cautions and contraindications. In the USA, a 250 mg tablet of mefloquine contains 228 mg of base; outside the USA, each 275 mg tablet contains 250 mg of base. Mefloquine is hazardous with quinine, quinidine, or halofantrine.
[12]The dosage is 500 mg (salt) every 6 hours for three doses and repeat in 1 week. A possible contraindication is the presence of cardiac conduction abnormalities. Do not use if mefloquine has been taken in previous 2–3 weeks.
[13]Not available in the USA but available in some other countries.
[14]To avoid potential severe toxicity, give parenteral chloroquine by low-dose intramuscular injection (maximum, 3.5 mg/kg [salt] every 6 hours).

lar damage. Theoretically, a total cumulative dosage of 100 g (base) may be critical in the development of ocular, ototoxic, and myopathic effects. However, with weekly long-term administration of chloroquine, serious eye damage has not been confirmed; therefore, periodic eye examinations may no longer be indicated. Chloroquine should be used with caution in patients who have histories of liver damage, alcoholism, or neurologic or hematologic disorders. It is contraindicated in patients with psoriasis. Chloroquine suppresses the immune response to the rabies vaccine.

Certain antacids and antidiarrheal agents (kaolin, calcium carbonate, and magnesium trisilicate) should not be taken within about 4 hours before or after chloroquine administration, since they interfere with its absorption.

2. Mefloquine hydrochloride–Mefloquine, a quinoline methanol derivative, is used for oral prophylaxis and treatment of chloroquine-resistant and multidrug-resistant *P falciparum* malaria. In treatment, it is used only for mildly to moderately ill patients; severely ill patients require parenteral treatment. Mefloquine has strong schizonticidal activity against *P falciparum* (except for resistant strains) and *P vivax*—and presumably against *P ovale* and *P malariae*—but it is not active against *P falciparum* gametocytes or the hepatic stages of *P vivax* or *P ovale,* which require a course of primaquine. With weekly doses of mefloquine, the steady state drug level is reached in about 7 weeks, and adverse reactions thus may not appear for 3–7 weeks. The steady state interval can be reduced to 4 days, revealing adverse reactions within a week, by giving an initial course of 250 mg daily for 3 days; this, however, is not standard practice.

With the lower doses used in prophylaxis, frequent minor and transient side effects (apparently no more frequent than those associated with chloroquine) include nausea, vomiting, epigastric pain, diarrhea, headache, dizziness, syncope, and extrasystoles. Severe neuropsychiatric symptoms are rare (estimated 1:10,000 to 1:1500). If prophylaxis is continued for more than a year, periodic liver function and ophthalmologic tests should be done. With treatment doses—particularly over 1000 mg—gastrointestinal symptoms and fatigue are more likely to occur, and the frequency of neuropsychiatric symptoms (dizziness, headache, visual disturbances, vertigo, tinnitus, insomnia, restlessness, anxiety, depression, confusion, disorientation, acute psychosis, or seizures) may be of the order of 1:1200. In experimental animals, the drug affects fertility and is teratogenic; it also causes degenerative changes in the epididymis in rats and in the lens and retina of some species. In human males, however, no deleterious effects on spermatozoa were found, and no effects have been noted in the human retina or lens.

Mefloquine is contraindicated in the presence of a cardiac conduction abnormality, liver impairment, or a history of a psychiatric or neurologic disorder, including epilepsy. Also contraindicated is concurrent administration of mefloquine with quinine, quinidine, or halofantrine. If these drugs precede use of mefloquine, 12 hours should elapse before mefloquine is started; however, because of the long elimination half-life of mefloquine (13–26 days), extreme caution is required because of arrhythmias if one of these drugs is used to treat malaria after mefloquine has been taken. Concurrent administration with tetracyclines or ampicillin results in increased mefloquine blood levels.

The development of neuropsychiatric symptoms during prophylaxis is an indication for stopping the drug. Patients taking anticonvulsant drugs (particularly valproic acid and divalproex sodium) may have breakthrough seizures. The drug is no longer contraindicated when beta-blockers and calcium channel blockers are taken. CDC has recently advised that mefloquine can be used throughout pregnancy; nevertheless, its use during the first trimester should be based on risk-benefit assessment. Women of childbearing potential who take mefloquine for antimalarial prophylaxis should preferably avoid conception for the duration of mefloquine usage and for 2 months after the last dose.

Note: The tablet formulation in the USA contains 250 mg of the salt (= 228 mg of base). However, in Canada and many other countries, the tablets contain 274 mg of the salt (= 250 mg of base). Mefloquine should not be taken on an empty stomach and should be taken with 8 oz of water.

3. Primaquine phosphate–Primaquine is used to prevent relapse by eliminating persistent liver forms of *P vivax* or *P ovale* in patients who have had an acute attack and for individuals returning from an endemic area who have probably been exposed to malaria. However, in persons with a low probability of exposure, it is preferable to avoid primaquine's potential toxicity by not giving the drug. Instead, such patients are advised to seek medical evaluation in the event of malaria-like symptoms, which usually occur within 2 years after infection but can occur up to 4 years after. Because primaquine is effective against the liver stages of all malarial parasites, it has been reevaluated recently for chemoprophylaxis when taken daily. Though effective, this new usage should be limited until there is additional study of its toxicity in long-term use. Primaquine is sometimes given as a single 45 mg (base) dose to eliminate *P falciparum* gametocytes.

Primaquine is generally well tolerated. Occasional side effects of the drug are gastrointestinal disturbances, headache, dizziness, or neutropenia. Primaquine should not be used in pregnancy (risk of hemolytic disease in the fetus), in autoimmune disorders, or concurrently with quinine.

All patients should be tested for glucose-6-phosphate dehydrogenase (G6PD) deficiency before therapy is begun and followed carefully during treatment; this is because primaquine may cause mild, self-limited hemolysis or marked hemolysis (pallor, weakness, abdominal pain, dark urine) or methemoglobinemia. G6PD deficiency is most common among persons of Mediterranean, African, or certain East Asian extractions. Patients with severe G6PD deficiency (< 10% residual enzyme activity) should not receive primaquine. For individuals with 10–60% residual activity, it is generally safe to give combined primaquine phosphate, 78.9 mg (45 mg base), and chloroquine phosphate, 0.5 g (0.3 g base), weekly for 8 weeks. However, for persons suspected of having the Mediterranean or Canton forms of G6PD deficiency, it may be preferable not to give primaquine but to treat attacks of malaria with chloroquine as they occur.

4. Quinine–Oral quinine sulfate in conjunction with another drug (see Table 35–3) is used to treat malaria due to multidrug-resistant strains of *P falciparum;* however, compliance with the 7-day course is poor because of quinine side effects.

Because quinine is an irritant to the gastric mucosa, it should be taken with food. Mild to moderate quinine toxicity (cinchonism) is manifested by headache, nausea, slight visual disturbances, dizziness, and mild tinnitus. These symptoms may abate as treatment continues and usually do not require discontinuation of treatment. Where available, quinine blood levels can be monitored; desired plasma levels are 5–10 μg/mL. Severe cinchonism requiring temporary or permanent discontinuation of therapy is rare and begins to appear at plasma levels greater than 7 μg/mL; findings include fever, skin eruptions, deafness, marked visual abnormalities (scotomas, diplopia, contracted visual fields, retinal vessel spasticity, optic atrophy, blindness), other central nervous system abnormalities (vertigo, somnolence, confusion, seizures), disturbances in cardiac rhythm or conduction, massive intravascular hemolysis with renal failure (blackwater fever), agranulocytosis, and thrombocytopenia.

Parenteral quinine dihydrochloride is used in the treatment of severe attacks of malaria due to *P falciparum* strains sensitive or resistant to chloroquine. The drug is given intravenously at a slow rate (Table 35–3); rapid infusions may be severely toxic. The drug should be used with extreme caution and only for patients who cannot take the medication orally; appropriate oral therapy should be started as soon as possible. Infusions may cause thrombophlebitis. In the USA, parenteral quinine is no longer available and parenteral quinidine gluconate is used instead.

See references and manufacturers' recommendations for drug interactions (including aluminum-containing antacids, digoxin, anticoagulants, and cimetidine). Quinine is safe to use in pregnancy. Systemic clearance of quinine slows in proportion to the severity of the disease.

5. Quinidine gluconate–Quinidine is the dextrorotatory diastereoisomer of quinine. The two drugs are equally efficacious in parenteral treatment of severe malaria (Table 35–3). The two drugs are also similar with regard to toxicity and drug interactions, but quinidine has a greater cardiosuppressant effect. The principal adverse effect of quinine and quinidine in severe malaria is hypoglycemia, which usually develops after 24 hours of treatment; it is a particular problem in pregnancy.

6. Halofantrine–Halofantrine is a schizonticide for all four malaria species, including multidrug-resistant *P falciparum.* The drug is not active against hepatic stages or gametocytes. It is used only in oral treatment. Infrequent to rare, minor side effects are abdominal pain, diarrhea, cough, rash, and pruritus. The drug should not be given from 1 hour before to 3 hours after a meal, because fatty food enhances and results in irregular absorption. Halofantrine is not used for prophylaxis or standby treatment because of this variable bioavailability; because the standard dose prolongs the QT_c interval; and because there have been rare reports of ventricular arrhythmias, sometimes fatal. The drug should not be used in the presence of preexisting cardiac conduction defects, long QT intervals, recent (4 weeks) usage of or concomitant treatment with mefloquine, or treatment with other drugs that prolong the QT interval (ie, quinine, quinidine, chloroquine, tricyclic antidepressants, neuroleptic drugs, terfenadine, astemizole). Because halofantrine is embryotoxic in animals, it should not be given to pregnant women. Halofantrine is widely available abroad; in the USA, however, although approved by the FDA, it has not been marketed.

7. Pyrimethamine-sulfadoxine (Fansidar)– Fansidar is supplied as tablets that contain pyrimethamine (25 mg) and sulfadoxine (500 mg). Fansidar's limitations are that it is effective only against susceptible strains of *P falciparum* (see above); its low efficacy against *P vivax, P ovale,* or *P malariae* and that it is slow-acting. Fansidar is no longer used for weekly prophylaxis because of rare reports of severe cutaneous toxicity and death. However, in single-dose treatment, Fansidar is generally well tolerated. Cutaneous reactions are more common in persons who are HIV-positive.

Current indications for Fansidar are (1) as a single dose (slow-acting) in conjunction with quinine (rapid-acting) in treatment of sensitive strains of acute chloroquine-resistant falciparum malaria and (2) in presumptive self-treatment of malaria (see above).

Fansidar is contraindicated for individuals with known sulfonamide sensitivity and those in the last month of pregnancy (the sulfadoxine component, which has a long half-life, can cause kernicterus in the newborn). The drug should be used with caution in the presence of impaired renal or hepatic function, in patients with G6PD deficiency (hemolysis occurs in some), and in those with severe allergic disorders or bronchial asthma. If folic acid is needed, ingestion should be delayed 1 week to avoid an inhibitory effect on the antimalarial action of Fansidar.

8. Doxycycline–Doxycycline is effective against chloroquine-sensitive and chloroquine-resistant *P falciparum, P vivax,* and (apparently) against *P ovale* and *P malariae*. It is used prophylactically against chloroquine-resistant and mefloquine-resistant falciparum malaria in Thailand and adjacent countries and elsewhere for patients who cannot tolerate mefloquine (Table 35–2). Doxycycline is also used as an adjunct drug with quinine for the treatment of resistant falciparum malaria (Table 35–3). Side effects include infrequent gastrointestinal symptoms (take with meals plus copious amounts of water to avoid esophageal irritation; avoid milk, which reduces absorption); candidal vaginitis (advise carrying a self-treatment antifungal regimen, either vaginal suppositories or cream); and rare photosensitivity (prevention may be achieved by use of sunscreens that absorb ultraviolet radiation and by avoidance of exposure to direct sunlight as much as possible). The drug is contraindicated in pregnancy, in nursing mothers, in children under 8 years of age, and in persons with hepatic dysfunction. No data are available on the long-term use of the drug.

9. Artemisinin (qinghaosu) and its derivatives–Artemisinin and its derivatives are available in some countries but not in the USA. Artemether is administrated intramuscularly, whereas artesunate is given either orally, by intravenous infusion, or by rectal suppository. The drugs are effective against all malarial parasites. No drug resistance has been reported except for a degree of reduced effectiveness in falciparum malaria resistant to mefloquine. The artemisinin drugs are used only to treat acute malaria, for which they are the most rapidly acting of all schizonticides. They are the only drugs that remain reliably effective against *P falciparum* strains resistant to quinine. They are not effective against the liver stage of vivax and malariae malaria, and because of their short half-lives they cannot be used in prophylaxis. Recrudescences are common, however (up to 50%), when the artemisinin drugs are used alone; therefore, they are usually given with another drug (eg, mefloquine). Mild adverse events—symptoms that also occur in malaria—are headache, gastrointestinal symptoms, pruritus, and fever. Animal studies suggest a potential for embryotoxicity (the drug should be avoided in pregnancy when possible) and central nervous system toxicity (in humans, this has not been documented in prospective studies in more than 10,000 patients).

10. Proguanil–Proguanil (chlorguanide, paludrine; not available in the USA), 200 mg/d, is a schizonticide against three of the malaria parasites (unknown degree against *P malariae*) and has some causal prophylactic action. It is used in prophylaxis in combination with chloroquine (0.5 g/wk) in areas with no or low-intensity chloroquine-resistant *P falciparum.* It is not used in treatment, either alone or in combination. Rarely reported side effects are nausea, vomiting, hair loss, and mouth ulcers. The drug is safe to use in pregnancy; it should not be used in persons with hepatic or renal dysfunction.

11. Atovaquone–Atovaquone, active against the liver and blood stages of *P falciparum,* is used in malaria prevention and in treatment of uncomplicated *P falciparum* malaria, resistant or not resistant to chloroquine. Because frequent failures occur (30%) when atovaquone is used alone, it is now combined with other drugs—atovaquone/proguanil (Malarone), 250 mg/100 mg; or atovaquone/doxycycline, 250 mg/100 mg—which results in synergistic antimalarial activity even against proguanil-resistant parasites. Atovaquone's suppressive efficacy against the other malarial parasites is not yet determined; primaquine will be needed to eliminate the liver stages of *P vivax* and *P ovale.* Atovaquone is approved for use in the USA for the treatment of *Pneumocystis carinii* infections but not for malaria. Malarone and proguanil are not available in the USA but are marketed in many countries.

Chemoprophylaxis for Nonimmune Populations

See Table 35–2 for methods and dosages and under the individual drugs (above) for details on cautions, contraindications, and toxicities.

Antimalarials should be taken with water at mealtime. The selected drug should be tested for side effects in advance of departure (to allow time for selection of an alternative drug if necessary) and started sufficiently in advance of exposure that a satisfactory prophylactic blood level is achieved. On returning home, primaquine is given to eradicate persistent liver stages of *P vivax* or *P ovale* if there has been significant exposure to these parasites (see above under Primaquine).

A. Chemoprophylaxis in Regions Where *P falciparum* and *P vivax* Are Sensitive to Chloroquine:

1. Drug of choice–Chloroquine prevents attacks for all forms of malaria and is curative for *P falciparum* and *P malariae* when taken for 4 weeks after leaving the endemic area.

2. Alternative drugs–For persons who cannot tolerate chloroquine, hydroxychloroquine sulfate (400 mg [salt]) can be tried. Other alternative drugs are those used in regions where *P falciparum* is resistant to chloroquine.

Schizonticides *not used for chemoprophylaxis* are halofantrine (erratic absorption and variable bioavailability), Fansidar (hypersensitivity reactions with rare deaths), amodiaquine (agranulocytosis and toxic hepatitis), pyrimethamine (widespread resistance of both *P falciparum* and *P vivax*), artemisinin and related drugs (short duration of action), proguanil (resistance, except in combination with chloroquine or atovaquone), and generally quinine (toxicity).

B. Chemoprophylaxis in Regions Where *P falciparum* Is Resistant to Chloroquine:

1. Drug of choice–Mefloquine is the drug of choice.

2. First alternative–Doxycycline.

3. Second alternative–Newly available for prophylaxis is atovaquone/proguanil (Malarone), 250 mg/100 mg. The combined drug is marketed in some countries but not in the USA.

4. Other alternatives–When daily proguanil (200 mg) is added to weekly chloroquine (0.5 g), more protection is obtained than when chloroquine is used alone. The combination is recommended by some authorities for some countries where chloroquine resistance is uncommon, such as the Indian subcontinent and the Philippines; the combination may still be useful in sub-Saharan Africa, but mefloquine is more reliable. The combination should not be used in Southeast Asia or Papua New Guinea. Continuing under evaluation for prophylaxis and not approved for this indication by FDA in the USA is primaquine taken daily.

C. Chemoprophylaxis in Southeast Asia: Multidrug *P falciparum* resistance is extensive in Southeast Asia. Chloroquine cannot be used throughout the region. Fansidar is not effective in Thailand,

Cambodia, and Myanmar and probably in other areas. Additionally, because of the increasing frequency of mefloquine resistance, doxycycline (100 mg daily) is recommended instead in Thailand, Cambodia, Myanmar, and Papua New Guinea.

D. Prophylaxis for Pregnant Women: Pregnant women should be protected; malaria infection during pregnancy may be particularly severe. Drugs contraindicated in pregnancy are doxycycline and primaquine. Therefore, the best course is weekly chloroquine (or hydroxychloroquine) with or without proguanil. In areas of chloroquine-resistant malaria, mefloquine can be used except in the first trimester.

E. Emergency Self Treatment: In selected instances, medication should be provided for emergency self-treatment of breakthrough attacks (see above).

Treatment of Acute Attacks

See under individual drugs and Table 35–3 for dosages.

A. General Considerations: It is important to determine whether a patient has been treated with antimalarials in the previous 1–2 days (3 weeks for mefloquine because of its slow excretion) to avoid the risk of overdose or adverse drug interactions. In the event of mefloquine prophylaxis or treatment failure, it is hazardous—although it may be essential—to use quinine, quinidine, or halofantrine (Table 35–3); under these circumstances, apparently the safest drug to use is artemisinin or one of its derivatives, which are available in some countries.

In falciparum malaria, indications for parenteral treatment are (1) failure to retain ingested drugs, (2) cerebral malaria, (3) multiple complications, and (4) a peripheral asexual parasitemia of 5% (250,000/μL) or higher. Patients with falciparum malaria should be hospitalized to observe for therapeutic response. As frequently as possible, the following should be monitored: vital signs, coma score, glucose level, lactate level, arterial pH, blood gases, urine output, and blood urea nitrogen. It is essential to determine the density of parasites on the blood smear (as a measure of severity of infection) and to recheck at least twice daily. Within 48–72 hours after start of treatment, patients usually become afebrile and improve clinically; within 48 hours, parasitemia is generally reduced by about 75% (though there may be an initial increase during the first 6–12 hours). If there is no improvement within 48–72 hours for mild infections or 24 hours for severe ones or if there is increasing asexual parasitemia after 1–2 days (in the presence of adequate drug ingestion and retention), parasite resistance to the drug must be assumed and treatment changed.

B. Treatment of All Forms of Malaria Except *P falciparum* and *P vivax* Strains Resistant to Chloroquine: (Table 35–3)

1. Elimination of asexual erythrocytic parasites–Infection by all four species of malaria is treated with oral chloroquine. Alternative oral drugs if chloroquine cannot be tolerated—or if the *P vivax* strain is resistant to chloroquine—are mefloquine, quinine sulfate (plus doxycycline, clindamycin, or Fansidar), atovaquone (plus doxycycline or proguanil*), halofantrine*, or artemisinin or its derivatives*. For *P vivax* and *P ovale* infections, a course of primaquine must follow to eliminate the liver stages.

If the patient is severely ill, treat with intravenous quinine dihydrochloride* or quinidine gluconate, parenteral preparations of artemisinin derivatives*, or parenteral chloroquine. Start oral therapy with chloroquine as soon as possible.

2. Eradication of *P vivax* or *P ovale* infections–This is accomplished with a standard course of primaquine (Table 35–3) except in regions of rare partial resistance, where a higher dosage or longer course of treatment is needed (see above).

3. Elimination of persistent gametocytemia–Gametocytes of *P vivax*, *P ovale*, and *P malariae* can be eliminated by chloroquine. Gametocytes of *P falciparum* are eliminated by a single dose of 26.3 mg of primaquine salt.

4. Treatment of semi-immunes–Treatment of attacks in semi-immune patients generally requires shorter courses of drug treatment.

C. Treatment of Falciparum Malaria Acquired in Areas Where *P falciparum* Is Resistant to Chloroquine: Start treatment with oral quinine sulfate and a second drug (Table 35–3) (but not Fansidar if the infection was acquired in an area with Fansidar resistance). Alternative drugs are mefloquine, halofantrine*, artesunate* (followed by mefloquine), or atovaquone (combined with proguanil or doxycycline). In Southeast Asia, mefloquine and halofantrine cannot be used because of multidrug resistance.

If the patient is severely ill, treat with intravenous quinine or quinidine (Table 35–3). A second drug (doxycycline or clindamycin) should also be given parenterally. Oral treatment with quinine plus the antibiotic should be started as soon as possible. An alternative approach is parenteral artesunate* followed by mefloquine (not effective in Southeast Asia).

D. Special Measures for Treatment of Severe *P falciparum* Malaria: (See references for further details.) Severe and complicated falciparum malaria is a medical emergency that requires hospitalization, intensive care and the initiation of intravenous chemotherapy as rapidly as possible. In patients requiring more than 48 hours of parenteral therapy, reduce the quinine or quinidine dose by one-third to one-half. Rehydration of the patient should be done with great caution, particularly in the first 24 hours, since overhydration may precipitate noncardiogenic pulmonary edema. Fluid, electrolyte, and

*Not available in the USA but available in some countries.

acid-base balance must be monitored. In general, 2–3 L of fluid is required the first day, followed by 10–20 mL/kg/d; intake and output should be carefully recorded. After rehydration, the central venous pressure should be maintained at approximately 5 cm of water (pulmonary artery occlusion pressure < 15 mm Hg). Early dialysis may be necessary for renal failure and then sustained for 4–7 days or longer. Blood glucose levels should be monitored every 6 hours during the acute and early convalescent period, since hypoglycemia may be severe, either as a result of the malaria infection or the use of quinine or quinidine; treatment is with 50% dextrose (1–2 mL/kg) followed by maintenance infusion of 5–10% dextrose. Patients with clinically significant disseminated intravascular coagulation should be treated with fresh whole blood. Hematocrit levels below 20% require transfusion. Anticonvulsants (eg, phenobarbital, diazepam) are used for seizures; the temperature is maintained below 38.5 °C. Bacterial infections are common (eg, pneumonia, cystitis, salmonellosis); acetaminophen can be used as an antipyretic. Exchange transfusion (5–10 L for adults) is used when more than 15% of red blood cells are parasitized (5% if severe dysfunction of other organs is present), but there is no evidence that exchange transfusion increases survival. Corticosteroids, heparin, and aspirin have been shown to be deleterious in cerebral malaria and should not be used.

Follow-Up for *P falciparum* Malaria

Blood films should be checked daily until parasitemia clears; check weekly thereafter for 4 weeks to observe for recrudescence of infection.

Prognosis

The uncomplicated and untreated primary attack of *P vivax, P ovale,* or *P falciparum* malaria usually lasts 2–4 weeks; that of *P malariae* about twice as long. Attacks of each type of infection may subsequently recur (once or many times) before the infection terminates spontaneously. With prompt antimalarial therapy, the prognosis is generally good, but in *P falciparum* infections, when severe complications such as cerebral malaria develop, the prognosis is poor even with treatment. It is now recognized that after cerebral malaria, residual neurologic deficits can occur.

Baird JK et al: Prevention of malaria in travelers. Med Clin North Am 1999;83:923. [NLM Cit ID: 99382629]

Fradin MS: Mosquitoes and mosquito repellent: A clinician's guide. Ann Intern Med 1998;128:931. [NLM Cit ID: 98285338]

Health information for international travel. 1999–2000. HHS Publication. For sale from the Superintendent of Documents, U.S. Government Printing Office, Washington, DC 20402. Telephone: 202-512-1800.

International Travel and Health: *Vaccination Certificate Requirements and Health Advice.* WHO, 2000.

McIntosh HM et al: Treatment of uncomplicated malaria with artemisinin derivatives. A systematic review of randomised controlled trials. Med Trop (Mars) 1998;58(3 Suppl):57. [NLM Cit ID: 99229370] (A review of the evidence for this herb turned prescription drug.)

Newton P et al: Malaria: new developments in treatment and prevention. Ann Rev Med 1999;50:179. [NLM Cit ID: 99172926]

Prevention of malaria. Med Lett Drugs Ther 2000;42:8. [NLM Cit ID: 20161222]

Price R et al: Adverse effects in patients with acute falciparum malaria treated with artemisinin derivatives. Am J Trop Med Hyg 1999;60:547. [NLM Cit ID: 99275983]

Schlagenhauf P: Mefloquine for malaria chemoprophylaxis 1992–1998: a review. J Travel Med 1999;6:122. [NLM Cit ID: 99316447]

Shanks GD et al: Efficacy and safety of atovaquone/proguanil as suppressive prophylaxis for *Plasmodium falciparum* malaria. Clin Infect Dis 1998;27:494. [NLM Cit ID: 99842282]

Soto J et al: Primaquine prophylaxis against malaria in nonimmune Colombian soldiers: Efficacy and toxicity. A randomized double-blind placebo controlled trial. Ann Intern Med 1998;129:241. [NLM Cit ID: 98348299]

van Vugt M et al: The treatment of chloroquine-resistant malaria. Trop Doct 1999;29:176. [NLM Cit ID: 99377358]

TOXOPLASMOSIS

Essentials of Diagnosis

Acute primary infection:

- Fever, malaise, headache, lymphadenopathy (especially cervical), myalgia, arthralgia, stiff neck, sore throat; occasionally, rash, hepatosplenomegaly, retinochoroiditis, confusion; in various combinations.
- Positive serologic tests with high and rising IgG and IgM.
- Isolation of *Toxoplasma gondii* from blood or body fluids; tachyzoites in histologic sections of tissue or cytologic preparations of body fluids.

Acute primary or recrudescent infection in immunocompromised patients:

- Central nervous system mass lesions; retinochoroiditis, pneumonitis, myocarditis less common; sometimes other findings as above.
- Positive IgG titers moderately high; IgM antibody usually absent. Tissue diagnosis as above.

General Considerations

T gondii, an obligate intracellular protozoan, is found worldwide in humans and in many species of animals and birds. The parasite is a coccidian of cats, the definitive host, and exists in three forms: The *trophozoite* (tachyzoite) (3 × 7 µm) is the rapidly proliferating form in tissues and body fluids that causes acute disease. The trophozoites can enter and multiply in most mammalian nucleated cells. The *cyst,* containing viable bradyzoites, is the latent form that can persist indefinitely as a chronic infection and is found particularly in muscle and nerve tissue. The *oocyst* is the form passed only in the feces of the cat family. In the intestinal epithelium of cats, a sexual cycle occurs, with subsequent release of oocysts for 3–14 days; cats may, however, become reinfected and excrete oocysts multiple times. The oocysts, which contain infective sporozoites, are infectious within 12 hours to several days after passage and can remain infective in moist soil for weeks or months.

Human infection results (1) from ingestion of cysts in raw or undercooked meat; (2) from ingestion of oocysts in contaminated food or water, by careless handling of contaminated cat litter, or from soil by soil-eating children; (3) from transplacental transmission of trophozoites; or (4) rarely , from direct inoculation of trophozoites, as in blood transfusion. Reservoirs of human infection are rodents and birds eaten by cats and infected domestic animals used for food. Antibody prevalence rates range from less than 5% in some parts of the world (absence of cats and minimal ingestion of meat) to 3–55% in the USA and over 80% in France.

On ingestion, bradyzoites (from cysts) or sporozoites (from oocysts) invade multiple cells types and propagate as trophozoites; cell death and inflammation follow, but true granulomas do not form.

Clinical Findings

A. Symptoms and Signs: Over 80% of primary infections are asymptomatic. The incubation period for symptomatic persons is 1–2 weeks. Generally, on recovery, both asymptomatic and symptomatic infections persist as chronic latent (cyst) infections. Reactivation occurs almost exclusively in severely immunocompromised patients.

The clinical manifestations of toxoplasmosis may be grouped into four syndromes:

1. Primary infection in the immunocompetent host–Most symptomatic infections are acute, mild, febrile multisystem illnesses that resemble infectious mononucleosis. Lymphadenopathy, usually nontender, particularly of the head and neck, is the most common finding. Other features in various combinations are malaise, myalgia, arthralgia, headache, sore throat, and maculopapular or urticarial rash. Hepatosplenomegaly may occur. Rarely, severe cases are complicated by pneumonitis, meningoencephalitis, hepatitis, myocarditis, and retinochoroiditis. Symptoms may fluctuate, but most patients recover spontaneously within a few months.

2. Congenital infection–Congenital transmission occurs only as a result of infection (generally asymptomatic) in a nonimmune woman during pregnancy. Infection has been detected in up to 1% of women during pregnancy; 15–60% of such infections, the incidence varying by trimester, are transmitted to the fetus, but only a small percentage result in abortions or stillbirths or in active disease in premature or full-term, live-born infants. Though fetal infection may occur in any trimester, it is more severe early in pregnancy. Among all congenital infections, less than 15% show severe brain or eye damage at birth; however, of the apparently normal newborns, more than 85% will develop brain or eye sequelae later in life. Treatment of the mother reduces the congenital infection rate by about 60%. See specialized sources for clinical manifestations and approach to diagnosis.

3. Retinochoroiditis–This develops gradually weeks to years after congenital infection (the preponderant form, which is generally bilateral) or rarely after an acquired infection in a young child (generally unilateral). Acquired infections in older children and adults rarely progress to retinochoroiditis. The inflammatory process persists for weeks to months as focally necrotic retinal lesions (yellow or white patches with blurred margins). Visual defects, which include blurring, central defects, and scotomas, are accompanied by pain and photophobia. Rarely, progression may result in glaucoma and blindness. With healing, white or dark-pigmented scars may result. Panuveitis may accompany retinochoroiditis.

4. Reactivated disease in the immunologically compromised host–Reactivated toxoplasmosis occurs in patients with AIDS, cancer, or those given immunosuppressive drugs. The infection may present in specific organs (brain, lungs, and eye most commonly, but also heart, skin, gastrointestinal tract, and liver) or as disseminated disease. Between 30% and 50% of AIDS patients seropositive for past toxoplasma infection will develop focal or (less often) diffuse intracerebral toxoplasma lesions, associated with clinical findings of fever, headache, altered mental status, seizures, and focal (or, infrequently, nonfocal) neurologic deficits (see also Chapter 31).

B. Laboratory Findings: Diagnosis depends principally on serologic tests, which are sensitive and reliable. However, diagnosis is occasionally made from tissue (blood, bone marrow aspirates, cerebrospinal fluid sediment, sputum, and other tissues or body fluids or placental tissue) either histologically (demonstration of trophozoites or characteristic histology) or by isolation of the organism in mice or tissue culture.

1. Histology–Cysts or trophozoites may be directly identified in blood (buffy coat from centrifuged heparinized blood), other tissues, or body fluids by staining with standard stains or with specific antibody marked with fluorescein or enzyme. Demonstration of cysts does not establish a causal relationship to clinical illness, since cysts may be found in both acute and chronic infections. However, finding tachyzoites confirms active infection. In the placenta, fetus, or newborn, the presence of cysts does indicate congenital infection.

2. Serologic tests–The Sabin-Feldman dye test, indirect hemagglutination, indirect immunofluorescence (IFA), ELISA, and other tests can be done on blood, cerebrospinal fluid, aqueous humor, and other body fluids. The dye test is the standard but is rarely used because of laboratory safety factors; though extremely sensitive and specific, it does not separate IgM from IgG antibody. The ELISA, immunosorbent, and IFA tests do separate IgM and IgG antibody. In the IFA test for IgM, antibody appears 1–2 weeks after start of infection, reaches a peak at 6–8 weeks, and then gradually declines over 6 months. However, in the IgM capture test, IgM persists up to 6 years. IgM is absent in chronic infection. Maternal IgM is normally unable to cross the intact placenta; antibody which does pass through a leak has a half-life of only 3–5 days. IgG antibody persists for life in most patients. False-positive and false-negative tests can occur with the IFA test; the former can be avoided by use of IgM capture tests. Other tests that may be useful for patients who, after 3 months, continue to have low-positive, equivocal, or negative IgM titers are the IgA-ELISA and IgE tests by ELISA and immunosorbent agglutination assay. Using various body fluids, diagnosis by polymerase chain reaction or by detection of antigen or of nucleic acid sequences specific for *T gondii* is highly promising, especially for early diagnosis and to avoid invasive procedures.

The following are selected serologic and other findings in specific toxoplasmosis syndromes:

a. Acute infection in immunocompetent persons–The diagnosis is established by seroconversion from negative to positive, by a fourfold rise in serologic titers by any test, or by a single high titer (1:160) of IgM antibody. A presumptive diagnosis is based on a single IgM titer of over 1:64 and a very high IgG titer (> 1:1000). The diagnosis of acute toxoplasmosis is excluded if the dye test and an IgM test are negative for 3 months after onset of symptoms.

b. Recrudescent infection in immunosuppressed patients–In AIDS patients, toxoplasma can sometimes be isolated from the blood. Alternatively, definitive diagnosis is only by finding toxoplasma organisms in cerebrospinal fluid (Wright-Giemsa stain) or by brain biopsy. To avoid the latter, empirical antibiotic treatment is generally started after presumptive evidence is obtained by MRI (the more sensitive test) or CT scan (typically: multiple, isodense or hypodense, ring-enhancing mass lesions). Antibody titers cannot be depended on, since most patients have IgG titers that reflect past infection, significant rises are infrequent, and IgM antibody is rare. Absence of IgG does not rule out the diagnosis of central nervous system toxoplasmosis. The cerebrospinal fluid may show mild pleocytosis (predominantly lymphocytes and monocytes), elevated protein, and normal glucose. (See also Chapter 31.)

c. Toxoplasmic retinochoroiditis–This is usually associated with stable, usually low IgG titers and no IgM antibody. If IgG antibody in aqueous humor is higher than in the serum, the diagnosis is supported.

d. Congenital infection–The most useful tests for confirmation of fetal infection are ultrasound examination, amniocentesis for detection of toxoplasma DNA in amniotic fluid, and cordocentesis for detection of IgM-specific antibody. A negative result for IgM antibody does not exclude the diagnosis. IgG-specific antibody is nearly always present if the mother is positive, but that passively transferred antibody disappears in 6–12 months.

3. Other laboratory findings–Leukocyte counts are normal or reduced, often with lymphocytosis or monocytosis with rare atypical cells, but there is no heterophil antibody. Chest radiographs may show interstitial pneumonia. In cerebral imaging studies in HIV-infected persons, toxoplasmosis typically appears as multiple lesions with a predilection for the basal ganglion.

Differential Diagnosis

In acute febrile disease, consider cytomegalovirus infection, infectious mononucleosis, and other causes of pneumonitis, myocarditis, myositis, hepatitis, and splenomegaly. With lymphadenopathy, possibilities include sarcoidosis, tuberculosis, tularemia, lymphoma, cat-scratch disease, and metastatic carcinoma. With brain lesions in the immunosuppressed host, consider lymphoma, tuberculoma, brain abscess, metastatic carcinoma, and fungal lesions.

Treatment

A. Approach to Treatment: In immunocompetent hosts, asymptomatic infections are not treated except in children under 5 years of age. Symptomatic patients should be treated until manifestations of the illness have subsided and there is serologic evidence that immunity has been acquired.

Since most episodes of retinochoroiditis are self-limited, opinions vary on indications for and type of treatment. (See specialized texts.)

Immunocompromised patients with active infection (primary or recrudescent) must be treated. Therapy should continue for 4–6 weeks after cessation of symptoms—which may require up to a 6-month course, to be followed by drug prophylaxis as long as immunosuppression persists. In HIV-infected persons, acute toxoplasmosis must be treated followed by continued prophylaxis; in patients who have a positive IgG toxoplasma serology but are asymptomatic for the infection, toxoplasmosis prophylaxis is desirable. (See Chapter 31 for treatment.)

During pregnancy, because early treatment reduces (but does not eliminate) the incidence of fetal infection, most workers feel that treatment is justified in spite of the potential for drug toxicity on the fetus.

Congenitally infected newborns should be treated. For details on management of congenital infections and infections in pregnancy, see specialized sources.

B. Choice of Drugs: The treatment of choice in nonimmunocompromised patients is pyrimethamine, 25–100 mg once daily, plus either trisulfapyrimidines (4–6 g/d in four divided doses) or sulfadiazine, 1–1.5 g four times daily; continue this treatment for 3–4 weeks. Patients should be screened for a history of sulfonamide sensitivity (skin rashes, gastrointestinal symptoms, hepatotoxicity); to prevent crystal-induced nephrotoxicity, good urine output should be maintained (alkalinization with sodium bicarbonate may also be useful). Pyrimethamine side effects include headache and gastrointestinal symptoms; folinic acid (calcium leucovorin), 10 mg/d in two divided doses, is given to avoid the hematologic effects of pyrimethamine-induced folate deficiency. Platelet and white blood cell counts should be performed at least twice weekly. Clindamycin (600 mg four times daily) may be a useful alternative drug; because it concentrates in the choroid, it is also used in the treatment of ocular disease. Other macrolides, atovaquone (750 mg three or four times daily), and immunotherapy are under evaluation.

In toxoplasmosis in pregnancy, spiramycin is given at a dosage of 3–4 g in four divided doses for 4–6 weeks. The drug is not effective in other forms of the infection. In the USA, the drug is available from the manufacturer.

For the treatment of central nervous system toxoplasmosis in HIV-infected persons, see Chapters 24 and 31.

Prevention

Freezing of meat to –20 °C for 2 days or heating to 60 °C for 4 minutes kills cysts in tissues. Under appropriate environmental conditions, oocysts passed in cat feces can remain infective for a year or more. Thus, children's play areas, including sandboxes, should be protected from cat (and dog) feces; hand washing is indicated after contact with soil potentially contaminated by animal feces. Indoor cats should be fed only dry, canned, or cooked meat. Litter boxes should be changed daily, as freshly deposited oocysts are not infective for 48 hours.

Pregnant women should have their serum examined for toxoplasma antibody. If the IgM test is negative but an IgG titer is present and less than 1:1000, no further evaluation is necessary. Those with negative titers should take measures to prevent infection—preferably by having no further contact with cats and cat litter, by thoroughly cooking meat, and by hand washing after handling raw meat and before eating or touching the face. For seronegative women who continue to have significant environmental exposure, serologic screening should be conducted several times during pregnancy.

Prognosis

The outlook for acute toxoplasmosis in adults is excellent as long as the patient is immunocompetent. In immunosuppressed patients, the disease is usually fatal if untreated; improvement results if treatment is started early, but recrudescence is common. Chronic asymptomatic infection is usually benign.

Beazley DM et al: Toxoplasmosis. Semin Perinatol 1998;22:332. [NLM Cit ID: 98409378] (Review of toxoplasmosis in pregnancy.)

Bou G et al: Value of PCR for detection of *Toxoplasma gondii* in aqueous humor and blood samples from immunocompetent patients with ocular toxoplasmosis. J Clin Microbiol 1999;37:3465. [NLM Cit ID: 99454829]

Holland GN: Reconsidering the pathogenesis of ocular toxoplasmosis. Am J Ophthalmol 1999;128:502. [NLM Cit ID: 20043525]

Roberts F et al: Pathogenesis of toxoplasmic retinochoroiditis. Parasitol Today 1999;15:51. [NLM Cit ID: 20038366]

Torre D et al: Randomized trial of trimethoprim-sulfamethoxazole versus pyrimethamine-sulfadiazine for therapy of toxoplasmic encephalitis in patients with AIDS. Antimicrob Ag Chemother 1998;42:1346. [NLM Cit ID: 98287569]

Vergani P et al: Congenital toxoplasmosis: Efficacy of maternal treatment with spiramycin alone. Am J Reprod Immunol 1998 39:335. [NLM Cit ID: 98264962]

II. HELMINTHIC INFECTIONS

TREMATODE (FLUKE) INFECTIONS

SCHISTOSOMIASIS (Bilharziasis)

Essentials of Diagnosis

- Exposure to infection in an endemic area.
- Acute phase: Abrupt onset (2–6 weeks postexposure) of abdominal pain, weight loss, headache, malaise, chills, fever, myalgia, diarrhea (sometimes bloody), dry cough, hepatomegaly, and eosinophilia
- Chronic phase: Either (1) diarrhea, abdominal pain, blood in stool, hepatomegaly or hepatosplenomegaly, and bleeding from esophageal varices (*Schistosoma mansoni* or *Schistosoma japonicum* infection); or (2) terminal hematuria, urinary frequency, and urethral and bladder pain (*Schistosoma haematobium* infection).
- Depending on species, characteristic eggs in feces, urine, or scrapings or biopsy of rectal or bladder mucosa.

General Considerations

Schistosomiasis, which infects more than 200 million persons worldwide, induces severe consequences in 20 million persons annually, resulting in up to 200,000 deaths. The disease is caused mainly by three blood flukes (trematodes). *S mansoni,* which causes intestinal schistosomiasis, is widespread in Africa and occurs in the Arabian peninsula, South America (Brazil, Venezuela, Suriname), and the Caribbean (including Puerto Rico but not Cuba). Vesical (urinary) schistosomiasis, caused by *S haematobium*, is found throughout the Middle East and Africa. Asiatic intestinal schistosomiasis, due to *S japonicum,* is important in China and the Philippines, and a small focus is present in Sulawesi, Indonesia, but transmission in Japan has been interrupted. A number of schistosome species of animals sometimes infect humans, including *Schistosoma intercalatum* in central Africa and *Schistosoma mekongi* in the Mekong delta in Thailand, Cambodia, and Laos. In the USA, an estimated 400,000 immigrants are infected, but transmission does not occur.

Mammals are important reservoirs for *S japonicum.* Humans are the main reservoir for *S mansoni* and *S haematobium;* the few animal species infected with *S mansoni* are not epidemiologically important.

In the life cycle involving humans, the adult worms live in terminal venules of the bowel *(S mansoni, S japonicum)* or bladder *(S haematobium).* When eggs passed in feces or urine reach fresh water, a larval form is released that subsequently infects snails, the intermediate host. After development, infective larvae (cercariae) leave the snails, enter water, and infect exposed persons through the skin or mucous membranes. After penetration, the cercariae become schistosomula larvae that reach the portal circulation in the liver, where they rapidly mature. After a few weeks, adult worms pair, mate, and migrate mainly to terminal venules of specific veins, where females deposit their eggs. By means of lytic secretions, some eggs reach the lumen of the bowel or bladder and are passed with feces or urine. Others are retained in the bowel or bladder wall, while still others are carried in the circulation to the liver, lung, and (less often) to other tissues.

Except for the allergic response in the acute syndrome (see below), disease is primarily due to delayed hypersensitivity. Antigens released by the eggs stimulate a local T cell-dependent granulomatous response, followed by a strong fibrotic reaction. Live worms produce no lesions and rarely cause symptoms. The type or degree of tissue damage and symptoms varies with the intensity of infection (worm burden), host genetic factors, site of egg deposition, concurrent infection (eg, hepatitis B), and duration of infection.

S mansoni adults migrate to the inferior mesenteric veins of the large bowel and *S japonicum* to the superior and inferior mesenteric veins in the large and small bowel. Ulcers and polyps (common only in Egypt) result from granuloma formation and fibrosis in the bowel wall. Egg accumulation in the liver may result in periportal fibrosis and portal hypertension of the presinusoidal type, but liver function typically remains intact even in advanced disease. Portal-systemic collateralization due to portal hypertension can result in embolization of eggs to the lungs, with subsequent endarteritis, pulmonary hypertension, and cor pulmonale. Because greater numbers of eggs are produced by *S japonicum,* the resulting disease is often more severe.

Adult *S haematobium* mature in the venous plexus of the bladder, ureters, rectum, prostate, and uterus. Ulcers and polyps result from granuloma formation and fibrosis in the bladder wall, and eggshell remnants may calcify. Stricture or distortion of the ureteral orifices or terminal ureters may result in hydroureter, hydronephrosis, and ascending infection. Lesions in the pelvic organs rarely progress to extensive fibrosis and infection. Eggs are carried to the liver or lungs, but severe pathologic changes in these organs are less frequent than in *S mansoni* and *S japonicum* infections.

In size, adult *S mansoni* are 6–13 × 1 mm. The prepatent period—from cercarial penetration until appearance of eggs in feces—is about 50 days. The life span of the worms ranges from 5 to 30 years or more.

Clinical Findings

A. Symptoms and Signs: Although a large proportion of infected persons have light infections (< 100 eggs per gram of feces) and are asymptomatic, an estimated 50–60% have symptoms and 5–10% advanced organ damage. In children, schistosomal infections may contribute to decreased nutritional status and growth retardation. Persons with concomitant AIDS and schistosomiasis can be treated effectively and safely for the latter infection.

1. Cercarial dermatitis–Following cercarial penetration, clinical findings progress from a localized itchy erythematous or petechial rash to macules and papules that last up to 5 days. Most cases occur in fresh or marine water (worldwide) and are due to skin invasion by bird schistosome cercariae, parasites that do not mature in humans and do not cause systemic symptoms. The syndrome is uncommon with human schistosome infections.

2. Acute schistosomiasis (Katayama fever)– This syndrome, primarily an allergic response to the developing schistosomes, may occur with the three schistosomes (rare with *S haematobium*) and usually is not seen in natives. The incubation period is 2–7 weeks; the severity of illness ranges from mild to (rarely) life-threatening. In addition to fever, malaise, urticaria, diarrhea (sometimes bloody), myalgia, dry cough, leukocytosis, and marked eosinophilia, the liver and spleen may be temporarily enlarged. The patient again becomes asymptomatic in 2–8 weeks.

Early in the infection, stool examination may be negative (examinations should be repeated for at least 6 months) but serologic tests positive. Controversy continues about whether praziquantel plus corticosteroids are safe and effective in treatment of acute disease.

3. Chronic schistosomiasis–This stage begins 6 months to several years after infection. In *S mansoni* and *S japonicum* infections, findings include diarrhea, abdominal pain, irregular bowel movements, blood in the stool, a hard enlarged liver, and splenomegaly. With subsequent slow progression over 5–15 years or longer, the following may appear: anorexia, weight loss, weakness, polypoid intestinal tumors, and features of portal and pulmonary hypertension. Immune complex glomerulonephritis may also occur.

In *S haematobium* infection, early symptoms of urinary tract disease are frequency and dysuria, followed by terminal hematuria and proteinuria. Frank hematuria may be recurrent. Sequelae may include bladder polyp formation, cystitis, chronic salmonella infection, pyelitis, pyelonephritis, urolithiasis, hydronephrosis due to ureteral obstruction, renal failure, and death. Severe liver, lung, genital, or neurologic disease is rare. Bladder cancer has been associated with vesicular schistosomiasis.

4. Other complications–Portal hypertension may result in a contracted liver, splenomegaly, pancytopenia, esophageal varices, and variceal bleeding. Abnormal liver function, jaundice, ascites, and hepatic coma are end-stage findings. Pulmonary hypertension with cor pulmonale and edema due to right heart failure may supervene. Other large bowel complications include stricture, granulomatous masses, and persistent salmonella infection; colonic polyposis is manifested by bloody diarrhea, anemia, hypoalbuminemia, and clubbing. Transverse myelitis, epilepsy, or optic neuritis may result from collateral circulation of eggs or ectopic worms.

B. Laboratory Findings: Screening is by testing for eggs (ova) and occult blood in feces and urine (the excretion of which may be irregular and require repeated testing), for protein and leukocytes in urine, and by serology. Ova must be examined for internal detail or by the hatching test to determine that some are alive and that the infection therefore warrants treatment.

1. Eggs–Definitive diagnosis is by finding characteristic live eggs in excreta or mucosal biopsy.

In *S haematobium* infection, eggs may be found in the urine or, less frequently, in the stools. Eggs are sought in urine specimens collected between 9 AM and 2 PM or in 24-hour collections. They are processed either by examination of the sediment or preferably by membrane filtration. Occasionally, eggs are sought by vesical mucosa biopsy.

In *S mansoni* and *S japonicum* infections, eggs may be found in stool specimens by direct examination, but some form of concentration is usually necessary; the Kato-Katz quantitative method is preferred over formal ether concentration. One stool examination can reach 70% sensitivity and four, 92%. If results are negative, rectal mucosal biopsy of inflamed or granulomatous lesions or random biopsy specimens at two or three sites of normal mucosa may yield the diagnosis. Biopsy specimens should be examined as crush preparations between two glass slides and also examined histologically. If eggs are found, a quantitative test should be done after collecting a 24-hour urine or stool; heavy infections are those with counts over 400 eggs per gram.

2. Serologic tests–ELISA, immunoblot, and other tests are used in screening and may detect some egg-negative or ectopic infections. Deficiencies of the tests are that they are commonly negative early in infection and, as they remain positive for long periods of time, do not distinguish active from past infection. The Centers for Disease Control and Prevention uses a "fast ELISA" for screening (sensitivity and specificity = 99%) and a Western blot (specificity = 100%) for confirmation and speciation. Evidence is increasing that detection of antigen in blood and urine is a sensitive test, can distinguish old from new infection, and that loss of circulating antigen 5–10 days after treatment is indicative of cure. Skin testing is no longer recommended.

3. Other tests–Anemia is common. Eosinophilia, common during the acute stage, usually is absent in the chronic stage. In *S mansoni* and *S japonicum* infections, barium swallow, esophagoscopy, barium enema or colonoscopy, chest x-ray, or an ECG may be indicated. Ultrasound examination of the liver may show the pathognomonic pattern of periportal fibrosis and replaces the need for liver biopsy. The clinical settings in which ultrasonography is most useful are (1) early detection of hepatic lesions, (2) evaluation of portal hypertension, (3) distinguishing schistosomiasis from cirrhosis, and (4) documenting regression of lesions following treatment.

In *S haematobium* infection, occult hematuria can often be detected either microscopically or by reagent strip test, particularly if the first portion of the urine specimen is evaluated. In advanced disease, cystoscopy may show "sandy patches," ulcers, and areas of squamous metaplasia; lower abdominal plain films may show calcification of the bladder wall or ureters. Sonography is considered the imaging technique of choice but may fail to show the calcification. CT—which may demonstrate pathognomonic "turtleback" calcifications—intravenous pyelography, and retrograde cystography and pyelography may be useful.

Differential Diagnosis

Early intestinal schistosomiasis may be mistaken for amebiasis, bacillary dysentery, or other causes of diarrhea and dysentery. Later, the various causes of portal hypertension or of bowel polyps must be considered. In endemic areas, vesical schistosomiasis must be differentiated from other causes of urinary symptoms such as genitourinary tract cancer, bacterial infections of the urinary tract, nephrolithiasis, and the like.

Treatment

A. Medical Treatment: Treatment should be given only if live ova are identified. The safety and effectiveness of current drugs make it possible to treat all active infections orally, including advanced disease, and without concern for serious side effects. Praziquantel can be used to treat all species; alternative drugs of choice are oxamniquine for *S mansoni* and metrifonate for *S haematobium.* Under study are the use of artemisinin and its derivatives for prophylaxis and treatment of acute attacks. Instances of both oxamniquine and praziquantel resistance have been recognized in some localities.

After treatment, periodic laboratory follow-up for continued passage of eggs is essential, starting at 3 months and continuing at intervals for 1 year; if found, viability should be determined, since dead eggs are passed for some months.

1. Praziquantel–Cure rates at 6 months for *S haematobium, S mansoni,* and *S japonicum* infections are 95%, 90%, and 80%, respectively, with marked reduction in egg counts in those not cured. Immature schistosomes (2–5 weeks) are largely insensitive to praziquantel.

The praziquantel dosage is 20 mg/kg—give twice in 1 day for *S haematobium* and *S mansoni* and three times in 1 day for *S japonicum.* The dosages should be given at 4- to 6-hour intervals with water after a meal; the tablets should not be chewed.

Mild and transient side effects persisting for hours to 1 day are common and include malaise, headache, dizziness, and anorexia. Less frequent are fatigue, drowsiness, nausea, vomiting, generalized abdominal pain, loose stools, pruritus, urticaria, arthralgia and myalgia, and low-grade fever. Minimal elevations of liver enzymes have occasionally been reported. The drug should not be used in pregnancy, and because of drug-induced dizziness, patients should not drive and should be cautioned if their work requires physical coordination or alertness. In areas where cysticercosis may coexist with a schistosomal infection being treated with praziquantel, treatment is best conducted in a hospital to monitor for death of cysticerci, which may be followed by neurologic complications. Recently reported for praziquantel are comutagenic effects with several mutagens and carcinogens; the authors conclude that the import of these findings needs further study.

2. Metrifonate–Metrifonate is a highly effective alternative drug for the treatment of *S haematobium* infections only. The dosage is 7.5–10 mg/kg (maximum 600 mg) once and then repeated twice at 2-week intervals. Cure rates range from 44% to 93%. Those not cured show marked reduction in egg counts. Side effects range from none to mild and transient findings, including gastrointestinal symptoms, headache, bronchospasm, weakness, and vertigo. Metrifonate is not available in the USA.

3. Oxamniquine is highly effective only in *S mansoni* infections. For strains in the western hemisphere and western Africa, a dose of 12–15 mg/kg is given once. In Africa and the Arabian peninsula, some experts recommend 40–60 mg/kg/d in two or three divided doses for 2–3 days. The drug is administered with food; when divided doses are needed, they are separated by 6–8 hours. Cure rates are 70–95%, with marked reduction in egg counts in those not cured. Side effects occur within hours: dizziness is most common; less frequent are drowsiness, nausea and vomiting, diarrhea, abdominal pain, and headache. An orange or red discoloration of the urine may occur. Rarely reported is central nervous system stimulation with behavioral changes, hallucinations, or seizures; patients should be observed for 2 hours after ingestion of the drug for appearance of these findings. Since the drug makes some patients dizzy or drowsy, it should be used with caution in patients whose work or activity requires mental alertness. Instances of parasite resistance to the drug have been reported. Because the drug has shown mutagenic and embryotoxic effects, it is contraindicated in pregnancy.

B. Surgical Measures: In selected instances, surgery may be indicated for removal of polyps and for obstructive uropathy. For bleeding esophageal varices, sclerotherapy is the treatment of choice. Whether some patients may benefit from propranolol treatment is under evaluation. As a last resort in patients who have repeated bleeding, shunting procedures (esophagogastric devascularization with splenectomy or distal—but not proximal—splenorenal shunt) are used, though their effectiveness and relative usefulness are not well established. Severe pancytopenia is an indication for splenectomy.

Prognosis

With treatment, the prognosis is excellent in early and light infections. There may be shrinkage or elimination of bladder and bowel ulcerations, granulomas, and polyps and reduction in fibrosis by sonography. In advanced disease with extensive involvement of the intestines, liver, bladder, or other organs, the outlook is poor even with treatment. In endemic areas, mass treatment of children diminishes the risk of developing severely diseased organs, even though reinfection may occur.

Cioli D: Chemotherapy of schistosomiasis: An update. Parasitology Today 1998;14:418.

Cummings JF: Metrifonate: Overview of safety and efficacy. Pharmacotherapy 1998;18:43. [NLM Cit ID: 98202466]

El-Garem AA: Schistosomiasis. Digestion 1998;59:589. [NLM Cit ID: 98370943]

Feldmeier H et al: Therapeutic and operational profiles of metrifonate and praziquantel in *Schistosoma haematobium* infection. Arzneimittelforschung 1999;49:557. [NLM Cit ID: 99370789]

Mostafa MH et al: Relationship between schistosomiasis and bladder cancer. Clin Microbiol Rev 1999;12:97. [NLM Cit ID: 99123070]

Richter J et al: Sonographic prediction of variceal bleeding in patients with liver fibrosis due to *Schistosoma mansoni.* Trop Med Int Health 1998;3:728. [NLM Cit ID: 98425639]

Stelma FF et al: Oxamniquine cures *Schistosoma mansoni* infection in a focus in which cure rates with praziquantel are unusually low. J Infect Dis 1997;176:304. [NLM Cit ID: 97351013]

Tsang VC et al: Immunodiagnosis of schistosomiasis. Immunol Invest 1997;26:175. [NLM Cit ID: 9718936]

FASCIOLOPSIASIS

The large intestinal fluke, *Fasciolopsis buski,* is a common parasite of humans and pigs in central and southern China, Taiwan, Southeast Asia, Indonesia, eastern India, and Bangladesh. When eggs shed in stools reach water, they hatch to produce free-swimming larvae that penetrate and develop in the flesh of snails. Cercariae subsequently escape from the snails and encyst on various water plants. Humans are infected by eating these plants uncooked (usually water chestnuts, bamboo shoots, or caltrops). Adult flukes (length 2–7.5 cm) mature in about 3 months and live in the small intestine attached to the mucosa or buried in mucous secretions. The number of parasites ranges from a few to several thousand.

After an incubation period of 2–3 months, manifestations of gastrointestinal irritation appear in all but light infections. Symptoms in severe infections include nausea, anorexia, upper abdominal pain, and diarrhea, sometimes alternating with constipation. Ascites and edema of the face and lower extremities may occur later; the physiologic mechanism is not understood. Intestinal obstruction, ileus, cachexia, and extreme prostration have been described.

Diagnosis depends on finding characteristic eggs or, occasionally, flukes in the stools. Leukocytosis with moderate eosinophilia is common. No serologic test is available. Because the adult worms live for only 6 months, absence from the endemic area for a longer period makes the diagnosis unlikely.

The drug of first choice is praziquantel, given as a single 15 mg/kg dose after an evening meal. The alternative drug is niclosamide, administered as for taeniasis but given every other day for three doses.

In light infections—even without treatment—the prognosis is good; generally, spontaneous cure occurs within 1 year. In rare cases—particularly in children—heavy infections with severe toxemia have resulted in death from cachexia or intercurrent infection.

Liu LX et al: Liver and intestinal flukes. Gastroenterol Clin North Am 1996;25:627. [NLM Cit ID: 97016408]

FASCIOLIASIS

Infection by *Fasciola hepatica,* the sheep liver fluke, results from ingestion of encysted metacercariae on watercress or other aquatic vegetables or in water. A wide range of herbivorous mammals are reservoir hosts. The disease in humans probably occurs worldwide but is most prevalent in sheep-raising countries, particularly where raw salads are eaten. The infection has been reported from Europe, mainland USA, Hawaii, the West Indies, the Middle East, China, Siberia, and North, East and South Africa. Eggs of the worm, passed in host feces into fresh water, release a miracidium that infects snails; the snails subsequently release cercariae that in turn encyst as metacercariae on vegetation (some cercariae become metacercariae directly in the water) to complete their life cycle. The leaf-shaped adult flukes measure 3×1.5 cm.

In humans, metacercariae excyst, penetrate and migrate through the liver, and mature in the bile ducts, where they cause local parenchymal necrosis and abscess formation. Although the infection is usually mild, three clinical syndromes can develop: acute, chronic latent, and chronic obstructive. The acute illness, associated with migration of immature larvae through the liver, shows an enlarged and tender liver, high fever, leukocytosis, and marked eosinophilia (to 90%). Pain may be present in the epigastrium or right upper quadrant, and the patient may experience headache, anorexia, and vomiting, myalgia, urticaria, and other allergic reactions. Jaundice, cachexia, and prostration may appear in severe illness Anemia and hypergammaglobulinemia are common; other liver function tests may be abnormal. Early diagnosis is difficult in the acute phase, because eggs are not found in the feces for 3–4 months. The chronic latent phase may be asymptomatic or characterized by hepatomegaly and other acute findings. The chronic obstructive phase takes place if the extrahepatic bile ducts are occluded, producing a clinical picture similar to that of sclerosing cholangitis, biliary cirrhosis, or choledocholithiasis. Occasionally, adult flukes migrate and produce lesions and symptoms in ectopic sites.

Diagnosis is established by detecting characteristic eggs in the feces; repeated examinations may be necessary. Sometimes the diagnosis can only be made by finding eggs in biliary drainage and, in rare instances, only after liver biopsy or at surgical exploration. Exogenous transient fecal carriage can occur as a result of ingestion of egg-containing cow or sheep liver. Eosinophilia is characteristic. Liver imaging and cholangiography may be useful. Serologic tests are often useful in presumptive diagnosis, particularly in the acute phase (before eggs have appeared) or in ectopic infection. The ELISA is highly sensitive and specific in detection of both antibody and antigen, particularly in acute infections, but cross-reactions have occurred with schistosomiasis. Successful treatment appears to correlate with a decline in antibody titer. A fecal ELISA is promising.

Evidence is increasing that triclabendazole, a veterinary fasciolicide, is the drug of choice. At present, it is used in humans only on an experimental basis; 10 mg/kg given for 1–2 days with food achieves an 80% cure rate with an absence of side effects. The drug should be administered with food. Bithionol is the alternative drug of choice; its deficiencies are its long course (given as for paragonimiasis), failure rates of up to 50%, and frequent adverse reactions. Albendazole trials continue, but that drug also has shown high failure rates. An initial report suggests high effectiveness with low side-effects for nitazoxanide, a veterinary anthelmintic.

Reports on praziquantel have been variable; generally, it is ineffective even when used for up to 7 days at a dose of 25 mg/kg three times daily with a 4- to 6-hour interval between doses. If triclabendazole, bithionol, or praziquantel is not effective, dehydroemetine or emetine hydrochloride in dosages used for amebic liver abscess may help; both drugs are potentially toxic, but dehydroemetine may be less so. For any of the drugs, the destruction of parasites followed by release of antigen in sensitized patients may evoke symptoms.

Bithionol and dehydroemetine are available in the USA only from the Parasitic Disease Drug Service, Centers for Disease Control, Atlanta, GA 30333.

In endemic areas, aquatic plants should not be eaten raw; washing does not destroy the metacercariae, but cooking will. Drinking water must be boiled (1 minute) or purified.

Dowidar N et al: Endoscopic therapy of fascioliasis resistant to oral therapy. Gastrointest Endosc 1999;50:345. [NLM Cit ID: 99393948]

Espino AM et al: Dynamics of antigenemia and coproantigens during a human *Fasciola hepatica* outbreak. J Clin Microbiol 1998;36:2723. [NLM Cit ID: 98371121]

Liu LX et al: Liver and intestinal flukes. Gastroenterol Clin North Am 1996;25:627. [NLM Cit ID: 97016408]

Lopez-Velez R et al: Successful treatment of human fascioliasis with triclabendazole. Eur J Clin Microbiol Infect Dis 1999;18:526. [NLM Cit ID: 99408761]

Richter J et al: Fascioliasis: sonographic abnormalities of the biliary tract and evolution after treatment with triclabendazole. Trop Med Int Health 1999;4:774. [NLM Cit ID: 20056478]

CLONORCHIASIS & OPISTHORCHIASIS

Infection by *Clonorchis sinensis,* the Chinese liver fluke, is endemic in areas of Japan, Korea, China, Taiwan, Southeast Asia, and the far eastern part of Russia. Over 20 million people are affected. Opisthorchiasis is caused by worms of the genus opisthorchis, generally either *O felineus* (central, eastern, and southern Europe, eastern Asia, Southeast Asia, India) or *O viverrini* (Thailand, Laos, Vietnam). Clinically and epidemiologically, opisthorchiasis and clonorchiasis are identical.

Certain snails are infected when they ingest eggs shed into water in human or animal feces. Larval forms escape from the snails, penetrate the flesh of various freshwater fish, and encyst as metacercariae. Fish-eating wild and domestic mammals—including dogs, cats, and pigs—and humans maintain the life cycle. Human infection results from eating such fish, either raw or undercooked. Pickling, smoking, or drying may not suffice to kill the metacercariae. In humans, the ingested parasites excyst in the duodenum and ascend the bile ducts into the medium and small biliary radicals, but also into the larger ducts and the gallbladder, where they mature and remain throughout their lives (15–25 years), shedding eggs in the bile. In size, the worms are 7–20 × 1.5–3 mm. In the chronic stage of infection, there is progressive bile duct thickening, periductal fibrosis, dilation, biliary stasis, and secondary infection. Little fibrosis occurs in the portal tracts.

Most patients harbor few parasites and are asymptomatic. Among symptomatic patients, an acute and chronic syndrome occurs. Acute symptoms follow entry of immature worms into the biliary ducts and may persist for several weeks. Findings include malaise, low-grade fever, an enlarged, tender liver, pain in the hepatic area or epigastrium, urticaria, arthralgia, leukocytosis, eosinophilia, an elevated serum alanine aminotransferase, and jaundice. The acute syndrome is difficult to diagnose, since ova may not appear in the feces until 3–4 weeks after onset of symptoms.

In chronic infections, findings include weakness, anorexia, epigastric pain, diarrhea, prolonged low-grade fever, intermittent episodes of right upper quadrant pain, localized hepatic area tenderness, and progressive hepatomegaly; liver function tests are normal except in severe cases.

Complications include intrahepatic bile duct calculi that may lead to recurrent pyogenic cholangitis, biliary abscess, or endophlebitis of the portal-venous branches. Although focal initially, this may gradually result in destruction of the liver parenchyma, fibrosis, and, in a few patients, cirrhosis with jaundice and ascites. Chronic cholecystitis, cholelithiasis, and a nonfunctional, enlarged gallbladder may occur. Flukes may also enter the pancreatic duct, causing acute pancreatitis or cholelithiasis. Cholangiocarcinoma has been causally linked with prolonged clonorchis and opisthorchis infection.

Diagnosis is made by finding characteristic eggs in stools (repeated tests may be necessary) or duodenal aspirate (sensitivity approaches 100%). During the chronic stage, leukocytosis varies according to the intensity of infection; eosinophilia may be present. In severe infection, the number of eggs per gram of feces may not reflect the heavy worm burden. In the advanced chronic disease, (1) liver function tests will indicate parenchymal damage; (2) CT and sonography may show diffuse dilation of small intrahepatic bile ducts with no or minimal dilation of the large intra- and extrahepatic ducts; and (3) transhepatic cholangiograms may show alternating stricture and dilation of the biliary tree, with worms visualized as filling defects. In patients with biliary obstruction, eggs can be recovered in bile only by needle aspiration or at surgery. Where available, of the several evaluated serologic tests, the ELISA is preferred (sensitivity, 77%); however, unless a specific monoclonal antibody is used, cross-reactions are common with other trematode and cestode infections, tuberculosis, and liver cancer.

The drug of choice is praziquantel. With a dosage of 25 mg/kg three times daily for 2 days (with a 4- to 6-hour interval between doses), cure rates over 95% can be anticipated for clonorchis infections. One day of treatment may be sufficient for opisthorchis infections. (For side effects, see Schistosomiasis, above.) Albendazole, at a dosage of 10 mg/kg twice daily for 7 days, appears to be less effective and requires a longer course of treatment. Mebendazole, at a dosage of 30 mg/kg for 20–30 days, has sometimes been effective.

The disease is rarely fatal, but patients with advanced infections and impaired liver function may succumb more readily to other diseases. The prognosis is good for light to moderate infections.

Chiu A et al: Late complications of infection with *Opisthorchis viverrini.* West J Med 1996;164:174. [NLM Cit ID: 96371916]

Hong ST et al: Control of clonorchiasis by repeated praziquantel treatment and low diagnostic efficacy of sonography. Korean J Parasitol 1998;36:249. [NLM Cit ID: 99085781]

Liu LX et al: Liver and intestinal flukes. Gastroenterol Clin North Am 1996;25:627. [NLM Cit ID: 97016408]

Pungpak S et al: *Opisthorchis viverrini* infection in Thailand: Studies on the morbidity of the infection and resolution following praziquantel treatment. Am J Trop Med Hyg 1997;56:311. [NLM Cit ID: 97275764]

PARAGONIMIASIS

Paragonimus westermani, the lung fluke, commonly infects humans (estimated 20 million) throughout the Far East (prevalence in Korea reached 4%); foci are also present in West Africa, South and Southeast Asia, the Pacific Islands, Indonesia, and New Guinea. Many carnivores and omnivores in addition to humans serve as reservoir hosts for the adult fluke (8–16 × 4–8 × 3–5 mm). About a dozen other paragonimus species also infect humans in China, Japan, Mexico, and Central and South America.

Eggs reaching water, either in sputum or feces, hatch in 3–6 weeks. Released miracidia penetrate and develop in snails. Emergent cercariae encyst as metacercariae in the tissues of crabs and crayfish. Human infection results if metacercariae are ingested when the crustaceans are eaten raw or pickled or are crushed and food, vessels, drinking water or fingers become contaminated. The metacercariae excyst in the small intestine and penetrate the peritoneal cavity. Most migrate through the diaphragm and enter the peripheral lung parenchyma; some may lodge in the brain (about 1% of all cases) or at other ectopic sites. In the lungs, the parasite becomes encapsulated by granulomatous fibrous tissue, reaching up to 2 cm in diameter. The lesion, which usually opens into a bronchiole, may subsequently rupture, resulting in expectoration of eggs, blood, and inflammatory cells. Rarely, the eggs may also enter the general circulation and produce ectopic lesions in any tissue. The prepatent period until appearance of expectorated eggs is about 6 weeks. *P szechuanensis* in China has a propensity to migrate and produce subcutaneous nodules.

In pulmonary infections, most persons have light to moderate worm burdens and are asymptomatic. In symptomatic cases, low-grade fever and dry cough are present initially; subsequently, pleuritic pain is common, and a rusty, blood-flecked, viscous sputum or frank hemoptysis may occur. Following slow progression, complications of bronchitis, bronchiectasis, bronchopneumonia, lung abscess, fibrosis, and pleural thickening or effusion may appear.

Only a minority of patients with cerebral infections present with acute disease, usually manifested by meningitis. In chronic central nervous system disease, seizures, cranial neuropathies, or meningoencephalitis may occur; death can follow. Parasites in the peritoneal cavity or the intestinal wall may cause abdominal pain, diarrhea or dysentery, and a palpable tumor mass. Migratory subcutaneous nodules (a few millimeters to 1 cm in diameter) occur with about 10% of *P westermani* infections and up to 60% of *Paragonimus skrjabini* infections.

Pulmonary disease is diagnosed by finding (1) characteristic eggs in sputum (rusty sputum is nearly pathognomonic), feces, bronchoscopic washings, biopsy specimens, or pleural fluid; or (2) adult flukes in subcutaneous nodules or other surgical specimens. If eggs are not found after multiple direct sputum examinations, they may be detectable in a 24-hour sputum collection processed by alkaline sodium hypochlorite concentration. Stool examination for eggs has low sensitivity. Serum and cerebrospinal fluid serologic tests (ELISA, 99% sensitivity, 97% specificity; and immunoblot, 96% sensitivity and 99% specificity) are available but do not differentiate active from prior infection. An antigen detection assay is promising. Eosinophilia (sometimes to a high level) and low-grade leukocytosis are common. Chest films may show infiltrates, fibrosis, nodules, cavitary lesions, pleural thickening or effusion, or calcifications. By CT, round, low-attenuation cystic lesions (5–15 mm) filled with fluid or gas are seen within the consolidation. In acute cerebral disease, CT shows multilocular, ring-like enhancement with surrounding low-density areas. In chronic cerebral disease, plain skull films often show round or oval-shaped calcifications, sometimes surrounded by low-density areas. Cerebrospinal fluid may be turgid or bloody, with numerous eosinophils. The EEG is almost always abnormal.

Paragonimiasis and tuberculosis must be differentiated, though chest x-ray appearance alone does not make the distinction. Since paragonimus ova are destroyed by Ziehl-Neelsen stain for acid-fast bacilli, the sputum should first be examined for the eggs. The presence of a large number of eosinophils or Charcot-Leyden crystals in sputum suggests paragonimiasis.

In pulmonary paragonimiasis, praziquantel is the drug of choice (25 mg/kg after meals three times daily for 3 days, with a 4- to 6-hour interval between doses). (For side effects, see above under Schistosomiasis.) Bithionol is the alternative drug (30–50 mg/kg, given on alternate days for 10–15 doses [20–30 days]; the daily dose should be divided into a morning and evening dose). Side effects are frequent but generally mild and transient. Gastrointestinal side effects, particularly diarrhea, occur in most patients. Liver function should be tested serially. Bithionol is available in the USA only from the Parasitic Disease Drug Service, Centers for Disease Control, Atlanta, GA 30333. Antibiotics may be necessary for secondary pulmonary infection. Cure rates of over 90% can be anticipated for both praziquantel and bithionol. Triclabendazole, a veterinary fasciolicide, is under investigation at a dosage of 5 mg/kg once daily for 3 days.

In the acute stage of cerebral paragonimiasis, particularly meningitis, praziquantel or bithionol may be effective. With death of parasites, severe local reactions may occur; corticosteroids should therefore be given as in cerebral cysticercosis. In the chronic stage, both surgical removal of the parasites and drug usage are likely to be ineffective in diminishing neurologic symptoms.

Blair D et al: Paragonimiasis and the genus *Paragonimus.* Adv Parasitol 1999;42:113. [NLM Cit ID: 99159180]

Calvopina M et al: Treatment of human pulmonary paragonimiasis with triclabendazole: Clinical tolerance and drug efficacy. Trans R Soc Trop Med Hyg 1998;92:566. [NLM Cit ID: 99078376]

Kagawa FT: Pulmonary paragonimiasis. Semin Respir Infect 1997;12:149. [NLM Cit ID: 97339125]

Nomura M et al: MRI findings of cerebral paragonimiasis in chronic stage. Clin Radiol 1999;54:622. [NLM Cit ID: 99433819]

CESTODE INFECTIONS

TAPEWORM INFECTIONS (See also Cysticercosis and Echinococcosis, below.)

Classification

Six tapeworms infect humans frequently. The large tapeworms are *Taenia saginata* (the beef tapeworm, up to 25 m in length), *Taenia solium* (the pork tapeworm, 7 m), and *Diphyllobothrium latum* (the fish tapeworm, 10 m). The small tapeworms are *Hymenolepis nana* (the dwarf tapeworm, 25–40 mm), *Hymenolepis diminuta* (the rodent tapeworm, 20–60 cm), and *Dipylidium caninum* (the dog tapeworm, 10–70 cm). Four of the six tapeworms occur worldwide; the pork and fish tapeworms have more limited distribution. Humans are the only definitive host of *T saginata* and *T solium.*

An adult tapeworm consists of a head (scolex), a neck, and a chain of individual segments (proglottids) in which eggs form in mature segments. The scolex is the attachment organ and generally lodges in the upper part of the small intestine.

Multiple infections are the rule for small tapeworms and may occur for *D latum;* however, it is rare for a person to harbor more than one or two of the taeniae.

A. Beef Tapeworm: The infection occurs in most countries with beef husbandry but is highly endemic in parts of the Far East, central and eastern Africa, and the central Asian area of the former Soviet Union. Gravid segments of *T saginata* in the human intestine detach themselves from the chain and are passed in feces to soil. When proglottids or eggs are ingested by grazing cattle or other domesticated bovines, the eggs hatch to release embryos that encyst in muscle as cysticerci. Humans are infected by eating raw or undercooked beef containing viable cysticerci, *Cysticercus bovis.* In the human intestines, the cysticercus develops into an adult worm.

B. Pork Tapeworm: This tapeworm is particularly prevalent in Mexico, Latin America, the Iberian Peninsula, the Slavic countries, Africa, Southeast Asia, India, and China. In the USA and Canada, human infection is rare, usually encountered in persons infected abroad; cysticercosis in hogs is uncommon. The infection is no longer found in northwestern Europe. The life cycle of *T solium* is similar to that of *T saginata* except that pigs ingest human feces containing proglottids and eggs to become the host of the larval stage. Humans become infected when they eat undercooked pork containing viable *C cellulosae.* Humans are also the intermediate host when they become infected with the larval stage (see Cysticercosis, below) by accidentally ingesting eggs in human feces; the eggs are immediately infectious. Transmission of eggs may occur as a result of autoinfection (hand to mouth), direct person-to-person transfer, ingestion of food or drink contaminated by eggs, or (rarely) regurgitation of proglottids into the stomach.

C. Fish Tapeworm: *D latum* is found in temperate and subarctic lake regions in many areas of the world, including northern Europe, Canada, Alaska, the Pacific Coast of the USA (the infection may no longer be present in the Great Lakes areas), Japan, Taiwan, Siberia, Manchuria, Australia, and southern South America and southern Africa. Eggs passed in human feces that reach fresh water are taken up first by crustaceans that in turn are eaten by fish, both of which are intermediate hosts. Human infection results from eating raw or inadequately cooked brackish or freshwater fish, including salmon. Nonhuman reservoir hosts include dogs, bears, and other fish-eating mammals.

D. Dwarf Tapeworm: *H nana* is the most common cestode. It can reach high prevalence, particularly in children, in regions of the world with poor fecal hygiene and in closed institutions worldwide. Humans are the definitive host of the human strain of the parasite; rodent-adapted strains occur in rodents. The life cycle is unusual in that both larval and adult stages are found in the human intestine, internal autoinfection can occur, and generally there is no intermediate host. Transmission usually results from eggs transferred directly from human to human (the eggs are immediately infective) but sometimes involves fomites, water, or food or the swallowing of fleas or beetles infected with the larval stage. *H nana* infections in children are usually lost spontaneously in adolescence.

E. Rodent Tapeworm: *H diminuta* is a common parasite of rodents. Many arthropods (eg, rat fleas, beetles, and cockroaches) serve as intermediate hosts. Humans—most commonly young children—are infected by accidentally swallowing the infected arthropods, usually in cereals or stored products.

F. Dog Tapeworm: *D caninum* infection generally occurs in young children in close association with infected dogs or cats. Transmission results from swallowing the infected intermediate hosts, ie, fleas or lice.

Clinical Findings

A. Signs and Symptoms:

1. Large tapeworms–Large tapeworm infections are generally asymptomatic. Occasionally, vague gastrointestinal symptoms (eg, nausea, diarrhea, abdominal pain) and systemic symptoms (eg, fatigue, hunger, dizziness) have been attributed to the infections. Vomiting of proglottid segments or obstruction of the bile duct, pancreatic duct, or appendix is rare.

Some persons (mostly Scandinavian residents) who harbor the fish tapeworm develop a macrocytic megaloblastic anemia accompanied by thrombocytopenia and mild leukopenia. Gastric acidity is normal. The anemia is a result of the worm's competing with the host for vitamin B_{12}. Clinical findings are indistinguishable from those of pernicious anemia and include glossitis, dyspnea, tachycardia, and neurologic findings (numbness, paresthesias, disturbances of coordination, impairment of vibration and position sense, and dementia).

2. Small tapeworms–Light infections are generally asymptomatic. Heavy infections, particularly with *H nana*, may cause diarrhea, abdominal pain, anorexia, vomiting, weight loss, and irritability.

B. Laboratory Findings: Infection by a beef or pork tapeworm is often discovered by the patient finding segments in stool, clothing, or bedding. To determine the species, proglottid segments are either flattened between glass slides and examined microscopically for anatomic detail or differentiated by enzyme electrophoresis of glucose phosphate isomerase. Eggs are only infrequently present in stools, but the perianal cellophane tape test, as used to diagnose pinworm, is sometimes useful in detecting *T saginata* eggs. However, taenia eggs look alike and do not permit species differentiation except by specialized methods. Detection of taenia-specific antigens in stool, currently a research method, may become the most sensitive method for detecting infection.

Fish tapeworm is diagnosed by finding characteristic operculated eggs in stool; repeat examinations may be necessary. Proglottids are passed occasionally, and their internal morphology is also diagnostic. The presence of hydrochloric acid in the stomach differentiates the anemia from pernicious anemia; in both conditions, the Schilling test is abnormal.

H nana and *H diminuta* infections are diagnosed by finding characteristic eggs in feces; proglottids are usually not seen. *D caninum* infection is diagnosed by detection of proglottids (the size of melon seeds) in feces or after their active migration through the anus.

Serologic tests are not available for tapeworm infections; an ELISA for detection of coproantigens is under evaluation.

Treatment

A. Specific Measures: Although niclosamide and praziquantel are both drugs of choice for most tapeworm infections, praziquantel is more effective in hymenolepiasis, and some workers consider it to be somewhat more effective in taeniasis. In areas endemic for neurocysticercosis, a dose of praziquantel of 5 mg/kg or higher carries a small risk of activating the lesions.

1. *T saginata* and *D latum*–Praziquantel in a single dose of 10 mg/kg achieves cure rates of about 99%. At this dose, side effects (see under Schistosomiasis, above) are minimal. With a single dose of four tablets (2 g) of niclosamide, cure rates over 90% can be anticipated. The drug is given in the morning before the patient has eaten. The tablets *must be chewed thoroughly* and swallowed with water. Eating may be resumed in 2 hours. Niclosamide usually produces no side effects.

Pre- and posttreatment purges are not used for either drug. The anemia and neurologic manifestations of *D latum* respond to vitamin B_{12} as used in treatment of pernicious anemia.

2. *T solium*–The choice of drugs and methods of treatment are as above. Neither drug kills eggs released from disintegrating segments; therefore, to avoid the theoretical possibility of cysticercosis from hatching eggs, give a moderate purgative 2–3 hours after treatment to rapidly eliminate segments and eggs from the bowel. The patient must be instructed about the need after defecation for careful washing of the hands and perianal area and for safe disposal of feces for 4 days following therapy.

3. *H nana*–Praziquantel, the drug of choice, produces 95% cure rates with a single 25 mg/kg dose. Niclosamide, the alternative drug, produces cure rates of 75% when given at the above dosage for 5–7 days; some workers repeat the course 5 days later.

4. *H diminuta* and *D caninum*–Treatment is with niclosamide or praziquantel in dosages as for *H nana.* Cure rates are not established.

B. Follow-Up Care: In treatment of large tapeworm infections, a disintegrating worm is usually passed within 24–48 hours of treatment. Since efforts are not generally made to recover and identify the scolex, cure can be presumed only if regenerated segments have not reappeared 3–5 months later. If it is preferred that parasitic cure be established immediately, the head (scolex) must be found in posttreatment stools; a laxative is given 2 hours after treatment, and stools must be collected in a preservative for 24 hours. To facilitate examination, toilet paper must be disposed of separately.

Prevention & Prognosis

C cellulosae is killed by cooking at 65 °C or freezing at –20 °C for 12 hours; *C bovis* at 56 °C or –10 °C for 5 days. Pickling is not adequate. Because the prognosis is often poor in cerebral cysticercosis (see below), *T solium* infections must be immediately eradicated.

Hutchinson JW et al: Diphyllobothriasis after eating raw salmon. Hawaii Med J 1997;56:176. [NLM Cit ID: 97409881]

Ing MB et al: Human coenurosis in North America: Case reports and review. Clin Infect Dis 1998;27:519. [NLM Cit ID: 98442287]

Shantz P: Tapeworms (cestodiasis). Gastroenterol Clin North Am 1996;25:637. [NLM Cit ID: 97016409]

Wilkins PP et al: Development of a serologic assay to detect *Taenia solium* taeniasis. Am J Trop Med Hyg 1999;60:199. [NLM Cit ID: 99170352]

CYSTICERCOSIS

Essentials of Diagnosis

- History of exposure to *Taenia solium* in an endemic region; concomitant or past intestinal infection.
- Seizures and other symptoms and signs of a focal space-occupying central nervous system lesion.
- Subcutaneous or muscular nodules (5–10 mm); calcified lesions on x-rays of soft tissues.
- Calcified or uncalcified cysts by CT scan or MRI; positive serologic tests.

General Considerations

Human cysticercosis is infection by the larval (cysticercus) stage of the tapeworm *T solium* (see above). Prevalence rates to 10% are recognized in some endemic areas.

The natural history of the infection is incompletely known. Cysticerci complete their development within 2–4 months after larval entry and live for months to years. Several factors give rise to symptomatology: Initially, the live larva within a thin-walled cyst (vesicular cyst) is minimally antigenic. When the host immune response or chemotherapy results in gradual death of the cyst, there may be cyst enlargement (colloidal cyst) with mechanical compression, inflammation with pericyst edema, and (sometimes) vasculitis that can result in small cerebral infarcts; increased intracranial pressure and cerebrospinal fluid changes may follow. Subsequently, as the cyst degenerates over 2–7 years, it may disappear or be replaced by a granuloma, calcification, or residual fibrosis. Cysts at different life cycle stages—active (live), transitional, and inactive (dead)—may be present in the same organ. Although some patients develop an intense immune response to the parasite, others show a remarkable tolerance.

Locations of cysts in order of frequency are the central nervous system, subcutaneous tissues and striated muscle, globe of the eye, and, rarely, other tissues. Cysts reach 5–10 mm in soft tissues but may be larger (up to 5 cm) in the central nervous system. Attached to the inner wall of the cyst is an invaginated protoscolex with four suckers and a crown of hooks.

Clinical Findings

A. Signs and Symptoms:

1. Neurocysticercosis–In many patients, cysts remain asymptomatic. When symptomatic, the incubation period is highly variable (usually from 1 to 5 years but sometimes shorter). Manifestations are due to mass effect, inflammatory response, or obstruction of the brain foramina and ventricular systems. Neurologic findings are varied and nonspecific, in large part determined by the number and location of the cysts.

a. Acute invasive stage–This rare event, occurring shortly after invasion, results from extensive acute spread of cysticerci to the brain parenchyma. Fever, headache, myalgia, marked eosinophilia, and coma may occur.

b. Parenchymal cysts–Cysticerci can present singly or multiply and may be scattered or in clumps. Findings include epilepsy (focal or generalized), focal neurologic deficits, intracranial hypertension (intense headache, vomiting, papilledema, visual loss), and altered mental status. Seizures usually do not occur until the cyst or cysts have begun to die.

c. Subarachnoid space cysts and meningeal cysts–Small to large cysts are generally located in the cortical sulci or basal cisterns. The arachnoid is the principal basal membrane affected. Adhesive arachnoiditis may result in obstructive hydrocephalus, intracranial hypertension, arterial thrombosis leading to transient ischemia or stroke, and cranial nerve dysfunction (most often of the optic nerve).

d. Ventricular cysts may float freely (usually singly) within the ventricles or cerebral aqueduct or may be attached to the ventricular wall. They are usually asymptomatic but can cause increased intracranial pressure as a result of intermittent or total blockage.

e. Racemose cysts are rare aberrant forms that are multiple-branched, nonencysted, and lack a scolex; they present as grape-like irregular clusters and may reach over 10 cm in diameter. They generally are found in the ventricular and basal subarachnoid spaces, where they cause marked adhesive arachnoiditis and often obstructive hydrocephalus.

f. Spinal cord cysts can be extraspinal or intraspinal and cause arachnoiditis (meningitis, radiculopathy) or pressure symptoms.

2. Ophthalmocysticercosis–Usually there is a single cyst, free-floating in the vitreous or under the retina. Presenting symptoms include periorbital pain, scotomas, and progressive deterioration of visual acuity. Findings may include disk hemorrhage and edema, retinal detachment, iridocyclitis, and chorioretinitis. MRI but not CT may assist in diagnosis; immunologic tests are negative.

3. Subcutaneous and striated muscle cysticercosis–Subcutaneous cysts present as nodules that tend to appear, collapse and disappear, and then reappear in other sites after variable periods of time. They are usually asymptomatic.

B. Laboratory Tests: Definitive diagnosis of neurocysticercosis requires finding the parasite on histologic section of specimens removed by excisional biopsy of skin or subcutaneous tissues (not of brain tissue). Patients should be thoroughly examined by palpation for pea-sized nodules. Presumptive diagnosis may be made by the following tests.

1. Imaging–Plain radiographs of muscle may detect oval or linear calcified lesions (4–10 × 2–5 mm). The lesions are usually multiple, sometimes in the hundreds, and the long axes of the cysts are nearly always in the plane of the surrounding muscle fibers. Plain skull films may demonstrate one or more cerebral calcifications (generally 5–10 mm; sometimes 1–2 mm when only the scolex is calcified).

The most useful procedures for examining the skull are imaging initially by CT and then by MRI if CT is not conclusive. CT patterns include (1) vesicular cysts (viable cysts with no host immune reaction), which are rounded areas of low density with little or no enhancement after contrast medium; (2) colloidal cysts (dead or dying cysts with host immune reaction), which are hypodense or isodense lesions surrounded by edema associated with ring-like or nodular enhancement; and (3) granuloma or calcifications (dead cysts), which are often several millimeters in diameter but variable in size. Signs of increased intracranial pressure and diffuse brain edema may also be seen. A combination of images is often found, owing to different developmental stages. As compared with CT, MRI has superior resolution for vesicular cysts (isodense, similar to cerebrospinal fluid) and for colloidal cysts (hyperdense). However, CT is superior for granulomas and calcifications, the most frequent presentations of cysticercosis, which MRI may miss. The MRI sometimes detects pathognomonic 2- to 4-mm nodules (protoscoleces) within cyst fluid. Intraventricular cysts (isodense) are not seen on routine CT but require intraventricular contrast medium. Spinal cysticercosis is evaluated by CT myelography or MRI.

2. Immunologic tests–With serum, the new immunoelectrotransfer blot test appears to reach nearly 100% specificity and 95% sensitivity (sensitivity declines if only one or two cysts are present), whereas the ELISA showed, respectively, 63% and 65%. Hydatid disease and *H nana* infections cross-react in the ELISA. Sensitivity using cerebrospinal fluid was 86% by immunoblot and 62% by ELISA. Patients presenting with only calcified lesions or granulomas are generally serologically negative. The serologic tests do not distinguish between active and inactive infections.

3. Other tests–The cerebrospinal fluid in neurocysticercosis should be evaluated for IgM (by ELISA) and IgG antibody; the fluid typically shows increased protein, decreased glucose, and a cellular reaction of mainly lymphocytes and eosinophils; eosinophilia over 20% is diagnostically important. Lumbar puncture is contraindicated in case of increased intracerebral pressure. The EEG may be abnormal. Though the patient usually no longer harbors a tapeworm, stools from both the patient and family members should be examined over several days by each individual for the passage of proglottids and by the laboratory for proglottids and eggs.

Differential Diagnosis

The differential diagnosis includes tuberculoma, tumor, hydatid disease, vasculitis, chronic fungal disorders, toxoplasmosis and other parasitic diseases, and neurosyphilis.

Treatment

Medical treatment, which is usually preferable to surgery, is most effective for parenchymal cysts; less effective for intraventricular, subarachnoid, or racemose cysts; and has no effect on and is not needed for granulomatous or calcified cysts. It remains to be fully established that medical treatment is preferable to symptomatic treatment followed by normal death of the parasites. Some clinicians wait 3 months, with selected patients, to see if cysts will spontaneously disappear without treatment. Drug treatment is withheld but corticosteroids are used during the acute phase of cysticercotic encephalitis if intracranial hypertension is present.

Albendazole and praziquantel are both effective in treatment. Albendazole is preferred because its course of treatment is shorter (1 week) than that of praziquantel (2 weeks); because albendazole is less expensive; and because coadministration of albendazole and a steroid (to treat inflammation) results in increased albendazole absorption, whereas combined use of praziquantel and a steroid greatly decreases plasma levels of praziquantel. Both drugs are given with fatty meals which increases absorption fourfold to fivefold. Treatment should be conducted in hospital. In less than a week after starting treatment, inflammatory reactions around dying parasites may be manifested by meningismus, headache (analgesics may be sufficient for mild symptoms), vomiting, hyperthermia, mental changes, and convulsions; decompensation with death is very rare. It remains controversial whether to give steroids concomitantly to avoid or diminish this reaction or to use them only if marked symptoms appear or increase. Even when steroids are given prospectively, the inflammatory reaction may occur. Prednisone, 30 mg/d in two or three divided doses, starting 1–2 days before use of the drug and continuing at diminishing doses for about 14 days afterward, is one regimen. The reaction usually subsides in 48–72 hours, but continuing severity may require steroids in higher dosage and mannitol. Anticonvulsants should be given during drug treatment and probably for an indefinite time afterward.

Cure rates following treatment (disappearance of cysts and clearing of symptoms) ranged up to 88% for albendazole and 50–60% for praziquantel. Of the remaining patients, many have amelioration of symptoms, including intracranial hypertension and seizures.

An ophthalmologic examination should be done; if cysticercocidal drugs are used in treatment, irreparable damage can occur in the presence of ocular or spinal cysts.

A. Medical Measures:

1. Albendazole–The dosage is 15 mg/kg in divided doses with a fatty meal. The duration of treatment is controversial. Eight days may be sufficient for some patients, but a longer course (up to 28 days) is advisable at present; it can be repeated as necessary.

2. Praziquantel–Give 50 mg/kg/d for 15 days in three divided doses. Phenytoin, phenobarbital, and corticosteroids, when administered with praziquantel, reduce serum levels of the latter; high doses of praziquantel have been tried in these circumstances.

B. Surgical Measures: Surgery has successfully removed orbital, cisternal, and ventricular cysts and, if accessible, cerebral, meningeal, or spinal cord cysts. When hydrocephalus is present, surgical shunt is required even when the parasites have been destroyed.

Prognosis

The fatality rate for untreated neurocysticercosis is about 50%; survival time from onset of symptoms ranges from days to many years. Drug treatment has reduced the mortality rate to about 5–15%. Surgical procedures to relieve intracranial hypertension along with use of steroids to reduce edema improve the prognosis for those not effectively treated with the drugs.

Carpio A et al: Cysticercosis and epilepsy: A critical review. Epilepsia 1998;39:1025. [NLM Cit ID: 98447217]

Del Brutto OH, Sotelo J, Roman GC: *Neurocysticercosis: A Clinical Handbook.* Swets and Zeitlinger, 1998.

Noujaim SE et al: CT and MR imaging of neurocysticercosis. AJR Am J Roentgenol 1999;173:1485. [NLM Cit ID: 20049482]

Salinas R et al: Treating neurocysticercosis medically: a systematic review of randomized, controlled trials. Trop Med Int Health 1999;4:713. [NLM Cit ID: 20056470]

Sotelo J et al: Pharmacokinetic optimization of the treatment of neurocysticercosis. Clin Pharmacokinet 1998; 34:503. [NLM Cit ID: 98309979]

White AC: Neurocysticercosis: A major cause of neurologic disease worldwide. Clin Infect Dis 1997;24:101. [NLM Cit ID: 97268783]

ECHINOCOCCOSIS (Hydatid Disease, Hydatidosis)

Human echinococcosis results from parasitism by the larval stage of four echinococcus species of which *E granulosus* (cystic hydatid disease) and *E multilocularis* (alveolar hydatid disease) are the most important. Minor species are the polycystic species, *E vogeli* (polycystic hydatid disease) and *E oligarthrus,* both from Central and South America. Echinococcosis is a zoonosis in which humans are an intermediate host of the larval stage of the parasite. The definitive host is a carnivore (all of which, except for the lion, are Canidae) that harbors the adult tapeworm in the small intestine; the carnivore becomes infected by ingesting the larval form in tissue of the intermediate host. The intermediate hosts, chiefly herbivorous mammals but also humans, become infected by ingesting tapeworm eggs passed in carnivore feces. The larval stage is referred to as a hydatid cyst.

1. CYSTIC HYDATID DISEASE (Unilocular Hydatid Disease)

Essentials of Diagnosis

- History of exposure to dogs associated with livestock in a hydatid-endemic region.
- Avascular cystic tumor of liver, lung, or, infrequently, bone, brain, or other organs as detected by imaging procedures.
- Symptoms and signs of a space-occupying mass.
- Positive serologic tests.

General Considerations

Human infection with *E granulosus* is common throughout southern South America, the Mediterranean littoral and the Middle East, central Asia, and East Africa. Endemic foci are in eastern Europe, Russia, Australia, New Zealand, India, and the United Kingdom; in North America, foci have been reported from the western USA, the lower Mississippi valley, Alaska, and northwestern Canada.

The pastoral strain—which is more pathogenic to humans—has a transmission cycle in which dogs are the definitive host, and sheep (usually) but also cattle and other domestic livestock are intermediate hosts. However, the strain in horses, pigs, and camels may be of low or no infectivity for humans. The sylvatic, or northern, strain is maintained in wolves and wild ungulates (moose and reindeer) in northern Alaska, Canada, Scandinavia, and Eurasia.

Human infection occurs when eggs passed in dog feces are accidentally swallowed. Liberated embryos penetrate the intestinal mucosa, enter the portal bloodstream, and are carried to the liver where they become hydatid cysts (65% of all cysts). Some larvae reach the lung (25%) and develop into pulmonary hydatids. Infrequently, cysts form in the brain, bones, skeletal muscles, kidneys, spleen, or other tissues. Cysts of the sylvatic strain tend to localize in the lungs.

The cyst wall has three layers: an inner germinal layer that gives rise within the cyst to germinal elements, a supporting intermediate layer, and an outer layer produced by the host. In the liver, cysts may increase in size 1–30 mm in diameter per year and become enormous, but symptoms generally do not develop until they reach about 10 cm. Some cysts die spontaneously; others may persist unchanged for years. Part or all of the inner layer of hepatic and splenic cysts may calcify, which does not necessarily mean cyst death.

Clinical Findings

A. Symptoms and Signs: A liver cyst may remain silent for 10–20 or more years until it becomes large enough to be palpable, to be visible as an abdominal swelling, to produce pressure effects, or (rarely) to produce symptoms due to leakage or rupture. There may be right upper quadrant pain, nausea, and vomiting. The effects of pressure may result in biliary obstruction with secondary bacterial cholangitis, cirrhosis, and portal hypertension. If a cyst ruptures suddenly, anaphylaxis and death may occur. If fluid and hydatid particles escape slowly, allergic manifestations may result, including a rise in the eosinophil count. Rupture can occur into the pleural, pericardial, or peritoneal space or into the duodenum, colon, or renal pelvis. Dissemination of germinal elements may be followed by the development of multiple secondary cysts. A characteristic clinical syndrome may follow intrabiliary extrusion of cyst contents—jaundice, biliary colic, and urticaria.

Pulmonary cysts cause no symptoms until they leak; become large enough to obstruct a bronchus, causing segmental collapse; or erode into a bronchus and rupture. Brain cysts produce symptoms earlier and may cause seizures or symptoms of increased intracranial pressure. Cysts in the bone marrow or spongiosa do not have a host layer, are irregular in shape, erode osseous tissue, and may present as pain or as spontaneous fracture. The bones most often affected are the vertebrae; many of these patients develop epidural extension with compression of the spinal cord and paraplegia. Because 20% of patients have multiple cysts, upon diagnosis each patient should be screened for cysts in the liver, spleen, kidneys, lungs, brain, bones, skin, tongue, vitreous, and other tissues.

B. Imaging: Sonography and CT scan are most commonly used to detect a cystic mass in the liver. Nearly pathognomonic is the presence within a hydatid cyst of daughter cysts; they must be distinguished, however, from blood clots within the cavity of simple cysts. The mass can also be defined by MR imaging, scintillation scan, or by angiography (rarely used). Spotty calcified densities or a calcified cyst wall may be seen in the liver or spleen. Chest films, CT, and MRI may show pulmonary lesions, but calcification of the walls is rare. An intravenous urogram or bone scan may detect cysts at other sites.

C. Laboratory Findings: The immunoblot test, where available, is the test of choice (95% specific and 91% sensitive for liver cysts); the arc 5 test is also diagnostic. In both tests, cross-reactions can occur in 5–10% of patients with *T solium* cysticercosis infections. Several other serologic tests (ELISA and indirect hemagglutination and immunofluorescence) are useful for screening, but both false-negative and false-positive results are common. Persons from whom cysts have been completely removed and carriers of dead cysts may become seronegative. In patients with solitary lung cysts, false-negative results occur in up to 50% of infections. Testing for antigen in serum or cyst fluid (not available in the

USA) can be utilized, but the sensitivity of the test for detecting circulating antigen is lower than that for antibody. The Casoni intracutaneous skin test has been abandoned because of poor specificity.

Eosinophilia is uncommon except after cyst rupture. Liver function tests are usually normal. Confirmation of the diagnosis is possible by examination of cyst contents after surgical removal or cyst aspiration. Although in the past the procedure was contraindicated, ultrasonic-guided percutaneous aspiration of hydatid cysts followed by injection of a scolicidal agent and use of oral albendazole is now being used for diagnosis at some centers (see below).

Differential Diagnosis

Noninfected hydatid cysts of the liver need to be differentiated from simple epithelial cysts and bacterial and amebic abscesses. Hydatid cysts in any site may be mistaken for a variety of malignant and nonmalignant tumors and cysts. In the lung, a cyst may be confused with cavitary tuberculosis. Allergic symptoms arising from cyst leakage may resemble those associated with many other diseases.

Treatment & Prevention

Surgery was formerly the definitive approach to therapy but has now been partially supplanted by anthelmintic treatment. Decision-making between the two modes of treatment must take into account (1) current surgical mortality rates (2% or less), postoperative complications (10–25%), and recurrence rates after surgery (2–25%); and (2) cure rates after albendazole treatment of 30–40%. One approach is to give a course of albendazole to selected asymptomatic patients whose cysts are small and not in danger of rupture. If, after 6–9 months, the cyst has not disappeared or clearly died, it can then be removed surgically.

A. Surgical Treatment: Operative treatment of liver cysts involves several problems: total removal of all infective components of the cyst, avoiding cyst content spillage, selection of a scolicidal agent to be placed within the cyst, management of communications between the cyst and biliary tract (if present), management of the residual cavity, and minimizing the risk of operation. The main surgical options available for liver cysts are partial hepatic resection, pericystectomy, and cystectomy. Surgery for pulmonary cysts includes extrusion of cysts (Barrett's technique), pericystectomy, and lobectomy. Scolicidal solutions, which include cetrimide (5%), hypertonic saline (20%), silver nitrate (0.5%), ethanol (70–95%), and sodium hypochlorite (3.75%), have come under criticism because of their potential for direct and indirect toxicity (an estimated 20% of cysts are thought to communicate with the biliary tract). Preoperatively, to reduce the risk of recurrence due to spillage, two drugs (taken with meals) are used for 1 month: albendazole, 10 mg/kg/d in two divided doses, and praziquantel, 25 mg/kg/d. Postoperatively, albendazole should be continued for 1 month; the additional use of praziquantel is under evaluation. The treatment of bone cysts is by combined curettage, lavage, instillation of sterilization substances, and chemotherapy.

B. Drug Treatment: Albendazole is the drug of choice; in comparative studies, it is more effective than mebendazole and requires a smaller intake of pills.

1. Albendazole–Albendazole is more readily absorbed than mebendazole; this permits a lower dosage of albendazole to be used, yet its active metabolite, the sulfoxide, reaches effective concentrations in cyst wall and fluid. A current regimen is four tablets (800 mg) daily in divided doses with meals for 3 months, and longer if there is evidence of a response. Patients who relapse after a course of therapy should have one or more repeat courses. Among 253 patients treated in multiple studies, the outcomes for liver and lung cysts were, respectively, as follows: cured (33%, 40%), improved (44%, 37%), no change (21%, 22%), and worse (2%, 1%). In another study, findings for 59 patients with liver cysts (< 10 cm) followed for 3–7 years were as follows: cured (41%), improved (41%), no change (15%), worsened (none), and recurrences (two cases, or 3%). Bone cysts are more refractory and may require a year of treatment. In the 3-month courses, drug side effects include reversible low-grade aminotransferase elevations (17%), leukopenia to 2900/μL (2%), rare gastrointestinal symptoms (including pain at cyst sites), dizziness or headache, alopecia, rash, and pruritus. Anaphylaxis has been reported once and eosinophilia rarely, probably related to cyst fluid leakage. Liver function tests and complete blood counts should be monitored weekly. The drug is contraindicated in pregnancy.

2. Mebendazole–When mebendazole was used at high doses for several months, marked regression and apparent death of cysts occurred in some patients. In others, cysts were either stable or continued to grow and if removed were viable. The dosage is 50 mg/kg/d in three divided doses for 3 months, with many patients requiring repeated courses. The drug is taken with fatty meals. When possible, mebendazole levels should be monitored; serum levels in excess of 74 ng/mL 1–2 hours after an oral dose may be necessary for parasite killing. Occasional side effects with treatment include pruritus, rash, alopecia, reversible leukopenia, gastric irritation, musculoskeletal pain, fever, and acute pain in the cyst area; six cases of glomerulonephritis and three of agranulocytosis (with one death) have been reported.

3. Praziquantel–Praziquantel kills protoscoleces within hydatid cysts but does not affect the germinal membrane. The drug is being evaluated as adjunctive therapy with albendazole both pre- and postsurgery to protect against cyst spillage.

C. Percutaneous Aspiration and Injection of a Scolicidal Agent: Under ultrasonic guidance, this approach is indicated in the treatment of accessible cysts in patients who are inoperable or refuse surgery and are not candidates for a chemotherapeutic trial. The procedure's complications are infection and leakage at the aspiration site followed by an allergic reaction or dissemination of the infection. Several thousand patients have now had the procedure diagnostically while covered by oral albendazole. One case of anaphylaxis has been reported. Follow-up for spillage has not been sufficiently long to permit assessment of this risk.

D. Prevention: In endemic areas, prevention is by prophylactic treatment of pet dogs with 5 mg/kg of praziquantel at monthly intervals to remove adult tapeworms and by health education to prevent feeding of offal to dogs.

Prognosis

About 15% of untreated patients eventually die because of the disease or its complications.

2. ALVEOLAR HYDATID DISEASE (Multilocular Hydatid Disease)

Alveolar hydatid disease results from infection by the larval form of *Echinococcus multilocularis* and occurs only in the northern hemisphere. The life cycle involves foxes as definitive host and microtine rodents as intermediate host. Domestic dogs and cats can also become infected with the adult tapeworm when they eat infected wild rodents. Human infection is by accidental ingestion of tapeworm eggs passed in fox or dog feces. The disease in humans has been reported in parts of central Europe, much of Siberia, northern Japan, northwestern Canada, and western Alaska. Recent information has extended the Old World range southward to Iran and northern India and China. Increasing numbers of cases have been reported from central North America (eleven USA states and four Canadian provinces). The primary localization of alveolar cysts is in the liver, where they may extend locally or metastasize to other tissues. The larval mass has poorly defined borders and behaves like a neoplasm; it infiltrates and proliferates indefinitely by exogenous budding of the germinative membrane, producing an alveolus-like pattern of microvesicles. Pulmonary involvement is rare, usually occurring by direct extension from the liver. X-rays show hepatomegaly and characteristic scattered areas of radiolucency often outlined by 2- to 4-mm calcific rings. The serologic tests (ELISA and Western blot) are usually positive at high titer and differentiate *E granulosa* from *E multilocularis.* Treatment is by surgical removal of the entire larval mass when possible, accompanied by drug treatment. Ninety percent of patients with nonresectable masses die within 10 years. Long-term drug therapy (5 years to life) is with albendazole (preferred) (800 mg/d in divided doses) or with mebendazole (40 mg/kg/d in divided doses with fatty meals); the drugs inhibit growth of the parasite and have extended patient survival, but larval tissue is not completely destroyed.

Akhan O et al: Percutaneous treatment of liver hydatid cysts. Eur J Radiol 1999;32:76. [NLM Cit ID: 20046269]

Ammann RW et al: Long-term mebendazole may be parasitocidal in alveolar echinococcosis. J Hepatol 1998; 29:994. [NLM Cit ID: 99090826]

Cobo F et al: Albendazole plus praziquantel versus albendazole alone as a preoperative treatment in intra-abdominal hydaticosis caused by *Echinococcus granulosus.* Trop Med Int Health 1998;3:462. [NLM Cit ID: 98319613]

Cobo F et al: Albendazole plus praziquantel versus albendazole alone as a pre-operative treatment in intra-abdominal hydatidosis caused by *Echinococcus granulosus.* Trop Med Int Health 1998;3:462. [NLM Cit ID: 98319613]

Franchi C et al: Long-term evaluation of patients with hydatidosis treated with benzimidazole carbamates. Clin Infect Dis 1999;29:304. [NLM Cit ID: 99404382]

Horton RJ: Albendazole in treatment of human cystic echinococcosis: 12 years of experience. Acta Trop 1997;64:79. [NLM Cit ID: 97249404]

Mohamed AE et al: Combined albendazole and praziquantel versus albendazole alone in the treatment of hydatid disease. Hepatogastroenterology 1998;45:1690. [NLM Cit ID: 99053865]

Salih OK et al: Surgical treatment of hydatid cysts of the lung: Analysis of 405 patients. Can J Surg 1998;41:131. [NLM Cit ID: 98377025]

Shantz PM: Advances in clinical management of cystic echinococcosis. Acta Trop 1997;64:1. [NLM Cit ID: 97249398]

Taylor BR et al: Current surgical management of hepatic cystic disease. Adv Surg 1997;31:127. [NLM Cit ID: 98072771]

Venkatesan P: Albendazole. J Antimicrob Chemother 1998;41:145. [NLM Cit ID: 98192125]

NEMATODE (ROUNDWORM) INFECTIONS

ANISAKIASIS

Anisakiasis is larval invasion of the stomach or intestinal wall by anisakid nematodes. In the acute form, the infection may mimic surgical abdomen; in the chronic form, mild symptoms may persist for weeks to years.

Definitive hosts are marine mammals, including whales, seals, and dolphins. Eggs discharged with feces are ingested by crustaceans, in which larvae develop that are infective for squids, mackerel, herring, cod, halibut rockfish, salmon, tuna, and other marine fish. In the fish, in which infection rates can reach 80%, the larvae pass to the musculature and are able to transfer from fish to fish along the food chain, eventually reaching a marine mammal, where they mature into the adult stage.

Humans are infected when they ingest larvae in marine fish or squid eaten raw, undercooked, salted, or lightly pickled. Larvae liberated in the stomach attach to or partially penetrate the gastric or intestinal mucosa (small bowel is more common; colon is rare), resulting in localized ulceration, edema, and eosinophilic granuloma formation; eventually, the parasite dies. Rarely, worms are coughed up and expectorated or penetrate the gut wall, enter the peritoneal cavity, and migrate. Most larvae, however, probably fail to cause infection and are passed in feces. Although the larvae sometimes develop to the adult stages, gravid females are not found in humans.

The infection occurs worldwide, but most cases have been reported in Japan and the Netherlands, with a few in the United States, Scandinavia, Chile, and other fish-eating countries. Regional foods eaten raw such as sashimi in Japan, pickled herring in the Netherlands, and ceviche (seviche) in Latin America are common vehicles of infection.

Clinical Findings

A. Symptoms and Signs: The majority of acute cases present as gastric anisakiasis. Occasionally, acute infection is followed by a chronic course.

1. Acute gastric anisakiasis–Within hours after larval ingestion, the patient experiences nausea, vomiting, and epigastric pain that progressively becomes more severe. Allergic reactions, including rare anaphylaxis, can occur; chest pain and hematemesis are rare.

2. Acute intestinal anisakiasis–Within 1–7 days, colicky pain appears in the lower abdomen, often localized at the ileocecal region, accompanied by diarrhea, nausea, vomiting, diffuse abdominal tenderness, and mild fever.

3. Chronic disease–For weeks to several years, symptoms may continue that mimic gastric ulcer, gastritis, gastric tumor, bowel obstruction, or inflammatory bowel disease.

B. Laboratory Findings: Stools may show occult blood, but eggs are not produced. Mild leukocytosis and eosinophilia may be present. ELISA and RAST serologic tests may be helpful but are not reliable in chronic disease.

C. Imaging and Endoscopy: In acute infection, gastroscopy is preferred because the larvae sometimes can be seen and removed from the stomach. X-rays of the stomach may show a localized edematous, ulcerated area with an irregularly thickened wall, decreased peristalsis, and rigidity. Double contrast technique may show the threadlike larvae. Small bowel x-rays may show thickened mucosa and segments of stenosis with proximal dilation. Ultrasound examination of gastric and intestinal lesions may also be useful.

In the chronic stage, x-rays and endoscopy of the stomach—but not of the bowel—may be helpful. The diagnosis is often made only at laparotomy with surgical removal of the parasite.

Prevention & Treatment

Prevention is by avoidance of ingestion of raw or incompletely cooked squid or marine fish, especially salmon, rockfish, herring, and mackerel; early evisceration of fish is recommended. Larvae within fish may with difficulty be seen as colorless, tightly coiled or spiraled worms in 3-mm whorls or as reddish or pigmented larvae lying open in muscles or viscera. The larvae are killed by temperatures above 60 °C or by freezing at –20 °C for 24 hours (7 days is advised by some workers). Smoking procedures that do not bring the temperature to 60 °C, marinating in vinegar, and salt-curing are not reliable.

There is no drug treatment. Except where larvae can be removed by fiberoptic gastroscopy or colonoscopy, treatment of acute and chronic lesions is limited to symptomatic measures; symptoms generally improve in 1–2 weeks. Surgical excision of the worm may be necessary in severe cases.

Buendia E: Anisakis, anisakidosis, and allergy to Anisakis. (Editorial.) Allergy 1997;52:481. [NLM Cit ID: 97344991]

Ido K et al: Sonographic diagnosis of small intestinal anisakiasis. J Clin Ultrasound 1998;26:125. [NLM Cit ID: 98162765]

Moreno-Ancillo A et al: Allergic reactions to *Anisakis simplex* parasitizing seafood. Ann Allergy Asthma Immunol 1997;79:246. [NLM Cit ID: 97450244]

Muraoka A et al: Acute gastric anisakiasis: 28 cases during the past 10 years. Dig Dis Sci 1996;41:2362. [NLM Cit ID: 97148640]

ANGIOSTRONGYLIASIS

1. ANGIOSTRONGYLIASIS CANTONENSIS (Eosinophilic Meningoencephalitis)

A nematode of rats, *Angiostrongylus cantonensis,* is the causative agent of a form of eosinophilic meningoencephalitis. It has been reported from Hawaii and other Pacific islands, Southeast Asia, Japan, China, Taiwan, Hong Kong, Australia, Egypt, Madagascar, Nigeria, Bombay, Cuba, Puerto Rico, Bahamas, Brazil, and New Orleans.

Human infection results from the ingestion of infective larvae contained in uncooked food—either the intermediate mollusk hosts (snails, slugs, planarians) or transport hosts that have ingested mollusks (crabs, shrimp, fish). Leafy vegetables contaminated by small mollusks or by mollusk slime may also be the source of infection, as can fingers during collection and preparation of snails for cooking. The mollusks become infected by ingesting larvae excreted in feces of infected rodents, the definitive host.

The incubation period in humans is 1–3 weeks. Ingested larvae (0.5 × 0.025 mm) invade the central nervous system, where, during migration, they may cause extensive tissue damage; at their death, a local inflammatory reaction ensues. The usual clinical findings are those of meningoencephalitis, including severe headache, fever, neck stiffness, nausea and vomiting, and multiple neurologic findings, particularly asymmetric transient cranial neuropathies. Worms in the spinal cord may result in sensory abnormalities in the trunk or extremities; worms have also been seen in the eye.

The spinal fluid characteristically shows elevated protein, eosinophilic pleocytosis, and normal glucose. Occasionally, the parasite can be recovered from spinal fluid. Peripheral eosinophilia with a low-grade leukocytosis is common. A serologic test is available from the Centers for Disease Control and Prevention. CT and MRI may show a central nervous system lesion.

The differential diagnosis includes tuberculosis, coccidioidal or aseptic meningitis, syphilis, lymphoma, gnathostomiasis, cysticercosis, paragonimiasis, echinococcosis, and schistosomiasis japonicum.

No specific treatment is available; however, levamisole, albendazole, thiabendazole (25 mg/kg three times daily for 3 days), mebendazole (100 mg twice daily for 5 days), or ivermectin can be tried. Theoretically, parasite deaths may exacerbate central nervous system inflammatory lesions. Symptomatic treatment with analgesics or corticosteroids may be necessary. The illness usually persists for weeks to months, the parasite dies, and the patient then recovers spontaneously, usually without sequelae. However, fatalities have been recorded.

Prevention is by rat control; by cooking of snails, prawns, fish, and crabs for 3–5 minutes or by freezing them (–15 °C for 24 hours); and by examining vegetables for mollusks before eating. Washing contaminated vegetables to eliminate larvae contained in mollusk mucus is not always successful.

Chye SM et al: Detection of circulating antigen by monoclonal antibodies for immunodiagnosis of angiostrongyliasis. Am J Trop Med Hyg 1997;56:408. [NLM Cit ID: 97301648]

Noskin GA et al: Eosinophilic meningitis due to *Angiostrongylus cantonensis.* Neurology 1992;42:1423. [NLM Cit ID: 92319310]

2. ANGIOSTRONGYLIASIS COSTARICENSIS

Angiostrongylus costaricensis, which causes an eosinophilic ileocolitis, has been identified in humans (predominantly children) in Mexico, Central America, Venezuela, Brazil, and the USA (Texas). The known geographic range of the parasite in rodents (the definitive host) extends from northern South America to Texas. Infection occurs from ingestion of the larvae in the intermediate host (slugs, snails) or from food contaminated by larvae in slug or snail mucus. In humans, the larvae mature in the mesenteric vessels. The inflammatory response to adult worms, larvae, and eggs can be severe, resulting in a marked eosinophilic granulomatous reaction and vasculitis and ischemic necrosis of the intestine. Most cases involve the ileocecal region, appendix, ascending colon, and regional nodes, but other organs can be affected, including the liver and testes. Findings include fever, right lower quadrant abdominal pain and a mass, leukocytosis, and eosinophilia. Some patients have relapsing symptoms that can continue for months. Bowel complications include perforation, bleeding, incomplete or complete obstruction, and infarction. Neither eggs or larvae are passed in stool; a latex agglutination serologic test has been devised. The intra-abdominal mass can mimic tumor. There is no specific treatment; albendazole, thiabendazole, or mebendazole can be tried. Operative treatment is frequently necessary.

Kramer MH et al: First reported outbreak of abdominal angiostrongyliasis. Clin Infect Dis 1998;26:365. [NLM Cit ID: 98161562]

ASCARIASIS

Essentials of Diagnosis

- Pulmonary phase: Transient cough, dyspnea, wheezing, urticaria, with eosinophilia and transient pulmonary infiltrates.
- Intestinal phase: Vague upper abdominal discomfort; occasional vomiting, abdominal distention.
- Eggs in stools; worms passed per rectum, nose, or mouth.

General Considerations

Ascaris lumbricoides is the most common of the intestinal helminths; an estimated 1 billion people are infected worldwide. It is cosmopolitan in distribution and is found in high prevalence wherever there are low standards of hygiene and sanitation (including focally in southeastern USA) or where human feces are used as fertilizer. The infection is specific for humans and occurs in all age groups. Heavy worm burdens, however, are usually seen only in children, in whom there may be reduced nitrogen, fat, and D-xylose absorption and reduced mucosal lactate activity resulting in decreased growth rates.

Adult worms live in the upper small intestine. After fertilization, the female produces enormous numbers of eggs that pass in feces. Direct transmission between humans does not occur, as the eggs must remain on the soil for 2–3 weeks before they become infective. Thereafter, they can survive for years. Infection occurs through ingestion of mature eggs in fecally contaminated food and drink. The eggs hatch in the small intestine, releasing motile larvae that penetrate the wall of the small intestine and reach the right heart via the mesenteric venules and lymphatics. From the heart they move to the lung, burrow through the alveolar walls, and migrate up the bronchial tree into the pharynx, down the esophagus, and back to the small intestine. Egg production begins 60–75 days after ingestion of infective eggs. Adult worms (20–40 cm × 3–6 mm) live for 1 year or more.

Clinical Findings

A. Symptoms and Signs: As a result of their migration and induction of hypersensitivity, larvae in the lung cause capillary and alveolar damage, which may result in low-grade fever, nonproductive cough, blood-tinged sputum, wheezing, dyspnea, and substernal pain. There may be urticaria and localized rales. Rarely, larvae lodge ectopically in the brain, kidney, eye, spinal cord, etc, and may cause symptoms referable to those organs.

Small numbers of adult worms in the intestine usually produce no symptoms. With heavy infection, peptic ulcer-like symptoms or vague pre- or postprandial abdominal discomfort may be seen. Adult worms may also migrate with heavy infections; they may be coughed up, vomited, or emerge through the nose or anus. They may also force themselves into the common bile duct, pancreatic duct, appendix, diverticula, and other sites, which may lead to cholangitis, cholecystitis, pyogenic liver abscess, pancreatitis, or obstructive jaundice. With very heavy infestations, masses of worms may cause intestinal obstruction, volvulus, intussusception, or death. During typhoid fever, worms may penetrate the weakened bowel wall. Rare cases of lung abscess or laryngeal obstruction with suffocation have been described. Moderate to high worm loads have been associated with stunting of growth in children. Periodic treatment of children with albendazole for multiple intestinal parasitism has resulted in improved nutrition.

B. Imaging: During the larval migratory phase, chest radiographs may show transitory, patchy, ill-defined asymmetric infiltrations (Löffler's syndrome). Intestinal infection is sometimes established by chance, when radiologic examination of the abdomen (with or without barium) shows the presence of worms. The diagnosis of biliary ascariasis can be made by endoscopic retrograde cholangiopancreatography, which has the therapeutic potential of removing the worms, and by ultrasonography. In intestinal obstruction, plain abdominal films show air-filled levels and multiple linear images of ascarides in dilated bowel loops; ultrasonography can also demonstrate the dilated bowel and worm mass.

C. Laboratory Findings: During the pulmonary phase, eosinophils may reach 30–50% and remain high for about a month; larvae are occasionally found in sputum. During the intestinal phase, diagnosis usually depends upon finding the characteristic eggs in feces. Occasionally, an adult worm spontaneously passed per rectum or orally reveals an unsuspected infection. Serologic tests are not useful, and there is no eosinophilia.

Differential Diagnosis

Pulmonary ascariasis with eosinophilia must be differentiated from nonparasitic causes (asthma, Löffler's syndrome, eosinophilic pneumonia, allergic bronchopulmonary aspergillosis), and parasitic causes (tropical pulmonary eosinophilia, toxocariasis, strongyloidiasis, hookworm, paragonimiasis). Ascaris-induced pancreatitis, appendicitis, diverticulitis, etc, must be differentiated from other causes of inflammation of these tissues. Postprandial dyspepsia may simulate duodenal ulcer, hiatal hernia, gallbladder disease, or pancreatic disease.

Treatment

Albendazole and pyrantel pamoate are the treatments of choice. None of the drugs listed below require pre- or posttreatment purges. Stools should be rechecked at 2 weeks and patients re-treated until all ascarids are removed. Ascariasis, hookworm, and trichuriasis infections, which often occur together, may be treated simultaneously by albendazole, mebendazole, or oxantel-pyrantel pamoate.

Treatment with anthelmintics can cause worms to migrate before they die. Because anesthesia stimulates worms to hypermotility, they should be removed in advance in infected patients undergoing elective surgery. In pregnancy, ascariasis should be treated after the first trimester.

Drug treatment should not be used in the migratory phase. In intestinal obstruction or biliary ascariasis, surgery may be avoided by nasogastric suction followed by a standard dose of an anthelmintic given via the tube. In biliary ascariasis, endoscopic removal of the worm under ultrasonographic guidance is often successful; treatment by injection of a solution of albendazole or piperazine into the common duct followed by systemic treatment has also been effective.

A. Albendazole: In light infections, a single dose of albendazole (400 mg) results in cure rates over 95%; in heavy infections, however, a 2- to 3-day course is indicated. Side effects, including migration of ascaris through the nose or mouth, are rare. Albendazole is available in the USA though not approved for this indication. The drug is contraindicated in pregnancy.

B. Pyrantel Pamoate: Pyrantel pamoate as a single oral dose of 10 mg base/kg (maximum, 1 g) results in 85–100% cure rates. It may be given before or after meals. Infrequent and mild side effects include vomiting, diarrhea, headache, dizziness, and drowsiness.

C. Mebendazole: Mebendazole is highly effective when given in a dosage of 100 mg twice daily before or after meals for 3 days. Gastrointestinal side effects are infrequent. The drug is contraindicated in pregnancy.

D. Piperazine: The dosage for piperazine (as the hexahydrate) is 75 mg/kg body weight (maximum, 3.5 g) for 2 days in succession, giving the drug orally before or after breakfast. For heavy infestations, treatment should be continued for 4 days in succession or the 2-day course should be repeated after 1 week.

Gastrointestinal symptoms and headache occur occasionally; central nervous system symptoms (temporary ataxia and exacerbation of seizures) are rare. Allergic symptoms have been attributed to piperazine. The drug should not be used for patients with hepatic or renal insufficiency or in those with a history of seizures or chronic neurologic disease.

E. Levamisole: Levamisole, available in the USA but not approved for this indication, is highly effective as a single oral dose of 150 mg. Occasional mild and transient side effects are nausea, vomiting, abdominal pain, headache, and dizziness.

Prognosis

The complications caused by wandering adult worms require that all ascaris infections be treated and eradicated.

Akata D et al: Radiological findings of intraparenchymal liver *Ascaris* (hepatobiliary ascariasis). Eur Radiol 1999;9:93. [NLM Cit ID: 99132492]

al-Karawi M et al: Biliary strictures and cholangitis secondary to ascariasis: endoscopic management. Gastrointest Endosc 1999;50:695. [NLM Cit ID: 20007089]

Beckingham IJ et al: Management of hepatobiliary and pancreatic *Ascaris* infestation in adults after failed medical treatment. Br J Surg 1998;85;907. [NLM Cit ID: 98355289]

Osman M et al: Biliary parasites. Digest Surg 1998;15:287. [NLM Cit ID: 99062138]

Sarinas PS et al: Ascariasis and hookworm. Semin Respir Infect 1997;12:130. [NLM Cit ID: 97339123]

CUTANEOUS LARVA MIGRANS (Creeping Eruption)

Cutaneous larva migrans, prevalent throughout the tropics and subtropics, including southeastern USA, is caused by larvae of the dog and cat hookworms, *Ancylostoma braziliense* and *Ancylostoma caninum.* A number of other animal hookworms, gnathostomiasis, and strongyloidiasis are rarely also causative agents. Moist sandy soil (eg, beaches, children's sand piles) contaminated by dog or cat feces is a common site of infection. The infection is also reported in travelers to tropical beaches, among whom delayed onset beyond several weeks has been described.

At the site of larval entry, particularly on the hands or feet, up to several hundred minute, intensely pruritic erythematous papules appear. Two to 3 days later, serpiginous eruptions appear as the larvae migrate at a rate of several millimeters a day; the parasite lies slightly ahead of the advancing border. The process may continue for weeks; the lesions may become severely pruritic, vesiculate, encrusted, or secondarily infected. Without treatment, the larvae eventually die and are absorbed.

The diagnosis is based on the characteristic appearance of the lesions and the frequent presence of eosinophilia. Biopsy is usually not indicated.

Mild transient cases may not require treatment. For mild cases, thiabendazole, if available, can be applied topically three times daily for 5 or more days as a 15% cream, which can be formulated in a hygroscopic base using crushed 500 mg tablets. For more severe cases, oral treatment is indicated. Highly effective and nearly free of side effects are ivermectin as a single dose (150–200 μg/kg; a single 12 mg dose was curative in 49 of 50 patients) and albendazole (400 mg twice daily for 3–5 days or 400 mg daily for 7 days). Thiabendazole, given orally as for strongyloidiasis, is a less satisfactory alternative drug because it has significant side effects in about one-third of patients. With treatment, progression of the lesions and itching are usually stopped within 48 hours. Antihistamines are helpful in controlling pruritus; antibiotic ointments may be necessary to treat secondary infections.

Veraldi S et al: Effectiveness of a new therapeutic regimen with albendazole in cutaneous larva migrans. Eur J Dermatol 1999;9:352. [NLM Cit ID: 99348613] (Demonstrates the effectiveness of albendazole 400 mg/d for 7 days.)

Van den Enden E et al: Treatment of cutaneous larva migrans. N Engl J Med 1998;339:1246. [NLM Cit ID: 98442908]

DRACUNCULIASIS (Guinea Worm Infection, Dracunculosis, Dracontiasis)

Dracunculiasis is an infection of connective and subcutaneous tissues by the nematode *Dracunculus medinensis.* It occurs only in humans and is a major cause of disability. Since the start of the WHO eradication program, the number of infected persons has declined about 97% from over 3 million to 100,000. Endemic areas have been the Indian subcontinent; West and Central Africa north of the equator (Cameroon to Mauritania, Uganda, and southern Sudan); and Saudi Arabia, Iran, and Yemen. Almost all remaining cases are reported from Africa—75% from Sudan. All ages are affected, and prevalence may reach 60%.

Infection occurs by swallowing water containing the infected intermediate host, the crustacean *Cyclops* (copepods, water fleas). In the stomach, larvae escape from the crustacean and mature in subcutaneous connective tissue. After mating, the male worm dies and the gravid female (60–80 cm × 1.7–2.0 mm) moves to the surface of the body, where its head reaches the dermis and provokes a blister that ruptures on contact with water. Intermittently over 2–3 weeks, whenever the ulcer comes in contact with water, the uterus discharges great numbers of larvae, which are ingested by copepods. Most adult worms are gradually extruded; some worms retract and reemerge; and others die in the tissues, disintegrate, and may provoke a severe inflammatory reaction. Infection does not induce protective immunity.

Clinical Findings

A. Symptoms and Signs: Infection may be at several sites. Patients are asymptomatic during the 9- to 14-month incubation period except in the last 1–2 weeks, when the worm reaches and becomes palpable in the skin and a blister develops around its anterior end. Several hours before the head appears at the skin surface, local erythema, burning, pruritus, and tenderness often develop at the site of emergence. There may also be a 24-hour systemic allergic reaction (pruritus, fever, nausea and vomiting, dyspnea, periorbital edema, and urticaria). After rupture, the tissues surrounding the ulceration frequently become indurated, reddened, and tender. Because most lesions appear on the leg or foot, patients often must give up walking and working for days to several months. Uninfected ulcers heal in 4–6 weeks. The worm rarely reaches ectopic sites.

Secondary infections, including tetanus, are common. Deep "cold" abscesses may result at the sites of dying, nonemergent worms. Ankle and knee joint infections with resultant deformity are common complications.

B. Laboratory Findings: When an emerging adult worm is not visible in the ulcer or under the skin, the diagnosis may be made by detection of larvae in smears from discharging sinuses. Immersion of an ulcer in cold water stimulates larval expulsion. Eosinophilia is usually present. Skin and serologic tests are not useful. Calcified worms can be recognized on radiographs.

Treatment

All persons in an endemic area should be actively immunized against tetanus.

A. General Measures: The patient should be at bed rest with the affected part elevated. Cleanse the lesion, control secondary infection with topical antibiotics, and change dressings twice daily.

B. Manual Extraction: Traditional extraction of emerging worms by gradually rolling them out a few centimeters each day on a small stick is still useful, especially when done along with chemotherapy and use of aseptic dressings. The process appears to be facilitated by placing the affected part in water several times a day. If the worm is broken during removal, however, secondary infection almost always results, leading to cellulitis, abscess formation, or septicemia.

C. Anthelmintic Therapy: Metronidazole and thiabendazole are sometimes useful in alleviating symptoms and in reducing the duration of infection (by expediting spontaneous extrusion of worms or facilitating their manual extraction). The drugs have an anti-inflammatory effect but do not kill the adult or larvae.

1. Metronidazole, 250 mg three times daily for 10 days, causes only minimal toxicity. (See under Amebiasis.)

2. Thiabendazole, 25 mg/kg twice daily for 2–3 days after meals, frequently causes side effects, sometimes severe (see under Strongyloidiasis, below).

3. Mebendazole, 400–800 mg daily for 6 days, can be tried.

D. Surgical Removal: Preemergent female worms can be surgically removed intact under local anesthesia if not firmly embedded in deep fascia or around tendons.

Prevention & Control

The disease is readily prevented by use of only noncontaminated drinking water. This can be accomplished either (1) by preventing contamination of community water supplies through use of tube wells, hand pumps, or cisterns or treating water sources with temephos; or (2) by filtering water through nets (eg, nylon nets of 100 μm pore size) or by boiling water. As a result of the WHO-sponsored campaign, eradication of dracunculiasis is increasingly imminent; worldwide, the number of infected persons has declined about 97% from over 3 million to 100,000. Eradication remains to be achieved in Yemen, India, and parts of Africa south of the Sahara, particularly in Sudan, Ghana, and Nigeria.

Hopkins DR: Perspectives from the dracunculiasis eradication programme. Bull WHO 1998;76(Suppl 2):38. [NLM Cit ID: 99163159]

Rohde JE et al: Surgical extraction of guinea worm: Disability reduction and contribution to disease control. Am J Trop Med Hyg 1993;48:71. [NLM Cit ID: 93151379]

ENTEROBIASIS (Pinworm Infection)

Essentials of Diagnosis

- Nocturnal perianal and vulvar pruritus, insomnia, irritability, restlessness.
- Vague gastrointestinal symptoms.

- Eggs demonstrable by cellulose tape test; worms visible on perianal skin or in stool.

General Considerations

Enterobius vermicularis (8–13 × 0.5 mm) is common worldwide. Humans, the only host, can harbor a few to hundreds of worms. Young children are affected more often than adults, and multiple infections occur in households and institutions with young children. High rates have been recorded in homosexual men, but the infection does not become opportunistic in HIV. A second species, *Enterobius gregorii,* has been described in England.

The adult worms inhabit the cecum and adjacent bowel areas, lying loosely attached to the mucosa. Gravid females migrate through the anus to the perianal skin and deposit eggs in large numbers. The eggs become infective in a few hours and may then infect others or be autoinfective if transferred to the mouth by contaminated food, drink, fomites, or hands. After being swallowed, the eggs hatch in the duodenum, and the larvae migrate down to the cecum. Retroinfection occasionally occurs when the eggs hatch on the perianal skin and the larvae migrate through the anus into the large intestine. The development of a mature ovipositing female from an ingested egg requires about 3–4 weeks. Eggs remain viable for 2–3 weeks outside the host. The life span of the worm is 30–45 days.

Clinical Findings

A. Symptoms and Signs: Many patients are asymptomatic. The most common and important symptom is perianal pruritus (particularly at night), due to the presence of the female worms or deposited eggs. Insomnia, restlessness, enuresis, and irritability are common symptoms, particularly in children. Many mild gastrointestinal symptoms have also been attributed to enterobiasis, but the association is difficult to prove. At night, worms may occasionally be seen near the anus. Perianal scratching may result in excoriation and impetigo. Adults sometimes report a "crawling" sensation in the anal area. Rarely, worm migration—including migration through the female genital tract or into the urethra—results in ectopic inflammation (vulvovaginitis, diverticulitis, appendicitis, cystitis) or granulomatous reactions (colon, genital tract, peritoneum, and elsewhere). Colonic ulceration and eosinophilic colitis have been reported.

B. Laboratory Findings: Diagnosis is made by finding eggs on the perianal skin (eggs are seldom found on stool examination). The most reliable method is by applying a short strip of sealing cellulose pressure-sensitive tape (eg, Scotch Tape) to the perianal skin and then spreading the tape on a slide for low-power microscopic study; toluene is used to clear the preparation. Three such preparations made on consecutive mornings before bathing or defecation will establish the diagnosis in about 90% of cases. Before the diagnosis can be ruled out, five to seven such examinations are necessary. Nocturnal examination of the perianal area or gross examination of stools may reveal adult worms, which should be placed in preservative, alcohol, or saline for laboratory examination. The worms can sometimes be seen on anoscopy. Eosinophilia is rare.

Differential Diagnosis

Pinworm pruritus must be distinguished from similar pruritus due to mycotic infections, allergies, hemorrhoids, proctitis, fissures, strongyloidiasis, and other conditions.

Treatment

A. General Measures: Symptomatic patients should be treated, and in some situations all members of the patient's household should be treated concurrently, since for each overt case there are usually several inapparent cases. Generally, however, treatment of all nonsymptomatic cases is not necessary. Careful washing of hands with soap and water after defecation and again before meals is important. Fingernails should be kept trimmed close and clean and scratching of the perianal area avoided. Ordinary washing of bedding will usually kill pinworm eggs; some workers recommend daily washing.

B. Specific Measures: Treatment with the following drugs should be repeated at 2 and 4 weeks. Albendazole, mebendazole, and pyrantel pamoate are the drugs of choice and can be given with or without food. Albendazole and mebendazole should not be used in pregnancy.

1. **Albendazole** is available in the USA though not approved for this indication. It may reach a 100% cure rate when given as a single 400 mg dose. Abdominal pain and diarrhea are rare.
2. **Mebendazole** as a single 100 mg dose is also highly effective. It should be chewed for best effect. Gastrointestinal side effects are infrequent.
3. **Pyrantel pamoate** is highly effective, with cure rates of over 95%. It is administered as a 10 mg (base)/kg (maximum, 1 g) dose. Infrequent side effects include vomiting, diarrhea, headache, dizziness, and drowsiness. In the USA, pyrantel is available as self-medication for pinworm infection.
4. **Other drugs**–Piperazine, although effective, is not recommended because treatment requires 1 week. Thiabendazole is not recommended, because it causes frequent side effects which rarely are severe and life-threatening.

Prognosis

Although annoying, the infection is benign. Cure is readily attainable with one of several effective drugs. Reinfection is common, especially in children, because of continued exposure outside the home.

Avolio L et al: Perianal granuloma caused by *Enterobius vermicularis:* Report of a new observation and review of the literature. J Pediatr 1998;132:1055. [NLM Cit ID: 98291076]

Grencis RK et al: Enterobius, trichuris, capillaria, and hookworm including ancylostoma caninum. Gastroenterol Clin North Am 1996;25:579. [NLM Cit ID: 97016406]

Hugot JP et al: Human enterobiasis in evolution: origin, specificity and transmission. Parasite 1999;6:201. [NLM Cit ID: 99441638]

FILARIASIS

More than 80 million people are infected with lymphatic filariasis, which is caused by three filarial nematodes: *Wuchereria bancrofti, Brugia malayi,* or *Brugia timori. W bancrofti* is widely distributed in the tropics and subtropics of both hemispheres and on Pacific islands and is transmitted by *Culex, Aedes,* and *Anopheles* mosquitoes. *B malayi* is transmitted by *Mansonia* and *Anopheles* mosquitoes of South India, Sri Lanka, Southeast Asia, South China, the northern coastal areas of China, and South Korea. *B timori* is found on the southeastern islands of Indonesia.

No animal reservoir hosts are known for *W bancrofti* or *B timori*; cats, monkeys, and other animals may harbor *B malayi.* Mosquitoes become infected by ingesting microfilariae with a blood meal; at subsequent feedings, they can infect new susceptible hosts. Over months, adult worms (females, 8–9 cm × 0.2–0.3 mm) mature and live in or near superficial and deep lymphatics and lymph nodes and produce large numbers of viviparous circulating microfilariae, which may be seen in the blood starting 6–12 months after infection.

Pathologic changes in lymph vessels are due to host immunologic reactions to developing and mature worms. Living microfilariae generally cause no lesions, with the exception of tropical pulmonary eosinophilia. Rapid death of microfilariae, however, does produce findings, and an abscess may form at the site of a dying adult worm.

Dirofilariasis, infection by *Dirofilaria immitis,* the dog heartworm, has been reported in the USA, Japan, and Australia. Nodules have been found in the skin or as solitary 1–4.5 cm (usually 2 cm) "coin" lesions in the periphery of the lungs; they are rarely calcified. The serologic test for filariasis is positive, but there is no microfilaremia. Eosinophilia is seen in 15% of patients.

Other filarial worms. Several other species infect humans—*Mansonella perstans, Mansonella streptocerca,* and *Mansonella ozzardi*—but usually without causing important findings.

Clinical Findings

A. Symptoms and Signs: The incubation period is generally 8–16 months in expatriates but may be longer in indigenous persons. Many infections remain asymptomatic, with or without microfilariae.

1. Acute disease–Episodes of fever (filarial fever), with or without inflammation of lymphatics and nodes, occur at irregular intervals and last for several days. Characteristically, the adenolymphangitis presents as retrograde extension from the affected node. With disease progression, epididymitis and orchitis as well as involvement of pelvic, abdominal, or retroperitoneal lymphatics may also occur intermittently. Lymph node enlargement may persist. In travelers, allergic-like findings (hives, rashes, eosinophilia) and lymphangitis and lymphadenitis are more likely to be present.

2. Chronic disease–Obstructive phenomena occur as a result of interference with normal lymphatic flow; this includes hydrocele, scrotal lymphedema, lymphatic varices and elephantiasis, particularly of the extremities, genitals, and breasts. Chyluria may result from rupture of distended lymphatics into the urinary tract. Extrapulmonary manifestations seen in some patients include lymphadenopathy or moderate hepatomegaly or splenomegaly.

3. Occult disease–A small proportion of infected persons develop occult disease, in which the classic clinical manifestations and microfilaremia are not present but microfilariae are present in the tissues.

In **tropical pulmonary eosinophilia,** microfilariae of *W bancrofti* or *B malayi* are sequestered in the lungs but not found in the blood. The condition is characterized by episodic nocturnal coughing or wheezing, dyspnea, low-grade fever, scant expectoration, hypereosinophilia, high filarial antibody titers and IgE levels, diffuse miliary lesions or increased bronchovascular markings on chest films, and a response to diethylcarbamazine treatment (6 mg/kg daily for 21 days). Relapses (in 20%) require re-treatment with up to 12 mg/kg daily for up to 30 days. If untreated, the condition can progress to chronic pulmonary fibrosis.

B. Laboratory Findings: Diagnosis is established by finding microfilariae in the blood. In indigenous persons, they are rare in the first 2–3 years, abundant as the disease progresses, and again rare in the obstructive stage. In persons from nonendemic areas, inflammatory reactions may be prominent in the absence of microfilariae. Microfilariae of *W bancrofti* are found in the blood chiefly at night (nocturnal periodicity 10 PM to 2 AM), except for a nonperiodic variety in the South Pacific. *B malayi* microfilariae are usually nocturnally periodic but in Southeast Asia may be present at all times, with a slight nocturnal rise. Anticoagulated blood specimens are collected at times related to the periodicity of the local strain. Specimens may be stored at ambient temperatures until examined in the morning by wet film for motile larvae and by Giemsa-stained smears—thick for sensitivity and thin for specific morphology. A formalin-anionic detergent preservative can also be used. If these are negative, the blood specimens should be concentrated by the Knott concentration or membrane filtration technique. If all are negative, oral administration of 50 mg of diethylcarbamazine often results in positive blood specimens (within minutes to an hour) or a systemic reaction (itching, papular rash, myalgia). If negative, repeat with 200 mg. When onchocerciasis or loiasis may be present, this test must be done with extreme caution.

Serologic tests may be helpful in diagnostic screening, but false-positive (other filarial and helminthic infections) and false-negative reactions occur. An indirect hemagglutination titer of 1:128 and a bentonite flocculation titer of 1:5 in combination are considered minimum significant titers. ELISA-IgG and IgE tests are available. A PCR test has been effective in amicrofilaremic persons both with blood and with urine samples. Eosinophil counts may be elevated. Testing for antigenemia is proving useful in diagnosis (examining daytime blood specimens and detecting some amicrofilaremic infections) and in monitoring efficacy of treatment; a commercial test is now available. In differential diagnosis, lymphangiography (potentially damaging to the lymphatics) and radionuclide lymphoscintigraphy may be useful lymphatic imaging methods. As live adult worms can be detected by ultrasonography, the method, when applied to scrotal examination, can be useful in detecting adult worms in amicrofilaremic persons.

Treatment, Prevention, & Prognosis

Diethylcarbamazine, the drug of choice, rapidly kills blood microfilariae but only slowly kills or injures adult worms. Cure may require multiple 3-week courses (2 mg/kg three times a day after meals, starting with small doses, and gradually increasing over 3–4 days). At this dose, the drug rarely produces direct toxicity. However, adverse immunologic reactions to dying microfilariae and adult worms are common—more so with brugian than with bancroftian filariasis. Reactions are local (lymphadenitis, abscess, ulceration) and systemic (fever, headache, myalgia, dizziness, malaise, and other allergic responses). Antipyretics and analgesics may be helpful. In areas where onchocerciasis or loiasis is also prevalent, special care must be taken not to provoke severe reactions to dying microfilariae of these parasites. Diethylcarbamazine has also been extensively used in mass treatment programs and is being evaluated for prophylaxis. In the USA, the drug is available only from the Parasitic Diseases Drug Service, Centers for Disease Control and Prevention, Atlanta, GA 30333; phone 404-639-3670.

During acute inflammatory episodes, it is controversial whether to treat and whether drug usage will shorten the attack. General measures include bed rest, antibiotics for secondary infections, use of elastic stockings and pressure bandages for leg edema, and suspensory bandaging for orchitis and epididymitis.

Small hydroceles may benefit from a locally injected sclerosing agent, or surgery may be indicated. To manage elephantiasis, lymphovenous shunt procedures may be useful, combined with removal of excess subcutaneous fatty and fibrous tissue, postural drainage, and physiotherapy.

Ivermectin, a microfilaricide, continues under evaluation as a single 200–400 μg/kg dose, which is repeated in 6 months; recent findings are that albendazole 400 mg when combined with ivermectin is better than ivermectin alone. Ivermectin combined with diethylcarbamazine is also being evaluated. However, diethylcarbamazine is still needed to kill the adult worms, which are the cause of the pathologic manifestations of the disease. Diethylcarbamazine and ivermectin appear to be equally efficacious in reducing microfilarial burdens; mild side effects (myalgia, headache, fever) are similar in some studies but less so for ivermectin in others.

The prognosis is good with treatment of early and mild cases (including low-grade lymphedema, chyluria, small hydrocele), but in advanced infection the prognosis is poor.

Abbasi I et al: Diagnosis of *Wuchereria bancrofti* infection by the polymerase chain reaction employing patients' sputum. Parasitol Res 1999;85:844. [NLM Cit ID: 99423003]

Chitkara RK et al: Dirofilaria, visceral larva migrans, and tropical pulmonary eosinophilia. Semin Respir Infect 1997;12:138. [NLM Cit ID: 97339124]

Haarbrink M et al: Adverse reactions following diethylcarbamazine (DEC) intake in "endemic normals," microfilaremics and elephantiasis patients. Trans R Soc Trop Med Hyg 1999;93:91. [NLM Cit ID: 99422468]

Ismail MM et al Efficacy of single dose combinations of albendazole, ivermectin, and diethylcarbamazine for the treatment of bancroftian filariasis. Trans R Soc Trop Med Hyg 1998;92:94. [NLM Cit ID: 98357195]

Ottesen EA et al: The role of albendazole in programs to eliminate lymphatic filariasis. Parasitol Today 1999;15:382. [NLM Cit ID: 20038480]

Plaisier AP et al: Efficacy of ivermectin in the treatment of *Wuchereria bancrofti* infection: a model-based analysis of trial results. Parasitology 1999;119(Part 4):385. [NLM Cit ID: 20048318]

Rajan TV et al: Lymphatic filariasis. Chem Immunol 1997;66:125. [NLM Cit ID: 97256968]

Witte CL et al: Diagnostic and interventional imaging of lymphatic disorders. Int Angiol 1999;18:25. [NLM Cit ID: 99319648]

GNATHOSTOMIASIS

Gnathostomiasis, due for the most part to infection by the larval stage of the nematode *Gnathostoma spinigerum,* is rarely caused by other gnathostoma species. Infection is most common in Thailand and Japan but is also reported from Southeast Asia, China, India, Ecuador, Israel, and East Africa. In Mexico, where the gnathostoma species has not been identified, the number of cases is increasing; more than 1000 have been reported in the past 10 years, commonly associated with increased eating of raw fresh-water fish, especially a preparation called ceviche. In the USA, though *G spinigerum* has rarely been seen in minks, it has not been reported in humans. Eggs passed in feces of the definitive hosts, wild and domestic dogs and cats, are infective for copepods (water fleas). Ingestion of copepods by secondary hosts results in encysted larvae in their tissues; humans are infected when these larvae are ingested in raw, marinated, or inadequately cooked freshwater fish, chicken or other fowl, frogs, or pork. Infection has also been attributed to ingestion of infected copepods in water.

Within 24–48 hours, larval migration through the intestinal wall can cause acute epigastric pain, vomiting, urticaria, and eosinophilia. The worm then migrates to subcutaneous and other tissues but is unable to mature. Most common is a pruritic subcutaneous swelling up to 25 cm across, occasionally accompanied by stabbing pain. Over weeks to years, the swelling may remain in one area for days or weeks, or move continuously. Occasionally the worm becomes visible under the skin.

Internal organs and the eye may also be invaded. Spontaneous pneumothorax, leukorrhea, hematemesis, hematuria, hemoptysis, paroxysmal coughing, and edema of the pharynx with dyspnea have been reported as complications. Invasion of the brain can result in an eosinophilic meningoencephalitis or subarachnoid hemorrhage. Spinal cord invasion can lead to myelitis or radiculopathy.

Definitive diagnosis is sometimes possible by surgical removal of the worm when it appears close to the skin. Marked eosinophilia is common, except for parasites in the central nervous system. Serodiagnosis by immunoblot assay or ELISA is promising. Skin and other serologic tests are unsatisfactory.

Treatment with albendazole may be effective. Among presumptively diagnosed cases, 94 of 100 persons were apparently cured after a dosage of 400 mg or 800 mg (in divided doses) of the drug daily for 21 days. Larval death appeared to occur slowly over 1–2 weeks. Ivermectin has been reported to be effective in animals. Courses of prednisolone have provided temporary relief of symptoms.

Diaz Camacho SP et al: Clinical manifestations and immunodiagnosis of gnathostomiasis in Culiacan, Mexico. Am J Trop Med Hyg 1998;59:908. [NLM Cit ID: 99101290]

Ogata K et al: Short Report: Gnathostomiasis in Mexico. Am J Trop Med Hyg 1998;58:316. [NLM Cit ID: 98206486]

Ruiz-Maldonado R et al: Human gnathostomiasis. Int J Dermatol 1999;38:56. [NLM Cit ID: 99163496] (A review of nodular migratory eosinophilic panniculitis.)

HOOKWORM DISEASE

Essentials of Diagnosis

Early findings (not commonly recognized):

- Dermatitis: pruritic, erythematous, papulovesicular eruption at site of larval invasion.
- Pulmonary migration of larvae: transient episodes of coughing, asthma, fever, blood-tinged sputum, marked eosinophilia.

Later findings:

- Intestinal symptoms: anorexia, diarrhea, abdominal discomfort.
- Anemia (iron deficiency): fatigue, pallor, dyspnea on exertion, poikilonychia, heart failure.
- Characteristic eggs and occult blood in the stool.

General Considerations

Hookworm disease, widespread in the moist tropics and subtropics and sporadically in southeastern USA, is caused by *Ancylostoma duodenale* and *Necator americanus.* Probably a quarter of the world's population is infected, and in many areas the infection is a major cause of general debility, retardation of growth and development of children, and increased susceptibility to infection. Prevalence rates can reach 80% in the humid tropics under unsanitary conditions.

In the Western Hemisphere and tropical Africa, necator was the prevailing species, and in the Far East, India, China, and the Mediterranean area, ancylostoma was prevalent, but both species have now become widely distributed. Infection is rare in regions with less than 40 inches of rainfall annually. Humans are the only host for both species.

The adult worms are approximately 1 cm long. Eggs produced by females are passed in the stool and must fall on warm, moist soil if hatching followed by larval development is to take place. Larvae remain infective for hours to about a week, depending on environmental conditions. Following skin penetration, the larvae migrate in the bloodstream to the pulmonary capillaries, break into alveoli, and then are carried by ciliary action upward to the bronchi, trachea, and mouth. After being swallowed, they reach and attach to the mucosa of the upper small bowel; maturation and release of eggs occurs in 6–8 weeks. Ancylostoma infection can also be acquired by ingestion of the larvae in food or water. Adult ancylostomae survive about a year; necator, about 3–5 years.

The worms suck blood at their attachment sites. Blood loss is proportionate to the worm burden. A light infection is approximately 1000 eggs per gram of feces (equivalent to about 11 ancylostoma and 32 necator adults); a moderate worm load is 2000–8000 eggs per gram of feces. Iron loss with moderate infection is 1.1 mg/d for *N americanus* and 2.3 mg/d for *A duodenale,* which compares with a basal intake requirement of 0.72 mg/kg/day of iron for a typical woman. Over years—and depending upon the host's dietary intake of iron—iron reserves can be depleted and severe anemia can result from moderate infections with 30 or more ancylostoma or 100 or more necator worms.

Clinical Findings

A. Symptoms and Signs: Ground itch, the first manifestation of infection, is a pruritic erythematous dermatitis, either maculopapular or vesicular, that follows skin penetration of the infective larvae. Severity is a function of the number of invading larvae and the sensitivity of the host. Scratching may result in secondary infection. Strongyloidiasis and cutaneous larva migrans must be considered in the differential diagnosis at this stage.

The pulmonary stage, in which there is larval migration through the lungs, may show dry cough, wheezing, blood-tinged sputum, and low-grade fever. The pulmonary migration of ascaris and strongyloides larvae can produce similar findings.

After 2 or more weeks, maturing worms attach to the mucosa of the duodenum and upper jejunum. In heavy infections, worms may reach the ileum. Patients who have light infections and adequate iron intake often remain asymptomatic. In heavy infections, however, there may be anorexia, diarrhea, vague abdominal pain, and ulcer-like epigastric symptoms. Severe anemia may result in pallor, deformed nails, pica, and cardiac decompensation. Marked protein loss may also occur, resulting in hypoalbuminemia, with edema and ascites. There are conflicting reports of malabsorption in some severe infections.

Reduction in worm loads and symptoms after the first decade of life suggests that a moderate degree of immunity develops.

B. Laboratory Findings: Diagnosis depends upon demonstration of characteristic eggs in feces; a concentration method may be needed. The two species cannot be differentiated by the appearance of their eggs. The stool usually contains occult blood. Hypochromic microcytic anemia can be severe, with hemoglobin levels as low as 2 g/dL, a low serum iron and a high iron-binding capacity, and low serum ferritin. Eosinophilia (as high as 30–60% of a total white blood count reaching 17,000/μL) is usually present in the pulmonary migratory stage of infection but is not marked in the chronic intestinal stage.

Treatment

A. General Measures: The availability of safe anthelmintics makes it possible to treat all patients initially, irrespective of the intensity of infection; nevertheless, it may not be necessary or beneficial to treat light infections. Re-treatment may be necessary at 2-week intervals until the worm burden is reduced to a low level as estimated by semiquantitative egg counts. Eradication of infection is not essential, since light infections do not injure the well-nourished patient and iron loss is replaced if the patient is receiving adequate dietary iron.

If anemia is present, oral ferrous sulfate and a diet high in protein and vitamins are required for at least 3 months after the anemia has been corrected in order to replace iron stores. A dosage schedule for ferrous sulfate tablets (200 mg) is one tablet three times daily for 2 months followed by one tablet daily for 4 months. Parenteral iron is rarely indicated. Blood transfusion may be necessary if anemia is severe.

B. Specific Measures: Mebendazole, pyrantel, and albendazole are highly effective drugs for treatment of both hookworm species; mebendazole or albendazole can be used to treat concurrent trichuriasis, and all three drugs can be used to treat concurrent ascariasis. The drugs are given before or after meals, without purges. For the three drugs, mild gastrointestinal side effects are rare; none should be used in pregnancy. Albendazole and mebendazole should not be given to children under about 1 year of age.

1. Pyrantel pamoate–In *A duodenale* infections, pyrantel given as a single dose, 10 mg (base)/kg (maximum 1 g), produces cures in 76–98% of cases and a marked reduction in the worm burden in the remainder. For *N americanus* infections, a single dose may give a satisfactory cure rate in light infection, but for moderate or heavy infection a 3-day course is necessary. If the species is unknown, treat as for necatoriasis. Mild and transient drowsiness and headache may occur.

2. Mebendazole–When mebendazole is given at a dosage of 100 mg twice daily for 3 days, reported cure rates for both hookworm species range from 35% to 95%.

3. Albendazole, given orally once only at a dosage of 400 mg, results in the cure of 85–95% of patients with ancylostoma infection and markedly reduces the worm burden in those not cured. Because cure rates for single-dose treatments of necator infection were 33–90%, treatment should be continued for 2–3 days, especially in heavy infections. Albendazole is available in the USA, though it is not FDA-approved for this indication.

Prognosis

If the disease is recognized before serious secondary complications appear, complete recovery is the rule following treatment.

Eosinophilic Enteritis

In Australia. *Ancylostoma caninum,* the dog hookworm, has been found to cause abdominal pain, diarrhea, and peripheral eosinophilia.

Georgiev VS: Parasitic infections. Treatment and developmental therapeutics. 1. Necatoriasis. Curr Pharm Des 1999;5:545. [NLM Cit ID: 99370325]

Grencis RK et al: Enterobius, trichuris, capillaria, and hookworm including *Ancylostoma caninum.* Gastroenterol Clin North Am 1996;25:579. [NLM Cit ID: 97016406]

Prociv P et al: Human enteric infection with *Ancylostoma caninum:* Hookworm reappraised in the light of a "new" zoonosis. Acta Trop 1996;62:23. [NLM Cit ID: 97126361]

Reynoldson JA et al: Failure of pyrantel in treatment of human hookworm infections. Acta Tropica 1997;68:301. [NLM Cit ID: 98153935]

LOIASIS

Loiasis is a chronic filarial disease caused by infection with *Loa loa.* The infection occurs in humans and monkeys in rain and swamp forest areas of West Africa from Nigeria to Angola and throughout the Congo river watershed of central Africa eastward to southwestern Sudan and western Uganda. An estimated 3–13 million persons are infected.

The adult worms live in the subcutaneous tissues for up to 12 years. Gravid females release microfilariae into the bloodstream which subsequently are ingested in a blood meal by the vector-intermediate host, female *Chrysops* species, day-biting flies. When the fly feeds again, the larval stage can infect a new host or cause superinfection. The time to worm maturity and detection of new microfilariae is 6 months to several years.

Clinical Findings

A. Symptoms and Signs: Many infected persons are asymptomatic. In symptomatic persons, the worms (females, 4–7 cm × 0.5 mm) are evidenced by their temporary appearance beneath the skin or conjunctiva, by unilateral edema of an extremity, or by Calabar swellings. The latter are subcutaneous edematous reactions, 3–10 cm in diameter, nonpitting and nonerythematous, and at times associated with low-grade fever, local pain, and pruritus. The swellings may migrate a few centimeters for 2–3 days or stay in place before they subside. At irregular intervals, they recur at the same or different sites, but only one appears at a time. When near joints, they may be temporarily disabling. Migration across the eye may be asymptomatic or may produce pain, intense conjunctivitis, and eyelid edema. Dying adult worms may elicit small nodules or local sterile abscesses, and dead worms may result in radiologically detectable calcification.

Microfilariae in the blood do not induce symptoms. Rarely, however, they enter the central nervous system and may cause encephalitis, myelitis, or jacksonian seizures; the larvae can also induce lesions and complications in the retina, heart, lungs, and other tissues.

Natives generally have a mild form of the infection or are asymptomatic but are microfilaremic and serologically positive. The disease among visitors, however, is often characterized by more pronounced immunologically mediated symptoms (frequent and debilitating Calabar swellings, elevated leukocyte and eosinophil counts, hypergammaglobulinemia, increased polyclonal IgE) and frequently a positive serologic test but nondetectable microfilaremia.

B. Laboratory Findings: Specific diagnosis is made by finding characteristic microfilariae in daytime (10 AM to 4 PM) blood specimens by concentration methods; in order of increasing sensitivity, they are (1) thick films, (2) Knott's concentration, and (3) Nuclepore filtration. Presumptive diagnosis that permits treatment is based on Calabar swellings or eye migration, a history of residence in an endemic area, and marked eosinophilia (40% or greater). Serologic tests may be positive, but cross-reactions occur with other filarial diseases and sometimes with nematode infections.

Treatment & Prognosis

See specialized sources and references for details on proper use of diethylcarbamazine (drug of choice both as a micro- and macrofilaricide), since side effects to dying microfilariae may be severe, and life-threatening encephalitis can occur rarely. The dosage is 50 mg once (day 1), 50 mg three times daily (day 2), 100 mg three times daily (day 3), and 3 mg/kg three times daily (days 4–21). One course of treatment cures about 50% of patients; three courses, 90%. Reactions are more likely with pretreatment microfilaria counts greater than 25/μL. Cytapheresis has been used to reduce parasite loads before starting diethylcarbamazine. Prednisone is sometimes indicated to minimize reactions. Surgical removal of adult worms from the eye or skin is not recommended. When ivermectin was used in treatment of 1.1 million persons with onchocerciasis in the presence of endemic loiasis, 28 neurologic reactions occurred (some severe) from death of *Loa loa* microfilariae. The risk of these reactions was high when the *L loa* microfilaria load exceeded 8/μL and very high above 50/μL. Albendazole at a dosage of 200 mg twice daily for 3 weeks is being evaluated as a safe way to reduce the level of *L loa* microfilariae.

In the USA, diethylcarbamazine is available only from the Parasitic Diseases Drug Service, Centers for Disease Control and Prevention, Atlanta, GA 30333, telephone 404-639-3670.

Individual protection is facilitated by daytime use of insect repellent and by wearing light-colored clothing with long sleeves and trousers. Diethylcarbamazine prophylaxis, 300 mg weekly, may be useful if the risk of exposure is high. It is not indicated, however, for the casual traveler or for persons who might previously have acquired any of the filarial infections.

Most infections run a benign course, but some are

accompanied by severe and temporarily disabling symptoms. The prognosis is excellent with treatment.

Boussinesq M et al: Three probable cases of *Loa loa* encephalitis following ivermectin treatment for onchocerciasis. Am J Trop Med Hyg 1998;58:461. [NLM Cit ID: 98233980]

Chippaux JP et al: Impact of repeated large scale ivermectin treatments on the transmission of *Loa loa.* Trans R Soc Trop Med Hyg 1998;92:454. [NLM Cit ID: 99067394]

Churchill DR et al: Clinical and laboratory features of patients with loiasis (*Loa loa* filariasis) in the U.K. J Infect 1996;33:103. [NLM Cit ID: 97044926]

Klion AD et al: Albendazole therapy for loiasis refractory to diethylcarbamazine treatment. Clin Infect Dis 1999;29:680. [NLM Cit ID: 99458050]

ONCHOCERCIASIS

Onchocerciasis is a chronic filarial disease caused by *Onchocerca volvulus.* The advent of the safe and effective drug ivermectin has led to effective treatment and control of the disease. Primary findings are subcutaneous nodules that contain adult worms and skin and eye changes that result from dead or dying microfilariae. Heavy infection leads to chronic pruritus, disfiguring skin lesions, visual impairment, and debility. An estimated 18 million persons are infected, of whom 3–4 million have skin disease, 0.3 million are blinded, and 0.5 million severely visually impaired. In hyperendemic areas, more than 40% of inhabitants over 40 years of age are blind. The infection, predominant in West Africa, also occurs in many other parts of tropical Africa and in localized areas of the southwestern Arabian peninsula, southern Mexico, Guatemala, Venezuela, Colombia, and northwestern Brazil. The West African savanna strain is especially associated with severe blinding eye lesions.

Humans are the only important host. The vector and intermediate host are *Simulium* flies, day biters that breed in rivers and fast-flowing streams and become infected by ingesting microfilariae with a human blood meal; at subsequent feedings, they can infect new susceptible hosts.

Clinical Findings

A. Symptoms and Signs: Adult worms, which can live for up to 14 years, typically are in fibrous subcutaneous nodules that are painless, freely movable, and 0.5–1 cm in diameter. Many nodules, however, are deep in the connective and muscular tissues and nonpalpable. The interval from exposure to onset of symptoms can be as long as 1–3 years. Female worms release motile microfilariae into the skin, subcutaneous tissues, lymphatics, and eyes; microfilariae are occasionally seen in the urine but rarely in blood or cerebrospinal fluid. Skin manifestations are localized or cover large areas. Pruritus may be severe, leading to skin excoriation and lichenification; other findings include pigmentary changes, papules, scaling, atrophy, pendulous skin, and acute inflammation. Pruritus may occur in the absence of skin lesions. There may be marked enlargement of femoral and inguinal nodes and generalized lymph node enlargement. Microfilariae in the eye may lead to visual impairment and blindness; findings include itching, photophobia, anterior segment changes (limbitis, punctate and sclerosing keratitis, iritis, secondary glaucoma, cataract), and posterior segment changes (optic neuritis, optic atrophy, chorioretinitis, and other retinal and choroidal findings). Infected visitors, as compared with indigenous persons, may show a more prominent dermatitis despite a low to nondetectable microfiladerma or eosinophilia and an absence of nodules and eye disease.

B. Laboratory Findings: Diagnosis is by demonstrating microfilariae in skin snips (usually obtained with a punch biopsy instrument), identifying them in the cornea or anterior chamber by slitlamp examination (after the patient has sat with head lowered between knees for 2 minutes) or by nodule aspiration or excision. Skin snips are placed in saline and incubated overnight before examination. Adult worms may be recovered in excised nodules, whereas ultrasound has been used to detect nonpalpable onchocercomas and to distinguish them from other lesions (lipomas, fibromas, lymph nodes, foreign body granulomas). Traditional serologic tests are usually positive, but cross-reactions occur with other forms of filariasis, and the tests do not distinguish current from past infection. Immunoblot analysis of IgG4 antibodies and an ELISA appear to be more sensitive than skin snips early in infection, but occasional cross-reactions also occur with other filarial infections. Diagnosis by polymerase chain reaction on skin snips may prove to be the most sensitive test for diagnosis and for assessing posttreatment status. Eosinophilia (15–50%), polyclonal hypergammaglobulinemia, and elevated IgE levels are common. The Mazzotti skin test is no longer recommended because of the potential for dangerous reactions.

Treatment & Prognosis

Drug treatment is with ivermectin (a microfilaricide) as a single oral dose of 150 μg/kg given with water on an empty stomach; the patient should remain fasting for 2 more hours. The number of microfilariae in the skin diminishes markedly within 2–3 days, remains low for about 6 months, and then gradually increases; microfilariae in the anterior chamber of the eye decrease slowly in number over months, eventually disappear, and then gradually return. The optimum frequency of treatment to control symptoms and prevent disease progression remains to be determined. To initiate treatment, three schedules have been proposed: (1) an initial and repeat dose at 6 months, (2) repeated doses at 3-month intervals for a year, or (3) repeated doses at monthly intervals for a total of three doses. Thereafter, treatment is repeated at intervals of 6 months for 2 years and yearly thereafter until the adult worms die, which may take 12–15 years or longer. With the initial treatment only, patients with microfilariae in the cornea or anterior chamber may benefit from several days of prednisone treatment (1 mg/kg/d) to avoid inflammatory eye reactions. Although single-dose ivermectin does not kill the adult worms, with repeated doses, increasing evidence suggests that the drug has a low-level macrofilaricidal action. Adverse reactions, which are more marked with the first dose, are mild in 9% of patients and severe in 0.2%; these include edema (face and limbs), fever, pruritus, lymphadenitis, malaise, and hypotension. Ivermectin does not cause a severe reaction in the eyes or skin as does occur with diethylcarbamazine. Ivermectin should be used with great caution in the presence of concurrent infections with *Loa loa* (see that section); it should not be used in pregnancy. In developing countries, ivermectin is available on a compassionate basis from the manufacturer, Merck & Co. In Latin America only, nodulectomy continues to be used for nodules on or near the head. See specialized sources for further details concerning its use.

In comparison studies, ivermectin was as effective as diethylcarbamazine in reducing the number of microfilariae but did so with significantly fewer systemic and ocular adverse reactions. Diethylcarbamazine is no longer recommended by WHO in onchocerciasis therapy. For selected patients in whom repeated ivermectin treatments do not control symptoms, suramin can be given for its macrofilaricidal action; however, because of suramin's toxicity and complex administration, it should only be administered by experts. Amocarzine is under evaluation for its macro- and microfilaricidal actions.

With treatment, some skin and ocular lesions improve and ocular progression is prevented. The prognosis is unfavorable only for those patients who are seen for the first time with already far-advanced ocular onchocerciasis.

Awadzi K et al: The effects of high-dose ivermectin regimens on *Onchocerca volvulus* in onchocerciasis patients. Trans R Soc Trop Med Hyg 1999;93:189. [NLM Cit ID: 99378942]

Burnham G: Onchocerciasis. Lancet 1998;351:1341. [NLM Cit ID: 98305964]

Chippaux JP et al: Effect of repeated ivermectin treatments on ocular onchocerciasis: evaluation after six to eight doses. Ophthalmic Epidemiol 1999;6:229. [NLM Cit ID: 20013236]

Cousens SN et al: Impact of annual dosing with ivermectin on progression of onchocercal visual field loss. Bull World Health Organ 1997;75:229. [NLM Cit ID: 97422945]

Hall LR et al: Pathogenesis of onchocercal keratitis (river blindness). Clin Microbiol Rev 1999;12:445. [NLM Cit ID: 99328848]

STRONGYLOIDIASIS

Essentials of Diagnosis

- Pruritic dermatitis at sites of larval penetration.
- Diarrhea, epigastric pain, nausea, malaise, weight loss.
- Cough, rales, transient pulmonary infiltrates.
- Eosinophilia; characteristic larvae in stool specimens, duodenal aspirate, or sputum.
- Hyperinfection syndrome: Severe diarrhea, bronchopneumonia, ileus.

General Considerations

Strongyloidiasis is caused by infection with *Strongyloides stercoralis* (2–2.5 × 30–50 mm). Major symptoms result from adult parasitism, principally in the duodenum and jejunum, or from larval migration through pulmonary and cutaneous tissues. The primary host is humans, but dogs, cats, and primates have been found infected with strains indistinguishable from those of humans.

The disease is endemic in tropical and subtropical regions; although the prevalence is generally low, in some areas disease rates exceed 25%. An estimate of total world prevalence is 60 million. In temperate areas, the disease occurs sporadically. In the USA, highest infection rates are found in immigrants from endemic areas, in parts of Appalachia (up to 4%), and in southeastern areas; Puerto Rico is also an endemic area. Multiple infections in households are common, and prevalence may be high in institutions, particularly mental institutions (2–4%). The infection is also prevalent among immunosuppressed persons (see below).

The parasite is uniquely capable of maintaining its life cycle both within the human host and in soil. Infection occurs when filariform larvae in soil penetrate the skin, enter the bloodstream, and are carried to the lungs, where they escape from capillaries into alveoli and ascend the bronchial tree to the glottis. The larvae are then swallowed and carried to the duodenum and upper jejunum, where maturation to the adult stage takes place. The parasitic female, generally held to be parthenogenetic, matures and lives embedded in the mucosa, where its eggs are laid and hatch. Rhabditiform larvae, which are noninfective, emerge, and migrate into the intestinal lumen to leave the host via the feces. The life span of the adult worm may be as long as 5 years.

In the soil, the rhabditiform larvae metamorphose into the infective (filariform) larvae. However, the parasite also has a free-living cycle in soil, in which some rhabditiform larvae develop into adults that produce eggs from which rhabditiform larvae emerge to continue the life cycle.

Autoinfection in humans, which probably occurs at a low rate in most infections, is an important factor in determining worm burden and is responsible for the persistence of infections. Internal autoinfection takes place in the lower bowel when some rhabditiform larvae develop into filariform larvae that penetrate the intestinal mucosa, enter the intestinal lymphatic and portal circulation, are carried to the lungs, and return to the small bowel to complete the cycle. This process is accelerated by achlorhydria, constipation, diverticula, and other conditions that reduce bowel motility. In addition, an external autoinfection cycle can occur as a result of fecal contamination of the perianal area.

Recrudescence of a chronic asymptomatic infection may occur with the immunosuppression accompanying severe infections, corticosteroid treatment, metabolic diseases, severe malnutrition, or malignancy; exacerbation may lead to the hyperinfection syndrome. In the hyperinfection syndrome, autoinfection is greatly increased, resulting in a marked increase in the intestinal worm burden and in massive dissemination of filariform larvae to the lungs and most other tissues, where they can cause local inflammatory reactions and granuloma formation. Occasionally, in the lungs and elsewhere, larvae metamorphose into adults. Penetration of the bowel wall by filariform larvae can result in bacterial or fungal sepsis or meningitis. Hyperinfection is generally initiated under conditions of depressed host cellular immunity, especially in debilitated, malnourished persons and in patients with leukemia or lymphoma or those receiving immunosuppressive therapy, particularly chemotherapy or corticosteroids. Although the hyperinfection syndrome is rare in AIDS, these patients do have a protracted course that is difficult to cure.

Clinical Findings

A. Symptoms and Signs: Up to 30% of infected persons are asymptomatic. The time from larval penetration of the skin by filariform larvae until their appearance in the feces is 3–4 weeks. An acute syndrome can sometimes be recognized in which cutaneous symptoms, usually of the feet, are followed by pulmonary and then intestinal symptoms. Patients usually present, however, with chronic symptoms (continuous or with irregular exacerbations) that can persist for years or for life.

1. Cutaneous manifestations–In acute infection in sensitized patients, there may be focal edema, inflammation, petechiae, serpiginous or urticarial tracts, and intense itching. In chronic infections, there may be both stationary urticaria and larva currens, the latter characterized by transient eruptions that migrate in serpiginous tracts.

2. Intestinal manifestations–Symptoms range from mild to severe, the most common being diarrhea, abdominal pain, and flatulence. Anorexia, nausea, vomiting, epigastric tenderness, and pruritus ani may be present; with increasing severity, fever and malaise may appear. Diarrhea may alternate with constipation, and in severe cases the feces contain mucus and blood. The pain is often epigastric in location and may mimic duodenal ulcer. Malabsorption or a protein-losing enteropathy can result from a large intestinal worm burden.

3. Pulmonary manifestations–With migration of larvae through the lungs, bronchi, and trachea, symptoms may be limited to a dry cough and throat irritation or low-grade fever, dyspnea, wheezing, and hemoptysis may occur; asthma is rare. Bronchopneumonia, bronchitis, pleural effusion, progressive dyspnea, and miliary abscesses can develop; the cough may become productive of an odorless, mucopurulent sputum.

4. Hyperinfection syndrome–Intense dissemination of filariform larvae to the lungs and other tissues can result in additional complications, including pleural effusion, pericarditis and myocarditis, hepatic granulomas, cholecystitis, purpura, ulcerating lesions at all levels of the gastrointestinal tract, central nervous system involvement, paralytic ileus, perforation and peritonitis, gram-negative septicemia and meningitis (due to larval carriage of enterobacteria from the colon), cachexia, shock, and death. A nephrotic syndrome has been implicated.

B. Laboratory Findings:

1. Detection of eggs and larvae–Eggs are seldom found in feces. Diagnosis, which may be difficult, requires finding the larval stages in feces or duodenal fluid. Rhabditiform larvae may be found in recently passed stool specimens; filariform larvae will be present in specimens held in the laboratory for some hours. Four to six specimens, some unpreserved, should be collected at 2-day intervals or longer (the number of larvae in feces varies from day to day). Since the sensitivity of direct microscopic examination of one specimen is about 30%, it is essential that one-half of the specimens be processed, unpreserved, in the Baermann concentration or agar plate culture methods, the sensitivity of which are 90% and higher.

The diagnosis can sometimes be made by finding rhabditiform larvae or ova in mucus obtained by means of the duodenal string test or by duodenal intubation and aspiration. Duodenal biopsy is seldom indicated but will confirm the diagnosis in most patients. Occasionally, filariform or rhabditiform larvae can be detected in sputum or bronchial washings during the pulmonary phase of the disease.

2. Serologic and hematologic findings–In chronic low-grade intestinal strongyloidiasis, the white blood cell count is often normal, with a slightly elevated percentage of eosinophils. However, with increasing larval migration, eosinophilia may reach 50% and leukocytosis 20,000/μL. Mild anemia may be present. Serum IgE immunoglobulins may be elevated. An ELISA is sensitive (85%) and specific (97%), but cross-reactions can occur with the filaria and other helminthic infections. A positive test indicates current or past infection.

3. Hyperinfection–In the hyperinfection syndrome, there may also be findings of hypoproteinemia, malabsorption, abnormal liver function, and extensive pulmonary opacities. Filariform larvae may appear in the urine. Eosinopenia, when present, is thought to be an unfavorable prognostic sign.

C. Imaging: Small bowel x-rays may show inflammation, irritability, and prominent mucosal folds; there may also be bowel dilation, delayed emptying, and ulcerative duodenitis. In chronic infections, the findings can resemble those in nontropical and tropical sprue, or there may be narrowing, rigidity, and diminished peristalsis. During pulmonary migration of larvae, chest films are normal or show fine miliary nodules or irregular changing patches of pneumonitis, abscess, or pleural effusion.

Differential Diagnosis

Because of varied signs and symptoms, the diagnosis of strongyloidiasis is often difficult. Eosinophilia plus one or more of the following factors should further enhance consideration of the diagnosis: endemic area exposure, duodenal ulcer-like pain, persistent or recurrent diarrhea, or malabsorption, recurrent coughing or wheezing, and transient pulmonary infiltrates. The duodenitis and jejunitis of strongyloidiasis can also mimic giardiasis, cholecystitis, and pancreatitis. Transient pulmonary infiltrates must be differentiated from tropical pulmonary eosinophilia and Löffler's syndrome. The diagnosis should be considered among the many causes of malabsorption in the tropics and in immunocompromised persons, including HIV-infected patients.

Treatment

Since strongyloides can multiply in humans, treatment should continue until the parasite is eradicated. In follow-up, multiple stool examinations should be done at weekly intervals, preferably by the Baermann concentration method. Patients receiving immunosuppressive therapy should be examined for strongyloidiasis before and at intervals during that treatment. In concurrent infection with strongyloidiasis and ascariasis or hookworm (which is common), eradicate the latter infections first.

The drug of choice in treatment is ivermectin, which appears to be equal in effectiveness to thiabendazole but has far fewer side effects.

A. Ivermectin: The dosage is 200 μg/kg; since cure is essential in this disease, a second dose is recommended the next day. Cure rates reported in several studies ranged from 82% to 95%. In the hyperinfection syndrome in immunocompromised patients with or without AIDS, it may be necessary to prolong treatment or change to thiabendazole.

B. Thiabendazole: An oral dose of 25 mg/kg (maximum, 1.5 g per dose) is given after meals twice daily for 2–3 days. Repeat the course in 2 weeks. A 5- to 7-day course is needed for disseminated infections. Tablet and liquid formulations are available; tablets should be chewed. Side effects, including headache, weakness, vomiting, vertigo, and decreased mental alertness, occur in as many as 30% of patients and may be severe. These symptoms are lessened if the drug is taken after meals. Other potentially serious side effects occur rarely. Erythema multiforme and the Stevens-Johnson syndrome have been associated with thiabendazole therapy; several fatalities have occurred in children.

C. Albendazole: Albendazole is given at a dosage of 400 mg twice daily for 3–7 days and repeated in 1 week; cure rates in several studies ranged from 38% to 95%. In comparative studies, albendazole is less effective than ivermectin.

Prognosis

The prognosis is favorable except in the hyperinfection syndrome and in infections associated with emaciation, advanced liver disease, cancer, immunologic disorders, or the use of immunosuppressive drugs. In selected instances, to control infections that cannot be eradicated, once-monthly treatments can be tried with a 1-day dose of ivermectin or 2-day course of thiabendazole.

Al Samman M et al: Strongyloidiasis colitis: a case report and review of the literature. J Clin Gastroenterol 1999;28:77. [NLM Cit ID: 99113714]

Dreyer G et al: Patterns of detection of *Strongyloides stercoralis* in stool specimens: Implications for diagnosis and clinical trials. J Clin Microbiol 1996;34:2569. [NLM Cit ID: 97034865]

Link K et al: Bacterial complications of strongyloidiasis: *Streptococcus bovis* meningitis. South Med J 1999; 92:728. [NLM Cit ID: 99341436]

Marti H et al: A comparative trial of a single-dose ivermectin versus three days of albendazole for the treatment of *Strongyloides stercoralis* and other soil-transmitted helminth infections in children. Am J Trop Med Hyg 1996;55:477. [NLM Cit ID: 97095952]

Schneider JH et al: Strongyloidiasis. The protean parasitic infection. Postgrad Med 1997;102:177. [NLM Cit ID: 97445037]

TRICHINOSIS (Trichinelliosis, Trichinellosis)

Essentials of Diagnosis

- History of ingestion of raw or inadequately cooked pork, boar, or bear.
- First week: diarrhea, cramps, malaise.
- Second week to 1–2 months: muscle pain and tenderness, fever, periorbital and facial edema, conjunctivitis.
- Eosinophilia and elevated serum enzymes; positive serologic tests; larvae in muscle biopsy.

General Considerations

Trichinosis is caused worldwide by *Trichinella spiralis.* The disease is present wherever pork is eaten but is a greater problem in many temperate areas than in the tropics. In the USA, there has been a marked reduction in prevalence in pigs (rates in commercial pork are nil to 0.01%) and humans (fewer than 35 cases are reported yearly). Four other species of trichinella have been recognized in humans: *T nativa* appears to be restricted to Arctic and sub-Arctic regions and *T nelsoni* to tropical Africa. *T pseudospiralis,* reported rarely worldwide, occurs as a persistent muscular infection accompanied by prolonged myalgia, muscular weakness and swelling, elevated muscle enzymes, and asthenia. *T britovi* occurs in temperate areas of Europe.

Human infections occur sporadically or in outbreaks. Infection is usually acquired by eating viable encysted larvae in raw or uncooked pork or pork products. Ground beef has also been a source of infection when adulterated with pork or inadvertently contaminated in a common meat grinder. In some cases, the source of infection is the flesh of dogs (East Asia), horses (France), or wild animals, particularly bears, walruses, bush pigs, foxes, or cougars (USA).

Gastric juices liberate the encysted larvae. They rapidly mature and mate, and the adult female then burrows into the mucosa of the small intestine. Within 4–5 days, the female begins to discharge viviparous larvae (100 × 6 μm) that are disseminated via the lymphatics and bloodstream to most body tissues. Larvae that reach striated muscle encyst and remain viable for months to years; those that reach other tissues are rapidly destroyed. The adult worms (2–3.6 mm × 75–90 μm) survive for up to about 6 weeks.

In the natural cycle, larvae develop into adult worms in the intestines when a carnivore or omnivore ingests parasitized muscle. Pigs generally become infected by feeding on uncooked food scraps or, less often, by eating infected rats. Other reservoir hosts include swine, dogs, cats, rats, and many wild animals, including the wolf, bear, and boar; marine animals in the Arctic; and the hyena, jackal, and lion in the tropics.

Clinical Findings

A. Symptoms and Signs: The incubation period is 2–7 days (range: 12 hours to 28 days). Severity depends upon intensity of infection, tissues invaded, immune status and age of the host (children have less severe infections), and perhaps the strain of the parasite. Findings range from asymptomatic to a mild febrile illness with short-lasting symptoms to a severe progressive illness with multiple system involvement that in rare cases is fatal.

1. Intestinal stage–When present, intestinal symptoms persist for 1–7 days: diarrhea, abdominal cramps, and malaise are the major findings; nausea and vomiting occur less frequently; and constipation is uncommon. Fever, eosinophilia, and leukocytosis are rare during the first week.

2. Muscle invasion stage–This begins at the end of the first week and lasts about 6 weeks. Parasitized muscles show an intense inflammatory reaction. Findings include fever (low-grade to marked); muscle pain and tenderness, edema, and spasm; periorbital and facial edema; sweating; photophobia and conjunctivitis; weakness or prostration; pain on swallowing; dyspnea, coughing, and hoarseness; subconjunctival, retinal, and nail splinter hemorrhages; and rashes and formication. The most frequently parasitized muscles and sites of findings are the masseters, the tongue, the diaphragm, the intercostal muscles, and the extraocular, laryngeal, paravertebral, nuchal, deltoid, pectoral, gluteus, biceps, and gastrocnemius muscles. Inflammatory reactions around larvae that reach tissues other than muscle may result in a broad range of findings, including the development of meningitis, encephalitis, myocarditis, bronchopneumonia, nephritis, and peripheral and cranial nerve disorders.

3. Convalescent stage–This generally begins in the second month but in severe infections may not begin before 3 months or longer. Vague muscle pains and malaise may persist for several more months. Permanent muscular atrophy has been reported.

B. Laboratory Findings: The diagnosis is supported by findings of eosinophilia, elevated serum muscle enzymes, and positive serologic tests. There may be a marked hypergammaglobulinemia with reversal of the albumin-globulin ratio. Absence of an elevated sedimentation rate is a useful diagnostic clue. Confirmation of the diagnosis is by detection of larvae in muscle biopsy specimens.

Leukocytosis and eosinophilia appear during the second week. The proportion of eosinophils rises to a maximum of 20–90% in the third or fourth week and then slowly declines to normal over the next few months.

Serologic tests can detect most clinically manifest cases but are not sufficiently sensitive to detect low-level infections (ie, a few larvae per gram of ingested muscle). More than one test should be used and then repeated to observe for seroconversion or for a rising titer. A qualitative latex agglutination test is available for screening. The bentonite flocculation (BF) test (positive titer, ≥ 1:5) is highly sensitive and is considered nearly 100% specific. It becomes positive in the third or fourth week, and reaches a maximum titer at about 2 months and generally reverts to negative in 2–3 years. The immunofluorescence test (positive titer > 16) is also highly sensitive, though less specific than the BF test; it may become positive in the second week. The IgM and IgG ELISAs are also showing high sensitivity and specificity for antibody and detection of circulating antigens. The intradermal test is no longer recommended, as it may remain positive for years and batches of antigen vary in potency.

Adult worms may be looked for in feces, though they are seldom found. In the second week, there are occasional larvae in blood, duodenal washings, and, rarely, in centrifuged spinal fluid. In the third to fourth weeks, biopsy of skeletal muscle may be definitive (particularly gastrocnemius and pectoralis), preferably at a site of swelling or tenderness or near tendinous insertions. Portions of the specimen should be examined microscopically by compression between glass slides, by digestion, and by preparation of multiple histologic sections. If the biopsy is done too early, larvae may not be detectable. Myositis even in the absence of larvae is a significant finding.

C. Imaging: Chest films during the acute phase may show disseminated or localized infiltrates. Late calcification of muscle cysts cannot be detected radiologically.

Complications

The more important complications are granulomatous pneumonitis, encephalitis, and cardiac failure.

Differential Diagnosis

Because of its protean manifestations, trichinosis may resemble many other diseases. Eosinophilia, muscle pain and tenderness, and fever should lead the physician to consider collagen vascular disorders such as dermatomyositis or polyarteritis nodosa, which is generally accompanied by an elevated sedimentation rate.

Prevention

The frequency and intensity of infection in the USA and other countries have been significantly reduced by public health measures to prevent feeding of uncooked garbage to hogs and by animal inspection (not in the USA). The chief safeguard against trichinosis is adequate cooking of pork to 77 °C or by freezing meat at –17 °C for 20 days (longer if meat is over 15 cm thick). *T spiralis* in game is often relatively resistant to freezing. Low doses of gamma irradiation are also effective in killing larvae.

Treatment

Treatment is principally supportive, since in most cases recovery is spontaneous without sequelae.

A. Intestinal Phase: Though supporting evidence for efficacy is limited, albendazole, because of its relatively high absorption and freedom from adverse reactions, is proposed as the drug of choice in a dosage of 400 mg twice daily for 10 days. Mebendazole is an alternative drug at a dosage of 200–400 mg three times daily for 3 days, followed by 400–500 mg three times daily for 10 days. A second alternative drug is thiabendazole at a dosage of 25 mg/kg (maximum, 1.5 g per dose) twice daily after meals for 3–7 days; side effects, sometimes severe, are common (see Strongyloidiasis, above). Corticosteroids are contraindicated in the intestinal phase.

B. Muscle Invasion Phase: In this stage, severe infections require hospitalization and high doses of corticosteroids for 24–48 hours, followed by lower doses for several days or weeks to control symptoms. However, because corticosteroids may suppress the inflammatory response to adult worms, they should be used only when symptoms are severe. Thiabendazole has been tried in the muscle stage with equivocal relief of muscle pain or tenderness or lysis of fever; further trials are recommended. Mebendazole and albendazole may also be tried.

Prognosis

Death is rare—sometimes within 2–3 weeks in overwhelming infections, more often in 4–8 weeks from a major complication such as cardiac failure or pneumonia.

Cabie A et al: Albendazole versus thiabendazole as therapy for trichinosis: A retrospective study. Clin Infect Dis 1996;22:1033. [NLM Cit ID: 96377930]

Capo V et al: Clinical aspects of infection with *Trichinella* spp. Clin Microbiol Rev 1996;9:47. [NLM Cit ID: 96263586]

Jongwutiwes S et al: First outbreak of human trichinellosis caused by *Trichinella pseudospiralis.* Clin Infect Dis 1998;26:111. [NLM Cit ID: 98116696]

Moorhead A et al: Trichinellosis in the United States, 1991–1996: declining but not gone. Am J Trop Med Hyg 1999;60:66. [NLM Cit ID: 99140824]

TRICHURIASIS (Trichocephaliasis, Whipworm)

Trichuris trichiura is a common intestinal parasite of humans throughout the world, particularly in the subtropics and tropics. Persons of all ages are affected, but infection is heaviest and most frequent in children. The slender worms, 30–50 mm in length, attach by means of their anterior whip-like end to the mucosa of the large intestine, particularly to the cecum. Eggs are passed in the feces but require 2–4 weeks for larval development after reaching the soil before becoming infective; thus, person-to-person transmission is not possible. Infections are acquired by ingestion of the infective egg. The larvae hatch in the small intestine and mature in the large bowel but do not migrate through the tissues.

Clinical Findings

A. Symptoms and Signs: Light (fewer than 10,000 eggs per gram of feces) to moderate infections rarely cause symptoms. Heavy infections (30,000 or more eggs per gram of feces) may be accompanied by abdominal cramps, tenesmus, diarrhea, distention, flatulence, nausea, vomiting, and weight loss. Rectal prolapse and hematochezia or chronic occult blood loss may also occur, most often in malnourished young children. Sometimes, adult worms are seen in stools. Invasion of the appendix, with resulting appendicitis, is rare.

B. Laboratory Findings: Diagnosis is by identification of characteristic eggs and, sometimes, adult worms in stools. Eosinophilia (5–20%) is common with all but light infections. Severe iron deficiency anemia may be present with heavy infections.

Treatment

Patients with asymptomatic light infections do not require treatment. For those with heavier or symptomatic infections, give mebendazole, albendazole, or oxantel. Thiabendazole should *not* be used, because it is not effective and is potentially toxic.

A. Mebendazole: The dosage is 100 mg twice daily before or after meals for 3 days. It may be therapeutically advantageous for the tablets to be chewed before swallowing. Cure rates of 60–80% and higher are reported after one course of treatment, with marked reduction in ova counts in the remaining patients. For severe trichuriasis, a longer course of treatment (up to 6 days) or a repeat course will often be necessary. Gastrointestinal side effects from the drug are rare. The drug is contraindicated in pregnancy.

B. Albendazole: Albendazole, given orally at a single dose of 400 mg, has resulted in cure rates of 33–90%, with marked reduction in egg counts in those not cured. An appropriate dosage to achieve higher cure rates in moderate to heavy infections remains to be determined, but daily treatment for 2–3 days can be tried. Albendazole (available in the USA) should not be used in pregnancy.

C. Oxantel Pamoate: Oxantel pamoate is an analogue of pyrantel pamoate and acts only on *T trichiura.* Cure rates of 57–100% have been reported in various trials. One treatment schedule is 15 mg/kg (base) daily for 2 days for patients with mild to moderate intensity of infection. For patients with severe infection, give 10 mg/kg (base) daily for 5 days. Oxantel is not available in the USA. Safety in pregnancy is not established.

Chandra B et al: Diagnosis of *Trichuris trichiura* (whipworm) by colonoscopic extraction. J Clin Gastroenterol 1998;27:152. [NLM Cit ID: 98425774]

Forrester JE et al: Randomized trial of albendazole and pyrantel in symptomless trichuriasis in children. Lancet 1998;352:1103. [NLM Cit ID: 99012930]

Jackson TF et al: A comparison of mebendazole and albendazole in treating children with *Trichuris trichiura* infection in Durban, South Africa. S Afr Med J 1998;88:880. [NLM Cit ID: 98363873]

VISCERAL LARVA MIGRANS (Toxocariasis)

Most visceral larva migrans cases are due to *Toxocara canis,* an ascarid of dogs and other canids; *Toxocara cati* in domestic cats has occasionally been implicated and rarely *Belascaris procyonis* of raccoons. The adult worms live in the intestinal tracts of their respective hosts and release large numbers of eggs in the stool.

The reservoir mechanism for *T canis* is latent infection in female dogs which is reactivated during pregnancy. Transmission from mother to puppies is via the placenta and milk. Most eggs passed to the environment are from puppies (2 weeks to 6 months) and lactating bitches (up to 6 months after parturition). The life cycle of *T cati* is similar, but transplacental transmission does not occur.

Human infections are sporadic and probably occur worldwide. In the USA, antibody seroprevalence is 5–7%. Infection is generally in dirt-eating young children who ingest *T canis* or *T cati* eggs from soil or sand contaminated with animal feces, most often from puppies. Direct contact with infected animals does not produce infection, as the eggs require a 3- to 4-week extrinsic incubation period to become infective; thereafter, eggs in soil remain infective for months to years.

In humans, hatched larvae are unable to mature but continue to migrate through the tissues for up to 6 months. Eventually they lodge in various organs, particularly the lungs and liver and less often the brain, eyes, and other tissues, where they produce eosinophilic granulomas up to 1 cm in diameter.

Clinical & Laboratory Findings

A. Acute Infection: Migrating larvae may induce fever, cough, wheezing, hepatosplenomegaly, and lymphadenopathy. A variety of other findings may occur when other organs are invaded, including myelitis, encephalitis, and carditis. The acute phase may last 2–3 weeks, but resolution of all physical and laboratory findings may take up to 18 months.

Leukocytosis is marked (may exceed 100,000/μL), with 30–80% due to eosinophils. Hyperglobulinemia occurs when the liver is extensively invaded and is a useful clue in diagnosis. An ELISA test is the most specific (92%) and sensitive (78%) serologic test and may permit a presumptive diagnosis, although it does not distinguish acute from prior infection. Nonspecific isohemagglutinin titers (anti-A and anti-B) are usually greater than 1:1024. Chest radiographs may show infiltrates. With central nervous system involvement, the cerebrospinal fluid may show eosinophils. No parasitic forms can be found by stool examination.

Ultrasonography has been used to detect 1-cm hypoechoic lesions in the liver, each with a thread-like hyperechoic line. Specific diagnosis can only be made by percutaneous liver biopsy or by direct biopsy of a granuloma at laparoscopy, but these procedures are seldom justified.

B. Ocular Toxocariasis: Most cases occur in children, most commonly 5–10 years old, who present with visual impairment in one eye and sometimes leukocoria, squint, and red eye. The principal pathologic entity is eosinophilic granuloma of the retina that resembles retinoblastoma. Until the recent development of the ELISA test, this resulted in the enucleation of many eyes. Other common clinical findings are a diffuse, painless endophthalmitis; posterior pole granuloma; and a peripheral inflammatory mass. Uncommonly seen are an iris nodule, optic nerve granuloma, uniocular pars planitis, and a migrating retinal nematode. Ocular toxocariasis, which is generally recognized years after the acute infection, is generally not associated with peripheral eosinophilia, hypergammaglobulinemia, or isohemagglutinin elevation. Serum ELISA tests may be positive, but a negative test does not rule out the diagnosis. If doubt exists about whether a patient with a positive serum ELISA test has retinoblastoma, examination of the vitreous humor for ELISA antibody and eosinophils can be helpful. High-resolution CT scanning of the orbit should be done.

Prevention, Treatment, & Prognosis

Disease in humans is best prevented by periodic treatment of puppies, kittens, and nursing dog and cat mothers, starting at 2 weeks postpartum, repeating at weekly intervals for 3 weeks and then every 6 months.

A. Acute Infection: There is no proved specific treatment, but mebendazole (200–400 mg in divided doses for 21 days), albendazole (400 mg twice daily for 21 days), diethylcarbamazine (6 mg/kg in divided doses for 21 days), ivermectin, or thiabendazole (as used in strongyloidiasis) should be tried. Theoretically, release of antigens from dying parasites may exacerbate clinical findings. Corticosteroids, antibiotics, antihistamines, and analgesics may be needed to provide symptomatic relief. Symptoms may persist for months but generally clear within 1–2 years. The ultimate outcome is usually good, but permanent neuropsychologic deficits have been seen.

B. Ocular Toxocariasis: Treatment includes corticosteroids (subconjunctival applications may be preferable to oral usage), vitrectomy for vitreous traction, laser photocoagulation, and an anthelmintic drug. Partial or total permanent visual impairment is rare.

Arango CA: Visceral larva migrans and the hypereosinophilia syndrome. South Med J 1998;91:882. [NLM Cit ID: 98413999]

Beiran I et al: "Silent" ocular toxocariasis. Eur J Ophthalmol 1998;8:195. [NLM Cit ID: 99010192]

Chitkara RK et al: Dirofilaria, visceral larva migrans, and tropical pulmonary eosinophilia. Semin Respir Infect 1997;12:138. [NLM Cit ID: 97339124]

Kaushik SP et al: *Toxocara canis* infection and granulomatous hepatitis. Am J Gastroenterol 1997;92:1223. [NLM Cit ID: 97363514]

Kayes SG: Human toxocariasis and the visceral larva migrans syndrome: Correlative immunopathology. Chem Immunol 1997;66:99. [NLM Cit ID: 97256967]

RELEVANT WORLD WIDE WEB SITES

[Amebic Abscess]
http://www.brighamrad.harvard.edu/Cases/bwh/hcache/24/full.html

[Malaria Case Study]
http://path.upmc.edu:80/cases/case43.html

Infectious Diseases: Mycotic*

36

See http://www.current-med.com/ch36.html for updated addresses of Web sites referenced in this chapter.

Richard J. Hamill, MD

Fungal infections have assumed an increasingly important role as use of broad-spectrum antimicrobial agents has increased and the number of immunodeficient patients has risen. Some pathogens (eg, cryptococcus, candida, pneumocystis, fusarium) virtually never cause serious disease in normal hosts. Other endemic fungi (eg, histoplasma, coccidioides, paracoccidioides) commonly cause disease in normal hosts but tend to be more aggressive in immunocompromised ones.

[Medical Mycology Research Center]
http://fungus.utmb.edu/
(Comprehensive medical mycology Web site at the University of Texas Medical Branch that contains a glossary of medical mycology terms, laboratory procedures, images of clinically relevant fungi, and antifungal susceptibility information about various fungi. Links to other useful sites as well.)

CANDIDIASIS

Essentials of Diagnosis

- Common normal flora but opportunistic pathogen.
- Gastrointestinal mucosal disease, particularly esophagitis, most common; catheter-associated fungemia occurs in hospitalized patients.
- Diagnosis of invasive systemic disease requires tissue biopsy or evidence of retinal disease.

General Considerations

Candida albicans can be cultured from the mouth, vagina, and feces of most people. Cutaneous and oral lesions are discussed in Chapters 6 and 8, respectively. The risk factors for invasive candidiasis include prolonged neutropenia, recent surgery, broad-spectrum antibiotic therapy, the presence of intravascular catheters (especially when providing total parenteral nutrition), and intravenous drug use. Cellular immunodeficiency predisposes to mucocutaneous disease. When no other underlying cause is found, persistent oral or vaginal candidiasis should arouse a suspicion of HIV infection; over the course of their disease, AIDS patients will almost without exception have mucosal candidiasis as a complication.

Clinical Findings & Treatment

A. Mucosal Candidiasis: Esophageal involvement is the most frequent type of invasive mucosal disease. Individuals present with substernal odynophagia, gastroesophageal reflux, or nausea without substernal pain. Oral candidiasis, though often associated, is not invariably present. Diagnosis is best confirmed by endoscopy with biopsy and culture, since radiographically the condition may be difficult to distinguish from esophagitis caused by infection with cytomegalovirus or herpes simplex virus. Therapy depends upon the severity of disease. If patients are able to swallow and take adequate amounts of fluid orally, fluconazole, 100 mg/d (or itraconazole, 100 mg/d) for 10–14 days will usually suffice. In the individual who is more ill or has developed esophagitis while taking fluconazole, a 10- to 14-day course of amphotericin B at a dose of 0.3 mg/kg/d intravenously usually results in resolution. Relapse is common when there is underlying HIV infection.

Vulvovaginal candidiasis occurs in an estimated 75% of women during their lifetime. Risk factors include pregnancy, uncontrolled diabetes mellitus, broad-spectrum antimicrobial treatment, corticosteroid use, and AIDS. In women with AIDS, vaginal candidiasis is usually the first and most frequent opportunistic infection. Common symptoms include acute vulvar pruritus, burning vaginal discharge, and dyspareunia. Various topical azole preparations (eg, clotrimazole, 100 mg vaginal tablet for 7 days, or miconazole, 200 mg vaginal suppository for 3 days) are effective. One 150 mg oral dose of fluconazole has been shown to have equivalent efficacy with better patient acceptance.

B. Candidal Funguria: Candidal funguria usually resolves with discontinuance of antibiotics or removal of bladder catheters. Clinical benefit from treatment of asymptomatic candiduria has not been demonstrated. When symptomatic funguria persists,

*Superficial mycoses are discussed in Chapter 6.

oral fluconazole, 100 mg/d for 7–10 days, can be used if renal function is normal. If creatinine clearance is less than 10 mL/min, irrigation for 5 days with 50 mg/d of amphotericin B mixed in 1 L of D_5W may be necessary. Rare complications of candidal urinary tract infections are ureteral obstruction and dissemination.

C. Candidal Fungemia: Candidal fungemia may represent a benign, self-limited process, but until proved otherwise it should be considered a sign of serious disseminated disease. If fungemia resolves with removal of intravascular catheters, there are often no further complications. The incidence of endophthalmitis may be higher than previously recognized, and a short course of intravenous amphotericin B to a total dose of 200 mg appears to lower this incidence. Such an approach is strongly recommended for patients with candidal fungemia. (See Amphotericin B, Chapter 37.)

If fungemia is documented, if retinal lesions are identified, or if candida is isolated from other sites, the patient is considered to have disseminated disease. Important clinical findings in disseminated candidiasis are fluffy white retinal infiltrates that extend into the vitreous and raised, erythematous skin lesions that may be painful. However, though characteristic, these are seen in less than 50% of cases. Other organ system involvement in disseminated disease may include the brain, meninges, and myocardium. Amphotericin B to a total dose of 1 g is the agent of choice. Flucytosine, 150 mg/kg/d orally in four divided doses, is added if central nervous system involvement occurs until clinical improvement results. Individuals who do not tolerate amphotericin B may be given fluconazole, 200–400 mg/d intravenously, with equivalent efficacy. Serologic tests for candida have not proved helpful in differentiating transient fungemia from disseminated disease.

Another form of disseminated disease is hepatosplenic candidiasis. This results from aggressive chemotherapy and prolonged neutropenia in patients with underlying hematologic cancers. Patients typically present with fever and variable abdominal pain weeks after chemotherapy, when neutrophil counts have recovered. Blood cultures are generally negative. Hepatic enzymes reveal an alkaline phosphatase elevation that may be marked. CT scanning of the abdomen shows hepatosplenomegaly, most often with multiple low-density defects in the liver. Diagnosis is established by liver biopsy, histopathology, and culture. Amphotericin B is given to a total dose of 1 g intravenously but often works poorly; fluconazole, 400 mg daily, or liposomal preparations of amphotericin B may be better. Therapy is continued until clinical and radiographic improvement occurs.

D. Candidal Endocarditis: Candidal endocarditis rarely is a complication of transient fungemia. It usually results from direct inoculation at the time of valvular heart surgery or repeated inoculation with intravenous drug use. Candidal endocarditis occurs with increased frequency on prosthetic valves in the first few months following surgery. Splenomegaly and petechiae are common, and there is a predilection for large-vessel embolization. Non-albicans species such as *Candida parapsilosis* and *Candida tropicalis* are more often important etiologic agents in endocarditis than in fungemia, when *C albicans* is usual. The diagnosis is established definitively by culturing candida from emboli or from vegetations at the time of valve replacement. Valve destruction (usually aortic or mitral) is common, and surgical therapy is necessary in addition to a prolonged course of amphotericin therapy, usually to a total dose of 1–1.5 g intravenously.

It is important to note that non-albicans species of candida now account for over 50% of clinical bloodstream isolates and are often resistant to imidazole antibiotics such as fluconazole. The widespread use of these agents for prophylaxis in immunocompromised patients can lead to the emergence of pathogens such as *Candida krusei.* Dissemination of this organism has been reported in patients undergoing bone marrow transplantation for leukemia. Imidazole-resistant *C albicans* has increased in frequency in immunocompromised patients, particularly in patients with late-stage AIDS receiving chronic suppressive fluconazole.

In all forms of invasive candidiasis, an important element of therapy is reversal of the underlying predisposing factor when possible.

Powderly WG et al: Diagnosis and treatment of oropharyngeal candidiasis in patients infected with HIV: a critical reassessment. AIDS Res Hum Retroviruses 1999; 15:1405. [NLM Cit ID: 20021573] (In order to minimize the risk of the development of resistance, topical therapies should be considered first-line candidates for treatment of initial or recurrent cases of uncomplicated oropharyngeal candidiasis.)

Sobel JD et al: Candiduria: a randomized, double-blind study of treatment with fluconazole and placebo. Clin Infect Dis 2000;30:19. [NLM Cit ID: 20086530] (Oral fluconazole was safe and effective for short-term eradication of candiduria, especially following urinary catheter removal; however, long-term eradication rates were disappointing and not associated with clinical benefits.)

HISTOPLASMOSIS

Essentials of Diagnosis

- Epidemiologically linked to bird droppings and bat exposure; common along river valleys.
- Most patients asymptomatic; respiratory illness most common clinical problem.
- Rare patients with normal immune function develop dissemination, with hepatosplenomegaly, lymphadenopathy, and oral ulcers.
- Widespread disease especially common in AIDS or other immunosuppressed states, with poor prognosis.

- Skin test and serology seldom diagnostic; biopsy of affected organs with culture, or urinary polysaccharide antigen most useful in disseminated disease.

General Considerations

Histoplasmosis is caused by *Histoplasma capsulatum,* a dimorphic fungus that has been isolated from soil in endemic areas (central and eastern USA, eastern Canada, Mexico, Central America, South America, Africa, and southeast Asia). Infection presumably takes place by inhalation of conidia. These convert into small budding cells that are engulfed by phagocytic cells in the lungs. The organism proliferates and is carried hematogenously to other organs.

Clinical Findings

A. Symptoms and Signs: Most cases of histoplasmosis are asymptomatic or mild and so are unrecognized. Past infection is recognized by the development of a positive histoplasmin skin test and occasionally by pulmonary and splenic calcification noted on incidental x-rays. Symptoms and signs of pulmonary involvement are usually absent even in patients who subsequently show areas of calcification on chest x-ray. Symptomatic infection may present with mild influenza-like illness, often lasting 1–4 days. Moderately severe infections are frequently diagnosed as atypical pneumonia. These patients have fever, cough, and mild chest pain lasting 5–15 days. Physical examination is usually negative. Radiographic findings during acute illness are variable and nonspecific.

Clinically evident infections arise also in several forms: (1) **Acute histoplasmosis** frequently occurs in epidemics. It is a severe disease manifested by marked prostration, fever, and relatively few pulmonary complaints even when x-rays show pneumonia. The illness may last from 1 week to 6 months but is almost never fatal. (2) **Progressive disseminated histoplasmosis** is usually fatal within 6 weeks or less. Symptoms usually consist of fever, dyspnea, cough, loss of weight, and prostration. Ulcers of the mucous membranes of the oropharynx may be present. The liver and spleen are nearly always enlarged, and all the organs of the body are involved, particularly the adrenal glands. (3) **Chronic progressive pulmonary histoplasmosis** is usually seen in older patients with chronic obstructive lung disease. The lungs show chronic progressive changes, often with apical cavities. (4) **Disseminated disease in the profoundly immunocompromised host** often represents reactivation of prior infectious foci or may reflect acute infection. This form is commonly seen in patients with underlying HIV infection and is characterized by fever and multiple organ system involvement. Chest x-rays may show a miliary pattern. Presentation may be fulminant, simulating septic shock, with death ensuing rapidly unless treatment is provided.

B. Laboratory Findings: Most patients with progressive pulmonary disease show anemia of chronic disease. Bone marrow involvement may be prominent in disseminated forms with occurrence of pancytopenia. Alkaline phosphatase and marked LDH and ferritin elevations are also common.

In pulmonary disease, sputum culture is rarely positive except in chronic disease; in contrast, blood or bone marrow cultures from immunocompromised patients with acute disseminated disease are positive more than 80% of the time. A urine antigen assay has a sensitivity of greater than 90% for disseminated disease in AIDS patients and can be used to diagnose relapse. The sensitivity of screening immunodiffusion is 50% in acute pulmonary histoplasmosis, and complement fixation titers are positive in about 80% of cases. Combined results in immunodeficient patients approach 80%.

Treatment

For progressive localized disease and for mild to moderately severe nonmeningeal disseminated disease in immunocompetent or immunocompromised patients, itraconazole, 200–400 mg/d orally is the treatment of choice with an overall response rate of approximately 80%. Duration of therapy ranges from weeks to several months depending upon the severity of illness. Amphotericin B is reserved for individuals who cannot take oral medications; for those who have failed itraconazole therapy; for those with meningitis; and for management of severe disseminated disease in an immunocompromised host. Up to 2.5 g total may need to be given in the latter two situations, though this course of treatment can be abbreviated and oral itraconazole instituted once clinical stabilization has occurred. (See Amphotericin B, Chapter 37.) Patients with AIDS-related histoplasmosis require lifelong suppressive therapy with itraconazole, 200–400 mg/d orally.

COCCIDIOIDOMYCOSIS

Essentials of Diagnosis

- Influenza-like illness with malaise, fever, backache, headache, and cough.
- Arthralgia and periarticular swelling of knees and ankles.
- Erythema nodosum common.
- Dissemination may result in meningitis, bony lesions, or skin and soft tissue abscesses.
- Chest x-ray findings vary widely from pneumonitis to cavitation.
- Serologic tests useful; spherules containing endospores demonstrable in sputum or tissues.

General Considerations

Coccidioidomycosis should be considered in the diagnosis of any obscure illness in a patient who has lived in or visited an endemic area.

Infection results from the inhalation of arthroconidia of *Coccidioides immitis,* a mold that grows in soil in certain arid regions of the southwestern USA, in Mexico, and in Central and South America.

About 60% of infections are subclinical and unrecognized other than by the subsequent development of a positive coccidioidin skin test. In the remaining cases, symptoms may be of severity warranting medical attention. Fewer than 1% of immunocompetent hosts show dissemination, but among these patients the mortality rate is high.

In HIV-infected people in endemic areas, coccidioidomycosis is now a common opportunistic infection, occurring in approximately 25% of patients over the course of HIV disease.

Clinical Findings

A. Symptoms and Signs: Symptoms of primary coccidioidomycosis occur in about 40% of infections. The onset (after an incubation period of 10–30 days) is usually that of a respiratory tract illness with fever and occasionally chills. Pleuritic pain is common. Nasopharyngitis may be followed by bronchitis accompanied by a dry or slightly productive cough.

Arthralgia accompanied by periarticular swellings, often of the knees and ankles, is common. Erythema nodosum may appear 2–20 days after onset of symptoms. Erythema multiforme may also occur rarely. Persistent pulmonary lesions, varying from cavities and abscesses to parenchymal nodular densities or bronchiectasis, occur in about 5% of diagnosed cases.

About 0.1% of white and 1% of nonwhite patients develop disseminated disease due to *C immitis;* Filipinos and blacks are especially susceptible, as are pregnant women of all races. Symptoms in progressive coccidioidomycosis depend upon the site of dissemination. Any organ may be involved. Pulmonary findings usually become more pronounced, with mediastinal lymph node enlargement, cough, and increased sputum production. Lung abscesses may rupture into the pleural space, producing an empyema. Extension to bones and skin may take place, and pericardial and myocardial extension has been occasionally observed. Dissemination may be associated with fungemia, characterized clinically by a diffuse miliary pattern on chest x-ray and by early death. The course may be particularly rapid in immunosuppressed patients. HIV-infected persons with disseminated disease have a higher incidence of miliary infiltrates, lymphadenopathy, and meningitis, but skin lesions are uncommon.

Bone lesions most often occur at bony prominences. Meningitis occurs in 30–50% of cases of dissemination. Subcutaneous abscesses and verrucous skin lesions are especially common in fulminating cases. Lymphadenitis may occur and may progress to suppuration. Mediastinal and retroperitoneal abscesses are not uncommon.

B. Laboratory Findings: In primary coccidioidomycosis, there may be moderate leukocytosis and eosinophilia. Serologic testing is useful for both diagnosis and prognosis. The immunodiffusion test (CIE) and the tube precipitin test are useful for screening, and IgG and IgM by immunodiffusion are also adequate for diagnosis. Historically, a persistent rising complement fixation titer (≥ 1:16) has been considered suggestive of disseminated disease. Serum complement fixation titer may be low when there is meningitis but no other disseminated disease. In patients with HIV-related coccidioidomycosis, the false-negative rate may be as high as 30%. Demonstrable antibodies in spinal fluid are diagnostic of coccidioidal meningitis. These are found in over 90% of cases. Spinal fluid findings include increased cell count with lymphocytosis and reduced glucose. Spherules filled with endospores may be found in biopsy specimens; though they are not infectious, they convert to the highly contagious arthroconidia when grown in culture media. Exoantigen testing is in widespread use and substantially reduces the risk to laboratory personnel. Blood cultures in appropriate media are only rarely positive in disseminated disease. Spinal fluid culture is positive in approximately 30% of meningitis cases.

C. Imaging: Radiographic findings vary, but patchy, nodular pulmonary infiltrates and thin-walled cavities are most common. Hilar lymphadenopathy may be visible and is seen in localized disease; mediastinal lymphadenopathy suggests dissemination. There may be pleural effusions and lytic lesions in bone.

Treatment

General symptomatic therapy is given as needed for disease limited to the chest with no evidence of progression. For progressive pulmonary or extrapulmonary disease, amphotericin B intravenously has proved effective in some patients (see Chapter 37). Therapy should be continued to a total dose of 2.5–3 g. For meningitis, treatment consists of the intrathecal administration of amphotericin B daily in increasing doses up to 1–5 mg/d until the patient is clinically stable. The drug can then be tapered to once every 6 weeks for several years thereafter. Systemic therapy with amphotericin B, 0.6 mg/kg/d intravenously, is generally given concurrently with intrathecal therapy. Once the patient is clinically stable, oral therapy with an azole for an indefinite period, in dosages as discussed below, is an alternative to intrathecal amphotericin B therapy.

Results with fluconazole at a dose of 400 mg/d suggest that it may be possible to treat approximately 75% of selected patients with mild coccidioidal meningitis with oral fluconazole. Such therapy is suppressive only and must be continued indefinitely.

Ketoconazole, 200–800 mg orally daily 1–2 hours before breakfast, fluconazole, 200–400 mg orally daily, and itraconazole, 400 mg orally daily, are alternative regimens for disease in the chest, bones, and soft tissues; however, therapy must be continued for 6 months or longer after the disease is inactive in order to prevent relapse. Response to therapy should be monitored by following the decrease in serum complement fixation titers.

Thoracic surgery is occasionally indicated for giant, infected, or ruptured cavities. Surgical drainage is also useful for soft tissue abscesses and bone disease. Amphotericin B, 1 mg/kg/d intravenously, is advisable following extensive surgical manipulation of infected tissue until the disease is inactive, whereupon therapy may be continued with an azole.

Prognosis

The prognosis in the case of limited disease is good, but persistent pulmonary cavities may cause complications. Nodules, cavities, and fibrotic residuals may rarely progress after long periods of stability or regression. Serial complement fixation titers should be performed after therapy for patients with coccidioidomycosis; rising titers warrant reinstitution of therapy because relapse is likely. Disseminated and meningeal forms still have mortality rates exceeding 50%.

Galgiani JN: Coccidioidomycosis: a regional disease of national importance. Rethinking approaches for control. Ann Intern Med 1999;130:293. [NLM Cit ID: 99149966] (Coccidioidomycosis is an increasingly important health problem because of travel and migration of large numbers of individuals to endemic areas of the United States. Early diagnosis is important to allay patient anxiety, to lessen the need for further diagnostic studies, and to decrease the empirical use of antimicrobials.)

PNEUMOCYSTOSIS (*Pneumocystis carinii* Pneumonia)

Essentials of Diagnosis

- Fever, dyspnea, nonproductive cough.
- Bilateral diffuse interstitial disease without hilar adenopathy by chest x-ray.
- Bibasilar crackles on auscultation in many cases; others have no findings.
- Reduced partial pressure of oxygen.
- *P carinii* in sputum, bronchoalveolar lavage fluid, or lung tissue.

General Considerations

It is now generally accepted that *Pneumocystis carinii* is a fungus. The organism has been found in the lungs of a variety of domesticated and wild mammals and is distributed worldwide in humans. Although symptomatic *P carinii* disease is rare in the general population, serologic evidence indicates that asymptomatic infections have occurred in most persons by a young age. The overt infection is an acute interstitial plasma cell pneumonia that occurs with high frequency among two groups: (1) as epidemics of primary infections among premature or debilitated or marasmic infants on hospital wards in underdeveloped parts of the world, and (2) as sporadic cases among older children and adults who have an abnormal or altered cellular immune status. Cases occur generally in patients with cancer or severe malnutrition and debility, in patients treated with immunosuppressive or cytotoxic drugs or irradiation for the management of organ transplants and cancer, and, most commonly, in patients with AIDS (see Chapter 31).

The mode of transmission in primary infection is unknown, but the evidence suggests airborne transmission. Following asymptomatic primary infection, latent and presumably inactive organisms are sparsely distributed in the alveoli. Unsettled, however, is whether acute infection in older children and adults results from de novo infection or from reactivation of latent infection.

In AIDS, without specific prophylaxis, pneumocystis pneumonia occurs in up to 80% of patients and is a major cause of death. Its incidence increases in direct proportion to the fall in CD4 cells, with most cases occurring when the cells are below 200/μL. Dissemination of the infection to tissues other than the lung is rare, except in those who have received prophylactic aerosolized pentamidine. In non-AIDS patients receiving immunosuppressive therapy, symptoms frequently begin after corticosteroids have been tapered or discontinued.

Clinical Findings

A. Symptoms and Signs: Findings are usually limited to the pulmonary parenchyma; extrapulmonary disease is reported occasionally. In the sporadic form of the disease associated with deficient cell-mediated immunity, the onset is abrupt, with fever, tachypnea, shortness of breath, and usually nonproductive cough. Pulmonary physical findings may be slight and disproportionate to the degree of illness and to the radiologic findings; many patients have bibasilar crackles, but others do not. Without treatment, the course is usually one of rapid deterioration and death. In adult disease, patients may present with spontaneous pneumothorax, usually in patients with previous episodes or those receiving aerosolized pentamidine prophylaxis. In the infantile form of the disease, the patient is generally free of fever and may show eosinophilia. Patients with AIDS will usually have other evidence of HIV-associated disease, including fever, fatigue, and weight loss, for weeks or months preceding the illness.

B. Laboratory Findings: Chest radiographs most often show diffuse "interstitial" infiltration, which may be heterogeneous or miliary or patchy early in infection. There may also be diffuse or focal consolidation, cystic changes, nodules, or cavitation within nodules; pleural effusions are not seen; 5–10% of patients with pneumocystis pneumonia have normal chest films. Chest films are more often atypical in patients who have received prophylaxis with aerosolized pentamidine, demonstrating upper lobe infiltrates.

Typically, there is reduction in vital and total lung capacity, and the single-breath diffusing capacity for carbon monoxide shows impaired diffusion. The blood gases usually show hypoxemia with hypocapnia. Gallium lung scanning (sensitivity > 95%, specificity 20–40%) shows diffuse uptake; the test should be reserved for those with normal chest films and normal pulmonary function in whom the disease is suspected. Isolated elevation or rising levels of serum LDH are very sensitive but not specific findings for *P carinii.* Lymphopenia with depleted CD4 lymphocytes is common. Serologic tests, including tests to detect antigenemia, are not helpful in diagnosis.

Specific diagnosis depends on morphologic demonstration of the organisms in clinical specimens using specific stains. The organism cannot be cultured. Although patients rarely spontaneously produce sufficient sputum for examination, adequate specimens can be obtained with induced sputum by having patients inhale an aerosol of hypertonic saline (3%) produced by an ultrasonic nebulizer. Specimens are then stained with Giemsa's stain or methenamine silver, either of which allows detection of cysts. The use of monoclonal antibody with immunofluorescence has increased the sensitivity of diagnosis. Additional techniques for obtaining specimens include bronchoalveolar lavage (sensitivity 86–97%) followed if necessary by transbronchial lung biopsy (85–97%). Open lung biopsy and needle lung biopsy are infrequently done. Although conclusions are still preliminary, the polymerase chain reaction (PCR) test for the detection of *P carinii* appears to be sensitive but does not provide more rapid diagnosis.

Treatment (See Table 31–4.)

Treatment should be based on a proved diagnosis because of the toxicity of therapy and the possible coexistence of other infections. Trimethoprim-sulfamethoxazole (TMP-SMZ) and pentamidine isethionate are equally effective, but severe adverse reactions can occur in up to 50% of patients receiving either drug. In non-AIDS patients, the former drug is preferred because of its lower incidence of side effects. For most AIDS patients with mild to moderately severe disease, oral TMP-SMZ is the preferred agent because of its low cost and excellent bioavailability. Patients suffering from nausea and vomiting or intractable diarrhea should be given intravenous TMP-SMZ. Pentamidine is used if fluid must be restricted or if there is a history of sulfonamide drug sensitivity. Therapy should be continued with the selected drug for at least 5–10 days before one considers changing agents, as fever, tachypnea, and pulmonary infiltrates persist for 4–6 days after starting treatment; some patients have a transient worsening of their disease during the first 3–5 days, which may be related to an inflammatory response secondary to the presence of dead or dying organisms. See below and Chapter 31 for a discussion of the role of corticosteroids in treatment. Some clinicians prefer to treat episodes of AIDS-associated pneumocystis pneumonia for 21 days rather than the usual 14 days recommended for non-AIDS cases.

A. Trimethoprim-Sulfamethoxazole: The dosage is TMP 20 mg/kg (12–15 mg/kg may decrease side effects without decreasing efficacy) and SMZ 100 mg/kg given orally or intravenously daily in three or four divided doses for 14–21 days. Adverse reactions are generally those of the sulfonamide component. Patients with AIDS have a high frequency of hypersensitivity reactions—fever, rashes (sometimes severe), malaise, neutropenia, hepatitis, nephritis, thrombocytopenia, and hyperbilirubinemia.

B. Pentamidine Isethionate: This drug is administered intravenously (preferred) or intramuscularly as a single dose of 3 mg (salt) per kilogram per day for 14–21 days. To avoid injection site pain or sterile abscesses, most workers administer the drug only intravenously by diluting it in 250 mL of 5% dextrose in water and giving it slowly over 1 hour. Pentamidine causes side effects in nearly 50% of patients. Occasional reactions include rash, neutropenia, abnormal liver function tests, serum folate depression, hyperkalemia, and hypocalcemia. Hypoglycemia (often clinically inapparent), hyperglycemia, hyponatremia, and delayed nephrotoxicity with azotemia may occur. Rarely, a variety of other severe adverse reactions may occur, including anemia, thrombocytopenia, ventricular arrhythmias, and fatal pancreatitis. Blood glucose levels should be monitored. Inadvertent rapid intravenous infusion may cause precipitous hypotension.

C. Atovaquone: Atovaquone is a hydroxynaphthoquinone that has been FDA-approved for patients with mild to moderate disease who cannot tolerate TMP-SMZ or pentamidine, but failure is reported in 15–30% of cases. Mild side effects are common, but no serious reactions have been reported. The dosage is 750 mg three times daily for 21 days. Because absorption can be a problem leading to low serum concentrations and treatment failure, the drug should be taken with food, especially a fatty meal.

D. Other Drugs: Clindamycin, 600 mg three times daily, plus primaquine, 15 mg/d; and dapsone, 100 mg/d, plus trimethoprim 15 mg/kg/d, in three divided doses daily, are alternative oral regimens for mild to moderate disease or for continuation of therapy after intravenous therapy is initiated. Trimetrexate, 45 mg/m^2/d intravenously, plus high-dose leucovorin has been approved for salvage use in patients not responding to other therapies, but the success rate is less than 25%.

E. Prednisone: In conjunction with antimicrobials, prednisone is given when PaO_2 on admission is < 70 mm Hg; its use improves the prognosis in severe pneumocystis pneumonia. For dosages and durations of therapy, see the section on corticosteroids in Chapter 31 and the footnote in Table 31–4.

F. Supportive Care: Because of the hypoxia usually associated with this disease, oxygen therapy is indicated to maintain the oxygen saturation over 90% by pulse oximeter.

Prevention

See Chapter 31 and Table 31–6.

Prognosis

In the absence of early and adequate treatment, the fatality rate for the endemic infantile form of pneumocystis pneumonia is 20–50%; for the sporadic form in immunodeficient persons, the fatality rate is nearly 100%. Early treatment reduces the mortality rate to about 3% in the former and 25% in the latter forms of infection. In immunodeficient patients who do not receive prophylaxis, recurrences are common (30% in AIDS).

Toma E et al: Clindamycin with primaquine vs. trimethoprim-sulfamethoxazole therapy for mild and moderately severe *Pneumocystis carinii* pneumonia in patients with AIDS: A multicenter, double-blind, randomized trial (CTN 004). CTN-PCP Study Group. Clin Infect Dis 1998;27:524. [NLM Cit ID: 98442288] (Clindamycin with primaquine was equally effective compared with trimethoprim-sulfamethoxazole for therapy of *P carinii* infection and was associated with fewer adverse events.)

CRYPTOCOCCOSIS

Essentials of Diagnosis

- Most common cause of fungal meningitis.
- Predisposing factors: Hodgkin's disease, corticosteroid therapy, HIV infection.
- Symptoms of headache, abnormal mental states; meningismus seen occasionally, though rarely in HIV-infected patients.
- Demonstration of capsular polysaccharide antigen in cerebrospinal fluid diagnostic; 95% of HIV-infected patients also have a positive serum antigen.

General Considerations

Cryptococcosis is caused by *Cryptococcus neoformans,* an encapsulated budding yeast that has been found worldwide in soil and on dried pigeon dung.

Infections are acquired by inhalation. In the lung, the infection may remain localized, heal, or disseminate. Immunocompetent hosts rarely develop clinically apparent cryptococcal pneumonia. Progressive lung disease and dissemination most often occur in the setting of cellular immunodeficiency, including underlying hematologic cancer under treatment, Hodgkin's disease, long-term corticosteroid therapy, or HIV infection.

Clinical Findings

A. Symptoms and Signs: Disseminated disease may involve any organ, but central nervous system disease predominates. Headache is usually the first symptom of meningitis. Confusion and other mental status changes as well as cranial nerve abnormalities, nausea, and vomiting may be seen as the disease progresses. Nuchal rigidity and meningeal signs occur about 50% of the time but are uncommon in HIV-infected patients with this complication. Intracerebral mass lesions (cryptococcomas) are rarely seen. Obstructive hydrocephalus may complicate the course.

B. Laboratory Findings: Spinal fluid findings include increased pressure, variable pleocytosis, budding encapsulated fungus cells, increased protein, and decreased glucose, though as many as 50% of AIDS patients have no pleocytosis. Cryptococcal antigen in cerebrospinal fluid and culture establish the diagnosis over 90% of the time. Patients with AIDS often have the antigen in both cerebrospinal fluid and serum, and extrameningeal disease (lungs, blood, urinary tract) is common.

Treatment

In AIDS-related cryptococcal meningitis, oral fluconazole, 400 mg/d for a minimum of 10 weeks, has reasonable efficacy for acute therapy in patients with mild disease. Candidates for initial fluconazole therapy are patients with an intact level of consciousness and a spinal fluid cryptococcal antigen titer of less than 1:128. Higher-risk patients should receive amphotericin B initially, but it may be possible to shorten the course to 14 days and change to fluconazole once clinical stability has been achieved as assessed by a favorable clinical response and improvement in cerebrospinal fluid parameters, including conversion to negative culture and decreased cryptococcal antigen titers.

There has been a trend away from regimens based on prolonged amphotericin B therapy, particularly in HIV-infected patients. However, this agent remains important, especially in severe disease. Amphotericin B, 0.7–1 mg/kg/d intravenously for 14 days, followed by an additional 8 weeks of fluconazole, 400 mg/d orally, have been quite effective, achieving clinical responses and cerebrospinal fluid sterilization in about 70% of patients. It does not appear that the addition of flucytosine substantially contributes to improved cure rates, but adding flucytosine at this early stage does prevent late relapses. Flucytosine is administered orally at a dose of 100 mg/kg/d divided into four equal doses and given every 6 hours. Repeated lumbar punctures or ventricular shunting should be performed to relieve high cerebrospinal fluid pressures or if hydrocephalus is a complication. The end points for amphotericin B therapy are clinical response (decrease in temperature, improvement in headache, nausea, vomiting and mini-mental status scores) and culture negativity of the cerebrospinal fluid.

A similar approach is reasonable for patients with cryptococcal meningitis in the absence of AIDS, though the mortality rate is considerably higher. Because of serious underlying illnesses and generally greater age, this group of patients does not tolerate the higher doses of amphotericin B as well as patients with AIDS. Lipid amphotericin B preparations appear to have equivalent efficacy with reduced nephrotoxicity. Therapy is generally continued until cerebrospinal fluid cultures become negative and cerebrospinal fluid antigen titers are below 1:8.

A preliminary study in patients with AIDS suggests that fluconazole plus flucytosine is efficacious for mild cases, but this regimen has not been compared with fluconazole alone.

Maintenance antifungal therapy is important after treatment of an acute episode in HIV-related cases, since otherwise the rate of relapse is greater than 50%. Fluconazole, 200 mg/d, is the maintenance therapy of choice, decreasing the relapse rate approximately tenfold compared with placebo and threefold compared with weekly amphotericin B in patients whose cerebrospinal fluid has been sterilized by the induction therapy. There has been a trend among practitioners in recent years treating patients without AIDS to prescribe a brief course (eg, 3 months) of fluconazole as maintenance therapy following successful therapy for acute illness.

Prognosis

Factors that indicate a poor prognosis include the activity of the predisposing conditions, lack of spinal fluid pleocytosis, high initial antigen titer in either serum or cerebrospinal fluid, decreased mental status, and the presence of disease outside the nervous system.

Aberg JA et al: Pulmonary cryptococcosis in patients without HIV infection. Chest 1999;115:734. [NLM Cit ID: 99181976] (In the majority of patients, the lung was the sole organ involved. Therapy should be reserved for symptomatic patients, those with a positive serum antigen, and those with immunosuppressive illnesses.)

Graybill JR et al: Diagnosis and management of increased intracranial pressure in patients with AIDS and cryptococcal meningitis. Clin Infect Dis 2000;30:47. [NLM Cit ID: 20086535] (Patients with AIDS and acute cryptococcal meningitis who have lumbar punctures with opening pressures ≥ 250 mm H_2O should be treated with large-volume cerebrospinal fluid drainage.)

Saag MS et al: A comparison of itraconazole versus fluconazole as maintenance therapy for AIDS-associated cryptococcal meningitis. Clin Infect Dis 1999;28:291. [NLM Cit ID: 99162009] (Fluconazole remains the treatment of choice for maintenance therapy of AIDS-associated cryptococcal disease. Flucytosine may contribute to the prevention of relapse if used during the first 2 weeks of primary therapy.)

van der Horst CM et al: Treatment of cryptococcal meningitis associated with the acquired immunodeficiency syndrome. N Engl J Med 1997;337:15. [NLM Cit ID: 97330766] (The use of higher dose amphotericin B was associated with an increased rate of cerebrospinal fluid sterilization and decreased mortality at 2 weeks. Addition of flucytosine decreased late relapses.)

ASPERGILLOSIS

Aspergillus fumigatus is the usual cause of aspergillosis, though many species of aspergillus may cause a wide spectrum of disease. Burn eschar and detritus in the external ear canal are often colonized by these fungi. Clinical illness results either from an aberrant immunologic response or tissue invasion.

Allergic bronchopulmonary aspergillosis occurs in patients with preexisting asthma who develop worsening bronchospasm and fleeting pulmonary infiltrates accompanied by eosinophilia, high levels of IgE, and aspergillus precipitins in the blood. It also may complicate cystic fibrosis. The disease characteristically pursues a waxing and waning course with gradual improvement over time, but it may result in saccular bronchiectasis and end-stage fibrotic lung disease. For acute exacerbations, oral prednisone is begun at a dose of 1 mg/kg/d and then tapered slowly over several months. Itraconazole at a dose of 200 mg daily for 16 weeks appears to improve pulmonary function and decrease steroid requirements in these patients.

Invasive manifestations may be seen in immunocompetent adults. These include chronic sinusitis and colonization of preexisting pulmonary cavities (**aspergilloma**). Sinus disease may require long courses of antibiotics (itraconazole, 200 mg twice daily, for weeks to months) as well as surgical debridement. Aspergillomas of the lung may be found by incidental radiographic studies but may also present with significant hemoptysis. Intracavitary instillation of amphotericin B and bronchoscopic removal have been tried with little success; several uncontrolled trials have suggested some benefit from itraconazole. The most effective therapy for symptomatic aspergilloma remains surgical resection.

Life-threatening **invasive aspergillosis** most commonly occurs in profoundly immunodeficient patients, particularly those with prolonged severe neutropenia. Patients with very advanced HIV disease may also be at risk for invasive aspergillosis, particularly if they have other risk factors for the disease. Pulmonary disease is most common, with patchy infiltration leading to a severe necrotizing pneumonia. There is often tissue infarction as the organism grows into blood vessels; clues to this are the development of pleuritic chest pain and elevation of serum LDH. AIDS patients are also predisposed to a unique ulcerative tracheobronchitis that may coexist with parenchymal pulmonary disease. At any time, there may be hematogenous dissemination to the central nervous system, skin, and other organs. Early diagnosis and reversal of any correctable immunosuppression are essential. Blood cultures have very low yield. In contrast to allergic aspergillosis, serologic tests and antigen detection have low sensitivities for invasive disease but does identify a subset of patients at higher risk for developing invasive disease. Isolation of aspergillus from pulmonary secretions does not necessarily imply invasive disease. Therefore, the mainstay of diagnosis is demonstration of aspergillus in tissue. Histologically, one sees branched septate hyphae. Biopsy specimens will not invariably grow the organism.

When severe invasive aspergillosis is considered clinically likely or is demonstrable by biopsy, rapid institution of high doses of amphotericin B may be life-saving (see Chapter 37). The total daily dose is rapidly increased to 0.8–1.5 mg/kg/d intravenously as tolerated for the first several weeks of therapy. Thereafter, more traditional doses of 0.6 mg/kg/d are continued until a total dose of at least 2 g has been reached. Itraconazole orally or intravenously at a dosage of 200–400 mg/d has activity against aspergillus, and initial clinical experience is favorable for less severe disease. Until more data accumulate, amphotericin B should remain the first-line drug for invasive disease. Some experts believe that lipid preparations of amphotericin B should be used preferentially in this setting because they are better tolerated and can be given at higher doses. Based on promising results in neutropenic patients with invasive pulmonary aspergillosis, surgical resection warrants further study. The mortality rate of pulmonary or disseminated disease in the immunocompromised patient remains well above 50%, however.

Latge JP: *Aspergillus fumigatus* and aspergillosis. Clin Microbiol Rev 1999;12:310. [NLM Cit ID: 99212051] (Drug therapy for invasive aspergillosis should be viewed as a sequential process beginning with conventional amphotericin B and replacing it with a lipid-based formulation if renal dysfunction ensues. Itraconazole is an option when disease progression has been stabilized.)

Stevens DA et al: A randomized trial of itraconazole in allergic bronchopulmonary aspergillosis. N Engl J Med 2000;342:756. [NLM Cit ID: 20166592] (The addition of itraconazole to patients with corticosteroid-dependent allergic bronchopulmonary aspergillosis leads to a decrease in corticosteroid use, increase in exercise tolerance, and improvement in some pulmonary function tests.)

MUCORMYCOSIS

The term "mucormycosis" (zygomycosis, phycomycosis) is applied to opportunistic infections caused by members of the genera rhizopus, mucor, absidia, and cunninghamella. Predisposing conditions include diabetic ketoacidosis, chronic renal failure, and treatment with steroids or cytotoxic drugs. These organisms appear in tissues as broad, branching nonseptate hyphae. Biopsy with histologic examination is almost always required for diagnosis; cultures are frequently negative. Invasive disease of the sinuses, orbits, and the lungs may occur. Widely disseminated disease has been more commonly seen recently in patients who have received aggressive chemotherapy. The diagnosis should be considered in acidotic diabetic patients with black necrotic lesions of the nose or sinuses or with new cranial nerve abnormalities. Without treatment, cerebral invasion may ensue. A prolonged course of high-dosage amphotericin B (1–1.5 mg/kg/d intravenously) should be started early. Control of diabetes and other underlying conditions, along with extensive repeated surgical removal of necrotic, nonperfused tissue, are essential. Even when these measures are introduced in a timely fashion, the prognosis is poor, with a 30–50% mortality rate for localized disease and higher rates in disseminated cases.

Jiang RS et al: Endoscopic sinus surgery for rhinocerebral mucormycosis. Am J Rhinol 1999;13:105. [NLM Cit ID: 99236178] (When used in the management of rhinocerebral mucormycosis, endoscopic sinus surgery produces less operative morbidity.)

Lee FYW et al: Pulmonary mucormycosis. The last 30 years. Arch Intern Med 1999;159:1301. [NLM Cit ID: 99313077] (The main risk factors for disease were diabetes mellitus, hematologic cancers, renal insufficiency, and organ transplantation. Optimal therapy requires systemic antifungal therapy, surgical resection, and control of the patient's underlying disease.)

BLASTOMYCOSIS

Blastomycosis occurs more often in men infected during occupational or recreational activities out of doors and in a geographically limited area of the south central and midwestern USA and Canada. A few cases have been found in Mexico and Africa.

Pulmonary infection may be asymptomatic. When dissemination takes place, lesions are most frequently seen on the skin, in bones, and in the urogenital system.

Cough, moderate fever, dyspnea, and chest pain are evident in symptomatic patients. These may resolve or progress, with bloody and purulent sputum production, pleurisy, fever, chills, loss of weight, and prostration. Radiologic studies usually reveal infiltrates and enlarged regional lymph nodes, though less commonly than in histoplasmosis or coccidioidomycosis. Raised, verrucous cutaneous lesions that have an abrupt downward sloping border are usually present in disseminated blastomycosis. The border extends slowly, leaving a central atrophic scar. These lesions persist untreated for long periods, mimicking skin cancer. Bones—often the ribs and vertebrae—are frequently involved. Lesions appear to be both destructive and proliferative on radiography. Epididymitis, prostatitis, and other involvement of the male urogenital system may occur. Central nervous system involvement is uncommon. Cases in HIV-infected persons may progress rapidly, with dissemination common.

Laboratory findings usually include leukocytosis and anemia, though these are not specific. The organism is found in clinical specimens as a thick-walled cell 5–20 μm in diameter that may have a single broad-based bud. It grows readily on culture. Serologic tests are not well standardized.

Itraconazole, 100–200 mg/d orally for at least 2–3 months, is now the therapy of choice for nonmeningeal disease, with a response rate of over 80%. Amphotericin B, 0.3–0.6 mg/kg/d intravenously for a total dose of 1.5–2.5 g, is given for treatment failures or cases with central nervous system involvement.

Follow-up for relapse should be regularly made for several years so that therapy may be resumed or another drug instituted.

Bradsher RW: Therapy of blastomycosis. Semin Respir Infect 1997;12:263. [NLM Cit ID: 97458478] (Amphotericin B is the drug of choice for life-threatening or central nervous system blastomycosis. Itraconazole is the preferred drug for other forms.)

Patel RG et al: Clinical presentation, radiographic findings, and diagnostic methods of pulmonary blastomycosis: a review of 100 consecutive cases. South Med J 1999;92: 289. [NLM Cit ID: 99192082] (Patients with pulmonary blastomycosis had symptomatic disease. Air space or interstitial infiltrates or mass-like lesions were demonstrated radiographically. Response to therapy was generally good.)

PARACOCCIDIOIDOMYCOSIS (South American Blastomycosis)

Paracoccidioides brasiliensis infections have been found only in patients who have resided in South or Central America or Mexico. Long asymptomatic periods enable patients to travel far from the endemic areas before developing clinical problems. Ulceration of the naso- and oropharynx is usually the first symptom. Papules ulcerate and enlarge both peripherally and deeper into the subcutaneous tissue. Differential diagnosis includes mucocutaneous leishmaniasis and syphilis. Extensive coalescent ulcerations may eventually result in destruction of the epiglottis, vocal cords, and uvula. Extension to the lips and face may occur. Eating and drinking are extremely painful. Skin lesions may occur, usually on the face. Variable in appearance, they may have a necrotic central crater with a hard hyperkeratotic border. Lymph node enlargement may follow mucocutaneous lesions, eventually ulcerating and forming draining sinuses; in some patients, it is the presenting symptom. Hepatosplenomegaly may be present as well. Cough, sometimes with sputum, indicates pulmonary involvement, but the symptoms and signs are often mild, even though radiographic findings indicate severe parenchymatous changes in the lungs. The extensive ulceration of the upper gastrointestinal tract may prevent caloric intake and result in cachexia.

Laboratory findings are nonspecific. Serology by immunodiffusion is positive in 98% of cases. Complement fixation titers correlate with progressive disease and fall with effective therapy. The fungus is found in clinical specimens as a spherical cell that may have many buds arising from it. If direct examination does not reveal the organism, biopsy with Gomori staining may be helpful.

Itraconazole, 100–200 mg orally daily, is the treatment of choice and generally results in a clinical response within 1 month and effective control after 2–6 months.

Bethlem EP et al: Paracoccidioidomycosis. Curr Opin Pulm Med 1999;5:319. [NLM Cit ID: 99390639] (Primary pulmonary infection occurs commonly in the first and second decades of life and usually has a benign, self-limited course. Adult chronic manifestations are usually the result of reactivation of quiescent lesions with diffuse lung infiltrates, with or without systemic disease.)

SPOROTRICHOSIS

Sporotrichosis is a chronic fungal infection caused by *Sporothrix schenckii*. It is worldwide in distribution; most patients have had contact with soil, plants, or decaying wood. Infection takes place when the organism is inoculated into the skin—usually on the hand, arm, or foot.

The most common form of sporotrichosis begins with a hard, nontender subcutaneous nodule. This later becomes adherent to the overlying skin and ulcerates. Within a few days to weeks, similar nodules usually develop along the lymphatics draining this area, and these may ulcerate as well. The lymphatic vessels become indurated and are easily palpable.

Disseminated sporotrichosis is rare in the immunocompetent host but may present with widespread cutaneous, lung, bone, joint, and central nervous system involvement in immunocompromised patients, especially those with AIDS.

Cultures are needed to establish diagnosis. Antibody tests may be useful for diagnosis of disseminated disease, especially meningitis.

Itraconazole, 200–400 mg orally daily for several months, is now the treatment of choice for localized disease and some milder cases of disseminated disease. Amphotericin B intravenously, 1.5–2 g (see Chapter 37), is used for severe systemic infection. Surgery is usually contraindicated except for simple aspiration of secondary nodules. Joint involvement may require arthrodesis.

The prognosis is good for lymphocutaneous sporotrichosis; pulmonary, joint, and disseminated disease respond less favorably.

Kauffman CA: Sporotrichosis. Clin Infect Dis 1999;29:231. [NLM Cit ID: 99404368] (Itraconazole has become the drug of choice for lymphocutaneous and osteoarticular sporotrichosis. Pulmonary and disseminated disease are more difficult to treat; amphotericin B is the initial drug of choice for these severe manifestations.)

PENICILLIUM MARNEFFEI INFECTIONS

Penicillium marneffei is a dimorphic fungus, endemic in southeast Asia, that causes systemic infection in both healthy and compromised hosts. There have been increasing reports of patients with advanced AIDS presenting with disseminated infections, including travelers returning from southeast Asia. Clinical manifestations include fever, generalized umbilicated papular rash, lymphadenopathy, cough, and diarrhea. The best sites for isolation of the fungus include the skin, blood, bone marrow, respiratory tract, and lymph nodes. Patients with mild to moderate infection can be treated with itraconazole, 400 mg daily for 8 weeks. Amphotericin B, 0.5–0.7 mg/kg/d, is the drug of choice for severe disease. Because the relapse rate after successful treatment is 30%, maintenance therapy with itraconazole, 200–400 mg daily, is indicated.

Sirisanthana T et al: Amphotericin B and itraconazole for treatment of disseminated *Penicillium marneffei* infection in human immunodeficiency virus-infected patients. Clin Infect Dis 1998;26:1107. [NLM Cit ID: 98259525] (A response rate of 97.3% was seen in 72 AIDS patients with disseminated *P marneffei* infection treated with 2 weeks of amphotericin B at a dosage of 0.6 mg/kg/d followed by 10 weeks of itraconazole, 400 mg/d.)

Supparatpinyo K et al: A controlled trial of itraconazole to prevent relapse of *Penicillium marneffei* infection in patients infected with the human immunodeficiency virus. N Engl J Med 1998;339:1739. [NLM Cit ID: 99049886] (Secondary prophylaxis with oral itraconazole is well tolerated and prevents relapses of *P marneffei*.)

CHROMOBLASTOMYCOSIS (Chromomycosis)

Chromoblastomycosis is a chronic, principally tropical cutaneous infection usually affecting men who are agricultural workers and caused by several species of closely related black molds (fonsecaea species and phialophora species).

Lesions are slowly progressive and occur most frequently on a lower extremity. The lesion begins as a papule or ulcer. Over months to years, papules enlarge to become vegetating, papillomatous, verrucous elevated nodules. Satellite lesions may appear along the lymphatics. There may be secondary bacterial infection. Elephantiasis may result.

The fungus is seen as brown, thick-walled, spherical, sometimes septate cells in pus. The type of reproduction found in culture determines the species. *Fonsecaea pedrosoi* is the responsible pathogen in the vast majority of cases.

Itraconazole, 100–400 mg/d orally for 6–18 months, has resulted in a response rate of 65%. Response rates may be improved by the addition of flucytosine to itraconazole.

Elgart GW: Chromoblastomycosis. Dermatol Clin 1996; 14:77. [NLM Cit ID: 96418375]

Silva JP et al: Chromoblastomycosis: a retrospective study of 325 cases on Amazonic Region (Brazil). Mycopathologia 1998–99;143:171. [NLM Cit ID: 99281481] (Most patients are agricultural workers with disease in the lower limbs. *Fonsecaea pedrosoi* is responsible for most of the culturable cases.)

MYCETOMA (Maduromycosis & Actinomycetoma)

Maduromycosis is the term used to describe mycetoma caused by the true fungi. Actinomycotic mycetoma is caused by nocardia and actinomadura species. The disease begins as a papule, nodule, or abscess that over months to years progresses slowly to form multiple abscesses and sinus tracts ramifying deep into the tissue. Secondary bacterial infection may result in large open ulcers. Radiographs may show destructive changes in the underlying bone. The agents occur as white, yellow, red, or black granules in tissue or pus. Microscopic examination assists in the diagnosis.

The prognosis is good for patients with actinomycetoma, since they usually respond well to sulfonamides and sulfones, especially if treated early. Trimethoprim-sulfamethoxazole, 160/800 mg orally twice a day, or dapsone, 100 mg twice daily after meals, has also been reported to be effective. Streptomycin, 14 mg/kg/d intramuscularly, may be useful during the first month of therapy. All other medications must be taken for months and continued for several months after clinical cure to prevent relapse. Debridement assists healing.

The prognosis for maduromycosis is poor, though surgical debridement along with prolonged ketoconazole or itraconazole therapy may result in a response rate of 70%. Amputation is necessary in far-advanced cases.

McGinnis MR: Mycetoma. Dermatol Clin 1996;14:97. [NLM Cit ID: 96418377] (Review of the biology, clinical aspects, and treatment of mycetoma due to the true fungi.)

Table 36–1. Agents for systemic mycoses.

Drug	Dosing	Renal Clearance?	CSF Penetration?	Toxicities	Spectrum of Activity
Amphotericin B	0.3–1.5 mg/kg/d IV	No	Poor	Rigors, fever, azotemia, hypokalemia, hypomagnesemia, renal tubular acidosis, anemia	All major pathogens except *Pseudallescheria*
Amphotericin B lipid complex	5 mg/kg/d IV	No	Poor	Fever, rigors, nausea, hypotension, anemia, azotemia, tachypnea	Same as amphotericin B, above
Amphotericin B colloidal suspension	3–6 mg/kg/d IV	No	Poor	Fever, rigors, nausea, hypotension, azotemia, hypomagnesemia, anemia, tachypnea, thrombophlebitis	Same as amphotericin B, above
Liposomal amphotericin B	3–6 mg/kg/d IV	No	Poor	Fever, rigors, nausea, hypotension, azotemia, anemia, tachypnea, chest tightness	Same as amphotericin B, above
Flucytosine (5-FC)	100–150 mg/kg/d orally in four divided doses	Yes	Yes	Leukopenia,[1] rash, diarrhea, hepatitis, nausea, vomiting	Cryptococcosis,[2] candidiasis,[2] chromomycosis
Ketoconazole	200–800 mg/d orally in one or two doses	No	Poor	Anorexia, nausea, suppression of testosterone and cortisol, rash, headache, hepatic enzyme elevations, hepatic failure[3]	Nonmeningeal histoplasmosis and coccidioidomycosis, blastomycosis, paracoccidioidomycosis, mucosal candidiasis (except urinary)
Fluconazole	100–400 mg/d in one or two doses IV or orally	Yes	Yes	Nausea, rash, alopecia, headache, hepatic enzyme elevations[4]	Mucosal candidiasis (including urinary tract), cryptococcosis, histoplasmosis, coccidioidomycosis
Itraconazole	100–400 mg/d orally as single dose or 200–400 mg/d IV in one or two doses	No	Variable	Nausea, hypokalemia, edema, hypertension[3]	Same as ketoconazole plus sporotrichosis, aspergillosis, chromomycosis

[1]Use should be monitored with blood levels to prevent this or the dose adjusted according to creatinine clearance.
[2]In combination with amphotericin B.
[3]Drug interaction with terfenadine, astemizole, or cisapride may produce prolongation of the QT interval, ventricular arrhythmias, and torsade de pointes.
[4]Drug interaction with cisapride may produce prolongation of the QT interval, ventricular arrhythmias, and torsade de pointes.

OTHER OPPORTUNISTIC MOLD INFECTIONS

Fungi previously considered to be harmless colonizers, including *Pseudallescheria boydii (Scedosporium apiospermum),* fusarium, paecilomyces, and trichosporon, are emerging as significant pathogens in immunocompromised patients. This occurs most often in patients being treated for hematopoietic malignancies. Infection may be localized in the skin, lungs, or sinuses, or widespread disease may appear with lesions in multiple organs. Colonization of old cavitary disease may cause minimal symptoms or may precede dissemination with meningitis or brain abscesses. Endocarditis occurs more commonly in intravenous drug abusers. Sinus infection may cause bony erosion. Infection in subcutaneous tissues following traumatic implantation may develop as a well-circumscribed cyst or as an ulcer.

Nonpigmented septate hyphae are seen in tissue and are indistinguishable from those of aspergillus when infections are due to *Pseudallescheria boydii* or species of fusarium, paecilomyces, penicillium, or other hyaline molds. Spores or mycetoma-like granules are rarely present in tissue.

Infection by any of a number of black molds is designated as **phaeohyphomycosis.** These black molds (eg, exophiala, bipolaris, cladophialophora, curvularia, alternaria) are common in the environment, especially on decaying vegetation, and do not cause infection in the normal host, although some black molds, as well as some hyaline molds, are allergens. In tissues of patients with phaeohyphomycosis, the mold is seen as black or faintly brown hyphae, yeast cells, or both. Culture on appropriate medium is needed to identify the agent. Histologic demonstration of these organisms is definitive evidence of invasive infection; positive cultures must be interpreted cautiously and not assumed to be contaminants in immunocompromised hosts. Some isolates are sensitive to antifungal antibiotics. The differentiation of *Pseudallescheria boydii* and aspergillus is particularly important, since the former is uniformly resistant to amphotericin B but may be sensitive to imidazole antibiotics.

Fothergill AW: Identification of dematiaceous fungi and their role in human disease. Clin Infect Dis 1996; 22(Suppl 2):S179. [NLM Cit ID: 96302595] (Emphasizes the difficulty of identifying the phaeohyphomycoses that occur in patients who are not overtly immunocompromised.)

Perfect JR et al: The new fungal opportunists are coming. Clin Infect Dis 1996;22(Suppl 2):S112. [NLM Cit ID: 96302585] (Review of recently recognized fungal opportunists and suggestions for therapy.)

ANTIFUNGAL THERAPY

Table 36–1 summarizes the major properties of currently available antifungal agents. In addition to the newer antimicrobial agents that have been introduced over the past several years, there are several other important developments in the treatment of invasive fungal disease. A number of lipid-based amphotericin B formulations have recently become available. In early noncomparative studies, these agents have shown promise in the treatment of systemic candidiasis, invasive aspergillosis, and cryptococcal meningitis. Their principal advantage appears to be substantially reduced nephrotoxicity, allowing administration of much higher doses. Because of their expense, use of these agents should be reserved for individuals who develop significant nephrotoxicity during amphotericin B therapy. Cytokine therapy (such as with interferon-γ) and use of growth factors such as GM-CSF (sargramostim or molgramostim) have been shown in animal models to increase clearance of fungi and result in better clinical outcomes.

Patel R: Antifungal agents. Part I. Amphotericin B preparations and flucytosine. Mayo Clin Proc 1998;73:1205. [NLM Cit ID: 99085314] (Concise review of amphotericin B, the newer amphotericin B lipid preparations, and flucytosine.)

Sheehan DJ et al: Current and emerging azole antifungal agents. Clin Microbiol Rev 1999;12:40. [NLM Cit ID: 99123068] (Thorough review of the available azole antifungal agents and their various indications. Investigational agents are discussed.)

RELEVANT WORLD WIDE WEB SITES

[Athelete's Foot Information]
http://www.apma.org/topics/athfoot.htm
[Disseminated Aspergillus Sepsis Case Study]
http://path.upmc.edu:80/cases/case54.html
[Disseminated Cryptococcosis Case Study]
http://path.upmc edu:80/cases/case57.html
[Invasive Aspergillosis With Air Crescent]
http://www.brighamrad.harvard.edu/Cases/bwh/hcache/180/full.html
[Onychomycosis Information]
http://www.apma.org/topics/fungal.htm
[Reviews of Candidiasis]
http://www.iapac.org/clinmgt/diseases/fungal/candid.html
[Reviews of Cryptococcosis]
http://hivinsite.ucsf.edu/akb/1998/06crypt/index.html
http://www.iapac.org/clinmgt/diseases/fungal/crypto.html
[Cryptococcal Meningitis Case Study]
http://www.bcm.tmc.edu/neurol/challeng/pat4/history.html
[Reviews of Histoplasmosis]
http://hivinsite.ucsf.edu/akb/1998/06histo/index.html
http://www.iapac.org/clinmgt/diseases/fungal/histo.html
[Reviews of Coccidioidomycosis]
http://hivinsite.ucsf.edu/akb/1998/06cocci/index.html
http://www.iapac.org/clinmgt/diseases/fungal/cocc.html
[Review of *Pneumocystis carinii* Pneumonia]
http://hivinsite.ucsf.edu/akb/1998/06pcp/index.html

37 Anti-infective Chemotherapeutic & Antibiotic Agents

See http://www.current-med.com/ch37.html for updated addresses of Web sites referenced in this chapter.

Richard A. Jacobs, MD, PhD, & B. Joseph Guglielmo, PharmD

Some Principles of Antimicrobial Therapy

The proper use of antibiotics can result in favorable therapeutic results. However, indiscriminate use may result in the emergence of resistant organisms. In addition, antibiotics are associated with serious adverse reactions. Thus, the decision to use these drugs should be based on evidence that a treatable infection is present.

Drugs of first choice and alternative drugs are presented in Table 37–1.

The following steps are required in each patient considered for antibiotic therapy.

A. Etiologic Diagnosis: Based on the organ system involved, the organism causing infection can usually be predicted. See Tables 37–2 and 37–3.

B. "Best Guess": One selects a specific antimicrobial drug on the basis of past experience with empirical therapy. The clinician chooses a drug or combination of drugs that is likely to be effective against the suspected pathogens.

C. Laboratory Control: Specimens for laboratory examination are commonly obtained before institution of therapy to determine susceptibility.

D. Clinical Response: Based on the clinical response of the patient, evaluate the laboratory reports and consider the desirability of changing the antimicrobial drug regimen. If the specimen was obtained from a normally sterile site (eg, blood, cerebrospinal fluid, pleural fluid, joint fluid), the recovery of a microorganism in significant amounts is a meaningful finding even if the organism recovered is different from the clinically suspected agent, and this may force a change in treatment. On the other hand, isolation of unexpected microorganisms from the respiratory tract, gastrointestinal tract, or surface lesions (sites that have a complex flora) may represent colonization or contamination, and cultures must be critically evaluated before drugs are abandoned that were judiciously selected on a "best guess" basis.

E. Drug Susceptibility Tests: Some microorganisms are fairly uniformly susceptible to certain drugs; if such organisms are isolated, they need not be tested for drug susceptibility. For example, most group A hemolytic streptococci and clostridia respond predictably well to penicillin. On the other hand, some organisms (eg, enteric gram-negative rods) are variably susceptible and require drug susceptibility testing whenever they are isolated. Organisms that once had predictable antibiotic susceptibility patterns have now become resistant and require susceptibility testing. Examples include the pneumococcus, which may be resistant to multiple agents, including penicillin, and the enterococci, which may be resistant to penicillin, aminoglycosides, and vancomycin.

Antimicrobial drug susceptibility tests may be performed on solid media as "disk tests," in broth in tubes, or in wells of microdilution plates. The latter two methods yield results expressed as MIC (minimal inhibitory concentration), and the technique can be modified to give MBC (minimal bactericidal concentration) results. In most infections, the MIC is the appropriate in vitro test to guide selection of an antibacterial agent. When there appear to be marked discrepancies between susceptibility testing and clinical response, the following possibilities must be considered:

1. Selection of an inappropriate drug or drug dosage or route of administration.

2. Failure to drain a collection of pus or to remove a foreign body.

3. Failure of a poorly diffusing drug to reach the site of infection (eg, central nervous system) or to reach intracellular phagocytosed bacteria.

4. Superinfection in the course of prolonged chemotherapy. After suppression of the original infection or of normal flora, a second microorganism may establish itself against which the originally selected drug is ineffective.

5. Emergence of drug-resistant or tolerant organisms.

6. Participation of two or more microorganisms in the infectious process, of which only one was originally detected and used for drug selection.

Table 37–1. Drugs of choice for suspected or proved microbial pathogens, 1999.[1] (± = alone or combined with)

Suspected or Proved Etiologic Agent	Drug(s) of First Choice	Alternative Drug(s)
Gram-negative cocci		
Moraxella catarrhalis	TMP-SMZ[2]	Cefuroxime, cefotaxime, ceftizoxime, ceftriaxone, cefepime, cefuroxime axetil, an erythromycin,[3] a tetracycline,[4] azithromycin, amoxicillin-clavulanic acid, clarithromycin, a fluoroquinolone[5]
Neisseria gonorrhoeae (gonococcus)	Cefixime, ciprofloxacin, or ofloxacin	Ceftriaxone, spectinomycin, cefpodoxime proxetil
Neisseria meningitidis (meningococcus)	Penicillin[6]	Cefotaxime, ceftizoxime, ceftriaxone, ampicillin, chloramphenicol
Gram-positive cocci		
Streptococcus pneumoniae[8] (pneumococcus)	Penicillin[6]	An erythromycin,[3] a cephalosporin,[7] vancomycin, TMP-SMZ, chloramphenicol, clindamycin, azithromycin, clarithromycin, a tetracycline,[4] imipenem, meropenem, cuinupristin-dalfopristin, certain fluoroquinolones,[5] linezolid
Streptococcus, hemolytic, groups A, B, C, G	Penicillin[6]	An erythromycin,[3] a cephalosporin,[7] vancomycin, clindamycin, azithromycin, clarithromycin
Viridans streptococci	Penicillin[6] ± gentamicin	Cephalosporin,[7] vancomycin
Staphylococcus, methicillin-resistant	Vancomycin ± gentamicin ± rifampin	TMP-SMZ,[2] minocycline, a fluoroquinolone[5]
Staphylococcus, non-penicillinase-producing	Penicillin[6]	A cephalosporin,[3] vancomycin, imipenem, meropenem, a fluoroquinolone,[5] clindamycin
Staphylococcus, penicillinase-producing	Penicillinase-resistant penicillin[9]	Vancomycin, a cephalosporin,[7] clindamycin, amoxicillin-clavulanic acid, ticarcillin-clavulanic acid, ampicillin-sulbactam, piperacillin-tazobactam, imipenem, meropenem, a fluoroquinolone,[5] TMP-SMZ[2]
Enterococcus faecalis	Ampicillin – gentamicin[10]	Vancomycin + gentamicin
Enterococcus faecium	Vancomycin + gentamicin[10]	Quinupristin-dalfopristin, linezolid
Gram-negative rods		
Acinetobacter	Imipenem or meropenem	Minocycline, TMP-SMZ,[2] doxycycline, aminoglycosides,[11] piperacillin, ceftazidime, a fluoroquinolone[5]
Prevotella, oropharyngeal strains	Clindamycin	Penicillin,[3] metronidazole, cefoxitin, cefotetan
Bacteroides, gastrointestinal strains	Metronidazole	Cefoxitin, chloramphenicol, clindamycin, cefotetan, cefmetazole, imipenem, meropenem, ticarcillin-clavulanic acid, ampicillin-sulbactam, piperacillin-tazobactam
Brucella	Tetracycline[4] + gentamicin	TMP-SMZ[2] ± gentamicin; chloramphenicol ± gentamicin; doxycycline + rifampin
Campylobacter jejuni	A fluoroquinolone[5]	Tetracycline,[4] erythromycin[3] or azithromycin
Enterobacter	TMP-SMZ,[2] imipenem, meropenem	Aminoglycoside, aztreonam, a fluoroquinolone,[5] cefepime
Escherichia coli (sepsis)	Cefotaxime, ceftizoxime, ceftriaxone, ceftazidime, cefepime	Imipenem or meropenem, aminoglycosides,[11] a fluoroquinolone[5]
Escherichia coli (uncomplicated urinary infection)	Fluoroquinolones, nitrofurantoin	Sulfonamide, TMP-SMZ,[2] oral cephalosporin, fosfomycin
Haemophilus (meningitis and other serious infections)	Cefotaxime, ceftizoxime, ceftriaxone, ceftazidime	Chloramphenicol, meropenem
Haemophilus (respiratory infections, otitis)	TMP-SMZ[2]	Ampicillin, amoxicillin, doxycycline, azithromycin, clarithromycin, cefotaxime, ceftizoxime, ceftriaxone, cefepime, cefuroxime, cefuroxime axetil, ampicillin-clavulanate
Helicobacter pylori	Amoxicillin + clarithromycin + omeprazole	Clarithromycin + omeprazole or bismuth subsalicylate (Pepto Bismol) + metronidazole + tetracycline
Klebsiella	A cephalosporin	TMP-SMZ,[2] aminoglycoside,[11] imipenem or meropenem, a fluoroquinolone,[5] piperacillin, mezlocillin, aztreonam
Legionella species (pneumonia)	Erythromycin[3] or clarithromycin or azithromycin, or ciprofloxacin ± rifampin	TMP-SMZ,[2] doxycycline ± rifampin
Proteus mirabilis	Ampicillin	An aminoglycoside,[11] TMP-SMZ,[2] a fluoroquinolone,[5] a cephalosporin[7]
Proteus vulgaris and other species (morganella, providencia)	Cefotaxime, ceftizoxime, ceftriaxone, ceftazidime, cefepime	Aminoglycoside,[11] imipenem, TMP-SMZ,[2] a fluoroquinolone[5]
Pseudomonas aeruginosa	Aminoglycoside[11] + antipseudomonal penicillin[12]	Ceftazidime ± aminoglycoside; imipenem or meropenem ± aminoglycoside; aztreonam ± aminoglycoside; ciprofloxacin ± piperacillin; ciprofloxacin ± ceftazidime; ciprofloxacin ± cefepime

(continued)

Table 37–1. Drugs of choice for suspected or proved microbial pathogens, 1998.[1] (± = alone or combined with) (continued)

Suspected or Proved Etiologic Agent	Drug(s) of First Choice	Alternative Drug(s)
Pseudomonas pseudomallei (melioidosis)	Ceftazidime	Chloramphenicol, tetracycline,[4] TMP-SMZ,[2] amoxicillin-clavulanic acid, imipenem or meropenem
Pseudomonas mallei (glanders)	Streptomycin + tetracycline[4]	Chloramphenicol + streptomycin
Salmonella (bacteremia)	Ceftriaxone, a fluoroquinolone[5]	TMP-SMZ,[2] ampicillin, chloramphenicol
Serratia	Cefotaxime, ceftizoxime, ceftriaxone, ceftazidime, cefepime	TMP-SMZ,[2] aminoglycosides,[11] imipenem or meropenem, a fluoroquinolone[5]
Shigella	A fluoroquinolone[5]	Ampicillin, TMP-SMZ,[2] ceftriaxone
Vibrio (cholera, sepsis)	Tetracycline[4]	TMP-SMZ,[2] a fluoroquinolone[5]
Yersinia pestis (plague, tularemia)	Streptomycin ± a tetracycline[4]	Chloramphenicol, TMP-SMZ[2]
Gram-positive rods		
Actinomyces	Penicillin[6]	Tetracycline,[4] clindamycin
Bacillus (eg, anthrax)	Penicillin[6]	Erythromycin,[3] tetracycline,[4] a fluoroquinolone[5]
Clostridium (eg, gas gangrene, tetanus)	Penicillin[6]	Metronidazole, chloramphenicol, clindamycin, imipenem or meropenem
Corynebacterium diphtheriae	Erythromycin[3]	Penicillin[6]
Corynebacterium jeikeium	Vancomycin	Ciprofloxacin, penicillin + gentamicin
Listeria	Ampicillin ± aminoglycoside[11]	TMP-SMZ[2]
Acid-fast rods		
Mycobacterium tuberculosis[13]	INH + rifampin + pyrazinamide ± ethambutol or streptomycin	Other antituberculous drugs
Mycobacterium leprae	Dapsone + rifampin ± clofazimine	Minocycline, ofloxacin, clarithromycin
Mycobacterium kansasii	INH + rifampin ± ethambutol	Ethionamide, cycloserine
Mycobacterium avium complex	Clarithromycin or azithromycin + one or more of the following: ethambutol, rifampin or rifabutin, ciprofloxacin	Other antituberculous drugs
Mycobacterium fortuitum-cheilonei	Amikacin + clarithromycin	Cefoxitin, sulfonamide, doxycycline
Nocardia	TMP-SMZ[2]	Minocycline, imipenem or meropenem, sulfisoxazole
Spirochetes		
Borrelia burgdorferi (Lyme disease)	Doxycycline	Amoxicillin, ceftriaxone, cefuroxime axetil, penicillin
Borrelia recurrentis (relapsing fever)	Tetracycline[4]	Penicillin[6]
Leptospira	Penicillin[6]	Tetracycline[4]
Treponema pallidum (syphilis)	Penicillin[6]	Tetracycline,[4] ceftriaxone
Treponema pertenue (yaws)	Penicillin[6]	Tetracycline[4]
Mycoplasmas	Erythromycin[3] or tetracycline[4]	Clarithromycin, azithromycin, a fluoroquinolone[5]
Chlamydiae		
C psittaci	Tetracycline[4]	Chloramphenicol
C trachomatis (urethritis or pelvic inflammatory disease)	Doxycycline or azithromycin	Ofloxacin
C pneumoniae	Tetracycline[4]	Erythromycin,[3] clarithromycin, azithromycin, a fluoroquinolone
Rickettsiae	Tetracycline[4]	Chloramphenicol, a fluoroquinolone

[1]Adapted from Med Lett Drugs Ther 1999;41:95.
[2]TMP-SMZ is a mixture of 1 part trimethoprim and 5 parts sulfamethoxazole.
[3]Erythromycin estolate is best absorbed orally but carries the highest risk of hepatitis; erythromycin stearate and erythromycin ethylsuccinate are also available.
[4]All tetracyclines have similar activity against most microorganisms. Minocycline and doxycycline have increased activity against *S aureus.* Dosage is determined by rates of absorption and excretion of various preparations.
[5]Fluoroquinolones include ciprofloxacin, ofloxacin, levofloxacin, sparfloxacin, moxifloxacin, gatifloxacin, and others (see text). Levofloxacin and sparfloxacin have the best activity against gram-positive organisms, including penicillin-resistant *S pneumoniae* and methicillin-sensitive *S aureus.* Activity against enterococci and *S epidermidis* is variable. Clinafloxacin is active against anaerobes and ciprofloxacin and clinafloxacin have the best activity against *P aeruginosa.*
[6]Penicillin G is preferred for parenteral injection; penicillin V for oral administration—to be used only in treating infections due to highly sensitive organisms.
[7]Most intravenous cephalosporins (with the exception of ceftazidime) have good activity against gram-positive cocci.
[8]Intermediate and high-level resistance to penicillin has been described. Infections caused by strains with intermediate resistance may respond to high doses of penicillin, cefotaxime, or ceftriaxone. Infections caused by highly resistant strains should be treated with vancomycin ± rifampin. Many strains of penicillin-resistant pneumococci are resistant to erythromycin, macrolides, TMP-SMZ, and chloramphenicol.
[9]Parenteral nafcillin or oxacillin; oral dicloxacillin, cloxacillin, or oxacillin.
[10]Addition of gentamicin indicated only for severe enterococcal infections (eg, endocarditis, meningitis).
[11]Aminoglycosides—gentamicin, tobramycin, amikacin, netilmicin—should be chosen on the basis of local patterns of susceptibility.
[12]Antipseudomonal penicillins: ticarcillin, mezlocillin, piperacillin.
[13]Resistance may be a problem, and susceptibility testing should be done.

Table 37–2. Examples of initial antimicrobial therapy for acutely ill adults pending identification of causative organism.

	Suspected Clinical Diagnosis	Likely Etiologic Diagnosis	Drugs of Choice
(A)	Meningitis, bacterial	Pneumococcus,[1] meningococcus	Cefotaxime,[2] 2–3 g IV every 6 hours, or ceftriaxone, 2 g IV every 12 hours plus vancomycin, 10 mg/kg every 8 hours
(B)	Meningitis, bacterial, age > 50	Pneumococcus, meningococcus, *Listeria monocytogenes*,[3] gram-negative bacilli	Ampicillin, 2 g IV every 4 hours, plus cefotaxime or ceftriaxone and vancomycin as in (A)
(C)	Meningitis, postoperative (or posttraumatic)	*S aureus*, gram-negative bacilli (pneumococcus, posttraumatic)	Vancomycin, 10 mg/kg every 8 hours, plus ceftazidime, 3 g IV every 8 hours
(D)	Brain abscess	Mixed anaerobes, pneumococci, streptococci	Penicillin G, 4 million units IV every 4 hours, or metronidazole, 500 mg IV every 8 hours, plus cefotaxime or ceftriaxone as in (A)
(E)	Pneumonia, acute, community-acquired, severe	Pneumococci, *M pneumoniae*, legionella, *C pneumoniae*	Erythromycin,[4] 0.5 g orally or IV four times daily, or doxycycline, 100 mg IV or orally every 12 hours, plus cefotaxime, 1–2 g IV every 12 hours (or ceftriaxone, 1 g IV every 24 hours)
(F)	Pneumonia, postoperative or nosocomial	*S aureus*, mixed anaerobes, gram-negative bacilli	Cefotaxime or ceftriaxone or cefipime, 2 g IV every 8 hours, or piperacillin-tazobactam, 4–5 g IV every 6 hours, with or without tobramycin or ciprofloxacin
(G)	Endocarditis, acute (including IV drug user)	*S aureus*, *E faecalis*, gram-negative aerobic bacteria, viridans streptococci	Vancomycin, 15 mg/kg every 12 hours, plus gentamicin, 2 mg/kg every 8 hours
(H)	Septic thrombophlebitis (eg, IV tubing, IV shunts)	*S aureus*, gram-negative aerobic bacteria	Nafcillin, 2 g IV every 4 hours, plus gentamicin,[5] 2 mg/kg every 8 hours
(I)	Osteomyelitis	*S aureus*	Nafcillin, 2 g IV every 4 hours, orcefazolin, 2 g IV every 8 hours
(J)	Septic arthritis	*S aureus*, *N gonorrhoeae*	Ceftriaxone, 1–2 g IV every 4 hours
(K)	Pyelonephritis with flank pain and fever (recurrent UTI)	*E coli*, klebsiella, enterobacter, pseudomonas	Ciprofloxacin, 400 mg IV every 12 hours, or levofloxacin, 500 mg IV once daily
(L)	Suspected sepsis in neutropenic patient receiving cancer chemotherapy	*S aureus*, pseudomonas, klebsiella, *E coli*	Ceftazidime, 2 g IV every 8 hours, or cefepime, 2 g IV every 8 hours
(M)	Intra-abdominal sepsis (eg, post-operative, peritonitis, cholecystitis)	Gram-negative bacteria, bacteroides, anaerobic bacteria, streptococci, clostridia	Ampicillin, 1–2 g every 6 hours, or gentamicin, 2 mg/kg every 8 hours, plus metronidazole, 500 mg IV every 8 hours, or piperacillin or tazobactam as in (F) or ticarcillan-clavulanate, 3.1 g IV every 6 hours

[1]Some strains may be resistant to penicillin, vancomycin should be used with or without rifampin.
[2]Cefotaxime, ceftriaxone, ceftazidime, or ceftizoxime can be used. Most studies on meningitis have been done with cefotaxime or ceftriaxone (see text).
[3]TMP-SMZ can be used to treat *Listeria monocytogenes* in patients allergic to penicillin in a dosage of 15–20 mg/kg of TMP in three or four divided doses.
[4]Other macrolides such as azithromycin or clarithromycin can be used.
[5]Depending on local drug susceptibility pattern, use tobramycin, 5 mg/kg/d, or amikacin, 15 mg/kg/d, in place of gentamicin.

7. Inadequate host defenses, including immunodeficiencies and diabetes.

8. Noninfectious causes, including drug fever, malignancy, and autoimmune disease.

F. Promptness of Response: Response depends on a number of factors, including the host (immunocompromised patients respond slower than immunocompetent patients), the site of infection (deep-seated infections such as osteomyelitis and endocarditis respond more slowly than superficial infections such as cystitis or cellulitis), the pathogen (virulent organisms such as *Staphylococcus aureus* respond more slowly than viridans streptococci; mycobacterial and fungal infections respond slower than bacterial infections), and the duration of illness (in general, the longer the symptoms are present, the longer it takes to respond). Thus, depending on the clinical situation, persistent fever and leukocytosis several days after initiation of therapy may not indicate improper choice of antibiotics but may be due to the natural history of the disease being treated. In most infections, either a bacteriostatic or a bactericidal agent can be used. In some infections (eg, infective endocarditis and meningitis), one must kill the infecting organism to achieve a cure. When potentially toxic drugs (eg, aminoglycosides, flucytosine) are used, the serum levels of the drug

Table 37–3. Examples of empirical choices of antimicrobials for adult outpatient infections.

Suspected Clinical Diagnosis	Likely Etiologic Agents	Drugs of Choice	Alternative Drugs
Erysipelas, impetigo, cellulitis, ascending lymphangitis	Group A streptococcus	Phenoxymethyl penicillin, 0.5 g orally four times daily.	Erythromycin, 0.5 g orally four times daily, or cephalexin, 0.5 g orally four times daily for 7–10 days; azithromycin, 500 mg on day 1, and 250 mg on days 2–5.
Furuncle with surrounding cellulitis	*Staphylococcus aureus*	Dicloxacillin, 0.5 g orally four times daily for 7–10 days.	Cephalexin, 0.5 g orally four times daily for 7–10 days.
Pharyngitis	Group A streptococcus	Phenoxymethyl penicillin, 0.5 g orally four times daily for 10 days.	Erythromycin, 0.5 g orally four times daily for 10 days; azithromycin, 500 mg on day 1 and 250 mg on days 2–5, or clarithromycin, 500 mg twice daily daily for 10 days.
Otitis media	*Streptococcus pneumoniae, Haemophilus influenzae, Moraxella catarrhalis*	Amoxicillin, 0.5 g orally three times daily; or TMP-SMZ, one double-strength tablet twice daily for 10 days.	Augmentin,[2] 0.5 g orally three times daily; cefuroxime, 0.5 g orally twice daily; or cefpodoxime, 0.2–0.4 g daily, or doxycycline, 100 mg twice daily or TMP-SMZ, one double-strength tablet twice daily for 10 days.
Acute sinusitis	*S pneumoniae, H influenzae, M catarrhalis*	Amoxicillin, 0.5 g orally three times daily; or TMP-SMZ, one double-strength tablet twice daily for 10 days.	Augmentin,[2] 0.5 g orally three times daily; cefuroxime, 0.5 g orally twice daily; or cefpodoxime, 0.2–0.4 g daily, or doxycycline, 100 mg twice daily for 10 days.
Aspiration pneumonia	Mixed oropharyngeal flora, including anaerobes	Clindamycin, 0.3 g orally four times daily for 10–14 days.	Phenoxymethyl penicillin, 0.5 g orally four times daily for 10–14 days.
Pneumonia	*S pneumoniae, Mycoplasma pneumoniae, Legionella pneumophila, Chlamydia pneumoniae*	Doxycycline, 100 mg twice daily, or erythromycin, 0.5 g four times daily, or clarithromycin, 0.5 g twice daily, for 10–14 days; or azithromycin, 0.5 g on day 1 and 0.25 g on days 2–5.	Amoxicillin, 0.5 g four times daily, or a fluoroquinolone.[5]
Cystitis	*Escherichia coli, Klebsiella pneumoniae,* proteus species, *Staphylococcus saprophyticus*	Fluoroquinolones,[4] nitrofurantoin.	TMP-SMZ,[1] one double-strength tablet twice daily for 3 days; cephalexin, 0.5 g orally four times daily for 7 days.
Pyelonephritis	*E coli, K pneumoniae,* proteus species, *S saprophyticus*	Fluoroquinolones.[4]	TMP-SMZ,[1] one double-strength tablet twice daily.
Gastroenteritis	Salmonella, shigella, campylobacter, *Entamoeba histolytica*	See Note 3.	
Urethritis, epididymitis	*Neisseria gonorrhoeae, Chlamydia trachomatis*	Cefixime, 400 mg orally once, or ciprofloxacin, 500 mg orally once, for *N gonorrhoeae;* doxycycline, 100 mg twice daily for 10 days, or ofloxacin, 300 mg orally twice daily for 10 days for *C trachomatis.*	Ceftriaxone, 250 mg IM once, for *N gonorrhoeae*; plus doxycycline, 100 mg twice daily for 10 days, for *C trachomatis.*
Pelvic inflammatory disease	*N gonorrhoeae, C trachomatis,* anaerobes, gram-negative rods	Ceftriaxone, 250 mg IM once, followed by doxycycline, 100 mg orally twice daily for 14 days.	Cefoxitin, 2 g IM, with probenecid, 1 g orally, followed by doxycycline, 100 mg orally twice daily for 14 days; or ceftriaxone, 250 mg IM once, followed by by doxycycline, 100 mg orally twice daily for 14 days.
Syphilis			
Early syphilis (primary, secondary, or latent of < 1 year's duration)	*Treponema pallidum*	Benzathine penicillin G, 2.4 million units IM once.	Doxycycline, 100 mg orally twice daily for for 2 weeks.
Latent syphilis of > 1 year's duration or cardiovascular syphilis	*Treponema pallidum*	Benzathine penicillin G, 2.4 million units IM once a week for 3 weeks (total: 7.2 million units).	Doxycycline, 100 mg orally twice daily, for 4 weeks.

(*continued*)

Table 37–3. Examples of empirical choices of antimicrobials for adult outpatient infections. (continued)

Suspected Clinical Diagnosis	Likely Etiologic Agents	Drugs of Choice	Alternative Drugs
Neurosyphilis	*Treponema pallidum*	Aqueous penicillin G, 12–24 million units/d IV for 10–14 days.	Procaine penicillin G, 2–4 million units/d IM, plus probenecid, 500 mg orally four times daily, both for 10–14 days.

[1]TMP-SMZ is a fixed combination of 1 part trimethoprim and 5 parts sulfamethoxazole Single-strength tablets: 80 mg TMP, 400 mg SMZ; double-strength tablets: 160 mg TMP, 800 mg SMZ.

[2]Augmentin is a combination of amoxicillin, 250 mg, 500 mg, or 875 mg, plus 125 mg of clavulanic acid.

[3]The diagnosis should be confirmed by culture before therapy. Salmonella gastroenteritis does not require therapy. For sensitive shigella, give TMP-SMZ double-strength tablets twice daily for 5 days; or ampicillin, 0.5 g orally four times daily for 5 days; or ciprofloxacin, 0.5 g orally twice daily for 5 days. For campylobacter, give erythromycin, 0.5 g orally four times daily for 5 days; or ciprofloxacin, 0.5 g orally twice daily for 5 days. For *E histolytica*, give metronidazole, 750 mg orally three times daily for 5–10 days, followed by diiodohydroxyquin, 600 mg three times daily for 3 weeks.

[4]Fluoroquinolones and dosages include ciprofloxacin, 500 mg orally twice daily; ofloxacin, 400 mg orally twice daily; levofloxacin, 500 mg daily; and sparfloxacin, 500 mg as loading dose and then 200 mg once daily. For others see text.

[5]Fluoroquinolones with activity against *S pneumoniae*, including penicillin-resistant isolates, include levofloxacin (500 mg once daily), gatifloxacin (400 mg once daily), sparfloxacin (400 mg on day 1 and then 200 mg once daily), and moxifloxacin (400 mg once daily).

should be measured to avoid toxicity and ensure appropriate dosage. In patients with altered clearance of drugs, the dosage or frequency of administration must be adjusted. Especially in elderly, morbidly obese patients or those with altered renal function, it is best to measure levels directly and adjust therapy accordingly.

In renal or hepatic failure, the dosage must be adjusted as shown in Table 37–4.

G. Duration of Antimicrobial Therapy: Generally, effective antimicrobial treatment results in reversal of the clinical and laboratory parameters of active infection and marked clinical improvement. However, varying periods of treatment may be required for cure. Key factors include (1) the type of infecting organism (bacterial infections can be cured more rapidly than fungal or mycobacterial ones), (2) the location of the process (eg, endocarditis and osteomyelitis require prolonged therapy), and (3) the immunocompetence of the patient. It is noteworthy that very few studies have examined appropriate length of treatment to effect a cure, and duration of therapy is often arbitrary.

H. Adverse Reactions and Toxicity: All antimicrobials can cause adverse effects. Most commonly these are (1) hypersensitivity reactions (eg, fever, rashes, anaphylaxis), (2) direct adverse effect or toxicity (eg, diarrhea, vomiting, impairment of renal or hepatic function, neurotoxicity), (3) superinfection by drug-resistant microorganisms, or (4) drug interactions such as the increased INR associated with trimethoprim-sulfamethoxazole added to warfarin.

If the infection is life-threatening and treatment cannot be stopped, the reactions may be managed symptomatically (especially if mild) or another drug may be chosen that does not cross-react with the offending one (Table 37–1). If the infection is less severe, it may be possible to stop all antimicrobials and follow the patient carefully.

I. Route of Administration: Parenteral therapy is preferred for acutely ill patients with serious infections (eg, endocarditis, meningitis, sepsis, severe pneumonia) when high levels of antibiotics are required for successful therapy. Certain drugs (eg, fluconazole, rifampin, metronidazole, and fluoroquinolones) are so well absorbed that they can be administered orally even in seriously ill patients.

Food does not significantly influence the bioavailability of most oral antimicrobial agents. Exceptions include the tetracyclines and the quinolones, which are chelated by heavy metals. Azithromycin capsules are associated with decreased bioavailability when taken with food and should be given 1 hour before or 2 hours after meals.

A major complication of intravenous antibiotic therapy is catheter infections. To minimize infections, peripheral Teflon catheters are routinely changed every 48–72 hours to prevent phlebitis, and antimicrobial-coated central venous catheters (minocycline and rifampin, chlorhexidine and sulfadiazine) have been associated with a decreased incidence of catheter-related infections Most catheter-related infections present with local signs of infection (erythema, tenderness) at the insertion site; in some, there is a normal-appearing insertion site. In the evaluation of a patient with fever who is receiving intravenous therapy, the catheter must always be considered as a potential source. Some small-gauge (20–23F) peripherally inserted silicone or polyurethane catheters (Per Q Cath, A-Cath, Ven-A-Cath, and others) are associated with a very low infection rate and can be maintained for 3–6 months without replacement. Such catheters are ideal for long-term outpatient antibiotic therapy.

J. Cost of Antibiotics: Because of the widespread use of antibiotics, the cost of these agents can be substantial both to institutions and to individuals. In addition to the direct cost of purchasing a drug, one must consider the costs of monitoring for toxicity (drug levels, liver function tests, electrolytes, etc), the cost of treating adverse reactions, the cost of treat-

Table 37–4. Use of antimicrobials in patients with renal failure[1] and hepatic failure.

	Principal Mode of Excretion or Detoxification	Approximate Half-Life in Serum		Proposed Dosage Regimen in End-Stage Renal Failure		Removal of Drug by Hemodialysis	Dose After Hemodialysis	Dosage in Hepatic Failure
		Normal	Renal Failure[2]	Initial Dose[3]	Maintenance Dose			
Acyclovir	Renal	2.5–3.5 hours	20 hours	2.5 mg/kg	2.5 mg/kg q24h	Yes	2.5 mg/kg	No change
Ampicillin-sulbactam	Renal	0.5–1 hour	8–12 hours	3 g	1.5 g q8–12h	Yes	1.5 g	No change
Amphotericin B	Unknown	360 hours	360 hours	No change	No change	No	None	No change
Ampicillin	Tubular secretion	0.5–1 hour	8–12 hours	1 g	1 g q8–12h	Yes	1 g	No change
Azithromycin	Renal 20%; hepatic 35%	3–4 hours	Not known	500 mg	250 mg q24h	No	None	Not known[4]
Aztreonam	Renal	1.7 hours	6 hours	1–2 g	0.5–1 g q6–8h	Yes	0.5–1 g	No change
Chloramphenicol	Mainly liver	3 hours	4 hours	0.5 g	0.5 g q6h	Yes	0.5 g	0.25–0.5 g q12h
Clarithromycin	Renal 30%; hepatic > 50%	3–4 hours	15 hours	500 mg	250 mg q12h	No	None	Not known[4]
Clindamycin	Liver	2–4 hours	2–4 hours	0.6 g IV	0.6 g q8h	No	None	0.3–0.6 g q8h
Doxycycline	Renal	15–24 hours	15–24 hours	100 mg	100 mg q12h	No	None	Not known[4]
Erythromycin	Mainly liver	1.5 hours	1.5 hours	0.5–1 g	0.5–1 g q6h	No	None	0.25–0.5 g q6h
Famciclovir[5]	Renal	2.5 hours	13–20 hours	500 mg	500 mg q24h	Yes	500 mg	No change
Fluconazole	Renal	30 hours	98 hours	0.2 g	0.1 g q24h	Yes	Give q24h dose	No change
Flucytosine	Renal	3–6 hours	30–250 hours	37.5 mg/kg	25 mg/kg q24h	Yes	25 mg/kg	No change
Foscarnet	Renal	3–8 hours	Not known	90–120 mg	Not known[6]	No	None	No change
Fosfomycin	Renal	6 hours	11–50 hours	NA	NA	NA	NA	No change
Ganciclovir[7]	Renal	3 hours	11–28 hours	1.25 mg/kg	1.25 mg/kg q24h	Yes	Give q24h dose	No change
Imipenem	Glomerular filtration	1 hour	3 hours	0.5 g	0.25–0.5 g q12h	Yes	0.25–0.5 g	No change
Isoniazid	Renal	1–5 hours	2.5 hours	300 mg	300 mg q24h	Yes	None	Not known[4]
Itraconazole	Hepatic	21 hours	25 hours	50–200 mg	50–200 mg q24h	No	None	Not known[4]
Ketoconazole	Hepatic	8 hours	8 hours	200 mg	200–400 mg q24h	No	None	Not known[4]
Meropenem	Renal	1 hour	5–10 hours	1 g	0.5–1 g q24h	Yes	0.5 g	No change
Metronidazole	Liver	6–10 hours	6–10 hours	0.5 g IV	0.5 g q8h	Yes	0.25 g	0.25 g q12h
Mezlocillin	Renal 50–70%; biliary 20–30%	1 hour	3–6 hours	3 g	2 g q6–8h	Yes	1 g	1–2 g q8h
Nafcillin	Liver 80%; kidney 20%	0.75 hours	1.5 hours	1.5 g	1.5 g q4h	No	None	2–3 g q12h
Penicillin G	Tubular secretion	0.5 hours	7–10 hours	1–2 million units	1 million units q8h	Yes	500,000 units	No change

Pentamidine	Not known	6–9 hours	6–9 hours	4 mg/kg	4 mg/kg q24h	No	None needed	No change
Piperacillin and piperacillin + tazobactam	Renal 50–70%; biliary 20–30%	1 hour	3–6 hours	3 g	2 g q6–8h	Yes	1 g	1–2 g q8h
Rifampin	Hepatic	2–3 hours	3–5 hours	600 mg	600 mg q24h	No	None	Not known[4]
Ticarcillin	Tubular secretion	1.1 hour	15–20 hours	3 g	2 g q6–8h	Yes	1 g	No change
Trimethoprim-sulfamethoxazole	Some liver	TMP 10–12 hours; SMZ 8–10 hours	TMP 24–48 hours; SMZ 18–24 hours	320 mg TMP + 1600 mg SMZ	80 mg TMP + 400 mg SMZ every 12 hours	Yes	80 mg TMP + 400 mg SMZ	No change
Trimetrexate	Hepatic	15 hours	Not known	45 mg/m^2	40 mg/m^2 q24h	No	None	Not known
Vancomycin	Glomerular filtration	6 hours	6–10 days	1 g	1 g q6–10d based on serum levels[8]	No	None	No change

[1]For cephalosporins, see text and Table 37–7; for aminoglycosides, see Table 37–8.
[2]Considered here to be marked by creatinine clearance of 10 mL/min or less.
[3]For a 70-kg adult with a serious systemic infection.
[4]Dose adjustment in hepatic failure has not been studied, but because clearance of the drug is principally hepatic, dose reduction may be required.
[5]Pharmacokinetics and dosing are in reference to the active agent, penciclovir.
[6]When creatinine clearance is 30 mL/min, a dose of 60 mg/kg is given once daily. For clearances less than 30 mL/min, the dose has not been established.
[7]Oral ganciclovir is same as IV ganciclovir except that the initial dose is 1000 mg, maintenance dose is 500 mg daily, and dose after hemolysis is 500 mg.
[8]When serum levels reach 5–10 μg/mL, another dose should be given.

ment failure, and the costs associated with the time required for administering drugs that are given at frequent intervals. Although cost should not be the only determinant in choosing antibiotics, if several drugs with equal efficacy and toxicity are available, one should choose the least expensive. Table 37–5 lists the costs of commonly used antibiotics.

The Choice of Antibacterial Drugs. Med Lett Drugs Ther 1999;41:95. (Current recommendations.)

JAMA patient page: Antibiotic resistance. JAMA 1998; 280:1288. [NLM Cit ID: 99000349]

Jorgensen JH: Antimicrobial susceptibility testing: General principles and contemporary practices. Clin Infect Dis 1998;26:973. [NLM Cit ID: 98225672] (Review of tests available.)

Lampiris HW et al: Clinical use of antimicrobial agents. In: *Basic & Clinical Pharmacology,* 7th ed. Katzung BG (editor). Appleton & Lange, 1998.

Mermel LA: Prevention of catheter-associated infection. Ann Intern Med 2000;132:391. [NLM Cit ID: 20143062] (Literature review of preventive methods with recommendations.)

PENICILLINS

The penicillins are a large group of antimicrobial substances, all of which share a common chemical nucleus (6-aminopenicillanic acid) that contains a β-lactam ring essential to their biologic activity. All β-lactam antibiotics inhibit formation of microbial cell walls.

Penicillins fall into four major categories, discussed below.

Antimicrobial Action & Resistance

The initial step in penicillin action is the binding of the drug to receptors—penicillin-binding proteins—some of which are transpeptidation enzymes. The penicillin-binding proteins of different organisms differ in number and in affinity for a given drug. After penicillins have attached to receptors, peptidoglycan synthesis is inhibited because the activity of transpeptidation enzymes is blocked. The final bactericidal action is the removal of an inhibitor of the autolytic enzymes in the cell wall, which activates the enzymes and results in cell lysis. Organisms that are defective in autolysin function are inhibited but not killed by β-lactam antibiotics ("tolerance"). Organisms that produce β-lactamases (penicillinases) are resistant to some penicillins because the β-lactam ring is broken and the drug is inactivated. Only organisms that are actively synthesizing peptidoglycan (in the process of multiplication) are susceptible to β-lactam antibiotics. Nonmultiplying organisms or those lacking cell walls are not susceptible.

Microbial resistance to penicillins is caused by four factors:

(1) Production of β-lactamases, eg, by staphylococci, gonococci, haemophilus species, and coliform organisms.

(2) Lack of penicillin-binding proteins or decreased affinity of penicillin-binding protein for β-lactam antibiotic receptors (eg, resistant pneumococci, methicillin-resistant staphylococci, enterococci) or impermeability of cell envelope, so that penicillins cannot reach receptors (eg, metabolically inactive bacteria).

(3) Failure of activation of autolytic enzymes in the cell wall; "tolerance," eg, in staphylococci, group B streptococci.

(4) The presence of cell wall-deficient (L) forms or mycoplasmas, which do not synthesize peptidoglycans.

1. NATURAL PENICILLINS

The natural penicillins include forms of penicillin G for parenteral administration (aqueous crystalline, procaine, and benzathine penicillin G) or for oral administration (penicillin G and phenoxymethyl penicillin [penicillin V]). They are most active against gram-positive organisms, less active against gram-negatives, and susceptible to hydrolysis by β-lactamases. They are used for infections caused by susceptible and moderately susceptible pneumococci depending upon the site of infection (however, up to 30–35% of strains now demonstrate intermediate- or high-level resistance to penicillin), streptococci (including anaerobic streptococci), meningococci, non-β-lactamase-producing staphylococci, *Treponema pallidum* and other spirochetes, *Bacillus anthracis* and other gram-positive rods, clostridia, actinomyces, and most anaerobes except β-lactamase-producing strains, eg, *Bacteroides fragilis* (Table 37–1).

Pharmacokinetics & Administration

After parenteral administration, penicillin is widely distributed in tissues. Levels equal to those in serum occur in many tissues, but lower levels are present in the eye, prostate, and central nervous system. However, with acute inflammation of the meninges (eg, in bacterial meningitis) and with appropriate dosing, adequate penetration into the cerebrospinal fluid takes place, allowing for treatment of susceptible organisms.

Special dosage forms of penicillin permit delayed absorption to yield low blood and tissue levels for long periods, eg, benzathine penicillin G and procaine penicillin G.

Phenoxymethyl penicillin (penicillin V) is the oral penicillin of choice. It is more acid-stable than oral penicillin G, is better absorbed, and gives higher serum levels.

Most of the absorbed penicillin is rapidly excreted by the kidneys into the urine; small amounts are excreted by other routes. About 10% of renal excretion is by glomerular filtration and 90% by tubular secretion. Tubular secretion can be partially blocked by probenecid, 0.5 g (10 mg/kg) every 6 hours orally, to achieve higher systemic levels. Individuals with im-

Table 37–5. Approximate costs of antimicrobials.

Drug	Dose per Day[1]	Cost per Unit[2]	Daily Cost of Therapy[3]
	INTRAVENOUS PREPARATIONS		
Acyclovir	15 mg/kg (mucocutaneous herpes)	$42.60/1 g	$42.60
Acyclovir	30 mg/kg (CNS herpes)	$42.50/1 g	$85.20
Amikacin (Amikin, others)	15 mg/kg	$99.30/0.5 g	$198.60
Ampicillin	100 mg/kg	$2.50/2 g	$10.00
Ampicillin plus sulbactam (Unasyn)	3 g q8h	$15.25/3 g (IV)	$45.75
Aztreonam (Azactam)	50 mg/kg	$16.00/1 g	$48.00
Cefazolin (Ancef, others)	50 mg/kg	$1.75/1 g (IV)	$5.25
Cefepime (Maxipime)	500 mg/kg	$16.00/1 g	$48.00
Cefoxitin (Mefoxin)	80 mg/kg	$10.50/1 g	$31.50
Ceftazidime (Fortaz, others)	50 mg/kg	$14.50/1 g	$43.50
Ceftizoxime (Cefizox)	50 mg/kg	$12.00/1 g	$36.00
Ceftriaxone (Rocephin)	30 mg/kg	$45.50/1 g	$91.00
Cefuroxime (Zinacef, others)	60 mg/kg	$24.00/1.5 g	$72.00
Ciprofloxacin (Cipro IV)	0.8 g	$15.60/0.2 g	$62.40
Clindamycin (Cleocin, others)	2400 mg	$23.75/0.6 g	$95.00
Fluconazole (Diflucan IV)	0.2–0.4 g	$88.25/0.2 g $129.00/0.4 g	$88.25–129.00
Foscarnet (Foscavir)	180 mg/kg (induction) 90–120 mg/kg (maintenance)	$73.00 (24 mg/mL × 250 mL = 6000 mg)	$146.00 $73.00–102.00
Ganciclovir (Cytovene IV)	10 mg/kg	$36.00/0.5 g	$72.00
Gatifloxacin (Tequin)	400 mg	$38.00/400 mg	$38.00
Gentamicin	5 mg/kg	$1.00/80 mg	$5.00
Imipenem (Primaxin IV)	50 mg/kg	$30.00/0.5 g	$120.00
Meropenem (Merrem IV)	500 mg/kg	$26.00/0.5 g	$78.00–104.00
Metronidazole (Flagyl, others)	1500 mg	$10.00/0.5 g	$30.00
Mezlocillin (Mezlin)	250 mg/kg	$14.50/3 g	$58.00
Nafcillin	100 mg/kg	$4.50/2 g	$18.00
Ofloxacin (Floxin)	400 mg twice daily	$27.60/0.4 g	$55.20
Penicillin	12 million units	$1.00/1 million units	$12.00
Piperacillin (Pipracil)	250 mg/kg	$19.00/3 g	$76.00
Piperacillin plus tazobactam (Zosyn)	3.75 g q6–8h	$16.00/3.375 g	$64.00
Ticarcillin (Ticar)	250 mg/kg	$13.00/3 g	$52.00

(*continued*)

Table 37–5. Approximate costs of antimicrobials. (continued)

Drug	Dose per Day[1]	Cost per Unit[2]	Daily Cost of Therapy[3]
INTRAVENOUS PREPARATIONS			
Ticarcillin-potassium clavulanic acid (Timentin)	3.1 g q6h	$15.00/3.1 g	$60.00
Tobramycin	5 mg/kg	$3.50/80 mg	$17.50
Trimethoprim-sulfamethoxazole (Bactrim, Septra)	15 mg/kg TMP	$35.00 (0.48 g TMP in 30 mL)	$70.00
Trimetrexate (Neutrexin)	45 mg/m^2	$73.50/25 mg	(Depends on surface area.)
Vancomycin	20–30 mg/kg	$11.00/0.5 g	$44.00
ORAL PREPARATIONS			
Acyclovir	1000 mg (therapy of herpes)	$1.00/0.2 g	$5.00
Acyclovir	800 mg three times daily (herpes suppression for immunocompromised patient)	$4.00/0.8 g	$12.00
Amoxicillin	20–30 mg/kg	$0.25/0.5 g	$0.75
Ampicillin	20–30 mg/kg	$0.25/0.5 g	$0.75
Augmentin (0.5 g amoxicillin plus 0.125 g clavulanic acid)	30 mg/kg	$3.75/0.5 g	$7.50
Azithromycin (Zithromax)	500 mg as loading dose, then 250 mg/d for 4 days	$7.00/0.25 g	$14.00 load, then $7.00
Azithromycin (Zithromax)	1 g as single dose for *C trachomatis* infection	$21.00/1 g packet	$21.00/1 g packet
Cefaclor (Ceclor)	20–30 mg/kg	$4.50/0.5 g	$13.50
Cefixime (Suprax)	400 mg	$7.50/0.4 g	$7.50
Cefpodoxime proxetil (Vantin)	400 mg	$4.25/0.2 g	$8.50
Cefprozil (0.5 g) (Cefzil)	15 mg/kg	$6.50/0.5 g	$13.00
Cefuroxime (0.5 g) (Ceftin)	0.5 g twice daily	$7.40/0.5 g	$14.80
Cephalexin (0.5 g) (Keflex, others)	30 mg/kg	$1.00/0.5 g	$4.00
Ciprofloxacin (0.5 g) (Cipro)	0.5–0.75 g twice daily	$4.15/0.5 g	$8.30
Ciprofloxacin (0.75 g) (Cipro)		$4.15/0.75 g	$8.30
Clarithromycin (0.25 or 0.5 g) (Biaxin)	250–500 mg twice daily	$3.75/0.5 g	$7.50
Clindamycin (0.3 g) (Cleocin, others)	15 mg/kg	$3.60/0.3 g	$14.40
Doxycycline (0.1 g)	3 mg/kg	$0.50/0.1 g	$1.00
Erythromycin (0.5 g)	30 mg/kg	$0.30/0.5 g	$0.90
Famciclovir (0.5 g) (Famvir)	500 mg three times daily	$7.40/0.5 g	$22.20
Fluconazole (0.1 g) Fluconazole (0.2 g) (Diflucan)	0.1–0.2 g daily	$7.50/0.1 g $12.25/0.2 g	$7.50 $12.25
Flucytosine (0.5 g) (Ancobon)	150 mg/kg	$7.00/0.5 g	$147.00
Ganciclovir (0.25 g) (Cytovene)	1 g three times daily	$4.00/0.25 g	$48.00

(*continued*)

Table 37–5. Approximate costs of antimicrobials (continued).

Drug	Dose per Day[1]	Cost per Unit[2]	Daily Cost of Therapy[3]
ORAL PREPARATIONS			
Gatifloxacin (400 mg) (Tequin)	400 mg	$7.25/400 mg	$7.25
Itraconazole (0.1 g) (Sporanox)	200–400 mg	$7.00/0.1 g	$14.00–28.00
Ketoconazole (0.2 g) (Nizoral)	0.2–0.4 g	$3.50/0.2 g	$3.50–7.00
Levofloxacin (0.5 g) (Levaquin)	0.5 g daily	$8.50/0.5 g	$8.50
Lomefloxacin (0.4 g) (Maxaquin)	400 mg	$6.60/0.4 g	$6.60
Loracarbef (0.4 mg) (Lorabid)	800 mg	$5.60/0.4 g	$11.20
Metronidazole (0.5 g) (Flagyl)	2 g (trichomonas) 20 mg/kg	$0.50/0.5 g	$2.00 $1.50
Moxifloxacin (400 mg) (Avelox)	400 mg	$8.70/400 mg	$8.70
Ofloxacin (0.4 g) (Floxin)	400 mg twice daily	$5.00/0.4 g	$10.00
Penicillin VK (0.5 g)	30 mg/kg	$0.15/0.5 g	$0.60
Sparfloxacin (0.2 g) (Zagam)	0.2 g daily	$6.75/0.2 g	$13.50 day 1, then $6.75/daily
Tetracycline (0.5 g)	30 mg/kg	$0.10/0.5 g	$0.40
Trimethoprim-sulfamethoxazole (Bactrim, Septra)	5 mg/kg TMP	$0.40/160 mg TMP and 800 mg SMZ	$0.80
Valacyclovir (0.5 g) (Valtrex)	0.5–1 g three times daily	$3.30/0.5 g	$9.90–19.80
Vancomycin (Vancocin)	125 mg 3 times daily	$5.40/125 mg	$16.20

[1]Doses based on a 70-kg individual with normal renal function.
[2]Approximate (for this table only) cost to pharmacist (average wholesale price, generic when possible) for quantity listed. Source: *Drug Topics Red Book*, March 2000; Vol. 19, No. 3.
[3]Daily cost for intravenous antibiotics includes acquistion cost only and not preparation and administration costs.

paired renal function likewise tend to maintain higher penicillin levels longer, and the dose should be reduced in moderate to severe renal failure. One commonly used formula for calculating the maximum daily dose of penicillin in millions of units in patients with a creatinine clearance of less than 40 mL/min is as follows (see also Table 37–4):

$$\frac{\text{Dosage}}{(\text{millions of units/d})} = 3.2 + \frac{\text{Creatinine clearance (mL/min)}}{7}$$

Clinical Uses

Most infections caused by organisms sensitive to penicillin will respond to aqueous penicillin G in daily doses of 1–2 million units administered intravenously every 4–6 hours. For severe or life-threatening infections (meningitis, endocarditis), much larger daily doses (18–24 million units) should be given by intermittent intravenous infusion every 4–6 hours in equally divided doses.

Penicillin V is indicated only in minor disorders such as mild respiratory infections, pharyngitis, and skin and soft tissue infections. The usual dose is 1–2 g/d in four equally divided doses.

A single injection of 1.2 million units of benzathine penicillin intramuscularly is satisfactory for treatment of β-hemolytic streptococcal pharyngitis. An injection of 1.2–2.4 million units every 3–4 weeks provides satisfactory prophylaxis for rheumatics against reinfection with group A streptococci. Syphilis is usually treated with benzathine penicillin, 2.4 million units intramuscularly weekly for 1–3 weeks, depending on the stage of the disease (see Table 37–3).

Procaine penicillin is rarely used but is still recommended as an alternative drug for neurosyphilis (Table 37–3).

2. EXTENDED-SPECTRUM PENICILLINS

The extended-spectrum group of penicillins includes the aminopenicillins: ampicillin and amoxicillin; the carboxypenicillins: ticarcillin; and the ureidopenicillins: piperacillin and mezlocillin. These drugs are all susceptible to destruction by staphylococcal (and other) β-lactamases. They tend to be active against many gram-negative rods and have the same activity as natural penicillins against gram-positive bacteria.

Antimicrobial Activity

Ampicillin and amoxicillin are active against most strains of *Proteus mirabilis,* listeria, and non-β-lactamase-producing strains of *Haemophilus influenzae* but inactive against most strains of klebsiella, pseudomonas, serratia, enterobacter, and indole-positive proteus. Activity against salmonella and shigella species is variable. While amoxicillin is equal to penicillin in its activity against the pneumococcus, ampicillin is generally one to two dilutions less active; both drugs are more active than penicillin against *Enterococcus faecalis.*

Ticarcillin extends the activity of ampicillin to include many strains of pseudomonas, serratia, and indole-positive proteus, but it has poor activity against most strains of klebsiella and enterococci.

The ureidopenicillins are similar to ticarcillin but exhibit slight differences in activity against gram-negative organisms. Piperacillin is more active than ticarcillin against *Pseudomonas aeruginosa* and klebsiella, but otherwise its gram-negative spectrum of activity is similar to that of ticarcillin. Mezlocillin is similar in activity to piperacillin but slightly less active against *P aeruginosa.* Similar to ampicillin, mezlocillin and piperacillin are active against *E faecalis.* The extended-spectrum penicillins are active against most anaerobes. Ampicillin and amoxicillin are not active against β-lactamase-producing strains of *B fragilis*—in contrast to the other drugs in this class which are active at high concentrations.

Pharmacokinetics & Administration

Ampicillin can be given orally or parenterally. The usual oral dose is 1–2 g/d (15–50 mg/kg/d), resulting in serum levels of 4–6 μg/mL. Intravenous dosages range from 20 to 200 mg/kg/d (the higher dosages required in meningitis), resulting in serum levels of up to 40 μg/mL. Amoxicillin is given orally only, in dosages of 25–100 mg/kg/d, usually as 250 or 500 mg tablets three times daily, and is absorbed better than ampicillin, resulting in serum levels twice as high as those achieved with ampicillin.

The carboxy- and ureidopenicillins are given intravenously (200–300 mg/kg/d) in dosages of 3–4 g every 4–6 hours when treating infection due to *P aeruginosa,* resulting in serum levels of 250–300 μg/mL.

Dosage adjustments in renal failure are required for the extended-spectrum penicillins and are summarized in Table 37–4.

Clinical Uses

Ampicillin and amoxicillin are given orally for minor infections, such as acute exacerbations of chronic bronchitis, sinusitis, or otitis. Ampicillin is given intravenously for pneumonia, meningitis, bacteremia, or endocarditis. In meningitis in the neonate or elderly, ampicillin is given to cover listeria.

Amoxicillin is also used as antibacterial prophylaxis to prevent endocarditis. Because of the increased serum and respiratory secretion levels, this agent is valuable in the treatment of moderately penicillin-susceptible pneumococcus. In general, if amoxicillin levels remain above the MIC of the pneumococcus more than 40% of the dosing interval, bacteriologic cure rates approach 85–100%. Although ticarcillin, mezlocillin, and piperacillin have been used as single drugs, they are commonly administered in combination with an aminoglycoside or a quinolone to treat serious pseudomonas infections and as empirical therapy in the febrile neutropenic patient.

3. PENICILLINS COMBINED WITH β-LACTAMASE INHIBITORS

The addition of β-lactamase inhibitors (clavulanic acid, sulbactam, tazobactam) can prevent inactivation of the parent penicillin by bacterial β-lactamases. Augmentin (amoxicillin, 250 mg, 500 mg, or 875 mg, plus 125 mg of clavulanic acid), Timentin (ticarcillin, 3 g, plus 100 mg of clavulanic acid), Unasyn (ampicillin 1 g plus sulbactam 0.5 g, and ampicillin 3 g plus sulbactam 1.5 g), and Zosyn (piperacillin 3 g plus tazobactam 0.375 g, and piperacillin 4 g plus tazobactam 0.5 g) are available. Augmentin is given orally and the others intravenously. In general, the β-lactamase inhibitors effectively inactivate β-lactamases produced by *S aureus, H influenzae, Moraxella catarrhalis,* and *Bacteroides fragilis,* thus making Augmentin, Timentin, Unasyn, and Zosyn effective agents for infections with these organisms. In contrast, the β-lactamase inhibitors are variably and unpredictably effective against certain β-lactamases produced by certain aerobic gram-negative bacilli, such as enterobacter, and thus cannot be relied upon to treat these organisms unless specific sensitivity testing is done. Of the available parenteral drugs, Zosyn has the broadest spectrum of activity. Like Unasyn (but not Timentin) it is active against ampicillin-susceptible enterococci. It has greater in vitro activity against *P aeruginosa* than Timentin and is more active than either Timentin or Unasyn against serratia and klebsiella species.

Augmentin, because of its high cost and gastrointestinal intolerance, is limited to the treatment of refractory cases of sinusitis and otitis that have not responded to less costly agents and is used for therapy and prophylaxis of infections resulting from animal and human bites. The roles of Timentin, Unasyn, and Zosyn include the treatment of polymicrobial infections such as peritonitis from a ruptured viscus, osteomyelitis in a diabetic patient, or traumatic osteomyelitis.

The dosage regimens of these drugs are the same as those of the parent drugs. When Timentin or Zosyn is used to treat pseudomonas infections, dosages of 200–300 mg/kg/d are used. Nonpseudomonal infection can be treated with lower doses (100–200 mg/kg/d).

4. PENICILLINASE-RESISTANT PENICILLINS

Methicillin, oxacillin, cloxacillin, dicloxacillin, nafcillin, and others are relatively resistant to destruction by β-lactamases produced by staphylococci and are limited to the treatment of infections with such organisms. They are less active than natural penicillins against gram-positives; however, they are still adequate in streptococcal infections.

Oxacillin, cloxacillin, and dicloxacillin are given orally in dosages of 0.25–0.5 g every 6 hours in mild or localized staphylococcal infections.

For serious systemic staphylococcal infections, nafcillin, 6–12 g/d, is given intravenously in four to six divided doses. Eighty percent of administered nafcillin is excreted into the biliary tract and only 20% by renal tubular secretion.

5. ADVERSE EFFECTS OF PENICILLINS

Allergy

All penicillins are cross-sensitizing and cross-reacting. In general, sensitization occurs in proportion to the duration and total dose of penicillin received in the past. The responsible antigenic determinants appear to be degradation products of penicillins, particularly penicilloic acid and products of alkaline hydrolysis (minor antigenic determinants) bound to host protein. Skin tests with penicilloyl-polylysine, with minor antigenic determinants, and with undegraded penicillin can identify most hypersensitive individuals. Among positive reactors to skin tests, the incidence of subsequent immediate severe penicillin reactions is high. Although many persons develop IgG antibodies to antigenic determinants of penicillin, the presence of such antibodies is not correlated with allergic reactivity (except for rare instances of hemolytic anemia), and serologic tests have little predictive value. A history of a penicillin reaction in the past is not reliable. Only one-fourth of patients with a history of penicillin allergy have an adverse reaction when challenged with the drug. The decision to administer penicillin or related drugs (other β-lactams) to patients with an allergic history depends upon the severity of the reported reaction, the severity of the infection being treated, and the availability of alternative drugs. For patients with a history of severe reaction (anaphylaxis), alternative drugs should be used. In the rare situations when there is a strong indication for using penicillin (eg, syphilis in pregnancy) despite a history of severe reaction, desensitization can be performed. If the history is unclear or the reaction mild (rash), the patient may be rechallenged with penicillin or may be given another β-lactam antibiotic. (See Chapter 30 for discussion and methods of desensitization.)

Allergic reactions include anaphylaxis, serum sickness (urticaria, fever, joint swelling, angioneurotic edema 7–12 days after exposure), and a variety of skin rashes, oral lesions, fever, interstitial nephritis, eosinophilia, hemolytic anemia, other hematologic disturbances, and vasculitis. The incidence of hypersensitivity to penicillin is estimated to be 1–5% among adults in the USA. Life-threatening anaphylactic reactions are very rare (0.05%). Ampicillin produces maculopapular skin rashes more frequently than other penicillins, but some ampicillin rashes are not allergic in origin. The nonallergic ampicillin rash usually occurs after 3–4 days of therapy, is maculopapular, is more common in patients with coexisting viral illness (especially Epstein-Barr infection), and resolves with continued therapy. Penicillins can induce nephritis with primary tubular lesions association with anti-basement membrane antibodies.

Toxicity

Since the action of penicillin is directed against a unique bacterial structure, the cell wall, it is virtually without effect on animal cells. The toxic effects of penicillin G are due to irritation caused by intramuscular or intravenous injection and include local pain, induration, thrombophlebitis, or degeneration of an accidentally injected nerve. All penicillins are irritating to the central nervous system, and excessive doses have been associated with seizures. There is no indication for intrathecal administration since they sufficiently cross the blood-brain barrier with inflamed meninges. In rare cases, a patient with renal insufficiency receiving large doses may exhibit signs of cerebrocortical irritation as a result of passage of unusually large amounts of penicillin into the central nervous system.

Of the oral penicillins, Augmentin is most commonly associated with diarrhea. Nafcillin administered at high doses is associated with a modest leukopenia. High doses of ticarcillin, mezlocillin, or piperacillin can produce hypokalemic alkalosis and elevation of serum aminotransferases and can inhibit platelet aggregation.

Craig WA: Pharmacokinetics/pharmacodynamics parameters: Rationale for antibacterial dosing of mice and men. Clin Infect Dis 1998;26:1. [NLM Cit ID: 98116680] (Review of pharmacologic principles with application of principles to rational dosing.)

Wright AJ: The penicillins. Mayo Clin Proc 1999;74:290. [NLM Cit ID: 99189870] (Review of activity, clinical uses, and adverse effects of this class of drugs.)

CEPHALOSPORINS (Tables 37–6 and 37–7)

The cephalosporins are structurally related to the penicillins. They consist of a β-lactam ring attached to a dihydrothiazoline ring. Substitutions of chemical groups at various positions on the basic structure have resulted in a proliferation of drugs with varying pharmacologic properties and antimicrobial activities.

The mechanism of action of cephalosporins is analogous to that of the penicillins: (1) binding to specific penicillin-binding proteins that serve as drug receptors on bacteria, (2) inhibition of cell wall synthesis, and (3) activation of autolytic enzymes in the cell wall that result in bacterial death. Resistance to cephalosporins may be due to poor permeability of the drug into bacteria, lack of penicillin-binding proteins, or degradation by β-lactamases.

Cephalosporins have been divided into four major groups or "generations" (Table 37–6) based mainly on their antibacterial activity: First-generation cephalosporins have good activity against aerobic gram-positive organisms and some community-acquired gram-negative organisms (*P mirabilis, E coli,* klebsiella species); second-generation drugs have a slightly extended spectrum against gram-negative bacteria, and some are active against anaerobes; and third-generation cephalosporins have less activity against gram-positives but are extremely active against most gram-negative bacteria (except enterobacter and citrobacter). Not all cephalosporins fit neatly into this grouping, and there are exceptions to the general characterization of the drugs in the individual classes; however, the generational classification of cephalosporins is useful for discussion purposes. Cefepime is considered a fourth-generation agent because it is more stable against plasmid-mediated β-lactamase and has little or no β-lactamase-inducing capacity. Cefepime compares favorably with ceftazidime with respect to its gram-negative activity; however, its stability versus plasmid-mediated β-lactamase results in improved coverage against enterobacter and citrobacter species.

Table 37–6. Major groups of cephalosporins.

First Generation	Second Generation	Third Generation	Fourth Generation
Cephalothin	Cefamandole	Cefotaxime	Cefepime
Cephapirin	Cefuroxime	Ceftizoxime	
Cefazolin	Cefonicid	Ceftriaxone	
Cephalexin[1]	Ceforanide	Ceftazidime	
Cephradine[1]	Cefaclor[1]	Cefoperazone	
Cefadroxil	Cefoxitin	Cefixime[1]	
	Cefotetan	Cefpodoxime proxetil[1]	
	Cefprozil[1]	Ceftibuten[1]	
	Cefuroxime axetil[1]	Cefdinir[1]	
	Cefmetazole		

[1]Oral agents.

The gram-positive coverage of cefepime approaches that of cefotaxime or ceftriaxone.

Both parenteral and oral cephalosporins—especially second- and third-generation agents—are somewhat costly (Table 37–5). Because of their broad spectrum of activity and low toxicity, these drugs are used to treat many infections.

1. FIRST-GENERATION CEPHALOSPORINS

Antimicrobial Activity

These drugs are very active against gram-positive cocci, including penicillin-sensitive pneumococci, viridans streptococci, group A hemolytic streptococci, and *S aureus.* Like all cephalosporins, they are inactive against enterococci and methicillin-resistant staphylococci. Activity against *H influenzae* is poor, and many strains of penicillin-resistant streptococci (both intermediately and highly resistant) are resistant also to first-generation cephalosporins. Among gram-negative bacteria, *E coli, K pneumoniae,* and *P mirabilis* are usually sensitive except for some hospital-acquired strains. There is very little activity against such gram-negatives as *P aeruginosa,* indole-positive proteus, enterobacter, *H influenzae, Serratia marcescens,* citrobacter, and acinetobacter. Anaerobic cocci are usually sensitive, but *B fragilis* is not.

Pharmacokinetics & Administration

A. Oral: Cephalexin, cephradine, and cefadroxil are variably absorbed. Urine levels of these drugs are several hundred times higher than serum levels, but concentrations in other tissues are variable and usually lower than in the serum. Cefadroxil, because of its longer half-life, can be given twice daily. Dosage adjustment is required in renal insufficiency.

B. Intravenous: Cefazolin is preferred over cephalothin and cephapirin because it has a longer half-life, requires less frequent dosing, and achieves higher serum levels. In renal insufficiency, all of these agents require dosage adjustments.

C. Intramuscular: Both cephapirin and cefazolin can be given intramuscularly, but pain on injection is less with cefazolin.

Clinical Uses

Oral drugs are sometimes used for treatment of urinary tract infections in patients who are allergic to sulfonamides, and they can be used for minor staphylococcal infections. Oral cephalosporins may also be preferred for minor polymicrobial infections (eg, cellulitis, soft tissue abscess).

Intravenous first-generation cephalosporins penetrate most tissues well and are the drugs of choice for surgical prophylaxis in many cases. More expensive second- and third-generation cephalosporins offer no advantage over the first-generation drugs for surgical prophylaxis except where anaerobes play an impor-

Table 37–7. Pharmacology of the cephalosporins.

Drug	Peak Serum Level (μg/mL) After 1 g IV	Serum Half-Life (min)	Total Daily Dose (mg/kg)	Dosage Interval (hours)	Dosage Adjustments in Renal Failure: Moderate (Cl_{cr} 10–50 mL/min)	Severe (Cl_{cr} < 10 mL/min)	Post-Hemodialysis Dose
Cephalothin, cephapirin	40–60	40	50–200	4–6	1–2 g q6–12h	1 g q12h	1 g
Cefazolin	90–120	90	25–100	8	0.5–1 g q6–12h	0.5 g daily	0.5 g
Cephalexin, cephradine[1]	15–20	50–60	15–30	6	0.25–0.5 g q8–12h	0.25–0.5 g daily	0.5 g
Cefadroxil[1]	15	75	15–30	12–24	1 g daily	0.5 g daily	0.5 g
Cefamandole	60–80	45	75–200	6–8	1 g q12h	1–2 g daily	0.5 g
Cefepime	60–70	120	50–75	8–12	1 g q12h	1 g q24h	1 g
Ceftibuten[1]	20	120	9	12–24	0.4 g daily	0.1–0.2 g daily	0.7 g
Cefuroxime	80–100	80	50	6–12	1 g q12h	1–2 g daily	0.5 g
Cefuroxime axetil[1]	6–8	75	5–15	12	0.5 g q24h	0.25 g daily	0.25 g
Cefonicid	200–250	240	15–30	24	0.5 g daily	1 g q72h	0.25 g
Ceforanide	125	180	15–30	12	1 g daily	1 g q48h	0.25 g
Cefaclor[1]	15–20	50	20–40 children, 10–15 adults	6–8	0.5 g q8–12h	0.25–0.5 g q12–24h	0.25–0.5 g
Cefixime	3–5	180–240	8 (with maximum of 0.4 g/d total)	12–24	0.4 g daily	0.1 g daily	None
Cefpodoxime proxetil[1]	2	150	5	12	0.2 g q24h	0.2 g 3 times/wk after dialysis	0.2 g
Cefprozil[1]	10	90	10–15	12	0.5 g q12–24h	0.25–0.5 g q12–24h	0.5 g
Cefotetan	60–80	150	50–100	8–12	1 g q8–12h	0.5–1 g daily	0.5 g
Cefotaxime	40–60	60	50–75	6–8	1–2 g q6–8h	1–2 g q24h	1–2 g
Cefoxitin	60–80	60	50–100	6–8	1 g q12h	1–2 g daily	0.5 g
Cefmetazole	70–100	60–80	50–100	6–8	1 g q12–24h	1–2 g q24–48h	1 g
Ceftizoxime	80–100	100	50–75	8–12	0.5–1 g q8–12h	0.25–0.5 g q12–24h	0.5 g
Ceftriaxone	150	480	30–50	12–24	1–2 g daily	1–2 g daily	None
Ceftazidime	100–120	120	50–75	8–12	1 g q12h	0.5–1 g daily	0.5 g
Cefoperazone	150	120	30–200	8–12	1–2 g q12h	1–2 g q12h	None
Loracarbef[1]	10	60	10–15	12	0.2 g q24h	0.2 g 3 times/wk after dialysis	0.2 g

[1]Oral agents. Serum levels based on 0.5 g oral dose.

tant role, such as for colorectal surgery or for hysterectomy.

First-generation cephalosporins do not penetrate the cerebrospinal fluid and cannot be used to treat meningitis.

2. SECOND-GENERATION CEPHALOSPORINS

Second-generation cephalosporins are a heterogeneous group with marked individual differences in activity, pharmacokinetics, and toxicity. In general, all are active against organisms also covered by first-generation drugs, but they have an extended gram-negative coverage. Indole-positive proteus and klebsiella (including cephalothin-resistant strains) as well as *Moraxella catarrhalis* and neisseria species are usually sensitive. Cefamandole, cefuroxime, cefonicid, ceforanide, cefuroxime axetil, and cefprozil are active against *H influenzae,* including β-lactamase-producing strains, but have little activity against serratia and *B fragilis.* In contrast, cefoxitin and cefotetan are active against most strains of *B fragilis* and some strains of serratia. Cefmetazole is similar in activity to cefoxitin and cefotetan but has more activity against *H influenzae.* Against gram-positive organisms, these drugs are generally less active than the first-generation cephalosporins (cefuroxime and cefamandole are exceptions). Second-generation agents have no activity against *P aeruginosa* or enterococci.

Pharmacokinetics & Administration

A. Oral: Only cefaclor, cefuroxime axetil, and cefprozil can be given orally. All are available as capsules (0.25 or 0.5 g) and in suspension (0.125 or 0.25 g/5 mL). Cefuroxime axetil is deesterified to cefuroxime after absorption. Its longer half-life permits twice-daily dosing, and absorption is enhanced when it is taken with food (as is not the case with many other oral antibiotics).

B. Intravenous and Intramuscular: Because of differences in drug half-life and protein binding, peak serum levels achieved and dosing intervals vary greatly for this group of drugs (Table 37–7). Drugs with shorter half-lives (cefoxitin, cefamandole) require higher doses and more frequent dosing than drugs with longer half-lives (cefuroxime, cefonicid, cefotetan). Dosage adjustments are required with renal impairment.

Clinical Uses

Because of their activity against β-lactamase-producing *H influenzae* and *M catarrhalis,* cefprozil and cefuroxime axetil can be used to treat sinusitis and otitis media in patients with mild allergy to ampicillin or amoxicillin or have not responded to treatment with those drugs.

Because of their activity against *B fragilis,* cefoxitin, cefmetazole, and cefotetan can be used to treat mixed anaerobic infections, eg, peritonitis and diverticulitis. However, since 10–15% of *B fragilis* and many enteric gram-negative organisms are resistant to these drugs, for severe life-threatening intra-abdominal infections metronidazole plus an aminoglycoside or a third-generation cephalosporin is preferred. Cefoxitin and cefotetan are useful as prophylaxis in colorectal surgery, vaginal or abdominal hysterectomy, and appendectomy because of their activity against *B fragilis.* Cefonicid and ceforanide have also been promoted for surgical prophylaxis, but there is no evidence that they are more effective than first-generation cephalosporins, and they tend to be more expensive.

3. THIRD- & FOURTH-GENERATION CEPHALOSPORINS

Antimicrobial Activity

Most of these drugs are active against staphylococci (not methicillin-resistant strains) but less so than first-generation cephalosporins. Ceftazidime, however, has notably weak activity against *S aureus* and pneumococci. They have no activity against enterococci but do inhibit most streptococci. A major advantage of these cephalosporins is their expanded gram-negative coverage. In addition to organisms inhibited by other cephalosporins, they are consistently active against *S marcescens,* providencia, haemophilus, and neisseria, including β-lactamase-producing strains. Ceftazidime has good activity against *P aeruginosa.* Acinetobacter, citrobacter, enterobacter, and non-aeruginosa strains of pseudomonas are variably sensitive to third-generation cephalosporins, and listeria is uniformly resistant. Activity against *B fragilis* is variable, and these agents should not be relied upon to treat serious infections with this organism. In contrast to the third-generation agents, cefepime—the only currently available fourth-generation cephalosporin—is active against enterobacter and citrobacter, has activity comparable to that of ceftazidime against *P aeruginosa,* and has gram-positive activity similar to that of ceftriaxone.

Cefixime, cefpodoxime proxetil, cefdinir, and ceftibuten, the only oral agents in this group, are more active than cefuroxime axetil but are not as active as parenteral third-generation cephalosporins against gram-negative organisms such as pseudomonas, enterobacter, morganella, and *S marcescens.* The major difference in these drugs is activity against gram-positive bacteria. All are active against *Streptococcus pyogenes* (group A streptococcus). Cefpodoxime proxetil and cefdinir are active against methicillin-sensitive *S aureus,* whereas cefixime and ceftibuten have little activity (none are active against methicillin-resistant strains). Cefdinir, cefixime, and cefpodoxime proxetil are active against penicillin-sensitive strains of *Streptococcus pneumoniae* (the pneumococcus), but ceftibuten has marginal activity. None of the oral cephalosporins are reliable against intermediately susceptible or penicillin-resistant *S pneumoniae.* Like other members of this class, these drugs are inactive against enterococci and *Listeria monocytogenes.*

Pharmacokinetics & Administration

The intravenous agents penetrate well into body fluids and tissues and—except for cefoperazone—reach levels in the cerebrospinal fluid that exceed those needed to inhibit most pathogens, including gram-negative rods. The half-lives of these drugs are variable, which accounts for the differences in dosing intervals (Table 37–7). Cefoperazone and ceftriaxone are eliminated primarily by biliary excretion, and no dosage adjustment is required in renal insufficiency. The other drugs are eliminated primarily by the kidney and thus require dosage adjustments in renal insufficiency.

Clinical Uses

Because of their penetration into the cerebrospinal fluid, third-generation cephalosporins—except cefoperazone—can be used to treat meningitis. Meningitis due to susceptible pneumococci (strains that are resistant to penicillin may have high MICs to third-generation cephalosporins, and these agents should not be used to treat meningitis caused by highly penicillin-resistant pneumococci), meningococci, *H influenzae,* and susceptible enteric gram-negative rods has been successfully treated. In meningitis in the elderly, third-generation cephalosporins should be combined with ampicillin until *L monocytogenes* has been excluded as the etiologic agent. Ceftazidime has been used to treat pseudomonas meningitis. The dosage for meningitis should be at the upper limits of the recommended range, because cerebrospinal fluid levels of these drugs are only 10–20% of serum levels. Ceftazidime or cefepime is frequently administered empirically in the febrile neutropenic patient. Ceftriaxone is indicated for gonorrhea, chancroid, and more serious forms of Lyme disease (see Chapter 34). Because of its long half-life and once-daily dosing requirement, ceftriaxone is an attractive option for the outpatient parenteral therapy of infections due to susceptible organisms.

Cefepime is useful for indications similar to those of ceftazidime, including treatment of the febrile neutropenic patient. It is also indicated for therapy of susceptible strains of enterobacter and citrobacter.

Cefixime, because of its long half-life, can be given once daily. Ceftibuten also can be given once daily, 400 mg. Although approved for use in otitis media and acute exacerbations of chronic bronchitis, its limited activity against *Moraxella catarrhalis* and *Streptococcus pneumoniae,* frequent pathogens in these entities, makes it a poor choice for these infections. Cefdinir has poor bioavailability (about 20% absorption) but is effective for therapy of acute sinusitis and uncomplicated skin and soft tissue infections. The usual dose is 300 mg twice daily. Cefixime (400 mg as a single dose) and cefpodoxime proxetil (200 mg as a single dose) are as effective as ceftriaxone (125 mg intramuscularly) for the therapy of genital, rectal, and pharyngeal gonorrhea.

4. ADVERSE EFFECTS OF CEPHALOSPORINS

Allergy

Cephalosporins are sensitizing, and a variety of hypersensitivity reactions occur, including anaphylaxis, fever, skin rashes, nephritis, granulocytopenia, and hemolytic anemia. The frequency of IgE cross-allergy between cephalosporins and penicillins approximates 5–10%. Persons with a history of anaphylaxis to penicillins should not receive cephalosporins.

Toxicity

Local pain can occur after intramuscular injection, or thrombophlebitis after intravenous injection. Hypoprothrombinemia is a frequent adverse effect (40–68%) of cephalosporins that have a methylthiotetrazole group (eg, cefamandole, cefmetazole, cefoperazone, cefotetan). Prophylactic administration of vitamin K, 10 mg twice weekly, can prevent this complication. Drugs containing the methylthiotetrazole ring can also cause severe disulfiram-like reactions, and use of alcohol or medications containing alcohol (eg, theophylline elixir) must be avoided. Ceftriaxone has been associated with a dose-dependent biliary sludging syndrome and cholelithiasis due to precipitation of drug when its solubility in bile is exceeded. Long term administration of 2 g/d or more is a risk factor for this complication. All β-lactams have been associated with leukopenia, and this adverse effect may occur more frequently in those who have severe hepatic dysfunction.

Superinfection

Third- and fourth-generation cephalosporins have little activity against gram-positive organisms, particularly methicillin-resistant staphylococci and enterococci. Superinfection with these organisms—as well as with fungi—may occur.

Marshall WF et al: The cephalosporins. Mayo Clin Proc 1999;74:187. [NLM Cit ID: 99166889] (Review of spectrum of activity, clinical use, adverse effects, and mechanisms of resistance.)

OTHER β-LACTAM DRUGS

Monobactams

These are drugs with a monocyclic β-lactam ring that are resistant to β-lactamases and active against gram-negative organisms (including pseudomonas) but have no activity against gram-positive organisms or anaerobes. Aztreonam resembles ceftazidime in its gram-negative activity. The usual dosage is 1–2 g intravenously every 6–8 hours. Clinical uses of aztreonam are limited because of the availability of third-generation cephalosporins with a broader spectrum of activity and minimal toxicity. Despite the structural similarity of aztreonam to penicillin, cross-reactivity is limited, and it can therefore be used in most patients with penicillin allergy.

Carbapenems

This class of drugs is structurally related to β-lactam antibiotics. Imipenem, the first drug of this type, has a wide spectrum of activity that includes most gram-negative rods (including *P aeruginosa*) and gram-positive organisms and anaerobes, with the exception of *Pseudomonas cepacia, Stenotrophomonas maltophilia, E faecium,* and most methicillin-resistant *S aureus* and *S epidermidis*. It is resistant to β-lactamases but is inactivated by dipeptidases in renal tubules. Consequently, it must be combined with cilastatin, a dipeptidase inhibitor, for clinical use.

The half-life of imipenem is 1 hour. Penetration into body tissues and fluids is good. The usual dosage is 0.5–1 g intravenously every 6 hours (maximum dose 50 mg/kg/d). Dosage adjustment is required in renal insufficiency.

Meropenem is similar to imipenem in spectrum of activity and pharmacology but is not inactivated by dipeptidase. It is less likely to cause seizures than imipenem, though the risk of seizures is low with imipenem if dosage is appropriately adjusted for renal insufficiency. Meropenem is associated with less nausea and vomiting than imipenem, a feature of importance when high doses must be used, as in the treatment of pseudomonas infection in patients with cystic fibrosis. The usual dose is 1–2 g every 8 hours. Dosage adjustment in renal insufficiency is required.

Imipenem and meropenem should not be routinely used as first-line therapy unless the organism causing infection is multidrug-resistant and is known to be sensitive to these agents. In patients hospitalized for a prolonged period who may have infection with a multidrug-resistant organism, empirical use of imipenem or meropenem while awaiting culture results is reasonable. Pseudomonas may rapidly develop resistance to these drugs. In cystic fibrosis, doubling of the rate of resistance every 5–7 days of treatment has been documented. The use of imipenem or meropenem alone appears to be as effective as combination therapy in the febrile neutropenic patient and as effective as combination therapy in certain polymicrobial infections such as peritonitis and obstetric pelvic infections.

The most common adverse effects of imipenem and meropenem are nausea, vomiting, diarrhea, reactions at the infusion site, and skin rashes. Seizures are more commonly observed with imipenem. Patients allergic to penicillins may be allergic to imipenem and meropenem as well.

Carbacephems

Loracarbef is a β-lactam antibiotic that is structurally similar to cefaclor except that a methylene group has replaced the sulfur in the dihydrothiazine ring. This structural change adds chemical stability to the drug but does not greatly enhance its antibacterial activity, which is essentially the same as that of cefaclor, cefuroxime axetil, and cefprozil. Loracarbef should be reserved for the therapy of sinusitis, otitis media, bronchitis, and urinary tract infections in patients who have failed therapy with less expensive agents (eg, ampicillin, amoxicillin, trimethoprim-sulfamethoxazole). The usual dosage is 200–400 mg orally every 12 hours.

Edwards JR et al: Carbapenems: the pinnacle of the beta-lactam antibiotics or room for improvement? J Antimicrob Chemother 2000;45:1. [NLM Cit ID: 20094813]

Hellinger WC et al: Carbapenems and monobactams: Imipenem, meropenem, and aztreonam. Mayo Clin Proc 1999;74:420. [NLM Cit ID: 99236661] (Review of activity, indications and adverse effects.)

Iaconis JP et al: Comparison of antibacterial activities of meropenem and six other antimicrobials against *Pseudomonas aeruginosa* isolates from North American studies and clinical trials. Clin Infect Dis 1997;24(Suppl 2):S191. [NLM Cit ID: 97271783]

ERYTHROMYCIN GROUP (Macrolides)

The erythromycins are a group of closely related compounds characterized by a macrocyclic lactone ring to which various sugars are attached.

Antimicrobial Activity

Erythromycins inhibit protein synthesis by binding to the 50S subunit of bacterial ribosomes. They generally are bacteriostatic and sometimes bactericidal for gram-positive organisms, including most pneumococci, streptococci, and corynebacteria in a concentration of 0.02–2 μg/mL. Similar to penicillin, macrolide-resistant *S pneumoniae* is being reported with increased frequency (15–30%), and group A streptococci also can be resistant. Erythromycin-resistant pneumococci are azalide-resistant as well (azithromycin, clarithromycin). Chlamydiae, mycoplasmas, legionella, and campylobacter are susceptible.

Pharmacokinetics & Administration

Preparations for oral use include erythromycin base, erythromycin stearate, estolate, and ethyl succinate. The base is most acid-stable, and the estolate is the best-absorbed; none of the oral preparations have any advantage over others. The usual adult oral dose is 250–500 mg four times daily. Erythromycins are excreted largely in the bile; only 5% is excreted in the urine, and no adjustment is therefore required in renal failure.

Erythromycin lactobionate and gluceptate are available for intravenous use. The usual dosage is 250–500 mg every 6 hours, but higher dosages (1 g every 6 hours) are sometimes used initially in the treatment of Legionnaires' disease.

Clinical Uses

Erythromycins are drugs of choice for infections caused by legionella, mycoplasma, ureaplasma, corynebacterium (including diphtheria and bacteremia), and chlamydia (including ocular and respiratory infections). They are effective in streptococcal and pneumococcal disease in penicillin-allergic patients, though increasing resistance is becoming a problem. They can also be used in combination with sulfisoxazole for acute otitis media and with neomycin in prophylaxis for bowel surgery. When administered early, erythromycin may shorten the course of campylobacter enteritis. Erythromycins are effective against certain bartonella species (bacillary angiomatosis) and rhodococcus species. In vitro data suggest that macrolides have a direct effect on neutrophil function and the production of cytokines associated with inflammation. Thus, these agents are being evaluated for their anti-inflammatory effects in infectious diseases as well.

Adverse Effects

Nausea, vomiting, and diarrhea may occur after oral intake. Erythromycins—particularly the estolate—can produce acute cholestatic hepatitis (fever, jaundice, impaired liver function), probably as a hypersensitivity reaction. Most patients recover, but hepatitis recurs if the drug is readministered. Reversible auditory impairment occurs with large doses (4 g/d or more), particularly in patients with impaired renal or hepatic function. Ototoxicity has been reported with high doses of all agents. Intravenous erythromycin has been associated with prolongation of the QT interval and torsade de pointes—seen more commonly in women than in men. Erythromycins can increase the effects of oral anticoagulants, digoxin, theophylline, and cyclosporine by inhibiting cytochrome P450. Patients taking these medications who are treated with erythromycin should have levels monitored and dosages adjusted appropriately.

AZALIDES

Azalides (azithromycin, clarithromycin, dirythromycin, and others) are a group of antibiotics closely related structurally to the macrolides. Like erythromycin, they are active against *Streptococcus pneumoniae,* group A streptococcus, viridans streptococci, *M catarrhalis,* legionella, *Mycoplasma pneumoniae,* and *Chlamydia pneumoniae* and are slightly more active in vitro than erythromycin against *H influenzae* (with azithromycin having better activity than clarithromycin and dirythromycin having activity equivalent to that of erythromycin). They are also active against *Chlamydia trachomatis, N gonorrhoeae, Ureaplasma urealyticum,* and *Haemophilus ducreyi.* In addition, these drugs have in vitro activity against a number of unusual pathogens. including atypical mycobacteria *(Mycobacterium avium-intracellulare, Mycobacterium chelonei, Mycobacterium fortuitum, Mycobacterium marinum), Toxoplasma gondii, Campylobacter jejuni, Helicobacter pylori,* and *Borrelia burgdorferi.*

The azalides are more acid-stable than erythromycin, penetrate tissues well, and have a long terminal half-life, with high tissue concentrations that persist for days. Azithromycin, clarithromycin, and dirythromycin are approved for treatment of streptococcal pharyngitis, uncomplicated skin infections, and acute bacterial exacerbations of chronic bronchitis. Because of the long half-life, treatment with azithromycin is with once-daily dosing for a total of 5 days (500 mg on day 1 and then 250 mg on days 2–5). Clarithromycin is usually administered in a dosage of 250–500 mg twice daily, though an extended-release formulation that is given as a single daily 1000 mg dose has been approved for acute sinusitis and acute exacerbation of chronic bronchitis. Dirythromycin is given as a single daily dose of 500 mg.

The azalides are more expensive than erythromycin. Whether the decreased gastrointestinal distress that occurs and the less frequent dosing that is required outweigh the increased cost is not yet determined.

Azithromycin has also been approved as single-dose therapy (1 g) for chlamydial genital infections. This is much more expensive than 7 days of treatment with doxycycline (Table 37–5), but the assurance of adequate supervised therapy for this infection makes azithromycin preferred therapy in some patients. Azithromycin can also be used as single-dose therapy (1 g) for chancroid, and a single-dose of 1 g is as efficacious as 7 days of doxycycline for nongonococcal urethritis in men and is effective also for incubating syphilis. While a 2 g dose of azithromycin is used for the treatment of gonorrhea, its efficacy is less than that observed with quinolones or ceftriaxone Furthermore, the incidence of upper gastrointestinal side effects is increased with this dose. The spectrum of activity of erythromycin and the macrolides suggests that they might be useful for community-acquired pneumonia and that they can be used for mild to moderate cases that are appropriate for oral therapy; however, penicillin-resistant strains are often resistant to these agents as well. Weekly 1200 mg doses of azithromycin are effective in preventing *Mycobacterium avium* complex infections in HIV-positive patients and in doses of 500 mg daily may be effective in *M avium* complex pulmonary infections in non-HIV-positive patients. Azithromycin may be considered for therapy of dysentery caused by multidrug-resistant shigella. Used as prophylaxis, azithromycin (500 mg weekly) is as effective as benzathine penicillin in preventing upper respiratory tract infections in military recruits, and at a dose of 250 mg daily it is adequate as prophylaxis for malaria (though inferior to doxycycline for multidrug-resistant *P falciparum*). Clarithromycin has been used for the therapy of *M avium* complex infections, usually in combination with other drugs (eg, rifabutin and ethambutol), and can be given daily (500 mg twice daily) or three times weekly (1000 mg) as intermittent therapy. Clarithromycin (500 mg twice daily for 6 months) is very effective therapy for disseminated *Mycobacterium chelonei* infections and may be the drug of choice for use against this pathogen. Clarithromycin has also been used in combination regimens for the therapy of *Helicobacter pylori* infections. When clarithromycin is given with omeprazole and amoxicillin or metronidazole, cure rates in excess of 80–90% have been achieved.

Adverse effects of these agents are similar to those of erythromycin, but gastrointestinal upset, the major side effect, occurs about 50% less often with the azalides. Hepatic enzyme elevations, interstitial nephritis, headache, and dizziness have been reported rarely. Similar to erythromycin, azithromycin and clarithromycin have been associated with dose-dependent ototoxicity. Clarithromycin is similar to erythromycin in its effect on the cytochrome P450 system. Azithromycin appears to affect metabolism of other drugs only minimally.

Alvarez-Elcoro S et al: The macrolides: erythromycin, clarithromycin and azithromycin. Mayo Clin Proc 1999; 74:613. [NLM Cit ID: 99305702] (Review of spectrum of activity, clinical uses, and adverse effects.)

McConnell SA et al: Review and comparison of advanced-generation macrolides clarithromycin and dirithromycin. Pharmacotherapy 1999;18:404. [NLM Cit ID: 99226993]

TETRACYCLINE GROUP

The tetracyclines are a large group of drugs with common basic chemical structures, antimicrobial activity, and pharmacologic properties. Microorganisms resistant to this group show extensive cross-resistance to all tetracyclines.

Antimicrobial Activity

Tetracyclines are inhibitors of protein synthesis and are bacteriostatic for many gram-positive and gram-negative bacteria. They are strongly inhibitory for the growth of mycoplasmas, rickettsiae, chlamydiae, spirochetes, and some protozoa (eg, amebas). Their antipneumococcal activity approaches that of the macrolides; almost all *H influenzae* are inhibited. Tetracyclines also have moderate activity against some vancomycin-resistant enterococci. There are great differences in the susceptibility of different strains of a given species of microorganism. Because of the emergence of resistant strains—particularly gram-negative organisms—tetracyclines have lost most of their former usefulness. Proteus and pseudomonas are regularly resistant; bacteroides, streptococci, shigellae, and vibrios are increasingly so.

Pharmacokinetics & Administration

Tetracyclines are absorbed irregularly from the gastrointestinal tract. Absorption is impaired by dairy products, aluminum hydroxide gels (antacids), and chelation with divalent cations, eg, Ca^{2+} or Fe^{2+}. Absorption is moderate with tetracycline and highest with doxycycline and minocycline (95% or more). Tetracyclines are widely distributed, and low levels can be found in many tissues. Lipid solubility of minocycline and doxycycline probably accounts for their penetration into the cerebrospinal fluid, tears, and saliva.

The usual dosage of tetracyclines is 250–500 mg four times daily. Doxycycline and minocycline are given as 100 mg twice daily and demeclocycline and methacycline as 150 mg four times daily or 300 mg twice daily.

Tetracyclines are primarily metabolized in the liver and concentrated in bile. Excretion is mainly through bile and urine. All tetracyclines except doxycycline accumulate in renal insufficiency and are antianabolic in high doses. Doxycycline requires no dosage adjustment in renal failure; the other tetracyclines should be avoided or given in reduced dosage.

For patients unable to take oral medication, some tetracyclines (doxycycline, minocycline) are formulated for parenteral administration in doses similar to the oral ones. A 1% topical tetracycline ointment is available for conjunctival infections.

Clinical Uses

Tetracyclines are the drugs of choice for infections with chlamydiae, mycoplasmas, rickettsiae, ehrlichia, and vibrio and for some spirochetal infections. Sexually transmitted diseases in which chlamydiae often play a role—endocervicitis, urethritis, proctitis, and epididymitis—should be treated with a tetracycline for 7–14 days. Pelvic inflammatory disease is often treated with doxycycline plus cefoxitin or cefotetan. Other chlamydial infections (psittacosis, lymphogranuloma venereum, trachoma) and sexually transmitted diseases (granuloma inguinale) also respond to tetracyclines. Other uses include treatment of acne, respiratory infections, Lyme disease and relapsing fever, brucellosis, glanders, tularemia (often in combination with streptomycin), cholera, mycoplasmal pneumonia, actinomycosis, nocardiosis, malaria, infections caused by *M marinum* and *Pasteurella multocida* (often after an animal bite), and as malaria prophylaxis (including multidrug-resistant *P falciparum*). Tetracycline has also been used in combination with other drugs for amebiasis, falciparum malaria, and recurrent ulcers due to *H pylori.* Because of generally good activity against pneumococci, *Haemophilus influenzae,* chlamydia, legionella, and mycoplasma, doxycycline should be considered as empirical therapy for outpatient pneumonia.

Minocycline achieves a high concentration in the saliva and can be used for eradication of meningococci in carriers who cannot tolerate rifampin. Minocycline is equally as efficacious as doxycycline for the therapy of nongonococcal urethritis and cervicitis.

Adverse Effects

A. Allergy: Hypersensitivity reactions with fever or skin rashes are uncommon.

B. Gastrointestinal Side Effects: Gastrointestinal side effects, especially diarrhea, nausea, and anorexia, are common. These can be diminished by reducing the dose, but sometimes they force discontinuance of the drug.

C. Bones and Teeth: Tetracyclines are bound to calcium deposited in growing bones and teeth, causing fluorescence, discoloration, enamel dysplasia, deformity, or growth inhibition. Therefore, tetracyclines should not be given to pregnant women or children under 6 years of age.

D. Liver Damage: Tetracyclines can impair hepatic function or even cause liver necrosis, particularly during pregnancy or in the presence of preexisting liver damage.

E. Kidney Effects: Demeclocycline can cause nephrogenic diabetes insipidus and has been used therapeutically to treat inappropriate antidiuretic hormone secretion. Tetracyclines may increase blood urea nitrogen when diuretics are administered.

F. Other: Tetracyclines—principally demeclocycline—may induce photosensitization, especially in fair-skinned individuals. Minocycline induces vestibular reactions (dizziness, vertigo, nausea, vomiting), with a frequency of 35–70% after doses of 200 mg daily and has also been implicated as a cause of hypersensitivity pneumonitis.

Smilack JD: The tetracyclines. Mayo Clin Proc 1999; 74:727. [NLM Cit ID: 99334177] (Review of clinical indications and adverse effects.)

CHLORAMPHENICOL

Antimicrobial Activity

Chloramphenicol is active against certain rickettsiae. It binds to the 50S subunit of ribosomes and inhibits protein synthesis. It is bacteriostatic for most organisms but is often bactericidal for *S pneumoniae, H influenzae,* and *Neisseria meningitidis.* Of currently available agents, it is one of the few with any activity against some vancomycin-resistant enterococci.

Pharmacokinetics & Administration

For most systemic infections, chloramphenicol, 30 mg/kg/d, is given intravenously, but meningitis in adults may require 50 mg/kg/d in four divided doses. Since the intravenous preparation—chloramphenicol sodium succinate—must be hydrolyzed to active drug by nonspecific plasma esterases, it yields somewhat lower levels than the oral form.

Chloramphenicol is widely distributed in tissues, including the eye and central nervous system. Cerebrospinal fluid levels are 70–80% of peak serum levels, and the levels in brain tissue may even exceed those in serum.

Chloramphenicol is metabolized in the liver, and less than 10% is excreted unchanged in the urine. Thus, no dosage adjustment is needed in renal insufficiency. Patients with liver disease may accumulate the drug, and levels should be monitored.

Clinical Uses

Chloramphenicol is a possible choice in the following circumstances: (1) Meningococcal, *H influenzae,* or pneumococcal infections of the central nervous system in patients with a history of anaphylaxis to β-lactam drugs. (2) Anaerobic or mixed infections in the central nervous system, eg, brain abscess. (3) As an alternative to tetracyclines in rickettsial infections, especially in pregnant women in whom tetracycline is contraindicated. (4) For treatment of vancomycin-resistant enterococcal infections if susceptibility has been demonstrated.

Adverse Effects

Nausea, vomiting, and diarrhea occur infrequently. The most serious adverse effects pertain to the hematopoietic system. Adults taking chloramphenicol in excess of 50 mg/kg/d regularly exhibit disturbances in red cell maturation within 1–2 weeks. There is anemia, hyperferremia, reticulocytopenia, and the appearance of vacuolated nucleated red cells in the bone marrow. These changes regress when the drug is stopped and are not related to aplastic anemia. The latter is an irreversible consequence of chloramphenicol administration and represents a specific, probably genetically determined individual defect. It occurs in 1:40,000–1:25,000 courses of chloramphenicol treatment.

Chloramphenicol inhibits the metabolism of certain drugs. Thus, it may prolong the action and raise the blood concentration of tolbutamide, phenytoin, chlorpropamide, and warfarin sodium.

Chloramphenicol is specifically toxic for newborns, particularly premature infants. Because these patients lack the mechanism for detoxification of chloramphenicol in the liver, the drug may accumulate, producing the highly fatal "gray baby syndrome," with vomiting, flaccidity, hypothermia, and hypotension.

Kasten MJ: Clindamycin, metronidazole and chloramphenicol. Mayo Clin Proc 1999;74:825. [NLM Cit ID: 99400341] (Review of clinical uses and adverse effects.)

Lautenbach E et al: The role of chloramphenicol in the treatment of bloodstream infection due to vancomycin-resistant enterococcus. Clin Infect Dis 1998;27:1259. [NLM Cit ID: 99044529]

AMINOGLYCOSIDES

Aminoglycosides are a group of bactericidal drugs sharing chemical, antimicrobial, pharmacologic, and toxic characteristics. At present, the group includes streptomycin, neomycin, kanamycin, amikacin, gentamicin, tobramycin, sisomicin, netilmicin, paromomycin, and spectinomycin. All these agents inhibit protein synthesis in bacteria by attaching to and inhibiting the function of the 30S subunit of the bacterial ribosome. Resistance is based on (1) a deficiency of the ribosomal receptor (chromosomal mutant); (2) the enzymatic destruction of the drug (plasmid-mediated transmissible resistance of clinical importance) by acetylation, phosphorylation, or adenylylation; or (3) a lack of permeability to the drug molecule or failure of active transport across cell membranes. (This can be chromosomal, eg, streptococci are relatively impermeable to aminoglycosides; or plasmid-mediated, eg, in gram-negative enteric bacteria.) Anaerobic bacteria are resistant to aminoglycosides because transport across the cell membrane is an oxygen-dependent energy-requiring process.

All aminoglycosides are more active at alkaline than at acid pH. All are potentially ototoxic and nephrotoxic, though to different degrees. All can accumulate in renal insufficiency; therefore, dosage adjustments must be made in patients with renal dysfunction (see Table 37–8).

Because of their considerable toxicity and the availability of other antibiotics with broad spectrums of activity and fewer adverse effects (eg, third-generation cephalosporins, quinolones, imipenem, meropenem), aminoglycosides have been used less often in recent years. They are most commonly used to treat resistant gram-negative organisms that are sensitive only to aminoglycosides, or in low doses in combination with β-lactam drugs for their synergistic effect (eg, enterococci, penicillin-resistant viridans streptococci, right-sided *S aureus* endocarditis, *S aureus* and *S epidermidis* prosthetic valve infection). Although aminoglycosides demonstrate in vitro activity against many gram-positive bacteria, they should never be used alone to treat infections caused by these organisms—both because there is no clinical experience with the treatment of such infections and because less toxic alternatives are available.

General Properties of Aminoglycosides

Because of the similarities of the aminoglycosides, a summary of properties is presented briefly.

A. Absorption, Distribution, Metabolism, and Excretion: Aminoglycosides are well absorbed after intramuscular or intravenous injection, but they are not absorbed from the gastrointestinal tract. They are distributed widely in tissues and penetrate into pleural, peritoneal, and joint fluid in the presence of inflammation. They diffuse poorly into the eye, prostate, bile, central nervous system, and spinal fluid after parenteral injection.

There is no significant metabolic breakdown of aminoglycosides. The serum half-life is 2–3 hours in patients with normal renal function. Excretion is almost entirely by glomerular filtration. Urine levels usually are 10–50 times higher than serum levels. Aminoglycosides are removed fairly effectively by hemodialysis but irregularly by peritoneal dialysis. Continuous arteriovenous hemofiltration is associated with significant aminoglycoside clearance.

B. Dosage and Effect of Impaired Renal Function: In persons with normal renal function, the dosage of amikacin is 15 mg/kg/d in a single daily dose; that for gentamicin, tobramycin, or netilmicin is 5 mg/kg injected once daily. A single large daily dose of gentamicin, tobramycin, netilmicin, or amikacin is just as efficacious as—and no more nephrotoxic than—traditional dosing every 8–12 hours. Trough aminoglycoside levels should be undetectable in patients with normal body composition and renal function receiving once-daily dosing. Some clinicians recommend serum level monitoring 12–18 hours after the dose and extending the interval to every 48–72 hours for patients with elevated aminoglycoside levels. Others have suggested maintaining the dosage interval but decreasing the dose. Patients with renal failure, volume overload, or obesity have altered antibiotic clearance or volume of distribution. In patients with abnormal renal function or body composition, once-daily dosing is not recommended and aminoglycoside levels are recommended to guide dosing. In general, peak levels greater than 6 μg/mL are necessary for optimal outcome in the treatment of serious gram-negative infection, including pneumonia. Trough levels of more

Table 37–8. Dosing of aminoglycosides.[1]

	Creatinine Clearance				
	> 80	60–80	40–60	20–40	< 20
Gentamicin, tobramycin, netilmicin	5 mg/kg q24h	1.5–2.5 mg/kg q12h	1.2–1.5 mg/kg q24h	1.2–1.5 mg/kg q12–24h	2 mg/kg as loading dose and then 1–1.5 mg/kg q24–48h
Amikacin	15 mg/kg q24h	4.5–7.5 mg/kg q12h	3.5–4.5 mg/kg q12h	3.5–4.5 mg/kg q12–24h	7.5 mg/kg as loading dose and then 3–4.5 mg/kg q24–48h

[1]Additional dosing should be guided by serum level measurements (peaks 30 minutes after the end of intravenous infusion and troughs ≤ 30 minutes before the next dose). When a single large daily dose is given, peak levels are not required. Trough levels should be undetectable with high dose (5 mg/kg) once daily gentamicin or amikacin. For those patients with creatinine clearances less than 80 mL/min, the dosage ranges in the table are those used to treat gram-negative infections are intended to achieve, for gentamicin, tobramycin, and netilmicin, peak levels of 6–10 mg/L and trough levels of ≤ 2 mg/L; for amikacin, peak levels of 20–30 mg/L and trough levels of ≤ 5 mg/L.

than 2 μg/mL have been associated with an increased incidence of nephrotoxicity. In patients with normal body composition, once-daily dosing regimens as set forth in Table 37–8 should be followed. Reduced gentamicin doses (1 mg/kg every 8 hours) are recommended when used synergistically with β-lactams or vancomycin in the treatment of serious gram-positive infection (eg, enterococcal endocarditis).

C. Adverse Effects: All aminoglycosides can cause ototoxicity and nephrotoxicity. Ototoxicity is worrisome because it can be irreversible and is cumulative. Ototoxicity presents as hearing loss (cochlear damage), noted first with high-frequency tones, or as vestibular damage, manifested by vertigo and ataxia. Amikacin appears to be more ototoxic than gentamicin, tobramycin, or netilmicin. Nephrotoxicity, which is more frequent than ototoxicity, is accompanied by rising serum creatinine levels or reduced creatinine clearance. Nephrotoxicity is usually reversible and occurs with similar frequency with gentamicin, tobramycin, amikacin, and netilmicin.

In very high doses, particularly with irrigation of an inflamed peritoneum, aminoglycosides can be neurotoxic, producing a curare-like effect with neuromuscular blockade that results in respiratory paralysis. Calcium gluconate or neostigmine can serve as an antidote to this reaction.

1. STREPTOMYCIN

The usual dosage of streptomycin is 15–25 mg/kg/d (about 1 g/d) injected in one or two divided doses intramuscularly. Streptomycin exhibits all the adverse effects typically associated with the aminoglycosides; however, it has greater vestibular toxicity and probably less nephrotoxicity when compared with gentamicin.

Resistance emerges so rapidly and has become so widespread that only a few specific indications for this drug remain:

(1) Plague and tularemia.

(2) Endocarditis caused by *Enterococcus faecalis* or viridans streptococci (use in conjunction with penicillin or vancomycin) in strains that are susceptible to high levels of streptomycin (ie, ≤ 2000 μg/mL). Gentamicin is often substituted for streptomycin in this setting.

(3) Serious active tuberculosis when other less toxic drugs cannot be used.

(4) Acute brucellosis (in combination with tetracycline).

2. NEOMYCIN, KANAMYCIN, & PAROMOMYCIN

These aminoglycosides are closely related, with similar activity and complete cross-resistance. Systemic use has been abandoned because of oto- and nephrotoxicity.

Ointments containing 1–5 mg/g of neomycin, often combined with bacitracin and polymyxin, can be applied to infected superficial skin lesions. The drug mixture covers most staphylococci, streptococci, and gram-negative bacteria likely to be present, but the efficacy of topical application is questionable. Solutions of neomycin, 2.5–5 mg/mL, have been used for irrigation of infected joints or wounds. The total amount of drug must be kept below 15 mg/kg/d, since absorption may lead to systemic toxicity.

In preparation for elective bowel surgery, 1 g of neomycin is given orally every 6–8 hours for 1–2 days (often combined with erythromycin, 1 g) to reduce aerobic bowel flora. Action on gram-negative anaerobes is negligible. In hepatic coma, the coliform bacteria can be suppressed for prolonged periods by oral neomycin or kanamycin, 1 g every 6–8 hours, during reduced protein intake, resulting in diminished ammonia production.

In addition to oto- and nephrotoxicity, which can result from systemic absorption, neomycin or kanamycin can give rise to allergic reactions when applied topically to skin or eye. Respiratory arrest has followed the instillation of 3–5 g of kanamycin into the peritoneal cavity after colonic surgery; this is treated with neostigmine.

Paromomycin, closely related to neomycin and kanamycin, is poorly absorbed after oral administration and has been used mainly to treat asymptomatic intestinal amebiasis and in doses of 25–30 mg/kg/d in three divided doses for 7 days to treat giardiasis in pregnancy. A dosage of 500 mg orally three or four times daily is somewhat effective for cryptosporidiosis in AIDS.

3. AMIKACIN

Amikacin is a semisynthetic derivative of kanamycin. It is relatively resistant to several of the enzymes that inactivate gentamicin and tobramycin, and bacterial resistance is increasing only slowly. Many gram-negative enteric bacteria—including many strains of proteus, pseudomonas, enterobacter, and serratia—are inhibited. After injection of 500 mg of amikacin intramuscularly every 12 hours (15 mg/kg/d), peak levels in serum are 10–30 μg/mL. Some infections caused by Enterobacteriaceae resistant to gentamicin respond to amikacin. In addition to therapy for serious gram-negative infections, amikacin is often included with other drugs for therapy of *M avium* complex and *Mycobacterium fortuitum* complex.

Like all aminoglycosides, amikacin is nephrotoxic and ototoxic (particularly for the auditory portion of the eighth nerve). Its levels should be monitored in patients with renal failure.

4. GENTAMICIN

With doses of 5 mg/kg/d of this aminoglycoside, serum levels are sufficient for bactericidal effect against many strains of staphylococci, coliforms, and other gram-negative organisms. Enterococci are resistant unless a penicillin or vancomycin is also given. Gentamicin may be synergistic with penicillins active against pseudomonas, proteus, enterobacter, klebsiella, and other gram-negatives. Sisomicin resembles the C1a component of gentamicin.

Indications, Dosages, & Routes of Administration

Gentamicin is used in serious infections caused by gram-negative bacteria. Included are sepsis, infected burns, pneumonia, pyelonephritis, and other serious infections. The usual dosage is 5 mg/kg/d intravenously administered once daily. In endocarditis due to viridans streptococci or *E faecalis,* gentamicin in lower synergistic doses (3 mg/kg/d) is combined with penicillin or ampicillin. Historically, when used synergistically, gentamicin has been administered in three divided doses (ie, 1 mg/kg every 8 hours), but recent data suggest that a single daily dose of 3 mg/kg is equally as efficacious in the synergistic treatment of endocarditis due to viridans streptococci. In renal insufficiency, the dose should be adjusted as noted above. For infected burns or skin lesions, creams containing 0.1% gentamicin are used. Such topical use should be restricted to avoid favoring the development of resistant bacteria in hospitals.

5. TOBRAMYCIN

Tobramycin closely resembles gentamicin in antibacterial activity, toxicity, and pharmacologic properties and exhibits partial cross-resistance. Tobramycin may be effective against some gentamicin-resistant pseudomonads but is not used synergistically with penicillin for enterococcal endocarditis. Dosing is the same as for gentamicin. Tobramycin has also been given by aerosol (300 mg twice daily) to patients with cystic fibrosis. It was effective in improving pulmonary function and decreasing colonization with pseudomonas without toxicity and without selecting for resistant strains.

Netilmicin shares many characteristics with gentamicin and tobramycin and can be given in a similar dosage. It may be less ototoxic and less nephrotoxic than the other aminoglycosides.

6. SPECTINOMYCIN

Spectinomycin is an aminocyclitol antibiotic (related to aminoglycosides) for intramuscular administration. Its sole application is in the treatment of uncomplicated urogenital and anorectal gonorrhea in persons who are hypersensitive to penicillin and who cannot tolerate fluoroquinolones. It is not effective for pharyngeal gonorrhea. One injection of 2 g (40 mg/kg) is given. About 5–10% of gonococci are probably resistant. There is usually pain at the injection site, and there may be nausea and fever.

Ali MZ et al: A meta-analysis of the relative efficacy and toxicity of single daily dosing versus multiple daily dosing of aminoglycosides. Clin Inf Dis 1997;24:796. [NLM Cit ID: 97287644]

Edson RS et al: The aminoglycosides. Mayo Clin Proc 1999;74:519. [NLM Cit ID: 99252664]

Mingeot-Leclercq MP et al: Aminoglycosides: activity and resistance. Antimicrob Ag Chemother 1999;43:727. [NLM Cit ID: 99216878]

POLYMYXINS

The polymyxins are basic polypeptides that are bactericidal for most gram-negative aerobic rods, including pseudomonas. Because of poor distribution into tissues and substantial toxicity (primarily nephrotoxicity and ototoxicity), systemic use of these agents is limited to infections caused by multidrug-resistant gram-negative organisms that are sensitive only to the polymyxins. Polymyxins B and E (colistin) are the only parenteral agents available. Polymyxin B can be given intravenously in a dose of 1.5–2.5 mg/kg/d in four divided doses or intramuscularly in a dose of 2.5–3 mg/kg/d. Colistin is given intramuscularly or intravenously in a dosage of 2.5–5 mg/kg/d in two divided doses. Dosage adjustments are required with renal insufficiency.

Topical preparations are used more commonly but with unproved efficacy. Solutions of polymyxin B sulfate, 1 mg/mL, can be applied to infected surfaces; injected into joint spaces, the pleural cavity, or subconjunctivally; or inhaled as aerosols. Ointments containing 0.5 mg/g of polymyxin B sulfate in a mixture with neomycin or bacitracin (or both) are often applied to superficial infected skin lesions. Polymyxins are inactivated by purulent exudates. They rarely cause local sensitization.

ANTITUBERCULOUS DRUGS

Singular problems exist in the treatment of tuberculosis and other mycobacterial infections. The organisms are intracellular, have long periods of metabolic inactivity, and tend to develop resistance to any one drug. Therefore, combined drug therapy is employed to delay the emergence of this resistance. First-line drugs, increasingly used together in all tuberculosis, are isoniazid, ethambutol, rifampin, and pyrazinamide.

1. ISONIAZID

Isoniazid is the hydrazide of isonicotinic acid (INH), the most active antituberculosis drug. However, some atypical mycobacteria as well as some strains of *M tuberculosis* are resistant. In susceptible large populations of *M tuberculosis,* isoniazid-resistant mutants occur at a rate of one in 10^6 organisms, and emergence of resistance is delayed in the presence of a second drug. There is no cross-resistance between isoniazid and other antituberculosis drugs.

Isoniazid is well absorbed from the gastrointestinal tract and diffuses readily into all tissues, including the central nervous system. The inactivation of isoniazid—particularly its acetylation—is under genetic control. However, the speed of isoniazid acetylation has little influence over the selection of drug regimens. Isoniazid and its conjugates are excreted mainly in the urine.

Indications, Dosages, & Routes of Administration

Isoniazid should not be given as the sole drug in active tuberculosis, because resistant organisms will emerge, but it is used alone for prophylaxis (see Chapter 9). The usual oral adult dose is 300 mg/d. In directly observed therapy, it can be given twice weekly in a dosage of 15 mg/kg/dose (maximum, 900 mg/dose). In addition to capsules, a solution for parenteral injection is available.

Toxic reactions to isoniazid include insomnia, restlessness, fever, myalgia, hyperreflexia, and even convulsions and psychotic episodes. Some of these are attributable to a relative pyridoxine deficiency and along with peripheral neuropathy can be prevented by the administration of pyridoxine, 25–50 mg/d. Isoniazid causes hepatitis. Progressive liver damage occurs rarely in patients under age 20; in 1.5% of persons between 30 and 50 years of age; and in 2.5% of older individuals. The risk of hepatitis is greater in alcoholics. Mild elevations (two to three times normal) of aminotransferases are common, occurring in 10–20% of patients taking isoniazid. If they are elevated more than three to five times normal or if hepatitis occurs, the drug should be discontinued. Isoniazid can reduce the metabolism of phenytoin, increasing its blood level and toxicity.

Nolan CM et al: Hepatotoxicity associated with isoniazid preventive therapy: a 7-year survey from a public health tuberculosis clinic. JAMA 1999;281:1014. [NLM Cit ID: 99184240]

2. ETHAMBUTOL

Ethambutol is a synthetic, water-soluble, heat-stable compound, dispensed as the hydrochloride.

Many strains of *M tuberculosis* and of "atypical" mycobacteria are inhibited in vitro by ethambutol. The mechanism of action is not known.

Ethambutol is well absorbed from the gastrointestinal tract. About 20% of the drug is excreted in feces and 50% in the urine, in unchanged form. Excretion is delayed and dosage adjustment is required in renal insufficiency. Ethambutol penetrates the cerebrospinal fluid sufficiently to be used in the treatment of meningitis.

Resistance to ethambutol emerges fairly rapidly among mycobacteria when the drug is used alone. Therefore, ethambutol, 15 mg/kg, is given as a single daily dose in combination with other antituberculosis drugs.

Hypersensitivity to ethambutol is uncommon. It may cause a rise in the serum uric acid. The commonest side effects are visual disturbances: Reduction in visual acuity, optic neuritis, and perhaps retinal damage occur in some patients receiving ethambutol, 25 mg/kg/d for several months. Most changes are reversible, but periodic visual acuity testing is mandatory when doses above 15 mg/kg/d are used. At lower doses, side effects are rare.

3. RIFAMPIN, RIFABUTIN, & RIFAPENTINE

Rifampin is a semisynthetic derivative of rifamycin that inhibits many gram-positive cocci, meningococci, and mycobacteria in vitro. Gram-negative organisms are often more resistant. Highly resistant mutants occur frequently in susceptible microbial populations (one in 10^6–10^8 bacteria).

Rifampin binds strongly to DNA-dependent bacterial RNA polymerase and thus inhibits RNA synthesis in bacteria. Rifampin penetrates well into phagocytic cells and can kill intracellular organisms.

Rifampin given orally is well absorbed and widely distributed in tissues, including the central nervous system. Levels in cerebrospinal fluid are 50% of those in serum. The drug is excreted mainly through the liver and thus no adjustment is needed in renal insufficiency. A solution for intravenous administration is available.

In the treatment of tuberculosis, a single oral dose of 600 mg (10–20 mg/kg) is given daily or, in directly observed therapy, 600 mg twice weekly. In order to delay the rapid emergence of resistant microorganisms, combined treatment with other antituberculous drugs is required. Rifampin is effective for treatment of leprosy (see below), and 600 mg twice daily for 2 days can terminate the meningococcal carrier state; rifampin-resistant strains emerge in 10% of subjects. Close contacts of children with *H influenzae* infection (eg, in the family or in day care centers) can receive rifampin, 20 mg/kg/d for 4 days, as prophylaxis. Rifampin combined with trimethoprim-sulfamethoxazole can eradicate staphylococcal carriage in the nasopharynx. Combination of rifampin with either penicillin or clindamycin is effective in eradication of group A β-hemolytic streptococci from the pharynx of chronic carriers. Synergistic action of rifampin with nafcillin and vancomycin against staphylococci in vitro is of uncertain clinical significance. However, in patients with *S aureus* or *S epidermidis* prosthetic valve endocarditis, rifampin at a dose of 300 mg every 8 hours for 6 weeks is recommended along with nafcillin or vancomycin for 6 weeks and gentamicin for 2 weeks. Ciprofloxacin in combination with rifampin has been associated with favorable outcomes in the treatment of orthopedic implant-related staphylococcal infections. With the exception of prophylaxis, rifampin should never be used alone.

Rifampin imparts an orange color to urine, sweat, and contact lenses. Occasional adverse effects include rashes, thrombocytopenia, impaired liver function, light-chain proteinuria, and rare, mild impairment of immune response. In intermittent administration, rifampin must be given at least twice weekly to avoid a "flu syndrome" and anemia. Rifampin increases the metabolism of oral anticoagulants and contraceptives and lowers serum levels of methadone, ketoconazole, chloramphenicol, oral hypoglycemic drugs, some antiarrhythmic agents, and cyclosporine.

Rifabutin is structurally similar to rifampin but is slightly more active against *M avium* complex. In a dose of 300 mg/d, it is effective for prophylaxis against *M avium* complex in HIV-infected patients with CD4 counts less than 100/μL. Once weekly azithromycin is as efficacious as rifabutin in the prevention of *M avium* complex infection. When rifabutin is used as part of a multidrug regimen to treat *M avium* complex pulmonary infections, adverse effects (leukopenia, nausea, vomiting, polyarthralgia, uveitis) occur commonly—particular when clarithromycin is in the regimen; in such circumstances, doses of rifabutin should not exceed 300 mg/d. When compared with rifabutin, rifampin is a more potent inducer of cytochrome P450. Uveitis can also occur with rifabutin.

Rifapentine is similar to rifampin in adverse effects and drug interactions. However, owing to its long half-life, it can be administered less frequently. Rifapentine is given twice-weekly for 2 months and then once-weekly for 4 months. Its use is limited to the therapy of tuberculosis, and it is always given in combination with other active drugs against *M tuberculosis.*

4. STREPTOMYCIN

The general pharmacologic features and toxicity of streptomycin are described above in the section on aminoglycosides. Streptomycin is inhibitory and bactericidal for most tubercle bacilli, whereas most atypical mycobacteria are resistant. All large populations of tubercle bacilli contain some streptomycin-resistant mutants. Therefore, streptomycin is employed only in combination with other antituberculosis drugs.

Streptomycin penetrates poorly into cells and exerts its action mainly on extracellular organisms. Since at any moment 90% of tubercle bacilli are intracellular and thus unaffected by streptomycin, treatment for many months is required.

For combination therapy in tuberculous meningitis, miliary dissemination, and severe organ tuberculosis, streptomycin is given intramuscularly, 0.5–1 g daily (30 mg/kg/d for children) for weeks or months. This is followed by streptomycin, 1 g intramuscularly two or three times a week for months.

Prolonged streptomycin treatment may impair eighth nerve function. A total cumulative dose of 120 g should not be exceeded, and the drug should be used with caution in persons over 60 years of age since they are more prone to oto- and nephrotoxicity.

5. PYRAZINAMIDE

Pyrazinamide is bactericidal for most *M tuberculosis* strains and also for many "atypical" mycobacteria. It is well absorbed after oral administration and is widely distributed in tissues. It penetrates well into the cerebrospinal fluid and achieves levels equal to those in serum. The usual oral dose is 20–30 mg/kg (1.5–2 g) given once daily. In directly observed therapy regimens, 50 mg/kg (not to exceed 3 g) can be given twice weekly. Pyrazinamide is commonly used in the therapy of tuberculosis because of its demonstrated efficacy in short-course therapy regimens.

When pyrazinamide is used at recommended doses of 20–30 mg/kg/d, the drug is well tolerated. When higher doses are given, hepatic toxicity can be seen in up to 5% of patients. Nausea, vomiting, drug fever, and hyperuricemia can occur.

6. FIXED-DOSE COMBINATIONS

Two fixed-dose combinations are available in the United States. **Rifamate** contains rifampin 300 mg and isoniazid 150 mg. The usual adult dose is two tablets each day. **Rifater** contains a combination of rifampin 120 mg, isoniazid 50 mg, and pyrazinamide 300 mg. Dosage varies by weight (ie, four tablets for those weighing < 44 kg, five tablets for those weighing 45–54 kg, and six tablets for those weighing > 55 kg). These combinations prevent selecting for resistance, which may occur with monotherapy. Such combinations are rational and should be encouraged.

7. ALTERNATIVE DRUGS IN TUBERCULOSIS TREATMENT

The drugs listed alphabetically below are usually considered only in cases of drug resistance (clinical or laboratory) to first-line drugs.

Aminosalicylic acid (PAS), closely related to *p*-aminobenzoic acid, inhibits most tubercle bacilli but has no effect on other bacteria.

Aminosalicylic acid is readily absorbed from the gastrointestinal tract, and the usual dosage is 8–12 g/d orally. The drug is widely distributed in tissues (except the central nervous system) and rapidly excreted into the urine.

Common side effects include anorexia, nausea, diarrhea, and epigastric pain. Sodium aminosalicylate may be given parenterally. Hypersensitivity reactions include fever, skin rashes, granulocytopenia, lymphadenopathy, and arthralgias.

Clofazimine is a phenazine dye used in the treatment of leprosy and is active in vitro against *M avium* complex and *M tuberculosis.* It is given orally as a single daily dose of 100 mg for treatment of *M avium* complex disease. Its clinical efficacy for the therapy of tuberculosis has not been established. Adverse effects include nausea, vomiting, abdominal pain, and skin discoloration from red-brown to black.

Capreomycin is an injectable agent given intramuscularly in doses of 15–30 mg/kg/d (maximal dose 1 g). Major toxicities include ototoxicity (both vestibular and cochlear) and nephrotoxicity. If the drug must be used in older patients, the dose should not exceed 750 mg.

Cycloserine, a bacteriostatic agent, is given in doses of 15–20 mg/kg (not to exceed 1 g) orally and has been used in re-treatment regimens and for primary therapy of highly resistant *M tuberculosis.* It can induce a variety of central nervous system dysfunctions and psychotic reactions. These may be controlled by phenytoin, 100 mg/d orally, or pyridoxine, 50–100 mg daily.

Ethionamide, like cycloserine, is bacteriostatic and is given orally in a dose of 15–20 mg/kg (maximal dose 1 g). It has been used in combination therapy but produces marked gastric irritation and is the least well tolerated antimycobacterial agent.

The **fluoroquinolones** ofloxacin, ciprofloxacin, and sparfloxacin are active in vitro against *M tuberculosis,* with MICs of 0.25–2 μg/mL. Limited data suggest that these drugs are efficacious in therapy of tuberculosis, particularly in re-treatment regimens. In re-treatment schedules or for infection with resistant organisms, high doses should be used (ciprofloxacin, 750 mg orally twice daily; ofloxacin, 400 mg orally twice daily).

Telenti A et al: Drug-resistant tuberculosis: What do we do now? Drugs 2000;59:171. [NLM Cit ID: 20192786]

Van Scoy RE et al: Antimycobacterial therapy. Mayo Clin Proc 1999;74:1038.

SULFONAMIDES & ANTIFOLATE DRUGS

More than 150 different sulfonamides have been marketed at one time or another, the modifications being designed principally to achieve greater antibacterial activity, a wider antibacterial spectrum, greater solubility, or more prolonged action. Because of their low cost and relative efficacy in many infections, sulfonamides are still used widely.

Antimicrobial Activity

Sulfonamides are structural analogs of *p*-aminobenzoic acid (PABA) and compete with PABA to block its conversion to dihydrofolic acid. Organisms that utilize PABA in the synthesis of folates and pyrimidines are inhibited. Animal cells and some resistant microorganisms use exogenous folate and thus are not affected by sulfonamides.

Trimethoprim, pyrimethamine, and trimetrexate are compounds that inhibit the conversion of dihydrofolic acid to tetrahydrofolic acid by blocking the enzyme dihydrofolate reductase. These agents have been used alone or (more commonly) in combination with other drugs (usually sulfonamides) to prevent or treat a number of bacterial and parasitic infections. Trimetrexate is the most potent agent and is about 1500 times more active than trimethoprim. At high doses, all can inhibit mammalian dihydrofolate reductase, but clinically this is a problem only with pyrimethamine and trimetrexate. Folinic acid (leucovorin) is given concurrently with pyrimethamine and trimetrexate to prevent bone marrow suppression.

Sulfonamides inhibit many gram-positive (including nocardia) and gram-negative organisms. Emerging resistance, particularly among pneumococci, gonococci, meningococci, and enteric gram-negative organisms, has limited their use. Sulfonamides are also active against some strains of chlamydia and such organisms as toxoplasma, plasmodium, and *Pneumocystis carinii.*

The combination of trimethoprim (TMP) (one part) plus sulfamethoxazole (SMZ) (five parts) is bactericidal for such gram-negative organisms as *E coli,* klebsiella, enterobacter, salmonella, and shigella, though resistance has emerged. It is also active against many strains of serratia, providencia, *Stenotrophomonas maltophilia, Burkholderia cepacia* (formerly *Pseudomonas cepacia*), and *P pseudomallei,* but not against *P aeruginosa.* It is inactive against anaerobes and enterococci but inhibits *S aureus* and about 50% *S epidermidis. M catarrhalis, H influenzae, H ducreyi, L monocytogenes,* and some atypical mycobacteria, eg, *M marinum, M kansasii,* and *M scrofulaceum,* are also inhibited by this combination.

Pharmacokinetics & Administration

Trimethoprim-sulfamethoxazole is well absorbed from the gastrointestinal tract and widely distributed in tissues. For patients who are unable to take oral drugs, intravenous trimethoprim-sulfamethoxazole is available. Each vial contains 80 mg TMP + 400 mg SMZ in a volume of 5 mL, which must be diluted in 125 mL of 5% dextrose in water. For many bacterial infections, the dose is 10 mg TMP + 50 mg SMZ/kg/d in two doses; for pneumocystis infections, 15–20 mg TMP + 75–100 mg SMZ/kg/d is given in three or four doses. Dosage adjustment is required for significant renal impairment (creatine clearance ≤ 50 mL/min).

Topical uses of sulfonamides include the application of sodium sulfacetamide solution (30%) or ointment (10%) to the conjunctiva and mafenide acetate cream or silver sulfadiazine to burn wounds.

Clinical Uses

Present indications for sulfonamides include the following.

A. Urinary Tract Infections: Coliform bacteria, the commonest cause of urinary tract infections, generally remain susceptible to sulfonamides. Short-course therapy (3 days) with double-strength TMP-SMZ (160 mg TMP + 800 mg SMZ) given twice daily is effective therapy for lower urinary tract infections in women who are symptomatic for less than a week. Since TMP is concentrated in the prostate, TMP-SMZ, one double-strength tablet twice daily for 14–21 days, is effective in acute prostatitis. In chronic prostatitis, treatment for 6–12 weeks is indicated. *E coli,* the most common urinary pathogen, has become progressively more resistant to TMP-SMZ over the years. Considering this trend, the routine use of TMP-SMZ for empirical therapy of urinary tract infections has been questioned. In those areas where resistance of *E coli* is greater than 20%, alternative agents should be used as empirical therapy.

B. Parasitic Infections: TMP-SMZ is effective for prophylaxis and treatment of pneumocystis pneumonia, cyclospora infection, and *Isospora belli* infection. For therapy of pneumocystis pneumonia, 15–20 mg/kg/d of trimethoprim and 75–100 mg/kg/d of sulfamethoxazole in three or four divided doses is administered intravenously or orally—depending upon the severity of disease—for 3 weeks. The dose for prophylaxis is 160 mg TMP + 800 mg SMZ daily or three times per week. (When given daily, it is also effective prophylaxis against toxoplasmal encephalitis.) *I belli* infection in AIDS has been successfully treated with 160 mg TMP + 800 mg SMZ orally four times daily for 10 days followed by twice-daily administration for 3 weeks. Treatment with 160 mg TMP + 800 mg SMZ three times a week or 500 mg sulfadoxine with 25 mg pyrimethamine once a week has prevented recurrences. Cyclosporiasis is successfully treated with 160 mg TMP and 800 mg SMZ twice daily for 7–10 days. Sulfadiazine with pyrimethamine is also used to treat and prevent recurrence of toxoplasmosis and sulfadoxine plus pyrimethamine is used to treat chloroquine-resistant falciparum malaria.

C. Bacterial Infections: Sulfonamides are the drugs of choice for nocardia infections. TMP-SMZ is widely distributed in tissues, penetrates into the cerebrospinal fluid and has been used to treat meningitis caused by gram-negative rods, though third-generation cephalosporins are now preferred. TMP-SMZ is a frequent choice for management of acute sinusitis, otitis media, and infection with susceptible strains of shigella. The usual dose for adults is 160 mg TMP + 800 mg SMZ twice daily for 10 days.

TMP-SMZ is effective also for infections with enterobacter, *Pseudomonas pseudomallei* (melioidosis), *Stenotrophomonas maltophilia,* or *Burkholderia cepacia;* in combination with rifampin, for eradication of nasopharyngeal carriage of staphylococci; for prophylaxis against meningococcal disease when susceptible strains predominate; for antibacterial prophylaxis in organ transplant recipients or patients with chronic granulomatous disease; for treatment of *Listeria monocytogenes* meningitis; and perhaps also for management of Wegener's granulomatosis.

D. Leprosy: Certain sulfones are widely used (see below).

Adverse Effects

Adverse reactions to sulfonamides occur in 10–15% of non-AIDS patients (usually a minor rash or gastrointestinal disturbance) and in up to 50% of patients with AIDS (predominantly rash, fever, neutropenia, and thrombocytopenia, often severe enough to require discontinuation of therapy). These drugs are capable of producing a wide variety of side effects—due partly to hypersensitivity, partly to direct toxicity—that must be considered whenever unexplained symptoms or signs occur in a patient who may have received these drugs.

A. Systemic Side Effects: Fever, skin rashes, urticaria; nausea, vomiting, or diarrhea; stomatitis, conjunctivitis, arthritis, aseptic meningitis, exfoliative dermatitis; bone marrow depression, thrombocytopenia, hemolytic (in G6PD deficiency) or aplastic anemia, granulocytopenia, leukemoid reactions; hepatitis, polyarteritis nodosa, vasculitis, Stevens-Johnson syndrome; reversible hyperkalemia; and many others.

HIV-positive patients intolerant to TMP-SMZ can often be desensitized. A 70% success rate has been reported after giving 0.004 mg TMP/0.02 mg SMZ as oral suspension and increasing the dose tenfold each hour to achieve a final dose of 160 mg TMP/500 mg SMZ.

B. Urinary Tract Disturbances: Older sulfonamides were relatively insoluble and would precipitate in urine. The most commonly used sulfonamides presently (sulfisoxazole and sulfamethoxazole) are quite soluble, and the old admonition to force fluids is no longer warranted. Sulfonamides have been implicated in interstitial nephritis. HIV-positive patients receiving high-dose sulfadiazine therapy are predisposed to crystalluria.

SULFONES USED IN THE TREATMENT OF LEPROSY

A number of drugs closely related to the sulfonamides (eg, dapsone; diaminodiphenylsulfone, DDS) have been used effectively in the long-term treatment of leprosy. The clinical manifestations of both lepromatous and tuberculoid leprosy can often be suppressed by treatment extending over several years. At least 5–30% of *Mycobacterium leprae* organisms are resistant to dapsone, so initial combined treatment with rifampin is advocated. Dapsone, 100 mg daily, is effective therapy for mild to moderate pneumocystis pneumonia in AIDS when combined with trimethoprim, 20 mg/kg/d in four divided doses. At a dose of 50–100 mg daily or 100 mg two or three times a week, it is effective prophylaxis for *P carinii* infection and, when combined with pyrimethamine, 50 mg per week, also prevents toxoplasma encephalitis in HIV-infected patients.

Absorption, Metabolism, & Excretion

All sulfones are well absorbed from the intestinal tract, are distributed widely in all tissues, and tend to be retained in skin, muscle, liver, and kidney. Skin involved by leprosy contains ten times more drug than normal skin. Sulfones are excreted into the bile and reabsorbed by the intestine. Consequently, blood levels are prolonged. Excretion into the urine is variable, and the drug occurs in urine mostly as a glucuronic acid conjugate. Some persons acetylate sulfones slowly and others rapidly; this requires dosage adjustment.

Dosages & Routes of Administration

See Leprosy, Chapter 35, for recommendations.

Adverse Effects

The sulfones may cause any of the side effects listed above for sulfonamides. Anorexia, nausea, and vomiting are common. Hemolysis, methemoglobinemia, or agranulocytosis may occur. G6PD levels should be determined prior to initiation of dapsone therapy. If sulfones are not tolerated, clofazimine can be substituted.

SPECIALIZED DRUGS USED AGAINST BACTERIA

1. BACITRACIN

This polypeptide is selectively active against gram-positive bacteria. Because of severe nephrotoxicity upon systemic administration, its use has been limited to topical application on surface lesions, usually in combination with polymyxin or neomycin. Occasionally it is given orally for pseudomembranous colitis caused by toxin-producing *C difficile;* however, it is inferior to oral vancomycin or metronidazole.

2. MUPIROCIN

Mupirocin (formerly pseudomonic acid) is a naturally occurring antibiotic produced by *Pseudomonas fluorescens* that is active against most gram-positive cocci, including methicillin-sensitive and methicillin-resistant *S aureus* and most streptococci (but not enterococci). It is used topically. It is effective in eliminating staphylococcal nasal carriage in the majority of patients for up to 3 months after application to the anterior nares twice daily for 5 days. However, recurrent colonization can occur (53% are recolonized at the end of 1 year) and when mupirocin is used chronically over months, resistant organisms can emerge. Monthly application for 5 days each month for up to a year decreases staphylococcal colonization, which in turn lowers the risk of recurrent staphylococcal skin infections. Whether it is more effective than trimethoprim-sulfamethoxazole or dicloxacillin plus rifampin for eradication of staphylococcal nasal carriage is unknown. The other major use of mupirocin is for therapy of impetigo; it is useful in mild disease.

3. CLINDAMYCIN

Clindamycin resembles erythromycin (though different in structure) and is active against gram-positive organisms including *S pneumoniae,* viridans streptococci, group A streptococci, and *S aureus,* though resistance has been described in all of these organisms. Enterococci, methicillin-resistant *S aureus,* and most *S epidermidis* isolates are resistant. A dosage of 0.15–0.3 g orally every 6 hours generally is used. It is widely distributed in tissues but not in cerebrospinal fluid. Excretion is primarily nonrenal. Clindamycin is an alternative to erythromycin as a substitute for penicillin. Clindamycin is currently recommended as an alternative drug for prophylaxis against endocarditis following oral procedures in patients allergic to amoxicillin. Clindamycin, 300 mg orally twice daily for 7 days, can be used as an alternative to metronidazole for the therapy of bacterial vaginosis. Topical application of a 2% vaginal cream once or twice daily for 7 days is also effective. Clindamycin is active against most anaerobes, including bacteroides, prevotella, clostridium, peptococcus, peptostreptococcus, and fusobacterium. However, resistance has been described in 10–20% of these isolates, and alternative agents should be considered for serious life-threatening anaerobic infections due to these organisms. It is frequently used to treat less severe infections in which anaerobes are significant pathogens (eg, aspiration pneumonia, pelvic and abdominal infections), often in combination with other drugs (aminoglycosides, cephalosporins, aztreonam). In patients with necrotizing pneumonia or lung abscess following aspiration, clindamycin appears to be superior to penicillin. Seriously ill patients are given clindamycin, 600–900 mg (20–30 mg/kg/d) intravenously every 8 hours. Success has also been reported in staphylococcal osteomyelitis. Because tissue models document that clindamycin significantly decreases toxin production of a number of organisms, the addition of clindamycin to penicillin for therapy of group A streptococcus toxic shock syndrome has been suggested. In the sulfonamide-allergic patient, high-dose clindamycin therapy (600–1200 mg intravenously every 6 hours or 600 mg orally every 6 hours) in conjunction with pyrimethamine has been used to treat toxoplasmosis of the central nervous system and appears to be as effective as pyrimethamine and sulfadiazine. Clindamycin in combination with primaquine has been reported to be effective in the therapy of pneumocystis pneumonia in patients with AIDS, and clindamycin with quinine is effective therapy for falciparum malaria. These drugs are ineffective in meningitis.

Common side effects are diarrhea, nausea, and skin rashes. Bloody diarrhea with pseudomembranous colitis has been associated with the administration of clindamycin and other antibiotics. This antibiotic-associated colitis is due to a necrotizing toxin produced by *C difficile*. The organism is resistant to the antimicrobial, is selected out by its presence, and is favored in its growth and toxin production. *C difficile* is usually susceptible to—and can be treated with—vancomycin or metronidazole given orally, though metronidazole is the drug of choice (see below).

4. METRONIDAZOLE

Metronidazole is an antiprotozoal drug (see Chapter 35) that also has striking antibacterial effects against most anaerobic gram-negative bacilli (bacteroides, prevotella, fusobacterium) and clostridium species but has minimal activity against other anaerobic gram-positive and microaerophilic organisms. It is well absorbed after oral administration, and is widely distributed in tissues. It penetrates well into the cerebrospinal fluid, yielding levels similar to those in serum. The drug is metabolized in the liver, and dosage reduction is required in severe hepatic insufficiency or biliary dysfunction.

Metronidazole is employed in amebiasis and giardiasis (see Chapter 35) and in the following circumstances:

(1) Trichomonas vaginitis responds to either a single dose (2 g) or to 250 mg orally three times daily for 7–10 days. Bacterial vaginosis responds to a single 2 g dose or to 500 mg twice daily for 7 days. Metronidazole vaginal cream (0.75%) applied twice daily for 5 days is also effective.

(2) In anaerobic infections, metronidazole can be given orally or intravenously, 500 mg three times daily (30 mg/kg/d). It is more predictable against *B fragilis* than clindamycin or second-generation cephalosporins with anaerobic activity.

(3) Metronidazole is less expensive and equally as efficacious as oral vancomycin for the therapy of *C difficile* colitis and is the drug of choice for the disease. A dosage of 500 mg orally three times daily is recommended. If oral medication cannot be tolerated, intravenous metronidazole can be tried at the same dose; however, this route is unproved and may be less effective than the oral one. Because of the emergence of vancomycin-resistant enterococci as a major pathogen and the role of oral vancomycin in selecting for these resistant organisms, metronidazole should always be used as first-line therapy for *C difficile* disease.

(4) Preparation of the colon before bowel surgery.

(5) Therapy of brain abscess, often in combination with penicillin or a third-generation cephalosporin.

(6) In combination with clarithromycin and omeprazole for therapy of some *H pylori* infections.

Adverse effects include stomatitis, nausea, and diarrhea. Ingestion of alcohol while taking metronidazole can result in a disulfiram reaction. With prolonged use at high doses, reversible peripheral neuropathy can develop. Metronidazole can decrease the metabolism of warfarin and increase the prothrombin time, necessitating careful monitoring of the prothrombin time and dosage adjustment of warfarin when both drugs are used together. Metronidazole has been shown to be carcinogenic in certain animal models and mutagenic for certain bacteria. To date, human studies have not confirmed an increased incidence of malignancy.

Kasten MJ: Clindamycin, metronidazole, and chloramphenicol. Mayo Clin Proc 1999;74:825. [NLM Cit ID: 99400341] (Clinical review.)

Smilack JD: Trimethoprim-sulfamethoxazole. Mayo Clin Proc 1999;74:730. [NLM Cit ID: 99334178] (Review of clinical indications and adverse effects.)

5. VANCOMYCIN

This drug is bactericidal for most gram-positive organisms, particularly staphylococci and streptococci, and is bacteriostatic for most enterococci. While active against staphylococci, vancomycin kills more slowly when compared with nafcillin. Although vancomycin has retained activity against staphylococci and streptococci, vancomycin-resistant strains of enterococci (particularly *Enterococcus faecium*) have become a major problem. *Staphylococcus aureus* only intermediately sensitive to the drug has been observed in patients receiving long-term vancomycin therapy. Vancomycin is not absorbed from the gastrointestinal tract. It is given orally only for the treatment of antibiotic-associated enterocolitis. For systemic effect the drug must be administered intravenously (20–30 mg/kg/d in two or three divided doses). An intravenous injection of 10 mg/kg over a period of 20 minutes yields blood levels of 20–30 μg/mL. Vancomycin is excreted mainly via the kidneys. In renal insufficiency, the half-life may be up to 8 days. Thus, only one dose of 0.5–1 g may be given every 4–8 days to a uremic individual undergoing chronic hemodialysis. Patients receiving continuous arteriovenous hemofiltration (CAVH) require more frequent maintenance dosing. In patients with impaired renal function, the dosing interval is determined by measuring serum levels. When levels decline to 5–15 μg/mL, repeat dosing is required to maintain therapeutic levels.

Indications for parenteral vancomycin include the following: (1) Severe staphylococcal infections in penicillin-allergic patients; it is the drug of choice for methicillin-resistant *S aureus* and *S epidermidis* infections and for serious infections (pneumonia, meningitis) due to highly resistant *S pneumoniae.* (2) Severe enterococcal infections in the penicillin-allergic patient, usually in combination with an aminoglycoside. (3) Other gram-positive infections in penicillin-allergic patients, eg, viridans streptococcal endocarditis. (4) Surgical prophylaxis in penicillin-allergic patients. (5) For gram-positive infections due to organisms that are multidrug-resistant, ie, *Corynebacterium jeikeium.* (6) Endocarditis prophylaxis in the penicillin-allergic patient undergoing certain genitourinary and gastrointestinal procedures (in combination with an aminoglycoside). (See Table 33–3.)

In antibiotic-associated enterocolitis, vancomycin, 0.125 g, is given orally four times daily.

Vancomycin is irritating to tissues; thrombophlebitis sometimes follows intravenous injection. The drug is infrequently ototoxic and potentially nephrotoxic when administered with aminoglycosides. Rapid infusion or high doses (1 g or more) may induce diffuse hyperemia ("red man syndrome") and can be avoided by extending infusions over 1–2 hours or by pretreating with a histamine antagonist such as hydroxyzine.

Smith TL et al: Emergence of vancomycin resistance in *Staphylococcus aureus.* Glycopeptide-Intermediate *Staphylococcus aureus* Working Group. N Engl J Med 1999; 340:493. [NLM Cit ID: 99134018]

Wilhelm MP et al: Vancomycin. Mayo Clin Proc 1999;74:928. [NLM Cit ID: 99416901] (Review.)

STREPTOGRAMINS

Streptogramins are structurally similar to macrolides but do not share cross-resistance with that class. **Pristinamycin** is an oral streptogramin marketed in France for treatment of gram-positive infections. **Synercid** is a combination of two synthetic derivatives of pristinamycin—quinupristin and dalfopristin—in a 30:70 ratio that is administered intravenously. It is bactericidal and inhibits protein synthesis by binding to bacterial ribosomes. In vitro, it has activity against *Moraxella catarrhalis, Haemophilus influenzae,* clostridium, peptostreptococcus, mycoplasma, legionella, and chlamydia. It has no activity against enteric gram-negative bacilli. However, its major clinical use is in the therapy of gram-positive infections, including those due to streptococci (including penicillin-resistant pneumococci) staphylococci (including methicillin-sensitive and methicillin-resistant *S aureus* and *S epidermidis*) and enterococci, including vancomycin-resistant *Enterococcus faecium.* The drug is generally bacteriostatic against the enterococcus. The recommended dose is 7.5 mg/kg intravenously every 8 hours. In addition to phlebitis with peripheral administration, the major adverse effect is arthralgias and myalgias that resolve with discontinuation of the drug. It is primarily cleared via the liver; streptogramins inhibit the cytochrome P450 system, resulting in increased levels of cyclosporine and other agents.

Wood MJ (editor): Quinupristin/dalfopristin—A novel approach for the treatment of serious Gram-positive infections. J Antimicrob Chemother 1999;44 (Topic A). [Entire issue.]

QUINOLONES

The quinolones are synthetic analogs of nalidixic acid that have an exceedingly broad spectrum of activity against many bacteria. The mode of action of all quinolones involves inhibition of bacterial DNA synthesis by blocking the enzyme DNA gyrase.

The earlier quinolones (nalidixic acid, oxolinic acid, cinoxacin) did not achieve systemic antibacterial levels after oral intake and thus were useful only as urinary antiseptics. The newer fluorinated derivatives (norfloxacin, ciprofloxacin, ofloxacin, lomefloxacin, levofloxacin, gatifloxacin, moxifloxacin, and sparfloxacin) have greater antibacterial activity, achieve clinically useful levels in blood and tissues, and have low toxicity.

Antimicrobial Activity

A number of fluoroquinolones are currently available. Most have quite similar spectrums of activity. In general, these drugs have superb activity against Enterobacteriaceae but are also active against other gram-negative bacteria such as haemophilus, neisseria, moraxella, brucella, legionella, salmonella, shigella, campylobacter, yersinia, vibrio, and aeromonas. Ciprofloxacin has slightly better activity against *P aeruginosa* than the other fluoroquinolones, and none of these agents have reliable activity against *S maltophilia* or *P cepacia.* Against genital tract pathogens such as *Mycoplasma hominis, Ureaplasma urealyticum,* and *C pneumoniae,* the newer agents possess more activity than the others, and against *Gardnerella vaginalis* ciprofloxacin and ofloxacin are the most active. *M tuberculosis* is sensitive to the quinolones, as is *M fortuitum* and *Mycobacterium kansasii.* Although most *M avium* complex organisms are resistant to fluoroquinolones when combined with other agents (ethambutol, rifabutin, and amikacin), ciprofloxacin appears to be effective in treating infections caused by this organism.

In general, the fluoroquinolones are less active against gram-positive than gram-negative organisms, with norfloxacin and lomefloxacin having less activity than ciprofloxacin and ofloxacin—and levofloxacin, gatifloxacin, moxifloxacin, and sparfloxacin having the greatest activity. Ciprofloxacin and ofloxacin are active against some strains of *S aureus* and *S epidermidis,* including some methicillin-resistant strains. However, recent reports of the emergence of ciprofloxacin-resistant strains of staphylococci have limited the use of these drugs as monotherapy of infections caused by these organisms. Enterococci, including *E faecalis, S pneumoniae,* group A, B, and D streptococci, and viridans streptococci, are only moderately sensitive to the older quinolones. Anaerobic bacteria, *T pallidum,* and nocardia are resistant to the earlier fluoroquinolones.

Levofloxacin, sparfloxacin, gatifloxacin, and moxifloxacin are very similar to the previously described fluoroquinolones with the notable exception of improved activity against streptococci, including penicillin-resistant pneumococci. Gatifloxacin and moxifloxacin also demonstrate activity against many of the significant anaerobic pathogens, including *Bacteroides fragilis* and mouth anaerobes.

Pharmacokinetics & Administration (Table 37–9)

After oral administration, the fluoroquinolones are well absorbed and widely distributed in body fluids and tissues and are concentrated intracellularly. Fluoroquinolones are bound by some heavy metals, and absorption is inhibited when they are given with iron, calcium, and other multivalent cations. Optimal oral bioavailability is achieved if they are given about 1 hour before or 2 hours after meals. Ofloxacin appears to penetrate into the cerebrospinal fluid better than other fluoroquinolones. The serum half-life ranges from 4 hours (ciprofloxacin) to 20 hours (sparfloxacin). After ingestion of 500 mg, the peak serum level of ciprofloxacin is 2.5 μg/mL and is lower than that of the other quinolones (4–6 μg/mL), but this is offset by ciprofloxacin's slightly greater in vitro activity against most gram-negative organisms. A number of the fluoroquinolones can be administered intravenously, resulting in peak serum levels ranging

Table 37–9. Pharmacology of the quinolones.

Drug	Peak Serum Levels (μg/mL)	Serum Half-Life (h)	Total Daily Dose	Dosage Interval (h)	Dosage Adjustments in Renal Failure: Moderate (Cl_{cr} 10–50 mL/min)	Severe (Cl_{cr} < 10 mL/min)	Posthemodialysis Dose
Ciprofloxacin	3–4 (400 mg IV, 500–750 mg PO)	3–6	800–12 mg (IV) 0.5–1.5 g (PO)	8–12	400 mg q12h	200 mg q12h	None
Gatifloxacin	4–5 (400 mg PO or IV)	7	400 mg	24	200 mg q24h	200 mg q24h	200 mg
Levofloxacin	5–7 (500 mg PO or IV)	6–8	250–500 mg	24	250 mg q24–48h	250 mg q48h	None
Moxifloxacin	3–4 (400 mg PO)	12	400	24	400 mg q24h	250 mg q48h	None
Ofloxacin	5–7 (400 mg PO or IV)	6–8	400–800 mg	12	200–400 mg q24h	200 mg q24h	None
Sparfloxacin	1 (200 mg PO)	20	200 mg	24	200 mg q24h	200 mg q24h	None

from 4 to 9 μg/mL. Most of the quinolones are eliminated via mixed renal and nonrenal pathways. As a result, only modest accumulation takes place in the presence of renal insufficiency. Exceptions are ofloxacin, levofloxacin, lomefloxacin, and gatifloxacin, which are primarily dependent upon the kidney for elimination.

Clinical Uses

Because of their broad spectrum of activity and a tendency for some organisms (eg, *P aeruginosa,* staphylococcal species) to develop resistance, these agents should not be routinely used as first-line therapy when less expensive agents with narrower spectrums are available.

Urinary tract infections caused by trimethoprim-sulfamethoxazole-resistant gram-negative organisms that are sensitive to quinolones can be treated with any of the available agents.

Because of good penetration into prostatic tissue, quinolones are effective in treating bacterial prostatitis and are alternatives to trimethoprim-sulfamethoxazole (doses for prostatitis are the same as for urinary tract infection, but the duration should be 6–12 weeks).

Quinolones have been approved for use in therapy of certain sexually transmitted diseases. Ofloxacin, 300 mg twice daily for 7 days, is as effective as doxycycline, 100 mg twice daily for 7 days, for the therapy of *C trachomatis* cervicitis, urethritis, and proctitis. It is also effective for nongonococcal urethritis caused by *U urealyticum.* Ciprofloxacin and norfloxacin are not effective for the therapy of chlamydial infections or nongonococcal urethritis. In general, the use of quinolones for the therapy of any sexually transmitted disease will be limited by their lack of efficacy in concomitant syphilis. Gonococcal urethritis, cervicitis, pharyngitis, and proctitis can be treated with a single dose of 500 mg of ciprofloxacin, 400 mg of ofloxacin, or 400 mg of enoxacin. While not currently common in the United States, the increased worldwide prevalence of *N gonorrhoeae* resistant to fluoroquinolones may limit their usefulness for this infection in the future.

Pelvic inflammatory disease is usually caused by *Chlamydia trachomatis, N gonorrhoeae,* Enterobacteriaceae, or anaerobes. Oral outpatient treatment with ofloxacin, 400 mg twice daily for 14 days, in addition to clindamycin, 450 mg orally four times daily for 14 days, or metronidazole, 500 mg orally twice daily for 14 days, can be used. Epididymitis in young men (< 35 years of age) is caused most commonly by chlamydia and the gonococcus, and outpatient therapy with single-dose ciprofloxacin (500 mg) or ofloxacin (400 mg) followed by doxycycline, 100 mg twice daily for 10 days, is adequate therapy. Alternatively, ofloxacin, 300 mg twice daily for 10 days, can be used. *H ducreyi,* the agent that causes chancroid, is sensitive to quinolones, and ciprofloxacin, 500 mg twice daily, or enoxacin, 400 mg daily for 3 days, can be used as an alternative to erythromycin, azithromycin, or ceftriaxone as therapy for this disease.

Ciprofloxacin and ofloxacin have been successfully used to treat complicated skin and soft tissue infections and osteomyelitis caused by gram-negative organisms. Ciprofloxacin, 500–750 mg twice daily for at least 6 weeks, has been effective therapy for malignant otitis externa.

Because quinolones are the only available oral agents active against campylobacter in addition to the other major bacterial pathogens associated with diarrhea (salmonella, shigella, toxigenic *E coli*), they have been used for the therapy of traveler's diarrhea as well as domestically acquired acute diarrhea. Norfloxacin, ciprofloxacin, and ofloxacin may be effective in eradicating the chronic carrier state of salmonella when therapy is continued for 4–6 weeks.

Ciprofloxacin has been used to eradicate meningococci from the nasopharynx of carriers.

Norfloxacin, ciprofloxacin, and ofloxacin are effective for prophylaxis against gram-negative infections in the neutropenic patient, and intravenous ciprofloxacin in combination with aminoglycosides or β-lactam antibiotics has been used successfully to treat the febrile neutropenic patient.

Although some clinical studies have suggested that ciprofloxacin is efficacious in the therapy of lower respiratory tract infections, caution should be exercised since the drug has only marginal activity against *S pneumoniae* and *M pneumoniae,* and failures in treating pneumococcal pneumonia have been reported. Newer agents such as levofloxacin, sparfloxacin, gatifloxacin, and moxifloxacin are more active against the pneumococci, including penicillin resistant strains, and are useful in the treatment of infections due to these organisms. However, their broad spectrum of activity against resistant aerobic gram-negative pathogens suggests that they should be reserved for the treatment of refractory infections. One setting in which ciprofloxacin is indicated for the therapy of lower respiratory tract infections is in cystic fibrosis, where *P aeruginosa* is the predominant pathogen.

As noted above, ciprofloxacin in combination with other agents has been used to treat *M avium* complex infections, and ciprofloxacin and ofloxacin may be efficacious in the therapy of multidrug-resistant tuberculosis.

Adverse Effects

The most prominent adverse effects of the quinolones are nausea, vomiting, and diarrhea. Occasionally, headache, dizziness, seizures, insomnia, impaired liver function, and skin rashes have been observed as well as more serious reactions such as acute renal failure and anaphylaxis. Photosensitivity reactions are most common with sparfloxacin. Central nervous system adverse effects are common with enoxacin and trovafloxacin. Severe hepatotoxicity, including liver failure and the need for liver transplantation, has been reported with trovafloxacin use. Although the drug has not been withdrawn, a warning by the FDA has been issued, and trovafloxacin should not be used unless there are no other alternatives. Some agents, including grepafloxacin, maxifloxacin, and sparfloxacin, have been documented to prolong the QT interval; grepafloxacin has been withdrawn from the market as a result of this effect. Superinfections with enterococci and yeasts can develop. Clearance of theophylline may be inhibited by fluoroquinolones (especially enoxacin), and drug levels should be monitored in patients receiving both drugs. Prolongation of the prothrombin time has been observed in some patients receiving stable doses of warfarin after ciprofloxacin has been given, but this interaction is unpredictable and modest. Tendonitis and tendon rupture have been reported with quinolone agents, especially pefloxacin. Risk factors include concomitant glucocorticoid use and hepatic and renal failure. Patients experiencing musculoskeletal symptoms while receiving fluoroquinolones should discontinue therapy.

Gatifloxacin and moxifloxacin: two new fluoroquinolones. Med Lett Drugs Ther 2000;432:15. [NLM Cit ID: 20170069]

Hooper DC: New uses for new and old quinolones and the challenge of resistance. Clin Infect Dis 2000;30:243. [NLM Cit ID: 20137765]

Walker RC: The fluoroquinolones. Mayo Clin Proc 1999; 74:1030.

PENTAMIDINE & ATOVAQUONE

Pentamidine and atovaquone are antiprotozoal agents that are primarily used to treat pneumocystis pneumonia. Pentamidine is discussed in Chapters 31 and 35. Atovaquone inhibits mitochondrial electron transport and probably also folate metabolism. It is poorly absorbed and should be given with food to maximize bioavailability. The suspension is significantly better absorbed than the tablet formulation and thus should be used preferentially, especially in high-risk patients (those with diarrhea, malabsorption). It has moderate activity against *P carinii.* In comparative trials with trimethoprim-sulfamethoxazole and pentamidine in the therapy of pneumocystis pneumonia in AIDS, atovaquone, 750 mg orally three times daily for 3 weeks, was less effective than both agents but better tolerated. It has also been used as prophylaxis in AIDS patients at a dosage of 1500 mg daily. Major adverse effects include rash, nausea, vomiting, diarrhea, fever, and abnormal liver function tests. The use of atovaquone is limited to patients with mild to moderate pneumocystis infections who have failed or cannot tolerate other therapies.

URINARY ANTISEPTICS

These drugs exert antimicrobial activity in the urine but have little or no systemic antibacterial effect. Their usefulness is limited to therapy and prevention of urinary tract infections.

1. NITROFURANTOIN

Nitrofurantoin is active against the common gram-positive urinary pathogens *Enterococcus faecalis* and *Staphylococcus saprophyticus,* but the drug inhibits only about 50% of *Enterococcus faecium.* It is also used against *E coli* and citrobacter, but activity against proteus, serratia, and pseudomonas is poor. Following oral administration, about 50% of the drug is absorbed, but serum concentrations are very low and tissue levels are undetectable. Levels in the urine reach concentrations of 200–400 μg/mL, which are well above the MICs of susceptible organisms. Because clearance is primarily via the kidney, the amounts of these drugs in the urine are proportionate to the creatinine clearance, and with severe renal insufficiency subtherapeutic levels are present. Given low serum levels, poor tissue penetration, and renal elimination, the use of nitrofurantoin is limited to therapy or prophylaxis of cystitis in patients with normal renal function. Nitrofurantoin should not be used to treat pyelonephritis or prostatitis.

The average daily dose in urinary tract infections is 100 mg orally four times daily, taken with food. The macrocrystal preparation can be given at a dosage of 100 mg twice daily. A single daily dose of 50–100 mg can prevent recurrent urinary tract infections in women.

Oral nitrofurantoin often causes nausea and vomiting. The crystalline formulation is better tolerated than older preparations. Hemolytic anemia may occur in G6PD deficiency. Other side effects are skin rashes, pulmonary infiltrates, and, uncommonly, peripheral neuropathy. Acute and chronic pulmonary hypersensitivity reactions may occur, and pulmonary fibrosis has occurred with prolonged use.

2. FOSFOMYCIN

Fosfomycin tromethamine is a phosphonic acid derivative useful in the treatment of uncomplicated urinary tract infection. The spectrum of activity includes *E coli, E faecalis,* and other gram-negative aerobic urinary pathogens, but not *P aeruginosa.* Available as a 3 g sachet, fosfomycin may be useful for the single-dose treatment of the above organisms. Like nitrofurantoin, fosfomycin should not be used for systemic infection. However, the increased concentrations in urine allow for its use in uncomplicated bacteriuria. The most frequently reported adverse effects include diarrhea, headache, and nausea.

3. ACIDIFYING AGENTS

Urine with a pH below 5.5 tends to be antibacterial. Many substances have been used in an attempt to acidify urine, including ammonium chloride, ascorbic acid, methionine, and mandelic acid. In general, large doses are required and none are consistently effective. In view of the plethora of antibiotics that are available for therapy and prophylaxis of urinary tract infections, acidifying agents are of limited value.

Gupta K et al: Increasing prevalence of antimicrobial resistance among uropathogens causing acute uncomplicated cystitis in women. JAMA 1999;281:736. [NLM Cit ID: 99159809]

SYSTEMICALLY ACTIVE DRUGS IN URINARY TRACT INFECTIONS

Many antimicrobial drugs are excreted in the urine in high concentrations. For this reason, low and relatively nontoxic dosages of penicillins, cephalosporins, aminoglycosides, quinolones, and trimethoprim-sulfamethoxazole can reach high urinary concentrations and are effective in urinary tract infections.

ANTIFUNGAL DRUGS

Empirical antifungal therapy is rarely instituted except for febrile neutropenic patients. Therapy is reserved for situations in which yeast or mold is seen on KOH preparation or when isolated organisms are thought to be pathogenic. Antifungal sensitivity testing recently has been standardized for yeasts but not for molds and is not routinely recommended. Thus, therapy generally is based on experience and clinical trials and not on susceptibility tests.

1. AMPHOTERICIN B

Amphotericin B in vitro inhibits several organisms producing systemic mycotic disease in humans, including aspergillus, histoplasma, cryptococcus, coccidioides, candida, blastomyces, sporothrix, and others. This drug can be used for treatment of these systemic fungal infections. Intraventricular administration is necessary for the treatment of coccidioides meningitis and may be required in meningitis caused by other fungi if systemic therapy fails. *Pseudallescheria boydii* and fusarium are often resistant to amphotericin B.

There is no consensus on how amphotericin B should be administered or on the dosage and the duration of therapy. The first few milliliters of the initial dose was at one time administered over 10–20 minutes to test for anaphylaxis. However, most centers no longer use the "test dose," since anaphylaxis is extremely rare. The daily dose of amphotericin B for most fungal infections varies from 0.3 mg/kg to 1 mg/kg, though infections caused by aspergillus and mucor are often treated with 1–1.5 mg/kg daily. Full doses are reached by increasing the dose incrementally over several days.

In fungal meningitis, amphotericin B, 0.5 mg, is injected intraventricularly three times weekly; continuous treatment (many weeks) with an Ommaya reservoir is generally required. The dose is slowly increased over several weeks to improve tolerance. Relapses of fungal meningitis (especially coccidioides meningitis) occur commonly and can be seen years after completion of therapy. Thus, when treating meningitis due to *Coccidioides immitis,* intraventricular therapy is given three times a week for 8–10 weeks initially, and the frequency is then decreased to once-weekly doses for 6 months. Subsequent therapy is dictated by cerebrospinal fluid titers. In meningitis due to other fungi, long-term therapy beyond the initial 8–10 weeks is rarely needed. Combined treatment with flucytosine is beneficial in cryptococcal meningitis and possibly systemic candidiasis. Amphotericin B may have some benefit in naegleria meningoencephalitis.

Amphotericin B in low doses (0.1–0.25 mg/kg/d) has been used prophylactically to prevent invasive fungal infections in bone marrow transplant recipients and may be beneficial in this setting. Whether prophylactic administration is better than early empirical therapy in febrile patients who have not responded to broad-spectrum antibiotics has not been determined.

In patients with Foley catheters in place who have candiduria, amphotericin B bladder irrigations have been used to decrease colony counts. Although the procedure is widely used, the efficacy of amphotericin B bladder irrigation is unproved, and long-term eradication of candiduria following amphotericin B bladder irrigation rarely occurs.

In impaired renal function, the dose of amphotericin B need not be reduced initially. However, if the serum creatinine reaches 2.5–3 mg/dL, either a less nephrotoxic liposomal formulation of amphotericin can be used (see below) or the dose can be temporarily lowered (or even stopped for a few days) until renal function recovers. Amphotericin B is then resumed at about one-half the previous dosage and increased in increments as tolerated. The drug is not removed by hemodialysis, so that no additional drug is needed after dialysis.

The intravenous administration of amphotericin B often produces chills, fever, vomiting, and headache. As a rule, infusions given over 1–2 hours are as well tolerated as those given over 4–6 hours. However, patients who experience infusion-related adverse effects may benefit from slowing the rate of administration. Tolerance may be enhanced by temporary lowering of the dose or premedication with acetaminophen and diphenhydramine. Addition of 25 mg of hydrocortisone to the infusion decreases the incidence of rigors, and meperidine, 25–50 mg, is effective in arresting rigors once they start. Central intravenous administration eliminates the likelihood of thrombophlebitis. Amphotericin B commonly impairs kidney function and produces anemia (impaired iron utilization by bone marrow). Electrolyte disturbances (hypokalemia, hypomagnesemia, distal renal tubular acidosis) also occur. Renal insufficiency commonly seen with amphotericin B administration can be prevented with salt supplementation. As a result, administration of 0.5–1 L of 0.9% saline prior to infusion of amphotericin B may prevent nephrotoxicity.

The nephrotoxicity of amphotericin has resulted in the development of lipid-based amphotericin B products. Three such products are available: amphotericin B lipid complex (ABLC; Abelcet), amphotericin B colloidal dispersion (ABCD; Amphotec), and liposomal amphotericin B (L-AmB; AmBisome). Complexing amphotericin B with lipid allows larger doses to be administered (1–6 mg/kg, depending on the preparation and the fungal species). All three preparations are associated with less nephrotoxicity (about 5% of patients) than conventional amphotericin B and thus offer benefit for patients who develop renal insufficiency while receiving amphotericin B. Infusion-related adverse effects are variable, with liposomal amphotericin being associated with the lowest incidence of fevers and chills even when infused over 30–60 minutes. ABCD is associated with the highest rate of infusion toxicity and requires slow administration over 2.5–3 hours. ABLC is comparable to conventional amphotericin B. All three have significant differences in serum levels, half-life, and tissue penetration. Most of the data on efficacy are gleaned from open-label trials in patients who failed or were intolerant of conventional amphotericin B and who were infected with aspergillus or candida. Most clinical experience has been with L-Am B, largely because it has been licensed in Europe for several years. L-Am B is approved for therapy in the febrile neutropenic patient, with efficacy equal to that of conventional amphotericin B in success of therapy and prevention of emergent fungal infections. Direct comparative trials between liposomal preparations are limited.

Drug acquisition costs for all three products are much higher than for conventional amphotericin B. Whether decreased toxicity and the decreased need to monitor for adverse effects offset these cost differences is not known. At present, however, lipid-based preparations should be reserved for patients who fail conventional amphotericin B or those who develop renal insufficiency (serum creatinine 2.5–3 mg/dL). The lipid formulations are particularly effective for therapy of visceral leishmaniasis. Short courses (5–10 days) with low doses (2–24 mg/kg depending on which preparation is used) are very effective in eradicating the parasite, probably because of distribution of the drug to the reticuloendothelial system, the major site of parasite invasion.

Johansen HK et al: Problems in the design and reporting of trials of antifungal agents encountered during meta-analysis. JAMA 1999;282:1752. [NLM Cit ID: 20033296]

Patel R: Antifungal agents. Part I. Amphotericin B preparations and flucytosine. Mayo Clin Proc 1998;73:1205. [NLM Cit ID: 990085314]

Wong-Beringer A et al: Lipid formulations of amphotericin B: Clinical efficacy and toxicities. Clin Infect Dis 1998;27:603. [NLM Cit ID: 98442299]

2. GRISEOFULVIN

Griseofulvin is an agent that can inhibit the growth of some dermatophytes but has no effect on bacteria or on the fungi that cause deep mycoses. The absorbed drug has an affinity for skin and is deposited there, bound to keratin. Thus, it makes keratin resistant to fungal growth, and the new growth of hair or nails is free of infection. As keratinized structures are shed, they are replaced by uninfected ones. The bulk of ingested griseofulvin is excreted in the feces.

Oral doses of 0.5–1 g/d for 3–5 weeks are given if only the skin is involved and for 3–6 months or longer if the hair and nails are involved. Griseofulvin is most successful in severe dermatophytosis, particularly if caused by *Trichophyton rubrum,* though some strains are resistant.

An ultramicrosize particle formulation (Gris-PEG) is better absorbed. The dosage is 0.33–0.66 g orally daily.

Griseofulvin is relatively nontoxic and has a long history of clinical safety. Headache, nausea, vomiting, diarrhea, photosensitivity, and leukopenia have all been reported but are reversible and often will resolve without interruption of therapy. Routine monitoring for adverse effects is not required.

Major indications for use of this drug include tinea capitis, widespread tinea corporis, and tinea unguium (onychomycosis), though success rates in the latter are only 25–30%. Preferred agents in the treatment of onychomycosis include itraconazole and terbinafine. Preliminary data suggest that these drugs are at least as effective as griseofulvin; however, failures are reported in 30–50% of cases.

3. NYSTATIN

Nystatin has a wide spectrum of antifungal activity but is used almost exclusively to treat superficial candidal infections. It is too toxic for systemic administration, and the drug is not absorbed from mucous membranes or the gastrointestinal tract. Several preparations are available, including oral suspension (100,000 units/mL) and ointments, gels, and creams (100,000 units/g). For oral candidiasis, 500,000 units of suspension is used to rinse the mouth and is retained in the mouth as long as possible before it is swallowed. This is repeated four times a day for at least 2 days after resolution of the infection. Infections of skin are treated with cream or ointment, 100,000 units applied to the affected area twice daily until resolution of the infection. Nystatin is less effective than miconazole and clotrimazole for therapy of vaginal candidiasis.

4. FLUCYTOSINE

Flucytosine inhibits some strains of candida, cryptococcus, aspergillus, and other fungi. Dosages of 3–8 g daily (100–150 mg/kg/d) orally produce good levels in serum and cerebrospinal fluid. Clinical remissions of meningitis or sepsis due to yeasts have occurred. However, resistant organisms are selected out rapidly, and flucytosine is therefore not employed as a single drug except in urinary tract infections.

In renal insufficiency, flucytosine may accumulate to toxic levels, and dosage adjustments are needed. Because patients with HIV infection and normal renal function do not tolerate the normal doses of flucytosine (150 mg/kg/d in four divided doses), 75–100 mg/kg/d is recommended. The drug is effectively removed by hemodialysis. Toxic effects include bone marrow depression, abnormal liver function, loss of hair, and others. Bone marrow suppression is caused by conversion of flucytosine to fluorouracil. Combined use of flucytosine and amphotericin B in systemic candidiasis and cryptococcal meningitis has been shown to be of value.

5. NATAMYCIN

Natamycin is a polyene antifungal drug effective against many different fungi in vitro. When it is combined with appropriate surgical measures, topical application of 5% ophthalmic suspension may be beneficial in the treatment of keratitis caused by fusarium, acremonium (cephalosporium), or other fungi. The drug may also be effective in the treatment of oral or vaginal candidiasis. The toxicity after topical application appears to be low.

6. TERBINAFINE

Terbinafine, an allylamine, inhibits fungal cell membrane function by blocking ergosterol synthesis. Terbinafine is now available topically as well as in 250 mg tablets for oral administration. The recommended dosage is 250 mg daily for 12 weeks for toenail infections and 250 mg daily for 6 weeks for fingernail infections (success rate about 70%). Terbinafine is well tolerated. Most adverse effects are minor (diarrhea, dyspepsia) or transient (taste disturbance). Rare cases of hepatic injury have been reported.

7. ANTIFUNGAL IMIDAZOLES & TRIAZOLES

These antifungal drugs also inhibit synthesis of ergosterol, resulting in inhibition of membrane-associated enzyme activity, cell wall growth, and replication.

Clotrimazole, taken orally in the form of 10 mg troches five times daily, can prevent and treat oral candidiasis. Vaginal tablets (200 mg) inserted daily for 3 days are effective for vaginal candidiasis. Topical preparations for treatment of cutaneous dermatophytes are also available. Toxicity precludes systemic use.

Miconazole is active in vitro against coccidioides, candida, histoplasma, cryptococcus, paracoccidioides, pseudallescheria, sporothrix, and other fungi. However, it has substantial toxicity and little clinical activity and is rarely used intravenously. It is a drug that can be used for *P boydii* infections in a dosage of 30 mg/kg/d in three divided doses. However, itraconazole can also be used, and because it is associated with fewer adverse effects it is now considered the drug of choice. Its major use is as a 2% cream for dermatophytosis and as a 200 mg vaginal suppository for vaginal candidiasis.

Ketoconazole, an imidazole, can be given orally as a single daily dose of 200–600 mg, preferably with food. The dosage remains the same in renal or hepatic failure. Absorption is impaired by antacid and H_2-blockers; coadministration of phenytoin, isoniazid, and rifampin can cause enhanced metabolism of ketoconazole and lower plasma levels. The reduction in achievable serum levels in achlorhydria patients has been associated with decreased efficacy in the treatment of HIV-positive patients with esophageal candidiasis.

Ketoconazole is primarily used to treat superficial infections caused by candida, including oral, vaginal, and esophageal candidiasis. It dramatically improves lesions of chronic mucocutaneous candidiasis. Ketoconazole is also effective therapy for some deep-seated fungal infections such as blastomycosis, paracoccidioidomycosis, and nonmeningeal, localized histoplasmosis. However, this drug has been disappointing in the treatment of deep-seated candidal and coccidioidal infections (other than cutaneous lesions) and cryptococcal meningitis, where amphotericin B remains the drug of choice.

Adverse effects include nausea, vomiting, skin rashes, and occasional elevations in aminotransferase levels. Although most elevations of liver enzymes are asymptomatic, on rare occasions symptomatic and even fatal hepatitis can occur. All patients receiving azoles should be informed of the potential toxicity. Ketoconazole blocks the synthesis of adrenal steroids and testosterone and can cause gynecomastia and impotence. Ketoconazole can also cause increased levels of cyclosporine when administered with this drug, and careful monitoring of serum levels is needed to avoid toxicity.

Fluconazole, a bis-triazole with activity similar to that of ketoconazole, is water-soluble and can be given both orally and intravenously. Absorption of the drug after oral administration is not pH-dependent, in contrast to ketoconazole, and therapeutic serum levels are obtained even when H_2 receptor antagonists are given simultaneously. It penetrates well into the cerebrospinal fluid and eye and reaches therapeutically significant levels in the urine. The drug has been shown to be effective primarily in therapy of infections with candida, cryptococcus, and blastomyces. *Candida albicans* is usually sensitive to fluconazole, but other species of candida (*C tropicalis, C krusei, C glabrata,* etc) are often resistant. Fluconazole-resistant strains of *C albicans* have been reported and are usually seen in HIV-positive patients on long-term therapy. With the advent of highly active antiretroviral therapy, the rate of fluconazole resistance in *C albicans* has been decreased. The drug is inactive against aspergillus, mucor, and pseudallescheria. Fluconazole (50–100 mg) is as efficacious as ketoconazole (200 mg/d) and clotrimazole troches in the therapy of oropharyngeal candidiasis and is superior to ketoconazole for therapy of candidal esophagitis in immunosuppressed patients. It is also effective therapy for vaginal candidiasis, where a single oral dose of 150 mg is 80–90% effective, and chronic mucocutaneous candidiasis. Response to fluconazole in leukemic patients with hepatosplenic candidiasis has also been observed, as have other invasive infections such as peritonitis, wound infection, and pyelonephritis. Fluconazole, 400 mg daily, has been shown to be as effective as amphotericin B, 0.5–0.6 mg/kg/d, for candidemia in both neutropenic and nonneutropenic patients. Most of these infections were line-related, and removal of the line was critical to successful therapy. Fluconazole (200 mg/d) is effective as chronic suppressive therapy of cryptococcal meningitis in patients with AIDS and is the drug of choice in this setting. Its use as initial therapy is not established. At a dose of 200 mg/d, response rates and overall mortality rates are the same in patients treated with oral fluconazole and with amphotericin B. However, the mortality rate in the first 2 weeks is higher—and it takes longer to sterilize the cerebrospinal fluid—among patients treated with fluconazole than among patients treated with amphotericin. Higher dosages (400–800 mg daily) may be more effective but have not been studied. Most clinicians would initiate therapy with amphotericin B for 2 weeks and then switch to oral fluconazole. A dosage of 400 mg of fluconazole daily is effective therapy for coccidioidal meningitis (80% response), but improvement is slow, taking as long as 4–8 months; efficacy has been observed in both non-HIV-infected and HIV-infected individuals. Higher doses (800–1200 mg/d) have been used; however, it is unclear whether they are superior to usual doses. Fluconazole, 400 mg daily, has been shown to be effective as prophylaxis against superficial and invasive fungal infections in bone marrow and liver transplant recipients, but concern has been raised about superinfection with resistant organisms (*Candida krusei, C glabrata,* aspergillus). The same dose of fluconazole has not reduced the incidence of invasive fungal disease in leukemic patients undergoing intensive chemotherapy and has not reduced the need to use amphotericin B. Thus, the use of fluconazole as prophylaxis in the neutropenic patient remains controversial. In advanced HIV disease, prophylactic fluconazole has been more convincingly shown to be effective in preventing invasive fungal disease. Fluconazole, 200 mg daily, is more effective than clotrimazole troches, 10 mg five times daily, in preventing cryptococcal disease, candidal esophagitis, and superficial fungal infections, especially in those with 50 or less CD4 lymphocytes. Doses as low as 200 mg weekly have been effective in preventing oropharyngeal and vaginal candidiasis (but not esophageal disease) in HIV-positive women. Because the overall incidence of invasive fungal disease is low, universal prophylaxis to prevent disease in a few should be discouraged, especially with the advent of more potent antiretroviral therapy.

Fluconazole is well absorbed after oral administration (80% bioavailability), and serum levels approach those seen after administering the same dose intravenously. In addition, the intravenous preparation is about ten times more expensive than the oral medication. Thus, unless the patient cannot take medication by mouth or has an overwhelming infection, the preferred route of administration is orally.

Itraconazole is an oral triazole with antifungal and pharmacologic properties similar to those of ketoconazole. It is moderately well absorbed from the gastrointestinal tract (food increases absorption from 30% to 60%; antacids and H_2 receptor antagonists decrease absorption) and widely distributed in tissues with the notable exception of the central nervous system, where levels in spinal fluid are undetectable. Itraconazole solution is more predictably absorbed than the tablets. However, this preparation also is somewhat affected by elevated gastric pH. While the tablet formulation should be administered with food, the solution is best absorbed on an empty stomach. A parenteral formulation is now available, but it is not approved for patients with renal insufficiency (creatinine clearance < 30 mL/min) because of the risk of pancreatic adenocarcinoma. The drug is metabolized by the liver, and no dosage adjustment is needed in renal insufficiency. Itraconazole is very active against most strains of *Histoplasma capsulatum, Blastomyces dermatitidis, Cryptococcus neoformans, Sporotrichum schenkii,* and various dermatophytes. It is also active against some fluconazole-resistant strains of candida, especially *C albicans,* and aspergillus species but inactive against fusarium and zygomycetes. Itraconazole in doses of 200–400 mg/d is effective and approved therapy for localized or disseminated histoplasmosis and is more effective than ketoconazole in AIDS patients with histoplasmosis. It is also effective prophylaxis against recurrent histoplasmosis in these patients and is also effective as secondary prophylaxis against *P marneffei* infection in AIDS patients. Itraconazole is preferred over ketoconazole for therapy of blastomycosis because it is more efficacious and better tolerated. It is also effective in sporotrichosis, dermatophytic infections (including those of the nails), and oral and esophageal candidiasis. Noncomparative clinical trials indicate efficacy in therapy of invasive aspergillosis (55–80%) and coccidioidomycosis (57–94%). In the absence of comparative trials with other agents active against *C immitis* and aspergillus, it is difficult to know if itraconazole should be used as a first-line drug against these organisms, but the oral route of administration makes the drug attractive, particularly in patients who are not critically ill. At doses of 200 mg twice daily, itraconazole increases exercise tolerance and decreases steroid requirements in patients with allergic bronchopulmonary aspergillosis. Itraconazole has been shown to decrease superficial and invasive fungal infections compared with placebo when used as prophylaxis in neutropenic patients. Itraconazole has been approved for onychomycosis. Pulse therapy with 200 mg twice daily for 1 week each month, repeated for 4 consecutive months, is effective in 70% of cases.

Adverse effects are similar to those of ketoconazole and fluconazole, with anorexia, nausea, vomiting, and abdominal pain occurring most commonly. Skin rash has been reported in up to 8% of patients. Hepatitis and hypokalemia occur uncommonly. Drugs that increase hepatic drug-metabolizing enzymes (isoniazid, rifampin, phenytoin, phenobarbital) may increase itraconazole metabolism, and higher doses may be needed when these drugs are administered concurrently with itraconazole. Itraconazole also impairs the metabolism of cyclosporine and can result in toxic levels unless the dosage is adjusted. Like ketoconazole, itraconazole can increase blood levels of digoxin and warfarin.

The usual dosage is 200 mg once or twice daily with meals. Higher dosages (400–600 mg/d) may be required in patients who are immunocompromised and those with severe disease, especially that due to aspergillus. In patients with life-threatening infections, a 600 mg loading dose is given for 3 or 4 days.

Martin MV: The use of fluconazole and itraconazole in the treatment of *Candida albicans* infection: a review. J Antimicrob Chemother 1999;44:429. [NLM Cit ID: 20053523]

Summers KK et al: Therapeutic drug monitoring of systemic antifungal therapy. J Antimicrob Chemother 1997;40:753. [NLM Cit ID: 98122258]

Systemic antifungal drugs. Med Lett Drugs Ther 1997; 39:86. [NLM Cit ID: 97450304] (Activity, adverse effects, and clinical trials.)

Terrell CL: Antifungal agents. Part II: The azoles. Mayo Clin Proc 1999;74:78. [NLM Cit ID: 99142012]

ANTIVIRAL CHEMOTHERAPY

Several compounds can influence viral replication and the development of viral disease.

Amantadine is active against influenza A (but not influenza B) and has efficacy both in prophylaxis and therapy of this infection. Yearly immunization against influenza is recommended (see Chapter 30) for disease prevention, but in certain select situations amantadine can be used for this purpose. Amantadine prophylaxis is 70–90% effective and is suggested for the influenza season (6–8 weeks) in patients who cannot be immunized who are at increased risk of developing complications of influenza (those with chronic pulmonary and cardiac diseases, persons over 65 years of age, persons with chronic metabolic diseases such as diabetes mellitus, and chronic renal failure); in medical personnel who cannot receive vaccine but are capable of transmitting influenza to high-risk patients; if vaccine is not available; and if vaccine strains differ from the strain causing an epidemic. Short-term prophylaxis (2 weeks) is indicated if an outbreak occurs before vaccination has been given. In this setting, amantadine will protect against disease while antibody production is induced and will not interfere with antibody production. Because of its modest therapeutic benefit, high-risk patients and others with influenza A may benefit from treatment with amantadine if it is instituted within 48 hours after the onset of symptoms and continued for 1 week. The usual adult dosage is 200 mg orally per day (in persons over 65 years of age, 100 mg). Emergence of influenza A resistant to amantadine and rimantadine has been observed in patients receiving therapy. The most marked untoward effects are insomnia, nightmares, and ataxia, especially in the elderly. Amantadine may accumulate and be more toxic in patients with renal insufficiency, and the dosage should be reduced.

Rimantadine, an analog of amantadine, is as effective as amantadine and is associated with fewer central nervous system adverse effects. It is considerably more expensive than amantadine and thus should be considered only in the elderly, in whom central nervous system side effects occur more commonly.

Neuraminidase inhibitors. Zanamivir inhalation and oseltamivir tablets are available for prevention and treatment of influenza A and B. Like amantadine and rimantadine, they must be administered soon (within 48 hours) after the onset of symptoms to be effective. Zanamivir inhalers are difficult to use for some patients, especially those with asthma and chronic obstructive pulmonary disease, in whom bronchospasm has been reported. Oseltamivir is of limited application because of its gastrointestinal side effects. Both drugs are administered twice daily for 5 days when used for therapy. Both agents are significantly more expensive than amantadine and reduce the duration of symptoms by only 1 day and viral shedding by 2 days.

Acyclovir is useful in infections due to herpes simplex and in herpes zoster-varicella infections. In herpes-infected cells, it is selectively active against viral DNA polymerase and thus inhibits virus proliferation. Given intravenously (15 mg/kg/d in three divided doses), it can promote healing of mucocutaneous herpes simplex in immunocompromised patients. It can reduce pain, accelerate healing, and prevent dissemination of herpes zoster and varicella in immunocompromised patients. The usual dosage for varicella-zoster infections is 30 mg/kg/d intravenously in three equal doses. The drug has no effect on establishment of latency, frequency of recurrence, or incidence of postherpetic neuralgia. Acyclovir (30 mg/kg/d intravenously in three equal doses) is the drug of choice for herpes encephalitis. Intravenous or oral acyclovir is effective prophylaxis against recurrent mucocutaneous and visceral herpes infections in transplant and other severely immunosuppressed patients. Investigation of the role of intravenous acyclovir in the prevention of cytomegalovirus disease in transplant recipients has yielded conflicting data. Acyclovir appears to be effective in some transplant settings (renal and perhaps bone marrow) but not in others (liver).

Oral acyclovir, 400 mg three times daily, is effective in primary genital herpes simplex infections. Oral acyclovir for recurrent genital herpes reduces viral shedding but has marginal effects on symptoms and is less effective than in primary disease. Suppressive therapy (400 mg twice daily) for 4–6 months reduces the frequency and severity of recurrent genital herpetic lesions. Acyclovir minimally affects symptoms or viral shedding in recurrent herpes labialis and is not generally used for this disease. However, in a dose of 400 mg twice daily, it is effective in preventing recurrent herpes labialis in those with frequent relapses and in preventing sun-induced relapses.

Other uses of oral acyclovir include (1) therapy of acute herpetic keratitis and prevention of recurrences, (2) prevention and treatment of herpetic whitlow, (3) acceleration of healing of herpes zoster in immunocompetent patients if initiated within 48 hours after onset (800 mg five times daily for 7 days), (4) more rapid healing of rash and lessened clinical symptoms of primary varicella in adults and children if instituted within 24 hours after onset of rash and continued for 5–7 days, (5) therapy of herpes proctitis (400 mg five times daily for 10 days), (6) prevention of herpes simplex and cytomegalovirus infections in transplant recipients (in doses of 800 mg four or five times daily), (7) prevention of erythema multiforme that is herpes simplex-related, and (8) prophylaxis against varicella in susceptible household contacts.

Topical 5% acyclovir ointment can shorten the period of pain and viral shedding in herpes simplex mucocutaneous oral lesions in immunosuppressed patients but not in patients with normal immunity. In contrast (see famciclovir), penciclovir ointment appears to reduce the duration of pain and viral shedding by approximately 1 day in immunocompetent patients. Oral acyclovir generally has been found to be significantly more efficacious than topical therapy.

The absolute oral bioavailability of acyclovir is 10–30%. Newer agents (famciclovir, valacyclovir; see below) are significantly better absorbed than oral acyclovir and generally can be administered less frequently. Dosage reduction in renal insufficiency is required. For most herpes simplex infections except encephalitis, the dose is 5 mg/kg every 8 hours. Since hemodialysis reduces serum levels significantly, the daily dose should be given after hemodialysis.

Acyclovir is relatively nontoxic. Precipitation of drug in renal tubules has been described and can best be avoided by maintaining adequate hydration and urine flow. Central nervous system toxicity manifested by confusion, agitation, tremors, and hallucinations has been reported. Resistance has been described, usually in immunosuppressed patients who have received multiple courses of therapy.

Famciclovir is a prodrug of penciclovir. After oral administration, 75–80% of the famciclovir is absorbed and is deacetylated in the intestinal wall to the active drug, penciclovir. Penciclovir, like acyclovir, inhibits viral replication by interfering with viral DNA polymerase. Acyclovir-resistant strains of herpes simplex and varicella-zoster virus are also resistant to famciclovir. Famciclovir in a dose of 500 mg three times daily for 7 days accelerates healing of lesions in acute herpes zoster if started within 72 hours after the onset of rash. At a dose of 125 mg twice daily, famciclovir is effective suppressive therapy of recurrent genital herpes.

Valacyclovir is a prodrug of acyclovir that has significantly increased oral bioavailability when compared with acyclovir. After absorption, it is converted to acyclovir and serum levels are three to five times higher than those achieved with acyclovir. Valacyclovir at a dosage of 1 g three times daily is effective therapy for herpes zoster when started within 72 hours after onset of rash and is slightly more effective than acyclovir in relieving zoster-associated pain. It shortens the course of initial episodes of genital herpes (1 g twice daily for 10 days) and is effective prophylaxis for recurrent genital herpes when given as a single 1 g daily dose. At doses of 2 g four times daily, valacyclovir is more effective than placebo in preventing cytomegalovirus infections in seronegative recipients of a kidney from a seropositive donor. The adverse effect profile of valacyclovir is comparable to that of acyclovir. However, HIV-positive patients receiving long-term valacyclovir (8 g/d) for prevention of cytomegalovirus disease have been found to have an increased incidence of thrombocytopenic purpura-hemolytic anemic syndrome.

Foscarnet (trisodium phosphonoformate) is a pyrophosphate analog that inhibits viral DNA polymerase of human herpesviruses (CMV, herpes simplex, varicella-zoster) and the reverse transcriptase of human immunodeficiency virus. The drug is more expensive than ganciclovir, less well tolerated, and more difficult to administer. Therefore, its use is largely limited to patients who do not respond to ganciclovir or cannot tolerate it. Isolates of CMV resistant to ganciclovir and herpes simplex and varicella-zoster resistant to acyclovir are sensitive to foscarnet. Foscarnet appears to be effective for CMV retinitis and has been used successfully in patients who have failed to respond to ganciclovir. Once therapy is stopped, recurrences develop, and lifelong suppressive therapy is required for AIDS patients not receiving highly active antiretroviral therapy. Combination therapy with ganciclovir and foscarnet has been associated with improved efficacy over monotherapy in the treatment of CMV retinitis. While combination therapy reduced progression of disease (eg, retinal changes), no improvement of visual acuity was observed over either drug used alone. Foscarnet has also been used to treat acyclovir-resistant mucocutaneous herpes simplex in AIDS patients as well as varicella cutaneous lesions in AIDS patients who failed to respond to acyclovir. Uncontrolled trials suggest efficacy in CMV gastrointestinal disease, therapy of CMV infection following bone marrow and renal transplantation, and prevention of CMV disease when the drug is given prophylactically to seropositive bone marrow transplant recipients. Oral absorption is poor, and the drug must be given intravenously. The half-life is 3–5 hours, and this is prolonged with renal insufficiency. The usual induction dose is 60 mg/kg every 8 hours, and the dose for maintenance therapy is 120 mg/kg once daily. Adjustments are required for even minimal impairment in renal function (see package insert).

Toxicity is a major drawback to widespread use of foscarnet. The drug can cause severe phlebitis and must be diluted to a concentration of 12 mg/mL to be given peripherally. At higher concentrations, it must be given centrally. Nephrotoxicity, which is dose-dependent and reversible, is its major toxicity. Prehydration with 2.5 L of 0.9% saline may protect against nephrotoxicity. Foscarnet binds divalent cations and hypocalcemia with peripheral neuropathy, seizures and arrhythmias, hypomagnesemia, and hypophosphatemia can occur. Monitoring of electrolytes and renal function is required during therapy. Anemia (20–50%) and nausea and vomiting (20–30%) are other common adverse effects.

Resistance of herpes simplex virus to foscarnet has been described. Resistance is usually seen in patients who are infected with HIV and either have received foscarnet previously or were receiving suppressive therapy. Isolates may be sensitive to acyclovir.

Cidofovir is a nucleotide analog that is active against all human herpesviruses. The drug has a prolonged pharmacokinetic intracellular half-life, allowing for administration every 1–2 weeks. Phosphorylation of cidofovir to its active form does not depend on viral enzymes. Thus, strains of cytomegalovirus, herpes simplex virus, and herpes zoster virus that are resistant to ganciclovir or acyclovir often are sensitive to cidofovir. Cidofovir delays progression of CMV retinitis in newly diagnosed disease (5 mg/kg weekly for 2 weeks, followed by maintenance of 3–5 mg/kg every other week) and is effective therapy in relapsed disease or in patients who are intolerant of traditional therapy (5 mg/kg every other day). Limited data suggest that direct intravitreal injection (20 μg every 5–6 weeks) of cidofovir is also effective for initial and maintenance therapy. Cidofovir gel (as 3% or 1%) topically applied to mucocutaneous herpetic lesions in AIDS patients unresponsive to oral or intravenous acyclovir provides benefit in healing. Cidofovir is associated with a high incidence of nephrotoxicity, sometimes severe. To avoid nephrotoxicity, probenecid and intravenous saline must be administered with each dose.

Ribavirin aerosol is potentially useful in the treatment of respiratory syncytial virus infections in bone marrow transplant patients. It is not known whether the addition of immune globulin provides additional benefit. Intravenous ribavirin can significantly lower the fatality rate of Lassa fever and has been used as a therapeutic agent for hantavirus pneumonia. However, the benefit in hantavirus infection is unclear. The drug is teratogenic in animals, and pregnant women should not take care of patients receiving the aerosol.

Ganciclovir is an analog of acyclovir that has broad antiviral activity, including activity against CMV. The drug is efficacious in the therapy of CMV retinitis in AIDS patients, but once therapy is stopped, the relapse rate is high, and long-term maintenance suppressive therapy is required. Direct intravitreal injection of ganciclovir (400 mg) weekly is as efficacious as systemic therapy for maintenance. Ganciclovir has a modest effect on CMV colitis in AIDS patients. Ganciclovir at a dosage of 5 mg/kg every 12 hours for 14 days decreases the incidence of positive cultures and improves the appearance of the colon compared with placebo, but diarrhea, weight loss, and fever are unaffected. In bone marrow transplant recipients with CMV gastroenteritis (esophagitis, gastritis, duodenitis), ganciclovir is no better than placebo in relief of symptoms. Therapy of CMV pneumonitis with this agent has been disappointing. Studies of small numbers of patients have suggested that the addition of intravenous immunoglobulin or CMV immune globulin to ganciclovir may improve CMV pneumonitis. CMV viremia and hepatitis are often self-limited diseases, and the role of ganciclovir in treating these syndromes awaits clarification. However, because CMV viremia often predicts the presence of invasive disease, it is usually treated when it occurs. Ganciclovir is most efficacious as a prophylactic agent. Administration of ganciclovir for 100–120 days to seropositive bone marrow transplant recipients decreases the incidence of CMV disease. Similar results have been demonstrated in heart and liver transplant recipients treated for 28 days. In renal transplant patients, ganciclovir during periods of maximum immunosuppression (ie, when antilymphocyte antibody therapy is administered for rejection) prevents development of disease in seropositive individuals. Although ganciclovir alone is not effective in the therapy of CMV pneumonia, if the drug is initiated when asymptomatic viral excretion occurs (as determined by a positive culture in bronchoalveolar lavage) in bone marrow transplant patients, there is a marked reduction in the subsequent development of pneumonia. It should be emphasized that regimens employing high-dose intravenous and oral acyclovir have also been shown to be effective in preventing CMV disease following bone marrow, liver, and renal transplants. In practice, most high-risk solid organ transplant recipients receive ganciclovir intravenously for 10–14 days posttransplant followed by high-dose acyclovir therapy (800 mg four or five times daily adjusted for renal insufficiency) for 3–4 months or oral ganciclovir (1 g three times daily in donor-positive, recipient-negative transplant patients; see below). Because of the profound immunosuppression associated with bone marrow transplantation, following engraftment (usually at 1 month), intravenous ganciclovir, 5 mg/kg/d three times a week, is given for the first 100–120 days posttransplant, at which time high-dose acyclovir is given for an additional year. An alternative approach in the marrow transplant patient is to follow patients without therapy and to do surveillance cultures of blood (buffy coat) every 2–4 weeks or assay the blood for the presence of CMV DNA by antigen detection or PCR. If cultures are positive or CMV DNA is detected, therapy with ganciclovir, 5 mg/kg twice daily, is initiated.

The major adverse effect is neutropenia, which is reversible but requires dosage reduction. Thrombocytopenia, disorientation, nausea, rash, and phlebitis occur less commonly.

Oral ganciclovir has poor bioavailability, with maximum absorption of only 6–9% when taken with food. After a dose of 1 g, peak serum levels are about 1 μg/mL (clinical isolates of CMV are inhibited by 0.02–3.5 μg/mL). Controlled clinical studies indicate that the oral drug in a dose of 1 g three times a day is slightly less effective than intravenous ganciclovir, 5 mg/kg daily as maintenance therapy for CMV retinitis (time to progression is 5–12 days shorter in those treated with the oral drug). Thus, in selected populations with peripheral non-sight-threatening lesions, oral ganciclovir maintenance may be convenient and effective therapy compared with long-term intravenous therapy. Because of its poor bioavailability, oral ganciclovir is unlikely to be effective as primary therapy for active CMV infection. An esterified ganciclovir preparation currently under investigation is associated with significantly improved oral bioavailability. The role of oral ganciclovir in prevention of CMV infection following bone marrow or solid organ transplantation has not been well studied, but preliminary data in liver transplant recipients suggest that oral ganciclovir, 1 g three times daily for 3 months, was efficacious in preventing CMV disease when compared with placebo (4% versus 17%).

Vitrasert is a polymer impregnated with 6 mg of ganciclovir that has been designed to allow for the slow release of 1 or 2 mg per hour. The 2.5 mm disk is implanted into the affected eye in a minor outpatient surgical procedure. Limited studies in HIV-positive individuals with CMV retinitis have indicated that the device is about 90% effective in preventing disease progression when used as initial therapy or when used in those who have previously failed intravenous therapy. Implants last about 4–8 months depending upon rate of release of drug. Complications can occur. The most common is blurred vision, which usually only lasts 2–4 weeks after implantation. Other less common complications include retinal detachment, vitreal hemorrhage, and endophthalmitis secondary to the surgical procedure. The obvious advantage of not requiring intravenous therapy may be offset by the local delivery of drug and the risk of developing disease in the contralateral eye, which occurred in 67% of patients in one study. In patients not receiving highly active antiretroviral therapy, addition of oral ganciclovir reduces the incidence of new disease and delays the progression of retinitis.

Lamivudine (3TC), a well-tolerated oral antiviral nucleoside analog used in treatment of HIV infection, is effective against hepatitis B. Once-daily therapy (100 mg) for a year results in clinical, serologic, and histologic improvement in approximately 50% of patients. Therapy post liver transplantation is associated with a reduced risk of reinfection with hepatitis B.

Human interferons. Interferons have been prepared from stimulated lymphocytes and more recently by DNA recombinant technology. These agents have antiviral, antitumor, and immunoregulatory properties. The most common uses of these agents include therapy of chronic hepatitis due to hepatitis B, C, and D (see Chapter 15). Ribavirin in combination with interferon is more effective than interferon monotherapy in the treatment of chronic hepatitis C infection. Interferons are also efficacious in condyloma acuminatum, as prophylaxis against infection in patients with chronic granulomatous disease, and for therapy of a number of malignancies such as hairy cell leukemia, Kaposi's sarcoma in AIDS, chronic myelogenous leukemia, multiple myeloma, renal cell carcinoma, and others, as well as in therapy for relapsing multiple sclerosis. Other potential uses are for therapy of certain intracellular pathogens such as leprosy, atypical mycobacterial infection, toxoplasmosis, and leishmaniasis. Relapse of the underlying disease after cessation of therapy is common but usually responds to reinstitution of drug. Adverse effects are common and include an influenza-like illness with fever, chills, nausea, vomiting, headache, arthralgia, and myalgias. Bone marrow suppression, especially with high-dose therapy, has also been reported.

Balfour HH: Antiviral drugs. N Engl J Med 1999;340:1255. [NLM Cit ID: 99211820] (Review of activity, dosing, clinical indications, and toxicity.)

Gubareva LV et al: Influenza virus neuraminidase inhibitors. Lancet 2000;355:827. [NLM Cit ID: 20175104]

Keating MR: Antiviral agents for non-human immunodeficiency virus infections. Mayo Clin Proc 1999;74:1266. [NLM Cit ID 20058930]

Whitley RJ et al: Herpes simplex viruses. Clin Infect Dis 1998;26:541. [NLM Cit ID: 98185509]

RELEVANT WORLD WIDE WEB SITES

[Drugs in Development WebDatabase]
http://www.phrma.org/webdb/help.htm

38 Disorders Due to Physical Agents

See http://www.current-med.com/ch38.html for updated addresses of Web sites referenced in this chapter.

Richard Cohen, MD, MPH, & Brent R.W. Moelleken, MD

DISORDERS DUE TO COLD

Cold tolerance varies considerably among individuals. Factors that increase the likelihood of injury from exposure to cold include poor general physical conditioning, nonacclimatization, advanced age, systemic illness, poor tissue oxygenation, wet or insufficient clothing, previous cold weather injury, and the use of alcohol or other sedative drugs. High wind velocity ("windchill factor") increases the severity of cold injury at low temperatures.

Cold Urticaria

Some persons have a familial or acquired hypersensitivity to cold and may develop urticaria upon even limited exposure to a cold wind. The urticaria usually occurs only on exposed areas, but in markedly sensitive individuals the response can be generalized. Immersion in cold water may result in severe systemic symptoms, including shock. Recognition of the disorder is important because it has been responsible for deaths from swimming in cold water. Familial cold urticaria, manifested as a burning sensation of the skin occurring about 30 minutes after exposure to cold, does not seem to be a true urticarial disorder. In some patients with acquired cold urticaria, the disorder may be associated with the administration of drugs such as griseofulvin or with infections such as infectious mononucleosis. Cold urticaria may occur secondarily to cryoglobulinemia. Cold urticaria may be associated with cold hemoglobinuria as a complication of syphilis. In most cases of acquired cold urticaria, the cause is not known. For diagnosis, an ice cube is usually applied to the skin of the forearm for 4–5 minutes, then removed, and the area is observed for 10 minutes. As the skin rewarms, an urticarial wheal appears at the site and may be accompanied by itching. Histamine and other mediators released in the cold urticaria response are similar to those found in allergic reactions. Cyproheptadine, 16–32 mg/d in divided doses, is the drug of choice for cold urticaria. As an alternative, a combination of terbutaline, 5 mg three times daily, and aminophylline, 150 mg three times daily, has been recommended.

Raynaud's Phenomenon

See Chapter 12.

ACCIDENTAL SYSTEMIC HYPOTHERMIA

Systemic hypothermia may result from exposure (atmospheric or immersion) to prolonged or extreme cold. The condition may arise in otherwise healthy individuals in the course of occupational or recreational exposure or in victims of accidents.

Systemic hypothermia may follow exposure even to cool but not cold temperatures when there is altered homeostasis due to debility or disease. In colder climates, elderly and inactive individuals living in inadequately heated housing are particularly susceptible. Acute alcoholism is commonly a predisposing cause. Patients with cardiovascular or cerebrovascular disease, mental retardation, malnutrition, myxedema, and hypopituitarism are more vulnerable to accidental hypothermia. The use of sedative and tranquilizing drugs may be a contributing factor. Prolonged postoperative hypothermia with increased mortality rates after surgery has been reported, especially in elderly patients. Administration of large amounts of refrigerated stored blood (without rewarming) can cause systemic hypothermia.

Pathogenesis

Systemic hypothermia is a reduction of core (rectal) body temperature below 35 °C. It causes reduced physiologic function—with decreased oxygen consumption and slowed myocardial repolarization, peripheral nerve conduction, gastrointestinal motility, and respirations—as well as hemoconcentration and pancreatitis. The body defends itself against cold exposure by superficial blood vessel constriction and increased metabolic heat production.

Clinical Findings

Early manifestations of hypothermia are not specific. There may be weakness, drowsiness, lethargy, irritability, confusion, shivering, and impaired coordination. A lowered body temperature may be the sole finding; the skin may appear blue or puffy.

The internal (core) body temperature in accidental hypothermia may range from 25 to 35 °C. Oral temperatures are useless, so an esophageal or rectal probe that reads as low as 25 °C is required. At core temperatures below 35 °C, the patient may become delirious, drowsy, or comatose and may stop breathing. Indeed, the pulse and blood pressure may be unobtainable, leading clinicians to believe the patient is dead. Metabolic acidosis, hyperkalemia, pneumonia, pancreatitis, ventricular fibrillation, hypoglycemia or hyperglycemia, coagulopathy, and renal failure may occur. Abnormalities in cardiac rhythm are directly related to the lowering of core temperature; cardiac arrhythmias may occur, especially during the rewarming process. Progression of electrocardiographic abnormalities can also occur, including the pathognomonic J wave of Osborn—a second upward wave immediately following the S wave, which has been well described in lead II (Figure 38–1). Death in systemic hypothermia usually results from cardiac asystole or ventricular fibrillation.

Treatment (Figure 38–2)

Patients with mild hypothermia (rectal temperature > 33 °C) who have been otherwise healthy usually respond well to a warm bed or to rapid passive rewarming with a warm bath or warm packs and blankets. A conservative approach is also usually employed in treating elderly or debilitated patients, using an electric blanket kept at 37 °C. Gentle handling and movement of the patient are essential to avoid triggering arrhythmias.

Patients with moderate or severe hypothermia (core temperatures of < 33 °C) do not have the thermoregulatory shivering mechanism and so require active rewarming with individualized supportive care. Adequate cardiovascular support, acid-base balance, arterial oxygenation, and adequate intravascular volume should be established prior to rewarming to minimize the risk of organ infarction and "afterdrop" (recurrent hypothermia). The methods and rate of active rewarming are controversial. Successful treatment usually includes a combination of active external and internal methods (see below). Aggressive rewarming should be attempted only by those experienced in the methods. *Once begun, CPR should continue until the patient has been rewarmed to at least 32 °C.* The need for oxygen therapy, endotracheal intubation, controlled ventilation, warmed intravenous fluids, and treatment of metabolic acidosis should be dictated by careful clinical and laboratory monitoring during the rapid rewarming process. Essential laboratory tests include complete blood count, prothrombin time, partial thromboplastin time, electrolytes, blood urea nitrogen, serum creatinine, liver function tests,

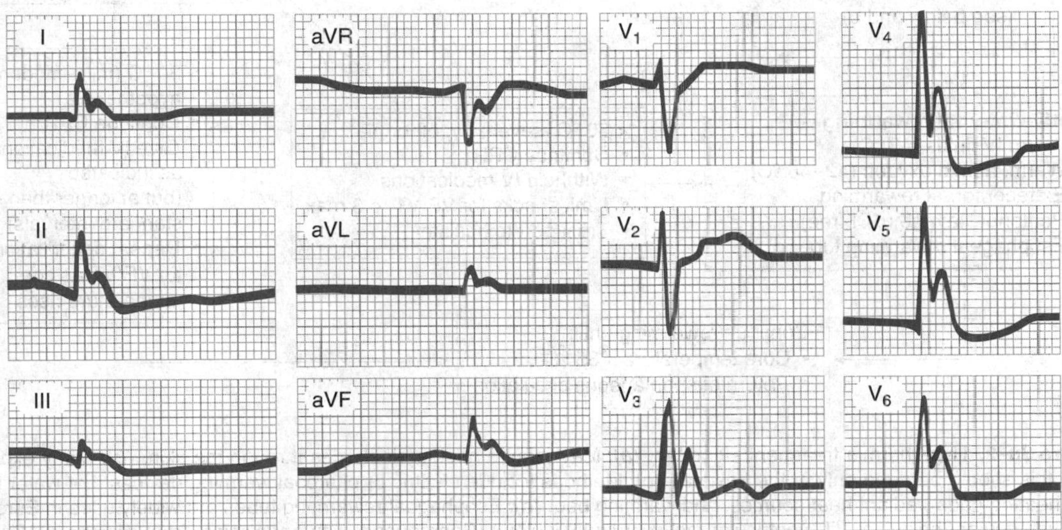

Figure 38–1. Hypothermia. The ventricular rate is 50/min. Atrial activity is not seen. The QRS complexes are narrow and are deformed at their terminal portions by a slurred wave occurring prior to the inscription of the ST–T waves; this is the J wave. The QT interval is prolonged. (Courtesy of R Brindis. Reproduced, with permission from Goldschlager N, Goldman MJ: *Principles of Clinical Electrocardiography,* 13th ed. Originally published by Appleton & Lange. Copyright © 1989 by The McGraw-Hill Companies, Inc.)

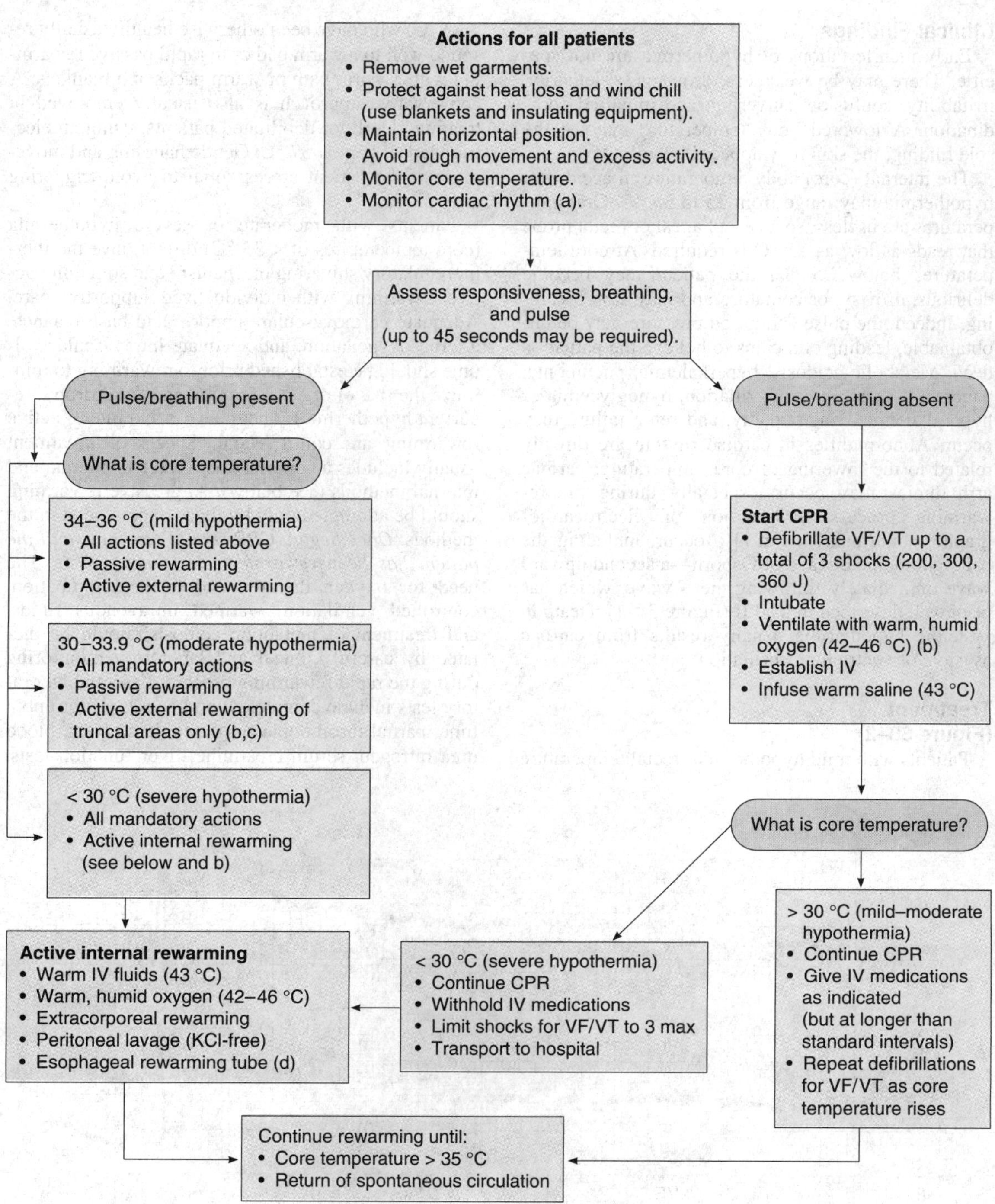

Figure 38–2. Hypothermia treatment algorithm. ***(a):*** May require needle electrodes through the skin. ***(b):*** Many experts think this should be done only in the hospital. ***(c):*** Methods include electric or charcoal warming devices, hot water bottles, heating pads, radiant heat sources, and warming bed. ***(d):*** Esophageal rewarming tubes are widely used in Europe. (VF, ventricular fibrillation; VT, ventricular tachycardia; J, joules.) (Reproduced, with permission, from Weinberg AD: Hypothermia. Ann Emerg Med 1993;22:370.)

amylase, glucose, pH, blood gases, urinalysis, and urine volume. Cardiac rhythm should be monitored, and cardiac, central vascular, or chest trauma or stimulation (catheter, cannulas, etc) should be avoided unless essential because of the risk of inducing ventricular fibrillation. However, patients who are comatose or in respiratory failure should be tracheally intubated. The patient should be evaluated for trauma and peripheral cold injury (eg, frostbite). Antibiotics are not routinely given and should be used only if indicated (neonate, elderly, or immunocompromised patient). Core temperature (esophageal preferred over rectal) should be monitored frequently during and after initial rewarming because of reports of recurrent hypothermia.

A. Active External Rewarming Methods: Heated blankets, forced hot air, radiant heat cradles, or warm baths may be used for active external rewarming. Rewarming by a warm bath is best done in a tub of moving water at 40–42 °C, with a rate of rewarming of about 1–2 °C/h. It is easier, however, to monitor the patient and to perform diagnostic and therapeutic procedures when heated blankets are used for active rewarming. Although relatively simple and generally available, active external warming methods may cause marked peripheral dilation that predisposes to ventricular fibrillation and hypovolemic shock and should be accompanied by core rewarming in moderate to severe hypothermia.

Forced air rewarming (38–43 °C) is recommended for clinic or field use when extracorporeal blood rewarming is not available.

B. Active Internal (Core) Rewarming Methods: Internal rewarming is essential for patients with severe hypothermia; extracorporeal blood rewarming (cardiopulmonary, venovenous, or femorofemoral bypass) is the treatment of choice, especially in the presence of cardiac arrest. Repeated peritoneal dialysis may be employed with 2 L of warm (43 °C) potassium-free dialysate solution exchanged at intervals of 10–12 minutes until the core temperature is raised to about 35 °C. Parenteral fluids (D_5 normal saline) should be warmed to 43 °C prior to administration. Heated, humidified air warmed to 42 °C through a face mask or endotracheal tube may be administered. Warm colonic and gastrointestinal irrigations are of less value.

Prognosis

With proper early care, more than 75% of otherwise healthy patients may survive moderate or severe systemic hypothermia. Prognosis is directly related to the severity of metabolic acidosis; if the pH is 6.6 or less, the prognosis is poor. The risk of aspiration pneumonia is great in comatose patients. The prognosis is grave if there are underlying predisposing causes or if treatment is delayed.

HYPOTHERMIA OF THE EXTREMITIES

Exposure of the extremities to cold produces immediate localized vasoconstriction followed by generalized vasoconstriction. When the skin temperature falls to 25 °C, tissue metabolism is slowed, but the demand for oxygen is greater than the slowed circulation can supply, and the area becomes cyanotic. At 15 °C, tissue metabolism is markedly decreased and the dissociation of oxyhemoglobin is reduced; this gives a deceptive pink, well-oxygenated appearance to the skin. Tissue damage occurs at this temperature. Tissue death may be caused by ischemia and thromboses in the smaller vessels or by actual freezing. Freezing (frostbite) does not occur until the skin temperature drops to –4 to –10 °C or even lower, depending on such factors as wind, mobility, venous stasis, malnutrition, and occlusive arterial disease. Neuropathic sequelae such as pain, numbness, tingling, hyperhidrosis, cold sensitivity of the extremities, and nerve conduction abnormalities may persist for many years after the cold injury.

Prevention

"Keep warm, keep moving, and keep dry." Individuals should wear warm, dry clothing, preferably several layers, with a windproof outer garment. Wet clothing, socks, and shoes should be replaced with dry ones. Extra socks, mittens, and insoles should always be carried in a pack in cold or icy areas. Cramped positions, constricting clothing, and prolonged dependency of the feet are to be avoided. Arms, legs, fingers, and toes should be exercised to maintain circulation. Wet and muddy ground and exposure to wind should be avoided. Tobacco and alcohol should be avoided when the danger of frostbite is present.

CHILBLAIN (Erythema Pernio)

Chilblains are red, itching skin lesions, usually on the extremities, caused by exposure to cold without actual freezing of the tissues. They may be associated with edema or blistering and are aggravated by warmth. With continued exposure, ulcerative or hemorrhagic lesions may appear and progress to scarring, fibrosis, and atrophy. Chilblain lupus erythematosus, while clinically similar to ordinary chilblain, can be differentiated by an association with other lupus manifestations or by biopsy.

Treatment consists of elevating the affected part slightly and allowing it to warm gradually at room temperature. Do not rub or massage injured tissues or apply ice or heat. Protect the area from trauma and secondary infection. Prazosin, 1 mg daily, has been recommended for treatment and prevention of recurrence.

FROSTBITE

Frostbite is injury due to freezing and formation of ice crystals within tissues. In mild cases, only the skin and subcutaneous tissues are involved; the symptoms are numbness, prickling, and itching. With increasing severity, deep frostbite involves deeper structures, and there may be paresthesia and stiffness. Thawing causes tenderness and burning pain. The skin is white or yellow, loses its elasticity, and becomes immobile. Edema, blisters, necrosis, and gangrene may appear. MRI with magnetic resonance angiography and triple-phase bone scanning have been used to assess the degree of involvement in severe frostbite and to distinguish viable from nonviable tissue.

Treatment

A. Immediate Treatment: Treat the patient for associated systemic hypothermia.

1. Rewarming–Superficial frostbite (frostnip) of extremities in the field can be treated by firm steady pressure with the warm hand (without rubbing), by placing fingers in the armpits, and, in the case of the toes or heels, by removing footwear, drying feet, rewarming, and covering with adequate dry socks or other protective footwear.

Rapid thawing at temperatures slightly above body heat may significantly decrease tissue necrosis. If there is any possibility of refreezing, the frostbitten part should not be thawed, even if this might mean prolonged walking on frozen feet. Refreezing results in increased tissue necrosis. Rewarming is best accomplished by immersing the frozen portion of the body for several minutes in a moving water bath heated to 40–42 °C until the distal tip of the part being thawed flushes. Water in this temperature range feels warm but not hot to the normal hand. Dry heat (eg, stove or open fire) is more difficult to regulate and is not recommended. After thawing has occurred and the part has returned to normal temperature (usually in about 30 minutes), discontinue external heat. Victims and rescue workers should be cautioned not to attempt rewarming by exercise or thawing of frozen tissues by rubbing with snow or ice water.

A protocol for treatment of frostbite is presented in Figure 38–3.

2. Protection of the part–Pressure or friction is avoided and physical therapy contraindicated in the early stage. The patient is kept at bed rest with the affected parts elevated and uncovered at room temperature. Casts, dressings, or bandages are not applied. A combination of ibuprofen, 200 mg four times daily, and aloe vera has been used to prevent dermal ischemia.

3. Anti-infective measures–Consider tetanus prophylaxis; frostbite increases susceptibility. Protect skin blebs from physical contact. Local infections may be treated with mild soaks of soapy water or povidone-iodine. Whirlpool therapy at 37–40 °C twice daily for 15–20 minutes for a period of 3 or more weeks helps cleanse the skin and debrides superficial sloughing tissue. Antibiotics may be required for deep infections.

B. Follow-Up Care: Gentle, progressive physical therapy to promote circulation should be instituted as soon as tolerated.

C. Surgery: Early regional sympathectomy (within 36–72 hours) has been reported to protect against the sequelae of frostbite, but the value of this measure is controversial. In general, other surgical intervention is to be avoided. *Amputation should not be considered until it is definitely established that the tissues are dead.* Tissue necrosis (even with black eschar formation) may be quite superficial, and *the underlying skin may sometimes heal spontaneously even after a period of months.*

Prognosis

Recovery from frostbite is most often complete, but there may be increased susceptibility to discomfort in the involved extremity upon reexposure to cold.

IMMERSION SYNDROME (Immersion Foot or Trench Foot)

Immersion foot (or hand) is caused by prolonged immersion in cool or cold water or mud, usually less than 10 °C. The affected parts are first cold and anesthetic (prehyperemic stage). They become hot with intense burning and shooting pains during the hyperemic stage and pale or cyanotic with diminished pulsations during the vasospastic period (posthyperemic stage); blistering, swelling, redness, heat, ecchymoses, hemorrhage, necrosis, peripheral nerve injury, or gangrene and secondary complications such as lymphangitis, cellulitis, and thrombophlebitis can occur later.

Treatment is best instituted during the stage of reactive hyperemia. Immediate treatment consists of air drying, protecting the extremities from trauma and secondary infection, and gradual rewarming by exposure to air at room temperature (not ice or heat) without massaging or moistening the skin or immersing it in water. Bed rest is required until all ulcers have healed. Affected parts are elevated to aid in removal of edema fluid, and pressure sites (eg, heels) are protected with pillows. Later treatment is as for Buerger's disease (see Chapter 12).

Hanania NA et al: Accidental hypothermia. Crit Care Clin 1999;15:235. [NLM Cit ID: 99261511] (Diagnosis and treatment of systemic hypothermia.)

Koller R et al: Deep accidental hypothermia and cardiac arrest: Rewarming with forced air. Acta Anaesthesiol Scand 1997;41:1359. [NLM Cit ID 98082769] (Resuscitation and rewarming.)

Mair P et al: Case 5–1997. Successful resuscitation of a patient with severe accidental hypothermia and prolonged

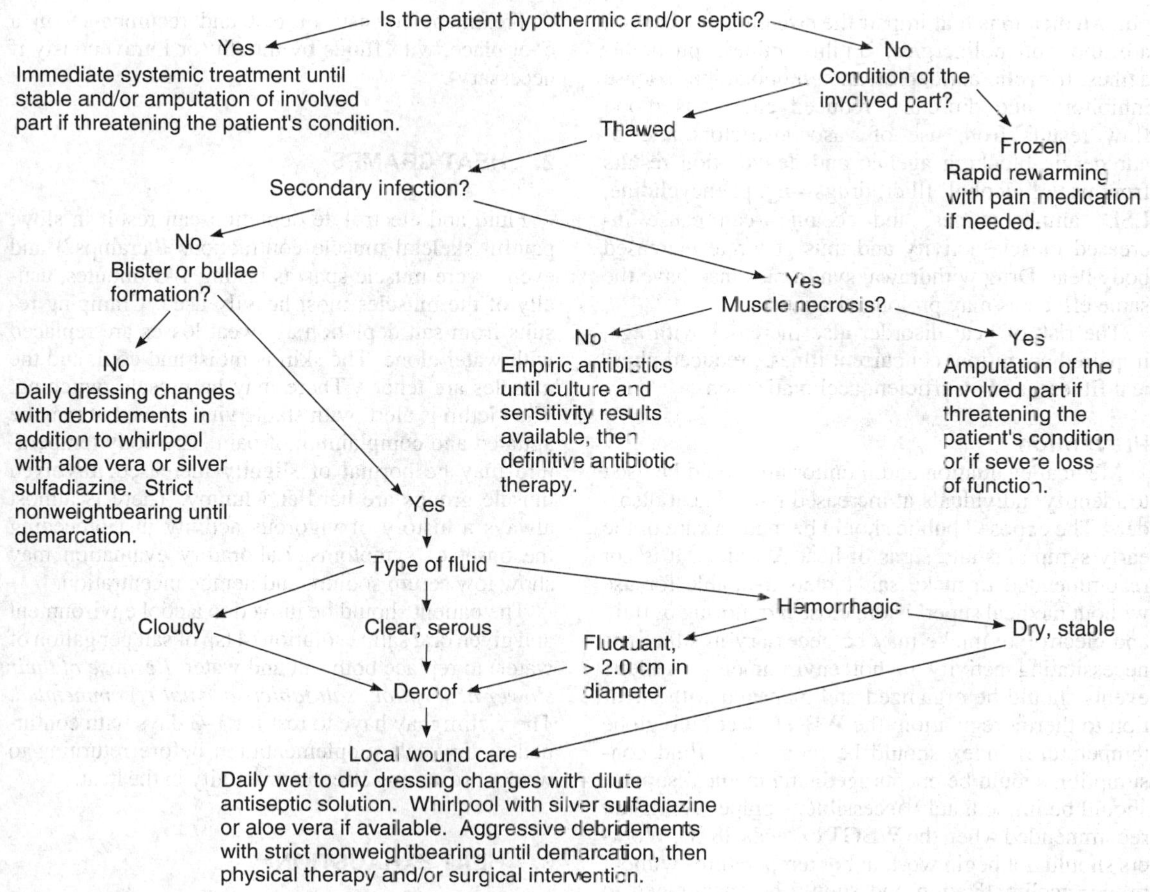

Figure 38–3. Treatment protocol for frostbite. (Modified and reproduced, with permission, from Pulla RJ et al: Frostbite: An overview with case presentations. J Foot Ankle Surg 1994;33:56.)

cardiocirculatory arrest using cardiopulmonary bypass. J Cardiothoracic Vasc Anesthesia 1997;11:901. [NLM Cit ID: 98074375] (Description of rewarming procedures.)

Reamy BV: Frostbite: Review and current concepts. J Am Board Fam Pract 1998;11:34. [NLM Cit ID: 98117561] (Pathophysiology, diagnosis, and treatment.)

DISORDERS DUE TO HEAT

Four medical disorders (listed here in order of increasing severity) comprise a spectrum of illness that can result from excessive exposure to hot environments: heat syncope, heat cramps, heat exhaustion, and heat stroke. A stable internal temperature requires a balance between heat production and heat loss, which the hypothalamus regulates by initiating changes in muscle tone, vascular tone, and sweat gland function.

Etiology

Sweat production and evaporation is a major mechanism of heat removal. Conduction (convection)—the direct transfer of heat from the skin to the surrounding air—also occurs, but with diminished efficiency as the ambient temperature rises. The passive transfer of heat from a warmer to a cooler object by radiation accounts for 65% of body heat loss under normal conditions. Radiant heat loss decreases as the temperature of the surrounding environment increases up to 37.2 °C, the point at which heat transfer reverses direction. At normal temperatures, evaporation accounts for approximately 20% of the body's heat loss, but at high temperatures it becomes the major mechanism for dissipation of heat; with vigorous exertion, sweat loss can be as much as 2.5 L/h. This mechanism is also limited as humidity increases.

Health conditions that inhibit sweat production or evaporation and increase susceptibility to heat disorders include obesity, generalized skin diseases (miliaria), diminished cutaneous blood flow, dehydration, malnutrition, hypotension, and reduced cardiac output. Medications that impair the sweating mechanism are the anticholinergics, antihistamines, phenothiazines, tricyclic antidepressants, monoamine oxidase inhibitors, and diuretics; reduced cutaneous blood flow results from use of vasoconstrictors and β-adrenergic blocking agents; and dehydration results from use of alcohol. Illicit drugs—eg, phencyclidine, LSD, amphetamines, and cocaine—can cause increased muscle activity and thus generate increased body heat. Drug withdrawal syndromes may have the same effect, as may prolonged seizures.

The risk of heat disorder also increases with age, impaired cognition, concurrent illness, reduced physical fitness, and insufficient acclimatization.

Prevention

Medical evaluation and monitoring should be used to identify individuals at increased risk of heat disorders. The exposed public should be made aware of the early symptoms and signs of heat disorders. It is not recommended to make salt tablets available for use without medical supervision; close monitoring of fluid and electrolyte intake may be necessary in situations necessitating activity in hot environments. Athletic events should be organized and managed with attention to thermoregulation: the WBGT (wet bulb globe temperature) Index should be monitored, fluid consumption should be encouraged, and medical support should be immediately accessible. Competition is not recommended when the WBGT exceeds 28 °C. Workers should not begin work in hot temperatures without proper acclimatization and should be encouraged to drink water or balanced electrolyte fluids frequently.

Protective cooled suits have been used successfully in industry for prolonged work in environments up to 60 °C.

Acclimatization is achieved by scheduled regulated exposure to hot environments and by gradually increasing the duration of exposure and the work load until the body adjusts by starting to produce sweat of lower salt content in greater amounts at lower ambient temperatures. Acclimatization is accompanied by increased plasma volume, cardiac output, and cardiac stroke volume and a slower heart rate.

SPECIFIC SYNDROMES DUE TO HEAT EXPOSURE

1. HEAT SYNCOPE

Sudden unconsciousness can result from cutaneous vasodilation with consequent systemic and cerebral hypotension. Systolic blood pressure is usually less than 100 mm Hg, and there is typically a history of vigorous physical activity for 2 hours or more just preceding the episode. The skin is typically cool and moist, and the pulse is weak.

Treatment consists of rest and recumbency in a cool place, with fluids by mouth (or intravenously if necessary).

2. HEAT CRAMPS

Fluid and electrolyte depletion can result in slow, painful skeletal muscle contractions ("cramps") and even severe muscle spasms lasting 1–3 minutes, usually of the muscles most heavily used. Cramping results from salt depletion as sweat losses are replaced with water alone. The skin is moist and cool, and the muscles are tender. There may be muscle twitching. The victim is alert, with stable vital signs, but may be agitated and complaining of pain. The body temperature may be normal or slightly increased. Involved muscle groups are hard and lumpy. There is almost always a history of vigorous activity just preceding the onset of symptoms. Laboratory evaluation may show low serum sodium and hemoconcentration.

The patient should be moved to a cool environment and given oral saline solution (4 tsp of salt per gallon of water) to replace both salt and water. *Because of their slower absorption, salt tablets are not recommended.* The victim may have to rest for 1–3 days with continued dietary salt supplementation before returning to work or resuming strenuous activity in the heat.

3. HEAT EXHAUSTION

Heat exhaustion results from prolonged heavy activity with inadequate salt intake in a hot environment and is characterized by dehydration, sodium depletion, or isotonic fluid loss with accompanying cardiovascular changes.

The diagnosis is based on prolonged symptoms and a rectal temperature over 37.8 °C, increased pulse rate—usually more than half again the patient's normal rate—and moist skin. Symptoms associated with heat syncope and heat cramps may also be present. The patient may be quite thirsty and weak, with central nervous system symptoms such as headache, fatigue, and, in cases due chiefly to water depletion, anxiety, paresthesias, impaired judgment, hysteria, and occasionally psychosis. Hyperventilation secondary to heat exhaustion can lead to respiratory alkalosis. Heat exhaustion may progress to heat stroke if sweating ceases.

Treatment consists of patient location in a shaded, cool environment, providing adequate hydration (1–2 L over 2–4 hours), salt replenishment—orally, if possible—and active cooling (fans, ice packs, etc) if necessary. Physiologic saline or isotonic glucose solution can be administered intravenously in severe cases or when oral administration is not appropriate. Intravenous 3% (hypertonic) saline may be necessary if sodium depletion is severe. At least 24 hours of rest is recommended.

4. HEAT STROKE

Heat stroke is a life-threatening medical emergency resulting from failure of the thermoregulatory mechanism. Heat stroke is imminent when the core (rectal) temperature approaches 41 °C. It presents in one of two forms: Classic heat stroke occurs in patients with compromised homeostatic mechanisms; exertional heat stroke occurs in previously healthy persons undergoing strenuous exertion in a thermally stressful environment. Morbidity or even death can result from cerebral, cardiovascular, hepatic, or renal damage.

The hallmarks of heat stroke are cerebral dysfunction with impaired consciousness, high fever, and absence of sweating. Persons at greatest risk are the very young, the elderly (> age 65) or chronically infirm, and patients receiving medications (eg, anticholinergics, antihistamines, phenothiazines) that interfere with heat-dissipating mechanisms.

Exertional heat stroke and exertion-related illnesses, including rhabdomyolysis, are appearing more frequently as complications of participation by unconditioned amateurs in strenuous athletic activities such as marathon running and triathlon competition.

Clinical Findings

A. Symptoms and Signs: Failure of the heat dissipation mechanism for any reason results in dizziness, weakness, emotional lability, nausea and vomiting, diarrhea, confusion, delirium, blurred vision, convulsions, collapse, and unconsciousness. The skin is hot and initially covered with perspiration. Later it dries. The pulse is strong initially. Blood pressure may be slightly elevated at first, but hypotension develops later. The core temperature is usually over 41 °C. As with heat exhaustion, hyperventilation can occur, leading to respiratory alkalosis.

Exertional heat stroke may present with sudden collapse and loss of consciousness followed by irrational behavior. Anhidrosis may not be present. Twenty-five percent of heat stroke victims have prodromal symptoms for minutes to hours that may include dizziness, weakness, nausea, confusion, disorientation, drowsiness, and irrational behavior.

B. Laboratory Findings: Laboratory evaluation may reveal dehydration, leukocytosis, elevated BUN, hyperuricemia, hemoconcentration, acid-base abnormalities (eg, lactic acidosis), and decreased serum potassium, sodium, calcium, and phosphorus; urine is concentrated, with elevated protein, tubular casts, and myoglobinuria. Thrombocytopenia, increased bleeding and clotting times, fibrinolysis, and consumption coagulopathy may also be present. Rhabdomyolysis and myocardial, hepatic, or renal damage may be identified by elevated serum creatine kinase and aminotransferase levels and BUN and by the presence of anuria, proteinuria, and hematuria. Electrocardiographic findings may include ST–T changes consistent with myocardial ischemia.

Treatment

Treatment is aimed at reducing the core temperature rapidly (within 1 hour) and controlling the secondary effects. Evaporative cooling is rapid and effective and is easily performed in most emergency settings. The patient's clothing should be removed and the entire body sprayed with water (15 °C) while cooled or ambient air is passed across the patient's body with large fans or other means at high velocity (100 ft/min). The patient should be in the lateral recumbent position or supported in a hands-and-knees position to expose as much skin surface as possible to the air. Other alternatives include use of cold wet sheets accompanied by fanning or immersion in chilled water. Cardiopulmonary bypass provides rapid cooling but is often not practical.

Immersion in an ice-water bath as initial treatment is no longer preferred because of its greater potential for complications of hypotension and shivering. However, it should be considered if core temperature is not decreased rapidly in response to other treatment. Alternatives include hand and forearm immersion in cold water, ice packs (groin, axillas, neck), and iced gastric lavage, though these are much less effective than evaporative cooling.

Treatment should be continued until the rectal temperature drops to 39 °C. The temperature remains stable in most cases, but it should continue to be monitored for 24 hours. Chlorpromazine (25–50 mg intravenously) or diazepam (5–10 mg intravenously) can be given initially and then every 4 hours to control shivering and other muscular activity associated with increased heat load. Antipyretics (aspirin, acetaminophen) have no effect on environmentally induced hyperthermia and are contraindicated.

Hypovolemic and cardiogenic shock must be carefully distinguished, as either or both may occur. Central venous or pulmonary artery wedge pressure should be monitored. Five percent dextrose in half-normal or normal saline should be administered for fluid replacement.

The patient should also be observed for renal failure due to rhabdomyolysis, hypokalemia, cardiac arrhythmias, disseminated intravascular coagulation, and hepatic failure. Hypokalemia frequently accompanies heat stroke but may not appear until rehydration. Maintenance of extracellular hydration and electrolyte balance should reduce the risk of renal failure due to rhabdomyolysis. Fluid administration to ensure a high urine output (> 50 mL/h), mannitol administration (0.25 mg/kg), and alkalinizing the urine (intravenous bicarbonate administration, 250 mL of 4%) are recommended. Corticosteroids have not been shown to be of value.

Fluid output should be monitored through the use of an indwelling urinary catheter.

Because sensitivity to high environmental temperature continues in some patients for prolonged periods following an episode of heat stroke, immediate reexposure should be avoided.

Dehydration, rehydration and exercise in the heat. Int J Sports Med 1998;19(Suppl 2):S89. [NLM Cit ID: 98433722] (Proceedings of an International Conference. Pathophysiology, diagnosis and treatment of exercise related heat disorders.)

Khosla R et al: Heat-related illnesses. Crit Care Clin 1999;15:251. [NLM Cit ID: 99261512] (Etiology, pathophysiology, diagnosis, and treatment of heat disorders.)

Montain SJ et al: Fluid replacement recommendations for training in hot weather. Mil Med 1999;164:502. [NLM Cit ID: 99342471] (Fluid replacement guidelines.)

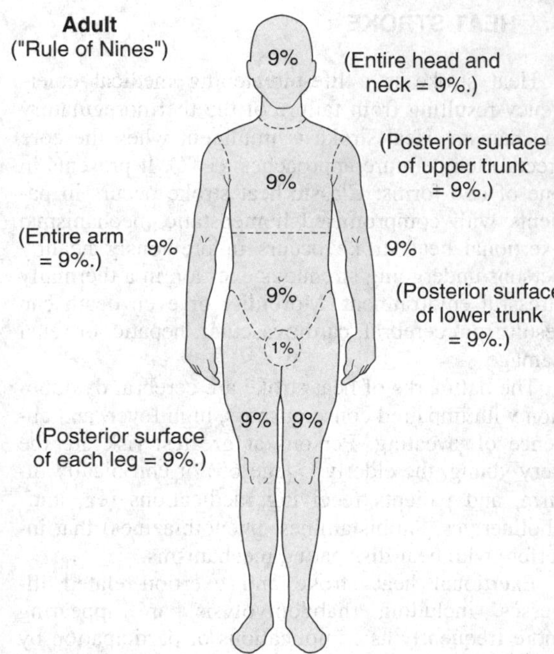

Figure 38–4. Estimation of body surface area in burns.

BURNS

The incidence and severity of burn injuries has been declining, with both deaths and acute hospitalizations attributable to burns down about 50%. Over three-fourths of burns involve less than 10% of total body surface area. Aggressive, early (24–72 hours postburn) excision of deeply burned tissues and skin grafting, early enteral feeding—and improved infection control—have contributed to significantly lower mortality rates and shorter hospitalizations. Nonetheless, an estimated 1.25 million burn injuries and 51,000 acute hospitalizations occur each year in the USA. Severe burns cause problems in the initial phase from hemodynamic compromise, related injuries such as smoke inhalation or fractures, and associated multiorgan failure and sepsis. Later, secondary scarring and constrictive wounds occur.

Significant quality of life and social functionality can be expected even for severely burned patients.

CLASSIFICATION

Burns are classified by extent, depth, patient age, and associated illness or injury.

Extent

The "rule of nines" (Figure 38–4) is useful for rapidly assessing the extent of a burn. More detailed charts based on age are available when the patient reaches the burn unit. Therefore, it is important to view the entire patient after cleaning soot to make an accurate assessment, both initially and on subsequent examinations. Only second- and third-degree burns are included in calculating the total burn surface area (TBSA), since first-degree burns usually do not represent significant injury in terms of prognosis or fluid and electrolyte management. However, first- or second-degree burns may convert to deeper burns, especially if treatment is delayed or bacterial colonization or superinfection occurs.

Depth

Judgment of depth of injury is difficult. The **first-degree burn** may be red or gray but will demonstrate excellent capillary refill. First-degree burns are not blistered initially. If the wound is blistered, this represents a partial-thickness injury to the dermis, or a **second-degree burn.** As the degree of burn is progressively deeper, there is a progressive loss of adnexal structures. Hairs can be easily extracted or are absent, sweat glands become less visible, and the skin appears smoother. The distinction between second- and third-degree burns is unclear and in a sense artificial. Deep second-degree burns are generally treated as full-thickness (third-degree) burns and excised and grafted earlier because of the long time necessary for reepithelialization and the thin, poor quality of the resultant skin. More accurate depth measurement is possible with immunohistochemical analysis.

Age of the Patient

The survival from major burn injury has dramatically increased in the last 20 years. In a large population, the average burn size was 14% of total body surface area, from which 96% of patients survived. Consistently, the three major risk factors for mortality were age greater than 60 years, burn area greater than 40% of total body surface area, and inhalation injury. A simple mortality formula indicates that mortality rates are 0.3%, 3%, 33%, or 90%, depending on whether 0, 1, 2, or 3 of these risk factors are present in the burned patient.

Associated Injuries or Illnesses

An injury commonly associated with burns is smoke inhalation (see Chapter 9). Suspicion of inhalation injury is aroused when the nasal hairs are singed, the mechanism of burn involves closed spaces, the sputum is carbonaceous, or the carboxyhemoglobin level exceeds 5% in nonsmokers. This suspicion should lead the clinician to institute early intubation before airway edema supervenes. The products of combustion, not heat, are responsible for lower airway injury. Electrical injury that causes burns may also produce cardiac arrhythmias that require immediate attention. Pancreatitis occurs in severe burns. Development of hyperamylasemia or hyperlipasemia may signal the development of pancreatic inflammation and subsequent pseudocyst or abscess formation. Prior alcohol exposure may exacerbate the pulmonary components of burn injury.

Toxic epidermal necrolysis (TEN) occasionally occurs following sulfonamide or phenytoin administration (see Chapter 6). If TEN is severe, patients are best transferred to a burn unit and treated as having severe burn injury. Corticosteroid therapy should be avoided.

SYSTEMIC REACTIONS TO BURN INJURY

The actual burn injury is only the incipient event in a cascade of deleterious local tissue and systemic inflammatory reactions leading to multiorgan system failure in the severely burned patient. Locally, substance P, serotonin, prostaglandins E_2 and $F_{2\alpha}$, histamine, platelet-activating factor, nitric oxide, bradykinin, and leukotrienes B_4 and D_4 play a role in the increased local capillary permeability and initiation of the systemic inflammatory cascade. Systemically, levels of interleukin-2, -4, -6, and interferon-gamma (IFN-γ) are elevated in proportion to the severity of the burn injury, perhaps as part of a generalized systemic release of inflammatory mediators. There is often an altered CD4/CD8 (T helper/T suppressor) cell ratio. In addition, in the first 24 hours following a significant burn, there is production of tumor necrosis factor (TNF) and IFN-γ, which in turn stimulate production of the enzyme nitric oxide synthetase in hepatocytes. After 24 hours, lipopolysaccharide (LPS) plays a dominant role in its production. Nitric oxide has been proposed as a mediator of the acute inflammation. Clinical attempts to modify these factors have had mixed success.

INITIAL MANAGEMENT

Airway

The physician or emergency medical technician should proceed as with any other trauma using standard Advanced Trauma Life Support (ATLS) guidelines. The priorities are first to establish an airway, recognizing the frequent necessity to intubate a patient who may appear to be breathing normally but who has sustained an inhalation injury; next, to evaluate the cervical spine and head injuries; and finally, to stabilize fractures. Fluid resuscitation by the Parkland formula (see below) may be instituted simultaneously with initial resuscitation. Endotracheal intubation should be considered for major burn cases regardless of the area of the body involved, because as fluid resuscitation proceeds generalized edema develops, including edema of the soft tissues of the upper airway and perhaps the lungs as well. Chest radiographs are typically normal initially but may develop an acute respiratory distress syndrome picture in 24–48 hours with severe inhalation injury. Supplemental oxygen should be administered. Inhalation injuries should be followed by serial blood gas determination and bronchoscopy. The use of corticosteroids is contraindicated because of the potential for immunosuppression.

Vascular Access

All clothing and jewelry should be removed and an expedient physical examination performed to assess the extent of burn and associated injuries. Simultaneously with the above procedures, venous access must be sought, since the victim of a major burn may develop hypovolemic shock. A percutaneous large-bore (14 or 16 gauge) intravenous line through nonburned skin is preferred. Subclavian lines are avoided in the emergency setting because of the risk of pneumothorax and subclavian vein laceration when such a line is placed in a volume-depleted patient. Femoral lines provide good temporary access during resuscitation. *All lines—without exception—placed in the emergency department should be changed within 24 hours because of the high risk of nonsterile placement.* Distal saphenous cutdown is occasionally necessary. An arterial line is useful for monitoring mean arterial pressure and drawing blood.

FLUID RESUSCITATION

Crystalloids

Generalized capillary leak results from burn injury over more than 25% of total body surface area. This often necessitates replacement of a large volume of fluid.

There are many guidelines for fluid resuscitation. The **Parkland formula** relies upon the use of lactated Ringer's injection. The fluid requirement in the first 24 hours is estimated as 4 mL/kg body weight per percent of body surface area burned. Deep electrical burns and inhalation injury increase the fluid requirement. Adequacy of resuscitation is determined by clinical parameters, including urine output and specific gravity, blood pressure, and central venous catheter or, if necessary, Swan-Ganz catheter readings.

Half the calculated fluid is given in the first 8-hour period. The remaining fluid, divided into two equal parts, is delivered over the next 16 hours. An extremely large volume of fluid may be required. For example, an injury over 40% of the total body surface area in a 70-kg victim may require 13 L *in the first 24 hours.* The first 8-hour period is measured from the hour of injury.

Because it may contribute to renal failure and death, use of hypertonic sodium in resuscitation of burn patients, once thought to be reasonable, has been abandoned in favor of conventional Ringer's lactate.

Colloids

Overly aggressive crystalloid administration must be avoided in patients with pulmonary injury, since significant pulmonary edema can develop in patients with normal pulmonary capillary wedge and central venous pressures. In addition, routine colloid administration, commonplace 5 years ago, must now be considered suspect in routine burn resuscitation in view of its deleterious effect on glomerular filtration and its association with pulmonary edema.

Monitoring Fluid Resuscitation

A Foley catheter is essential for monitoring urinary output. *Diuretics have no role in this phase of patient management unless fluid overload has occurred or mannitol diuresis is performed in the case of rhabdomyolysis.*

Escharotomy

As edema fluid accumulates, ischemia may develop under any constricting eschar of an extremity, neck, or trunk if the full-thickness burn is circumferential. Escharotomy incisions through the anesthetic eschar can save life and limb and can be performed in the emergency department or operating room.

Fasciotomy in Electrical Burns & Associated Crush Injuries

When high-voltage electrical injury occurs, extensive deep tissue necrosis is almost invariably present. Deep tissue necrosis leads to profound tissue swelling. Because deep tissue compartments in the arms and legs are contained by unyielding fascia, these compartments must be opened by surgical fasciotomy to prevent further soft tissue, vascular, and nerve death.

Electrical burn injuries remain the most devastating and underrecognized burn injuries, causing amputations (often because of unrecognized compartment syndromes) and acute renal failure, resulting in part from rhabdomyolysis. Prompt recognition of the severity of electrical burns, with early fasciotomy and debridement, may reduce the incidence of such complications.

THE BURN WOUND

Treatment of the burn wound is based on several principles: (1) Protection from desiccation and further injury of those burned areas that will spontaneously reepithelialize in 7–10 days by application of topical antibiotic such as silver sulfadiazine or mafenide acetate. Silver sulfadiazine is currently the most popular topical agent. It is painless, easy to apply, and effective against most strains of pseudomonas. (2) Regular and thorough cleansing of burned areas is a critically important intervention in burn units. Debridement of burn wounds may be aided by application of collagenase; such treatment may be more effective than silver sulfadiazine treatment alone. (3) Early excision and grafting of burned areas as soon as 24 hours after burn injury or when the patient will hemodynamically tolerate the excision and grafting procedure. Hyperbaric oxygen therapy has not gained wide acceptance.

Systemic infection remains a leading cause of morbidity among major burn patients, with nearly all burn patients having one or more septicemic episodes during their hospital course. Methicillin-resistant *Staphylococcus aureus,* pseudomonas species, klebsiella species, proteus species, methicillin-resistant *S epidermidis,* and acinetobacter remain commonly cultured microorganisms. Typically, gram-positive organisms predominate early in the clinical course, followed later by gram-negative organisms. Continuous microbiologic surveillance is necessary. There is an increasing trend toward use of prophylactic antibiotics in burn patients. Prophylactic administration of trimethoprim-sulfamethoxazole may help to prevent methicillin-resistant *Staphylococcus aureus* (MRSA) infection in ventilator-dependent burn patients. Systemic infections are manifestations of a globally suppressed immune system. Nitric oxide has been implicated in the depressed lymphoproliferative state in experimental animals. Increasingly, sterile multiple organ failure is regarded as a leading cause of death among severely burned patients. Clinicians must be vigilant for the development of squamous cell carcinoma and keratoacanthoma in burn scars.

Wound Closure

The goal of therapy after fluid resuscitation is closure of the wound. Nature's own blister is the best cover to protect wounds that spontaneously epithelialize in 7–10 days (ie, superficial second-degree burns). Where the blister has been disrupted, silver sulfadiazine, porcine heterografts (preferably fresh, or frozen and meshed), or collagen composite dressings (Biobrane) can be used as skin substitutes. In patients with scald burns—usually no more than superficial partial thickness (first or superficial second-degree) burns—use of Biobrane dressing is recommended. However, in medium partial thickness burn wounds treated by Biobrane dressing, there is a high rate of wound infection. These dressings are temporary and not indicated in deep partial or full-thickness burns or in burns that are heavily colonized or infected. Cadaver homografts can also serve this purpose if available.

Wounds that will not heal spontaneously in 7–10 days (ie, deep second-degree or third-degree burns) are best treated by excision and autograft; otherwise, granulation and infection may develop, and the quality of the skin in regenerated deep partial thickness burns is marginal because of the very thin dermis that emerges. Cultured keratinocytes remain an experimental modality owing to the lack of dermis. Although research is continuing, clinical results have been largely disappointing owing to the poor quality of reconstructed skin. The main usefulness of keratinocytes may be as a temporary dressing.

PATIENT SUPPORT

Burn patients require extensive support. An attempt must be made to maintain normal core body temperature in patients with burns over more than 20% of total body surface area, since the hypermetabolic state of burns is exacerbated by subnormal temperatures. Respiratory injury, sepsis, and multiorgan failure are common. Enteral feedings may be started once the ileus of the resuscitation period has resolved, usually the day after the injury. There is often a markedly increased metabolic rate after burn injury, due in large part to whole body synthesis and increased fatty acid substrate cycles. If the patient does not tolerate low-residue tube feedings, TPN should be started without delay through a central venous catheter. As much as 4000–6000 kcal/d may be required in the postburn period. The metabolic demands are immense. A useful guide is to provide 25 kcal/kg body weight plus 40 kcal per percent of burn surface area. Fat emulsions (Intralipid) given intravenously are useful during the resuscitation period to span the period of ileus. This ileus may be due to mesenteric ischemia mediated by thromboxane A_2. Human growth hormone administration may reduce both nitrogen loss and weight loss in burn patients, though it may cause hyperglycemia and a hypermetabolic state.

Occasionally, burn patients may develop acute respiratory distress syndrome or respiratory failure unresponsive to maximal ventilatory support. Heroic resuscitative measures are sometimes successfully employed, with use of extracorporeal life support (ECLS), in children who would otherwise die of ARDS, inhalation injury, or pneumonia in the postburn period. Early pulmonary dysfunction after severe burn injury is widely recognized. It is now apparent in children that late and permanent pulmonary dysfunction with later obstructive and restrictive lung disease can result from major burn injury.

Prevention of long-term scars remains a formidable problem in seriously burned patients. The tunable pulse-dye laser is emerging as an adjunctive treatment to the usual regimen of steroid injections, silicone patches, compression, and scar revision. Its efficacy is as yet unproved, however—the question remains whether laser therapy to the new vessels that characterize early burn wounds helps in the eventual scars. The role of TGF-β_2 is increasingly implicated as a cytokine that plays a significant role in hypertrophic scar formation.

Early burn care and grafting, splinting, and hand therapy are the result of coordinated care by general, hand, and plastic surgeons, therapists, and nurses. Late burn reconstruction is best dealt with by a plastic and reconstructive surgeon. Recent advances in reconstructive burn surgery include the use of microsurgery to perform muscle and fasciocutaneous flaps and tissue expansion. However, complex reconstructive options such as free tissue transfer involve much higher than normal complication rates when performed in the acutely burned patient. In late reconstruction of burns involving the head and neck, tissue expansion is sometimes used instead of conventional skin grafting, since this technique provides skin most similar to that lost because of the burn. After severe hand burns, function may be aided by expedient splinting or axial pin fixation to prevent flexion contractures and facilitate prompt skin grafting and physical therapy.

Patients who have suffered severe burn injuries can recover to a general health status slightly lower than that of the general population but still have very significant vocational and psychologic problems.

There is research interest in a possible role of antioxidants in early fluid resuscitation in order to prevent free radical-induced tissue damage. Monoclonal antibodies against offending pathogens and growth factors continue to be investigated. Dermal matrix substitutes continue to be developed but remain experimental.

Bang RL et al: Beta-haemolytic Streptococcus infection in burns. Burns 1999;25:242. [NLM Cit ID: 99255209]

Chrysopoulos MT et al: Growth hormone attenuates tumor necrosis factor alpha in burned children. Arch Surg 1999;134:283. [NLM Cit ID: 99186430]

Demling RH et al: Management of partial thickness facial burns: comparison of topical antibiotics and bio-engineered skin substitutes. Burns 1999;25:256. [NLM Cit ID: 99255205]

Demling RH: Comparison of the anabolic effects and complications of human growth hormone and the testosterone analog, oxandrone, after severe burn injury. Burns 1999;25:215. [NLM Cit ID: 99255211]

Ho-Asjoe M et al: Immunohistochemical analysis of burn depth. J Burn Care Rehabil 1999;20:207. [NLM Cit ID: 99271900]

Kimura A et al: Trimethoprim-sulfamethoxazole for the prevention of methicillin-resistant *Staphylococcus aureus* pneumonia in severely burned patients. J Trauma 1998;45:383. [NLM Cit ID: 98380933]

Masson I et al: Role of nitric oxide in depressed lymphoproliferative responses and altered cytokine production following thermal injury in rats. Cell Immunol 1998;186:121. [NLM Cit ID: 98330577]

Patel PJ et al: Elevation in pulmonary neutrophils and prolonged production of pulmonary macrophage inflammatory protein-2 after burn injury with prior alcohol exposure. Am J Respir Cell Mol Biol 1999;20:1229. [NLM Cit ID: 99272464]

Ryan CM et al: Objective estimates of the probability of death from burn injuries. N Engl J Med 1998;338:362. [NLM Cit ID: 98112307]

Saffle JR: Predicting outcomes of burns. N Engl J Med 1998;338:387. [NLM Cit ID: 98112313]

Sheridan RL et al: Death in the burn unit: sterile multiple organ failure. Burns 1998;24:307. [NLM Cit ID: 98351480]

Sheridan RL et al: Long-term outcome of children surviving massive burns. JAMA 2000;283:69. [NLM Cit ID: 20096143]

Yu YM et al: The metabolic basis of the increase in energy expenditure in severely burned patients. JPEN J Parenter Enteral Nutr 1999;23:160. [NLM Cit ID: 99268546]

ELECTRIC SHOCK

The possibility of life-threatening electrical injury exists wherever there is electric power or lightning. The amount and type of current, the duration and area of exposure, and the pathway of the current through the body determine the degree of damage. If the current passes through the heart or brain stem, death may occur immediately owing to ventricular fibrillation or apnea. Current passing through skeletal muscle can cause muscle necrosis and contractions severe enough to result in bone fracture. Current traversing peripheral nerves can cause acute or delayed neuropathy. Delayed effects can include damage to the spinal cord, peripheral nerves, bone, kidneys, and gastrointestinal tract as well as cataracts.

Direct current is less dangerous than alternating current. With alternating currents of 25–300 Hz, low voltages (< 220 Hz) tend to produce ventricular fibrillation; high voltages (> 1000 Hz), respiratory failure; intermediate voltages (220–1000 Hz), both. More than 100 mA of domestic house current (AC) of 110 volts at 60 Hz is, accordingly, dangerous to the heart, since it can cause ventricular fibrillation. DC current contact is more likely to cause asystole.

Lightning injuries differ from high-voltage electric shock injuries in that lightning usually involves higher voltage, briefer duration of contact, asystole rather than ventricular fibrillation, nervous system injury, a shock wave characteristic, and multisystem pathologic involvement.

Electrical burns are of three distinct types: flash (arcing) burns, flame (clothing) burns, and the direct heating effect of tissues by the electric current. The latter lesions are usually sharply demarcated, round or oval, painless yellow-brown areas (Joule burn) with inflammatory reaction. Significant subcutaneous damage can be accompanied by little skin injury, particularly with larger skin surface area electrical contact.

Electric shock may produce loss of consciousness. With recovery there may be muscular pain, fatigue, headache, and nervous irritability. The physical signs vary according to the action of the current. Ventricular fibrillation or respiratory failure (or both) can occur; the patient may be unconscious, pulseless, hypotensive, cold and cyanotic, and without respirations.

Electric shock may be a hazard in equipment that is usually considered to be harmless (eg, home appliances and medical equipment). Proper installation, utilization, and maintenance of equipment by qualified personnel should minimize this hazard.

Treatment

A. Emergency Measures: The victim must be freed from the electric current prior to initiation of CPR or other treatment; the rescuer must be protected. Turn off the power, sever the wire with a dry wooden-handled axe, make a proper ground to divert the current, or drag the victim carefully away by means of dry clothing or a leather belt.

Lightning injury. Victims of lightning injury, in whom coma may last for a few minutes to several days, should receive prompt and sustained artificial resuscitation. This should be continued as long as there is no clinical evidence of brain death.

B. Hospital Measures: Lightning or unstable electric shock victims should be hospitalized when revived and observed for shock, arrhythmia, thrombosis, infarction, sudden cardiac dilation, hemorrhage, and myoglobinuria. A urinalysis, serum CK and CK-MB, and an electrocardiogram should be obtained immediately. Victims should also be evaluated for blunt trauma, dehydration, skin burns, hypertension, posttraumatic stress, acid-base disturbances, and neurologic damage. Indications for hospitalization include significant arrhythmia or electrocardiographic changes, large burn, loss of consciousness, pulmonary or cardiac symptoms, or evidence of significant deep tissue or organ damage. Extra caution is indicated when the electroshock current has followed a transthoracic route (hand to hand or hand to foot).

To counteract fluid losses and myoglobinuria due to electric shock (not lightning) burns, aggressive hydration with Ringer's lactate should seek to achieve a urine output of 50–100 mL/h.

Prognosis

Complications may occur in almost any part of the body but most commonly include sepsis, gangrene requiring limb amputation, or neurologic, cardiac, cognitive, or psychiatric dysfunction.

Buniak B et al: Alteration in gastrointestinal and neurological function after electrical injury: a review of four cases. Am J Gastroenterol 1999;94:1532. [NLM Cit ID: 99290688]

Fish RM: Early predictors of myoglobinuria and acute renal failure following electrical injury. J Emerg Med 1999; 17:783. [NLM Cit ID: 20061332]

Fish RM: Electric injury, Part I: Treatment priorities, subtle diagnostic factors and burns. J Emerg Med 1999;17:977. [NLM Cit ID: 20061332]

Fish RM: Electric injury, Part II: Specific injuries. J Emerg Med 2000;18:27. [NLM Cit ID: 20108431] (Diagnosis and treatment of complications and secondary injuries.)

Jain S et al: Electrical and lightning injuries. Crit Care Clin 1999;15:319. [NLM Cit ID: 99261516] (Epidemiology, pathophysiology, diagnosis, and treatment.)

Rosen CL et al: Early predictors of myoglobinuria and acute renal failure following electrical injury. J Emerg Med 1999;17:783. [NLM Cit ID: 99428036]

IONIZING RADIATION REACTIONS

The effects of ionizing radiation on the body have been observed in clinical use of x-rays and radioactive agents, after occupational or accidental exposure, and following the use of atomic weaponry. The extent of damage due to radiation exposure depends on the quantity of radiation delivered to the body, the dose rate, the organs exposed, the type of radiation (x-rays, neutrons, gamma rays, alpha or beta particles), the duration of exposure, and the energy transfer from the radioactive wave or particle to the exposed tissue. The Chernobyl experience suggests that the best biologic indicators of dose are the duration of the asymptomatic latent period (particularly for nausea or emesis), the severity of early symptoms, the rate of decline of the lymphocyte count, and the number and distribution of dicentric chromosomes in peripheral lymphocytes.

The National Committee on Radiation Protection has established the maximum permissible radiation exposure for occupationally exposed workers over age 18 as 0.1 rem* per week for the whole body (but not to exceed 5 rem per year) and 1.5 rem per week for the hands. (For purposes of comparison, routine chest x-rays deliver from 0.1–0.2 rem.) The FDA has recommended 1 Gy as a threshold for skin-absorbed dose from medical fluoroscopy.

Death after acute lethal radiation exposure is usually due to hematopoietic failure, gastrointestinal mucosal damage, central nervous system damage, widespread vascular injury, or secondary infection. The acute radiation syndrome may be dominated by central nervous system, gastrointestinal, or hematologic manifestations depending on dose and survival. Four hundred to 600 cGy of x-ray or gamma radiation applied to the entire body at one time may be fatal within 60 days; death is usually due to hemorrhage, anemia, and infection secondary to hematopoietic injury. Levels of 1000–3000 cGy to the entire body destroy gastrointestinal mucosa; this leads to toxemia and death within 2 weeks. Total body doses above 3000 cGy cause widespread vascular damage, cerebral anoxia, hypotensive shock, and death within 48 hours.

ACUTE (IMMEDIATE) IONIZING RADIATION EFFECTS ON NORMAL TISSUES

Clinical Findings

A. Injury to Skin and Mucous Membranes: Irradiation may cause erythema, epilation, destruction of fingernails, or epidermolysis.

B. Injury to Deep Structures:

1. Hematopoietic tissues–Injury to the bone marrow may cause diminished production of blood

*In radiation terminology, a rad is the unit of absorbed dose and a rem is the unit of any radiation dose to body tissue in terms of its estimated biologic effect. Roentgen (R) refers to the amount of radiation dose delivered to the body. For x-ray or gamma ray radiation, rems, rads, and roentgens are virtually the same. For particulate radiation from radioactive materials, these terms may differ greatly (eg, for neutrons, 1 rad equals 10 rems). In the Système International (SI) nomenclature, the rad has been replaced by the gray (Gy), and 1 rad equals 0.01 Gy = 1 cGy. The SI replacement for the rem is the Sievert (Sv), and 1 rem equals 0.01 Sv.

elements. Lymphocytes are most sensitive, polymorphonuclear leukocytes next most sensitive, and erythrocytes least sensitive. Damage to the blood-forming organs may vary from transient depression of one or more blood elements to complete destruction.

2. Cardiovascular system–Pericarditis with effusion or constrictive pericarditis may occur after a period of months or even years. Myocarditis is less common. Smaller vessels (the capillaries and arterioles) are more readily damaged than larger blood vessels.

3. Reproductive effects–In males, small single doses of radiation (200–300 cGy) cause temporary aspermatogenesis, and larger doses (600–800 cGy) may cause permanent sterility. In females, single doses of 200 cGy may cause temporary cessation of menses, and 500–800 cGy may cause permanent castration. Moderate to heavy irradiation of the embryo in utero results in injury to the fetus (eg, mental retardation) or in embryonic death and abortion.

4. Respiratory tract–High or repeated moderate doses of radiation may cause pneumonitis, often delayed for weeks or months.

5. Mouth, pharynx, esophagus, and stomach–Mucositis with edema and painful swallowing of food may occur within hours or days after onset of irradiation. Gastric secretion may be temporarily (occasionally permanently) inhibited by moderately high doses of radiation.

6. Intestines–Inflammation and ulceration may follow moderately large doses of radiation.

7. Endocrine glands and viscera–Hepatitis and nephritis may be delayed effects of therapeutic radiation. The normal thyroid, pituitary, pancreas, adrenals, and bladder are relatively resistant to low or moderate doses of radiation; parathyroid glands are especially resistant.

8. Nervous system–The brain and spinal cord are much more sensitive to acute exposures than the peripheral nerves.

C. Systemic Reaction (Radiation Sickness): The basic mechanisms of radiation sickness are not known. Anorexia, nausea, vomiting, weakness, exhaustion, lassitude, and in some cases prostration may occur, singly or in combination. Dehydration, anemia, and infection may follow. Radiation sickness associated with x-ray therapy is most likely to occur when the therapy is given in large dosage to large areas over the abdomen, less often when given over the thorax, and rarely when therapy is given over the extremities.

Prevention

Persons handling radiation sources can minimize exposure to radiation by recognizing the importance of time, distance, and shielding. Areas housing x-ray and nuclear materials must be properly shielded. X-ray equipment should be periodically checked for reliability of output, and proper filters should be employed. When feasible, it is advisable to shield the gonads, especially of young persons. Fluoroscopic examination should be performed as rapidly as possible, using an optimal combination of beam characteristics and filtration, and the beam size should be kept to a minimum required by the examination. Special protective clothing may be necessary to protect against contamination with radioisotopes. In the event of accidental contamination, all clothing should be removed and the body vigorously bathed with soap and water. This should be followed by careful instrument (Geiger counter) check to localize the ionizing radiation.

Emergency Treatment for Radiation Accident Victims

The proliferation of radiation equipment and nuclear energy plants and the increased transportation of radioactive materials necessitate hospital plans for managing patients who are accidentally exposed to ionizing radiation or are contaminated with radioisotopes. The plans should provide for effective emergency care and disposition of victims and materials with the least possible risk of spreading radioactive contamination to health care personnel and facilities.

Treatment

The success of treatment of local radiation effects depends upon the extent, degree, and location of tissue injury. Particulate or radioisotope exposures should be decontaminated in designated confined areas. Serial lymphocyte counts are useful for dose estimation and monitoring of the clinical impact of exposure. For many radioisotopes, chelation, blocking, or dilution therapy is indicated (see NCRP No. 65 reference, below). Treatment of systemic reactions is symptomatic and supportive. Ondansetron, 8 mg orally twice or three times daily, has been recommended for nausea and vomiting. Alternatives include chlorpromazine, 25–50 mg given deeply intramuscularly every 4–6 hours as necessary or 10–25 mg orally every 4–6 hours as necessary; and dimenhydrinate, 50–100 mg, or perphenazine, 4–8 mg, 1 hour before and 1 and 4 hours after radiation therapy has been recommended. Simple, palatable foods and emotional support may help.

When radiation dosage levels are sufficient to cause damage to gastrointestinal mucosa, bone marrow, and other important tissues, good medical and nursing care may be lifesaving. Blood and platelet transfusions, blood stem cell transplantation, bone marrow transplants, antibiotics, fluid and electrolyte maintenance, and other supportive measures may be useful. Recombinant hematopoietic growth factors (filgrastim and sargramostim or molgramostim) have been effective in accelerating hematopoietic recovery.

CHRONIC (DELAYED) EFFECTS OF EXCESSIVE DOSES OF IONIZING RADIATION

These disorders may occur following excessive ionizing radiation exposure: skin scarring, atrophy, and telangiectasis; cataract, dry eye syndrome, retinopathy; neuropathy, myelopathy, cerebral injury; obliterative endarteritis, coronary artery disease, pericarditis; hypothyroidism; pulmonary fibrosis, hepatitis, intestinal stenosis, and nephritis. Neoplastic disease, including leukemia and cancers of the breast, lung, and thyroid, is increased in persons exposed to radiation at relatively low doses (< 0.2 Gy). High-dose radon exposure is associated with an increased risk of lung cancer. Association of ionizing radiation with several other cancers has been reported but not well quantified (salivary glands, skin, stomach, colon, bladder, ovary, and central nervous system). Prenatal irradiation may increase the risk of childhood cancer.

Microcephaly and other congenital abnormalities may occur in children exposed in utero, especially if the fetus was exposed during early pregnancy. Carcinogenesis from low-dose (< 10 rem) exposure to adults has not been demonstrated. However, because of age-related differences in sensitivity to radiation, carcinogenesis following childhood exposures has been observed (eg, Chernobyl and childhood thyroid cancer).

Bishop MR: Potential use of hematopoietic stem cells after radiation injury. Stem Cells 1997;15(Suppl 2):305. [NLM Cit ID: 98034687].

National Council on Radiation Protection and Measurement (NCRP): *Management of Persons Accidentally Contaminated With Radionuclides.* Report No. 65. NCRP, 1985. (Treatment recommendations for exposure to specific isotopes.)

Reeves GI: Radiation injuries. Crit Care Clin 1999;15:457. [NLM Cit ID: 99261522] (Pathophysiology and treatment.)

Ron E: Ionizing radiation and cancer risk: Evidence from epidemiology. Radiat Res 1998;150(Suppl):S30. [NLM Cit ID: 99021444].

DROWNING

Drowning is the fifth leading cause of accidental death in the USA. The number of deaths due to drowning could undoubtedly be significantly reduced if adequate preventive and first aid instruction programs were instituted.

The asphyxia of drowning is usually due to aspiration of fluid, but it may result from airway obstruction caused by laryngeal spasm while the victim is gasping under water. About 10% of victims develop laryngospasm after the first gulp and never aspirate water ("dry drowning"). The rapid sequence of events after submersion—hypoxemia, laryngospasm, fluid aspiration, ineffective circulation, brain injury, and brain death—may take place within 5–10 minutes. This sequence may be delayed for longer periods if the victim, especially a child, has been submerged in very cold water or if the victim has ingested significant amounts of barbiturates. Immersion in cold water can also cause a rapid fall in the victim's core temperature, so that systemic hypothermia and death may occur before actual drowning.

The primary effect is hypoxia due to perfusion of poorly ventilated alveoli, intrapulmonary shunting, and decreased compliance. *The first requirement of rescue is immediate cardiopulmonary resuscitation.*

A number of circumstances or primary events may precede near drowning and must be taken into consideration in management: (1) use of alcohol or other drugs (a contributing factor in an estimated 25% of adult drownings), (2) extreme fatigue, (3) intentional hyperventilation, (4) sudden acute illness (eg, epilepsy, myocardial infarction), (5) head or spinal cord injury sustained in diving, (6) venomous stings by aquatic animals, and (7) decompression sickness in deep water diving.

When first seen, the near-drowning victim may present with a wide range of clinical manifestations. Spontaneous return of consciousness often occurs in otherwise healthy individuals when submersion is very brief. Many other patients respond promptly to immediate ventilation. Other patients, with more severe degrees of near drowning, may have frank respiratory failure, pulmonary edema, shock, anoxic encephalopathy, cerebral edema, and cardiac arrest. A few patients may be deceptively asymptomatic during the recovery period—only to deteriorate or die as a result of acute respiratory failure within the following 12–24 hours.

Clinical Findings

A. Symptoms and Signs: The patient may be unconscious, semiconscious, or awake but apprehensive, restless, and complaining of headaches or chest pain. Vomiting is common. Examination may reveal cyanosis, trismus, apnea, tachypnea, and wheezing. A pink froth from the mouth and nose indicates pulmonary edema. Cardiovascular manifestations may include tachycardia, arrhythmias, hypotension, cardiac arrest, and circulatory shock. Hypothermia may be present.

B. Laboratory Findings: Urinalysis shows proteinuria, hemoglobinuria, and acetonuria. Leukocytosis is usually present. The PaO_2 is usually decreased and the $PaCO_2$ increased or decreased. The blood pH is decreased as a result of metabolic acidosis. Chest x-rays may show pneumonitis or pulmonary edema.

Prevention

Prevention consists of avoidance of alcohol during recreational swimming or boating, close supervision of toddlers, swimming lessons early in life, and use of personal flotation devices when boating. All swimming pools should be fenced.

Treatment

A. First Aid: Immediate measures to combat hypoxemia at the scene of the incident—with sustained effective ventilation, oxygenation, and circulatory support—are critical to survival with complete recovery. Hypothermia and cervical spine injury should always be suspected.

1. Standard CPR is initiated if pulse and respirations are absent.

2. *Do not* waste time attempting to drain water from the victim's lungs, since this measure is most often of no value. The Heimlich maneuver (subdiaphragmatic pressure) should be used only if airway obstruction by a foreign body is suspected. The cervical spine should be immobilized if neck injury is possible.

3. *Do not* discontinue basic life support for seemingly "hopeless" patients until core temperature reaches 32 °C. Complete recovery has been reported after prolonged resuscitation of hypothermic patients.

B. Hospital Care: Careful observation of the patient; continuous monitoring of cardiorespiratory function; serial determination of arterial blood gases, renal function (serum creatinine), pH, and electrolytes; and measurement of urinary output are required. Pulmonary edema may not appear for 24 hours.

1. Ensure optimal ventilation and oxygenation–The danger of hypoxemia exists even in the alert, conscious patient who appears to be breathing normally. Oxygen should be administered immediately at the highest available concentration. Endotracheal intubation and mechanical ventilation are necessary for patients unable to maintain an open airway or normal blood gases and pH. Nasogastric intubation will allow removal of swallowed water and prevention of aspiration. If the victim does not have spontaneous respirations, intubation is required. Oxygen saturation should be maintained at 90% or higher. Continuous positive airway pressure (CPAP) is the most effective means of reversing hypoxia in patients with spontaneous respirations and patent airways. Positive end-expiratory pressure (PEEP) is also effective for treating pulmonary insufficiency. Assisted ventilation may be necessary with pulmonary edema, respiratory failure, aspiration, pneumonia, or severe central nervous system injury. Serial physical examinations and chest x-rays should be carried out to detect possible pneumonitis, atelectasis, and pulmonary edema. Bronchospasm due to aspirated material may require use of bronchodilators. Antibiotics should be given only when there is clinical evidence of infection—not prophylactically.

2. Cardiovascular support–Central venous pressure (or, preferably, pulmonary artery wedge pressure) may be monitored as a guide to determining whether vascular fluid replacement and pressors or diuretics are needed. If low cardiac output persists after adequate intravascular volume is achieved, pressors should be given. Otherwise, standard therapy for pulmonary edema, cardiogenic or not, is administered.

3. Correction of blood pH and electrolyte abnormalities–Metabolic acidosis is present in 70% of near-drowning victims, but it is usually of minor importance and corrected through adequate ventilation and oxygenation. While controversial, bicarbonate administration (1 meq/kg) has been recommended for comatose patients (see Chapter 21).

4. Cerebral injury–Some near-drowning patients may progress to irreversible central nervous system damage despite apparently adequate treatment of hypoxia and shock. Mild hyperventilation to achieve a $PaCO_2$ of approximately 30 mm Hg is recommended to lower intracranial pressure.

5. Hypothermia–Core temperature should be measured and managed as appropriate (see Systemic Hypothermia, above).

Course & Prognosis

Victims of near drowning who have had prolonged hypoxemia should remain under close hospital observation for 2–3 days after all supportive measures have been withdrawn and clinical and laboratory findings have been stable. Residual complications of near drowning may include intellectual impairment, convulsive disorders, and pulmonary or cardiac disease.

Golden FS et al: Immersion, near-drowning and drowning. Br J Anaesth 1997;79:214. [NLM Cit ID: 98009845] (Assessment and treatment.)

Sachdova RC: Near drowning. Crit Care Clin 1999;15:281. [NLM Cit ID: 99261514] (Pathophysiology and treatment.)

OTHER DISORDERS DUE TO PHYSICAL AGENTS

DECOMPRESSION SICKNESS & DYSBARIC ILLNESS

Decompression sickness and other disorders related to rapid changes in environmental pressure are occupational hazards for fliers and professional divers who are involved in deep-water exploration, rescue, salvage, or construction. In recent years, the sport of scuba diving has exposed amateurs to the hazards of decompression sickness.

At low depths the greatly increased pressure (eg, at 30 meters [100 ft] the pressure is four times greater than at the surface) compresses the respiratory gases into the blood and other tissues. During ascent from depths greater than 9 meters, gases dissolved in the blood and other tissues escape as the external pressure decreases. The appearance of symptoms depends on the depth and duration of submersion; the degree of physical exertion; the age, weight, and physical condition of the diver; and the rate of ascent. The size and number of gas bubbles (notably nitrogen) escaping from the tissues depend on the difference between the atmospheric pressure and the partial pressure of the gas dissolved in the tissues. The release of gas bubbles and (particularly) the location of their release determine the symptoms.

Decompression sickness also occurs among fliers during rapid ascent from sea level to high altitudes when there is no adequate pressurizing protection. Deep-sea and scuba divers may be vulnerable to air embolism if airplane travel is attempted too soon (within a few hours) after diving.

The range of clinical manifestations includes gas bubble formation in the joints ("bends"), cerebral or pulmonary decompression sickness, arterial gas embolism (cerebral, pulmonary), ear and sinus barotrauma, and dysbaric osteonecrosis.

Predisposing factors include exercise, injury, obesity, dehydration, alcoholic excess, hypoxia, some medications (eg, narcotics, antihistamines), and cold. Reported sequelae include hemiparesis, neurologic dysfunction, and bone damage. Asthma, pneumothorax, low results on pulmonary function testing, lung cysts, or thoracic trauma may contraindicate diving.

The onset of acute decompression symptoms occurs within 30 minutes in half of cases and almost invariably within 6 hours. Symptoms, which are highly variable, include pain (largely in the joints), headache, fatigue, numbness, confusion, pruritic rash, visual disturbances, nausea, vomiting, loss of hearing, weakness or paralysis, dizziness or vertigo, dyspnea, paresthesias, aphasia, and coma.

Pulmonary decompression sickness ("chokes") presents with burning, pleuritic substernal pain, cough, and dyspnea.

Early recognition and prompt treatment are extremely important. Continuous administration of oxygen is indicated as a first aid measure whether or not cyanosis is present. Aspirin may be given for pain, but narcotics should be used very cautiously, since they may obscure the patient's response to recompression. Rapid transportation to a treatment facility for recompression, hyperbaric oxygen, hydration treatment of plasma deficits, and supportive measures is necessary not only to relieve symptoms but also to prevent permanent impairment. It has been recommended, however, that decompression symptoms be treated whenever they are seen—even up to 2 weeks postinjury—since it is still possible to completely alleviate symptoms. The clinician should be familiar with the nearest compression center. The local public health department or nearest naval facility should be able to provide such information. The National Divers Alert Network (DAN) (919-684-8111) provides assistance in the management of underwater diving accidents.

Moon RE: Treatment of diving emergencies. Crit Care Clin 1999;15:429. [NLM Cit ID: 99261521] (Diagnosis and treatment of barotrauma and decompression disorders.)

Van Meter K: Medical field management of the injured diver. Respir Care Clin North Am 1999;5:137. [NLM Cit ID: 99222547] (Emergency assessment, decompression and equipment guidelines.)

MOUNTAIN SICKNESS

Lack of sufficient time for acclimatization, increased physical activity, and varying degrees of health may be responsible for the acute, subacute, and chronic disturbances that result from hypoxia at altitudes greater than 2000 meters (6560 ft). Marked individual differences in tolerance to hypoxia exist. Patients with sickle cell disease are at high risk of painful crises from altitude-induced hypoxemia.

Acute Mountain Sickness

The severity of acute mountain sickness correlates with altitude and rate of ascent. Initial manifestations include headache (most severe and persistent symptom), lassitude, drowsiness, dizziness, chilliness, nausea and vomiting, facial pallor, dyspnea, and cyanosis. Later, there is facial flushing, irritability, difficulty in concentrating, vertigo, tinnitus, visual disturbances, auditory disturbances, anorexia, insomnia, increased dyspnea and weakness on exertion, increased headaches (due to cerebral edema), palpitations, tachycardia, Cheyne-Stokes breathing, and weight loss. More severe manifestations include pulmonary edema and encephalopathy (see below). Voluntary periodic hyperventilation may relieve symptoms. In most individuals, symptoms clear within 24–48 hours, but in some instances, if the symptoms are sufficiently persistent or severe, the patient must be returned to lower altitudes. Definitive treatment is immediate descent, which must be managed if reduced consciousness, ataxia, or pulmonary edema is present. Administration of oxygen, 1–2 L/min, will often relieve acute symptoms. Acetazolamide, 125–250 mg every 12 hours, or dexamethasone, 8 mg initially followed by 4 mg every 6 hours, for as long as symptoms persist, is recommended therapy; they may be used together in severe cases. Portable hyperbaric chambers can provide limited short-term symptom relief.

Preventive measures include slow ascent—300 meters (984 feet) per day—adequate rest and sleep the day before travel, reduced food intake, and avoidance of alcohol, tobacco, and unnecessary physical activity during travel. Acetazolamide, 125–250 mg every 12 hours, beginning the day before ascent and continuing for 48–72 hours at altitude, may be used as prophylaxis. Dexamethasone, 4 mg every 12 hours beginning on the day of ascent, continuing for 3 days at the higher altitude, and then tapering over 5 days, is an alternative.

Acute High-Altitude Pulmonary Edema

This serious complication usually occurs at levels above 3000 meters (9840 ft). Early symptoms of pulmonary edema may appear within 6–36 hours after arrival at a high-altitude area: incessant dry cough, shortness of breath disproportionate to exertion, headache, decreased exercise performance, fatigue, dyspnea at rest, and chest tightness. Later, wheezing, orthopnea, and hemoptysis may occur. Recognition of the early symptoms may enable the patient to descend before incapacitating pulmonary edema develops, but strenuous exertion should be avoided. An early descent of even 500 or 1000 meters may result in improvement of symptoms. Physical findings include tachycardia, mild fever, tachypnea, cyanosis, prolonged respiration, and rales and rhonchi. The patient may become confused or even comatose, and the entire clinical picture may resemble severe pneumonia. The white count is often slightly elevated, but the erythrocyte sedimentation rate is usually normal. Chest x-ray findings vary from irregular patchy infiltration in one lung to nodular densities bilaterally or with transient prominence of the central pulmonary arteries. Transient nonspecific electrocardiographic changes, occasionally showing right ventricular strain, may occur. Pulmonary arterial blood pressure is elevated, whereas wedge pressure is normal.

Treatment, which must often be given under field conditions, consists of rest in the semi-Fowler position (head raised) and administration of 100% oxygen by mask at a rate of 4–6 L/min for 15–30 minutes. *Immediate descent (at least 610 m [2000 ft]) is essential.* Recompression in a portable hyperbaric bag will temporarily reduce symptoms if rapid or immediate descent is not possible. To conserve oxygen, lower flow rates (2–4 L/min) may be used until the victim recovers or can be evacuated to a lower altitude. Treatment for acute respiratory distress syndrome (see Chapter 9) may be required for some patients who have a prolonged course of pulmonary edema. Nifedipine, 10 mg every 4 hours, may provide symptomatic relief. Dexamethasone, 4 mg every 6 hours, has been recommended if central nervous system symptoms are present. Acetazolamide, 125–250 mg every 12 hours, should be administered if acute mountain sickness is suspected. If bacterial pneumonia exists, appropriate antibiotic therapy should be given.

Preventive measures include education of prospective mountaineers regarding the possibility of serious pulmonary edema, optimal physical conditioning before travel, gradual ascent to permit acclimatization, and a period of rest and inactivity for 1–2 days after arrival at high altitudes. Prompt medical attention with rest and high-flow oxygen if respiratory symptoms develop may prevent progression to frank pulmonary edema. Persons with a history of high-altitude pulmonary edema should be hospitalized for further observation if possible. Pulmonary embolism and high-altitude bronchitis can also occur. Mountaineering parties at levels of 3000 meters (9840 ft) or higher should carry a supply of oxygen and equipment sufficient for several days. Persons with symptomatic cardiac or pulmonary disease should avoid high altitudes.

Acute High-Altitude Encephalopathy

High-altitude encephalopathy appears to be an extension of the central nervous system symptoms of acute mountain sickness (see above). It usually occurs at elevations above 2500 meters (8250 ft) and is more common in unacclimatized individuals. Clinical findings are due largely to hypoxemia and cerebral edema. Severe headaches, confusion, truncal ataxia, staggering gait, focal deficits, nausea and vomiting, and seizures may progress to obtundation and coma. Papilledema and retinal hemorrhages may be observed in about 50% of patients.

Treatment is immediate descent for at least 610 m (2000 ft), continuing until symptoms improve. Oxygen (2–4 L/min) should be administered by mask. Dexamethasone, 4–8 mg every 6 hours, is recommended thereafter. If immediate descent is impossible, a portable hyperbaric chamber should be used until symptomatic improvement occurs.

Subacute Mountain Sickness

This occurs most frequently in unacclimatized individuals and at altitudes above 4500 meters (14,764 ft). Symptoms, which are probably due to central nervous system anoxia without associated alveolar hyperventilation, are similar to but more persistent and severe than those of acute mountain sickness. There are additional problems of dehydration, skin dryness, and pruritus. The hematocrit may be elevated, and there may be electrocardiographic and chest x-ray evidence of right ventricular hypertrophy. Treatment consists of rest, oxygen administration, and return to lower altitudes.

Chronic Mountain Sickness (Monge's Disease)

This uncommon condition, consisting of chronic hypoxia in residents of high-altitude communities who have lost their acclimatization to such an environment, is difficult to differentiate from chronic pulmonary disease. The disorder is characterized by somnolence, mental depression, hypoxemia, cyanosis, clubbing of fingers, hemoglobin > 22 g/dL, polycythemia (hematocrit often > 75%), signs of right ventricular failure, electrocardiographic evidence of right axis deviation and right atrial and ventricular hypertrophy, and x-ray evidence of right heart enlargement and central pulmonary vessel prominence. There is no x-ray evidence of structural pulmonary disease. Pulmonary function tests usually disclose alveolar hypoventilation and elevated PCO_2 but fail to reveal defective oxygen transport. There is a diminished respiratory response to CO_2. Almost complete disappearance of all abnormalities eventually occurs when the patient returns to sea level.

Harris MD et al: High altitude medicine. Am Fam Physician 1998;57:1907. [NLM Cit ID: 98236240] (Pathophysiology, diagnosis and treatment, and frequently asked questions [FAQs] for patients.)

Krieger BP et al: Altitude related pulmonary disorders. Crit Care Clin 1999;15:265. [NLM Cit ID: 99261513] (Pathophysiology, diagnosis, and treatment.)

Zafren K et al: High-altitude medicine. Emerg Med Clin North Am 1997;15:191. [NLM Cit ID: 97209276] (Pathophysiology, diagnosis, and treatment of acute disorders.)

MEDICAL EFFECTS OF AIR TRAVEL & SELECTION OF PATIENTS FOR AIR TRAVEL

The decision about whether or not it is advisable for a patient to travel by air depends not only upon the nature and severity of the illness but also upon such factors as the duration of flight, the altitude to be flown, pressurization, the availability of supplementary oxygen and other medical supplies, the presence of attending physicians and trained nursing attendants, and other special considerations. Air carriers in the USA cannot legally allow the use of personal (passenger-supplied) oxygen containers, but most major airlines will supply oxygen upon advance written request from the passenger's physician. Airline policies, charges, and other details must be checked with each carrier. Medical hazards or complications of modern air travel are remarkably uncommon; unless there is some specific contraindication, air transportation may actually be the best means of moving patients. The medical hazard most likely to be realized is hypoxia. The most common in-flight emergencies are cardiovascular, syncopal, neuropsychiatric, and abdominal. The Air Transport Association of America defines an incapacitated passenger as "one who is suffering from a physical or mental disability and who, because of such disability or the effect of the flight on the disability, is incapable of self-care; would endanger the health or safety of such person or other passengers or airline employees; or would cause discomfort or annoyance of other passengers."

All commercial airlines retain medical consultants to assist their personnel in making decisions regarding the transportation of passengers with noticeable symptoms of sickness or injury. Clinicians may contact these medical consultants by calling or writing the medical departments of major airlines.

Pretravel clinician evaluation is advisable for patients with hospitalization, surgery, emergency care, or medication change within the past 4 weeks. Listed below are the more common contraindications to air travel.

Cardiovascular Disease

A. Cardiac Decompensation: Patients in congestive failure should not fly until they are stable or compensated by appropriate treatment; 100% oxygen should be available during the flight.

B. Compensated Valvular or Other Heart Disease: Patients should not fly above 2400–2800 meters (7874–9187 ft) unless the aircraft is pressurized and oxygen is administered at altitudes of 2400 meters (7874 ft) or higher.

C. Acute Myocardial Infarction, Convalescent and Asymptomatic: At least 3 weeks of convalescence is recommended even for asymptomatic patients; a negative exercise ECG is desirable. Unstable postinfarction patients should not fly. Post PTCA and post CABG patients should not fly until stable and at least 2 weeks after the procedure. Coronary disease patients with severe or poorly controlled hypertension or ventricular ectopy should not fly. Ambulatory, stabilized, and compensated patients tolerate air travel well. Oxygen should be available.

D. Angina Pectoris: Air travel is inadvisable for patients with new-onset severe or unstable angina. In mild to moderate cases of angina, air travel may be permitted, especially in pressurized planes. Oxygen should be available.

E. Deep Venous Thrombosis: Patients with deep venous thrombosis should not fly until their anticoagulant therapy is stable and they have no evidence of pulmonary complications. Long flights increase the risk of deep vein thrombosis and resulting embolic disease. Prevention includes avoidance of smoking and alcohol, low-dose aspirin, support hose, and leg exercises and walking during the flight.

Respiratory Disease

A. Nasopharyngeal Disorders: Nasal allergies and infections predispose to development of aerotitis. Chewing gum, nasal decongestants (pseudoephedrine timed-release, one 120 mg capsule 30 minutes before departure), appropriate anti-infective treatment, and avoiding sleep on descent may prevent barotitis. (See Barotrauma, Chapter 8.)

B. Asthma: Patients with mild asthma can travel without difficulty. Patients in status asthmaticus should not be permitted to fly.

C. Congenital Pulmonary Cysts: Patients should not travel unless cleared by a physician.

D. Tuberculosis: Patients with active, communicable tuberculosis or pneumothorax should not be permitted to travel by air.

E. Other Pulmonary Disorders: Breathlessness at rest is a contraindication to air travel. The degree of hypoxemia and hypercapnia should be assessed, and vital capacity should be evaluated. Patients should be able to walk 50 m (164 ft) or climb one flight of stairs without becoming severely dyspneic.

Anemia

Patients with severe anemia (hemoglobin < 8.5 g/dL or red cell count < 3 million/μL) should not travel by air. If hemoglobin is less than 8–9 g/dL, oxygen should be available. Patients with sickle cell disease appear to be particularly vulnerable.

Diabetes Mellitus

Diabetics who do not need insulin or who can administer their own insulin during flight may fly safely. Adjustment of the insulin administration schedule should be discussed prior to travel across time zones.

Patients With Surgical Problems

Patients convalescing from thoracic or abdominal surgery should not fly until 10 days (abdominal) to 21 days (thoracic) after surgery, and then only if the wound is healed and there is no drainage.

Colostomy patients may be permitted to travel by air providing they are nonodorous and colostomy bags are emptied before flight.

Patients with large hernias unsupported by a truss or binder should not be permitted to fly in nonpressurized aircraft because of an increased danger of strangulation of the herniated bowel.

Postsurgical or posttraumatic eye cases require pressurized cabins and oxygen therapy to avoid retinal damage due to hypoxia and intraocular gas bubbles.

Psychiatric Disorders

Severely psychotic, agitated, or disturbed patients should not be permitted to fly on scheduled airlines even when accompanied by a medical attendant.

Extremely nervous or apprehensive patients may travel by air if they receive adequate sedation before and during flight.

Motion Sickness

Patients subject to motion sickness can be given sedatives or antihistamines (eg, dimenhydrinate, 50 mg every 4–6 hours; promethazine, 25 mg every 6 hours; or meclizine, 25–50 mg every 24 hours) before and during the flight. Small meals of easily digested food before and during the flight may reduce the tendency to nausea and vomiting.

Pregnancy

Pregnant women may be permitted to fly during the first 8 months of pregnancy unless there is a history of complications of pregnancy or premature birth. During the ninth month of pregnancy, air travel is not recommended; if travel is essential, a physician's authorization is required. Infants less than 1 week old should not be flown at high altitudes or for long distances.

Jagoda A et al: Medical emergencies in commercial air travel. Emerg Med Clin North Am 1997;15:251. [NLM Cit ID: 97209279]

Lien D et al: Recommendations for patients with chronic respiratory disease considering air travel: A statement of the Canadian Thoracic Society. Can Respir J 1998;5:95. [NLM Cit ID: 98374207] (Assessment guidelines.)

Medical Guidelines for Airline Travel. Aerospace Medical Association, 1997, Alexandria, Virginia.

RELEVANT WORLD WIDE WEB SITES

[National Institute for Occupational Safety and Health]
http://www.cdc.gov/niosh/homepage.html

[Radiation Health Effects Resource: Ionizing Radiation Health Effects (RadEFX)]
http://radefx.bcm.tmc.edu/ionizing/ionizing.htm

Poisoning

39

See http://www.current-med.com/ch39.html for updated addresses of Web sites referenced in this chapter.

Kent R. Olson, MD

INITIAL EVALUATION OF THE PATIENT WITH POISONING OR DRUG OVERDOSE

Patients with drug overdoses or poisoning may initially present with no symptoms or with varying degrees of overt intoxication. The asymptomatic patient may have been exposed to or may have ingested a lethal dose of a poison but not yet have any manifestations of toxicity. It is always important to (1) quickly assess the potential danger, (2) perform gut decontamination to prevent absorption, and (3) observe the patient for an appropriate interval.

Assess the Danger

If the toxin is known, the danger can be assessed by consulting a text or computerized information resource (eg, Poisindex) or by calling a regional poison control center (Table 39–1). Assessment will usually take into account the dose ingested (in milligrams per kilogram of body weight), the time interval since ingestion, the presence of any clinical signs, preexisting cardiac, respiratory, renal, or liver disease, and, occasionally, specific serum drug or toxin levels. Be aware that the history given by the patient or family may be incomplete or unreliable.

The manufacturer or its local representative may be able to provide information over the phone concerning the toxic ingredients in question and can be contacted directly or via the regional poison control center (Table 39–1).

Gut Decontamination

The choice of gut decontamination procedure depends on the toxin and the circumstances. (See below for more discussion of methods.)

Observation of the Patient

Asymptomatic or mildly symptomatic patients should be observed for at least 4–6 hours. Longer observation is indicated if the ingested substance is a sustained-release preparation or is known to slow gastrointestinal motility or if there may have been exposure to a poison with delayed onset of symptoms (such as acetaminophen, colchicine, or hepatotoxic mushrooms). After that time, the patient may be discharged if no symptoms have developed and adequate gastric decontamination has been provided. Before discharge, psychiatric evaluation should be performed to assess suicidal risk. Intentional ingestions in adolescents should raise the possibility of unwanted pregnancy or sexual abuse.

THE SYMPTOMATIC PATIENT

In symptomatic patients, treatment of life-threatening complications takes precedence over in-depth diagnostic evaluation. Patients with mild symptoms may deteriorate rapidly, which is why all potentially significant exposures should be observed in an acute care facility. The following complications may occur, depending on the type of poisoning.

COMA

Assessment & Complications

Coma is commonly associated with ingestion of large doses of antihistamines, barbiturates, benzodiazepines and other sedative-hypnotic drugs, γ-hydroxybutyrate (GHB), ethanol, opioids, phenothiazines, or antidepressants. The most common cause of death in comatose patients is respiratory failure, which may occur abruptly. Aspiration of gastric contents may also occur, especially in victims who are deeply obtunded or convulsing. Hypoxia and hypoventilation may cause or aggravate hypotension, arrhythmias and seizures. Thus, protection of the airway and assisted ventilation are the most important treatment measures for any poisoned patient.

Table 39–1. Regional poison control centers.

Regional poison centers operate 24 hours a day, utilizing specially trained and dedicated staff with access to a variety of texts, files, and computerized information resources. They can also provide immediate telephone consultation with a physician specializing in medical toxicology.

State or City	Public Number	Other Numbers
ALABAMA		
Birmingham	800-292-6678 (AL only)	205-933-4050
Tuscaloosa	800-462-0800 (AL only)	205-345-0600
ARIZONA		
Phoenix	602-253-3334	
Tucson	520-626-6016	
CALIFORNIA	800-876-4766 (CA only)	800-411-8080 (CA only) (Health professionals)
COLORADO	800-332-3073 (CO only)	303-739-1123
CONNECTICUT	800-343-2722 (CT only)	860-679-3456
DELAWARE	800-722-7112	215-386-2100
DISTRICT OF COLUMBIA	202-625-3333	
FLORIDA	800-282-3171 (FL only)	
GEORGIA	800-282-5846	404-616-9000
IDAHO	800-860-0620 (ID only)	
ILLINOIS	800-942-5969 (IL only)	
INDIANA	800-382-9097 (IN only)	317-929-2323
KENTUCKY	502-589-8222	
LOUISIANA	800-256-9822 (LA only)	
MARYLAND	410-706-7701	
MASSACHUSETTS	800-682-9211 (MA and RI only)	617-232-2120
MICHIGAN		
Detroit	800-764-7661 (MI only)	313-745-5711
Grand Rapids	800-764-7661 (MI only)	
MINNESOTA	800-764-7661 (MN and SD only)	612-347-3141
MISSOURI	800-366-8888	314-772-5200
MONTANA	800-525-5042 (MT only)	
NEBRASKA	800-955-9119 (NE and WY only)	402-354-5555
NEVADA	503-494-8968	800-446-6179 (NV only)
NEW JERSEY	800-764-7661 (NJ only)	
NEW MEXICO	800-432-6866 (NM only)	505-272-2222
NEW YORK		
Buffalo	800-888-7655 (NY only)	716-878-7654
Hudson Valley	800-336-6997 (NY only)	914-366-3030
Long Island	516-542-2323	516-663-2650
New York City	800-210-3985	212-340-4494
Rochester	800-333-0542 (NY only)	716-275-3232
Syracuse	800-252-5655 (NY only)	315-476-4766
NORTH CAROLINA	800-848-6946 (NC only)	704-355-4000

(continued)

Table 39–1. Regional poison control centers (continued).

State or City	Public Number	Other Numbers
OHIO		
Cincinnati	513-558-5111	
Columbus	614-228-1323	
OREGON	503-494-8968	
PENNSYLVANIA		
Hershey	800-521-6110	
Philadelphia	800-722-7112	
Pittsburgh	412-681-6669	
RHODE ISLAND	800-682-9211 (RI & MA only)	617-232-2120
SOUTH DAKOTA	800-764-7661 (SD & MN only)	612-347-3141
TENNESSEE	800-288-9999 (TN only)	615-936-2034
TEXAS	800-764-7661 (TX only)	
UTAH	800-456-7707 (UT only)	
VIRGINIA		
Charlottesville	804-924-5543	
Richmond	800-552-6337	804-828-9123
WASHINGTON	800-732-6985	206-526-2121
WYOMING	800-955-9119	

Source: American Association of Poison Control Centers (http://www.aapcc.org)

Treatment

A. Emergency Management: The initial emergency management of coma can be remembered by the mnemonic *ABCD,* for *A*irway, *B*reathing, *C*irculation, and *D*rugs (dextrose, thiamine, and naloxone or flumazenil), respectively (Table 39–2).

1. Airway–Establish a patent airway by positioning, suction, or insertion of an artificial nasal or oropharyngeal airway. If the patient is deeply comatose or if there is no gag or cough reflex, perform endotracheal intubation. These airway interventions may not be necessary if the patient is intoxicated by an opioid or a benzodiazepine and responds rapidly to intravenous naloxone or flumazenil (see below).

Table 39–2. Initial management of coma.

A	Airway control
B	Breathing
C	Circulation
D	Drugs (give all three): Dextrose 50%, 50–100 mL IV Thiamine, 100 mg IM or IV Naloxone, 0.45–2 mg IV[1] And consider flumazenil, 0.2–0.5 mg IV[2]

[1]Repeated doses, up to 5–10 mg, may be required.
[2]Do not give if patient has coingested a tricyclic antidepressant or other convulsant drug or has a seizure disorder.

2. Breathing–Clinically assess the quality and depth of respiration, and provide assistance if necessary with a bag-valve-mask device or mechanical ventilator. Provide supplemental oxygen. The arterial blood CO_2 tension is useful in determining the adequacy of ventilation. The arterial blood Po_2 determination may reveal hypoxemia, which may be caused by respiratory arrest, bronchospasm, pulmonary aspiration, or noncardiogenic pulmonary edema. Pulse oximetry provides an assessment of oxygenation but is not reliable in patients with methemoglobinemia or carbon monoxide poisoning.

3. Circulation–Measure the pulse and blood pressure, and estimate tissue perfusion (eg, by measurement of urinary output, skin signs, arterial blood pH). Place the patient on continuous electrocardiographic monitoring. Insert an intravenous line, and draw blood for complete blood count, glucose, electrolytes, serum creatinine and liver tests, and possible toxicologic testing.

4. Drugs–

a. Dextrose and thiamine–Unless promptly treated, severe hypoglycemia can cause irreversible brain damage. Therefore, in all comatose or convulsing patients, give 50% dextrose, 50–100 mL by intravenous bolus, unless a rapid bedside blood sugar test is available and rules out hypoglycemia. In alcoholic or very malnourished patients who may have marginal thiamine stores, give thiamine, 100 mg intramuscularly or over 2–3 minutes intravenously.

b. Narcotic antagonists–Naloxone, 0.4–2 mg intravenously, may reverse opioid-induced respiratory depression and coma. If opioid overdose is strongly suspected, give additional doses of naloxone (up to 5–10 mg may be required to reverse potent opioids). ***Caution:*** Naloxone has a much shorter duration of action (2–3 hours) than most common opioids; repeated doses may be required, and continuous observation for at least 3–4 hours after the last dose is mandatory. Nalmefene, a recently introduced opioid antagonist, has a duration of effect longer than that of naloxone but still shorter than that of the opioid methadone.

c. Flumazenil–Flumazenil, 0.2–0.5 mg intravenously, repeated every 30 seconds as needed up to a maximum of 3 mg, may reverse benzodiazepine-induced coma. ***Caution:*** Flumazenil has a short duration of effect (2–3 hours), and resedation requiring additional doses is common. Furthermore, flumazenil should not be given if the patient has coingested a tricyclic antidepressant, is a user of high-dose benzodiazepines, or has a seizure disorder—because its use in these circumstances may precipitate seizures.

HYPOTHERMIA

Assessment & Complications

Hypothermia commonly accompanies coma due to opioids, ethanol, hypoglycemic agents, phenothiazines, barbiturates, benzodiazepines, and other sedative-hypnotics and depressants. Hypothermic patients may have a barely perceptible pulse and blood pressure and often appear to be dead. Hypothermia may cause or aggravate hypotension, which will not reverse until the temperature is normalized.

Treatment

Hypothermia treatment is discussed in Chapter 38. Gradual rewarming is preferred unless the patient is in cardiac arrest.

HYPOTENSION

Assessment & Complications

Hypotension may be due to poisoning by many different drugs and poisons. The most common drugs causing hypotension are antihypertensive drugs, beta-blockers, calcium channel blockers, iron, theophylline, phenothiazines, barbiturates, and tricyclic antidepressants. Poisons causing hypotension include cyanide, carbon monoxide, hydrogen sulfide, arsenic, and certain mushrooms.

Hypotension in the poisoned or drug-overdosed patient may be caused by venous or arteriolar vasodilation, hypovolemia, depressed cardiac contractility, or a combination of these effects. The only certain way to determine the cause of hypotension in any individual patient is to insert a pulmonary artery catheter and calculate the cardiac output and peripheral vascular resistance. Alternatively, a central venous pressure (CVP) monitor may indicate a need for further fluid therapy.

Treatment

Most patients respond to empirical treatment (200 mL intravenous boluses of 0.9% saline or other isotonic crystalloid up to a total of 1–2 L in an adult, or 20 mL/kg in children). If fluid therapy is not successful, give dopamine, 5–15 μg/kg/min by intravenous infusion in a large peripheral or central line. Consider pulmonary artery catheterization if hypotension persists.

Hypotension caused by certain toxins may respond to specific treatment. For hypotension caused by overdoses of tricyclic antidepressants or related drugs, administer sodium bicarbonate, 1–2 meq/kg by intravenous bolus injection. Norepinephrine is more effective than dopamine in some patients with tricyclic overdose. For beta-blocker overdose, glucagon (5–10 mg intravenously) may be of value. For calcium channel blocker overdose, administer calcium chloride, 15–20 mg/kg intravenously (repeated doses may be necessary; doses of 5–10 g and more have been given in some cases).

HYPERTENSION

Assessment & Complications

Hypertension may be due to poisoning with amphetamines, anticholinergics, cocaine, phenylpropanolamine, or monoamine oxidase inhibitors.

Severe hypertension (eg, diastolic blood pressure > 105–110 mm Hg in a person who does not have chronic hypertension) can result in acute intracranial hemorrhage, myocardial infarction, or aortic dissection. Patients often present with headache, chest pain, or encephalopathy.

Treatment

Treat hypertension if the patient is symptomatic or if the diastolic pressure is greater than 105–110 mm Hg—especially if there is no prior history of hypertension.

Hypertensive patients who are agitated or anxious may benefit from a sedative such as lorazepam, 2–3 mg intravenously. For persistent hypertension, administer phentolamine, 2–5 mg intravenously, or nitroprusside sodium, 0.25–8 μg/kg/min intravenously. If excessive tachycardia is present, add propranolol, 1–5 mg intravenously, or esmolol 25–100 μg/kg/min intravenously. ***Caution:*** Do not give beta-blockers alone, since doing so may paradoxically worsen hypertension.

ARRHYTHMIAS

Assessment & Complications

Arrhythmias may occur with a variety of drugs or toxins (Table 39–3). They may also occur as a result of hypoxia, metabolic acidosis, or electrolyte imbalance (eg, hyper- or hypokalemia, hypocalcemia), or following exposure to chlorinated solvents or chloral hydrate overdose.

Treatment

Arrhythmias are often caused by hypoxia or electrolyte imbalance, and these conditions should be sought and treated. If ventricular arrhythmias persist, administer lidocaine at usual antiarrhythmic doses. ***Caution:*** Avoid class Ia agents (quinidine, procainamide, disopyramide), which may aggravate arrhythmias caused by tricyclic antidepressants, calcium channel blockers, or beta-blockers. Wide QRS complex tachycardia in the setting of tricyclic antidepressant overdose (or quinidine and other class Ia drugs) should be treated with sodium bicarbonate, 50–100 meq intravenously by bolus injection. (See discussion of tricyclic antidepressant poisoning.)

For tachyarrhythmias induced by chlorinated solvents, chloral hydrate, or sympathomimetic agents, use propranolol or esmolol (see doses given above in hypertension section).

CONVULSIONS

Assessment & Complications

Convulsions may be due to poisoning with many drugs and poisons, including amphetamines, antihistamines, camphor, cocaine, isoniazid, lindane, phencyclidine (PCP), phenothiazines, theophylline, tricyclic antidepressants, and some newer antidepressants (eg, bupropion, venlafaxine).

Convulsions may also be caused by hypoxia, hypoglycemia, hypocalcemia, hyponatremia, withdrawal from alcohol or sedative-hypnotics, head trauma, central nervous system infection, or idiopathic epilepsy.

Prolonged or repeated convulsions commonly lead to hypoxia, metabolic acidosis, hyperthermia, and rhabdomyolysis.

Treatment

Administer lorazepam, 2–3 mg intravenously over 2 minutes, or—if intravenous access is not immediately available—midazolam, 5–10 mg intramuscularly. If convulsions continue, administer phenobarbital, 15–20 mg/kg slowly intravenously over no less than 30 minutes; or phenytoin, 15 mg/kg intravenously over no less than 30 minutes (maximum infusion rate, 50 mg/min). The drugs may be used together if necessary. Maintenance doses may be required if drug toxicity is expected to last more than 18–24 hours.

Convulsions due to a few drugs and toxins may require antidotes or other specific therapies (as listed in Table 39–4).

HYPERTHERMIA

Assessment & Complications

Hyperthermia may be associated with poisoning by amphetamines, atropine and other anticholinergic drugs, cocaine, dinitrophenol and pentachlorophenol,

Table 39–3. Common toxins or drugs causing arrhythmias.

Arrhythmia	Common Causes
Sinus bradycardia	Beta-blockers, calcium channel blockers, organophosphates, digitalis glycosides, opioids, clonidine, sedative-hypnotics.
Atrioventricular block	Beta-blockers, digitalis glycosides, calcium channel blockers, tricyclic antidepressants, quinidine and other class Ia drugs, lithium.
Sinus tachycardia	Theophylline, caffeine, cocaine, amphetamines, phencyclidine, beta-agonists (eg, albuterol), iron, anticholinergics, tricyclic antidepressants, antihistamines.
Wide QRS complex	Tricyclic antidepressants, quinidine and class Ia antiarrhythmics, class Ic antiarrhythmics, phenothiazines (eg, thioridazine), potassium (hyperkalemia).
QT interval prolongation	Lithium, quinidine and other class Ia drugs, class III antiarrhythmic drugs, terfenadine, astemizole

Table 39–4. Convulsions related to toxins or drugs requiring special consideration.[1]

Toxin or Drug	Comments
Isoniazid (INH)	Administer pyridoxine.
Lithium	May indicate need for hemodialysis.
Organophosphates	Administer pralidoxime (2-PAM) and atropine.
Strychnine	"Convulsions" are actually spinally mediated muscle spasms and usually require neuromuscular paralysis.
Theophylline	Convulsions indicate need for hemodialysis or charcoal hemoperfusion.
Tricyclic antidepressants	Hyperthermia and cardiotoxicity are common complications of repeated convulsions; paralyze early with neuromuscular blockers to reduce muscular hyperactivity.

[1]See text for dosages.

phencyclidine (PCP), salicylates, strychnine, tricyclic antidepressants, and various other medications. Use of serotonin reuptake inhibitors (eg, fluoxetine, paroxetine, sertraline) in a patient taking a monoamine oxidase inhibitor may cause agitation, hyperactivity, and hyperthermia ("serotonin syndrome"). Haloperidol and other antipsychotic agents can cause rigidity and hyperthermia (neuroleptic malignant syndrome [NMS]). Malignant hyperthermia is a rare disorder associated with general anesthetic agents.

Hyperthermia is a rapidly life-threatening complication. Severe hyperthermia (temperature > 40–41 °C) may rapidly cause brain damage and multiorgan failure, including rhabdomyolysis, renal failure, and coagulopathy (see Chapter 38).

Treatment

Treat hyperthermia aggressively by removing all clothing, spraying with tepid water, and fanning the patient. If this is not rapidly effective, as shown by a normal rectal temperature within 30–60 minutes, or if there is significant muscle rigidity or hyperactivity, induce neuromuscular paralysis with a nondepolarizing neuromuscular blocker (eg, pancuronium, vecuronium). Once paralyzed, the patient must be intubated and mechanically ventilated. Absence of visible muscular convulsive movements may give the false impression that brain seizure activity has ceased; however, this must be confirmed by electroencephalography.

Dantrolene (2–5 mg/kg intravenously) may be effective for hyperthermia associated with muscle rigidity that does not respond to neuromuscular blockade (ie, malignant hyperthermia). Bromocriptine, 2.5–7.5 mg orally daily, has been recommended for neuroleptic malignant syndrome. Cyproheptadine, 4 mg orally every hour for three or four doses, has been used to treat serotonin syndrome.

Table 39–5. Some toxic agents for which there are specific antidotes.[1]

Toxic Agent	Specific Antidote
Acetaminophen	Acetylcysteine
Anticholinergics (eg, atropine)	Physostigmine
Anticholinesterases (eg, organophosphate pesticides)	Atropine and pralidoxime (2-PAM)
Benzodiazepines	Flumazenil
Carbon monoxide	Oxygen
Cyanide	Sodium nitrite, sodium thiosulfate
Digitalis glycosides	Digoxin-specific Fab antibodies
Heavy metals (eg, lead, mercury, iron) and arsenic	Specific chelating agents
Isoniazid	Pyridoxine (vitamin B_6)
Methanol, ethylene glycol	Ethanol (ethyl alcohol) or fomepizole (4-methylpyrazole)
Opioids	Naloxone, nalmefene
Snake venom	Specific antivenin

[1]See text for indications and dosages.

ANTIDOTES & OTHER TREATMENT

ANTIDOTES

Give an antidote (if available) when there is reasonable certainty of a specific diagnosis (Table 39–5). Antidotes themselves may have serious side effects. The indications and dosages for specific antidotes are discussed in the respective sections for specific toxins.

DECONTAMINATION OF THE SKIN

Corrosive agents rapidly injure the skin and eyes and must be removed immediately. In addition, many toxins are readily absorbed through the skin, and systemic absorption can be prevented only by rapid action.

Wash the affected areas with copious quantities of lukewarm water or saline. Wash carefully behind the ears, under the nails, and in skin folds. For oily substances (eg, pesticides), wash the skin at least twice with plain soap and shampoo the hair. Specific decontaminating solutions or solvents (eg, alcohol) are rarely indicated and in some cases may paradoxically enhance absorption.

DECONTAMINATION OF THE EYES

Act quickly to prevent serious damage. Flush the eyes with copious amounts of saline (preferred) or water. (If available, instill local anesthetic drops in the eye before beginning irrigation.) Remove contact lenses if present. Direct the irrigating stream so that it will flow across both eyes after running off the nasal bridge. Lift the tarsal conjunctiva to look for undissolved particles and to facilitate irrigation. Continue irrigation for 15 minutes or until each eye has been irrigated with at least 1 L of solution. If the toxin is an acid or a base, check the pH of the tears after irrigation, and continue irrigation until the pH is between 6.5 and 7.5.

After irrigation is complete, perform a careful examination of the eye, using fluorescein and a slitlamp or Wood's lamp to identify areas of corneal injury. Patients with serious conjunctival or corneal injury should be immediately referred to an ophthalmologist.

GASTROINTESTINAL DECONTAMINATION

Removal of ingested poisons is a traditional part of emergency treatment. However, studies indicate that if more than 60 minutes has passed, induced emesis and gastric lavage are relatively ineffective. For small or moderate ingestions of most substances, toxicologists generally recommend activated charcoal alone without prior gastric emptying. Exceptions are large ingestions of anticholinergic compounds and salicylates, which often delay gastric emptying, and ingestion of sustained-release or enteric-coated tablets, which may remain intact for several hours.

Gastric emptying is not generally used for ingestion of corrosive agents or petroleum distillates, because further esophageal injury or pulmonary aspiration may result. However, in certain cases, removal of the toxin may be more important than concern over possible complications. Consult a medical toxicologist or regional poison control center (Table 39–1) for advice.

Emesis

Emesis using syrup of ipecac is a convenient and fairly effective way to evacuate gastric contents if given very soon after ingestion (eg, at work or at home). However, it may delay or prevent use of oral activated charcoal and is not generally used in the hospital management of ingestions.

A. Indications: For removal of poison in conscious, cooperative patients and for promptness, ipecac can be given in the home or at work in the first few minutes after poisoning.

B. Contraindications: Induced emesis is contraindicated for drowsy, unconscious, or convulsing patients and for patients who have ingested kerosene or other hydrocarbons (danger of aspiration of stomach contents), corrosive poisons, or rapidly acting convulsants (eg, tricyclic antidepressants, strychnine, camphor).

C. Technique: Give syrup of ipecac, 30 mL (15 mL in children), followed by an 8-oz glass of water. Repeat in 20 minutes if necessary.

Gastric Lavage

Gastric lavage is more effective for liquid poisons or small pill fragments than for intact tablets or pieces of mushroom. It is most effective when started within 60 minutes after ingestion. The lavage procedure may delay administration of activated charcoal and may hasten passage of pills and other toxic material into the small intestine.

A. Indications: Gastric lavage is indicated for removal of ingested poisons when emesis is refused, contraindicated, or unsuccessful; for collection and examination of gastric contents for identification of poison; and for convenient administration of charcoal and antidotes.

B. Contraindications: Do *not* use lavage for stuporous or comatose patients with absent gag reflexes unless they are endotracheally intubated beforehand. Some authorities advise against lavage when caustic material has been ingested; others regard it as essential to remove liquid corrosives from the stomach.

C. Technique: In obtunded or comatose patients, the danger of aspiration pneumonia is reduced by placing the patient in a head down, left lateral decubitus position and, if necessary, protecting the airway with endotracheal intubation. Gently insert a lubricated, soft but noncollapsible stomach tube (at least 37–40F) through the mouth or nose into the stomach. Aspirate and save the contents, and then lavage repeatedly with 50–100 mL of fluid until the return fluid is clear. Use lukewarm tap water or saline.

Activated Charcoal

Activated charcoal effectively adsorbs almost all drugs and poisons. Poorly adsorbed substances include iron, lithium, potassium, sodium, cyanide, mineral acids, and alcohols.

A. Indications: Activated charcoal should be used for prompt adsorption of drugs or toxins in the stomach and intestine. Studies show that activated charcoal given alone may be as effective as or more effective than ipecac-induced emesis or gastric lavage.

B. Contraindications: Activated charcoal should not be used for stuporous, comatose, or convulsing patients unless it can be given by gastric tube and the airway is first protected by cuffed endotracheal tube. This substance is contraindicated also for patients with ileus or intestinal obstruction or those who have ingested corrosives for whom endoscopy is planned.

C. Technique: Administer activated charcoal, 60–100 g orally or via gastric tube, mixed in aqueous slurry. Repeated doses may be given to ensure gastrointestinal adsorption or to enhance elimination of some drugs (see below).

Catharsis

A. Indications: Cathartics are used by some toxicologists for stimulation of peristalsis to hasten the elimination of unabsorbed drugs and poisons and the activated charcoal slurry.

B. Contraindications and Cautions: Do not use mineral oil or other oil-based cathartics. Avoid sodium-based cathartics in patients with hypertension, renal failure, and congestive heart failure and magnesium-based cathartics in those with renal failure.

C. Technique: Magnesium sulfate 10%, 2–3 mL/kg; or sorbitol 70%, 1–2 mL/kg. Sorbitol is commonly used in prepackaged charcoal slurry products.

Whole Bowel Irrigation

Whole bowel irrigation utilizes large volumes of balanced polyethylene glycol-electrolyte solution to mechanically cleanse the entire intestinal tract. Because of the composition of the irrigating solution, there is no significant gain or loss of systemic fluids or electrolytes.

A. Indications: Whole bowel irrigation is particularly effective for massive iron ingestion in which intact tablets are visible on abdominal x-ray. It has also been used for ingestions of sustained-release and enteric-coated tablets as well as drug-filled packets.

B. Contraindications: Same as for cathartics.

C. Technique: Administer the balanced polyethylene glycol-electrolyte solution (CoLyte, GoLYTELY) into the stomach via gastric tube at a rate of 1–2 L/h until the rectal effluent is clear. It is most effective when patients are able to sit on a commode to pass the intestinal contents.

Increased Drug Removal

A. Urinary Manipulation: Forced diuresis is hazardous; the risk of complications (pulmonary edema, electrolyte imbalance) usually outweighs its benefits. Acidic drugs (eg, salicylates, phenobarbital) are more rapidly excreted with an alkaline urine. Acidification (sometimes promoted for amphetamines, phencyclidine) is *not* very effective and is contraindicated in the presence of rhabdomyolysis or myoglobinuria.

B. Dialysis (Hemodialysis or Hemoperfusion): The indications for dialysis are as follows: (1) Known or suspected potentially lethal amounts of a dialyzable drug (Table 39–6). (2) Poisoning with deep coma, apnea, severe hypotension, fluid and electrolyte or acid-base disturbance, or extreme body temperature changes that cannot be corrected by conventional measures. (3) Poisoning in patients with severe renal, cardiac, pulmonary, or hepatic disease who will not be able to eliminate the toxin by usual mechanisms.

Many of the substances that cannot be removed effectively by aqueous dialysis can be removed by hemoperfusion through specially designed coated charcoal columns. Indications are the same as for dialysis. Peritoneal dialysis may occasionally be employed for acute poisonings when hemodialysis is not available, but it is very inefficient. Dialysis should usually augment rather than replace well-established emergency and supportive measures. Continuous arteriovenous and venovenous hemodiafiltration is of uncertain benefit for elimination of poisons.

Table 39–6. Recommended use of hemodialysis (HD) and hemoperfusion (HP) in poisoning.

Poison	Procedure[1]	Indications[2]
Carbamazepine	HP	Seizures, severe cardiotoxicity.
Ethylene glycol	HD	Acidosis, serum level > 50 mg/dL.
Lithium	HD	Severe symptoms; level > 4 meq/L more than 12 hours after last dose.
Methanol	HD	Acidosis, serum level > 50 mg/dL.
Phenobarbital	HP	Intractable hypotension, acidosis despite maximal supportive care.
Salicylate	HD	Severe acidosis, CNS symptoms, level > 100 mg/dL (acute overdose) or > 60 mg/dL (chronic intoxication).
Theophylline	HP or HD	Serum level > 90–100 mg/L (acute) or seizures and serum level > 40–60 mg/L (chronic).
Valproic acid	HD	Serum level > 900–1000 mg/L or deep coma, severe acidosis.

[1]Contact a regional poison control center or a clinical toxicologist before undertaking these procedures.
[2]See text for further discussion of indications.

C. Repeat-Dose Charcoal: Repeated doses of activated charcoal, 20–30 g every 3–4 hours, may hasten elimination of some drugs (eg, digitoxin, theophylline, phenobarbital) by adsorbing drug excreted into the gut lumen ("gut dialysis"). However, no clinical studies have documented improved outcome using multiple-dose charcoal. Sorbitol or other cathartics should *not* be used with each dose, or resulting large stool volumes may lead to dehydration or hypernatremia.

Chan TC et al: Drug-induced hyperthermia. Crit Care Clin 1997;13:785. [NLM Cit ID: 97471900] (Review of pathophysiology, presentation, and treatment of the drug-induced hyperthermia syndromes: malignant hyperthermia, neuroleptic malignant syndrome, sympathomimetic poisoning and anticholinergic toxicity.)

Krenzelok EP et al: Position statement: ipecac syrup. Am Acad Clin Toxicology; European Association of Poisons Centres and Clinical Toxicologists. J Toxicol Clin Toxicol 1997;35:699. [NLM Cit ID: 98141529] (There is no evidence from clinical studies supporting the use of ipecac in the management of poisoned patients in the emergency department.)

Tenenbein M: Position statement: whole bowel irrigation. American Academy of Clinical Toxicology; European

Association of Poisons Centres and Clinical Toxicologists. J Toxicol Clin Toxicol 1997;35:753. [NLM Cit ID: 98141533] (Whole bowel irrigation may be considered for toxic ingestions of sustained-release or enteric-coated drugs. If done after the administration of activated charcoal, the binding capacity of charcoal and the osmotic properties of whole bowel irrigations appear to be unchanged.)

Wax PM et al: Prehospital gastrointestinal decontamination of toxic ingestions: a missed opportunity. Am J Emerg Med 1998;16:114. [NLM Cit ID: 98176860] (Retrospective review of adult ambulance transports for drug overdose found that 30 out of 43 patients who were suitable candidates for oral activated charcoal received it in the ER rather than in the ambulance, which delayed this valuable medical treatment by 82 minutes.)

DIAGNOSIS OF POISONING

The identity of the ingested substance or substances is usually known, but occasionally a comatose patient is found with an unlabeled container or refuses or otherwise fails to give a coherent history. By performing a directed physical examination and ordering common clinical laboratory tests, the clinician can often make a tentative diagnosis that may allow empirical interventions or may suggest specific toxicologic tests.

PHYSICAL EXAMINATION

Important diagnostic variables in the physical examination include blood pressure, pulse rate, temperature, pupil size, sweating, and the presence or absence of peristaltic activity. Poisonings with many drugs fit into one of four common syndromes.

Sympathomimetic Syndrome

The blood pressure and pulse rate are elevated, though with severe hypertension reflex bradycardia may occur. The temperature is often elevated, pupils are dilated, and the skin is sweaty, though mucous membranes are dry. Patients are usually agitated, anxious, or frankly psychotic.

Examples: Amphetamines, cocaine, ephedrine and pseudoephedrine, phencyclidine (pupils normal or small), phenylpropanolamine (bradycardia common).

Sympatholytic Syndrome

The blood pressure and pulse rate are decreased and body temperature is low. The pupils are small or even pinpoint. Peristalsis is usually decreased. Patients are usually obtunded or comatose.

Examples: Barbiturates, benzodiazepines and other sedative hypnotics, γ-hydroxybutyrate (GHB), clonidine and related antihypertensives, ethanol, opioids.

Cholinergic Syndrome

Stimulation of muscarinic receptors causes bradycardia, miosis, sweating, and hyperperistalsis as well as bronchorrhea, wheezing, excessive salivation, and urinary incontinence. Nicotinic receptor stimulation may produce initial hypertension and tachycardia as well as fasciculations and muscle weakness. Patients are usually agitated and anxious.

Examples: Carbamates, nicotine, organophosphates, physostigmine.

Anticholinergic Syndrome

Tachycardia with mild hypertension is common, and the body temperature is often elevated. Pupils are widely dilated. The skin is flushed, hot and dry. Peristalsis is decreased, and urinary retention is common. Patients may have myoclonic jerking or choreoathetoid movements. Agitated delirium is frequently seen, and severe hyperthermia may occur.

Examples: Atropine, scopolamine, other naturally occurring and pharmaceutical anticholinergics, amantadine, antihistamines, phenothiazines (hypotension, small pupils), tricyclic antidepressants.

CLINICAL LABORATORY TESTS IN MANAGEMENT OF POISONING

The following clinical laboratory tests are recommended for screening of the overdosed patient: measured serum osmolality and osmolar gap, electrolytes, glucose, creatinine, BUN, urinalysis (eg, oxalate crystals with ethylene glycol poisoning, myoglobinuria with rhabdomyolysis), and electrocardiography. Serum acetaminophen and ethanol levels should be determined in all patients with drug overdoses.

OSMOLAR GAP

The osmolar gap is defined and calculation of the gap is described in Table 39–7. It is increased in the presence of large quantities of low-molecular-weight substances, most commonly ethanol. Common poisons associated with increased osmolar gap are acetone, ethanol, ethylene glycol, isopropyl alcohol, methanol, and propylene glycol. ***Note:*** Severe alcoholic ketoacidosis and diabetic ketoacidoses can cause an elevated osmolar gap resulting from the production of ketones and other low-molecular-weight substances.

ANION GAP

Metabolic acidosis associated with an elevated anion gap is usually due to an accumulation of lactic

Table 39–7. Use of the osmolar gap in toxicology.[1]

The osmolar gap (Δosm) is determined by subtracting the calculated serum osmolality from the measured serum osmolality.

$$\text{Calculated osmolality (osm)} = 2\,[\text{Na}^+(\text{meq/L})] + \frac{\text{Glucose (mg/dL)}}{18} + \frac{\text{BUN (mg/dL)}}{2.8}$$

$$\Delta\text{osm} = \text{Measured osmolality} - \text{Calculated osmolality}$$

Serum osmolality may be increased by contributions of circulating alcohols and other low-molecular-weight substances. Since these substances are not included in the calculated osmolality, there will be a gap proportionate to their serum concentration and inversely proportionate to their molecular weight:

$$\text{Serum concentration (mg/dL)} = \Delta\text{osm} \times \frac{\text{Molecular weight}}{10}$$

	Molecular Weight	Toxic Concentration	Approximate Corresponding Δosm (mosm/L)
Ethanol	46	300	65
Methanol	32	50	16
Ethylene glycol	60	100	16
Isopropanol	60	150	25

[1]Modified from Saunders CE, Ho MT (editors): *Current Emergency Diagnosis & Treatment,* 4th ed. Originally published by Appleton & Lange. Copyright © 1992 by The McGraw-Hill Companies, Inc.

Note: Most laboratories use the freezing point method for calculating osmolality. If the vaporization point method is used, alcohols are driven off and their contribution to osmolality is lost.

acid or other acids (see Chapter 21). Common causes of elevated anion gap in poisoning include carbon monoxide, cyanide, ethylene glycol, medicinal iron, isoniazid, methanol, phenformin, and salicylates.

One should also check the osmolar gap; combined elevated anion and osmolar gap suggests poisoning by methanol or ethylene glycol, though this may also occur in patients with diabetic ketoacidosis and alcoholic ketoacidosis.

TOXICOLOGY LABORATORY EXAMINATION

The routine toxicology screen (Table 39–8) is of little value in the initial care of the poisoned patient—on the contrary, it is time-consuming, expensive, and frequently erroneous. Specific quantitative levels of certain drugs may be extremely helpful (Table 39–9), however, especially if specific antidotes or interventions (eg, dialysis) would be indicated based upon the results.

Table 39–8. Examples of common drugs screened for in blood and urine in a reference toxicology laboratory.[1,2]

Blood	
Acetaminophen	Ethchlorvynol
Alcohols	Glutethimide
Barbiturates	Meprobamate
Benzodiazepines	Phenytoin
Carbamazepine	Salicylates
Carisoprodol	
Urine	
Acetaminophen	Meperidine
Alcohols	Meprobamate
Amphetamines	Methadone
Barbiturates	Morphine
Chlorpheniramine	Pentazocine
Cocaine	Phencyclidine
Codeine	Phenothiazines
Dextromethorphan	Propoxyphene
Diphenhydramine	Salicylates
Lidocaine	Tricyclic antidepressants

[1]The urine screen is usually more comprehensive, detecting drugs of abuse (opioids, stimulants), antihistamines, and, in many cases, drugs also found in serum.
[2]Many drugs and poisons are not screened for (eg, limited screens; newer drugs; a variety of drugs and poisons such as cyanide, digitalis, ethylene glycol, isoniazid, theophylline).

If a toxicology screen is required, urine is the best specimen for broad qualitative screening. Blood samples may be saved for possible quantitative testing, but blood is not generally used for screening purposes since it is relatively insensitive for many common drugs, including psychotropic agents, opioids, and stimulants.

ABDOMINAL X-RAYS

A plain film of the abdomen may reveal radiopaque iron tablets, drug-filled condoms, or other toxic material. Studies suggest that few tablets are predictably visible (eg, ferrous sulfate, sodium chloride, calcium carbonate, and potassium chloride). Thus, the x-ray is useful only if positive.

Goldfrank LR (editor): *Goldfrank's Toxicologic Emergencies,* 6th ed. Appleton & Lange, 1998.

Olson KR (editor): *Poisoning and Drug Overdose,* 3rd ed. Appleton & Lange, 1999.

Sporer KA et al: Acetaminophen and salicylate serum levels in patients with suicidal ingestion or altered mental status. Am J Emerg Med 1996;14:443. [NLM Cit ID: 96350122] (Retrospective study of 1820 patients supporting the utility of universal screening for acetaminophen but not salicylates in patients presenting with a history of suicidal ingestion or an altered mental status with a strong suspicion of ingestion.)

Table 39–9. Specific quantitative levels and potential therapeutic interventions.[1]

Drug or Toxin	Treatment
Acetaminophen	Specific antidote (acetylcysteine) based on serum level
Carbon monoxide	High carboxyhemoglobin level indicates need for 100% oxygen, consideration of hyperbaric oxygen
Carbamazepine	High level may indicate need for hemoperfusion
Digoxin	On basis of serum digoxin level and sevrity of clinical presentation, treatment with Fab antibody fragments (Digibind) may be indicated
Ethanol	Low serum level may suggest nonalcoholic cause of coma (eg, trauma, other drugs, other alcohols). Serum ethanol may also be useful in monitoring ethanol therapy for methanol or ethylene glycol poisoning.
Iron	Level may indicate need for chelation with deferoxamine
Lithium	Serum levels can guide decision to institute hemodialysis
Methanol, ethylene glycol	Acidosis, high levels indicate need for hemodialysis, therapy with ethanol or fomepizole
Methemoglobin	Methemoglobinemia can be treated with methylene blue intravenously
Salicylates	High level may indicate need for hemodialysis, alkaline diuresis
Theophylline	Immediate hemodialysis or hemoperfusion may be indicated based on serum level
Valproic acid	Elevated levels may indicate need to consider hemodialysis

[1]Some drugs or toxins may have profound and irreversible toxicity unless rapid and specific management is provided outside of routine supportive care. For these agents, laboratory testing may provide the serum level or other evidence required for administering a specific antidote or arranging for hemodialysis.

TREATMENT OF COMMON SPECIFIC POISONINGS (Alphabetical Order)

ACETAMINOPHEN

Acetaminophen is a common analgesic found in many nonprescription and prescription products. After absorption, it is metabolized mainly by glucuronidation and sulfation, with a small fraction metabolized via the P450 mixed-function oxidase system to a highly toxic reactive intermediate. This toxic intermediate is normally detoxified by cellular glutathione. With acute acetaminophen overdose (> 140 mg/kg, or 7 g in an average adult), hepatocellular glutathione is rapidly depleted and the reactive intermediate attacks other cell proteins, causing necrosis. Patients with enhanced P450 activity, such as chronic alcoholics and patients taking anticonvulsants, are at increased risk of developing hepatotoxicity. Hepatic toxicity may also occur after chronic accidental overuse of acetaminophen—eg, as little as 1 g of acetaminophen every 4–6 hours for 1–2 days in a patient with chronic excessive alcohol use.

Clinical Findings

Shortly after ingestion, patients may have nausea or vomiting, but there are usually no other signs of toxicity until 24–48 hours after ingestion, when hepatic aminotransferase levels begin to increase. With severe poisoning, massive hepatic necrosis may occur, resulting in jaundice, hepatic encephalopathy, renal failure, and death.

The diagnosis of severe poisoning after acute overdose is based on measurement of the serum acetaminophen level. Plot the serum level versus the time since ingestion on the acetaminophen nomogram shown in Figure 39–1. Ingestion of sustained-release products, such as Tylenol Extended Relief, or coingestion of an anticholinergic agent, salicylate, or opioid drug may cause delayed elevation of serum levels.

Treatment

A. Emergency and Supportive Measures: Empty the stomach by emesis (at home) or gastric lavage (within 1 hour after ingestion). (If more than 1–2 hours have passed since ingestion, do not attempt gut emptying procedures.) Administer activated charcoal. Although charcoal may bind the oral antidote acetylcysteine, this is not considered clinically significant.

B. Specific Treatment: If the serum acetaminophen level is higher than the upper toxic line on the nomogram (Figure 39–1), begin treatment with a loading dose of acetylcysteine, 140 mg/kg orally, followed by 70 mg/kg every 4 hours. Dilute the solution to 5% with water, juice, or soda. If vomiting interferes with oral acetylcysteine administration, give the dose by gastric tube and use metoclopramide, 1–2 mg/kg intravenously. The most widely used protocol in the USA continues treatment for 72 hours. However, other regimens have demonstrated equivalent success with 20–48 hours of treatment. Treatment with acetylcysteine is most effective if started within 8–10 hours after ingestion. If the precise time of ingestion is unknown or if the patient is at higher risk of hepatotoxicity (eg, alcoholic, liver disease, chronic

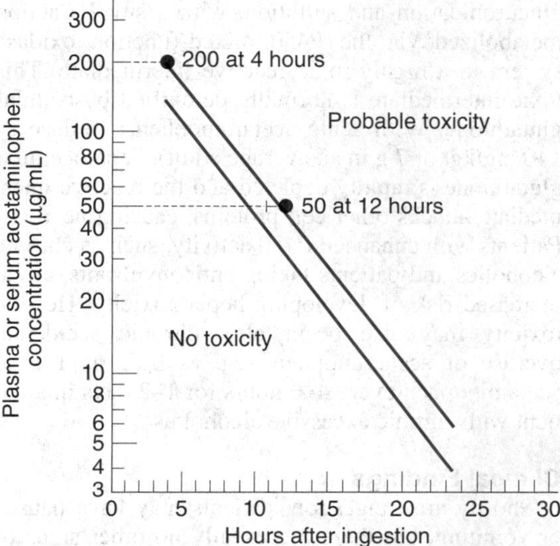

Figure 39–1. Nomogram for prediction of acetaminophen hepatotoxicity following acute overdosage. The upper line defines serum acetaminophen concentrations known to be associated with hepatotoxicity; the lower line defines serum levels 25% below those expected to cause hepatotoxicity. To give a margin for error and for patients at higher risk for hepatotoxicity, the lower line should be used as a guide to treatment. (Modified and reproduced, with permission, from Rumack BH, Matthew H: Acetaminophen poisoning and toxicity. Pediatrics 1975;55:871.)

use of P450-inducing drugs), then use a lower threshold for initiation of acetylcysteine (ie, the lower nomogram line; in some case reports, a level of 100 mg/L at 4 hours was suggested in very high-risk patients).

Acetylcysteine may also be given intravenously; this is the preferred method in Europe and Canada, but there is no approved parenteral formulation or dosing schedule in the United States. If the patient cannot tolerate acetylcysteine despite antiemetics and administration via a gastric tube, the United States formulation may be given intravenously. Call a regional poison control center or medical toxicologist for assistance.

Jones AL: Mechanism of action and value of *N*-acetylcysteine in the treatment of early and late acetaminophen poisoning: a critical review. J Toxicol Clin Toxicol 1998;36:277. [NLM Cit ID: 98377051] (A very good review of the rationale and evidence for the use of *N*-acetylcysteine in patients with acetaminophen poisoning. Highlights the need for lower treatment thresholds in chronic alcoholics and those who take anticonvulsants.)

Vale JA et al: Paracetamol (acetaminophen) poisoning. Lancet 1995;346:547. [NLM Cit ID: 95387731] (An excellent review of the pathophysiology, diagnosis, and treatment of acetaminophen poisoning.)

ACIDS, CORROSIVE (Table 39–10)

The strong mineral acids exert primarily a local corrosive effect on the skin and mucous membranes. Symptoms include severe pain in the throat and upper gastrointestinal tract; bloody vomitus; difficulty in swallowing, breathing, and speaking; discoloration and destruction of skin and mucous membranes in and around the mouth; and shock. Severe systemic metabolic acidosis may occur both as a result of cellular injury and from systemic absorption of the acid.

Severe deep destructive tissue damage may occur after exposure to hydrofluoric acid because of the penetrating and highly toxic fluoride ion. Systemic hypocalcemia and hyperkalemia also may occur after fluoride absorption, even following skin exposure.

Inhalation of volatile acids, fumes, or gases such as chlorine, fluorine, bromine, or iodine causes severe irritation of the throat and larynx and may cause upper airway obstruction and noncardiogenic pulmonary edema.

Treatment

A. Ingestion: Do *not* induce emesis. Dilute immediately by giving a glass (4–8 oz) of milk or water to drink. Do *not* give bicarbonate or other neutralizing agents. Some experts recommend immediate gastric lavage.

Perform flexible endoscopic esophagoscopy promptly to determine the presence and extent of injury. X-rays of the chest and abdomen may reveal the presence of free air in patients with esophageal or

Table 39–10. Common corrosive agents.[1]

Category and Examples	Injury Caused
Concentrated alkalies	
Clinitest tablets Drain cleaners Industrial-strength ammonia Lye Oven cleaners	Penetrating liquefaction necrosis
Concentrated acids	
Pool disinfectants Toilet bowl cleaners	Coagulation necrosis
Weaker cleaning agents	
Cationic detergents (dishwasher detergents) Household ammonia Household bleach	Superficial burns and irritation; deep burns (rare)
Other	
Hydrofluoric acid	Penetrating, delayed, destructive injury

[1]Reproduced, with permission, from Saunders CE, Ho MT (editors): *Current Emergency Diagnosis & Treatment,* 4th ed. Originally published by Appleton & Lange. Copyright © 1992 by The McGraw-Hill Companies, Inc.

gastric perforation. Perforation, peritonitis, and major bleeding are indications for surgery.

B. Skin Contact: Flood with water for 15 minutes. Use no chemical antidotes; the heat of the reaction may cause additional injury.

For hydrofluoric acid burns, soak the affected area in magnesium sulfate solution or apply 2.5% calcium gluconate gel (prepared by adding 3.5 g calcium gluconate to 5 oz of water-soluble surgical lubricant, eg, K-Y Jelly); then arrange immediate consultation with a plastic surgeon or other specialist. Binding of the fluoride ion may be achieved by injecting 0.5 mL of 5% calcium gluconate per square centimeter under the burned area. (***Caution:*** *Do not use calcium chloride.*)

C. Eye Contact: Anesthetize the conjunctiva and corneal surfaces with topical local anesthetic drops. Flood with water for 15 minutes, holding the eyelids open. Check pH with pH 6.0–8.0 test paper, and repeat irrigation, using 0.9% saline, until pH is near 7.0. Check for corneal damage with fluorescein and slitlamp examination; consult an ophthalmologist about further treatment.

D. Inhalation: Remove from further exposure to fumes or gas. Check skin and clothing. Treat pulmonary edema.

Andreoni B et al: Esophageal perforation and caustic injury: Emergency management of caustic ingestion. Dis Esophagus 1997;10:95. [NLM Cit ID: 97322987] (Prospective observation of 58 adult patients. Study recommends early staging of lesions by endoscopy.)

Hugh TB et al: Corrosive ingestion and the surgeon. J Am Coll Surg 1999;189:508. [NLM Cit ID 20015933] (Pathophysiology, presentation, and clinical management of patients with corrosive ingestion injuries.)

ALKALIES (Table 39–10)

The strong alkalies are common ingredients of some household cleaning compounds and may be suspected by their "soapy" texture. Those with alkalinity above pH 12.0 are particularly corrosive. Clinitest tablets and disk batteries are also a source. Alkalies cause liquefactive necrosis, which is deeply penetrating. Symptoms include burning pain in the upper gastrointestinal tract, nausea, vomiting, and difficulty in swallowing and breathing. Examination reveals destruction and edema of the affected skin and mucous membranes and bloody vomitus and stools. X-ray may reveal the presence of disk batteries in the esophagus or lower gastrointestinal tract.

Treatment

A. Ingestion: Do *not* induce emesis. Dilute immediately with a glass of water. Some gastroenterologists recommend immediate gastric lavage after ingestion of liquid caustic substances to remove residual material.

Immediate endoscopy is recommended to evaluate the extent of damage. If x-ray reveals the location of ingested disk batteries in the esophagus, immediate endoscopic removal is mandatory.

The use of corticosteroids to prevent stricture formation is of no proved benefit and is definitely contraindicated if there is evidence of esophageal perforation.

B. Skin Contact: Wash with running water until the skin no longer feels soapy. Relieve pain and treat shock.

C. Eye Contact: Anesthetize the conjunctival and corneal surfaces with topical anesthetic. Irrigate with water or saline continuously for 20–30 minutes, holding the lids open. Check pH with pH test paper, and repeat irrigation, using 0.9% saline, for additional 30-minute periods until the pH is near 7.0. Check for corneal damage with fluorescein and slitlamp examination; consult an ophthalmologist for further treatment.

Gunnarsson M: Local corticosteroid treatment of caustic injuries of the esophagus. A preliminary report. Ann Otol Rhinol Laryngol 1999;108:1088. [NLM Cit ID: 20043838] (Case report of topical application of steroid solutions in two patients. Although controlled studies of parenteral steroids have shown no benefit, this method of treatment deserves further study.)

Hugh TB et al: Corrosive ingestion and the surgeon. J Am Coll Surg 1999;189:508. [NLM Cit ID 20015933] (An excellent, well-written review of the pathophysiology, presentation, and clinical management of patients with corrosive ingestion injuries.)

AMPHETAMINES & COCAINE

Amphetamines and cocaine are widely abused for their euphorigenic and stimulant properties. Both drugs may be smoked, snorted, ingested, or injected. Amphetamines and cocaine produce central nervous system stimulation and a generalized increase in central and peripheral sympathetic activity. The toxic dose of each drug is highly variable and depends on the route of administration and individual tolerance. The onset of effects is most rapid after intravenous injection or smoking. Amphetamine derivatives and related drugs include methamphetamine ("crystal meth," "crank"), methylenedioxymethamphetamine (MDMA, "ecstasy"), ephedrine ("herbal ecstasy"), and methcathinone ("cat").

Clinical Findings

Patients may present with anxiety, tremulousness, tachycardia, hypertension, diaphoresis, dilated pupils, agitation, muscular hyperactivity, and psychosis. Metabolic acidosis may occur. In severe intoxication, seizures and hyperthermia may occur. Sustained or severe hypertension may result in intracranial hemorrhage, aortic dissection, or myocardial infarction.

The diagnosis is supported by finding amphetamines, cocaine, or the cocaine metabolite benzoylecgonine in the urine. Blood screening is not sensitive enough to detect these drugs.

Treatment

A. Emergency and Supportive Measures: Maintain a patent airway and assist ventilation, if necessary. Treat coma or seizures as described at the beginning of this chapter. Rapidly lower the body temperature (see p 1564) in patients who are hyperthermic (40 °C). Treat agitation or psychosis with a benzodiazepine such as diazepam, 5–10 mg intravenously (repeated as needed up to 20 mg), or midazolam, 0.1–0.2 mg/kg intramuscularly.

For poisoning by ingestion, perform gastric lavage and administer activated charcoal, or administer activated charcoal alone without prior gut emptying (see p 1565). Do *not* induce emesis, because of the risk of seizures.

B. Specific Treatment: Treat agitation with a sedative such as lorazepam, 2–3 mg intravenously. Treat hypertension with a vasodilator drug such as phentolamine (1–5 mg intravenously) or nifedipine (10–20 mg orally) or a combined α- and β-adrenergic blocker such as labetalol (10–20 mg intravenously). Do *not* administer a pure beta-blocker such as propranolol alone, as this may result in paradoxic worsening of the hypertension as a result of unopposed α-adrenergic effects.

Treat tachycardia or tachyarrhythmias with a short-acting beta-blocker such as esmolol (25–100 μg/kg/min by intravenous infusion).

Albertson TE et al: Methamphetamine and the expanding complications of amphetamines. West J Med 1999;170: 214. [NLM Cit ID: 99275643] (Review of effects and treatment options for methamphetamine toxicity.)

Boghdadi MS et al: Cocaine: Pathophysiology and clinical toxicology. Heart Lung 1997;26:466. [NLM Cit ID: 98093538] (Review of the medical complications of cocaine abuse.)

Callaway CW et al: Hyperthermia in psychostimulant overdose. Ann Emerg Med 1994;24:68. [NLM Cit ID: 94279932] (Pathophysiology and management of hyperthermia induced by amphetamines and cocaine.)

ANTICOAGULANTS

Warfarin and related compounds (including ingredients of many commercial rodenticides) inhibit the clotting mechanism by blocking hepatic synthesis of vitamin K-dependent clotting factors.

Anticoagulants may cause hemoptysis, gross hematuria, bloody stools, hemorrhages into organs, widespread bruising, and bleeding into joint spaces. The prothrombin time is increased within 12–24 hours (peak 36–48 hours) after a single overdose. After ingestion of brodifacoum and indanedione rodenticides (so-called superwarfarins), inhibition of clotting factor synthesis may persist for several weeks or even months after a single dose.

Treatment

A. Emergency and Supportive Measures: Discontinue the drug at the first sign of gross bleeding, and determine the prothrombin time. If the patient has ingested an acute overdose, empty the stomach by emesis (at home) or lavage and administer activated charcoal (see p 1565).

B. Specific Treatment: Do not treat prophylactically—wait for the evidence of anticoagulation (elevated prothrombin time). If the prothrombin time is elevated, give phytonadione (vitamin K_1), 5–10 mg subcutaneously or 10–25 mg orally, and additional doses as needed to restore the prothrombin time to normal. Give fresh-frozen plasma as needed to rapidly correct the coagulation factor deficit if there is serious bleeding. If the patient is chronically anticoagulated and has strong medical indications for being maintained in that status (eg, prosthetic heart valve), give much smaller doses of vitamin K (1 mg) and fresh-frozen plasma (or both) to titrate to the desired prothrombin time.

If the patient has ingested brodifacoum or a related superwarfarin, prolonged observation (over weeks) and repeated administration of large doses of vitamin K may be required.

Chua JD et al: Superwarfarin poisoning. Arch Intern Med 1998;158:1929. [NLM Cit ID: 98430490] (Case series and literature review.)

ANTICONVULSANTS (Carbamazepine, Phenytoin, Valproic Acid)

These drugs are widely used in the management of seizure disorders. In addition, carbamazepine and valproic acid are increasingly used for treatment of mood disorders.

Phenytoin can be given orally or intravenously. Rapid intravenous injection of phenytoin can cause acute myocardial depression and cardiac arrest owing to the solvent propylene glycol; a newer form of phenytoin (fosphenytoin) is available that does not contain this diluent. Phenytoin intoxication can occur with only slightly increased doses because of the small toxic-therapeutic window. Phenytoin intoxication can also occur following acute intentional or accidental overdose. The overdose syndrome is usually mild even with high serum levels. The most common manifestations are ataxia, nystagmus, and drowsiness. Choreoathetoid movements have been described.

Carbamazepine was first used for the treatment

of trigeminal neuralgia. It has since become a first-line agent for temporal lobe epilepsy and other seizure disorders. Intoxication causes drowsiness, stupor, and, with high levels, coma and seizures. Dilated pupils and tachycardia are common. Toxicity may be seen with serum levels greater than 20 mg/L, though severe poisoning is usually associated with concentrations greater than 30–40 mg/L. Because of erratic and slow absorption, intoxication may progress over several hours to days.

Valproic acid intoxication produces a unique syndrome consisting of hypernatremia (from the sodium component of the salt), metabolic acidosis, hypocalcemia, elevated serum ammonia, and mild liver aminotransferase elevation. Hypoglycemia may occur as a result of hepatic metabolic dysfunction. Coma with small pupils may be seen and can mimic opioid poisoning. Encephalopathy and cerebral edema can occur.

Treatment

A. Emergency and Supportive Measures: For recent ingestions, give activated charcoal orally or by gastric tube. For large ingestions of carbamazepine or valproic acid—especially of sustained-release formulations—consider whole bowel irrigation (see p 1566). Multiple-dose activated charcoal may be beneficial in ensuring gut decontamination for large ingestions and may enhance elimination of absorbed drugs.

B. Specific Treatment: There are no antidotes. Naloxone was reported to have reversed valproic acid overdose in one anecdotal case. Consider hemodialysis (valproic acid) or hemoperfusion (carbamazepine) for massive intoxication (eg, carbamazepine levels > 100 mg/L or valproic acid poisoning with levels > 1000 mg/L).

Franssen EJ et al: Valproic acid toxicokinetics: Serial hemodialysis and hemoperfusion. Ther Drug Monit 1999;21:289. [NLM Cit ID: 99291760] (Case report of coma, hypernatremia, and respiratory failure in a 27-year-old man with a serum valproic acid level of 1414 μg/mL. Hemodialysis clearance was 80 mL/min, compared with 40 mL/min for hemoperfusion.)

Johnson LZ et al: Successful treatment of valproic acid overdose with hemodialysis. Am J Kidney Dis 1999;33:786. [NLM Cit ID: 99211860] (Case report of effective hemodialysis in the treatment of a patient with a serum valproic acid level of 1380 μg/mL associated with metabolic acidosis, thrombocytopenia, refractory hypotension and coma.)

Schmidt S et al: Signs and symptoms of carbamazepine overdose. J Neurol 1995;242:169. [NLM Cit ID: 95271236] (Retrospective study of 427 patients that describes the clinical manifestations and prognosis of carbamazepine overdose.)

ARSENIC

Arsenic is found in pesticides and industrial chemicals. Symptoms of poisoning usually appear within 1 hour after ingestion but may be delayed as long as 12 hours. They include abdominal pain, vomiting, watery diarrhea, and skeletal muscle cramps. Profound dehydration and shock may occur. In chronic poisoning, symptoms can be vague but often include those of peripheral sensory neuropathy. Urinary arsenic levels may be misleading and are falsely elevated after certain meals (eg, seafood) that contain large quantities of relatively nontoxic organic arsenic.

Treatment

A. Emergency Measures: Induce vomiting or perform gastric lavage, and administer 60–100 g of activated charcoal (see p 1565).

B. Antidote: For symptomatic patients or those with massive overdose, give dimercaprol injection (BAL), 10% solution in oil, 3–5 mg/kg dimercaprol intramuscularly every 4–6 hours for 2 days. The side effects include nausea, vomiting, headache, and hypertension. Follow dimercaprol with oral penicillamine, 100 mg/kg/d in four divided doses (maximum, 2 g/d), or succimer (DMSA), 10 mg/kg every 8 hours, for 1 week. Consult a medical toxicologist or regional poison control center (Table 39–1) for advice regarding chelation.

Graeme KA et al: Heavy metal toxicity, Part I: arsenic and mercury. J Emerg Med 1998;16:45. [NLM Cit ID: 98132102] (Review of both acute and chronic arsenic and mercury toxicity with recommendations for diagnosis and management.)

Piamphongsant T: Chronic environmental arsenic poisoning. Int J Dermatol 1999;38:401. [NLM Cit ID: 99323707] (Dermatologic complications of chronic arsenic poisoning.)

ATROPINE & ANTICHOLINERGICS

Atropine, scopolamine, belladonna, diphenoxylate with atropine, *Datura stramonium, Hyoscyamus niger,* some mushrooms, tricyclic antidepressants, and antihistamines are antimuscarinic agents with variable central nervous system effects. The patient complains of dryness of the mouth, thirst, difficulty in swallowing, and blurring of vision. The physical signs include dilated pupils, flushed skin, tachycardia, fever, delirium, myoclonus, ileus, and flushed appearance. Antidepressants and antihistamines may induce convulsions.

Antihistamines are commonly available with or without prescription. Diphenhydramine commonly causes delirium, tachycardia, and seizures. Massive overdose may mimic tricyclic antidepressant poisoning. The nonsedating agents terfenadine and astemizole have caused QT interval prolongation and torsade de pointes (atypical ventricular tachycardia). Loratidine has not caused this problem.

Treatment

A. Emergency and Supportive Measures: Perform gastric lavage, and administer activated charcoal (see p 1565). Do *not* induce emesis in patients who have ingested antihistamines or antidepressants, because seizures may occur abruptly. Tepid sponge baths and sedation are indicated to control high temperatures (see p 1564).

B. Specific Treatment: For pure atropine or related anticholinergic syndrome, if symptoms are severe (eg, hyperthermia or excessively rapid tachycardia), give physostigmine salicylate, 0.5–1 mg slowly intravenously over 5 minutes, with electrocardiographic monitoring, until symptoms are controlled. Bradyarrhythmias and convulsions are a hazard with physostigmine administration, and it should not be used in patients with tricyclic antidepressant overdose.

Beaver KM et al: Treatment of acute anticholinergic poisoning with physostigmine. Am J Emerg Med 1998;16:507. [NLM Cit ID: 98394017] (Case series of five patients with acute anticholinergic toxicity successfully treated with intravenous physostigmine.)

Greene GS et al: Ingestion of angel's trumpet: An increasingly common source of toxicity. South Med J 1996;89:365. [NLM Cit ID: 961851121] (Case report of three patients. Reviews the literature on diagnosis, treatment, and sequelae.)

Scopolamine poisoning among heroin users—New York City, Newark, Philadelphia, and Baltimore, 1995 and 1996. MMWR Morb Mortal Wkly Rep 1996;45:457. [NLM Cit ID: 96224219] (Review of epidemiology and clinical manifestations of heroin overdoses contaminated with anticholinergic drugs.) (Published erratum appears in MMWR Morb Mortal Wkly Rep 1996 Jun 14;45:495.)

Weiner AL et al: Anticholinergic poisoning with adulterated intranasal cocaine. Am J Emerg Med 1998;16:517. [NLM Cit ID: 98394021] (Case report.)

BETA-ADRENERGIC BLOCKERS

There are a wide variety of β-adrenergic blocking drugs, with varying pharmacologic and pharmacokinetic properties (see Table 11–6). The most commonly used and most toxic beta-blocker is propranolol. Propranolol competitively blocks β_1 and β_2 adrenoceptors and also has direct membrane-depressant and central nervous system effects.

Clinical Findings

The most common findings with mild or moderate intoxication are hypotension and bradycardia. Cardiac depression from more severe poisoning is often unresponsive to conventional therapy with β-adrenergic stimulants such as dopamine and norepinephrine. In addition, with propranolol and other lipid-soluble drugs, seizures and coma may occur.

The diagnosis is based on typical clinical findings. Routine toxicology screening does not usually include beta-blockers.

Treatment

A. Emergency and Supportive Measures: Initially, treat bradycardia or heart block with atropine (0.5–2 mg intravenously), isoproterenol (2–20 μg/min by intravenous infusion, titrated to the desired heart rate), or an external transcutaneous cardiac pacemaker. Specific antidotal treatment may be necessary (see below).

For ingested drugs, empty the stomach by gastric lavage and administer activated charcoal (see p 1565). Do *not* induce emesis because of the risk of seizures.

B. Specific Treatment: If the above measures are not successful in reversing bradycardia and hypotension, give glucagon, 5–10 mg intravenously, followed by an infusion of 1–5 mg/h. Glucagon is an inotropic agent that acts at a different receptor site and is therefore not affected by beta-blockade.

Love JN et al: Characterization of fatal beta blocker ingestion: A review of the American Association of Poison Control Centers data from 1985 to 1995. J Toxicol Clin Toxicol 1997;35:353. [NLM Cit ID: 97348027] (Retrospective review of 52,156 cases of beta-blocker poisoning. Propranolol was implicated as the cause of death in a disproportionately high percentage of fatalities.)

Love JN et al: A potential role for glucagon in the treatment of drug-induced symptomatic bradycardia. Chest 1998;114:323. [NLM Cit ID: 98337245] (Case series highlighting the effectiveness of glucagon in the treatment of drug-induced symptomatic bradycardia refractory to atropine.)

Reith DM et al: Relative toxicity of beta blockers in overdose. J Toxicol Clin Toxicol 1996;34:273. [NLM Cit ID: 96248147] (Study of 58 patients with beta-blocker poisoning suggests that propranolol is associated with the most instances of poisoning.)

CALCIUM CHANNEL BLOCKERS

Calcium channel blockers used in the United States include verapamil, diltiazem, nifedipine, nicardipine, amlodipine, felodipine, isradipine, nisoldipine, and nimodipine. These drugs share the ability to cause arteriolar vasodilation and depression of cardiac contractility, especially after acute overdose. Patients may present with bradycardia, AV nodal block, hypotension, or a combination of these effects. With severe poisoning, cardiac arrest may occur.

Treatment

A. Emergency and Supportive Measures: Maintain a patent airway and assist ventilation, if necessary. Treat coma, hypotension, and seizures as described at the beginning of this chapter. Treat bradycardia with atropine (0.5–2 mg intravenously), isoproterenol (2–20 μg/min by intravenous infusion), or a transcutaneous or internal cardiac pacemaker.

For ingested drugs, perform gastric lavage and administer activated charcoal (see p 1565). In addition, whole bowel irrigation should be initiated as soon as possible if the patient has ingested a sustained-release product. Because of the risk of hypotension and seizures, *do not* induce emesis.

B. Specific Treatment: If bradycardia and hypotension are not reversed with these measures, administer calcium chloride intravenously. Start with calcium chloride 10%, 10 mL, or calcium gluconate, 20 mL. Repeat the dose every 3–5 minutes. The optimum (or maximum) dose has not been established, but there are reports of success after as much as 10–12 g of calcium chloride. Calcium is most useful in reversing negative inotropic effects and is less effective for AV nodal blockade and bradycardia. Epinephrine infusion (1–4 μg/min initially) and glucagon, 5–10 mg intravenously, have also been recommended.

Adams BD et al: Amlodipine overdose causes prolonged calcium channel blocker toxicity. Am J Emerg Med 1998;16:527. [NLM Cit ID: 98394025] (Case report of severe hemodynamic compromise that persisted for 10 days—treated with calcium, glucagon, and other vasopressors.)

Yuan TH et al: Insulin-glucose as adjunctive therapy for severe calcium channel antagonist poisoning. J Toxicol Clin Toxicol 1999;37:463. [NLM Cit ID: 99392912] (Case series of 5 patients with hypodynamic circulatory shock despite conventional treatment who responded to high-dose insulin plus glucose infusion. This novel treatment is now undergoing a multi-center study.)

CARBON MONOXIDE

Carbon monoxide is a colorless, odorless gas produced by the combustion of carbon-containing materials. Poisoning may occur as a result of suicidal or accidental exposure to automobile exhaust, smoke inhalation in a fire, or accidental exposure to an improperly vented gas heater or other appliance. Carbon monoxide avidly binds to hemoglobin, with an affinity approximately 250 times that of oxygen. This results in reduced oxygen-carrying capacity and altered delivery of oxygen to cells (see also Smoke Inhalation in Chapter 9).

Clinical Findings

At low carbon monoxide levels (carboxyhemoglobin saturation 10–20%), victims may have headache, dizziness, abdominal pain, and nausea. With higher levels, confusion, dyspnea, and syncope may occur. Hypotension, coma, and seizures are common with levels greater than 50–60%. Survivors of acute severe poisoning may develop permanent neurologic deficits. The fetus and newborn may be more susceptible because of high carbon monoxide affinity for fetal hemoglobin.

Carbon monoxide poisoning should be suspected in any person with severe headache or acutely altered mental status, especially in cold weather, when improper heating systems may have been used. Diagnosis depends on specific measurement of the arterial or venous carboxyhemoglobin saturation, although the level may have declined if high-flow oxygen therapy has already been administered. Routine arterial blood gas testing and pulse oximetry are not useful because they may give falsely normal oxyhemoglobin saturation determinations.

Treatment

A. Emergency and Supportive Measures: Maintain a patent airway and assist ventilation, if necessary. Remove the victim from exposure. Treat patients with coma, hypotension, or seizures, as described at the beginning of this chapter.

B. Specific Treatment: The half-life of the carboxyhemoglobin complex is about 4–5 hours in room air but is reduced dramatically by high concentrations of oxygen. Administer 100% oxygen by tight-fitting high-flow reservoir face mask or endotracheal tube. Hyperbaric oxygen (HBO) can provide 100% oxygen under higher than atmospheric pressures, further shortening the half-life; it may be useful if immediately available for patients with coma or seizures and in pregnant women, though controlled studies have failed to prove that HBO is superior to high-flow oxygen at normal pressure.

Scheinkestel CD et al: Hyperbaric or normobaric oxygen for acute carbon monoxide poisoning: a randomised controlled clinical trial. Med J Aust 1999;170:203. [NLM Cit ID: 99192876] (Randomized trial demonstrating that hyperbaric oxygen treatment compared with normobaric oxygen treatment provided no benefit and may have worsened the outcome of patients with carbon monoxide poisoning.)

Weaver LK: Carbon monoxide poisoning. Crit Care Clin 1999;15:297. [NLM Cit ID: 99261515]

CHEMICAL WARFARE AGENTS

Nerve agents used in chemical warfare work by cholinesterase inhibition and are most commonly organophosphates. Agents such as **tabun** (dimethylphosphoramidocyanidic acid ethyl ether) and **sarin** (methylphosphonofluoridic acid 1-methylethyl ester) are similar to insecticides such as malathion but are vastly more potent. They may be inhaled or absorbed through the skin. Systemic effects due to unopposed action of acetylcholine include miosis, salivation, abdominal cramps, diarrhea, and muscle paralysis producing respiratory arrest. Inhalation also produces severe bronchoconstriction and copious nasal and tracheobronchial secretions.

Treatment

A. Emergency and Supportive Measures: Perform thorough decontamination of exposed areas with repeated soap and shampoo washing. Personnel caring for such patients must wear protective clothing and gloves, since cutaneous absorption may occur through normal skin.

B. Specific Treatment: Give atropine in an initial dose of 2 mg intravenously, and repeat as needed to reverse signs of acetylcholine excess. (Some victims have required several hundred milligrams.) Treat also with the cholinesterase-reactivating agent pralidoxime, 1–2 g intravenously initially followed by 200–400 mg/h. United States military personnel in the Persian Gulf war were equipped with autoinjectable units containing 2 mg of atropine plus 600 mg of the cholinesterase-reactivating agent pralidoxime.

Brennan RJ et al: Chemical warfare agents: emergency medical and emergency public health issues. Ann Emerg Med 1999;34:191. [NLM Cit ID: 99353773] (Overview of the risk that chemical warfare agents pose to civilians and the necessary preparedness of emergency medical and public health services.)

Okumura T et al: Report on 640 victims of the Tokyo subway sarin attack. Ann Emerg Med 1996;28:223. [NLM Cit ID: 96322268]

Okumura T et al: The Tokyo subway sarin attack: Disaster management. Part 2: Hospital response. Acad Emerg Med 1998;5:618. [NLM Cit ID: 98321727] (Review of hospital planning for chemical disasters based on the author's experience with the Tokyo subway attack.)

Smith KJ: The prevention and treatment of cutaneous injury secondary to chemical warfare agents. Application of these findings to other dermatological conditions and wound healing. Dermatol Clin 1999;17:41. [NLM Cit ID: 99141428]

CHLORINATED INSECTICIDES (Chlorophenothane [DDT], Lindane, Toxaphene, Chlordane, Aldrin, Endrin)

Lindane (Kwell) and other chlorinated insecticides are central nervous system stimulants that can cause poisoning by ingestion, inhalation, or direct contact. The estimated lethal dose is about 20 g for DDT, 3 g for lindane, 2 g for toxaphene, 1 g for chlordane, and less than 1 g for endrin and aldrin. The manifestations of poisoning are nervous irritability, muscle twitching, convulsions, and coma. Arrhythmias may occur. Hepatic and renal damage are reported.

Treatment

Do *not* induce emesis, since seizures may occur abruptly. Perform lavage, and give activated charcoal (see p 1565). Repeat-dose activated charcoal may be effective for large ingestions. For convulsions, give diazepam, 5–10 mg slowly intravenously, or other anticonvulsants as described on p 1563.

Perform thorough decontamination of exposed areas with repeated soap and shampoo washing. Personnel caring for such patients must be wear protective clothing and gloves, since cutaneous absorption may occur through normal skin.

Aks S et al: Acute accidental lindane ingestion in toddlers. Ann Emerg Med 1995;26:647. [NLM Cit ID: 96060819] (Case reports of seizures, respiratory depression after ingestion.)

O'Malley M: Clinical evaluation of pesticide exposure and poisonings. Lancet 1997;349:1161. [NLM Cit ID: 97267694] (Review of pesticide exposure ranging from topical irritant reactions to severe systemic illness.)

CLONIDINE & OTHER SYMPATHOLYTIC ANTIHYPERTENSIVES (Clonidine, Guanabenz, Guanfacine, Methyldopa)

Overdosage with these agents causes bradycardia, hypotension, miosis, respiratory depression, and coma. (Hypertension occasionally occurs after clonidine overdosage, a result of peripheral alpha-adrenergic effects of this drug in high doses.) Symptoms are usually resolved in less than 24 hours, and deaths are rare. Similar symptoms may occur after ingestion of topical nasal decongestants chemically similar to clonidine (oxymetazoline, tetrahydrozoline, naphazoline).

Treatment

A. Emergency and Supportive Measures: Give activated charcoal and a cathartic (see p 1565). Maintain the airway and support respiration if necessary. Symptomatic treatment is usually sufficient even in massive overdose. Maintain blood pressure with intravenous fluids. Dopamine can also be used. Atropine is usually effective for bradycardia.

B. Specific Treatment: There is no specific antidote. Although tolazoline has been recommended for clonidine overdose, its effects are unpredictable and it should not be used. Naloxone has been reported to be successful in a few anecdotal and poorly substantiated cases.

Broderick-Cantwell JJ: Case study: accidental clonidine patch overdose in attention-deficit/hyperactivity disorder patients. J Am Acad Child Adolesc Psychiatry 1999;38:95. [NLM Cit ID: 99109300]

COCAINE

See Amphetamines & Cocaine, above.

CYANIDE

Cyanide is a highly toxic chemical used widely in research and commercial laboratories and many industries. Its gaseous form, hydrogen cyanide, is an important component of smoke in fires. Cyanide-generating glycosides are also found in the pits of apricots and other related plants. Cyanide is generated by the breakdown of nitroprusside, and poisoning can result from rapid high-dose infusions. Cyanide is also formed by metabolism of acetonitrile, found in some over-the-counter fingernail glue removers. Cyanide is rapidly absorbed by inhalation, skin absorption, or ingestion. It disrupts cellular function by inhibiting cytochrome oxidase and preventing cellular oxygen utilization.

Clinical Findings

The onset of toxicity is nearly instantaneous after inhalation of hydrogen cyanide gas but may be delayed for minutes to hours after ingestion of cyanide salts or cyanogenic plants or chemicals. Effects include headache, dizziness, nausea, abdominal pain, and anxiety, followed by confusion, syncope, shock, seizures, coma, and death. The odor of "bitter almonds" may be detected on the victim's breath or in vomitus, though this is not a reliable finding. The venous oxygen saturation may be elevated (> 90%) in severe poisonings because tissues have failed to take up arterial oxygen.

Treatment

A. Emergency and Supportive Measures: Remove the victim from exposure, taking care to avoid exposure to rescuers. For suspected cyanide poisoning due to nitroprusside infusion, stop or slow the rate of infusion. (Metabolic acidosis and other signs of cyanide poisoning usually clear rapidly.)

For cyanide ingestion, empty the stomach by gastric lavage and administer activated charcoal. At the scene, induce emesis if charcoal is not immediately available (see p 1565). Although charcoal has a low affinity for cyanide, the usual doses of 60–100 g are adequate to bind typically ingested lethal doses (100–200 mg).

B. Specific Treatment: In the United States, the cyanide antidote package (Taylor Pharmaceuticals) (Table 39–11) contains nitrites (to induce methemoglobinemia, which binds free cyanide) and thiosulfate (to promote conversion of cyanide to the less toxic thiocyanate). Administer amyl nitrite by crushing an ampule under the victim's nose or at the end of the endotracheal tube, and administer 3% sodium nitrite solution, 10 mL intravenously. ***Caution:*** Nitrites may induce hypotension and dangerous levels of methemoglobin. Also administer 25% sodium thiosulfate solution, 50 mL intravenously (12.5 g).

Table 39–11. Currently available (prepackaged) cyanide antidotes.[1,2]

Antidote	How Supplied	Dose
Amyl nitrite	0.3 mL (aspirol inhalant)	Break one or two aspirols under patient's nose.
Sodium nitrite	3 g/dL (300 mg in 10 mL vials)	6 mg/kg IV (0.2 mL/kg)
Sodium thiosulfate	25 g/dL (12.5 g in 50 mL vials)	250 mg/kg IV (1 mL/kg)

[1]Reproduced, with permission, from Saunders CE, Ho MT (editors): *Current Emergency Diagnosis & Treatment,* 4th ed. Originally published by Appleton & Lange. Copyright © 1992 by The McGraw-Hill Companies, Inc.
[2]In the United States, manufactured by Taylor Pharmaceuticals.

Beasley DM et al. Cyanide poisoning: pathophysiology and treatment recommendations. Occup Med 1998;48:427. [NLM Cit ID: 99148879] (Review of the available antidotes for cyanide toxicity.)

Suchard JR et al: Acute cyanide toxicity caused by apricot kernel ingestion. Ann Emerg Med 1998;32:742. [NLM Cit ID: 9832674] (Severe cyanide poisoning after ingestion of apricot kernels purchased in a health food store.)

DIGITALIS & OTHER CARDIAC GLYCOSIDES

Cardiac glycosides are derived from a variety of plants and are widely used to treat heart failure and supraventricular arrhythmias. These drugs paralyze the Na^+-K^+ ATPase pump and have potent vagotonic effects. Intracellular effects include enhancement of calcium-dependent contractility and shortening of the action potential duration. Digoxin and ouabain are highly tissue-bound, but digitoxin has a volume of distribution of just 0.6 L/kg, making it the only cardiac glycoside accessible to enhanced removal procedures such as hemoperfusion or repeated doses of activated charcoal.

Clinical Findings

Intoxication may result from acute single exposure or chronic accidental overmedication. After acute overdosage, patients frequently develop nausea and vomiting, bradycardia, hyperkalemia, and atrioventricular block. Patients who develop toxicity gradually during chronic therapy are often hypokalemic and hypomagnesemic owing to concurrent diuretic treatment and more commonly present with ventricular arrhythmias (eg, ectopy, bidirectional ventricular tachycardia, or ventricular fibrillation).

Treatment

A. Emergency and Supportive Measures: Maintain a patent airway and assist ventilation, if necessary. Monitor potassium levels and cardiac rhythm closely. Treat ventricular arrhythmias initially with lidocaine (2–3 mg/kg intravenously) or phenytoin (10–15 mg/kg intravenously slowly over 30 minutes) and treat bradycardia initially with atropine (0.5–2 mg intravenously), isoproterenol (1–5 μg/min initially), or a transcutaneous external cardiac pacemaker.

After acute ingestion, perform gastric lavage and administer activated charcoal (see p 1565). Emesis is not recommended because it may enhance vagotonic effects such as bradycardia and AV block.

B. Specific Treatment: For patients with severe intoxication (eg, marked bradycardia or AV block unresponsive to atropine, or ventricular arrhythmias unresponsive to lidocaine or phenytoin), administer digoxin-specific antibodies (digoxin immune Fab [ovine]; Digibind). Estimation of the Digibind dose is based on the body burden of digoxin calculated from the ingested dose or the steady-state serum digoxin concentration:

1. From the ingested dose–Number of vials = approximately 1.5 × ingested dose (mg).

2. From the serum concentration–Number of vials = serum digoxin (ng/mL) × body weight (kg) × 10^{-2}. ***Note:*** This is based on the equilibrium digoxin level; after acute overdose, serum levels are falsely high before tissue distribution is complete, and overestimation of the Digibind dose is likely.

3. Empirical dosing of Digibind may be utilized if the patient's condition is relatively stable and an underlying condition (eg, atrial fibrillation) suggests a residual level of digitalis activity. Start with one or two vials and reassess the clinical condition after 20–30 minutes.

Note: After administration of Digibind, serum digoxin levels may be falsely elevated depending on the assay technique.

Borron SW et al: Advances in the management of digoxin toxicity in the older patient. Drugs Aging 1997;10:18. [NLM Cit ID: 97265846]

Nordt SP et al: Clarithromycin induced digoxin toxicity. J Accid Emerg Med 1998;15:194. [NLM Cit ID: 98301058] (Case report of digoxin toxicity due to coadministration of clarithromycin.)

ETHANOL, BARBITURATES, BENZODIAZEPINES, & OTHER SEDATIVE-HYPNOTIC AGENTS

The group of agents known as sedative-hypnotic drugs includes a variety of products used for the treatment of anxiety, depression, insomnia, and epilepsy. Ethanol and other selected agents are also popular recreational drugs. All of these drugs depress the central nervous system reticular activating system, cerebral cortex, and cerebellum.

Clinical Findings

Mild intoxication produces euphoria, slurred speech, and ataxia. Ethanol intoxication may produce hypoglycemia, even at relatively low concentrations. With more severe intoxication, stupor, coma, and respiratory arrest may occur. Death or serious morbidity is usually the result of pulmonary aspiration of gastric contents. Bradycardia, hypotension, and hypothermia are common. Patients with massive intoxication may appear to be dead, with no reflex responses and even absent electroencephalographic activity. Diagnosis and assessment of severity of intoxication are usually based on clinical findings. Ethanol serum levels greater than 300 mg/dL (0.3 g/dL; 65 mmol/L) usually produce coma in persons who are not chronically abusing the drug, but regular users may remain awake at much higher levels. Phenobarbital levels greater than 80–100 mg/L usually cause coma.

Treatment

A. Emergency and Supportive Measures: Empty the stomach by gastric lavage and administer activated charcoal (see p 1565). Repeat-dose charcoal may enhance elimination of phenobarbital, and hemoperfusion may be necessary for patients with severe phenobarbital intoxication, but these procedures are not effective for most other drugs in this group.

B. Specific Treatment: Flumazenil is a benzodiazepine receptor-specific antagonist; it has no effect on ethanol, barbiturates, or other sedative-hypnotic agents. Flumazenil is given slowly intravenously, 0.2 mg over 30–60 seconds, repeated in 0.5 mg increments as needed up to a total dose of 3–5 mg. ***Caution:*** Flumazenil may induce seizures in patients with preexisting seizure disorder, benzodiazepine addiction, or concomitant tricyclic antidepressant overdose. If seizures occur, diazepam and other benzodiazepine anticonvulsants will not be effective. As with naloxone, the duration of action of flumazenil is short (2–3 hours) and resedation may occur, requiring repeated doses.

Barnett R et al: Flumazenil in drug overdose: randomized, placebo-controlled study to assess cost effectiveness. Crit Care Med 1999;27:78. [NLM Cit ID: 99131596] (Randomized trial of flumazenil in the empiric treatment of adults with suspected drug overdose and Glasgow Coma Scale score less than 13 failed to demonstrate its cost-effectiveness.)

Church AS et al: Laboratory testing in ethanol, methanol, ethylene glycol, and isopropanol toxicities. J Emerg Med 1997;15:687. [NLM Cit ID: 98006283] (Review of the indications and methods for both direct and indirect testing for ethanol, methanol, ethylene glycol, and isopropanol toxicity.)

Goldfrank LR: Flumazenil: A pharmacologic antidote with limited medical toxicology utility, or . . . an antidote in search of an overdose. Acad Emerg Med 1997;4:935. [NLM Cit ID: 97473779] (Editorial comment.)

GAMMA HYDROXYBUTYRATE

Gamma hydroxybutyrate (GHB) has become a popular drug of abuse. It originated as a short-acting general anesthetic and is occasionally used in the treatment of narcolepsy. It gained popularity among bodybuilders for its alleged growth hormone stimulation and found its way into social settings, where it is consumed as a liquid. Symptoms after ingestion include drowsiness and lethargy followed by coma with respiratory depression. Muscle twitching and seizures are sometimes observed. Recovery is usually rapid, with patients awakening within a few hours. Other related chemicals with similar effects include butanediol and gamma-butyrolactone (GBL).

Treatment

For recent ingestions, give activated charcoal orally or by gastric tube. There is no specific treatment. Most patients recover rapidly with supportive care.

Adverse events associated with ingestion of gamma-butyrolactone—Minnesota, New Mexico, and Texas 1998–1999. MMWR Morb Mortal Wkly Rep 1999;48:137. [NLM Cit ID: 10077458] (GBL is a liquid solvent chemical precursor to GHB; after ingestion, it produces similar effects.)

Chin RL et al: Clinical course of gamma-hydroxybutyrate overdose. Ann Emerg Med 1998;31:716. [NLM Cit ID: 98287394] (Retrospective review of 88 patients with GHB overdose. Although these patients presented with markedly decreased levels of consciousness, most had spontaneous recovery of consciousness within 5 hours after ingestion. Common findings included coingestion of ethanol and amphetamines, bradycardia, hypothermia, respiratory acidosis, and emesis.)

Li J et al: A tale of novel intoxication: a review of the effects of gamma-hydroxybutyric acid with recommendations for management. Ann Emerg Med 1998;31:729. [NLM Cit ID: 98287396]

IRON

Iron is widely used therapeutically for the treatment of anemia and as a daily supplement in multiple vitamin preparations. Most children's preparations contain about 12–15 mg of elemental iron (as sulfate, gluconate, or fumarate salt) per dose, compared with 60–90 mg in most adult-strength preparations. Iron is corrosive to the gastrointestinal tract and, once absorbed, has depressant effects on the myocardium and on peripheral vascular resistance. Intracellular toxic effects of iron include disruption of Krebs cycle enzymes.

Clinical Findings

Ingestion of less than 30 mg/kg of elemental iron usually produces only mild gastrointestinal upset. Ingestion of more than 40–60 mg/kg may cause vomiting (sometimes with hematemesis), diarrhea, hypotension, and acidosis. Death may occur as a result of profound hypotension due to massive fluid losses and bleeding metabolic acidosis, peritonitis from intestinal perforation, or sepsis. Fulminant hepatic failure may occur. Survivors of the acute ingestion may suffer permanent gastrointestinal scarring.

Serum iron levels greater than 350–500 μg/dL are considered toxic, and levels over 1000 μg/dL are usually associated with severe poisoning. A plain abdominal x-ray may reveal radiopaque tablets.

Treatment

A. Emergency and Supportive Measures: Maintain a patent airway and assist ventilation if necessary. Treat hypotension aggressively with intravenous crystalloid solutions (0.9% saline or lactated Ringer's solution). Fluid losses may be massive owing to vomiting and diarrhea as well as third-spacing into injured intestine.

Perform whole bowel irrigation to remove unabsorbed pills from the intestinal tract (see p 1565). Activated charcoal is not effective but may be used if other ingestants are suspected.

B. Specific Treatment: Deferoxamine is a selective iron chelator. It is not useful as an oral binding agent. For patients with established manifestations of toxicity—and particularly those with markedly elevated serum iron levels (eg, greater than 800–1000 μg/dL)—administer 10–15 mg/kg/h by constant intravenous infusion; higher doses (up to 40–50 mg/kg/h) have been used in massive poisonings. Hypotension may occur. The presence of iron-deferoxamine complex in the urine may give it a "vin rosé" appearance. Deferoxamine is safe for use in pregnant women with acute iron overdose. ***Caution:*** Prolonged infusion of deferoxamine (> 36–48 hours) has been associated with development of acute respiratory distress syndrome (ARDS)—the mechanism is not known.

Nordt SP et al: Comparison of the toxicities of two iron formulations in a swine model. Acad Emerg Med 1999;6:1104. [NLM Cit ID: 10569381] (Solid iron tablets caused more corrosive esophageal and gastric injures compared with chewable multivitamins, though the latter formulation type produced greater systemic iron absorption.)

Siff JE et al: Usefulness of the total iron building capacity in the evaluation and treatment of iron overdose. Ann Emerg Med 1999;33:73. [NLM Cit ID: 99084912] (Review article, points out the pitfalls of the total iron-binding capacity and recommends it not be used in the estimation of "free iron.")

Tenenbein M: Benefits of parenteral deferoxamine for acute iron poisoning. J Toxicol Clin Toxicol 1996;34:485. [NLM Cit ID: 96393398] (Review of the literature on deferoxamine.)

ISONIAZID

Isoniazid (INH) is an antibacterial drug used mainly in the treatment and prevention of tuberculosis. It may cause hepatitis in certain patients with chronic use. It produces acute toxic effects by competing with pyridoxal 5-phosphate, resulting in lowered brain γ-aminobutyric acid (GABA) levels. Acute ingestion of as little as 1.5–2 g of isoniazid can cause toxicity, and severe poisoning is likely to occur after ingestion of more than 80–100 mg/kg.

Clinical Findings

Confusion, slurred speech, and seizures may occur abruptly after acute overdose. Severe lactic acidosis—out of proportion to the severity of seizures—is probably due to inhibited metabolism of lactate.

Diagnosis is based on a history of ingestion and the presence of severe acidosis associated with seizures. Isoniazid is not usually included in routine toxicologic screening, and serum levels are not readily available.

Treatment

A. Emergency and Supportive Measures: Seizures may require higher than usual doses of benzodiazepines (eg, lorazepam, 3–5 mg intravenously) or administration of pyridoxine as an antidote (see below).

Empty the stomach by gastric lavage and administer activated charcoal (see p 1565). Do *not* induce emesis, because of the risk of abrupt onset of seizures.

B. Specific Treatment: Pyridoxine (vitamin B_6) is a specific antagonist of the acute toxic effects of isoniazid and is usually successful in controlling convulsions that do not respond to benzodiazepines. Give 5 g intravenously over 1–2 minutes or, if the amount ingested is known, give a gram-for-gram equivalent amount of pyridoxine.

Romero JA et al: Isoniazid overdose: recognition and management. Am Fam Physician 1998;57:749. [NLM Cit ID: 98151697]

Santucci KA et al: Acute isoniazid exposures and antidote availability. Pediatr Emerg Care 1999;15:99. [NLM Cit ID: 99235483] (A survey of teaching hospitals with emergency medicine or pediatric emergency medicine training programs found that one-third to one-half had insufficient supplies of the antidote pyridoxine.)

Sullivan EA et al: Isoniazid poisonings in New York City. J Emerg Med 1998;16:57. [NLM Cit ID: 98132103] (Review of 41 patients, 22 of whom presented with seizures. Treatment with pyridoxine is emphasized.)

LEAD

Lead is used in a variety of industrial and commercial products, such as storage batteries, solders, paints, pottery, plumbing, and gasoline and is found in some traditional ethnic medicines. Lead toxicity usually results from chronic repeated exposure and is rare after a single ingestion. Lead produces a variety of adverse effects on cellular function and primarily affects the nervous system, gastrointestinal tract, and hematopoietic system.

Clinical Findings

Lead poisoning often goes undiagnosed initially because presenting symptoms and signs are nonspecific and exposure is not suspected. Common symptoms include colicky abdominal pain, constipation, headache, and irritability. Severe poisoning may cause coma and convulsions. Chronic intoxication can cause learning disorders (in children) and motor neuropathy (eg, wrist drop).

Diagnosis is based on measurement of the blood lead level. Whole blood lead levels less than 10 μg/dL are usually considered nontoxic. Levels between 10 and 25 μg/dL have been associated with impaired neurobehavioral development in children. Levels of 25–50 μg/dL may be associated with headache, irritability, and subclinical neuropathy. Levels of 50–70 μg/dL are associated with moderate toxicity, and levels greater than 70–100 μg/dL are often associated with severe poisoning. Other laboratory findings of lead poisoning include microcytic anemia with basophilic stippling and elevated free erythrocyte protoporphyrin.

Treatment

A. Emergency and Supportive Measures: For patients with encephalopathy, maintain a patent airway and treat coma and convulsions as described at the beginning of this chapter.

For recent acute ingestion, give activated charcoal and a cathartic (see p 1565). If a large lead-containing object (eg, fishing weight) is still visible in the stomach on abdominal x-ray, repeated cathartics, whole bowel irrigation, endoscopy, or even surgical removal may be necessary to prevent subacute lead poisoning. (The acidic gastric contents may corrode the metal surface, enhancing lead absorption. Once the object passes into the small intestine, the risk of toxicity declines.)

Conduct an investigation into the source of the lead exposure. Workers with a single lead level greater than 60 μg/dL (or three successive monthly levels greater than 50 μg/dL) or construction workers with any single blood lead level greater than 50 μg/dL must by federal law be removed from the site of exposure. Contact the regional office of the United States Occupational Safety and Health Administration (OSHA) for more information. Several states mandate reporting of cases of confirmed lead poisoning.

B. Specific Treatment: The indications for chelation depend on the blood lead level and the patient's clinical state. A medical toxicologist or regional poison control center (Table 39–1) should be consulted for advice about selection and use of these antidotes.

Note: It is impermissible under the law to treat asymptomatic workers with elevated blood lead levels in order to keep their levels under 50 μg/dL rather than remove them from the exposure.

1. Severe toxicity–Patients with severe intoxication (encephalopathy or levels greater than 70–100 μg/dL) should receive edetate calcium disodium (EDTA), 1500 mg/m^2/kg/d (approximately 50 mg/kg/d) in four to six divided doses or as a continuous intravenous infusion. Some clinicians also add dimercaprol (BAL), 4–5 mg/kg intramuscularly every 4 hours for 5 days.

2. Less severe toxicity–Patients with less severe symptoms and asymptomatic patients with blood lead levels between 55 and 69 μg/dL may be treated with edetate calcium disodium alone in dosages as above. An oral chelator, succimer (dimercaptosuccinic acid, DMSA), is available for use in patients with mild to moderate intoxication. The usual dose is 10 mg/kg orally every 8 hours for 5 days, then every 12 hours for 2 weeks.

Graeme KA et al: Heavy metal toxicity, part II: lead and metal fume fever. J Emerg Med 1998;16:171. [NLM Cit ID: 98202399] (Review of clinical presentation and management of lead toxicity.)

Jongnarangsin K et al: An unusual cause of recurrent abdominal pain. Am J Gastroenterol 1999;94:3620. [NLM Cit ID:10606329] (Case report of lead poisoning from stripping old paint from a Victorian house.)

Lin JL et al: Chelation therapy for patients with elevated body lead burden and progressive renal insufficiency. A randomized, controlled trial. Ann Intern Med 1999; 130:7. [NLM Cit ID: 99087455] (Randomized study demonstrating possible role for lead chelation therapy in patients with chronic renal insufficiency and mildly elevated body lead burden.)

Porru S et al: The use of chelating agents in occupational lead poisoning. Occup Med 1996;46:41. [NLM Cit ID: 96271905] (Review of the indications, contraindications, and side-effects of the chelating agents dimercaprol, penicillamine, CANA2EDTA, and dimercaptosuccinic acid.)

Staudinger KC et al: Occupational lead poisoning. Am Fam Physician 1998;57:719. [NLM Cit ID: 98151695] (Review of lead poisoning with a special emphasis on the implications of occupational exposures.)

LSD & OTHER HALLUCINOGENS

A variety of substances—ranging from naturally occurring plants and mushrooms to synthetic substances such as phencyclidine (PCP), toluene and other solvents, and LSD—are abused for their hallucinogenic properties. The mechanism of toxicity and the clinical effects vary for each substance.

Many hallucinogenic plants and mushrooms produce anticholinergic delirium (see p 1573), characterized by flushed skin, dry mucous membranes, dilated pupils, tachycardia, and urinary retention. Some plants and mushrooms may contain hallucinogenic indoles such as mescaline and lysergic acid diethylamide (LSD), which typically cause marked visual hallucinations and perceptual distortion, widely dilated pupils, and mild tachycardia. Phencyclidine (PCP), a dissociative anesthetic agent similar to ketamine, can produce fluctuating delirium and coma, often associated with vertical and horizontal nystagmus. Toluene and other hydrocarbon solvents (butane, trichloroethylene, "chemo," etc) cause euphoria and delirium and may sensitize the myocardium to the effects of catecholamines, leading to fatal dysrhythmias.

Treatment

A. Emergency and Supportive Measures: Maintain a patent airway and assist respirations if necessary. Treat coma, hyperthermia, and seizures as outlined at the beginning of this chapter. For recent large ingestions, consider giving activated charcoal orally or by gastric tube.

B. Specific Treatment: Patients with anticholinergic delirium may benefit from a dose of physostigmine (see p 1574). However, this drug should not be used if poisoning by tricyclic antidepressants is suspected. Dysphoria, agitation, and psychosis associated with LSD or mescaline intoxication may respond to benzodiazepines (eg, lorazepam, 1–2 mg orally or intravenously) or haloperidol (2–5 mg orally or intravenously). Monitor patients who have sniffed solvents for cardiac dysrhythmias (most commonly premature ventricular contractions, ventricular tachycardia, ventricular fibrillation); treatment with beta-blockers such as propranolol (1–5 mg intravenously) or esmolol (250–500 μg/kg intravenously, then 50 μg/kg/min by infusion) may be more effective than lidocaine.

Dewitt MS et al: The dangers of jimson weed and its abuse by teenagers in the Kanawha Valley of West Virginia. West Virginia Med J 1998;93:182. [NLM Cit ID: 97419635] (Nine patients treated for ingestion of jimson weed [*Datura stramonium*].)

Einav S et al: Bradycardia in toluene poisoning. J Toxicol Clin Toxicol 1997;35:295. [NLM Cit ID: 97285051] (Case reports of patients with toluene ingestion demonstrating that bradyarrhythmias can occur as opposed to the more typical cardiotoxicity-associated tachyarrhythmias.)

Nelson LS et al: Dangerous form of marijuana (letter). Ann Emerg Med 1999;34:115. [NLM Cit ID: 99334680] (Phencyclidine is sometimes added to marijuana.)

MERCURY

Acute mercury poisoning usually occurs by ingestion of inorganic mercuric salts or inhalation of metallic mercury vapor. Ingestion of the mercuric salts causes a metallic taste, salivation, thirst, a burning sensation in the throat, discoloration and edema of oral mucous membranes, abdominal pain, vomiting, bloody diarrhea, and shock. Direct nephrotoxicity causes acute renal failure. Inhalation of high concentrations of metallic mercury vapor may cause acute fulminant chemical pneumonia. Chronic mercury poisoning causes weakness, ataxia, intention tremors, irritability, and depression. Exposure to alkyl (organic) mercury derivatives from contaminated fish or fungicides used on seeds has caused ataxia, tremors, convulsions, and catastrophic birth defects.

Treatment

A. Acute Poisoning: There is no effective specific treatment for mercury vapor pneumonitis. Remove ingested mercuric salts by lavage, and administer activated charcoal (see p 1565). For acute ingestion of mercuric salts, give dimercaprol (BAL) at once, as for arsenic poisoning. Unless the patient has severe gastroenteritis, consider succimer (DMSA), 10 mg/kg orally every 8 hours for 5 days and then every 12 hours for 2 weeks. Maintain urine output. Treat oliguria and anuria if they occur.

B. Chronic Poisoning: Remove from exposure. Neurologic toxicity is not considered reversible with chelation, though some authors recommend a trial of succimer.

Graeme KA et al: Heavy metal toxicity. Part I: Arsenic and mercury. J Emerg Med 1998;16:45. [NLM Cit ID: 98132102] (Review of mercury toxicity, including exposure, clinical manifestations, diagnosis, and treatment.)

Risher JF et al: Summary report for the expert panel review of the toxicological profile for mercury. Toxicol Ind Health 1999;15:483. [NLM Cit ID: 99415301]

METHANOL & ETHYLENE GLYCOL

Methanol (wood alcohol) is commonly found in a variety of products, including solvents, duplicating fluids, record cleaning solutions, and paint removers. It is sometimes ingested intentionally by alcoholics as a substitute for ethanol and may also be found as a contaminant in bootleg whiskey. Ethylene glycol is the major constituent in most antifreeze compounds. The toxicity of both agents is caused by metabolism to highly toxic organic acids—methanol to formic acid; ethylene glycol to glycolic and oxalic acids.

Clinical Findings

Shortly after ingestion of either of these agents, patients usually appear "drunk." The serum osmolality (measured with the freezing point device) is usually increased, but acidosis is often absent early. After several hours, metabolism to toxic organic acids leads to a severe anion gap metabolic acidosis, tachypnea, confusion, convulsions, and coma. Methanol intoxication frequently causes visual disturbances, while ethylene glycol often produces oxalate crystalluria and renal failure.

Treatment

A. Emergency and Supportive Measures: For patients presenting within 30–60 minutes after ingestion, empty the stomach by emesis or gastric lavage and administer activated charcoal (see p 1565). (***Note:*** Charcoal is not very effective.)

B. Specific Treatment: Patients with significant toxicity (manifested by severe metabolic acidosis, altered mental status, serum methanol or ethylene glycol level > 50 mg/dL, or osmolar gap > 10 mosm/L) should undergo hemodialysis as soon as possible to remove the parent compound and the toxic metabolites.

Ethanol blocks metabolism of the parent compounds by competing for the enzyme alcohol dehydrogenase. The desired serum ethanol concentration is 100 mg/dL. To achieve this, administer a loading dose of approximately 750 mg/kg orally or in a dilute intravenous solution (available from the pharmacy in 5% and 10% solution), and then provide a maintenance infusion of 100–150 mg/kg/h. The infusion will have to be increased to about 175–250 mg/kg/h during hemodialysis to replace dialysis elimination of ethanol. A new antidote, fomepizole (4-methypyrazole), blocks alcohol dehydrogenase and can be used instead of ethanol. A regional poison control center (Table 39–1) should be contacted for indications and dosing.

Barceloux DG et al: American Academy of Clinical Toxicology Practice Guidelines on the Treatment of Ethylene Glycol Poisoning. Ad Hoc Committee. J Toxicol Clin Toxicol 1999;37:537. [NLM Cit ID: 99427283] (Clinical manifestations, diagnosis, and treatment.)

Brent J et al: Fomepizole for the treatment of ethylene glycol poisoning. N Engl J Med 1999;340:832. [NLM Cit ID: 99165316] (Fomepizole was effective in preventing renal failure if given early.)

Jacobsen D et al: Antidotes for methanol and ethylene glycol poisoning. J Toxicol Clin Toxicol 1997;35:127. [NLM Cit ID: 97238138]

Liu JJ et al: Prognostic factors in patients with methanol poisoning. J Toxicol Clin Toxicol 1998;36:175. [NLM Cit ID: 98321128]

METHEMOGLOBINEMIA-INDUCING AGENTS

A large number of chemical agents are capable of oxidizing ferrous hemoglobin to its ferric state (methemoglobin), a form that cannot carry oxygen. Drugs and chemicals known to cause methemoglobinemia include benzocaine (a local anesthetic found in a variety of nonprescription products), aniline, nitrites, nitrogen oxide gases, nitrobenzene, dapsone, pyridium, and many others. Dapsone has a long elimination half-life and may produce prolonged or recurrent methemoglobinemia.

Clinical Findings

Methemoglobinemia reduces oxygen-carrying capacity and may cause dizziness, nausea, headache, dyspnea, confusion, seizures, and coma. The severity of symptoms depends on the percentage of hemoglobin oxidized to methemoglobin; severe poisoning is usually present when methemoglobin fractions are greater than 40–50%. Even at low levels (15–20%), victims appear cyanotic because of the "chocolate brown" color of methemoglobin, but they have normal Po_2 results on arterial blood gas determinations. Pulse oximetry gives inaccurate oxygen saturation measurements. Severe metabolic acidosis may be present. Hemolysis may occur, especially in patients susceptible to oxidant stress (ie, those with glucose-6-phosphate dehydrogenase deficiency).

Treatment

A. Emergency and Supportive Measures: Administer high-flow oxygen. If the causative agent was recently ingested, empty the stomach by gastric lavage and administer activated charcoal (see p 1565). For dapsone ingestion, repeat-dose activated charcoal may enhance dapsone elimination (see p 1565).

B. Specific Treatment: Methylene blue enhances the conversion of methemoglobin to hemoglobin by increasing the activity of the enzyme methemoglobin reductase. For symptomatic patients, administer 1–2 mg/kg (0.1–0.2 mL/kg of 1% solution) intravenously. The dose may be repeated once in 15–20 minutes if necessary. Patients with hereditary methemoglobin reductase deficiency or glucose-6-phosphate dehydrogenase deficiency may not respond to methylene blue treatment.

Coleman MD et al: Drug-induced methaemoglobinaemia. Treatment issues. Drug Saf 1996;14:394. [NLM Cit ID: 96425675] (Clinical manifestations and treatment.)

Ward KE et al: Dapsone-induced methemoglobinemia. Ann Pharmacother 1998;32:549. [NLM Cit ID: 98269321]

MONOAMINE OXIDASE INHIBITORS (Isocarboxazid, Phenelzine)

Overdoses cause ataxia, excitement, hypertension, and tachycardia, followed several hours later by hypotension, convulsions, and hyperthermia.

Ingestion of tyramine-containing foods may cause a severe hypertensive reaction in patients taking monoamine oxidase inhibitors. Foods containing tyramine include aged cheese and red wines. Hypertensive reactions may also occur with any sympathomimetic drug. Severe or fatal hyperthermia (serotonin syndrome) may occur if patients receiving monoamine oxidase inhibitors are given meperidine, fluoxetine, paroxetine, fluvoxamine, venlafaxine, tryptophan, dextromethorphan, or other serotonin-enhancing drugs. This reaction can also occur with the newer selective MAO inhibitor moclobemide.

Treatment

Remove ingested drug by gastric lavage, and administer activated charcoal and a cathartic (see p 1565). Treat severe hypertension with nitroprusside, phentolamine, or other rapid-acting vasodilators (see p 1562). Treat hypotension with fluids and positioning, but avoid use of pressor agents if possible. Observe patients for at least 24 hours, since hyperthermic reactions may be delayed. Treat hyperthermia with aggressive cooling; neuromuscular paralysis may be required (see p 1564). Cyproheptadine, 4 mg orally (or by gastric tube) every hour for three or four doses, has been reported to be effective against serotonin syndrome.

Brown TM et al: Pathophysiology and management of the serotonin syndrome. Ann Pharmacother 1996;30:527. [NLM Cit ID: 96309758]

Chan BS et al: Serotonin syndrome resulting from drug interactions. Med J Aust 1998;169:523. [NLM Cit ID: 99078902] (Series of six patients with serotonin syndrome after exposure to combinations of tricyclic antidepressants, selective serotonin uptake inhibitors, selective norepinephrine reuptake inhibitors, or monoamine oxidase inhibitors.)

Mills KC: Serotonin syndrome. A clinical update. Critic Care Clin 1997;13:763. [NLM Cit ID: 97471899] (Retrospective review of 127 patients.)

MUSHROOMS

There are thousands of mushroom species that cause a variety of toxic effects. The most dangerous species of mushrooms are *Amanita phalloides, Amanita verna, Amanita virosa, Gyromitra esculenta,* and the *Galerina* species, all of which contain amatoxin, a potent cytotoxin. Ingestion of even a portion of one mushroom of a dangerous species may be sufficient to cause death.

The characteristic pathologic finding in fatalities from amatoxin-containing mushroom poisoning is acute massive necrosis of the liver.

Clinical Findings (Table 39–12)

A. Symptoms and Signs:

1. Amatoxin-type cyclopeptides–(*Amanita phalloides, Amanita verna, Amanita virosa,* and *Galerina* species.) After a latent interval of 8–12 hours, severe abdominal cramps and vomiting begin and progress to profuse diarrhea, followed in 1–2 days by

Table 39–12. Poisonous mushrooms.

Toxin	Genus	Symptoms and Signs	Onset	Treatment
Amanitin	*Amanita (A phalloides, A verna, A virosa)*	Severe gastroenteritis followed by delayed hepatic and renal failure after 48–72 hours	6–24 hours	Supportive. Correct dehydration. Give repeated doses of activated charcoal orally. Penicillin, thioctic acid, and silibinin are unproved antidotes.
Muscarine	*Inocybe, Clitocybe*	Muscarinic (salivation, miosis, bradycardia, diarrhea)	30–60 minutes	Supportive. Give atropine, 0.5–2 mg intravenously, for severe cholinergic symptoms and signs.
Ibotenic acid, muscimol	*Amanita muscaria* ("fly agaric")	Anticholinergic (mydriasis, tachycardia, hyperpyrexia, delirium)	30–60 minutes	Supportive. Give physostigmine, 0.5–2 mg intravenously, for severe anticholinergic symptoms and signs.
Coprine	*Coprinus*	Disulfiram-like effect occurs with ingestion of ethanol	30–60 minutes	Supportive. Abstain from ethanol for 3–4 days.
Monomethylhydrazine	*Gyromitra*	Gastroenteritis; occasionally hemolysis, hepatic and renal failure	6–12 hours	Supportive. Correct dehydration. Pyridoxine, 2.5 mg/kg intravenously, may be helpful.
Orellanine	*Cortinarius*	Nausea, vomiting; renal failure after 1–3 weeks	2–14 days	Supportive.
Psilocybin	*Psilocybe*	Hallucinations	15–30 minutes	Supportive.
Gastrointestinal irritants	Many species	Nausea and vomiting, diarrhea	½–2 hours	Supportive. Correct dehydration.

hepatic necrosis, hepatic encephalopathy, and frequently renal failure. The fatality rate is about 20%. Cooking the mushrooms does not prevent poisoning.

2. Gyromitrin type–(*Gyromitra* and *Helvella* species.) Toxicity is more common following ingestion of uncooked mushrooms. Vomiting, diarrhea, hepatic necrosis, convulsions, coma, and hemolysis may occur after a latent period of 8–12 hours. The fatality rate is probably less than 10%.

3. Muscarinic type–(*Inocybe* and *Clitocybe* species.) Vomiting, diarrhea, bradycardia, hypotension, salivation, miosis, bronchospasm, and lacrimation occur shortly after ingestion. Cardiac arrhythmias may occur. Fatalities are rare.

4. Anticholinergic type–(Eg, *Amanita muscaria, Amanita pantherina*.) This type causes a variety of symptoms that may be atropine-like, including excitement, delirium, flushed skin, dilated pupils, and muscular jerking tremors, beginning 1–2 hours after ingestion. Fatalities are rare.

5. Gastrointestinal irritant type–(Eg, *Boletus, Cantharellus*.) Nausea, vomiting, and diarrhea occur shortly after ingestion. Fatalities are rare.

6. Disulfiram type–(*Coprinus* species.) Disulfiram-like sensitivity to alcohol may persist for several days. Toxicity is characterized by flushing, hypotension, and vomiting after coingestion of alcohol.

7. Hallucinogenic–(*Psilocybe* and *Panaeolus* species.) Mydriasis, nausea and vomiting, and intense visual hallucinations occur 1–2 hours after ingestion. Fatalities are rare.

8. *Cortinarius orellanus*–This mushroom may cause acute renal failure due to tubulointerstitial nephritis.

Treatment

A. Emergency Measures: After the onset of symptoms, efforts to remove the toxic agent are probably useless, especially in cases of amatoxin or gyromitrin poisoning, where there is usually a delay of 12 hours or more before symptoms occur and patients seek medical attention. However, induction of vomiting or administration of activated charcoal is recommended for any recent ingestion of an unidentified or potentially toxic mushroom (see p 1565).

B. General Measures:

1. Amatoxin-type cyclopeptides–A variety of antidotes (eg, thioctic acid, silibinin, penicillin, corticosteroids) have been suggested for amatoxin-type mushroom poisoning, but controlled studies are lacking and experimental data in animals are equivocal. Aggressive fluid replacement for diarrhea and intensive supportive care for hepatic failure are the mainstays of treatment.

Interruption of enterohepatic circulation of the amatoxin by the administration of activated charcoal and laxatives may be of value. However, by the time this method is employed, most of the amatoxin has already caused cellular damage and has already been excreted. Charcoal hemoperfusion has been recommended but is of unproved value.

Liver transplant may be the only hope for survival in gravely ill patients—contact a liver transplant center early.

2. Gyromitrin type–For gyromitrin poisoning, give pyridoxine, 25 mg/kg intravenously.

3. Muscarinic type–For mushrooms producing predominantly muscarinic-cholinergic symptoms, give atropine, 0.005–0.01 mg/kg intravenously, and repeat as needed.

4. Anticholinergic type–For anticholinergic type, physostigmine, 0.5–1 mg intravenously, may calm extremely agitated patients and reverse peripheral anticholinergic manifestations, but it may also cause bradycardia, asystole, and seizures.

5. Gastrointestinal irritant type–Treat with antiemetics and intravenous or oral fluids.

6. Disulfiram type–For *Coprinus* ingestion, avoid alcohol. Treat alcohol reaction with fluids and supine position.

7. Hallucinogenic type–Provide a quiet, supportive atmosphere. Diazepam or haloperidol may be used for sedation.

8. *Cortinarius*–Provide supportive care and hemodialysis as needed for renal failure.

Leathem AM et al: Renal failure caused by mushroom poisoning. J Toxicol Clin Toxicol 1997;35:67. [NLM Cit ID: 97174995] (Case reports of four patients.)

Yameda EG et al: Mushroom poisoning due to amatoxin. Northern California, winter 1996–1997. West J Med 1998;169:380. [NLM Cit ID: 99083676] (Case reports of illness and death after *Amanita phalloides* ingestion.)

OPIOIDS (Morphine, Heroin, Codeine, Propoxyphene, Etc)

Prescription and illicit opioids are popular drugs of abuse and the cause of frequent hospitalizations for overdose. These drugs have widely varying potencies and durations of action; for example, some of the illicit fentanyl derivatives are up to 2000 times more potent than morphine. All of these agents decrease central nervous system activity and sympathetic outflow by acting on opiate receptors in the brain. Tramadol is a newer analgesic that is unrelated chemically to the opioids but acts on opioid receptors.

Clinical Findings

Mild intoxication is characterized by euphoria, drowsiness, and constricted pupils. More severe intoxication may cause hypotension, bradycardia, hypothermia, coma, and respiratory arrest. Pulmonary edema may occur. Death is usually due to apnea or pulmonary aspiration of gastric contents. Propoxyphene may cause seizures and prolongation of the QRS interval. Tramadol, dextromethorphan, and meperidine also occasionally cause seizures. With meperidine, the metabolite normeperidine is probably the cause of seizures and is most likely to accumulate with repeated dosing in patients with renal insufficiency. While the duration of effect for heroin is usually 3–5 hours, methadone intoxication may last for 48–72 hours or longer. Most opioids, with the exception of illicit newer fentanyl derivatives, tramadol, and methadone, are detectable on routine urine toxicology screening

Treatment

A. Emergency and Supportive Measures: If the patient arrives for medical care shortly after ingestion, empty the stomach by emesis or gastric lavage and administer activated charcoal (see p 1565).

B. Specific Treatment: Naloxone is a specific opioid antagonist that can rapidly reverse signs of narcotic intoxication. Although it is structurally related to the opioids, it has no agonist effects of its own. Administer 0.4–2 mg intravenously, and repeat as needed to awaken the patient and maintain airway protective reflexes and spontaneous breathing. Very large doses (10–20 mg) may be required for patients intoxicated by some opioids (eg, propoxyphene, codeine, fentanyl derivatives). ***Caution:*** The duration of effect of naloxone is only about 2–3 hours; repeated doses may be necessary for patients intoxicated by long-acting drugs such as methadone. Continuous observation for at least 3 hours after the last naloxone dose is mandatory.

Kaplan JL et al: Double-blind, randomized study of nalmefene and naloxone in emergency department patients with suspected narcotic overdose. Ann Emerg Med 1999;34:42. [NLM Cit ID: 99315124] (Similar efficacy and safety.)

Passaro DJ et al: Wound botulism associated with black tar heroin among injecting drug users. JAMA 1998;279:859. [NLM Cit ID: 98175756] (Case series of 26 patients.)

Sporer KA: Acute heroin overdose. Ann Intern Med 1999;130:584. [NLM Cit ID: 99188833] (Review article.)

PARAQUAT

Paraquat is used as a herbicide. Concentrated solutions of paraquat are highly corrosive to the oropharynx, esophagus, and stomach. The fatal dose after absorption may be as small as 4 mg/kg. If ingestion of paraquat is not rapidly fatal because of its corrosive effects, the herbicide may cause progressive pulmonary fibrosis, with death ensuing after 2–3 weeks. Patients with plasma paraquat levels above 2 mg/L at 6 hours or 0.2 mg/L at 24 hours are likely to die.

Treatment

Remove ingested paraquat by immediate induced emesis, or by gastric lavage if the patient is already in a health care facility. Clay (bentonite or fuller's earth) and activated charcoal are effective adsorbents. Administer repeated doses of 60 g of activated charcoal by gastric tube every 2 hours for at least three or four doses. Charcoal hemoperfusion, 8 hours per day for 2–3 weeks, has been anecdotally reported to be lifesaving, but clinical and animal studies are equivocal. Supplemental oxygen should be withheld unless the PO_2 is less than 70 mm Hg because oxygen may contribute to the pulmonary damage, which is mediated through lipid peroxidation.

Walder B et al: Successful single-lung transplantation after paraquat intoxication. Transplantation 1997;64:789. [NLM Cit ID: 97456411] (Forty-four days after poisoning.)

Wesseling C et al: Unintentional fatal paraquat poisonings among agricultural workers in Costa Rica: Report of 15 cases. Am J Ind Med 1997;32:433. [NLM Cit ID: 97467889]

PESTICIDES: CHOLINESTERASE INHIBITORS (Organophosphates: Parathion, Malathion, etc; Carbamates: Carbaryl, Aldicarb, Etc)

Organophosphate and carbamate insecticides are widely used in commercial agriculture and home gardening and have largely replaced older, more environmentally persistent organochlorine compounds such as DDT and chlordane. The organophosphates and carbamates—also called anticholinesterases because they inhibit the enzyme acetylcholinesterase—cause an increase in acetylcholine activity at nicotinic and muscarinic receptors and in the central nervous system. There are a variety of chemical agents in this group, with widely varying potencies. Most of them are poorly water-soluble and are formulated with an aromatic hydrocarbon solvent such as xylene. Most of them are well absorbed through intact skin. Most chemical warfare "nerve agents" (see p 1575) are organophosphates.

Clinical Findings

Inhibition of cholinesterase results in abdominal cramps, diarrhea, vomiting, excessive salivation, sweating, lacrimation, miosis (constricted pupils), wheezing and bronchorrhea, seizures, and skeletal muscle weakness. Initial tachycardia is usually followed by bradycardia. Profound skeletal muscle weakness, aggravated by excessive bronchial secretions and wheezing, may result in respiratory arrest and death. Signs and symptoms of poisoning may persist or recur over several days, especially with highly lipid-soluble agents such as fenthion or dimethoate.

The diagnosis should be suspected in patients who present with miosis, sweating, and hyperperistalsis. Serum and red blood cell cholinesterase activity can be measured in the laboratory and is usually depressed at least 50% below baseline in those victims who have severe intoxication.

Treatment

A. Emergency and Supportive Measures: If the agent was recently ingested, empty the stomach by gastric lavage and administer activated charcoal (see p 1565). Do not induce emesis because of the risk of abrupt onset of seizures. If the agent is on the victim's skin or hair, wash repeatedly with soap or shampoo and water. Providers must take care to avoid skin exposure by wearing gloves and waterproof aprons.

B. Specific Treatment: Atropine reverses excessive muscarinic stimulation and is effective for treatment of salivation, wheezing, abdominal cramping, and sweating. However, it does not interact with nicotinic receptors at autonomic ganglia and at the neuromuscular junction and has no effect on muscle weakness. Administer 2 mg intravenously, and give repeated doses as needed to dry bronchial secretions and decrease wheezing; as much as several hundred milligrams of atropine have been given to treat severe poisoning.

Pralidoxime (2-PAM, Protopam) is a specific antidote that reverses organophosphate binding to the cholinesterase enzyme; therefore, it is effective at the neuromuscular junction as well as other nicotinic and muscarinic sites. It should be started as soon as possible, to prevent permanent binding of the organophosphate to cholinesterase. Administer 1–2 g intravenously, and begin a continuous infusion (200–400 mg/h). Constant infusion is more effective because of the short duration of action of single doses. Continue to give pralidoxime as long as there is any evidence of acetylcholine excess. Pralidoxime is of questionable benefit for carbamate poisoning, because carbamates have only a transitory effect on the cholinesterase enzyme.

O'Malley M: Clinical evaluation of pesticide exposure and poisonings. Lancet 1997;349:1161. [NLM Cit ID: 97267694] (Review ranging from topical irritant reactions to severe systemic illness.)

Saadeh AM et al: Cardiac manifestations of acute carbamate and organophosphate poisoning. Heart 1997; 77:461. [NLM Cit ID: 97339864] (Retrospective study highlighting the frequency, extent, and management of poisoning.)

PETROLEUM DISTILLATES & SOLVENTS

Petroleum distillate toxicity may occur from inhalation of the vapor or as a result of pulmonary aspiration of the liquid during or after ingestion. Acute manifestations of aspiration pneumonitis are vomiting, coughing, and bronchopneumonia. Some hydrocarbons—ie, those with aromatic or halogenated subunits—can also cause severe systemic poisoning after oral ingestion (Table 39–13). Hydrocarbons can also cause systemic intoxication by inhalation. Vertigo, muscular incoordination, irregular pulse, myoclonus, and convulsions occur with serious poisoning and may be due to hypoxemia or the systemic effects of the agents. Chlorinated and fluorinated hydrocarbons (trichloroethylene, freons, etc) and many other hydrocarbons can cause ventricular arrhythmias due to increased sensitivity of the myocardium to the effects of endogenous catecholamines.

Treatment (Table 39–13)

Remove the patient to fresh air. Since aspiration is the primary danger after ingestion of many common products, use of lavage or emesis is controversial; removal of ingested hydrocarbon is usually suggested only if the preparation contains toxic solutes (eg, an insecticide) or is an aromatic or halogenated product. Observe the victim for 6–8 hours for signs of aspiration pneumonitis (cough, localized rales or rhonchi, tachypnea, and infiltrates on chest radiograph). Corticosteroids are not recommended. If fever occurs, give a specific antibiotic only after identification of bacterial pathogens by laboratory studies. Because of the risk of arrhythmias, use bronchodilators only with caution in patients with chlorinated or fluorinated solvent intoxication.

Chang YL et al: Diverse manifestations of oral methylene chloride poisoning: report of 6 cases. J Toxicol Clin Toxicol 1999;37:497. [NLM Cit ID: 99392917] (Toxic effects included central nervous system depression, tachypnea, and corrosive gastrointestinal injury. Two patients had mild to moderate elevation of blood carboxyhemoglobin levels.)

Gerkin RD Jr et al: Rapid reversal of life-threatening toluene-induced hypokalemia with hemodialysis. J Emerg Med 1998;16:723. [NLM Cit ID: 9752945] (Unusual complication of toluene poisoning.)

PHENOTHIAZINES & OTHER ANTIPSYCHOTIC AGENTS (Chlorpromazine, Promazine, Haloperidol, Prochlorperazine, Risperidone, Clozapine, Etc)

Chlorpromazine and related drugs are used as antiemetics and antipsychotic agents and as potentiators of analgesic and hypnotic drugs.

Small doses of phenothiazines induce drowsiness and mild orthostatic hypotension in as many as 50% of patients. Larger doses can cause obtundation, miosis, severe hypotension, tachycardia, convulsions, and coma. Abnormal cardiac conduction may occur (particularly with thioridazine), resulting in prolongation of QRS or QT intervals (or both) and ventricular arrhythmias.

With therapeutic or toxic doses, some patients develop an acute extrapyramidal dystonic reaction similar to Parkinson's disease, with spasmodic contractions of the face and neck muscles, extensor rigidity of the back muscles, carpopedal spasm, and motor restlessness. Severe rigidity accompanied by hyperthermia and metabolic acidosis ("neuroleptic malignant syndrome") may occasionally occur and is life-threatening (see Chapters 1 and 25).

Table 39–13. Clinical features of hydrocarbon poisoning.[1]

Type	Examples	Risk of Pneumonia	Risk of Systemic Toxicity	Treatment
High-viscosity	Vaseline[2] Motor oil	Low	Low	None.
Low-viscosity, nontoxic	Furniture polish Mineral seal oil Kerosene Lighter fluid	High	Low	Observe for pneumonia. *Do not* induce emesis. *Do not* administer activated charcoal.
Low-viscosity, unknown systemic toxicity	Turpentine Pine oil	High	Variable	Observe for pneumonia. Consider activated charcoal.
Low-viscosity, known systemic toxicity	Camphor Phenol Chlorinated insecticides Aromatic hydrocarbons (benzene, toluene, etc)	High	High	Observe for pneumonia. Give activated charcoal.

[1]Reproduced, with permission, from Saunders CE, Ho MT (editors): *Current Emergency Diagnosis & Treatment*, 4th ed. Originally published by Appleton & Lange. Copyright © 1992 by The McGraw-Hill Companies, Inc.
[2]"Vaseline" is one of several proprietary names for petrolatum (petroleum jelly, paraffin jelly).

successful treatment of severe neurologic symptoms with mannitol, 1 g/kg intravenously.

2. Scombroid–Antihistamines such as diphenhydramine, 25–50 mg intravenously, and the H_2 blocker cimetidine, 300 mg intravenously, are usually effective. For severe reactions, give also epinephrine, 0.3–0.5 mL of a 1:1000 solution subcutaneously.

Ciguatera fish poisoning—Texas, 1997. MMWR Morb Mortal Wkly Rep 1998;47:692. [NLM Cit ID: 98402252] (A contaminated barracuda caused 17 cases of ciguatera poisoning.)

Clark RF et al: A review of selected seafood poisonings. Undersea Hyperb Med 1999;26:175. [NLM Cit ID: 99413529] (Review of the pathophysiology, clinical presentation, and treatment of the most common varieties of seafood poisoning resulting from toxins.)

Field J: Puffer fish poisoning. J Accid Emerg Med 1998;15:334. [NLM Cit ID: 99001344] (The deadly toxin in this fish can cause rapid onset of muscular paralysis and respiratory arrest.)

Mines D et al: Poisonings: food, fish, shellfish. Emerg Med Clin North Am 1997;15:157. [NLM Cit ID: 97209274] (Review of scombroid, ciguatera, pufferfish, and shellfish poisoning.)

SNAKE BITES

The venom of poisonous snakes and lizards may be predominantly neurotoxic (coral snake) or predominantly cytolytic (rattlesnakes, other pit vipers). Neurotoxins cause respiratory paralysis; cytolytic venoms cause tissue destruction by digestion and hemorrhage due to hemolysis and destruction of the endothelial lining of the blood vessels. The manifestations of rattlesnake envenomation are mostly local pain, redness, swelling, and extravasation of blood. Perioral tingling, metallic taste, nausea and vomiting, hypotension, and coagulopathy may also occur. Neurotoxic envenomation may cause ptosis, dysphagia, diplopia, and respiratory arrest.

Treatment

A. Emergency Measures: Immobilize the patient and the bitten part in a neutral position. Avoid manipulation of the bitten area. Transport the patient to a medical facility for definitive treatment. Do *not* give alcoholic beverages or stimulants; do *not* apply ice; do *not* apply a tourniquet. The trauma to underlying structures resulting from incision and suction performed by unskilled people is probably not justified in view of the small amount of venom that can be recovered.

B. Specific Antidote and General Measures:

1. Pit viper (eg, rattlesnake) envenomation–With local signs such as swelling, pain, and ecchymosis but no systemic symptoms, give 5–10 vials of polyvalent crotalid antivenin by slow intravenous drip in 250–500 mL saline. (This should be preceded by skin testing for horse serum sensitivity with the kit supplied.) For more serious envenomation with marked local effects and systemic toxicity (eg, hypotension, coagulopathy), 10–20 vials may be required. Epinephrine should be available for immediate use in the event of an allergic reaction. Monitor vital signs and the blood coagulation profile. Type and cross-match blood. The adequacy of venom neutralization is indicated by improvement in signs and symptoms, and the rate of swelling slows. Serum sickness reactions are common after antivenin use, usually occur 5–10 days after antivenin administration, and may be treated with prednisone, 45–60 mg daily with tapering doses.

2. Elapid (coral snake) envenomation–Give 1–2 vials of specific antivenom as soon as possible. To locate antisera for exotic snakes, call a regional poison control center (see Table 39–1).

Gibley RL et al: Intravascular hemolysis associated with North American crotalid envenomation. J Toxicol Clin Toxicol 1998;36:337. [NLM Cit ID: 9711200] (Case report.)

Theakston RD: An objective approach to antivenin therapy and the assessment of first-aid measures in a snake bite. Ann Trop Med Parasitol 1997;91:857. [NLM Cit ID: 98289183]

Walter F et al: Envenomations. Crit Care Clin 1999;15:353. [NLM Cit ID: 99261518] (Review of envenomations caused by snakes, spiders and scorpions.

SPIDER BITES & SCORPION STINGS

The toxin of most species of spiders in the USA causes only local pain, redness, and swelling. That of the more venomous black widow spiders *(Latrodectus mactans)* causes generalized muscular pains, muscle spasms, and rigidity. The brown recluse spider *(Loxosceles reclusa)* causes progressive local necrosis as well as hemolytic reactions (rare). Stings by most scorpions in the USA cause only local pain. Stings by the more toxic *Centruroides* species (found in the southwestern USA) may cause muscle cramps, twitching and jerking, and occasionally hypertension, convulsions, and pulmonary edema.

Treatment

A. Black Widow Spider Bites: Pain may be relieved with parenteral narcotics or muscle relaxants (eg, methocarbamol, 15 mg/kg). Calcium gluconate 10%, 0.1–0.2 mL/kg intravenously, may relieve muscle rigidity, though its effectiveness is questionable. Antivenin is rarely indicated, usually only for the very young or elderly patients or those who do not respond to the above measures. Horse serum sensitivity testing is required. (Instruction and testing materials are included in the antivenin kit.)

B. Brown Recluse Spider Bites: Because bites occasionally progress to extensive local necrosis, some authorities recommend early excision of the bite site, whereas others use oral corticosteroids. Anecdotal reports have claimed success with dapsone and colchicine. An antivenin is being developed. All of these treatments remain of unproved value.

C. Scorpion Stings: No specific treatment is available. For *Centruroides* stings, some toxicologists use a specific antivenom developed in Arizona, but this is neither FDA-approved nor widely available.

Heard K et al: Antivenom therapy in the Americas. Drugs 1999;58:5. [NLM Cit ID: 99368799] (Review of the indications, method of administration, and incidence of adverse reactions for antivenoms in the treatment of envenomations from snakes, spiders, and scorpions.)

Hobbs GD et al: Comparisons of hyperbaric oxygen and dapsone therapy for *Loxosceles* envenomation. Acad Emerg Med 1996;3:758. [NLM Cit ID: 97006377] (Animal study showed no benefit with either of these treatments compared with controls.)

Premawardhena AP et al: Low dose subcutaneous adrenaline to prevent acute adverse reactions to antivenom serum in people bitten by snakes: randomised, placebo controlled trial. BMJ 1999;318:1041. [NLM Cit ID: 99221567] (Prospective, double-blind, randomized, placebo-controlled trial in 105 patients demonstrating the reduction of acute adverse reactions to antivenom serum by the administration of 0.25 mL of 1:1000 epinephrine subcutaneously.)

Wright SW et al: Clinical presentation and outcome of brown recluse spider bite. Ann Emerg Med 1997;30:28. [NLM Cit ID: 97352963] (Retrospective case series of 111 patients with brown recluse spider bites. Three of 11 required skin grafting. Study recommends supportive care alone.)

THEOPHYLLINE

Theophylline is used in the treatment of bronchospasm due to asthma, chronic lung disease, and congestive heart failure. Its toxicity may be caused by several of its pharmacologic effects, including inhibition of phosphodiesterase and adenosine and release of catecholamines. Theophylline may cause intoxication after an acute single overdose, or intoxication may occur as a result of chronic accidental repeated overmedication or reduced elimination resulting from hepatic dysfunction or interacting drug (eg, cimetidine, erythromycin). The usual serum half-life of theophylline is 4–6 hours, but this may increase to more than 20 hours after overdose.

Clinical Findings

Mild intoxication causes nausea, vomiting, tachycardia, and tremulousness. Severe intoxication is characterized by ventricular and supraventricular tachyarrhythmias, hypotension, and seizures. Status epilepticus is common and often intractable to usual anticonvulsants. After acute overdose (but not chronic intoxication), hypokalemia, hyperglycemia, and metabolic acidosis are common. Seizures and other manifestations of toxicity may be delayed for several hours after acute ingestion, especially if a sustained-release preparation such as Theo-Dur was taken.

Diagnosis is based on measurement of the serum theophylline concentration. Acute overdose patients with serum levels greater than 100 mg/L are likely to develop seizures and hypotension. Patients with chronic intoxication may develop serious toxicity at lower levels (ie, 40–60 mg/L).

Treatment

A. Emergency and Supportive Measures: After acute ingestion, administer activated charcoal and a cathartic (see p 1565). Repeated doses of activated charcoal may enhance theophylline elimination by "gut dialysis" (see p 1565). Addition of whole bowel irrigation (see p 1566) should be considered for massive ingestions involving sustained-release preparations.

Hemodialysis (or hemoperfusion) is effective in removing theophylline and is indicated for patients with status epilepticus or markedly elevated serum theophylline levels (eg, > 100 mg/L after acute overdose or > 60 mg/L with chronic intoxication).

B. Specific Treatment: There is no antidote for seizures, but hypotension and tachycardia—which are mediated through excessive beta-adrenergic stimulation—may respond to beta-blocker therapy even in low doses: Administer esmolol, 25–50 μg/kg/min by intravenous infusion, or propranolol, 0.5–1 mg intravenously.

Minton NA et al: Treatment of theophylline overdose. Am J Emerg Med 1996;14:506. [NLM Cit ID: 97010784]

Shannon MW: Comparative efficacy of hemodialysis and hemoperfusion in severe theophylline intoxication. Acad Emerg Med 1997;4:674. [NLM Cit ID: 97366876] (Hemoperfusion provides a higher theophylline clearance rate than hemodialysis; however, hemodialysis appears to have comparable efficacy in reducing morbidity.)

Shannon M: Life-threatening events after theophylline overdose: a 10-year prospective analysis. Arch Intern Med 1999;159:989. [NLM Cit ID: 99256873] (Review of 356 patients with theophylline intoxication highlighting the substantial morbidity and mortality.)

TRICYCLIC ANTIDEPRESSANTS

Tricyclic and related cyclic antidepressants are among the most dangerous drugs involved in suicidal overdose. These drugs have anticholinergic and cardiac depressant properties ("quinidine-like" sodium channel blockade). Tricyclic antidepressants produce more marked membrane-depressant cardiotoxic effects than the phenothiazines.

Newer antidepressants such as trazodone, fluoxetine, paroxetine, sertraline, bupropion, venlafaxine,

mosome is a complex of protein and nucleic acid in which an unbroken double helix of DNA is coiled and supercoiled into a space many orders of magnitude less than the extended length of the DNA. Within the chromosome there occur highly complicated and integrated processes, including DNA replication, recombination, and transcription. In the nucleus of each somatic cell, humans normally have 46 chromosomes, which are arranged in 23 pairs. One of these pairs, the **sex chromosomes** X and Y, determines the sex of the individual; females have the pair XX and males the pair XY. The remaining 22 pairs are called **autosomes** (Figure 40–1).

In all somatic cells, the 44 autosomes and one of the X chromosomes are transcriptionally active. In males, the active X is the only X; portions of the Y chromosome are also active. In females, the requirement for **dosage compensation** (to be equivalent to the situation in males) is satisfied by inactivation of most of one X chromosome early in embryogenesis. This process of X chromosomal inactivation, while incompletely understood, is known to be random, so that on average, in 50% of a female's cells, one of the X chromosomes will be active, and in the other 50% the **homologous** member of the pair will be active. The phenotype of the cell is determined by which genes on the chromosomes are active in producing mRNA at any given time.

GENES & CHROMOSOMES

In all genes, information is contained in parcels called **exons,** which are interspersed with stretches of DNA called **introns** that do not encode any information about the protein sequence. However, introns may contain genetic regulatory sequences, and some introns are so large that they encode an entirely distinct gene.

The exact location of a gene on a chromosome is its **locus,** and the array of loci constitutes the **human gene map.** Currently, the chromosomal sites of more than 6000 genes (for which normal or abnormal function has been identified) are known, often to a high degree of resolution. A variation of this map, identifying selected loci known to be involved in human disease, is shown in Figure 40–2. The difference in the higher resolution of the ordering of genes achievable by molecular techniques (such as linkage analysis) compared to cytogenetic techniques (such as vi-

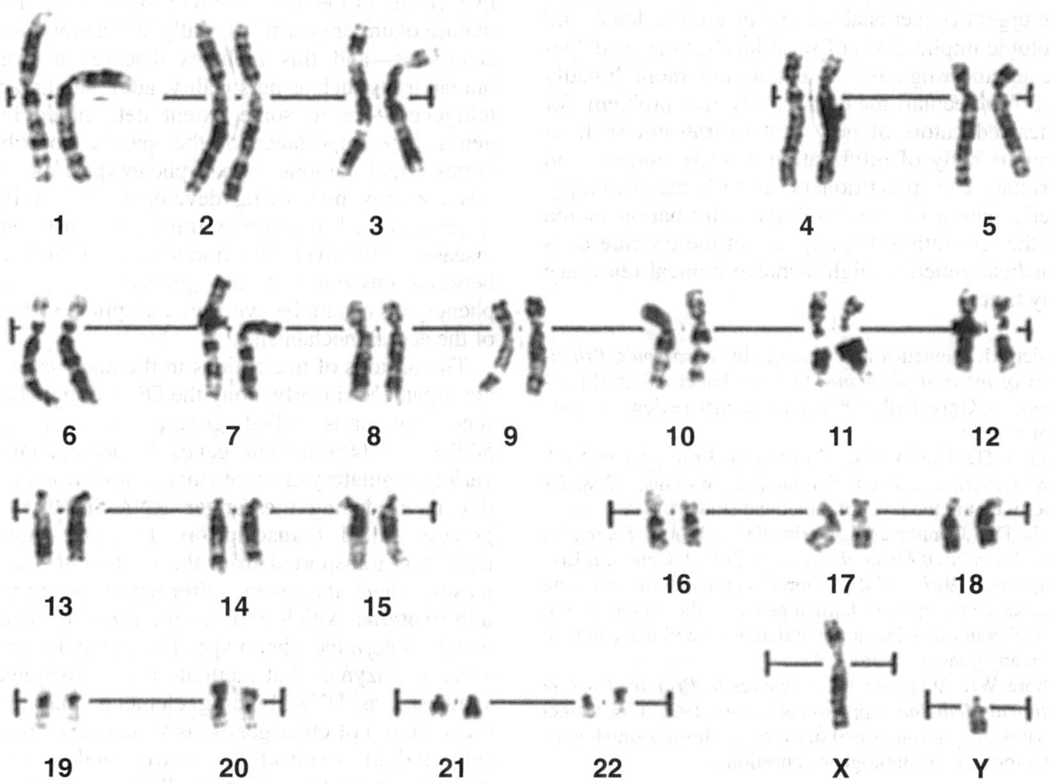

Figure 40–1. Normal karyotype of a human male. Prepared from cultured amniotic cells and stained with Giemsa's stain. About 400 bands are detectable per haploid set of chromosomes.

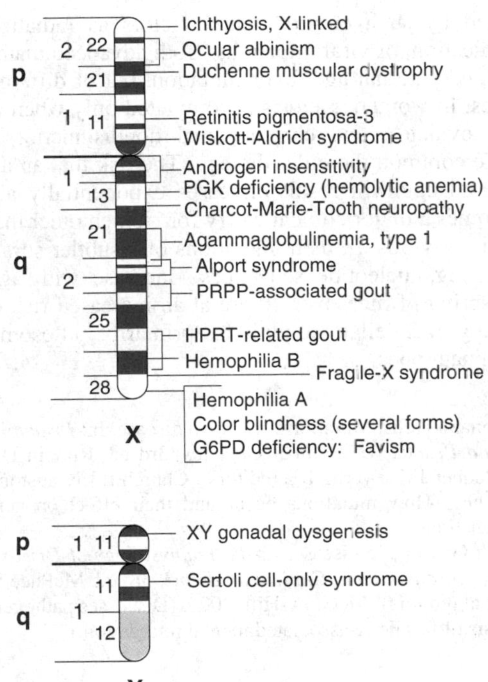

Figure 40–2. A partial "morbid map" of the human genome. Shown next to the ideogram of the human X and Y chromosomes are representative mendelian disorders caused by mutations at that locus. Over 400 genes and phenotypes have been mapped to the X chromosome and 25 to the Y chromosome. (Courtesy of V McKusick and J Strayer.)

sualization of small defects) is substantial, though the gap is narrowing. The chromosomes in the "standard" karyotype shown in Figure 40–1 have about 450 visible bands; under the best of cytologic and microscopic conditions, a total of about 1600 bands can be seen. But even in this extended configuration, each band contains dozens—sometimes hundreds—of individual genes. Thus, loss **(deletion)** of a small band will involve loss of many coding sequences and will have diverse effects on the phenotype.

The number and arrangement of genes on homologous chromosomes are identical even though the actual coding sequences of homologous genes may not be. Homologous copies of a gene are termed **alleles.** In comparing alleles, it must be specified at what level of analysis the comparison is being made. When alleles are truly identical—in that their coding sequences are invariant—the individual is **homozygous** at that locus. At a coarser level, the alleles may be functionally identical despite subtle variations in nucleotide sequence—with the result either that the proteins produced from the two alleles are identical or that whatever differences there may be in amino acid sequence will have no bearing on the function of the protein. If the individual is being analyzed at the level of the protein phenotype, allelic homozygosity would again be an apt descriptor. However, if the analysis were at the level of the DNA—as occurs in restriction enzyme examination or nucleotide sequencing—then, despite functional identity, the alleles would be viewed as different and the individual would be **heterozygous** for that locus. Heterozygosity based on differences in the protein products of alleles has been detectable for decades and was the first hard evidence concerning the high degree of human biologic variability. In the past decade, analysis of DNA sequences has shown this variability to be much more remarkable—differences in nucleotide sequence between individuals occur about once every 400 nucleotides.

Cantor CR: How will the Human Genome Project improve our quality of life? Nat Biotechnol 1998;16:212. [NLM Cit ID: 98188410] (Perspective on improved diagnostics, more efficient clinical trials, and gene therapy.)

Collins FS et al: New goals for the U.S. Human Genome Project: 1998–2003. Science 1998;282:682. [NLM Cit ID: 99000794] (The official enumeration of the plans to sequence the human genome by 2003 (subsequently advanced to 2001, and then to 2000), to catalogue sequence variation to assist in mapping the genes involved in complex traits, and to continue to study the ethical, legal, and social implications of genetics.)

Collins FS: Shattuck lecture—medical and societal consequences of the Human Genome Project. N Engl J Med 1999;341:28. [NLM Cit ID: 99294368] (What knowing the sequence of the human genome may mean for understanding, diagnosing, and managing disease.)

Reilly PR et al: We're off to see the genome. Nat Genet 1998;20:15. [NLM Cit ID: 98400249] (Some of the legal and societal implications of the "human genetics revolution.")

MUTATION

Allelic heterozygosity most often results when different alleles are inherited from the egg and the sperm, but it also occurs as a consequence of spontaneous alteration in nucleotide sequence **(mutation).** Genetic change occurring during formation of an egg or a sperm is called a **germinal mutation.** When the change occurs after conception—from the earliest stages of embryogenesis to dividing cells in the body of the oldest adult—it is termed a **somatic mutation.** As is discussed below, the role of somatic mutation in the etiology of human disease is now increasingly recognized.

The coarsest type of mutation is alteration in the number or physical structure of chromosomes. For example, **nondisjunction** (failure of chromosome pairs to separate) during **meiosis**—the reduction division that leads to production of mature ova and sperms—causes the embryo to have too many or too few chromosomes, a situation called **aneuploidy.** Rearrangement of chromosome arms, such as occurs in **translocation** or **inversion,** is a mutation even if breakage and reunion does not disrupt any coding sequence. Thus, the phenotypic effect of gross chromosomal mutations can range from profound (as in aneuploidy) to nil.

A bit less coarse, but still detectable cytologically, are **deletions** of part of a chromosome. Such mutations almost always alter phenotype, because a number of genes are lost; however, a deletion may involve only a single nucleotide, whereas about 1–2 million nucleotides (1–2 megabases) must be lost before the defect can be visualized by the most sensitive cytogenetic methods short of in situ hybridization. Molecular biologic techniques are needed to detect smaller losses.

Mutations of one or a few nucleotides in exons have several potential consequences. Changes in one nucleotide can alter which amino acid is encoded; if the amino acid is in a critical region of the protein, function might in this way be severely deranged (eg, sickle cell disease). On the other hand, some amino acid substitutions have no detectable effect on function, and the phenotype is therefore unaltered by the mutation. Similarly, because the genetic code is **degenerate** (two or more different three-nucleotide sequences called **codons** encode the same amino acids), nucleotide substitution does not necessarily alter the amino acid sequence of the protein. Three specific codons signal termination of translation; thus, a nucleotide substitution in an exon that generates one of the stop codons usually causes a truncated protein, which is nearly always dysfunctional. Other nucleotide substitutions can disrupt the signals that direct splicing of the mRNA molecule and grossly alter the protein product. Finally, insertions and deletions of one or more nucleotides can have dramatic effects—any change that is not a multiple of three nucleotides disrupts the reading frame of the remainder of the exon—or potentially minimal effects (if the protein can tolerate the insertion or loss of an amino acid).

Mutations in introns may disrupt mRNA splicing signals or may be entirely silent with respect to the phenotype. A great deal of variation in nucleotide sequences among individuals (averaging one difference every few hundred nucleotides) resides within introns. Mutations in the DNA between adjacent genes may also be silent or may have a profound effect on phenotype if regulatory sequences are disrupted. A novel mechanism for mutation, which also helps explain clinical variation among relatives, has been discovered in myotonic dystrophy, Huntington's disease, fragile X mental retardation syndrome, Friedreich's ataxia, and other disorders. A region of repeated trinucleotide sequences close to or within a gene can be unstable in some families; expansion of the number of repeated units within this segment beyond a critical threshold is associated with a more severe phenotype.

Mutations may occur spontaneously or may be induced by such environmental factors as radiation, medication, or viral infections. Both advanced maternal and paternal age favor mutation, but of different types. In women, meiosis is completed only when an egg ovulates, and chromosomal nondisjunction is more common the older the egg. The risk that an aneuploid egg will result increases exponentially and becomes a major clinical worry for women older than their early 30s. In men, mutations of a subtler sort—affecting nucleotide sequences—increase with age. Offspring of men over 40 are at an increased risk of having mendelian conditions, primarily autosomal dominant ones.

Antonarakis SE: Mutations in human disease. In: *Principles and Practice of Medical Genetics,* 3rd ed. Rimoin DL, Conner JM, Pyeritz RE (editors). Churchill Livingstone, 1997. (How mutations occur and their effect on gene function.)

Barsh G: Genetic disease. In: *Pathophysiology of Disease: An Introduction to Clinical Medicine,* 3rd ed. McPhee SJ et al (editors): McGraw-Hill, 2000. (Discusses pathogenesis of fragile X-associated mental retardation.)

GENES IN INDIVIDUALS

For some quantitative traits such as adult height or serum glucose concentration in normal individuals, it is virtually impossible to distinguish the contributions of individual genes; this is because in general, phenotypes are the products of multiple genes acting in concert. However, if one of the genes in the system is aberrant, a major departure from the "normal" or expected phenotype might arise. Whether the aberrant phenotype is serious (ie, a disease) or even recognized will depend on the nature of the defective gene product and how resilient the system is to disruption. The latter point emphasizes the importance of homeostasis in both physiology and development—many mutations go unrecognized because the system can cope, even though tolerances for further perturbation might be narrowed.

In other words, virtually all human characteristics are **polygenic,** while many of the disordered phenotypes thought of as "genetic" are **monogenic** but still influenced by other loci in a person's genome.

Phenotypes due to alterations at a single gene are also characterized as **mendelian,** after the monk and part-time biologist who studied the reproducibility and recurrence of variation in garden peas. Gregor Mendel showed that some traits were **dominant** to others, which he called **recessive.** The dominant traits required only one copy of a "factor" to be expressed, regardless of what the other copy was, whereas the recessive traits required two copies before expression occurred. In modern terms, the mendelian factors are genes, and the alternative copies of the gene are alleles. Let *A* be the common (normal) allele and let *a* be a mutant allele at a locus: If the same phenotype is present no matter whether the genotype is *A/a* or *a/a*, the phenotype is dominant, whereas if the phenotype is present only when the genotype is *a/a*, it is recessive.

In medicine, it is important to keep two considerations in mind: First, dominance and recessiveness are attributes of the phenotype, not the gene; and second, the concepts of dominance and recessiveness depend on how one defines the phenotype. To illustrate both points, consider sickle cell disease. This condition occurs when a person inherits two alleles for β^S-globin, in which the normal glutamate at position 6 of the protein has been replaced by valine; the genotype for the β-globin locus is *HbS/HbS*, compared to the normal *HbA/HbA*. When the genotype is *HbS/HbA*, the individual does not have sickle cell disease, so this condition satisfies the criteria for being a recessive phenotype. But now consider the phenotype of sickled erythrocytes. Red cells with the genotype *HbS/HbS* clearly sickle—but, if the oxygen tension is reduced, so do cells with the genotype *HbS/HbA*. Therefore, sickling is a dominant trait.

A mendelian phenotype is characterized not only in terms of dominance and recessiveness but also according to whether the determining gene is on the X chromosome or on one of the 22 pairs of autosomes. Traits or diseases are therefore called autosomal dominant, autosomal recessive, X-linked recessive, and X-linked dominant.

Beaudet AL: Making genomic medicine a reality. Am J Hum Genet 1999;64:1. [NLM Cit ID: 99115074] (An enthusiastic perspective on how genetics does and can influence medical care.)

Mueller R, Cook J: Mendelian inheritance. In: *Principles and Practice of Medical Genetics,* 3rd ed. Rimoin DL, Connor JM, Pyeritz RE (editors): Churchill Livingstone, 1997.

GENES IN FAMILIES

Since the first decade of this century, the patterns of recurrence of specific human phenotypes have been explained in terms of principles first described by Mendel in the garden pea plant. Mendel's second principle—usually referred to as his first*—is called the **law of segregation** and states that a pair of factors (alleles) that determines some trait separates (segregates) during formation of gametes. In simple terms, a heterozygous *(A/a)* person will produce two types of gametes with respect to this locus—one containing only *A* and one containing only *a*, in equal proportions. Offspring of this person will have a 50–50 chance of inheriting the *A* allele and a similar chance of inheriting the *a* allele.

The concepts of genes in individuals and in families can be combined to specify how mendelian traits will be inherited.

Autosomal Dominant Inheritance

The characteristics of autosomal dominant inheritance in humans can be summarized as follows:

(1) There is a vertical pattern in the pedigree, with multiple generations affected (Figure 40–3).

(2) Heterozygotes for the mutant allele show an abnormal phenotype.

(3) Males and females are affected with equal frequency and severity.

(4) Only one parent must be affected for an offspring to be at risk for developing the phenotype.

(5) When an affected person mates with an unaffected one, each offspring has a 50% chance of inheriting the affected phenotype. This is true regardless of the sex of the affected parent—specifically, male-to-male transmission occurs.

(6) The frequency of sporadic cases is positively associated with the severity of the phenotype. More precisely, the greater the **reproductive fitness** of affected persons, the less likely it is that any given case resulted from a new mutation.

(7) The average age of fathers is advanced in the case of isolated (sporadic or new mutation) cases.

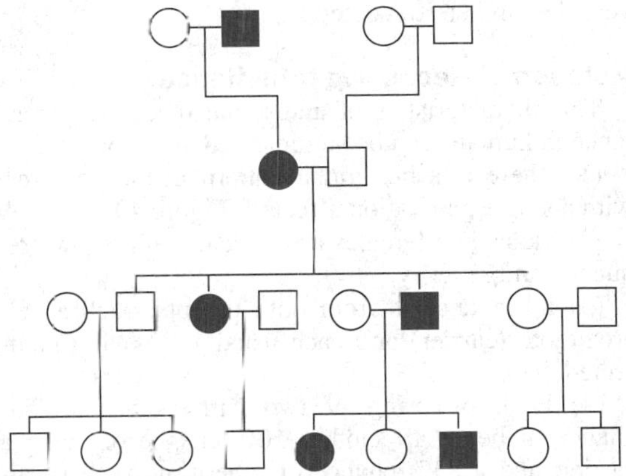

Figure 40–3. A pedigree illustrating autosomal dominant inheritance. Square symbols indicate males and circles females; open symbols indicate that the person is phenotypically unaffected, and filled symbols indicate that the phenotype is present to some extent.

*Mendel's first law stated that—from the perspective of the phenotype—it mattered not from which parent a particular mutant allele was inherited. For years this principle was thought to be too obvious to be codified as anybody's "law" and was therefore ignored. In fact, however, recent evidence from studies of human disorders suggests that certain genes are "processed" **(imprinted)** as they move through the gonad and that processing in the testis is different from that in the ovary. Thus, not only is this first mendelian principle important, it was incorrect as originally formulated from observations in peas.

Autosomal dominant phenotypes are often age-dependent, less severe than autosomal recessive ones, and associated with malformations or other physical features. They are **pleiotropic** in that multiple, even seemingly unrelated clinical manifestations derive from the same mutation; and **variable** in that expression of the same mutation among people will differ.

Penetrance is a concept often associated with mendelian conditions—especially dominant ones—and the term is often misused. It should be defined as an expression of the frequency of appearance of a phenotype (dominant or recessive) when one or more mutant alleles are present. For individuals, penetrance is an all-or-none phenomenon—the phenotype is either present (penetrant) or not (nonpenetrant). The term **variability**—not "incomplete penetrance"—should be used to denote differences in expression of an allele.

The most frequent cause of apparent nonpenetrance is insensitivity of the methods for detecting the phenotype. If an apparently normal parent of a child with a dominant condition were in fact heterozygous for the mutation, the parent would have a 50% chance at each subsequent conception of having another affected child. A common cause of nonpenetrance in adult-onset mendelian diseases is death of the affected person before the phenotype becomes evident but after transmission of the mutant allele to offspring. Thus, accurate genetic counseling demands careful attention to the family medical history and high-resolution scrutiny of both parents of a child with a condition known to be a mendelian dominant trait.

When both alleles are expressed in the heterozygote, as in blood group AB, in sickle trait (HbS/HbA), in the major histocompatibility antigens (eg, A2B5/A3B17), or in sickle-C disease (HbS/HbC), the phenotype is called **codominant.**

In human dominant phenotypes, the homozygous state for the mutant allele is almost always more severe than in heterozygotes.

Autosomal Recessive Inheritance

The characteristics of autosomal recessive inheritance in humans can be summarized as follows:

(1) There is a horizontal pattern in the pedigree, with a single generation affected (Figure 40–4).

(2) Males and females are affected with equal frequency and severity.

(3) Inheritance is from both parents, each a heterozygote (carrier) and each usually clinically unaffected.

(4) Each offspring of two carriers has a 25% chance of being affected, a 50% chance of being a carrier, and a 25% chance of inheriting neither mutant allele. Thus, two-thirds of all clinically unaffected offspring are carriers.

(5) In matings between individuals, each with the same recessive phenotype, all offspring will be affected.

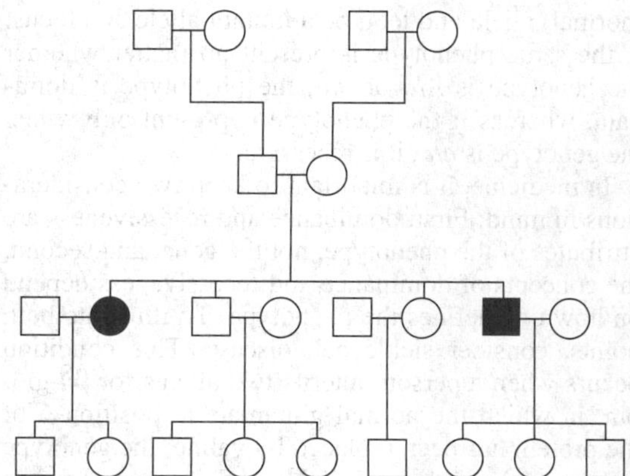

Figure 40–4. A pedigree illustrating autosomal recessive inheritance. (Symbols as in Figure 40–3.)

(6) Affected individuals who mate with unaffected individuals who are not carriers have only unaffected offspring.

(7) The rarer the recessive phenotype, the more likely it is that the parents are **consanguineous** (related).

Autosomal recessive phenotypes are often associated with deficient activity of enzymes and are thus termed **inborn errors of metabolism.** Such disorders include phenylketonuria, Tay-Sachs disease, and the various glycogen storage diseases and tend to be more severe, less variable, and less age-dependent than dominant conditions.

When an autosomal recessive condition is quite rare, the chance that the parents of affected offspring are consanguineous is increased. As a result, the prevalence of rare recessive conditions is high among inbred groups such as the Old Order Amish. On the other hand, when the autosomal recessive condition is common, the chance of consanguinity between parents of cases is no higher than in the general population (about 0.5%).

Two different *mutant* alleles at the same locus, as in HbS/HbC, form a **genetic compound.** The phenotype usually lies between those produced by either allele present in the homozygous state. Because of the large number of mutations possible in a given gene, many autosomal recessive phenotypes are probably due to genetic compounds. Sickle cell disease is an exception. Consanguinity is strong presumptive evidence for true homozygosity of mutant alleles and against a genetic compound.

X-Linked Inheritance

The general characteristics of X-linked inheritance in humans can be summarized as follows:

(1) There is no male-to-male transmission of the phenotype (Figure 40–5).

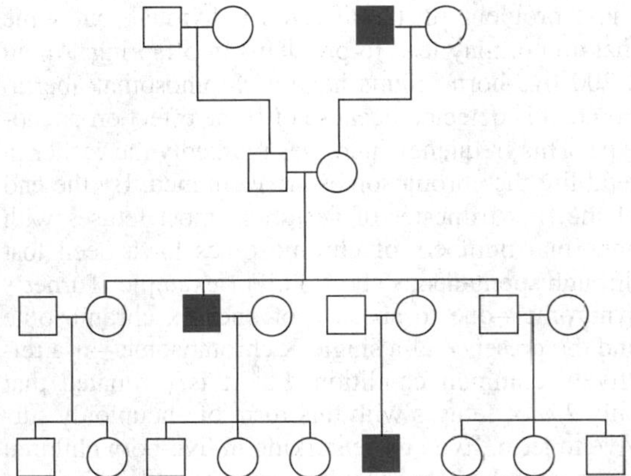

Figure 40–5. A pedigree illustrating X-linked inheritance. (Symbols as in Figure 40–3.)

(2) Unaffected males do not transmit the phenotype.

(3) All of the daughters of an affected male are heterozygous carriers.

(4) Males are usually more severely affected than females.

(5) Whether a heterozygous female is counted as affected—and whether the phenotype is called "recessive" or "dominant"—depends often on the sensitivity of the assay or of the examination.

(6) Some mothers of affected males will not themselves be heterozygotes (ie, they will be homozygous normal) but will have a germinal mutation. The proportion of heterozygous (carrier) mothers is negatively associated with the severity of the condition.

(7) Heterozygous women transmit the mutant gene to one-half of sons, who are affected, and to one-half of daughters, who are heterozygotes.

(8) If an affected male mates with a heterozygous female, half of the male offspring will be affected, giving the false impression of male-to-male transmission. One-half of the female offspring of such matings will be affected as severely as the average hemizygous male; in small pedigrees, this pattern may simulate autosomal dominant inheritance.

The characteristics of X-linked inheritance depend on phenotypic severity. For some disorders, affected males do not survive to reproduce. In such cases, about two-thirds of affected males have a carrier mother; in the remaining third, the disorder arises by new germinal mutation in an X chromosome of the mother. When the disorder is nearly always manifest in heterozygous females (X-linked dominant inheritance), females tend to be affected about twice as often as males; and on average an affected female transmits the phenotype to half of her sons and half of her daughters.

X-linked phenotypes are often clinically variable—particularly in heterozygous females—and suspected of being autosomal dominant with nonpenetrance. For example, Fabry's disease (α-galactosidase A deficiency) may be clinically silent in carrier women or may cause stroke, renal failure, or myocardial infarction by middle age.

Germinal mosaicism occurs in mothers of boys with X-linked conditions. The chance of such a mother having a second affected son or a heterozygous daughter depends on the fraction of her oocytes that carries the mutation. Currently, this fraction is impossible to determine. However, the presence of germinal mosaicism can be detected in some conditions (eg, Duchenne's muscular dystrophy) in a family by analysis of DNA, and this knowledge becomes crucial for genetic counseling.

Nearly 10,500 human genes have been identified through their phenotypes and inheritance patterns in families. This total represents 10–15% of all genes thought to be encoded by the 22 autosomes and 2 sex chromosomes. Victor McKusick coordinates an international effort to catalogue human mendelian variation.

Hall JG: Genomic imprinting: Nature and clinical relevance. Annu Rev Med 1997;48:35. [NLM Cit Id: 97198968 (A review of how clinicians can detect situations in which it makes a difference if a particular allele is passed—or is not passed—from one parent or the other to their offspring.)

McKusick VA: *Mendelian Inheritance in Man,* 12th ed. Johns Hopkins Univ Press, 1998. (A catalogue consisting, for each phenotype, of a six-digit identification number—used extensively in the medical literature—a summary statement, and a list of pertinent references. Editions are published periodically, but the catalogue is updated continuously and is computer-accessible as Online Mendelian Inheritance in Man [OMIM], accessible through the National Center for Biotechnology Information [http://www.ncbi.nlm.nih.gov/omim]. For information, contact OMIM User Support, FAX 410-955-4999.)

DISORDERS OF MULTIFACTORIAL CAUSATION

Many disorders cluster in families but are not associated with evident chromosomal aberrations or mendelian inheritance patterns. Examples include congenital malformations such as cleft lip, pyloric stenosis, and spina bifida; coronary artery disease; type 2 diabetes mellitus; and various forms of neoplasia. They are often characterized by varying frequencies in different racial or ethnic groups, disparity in sexual predilection, and greater frequency (but less than full concordance) in monozygotic than in dizygotic twins. This inheritance pattern is called "multifactorial" to signify that multiple genes interact with various environmental agents to produce the phenotype. The familial clustering is assumed to be due to sharing of both alleles and environment.

For most multifactorial conditions, there is little understanding of which particular genes are involved, how they and their products interact, and in what way different nongenetic factors contribute to the phenotype. For some disorders, biochemical and genetic studies have identified mendelian conditions within the coarse phenotype: Defects of the low-density lipoprotein receptor account for a small fraction of cases of ischemic heart disease (a larger fraction if only patients under age 50 are considered); familial polyposis of the colon predisposes to adenocarcinoma; and some patients with emphysema have inherited deficiency of α_1-proteinase inhibitor. Despite these notable examples, this reductionistic preoccupation with mendelian phenotypes is unlikely to explain the great majority of human disease; but even so, in the last analysis, much of human pathology will prove to be associated with genetic factors in cause, pathogenesis, or both.

Our ignorance about fundamental genetic mechanisms in development and physiology has not completely restricted practical approaches to the genetics of multifactorial disorders. For example, recurrence risks are based on empirical data derived from observation of many families. The risk of recurrence of multifactorial disorders is increased in several instances: (1) in close relatives (sibs, offspring, and parents) of an affected individual; (2) when two or more members of a family have the same condition; (3) when the first case in a family is in the less commonly affected sex (eg, pyloric stenosis is five times more common in boys; an affected woman has a three- to fourfold greater risk of having a child with pyloric stenosis); and (4) in ethnic groups in which there is a high incidence of a particular condition (eg, spina bifida is 40 times more common in Caucasians—and even more frequent among the Irish—than in Asians).

For many apparently multifactorial disorders, enough families have not been examined to have established empirical risk data. A useful approximation of recurrence risk in close relatives is the square root of the incidence. For example, many common congenital malformations have an incidence of 1:2500 to 1:400 live births; the calculated recurrence risks are thus in the 2–5% range—values that correspond closely to experience.

Childs B: *Genetic Medicine.* Johns Hopkins Univ Press, 1999. (An approachable book that lays out a life's perspective on the role of genetics in health and disease.)

CHROMOSOMAL ABERRATIONS

Any deviation from the structure and number of chromosomes as displayed in Figure 40–1 is, technically, a chromosomal aberration. Not all aberrations cause problems in the affected individual, but some that do not may lead to problems in offspring. About 1:200 live-born infants have a chromosomal aberration that is detected because of some effect on phenotype. This frequency increases markedly the earlier in fetal life the chromosomes are examined. By the end of the first trimester of gestation, most fetuses with abnormal numbers of chromosomes have been lost through spontaneous abortion. For example, Turner's syndrome—due to absence of one sex chromosome and the presence of a single X chromosome—is a relatively common condition, but it is estimated that only 2% of fetuses with this form of aneuploidy survive to term. Even more striking in live-born children is the complete absence of most autosomal trisomies and monosomies despite their frequent occurrence in young fetuses.

Types of Chromosomal Abnormalities

Major structural changes occur in either **balanced** or **unbalanced** form. In the latter, there is a gain or loss of genetic material; in the former, there is no change in the amount of genetic material but only a rearrangement of it. At the sites of breaks and new attachments of chromosome fragments, there may be permanent structural or functional damage to one gene or to only a few genes. Despite no visible loss of material, the aberration may nonetheless be recognized as unbalanced through an abnormal phenotype and the chromosomal defect confirmed by molecular analysis of the DNA.

Aneuploidy results from nondisjunction—the failure of a chromatid pair to separate in a dividing cell. Nondisjunction in either the first or second division of meiosis results in gametes with abnormal chromosomal constitutions. In aneuploidy, more or fewer than 46 chromosomes are present (Table 40–1). The following are all forms of aneuploidy: (1) **monosomy,** in which only one member of a pair of chromosomes is present; (2) **trisomy,** in which three

Table 40–1. Clinical phenotypes resulting from aneuploidy.

Condition	Karyotype	Incidence at Birth
Trisomy 13	47,XX or XY,+13	1:15,000
Trisomy 18	47,XX or XY,+18	1:11,000
Trisomy 21 (Down's syndrome)	47,XX or XY,+21	1:900
Klinefelter's syndrome	47,XXY	1:600 males
XYY	47,XYY	1:1000 males
Turner's syndrome	45,X	1:2500 females
XXX syndrome	47,XXX	1:1200 females

chromosomes are present instead of two; and (3) **polysomy,** in which one chromosome is represented four or more times.

If nondisjunction occurs in mitosis, **mosaic** patterns occur in somatic tissue, with some cells having one karyotype and other cells of the same organism another karyotype. Patients with a mosaic genetic constitution often have manifestations of each of the genetic syndromes associated with the various abnormal karyotypes.

Translocation results from an exchange of parts of two chromosomes.

Deletion is loss of chromosomal material.

Duplication is the presence of two or more copies of the same region of a given chromosome. The redundancy may occur in the same chromosome or in a nonhomologous chromosome. In the latter case, a translocation will also have occurred.

An **isochromosome** is one in which the arms on either side of the centromere have the same genetic material in the same order—ie, the chromosome has at some time divided in such a way that it has a double dose of one arm and absence of the other.

In an **inversion,** a chromosomal region becomes reoriented 180 degrees out of ordinary phase. The same genetic material is present, but in a different order.

Ferguson-Smith MA, Andrews T: Cytogenetic analysis. In: *Principles and Practice of Medical Genetics,* 3rd ed. Rimoin DL, Connor JM, Pyeritz RE (editors). Churchill Livingstone, 1997. (A review of the indications for and techniques of clinical cytogenetics.)

THE TECHNIQUES OF MEDICAL GENETICS

Hereditary disorders affect multiple organ systems and people of all ages. Many disorders are chronic ones, but often there are acute crises. The concerns of patients and families span a wide range of medical, psychologic, social, and economic issues. These characteristics emphasize the need for pediatricians, internists, obstetricians, and family practitioners to provide medical genetics services for their patients. This section reviews the laboratory and consultative services available from clinical geneticists and the indications for their use.

CYTOGENETICS

Cytogenetics is the study of chromosomes by light microscopy. The chromosomal constitution of a single cell or an entire individual is specified by a standardized notation. The total chromosome count is determined first, followed by the sex chromosome complement and then by any abnormalities. The autosomes are all designated by numbers from 1 to 22. A plus (–) or minus (–) sign indicates, respectively, a gain or loss of chromosomal material. For example, a normal male is 46,XY, while a girl with Down's syndrome caused by trisomy 21 is 47,XX,+21; a boy with Down's syndrome caused by translocation of chromosome 21 to chromosome 14 in a sperm or an egg is 46,XY,–14,+t(14;21).

Chromosomal analyses are done by growing human cells in tissue culture, chemically inhibiting mitosis, and then staining, observing, photographing, sorting, and counting the chromosomes. The display of all of the chromosomes is termed the **karyotype** (Figure 40–1) and is the end result of the technical aspect of cytogenetics.

Specimens for cytogenetic analysis can be obtained for routine analysis from the peripheral blood, in which case T lymphocytes are examined; from amniotic fluid for culture of amniocytes; from trophoblastic cells from the chorionic villus; from bone marrow; and from cultured fibroblasts, usually obtained from a skin biopsy. Enough cells must be examined so that the chance of missing a cytogenetically distinct cell line (a situation of mosaicism) is statistically low. For most clinical indications, 20 mitoses are examined and counted under direct microscopic visualization, and two are photographed and karyotypes prepared. Observation of aberrations usually prompts more extended scrutiny and in many cases further analysis of the original culture.

A variety of methods can be used to reveal banding patterns—unique to each pair of chromosomes—in the analysis of aberrations. The number of bands that can be visualized is a function of how "extended" the chromosomes are, which in turn depends chiefly on how early in metaphase (or even in prophase for the most extensive banding) mitosis was arrested. The "standard" karyotype reveals about 400 bands per haploid set of chromosomes, whereas a prophase karyotype might reveal four times that number. As invaluable as extended karyotypes are in certain clinical circumstances, their interpretation is often difficult—in terms of the time and effort required and of ambiguity about what is abnormal, what is a normal variation, and what is a technical artifact. In situ hybridization with DNA probes for specific chromosomes or regions of chromosomes can be labeled and used to identify subtle aberrations. Given proper technique, fluorescent in situ hybridization (FISH) yields sensitivities and specificities of virtually 100%. Some applications are being used routinely and marketed commercially, though the FDA has only recently begun to approve probes for clinical use.

risk. Some states have enacted legislation to protect people identified as having a heightened genetic risk of disease.

Logistics of DNA Diagnosis

Lymphocytes are a ready source of DNA; 10 mL of whole blood yields up to 0.5 mg of DNA, enough for dozens of analyses based on hybridization, each of which requires only 5 μg. If the analysis is quite narrowly focused on a specific mutation (such as in a family study, in which only one specific nucleotide change is addressed), PCR analysis can often be used and the amount of DNA needed is truly infinitesimal—a few hair bulbs or sperm are adequate. Once isolated, the DNA sample can be divided into aliquots and frozen. Alternatively, lymphocytes can be transformed with viruses into lymphoblasts; these cells are immortal, can be frozen, and—whenever DNA is required—can be thawed, propagated, and their DNA isolated. These stored specimens provide access to a person's genome long after the individual dies. This is such an important advantage that many clinical genetics centers and commercial laboratories "bank" DNA from patients and informative relatives even if the samples cannot be put to use immediately. The specimens may later prove invaluable to relatives or to other patients being evaluated. DNA in some instances has become more reliable than the medical record and even more readily retrievable!

Blood for DNA isolation should be drawn in EDTA anticoagulant (lavender-top tubes); blood for lymphoblast culture should be drawn in heparin (green-top tubes). Neither should be frozen. Specimens for DNA isolation can be stored or shipped at room temperature over a period of a few days. Lymphoblast cultures should be established within 48 hours, so prompt shipment is essential. For one or a few specific DNA analyses, some laboratories accept a cotton swab that has been placed between the cheek and gum for a minute (buccal swab); enough cells adhere to the fibers that DNA from the subject can be isolated.

Fetal DNA can be isolated from amniotic cells, from trophoblastic cells taken by chorionic villus sampling, or from either cell type grown in culture. Samples need to be processed promptly but can be shipped by overnight mail and *must not be frozen.*

American Society of Human Genetics: Professional disclosure of familial genetic information. Am J Hum Genet 1998;62:474. [NLM Cit ID: 98196478] (Guidelines for dealing with the unavoidable conflicts between confidentiality, opportunities to diagnose relatives, and the law.)

Geller G et al: Genetic testing for susceptibility to adult-onset cancer: The process and content of informed consent. JAMA 1997;277;1467. [NLM Cit ID: 97291106] (The impact of testing on patients and families, emphasizing educating patients.)

Gregg JP et al: Diagnostic molecular genetics: Current applications and future technologies. Pediatr Ann 1997; 26:553. [NLM Cit ID: 97448308] (A concise review of how the tests are performed and the data that result.)

Grody WW et al: Report card on molecular testing: Room for improvement? JAMA 1999;281:845. [NLM Cit ID: 99168556] (An editorial that addresses the quality and proficiency aspects of DNA diagnostics in the United States.)

Gupta GK et al: DNA diagnosis for the practicing obstetrician. Obstet Gynecol Clin North Am 1997;24:123. [NLM Cit ID: 97241123]

Maron BJ et al: Impact of laboratory molecular diagnosis on contemporary diagnostic criteria for genetically transmitted cardiovascular diseases: hypertrophic cardiomyopathy, long QT syndrome and Marfan syndrome. Circulation 1998;98:1460. [NLM Cit ID 99008266] (A consensus panel concludes that DNA diagnosis has limited applicability for these relatively common hereditary disorders of the cardiovascular system, mainly because the genes are so large and so many mutations cause the disorders.)

PRENATAL DIAGNOSIS

It is possible to diagnose in utero, before the middle of the second trimester, several hundred mendelian disorders, all chromosome aberrations, and a number of congenital malformations that are not mendelian. The first step toward prenatal diagnosis is taken when the expecting couple, the primary care provider, or the obstetrician thinks of the need for it. Recent surveys suggest that even for the most common indication for such service—advanced maternal age—less than half of all women 35 years and older in the United States are offered prenatal testing.

Techniques Used in Prenatal Diagnosis

Prenatal diagnosis depends on the ability to assay the fetus directly (fetal blood sampling, fetoscopy), indirectly (analysis of amniotic fluid, amniocytes or trophoblastic cells, ultrasound), or remotely (analysis of maternal serum). Some of these techniques satisfy the requirements for screening (Table 40–4) and should be offered to all pregnant women; others carry considerable risk and should be reserved for specific circumstances. A few centers are developing preimplantation diagnosis of the embryo; a single cell is plucked from the six- to eight-cell blastocyst, which has been cultured after in vitro fertilization, without harming future development. The chromosomes of the cell can be studied by FISH or the genes by PCR. Another new approach, with considerable potential, is isolation of fetal cells that are circulating in minute numbers in the maternal circulation.

Ultrasound scanning of the fetus is a safe, noninvasive procedure that can diagnose gross skeletal malformations as well as nonbony malformations known to be associated with specific diseases. Some obstetricians routinely perform fetal ultrasound at least once between 12 and 20 weeks of gestation.

Other prenatal diagnostic procedures—fetoscopy, fetography, and amniography—are more invasive and a definite risk to the mother and fetus. They are indicated only if the risk of the suspected abnormality is high and the information cannot be obtained by other means.

All of the cytogenetic, biochemical, and DNA analytic techniques discussed above can be applied to specimens from the fetus. Aside from screening for α-fetoprotein in maternal serum to detect neural tube defects, analysis of fetal chromosomes is the most frequently performed test. Chromosomal analysis can be performed on amniotic cells and on trophoblastic cells grown in culture and directly on any trophoblastic cells that happen to be undergoing mitosis. Amniotic fluid cells are derived chiefly from the fetal urinary system. Amniocentesis can be performed during gestational weeks 16–18 to permit unhurried sample analysis, transmission of results, and reproductive decisions. The time from obtaining the sample to a final reading of the karyotype has now been shortened to an average of 10–14 days, and automated methods may reduce the time a bit further. Sampling the chorionic villus (CVS) for trophoblastic cells (derived embryologically from the same fertilized egg as the fetus) is usually done during gestational weeks 11–13. If the tissue can be analyzed directly, cytogenetic results can be obtained within a few hours; however, the quality of the karyotypes is inferior to that from cultured cells, and most laboratories routinely culture cells and reexamine any suspected abnormalities. The advantage of CVS is that the results are available early in pregnancy, so that termination, if elected, can occur earlier in the pregnancy and the obstetric complications of termination are fewer.

The risk of CVS is somewhat higher than that of amniocentesis, though both are relatively safe. Between 0.5% and 1% of pregnancies are lost as a complication of CVS, whereas less than one in 300 amniocenteses result in fetal loss. Some centers offer "early amniocentesis," performed during gestational weeks 12–14; the magnitude of the risks is similar to that of CVS. These figures are lower than—but are in addition to—the 2–3% spontaneous abortion rate after the first trimester ends.

Indications for Prenatal Diagnosis

The indications for prenatal diagnosis are listed in Table 40–7. A few deserve comment.

Most studies done for advanced maternal age will detect no chromosomal aberration, and the couple will be reassured by this news. However, it is always appropriate to emphasize that the average risk of producing a child with a defect evident at birth, such as a physical malformation or some inborn error of metabolism, is about 3%, and that the risk increases with the age of either parent. Simply examining the chromosomes reduces this risk minimally. On the other hand, unless one of the other indications is present, it is simply not possible to "screen" a pregnancy for most birth defects (neural tube defects being an exception).

Table 40–7. Indications for prenatal diagnosis.

Indications	Methods
Advanced maternal age, previous child with chromosome aberration, intrauterine growth delay	Cytogenetics (amniocentesis, chorionic villus sampling)
Biochemical disorder	Protein assay, DNA diagnosis
Congenital anomaly	Ultrasound, fetoscopy
Screening for neural tube defects and trisomy	Maternal serum α-fetoprotein

Individuals contemplating pregnancy—especially those of Ashkenazic Jewish or other Caucasian ethnicity—should be offered screening for the most common mutations in the *CFTR* gene that cause cystic fibrosis. If both partners are detected as being carriers, prenatal diagnosis of a fetus would be an option for them.

A history for cytogenetic aberrations emphasizes a chromosomal defect in a parent, a family history of a chromosomal defect, or a previous child or conceptus with a defined or undefined chromosomal defect. The factors that render some couples susceptible to repeated episodes of aneuploidy are unclear, and routine prenatal testing is warranted once a defect has occurred.

Cytogenetic analysis of the fetus will of course give information about the sex chromosomes. Some couples do not desire advance knowledge of the sex of their child, and the person transmitting the results to the couple should always address this issue first. On the other hand, some couples *only* want to know the sex of the fetus and plan to terminate the pregnancy if the undesired sex is detected. Virtually no centers in the United States consider sex selection to be an appropriate indication for prenatal diagnosis.

The level of α-fetoprotein in maternal serum changes with gestational age, with the mother's medical status, and with abnormalities of the fetus. If the first two factors can be well controlled, the assay can be used to provide information about the fetus. Levels are expressed as multiples of the median value for a particular gestational age. Higher than normal levels are associated with open neural tube defects (the conditions for which the test was developed), recent or impending fetal demise, gastroschisis, and fetal renal disease. Extremely high levels are highly specific for fetal anomalies—a level three times the median increases 20-fold the risk of meningomyelocele or anencephaly. Low α-fetoprotein levels in maternal serum are associated with fetal trisomy, especially

notypic females have a heightened risk of developing ovarian cancer, primarily gonadoblastoma.

The indications for cytogenetic analysis of neoplasia continue to evolve. Not all tumors require study. However, in cases of tumors of unclear type (especially leukemias and lymphomas), with a strong family history of early neoplasia, or for certain tumors associated with potential generalized chromosomal defects (present in nonneoplastic cells), cytogenetic analysis should be strongly considered.

American Society of Clinical Oncology: Genetic testing for cancer susceptibility. J Clin Oncol 1996;14:1730. [NLM Cit ID: 96208855] (One professional society's guidelines on when to order DNA tests.)

Burke W et al: Recommendations for follow-up care of individuals with an inherited predisposition to cancer: I. Hereditary nonpolyposis colon cancer. JAMA 1997;277:915. [NLM Cit ID: 97216041] (Review of increased risks and implications for the patient.)

Dunlop MG et al: Cancer risk associated with germline DNA mismatch repair gene mutations. Hum Molec Genet 1997;6:105. [NLM Cit ID: 97156217] (Useful in families with a history of colon cancer.)

Fearon E, Cho KR: The molecular biology of cancer. In: *Principles and Practice of Medical Genetics,* 3rd ed. Rimoin DL, Connor JM, Pyeritz RE (editors): Churchill Livingstone, 1997.

Glassman AB: Cytogenetics: An evolving role in the diagnosis and treatment of cancer. Clin Lab Med 1997;17:21. [NLM Cit ID: 97227198] (When to order chromosome studies in patients with cancer.)

Lindor NM et al: The concise handbook of family cancer syndromes. J Natl Cancer Inst 1998;90:1040. [NLM Cit ID: 98335998] (Short descriptions of the 35 syndromes involving one or more benign or malignant tumors.)

Mitelman F et al: A breakpoint map of recurrent chromosomal rearrangements in human neoplasia. Nat Genet 1997;15:417. [NLM Cit ID: 97285136] (A compilation of cytogenetic changes in all types of cancer.)

Offit K: *Clinical Cancer Genetics: Risk Counseling and Management.* Wiley, 1998. (Current state of knowledge and how to apply it in everyday clinical situations.)

Struewing JP et al: The risk of cancer associated with specific mutations of *BRCA1* and *BRCA2* among Ashkenazi Jews. N Engl J Med 1997;336:1401. [NLM Cit ID: 97274028] (A study, unbiased by ascertainment, that reduced the lifetime risk in one ethnic group of carrying a mutation in a gene predisposing to cancer.)

SELECTED GENETIC DISORDERS

ACUTE INTERMITTENT PORPHYRIA

Essentials of Diagnosis

- Unexplained abdominal crisis, generally in young women.
- Acute peripheral or central nervous system dysfunction.
- Recurrent psychiatric illnesses.
- Hyponatremia.
- Porphobilinogen in the urine during an attack.

General Considerations

Though there are several different types of porphyrias, the one with the most serious consequences and the one that usually presents in adulthood is acute intermittent porphyria, which is inherited as an autosomal dominant, though it remains clinically silent in the majority of patients who carry the trait. Those who develop clinical illness are usually women, with symptoms beginning in the teens or 20s, but in rare cases onset can begin after menopause. The disorder is caused by deficiency of porphobilinogen deaminase activity, leading to increased excretion of aminolevulinic acid and porphobilinogen in the urine. The diagnosis may be elusive if not specifically considered. The characteristic abdominal pain may be due to abnormalities in autonomic innervation in the gut. In contrast to other forms of porphyria, cutaneous photosensitivity is absent in acute intermittent porphyria. Attacks are precipitated by numerous factors, including drugs and intercurrent infections. Harmful and relatively safe drugs for use in treatment are listed in Table 40–10. Hyponatremia may be seen, due in part to inappropriate release of antidiuretic hormone, though gastrointestinal loss of sodium in some patients may contribute.

Clinical Findings

A. Symptoms and Signs: Patients show intermittent abdominal pain of varying severity, and in some instances it may so simulate acute abdomen as to lead to exploratory laparotomy. Since the origin of the abdominal pain is neurologic, there is absence of fever and leukocytosis. Complete recovery between attacks is usual. Any part of the nervous system may be involved, with evidence for autonomic and peripheral neuropathy. Peripheral neuropathy may be symmetric or asymmetric and mild or profound; in the latter instance, it can even lead to quadriplegia with respiratory paralysis. Other central nervous system manifestations include seizures, psychosis, and abnormalities of the basal ganglia. Hyponatremia may further cause or exacerbate central nervous system manifestations.

B. Laboratory Findings: Often there is profound hyponatremia. The diagnosis can be confirmed by demonstrating an increased amount of porphobilinogen in the urine during an acute attack. Freshly voided urine is of normal color but may turn dark upon standing in light and air.

Most families have a different mutation in the porphobilinogen deaminase gene causing acute intermittent porphyria. With some effort in research laborato-

Table 40–10. Some of the "unsafe" and "probably safe" drugs used in the treatment of acute porphyrias.

Unsafe	Probably Safe
Alcohol	Acetaminophen
Alkylating agents	β-Adrenergic blockers
Barbiturates	Amitriptyline
Carbamazepine	Aspirin
Chlorpropamide	Atropine
Chloroquine	Chloral hydrate
Clonidine	Chlordiazepoxide
Dapsone	Diazepam
Ergots	Digoxin
Erythromycin	Diphenhydramine
Estrogens, synthetic	Guanethidine
Food additives	Glucocorticoids
Glutethimide	Hyoscine
Griseofulvin	Ibuprofen
Hydralazine	Imipramine
Ketamine	Insulin
Meprobamate	Lithium
Methyldopa	Naproxen
Metoclopramide	Nitrofurantoin
Nortriptyline	Opioid analgesics
Pentazocine	Penicillamine
Phenytoin	Penicillin and derivatives
Progestins	Phenothiazines
Pyrazinamide	Procaine
Rifampin	Streptomycin
Spironolactone	Succinylcholine
Succinimides	Tetracycline
Sulfonamides	Thiouracil
Theophylline	
Tolazamide	
Tolbutamide	
Valproic acid	

ries, mutations can be discovered and used for presymptomatic and prenatal diagnosis.

Prevention

Avoidance of factors known to precipitate attacks of acute intermittent porphyria—especially drugs (sulfonamides and barbiturates, or drugs listed in Table 40–10)—can reduce morbidity. Starvation diets also cause attacks and so must be avoided.

Treatment

Treatment with a high-carbohydrate diet diminishes the number of attacks in some patients and is a reasonable empirical gesture considering its benignity. Acute attacks may be life-threatening and require prompt diagnosis, withdrawal of the inciting agent (if possible), and treatment with analgesics and intravenous glucose and hematin. A minimum of 300 g of carbohydrate per day should be provided orally or intravenously. Electrolyte balance requires close attention. Hematin therapy is still evolving and should be undertaken with full recognition of adverse consequences, especially phlebitis and coagulopathy. The intravenous dosage is up to 4 mg/kg once or twice daily.

Grandchamp B: Acute intermittent porphyria. Semin Liver Dis 1998;18:17. [NLM Cit ID: 98177317] (A succinct review of the clinical and biochemical features and guidelines for DNA diagnosis.)

Jeans JB et al: Mortality in patients with acute intermittent porphyria requiring hospitalization: A United States case series. Am J Med Genet 1996;65:269. [NLM Cit ID: 97082697] (Threefold increased risk of mortality in patients recognized to have the disorder.)

McGovern MM et al: Inherited porphyrias. In: *Principles and Practice of Medical Genetics,* 3rd ed. Rimoin DL, Conner JM, Pyeritz RE (editors). Churchill Livingstone, 1997. (Diagnosis and management are stressed.)

ALKAPTONURIA

Alkaptonuria is caused by a recessively inherited deficiency of the enzyme homogentisic acid oxidase. This acid derives from metabolism of both phenylalanine and tyrosine and is present in large amounts in the urine throughout the patient's life. An oxidation product accumulates slowly in cartilage throughout the body, leading to degenerative joint disease of the spine and peripheral joints. Indeed, examination of patients in the third and fourth decades shows a slight darkish blue color below the skin in areas overlying cartilage, such as in the ears, a phenomenon called "ochronosis." In some patients, a more severe hyperpigmentation can be seen in the sclera, conjunctiva, and cornea. Accumulation of metabolites in heart valves can lead to aortic or mitral stenosis. A predisposition to coronary artery disease may also be present. While the syndrome causes considerable morbidity, life expectancy is reduced only modestly. Symptoms are more often attributable to spondylitis with back pain, leading to a clinical picture difficult to distinguish from that of ankylosing spondylitis, though on radiographic assessment the sacroiliac joints are not fused in alkaptonuria.

The diagnosis is established by demonstrating homogentisic acid in the urine, which turns black spontaneously on exposure to the air; this reaction is particularly noteworthy if the urine is alkaline or when alkali is added to a specimen. Molecular analysis of the homogentisic acid oxidase gene, recently mapped to chromosome 3, is not necessary for diagnosis. Treatment of the arthritis is similar to that for other arthropathies. Though in theory rigid dietary restriction might reduce accumulation of the pigment, this has not proved to be of practical benefit.

La Du BN: Alcaptonuria. In: *The Metabolic Bases of Inherited Disease,* 7th ed. Scriver CR et al (editors). McGraw-Hill, 1995. (Clinical and biochemical aspects of one of Garrod's original inborn errors of metabolism.)

Scriver CR: Alkaptonuria: Such a long journey. Nat Genet 1996:14:5. [NLM Cit ID: 96376959] (An instructive editorial about the history of the disorder and the importance of mapping the causative gene.)

DOWN'S SYNDROME

Down's syndrome is usually diagnosed at birth on the basis of the typical facial features, hypotonia, and single palmar crease. Several serious problems that may be evident at birth or may develop early in childhood include duodenal atresia, congenital heart disease (especially atrioventricular canal defects), and leukemia. The intestinal and cardiac anomalies usually respond to surgery, and the leukemia generally responds to conservative management. Intelligence varies across a wide spectrum. Many people with Down's syndrome do well in sheltered workshops and group homes, but few achieve full independence in adulthood. An Alzheimer-like dementia usually becomes evident in the fourth or fifth decade and, for those who survive childhood, accounts for a reduced life expectancy. Studies addressing the risk and severity of dementia in relation to the apolipoprotein E genotype have had conflicting results. Cytogenetic analysis should always be performed—even though most patients will have simple trisomy for chromosome 21—to detect unbalanced translocations; such patients may have a parent with a balanced translocation, and there will be a substantial recurrence risk of Down's syndrome in future offspring.

Many pregnancies carrying a fetus with Down's syndrome can be detected in the early second trimester through screening maternal serum for α-fetoprotein and certain hormones ("triple screen") and by detecting increased nuchal thickness on fetal ultrasound.

The risk of bearing a child with Down's syndrome increases exponentially with the age of the mother at conception and begins a marked rise after age 35. By age 45 years, a mother has one chance in 40 of having an affected child. The risk of other conditions associated with trisomy also increases, because of the increased predisposition of older oocytes to nondisjunction during meiosis. There is virtually no risk of trisomy associated with increased paternal age. However, older men do have an increased risk of fathering a child with a new autosomal dominant condition. But because there are so many distinct conditions, the chance of fathering an offspring with any given one is extremely small.

Barsh G: Genetic disease. In: *Pathophysiology of Disease: An Introduction to Clinical Medicine,* 3rd ed. McPhee SJ et al (editors): McGraw-Hill, 2000. (Discusses pathogenesis of Down's syndrome.)

Tolmie JL: Down syndrome and other autosomal trisomies. In *Principles and Practice of Medical Genetics,* 3rd ed. Rimoin DL, Conner JM, Pyeritz RE (editors). Churchill Livingstone, 1997.

Wyllie JP et al: Strategies for antenatal detection of Down's syndrome. Arch Dis Child 1997;76:F26. [NLM Cit ID: 97212326] (The limits of prenatal screening given current technology.)

FRAGILE X MENTAL RETARDATION

This X-linked condition accounts for more cases of mental retardation in males than any condition except Down's syndrome; about one in 2000 males is affected. The first marker for this condition was a small gap, or fragile site, evident near the tip of the long arm of the X chromosome. Subsequently, the condition was found to be due to expansion of a trinucleotide repeat (CGG) near a gene called *FMR1.* All individuals have some CGG repeats in this location, but as the number increases beyond 52, the chances of further expansion during spermatogenesis or oogenesis increase. Being born with one *FMR1* allele with 200 or more repeats results in mental retardation in virtually all men and about 60% of women. The more repeats, the greater the likelihood that further expansion will occur during gametogenesis; this results in **anticipation,** in which the disorder can worsen from one generation to the next.

Affected (heterozygous) women show no physical signs other than early menopause, but they may have learning difficulties or frank retardation. Affected males show macroorchidism (enlarged testes) after puberty, large ears and a prominent jaw, a high-pitched voice, and mental retardation. Some show evidence of a mild connective tissue defect, with joint hypermobility and mitral valve prolapse.

DNA diagnosis for the number of repeats has supplanted cytogenetic analysis for both clinical and prenatal diagnosis. This should be done on any male or female who has unexplained mental retardation.

Barsh G: Genetic disease. In: *Pathophysiology of Disease: An Introduction to Clinical Medicine,* 3rd ed. McPhee SJ et al (editors): McGraw-Hill, 2000. (Discusses pathogenesis of fragile X mental retardation.)

Holden JJ et al: Eighth International Workshop on the fragile X syndrome and X-linked mental retardation, August 16–22, 1997. Am J Med Genet 1999;83:221. [NLM Cit ID: 99222835] (A review of the considerable advances reported in diagnosis, pathogenesis, and management at the most recent meeting of the experts.)

Sutherland GR, Mulley JC: Fragile X syndrome and other causes of X-linked mental handicap. In: *Principles and Practice of Medical Genetics,* 3rd ed. Rimoin DL, Conner JM, Pyeritz RE (editors). Churchill Livingstone, 1997.

GAUCHER'S DISEASE

Gaucher's disease is inherited as an autosomal recessive. A deficiency of β-glucocerebrosidase causes an accumulation of sphingolipid within phagocytic cells throughout the body. Anemia and thrombocytopenia are common and may be symptomatic; both are due primarily to hypersplenism, but marrow infiltration with Gaucher cells may contribute. Cortical erosions of bones, especially the vertebrae and femur, are due to local infarctions, but the mechanism is unclear. Episodes of bone pain (termed "crises") are reminiscent of those in sickle cell disease. A hip fracture in a patient with a palpable spleen—especially in a Jewish person of Eastern European origin—suggests the possibility of Gaucher's disease. Bone marrow aspirates reveal typical Gaucher cells, which have an eccentric nucleus and PAS-positive inclusions, along with wrinkled cytoplasm and inclusion bodies of a fibrillar type. In addition, the serum acid phosphatase is elevated. Definitive diagnosis requires the demonstration of deficient glucocerebrosidase activity in leukocytes.

Until recently, treatment has been supportive and has included splenectomy for thrombocytopenia secondary to platelet sequestration. The purification of sufficient quantities of alglucerase (glucocerebrosidase-β-glucosidase) to permit intravenous administration on a regular basis now permits a reduction in total body stores of glycolipid and improvement in orthopedic and hematologic manifestations. The major drawback is the exceptional cost of alglucerase, which can exceed $350,000 per year, though recent studies suggest that more frequent administration of less enzyme (30 units/kg per month) is just as effective and reduces the cost to about $100,000 annually for an adult.

Beutler E: Gaucher disease. Curr Opin Hematol 1997;4:19. [NLM Cit ID: 97196354] (Concise overview.)

Beutler E, Grabowski GA: Gaucher disease. In: *The Metabolic and Molecular Bases of Inherited Disease,* 7th ed. Scriver CR et al (editors). McGraw-Hill, 1995. (A comprehensive review.)

Charrow J et al: Gaucher disease: Recommendations on diagnosis, evaluation, and monitoring. Arch Intern Med 1998;158:1754. [NLM Cit ID 98408984] (Recommendations, developed by consensus, on the major issues involved in managing a person with this highly variable disorder.)

HOMOCYSTINURIA

Homocystinuria in its classic form is caused by cystathionine β-synthase deficiency and exhibits an autosomal recessive pattern of inheritance. This results in extreme elevations of plasma and urinary homocystine levels, a basis for diagnosis of this disorder. Homocystinuria is similar in certain superficial aspects to Marfan's syndrome, since patients may show a similar body habitus and ectopia lentis is almost always present. However, mental retardation is often present, and the cardiovascular events are those of repeated venous and arterial thromboses whose precise cause remains obscure. Life expectancy is reduced, especially in untreated and pyridoxine-unresponsive patients; myocardial infarction, stroke, and pulmonary embolism are the most common causes of death. This condition is diagnosed in some states by newborn screening for hypermethioninemia; however, pyridoxine-responsive infants may not be detected. The diagnosis should be suspected in patients in the second and third decades of life who show evidence of arterial or venous thromboses and have no other risk factors. Although many mutations have been identified in the cystathionine β-synthase gene, amino acid analysis of plasma remains the most appropriate diagnostic test. Patients should be studied after they have been off folate or pyridoxine supplementation for at least 1 week. The plasma should be separated promptly from the fresh venous blood specimen.

About one-half of patients have a form of cystathionine β-synthase deficiency that improves biochemically and clinically through pharmacologic doses of pyridoxine and folate. For these patients, treatment from infancy can prevent retardation and the other clinical problems. Patients who are pyridoxine-nonresponders must be treated with dietary reduction in methionine and supplementation of cysteine, also from infancy. The vitamin betaine is also useful in reducing plasma methionine levels by facilitating a metabolic pathway that bypasses the defective enzyme. Patients who have suffered venous thrombosis should be anticoagulated, but there are no studies to support prophylactic use of warfarin or antiplatelet agents.

Mudd H, Levy HL, Skovby F: Disorders of transsulfuration. In: *The Metabolic and Molecular Bases of Inherited Disease,* 7th ed. Scriver CR et al (editors). McGraw-Hill, 1995. (A comprehensive review of the genetics and clinical features of all of the disorders associated with elevated homocysteine, including the risk of vascular disease in heterozygotes.)

Pyeritz RE: Homocystinuria. In: *McKusick's Heritable Disorders of Connective Tissue,* 5th ed. Mosby, 1993. (Clinical, genetic, and biochemical aspects of an inborn error of metabolism with extensive effects on the extracellular matrix.)

HOMOCYSTEINE & ARTERIAL OCCLUSIVE DISEASE

Over the past 5 years, considerable evidence has accumulated to support the 20-year-old observation that patients with clinical and angiographic evidence of coronary artery disease tend to have higher levels of plasma homocysteine than controls without coronary artery disease. The relationship has been extended to cerebrovascular and peripheral vascular diseases. Although this effect was initially thought to be due at least in part to heterozygotes for cystathionine β-synthase deficiency (see above), in fact there is little evidence for this. Rather, the major factor leading to hyperhomocysteinemia is folate deficiency. Pyridoxine (vitamin B_6) and vitamin B_{12} are also important in the metabolism of methionine, and deficiency of any of these vitamins can lead to accumulation of homocysteine. A number of genes influence utilization of these vitamins and can predispose to deficiency. For example, having one—and especially two—copies of an allele that causes thermolability of methylene tetrahydrofolate reductase predisposes to elevated fasting homocysteine levels. However, both nutritional and most genetic deficiencies of these vitamins can be corrected by dietary supplementation of folic acid and, if serum levels are low, vitamins B_6 and B_{12}. In the United States, cereal grains are now fortified with folic acid. Studies are ongoing to determine the long-term utility of routine vitamin supplementation in people at risk for arterial occlusive disease, but many workers in this field recommend, at a minimum, taking 1 mg of folic acid per day. Because patients with end-stage renal disease tend to have marked hyperhomocysteinemia and low serum folate, 5 mg of folic acid per day seems warranted.

Relatively few laboratories currently provide highly reliable assays for homocysteine. Processing of the specimen is crucial to obtain accurate results. The plasma must be separated within 30 minutes; otherwise, blood cells release the amino acid and the measurement will then be artificially elevated.

Graham IM et al: Plasma homocysteine as a risk factor for vascular disease. JAMA 1997;277:1775. [NLM Cit ID: 97322136] (A multinational study that confirmed homocysteine as an independent risk factor for vascular disease and a potentiator of the effects of smoking and hypertension.)

Nygard O et al: Plasma homocysteine levels and mortality in patients with coronary artery disease. N Engl J Med 1997;337:230. [NLM Cit ID: 97357244] (The higher the homocysteine level, the greater the risk of dying of coronary artery disease.)

Rimm EB et al: Folate and vitamin B_6 from diet and supplements in relation to risk of coronary heart disease among women. JAMA 1998;279:359. [NLM Cit ID: 98119556] (Healthy women had lower homocysteine levels and less risk of coronary artery disease if they consumed more than 400 μg of folate and 3 mg of vitamin B_6 per day.)

Stein JH et al: Hyperhomocysteinemia and atherosclerotic vascular disease. Arch Intern Med 1998;158:1301. [NLM Cit ID 98307755] (A brief review of the causes of elevated homocysteine.)

KLINEFELTER'S SYNDROME

Boys with an extra X chromosome are normal in appearance before puberty; thereafter, they have disproportionately long legs and arms, a female escutcheon, gynecomastia, and small testes. Infertility is due to azoospermia; the seminiferous tubules are hyalinized. The diagnosis is often not made until a couple is evaluated for inability to conceive. Mental retardation is somewhat more common than in the general population. Many men with Klinefelter's syndrome have learning problems. The risk of breast cancer is much higher in men with Klinefelter's syndrome than in 46,XY men, as is the risk of diabetes mellitus.

Treatment with testosterone after puberty is advisable but will not restore fertility. However, men with Klinefelter's syndrome have had mature sperm aspirated from their testes and injected into oocytes, resulting in fertilization. After the blastocysts were implanted into the uterus of a partner, "natural" children resulted.

Palermo GD et al: Births after intracytoplasmic injection of sperm obtained by testicular extraction from men with nonmosaic Klinefelter's syndrome. N Engl J Med 1998;338:588. [NLM Cit ID 98129152] (A reproductive option for men previously termed "infertile.")

Robinson A, de la Chapelle A: Sex chromosome abnormalities. In: *Principles and Practice of Medical Genetics,* 3rd ed. Rimoin DL, Connor JM, Pyeritz RE (editors). Churchill Livingstone, 1997.

Smyth CM et al: Klinefelter syndrome. Arch Intern Med 1998;158:1309. [NLM Cit ID 98307756] (A concise review of the diagnosis and associated clinical abnormalities of this chromosomal disorder.)

MARFAN'S SYNDROME

Essentials of Diagnosis

- Disproportionately tall stature, thoracic deformity, and joint laxity or contractures.
- Ectopia lentis and myopia.
- Aortic dilation and dissection.
- Mitral valve prolapse.

General Considerations

Marfan's syndrome, a systemic connective tissue disease, is inherited as an autosomal dominant. It is characterized by abnormalities of the skeletal system, ocular system, and cardiovascular system. Spontaneous pneumothorax, dural ectasia, and striae atrophicae can also occur. Of most concern is disease of the ascending aorta, which is associated with a dilated aortic root. Histology of the aorta shows diffuse medial abnormalities. Aortic and mitral valve leaflets are also abnormal and mitral regurgitation may be present as well, often with elongated chordae tendineae, which on occasion may rupture.

Clinical Findings

A. Symptoms and Signs: Affected patients are typically tall, with particularly long arms, legs, and digits (arachnodactyly). However, there can be wide variability in the clinical presentation. Commonly, joint dislocations and pectus excavatum are found. Ectopia lentis may lead to severe myopia and retinal detachment. Mitral valve prolapse is seen in about 85% percent of patients. Aortic root dilation with aortic regurgitation or dissection with rupture can occur. To diagnose Marfan's syndrome, people with an affected relative need features in at least two systems. People with no family history need features in the skeletal system, two other systems, and one of the major criteria of ectopia lentis, dilation of the aortic root, or aortic dissection. Patients with homocystinuria due to cystathionine synthase deficiency also have dislocated lenses; tall, disproportionate stature; and thoracic deformity. They tend to have below normal intelligence, stiff joints, and a predisposition to arterial and venous occlusive disease. Males with Klinefelter's syndrome do not show the typical ocular or cardiovascular features of Marfan's syndrome and are generally sporadic occurrences in the family.

B. Laboratory Findings: Mutations in the fibrillin gene on chromosome 15 cause Marfan's syndrome. Nonetheless, no simple laboratory test is available to support the diagnosis in questionable cases because related conditions may also be due to defects in fibrillin.

Prevention

There is prenatal and presymptomatic diagnosis for patients in whom the molecular defect in fibrillin has been found and for large enough families in whom linkage analysis using polymorphic markers around the fibrillin gene can be performed.

Treatment

Children with Marfan's syndrome require regular ophthalmologic surveillance to correct visual acuity and thus prevent amblyopia, and annual orthopedic consultation for diagnosis of scoliosis at an early enough stage so that bracing might delay progression. Patients of all ages require echocardiography at least annually to monitor aortic diameter and mitral valve function. All patients should use standard endocarditis prophylaxis. Chronic β-adrenergic blockade, titrated to individual tolerance but enough to produce a negative inotropic effect (atenolol, 1–2 mg/kg), retards the rate of aortic dilation. Restriction from vigorous physical exertion protects from aortic dissection. Prophylactic replacement of the aortic root with a composite graft when the diameter reaches 50–55 mm (normal: < 40 mm) prolongs life. A procedure to spare the patient's aortic valve and replace just the aneurysmal sinuses of Valsalva is showing promise and would also avoid the need for life-long anticoagulation.

Prognosis

People with Marfan's syndrome who are untreated commonly die in the fourth or fifth decade from aortic dissection or congestive heart failure secondary to aortic regurgitation.

Deitz HC et al: Mutations in the human gene for fibrillin-1 *(FBN1)* in the Marfan syndrome and related disorders. Hum Mol Genet 1995;4:1799. [NLM Cit ID: 96121575] (A review of the molecular biology of microfibrils and an important group of connective tissue disorders.)

DePaepe A et al: Revised diagnostic criteria for the Marfan syndrome. Am J Med Genet 1996;62:417. [NLM Cit ID: 96298350] (A matrix for assigning the diagnosis based on clinical findings, family history, and molecular biology.)

Gott VL et al: Replacement of the aortic root in patients with Marfan's syndrome. N Engl J Med 1999;340:1307. [NLM Cit ID: 99219764] (The largest published series, demonstrating excellent long-term results from prophylactic surgery.)

Pyeritz RE: The Marfan syndrome. Ann Rev Med 2000;51:481. [NLM Cit ID: 20236293] (A comprehensive survey of Marfan's syndrome and related conditions.)

Rossiter JP et al: A prospective longitudinal evaluation of pregnancy in the Marfan syndrome. Am J Obstet Gynecol 1995;173:1599. [NLM Cit ID: 96081799] (Pregnancy is not that dangerous for the Marfan woman with an aortic diameter less than 40 mm.)

Shores J et al: Progression of aortic dilatation and the benefit of long-term beta-adrenergic blockade in Marfan's syndrome. N Engl J Med 1994;330:1335. [NLM Cit ID: 94203239]

RELEVANT WORLD WIDE WEB SITES

[National Marfan Foundation]
http://www.marfan.org

[GeneSage: Genetic resource site for professionals]
http://www.genesage.com

[Alliance of Genetic Support Groups]
http://www.genticalliance.org

[Blazing a Genetic Trail]
http://www.hhmi.org/GeneticTrail

[CDC Genetics Mailing List]
genetics@listserv.cdc.gov

[Genetic Conditions/Rare Conditions Support Group and Information]
http://www.kumc.edu/gec/support/

[GeneClinics: Medical Genetics Knowledge Base]
http://www.geneclinics.org/

[Helix]
http://www.genetests.org

[List of Biochemical Genetics Tests by Diseases]
http://biochemgen.ucsd.edu/wbgtests/dz-tst.htm

[March of Dimes Genetics Site]
http://www.modimes.org/HealthLibrary2/portal.htm

[Understanding Gene Testing]
http://www.accessexcellence.org/AE/AEPC/NIH/index.html

[US Department of Energy—Human Genome Information]
http://www.ornl.gov/TechResources/Human_Genome/publicat/publications.html

[Alzheimer's Disease—GeneClinics]
http://www.geneclinics.org/profiles/alzheimer

[Down's Syndrome]
http://www.nas.com/downsyn/index.html

[Gaucher's Disease Case Study]
http://path.upmc.edu:80/cases/case39.html

[Huntington's Disease—GeneClinics]
http://www.geneclinics.org/profiles/huntington

Table 41–1. Criteria for use of screening procedures.

Characteristics of population
1. Sufficiently high prevalence of disease.
2. Likely to be compliant with subsequent tests and treatments.

Characteristics of disease
1. Significant morbidity and mortality.
2. Effective and acceptable treatment available.
3. Presymptomatic period detectable.
4. Improved outcome from early treatment.

Characteristics of test
1. Good sensitivity and specificity.
2. Low cost and risk.
3. Confirmatory test available and practical.

properly conducted laboratory test is an appropriate specimen.

Patient Preparation

Preparation of the patient is important for certain tests—eg, a fasting state is needed for optimal glucose and triglyceride measurements; posture and sodium intake must be strictly controlled when measuring renin and aldosterone levels; and strenuous exercise should be avoided before taking samples for creatine kinase determinations, since vigorous muscle activity can lead to falsely abnormal results.

Specimen Collection

Careful attention must be paid to patient identification and specimen labeling. Knowing when the specimen was collected may be important. For instance, aminoglycoside levels cannot be interpreted appropriately without knowing whether the specimen was drawn just before ("trough" level) or after ("peak" level) drug administration. Drug levels cannot be interpreted if they are drawn during the drug's distribution phase (eg, digoxin levels drawn during the first 6 hours after an oral dose). Substances that have a circadian variation (eg, cortisol) can be interpreted only in the context of the time of day the sample was drawn.

During specimen collection, other principles should be remembered. Specimens should not be drawn above an intravenous line, as this may contaminate the sample with intravenous fluid. Excessive tourniquet time will lead to hemoconcentration and an increased concentration of protein-bound substances such as calcium. Lysis of cells during collection of a blood specimen will result in spuriously increased serum levels of substances concentrated in cells (eg, lactate dehydrogenase and potassium). Certain test specimens may require special handling or storage (eg, blood gas specimens). Delay in delivery of specimens to the laboratory can result in ongoing cellular metabolism and therefore spurious results for some studies (eg, low blood glucose).

TEST CHARACTERISTICS

Table 41–2 lists the general characteristics of useful diagnostic tests. Most of the principles detailed below can be applied not only to laboratory and radiologic tests but also to elements of the history and physical examination.

Accuracy

The accuracy of a laboratory test is its correspondence with the true value. An inaccurate test is one that differs from the true value even though the results may be reproducible (Figures 41–1A and 1B). In the clinical laboratory, accuracy of tests is maximized by calibrating laboratory equipment with reference material and by participation in external quality control programs.

Precision

Test precision is a measure of a test's reproducibility when repeated on the same sample. An imprecise test is one that yields widely varying results on repeated measurements (Figure 41–1B). The precision of diagnostic tests, which is monitored in clinical laboratories by using control material, must be good enough to distinguish clinically relevant changes in a patient's status from the analytic variability of the test. For instance, the manual white blood cell differential count is not precise enough to detect important changes in the distribution of cell types, because it is calculated by subjective evaluation of a small sample (100 cells). Repeated measurements by different technicians on the same sample result in widely different results. Automated differential counts are more precise because they are obtained from machines that use objective physical characteristics to classify a much larger sample (10,000 cells).

Table 41–2. Properties of useful diagnostic tests.

1. Test methodology has been described in detail so that it can be accurately and reliably reproduced.
2. Test accuracy and precision have been determined.
3. The reference range has been established appropriately.
4. Sensitivity and specificity have been reliably established by comparison with a gold standard. The evaluation has used a range of patients, including those who have different but commonly confused disorders and those with a spectrum of mild and severe, treated and untreated disease. The patient selection process has been adequately described so that results will not be generalized inappropriately.
5. Independent contribution to overall performance of a test panel has been confirmed if a test is advocated as part of a panel of tests.

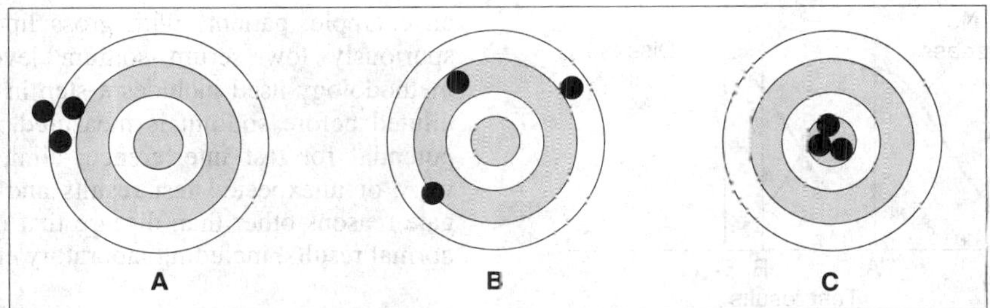

Figure 41–1. Relationship between accuracy and precision in diagnostic tests. The center of the target represents the true value of the substance being tested. Figure "A" represents a diagnostic test which is precise but inaccurate; on repeated measurement, the test yields very similar results, but all results are far from the true value. Figure "B" shows a test which is imprecise and inaccurate; repeated measurement yields widely different results, and the results are far from the true value. Figure "C" shows an ideal test, one that is both precise and accurate.

Reference Range

Reference ranges are method- and laboratory-specific. In practice, they often represent test results found in 95% of a small population presumed to be healthy; by definition, then, 5% of healthy patients will have a positive (abnormal) test (Figure 41–2). As a result, slightly abnormal results should be interpreted critically—they may be either truly abnormal or falsely abnormal. The practitioner should be also aware that the more tests ordered, the greater the chance of obtaining a falsely abnormal result. For a healthy person subjected to 20 independent tests, there is a 64% chance that one test result will lie outside the reference range (Table 41–3). Conversely, values within the reference range may not rule out the actual presence of disease since the reference range does not establish the distribution of results in patients with disease.

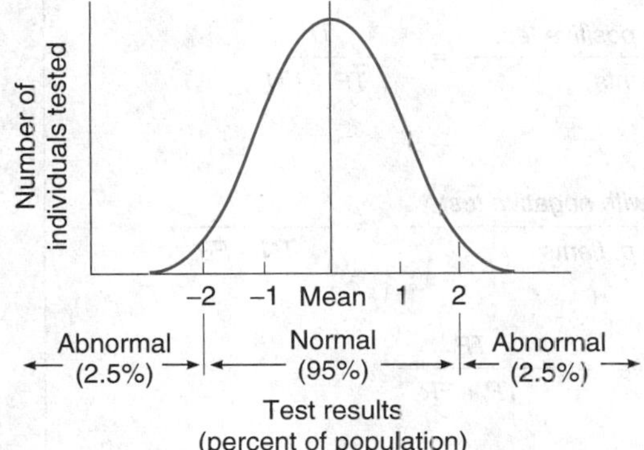

Figure 41–2. The reference range is usually defined as within 2 SD of the mean test result (shown as −2 and 2) in a small population of healthy volunteers. Note that in this example, test results are normally distributed; however, many biologic substances will have distributions that are skewed.

It is important to consider also whether published reference ranges are appropriate for the patient being evaluated, since some ranges depend on age, sex, weight, diet, time of day, activity status, or posture. For instance, the reference ranges for hemoglobin concentration are age- and sex-dependent. Table 2 of the Appendix contains the reference ranges for commonly used chemistry and hematology tests. Test performance characteristics such as sensitivity and specificity are needed to interpret results and are discussed below.

Interfering Factors

The results of diagnostic tests can be altered by external factors, such as ingestion of drugs; and internal factors, such as abnormal physiologic states.

External interferences can affect test results in vivo or in vitro. In vivo, alcohol increases γ-glutamyl transpeptidase, and diuretics can affect sodium and potassium concentrations. Cigarette smoking can induce hepatic enzymes and thus reduce levels of substances such as theophylline that are metabolized by the liver. In vitro, cephalosporins may produce spurious serum creatinine levels due to interference with a common laboratory method.

Internal interferences result from abnormal physiologic states interfering with the test measurement. As

Table 41–3. Relationship between the number of tests and the probability that a healthy person will have one or more abnormal results.

Number of Tests	Probability That One or More Results Will Be Abnormal
1	5%
6	26%
12	46%
20	64%

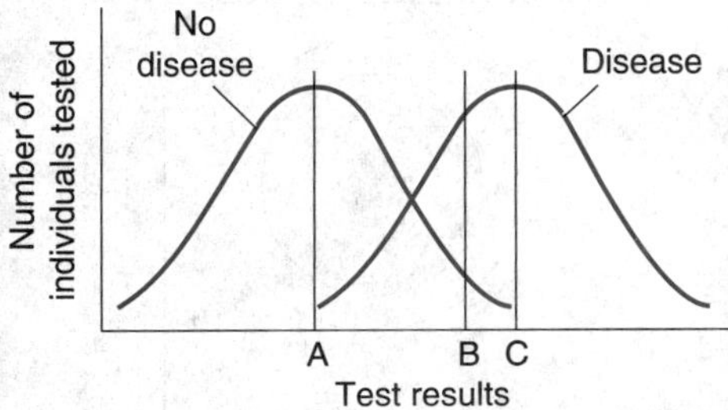

Figure 41–3. Hypothetical distribution of test results for healthy and diseased individuals. The position of the "cutoff point" between "normal" and "abnormal" (or "negative" and "positive") test results determines the test's sensitivity and specificity. If point "A" is the cutoff point, the test would have 100% sensitivity but low specificity. If point "C" is the cutoff point, the test would have 100% specificity but low sensitivity. For many tests, the cutoff point is determined by the reference range, ie, the range of test results that are within 2 SD of the mean of test results for healthy individuals (point "B"). In some situations, the cutoff is altered to enhance either sensitivity or specificity.

an example, patients with gross lipemia may have spuriously low serum sodium levels if the test methodology used includes a step in which serum is diluted before sodium is measured. Because of the potential for test interference, clinicians should be wary of unexpected test results and should investigate reasons other than disease that may explain abnormal results, including laboratory error.

Sensitivity & Specificity

Clinicians should use measures of test performance such as sensitivity and specificity to judge the quality of a diagnostic test for a particular disease. Test **sensitivity** is the likelihood that a diseased patient has a positive test. If all patients with a given disease have a positive test (ie, no diseased patients have negative tests), the test sensitivity is 100%. A test with high sensitivity is useful to exclude a diagnosis because a highly sensitive test will render few results that are falsely negative. To exclude infection with the AIDS virus, for instance, a clinician might choose a highly sensitive test such as the HIV antibody test.

A test's **specificity** is the likelihood that a healthy patient has a negative test. If all patients who do not

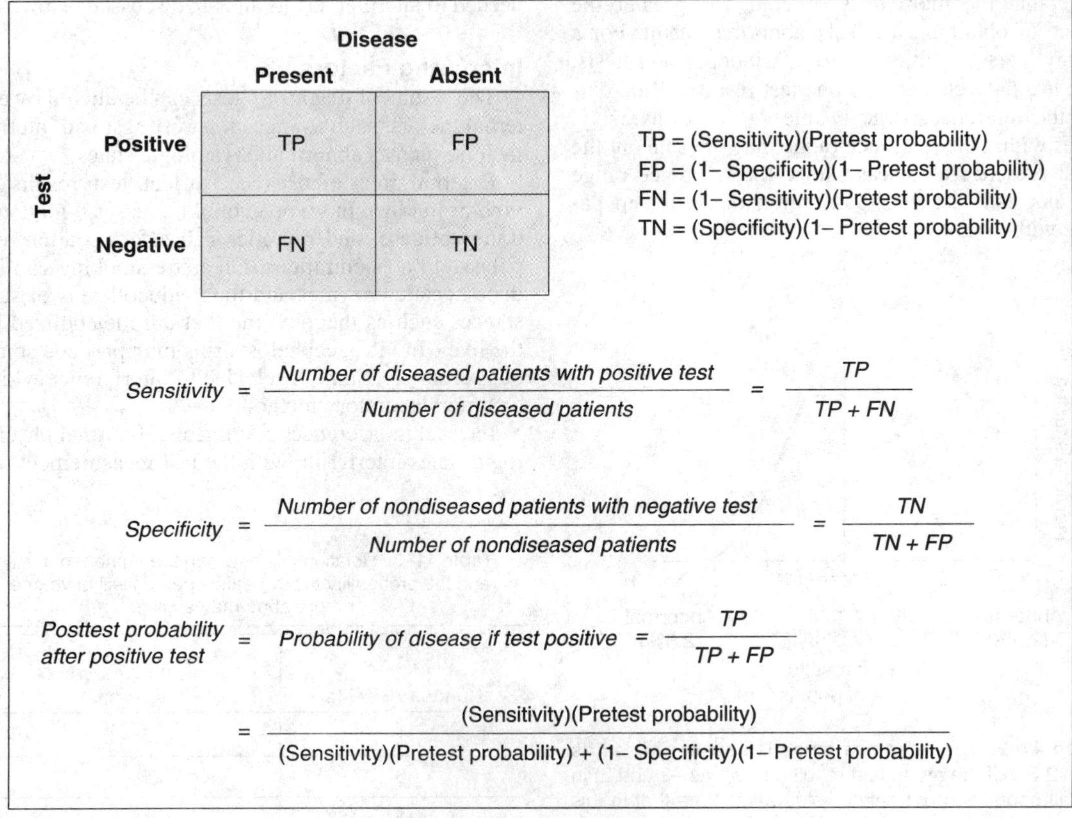

Figure 41–4. Calculation of sensitivity, specificity, and probability of disease after a positive test (posttest probability). (TP, true positive; FP, false positive; FN, false negative; TN, true negative.)

have a given disease have negative tests (ie, no healthy patients have positive tests), the test specificity is 100%. A test with high specificity is useful to confirm a diagnosis, because a highly specific test will have few results that are falsely positive. For instance, to make the diagnosis of gouty arthritis, a clinician might choose a highly specific test, such as the presence of negatively birefringent needle-shaped crystals within leukocytes on microscopic evaluation of joint fluid.

To determine test sensitivity and specificity for a particular disease, the test must be compared against a "gold standard," a procedure that defines the true disease state of the patient. For instance, the sensitivity and specificity of the ventilation/perfusion scan for pulmonary embolus are obtained by comparing the results of scans with the gold standard, pulmonary arteriography. Application of the gold standard examination to patients with positive scans establishes specificity. Failure to apply the gold standard examination following negative scans may result in an overestimation of sensitivity, since false negatives will not be identified. However, for many disease states (eg, pancreatitis), such a gold standard either does not exist or is very difficult or expensive to apply. Therefore, reliable estimates of test sensitivity and specificity are sometimes difficult to obtain.

Sensitivity and specificity can also be affected by the population from which these values are derived. For instance, many diagnostic tests are evaluated first using patients who have severe disease and control groups who are young and well. Compared with the general population, this study group will have more results that are truly positive (because patients have more advanced disease) and more results that are truly negative (because the control group is healthy). Thus, test sensitivity and specificity will be higher than would be expected in the general population, where more of a spectrum of health and disease are found. Clinicians should be aware of this **spectrum bias** when generalizing published test results to their own practice.

Test sensitivity and specificity depend on the threshold above which a test is interpreted to be abnormal (Figure 41–3). If the threshold is lowered, sensitivity is increased at the expense of lowered specificity, or vice versa.

Figure 41–4 shows how test sensitivity and specificity can be calculated using test results from patients previously classified by the gold standard as diseased or nondiseased.

The performance of two different tests can be compared by plotting the sensitivity and (1 minus the specificity) of each test at various reference range cutoff values. The resulting **receiver operator characteristic (ROC) curve** will often show which test is better; a clearly superior test will have an ROC curve that always lies above and to the left of the inferior test curve, and, in general, the better test will have a larger area under the ROC curve. For instance, Figure 41–5 shows the ROC curves for prostate-specific antigen (PSA) and prostatic acid phosphatase (PAP) in the diagnosis of prostate cancer. PSA is a superior test because it has higher sensitivity and specificity for all cutoff values.

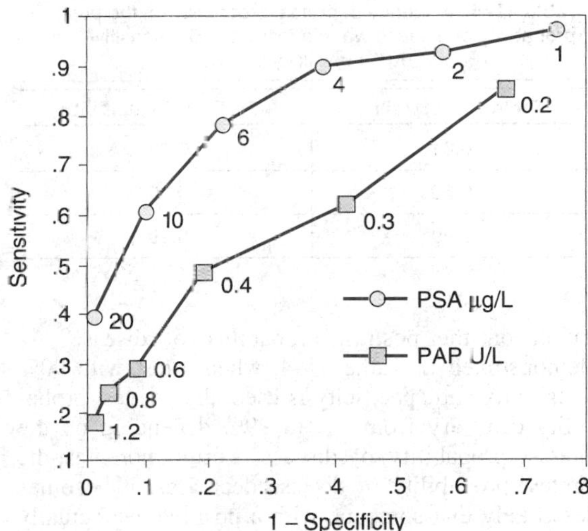

Figure 41–5. Receiver operator characteristic (ROC) curves for prostate-specific antigen (PSA) and prostatic acid phosphatase (PAP) in the diagnosis of prostate cancer. For all cutoff values, PSA has higher sensitivity and specificity; therefore, it is a better test based on these performance characteristics. (Modified and reproduced, with permission, from Nicoll D et al: Routine acid phosphatase testing for screening and monitoring prostate cancer no longer justified. Clin Chem 1993;39:2540.)

Sox HC: The evaluation of diagnostic tests: Principles, problems, and new developments. Annu Rev Med 1996;47:463. [NLM Cit ID: 96226658]

USE OF TESTS IN DIAGNOSIS & MANAGEMENT

The value of a test in a particular clinical situation depends not only on the test's sensitivity and specificity but also on the probability that the patient has the disease before the test result is known **(pretest probability)**. The results of a valuable test will substantially change the probability that the patient has the disease **(posttest probability)**. Figure 41–4 shows how posttest probability can be calculated from the known sensitivity and specificity of the test and the estimated pretest probability of disease (or disease prevalence).

The pretest probability of disease has a profound

Table 41–4. Influence of pretest probability on the posttest probability of disease when a test with 90% sensitivity and 90% specificity is used.

Pretest Probability	Posttest Probability
0.01	0.08
0.50	0.90
0.99	0.999

effect on the posttest probability of disease. As demonstrated in Table 41–4, when a test with 90% sensitivity and specificity is used, the posttest probability can vary from 1% to 99% depending on the pretest probability of disease. Furthermore, as the pretest probability of disease decreases, it becomes less likely that someone with a positive test actually has the disease and more likely that the result represents a false positive.

As an example, suppose the clinician wishes to calculate the posttest probability of prostate cancer using the PSA test and a cut-off value of 4 ng/mL. Using the data shown in Figure 41–5, sensitivity is 90% and specificity is 60%. The clinician estimates the pretest probability of disease given all the evidence and then calculates the posttest probability using the approach shown in Figure 41–5. The pretest probability that an otherwise healthy 50-year-old man has prostate cancer is equal to the prevalence of prostate cancer in that age group (probability = 10%) and the posttest probability is only 20%—ie, even though the test is positive, there is still an 80% chance that the patient does not have prostate cancer (Figure 41–6A). If the clinician finds a prostate nodule on rectal examination, the pretest probability of prostate cancer rises to 50% and the posttest probability using the same test is 69% (Figure 41–6B). Finally, if the clinician estimates the pretest probability to be 98% based on a prostate nodule, bone pain, and lytic lesions on spine x-rays, the posttest probability using PSA is 99% (Figure 41–6C). This example illustrates that pretest probability has a profound effect on posttest probability and that tests provide more information when the diagnosis is truly uncertain (pretest probability about 50%) than when the diagnosis is either unlikely or nearly certain.

ODDS-LIKELIHOOD RATIOS

Another way to calculate the posttest probability of disease is to use the odds-likelihood approach. Sensitivity and specificity are combined into one entity called the likelihood ratio (LR).

$$\text{LR} = \frac{\textbf{Probability of result in diseased persons}}{\textbf{Probability of result in nondiseased persons}}$$

When test results are dichotomized, every test has two likelihood ratios, one corresponding to a positive test (LR^+) and one corresponding to a negative test (LR^-):

$$LR^+ = \frac{\text{Probability that test is positive in diseased persons}}{\text{Probability that test is positive in nondiseased persons}} = \frac{\text{Sensitivity}}{1-\text{Specificity}}$$

$$LR^- = \frac{\text{Probability that test is negative in diseased persons}}{\text{Probability that test is negative in nondiseased persons}} = \frac{1-\text{Sensitivity}}{\text{Specificity}}$$

For continuous measures, multiple likelihood ratios can be defined to correspond to ranges of results. (See Table 41–5 for an example.)

Lists of likelihood ratios can be found in some textbooks, journal articles, and computer programs (see Table 41–6 for sample values). Likelihood ratios can be used to make quick estimates of the usefulness of a contemplated diagnostic test in a particular situation. The simplest method for calculating posttest probability from pretest probability and likelihood ratios is to use a nomogram (Figure 41–7). The clinician places a straightedge through the points that represent the pretest probability and the likelihood ratio and then reads the posttest probability where the straightedge crosses the posttest probability line.

A more formal way of calculating posttest probabilities uses the likelihood ratio as follows:

$$\text{Pretest odds} \times \text{Likelihood ratio} = \text{Posttest odds}$$

To use this formulation, probabilities must be converted to odds, where the odds of having a disease are expressed as the chance of having the disease divided by the chance of not having the disease. For instance, a probability of 0.75 is the same as 3:1 odds (Figure 41–8).

To estimate the potential benefit of a diagnostic test, the clinician first estimates the pretest odds of disease given all available clinical information and then multiplies the pretest odds by the positive and negative likelihood ratios. The results are the **posttest odds,** or the odds that the patient has the disease if the test is positive or negative. To obtain the posttest probability, the odds are converted to a probability (Figure 41–8).

For example, if the clinician believes that the patient has a 60% chance of having a myocardial infarction (pretest odds of 3:2) and the creatine kinase MB test is positive ($LR^+ = 32$), then the posttest odds of having a myocardial infarction are

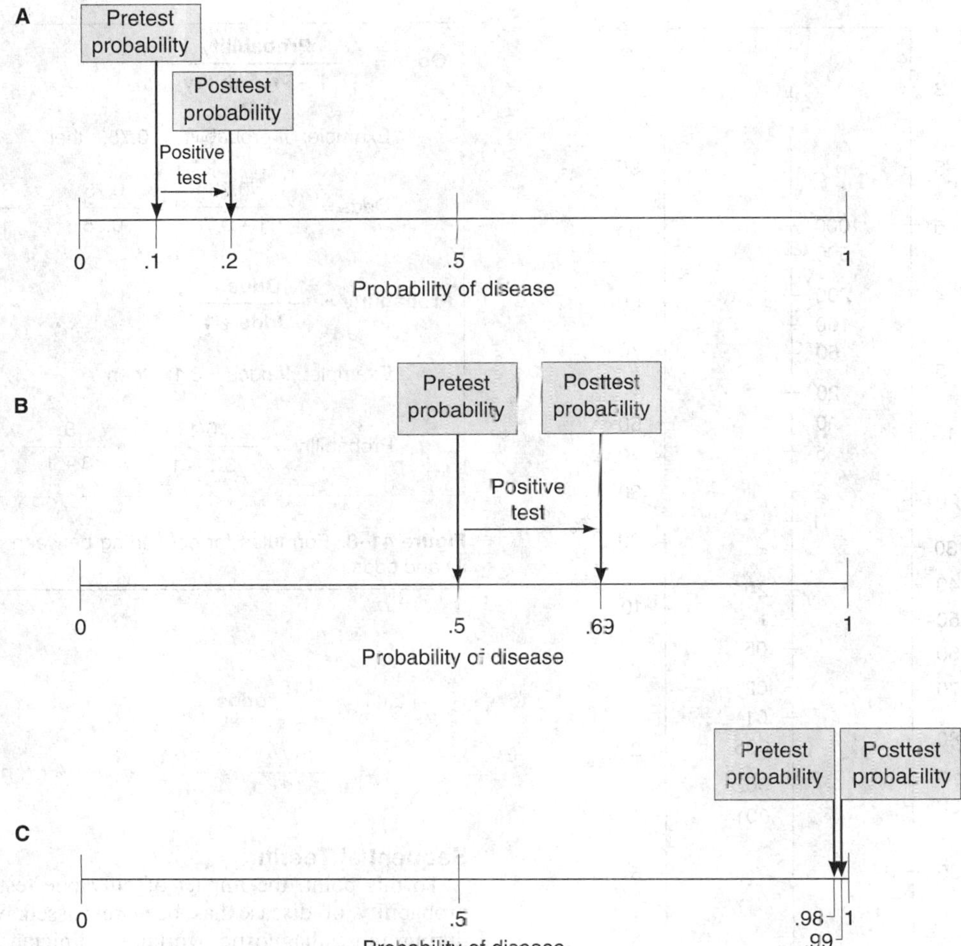

Figure 41–6. Effect of pretest probability and test sensitivity and specificity on the posttest probability of disease. (See text for explanation.)

Table 41–5. Examples of likelihood ratios.[1]

Target Disease	Test	LR+	LR−
Abscess	Abdominal CT	9.5	0.06
Coronary artery disease	Exercise ECG (1 mm depression)	3.5	0.45
Lung cancer	Chest x-ray	15	0.42
Left ventricular hypertrophy	Echocardiography	18.4	0.08
Myocardial infarction	CK-MB	32	0.05
Prostate cancer	Digital rectal examination	21.3	0.37

[1]From: http://www.med.unc.edu/medicine/edursrc/lrdis.htm

Table 41–6. Likelihood ratios of serum ferritin in the diagnosis of iron deficiency anemia.[1]

Serum Ferritin (μg/L)	LR for Iron Deficiency Anemia
≥ 100	0.08
45–99	0.54
35–44	1.83
25–34	2.54
15–24	8.83
< 15	51.85

[1]From Guyatt G: Laboratory diagnosis of iron deficiency anemia. J Gen Intern Med 1992;7:145.

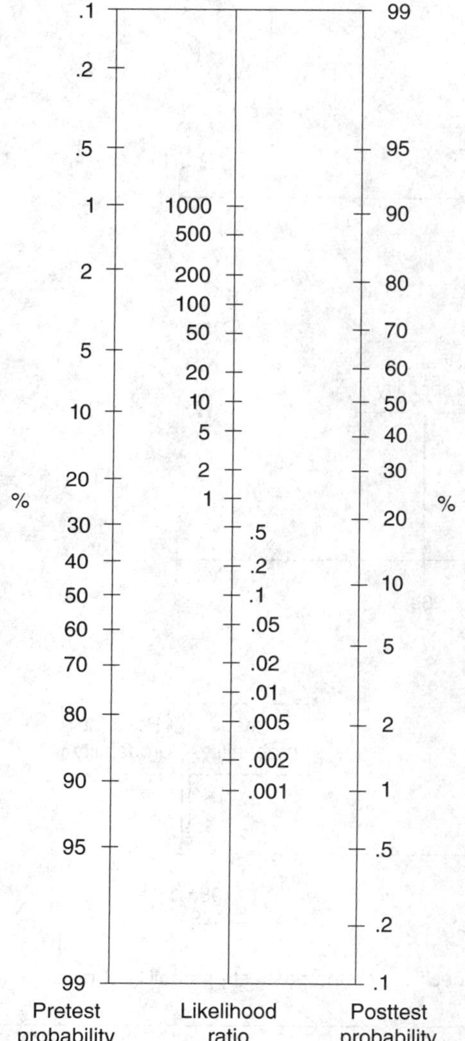

Figure 41–7. Nomogram for determining posttest probability from pretest probability and likelihood ratios. To figure the posttest probability, place a straightedge between the pretest probability and the likelihood ratio for the particular test. The posttest probability will be where the straightedge crosses the posttest probability line. (Adapted and reproduced, with permission, from Fagan TJ: Nomogram for Bayes's theorem. N Engl J Med 1975;293:257.)

$$\frac{3}{2} \times 32 = \frac{96}{2} \text{ or 48:1 odds}$$

$$\left(\frac{48/1}{48/1+1} = \frac{48}{48+1} = 98\% \text{ probability}\right)$$

If the CKMB test is negative ($LR^- = 0.05$), then the posttest odds of having a myocardial infarction are

$$\text{Odds} = \frac{\text{Probability}}{1 - \text{Probability}}$$

Example: If probability = 0.75, then

$$\text{Odds} = \frac{0.75}{1 - 0.75} = \frac{0.75}{0.25} = \frac{3}{1} = 3{:}1$$

$$\text{Probability} = \frac{\text{Odds}}{\text{Odds} + 1}$$

Example: If odds = 3:1, then

$$\text{Probability} = \frac{3/1}{3/1 + 1} = \frac{3}{3 + 1} = 0.75$$

Figure 41–8. Formulas for converting between probability and odds.

$$\frac{3}{2} \times 0.05 = \frac{0.15}{2} \text{ odds}$$

$$\left(\frac{0.15/2}{0.15/2+1} = \frac{0.15}{0.15+2} = 7\% \text{ probability}\right)$$

Sequential Testing

To this point, the impact of only one test on the probability of disease has been discussed, whereas during most diagnostic workups, clinicians obtain clinical information in a sequential fashion. To calculate the posttest odds after three tests, for example, the clinician might estimate the pretest odds and use the appropriate likelihood ratio for each test:

$$\text{Pretest odds} \times LR_1 \times LR_2 \times LR_3 = \text{Posttest odds}$$

When using this approach, however, the clinician should be aware of a major assumption: the chosen tests or findings must be **conditionally independent.** For instance, with liver cell damage, the aspartate aminotransferase (AST) and alanine aminotransferase (ALT) enzymes may be released by the same process and are thus not conditionally independent. If conditionally dependent tests are used in this sequential approach, an overestimation of posttest probability will result.

Black ER et al (editors): *Diagnostic Strategies for Common Medical Problems,* 2nd ed. ACP-ASIM, 1999.

Threshold Approach to Decision Making

A key aspect of medical decision making is the selection of a treatment threshold, ie, the probability of disease at which treatment is indicated. Figure 41–9 shows a possible way of identifying a treatment threshold by considering the value (utility) of the four possible outcomes of the treat/don't treat decision.

A diagnostic test is useful only if it shifts the disease probability across the treatment threshold. For example, a clinician might decide to treat with antibiotics if the probability of streptococcal pharyngitis in a patient with a sore throat is greater than 25% (Figure 41–10A). If, after reviewing evidence from the history and physical examination, the clinician estimates the pretest probability of strep throat to be 15%, then a diagnostic test such as throat culture ($LR^+ = 7$) would be useful only if a positive test would shift the posttest probability above 25%. Use of the nomogram shown in Figure 41–7 indicates that the posttest probability would be 55% (Figure 41–10B); thus, ordering the test would be justified as it affects patient management. On the other hand, if the history and physical examination had suggested that the pretest probability of strep throat was 60%, the throat culture ($LR^- = 0.33$) would be indicated only if a negative test would lower the posttest probability below 25%. Using the same nomogram, the posttest probability after a negative test would be 33% (Figure 41–10C). Therefore, ordering the throat culture would not be justified.

This approach to decision making is now being applied in the clinical literature.

Pauker SG et al: The threshold approach to clinical decision making. N Engl J Med 1980;301:1109. [NLM Cit ID: 80165393]

Tugwell P et al: Laboratory evaluation in the diagnosis of Lyme disease. Ann Intern Med 1997;127:1109. [NLM Cit ID: 98049722] (Sensitivity, specificity, likelihood ratios, and pretest and posttest probabilities used to formulate guidelines for clinical diagnosis of Lyme disease.)

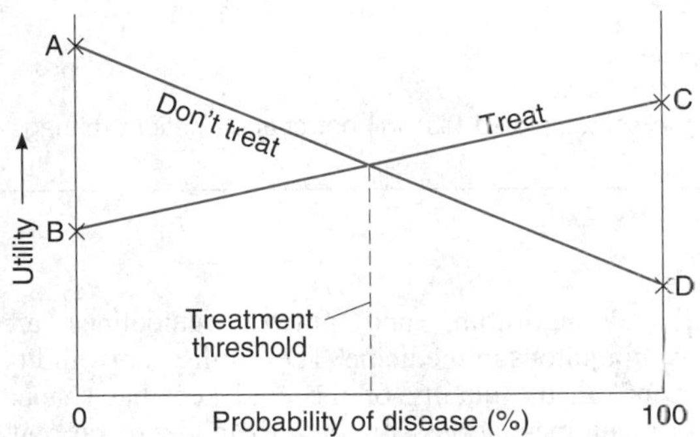

Figure 41–9. The "treat/don't treat" threshold. ***A:*** Patient does not have disease and is not treated (highest utility). ***B:*** Patient does not have disease and is treated (lower utility than A). ***C:*** Patient has disease and is treated (lower utility than A). ***D:*** Patient has disease and is not treated (lower utility than C).

Decision Analysis

Up to this point, the discussion of diagnostic testing has focused on test characteristics and methods for using these characteristics to calculate the probability of disease in different clinical situations. Although useful, these methods are limited because they do not incorporate the many outcomes that may occur in clinical medicine or the values that patients and clinicians place on those outcomes. To incorporate outcomes and values with characteristics of tests, decision analysis can be used.

The basic idea of decision analysis is to model the options in a medical decision, assign probabilities to the alternative actions, assign values (utilities) to the various outcomes, and then calculate which decision gives the greatest value. To complete a decision analysis, the clinician would proceed as follows:

(1) Draw a decision tree showing the elements of the medical decision.

(2) Assign probabilities to the various branches.

(3) Assign values (utilities) to the outcomes.

(4) Determine the expected utility (the product of probability and utility) of each branch.

(5) Select the decision with the highest expected utility.

Figure 41–11 shows a decision tree where the decision to be made is whether to treat without testing, perform a test and then treat based on the test result, or perform no tests and give no treatment. The clinician begins the analysis by building a decision tree showing the important elements of the decision. Once the tree is built, the clinician assigns probabilities to all the branches. In this case, all the branch probabilities can be calculated from (1) the probability of disease before the test (pretest probability), (2) the chance of a positive test if the disease is present (sensitivity) and (3) the chance of a negative test if the disease is absent (specificity). Next, the clinician assigns utility values to each of the outcomes.

After the expected utility is calculated for each branch of the decision tree, by multiplying the utility of the outcome by the probability of the outcome, the clinician can identify the alternative with the highest expected utility.

Although time-consuming, decision analysis can help to structure complex clinical problems and to make difficult clinical decisions.

Dekay ML et al: Is the defensive use of diagnostic tests good for patients, or bad? Med Decis Making 1998;18:19. [NLM Cit ID: 98115737]

Detsky AS et al: Primer on medical decision analysis. (Five parts.) Med Decis Making 1997;17:123. [NLM Cit ID: 96261683]

Evidence-Based Medicine

The focus over the past decade on evidence-based medicine stresses the examination of evidence from

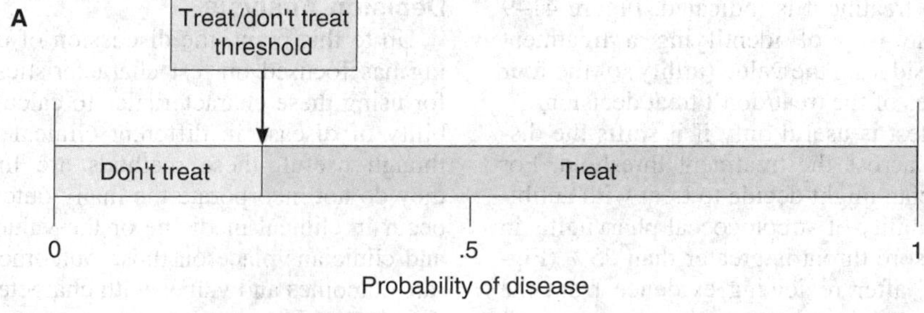

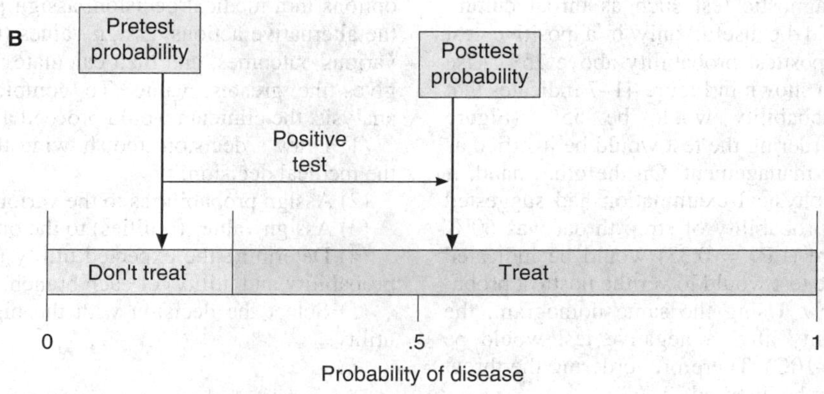

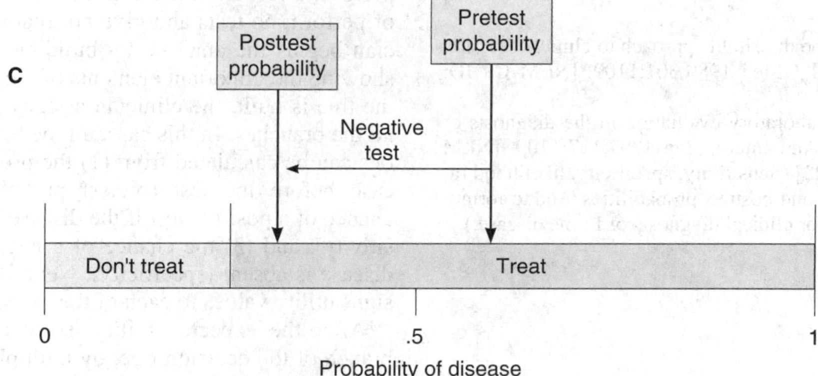

Figure 41–10. Threshold approach applied to test ordering. If the contemplated test will not change patient management, the test should not be ordered. (See text for explanation.)

clinical research—rather than intuition and pathophysiologic reasoning—as a basis for clinical decision making. Evidence-based medicine relies on systematic reviews of the medical literature to inform clinical practice. Meta-analysis uses statistical techniques to combine evidence from different studies.

Clinical practice guidelines are systematically developed statements intended to assist practitioners and patients in making decisions about health care. Clinical algorithms and practice guidelines are now ubiquitous in medicine. Their utility and validity depend on the quality of the evidence that shaped the recommendations, on their being kept current, and on their acceptance and appropriate application by clinicians. While clinicians are concerned about the effect of guidelines on professional autonomy, many organizations are trying to use compliance with practice guidelines as a measure of quality of care.

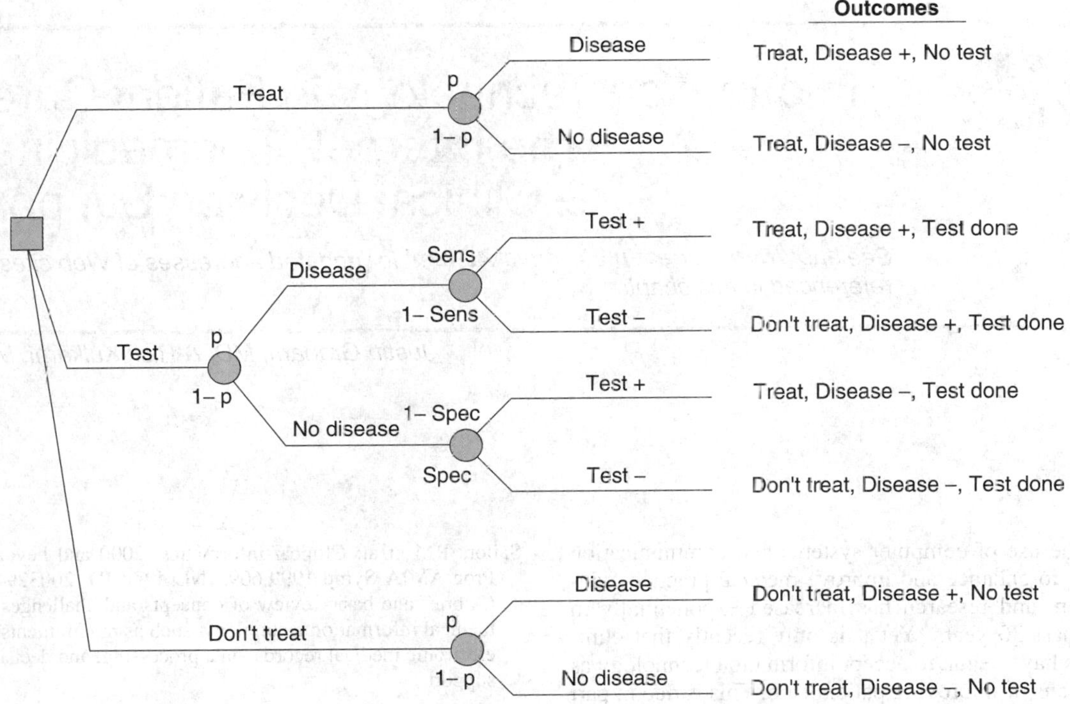

Figure 41–11. Generic tree for a clinical decision where the choices are (1) to treat the patient empirically, (2) to do the test and then treat only if the test is positive, or (3) to withhold therapy. The square node is called a decision node, and the circular nodes are called chance nodes. (p, pretest probability of disease; Sens, sensitivity; Spec, specificity.)

Jadad AR et al: The Cochrane collaboration: Advances and challenges in improving evidence-based decision making. Med Decis Making 1998;18:2. [NLM Cit ID: 98115735]

Maynard A: Evidence-based medicine: An incomplete method for informing treatment choices. Lancet 1997;349:126. [NLM Cit ID: 97149627]

Sackett DL et al: *Clinical Epidemiology. A Basic Science for Clinical Medicine,* 2nd ed. Little, Brown, 1991.

Computer Access to Medical Information

The development of medical information science and computer technology now offer a vast amount of clinical information on CD-ROM or over the World Wide Web.

RELEVANT WORLD WIDE WEB SITES

[Artificial Intelligence Systems in Routine Clinical Use]
http://www.coiera.com/ailist/list.html
[Cochrane Collaboration]
http://hiru.mcmaster.ca/ebm/default.htm
[CenterWatch Clinical Trials Listing Service]
http://www.centerwatch.com
[Evidence-Based Practice on the Internet]
http://www.shef.ac.uk/~scharr/ir/netting.html

42 Information Technology in Patient Care: The Internet, Telemedicine, & Clinical Decision Support

See http://www.current-med.com/ch42.html for updated addresses of Web sites referenced in this chapter.

Justin Graham, MD, & Rick Kulkarni, MD

The use of computer systems and communication tools to enhance and improve medical practice, education, and research has increased exponentially in the past 30 years. Yet it is only recently that clinicians have begun to accept information technology as a means of improving patient care. This is due in part to substantial advances in component technologies: processors and memory, networks, and software. But perhaps more importantly, health care workers and their patients have grown more familiar with computers in other occupational, commercial, and recreational applications. Therefore, an increasing number of clinicians seek to apply these tools to the practice of medicine.

Modern medicine is very information-intensive. Clinicians regularly synthesize the vast, growing body of medical literature with detailed, ongoing patient evaluations. They must communicate the resulting reams of data to their patients and to other clinicians. Never before in human history has information technology been better suited to assist in these tasks. Modern information systems offer the promise of unprecedented quality, innovation, and efficiency in the delivery of health care. But—as happens with any new medical device or technologic innovation—there are both old pitfalls and new perils to be sedulously avoided.

The complex technical and theoretical details underlying medical informatics and computer science are beyond the scope of this chapter. What follows is a brief introduction to topics and resources of general interest in this field, offered to help clinicians care for their patients as information technology becomes an integral part of the patient-clinician relationship.

Coiera E: *Guide to Medical Informatics, the Internet, and Telemedicine.* Chapman & Hall Medical, 1997. (Introductory text describing the information science and logic behind medical informatics.)

Sailors RM et al: Clinical informatics: 2000 and beyond. Proc AMIA Symp 1999:609. [NLM Cit ID: 20032941] (A brief and basic review of concepts and challenges in medical information technology, such as requirements of electronic medical records, data processing, and decision support.)

THE INTERNET IN CLINICAL PRACTICE

An overview of basic concepts related to the Internet is presented in this section to allow the practicing physician to fully exploit the communication medium's resources. Several individual components of the communication technology when taken together comprise the contemporary Internet. The dominant form of communication since its popularization several years ago has continued to be the World Wide Web. The Web's popularity derives from its ability to rapidly transmit both text and graphics to a user's computer screen through browsers (eg, Microsoft Internet Explorer, Netscape Navigator). Rapid transmission of large amounts of data is achieved by omitting redundancies in code via higher generation programming languages (eg, Hypertext Markup Language, HTML).

Despite the Web's dominance, other forms of communication on the Internet continue to be vital to the medium's success in facilitating communication. Electronic mail (e-mail) is a text-based form of communication employed by most Internet users in a "store-and-forward" fashion (ie, not processed immediately by the recipient). File transfer protocol (FTP) permits rapid transfer of files from one computer to another through the Internet. Usegroups make possible congregation and communication between individuals with similar interests.

The individual physician's interaction with the Internet depends on his or her personal requirements and expectations. Simple store-and-forward modes of communication such as e-mail simplify exchanges with patients and colleagues. Most academic institutions offer to faculty and staff e-mail accounts that can be used without charge. Several online organizations offer free e-mail accounts to the general public.

Activities such as keeping up to date with current events in medicine, learning from electronic journals, and interacting with an institution's Web site for professional activities all require the use of browser software in order to access the Web. Several high-quality medical news Web sites (eg, CNN Interactive—Health; BBC News—Health) and an increasing number of online medical journals offering direct access to current and archived issues have made the Internet a valuable resource for physicians. Clinicians actively participate in online medical communities providing access to searchable reference material and discussion groups (eg, Physicians' Online, MDConsult).

With increasing confidence with the medium, the clinician may consider taking further advantage of the power of the Web by constructing a personal Web site. Although the details of programming and implementing a Web site are beyond the scope of this chapter, the process itself can be straightforward and achievable if the legal implications and the scope of the project are appropriately addressed. While family-oriented Web sites are shielded from liability issues, offering clinical information to patients on the Web requires some consideration of the potential legal pitfalls of providing knowledge that can be construed as formal medical advice. General patient education material and online recommendations should be followed by instructions directing patients to first discuss any suggested lifestyle or medication changes with a physician prior to adoption. In addition, the prudent physician should review previously published guidelines on responding to unsolicited e-mail requests for medical guidance (refer to the section on Patient-Clinician E-mail Communication, below). The provision of direct physician e-mail access to patients and the general Internet community can quickly result in a significant volume of such requests.

The scope of the personal Web site should also be established prior to embarking on its construction. Programming a small Web site composed of several standard HTML "Web pages" can be accomplished by the individual physician without a significant expenditure of time spent in learning computer code. HTML editors such as Microsoft FrontPage and Adobe PageMill have greatly simplified HTML programming by providing intuitive, user-friendly work environments. The actual installation of the Web pages onto a computer that "serves" content to the general Internet community can be accomplished by locating an Internet Service Provider (ISP). Professional assistance is recommended for advanced Web activities such as interacting with online databases and implementing interactive Web pages (eg, submission forms, online applications). The commitment of time that is necessary to achieve facility with these advanced activities is an impractical investment for the busy practicing clinician.

[BBC News—Health]
http://news.bbc.co.uk/hi/english/health/default.htm. (Current health-related news from a trusted source.)

[CNN Interactive—Health]
http://www.cnn.com/HEALTH. (Another reliable source.)

[MDConsult]
http://www.mdconsult.com/ (A comprehensive, fee-based medical information service providing access to fully searchable online medical textbooks, full-text medical journals, patient education material, practice guidelines, drug information, and access to online discussion groups.)

[Physicians' Online]
http://www.po.com/ (An online community of clinicians actively engaged in clinical discussion. The service also offers access to current medical news stories and Internet access services.)

JAMA patient page: Health and the Internet. JAMA 1998;280:1380. [NLM Cit ID: 99008454]

Peters RN et al: Building your own: A physician's guide to creating a Web site. JAMA 1998;280:1365. [NLM Cit ID: 99008452]

INFORMATION RELIABILITY & QUALITY ASSESSMENT

The contemporary Internet contains a vast collection of Web sites devoted to the dissemination of health-related information. These Web sites provide a constantly expanding repository of information that previously was inaccessible to most physicians and their patients. Unfortunately, owing to the lack of control over the posted content and the speed with which new information is incorporated into both existing Web sites and new health-related Internet endeavors, a lot of the information "out there" is either incomplete, outdated, or otherwise inaccurate.

Finding useful health-related information on the Internet can become prohibitively time-consuming for the physician unfamiliar with Internet search strategies. Even for the Internet veteran, location of reliable and useful information depends on one's ability to first assemble a short list of potentially useful Web sites and then navigate to those Web sites and assess their value.

A better alternative is to use Internet health information meta-Web sites that have already rated and reviewed the content. It is the function of meta-Web sites to apply a core set of reviewing criteria to all the primary Web sites they review and rate. The criteria should be based on primary publisher accountability and should be applied to all health content Web sites. Table 42–1 sets forth an example of a core set of

Table 42–1. Core standards for information reliability and quality assessment.

Authorship: The relevant credentials and affiliations of the editors, authors, and contributors should be easily accessible.
Attribution: Detailed reference information for information content should be clearly listed on the entry page of the Web site.
Disclosure: All sponsorships, advertising sources, underwriting, and any other potential conflicts of interest should be prominently and fully disclosed.
Dating: The date of the last critical internal review of the content should be available to the user for review.

standards. The weakness of this model is the potential for error if the reviewing meta-Web site uses a flawed rating method.

Efforts to better assess and summarize the quality of the information provided on the Web are currently under way. Several review services have in the past few years provided rating criteria as well as "seals of approval" that individual Web sites can apply for and display to indicate compliance with established codes of conduct. Examples include the Geneva-based Health on the Net Foundation and the OncoLink's Editor's Choice Awards. Other Web sites such as the Current Medical Diagnosis & Treatment Companion Web Page (CMDT-CWP) offer stand-alone reviews and categorical ratings of hundreds of health care-related Web sites without requiring any display of seals of approval. Table 42–2 is an example of a well-constructed rating system currently in use on the CMDT-CWP.

[Current Medical Diagnosis and Treatment—Companion Web Page]
http://www.current-med.com (The CMDT-CWP offers physicians and patients direct access to a large collection of physician-reviewed health-related Web sites. In addition to concise and informative reviews, a rating based on a six-category instrument also follows each Web site. The Web sites are organized by the textbook's 43 chapters.)

Table 42–2. An example of a well-constructed rating system.

Peer-reviewed	Web page claims that other experts in the field have critically evaluated material presented.
MD-oriented	Presentation explicitly designed for health-care professionals.
Patient resources	Substantial material presented here suitable for motivated patients.
Noncommercial	Corporate or for-profit sponsor does not exclusively support Web site. These sites may contain some advertising, however.
Multimedia-enhanced	Easy access to video, audio, animation, high-quality images and other multimedia teaching tools.
Updated regularly	Content was updated within 6 months of researching this guide.

[Health on the Net Foundation Code of Conduct]
http://www.hon.ch/HONcode/Conduct.html (A Geneva-based organization offering health-related Web sites an opportunity to earn a symbol of good conduct if certain criteria are adhered to, including provision of medical information only from medically trained professionals, the precept that all information be provided only as an adjunct to the relationship between a physician and a patient, and the clear identification of all reference sources, funding sources, and "last-modified" details.)

[OncoLink's Editors' Choice Awards]
http://nisc8a.upenn.edu/ed_choice/ (A rating instrument for health-related Web sites that uses the following criteria [among others]: quality of material, accessibility of information, ability to access and identify authors and editors, clear statement of mission, frequency of updates, and editorial oversight.)

Eysenbach G et al: Towards quality management of medical information on the Internet: Evaluation, labeling, and filtering of information. BMJ 1998;317:1496. [NLM Cit ID: 99051215] (Guide for overcoming the potential inaccuracy of health-related material on the Internet.)

Jadad AR et al: Rating health information on the Internet: navigating to knowledge or to Babel? JAMA 1998;279:611. [NLM Cit ID: 98146162]

Silberg WM et al: Assessing, controlling, and assuring the quality of medical information on the Internet: Caveant lector et viewor—Let the reader and viewer beware. JAMA 1997;277:1244. [NLM Cit ID: 97256510]

HEALTH INFORMATION SECURITY

Today's health care environment includes electronic medical records (EMRs), intranets connecting affiliated health care organizations for sharing patient information, and off-site access protocols for making patient information available to providers. One consequence of these rapidly proliferating technologies is that the confidentiality of sensitive patient information may be compromised. Although significant strides toward acceptable levels of security have been made in the past several years, recent surveys have raised questions regarding the integrity of existing privacy and security measures at both government and third-party institutional levels.

The burden of maintaining a secure electronic health information environment and complying with federally mandated regulations for the secure transmission of patient-related health care information between health care providers and other third-party organizations (eg, Health Insurance Portability and Accountability Act; HIPAA) falls primarily on the health information management specialists at the hospital. However, the individual physician must become familiar with the general principles of electronic security to prevent accidental compromise of sensitive information. Most hospital health information systems use a comparable collection of security tools (Table 42–3). Further information can be found in the Web sites listed below.

[Consumer Project on Technology—Medical Records Privacy]
http://www.cptech.org/privacy/medical.html (A not-for-profit organization providing direct links to recently published government and public policy institution reports on the protection of health information privacy. Also included are e-mail links to persons actively involved in the debate as well as a method to join a listserve on the topic.)

[Current Medical Diagnosis and Treatment—Companion Web Page]
http://www.books.mcgraw-hill.com/medical/lange/cmdt (The CMDT-CWP offers physicians and patients direct access to a large collection of physician-reviewed health-related Web sites. In addition to concise and informative reviews, a rating based on a six-category instrument also follows each Website. The Web sites are organized by the textbook's 43 chapters.)

[Electronic Privacy Information Center—Medical Record Privacy]
http://www.epic.org/privacy/medical/. (An online resource for recent legislative and judicial reports on the topic of medical records privacy. The Web page provides direct links to congressional reports, recent publications in medical and legislative journals, and landmark white papers on the topic.)

[Health Insurance Portability and Accountability Act (HIPAA), Department of Health and Human Services]
http://aspe.os.dhhs.gov/admnsimp/
http://www.hcfa.gov/regs/hipaacer.htm
(Act intended to reduce the cost and administrative burdens of health care by making the standardized electronic transmission of many administrative and financial transactions possible. Contains a patient privacy section mandating that all participating providers and organizations that store, maintain, or transmit patient health information adhere to basic security standards, policies, and practices.)

Clayton PD, Boebert WE, DeFriese GH: *For The Record: Protecting Electronic Health Information.* Committee on Maintaining Privacy and Security in Health Care Applications of the National Information Infrastructure, National Research Council, 1997.

O'Brien DG et al: Privacy, confidentiality, and security in information systems of state health agencies. Am J Prev Med 1999;16:351. [NLM Cit ID: 99421038] (Overview of specific deficiencies in patient information security and privacy standards at the state health agency level.)

Table 42–3. Specific methods commonly used to ensure security of electronic patient information.

Authentication: The process of verifying the identity of a user requesting data from the health care information system. Authentication is usually achieved by requesting private information from the user, such as a password or a personal ID number.
Access control: The process of determining the privileges a user has in terms of accessing information and services on the health care information system.
Encryption: Transformation of information into unintelligible data that is only interpretable with a private decryption key.
Audit trails: A record of information access events that is commonly used in health care information systems to deter individual users from system abuses.
Sessions: Persistence of user information designed to ensure user validation and automatic termination at time-outs.

PATIENT-CLINICIAN E-MAIL COMMUNICATION

Electronic mail is a communication tool currently used by hundreds of millions of people worldwide. Although physicians have been communicating with their patients by e-mail for over 5 years, it is only recently that this aspect of the patient-provider relationship has come under careful scrutiny. Electronic communication can extend and complement personal encounters, improve compliance and access to care, and increase the involvement of patients in their own care. However, the very nature of e-mail creates legal, ethical, and practical considerations that must be respected by patients and physicians alike.

E-mail is more permanent than oral communication and more spontaneous than letters and other written communications. It is by its nature self-documenting. E-mail can be duplicated or forwarded with the press of a button, and copies may linger on intermediate or back-up computer systems long after both the sender and receiver have deleted the originals. It can be easily altered, with or without attribution, by the sender, the recipient, or a third party. E-mail lends itself readily to detailed instructions as well as attachments and links to other information sources.

Electronic communication is well suited for communicating administrative information. medication or dressing instructions, patient education materials, routine laboratory results, appointment reminders, and prescription refills. It can augment home monitoring of a variety of treatment plans, such as diabetic diets or smoking cessation programs. Providers can easily make general announcements to an entire patient practice about issues such as vacation coverage, influenza vaccine availability, or changes in referral procedures (Table 42–4).

E-mail imposes the same legal and ethical obligations that inform other kinds of doctor-patient communication. Providers have a duty to respond promptly to patient inquiries and to maintain strict confidentiality regardless of the technology involved. The very nature of e-mail complicates these issues and presents unfamiliar considerations such as source verification and technical failure. Thus, some experts have advocated obtaining formal informed consent from patients before exchanging e-mails. Providers ought at least come to agreement with their patients about basic policies for exchanges of e-mail messages (Tables 42–5 and 42–6).

Some physicians have expressed concern that once

Table 42–4. Some suggested uses of patient-provider e-mail.

Patient education
Medication, diet, or dressing instructions
Multimedia disease education presentations
References to appropriate Internet resources
Disease monitoring
Home glucose, blood pressure, weight, or peak flow measurements
Progress towards smoking cessation
Administrative information
Referral requests
Vacation coverage
Changes in demographic data
Patient requests for prescription refills
Normal laboratory test results and interpretation
Reminders
Scheduled appointments
Vaccines or screening tests due
Clarifications, follow-ups, or reinforcement of issues discussed in person

their e-mail addresses become widely available, they will be deluged by messages from individuals with whom they have no preexisting relationship. Recent small studies have not found e-mail from unfamiliar patients to be burdensome. However, there is currently no consensus on the physician's duty in this situation or the legal consequences of providing advice to unknown patients perhaps beyond the scope of the physician's license. At the very least, physicians should post electronic communication policies addressing unsolicited communication wherever their e-mail addresses can be found.

Table 42–5. Provider strategies for management of electronic communication.[1]

Use password-protected workstations and encryption for all messages when readily available.
Print all messages, with replies and confirmation of receipt, and place in patient's permanent medical record.
Double-check all "To:" fields prior to sending messages.
Configure automatic reply to acknowledge receipt of messages.
Send a new message to inform patient of completion of request.
Maintain a mailing list of patients, but do not send group mailings where recipients are visible to each other. Use blind copy feature in software.
Create template banner headings and footers giving explicit instructions about how to escalate communication to telephone calls and office visits.
Never forward a patient's message or patient-identifiable information to a third party without the express permission of the patient.
Perform at least weekly backups of mail onto long-term storage.
Commit policy decisions to writing and electronic form.
Avoid anger, sarcasm, harsh criticism, and libelous references to third parties in messages.

[1]Adapted, with permission, from Kane B, Sands DZ: Guidelines for the clinical use of electronic mail with patients. J Am Med Inform Assoc 1998;5:104.

Table 42–6. Suggested elements of a patient-provider agreement for electronic communication.[1]

Establish turnaround time for messages and expressly state that e-mail is not for urgent matters or emergencies.
Provide instructions on how and when to escalate to phone calls, office appointments, and emergency room visits.
Agree on privacy issues and who, besides the addressee, will read messages. Make specific reference to office staff, covering providers, and third-party consultations.
Inform patients about the possibility of electronic eavesdropping by patients' own employers, Internet service providers, and others, such as family, who have access to the same computers or e-mail account.
Establish types of transactions (prescription refill, appointment scheduling, etc) and sensitivity of subject matter (HIV, mental health, etc) permitted over e-mail.
Instruct patients to put category of transaction in subject line of message for filtering: "prescription," "appointment," "medical advice," "billing question."
Request that patients put their name and patient identification number in the body of the message.
Ask that patients use autoreply feature to acknowledge reading provider's message.
Describe how messages will be incorporated into the permanent medical record.

[1]Adapted, with permission, from Kane B, Sands DZ: Guidelines for the clinical use of electronic mail with patients. J Am Med Inform Assoc 1998;5:104.

Kane B et al: Guidelines for the clinical use of electronic mail with patients. J Am Med Inform Assoc 1998;5:104. [NLM Cit ID: 98115079]

Mandl KD et al: Electronic patient-physician communication: problems and promise. Ann Intern Med 1998; 129:495. [NLM Cit ID: 98396874]

Spielberg AR: On call and online: Sociohistorical, legal, and ethical implications of e-mail for the patient-physician relationship. JAMA 1998;280:1353. [NLM Cit ID: 99008448]

Spielberg AR: Online without a net: physician-patient communication by electronic mail. Am J Law Med 1999;25:267. [NLM Cit ID: 99405246] (Legal analysis of confidentiality, reimbursement, and malpractice issues.)

INTERACTIVE FORUMS

Informal consultations among clinicians are common, but until recently they have been limited to the offices and conference rooms of specific health care settings or, periodically, academic meetings. With the advent of the Internet and the dramatic reduction in barriers to communication, discussions among health care providers can be continuous and far-reaching.

Many on-line discussion groups are currently available for health care providers with similar interests (Table 42–7). Almost all function as electronic bulletin boards, where individuals leave new messages or comments germane to ongoing discussion threads in a series of static postings.

Newsgroups (also called Usenet newsgroups) are one of the oldest applications of the Internet, predat-

Table 42–7. Examples of interactive forums.

Newsgroups (accessible at http://deja.com/usenet)
- Sci.Med.Cardiology
- Alt.Support.Lupus

Web-based forums
- Journal Club on the Web (http://www.journalclub.org/)
- Medical Studies Seminars (http://www.mdsem.com/index.html)
- Clinical Discussions (http://www.medscape.com/Medscape/features/spotlight/ClincalDiscussions.html)

Mailing lists
- Clinical Q&A Discussions (http://www.cma.ca/clinical/groups/clinical.htm)
- Program for Monitoring Emerging Diseases (ProMED) (http://www.healthnet.org/programs/promed.html)
- NEPHRO-L Nephrology Mailing List (send mail to majordomo@majordomo.srv.ualberta.ca)
- CARDIO-CONSULT (http://www.lstoft.com/scripts/wl.exe?SL1=CARDIOCONSULT&H=SHRSYS.HSLC.ORG)

Chatrooms
- Weekly Webdoctor Chat (http://www.gretmar.com/Webdoctor/FrameChat.html
- The Medical Studies Seminar http://www.mdsem.com/

ing the World Wide Web, though today the Web provides a convenient Usenet interface. There are tens of thousands of newsgroups organized in nested series with names like "sci.med.prostate.bph" or "http://www.deja.com/group/alt.support.crohns-colitis." Newsgroups are open to the general public, are unmoderated, and are subject to little or no information quality control.

Web-based forums are usually adjuncts to specific Web sites. They frequently require registration demonstrating appropriate credentials (eg, medical license number), and moderators often monitor postings for veracity and relevance. Thus, Web-based forums generally carry discussions of higher quality among fewer participants.

Mailing lists are discussions delivered directly by e-mail. Any comment posted to the ongoing dialogue is instantly sent to every subscriber throughout the world. Mailing lists can be moderated or unmoderated, private or public, and may have as few as two or as many as tens of thousands of subscribers. High-volume lists, which can average hundreds of postings each day, can be received using digest mode, which gathers the day's postings into a single e-mail message. Subscribing usually involves sending an e-mail message to an address containing "listserve" or "majordomo" with the text containing "Subscribe" followed by the name of the list in question (eg, Stroke-L or Lymenet-L).

The Internet's closest approximation to a face-to-face conversation takes place in chatrooms, where participants take turns typing text visible to the whole group as the discussion unfolds. More advanced chatrooms allow participants to "whisper" private messages to one another. Although—as with everywhere on the Internet—it is impossible to verify the identities of those you are communicating with, quality chatrooms provide moderators, discussants, or attendants responsible for guiding discussions and weeding out noncontributing participants. Most chatrooms of interest to health care providers are hosted by medical Web sites.

TELEMEDICINE

Telemedicine has been defined as "the use of electronic information and communications technologies to provide and support health care when distance separates the participants." The first widely used tool of telemedicine was the telephone.

Telemedicine applications of the past 20 years have relied mainly on interactive video to connect patients and referring clinicians in remote locations with specialists in urban tertiary care centers. Using studio or home video recording equipment, visual and audio information is conveyed either by physical transportation of videotape or other recording media or by more sophisticated, specially designed video conferencing networks.

More recently, as broad-bandwidth (high transmission rate) networks have become increasingly available, "store-and-forward" telemedicine has become more commonplace, using multimedia e-mail and Web technology to forward medical images, audio, medical records, and laboratory results. By combining these data with real-time synchronous consultations, consultants can now provide comprehensive evaluations from anywhere in the world.

The next generation of telemedicine applications will expand the remote clinician's capabilities beyond diagnosis to therapeutic interventions. Telesurgery, remote psychotherapy, and virtual "home visits" to manage chronic medical problems are all in early development. Multiple Web sites attest to these and even more innovative uses of telemedicine for clinicians to explore (Table 42–8).

Table 42–8. Examples of current telemedicine applications.

- In-flight emergency resuscitation guidance on commercial aircraft
- Home fetal monitoring during complicated pregnancies
- Monitoring compliance with home drug dispensers
- Preoperative screening and postoperative follow-up of patients of surgeons on service missions to developing nations
- Remote dermatologic, pathologic, or radiographic consultations
- The Visible Human Project
- Teleproctoring laparoscopic surgery

Telemedicine applications have several limitations. Given the ease of transmission and duplication of digital information, confidentiality and security need to be safeguarded. Although information transfer ignores geographic boundaries, medical licensure does not—especially in the United States, where several states have limited the interstate practice of medicine. Liability and malpractice are thorny and untested issues, as the practice of telemedicine presents a new form of the patient-caregiver relationship and new potential hazards, such as technical failures leading to altered or suboptimal data. Finally, health care payer policy is lagging behind the technology. Most insurers will not yet provide reimbursement to physicians for telemedicine consultations. Medicare will reimburse teleconsultations that meet a very restrictive set of criteria: the patient must be in an underserved rural area; the referring practitioner, who must be present, earns 25% of the consultation fee; and only teleradiology—and no other form of store-and-forward technology—is used in the consultation.

[Department of Defense Comprehensive Telemedicine Site] http://www.matmo.org

[Telemedicine Internet Exchange] http://208.129.211.51/

Grigsby J et al: Telemedicine: Where it is and where it's going. Ann Intern Med 1998;129:123. [NLM Cit ID: 98318192]

Kuszler PC: Telemedicine and integrated health care delivery: compounding malpractice liability. Am J Law Med 1999;25:297. [NLM Cit ID: 99405247] (Legal issues raised by telemedicine.)

Strode SW et al: Technical and clinical progress in telemedicine. JAMA 1999;281:1066. [NLM Cit ID: 99202525]

CLINICAL DECISION SUPPORT SYSTEMS

Computers and artificial intelligence systems have played a role in improving the quality of health care delivery to patients for several decades. One specific aspect of their contribution has been in the area of clinical decision support. Recent advances in enabling technology (eg, the Internet) have led to the dissemination of clinical decision support modalities into the individual practitioner's clinical environment. Two examples are the production of electronic, up-to-date versions of clinical references (ie, medical journals and textbooks) and development of efficient search tools for large bibliographic databases such as Medline.

In contrast to the general clinical modalities outlined above, computer-based decision support systems directly assist the clinician in making a clinical decision about a specific patient. These applications incorporate individual patient characteristics into a computerized knowledge base to generate patient-specific assessments or recommendations.

Clinical decision support systems perform a variety of functions from providing feedback to actions taken by clinicians to initiating communication between providers upon encountering unusual data. Specific examples of the types of logic used by clinical decision support systems in addition to topical examples are provided in Table 42–9.

Clinical decision support systems save lives and reduce costs. Inpatient order entry systems routinely result in double-digit percentage reductions in costs of patient care without negative effects on outcomes. Drug family checking systems reduce the frequency of adverse drug events by up to 55%. Time-based reminders for preventive care activities increase the percentage of patients who are up-to-date with recommended adult preventive testing schedules, and automated e-mails increase interprovider satisfaction. Hospital-based physicians have accepted use of clinical decision support systems in their daily practice, and such systems are moving also into mainstream clinical practice. Physicians must investigate how these innovative and rationally developed technologies can be most effective for their specific situations.

Classen DC: Clinical decision support systems to improve clinical practice and quality of care. JAMA 1998;280: 1360. [NLM Cit ID: 99008449]

Grundmeier R et al: House staff attitudes toward computer-based clinical decision support. Proc AMIA Symposium 1999:266. [NLM Cit ID: 20032872]

Hunt DL et al: Effects of computer-based clinical decision support systems on physician performance and patient outcomes: A systematic review. JAMA 1998;280:1339. [NLM Cit ID: 99008446]

Teich JM et al: Clinical decision support systems come of age. MD Computing 2000;17:43. (Structured overview and categorization of clinical decision support systems.)

PALM DIGITAL ASSISTANTS (Handhelds)

Most clinicians purchase and use palm digital assistants for access to personal information. Handheld devices are convenient for keeping track of schedules, to-do lists, and contact information. The devices vary widely in the number of entries and amount of detail they can accommodate, but a defining feature of all handhelds is their ability to synchronize directly with a conventional PC to maintain up-to-date data on both devices. The utility and functionality of handhelds is significantly extended for physicians through specifically designed third-party software.

However, limited storage, less than full-size keyboards, and less than full-featured software restrict the clinician's ability to do much work. Instead, these devices are designed for limited data handling, particularly for data reference and minor data creation tasks such as recording expenses and writing notes, memos, and e-mail. Handheld devices also often in-

Table 42–9. Functional classes and examples of clinical decision support systems.

Class	Function	Examples
Feedback	Provide feedback by responding to an action taken by the clinician or to new data entered into the system	Drug family checking results in alerts on allergies, drug-drug interactions, and other patient-specific conflicts Parameter checking looks for dosing errors and other parameter discrepancies in patient-specific scenarios (eg, gentamicin dosing in renal failure) Redundant utilization checking alerts physicians to duplicate test orders
Data organization	Organization and presentation of disparate data into logical, intuitive schemas at the point-of-need	Aggregate data trending observe key indicators for large numbers of patients over time (eg, emergence of antibiotic resistance patterns)
Proactive information	Provision of information to the clinician at the point-of-need (eg, clinical pathway on pneumonia when patient with pneumonia being admitted to hospital)	Template and order sets can be provided appropriate to given situations
Intelligent actions	Automation of routine and repeated tasks for the clinician on a regular time schedule (eg, provision of all new laboratory values on current patient list every morning)	Rule-based event detection allows users to create logical rules to be checked when triggering events occur (eg, check glucose level in hyponatremia) Time-based checks post reminders when expected transactions have not occurred (eg, warfarin order not filled by 8:00 PM)
Communication	Alert clinician and other providers who need to know about unusual data (eg, test results) or communications regarding specific patients	Parameter alerts provide clinicians with key information on panic values Automated e-mails send information to clinicians when provider-patient encounters occur (eg, e-mail to primary doctor when patient evaluated in the emergency department)

clude software that can import and read word processing, spreadsheet, and limited database files and to display (but not to edit) slide presentations.

Communication through standard telephone line, wireless modems, or networks is also possible. However, most models do not come with internal modems; rather, they require the user to purchase an external modem. Though still in their infancy, wireless services enable the clinician to send and receive e-mail, pages, and to access Web-based information with a handheld device when away from a telephone line.

All handheld devices include at least rudimentary personal-information-management programs to help the busy clinician keep track of his or her schedule, tasks, to-do lists, and contact information. Synchronization software for updating the data and coordinating it with information on a PC is standard. Additional capabilities of handheld devices include file-transfer utilities; backup utilities; personal financial applications including budget utilities, expense trackers, investment programs, and security programs; communications programs; and mapping and navigation programs. Some devices also offer digital imagery programs and spoken and music audio software. Some handheld devices have voice-recording capability, including an internal microphone and speaker and software packaged in the base models. This functionality may be useful for dictation and voice messaging. Currently, however, no software is available to convert voice to text using a handheld device. Vertical applications are available for medicine. Applications specific to medical productivity exist in abundance and are outlined in Table 42–10.

Clinical calculators perform a variety of pertinent clinical functions such as medication calculations

Table 42–10. Categorization of medicine-specific palm digital assistant applications.

Category	Example Applications
Clinical calculators	Intravenous antibiotic and pressor drip calculator Fractional excretion of sodium Caloric converter Estimated date of confinement
Medical databases	Microbes, diseases Pediatric immunization schedule Laboratory tests Differential diagnosis generators
Drug references	Adult and pediatric drug dosing guides
Information management	Patient charting and clinical management Procedure and case logs Prescription generators

(eg, intravenous antibiotic and pressor drip calculations), clinical parameter calculations (eg, fractional excretion of sodium and free water deficit) and physiology calculators (eg, caloric converters, pregnancy estimated date of confinement). Medical databases include collections of useful information on such topics as microbial diseases, immunization schedules, and interpretation of laboratory tests. Drug references provide easy access to comprehensive databases on adult and pediatric drug dosing, regimens, contraindications, adverse reactions, pregnancy and lactation, and mode of metabolism or excretion. Finally, information management applications provide extended functionality through innovative patient charting and clinical management software, procedure and case log, and electronic prescription generators.

[ePocrates]

http://www.epocrates.com (A commercial Web site offering a free drug database for the Palm OS. The database provides adult and pediatric drug dosing schedules in addition to information on adverse effects, drug interactions, and contraindications.)

MEDICAL CODING & TERMINOLOGY

Medical classification systems are tools used for bringing semantic and conceptual order to the chaos inherent in the enormously complex practice of medicine. Once thought to be the exclusive domain of data analysts and bureaucrats, disease coding and classification have increasingly become important for clinicians to understand. Many large epidemiologic studies published in major medical journals rely exclusively on disease coding for patient selection and stratification. Political and economic public health decisions are frequently made on the basis of data collected via specialized classification systems. And unfortunately, disease coding can intrude on the patient-physician relationship if it is allowed to dictate reimbursements, elements of the clinical encounter, documentation, and appropriateness of testing and treatment.

One of the most influential classification systems in use today is the World Health Organization's International Classification of Diseases (Table 42–11). It is currently in its tenth formal revision (ICD-10), though many institutions have not yet upgraded from ICD-9. It divides all of medicine into 21 "chapters," with titles like Diseases of the Digestive System, or External Causes of Morbidity and Mortality. Each chapter is subdivided into blocks, categories, and subcategories, to allow increasing level of detail—nearly 8000 in all. Categorization is inconsistent and incomplete: code outlines can be derived from anatomy, etiology, or epidemiology and frequently end with the category "not elsewhere classified" (NEC) or "not otherwise specified" (NOS). Although ICD was originally designed for epidemiology and health statistics, clinical modifications (ICD-10-CM) have been created that contain more clinical detail for use with billing, medical review, and reimbursement, raising the number of categories to 50,000. So, for example, while ICD-10 may have categories that correspond loosely to the level of information found on a death certificate, ICD-10-CM would be able to categorize the fine detail found in that patient's hospital chart.

In an attempt to correlate diagnosis with cost of treatment, the United States Health Care Finance Administration created Diagnosis Related Groups (DRG) (Table 42–11). There are about 500 DRG codes in 23 Major Diagnostic Categories, derived to simplify adult inpatient Medicare billing, each corresponding to a patient's principal diagnosis or procedure and associated with a standardized cost. These correlations can be used to help determine an institution's case-mix or a population's relative severity of illness. Many different ICD codes may fall under a single DRG code—as long as the diseases they represent incur similar inpatient expenses.

Table 42–11. Examples of medical coding and terminology classification systems.

ICD-9	786.52 Painful respiration
SNOMED	F-37070 Crushing chest pain & F-37022 & Substernal chest pain & (G-CO40 T-D8 200) & radiating to the left arm
DRG	247, Circulatory disease with MI, w/o invasive investigation or procedure, died
CPT	58150, Total abdominal hysterectomy (corpus and cervix), with or without removal of tube(s), with or without removal of ovary(ies)
MeSH	Cardiovascular diseases [C14] Heart diseases [C14.280] Myocardial ischemia [C14.280.647] Coronary disease [C14.280.647.250] Angina pectoris [C14.280.647.250.125] Angina, unstable [C14.280.647.250.125.150]

There are many other coding systems, each designed for a different purpose (Table 42-11). Current Procedural Terminology (CPT) is a listing of descriptive terms and identifying codes created by the American Medical Association for reporting medical services and procedures—again for billing. The Systematized Nomenclature of Medicine (SNOMED) is a general purpose nomenclature designed to encompass all of the events in the medical record; unlike CPT, it is intended not for billing but for the standardization of databases, trials, and comparative information. Medical Subject Headings (MeSH) are devised by librarians at the National Library of Medicine to create a loose hierarchy for structuring the medical literature.

Most coding systems are created with very specific purposes in mind, and they usually succeed. However, problems occur when coding systems are applied to tasks for which they were not originally intended.

[Duke Healthcare Informatics Links to Coding Systems]
http://www.mcis.duke.edu/standards/termcode/codehome.htm

[EICD.com]
http://www.eicd.com/ (Online resource for looking up ICD-9 and CPT codes.)

Brett AS: New guidelines for coding physicians' services—a step backward. N Engl J Med 1998;339:1705. [NLM Cit ID: 99041185] (A strongly worded critique of the inappropriate practice of applying a coding system created for billing to patient encounters.)

RELEVANT WORLD WIDE WEB SITES

[American Medical Informatics Association]
http://www.amia.org

[American Medical Informatics Management Association]
http://www.ahima.org

[Handbook of Medical Informatics]
http://www.mihandbook.stanford.edu/handbook/home.htm

[Health on the Net Foundation Code of Conduct]
http://www.hon.ch/HONcode/Conduct.html

[MedHunt]
http://www.hon.ch/MedHunt

[Medical Informatics Taxonomy]
http://www.med.usf.edu/CLASS/ovrview2.htm

[National Academy Press Reading Room—Medical Technologies]
http://www.nap.edu/readingroom/enter2.cgi?MS.html

[National Center for Emergency Medicine Informatics]
http://www.ncemi.org

[On-line Lessons in Clinical Informatics]
http://www.informatics-review.com/lessons.html

[OncoLink's Editors' Choice Awards]
http://nisc8a.upenn.edu/ed_choice

43 Complementary & Alternative Medicine

See http://www.current-med.com/ch43.html for updated addresses of Web sites referenced in this chapter.

Bradly Jacobs, MD, & Brian Berman, MD

The use of complementary and alternative medicine has become common in the United States. To maintain effective clinician-patient communication and ensure responsible clinical practice, it is important that clinicians learn the theory, practice, and scientific evidence associated with these therapies. This chapter provides an overview of four alternative medicine therapies: herbal medicine, nonherbal dietary supplements, acupuncture, and homeopathy.

Background

In the United States, a 1998 survey by Eisenberg estimated that over 40% of the general population made over 629 million visits to alternative medicine practitioners and spent over $27 billion in out-of-pocket expenditures for their services and therapies. These figures exceeded the total number of visits to all United States primary care physicians and approximate the out-of-pocket expenditures for all physician services.

Common indications for seeking this care include acute musculoskeletal strain and chronic conditions such as back pain, anxiety, depression, insomnia, chronic pain, and addiction. A 1998 survey by Astin identified the following predictors for Americans who use this category of care: higher education, poorer health status, having had an experience that caused a change in worldview, a holistic orientation toward life, and identification with a cultural group that has a commitment to women's rights, environmentalism, spirituality, and personal growth psychology. Of patients using alternative medicine, only 4% used it exclusively, rejecting conventional medicine.

Within the conventional medical paradigm, efforts are being made to understand this phenomenon. A significant minority of medical schools offer elective courses. Special interest groups to discuss the role of alternative medicine have been organized in the Association of American Medical Colleges, the Society of Teachers of Family Medicine, and the American Public Health Association. Private and public hospitals are providing outpatient and inpatient clinical services for people seeking such care. Funding for biomedical research in this field has increased dramatically. The National Institutes of Health established the Office of Alternative Medicine in 1992 with an annual budget of $2 million; in 2000, its role was expanded as the National Center for Complementary and Alternative Medicine with an annual budget of $68.7 million and with its own peer review committee. As recipients of both NIH and private funding, several medical universities now conduct research, educate students, and provide clinical alternative medicine services. In 1998, JAMA and its ten affiliated Archives journals published theme issues including more than 80 articles pertaining to the field.

In 1996, Washington State passed legislation requiring insurance companies to reimburse policy holders for all treatments provided as alternative medicine. Across the United States, recognizing the large public outcry for these services, many health insurance companies have voluntarily expanded benefit packages—for an additional charge—to include a limited number of treatments.

As of 1998, statutory licensure of practitioners exists for chiropractors in all 50 states, for acupuncturists in 35 states, for massage therapists in 27 states, for practitioners of naturopathic medicine in 14 states, and for homeopathic practitioners in 4 states. Insurance coverage is mandated for the costs of chiropractic medicine in 42 states and for costs of acupuncture in 7 states.

The National Institutes of Health divides this field into six major categories: mind-body medicine, alternative medical systems, lifestyle modification and disease prevention, biologically based therapies, manipulative and body-based systems, and bioelectromagnetics. Herbs and nonherbal dietary supplements, which are classified as biologically based therapies, and acupuncture and homeopathy, which are classified under alternative medical systems, will be the focus of this chapter.

Astin JA: Why patients use alternative medicine: results of a national study. JAMA 1998;279:1548. [NLM Cit ID: 98266936]

Eisenberg DM et al: Trends in alternative medicine use in the United States, 1990–1997. JAMA 1998;280;1569. [NLM Cit ID: 99036143]

Levin J, Jonas W: *Essentials of Complementary and Alternative Medicine.* Lippincott Williams & Wilkins, 1999.

HERBAL MEDICINES

Epidemiology

The use of herbs for medicinal purposes has dramatically increased over the past decade in the United States. Annual sales for herbal medicines totaled $350 million in 1980 and have increased to $4 billion dollars in 1998, averaging a 30% increase in sales annually. In Germany, herbs comprise about 30% of all drugs sold in pharmacies, with two-thirds of physicians prescribing one-third of these products. St. John's wort is used seven times more frequently than fluoxetine to treat depression in Germany.

In the 1850s, 80% of medicines in the *United States Pharmacopeia* derived from plants. Today, roughly 20–30% of the pharmacopeia originates from plants—examples are atropine, colchicine, digoxin, emetine, and many antineoplastic agents. Although many medicinal herbs are relatively safe, some can have significant toxicity. For example, chaparral, with purported anticancer effects, can be hepatotoxic. Ma-huang contains ephedrine and related alkaloids and is sold in many formulations, including weight loss products such as "herbal fen-phen" or as a euphoriant called "herbal ecstasy." Over 800 cases of adverse events associated with this product have been reported to the FDA. Sympathomimetic effects include tremors, severe hypertension, seizures, and arrhythmias. These may lead to myocardial infarction, stroke, and death. In response, the FDA has proposed dosage limits and advised patients with hypertension, glaucoma, seizure disorders, and coronary artery disease to avoid using this product.

Only a minority of herbs have been tested in controlled clinical studies. Recent technologic advances and commercial enthusiasm have modified the traditional manufacturing process. Traditionally, herbalists were intimately involved with the cultivation, preparation, and prescribing process and could readily verify plant speciation and potency. Herbal products today are cultivated and processed in unregulated environments with varying quality assurance protocols. These products are then packaged into capsules or tablets, making quality assurance for species identification, potency, contaminants, adulterants, and heavy metals impossible without expensive laboratory testing. They are then marketed directly to the consumer, bypassing the participation of the health care provider. Therefore, despite abundant historical accounts of experience with these agents supervised by herbalists, unsupervised use of unregulated over-the-counter botanicals by the public is a new phenomenon.

Regulatory Issues

In response to FDA discussions about the possible benefits of regulating herbal medicines, the United States Congress passed the Dietary Supplement and Health Education Act (DSHEA) in 1994. This act limited the FDA's regulatory control over dietary supplements and herbs. Items defined within this act include vitamins, herbs, minerals, amino acids, and any article said to "supplement" the diet. Prior to enactment of DSHEA, these substances were considered foods or food additives, and manufacturers were allowed to make health claims based only on the nutritive value of their products. The Act permitted manufacturers to make "structure and function" claims about these items not based on their nutritive value. As a result, they were no longer considered food additives, and no premarketing screening for product safety, effectiveness, and quality is required. Premarketing screening for articles such as drugs takes approximately 17 years and costs $500 million per product. Since passage of DSHEA, manufacturers increasingly utilize direct consumer advertising to promote the health claims of their products. Herbs are primarily purchased in a health food store, grocery store, pharmacy, or on the Internet without supervision from a health care provider.

Manufacturers can claim that a product enhances the normal structure and function of the body or any of its constituent parts without submitting supporting evidence to the FDA or any other regulatory body. For example, a manufacturer can claim that Choleston promotes "cholesterol health" but cannot claim that the product reduces elevated cholesterol levels or prevents myocardial infarction.

Unlike drugs, these articles do not require the manufacturer to provide sufficient evidence of safety and efficacy to justify their health claims. To disprove health claims made by the manufacturers, the FDA must prove that these substances impose an unreasonable risk of illness or injury.

Legislation now pending may regulate manufacturers and give them the option of obtaining 7-year patents for herbal compounds, thus creating incentives for manufacturers to conduct research for safety and efficacy. In Germany, for example, herbal medicines are regulated. The German Federal Health Agency Commission E was formed in the 1970s to investigate these products and publish an opinion about their safety and effectiveness. Over 400 monographs have been produced on over 350 herbal preparations. Since the United States has no such regulatory system, patients are advised to follow certain guidelines when considering whether to use herbal medicines (Table 43–1).

Quality Assurance

Quality assurance entails upholding standards for microbiologic content, heavy metal content, moisture content, potency, toxic residues, chemical analysis, and ash levels. Since there are few quality assurance regulations or guidelines for these products in the United States, the Corporate Alliance for Integrative Medicine (CAIM) was formed to provide seed moneys for research in this emerging industry. This group is made up of ten manufacturers and suppliers interested in cooperating with academic institutions to perform basic research in this field. The European Scientific Cooperative for Phytotherapy (ESCOP) pursues similar goals.

Product Standardization

The European scientific community has played a significant role in identifying active ingredients in herbal products and in determining their mechanisms of action. This work has laid the foundation for developing guidelines for standardization of active ingredients and conducting phase II and phase III clinical trials. Standardization of herbs ensures a consistent percentage of the primary active ingredients across batches and brand names. Investigators can combine historical documentation of safety with proposed active ingredients and mechanisms of action to develop a rational approach to studying several promising herbal preparations using randomized controlled clinical trial methodology.

Since multiple constituents may have pharmacologic activity, determining the active ingredient for standardization purposes may be difficult in some cases. Variability in clinical outcomes or toxic effects between studies for a given intervention may result from inconsistent potency due to regional and seasonal variability, inappropriate harvesting and preparation methods, or misidentification of plant species.

Herbal formulations available include liquids (extracts, tinctures, infusions, and decoctions) and fresh, dried, and powdered preparations. More recently, standardized extracts have been developed to provide a standard potency that will ensure consistency in dose. This requires identification of the active ingredients, which are extracted and processed. However, the active ingredients have been identified for only a select group of herbs. Furthermore, although concentration of the product can be guaranteed, there is great inconsistency of herb potency within a single herb farm from year to year as a result of changes in growing conditions. To verify correlation between dosage and potency, one must perform bioassay testing.

Table 43–1. Advice to patients using herbal medicines.

Communication
- Discuss use of all therapies with your primary care provider.

Product Quality
- There is no regulatory body looking out for your best interest.
- Be skeptical of manufacturer health claims.
- Manufacturers are not required to submit evidence to the FDA or any regulatory body to demonstrate product safety, effectiveness, or quality.
- Ask your primary care provider, a pharmacist, or a trained herbalist regarding the specific herbs you are using.
- Use herbs that are standardized to contain a specific quantity of the active ingredients.
- Preferentially select herbs that are produced by larger companies. They are more likely to ensure product quality in order to protect their reputation.

Labeling
- It should state the common and scientific names of herb(s).
- It should state the concentration or dose of the herb(s) and provide instructions on dose and frequency.
- It should state that the product is "standardized" to contain a certain amount of the active ingredient(s).
- It should state the methods used to ensure product quality.
- It should state the name and address of the manufacturer.
- It should state the batch or lot number and the expiration date.
- It should list potential side effects and interactions.

Pregnancy
- Few herbs have been studied for safety during pregnancy.
- Seek advice from your primary care provider before using herbs during pregnancy.

Interactions
- Discuss with your primary care provider the safety profile and interactions that may occur when combining herbs and when taking herbs plus drugs.

Reporting
- Report any adverse reactions to your state poison control program or the FDA.

REVIEW OF THE EVIDENCE FOR SELECTED HERBAL MEDICINES

Table 43–2 provides an overview of selected herbal medicines.

Barrett B et al: Assessing the risks and benefits of herbal medicine: Overview of scientific evidence. Altern Ther Health 1999;5:40. [NLM Cit ID: 99322977]

Blumenthal M: *The Complete German Commission E Monographs. Therapeutic Guide to Herbal Medicines.* American Botanical Council. Integrative Medicine Communications, 1998.

Fetrow C, Avila J: *Professional's Handbook of Complementary and Alternative Medicine.* Springhouse Publications, 1999.

Klepser TB et al: Unsafe and potentially safe herbal therapies. Am J Health Syst Pharm 1999;56:125. [NLM Cit ID: 99153600]

O'Hara M et al: A review of 12 commonly used medicinal herbs. Arch Fam Med 1998;7:523. [NLM Cit ID: 99037588]

Shulz V, Hansel R, Tyler VE: *Rational Phytotherapy: A Physician's Guide to Herbal Medicine.* Springer, 1998.

Table 43–2. Overview of selected herbal medicines.

	Leading Indications	Active Constituents	Mechanism of Action	Standardized Complex	Dosage	Efficacy:[1] Size of Effect	Safety[2]	Interaction; Side Effects	Comments	Cost per Day[3]
Echinancea (purple cone-flower)	Treatment and prevention of URIs	Isobutyl-amides, chichoric acid, polyenes, alkaloids, and alkylamides	Immunostimulant, phagocytosis, cytokines (IL-1, TNF, IFN)	Fresh-pressed juice of *E purpurae* with 2.4% β-1,2- fructo-furanosides, in 20% ethanol solute.	300 mg, or 3 mL q3–4 h	C: minimal	A	None known; rash, pruritis, nausea.	Avoid in immuno-compromised patients; avoid use > 4 weeks	$1.25–2.00
Garlic *(Allium sativum)*	1. Hypercholesterolemia 2. Hypertension 3. Coronary artery disease	Allicin	1. HMG CoA-reductase, 14α-demethylase 2. Unclear 3. Antiplatelet effects	Allicin 0.6–1.3%	600–900 mg qd	1. A: small 2. B: absent 3. C	A	None known; bloating, flatulence		$0.04–0.12
Ginkgo biloba (EGB 761, GBE)	Dementia, claudication	Flavonoid glycosides, terpenes such as ginkgolide B	PAF inhibition, antioxidant, reduction of capillary fragility	24% flavonoid glycoside	40 mg tid	A: Moderate. Several studies with positive results.	B	Anticoagulants; may have anticoagulant effect.	Use caution if allergic to urusiols (mango rind, sumac-poison ivy, cashew nuts)	$0.30–0.50
Asian ginseng *(Panax ginseng)*	Stamina, aphrodisiac, fertility, "tonic," "energy-booster"	Ginsenosides	Unclear	> 2% ginsenosides	200–600 mg qd extract; 1–2 g crude drug	D: mixed. Multiple studies but few for any given indication.	A		Take no longer than 12 weeks (potential hormone-inducing effects). Previous reports of toxicity have been attributed to aldulterants.	$0.30–2.00

(*continued*)

Table 43–2. Overview of selected herbal medicines (continued).

	Leading Indications	Active Constituents	Mechanism of Action	Standardized Complex	Dosage	Efficacy:[1] Size of Effect	Safety[2]	Interaction; Side Effects	Comments	Cost per Day[3]
Milk thistle (silymarin)	1. Chronic liver disease 2. Acute hepatic failure	Silymarin complex (silybin, silychristin, and silydianin)	Antioxidant, antifibrotic, protein synthesis, toxin blockade	Silymarin 70–80%	140 mg tid	A–: survival benefit	A	None known; no greater than placebo (gastrointestinal, headache, skin).	No antiviral effect	\$0.40–1.00
St. John's wort *(Hypericum perforatum)*	Depression	Napthodianthrones (such as hypericum), flavonoids, and xanthones	Unclear; SSRI, GABA, MAO effects in vitro	Hypericin 0.3% 0.5–3 mg hypericin	300 mg tid 2–4 g powdered herb	A–: moderate; NIH-funded multicenter randomized controlled trial ongoing.	A	Cyclosporine, protease inhibitors, oral contraceptives, warfarin, digoxin		\$0.50–1.00
Saw palmetto *(Serenoa repens)*	Benign prostatic hyperplasia	Sterols, free fatty acids	5α-Reductase inhibition; inhibition of DHT binding to androgen receptor	85–95% sterols and fatty acids	160 mg bid	B+: moderate; NIH-funded randomized controlled trial ongoing.	A	Mild gastrointestinal disturbances and headaches (each rare)	May alter PSA levels	\$0.30–0.60

[1]Efficacy: A, good evidence; B, some evidence; C, insufficient evidence; D, some evidence showing no effect; E, significant evidence showing no effect; F, evidence showing contrary effect.
[2]Safety: A, generally safe; B, relatively safe; C, insufficient evidence; D, may be harmful; E, clear evidence of harm.
[3]Average range of costs in retail drug stores.

Garlic

Garlic is one of the most popular herbal remedies and is readily available in fresh, dried, and powdered forms. The German Federal Health Agency Commission E and the European Scientific Cooperative on Phytotherapy have approved garlic for the treatment of hyperlipidemia and atherosclerosis. Allicin, the active ingredient associated with garlic's therapeutic benefit, is highly unstable and odoriferous. Both heat and acid destroy the enzyme, allinase, which is necessary to produce allicin, and for that reason garlic is best ingested raw. Garlic is also available over the counter in multiple formulations; the most active form is the enteric-coated capsule of dehydrated garlic. The coating permits allicin to be released in the small intestine, thereby enhancing release and absorption and reducing the breath odor. Dehydrated preparations retain most of the active constituents found in the raw form. Over-the-counter preparations frequently are standardized as to dosage.

Garlic appears to have modest effects on cholesterol and on blood flow and minimal to no effect on blood pressure and glucose levels. The mechanisms of action thought to underlie the lipid-lowering effects include HMG-CoA reductase and 14α-demethylase inhibitors. Garlic is well tolerated and apparently safe for chronic use. In addition to the well-known breath and body odor associated with garlic, adverse events reported have included flatulence, esophageal and abdominal pain, small intestinal obstruction, dermatitis, rhinitis, asthma, and increased risk of bleeding, but there is insufficient evidence to determine a causal association. A recent systematic review by Ackerman funded by the Agency for Health Care Policy and Research identified thirty-six randomized controlled trials on the use of garlic for the treatment of cardiovascular risk factors. Among the 26 trials evaluating hyperlipidemia, small but statistically significant reductions (16 mg/dL) were found for total cholesterol at 3 months among patients treated with garlic compared with placebo. Among the eight trials with outcomes at 6 months, no significant reductions in lipids were seen with garlic compared with placebo. In a qualitative review of antithrombotic effects, a modest and short-term effect was identified. Effects on glucose and blood pressure were none to minimal in studies reviewed.

Silagy and Neil reviewed 16 randomized controlled clinical trials representing 952 patients for the treatment of hyperlipidemia with garlic and found approximately 12% total cholesterol and triglyceride reductions. They also performed a meta-analysis of garlic for the treatment of hypertension and found a pooled mean blood pressure reduction of 8 mm Hg systolic and 5 mm Hg diastolic between groups. Warshafsky performed a meta-analysis of garlic's effect on hyperlipidemia with more restricted inclusion criteria which identified only five trials and found a 23 mg/dL lower total cholesterol among patients treated with garlic compared with those receiving placebo.

Neil H et al : Garlic powder in the treatment of moderate hyperlipidaemia: a controlled trial and meta-analysis. J R Coll Physicians Lond 1996;30:329. [NLM Cit ID: 97029368]

Silagy C et al: Garlic as a lipid lowering agent: a meta-analysis. J R Coll Physicians Lond 1994;28 39. [NLM Cit ID: 94223605]

Warshafsky S et al Effect of garlic on total serum cholesterol. A meta-analysis. Ann Intern Med 1993;119:599. [NLM Cit ID: 93370791]

St. John's Wort (*Hypericum perforatum*)

St. John's wort is commonly used in Europe for the treatment of depression. It also has purported usefulness when applied topically to promote healing of wounds and burns. The German Federal Health Agency Commission E approved it for the treatment of mild to moderate depression and anxiety. Multiple constituents identified as potential active ingredients include naphthodianthrones, flavonoids, and xanthones. Most preparations are standardized to hypericin content (a naphthodianthrone). Recent data indicate that there are multiple other active ingredients as well. The highest potency can be found in the flowering tops. The mechanism of action is not known. Irreversible MAO-inhibitory properties noted in vitro have not been observed in vivo. Other postulated mechanisms include serotonin reuptake inhibition, synaptic uptake of GABA, and binding to GABA receptors.

St. John's wort appears as effective as and better tolerated than tricyclic antidepressants at low to moderate doses for the treatment of mild to moderate depression. Duke University is currently conducting a multicenter randomized controlled trial funded by the National Institutes of Health that will address some of the methodologic issues raised in earlier studies, including long-term effectiveness and relative efficacy compared with the newer SSRIs. Side effects include mild photosensitivity, gastrointestinal irritation, and restlessness. Because of its abortifacient properties, St. John's wort should not be taken during pregnancy. Patients are advised to avoid concurrent ingestion with MAO inhibitors, serotonin reuptake inhibitors, and tyramine-containing foods because of the drug's postulated MAO-inhibitory activity.

Linde et al reviewed 23 randomized controlled trials totaling 1757 subjects with mild to moderate depression comparing St. John's wort with placebo or tricyclic antidepressants; inclusion criteria required the use of validated depression scales as the primary outcome measurement. Treatment response was defined as a 50% improvement, or less than 10 points scored at study end. Results indicated that hypericin 0.5–2.7 mg daily (350–1000 mg/d hypericum extract) was superior to placebo in achieving this response

(OR = 2.7; 95% CI, 1.8–4.0) and was equivalent to tricyclic antidepressants such as imipramine 50–75 mg/d, maprotiline 75 mg/d, desipramine 100–150 mg/d, and amitriptyline 30 mg/d (OR = 1.1; 95% CI, 0.9–1.3). Side effects occurred in over 50% of patients taking conventional antidepressants compared with 20% of patients taking St. John's wort. Subsequent studies found equal efficacy of St. John's wort compared with tricyclic antidepressants, with better tolerance.

Gaster B et al: St. John's wort for depression: A systematic review. Am J Med 2000;160:152. [NLM Cit ID: 20112278]

Linde K et al: St John's wort for depression: an overview and meta-analysis of randomised clinical trials. BMJ 1996;313:253. [NLM Cit ID: 96322668]

Vorbach EU et al: Effectiveness and tolerance of the hypericum extract LI 160 in comparison with imipramine: randomized double blind study of 135 outpatients. J Geriatr Psychiatry Neurol 1994;7:S19. [NLM Cit ID: 95160914]

Wheatley D: LI 160, an extract of St John's wort, versus amitriptyline in mildly to moderately depressed outpatients: a controlled 6-week clinical trial. Pharmacopsychiatry 1997;30:77. [NLM Cit ID: 98002171]

Ginkgo

Ginkgo ranks first in sales among herbal medications sold in health food stores. Its use for medicinal purposes can be traced to the Chinese *Materia Medica* more than 2000 years ago. Ginkgo is derived from the dried green leaves of the *Ginkgo biloba* tree. The German Federal Health Agency Commission E has approved a standardized form of ginkgo leaf extract (Egb 761) for the treatment of cognitive impairment and intermittent claudication. In Germany, more than 5 million prescriptions for ginkgo are written annually. Several ingredients are considered pharmacologically active, including the flavonoid glycosides, which are thought to have antioxidant activity and to reduce capillary fragility; and a terpene called ginkgolide B, which is considered to have potent platelet-activating factor antagonist effect on platelet aggregation. The extract has been standardized to contain 24% flavonoid glycosides, 6% terpene lactones, and less than 5 parts per million of ginkgolic acids.

Ginkgo is effective in treating mild to moderate dementia and has modest efficacy in treating intermittent claudication. The NIH has recently funded at the University of Pittsburgh a study of the effect of ginkgo for the prevention of dementia among patients 75 years or older. In general, this herb is well tolerated. Allergic skin reactions, gastrointestinal disturbances, and headache occur infrequently. Allergic skin reactions from the ginkgolic acids do occur rarely; since these acids have properties similar to those of the urushiols, which are found in the sumac-poison ivy family, mango rinds, and cashew nuts, patients allergic to these compounds should use ginkgo with caution. Because of a reported increased risk of bleeding among patients using ginkgo, caution should be exercised when combining this herb with anticoagulants such as warfarin, aspirin, and NSAIDs.

A 1998 review identified 50 trials that assessed ginkgo's efficacy on cognitive function in the elderly; however, the vast majority did not require a definitive diagnosis of dementia or Alzheimer's disease. Consequently, only four trials involving 424 patients met study entry criteria for meta-analysis (Table 43–3), with results showing a modest effect on cognitive function when compared with the placebo group. This effect is considered comparable to the effect of donepezil on dementia.

Pittler and Ernst recently performed a meta-analysis on eight randomized, placebo-controlled, double-blinded trials involving 418 patients to evaluate the efficacy of ginkgo for the treatment of intermittent claudication. They found a modest treatment difference in the increase of pain-free walking distance in favor of ginkgo over placebo. No significant adverse events were reported.

Jacobs BP et al: Ginkgo biloba: A living fossil. Am J Med 2000;108:341.

Kleijnen J et al: Ginkgo biloba for cerebral insufficiency. Br J Clin Pharmacol 1992;34:352. [NLM Cit ID: 93090574]

Table 43–3. Individual and summary estimates of effect size for trials evaluating the efficacy of ginkgo for the treatment of Alzheimer's disease and dementia.[1]

Source	Daily Dose	Duration	Sample Size	Effect Size[2]	95% Confidence Interval	*p* Value
Wesnes et al, 1987	120 mg	12 wks	52	0.11	−0.44 to +0.65	.69
Hofferberth et al, 1994	240 mg	12 wks	40	1.12	0.45 to 1.78	.001
Kanowski et al, 1996	240 mg	24 wks	125	0.52	0.16 to 0.87	.005
LeBars et al, 1997	120 mg	26 wks	207	0.31	0.04 to 0.59	.03
Overall			424	0.41	0.22 to 0.61	< .0001

[1]Modified with permission from Oken BS et al: The efficacy of Ginkgo biloba on cognitive funtion in Alzheimer disease. Arch Neurol 1998;55:1409.

[2]Effect on cognitive subtest of Alzheimer Disease Assessment Scale.

Oken B et al: The efficacy of ginkgo biloba on cognitive function in Alzheimer disease. Arch Neurol 1998;55:1409. [NLM Cit ID: 99039429]

Echinacea

Echinacea ranks in the top three herbs in the United States, accounting for more than $300 million in sales annually. It is known as the purple coneflower and is native to North America. In the 1920s, echinacea tincture was a popular anti-infective until the discovery of antibiotics. Currently, it is used for the treatment and prevention of upper respiratory infections. Above-ground parts and roots of *Echinacea pallida, E angustifolia,* and, most commonly, *E purpurea* are used for medicinal purposes. Choice of plant part, active compounds for standardization, and dosage are not well defined. Several active ingredients have been identified, including isobutylamides, chicoric acid, polyenes, alkaloids, and alkylamides. Postulated mechanisms of action from in vitro and animal studies suggest that active ingredients cause stimulation of natural killer cells, macrophages, and cytokine activity.

Most of the published laboratory and clinical research about echinacea has been performed in Germany. The overall study quality of clinical trials has been fair. Many trials did not employ randomized, placebo-controlled, double-blind methodology, and others have studied echinacea as part of a combination of herbs. Overall, there is inconclusive evidence to support the use of echinacea for the prevention or treatment of upper respiratory infections. In general, it is well tolerated, with few reported adverse events.

Brinkeborn RM et al: Echinaforce and other Echinacea fresh plant preparations in the treatment of the common cold. A randomized, placebo controlled, double-blind clinical trial. Phytomedicine 1999;6:1. [NLM Cit ID: 99245288]

Grimm W et al: A randomized controlled trial of the effect of fluid extract of *Echinacea purpurea* on the incidence and severity of colds and respiratory infections. Am J Med 1999;106:138. [NLM Cit ID: 99245772]

Melchart D et al: Echinacea for the prevention and treatment of the common cold. Cochrane Review Issue 1 ed: The Cochrane Library. Oxford: Update Software; 1999.

Melchart D et al: Echinacea root extracts for the prevention of upper respiratory tract infections: a double-blind, placebo-controlled randomized trial. Arch Fam Med 1998;7:541. [NLM Cit ID: 99037590]

Milk Thistle

In the first century, Dioscorides and Pliny the Elder described using milk thistle "for those bitten by serpents" and for "carrying off the bile." Currently, this herb is used in oral form to treat chronic liver disease of various causes. In Europe, based on case series evidence, it has been given parenterally to treat acute hepatic failure from amanita mushroom poisoning. Silymarin, the active complex, is extracted from the seeds of the plant to create a product which is standardized to 70–80% silymarin content. Silymarin is composed of three isomers: silybin (the most active compound), silychristin, and silydianin. Postulated mechanisms of action include antioxidant activity, antifibrotic activity, toxin blockade, and enhanced protein synthesis.

A systematic review identified 15 randomized controlled trials using milk thistle in the treatment of acute and chronic liver disease. Fourteen out of 15 trials evaluated patients with chronic liver disease. Three trials assessed survival and found a one-third lower mortality rate over the 4- to 5-year follow-up period in the milk thistle group compared with placebo. Milk thistle was well tolerated. There was inconclusive evidence for its effects on liver biopsy specimens, and it appeared to have little or no effect on aminotransferase levels.

Flora K et al: Milk thistle *(Silybum marianum)* for the therapy of liver disease. Am J Gastroenterol 1998;93:139. [NLM Cit ID: 98127747]

Ginseng

Ginseng root has been used for medicinal purposes in Asia for over 2000 years. There are three forms of ginseng in use today. *Panax ginseng,* which is known as Asian ginseng, is commonly used in the United States. It is a perennial herb with multibranched roots and a fragrant odor. *Panax quinquefolius* is cultivated in the United States and exported to China. *Eleutherococcus senticosus,* or Siberian ginseng, is not a member of the panax genus. The German Federal Health Agency Commission E monograph on ginseng root approves its use as "a tonic to counteract weakness and fatigue, as a restorative for declining stamina and impaired concentration, and as an aid to convalescence." The extracts are made from dried roots, which contain ginsenosides. Over 25 ginsenosides have been isolated, each with unique and sometimes oppositional effects on the cardiovascular system, central nervous system, and immune system. The mechanisms of action have not been clearly delineated.

There is an extensive body of scientific literature on this subject, with over 400 books and papers published. Multiple indications have been studied using a variety of plant species with variable methodologic rigor. Insufficient evidence is available to support or refute the use of ginseng for any of the purported indications. Ginseng is well tolerated, with few adverse effects, and earlier reports of "ginseng abuse syndrome" and other toxicities which were secondary to identified adulterants found in the over-the-counter unregulated ginseng products have been discredited.

Ong YC et al: Panax (ginseng)—panacea or placebo? Molecular and cellular basis of its pharmacological activity.

Ann Acad Med Singapore 2000;29:42. [NLM Cit ID: 20212451]
Vogler BK et al: The efficacy of ginseng. A systematic review of randomised clinical trials. Eur J Clin Pharmacol 1999; 55:567. [NLM Cit ID: 20009422]

Saw Palmetto

Use of saw palmetto *(Serenoa repens)* for the treatment of benign prostatic hyperplasia can be traced to the early 1900s. The herb is prepared as a lipophilic extract from the berries of this short, scrubby palm. The German Federal Health Agency Commission E has approved saw palmetto for the treatment of stage I and stage II benign prostatic hyperplasia. The principal active ingredients are sterols and free fatty acids. The mechanism of action is unclear; however, there is good evidence for 5α-reductase inhibition and inhibition of dihydrotestosterone binding at the androgen receptor.

A recent systematic review of saw palmetto extracts for the treatment of benign prostatic hyperplasia identified 18 randomized controlled trials involving 2939 patients with mean study duration of 9 weeks (range, 4–48 weeks). Investigators found that saw palmetto was superior to placebo and equal to finasteride on multiple outcomes. Adverse events included gastrointestinal symptoms but were rare and mild; erectile dysfunction was more prevalent among persons using finasteride compared with saw palmetto (4.9% versus 1.1%; $p < .01$). The University of California at San Francisco is conducting a randomized controlled trial funded by the NIH to evaluate the long-term efficacy of this herb.

Wilt TW et al: Saw palmetto extracts for treatment of benign prostatic hyperplasia. JAMA 1998;280:1604. [NLM Cit ID: 99036150]

DIETARY SUPPLEMENTS

Sales of dietary supplements have increased dramatically over the past decade. The Dietary Supplement Health Education Act of 1994 has made it possible for manufacturers to sell dietary supplements directly to the public without FDA approval or oversight. Consequently, in the United States, there are no quality assurance regulations that pertain to these products. Reports of adulteration and contamination are available, but the magnitude of this problem remains unknown. Furthermore, there have been several reports of the dose printed on the label being different from the actual dose provided. (See section on herbal medicines for further details on regulatory and quality assurance issues and advice for patients to follow when purchasing these products.) Table 43–4 provides an overview of selected dietary supplements commonly used in the United States today.

S-Adenosylmethionine (SAMe; Adenometionine)

S-Adenosylmethionine is an endogenous compound that serves as a methyl group donor for hundreds of compounds, including neurotransmitters, fatty acids, nucleic acids, proteins, and membrane phospholipids. Endogenous production is dependent on vitamin B_{12} and folic acid metabolism. Primary uses of the drug include depression, osteoarthritis, fibrositis, alcoholic liver disease, and migraine headaches. Originally discovered in the 1950s, SAMe was not synthesized as a stable compound that could be made commercially available until the 1970s. SAMe is available by prescription throughout Europe. The mechanism of action is unclear for most conditions. Based on clinical trial data from over 22,000 patients, SAMe is well tolerated and safe. A phase IV open-label clinical trial involving over 20,000 patients followed for 8 weeks found 87% of the cohort reported good to very good tolerance with SAMe. There are no known drug interactions.

In the treatment of depression, SAMe may affect multiple neurotransmitters; there is evidence suggesting increased levels of serotonin, 5-hydroxyindoleacetic acid, and dopamine as well as inhibition of norepinephrine reuptake after SAMe administration. A meta-analysis published in 1994 identified 11 trials comparing SAMe with tricyclic antidepressants and 13 trials comparing either oral or parenteral formulations of SAMe with placebo. SAMe was found to be as effective as tricyclic antidepressants and superior to placebo in the treatment of depression. Furthermore, SAMe was better tolerated and had a more rapid onset of clinical effect than tricyclic antidepressants. Overall, there is moderate evidence to support the use of SAMe for the treatment of depression.

In the treatment of osteoarthritis, SAMe appears to have analgesic and anti-inflammatory properties. The mechanism of action for these effects is unknown. SAMe appears to enhance native proteoglycan production in vitro, and in animal studies SAMe is associated with higher proteoglycan content in cartilage and a reduction in surgically induced osteoarthritis following partial meniscectomy. A multicenter randomized, double-blind, placebo-controlled trial involving over 734 patients compared treatment with naproxen (750 mg daily), SAMe (1200 mg daily), and identical placebo over 30 days. Investigators found that SAMe was as effective as naproxen and superior to placebo. Patient lack of tolerability, number of patients reporting side effects, and frequency of occult blood identified in stool were higher in the naproxen-treated group compared with the SAMe or placebo groups. Other studies have shown similar efficacy when SAMe is compared with piroxicam 20

Table 43–4. Overview of selected dietary supplements

	Leading Indications	Mechanism of Action	Dosage	Efficacy[1]: Size of Effect	Safety[2]	Interactions; Side Effects
S-Adenosylmethionine (SAMe, SAM, Adomet)	1. Depression 2. Osteoarthritis 3. Alcohol-related liver cirrhosis	Unknown	200–800 mg bid	1. B– (moderate) 2. B+ (moderate to large) 3. B (survival benefit)	A	None; may precipitate mania in persons with bipolar disorder
Dehydroepiandrosterone (DHEA, DHEAS)	Depression, dysthymia, lupus, adrenal insufficiency	Unknown	50 mg qd	B– Moderate	D Long-term concerns for development of hormone-dependent malignancies	None reported; androgenic effects
Glucosamine sulfate and chondroitin (Arth-X Plus, Flexi-Factors, Glucosamine Mega)	Osteoarthritis	Proteoglycan production	Glucosamine 500 mg tid; chondroitin 400 mg tid	B+ Moderate to large	A	None reported; rare reports of constipation, diarrhea, drowsiness
Coenzyme Q10[3] (ubiquinone, ubidecarenone, Co-Q10 Heartcin)	Congestive heart failure, angina pectoris, acute myocardial infarction, periodontal disease	ATP production, membrane stabilization	50–100 mg bid; goal is to achieve serum level of 2.1 μg/mL	C	A	Use with HMG-CoA reductase inhibitors is associated with reduced endogenous coenzyme-Q10 levels; rare reports of nausea, insomnia

[1]Efficacy: A—good evidence; B—some evidence; C—insufficient evidence; D—some evidence showing no effect; E—significant evidence of contrary effect
[2]Safety: A—generally safe; B—relatively safe; C—insufficient evidence; D—may be harmful; E—clear evidence of harm
[3]Found in meat and seafood. Combined with lipid-base suspension.

mg/d, ibuprofen 1200 mg/d, and indomethacin 150 mg/d. Overall, SAMe appears to be better tolerated than and as effective as NSAIDs; however, SAMe requires a longer course of treatment to obtain desired clinical effects. Thus, there is some evidence to support the use of SAMe for the treatment of osteoarthritis.

Studies of alcohol-fed baboons suggest that SAMe increases glutathione levels and attenuates liver injury. There is some evidence that SAMe increases glutathione levels in humans as well. In liver cirrhosis, SAMe synthesis is markedly reduced. Based on this information, investigators performed a multicenter clinical randomized, double-blind, placebo-controlled trial involving 123 patients with alcoholic liver cirrhosis treated with SAMe or placebo over 2 years. They reported that the combined mortality and liver transplantation rate was 30% in the placebo group compared with 16% in the SAMe group (p = .08). When Child class C subjects (n = 8) were excluded, respective rates were 29% and 12% (p = .03). This study provides support for SAMe supplementation in alcoholic liver disease.

Berger R et al: A new medical approach to the treatment of osteoarthritis. Report of an open phase iv study with ademetionine (Gumbaral). Am J Med 1987;83:84. [NLM Cit ID: 88074427]

Caruso I et al: Italian double-blind multicenter study comparing *S*-adenosylmethionine, naproxen and placebo in the treatment of degenerative joint disease. Am J Med 1987;83:66. [NLM Cit ID: 88074423]

Mato JM et al: *S*-Adenosylmethionine in alcoholic liver cirrhosis: a randomized, placebo-controlled, double-blind, multicenter clinical trial. J Hepatol 1999;30:1081. [NLM Cit ID: 99332820]

Dehydroepiandrosterone (DHEA)

DHEA and its sulfate ester, DHEAS, are produced mainly by the adrenal cortex. In healthy individuals, there is an age-related decline of DHEA secretion, most notably during the fifth and sixth decades, and by age 70 the DHEA levels are 20–30% of lifetime peak levels. Low DHEA levels have been identified in people who are critically ill, suffering from major burns, or depressed and in premenopausal women with breast cancer. Low levels with advanced age and in conditions of stress have been touted in the popular press as evidence that DHEA supplementation would be beneficial.

The mechanism of action of DHEA remains unknown. Evidence regarding therapeutic efficacy from clinical trials is provocative but preliminary. There are neither large multicenter trials nor randomized double-blinded trials with independent validation; nonetheless, there are a few conditions—depression, dysthymia, systemic lupus erythematosus, and adrenal insufficiency—for which clinical evidence for DHEA supplementation appears promising.

Animal studies suggest that DHEA may be an agonist of the *N*-methyl-D-aspartate (NMDA) receptor, and DHEAS—and, to a lesser extent, DHEA—may be an antagonist of the γ-aminobutyric acid-benzodiazepine receptor complex. Both of these effects suggest that DHEA and DHEAS have excitatory effects on the central nervous system, which may account for their possible effectiveness in influencing mood and well-being. A randomized, double-blind, placebo-controlled pilot study of 22 subjects with major depression treated with DHEA or placebo for 6 weeks found DHEA to be superior to placebo as measured by a 50% reduction from baseline using the Hamilton Depression Scale. Another study by Bloch found similar improvements using multiple well-validated instruments for the treatment of midlife dysthymia in a randomized, double-blind crossover pilot study involving 15 patients.

Low DHEA levels have been identified in men and women with systemic lupus erythematosus. It is hypothesized that sex steroids such as DHEA play a causative role in the pathogenesis of this disorder. Results from a randomized, double-blind, placebo-controlled pilot study involving 28 subjects with mild to moderate disease treated for 3 months with DHEA or placebo identified reductions in observer-blinded "lupus flare" episodes and improvements in patient assessment of overall disease severity using a visual analog scale.

Since women do not have alternative sources for DHEA secretion aside from the adrenal glands, women with adrenal insufficiency will have unmeasurable DHEA serum levels. A recent study assessed the effects of DHEA on biochemical markers and psychologic states in a 4-month randomized, double-blinded, placebo-controlled crossover study. DHEA was associated with improvements in mood, well-being, and libido. Many endocrinologists now include DHEA as part of the replacement therapy regimen for women with adrenal insufficiency.

DHEA supplementation for the treatment of depression, dysthymia, systemic lupus erythematosus, and adrenal insufficiency appear promising. However, the majority of these results are from small to moderate-sized trials without independent validation. Side effects included acne, deepening of the voice, and facial hair growth, but no more serious adverse events were reported. However, the long-term effects of DHEA supplementation remain unknown. The safety issue of most concern is that DHEA, as a potent precursor of sex steroids, may increase the risk of estrogen- or androgen-dependent malignancies. Therefore, if supplementation is used, patients should be monitored closely. Furthermore, patients at high-risk for prostate, ovarian, breast, or uterine cancer should be counseled against DHEA supplementation.

Arlt W et al: Dehydroepiandrosterone replacement in women with adrenal insufficiency. N Engl J Med 1999; 341:1013. [NLM Cit ID: 99417078]

Barrett-Connor E et al: A prospective study of dehydroepiandrosterone sulfate, mortality and cardiovascular disease. N Engl J Med 1986;315:1519. [NLM Cit ID: 87064909]

Bloch M et al: Dehydroepiandrosterone treatment of midlife dysthymia. Biol Psychiatry 1999;45:1533. [NLM Cit ID: 99304401]

Ebeling P et al: Physiological importance of dehydroepiandrosterone. Lancet 1994;343:1479. [NLM Cit ID: 94260791]

Kroboth PD et al: DHEA and DHEA-S: A review. J Clin Pharmacol 1999;39:327. [NLM Cit ID: 99213041]

Van Vollenhoven R et al: Dehydroepiandrosterone in systemic lupus erythematosus. Arthritis Rheum 1995;38: 1826. [NLM Cit ID: 96110687]

Wolkowitz O et al: Double-blind treatment of major depression with dehydroepiandrosterone. Am J Psychiatry 1999;156:646. [NLM Cit ID: 99216758]

Glucosamine & Chondroitin

Glucosamine and chondroitin have been used in Europe for the treatment of osteoarthritis since the 1980s. These compounds can be extracted from animal products and have been observed to increase proteoglycan production of articular cartilage in vitro and in animals. Glucosamine sulfate, the compound commonly used in supplements, is synthetically manufactured. It has anti-inflammatory properties in animal models. It is frequently combined with chondroitin sulfate, which is a glycoaminoglycan. Research suggests that chondroitin may influence articular fluid viscosity, inhibit breakdown of cartilage, and stimulate cartilage repair.

A recent meta-analysis by McAlindon et al identified 15 randomized, double-blind, placebo-controlled trials involving 1710 patients with knee or hip osteoarthritis. Summary estimates found glucosamine and chondroitin to have moderate to large effects for treating osteoarthritis symptoms. Most trials were of poor to fair quality, and publication bias probably exaggerated the benefits. However, at least a modest degree of efficacy can perhaps be assumed. Investigators at the University of Utah are conducting a multicenter trial, funded by the NIH, to evaluate these compounds under rigorous conditions to determine their long-term effectiveness. In the interim, glucosamine and chondroitin appear to be safe and well tolerated. The clinical trial literature suggests that these compounds are moderately effective in the treatment of osteoarthritis.

McAlindon RE et al: Glucosamine and chondroitin for the treatment of osteoarthritis: A systematic quality assessment and meta-analysis. JAMA 2000;283:1469. [NLM Cit ID: 20195075]

Coenzyme Q10 (Ubidecarenone)

Coenzyme Q10 (Co-Q10), also known as ubiquinone-10, is a lipid-soluble endogenous provitamin. The compound resides in the lipid layer of the mitochondria and plays a crucial role in the two-electron transfer activities during oxidative phosphorylation for ATP production. Lipid vehicles are used to enhance its bioavailability. It has also been observed to have effects on membrane stabilization, free radical scavenging, and calcium-dependent slow channels. Deficiencies in coenzyme Q10 have been observed among patients with congestive heart failure, renal failure, male infertility, and periodontal disease. No serious adverse events have been reported with its use, and it is generally well tolerated. Interestingly, use of HMG-CoA reductase inhibitors is associated with reduced levels of endogenous coenzyme Q10 in serum.

Based on observations that coenzyme Q10 appears to have an important role in ATP production and to have antioxidant effects, investigators have postulated that supplementation in patients with known deficiencies may lead to better clinical outcomes. Within the cardiovascular disease literature, results have been mixed. Earlier trials studying patients with congestive heart failure demonstrated positive results using outcomes such as disease exacerbations, hospitalizations, ejection fraction by echocardiography, and quality of life measurements. Morisco and colleagues in 1993 reported the results of a yearlong multicenter randomized, double-blind, placebo-controlled study of 651 patients with class III and class IV congestive heart failure—finding fewer hospitalizations and episodes of congestive heart failure. A methodologically more rigorous study performed by Watson et al in 1999 showed that coenzyme Q10 had no effect on ejection fraction, hemodynamic parameters, or quality of life. Other studies have evaluated coenzyme Q10 for acute myocardial infarction, angina, diabetes, and periodontal disease. There is convincing evidence that several medical conditions are associated with coenzyme Q10 deficiency. However, there is insufficient evidence to support or refute the use of coenzyme Q10 to improve outcomes for a particular condition. Although coenzyme Q10 supplementation is safe, it is relatively expensive.

Morisco C et al: Effect of coenzyme Q10 therapy on patients with congestive heart failure: a long-term multicenter randomized study. Clin Investig 1993;71(8 Suppl):S134. [NLM Cit ID: 94060607]

Watson P et al: Lack of effect of Coenzyme Q10 on left ventricular function with congestive heart failure. J Am Coll Cardiol 1999;33:1549. [NLM Cit ID: 99265591]

ACUPUNCTURE

Acupuncture is the stimulation of certain points on the surface of the body using needles to treat illness and promote health. Practitioners trained in Chinese medicine believe that a vital energy called "Qi" (pronounced "chee") circulates in the body through 12 main pathways called meridians. Each meridian is named after a particular organ or "official," but the term actually relates to the energetic function more than the structure or anatomy of the organ. There are both surface and internal projections for each meridian. The surface projections contain sites called acupuncture points. Chinese medicine practitioners insert needles into these points to influence the body's Qi to restore health.

Practitioners trained as Western acupuncturists believe that needling provides a neurologic input and thus will select points according to the patient's anatomic and physiologic presentation, which is based on a conventional diagnosis. Depending on the depth and school of training of the practitioner, there is significant overlap between these two schools in clinical practice.

History

The earliest reference to acupuncture can be traced to a text on Chinese medicine called *The Yellow Emperor's Classic of Internal Medicine* (the *Huang Ti Nei Ching*), which dates to the second century BC. This text is often referenced to support the authenticity of a particular practice or theory and is used as part of the curriculum in training colleges. Acupuncture spread through much of Asia and by the sixteenth century Jesuit missionaries had brought the practice to Europe. As early as 1912, William Osler described its use in the first edition of *The Principles and Practice of Medicine.* "For lumbago," he wrote, "acupuncture is, in acute cases, the most efficient treatment." Research and enthusiasm in the United States grew dramatically in 1971 when James Reston wrote an article describing his experience with acupuncture for postoperative analgesia after undergoing an appendectomy while in China.

Mechanism of Action

Acupuncture for analgesia stimulates the small-diameter nerve fibers in muscles that enter the dorsal horn of the spinal cord. An impulse is then sent to other levels within the spinal cord, the midbrain, and the hypothalamic-pituitary system, which then release neurotransmitters that cause analgesia. The spinal cord releases enkephalin, dynorphin, and other endorphins; the midbrain releases enkephalin to activate the raphe descending system, which stimulates release of monoamines, serotonin, and norepinephrine; and the hypothalamic-pituitary system, which releases beta-endorphins. Therefore, when practitioners place a needle in the region of pain, all three centers are activated to provide an analgesic effect. When practitioners place needles in locations distant from the pain site, only the midbrain and hypothalamic-pituitary systems are activated. This suggests that noxious stimulation of heterotopic regions of the body will modulate pain experience in the original location. Although this theory implies that sham acupuncture may be as effective as real acupuncture, experimentally induced acute pain studies in animals and humans have consistently shown that real point stimulation is far superior to sham. Chronic pain studies, however, have shown less consistent results. Despite extensive histologic studies, investigators have been unable to identify unique anatomic structures or physiologic effects at acupuncture points. Despite these shortcomings, our understanding of the mechanisms of action of acupuncture for the treatment of pain is superior to our understanding of the mechanisms of action of many drugs in widespread use today.

Clinical Practice

In the United States and Europe, Chinese medicine-trained practitioners will conduct a 1-hour comprehensive multisystem history, observation, and physical examination during the initial consultation. Examination consists of palpation of the abdomen and selected acupuncture points, examination of the tongue to assess color, shape, and coating, and palpation of the pulse along the wrist at three locations on both arms to assess its quality, rhythm, and strength. Treatment by the **classic acupuncture method** is based on the belief that each patient presents with a unique constellation of symptoms and signs. What this means is that ten patients presenting with migraine headaches may receive ten different treatments. Western-style practitioners will conduct a conventional examination and include variable components of the Chinese medicine approach depending on the depth and school of training. Treatment based on the **formula acupuncture method** relies on the signs and symptoms obtained from the Western-based diagnostic paradigm. What this means is that a cohort of migraine sufferers will be treated in the same way.

Treatment involves inserting four to fifteen needles at selected acupuncture points for 10–30 minutes—though certain schools leave the needles in place for only a few seconds to minutes. Needles are approximately 37 gauge, stainless steel, and disposable. Needles are manipulated with electricity, heat, or manually. Follow-up consultations last from 20 minutes to 45 minutes.

Patients can expect to see the practitioner weekly or bimonthly for 4–10 weeks, followed by less frequent visits as the condition improves.

Adverse Events

In current practice in the United States and Europe, acupuncture is generally considered safe, associated with a very low incidence of adverse events. Precautions for avoiding serious adverse events are listed in Table 43–5. The most frequent adverse events include vasovagal or sedating reactions such as presyncope, syncope, and drowsiness. These are easily prevented by having the patient lie flat on the table, monitoring patients during the initial visit, and permitting the patient to remain in the office until a normal state of awareness is achieved. Serious adverse events in the literature over the past 30 years have been due to the reuse of needles between patients, leading to transmission of infection such as hepatitis B and C or HIV, and needling the thorax in patients with emphysema, leading to pneumothorax. There have also been case reports of unusual serious adverse events, including endocarditis in patients with prosthetic heart valves who had small indwelling needles in place for several days, cardiac tamponade after needling directly over the heart, spinal cord trauma from deep insertion or migration of cut or broken retained needles, and pacemaker malfunction during acupuncture with electrical stimulation.

Most surveys estimate that the frequency of adverse events is 1:100,000 to 1:10,000. A 14-year review of the world literature identified 193 complications and concluded that acupuncture is generally safe except for patients with emphysema, in whom the risk of pneumothorax is of significant consequence. Another review identified 300 complications reported in the literature over a 30-year period. With more than 10 million acupuncture visits in the United

Table 43–5. How to avoid preventable adverse events associated with acupuncture.[1]

Make certain that only sterile disposible needles are used.
When press-in needles are used, make certain that sterile technique is employed.
Make certain that the patient is lying flat during the treatment.
Make certain that the practitioner counts the number of needles used before and after treatment.
Exert caution when patients are taking anticoagulants.
Avoid electrical stimulation in patients with pacemakers.
Exert caution when needling the thorax in patients with emphysema.

[1]Modified, with permission, from Rampes H: Adverse reactions to acupuncture. In: *Medical Acupuncture: A Western Scientific Approach.* Filshie J, White A (editors). Churchill Livingstone, 1998.

States annually, the frequency approximates one per million visits.

CLINICAL USES OF ACUPUNCTURE

In the United States, acupuncture is frequently used to treat acute non-life-threatening conditions or chronic conditions that conventional medicine is unable to treat effectively (Table 43–6). What follows is a survey of some conditions for which patients frequently seek acupuncture care.

Chronic Pain

A 1989 meta-analysis of randomized controlled trials of acupuncture for chronic pain identified 14 trials meeting study entry criteria with five studies on low back pain, five studies on head and neck pain, and three studies on other types of chronic pain. Only two studies used inert medical placebo, with the remainder using sham acupuncture, transcutaneous electrical nerve stimulation (TENS), or continued standard medical care. Heterogeneity was present across trials as well as in all subgroups. With this limitation, the overall risk difference was statistically significant in favor of acupuncture ($p < .01$). In sensitivity analyses, individualized treatments (classic acupuncture) were superior to placebo; however, standardized treatments (formula acupuncture) were no different from placebo. The summary estimate from trials reporting at least partial blinding was no different from the estimate from control groups. Overall, although this review found acupuncture superior to control group intervention, serious methodologic issues were present. A criterion-based review of 51 controlled trials of acupuncture for the treatment of chronic pain found 24 trials reporting results favoring acupuncture. Using a 100-point quality scale, only 11 trials scored at least 50 points. Heterogeneity across studies precluded pooled analysis, and the investigators concluded that poor study quality made it impossible to arrive at definitive conclusions.

Overall, there is some evidence suggesting benefit of acupuncture for persons with chronic pain when compared with placebo and insufficient evidence to suggest benefit of acupuncture when compared with standard medical care or sham acupuncture. The ability to make definitive recommendations regarding efficacy for chronic pain is hampered by poor methodologic study quality and potential inadequate "dosing" (frequency and duration) of acupuncture in the current literature.

Ezzo J: Is acupuncture effective for the treatment of chronic pain? A systematic review. Pain 2000;86:217. [NLM Cit ID: 20274062]

Patel M et al: A meta-analysis of acupuncture for chronic pain. Int J Epidemiol 1989;18:900. [NLM Cit ID: 90153032]

ter Riet G et al: Acupuncture and chronic pain: a criteria-based meta-analysis. J Clin Epidemiol 1990;43:1191. [NLM Cit ID: 91055347]

Low Back Pain

Ernst et al performed a meta-analysis on acupuncture in the treatment of low back pain and identified 30 trials, of which nine met inclusion criteria involving 377 patients The summary odds ratio was 2.3 (95% CI, 1.3–4.1) favoring acupuncture compared with various control groups. Heterogeneity was not present. Subgroup analysis limited to four trials using sham acupuncture as the control group found real and sham acupuncture to have similar effectiveness. Investigators concluded that acupuncture is an effective treatment for low back pain; however, larger studies using sham acupuncture are needed to distinguish between the specific effects of treatment at correct acupuncture points and the nonspecific effects of needling.

Van Tulder et al performed a systematic review using 11 randomized controlled trials on acupuncture for low back pain—none of which studied acute back pain. The quality of the studies was poor, and pooled analyses were not performed because of heterogeneity across trials. Overall, the reviewers did not find evidence that acupuncture was superior to no treatment; there was moderate evidence that acupuncture was equal in effectiveness to trigger point injection or TENS, and there was limited evidence that acupuncture was similar to sham or placebo acupuncture.

In summary, the literature is contradictory, with results from a meta-analysis favoring acupuncture and results from a systematic review finding no clear evidence for effectiveness. There is limited evidence that acupuncture may be more effective in the treatment of low back pain than inert placebo or standard medical care.

Ernst E et al: Acupuncture for back pain: a meta-analysis of randomized controlled trials. Arch Intern Med 1998;158:2235. [NLM Cit ID: 99034112]

van Tulder MW et al: The effectiveness of acupuncture in the treatment of acute and chronic low back pain. A systematic review within the framework of the Cochrane Collaboration Back Review Group. Spine 1999;24:1113. [NLM Cit ID: 99290012]

Osteoarthritis

A systematic review performed by Ernst in 1997 found 13 trials that met study entry criteria. Pooled analysis was not done because of heterogeneity in outcome measures, diagnostic criteria, affected joints, and style of acupuncture. The great majority of trials used formula acupuncture. Seven of the 13 trials reported positive results; however, overall the methodologic quality was poor. Among randomized trials, five out of ten were positive. When sham acupuncture was used as the control group, only one

Table 43–6. Overview of acupuncture literature for selected medical conditions.

First Author, Year	Condition	Study Type	Inclusion Criteria	No. of Studies	No. of Patients	Measures	Results
Patel, 1989	Chronic pain	Meta-analysis	RCTs published in English from 1970 to 1989 listed in Index Medicus	14	558 plus 182 in cross-over studies	Positive report of pain relief; otherwise, not specified	Positive result overall and for head-neck pain. Heterogeneity across trials was present. However, inconclusive due to potential for bias resulting from poor study quality.
ter Riet, 1990	Chronic pain	Systematic review	Controlled trials. Needles used. "Chronic" mentioned in title or abstract or pain > 6 months	51	N/A	Positive report of pain relief; otherwise, not specified	No pooled analysis due to heterogeneity. 24/51 trials favoring acupuncture compared with control. However, inconclusive because of poor study quality.
Ezzo, 2000	Chronic pain	Systematic review	RCTs published in English. Pain > 3 months.	47	N/A	Positive report of pain relief; otherwise not specified	Inconclusive
van Tulder, 1999	Low back pain	Systematic review	RCTs, acute or chronic low back pain.	11	542	Pain relief	Inconclusive
Ernst, 1998	Low back pain	Meta-analysis	RCTs, any type of low back pain.	9	377	Pain relief	Overall, acupuncture was superior to control. However, subgroup analysis found no difference between real and sham acupuncture.
Ernst, 1997	Osteoarthritis	Systematic review	Controlled trials, symptomatic disease.	13	437	Pain relief	Inconclusive. Overall, the literature is conflicting. There is limited evidence to suggest real acupuncture is not more effective than sham acupuncture.

Ernst, 1998	Acute dental pain	Systematic review	Controlled trials.	16	941	Pain relief	Definitive conclusion that acupuncture is superior to sham and placebo-controlled acupuncture. Evidence for use as adjunctive therapy.
Vickers, 1996	Nausea and vomiting from surgery, cancer chemotherapy, and pregnancy	Systematic review	Trials stimulating P6 acupuncture point by needling, manual pressure, or electricity. Controlled trials.	33	2456	Number and duration of vomiting episodes. Symptom-free days. Nausea score.	Clear evidence of benefit for all conditions excluding subjects under anesthesia.
Kleijnen, 1991	Asthma	Systematic review	Needles used. Reference group used.	13	N/A	Severity of symptoms, lung function.	Results conflicting and poor study quality.
Melchart, 1999	Recurrent headache	Systematic review	RCTs, quasi-RCTs.	22	1032	Any one clinical outcome related to headache, eg, pain intensity, global assessment.	Positive trend favoring real over sham acupuncture. Inconclusive for real vs. other forms of therapy. Suggestive of effect and warrants further investigation.
White, 1999	Tobacco addiction	Meta-analysis	RCTs.	16	N/A	Abstinence at first treatment, 6 months, 12 months.	Negative at all time intervals.
ter Riet, 1990	Addiction to tobacco, heroin, and alcohol.	Systematic review	Controlled trials.	22	N/A	Statement of efficacy.	Inconclusive due to poor study quality.

RCT = randomized controlled trial.

out of five trials were positive. The reviewers concluded that acupuncture was not clearly superior to control interventions and that the literature was of poor quality.

A recent methodologically rigorous randomized controlled trial involved 73 patients treated for 12 weeks with acupuncture or conventional care. Subjective scores were recorded using the Western Ontario and McMaster Universities Osteoarthritis Index (WOMAC) and theLequesne Index. Acupuncture was superior to control intervention based on the WOMAC and Lequesne scores. No adverse events were reported. Investigators concluded that acupuncture for osteoarthritis appeared safe and effective when compared with standard care.

In conclusion, there is limited evidence suggesting that acupuncture is more effective than conventional care alone. An NIH-funded multicenter randomized, controlled trial currently under way at the University of Maryland will more definitively assess efficacy and long-term outcomes.

Berman BM et al: A randomized trial of acupuncture as adjunctive therapy in osteoarthritis of the knee. Rheumatology (Oxford) 1999;38:346.

Ernst E: Acupuncture as a symptomatic treatment of osteoarthritis. A systematic review. Scand J Rheumatol 1997;26:444. [NLM Cit ID: 98094990]

Acute Dental Pain

The NIH consensus development statement on acupuncture states, "There is evidence of efficacy for postoperative dental pain." A review in 1999 identified 16 controlled trials of acupuncture for the treatment of acute dental pain. Among the eight randomized and at least partially blinded trials, seven showed benefit. Among the seven trials using sham control, six showed benefit. Subsequent to this review, a randomized, double-blind, placebo acupuncture-controlled trial involving 39 patients evaluated acupuncture for the treatment of postsurgical dental pain. Controls experienced a similar tap sensation next to the acupuncture sites to produce a noticeable sensation; however, needle insertion was not performed. Patients receiving acupuncture scored more favorably than controls on multiple outcomes. There is thus sufficient evidence to recommend the use of acupuncture as effective adjunctive treatment for the treatment of acute dental pain. Multiple studies have demonstrated its efficacy when compared with sham acupuncture.

Ernst E et al: The effectiveness of acupuncture in treating acute dental pain: a systematic review. Br Dent J 1998;184:443. [NLM Cit ID: 98279986]

Lao L et al: Evaluation of acupuncture for pain control after oral surgery: a placebo-controlled trial. Arch Otolaryngol Head Neck Surg 1999;125:567. [NLM Cit ID: 99256748]

Headache

There is insufficient evidence on which to form an opinion for the efficacy of acupuncture in the treatment of recurrent headaches. Melchart et al performed a systematic review in 1999 to evaluate the treatment of acupuncture for recurrent headaches. That group identified 22 randomized and quasi-randomized trials involving 1042 subjects in which 15 trials studied migraine headaches, six studied tension headaches, and one studied mixed headaches. Of the 14 trials that used sham acupuncture, investigators reported a trend in favor of real acupuncture. In the remaining eight trials, in which control groups varied, conflicting results were reported. Overall, investigators felt there was evidence that acupuncture may be effective in the treatment of recurrent headaches; however, more research is needed to ascertain which headaches would be most responsive to such treatment. Furthermore, owing to the variable quality of the studies, methodologic rigor is warranted to better quantify the magnitude of effect.

Melchart D et al: Acupuncture for recurrent headaches: a systematic review of randomized controlled trials. Cephalalgia 1999;19:779. [NLM Cit ID: 20061661]

Asthma

Kleijnen et al performed a systematic review of 13 trials of acupuncture for the treatment of asthma, with eight studies finding that acupuncture was superior to control. Among high-quality trials, acupuncture was superior to controls in three out of eight studies. This group concluded that owing to the poor study quality and conflicting results, any claims that acupuncture is effective in the treatment of asthma are not supported by clinical trials. No research has evaluated the efficacy of acupuncture as part of a comprehensive treatment program. Investigators have focused their research on comparing the efficacy of real acupuncture with sham acupuncture for this condition. Among trials reporting positive results, benefit was primarily identified in subjective rather than objective measures. Since asthma can be a life-threatening condition and effective standard medical therapy exists, acupuncture should only be used as an adjunct to conventional therapy.

Jobst KA: Acupuncture in asthma and pulmonary disease: an analysis of efficacy and safety. J Altern Complement Med 1996;2:179. [NLM Cit ID: 98051836]

Kleijnen J et al: Acupuncture and asthma: a review of controlled trials. Thorax 1991;46:799. [NLM Cit ID: 92124401]

Nausea & Vomiting

Based on multiple randomized controlled trials, there is strong evidence demonstrating effectiveness of acupuncture in the treatment of pregnancy-induced, chemotherapy-induced, and postoperative nausea and vomiting. One review identified 33 trials using a particular acupuncture point (P6) for treatment of nausea and vomiting. None of the four trials in which acupuncture was given while the patient was under general anesthesia demonstrated a positive effect. Among the remaining 29 trials, 27 identified real acupuncture as being more effective than sham acupuncture or inert placebo control. In subgroup analyses, all five studies evaluating acupuncture for cancer chemotherapy-induced nausea and vomiting were positive. Six out of seven studies for pregnancy-induced symptoms were positive. Among trials in which acupuncture was performed while the subjects were not under general anesthesia, 16 out of 17 studies of treatment for postoperative nausea and vomiting were positive. In sensitivity analyses, 11 out of the 12 high-quality trials involving over 2000 patients identified acupuncture as superior to control. The NIH consensus development panel on acupuncture stated, "There is clear evidence that needle acupuncture is efficacious for adult postoperative and chemotherapy induced nausea and vomiting and probably for the nausea of pregnancy."

Vickers AJ: Can acupuncture have specific effects on health? A systematic review of acupuncture antiemesis trials. J R Soc Med 1996;89:303. [NLM Cit ID: 96318223]

Nicotine, Heroin, & Alcohol Addiction

There is good evidence suggesting that acupuncture is not effective in maintaining abstinence from nicotine addiction. Systematic reviews have identified multiple trials of sufficient quality to determine that there is no evidence to support its use. In one review, only three out of fifteen studies identified acupuncture as superior to control; however, all were rated as low-quality studies. In a recent randomized trial comparing electroacupuncture and sham control for nicotine withdrawal symptoms, there was no difference in nicotine withdrawal symptoms or abstinence rates at day 14. The NIH consensus development statement on acupuncture states, "There is evidence that acupuncture does not demonstrate efficacy for cessation of smoking."

Although heroin and alcohol addiction studies have frequently reported positive outcomes, serious methodologic flaws are present. Until further research can demonstrate efficacy, acupuncture should not be used as monotherapy in the treatment of these addictions.

Ernst E, White A: *Acupuncture: A Scientific Appraisal.* Butterworth-Heinemann, 1999.

Kaptchuk T: *The Web That Has No Weaver: Understanding Chinese Medicine.* NTC/Contemporary Publishing Book, 2000.

Stux G, Hammerschlag R (editors): *Scientific Basis of Acupuncture.* [In press.]

Stux G, Pomeranz B: *Basics of Acupuncture,* 4th ed. Springer, 1998.

ter Riet G et al: A meta-analysis of studies into the effect of acupuncture on addiction. Br J Gen Pract 1990;40:379. [NLM Cit ID: 91090957]

White AR et al: A meta-analysis of acupuncture techniques for smoking cessation. Tob Control 1999;8:393. [NLM Cit ID: 20096830]

HOMEOPATHY

Christian F.S Hahnemann is credited with devising the system of homeopathy in 1790. Three main principles of homeopathy include the "law of similars," the use of dilute concentrations of medicines, and "potentization." The second and third principles remain the most controversial for many scientists and conventionally trained physicians. The law of similars is also known as the principle of "like cures like"; it is derived from the observation that a homeopathic medicine when given to a healthy volunteer will produce a constellation of symptoms similar to those it will cure in an ill patient. Since the 1800s, the process of testing medicines on healthy volunteers to record the symptoms provoked (known as "provings") has been recorded and compiled to create the *Homeopathic Pharmacopoeia* and several materia medicas.

The second principle, the use of dilute concentrations of medicine, entails serially diluting and "succussing" (shaking) a substance to concentrations in which there is little probability of any molecules remaining in solution. Yet homeopathic physicians affirm that these remedies remain pharmacologically active and allude to allergy desensitization and immunization as sharing similar approaches to homeopathy, ie, in that both use low doses of potentially toxic substances to achieve beneficial clinical effects. Potentization is based on the claim that once a medicine is at low concentration, the more dilute the solute the more potent the effect.

The World Health Organization states that homeopathy is the second most used medical system internationally, with over $1 billion in expenditures for such therapy. Twenty to 30 percent of French and German physicians use homeopathy in clinical practice. In Great Britain, five homeopathic hospitals are part of the National Health System, and over 30% of generalists use homeopathy. In the United States, there are more than 500 physicians and 5000 nonphysicians using homeopathy in clinical practice, and 2.5 million Americans currently use homeopathic medicines—of which two-thirds are self-prescribed—spending more than $250 million annually.

Mechanisms of Action

Although there are several mechanisms under investigation, none are well validated.

Adverse Events

Given the low concentration of homeopathic medicines, the probability of adverse events is remote. However, adverse events have been reported from ingestion of large quantities of remedies containing heavy metals. Indirect adverse events may occur—eg, if children are not given immunizations because certain homeopathic physicians advise parents against this practice.

Training, Licensure, & Regulation

Homeopathic educational programs are accredited by the Council for Homeopathic Education. There are two levels of training for homeopaths. The Primary Care Certificate in Homeotherapeutics requires 60–100 hours of course work and passage of a written examination. The more advanced level, The Diplomate in Homeotherapeutics (DHt), requires an additional 3 years of clinical practice. There is comprehensive homeopathic training which involves 3 or more years of part-time to full-time study. Nonphysicians may practice homeopathy within the scope of practice of their specific profession. The American Board of Homeotherapeutics governs certification for physicians; the Homeopathic Association of Naturopathic Physicians governs naturopaths; and the Council for Homeopathic Certification governs all others practitioners.

The *Homeopathic Pharmacopoeia* was included in the original Food and Drug Act of 1938, which classified these medicines as drugs. Currently, the Food and Drug Administration considers these medicines as nonprescription products. Unlike preparations in Great Britain and Europe, there is little oversight of the manufacturing of these products.

Clinical Encounter

The initial consultation takes about 1–1½ hours, with significant time spent on obtaining a detailed history. Attention is given to the physical, mental, and emotional symptoms, overall personality type, and any internal or external factors that influence the presenting symptoms, such as emotions, wind, season of the year, and reactions to different foods. The symptom inventory is then matched to an appropriate remedy taken from the Materia Medica. Follow-up visits may last for a few minutes to 40 minutes. During the follow-up visit, the practitioner determines if there has been improvement in symptoms, no change, or aggravation of symptoms. The latter scenario, if transient, is viewed as the first sign of recovery.

Clinical Uses

Homeopathic physicians are trained to treat a broad range of conditions in the primary care and specialty setting. In clinical practice, however, practitioners frequently treat patients with chronic conditions that conventional medicine cannot adequately address, including arthritis, allergies, autoimmune diseases, or non-life-threatening acute conditions such as viral infections or minor trauma. Parents may take their children to homeopathic physicians for recurrent conditions such as otitis media and allergies with the goal of avoiding repetitive antibiotic, steroid, or chronic conventional medications.

Research

Over 180 controlled trials and over ten reviews have been published on the effects of homeopathy compared with placebo. The majority of trials are published in non-English language journals and are frequently not listed in Medline. A few methodologically rigorous reviews have been published in English (Table 43–7). The majority of systematic reviews have pooled trials on homeopathy regardless of the medical condition being treated. These reviews have found that patient outcomes in homeopathic treatment groups were superior to placebo group outcomes. Since many of the trials do not provide in-depth reports on the treatment encounter, it remains unclear whether these positive effects are specific to the homeopathic remedy itself or to nonspecific effects that occur as part of the treatment encounter. Since few trials have been independently replicated, there is insufficient evidence to determine if treatment effects found for a single medical condition are reproducible by independent investigators.

A 1991 systematic review identified 107 controlled clinical trials and found 77% reported a positive result. Since 84 out of 107 trials scored < 55 points on a 100-point quality scale, high-quality studies were analyzed separately. Sixty-eight percent of high-quality trials favored patients in the homeopathy-treated group compared with placebo. A 1997 systematic review identified 89 double-blind or randomized placebo-controlled trials and found the overall combined odds ratio was 2.45 (95% CI, 2.0–2.9) favoring patients in the homeopathy-treated group. Analyses restricted to high-quality studies found similar statistically significant results with an odds ratio of 1.66 (95% CI, 1.3–2.1), and no change of effect was identified after adjustment for publication bias. This review attempted to assess whether these positive findings were reproducible for a specific condition but were unable to identify condition-specific trials performed by independent investigators. Pooled analysis of four multicenter trials by the same investigator evaluating the effects of *Galphimia glauca* for seasonal allergies found an odds ratio 2.0 (95% CI, 1.5–2.7) for improvement in ocular and nasal symptoms at 4 weeks.

Chapman E: Homeopathy. In: *Essentials of Complementary and Alternative Medicine.* Jonas W, Levin J (editors). Lippincott Williams & Wilkins, 1999.

Table 43–7. Overview of English language homeopathy systematic reviews.

First Author, Year	Indication	Inclusion Criteria	No. of Studies	Measures	Results	Conclusions
Kleijnen, 1991	No limitation	Controlled trials	107	Vote-count	All trials: 81/107 positive High quality: 15/22 positive Majority of trials received low-quality scores, but effect remained after adjustment.	Positive findings; however, no definitive conclusions due to poor study quality of majority of trials
Linde, 1997	No limitation	Double-blind or randomized placebo-controlled	89	Pooled summary estimates	Overall: OR = 2.45 (95% CI 2.0–2.9) High-quality: OR = 1.7 (95% CI 1.3–2.1) Publication-bias correction: OR = 1.8 (95% CI 1.0–3.1) Seasonal allergies[1]: OR = 2.0 (95% CI 1.5–2.7) Postoperative ileus[2]: effect-size difference = −0.22 SD (95% CI −0.33 to −0.03)	Rejection of hypothesis that treatment effect of homeopathy is attributable to placebo effects. Unable to determine if homeopathy is effective for any single clinical condition under a priori defined criteria.
Barnes, 1997	Postoperative ileus	Randomized controlled clinical trials	6	Pooled summary estimates	Time to first flatus: 7.4 hours earlier favoring homeopathy ($p < .05$). Effect remained after adjustment for study quality.	Clincally meaningful effect with reservation due to variable study quality of trials

[1]Not independent investigators.
[2]Different remedies used.
[3]OR = odds ratio; CI = confidence interval.

Ernst E et al: Homeopathy revisited. Arch Intern Med 1996;156:2162. [NLM Cit ID: 97040500]

Eskinazi D: Homeopathy re-revisited. Arch Intern Med 1999;159:1981.

Jacobs J et al: Treatment of acute childhood diarrhea with homeopathic medicine: a randomized clinical trial in Nicaragua. Pediatrics 1994;93:719. [NLM Cit ID: 94218172]

Kleijnen J et al: Trials of homeopathy. BMJ 1991;302:316. [NLM Cit ID: 91159730]

Linde K et al: Are the clinical effects of homeopathy placebo effects? A meta-analysis of placebo-controlled trials. Lancet 1997;350:834. [NLM Cit ID: 97456644]

Linde K et al: Critical review and meta-analysis of serial agitated dilutions in experimental toxicology. Hum Exp Toxicol 1994;13:481. [NLM Cit ID: 95000906]

Reilly D et al: Is evidence for homoeopathy reproducible? Lancet 1994;344:1601. [NLM Cit ID: 95075184]

Reilly D et al: Is homoeopathy a placebo response? Controlled trial of homoeopathic potency, with pollen in hayfever as model. Lancet 1986;2:881. [NLM Cit ID: 87013672]

RELEVANT WORLD WIDE WEB SITES

Introduction and Background

http://nccam.nih.gov/ (NIH National Center for Complementary and Alternative Medicine)

http://cpmcnet.columbia.edu/dept/rosenthal/ (Center for CAM Research in Aging and Women's Health, Columbia University College of Physicians and Surgeons)

http://www.c3r.org (Consortial Center for Chiropractic Research)

http://www.ohsu.edu/orccamind/ (Oregon Center for Complementary and Alternative Medicine in Neurological Disorders, Oregon Health Sciences University)

http://www.crc.arizona.edu/ (University of Arizona Health Sciences Center, Pediatric Center for Complementary and Alternative Medicine, Department of Pediatrics)

http://www.compmed.ummc.umaryland.edu/compmed/Cochrane/Cochranefr.htm (University of Maryland School of Maryland Cochrane Collaboration Complementary Medicine Field)

http://www.naturalhealthvillage.com (Legislation, reports, congressional information, and recent clinical studies)

http://dtp.nci.nih.gov (Natural Products Branch of National Cancer Institute)

Herbal Medicines

http://www.herbalgram.org (American Botanical Society)

http://www.herbalgram.org (Herbal Research Foundation)

http://www.herbal-ahp.org (American Herbal Pharmacopoeia)

http://www.amfoundation.org (The Alternative Medicine Foundation)

http://www.ex.ac.uk/phytonet/escop.html (European Scientific Cooperative on Phytotherapy)

Dietary Supplements

http://web.health.gov/dietsupp/ (Commission on Dietary Supplement Labels)

http://www.fda.gov/medwatch/index.html (FDA Medwatch)

http://vm.cfsan.fda.gov/~dms/supplmnt.html (U.S. Food and Drug Administration dietary supplement information)

Acupuncture

http://acupunctureresearch.homestead.com/ (Society for Acupuncture Research)

http://odp.od.nih.gov/consensus/cons/107/107_intro.htm (NIH Consensus Development Statement)

http://www.compmed.ummc.umaryland.edu (University of Maryland Center for Complementary and Alternative Medicine)

http://www.medicalacupuncture.org (American Academy of Medical Acupuncture)

http://www.aaom.org (American Association for Oriental Medicine)

Appendix: Therapeutic Drug Monitoring & Laboratory Reference Ranges

C. Diana Nicoll, MD, PhD

Table 1. Therapeutic drug monitoring.[1,2]

Drug	Effective Concentrations	Half-Life (hours)	Dosage Adjustment	Comments
Amikacin	Peak: 20–30 μg/mL; trough: < 10 μg/mL	2–3 ↑ in uremia	↓ in renal dysfunction	Concomitant kanamycin or tobramycin therapy may give falsely elevated amikacin results by immunoassay.
Amitriptyline	160–240 ng/mL	9–46		Drug is highly protein-bound. Patient-specific decrease in protein binding may invalidate quoted range of effective concentration.
Carbamazepine	4–12 μg/mL	10–15		Induces its own metabolism. Metabolite 10,11-epoxide exhibits 13% cross-reactivity by immunoassay.
Cyclosporine	150–400 mg/mL (ng/L) whole blood	6–12	Need to know specimen and methodology used	Cyclosporine is lipid-soluble (20% bound to leukocytes; 40% to erythrocytes; 40% in plasma, highly bound to lipoproteins). Binding is temperature-dependent, so whole blood is preferred to plasma or serum as specimen. High-performance liquid chromatography (HPLC) or monoclonal fluorescence polarization immunoassay measures cyclosporine reliably; polyclonal fluorescence polarization immunoassays cross-react with metabolites, so the therapeutic range used with those assays is higher. Anticonvulsants and rifampin increase metabolism. Erythromycin, ketoconazole, and calcium channel blockers decrease metabolism.
Desipramine	100–250 ng/mL	13–23		Drug is highly protein-bound. Patient-specific decrease in protein binding may invalidate quoted range of effective concentration.
Digoxin	0.8–2 ng/mL	42 ↑ in uremia, CHF	↓ in renal dysfunction, CHF, hypothyroidism ↑ in hyperthyroidism	Bioavailability of digoxin tablets is 50–90%. Specimen must not be drawn within 6 hours of dose. Dialysis does not remove a significant amount. Hypokalemia potentiates toxicity. Digitalis toxicity is a clinical and *not* a laboratory diagnosis. Digibind (digoxin-specific antibody) therapy of digoxin overdose can interfere with measurement of digoxin levels depending on the digoxin assay. Elimination reduced by quinidine, verapamil, and amiodarone.
Ethosuximide	40–100 μg/mL	Child: 30 Adult: 50		Levels used primarily to assess compliance. Toxicity is rare and does not correlate well with plasma concentrations.
Gentamicin	Peak: 4–8 μg/mL; trough: < 2 μg/mL	2–5 ↑ in uremia (7.3 on dialysis)	↓ in renal dysfunction	Draw peak specimen 30 minutes after end of infusion. Draw trough just before next dose. In uremic patients, carbenicillin may decrease gentamicin half-life from 46 hours to 22 hours.

(continued)

Table 1. Therapeutic drug monitoring.[1,2] (continued)

Drug	Effective Concentrations	Half-Life (hours)	Dosage Adjustment	Comments
Imipramine	180–350 ng/mL	10–16		Drug is highly protein-bound. Patient-specific decrease in protein binding may invalidate quoted range of effective concentration.
Lidocaine	1–5 µg/mL	1.8 ↔ in uremia, CHF; ↑ in cirrhosis	↓ in CHF, liver disease	Levels increased with cimetidine therapy. CNS toxicity common in the elderly.
Lithium	0.7–1.5 meq/L	22 ↑ in uremia	↓ in renal dysfunction	Thiazides and loop diuretics may increase serum lithium levels.
Methotrexate		8.4 ↑ in uremia	↓ in renal dysfunction	7-Hydroxymethotrexate cross-reacts 1.5% in immunoassay. To minimize toxicity, leucovorin should be continued if methotrexate level is > 0.1 µmol/L at 48 hours after start of therapy. Methotrexate > 1 µmol/L at > 48 hours requires an increase in leucovorin rescue therapy.
Nortriptyline	50–140 ng/mL	18–44		Drug is highly protein-bound. Patient-specific decrease in protein binding may invalidate quoted range of effective concentration.
Phenobarbital	10–30 µg/mL	86 ↑ in cirrhosis	↓ in liver disease	Metabolized primarily by the hepatic microsomal enzyme system. Many drug-drug interactions.
Phenytoin	10–20 µg/mL; 5–10 µg/mL in uremia, hypoalbuminemia	Dose-dependent		Metabolite cross-reacts 10% in immunoassay. Metabolism is capacity-limited. Increase dose cautiously when level approaches therapeutic range, since new steady-state level may be disproportionately higher. Drug is very highly protein-bound; protein binding is decreased in uremia and hypoalbuminemia.
Primidone	5–10 µg/mL	8		Phenobarbital cross-reacts 0.5%. Metabolized to phenobarbital. Primidone/phenobarbital ratio > 1:2 suggests poor compliance.
Procainamide	4–8 µg/mL	3 ↑ in uremia	↓ in renal dysfunction	30% of patients with plasma levels of 12–16 µg/mL have electrocardiographic changes; 40% of patients with plasma levels of > 16 µg/mL have severe toxicity.
Quinidine	1–4 µg/mL	7 ↔ in CHF; ↑ in liver disease	↓ in liver disease, CHF	Effective concentration is lower in chronic liver disease and nephrosis, where binding is decreased.
Salicylate	150–300 µg/mL	Dose-dependent		
Theophylline	5–20 µg/mL	9	↓ in CHF, cirrhosis, and with cimetidine	Caffeine cross-reacts 10%. Elimination is increased 1½–2 times in smokers. 1,3-Dimethyl uric acid metabolite increased in uremia and, because of cross-reactivity, may cause an apparent slight increase in serum theophylline.
Tobramycin	Peak: 5–10 µg/mL; trough: < 2 µg/mL	2–3; ↑ in uremia	↓ in renal dysfunction	Tobramycin, kanamycin, and amikacin may cross-react in immunoassay.
Valproic acid	55–100 µg/mL	13–19		95% protein-bound. Decreased binding in uremia and cirrhosis.
Vancomycin	Trough: 5–15 µg/mL	6 ↑ in uremia	↓ in renal dysfunction	Toxicity in uremic patients leads to irreversible deafness. Keep peak level < 30–40 µg/mL to avoid toxicity.

↔ = unchanged; ↑ = increase(d); ↓ = decrease(d); CHF = congestive heart failure.
[1]Modified and reproduced, with permission, from Nicoll D et al: *Pocket Guide to Diagnostic Tests,* 3rd ed. McGraw-Hill, 2000.
[2]Use red-topped tube (not marbled) for therapeutic drug monitoring. In general, the specimen should be drawn just before the next dose (trough).

Table 2. Reference ranges for commonly used tests.[1,2]
Current metric units × Conversion factor = SI units
SI units ÷ Conversion factor = Current metric units

Test	Specimen	Conventional Units	Conversion Factor	SI Units[2]	Collection
Acetaminophen	Serum	10–20 mg/L **Panic:** > 50 mg/L	66.16	66–132 μmol/L	Marbled
Acetoacetate	Serum or urine	Negative		Negative	Marbled or urine container
Adrenocorticotropic hormone (ACTH)	Plasma	20–100 pg/mL (laboratory-specific)	0.22	4–22 pmol/L	Heparinized plastic container
Alanine aminotransferase (ALT, SGPT, GPT)	Serum	0–35 units/L (laboratory-specific)	0.02	0–0.58 μkat/L (laboratory-specific)	Marbled
Albumin	Serum	3.4–4.7 g/dL	10.00	34–47 g/L	Marbled
Aldosterone	Plasma	Salt-loaded (120 meq Na^+/d): Supine: 3–10 ng/dL Upright: 5–30 ng/dL Salt-depleted (20 meq Na^+/d): Supine: 12–36 ng/dL Upright: 17–137 ng/dL	27.74	 83–277 pmol/L 139–831 pmol/L 332–997 pmol/L 471–3795 pmol/L	Lavender or green
Alkaline phosphatase	Serum	41–133 units/L (method- and age-dependent)	0.02	0.7–2.2 μkat/L (method- and age-dependent)	Marbled
Ammonia (NH_3)	Plasma	18–60 μg/dL	0.59	11–35 μmol/L	Green
Amylase	Serum	20–110 units/L (laboratory-specific)	0.02	0.33–1.83 μkat/L (laboratory-specific)	Marbled
Angiotensin-converting enzyme (ACE)	Serum	12–35 units/L (method-dependent)	16.67	< 590 nkat/L (method-dependent)	Marbled
Antithrombin III (AT III)	Plasma	84–123% (qualitative) 22–39 mg/dL (quantitative)			Blue
α_1-Antitrypsin[3]	Serum	110–270 mg/dL	0.01	1.1–2.7 g/L	Marbled
Aspartate aminotransferase (AST, SGOT, GOT)	Serum	0–35 units/L (laboratory-specific)	0.02	0–0.58 μkat/L (laboratory-specific)	Marbled
Basophil count	Whole blood	0.01–0.12 × 10^9/L			Lavender
Bilirubin	Serum	Total: 0.1–1.2 mg/dL Direct (conjugated to glucuronide): 0.1–0.4 mg/dL Indirect (unconjugated): 0.1–0.7 mg/dL	17.10	2–21 μmol/L < 7 μmol/L < 12 μmol/L	Marbled
Blood urea nitrogen (BUN)	Serum	8–20 mg/dL	0.36	2.9–7.1 mmol/L	Marbled
C-peptide	Serum	0.8–4.0 ng/mL	1.00	0.8–4.0 μg/L	Marbled (fasting)
Calcitonin	Plasma	Male: < 90 pg/mL Female: < 70 pg/mL	1.00	Male: < 90 ng/L Female: < 70 ng/L	Green
Calcium (Ca^{2+})	Serum	8.5–10.5 mg/dL **Panic:** < 6.5 or > 13.5 mg/dL	0.25	2.1–2.6 mmol/L	Marbled
Calcium (ionized)	Serum	4.6–5.3 mg/dL	0.25	1.15–1.32 mmol/L	Marbled
Calcium (U_{Ca})	Urine	100–300 mg/d	0.025	2.5–7.5 mmol/d	Urine bottle containing hydrochloric acid

(*continued*)

Table 2. Reference ranges for commonly used tests.[1,2] (continued)

Test	Specimen	Conventional Units	Conversion Factor	SI Units[2]	Collection
Carbon dioxide, partial pressure (P_{CO_2})	Whole blood	32–48 mm Hg	0.13	4.26–6.38 kPa	Heparinized syringe
Carbon dioxide (CO_2), total (bicarbonate)	Serum	22–28 meq/L **Panic:** < 15 or > 40 meq/L	1.00	22–28 mmol/L **Panic:** < 15 or > 40 mmol/L	Marbled
Carboxyhemoglobin (HbCO)	Whole blood	< 9% of total hemoglobin (Hb)	0.01	< 0.09 fraction of total hemoglobin	Lavender
Carcinoembryonic antigen (CEA)	Serum	0–2.5 ng/mL	1.00	0–2.5 μg/L	Marbled
CD4 T cell count	Whole blood	359–1725 cells/μL			Lavender (CBC and differential and % CD4 required)
Ceruloplasmin	Serum	20–35 mg/dL (laboratory-specific)	10.00	200–350 mg/L	Marbled
Chloride (Cl^-)	Serum	98–107 meq/L	1.00	98–107 mmol/L	Marbled
Cholesterol	Serum	Desirable: < 200 mg/dL Borderline: 200–239 mg/dL High risk: > 240 mg/dL	0.03	Desirable: < 5.2 mmol/L Borderline: 5.2–6.1 mmol/L High risk: > 6.2 mmol/L	Marbled
Chorionic gonadotropin, β-subunit (β-hCG), quantitative	Serum	Males and nonpregnant females: undetectable or < 5 mU/mL	1.00	Males and nonpregnant females: undetectable or < 5 units/L	Marbled
Complement C3	Serum	64–166 mg/dL	10.00	640–1660 mg/L	Marbled
Complement C4	Serum	15–45 mg/dL	10.00	150–450 mg/L	Marbled
Complement CH50	Plasma or serum	22–40 units/mL (laboratory-specific)			Marbled
Cortisol	Plasma or serum	8:00 AM: 5–20 μg/dL	27.59	140–550 nmol/L	Marbled, lavender, or green
Cortisol (urinary free)	Urine	10–110 μg/24 h	2.76	30–300 nmol/d	Urine bottle containing boric acid
Creatine kinase (CK)	Serum	32–267 units/L (method-dependent)	0.02	0.53–4.45 μkat/L (method-dependent)	Marbled
Creatine kinase MB (CKMB)	Serum	< 16 units/L or < 4% of total CK (laboratory-specific) Mass units: 0–7 μg/L	0.04	< 0.27 μkat/L	Marbled
Creatinine (Cr)	Serum	0.6–1.2 mg/dL	83.3	50–100 μmol/L	Marbled
Creatinine clearance (Cl_{Cr})	See Collection column.	Adults: 90–140 mL/min/1.73 m^2 BSA	0.017	1.5–2.3 mL/s/1.73 m^2 BSA	Carefully timed 24-hour urine and simultaneous serum or plasma creatinine sample
Cryoglobulins	Serum	< 0.12 mg/dL			Marbled at 37 °C
Eosinophil count	Whole blood	0.4–0.5 × 10^9/L			Lavender
Erythrocyte count (RBC count)	Whole blood	4.2–5.6 × 10^6/μL	1.00	4.2–5.6 × 10^{12}/L	Lavender
Erythrocyte sedimentation rate	Whole blood	Male: < 10 mm/h Female: < 15 mm/h (laboratory-specific)		Same	Lavender
Erythropoietin (EPO)	Serum	5–20 mU/mL	1.00	5–20 units/L	Marbled

(*continued*)

Table 2. Reference ranges for commonly used tests.[1,2] (continued)

Test	Specimen	Conventional Units	Conversion Factor	SI Units[2]	Collection
Ethanol	Serum	mg/dL Legal "driving under the influence" in many states is defined as > 80 mg/dL (> 17 mmol/L)	0.217	mmol/L	Marbled
Factor VIII assay	Plasma	40–150% of normal (varies with age)			Blue
Fecal fat	Stool	Random: < 60 droplets of fat per high-power field 72-hour: < 7 g/d			Qualitative: Random stool sample Quantitative: 72-hour collection following 2-day dietary fat regimen
Ferritin	Serum	Male: 16–300 ng/mL Female: 4–161 ng/mL	1.00	Male: 16–300 μg/L Female: 4–161 μg/L	Marbled
α-Fetoprotein (AFP)	Serum	0–15 ng/mL	1.00	0–15 μg/L	Marbled
Fibrin D-dimers	Plasma	Negative			Blue
Fibrinogen (functional)	Plasma	175–433 mg/dL **Panic:** < 75 mg/dL	0.01	1.75–4.3 g/L	Blue
Folic acid (red cells)	Whole blood	165–760 ng/mL	2.27	370–1720 nmol/L	Lavender
Follicle-stimulating hormone (FSH)	Serum	Female: Follicular phase 4–13 mU/mL Luteal phase 2–13 mU/mL Midcycle 5–22 mU/mL Postmenopausal 30–138 mU/mL Male: 1–10 mU/mL (laboratory-specific)	1.00	Female: 4–13 units/L 2–13 units/L 5–22 units/L 30–138 units/L Male: 1–10 units/L (laboratory-specific)	Marbled
Free erythrocyte protoporphyrin (FEP)	Whole blood	< 35 μg/dL (method-dependent)			Lavender
Gamma-glutamyltranspeptidase (GGT)	Serum	9–85 units/L (laboratory-specific)	0.02	0.15–1.42 μkat/L (laboratory-specific)	Marbled
Gastrin	Serum	< 100 pg/mL (laboratory-specific)	1.00	< 100 ng/L	Marbled
Glucose	Serum	60–115 mg/dL **Panic:** < 40 or > 500 mg/dL	0.06	3.3–6.3 mmol/L	Marbled (fasting)
Glucose-6-phosphate dehydrogenase (G6PD) screen	Whole blood	5–14 units/g Hb	0.02	0.1–0.28 μkat/L	Green or blue
Glutamine	CSF	6–16 mg/dL **Panic:** > 40 mg/dL	0.07	0.1–0.28 mmol/L	Collect CSF in a plastic tube
Glycated (glycosylated) hemoglobin (HbA_{1c})	Serum	3.9–6.9% (method-dependent)			Lavender
Growth hormone (GH)	Serum	0–5 ng/mL	1.00	0–5 μg/L	Marbled
Haptoglobin	Serum	46–316 mg/dL	0.01	0.5–3.2 g/L	Marbled
HDL cholesterol	Serum	Male: 27–67 mg/dL Female: 34–88 mg/dL	0.026	0.7–1.73 mmol/L 0.88–2.28 mmol/L	Marbled

(*continued*)

Table 2. Reference ranges for commonly used tests.[1,2] (continued)

Test	Specimen	Conventional Units	Conversion Factor	SI Units[2]	Collection
Helicobacter pylori antibody	Serum	Negative			Marbled
Hematocrit (Hct)	Whole blood	Male: 39–49% Female: 35–45% (age-dependent)	0.01	Male: 0.39–0.49 Female: 0.35–0.45	Lavender
Hemoglobin A_2 (HbA_2)	Whole blood	1.5–3.5% of total hemoglobin	0.01	0.015–0.035	Lavender
Hemoglobin electrophoresis	Whole blood	HbA: > 95% HbA_2: 1.5–3.5%			Lavender, blue, or green
Hemoglobin, fetal (HbF)	Whole blood	Adult: < 2% (varies with age)			Lavender, blue, or green
Hemoglobin, total (Hb)	Whole blood	Male: 13.6–17.5 g/dL Female: 12.0–15.5 g/dL **Panic:** ≤ 7 g/dL (age-dependent)	10.00	Male: 136–175 g/L Female: 120–155 g/L	Lavender
Hemosiderin	Urine	Negative			Urine container
HIV viral load	Plasma	Negative			Lavender
β-Hydroxybutyrate	Serum	0.5–3 mg/dL	0.096	0.05–0.3 mmol/L	Marbled
5-Hydroxyindoleacetic acid (5-HIAA)	Urine	2–8 mg/24 h	5.23	10–40 μmol/d	Urine bottle containing hydrochloric acid
IgG index	Serum and CSF	0.29–0.59 ratio			Marbled and glass or plastic tube for CSF
Immunoglobulins (Ig)	Serum	IgA: 78–367 mg/dL IgG: 583–1761 mg/dL IgM: 52–335 mg/dL	0.01	IgA: 0.78–3.67 g/L IgG: 5.83–17.6 g/L IgM: 0.52–3.35 g/L	Marbled
Insulin, immunoreactive	Serum	6–35 μU/mL	7.18	42–243 pmol/L	Marbled
Insulin-like growth factor-1	Plasma	123–463 ng/mL (age- and sex-dependent)	1.0	123–463 μg/L	Lavender
Iron (Fe^{2+})	Serum	50–175 μg/dL	0.18	9–31 μmol/L	Marbled
Iron-binding capacity, total (TIBC)	Serum	250–460 μg/dL	0.18	45–82 μmol/L	Marbled
Lactate dehydrogenase (LDH)	Serum	88–230 units/L (laboratory-specific)	0.02	1.46–3.82 μkat/L (laboratory-specific)	Marbled
Lactate dehydrogenase (LDH) isoenzymes	Serum	LDH_1/LDH_2: < 0.85			Marbled
Lactic acid (lactate)	Venous blood	0.5–2.0 meq/L	1.00	0.5–2.0 mmol/L	Gray
LDL cholesterol	Serum	< 130 mg/dL	0.026	< 3.37 mmol/L	Marbled
Lead (Pb)	Whole blood	Child: < 25 μg/dL Adult: < 40 μg/dL	0.05	Child: < 1.21 μmol/L Adult: < 1.93 μmol/L	Navy
Lecithin/sphingomyelin (L/S) ratio	Amniotic fluid	> 2.0 (method-dependent)			Collect in a plastic tube
Leukocyte alkaline phosphatase (LAP)	Whole blood	40–130 Based on 0 to 4+ rating of 100 PMNs stained for alkaline phosphatase			Green
Leukocyte (white blood cell) count, total (WBC count)	Whole blood	3.4–10 × 10^3/μL **Panic:** < 1.5 × 10^3/μL	1.00	3.4–10 × 10^9/L	Lavender

(*continued*)

Table 2. Reference ranges for commonly used tests.[1,2] (continued)

Test	Specimen	Conventional Units	Conversion Factor	SI Units[2]	Collection
Lipase	Serum	0–160 units/L (laboratory-specific)	0.02	0–2.66 μkat/L (laboratory-specific)	Marbled
Luteinizing hormone (LH)	Serum	Female: Follicular phase 1–18 mU/mL Luteal phase 0.4–20 mU/mL Midcycle 24–105 mU/mL Postmenopausal 15–62 mU/mL Male: 1–10 mU/mL (laboratory-specific)	1.00	1–18 units/L 0.4–20 units/L 24–105 units/L 15–62 units/L Male: 1–10 units/L (laboratory-specific)	Marbled
Lymphocyte count	Whole blood	$0.8–3.5 \times 10^9/L$			Lavender
Magnesium (Mg^{2+})	Serum	1.8–3.0 mg/dL **Panic:** < 0.5 or > 4.5 mg/dL	0.41	0.75–1.25 mmol/L	Marbled
Mean corpuscular hemoglobin (MCH)	Whole blood	26–34 pg			Lavender
Mean corpuscular hemoglobin concentration (MCHC)	Whole blood	31–36 g/dL	10.00	310–360 g/L	Lavender
Mean corpuscular volume (MCV)	Whole blood	80–100 fL			Lavender
Metanephrines	Urine	0.3–0.9 mg/24 h	5.46	1.6–4.9 μmol/d	Urine bottle containing hydrochloric acid
Methemoglobin (MetHb)	Whole blood	< 1% of total hemoglobin	0.01	< 0.01 fraction of total hemoglobin	Lavender
Monocyte count	Whole blood	$0.2–0.8 \times 10^9/L$			Lavender
Neutrophil count	Whole blood	$2.2–8.6 \times 10^9/L$			Lavender
Osmolality	Serum	275–293 mosm/kg H_2O **Panic:** < 240 or > 320 mosm/kg H_2O	1.00	275–293 mmol/kg H_2O	Marbled
	Urine	Random: 100–900 mosm/kg H_2O	1.00	Random: 100–900 mmol/kg H_2O	Urine container
Oxygen, partial pressure (Po_2)	Whole blood	83–108 mm Hg	0.13	11.04–14.36 kPa	Heparinized syringe
Parathyroid hormone (PTH)	Serum	Intact PTH: 11–54 pg/mL (laboratory-specific)	0.11	Intact PTH: 1.2–5.7 pmol/L (laboratory-specific)	Marbled
Partial thromboplastin time, activated (PTT)	Plasma	25–35 seconds (range varies) **Panic:** ≥ 60 seconds			Blue
pH	Whole blood	Arterial: 7.35–7.45 Venous: 7.31–7.41			Heparinized syringe
Phosphorus	Serum	2.5–4.5 mg/dL **Panic:** < 1.0 mg/dL	0.32	0.8–1.45 mmol/L	Marbled
Platelet count (Plt)	Whole blood	$150–450 \times 10^3/\mu L$ **Panic:** $< 25 \times 10^3/\mu L$	1.00	$150–450 \times 10^9/L$ **Panic:** $< 25 \times 10^9/L$	Lavender
Platelet-associated IgG	Whole blood	Negative			Yellow (17 mL of blood)

(continued)

Table 2. Reference ranges for commonly used tests.[1,2] (continued)

Test	Specimen	Conventional Units	Conversion Factor	SI Units[2]	Collection
Porphobilinogen (PBG)	Urine	Negative			
Potassium (K^+)	Serum	3.5–5.0 meq/L **Panic:** < 3.0 or > 6.0 meq/L	1.00	3.5–5.0 mmol/L	Marbled
Prolactin (PRL)	Serum	< 20 ng/mL	1.00	< 20 μg/L	Marbled
Prostate-specific antigen (PSA)	Serum	0–4 ng/mL	1.00	0–4 μg/L	Marbled
Protein C	Plasma	71–176%			Blue
Protein electrophoresis	Serum	Adults: Albumin: 3.3–4.7 g/dL α_1: 0.1–0.4 g/dL α_2: 0.3–0.9 g/dL β_2: 0.7–1.5 g/dL γ: 0.5–1.4 g/dL	10.00	 33–47 g/L 1–4 g/L 3–9 g/L 7–15 g/L 5–14 g/L	Marbled
Protein S (antigen)	Plasma	76–178%			Blue
Protein, total	Plasma or serum	6.0–8.0 g/dL	10.00	60–80 g/L	Marbled
Prothrombin time (PT)	Whole blood	11–15 seconds **Panic:** ≥ 30 seconds (laboratory-specific) INR (international normalized ratio): 2–3.5 **Panic:** > 6			Blue
Red blood cell count	Whole blood	4.7–6.1 × 10^9/L			Lavender
Red cell volume	Whole blood	25–35 mL/kg			Green
Renin activity (PRA)	Plasma	High-sodium diet ($75–150$ meq Na^+/d): Supine: 0.2–2.3 ng/mL/h Standing: 1.3–4.0 ng/mL/h Low-sodium diet ($30–75$ meq Na^+/d): Standing: 4.0–7.7 ng/mL/h			Lavender
Reptilase clotting time	Plasma	13–19 seconds			Blue
Reticulocyte count	Whole blood	33–137 × 10^3/μL	1.00	33–137 × 10^9/L	Lavender
Russell's viper venom clotting time (dilute) (RVVT)	Plasma	24–37 seconds			Blue
Salicylate (aspirin, others)	Serum	20–30 mg/dL **Panic:** > 35 mg/dL	10.00	200–300 mg/L	Marbled
Sodium (Na^+)	Serum	135–145 meq/L **Panic:** < 125 or > 155 meq/L	1.00	135–145 mmol/L	Marbled
Testosterone	Serum	Male: 3.0–10.0 ng/mL Female: 0.3–0.7 ng/mL	3.47	Male: 10–35 nmol/L Female: 1.0–2.4 nmol/L	Marbled
Thrombin time	Plasma	24–35 seconds (laboratory-specific)			Blue
Thyroglobulin	Serum	3–42 ng/mL	1.00	3–42 μg/L	Marbled
Thyroid-stimulating hormone (TSH)	Serum	0.4–6 μU/mL	1.00	0.4–6 mU/L	Marbled

(*continued*)

Table 2. Reference ranges for commonly used tests.[1,2] (continued)

Test	Specimen	Conventional Units	Conversion Factor	SI Units[2]	Collection
Thyroid-stimulating hormone receptor antibody (TSH-R Ab [stim])	Serum	< 130% of basal activity. Based on cAMP generation in thyroid cell tissue culture.			
Thyroxine, free (FT_4)	Serum	9–24 pmol/L (varies with method)			Marbled
Thyroxine (T_4), total	Serum	5–11 μg/dL	12.80	64–142 nmol/L	Marbled
Thyroxine index, free (FT_4I)	Serum	6.5–12.5			Marbled
Transferrin	Serum	190–375 mg/dL	0.01	1.9–3.75 g/L	Marbled
Triglycerides	Serum	< 165 mg/dL	0.01	< 1.65 g/L	Marbled (fasting)
Triiodothyronine (T_3), total	Serum	95–190 ng/dL	0.015	1.5–2.9 nmol/L	Marbled
Troponin-I (cTnI)	Serum	< 1.5 ng/mL			Marbled
Uric acid	Serum	Male: 2.4–7.4 mg/dL Female: 1.4–5.8 mg/dL	59.48	Male: 140–440 μmol/L Female: 80–350 μmol/L	Marbled
Vanillylmandelic acid (VMA)	Urine	2–7 mg/24 h	5.05	10–35 μmol/d	Urine bottle containing hydrochloric acid
Vitamin B_{12}	Serum	140–820 pg/mL	0.74	100–600 pmol/L	Marbled
Vitamin B_{12} absorption test (Schilling test)	24-hour urine	Excretion of > 8% of administered dose			Urine bottle
Vitamin D, 25-hydroxy (25[OH]D)	Serum or plasma	10–50 ng/mL	2.5	25–125 nmol/L	Marbled or green
Vitamin D, 1,25-dihydroxy ($1,25[OH]_2D$)	Serum or plasma	20–76 pg/mL	2.4	48–182 pmol/L	Marbled or green
White blood cell count	Whole blood	$4.8–10.8 \times 10^9$/L			Lavender

[1]The reference ranges given here in conventional units and in SI units are from several large medical centers. Always use the reference ranges provided by your clinical laboratory, since ranges may be method-dependent.
[2]Reference: Young DS: Implementation of SI units for clinical laboratory data. Ann Intern Med 1987;106:114; JAMA Instructions for Authors, JAMA 1997;278:74.
[3]Also called α_1-antiprotease in some clinical contexts.

Commonly Used Specimen Collection Tubes

Tube Color	Tube Contents	Typical Use
Lavender	EDTA	Complete blood count
Marbled	Serum separator	Serum chemistry tests
Red	None	Blood banking (serum); therapeutic drug monitoring
Blue	Citrate	Coagulation studies
Gray	Inhibitor of glycolysis (sodium fluoride)	Lactic acid
Green	Heparin	Plasma studies
Yellow	Acid citrate	HLA typing
Navy	Trace metal free	Trace metals (eg, lead)

Index

NOTE: Page numbers in **bold face** type indicate a major discussion. A *t* following a page number indicates tabular material and an *f* following a page number indicates a figure. Drugs are listed under their generic names. When a drug trade name is listed, the reader is referred to the generic name.